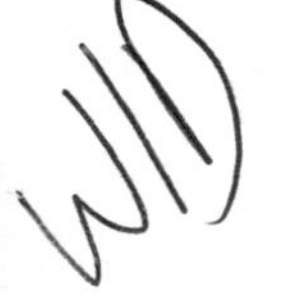

O. BRAUN-FALCO • G. PLEWIG
H.H. WOLFF • W.H.C. BURGDORF

DERMATOLOGY

Second, Completely Revised Edition

With 1038 Color Figures
and 281 Tables

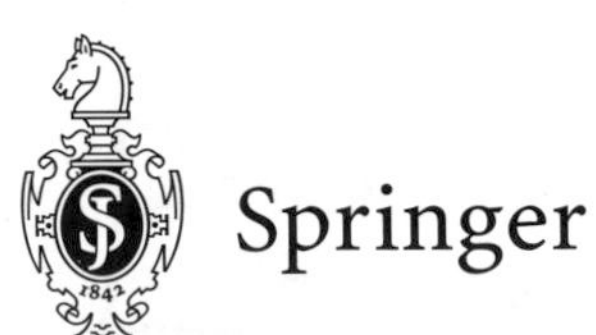

Springer

Prof. Dr. med. Dr. h.c.mult. OTTO BRAUN-FALCO
Emeritus Professor and Chairman
Department of Dermatology
and Allergology
Ludwig Maximilians University
Frauenlobstraße 9–11
D-80337 Munich, Germany

Prof. Dr. med. HELMUT H. WOLFF
Professor and Chairman
Department of Dermatology
and Venerology
University of Lübeck
Ratzeburger Allee 160
D-23562 Lübeck, Germany

Prof. Dr. med. GERD PLEWIG
Professor and Chairman
Department of Dermatology
and Allergology
Ludwig Maximilians University
Frauenlobstraße 9–11
D-80337 Munich, Germany

WALTER H.C. BURGDORF, M.D.
Clinical Lecturer
Department of Dermatology
and Allergology
Ludwig Maximilians University
Frauenlobstraße 9–11
D-80337 Munich, Germany

Based on: O. Braun-Falco, G. Plewig, H. H. Wolff: Dermatologie und Venerologie, 4th revised edition. © Springer-Verlag Berlin Heidelberg 1996

ISBN 3-540-59452-3 2nd Edition Springer-Verlag Berlin Heidelberg New York

ISBN 3-540-16672-6 1st Edition Springer-Verlag Berlin Heidelberg New York

Library of Congress Cataloging-in-Publication Data
Dermatologie und Venerologie. English, Dermatology / O. Braun-Falco ... [et al.]. – 2nd, completely rev. ed. p. ; cm. Includes bibliographical references and index.
ISBN 3-540-59452-3 (alk. paper)
1. Skin – Diseases – Diagnosis. 2. Sexually transmitted diseases – Diagnosis. I. Braun-Falco, Otto. II. Title.
[DNLM: 1. Skin Diseases. 2. Sexually Transmitted Diseases. WR 140 D4354 2000a] RL105 .45413 2000

Springer-Verlag Berlin Heidelberg New York
a member of BertelsmannSpringer Science+Business Media GmbH

Printed in Italia

Production editor: W. Bischoff, Heidelberg
Cover design: de'blik Konzept & Gestaltung, Berlin
Illustrations: R. Darroll, Hamburg
Reproduction of figures: Schneider Repro, Heidelberg
Data conversion: Fotosatz-Service Köhler GmbH, Würzburg
Printing and binding: Printer Trento S.r.l.

SPIN 10503068 22/3130 – 5 4 3 2 1 0 Printed on acid-free paper

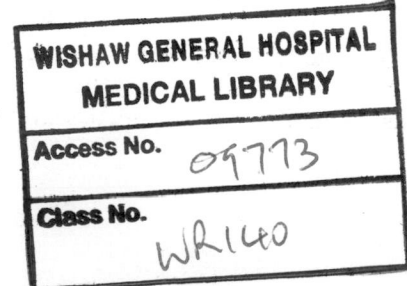

Preface

This text book has a long history. The first two German editions of *Dermatologie und Venerologie* were written by Egon Keining and Otto Braun-Falco and appeared in 1961 and 1969. Otto Braun-Falco invited two of his protégés, Gerd Plewig and Helmut H. Wolff, to assist him in writing the third German edition, which was published in 1984. These authors, along with Richard K. Winkelmann, joined together, in 1991, to create the first English edition. The fourth German edition appeared in 1996 and now the second English edition is ready.

This second English edition is quite different from both the fourth German edition and the first English edition. The fourth German edition was used as the framework for an entirely new translation; this work is not based on the first English edition. Many new topics have been introduced and much of the material has been reorganized. Two new chapters, on diseases of black skin and operative dermatology, have been added. Every chapter has been checked by at least two of the German authors; most have been revised several times.

This book is designed for a wide variety of readers. Dermatology residents will find it valuable both in their daily work and when reviewing for specialty board examinations. Experienced dermatologists should be able to update their knowledge, as well as refer to the chapters on specific diseases for therapeutic options. Ambitious medical students may want to use our book as an introduction to dermatology, for it will stand them in good stead as they pursue training in other specialties. Finally, for the increasing number of primary care physicians, be they family doctors, pediatricians, internists, gynecologists or emergency room physicians, caring for patients with skin diseases, we hope that this book will be a helpful source of information that can be used in daily practice.

Dermatology remains a highly visual specialty, and in this respect the major strengths of this book are unchanged. We have concentrated on providing detailed clinical and morphological descriptions and excellent clinical photographs. Many new photographs have been added or have replaced older ones. To be more representative, we have also included photographs of black and Hispanic patients. In addition, all of the illustrations in the book have been redrawn. While a correlation between the clinical findings and the histology remains a cornerstone of dermatologic diagnosis, we have once again not included photomicrographs. Instead, the histological descriptions are designed to orient the reader and not to be exhaustive. Many excellent dermatopathology books are available; some are almost as long as this book. We refer the reader to these sources for more detailed information.

The changes since the last English edition have been immense. The pathogenesis of many diseases is better understood because of advances in immunology, molecular biology and molecular genetics. We have tried to distill these advances into a form understandable to the student, resident or practicing physician. In the process, we have undoubtedly oversimplified and introduced mistakes, for which we apologize in advance. Finally, the HIV/AIDS epidemic has once again made the sexually transmitted diseases and other infectious diseases such as syphilis and tuberculosis critically important, so we have retained the extensive sections on these disorders.

Many friends and colleagues helped with this book. Several colleagues took complete responsibility for a chapter: Roselyn E. Epps and John A. Kenney, Jr., (Chapter 66 Diseases of Black Skin), Hans Wolff and Wolf-Bernhard Schill (Chapter 68 Andrology) and Rainer Rompel (Chapter 72 Operative Dermatology). Other colleagues provided particular input into either new sections or ones that received extensive revision: Wybo Bruinsma (drug reactions), Rudolf Happle (genetics and epidermal nevi), Axel Hauschild (malignant melanoma), Ulrich Hohenleutner (stump dermatoses), Thomas Jansen (acne and rosacea), Michael Landthaler (lasers), Gerald Messer (bullous and connective tissue diseases), Maja Mockenhaupt (severe skin reactions), Bernhard Ortel (phototherapy equipment), Martin Röcken (immunology), Franziska Ruëff (allergy), Christian Sander (malignant lymphoma), Martin Schaller (infectious diseases), Eva-Regina Thoma-Greber (AIDS) and Franz Trautinger (phototherapy). Elke Bornhövd attempted to identify as many original reference citations as possible and helped extensively with checking of other references and responding to copy editing queries. Anette Bonowitz and Tilmann Oppel helped with the index. Other colleagues provided figures, including Jürg Hafner, Rebat M. Halder, Michael Landthaler, Juan J. Ochoa, Johannes Ring, Thomas Ruzicka, Robert H. Schosser and Robert Swerlick.

Once again many co-workers from the Department of Dermatology, Ludwig Maximilian University, Munich, reviewed chapters and helped with references. They include: Hans Peter Bertsch, Ursula Böhmer, Susanne Breit, Elke Bornhövd, René Chatelain, Klaus Degitz, Michael Flaig, Kamran Ghoreschi, Marc Heckmann, Thomas Herzinger, Thomas Jansen, Peter Kaudewitz, Gerold Kick, Hans Christian Korting, Christian Kunte, Dagmar Ludolph-Hauser, Gerald Messer, Silke Michelsen, Uwe Neubert, Bettina Prinz, Jörg Prinz, Martin Röcken, Ricardo Romiti, Franziska Ruëff, Rudolf Rupec, Arne Sakrauski, Christian Sander, Martin Schaller, Monika-Hildegard Schmid-Wendtner, Kathrin Schuhmann, Eva-Regina Thoma-Greber, Peter Thomas, Beata Trautner, Sabine Werfel, Ralf Wienecke, Hans Wolff, Andreas Wollenberg and Sabine Zenker.

Finally, the following colleagues helped with the fourth German edition, and thus some of their work has been carried over into this translation. Their titles and addresses are given in the German text. They include: Dietrich Abeck, Ulrich Amon, Thomas Bergner, Thomas Bieber, Leena Bruckner-Tuderman, Friedemann Enders, Peter Frosch, Günter Goerz (†), Wolfgang Hartschuh, Conrad Hauser, Stefan Hödl, Erhard Hölzle, Heiko Iven, Thomas Jansen, Peter Kaudewitz, Martina Kerscher, Peter Kind, Peter Karl Kohl, Hans Christian Korting, Jürgen Kreusch, Thomas Krieg, Wolfgang Küster, Michael Landthaler, Bodo Melnik, Michael Meurer, Helmut Näher, Uwe Neubert, Jörg Prinz, Bernhard Przybilla, Johannes Ring, Martin Röcken, Thomas Ruzicka, Christian Sander, Martin Schaller, Rüdiger Scharf, Wolf-Bernhard Schill, Carl-Georg Schirren, Wilfried Schmeller, Eva-Regina Thoma-Greber and Michael Tronnier.

Many other thanks are also due. Once again Peter Bilek, our clinic photographer in Munich, provided invaluable aid, as did his assistants Claudia Jakobec and Diana Kellermeier. Robert Darroll, a free-lance medical illustrator, executed the new drawings. Claudia Tielkes managed the entire process of transferring material back and forth between authors, colleagues and the publishers without a glitch. Springer-Verlag, and especially Willi Bischoff, was very patient with the slow writing process and provided their usual excellent support in terms of editorial advice, design and production.

We suspect this will be one of the last textbooks of this size to be typed by a single physician, as WB transcribed each chapter, translating and modifying the German text. This approach has resulted in a uniform style and hopefully kept replications and contradictions to a minimum. Finally, we thank a most unusual helper – an aging, red Manx cat named Boris who sat by WB's side for almost all of the computer time required to produce this text. If one can learn by proximity, then he is a feline master of dermatology.

Munich and Lübeck, 2000

Otto Braun-Falco
Gerd Plewig
Helmut H. Wolff
Walter H.C. Burgdorf

Contents

Contributing Autors

Roselyn E. Epps, M.D.
Chairperson
Department of Pediatric Dermatology
Children's National Medical Center
111 Michigan Avenue NW
Washington, D.C. 20010, USA
(Chapter 66)

John A. Kenney, Jr., M.D.
Emeritus Professor and Chairman
Department of Dermatology
Howard University School of Medicine
2041 Georgia Avenue NW
Washington, D.C. 20060, USA
(Chapter 66)

Privatdozent Dr. med. Rainer Rompel
Director
Department of Dermatology
Klinikum Kassel
Mönchebergstraße 41–43
D-34125 Kassel, Germany
(Chapter 72)

Prof. Dr. med. Wolf-Bernhard Schill
Professor and Chairman
Center for Dermatology and Andrology
Justus Liebig University
Gaffkystraße 14
D-35385 Giessen, Germany
(Chapter 68)

Privatdozent Dr. med. Hans Wolff
Department of Dermatology and Allergology
Ludwig Maximilians University
Frauenlobstraße 9–11
D-80337 Munich, Germany
(Chapter 68)

CHAPTER 1

Basic Science and Principles of Dermatologic Diagnosis

Contents

Structure and Function of the Skin

In contrast to other dermatology textbooks, we have not devoted a single chapter to the embryology, anatomy and physiology of the skin. Since this text is conceived as a clinical text, basic science information is placed with the clinically related diseases. For example, the anatomy and physiology of the sebaceous glands is considered along with acne. Here we will briefly review the fundamental aspects of skin structure and function, with many cross-references to the chapters where topics are expanded upon.

Embryology

The skin arises from both the ectoderm and the mesoderm. The superficial or outer layer, the epidermis, is ectodermal, while the dermis, subcutaneous fat, nerves and vessels are all mesodermal. Initially the embryo is covered by a single layer of simple epithelium known as ectoderm. The most primitive epidermal cell is the so-called epidermal stem cell, from which epidermis, sweat gland epithelium and hair epithelium derive. In about the 2nd month of gestation, the ectoderm differentiates into the outer flattened periderm and the cuboidal basal layer. As the embryo elongates and develops a humanoid shape, the cells of the epidermis migrate in elongated dorsally sweeping swirls that produce Blaschko lines. By birth all the layers of the epidermis are present. Shed scales, hair and sebum combine to form the protective vernix caseosa.

The primitive dermis is more cellular than that of an adult, but relatively amorphous. At about 2 months of age, the cellular fibroblasts begin manufacturing collagen, so that the dermis becomes more fibrous. The fat layer begins to form, as do islands of primitive endothelial cells (blood islands). These develop into tubular structures; often similar lobular islands of new vessels are seen at the edge of vascular tumors in adults. Nerves begin to migrate into the dermis at about 4 months.

The ectodermal and mesenchymal elements interact extensively. The epidermal-dermal junction appears in the first trimester, while all of its elements present by the end of this period. This is of particular importance in the prenatal diagnosis of epidermolysis bullosa, a group of diseases with inherited defects in different components of this junction.

In addition, the epidermal appendages develop as a result of the interaction between epidermal buds or invaginations and dermal elements. The hairs, sebaceous glands and apocrine glands form as a result of the interaction between a cluster of basal epidermal cells (hair germ) and specialized mesenchymal cells (hair papillae). While apocrine glands are widespread in fetal skin, most become very small and insignificant, except in apocrine-rich areas such as the axilla and groin. The arrector pili muscles form between the hair follicle and the dermal connective tissue and the hair follicle. When they contract, the hair is pulled into the vertical position, important for temperature control in furry mammals but only producing goose bumps (cutis anserina) in humans. Eccrine glands develop from separate epidermal buds. The nail anlagen are initially seen at about the 3rd month; they arise on the finger and then toe tips, but slowly migrate to their final dorsal position and then form nails.

The epidermis is also populated by three groups of cells that migrate in during the first few months of life. Langerhans cells are bone-marrow-derived antigen-processing cells. The neural crest provides melanocytes, which are responsible for melanin production and transfer. Merkel cells are neuroendocrine cells that also probably arise in the neural crest.

Anatomy of the Skin

Epidermis and Associated Structures

The epidermis is a multilayered self-renewing sheet of cells. The cells of the basal layer divide, and then the new keratinocytes undergo terminal differentiation as they migrate towards the skin surface. Some cells in the basal layer are designated epidermal stem cells. They divide giving rise to keratinocytes capable of differentiation and to additional primitive stem cells. Exactly how these self-generating basal layer cells relate to the precursor cells of hair follicle and sweat gland epithelium is unclear. They may develop from even more primitive cells. Good markers or labels are unavailable. Epidermal stem cells are attractive when considering the possibility of skin replacement, as in patients with widespread burns. If they can be identified and enhanced, then epidermal stem cells should offer the best way of generating new nearly normal epidermis rapidly.

The epidermal turnover time is about 1 month. The keratinocytes reach the interface of the granular layer and the stratum corneum after about 2 weeks; the empty shell of the keratinocyte is known as a corneocyte. Another 2 weeks are normally required for the corneocytes to reach the surface of the stratum corneum and be shed into the environment. In psoriasis (Chap. 14) this turnover time is dramatically decreased. Derangements in the process of keratinization are responsible for a wide variety of disorders, including ichthyoses and palmoplantar keratoderma (Chap. 17). The keratinocytes are held together by complex structures known as desmosomes. When the desmosomes are damaged, as in a variety of autoimmune disorders, then the keratinocytes become separated, in a process known as acantholysis (Chap. 15).

The skin surface is characterized by many fine and coarse lines. Sometimes, if the skin is rubbed, these marking become accentuated as in lichenification. The skin lines on the palms (and soles) are quite distinctive, forming the basis for finger printing. Patients with atopic dermatitis have increased markings on their palms and soles. Alterations of the skin surface are prominent in the skin of older individuals. One must distinguish between intrinsic aging and photo-aggravated aging. In intrinsic aging, there is thinning of the skin and fine wrinkling as seen on the buttocks. In photo-aged skin, as seen on the face, there are typically far coarser changes in the skin markings with deeper furrows and dermal alterations.

The hair follicles become quite complex, acquiring multiple layers with delicate epithelial-mesenchymal interactions controlling the cyclic pattern of hair growth. They change from infantile lanugo hairs to vellus and terminal hairs, such as those on the scalp. Later, under primarily hormonal influence, terminal hairs develop in other regions, such as the axilla, the groin, the male beard region and on the trunk and limbs (Chap. 31).

The sebaceous glands are large at birth, then involute but become prominent once again in puberty. The main function of the sebaceous glands is to provide lipids, which lubricate the hair shaft and, along with lipids produced by the epidermal cells, maintain a lipid film on the skin surface. In adolescence the sebaceous follicles are the site of action for acne (Chap. 28).

The role of the apocrine glands is unclear. In some mammals they serve as a source of pheromones, secreted products that influence the behavior of others via olfactory networks. In humans apocrine glands are concentrated in the axillae, perianal region and genitalia (Chap. 29).

The eccrine glands are primarily temperature control glands. They are under extensive neural regulation and excrete sweat, as a result of physical activity, excess temperature or emotional stress. Wetting the skin surface also improves one's grip, as often needed in sports or manual labor. Some medications are concentrated in eccrine sweat and reach the skin through this route, in a sprinkler effect (Chap. 30).

The nails formerly served as tools and to protect and support the distal digits. Today they also have a significant cosmetic role. Their keratin is much more compactly bound together than that of the skin or hairs, producing thick, relatively unyielding structures (Chap. 32).

A number of mucosal surfaces are also of interest to dermatologists, including the oral mucosa (Chap. 33), the genital mucosa (Chaps. 34, 35) and the anal mucosa (Chap. 66). Mucosal surfaces tend to be moist and either not to be keratinized or to have very different patterns of keratinization. Technically, one should speak of the epithelium and lamina propria, not the epidermis and dermis, when discussing the tissues.

Melanin in the epidermis is the main determinant of skin color, distinguishing between skin types I–VI in whites, Orientals and blacks. Melanocytes manufacture melanin and transfer it to adjacent keratinocytes. The packaging of the melanin, rather than the number of melanocytes, determines the skin color. Some individuals lack enzymes needed to manufacture melanin and thus have pale skin; they are known as albinos. In other instances, melanocytes are either absent at birth or later disappear from an area of skin, causing depigmentation (Chap. 26).

Epidermal-Dermal Junction

The epidermis and dermis are held together by a very complex region known as the epidermal-dermal junction. It consists of contributions from both keratinocytes and fibroblasts. Congenital lack of some of the elements leads to fragile skin; epidermolysis bullosa or mechanobullous disease results. In addition, in adults, there may be damage to the epidermal-dermal junction because of the production of autoantibodies against various component structures (Chap. 15) or because of intense inflammation in the region, as can be seen with lichen planus (Chap. 14) or lupus erythematosus (Chap. 18).

Dermis

The dermal connective tissue consists primarily of collagen fibers with some elastic fibers added. The dermis is responsible for the bulk of the skin, as it is far thicker than the epidermis. In tanning the dermis is converted into leather, hence the German name for the dermis is *Lederhaut* (leather skin). There are many congenital and acquired disorders that result in defects in collagen or elastin. There may be overproduction of normal fibers, manufacture of abnormal fibers or marked destruction. The term connective tissue disorders is often employed (Chap. 18), although it is not entirely correct.

The dermis is served by a complex series of blood vessels, bringing nutrients and removing waste products. The vessels serve as the site of many inflammatory reactions, as the host immune cells migrate into the dermis and encounter invaders, whether they be organisms, foreign antigens or other factors (Chap. 22). Blood may leak into the skin, either as a result of blood vessel damage or because of defects in the clotting mechanism, leading to a variety of types of hemorrhage (Chap. 23). The venous system is particularly stressed in the legs, the price man pays for standing erect. Impaired venous circulation leads to swelling and a variety of skin changes; for this reason, in Germany dermatologists are primarily responsible for the treatment of chronic venous insufficiency (Chap. 22). The lymphatics help the venous system drain the skin and subcutaneous tissue, removing larger molecules and protein-rich exudates; they too may be defective, because of either congenital variations or inflammatory changes (Chap. 24).

Subcutaneous Tissue

The subcutaneous fat serves as protective padding and a reservoir of energy. In addition, it is a major cosmetic factor, responsible for both attractive curves and unsightly bulges. Inflammation of the fat is known as panniculitis; it is typically seen on the legs and may be associated with trauma, vascular disease or underlying disorders such as pancreatitis or tumors (Chap. 21).

Cartilage is also responsible for some subcutaneous support and modeling, as in the ears and nose primarily. Inflammation and injuries to cartilage are slow to heal because of the limited vascular supply (Chap. 20).

Functional Aspects

The skin serves as the interface between humans and their environment. Thus, elaborate neural and immunologic mechanisms have been developed for protective purposes. A wide variety of nerves serve the skin, allowing for perception of touch, pain, warmth, cold and other modalities. Nerves also regulate cutaneous blood flow and control sweat gland function. Dysregulation is responsible for many disorders, including Raynaud phenomenon (Chap. 22) and hyperhidrosis (Chap. 30). A feature unique to the skin is the presence of itch, a phenomenon not described in internal organs. It probably initially was protective, to encourage one to scratch away a biting or burrowing insect, but today itch is responsible for much misery (Chap. 25).

The protective keratin and lipid layers combine to shield the skin against external insults. The Langerhans cells take up materials that penetrate into the epidermis and then present them to the immune system so an immunologic response can be mounted. The most acute reaction involves the presence of immunoglobulin E (IgE) antibodies on mast cells; when an appropriate antigen rechallenge occurs, there is mast cell degranulation and a type I reaction of Gell and Coombs (Chap. 11). In addition, a number of other dermal cells are available to take up foreign material; most are bone-marrow-derived monocytes, which are called macrophages once they settle in peripheral tissues. Sometimes the macrophages combine with other inflammatory cells to produce a chronic inflammatory response known as a granuloma (Chap. 50). Sometimes eosinophils are the dominant cell in the cutaneous reaction; this is seen not only in allergic reactions but also in response to infections, especially parasitic diseases. In other instances, the presence of the eosinophils remains unexplained (Chap. 51).

A number of metabolic processes are reflected in the skin. For example, patients with disturbances in triglyceride and cholesterol metabolism often have lipid deposits in the skin known as xanthomas (Chap. 37). Many systemic metabolic disorders, involving a wide range of proteins, lipids and amino acids, also have cutaneous findings (Chaps. 38, 39, 42). A variety of materials may accumulate in the dermis, including immunoglobulins (Chap. 40), amyloid (Chap. 41), mucins (Chap. 43), calcium salts (Chap. 45) and urate crystals (Chap. 47). Abnormalities in hemoglobin metabolism lead to the production of porphyrins, chemicals which in the skin are often photosensitizing (Chap. 44). Metals and metal salts may also be deposited in the dermis, producing a variety of pigmentary changes (Chap. 46). Vitamins (Chap. 49) and other nutritional factors (Chap. 48) also have marked effects on the skin, as do endocrine diseases (Chap. 48).

Cellular Proliferations

Nevi or hamartomas are congenital abnormalities in which a given cell type is present in excess, such as a vascular malformation consisting of too many blood vessels (Chap. 52). A variety of benign and malignant tumors can develop in the skin and subcutaneous tissue reflecting virtually all of the tissue types, including epidermal cells (Chaps. 54–56), adnexal structures (Chaps. 53, 57), melanocytes (Chap. 58) and mesenchymal elements (blood vessels, nerves, muscles, connective tissue) (Chap. 59).

Many other cell types may also produce cutaneous disease. Lymphocytes may also proliferate in the cutaneous compartment, either as a reactive process known as pseudolymphoma (Chap. 60) or as a malignant lymphoma, either primary in the skin or secondary to nodal disease (Chap. 61). Leukemic cells may also infiltrate the skin, and rarely leukemia presents as a cutaneous tumor known as a chloroma (Chap. 62). Mast cell proliferations may be benign or in rare cases quite aggressive (Chap. 63). Histiocytoses refer to proliferations of either Langerhans cells or macrophages; the skin is frequently involved (Chap. 64). Finally, the skin may reflect underlying malignancies; such changes are known as paraneoplastic phenomena (Chap. 65).

The Dermatologic Patient

Prevalence of Skin Diseases

In a general medical practice, about 20–25% of patients have skin complaints. In the tropics, skin disorders are the most common presenting problem. Thus, every physician must be capable of identifying and treating skin disorders.

Age Distribution

Many skin disorders are typical for certain age groups.

Infants. Congenital malformations (including melanocytic nevi, epidermal nevi and hemangiomas), diaper dermatitis and atopic dermatitis are the most common problems. Many genodermatoses also manifest themselves in early life; two examples are the ichthyoses and the epidermolysis bullosa family.

Children. Atopic dermatitis, warts, molluscum contagiosum, impetigo, scabies and head lice are common in this group.

Adolescents. Acne vulgaris is the dominant disease in teenagers. Teenagers may worry about the possibility of venereal diseases and present with skin lesions or problems in the genital area, requiring reassurance.

Adults. Almost all the disorders discussed in this book can present in adults. Rosacea is often cited as a disease generally limited to people in middle age. Many patients present with problems that may be work-related. Cosmetic problems take on increased importance. Concern about malignancy will also prompt many visits, as will widespread disease or intense itching.

The Elderly. Dry skin and signs of actinic and intrinsic aging are the main problems, as well as an increased incidence of malignant tumors.

Inpatient Versus Outpatient Treatment

In the USA, almost all care, including extensive cutaneous surgery, is provided in the ambulatory setting. Nonetheless, there are dermatologic patients who deserve hospitalization. Included in this group are patients with widespread blistering disease, severe connective tissue disease, pustular psoriasis, widespread atopic dermatitis, erythroderma and similar conditions. More important, patients in whom ambulatory treatment has failed or is extremely difficult also benefit from hospitalization. Many patients with metastatic malignant melanoma are still treated by dermatologists in Germany; these individuals are admitted for chemotherapy and immunotherapy. Patients requiring operations too large for the ambulatory arena or for whom home care of the postoperative wound would be a burden should also be admitted, a service still available in Germany. Similarly, patients with severe leg ulcers usually need hospitalization, especially when skin grafting or other surgery is required. In Germany they are almost always treated by dermatologists; in the USA, this is not the case.

Patient Evaluation

History

Family History

Genetically determined diseases of the skin or genodermatoses can be identified from the history. A pedigree can be constructed to help identify the pattern of inheritance. In addition, many multifactorial diseases such as psoriasis and atopic dermatitis tend to run in families, even if an exact pattern of inheritance is not apparent. Syphilis or HIV infection may be transferred from mother to child during pregnancy or at birth. Finally, infectious diseases such as impetigo or scabies may be present in other family members.

General History

While the dermatologist can often make a rapid and correct diagnosis simply by looking at the patient, in more puzzling cases a detailed history may unearth valuable clues, just as it does in internal medicine or pediatrics. A more exact history requires time and patience, but helps seal a positive doctor-patient relationship.

Occupational History. Patients with dermatitis, especially hand dermatitis, should be questioned about their occupational exposure. Work-related skin disorders tend to improve on weekends, during sick leave or while the patient is on vacation. They may be sharply localized to specific areas. Dermatologic problems and hearing loss are the two most common occupational diseases in Germany.

The dermatologist must take a careful history, keeping in mind that every hand dermatitis case and many other innocent-appearing problems may reappear as worker's compensation cases, at which time clear and legible notes will be invaluable. One may need to contact the employer or company health office; this is best done with the patient's permission.

Other Exposures. Hobbies and routine household activities can also influence the skin. The patient should be asked about household chemicals, sun exposure, soaps, cosmetics, and other possible exposures. Often the localization of the skin problem will guide the questioning.

Animal Contact. Patients may acquire infectious diseases such as tinea from pets. In addition, they may have rhinitis, conjunctivitis or asthma related to animal dander or in the case of cats, saliva.

Diet History. Patients should be asked whether their skin disease flares with any given food. Sometimes urticaria or even atopic dermatitis in infants may be clearly related to ingestion. In addition, one should inquire about unusual diets or eating disorders. Many patients suspect that diet is responsible for their skin disease, so a few simple questions offer a chance to reassure them.

Seasonal Variation. Some disorders, such as polymorphic light eruption and other photosensitive disorders, have a typical seasonal pattern, flaring in the spring and summer. Lupus erythematosus may severely flare following intensive sun exposure during a holiday. Miliaria or heat rash is a disease of sweaty summer months. In contrast, pernio or frostbite is obviously more likely in the winter. Yet other diseases, perhaps because they are triggered by infectious agents, seem more common in spring and fall; one example is pityriasis rosea.

Association with Menses/Pregnancy. Both acne and herpes simplex may flare just before the menses. Some patients may take pain medication during this period and thus have recurrent drug-induced exanthems or even fixed drug reactions.

Other diseases, such as melasma, often start or worsen during pregnancy, as do the extremely rare disorders of pregnancy, such as herpes gestationis. In addition, it is crucial to know whether a patient is pregnant or nursing before prescribing medications such as the systemic retinoids or tetracycline.

Past History

A history of flexural dermatitis as a child supports the adult diagnosis of atopic dermatitis. Patients who have had chicken pox, measles or other viral exanthems are extremely unlikely to develop them a second time, unless they are severely immunosuppressed. A variety of systemic disorders may be reflected in the skin, as will become clear throughout this book. Sometimes, the cutaneous changes point the way towards systemic disease; for example, a patient with xanthomas should be evaluated for lipid abnormalities. Similarly, the new onset of acanthosis nigricans in an adult strongly suggests an internal carcinoma. Surely a patient with cutaneous lupus erythematosus should be evaluated for systemic disease. Finally, one needs to know about other systemic problems of the patient; a history of breast cancer instantly changes the differential diagnosis for a scalp nodule in a middle-aged female.

History of Present Illness

The time course of a skin problem is useful in making the diagnosis. If a solitary lesion is present, one should establish whether it was present at birth, and if not, when it appeared and how it has changed. When dealing with a dermatitis, once again the physician needs to know whether the skin changes appeared suddenly or gradually, and whether the patient has had previous problems. For example, a diffuse pruritic macular exanthem is usually the result of a drug allergy or viral infection. Sunburn, allergic or irritant contact dermatitis and impetigo are also usually of acute onset. Tinea pedis, seborrheic dermatitis or major systemic disorders such as sarcoidosis or lupus erythematosus tend to be chronic.

The subjective symptoms are also helpful. The classic cutaneous complaint is pruritus. Some diseases almost always itch, such as scabies. Others rarely itch, such as pityriasis rosea, and yet others, such as syphilis, never itch. How the patient responds to the pruritus also offers clues to the diagnosis: atopic dermatitis is usually scratched, lichen planus rubbed, and scabies picked at or excoriated.

Medication History

A history of drug allergies should be documented in the patient record, for both medical and medicolegal reasons. Patients should be questioned about all medications, including over-the-counter products. All too often an agent such as a laxative, pain reliever or tranquilizer is not considered a medication by the patient. Obviously, one takes a longer medication history in a 70-year-old patient with an unclear exanthem than in a teenager with acne, but even in the latter case one may unearth a history of corticosteroid use, anabolic hormone abuse for bodybuilding or excessive iodine ingestion. Similarly, topical products such as sunburn remedies are often responsible for allergic contact dermatitis, although the patient considers them harmless. In complex cases, the patient should be asked to bring all medications to the next visit.

The next step is to inquire in detail how the current cutaneous disorder has been treated – what has worked and what has not. One should profit from the efforts of the previously consulted physicians. Sometimes the cutaneous picture is so altered by therapy that one must stop everything and reevaluate the patient a few days later. In addition the past treatment may interfere with diagnostic evaluation. For example, a fungal culture may be negative if the suspected lesion has been recently treated with an antifungal agent. Similarly, antibiotics may interfere with cultures or serologic tests.

Physical Examination

It is wisest to examine the entire skin of every new patient, and sporadically to reexamine the entire skin of long-standing patients. In practice, this usually translates to offering a complete examination to each patient. Acne patients may not want to be entirely examined, or a patient with a single wart on the hand may find the request to disrobe absurd. But one should make the offer, for a complete examination may produce a variety of clues and serves as effective skin cancer screening, especially for dysplastic nevi and malignant melanomas. If a patient refuses a complete examination, it is wise to document this fact. A total examination should include the hair, nails, mouth, genitalia, anal region and the feet, including between the toes. Often a lesion on the forearm, which the patient offers for view, may be nondiagnostic, while typical pityriasis rosea is seen on the back or classic lichen planus found in the mouth.

In cases where systemic complaints are present, a complete or modified general physical examination may be needed.

Localization of Diseases

Both structural and functional variations in the skin may be responsible for localization of various disease processes.

Scalp. Not surprisingly, most disorders of hair are seen on the scalp. However, many inflammatory dermatoses involve the scalp and scalp hairs but spare hairs in other areas.

Sebaceous Regions. The face, upper aspect of the chest and back are rich in hair follicles with large sebaceous glands and relatively small hairs. Acne vulgaris is limited almost exclusively to these areas.

Palms and Soles. The palms and soles are rich in eccrine sweat glands and have a thick protective stratum corneum. Dyshidrotic dermatitis occurs only at these sites. Disorders that involve hair follicles never appear.

Apocrine Regions. The axillae and groin are rich in apocrine glands. Hidradenitis suppurativa has been classically described as an apocrine infection but appears to be a variant of acne known as acne inversa starting in the hair follicles. While it is limited to the apocrine regions, the glands themselves are innocent bystanders.

Intertriginous Regions. Areas where skin touches skin, such as in the groin, under pendulous breasts or in fatty abdominal folds, are inevitably moist and somewhat macerated. This change is known as intertrigo. Such regions are particularly predisposed to infections by *Candida albicans* and dermatophytes. In addition, papillomatous changes are common here, be it skin tags or warty changes in pemphigus vegetans.

Mucosal Surfaces. Some diseases, such as pemphigus vulgaris, often involve mucosal surfaces; other not too dissimilar disorders, such as dermatitis herpetiformis, rarely do. The transitional zone between skin and mucosa is a common site for herpes simplex, erythema multiforme and fixed drug eruptions.

Dry Versus Oily Skin. European dermatologists attach considerable importance to whether a patient has sebostasis (reduced sebum flow and thus dry skin) or seborrhea (increased sebum flow and thus oily skin). Many Americans feel that the connection between sebum output and dry or oily skin is less well defined. In any event, all agree that patients with atopic dermatitis are likely to have dry skin. The oily skin seen in acne represents increased sebum flow. The skin type is crucial when choosing topical medications; a patient with dry skin will not tolerate a drying solution, and a patient with oily skin will reject a thick ointment.

Peripheral Circulation. Patients, especially smokers, who have continuously cold clammy feet may be more likely to have warts or tinea pedis. They clearly are at greater risk for cold injury, such as pernio and Raynaud phenomenon, and for complications if affected with systemic sclerosis.

Types of Skin Lesions

The entire patient should first be viewed from a distance; their facies, habitus and general condition should be assessed. The pattern of distribution of the individual skin lesions can also be viewed; asymmetric involvement suggests exogenous causes, while a symmetric pattern speaks for a systemic problem. A widespread cutaneous eruption is described as an exanthem; when mucosal surfaces are involved, one speaks of an enanthem. Both are composed of individual lesions, often localized to specific areas or arranged in definite patterns. The combination of lesion type, localization and pattern usually allows the dermatologist to make a working or specific diagnosis. The size of an individual lesion should be documented in millimeters or centimeters, as discussed below.

Lesion analysis is one of the true specialties of the dermatologist. It initially appears befuddling to the student, but the ability to precisely describe and document lesions has two essential roles: it allows dermatologists to communicate precisely with one another and with other colleagues, and it often makes the diagnostic process more precise. One traditionally speaks of primary and secondary lesions. In principle, a primary lesion such as a papule may over time develop a crust or heal with a scar; the latter are secondary lesions. This distinction is somewhat artificial, however, as a burn may evolve into a blister (a primary lesion) or a patient may create an excoriation (a secondary lesion) primarily.

In addition, as crucial as the language of lesions is, one should choose normal English in preference to misusing "lesion talk". For example, if a patient presents with a flat, irregularly bordered brown spot on the cheek, one should use the term macule when describing the lesion. If one is unsure of the correct lesion designation, it is better to say flat spot, which will be understood by all.

Macule

A macule is a flat circumscribed lesion. In other words, it represents a change in skin color (Fig. 1.1). A macule cannot be identified by mere touch. The macule may have a sharp or indistinct border; it should be described based on its measured size and color. In some systems, a macule is defined as less than 1.0 cm; a larger lesion is a patch. Using descriptions such as "the size of a silver dollar" or "ash-leaf macule" is colorful, but often confusing. Causes for changes in cutaneous color, summarized in Table 1.1, include the following.

Table 1.1. Macules and patches: color changes at skin level and their causes

Color	Cause
Red	Hyperemia (erythema) Extravasation of blood (purpura) Telangiectasia
Blue	Cyanosis Hematoma (older or deeper extravasation) Melanin in the dermis
Brown	Melanin Hemosiderin
White	Absence of melanin (depigmentation) Reduced melanin (hypopigmentation) Anemia Vascular spasm Pseudoleukoderma (surrounding skin is darker, as in psoriasis treated with anthralin)
Orange	Carotene
Yellow	Lipids Bile pigments Excess or damaged dermal elastic tissue
Gray, black	Melanin Arsenic Silver Mercury Dirt, coal dust, gunpowder, metal fragments, pencil lead, tar Anthralin Amiodarone
Mixed colors	Tattoos

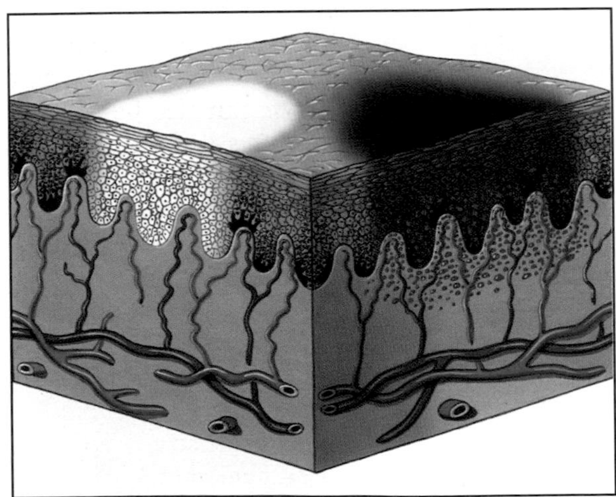

Fig. 1.1. Macules. On the *left* is a hypopigmented macule lacking melanin, as might be seen in vitiligo, while on the *right* the macule is hyperpigmented with excess melanin, as seen in a freckle

Exogenous Pigment. Decorative tattoos, accidental tattoos (pencil lead, gunpowder), externally applied medications (silver nitrate, potassium permanganate) and systemic medications (silver, gold, antimalarials, amiodarone) may all discolor the skin.

Endogenous Pigment. Hemosiderin, bile pigments, lipids and carotene (which could also be considered exogenous) may be deposited.

Extravasation of Blood. Deep extravasations of blood tend to be blue; more superficial ones, red. The color shifts from red to blue-red to yellow-brown as hemoglobin is converted to hemosiderin.

When pressure is applied with a transparent glass or plastic spatula (diascopy) extravasated blood does not disappear, while that in a vessel does.

Purpura is a general term used when widespread areas, such as both legs, are marked by diffuse extravasation of blood. Tiny lesions are designated petechiae; larger ones, suggillations (a rarely used term); and yet larger, ecchymoses. Hematoma refers to more extensive bleeding in the skin or subcutaneous tissue producing a painful, palpable mass.

Melanin. When excess melanin is present, one speaks of hyperpigmentation; reduced melanin is described as hypopigmentation and total absence of melanin (such as in vitiligo) as depigmentation. Leukoderma is another term for secondary hypopigmentation. Pseudoleukoderma refers to a spot that has a lighter color but not less pigment. Vascular anomalies can cause focal blanching. The surrounding skin can be darker, for example following sun exposure or treatment with tar products.

Lupoid Infiltrate. Accumulation of inflammatory granulomas in the dermis may produce an apple-jelly color, when examined with diascopy. While this phenomenon is typical for lupus vulgaris, hence its name, it also occurs in lupoid rosacea, sarcoidosis and lymphocytic infiltrates. In general, the lesions are palpable, but early lesions may be macular and still have the characteristic color change.

Active Hyperemia or Vasodilatation. Increased blood flow produces a red color (erythema) and warmth. This color disappears with diascopy. Acute inflammation, such as a viral exanthem or erysipelas, may cause erythema. In addition, a physiologic increase in blood flow, such as in blushing, also produces erythema and warmth.

Passive Hyperemia or Venous Congestion. Cyanosis, or a blue coloration, occurs in areas with decreased venous blood flow. Cyanotic areas are cold and also disappear with diascopic pressure. Typical causes of cyanosis include simply a physiologic response to cold. Cyanosis is most common on the legs. Sometimes the same disease process will appear erythematous on the trunk and cyanotic on the feet.

Arterial Vasoconstriction. Absence of blood produces a white color and cold skin. An interesting example is nevus anemicus, an area of structurally normal skin with persistent vasoconstriction. Vessel spasm may produce similar changes, following cold injury or emboli.

Urticaria

Urticaria or hives are both a type of lesion and a disease diagnosis. In German, the terminology is less confusing as *Urtica* (plural *Urticae*) refers to the individual lesion, while the disease state is *Urticaria*. The only use of the word *Urtica* in English is as the genus name for the stinging nettle plants that cause urticaria. The lesions, also known as wheals, arise when fluid escapes from a blood vessel, causing localized edema or swelling. Thus they are sharply circumscribed, raised, highly pruritic transitory lesions (Fig. 1.2). By definition, individual hives last less than 24 h as the edema fluid is resorbed. More persistent lesions suggest the diagnosis of urticarial vasculitis. This is not to say that an attack of hives usually lasts less than 24 h. The vascular dilatation can produce erythema, or the swelling can compress the capillaries producing a white lesion. Hives range in size from tiny 2- to 5-mm lesions of cholinergic urticaria through typical wheals several centimeters in diameter to much larger lesions. Typically hives are not scratched, just rubbed.

Angioedema is similar to urticaria but develops in the subcutaneous tissues. Thus instead of wheals there is simply massive swelling, as seen in angioneurotic edema. Rapid resolution is also the rule. Seropapules are another urticarial variant, seen

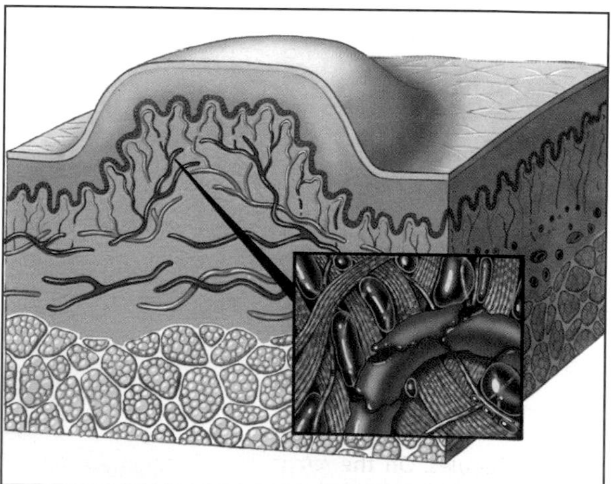

Fig. 1.2. Hive with dilated leaking vessels; the resulting edema causes surface blanching with an inflammatory halo

in insect-bite reactions, cholinergic urticaria and prurigo. They consist of a small urticarial lesion with a central vesicle. The edema is so superficial and localized that it produces a tiny blister.

Papule, Nodule, and Plaque

These are raised nontransitory lesions that are produced by epidermal, dermal or combined changes. They are distinguished by their size.

Papule. An elevated lesion less than 1.0 cm in diameter (Fig. 1.3). An epidermal papule results from epidermal thickening or hyperkeratosis, as in a wart. A dermal papule is produced by changes in the dermis, either through increased collagen production (connective tissue nevus), a cellular infiltrate, or proliferation of adnexal elements (syringoma), vessels (hemangioma), neural tissues (neurofibroma) or melanocytes (melanocytic nevus). A mixed papule combines dermal and epidermal changes; one example is hypertrophic lichen planus. In some systems, "papule" refers only to inflammatory or reactive processes that are capable of resolution. When abnormal structures are present, as in a hemangioma, one can also speak of a papular tumor.

Nodule. An elevated lesion greater than 1.0 cm in diameter. Sometimes nodules are also referred to as tumors, but tumor is imprecise and usually suggests malignancy to the patient. Nodules can be inflammatory, as in rheumatoid nodule, but often represent proliferations of the same elements discussed under papules (Fig. 1.4).

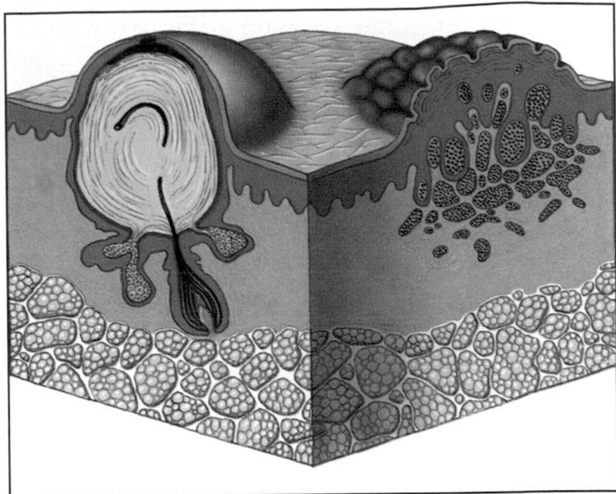

Fig. 1.4. Nodules. On the *left* is an epidermoid cyst centered around a hair follicle, while on the *right* the mass of the lesion is contributed by a proliferation of melanocytes

Plaque. A flat-topped nodule. In the western USA, it suffices to call a plaque a mesa, a flat-topped mountain. Plaques usually result from diffuse dermal accumulations, as in mycosis fungoides. Even more diffuse areas are simply described as infiltrations.

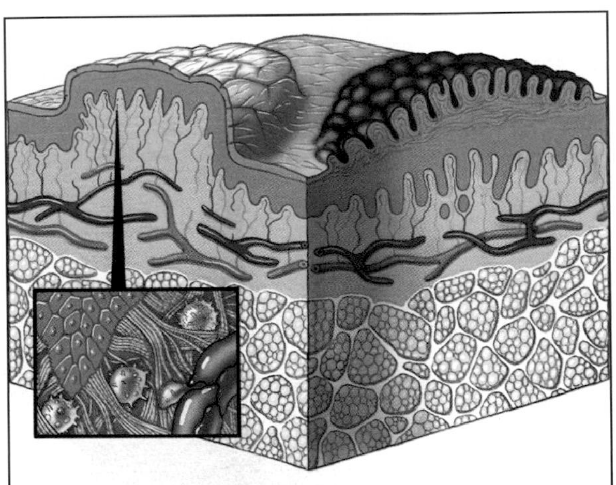

Fig. 1.3. Papules. On the *left* is an inflammatory dermal papule, as might be seen in lichen planus, while on the *right* the change in elevation is caused by epidermal proliferation, as seen in an epidermal nevus

Lichenification

Grouped papules associated with exaggerated skin markings and thickening that result from chronic rubbing and scratching of an inflammatory dermatosis such with lichen planus or atopic dermatitis (Fig. 1.5).

Several older terms also refer to nodules. They include phyma, which usually describes a protuberance in rosacea and tuber, which in older systems described a papule that was likely to ulcerate and scar, as in some forms of syphilis or tuberculosis.

Blister

Blisters are fluid-filled lesions. Vesicles are less than 1.0 cm in diameter, while bullae are larger. Blisters can be subdivided in a number of ways.

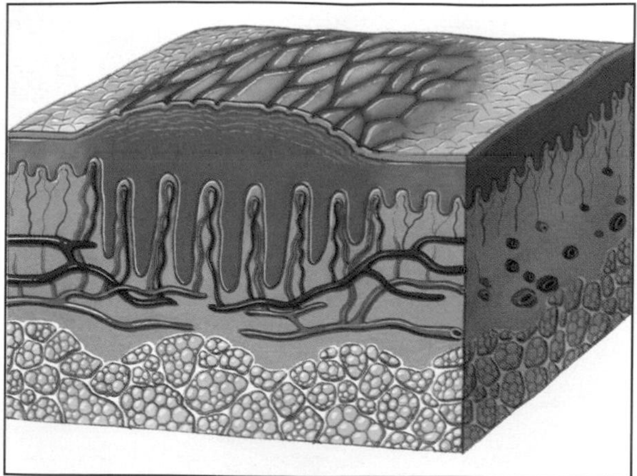

Fig. 1.5. Lichenification with prominent epidermal skin markings, acanthosis or thickening of the epidermis and increased vascularity in the dermal papillae

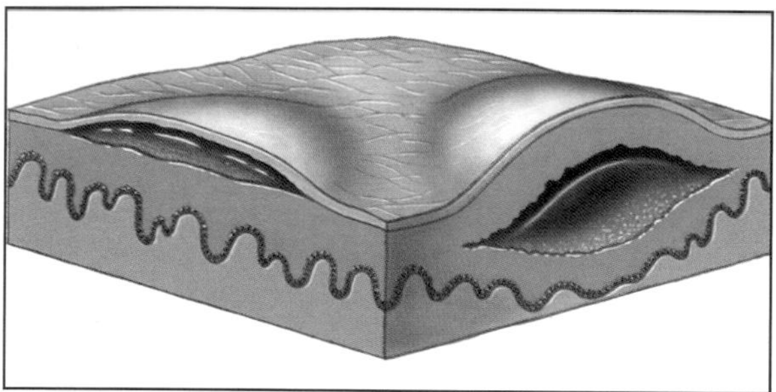

Fig. 1.6. Intraepidermal blisters. On the *left* the lesion is subcorneal, while on the *right* it is somewhat deeper

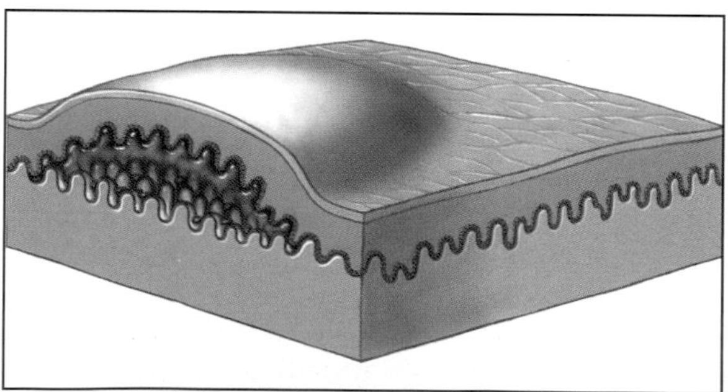

Fig. 1.7. Subepidermal blister

Location. Blisters can be subcorneal (impetigo), intraepidermal (pemphigus vulgaris), subepidermal (bullous pemphigoid) or dermal (dystrophic epidermolysis bullosa) (Figs. 1.6, 1.7).

Contents. Blisters may contain fluid (spongiotic dermatitis, pemphigus vulgaris), pus (impetigo) or blood (bullous pemphigoid).

Pathogenesis. The epidermal cells can come apart because of intracellular edema (balloon degeneration in herpes simplex), intercellular edema (spongiosis in an acute contact dermatitis) or acantholysis (dissolution of intercellular adhesion structures as in pemphigus vulgaris). Subepidermal blisters can develop because of changes in the basal keratinocytes (lichen planus), alterations in the epidermal-dermal junction (bullous pemphigoid) or in the upper dermis (epidermolysis bullosa acquisita).

Etiology. Many factors can produce blisters, including genetic defects (epidermolysis bullosa group), immunologic phenomena (pemphigus vulgaris, bullous pemphigoid), physical damage (sunburn or mechanical pressure, e.g., following a long hike), chemical damage (caustic burn), infections (impetigo, herpes simplex) and still unexplained factors (bullous lichen sclerosus et atrophicus).

Pustule

A pustule is a blister filled with pus. While pustules are most often associated with an infection, such as impetigo or folliculitis (Fig. 1.8), they can contain nonpyogenic bacteria, as in acne, or be sterile, as in pustular psoriasis. Often, vesicles and bullae evolve into pustules. At other times pustules are primary; once again, pustular psoriasis is an example. The secondary infection of inflammatory dermatoses such as atopic dermatitis is known as impetiginization. Here, too, pustules may be seen, especially at the border of the lesion.

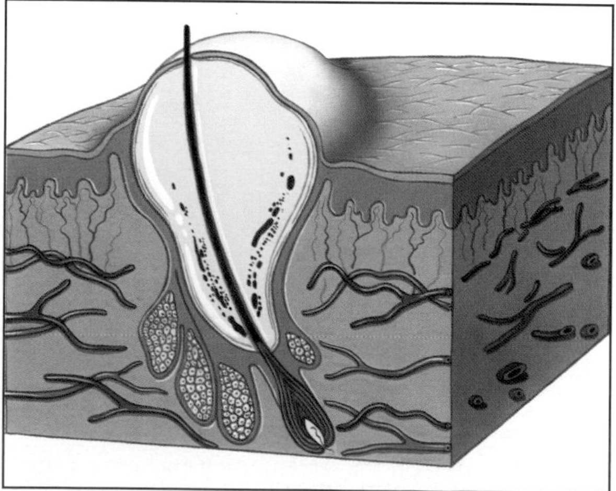

Fig. 1.8. Pustule involving hair follicle, clinically known as folliculitis

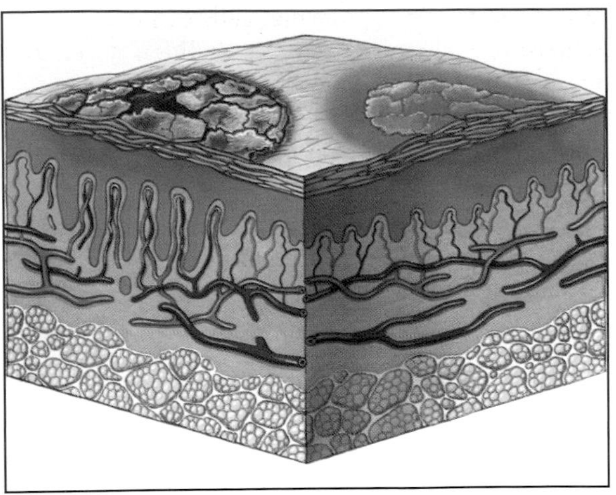

Fig. 1.9. Scales. On the *left* is psoriasiform scale with epidermal thickening and prominent dermal vessels, while on the *right* is more pityriasiform change with central scales, peripheral erythema and few deeper changes. In both situations the stratum corneum is less cohesive than normal

Scale

Scales are cornified epithelial cells often mixed with serum, bacteria, extravasated white or red blood cells and other debris (Fig. 1.9). Every person loses innumerable scales daily; dandruff, for example, is the shedding of scales from the scalp. A single corneocyte is invisible to the naked eye; conglomerations of approximately 20–50 corneocytes make up a scale that is barely visible.

Some diseases are distinguished by certain types of scaling:

- Pityriasiform: fine, bran-like (dandruff)
- Psoriasiform: white, noncoherent (psoriasis)
- Ichthyosiform: large, discrete (ichthyosis)
- Exfoliative: widespread, large (following scarlet fever)
- Collarette: scales surround lesion (pityriasis rosea)

These scale types overlap to a great extent. Scales may be mixed with blood or pus; this produces is a crust.

Keratosis

Keratosis is a generic term for any attached adherent mass of keratin, known as a *Horn* in German. Typical examples include genetic disorders (palmoplantar keratoderma), viral infections (warts), sun-damaged skin (actinic keratosis) and disorders of unknown etiology (seborrheic keratosis). Some keratoses are limited to follicular openings. These are distinguished by their small size and pattern of distribution; the most common example is keratosis pilaris.

Erosion, Ulcer and Wound

These terms refer to different types of tissue loss, varying in their depth and breadth.

Erosion. Superficial loss of tissue, much wider than it is deep (Fig. 1.10). An erosion affects primarily the epidermis, so it heals without scarring. Typical causes include maceration, friction, rupture of a blister or pustule and mild sunburn or second-degree burn.

Ulcer. A larger defect, involving the dermis or subcutaneous tissues, and often deeper than it is wide (Fig. 1.10). It develops in damaged skin (such as in areas of chronic venous insufficiency), is slow to heal, and leaves a scar. There are many causes, including more extensive external damage (X-rays, third-degree burns, frostbite, chemical injuries), deep infections (ecthyma), inadequate tissue blood supply, pressure (decubitus ulcer) or simply necrotic tissue (known in German as *Schorf*) associated with a granulomatous or malignant process.

Ulcers heal from the edge by growth of epithelial elements and from the base through the formation of granulation tissue. The final scar lacks some ap-

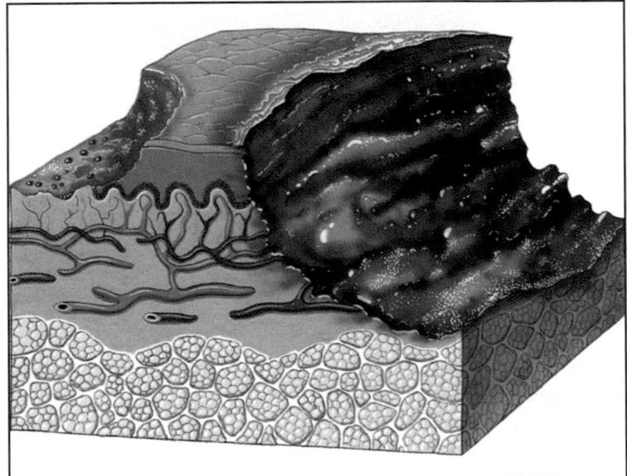

Fig. 1.10. Tissue destruction. On the *left* is an erosion involving just the epidermis, while on the *right* is a more extensive ulcer extending in areas into the subcutaneous fat

pendageal structures, may be hypo- or hyperpigmented, and is usually depressed.

Ulcers can be subdivided clinically to some extent, aiding in the differential diagnosis:

- Location and number
- Size, depth and shape (round, oval, irregular: it is always wise to measure an ulcer in order to be able to document its course)
- Base (granulation tissue, pus, exposed structures)
- Margins (undermined, sharply defined)
- Nature of adjacent skin (indurated, inflamed, signs of chronic venous insufficiency, normal)

Wound. Traumatic defect in normal skin, as produced by an injury or operation. Wounds also heal more rapidly and generally with less scarring than ulcers.

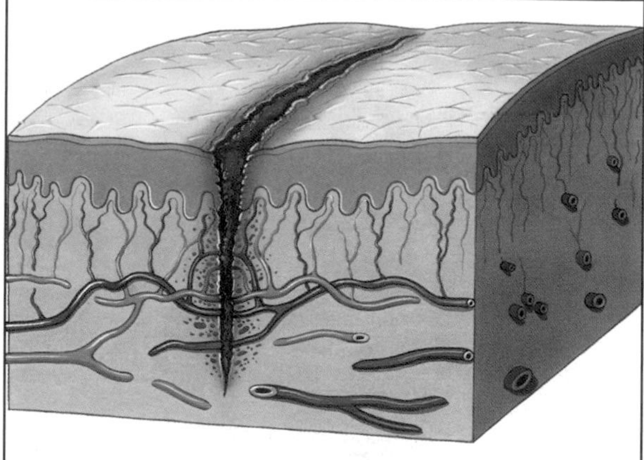

Fig. 1.11. Fissure

Excoriation, Rhagade and Fissure

These terms also describe special types of tissue loss with unique configurations:

Excoriation. A small superficial defect, involving the epidermis and papillary dermis. It results from localized trauma through picking or scratching, such as seen in acne excoriée.

Rhagade. A superficial linear crack or tear, radiating out from a skin fold, such as at the corner of the mouth, in the perianal region, between the fingers or coursing through a callused heel.

Fissure. A deep linear lesion – in essence a deep rhagade. Fissures most commonly radiate from circular structures, such as perianal fissures (Fig. 1.11).

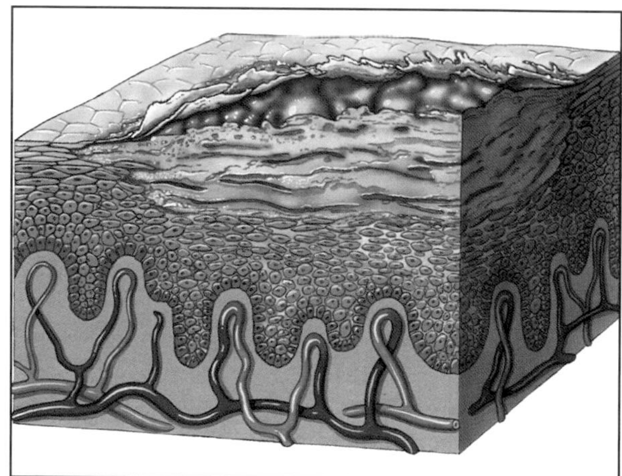

Fig. 1.12. Crust with loss of epidermis coupled with accumulation of pus and scales

Crust

“Crust” is the elegant term for what every patient calls a scab (Fig. 1.12). Crusts develop as a pustule dries out or as an excoriation or ulcer heals. Depending on the fluid present, the crusts may vary: serum yields a relatively clear crust (superficial erosion or superficial basal cell carcinoma); blood, a dark-red to black hemorrhagic crust (bullous pemphigoid, erythema multiforme on the vermilion); and pus, a honey-colored or yellow crust (impetigo). Extremely thick crusts are described as rupial, as in rupial psoriasis. Sometimes crusts must be softened by soaking and keratolytic agents; only then can the underlying lesion be evaluated. Since a basal cell carcinoma is often covered by crust as it becomes larger, it is essential to determine what lies at the base of every crust, either through examination or biopsy.

Necrosis goes under a variety of names, including mummification when the tissue is dry and gangrene when it remains moist. Most necrotic tissue is dark. Causes of necrosis include impaired blood supply and exogenous trauma, such as burn or frostbite.

Scar

Scars are permanent skin changes that result when a defect heals (Fig. 1.13). They lack the normal skin

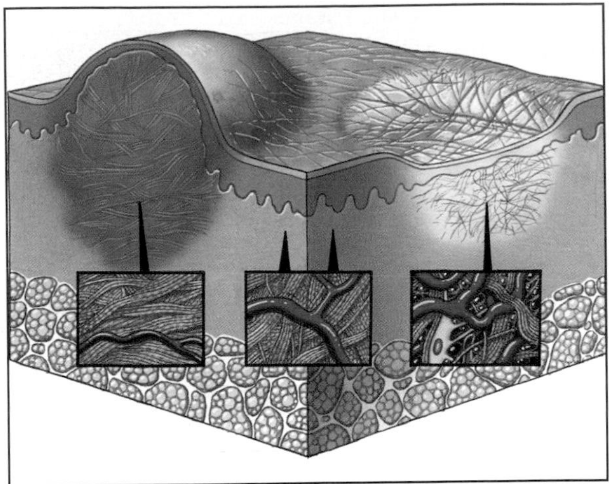

Fig. 1.13. Scars. On the *left* is a hypertrophic scar with increased dermal collagen, while on the *right* is an atrophic scar with prominent vessels. The central *insert* shows normal dermis

markings. Initially scars are red but after many years they may become skin-colored, hypo- or hyperpigmented. Scars may be perfectly flat and smooth (e.g. following a totally successful surgical procedure), but usually they are either depressed (atrophic, as when ulcers heal) or elevated (hypertrophic scars and keloids). Histologically most appendageal structures are absent. The collagen fibers are arranged parallel to the skin surface rather than interdigitating. Elastic fibers are reduced to absent. Increased numbers of vessels may be seen, especially in new scars. Scars represent the end of a process and generally offer few clues as to their origin. There are some exceptions. Acne scars, for example, typically involve the face, chest and back in a distinctive pattern. Chicken pox scars are typically small and depressed. Those of zoster are arranged in a dermatomal pattern. Scars with communicating sinuses usually suggested acne inversa or a chronic infection.

Atrophy and Poikiloderma

Atrophy. Thinning of the skin, including both epidermis and dermis. Vessels can often be visualized through atrophic skin. Probably the best known atrophy is the thin skin on the back of the hands in elderly patients. Some atrophic skin is slack, so that is can be pinched together or rolled about; such skin is described as cigarette paper-like. Such slack atrophy is epitomized by acrodermatitis chronica atrophicans. Other atrophic skin may be shiny, lack surface markings and be tightly bound to underlying structures; such changes are seen for example in systemic sclerosis.

Poikiloderma. Combination of atrophy, hyper- and hypopigmentation and telangiectases. The prototype is chronic radiation damage, but there are congenital poikilodermas and mycosis fungoides may present with poikiloderma.

Pseudoatrophy. Skin that clinically appears wrinkled and thinned, but histologically is normal. The most common example is the early lesions of some types of parapsoriasis.

Hypertrophy or Thickened Skin

There is no one single acceptable term for the opposite of atrophy; neither of the above terms is correct. Technically hypertrophy means a homogeneous overgrowth of a normal structure, such as hypertrophied muscles in an athlete; it is impossible to manipulate the skin to produce hypertrophy of the epidermis or dermis. When the skin is thickened, it may be a result of scar formation, fibrosis (which also lacks specificity and usually means a scar), sclerosis (which suggests increased collagen, often associated with epidermal atrophy), accumulation of fluid (chronic venous insufficiency), deposition of material (amyloidosis) or any of many other processes. Epidermal changes, such as lichenification, also cause thickening of skin. Pachyderma refers to a thickened dermis associated with reactive epidermal changes, as is seen in extreme variants of chronic venous insufficiency and in some congenital disorders. In sum, there is no single unified way to describe either an increase or a decrease in skin thickness.

Distribution of Lesions

In addition to identifying individual lesions, one must pay attention to how they are dispersed on the skin.

Distribution. Lesions may be confined to a small area, be widespread or disseminated, or be diffuse, involving wide areas with no intervening normal skin. Chicken pox, for example, is disseminated, while erysipelas is diffuse.

Arrangement. Solitary or circumscript lesions are single lesions. Multiple lesions can be grouped or randomly arranged. Grouped lesions may be arranged in a linear fashion, such as an epidermal nevus, or a segmental pattern, such as zoster confined to a dermatome. Some lesions, typically pityriasis rosea, follows the skin creases or folds, especially on the trunk (Christmas tree pattern). Grouped blisters are described as herpetiform, because of the characteristic pattern of herpes simplex.

Some lesions are arranged in peculiar swirls and stripes such as the pigmentary changes in incontinentia pigmenti; such changes are usually the result of mosaicism in the skin reflecting migration of different cell populations during development. This pattern is known as Blaschko lines and is discussed further below. Less often a linear distribution may reflect underlying vascular and nervous patterns. Follicular lesions are limited to the follicle openings, so that have a typical arrangement and are not seen on nonhairy surfaces.

Size. Many nonmedical terms are used to describe lesion size, e.g., foodstuffs (barley, pea, walnut, hazelnut) to coins (nickel, dime, quarter; *Pfennig, Mark*). Such terms are inexact and do not cross cultural lines well. Individual lesions, such as pigmented lesions or ulcers, should be measured and their size expressed in millimeters or centimeters. When describing a basal cell carcinoma, malignant melanoma or leg ulcer, two perpendicular diameters are given, one representing the maximum lesion size. The size is essential for planning treatment, following the disease course, and, in many countries, for billing purposes.

Margins. The border of a lesion is either sharp or indistinct. A burn has a sharp exact margin; a patch of atopic dermatitis does not. Scale at the margin may suggest a fungal infection; scale just central to the margin (collarette or inward-pointing scale) suggests pityriasis rosea or erythema annulare centrifugum. A ring-like margin is typical for porokeratosis. A boggy, inflamed, often undermined margin is one hallmark of pyoderma gangrenosum.

Shape. Most lesions are round or oval, as presumably whatever is triggering the disease spreads out radially from its initial site of action. Annular or circular lesions result from a peripheral spread associated with central healing (granuloma annulare). Multiple such stages can produce target or iris lesions, as seen in erythema multiforme. Intersecting incomplete rings produce gyrate (flowing curved lines) or serpiginous (wavy or snake-like) patterns, such as in tinea corporis or psoriasis. Many small circular lesions coming together are described as polycyclic.

The Skin and Systemic Disorders

Disorders Confined to the Skin. One of the attractions of dermatology is that many lesions can be identified by physical examination without additional evaluation of the patient. For example, if a patient has a wart on the finger, one can proceed to treatment, although we favor offering a general skin evaluation at the first visit.

Systemic Disorders Involving the Skin. Many diseases, particularly the connective tissue disorders, involve the skin and other organs simultaneously. Examples include lupus erythematosus with renal disease and photosensitivity or dermatomyositis with muscle weakness and poikiloderma. Similarly, malignant lymphomas may involve the skin and lymph nodes, or a metastatic malignant melanoma may be found almost anywhere. Such patients are best followed together by dermatologists and internists.

Skin Diseases as Signs of Systemic Diseases. This category differs only in degree from that discussed above. Often cutaneous findings suggest an underlying disorder that has not been diagnosed. Here the dermatologist is obliged to either pursue the systemic problem or refer the patient to another physician. Examples include xanthomas as a sign of serum lipid abnormalities and necrobiosis lipoidica diabeticorum as a marker of diabetes mellitus. Many metastatic tumors appear in the skin and are identified by the dermatologist. On the bright side, patients can be identified who are at risk of internal malignancies but who can be treated prior to developing frank tumors (Gardner syndrome and many other paraneoplastic syndromes).

Systemic Manifestations of Cutaneous Disease. This aspect of dermatology is often overlooked. Patients with widespread cutaneous disease, such as erythroderma or widespread blistering diseases, have electrolyte disturbances, become hypothermic, lose proteins through both their skin and gastrointestinal system and suffer many other problems. In a similar vein, some dermatologic medications cause significant systemic problems. The main offenders are corticosteroids; when one uses systemic corticosteroids, one usually anticipates the problems of fluid retention, gastric distress and hypertension, to name but a few; patients using excessive amounts of topical corticosteroids can also have systemic problems that may be overlooked.

We will expand on all of these topics when we deal with individual diseases. Our intention here is to highlight the numerous interactions between dermatology and other medical specialties and to encourage readers view our specialty as an interactive one, rather than a dead end where only skin problems are treated without regard for the entire patient.

Quality of Life Measurements

Many other specialties have long used quality of life measurements to document how disabling a given disorder is or how much suffering it causes. Examples include cardiac, orthopedic and mental illness rating scales. Dermatologists have been slow to adopt such measurements, even though it has long been clear that many skin disorders severely hamper the quality of life of the individuals they affect. A variety of rating systems are now available that can document just how disabling diseases such as psoriasis, atopic dermatitis, ichthyosis, epidermolysis bullosa and acne can be.

Diagnostic Tests

A wide variety of tests may be employed to expand the dermatologic diagnosis. In Germany, most of these tests are carried out in dermatology clinics or departments; in the USA, other specialties have to some extent taken them over. Useful procedures include the following:

- Patch tests are essential for diagnosing allergic contact dermatitis, while photopatch testing is used to study patients with photosensitivity disorders.
- Allergy or prick tests are useful for evaluating patients with atopic dermatitis and essential if the patient has seasonal rhinitis; they can be combined with RAST or other in vitro identification of allergens or antibodies.
- Routine microscopic procedures. Almost every dermatologist performs KOH examination to identify fungi, hair mounts to study structural abnormalities, scrapings for scabies and similar procedures.
- Dark-field examination can be performed to identify *Treponema pallidum* in moist lesions of primary and secondary syphilis. In a dark-field microscope the ordinary condenser is exchanged for a special dark-field condenser. The microscope is not otherwise changed. The principle is that only the light rays that are bent by the object under observation are seen. Thus the spirochetes are white on a dark background and can be seen to move in their spiral fashion. Further details are givenin Chapter 5.
- Histopathologic evaluation of skin specimens, including routine histology, immunofluorescent microscopy, immunohistochemistry and electron microscopy. Immunofluorescent microscopy is essential for diagnosing the bullous diseases and is applied in many other settings. Transmission electron microscopy was formerly essential in tumor diagnosis but today has been replaced to a great extent by monoclonal antibody techniques. Identification of the Birbeck granules in Langerhans cell histiocytosis or rapid identification of viral particles with shadowing techniques remains quite useful. Scanning electron microscopy is best suited to define structural hair shaft defects; it produces many intriguing almost three-dimensional pictures.
- Direct identification of organisms, ranging from bacteria to parasites, as well as mycological, viral and bacterial cultures.
- Serologic evaluation of infectious and autoimmune diseases.
- General clinical laboratory tests.
- Specialized clinical evaluation; most German clinics also have special expertise in angiology, proctology and andrology so that such patients need not be referred elsewhere.

A typical American dermatologic practice (if such a creature exists) probably only offers patch testing, routine microscopic evaluations, fungal cultures and perhaps histopathology. Recent federal regulations, notably the CLIA (Clinical Laboratory Improvement Act) have restricted even these simple services and added layers of bureaucracy. The "improvement" has proven hard to find.

Specialized Procedures

Dermatoscopy

The dermatoscope or skin-surface microscope allows the physician to examine the skin more closely. Another commonly employed term is epiluminescence microscopy, but this is technically not entirely correct as no luminescence is involved. The simplest and most widely used instrument is hand-held and monocular, resembling an otoscope. To reduce reflection from the stratum corneum, fluid, disinfectant solution or oil is applied to a glass disc in the front of the instrument. The examiner can then focus to magnify the skin up to 10-fold with the simple instrument. Higher magnifications are available with more elaborate equipment, including both larger optical systems and videoscopes with computer-enhanced images.

Dermatoscopy is most often used to analyze pigmented lesions; specific criteria are available in specialized textbooks and taught at seminars. The experienced physician can identify 90–95% of malignant melanomas with the dermatoscope, against a clinical diagnostic success rate of about 70–80%. In our clinics, dermatoscopic evaluation of suspicious pigmented lesions has become standard; insurance companies have gradually come to see the utility of this procedure and to offer reimbursement. In some instances one can estimate the tumor thickness, but preoperative ultrasonography is superior in this respect. The increased accuracy aids in planning the operative approach to a suspicious pigmented lesion. In addition, one can often totally exclude a malignant melanoma, when for example a vascular lesion or seborrheic keratosis is present, avoiding unnecessary procedures. The dermatoscope can also be employed to identify the scabies mite in its burrow, to recognize foreign objects, to examine the vascular pattern of the nail fold in connective tissue disorders and to evaluate nail pigmentation and hair-shaft anomalies (Figs. 1.14, 1.15). Patients like the dermatoscopic examination as it reassures them that their skin lesions are being studied in detail.

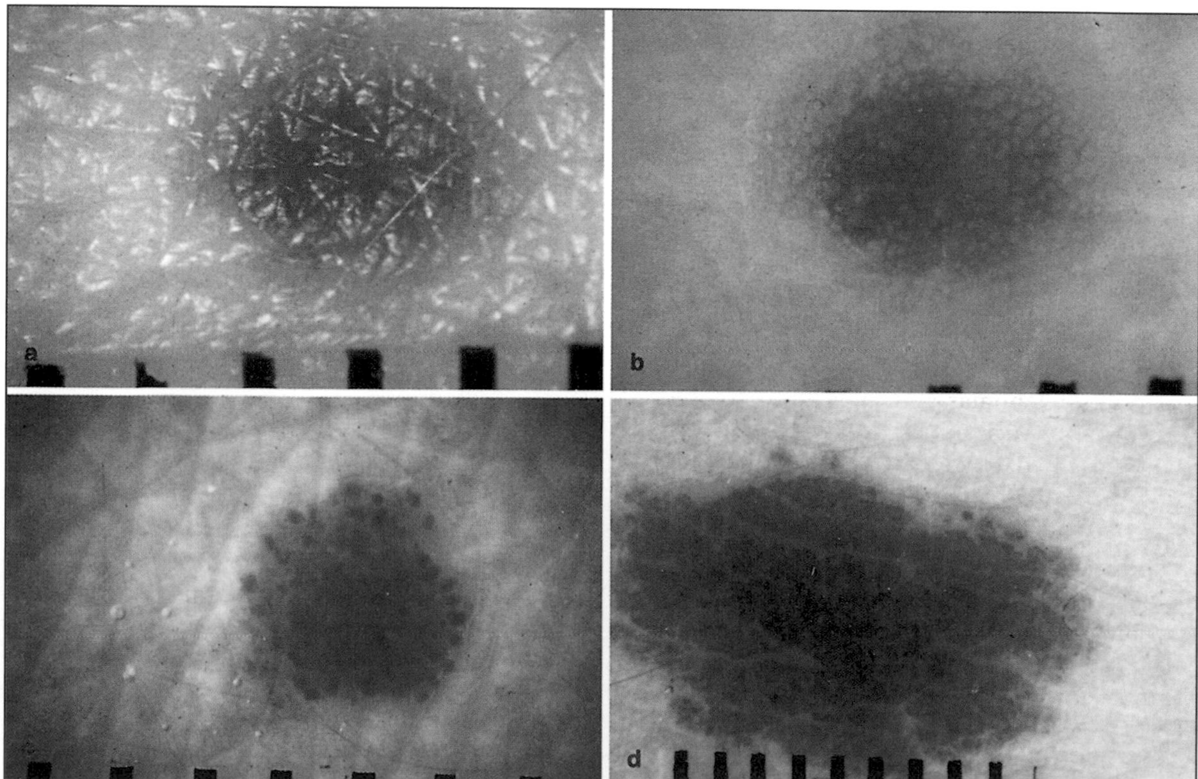

Fig. 1.14 a–d. Dermatoscopy. **a** Junctional nevus viewed without immersion oil; **b** same nevus under oil showing the reticular pattern; **c** compound nevus; **d** dermal nevus showing the uniform globular nature of the pigment

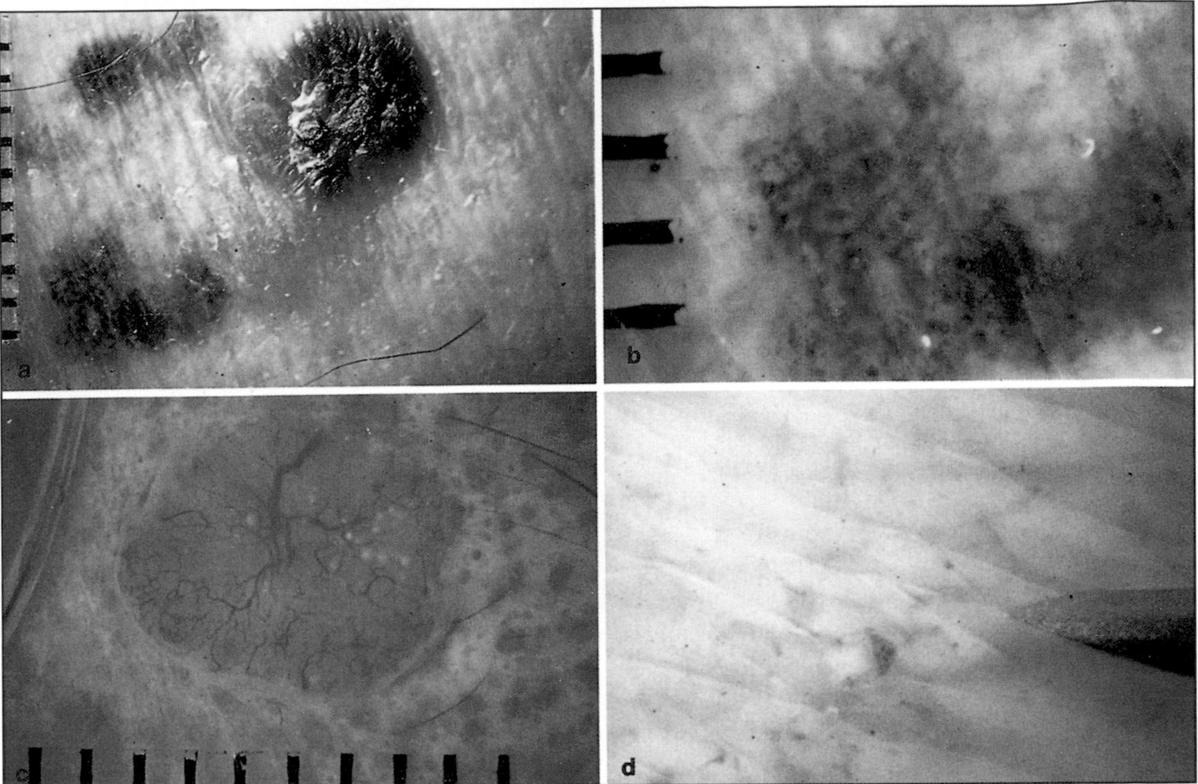

Fig. 1.15 a–d. Dermatoscopy. **a** Malignant melanoma with nodular areas and regression; **b** the same malignant melanoma under oil immersion showing the melanophages in the regression zone; **c** telangiectases in a basal cell carcinoma; **d** scabies mite at 60 × magnification, shown together with the tip of a needle

Ultrasonography

Ultrasound examination of the skin is usually accomplished with high-frequency 20-MHz units. These units can penetrate to about 2–3 mm and offer good resolution. Color-coded B-mode images are usually produced. In our clinics, ultrasound is used for preoperative assessment of the depth of malignant melanomas and other tumors. The resolution is not such that different types of tumors can be identified. In addition, the skin thickness in scleroderma can be quantified and used to follow the course of the disease or assess therapeutic measures. Skin thickness can also be measured to assess the effect of systemic or topical corticosteroids, which may cause skin atrophy.

Another standard use of ultrasonography involves the 7.5-MHz device, which penetrates about 50 mm and is routinely employed to search for lymph node involvement with malignant melanoma and other tumors. We routinely employ 7.5-MHz ultrasonography in the follow-up of patients with malignant melanoma, evaluating both the operative site and the appropriate regional lymph nodes. A variety of ultrasound techniques are also essential in assessing venous flow and function (Chap. 22). Continuous wave (CW) Doppler can assess the direction and speed of blood flow, while duplex sonography combines CW Doppler with a B-mode picture of the vessels. Longitudinal, diagonal and transverse sections of vessels can be obtained and the flow in individual vessels studied.

Photography

Clinical photographs have long been an essential part of dermatology, useful for teaching and documentation. For over two decades, varieties of whole-body photographs coupled with close-up views of individual lesions have been employed to follow up patients with multiple atypical melanocytic nevi. Today computerized storage of visual images has revolutionized this field. Routine clinical photographs can be conveniently stored in a personal computer and used to follow up a patient or to document operative procedures. Not only can multiple melanocytic nevi be more easily and conveniently documented, but programs are available to analyze the changes between two photographs of the same lesion to quantify alterations. Similarly, most dermatoscopic images today are both stored in a computer and subjected to some form of computerized analysis.

Other Physical Measuring Tools

An almost endless list of noninvasive devices designed to assist in measuring skin function have become relatively widely available in recent years. Most have personal computer interfaces so that data can be analyzed and stored efficiently. To cite but a few examples, the following parameters can be assessed: stratum corneum moisture, dermal elasticity, sebum flow, skin color (usually combining measurements of melanin and blood) and skin-surface evaporation rate. In addition, wrinkling can be measured by taking impressions of the skin with a variety of rubber and plastic materials and then analyzing the surface with a laser reading device. All such techniques are used primarily to evaluate the effects of drugs and cosmetics on normal or diseased skin.

Biopsy and Histopathologic Examination

Dermatologists have the opportunity to observe lesions macroscopically, then perform a skin biopsy and evaluate the lesion microscopically. Many prominent dermatologists have made major contributions to cutaneous histopathology. Both university programs and private physicians have specialized dermatopathology laboratories that process and interpret slides from practitioners. In the USA dermatopathology is a subspecialty available to both dermatologists and pathologists who avail themselves of additional training.

Indications for Skin Biopsy

All tissue that is removed from a patient must be submitted for histologic interpretation. In many hospitals, this is a rule that cannot be ignored. While exceptions are occasionally made, they should be part of a formal written policy. For example, one can agree not to submit skin tags or warts. Mistaken diagnoses are always possible, and it is simplest to submit everything.

All tumors should be histologically evaluated prior to therapy to provide an exact diagnosis. When a tumor is then treated by excision, the adequacy of the procedure can be evaluated by a variety of techniques. In complex cases, some dermatologists prefer to employ micrographic surgery, in which the margins are carefully evaluated with multiple sections and the tumor reconstructed three-dimensionally to insure complete removal (Chap. 72). The histopathology may be of prognostic value. Malignant melanomas are evaluated by measuring the Breslow tumor thickness, the distance in millimeters from the granular layer to the base of the tumor. This number correlates well with patient survival, although many other variables also play a role.

Clearly not every benign tumor needs to be excised. There are reliable criteria that allow the clinician to identify pigmented lesions that need microscopic evaluation. Dermatoscopy helps greatly in this area. Dermatofibromas, seborrheic keratoses, warts, angiomas and a whole host of other lesions can be identified with almost 100% certainty by clinical examination. However, if such a lesion strikes the clinician as unusual for any reason, then complete excision, or occasionally biopsy, is appropriate. The diagnosis of amelanotic malignant melanoma or desmoplastic malignant melanoma is often a surprise, as the clinician usually has not considered a malignant melanoma. In addition, a histologic diagnosis is usually a definitive document, essential to planning therapy and suggesting the prognosis for many cutaneous malignancies, especially malignant melanoma.

With inflammatory dermatoses, recommendations are harder to make. Biopsy is often useful to exclude a more serious problem (chronic dermatitis versus mycosis fungoides), to make an unequivocal diagnosis (lichenified atopic dermatitis versus lichen planus) or to reassure the clinician treating a puzzling rash that he is not missing anything. Consecutive biopsies of inflammatory dermatoses often help to track the disease and to assess therapeutic efforts.

Choice of Biopsy Site

When dealing with a dermatitis, one must select a fresh lesion. Areas with excoriations, crusts or similar damage are usually not suitable for pathologic evaluation. If a rash is widespread, it is wise to obtain a specimen from an area where healing is good, thus avoiding elective biopsies below the knee. In addition, areas where keloids are common, such as over the sternum or over joints, should not be chosen. Biopsies in the skin lines usually heal with the best cosmetic results.

Biopsy Techniques

The many appropriate ways to perform a skin biopsy incude the following.

Simple Excision

A simple elliptical excision is nearly always appropriate. In a larger lesion, an incisional biopsy is reasonable. A carefully placed excisional biopsy provides an ideal specimen and minimum scar. Whenever possible, the long axis of the ellipse should follow the relaxed skin tension lines (Chap. 72).

Punch Biopsy

A sharpened cylindrical punch is rotated to create a circular defect. Typical punch diameters range from 2 mm to 6 mm, but 3–4 mm is standard. Both disposable punches and instruments that can be sterilized and reused are available. If the skin is stretched during the cutting phase, an elliptical wound is created. The biopsy site can be closed with a suture; if a tumor such as a basal cell carcinoma is being biopsied prior to treatment, no closure is needed.

Tangential Biopsy

Here a lesion is cut off at its base parallel to the skin surface. In the USA such a procedure is called a shave biopsy. Either a scalpel or a flexible, double-edged razor blade can be used. Pedunculated or exophytic lesions can be easily removed in this way. There are both cosmetic and scientific problems. There is always a risk of cutting through a tumor, rather than below its base. Therefore tangential biopsies should not be performed for pigmented lesions when there is even the slightest possibility of a malignant melanoma being present. If the tumor is a malignant melanoma, one has usually lost a chance to accurately measure its thickness. If the lesion is benign but incompletely removed, a less than desirable cosmetic appearance may result. In addition, recurrences may be clinically atypical and histologically resemble a malignant melanoma. Some physicians speak of saucer excisions, which are deep tangential excisions. They invariably leave an unacceptable scar and may still not reach the base of the tumor.

Curettage

Many lesions are removed with a curette; warts, seborrheic keratoses and actinic keratoses are typically treated in this way. In addition, some basal cell carcinomas are treated by curettage, usually combined with cautery or electrodesiccation and often repeated three times in the same sitting. Such specimens are less than ideal, but a diagnosis can be made. Of course, no conclusions can be drawn about completeness of removal.

Electrosurgery

When material is removed by electrosurgery alone, the tissue damage is such that an accurate histologic diagnosis is often difficult. We rarely perform electrosurgery, except in the case of condylomata acuminata when laser equipment is not available.

Size and Depth of Biopsy Specimen

One must go deep enough to reveal the pathology. Thus, a tangential biopsy is adequate for a skin tag and a punch biopsy deep enough for a superficial dermatitis such as lichen planus, but a full-thickness excision including fat is needed for panniculitis. As obvious as this seems, in the rush of a busy practice biopsies are occasionally inadequate.

The myth is often recounted that one should include normal skin for the pathologist. In fact, most of the time normal skin is not needed, but there are exceptions. When diagnosing a dermal process, such as morphea or an elastic fiber defect, it is very helpful to take two mirror biopsies, one of diseased skin and the other of normal skin from roughly the same region. Other diseases, few in number, are diagnosed by their border; thus, in porokeratosis, atrophoderma (atrophic morphea) and similar disorders an ellipse whose long axis transacts the border must be obtained.

Submission of Specimen

The biopsy specimen should immediately be placed in the appropriate fixative. Most routine material is submitted in formaldehyde solution. One should simply use the standard fixative from the service laboratory. In cold weather, formaldehyde solutions may freeze in the mail. One should let specimens fix for at least 6 h prior to mailing or add alcohol to the fixative. One needs at least 20 times as much fixative as the volume of the specimen. A large ellipse should not be jammed into a small bottle. Tissue can be marked with special inks, or sutures used to identify specific ends of a specimen. Unless arrangements have been made with the dermatopathologist, the clinician should not cut or trim the tissue. The specimen bottle should be labeled immediately.

The name on the bottle should be matched with that on the submission slip. While all of us have at one time or another scribbled an indistinct note on a requisition slip, one should strive to avoid this terrible habit. Every effort should be made to communicate the pertinent details to the pathologist. Essential facts include the history, clinical description, differential diagnosis, previous treatment and site of biopsy. Obviously one will not provide all this information when submitting fragments of a curetted seborrheic keratosis, but for an inflammatory dermatosis or unusual tumor it is mandatory. If a specimen is marked, that can be shown with a drawing. Findings of previous biopsies, from the same or other laboratories, should be noted. The patient's age and sex are essential details, although today most patient data are entered by computer, eliminating this problem. If there are specimen-handling issues, such as an ellipse that should be cut along its long axis, this should be written prominently or highlighted on the request.

In some situations, tissue should be submitted frozen or in Michel medium for immunofluorescent examination, or in special fixative for electron microscopy or specialized procedures. When a special biopsy is being performed, the clinician should call the laboratory to ensure the correct medium is used. All too often immunofluorescent specimens are inadvertently submitted in formaldehyde, making them worthless.

Limitations of Histologic Diagnosis

The worst nightmare for the pathologist is an inadequate specimen. Typically the specimen is too small, too superficial, damaged by electrosurgery or crushed by the tissue forceps. Most biopsy specimens are small enough to be removed without even using a forceps; they can simply be freed and lifted out with scissors. In other cases, the biopsy is technically perfect but the specimen is not representative. A punch biopsy of an annular infiltrate may miss the necrobiotic dermal foci of granuloma annulare, or a biopsy of a facial rash may simply show increased vascularity but no signs of lupus erythematosus or rosacea.

When dealing with tumors, a diagnosis is usually obtainable. When evaluating rashes, the situation is different. Sometimes one cannot distinguish with certainty between various types of dermatitis. In such cases, when possible, it is helpful for the clinician and pathologist to view the patient together.

Finally, our level of knowledge is not always sufficient to distinguish two processes. Sometimes, for example, keratoacanthoma and squamous cell carcinoma cannot be told apart histologically. When an experienced clinician and histopathologist work together, such borderline cases should be infrequent but nevertheless occur.

Basic Terminology of Dermatopathology

Knowledge of the basic nomenclature of dermatopathology is essential in understanding the descriptions throughout this book and appreciating the pathophysiology of cutaneous disease. Changes can occur in the epidermis, adnexal structures, dermis and subcutaneous fat. A sound knowledge of normal skin structure and its regional variation is essential to understand pathologic changes. Lentigo maligna and actinic keratosis are poor diagnoses if there is no evidence of photoaged skin; hundreds of other examples could be cited.

Epidermal Changes

Hyperkeratosis. Thickening of the stratum corneum. One speaks of retention hyperkeratosis, with a thin granular layer and reduced shedding of corneocytes, and proliferative hyperkeratosis, with a prominent granular layer and increased production of corneocytes. In practice, these two phenomena frequently overlap.

Hypokeratosis. Thinning of the stratum corneum. This is rarely a primary diagnosis but instead is usually associated with epidermal thinning in atrophic skin, e.g., in the elderly or those undergoing corticosteroid treatment.

Orthokeratosis. Orderly production of stratum corneum. Often subdivided into basket-weave or loose orthokeratosis and compact orthokeratosis.

Parakeratosis. Retention of nuclei in stratum corneum, often combined with a reduced to absent granular layer. May be normal in parts of the mouth (hard palate) but reflects disturbed keratinization in skin.

Dyskeratosis. Premature or individual cell keratinization. Typically seen in Darier disease, but also in actinic keratoses and squamous cell carcinoma.

Apoptosis. Programmed individual cell death, as found in remodeling of tissues or in the intrinsic control of some tumors. Apoptosis is a troublesome microscopic concept, as it is either the same as necrosis or a variant thereof. The eosinophilic necrotic keratinocytes known as Civatte bodies in lichen planus are one example of apoptotic cells.

Hypergranulosis. Thickening of the granular layer. The prototype of this change is lichen planus, where focal thickening of the granular layer is almost always seen.

Acanthosis. Thickening of the growing or mid-epidermis (stratum spinosum) by an increased number of cell layers produced by either a thickened epidermis or elongated and thickened rete ridges.

Hyperplasia. Thickening of the epidermis by increase in size of the individual cells. Presumably more often reactive, but the distinction between acanthosis and hyperplasia is of little practical value. We view the two terms as virtually interchangeable.

Atrophy. Thinning of the epidermis by a decrease in cells layers of stratum spinosum, leading to flattening of the rete ridges and thinning of the stratum corneum, also commonly seen in corticosteroid-treated skin.

Spongiosis. Intercellular edema in the epidermis, usually the result of inflammation, typical of acute dermatitis.

Exocytosis. Accumulation of inflammatory cells in the epidermis. While common in most types of dermatitis, exocytosis is of diagnostic importance in psoriasis, where small accumulations of neutrophils form in the stratum corneum (Munro microabscesses) and in mycosis fungoides, where atypical T cells and dendritic cells are involved (Pautrier microabscesses).

Spongiform Pustule. In the upper layers of the epidermis, accumulations of neutrophils are situated in a sponge-like network of shrunken keratinocytes. This is known as the spongiform pustule of Kogoj and is typical of pustular psoriasis.

***Altération Cavitaire*, Ballooning Degeneration and Reticular Degeneration.** *Altération cavitaire* describes intracellular edema of epidermal cells. Ballooning degeneration is very similar, but the term is used to describe the changes in herpes simplex and zoster, when the cells are greatly expanded with the nucleus pushed to one side. Reticular degeneration is the end result, after the balloons have burst leaving behind cell wall remnants.

Acantholysis. Dissolution of the desmosomal contacts in the epidermis, producing almost round, epidermal cells in blister spaces. Acantholysis has many causes, including autoimmune disease (pemphigus vulgaris), infections (herpes simplex virus or impetigo) and genetic disturbances (Darier disease, Hailey-Hailey disease).

Hydropic or Vacuolar Change. Alterations in the cells of the basal layer are typical of lupus erythematosus and lichen planus. Typically the cells may be swollen or completely disrupted, then producing a subepidermal blister. Some groups distinguish between lupus erythematosus, where there is less inflammation, and lichen planus, where the damage is usually associated with a thick band-like lymphocytic infiltrate (lichenoid infiltrate)

Incontinence of Pigment. Dropping of melanin into the papillary dermis. Anytime the basal layer is damaged, melanin from the basal cells may wind up in the upper dermis, where it is engulfed by macrophages, which are then known as melanophages. Typically this is seen in fixed drug eruptions and lichen planus.

Dermal Changes

Papillomatosis. Combination of epidermal and dermal changes including elongation of the rete ridges and dermal papillae and thickening of the papillary dermis. The result is an undulating epidermal surface, most common in warts and fleshy nevi.

Solar or Actinic Elastosis. Sun-damaged skin, particularly facial skin, shows changes in the collagen. The usual eosinophilic collagen acquires a bluish tint and may form larger clumped fibers (basophilic degeneration). This altered collagen stains positively with elastic fiber stains and is called elastotic. Whether it is damaged collagen or peculiar elastin remains unclear.

Inflammation. Inflammatory infiltrates can be described on the basis of their pattern, which includes the distribution of the cells, the cell type and the parallel changes in the epidermal, adnexal and dermal structures.

- Distribution of Cells. Many different arrangements are seen, including perivascular (involving superficial vessels, deeper vessels or both), periappendageal, lichenoid (along the epidermal-dermal junction) or diffuse. Sometimes the subcutaneous fat is involved, as in panniculitis.
- Cell Type. Lymphocytes, neutrophils, eosinophils, plasma cells, mast cells, dendritic cells and any combination thereof may be involved. Sometimes the infiltrate is relatively homogeneous; in other instances, it is quite mixed. Malignant or atypical cells can be found in the infiltrates of malignant lymphoma and leukemia.

Cells can undergo considerable change in the dermis. Cells of the monocyte/macrophage lineage may form granulomas, develop into giant cells of various types, or phagocytose lipids, melanin, hemosiderin or foreign materials. They may also cluster into granulomas, once again of many types, including sarcoidal, tuberculoid and foreign body. Foreign bodies in granulomas can often be identified with polarization microscopy.

Many traditional methods of identifying inflammatory cells are available, including the Giemsa stain for mast cells and various enzymatic stains for neutrophils. Today, most cell identification is achieved by means of monoclonal antibodies, with which lymphocytic infiltrates can be accurately typed and eosinophilic basic protein identified. In addition, electron microscopy may be used to identify Langerhans cells.

Basement Membrane Zone Thickening. Amorphous condensation of material just beneath the basal cell layer. Most often seen in lupus erythematosus and porphyria cutanea tarda.

Other Changes in Collagen and Elastin. Disruption and calcification of elastin fibers is seen in a rare genodermatosis, pseudoxanthoma elasticum. Elastic fibers are lacking in scars. Special stains are available to identify elastin fibers, so their pattern can be assessed. Evaluation of thickening, thinning or qualitative changes in collagen is far more subjective. Scars can be identified because the fibers tend to be rearranged parallel to the skin surface. A variety of foreign materials can be deposited in the dermis; most are identified by special stains. Included in the group are amyloid, hyaline, mucin, lipids, calcium and many others.

Vessels. Vasculitis refers to damage to the vessel walls. One should specify whether the small vessels of the papillary dermis or the larger arteries of the deep dermis and subcutaneous fat are inflamed. Features of vasculitis include inflammatory cells in the vessel wall, necrosis, fibrin deposition and fragments of neutrophils in the adjacent tissue. Damage to the vessel wall and obstruction lead to the extravasation of erythrocytes. True vessel destruction is rarely a feature of lymphocytic infiltrates but is almost entirely restricted to neutrophilic and eosinophilic processes. Vessel wall swelling or thickening may also be seen.

Subcutaneous Changes

Panniculitis is a challenging diagnosis which is more easily made clinically than histologically (Chap. 21). In general, inflammation may involve the fat septa or lobules and be associated with vasculitis or not. In addition, one should always search for foreign objects, as some panniculitis is artifactual.

Approach to Histologic Diagnosis

Inflammatory Dermatoses

Ackerman, in his classic textbook *Histologic Diagnosis of Inflammatory Skin Diseases*, revolutionized how most dermatopathologists approach inflammatory diseases. He described nine patterns:

- Superficial perivascular dermatitis
- Both superficial and deep perivascular dermatitis
- Nodular and diffuse dermatitis
- Vasculitis
- Intraepidermal vesicular and pustular dermatitis
- Subepidermal vesicular dermatitis
- Folliculitis and perifolliculitis
- Fibrosing dermatitis
- Panniculitis

Employing these patterns and looking for additional helpful signs, such as type of inflammatory cell, presence or absence of spongiosis, acantholysis, psoriasiform hyperplasia and many others, one can often reach a differential diagnosis which, combined with the clinical history, produces a diagnosis.

Tumors

The distinction between benign and malignant tumors is usually made on silhouette. Factors such as tumor size, depth, symmetry, border and interaction with epidermis, stroma and inflammatory infiltrate are essential. In addition, one must carefully study the cells, describing their morphology (epithelioid, spindle, mixed), their arrangement (nests, glands, cysts) and their cytologic features (mitoses, nucleoli).

Special Stains and Techniques

A skeptic once said, "A special stain allows you to see what you don't know in a different color." On the other hand, Hermann Pinkus, one of the greatest names in dermatopathology, insisted on having every specimen stained not only with hematoxylineosin but also with acid-orcein. The truth lies somewhere in between. While most diagnoses can be made on routine hematoxylin-eosin sections, sometimes special stains are helpful. Table 1.2 lists some of the useful stains.

Today the standard special stains are complemented by monoclonal antibodies, which allow one to identify inflammatory infiltrates and tumors, even poorly differentiated ones, with great precision. Monoclonal antibodies have to a great extent replaced electron microscopy in tumor diagnosis. Useful examples are shown in Table 1.3.

Table 1.2. Useful special stains

Stain	Material identified
PAS	Fungi, thickened basement membrane, carcinoma cells in Paget disease
Methenamine silver (Grocott)	Fungi, other organisms
Hale, colloidal iron, alcian blue	Mucin
Giemsa, toluidine blue	Mast cells
Von Kossa	Calcium
Elastin stains (many)	Elastic fibers
Gram, Brown-Brenn	Bacteria
Fite, Ziehl-Neelsen	Acid-fast bacilli

Table 1.3. Useful monoclonal antibodies

Antibody against	Material identified
Vimentin	Mesenchymal cells
Desmin	Muscle cells
Actin	Smooth muscle cells
Factor VIII	Endothelial cells
Neurofilaments	Nerve cells
CEA (carcino-embryonic antigen)	Carcinoma cells in Paget disease
S100	Melanocytes, neural cells, Langerhans cells
HMB-45	Melanocytes, often abnormal
Cytokeratins	Squamous cell carcinoma, appendageal tumors, Merkel cell tumors
Leukocyte markers (CD antigens)	T cells, B cells, differentiation and proliferation antigens, Langerhans cells

In Situ Hybridization and Polymerase Chain Reaction

These techniques have taken special stains to a new level of exactitude and are being continuously refined. Both identify specific DNA sequences in tissue, offering a very precise diagnosis. In in situ hybridization, tissue sections are heated and then layered with radioactive labeled DNA probes that are complementary to the sequence under investigation. If the antigen under study is present in the sections, the two strands hybridize. Autoradiography is then used to identify the localization of the DNA. Usually very small amounts of DNA are present in the tissue, so the technique is tricky, but the DNA can be localized to a specific structure, such as the vessel wall or epidermis.

The polymerase chain reaction (PCR) corrects the problem of limited amounts of DNA by multiplying it million-fold. Under appropriate conditions, cyclic changes in temperature lead to DNA replication and splitting. Thus, even a single strand of DNA can be multiplied enough to be identified. Obviously, such a technique is at risk of being contaminated. PCR is usually performed on digested tissue, but it too can be done in situ in specialized laboratories.

PCR has enabled dermatologists to acquire many new insights into disease. Two from the Munich clinic are the identification of *Mycobacterium tuberculosis* in erythema induratum, a type of vasculitis/panniculitis that was clinically connected with tuberculosis but in which organisms could not be cultured, and identification of various subtypes of *Borrelia burgdorferi*, the causative agent of Lyme disease, in different clinicopathologic settings.

Introduction to Immunology

The immune system is the body's protective mechanism against infectious agents, foreign objects and other intruders. There are two types of immunity – innate and adaptive. Innate reactions are effective against many pathogens, while adaptive responses are highly specific for single pathogens and involve memory and recall. Through the window of the skin one can watch many immuno-

Table 1.4. Brief definitions of important immunologic terms

Term	Abbreviation	Definition
Antibody		Immunoglobulin produced during immune response, capable of combining with antigen
Antigen		Any substance capable of inducing immune response
Antigen-presenting cell	APC	Cell capable of presenting antigen to T cells. Most are dendritic cells, such the Langerhans cell in the skin
Cluster designation	CD	Surface marker proteins that are identified by monoclonal antibodies and used to characterize hematopoietic cells
Cytokines		Soluble molecules that mediate reactions between cells
Cytotoxic T cells	TC cells	T cells that can kill targeted cells expressing peptides presented by class I MHC molecules
Helper T cells	TH cells	T cells that recognize antigen in association with class II MHC molecules and cooperate with B cells in antibody responses
	TH1	Helper T cells that support cell-mediated immunity
	TH2	Helper T cells that support antibody-mediated immunity
Human leukocyte antigen	HLA	Major human histocompatibility system
Natural killer cell	NK cells	Lymphocytes that have intrinsic ability to destroy some cells, such as tumor cells and virally infected cells
Interferon	IFN	Cytokine first discovered to protect against (interfere with) viral infections
Interleukin	IL	Another group of cytokines with many different properties
Major histocompatibility complex	MHC	Series of linked genetic loci coding for cell-surface antigens primarily responsible for tissue graft rejection
T cells		Lymphocytes that differentiate in thymus and are primarily responsible for directing immune response
T cell receptor	TCR	Immunoglobulin-like molecule on T cells that interacts with presented antigen and with CD3 to activate the T cell
Tumor necrosis factor	TNF	Cytokines released by macrophages, many having antitumor properties; similar to lymphotoxin released by T cells

logic processes. Some of the most common dermatologic disorders, such as atopic dermatitis and psoriasis, have an immune background. Medications or viruses, such as HIV, may block the body's immune response, leading to disastrous problems. Misguided immune responses are responsible for many diseases; allergic disorders include allergic rhinitis and some forms of asthma, while delayed hypersensitivity is associated with such diverse problems as allergic contact dermatitis and graft-versus-host disease. Immunologic concepts today allow one to begin to explain the pathogenesis of many skin diseases and more rationally approach therapy.

In discussing the immune system, there are a number of problems. The first is the enormous complexity. Everything is interwoven, so starting and finishing points are hard to find, leading to circular definitions. For this reason, in Table 1.4 we have listed some of the basic definitions for immunologic terms that appear in the text without proper introduction. Furthermore, nothing is static; immune responses change with time, age, activation of various cells and countless other factors. Very few cells or mediators have only one role, and none act in isolation. We present a brief overview, designed to bring colleagues of our generation more up-to-date and to remind younger physicians where the immunology they learned in medical school fits into the dermatologic picture. One price for such over-simplification is mistakes; we beg the indulgence of our immunologically sophisticated readers.

Cells of the Immune System

Almost all the cells of the immune system are bone marrow derived. They can be divided into several major groups. The hematopoietic stem cell differentiates into a common lymphoid progenitor that gives rise to T cells, B cells and natural killer cells. The B cells may evolve into plasma cells. The common myeloid progenitor forms granulocytes, including neutrophils and eosinophils; monocytes, which develop into tissue macrophages, mast cells and the closely related granulocytic basophilic cells; and megakaryocytes, which yield platelets. The dendritic antigen-presenting cells, such as the cutaneous Langerhans cell, are also bone marrow-derived and related to the monocyte lineage.

Lymphocytes

This heterogeneous group of mononuclear cells is classified primarily based on function (Fig. 1.16). The main members of the group are B cells, T cells and natural killer cells. The adaptive ability of the immune system to recognize antigens is provided by lymphocytes. While lymphocytes originate in the bone marrow and thymus, the main lymphoid organs include the spleen, lymph nodes and mucosa-associated lymphoid tissue (MALT). The skin is also a major site of lymphocyte activity; some speak of skin-associated lymphoid tissue or SALT.

Lymphocyte classification is extremely complex. When morphologists look at normal lymphocytes in peripheral blood smears, they cannot identify many different cell types. When lymphocytes are separated via surface markers into T cells and B cells, the situation becomes more complex. T cells are further divided into helper T cells (TH) and cytotoxic T cells (TC). Most TH cells, TC cells and B cells are small nondistinctive lymphocytes. Some cells have no surface markers; they were formerly

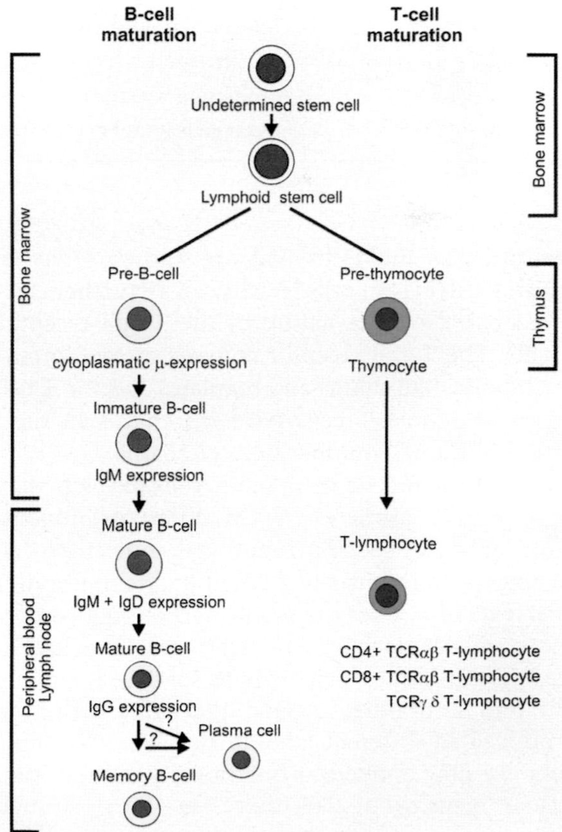

Fig. 1.16. Developmental classification of lymphocytes

Table 1.5. Cluster designations of importance in dermatology

Cluster designation	Corresponding cell and function
CD2	Pan T cell marker that interacts with antigen-presenting cell
CD3	T cell; constant part of T cell receptor complex involved in signaling
CD4	Helper T cell; responsible for interaction of T cell receptor with class II MHC molecule
CD7	Antigen present in most peripheral T cells; often lost in mycosis fungoides
CD8	Cytotoxic T cell marker; responsible for interaction of T cell receptor with class I MHC molecule
CD10	Endopeptidase expressed on immature and activated B cells, T cells and neutrophils; also known as CALLA (common acute lymphoblastic leukemia antigen)
CD15	Carbohydrate moiety present on macrophages, monocytes and neutrophils
CD16	IgG receptor present on macrophages, monocytes and NK cells
CD19	B cell antigen; part of B cell coreceptor for activation by antigen
CD20	B cell antigen; involved with calcium channel
CD22	B cell antigen; another adhesion molecule
CD23	B cell antigen; low-affinity IgE receptor (FCεRII)
CD25	Activation marker, IL-2 receptor
CD30	Activation marker for a subset of T cells, TNF receptor involved in apoptosis
CD41	Platelet adhesion factor
CD45	Common leukocyte antigen expressed on hematopoietic cells except mature erythrocytes
CD45RO CD45RA	Isoforms of CD45 created by differential RNA splicing that are involved in lymphocyte activation; CD45RO refers to naive and CD45RA to activated T cells
CD56	NK cell marker, adhesion molecule
CD79a, CD79b	Igα and Igβ, both associated with surface immunoglobulins on B cells
CD103	Integrin molecule, best expressed on activated T cells
Ki-67	Proliferation marker
CLA	Cutaneous lymphocyte-associated antigen; expressed by T cells homing to skin

identified as null cells and are known today as natural killer (NK) cells. T cells can be further classified based on the nature of the T cell receptor (TCR). The T cell receptor consists of two immunoglobulin-like chains and regulates specific T cell activation. Most T cells have $\alpha\beta$ chains in their receptor; a small number have $\gamma\delta$ chains.

As the various hematopoietic cells develop, they acquire and lose a variety of different antigens. Most of these specific functional molecular cell structures were initially defined by the antibodies that reacted against them. At international conferences, cluster designations (CD) were attached to various antibodies, primarily to sort out the many different antibodies against the same structure produced in different laboratories. The CD numbers are now applied to functionally distinct surface antigens. As of 2000, there were over 150 such designations; some of importance in dermatology are listed in Table 1.5.

One can scarcely discuss lymphocytes without using CD designations. T cell precursors go from the bone marrow to the thymus, where they develop. Various markers are present in the bone marrow (prethymic), others only in the thymus, and yet others in circulating T cells. An early and important developmental marker in the thymus is the rearrangement of the α and β chain of the TCR, along with the expression of CD3. Later the cells become positive for both CD4 and CD8, but after leaving the thymus, mature T cells express only one of these antigens. B cells develop in the fetal liver and in the bone marrow; birds have a special lymphoid organ in their hindgut known as the bursa of Fabricius where B cells develop and from where their name comes. Important B cell markers are surface immunoglobulins as well as CD79 a and b (Igα and Igβ). There are also a series of other B cell markers. The diagnosis and classification of malignant lymphoma would be inconceivable without antibodies against various CDs (Chap. 61).

T Cells. The main roles of these cells are the modulation of both cell-mediated and humoral immunity and the direct destruction of infected cells. The variable regions of the TCR project from the surface of the cell and determine its antigenic specificity. The constant region is anchored to the cell membrane in association with CD3, a series of five proteins also known as the T cell signaling complex. T cells can recognize antigen only when it is presented to the TCR by an MHC molecule.

Helper T Cells (TH). These cells are defined by the presence of CD4 and have been called the conductors of the immune response. They recognize antigen only when it is presented by MHC class II molecules (HLA-DQ, -DP, -DR). The stimulated TH then express new surface molecules and secrete an array of cytokines that both have direct effects and help steer the entire immune response. CD4 is responsible for interacting with antigen-presenting cells and serves as one attachment site for HIV (human immunodeficiency virus).

Two subtypes of helper T cells have been identified based on their pattern of secretion. TH1 cells secrete primarily interleukin (IL)-2, interferon (IFN)-γ and lymphotoxin, support cell-mediated immunity and inhibit TH2 cell functions, while TH2 cells produce IL-4, IL-5, IL-9, and IL-13, support humoral responses and inhibit TH1 cell functions.

Cytotoxic T Cells (TC). These cells are defined by the presence of CD8 and recognize antigen presented in association with MHC class I molecules (HLA-A,-B,-C). They identify and then destroy cells with altered "peptides" presented by the MHC class I molecules, such as virally infected and tumor cells. TC secrete a variety of proteins capable of damaging cells, the most important of which are perforin and granzymes. They also express the Fas ligand (FasL), which attaches to the Fas molecule on other cells, triggering apoptosis.

Suppressor T Cells. There is apparently not a single distinct suppressor T cell. Instead, both TC and TH cells can suppress immune responses.

B Cells. Naive B cells express immunoglobulins, primarily IgD and monomeric IgM, on their surface. When B cells in lymph nodes encounter the appropriate antigen and receive the needed TH support, they are transformed into either long-lived memory cells or immunoglobulin-producing plasma cells. Plasma cells secrete immunoglobulins that have almost exactly the same antigenic specificity as the surface molecules expressed in the naive state. They are also capable of presenting antigen to a T cell.

Natural Killer Cells. NK cells do not express either B or T cell markers. There is no unique marker for this lineage, although CD16, one of the Fc receptors, and CD56, a neural cell adhesion molecule (NCAM) are often used. CD3 is absent, as there is no TCR. NK cells can kill tumor cells and virally infected cells, thus playing a major role in innate immunity. In addition, they serve in adaptive immunity as one of the effectors of antibody-dependent cell-mediated cytotoxicity (ADCC), attaching to cells coated with IgG via Fc domains (CD16) and destroying them.

Phagocytes

Phagocytes take up antigens and pathogenic organisms which they then destroy or degrade. Some may also present antigen to lymphocytes. The two main classes of phagocytes are neutrophils and monocytes.

Neutrophils. Also known as polymorphonuclear neutrophils or "polys", these short-lived circulating cells may migrate to sites of inflammation or infection. They are attracted by a variety of chemotactic agents and go through a complex process of attachment and then migration through vessel walls and into tissues. They account for about 70% of the leukocytes in adults. They are capable of ingesting bacteria and other smaller organisms. They have an arsenal of weapons in their granules, including destructive enzymes, lactoferrin (to deprive organisms of iron), antibiotics such as defensins and other enzymes to create highly active nitrogen and oxygen molecules.

Monocytes. These bone-marrow-derived cells settle in tissues, including the skin, where they are then known as macrophages. Macrophages are phagocytes responsible for taking up and processing foreign materials, but with relatively poor antigen-presenting function compared with dendritic cells. They are involved in the granulomatous response directed against many foreign objects and numerous infectious agents. There are no specific monocyte/macrophage markers. Fc receptors, complement receptors (CR) and a series of other CDs are employed.

Histiocyte is an old term referring collectively to monocytes, macrophages and perhaps phagocytic cells derived from mesenchymal elements. Immunologists no longer employ the term, but it remains in use to describe a collection of disorders – the histiocytoses (Chap. 64)

Antigen-Presenting Cells. These cells, probably derived from monocytic precursors, take up foreign materials and produce small peptide fragments that serve as antigens. They are also called dendritic cells because of their long cellular dendrites, which presumably aid in bringing antigens into the cell. The Langerhans cell is the cutaneous dendritic cell residing in the epidermis. It is $S100^+$, $CD1^+$ and has characteristic Birbeck granules. There is a reseeding of the epidermis by bone-marrow-derived Langerhans cells. About 100 days after bone-marrow transplantation, many cutaneous Langerhans cell carry the markers of the donor.

After taking up antigen, the Langerhans cells migrate into the dermis, where they are known as veiled cells, and then into the lymph nodes. Here, antigen is presented on the cell surface by MHC class II molecules to T cells. A T cell receptor recognizes the antigen, a fundamental step in antigen-specific T cell activation. While the primary antigen-presenting cells are the dendritic cells, macrophages and B cells can also perform this task, albeit far less effectively.

Other Cells

Eosinophils. Eosinophils are granulocytes whose granules stain red with eosin. They normally account for 2–4% of leukocytes in healthy nonallergic individuals. In such individuals eosinophils seem to be primarily involved in downregulating mast cell products and protecting against parasitic worms; they can release the contents of their granules, such as major basic protein, eosinophilic cationic protein and many others. Eosinophils play a major role in type I immune responses; their levels are elevated in patients with atopy (Chap. 12). Other diseases with hypereosinophilia are discussed in Chapter 51.

Mast Cells. Mast cells (Chap. 63) release a variety of inflammatory mediators upon appropriate stimuli. Often this is an allergen that interacts with IgE bound to the mast cell surface (Chap. 11). The basophil is an uncommon circulating granulocyte that has properties similar to those of the mast cell.

Platelets. Platelets and their role in clotting are discussed in detail in Chapter 23. They are also involved in inflammatory reactions, secreting a variety of mediators; they are the main source of serotonin. Platelets also express class I MHC proteins, carrying immunoglobulin receptors and a number of adhesion factors. CD41 is a complex cytoadhesin; monoclonal antibodies against it inhibit platelet aggregation and are in clinical use.

Antigens

Antigens are substances that can trigger an immune response. Most antigens are glycoproteins that can be recognized by lymphocytes. There are foreign antigens that may or may not elicit a clinically relevant immune response. For example, most foods do not serve as antigens, while many microbes do. Self antigens are all the proteins of an individual. They should not trigger a harmful immune response, although many do elicit clinically inapparent responses, as shown by the presence of antinuclear antibodies in many healthy individuals.

Both T cells and B cells can recognize antigens. B cells recognize small regions known as epitopes on intact antigens, while T cells identify small digested fragments of larger antigens presented to them on the surface of antigen-presenting cells by the MHC molecules. T cell receptors recognize 10- to 20-amino-acid polypeptide fragments of these glycoproteins. Haptens are small molecules that are immunogenic only if bound to a carrier group. TH cells recognize the carrier, while B cells identify the hapten; this discovery was one of the first clues to the complex interactions between T cells and B cells. Adjuvants are totally different; they are substances that are administered with an antigen and stimulate innate immunity. This activates the antigen-presenting cells and lymphocytes, enhancing the adaptive response.

Major Histocompatibility Complex

The genes involved in the rejection of nonself tissues form a region on chromosome 6 known as the major histocompatibility complex (MHC), which in humans is also known as the human leukocyte antigen (HLA) system. Although these structures are known as antigens, they serve in this capacity only when exposed to a foreign immune system, such as in transplantation. In addition, there are minor or host-specific histocompatibility antigens located away from chromosome 6 that possess no antigen-presenting properties.

There are three types of MHC proteins:

- Class I MHC includes HLA-A, -B and -C antigens. Each consists of a heavy chain that is folded to expose two variable regions and $\beta 2$ microglobulin, a small chain coded on chromosome 15 that is one of the precursor proteins of amyloid (Chap. 41). Class I antigens are present on almost all cells and present intracellular peptides, including viral and tumor products, to T cells.
- Class II MHC includes the HLA-DP, -DQ and -DR antigens, which are found only on antigen-presenting cells and some other activated cells. They are made up of two immunoglobulin-like heavy chains and present exogenous peptides such as haptens and allergens to T cells.
- Class III MHC genes include a variety of complement genes, cytokines and enzymes. They do not play a role in histocompatibility.

The main function of HLA antigens is antigen presentation, as most individuals do not ever have to reject a foreign graft or have their immune response altered so that they can receive a life-saving kidney, heart or bone-marrow transplantation. There are a variety of disease associations with different HLA loci. Throughout the book, we will mention various HLA genes associated with psoriasis, lupus erythematosus, dermatitis herpetiformis and many other disorders. Several explanations have been proposed for these associations.

- Molecular mimicry suggests that immune responses directed against an infectious agent could cross-react with self peptides presented by HLA antigens, triggering an autoimmune disease.
- Linkage means that the HLA antigen is closely linked to another gene responsible for a given disease, such as one of the class III genes.
- Antigen presentation is so dependent on the HLA structure that there may be situations where only patients with certain variations in HLA can produce antibodies against a given structure. This has been suggested as part of the mechanism of pemphigus vulgaris.
- Receptor function may also be important. Just as HIV uses CD4, other agents may attach selectively to certain HLA molecules.

Adaptive Immunity

There are a series of steps in adaptive immunity, including antigen presentation, selection of the appropriate responding T cell or B cell, clonal expansion of the selected cells with associated differentiation, and development of memory, so that if the antigen is encountered again the immune response can be prompter and greater. While classically adaptive immunity is divided into humoral or B cell and cell-mediated or T cell responses, this is inaccurate because of the essential role that T cells play in both types of immunity.

When the body is confronted with an antigen, it takes several days before an immune response is in full swing. Thus it is impossible to have an allergic reaction on first contact with an antigen, unless one has been sensitized to a cross-reacting molecule previously. The second time the body is exposed to an antigen the recognition is prompter and greater. The same is true whether speaking of a cellular response following topical sensitization or an antibody response. This recall response is utilized in immunization.

Antigen Presentation

Endogenous Antigens. MHC class I antibodies present antigen to $CD8^+$ TC cells. The antigen is typically a viral, tumor or self antigen that is broken down to a small peptide in an infected cell or macrophage. Once a TC cell has been activated by an antigen-presenting cell, it identifies infected or damaged cells and destroys them with perforin and granzymes, enzymes that lyse cells, as well as Fas ligand, which triggers the Fas or apoptosis gene.

Exogenous Antigens. Only antigen-presenting cells present antigen with MHC class II molecules to $CD4^+$ TH cells (Fig. 1.17). There is selection in the thymus for cells whose TCR have intermediate affinity for the class II antigens. If affinity were too high, autoimmune reactions would be more common. The TCR is attached to CD3 at its base. There is considerable diversity in the variable regions of the TCR. The variable region forms a groove where peptides with about 10–20 amino acids are recognized, when presented by MCH class II molecules. A complex series of signals that also requires CD4 then specifically activates TH cells.

The activated cell clonally expands, enters the circulation and tends to home to the initial contact site. Thus, when a cutaneous Langerhans cell pre-

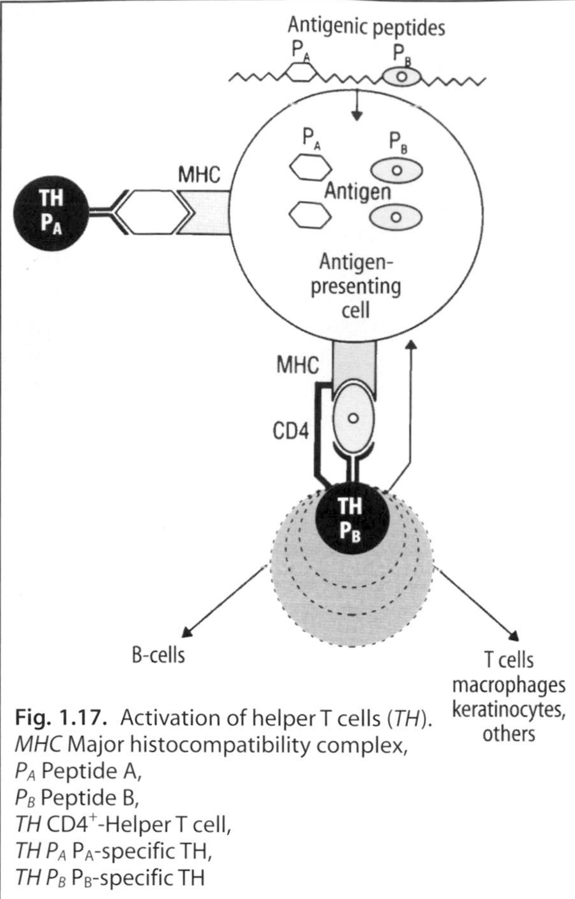

Fig. 1.17. Activation of helper T cells (*TH*). *MHC* Major histocompatibility complex, *P_A* Peptide A, *P_B* Peptide B, *TH* $CD4^+$-Helper T cell, *TH P_A* P_A-specific TH, *TH P_B* P_B-specific TH

sents antigen in a regional lymph node, a population of sensitized antigen-specific T cells is generated, armed with special adhesion molecule profiles, known as addressins, that allow them to migrate specifically to the skin. The cells leave the circulation at what are called high endothelial venues, areas where the endothelial cells are activated and more cuboidal. Irritation in the skin, e.g., from an ulcer, may induce such changes in vessels, enhancing cell-mediated immunity. If the activated cell finds the antigen, there is a massive cascade of recruited cells and cytokines causing inflammation and destruction.

The classical antigens activate T cells with the $\alpha\beta$ chains. T cells with $\gamma\delta$ chains tend to be activated by heat shock proteins and are often found on mucosal surfaces. They are also capable of interacting with CD1 on Langerhans cells. While $\gamma\delta$ T cells are common in mouse skin, they are almost absent in human skin, but may be present in some lymphomas.

Antibody Production

B cell activation requires presentation of antigen and in most cases stimulation by TH cells (Fig. 1.18). It usually occurs in the germinal centers of lymph nodes or the spleen. The antigen receptors on B cells are surface-bound immunoglobulins, primarily IgD and monomeric IgM. The variable regions of immunoglobulins create a great amount of diversity. B cells tend to recognize epitopes or small three-dimensional structures. Thus the old analogy of lock and key fits well for recognition by immunoglobulins. Any antigen can find an immunoglobulin that fits it. Once the antigen binds to the B cell, a series of complex steps occur to improve the fit and at the same time cause a clonal proliferation of the cells. Some B cells seem to remain in the germinal centers and there establish B cell memory. The vast bulk of activated B cells evolve into circulating plasma cells that secrete about 90% of their immunoglobulin into the serum. Except for minor alterations improving fit, the serum immunoglobulin has the same conformation as the initial surface receptor. The role of TH cells is often crucial. They are activated by another part of the same antigen as the B cell and secrete cytokines that steer the immunoglobulin response. In rare instances B cells can respond to antigen without the help of T cells. These T cell-independent antigens are usually polysaccharides, and the antibody response is generally modest.

Immunoglobulins

Structure

Immunoglobulins come in many forms, as shown in Table 1.6. They are chains of polypeptides manufactured by B cells that are either expressed as a membrane-bound molecule or secreted. Each B cell manufactures only a single specific immunoglobulin. Immunoglobulins consist of two light chains and two heavy chains. The antigen-binding region or Fab is formed by the variable regions of a light and heavy chain. Each immunoglobulin has two such regions. The constant tail (Fc) of the heavy chain provides attachment to the B cell membrane bound, and once soluble mediates the biologic effects of the circulating antibodies. A number of events determine the specificity and type of immune responses provided by immunoglobulins.

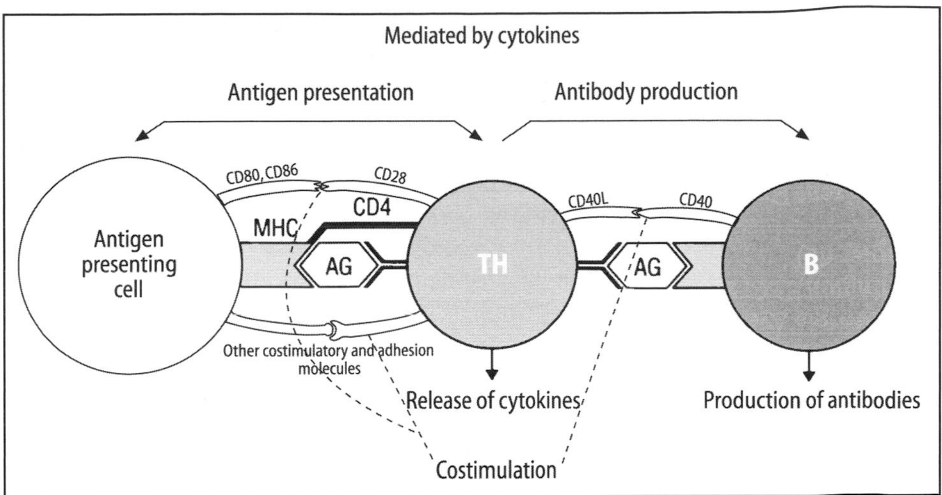

Fig. 1.18. The immune response cascade. *AG* Antigen, *B* B cell, *MHC* Major histocompatibility complex, *TH* $CD4^+$-Helper T cell

Table 1.6. Types of immunoglobulins

Type	Proportion in Serum (%)	Molecular weight (kDa)	Comments
IgG	75–80%	145–170,000	Main immunoglobulin in adaptive responses; several subclasses
IgA			Two forms and two subclasses
Monomer	15–20%	160,000	Usually found in external body fluids such as tears, saliva and gastrointestinal secretions
Dimer	< 1	385,000	J chain joins the two units, while secretory piece facilitates transfer across epithelial surfaces
IgM	5–10	970,000	In serum as pentamer with J chain
IgD	< 1	160,000	Mainly membrane-bound; function unclear
IgE	< 0.001	190,000	Bound to mast cells; interacts with allergens leading to immediate-type hypersensitivity

Organization of the Immunoglobulin Light Chain. The constant regions are of two types, κ and λ. When evaluating a B cell infiltrate in the skin, presence of only one type of light chain is a simple sign of monoclonality.

Organization of the Immunoglobulin Heavy Chain. There are five different classes, determining the five types of immunoglobulins. They carry the Greek names corresponding to the Roman names for the immunoglobulin classes, i.e., IgG has a γ heavy chain. There are four subclasses of γ chains, leading to IgG1, IgG2, IgG3 and IgG4. While all are similar, IgG3 is a more elongated molecule that is more effective at fixing complement than its colleagues. There are also two IgA subtypes.

Recombination. The heavy chains and the κ and λ light chains are encoded on chromosomes 14,2 and 22. The light chains are encoded by variable (V), joining (J) and constant (C) regions, while the heavy chains also have a diversity (D) segment. These fragments are shuffled to create mRNA for the respective immunoglobulin chains.

Class Switching. Often IgM is first produced against a given antigen. The production may be shifted to IgG by splicing a different constant region onto the antigen-specific variable region.

Somatic Mutations. As class switching is occurring, somatic mutations occur in the germinal centers of lymph nodes and there is a selection process to favor the progeny that produce higher-affinity antibodies.

There are two major forms of variation between different immunoglobulins.

Isotypic. The presence of the κ and λ chains and the presence of different classes of IgG and IgA are examples of isotypic variation, seen in all members of a species.

Idiotypic. The variations in the highly variable regions that determine the binding specificity of immunoglobulins and TCR are usually unique and known as idiotypes.

Function

Immunoglobulins play a wide variety of roles. IgM is usually the first immunoglobulin manufactured upon exposure to an antigen. The bulk of the humoral immune response is mediated by IgG, which is also capable of crossing the placenta and, in most cases, of fixing complement. IgG1 is the major immunoglobulin, while IgG3 is especially flexible and capable of activating complement. IgG4 is specifically activated by TH2 responses such as seen in pemphigus vulgaris. IgA is the main antibody in mucosal secretions. It forms a dimer and is transported across mucosal surfaces by a secretory piece manufactured locally by the epithelial cells. IgA1 is made in the bone marrow, while IgA2 is the main form in the gastrointestinal and respiratory tracts. IgE is primarily associated with immediate hypersensitivity reactions and plays a positive role in dealing with parasitic infestations. IgD still is a mystery molecule; it is found primarily fixed to naive B cells, where it probably binds antigens and helps in activation.

Measurement

Serum protein electrophoresis is not a satisfactory way to study the different immunoglobulin types. It is the best approach for identifying a gammopathy. When assessing humoral immune status, the individual levels of the various immunoglobulins should be measured. A wide variety of methods are available.

Cell Migration

There is steady trafficking in leukocytes throughout the body. Neutrophils and monocytes leave the bone marrow and migrate to sites of inflammation. For neutrophils, it is a one-way trip. They attack invaders, phagocytose what they can and die. Monocytes differentiate into macrophages and dendritic cells and may return to lymph nodes to present antigen. They also help locally to establish chronic granulomatous inflammation with fibrosis.

Lymphocytes have a more sophisticated pattern. Naive B cells and T cells are primarily found in lymph nodes, although they are found in the blood migrating to the nodes and perhaps occasionally scavenging. Activated or memory B cells wait in the germinal center for antigen to come to them. In contrast, activated T cells tend to return to the home address, the tissue where they encountered antigen, be it the gut, respiratory tract or skin. Complex interactions between endothelial and T cell adhesion molecules make this precise return possible. To return to the skin, T cells express a cutaneous lymphocyte-associated antigen (CLA) which seems to be essential for specific recirculation to sites of cutaneous inflammation. This provides a plausible explanation why some pseudolymphomas and lymphomas are restricted to the skin for long periods of time.

Cytokines

Cytokines are small, biologically highly active proteins that regulate the growth, function and differentiation of cells and help steer the immune response and resultant inflammation. They may act on the cell that produces them or on cells nearby. Not only the cells of the immune system are involved; any cell is capable of producing a certain set of cytokines. For example, keratinocytes secrete a number of cytokines and chemokines that either activate or suppress immune responses. Thus keratinocytes are immunologically active cells, not just cells designed to die and be shed. Well over 100 human cytokines have been identified. In addition to the great number, the situation is made more confusing because most cytokines have a variety of different roles.

Cytokines bind to receptors in order to act upon cells. Increased expression of these receptor molecules, or changes in them to increase binding affinity, also modulate cell activity. Most receptors are transmembrane proteins that can activate intracellular kinase pathways, producing transcription factors that then induce transcription of a selected gene.

The major families of cytokines include the following:

Interleukins (IL). These agents are secreted by lymphocytes or macrophages and mainly regulate lymphocyte differentiation and function. For example, when the TCR and CD3 are appropriately stimulated, a high-affinity receptor for IL-2 is created. IL-2, released by T cells, plays a central role in T cell activation and proliferation. Other interleukins play key roles in regulating the development of T cells towards TH1 or TH2 phenotypes. IL-4, secreted by T cells and some other cell types, directs the development of activated T cells towards TH2 phenotypes. IL-12 and IFN-α, secreted by macrophages, direct T cell differentiation towards TH1 phenotype.

Interferons (IFN). Interferons were initially identified as agents produced by one virally infected cell to protect adjacent cells from infection. IFN-α and IFN-β are produced by leukocytes and fibroblasts and form one of the earliest recognized lines of defense against viral infections. IFN-γ, also known as macrophage-activating factor, has quite different roles, as it increases the expression of MHC molecules, activates macrophages, stimulates NK cells and some B cells and inhibits TH2 cell functions.

Tumor Necrosis Factor (TNF). TNF-α is made by macrophages, often in response to infection, and plays a role in endotoxin shock and the purpuric rash associated with *Neisseria meningitidis*. TNF-β, also known as lymphotoxin, is an important part of the TH1 secretory pattern. Both also bind to a receptor that is capable of triggering cell death.

Transforming Growth Factor (TGF). TGFβ is a potent immunosuppressive agent inhibiting T cell and macrophage activation and function. Many of the other growth factors are of primarily endocrine importance.

Adhesion Molecules

Intercellular adhesion molecules are membrane-bound proteins that facilitate the interaction between cells. The list of cell adhesion molecules is long. Many can react with a variety of ligands. Cells can alter their ability to interact with other cells, either by increasing the number of adhesion molecules or by altering the molecule to increase affinity. There are four major families of adhesion molecules; the process of cell migration offers a chance to review them.

Immunoglobulin Supergene Family. Members of this group have immunoglobulin-like domains. Examples include intercellular adhesion molecules (ICAM-1, ICAM-2), vascular adhesion molecule (VCAM-1) and mucosal adhesion molecule (MAd-CAM-1).

Integrins. Members of this large group have two polypeptides (α and β), which traverse the cell membrane. The β-chains determine the general properties of integrins:

- β_1-integrins link cells to the extracellular matrix. They are known as very late antigens (VLAs), as they facilitate the migration of leukocytes through connective tissue.
- β_2-integrins interact with CAMs to facilitate the attachment of leukocytes to endothelium. Examples include lymphocyte functional antigen (LFA-1).
- β_3-integrins are primarily involved in platelet-neutrophil interactions.

Selectins. There are three major types of selectins; all have terminal lectin domains and bind carbohydrates. E-selectins are expressed on endothelial cells and bind to leukocytes, while L-selectins are found on leukocytes and binds to endothelium. P-selectin may be on either platelets or endothelial cells and then binds to the other.

Carbohydrate Ligands. These structures bind to selectins. For example, P- and E-selectins expressed on activated endothelial cells bind to CD15, a carbohydrate on many leukocytes, and slow them down prior to migration.

The process of cell migration in inflammation consists of several steps:

- Tethering. The interaction between E-selectin and CD 15 slows down the leukocyte. Expression of E-selectin by endothelial cells is increased by various cytokines.

- Triggering. The leukocytes are activated, often by chemokines, small cytokines that bind to heparin groups present on endothelium and signal tethered cells to increase the avidity of their integrins.
- Strong Adherence or Latching. This step involves the interaction between integrins and CAMs to firmly attach the cell.
- Migration. Cells pass between endothelial cells, through the basement membrane and into the extracellular matrix. Here the β_1-integrins (VLAs) allow interactions with collagen, laminin and fibronectin.

Innate Immunity

Many of the aspects of innate immunity are taken for granted. Included in this group are exterior defenses, inflammation, parts of the complement system, chemotaxis, phagocytosis, and destruction by NK cells. All have in common that they can be directed against any invader and require no priming or prior exposure.

Exterior Defenses

The skin is an extremely important part of the exterior defense mechanisms of the body. Protective factors include the stratum corneum, the fatty acids in the epidermal lipid layer, the surface pH (acid mantle) and the many normal or commensal bacteria that colonize the skin. Few bacteria, viruses or fungi penetrate intact skin to cause disease. Additional protection is provided by nonspecific antibacterial chemicals on the skin surface. Magainins are such biocidal agents secreted in frogs and effective against bacteria, fungi and protozoa, as well as showing antitumor properties in the laboratory. The closely related defensors have been detected in human skin.

Inflammation

Inflammation is the response that brings white blood cells and serum molecules to sites or infection or injury. The classic cutaneous signs of inflammation are erythema, swelling, warmth and pain. All result from the increased blood flow, dilation of small vessels, leakage of inflammatory mediators into the skin and enhanced cell migration through the vessel wall. The early cells are usually nonspecific phagocytes but later cells involved in the adaptive immune response arrive.

Mediators of Inflammation

Several complex systems are essential in inflammation.

Complement. Complement is a series of proteins that interact to mediate inflammation. They form a mainstay of the innate immune system but are also linked to the adaptive system. The central molecule is C3, which can be activated by either the alternate or classical pathway. The alternate pathway can be activated directly by microbes, while the classical pathway is usually triggered by immunoglobulin complexes. There are a number of effector mechanisms in the complement system.

- C5a is a potent chemotactic agent for neutrophils, which it also activates. It has been caused by an anaphylotoxin, because excessive levels of C5a, as occurs in Gram-negative sepsis, can produce cardiovascular collapse.
- C5b is a potent opsonin coating microorganisms and immune complexes to facilitate phagocytosis.
- Components C5-C9 are capable of directly lysing target cells.
- Activation of B cells. There are actually several fragments of C3 and they may attach to four different complement receptors (CR).

Patients with defects in the activation part of the classical pathway often have autoimmune diseases, such as systemic lupus erythematosus. Those with defects in the later stages are unable to handle *Neisseria* appropriately.

Other Enzyme Systems. The clotting system generates fibrin and fibrinopeptides, which are chemotactic and increase vascular permeability. In addition, activated factor XII (Hageman factor) breaks down kininogen to produce bradykinin, a nonapeptide capable of vasodilatation, increased vascular permeability and smooth muscle contraction. The fibrinolysis pathway produces plasmin, which generates kallidin or lysyl-bradykinin.

Vasoactive Amines. Mast cells release a wide variety of mediators, including histamine. Platelets contain 5-hydroxytryptamine or serotonin. Both lead to vasodilatation and smooth muscle contraction.

Reactive Oxygen and Nitrogen Products. Reactive oxygen intermediates such the superoxide anion are produced by phagocytic cells to kill bacteria.

Patients with chronic granulomatous disease (Chap. 4) have defects in this system. Nitric oxide is also made by phagocytes, as well as released by endothelial cells as a potent vasodilator. Both of these families of agents cause inflammation when they are released into tissues.

Arachidonic Acid Products. Arachidonic acid is a common component of cell membranes that can be used to synthesize a befuddling number of mediators. In mast cell activation, phospholipases are stimulated to produce arachidonic acid from phospholipids. At this point, the pathway diverges. Cyclooxygenase acts on arachidonic acid to synthesize prostaglandins and thromboxane. The prostaglandins are potent vasodilators that also increase vessel permeability. Prostacylin, one of the prostaglandins, prevents platelet aggregation and is used therapeutically for this purpose. Prostaglandins mediate the erythema and pain associated with sunburn. In contrast, thromboxane is a vasoconstrictor and causes platelet aggregation. In the other pathway, 5-lipoxygenase manufactures the leukotrienes, primarily in neutrophils and mast cells. The leukotrienes also play a variety of roles, including chemotaxis and smooth muscle contraction, as in bronchial asthma. Specific leukotriene inhibitors are now available in asthma therapy. The nonsteroidal antiinflammatory drugs act primarily by inhibiting cyclooxygenase or 5-lipoxygenase and blocking mediator production.

Chemotaxis

Chemotaxis refers to the directed migration of a cell along a concentration gradient of the chemotactic agent. Many of the signaling molecules that trigger migration are also chemotactic. Included in the list are C5a, LTB_4 (a leukotriene) and the amino-acid sequence Met-Leu-Phe. Formylated Met-Leu-Phe is found only in bacteria and is a convenient signal for both macrophages and neutrophils. An increasingly important group of molecules that help control the influx of different cell types into sites of inflammation is the chemokines. These small molecules with a characteristic structure direct migration of selected leukocyte populations; RANTES (regulated on activation, normal T expressed and secreted) is chemotactic for monocytes and T cells, while IL-8 only affects neutrophils. Chemokinesis is the stimulation of undirected motion.

Clearance

Once neutrophils or macrophages have contacted an invader, they must attempt to destroy it. By pinocytosis or phagocytosis, they take up the microorganisms or other antigens; they then release enzymes that decompose the foreign material in lysosomes. Neutrophils then die, but macrophages may go on to form a granulomatous or giant cell response, particularly if they are unable to kill the intracellular organisms. Under certain conditions macrophages can also manufacture vitamin D, which blocks TH1 cell development and may change a chronic failing granulomatous response into an antibody-mediated TH2 response. Enough vitamin D can spill out to cause the hypercalcemia of sarcoidosis. Eosinophils are called into action when parasitic worms or some fungi (notably *Aspergillus*) are present. They tend to discharge their granules rather than engaging in effective phagocytosis.

NK cells and TC cells can recognize virally infected cells and destroy them. TC cells recognize only antigens presented by MHC class I molecules, while NK cells exclusively kill MHC class I-deficient cells. Both are dependent on appropriate costimulation and cytokine activation.

Tolerance

In this state the immune response does not destructively act against self. Some antigens elicit no clinically significant immune response; the body is said to be tolerant of these molecules. Tolerance is the expected relation to self antigens, but in hyposensitization, tolerance to foreign antigens can be induced. Manipulation of tolerance is a goal of transplantation medicine. Mice can be conditioned to accept skin grafts if grafts are performed early in their life. Today many more sophisticated methods are used to induce tolerance.

The route of antigen administration is important. Sulzberger and Chase demonstrated long ago that oral exposure to an antigen often made it difficult to sensitize the individual later with topical measures. Many tumors induce an undesirable tolerance; attempts to activate NK and perhaps TC cells with cytokines are designed to reduce tolerance, although the cytokines have many other roles. Modern approaches use the lessons from tumors and try to generate tolerogenic antigen-presenting cells that should protect against autoimmune disease.

Immunologic Diseases

There are four basic ways in which the immune system can go wrong – immunodeficiency, autoimmune disease, hypersensitivity reactions and providing the wrong type of immune response.

Immunodeficiency

In immunodeficiency, be it primary or secondary, the immune response fails. There are many inherited forms of immunodeficiency with defects in such varied factors as response to chemotaxis, poor neutrophil killing and faulty T cell maturation or stimulation. Those with cutaneous findings are reviewed briefly at the end of Chapter 4. The most dramatic acquired form of immunodeficiency is HIV/AIDS (Chap. 2), but iatrogenic immunosuppression is also a common problem.

Autoimmune Disease

In humans there is a wide discrepancy between the casual way in which we refer to diseases as autoimmune and our understanding of the mechanisms. There are many possible explanations for the development of autoimmune disease. They include anatomic sequestration so that the immune system is not exposed to an antigen during the early days of life when tolerance is established, loss of tolerance in later life and alteration of self antigens by infectious agents.

Faulty Differentiation

In many different disease settings, such as allergies and autoimmune diseases, development of an inappropriate phenotypic response, i.e., TH1 instead of TH2, may result in severe damage. Other examples include infectious diseases such as leprosy, leishmaniasis and tuberculosis, where the immune response is often more threatening than any other aspect of the infection.

Hypersensitivity Reactions

The difference between immunity and hypersensitivity is the degree of the immune response. Table 1.7 shows the four major classes of hypersensitivity reactions identified by Gell and Coombs many years ago. Figure 1.19 demonstrates the time scale of these reactions. When the body reacts to a usually nonpathogenic natural substance such as a tree pollen or reacts too vehemently to a known toxic substance such as a wasp sting, we speak of allergy, which in its most restricted sense is a type I reaction featuring an excessive TH2 response. Delayed hypersensitivity or a type IV reaction to exogenous allergens is also described as an allergy, as in allergic contact dermatitis, in which there is an exaggerated TH1 response. One of the most common types of hypersensitivity is drug reactions, as discussed in Chap. 10. Any of the four immunologic mechanisms can be responsible.

Anaphylaxis

A prototypic type I reaction is anaphylaxis, as discussed in Chap. 11. Antigen-specific IgE is attached to mast cells via specific receptors, primarily the high-affinity form FCεRI. When antigen binds to the IgE on the mast cell, degranulation occurs and all the mast cell mediators, together with a complex immune cascade, produce the well-known clinical picture. Patients with atopy or the atopic diathesis tend to have marked problems with type I reactions, such as allergic rhinitis, conjunctivitis and asthma. Atopic dermatitis (Chap. 12) has more complex mechanisms and is not clearly a type I reaction. Most cases of urticaria also are not type I reactions; instead, the mast cell degranulation is caused by other, often poorly understood mechanisms.

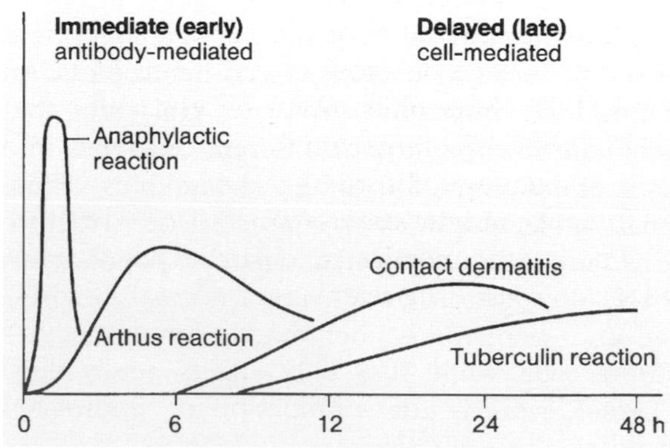

Fig. 1.19. Time course of immune reactions

Table 1.7. Types of hypersensitivity reactions (Gell and Coombs)

Type	I	II	III	IV
Name	**Anaphylaxis**	**Antibody-dependent cytotoxity**	**Immune complex disease**	**Delayed-type hypersensitivity**
Antigens	Allergens, usually soluble (drugs, foods arthropod toxins, pollens)	Blood cells, drugs, tissue antigens	Drugs, serum, microbial antigens, tissue antigens, inhaled antigens	Drugs, contact allergens, microbial antigens
Effectors	IgE on mast cells	IgG, IgM	Primarily IgG, forming immune complexes with antigens	Sensitized T cells
Mediators	Mast cell products	Complement, NK cells	Complement, neutrophils are attracted, cannot ingest complexes, discharge granules	Macrophages activated by T cell cytokines
Tissue reaction	Vasodilatation, increased vessel permeability, edema, smooth muscle contraction	Cytolysis, tissue destruction	Acute necrosis	Variable, ranging from acute dermatitis to granulomatous responses
Time	Usually seconds to minutes	Hours	Minutes to hours (serum sickness starts at about 9 days)	Usually 24–48 h
Clinical examples	Anaphylaxis, angio-edema, allergic rhinitis, conjunctivitis asthma	Transfusion reactions, hemolytic disease of newborn, Goodpasture syndrome	Serum sickness, lupus erythematosus, Arthus reaction, farmer's lung, many persistent infections	Allergic contact dermatitis, tuber-culin reaction

Antibody-Dependent-Cell-Mediated Cytotoxicity

In the type II reaction, IgG or IgM antibodies bind to cell surfaces and their Fc portions react with complement or effector cells to bring about tissue damage. The generation of complement can cause lytic cell damage or, more often, allow NK cells, neutrophils, eosinophils, macrophages and other cells to bind to the target where they are activated. Many hematologic disorders, such as transfusion reactions, hemolytic disease of the newborn and other hemolytic anemias, involve this type of reaction, as do some drug reactions.

Immune Complex Disease

In type III reaction immune complexes settle in tissue or circulate, rather than being destroyed by phagocytes. Immune complexes may arise as a result of persistent infection or in autoimmune diseases with production of antibodies. The kidney is a common site for the deposition of immune complexes. A special example is farmers' lung, in which immune complexes form in the alveoli as circulating antibodies meet inhaled antigens. The immune complexes are usually broken down by complement and then removed by phagocytes. If the complexes are difficult to break down, then both complement and effector cells may cause significant tissue damage, as is the case in some forms of vasculitis.

The Arthus reaction is a special type of type III process. An individual can be sensitized to an antigen by repeated injections. Then, if the antigen is injected into the skin or subcutaneous tissue, a diffuse swelling and erythema is produced after several hours and fades after about 48 h. The presence of antigen, antibodies and complement in the dermal vessels can be shown.

In serum sickness, a foreign protein is injected into the patient and persists. After about 9–10 days, the patient may develop antibodies against the antigen, leading to distinctive erythematous skin lesions, arthritis and glomerulonephritis. Serum sickness today may be seen with long-lasting parenteral antibiotics, as horse serum is rarely employed therapeutically. The antilymphocyte serum prepared from horses and used in transplantation was formerly an almost invariable cause of serum sickness, as were other antisera.

Delayed-Type Hypersensitivity

The type IV reaction or delayed type hypersensitivity is often seen by a dermatologist. Allergic contact dermatitis (Chap. 12) is a prototypical type IV reaction. A wide variety of substances when applied topically to the skin can induce cell-mediated immunity. The Langerhans cell is the antigen-presenting cell in the skin, but the keratinocytes produce a wide range of cytokines to modulate the reaction. The initial sensitization phase takes about 10–14 days. This means that allergic contact dermatitis cannot be developed upon first exposure to a substance, unless the patient is already sensitized to a cross-reacting material. When the antigen is applied again, the elicitation phase involves the recruitment of TH cells to the skin, with a cytokine cascade triggering the inflammation. Patients with already inflamed skin, such as those with leg ulcers, are more likely to develop allergic contact dermatitis because their antigen-presenting cells are activated and better able to participate in sensitization.

The tuberculin test is another example of delayed-type hypersensitivity. Here there is a response to a soluble antigen previously encountered during the course of the infection. Thus the pattern of cellular response is slightly different, as the sensitized T cells secrete cytokines and trigger a predominantly dermal monocytic response.

Granulomatous inflammation is also a major part of many infectious diseases, such as tuberculosis and leprosy (Chap. 4). In leprosy, the tuberculoid form is dominated by TH1-mediated type IV reactions, while the lepromatous form reflects an inefficient TH2-type immune response which resembles anaphylaxis. There are other granulomatous diseases, such as sarcoidosis (Chap. 50), in which type IV mechanisms also appear important, although the immunologic mechanisms are less clear.

Superantigens

Both staphylococci and streptococci make toxins that are capable of serving as superantigens. This means they can activate the TCR via its β chain without MHC restriction. Such a toxin is capable of activating 10–30% of the T cells, thus stimulating the release of a massive outpouring of cytokines and leading to shock and related symptoms (Chap. 4).

Immune Therapy

There are many ways in which modern immunology plays a role in therapy.

Immunization

Immunization is the oldest and most elegant immunology therapy. Antigens that are very similar to or identical with antigens from a pathogenic virus or bacteria are injected into the body. This may establish an immunologic memory, which is stimulated when the individual has contact with the real antigen. Then the immune system reacts both faster and more effectively than in a naive individual, thus efficiently protecting against the invading agent.

Immune Mediators

Some of the cytokines alluded to in the text are used as therapeutic agents. Most widely used are IFN-α and IL-2. While several different interferons are approved for treating human papilloma virus infections, IFN-α appears most effective. Both IFN-α and IL-2 are used in treating patients with malignant melanoma (Chap. 58). IL-10 has shown some promise in treating psoriasis. Blocking TNF with antibodies, receptor inhibitors or drugs like thalidomide are effective in suppressing severe aphthae, systemic lupus erythematosus and some leprosy reactions. Many of the mediators of innate immunity, such as the prostaglandins, can be used for therapy or inhibited, as the clinical setting dictates.

Immunosuppressive Therapy

Other manipulations of the immune system are less specific and usually less effective (Fig. 1.20).

Corticosteroids. The mainstay of immunosuppressive therapy is systemic corticosteroids that have a broad palette of effects on the immune system as well as a panoply of side effects. They are also the most important natural hormonal regulators of the immune response. Among other effects corticosteroids inhibit cell trafficking, reduce leukocyte migration, block T cell activation at the antigen presenting cell level and interfere with cytokine production and metabolism.

Cyclophosphamide and Chlorambucil. These alkylating agents primarily affect lymphocytes, reducing their number and function. B cells are more sensitive than T cells, and TC more than TH, but at the usual therapeutic levels the effects are profound and affect all lymphocytes.

Azathioprine. This drug inhibits purine metabolism and thus DNA synthesis. It is cytostatic and affects NK cells more than T cells and B cells, but all the effects are modest. Together with corticosteroids, azathioprine is well established in the treatment of immunoglobulin-mediated disease, especially bullous pemphigoid and pemphigus vulgaris.

Methotrexate. Despite its wide use in psoriasis and rheumatoid arthritis, the function of methotrexate is poorly understood. It too inhibits DNA synthesis via folic acid-dependent pathways. Methotrexate has a profound antiinflammatory effects independent of its cell-killing action, which may explain its effectiveness in the above disorders. Activated T cell subsets seem to be very sensitive to methotrexate, for it is effective in very low dosages in some patients with pityriasis lichenoides et varioliformis acuta and lymphomatoid papulosis.

Mycophenolate Mofetil. This drug blocks a pathway in purine synthesis of particular importance when lymphocytes are responding to antigenic

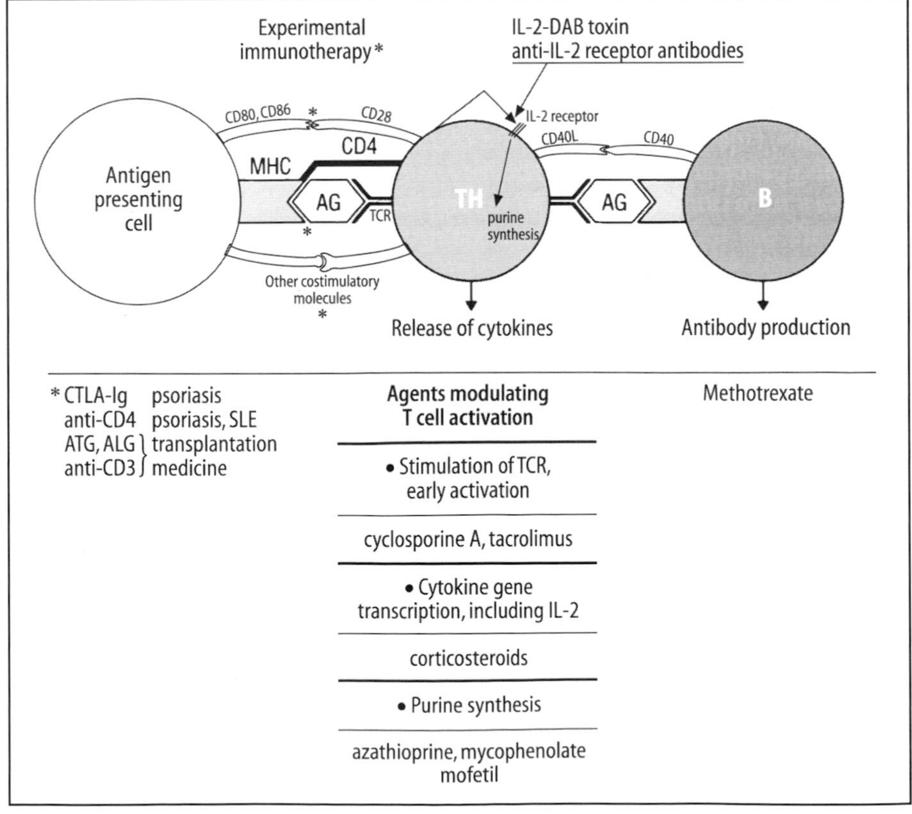

Fig. 1.20. Sites of action of immunosuppressive therapy. *AG* Antigen, *B* B cell, *MHC* Major histocompatibility complex, *TH* Helper T cell, *TCR* T cell receptor

challenge. Thus it appears to impair T cell and B cell proliferation with few side effects.

Cyclosporine and Tacrolimus (FK-506). These drugs both block signal transduction pathways in T cells. Thus they inhibit the transcription of genes needed for T cell activation and proliferation as well as for the production of cytokines.

Introduction to Genetics

The standard molecular genetic textbooks are longer and far more detailed than this book. Similarly, the bibles of dysmorphology are equally large and only handy when approached with a computer. Thus we will not attempt to tackle either molecular genetics or syndromes but only mention enough to allow residents and practicing dermatologists to understand the important clinical points.

Patterns of Inheritance

Lengthy discussions of "Is this disease inherited in an autosomal dominant or autosomal recessive pattern?" have lulled generations of dermatologists to sleep. Nonetheless, when confronted with a given syndrome or disease, one should consider a possible genetic basis. Most recent estimates from *On-line Mendelian Inheritance in Man* suggest that there are perhaps 9000 diseases inherited in autosomal fashion, 500 in an X-linked pattern, about 25 in a Y-linked pattern and perhaps 60 in a mitochondrial pattern.

Autosomal Dominant Inheritance

The trademark of autosomal dominant inheritance is diseases running through many generations if a family is large enough. One abnormal gene is sufficient to cause the disease. An example is neurofibromatosis type 1 or von Recklinghausen disease. The children of an affected patient have a 50% chance of developing the disease. Children of an unaffected member of the pedigree have no risk. In most instances, if the parents are not affected the child has a sporadic mutation and his future siblings have little risk. The frequency of mutations at the gene locus and the reduction in reproductive potential determine the relative proportions of new mutations and familial cases. For example, in neurofibromatosis the ratio is about 50 : 50, while in tuberous sclerosis more sporadic mutations or new patients are seen. Homozygotes for such genes are only rarely identified, but typically are more severely affected. In many instances the homozygous state may be lethal.

Some very large pedigrees have been traced; in one for variegate porphyria, in South Africa, all the patients appear to be related to a single affected Boer settler; this is known as the founder effect. If a grandparent and grandchild are affected, then the intervening father or mother must also be affected. If this is not clinically apparent, one speaks of incomplete penetrance. If the intervening member is more or less severely involved than the proband (first patient to be identified in a pedigree), the explanation is variable expressivity. Penetrance and expressivity have little intrinsic value; they are ways to explain a puzzling situation.

In general, dominant genes affect structural proteins so that if 50% of the protein made is abnormal, the function will be abnormal. While some enzymatic disorders, such as some of the porphyrias, are also inherited in an autosomal dominant fashion, it is rare for reduced enzyme levels to be so critical. Many disorders with an increased incidence of malignancy are inherited in an autosomal dominant fashion. Possible mechanisms are discussed below.

Autosomal Recessive Inheritance

The hallmarks of autosomal recessive inheritance are consanguinity and involvement of multiple offspring of the same parents. Thus, when confronted with a new syndrome in a family, one should always inquire about inbreeding and about the family's background, i.e., do they come from a small racial isolate. Both parents have one abnormal gene for a given structure, usually an enzyme, and are designated carriers. Their children each have an independent 25% risk of receiving two abnormal genes and being affected, as well as a 50% risk of being carriers; only 25% of their children are free of the abnormal gene. Children of an affected person have a low risk of being affected, as both parents must carry the same abnormal gene. Often a heterozygotic carrier has some sort of selective advantage to compensate for the disadvantage of an affected homozygote and help maintain the gene. The best example is sickle cell anemia, where carriers have increased resistance against malaria.

Codominant Inheritance

In many instances, one cannot convincingly speak of autosomal dominant or autosomal recessive inheritance. The classic example is the ABO blood group, in which both genes are expressed. In addition, often when one speaks of autosomal dominant inheritance, one could argue that the affected patient is merely a heterozygote and that if both abnormal genes were present, then the true clinical picture would be seen. Thus, autosomal dominant inheritance really means that the presence of one abnormal gene is enough to produce a given clinical picture. Conversely, so-called heterozygous carriers in autosomal recessive disorders are often not entirely normal; carriers of sickle cell disease have resistance against malaria but may suffer sickle crises when ill or at high latitudes. In essence, an abnormal gene makes abnormal products or fails to make normal ones; the body's dependence on these products determines how we interpret the inheritance.

X-Linked Recessive Inheritance

If a gene is located on the X chromosome, the pedigree becomes more confusing. Men have an XY karyotype, while women have two X chromosomes. If a given mutation is sufficient to cause disease in an XY man, then we speak of X-linked recessive inheritance. Women typically are not affected; they are heterozygous carriers with one normal and one abnormal X gene. The best known pedigree of this type involves the relatives of Queen Victoria, who was a carrier for hemophilia. Her gene wound up in the Russian and other European royal families, causing the hemophilia of the young Romanov princes. If a man is affected, all his daughters will be carriers and none of his sons will be affected. If a women is a carrier, 50 % of her sons will be affected and 50 % of her daughters will be carriers. Because of female carriers, skipped generations are the rule. If a women should receive two abnormal genes, she will be affected and the pedigree will become very confusing.

X-Linked Dominant Inheritance

This is a rare pattern but of special interest to dermatologists. In this situation a gene located on the X chromosome causes disease in a women with one abnormal gene. Since women are mosaics for the X chromosome, such diseases provide the most dramatic example of cutaneous mosaicism, as discussed below. The skin involvement is often linear or blotchy, following Blaschko lines, and may stop abruptly at the midline. Because of random inactivation of the X chromosome, the severity of the cutaneous and systemic disease can be highly variable in an affected women, depending on the proportion of active normal and defective genes. Affected males are very rare; most die in utero. Often there is a history of a number of stillborn male children. Some affected males have Klinefelter syndrome with two X chromosomes. Some males may be the result of gametic half-chromatid mutation, i.e., a mutation in the second meiotic division. Half the daughters of an affected women will be affected; half the sons will die in utero and the other half will be entirely normal. A mildly affected mosaic father can have a severely affected daughter.

Y-Linked Inheritance

The most obvious trait inherited on the Y chromosome is maleness. The sex-determining region of the Y chromosome (SRY) encodes the testis-determining factor, which is responsible for maleness. Many other genes on both the X chromosome and autosomes modify the sex of the individual. In addition, other genes are found on both the X and Y chromosomes; the traits that they determine are inherited in a pseudoautosomal fashion. No dermatologic diseases have been identified on the Y chromosome, although a knowledge of its function is essential in andrology (Chap. 68).

Mitochondrial Inheritance

Mitochondrial defects are responsible for a wide range of disorders. They are always inherited from the mother because the sperm does not transfer mitochondria. Thus an unusual pedigree is produced where an affected man cannot transmit the disease but an affected women often does. A variety of muscular and ocular disorders are inherited in this fashion; renal tubular disease, myopathy, growth retardation and seizures may also be seen. An association of symmetric lipomas of the neck and myoclonic seizures has been described, as have patients with poikiloderma and anhidrosis.

Unusual Patterns of Inheritance

There are many apparent exceptions to the rules outlined above. We will mention only briefly those that play a role in various genodermatoses.

Sex Limitation. Some diseases are only expressed in one sex even though the gene is located on an autosome. There is a gene for precocious puberty that affects young boys but not young girls. In other instances, the expression occurs more severely in one sex. For example, hemochromatosis (bronze diabetes) is seen earlier and more severely in men, presumably because menstruation provides treatment for affected women.

Age at Onset. Several serious diseases, most notably Huntington chorea, amyotrophic lateral sclerosis (Lou Gehrig disease) and myotonic dystrophy (of interest to dermatologists because of the presence of multiple pilomatricomas or hair follicle tumors), first become clinically apparent in adult life. This is particularly disturbing because frequently affected individuals have already founded a family by the time they are aware of the diagnosis. In most instances, early genetic diagnosis is now available. Sometimes the disease appears earlier in subsequent generations; this is known as anticipation. In some instances, anxiety and closer medical supervision may lead to an earlier diagnoses. In the cases of myotonic dystrophy and Huntington chorea, however, the answer lies in the phenomenon of trinucleotide repeats, pieces of DNA coding for three amino acids. While a normal individual may have 20–40 of these repeats in a given gene, an affected individual may have many hundred. In the next generation, the affected gene may have even more repeated material and the symptoms become more apparent.

Genomic Imprinting. Sometimes it makes a difference whether a gene comes from one parent or the other. The best known example concerns chromosome 15q11–13, in which if the paternal gene is missing Prader-Willi syndrome (Chap. 14) develops, while if the maternal gene is not expressed Angelman or happy puppet syndrome occurs. The two disorders are so different that one's imagination is challenged.

Genes and Cancers

The role of genes in cancer has become both clearer and simultaneously infinitely more complex in recent years. There are many ways in which a genetic mutation can predispose to the development of a malignancy. Three major categories of genes are involved.

Tumor Suppressor Genes. In disorders such as Gardner syndrome (Chap. 65), a gene is damaged that normally serves to downregulate or modulate cell growth. When this gene product is loss, cell growth is less well controlled.

Oncogenes. Despite their name, oncogenes are part of the normal cellular growth control pattern. When they suffer a mutation, they then overexpress their gene product or are not longer controllable by the usual cellular mechanisms, resulting in unrestricted growth. An example of an dermatologic disease with overexpression of an oncogene is MEN IIB (Chap. 65).

DNA Repair Genes. A wide variety of genes are responsible for repairing defects in DNA. Mutations in specific enzymes that repair DNA defects lead to the family of diseases known as xeroderma pigmentosum (Chap. 13). In the Muir-Torre syndrome (Chap. 65), mutations in a number of different DNA repair genes lead to microsatellite instability, may affect growth genes and predispose to cancer.

In many examples relating to all three types of cancer-related genes, autosomal dominant inheritance is the rule. The two-hit hypothesis of Knudsen best explains this phenomenon. He noticed that there were two different clinical settings for retinoblastoma. Some infants developed bilateral retinoblastomas early in life, while others acquired a solitary lesion later in life. In a normal individual, every cell has two functioning tumor suppressor genes; for such a cell to go astray, two mutations or hits are required. In an affected individual, each cell has only one functioning cancer control gene (regardless of type) and only a single mutation is required to produce a cell lacking adequate growth control or repair mechanisms and likely to become a tumor. Loss of heterozygosity also plays a role. A cell may have one functioning gene and one aberrant gene; the chromosome with the normal gene may be lost as a somatic mutation, producing a cell with only an aberrant tumor control gene.

Cell Immortalization

There is another genetic aspect of cancer development with dermatologic implications. All of the above defects involve a loss of regulation of growth or a failure to repair genetic damage. Human fibroblasts in culture typically go through about 50 divisions before their growth rate slows; they go through another 15–20 divisions in senescence and then eventually die off. A small proportion of cells escape senescence and continue to grow; such cells are immortalized. Malignant cell lines in culture are also often immortalized.

One explanation for immortalization may reside in the telomeres. Every chromosome has protective pieces at its ends known as telomeres. Each time DNA replication occurs a few telomeres are lost. Chromosomes without telomeres tend to fuse with other chromosomes or fragments, and the cell loses its ability to divide accurately. Many immortalized cells have an enzyme known as telomerase, so they can synthesize new telomeres and stabilize their chromosomes. One theoretical approach to treating cancers would be selective inhibition of telomerase.

Cytogenetic Defects

While cytogenetics or the analysis of chromosome number and structure has taken something of a back seat to molecular genetics in recent years, chromosomal abnormalities are still an important cause of disease. They are found in over 50% of first-trimester spontaneous abortions and in about 10% of stillborn infants and play a significant role in abnormal sexual development, primary amenorrhea and infertility. The most dramatic changes are the presence of an extra chromosome or the loss of a chromosome. In other instances, through complex errors in cell division, part of a chromosome may be lost or duplicated. Finally, two genes may be placed together through the process of translocation, where pieces of two chromosomes are exchanged. Such abnormal crossing over may place a growth control gene next to a structural gene. The classic example is Burkitt lymphoma, in which the *myc* oncogene on chromosome 8 is placed in contiguity with an immunoglobulin gene, usually the heavy chain gene on chromosome 14. As a result, the *myc* oncogene loses its control elements and is overexpressed, leading to a lymphoma. The Epstein-Barr virus appears to play a role in this change. Many other such examples are found, especially in hematologic malignancies; in the cases of many types of leukemia, the nature of the translocation helps determine therapy and predict prognosis.

A number of syndromes well known to dermatologists are caused by chromosomal defects; they are reviewed in Chapter 19.

Contiguous Gene Syndromes

There are a number of syndromes caused by highly specific deletions of small areas of chromosomes, causing a functional monosomy for one or more connected genes. Thus sometimes a series of single gene disorders are coupled. We have already mentioned the Prader-Willi and Angelman syndromes, caused by the deletion of paternal and maternal 15q11–13 segments respectively. DiGeorge syndrome, a primary immunodeficiency syndrome with thymic defects, is caused by a deletion of 22q11.21-q11.23 (Chap. 4). Retinoblastomas are caused by a deletion at 13q14 of a tumor suppressor gene, Rb1.

Multifactorial Inheritance

In a number of common disorders, there is no clear pattern of single gene inheritance, but nonetheless a definite familial tendency. Two excellent examples from dermatology are atopic dermatitis and psoriasis. Here a number of genes as well as a variety of environmental factors are felt to combine to determine the likelihood of an individual having the disease. The risk for children or other relatives to be affected is determined in a statistical sense, rather than as a simple proportion.

Mutations

While the ability of chromosomes to duplicate themselves exactly is crucial, a certain degree of variability is also essential, for without this we would all be identical and no species of animal would be able to adapt well to environmental or population changes. In every generation, there is a shuffling of the genetic material, technically known as recombination, putting different alleles of two adjacent genes together. Mutations may occur in the germ line, in which case they first appear in the offspring of the affected individual, or they may appear in somatic cells, often leading to malformations and tumors. Mutations that occur in early embryonic life cause both germ-line and somatic damage, as in the 8–16-cell embryo the distinctions between the two tissues are not yet clear. Somatic cell mutations lead to mosaicism and are discussed at greater length under that heading.

More important is the development of spontaneous mutations. These may take several forms.

Gene Mutation. In this instance change in a given gene, often in just one base pair, leads to a functionally abnormal protein that produces a change in the phenotype. These changes usually occur in the gametes or very early embryos and lead to the Mendelian traits with single gene inheritance. For every disorder, there is a spontaneous mutation rate that can be estimated; for neurofibromatosis 1, for example, it is 6×10^{6}.

Chromosome Mutation. A variety of gross structural changes can occur. They include loss or duplication of a segment of a chromosome, inversion of a segment, insertion of a loose segment into the false site, or translocation in which one or more segments exchange places. Chromosomal mutations cause a variety of congenital syndromes, as well as playing a role in many malignancies, especially hematologic ones. If they arise in the germline they produce congenital defects, and if they arise later they may cause tumors.

Genomic Mutations. One or more chromosomes can either be missing or present in excess. This is known as aneuploidy. When three of a given chromosome are found, one speaks of trisomy, such as in Down syndrome or trisomy 21. Rare fetuses have three sets of chromosomes, being either 69 XX or 69 XY; almost all die in utero.

In addition to spontaneous mutations, there may be acquired mutations. These may also be of evolutionary advantage but in many instances they are deleterious. Among the best known mutagens are:

Ionizing Radiation (Chaps. 13, 71). The mutagenic region stretches from ultraviolet radiation into X-rays and gamma rays. Exposure to ionizing radiation can be the result of a nuclear explosion, as in survivors of Hiroshima and Nagasaki; in some areas there is low-grade spontaneous background radiation, e.g., from radon; and, of special interest to dermatologists, mutations may be caused by therapeutic intervention with both X-rays and ultraviolet radiation. Ultraviolet radiation only affects the skin, as it does not penetrate into the body. The induction of actinic keratoses and perhaps even some squamous cell carcinomas depends on UV-induced mutations coupled with the immunosuppressive effects of the same radiation. X-rays and gamma rays can penetrate the body, causing both germ-line and somatic mutations. The latter may lead to a variety of malignancies, especially involving the hematopoietic system.

Chemicals. Many agents used for cancer chemotherapy are mutagens. The genetic damage they cause to the tumor cells is often the reason for their clinical effectiveness, but they also damage the DNA of other cells and the germ line. Thus both later or second tumors as well as genetic aberrations in offspring are possible sequelae.

Viruses. Some viruses alter the genetic material of the host cell. The translocations so characteristic of Burkitt lymphoma appear to be induced by Epstein-Barr virus.

Mosaicism

Mosaicism refers to the presence in an organism of at least two populations of genetically distinct cells arising from the same zygote or fertilized egg. A chimera results when an organism contains cells from two different zygotes, e.g., after a bone-marrow transplant or in complex twin situations. Mosaicism is actually quite common; all women are mosaic for the X chromosome, and all organisms are mosaic for a series of genes.

X Chromosome Mosaicism and the Lyon Hypothesis

To understand mosaicism one must consider the role of the X chromosome in some detail. The X chromosome carries a considerable amount of genetic information, perhaps 5% of the genome, while the Y chromosome contains the sex-determining region and little else. Thus, one could imagine that if an enzyme were encoded on the X chromosome, a XX women would have twice as much of the enzyme as an XY male. In most instances this is not the case.

To explain this paradox, Mary Lyon (1961) proposed a hypothesis of X chromosome inactivation. It states that in early embryonic life one of the two X chromosomes in each female cell is randomly inactivated. All progeny of that cell have the same X chromosome inactivated. Thus a normal women is a mosaic consisting of some cells with one X chromosome functioning and some with the other active. Because the inactivation is random, the number of cells with a given X chromosome active follows a Gaussian distribution. While in most individuals there is about a 50:50 split, some patients carry a given chromosome in almost all their cells or in virtually none. The inactivated X chromosome condenses in the periphery of the nucleus; it is known as a Barr body and can be most easily seen on mucosal smears or as drumsticks in leukocytes.

There are exceptions to the Lyon hypothesis. In some instances, the inactivation is not random. In Wiskott-Aldrich syndrome (Chap. 23), for example, in lymphocytes the normal X chromosome is active, while in mucosal cells the inactivation is random. Moreover, sometimes in very early embryogenesis the paternal X chromosome may be selectively inactivated. Furthermore, a small area of the X chromosome is not completely inactivated; it is known as the pseudoautosomal region 1 (PAR1) and contains several genes of interest to dermatologists, including the steroid sulfatase gene for X-linked recessive ichthyosis. Thus a carrier female will have half the levels of a normal female.

The clonality of X chromosome inactivation is seen in many clinical examples. Blood group antigens or enzyme variations can be studied in women. For example, uterine leiomyomas (fibroids) are a common tumor in women; the neoplasms are often clonal. In the most common form of chronic granulomatous disease, inherited in an X-linked recessive pattern, the carrier mothers have two populations of leukocytes, those with normal and those with abnormal bactericidal function (Chap. 4). Finally, with Duchenne-type muscular dystrophy, the mothers of affected males have a patchwork pattern of normal and dystrophic muscle cells.

The Lyon hypothesis and mosaicism are intimately involved in diseases inherited in an X-linked dominant pattern. Almost all such patients are female, as males are generally too severely affected to survive. If a gene on the X chromosome is involved that produces abnormal skin, then an affected female will have a patchwork of normal and abnormal skin. The unifying cutaneous feature is the unique distribution of the lesions. Blaschko (1901) described the patterns seen with epidermal nevi. He thought the distribution of nerves played a role in the changes but his lines actually have nothing to do with dermatomes. They reflect the migration of cells as the embryo elongates and becomes more complex.

Today four patterns of mosaicism in the skin are identified (Happle 1993):

- Blaschko Lines. Starting at the dorsal midline, these lines arch towards the head and form a bow, dropping off to the side. On the flank and abdomen, they have a more S-shaped form. They may be either relatively thin, as in hypomelanosis of Ito (Chap. 26), or much thicker, as in McCune-Albright syndrome (Chap. 26).
- Checkerboard Pattern. Large rectangular areas are produced, typically ending abruptly at the midline. The best example is CHILD syndrome (Chap. 17).
- Phylloid Pattern. Phylloid means leaf-like. Large irregular leafy structures are distributed much like a Jugendstil painting but with the midline respected.
- Patchy Pattern. Perhaps because of very early inactivation or failure of some clones to survive, very large patches crossing the midline are found. Giant hairy melanocytic nevi, especially those associated with leptomeningeal melanosis (Chap. 58), are a good example.

The classic X-linked dominant disorders include focal dermal hypoplasia (Chap. 19), oral-facial-digital syndrome type 1 (Chap. 19), incontinentia pigmenti (Chap. 26), CHILD syndrome (Chap. 17) and X-linked dominant chondrodysplasia punctata or Conradi-Hünermann syndrome (Chap. 17). In focal dermal hypoplasia, the bones show peculiar linear streaks which are also felt to represent clonal inactivation, as is the case for the cartilage defects in chondrodysplasia punctata. The pigmentary changes of hypomelanosis of Ito, linear and whorled nevoid hypomelanosis and nevus depigmentosus (Chap. 26) also follow Blaschko lines. Sometimes the Blaschko lines can be more subtle; in X-linked recessive hypohidrotic ectodermal dysplasia (Chap. 30), affected patients are males. Their mothers, as female carriers, show areas of normal sweating and of hypohidrosis which also follow Blaschko lines.

Autosomal Mosaicism

A somatic mutation can produce autosomal mosaicism. In most instances, such a mutation is a dead-end street; it cannot be transmitted. If a mutation occurs very early in embryonic life, it may involve the germ line as well as somatic cells. In this situation, a person with somatic mosaicism is a potential carrier for a systemic malformation.

For dermatologists, the best example of somatic mutations is provided by epidermal nevi (Chap. 52). These lesions follow Blaschko lines; indeed, they stimulated Blaschko to suggest the lines. They represent mutations in genes concerning with keratinization, such as the gene for Darier disease (Chap. 17). What has been called linear Darier disease is nothing more than an individual who is mosaic for the Darier gene as a result of a somatic mutation. Another common pattern in epidermal nevi is epidermolytic hyperkeratosis (Chap. 17). In several instances individuals with mosaicism for a mutation in keratin 1 or 10 and an epidermal nevus have had children with bullous ichthyosiform erythroderma, a disorder of keratinization inherited in an autosomal dominant pattern. The best explanation is that the parent with the mosaic skin lesion also carried the abnormal gene in his gametes. The abnormal keratin gene is inherited, not the epidermal nevus.

Inflammatory diseases may also follow the distribution of Blaschko lines. The term blaschkitis or *blaschkite de l'adulte* (Grosshans and Marot 1990) has been proposed for this change, but it is slightly misleading. Blaschkitis is not one disease, but probably many. The best example is lichen striatus (Chap. 14), but lichen planus, psoriasis and many other forms of dermatitis have been seen in the same distribution following Blaschko lines.

A second genetic mechanism can lead to segmental epidermal nevi or other changes. There may be loss of heterozygosity. This is a common mechanism in the development of tumors, but may also cause cutaneous mosaicism. In many diseases, including both Darier disease (Chap. 17) and neurofibromatosis 1 (Chap. 19), patients have been identified with the disease who also had a epidermal nevus or localized increase in neurofibromas respectively. Either the normal gene is lost, as is usually the case, or a second mutation creates a cell line homozygous for the mutation.

Mosaicism with Lethal Mutations

Some autosomal gene mutations are so deleterious to cell function that abnormal cells can exist only in a mosaic with normal cells. If a germ-line mutation occurs involving such a gene, the embryo does not survive. Thus such diseases almost always occur in a sporadic fashion. In the case of Proteus syndrome (Chap. 19) and McCune-Albright syndrome (Chap. 26), this hypothesis has been fairly well supported. It also may explain neurocutaneous melanosis, hypomelanosis of Ito and some vascular malformations, such as Klippel-Trénaunay-Weber and Sturge-Weber syndromes. In addition, some of the epidermal nevus syndromes (Chap. 52) may also be caused by lethal dominant genes.

Paradominant Inheritance

Paradominant inheritance has been proposed to explain the occurrence of a variety of lesions that suggest somatic mosaicism but appear in families, such as Klippel-Trénaunay-Weber syndrome and Becker nevus. Imagine that an individual is heterozygous for a gene capable of causing a vascular malformation yet is clinically completely normal. The gene can thus be passed through many generations without producing any clinical signs. But if a second mutation or loss of heterozygosity occurs in an early embryologic stage, a somatic mutation is produced. If the same event occurs in a descendant several generations later, then the picture of autosomal dominant inheritance with skipped generations is produced.

Twin Spotting

Twin spotting is an unusual form of allelic loss that is well established in plants and may explain vascular twin nevi, phakomatosis pigmentovascularis and phakomatosis pigmentokeratotica (Chap. 19). If a patient is heterozygous for two different recessive mutations, somatic recombination (also known as sister chromatid exchange) may produce closely related clones that are homozygous for the defects. Imagine a gene for vascular tone – one gene causes dilated vessels; the other, constricted vessels. Thus heterozygous cells have a balance between dilation and constriction. But if recombination occurs, then there may be two adjacent patches, one of which has widely dilated and the other firmly constricted vessels. If yet another gene is closely linked to the vascular tone gene, then more complex recombination could produce three lesions, as seen in phakomatosis pigmentovascularis.

Identification of Genes

The Human Genome Project is in full swing as we write. It involves using complicated automated devices to identify all the genes in the human genome. This will have many benefits for man. It should be possible to find the responsible gene and protein for virtually every genetic disease. Many new proteins, such as fibrillin in Marfan syndrome and neurofibromin in neurofibromatosis type 1, were first identified via reverse genetics; first the gene was identified, then the responsible protein found. The techniques of localizing genes, identifying proteins and exploring their functions both in mouse models and humans are a fascinating story beyond our scope.

Genetic Counseling

Our advice regarding genetic counseling can be easily summed up: Be careful. Considerable intellectual, emotional and legal problems are associated with advising patients about the risk of possible genetic disease. There are two typical situations:

- Parents with one affected child want to know the risk of a second affected child.
- A parent with a given disease wants to know the risk for a child.

The main role of the dermatologist is to ensure an absolutely correct and precise diagnosis. Diagnoses such as poikiloderma, ichthyosis or epidermolysis bullosa are of no benefit to the family or genetic counselor. Because many genodermatoses are so rare, the practicing physician should make use of national and even international experts whenever appropriate.

Once the diagnosis has been made, in many instances the pattern of inheritance is known and the risk can be estimated. For example, a parent with autosomal dominant dystrophic epidermolysis bullosa has a 50% chance of having affected children, while one with autosomal recessive epidermolysis bullosa has almost no chance of passing the disease on. In the case of X-linked disorders, an affected male cannot transmit the disease. His daughters will all be carriers; his sons, all normal.

In the other setting, when two apparently normal parents have an affected child, one must first decide on the pattern of transmission. The parents should be carefully examined for mild signs of an autosomal dominant disease. For example, in tuberous sclerosis one might find a connective tissue nevus and ash-leaf macules in an otherwise normal parent. The risk for subsequent children is 50% if a parent is involved. If the child's disease represents a new mutation, then the risk of a second affected child is the same as in the general population. If the new disorder is inherited in an autosomal recessive pattern, then the risk for each subsequent child is 25%. If the mother is a carrier for a disorder inherited in an X-linked recessive pattern, then boys have a 50% risk of being affected and girls a 50% risk of being carriers.

In both Germany and the USA, physicians receive special training and certification in human genetics and genetic counseling. If someone without this training performs genetic counseling, their medicolegal position is weakened. In addition, many studies have shown that special skills are required to convey such sensitive information to parents. Simply stating a 25% risk for a second child with a syndrome inherited in an autosomal recessive pattern is inadequate; many parents understand this to mean that their risk is small as they have already had one affected child and can expect three normal ones. The information must be repeated many times, questions repeatedly answered and documentation made precise. In some series, even immediately after a session only about 50% of the counseled individuals can remember their diagnosis or their estimated risk.

Genetic counseling also cannot be separated from the very emotional issue of abortion. In many instances following prenatal diagnosis, all that can be said to the parents is that they can either opt for an abortion or expect a child with the disorder concerned. Thus one is both morally and medically required to strive for the lowest possible false-positive rate, to avoid recommending abortion for healthy fetuses; at the same time, however, any false-negative diagnosis is likely to result in a confrontation, often in the legal system.

Prenatal Diagnosis

When a couple at risk has conceived a child and wish to know whether their child is affected, the many tools of prenatal diagnosis come into play. Couples who benefit from prenatal diagnosis include older parents (usually mothers older than 35 years), parents with a genetic disorder and those with a documented family history of such a disorder. The possibility of in utero or early therapy, the accuracy of the test method and the severity of the suspected disorder must all be balanced against the risk to the mother and child. We intentionally have not listed all the genetic disorders for which prenatal diagnosis is possible because the list and the methods are changing rapidly as more and more genes are identified. Once a clinical diagnosis has been made, even an experienced genetic counselor will consult on-line sources for information about the latest possibilities in diagnosis. In most cases, positive prenatal identification of a disorder will lead to the recommendation for an abortion.

There are both noninvasive and invasive methods of prenatal diagnosis. The noninvasive methods include the following:

- Ultrasound can observe many defects, such as cardiac rhabdomyoma in tuberous sclerosis, nuchal thickening in Down syndrome and Turner syndrome and missing patellas in nail-patella syndrome.
- Maternal blood screening can identify fetal cells and has been employed to diagnosis Down syndrome. This very powerful technique remains experimental. Often the α-fetoprotein is measured to asses the risk of neural tube defects.

The invasive methods are used to obtain fetal cells for chromosomal analysis, biochemical tests to identify enzyme defects and DNA tests to identify candidate gene mutations. The sex of the fetus can also be determined. In the past, if a carrier of an X-linked recessive disorder became pregnant, sometimes she was advised to abort male fetuses. Today usually one can determine whether the boy has the disorder concerned. Possibilities include the following:

- Preimplantation analysis can be used to study eight-cell blastocysts prior to implantation. A single cell is removed, cloned and studied for mutations in the candidate gene. Only blastocysts without the mutation are implanted. The loss of a single cell at the eight-cell stage does not produce fetal defects.
- Chorionic villus sampling is can be performed as early as 8–12 weeks. It offers the earliest diagnosis of the standard techniques, but bears a slightly higher risk for the fetus.
- Amniocentesis yields not only cells for the genetic tests, but also amniotic fluid, which can be analyzed for α-fetoprotein and other biochemical parameters. It is performed after the 14th week, so when cells must be cultured the diagnosis may not be available before the 18th week and a repeat study becomes difficult.
- Umbilical vein catheterization is usually used to search for infections but is also used for some hematologic disorders and as an avenue for fetal transfusion or treatment. It is performed after the 18th week.
- Fetal skin biopsy is of great interest to dermatologists. Carried out between 18 and 20 weeks, it can diagnose some genodermatoses with distinctive histologic appearances, such as some types of ichthyosis and epidermolysis bullosa. Light-microscopic, electron-microscopic or immunohistochemical features can be utilized to make a diagnosis. In the case of trichothiodystrophy, the characteristic changes first appear in the 24th week, necessitating a delay. Other diseases that have been diagnosed include X-linked hypohidrotic ectodermal dysplasia, Chédiak-Higashi syndrome, tyrosinase-negative albinism and incontinentia pigmenti. Because of the mosaicism in incontinentia pigmenti, a negative biopsy here is of no meaning.

Genetic Therapy

Fortunately the black hole of genetic therapy taken in its broadest sense is becoming smaller. For example, with appropriate prenatal diagnosis, prenatal transfusions, administration of medications and even surgery (such as closing a neural tube defect) are possible. The replacement of defective genes has been attempted in a number of disorders, but has not functioned perfectly. The skin is seen as a possible site of therapy not only for cutaneous diseases but also for other disorders, because cultured, genetically modified keratino-cytes or fibroblasts can be regrafted in a patient where they can produce needed proteins, not just for skin disorders but perhaps for other problems.

Bibliography

General Textbooks

Arndt KA, Robinson JK, Leboit PE et al. (eds) (1994) Cutaneous medicine and surgery. An integrated program in dermatology. Saunders, Philadelphia

Champion RH, Burton JL, Burns AD et al. (eds) (1998) Textbook of dermatology, 6th edn. Blackwell, Oxford

Fitzpatrick TB, Eisen AZ, Wolff K et al. (eds) (1999) Dermatology in general medicine, 5th edn. McGraw-Hill, New York

Basic Biology of Skin

Bereiter-Hahn J, Matoltsy AG, Richards KS (eds) (1986) Biology of the integument, vol 2. Vertebrates. Springer, Berlin

Breathnach AS (ed) (1971) An atlas of the ultrastructure of human skin. Churchill, London

Goldsmith LLA (ed) (1992) Physiology, biochemistry and molecular biology of the skin. Oxford University Press, New York

Dermatoscopy

Krahn G, Gottlober P, Sander C et al. (1998) Dermatoscopy and high frequency sonography: two useful non-invasive methods to increase preoperative diagnostic accuracy in pigmented skin lesions. Pigment Cell Res 11(3):151–154

Stolz W, Braun-Falco O, Bilek P et al. (eds) (1994) Color atlas of dermatoscopy. Blackwell, Berlin

Ultrasonography

Korting HC, Gottlöber P, Schmid-Wendtner MH et al. (eds) (1999) Ultraschall in der Dermatologie. Blackwell, Berlin

Dermatopathology

Ackerman AB (ed) (1997) Histologic diagnosis of inflammatory skin diseases, 2nd edn. Williams and Wilkins, Baltimore

Maize JC, Burgdorf WHC, Hurt MA et al. (eds) (1998) Cutaneous pathology. Churchill Livingstone, Philadelphia

Elder D, Elenitsas R, Jaworsky C et al. (eds) (1997) Lever's histopathology of the skin, 8th edn. Lippincott-Raven, Philadelphia

Weedon D (ed) (1997) Skin pathology. Churchill-Livingstone, Edinburgh

Immunology

Abbas AK, Lichtman AH, Pober JS (eds) (1997) Cellular and molecular immunology, 3rd edn. Saunders, Philadelphia

Bos JD (ed) (1995) Skin immune system, 2nd edn. CRC Press, Boca Raton

Dahl MV (ed) (1996) Clinical immunodermatology, 3rd edn. Mosby, St. Louis

Janeway CA, Travers P (1997) Immunobiology – the immune system in health and disease, 3rd edn. Garland, New York

Roitt I (ed) (1998) Essential immunology, 9th edn. Blackwell, Oxford

Roitt I, Brostoff J, Male D (eds) (1998) Immunology, 5th edn. Mosby, London

Genetics

Blaschko A (1901) Die Nervenverteilung in der Haut in ihrer Beziehung zu den Erkrankungen der Haut. In: Braumüller (ed) Beilage zu den Verhandlungen der Deutschen Dermatologischen Gesellschaft: VII. Congress zu Breslau, May 1901, Vienna, Austria

Grosshans E, Marot L (1990) Blaschkite de l'Adulte. Ann Dermatol Venereol 117:9–15

Happle R (1999) Loss of heterozygosity in human skin. J Am Acad Dermatol 41:143–161

Moss C, Savin J (eds) (1995) Dermatology and the new genetics. Blackwell, Oxford

Novice FM, Collison DW, Burgdorf WHC et al. (eds) (1994) Handbook of genetic skin disorders. Saunders, Philadelphia

Sybert VP (ed) (1997) Genetic skin disorder. Oxford University Press, New York

Viral Diseases

Contents

A wide variety of skin diseases are caused by viruses. Cutaneous lesions may either reflect a direct skin infection by an epidermotropic virus, such as in molluscum contagiosum or verrucae, or may be a reflection of a widespread viral infection, such as in measles or chicken pox. Finally, the human immunodeficiency virus (HIV) causes an almost endless list of skin findings primarily through the acquired immunodeficiency syndrome (AIDS).

Warts

Synonym: Verrucae (singular, verruca)

Definition. Cutaneous tumors caused by epidermotropic viruses which tend to spontaneously regress but may rarely progress into cutaneous malignancies.

Causative Organism. Human papilloma virus

Epidemiology. Warts are extremely common because of the multiplicity of human papilloma viruses (HPVs), their worldwide distribution and the ease with which humans are infected. Immunosuppressed patients are likely to develop large, unusual and therapy-resistant warts. Some wart infections are occupational in nature, particularly in butchers and slaughterhouse workers. Of special interest are the oncogenic viruses, such as HPV-16, in genital infections. Patients with cervical infections in whom this HPV is identified are at a greater risk of cervical carcinoma than women in whom other HPVs are found.

HPVs are transferred between humans, from animals to humans, and presumably from humans to animals. Papilloma viruses have been identified in virtually all animals, including cats, dogs, cows and horses; even cases involving giraffes have been reported. The incubation time is highly variable ranging from weeks to years. In addition, autoinoculation is the rule, not the exception. Most typical is the child with warts on his hands who chews them and then develops oral warts. Warts may also appear in scratches.

Etiology and Pathogenesis. Human papilloma virus contains closed, circular double-stranded DNA of about 7.9 kilobases (kb). A long list of HPV types have been identified. Each type shows less than 50% homology to the others. Different HPVs are found in different clinical settings, such as common warts, genital lesions and epidermodysplasia verruciformis. Many different HPVs cause the same types of clinical lesions, as Table 2.1 shows. Sometimes more than one HPV will be found in a given wart.

A variety of possibilities exist to detect HPV. Each has its strengths and weaknesses.

- Direct immunofluorescence. Specific antigens, usually related to a group of HPVs, can be detected in well-differentiated cells which contain

Table 2.1. Human papilloma virus (HPV) types in various clinical lesions of the skin, genitalia and head and neck region

Lesions	Virus type
Skin lesions	
Verruca vulgaris	1–4, 26–29, 38, 41, 49, 57, 63, 65, 75, 76, 77
Butchers' warts	2, 7
Epidermodysplasia verruciformis	2, 3, 5, 8–10, 12, 14, 15, 17, 19, 20–25, 37, 47, 50
Bowen disease	16, 34, 35, 555
Squamous cell carcinoma	5, 8, 14, 17, 20, 41, 47
Actinic keratosis	36
Keratoacanthoma	37 (single case)
Malignant melanoma	38 (single case)
Genital lesions	
Condylomata acuminata	6, 11, 42, 44, **51**, 54, 55, 69
Carcinoma in situ	6, 11, **16, 18, 30, 31, 33, 35, 39**, 40, 42, 43, **45, 51, 52, 56**, 57, **58**, 59, 61, 62, 64, **66**, 67, 68, 69, 70
Anal intraepithelial neoplasia	**16, 18, 30, 31, 33, 35, 39, 45, 51, 52, 56, 58, 66, 69**, many others not high risk
Carcinoma	6, 11, **16, 18, 31, 33, 35, 39, 45, 51, 52**, 54, **56, 66, 69**
Oropharyngeal lesions	
Papillomas	6, 7, 11, 32, 57, 72, 73
Focal epithelial hyperplasia	13, 32
Carcinoma	2, 6, 11, 16, 18, **30**

HPVs in **boldface** have a high risk of causing malignancy. Modified from de Villiers 1994.

large amounts of virus, such as HPV in common warts. Commercially available but not sensitive or specific.
- Serologic tests. Primarily available as research tool for a limited number of HPVs.
- DNA hybridization. The standard for identifying new types but not easily applicable to screening and not sensitive.
- Polymerase chain reaction. Readily available and able to identify very small amounts of virus even in fixed tissue; in some instances perhaps too sensitive.

While HPV can readily be identified in all types of warts, exactly how it alters the infected keratinocytes to produce a clinical lesion is not entirely understood. One interesting phenomenon is that, as HPV infected lesions evolve into carcinomas, the HPV becomes harder to identify. We will consider warts based on their clinical appearance, rather than their HPV type.

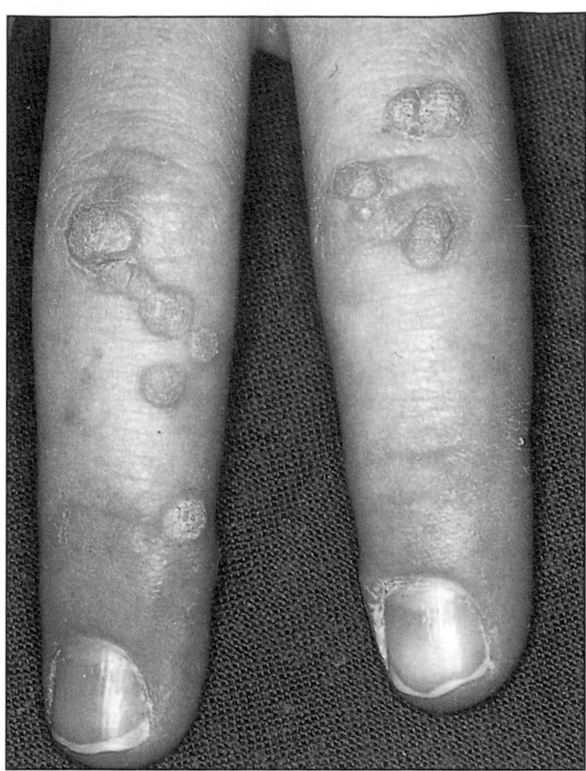

Fig. 2.1. Common warts

Common Wart

Synonym: verrucae vulgares (verruca vulgaris)

Clinical Findings. Common warts are usually multiple. Cool acrocyanotic areas are more likely to be infected, and children with atopic dermatitis seem to be more susceptible. An initial wart is a small smooth-domed papule, not much larger than the head of a pin. It can usually be distinguished from adjacent skin because it interrupts the normal skin lines. As warts grow, they tend to become darker and have a rougher surface. This reflects the convoluted epidermal surface (papillomatosis), hyperkeratosis and often punctate bleeding into the stratum corneum. Often the initial or mother wart will become considerably larger than the adjacent daughter warts. Sometimes warts which have been frozen in cryotherapy will clear centrally but expand as a ring, resembling a Pacific atoll.

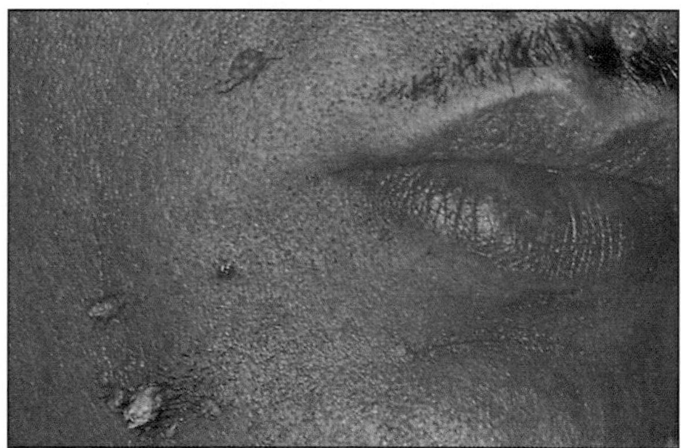

Fig. 2.2. Filiform warts

Regional localization also plays a role in determining the nature of the wart.

- Fingers and back of hands: Papular warts are the rule (Fig. 2.1).
- Eyelids: Long thin, filiform warts are most common.
- Beard area:. Both flat and filiform warts; often large numbers spread through shaving (Fig. 2.2). The same pattern is seen on the legs of women who shave.
- Scalp: Warts tend to be large and often exophytic, sometimes called digitate warts.
- Interdigital space: Warts are somewhat protected here, tending to become more papillomatous.
- Palms, volar surfaces of fingers: Warts usually smooth and sharply bordered; after mechanical debridement, the punctate hemorrhages are often easily seen.
- Soles: Warts are flat and often grow into the skin, much like a thorn, or spread like a tile mosaic.

- Periungual region: Warts in this area are common; while they are usually along the lateral nail fold, they may also grow under the distal nail fold (Fig. 2.3).
- Nail bed: Warts of the nail bed are most uncommon; they present as painful discolored spots or nodules which are generally diagnosed as "guilt by association." If the patient has many warts, the change under the nail may also be a wart.
- Vermilion: Warts are white and either papillomatous or filiform.
- Mucosa: Lesions tend to be white and moist.
- Penis and labia majora: Warts often broad-based and flat, occasionally hyperpigmented. When cytological atypia is found, one speaks of Bowenoid papulosis.
- Miscellaneous: Any body surface can be infected; other sites include the nasal mucosa, the nasal orifice and the conjunctivae.
- Immunosuppressed patients: Patients with congenital immunodeficiencies, HIV/AIDS and immunosuppression through chemotherapy may develop widespread, almost uncontrollable, warts. Similarly some patients with atopic dermatitis, especially those treated with topical corticosteroids for long periods, may also wind up covered with warts (Fig. 2.4).

Histopathology. The histologic picture of the common wart is distinctive. The overall pattern is a protuberant growth with epidermal hyperplasia and lateral epidermal strands enveloping the dermal base of the lesion. There is acanthosis or epidermal thickening, elongated rete ridges and papillae (papillomatosis) and prominent dilated vessels in the upper dermis. The latter are responsible for the leaking of blood into the stratum corneum where it can be clinically and histologically detected. The outer layers of the epidermis typically show vacuolar or ballooning degeneration with basophilic inclusions. The stratum corneum contains parakeratotic nuclei as well as hemorrhage.

Electron microscopic examination often allows one to identify viral particles. This is most easily achieved in new warts; in old lesions, particles may not be found. The particles are typically found in the ballooned or koilocytic cells of the granular layer.

Course and Prognosis. Most warts tend to resolve spontaneously, usually without scarring. When scarring does occur, it is a result of therapy. Often the warts will first become inflamed, signaling that the host's immune response is active, before they disappear.

Differential Diagnosis. A long list of cutaneous lesions look like warts. The most realistic approach is to suspect that hyperkeratotic, hemorrhagic papules are warts and to worry about the differential diagnosis only if the lesions appear atypical, are present in the elderly, or do not respond to

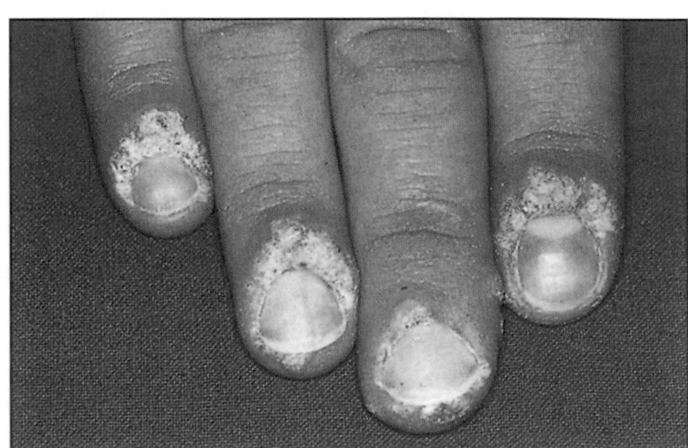

Fig. 2.3. Periungual warts

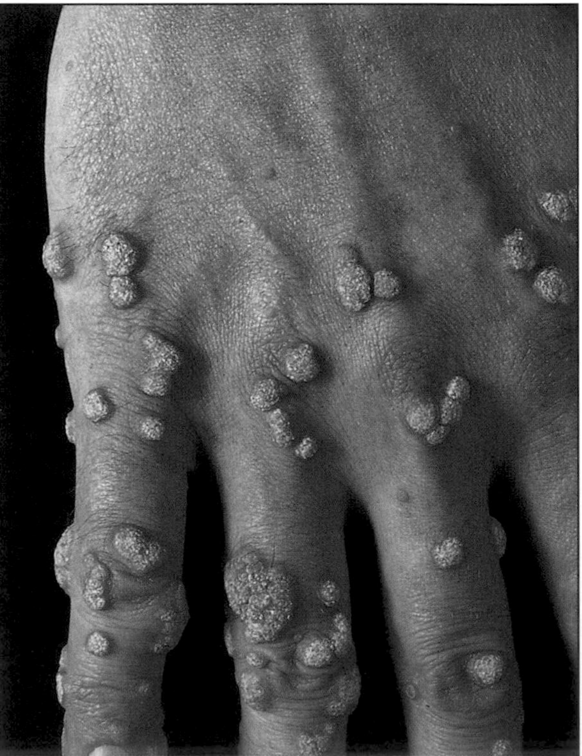

Fig. 2.4. Multiple warts in immunosuppressed patient

therapy. A partial list of verrucous lesions includes: keratoacanthoma and squamous cell carcinoma in sun-damaged skin or on the lip; warty dyskeratoma and trichilemmoma for solitary facial lesions; hypopigmented seborrheic keratosis on the face or trunk in older patients; hypertrophic lichen planus and clear cell acanthoma on the lower leg; punctate palmoplantar keratoderma and arsenical keratoses on the palms and soles; and tuberculosis cutis verrucosa on acral surfaces.

Plantar Warts

Epidemiology. The incidence of plantar warts seems to have increased in recent years. They are probably among the most contagious of warts, spread wherever large numbers of people go barefoot, as in swimming pools, gymnasiums, and group living situations (dormitories, prisons, and the like).

Clinical Findings. Plantar warts can either be solitary or widespread. The solitary form tends to be pushed into the skin or invaginated, presumably through the pressure and weight from walking. In addition, a reactive callus forms which often acts as a foreign object, much like having a stone in one's shoe. When the callus is trimmed, one can see the dilated capillaries and hemorrhage, producing black puncta. These are the "roots" of the wart, as so often described by the patient. They are helpful in distinguishing between a plantar wart, a clavus or corn, which has a central keratotic core, and a callus, which is simply hyperkeratotic. The most typical location is over the metacarpal heads. When plantar warts are not on weight-bearing areas, they tend to be less symptomatic and more exophytic (Fig. 2.5).

The second major category of plantar warts are mosaic warts. Here multiple warts coalesce together resembling a tile or mosaic floor. They tend to be flat and asymptomatic, which is just as well because they are almost impossible to treat. A much rarer variant is the giant plantar wart or epithelioma cuniculatum. The difference between a giant plantar wart of the heel, which is benign and reactive, and an epithelioma cuniculatum which is a verrucous carcinoma is one of degree and definition. If a large plantar wart on the heel of an adult does not respond to therapy, it should be biopsied.

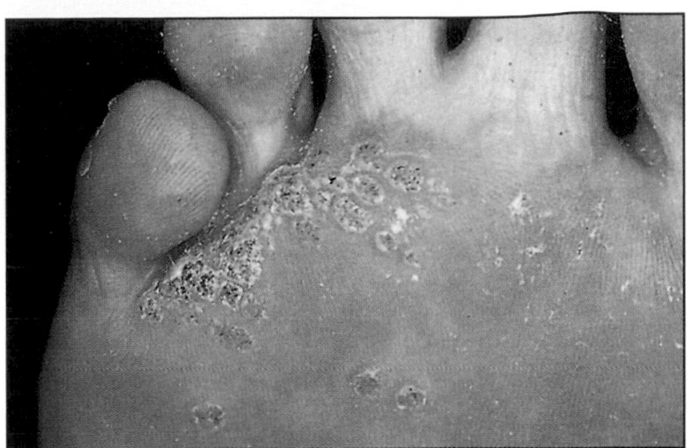

Fig. 2.5. Plantar warts

Histopathology. Plantar warts are notorious for being full of viral inclusions, showing striking granular layer changes. Usually the biopsy or curettage fragments do not allow one to appreciate the endophytic nature of the lesion, but clearly the papillary features of a common wart are missing. A verrucous carcinoma is typically bland without mitoses and also without viral changes, thus presenting a challenging diagnosis.

Plane Warts

(Besnier and Doyon 1881)

Clinical Findings. Plane warts are small flat papules, often slightly hyperpigmented and most commonly found on the face (Fig. 2.6). They are typically seen in children and young adults; similar lesions occur on the beard area and legs when spread by shaving. They may also be seen on the hands, arms and trunk. They may have a yellow or brown color, especially in darker individuals (Fig. 2.7); when inflamed, they are red. Frequently, plane warts disappear spontaneously. A herald of this event is the diffuse inflammation, suggesting that the body is beginning to recognize the wart as an invader and to mount a successful immunologic counterattack.

Histopathology. The changes are subtle. One sees a flat-topped papule with often minimal clear cell change in the granular layer. Other features of warts are absent.

Differential Diagnosis. When patients have many large, flat plane lesions, one should consider epidermodysplasia verruciformis. On the face other possibilities include syringomas and sebaceous

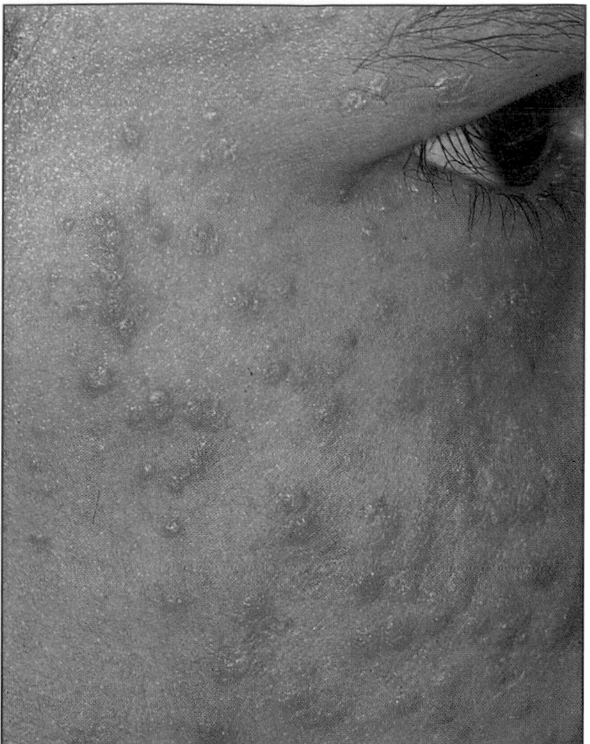

Fig. 2.6. Plane warts

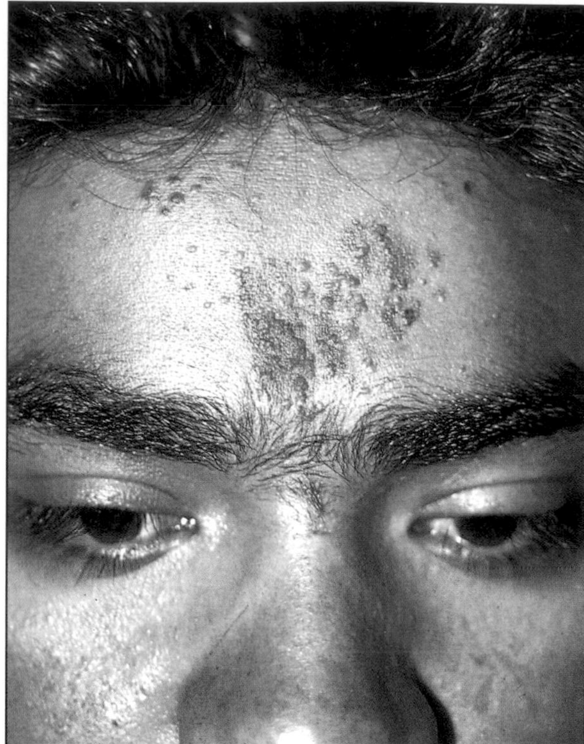

Fig. 2.7. Plane warts with marked hyperpigmentation in darker individual. (Courtesy of Juan J. Ochoa, MD, Chihuahua, Mexico)

gland hyperplasia, as well as dermatosis papulosa nigra in blacks. On the acral surfaces, the list is much longer. Lichen planus and lichen nitidus should be considered, but can be excluded histologically. Acrokeratosis verruciformis of Hopf is virtually identical, but generally occurs in patients with Darier's disease showing dyskeratosis histologically. Acrokeratoelastoidosis is limited to the sides of the hands and shows abnormal elastic fibers on biopsy.

Genital Warts

There are three relatively distinct variants of warts which arise on the genital and perianal mucosa, including the classical condylomata acuminata, the flat variant (condylomata plana) and the giant or destructive form.

Condylomata Acuminata

Epidemiology. Condylomata acuminata are highly contagious. The current epidemic of genital HPV disease has been somewhat overshadowed by the HIV/AIDS story, but it too is a major public health problem. In addition, several types of HPV found in the genital region, particularly HPV-16 and -18, appear to be oncogenic. Finally, perianal warts in children raise the possibility of child abuse, although usually autoinoculation is the case.

Clinical Findings. Genital warts grow best in a warm moist environment, such as under the foreskin, about the anus, and on the labia minora. Associated disorders such as a perianal dermatitis, chronic vaginal discharge or phimosis predispose the patient to HPV infection. Despite their disturbing clinical appearance, such warts rarely show malignant degeneration and often heal spontaneously.

The initial lesion is a tiny red papule, which may be white if hyperkeratotic and moist. Rapidly new lesions develop and all coalesce together, producing a cauliflower like picture. When such condylomata acuminata are examined, the lesions separate apart into many tiny pointed papillomas. When the lesions form in an area where they are under pressure, such as between the buttocks, in the inguinal folds and in the perineum, they became laterally flattened; such lesions are known as "rooster's comb warts" in German. Such large vegetating lesions are often macerated and foul-smelling.

The most typical locations are:

- Women. Labia minora reaching to the introitus, occasionally in the vagina. Lesions on the labia majora tend to be large, flat hyperkeratotic common warts.
- Men. The coronal sulcus is the most common site (Fig. 2.8); lesions may involve the glans and are also common in the urethral meatus, which may be overlooked in therapy. There is often a secondary balanitis, which may be symptomatic and obscure the clinical diagnosis. Large condylomata acuminata may ulcerate through the foreskin, creating an alarming clinical picture. Warts of the shaft are typically small, flat common warts.
- Perianal region. Here the condylomata acuminata have ample opportunity to grow, so that the cauliflower picture is most typical. Since HPV also thrives in the rectum, anoscopy or proctoscopy should be performed in all such patients to exclude foci which can lead to reseeding. Homosexual males are at particular risk for perianal warts (Fig. 2.9).
- Other sites. Rarely, moist regions such as under the breast or in the axillae will allow HPV to grow in the condylomata acuminata pattern.

Differential Diagnosis. Condylomata acuminata are fairly specific clinically. The distinction from condylomata lata is more linguistic than clinical. The latter are the broad, flat-based, moist genital patches of secondary syphilis, teeming with spirochetes. When enough maceration and inflammation is present, the primary diagnosis may be overlooked. Pemphigus vegetans presents with massive vegetating lesions which can be mistaken for macerated condylomata acuminata. Pustules at the periphery are a subtle clue to the correct diagnosis of the blistering disorder; in addition, it tends to involve other body areas, including the mouth.

Flat Genital Warts

Large flat warts or condylomata plana are typically found on the cervix and prepuce. They tend to

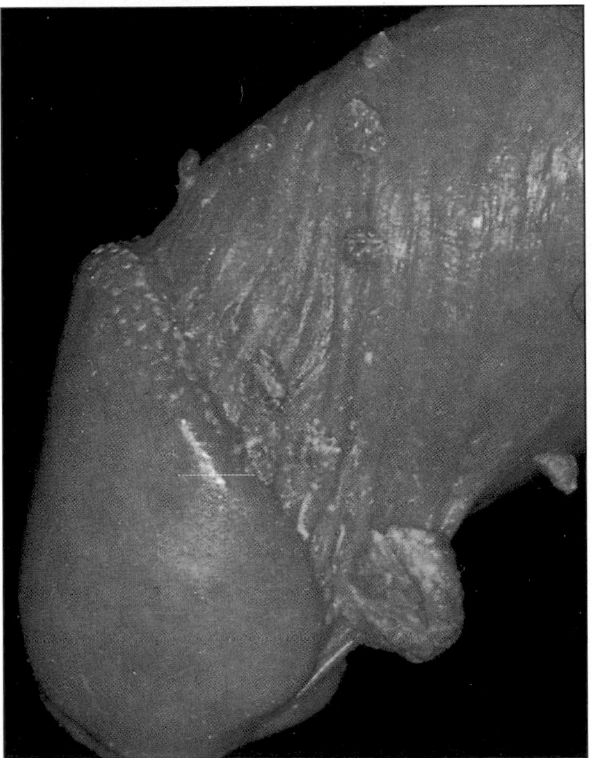

Fig. 2.8. Condylomata acuminata

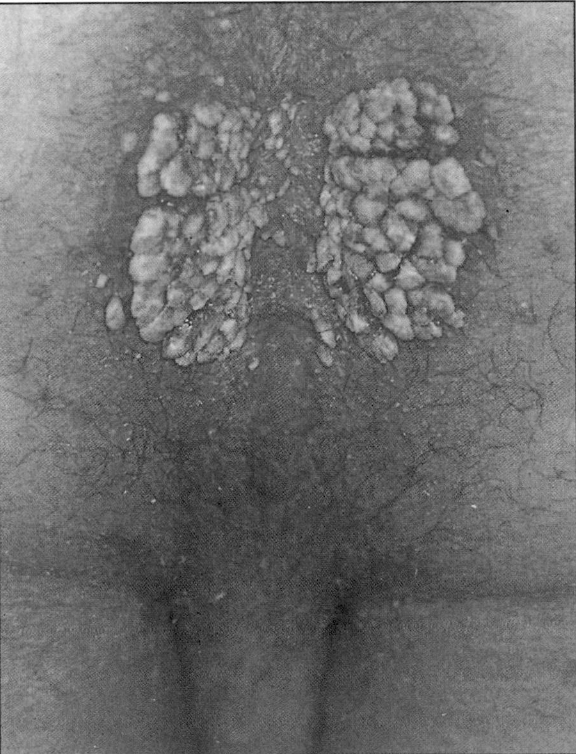

Fig. 2.9. Perianal condylomata acuminata

be HPV-16 or -18, types associated with cervical carcinoma. In silhouette they resemble condylomata lata, but the localization and clinical story are different.

Giant Genital Warts

(Buschke and Löwenstein 1925)

Clinical Findings. These large destructive tumors, usually called Buschke-Löwenstein tumors, are typically perianal or under the foreskin. They often ulcerate the foreskin, producing a buttonhole effect, and may also invade the corpora cavernosa leading to marked hemorrhage.

Histopathology. While most agree that such tumors begin as warts, they at some point become squamous cell carcinomas, most often of the verrucous type (Chap. 56). The time of transition is impossible to determine clinically, and often difficult under the microscope on small biopsies. Thus, a large, persistent penile or perianal wart, especially if it appears clinically destructive, should be generously biopsied or excised.

Mucosal Warts

As confusing as the terminology of cutaneous HPV infections is, it is lucid in comparison to the situation in the mouth. Oral pathologists speak of squamous papilloma and oral verruca vulgaris, which they agree may be identical, and then of oral condylomata acuminata. In addition, focal epithelial hyperplasia or Heck disease is also caused by HPV, usually type 13. Verrucous carcinoma was first described in the mouth; some such lesions have an HPV origin. Finally, florid oral papillomatosis, a vague and even more poorly defined disorder, is felt by some to represent diffuse oral HPV infection and by others to be a precursor of verrucous carcinoma.

Squamous Papilloma

Synonym. Oral verruca vulgaris

Etiology and Pathogenesis. Most such lesions are solitary oral verruca, probably transmitted to the oral mucosa from the hands. In some tissues, no HPV can be identified ; these lesions may represent old warts or a reactive phenomenon. Some oral pathologists diagnose oral verruca vulgaris when other warts are present on the skin and squamous papilloma for a solitary lesion.

Clinical Findings. These generally solitary, painless exophytic lesions are most commonly found on the tongue, floor of the mouth, palate, uvula and lips. They are typically present in children and young adults. The surface is usually white and, while they may be stalked, they are not pedunculated.

Condylomata Acuminata

Etiology and Pathogenesis. These lesions represent the oral equivalent of genital warts, usually caused by genital HPV types and often transmitted by oral-genital sex.

Clinical Findings. Generally, there are many, small pedunculated papules, usually white or pale because they are not strikingly hyperkeratotic. Such changes are far more common in immunosuppressed patients, especially those with HIV/AIDS.

Florid Oral Papillomatosis

Synonym. Disseminated oral verrucae

Clinical Findings. A few patients, occasionally immunosuppressed ones, have multiple, slowly spreading, therapy- resistant oral verruca. In some patients there are bilateral lesions on the buccal mucosa, usually close to the angle of the mouth. This problem is further discussed in Chapter 55.

Focal Epithelial Hyperplasia

(Archard et al. 1965)

Synonym. Heck disease

Etiology and Pathogenesis. This is a common infection of the oral mucosa by HPV-13 and occasionally other HPVs in American Indians, Eskimos and other racial groups. Heck was a dentist assigned to the Public Health Service in Gallup, New Mexico, where he described the disorder among Navajo patients. Initially, it was felt to be a genetic disorder because of the common occurrence in multiple members of different generations of a family; instead, the correct answer turned out to be vertical transmission of a virus within a family.

Clinical Findings. The disease usually presents in childhood. Typically, patients have hundreds of small papules, some skin-colored, others white, covering the lips, gingiva and labial and buccal mucosa. There is some tendency for improvement in adulthood. Histologically the lesions are typical condyloma acuminata.

Epidermodysplasia Verruciformis

(Lewandowsky and Lutz 1922)

Definition. A rare disorder in which patients are uniquely predisposed to infection with a wide range of otherwise nonpathogenic HPV.

Etiology and Pathogenesis. Most cases of epidermodysplasia verruciformis are sporadic, but about 25% of patients have been reported as displaying autosomal recessive inheritance, and some families show X-linked recessive inheritance. A long list of HPVs are found, most of which are extremely uncommon in the rest of the population and some of which are carcinogenic. Individual patients typically have lesions with several HPV types. Types HPV-5 and -8 are especially likely to lead to malignant transformation, which is described in over 50% of patients.

Clinical Findings. Two types of lesions are seen, appearing first in childhood. The broad, flat, often scaly lesions of the face and trunk resemble tinea versicolor, while the more acral lichenoid papules, especially in sun-exposed areas, resemble plane warts. The latter lesions are more likely to become carcinomas. Lesions may become confluent, especially on the knees, elbows and trunk, producing large patches of infection. While the mucosal surfaces are spared, almost any part of the body may be infected.

Histopathology. There are subtle differences between the two types of lesions, with more epidermal atypia seen in the papular lesions.

Therapy. Regular control examinations to detect changing or suspicious lesions, which can then be treated, are important. Cryotherapy, tangential excisions, curettage and laser ablation are all appropriate. Radiation therapy should be avoided, since it serves as a cocarcinogen in this subgroup. Oral retinoids show no convincing benefits.

Warts in Immunosuppressed Patients

Like many other infections, HPV can overwhelm immunocompromised hosts. Patients with organ transplants, Hodgkin disease, or HIV/AIDS as well as those requiring chemotherapy are at special risk. In these individuals, warts tend to be multiple, reach great size and not be amenable to therapy. Often, if the immune status improves, as with aggressive anti-viral therapy in HIV/AIDS, the warts may improve.

Therapy

A wide range of therapeutic measures are available for treating warts. Their multiplicity underscores the fact that no one regimen is highly effective. Since warts are an infection and in most cases self-limited, treatment should be designed to avoid scarring and should not be terribly aggressive or painful. Obviously, when dealing with warts which have the potential to turn into squamous cell carcinoma, such as Buschke-Löwenstein tumors and growing lesions in epidermodysplasia verruciformis and immunosuppressed patients, one must treat more aggressively.

The choice of methods is primarily based on the experience and skills of the physician; other factors include location, number, and size of the warts as well as previous therapeutic attempts by the patient, parents or other physicians. One should remember that, regardless of the method chosen, HPV will probably be left behind in the skin so the likelihood of recurrence is high.

Cryotherapy. Liquid nitrogen cryotherapy is probably the most widely used method of wart treatment. The liquid can be applied either with a spray applicator, metal sounds or cotton-tipped swabs. The spray applicator is faster, more precise and allows deeper freezing. One needs to freeze hard enough to produce a blister or at least some epidermal loss. The HPV themselves are not damaged by the cold temperature. The recommended freezing interval is every2 weeks; a range of 1–3 weeks is acceptable.

Surgery. Warts can be removed under local anesthesia, using a curette, scalpel or electrosurgical device. Even plantar warts can be enucleated, but the likelihood of recurrence and a painful scar is high. Surgery is best suited for a small number of warts on glabrous skin.

Lasers. Warts can be excised or vaporized with a CO_2 laser. Since the HPV particles are potentially infectious for the patient and operating room personnel, an exhaust system and double-masking are needed. Lasers are well-suited for periungual warts, since they allow better visualization, because of less bleeding, and facilitate removal of part or all the nail. Lasers are also convenient in other areas, such as when treating hundreds of perianal or intraanal warts.

Keratolytic Agents. A wide variety of topical keratolytic agents can be applied, often in conjunction with cryotherapy. Salicylic acid is the mainstay, available in solutions of flexible collodion, as 40–60% plasters and in special gel patches. The patient should change the plasters after 3–5 days, or repeat the solution daily. Dead skin must be removed with a special callus plane, fine scissors, diamond nail file, pumice stone or similar device before repeating the treatment. A popular keratolytic ointment in Europe is:

Rx Anthralin ointment

Anthralin	0.5–1.0
Salicylic acid	12.5
Paraffin liq.	2.5
White petrolatum ad	50.0

Other ingredients such as lactic acid can also be combined with salicylic acid in the wart tinctures.

Tricholoracetic acid in solutions of 20–50% can be painted on warts. The wart surface then turns white, burns and later desquamates. While a degree of caution is required, this is a rapid way to treat genital warts. Much milder keratolytic agents can be employed for facial plane warts. Often, topical tretinoin is used; one can adjust the strength to induce erythema and inflammation. Similarly, salicylic acid, 1–5% solution in alcohol, can be used.

Cytostatic Agents. The main cytostatic agent employed is podophyllin, an inhibitor of the mitotic cytoskeleton derived from the may apple, *Podophyllum peltatum.* The large yellow fruit contains an emetic, while the rest of the large plant is rich in podophyllotoxin and peltatins, which have antimitotic action. Traditionally, podophyllin has been mixed as a 20–25% solution in tincture of benzoin. Since plant extracts are highly variable, the compounded products are also not uniform. Podophyllin is best suited for mucosal surfaces; for example, it works well on the glans penis but poorly on the shaft. Podophyllin should not be used in the mouth or on the urethral orifice (except by urologists) and is contraindicated in pregnancy. It is applied by the physician; the patient is instructed to wash the medication off after 4–6 h or immediately if marked burning or pain occurs. The treatment is repeated weekly.

A more standardized podophyllin mixture contains 1% podophyllotoxin (podofilox), known in the USA as Condylox. It is FDA-approved for home treatment of genital warts. It can be applied b.i.d. for 3 days, followed by 4 days of rest. Up to four cycles can be completed prior to reexamination by the physician. A 0.5% podofilox gel is also available, designed specifically for anogenital warts. Gynecologists often employ 5-fluorouracil cream, initially designed for actinic keratoses, to treat condylomata acuminata of the labia minora and introitus. While this approach is not officially approved in the USA, a mixture of 0.5% 5-fluorouracil and 10% salicylic acid is available in Germany for treating common warts.

Immunologic Therapy. Since the body eventually clears warts by cell-mediated immunity, there has long been a search to treat warts in this way. Today, several different interferons are approved for therapy of difficult to treat warts. They can be used for intralesional injection, often combined with mechanical debulking. In other instances, interferons are injected subcutaneously when treating large numbers of warts. In Germany, a topical gel is also produced. Since interferons are very expensive and have not produced strikingly better results than traditional methods, they have not achieved widespread acceptance.

Imiquimod 5% cream is approved for external anogenital warts. The imidazoquinolines are heterocyclic amines that act as immune response modifiers, inducing production of interferon-α. The cream is applied three times weekly. Lengthy treatment periods of up to 16 weeks are a major disadvantage, both for the patient and in assessing efficacy.

Other Approaches. Since warts are self-limited, especially in children, often no therapy is a wise approach. Since parents and insurers are unlikely to pay for a visit to the physician that results in no therapy, a wide range of harmless or placebo approaches have been employed, including colored or fluorescent dyes, special elixirs or even well-known folk remedies such as touching the wart with a frog.

One should work with the appropriate clinical specialist when treating urethral, perianal or genital warts to insure that seeding from internal sources is excluded or controlled. When warts are in moist areas, this predisposing factor must also be addressed. Patients with condylomata acuminata should be evaluated for other sexually transmitted disease. Children with condylomata acuminata should be referred for social service evaluation regarding the possibility of child abuse. Women with genital warts should be reminded to have yearly Papanicolau smears. Partners of patients with genital warts should be advised to be examined and treated, if needed.

Prophylaxis

Several vaccines against HPV are in development with early clinical testing now in progress. Initially they will be aimed against the types of HPV that are found in premalignant cervical lesions.

Herpes Viruses

There are at least eight human herpes viruses (HHV), all which have been associated with cutaneous disease, as shown in Table 2.2. The herpes viruses are DNA viruses with an icosahedral structure containing 162 capsomeres. This capsid is surrounded by a lipid coat with spikes of glycoproteins. The herpes viruses remain in the host for a lifetime, despite the development of antibodies or cellular immune responses. They can be subdivided on DNA sequencing and separated by PCR, culture and immunohistochemical tests, although most appear identical by electron microscopy. While humans are the only host for these eight viruses, monkeys and apes harbor a variety of simian herpes viruses which can infect and kill humans.

Herpes Simplex Viruses

The herpes simplex viruses (HSVs) are neurotropic and epidermotropic. They cause a wide range of clinical disorders, depending on the age and immune status of the patient, as well as whether the viral infection is primary or secondary. In newborns, HSV may cause sepsis and encephalitis; in young children, severe primary herpetic gingivostomatitis; in older individuals recurrent oral or genital infections; and in the elderly or immunosuppressed disseminated infections. Often there is a trigger such as fever, sunlight, trauma or stress involved in the recurrent attack. Grouped blisters or erosions frequently appear; this arrangement is referred to as herpetiform.

Causative Organism. Two types of HSV have been identified. HSV type 1 (HSV-1) is typically found above the waistline, usually on the lips, oral mucosa and head and neck. HSV type 2 (HSV-2) occurs most often on the genitalia.

Epidemiology. Both types of HSV are very widespread so that almost every individual harbors one or both of them. Either type can appear anywhere on the body. Tiny abrasions or defects in the skin, conjunctiva, oral mucosa or gastrointestinal tract serve as entry sites. The initial HSV-1 infection usually occurs in childhood. After a incubation period of about 1 week, the widespread oral mani-

Table 2.2. Herpes viruses

Virus	Diseases
Herpes simplex virus 1	Oral, labial, cerebral herpes simplex
Herpes simplex virus 2	Genital, neonatal herpes simplex
Varicella zoster virus	Chicken pox, zoster
Epstein-Barr virus	Infectious mononucleosis, Burkitt lymphoma, nasopharyngeal carcinoma lymphoproliferative diseases in immunocompromised patients
Cytomegalovirus	Neonatal infections, atypical mononucleosis, transfusion infections, chorioretinitis in HIV/AIDS
Human herpes virus-6	Exanthem subitum, pneumonia in immunocompromised patients
Human herpes virus-7	Hepatitis, infectious mononucleosis-like picture, exanthem subitum, pityriasis rosea
Human herpes virus-8	Kaposi sarcoma

festations appear. The source is usually an infected parent or sibling, often with a subclinical recurrent infection associated with viral shedding. About 90% of adults have antibodies against HSV-1 and may suffer from recurrent disease.

For HSV-2 the pattern is less clear; the primary infection usually occurs during adolescence or early adult life, presumably as sexual contact begins. The primary infection is often asymptomatic. With HSV-2, one speaks of the initial infection that brings the patient to medical attention but which may well not be the primary event. Many patients are asymptomatic shedders of the virus. On any given day, about 1% of infected patients experience reactivation of HSV-2. The percentage of adults with antibodies against HSV-2 has risen in recent years. In the USA about 20% of adults are infected. Not surprisingly, multiple sexual contacts and failure to use a condom are the major risk factors. In a large study of women who were not infected at the start of their pregnancy, about 2% acquired HSV-2 during pregnancy. Acquisition towards the end of pregnancy is associated with neonatal herpes simplex and perinatal morbidity. Primary infections late in pregnancy are far more dangerous than reactivation. Seroconversion completed before the onset of labor carries few risks.

Etiology and Pathogenesis. The patient's immune response plays a key role in HSV infection. In addition, one distinguishes between primary and recurrent infections (Table 2.3). In the initial infection, HSV enters a local defect and multiplies, producing local clinical changes and causing a viremia. Antibodies develop but do not lead to viral elimination. Instead the virus remains latent in nerve ganglia. Herpes viruses spread from cell to cell, as well as along nerves. The lack of effectiveness of herpes vaccines that produced significant antibody titers underscores the fact that the antibodies are an epiphenomenon and epidemiological marker, but not a form of protection.

Recurrences usually come from the reactivation of latent viruses in the nerves. Another possible explanation is that viral DNA, but not intact viruses, remain in the body. Recurrences often have an identifiable trigger. In the head and neck region, fever and sunlight are the main culprits. In the genital region, trauma (from sexual intercourse), menses, and stress are usually blamed.

HSV-2 may also be a co-carcinogen for cervical carcinoma. HSV-2 infections are more common in women with cervical carcinoma. Conversely, early cervical dysplasia and carcinoma in situ are about four times more common in HSV-2-positive individuals. The exact significance and mechanisms of carcinogenesis are unclear; HSV-2 may act as a cofactor with HPV-16 and -18.

Table 2.4 shows which diseases are most often associated with HSV-1 and HSV-2.

Laboratory Findings. The following methods are available to identify HSV.

- Tzanck smear. Blister contents are spread on a glass slide, stained with almost any contrast media, and examined for the typical multinucleated giant cells created, as HSV causes epithelial cells to fuse together. Normally, the Tzanck smear, despite its simplicity, offers the most definitive diagnosis.
- Electron microscopy. Negative staining of blister material can be examined quickly (within hours) to identify the viral bodies.
- Routine histology. While HSVs cause fairly typical microscopic changes of epidermal necrosis, multinucleated giant cells and a steel-gray cytoplasm in infected cells, detection of these changes is less specific than the above methods.

Table 2.3. Primary and secondary herpes simplex virus infections

Primary infections	Secondary infections
Herpetic gingivostomatitis	Recurrent (labial, genital, cutaneous) herpes simplex
Aphthoid Pospischill-Feyrter	Herpetic keratoconjunctivitis
Herpetic vulvovaginitis	Eczema herpeticum
Neonatal herpes with sepsis	Herpetic meningoencephalitis
Herpetic keratoconjunctivitis	Inoculation herpes infections
Eczema herpeticum	Recurrent erythema multiforme
Herpetic meningoencephalitis	
Inoculation herpes infections (herpetic whitlow, herpes gladiatorum)	

Table 2.4. Correlation between clinical disorder and herpes simplex virus (HSV) type

Location	Clinical disorder	HSV type
Skin	Recurrent herpes simplex (cold sore, fever blister)	1
	Herpetic whitlow	Usually 1
	Recurrent genital and buttocks herpes simplex	2
	Eczema herpeticum	1
Mucosa	Herpetic gingivostomatitis	1
	Aphthoid Pospischill-Feyrter	1
	Herpetic vulvovaginitis	2
Eyes	Herpetic keratoconjunctivitis	1 and 2
CNS	Herpetic meningoencephalitis	1 and 2
Sepsis	Neonatal herpes sepsis	2, rarely 1

None of these methods identify the HSV type nor can they separate HSV from varicella zoster virus (VZV). If this is needed, one must use one of the following, more sophisticated, techniques.

- PCR: In a matter of hours, the HSV type can be identified from virtually any tissue or fluid, fixed or fresh.
- Immunofluorescent examination: Tissue can be examined with antibodies against HSV-1, HSV-2 and VZV, allowing an exact and rapid discrimination.
- Viral culture: Culture takes up to 48 h and may not yield organisms if the source is not fresh. For example, a crusted blister may no longer contain living viruses.
- Serologic tests: These evaluations are of epidemiological interest but play no role in the prompt diagnosis of a clinical problem.

Therapy. While the therapy of the various types of herpes simplex and zoster infections is considered individually below, in the interest of space, we summarize the available antiviral agents here.

The mainstay of antiviral therapy is acyclovir, an acyclic purine nucleoside analogue. It is phosphorylated by viral thymidine kinase and then interferes with viral DNA synthesis. Thus it is able to inhibit viral reproduction without significantly affecting the host cells, since they lack the appropriate enzymes to phosphorylate and incorporate acyclovir. While acyclovir is available as a cream or gel, we find these forms ineffective. In general, oral acyclovir or similar products suffice for nonimmunosuppressed patients; in neonates and immunosuppressed patients, intravenous therapy is usually appropriate. Acyclovir can be used to treat initial infections, recurrences or it can be prescribed for many months to suppress infections. Acyclovir is a very safe drug; the main consideration is to adjust dosage to reflect decreased renal function.

Several variants of acyclovir are available.

- Valacyclovir: This is a pro-drug of acyclovir that is converted rapidly to the parent drug following the first intestinal or hepatic passage. It can be used in b.i.d. or t.i.d. dosages and provides higher blood levels than acyclovir.
- Famciclovir: Another purine nucleoside analogue, famciclovir is converted to penciclovir in the gastrointestinal tract and liver. It is available very quickly but otherwise has a spectrum similar to that of acyclovir.
- Penciclovir: Only available as a cream, penciclovir is more effective topically than other drugs in the family but still is not comparable in efficacy to the oral forms.
- Bromvinyldeoxyuridine or brivudine: This is another modified nucleoside. It is available in Germany and several other countries.
- Foscarnet: This agent should be reserved for resistant herpes simplex infections in immunosuppressed hosts. It is a toxic drug which inhibits DNA polymerases and does not work through thymidine kinase. Foscarnet is also often employed as a second agent in cytomegalovirus (CMV) retinitis in HIV/AIDS patients. It may cause acute renal failure, cardiac problems, marrow toxicity and even produces cutaneous ulcerations which may resemble the condition for which it is being employed.

Table 2.5 includes dosage recommendations for all of the above mentioned agents.

Table 2.5. Recommended dosages of antiviral agents for herpes simplex virus

Disease form	Medication	Dosage
Primary episode	Acyclovir Valacyclovir	400 mg PO t.i.d. or 200 mg PO 5× daily for 7–10 days 1.0 g b.i.d.– t.i.d. for 7–10 days
Recurrence	Acyclovir Valacyclovir Famciclovir	400 mg PO t.i.d. for 5 days 500 mg PO b.i.d. for 5 days 125–250 mg PO b.i.d. for 5 days
Suppression	Acyclovir Valacyclovir Famciclovir	400 mg PO b.i.d. 500 mg PO b.i.d. 125 mg PO b.i.d
Immunosuppressed patient	Acyclovir[a]	5 mg/kg IV t.i.d. for 1–2 weeks (can switch to 400 mg PO 5× daily)
Neonatal infection	Acyclovir)[a]	10 mg/kg IV t.i.d. for 2–3 weeks

[a] Other agents can also be employed; the relevant literature should be consulted

Prophylaxis. A variety of herpes simplex vaccines have been available over the past 30 years. One was widely sold in Germany for many years before it was firmly established that efficacy was lacking. The latest attempt involves an interesting biological twist, using disabled infectious single cycle (DISC) viruses. These viruses can only complete a single replicative cycle in the vaccine recipient, but still stimulate both antibody and cell-mediated responses.

Differential Diagnosis. Angular cheilitis may initially have a similar appearance. Widespread oral candidiasis in an immunosuppressed patient can also be severe. Aphthae are uncommon in small children. Impetigo may appear similar in the perioral region, but does not involve the mucosa. Other viral enanthems such as herpangina are not as severe and do not spread to the skin.

Primary Herpes Simplex Virus Infections

Herpetic Gingivostomatitis

Definition. Initial infection with HSV-1, typically involving the oral mucosa of small children.

Clinical Findings. After an incubation period of 2–7 days, the child presents with fever, malaise and a painful mouth (Fig. 2.10). Often the first sign is refusal to eat. Typically there are oral erosions and ulcerations which spread to involve the perioral skin (Fig. 2.11). They are rarely deep and tend to spare the posterior mouth. Marked salivation and a foul odor are typical. Regional lymphadenopathy is almost always present. Since the disease is spread by direct contact or droplets, small epidemics may develop within families, kindergartens and even pediatric nursing stations. Usually healing is prompt, over a week or two. Occasionally herpetic whitlow (paronychia) may develop in the small patient, from sucking the fingers, or in the mother and health personnel, who are inoculated during feeding attempts. The outlook is good, as most patients recover uneventfully.

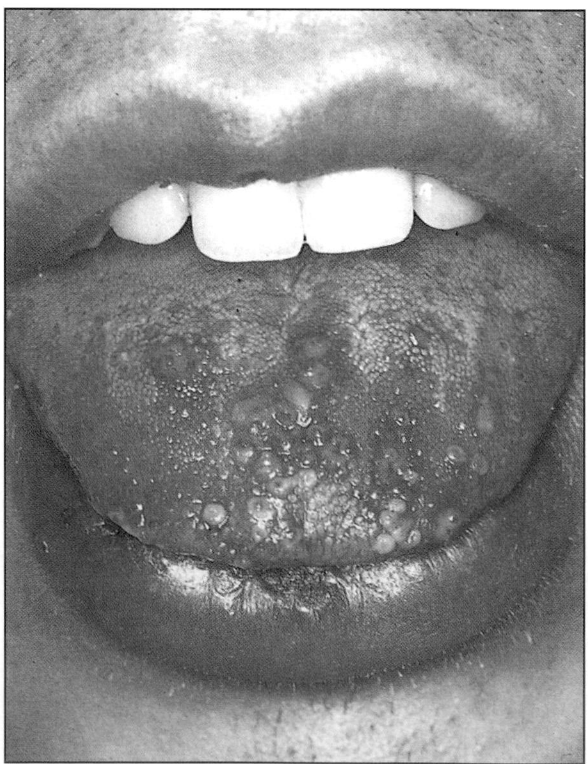

Fig. 2.10. Acute herpetic gingivostomatitis

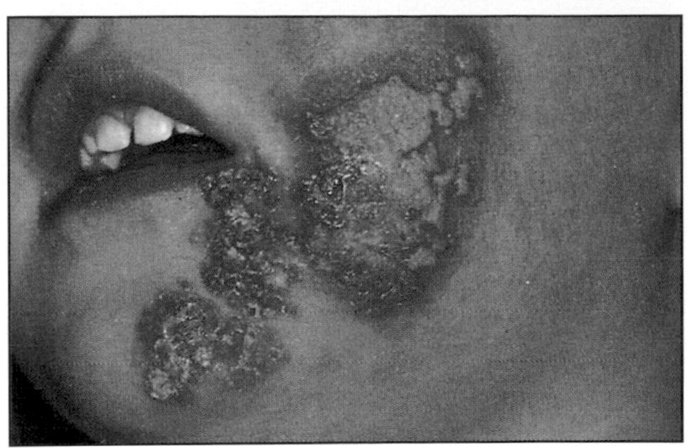

Fig. 2.11. Severe primary herpes simplex infection

Therapy

Systemic. Because of feeding difficulties, intravenous fluids are usually required. Young infants, immunosuppressed patients and perhaps patients with very severe disease should receive intravenous acyclovir or other antiviral agents. Systemic antibiotics may be used to treat or cover for secondary bacterial infection.

Topical. Usually supportive nursing care is all that is needed. Topical anesthetics may make eating more comfortable.

Aphthoid of Pospischill-Feyrter

(Pospischill 1921; Feyrter 1938)

Clinical Findings. Extremely severe, primary herpetic gingivostomatitis may develop in a child whose resistance has been reduced by a concomitant infection such as measles. The same pattern is seen in immunosuppressed children, especially those undergoing cancer chemotherapy. The young patient is quite ill and the findings spread beyond the mouth. Severe perioral erosions and ulcers are the rule, but genital and even acral lesions may be seen. The latter are called wandering aphthae in German. Such patients usually require intravenous antiviral therapy.

Herpetic Vulvovaginitis

Definition. First attack of genital herpes, often with severe inflammation of the female genitalia.

Epidemiology. While previously most cases of genital HSV infection were caused by HSV-2, today HSV-1 and HSV-2 are about equally common.

Clinical Findings. The patient, usually an adolescent or young adult, presents with severe genital pain, fever and malaise. The vulva is swollen and red; blisters and crust extend onto the adjacent skin. Internal spread may also occur, ascending the vagina and involving the cervix.

Differential Diagnosis. Behçet disease and genital aphthae may appear similar, but do not have as much internal involvement. While sexually transmitted diseases are often considered, none of the others present with such diffuse findings. Recurrent HSV infection in an immunosuppressed host may be equally severe.

Therapy

Systemic. Oral acyclovir or other antiviral therapy is given in primary and initial genital infections. This was the first setting in which the benefits of the drug were proven.

Topical. Drying measures such as zinc oxide lotions are helpful, as are sitz baths.

Other Primary Cutaneous Herpes Simplex Infections

Herpes simplex virus can be inoculated into other body sites, producing a confusing clinical picture. One common scenario is herpes gladiatorum, in which HSV is spread through a group of wrestlers. While the initial source usually has labial HSV, he spreads it to other body parts of opponents during wrestling and they in turn spread it further. Acyclovir has reduced the frequency and severity of such outbreaks.

Dentists and other people working in the mouth may be inoculated around the nail fold with HSV. Small barrier breaks lead to an acute, swollen painful digit known as a herpetic whitlow. The increased use of gloves because of hepatitis B and HIV has helped ameliorate this problem.

The third most common site of herpes is the buttocks – a fact often forgotten. Herpes of the buttocks is more common in women and gay men, suggesting that it is spread by spooning (front-to-back sexual contact). In the same groups, especially gay males, perianal HSV infection is another possible presentation.

All of these primary forms of HSV can be misdiagnosed because of their unusual locations. All tend to recur, just as do labial or genital HSV. Thus a recurrent blistering or ulcerated eruption on any body site is HSV until proven otherwise.

Neonatal Infections

Definition. Acute primary HSV infection of the newborn.

Etiology and Pathogenesis. Herpes simplex virus can be transferred from the cervical canal or external genitalia to the infant during delivery. Many studies have been performed to determine the most effective way to ameliorate this risk. Cesarean sections have been recommended for women with active genital HSV disease or a positive culture during pregnancy. If the membranes rupture in a mother at risk, section should be performed within 4–6 h. Unfortunately, the bulk of all neonatal HSV occurs in infants whose mothers are asymptomatic shedders. Most cases (about 75%) involve HSV-2. The problem is more common and severe in premature infants. HSV can also be transferred in the immediate postdelivery period if the mother or nursing personnel have active herpetic lesions, such as a herpetic whitlow.

Clinical Findings. The patient may present with grouped blisters or erosions on the scalp or buttocks, depending on the type of obstetric presentation. In at least half the patients, there are no cutaneous signs, just a septic newborn whose life is at risk. In about 75% of infected infants, the HSV disseminates. Such patients are likely to die, while the survivors are at risk for mental retardation and other severe problems.

Differential Diagnosis. Herpes simplex virus always enters into the differential diagnosis of neonatal sepsis, regardless of the cutaneous findings or maternal history. Other causes of blisters and pustules in neonates include staphylococcal infections, superficial candidiasis, erythema toxicum neonatorum, neonatal pustular melanosis, folliculitis and trauma.

Therapy

Systemic. The mainstay of therapy is intravenous acyclovir. In the past, other antivirals and immunoglobulins were also employed but they play less of a role today.

Topical. Mild drying measures are all that is needed.

Prophylaxis. Prevention is most important. Mothers at clear risk, such as those with a history of genital HSV infection or with a partner with such an infection, should be followed closely. Cultures every 7–14 days during the last 6–8 weeks of pregnancy have been recommended, but still miss many asymptomatic shedders. There is good evidence that treating mothers at risk with oral acyclovir during the last weeks of pregnancy is helpful. Even though acyclovir is not officially approved in pregnancy, the risks of neonatal HSV are so great that its use is recommended by many sources.

Central Nervous System Infections

Primary herpetic meningoencephalitis is usually caused by HSV-1. It is a feared complication of primary herpetic gingivostomatitis but may also appear in patients with minimal cutaneous findings. Rarely is meningoencephalitis associated with recurrences. The patient is critically ill with nausea, vomiting, seizures, lethargy and other problems. In contrast, HSV-2 usually causes an aseptic meningitis or peripheral neuropathy which is much milder. It can appear either as part of a primary infection or during a recurrence.

Eczema Herpeticum

(Juliusberg 1889)

Synonyms. Eczema herpeticatum, Kaposi varicelliform eruption

Definition. Generalized HSV infection in patients with atopic dermatitis and other widespread skin diseases. The same term may also be used for disseminated HSV infection in immunosuppressed hosts.

Etiology and Pathogenesis. Eczema herpeticum seems to be increasing in prevalence. This may relate to the increased use of topical corticosteroids, to the increased number of immunosuppressed patients or to a change in viral virulence. The problem can be associated with either a primary or recurrent HSV infection. It can result from autoinoculation, usually from labial HSV, or heteroinoculation from an infected contact. Many diseases with epidermal barrier defects, such as atopic dermatitis, Darier disease or Hailey-Hailey disease, facilitate the spread of HSV. In addition, systemic immune defects as in HIV/AIDS also predispose to systemic spread.

Clinical Findings. The patient presents with fever, malaise, tight-feeling skin and shortly thereafter a rapidly spreading blistering eruption. In some patients no blisters are seen but instead slit-like defects, clefts and superficial erosions. In such cases the initial diagnosis is often incorrect. Since labial infections are the most common source, the blisters usually start on the face and neck, but they spread rapidly to cover much of the body, evolving into large erosions and ulcers. Systemic involvement, such as diarrhea or pneumonia, may also occur. Prior to antiviral therapy the prognosis was guarded (Fig. 2.12).

Differential Diagnosis. In the past, the main concern was eczema vaccinatum, in which the same group of patients are infected by the smallpox virus. That disorder tended to be lethal. Today animal pox viruses, such as cowpox or monkeypox in zoo keepers or laboratory workers, can occasionally produce a similar picture.

Therapy

Systemic. Acyclovir and its relatives have revolutionized the care of eczema herpeticum. If a patient at risk develops a herpetic lesion, he should be treated with oral acyclovir (200 mg five times daily) for 5 days. If there are already signs of dissemination, then intravenous acyclovir is preferred. Usually hospitalization is needed and sometimes antibiotics are required for secondary bacterial infections.

Topical. Wet soaks and then application of a zinc lotion, such as one with 1.0% clioquinol, produces dryness and reduces bacterial secondary infections.

Secondary Herpes Simplex Virus Infections

Recurrent Mucocutaneous Herpes Simplex Virus

Synonyms. Cold sore, fever blister

Definition. Repeated HSV infections at the approximate site of the primary infection, often following a triggering event.

Etiology and Pathogenesis. Because of the widespread occurrence of primary oral HSV, recurrent labial HSV is a disease familiar to almost everyone. The most frequent triggers include sunlight and fever. In Germany, the lesions are known as glacier burns. They are also common among skiers, swimmers and sailors, although no catchy name exists. As mentioned earlier, the HSV lies dormant in peripheral nerve ganglia and then returns to the skin via the nerve tracts. In recurrent genital HSV, the triggers are less clear, but include menses, sexual intercourse and stress.

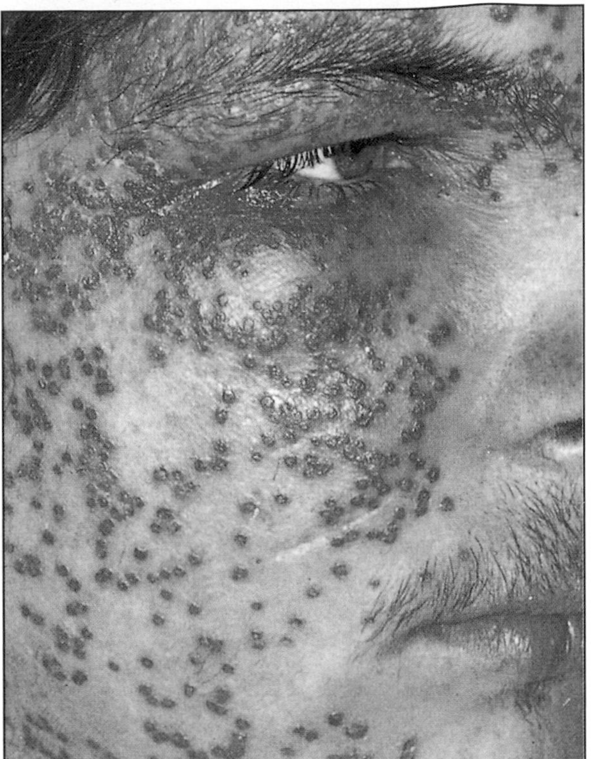

Fig. 2.12. Eczema herpeticum

Clinical Findings. While primary oral HSV is usually intraoral, with later spread to the lips and perioral skin, recurrent labial HSV typically involves only the lips and immediately adjacent skin. Recurrent intraoral HSV infections involving the hard palate, and occasionally the tongue or buccal mucosa, may occur. Attacks occur 2–5 days after the trigger; the patient almost always has a prodrome, whether it is tingling, burning or simply knowing something is coming (Figs. 2.13–2.15).

Blisters appear on a erythematous base, rupture and often crust. The disease course typically lasts 7–14 days. On the genitalia, the most common sites are the glans and prepuce, as well as labia minora, but any site can be involved. Other common sites for recurrent HSV include the perianal region, buttocks, and fingers. In gay males, persistent painful perianal ulcerations are HSV until proven otherwise. Sometimes the lesions are vegetative (herpes simplex vegetans) mimicking verrucous carcinoma.

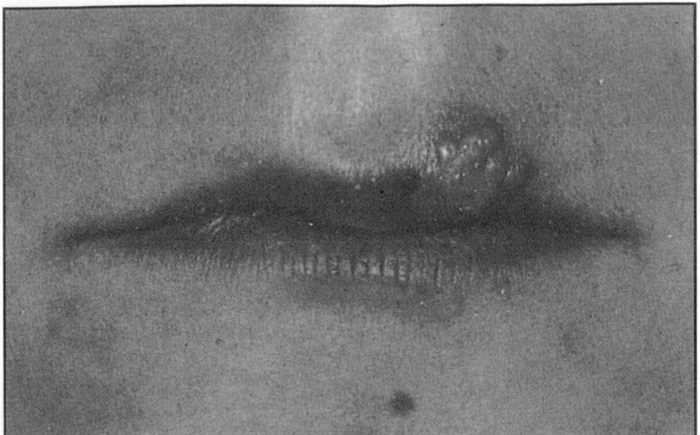

Fig. 2.13. Recurrent labial herpes simplex infection

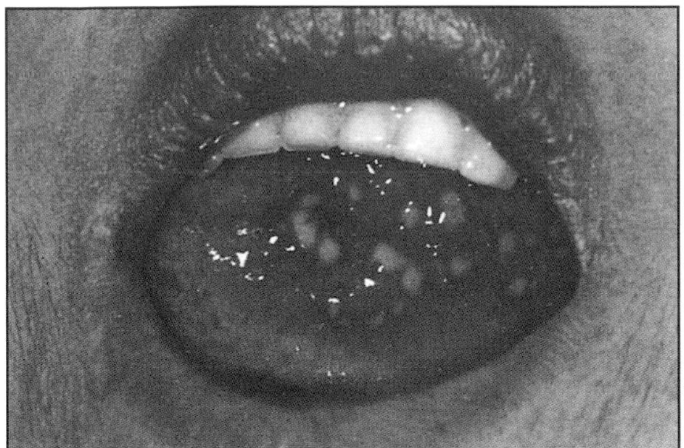

Fig. 2.14. Recurrent lingual herpes simplex infection

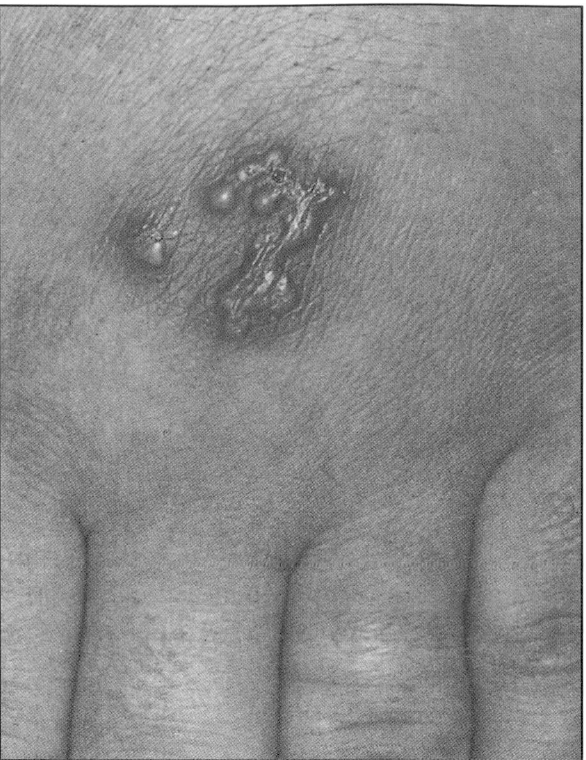

Fig. 2.15. Recurrent herpes simplex infection of glabrous skin

There may be mild lymphadenopathy, dysesthesias and secondary bacterial infections. Recurrent labial HSV combined with recurrent erysipelas may lead to a chronic swollen lip known as elephantiasis nostras. The streptococci enter the skin because of the damage from HSV and then themselves damage the lymphatics.

A very typical scenario is the development of recurrent labial HSV and then, 5–14 days later, the appearance of erythema multiforme. Surprisingly, it rarely follows recurrent genital HSV. A difficult clinical problem is the patient with erythema multiforme and labial lesions: Are they old herpes or new erythema multiforme lesions of the lips? HSV can be identified in the target lesions of erythema multiforme with PCR.

Differential Diagnosis. The differential diagnosis of recurrent HSV varies in different body sites. In the mouth, most recurrent lesions are aphthae. If one suspects HSV because the lesions are grouped or polycyclic, the virus must be identified with culture or PCR. On the lips, impetigo may occasionally have a similar appearance, but it is often combined with HSV. In the genital region, the overlap between aphthae, Behçet disease and HSV is less distinct, so in unusual cases viral identification is needed. Chancroid and chancriform pyoderma may also appear similar, as do the transient early lesions of lymphogranuloma venereum. Herpetic whitlows are usually misdiagnosed as bacterial paronychia. Zosteriform HSV can look exactly like zoster; if zoster develops a second time in the same dermatome, viral studies should be taken to clarify the diagnosis. Clinically the two conditions are identical.

Therapy

Systemic. Oral acyclovir therapy is expensive but is the therapy of choice for recurrent HSV. It can be used in two ways.

Interval: The patient is given 25 acyclovir 200 mg tablets and takes onetablet five times daily for 5 days, starting at the first warning of an attack. For most individuals, this approach suffices to abort or ameliorate attacks.

Suppressive: If interval therapy fails, one can use acyclovir 200 mg b.i.d.–t.i.d. or 400 mg b.i.d. for long periods of time, often for many months to years, to suppress recurrences. Every 6 or 12 months, the patient should abstain from the drug to see if the attacks have reduced in frequency. Even with extremely long treatment periods, resistance to acyclovir is uncommon, although it does develop in HIV/AIDS patients. The main indications for suppressive therapy are patients with severe erythema multiforme secondary to HSV, patients with continuous attacks, i.e., the typical disease course is such that new lesions start before the old ones heal, and immunosuppressed patients.

Topical. Most patients can simply use any one of a number of topical drying measures, all available over-the-counter. Corticosteroid creams applied early in the disease course may reduce the severity of the inflammation. Topical antiviral creams containing acyclovir and many other agents (tromantadine, vidarabine and idoxuridine) have proven to be minimally effective and may be associated with allergic contact dermatitis.

Keratoconjunctivitis

In primary herpetic gingivostomatitis, there may be ocular involvement but it tends to be overlooked because of the many other problems. Recurrent disease, however, may be limited to the eyes and threaten vision. Any dendritic corneal erosion in a patient older than 5 years of age is likely to be recurrent herpetic disease, as primary ocular disease only occurs in infants. Two pathophysiological processes dominate. HSV causes loss of cohesion of the corneal and conjunctival epithelia, producing usually painful erosions, blisters and ulcers. The host response may also be quite extreme, causing uveitis and other ocular inflammatory disease. For this reason, ophthalmologists view corticosteroids as a two-edged sword, effective against inflammation but perhaps capable of facilitating the spread of the virus. Topical treatments with a variety of antiviral agents are usually effective, although systemic medications are also employed.

Herpes Simplex Virus in HIV/AIDS

Clinical Findings. There are a number of unusual manifestations of HSV in patients with HIV/AIDS. They are discussed in greater detail later in this chapter. Patients in risk groups with severe or unusual HSV infections should be further questioned and tested. Perianal HSV in gay males is quite common; it may be very painful, persistent, ulcerated and locally destructive. Often a simultaneous infection with CMV occurs. Clinically persistent phagedenic ulcers can also develop about the mouth or in any other site where HSV is seen. Zosteriform HSV is often confusing in such patients. Systemic complications such as sepsis and cerebral infections may develop in AIDS patients, even when the cutaneous lesions are not dramatic.

Differential Diagnosis. One must simply remember that, as with so many infections, HSV tends to be atypical in HIV/AIDS. The grouped blisters on an erythematous base are depicted in textbooks, but are rarely found in the examining room. Thus, in HIV/AIDS patients, any erosive, ulcerative or blistering disease may represent HSV and should be evaluated with virological methods.

Therapy

Systemic. Acyclovir or similar derivatives are usually the answer. In mild cases in HIV/AIDS patients, oral medication may be acceptable, but in most instances the intravenous route is preferred. HSV resistant to acyclovir is usually sensitive to foscarnet.

Varicella Zoster Virus

Causative Organism. Varicella zoster virus, or human herpes virus-3, is another α-herpes virus, almost identical to HSV, but distinguishable with viral cultures, immunofluorescent studies and PCR.

Exactly the same virus causes varicella or chicken pox in children and immunosuppressed hosts and zoster in older patients. Thus varicella can be viewed as the primary infection and zoster as the secondary one. Patients with zoster can infect nonexposed children and immunosuppressed hosts, creating varicella. Conversely, exposure to varicella also very rarely triggers zoster, but here immunologic mechanisms rather than infection must be involved. The first infection with VZV leads to immunity, but the virus remains behind in neural ganglia. With age or immunosuppression, unknown trigger factors reactivate the virus which typically then involves a single sensory nerve and its dermatome. Patients with HIV/AIDS, lymphoma, especially Hodgkin disease, leukemia and iatrogenic immunosuppression, are likely to develop zoster at an early age, have more severe zoster which spreads beyond dermatomes, or present with a varicella-like picture with little or no dermatomal localization.

Varicella

Synonym. Chickenpox

Definition. Initial infection with VZV in an unprotected host.

Epidemiology. Varicella zoster virus is spread primarily by droplets; in Germany, the disease is known as windpox.

Chicken pox is an extremely common disease. In most countries, 90–95% of the population has had the infection by 15 years of age.

Etiology and Pathogenesis. Chicken pox is highly contagious and virtually every child is exposed and develops immunity, even the small percent who never develop clinical disease. Reinfection and a second clinical attack of varicella is unheard of in normal individuals. Sometimes infants exposed during the first months of life have partial protection from maternal immunoglobulins and never develop a full-blown, protective response.

Clinical Findings. After an incubation period of about 2 weeks, the child begins to develop fever, malaise and then widespread blisters typically on an erythematous base. The head is most often involved, but the disease spreads centripetally and covers most of the body but spares the palms and soles. The scalp is typically affected. Lesions in many different stages are found, ranging from red macules to blisters on a red base to erosions and crusts. Patients are generally infective for 1–2 days before their rash and then for about 5 days thereafter (Fig. 2.16).

The crusts are persistent and fall off after several weeks, usually without scars. However, lesions that have been secondarily infected or excoriated will often leave behind shallow scars, typically on the forehead and cheeks. They may be hypo- or hyperpigmented. Sometimes varicella lesions are limited to and more severe in areas of sunburn.

There is also almost always an enanthem. Small ulcers, also usually with a red base, are seen especially on the hard palate (Fig. 2.17). Thus, when varicella is considered, one should check the mouth. Conjunctival, pharyngeal, laryngeal and genital erosions may also appear.

While children are usually relatively symptom-free, the rare unlucky adult who never developed adequate immunity to VZV is often quite ill. Varicella pneumonia is the most dreaded complication in the group. Varicella meningitis may also occur, not only in adults but also in children. However, it is generally mild.

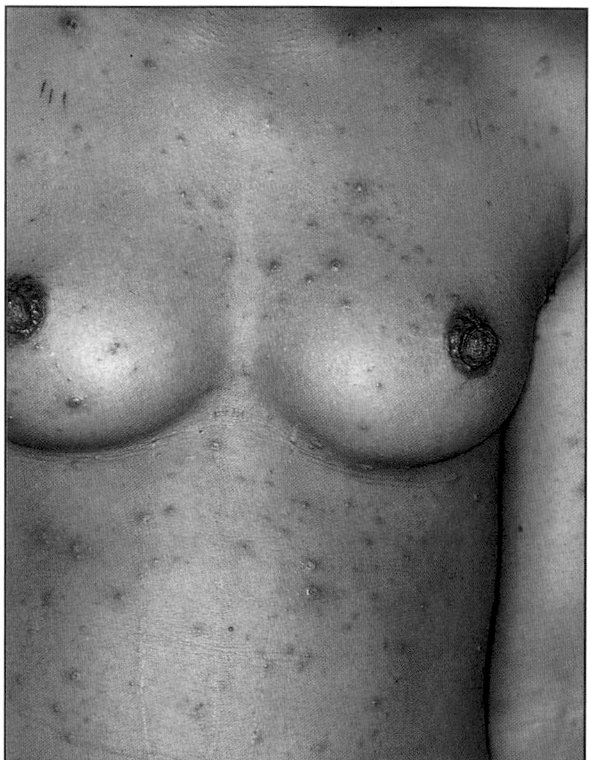

Fig. 2.16. Varicella

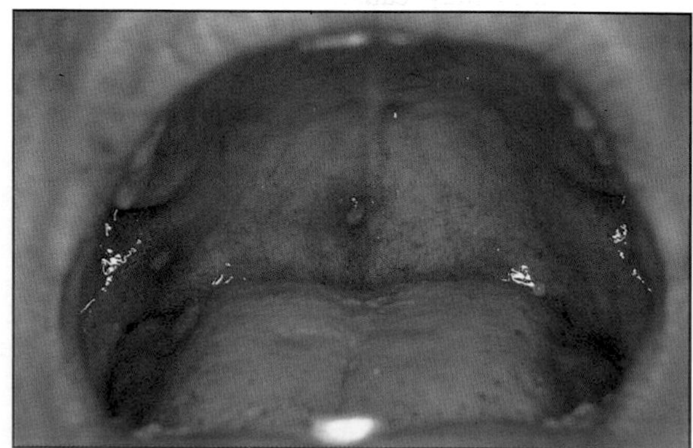

Fig. 2.17. Palatal lesions in varicella

Histopathology. The Tzanck smear and microscopic picture are indistinguishable from that of HSV. The two viruses are also identical upon electron microscopic examination. Thus one must rely on other techniques to distinguish the two viruses.

Epidemiology. Viral culture, immunofluorescent studies and PCR can be used to separate HSV and VZV. Serological testing is also available for epidemiological studies.

Course and Prognosis. The outlook in normal children is excellent. The mortality rate is about 2/100,000, rising to 30/100,000 in adults. The fatality rate in childhood leukemia patients may be as high as 10%. Chicken pox has also been associated with Reye syndrome.

Differential Diagnosis. In the past, the main question was smallpox vs chicken pox. Fortunately, this is no longer the case. The main difference was that the smallpox patient was extremely ill and typically had umbilicated blisters and pustules all of which were roughly at the same stage of evolution. A more difficult differential diagnostic problem was patients with partial immunity and a so-called variola minor or alastrim infection in whom the clinical features were less typical. Today an important challenge is diagnosing varicella or disseminated zoster in an immunosuppressed patient. It is a matter of definition, but if a prodromal dermatomal eruption has been seen, one diagnoses disseminated zoster; if not, varicella. The prognosis and treatment are identical.

Occasionally, a widespread insect bite reaction may look similar, but the lesions are urticarial, not vesicular, and no intraoral lesions occur. Herpangina may have a similar enanthem but no vesicular cutaneous lesions. Rarely, Coxsackie and ECHO viruses may cause a vesicular exanthem, but it is seldom as widespread or dramatic as in varicella. In such causes, the Tzanck smear will be negative.

Therapy

Systemic. Oral acyclovir reduces the severity of varicella and can be employed. It may reduce scarring, decrease the number of visits to the doctor and get the child back into school sooner, thus being cost-effective despite being expensive. Oral antibiotics should be used if secondary infection is suspected in order to reduce scarring. Table 2.6 shows the possible drugs that can be used for both varicella and zoster.

Topical. Drying measures such as zinc oxide lotion usually suffice.

Prophylaxis. A live attenuated VZV vaccine is available; in the USA it is known as Varivax and given once to susceptible children 1–12 years of age. The efficacy is estimated at 70–90% over 6 years. Different regimens are used in adults and immunosuppressed individuals. In addition, children with varicella should be kept away from immunosuppressed patients. They should not be admitted to the hospital, or, if admitted, they must be isolated. However, VZV is highly contagious and most nonimmune contacts will develop varicella.

Varicella in Pregnancy

Clinical Findings. Varicella zoster virus infection in pregnancy is worthy of special mention. Infection in the first trimester may lead to congenital varicella syndrome with a series of significant developmental anomalies including skin defects (papyrus infant), hydrocephalus, cataracts and chorioretinitis. The incidence of congenital varicella syndrome is low, probably less than 1%, and the disorder poorly documented. In the second trimester, VZV

Table 2.6. Recommended dosages of antiviral agents for varicella zoster virus

Disease form	Medication	Dosage
Chicken pox	Acyclovir	20 mg/kg (up to 800 mg) PO q.i.d. for 5 days
Zoster	Acyclovir	800 mg PO 5× daily for 7–10 days
	Valacyclovir	1.0 g PO t.i.d. for 7 days
	Famciclovir	500 mg PO t.i.d. for 7 days
Immunosuppressed patient	Acyclovir	10 mg/kg IV t.i.d. for 7 days[a]

[a] Pediatric dosages vary and are based on surface area

infection may lead to in utero varicella infection and then to an infant with modest immunity who may develop zoster upon reexposure during childhood. Third-trimester VZV infection becomes more serious the closer the infection coincides to the delivery date. Very specific recommendations are available from gynecologic and pediatric sources in different countries regarding the exact approach to a term mother with varicella. Newborns with varicella tend to have a severe course.

Therapy
Systemic. Acyclovir is frequently recommended, but adequate studies of safety for the child and effectiveness in preventing disease are not available. Close to birth, zoster immune globulin can be used for prophylaxis in the nonimmune mother if she is exposed but has no symptoms, or in the newborn to reduce the severity of the varicella.

Zoster

Synonyms. Zoster (from the Greek *zostrix* = belt), shingles (from the Latin *cingulus* = belt); in German, Gürtelrose (belt-rose or belt-exanthem)

Definition. Second infection with VZV, usually in adults and limited to a dermatome.

Epidemiology. Zoster is primarily a disease of the elderly and immunosuppressed. In Germany, the incidence is about 22/10,000, increasing with each decade and peaking in the eighth decade with an incidence of 65/10,000. Nonetheless, one must remember that zoster does occur in healthy adolescents and younger adults. While one should inquire about risk factors, the yield will greatly depend on the practice population. The incidence in homosexual men in New York is about 200/10,000.

Etiology and Pathogenesis. Varicella zoster virus remains in a neural ganglion while the patient has general immunity to the virus. Local factors such as trauma, radiation therapy, and even sunburn can trigger the outbreak of zoster, as can exposure to VZV. Other infections such as syphilis and smallpox have also been described to stimulate zoster. In addition, poisons such as arsenic and carbon monoxide have been implicated.

The most important factor is clearly immunosuppression, whether it be from HIV, leukemia, lymphoma or chemotherapy. An increase in zoster in young gay males preceded the recognized outbreak of AIDS in San Francisco by several years; Conant, a dermatologist with an interest in infectious diseases, studied these patients and saved serum from which later HIV was identified in some cases. In the vast bulk of patients, the only risk factor is increasing age, and no triggering factor is identified. Zoster is not a reliable marker of underlying malignancy or serious disease in the normal elderly population.

Clinical Findings. Zoster is generally a dermatomal disease (Figs. 2.18, 2.19). On the trunk, the dermatomes can be followed easily, but notice in Fig. 2.18 how at the shoulder the dermatomes blur together. On the face, the three branches of cranial nerve V, involving the forehead, mid-face and jaw line, are relatively clear (Fig. 2.20). Typically, the patient initially experiences pain without cutaneous findings. The pain may become quite intense and leads to a variety of embarrassing misdiagnoses ranging from a dental problem to a herniated disc. Any nerve can be involved. Occasionally there are prodromal signs and symptoms.

Within 24–48 h of the onset of pain, cutaneous lesions appear. Initially, erythematous infiltrated macules and plaques develop; they are often oval and follow skin lines. Over a period of days, tense initially clear blisters develop in the red areas and new lesions spread throughout the involved dermatome. The blisters are usually quite stable and develop into pustules before breaking. Adherent crusts then appear.

Usually new lesions continue to develop for 2–3 days. Some may be outside the immediate dermatome. Involvement of three dermatomes is considered normal. More than a handful of lesions outside the three adjacent dermatomes suggests dissemination, but the time course must also be considered. The appearance of extradermatomal lesions in the first 12–24 h is far more a matter for concern than are a few scattered lesions over the course of the disease. As mentioned above, there is a gradual transition between disseminated zoster and recurrent varicella; both suggest an immunosuppressed patient. The midline is almost invariably not crossed, except that a few lesions may appear just over the line, reflecting the paths of small nerve branches. Zoster involving two separate nerves simultaneously occurs rarely.

In some instances, cutaneous lesions may develop without any significant pain. Conversely, there may be intense unilateral pain without skin findings (zoster sine herpete). Such patients usually

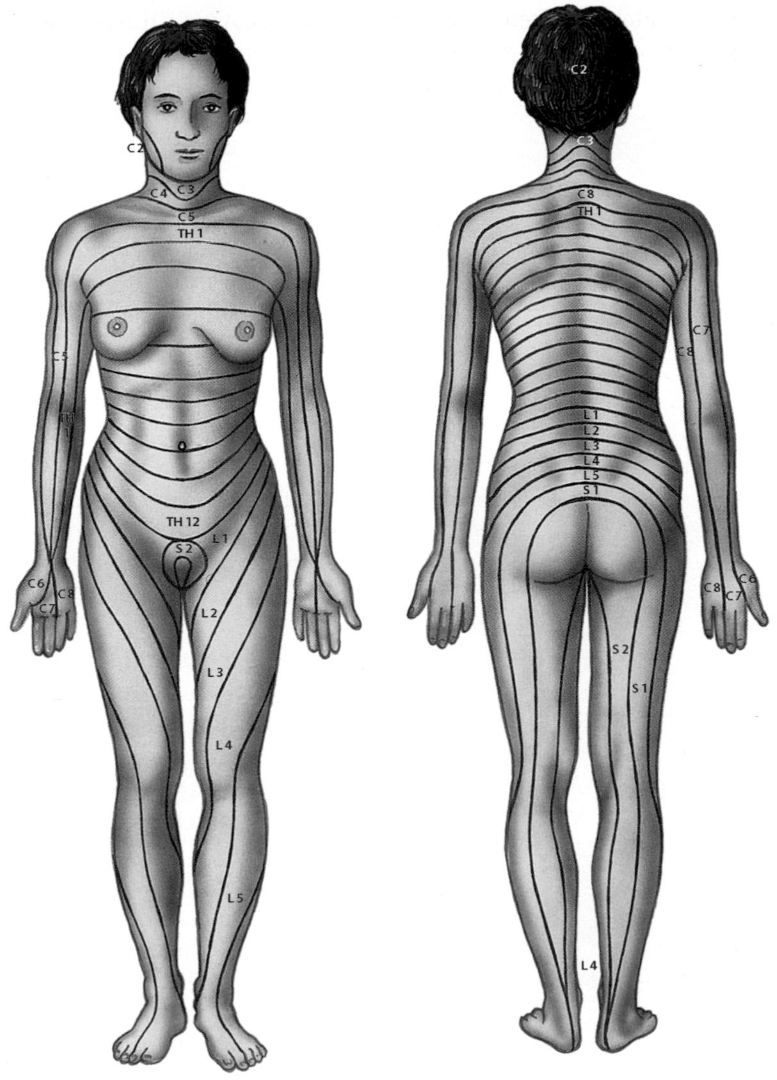

Fig. 2.18. Pattern of segmental innervation (dermatomes)

do not wind up in the dermatologist's office, but they present a diagnostic challenge for other physicians. Since sensory nerves are primarily involved, pain is the most common complaint. In addition to the intense acute pain, there may be persistent pain, known as postherpetic neuralgia, which may last for months to years and which may be disabling. Up to 30% of elderly patients develop some degree of neuralgia. Motor involvement may also be seen, involving muscles of ocular motion as well as those of the bladder, rectum, abdominal wall and other sites.

In addition to dissemination and pain, there are many other complications of zoster. Sometimes the lesions may be very hemorrhagic. In other instances, they become necrotic, perhaps through secondary infection, and then scar; the bizarre, often hypopigmented scars remain as a lifelong marker. Zoster may also recur, but it is most unusual and suggests an immunosuppressed patient.

Special Variants of Zoster

Ophthalmic Zoster. Involvement of the first branch of the trigeminal nerve leads to lesions of the forehead and eyelid. There is often lid edema and the lesions tend to be very painful and hemorrhagic. Preauricular lymphadenopathy is commonly present. In some patients, especially those in whom the tip of the nose is involved (via the nasociliary branch), there maybe ocular involvement, including keratitis, uveitis and muscle paralysis. Ophthalmologic consultation is mandatory, for one must carefully weigh the antiinflammatory benefits of corticosteroids against the potential for spread as a result of iatrogenic immunosuppression.

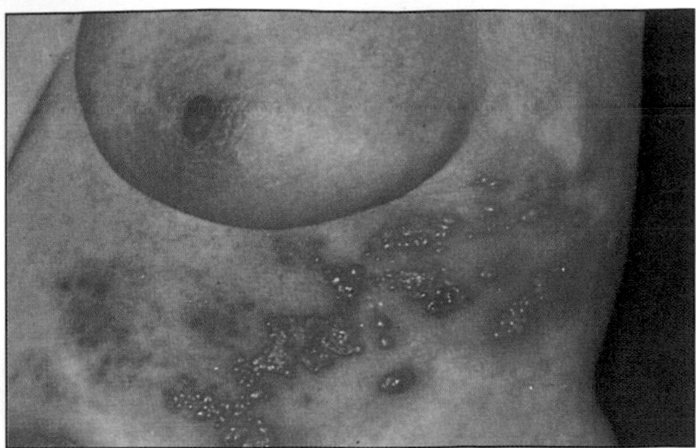

Fig. 2.19. Zoster

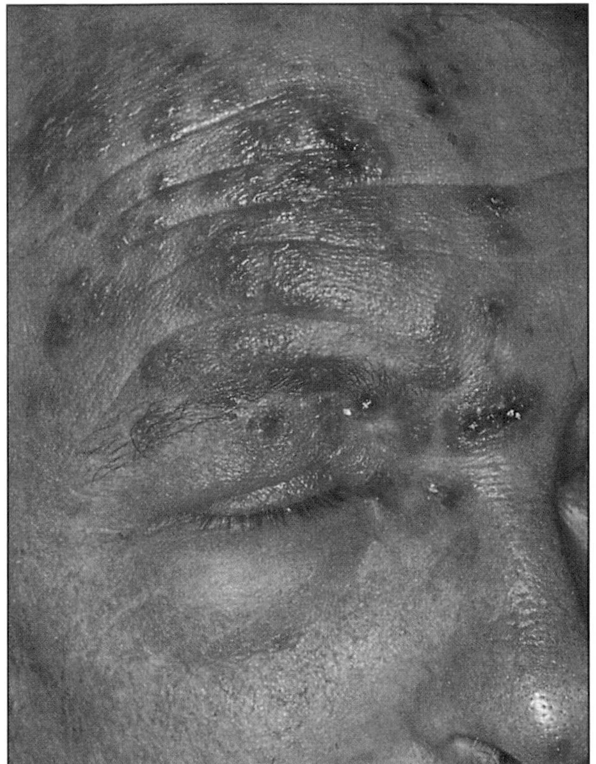

Fig. 2.20. Zoster involving first branch of trigeminal nerve

Oral Zoster. When the second and third branches of the trigeminal nerve are involved, there may be intraoral lesions involving the hard palate and maxilla (second branch) or tongue and mandible (third branch). Grouped erythematous erosions are seen. Such patients may present with a toothache and no skin or mucosal lesions.

Cranial Zoster. Patients with involvement of the nerves of the scalp and neck may present with headache, a stiff neck and lymphadenopathy. The dermatomal patterns are unclear and the localization to one side may also not be apparent. Such patients may be evaluated for meningitis and even have minor CSF abnormalities.

Otic Zoster (Ramsey-Hunt syndrome). Tiny erosions may be seen on the tympanic membrane or along the ear canal in patients with exquisite unilateral ear pain. Tinnitus and vertigo are also common. There is permanent hearing loss in about one-third of the patients.

Perineal Zoster. In this region, once again the dermatomal pattern is unclear and patients may present with pain, inability to urinate or constipation. Such patients, particularly if elderly, should be closely examined for a blister or two, which can go a long way in explaining puzzling symptoms.

Zoster Embryopathy. When a pregnant woman develops zoster, there is a risk to the infant which is theoretically similar to that discussed under varicella in pregnancy. However, zoster is rare in the childbearing age group and there is less viremia, so the risk is much less.

Zoster in HIV/AIDS. Zoster in a young adult should suggest an immunosuppressed patient, and thus HIV/AIDS. Zoster is more common when the patient has HIV and is asymptomatic. In addition, patients with more advanced infections tend to have more sever zoster, often hemorrhagic or necrotic, slow to heal and even recurrent with several attacks in a year. Dissemination is the main risk. Some patients fail to respond to acyclovir and require other antiviral therapy.

Histopathology. A lesion of zoster is identical to that of varicella and herpes simplex. There may be a vasculitis in more severe cases. The Tzanck smear is once again positive, revealing multinucleated giant cells.

Epidemiology. If more convincing proof is needed, or VZV must be separated from HSV, then viral cultures, PCR or serological studies can be employed.

Differential Diagnosis. The main differential diagnosis is zosteriform herpes simplex, which can only be diagnosed by identifying the virus or suspected when there are recurrent attacks, even though zoster too can recur. Zoster tends to have lesions in multiple stages of development and to be more hemorrhagic than herpes simplex. Other viruses such as Coxsackie have been described to cause zosteriform eruptions but such events are rare.

Therapy of Acute Zoster

Systemic. The exact role of acyclovir and other nucleosides in zoster is unclear. Antiviral therapy reduces the length of infectivity and pain, as well as producing some reduction in neuralgia. The main issue is a cost-benefit one. Antiviral medications should be used in immunosuppressed patients. Most HIV/AIDS patients are admitted for intravenous therapy; some chemotherapy patients are treated with oral regimens. Patients showing signs of dissemination early in the disease course should also be treated. The real question is whether all patients with zoster should be treated. VZV is much less sensitive to acyclovir than HSV so that a minimum, albeit expensive, regimen requires 800 mg five times daily for 1 week. Valacyclovir and brivudine are more convenient, but whether they are more effective in relieving pain or preventing dissemination or postherpetic neuralgia is unclear.

A second controversy is the role of systemic corticosteroids. While there is a theoretical risk of dissemination during the early phase, there may also be prompt improvement in the pain and inflammation when prednisone (60 mg/day), in tapering dosages over 3 weeks (for example 60 mg daily for 1 week, then 40 mg daily for 1 week, then 20 mg daily for 1 week), is employed. It is unclear if corticosteroids help prevent postherpetic neuralgia, with conflicting opinions in the literature.

Both nonsteroidal antiinflammatory drugs and analgesics may be used to treat the acute pain.

Topical. Most patients with zoster do fine with topical drying agents such as zinc oxide lotion or clioquinol lotion. Zinc oxide lotion should not be used around the eyes, because, as it dries, small oxide particles may reach the eyes causing irritation. As the lesions dry out, patients are more comfortable with a cream or ointment to help loosen the scales.

Therapy of Postherpetic Neuralgia

Systemic. Both corticosteroids and antiviral agents are recommended not only for acute problems, but also to reduce the incidence of postherpetic pain. Exactly how well either or both work has been the subject of numerous studies and remains unclear. A variety of psychotherapeutic agents have also been employed in this setting; none have distinguished themselves. It is often helpful to enlist the help of a neurologist or pain clinic, so that the patient has access to a wide range of approaches.

Topical. Topical capsaicin, other topical antipruritic agents and distracters may be tried, but postherpetic neuralgia reflects true nerve damage and is usually not influenced by topical measures.

Other Measures. Acupuncture seems to have a role, as do biofeedback techniques.

Epstein-Barr Virus

Epstein-Barr virus is responsible for a number of diseases. In addition to infectious mononucleosis, it is associated with Burkitt lymphoma, lymphoepithelial nasopharyngeal carcinoma, some cases of gastric carcinoma and a variety of other lymphoproliferative disorders, especially in HIV/AIDS patients and other immunocompromised individuals (Chap. 61). Epstein-Barr virus is also responsible for oral hairy leukoplakia in HIV/AIDS patients (Chap. 33), as well as leiomyosarcomas in HIV/AIDS patients and other immunocompromised hosts (Chap. 59).

Infectious Mononucleosis

(PFEIFFER 1889)

Synonyms. Glandular fever, Pfeiffer glandular fever, kissing disease, mono

Definition. Acute infectious illness with lymphadenopathy usually in young adults.

Causative Organism. Epstein-Barr virus, a γ-herpesvirus, also known as human herpes virus-4.

Epidemiology. Infectious mononucleosis usually occurs in small epidemics, most common in the spring. Young adults are most often infected. Droplet spread is the usual transfer, although close personal contact is also a likely method. In children less than 5 years of age, the infection is usually not apparent. Even in young adults, only about half have symptoms. By age 30 years almost everyone has had an infection.

Etiology and Pathogenesis. The Epstein-Barr virus initially multiplies in the oral mucosa and colonizes the salivary glands. Some individuals retain the virus in these glands and continue to secrete it in their saliva for many years. The main target however is B lymphocytes, which expand in a polyclonal manner during the infection. In the laboratory, lymphocytes infected with Epstein-Barr virus often achieve immortality.

Clinical Findings

Systemic Findings. The incubation period is variable, ranging over 4–14 days. The most striking finding is angina, as the tonsils are swollen and have a necrotic, pseudomembranous coating (Fig. 2.21). At the same time there is prominent lymphadenopathy, especially involving the posterior cervical nodes, as well as hepatosplenomegaly. Almost all patients have fever and malaise. Many simply have no energy without other dramatic signs and thus their disease is initially overlooked.

Cutaneous Findings. About 3–15% of patients have a generalized, often pruritic maculopapular exanthem (Fig. 2.22). If the patients are treated with ampicillin or amoxicillin, the likelihood of a rash is almost 100%. The legs are typically affected. Other features can include facial edema, palatal petechiae and genital ulcerations.

Epidemiology. Almost all patients have an elevated lymphocyte count, usually with a lymphocytosis >50% with more than 10% atypical cells. In addition, liver enzymes are elevated in almost all patients although jaundice is rare. The Paul-Bunnell or heterophile test is relatively nonspecific and may be negative in children. Immunofluorescent testing is available to identify both the early or viral capsid antigen and the Epstein-Barr virus nuclear antigen, which is absent during the acute phase. Both IgG and IgM tests are available.

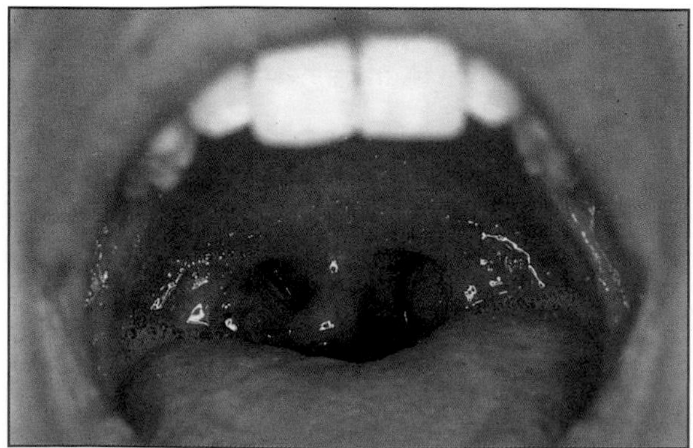

Fig. 2.21. Tonsillar lesions in infectious mononucleosis

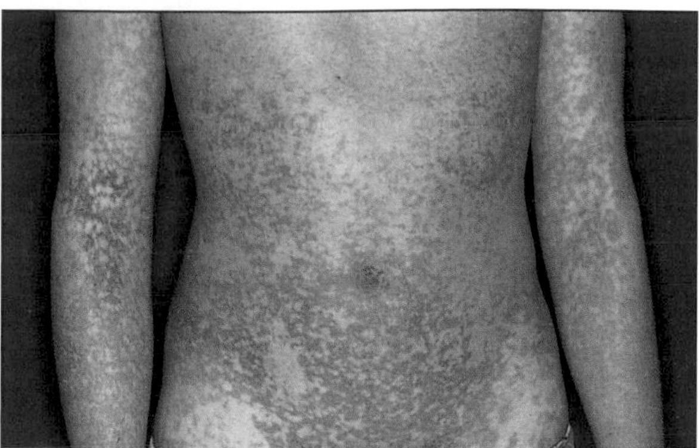

Fig. 2.22. Widespread exanthem in infectious mononucleosis

Course and Prognosis. The outlook is good in most cases. Reactivation during immunosuppression is the main problem. While patients with Epstein-Barr virus infections often have prolonged fatigue, no clear relationship has been shown between the chronic fatigue syndrome and persistent shedding of Epstein-Barr virus, which is usually asymptomatic.

Differential Diagnosis. The list is long. Most patients who clinically have infectious mononucleosis and are seronegative turn out still to have Epstein-Barr virus infections. The other common cause in adults is primarily CMV, but human herpes virus-6 and toxoplasmosis can produce similar changes. The exanthem is not specific and is usually first identified when other clinical findings become apparent. Often the presence of lymphadenopathy and an abnormal peripheral blood picture suggest leukemia but usually the patient can be rapidly reassured.

Therapy. No specific therapy is recommended.

Cytomegalovirus

Cytomegalovirus is also known as β-herpesvirus or human herpes virus-5. It plays little role in ordinary dermatologic practice, but causes a variety of problems including chorioretinitis and cutaneous ulcerations in HIV/AIDS patients and is a feared problem following intrauterine infection. In newborns it is one of the causes of sepsis along with cutaneous nodules of extramedullary hematopoiesis (TORCH syndrome). In adults, CMV may cause an infectious mononucleosis-like picture; it is responsible for about 10% of cases of infectious mononucleosis diagnosed clinically. Finally, CMV is a common cause of posttransfusion fever and its reactivation or transfer is a major complication of organ transplantation.

Exanthem Subitum

(Zahorsky 1910)

Synonyms. Sixth disease, roseola infantum, pseudorubella. The correct name is exanthema subitum but it has become bastardized in English.

Definition. Viral infection characterized by high fever which disappears just as a rubella-like exanthem appears.

Causative Organism. In most cases human herpes virus-6 is found; human herpes virus-7 and some ECHO and Coxsackie viruses may also cause the same or a very similar disease.

Epidemiology. Minor local epidemics are reported; either the virus is only moderately contagious or many cases are asymptomatic. By 3 years of age, over 90% of children have serological evidence of infection.

Clinical Findings. Only small children, ranging in age from a few months to several years, are affected. After a incubation period of 3–7 days, the patient suddenly develops a fever of 40 °C in the absence of other specific findings. The fever lasts for about 3 days, and then, as it is breaking, a rubella-like exanthem develops. Pale red macules, 3–5 mm in size, appear in a somewhat different pattern than rubella. Initially the trunk is involved and then the extremities; the face is usually spared. There is no enanthem. After 1–2 days, the rash clears rapidly.

Epidemiology. Serologic testing is still primarily a research tool; clinically, it is rarely needed. If there is any clinical question or if the patient is older, rubella titers should be obtained to rule out an atypical rubella with its more serious consequences.

Differential Diagnosis. The exanthem can be confused with a variety of other viral exanthems, such as measles, rubella and scarlet fever, but the patient is well even with the fever and lacks systemic signs.

Therapy. None is required other than antipyretic therapy. Because of the high temperature, febrile seizures are a possible complication.

Pox Viruses

Pox viruses are large brick-shaped DNA viruses. Three major groups affect humans: (1) orthopox viruses, including smallpox, vaccinia, monkeypox and cowpox; (2) parapox viruses, which cause milker's nodule and orf; (3) molluscum contagiosum virus.

Smallpox

Synonym. Variola

Definition. Severe, often fatal viral disease responsible for large epidemics and many deaths in the past, but today extinct in the wild.

Causative Organism. Variola vera virus, a DNA virus 150 × 260 nm in size, was discovered by Paschen in 1907.

History. Smallpox has a fascinating history. In the Middle Ages, it was responsible for many deaths as it was a scourge comparable to plague. Jenner, in 1796, developed the smallpox vaccination using cowpox virus; he had noticed that milkmaids who were exposed to cowpox had some immunity against smallpox. The vaccinia virus still available for smallpox vaccinations is biologically distinct from both cowpox and smallpox, probably through divergent evolution.

Smallpox has become extinct over the years through aggressive vaccination campaigns and isolation of infected individuals. The last patients in Bangladesh were identified in 1975; in Africa, the last case was in Somali in 1977. The last human to have smallpox was a laboratory worker in England in 1978. The USA and Russia still have laboratory stocks of the virus whose DNA has been sequenced. Opinions are divided as to whether the virus should be destroyed entirely or further studied to see why it was such an effective virus and if it can be employed in gene therapy.

Epidemiology. The smallpox virus was highly infective. It was spread primarily by droplets, but also through crusts, fomites and drinking water. Smallpox was a feared disease among travelers because of the likelihood of upper respiratory tract transmission prior to the presence of skin lesions. Major endemic areas were the Indian subcontinent and parts of Africa.

Etiology and Pathogenesis. Following respiratory transmission, there was about a 2-week incubation period. At this time, viremia as well as infectious droplets developed. The skin lesions were also highly infective.

Clinical Findings. The three main clinical hallmarks of smallpox were umbilication of individual lesions, all lesions in one stage of evolution (in contrast to chicken pox) and scarring.

The disease presented with a severe prodrome, then a short phase of false hope, and then the fulminant attack with widespread blisters and pustules, fluid loss, cardiac problems and often death. Hemorrhagic pustules, rapid confluence of pustules and large ecchymoses without pustules were life-threatening signs. The mortality rate was between 10% and 30%.

Two variants of smallpox included: (1) variola minor (variolois), a milder form of disease in patients with partial immunity due to vaccination; (2) alastrim (whitepox), also a milder form of disease caused by modified wild-type virus.

Histopathology. The virus wreaked considerable havoc with the skin, causing epidermal necrosis. Often, only a network of epidermal strands remained; this is known as reticular degeneration. In addition, characteristic cytoplasmic inclusions of viral products (Guarneri bodies) were seen. The viral bodies can also be identified by electron microscopy.

Differential Diagnosis. Early in the disease course, the exanthem was not very specific and isolated cases resembled chicken pox, secondary syphilis, drug reactions, pityriasis lichenoides et varioliformis acuta (PLEVA), and other viral exanthems. The widespread pustular eruption in a critically ill patient or the severe prodrome in an epidemic setting were both unmistakable.

Therapy. No specific therapy was available. Supportive measures, especially cardiac support, were essential.

Prophylaxis. Vaccination with the vaccinia virus was so effective that it eliminated the disease.

Other Orthopox Viruses

Vaccinia

Causative Organism. Vaccinia is a distinct pox virus which may have evolved from either the smallpox or the cowpox virus.

Epidemiology. Vaccinia was used for vaccination to induce immunity against smallpox. Vaccination was employed in the past as a nonspecific stimulator of immunity. In addition, the military services continued vaccinating patients long after the risk of smallpox was eliminated. In 1987 severe vaccinia was described in a military recruit who was HIV-positive. Because it is so large and readily enters the human host, the vaccine is still being investigated as a biologic carrier for immunizing antigens.

Clinical Findings. Vaccination was not an innocuous procedure. Most experienced a brisk local reaction and resultant scar, regarded as a sign of a successful procedure. Many patients developed fever and malaise. A variety of undesirable reactions occurred, ranging from an intense local reaction to autoinoculation (as of the eye) to erythema multiforme to widespread or generalized vaccinia.

Immunosuppressed patients were at risk for a progressive and often fatal case of vaccinia, as the disease spread from the site of vaccination to massively involve the trunk and upper extremities. Patients with atopic dermatitis, Darier disease, Hailey-Hailey disease and other epidermal defects occasionally developed eczema vaccinatum, in which the virus spread to involve wide areas of damaged skin. This could result from either vaccination or exposure to another individual with a vaccination site. While the risk of eczema vaccinatum is small, one must keep it in mind when dealing with acutely ill atopic dermatitis patients and ask the pertinent questions.

Therapy. Severe vaccinia reactions were treated with vaccinia immune globulin and a variety of antiviral regimens, as well as symptomatic measures.

Monkeypox

Monkeypox is found primarily in Zaire. Although it was isolated from captive monkeys, its natural history remains unclear. Monkeypox produces a disease picture identical to smallpox with a fatality of about 10 %. Human to human spread occurs but is uncommon. Tana pox is an even rarer pox virus from the Tana river region of Zaire that also causes a similar clinical picture. Both viruses possibly could also cause eczema vaccinatum. They can be identified by specialized laboratory techniques. Vaccination provides protection and is used in laboratory workers.

Cowpox

Cowpox is actually uncommon in cattle and better named catpox. It is a zoonosis in Europe, most commonly spread from the domestic cat. At the inoculation site, there is an intense local reaction with hemorrhage and necrosis, usually accompanied by lymphadenopathy and fever. The disease is self-limited and does not spread to other patients. In immunocompromised patients, potentially fatal generalized disease can develop. Treatment is symptomatic.

Parapox Viruses

Orf and milker's nodule are caused by two closely related parapox viruses and are clinically very similar; the name barnyard pox has been proposed as a unifying term. In both diseases, there is transfer from an infected animal to a human, usually a farmer, shepherd or veterinarian.

Milker's nodule

(Jenner 1798)

Synonym. Udder pox

Clinical Findings. The cow, usually a young animal, has vesicular lesions of the udder. The milker develops inflamed nodules on one or both hands that go on to ulcerate and may have a necrotic top. Sometimes there is an intense local inflammatory reaction. Some degree of immunity develops; the disease is not transferred to other humans (Fig. 2.23).

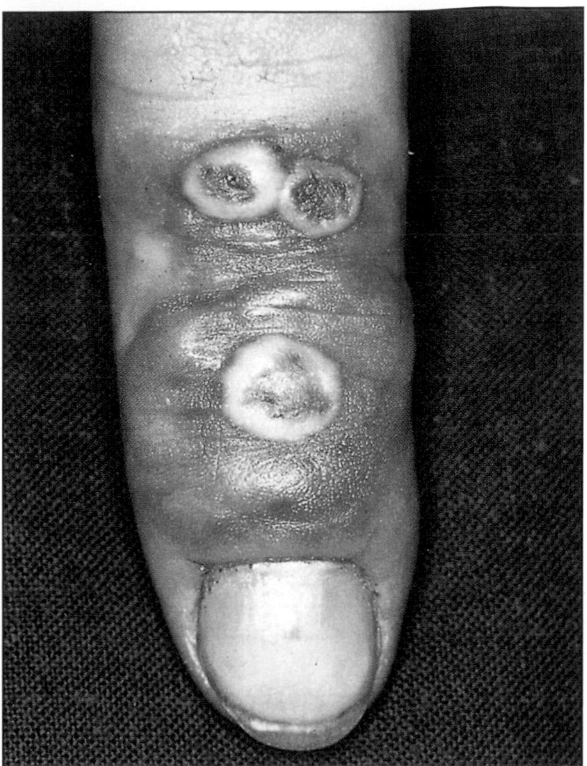

Fig. 2.23. Milker's nodule

Histopathology. There is marked epidermal damage, similar to smallpox, but without inclusion bodies or giant cells. Eosinophils may be prominent in the dermal infiltrate.

Differential Diagnosis. In most cases, the patient knows the correct diagnosis, because the problem is so well-known to those who work with cows. When needed, the virus can be identified by electron microscopy and speciated by special culture techniques. Milker's nodule is entirely different from cowpox; not only is it a different virus, but cowpox is usually from cats.

The main considerations are a bacterial paronychia or a herpetic whitlow. When there is a history of injury, pyogenic granuloma may be considered. The primary lesion of anthrax or tularemia may appear similar but the patient is more ill. Tuberculosis cutis verrucosa can also be transferred to the hands of milkers. Primary syphilitic chancres of the finger may appear similar, but there should be a different type of contact in the history.

In addition, there are several other types of noninfectious nodules seen in milkers. Depending on the milking technique, in the past, almost every milker developed some sort of callus. Today, with the widespread use of milking machines, this is no longer the case. In Europe, one popular milking technique was the Swiss method, in which the thumb strikes the palm of the hand, producing a callus on the tip of the thumb. In milker's granuloma, hairs may be driven into the skin between two fingers, producing an intense chronic inflammatory response. The same phenomenon is seen in barbers, in whom it is known as barber's granuloma. In either case, the granuloma is similar to a pilonidal sinus, except that the hairs are exogenous. Usually, removing the hairs results in a cure; in other cases, local excision is needed.

Therapy. Symptomatic drying measures are all that is needed.

Orf

Synonyms. Ecthyma contagiosum, bovine pustular stomatitis. Orf is an unusual word, probably derived from the old Icelandic word *hrufa* which occurs in present day German as *Schorf*, or crust.

Clinical Findings. Orf is a disease of sheep, primarily young lambs. The virus is quite resistant and may survive on fences, troughs and in stalls. The young animals develop inflamed nodules about the mouth. The most typical story is that, in the spring, the individual who cares for the runt of the litter develops orf. In the fall, with shearing and slaughter, the shepherd is more likely to be inoculated. Epidemics have been described in veterinary students exposed to sheep for the first time. Some religious ceremonies involving the sacrifice of live lambs have also led to multiple cases of orf.

The patient develops an erythematous nodule which goes on to ulcerate and heal with a firm necrotic crust (Fig. 2.24). There may be an intense local reaction and erythema multiforme has been described. Lymphangitis may occur. The histopathology, diagnosis, differential diagnosis and therapy are the same as for milker's nodule.

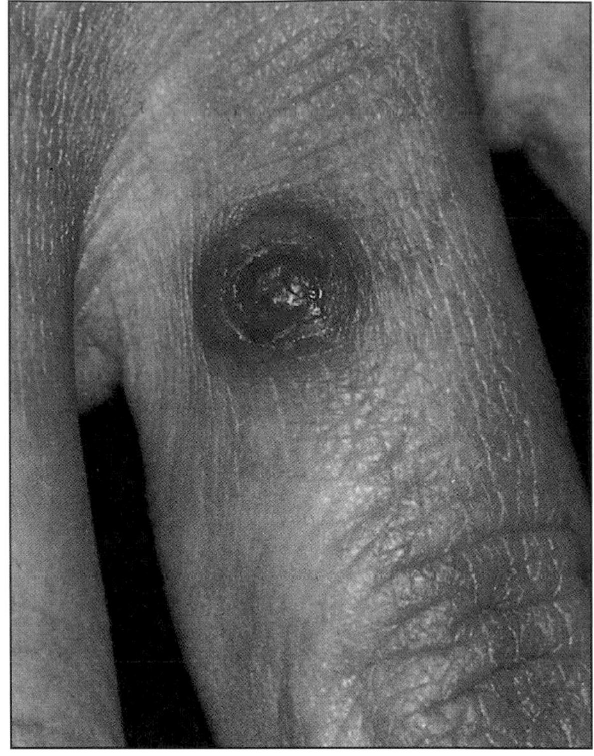

Fig. 2.24. Orf

Molluscum Contagiosum

(Batemann 1817)

Definition. Epidermotropic pox virus infection producing papular lesions with a central dell; often confused with warts.

Causative Organism. Molluscum contagiosum virus.

Epidemiology. Molluscum contagiosum is a common viral infection. In children, it is spread by casual contact, while in adults it is often transmitted during sexual intercourse.

Etiology and Pathogenesis. The molluscum contagiosum virus is a large pox virus which is highly epidermotropic. The virus is transferred by direct human to human contact and only infects the skin. The host response plays an important role; children with widespread molluscum contagiosum usually have atopic dermatitis, while in adults one should think of HIV.

Clinical Findings. Typically, one sees small flesh-colored papules with a central dell (Fig. 2.25). The lesions may be grouped together or arranged in lines of scratching – the pseudo-Köbner phenomenon, also seen with HPV. Typical sites are the inguinal, axillary and neck regions, although any body region may be infected. Often many lesions are present (Fig. 2.26). The eyelids are a troublesome site. In adults, the most likely site is the genital region. Occasionally, adults present with a single, flesh-colored facial papule; such lesions are often misdiagnosed until examined histologically. Often the papules are inflamed and even secondarily infected. Sometimes the lesions can be very large, pedunculated, limited to hair follicles or most unusually, limited to an area of atopic dermatitis (eczema molluscatum).

Histopathology. Molluscum contagiosum has a spectacular and diagnostic histologic appearance. There is epidermal hyperplasia and an invagination, representing the clinically seen dell. This pouch is filled with large, multicolored, virally infected epidermal cells – the molluscum bodies.

Differential Diagnosis. When multiple lesions are present, the diagnosis is usually clear; occasionally one may suspect warts. In adults with facial lesions, one may think of sebaceous hyperplasia, intradermal nevus, adnexal tumor or even basal cell carcinoma for solitary lesions, and of milia, hidrocystomas and syringomas for multiple lesions. Giant molluscum contagiosum, as seen in HIV/AIDS patients, is very difficult to identify; it is usually misdiagnosed as squamous cell carcinoma or regressing keratoacanthoma.

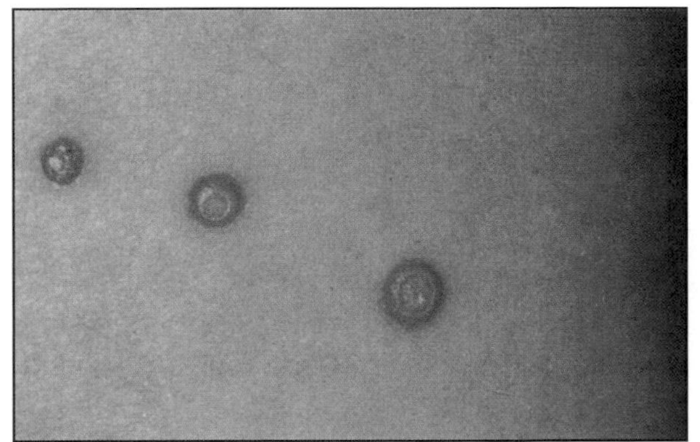

Fig. 2.25. Molluscum contagiosum with delled papules

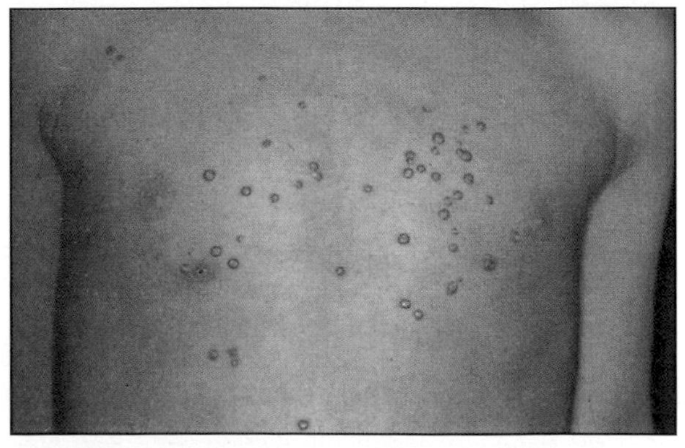

Fig. 2.26. Widespread molluscum contagiosum

Therapy. Any destructive measure is effective. In children, applying EMLA (eutectic mixture of local anesthetic) cream under plastic foil occlusion about 30 – 60 min prior to treatment offers effective anesthesia. In adults, usually no anesthesia is needed. One can then use a sharp curette; stubborn lesions can first be opened with a scalpel or large-bore needle. Others prefer a fine forceps. Alternative approaches include applying occlusive tape patches for 3 – 5 days or podophyllin tincture, sometimes combined with tape. Rarely, in small children with hundreds of molluscum contagiosum, general anesthesia and curettage are employed.

Picorna Viruses

Picorna viruses are small RNA viruses. Included in the family are the rhinoviruses, responsible many common colds, and the enteroviruses, including Coxsackie, ECHO, polio and other enteroviral species. The picorna viruses of most interest to dermatologists are those in the Coxsackie group, named after the town of Coxsackie, New York, where an epidemic was identified. Coxsackie viruses cause a number of diseases, as shown in Table 2.7.

Hand-Foot-and-Mouth Disease

(Robinson et al. 1958)

Synonym. Enteroviral vesicular stomatitis with exanthem

Definition. Acute viral infection with blisters on the hands, feet, buttocks and in the mouth.

Etiology and Pathogenesis. A wide number of Coxsackie viruses can cause hand-foot-and-mouth disease. The most common type is A-16, but many others have been identified. The virus is spread through respiratory secretions, and the disease

Table 2.7. Enteroviral diseases with cutaneous manifestations

Disease	Virus
Hand-foot-and-mouth disease	Most often group A16; also A4, 5, 9, 10; B2, 5; enterovirus-71 (rarely)
Herpangina	A1–10, 16, 22
Lymphonodular pharyngitis	A10
Rubelliform exanthem	Echovirus-9
Roseoliform exanthem (Boston exanthem)	Echovirus-16

tends to appear in small epidemics, most commonly in the summer months.

Clinical Findings. After an incubation period of 3–5 days, the patient simultaneously develops erosions in the mouth, especially on the palate, and more intact blisters on the palms, soles, and buttocks (Fig. 2.27). The blisters typically are deep, have a gray sheen, and may later erode (Fig. 2.28). Other regions are usually spared. The child may have a fever, but is generally well. The lesions heal without complications.

Histopathology. Intraepidermal vesicles are seen with reticular degeneration and balloon cells. No giant cells are present.

Differential Diagnosis. Herpes simplex infection with erythema multiforme may present a similar combination of oral and acral lesions, but there are clear clinical differences: The typical primary HSV lesion is far more severe and the patient is sick; recurrent HSV involves the lips, not the palate. In addition, erythema multiforme usually features iris- or target-shaped lesions on the hands. Herpangina favors the tonsillar pillars and does not have acral lesions.

Confusion arises because of two other viral infections. The vesicular stomatitis virus causes blisters of the mouth, tongue and nipples in horses and cattle. Humans can be infected, but usually get an influenza-like illness, only rarely accompanied by oral lesions. In sharp contrast, hoof-and-mouth disease is caused by a rhinovirus and only infects animals, although humans can inadvertently transfer it to other animals.

Therapy. Symptomatic therapy suffices.

Herpangina

(Zahorsky 1924)

Synonyms. Enteroviral vesicular pharyngitis, aphthous pharyngitis

Definition. Acute viral infection with fever and characteristic small gray oral ulcers.

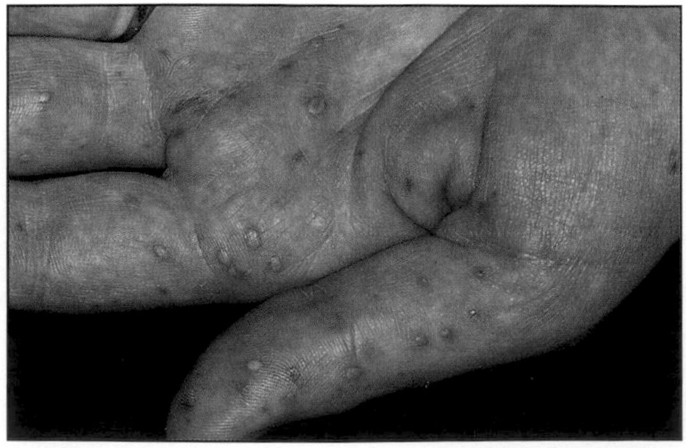

Fig. 2.27. Hand-foot-and-mouth disease

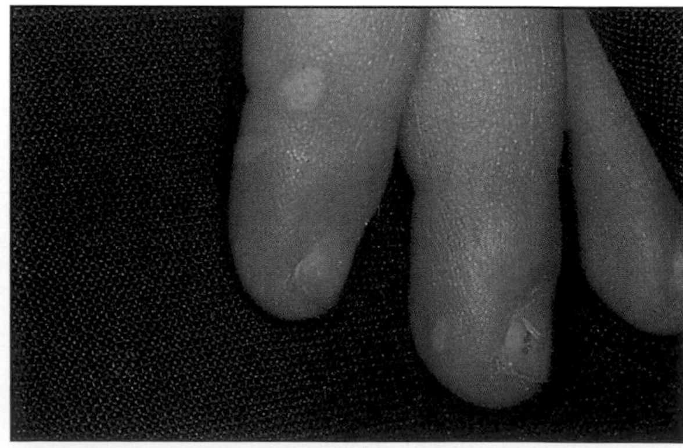

Fig. 2.28. Hand-foot-and-mouth disease with deep gray blisters

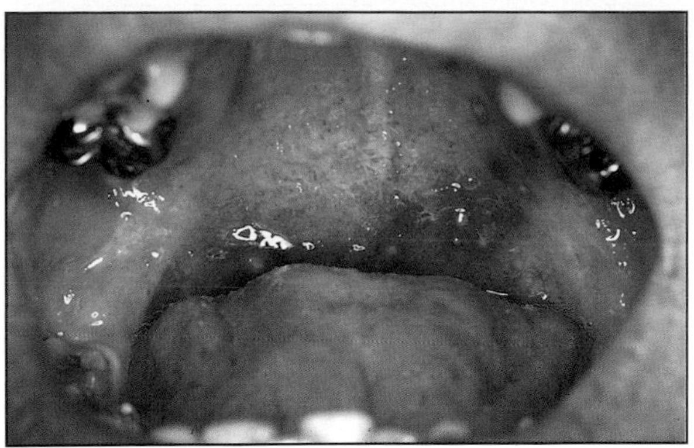

Fig. 2.29. Herpangina

Epidemiology. Herpangina also tends to present in small epidemics among children in the summer or fall months.

Clinical Findings. After an incubation period of 2–9 days, a high fever (up to 40 °C) develops, and the child is sick with nausea, vomiting and muscle pain. Tiny 1–2-mm blisters on a red base develop on the tonsillar pillars, uvula and extreme posterior aspect of the soft palate (Fig. 2.29). They evolve into ulcers with a gray top over a few days. Healing is spontaneous and complete. Up to 5% of patients may have febrile convulsions.

Differential Diagnosis. The main differential diagnostic point is acute lymphonodular pharyngitis, also an enteroviral disease. Here the lesions are 3–6 mm, firm yellow nodules, rather than tiny ulcers. The biopsy specimen shows a reactive lymphocytic infiltrate. Most clinicians no longer separate this entity and herpangina. Many misdiagnoses are made, including herpetic gingivostomatitis, Koplik spots of measles and bacterial pharyngitis, but all are quite distinct clinically.

Therapy. Symptomatic care suffices.

Other Coxsackie Infections

A wide range of other clinical patterns can be seen with Coxsackie viruses, including several clinically indistinct macular exanthems. They are generally separated into rubelliform rashes, usually caused by ECHO virus-9, and roseoliform exanthems, which tend to appear as the associated fever disappears. The rubelliform rash starts on the face with pale tiny pink macules not associated with pruritus or lymphadenopathy. Most epidemics occur in the summer and older children rarely have a rash. The first roseoliform rash to be described was caused by ECHO virus-16 and is known as the Boston exanthem. Diffuse salmon-colored macules and papules appear as the febrile child starts to improve, just as in roseola infantum. Purpuric exanthems have also been reported.

Some type B viruses cause aseptic meningitis and the so-called summer flu in Europe, while type A viruses are responsible for epidemic pleurodynia or Bornholm disease (named after the Swedish island of Bornholm in the Baltic Sea), myocarditis, pericarditis and aseptic meningitis. Acute hemorrhagic conjunctivitis is caused by enterovirus-70. Neonates are especially susceptible to enteroviral infections and may develop fulminant, frequently fatal disease.

The Six Diseases

Originally, six exanthems were identified and numbered before the turn of the century. They included: (1) measles, (2) German measles, (3) scarlet fever, (4) rubeola scarlatinosa or Dukes disease, (5) erythema infectiosum, and (6) exanthem subitum.

While the numbers today are unimportant, the six diseases cause clinical confusion and are often included on medical school examinations. Scarlet fever is covered in Chapter 4, while exanthem subitum is included above with herpes viruses.

Measles

Synonyms. Rubeola (in English), morbilli

Definition. Highly contagious viral disease of childhood, characterized by fever, cough, conjunctivitis, characteristic oral mucosa changes (Koplik [1898] spots) and diffuse exanthem.

Causative Organism. The measles virus is a paramyxovirus about 140 nm in size.

Epidemiology. Measles is highly contagious, spread primarily via droplets from the nose, throat and oral cavity. The incubation period is about 11 days between infection and the development of fever and other symptoms; the time until the rash appears is about 14 days. Patients are infectious several days before their rash appears; the virus disappears from the droplets at about the same time the rash clears. Previously, almost every individual had measles and thereby developed lifelong immunity. City children were invariably infected, while in more rural areas the disease occurred every several years. Immunizations have changed this picture, reducing the incidence of measles dramatically, but also creating individuals with partial immunity and placing nonimmunized patients at new risks.

Clinical Findings. The prodrome is characterized by fever up to 40 °C, rhinitis, conjunctivitis, photophobia, pharyngitis and often a dry cough. On the second or third day, the Koplik spots appear. These small white grains surrounded by a red rim appear on the buccal mucosa opposite the upper molars. They cannot be scraped away, in contrast to *Candida albicans*, and persist for several days. Although almost diagnostic for measles, they may be seen in other viral disorders. There may also be an erythematous enanthem on the gingivae, uvula and tonsils.

On about the third day, the exanthem starts. While the temperature may transiently drop, the fever rapidly returns. The rash consist of red macules that may be round or oval; initially they are pale red but they become darker and even hemorrhagic. Typically, the rash begins on the face and behind the ears, spreading to the neck, trunk and extremities. The macules enlarge and may coalesce. After about 4 days, the fever drops and the rash, by now often copper-colored, begins to desquamate, usually in the same sequence as it appeared (Fig. 2.30).

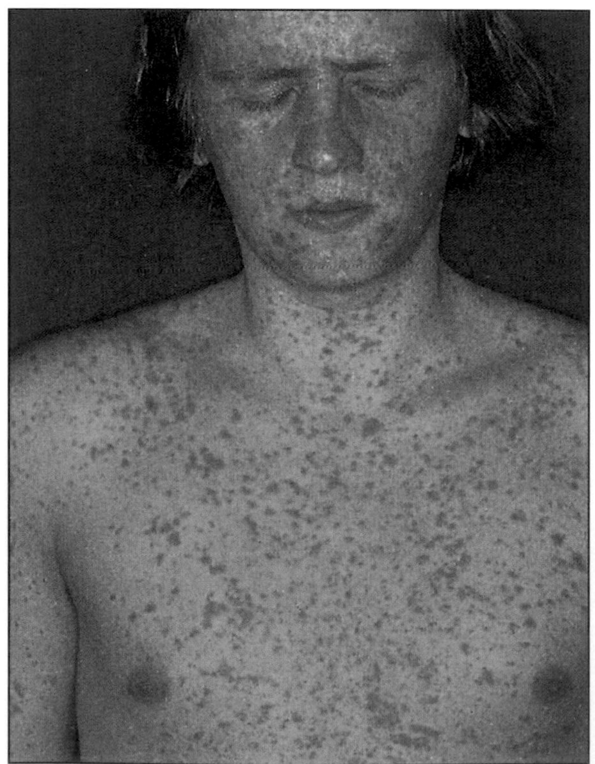

Fig. 2.30. Measles

The main complications are pneumonia and otitis media, both caused by secondary bacterial infections. The old diagnosis of measles pemphigoid described patients who developed widespread blisters; it probably represents staphylococcal scalded skin disease as a complication of measles. Streptococcal infections, however, are particularly common. There is also a transient reduction in cellular immunity so that reactivation and spread of tuberculosis or atypical mycobacterial infections may occur. Rarer complications include thrombocytopenic purpura, encephalitis (incidence of 1:100,000) and subacute sclerosing panencephalitis, a fatal disorder which occurs months to years after acute measles. Some patients may have fulminant measles with very high fever, hemorrhage, cardiopulmonary collapse, seizures and death.

The use of vaccines has created several other clinical patterns which are less distinct. They include:

- Atypical measles syndrome. The old, killed vaccines and inadvertently inactivated, current live vaccines fail to prevent infection by the wild-type virus but alter clinical expression of the disease. Typically, patients have fever, headache and abdominal pain and then, after 2 days, develop an acral petechial or urticarial rash associated with edema of the hands and feet. Pneumonia frequently occurs.
- Modified measles. Children with diminishing maternal immunity and those in whom vaccination has produced only partial immunity may have a milder variant of the disease with less dramatic skin findings. Koplik's spots may be absent.
- Vaccine exanthem. About 20 % of vaccinated individuals develop a faint rash but are not infectious.

Histopathology. While measles is never diagnosed by biopsy, there are characteristic multinucleated giant cells present in the lymph nodes, known as Warthin-Finkeldey (1931) cells, and syncytial giant cells in the epidermis.

Epidemiology. Typically, there is a leukopenia with a relative lymphocytosis. The virus can be cultured from the nasopharynx or identified via serological testing. As always, an increase in titer of two dilutions between acute and convalescent serum is required to confirm a recent infection. The measles virus can be identified in the CSF in encephalitis.

Differential Diagnosis. Virtually every viral exanthem could remotely be considered, but actually measles is quite distinct. The involvement behind the ears and the coppery desquamation are typical. In rubella, the patient is less ill and there is typically lymphadenopathy of the nape and over the mastoids. In scarlet fever, the lesions are smaller and more punctate; the mid-face is often spared, while the patient has a glossitis (strawberry tongue) and angina. In addition, there is usually a leukocytosis in scarlet fever. Exanthem subitum may appear similar, but the children are usually very young and have a high fever at the time their rash appears. Drug eruptions, especially from sulfonamides or barbiturates, are often similar to measles, but typically the patient is less ill and the rash has a different distribution, involving the palms and soles.

Atypical measles may be confused with Rocky Mountain spotted fever or Kawasaki syndrome because of the acral changes; when hemorrhage is prominent, other such disorders must be excluded.

Therapy. No effective treatment is available, other than adequate supportive care and treatment of complications.

Prophylaxis. A wide variety of measles vaccines are available. Today, in the USA, MMR is usually recommended at age 15 months. It contains live measles, mumps and rubella vaccines; the various live vaccines do not interfere with one another and provide excellent immunity. Exposed individuals can also be vaccinated within 2 days of exposure with good protection. Immunosuppressed patients require special treatment with immune globulin; exact protocols should be consulted.

Rubella

Synonyms. Rubeola (in German), German measles

Definition. Viral illness with typical exanthem which causes a less severe illness than measles but is associated with congenital defects when pregnant mothers are infected.

Causative Organism. The rubella virus is a RNA Toga virus with a size of 60 nm and a folded coat, which allegedly resembles a Roman toga.

Epidemiology. Rubella is spread by airborne droplets, but apparently has a lower degree of infectivity than, for example, measles. Even though immunity after infection is lifelong, a significant number of young adults lacked immunity prior to the development of a vaccine. Rubella is more common in the spring; previously cycles of epidemics every 6–9 years were noted. Patients are infectious from about 1 week before the onset of a rash until 1 week after it has disappeared.

Clinical Findings. After an incubation period of 2–3 weeks, a prodrome period of several days may be seen in children. They typically have malaise and perhaps minimal lymphadenopathy. In adolescents and adults, there is often no prodrome. The rash suddenly appears and rapidly progresses, lasting only about 3 days. It usually starts in a butterfly pattern on the cheeks, spreads to the retroauricular region and then soon involves the trunk and extremities. The individual lesions are small, minimally elevated red papules, often with peripheral blanching (Fig. 2.31). There is almost always cervical and occipital lymphadenopathy at this stage. Occasionally, adults may have a mild arthritis or testicular pain. Rarely, encephalitis

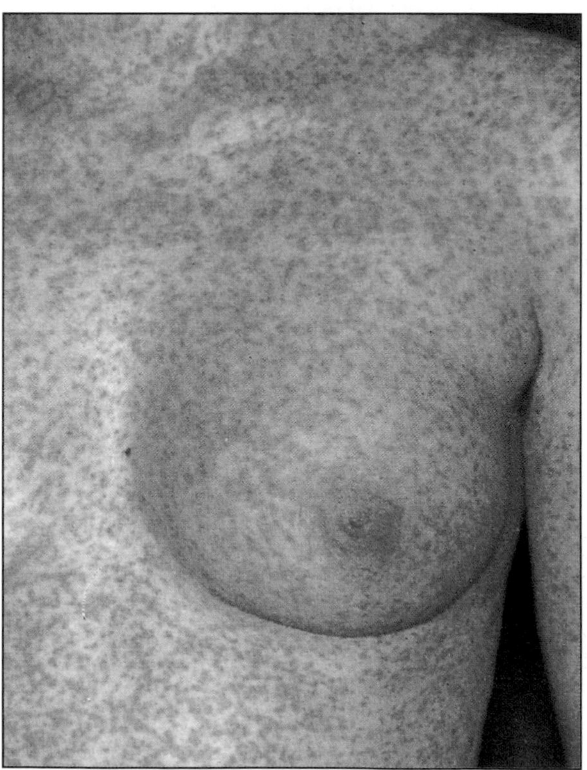

Fig. 2.31. Rubella

has been described, primarily among military recruits.

Problems with rubella begin when an infection occurs during pregnancy. Both the rate of transmission to the fetus and the likelihood of congenital defects are highest in the first 8 weeks of pregnancy, with little risk occurring after 20 weeks. The classic rubella syndrome is characterized by cardiac, ocular and hearing defects. Pregnant mothers suspected of possibly having rubella should be serologically diagnosed; offering a clinical opinion is hazardous, not only for medical but also for medicolegal reasons.

Epidemiology. The WBC count is usually normal. Serologic diagnosis can be performed; usually hemagglutination inhibition tests are preferred. The virus can also be cultured. Most of the complicated tests are reserved for pregnant mothers and newborn infants.

Differential Diagnosis. The main problems involve measles and scarlet fever. In measles, the patient is sicker and the rash eventually becomes more confluent and scaly. In scarlet fever, the WBC count is elevated and there should be oral changes. Secondary syphilis may also appear similar, so a serologic test for syphilis should be ordered. Infectious mononucleosis may also be clinically hard to distinguish but can be diagnosed serologically.

Therapy. No effective therapy is available and none is usually needed.

Prophylaxis. A live rubella vaccine, usually combined as MMR, is given at 15 months of age.

Rubeola Scarlatinosa

(Dukes 1881; Filatoff 1887)

Synonyms. Fourth disease, Dukes disease, Dukes-Filatoff disease, scarlatinella. It is actually unclear what Dukes was describing as fourth disease, when, in the 1880s, he described an epidemic at Rugby, a noted English public, i.e., private, school where he was the physician. In his 1881 paper, he discussed the incubation of scarlet fever, varicella, mumps and German measles. No repeatable clinical description has ever been offered and no etiologic agent cultured. The disorder is mentioned here only for completeness and historical accuracy; we do not pretend to suggest we can identify it.

Erythema Infectiosum

(Sticker 1899)

Synonyms. Fifth disease, slapped cheek disease

Definition. Mild viral disease characterized by gyrate erythemas.

Causative Organism. B19 parvovirus, a small DNA virus.

Epidemiology. The disease typically occurs as small outbreaks during the spring. Spread is through respiratory droplets and inapparent infections are quite common.

Etiology and Pathogenesis. B19 parvovirus causes aplastic crises in patients with sickle cell anemia and other hematologic disorders and may be responsible for hydrops fetalis and fetal death if maternal infection occurs in the first trimester.

Clinical Findings. After an incubation period of 6–14 days, the patient suddenly develops livedo-like or gyrate erythema on the cheeks, often coalescing to produce the slapped cheek sign. The eruption on the face may be transitory. On the arms, the eruption develops later and usually remains more lacy or even wreath-like. The cutaneous features resolve spontaneously over a week without significant desquamation. Other symptoms, such as fever, enanthems, or even malaise, are most uncommon (Figs. 2.32, 2.33).

Epidemiology. The infection can be confirmed by serologic studies; in pregnancy, maternal IgM against B19 can be measured. Prenatal diagnosis using PCR to identify the virus itself has also been

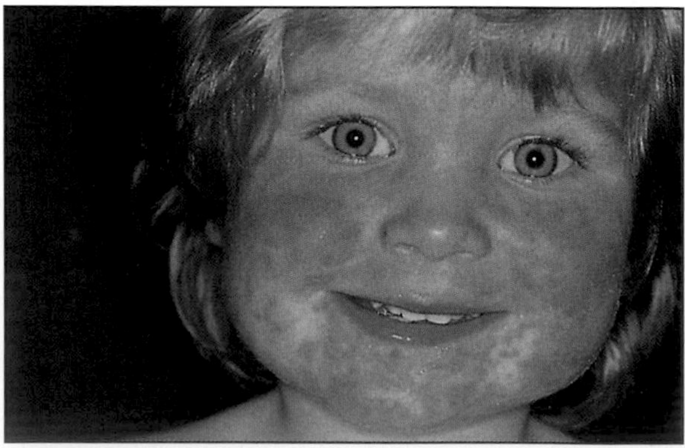

Fig. 2.32. Erythema infectiosum

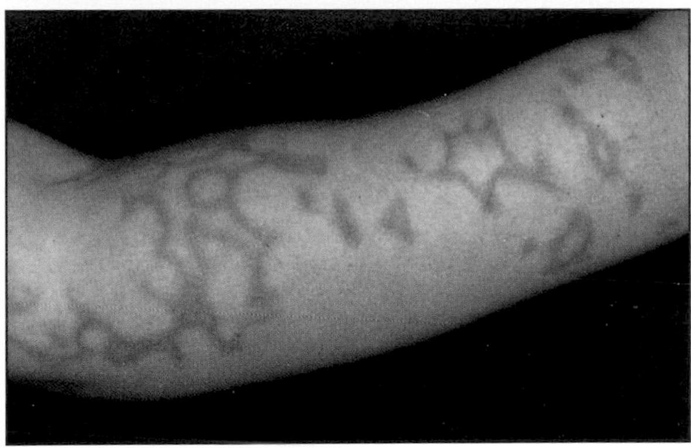

Fig. 2.33. Erythema infectiosum

described. While an ordinary case in a child can comfortably be diagnosed clinically, if a pregnant woman or her children present with likely erythema infectiosum, a serologic evaluation should be undertaken.

Differential Diagnosis. In the typical case, there is no serious differential diagnosis. Rarely, drug eruptions or other viral exanthems may appear somewhat similar.

Therapy. None is needed or available.

Other Viral Infections

Infective Dermatitis

(Sweet 1966)

Causative Organism. Human T cell leukemia virus (HTLV 1).

Infective dermatitis sounds nonspecific but refers to the skin findings associated with the primary infection by HTLV 1, the retrovirus responsible for adult T cell leukemia/lymphoma (Chap. 62). HTLV 1 infections are endemic in parts of the Caribbean and Japan. The clinical constellation of crusting and exudation around the nostrils, ears and scalp associated with a widespread, fine papular exanthem and lymphadenopathy usually allows identification in endemic areas. Resolution is prompt and spontaneous, but recurrences can be seen.

Flavivirus Infections

A number of flavivirus infections have cutaneous manifestations, although none are treated routinely by dermatologists. Included in the group are:

- Hepatitis C, which is discussed below separately.
- Tick-borne encephalitis, which in Europe may be transferred by the same ticks responsible for borreliosis.
- Dengue, which is arguably the most important arbovirus disease, transmitted primarily by *Aedes aegypti*, an urban mosquito. There are four closely related dengue viruses. Over half the world's population is at risk. Central and South America, Southeast Asia and parts of sub-Saharan Africa are the major areas today. The vector is found in the Southeastern USA and occasional cases have been seen in Texas. In ordinary dengue, the key features are fever, headache, retroocular pain and gastrointestinal distress. More than 50 % of patients have skin findings during their primary infection. These include facial erythema, a macular exanthem and petechiae. In the more severe form, known as dengue hemorrhagic fever, all patients have thrombocytopenia, petechiae and fluid leakage leading to edema and in some cases shock. Treatment is symptomatic. A vaccine is not currently available; it will have to cover all four types, since the presence of antibodies to one of the other types can enhance the severity of a given infection and lead to the hemorrhagic form.
- Yellow fever, which is also caused by a flavivirus, the yellow fever virus. It is transmitted in two patterns. Sylvatic transmission involves primates as the natural host and transmission occurs via forest mosquitoes; several hundred cases yearly are seen among outdoor workers, primarily in Bolivia and Peru. Controlling yellow fever was a major challenge in the building of the Panama Canal. Urban epidemics involving *Aedes aegypti* and human to human spread have not been described since World War II in the Americas, although an epidemic was seen in Nigeria in the 1980s. The clinical disease is biphasic. Early on there is the usual constellation of fever, chills, headache and malaise. Most patients recover uneventfully; some develop jaundice and hemorrhage. The mortality rate among the latter group is around 50 %. There is no specific treatment. Immunization is highly effective.

Papular Purpuric Socks-and-Gloves Syndrome

(Harms et al. 1990)

Synonym. Petechial glove-and-socks syndrome

Definition. Acute viral infection with distinctive edematous-hemorrhagic acral lesions.

Etiology and Pathogenesis. A number of viruses have been incriminated as causing this peculiar clinical constellation. In many cases, parvovirus B19 is responsible, but herpes human virus-6, the measles virus, hepatitis B and many others have been incriminated. Parvovirus B19 has been detected in skin lesions, adding credence to its role.

Clinical Findings. The clinical findings are somewhat indistinct, perhaps reflecting multiple etiologies. Patients generally are ill with fever, malaise, arthralgias and lymphadenopathy. There is a maculopapular purpuric exanthem which involves the hands and feet in a gloves and socks distribution, ending abruptly just above the wrists or ankles (Fig. 2.34). The extremities are often edematous. There may be an enanthem with oral erosions, petechiae or lesions resembling Koplik's spots.

Epidemiology. Viral serology can be performed; in at least some cases, no parvovirus B19 will be identified and one is left puzzled.

Differential Diagnosis. Since many viruses are probably responsible, the differential diagnosis is difficult to present. One must exclude hemorrhagic disorders and Henoch-Schönlein purpura.

Therapy. No therapy is needed.

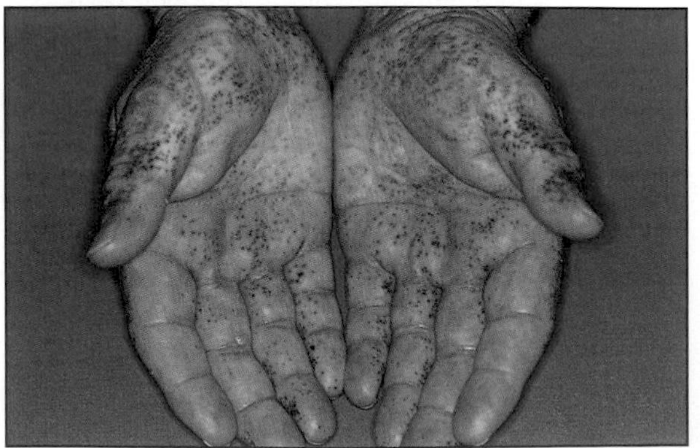

Fig. 2.34. Papular purpuric socks and gloves syndrome

Asymmetric Periflexural Exanthem of Childhood

(Brunner et al. 1962)

Synonym. Unilateral laterothoracic exanthem (Bodemer and de Prost 1992)

Etiology and Pathogenesis. This unique entity has not been proven to be viral in origin, but the evidence is quite suggestive. Several parainfluenza and adenoviruses have been implicated. Patients develop papules on the lateral aspect on their trunk, typically just on one side and near the axilla. While the papules increase in number and eventually involve both sides of the trunk, the asymmetry remains. The primary lesion is a tiny papule often surrounded by a pale halo. Occasionally the inner aspects of the arms and the groin are involved. There may be associated axillary lymphadenopathy. The minimally pruritic rash is more persistent than other viral exanthems, lasting 4–6 weeks. The histologic findings are not helpful in the diagnosis. The main differential diagnostic points include Gianotti-Crosti syndrome and inverse pityriasis rosea, but both are rarely so asymmetrical. Mild topical antipruritic measures suffice.

Eruptive Pseudoangiomatosis

Several patients with viral illnesses have developed multiple hemangioma-like papules which resolved spontaneously. In several cases, enteroviruses have been isolated but not from the vascular lesions. Both ECHO virus-25 and -32 have been incriminated. The patients typically develop blanchable red papules which disappear over 1–2 weeks.

Hepatitis Viruses

The advances made in recent years in understanding hepatitis and the many viruses associated with it have been overshadowed by the HIV/AIDS story but are nonetheless remarkable. At least five distinct viruses have been identified; in some cases they have complex interactions, combining forces to cause disease. In addition, there are still cases of infective hepatitis involving as yet unidentified viruses. The most common skin finding is jaundice, which depends on the severity of the liver disease, not the type of virus. Typically, jaundice is also detected in the sclerae, while the yellow skin color associated with carotenemia and drug reactions does not in-

Table 2.8. Hepatitis viruses

Virus	Transmission	Risk groups	Clinical features	Cutaneous features
A	Fecal/oral	Travelers, military personnel, children in day care	Usually mild, self-limited; no carriers or chronic hepatitis	None
B	Blood, sexual, perinatal	Drug abusers, homosexuals, Asians, health care providers, transfusion recipients	Mild to moderate disease, carriers and chronic disease occur; associated with hepato-cellular carcinoma	Gianotti-Crosti syndrome, serum sickness, urticaria, polyarteritis nodosa, cryoglobulinemia, lichen planus
C	Blood, sexual, perinatal, sporadic	Drug abusers, health care providers, transfusion recipients	Mild to moderate disease, carriers and chronic disease occur	Cryoglobulinemia, porphyria cutanea tarda, Sjögren syndrome, lichen planus
D	Blood, sexual, perinatal	Drug abusers, those with hepatitis B	Moderate to severe disease with frequent sequelae	None
E	Fecal/oral	Travelers	Mild to moderate, severe disease during pregnancy	None

clude eye deposits (Chap. 27). Nonspecific exanthems have also been described for most of the hepatitis viruses, but they are not clinically useful. Acute urticaria may also be associated with hepatitis.

Table 2.8 lists the common hepatitis viruses and their associated dermatologic disorders. All of the dermatologic disorders mentioned in the table are covered elsewhere in the text. The associations in some cases are difficult to sort out; for example, with porphyria cutanea tarda, is hepatitis C virus a direct cause or does it produce the disease indirectly via liver damage? Many problems blamed in the past on hepatitis B virus seem more likely related to hepatitis C virus. Included in this group are disorders such as cryoglobulinemia, porphyria cutanea tarda and polyarteritis nodosa.

Human Immunodeficiency Virus Infection and AIDS

Definition. Infection with HIV leads to AIDS, characterized by a variety of infections and tumors, some of which are almost specific for HIV infection and unusual in other settings.

Causative Organism. Human immunodeficiency virus is a retrovirus that belongs to the lentivirus group. Its genetic material is RNA; the genetic sequence is converted into DNA by reverse transcriptase and this DNA retroscript is incorporated into the host cell genome. This process is notoriously inaccurate leading to many mutations, so that many different HIV strains may appear in a given patient and population, often with strikingly different degrees of drug sensitivity.

The genome of HIV is well understood. In addition to structural genes, a number of regulatory genes are present, as well as those coding for reverse transcriptase and other enzymes. HIV-1 and HIV-2 show distinct differences, especially in their envelope proteins; they belong to the same group but are definitely different virus types. HIV-2 is more common in West Africa and may be associated with a milder course of disease. For the balance of the text, HIV will mean HIV-1. HIV can be serotyped; different serotypes suggest different routes of infection and degrees of virulence.

History. The first cases of AIDS were probably described between 1959 and 1970. The early cases were retrospectively identified and thus documented with varying degrees of completeness, depending on what archival material was available. Among the earliest cases were a British seaman in 1959 and a Norwegian family in 1966; both had been in Africa in the decade before their illness became apparent. In the late 1970s and early 1980s, new clinical features such as *Pneumocystis carinii* pneumonia, Kaposi sarcoma and other opportunistic infections were identified in homosexual men, initially in New York City, San Francisco and Los Angeles, and reported to the CDC (Centers for Disease Control). In 1982, the term AIDS was established and the risk groups identified: homosexual males, intravenous drug abusers, natives of certain endemic areas in Central Africa as well as Haiti, and recipients of transfusions, especially multiple transfusions, or hemophiliacs treated with Factor VIII . A year later Montagnier's group in Paris and then Gallo's group in Washington, D.C., identified the causative virus, now called HIV (human immunodeficiency virus). Within another year, standardized tests were available to identify the virus, so that the diagnosis could be based on proof of infection rather than on clinical criteria, allowing most patients to be identified earlier. HIV-2, a second subtype, was identified in West African patients. About the same time, antiretroviral therapy was introduced; it has dramatically expanded and increased both the life expectancy and quality of life for infected individuals. HIV infections have spread to cover most of the globe; currently they are most rapidly increasing in Africa, India, Southeast Asia and the former USSR. Newer victims include women and children, as no group of society has been spared. At this writing in 2000, the optimism produced by the successes of multiple drug antiretroviral therapy is counterbalanced by the relentless spread of the disease, especially in populations which cannot begin to afford therapy.

Epidemiology. As of January 2000, the World Health Organization (WHO) estimates that there are about 35 million people worldwide with HIV/AIDS. One in 100 adults around the world between the ages of 15 and 49 is infected. About 14 million people died from AIDS in 1997. There have been striking changes in the distribution of the disease. In the USA, the number of deaths from AIDS has begun to drop. In western Europe, there has been an even more dramatic drop. England, with its safe sex campaigns and free needles for drug addiction, achieved better results than countries such as the USA, where free needles are not widely available, or Spain and France, where open safe sex programs never gained momentum. In western countries, the epidemic has remained largely confined to homosexuals, prostitutes and drug addicts, with a measurable but minimal creep into the heterosexual population. The introduction of HAART (highly active antiretroviral therapy) has caused optimism, as many infected individuals are functioning at almost normal levels and some of the severe associated illnesses have become less common.

The story becomes grim when one considers the Third World, women and children. Of the 35 million individuals in the world with HIV/AIDS, 23 million live in sub-Saharan Africa and 7 million in India and Southeast Asia. Some 40% of the infected individuals are women; more than half are less than 25 years old and most are unaware that they are infected, with no possibility for treatment. In 1998; 3 million children died from AIDS, another 1.2 million were infected and about 8 million were orphans because of disease in their parent(s). Most of these people are unlikely to ever receive effective treatment and are very likely to continue to spread the virus. AIDS alone has wiped out most of the public health advances in the Third World since the end of World War II.

Etiology and Pathogenesis. Discussions of the pathogenesis of HIV infections consume entire textbooks and are beyond our scope. In briefest terms, HIV has an attraction for $CD4^+$ helper T cells, but other cellular receptors are also essential, as some patients are surprisingly resistant to HIV infection. Mutations in the CCR-5 receptor allele seem protective. HIV can also enter macrophages, such as the Langerhans cells in the skin. While in the past it was felt that HIV was relatively slow-growing, more sophisticated techniques have shown an unquestionably massive increase in virus load in untreated patients well before any clinical symptoms are present and an equally striking drop with appropriate antiretroviral therapy.

HIV can be found in all body fluids. The risk of spread correlates with the concentration of HIV in the bodily fluid, as well as with the resistance of the recipient. The most important means of spread is sexual contact, especially when semen comes in contact with mucosal surfaces. Damaged skin or mucosa, such as caused by HSV or syphilis, increases the risk of infection. Blood products are the second most important means of spread. While refined testing has almost eliminated the risk from transfusion products, the transfer of blood among drug abusers, as well as the risk through health care accidents, remains a serious problem. HIV has also been transferred during solid organ transplantation.

Transfer from mother to infant is another problem, one that is increasing in scope. HIV can be passed to the child during pregnancy, delivery or even during nursing. In western countries the risk is less than 15%, but it is apparently higher in some underdeveloped countries. Treatment of the pregnant patient with antiretroviral drugs has markedly reduced the risk of having an infected infant. Today in Munich it is around 3%.

Table 2.9. Simple clinical classification of HIV/AIDS

Acute infection
Seropositive latent stage
Lymphadenopathy syndrome
AIDS-related complex (ARC)
Full-blown AIDS

Clinical Findings. The classification of HIV/AIDS has involved the efforts of many groups. Tables 2.9–2.11 show three standard classification schemes. In general, the most usual parameters, as of this writing, are the HIV status, primarily the absolute viral count or load, and the $CD4^+$ count. Table 2.12 shows some of the opportunistic infections and unusual tumors that are also considered AIDS-defining illnesses. While such diseases are no longer so critical for the official diagnosis of AIDS, they are of immense importance in identifying patients at risk in order to determine appropriate testing. If a patient with an opportunistic infection or unusual tumor does not have evidence of HIV, other types of immunodeficiency should be sought and the patient's HIV status monitored.

In the often long course of HIV/AIDS, there may be a wide variety of cutaneous and mucosal findings. Frequently, the cutaneous changes are the first clinical sign of infection (diagnostic importance) or a clue to a worsening immune status (prognostic importance). There are few cutaneous changes which are unique to HIV/AIDS; instead the triad of unusual age distribution, atypical location and unusual morphological appearance may suggest the underlying problem. Ulceration, persistence and dissemination of cutaneous infections or tumors is often a poor prognostic sign, pointing towards progressive immune deficiency. All of the objective cutaneous findings, as discussed below, are complicated by the patient's logical and understandable fear of confronting the diagnosis of HIV/AIDS. Thus, when a patient in a possible risk group inquires if a lesion could be Kaposi sarcoma, one must not fail to get the message. Patient confidentiality is a crucial issue, but one that has hampered some public health measures.

Acute HIV Infection

Within 2–8 weeks after infection with HIV, individuals may develop an acute viral illness. This often resembles infectious mononucleosis, with fever and marked malaise; other findings may include

Table 2.10. Walter Reed classification of HIV/AIDS

Stage[a]	HIV	LAP	$CD4^+$	Recall	Thrush	OI
WR1	+	–	>400	N	–	–
WR2	+	+	>400	N	–	–
WR3	+	+	<400	N	–	–
WR4	+	+	<400	H	–	–
WR5	+	+	<400	A	+	–
WR6	+	+	<400	A/H	+/–	+

WR, Walter Reed stage; LAP, lymphadenopathy; $CD4^+$, number of cells/µl; recall, positive skin test for recall antigens (N: normal, H: hypergic, A: anergic); OI, opportunistic infections; K, Kaposi sarcoma

[a] Modifiers which can be applied to any stage include: CNS (evidence of brain involvement; encephalopathy), N (neoplasia), B (constitutional symptoms (night sweats, fever, >10% weight loss, diarrhea >4 weeks)

Table 2.11. Centers for Disease Control (CDC) classification

$CD4^+$	Stage	Clinical division A	B	C
>500	1	Stage 1	Stage 1	Stage 3 (AIDS)
200–499	2	Stage 1	Stage 2	Stage 3 (AIDS)
<200	3	Stage 2	Stage 2	Stage 3 (AIDS)

A, asymptomatic, acute retroviral syndrome, lymphadenopathy syndrome; B, HIV-associated but not AIDS-defining illnesses; C, AIDS-defining illnesses

Table 2.12. AIDS-associated illnesses

Protozoan infections	Fungal infections	Bacterial infections
Pneumocystis carinii pneumonia (also classified as fungal)	Candidal esophagitis, bronchitis, tracheitis and pneumonia	Recurrent salmonella sepsis
Cerebral toxoplasmosis	Extrapulmonary cryptococcosis, especially meningitis	Tuberculosis
Cryptosporidiosis lasting more than 1 month than 1 month	Aspergillosis, especially pneumonia and meningitis	Disseminated or extra -pulmonary infections with atypical myco-bacteria
Isosporidosis, especially chronic	Disseminated or extra-pulmonary histoplasmosis	Recurrent infections with *Haemophilus, Streptococcus pneumoniae*, other streptococci, *Staphylococcus aureus* within 2 years in patients > 13 years that lead to septicemia, meningitis, osteomyelitis, arthritis or internal abscesses (otitis media, skin and mucosal abscesses are excluded)

Viral infections	Tumors and others
Cytomegalovirus infections involving organs other than liver, kidneys or lymph nodes	Kaposi sarcoma
	Non-Hodgkin lymphoma, especially primary CNS B cell lymphoma
Herpes simplex virus infections which last > 1 month, especially when perianal, or cause bronchitis, pneumonia or esophagitis	Invasive cervical carcinoma
	HIV-wasting syndrome or slim disease
Progressive multi-focal leukoence-phalopathy (polyoma virus)	
Exaggerated or resistant human papilloma virus infections	

The CDC definitions were expanded in 1993 to include pulmonary tuberculosis, recurrent pneumonia and invasive cervical carcinoma, as well as all HIV-infected individuals with a $CD4^+$ count < 200, no matter what their clinical status.

lymphadenopathy, night sweats, joint and muscle pain and even gastrointestinal problems. The patient may also have a relatively nonspecific viral exanthem, consisting of small erythematous macules and papules primarily on the trunk. Tiny oral ulcerations may also be found.

The clinical diagnosis can only be suggested when a patient is in an at risk situation. Repeated evaluation for at least 12 weeks after a suspected exposure is essential; we rely primarily on PCR examination and viral load, but also measure p24 antigen and HIV-specific antibodies. Theoretically, an infection can be documented by PCR or viral load prior to seroconversion. We recommend control evaluations for a year. Any symptoms can be treated with general measures. If an infection is diagnosed, then early and aggressive multiple-drug therapy is started.

Malignancies

Kaposi Sarcoma

(Kaposi 1872)

History. Kaposi sarcoma was described in Vienna in 1872 by the Hungarian dermatologist Moritz Kaposi under the name "sarcoma idiopathicum mulitplex haemorrhagicum". The classic Kaposi sarcoma is primarily a disease of elderly men, often of Mediterranean or Jewish background, typically involves the legs and has an indolent course. The classic work of Templeton and co-workers outlined the different features of African Kaposi sarcoma, presenting as a lymphoma-like illness in children and as very destructive cutaneous and soft tissue tumors in adolescents and adults. The frequency of Kaposi sarcoma in some African populations first suggested the possibility of an infectious etiology. Then, as iatrogenic immunosuppression became common in the 1970s, patients were seen with widespread cutaneous Kaposi sarcoma usually consisting of small papules that waxed and waned with the degree of immunosuppression. The main scientific questions in the 1970s were: (1) Is Kaposi sarcoma a tumor or a reactive process? (2) Does it start in arterioles, veins or lymphatics?

With the AIDS epidemic, Kaposi sarcoma suddenly became a household word. Friedman-Kien and coworkers (Friedman-Kien et al. 1981)in New York, and soon thereafter other workers in Los Angeles and San Francisco, identified disseminated and aggressive Kaposi sarcoma in immunosuppressed homosexual males. The lesions tended to grow rapidly, facial and oral involvement was common and internal lesions (usually gastrointestinal tract or lymph nodes) were also frequently found. Initially, Kaposi sarcoma was one of the defining criteria for AIDS, until the virus was identified.

Epidemiology. Kaposi sarcoma is almost a marker for homosexual male HIV/AIDS patients; it is relatively uncommon in all other AIDS risk groups. While about 20% of homosexual males with HIV/AIDS develop Kaposi sarcoma, less than 5% of other AIDS patients do so. For example, in women with bisexual partners, the prevalence of Kaposi sarcoma is about 3%; in those with drug-abusing partners, it is only 0.7%. It is very rare in hemophiliacs and has not been reported in partners of hemophiliacs.

Etiology and Pathogenesis. The single most important factor is prior infection with human herpes virus-8. Evidence for this herpesvirus is more commonly found in homosexuals. Viral nucleic acids have been identified in Kaposi sarcoma tissue. Human herpes virus-8 has also been found in Kaposi sarcoma from patients without HIV/AIDS. While there is conflicting laboratory and clinical data, Kaposi sarcoma seems to be a widespread but monoclonal or oligoclonal tumor in most patients. The tissue of origin remains unclear.

Clinical Findings. About 3% of the HIV-positive patients who develop Kaposi sarcoma still have relatively intact immunity with normal CD4 counts. As the patient's immunity decreases, the likelihood of Kaposi sarcoma increases. The only absolutely typical site for AIDS-associated Kaposi sarcoma is the hard palate; such involvement is very common and almost unheard of in classic Kaposi sarcoma (Fig. 2.35). The lesions begin as very subtle red macules, but are generally identified as spindle-shaped, red-brown papules and nodules that follow the lines of skin tension. The course is quite unpredictable; some lesions regress, others remain small and a few enlarge dramatically, causing significant problems (Figs. 2.36, 2.37). The large tumors become very dark, because of hemosiderin deposits, especially on the legs. Some tumors grow rapidly, similar to a pyogenic granuloma, ulcerate and can be mutilating. Involvement of the hands, feet, genitalia and especially the mouth can lead to

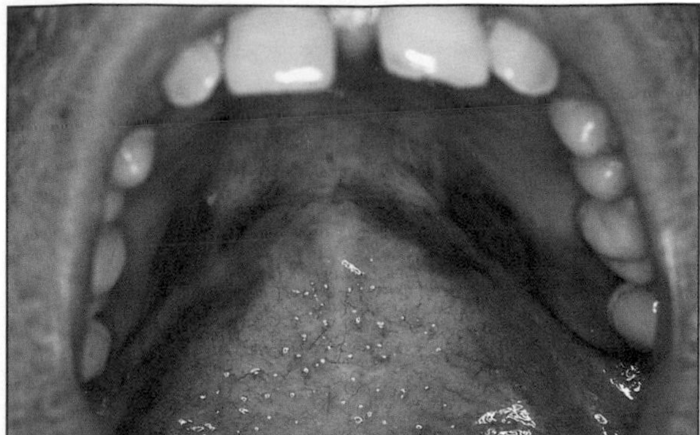

Fig. 2.35. Oral Kaposi sarcoma in HIV/AIDS

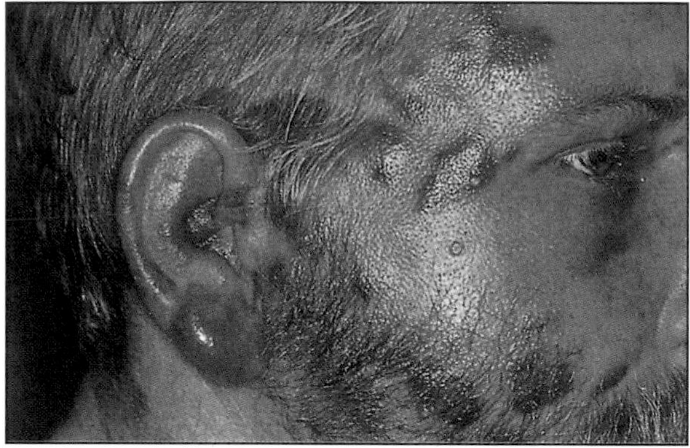

Fig. 2.36. Facial Kaposi sarcoma in HIV/AIDS

functional as well as cosmetic problems. The oral lesions may ulcerate and interfere with eating or feeding. Table 2.13 shows the classification we most often employ.

Histopathology. The mainstay of diagnosis of subtle lesions is microscopic examination (Chap. 59). Early macular lesions can be quite difficult to interpret; often there are only subtle dilated vessels about appendages or in the papillary dermis.

Differential Diagnosis. The differential diagnostic list is endless if one is dealing with a solitary small lesion or does not know that the patient has HIV/AIDS. Initially, other vascular lesions, pigmented purpuras, dermatofibromas and other malignant infiltrates can be considered. The oral lesions frequently are totally flat, mimicking purpura. More widespread disease can initially be mistaken for a variety of exanthems; in particular, secondary syphilis should be excluded. Larger ulcerated lesions can be confused with pyogenic granuloma or bacillary angiomatosis.

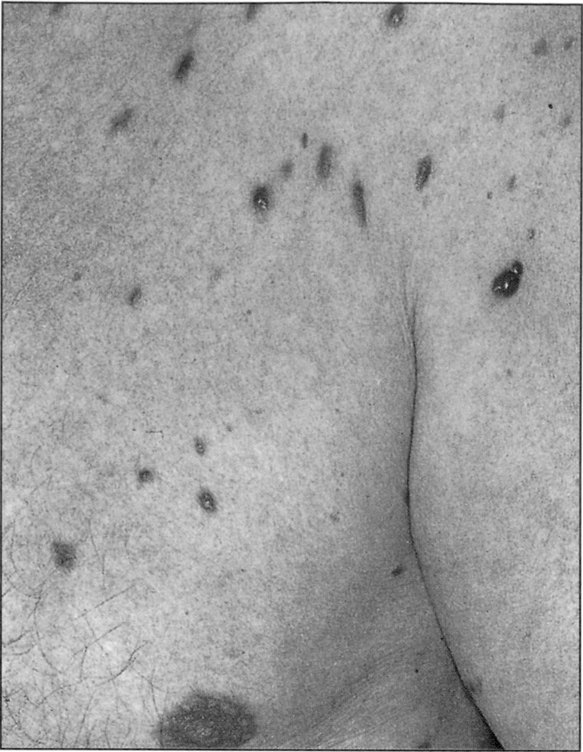

Fig. 2.37. Kaposi sarcoma on chest following skin lines in HIV/AIDS

Table 2.13. Stages of Kaposi sarcoma (from Mitsuyasu 1986)

Stage I	Minimal cutaneous involvement; fewer than ten lesions or involvement of just one anatomic region
Stage II	Widespread cutaneous disease; more than ten lesions or involvement of multiple anatomic regions
Stage III	Only visceral involvement (lymphadenopathy, gastrointestinal tract)
Stage IV	Cutaneous and visceral involvement, or pulmonary involvement: A (no systemic symptoms), B (fever and diarrhea >2 weeks, >10% weight loss

Therapy. As a general rule, one should not feel the need to treat Kaposi sarcoma aggressively in HIV/AIDS patients when there is only skin involvement and the lesions are not widespread, ulcerated or interfering with function. The risk of immunosuppression is probably greater than the benefit of having a "tumor-free" skin. Therapy should be planned with consideration of the patient's tumor load and immune status, as shown in Table 2.14.

Table 2.14. Therapy of HIV-associated Kaposi sarcoma

CD4 lymphocytes	Tumor stage[a]	Therapy
>500	I, II	Local therapy[b]
		Fractionated radiation Rx
	II (severe)	HAART and INF α-2
	III, IV	Vinca alkaloids
499–200	I, II	Local therapy[b]
		Fractionated radiation Rx
	II (severe)	HAART and INF α-2
	III, IV	Vinca alkaloids
<200	I, II	Local therapy[b]
		Fractionated radiation Rx
	II (severe), III, IV	Liposomal dauno- or doxorubicin
		Polychemotherapy

HAART, highly active antiretroviral therapy; INF, interferon
[a] From Mitsuyasu 1986
[b] Cryotherapy, laser destruction, intralesional vinca alkaloids

Systemic. When patients have widespread cutaneous disease or systemic involvement, systemic therapy should be considered. When the CD4 count is >200, monotherapy with vinca alkaloids (vincristine or vinblastine) or etoposide can be considered. Interferon α-2 can be used as a monotherapy (9–36 million units subcutaneously daily); typical problems include flu-like symptoms and mild hematological changes.

When more severe disease is present, polychemotherapy is usually recommended. Regimens typically include vincristine or vinblastine combined with bleomycin and adriamycin; this combination causes significant marrow depression, neurological toxicity and pulmonary fibrosis. A new approach is the use of doxorubicin (20 mg/m^2) or daunorubicin (40–60 mg/m^2) enclosed in a liposomal delivery system. The hope is that these agents can be delivered more specifically to the tumor, increasing effectiveness and reducing toxicity, especially hematological problems. The use of HAART has made severe Kaposi sarcoma much less commonly seen and reduced the need for these relatively drastic treatment regimens.

Topical. When the lesions are small and only present a cosmetic problem, simple camouflage make-up may suffice. Cryotherapy and intralesional vinca alkaloids can be used for small lesions. We use vincristine, trying to inject 0.1 mg into an already anesthetized lesion. We do not treat more than five lesions at one sitting. This approach is especially helpful for palatal lesions. The argon laser is particularly useful for large ulcerated or edematous tumors, especially on the face, about the eyes or mouth. All such destructive methods are associated with open, sometimes painful, wounds and prolonged healing.

The mainstay of local therapy is fractionated radiation, as Kaposi sarcoma is exquisitely radiosensitive. We employ 20–30 Gy total dosage, fractionated over ten sittings, with a half-value layer appropriate for the tumor thickness. Electron beam therapy can also be employed. Radiation therapy is ideal for facial and genital lesions; it is virtually independent of the patient's immune status and has few side effects. Ulceration may be seen, especially on the legs. Photodynamic therapy also seems effective.

Lymphomas

Most HIV-associated lymphomas are B cell lymphomas, in which Epstein-Barr virus appears to be an important cofactor. While the initial presentation is usually lymphadenopathy, the oropharynx is a typical site of presentation. Cutaneous T cell lymphomas are also seen, and patients present with erythroderma, ulcerated tumors or lymphadenopathy (Chap. 61).

Carcinomas

Both basal cell carcinomas and squamous cell carcinomas can be more aggressive in HIV/AIDS patients, especially as their immune status deteriorates. For example, basal cell carcinomas may infiltrate deeply into the subcutaneous tissues or become quitelarge. With squamous cell carcinoma, the role of HPV as a carcinogen seems well-established. Invasive cervical carcinoma is an AIDS-defining illness in which HPV clearly plays a role. Cloacogenic carcinoma of the rectum is HPV-related, while ordinary genital warts associated with carcinogenic HPV types can be very aggressive.

Infectious Diseases

While all of these infectious agents are discussed elsewhere in the book, they are repeated here to emphasize the special aspects of their diagnosis and therapy in HIV/AIDS.

Viral Infections

Herpes Simplex Virus

Clinical Findings. About 85–90% of adults carry either HSV-1, HSV-2 or both. As the CD4 counts drop below 200, persistent ulcerated lesions are typically seen about the anus, nose or mouth (Figs. 2.38, 2.39). The lesions are often polycyclic and crusted. Other sites, such as the trunk or extremities, can also be involved; occasionally disseminated lesions are found. While the oral mucosa is commonly affected, further spread in the gastrointestinal tract is unexpected. Often a mixed infection with HSV and CMV is present.

Epidemiology. The Tzanck smear is usually strikingly positive. Electron microscopy, immunofluorescent examination or PCR can also be used to definitely identify the virus. CMV can often be diagnosed on a smear or biopsy because of its characteristic inclusions.

Differential Diagnosis. A number of other infections must be considered. Primary CMV infections or mixed infections are common. In addition, syphilitic chancre, chancroid and chancriform pyoderma must be excluded. Two special problems are foscarnet-induced ulcerations and trimethoprim-sulfamethoxazole-induced erythema multiforme.

Therapy

Systemic. The same therapeutic agents discussed in the first part of the chapter are appropriate. Depending on the patient's other problems, one may elect oral or intravenous therapy.

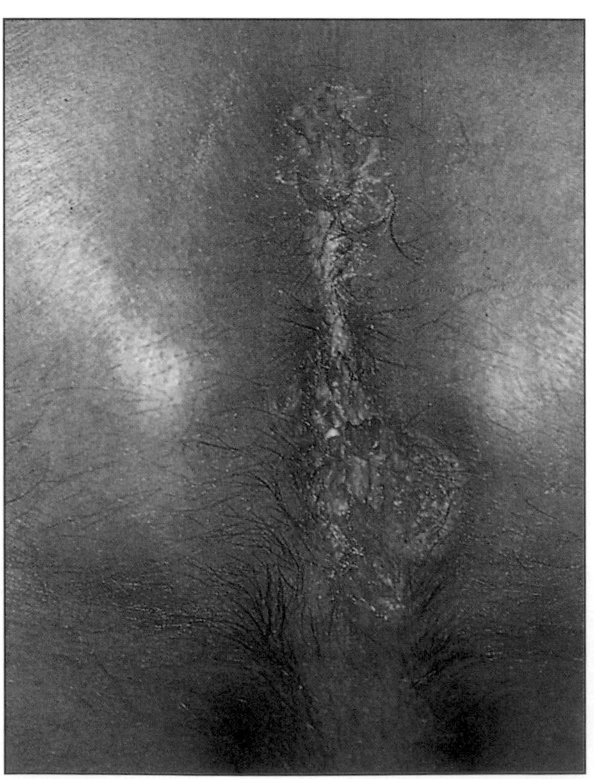

Fig. 2.38. Chronic perianal ulceration from herpes simplex virus in HIV/AIDS

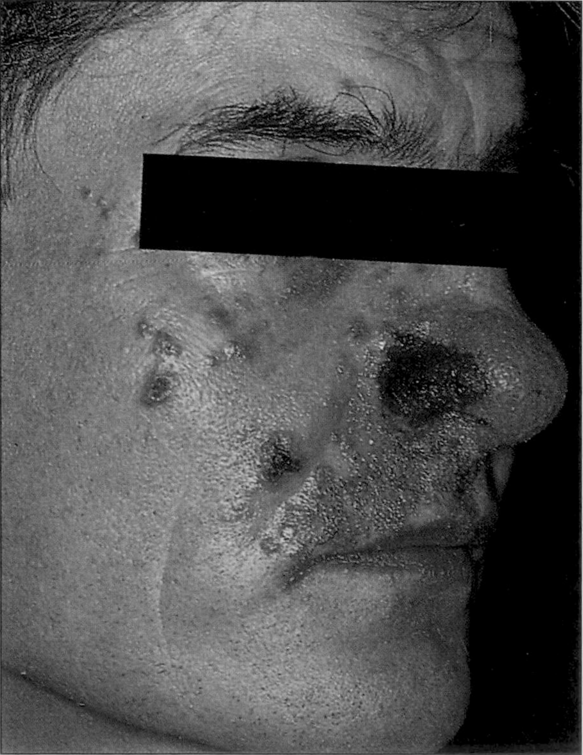

Fig. 2.39. Ulcerating facial herpes simplex infection in HIV/AIDS

Topical. External therapy alone is inappropriate in AIDS patients. Use of topical antiviral agents alone may lead to increased resistance. Standard drying measures can be used as an adjunct.

Varicella Zoster Virus

Over 90 % of patients carry VZV and reactivation is expected in HIV/AIDS. Often the presence of zoster in otherwise healthy young adults is the first sign of HIV/AIDS. This is especially true if the course is severe, in contrast to that expected in younger individuals. As the patient's immunity drops, more unusual forms of VZV appear, such as multisegmental, hemorrhagic or recurrent zoster and disseminated infection (identical to chickenpox). Least common but most typical for HIV/AIDS is the persistent, crusted hyperkeratotic variant, which is often missed.

Histopathology. The hyperkeratotic lesions are distinctive, with classical granular inclusions under a marked crust. Otherwise, the diagnosis is usually clinical.

Differential Diagnosis. Zoster is usually a straightforward diagnosis; the question may be what type of immunodeficiency is predisposing the patient. The later disseminated and crusted forms can be confused with disseminated HSV infections, pyodermas and syphilis.

Therapy

Systemic. High doses of intravenous acyclovir are usually preferred. Oral valacyclovir can also be used.

Topical. Standard drying measures should be used. Once again, topical antiviral agents should be avoided.

Cytomegalovirus

Clinical Findings. While about 50 % of the general population carries CMV, the numbers rise to about 90% in homosexuals and drug abusers. Cutaneous lesions are almost unheard of in the normal host. In immunodeficient patients, the most typical lesions are persistent genital or perioral ulcerations, often associated with HSV. A wide range of other findings has been described, including macular exanthems, nodules, verruciform plaques, blisters, petechiae and purpura. CMV involvement of the skin and mucosal surfaces often is a sign of disseminated infection, associated with an 85 % mortality rate over 6 months. The most common manifestation of CMV in HIV/AIDS is chorioretinitis.

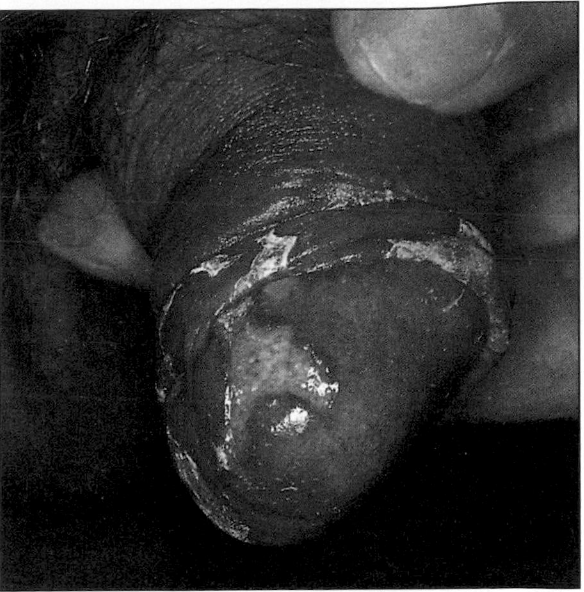

Fig. 2.40. Foscarnet-induced ulcerations in HIV/AIDS patient treated for cytomegalovirus infection

Histopathology. Cytomegalovirus can be identified histologically because of the "owl eye" inclusions. In the skin, they are usually found in endothelial cells as eosinophilic inclusions with a peripheral halo. Other histologic findings rarely help in the diagnosis.

Epidemiology. Standard techniques such as culture, immunofluorescent examination and PCR can be employed.

Differential Diagnosis. Herpes simplex, mixed ulcers, syphilis and foscarnet-induced ulcers (Fig. 2.40) are the main possibilities.

Therapy

Systemic. Ganciclovir 5 mg/kg intravenously b.i.d. is used until healing, and then 6 mg/kg five times weekly for maintenance therapy. Marrow toxicity is the main side effect. For ocular CMV, different regimens, including even intraocular therapy, are used. If the treatment fails, foscarnet is the next alternative – initially 90 mg/kg intravenously b.i.d. then 90–120 mg/kg i.v. daily. In addition to the ulcerations, foscarnet also causes nephrotoxicity and electrolyte changes.

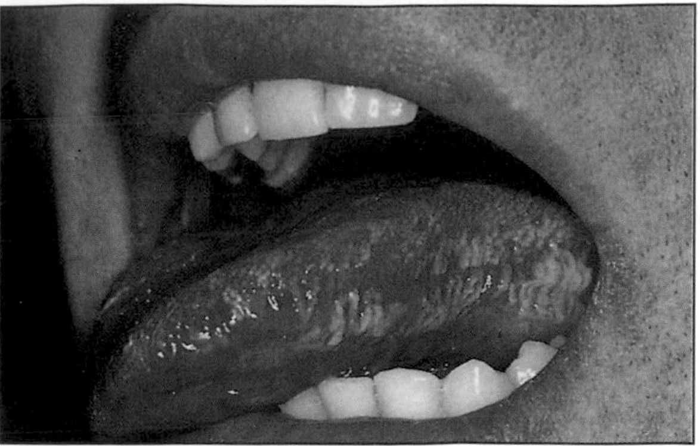

Fig. 2.41. Oral hairy leukoplakia

Oral Hairy Leukoplakia

Oral hairy leukoplakia is a distinctive finding in HIV/AIDS, although it has rarely been described in other settings. The typical persistent white growths along the side of the tongue can be seen early in the course of the disease, but usually reflect more advanced disease and are a poor prognostic sign (Fig. 2.41) While Epstein-Barr virus is the primary agent, secondary colonization with both HPV and *Candida albicans* is seen. The histologic picture is relatively distinctive, with pathognomonic balloon cells. The differential diagnosis includes candidiasis, lichen planus and frictional hyperkeratosis, but there is usually no question.

Therapy. There is no specific therapy. Oral hairy leukoplakia may improve during anti-viral therapy for HIV or even with systemic acyclovir or related drugs. Both ganciclovir and foscarnet produce striking improvement, although they are never used for this purpose. Topical therapy with retinoids or podophyllin may also be effective.

Human Papilloma Virus

The most serious problem with HPV in HIV/AIDS is the presence of carcinogenic types 16 and 18 and their role in cervical, genital and anal malignancies. Widespread condylomata acuminata may be found; on biopsy some show carcinoma in situ (bowenoid papulosis). In addition, cutaneous involvement may be very widespread and difficult to treatment. Typical for HIV/AIDS is the presence of multiple filiform warts of the face and neck as well as about the mouth.

Treatment should be aggressive to hopefully reduce the risk of malignant change. There are no specific approaches. For genital lesions, podophyllin or podophyllotoxin can be employed, along with cryotherapy. When laser or electrosurgical destruction is performed, the plume should be evacuated in such a way as to insure operator safety.

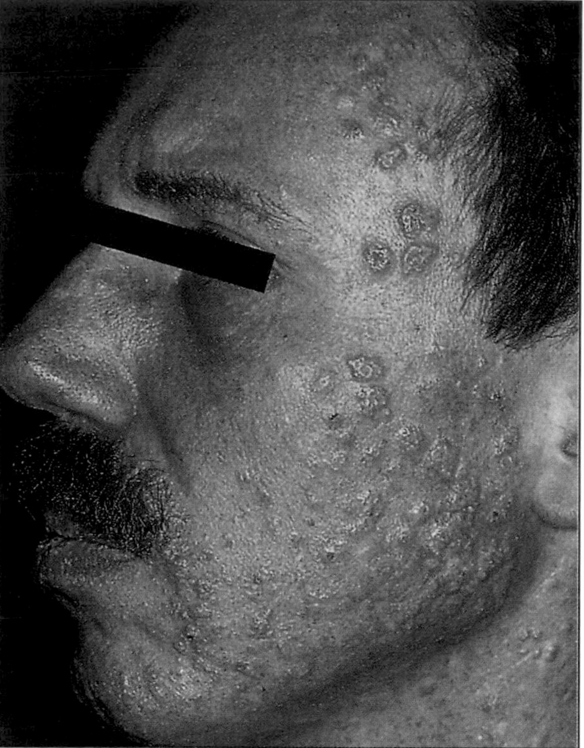

Fig. 2.42. Multiple giant mollusca contagiosa

Molluscum Contagiosum

Clinical Findings. Mollusca contagiosa take on a different clinical appearance in HIV/AIDS. They typically involve the face and the genital region, often becoming very large (Fig. 2.42) We have seen lesions 3–4 cm in diameter on the neck. Sometimes there are so many lesions that the infection resembles an exanthem. While the clinical diagnosis is usually easy, microscopic evaluation provides a quick definite answer.

Therapy. The individual lesions must be destroyed. Curettage and cryotherapy are the mainstays. In addition, podophyllin (25%), trichloracetic acid (up to 50%), pyruvic acid (95%), 5-fluorouracil (2–5% standard preparations) and retinoids can be tried. All must be used to the point of extreme irritation. Isolated reports have shown benefit from long-term oral use of retinoids, primarily acitretin.

Fungal and Yeast Infections

Candidiasis

Candidiasis is the most common infectious disease in HIV/AIDS. It may be an early sign of disease, may help to define AIDS and presents a very pleomorphic picture. Over 90% of the infections are caused by *Candida albicans*, but *C. tropicalis*, *C. krusei* and *Torulopsis glabrata* can also be found.

Clinical Findings. While patients with HIV/AIDS may have a variety of candidal infections, oral and esophageal involvement is most common. Almost all patients have such disease and in at least 80% of them treatment is required. Persistent oral candidiasis is very suggestive of HIV/AIDS when present in otherwise healthy individuals; involvement of the esophagus is an AIDS-defining disorder. Several different forms of oral candidiasis have been described in this patient group. They include:

- Thrush (acute pseudomembranous candidiasis)
- Angular cheilitis (perlèche)
- Acute erosive candidiasis with marked erythema, pain and erosions but no typical white deposits
- Chronic atrophic candidiasis with marked erythema of the buccal mucosa and a flat, smooth shiny tongue
- Chronic hypertrophic candidiasis with thick nodules or plaques especially on the hard palate and tongue

The diagnosis can be difficult, since almost everyone has *C. albicans* in the mouth at some time. Quantitative cultures and biopsies to show tissue invasion can help confirm the clinical diagnosis. Often a trial of therapy is the easiest way to show if *C. albicans* is involved. Any patient with oral candidiasis or with any symptoms of heartburn or dysphagia should be evaluated for candidal esophagitis.

Other problems associated with candidiasis are exaggerations of the disorders seen in other patient populations. Persistent, refractory genital infections, intertrigo, nail fold infections and, rarely, involvement of nonoccluded skin sites occur.

Differential Diagnosis. The differential diagnosis is endless. The main problem is that *C. albicans* is often present in association with other problems. One must exclude HSV infections, AIDS-associated gingivitis, aphthae, oral hairy leukoplakia and medication-induced ulcerations.

Therapy

Systemic. In most instances, systemic therapy is needed for treatment of active disease. The imidazoles are the mainstays of therapy; fluconazole (100 mg daily p.o.) or itraconazole (200–400 mg p.o.) for 1 week are acceptable. If esophageal involvement is documented, initial therapy should be for 2 weeks. With persistent or recurrent candidiasis in patients with CD4 counts <100, prophylaxis with fluconazole (50–100 mg thrice weekly) is appropriate, even though there is a chance of selecting resistant organisms. In severe infections, amphotericin B and flucytosine can be considered.

Topical. In early stages of HIV/AIDS, prophylaxis with imidazole trochees or lozenges may be sufficient.

Black Hairy Tongue

This is an uncommon harmless problem in the normal population, present in about 1% of individuals. It is felt to represent a mixed proliferation of nonpathogenic yeast and bacteria, perhaps on a background of elongated tongue papillae. In some patients, the accumulations are white or yellow, not black at all. The prevalence in HIV/AIDS patients is about 25%, supporting the importance of infectious agents in the disease's pathogenesis. Treatment consists of brushing the tongue with antibacterial washes or gels; retinoid solutions may also help but are rarely needed.

Pityrosporum ovale Infections

While *P. ovale* is common, present as part of the normal flora in most individuals, it flourishes in immunosuppressed hosts such as renal transplant patients or HIV/AIDS patients. The night sweats associated with type B symptoms may be another predisposing factor. In our experience, florid or excessive tinea versicolor is not a common finding in HIV/AIDS. In contrast *Pityrosporum* folliculitis is more of a problem in these patients. It presents as intensely pruritic papules, often excoriated, usually on the shoulder girdle and face; biopsy reveals a folliculitis with numerous organisms in the follicle. The differential diagnostic considerations include bacterial folliculitis, *Demodex* folliculitis and eosinophilic folliculitis, as well as all other papular exanthems. Topical imidazoles are usually sufficient for both tinea versicolor and *Pityrosporum* folliculitis; if they fail, especially in severely immunosuppressed patients, oral agents can be employed, such as itraconazole. Ketoconazole should be avoided as it cross-reacts with protease inhibitors.

Pityrosporum sepsis can also occur in immunocompromised patients. It is usually a result of contaminated hyperalimentation fluid, which is rich in lipids, the favorite food of the organisms. In rare occasions, improper disinfection of the subclavian area, where *P. ovale* is almost always present, has been blamed for inoculation of the organisms during a venous or arterial stick. If the sepsis is recognized, intravenous imidazole therapy is needed but usually fails to save the individual.

Dermatophyte Infections

Opinions about the nature of tinea corporis and onychomycosis in HIV/AIDS vary greatly. We have not been impressed by the severity of the problem, although in some patients tinea corporis is more severe or widespread. In addition, proximal subungual onychomycosis is very suggestive of HIV/AIDS, although uncommon in our practice. The patients present with white chalky nails and proximal nail fold inflammation, an unusual picture in immunocompetent hosts. Systemic imidazoles are required, often for longer periods of time than in the general population.

Deep Fungal Infections

The deep fungal infections can be a considerable cause of morbidity in HIV/AIDS but only rarely have cutaneous manifestations. The organisms often can be identified in a skin biopsy, sometimes with special stains; this is often very helpful since cultures require several weeks, time which many HIV/AIDS patients do not have.

Cryptococcosis

Cryptococcus neoformans is a worldwide fungus which usually is found in the lungs but can disseminate hematogenously to involve the meninges (the main problem in HIV/AIDS patients), bones, kidneys and skin. The skin lesions are often ulcerated papules or nodules that mimic molluscum contagiosum. Because of the urgency in diagnosing disseminated cryptococcosis, some authors recommend frozen section evaluation of mollusca in HIV/AIDS. If a patient is febrile, feels worse or has a rapid onset of multiple eroded papules, this is a wise precaution. But so many HIV/AIDS patients have mollusca that one must rely on clinical judgment in most cases. The treatment is complex; usually fluconazole, amphotericin B and flucytosine are all administered for at least 8 weeks. Once clinical healing has been attained, fluconazole is continued indefinitely as a suppressive therapy.

Histoplasmosis

Histoplasma capsulatum can also disseminate in HIV/AIDS patients, spreading from its primary pulmonary site. The cutaneous findings include eroded papules (once again resembling molluscum contagiosum), pustules, abscesses, deep inflamed nodules and persistent ulcerations. The mainstay of therapy is amphotericin B; itraconazole is employed for maintenance purposes.

Coccidioidomycosis

In the western USA, many patients are infected by the spores of *Coccidioides immitis*. The method of spread is airborne; the dry sand and dust of the Sonoran desert (parts of California, Arizona, New Mexico and northern Mexico) are ideal for the organism. Usually, the initial pulmonary infection is uneventful. In HIV/AIDS patients, it can be far more dramatic, but more often reactivation is the case, as with the other deep fungi. The main clinical problem is meningitis; the cutaneous lesions are once again nonspecific. Papules, pustules, nodules and ulcerated abscesses have been described. The treatment is amphotericin B, itraconazole and fluconazole; with CNS involvement, intrathecal amphotericin B is usually required. Ketoconazole and itraconazole may be employed for maintenance therapy.

Aspergillosis

In contrast to the other deep fungi, *Aspergillus fumigatus* is more likely to be an acquired infection during HIV/AIDS, rather than a reactivation. The reduced T cell counts as well as the neutropenia contribute to the patient's susceptibility. Contaminated venous lines are a major risk; inhalation and ingestion are other possibilities. Sepsis develops with multiple organ involvement, including the brain, heart, kidneys, bones, lymph nodes and skin. Once again, the cutaneous lesions are inflammatory papules, pustules and nodules, often ulcerated. Therapy is usually amphotericin B, flucytosine and itraconazole.

Bacterial Infections

Treatment is not discussed in detail here, as there are few differences between HIV/AIDS patients and other individuals in terms of response to antibiotics, so standard regimens can usually be employed. Exceptions are noted. Systemic therapy is almost always preferable.

Pyoderma

Bacteria play a surprisingly small role in adult HIV/AIDS. In children, staphylococcal infections are a significant factor. There are also differences among the various adult groups. Among homosexuals, folliculitis and perianal abscesses are the most common problems, but in drug abusers recurrent furuncles and other deep mixed infections are common. Those who are using methadone seem to be at greater risk. So-called chancriform pyoderma or blastomycotic-like pyoderma can also be seen; here, large ulcers develop with mixed flora. The nutritional deficiencies and lack of hygiene in this patient subset contribute greatly to the recurrent infections. As HIV/AIDS patients become more immunocompromised or develop medication-induced neutropenia, they are at greater risk.

Deeper infections, such as furuncles and abscesses, are usually caused by *Staphylococcus aureus*, but also by gram-negative agents such as *Escherichia coli*, *Haemophilus influenzae* and *Pseudomonas aeruginosa*. Deep ulcerated infections may be caused by viruses, deep fungi or any of a broad range of bacteria. Mixed infections are the rule, not the exception. Sepsis is unusual, although persistent and locally aggressive lesions may occur. Biopsy and tissue culture have a far higher yield than scrapings or swabs.

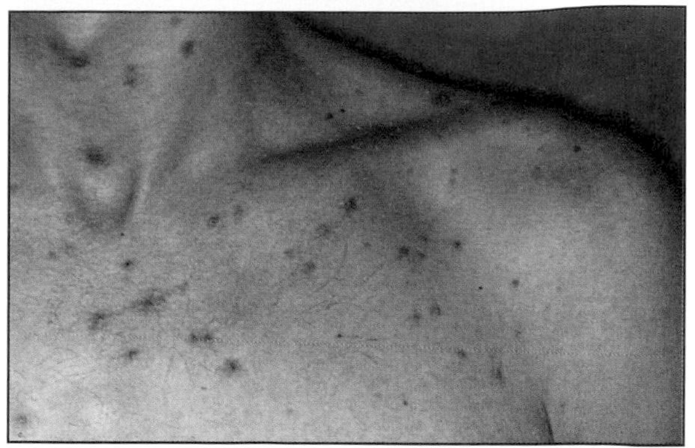

Fig. 2.43. Recurrent pruritic folliculitis in HIV/AIDS

Folliculitis

Bacterial folliculitis in HIV/AIDS is usually caused by *S. aureus*; occasionally *Propionibacterium acnes* is blamed. The most typical sites are the back, thighs and buttocks; irregularly distributed pustules with an erythematous periphery are seen (Fig. 2.43). Staphylococcal folliculitis is more common in children than adults. The differential diagnosis is shown in Table 2.15.

Table 2.15. Differential diagnosis of folliculitis and papular exanthems in AIDS

Type	Clinical features	Histology	Therapy
Staphylococcal	Usually pustules, associated pyodermas	Neutrophils involving follicle	Oral antibiotics
Demodex	Larger pustules, often facial	*Demodex* mites present	Lindane, sulfur-containing products
Pityrosporum	Smaller papules, trunk	Many *Pityrospora* (hard to quantify)	Antifungal agents (many patients on imidazoles for candidiasis)
Necrotizing	Necrotic lesions, similar to acne necrotica	Superficial necrosis, often deeper folliculitis	–
Eosinophilic	Very pruritic, face and trunk	Rich eosinophilic infiltrates	High-potency topical corticosteroids
Fungal	More likely on legs, genitalia	Also may have eosinophils; hyphae present	Oral antifungal agents
Scabies	Highly pruritic	Not follicular; mites may be found	Lindane, ivermectin, other scabicides
Idiopathic (papular eruption of AIDS)	Highly pruritic	Not follicular	High-potency topical corticosteroids, thalidomide

Bacillary Angiomatosis

This infection with *Bartonella henselae* was first identified in HIV/AIDS patients. It typically produces a pyogenic granuloma-like lesion which can be mistaken microscopically for Kaposi sarcoma. The infection is considered in Chap. 4.

Mycobacterial Infections

Both tuberculosis and atypical mycobacterial infections play a major role in HIV/AIDS, but neither is characterized by striking or specific skin involvement.

Tuberculosis

Reactivation of infection with *Mycobacterium tuberculosis* is a major problem in HIV/AIDS patients as their immunity drops. Studies in Africa have shown that tuberculosis prophylaxis provides as much prolongation of disease-free days as antiviral therapy and at lower cost. While this is clearly not true in western countries, it has emphasized the importance of this organism. Cutaneous tuberculosis usually takes the form of ulcerative local extension from a lymph node (lymphadenitis colliquativa), ulceration about orifices or disseminated papules and nodules. Tissue culture is the best diagnostic bet, but often the lesions are so rich in organisms that the Ziehl-Neelsen stain suffices. Monoclonal antibodies are also available for rapid identification, although cross-reactions are common. PCR can be employed, but it is most useful in the forms of cutaneous tuberculosis with few organisms. The cutaneous disease is treated with the appropriate multiagent systemic regimen, based on local resistance patterns and bacteriological results. In some regions, *M. tuberculosis* is resistant to all known treatment modalities and poses a major problem not only for patients but also for caregivers.

Atypical Mycobacteria

Etiology and Pathogenesis. *Mycobacterium avium-intracellulare complex* (MAI) has become a household word because of HIV/AIDS. Formerly the atypical mycobacteria were uncommon pathogens, usually acquired from soil or water and causing local infections. Their name is unfortunate, for there is nothing atypical about them; they fulfill all the taxonomic criteria for *Mycobacterium*. As the name suggests, MAI originally was identified in birds and bird droppings. While MAI is the most common atypical mycobacterium in HIV/AIDS, the other types may also be found.

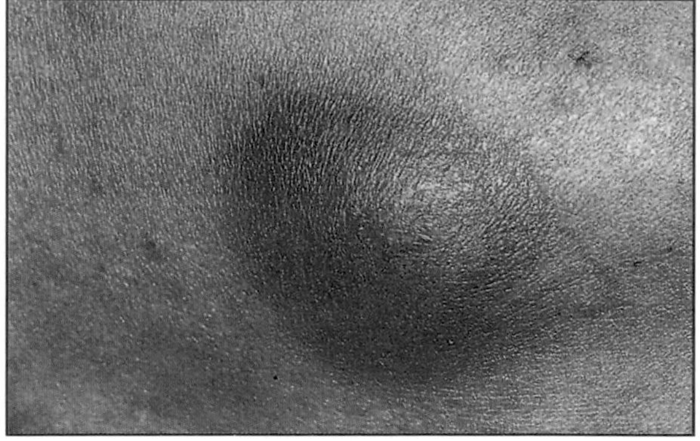

Fig. 2.44. Abscess caused by *Mycobacterium kansaii* in HIV/AIDS

Clinical Findings. Most often the patient presents with type B symptoms, including lymphadenopathy and weight loss, which are hardly uncommon in HIV/AIDS. Some may have hepatosplenomegaly or diarrhea. Most patients have a CD4 count <100 when they become symptomatic. The organism should be identified by culture; blood culture is most useful but bone marrow, lymph node, liver or stool culture may help.

Skin lesions are uncommon but reflect dissemination; papules, nodules and even cystic abscesses can be seen (Fig. 2.44). Today a high percentage of HIV/AIDS patients require prophylaxis for MAI following successful treatment of the initial infection.

Therapy. *Mycobacterium avium-intracellulare complex* is very difficult to treat. The standard regimens around the world include up to five drugs. Our usual protocol includes clarithromycin 500 mg b. i. d.; rifabutin 150 mg b. i. d.; and ethambutol 400 mg t. i. d. Patients with a CD4 <100 are candidates for prophylaxis; rifabutin 300 mg daily is most often used.

Syphilis

Epidemiology. The interrelationship between syphilis and HIV/AIDS is complex. Many patients have both diseases. In some groups of homosexual men with HIV/AIDS, over 40% have a positive syphilis serology. The presence of a chancre predisposes the patient to HIV/AIDS, presumably by providing an open entry site for HIV. For the same reason, chancroid and recurrent HSV infections are also risk factors.

Clinical Findings. Many patients with HIV/AIDS and syphilis have a clinical picture identical to that described in detail in Chap. 4. Because of the intricate relationship between immune status and expression of syphilis, some may have a more severe course. Primary syphilis may have a shorter incubation period, multiple primary lesions and persistent, painful, slowly expanding chancres. In secondary syphilis, lues maligna is more common, with both necrotic painful skin lesions and general symptoms such as fever and weight loss. Finally, the progression to tertiary syphilis, especially neurosyphilis, may be rapid.

Epidemiology. The diagnosis of syphilis can be difficult in HIV/AIDS because of the reduced immune response. Thus, many of the antibody-dependent tests may be hard to interpret. Ideally, the diagnosis should be based on identification of the organism, be it via dark field, Warthin-Starry stained sections or PCR. Cases are seen with positive identification of *Treponema pallidum* but a negative serology. In other instances, serological titers may be very high. Many groups recommend CSF examination in all cases of syphilis in HIV/AIDS patients. Here PCR and immunofluorescent examination can be helpful, along with serology.

Therapy. The therapy is also confusing. Public health authorities in many countries, including Germany, are skeptical of the efficacy of the CDC-recommended treatment of primary and secondary syphilis, which is benzathine penicillin, 2.4-million units IM weekly for 2–3 weeks. There is more rapid progression to neurosyphilis and treatment failures are more common in HIV/AIDS patients. One major study showed no significant differences in this disturbing trend whether the CDC regimen or more aggressive regimens were used. However, other studies have shown conflicting results, and we prefer to perhaps overtreat, employing clemizole penicillin, 1 million units IM daily for 2 weeks, or in the case of neurosyphilis, for 3 weeks.

Parasitic Infections

Scabies

While scabies is a frequent problem in HIV/AIDS patients, on occasion crusted scabies may be seen. Such patients have widespread thickened scales, especially on the hands and feet, erythroderma and surprisingly little pruritus. Often the diagnosis of scabies is not even suggested. On biopsy, many mites and their tunnels can be found in the hyperkeratotic scale. It is estimated that up to 10,000 mites can be found in a gram of scale. Thus the patients are highly contagious and their partners or caregivers should be investigated. The differential diagnosis may include atopic dermatitis, psoriasis and mycosis fungoides. In addition to standard topical therapy, one may want to consider oral ivermectin. Keratolytics help to remove the excess scales, speeding up resolution.

Protozoan Infections

Protozoa cause many problems for HIV/AIDS patients, but relatively few skin findings. A number of organisms are responsible for acute and chronic diarrhea (Table 2.12). *Pneumocystis carinii,* also classified as a fungus by some, causes pulmonary disease and is of interest to dermatologists primarily because the prophylactic treatment with trimethoprim-sulfamethoxazole so often causes drug eruptions. On rare occasions, there may be disseminated *P. carinii* infection, with erythematous papules primarily on the trunk and face. Two unusual findings have been outer ear abscesses and digital necrosis. Toxoplasmosis also occasionally disseminates, producing red papules that are not distinctive. In countries where leishmaniasis is a problem, the course of the disease is usually more aggressive in HIV/AIDS patients. In Europe, individuals are seen with nodular or ulcerated cutaneous leishmaniasis usually following vacations in the Mediterranean or Middle East. Their risk of systemic spread is far greater than for non-HIV/AIDS patients.

Noninfectious Dermatoses

Seborrheic Dermatitis

HIV/AIDS patients have given us insight into the nature of seborrheic dermatitis. While the incidence of the disorder in the general population is less than 10%, in this group it has been estimated at

20–70%. Severe sudden seborrheic dermatitis is one of the presenting signs of HIV/AIDS. The possible role of *P. ovale* in triggering the problem was dramatically suggested by the response of seborrheic dermatitis to the imidazoles used for other infections. Ketoconazole solution or shampoo forms a mainstay of treatment in all patient groups. Traditional measures are also helpful. In rare cases, intermittent therapy with oral imidazoles may be considered.

Psoriasis

HIV/AIDS has more convincingly demonstrated the importance of immunological factors in psoriasis. Patients with HIV/AIDS may experience a worsening of a preexisting psoriasis or present with severe psoriasis. Often there are dramatic overlaps between seborrheic dermatitis, psoriasis and Reiter syndrome. We suggest an HIV test in patients with rapid development of psoriasis or unexplained flares. The psoriasis may be more severe, often exudative, difficult to treat and evolve into erythroderma.

Therapy must also be adjusted as the patient's immune status declines. The routine topical measures should be tried first, but in many cases they are inadequate. We generally avoid immunosuppressive agents such as methotrexate or cyclosporine; the oral retinoids such as acitretin are more satisfactory. Often antiviral therapy produces improvement.

Both UVB and PUVA are effective; while there is a degree of phototherapy-related immunosuppression, it is probably less harmful than other measures. PUVA-bath therapy seems to be the best treatment, combing efficacy and a lack of systemic side effects.

Reiter Syndrome

Reiter syndrome is an uncommon disease, but is seen in about 0.5–1.0% of the HIV/AIDS population. It is viewed as a poor prognostic sign. Reiter syndrome may overlap clinically with psoriatic arthritis, but the standard differential diagnostic criteria should be applied. One speculation is that the initial immunosuppression in HIV/AIDS facilitates autoimmune phenomena that lead to Reiter syndrome, as well as psoriasis. Often the symptoms remit as the HIV/AIDS progresses. Treatment is problematic; we once again prefer oral retinoids, occasionally combined with short-term systemic corticosteroids. We screen all patients with Reiter syndrome for HIV infection prior to initiating therapy with immunosuppressive agents. The cutaneous findings can be treated just as in psoriasis.

Atopic Dermatitis

The nature of atopic dermatitis in HIV/AIDS patients is unclear. Some studies suggest an incidence of 50% in infected children. Other studies are more conservative and some doubt if the incidence is even increased. In patients with preexisting atopic dermatitis, it is not surprising that HIV/AIDS, with its associated infections, can trigger flares. One must exclude other causes of dermatitis and pruritus, such as scabies and even mycosis fungoides. Once again, we try to avoid immunosuppressive therapy, relying on topical measures and light therapy.

Xerosis and Acquired Ichthyosis

Although these two terms are often used as synonyms, they actually represent two different clinical problems. About 25–30% of our patients complain about dry skin and the associated pruritus, especially during the winter months. Reduced sebaceous secretions, altered skin lipids and perhaps hormonal changes have been blamed. The dry skin may be present early in the disease course and tends to worsen as the immune status declines. Xeroderma is most severe in patients with wasting. In acquired ichthyosis, the patients develop thick adherent scales often on the extensor aspects of the extremities or the trunk, sometimes associated with palmar-plantar keratoderma. HIV testing should be part of the evaluation of patients with acquired ichthyosis.

Papular Dermatitis

Synonyms. Papular eruption of AIDS, prurigo of AIDS

Etiology and Pathogenesis. Many HIV/AIDS patients suffer from pruritic papular eruptions. Despite the use of the term "papular dermatitis of AIDS", no single disorder is meant. Causes may include scabies, all forms of folliculitis including eosinophilic pustular folliculitis (Chap. 4), miliaria (associated with night sweats) and also some apparently idiopathic eruptions.

Clinical Findings. The patients have prurigo with marked pruritus, frequent excoriations but also occasional primary lesions, usually small seropapules (Chap. 25). Urticarial lesions may be seen. The upper aspects of the trunk and the limbs are most often involved. In our patients, this problem is far more common in the drier winter months.

Histopathology. Biopsy usually helps to exclude other diagnoses. The block should be sectioned carefully, searching for follicular involvement, possible mites, eosinophils and other perhaps specific features. In some cases, the follicles are filled with *Demodex folliculorum* or *P. ovale*, suggesting a proliferation of these saprophytes. In other instances there is simply a lymphocytic perivascular infiltrate with scattered eosinophils.

Therapy. If a cause is identified, then it should be treated. Otherwise, UVB irradiation or high potency topical corticosteroids offer the most promise.

Acne Vulgaris

During the early stages of HIV/AIDS, preexisting acne may flare or acne may appear for the first time. The patients are usually not in the typical acne age group, but otherwise the acne is fairly typical. Papulopustular lesions tend to dominate over comedones, and treatment should be so directed. Some patients have acneiform eruptions from taking massive dosages of B vitamins or so-called protein cocktails.

Photosensitivity

Porphyria Cutanea Tarda

Acquired porphyria cutanea tarda is much more common in HIV/AIDS patients. It is estimated that the prevalence is 20 times (2000%) that of the normal population. Chronic infections with hepatitis B and especially hepatitis C viruses are felt to be the major triggers. The patients are difficult to treat, as most are too anemic for blood letting and tolerate chloroquine poorly.

Chronic Actinic Dermatitis

In some patients, the development of chronic actinic dermatitis is one of the first signs of increasing immunodeficiency in HIV/AIDS. Most often UVB radiation is the trigger, although UVA radiation and combinations of both have also been implicated. Usually there is no history of using systemic or topical photosensitizers, in contrast to non-HIV/AIDS patients. The treatment guidelines are identical (Chap. 13).

Photosensitive Granuloma Annulare

Granuloma annulare is more common in the HIV/AIDS population. Its prevalence has been estimated at 2%. In some patients there are multiple lesions in sun-exposed areas, often associated with a documented increased sensitivity to UVB radiation. Photoprotection is the most reasonable treatment; troublesome lesions can be injected with corticosteroids.

UV-Induced Lichenoid Dermatitis

In general, lichenoid reactions are uncommon in HIV/AIDS. Some patients, however, develop lesions identical to lichen planus in sun-exposed skin. Often the time sequence fits with the ingestion of photosensitizing medications, especially trimethoprim-sulfamethoxazole. We suspect that most of these eruptions are lichenoid drug eruptions, which usually resolve when (or if) the triggering medication can be stopped.

UV-Induced Hyperpigmentation

Patients with dark skin (types V and VI) frequently develop hyperpigmentation in sun-exposed areas, often associated with increased UVB sensitivity. In some cases, zidovudine may be a cofactor.

Hair Disorders

Many HIV/AIDS patients have diffuse hair loss. Early in the disease, there may be a telogen effluvium, perhaps accounted for by the initial HIV infection. In the later stages of the illness, the hair loss is probably caused by malnutrition, zinc deficiency, medications and perhaps reduced hormone levels. Furthermore, androgenic alopecia may also be more severe. A much more distinctive change is trichomegaly of the eyelashes; patients with dramatically reduced CD4 counts not infrequently complain of having to trim their eyelashes (Fig. 2.45).

Pigmentary Changes

The most common changes are caused by zidovudine, which produces brown macules on the mucosal surfaces and linear or diffuse changes of the nails. Patients with severe wasting may acquire diffuse hyperpigmentation. Scattered reports

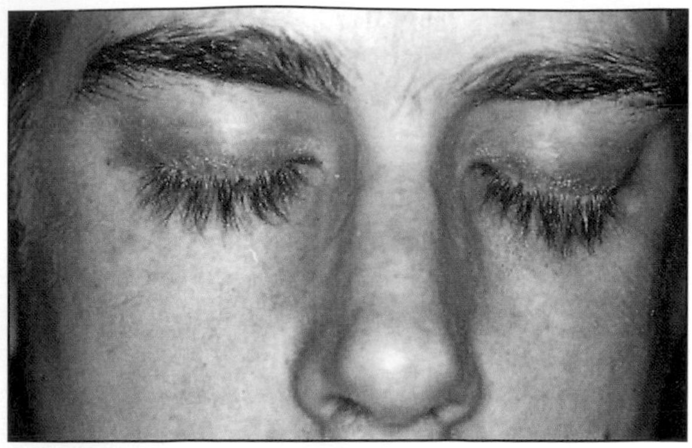

Fig. 2.45. Trichomegaly in HIV/AIDS

suggest more problems with vitiligo, melasma and even erythema dyschromicum perstans, but we have not found these changes to be clinically relevant.

Vascular and Hematological Problems

Disseminated Telangiectases

One of the earliest signs of HIV/AIDS is the proliferation of numerous small telangiectases, especially on the neck and thorax. In the early days of the epidemic, this was touted as a highly useful clinical pointer, but we have seen few examples in recent years.

Vasculitis

Small vessel vasculitis may be more common in HIV/AIDS but the situation is complex. Multiple viral and bacterial infections may lead to immune complex formation and resultant vasculitis. Lesions tend to be hemorrhagic, perhaps because of decreased platelets, and often ulcerate. Disseminated infections, especially with HSV, must be excluded. Hepatitis viruses may play a role in some cases, while in other instances drugs are a trigger.

Thrombocytopenia

HIV/AIDS patients often have markedly reduced platelet counts. Platelet-specific autoantibodies and immune complex formation, both with subsequent sequestration and destruction in the spleen, have been suggested as potential mechanisms. As the counts fall below 30,000/µl, petechiae can be seen, especially on the hard palate but also elsewhere on the body. Perifollicular hemorrhages, as in scurvy, may also be found. Other dermatoses may be complicated by hemorrhage.

If the platelet count drops below 30,000/µl, HAART and systemic corticosteroids (prednisone 1 mg/kg daily for many weeks) produce a dramatic response. Immunoglobulins (0.4 g/kg intravenously every 3 weeks) is another approach.

Autoimmune Disorders

One of the paradoxes of HIV/AIDS is the emergence of autoimmune disorders as the immune status declines. Presumably the initial changes are those of altered immunomodulation, leading to increased antibody formation. Both antinuclear antibodies and anticardiolipin antibodies are more common. Sicca syndrome is also relatively common, but only rarely are the appropriate anti-Ro and anti-La antibodies found. Vasculitis, myositis, arthralgias and autoimmune renal disease have all been reported.

Oral Changes

Sicca Syndrome

Dry mouth and dry eyes are major causes of morbidity. Even in those patients without serologic evidence for Sjögren syndrome, the problem can be severe. Artificial saliva and tears should be used generously. In patients with very dry mouths, radiation therapy for Kaposi sarcoma of the oral mucosa should be avoided if possible. The dryness often improves dramatically with HAART.

Acute Necrotizing Ulcerative Gingivitis

Clinical Findings. Almost every HIV/AIDS patient has gingivitis. Those with a relatively good immune status develop acute necrotizing ulcerative gingivitis (ANUG). This common disorder is more severe in HIV/AIDS and represents the collision of a combination of factors, including mixed bacterial infection featuring fusiform bacilli, *Spirella*, gram-negative bacteria, *Candida albicans* (uncommon in non-HIV/AIDS patients) and many other microorganisms, as well as inadequate oral hygiene and malnutrition. The key clinical features are initial necrosis of the interdental papillae, followed by more extensive destruction, pain, bleeding, halitosis, and later even fever and lymphadenopathy (Fig. 2.46). ANUG is similar to noma, as seen in malnourished Third World children (Chap. 33).

Differential Diagnosis. Two other conditions must be considered: (1) Marginal gingivitis with band-like erythema on the gingival margins is almost specific for HIV/AIDS and is caused by *C. albicans.* (2) Periodontitis is similar to ANUG but produces more pain, more extensive tissue destruction and involves the teeth and bones.

Therapy. Intensive dental care, both by a hygienist and by the patient or caregiver, is the mainstay. Despite the initial pain, the necrotic tissue must be debrided. Sometimes oral metronidazole or trimethoprim-sulfamethoxazole is useful for the short term, presumably because of their gram-negative spectrum. Chlorhexidine oral rinses are helpful during the acute phase and essential for prophylaxis. Oral anesthetic rinses may help to allow the patient to eat properly.

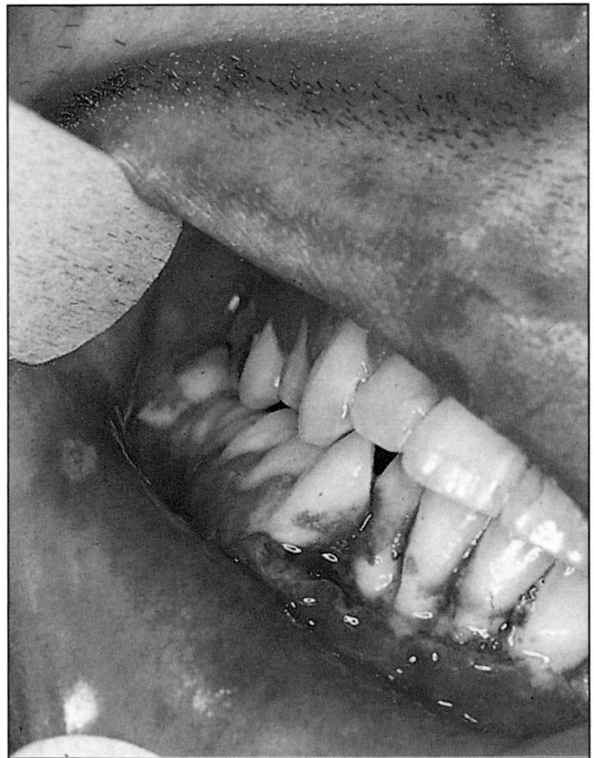

Fig. 2.46. Acute necrotizing ulcerative gingivitis in HIV/AIDS

Aphthae

Oral aphthae are a major problem in HIV/AIDS. They can range from ordinary small, self-limited lesions to large, necrotic slow-to-heal ulcerations that are quite painful. One must exclude HSV and CMV infections, as well as candidiasis. Sometimes leukopenia is a predisposing factor. On rare occasions, there are associated genital ulcerations or even other manifestations of Behçet syndrome. Treatment is very unsatisfactory. If routine measures fail, one should consider oral thalidomide, which seems extremely effective for HIV/AIDS-associated aphthae.

AIDS in Children

The clinical manifestations of HIV/AIDS in childhood are somewhat different. In the past some children were infected via blood or blood product transfusions; today almost all have an HIV-positive mother. In contrast to adults, infants may have many other, albeit rare, causes of immunodeficiency. Until HIV is unequivocally identified, one must consider the other causes of congenital immune defects (Chap. 4).

By 1 year, about 75 % of HIV-infected infants have symptoms, including recurrent severe bacterial infections, lymphadenopathy, hepatosplenomegaly, parotid gland swelling and lymphocytic interstitial pneumonia. They tend to have elevated immunoglobulins and falling CD4 counts. Neurological signs and symptoms are also often prominent, as well as *P. carinii* pneumonia.

Skin findings are rather different from those of adults. For example, Kaposi sarcoma is almost unheard of. Other neoplasms are also rare, but multiple leiomyomas and leiomyosarcomas have been described associated with Epstein-Barr virus. In contrast to adults, in whom rare infections have made a name for themselves, in children, common infections are severe, persistent and recurrent. *Streptococcus pneumoniae*, *Haemophilus influenzae* and *Staphylococcus aureus* are among the usual perpetrators. In addition, severe oral or diaper candidal infections, widespread mollusca and warts and chronic VZV and HSV infections are all seen and should raise the question of possible HIV/AIDS. Another finding is severe atopic dermatitis or seborrheic dermatitis.

While slightly different grading schemes are used, in general, the approach to the child with suspected HIV/AIDS is similar to that in the adult, although treatment differs somewhat.

Diagnostic Criteria

Table 2.16 lists the types of individuals in whom an HIV test is appropriate. Many other individuals will give a history of high-risk behavior and request testing. In addition, others will have frivolous indications, but should still be tested, as they may be hiding high-risk behavior. In general, since the confidentiality of HIV/AIDS testing is for the most part well-established, there should be no reluctance to evaluate a patient.

The major tests are shown in Table 2.17. If a test comes back positive, a number of rules must be observed. We inform a patient of a positive test only when two screening tests and a confirmatory test (ELISA × 2 and Western blot) are positive. If the initial screening test is positive, we redraw the blood and repeat the procedure, explaining to the patient that the initial test was questionable. If one orders or draws an HIV test, one must be prepared to compulsively follow up the results and provide the patient with appropriate counseling and referral. For this reason, we are not enthusiastic about the rapid test kits available for home testing. They may provide a false sense of security if negative and produce panic-stricken patients with inadequate access to counseling when positive. The quick tests are sometimes useful in emergency settings, but they should be coupled with confirmatory standard testing. If clinical suspicion is high and the testing is negative, it should be repeated in 6–12 weeks. There is a window during which the patient has negative serological tests following successful infection. On rare occasions, seroconversion may take as long as 1 year.

Table 2.17. Diagnosis of HIV infection

Direct methods: identification of HIV or its components
p24 antigen test[a]
Polymerase chain reaction (PCR)[a]
HIV culture
Electron microscopy
Indirect methods: identification of antibodies against HIV components
ELISA (screening test)[a]
Western blot (confirmatory test)[a]
Immunofluorescence examination
Radioimmunoprecipitation assay (RIPA)
Agglutination test
Dotblot assay

[a] Most widely used tests.

Once the diagnosis is established, the patient should be staged. The following factors should be considered.

History. The patient should be asked about the occurrence of fever, night sweats, weight loss, reduced activity, cough, difficulty in breathing, diarrhea, headache, visual problems.

Clinical Findings. The clinical examination should include: (1) an evaluation of the skin, mucous membranes and lymph nodes, (2) a directed internal and neurological evaluation, (3) an ophthalmologic examination, (4) a chest X-ray, (5) an abdominal ultrasound and (6), in women, a pelvic examination.

Laboratory Evaluation. We primarily rely on the identification of HIV, the CD4 and CD8 levels and

Table 2.16. Indications for HIV testing

Historical features
Homosexual or heterosexual with changing partners without protection
Sexually transmitted diseases such as syphilis or gonorrhea
Drug abuse, especially when intravenous with high risk behavior
Prostitute not using protective measures
Children of HIV-positive mother
Travelers from endemic region, especially if history of transfusion or sexual exposure
Hemophilia with replacement therapy prior to 1985
Blood transfusion prior to 1985 or while in high risk area
Clinical features
Lymphadenopathy of undetermined origin for more than 6 weeks
Increased number of infectious illnesses
Presence of HIV-associated skin diseases
Wasting

Table 2.18. Laboratory evaluation of HIV/AIDS patient

Primary tests
Viral load (b-DNA, PCR, NASBA methods)
Absolute CD4, CD8 counts and ratio
Secondary tests
Serum p24 antigen
Serum β2-microglobulin
Urine neopterin
Serum electrophoresis with quantitative immuno globulins
CBC with differential and platelet count
Erythrocyte sedimentation rate
Routine chemistry (LFT, BUN, creatinine, electrolytes)
Serological search for syphilis, toxoplasmosis, hepatitis, Epstein-Barr virus, cytomegalovirus and herpes simplex virus

the viral load (b-DNA, PCR, NASBA methods), as shown in Table 2.18. Additional tests which are frequently ordered include CBC, routine chemistries, serum protein electrophoresis, and serological evaluation for toxoplasmosis, syphilis, hepatitis, Epstein-Barr virus, CMV and HSV.

If the patient is HIV-positive, he or she should be evaluated two to four times yearly, concentrating on viral load and CD4 count. As the counts change, more frequent and individualized testing may be required. If the CD4 count is <50, repeated testing brings little additional information.

Therapy

During the first 10 years of an HIV infection, around 50% of the patients will have an AIDS-associated opportunistic infection or tumor. About 20% remain symptom-free over the decade The other 30% will have possibly AIDS-associated illnesses but not a definite diagnosis. Previously, the main tasks of the physician during early-stage HIV/AIDS were to monitor the course and be alert to the first signs of immunodeficiency. Today, HAART is the established approach in western countries. Most of our patients receive initial, aggressive antiretroviral therapy. The price of these medications is such that this therapy is not available for many HIV/AIDS victims in the Third World. In addition to antiretroviral therapy, one must consider primary and secondary prophylaxis of infections. The former refers to treating a patient for a possible infection, before clinical problems have arrived, while the latter means continuing some form of treatment after successfully treating an infection to prevent relapse.

Antiretroviral Therapy. The basic problem in antiretroviral therapy is the development or selection of resistant viruses. Intrinsic to the process of producing DNA from RNA via reverse transcriptase is a high rate of mistakes, leading to a high rate of mutations and thus resistant strains. The antiretroviral agents fall into three categories: reverse transcriptase inhibitors of two types, nucleoside analogues and nonnucleoside inhibitors, as well as protease inhibitors. An ever increasing number of agents is available in each of these categories. As of January 2000, the drugs listed in Table 2.19 were available in Germany. Table 2.20 gives rough guidelines for which patients should be treated. Our tendency is to treat all patients very early.

There is no one specific regimen which can be recommended. Many possible combinations are effective. We tend to use two reverse transcriptase inhibitors (RTIs) and a protease inhibitor. A typical regimen might be zidovudine, lamivudine (perhaps as Combivir) and indinavir. Many new agents are on the way. One must consider what is available, its side effects in relation to other problems of the patient, cross-reactions with other medications and, lastly, the cost.

Resistance can develop even with triple or quadruple drug therapy. This is especially likely if the viral load is >10,000/ml. Cross-resistance between drugs in the same group is not unusual. Resistance can be measured with two techniques. Usually the viral strain from a patient is analyzed for specific mutations which impart resistance; this is known as genotypic testing. The far more time-consuming and expensive phenotypic testing is similar to bacterial sensitivity testing, in that the patient's virus is exposed to the medications in question. If the viral load fails to respond to the initial combination, usually one switches to two new products simultaneously.

Treatment of Infants and Children. Aggressive therapy is also being used for infants and children. One must distinguish between the treatment of children exposed in utero to HIV, who are treated for 6 weeks with RTIs and then followed carefully, and those children who are known to be HIV-positive. Formerly, one had to wait for up to 18 months for serological testing to be positive, but with PCR and other sensitive measures of viral load an infec-

Table 2.19. Antiretroviral drugs

Drug	Daily dosage[a]	Major side effects
Nucleoside reverse transcriptase inhibitors (RTIs)		
Zidovudine AZT	250 mg b.i.d.	Nausea, vomiting, headache, anemia, fatigue
Didanosine ddI[b]	200 mg b.i.d.	Diarrhea, neuropathy, pancreatitis
Zalcitabine ddC	0.75 mg t.i.d.	Neuropathy, oral ulcerations
Stavudine d4T[b]	40 mg b.i.d.	Neuropathy, sleep disturbances, ↑ transaminase, myalgias
Lamuvidine 3TC	150 mg b.i.d.	Excessive gas, diarrhea, neuropathy, paronychiae
Abacavir ABC	300 mg b.i.d.	Hypersensitivity reaction (do not use again)
Combivir AZT 300 m, 3 TC 150 mg	One tablet b.i.d.	See above
Nonnucleoside RTI (NNRTI)		
Nevirapine NVP	For 14 days, 200 daily, then b.i.d.	Exanthem which requires discontinuation, fever, ↑ transaminase
Delaviridine DLV	400 mg t.i.d.	Exanthem, nausea, diarrhea
Efavirenz EFV	600 mg h.s.	Exanthem, nightmares, dizziness
Protease inhibitors		All cause lipid, glucose abnormalities (see text)
Saquinavir SQV	600 mg t.i.d.	Diarrhea, satiety
Indinavir IDV	800 mg t.i.d.	↑ Bilirubin, dry skin, pruritus, self-limited papular exanthem, paronychia, renal stones
Ritonavir RTV	600 mg b.i.d.	Nausea, diarrhea, circumoral numbness, ↑ triglycerides, ↑ transaminase
Nelfinavir NFV	750 mg t.i.d.	Diarrhea, exanthem
Amprenavir APV	1200 mg b.i.d.	Exanthem, headache, diarrhea

[a] Dosages are only rough guidelines
[b] ddI and d4T must be adjusted for patients weighing less than 50 and 60 kg, respectively

Table 2.20. Indications for anti-HIV therapy

Status	Recommendation
Symptomatic HIV infection	Treat all patients
Asymptomatic HIV infection, CD4 $<500/mm^3$	Treat all patients (some may wait if CD4 count is stable at 350–500 and viral load is <5000/ml
Asymptomatic HIV infection, CD4 $>500/mm^3$	Treat if viral load is $>30,000$/ml or CD4 is dropping rapidly; probably treat if viral load is $>5,000-10,000$/ml

tion can usually be excluded (or diagnosed) by 3 months.

If a child is HIV-positive, he is evaluated much like an adult and usually treated with at least three drugs. Many of the agents in Table 2.17 are available for children and almost all are employed, at least occasionally. Intravenous immunoglobulin infusions are widely used, in contrast to their limited role in adults. We personally do not treat children with HIV/AIDS, so the reader is encouraged to refer to specialized texts or knowledgeable colleagues for further information on this difficult topic.

Prophylaxis

Primary Prophylaxis. The recommended therapy will depend on the clinical picture and the CD4 count. Prophylaxis is less often needed when HAART is employed.

- CD4 <200
  - *Pneumocystis carinii*: Trimethoprim (80 mg)-sulfamethoxazole (400 mg) daily or pentamidine aerosol therapy (300 mg) once monthly-
- CD4 <100
  - *Toxoplasma gondii*: If the toxoplasmosis titer is positive, usually trimethoprim-sulfamethoxazole is employed. Most patients are already

on the agent for *Pneumocystis carinii* prophylaxis. As an alternative, dapsone and pyrimethamine plus folic acid can be considered.
 - *Mycobacterium avium-intracellulare complex*: Rifabutin (300 mg daily) is suggested but less well-proven.

Secondary Prophylaxis. The awkward term "secondary prophylaxis" refers to further treatment following a given infection to reduce risk of relapse or recurrence.

- *Pneumocystis carinii*: Same as primary prophylaxis.
- *Toxoplasma gondii*: Following encephalitis, pyrimethamine (50 mg daily) plus folic acid.
- Cytomegalovirus: Ganciclovir 6 mg/kg, or foscarnet 90–120 mg/kg, 5–7 days a week.
- *Candida albicans*: With CD4 <100 and oral or esophageal involvement, 300 mg fluconazole weekly. There is some increase in resistance to imidazoles.
- Herpes simplex virus: With persistent problems, acyclovir (200–400 mg t.i.d. permanently), although this is not uniformly accepted.

Prophylaxis for Vertical Transmission. Most studies have involved zidovudine to treat pregnant HIV-positive mothers. Using zidovudine in the third trimester, intravenously during delivery and for 6 weeks afterwards in the infant has reduced transmission from 25% to 8%. Zidovudine in combination with lamivudine seems even better; currently, in Munich, the transmission rate is about 3.5% but larger studies are needed. Protease inhibitors are not used in pregnancy. The delivery should be via Cesarean section.

Drug Eruptions

While drug eruptions are a major problem in HIV/AIDS, often the medications are so important that the patient must simply tolerate the reaction. In many cases, some degree of hardening occurs. A number of factors probably interact to explain why almost every patient experiences several cutaneous drug eruptions. Fist, patients take a large number of medications, often in high doses and in many instances life long. In addition, the likelihood of self-medication is very high. The chances for cross-reactions are great. Second, the metabolism of many medications is altered in HIV/AIDS. Finally, the immune defects probably also contribute to the problem. The range of drug eruptions is similar to that in the general population, extending from a single patch of fixed drug eruption to toxic epidermal necrolysis.

Sulfonamides. The most common drug reaction in HIV/AIDS is to trimethoprim-sulfamethoxazole. The key molecule is the sulfonamide portion of the combination. Over 50% of patients experience a reaction, and almost every patient receives the medication ether as a treatment or prophylaxis for *P. carinii* infection. When sulfadiazine is used in treating toxoplasmosis, the rate of cutaneous reactions is about 30%. Typically a maculopapular bright red exanthem develops 10–14 days after starting therapy. On occasion, it may begin after 2–3 days, perhaps in individuals with prior exposure to sulfonamides. While the trunk is usually the first site, the lesions extend to the extremities. Mucosal involvement is not uncommon, as oral erosions develop. While pruritus is minimal, the lesions may burn. In addition, there may be fever and malaise.

The diagnosis is often difficult, as one must exclude infectious exanthems and the patient is usually on many medications. Because of the altered immune status, immunologic investigations to document the drug allergy are even more difficult. Thus, one must make a clinical diagnosis in most cases. If the reaction is mild, systemic corticosteroids (prednisone 40–100 mg daily) and antihistamines can be employed, as well as topical antipruritic measures. In the presence of confluent cutaneous lesions, extensive oral ulcerations or increasing systemic problems, the medication must be stopped. Alternative medications such as pentamidine for *P. carinii* and atovaquone for *T. gondii* should be considered.

Other Antibiotics. Just as in the general population, antibiotics are a major cause of drug eruptions. Ampicillin and amoxicillin cause rashes in about 15% of patients, while the combination antituberculosis regimens have cutaneous side effects in over 25% of cases. Photosensitivity has been reported in association with ciprofloxacin.

Foscarnet. About 20% of those treated with foscarnet develop painful mucosal ulcerations. The glans penis is most commonly involved, but oral and even esophageal erosions have been reported. Foscarnet is used to treat resistant HSV infections; often it is hard to distinguish between a viral. and drug-induced ulceration. In addition, esophageal symptoms are usually blamed on candidiasis in this population. If the medication cannot be stopped, then fluids should be forced, the penis rinsed after each urination and either protective zinc oxide pastes or corticosteroid ointments used.

Antiretroviral Agents. The main problems associated with the various retroviral agents are summarized in Table 2.17. Several unusual problems occur. When the protease inhibitors are employed for 1 year, about 5% of patients develop abnormalities in lipid and carbohydrate metabolism. They may have elevated triglycerides, insulin-resistant diabetes mellitus and lipodystrophy, manifested as either a buffalo hump or centripetal lipodystrophy with sunken cheeks and skinny limbs but increased abdominal girth (Fig. 2.47). Indinavir causes a papular exanthem early during its use; one should continue the treatment as the papules will resolve. In contrast, nevirapine causes an early diffuse exanthem which frequently goes on to widespread skin loss, so the medication should be stopped. Indinavir also causes paronychia and pyogenic granuloma, most often involving the great toes.

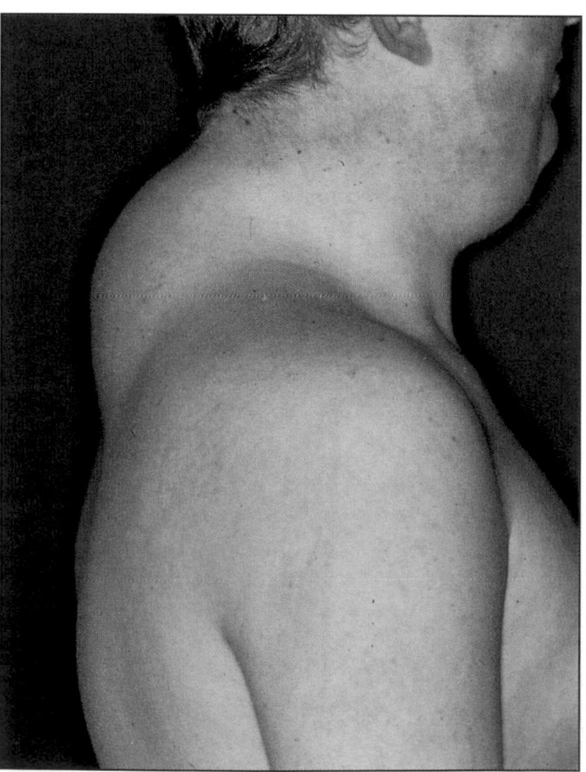

Fig. 2.47. Buffalo hump lipodystrophy in HIV/AIDS patient treated with protease inhibitor

Public Health Measures

AIDS is a reportable illness in some countries with organized public health systems. In most countries, however, an HIV infection is not likely to be reported because of the fear of discrimination at work, in obtaining insurance and in many other aspects of life. In Germany, AIDS reporting is totally confidential, without disclosure of the patient's name. This attitude has, of course, made traditional public health control, such as tracking contacts and counseling, difficult. Much of the public health counseling has been done on a community level, by peers or volunteers, or accomplished through the media. Countries such as England and Switzerland, or communities such as San Francisco, which have directed efforts towards safe sex and the availability of sterile needles, have achieved promising results.

Protection of Health Care Workers

After a period of near-hysteria when AIDS and then HIV were identified, there is now general acceptance of universal precautions. This simply means that, rather than worrying about which patient could have HIV/AIDS, one must regard all patients, their blood and their other body fluids as potentially infectious. This has led to a dramatic increase in the number of rubber gloves used and an almost parallel increase in latex sensitivity. During surgery two pairs of gloves are recommended. Following major abdominal surgery, 10–33% of all gloves show at least a pinprick leak; in orthopedic surgery, the rate is much higher. When a blood-coated needle penetrates a glove, 90% of the blood is wiped off by the glove. In addition to gloves, masks, eye protection and protective disposable robes are often appropriate. No attempt should be made to recap needles; in the USA there are fines for doing this, although they are rarely collected. Many new guidelines for disposal of contaminated material exist. Endoscopes and similar instruments have more rigorous sterilization rules or disposable instruments are employed. One possible exception to universal precautions is to pay particular attention to HIV status when considering laser destruction or dermabrasion, as there is little need to expose oneself to a contaminated spray or plume when alternate treatments are available.

Health care workers are at risk of acquiring HIV following accidental exposure to virus-contaminated blood and other body fluids. The major risk factor is exposure to significant amounts of blood from a patient with advanced disease (and presumably high viral levels). Thus a drop of saliva on intact skin poses almost no risk, but jabbing oneself with a contaminated blood-drawing syringe is dangerous. Recent studies have shown higher rates of seroconversion in individuals not receiving post-exposure antiretroviral therapy. All such studies only consider zidovudine, but today combination therapy is used. The risk of conversion in general is estimated at 1:200 to 1:400.

The following protocol is the one followed in our institution. Others may have slightly different approaches, but what is crucial is to have a plan in place, so that, if an accidental exposure occurs, the victim can be treated logically and efficiently. The following steps can be followed:

- Encourage bleeding from wound; consider excision or tourniquet even though neither has been proven to be effective.
- Disinfect with alcohol solution, at least 70%, for at least 3 min; with small puncture wounds, it may help to enlarge the entry site. Conjunctival exposure should be followed by intensive rinsing with water or physiological saline; oral exposure can be treated with up to 45% alcoholic mouth rinses.
- Serological evaluation of patient and health care victim to establish HIV status of both. If negative, no follow-up is needed unless the patient is suspected of having HIV despite negative testing. If the patient does have HIV, most health care workers are rechecked at 12 weeks, 6 months and even 1 year.
- Chemoprophylaxis with antiretroviral agents. Almost all studies only involve zidovudine, usually given as 250 mg five times daily for 2–6 weeks. Many recommend that the victim take the first capsule no matter what; they then have a period of 4–6 h in which to consider their further course. At these levels, gastrointestinal problems, headache and anemia are the main risks.

Today, almost every health care worker who is exposed is started on at least three drugs, two RTIs and a protease inhibitor. Protease inhibitors are not used in pregnancy. Many physicians prescribe a different set of drugs than those the HIV-positive individual is taking. In addition, the victim should practice protected sex until the entire issue is clarified.

Bibliography

Review

Memar O, Tyring SK (1995) Cutaneous viral infections. J Am Acad Dermatol 33:279–287

Warts

Archard HO, Heck JW, Stanley HR (1965) Focal epithelial hyperplasia: an unusual oral mucosal lesion found in Indian children. Oral Surg Oral Med oral Pathol 20:201

Baker GE, Tyring SK (1997) Therapeutic approaches to papillomavirus infections. Dermatol Clin 15:331–340

Benton EC (1997) Therapy of cutaneous warts. Clin Dermatol 15:449–455

Buschke A, Löwenstein L (1925) Über carcinomähnliche Condylomata acuminata des Penis. Klin Wochenschr 4:1726–1728

de Villiers EM (1994) Human pathogenic papillomavirus types: an update. In: zur Hausen H, ed. Human Pathogenic Papillomaviruses. Springer-Verlag Berlin Heidelberg

de Villiers EM (1997) Papillomavirus and HPV typing. Clin Dermatol 15(2):199–206

Drake LA, Ceilley RI, Cornelison RL et al. (1995) Guidelines of care for warts: human papillomavirus. Committee on Guidelines of Care. J Am Acad Dermatol 32:98–103

Edwards L, Ferenczy A, Eron L et al. (1998) Self-administered topical 5% imiquimod cream for external anogenital warts. HPV Study Group. Human Papilloma Virus. Arch Dermatol 134:25–30

Gross G, Rogozinski T, Schofer H et al. (1998) Recombinant interferon beta gel as an adjuvant in the treatment of recurrent genital warts: results of a placebo-controlled double-blind study in 120 patients. Dermatology 196: 330–334

Jablonska S, Majewski S, Obalek S et al. (1997) Cutaneous warts. Clin Dermatol 15:309–319

Lee AN, Mallory SB (1999) Contact immunotherapy with squaric acid dibutylester for the treatment of recalcitrant warts. J Am Acad Dermatol 41:595–599

Lewandowsky F, Lutz W (1922) Ein Fall einer bisher noch nicht beschriebenen Hauterkrankung (Epidermodysplasia verruciformis) Arch Dermatol Syph 41:193–202

Majewski S, Jablonska S (1995) Epidermodysplasia verruciformis as a model of human papillomavirus-induced genetic cancer of the skin. Arch Dermatol 131:1312–1318

Majewski S, Jablonska S (1997) Human papillomavirus-associated tumors of the skin and mucosa. J Am Acad Dermatol 36:659–685

Routh HB, Bhowmik KR, Parish LC (1997) Myths, fables and even truths about warts and human papillomavirus. Clin Dermatol 15:305–307

Wikstrom A (1995) Clinical and serological manifestations of genital human papillomavirus infection. Acta Derm Venereol Stockh [Suppl] 193:1–85

Herpes Viruses

Alrabiah FA, Sacks SL (1996) New antiherpesvirus agents. Their targets and therapeutic potential. Drugs 52: 17–32

Brugha R, Keersmaekers K, Renton A et al. (1997) Genital herpes infection: a review. Int J Epidemiol 26:698–709

Fricker J (1996) Herpes vaccines: spinning a new DISC. Lancet 348:1576
Goh CL, Khoo L (1998) A retrospective study on the clinical outcome of herpes zoster in patients treated with acyclovir or valaciclovir vs. patients not treated with antiviral. Int J Dermatol 37:544–546
Goodyear HM, McLeish P, Randall S et al. (1996) Immunological studies of herpes simplex virus infection in children with atopic eczema. Br J Dermatol 134:85–93
Pereira FA (1996) Herpes simplex: evolving concepts. J Am Acad Dermatol 35:503–520
Slomka MJ, Emery L, Munday PE et al. (1998) comparison of PCR with virus isolation and direct antigen detection for diagnosis and typing of genital herpes. J Med Virol 55:177–183
Tang WY, Lo JY, Yuen MK et al. (1997) Herpes simplex virus type 2 infection in a 5-year-old boy presenting with recurrent chest wall vesicles and a possible history of herpes encephalitis. Br J Dermatol 137:440–444
Wolf R, Wolf D, Ruocco V (1997) Antiviral therapy for recurrent herpes simplex reconsidered. Dermatology 194: 205–207

Varicella Zoster Virus

Arvin AM (1996) Varicella-zoster virus: overview and clinical manifestations. Semin Dermatol 15:4–7
Kakourou T, Theodoridou M, Mostrou G et al. (1998) Herpes zoster in children. J Am Acad Dermatol 39:207–210
Kost RG, Straus SE (1996) Postherpetic neuralgia – pathogenesis, treatment, and prevention. N Engl J Med 335: 32–42
Weller TH (1996) Varicella: historical perspective and clinical overview. J Infect Dis 174 [Suppl 3]:S306–S309
White CJ (1997) Varicella-zoster virus vaccine. Clin Infect Dis 24:753–761

Epstein-Barr Virus

Cruchley AT, Williams DM, Niedobitek G et al. (1997) Epstein-Barr virus: biology and disease. Oral Dis 3: S156–S163
Itin PH, Lautenschlager S (1997) Viral lesions of the mouth in HIV-infected patients. Dermatology 194:1–7
Sangueza OP (1997) Epstein-Barr virus. A serial killer or an innocent bystander? Arch Dermatol 133:1156–1157
Voog E (1996) Genital viral infections. Studies on human papillomavirus and Epstein-Barr virus. Acta Derm Venereol (Stockh) [Suppl] 198:1–55

Cytomegalovirus

Grimes PE, Sevall JS, Vojdani A (1996) Cytomegalovirus DNA identified in skin biopsy specimens of patients with vitiligo. J Am Acad Dermatol 35:21–26

Human Herpes Virus-6 and Exanthema Subitum

Agut H (1993) Puzzles concerning the pathogenicity of human herpesvirus 6. N Engl J Med 329:203–204
Asano Y, Yoshikawa T, Suga S et al. (1994) Clinical features of infants with primary human herpesvirus 6 infection (exanthem subitum, roseola infantum). Pediatrics 93: 104–108
Le Cleach L, Fillet AM, Agut H et al. (1998) Human herpesviruses 6 and 7. New roles yet to be discovered? Arch Dermatol 34:1155–1157
Linnavuori K, Peltola H, Hovi T (1992) Serology versus clinical signs or symptoms and main laboratory findings in the diagnosis of exanthema subitum (roseola infantum). Pediatrics 89:103–106
Zarhorsky J (1910) Roseola infantilis. Pediatrics 22:60–64

Human Herpes Virus-8

Kemeny L, Gyulai R, Kiss M et al. (1997) A Kaposi's sarcoma-associated herpesvirus/human herpesvirus-8: a new virus in human pathology. J Am Acad Dermatol 37:107–113
Kowalzick L, Hoffmann I, Neipel F et al. (1998) Detection of HHV-8 DNA in a German patient. Eur J Dermatol 8: 432–434
Porter SR, Di Alberti L, Kumar N (1998) Human herpes virus 8 (Kaposi's sarcoma herpesvirus). Oral Oncol 34:5–14

Variola, Monkeypox, Cowpox

Baxby D, Bennett M, Getty B (1994) Human cowpox 1969–1993: a review based on 54 cases. Br J Dermatol 131:598–607
Duffill MB (1993) Milkers' chilblains. N Z Med J 106:101–103
Stolz W, Gotz A, Thomas P, Ruzicka T, Suss R, Landthaler M, Mahnel H, Czerny CP (1996) Characteristic but unfamiliar – the cowpox infection, transmitted by a domestic cat. Dermatology 193:140–143

Milker's Nodule

Groves RW, Wilson-Jones E, MacDonald DM (1991) Human orf and milker's nodule: a clinicopathologic study. J Am Acad Dermatol 25:706–711
Hansen SK, Mertz H, Krogdahl A, Veien NK (1996) Milker's nodule – a report of 15 cases in the county of North Jutland. Acta Derm Venereol (Stockh) 76:88

Ecthyma Contagiosum (Orf)

Macfarlane AW (1997) Human orf complicated by bullous pemphigoid. Br J Dermatol 137:656–657
Murphy JK, Ralfs IG (1996) Bullous pemphigoid complicating human orf. Br J Dermatol 134:929–930
Roingeard P, Machet L (1997) Images in clinical medicine. orf skin ulcer. N Engl J Med 337:1131
Yirrell DL, Vestey JP, Norval M (1994) Immune responses of patients to orf virus infection. Br J Dermatol 130:438–443

Molluscum Contagiosum

Bugert JJ, Darai G (1997) Recent advances in molluscum contagiosum virus research. Arch Virol [Suppl] 13:35–47
Gottlieb SL, Myskowski PL (1994) Molluscum contagiosum. Int J Dermatol 33:453–461
Janniger CK, Schwartz RA (1993) Molluscum contagiosum in children. Cutis 52:194–196
Lewis EJ, Lam M, Crutchfield CE III (1997) An update on molluscum contagiosum. Cutis 60:29–34
Myskowski PL (1997) Molluscum contagiosum. New insights, new directions. Arch Dermatol 133:1039–1041
Nehal KS, Sarnoff DS, Gotkin RH et al. (1998) Pulsed dye laser treatment of molluscum contagiosum in a patient with acquired immunodeficiency syndrome. Dermatol Surg 24:533–535
Ogg GS, Coleman R, Rosbotham JL et al. (1997) Atypical molluscum contagiosum – a diagnostic problem. Acta Derm Venereol (Stockh) 77:77–78

Coxsackie and Herpangina
Bauer K (1997) Foot- and mouth-disease as zoonosis. Arch Virol [Suppl] 13:95–97
Modlin JF, Rotbart HA (1997) Group B coxsackie disease in children. Curr Top Microbiol Immunol 223:53–80
Resnick SD (1997) New aspects of exanthematous diseases of childhood. Dermatol Clin 15:257–266
Robinson CR, Doane FW, Rhodes AJ (1958) Report of an outbreak of febrile illness with pharyngeal lesions and exanthem: Toronto, summer 1957 – isolation of group A Coxsackie virus. Can Med Assoc J 79:615–621
Shelley WB, Hashim M, Shelley ED (1996) Acyclovir in the treatment of hand-foot-and-mouth disease. Cutis 57:232–234
Smith PT, Landry ML, Carey H et al. (1998) Papular-purpuric gloves and socks syndrome associated with acute parvovirus B19 infection: case report and review. Clin Infect Dis 27:164–168
Stolz W, Gotz A, Thomas P et al. (1996) Characteristic but unfamiliar – the cowpox infection, transmitted by a domestic cat. Dermatology 193:140–143
Zahorsky J (1924) Herpangina (a specific infectious disease). Arch Pediat 41:181–184

Measles
Atkinson WL (1995) Epidemiology and prevention of measles. Dermatol Clin 13:553–559
Bellini WJ, Rota JS, Rota PA (1994) Virology of measles virus. J Infect Dis 170:S15–S23
Dukes C (1881) The incubation period of scarlatina, varicella, parotis, and roetheln. Lancet 10:743–745
Garenne M, Glasser J, Levins R (1994) Disease, population and virulence. Thoughts about measles mortality. Ann N Y Acad Sci 740:297–302
Gellin BG (1994) Measles: state of the art and future directions. J Infect Dis 170 [Suppl 1]:S3–S14
Griffin DE, Ward BJ, Esolen LM (1994) Pathogenesis of measles virus infection: an hypothesis for altered immune responses. J Infect Dis 170 [Suppl 1]:S24–S31
James JM, Burks AW, Roberson PK et al. (1995) Safe administration of the measles vaccine to children allergic to eggs. N Engl J Med 332:1262–1266
Katz M (1995) Clinical spectrum of measles. In: ter Meulen V, Billeter MA (eds) Measles virus. Springer, Berlin, pp 1–12 (Current topics in microbiology and immunology, vol 191)
Liebert UG (1997) Measles virus infections of the central nervous system. Intervirology 40:176–184

Rubella
Arai M, Wada N, Maruyama K et al. (1995) Acute hepatitis in an adult with acquired rubella infection. J Gastroenterol 30:539–542
Cutts FT, Robertson SE, Diaz-Ortega JL et al. (1997) Control of rubella and congenital rubella syndrome (CRS) in developing countries, part 1: burden of disease from CRS. Bull World Health Organ 75:55–68
Frey TK(1997) Neurological aspects of rubella virus infection. Intervirolog 40:167–175
Murph JR (1994) Rubella and syphilis: continuing causes of congenital infection in the 1990s. Semin Pediatr Neurol 1:26–35
Robertson SE, Cutts FT, Samuel R et al. (1997) Control of rubella and congenital rubella syndrome (CRS) in developing countries, part 2: vaccination against rubella. Bull World Health Organ 75:69–80
Skendzel LP (1996) Rubella immunity. Defining the level of protective antibody. Am J Clin Pathol 106:170–174

Erythema Infectiosum, Rubeola Scarlatinosa, Papular-Purpuric Gloves and Socks Syndrome, and Other Viral Infections
Bodemer C, de Prost Y (1992) Unilateral laterothoracic exanthem in children: a new disease? J Am Acad Dermatol 27:693–696
Brunner MJ, Rubin L, Dunlap F (1962) A new papular erythema of childhood. Arch Dermatol 85:539–540
Carrascosa JM, Just M, Ribera M et al. (1998) Papular acrodermatitis of childhood related to poxvirus and parvovirus B19 infection. Cutis 61:265–267
Harms M, Feldmann R, Saurat JH (1990) Papular-purpuric "gloves and socks" syndrome. J Am Acad Dermatol 23:850–854
Manns A, Hisada M, La Grenade L (1999) Human T-lymphotropic virus type I infection. Lancet 353:1951–1958
McCuaig CC, Russo P, Powell J et al. (1996) Unilateral laterothoracic exanthem. J Am Acad Dermatol 34:979–984
Sticker G (1899) Die neue Kinderseuche in der Umgebung von Giessen (Erythema infectiosum). Zschr Prakt Ärzte 8:353–358
Sweet RD (1966) A pattern of eczema in Jamaica. Br J Dermatol 78:93–100
Vargas-Diez E, Buezo GF, Aragues M et al. (1996) Papular-purpuric gloves-and-socks syndrome. Int J Dermatol 35:626–632

Hepatitis
McElgunn PSJ (1983) Dermatologic manifestations of hepatitis B virus infection. J Am Acad Dermatol 8: 539–548
Ryder SD (1999) Viral hepatitis. In: Armstrong D, Cohen J (eds) Infectious diseases. Mosby, London, pp 1–12

AIDS
Allen JE (1993) Drug-induced photosensitivity. Clin Pharmacol 12:580–587
Balfour HH, Benson C, Braun J et al. (1994) Management of acyclovir-resistant herpes simplex and varicella zoster virus infections. J Acquir Immune Defic Syndr 7:254–260
Ballem PJ, Belzberg A, Devine PV et al. (1992) Kinetic studies of the mechanism of thrombocytopenia in patients with human immunodeficiency virus infection. N Engl J Med 327:1779–1784
Berger EA, Doms RW, Fenyö E-M et al. (1998) A new classification for HIV-1. Nature 391:240
Berger TG, Dhar A (1994) Lichenoid photoeruptions in human immunodeficiency virus infection. Arch Dermatol 140:609–613
Berry CD, Hooton TM, Collier AC (1987) Neurologic relapse after benzathine penicillin therapy for secondary syphilis in a patient with HIV infection. N Engl J Med 316: 1387–1389
BHIVA Guidelines Co-ordinating Commitee (1997) British HIV Association guidelines for antiretroviral treatment of HIV seropositive individuals. Consensus statement. Lancet 349:1086–1092

Bogner JR, Kronawitter U, Rolinski B et al. (1994) Liposomal doxoribicin in the treatment of advanced AIDS-related Kaposi sarcoma. J Acquir Immune Defic Syndr 7:453–569

Boisseau AM, Conzigou P, Forestier JF et al. (1991) Porphyria cutanea tarda associated with human immunodeficiency virus infection. Dermatologica 182:155–159

Bournèrias I, Biosnic S, Patey O et al. (1989) Unusual cutaneous cytomegalovirus involvment in patients with acquired immunodeficiency syndrome. Arch Dermatol 125:1243–1246

Bouscarat F, Bouchard C, Bouhour D (1998) Paronychia and pyogenic granuloma of the great toes in patients treated with indinavir. N Engl J Med 338:1776–1777

Brambilla L, Boneschi V, Beretta G et al. (1984) Intralesional chemotherapy for Kaposi's sarcoma. Dermatologica 169: 150–155

Broder S, Merigan TC Jr, Bolognesi D (1994) Textbook of AIDS medicine. Williams and Wilkins, Baltimore

Buchness MR, Lim HW, Hatcher VA et al. (1988) Eosinophilic pustular folliculitis in the acquired immunodeficiency syndrome. N Engl J Med 318:1183–1186

Carr A, Cooper DA (1995) Pathogenesis and management of HIV-associated drug hypersensitivity. AIDS Clin Rev 96:65–97

Carr A, Samaras K, Thorisdottir A et al. (1999) Diagnosis, prediction, and natural course of HIV-1 protease-inhibitor-associated lipodystrophy, hyperlipidaemia, and diabetes mellitus: a cohort study. Lancet 353:2093–2099

Casanova JM, Puig T, Rubio M (1987) Hypertrichosis of the eyelashes in acquired immuno-deficiency syndrome. Arch Dermatol 123:1599–1601

Caumes E, Guermonprez G, Lecomte C et al. (1997) Efficacy and safety of desensitization with sulfamethoxazole and trimethoprim in 48 previously hypersensitive patients infected with human immunodeficiency virus. Arch Dermatol 133:465–469

Cavert W, Notermans DW, Staskus K et al. (1997) Kinetics of response in lymphoid tissues to antiretroviral therapy of HIV-1 infection. Science 276:960–964

Center for Disease Control and Prevention MMWR (1993) Revised classification system for HIV infection and expanded surveillance case definition for AIDS among adolescents and adults. Arch Dermatol 129:287–290

Chun TW, Carruth L, Finzl D et al. (1997) Quantification of latent tissue reservoirs and total body viral load in HIV-1 infection. Nature 387:183–187

Cohen PR, Grossman ME, Silvers DN et al. (1990) Generalized granuloma anulare located in sunexposed areas in a human immunodeficiency virus-seropositive man with ultraviolet B photosensitivity. Arch Dermatol 126: 830–831

Conant MA (1987) Hairy leukoplakia. A new disease of the oral mucosa. Arch Dermatol 123:585–587

Coodley GO, Loveless MO, Merrill TM (1994) The HIV wasting syndrome: a review. J Acquir Immune Defic Syndr 7:681–694

Coopman SA, Johnson RA, Platt R et al. (1993) Cutaneous disease and drug reactions in HIV infection. N Engl J Med 328:1670–1674

Corbett EL, Crossley I, Holton J et al. (1996) Crusted ("Norwegian") scabies in a specialist HIV unit: successful use of ivermectin and failure to prevent nosocomial transmission. Genitourin Med 72:115–117

Coulman CU, Greene I, Archibald RWR (1987) Cutaneous pneumocystosis. Ann Intern Med 106:396–398

Deutsche AIDS-Gesellschaft (DAIG), Österreichische AIDS-Gesellschaft (ÖAG), Robert-Koch-Institut (RKI) et al. (1997) German-Austrian guidelines for antiretroviral therapy of HIV infection. Eur J Med Res 2:535–542

DeVita VT Jr, Hellmann S, Rosenberg SA et al. (1997) AIDS. Etiology, diagnosis, treatment and prevention, 4th edn. Lippincott-Raven, Philadelphia

Duvic M, Johnson TM, Rapini RP et al. (1987) Acquired immunodeficiency syndrome – associated psoriasis and Reiter's syndrome. Arch Dermatol 123:1622–1632

Fahey JL, Tailor JMG, Detels R et al. (1987/1990) The prognostic value of cellular and serologic markers in infection with human immunodeficiency virus type I. N Engl J Med 322:166–172

Frentz G, Niordson AM, Thomsen K (1989) Eosinophilic pustular dermatosis: an early skin marker of infection with human immunodeficiency virus? Br J Dermatol 121:271–274

Friedman-Kien AE, Saltzman BR (1990) Cilinical manifestations of classical, endemic African, and epidemic AIDS-associated Kaposi's sarcoma. J Am Acad Dermatol 22: 1237–1250

Friedman-Kien AE, Laubsenstein L, Marmor M et al. (1981) Kaposi's sarcoma and Pneumocystis pneumonia among homosexual men – New York and California MMWR 30:250–252

Gallant JE, Moore RD, Chaisson RE (1994) Prophylaxis for opportunistic infections in patients with HIV infection. Ann Intern Med 120:932–944

Gallo RC, Salahuddin SZ, Popovic M et al. (1984) Frequent detection and isolation of cytopathic retroviruses (HTLV-III) from patients with AIDS and at risk for AIDS. Science 224:500–503

Gaudreau A, Hill E, Balfour HH Jr et al. (1998) Phenotypic and genotypic characterization of acyclovir-resistant herpes simplex viruses from immunocompromised patients. J Infect Dis 178:297–303

Gazzard B, Moyle G (1997) Anti-infectives – to sequence or not to sequence? Exp Opin Invest Drugs 6:99–102

Glover R, Young L, Goltz RW (1987) Norwegian scabies in acquired immunodeficiency syndrome: report of a case resulting in death from associated sepsis. J Am Acad Dermatol 16:396–399

Goldstein B, Berman B, Sukenik E et al. (1997) Correlation of skin disorders with CD4 lymphocyte counts in patients with HIV/AIDS. J Am Acad Dermatol 36: 262–264

Greenberg RG, Berger TG (1990) Nail and mucocutaneous hyperpigmentation with azidothyidine therapy. J Am Acad Dermatol 22:327–330

Greenspan D, Greenspan JS, Hearst NG et al. (1987) Relation of oral hairy leukoplakia to infection with the human immunodeficiency virus and the risk of developing AIDS. J Infect Dis 155:475–481

Gregory N, Sanchez M, Buchness MR (1990) The spectrum of syphilis in patients with human immunodeficiency virus infection. J Am Acad Dermatol 22:1061–1067

Gürtler LG, Hauser PH, Eberle J et al. (1994) A new subtype of human immunodeficiency virus type 1 (MVP-5180) from Cameroon. J Virol 68:1581–1585

Guidelines for the management of health care worker exposures to HIV and recommendation for postexposure prophylaxis. MMWR (1998) 134:1317–1318; Arch Dermatol 134:1317–1318

Heng MCY, Heng SY, Allen SG (1994) Co-infection and synergy of human immunodeficiency virus-1. Lancet 343:255–258

Hengel RL, Watts NB, Lennox JL (1997) Benign symmetric lipomatosis associated with protease inhibitors. Lancet 350:1596

Hevia O, Jiminez-Acosta F, Ceballos PI et al. (1991) Pruritic papular eruption of the acquired immunodeficiency syndrome: a clinicopathologic study. J Am Acad Dermatol 24:231–235

Hirsch MS, D'Aquila RT (1993) Therapy for human immunodeficiency virus infection. N Engl J Med 328:1686–1695

Hoegl L, Thoma-Greber E, Röcken M et al. (1998) HIV protease inhibitors influence the prevalence of oral candidosis in HIV-infected patients: a 2-year-study. Mycoses 41:321–325

Inwald D, Nelson M, Cramp M et al. (1994) Cutaneous manifestations of mycobacterial infection in patients with AIDS. Br J Dermatol 130:111–114

Jaffe D, May LP, Sanchez M et al. (1991) Staphylococcal sepsis in HIV antibody seropositive psoriasis patients. J Am Acad Dermatol 24:970–972

Jasny B, Cohen G, Merson H et al. (1993) AIDS. The unanswered questions. Science 260:1253–1292

Kaposi M (1872) Idiopathisches multiples Pigmentsarkom der Haut. Arch Dermatol Syph 4:265–272

Katz DH (1993) AIDS: primarily a viral or an autoimmune disease? AIDS Res Hum Retroviruses 9:489–493

Kopelman RG, Zolla-Pazner S (1988) Association of human immunodeficiency virus infection and autoimmune phenomena. Am J Med 84:83–89

Krown SE, Gold JWM, Niedzwiecki D et al. (1994) Interferon-α with zidovudine: safety, tolerance and clinical and virologic effects in patients with Kaposi sarcoma associated with the acquired immunodeficiency syndrome (AIDS). Ann Intern Med 112:812–821

Lane HC, Laughton BE, Falloon J et al. (1994) Recent advances in the management of AIDS-related opportunistic infections. Ann Intern Med 120:945–955

Lo J, Mulligan K, Tai VW et al. (1998) "Buffalo hump" in men with HIV-1 infection. Lancet 351:867–870

Magro CMJ, Crowson AN (1994) Eosinophilic pustular folliculitis reaction: a paradigm of immune dysregulation. Int J Dermatol 33:172–178

Malone JL, Wallace MR, Hendrick BB et al. (1995) Syphilis and neurosyphilis in a human immunodeficiency virus type-1 seropositive population: evidence for frequent serologic relapse after therapy. Am J Med 1:55–63

McNeely MC, Yarchoan R, Broder S et al. (1989) Dermatologic complications associated with administration of 2′,3′-dideoxycytidine in patients with human immunodeficiency virus infection. J Am Acad Dermatol 21:213–217

Meola T, Soter NA, Ostreicher R et al. (1993) The safety of UVB phototherapy in patients with HIV infection. J Am Acad Dermatol 29:216–220

Mirowski GW, Hilton JF, Greenspan D et al. (1998) Association of cutaneous and oral diseases in HIV-infected men. Oral Dis 4:16–21

Mitsuyasu RT, Taylor JM, Glaspy J et al. (1986) Heterogeneity of epidemic Kaposi's sarcoma. Implications for therapy. Cancer 57 (8 Suppl): 1657–1661

Mole L, Ripich S, Margolis D et al. (1997) The impact of active herpes simplex infection on human immunodeficiency virus load. J Infect Dis 176:766–770

Palefsky JM, Holly EA, Ralston ML et al. (1998) Prevalence and risk factors for human papillomavirus infection of the anal canal in human immunodeficiency virus (HIV)-positive and HIV-negative homosexual men. J Infect Dis 177:361–367

Pantaleo G, Graziosi C, Fauci AS (1993) The immunopathogenesis of human immunodeficiency virus infection. N Engl J Med 328:327–332

Pechere M, Wunderli W, Trellu-Toutous L et al. (1998) Treatment of acyclovir-resistant herpetic ulceration with topical foscarnet and antiviral sensitivity analysis. Dermatology 197:278–280

Perelson AS, Essunger P, Cao Y et al. (1997) Decay characteristics of HIV-1-infected compartments during combination therapy. Nature 387:188–191

Perrin L, Schockmel GA (1997) Should clinicians watch for and treat primary HIV infection? HIV 7:17–23

Portu JJ, Santamaria JM, Zubero Z et al. (1996) Atypical scabies in HIV-positive patients. J Am Acad Dermatol 34:915–917

Presant CA, Scoriaro M, Kennedy P et al. (1993) Liposomal daunorubicin treatment of HIV-associated Kaposi's sarcoma. Lancet 341:1242–1243

Ranki A, Puska P, Mattinen S et al. (1991) Effect of PUVA on immunologic and virologic findings in HIV-infected patients. J Am Acad Dermatol 24:404–410

Rizzuto CD, Wyatt R, Hernández-Ramos N et al. (1998) A conserved HIV gp120 glyco-protein structure involved in chemokine receptor binding. Science 280:1949–1953

Rosenthal D, LeBoit PE, Klumpp L et al. (1991) Human immunodeficiency virus-associated eosinophilic folliculitis. A unique dermatotis associated with advanced human immunodeficiency virus infection. Arch Dermatol 127:206–209

Royce RA, Sena A, Cates W Jr et al. (1997) Sexual transmission of HIV. N Engl J Med 336:1072–1078

Ruzicka T, Fröschl M, Hohenleutner U et al. (1987) Treatment of HIV-induced retinoid-resistant psoriasis with zidovudine. Lancet 2:1469–1470

Samaranayake LP (1992) Oral mycoses in HIV infection. Oral Surg Med Oral Pathol 73:171–180

Schacker T, Zehl J, Hu HL et al. (1998) Frequency of symptomatic and asymptomatic herpes simplex virus type 2 reactivations among human immunodeficiency virus-infected men. J Infect Dis 178:1616–1622

Schaller M, Hube B, Ollert MW et al. (1999) In vivo expression and localization of Candida albicans secreted aspartyl proteinases during oral candidiasis in HIV-infected patients. J Invest Dermatol 112:383–386

Schlüpen EM, Schirren CG, Hoegl L et al. (1997) Molecular diagnosis of deep nodular bacillary angiomatosis and monitoring of therapeutic success. Br J Dermatol 136:747–751

Schöfer H, Ochsendorf FR, Helm EB et al. (1987) Treatment of oral "hairy" leukoplakia in AIDS patients with vitamin A acid (topically) or acyclovir (systemically). Dermatologica 174:150–153

Schöpfer H, Imhof M, Thoma-Greber E et al. (1996) Active syphilis in HIV infection: a multicentre retrospective survey. Genitourin Med 72:176–181

Segal BH, Engler HD, Little R et al. (1997) Early foscarnet failure in herpes simplex virus infection in a patients with AIDS. AIDS 11:552–553

Tappero JW, Conant MA, Wolfe SF et al. (1993) Kaposi's sarcoma. Epidemiology, pathogenesis, histology, clinical spectrum, staging criteria and therapy. J Am Acad Dermatol 28:371–395

Taylor JF, Templeton AC, Vogel CL et al. (1971) Kaposi's sarcoma in Uganda: a clinico-pathological study. Int J Cancer 8(1):122–135

Templeton AC (1981) Kaposi's sarcoma. Pathol Annu 16 (Pt 2):315–336

Toome BK, Bowers KE, Scott GA (1991) Diagnosis of cutaneous cytomegalovirus infection: a review of cutaneous cytomegalovirus infection: a review and report of a case. J Am Acad Dermatol 24:857–863

Williams CA, Winkler JR, Grassi M et al. (1990) HIV-associated periodontitis complicated by necrotizing stomatitis. Oral Surg Oral Med Oral Pathol 69:351–355

Wright S, Johnson RA (1997) Human immunodeficiency virus in women: mucocutaneous manifestations. Clin Dermatol 15:93–111

Rickettsial Diseases

Contents

Introduction

The rickettsiae are a group of fastidious bacteria that are intracellular parasites; therefore, they occupy a niche between traditional bacteria and viruses. In recent years, a number of new rickettsiae have been discovered – as many as seven new species have been found ranging from sites as exotic as Flinders Island (Australia) to California.

Most rickettsial diseases have an insect vector and a mammal reservoir. For some diseases reservoir is humans, as in epidemic typhus, although here flying squirrels provide a second reservoir. In some cases, the organism may also reproduce in the vector. And finally, for some rickettsiae, such as *Rickettsia rickettsii*, which causes Rocky Mountain spotted fever, the main mode of transmission is transovarial in ticks, thus the vector and reservoir are the same species.

Following infection, the most typical change is a diffuse exanthem, usually involving primarily the trunk. Rickettsialpox is vesicular, but the other rickettsial diseases are not. Q-fever has no skin findings, while Brill-Zinsser disease and trench fever only rarely show cutaneous changes. Many patients develop a necrotic dark eschar at the site of the initial bite and inoculation. All the members of the spotted fever group, except Rocky Mountain spotted fever, cause an eschar, as does scrub typhus.

Rickettsiae are difficult to culture because of their highly specific growth requirements. Only *Coxiella burnetii* survives for any time outside a living host. In the past serologic tests were used to detect infection – primarily the Weil-Felix reaction, which utilizes cross-reactivity between rickettsiae and *Proteus* species OX2,OX19 and OXK. Today, several, more specific serologic tests as well as molecular biologic techniques and direct immunofluorescent identification of the organismscan be employed.

Considerable cross-reactivity exists between related rickettsial groups, forming to some extent the basis for the classification in Table 3.1. More information on the various serologic methods can be found in specialized texts or obtained from the relevant reference laboratory. Serologic evidence of infection occurs after several weeks, so patients must be diagnosed and treated empirically in most cases. Direct immunofluorescent examination of a skin biopsy can provide a rapid answer in Rocky Mountain spotted fever.

Microscopic examination reveals surprisingly uniform findings. Usually, a vasculitis follows introduction of the organism into the skin. The rickettsiae can be identified in the same vessel walls in which they both proliferate and elicit an inflammatory response as they disseminate. Q-fever is different since the organisms are usually inhaled.

In general the rickettsiae are sensitive to tetracycline and chloramphenicol. In many instances, this is used as a diagnostic approach, but clearly it lacks both specificity and sensitivity.

Related Organisms

The larger family of Rickettsiaceae also includes the genus *Ehrlichia*, the members of which cause a variety of febrile illnesses in dogs. *Ehrlichia chaffeensis* (isolated near Fort Chaffee, Arkansas) causes human ehrlichiosis, which resembles Rocky Mountain spotted fever but lacks a rash. A related organism is *Erhlichia phagocytophilia*, which causes human granulocytic ehrlichiosis, another febrile illness but with characteristic leukocyte inclusions. Also related are *Bartonella quintana*, responsible for

Table 3.1. Rickettsial diseases

Group	Disease	Geographic distribution	Causative agent	Arthropod vector	Reservoir
Spotted fevers	Rocky Mountain spotted fever	USA (especially North Carolina, Oklahoma)	*Rickettsia rickettsii*	Tick	Ticks, wild rodents, dogs
	Boutonneuse	Mediterranean, Africa, India	*Rickettsia conori*	Tick	Ticks, dogs, wild rodents
	North Asian tick typhus	Siberia, Mongolia	*Rickettsia sibirica*	Tick	Ticks, wild rodents
	Queensland tick typhus	Australia	*Rickettsia australia*	Tick	Ticks, wild rodents, marsupials
	Rickettsialpox	USA, Russia, Korea, Africa	*Rickettsia akari*	Mite	Mouse
Typhus group	Murine (endemic) typhus	Worldwide, small foci	*Rickettsia typhi* (*Rickettsia mooseri*)	Rat flea	Rat
	Epidemic typhus	Small areas of South America, Africa, Asia, USA	*Rickettsia prowazekii*	Body louse	Humans, flying squirrels
	Brill-Zinsser disease	Worldwide	*Rickettsia prowazekii*	None	Humans (recurrence of epidemic typhus)
	Scrub typhus	Asia, Australia, South Pacific	*Rickettsia tsutsugamushi*	Mite	Mites, wild rodents
Others	Q-fever	Worldwide	*Coxiella burnetii*	Ticks?	Domestic mammals

trench fever, and *Bartonella henselae,* involved in cat-scratch fever and bacillary angiomatosis. The latter two organisms are discussed in Chap. 4.

The rickettsial diseases are summarized in Table 3.1 Because they only rarely come to the attention of dermatologists, we comment on the dermatologic aspects and other interesting features of each disease.

Rocky Mountain Spotted Fever

Synonyms. North American tick typhus, New World spotted fever, tick-borne typhus, São Paulo fever

Definition. Acute tick-borne illness, primarily found in North America, featuring fever, malaise and an exanthem which typically starts on the palms and soles.

Causative Organism. *Rickettsia rickettsii*

Epidemiology. While Rocky Mountain spotted fever was described initially in the Rocky Mountains, today the name is a misnomer. The two states with the most cases are North Carolina and Oklahoma. There are focal regions in Oklahoma City, such as golf courses, where a very high percentage of ticks are infected. Rocky Mountain spotted fever is also found in Mexico, Central and South America.

Etiology and Pathogenesis. The microbe is maintained in nature primarily in the *Dermacentor* species of hard-shelled ticks. Domestic dogs may be another reservoir. While *Rickettsia rickettsii* is found in a variety of small mammals, their role in the cycle is probably less important. The transmission to the human occurs via the tick bite, without formation of an eschar.

Clinical Findings. The incubation period is about 1 week. The patients usually presents with fever greater than 38.5 °C, myalgias and headache. Gastrointestinal complaints may also be present. The rash is very helpful in diagnosing Rocky Mountain spotted fever. It usually appears within the first 3 days following the fever, and is found in over 80% of patients. The most typical locations are the palms and soles (Fig. 3.1), with initial involvement usually on the extremities, not the trunk as in other rickettsial diseases. Because of the vessel involvement, the lesions are often purpuric or hemorrhagic. Lesions may coalesce, especially on the trunk. Spotless, i.e., no rash, Rocky Mountain spotted fever is more common in older and black patients. Occasionally the vascular damage is so severe that necrosis or even gangrene occurs.

Histopathology. Routine histopathology reveals a perivascular inflammatory infiltrate often associated with small thrombi. Direct immunofluorescent examination of a skin biopsy, ideally from the nape, can reveal the organisms early in the disease course.

Laboratory Findings. The serologic diagnosis is only made weeks after exposure and plays no role in therapy. The neutrophil count is usually normal, but there may be a shift to the left, thrombocytopenia and anemia. The CSF examination may reveal increased leukocytes or protein but is never diagnostic.

Course and Prognosis. Untreated, 15–25% of patients die. A recent series in the USA with relatively prompt treatment still show a 3–5% mortality.

Differential Diagnosis. The differential diagnostic list is very long and includes all the febrile diseases that present with headache and a rash. Meningococcemia, viral meningoencephalitis and infectious mononucleosis are usually high on the list, along with other viral and bacterial infections and hematologic disorders, if the hemorrhagic features predominate.

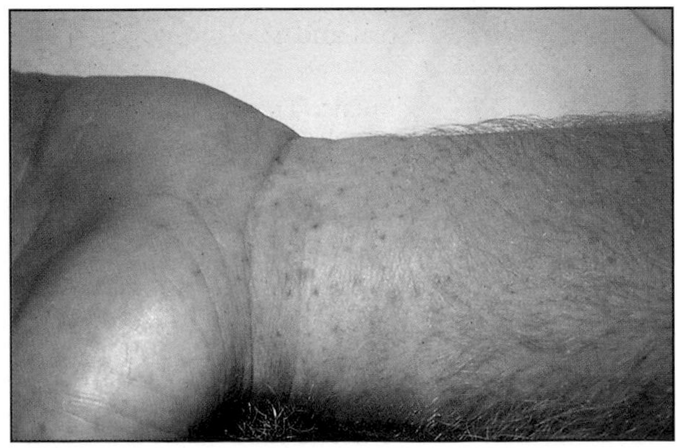

Fig. 3.1. Rocky Mountain spotted fever involving palms. (Courtesy of Robert H. Schosser, M.D., Lexington, Kentucky)

Therapy. Treatment must be started based on clinical features and local epidemiologic information. The two agents of choice are tetracycline and chloramphenicol. The latter is preferred for patients under the age of eight and in pregnancy. Doxycycline 100 mg b.i.d. is effective; oral tetracycline 25–50 mg/kg daily in four divided doses is standard. Treatment should be provided for 5–7 days; generally one treats for a minimum of 2 days after the patient is afebrile. When chloramphenicol is used, the dosage is 50–75 mg/kg daily in four divided dosages. The same treatment regimens are appropriate for all the rickettsial diseases.

Prophylaxis. No vaccine is available.

Public Health Measures. Rocky Mountain spotted fever is a reportable infection.

Boutonneuse Fever

Synonyms. Mediterranean tick fever, Marseilles fever, Kenya tick typhus, Africa tick typhus, India tick typhus

Causative Organism. *Rickettsia conorii*
This infection is much milder than Rocky Mountain spotted fever, with a fatality rate of less than 3% in untreated patients. It is widespread in Africa, Asia and the Mediterranean Basin. Cases are now appearing more often in Northern Europe due to mass tourism and because the disease and its vectors are moving north. Dogs that have been taken along on vacations in endemic areas are likely to be responsible for bringing the infected ticks back home with them.

The classic skin finding is an eschar; the rash is perhaps less acral than in Rocky Mountain spotted fever and appears later in the disease course.

Rickettsialpox

Causative Organism. *Rickettsia akari*
Rickettsialpox was first identified in a New York City housing project in 1946. The organism is transmitted from mice to humans by the mouse mite.

An eschar develops at the bite site and is accompanied by regional lymphadenopathy in the first week. After another week, fever, chills and headache appear, associated with a diffuse vesicular rash that heals with crusting. No oral lesions are seen. The disease course is mild and fatalities few. The main differential diagnostic consideration is chickenpox, but in chickenpox the lesions are larger and oral involvement is common.

Endemic Typhus

Synonym. Murine typhus, flea-borne typhus

Causative Organism. *Rickettsia typhi* (formerly known as *Rickettsia mooseri*)

Murine typhus can occur worldwide wherever humans and rats live in close contact. In the USA, most cases occur in Texas and the other Gulf Coast states. The organism does not make the host rat sick; the rat flea *Xenopsylla cheopis* takes up the pathogen and is also not harmed. Vertical transmission in the rat flea also occurs. When the rat flea bites a human, the rickettsiae are transmitted via flea fecal contamination of the bite wound. After an incubation period of 1–2 weeks, the victim develops fever, headache and myalgias. No eschar is found; about two-thirds of patients have a maculopapular, often fleeting truncal exanthem. The course is mild and the outlook good. When control measures are taken, it is wise to kill the fleas first and then the rats; otherwise the fleas move to the next host, a human, and the epidemic temporarily surges.

Public Health Measures. Endemic typhus is a reportable infection.

Epidemic Typhus

(Brill 1910; Ricketts 1910; Prowazek 1913)

Synonym. Louse-borne typhus

Definition. Acute febrile illness with marked toxicity and late onset of exanthem which typically spares palms and soles.

Causative Organism. *Rickettsia prowazekii.* Prowazek (1875–1915) was an Austrian zoologist who died as a result of inoculating himself with material from patients with epidemic typhus.

Epidemiology. Epidemic typhus fever has caused a number of disastrous epidemics. In Russia, between 1918 and 1922, it is estimated that 30 million people were affected with typhus, resulting in 3 million fatalities. Typhus fever was rampant in concentration and prison camps during World War II, accounting for untold numbers of victims. Crowded housing and poor sanitary conditions facilitate the proliferation of rats, lice and thus typhus, as Hans Zinsser (1935) so elegantly described in his classic book *Rats, Lice and History*. The last epidemic of louse-borne typhus occurred in the USA in 1921. Foci persist in rural highland areas of Central and South America, as well as Africa and Asia. Since the lice die from the infection, there is no vertical vector transmission. In addition to humans, flying squirrels in the Southeastern USA are a second reservoir. Rare cases of indigenous *Rickettsia prowazekii* infection transmitted from a flying squirrel to a human have been described.

Etiology and Pathogenesis. After inoculation, the organism proliferates and causes diffuse vascular inflammation involving the skin, CNS, heart, muscle and kidneys.

Clinical Findings. After an incubation period of about 1 week, the patient suddenly becomes ill with headache, chills and high fever up to 40 °C. There is no eschar. There rash begins on the trunk, most often in the axillary folds. The lesions are typically 2–4 mm, pale red macules that often have a central blue tint. Initially the lesions blanche on pressure, but later they become darker and nonblanching as extravasation occurs. They spread to the extremities, but generally spare the palms, soles and face. Considerable diversity among the lesions in a given area is typical for typhus. A variety of neurologic symptoms, pulmonary infiltrates and thrombotic events complicate the overwhelming malaise and discomfort.

Histopathology. Skin biopsy is not distinctive; perivascular inflammation and intravascular thrombi may be found.

Laboratory Findings. It is often important to separate flea-borne typhus from louse-borne typhus. The serologic cross-reactions are quite intricate, so specialized laboratories, such as the Centers for Disease Control (CDC) in the USA, should be involved.

Course and Prognosis. The prognosis in untreated cases is gloomy; fatality rates of 40 – 60 % have been reported, with the elderly and infirm at greater risk. The response to therapy, however, is prompt and dramatic.

Differential Diagnosis. All the various febrile illnesses associated with a rash must be considered. Thus epidemiologic suspicion is crucial.

Therapy. The same regimens of tetracycline and chloramphenicol recommended for Rocky Mountain spotted fever are appropriate.

Prophylaxis. A vaccine is available and recommended for people entering high-risk situations, such as soldiers, medical personnel, laboratory workers and other individuals who will be living in rat-infested areas in areas where typhus is endemic.

Public Health Measures. Epidemic typhus is a reportable infection.

Brill-Zinsser Disease

Brill-Zinsser disease is the recrudescence of epidemic typhus. In the USA, it has been mainly seen in Eastern European immigrants, many of whom experienced typhus during World War II. The course is milder and the rash, if present at all, not dramatic.

Scrub Typhus

Synonyms. Tsutsugamushi fever, akamushi disease, mite-borne typhus fever, Kedani disease and many more.

Causative Organism. *Rickettsia tsutsugamushi*

Epidemiology. Scrub typhus is found throughout eastern Asia and the western Pacific. It was a significant military problem in World War II, the Korean War and especially the Vietnam War. Rarely, the disease is brought home by travelers, but as Vietnam becomes an increasing tourist attraction this problem may increase. The vector is the larval stage of a variety of trombiculid mites; these mites are probably also the major reservoir, but wild rodents are also carriers. The larval mites, or chiggers, attach to low-lying vegetation (scrub) and then onto passersby.

Etiology and Pathogenesis. Scrub typhus is unusual in that there are many different serotypes; resistance to the given serotype is good, but reinfection with another one is common. When growing intracellularly, *Rickettsia tsutsugamushi* loses its cellular membrane, another quirk.

Clinical Findings. The incubation period is about 2 weeks. About half the patients have an eschar, which is usually on a leg and accompanied by inguinal lymphadenopathy. Headache, malaise and 40 °C temperatures complete the clinical picture. The rash is maculopapular and starts on the trunk after about 5 days of illness. Pulmonary and cardiac problems are the main threat; a small percentage of patients develop CNS problems.

Course and Prognosis. With treatment everyone survives. The mortality in untreated patients has been estimated as high as 30 %. Among troops with a missed diagnosis but adequate supportive care, deaths are an exception.

Therapy. Tetracyclines and chloramphenicol are effective. Doxycycline 200 mg in one dose is as good as a week of therapy.

Prophylaxis. Doxycycline 200 mg weekly offers promise. A vaccine is not available because of the many phenotypes.

Public Health Measures. Scrub typhus is a reportable infection.

Q-Fever

Synonym. Query fever (*not* Queensland fever)

Causative Organism. *Coxiella burnetii*

Epidemiology. Q-fever occurs worldwide. The best epidemiologic study was done in a slaughterhouse in Brisbane, Queensland, Australia, but the investigating physician named the disease query (or question) fever. The major source is domestic mammals, so that farmers, veterinarians, butchers and others with exposure are at greatest risk. In a Swiss epidemic, people living along a road where sheep were driven became infected. The organism is transmitted to humans via spores in the air and soil which are inhaled. Another major pathway is via infected milk. Spread among animals is due to a variety of ticks. Organisms can also be transmitted via blood and fomites, but person to person transmission is almost unheard of.

Etiology and Pathogenesis. *Coxiella burnetii* is a little different than the other rickettsiae. It must be phagocytosed by host cells as it has no means of active entry. It does not react with the Weil-Felix test. *Coxiella burnetii* spores are very resistant and long-lived. Since a single spore is enough to cause an infection, Q-fever has been of considerable interest in biological warfare.

Clinical Findings. There are no skin findings. Most patients have a limited febrile illness, but pneumonia, endocarditis and hepatitis are feared complications. While severe headache is common, other CNS findings are rare.

Therapy. Tetracyclines and chloramphenicol are effective. When endocarditis is present, modified regimens must be employed.

Prophylaxis. Anyone in contact with domestic animals, especially pregnant ones, must be extremely careful as the placenta is highly contagious. For such risk groups, an experimental vaccine is available, not coincidentally from Fort Detrick, Maryland, where the US Army conducts its germ warfare studies.

Public Health Measures. Q-fever is a reportable infection, in many jurisdictions as an emergency.

Other Rickettsial Diseases

At least six new rickettsial diseases have been described in the past decade, as sophisticated methods of both isolation and subclassification have become available. One example from central Europe is *Rickettsia slovaca*. The responsible tick is *Dermacentor marginatus*, a common arthropod in Central Europe. Most patients are children with a tick bite on the scalp and prominent cervical lymphadenopathy. In addition, there is a vesicular herpetic eruption about the site of attachment, sometimes combined with an erythematous band. As the lesion heals, alopecia may evolve.

Bibliography

General Reading

Mahon CR, Manuselis G (1995) Diagnostic microbiology. Saunders, Philadelphia

Poinar G Jr, Poinar R (1998) Parasites and pathogens of mites. Annu Rev Entomol 43:449–469

Raoult D, Roux V (1997) Rickettsioses as paradigms of new or emerging diseases. Clin Microbiol Rev 10:694–719

Shapiro ED (1997) Tick borne diseases. Adv Pediatr Infect Dis 13:187–218

Walker DH (1998) Tick transmitted infectious disease in the United States. Annu Rev Public Health 19:237–269

Rocky Mountain Spotted Fever

Akinbami L (1998) Rocky Mountain spotted fever. Pediatr Rev 19:171–172

Cale DF, McCarthy MW (1997) Treatment of Rocky Mountain spotted fever in children. Ann Pharmacother 31: 492–494

Boutonneuse Fever

Chaumentin G, Zenone T, Bibollet C et al. (1997) Malignant boutonneuse fever and polymyalgia rheumatica: a coincidental association? Infection 25:320–322

Miras Parra FJ, Gomez Jimenez FJ, Salvatierra Ossorio D et al. (1998) Pericarditis and Mediterranean spotted fever. Infection 26:61–62

Rickettsialpox

Angeloni VL, Keller RA, Walker DH (1997) Rickettsialpox like illness in a traveller. Mil Med 162:636–639

Boyd AS (1997) Rickettsialpox. Dermatol Clin 15:313–318

Kass EM, Szaniawski WK, Levy H et al. (1994) Rickettsialpox in a New York City hospital, 1980 to 1989. N Engl J Med 331:1612–1617

Endemic Typhus

Bernabeu Wittel M, Villanueva Marcos JL, de Alarcon Gonzalez A et al. (1998) Septic shock and multiorganic failure in murine typhus. Eur J Clin Microbiol Infect Dis 17:131–132

Scrub Typhus

Pai H, Sohn S, Seong Y et al. (1997) Central nervous system involvement in patients with scrub typhus. Clin Infect Dis 24(3):436–440

Olson JG, Church CJ, Corwin AL (1997) Seroepidemiologic evidence for murine and scrub typhus in Malang, Indonesia. Am J Trop Med Hyg 57:91–95

Richards AL, Soeatmadji DW, Widodo MA et al. (1997) Pregnancy with scrub typhus and vertical transmission: a case report. J Obstet Gynaecol Res 23:75–78

Thiebaut MM, Bricaire F, Raoult D (1997) Scrub typhus after a trip to Vietnam. N Engl J Med 336:1613–1614

Zinsser H (1935) Rats, lice and history. Little, Brown, New York

Q-Fever

Antony SJ, Schaffner W (1997) Q fever pneumonia. Semin Respir Infect 12:2–6

Ludlam H, Wreghitt TG, Thornton S et al. (1997) Q fever in pregnancy. J Infect 34:75–78

CHAPTER 4

Bacterial Diseases

Contents

Normal Flora of the Skin

Although the infant's skin is sterile in utero, it becomes contaminated in the birth canal. For the rest of an individual's life, varying types and numbers of microorganisms reside on the skin and mucous membranes. One distinguishes between resident flora, which are always present; temporary resident flora, which are established for a period of time; and transient flora, which only are found briefly. In addition, there are many different ecological niches on the human skin, ranging from moist to dry to oily (sebum-rich).

The skin surface pH plays a role in determining the microbial inhabitants. It usually has an acidic pH, the so-called acid mantle (Schade and Marchionini 1928), most often with a pH value of around 5.4–5.9 on free skin, such as the forehead. In general, the acidity of the skin favors relatively harmless bacteria and may thus protect somewhat from pathogenic strains. The pH value varies, being higher in the axillae and groin than on the forearm.

Exogenous influences can alter the acid mantle. Too frequent cleansing with alkaline soaps can both dry the skin and raise the pH. This leads to changes in the resident flora. On the forehead and forearm, an elevated pH leads to increased numbers of propionibacteria but unaltered levels of coagulase-negative staphylococci. The increase in propionibacteria, as measured by colony forming units per cm^2 (CFU), is of the order of magnitude 10^2-10^3.

Resident Flora

A wide range of bacteria are permanent residents of the skin. In general, they are organisms that grow best in the presence of oxygen, that is aerobic organisms. Other skin flora tolerate somewhat reduced oxygen levels and are known as microaerophilic. On a morphologic basis, one can distinguish between cocci (ball-shaped bacteria) and bacilli (rod-shaped bacteria). The main normal cocci are the *Micrococcaceae;* the main representatives are the coagulase-negative staphylococci. The main resident bacteria on the free, that is nonfollicular, skin is *Staphylococcus epidermidis.* In the region of the follicle opening, with reduced oxygen availability, propionibacteria are most common, primarily *Propionibacterium acnes* but also *P. granulosum* and

P. avidum. Other bacilli include the diphtheroids, whose taxonomy remains befuddling. Included are a variety of corynebacteria. Another normal inhabitant is the lipophilic yeast *Malassezia furfur*. Alternate names include *Pityrosporum ovale* and *P. orbiculare*; some subclassify this organism extensively. *Malessezia furfur* favors the face, upper chest and shoulders; the supraclavicular fossa is the ideal place to find it.

The most important method for determining the density of bacteria on skin is the detergent washing method of WILLIAMSON and KLIGMAN (1965). A defined volume of a tenside-containing washing fluid is placed in a glass cylinder of a specific diameter and placed on the skin, which is then scrubbed with a plastic spatula. The fluid is then diluted and plated onto appropriate culture plates under suitable atmospheric conditions. The resulting colonies are counted. On the dry forearm, *S. epidermidis* is the most prevalent; there are 10^2-10^3 CFU/cm^2. Propionibacteria and corynebacteria are present in only small numbers. In the moist axillae, the picture is different. In some individuals the coagulase-negative staphylococci dominate; in others, the corynebacteria are most common. On the forehead, which is rich in sebum, propionibacteria dominate but there are also a significant number of staphylococci. In the follicle itself, *Malessezia furfur* is found in the upper reaches, as are coagulase-negative staphylococci; propionibacteria, especially *P. acnes*, inhabit the entire follicle.

Removing the resident flora becomes an issue when preparing the skin for surgery. In general, one can only reduce the level of bacteria by about 10^2; the follicle openings are felt to be hiding places for bacteria which repopulate the epidermis. It usually takes 24–72 h for the normal flora to reconstitute itself.

Transient and Temporary Flora

When other bacteria come on the skin, they usually remain only for a couple of hours under normal conditions. *Staphylococcus aureus* is present in the nose and perianal region of some individuals and can then be spread to the skin. Gram-negative bacteria of the families Enterobacteriaceae and Pseudomonadaceae also appear on the skin. The former are part of the normal gut flora and can be spread to the skin by the hands; the latter are present in the environment, most often in moist places, such as flower vases, and can be picked up.

If the epidermal barrier is intact, these contacts do not lead to disease. Important factors include pH, water and fat content of the stratum corneum, degree of shedding, skin temperature and integrity of the normal flora. If the normal flora count is reduced, such as by repeated washing with antibacterial soaps, then increased numbers of *S. aureus* will appear. Additional important factors are those which determine the virulence of a given organism. Some strains of bacteria such as the streptococci secrete M-factors, which hinder phagocytosis, and also toxins that increase exfoliation. The presence of bacteriophages carrying viral genetic information also influences virulence, as seen with both staphylococci and *Corynebacterium diphtheriae*.

Clinical Aspects of Bacterial Skin Infections

One is faced with an impossible task when writing such a chapter. Is the material best organized along the lines of clinical lesions or causative organisms? We have chosen the latter for our framework but with frequent cross-referencing to indicate situations in which several organisms can be responsible for a given clinical picture. One reason for this choice is that therapy must be based on the organisms suspected or cultured, not just on the description of the disease. Cellulitis in an infant is different from cellulitis in the leg of a patient with chronic venous insufficiency and must be approached otherwise. Thus a degree of repetition is unavoidable.

Diagnosis of Bacterial Infections

There are a number of ways to diagnose a bacterial disease. While the clinical features often suggest the causative organism, they are almost never diagnostic by themselves. KOCH's postulates (1888) suggested that the following steps be followed to prove that a given organism causes a disease.

- The organism must be found in every case of the disease.
- It must be isolated and grown in pure culture.
- It must reproduce the disease when inoculated into an experimental animal.
- It must be identified in or recovered from the diseased animal.

While these criteria today are not rigidly applied, they still contain the basic elements of bacteriological diagnosis.

Direct Examination

Bacteria may be found in pus, blood, urine, sputum and almost every other body fluid, as well as in skin and many other tissues. Of particular relevance to dermatologists are skin smears and biopsies, while venereal disease experts also rely heavily on studying urethral, cervical, vaginal and anal discharges. The dark field examination is performed on unstained fluid from a suspected syphilitic lesion. Most often the material is examined on a glass slide following staining. The GRAM stain (1884), using a basic aniline dye such as gentian violet or crystal violet, is used not only to identify but also to classify bacteria. Gram-positive bacteria have a much thicker peptidoglycan cell wall than do gram-negative bacteria and thus are not decolorized as easily. When studying tissue sections modified Gram stains are usually employed. The ZIEHL-NEELSEN (1882) and FITE (1940) stains are usually employed to stain mycobacteria, while the WARTHIN-STARRY (1883) and Dieterle stains are used for spirochetes.

Many newer methods to identify organisms directly are available today. A polyclonal anti-*Mycobcaterium bovis* antibody shows marked interspecies cross-reactivity and is very useful for staining bacteria and fungi in formalin-fixed tissues. Some monoclonal antibodies are also available for use both on frozen and fixed tissue. For example, direct immunofluorescence is widely used in the diagnosis of *Chlamydia* urethritis (Chap. 5). In addition, PCR can be used to identify bacterial DNA, while in situ hybridization may also be applied.

Culture

The obtaining of material for a culture is of crucial importance. When studying cutaneous lesions, fluid from an intact blister is ideal. When a serous exudate is cultured, one usually identifies a number of contaminants. If an inflamed nodule, deeper cellulitis or abscess is studied, one can try aspirating material, but culturing tissue obtained by biopsy will often have a higher yield. The laboratory personnel should be provided with appropriate clinical information so they can choose the correct culture media, select the correct conditions (aerobic vs anaerobic) and observe the culture for the needed time period.

Serology

Most bacteria elicit an immune response so that a variety of serological approaches can be used to confirm the presence of an infection. In many instances, acute and convalescent titers are needed; thus, serological studies often have more epidemiological than clinical value. The various situations in which serological tests are helpful will be cited throughout the text.

Treatment

For the most part, we will only outline appropriate antibiotic therapy. Exact dosages usually depend on the age or weight of the patient and should be sought in appropriate reference sources, ideally ones which reflect local or regional patterns of antibiotic sensitivity. The increased bacterial resistance to antibiotics is a major problem today. Dermatologists have been accused of contributing to the problem by overusing antibiotics for noninfectious problems such as acne, but the evidence for this claim is controversial. Most of the *S. aureus* found in cutaneous infections are resistant to penicillin and worldwide about 50% are resistant to methicillin. There are marked regional variations but resistance to tetracycline and erythromycin is also common. When fewer antibiotics are prescribed in a given community, the resistance rates to many antibiotics tends to drop. Group A β-hemolytic streptococci are almost always sensitive to penicillin, but often resistant to erythromycin and tetracycline. In the course of acne treatment, *P. acnes* often becomes resistant to topical and systemic antibiotics. Those physicians treating skin diseases should take the development of resistance seriously and try to prescribe antibiotics only for specific indications and for short periods of time.

Gram-Positive Cocci

The gram-positive cocci are responsible for most skin infections. We will first briefly consider staphylococci and streptococci, and then some of the many clinical disorders they cause.

Staphylococci

Staphylococci produce a wide range of infections. While the traditional and most important pathogen is *S. aureus*, which is coagulase-positive, several coagulase-negative types also cause disease, as shown in Table 4.1. *S. aureus* is an aerobic spherical bacteria with a diameter of 0.7–1.2 µm. It may also be grown as a facultative anaerobe. The bacteria has bacteriophage receptors on its surface; subtyping is based on the resultant lysis induced by specific phages. Most *S. aureus* have protein A on their surface; this molecule binds with the Fc fragment of immunoglobulins, blocking phagocytosis. The bacteria produce a variety of destructive enzymes, such as coagulase, nucleases, catalases, proteases, hyaluronidase, and lysozyme. Coagulase activates prothrombin; its presence usually indicates *S. aureus*. Beta-lactamase, which inactivates penicillin, is produced as are penicillin-binding proteins, which provide resistance against the penicillinase-resistant penicillins and cephalosporins. Most staphylococcus species produce a variety of toxins including cytotoxins and leukocytolytic toxins, as well as the major toxins discussed below. The enterotoxin molecules cause staphylococcal food poisoning.

Laboratory Findings

The classic microscopic finding is gram-positive cocci arranged in grape-like clusters. For culture, pus from an intact pustule should be taken when available; otherwise a skin smear can be used. *Staphylococci* are easy to culture on blood agar; adding CO_2 facilitates growth. The presence or absence of coagulase is the main method for identifying *S. aureus* and can be done on a direct slide test.

Table 4.1. The gram-positive cocci

Organism	Clinical disorders
Staphylococcus	
Staphylococcus aureus (coagulase-positive)	Pyodermas Toxic epidermal necrolysis Osteomyelitis Pneumonia Endocarditis
With TSS toxin	Toxic shock syndrome
With enterotoxin	Food poisoning
Staphylococcus epidermidis (coagulase-negative)	Rarely pathogenic; immunosuppressed and hospitalized patients, indwelling catheters, sepsis
Staphylococcus saprophyticus (coagulase-negative)	Urinary tract infections
Streptococcus	
Group A *Streptococcus pyogenes* (β-hemolytic)	Pyodermas Erysipelas Cellulitis Scarlet fever Pharyngitis Acute glomerulonephritis Rheumatic fever
Group B *Streptococcus agalctiae*	Neonatal meningitis, endometritis
Group C *Streptococcus equi, Streptococcus dysgalactiae*	Pharyngitis
Group D	Endocarditis
Streptococcus bovis	Endocarditis
Viridans group (α-hemolytic)	Deep abscesses Other chronic infections

TSS, toxic shock syndrome

Therapy

The usual therapy of choice for staphylococcal infections is either a penicillinase-resistant penicillin, such as dicloxacillin or flucloaxacillin, or a second generation oral cephalosporin. Erythromycin is frequently used by dermatologists, but in most communities there is widespread resistance.

Methicillin-resistant *S. aureus* (MRSA) are mainly a problem in hospitals, especially in intensive care settings; vancomycin is the only available agent but strains resistant to vancomycin have now emerged. Further details on therapy are given under the individual infections.

Streptococci

The streptococci are gram-positive bacteria, with a diameter of 0.5 µm, which are frequently arranged in chains. Streptococci are classified in a number of ways. One is their ability to induce hemolysis on blood agar: β-hemolysis refers to a clear area, while α-hemolysis represent a green change; no hemolysis is described as γ-hemolysis. Another method is the LANCEFIELD (1928) groups, which divide the streptococci into five groups (A-D, G) based on serological characteristics of their cell walls.

The main skin pathogens are the group A *Streptococci*, also known as *Streptococcus pyogenes*, which are β-hemolytic. They cause a long list of cutaneous infections as well as pharyngitis, scarlet fever, rheumatic fever, glomerulonephritis, puerperal sepsis, and toxic shock syndrome. The varying clinical features are determined in part by the ability of the various streptococci to produce extracellular toxins, such as the erythrogenic toxin in scarlet fever. They also release many enzymes such as DNase B and streptokinase; measuring host antibodies to these enzymes is one way of documenting streptococcal infection. Immunological cross-reactions that occur with select rheumatogenic and nephritogenic strains lead to rheumatic fever and glomerulonephritis, respectively. Rheumatic fever has been on a surge around the world for the past 15 years, as have severe streptococcal infections in general. Different stains cause pharyngitis and renal disease, as compared to impetigo and renal disease. While glomerulonephritis often follows skin infections, rheumatic fever rarely, if ever, does. Cutaneous streptococcal infections also may trigger guttate psoriasis.

Laboratory Findings. Blister fluids and pus can be examined directly, searching for gram-positive cocci arranged in chains. The culture is done on blood agar. From the standpoint of dermatology, the anti DNase B titer is probably the most useful serologic test. The rapid Strep test identifies group A antigens in the saliva; it is very sensitive but not specific. Typing of the bacteria is useful for epidemiological studies, so that one is alert when organisms potentially causing cardiac or renal disease are common in the community.

Therapy. Streptococci have remained amazingly sensitive to penicillin. A number of alternatives are available including erythromycin, tetracycline and cephalosporins.

Toxin-Mediated Streptococcal and Staphylococcal Disease

There are a number of serious diseases which are caused by toxins manufactured by staphylococci and streptococci. Some have long been known, such as scarlet fever, while others have only been identified within the past two decades. The major toxins are shown in Table 4.2. Toxin-mediated disease has a number of distinctive features. First of all, the diseases are often quite severe. Some clinical findings are common, such as strawberry tongue, erythema with desquamation and prominent perineal involvement. Culture often fails to reveal the bacteria, or there may be a positive culture at an asymptomatic site while the disease elsewhere may be severe. There are marked overlaps between staphylococcal and streptococcal disorders, such as toxic shock syndrome and streptococcal toxic shock syndrome. A single toxin such as toxic shock syndrome toxin-1 (TSST-1) may lead to a number of clinical presentations. About 20% of *S. aureus* isolates have the gene for TSST-1. This toxin is structurally similar to the staphylococcal enterotoxins B

Table 4.2. Major staphylococcal and streptococcal toxins

Organism	Toxin
Group A β-hemolytic streptococci	Streptococcal pyrogenic exotoxins (SPE-A, SPE-B, SPE-C; formerly erythrogenic toxin SPE-A) Streptococcal superantigen (SAA) Mitogenic antigen
Other streptococci	Streptococcal pyrogenic exotoxins
Staphylococci	Toxic shock syndrome toxin-1 (TSST-1) Staphylococcal enterotoxins (SEA, SEB, SEC, SED, SEE, SEG) Exfoliative toxin A and B

and C, even though there are no amino acid homologies. Finally, many of these toxins serve as superantigens, activating massive number of T cells without following the conventional immunologic pathways. This can lead to marked cytokine release, especially of tumor necrosis factor (TNF)-α, interleukin (IL)-1, IL-6, and dramatic clinical signs including fever, hypotension, tissue destruction and even shock, along with an erythematous rash.

Bullous impetigo and its related diseases including staphylococcal scalded skin syndrome are also toxin-mediated but are considered below-under pyodermas, where they have been traditionally included.

Toxic Shock Syndrome

Synonym. TSS

Definition. Life-threatening multisystem disease with skin involvement caused by staphylococcal exotoxin.

Table 4.3. Diagnostic criteria for staphylococcal toxic shock syndrome

The following three findings must be present:
Fever > 38.8 °C
Diffuse macular exanthem with desquamation after 1–2 weeks, especially on the palms and soles
Hypotension, systolic < 90 mmHg
In addition, three of the following organs must be involved:
Gastrointestinal tract (nausea, vomiting, diarrhea)
Skeletal muscle (myalgias, elevated muscle enzymes)
Mucosal surfaces (conjunctivitis, vaginal or oral erythema)
Renal disease (decreased function, pyuria without documented infection)
CNS (disorientation, decreased level of consciousness)
Hepatic dysfunction
Hematologic disease (platelets < 100,000 µl)
Rocky Mountain spotted fever, leptospirosis and measles must be excluded

Epidemiology. The major outbreak of toxic shock syndrome occurred in the 1980s , involving almost exclusively women who were using superabsorbent tampons. Today less than 50% of cases are associated with menses. Other risk factors include using contraceptive sponges and diaphragms. In other cases, focal staphylococcal infection of the skin, bones or soft tissue may be responsible for the exotoxin, while in many other cases, a focus is never found.

Etiology and Pathogenesis. The staphylococci may produce local symptoms, but most often there is a silent infection with production of the 24 kDa protein TSST-1. This molecule is a superantigen which activates T cells, which in turn stimulate macrophages to produce TNF and various ILs, especially IL-1. Susceptible patients do not have adequate antibody levels against TSST-1. In about 25% of cases, the isolated bacteria do not produce TSST-1 but rather other staphylococcal enterotoxins that also act as superantigens.

Clinical Findings. The clinical features are best understood in the form of the diagnostic criteria, as used by the CDC for case definition (Table 4.3). As should be apparent, the patients are ill enough that they are rarely cared for by dermatologists, but two of the four major diagnostic points involve the skin.

The initial rash is a diffuse, blanching, nonpruritic macular exanthem which lasts several days and fades. It may have a rough sandpaper feel. Sometimes the erythema is diffuse, as in a sunburn; in other cases it remains macular. After about 2 weeks, there is desquamation, which is usually most prominent on the tips of the fingers and toes There may be periorbital edema. The conjunctival, vaginal or oral mucosa may be erythematous and have tiny ulcerations. The tongue is often red with hyperplastic papillae; it has been compared to the strawberry tongue of scarlet fever.

In general the patient is ill with fever, chills, malaise and headache. The hypotension is uncomfortable and mandates bed rest. As the disease evolves, multisystem problems become apparent.

Histopathology. Biopsy plays no role in diagnosing toxic shock syndrome.

Laboratory Findings. The vagina, mouth, eyes and any other possible sites of abscess formation should be cultured.

Course and Prognosis. The morbidity is less than 2% with aggressive intensive care.

Differential Diagnosis. The main differential diagnostic issue is streptococcal toxic shock syndrome. Scarlet fever also has similar skin findings, but lacks the multisystem disease, as do most other toxic erythemas.

Therapy. Systemic antistaphylococcal therapy must be combined with aggressive supportive care. If an abscess is identified, it should be opened and drained. If predisposing factors are identified, they should be corrected or changed.

Streptococcal Toxic Shock Syndrome

Synonym. STSS

Definition. Toxic shock syndrome-like clinical picture but produced by streptococcal toxins.

Causative Organism. β-hemolytic group A streptococci, usually phage types M1, M3, M5 and others. Occasionally other non-group A streptococci are identified.

Table 4.4. Diagnostic criteria for streptococcal toxic shock syndrome

- I. **Isolation of *Streptococcus pyogenes***
  - A. From a normally sterile site
  - B. From a normally unsterile site
- II. **Clinical findings**
  - A. Hypotension with systolic pressure ≤ 90 mmHg
  - B. Two or more of the following:
    - Renal involvement
    - Reduced platelets or disseminated intravascular coagulation
    - Liver involvement
    - Adult respiratory distress syndrome
    - Macular exanthem, often with later desquamation
    - Soft tissue necrosis, including necrotizing fasciitis or myositis

If IA, IIA and IIB are fulfilled, the diagnosis is definite
If IB, IIA and IIB are fulfilled, the diagnosis is probable

Epidemiology. Streptococcal toxic shock syndrome differs in some ways from staphylococcal or classical toxic shock syndrome. Patients are usually healthy adults who apparently lack immunity and experience the sudden onset of painful soft tissue damage and bacteremia. Most often, the site of the initial infection is the skin, often associated with surgical wounds. Vaginal and throat infections may also be the first sign. Other scenarios include STSS following varicella or a wound infection, as well as occurring in immunosuppressed patients. This pattern is in contrast to that in patients with staphylococcal toxic shock syndrome, whose primary infection is often subclinical.

Etiology and Pathogenesis. These highly destructive streptococci are relatively new, first identified in adults in the late 1980s and in children in the early 1990s. They have been called "flesh-eating bacteria" in the tabloid press. The bacteria produce a wide variety of toxins but streptococcal pyrogenic exotoxin A (SPE-A) is usually responsible. There are homologies between the streptococcal pyrogenic exotoxins and the staphylococcal enterotoxins, but TSST-1 is distinct.

Clinical Findings. The criteria for streptococcal toxic shock syndrome are slightly different, as shown in Table 4.4. The biggest difference is that there is a symptomatic streptococcal infection; in 80% of cases the skin is the portal of entry and there is soft tissue spread. One of the major causes of necrotizing fasciitis is these same streptococci, as discussed below. The patients rapidly develop fever, hypotension, multisystem disease and shock. The literature is somewhat divergent on the frequency of skin findings, but many patients have a diffuse erythema with perineal accentuation and, later, desquamation. Ocular and oral mucosal erythema may also be seen.

Laboratory Findings. Attempts should be made to culture any wound or skin lesion, as well as the throat, sputum and blood. Other attempts to identify streptococci, such as anti DNase B and rapid protein A testing, are also reasonable.

Course and Prognosis. The course can be extremely rapid, leading to death before any therapy has a chance to take hold. The mortality rate is around 30%.

Differential Diagnosis. The main differential diagnostic consideration is staphylococcal toxic shock syndrome, as well as other types of severe cellulitis.

Therapy. Aggressive intravenous penicillin therapy is required. Clindamycin may more rapidly shut down toxin production and is thus not only useful in therapy but for prophylaxis in contacts. Early studies showed that intravenous immunoglobulin is quite effective. If necrotizing fasciitis is present, debridement is also essential.

Scarlet Fever
(SYDENHAM 1664)

Synonym. Scarlatina

Definition. Streptococcal infection characterized by pharyngitis, fever, glossitis and a diffuse exanthem.

Causative Organism. Group A β-hemolytic streptococci.

Epidemiology. Scarlet fever is a worldwide infection caused by a group A, β-hemolytic streptococcus that produces an erythrogenic toxin; otherwise it is similar to an ordinary streptococcal pharyngitis (strep throat). The incidence of scarlet fever appears to be on the rise again. It is a disease of childhood, most common in the late fall and winter months and usually transferred by droplet spread, like any other upper airway infection. Rarely, streptococcal infections elsewhere, such as wound infections, burns and puerperal infection, can also cause scarlet fever. Asymptomatic carriers can also spread the disease.

Etiology and Pathogenesis. Most group A β-hemolytic streptococci produce one or more forms of pyrogenic (previously called erythrogenic) exotoxin, such as SPE-A, SPE-B and SPE-C. In scarlet fever, SPE-A is usually responsible. Occasionally other streptococci produce similar toxins. Patients form antitoxins which block the erythrogenic action of the toxin; these antitoxins last for life. In the SCHULTZ-CHARLTON (1918) test, antitoxin is injected into the skin and blanches the rash. This approach is no longer used for diagnosis because of obvious problems with injecting serum from another patient. A patient resistant to the toxin can still develop repeated attacks of pharyngitis.

Clinical Findings. After an incubation period of 2–5 days, the initial symptoms appear. They include fever, headache, vomiting and a sore throat. The pharynx is erythematous; there may be an enanthem on the palate, the tongue is coated and the cervical lymph nodes are usually swollen and tender. At this stage, the rash may begin. It is typically diffuse and erythematous, with the antecubital and popliteal fossa as well as the groin the usual initial sites. The erythema spreads to involve the chest and face, but only in extreme cases is the face involved. Even then the cheeks are flushed while the chin and perioral region remain spared, producing circumoral pallor. Depending on the patient's antitoxin status, the exanthem may appear later or be limited.

The lesions are centered around follicles and are usually described as resembling the head of a stick pin. When the skin is stroked, the many tiny papules give the impression of velvet. Other authors describe them as sandpaper-like. In black patients, the erythema cannot be appreciated, so they may present with many tiny bumps, which have been called goose skin (cutis anserina), although this clearly differs from the goose bumps produced by contraction of the arrector pili muscles. Occasionally, small blisters develop (miliaria scarlatinosa) or tiny hemorrhages. Streaks of petechiae, such as along the axillary lines, are called Pastia lines. Punctate palatal petechiae are known as Forscheimer spots. A RUMPEL (1909)-LEEDE (1911) test is often positive. When the skin is stroked, white dermographism occurs.

The white coating of the tongue is shed, leaving behind a red inflamed tongue with prominent papillae: the raspberry tongue in German but the strawberry tongue in English. As the fever drops, desquamation also occurs. It is so typical that it is often used to confirm the suspected clinical diagnosis. Initially scaling is found on the ears, neck, trunk and extremities. On the palms and soles, large sheets of skin are shed; sometimes the tips of the digits lose skin much as when one removes a glove. Later on the nails may show transverse ridges, Beau lines. Occasionally a patient may have a fever and no exanthem, but then undergo the characteristic desquamation.

Histopathology. Lesions are rarely biopsied but on occasion one may wish to exclude staphylococcal scalded skin syndrome. Typical for scarlet fever are tiny accumulations of exudate in the stratum corneum which may account for the clinical sandpaper feeling. In the dermis there are dilated vessels with scattered neutrophils.

Laboratory Findings. Usually there is a marked leukocytosis, up to 40,000 WBC/ml. The granulocytes may contain inclusion bodies (DÖHLE [1912] bodies). The sedimentation rate is elevated. Group A β-hemolytic streptococci can be cultured from the throat or other suspected sites and also identified directly in smears or tissues with a variety of immunofluorescent stains. In addition, the various streptococcal antibodies can be identified.

Course and Prognosis. Most patients do well. Rarely, patients may experience a more dramatic course, but this has become uncommon with antibiotic treatment. In the fulminant version, high fever, hemorrhage, seizures and shock occur and death is possible. In the past, cavernous sinus thrombosis and meningitis were described. In addition, secondary bacterial infections of many types can occur. More importantly, both rheumatic fever and glomerulonephritis can follow scarlet fever.

Differential Diagnosis. Some drug reactions are described as scarlatiniform and do resemble scarlet fever but the pharyngitis and tongue changes do not occur. Kawasaki disease is quite similar, but has more severe lymphadenopathy. Measles and rubella have some similarities but their exanthems are generally distinct. Staphylococcal scarlet fever is quite similar, but usually lacks the oral changes. The rash of infectious mononucleosis may seem similar and there is pharyngitis, but the throat culture is negative, the lymphadenopathy more pronounced, and the blood smear and serologic tests confirm the presence of Epstein-Barr virus. Other respiratory viruses may also produce a similar exanthem, but lack the other features of a streptococcal infection.

Therapy

Systemic. Once again oral or parenteral penicillin produces prompt improvement. A single injection of benzathine penicillin G (600,000–1,200,000 units) suffices; if the oral route is chosen, 10 days of therapy are recommended. Erythromycin is usually preferred in patients with allergies to penicillin. Good supportive care is essential, as for a short period of time the patients are quite ill.

Topical. The desquamation is disturbing, but can be treated with any bland cream.

Staphylococcal Scarlet Fever

(Stevens 1927)

A scarlet fever-like picture can also be produced by some phage group II staphylococci. Patients present with a diffuse erythema, often with a sandpaper-like texture and skin tenderness. There is no pharyngitis, throat cultures are negative, other streptococcal tests are negative and the typical desquamation of scarlet fever usually is lacking. Staphylococcal scarlet fever probably represents a mild variant of either toxic shock syndrome or staphylococcal scalded skin syndrome. Antistaphylococcal therapy is curative.

Recalcitrant Erythematous Desquamating Disorder

(Cone et al. 1992)

Recalcitrant erythematous desquamating disorder (REDD) is seen primarily in patients with HIV/AIDS. Most often, *S. aureus* is isolated, with TSST-1 the most commonly identified toxin. Occasionally toxins SEA and SEB have been found. Not surprisingly, REDD shares many features with the toxic shock syndrome, including fever, hypotension, diffuse erythema with desquamation, strawberry tongue and mucosal erythema. Nonetheless,there are marked differences including a prolonged course with frequent recurrences. Even though REDD has a less fulminant course, the mortality rate is higher, probably because of the HIV/AIDS. One explanation is that there are fewer T cells available in such patients for immediate activation and that control mechanism are impaired. Treatment consists of antistaphylococcal antibiotics and supportive measures.

Neonatal Toxic Shock Syndrome-Like Exanthematous Disease

(Takahashi et al. 1995)

Newborns who are carriers of *S. aureus* infection may develop a diffuse exanthem, thrombocytopenia and fever. In most cases the bacteria is resistant to methicillin and all produce TSST-1. Clonal expansion of T cell receptor Vβ has been demonstrated in such cases. Most infants have no signs of clinical staphylococcal infection and recover spontaneously. The macular exanthem tends to spread from the trunk to the face and extremities. The palms and soles may be involved. The macules tend to coalesce and may be accompanied by petechiae. Desquamation does not occur. Complications include patent ductus arteriosus, sclerema neonatorum (Chap. 21), and mucosal damage, all of which are more common in premature infants.

Recurrent Toxin-Mediated Erythema

(Manders et al. 1996)

Synonyms. Recurrent toxin-mediated perineal erythema

The typical case of toxin-mediated erythema features a diffuse, macular perineal erythema 24–48 h after a bacterial pharyngitis. Strawberry tongue, acral edema and desquamation may also occur, but the disease is self-limited and systemic toxicity does not occur; however, recurrences are the rule. Toxin-producing bacteria, both streptococci and staphylococci, are isolated from normal sterile sites, not just the pharynx. Since the initial description, it has become clear that areas other than the perineum may be affected. Treatment consists of antistaphylococcal antibiotics. This disorder is not the same as perianal streptococcal cellulitis which is a direct perianal infection.

Other Possibly Toxin Mediated Diseases

Kawasaki disease (Chap. 22) is a severe illness of infants and young children that has many features of a toxin-mediated disease. The self-limited nature, seasonal and geographic clustering, appearance almost exclusively in children, and clinical findings, such as perineal erythema, mucosal involvement and desquamation, all point towards a toxin mediator. Nonetheless, neither staphylococci nor streptococci have been isolated from patients. In the most convincing study *S. aureus* was isolated in 13 of 16 patients. If a toxin is responsible, TSST-1 is probably the best candidate, along with streptococcal pyrogenic exotoxins.

The role of streptococci in psoriasis (Chap. 14), especially guttate psoriasis, has long been appreciated. The T cell activation in early psoriatic lesions in the skin often shows clonal expansion of limited subsets, just as with toxin-mediated disease. Similarly, in atopic dermatitis (Chap. 12), colonization with *S. aureus* is almost the rule and staphylococcal toxins may serve to trigger flares of the dermatitis.

Pyoderma

Definition. Bacterial skin infection with pus involving either free skin or the adnexal structures.

The term pyoderma is not often employed in the USA but is useful as a cover term for a wide range of streptococcal and staphylococcal skin infections that classically produce pus. Other bacteria may also cause pyodermas, and one should be aware that sometimes pyoderma does not refer to an infection, as in "pyoderma gangrenosum." In addition to the primary pyoderma covered below, there are many situations in which the skin becomes secondarily infected, almost always by a mixture of both staphylococci and streptococci. Typical situations include atopic dermatitis, when one often speaks of impetiginization, viral infections such as herpes simplex and zoster, ulcers, ulcerated tumors and various injuries including abrasions and burns.

Impetigo

In the past one sharply distinguished between ordinary, nonbullous impetigo, caused by group A *Streptococcus*, and bullous impetigo, caused by *S. aureus*. Today this distinction is inaccurate, as *S. aureus* can also cause ordinary impetigo; in the USA, it is the usual organism. Since the lesions have clinical differences, we will consider them separately.

Nonbullous Impetigo

Synonyms. Impetigo

Definition. Common superficial skin infection characterized by small blisters that rapidly rupture and evolve into honey colored crusts.

Causative Organisms. *Staphylococcus aureus* and group A *Streptococcus*.

Epidemiology. Nonbullous impetigo (from here on referred to as impetigo) is most common among children and is quite contagious. Often several children in a family or classmates from a kindergarten will present simultaneously. The infection can also be transferred via wash clothes or towels. In adults, inadequate hygiene is a risk factor. Both *S. aureus* and *Streptococcus pyogenes* can be spread from the nares to the skin.

Etiology and Pathogenesis. In practice, many cultures from impetigo grow out both *S. pyogenes* and *S. aureus*. When early lesions are studied and pure cultures obtained, in the USA most often *S. aureus* is found, although in some instances only *S. pyogenes* grows. In other parts of the world, such as Germany, streptococci remain the most important cause, being responsible for up to 80 % of cases.

Clinical Findings. Initially, small red macules develop with tiny, pin-head sized, tense clear vesicles set amidst the erythematous background. It is very difficult to see the blisters since they rupture easily, evolving into a characteristic honey

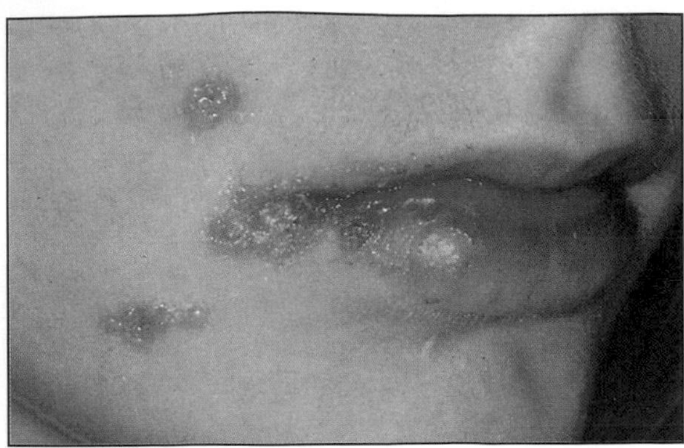

Fig. 4.1. Impetigo with crusting

colored thick crust (Fig. 4.1). While initially only a few, small asymmetrically scattered lesions are present, the lesions extend to expand and coalesce, producing arcuate patterns. Patients tend to spread the infection with their hands and wash clothes, inoculating new spots as they scratch. One well established scenario is scabies → impetigo → glomerulonephritis; this seems especially common on some Caribbean islands. The most typical sites are the face, especially about the nose and mouth, as well as the neck and hands. The perinasal location may be explained by carriage of the bacteria in the nose and their spread through nasal discharge and sneezing. Both perlèche and paronychia may be seen. There may be associated lymphadenopathy. The lesions usually heal without scarring.

Histopathology. Biopsies are rarely done. The blister is subcorneal, contains neutrophils, bacteria and fibrin, as well as occasional acantholytic cells. There is accompanying spongiosis and dermal inflammation. In more advanced cases, one only sees crusting.

Laboratory Findings. If possible, an intact blister should be cultured. Otherwise, one is likely to get mixed results. In our experience in Germany, cultures taken directly in the hospital and plated immediately are most likely to yield *Streptococcus.*

Course and Prognosis. The outlook for impetigo is good, with a prompt response to treatment. The main problem is the development of glomerulonephritis, if the infection is caused by a nephritogenic strain. While the incidence of this feared complication has been estimated at 4%, we suspect that is high. If any clinical suspicion exists, the child's urine should be evaluated.

Differential Diagnosis. The main differential diagnostic point is to exclude a secondarily infected herpes simplex virus (HSV) infection. Often, in later stages of the disease, this is impossible, as herpes simplex infections often become impetiginized. They are more likely to involve mucus membranes and tend to have a more polycyclic pattern. A very inflamed dermatophyte infection, such as that caused by an animal pathogen, may also be crusted and weep.

Therapy. The appropriate therapy depends on several factors, including the likelihood of either *S. aureus* or *S. pyogenes* in one's community, the prevalence of nephritogenic strains, the severity of the infection and perhaps the presence of underlying atopic dermatitis.

Systemic. When *S. pyogenes* is the usual cause, therapy can be begun with oral penicillin G, while if *S. aureus* is a consideration, then a penicillinase-resistant penicillin or a cephalosporin should be used. Erythromycin is a consideration when documented penicillin allergy is present. The main purpose of systemic therapy is to attempt to eliminate the spread of possibly nephritogenic strains in a population. In an individual patient, often the die has been cast as far as glomerulonephritis goes, but in the population, one can play a positive role with systemic antibiotics.

Topical. Topical antibiotics are effective in impetigo and can be used for patients with a limited number of lesions. Without question, mucopiricin ointment is the best, comparable to oral antibiotics in many studies. It should be applied four to five times daily. Bacitracin ointment is a second choice, far less expensive but also less effective. In addition, the crusts should be removed; wet compresses are helpful but the skin should not be allowed to become macerated, as this may spread the disease. Clioquinol ointments or creams can also be used.

Other Measures. The skin should be washed two to three times daily with a disinfectant soap to prevent spread. Each patient in a family should have his or her own wash cloth. One should always suspect that multiple children in a family may be infected and inquire about this possibility. Cutting the fingernails short helps to reduce autoinoculation.

Bullous Impetigo

Synonym. Impetigo (contagiosa) staphylogenes

Definition. An infection more common in children which features large flaccid blisters.

Causative Organism. *Staphylococcus aureus*

Epidemiology. Bullous impetigo is also a highly contagious disease, most often in moist, warm climates or in the summer months in temperate zones. Epidemics can be seen in kindergartens or even pediatric wards.

Etiology and Pathogenesis. The key factor is the produce of two exotoxins, exfoliatin A and B, both with a molecular weight of around 30 kDa, which cause superficial separation in the epidermis. The split develops in the stratum granulosum as the filaggrin in the desmosomes is destroyed. In the newborn mouse model, introduction of the toxin produces acantholysis and separation of the stratum corneum. In humans, there is a direct relationship between the age of the patient and the action of the toxin, with the disease being more widespread in newborns. In older infants, the process is localized, thus bullous impetigo. Rarely, older children and adults, perhaps immunosuppressed, may also develop staphylococcal scalded skin syndrome. Phage group II type 71 is the strain of *S. aureus* most likely to cause bullous impetigo and related disorders.

Clinical Findings. The key finding is the presence of flaccid blisters on an erythematous base; the fluid is initially clear, but later becomes white-gray and then yellow, forming pus. Typically the blister roof collapses and lies pressed upon the eroded blister base, much like a wet leaf on the street. The most common locations are the face, groin and acral regions (Fig. 4.2). Large intact blisters on dependent areas may show a fluid level, with the neutrophils sunken to the bottom of the fluid space. When the blister roof is shed, one sees a moist, glistening, varnish-like erosion with a collarette scale. Heavy crusting, as in nonbullous impetigo, generally does not develop. Lesions usually heal without scarring, but may leave behind erythema or hyperpigmentation. In most instances, the patient is surprisingly well; often there is an associated atopic dermatitis.

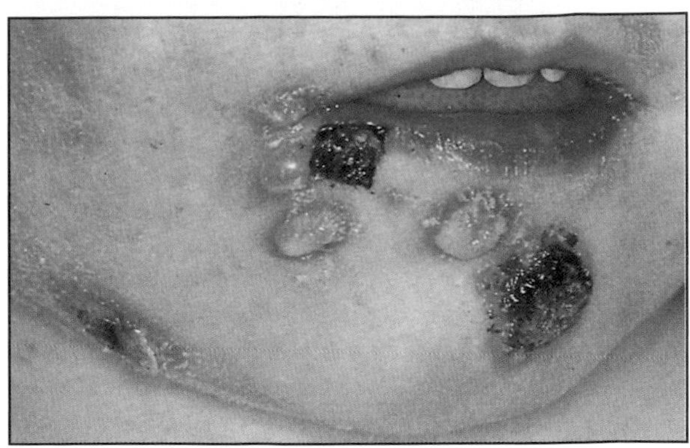

Fig. 4.2. Bullous impetigo

Histopathology. The key finding is the presence of a cleft or split high in the epidermis just beneath the stratum corneum. This is discussed further under staphylococcal scalded skin syndrome.

Laboratory Findings. An intact blister should be cultured and phage typing performed, as well as antibiotic sensitivity.

Course and Prognosis. The outlook is good in children. The major risk is that of developing staphylococcal scalded skin syndrome.

Therapy

Systemic. Appropriate antistaphylococcal therapy should be instituted.

Topical. The same topical measures discussed under nonbullous impetigo are appropriate.

Impetigo Neonatorum

Synonyms. Neonatal staphylococcal pustulosis

Definition. A variant of bullous impetigo seen in newborns.

One can argue whether *S. aureus* infection with exfoliation in a newborn should be considered bullous impetigo or staphylococcal scalded skin syndrome. In any event, the infection usually starts about the umbilical stump or circumcision site, although other traumatized areas, the rectum and conjunctiva also can be initially involved. The blisters spread very rapidly; in German they are described as peeling blisters. The intertriginous areas are prominently involved (Fig. 4.3). The patients experience problems with fluid loss and secondary infections. In the past, the mortality

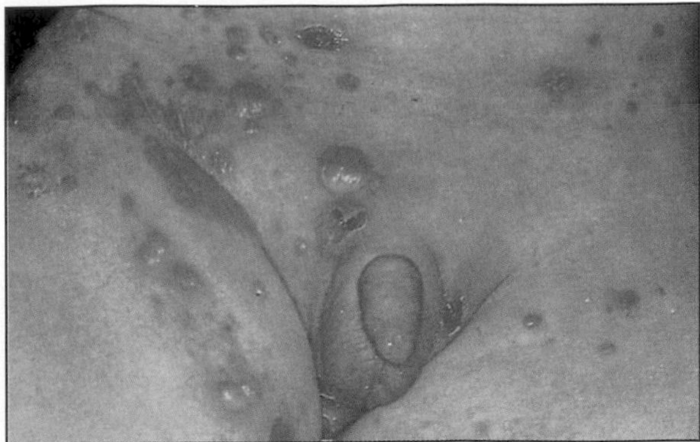

Fig. 4.3. Impetigo neonatorum

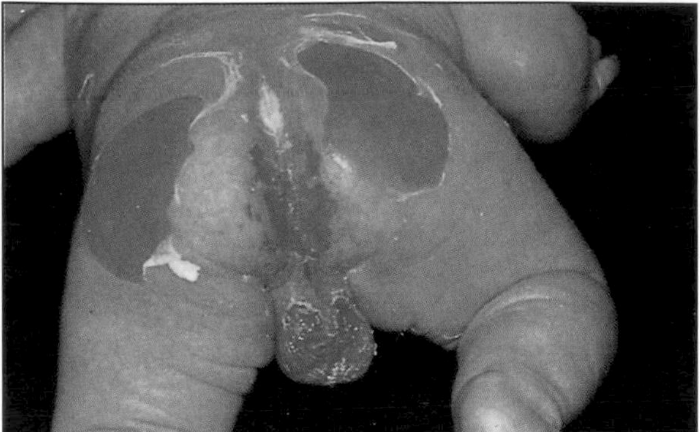

Fig. 4.4. Staphylococcal scalded skin syndrome

rate was high, but today almost all survive because of appropriate antistaphylococcal therapy. Often the infection is introduced by a nurse or parent who is a *S. aureus* carrier. Sometimes epidemics develop in newborn nurseries, causing considerable problems.

Staphylococcal Scalded Skin Syndrome

(LYELL 1956)

Synonyms. Dermatitis exfoliativa neonatorum (RITTER VON RITTERSHAIN 1878), Ritter disease, staphylococcal Lyell syndrome, toxic epidermal necrolysis, pemphigus neonatorum, SSSS

Definition. Widespread superficial skin loss caused by staphylococcal exfoliatin. We encourage use of the term staphylococcal scalded skin syndrome, saving toxic epidermal necrolysis for a widespread drug-induced skin loss with a different pathophysiology and prognosis.

Causative Organism. *Staphylococcus aureus*

Epidemiology. Usually infants or children up to age five are involved. Rarely, adults with renal disease or immunodeficiency may develop the disorder.

Etiology and Pathogenesis. The mechanisms are the same as in bullous impetigo. Infants are not able to neutralize the exfoliatins, perhaps because of an inadequate antibody response. Usually the *S. aureus* infection is in the oropharynx or vagina; the site is asymptomatic but allows excellent absorption of the toxin. In adults, there may be deep indolent abscesses or even osteomyelitis as a source of the bacteria and toxin.

Clinical Findings. Typically the patient has fever and is irritable, but otherwise looks well. Initially a subtle scarlatiniform rash develops with marked tenderness. The changes usually begin about the mouth and in the diaper area. They spread rapidly and the skin is easily separated by pressure (Nikolsky sign). Within 24–48 h, the entire body is covered by large, flaccid blisters that rupture easily and lie on the eroded skin (wet newspaper sign) (Fig. 4.4). Thus, the resemblance to a burn is striking, although the damage is never as deep as a burn, confined to the upper reaches of epidermis. The blister dries out and is shed in the form of large, irregular scales. Usually within 7–14 days, regeneration of the epidermis has begun and proceeds uneventfully without scarring. Despite the alarming clinical appearance, the patients are surprisingly healthy. In adults, the focal infection is more likely to be symptomatic than in children.

Histopathology. The biopsy at the edge of a blister shows a split high in the epidermis, just below the stratum corneum. This is in sharp contrast to toxic epidermal necrolysis, where full-thickness epidermal loss is seen. The balance of the epidermis and the dermis are normal. The quickest diagnosis can be made by studying frozen sections of such a biopsy. One can also freeze and section the blister roof, as shed by the patient, but occasionally false results are obtained, so that biopsy is usually preferable.

Laboratory Findings. One should culture the perineum, eyes and throat, looking for *S. aureus*, phage group II. The bacteria cannot be cultured from the skin.

Course and Prognosis. In infants and children, the mortality is less than 5%; in adults it approaches 50%, presumably because of more severe underlying disturbances.

Differential Diagnosis. Toxic epidermal necrolysis usually involves adults as part of a severe drug eruption, but it can be seen in children. The difference between severe bullous impetigo and staphylococcal scalded skin syndrome is one of degree. Scarlet fever can appear similar in the early stages, as can other toxic exanthems.

Therapy. Oral antistaphylococcal therapy is mandatory. Routine protective measures against secondary infection, replacement of fluids and temperature control are also important, although the young patients are relatively stable.

Nail Fold Infections

Paronychia

Synonym. Onychia periungualis. Paronychia is a word created from Greek roots meaning a condition (-ia) about (par-) the nail (-onych-). Panaritium is a deeper infection or felon.

Definition. Inflammation or infection of the nail fold.

Causative Organisms. *Staphylococcus aureus* is the most common cause of acute paronychia, while *Candida albicans* is responsible for many chronic lesions (Chap. 32).

Etiology and Pathogenesis. Paronychia usually involves some degree of cuticle or lateral nail fold damage or manipulation, offering access to microorganisms. The damage can lead to an acute infection or a chronic smoldering process.

Clinical Findings. There is erythema and swelling of the lateral or proximal nail fold, usually with associated cuticle damage, an ingrown nail or a history of trauma. Pus may ooze from the nail fold and crusts develop.

Laboratory Findings. Cultures should be taken and a smear performed. Biopsy is not helpful.

Differential Diagnosis. The main acute differential diagnostic point is a herpetic whitlow. With a history of recent or recurrent oral or labial HSV infections, repeated paronychia in the same location or an at-risk occupation such as dentistry, the chance of a viral infection is greater. Herpetic whitlow is usually more polycyclic and more likely to rupture. Fungal and candidal paronychiae are usually more chronic and have more obvious nail fold or nail involvement.

Therapy. Drainage and local disinfecting measures usually suffice. Because it is so hard to predict which cases will develop deeper involvement, many clinicians still prefer to use broad-spectrum antibiotic therapy.

Bulla Repens

Synonyms. Staphylococcal whitlow; *Umlauf* in German because the infection creeps under the sturdy acral stratum corneum around the nail.

Clinical Findings. Bulla repens is a bullous staphylococcal infection developing in the thick acral skin. It usually arises on the tip of the digit or on the volar surface as a firm well-circumscribed blister (Fig. 4.5). Because of its location, in an area with thick stratum corneum, the blister rarely ruptures. There is a slowly expanding erythema, and usually only one blister. Often the entire nail is surrounded, with involvement of the nail fold and bed, so that the nail becomes loose. The astonishingly tough blister may contain pus but more often has serious fluid. Once the blister is opened, there is an erosion and residual thick scale and crust. The lesion is often quite painful.

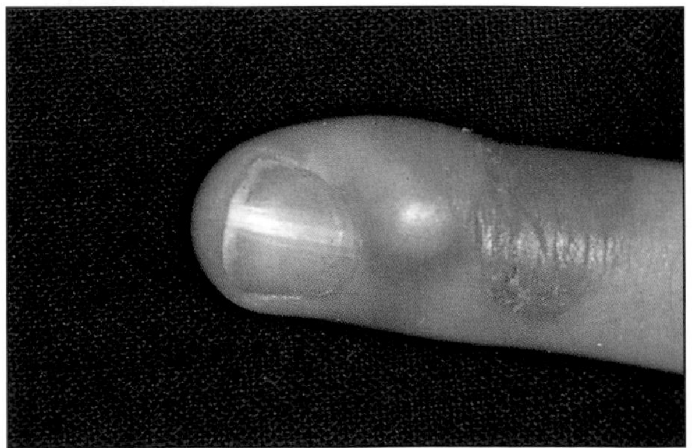

Fig. 4.5. Bulla repens

Differential Diagnosis. The differential diagnosis includes a herpetic whitlow and perhaps dermatitis repens (Chap. 16), which is localized pustular psoriasis of the finger tip.

Therapy. Superficial incision and drainage, as well as systemic antistaphylococcal therapy, are required.

Felon

Felon is another puzzling term, probably derived from the Latin term *fello*, meaning a wrongdoer. It refers to a deeper digital or closed space infection, with the potential to spread proximally along tendons and their sheaths causing infections of the deep tissues of the hands or feet. Patients also tend to be systemically ill with fever, leukocytosis and an elevated erythrocyte sedimentation rate. The distinction between bulla repens and felon is one of degree, although bulla repens is more superficial and bullous. Felons should be referred to a hand surgeon for appropriate drainage and also treated with systemic antistaphylococcal therapy.

Botryomycosis

Synonyms. Actinophytosis, bacterial pseudomycosis

Clinical Findings. Botryomycosis is a chronic infection of the skin which features sinus tracts and discharge of granules. Among the bacterial causes, *S. aureus* is the most common etiologic agent. Granules may be discharged from a usually solitary inflamed cystic area or deeper abscess. The most common location is the genital and perianal region; the hands and feet are also frequently involved. Often there has been a penetrating injury presumably inoculating the bacteria. The relative lack of oxygen may explain the unusual localized growth pattern with grain formation. Patients with HIV/AIDS and the hyper IgE syndrome are more likely to develop such infections and may have many other bacteria besides staphylococci. Botryomycosis is an uncommon complication of intramuscular corticosteroid injections.

Histopathology. Small granules are found in an abscess. They tend to be basophilic with an eosinophilic peripheral band, known as the SPLENDORE-HOEPPLI (1912) phenomenon, and probably representing deposits of host immunoglobulin. In contrast to actinomycosis and nocardiosis, no filaments are associated with the granules.

Differential Diagnosis. Clinically, botryomycosis presents as an infected cyst or small abscess. The histologic differential diagnosis includes actinomycosis, nocardiosis and mycetomas. The bacterial diseases are covered later in this chapter, while mycetomas are considered in Chap. 7.

Therapy. Debridement or excision is most essential. In a healthy host, no further treatment may be required. In immunosuppressed patients, long-term antistaphylococcal therapy has been recommended, but no large series are available.

Folliculitis

Definition. Inflammation of the hair follicle, usually clinically manifested as distinct papules or pustules. Table 4.5 indicates some of the different types of folliculitis.

Etiology and Pathogenesis. The hair follicle is an opening in the skin surface, inhibited by different microorganisms and with a different microenvironment. There are a long list of infectious causes of folliculitis, including bacteria, viruses, and fungi, as well as many noninfectious causes. Hyperhidrosis, maceration, friction from clothes, especially in the overweight, some medications such as corticosteroids and halogenated compounds, occlusive medications, skin care products and topical hydrocarbons, such as oils or tars (whether from medica-

Table 4.5. Types of folliculitis

Infectious
Bacterial (staphylococcal, gram-negative)
Fungal (dermatophytes, *Pityrosporum ovale*, *Candida albicans*)
Viral (herpes simplex virus)
Parasitic (*Demodex folliculorum*)
Inflammatory
Folliculitis decalvans
Eosinophilic folliculitis (infants, adults, HIV/AIDS)
Infundibulofolliculitis
Acne inversa (perifolliculitis capitis abscendens et suffodiens)
Mechanical
Chronic irritative (truck driver, blue jeans, acne mechanica)
Hot comb folliculitis
Pseudofolliculitis barbae
Acne keloidalis
Acne necroticans

tions or industrial exposures), are just a sampling of the predisposing factors in folliculitis. In addition, patients with reduced immunity, such as those with HIV/AIDS, have many different types of folliculitis (Chap. 2). Diabetes mellitus also seems to predispose to follicular infections. Typical sites for folliculitis include the scalp, face, neck and buttocks. The palms and soles are spared, as they bear no hair follicles.

Folliculitis is often not a self-contained disease. When the infection is high in the follicular canal, it can spread across the skin surface, producing a secondary pyoderma. When it is deeper, there is often perifollicular inflammation followed by destruction of the follicle wall. In Germany, this is called perifolliculitis; it represents an intermediate stage between folliculitis and furuncles or carbuncles. Many of the forms of folliculitis are considered below; while others are discussed throughout this book.

Suppurative Folliculitis

Synonym. Folliculitis; many subtypes are discussed below.

Causative Organism. Usually *Staphylococcus aureus*

Etiology and Pathogenesis. Infections of the terminal hairs are almost exclusively a disease of men. When women develop folliculitis, it involves the axilla, groin or legs, the three places where they have terminal hairs. Scalp folliculitis, for unclear reasons, is also more common in men.

Clinical Findings. The typical lesion of folliculitis is an inflamed papule or pustule. In contrast to superficial folliculitis, the lesions often itch. Typical locations include the scalp, especially the hairline (where excoriated folliculitis is sometimes called acne necrotica), face, axillae, buttocks and occasionally pubic hairs (Fig. 4.6). The lesions are often painful or pruritic, generally excoriated and usually have an erythematous periphery. There may be systemic symptoms such as fever or lymphadenopathy when the involvement is widespread.

Histopathology. Biopsies are occasionally done to help exclude fungal or viral folliculitis, or when the small red papules are not clinically distinct. There is infection of the entire follicle, usually with peri-

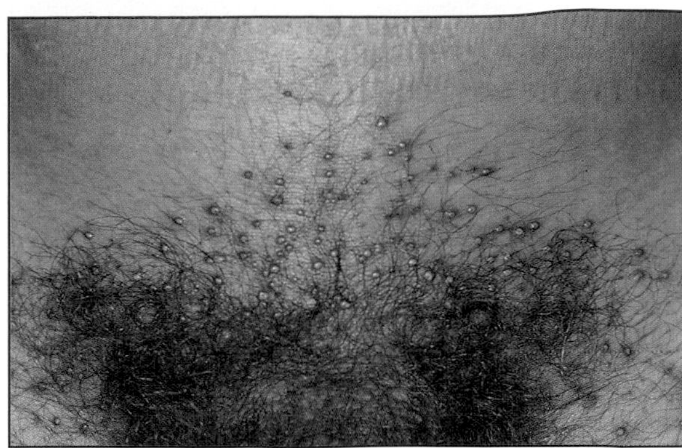

Fig. 4.6. Folliculitis

follicular edema, neutrophils in the dermis and usually some damage to the follicular wall. Multiple sections should be searched for fungi, yeast and *Demodex folliculorum*. The presence of bacteria can be demonstrated with special stains but is of little clinical benefit.

Laboratory Findings. Cultures are only useful if an intact pustule is found. Otherwise, one will invariably grow staphylococci and streptococci from the eroded, inflamed skin.

Course and Prognosis. Folliculitis in most cases is chronic and recurrent, indicating that local factors are just as important as eradication of infection. Patients with recurrent folliculitis may be carrying *S. aureus* in the nares or perineum; these regions should be cultured.

Differential Diagnosis. The differential diagnosis for folliculitis includes all the diseases discussed in this section.

Therapy

Systemic. Antistaphylococcal antibiotics produce a temporary improvement, but relapses are common and eventually resistant organisms appear. If nasal carriage is identified, it should be treated as discussed under furuncles.

Topical. We usually use antibiotic drying solutions or lotions, just as might be used for acne. If marked inflammation is present, a corticosteroid lotion can be used as an after-shave for a short period of time.

Folliculitis Simplex Barbae

Synonyms. Folliculitis of the beard, sycosis barbae

This is the most common variant of ordinary folliculitis. It involves the beard region and especially the side of the neck. In the latter region, the trauma of tight collars magnifies the problem of bacterial infection. On the neck, the lesions initially resemble superficial folliculitis with distinct pustules penetrated by hairs and surrounded by erythema. The infection may be spread by shaving, so disposable razors are recommended; patients often complain of burning and pain when shaving. A typical finding is the coalescence of multiple lesions on the upper lip, producing grouped erythematous papules most of which are penetrated by a hair. The differential diagnosis includes fungal folliculitis, rarely candidal folliculitis and in blacks, pseudofolliculitis barbae. Treatment includes topical disinfectants and occasionally corticosteroid lotions when marked inflammation is present. When the problem is chronic or systemic symptoms are present, oral antibiotics can be used, but they rarely produce a cure. Epilation of the hairs increases the inflammation and is probably best avoided. Patients are also advised not to trim their beard hairs too closely until the infection remits somewhat.

Folliculitis Eczematosa Barbae

Sometimes both dermatitis of the beard region and folliculitis occur simultaneously. Either problem can come first, but the usual scenario is folliculitis in a patient with atopic dermatitis. The infection usually begins on the upper lip and spreads to involve the entire perioral region and chin. The surface often has dried yellow secretions admixed with erosions; the hairs can be easily epilated. Deeper abscesses or sinus tracts are unusual, in contrast to fungal folliculitis which forms the main differential diagnostic question. Therapy is difficult, as both the folliculitis and the dermatitis must be treated. In this scenario, a search for staphylococcal carriage is mandatory.

Folliculitis Eczematosa Vestibuli Nasi

This awesome sounding tongue twister is actually a fairly common problem. Patients develop a staphylococcal infection of the vibrissae, or thick hairs of the nares. The typical complaint is of pain in the opening of the nostril. There are two features: dermatitic changes around the nostrils and painful papules or nodules within. Prior to antibiotics, such infections could spread internally into the CNS but today the problem is insignificant. Sometimes a follicle will rupture and perforate towards the outside; this is known as folliculitis narium perforans. Occasionally HSV can produce a similar picture. Systemic antistaphylococcal antibiotics as well as an antibiotic nasal ointment or cream are useful. Almost by definition the patients are staphylococcal carriers, so this should be pursued.

Tufted Hair Folliculitis

Some patients with folliculitis caused by *S. aureus* develop an unusual clinical condition, with scarring alopecia and tufts of hairs emerging from single follicular openings. This may be a variant of folliculitis decalvans but the relationship to staphylococci has been better established. Why multiple hairs emerge from the same follicle remains unclear. Antibiotic therapy is helpful in the early stages, but does not influence the scarring.

Perforating Folliculitis

All suppurative folliculitis is perforating, as the follicle wall is damaged and the infection moves into the adjacent dermis. Perforating folliculitis was identified as a unique disease by MEHREGAN and COSKEY (1968), but we do not accept it as a diagnosis, as discussed in Chap. 25.

Superficial Folliculitis

Synonyms. Ostiofolliculitis, BOCKHART (1887) folliculitis

Definition. Very superficial infection of the hair follicle presenting as tiny pustules.

Causative Organism. *Staphylococcus aureus* is usually identified, but other bacteria may be found. In some cases, no single agent is identified.

Epidemiology. This disease is more common in humid climates or in the summer months in temperate regions. Children are often affected with scalp lesions; among adults, men are more often involved then women.

Etiology and Pathogenesis. Maceration and occlusion are the most likely triggers of superficial

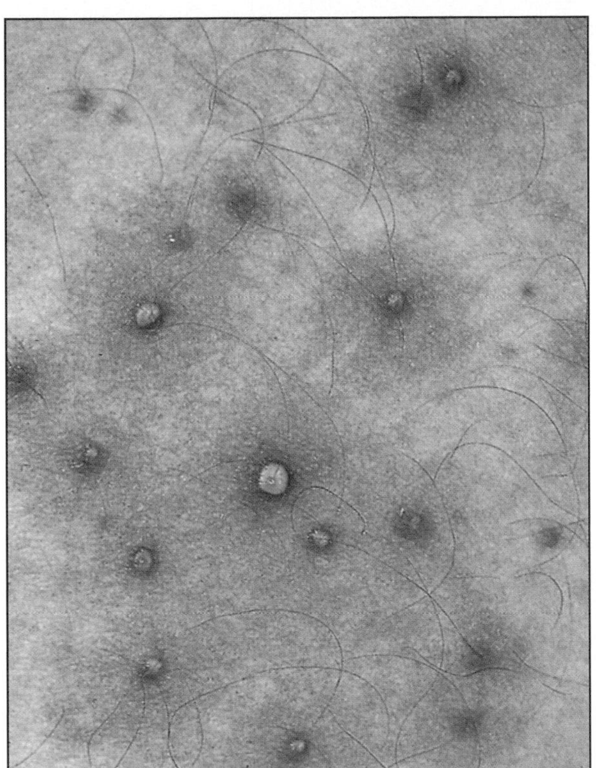

Fig. 4.7. Superficial folliculitis

folliculitis, which seems less dependent on systemic factors than does ordinary folliculitis.

Clinical Findings. The initial clinical finding is pustules in a follicular distribution often associated with hairs (Fig. 4.7). If vellus follicles are involved, the hairs are harder to see. The pustules are tense, yellow dome-shaped lesions, usually the size of a pin head. There is often a peripheral erythema. As the lesions burst, crust and erythema may obscure their follicular origin. In children, the scalp is the most common site. In adults, other frequent sites include the neck, face and axillae. Even without treatment, the course is usually self-limited. On occasion, in adults the folliculitis will become chronic.

Histopathology. Biopsy shows neutrophils in just the upper aspect of the follicle, the infundibulum. If the pustule is intact, it will be subcorneal, just as with impetigo.

Laboratory Findings. If systemic antibiotics are going to be used, a culture should be taken.

Differential Diagnosis. The acute lesions are almost unmistakable. Other forms of folliculitis should be excluded. Occasionally, candidal folliculitis about the mouth can appear similarly. Occlusion and follicular irritation, as through the use of tar products or corticosteroids, also produce superficial follicular pustules, as can acne, halogenoderma and even a syphilid.

Therapy

Systemic. Antistaphylococcal coverage should be provided if systemic antibiotics are used. They generally should be reserved for widespread or resistant disease.

Topical. Drying therapy with antibiotic or disinfectant solutions or shake lotions is usually sufficient. One can mechanically open the intact pustules. Occlusive topical products should be avoided. Hygiene should be meticulous to avoid transferring the bacteria to other body regions or family members.

Gram-Negative Folliculitis

(Fulton et al. 1968)

Definition. Chronic recurrent folliculitis of the mid-face caused by gram-negative bacteria primarily in acne patients.

Causative Organisms. Type 1: *Enterobacter, Klebsiella, Escherichia coli*; Type 2: *Proteus* species. Often several different organisms are present.

Epidemiology. Relatively common complication of acne or rosacea, almost exclusively limited to adult men with oily skin.

Etiology and Pathogenesis. The long-term use of oral or, less often, topical antibiotics can produce a microenvironment in which the normal bacteria are destroyed and gram-negative organisms move into the vacuum. The nares and genitourinary tract may harbor the same bacteria. In some situations, immunosuppressed patients are at increased risk of gram-negative folliculitis.

Clinical Findings. There are two clinical subtypes. In type 1, multiple papules and pustules are present, usually centered about the nose. In type 2, fewer but deeper nodules are present in the same distribution. In some patients, there is what clinically appears to be antibiotic-resistant acne without any distinguishing features. The lesions seem particularly likely to start on the upper lip and nasolabial

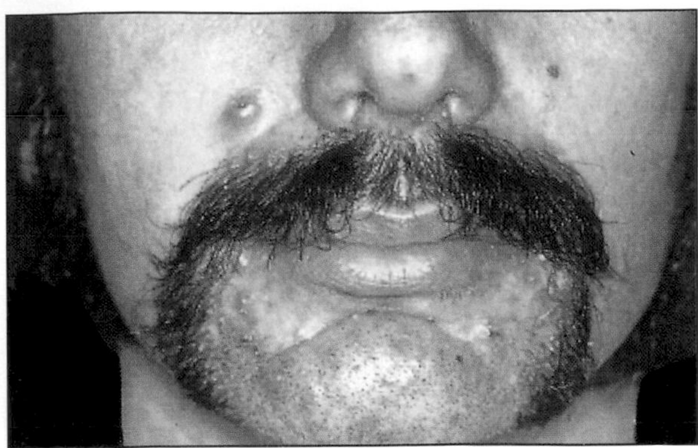

Fig. 4.8. Gram-negative folliculitis

fold and slowly spread (Fig. 4.8). Any given lesion is identical to typical gram-positive folliculitis.

Laboratory Findings. If an acne patient has large, painful or therapy-resistant pustules about the nose, cultures should be taken of an intact pustule's content and of the nares, looking especially for gram-negative organisms.

Differential Diagnosis. In addition to acne and rosacea, the differential diagnosis includes all the other forms of folliculitis, especially staphylococcal folliculitis.

Therapy

Systemic. The therapy of gram-negative folliculitis is difficult. In past, the main approach was systemic antibiotics with a gram-negative spectrum, such as cephalosporins, or more recently, quinolones such as ciprofloxacin. Systemic isotretinoin is the treatment of choice in our opinion. We use 0.5–1.5 mg/kg for 3–5 months; this is a somewhat higher dosage than our usual acne regimen. The retinoids eliminate the seborrhea, treat the acne and remove the microenvironment for the organisms, which then disappear without specific antibacterial therapy. Long-term remissions are the rule. If genitourinary tract infection is simultaneously present, then antibiotics and retinoids can be combined.

Topical. Benzoyl peroxide is probably the most helpful, but still not the answer. Topical antibiotics just exacerbate the problem. Shaving can spread the infection, so disposable razors should be considered.

Hot Tub Folliculitis

(McCausland and Cox 1975)

Synonyms. Hot tub dermatitis, whirl pool folliculitis or dermatitis. Skin diver's dermatitis or folliculitis is almost the same.

Definition. *Pseudomonas aeruginosa* folliculitis induced by warmth, maceration or a combination of both.

Causative Organism. *Pseudomonas aeruginosa*, often seroytpe 0:11.

Etiology and Pathogenesis. The epidemiology and the etiology are inseparable. Hot tub or whirlpool use is the key predisposing factor. Even with relatively meticulous disinfectant control of the water, contamination with *P. aeruginosa* can occur. Occasionally the water may be clouded or have an unpleasant smell, but this is usually not the case. When individuals use the facility, the warm water hydrates their stratum corneum and exposes tiny injuries, especially around follicles, easing access for the bacteria. Rates of infection among users of contaminated hot tubs have ranged from 7% to 100%, probably reflecting bacterial load and how extensively the facility was used.

Rarely, warm water boilers are contaminated, so that ordinary bathing or showering may lead to infection, or an entire load of wash may be contaminated. A similar condition can occur in skin divers, who may have small amounts of infected water trapped between their skin and their suit.

Clinical Findings. Tiny red macules, papules and pustules are found primarily on the trunk (Fig. 4.9). The usual complaint is pruritus. Sometimes larger abscesses evolve. Swelling of the breasts has been described, but is uncommon. Signs of systemic infection are equally rare, but ear infections and even sepsis have occurred. Usually the process is mild and self-limited, resolving after 7–10 days.

Laboratory Findings. Culture usually reveals *P. aeruginosa*. A biopsy is of little benefit.

Differential Diagnosis. Other forms of folliculitis, miliaria and swimmers' itch (among divers) are the main considerations.

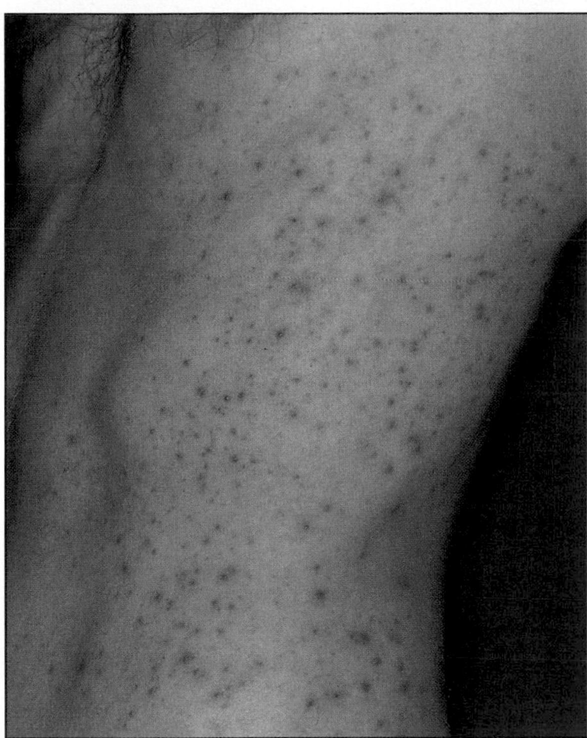

Fig. 4.9. Hot tub folliculitis

Therapy. Usually systemic antibiotic therapy is not needed. Topical drying measures suffice. If questions exist regarding systemic features, then a course of systemic antibiotics is appropriate.

Prophylaxis. The water should be maintained at the appropriate pH with the indicated level of chlorine or bromine. It is simplest to drain the hot tub or whirl pool and start again, rather than trying to shock or over-halogenate the water.

Other Infectious Types of Folliculitis

A number of other organisms can cause folliculitis.

- Herpetic folliculitis: Usually in men, herpetic folliculitis often is spread from a cold sore by shaving. Later it may recur as pruritic follicular vesicles and pustules which tend to become superficially eroded. If vesicles are seen or if there is evidence for simultaneous HSV infection elsewhere, always do a Tzanck smear.
- Candidal folliculitis: *C. albicans* is a rare cause of perioral folliculitis, often associated with perlèche and found in immunocompromised patients. The pustules are full of hyphae. The main differential diagnosis includes gram-negative folliculitis.
- Fungal folliculitis: Women with tinea pedis may inoculate the hair follicles of their legs with fungi; the resulting nodular inflammatory folliculitis is known as Majocchi granuloma. Occlusive corticosteroids applied erroneously to dermatophyte infections may induce a similar picture.
- *Pityrosporum ovale* folliculitis. While this problem can be seen in ordinary individuals, it is perhaps more common in those with HIV/AIDS. The lesions are primarily truncal and biopsy reveals large numbers of organisms.
- *Demodex folliculorum* folliculitis. An abnormal inflammatory response to *D. folliculorum* resembles rosacea, but is more pustular. It typically occurs on the face of elderly patients, but may cause truncal lesions mimicking ordinary folliculitis in HIV/AIDS.

Noninfectious Folliculitis

There are a number of disorders in which there are varying degrees of follicular inflammation and scarring. While bacteria may be cultured, none of the disorders appears to be strictly bacterial. We have included the diseases here rather than under disorders of hairs because they often enter the differential diagnosis of infectious folliculitis.

Folliculitis Decalvans

(Quinquand 1888)

Synonyms. Folliculitis spinulosa decalvans, folliculitis decalvans capilliti

Definition. Uncommon scarring folliculitis of scalp that leads to alopecia [decalvans (Latin) = making bald].

Epidemiology. Very uncommon disorder, primarily seen in adult men.

Etiology and Pathogenesis. The nature of folliculitis decalvans is unclear. Bacteria may be cultured, most often *S. aureus*, but antibacterial therapy brings little relief. Patients may be immunosuppressed, either with diabetes mellitus, chronic renal disease, gammopathy or due to iatrogenic immunosuppression.

Clinical Findings. The initial lesions are localized papules and nodules of folliculitis, with erythema, pus and almost always scale and crust

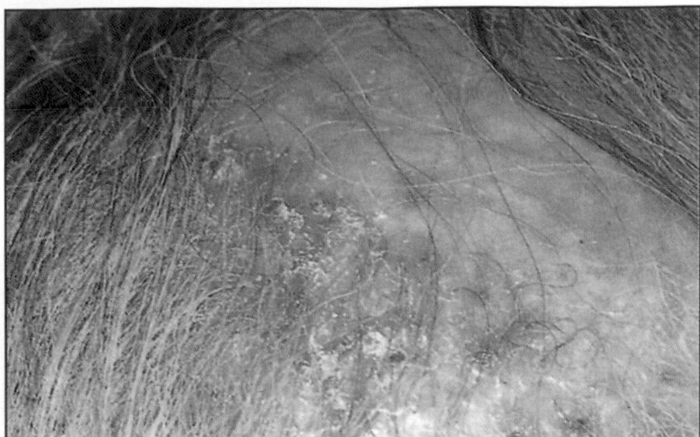

Fig. 4.10. Folliculitis decalvans

(Fig. 4.10). The inflamed follicles coalesce with the inflammation, extending deeply and laterally. Eventually a bald patch evolves, speckled with occasional residual hairs, sometimes as tufts of hairs. The skin becomes atrophic, resembling pseudopelade. At the periphery, follicular pustules continue to form. The disease is chronic and difficult to interrupt.

Histopathology. Biopsies from the early lesions show neutrophilic folliculitis. Frank abscesses can be seen within the follicles; the adjacent dermis may also contain plasma cells. Later on there is nonspecific scarring alopecia.

Differential Diagnosis. During the acute stage, a highly inflammatory tinea capitis is similar, but usually seen in children. The scarring stage resembles all other types of scarring alopecia, including discoid lupus erythematosus and lichen planus. Keratosis follicularis spinulosa decalvans affects only men and is usually most severe prior to puberty (Chap. 17); it lacks pustules.

Therapy

Systemic. We generally try systemic antibiotics, based on culture results, but the effects are temporary and often disappointing. In severe cases, short courses of systemic corticosteroids are indicated to reduce inflammation. Dapsone 100–150 mg daily for several months is worth trying. If the patient is a nasal carrier of *S. aureus*, this problem should be addressed.

Topical. Lotions or solutions containing antibiotics such as erythromycin can be tried, often combined with topical corticosteroids.

Facial Folliculitis Decalvans

Synonyms. Folliculitis sycosiformis atrophicans (Hoffmann 1931), ulerythema sycosiforme, lupoid sycosis (Brocq 1888)

Folliculitis decalvans can also affect the face, involving the eyelids or beard hair (Fig. 4.11). The clinical features are similar; central atrophy and alopecia with peripheral folliculitis. It seems that bacteria play a more central role in the facial form, at least in terms of response to therapy. As the synonyms suggest, the main differential diagnostic question was lupus vulgaris; today one thinks primarily of discoid lupus erythematosus. The treatment is just as for folliculitis decalvans of the scalp, listed above.

Infundibulofolliculitis

Synonym. Disseminate and recurrent infundibulofolliculitis

Some black men have multiple tiny papules, usually following the skin lines in a beaded pattern along

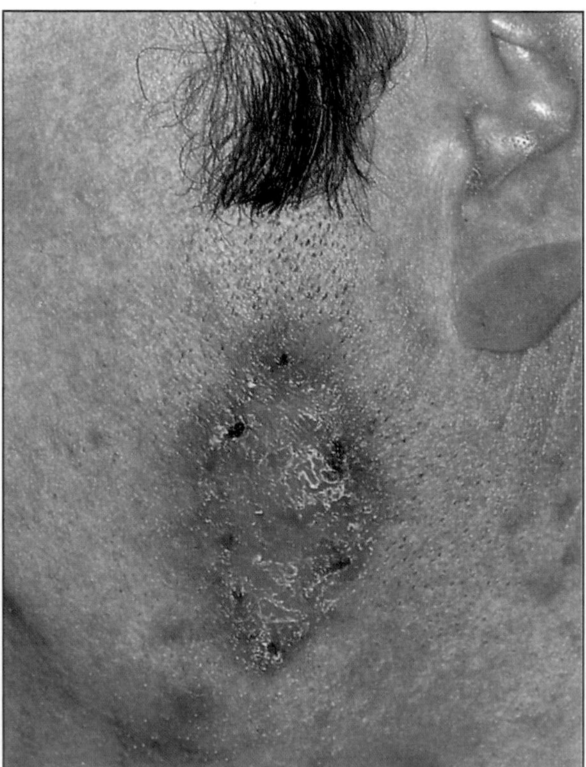

Fig. 4.11. Folliculitis decalvans faciei

the upper trunk. The distribution is similar to beaded juxtaclavicular lines but the lesions itch and may become inflamed. The problem is not bacterial, but biopsy reveals a very superficial folliculitis without a pustule. Treatment is difficult; antipruritic measures are the only hope, as antibiotics bring no improvement.

Actinic Superficial Folliculitis

(Nieboer 1985)

Synonym. Actinic folliculitis

Rare patients develop sterile follicular pustules 24–36 h following sunlight exposure. They probably represent part of the spectrum of acne aestivalis (Chap. 28). On biopsy there is suppurative folliculitis of the superficial aspect of the follicle, allowing separation from polymorphic light eruption. Lesions resolve spontaneously without scarring. Detailed photobiologic information is not available.

Eosinophilic Folliculitis

Eosinophilic folliculitis is a histologic description; not a diagnosis. There are at least three clinical settings in which it is regularly founded: eosinophilic pustular folliculitis of infancy, eosinophilic pustular folliculitis of adults (Ofuji disease) and eosinophilic folliculitis of HIV/AIDS. In addition, fungal folliculitis often features eosinophils, as can other infectious forms.

Eosinophilic Pustular Folliculitis of Infancy

Synonym. Eosinophilic pustulosis of the scalp

Definition. Uncommon pustular eruption of the scalp and forehead in first year of life.

Epidemiology. Boys are much more often involved than girls. Most patients are several months old; only a few cases have been present at birth.

Etiology and Pathogenesis. The etiology is unknown. There are similarities with erythema toxicum neonatorum, but it, by definition, fades after a few days. Microbial studies have all been negative. Many patients have atopic dermatitis. No association with HIV/AIDS or other immunodeficiencies has been shown.

Clinical Findings. The infants experience recurrent pustules on their scalp and forehead, only rarely involving other parts of the body, in contrast to the acral location of infantile acropustulosis. The lesions are small, tend to crust after a few days and resolve without scarring over weeks. Recurrences are the rule but the eruption tends to burn out.

Histopathology. Microscopic examination shows a folliculitis with abundant eosinophils that also enter the epidermis, producing either eosinophilic spongiosis or subcorneal pustules full of eosinophils, as well as diffusely involving the dermis.

Laboratory Findings. There may be elevated blood eosinophils.

Differential Diagnosis. The list is long and includes all forms of infectious folliculitis, miliaria, Langerhans cell histiocytosis, and scabies.

Therapy. Most pediatric cases have been treated with low- to mid-potency topical corticosteroids. Systemic corticosteroids have also been endorsed. The few patients we have followed required no therapy. Many of the approaches discussed under the adult form could probably be tried here in desperate cases.

Eosinophilic Pustular Folliculitis

(Ofuji 1970)

Synonyms. Ofuji disease, sterile eosinophilic pustulosis, eosinophilic pustular dermatosis, circinate eosinophilic dermatosis

Definition. Noninfectious folliculitis, most common among Japanese, with abundant eosinophilic infiltrates.

Epidemiology. Ofuji and colleagues first described eosinophilic pustular folliculitis among Japanese patients. In that population, it is primarily a disease of young adult men, but occasionally described in children and even at birth. Later cases were described in non Asian patients, but in the early 1980s the whole issue became confusing. HIV/AIDS patients also have a maddening pruritic eosinophilic folliculitis; after many years of debate, the consensus is now that this represents a different disorder than that described by Ofuji.

Etiology and Pathogenesis. The cause is unknown. A number of immune phenomena have been identified, including eosinophilic chemotactic factors and autoantibodies, but their roles are unclear.

Clinical Findings. The initial lesions are pruritic papules located on the face (Fig. 4.12) or trunk. They evolve into confluent polycyclic plaques with peripheral pustules and central clearing, producing a bizarre pattern. There may be residual hyperpigmentation. About 20% of patients show involve-

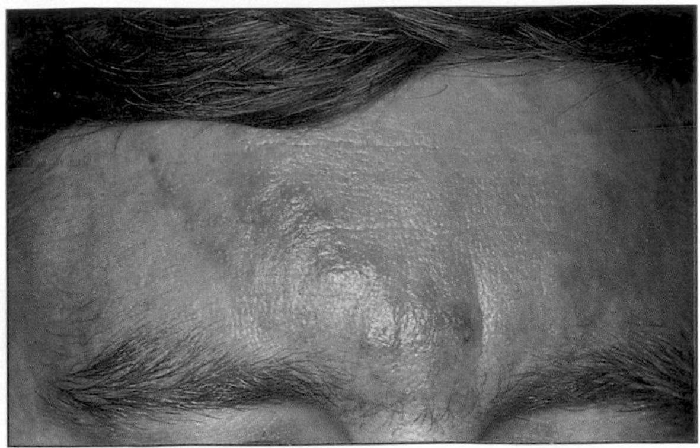

Fig. 4.12. Eosinophilic pustular folliculitis. (Courtesy of Reinhard Breit, M.D., Munich, Germany)

ment of the palms and soles, indicating that the process is not entirely follicular. In other patients, the ordinary pattern of folliculitis is seen, with scattered inflamed nodules.

Histopathology. On biopsy, there is an intense eosinophilic infiltrate involving both the follicles and the adjacent dermis. Usually the infiltrate is more intense in the upper parts of the follicle. Lesions on the palms and soles show subcorneal pustules. One should always do a PAS stain to exclude possible fungal folliculitis. In most instances, immunofluoresecent examination is negative.

Laboratory Findings. There may be elevated blood IgE and eosinophil levels. For safety's sake, HIV screening is probably indicated, but the connection is flimsy.

Course and Prognosis. Ofuji's patients showed a very chronic course, frequently waxing and waning. Often the lesions heal with hyperpigmentation or scarring.

Differential Diagnosis. The main differential diagnostic point is eosinophilic folliculitis of HIV/AIDS. In the latter disorder, the pruritus is overwhelming, the lesions tend to be more numerous and diffuse, not arranged in patterns, and there is usually not an elevated eosinophil count. How much these differences are intrinsic and how much thay reflect the underlying HIV/AIDS is a matter of discussion. Otherwise one must consider all the disorders in this chapter as well as early pustular psoriasis and impetiginized nummular dermatitis. On the scalp, tina capitis, folliculitis decalvans, and erosive pustular dermatosis may appear similar.

Therapy

Systemic. Dapsone (100–150 mg daily) appears to be the most effective agent; systemic corticosteroids have also been used, occasionally combined with erythromycin or other antibiotics. If pruritus is severe, antihistamines can be used. In some cases, nonsteroidal antiinflammatory drugs are useful.

Phototherapy. Phototherapy with PUVA or PUVA bath appears helpful.

Topical. Corticosteroid and antipruritic agents should be tried first. They often suffice.

Eosinophilic Folliculitis of HIV/AIDS

This entity is considered in Chapter 2. In short, the lesions are intensely pruritic and scattered over the trunk as typical lesions of ordinary folliculitis without any patterning.

Mechanical Folliculitis

Chronic Irritative Folliculitis

There are some settings in which mechanical trauma and maceration are more important factors than any one organism. Two common scenarios are "blue jean folliculitis" and "truck driver's folliculitis." In the former, individuals with hairy legs and too tight pants get many small irritated pustules. In the later, prolonged sitting with sweating and friction, whether it be in a truck or on a plastic-coated chair at work, lead to follicular irritation. Perhaps because of the anatomy of the buttocks, the lesions tend to be deeper and more painful. Another variant is acne mechanica, in which young athletes get a follicular irritation from the combination of excessive perspiration and friction. The best documented scenario is under the shoulder pads and on the nape in American football players, but any situation featuring friction and moisture can produce a folliculitis. While organisms can be cultured, there is no one single pathogen. In general, trying to correct the predisposing cause is the best approach. Topical disinfectants, such as antibiotic solutions, can be chosen to reduce the surface flora and perhaps ameliorate the problem somewhat.

Hot Comb Folliculitis

Blacks may use oils and heated combs when they wish to straighten their scalp hairs. The combination of tension and heat on the hair, tugging on the follicle, and perhaps hot oil dripping into the follicle can produce an intense scarring folliculitis. This unusual complication is considered in Chapter 66.

Pseudofolliculitis Barbae

This is primarily a problem of blacks, in which hairs reenter the skin inducing a perifollicular inflammation and often scarring. It is covered in Chapter 66.

Other Forms of Folliculitis

Perifolliculitis Capitis Abscedens et Suffodiens

(HOFFMANN 1908)

Definition. Severe destructive folliculitis leading to scarring alopecia; often associated with sinus tracts, fistulas and recurrent gram-negative infections.

Epidemiology. Perifolliculitis capitis abscedens et suffodiens is often part of the acne inversa spectrum (Chap. 28) and may be more common in blacks (Chap. 66). It is seen almost exclusively in young men.

Etiology and Pathogenesis. The cause is unknown. Tufted or bundled hairs may predispose to the problem, as when many hairs are grouped, the follicular opening may be widened and more easily infected.

Clinical Findings. The disease process can occur on the scalp or nape. Initially a severe deep folliculitis is observed. The persistent inflammation leads to destruction of follicles (Fig. 4.13). Often fluid-filled masses are present, representing subcutaneous liquefaction necrosis. As the hairs are lost, subcutaneous tracts may tunnel down to the galea. The skin may be covered with crusts and scales; when one presses on the scalp, pus often oozes out of multiple follicular openings. Later there is a "moth-eaten" scarring alopecia, usually with bridged scars jumping over a remnant of normal skin and keloids. Flare-ups are frequent and the disease is very chronic.

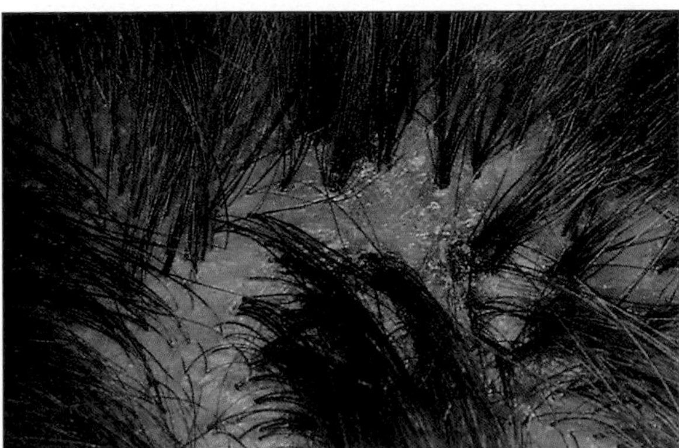

Fig. 4.13. Perifolliculitis capitis abscedens et suffodiens with tufted hairs

Histopathology. Microscopic evaluation brings little information, showing granulomatous inflammation, necrosis and scarring.

Laboratory Findings. Bacterial cultures are also of little help, as a wide variety of organisms can be found. Often, gram-negative bacteria prevail.

Differential Diagnosis. Acne keloidalis (Chap. 66) can be similar but is usually on the nape and rarely has pus or abscesses. Other forms of severe folliculitis are also similar but rarely so extreme.

Therapy. Perifolliculitis capitis abscedens et suffodiens is extremely difficult to treat.

Systemic. Acute flare-ups are best treated with broad-spectrum antibiotics, usually administered for 4–6 weeks. Systemic corticosteroids (40–60 mg daily of prednisone, tapered over 3 weeks) may interrupt the inflammatory response and allow more rapid healing. We have seen good results with subsequent treatment with isotretinoin 1 mg/kg daily for 12–20 weeks in an occasional patient.

Topical. Local care is important but rarely suffices. We generally employ disinfectant solutions such as chinosol. Epilation of involved follicles may reduce inflammation and spread.

Surgical. If the process quiets down, surgical excision of scarred areas is recommended.

Acne Necrotica

(BAUM 1910)

Synonyms. Acne varioliformis, necrotizing lymphocytic folliculitis

Definition. Chronic pruritic eruption of the hairline and scalp which heals with varioliform scars.

Etiology and Pathogenesis. This uncommon disorder may be nothing more than excoriated bacterial folliculitis, although there are some distinctive

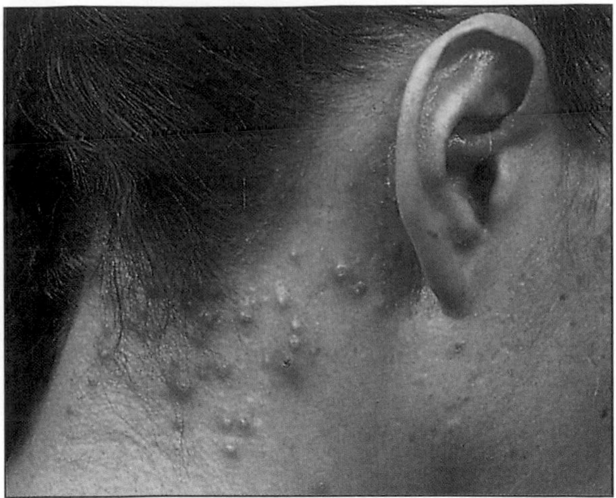

Fig. 4.14. Acne necrotica

clinical features. Most patients are adult women. Rarely herpes simplex virus is found. While bacteria can occasionally be cultured, the response to antibiotics is minimal. The primary lesion may be ordinary folliculitis, while individual differences in the inflammatory response lead to the distinctive clinical course.

Clinical Findings. The classic lesions are intensely pruritic papules that arise along the hair line (Fig. 4.14). The most common sites are the nape and the temporal region. The 2–4-mm, red firm papules usually lie very close to the hairline, whether they are on the free skin or the scalp. When the patient is a balding male, then the area of involvement follows the new hair border. The papules rapidly crust, forming a papulonecrotic lesion. This is where the controversy starts – does scratching produce the excoriation and crust, or is there a unique biologic process? In any event, the lesion is distinct; it often shows slight hemorrhage, a central yellow-brown crust and peripheral erythema. Over weeks it slowly involutes, leaving behind a varioliform scar.

Histopathology. Most biopsy reports describe more advanced crusted lesions, in which there is epidermal damage and a mixed dermal inflammatory infiltrate. Early lesions, however, show a lymphocytic infiltrate about the follicle but also involving other adnexal structures and sometimes causing spongiosis.

Differential Diagnosis. In the past, the main issue was papulonecrotic tuberculid. The individual lesions resemble hydroa vacciniforme but the overall picture is different. Occasionally leukocytoclastic vasculitis may appear similar, but the location along the hair line is almost unheard of. Another confusing disorder is acne necrotica miliaris; this is generally accepted to be excoriated folliculitis of the scalp in patients with atopic dermatitis.

Therapy

Systemic. Antibiotics are usually disappointing. We have treated a limited number of patients with isotretinoin, in the standard acne dosages, with good results. Corticosteroids often bring immediate improvement.

Topical. External applications are generally ineffective; high-potency topical corticosteroids may help reduce the pruritus. In other patients, benzoyl peroxide has been helpful.

Furuncle

Synonym. Boil

Definition. Deep inflammatory nodule with central pus that develops from a bacterial hair follicle infection.

Causative Organism. *Staphylococcus aureus*

Epidemiology. Furuncles are very common, especially under conditions of poor hygiene or reduced immune status. Most patients are perfectly healthy with no obvious reason for an infection. There may be autoinoculation from the nares or perineum by the patient, or transfer via close personal contact or even contaminated clothes or wash cloths. In hospitals, nursing personal and fomites are the usual means of spread. Close contact in sports, especially wrestling, has also been responsible for epidemics of furunculosis.

Etiology and Pathogenesis. The staphylococci enter the follicle from the outside and multiply, eliciting an intense inflammatory response. This probably contains many infections, but in the presence of corticosteroid or immunosuppressive therapy, diabetes mellitus, HIV/AIDS, other immune defects and wasting illnesses, the process may progress more rapidly. Many furuncles arise in patients with atopic dermatitis who have a heavy skin carriage of *S. aureus* and minor defects in their skin surface. Rubbing is also a factor, as furuncles are more common in areas of friction, e.g., under a bra strap, or worsened by drying with a towel. It is unclear why some individuals get furuncles and others, multiple lesions of superficial folliculitis.

Clinical Findings. Furuncles can be found on all body sites where hairs are present. Especially common locations are the nape, face, axilla, buttocks, arms and legs, as well as nasal vestibule and external ear canal. A furuncle starts with a small, yellow creamy pustule that rapidly evolves into a red nodule, often with a central yellow plug (Fig. 4.15). As the lesion expands, it becomes painful, tense and often associated with local edema, lymphangitis, regional lymphadenopathy and fever.

The inflammation and necrosis continue to advance. After a few days, the pustule is replaced by a yellow-brown crust. The involved hairs are usually destroyed. Eventually the central part of the nodule becomes soft and drains spontaneously. After an initial discharge of pus, there is a plug-like concentration which takes a little while to free itself up. Once the plug is out, the defect is closed by granulation tissue, evolving into a scar. Sometimes furuncles do not rupture, but simply heal after a longer period of time with a depressed scar.

Some furuncles are considered more dangerous than others. Traditionally those involving the midface have been feared because of the possibility of cavernous sinus thrombosis. Thus lesions about the nose, such as those involving the vibrissae, deserve close attention. Fortunately with effective antibiotics the risk is minimal. The upper lip is another troublesome location. The deep nature of the hairs and the loose structure of the dermis lead to deep infections with marked edema and little tendency to liquefaction and drainage. Any patient with fever, chills or lymphadenopathy associated with a furuncle is obviously septic or headed in that direction and should be regarded as such. Complications such as endocarditis and osteomyelitis have been associated with furuncles.

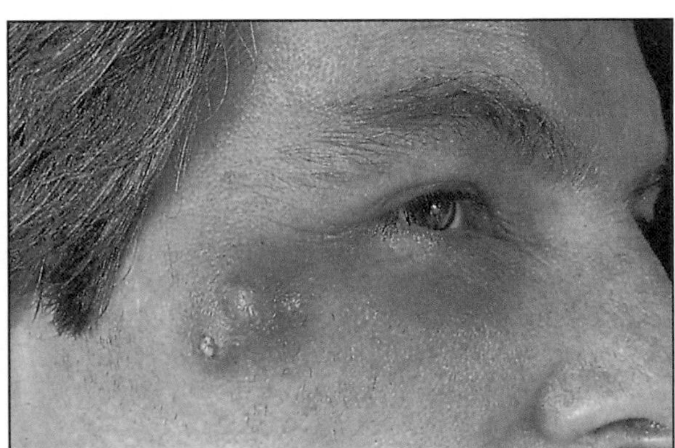

Fig. 4.15. Furuncle

Histopathology. Biopsies are of little value, but early on they show follicular-based neutrophilic infection. Later on there is granulomatous inflammation with giant cells, necrosis and eventually scarring.

Laboratory Findings. While *S. aureus* is usually found, it is worth doing a culture and assessing sensitivity to best guide therapy.

Differential Diagnosis. A given lesion of acne inversa in the axilla or groin can be identical. The distribution is different, and the scarring usually is associated with sinus tracts. Acne inversa lesions tend not to liquefy and rupture. In addition, large pustules in acne are also clinically identical to furuncles; the background usually tells the story, although acne patients seem prone to also develop furuncles, that is, to have both *S. aureus*-induced lesions and acne, especially when they are on systemic isotretinoin. Kerions and other inflammatory tinea infections look similar. Any organism can produce a furuncle under the right circumstances. In travelers, for example, one must consider myiasis and many other infections.

Therapy

Systemic. Appropriate antistaphylococcal therapy is required, based on local antibiotic sensitivity profiles and the patient's age and weight. In general, penicillinase-resistant penicillins or cephalosporins are used. If systemic symptoms are marked or the patient is immune-compromised, hospitalization and intravenous therapy should be considered.

Topical. Drawing ointments are popular in Germany, usually based on ichthyol, a concentrated shale oil similar to the tar family. They are generally not needed if systemic antibiotics are promptly started. Otherwise, a topical antibacterial lotion, such as povidone-iodine solution, can be used to clean the area and as a dressing.

Surgical. Whether or not to incise a furuncle is controversial. If the patient is not on systemic antibiotics, it is clearly unwise because of risk of systemic spread. Patients should be strongly encouraged not to manipulate their lesions. If the patient is on antibiotics anyway, then the question becomes cosmetic. In the past, there was much concern about spreading the infection internally, but antibiotics have removed this worry. A small puncture wound often gives less of a scar than allowing spontaneous rupture and also reduces the pain.

Furunculosis

Definition. Multiple recurrent furuncles.

Etiology and Pathogenesis. When a patient has an occasional boil, it probably just represents bad luck. When, on the other hand, the problem is persistent or recurrent, often with multiple lesions, one speaks of furunculosis. In this setting, one should search for predisposing factors such as atopic dermatitis and for nasal or perineal carriage of *S. aureus*.

Clinical Findings. The individual lesions are not unique. The problem is their multiplicity and chronicity. The face, neck and axillae are once again the most common sites, but with multiple lesions other parts of the body are more likely to be involved (Fig. 4.16).

Therapy. While individual lesions are treated as outlined above, one needs a strategy to prevent the recurrent lesions. The patients should be encouraged to keep their nails short, clean their skin with a synthetic detergent (syndet) or antibacterial soap, use fresh wash cloths, frequently change undergarments and bedding and in general stay clean. However, this advice, while sound, is rarely sufficient.

Systemic. One can use regimens of systemic antibiotics which are designed to reduce *S. aureus* carriage, for example, clindamycin (300 mg b.i.d.) or dicloxacillin (500 mg q.i.d.) with rifampicin (600 mg p.o.) for 14 days. Lower dosages of clindamycin for a longer period of time have also been suggested.

Topical. Applying mupirocin cream to the nares is occasionally effective. Initially it can be applied twice daily, and then later twice weekly for maintenance. Resistant strains of *S. aureus* have been described, but they are uncommon.

Other Measures. Colonization of the nares with non-pathogenic *S. aureus* has been used, especially in epidemics of furunculosis, such as in a wrestling team. There are problems with being sure the introduced organism is harmless for all concerned, and this technique is no longer widely recommended.

Carbuncle

Definition. A carbuncle is the worst form of a furuncle, with coalescence of lesions and marked inflammation.

Clinical Findings. Carbuncles are most common on the neck and trunk There is no sharp division between a large furuncle and a carbuncle. If multiple pustules are seen amidst an inflamed plaque, then one speaks of a carbuncle (Fig. 4.17). Typically the carbuncle is associated with marked inflammation, edema and fibrosis. If the neck is involved, mobility will be limited. Sometimes massive amounts of necrosis occur. Most patients have systemic symptoms.

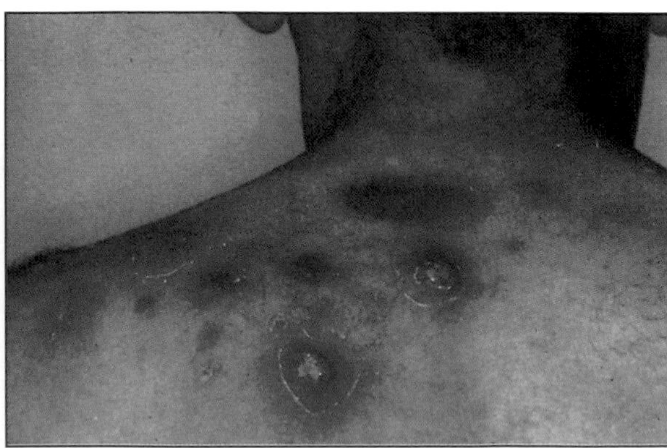

Fig. 4.16. Furunculosis

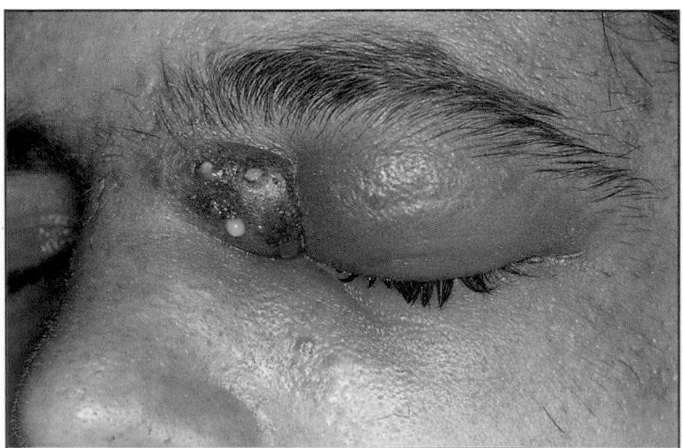

Fig. 4.17. Carbuncle

Therapy. Antistaphylococcal antibiotics are essential; often, hospitalization and initial intravenous therapy are wise. Drainage of large lesions should be discussed with the surgeons. Sometimes elderly patients are seen with a criss-cross scar on their nape, a dramatic documentation of the surgical drainage performed in the preantibiotic era.

Eyelid Infections

A number of primarily staphylococcal infections involve the eyelids. They require special attention because of their dramatic appearance, facilitated by the thin loose skin of the eyelid and their ability to impinge on a vital structure.

Hordeolum

Synonym. Sty

Definition. Acute infection of the modified apocrine or sebaceous glands in the eyelids.

Causative Organism. *Staphylococcus aureus*

Etiology and Pathogenesis. *Staphylococcus aureus* is usually responsible. Patients often have an associated blepharitis. The glands are infected via their openings to the exterior. The glands of Zeis are small sebaceous glands connected to the eyelashes, while the glands of Moll are apocrine glands of the lid. The glands of Meibom are large, modified sebaceous glands lying within the tarsal plate. All can be infected, producing varying clinical pictures.

Clinical Findings. An external hordeolum involves the more superficial glands of Zeis or Moll. Thus it presents as a painful red papule or pustule along the margin of the lid, often penetrated by an eyelash (Fig. 4.18). The upper lid is far more often involved than the lower. The patient initially has a foreign body sensation and later tearing and perhaps photophobia. Lid edema is usually present. Eventually the hordeolum ruptures spontaneously, discharging pus. While usually just one lesion is present, in patients with blepharitis and especially atopic dermatitis, multiple lesions (hordeolosis) may appear. Recurrences are common.

In contrast, an internal hordeolum involves the deeper lying glands of Meibom. It is considerably more painful and usually larger. When the conjunctival side of the lid is examined, a yellow-red swelling may be found roughly in the middle of the lid, not towards the margin. When spontaneous rupture occurs, drainage is usually to the conjunctival side. Recurrences are the rule rather than the exception.

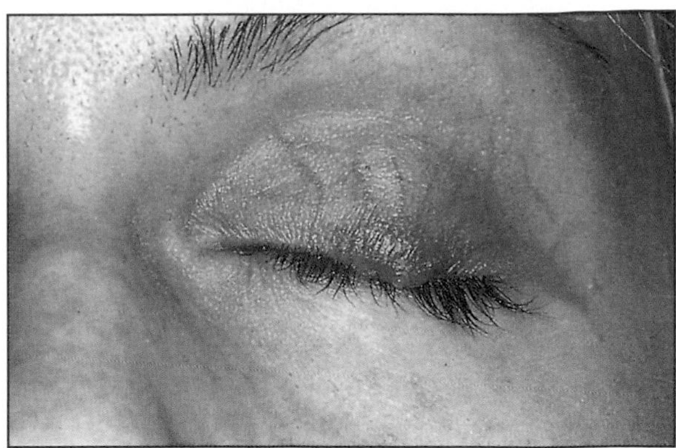

Fig. 4.18. External hordeolum

Differential Diagnosis. When an internal hordeolum is near the inner corner of the eye, dacryocystitis, an infection of the tear duct, must be excluded by an ophthalmologist. If the lesion is persistent, a sebaceous tumor or basal cell carcinoma of the lid margin should be considered.

Therapy. Warm compresses and topical antibiotics usually suffice. We often use bacitracin or erythromycin ophthalmic ointments; sulfacetamide ophthalmic drops are a reasonable adjunct to prevent spread to the adjacent structures. Despite the presence of increased numbers of resistant staphylococci, the response here is usually good. A pointing or succulent lesion on the lid can be incised; an internal lesion is best handled by an ophthalmologist.

Blepharitis

Definition. Inflammation of the lid margins, often with scales and crusts.

Etiology and Pathogenesis. In many cases *S. aureus* is responsible. In others, no microorganisms are found.

Clinical Findings. Blepharitis is usually bilateral with multiple lesions. Patients present with pruritus, burning and redness of the lids, and admit to frequent rubbing often to the point of removing their eyelashes. Multiple small pustules develop along the lid margin which ulcerate and crust. The secretions are marked and the lids may become glued together at night. When the crusts are removed, there is often bleeding. Ophthalmologists sometimes refer to staphylococcal blepharitis as ulcerative blepharitis. In addition to the loss of eyelashes, there may be scarring and even corneal abrasions and ulcerations as long-term sequelae.

Differential Diagnosis. The differential diagnosis is lengthy. The other common form of blepharitis is nonulcerative or seborrheic blepharitis. If the patient has obvious seborrheic dermatitis elsewhere, the diagnosis is easier. The scales in their condition are more easily removed and leave no ulcers or crusts behind. Some patients have associated atopic dermatitis, while others have rosacea. Many other bacteria may occasionally cause lid infections, as may molluscum contagiosum and HSV. In addition, *Phthirus pubis* can attach to the lids. The role of *D. folliculorum* in chronic blepharitis is disputed. Finally, allergic contact blepharitis may develop, caused by cosmetics or eye medications.

Therapy. Often it is unclear just what type of blepharitis is present, so empirical therapy is often instituted. Warm compresses are used to remove the crust; around the eyes, it may be wise to replace tap water compresses with a sterile solution. Erythromycin or bacitracin ophthalmic ointment should be applied to the lid margins three to four times daily; sulfacetamide drops should also be used. In some instances, corticosteroid-antibiotic drops are used to reduce inflammation; if this is done, the intraocular tension must be monitored. Treatment must be continued for several weeks, and relapses are common.

If the patient has obvious seborrheic dermatitis elsewhere, it should be treated by standard measures. Sometimes this treatment, coupled with shampooing of the eyelids, produces improvement in the seborrheic variant. Low-potency corticosteroids are also helpful, but the risk of glaucoma is such that one should be very hesitant to employ them over the long term. Allergic contact dermatitis particularly to antibiotics and preservatives should be excluded.

Chalazion

Definition. Chronic granulomatous inflammation of the gland of Meibom.

A chalazion is not an infection, but is discussed here because of the inevitable confusion. It is probably closest to a mucocele of the gland of Meibom; the duct is occluded and the gland becomes inflamed. As healing occurs, granulomatous inflammation develops. Thus an initial chalazion may resemble an internal hordeolum, but later on there is a nontender, often mobile mass. Most lesions point towards the conjunctival surface; they may rupture and produce a pyogenic granuloma. Chalazia usually resolve over a period of weeks. Treatment consists of warm compresses and topical antibiotics; occasionally surgical removal is needed. A persistent chalazion should also be biopsied to exclude a benign or malignant sebaceous tumor of the lid.

Infections of Sweat Glands

In contrast to the ease with which staphylococci and other bacteria infect hair follicles, they rarely involve eccrine sweat glands. When the glands are occluded, as in miliaria, there may be minor bacterial secondary infection. It is speculated that the high amounts of IgA secreted through the sweat glands are protective against infectious organisms.

Neutrophilic Eccrine Hidradenitis

Definition. Inflammation of eccrine glands, most often seen in chemotherapy patients.

In rare cases, there is inflammation of the eccrine glands without infection. The typical scenario is a cancer patient undergoing chemotherapy. Numerous cytotoxic agents are concentrated in the eccrine sweat and to an extent eliminated via this route. The patient may present with multiple pustules and erythematous plaques, usually on the trunk and extremities. Similar lesions have been described in both healthy adults and children, also on the palms and soles, where the eccrine glands are most concentrated. Finally, neutrophilic eccrine hidradenitis has been seen in HIV/AIDS patients. Biopsy shows neutrophilic inflammation around eccrine glands without an obvious follicular component. The main differential diagnosis is bacterial folliculitis. No treatment is required; resolution occurs over a period of weeks.

Multiple Sweat Gland Abscesses of the Newborn

Synonyms. Poritis, periporitis

Definition. Unusual infection of the eccrine sweat glands in neonates.

Poritis or periporitis most likely does not exist. It was formerly described in immunosuppressed or ill newborns as a diffuse widespread infection of the eccrine glands, presenting much like a furunculosis. Today, with many more premature babies with almost no defense mechanisms, the disease is no longer seen. There is a long list of pustular eruptions of the newborn, but none fit in this category and we have abandoned this term.

Erysipelas

Definition. Acute erythematous, rapidly spreading skin infection, usually associated with systemic symptoms.

Causative Organisms. Usually *S. pyogenes* (β-hemolytic group A streptococci); occasionally other streptococci are identified, as well as other bacteria, but in general one defines the disease by the presence of *S. pyogenes*.

Epidemiology. Erysipelas was formerly a common, feared and often fatal disease; with antibiotics, it is much less of a problem in most Western countries. In the past, erysipelas was usually facial, but today most lesions are on the legs. It tends to be a disease of the young and the elderly.

Etiology and Pathogenesis. The key to erysipelas is the presence of a defect in the skin barrier function. Thus it is often associated with HSV infection, interdigital tinea pedis, a leg ulcer or any other minor injury. About 30% of patients have *S. pyogenes* in their nares. Along with minor trauma, lymphatic obstruction is a second cofactor. The streptococci themselves cause further lymphatic damage, creating a vicious cycle facilitating recurrence.

Clinical Findings. The key finding is a warm painful erythema that rapidly spreads peripherally but always has a sharp border to the adjacent normal skin. Tongue-like or irregular extensions are common. The two most common sites are the cheeks and legs (Figs. 4.19, 4.20). On the face, the process usually starts on the bridge of the nose and spreads

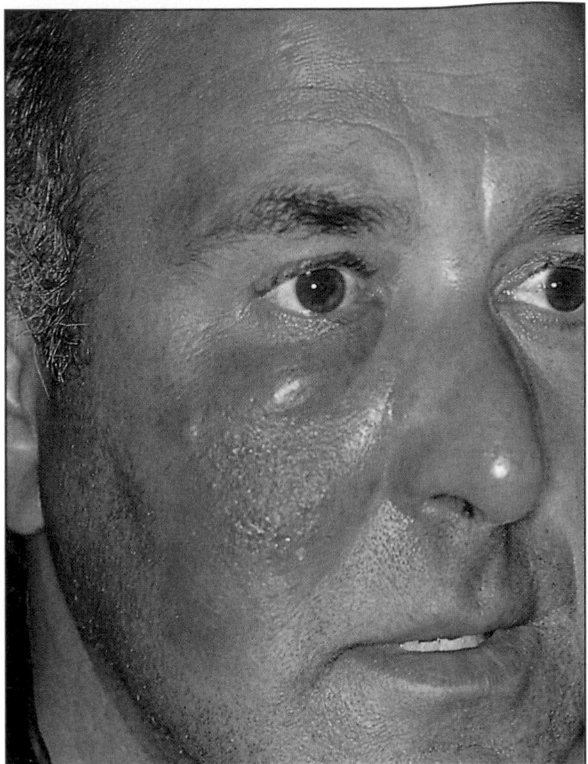

Fig. 4.19. Erysipelas

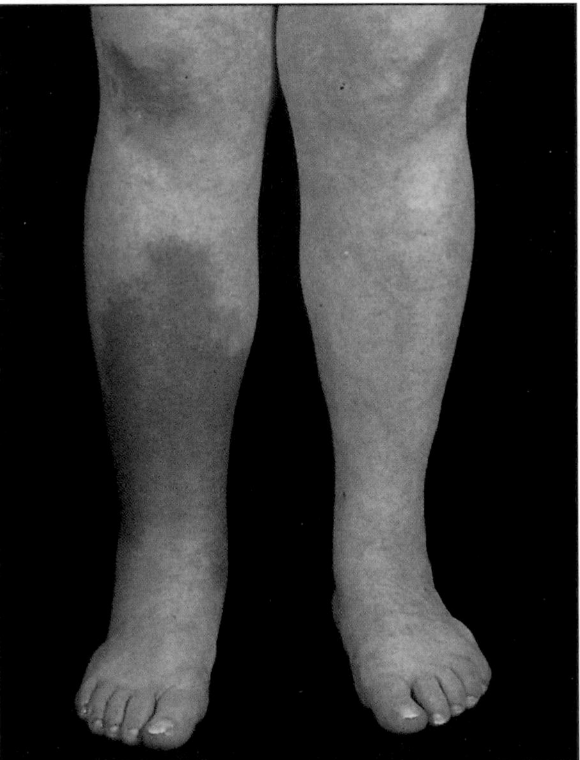

Fig. 4.20. Erysipelas

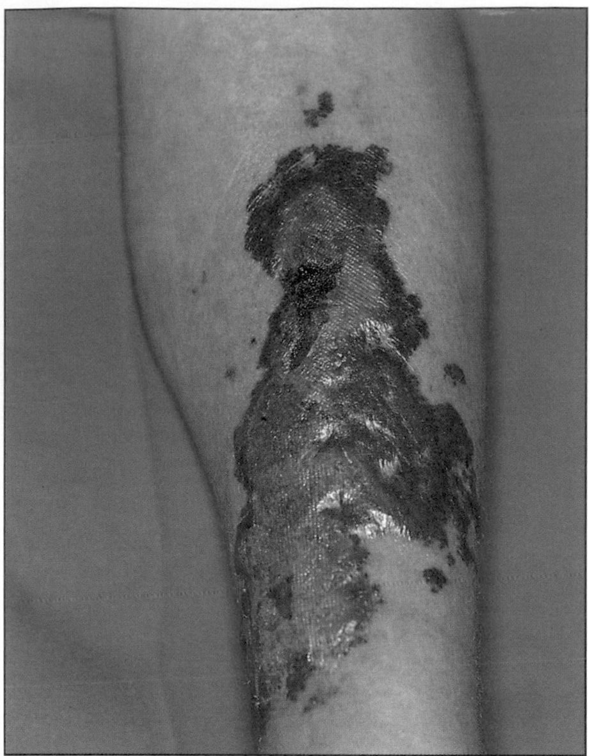

Fig. 4.21. Bullous erysipelas

bilaterally, associated with lid edema. On the legs, there is slower spread and less edema, but often lymphangitis and lymphadenopathy may be found. Another common site is in an edematous arm following mastectomy and lymph node dissection. Most patients are febrile and may have chills.

Erysipelas can have many variants. Most are no longer seen today because of the effectiveness of antibiotic therapy. In some instances vesicles and blisters are seen. On the legs, the blisters are often hemorrhagic (erysipelas vesiculosum et bullosum; Fig. 4.21). In other instances, there is necrosis (erysipelas gangraenosum), often in patients with reduced immune defenses, diabetes mellitus, or inadequate limb circulation. Necrosis of the eyelids can also occur. In the most extreme form (erysipelas phlegmonosum), there are underlying abscesses and involvement of the fascia, overlapping with necrotizing fasciitis. Once deeper tissues are involved, many prefer the diagnosis streptococcal cellulitis. In addition, the mucosa can be involved, producing marked swelling and destruction, be it in the larynx or genitalia.

Histopathology. Biopsy shows primarily dermal edema and dilated vessels. There is usually a sparse neutrophilic infiltrate. On occasion, the streptococci can be demonstrated with special stains.

Laboratory Findings. The *S. pyogenes* cannot be cultured from the skin and only rarely from fluid aspirated from the advancing edge. When a leg ulcer is present, streptococci are somewhat easier to find. Throat culture may also be positive. About 5% of cases have a positive blood culture.

Course and Prognosis. Because of the rapid response to antibiotics, the acute complications of erysipelas have become uncommon. Myo-, peri- and endocarditis has been described, as well as rare cases of glomerulonephritis. With those infections that start on the face, cavernous sinus thrombosis is a theoretical risk, as are descending airway infections and even pneumonia. Laryngeal involvement remains dangerous. Infants, immunosuppressed patients and the elderly deserve special attention.

The biggest problem is the well-document effect on the lymphatics, producing obstruction and increasing the likelihood of recurrent disease. There may be residual mid-facial swelling; when the upper lip is involved, one speaks of elephantiasis nostras or, less pleasantly, tapir lip. On the legs, patients with chronic venous insufficiency and recurrent ulcerations frequently suffer from multiple attacks of erysipelas.

Laboratory Findings. The diagnosis is usually made clinically, based on cutaneous findings, fever and elevated erythrocyte sedimentation rate. One can try to culture the throat and the wound, if a preexisting ulceration is present. A rise in the anti-DNase B titer is taken as supportive evidence, but does not help in the acute situation.

Differential Diagnosis. Acute contact dermatitis can appear similar, but does not spread rapidly and the patient is not ill. Early facial zoster may appear very similar; if a blister is present, a Tzanck smear should be done. Acute anterior tibial compartment syndrome is a painful swelling in the muscle compartment over the shin after unaccustomed exertion; the overlying skin may be red and mistaken for erysipelas. Erythema migrans has a slowly spreading circle but once again in a relatively healthy patient. Angioneurotic edema may present with mid-facial swelling but without erythema. Erysipeloid usually presents on the hands in a person with exposure to raw meat or fish. Patients with familial Mediterranean fever also have erysipelas-like lesions during their febrile attacks. Pseudoerysipelas is a type of mechanical cellulitis, not infectious, which occurs most often in patients with chronic venous insufficiency; it responds best to improved mechanical support and sometimes a short course of systemic corticosteroids.

Therapy
Systemic. Fortunately, streptococci have remained very sensitive to penicillin, so the approach is usually easy. Most patients are hospitalized and treated with intravenous penicillin G (600,000–2,000,000 units q.i.d.). In the USA early cases are frequently treated with oral or intramuscular penicillin. If deeper involvement appears to be present, one should consider the possibility of a different organism and provide broad-spectrum intravenous coverage until a definite bacteriological diagnosis is available. In the case of penicillin allergy, oral erythromycin is usually used. Treatment should be carried out for 2 weeks to reduce the likelihood of recurrence.

Prophylaxis. In Germany, selected patients are given benzathine penicillin G (1.2 million units intramuscularly) monthly for 6 months. If HSV infection is the source of the entry portal, acyclovir prophylaxis should be employed. Tinea pedis and onychomycosis should also be treated aggressively with topical or systemic antimycotic agents.

Blistering Dactylitis

Causative Organisms. Usually β-hemolytic streptococci; rarely, *Staphylococcus aureus*

Blistering dactylitis is a unique bullous eruption featuring tense stable blisters often with a dusky color involving the volar tips of the toes or fingers. There is surrounding and often proximally spreading erythema. Frequently the patients, mostly children, are healthy and the problem is initially diagnosed as a blister. Later they may become quite ill. The diagnosis can be made by Gram stain and culture of the blister. Positive results help exclude a herpetic whitlow. There is an overlap with staphylococcal bullous impetigo and bulla repens. Oral or intramuscular penicillin usually suffices; draining the lesion may offer pain relief.

Perianal Streptococcal Dermatitis
(Amren et al. 1966)

Synonym. Perianal streptococcal cellulitis

Definition. Streptococcal infection of the perianal skin in children.

Epidemiology. This is a relatively common type of group A β-hemolytic streptococcal infection involving primarily children. Boys are more often affected and most are preschoolers.

Etiology and Pathogenesis. In most cases, group A β-hemolytic streptococci can be isolated in the pharynx and there is probably hand transfer to the perineum. Most often, the patients do not have pharyngitis. Why the bacteria favor the perianal region is unclear.

Clinical Findings. Patients may present in a variety of ways. Most commonly there is a circumferential band of erythema about the anus, extending for perhaps a few centimeters. The skin is tender and the patient may complain of pain on defecation, or the parents may have noticed a reluctance to use the toilet. In other cases, there is an anal fissure with dried secretions or more massive inflammation with erosions and pustules. Lengthy delays in diagnosis have been described.

Laboratory Findings. Both a throat culture and perianal culture should be taken. The laboratory should be warned that the perianal culture should be studied for streptococci; otherwise they will only try to identify enteric organisms.

Differential Diagnosis. The differential diagnostic list is long, including pinworms, psoriasis, toxin-mediated perineal erythema, candidiasis, inflammatory bowel disease and child abuse. It is often easier to prove the presence of streptococci than to exclude some of the other problems.

Therapy. Oral penicillin is usually curative; a 10-day course should be given. Because of the likelihood of recurrence, some clinicians suggest using mupirocin ointment b.i.d. for another 10–14 days in the perianal region. Others suggest using the topical antibiotic once or twice weekly for prophylaxis following treatment.

Skin Findings Associated with Streptococcal Infections

A number of skin findings are associated with subacute bacterial endocarditis, which is most often caused by streptococci. They include:

- Petechiae
- Subungual splinter hemorrhages
- JANEWAY (1899) macules: Small hemorrhagic lesions on palms and soles, usually painless
- OSLER (1893) nodes: Erythematous, painful subcutaneous nodules, almost urticarial in nature, most common on finger and toe tips, as well as thenar and hypothenar pads

In all likelihood, these last two famous findings both represent small microemboli, but in different sized vessels at different skin levels.

In addition, a broad range of dermatologic reactions can be triggered by streptococci. The most interesting to dermatologists is the flares of psoriasis, known as guttate psoriasis, that often follow streptococcal pharyngitis. We do a throat culture on all patients with guttate psoriasis. Erythema nodosum, leukocytoclastic vasculitis and many other reactions also occasionally follow infections.

Ecthyma

Definition. Pyoderma with ulceration.

Causative Organism. Usually group A β-hemolytic streptococci

Epidemiology. Ecthyma is most common in children, especially those living in tropical countries. In industrialized countries, ecthyma may be seen in tourists returning from exotic vacations and in the homeless. It is also associated with poor hygiene and more common in debilitated or immunosuppressed patients. Ecthyma was apparently very common in the trenches of World War I; a synonym in German is trench ulcer.

Etiology and Pathogenesis. The organisms generally enter the skin through areas of minor trauma. Thus scabies, other arthropod bites and atopic dermatitis are common predisposing factors. Many lesions diagnosed in nontropical countries as tropical ulcers are ecthyma. Excoriation and manipulation by the patient also play a role.

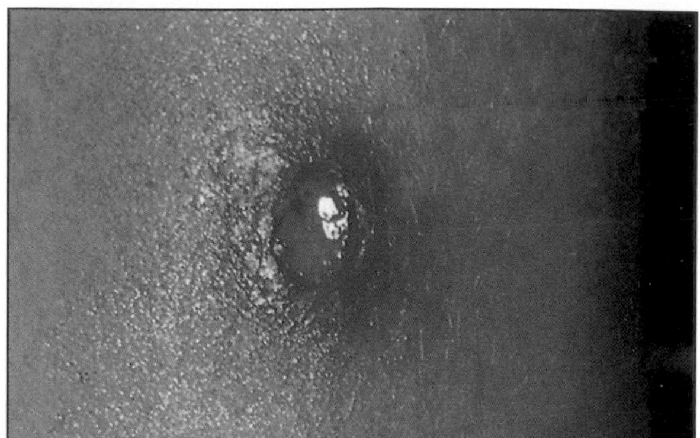

Fig. 4.22. Ecthyma

Clinical Findings. The initial lesion is similar to impetigo, as a large pustule on an erythematous base appears. Rather than spreading in the epidermis, the infection penetrates deeply, damaging the dermis and producing a dirty ulcer (Fig. 4.22). There is usually a thick yellow-gray crust. The lower parts of the extremities are the most common site. Associated lymphangitis and lymphadenopathy are frequent. The course is very chronic in the absence of appropriate therapy. Scarring always occurs. Glomerulonephritis may be a secondary complication.

Laboratory Findings. Ecthyma is usually a clinical diagnosis. In early lesions, one may succeed in culturing streptococcus. Later on, there is almost always a mixed flora present.

Differential Diagnosis. The entire list of leg ulcerations comes into question, including leukocytoclastic vasculitis, erythema induratum, secondary and tertiary syphilis and cutaneous diphtheria. Ecthyma gangrenosum refers to necrotic cutaneous lesions with *P. aeruginosa* sepsis and is an entirely different problem.

Therapy

Systemic. Usually oral antibiotics suffice, although in Germany parenteral administration is preferred. Even though streptococci most likely are involved, many physicians prefer a broader spectrum antibiotic than ordinary penicillin, choosing either a penicillinase-resistant penicillin or a cephalosporin.

Topical. Local care is crucial. Wet compresses with disinfectant solutions (povidone-iodine, 0.5–1% aqueous silver nitrate) should be used for debridement. Once the lesions are dry and crusted they should be left alone to heal in from the base. The patients must refrain from manipulating the crust as repeated removal will prolong the disease course. When deep lesions are present on the legs, the patient should be at bed rest with the limb elevated.

Cellulitis

Definition. Bacterial infection of the skin and soft tissue, often with involvement of underlying structures such as fascia, muscles and tendons.

Causative Organism. Most often group A β-hemolytic streptococci or *Staphylococcus aureus*.

Epidemiology. Cellulitis is not one disease but many; thus it is difficult to describe an epidemiological pattern.

Etiology and Pathogenesis. In most instances, the bacteria enter the skin from outside via a minor injury and proliferate. Surgical wound infections also rapidly evolve into cellulitis. On rare occasions, organisms may settle in the skin in a septic patient and then produce a cellulitis from within. Group A β-hemolytic streptococci are the most common cause; they secrete many enzymes which facilitate spread. *S. aureus* is only responsible when there is an obvious adjacent wound or skin defect; this type of cellulitis usually spreads more slowly. Other bacteria may cause cellulitis in immunosuppressed hosts. When unusual organisms are introduced, for example, via an animal bite or dirty wound, the list of possible causative agents is large.

Clinical Findings. The most typical location is the leg. Often there is a sign of tinea pedis, chronic venous insufficiency, a minor injury or surgery. There is erythema, swelling and tenderness, but without a sharp border of erysipelas. Pitting edema is prominent; the skin is sometimes slightly blanched because of the swelling. In addition to pain, there may be restriction of motion about a joint. While necrosis occurs, it is rarely superficial so that draining abscesses and new ulcerations are most common. Lymphangitis, lymphadenopathy and sepsis are logical sequelae.

There are several special types of cellulitis worthy of short notice.

- Postbypass cellulitis: When the saphenous vein(s) are harvested for coronary artery bypass, many patients develop a smoldering cellulitis just below the distal operative site. β-hemolytic streptococci are often responsible, although bacteriological studies are limited. Almost all affected individuals also have tinea pedis, which should be treated aggressively.
- Periorbital cellulitis: About the eye, cellulitis plays a slightly different role. In children *Haemophilus influenzae* is the most common cause, especially if no injury is present. Both sinusitis and bacteremia may seed the orbit. In patients with diabetes mellitus or immunosuppression, phycomycosis may be involved (Chap. 7).
- Ludwig angina: Cellulitis of the submandibular, sublingual and submaxillary spaces goes by the old name of Ludwig (1836) angina (angina Ludovici). Patients usually present with bilateral involvement, a brawny hard neck with pain on mastication and motion (Fig. 4.23). In over half the cases, the source of infection is dental. The risk of airway obstruction is considerable.

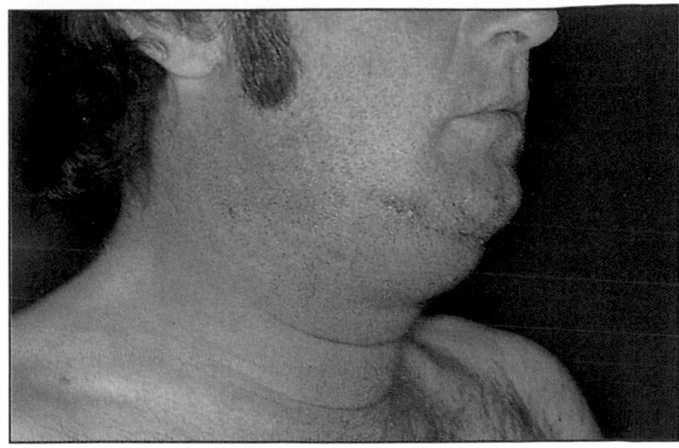

Fig. 4.23. Cellulitis

Histopathology. A biopsy is not helpful for routine cases, showing only edema and neutrophils. However, if the patient is immunosuppressed or has diabetic ketoacidosis, a tissue biopsy should be performed, both to search for fungal hyphae and to provide material for culture.

Laboratory Findings. In most cases, culture is not needed. The lesion can be aspirated and that material used for culture. As mentioned above, in complex cases, tissue for culture gives more reliable results.

Course and Prognosis. The outlook in immunosuppressed patients is guarded. In healthy individuals recovery is expected. The danger is to miss involvement of underlying structures, such as the fascia or muscle. Both necrotizing fasciitis and myonecrosis can lead to rapid death. In addition, sepsis is a threat.

Differential Diagnosis. The main differential diagnosis is the various types of cellulitis. The distinction between erysipelas and early cellulitis is often clouded. Deep vein thrombosis also sometimes causes confusion, but the latter features cool, pale skin with edema and should be easily recognized.

Therapy. For mild localized lesions with an obvious history in healthy patients, oral antibiotics can be used, usually penicillin or a cephalosporin. In febrile or otherwise ill patients, hospitalization and parenteral antibiotic therapy are usually required. The choice of antibiotics depends on the patient's medical status and background. Surgeons should be consulted regarding the wisdom of incision and drainage or debridement.

Necrotizing Infections

Definition. Group of somewhat related infections which are characterized by rapidly progressive cellulitis with extensive underlying tissue damage.

The severe necrotizing infections are not the province of the dermatologists, but they should at least be familiar with these disorders. Missing a progressive cellulitis has serious medical and legal consequences. While not everyone will agree with the groupings below, they provide a working framework to approach the problem. In all such cases, one should be alert to the roles of diabetes mellitus, HIV/AIDS and iatrogenic immunosuppression as predisposing factors. In all situations, appropriate antibiotic coverage, debridement and exclusion of specific infections, such as group A β-hemolytic streptococci, *P. aeruginosa* or deep fungi are crucial. Debridement is needed not only to remove revitalized tissue, but to examine the muscles; if they too are involved (myonecrosis), the course is grimmer and even more extensive mutilating therapy is needed.

Necrotizing Fasciitis

Synonyms. Streptococcal gangrene, streptococcal soft tissue infection

Definition. Severe, aggressive, potentially fatal soft tissue infection with streptococci.

Epidemiology. Of the estimates 10,000–15,000 severe cases of group A β-hemolytic streptococci that occur in the USA yearly, about 20% are estimated to advance to necrotizing fasciitis. These are the so-called meat eating bacteria of the tabloids, responsible for the death of the beloved puppeteer Jim Henson. Most patients are older or have other risk factors such as pre-existing vascular disease, alcohol or drug abuse, immunosuppression or even HIV/AIDS. Nonetheless totally healthy individuals can also be struck.

Etiology and Pathogenesis. Necrotizing fasciitis has traditionally been divided into type 1, which is a mixed bacterial infection, and type 2, caused by group A β-hemolytic streptococci. Today, the term is usually reserved just for the streptococcal disease, even though the mixed infections are more common. Group A β-hemolytic streptococci alone are isolated in about 20% of cases in Germany. Perineal cases are almost always mixed infections; when the extremities are involved, streptococci are a better bet. The major mechanisms of tissue destruction include deformation of erythrocytes and endothelial cell damage leading to thrombus formation, hemorrhage and tissue necrosis. The combination of kinin activation, coagulation and fibrinolysis leads to a disseminated intravascular coagulation-like picture (Chap. 22). The many streptococcal enzymes such as hyaluronidase, streptolysins and streptokinases also play a major role.

Clinical Findings. The infection usually follows minor trauma or surgery. Initially a small region of cellulitis is present, but expands rapidly, becomes dusky with bullae and a necrotic eschar, resembling a severe burn. Extensive soft tissue damage occurs, extending far beyond the lines indicated on the skin (Fig. 4.24). Crepitation may be present, but is more common in mixed infections. Lymphadenopathy is absent. The patient is very ill, with fever, extensive pain and possibly changes in mental status.. The pain decreases as the disease progresses because the neurons are destroyed. There may be overlaps with streptococcal toxic shock syndrome.

Histopathology. There is massive destruction of the soft tissue and fascia with thromboses and liquefaction. The muscle may be secondarily damaged.

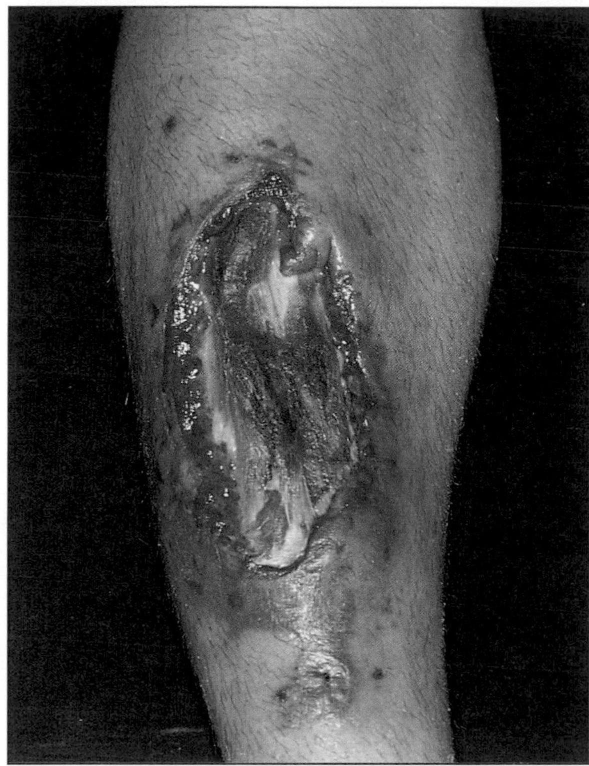

Fig. 4.24. Necrotizing fasciitis

Laboratory Findings. Group A β-hemolytic streptococci can be cultured from the skin, fascia and usually from the blood. Even when group A β-hemolytic streptococci are clearly the primary cause, other organisms may be cultured.

Course and Prognosis. The mortality rate ranges between 20% and 30% in large series. Some patients require amputations and most are left with significant scars.

Differential Diagnosis. Streptococcal myositis refer to a primary infection of the muscle, with muscle damage, often leading to a compartment syndrome and later fascial and soft tissue changes. The other necrotic processes discussed below are the main challenge.

Therapy
Surgical. The most important therapeutic approach is extensive surgical debridement. If surgery is delayed, the mortality rate jumps to over 75%. Complete removal of necrotic tissue is required; incision and drainage or partial debridement is ineffective. Later, surgical reconstruction is necessary with either secondary closure or, usually, mesh grafts or a flap closure.

Systemic. Penicillin G, 30 million units daily for at least 10 days, is often combined with clindamycin 600 mg t.i.d. for 1–2 days. The clindamycin inhibits the cellular metabolism of the streptococci more quickly than penicillin, which only blocks growth. Intravenous immunoglobulin is also recommended, as well as organ-specific supportive measures.

Prophylaxis. Careful isolation should be practiced. Clindamycin is probably the best choice for prophylaxis for those with direct exposure to an infected patient. Vaccines are under development using a variety of streptococcal proteins.

Synergistic Necrotizing Cellulitis

Synonym. Type 2 necrotizing fasciitis

When surgery is performed in the perineal area, the risk of mixed destructive infections is high. Involvement of the male genitalia is known as FOURNIER (1883) gangrene. Both aerobic and anaerobic organisms are present. They produce a foul-smelling draining ulcer that rapidly expands. The anaerobes produce gas so that crepitation is present. Treatment is similar to that for group A β-hemolytic streptococcal necrotizing fasciitis, except that the antibiotic regimen must be adjusted to the culture results.

Progressive Bacterial Synergistic Gangrene

Synonym. MELENEY (1924) ulcer

This disease may be identical to synergistic necrotizing cellulitis or fasciitis. The concept of synergistic gangrene is a puzzling one but real. A mixed bacterial infection develops following surgery or sometimes associated with a leg ulcer or sinus tract. There is a shaggy ulcer with a dusky periphery that expands more slowly than in streptococcal necrotizing fasciitis and in a less ill patient. Meleney produced similar lesions by injecting both staphylococci and non-group A streptococci simultaneously into experimental animals. Usually, cultures reveal these two organisms. When sinus tracts develop with drainage at distant sites, the term Meleney ulcer is often used.

Gas Gangrene

Inoculation of *Clostridium perfringens* into an often minor wound or bite can lead to disastrous consequences. The course is similar to necrotizing fasciitis but even more rapid, associated with more extensive necrosis and prominent crepitation. Gas can easily be seen on radiological films. Treatment consists of high-dose penicillin intravenously. Tetanus immunization or antitoxin administration is not helpful.

Rarely nonclostridial gas gangrene may be seen. Responsible organisms include *Escherichia coli, Enterococcus, Proteus, Bacteroides, Klebsiella* and some normally nonpathogenic streptococci. Because of this possibility in immunosuppressed patients or those with diabetes mellitus, some experts recommend initially using broader spectrum systemic antibiotics until culture results are available.

Miscellaneous Causes of Necrosis

- Pyoderma gangrenosum (Chap. 22)
- *P. aeruginosa* sepsis
- Phycomycosis or aspergillosis (Chap. 7), especially in immunosuppressed, burn or diabetes mellitus patients
- Necrosis secondary to peripheral vascular occlusion. True gangrene, usually has a much slower course and patient is not febrile (Chap. 22)
- Subcutaneous injections

Chronic Pyodermas

There are a number of disorders described which have features of a bacterial infection but also show marked epidermal reaction and often a prominent host response. While it is difficult to exactly classify these disorders, they enter into the differential diagnosis of cutaneous tuberculosis, fungal infections and halogenodermas, as well as being mistaken for carcinomas.

Pyoderma Vegetans
(NANTA and BASEX 1937)

Synonyms. Blastomycotic pyoderma, pyodermite végétante et verruqueuse

Definition. Chronic ulcerated skin infection with papillomatous changes at the wound edge.

Causative Organism. Many bacteria have been implicated, primarily streptococci, *S. aureus* and Enterobacteriaceae.

Etiology and Pathogenesis. The mechanism of pyoderma vegetans is unclear. Some patients are immunosuppressed, including those with HIV/AIDS. Usually there is a trivial skin infection or injury, but instead of healing, the wound becomes more inflamed and proliferates at its edges. In some instances, treatment with an ointment, rather than a more drying product, is probably responsible.

Clinical Findings. This rare problem occurs mostly on the extremities. Usually there is a solitary lesion, usually ranging in size from 3 cm to 10 cm, although occasionally larger areas are involved. The primary lesion gradually expands. Large, livid infiltrated nodules appear at the periphery, dotted with tiny pustules. In the center, there may be necrosis, ulceration, fistulae and sinus tracts. Eventually the lesion is marked by papillomatous and even warty excrescences which dominate the picture. At the same time there is drainage of pus from the sinus tracts and accumulation of yellow-brown crusts. As healing occurs, complex atrophic scars with sinus tracts evolve. The course is long, chronic and frustrating for patient and physician.

Histopathology. Microscopic examination reveals pseudoepitheliomatous hyperplasia and dermal abscesses.

Differential Diagnosis. Halogenoderma, deep fungal infections, actinomycosis, nocardiosis, tuberculosis and pyoderma gangrenosum should be excluded. With very chronic lesions, a squamous cell carcinoma also comes into question. The other lesions described in the section are also part of the differential diagnosis.

Therapy

Systemic. Appropriate systemic antibiotics are indicated, often for a several-week course, but they do not provide the entire solution. Sometimes a short course of systemic corticosteroids will reduce the inflammatory response.

Topical. We prefer drying measures, such as 1% aqueous silver nitrate or 0.5–1.0% aqueous aluminum chloride as wet to dry compresses. Castellani solution or 1.0% aqueous gentian violet can also be used.

Surgical. Debridement of the wound edge may be useful. In extreme cases, the entire lesion can be excised; the wound is allowed to granulate and then covered with a mesh graft.

Pyoderma Végétante

(Azua 1903)

In this case, the papillomatous changes predominate; thus, the disorder is virtually identical to papillomatosis cutis carcinoides of Gottron (Chap. 55). A low-grade squamous cell carcinoma, i.e., verrucous carcinoma, must be excluded.

Pyoderma Ulcerosa Serpiginosa

Sometimes immunosuppressed or debilitated patients develop large serpiginous ulcerated lesions on their trunk. Many such cases probably represent pyoderma gangrenosum.

Chancriform Pyoderma

In this variant, the intense inflammatory response dominates, producing a lesion that resembles a syphilitic chancre. The face is most often involved, especially the lower lip and eyebrows (Fig. 4.25) In other instances, lesions are found on the genitalia. There is a sharply defined ulcer with peripheral edema and erythema. Both syphilis and chancroid, as well as other specific infections, should be excluded via direct examination. cultures and serology. In addition to coverage with a broad-spectrum antibiotic, assuming no specific organism has been identified, it is often helpful to prescribe a short course of systemic corticosteroids. The same topical approach as for pyoderma vegetans is recommended.

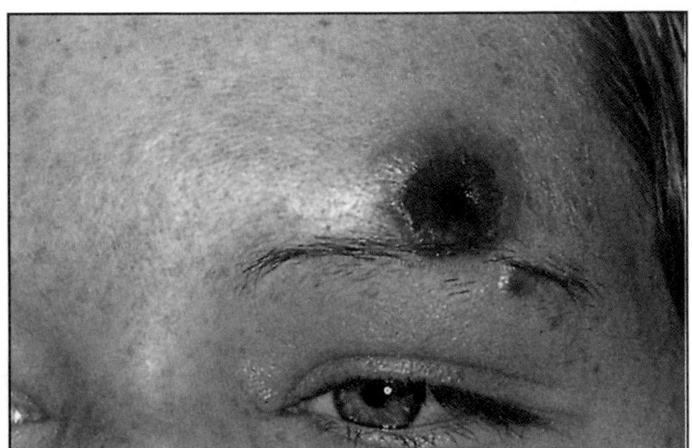

Fig. 4.25. Chancriform pyoderma

Gram-Positive Diphtheroid Bacilli

Diphtheroid bacilli or diphtheroids are gram-positive rods with clubbed ends. Many of them are part of the normal flora and not associated with any cutaneous disease. In many instances they are responsible for much of the body odor which develops in the axillae and groin, explaining the use of antimicrobial agents in deodorants. Table 4.6 lists some of the disease associations. *Propionibacterium acnes* plays an important role in acne but is not considered a direct cause. It may rarely cause cellulitis in immunosuppressed individuals. Other organisms cause a variety of relatively harmless problems. Finally, there is diphtheria itself, a potentially fatal disease which sometimes is limited to the skin.

Table 4.6. Diseases caused by diphtheroid bacilli

Organisms	Disease	Frequency
Corynebacterium minutissimum	Erythrasma	Common
*Corynebacterium tenuis*axillaris	Trichomycosis	Uncommon
Corynebacterium species	Pitted keratolysis	Common
Corynebacterium diphtheriae	Cutaneous diphtheria	Rare
Corynebacterium haemolyticum, Corynebacterium pyogenes	Skin ulcers	Rare, common in Thailand
Corynebacterium, group JK	Sepsis in immunosuppressed hosts	Common in oncology patients
Propionibacterium acnes, Propionibacterium granulosum	Acne vulgaris, acne conglobata, acne fulminans	Very common, but perhaps not causative
Propionibacterium acnes, Propionibacterium granulosum	Folliculitis	Rarely, if ever, pathogenic

Erythrasma

Definition. Bacterial infection of intertriginous areas, usually with asymptomatic red-brown macules.

Causative Organism. *Corynebacterium minutissimum*

Epidemiology. About 20% of the population is infected with *C. minutissimum*. The amount of clinical disease seen in a given region varies almost directly with the humidity. Thus erythrasma is common in Houston; rare in Albuquerque. Most patients are older men. Intertriginous sites are preferred; hyperhidrosis, obesity and diabetes mellitus are predisposing factors.

Etiology and Pathogenesis. The normally harmless bacteria can penetrate a stratum corneum damaged by moisture or trauma, but do not enter the living part of the epidermis. They manufacture porphyrins so that Wood light examination reveals a coral red fluorescence, which is very useful for diagnosis.

Clinical Findings. The most common sites are all intertriginous. In the groin, the bacteria is usually found where the scrotum touches the thigh or in the narrow contact zone between the labia majora and thigh. Other locations include the axilla, gluteal cleft, inframammary folds, umbilicus and toe web spaces. Initially small red-brown macules are seen; they tend to coalesce into larger patches with a sharp border (Fig. 4.26). Sometimes tiny punctate lesions are scattered about the periphery. The skin surface is smooth; occasional fine scale is seen. Often the lesion is asymptomatic; in other instances it is pruritic and may be excoriated or inflamed. Marked sweating, prolonged sitting and similar activities may trigger the pruritus. In some instances, nothing is seen, but the area fluoresces.

Histopathology. Erythrasma is an invisible dermatosis; the tiny bacteria in the stratum corneum are not identifiable. There may be a sparse, dermal perivascular infiltrate.

Laboratory Findings. The best way to make the diagnosis is Wood light examination. Using a double filter system, a Wood light releases almost exclusively UVA radiation. The porphyrins made by *C. minutissimum* have their absorption spectrum in this band, producinga coral red fluorescence (Fig. 4.27). In contrast, *Microsporum canis* shows a green fluorescence. Other dermatophytes commonly seen in the groin do not fluoresce. Wood light will also highlight the follicles in acne patients, as *P. acnes* also fluoresces pink-red, while tetracycline has a yellow hue.

C. minutissimum can be cultured under aerobic conditions with special media and then identified and subclassified among the diphtheroids, but the procedure is not practical or needed.

Course and Prognosis. Erythrasma is both chronic and frequently recurrent, despite therapy.

Differential Diagnosis. The main differential diagnostic point is tinea cruris, which usually has a more prominent scaly border, often with pustules, and may show central regression. Tinea versicolor

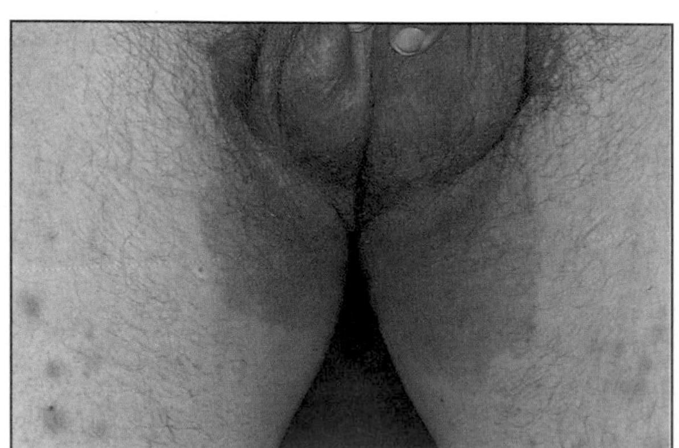

Fig. 4.26. Erythrasma

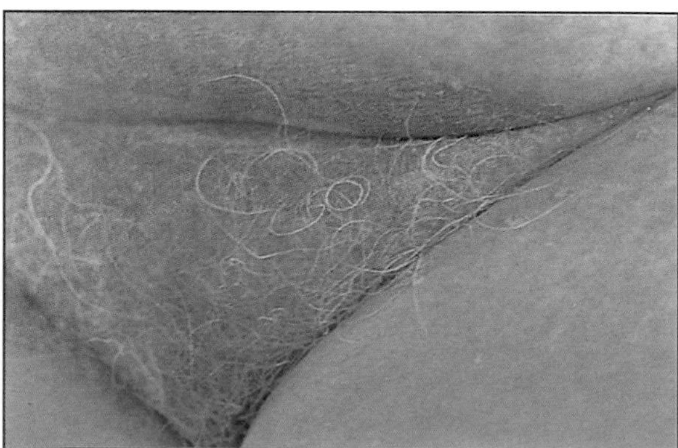

Fig. 4.27. Erythrasma with coral red fluorescence on Wood light examination

may also be seen in the groin, but usually there are lesions on the trunk. Intertrigo is identical to erythrasma; the Wood light examination is decisive. Early or treated psoriasis in the groin can also appear identical; one needs a history or evidence of psoriasis elsewhere.

Therapy

Systemic. A short course of systemic erythromycin is the easiest method; a total dose of 1.0 g can divided into two or four doses. Other clinicians prescribe 250 mg daily for 1 week. While the response is prompt, so is relapse.

Topical. Topical imidazole creams are also effective; one can treat b.i.d. for perhaps 1 week and then weekly for prophylaxis. This is our treatment of choice.

Other Measures. Eliminating the predisposing factors, such as obesity, sweating and maceration, is very important but hard to achieve. Frequent washing with antibacterial soaps may also help. The success of therapy can be monitored with Wood light examination.

Trichomycosis Axillaris

Synonyms. Trichomycosis palmellina, trichobacteriosis palmellina

Definition. Collections of bacteria forming concretions on hairs, usually in the axilla.

Causative Organism. *Corynebacterium tenuis*

Epidemiology. A relatively uncommon disorder, more frequently found in men.

Etiology and Pathogenesis. Hyperhidrosis and improper hygiene are the two predisposing factors. Corynebacteria are usually common in the axilla, but what stimulates the bacteria to form accumulations along the hair shaft has not been demonstrated.

Clinical Findings. Often the diagnosis can be made with the nose, not the eyes, even before the patient undresses. There is always a rancid acid smell, not only from the axillae but also from the clothing. The bacteria are able to metabolize testosterone found in the apocrine sweat into malodorous compounds. The axillary hairs are surrounded by white-yellow, red or black, dull difficult to remove accumulations that extend for several centimeters (Fig. 4.28). One speaks of trichomycosis axillaris flava, rubra or nigra, although the color is of no clinical importance. The synonym palmellina refers to the red dye from an algae, *Palmella cruenta*. Rarely, pubic hairs or other terminal hairs may be affected. The hairs look as if they are covered by hoar frost. The changes tend to be chronic. Clothing may also be discolored.

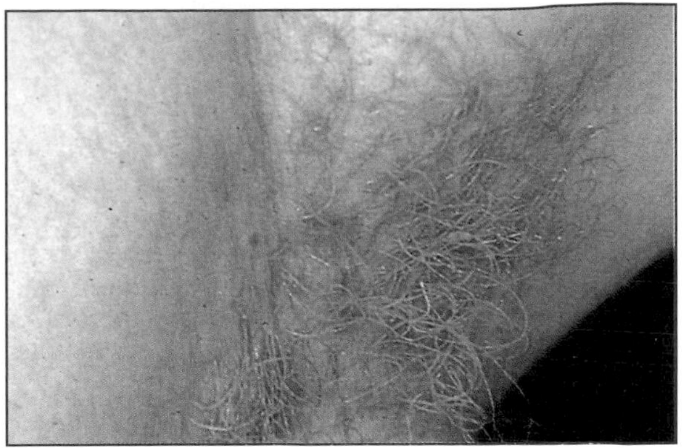

Fig. 4.28. Trichomycosis axillaris

Laboratory Findings. The hairs should examined under a microscope. The main differential question is hair casts, which are amorphous and do not show clumps of bacteria. Dark-field examination is a nice way to exaggerate the differences between the masses of bacteria and the hair shaft. *Corynebacterium tenuis* also fluoresces with Wood light; the differences in color reflect the type of porphyrin produced. The bacteria can be cultured but it is complicated and unnecessary.

Differential Diagnosis. The main differential diagnostic questions are hair casts and nits, but the latter are quite distinct.

Therapy. The easiest treatment is to shave the axillae and then treat the regrowing hairs with any topical disinfectant. Rubbing alcohol is fine; sometimes antibiotic washes, such as chlorhexidine, are sufficient. The rancid odor sticks to textiles so attention should also be paid to proper washing or dry cleaning.

Pitted Keratolysis
(Castellani 1910)

Synonym. Keratoma sulcatum

Definition. Pitted defect in thick horny layer of soles caused by moisture and bacterial overgrowth.

Causative Organism. Variety of *Corynebacterium* species.

Epidemiology. Pitted keratolysis is a common disorder among members of the military. The first descriptions concerned British troops in colonial India. Many American ground troops in Vietnam were affected. The disorder is a worldwide problem, far more common in the tropics and among men.

Etiology and Pathogenesis. The key factor is maceration, usually arising from hyperhidrosis, prolonged wearing of shoes and improper hygiene. Pitted keratolysis is thus common among athletes, those who must wear occlusive shoes (industrial workers, fishermen in rubber boots, soldiers in high boots); those working in water, such as rice field workers; and in Western countries in people who have easy access to swimming pools and spas. There is a general increase in the number of diphtheroids, which release various keratolytic enzymes that eat little holes or pits in the stratum corneum. In addition to *Corynebacterium* species, other unrelated bacteria such as *Dermatophilus congolensis* and *Micrococcus sedentarius* have been identified.

Clinical Findings. Most often, the thickest skin of the soles, that is the metatarsal region and heel, is involved. Rarely, the instep or the palms may be affected. The most typical finding is multiple small 2–5 mm pits which look as though cut out of the stratum corneum with a biopsy punch (Fig. 4.29). Sometimes the pits have a discolored or dark border which outlines the defect. The stratum corneum can also be white and swollen, typically involving areas several centimeters in size. There may be erythema at the periphery of the area. Lesions may coalesce forming larger erosions. While most often pitted keratolysis is asymptomatic, when the lesions are extensive or the patient is required to spend a lot of time walking or marching, the problem may become painful. In addition, the odor may be annoying.

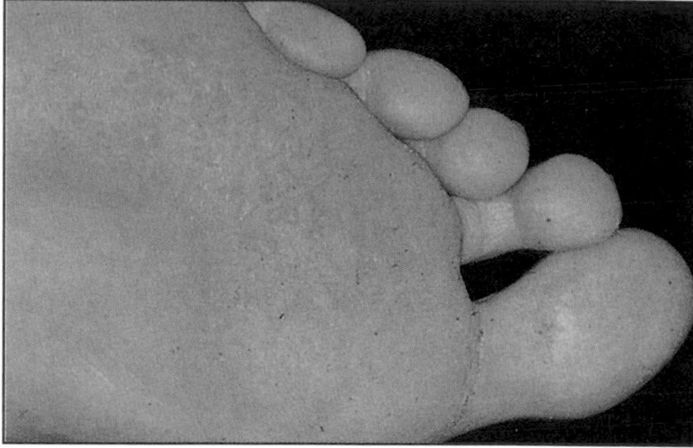

Fig. 4.29. Pitted keratolysis

Histopathology. The microscopic picture is striking. There are clearly defined pits in the stratum corneum associated with areas of pallor. The bottoms of the pits are lined with bacteria which can be identified with Gram stain or silver stain. Often the diphtheroids show filamentous forms.

Differential Diagnosis. Sometimes maceration and blistering can produce erosions but the tiny pits are pathognomonic.

Therapy. Reducing the moisture and mechanical pressure are most important. In addition, topical erythromycin solution or benzoyl peroxide gels can be applied once or twice daily. If the hyperhidrosis is severe, it can be treated (Chap. 30).

Cutaneous Diphtheria
(Bretonneau 1826)

Definition. Uncommon pyoderma which can progress to systemic diphtheria.

Causative Organism. *Corynebacterium diphtheriae*, usually type mitis

Epidemiology. Cutaneous diphtheria is an uncommon disorder. It is seen primarily in tropical areas, where a nonspecific synonym is jungle sore. In the USA, there is a focus of diphtheria among homeless alcoholic patients in the Seattle area and among Native Americans in the Pacific Northwest, with considerable overlap. In the 1970s there were over 1000 infections in Seattle, over 80 % of which were cutaneous. About five cases a year of systemic diphtheria are reported annually in the USA at this time. In the former Soviet Union, immunization has broken down and over 1000 people die yearly from diphtheria. The disease has spread into Western Europe, where many people do not have adequate immunity. In addition, there was a recent epidemic in Bolivia. Thus, physicians must once again be alert to the clinical spectrum of diphtheria.

Etiology and Pathogenesis. *Corynebacterium diphtheriae* is a strictly human pathogen that infects mucosal surfaces, usually the throat, and the skin. Most often, the pharyngitis comes first. The incubation period is very short, usually 1–4 days. Either via auto- or heteroinoculation the bacteria are transferred to an otherwise insignificant wound. The skin can be the primary entry site as well. Asymptomatic carriers of *C. diphtheriae* are common. There are three biotypes of *C. diphtheriae* (*mitis, intermedius* and *gravis*) determined on the basis of culture morphology, oxidization of tellurite and hemolytic potential. Only those bacteria infected by prophage β have the tox^+ gene, produce exotoxin and cause serious disease. The *intermedius* and *gravis* types are far more likely to produce toxin, which interferes with cellular NAD^+ metabolism. It can cause local damage to the skin or tonsils or spread through the system, where myocardial and neural damage are the most common complications.

Clinical Findings. There are two major types of cutaneous diphtheria. One is primary disease, when *C. diphtheriae* is inoculated into the skin and begins to grow locally. Usually a sharply bordered, punched out ulcer develops, often with a dirty, yellow leathery (diphtheria means leathery) pseudomembrane. In secondary disease, a preexisting wound is infected – this is the usual scenario in the USA. Most lesions are on the extremities. If a toxin is produced, the patient may become systemically ill. In the absence of toxin production, a smoldering dirty ulcer persists for a long period of time. *Streptococcus pyogenes* is often present in the same wound.

Histopathology. The necrotic membrane has no distinctive histologic features.

Laboratory Findings. On a smear, bipolar staining bacilli arranged in the so-called Chinese letter pattern are suggestive. Culture is done on Loeffler medium. The organism can be isolated from the throat in many patients with skin lesions so both should be checked. The now obsolete Schick (1913) test involves the injection of a small amount of diphtheria toxin into the skin; in a patient with immunity, nothing will happen; in the unprotected individual, the toxin produces necrosis.

Course and Prognosis. If the patient goes on to producing circulating exotoxins, the main acute risk is from myocarditis and bulbar paralysis. Prompt treatment reduces the risk of systemic complications; the cardiac damage is often permanent while the nerve damage is usually reversible.

Differential Diagnosis. Many skin lesions can be identical to diphtheria. One must be alert to the clinical setting, where the patient has traveled, what their immunization status is, and the risks in one's own area. In eastern Europe or perhaps the Seattle waterfront, a dirty cutaneous ulcer should be checked for diphtheria. The lesions of cutaneous diphtheria are not as deeply invasive, as are mixed bacterial infections (tropical ulcer). They have a membrane which is uncommon for ordinary impetigo.

Therapy

Systemic. Administration of antitoxin is the key. It must be given early before the toxin has had a chance to bind to cells. One cannot wait for the results of culture. Nonetheless, the equine antitoxin is not without risk, and the patient must be skin-tested prior to administration. Both intramuscular penicillin G and oral erythromycin are effective in killing the bacteria, but the antitoxin is far more crucial. The antibiotic treatment should last for 2 weeks.

Topical. Ordinary wound care suffices.

Public Health Measures. Diphtheria is a reportable disease. Patients should be isolated until cultures are negative. Contacts should be investigated and cultured, and anyone with symptoms should be treated. Carriers can be treated with a single dose of intramuscular penicillin. Food handlers should be kept away from work until cleared by culture, as milk has also served as a vehicle. Contacts should also receive either a diphtheria toxoid booster or immunization series depending on their status. All individuals should be encouraged to maintain appropriate immunization against *C. diphtheriae*.

Other Coryneform Bacteria

Corynebacterium pyogenes is an animal pathogen which may cause superficial ulcerations in humans, as well as a variety of opportunistic infections. An epidemic of leg ulcers among Thai school children was caused by this organism. *Corynebacterium* JK may cause sepsis in immunosuppressed individuals.

Closely related is *Arcanobacterium haemolyticum*, formerly *Corynebacterium haemolyticum*, which causes pharyngitis and skin ulcers. It was first identified as clinical problem among American soldiers in the South Pacific during World War II. The organism can only be cultured on blood agar, so it is easily overlooked in distinguishing between streptococcal and viral pharyngitis. The associated exanthem may be morbilliform or scarlatiniform, favoring the trunk and proximal extremities. Fortunately, antistreptococcal therapy usually eliminates this organism as well.

There are many other members of this family, whose classification remains befuddling. Some are common in animals and affect humans only as a zoonotic infection, while others are part of the normal flora of the oral mucosa, groin and toe webs.

Other Bacterial Diseases

Listeriosis

Epidemiology. *Listeria monocytogenes* is a motile, microaerophilic gram-positive bacillus. It infects many animals and is found in sewage and organic debris. While veterinarians and farmers may be infected directly, most humans are exposed via dairy and poultry products. Many individuals transiently carry the bacteria in their gastrointestinal tract for a period of time. Thus it assumes a position somewhere between a zoonotic and commensal infectious organism.

Clinical Findings. *Listeria monocytogenes* produces a variety of clinical pictures in humans including an infectious mononucleosis-like condition or gastrointestinal disease. Pregnant women are at increased risk; they may have a mild febrile illness but the risk of in utero infection is considerable. Here disseminated abscesses (granulomatosis infantiseptica) develop which have a very high mortality rate. There may be cutaneous abscesses, petechiae or extramedullary hematopoiesis (blueberry muffin syndrome). Other infants only have meningitis, with a somewhat better outlook. In immunosuppressed and chronically ill adults, especially HIV/AIDS patients, the organism may cause pneumonia, meningitis and sepsis, once again with a poor prognosis.

The situation in veterinarians and farmers is somewhat different, as they perhaps have some degree of immunity because of repeated exposures. Localized cutaneous lesions may develop following contact. They are typically red nodules which tend to become pustular and ulcerate. Thus they may be confused with more common pox and herpes virus infections.

Laboratory Findings. The diagnosis is made through culture, either from blood, stool or infected sites. The laboratory must be warned of the possible diagnosis, since special techniques including cold enhancement are needed.

Therapy. The agent of choice is ampicillin. In severe infections it is often combined with gentamicin.

Actinomycosis

(Bollinger 1877; Israel 1878)

Definition. Chronic granulomatous, often draining, infection caused by filamentous bacteria.

Causative Organism. *Actinomyces israelii* is a gram-positive, pleomorphic bacteria that forms filaments about 1 µm in thickness. It is anaerobic or microaerophilic and not acid-fast. Rarely, other organisms such as *Actinomyces naeslundi* or *Actinomyces viscosus* are isolated; the latter usually is associated with periodontal disease. Many accompanying bacteria can also be cultured, the most specific being *Actinobacillus actinomycetemcomitans*.

Epidemiology. Actinomycosis is a worldwide infection, more common among farmers than city dwellers. There is a strong male predominance.

Etiology and Pathogenesis. *Actinomyces israelii* is part of the normal oral mucosa and occasionally found in the intestinal flora. It alone is not a pathogen; for example, the bacteria are identified in over 50% of tonsillectomy specimens but not responsible for tonsillitis. Usually some sort of an injury and the presence of accompanying bacteria are required to produce a microenvironment with low oxygen favoring the growth of *A. israelii*. Dental problems, broken bones and traumatic injuries are the main predisposing factors. There are a large number of actinomyces species which are found in soil and plants, as well as in other animals, but they are not often human pathogens.

Clinical Findings. There are three classic types of actinomycosis.

- Cervicofacial infections are the most common form of actinomycosis. Decayed or damaged teeth offer a focus for the initial infection which involves the soft tissue of the oral cavity extending into the overlying skin; dental procedures are another trigger, as the harmless surface organisms may be introduced into deeper tissues. The subcutaneous swellings may enlarge, coalesce and break through to the skin surface, secreting pus and granular concretions known as sulfur bodies, which are simply masses of the bacteria. The neck is most often affected; the firm hardened end-product is known as woody neck (Fig. 4.30). As the disease progresses, multiple sinus tracts evolve. The skin tends to be red and warm. Usually there is no lymphadenopathy. Bones may also be infected producing osteomyelitis and periostitis.
- Gastrointestinal tract infection usually follows appendicitis with an appendectomy or ruptured viscera. The patient has a space-occupying mass or pseudotumor and presents with abdominal pain and other bowel complaints. Psoas abscesses can occur. Systemic complaints include-fever, chills and weight loss. Prominent anorectal involvement may result.
- Thoracic actinomycosis presumably results from the aspiration of *A. israelii* into the lungs, where in rare cases ideal growth circumstances arise and a pulmonary infection develops. Involvement of the chest wall with sinus tracts, drainage and rib destruction is common.

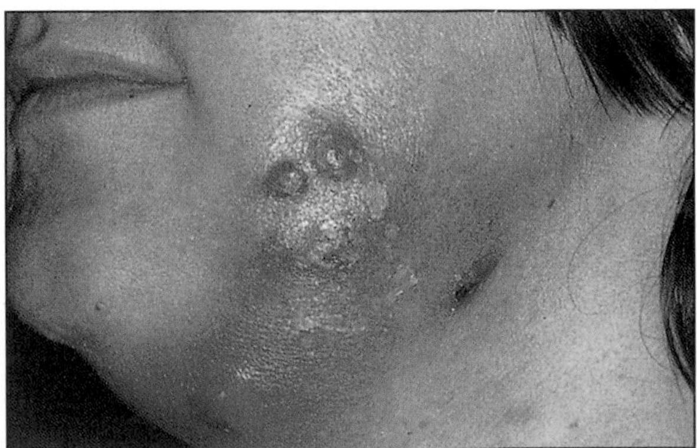

Fig. 4.30. Actinomycosis

Rarely, disseminated infection with multiple abscesses may develop. Pelvic actinomycosis is a complication of intrauterine contraceptive devices.

Histopathology. The sulfur granules or grains are identified amidst pockets of pus and chronic granulomatous inflammation. The granules tend to be gram-negative, but the fine filaments seen at the periphery are gram-positive, stain with PAS and silver methenamine, but are not acid-fast. These filaments are the reason why *A. israelii* was initially classified as a fungus. Grains are considered in more detail in Chapter 7, as they are a feature of mycetomas, actinomycosis, nocardiosis and botryomycosis.

Laboratory Findings. *Actinomyces israelii* is a fastidious organism which should be immediately inoculated into an anaerobic culture. Usually brain-heart dextrose agar culture is used, but specialized media are available. The culture plates are kept at 35–37°C. After 48 h spider-like mycelial colonies can be seen with a dissecting microscope. In about 10 days larger white colonies are formed. The organisms can be speciated using immunofluorescence techniques. It is important to isolate them from clinically infected tissue, as they are frequently identified in normal hosts.

Course and Prognosis. If untreated, the disease tends to spread diffusely and may damage adjacent structures, such as the eyes, great vessels or heart. The outlook depends on the degree of osteomyelitis and the speed with which the diagnosis is made.

Differential Diagnosis. Many different granulomatous infections may resemble actinomycosis. Early mandibular lesions are very similar to dental fistulas; this process should be excluded by dental evaluation and radiological examination. Nocardiosis must be excluded by culture; it can cause identical pulmonary and cutaneous changes. In addition, some forms of tuberculosis, tertiary syphilis, sporotrichosis and lymphogranuloma venereum should all be considered.

Therapy. The damaged tissue should be debrided or surgically managed, as once the microaerophilic environment is destroyed, treatment is far easier. The mainstay is penicillin; the usual recommendation is intravenous aqueous penicillin G (1.5–3.0 million units every 4 h) for at least 6 weeks, followed by oral penicillin VK (2.0–4.0 g daily) for one year. Some regimens incorporate intramuscular penicillin. In case of penicillin allergy, many alternate antibiotics are available, as discussed in infectious disease texts.

Nocardiosis

(Nocard 1888)

Definition. Chronic cutaneous and systemic infection which is most often seen in immunosuppressed individuals.

Causative Organism. *Nocardia asteroides* is the usual cause. Less often *Nocardia brasiliensis* and other nocardia species are identified.

Epidemiology. Nocardia species are found worldwide in the soil and on plants and other organic material.

Etiology and Pathogenesis. The bacteria are usually inoculated into the skin or inhaled, producing the two relatively different clinical patterns discussed below. About 85% of patients with nocardiosis are immunosuppressed, typically with HIV/AIDS, hematological or solid tumors, collagen vascular diseases and iatrogenic immunosuppression for organ transplantation. Preexisting pulmonary disease is also a predisposing factor.

Clinical Findings

- Systemic disease: Pulmonary disease is the most common form of nocardiosis with *N. asteroides* almost always responsible. Patients develop a chronic lung infection with systemic symptoms and nonspecific radiological changes. Secondary involvement is most common in the chest wall, overlying skin and CNS. Thus the presence of a therapy-resistant pneumonia with CNS findings in an immunosuppressed patient should always suggest nocardiosis.
- Sporotrichoid form: Inoculation via a rose thorn or other sharp plant material may produce a sporotrichoid pattern of infection (Chap. 7). Both *N. asteroides* and *N. brasiliensis* may be identified. A series of abscesses develop, advancing proximally along the lymphatic drainage of the limb. On the leg the initial lesion may evolve into an expanding leg ulcer. In some instances, the cutaneous infections remain superficial and localized without lymphatic spread.
- Oculoglandular form: *N. brasiliensis* can be rubbed into the eye, producing conjunctivitis with associated lymphadenopathy, just as with cat-scratch fever.
- Mycetomas are caused by *N. brasiliensis* and rarely *N. asteroides*. They are considered in Chapter 7.

Histopathology. The organisms cannot be seen on routine sections, where typically an abscess is revealed. The fine branched filaments are similar to *Actinomyces* but are weakly acid-fast, as well as positive with Gram, PAS and methenamine silver stains.

Laboratory Findings. Nocardiosis is a culture diagnosis. In contrast to actinomycosis, *Nocardia* are usually pathogenic. If they are isolated from skin, lung tissue or brain tissue, they are always pathogens. Occasionally they may be found in sputum cultures from healthy individuals. The laboratory must be notified that *Nocardia* is expected, as it can be very slow-growing. While small colonies are usually seen after 2–4 days, they may require up to 2 weeks. Routine bacterial and fungal media as well as Löwenstein-Jensen medium are all satisfactory. Speciation is difficult and is based on hydrolysis tests.

Course and Prognosis. In immunosuppressed hosts the mortality, even with prompt treatment, is about 25%, but approaches 40% when CNS disease is present. The cutaneous disease responds well to treatment and does not tend to generalize.

Differential Diagnosis. The differential diagnosis of the pulmonary form includes almost all infectious pneumonias. Extension to the chest wall is similar to that seen in actinomycosis. The sporotrichoid pattern should suggest sporotrichosis, deep fungi, atypical mycobacteria and the other causes discussed in Chapter 7.

Therapy. Once again debridement is important. The mainstay of therapy is long-term administration of sulfa-type antibiotics. Trimethoprim-sulfamethoxazole has become the treatment of choice for both cutaneous and systemic forms. In the later case, serum sulfa levels should be kept at around 15 mg/dl; when treating strictly cutaneous lesions, oral trimethoprim-sulfamethoxazole (160 mg–800 mg) b.i.d. is sufficient. Adjunctive local heat therapy may also be useful. In normal hosts therapy is continued for 2–3 months, while in immunosuppressed hosts, at least 1 year is recommended.

Cat-Scratch Disease

(Debré et al. 1930)

Synonyms. Cat-scratch fever, benign lymphoreticulosis

Definition. Chronic infection with marked regional lymphadenopathy usually associated with a skin defect and exposure to a cat.

Causative Organism. *Bartonella henselae* is a small, delicate gram-negative bacillus. Formerly known as *Rochalimaea henselae*, it is closely related to *Bartonella bacilliformis* but also shares features with rickettsiae. It is responsible for over 95% of cases of cat-scratch disease. *Afipia felis*, another gram-negative bacillus identified at the Armed Forces Institute of Pathology (AFIP) in lymph nodes from patients with cat-scratch disease, is responsible for less than 5% of cases.

Epidemiology. Cat-scratch disease involves primarily children and adolescents. Almost all have had direct contact with a cat, usually a kitten, and many have been scratched. The disease is not spread between humans. It is the most common cause of benign localized or regional lymphadenopathy in this age group. The incidence in the USA is around 4/100,000 yearly, making it all the more amazing that the causative organism has only been identified with certainty in the past decade. In immunosuppressed hosts, *B. henselae* causes bacillary angiomatosis, hepatic peliosis and bacteremia, as discussed in the next section.

Etiology and Pathogenesis. In most instances there is cutaneous inoculation coupled with bacterial proliferation in regional lymph nodes. Only rarely does disseminated disease occur.

Clinical Findings. Typically a papule develops as the primary lesion at the site of injury or inoculation, most often on the arm. Nail fold infections may also develop if the tip of a digit is bitten. The incubation period is usually about 10 days, but varies from 3 to 60 days. Patients often present with regional lymphadenopathy, most commonly involving the neck or axilla, and some have multiple areas of involvement. Spontaneous regression is the rule, but in up to 20% of patients suppuration may develop. About 75% of patients develop systemic complaints such as fever, chills and malaise. The most severe systemic complication is encephalitis; hepatosplenomegaly, facial nerve palsy and arthritis may also occur. The patients may also have transient nonspecific exanthems, erythema multiforme or erythema nodosum. Parinaud or oculoglandular syndrome is a special clinical form; inoculation occurs in the conjunctiva and the preauricular lymph nodes are involved. CNS and facial nerve involvement, as well as optic neuritis, may develop in these patients.

Histopathology. The primary inoculation site simply shows an abscess or ulcer. The organism can occasionally be found and is best seen with the Warthin-Starry stain. The lymph nodes contain *B. henselae* and typically show granulomatous inflammation and necrosis.

Laboratory Findings. *Bartonella henselae* cannot be reliably cultured. Diagnosis is usually made by identifying the organism in lymph nodes using either Warthin-Starry stain or PCR. Serological methods are also available; detection of an IgG antibody against a bacterial antigen is the most sensitive. Indirect immunofluorescent antibodies are also available. In the past, a skin test using suppurative material from an infected lymph node was employed, but it is no longer available and not recommended because of the risk of transferring HIV and viral hepatitis.

Course and Prognosis. The outlook is good in patients with normal immune status. Spontaneous resolution is the rule; even the encephalitis heals without sequelae. Lifelong immunity develops.

Differential Diagnosis. The differential diagnostic considerations are endless. The presence of lymphadenopathy and malaise may suggest infectious mononucleosis. Tularemia, brucellosis, plague, toxoplasmosis, tuberculosis and many other infections can produce similar changes in the lymph nodes.

Therapy. Generally no treatment is required. If a lymph node biopsy is performed, often suppuration and drainage develop. Aspiration may be helpful. Many antibiotics appear to be effective, but no clear first-choice agent exists. Many texts recommend ciprofloxacin 500 mg b.i.d., for use in patients who are immunosuppressed or ill. Erythromycin is clearly effective, as it is the agent of choice in treating the same organism when it causes bacillary angiomatosis.

Bacillary Angiomatosis

(Stoler et al. 1983; Weaver et al. 1983)

Definition. Infection is most common in HIV/AIDS patients ,causes endothelial proliferation and produces vascular tumors.

Causative Organism. *Bartonella henselae*

Etiology and Pathogenesis. Bacillary angiomatosis is an infection which was first identified in HIV/AIDS patients.

The main source of the organism is cats; in immunocompetent hosts, it causes cat-scratch disease. *B. henselae* causes cutaneous lesions, hepatic infections (peliosis) and often osteomyelitis in HIV/AIDS patients. Other organs, such as eyes, CNS and lymph nodes may also be infected. Some patients may present with fever of unknown origin. Rarely *Bartonella quintana*, the cause of trench fever, can be identified from lesions of bacillary angiomatosis or peliosis.

Clinical Findings. The typical skin lesions are edematous, relatively rapidly growing, pyogenic granuloma-like papules and nodules which often ulcerate (Fig. 4.31). Sometimes subcutaneous plaques and nodules develop, but usually the lesions are exudative, eroded and often ulcerated.

Histopathology. The diagnosis is made microscopically. In the dermis there is a proliferation of small vessels resembling an ordinary capillary hemangioma and associated with many neutrophils. The slits and hemosiderin associated with Kaposi sarcoma are usually not found, nor are mitoses present. Instead, blue gray clumps of necrotic bacteria are present; Warthin-Starry stain identifies the clumps and individual bacteria nicely. PCR, electron microscopy and culture can also be done.

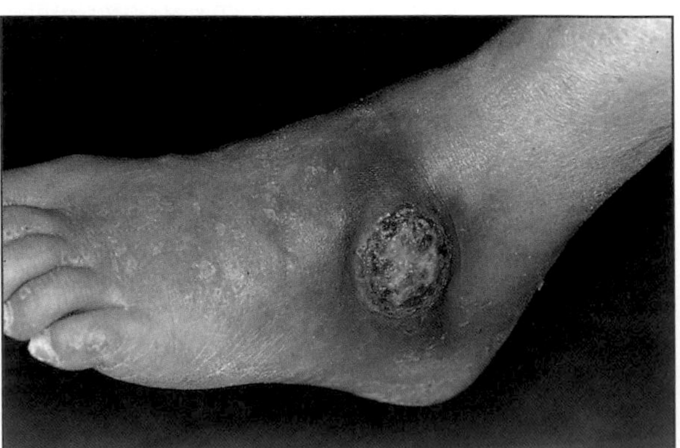

Fig. 4.31. Bacillary angiomatosis

Differential Diagnosis. The diagnosis of pyogenic granuloma should be made reluctantly in HIV/AIDS patients. *B. henselae* should always be excluded. Many cases were mistaken for Kaposi sarcoma initially, but the latter disease usually features more elongated or spindle-shaped lesions, ulcerates much later and has a different histology.

Therapy. The mainstay of treatment is erythromycin; 2.0–3.0 g daily for 4 weeks is the minimum therapy. Many alternative regimens are available; we have used doxycycline 200 mg daily for 4 weeks with good results. Some clinicians recommend ciprofloxacin 500 mg b.i.d., just as for cat-scratch disease.

Trench Fever

(Werner 1916; His 1916)

Synonyms. Werner-His disease, Wolhynia fever, Meuse fever, quintan fever, shin bone fever

Causative Organism. *Bartonella quintana.*

Epidemiology. Epidemics of trench fever were first described during World War I and then again during World War II. The crowded and unsanitary conditions favored the presence of lice (*Pediculus humanus corporis)* which transfers *B. quintana* from individual to individual. Today foci exist in Poland, Russia and parts of Africa, Central and South America. Outbreaks have been reported among the homeless in both Seattle and Marseilles in recent years.

Etiology and Pathogenesis. Humans are the only hosts. The bacteria is taken up from the blood by the louse during feeding; it develops in the arthropod gut and is then transmitted by infectious lice feces. No transovarian development occurs. Human to human transmission is not seen. The incubation period is about 1–3 weeks. A past history of trench fever is a permanent contraindication to blood donation because the organism may circulate in the blood of an asymptomatic carrier for months to years.

Clinical Findings. The patients present with fever, chills and tenderness, especially over the shins.

There is usually a transient macular exanthem. There may be relapsing fevers or a single peak of several days. The bacteremia persists for a long time and may or may not be associated with chronic symptoms.

Laboratory Findings. The diagnosis is made with blood culture on blood agar under 5% CO_2. Serological tests are available.

Differential Diagnosis. The differential diagnosis is endless, including all louse-borne fevers (Chap. 8).

Therapy. The lice infestation should be treated and the environment cleaned. Both tetracycline and chloramphenicol are effective, but no adequate studies are available.

Public Health Measures. This is a reportable infection, primarily because lice also transmit epidemic typhus (Chap. 3).

Bartonellosis

(Carrión 1885; Odriazola 1895)

Synonyms. Carrión disease, Carrión fever, Oroya fever, verruga peruana, Peruvian warts

Causative Organism. *Bartonella bacilliformis*, another small, delicate gram-negative bacillus

History. Daniel Carrión was a Peruvian medical student who inoculated himself with material from an infected patient and died of the bacteremic form of the disease in 1885 before he could write up his findings. Nonetheless he is usually credited as the discoverer of the infection.

Epidemiology. The natural history of bartonellosis is well-understood. The bacteria is transmitted by sandflies of the genus *Lutzomyia*, especially *L. verrucarum*. The arthropod only lives in the high mountain valleys of Peru, Ecuador and southwestern Colombia at elevations from 600 to 3000 m. The flies are active from dusk to dawn.

Etiology and Pathogenesis. The only known source is humans. In endemic areas, the asymptomatic carrier rate is about 5%. The disease is transmitted by the bites of the fly, but can also be transferred by blood transfusion. The incubation period is usually several weeks, but can be many months, a point of importance when evaluating travelers who have returned from the Andes.

Clinical Findings. *Bartonella bacilliformis* causes two clinically distinct diseases: a bacteremic toxic condition known as Oroya fever and chronic dermal nodules called verruga peruana. Oroya fever may occasionally precede verruga peruana, but most often the initial infection is asymptomatic.

In Oroya fever, the patient is seriously ill with fever, malaise, chills and a striking hemolytic anemia. Marked lymphadenopathy and hepatosplenomegaly are also present. Skin findings frequently include a petechial exanthem. The mortality in untreated patients is considerable, with estimates ranging from 10% to 90% in different studies. Secondary bacterial infections, most often *Salmonella* sepsis, are the usual cause of death, perhaps explaining the wide range of mortality.

Verruga peruana consists of dermal papules and nodules, some of which become pedunculated, verrucous or eroded. They may appear in crops and be clustered on a given body region, usually the face or limbs. Mucous membrane involvement has been described. While the lesions generally resolve spontaneously, they may persist for many years.

Histopathology. The verruga peruana are quite similar to bacillary angiomatosis with endothelial proliferation. Using Warthin-Starry stain, the bacteria can be identified in the tumors.

Laboratory Findings. In bacteremic patients, *B. bacilliformis* can be found in blood films adherent to erythrocytes. It can also be cultured from the blood during either stage, although it is more easily found in septic patients. The skin lesions can be cultured or studied with PCR to identify the bacteria. Serological testing is also available.

Differential Diagnosis. The differential diagnosis of the septic form is infections with hemolysis. The regional distribution offers the best clue; the exanthem is nonspecific. The verruga peruana can be mistaken for pyogenic granuloma, Kaposi sarcoma and bacillary angiomatosis, which can be viewed as the same tumor under a different name.

Therapy. For Oroya fever, the agent of choice is chloramphenicol, 2.0 g daily for 1 week, as this also covers the possibility of a *Salmonella* infection. *B. bacilliformis* responds to many antibiotics, such as tetracyclines, erythromycin and penicillin. Nonetheless, verruga peruana are less responsive to antibiotics than bacillary angiomatosis in HIV/

AIDS patients; usually one must await natural resolution.

Enterobacter Infections

Many different species of closely related gram-negative rods, both anaerobic and aerobic, are grouped together here. Some are always pathogenic, while others are part of the normal intestinal flora. They tend to produce clinical disease only in chronically ill or immunosuppressed individuals. Thus they are a feared cause of nosocomial infections.

The terminology is quite complex and will undoubtedly change again in the near future. The major enterobacteria will be considered briefly when they produce cutaneous manifestations. Only a few will be explored in detail, such as *Klebsiella pneumoniae rhinoscleromatis* which causes a distinct cutaneous disease. Treatment will be only be considered for those organisms of special interest to dermatologists.

Escherichia coli Infections

Escherichia coli causes genitourinary tract infections and sepsis. It is often a cause of wound infections or cellulitis in the perianal area or other sites where fecal contamination has occurred. Several variants of *E. coli* are obligate pathogens and cause more severe disease.

- Enterohemorrhagic *E. coli* (EHEC) of serotype O157:H7 produces potent cytotoxins that cause hemorrhagic colitis without fever. They are designed as verotoxins or shiga-like toxins. Patients may go on to develop hemolytic-uremic syndrome and thrombotic thrombocytopenic purpura (Chap. 23). Infection is usually transmitted by inadequately cooked or processed beef. Antibiotic therapy is of no benefit; supportive care is required, including renal dialysis.
- Enteropathogenic *E. coli* (EPEC) causes severe diarrhea. Transmission is usually fecal-oral. Infections are primarily a problem in developing countries.
- Enterotoxigenic *E. coli* (ETEC) causes diarrhea in small children and is responsible for most travelers' diarrhea or Montezuma's revenge.
- Enteroinvasive *E. coli* (EIEC) causes a bloody diarrhea with mucus, very similar to *Shigella.*

Klebsiella Infections

Klebsiella pneumoniae is associated primarily with lobar pneumonia in weakened patients. It produces an acute pneumonia (Friedländer 1882) which can be quite severe; in such cases the sputum is often rich in necrotic tissue and has been described as jelly-like. Urinary tract and wound infections in hospitalized patients may also be seen.

Klebsiella pneumoniae ozaenae causes upper respiratory tract infections. It has been linked with chronic atrophic rhinitis, but this connection is disputed as antibiotic therapy rarely helps the disorder.

Serratia and *Enterobacter* are closely related to *Klebsiella.* They may cause wound infections and cellulitis in appropriate hosts. *Serratia* is common among heroin addicts and may cause endocarditis and cutaneous abscesses. It has also caused skin and joint abscesses because of the use of contaminated benzalkonium solution to sterilize the skin for procedures.

Rhinoscleroma

(Hebra 1870)

Definition. Chronic progressive infection of the upper and lower airways.

Causative Organism. *Klebsiella pneumoniae rhinoscleromatis*

Epidemiology. Rhinoscleroma was formerly common in Central Europe, as it was described in Vienna and has been identified in moulages from other clinics. Today, focal endemic areas are found in Africa, South America, Scandinavia and New Guinea, but sporadic cases may appear anywhere. The disease is most often seen among young adults, mostly living in rural areas with lower standards of hygiene.

Etiology and Pathogenesis. The organism has a very low degree of infectivity. Transmission is presumably via droplets or fomites but with many inapparent infections. The granulomatous response is apparently inadequate, as the bacteria are phagocytosed but not destroyed. Their capsule is rich in mucopolysaccharides, which facilitate attachment and damage the respiratory mucosa of the posterior nares.

Clinical Findings. The infection usually starts with a chronic rhinitis, which may be characterized by foul odor, crusting and lack of response to ordinary therapy. Granulation tissue then appears on the nasal septum and slowly spreads. Later, nodules develop within the nostrils, on the upper lip and posteriorly into the pharynx and larynx. These firm, red-brown vegetating nodules slowly expand and distort the anatomy. The typical involvement of the nose and upper lip has been described as a Hebra nose, tapir lip or rhinoceros lip. Breathing is impaired and vocal chord changes alter the voice. Later, fibrosis occurs with bony destruction. The entire process is allegedly surprisingly painless.

Histopathology. The microscopic picture is dramatic. The dermis shows chronic inflammation rich in plasma cells, Russell bodies and the diagnostic Mikulicz cells, which are engorged large (up to 200 µm) histiocytes containing mucin and many bacteria, which can be seen with Giemsa or Gram stains. Mikulicz was the first to identify rhinoscleroma as an infectious disease; Hebra felt it was a malignancy.

Laboratory Findings. While *K. pneumoniae rhinoscleromatis* can be cultured, the microscopic picture usually suffices. If the bacteria is cultured, it must be separated from other related bacteria by using complex antigenic markers. It is also pathogenic for mice.

Differential Diagnosis. Mucocutaneous leishmaniasis, paracoccidioidomycosis and blastomycosis should all be considered. If the histology is not typical, then cultures for *Leishmania* and deep fungi should be employed. Malignant lymphomas can sometimes present with nasal destruction but their course is usually more rapid.

Therapy. Many different antibiotic regimens have been proposed. Tetracycline, ciprofloxacin and trimethoprim-sulfamethoxazole are all effective. While tetracycline has traditionally been used for an entire year (2.0 g daily for 6 months, then 1.0 g daily for the next 6 months), shorter regimens of 2–3 months appear satisfactory for the other antibiotics. Surgical debridement is also recommended.

Proteus Infections

Proteus typically causes genitourinary tract infections. The most common species is *P. mirabilis.* The bacteria are also frequently found in burns, decubitus ulcers, and peroneal abscesses. They may cause cellulitis in immunosuppressed hosts. *Proteus* species can be found in botryomycosis.

Typhoid Fever

Causative Organism. *Salmonella typhi*

Etiology and Pathogenesis. Typhoid fever has become uncommon in the USA, but it is estimated to cause over 500,000 deaths worldwide annually. The source of the bacteria is humans; individuals may be short-term carriers following a mild infection or chronic carriers. Transmission is via the food and water contaminated by the urine and feces of carriers.

Clinical Findings. Typical findings include fever, malaise, headache and, surprisingly, constipation, not usually diarrhea. The classic cutaneous finding is rose spots, found in over 50% of patients. After about 1 week of fever, the 2–3-mm tiny pink papules appear in crops generally on the abdomen. They are blanchable and spontaneously disappear, leaving behind brown postinflammatory hyperpigmentation. If the patient is not treated, new crops will develop.

Histopathology. The rose spots show widely dilated capillaries. It is unlikely that this is specific enough to suggest the diagnosis.

Laboratory Findings. The organisms can be cultured from the stool or blood. Serological testing is also available.

Therapy. Chloramphenicol remains the treatment of choice. Resistance to this reliable drug is becoming more common and alternative drugs such as ciprofloxacin may be advisable but are rarely affordable for the patient.

Other Salmonella Infections

Salmonella paratyphi may cause a disease identical to typhoid fever, but usually produces milder problems. Rose spots may occur and have even been reported on the face. Some patients with intestinal salmonella infections may present with vulvovaginitis. In other instances, subcutaneous abscesses may form as a result of vascular dissemination.

S. typhimurum, S. enteritidis and other species cause a food-borne gastroenteritis which may advance to sepsis in the weakened or elderly. The sources are numerous including contaminated milk, eggs, poultry and meat. The animal sources may be infected or the products can be infected during handling by an infected individual. Large epidemics have been seen; one with improperly pasteurized milk affected almost 300,000 individuals.

Direct contact with a wide variety of animal salmonella may produce lesions on the hands and forearms of veterinarians. Papules, nodules and pustules have been described. Rarely, salmonella can cause a gram-negative folliculitis.

Shigella Infections

The various species of *Shigella* cause severe diarrhea. *S. dysenteriae* may produce the hemolytic uremic syndrome. *S. flexneri* is one of the common gastrointestinal triggers of Reiter syndrome.

Yersinosis

(Yersin 1894; Kitasato 1894)

Causative Organism. *Yersinia enterocolitica* is a small gram-negative bacillus. Two other species are also pathogenic: *Y. pseudotuberculosis* causes zoonotic disease, with humans only rarely infected; *Y. pestis* is responsible for plague.

Epidemiology. *Yersinia enterocolitica* is most common in Scandinavia and northern Europe. It is difficult to culture, perhaps leading to underdiagnosis. *Y. enterocolitica* is spread from patient to patient, while swine serve as the usual reservoir. *Y. pseudotuberculosis* is usually found among rodents and other small mammals. The bacterium grows well at low temperatures so it is a potential food contaminant. Chocolate milk, tofu and improperly cooked pork have been implicated.

Etiology and Pathogenesis. The usual gastrointestinal infection with *Y. enterocolitica* or *Y. pseudotuberculosis* is not dramatic. However, this bacterium is one of the triggers of the whole spectrum of reactive arthritis, enthesopathies, iritis and many other problems associated with HLA-B27 positivity and a negative rheumatoid factor. Presumably some *Yersinia* antigen serves as a superantigen or as a basis for molecular mimicry.

Clinical Findings. Small children tend to present with diarrhea while older children are more likely to have mesenteric lymphadenitis, which mimics appendicitis. Rare patients develop bacteremia; those with iron overload (hemochromatosis and other disorders) and immunosuppression are at particular risk. Yersinia arthritis usually has no cutaneous features; it is most common in young adults. In older individuals there are several cutaneous manifestations.

- Erythema nodosum occurs in about 10% of adults with *Yersinia* infections. In Scandinavia, this infection is the most common identifiable cause of erythema nodosum. The combination of erythema nodosum and gastrointestinal symptoms should always suggest yersinosis. There is no correlation with HLA-B27.
- Sweet syndrome is another possible cutaneous manifestation of yersinosis (Chap. 14).

Laboratory Findings. The laboratory must be alerted to the need to look for *Yersinia*. The organism must be searched for with cold-enriched cultures; for example, the fecal material can be held in sterile saline for 10 days at 2–6 C. Selective media are also required. The final identification is usually done with serotyping. Serological testing is available for some serotypes but is not widely used except in epidemiological studies.

Differential Diagnosis. The differential diagnosis includes all the causes of acute gastroenteritis including *Salmonella, Shigella* and many viruses. When confronted with erythema nodosum or Sweet syndrome, the physician may wish to exclude the presence of yersinosis.

Therapy. Most often the bowel infection requires no therapy. If the patient is bacteremic, third generation cephalosporins alone or combined with fluoroquinolones are most effective. Tetracycline has been the traditional choice. Antibiotics play little role in treating the arthritis, which requires standard antiinflammatory measures.

Pneumococcal Infections

Causative Organism. *Streptococcus pneumoniae*

Etiology and Pathogenesis. Better known as pneumococcus or diplococcus, this α-hemolytic streptococcus is an important pathogen. The discovery of the transforming factor in this organism and its subsequent identification as DNA not only won the Nobel Prize for Avery, MacLeod and McCarty but also marked the beginning of molecular genetics. These bacteria are part of the normal flora of the throat in over 50% of individuals and it seems that most pneumococcal infections are endogenous, not acquired via droplets.

Clinical Findings. *Streptococcus pneumoniae* is a well-known as a cause of acute lobar pneumonia. It typically affects the chronically ill and immunosuppressed. In children it is also responsible for otitis media and meningitis, as well as orbital cellulitis. In addition, *S. pneumoniae* may cause cellulitis in immunosuppressed adults. Sometimes bullous lesions develop. In most instances the cellulitis follows an attack of pneumococcal pneumonia. Since most cellulitis is treated empirically to cover staphylococci and streptococci, many cases of cellulitis caused by *S. pneumoniae* are not identified but nonetheless treated.

Laboratory Findings. Paired gram-positive cocci can be identified in blister fluid or pus, but cultures are needed to identify the organism with certainty.

Therapy. The development of penicillin-resistant strains of *S. pneumoniae* has become a major public health problem. Alterations in the bacterial penicillin-binding proteins are responsible. For dermatological purposes, treatment with higher doses of penicillin is probably still the best approach. However, for life-threatening illnesses such as meningitis, infectious disease experts should be consulted. Immunization is available and recommended for high-risk individuals.

Meningococcemia

(Weichselbaum 1887)

Causative Organism. *Neisseria meningitidis*

Epidemiology. Meningococcal infections occur worldwide. In Germany they are most common in the late winter and spring. About 5% of the population are carriers of *N. meningitidis*; in crowded living conditions such as in military barracks the rates may rise dramatically. In Africa one speaks of the meningococcal belt – a broad path along the equator in which infections are extremely frequent. The usual type of spread is via droplets.

Etiology and Pathogenesis. Many different serogroups have been identified; their prevalence varies geographically. The bacteria attach to the respiratory mucosa with their pili and are taken up by phagocytes, but are usually protected by their capsule and wind up in endothelial cells. Here they release endotoxins which damage the vessels, producing the typical purpura and leading to more severe hemorrhagic complications such as disseminated intravascular coagulation (Chap. 23). Infections usually produce immunity; individuals with defects in the late components of complement (C6 – C9) or IgM are likely to have recurrent infections. Circulating immune complexes may develop leading to vasculitis, arthritis, episcleritis and other complications.

Clinical Findings. Most meningococcal infections are subclinical. Often the first clinical sign is petechiae. In other instances, tiny pink or red papules may first be seen. In any child with fever and petechiae, meningococci should be considered; if one searches carefully, most patients do have some cutaneous lesions. Most often the limbs and trunk are involved. The degree of cutaneous vascular damage correlates well with the severity of the systemic disease. Purpuric patches greater than 1 cm in diameter, bullae or ulceration suggest a poor outcome (Fig. 4.32). The Waterhouse-Friderichsen syndrome (Chap. 23) represents the most severe form of meningococcal sepsis, with cutaneous necrosis and disseminated intravascular coagulation. Patients without a spleen are at special risk of meningococcal sepsis. Sometimes vasculitis develops, either during the acute phase or even following adequate treatment. In this instance, nodular or palpable purpura appears along with

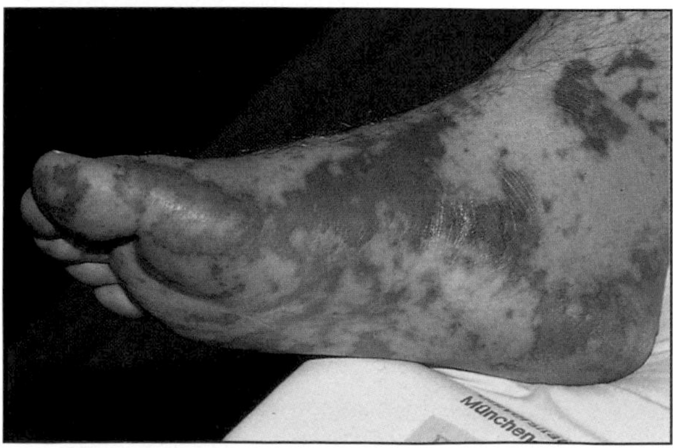

Fig. 4.32. Meningococcal purpura

the cutaneous hemorrhage. The vasculitis is part of the immune complex reaction.

Of special interest to dermatologists is chronic meningococcemia. Patients typically are military recruits or refugees living in crowded conditions with a high carrier rate of a not particularly aggressive strain of *N. meningitidis*. Other patients often have a smoldering meningococcal infection in the head and neck region. While the patients may have low-grade fever and feel ill, they do not develop meningitis but instead a pustular cutaneous vasculitis almost identical to that seen with disseminated gonococcal infection.

Histopathology. In acute lesions, vascular thrombi may be identified. Organisms are not usually found. Chronic meningococcal lesions show leukocytoclastic angiitis with increased amounts of neutrophils, often with pustules.

Laboratory Findings. If there is any suspicion of meningococcemia both CSF for direct examination and culture as well as a blood culture should be obtained. Often direct staining of the pus-laden spinal fluid provides a working diagnosis which is confirmed by the cultures. If purpura is more extensive, the patient's hemostatic parameters should be assessed.

Course and Prognosis. Untreated meningococcal meningitis has a mortality of over 80%. Prompt and appropriate treatment reduces this to less than 10%. The patients with Waterhouse-Friderichsen syndrome have a dismal outlook even with adequate care; the mortality rate is around 50%. The outlook for chronic meningococcemia is excellent.

Differential Diagnosis. The differential diagnosis of meningitis is lengthy and dependent on the age group and geographic location. The combination of fever and petechiae also suggests Rocky Mountain spotted fever, *Haemophilus influenzae* sepsis, enteroviral infections, subacute bacterial endocarditis and many other infections.

Therapy. Intravenous penicillin G in high doses is still the treatment of choice. Prior to definite diagnosis, the choice of therapy in children must also cover *H. influenzae* and *S. pneumoniae*. Regional resistance patterns will also determine treatment choices. In adults with chronic meningococcemia, intravenous and then oral penicillin is effective. When patients experience purpura fulminans and shock, standard therapy is often inadequate. Many new approaches have been tried including recombinant bactericidal/permeability-increasing protein, a combination of protein C and heparin, and monoclonal antibodies against TNF-α.

Prophylaxis. Rifampicin is recommended as prophylactic treatment for close contacts of patients with meningococcal infections.

Meningococcal vaccines are directed against the specific capsular polysaccharides. Currently, a quadrivalent vaccine is in use; no effective vaccination against group B *Neisseria meningitidis*, the most common type in Germany, is available. Vaccines are used in military personal, in patients without spleens and to control local epidemics. Travelers to areas where group A *N. meningitidis* are prevalent should also consider immunization.

Public Health Measures. Meningococcal infections are reportable.

Vibrio Infections

Cholera is the best know disease in this group, caused by *Vibrio cholerae*. Despite its immense public heath consequences, cholera has no specific cutaneous findings and will not be further considered.

Some other vibrios may cause severe cellulitis. The best known member of the group is *V. vulnificus*, which is found in warm sea water. In the USA it is a particular problem in the Gulf Coast states. Two patterns of infection may be seen following ingestion of raw or inappropriately cooked infected seafood or following a cutaneous injury. In both instances, patients who are immunosuppressed or have hemochromatosis or other forms of chronic liver disease are at greatest risk. The patients with sepsis develop hypotension, thrombocytopenia, hemorrhagic bullae and disseminated intravascular coagulation; the mortality rate is over 90% if hypotension occurs. The skin is almost always seeded when bacteremia develops. Following inoculation, painful, bullous, rapidly spreading cellulitis develops; underlying structures can be affected, producing necrotizing fasciitis, muscle necrosis, and sepsis. The treatment of choice is tetracycline; the challenge is to think of *V. vulnificus* and treat promptly.

Another pathogenic member of the family is *Aeromonas hydrophilia*, which is found in fresh and brackish water. While it usually causes gastroenteritis, the organism can also cause cellulitis with crepitation and subcutaneous abscesses. It may also infect muscles, mimicking severe group A β-hemolytic streptococcal infections.

Helicobacter Infections

Causative Organism. *Helicobacter pylori*

This gram-negative curved rod has been identified for less than two decades but has assumed an important place in the gastrointestinal literature. It is responsible for most cases of chronic atrophic gastritis, as well as gastric and duodenal ulcers. It can be identified on endoscopic biopsies, via serological testing or with carbon-labeled urea breath tests. The latter has become popular for the rapid office diagnosis of the infection. Complex therapy schemes have been designed for the eradication of *H. pylori;* they incorporate multiple antibiotics, bismuth compounds and omeprazole. *H. pylori* has been incriminated as a possible cause of chronic urticaria (Chap. 11) and rosacea (Chap. 28). In both diseases, some physicians recommend a trial of anti-*Helicobacter pylori* therapy.

Pseudomonas Infections

Many different species of *Pseudomonas* can be identified. *P. mallei* causes glanders, while *P. pseudomallei* is responsible for melioidosis. The most common species is *P. aeruginosa;* rarely other species will be isolated in the same clinical settings.

Etiology and Pathogenesis. Pseudomonas species are part of the normal flora in the groin, perianal region, axillae and between the toes. Usually they are only transiently present. Continued soaking of the feet, as can occur in military conditions, reduces the number of gram-positive bacteria and allows *P. aeruginosa* to flourish. There are a number of relatively harmless infections, all related somewhat to moisture, in which *P. aeruginosa* can be isolated but its pathogenicity is question. On the other hand, *P. aeruginosa* is a life-threatening pathogen in immunosuppressed or critically ill patients. Both reduced host defense mechanisms and altered levels of other primarily gram-positive bacteria are held responsible for its increased growth capacity. *P. aeruginosa* infections may be green in color because of pyocyanin and fluoresce with a Wood light because of pyoverdin (fluorescin). *Xanthomonas (Pseudomonas) maltophilia* may also cause infections in immunosuppressed patients, typically either erythematous nodules or cellulitis.

Clinical Findings. A number of distinct clinical settings may feature *P. aeruginosa* infections.

- Immunosuppressed patients are at risk for pseudomonas septicemia, especially those with granulocytopenia or indwelling catheters. As part of the sepsis, dramatic skin lesions may be produced. The best known is ecthyma gangrenosum. Here an indurated, often painless ulcer with a dark eschar develops, usually in the axilla or groin. In addition, vesicular and bullous lesions may be seen. They are often hemorrhagic and occasionally may have an erythematous halo. Early lesions are smaller papules and nodules. Finally, cellulitis may develop if the patient survives long enough.
- Burns are quite likely to be invaded. The eschar may acquire a green color and rest on a creamy base. If untreated, the infection evolves into a life-threatening sepsis.
- Infants may develop an umbilical infection which, if not treated, can disseminate.

In addition to these serious problems, *P. aeruginosa* causes a long list of almost nuisance infections.

- Gram-negative toe web infections frequently feature *P. aeruginosa*. Typically patients are soldiers or engaged in heavy manual labor, so they spend a long time in wet sweaty shoes. Those individuals with deformed toes with marked overlapping are also at risk. Secondary infection with *C. albicans* or dermatophytes is common.
- Hot tub folliculitis, also called swimming pool folliculitis, almost always involves a relatively nonpathogenic strain of *P. aeruginosa*. Heat and maceration are the main factors, as levels of chlorination adequate for a swimming pool may be insufficientin a hot tub or whirlpool.
- Gram-negative folliculitis in acne patients may feature *P. aeruginosa*. The smaller more superficial infections usually carry *Klebsiella*, while the deeper cystic or nodular lesions contains *Proteus* or *Pseudomonas.*
- Green nail syndrome refers to subungual pseudomonas infection producing a green nail and onycholysis. Wood light examination is confirmatory. Most often the patient spends much time with wet hands.
- Blastomycotic pyoderma may yield *P. aeruginosa*, *Proteus* or *S. aureus*. Here there is an overexuberant, verrucous epidermal reaction with multiple sinus tracts. In Australia this has been called coral reef granuloma, not because it is

acquired at a coral reef but because its gross morphology resembles that natural structure.
- Otitis externa is more complex. The typical swimmer's ear usually contains *P. aeruginosa;* the external canal is swollen, red, tender and drains. But the infection almost never develops spontaneously – there is usually a history of repeated exposure to water. In contrast, malignant otitis externa always involves *P. aeruginosa* as an aggressive pathogen in elderly patients with diabetes mellitus. If untreated, it spreads to destroy local tissue and cause sepsis and death.

Histopathology. Ecthyma gangrenosum shows necrosis of the epidermis and dermis with surprisingly little inflammation. Vessel thrombosis and destruction is seen at the periphery of the infarct, and gram-negative bacteria can be seen in the vessel walls and among the collagen, often providing a quicker diagnosis than culture in the appropriate setting.

Laboratory Findings. Identification of *P. aeruginosa* or other species in culture must always be matched with the clinical setting. A necrotic eschar in a leukemia patient that yields *P. aeruginosa* means the patient's life is at risk; a toe web erythema that grows out the same organisms says little.

Therapy. For the more superficial infection, simply drying out the folliculitis, ear or nail with acetic acid or similar solutions is often sufficient. In the case of gram-negative toe web infections, trimethoprim-sulfamethoxazole is often helpful but it may work by altering the flora rather than specifically attacking *P. aeruginosa.*

If a patient has pseudomonas sepsis, aggressive antibiotic therapy is required. Complicated and expensive regimens are necessary; infectious disease consultation is a must.

Actinetobacter, Moraxella and *Branhamella* Infections

All three of these closely related gram-negative species are part of the normal flora but may cause severe infections in immunosuppressed individuals. *Actinetobacter* species are the only true resident gram-negative bacilli on human skin and are found in the groin, perineum, axilla and toe webs, just like *Pseudomonas,* and may cause cellulitis, wound infections, sepsis and deeper infections. *Moraxella* usually causes ocular infections but can produce a septic vasculitis mimicking gonococcemia, as well as causing reactive arthritis similar to Reiter syndrome. *Branhamella catarrhalis* causes a pus-laden bronchitis.

Haemophilus influenzae Infections

Haemophilus influenzae is a common pathogen in childhood and causes meningitis and sepsis. Prior to the introduction of a vaccine against *H. influenzae* type b (Hib), it was the most common cause of life-threatening bacterial infections in children. Today, it is rarely encountered in developed lands. Orbital or buccal cellulitis was another common clinical feature of Hib; most such patients had meningeal signs along with their orbital swelling and erythema. Today *S. pneumoniae* is the most likely cause of orbital cellulitis, often extending from a maxillary sinus infection.

Pasteurella multocida Infections

A small gram-negative bacillus, *P. multocida* is part of the normal gastrointestinal and respiratory flora of many animals. It is occasionally identified in humans with chronic respiratory disease. The overwhelming bulk of human infections follow a cat or, less often, a dog bite.

Typically a painful, expanding red abscess develops, spreading laterally and deeply. The wound is typically quite painful and may break down, discharging pus. Both osteomyelitis and synovitis can occur because of the deep penetration achieved by cats' teeth. Rare patients may have pulmonary or abdominal disease without history of a bite; they presumably were carriers of the organism whose resistance dropped. Both tetracyclines and penicillin are effective therapy.

Whipple Disease

(Whipple 1907)

Causative Organism. *Tropheryma whippelii,* a poorly understood, anaerobic gram-positive rod in the *Actinomyces* family, also known as the Whipple bacillus.

Whipple described what was thought for almost a century to be a metabolic derangement. Most patients are middle-aged men with intermittent arthralgias, diarrhea, steatorrhea, abdominal pain, low-grade fever, weight loss, microcytic anemia and a slow downhill course. About half the patients have diffuse hyperpigmentation whose etiology has not been explained. The classic microscopic finding is xanthomatous macrophages filled with PAS-positive material in almost every organ; the diagnosis is usually made on small bowel biopsy. While the organism has proven difficult to culture, its DNA has been found in most patients and disappeared following antibiotic therapy. Treatment guidelines are confusing, but most experts recommend 2 weeks of parenteral penicillin G and streptomycin, followed by 1 year of trimethoprim-sulfamethoxazole.

Spirochetal Infections

Lyme Disease

Synonyms. Lyme borreliosis, erythema migrans borreliosis, tick-borne meningopolyneuritis. The dermatologic disorders erythema migrans and acrodermatitis chronica atrophicans are part of the spectrum and not truly synonyms.

Definition. Infection caused by *Borrelia burgdorferi sensu lato*, transferred to humans by hard ticks, and characterized by varying patterns of cutaneous, rheumatological, neurological and cardiac involvement.

History. The dermatologic disorders erythema migrans and acrodermatitis chronica atrophicans have been identified in Europe since the beginning of the twentieth century. While an infectious etiology was suspected and a connection with ticks well-established in the case of erythema migrans, the etiologic agent remained unknown. In the early 1970s there was a cluster of cases of peculiar "juvenile rheumatoid arthritis" in Connecticut near the mouth of the Lyme River. Steere, Malawista and colleagues from Yale University identified the features of the new disease, which became known as Lyme disease. These investigators also recognized the importance of tick bites and the search was on in earnest in both Europe and North America for the organisms. Since ticks carry primarily rickettsiae and borreliae, the search was headed in this direction. In 1981 Willy Burgdorfer, a Ph. D. entomologist from the Rocky Mountain Laboratories, discovered a new spirochete in Long Island ticks while searching for rickettsiae associated with Rocky Mountain spotted fever.

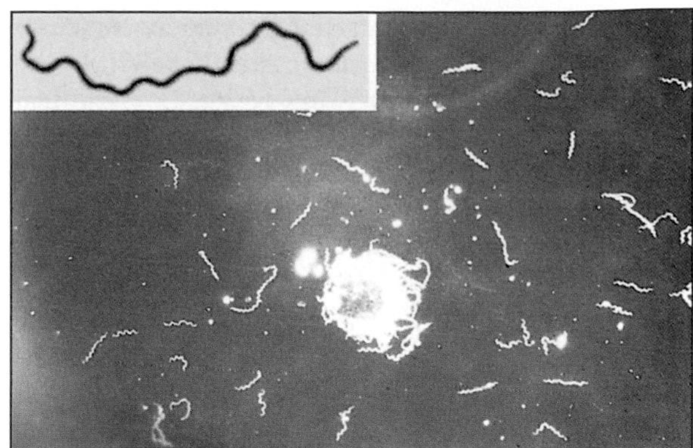

Fig. 4.33. *Borrelia burgdorferi* in culture. Inset: electron microscopic image

Causative Organism. *Borrelia burgdorferi sensu lato* belongs to the genus *Borrelia* in the family *Treponemataceae* (Fig. 4.33). Other pathogenic borreliae include *B. recurrentis*, the cause of louse-borne relapsing fever, and many different species that cause tick-borne relapsing fever. The three major subspecies are shown in Table 4.7.

Borrelia are corkscrew-like organisms ranging in length from 4 to 30 μm, with a thickness of 0.2–0.4 μm. The inner protoplasmic cylinder is enclosed by a cytoplasmic membrane. On its surface are 7–11 axial filaments or flagellae that are themselves enclosed by an outer membrane. *B. burgdorferi* is difficult to culture, but with Barbour-Stoenner-Kelly (BSK) media, the generation time is 8–24 h. Borrelia are gram-negative, but can be stained with aniline dyes or silver impregnation, or visualized with dark-field examination when found in the blood or culture medium.

B. burgdorferi has one long chromosome and four to nine linear or circular plasmids. Some of the plasmids code for the surface proteins OspA, OspB and OspC, but others have an unclear role. With repeated passages in culture, some plasmids are lost and the infectivity tends to diminish. Bacterio-

Table 4.7. Types of *Borrelia burgdorferi*

Organism	Disease association
Borrelia burgdorferi sensu stricto	North American Lyme disease
Borrelia garinii	Neurological disease (Bannwarth syndrome)
Borrelia afzelii	Erythema migrans and acrodermatitis chronica atrophicans

phages may also be integrated in the genome, both in spirochetes found in ticks and in the skin. The European forms of *B. burgdorferi* show a great deal of antigenic variability.

Etiology and Pathogenesis. Infection by *B. burgdorferi* is best explained by understanding the various vectors and their life cycles. It is difficult to separate pathogenesis from epidemiology, so we consider both together. Hard ticks are responsible for the transmission; they primarily belong to the genus *Ixodes* and include *I. ricinus* in Europe and *I. persulcatus* in Asia, as well as *I. pacificus* and *I. scapularis* in North America. With regional variations anywhere from 4% to 60% of the ticks contain *B. burgdorferi* in the mid-gut. The typical 24-month life cycle of an *Ixodes* tick is as follows: The female tick lays about 2000 eggs in the spring. The larvae hatch in the summer, feed from a variety of small mammals and birds and spend the winter as fed larva. In the next spring, the nymph hatch and seek hosts in May and June. Their main host are the white-footed deer mouse in the USA. The mice may infect the ticks not only with *B. burgdorferi* but also the piroplasma of *Babesia microti*, the cause of babesiosis or Nantucket fever, and *Ehrlichia phagocytophilia species*, the cause of human granulocytic ehrlichosis (Chap. 3). Humans may also be bitten at this stage. The nymphs molt and become adults in the fall; they then seek a new blood meal, often from a Virginia deer, but also from mice and humans. If they do not find a meal by the spring, they die; if successful, the female ticks lay eggs to start the cycle over.

Transmission is always through the saliva as the tick feeds. When the tick finds a host, the spirochetes must be activated before they can enter the host. This leaves a window of 48 h in the case of *B. burgdorferi*, during which transmission is unlikely. The majority of erythema migrans is seen in the early summer, suggesting that nymphs play a more important role than adults. The nymphs are quite small and the initial bite is usually painless so that frequently the bite is overlooked and the tick can feed as long as needed to become full and transfer disease. In any event, the acute stages of the disease are seen in the spring, summer and early fall when ticks are biting.

I. ricinus is very widespread in Europe, ranging from Scandinavia and Ireland to the Caspian Sea and North Africa. It has over 200 natural hosts; the nymphs feed primarily on small mammals, while the adults favor larger mammals. Birds may also be hosts and assist in the spread of ticks, as do domestic and animals house pets. In North America, the tendency towards suburban living on the East Coast put people, deer and mice in closer contact and is probably responsible for the upsurge of the disease. Studies on museum specimens have shown that *B. burgdorferi* has been around for a long time. In the upper Midwest and Northern California, the other two hotspots for Lyme disease, more cases are acquired on camping trips and other activities that are farther away from the home. In our area, gardening, golfing, hiking and hunting are the most usual ways of acquiring a tick bite.

Following inoculation, the course is highly variable. Steere identified three stages of Lyme disease, analogous to syphilis. In the first stage, there is a localized skin reaction. The second stage features widespread, but for the most part reversible, systemic disease, while in the third stage there are chronic changes.

Clinical Findings. There are significant differences between Lyme disease in the USA and the European variants. The most obvious example for a dermatologist is the occurrence of acrodermatitis chronica atrophicans in Europe, nearly always associated with *B. afzelii*. In contrast to the more variable species distribution in Europe, *B. burgdorferi sensu stricto* is clearly the dominating species in North American. American patients are more likely to have multiple lesions of erythema migrans, more severe arthritis and cardiac disease, while the acute neurologic symptoms are more common in Europe. The major dermatologic disorders associated with Lyme disease will be considered as separate entities below.

Stage I. The classic finding is erythema migrans. Some patients will either develop such a small reaction at their initial bite that they do not notice it, or it will be on a part of their body where they cannot see it. The number of patients with documented Lyme disease who notice erythema migrans is highly variable, so the absence in the history of such a reaction has little significance. Occasionally, a pseudolymphoma may develop at the site of the initial bite. Many patients heal after the primary stage.

Stage II. The following changes have been described during the acute systemic illness. Within weeks to months, neurological and cardiac problems may develop. The joint changes usually appear first after 6 months or more. The distinctions between stage II and stage III are even less clear than in syphilis.

Table 4.8. Clinical stages of Lyme borreliosis

Stage	Features
Stage I	**Early localized infection** Erythema migrans Flu-like symptoms
Stage II	**Early disseminated infection** Skin: secondary erythema migrans (uncommon); pseudolymphoma; panniculitis Neurologic: meningitis; encephalitis; cranial nerve paralysis, especially VII; polyneuritis Cardiac: myocarditis with AV block Rheumatologic: myalgias; arthralgias; arthritis
Stage III	**Persistent infection** Skin: acrodermatitis chronica atrophicans Neurologic: peripheral neuropathies; subacute encephalopathy; progressive encephalomyelitis Rheumatologic: recurrent or persistent arthritis; myositis; periostitis; joint subluxation, usually with acrodermatitis chronica atrophicans Ophthalmologic: keratitis

Table 4.8 shows some of the features of stage II disease. All of the problems are usually of relatively short duration. In the absence of treatment, they may either resolve or recur.

Stage III. Months to years after the secondary problems, chronic changes can develop, as shown in Table 4.8.

Infections During Pregnancy. Borrelia burgdorferi can cross the placenta. Fetal death, spontaneous abortions and congenital malformations may all occur, but are quite uncommon. This risk of fetal involvement is apparently greatest if the infection occurs early in pregnancy.

Laboratory Findings. Many relatively nonspecific parameters may be altered, including elevated erythrocyte sedimentation rate, hyperglobulinemia, hypocomplementemia, elevated liver enzymes, anemia, proteinuria and microscopic hematuria. When the central nervous system is involved, the CSF shows mononuclear pleocytosis and sometimes autochthonous antiborrelial antibodies.

Direct Examination. The organism is difficult to identify in tissue sections. The use of monoclonal antibodies and immunogold or immunoperoxidase staining remains a research technique.

Culture. Even using the special BSK medium, culturing *B. burgdorferi* is a task for specialized laboratories. Fresh skin biopsies, other fresh tissue and body fluids can be cultured. The yield is highest in erythema migrans.

Serology. The main tool in diagnosing Lyme disease is serological examination. It is also responsible for the misdiagnosis of the disorder, since many patients in endemic areas have some signs of seropositivity. While CSF titers can be performed, they are even less standardized than those done with blood. The most common screening tests are an indirect immunofluorescent test using cultured *B. burgdorferi* and serum preexposed to a nonpathogenic treponeme (*Treponema phagedenis*) to reduce cross-reactions, and an ELISA test commonly using sonicated *B. burgdorferi.* Both of these tests have been somewhat disappointing, as false-negative reactions are common early and may remain negative if the patient is treated promptly with antibiotics. False-positive reactions can occur with syphilis, relapsing fever, infectious mononucleosis and other disorders with activated B cells.

More specific tests are, however, available. Attempts to incorporate the use of IgM antibodies, as in syphilis, have been less successful. IgM rises early in the infection, after 3–6 weeks, mainly directed against OspC and a flagellar antigen. An IgM ELISA looking for antibodies against OspC seems most specific. Immunoblotting, or performing a western blot with the patient's serum and various *B. burgdorferi* antigens, is potentially more accurate but the antigens have not been standardized.

Antibody titers are also not useful in following the disease course. The absence of IgM antibodies does not mean a cure. While the IgG antibodies usually drop 2–3 months after treatment, the titers are not standardized. Patients with late manifestations may be serofast, despite treatment and absence of symptoms.

Another big problem with Lyme disease serology is the presence of positive titers in patients with vague symptoms, such as chronic fatigue syndrome. Such patients living in endemic areas may well have a positive titer but no evidence of active Lyme disease. Nonetheless, special "Lyme disease" clinics may treat patients based on serology alone for nonspecific complaints. In several studies, serum from patients in endemic areas was sent to multiple reference laboratories; the results showed an amazingly discordant diagnostic spectrum. In sum, the diagnosis of Lyme disease should never be based on serology alone, but must include clinical evaluation.

Other Methods. PCR can identify the organisms in skin, synovial fluid, CSF, blood and urine, as well as other tissues. PCR can also be used to subspeciate *B. burgdorferi*. For example, PCR studies have shown that, when a spirochete is found in acrodermatitis chronica atrophicans, it is always *B. afzelii*.

Differential Diagnosis. The differential diagnosis of Lyme disease is too long for a chapter. It includes all of medicine. In endemic areas, or in patients returning from endemic areas, one should take a careful history of a tick bite and be suspicious of musculoskeletal, neurologic or cardiovascular symptoms that are not easily explained.

Therapy. In early Lyme disease the preferred treatment is tetracycline 250–500 mg orally q. i. d. for 14–21 days or doxycycline 100 mg b. i. d. for 14–21 days. When patients have early acrodermatitis chronica atrophicans, most clinicians would choose the 21-day regimen.

Patients with neurologic or cardiovascular manifestations are best treated with parenteral antibiotics; both ceftriaxone, 2.0 g IV daily for 14 days, and crystalline penicillin G, 5 million units IV q. i. d. for 10 days, have been employed. The patients with AV block should be treated under cardiac monitoring. A 30-day course of doxycycline 100 mg orally b. i. d. is probably sufficient to treat the arthritis, although parenteral regimens can also be employed.

Patients with early signs such as erythema migrans, treated appropriately, still tend to develop some minor symptoms such as recurrent headache or muscle pain. Studies in our clinic have identified *B. burgdorferi* in the skin after treatment. The spirochetes interact with various connective tissue proteins and may hide or mask themselves. This skill may explain the persistent symptoms and occasional relapses.

Prophylaxis. A vaccine consisting of recombinant OspA from *B. burgdorferi* has been tested in the USA. It may be worthwhile for individuals in high-risk groups. While children stand to benefit the most, the vaccine has not been tested in that age group. Metaanalysis has not shown significant benefit for prophylactic antibiotic therapy following tick bites. Following patients with serological studies is neither accurate nor cost effective. Protective clothing, insect repellents and prompt removal of ticks are all more important.

Erythema Migrans

(Afzelius 1909; Lipschütz 1913)

Synonym. Erythema chronicum migrans

Definition. Peripherally spreading annular erythema following tick bite and transmission of *B. burgdorferi*. The presence of erythema migrans is a defining characteristic of Lyme disease; in most studies, the lesion's diameter must exceed 5 cm.

Causative Organism. *Borrelia burgdorferi sensu stricto* in USA and occasionally in Europe, *Borrelia afzelii* in Central Europe and *Borrelia garinii* throughout Europe.

Etiology and Pathogenesis. Following the bite of an *Ixodes* tick, the borrelia is introduced via the tick's saliva into the skin. There it slowly proliferates and migrates peripherally, producing an erythematous ring. Other ticks and rarely other arthropods have been incriminated but the overwhelming majority of erythema migrans are caused by *Ixodes*. *B. burgdorferi* needs about 48 h to be activated in the starving tick's gut and reach the saliva, so ticks removed within this time window are unlikely to produce erythema migrans. Other aspects are discussed under Lyme disease.

Clinical Findings. Erythema migrans can occur anywhere on the body and in patients of any age and either sex. The location is determined by the habits of the patients and the ticks. Thus, the most likely sites are the legs, where bites are common, and the back, where ticks are easily overlooked. While genital involvement is common, the distribution varies between the sexes. Men tend to have lesions on the penis or anterior groin, while women are affected on the buttocks, perhaps reflecting the ways they expose themselves when urinating in the woods. The incubation period is quite variable, but averages about 10 days. In some patients, there may be an interval of months, making the history difficult to obtain, and in others, the erythema migrans may surround a still attached tick. The history of a tick bite is intrinsically unreliable; only about 50% of patients with erythema migrans definitely remember a bite.

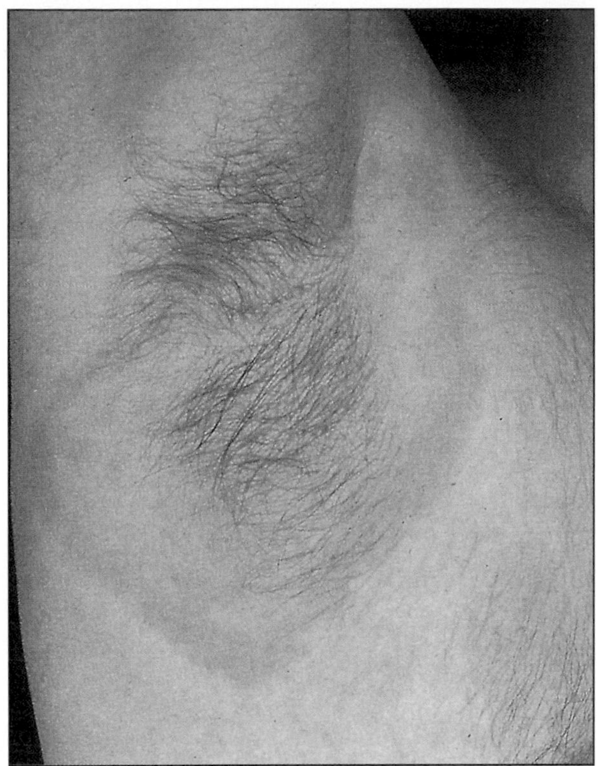

Fig. 4.34. Erythema migrans

The initial lesion is a homogenous erythematous patch that spreads peripherally from the bite site, which itself may appear as a small papule or a more diffuse, puffy blue-red swelling. In about 80% of patients there is central clearing as the erythematous border slowly expands. The border remains slightly indurated, red and irregularly shaped (Fig. 4.34).

There are many variations on the standard theme. Lesions may be quite large, obtaining diameters greater than 20 cm. Multiple lesions may develop (Fig. 4.35), although this usually occurs in the second stage of the disease and is associated with systemic complaints. Lesions on the face frequently do not show central clearing. Sometimes the periphery is sharply elevated; other lesions may be spotty rather than annular. Rare variants include scaly, vesicular and on the legs purpuric lesions. Spontaneous healing occurs in about 10 weeks, although recurrences are possible. About one-third of patients complain of pruritus or even pain or a sensation of warmth; this group is more likely to have problems in the later stages of Lyme disease.

Systemic problems are rarely present during the early stage with typical erythema migrans. Regional lymphadenopathy is present in 40% of patients

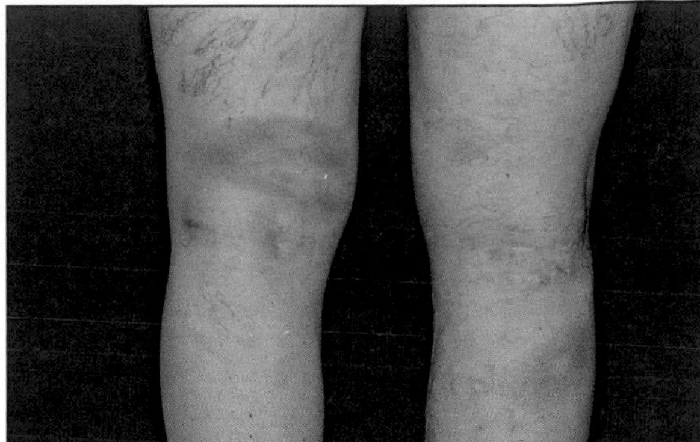

Fig. 4.35. Multiple lesions of erythema migrans

but rarely a presenting complaint. When questioned, two-thirds describe general complaints such as malaise or fever, but most often patients do not present with such troubles. Patients with multiple systemic complaints are also more likely to advance to later stages. Multiple erythema migrans are a certain sign of systemic spread and thus of the transition to stage II. About one-third of patients in North America develop multiple lesions of erythema migrans, as compared to 5% in Europe. The healing of erythema migrans should not be taken as a sign that the infection is cured. A typical scenario in Europe is the appearance of Bannwarth (1941) syndrome as the erythema migrans disappears. Bannwarth syndrome (lymphocytic meningitis and polyradiculopathies) is an acute polyneuropathy which is typically asymmetric, shows both meningeal and peripheral involvement and has associated pain. The CSF shows increased lymphocytic counts and borrelial antibodies are found.

Histopathology. The erythematous part of erythema migrans reveals a normal epidermis and a modest lymphocytic perivascular infiltrate in the upper dermis. A key feature is the tight perivascular cuffing. The infiltrate usually contains at least some plasma cells. Since many cases of erythema migrans have been studied microscopically at the same time that PCR identified *B. burgdorferi* in the tissue, it has become clear that the histologic spectrum is quite broad. Some biopsy specimens show spongiotic dermatitis; others, vasculitis; and yet others, almost nothing. If one is lucky and sees the initial bite site, there may be fibrosis associated with a plasma cell and eosinophilic infiltrate.

Differential Diagnosis. The chief question is: are all spreading erythemas associated with insect bites erythema migrans? This becomes a matter of definition, but other soluble materials injected by a wide variety of arthropods can produce a slowly expanding erythema. Thus, the 5 cm case definition is useful. Urticaria may appear similar but should have multiple lesions that change more rapidly. Erythema annulare centrifugum, despite its name, is usually more urticarial and does not form as definite a ring as does erythema migrans. Tinea should be excluded if scale is present. Occasionally erysipelas can appear similar in the early stages, but the patient is more ill and the annular pattern does not evolve.

Therapy. Tetracycline 500 mg orally q.i.d. for 14 days or doxycycline 100 mg orally b.i.d. for 14 days are the standard regimens. Longer periods of therapy, intravenous medications and more potent antibiotics are usually not needed if treatment is instituted promptly for erythema migrans.

Borrelial Pseudolymphoma

Synonyms. Borrelial lymphocytoma, lymphadenosis cutis benigna

Epidemiology. The distribution of borrelial pseudolymphoma follows that of *Ixodes* in Europe. It is quite uncommon in North America. Children, adolescents and women are more often affected. It may appear in the early stage as a reaction to the initial bite or later usually in association with acrodermatitis chronica atrophicans.

Etiology and Pathogenesis. When pseudolymphoma develops in a bite site, then it is unclear if the borrelial proliferation, other organisms or part of the tick has triggered the lymphocytic proliferation. However, the diffuse lymphadenopathy seen in Lyme disease and the presence of pseudolymphoma in areas where no tick was attached suggest a primary immunostimulatory role for *B. burgdorferi.*

Clinical Findings. The usual borrelial lymphocytoma is a solitary, relatively sharply circumscribed, soft deep red or blue-red nodule. The overlying skin may be thinned. The typical sites of predilection are ear lobes, nipples, areolae, nape, axillae, scrotum and back of the foot. Diascopy reveals a uniform yellow-gray infiltrate. About 25% of patients have an associated regional lymphadenopathy. There seems to be an increased incidence of neurological problems in patients with lymphocytoma. If untreated, the lesions can persist for months to years. Pseudolymphomas are illustrated in Chapter 60.

Histopathology. The microscopic picture is that of a pseudolymphoma. There is a polyclonal proliferation of lymphocytes associated with plasma cells, macrophages and occasionally eosinophils. Typically the uppermost dermis is spared, producing a Grenz zone. The balance is replaced by follicular lymphoid structures which must be separated from a follicular B cell lymphoma by immunohistochemical studies. There is extensive destruction of the elastic fibers and appendages.

Differential Diagnosis. Clinically a number of nodular changes must be differentiated from borrelial pseudolymphoma. Other arthropod bite reactions, foreign body granulomas, a variety of cysts, cystic adnexal tumors, cutaneous metastases, sarcoidosis and facial granuloma can all be confidently excluded histologically. Nonetheless, the histologic differential diagnosis is challenging, as not only follicular lymphoma but also other types of pseudolymphoma and lupus erythematosus appear similar.

Therapy. While the same regimens as used for erythema migrans are often recommended, we usually employ ceftriaxone, 2.0 g intravenously daily for 21 days.

Acrodermatitis Chronica Atrophicans

(Herxheimer and Hartmann 1902)

Synonym. Herxheimer disease

Epidemiology. Acrodermatitis chronica atrophicans is a mid- to late manifestation of a *B. afzelii* infection which is only seen in central and northern Europe. Rare reports from other countries have often not been well-documented. Over two-thirds of patients are women, usually in their forties to fifties.

Etiology and Pathogenesis. The role of *B. afzelii* is clear, but the rest of the story is a mystery. Why there is such extensive damage and atrophy of the epidermis and dermis is unclear. Perhaps the periarticular regions are favored because of reduced acral skin temperatures or reduced oxygen pressure. About 20% of patients have a history of erythema migrans, often involving the same limb, in the preceding months.

Clinical Findings. Acrodermatitis chronica atrophicans favors the knees, elbows and ankles, as well as the extensor surfaces of the arms and legs. Other sites can also be involved, including the trunk, face and even in rare cases the entire integument (dermatitis chronica atrophicans). On the arms and less often the legs, there may be erythematous stripes or cords – the so-called ulnar or tibial bands. The changes tend to move proximally to affect the contralateral structures and are often associated with regional or generalized lymphadenopathy.

In the early stage, there is a vague erythema with minimal swelling (Fig. 4.36). Usually the changes are sharply bordered, have a blue-red tint and slowly expand. Sometimes only one digit is involved initially (blue toe sign), or there may be localized redness over a tendon. Patients frequently overlook the early changes because they are so subtle. On occasion, only the swelling is appreciated, so that one thinks of lymphedema or even a thrombosis. A typically scenario is discovering one foot is larger when buying shoes.

Later on, the findings become far more dramatic and impossible to overlook (Figs. 4.37, 4.38). The skin becomes atrophic and white, so-called cigarette

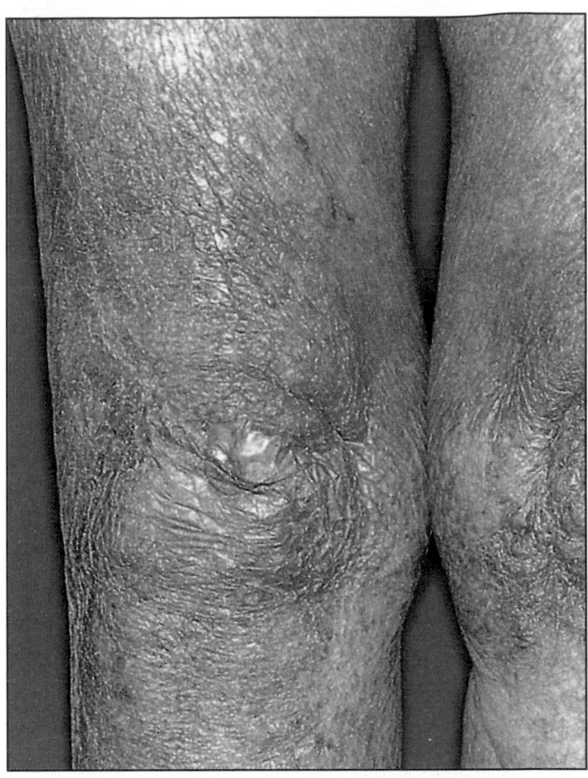

Fig. 4.37. More advanced acrodermatitis chronica atrophicans

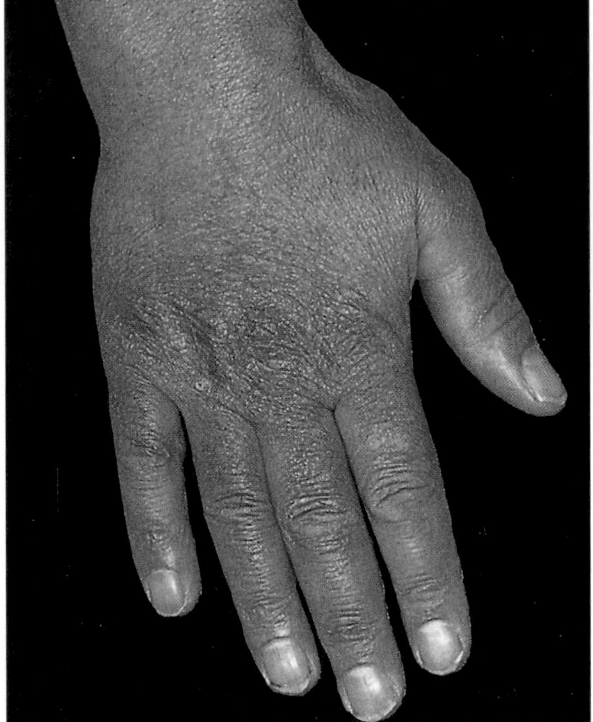

Fig. 4.36. Early acrodermatitis chronica atrophicans

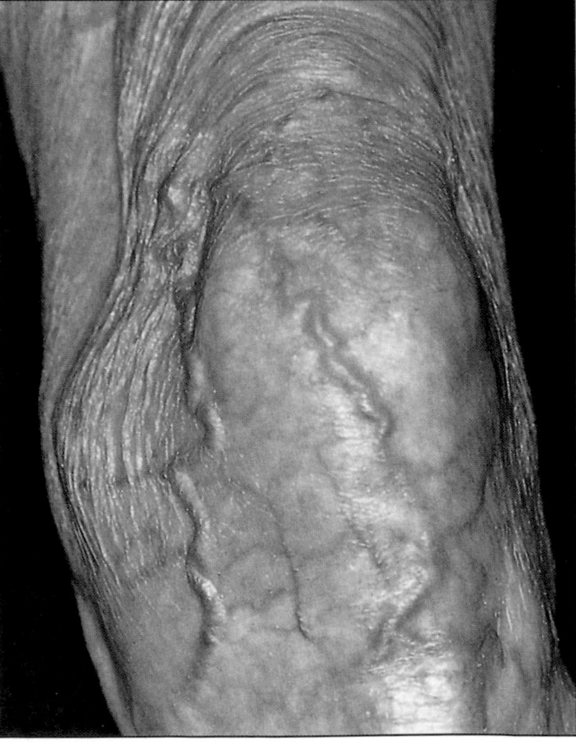

Fig. 4.38. Extreme skin thinning in acrodermatitis chronica atrophicans

paper skin, so that the vessels and other structures can be easily seen. The hairs are lost; telangiectases and focal hyperpigmentation may develop. At the same time, fibrosis may occur. The collagen appears to proliferate as the elastin is destroyed, producing thick ivory stripes and plaques within the lesions on the shins and backs of the feet. The joint capsules, especially of the digits, hands and ankles, can be involved. Fibrous nodules are the most exaggerated form of reactive proliferation; they occur primarily about the elbow and are hard subcutaneous nodules, often several centimeters in diameter, which lie beneath the atrophic skin.

In addition, lesions similar to both morphea and lichen sclerosus et atrophicus may appear on skin where no acrodermatitis chronica atrophicans is present. Furthermore, sometimes patients have many small lesions which are otherwise identical to acrodermatitis chronica atrophicans; this is known as dermatitis atrophicans maculosa and evolves into an anetoderma (Chap. 18). Herniations may also develop within larger atrophic plaques.

The atrophic skin lacks hair, sebaceous and often sweat glands. Thus it is very dry and poorly protected against the elements. Asteatotic dermatitis is a common sequelae. In addition, minor trauma may produce large, slow to heal ulcerations. The damaged skin is also a surprisingly fertile ground for malignant tumors, including squamous cell carcinomas, lymphomas and even sarcomas.

A variety of systemic problems, primarily neurological and musculoskeletal, have been described for acrodermatitis chronica atrophicans. Since acrodermatitis chronica atrophicans is but one manifestation of late Lyme disease, these changes are best considered as other manifestations of a late *B. burgdorferi* infection rather than specific changes of acrodermatitis chronica atrophicans. The exception is the involvement of the small joints of the hands and feet by the fibrotic reaction, which can frequently produce subluxation and is rarely seen in the absence of acrodermatitis chronica atrophicans.

Histopathology. In the early phase, there is dermal edema and perivascular lymphocytic infiltrates with prominent participation by plasma cells. Later, the epidermal atrophy becomes obvious and in the dermis the collagen fibers become swollen and homogenous as the elastic fibers disappear. In contrast, in morphea and scleroderma the elastic fibers are always preserved. The dermal pattern is zonal; the entire structure is thinned. Just below the epidermis is a normal Grenz zone, then an infiltrative band containing lymphocytes and plasma cells and, at the bottom, relatively normal tissue. The adnexal structures are often obliterated by the inflammatory infiltrate.

B. afzelii can be identified by PCR reaction, but both cultures and direct spirochetal stains are usually negative.

Course and Prognosis. When the early stage is treated, the outlook is good. In the late stage, many changes are only partially reversible and malignant degeneration remains a potential problem.

Differential Diagnosis. Early on, one typically thinks of pernio, acrocyanosis and venous insufficiency. Later on the atrophic lesions are distinctive. The periarticular nodules can be confused with rheumatoid nodules, while the focal fibrosis suggests morphea. The relationship of lichen sclerosus et atrophicus and morphea to *B. burgdorferi* remains controversial, but we doubt either disease has an infectious etiology.

Therapy. Doxycycline 100 mg orally b.i.d. for 21 day is the usual suggestion. Tetracycline and ampicillin can also be used. If there are extracutaneous manifestations, the recommendations given for Lyme disease are appropriate.

Leptospirosis

Synonyms. Hemorrhagic jaundice, Weil (1886) disease, canicola fever, Fort Bragg fever, pretibial fever, mud fever

Causative Organism. *Leptospira interrogans* is the only human pathogen but it has more than 200 serovars causing a variety of clinical patterns. *Leptospira* are in the same order as spirochetes; leptospira means gently spiraled while interrogans refers to a question mark – both describing the shape of *L. interrogans*, a gently twisted spirochete with a hooked end.

Epidemiology. Leptospirosis is a worldwide disease. The reservoir is a variety of wild and domestic animals including rats, pigs, cattle, dogs and raccoons – each of which carries a different serovar. In Europe, the badger is a common carrier. The organisms survive in the host's kidneys and are excreted in the urine. Contact with the urine and tissue of these animals or more often with water contaminated by their urine is the scenario for infection. Rice paddy and sugar cane field workers, miners, hunters and people in many other similar professions, as well as recreation seekers, are at risk. In Kauai, Hawaii, several large shallow ponds seen easily from the airport have been a frequent source of leptospirosis epidemics.

Etiology and Pathogenesis. Tiny skin injuries are necessary to allow penetration of the organism. They enter the blood, multiply and typically settle in an extracellular location in the liver or kidneys.

Clinical Findings. In the past, different serovars were associated with slightly different disease patterns but it has become clear that this distinction is somewhat artificial. Typically there is an incubation period of 1–2 weeks, followed by the sudden onset of fever, chills, headache and malaise. After about 1 week the fever disappears for several days. Then the second phase starts with meningeal signs; this later phase is known as the immune phase.

A variety of cutaneous findings develop. The most distinctive is painful pre-tibial plaques developing during the fist phase in what was formerly called Fort Bragg fever, because it was so often seen in US military recruits in training at Fort Bragg, North Carolina. Other patients may have a diffuse exanthem, conjunctival injection or jaundice. The latter is most common in the most severe form of leptospirosis, known as Weil disease, which includes hepatorenal involvement. There may also be hemolytic anemia and extensive hemorrhage including into the skin.

Laboratory Findings. The infection is diagnosed based on positive blood culture in the early phase or CSF culture later on. Serological testing is available, and both ELISA and immunofluorescent techniques can be used to identify the organism in clinical specimens. Hepatic and renal status should be assessed.

Course and Prognosis. The outlook is good with gradual resolution occurring over months. In elderly patients, the mortality of the Weil variant approaches 20 %, especially if renal dialysis and other supportive measures are not promptly instituted.

Differential Diagnosis. Many cases are misdiagnosed as influenza, meningitis or encephalitis without ever identifying the causative organism.

Therapy. Doxycycline appears to be the most effective treatment. In individuals at high risk, such as military recruits, once weekly doxycycline is an effective short-term prophylactic measure.

Relapsing Fever

Causative Organism. *Borrelia recurrentis* and many other *Borrelia* species.

Epidemiology. Louse-borne relapsing fever is caused by *B. recurrentis*; the reservoir is humans. In contrast, tick-borne relapsing fever is caused by a variety of *Borrelia* transferred from wild rodents by soft (argasid) ticks. Louse-borne disease was a major problem during World Wars I and II in eastern Europe. Today the highlands of central Africa are the hotspot, but foci are found in Asia and South America. Tick-borne disease is more scattered; sporadic cases are seen in the western USA and Canada, as well as in many other parts of the world. In Europe, small foci exist in Spain.

Etiology and Pathogenesis. For louse-borne disease, close unsanitary living conditions are required to favor a population of lice. One must crush the louse to contaminate a bite or scratch, as the spirochetes are not excreted in the saliva or feces. In the other form, exposure to the ticks of wild rodents is needed, thus suggesting camping or other outdoor activities; the tick saliva transfers the spirochete.

Clinical Findings. As the name suggests, the disease is characterized by episodes of fever lasting several days, followed by a symptom-free period and then a relapse. Usually there are two to three relapses, but sometimes as many as ten may recur. About 10 % of untreated patients die; the main cause of mortality is myocarditis. There are no specific cutaneous findings, not even a toxic exanthem is described. The disease is discussed only because one should be aware of its existence when evaluating patients with tick bites.

Laboratory Findings. The diagnosis is made by finding the organisms on a thick blood smear stained with Giemsa or Wright stain. Cultures and animal inoculation are also possible.

Differential Diagnosis. The differential diagnosis includes Lyme disease, Rocky Mountain spotted fever, tick-borne encephalitis and many other regional tick-borne diseases.

Therapy. Tetracyclines are the most effective therapy. In the case of louse-borne disease, the arthropods should be eliminated.

Clostridial Infections

Causative Organism. Clostridia are anaerobic gram-positive rods which produce spores.

Epidemiology. Clostridia are widespread in nature and cause a variety of severe infections. Their spores are found in soil, water and the gastrointestinal tract of many animals including humans.

Etiology and Pathogenesis. These bacteria usually cause trouble only when anaerobic conditions are produced, such as in a puncture, crush trauma or very dirty wound. In addition, they produce a wide variety of toxins, responsible for many of their effects.

Clinical Findings. A wide variety of clinical patterns may be seen.

- *Clostridium tetani* causes tetanus. It is usually found in the soil and introduced via puncture wounds, bites or foreign bodies. It does not produce changes at the wound but instead a toxin which inhibits the motor neuron synapses. Typical changes include trismus producing a silly or sardonic smile (risus sardonicus) and opisthotonos. The mortality is around 20%, rising in the elderly. Infections of the umbilicus in newborns because of exposure of the newly severed cord to fecal material are very dangerous. Heroin addicts also do poorly with tetanus; often they are misdiagnosed as having withdrawal symptoms. Each physician must be aware of the immunization status and public health recommendations for treating a patient with an unclean wound or bite. The primary immunization is accomplished via the DPT series in childhood. Additional tetanus toxoid injections are recommended every 10 years thereafter. Both tetanus toxoid and tetanus immune globulin may be required.

- *Clostridium difficile* causes diarrhea and pseudomembranous colitis in patients treated with antibiotics who have the organism in their gastrointestinal tracts. It is of special interest to dermatologists because this complication led to the discontinuation of clindamycin as an oral agent in treating acne. Other antibiotic regimens for acne may rarely produce the same problem. But the vast majority of such cases develop in hospitalized patients, who have a higher rate of colonization and are exposed to more aggressive antibiotic regimens. Metronidazole is used in moderate cases; in severe disease, vancomycin is recommended but resistance is becoming a grave problem and alternate agents are not available.

- *Clostridium botulinum* produces several toxins which inhibit the presynaptic release of acetylcholine. This produces a flaccid paralysis associated with cranial nerve impairment, visual difficulties and a dry mouth. In food-borne botulism, improperly canned or processed foods contain the preformed toxin. In contrast, in wound and infant botulism, the toxin is manufactured in vivo. The most common source of infant botulism is raw honey, which should not be fed to those less than 1 year of age. Botulinum A toxin is used to reduce wrinkling caused by muscular action and to block hyperhidrosis. It is also used in a variety of neurological and gastrointestinal disorders.

- *Clostridium perfringens* and several other species cause gas gangrene or clostridial myonecrosis. Following an outdoor injury, the spores are introduced into a wound. They rapidly develop, secreting a wide ranging of toxins which in a matter of days lead to severe pain, crepitation and shock in a very ill patient. The digested subcutaneous fat and muscle drains out of the wound as a foul-smelling serous discharge. Sometimes the infection is confined to the skin and subcutaneous tissue, in which case it is less severe. The main differential diagnoses are streptococcal infections and synergistic infections, both of which can also be very destructive. The treatment is extensive debridement and intravenous penicillin in high dosages. *C. perfringens* can also cause an equally devastating gas gangrene of the intestine.

Bites

Bites are a frequent clinical problem, accounting for about 1% of emergency room visits in the USA. Most patients are treated by emergency room or family doctors but it is essential for all physicians to be aware of the problem, for the opportunities for therapeutic errors are immense. All patients who suffer animal bites should be evaluated for the possible need for rabies and tetanus immunization.

Dog Bites

Most animal bites which present to physicians are dog bites, about 15–20% of which become clinically infected. The risk is greater if the hand is involved or if a crush or puncture wound is present. The most common organisms are α-hemolytic streptococci, *S. aureus* and *Pasteurella multocida*. Three rarer bacteria are *Eikenella corrodens*, *Weeksella zoohelcum* and *Capnocytophaga canimorsus* (also known as DF-2), which may cause fulminant sepsis in splenectomized bite victims.

It is difficult to predict which dog bite will be come infected, so most physicians treat all dog bite victims with oral antibiotics. Typically the organisms are very sensitive to antibiotics. Ampicillin-clavunate is the usual recommendation. When penicillin allergy is present, the choice is not clear. In severe bites, cultures should be taken and appropriate intravenous antibiotics employed. Wounds older than 24 h or obviously infected should not be closed. Fresh wounds on the face are generally closed because of the need for a good cosmetic result. Opinions vary about the wisdom of closing other fresh wounds.

Cat Bites

Cats have sharper canine teeth (despite the name) than dogs so puncture wounds are more likely. Often tendon sheaths or joint spaces are reached. The risk of infection is about 50%. Thus the need for antibiotic treatment is greater. The most common organism is *P. multocida* but the spectrum and therapeutic approach are similar as for dogs.

Exotic Bites

Inadequate data are available for most exotic species. In our area, feeding swans is a common activity for strollers along a lake shore. Swan bites and those of other animals living in the water seem more likely to transfer *P. aeruginosa* so ciprofloxacin should be employed. Monkey bites have often been described to transfer herpes virus B (herpes virus simiae).

Human Bites

Human bites are far more serious than animal bites. Prior to antibiotics about a quarter of all human bite injuries involving the hand resulted in amputation. The clenched fist injury, when a closed fist strikes the teeth of another individual is the most serious of all. In this instance deep space infections, ascending tendon space infections and even joint infections and osteomyelitis may occur. The range of organisms includes *S. aureus*, *E. corrodens*, *H. influenzae* and many oral anaerobes which often lead to synergistic infections. In the case of hand injury, anaerobic bacteria especially *E. corrodens* are expected.

Usually oral amoxicillin-clavunate is sufficient. In hospitalized patients, ampicillin-sulbactam may be used intravenously. Any patient with a significant clench fist injury should be hospitalized, with a hand surgeon directing the care.

Zoonoses

There are many methods of transmission of infection from animals to humans. They include direct contact, scratches, bites, inhalation, contact with urine or feces and ingestion of infected meat, eggs, dairy products or contaminated foods. In addition, many other infections are transmitted by arthropod hosts. In this section we discuss the traditional zoonoses, those bacterial infections which are generally restricted to animals but can be transferred to humans, causing significant human disease. Many of the organisms have already been alluded to above.

Erysipeloid

(Rosenbach 1909)

Synonyms. Fish-handler's disease, crab dermatitis, seal finger, blubber finger

Definition. Acute infection usually following a trivial hand injury in people who have contact with fresh fish, meat or poultry, such as butchers, fishermen and housewives.

Causative Organism. *Erysipelothrix rhusiopathiae* is an easily cultured short, nonmotile gram-positive rod.

Epidemiology. This agent is found in a wide range of marine animals, including fish, crabs, seals and even whales, as blubber finger suggests. Blubber is the thick fat layer in whales and other marine mammals; cutting it away apparently produces minor injuries and secondary infection. *E. rhusiopathiae* also causes skin and systemic infections in pigs, known as swine erysipelas, and may contaminate animal skins and bones. The infection is almost exclusively limited to individuals who have direct contact with animal material and is more common in the summer months. Epidemics have been described among crab fishermen and workers making bone buttons. Erysipeloid can also be transmitted by contaminated food.

Etiology and Pathogenesis. A minor injury is usually required. While *E. rhusiopathiae* does not appear to penetrate normal skin, individuals in the occupations involved have an extremely high rate of hand scrapes and scratches.

Clinical Findings. After an incubation time of 3–7 days, a painful reddish patch develops and begins to spread peripherally, just like erysipelas. The spreading edge is sharply marginated, while in the center clearing may occur. The changes are usually limited to a small area on the hand (Fig. 4.39). Occasionally larger, vesicular or multiple diffuse lesions may develop. Typically, adjacent joints become painful and swollen. While there are usually no other systemic signs or symptoms, erysipeloid can lead to sepsis and then endocarditis, which is life-threatening. Such patients may have a purpuric exanthem; only about one-third have the typical spreading lesion. The infection usually heals within several weeks even without treatment, but can wax and wane over months. No permanent immunity develops. The outlook is excellent for localized forms but serious for the rare patient with sepsis.

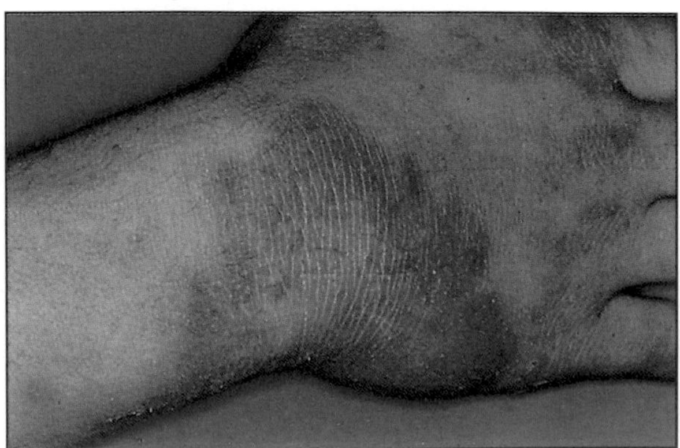

Fig. 4.39. Erysipeloid

Laboratory Findings. Culture of the organism from the skin is best made with a skin biopsy. Blood cultures identify patients with sepsis.

Differential Diagnosis. Erysipelas has a rapid course; not only do the skin lesions expand rapidly, but most patients are very ill. Erythema migrans usually involves the trunk or proximal aspects of the limbs and spreads far more slowly.

Therapy

Systemic. Oral penicillin remains the treatment of choice. Penicillin V-K 500 mg (800,000 IU) q.i.d. for 1 week is effective for local disease. In case of penicillin allergy, erythromycin 250 mg q.i.d. is an acceptable alternative. Hospitalization and intravenous therapy with penicillin G 12–20 million units/day are required for patients with signs of sepsis because of the risk of fatal endocarditis.

Prophylaxis. A vaccine for veterinarians and animal handlers is available, but of unclear effectiveness.

Glanders

Synonym. Malleus

Definition. Acute or chronic infection primarily of equines (horses, donkeys, mules) which can involve other domestic animals and may be spread to humans.

Causative Organism. *Pseudomonas mallei*, an easily cultured, nonmotile gram-negative bacterium which is an obligate mammalian parasite.

Epidemiology. Glanders is quite uncommon in both Europe and North America. The main risk is contact with sick horses. Stable boys, farmers, veterinarians and people disposing of dead animals are at particular risk, specially through contact with nasal secretions, sores, or the flesh of sick animals. While no sporadic cases have been seen in the USA since the 1930s, epidemics have been reported in laboratory workers in whom the spread occurred via aerosols.

Clinical Findings. Glanders may take either an acute or chronic course in humans. The site of entry may be the skin or respiratory mucosa. In either case, the patient may rapidly develop sepsis or contain the organism locally, but remain at risk for later sepsis. Many different variants of glanders have been described. The acute systemic form is almost always fatal; the other variants, distressing and possibly disfiguring.

Acute Cutaneous Glanders. Inoculation of the organism from an ill animal occurs via a minor skin injury. At the inoculation site, erythema and swelling first appear, followed by pustules and then a rapidly spreading undermined ulcer. This primary focus is accompanied by lymphangitis and regional lymphadenopathy. The disease may also disseminates in the skin, producing a macular exanthem which progresses to pustules, bullae and ulcers. The face and especially the nasal, ocular and oral mucosa are particularly likely to be involved.

Primary Nasal Glanders. Here inoculation occurs through the nose. The nasal mucosa becomes swollen and then ulcerated, while the infection can spread rapidly to the lungs.

Acute Systemic Glanders. Some 3–7 days after either local inoculation or inhalation, the patient may become septic with fever, chills, nausea and vomiting. Subcutaneous and systemic abscesses, especially involving muscles, joints and the kidneys, and pneumonia are usually the causes of death after 2–3 weeks in untreated patients.

Chronic Cutaneous Glanders. This rare form of glanders was responsible for the dermatologic interest in the disease. Some patients, presumably those with partial immunity, develop localized skin nodules, often without a history of a primary lesion, lymphatic involvement or illness. The nodules may spread, coalesce, undermine or ulcerate. Sometimes there may be a sporotrichoid pattern with progressive proximal lymphatic spread. The limbs are the most common sites of involvement. The ulcerated lesions may heal, but then recrudesce. The patient remains at risk for sepsis.

Chronic Mucosal Glanders. The local infection is once again contained, leading to ulceration, deep abscesses and disfigurement, since the face is most often involved. Once again, the course may wax and wane.

Laboratory Findings. The organism can be identified in pus, ulcer scraping or tissue, both directly with a Gram-stain and by culture. Blood cultures are negative. Serologic tests are positive after about 2 weeks.

Differential Diagnosis. The list is long. If the initial cutaneous lesions are not seen, all forms of sepsis must be considered and blood cultures relied upon. Chronic cutaneous lesions, especially when ulcerated, suggest tuberculosis. Melioidosis may also have recurrent multiple cutaneous abscesses. The sporotrichoid picture suggests a long range of bacterial and fungal infections.

Therapy

Systemic. Sulfonamides are still the most effective agent. Sulfadiazine 100 mg/kg per day for 3 weeks is usually recommended.

Topical. Wound debridement and standard ulcer care help supplement internal therapy. In chronic glanders, once the disease is treated, surgical reconstruction may be needed. Human to human spread in nursing situations has been reported, so extreme care is warranted.

Melioidosis

(Whitmore and Krishnaswami 1912)

Synonym. Whitmore disease

Definition. Acute septic or chronic granulomatous infection with *Burkholderia pseudomallei*. The name melioidosis means "similar to equine distemper or glanders."

Causative Organism. *Burkholderia pseudomallei*, formerly *Pseudomonas pseudomallei*, a bipolar, gram-negative aerobic bacillus with an affinity for the lungs.

Epidemiology. While most commonly found in southeast Asia, melioidosis occurs across wide bands of the tropical world. It is extremely rare in the western hemisphere. The organism is usually found in a moist environment, whether it be the ground, plants or small collections of water. While many domestic and wild animals are infected, they do not seem to serve as a reservoir for human disease. Instead, contamination of minor scrapes by infected soil or water is the usual route; ingestion and inhalation also occur. About one-third of the US soldiers with burns or open wounds during the Vietnam War had serological evidence of melioidosis. Drug abuse among troops furthered the spread via used injection needles.

Etiology and Pathogenesis. While infections can appear after a matter of days, there may be very long latent periods, making diagnosis a problem.

Clinical Findings. Melioidosis has protean manifestations but usually features pneumonia as well as fever and musculoskeletal pain. There may be an ulcerated nodule at the injury site, but often the patient fails to even notice the inoculation. This localized process often leads to sepsis. Typically the patient presents with pneumonia, either as a primary event or associated with sepsis. Occasionally diarrhea may be associated. Such patients may also have disseminated cutaneous disease. If chronic, the pulmonary picture may resemble tuberculosis. In this stage, there may be subcutaneous abscesses and sinus tracts. The disease may recrudesce after many years. Without therapy melioidosis is a progressive and potentially fatal disease.

Laboratory Findings. *Burkholderia pseudomallei* can be cultured from blood, sputum or infected tissue. Serological tests can help confirm the diagnosis.

Differential Diagnosis. Chronic melioidosis may resemble glanders, as the name of the organism suggests. Only for this reason is melioidosis included in this section, as it is not a zoonosis.

Therapy

Systemic. The antibiotic therapy is complex. In patients with localized skin or lung disease, tetracycline and trimethoprim-sulfamethoxazole are recommended; treatment protocols last from 2 to 6 months. The septic form requires more aggressive therapy.

Public Health Measures. Melioidosis is a reportable infection.

Anthrax

Synonyms. Malignant pustule, wool sorter's disease

Definition. Disease of domestic and wild animals which can accidentally be transmitted to humans.

Causative Organism. *Bacillus anthracis*, a gram-positive organism which forms spores both in nature and under culture conditions but not in tissue. In smears, the chains of bacilli are described as resembling boxcars.

Epidemiology. Anthrax is a dangerous disease because of the persistence of its spores in nature. They may exist for decades in pasture land, stables and even in animal products such as hides or fur. Cows, sheep, goats and to a lesser extent horses, swine and poultry are infected. New infections occur when animals ingest spores with their food and develop gastrointestinal symptoms. Fields are spoiled by anthrax spores for decades or centuries. Under the right weather conditions, the old spores suddenly multiply and reach a critical mass to infect grazing animals. Such anthrax fields have been found in some of the Great Plains states.

A wide range of humans are at risk. Direct contact with an ill animal can result in transfer to farmers, veterinarians, butchers and slaughterhouse workers. In addition, individuals handling furs, hides or other animal by-products may be exposed to spores; included in this group are such exotic jobs as shaving brush makers. Goat hair from the Middle East is particularly likely to be infected. Even harbor workers unloading shipped animal material are at significant risk. While vaccination programs and good animal health measures have reduced the risk of anthrax in western countries, it remains a worldwide problem. In recent years, anthrax has once again been in the public eye as a possible biological weapon; an accident at a probable biological weapons plant in Yekaterinburg, Russia, resulted in at least 60 deaths from anthrax in the local inhabitants.

Etiology and Pathogenesis. The spores can be inoculated by direct contact, ingested or inhaled. They begin to grow with appropriate moisture and release a series of plasmid-mediated exotoxins that are responsible for the dramatic clinical effects. The two major toxins are known as edema factor and lethal factor.

Clinical Findings. The type of anthrax is dependent on how the spores or organisms enter the patient. Cutaneous anthrax is probably most common. The organism is introduced into the skin from an infected animal via minor injury. After an incubation period of 3–8 days, the patient becomes ill with fever and malaise and develops a pustule at the

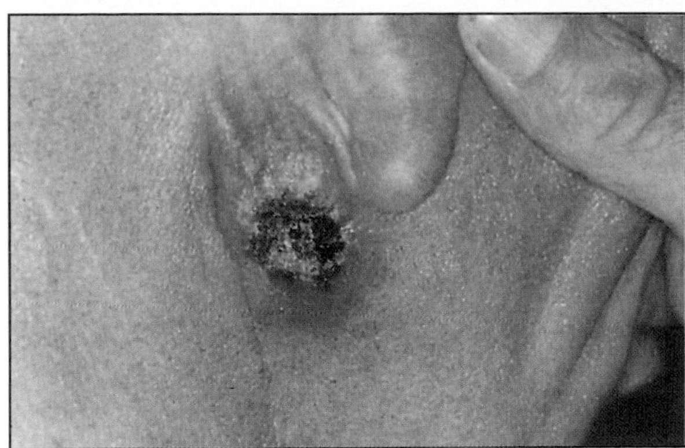

Fig. 4.40. Malignant pustule in anthrax

inoculation site. The pustule spreads, becomes a hemorrhage and blisters, then dries centrally. Anthrax is Latin for hard coal; the name reflects the dark hemorrhagic crust that develops in the malignant pustule (Fig. 4.40). The bacteria secrete toxins responsible for hemorrhage and edema. There may be lymphangitis or even a sporotrichoid picture, but usually the disease is self-limited and heals after 7–10 days with scarring. Some degree of permanent immunity develops.

Unfortunately not all patients do well. Two dreaded complications are anthrax edema and anthrax sepsis. The edema tends to develop more often in the head and neck region, as the swelling and hemorrhage seen with the malignant pustule simply becomes more extreme. Sepsis is more common in association with the edema but can develop directly from the primary inoculation site, especially in immunosuppressed patients. One characteristic of anthrax sepsis is splenic involvement. Meningitis may also develop.

Pulmonary anthrax or wool sorter's disease follows the inhalation of spores, such as from infected furs. It tends to be a biphasic disease, with mild systemic and respiratory symptoms initially, followed by a fulminant downhill course. Gastrointestinal anthrax (the usual disease form in animals) occurs when infected meat is eaten or spores are ingested. Both forms can evolve rapidly into sepsis.

Laboratory Findings. The organism can be identified most easily in smears from infected tissue, such as from a malignant pustule; the same material can be cultured. Blood cultures and serologic tests are less reliable.

Course and Prognosis. While cutaneous anthrax has a good prognosis, pulmonary anthrax is almost always fatal. Unfortunately, the physician can never know who will progress into sepsis.

Differential Diagnosis. One must consider ordinary staphylococcal furuncles and carbuncles but they rarely are as hemorrhagic or edematous as is the malignant pustule. Other inoculation diseases, as discussed throughout this chapter, may appear similar. The pulmonary form evokes the differential diagnosis of all types of severe pneumonia.

Therapy

Systemic. Penicillin is the mainstay of treatment; initially penicillin G should be given IM and after the edema has resolved one can switch to oral medication. Little data are available for the pulmonary form, for which there is almost no hope, but high dose IV penicillin appears the best bet.

Topical. The wound dressings may contain spores and must be considered dangerous biological waste. Unfortunately, often the early diagnosis is not anthrax and thus the spores can be spread about the hospital. Person to person spread in nursing situations has also been reported.

Prophylaxis. A vaccine is available for high-risk workers. Newer toxoid vaccines are also being employed.

Public Health Measures. Anthrax is areportable infection, in most jurisdictions as an emergency.

Other Bacillus Species

In addition to *B. anthracis*, several other *Bacillus* species can cause human disease. Most are found in decaying organic material; some are part of the normal flora. All can potentially form spores. Most patients have a significant risk factor, including burns, intravenous drug abuse, renal dialysis, immunosuppression and HIV/AIDS. *B. cereus* causes food poisoning, usually involving cereal products. *B. subtilis* is notorious for extensive ocular infections especially following ocular trauma or in intravenous drug abusers. Deep abscesses and necrotizing fasciitis are the main changes that are likely to be encountered by dermatologists.

Plague

Synonym. Black death

Definition. Severe, often fatal bacterial illness transmitted to human from infected rodents by fleas.

Causative Organism. *Yersinia pestis* is aerobic gram-negative organism which typically stains in a bipolar fashion, known as the safety pin sign. Yersin isolated the organism from lymph nodes during the Hong Kong plague epidemic in 1894.

Epidemiology. Epidemic plague or the black death of the Middle Ages was a great pestilence, killing enormous numbers of people and striking fear into the hearts of all. The then unknown "humor" was transferred from rats to humans by flea bites, and then spread among humans either once again by fleas or by pulmonary droplet transmission. The disease was spread primarily by rats aboard ships. The last major epidemic occurred in China in the last half of the nineteenth century. Plague still occurs in vast areas of Africa and Asia. An urban outbreak of plague occurred in India in 1994. In the USA, plaque is seen in the Southwest, both among hunters encountering infested animals and among suburbanites whose pets bring home infected fleas or become infected with the bacteria.

Etiology and Pathogenesis. *Yersinia pestis* is present in rodent populations in many parts of the world. For example, in the southwest United States, prairie dogs, ground squirrels and rock squirrels are often infected. In Asia, urban and rural rats remain the largest reservoir. Plague is transmitted to humans directly by flea bites from infected animals or via domestic animals that either bring home infected fleas or themselves develop plague. The flea's foregut is blocked by a clump of bacteria; each time the arthropod bites, it regurgitates bacteria into the wound. When plague is acquired sporadically from animal hosts, once speaks of endemic plague, in contrast to the epidemic plague of the past.

Clinical Findings. After an incubation period of 2–8 days, the patient suddenly develops fever, chills, gastrointestinal distress and a variety of other systemic complaints. The initial flea bite is usually not found or is simply a tiny nonspecific papule. The most dramatic physical finding is the bubo, which is a massive, painful eruptive lymphadenitis usually involving the inguinal, axillary or cervical nodes, since most bites are on the extremities.

Sometimes the disease course stops at this stage, but most often sepsis develops. Thus, it is somewhat of a misnomer to speak of bubonic plague; all patients are at risk for sepsis, whether they develop a bubo or not. If sepsis develops, the two most feared problems are pulmonary involvement and disseminated intravascular coagulation with widespread ecchymoses and necrosis (hence, black death). Patients with pulmonary involvement can transmit the disease directly via droplets, although this is unusual.

The outlook is grim in the absence of therapy. Plague stands out for its rapid fulminant course. A patient sent home with minor complaints may be brought back a few hours dying or dead.

Laboratory Findings. The organism must be identified either through direct examination or culture of blood, sputum or bubo aspirates. Serologic tests are of epidemiological interest only, for they take too long.

Therapy

Systemic. The treatment of choice is streptomycin 30 mg/kg per day IM for 10 days, with gentamicin as the best alternative. Chloramphenicol and doxycycline are also alternatives, but usually reserved for prophylaxis. While all the drugs have significant side effects, untreated plague is worse. Drug resistance has not been a major problem with plague, although a strain with plasmid-transferred multidrug resistance was recently identified in Madagascar. In endemic regions, patients with unexplained high fever and other symptoms who have had outdoor contact (or have pets who are exposed to wild animals, as in suburban or rural areas) should be treated while awaiting culture results.

Other Measures. The patient must be isolated; extreme care must be taken when pulmonary involvement is present.

Public Health Measures. Plague is a reportable infection, in most jurisdictions on an emergency basis.

Tularemia

(McCoy and Chapin 1912)

Synonyms. Rabbit fever, lemming fever

Definition. Endemic disease of many animals which causes epidemics among the animals and can be spread to humans in a variety of ways.

Causative Organism. *Francisella tularensis* is a small, pleomorphic, nonmotile gram-negative rod. It was identified by Francis shortly after the disease was recognized in Tulare, California, in the San Joaquin Valley, in 1912.

Epidemiology. While tularemia was identified in California, it is most common in Arkansas, Missouri, Oklahoma and north Texas. It also occurs in Europe, primarily in Scandinavia. Between 100 and 150 cases are reported yearly in the USA. Hunters are at greatest risk; likely hosts include rabbits, hares, foxes, squirrels, skunks and many other wild and domestic species. The organism is also transferred by bites from ticks, deerflies and other arthropods. In the USA, one speaks of rabbit-borne tularemia and tick-borne tularemia, since both ingestion of infected animals and tick bites are methods of infection.

Etiology and Pathogenesis. The organism is far more aggressive if inhaled or inoculated than if ingested. After local multiplication, it spreads to regional lymph nodes and induces a necrotic granulomatous response.

Clinical Findings. The pathogen can enter the human host in many ways, thus leading to a variety of clinical patterns.

Ulceroglandular Tularemia. In the most common form, the organism enters the skin through a minor injury, often incurred as the hunter skins the animal, usually a rabbit or hare. Infected ticks may also bite the hunter, transferring the disease. In rabbit-borne disease the primary lesion is on the hands, while in the tick-borne form it is on the legs. In either case, the inoculation site develops into an indurated papule which then ulcerates. Multiple primary lesions may be seen or sporotrichoid spread may occur. Lymphangitis develops rapidly, once again either axillary or inguinal depending on the type of exposure. It is usually quite prominent and associated with fever and malaise. After several weeks, the nodes tend to fuse and break down. Sometimes no primary lesion is seen and the patient presents with lymphatic involvement. Healing occurs over months. The lymph nodes can be biopsied to rule out lymphoma; they are effaced and have a typical necrotic pattern. About 15% of patients have pneumonia.

Mucosal Tularemia. Inoculation can also occur in the mouth; the primary lesion mimics an aphthous ulcer but the patient rapidly develops more severe ulceration and lymphadenopathy. Tonsillitis may also occur.

Ocular Tularemia. When the hunter inadvertently wipes his eye while skinning an infected animal, ocular mucosal inoculation is a possibility. Sequelae include striking lid edema and then lymphadenopathy, usually submandibular.

Typhoidal Tularemia. Some patients present with fever, malaise, weight loss and gastrointestinal symptoms without any history of injury or lymphadenopathy. Over half of them have pneumonia, often leading to respiratory distress. Any of these forms can evolve into the septic form with the main focus of damage being the lungs. There may also be gastrointestinal disease including splenomegaly and CNS involvement. During the course of typhoid tularemia, there may be secondary cutaneous findings. A variety of polymorphic exanthems may be seen, as well as erythema nodosum.

Patients with pulmonary involvement or the typhoid form are at great risk; the other variants are usually self-limited. Immunity develops, but reinoculation can lead to an exaggerated local reaction.

Histopathology. The lymph nodes in tularemia show a characteristic necrosis, but a lymph node biopsy frequently induces septicemia and is not desirable.

Laboratory Findings. The organism is difficult to identify directly and dangerous to culture. Immunofluorescent identification of the organism in tissue is a rapid, accurate diagnostic tool. In most cases, the diagnosis is made with serologic methods.

Differential Diagnosis

Primary lesion: Furuncle, herpetic whitlow, paronychia, anthrax (malignant pustule), sporotrichosis

Lymphadenopathy: Cat-scratch fever, melioidosis, glanders, infectious mononucleosis and many others
Sepsis: Rocky Mountain spotted fever, other rickettsial diseases, long list of bacterial diseases

Therapy

Systemic. Streptomycin 15 – 20 mg/kg per day IM for 7 – 14 days is usually recommended. Other regimens and agents have been suggested for the typhoidal form.

Prophylaxis. Insect repellents and the use of gloves when skinning animals would avoid most of the cases.

Public Health Measures. Tularemia is a reportable infection.

Brucellosis

(Bruce 1887)

Synonyms. Undulant fever, Malta fever, Mediterranean fever

Definition. Common disease of several domestic animals which can be spread from infected animals or animal products to humans.

Causative Organism. *Brucellae* are small, nonmotile, gram-negative coccobacillary organisms. Three different species are responsible for most human disease: *Brucella suis* (swine), *B. melitensis* (goats) and *B. abortus* (cattle). The latter causes Bang's disease or epidemic abortions in cattle herds.

Epidemiology. Brucellosis was first described by British Army physicians serving on Malta in the last half of the nineteenth century. Today farmers, butchers and veterinarians are most likely to be infected by direct contact with a sick animal. However, infected animals can also transfer the disease through their milk or meat. In both Germany and America (mainly Texas and California), about 100 human cases yearly are reported. Worldwide, the disease remains common and is often overlooked, about 10 % of the cases are from raw milk. Infected goat milk and cheese from Mexico represents a new source of infection. Workers in slaughtering plants are also at risk; the airborne particles created by sawing bones are highly infective. Vaccines and herd testing have reduced the problem in cattle.

Etiology and Pathogenesis. Brucellae have an affinity for the reticuloendothelial system and can survive for long periods of time in macrophages, lymph nodes and the spleen. Thus, if they evade the initial neutrophilic response, they can cause persistent problems. They also secrete exotoxins, which may partially explain their acute effects.

Clinical Findings. The source of entry may be inoculation, inhalation or ingestion. After 1 – 3 weeks, patients develop a low-grade fever and malaise. Often the fever has a cyclic pattern, leading to the name undulant fever. Cutaneous changes are uncommon and uncharacteristic. There may be a variety of transient, often purpuric exanthems. Virtually every organ system can be involved; the scope of brucellosis is beyond the range of this chapter.

Veterinarians appear at risk for two unusual problems. Contact with *Brucella abortus* during a delivery or when removing a dead fetus (usually performed without gloves, which tend to rip on the calf's sharp hoofs) may lead to an eruption on the forearms consisting of swollen red papules which may ulcerate. Similarly inadvertent inoculation with the vaccines designed for animal use usually leads to a severe reaction in the human victim. Presumably veterinarians are highly sensitized to the organisms and have an excessive immune response.

Laboratory Findings. Culture of tissue fluids or blood and serology all are helpful in identifying the organism.

Course and Prognosis. If treated, the outlook is good. Otherwise, brucellosis can evolve into a chronic disabling disease, often misdiagnosed for long periods of time. In the 1950s, it was proposed as one of the first "causes" of the chronic fatigue syndrome.

Differential Diagnosis. The list is endless; brucellosis is a great imitator.

Therapy

Systemic. Doxycycline 200 mg/day and rifampicin 600 – 900 mg/day for 6 weeks are currently recommended. Streptomycin is also effective and employed in severe or chronic cases.

Prophylaxis. The strain 19 vaccine is effective for cattle. Equally effective vaccines for pigs and goats are available, but they have not been as efficiently employed. No human vaccine is available in the USA.

Public Health Measures. Brucellosis is a reportable infection.

Rat Bite Fever

Synonym. Haverhill fever

Definition. Acute illness transferred to humans from rats, often through a bite.

Causative Organism. *Streptobacillus moniliformis* is as gram-negative pleomorphic bacillus which may appear filamentous in culture and mimic *Candida albicans.*

Epidemiology. The organism is present in the oropharynx of most wild or laboratory rats, who do not appear to suffer from the infection. Many other small mammals are involved, such as mice and squirrels. There was an epidemic in Haverhill, Massachusetts, in 1926 that was spread through milk infected by rat feces. Fecal contamination of grain has also led to epidemics.

Clinical Findings. The rat bite has often healed when after several days the patient develops fever, chills and malaise. Arthralgias are common; lymphadenopathy is rare. A nonspecific morbilliform rash then follows. Acral involvement is common; hemorrhage may develop. The Haverhill fever variant develops after ingestion and the patient typically presents with gastrointestinal signs and symptoms. It may eventuate into endocarditis, the most feared complication.

Laboratory Findings. Blood culture is most reliable. Serologic testing may also be helpful.

Differential Diagnosis. There is a second rat bite fever, more common in the Orient and known in Japan as soduku (rat-poison). It is caused by *Spirillum minor*, a gram-negative spirochete. Soduku is only spread by bites, not by the other routes. The initial bite usually heals; then after several weeks, the bite site becomes swollen, painful, ulcerates and forms an eschar. Massive lymphadenopathy occurs and there may be a widespread exanthem. Endocarditis is the most dangerous complication. The syphilis serology is false-positive in about 50% of cases. Serology and culture are not helpful; the organism must be identified by direct examination of blood or tissue.

Leptospirosis is the other common organism transmitted by rat bites. Clinically one should also consider Rocky Mountain spotted fever, syphilis, and other viral and rickettsial diseases; if the rash is hemorrhagic, meningococcemia should be excluded.

Therapy

Systemic. Fortunately the therapy for both types of rat bite fever is the same. Penicillin G, 600,000 IU b.i.d. IM for 14 days, is recommended. If endocarditis is diagnosed, higher IV doses are needed.

Other Zoonoses

There are many other zoonoses which are traditionally not included in this category. For example, many dermatophytoses are acquired from domestic or, less often, wild animals. Leptospirosis is also transmitted from animals, and one could view many food-borne infections as zoonoses.

In recent years, a new category of nosocomial or facultative zoonoses has emerged. One example will suffice. *Malassezia furfur* is a lipophilic yeast (Chap. 7) which causes tinea versicolor but can cause bloodstream infections in neonates receiving lipid emulsions. An epidemic of neonatal infections in a nursery was recently caused by *M. pachydermatis*, a usually harmless yeast first described in a rhinoceros with exfoliative dermatitis (hence, the name pachydermatis) but often found in dogs, either as a harmless commensal or as a cause of otitis externa. A nursery worker with pets introduced the yeast and it was then transmitted by other individuals as well.

Mycobacteria

The Mycobacteria are a family of bacteria with several special features. They are obligate aerobic organisms which grow very slowly and have abundant lipids in their cell wall. For this reason, they are very resistant to acids, bases and alcohols and are identified with special staining methods such as the Ziehl-Neelsen stain. The major members of the family include are shown in Table 4.9.

Table 4.9. Types of mycobacteria

Organism	Disease
Mycobacterium tuberculosis	Tuberculosis
Mycobacterium bovis	Tuberculosis (very rare in humans)
Mycobacterium leprae	Leprosy
Mycobacterium ulcerans	Buruli ulcer
Mycobacterium avium-intracellulare	Many infections in HIV/AIDS
Mycobacterium marinum	Swimming pool granuloma
Other atypical mycobacteria	Variety of infections, including skin

Tuberculosis

Definition. Chronic infection caused by *Mycobacterium tuberculosis* with usual primary involvement of the lungs and occasional skin changes.

History. Hippocrates used the tongue-twisting term phthisis to describe tuberculosis as a disease associated with the general demise or disappearance of the patient. Tuberculosis was the major cause of death in Europe between the sixteenth and eighteenth centuries but became even more of a problem during the Industrial Revolution. In some countries, the yearly death rate was as high as 1000/100,000. Schönlein first suggested the name tuberculosis, while three major contributions in the 19th century led to the identification of the disease. Laënnec (1819) noted that the many manifestations of tuberculosis were expressions of a single disease, while Villemin (1868) transferred tissue from a patient's lungs to a rabbit where the disease took hold. Koch's name is most often attached with tuberculosis; he identified the bacillus in 1882 and received the Nobel Prize for this work in 1905.

Just 2 years later Koch identified *M. tuberculosis* in lupus vulgaris, beginning the description of the various cutaneous aspects of tuberculosis. In 1891, he recognized the reactivity of the skin towards altered mycobacteria in individuals who had experienced an infection. Von Pirquet in 1906 interpreted this phenomenon as tuberculospecific allergy, the basis for all future tuberculosis skin testing. The host response was soon identified as crucial in tuberculosis; in the skin, tuberculids were described as widespread, symmetric, noncontagious cutaneous eruptions caused by an allergic response to *M. tuberculosis* rather than a direct infection. Modern PCR techniques have identified mycobacterial DNA in these lesions. The use of the Bacillus Calmette-Guérin (BCG), a passage-modified form of *M. bovis*, as an immunization against tuberculosis is also based on the development of marked delayed hypersensitivity.

Causative Organisms. *Mycobacterium tuberculosis*, *M. africanum*, *M. bovis* and other minor variants. *M. tuberculosis* is a 2.5–3.5 µm long and 0.3–0.6 µm wide, slightly curved gram-positive bacillus.

Epidemiology. While the incidence and prevalence of tuberculosis dropped markedly around the world after the end of World War II, in the past decade *M. tuberculosis* has become a scourge once again. The combination of better hygiene, immunizations and antibacterial agents led to a drop, but the explosion of HIV/AIDS infections, the development of drug-resistant bacteria and, in many countries, a general diminution in health care have led to an unfortunate renaissance for *M. tuberculosis*. About one-third of the world's people are infected with the bacteria. In developing countries, tuberculosis is still one of the most common infections, with an estimated 10 million new infections yearly worldwide and about 3 million deaths. Over 95% of all new cases and 98% of all deaths occur in the Third World. Three-quarters of the cases involve individuals between 15 and 50 years of age.

Concomitant HIV/AIDS is the biggest factor in the resurgence of tuberculosis. In many parts of sub-Saharan Africa, 70% of tuberculosis patients are HIV-positive; and about one-third of the HIV-infected people worldwide also have tuberculosis. Having HIV/AIDS increases the risk of tuberculosis tenfold. Among patients with HIV/AIDS, the lifetime risk of developing active tuberculosis has been estimated at over 50%, depending on the prevalence of the organism in the society. Patients treated with immunosuppressive agents, especially after solid organ transplantation, are also at risk for reactivation of latent disease.

In the USA, the incidence is about 10/100,000. In areas with relatively low rates, most cases represent reactivation of latent pulmonary infection. In Germany, the incidence is about twice as high, 20/100,000. Even though *M. tuberculosis* is not very infectious, there is about a 30% chance of household contacts becoming infected over 1 year. Major risk factors include patients with active, untreated pulmonary disease and contact with immunosuppressed individuals. For this reason, isolation was practiced in the past, and today prompt treatment, screening of contacts and prophylaxis all play a major role. In recent years, strains of *M. tuberculosis* resistant to multiple drugs have appeared, usually in hospitals, homeless shelters, prisons or AIDS hospices. These infections have a very high mortality rate, not only among the immunosuppressed patients but also among health-care workers unlucky enough to become infected.

Most infections today are caused by *M. tuberculosis*, the closely related *M. africanum* and other almost identical variants. We will use *M. tuberculosis* to discuss this entire group. In the past, tuberculosis was often transferred from cattle, usually via infected milk. *M. bovis* has disappeared in the USA and Germany because of programs to eliminate the organism and pasteurization of milk. About 0.1% of all infections in Germany today are traced back to cattle or milk, often in individuals who for health reasons unwisely drink nonpasteurized milk. One should be suspicious when tuberculosis is identified among farmers or veterinarians.

Etiology and Pathogenesis. Tuberculosis is a chronic infection with a primary infection and then a latency period with the risk of reactivation. While the entire sequence of events of systemic tuberculosis and the clinical manifestations are beyond the scope of this chapter, a slight review is needed in order to adequately understand the cutaneous manifestations. In well over 90% of cases, the airways are the site of initial infection, as *M. tuberculosis* is spread from an infected patient via droplets. In the lungs, a primary lesion develops, usually in a subpleural location. Macrophages engulf the bacilli but then die before they can kill the bacteria. Gradually, Langerhans giant cells form, along with central necrosis, producing a tubercle or granuloma, also known as a Ghon focus. The bacteria eventually reach the local lymphatics and spread to the regional lymph nodes. The primary lesion and the involved regional lymph nodes comprise the primary complex.

In most patients, the disease is arrested at this stage. In the USA and Germany, at least 90% of patients develop sufficient immunity. The primary complex calcifies and scars and the patient has a latent infection. Many patients do not even realize they have had a primary infection with *M. tuberculosis* and are identified later with skin tests or radiological examinations. In others the infection progresses. In the lungs, there may be more widespread disease leading to pneumonia, pleural effusions and even extensive necrosis, depending on the host status. Hematogenous spread may occur; the kidneys, spleen and epiphyses are favorite sites. In miliary tuberculosis, there is widespread hematogenous spread seeding many organs, including the liver, bone marrow and especially the meninges. Landouzy syndrome is the acute development of tuberculosis sepsis in especially weak patients, such as those with HIV/AIDS.

Postprimary pulmonary tuberculosis most closely corresponds to Hippocrates' phthisis. Patients tend to present with malaise, weight loss, night sweats, a productive cough and a variety of other pulmonary symptoms. The disease typically develops in the elderly, chronically ill or immunosuppressed, representing a reactivation of an apparently healed infection. Apparently only a small number of *M. tuberculosis* are needed for reactivation and they have an amazing capacity to bide their time in tissue, over decades.

Cutaneous tuberculosis can arise in many ways. Skin involvement may occur from direct inoculation, such as in a pathologist, from draining regional lymph nodes, from miliary spread or as part of the spectrum of reactivation. For clinical lesions to develop, the organisms must reach the skin and the local resistance must be impaired. All of these patterns will be considered in detail below.

Clinical Findings. The clinical features of tuberculosis can involve every organ and a description thereof should be sought in internal medicine textbooks. The skin findings are very pleomorphic and will be considered separately.

Histopathology. The characteristic lesion is the tubercle, with central necrosis, a wall of macrophages and Langerhans giant cells and a mantle of lymphocytes. Because the necrosis is often extreme, the material on gross inspection may appear cheesy, leading to the expression caseation necrosis. The bacteria are sparse and difficult to find in a granuloma.

A number of other diseases can cause tuberculoid granulomas in the skin, including tuberculoid leprosy, atypical mycobacterial infections, perioral dermatitis, rosacea, sarcoidosis, Melkersson-Rosenthal syndrome or deep fungi. Some foreign body granulomas are also tuberculoid.

The identification of *M. tuberculosis* requires special stains. Most widely used are Ziehl-Neelsen, fluorochrome and anti-BCG polyclonal antibody stains. In anergic forms of the disease with numerous organisms, the stains are abundantly positive. In granulomas and allergic forms, PCR can help to identify mycobacterial DNA. In a true tuberculid, intact organisms should not be present, although PCR sometimes reveals DNA. Positive PCR results should not be equated with the presence of living or potentially infective *M. tuberculosis.*

Laboratory Findings. The diagnosis of tuberculosis can usually be made by the following techniques:

- Direct identification in sputum, gastric fluids or tissue sections
- Positive sputum or tissue culture, which takes 4–6 weeks and then allows determination of antibiotic sensitivities
- Animal inoculation, often using guinea pigs – available but rarely needed
- Characteristic radiological findings
- Skin testing

The development of immunity and its assessment via skin testing is more important in screening and monitoring patients than it is in confirming the diagnosis of active infection. Koch viewed the immunity as a marker of resistance, while Conan Doyle (of Sherlock Holmes fame) was the first to suggest using it for diagnosis. Many different antigens have been used over the years including:

- Tuberculin pastes or ointments (Moro ointment) for screening school children in some countries.
- Tine tests for mass screening efforts.
- Purified protein derivative, a standardized form (PPD-S) of killed tuberculin calibrated in international units (IU). Some individuals still use old tuberculin (OT); first strength OT is roughly equal to intermediate PPD-S.

The Mantoux test using PPD-S is the most accurate form of skin testing. In the USA the standard intradermal dose is intermediate strength PPD containing 5 IU; a weaker material is available for highly sensitive individuals and a more concentrated one for nonreactors. The reaction is read after 48–72 h. In the past, greater than 10 mm induration was considered positive but this has been refined in recent years. Many schemes are employed such as the following.

- A 5 mm reaction is positive in patients with HIV/AIDS, other immunosuppression and a history of exposure.
- A 10 mm reaction is positive in high risk individuals, such as immigrants from endemic areas, prisoners and nursing home residents.
- A 15 mm reaction is positive in low risk individuals

Changes in reactivity can be more important than a single test, especially in trying to assess reactivation, when immunity may drop. In some instances the Mantoux test is not accurate. If a patient's immunity is impaired enough, he may become anergic. Thus when a patient with active tuberculosis no longer reacts, it is usually a bad sign. Some individuals have a hyperergic reaction, responding positively to very diluted forms of PPD, such as 1 IU. These patients are felt to be more likely to develop tuberculids.

Course and Prognosis. The usual outcome following primary infection, seen in over 90 % of healthy individuals, is a positive tuberculin skin test and no clinical disease. Some patients may have hypersensitivity reactions, such as erythema nodosum; other may have pulmonary complications and yet others may have disseminated disease. The latter is more likely in children and immunosuppressed individuals. Pulmonary tuberculosis may also be postprimary, resulting from reactivation. About 50 % of patients with pulmonary tuberculosis die within 5 years if untreated. One-quarter are cured by their strong immune response, while the balance have chronic active disease. Today, the presence of associated diseases and the development of drug resistance are the main complicating factors. In one African study, it was suggested that treating concurrent tuberculosis was the most cost-effective way of helping an HIV/AIDS patient.

Therapy The therapy of tuberculosis is beyond our scope. Table 4.10 shows the drugs recommended by the World Health Organization. In the USA, the usual initial treatment consists of four drugs: isoniazid, rifampicin, pyrazinamide and either ethambutol or streptomycin. Many other regimens are available; one should consult local health authorities. The major therapeutic principle is to use multiple drugs to avoid development of resistant strains. In addition, once culture and sensitivities are available, one must be sure that the strain is susceptible to at least two of the employed drugs. In settings in which compliance is unlikely, direct observation of ingestion is effective. Pulmonary tuberculosis is usually treated for

Table 4.10. Anti-tuberculosis medications

Drug	Mode of action	Potency	Recommended dose (mg/kg)		
			Daily	3×/week	2×/week
Isoniazid	Bactericidal	High	5	10	15
Rifampicin	Bactericidal	High	10	10	10
Pyrazinamide	Bactericidal	Low	25	35	50
Streptomycin	Bactericidal	Low	15	15	15
Ethambutol	Bacteriostatic	Low	15	?30[a]	?45[a]
Thiacetazone	Bacteriostatic	Low	3	–[b]	–[b]

[a] Ethambutol's efficacy in such protocols is unclear.
[b] Thiacetazone is not effective when given intermittently.
(Based on the table on page 84 of WHO 1996)

6–9 months; more advanced disease, such as bone involvement, requires 18 months or more of therapy. In HIV/AIDS patients, some type of therapy is usually required lifelong.

Public Health Measures. Tuberculosis is a reportable infection. There are many steps to be considered. Extensive case control work is needed and all individuals with contact should be screened. Isoniazid prophylaxis should be offered to all individuals who show signs of conversion or latent disease and are under 35 years of age and to those in high risk groups who are older. The limiting factor is the problem with isoniazid-induced hepatitis. Special attention should be paid to the above mentioned high risk settings, such as HIV/AIDS hospices, prisons and nursing homes.

Prophylaxes The use of bacillus Calmette-Guérin (BCG) for immunization is also effective. In Germany, the procedure is often carried out during infancy, just as it is in endemic areas and among high risk groups. Health care workers with a negative PPD test are also immunized in Germany. Infants receive 0.05 ml; older children and adults, 0.1 ml. About 90% of immunized patients show an increased cell-mediated immunity. The best clinical data are those indicating less tuberculous meningitis in infants; BCG probably offers little protection against pulmonary tuberculosis in adults. In most cases BCG is safe in HIV/AIDS patients, but the World Health Organization does not recommend vaccinating infants with signs or symptoms of HIV/AIDS.

Infants can be immunized in the first 6 weeks of life without checking their PPD status. Later on it is essential to be sure that the patient shows no skin reactivity. If a patient with immunity is immunized, an inflammatory reaction (Koch reaction) with ulceration at the site of injection, usually the hip, may develop (Fig. 4.41).

Normally after 2–6 weeks an inflamed red nodule develops and slowly evolves into a blue or livid plaque that clinically and histologically resembles lupus vulgaris. If such a site is biopsied, granulomas can be observed for up to 1 year. Regional lymphadenopathy may develop. The PPD test usually converts at about 12 weeks. Sometimes an injection site may ulcerate, even in a correctly identified nonreactive patient. The cause may be injecting the material too deeply into the subcutaneous fat, rather than the dermis. In other instances bacterial secondary infections or scratching may be responsible. The BCG organisms can be found in the ulcer or discharge. All the phenomena associated with primary pulmonary tuberculosis can develop, although rarely, including tuberculids. Although the reaction to BCG is viewed as protective, if cutaneous ulceration persists or there is draining

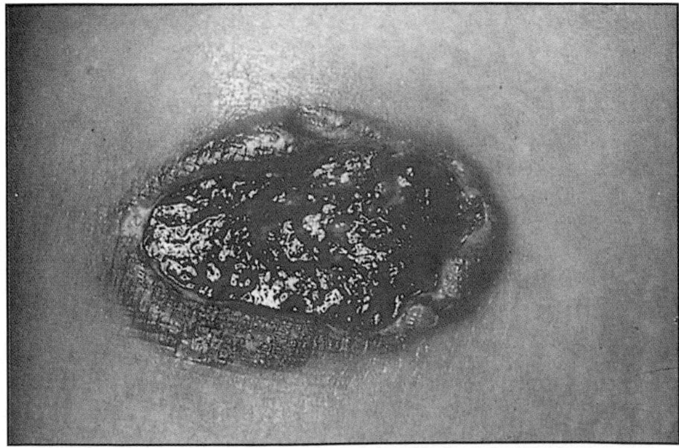

Fig. 4.41. Ulcer following Bacillus Calmette-Guérin immunization

lymphadenopathy, then systemic therapy should be considered. In children isoniazid is used, but in adults consideration should be given to a multidrug regimen.

Cutaneous Tuberculosis

Even though cutaneous tuberculosis is very rare, with a prevalence in Germany around 0.5–1.0/100,000, one must expect a resurgence around the world. Cutaneous tuberculosis is usually classified into anergic, reactive and hyperergic forms, as shown in Table 4.11. There is an inverse relationship between immune reactivity or PPD test and the presence of organisms. Anergic patients have a negative test and many organisms, reactive patients a positive test and fewer organisms, and hyperergic patients a strongly positive test and very few or no organisms.

Cutaneous Tuberculosis in Anergic Patients

These forms develop in patients with no prior exposure to *M. tuberculosis* and thus no immunity, or in people who have lost their immune response to the organism, usually as a sign of weakening overall immunity and impending disaster. The PPD test is negative, often even when the large 250 IU dose is used. The cutaneous and mucosal lesions are rich in bacteria and contagious.

Primary Cutaneous Complex

Synonyms. Tuberculosis primaria cutis, primary cutaneous tuberculosis, inoculation tuberculosis, tuberculoid chancre

Definition. Primary infection of a skin portal, often with associated regional lymphadenopathy, in a patient with no evidence of pulmonary tuberculosis.

Epidemiology. This form is extremely rare; almost all tuberculosis starts in the lungs.

Etiology and Pathogenesis. Three conditions must be met:

- No prior exposure
- Contact with *M. tuberculosis*
- Small skin defect or injury; the bacteria cannot penetrate normal intact skin.

The same process described for a Ghon focus occurs in the skin and subcutaneous tissue, as well as regional lymph nodes.

Clinical Findings. The inoculation lesion develops after an incubation period of 3–4 weeks. Typically there is a small, easily overlooked papule, which ulcerates and shows no tendency towards healing. This is the primary focus. In addition, there may be lymphangitis, and there is almost always lymphadenopathy with pain, swelling and frequently perforation to the exterior, producing an ulcer and sinus tracts. In most cases healing is spontaneous.

Table 4.11. Types of cutaneous tuberculosis

Host immune response	PPD test	Organisms	Cutaneous disease	Subcutaneous disease
Anergic				
First exposure	–	+++	Primary inoculation complex	–
Lost reactivity	–	+++	Tuberculosis cutis miliaris disseminata	–
			Tuberculosis miliaris ulcerosa cutis et mucosae	–
			Tuberculosis fungosa serpiginosa	–
Reactive	+	+	Lupus vulgaris	Tuberculosis cutis colliquativa
			Tuberculosis cutis verrucosa	–
Hyperergic	++	+/–	Lichen scrophulosorum	Erythema induratum
			Papulonecrotic tuberculid	–

Some patients may develop erythema nodosum. There are two variants of the primary complex.

- Primary cervical tuberculosis: Children who drink milk infected with *M. bovis* can develop a primary tonsillar infection with secondary involvement of the lymph nodes of the neck, usually unilaterally and anterior to the sternocleidomastoid muscle. The massive lymphadenopathy with erythema, swelling, draining sinus tracts and typical scars resembles scrofuloderma.
- Circumcision tuberculosis:. If the physician or individual performing the circumcision, such as the Jewish *moel*, has tuberculosis, there is a slight chance of infecting the wound. This has become extremely rare, if not extinct.

Histopathology. In the early stages, a granulomatous response is not seen. There may be an abscess; the necrotic material is rich in *M. tuberculosis*. After 3–6 weeks, as the PPD test becomes positive, granuloma formation may begin.

Laboratory Findings. The bacteria should also be cultured.

Differential Diagnosis. Among other forms of tuberculosis, in children tuberculosis cutis colliquativa or scrofuloderma may appear similar, but there is no primary focus in the skin and the bacteria are fewer in number. Other infections such as tularemia, actinomycosis, sporotrichosis and atypical mycobacteria, especially *M. marinum*, can produce a similar lesion. Culture is decisive.

Therapy. Despite the innocent nature of the findings and the tendency towards spontaneous resolution, the risk of dissemination and reactivation make full treatment mandatory.

Tuberculosis Cutis Miliaris Disseminata

Synonym. Miliary tuberculosis of the skin

Definition. Very rare hematogenous form of tuberculosis with seeding of the skin, as well as other organs in most cases, in anergic patients.

Etiology and Pathogenesis. Tuberculosis cutis miliaris disseminata is extremely rare, but most common in infants and markedly immunosuppressed patients. Most often the hematogenous spread involves multiple organs, but in some instances the skin may be dramatically affected. It is still felt that all such patients have bacteremia, even if it is silent in some cases. Concomitant infections such as measles may predispose an infant towards dissemination. Sometimes one or several larger abscesses may develop. Such a lesion is known as a tuberculous gumma and is most common on the scalp in children or immunosuppressed patients. Individuals with a small number of abscesses sometimes have slightly better immunity (a weakly positive PPD test) and are thus at the more favorable end of the anergic spectrum.

Clinical Findings. Usually there are numerous red-brown macules and papules which appear relatively suddenly, may be hemorrhagic and tend to ulcerate. They are not pruritic. They are rich in organisms. The mucosal surfaces may be similarly involved. The course is determined by the degree of internal organ involvement.

Differential Diagnosis. All of the disorders with red-brown nodules including Langerhans cell histiocytosis, pseudolymphoma, malignant lymphoma, leukemia, TORCH infections, secondary syphilis and pityriasis lichenoides et varioliformis acuta should be considered.

Therapy. Multidrug regimens for systemic tuberculosis are required.

Tuberculosis Cutis Orificialis

Synonyms. Tuberculosis miliaris ulcerosa mucosae et cutis, orificial tuberculosis

Definition. Direct infection of orificial mucosal and skin surfaces in anergic patient with fulminant pulmonary or gastrointestinal tuberculosis.

Etiology and Pathogenesis. This is another rare form of cutaneous tuberculosis, appearing in about 0.2% of infected patients. Most patients are older men with active pulmonary or gastrointestinal disease. The presence of numerous bacilli in sputum or saliva leads to infection of the oral mucosa and adjoining skin. In the case of gastrointestinal disease, the perianal tissues are at risk, as often seen in HIV/AIDS patients, while rarely renal tuberculosis will lead to urethral seeding. The patient's weakened immune status also aids the spread.

Clinical Findings. Tiny red papules appear, become pustular and then degenerate into very painful superficial ulcers. The ulcers are small, less than 2 cm, superficial, irregular and usually have a pus-covered base. Marked tissue destruction and swelling may occur so that a large part of a lip is destroyed. The tip of the tongue is commonly involved, as is the palate. Sometimes many tiny yellow dots are present on the floor of the ulcer, corresponding to tiny necrotic tubercles. Anal and perianal lesions are quite similar. There may be spread to the adjacent skin. The severe pain may interfere with eating, defecating or urinating. The lesions are highly contagious.

Histopathology. The ulcer is nonspecific and granulomas are uncommon, but many organisms can be found with Ziehl-Neelsen staining.

Course and Prognosis. The outlook is poor because the systemic tuberculosis is usually quite advanced and the patient's resistance very low.

Differential Diagnosis. Lues miliaris ulcerosa mucosae in tertiary syphilis is identical, but can be excluded because of the lack of systemic tuberculosis, the negative Ziehl-Neelsen stain and the positive syphilis serology. Severe herpes simplex and cytomegalovirus infections in immunosuppressed hosts can appear similar but viral cultures are positive. Aphthae usually heal quickly, but in HIV/AIDS patients may be persistent and larger. Large lip ulcers may suggest squamous cell carcinoma, but the latter is usually painless and hard. Histology is decisive.

Therapy. Standard multidrug regimens should be employed. A 2% aqueous lactic acid solution is helpful for locally treating the ulcerations. Topical anesthetics can be used for pain relief.

Tuberculosis Fungosa Serpiginosa

Definition. Extremely rare form of inoculation tuberculosis in older patients with relative anergy.

Etiology and Pathogenesis. The bacteria can reach the skin in many ways. There can be exogenous inoculation but this is less common than autoinoculation or even spread from involved bones or muscles.

Clinical Findings. The most common locations are the forearms and backs of the hands. Papules develop and rapidly ulcerate forming sinus tracts and draining a cloudy or pus-laden discharge. The inflammatory infiltrates continue to enlarge at the periphery but there may be central clearing and atrophic scars, causing the serpiginous pattern.

Histopathology. Tiny tuberculoid granulomas can occasionally be found in the inflammatory infiltrate and the organisms are numerous.

Course and Prognosis. The outlook depends on the clinical scenario. If there is accidental inoculation from a modest pulmonary tuberculosis, then usually treatment for both conditions is effective. When spread occurs from bone, the outlook is less favorable. The fact that the patient has some resistance, as manifested by the central healing, places this type at the better end of the anergic spectrum.

Differential Diagnosis. Tuberculosis cutis verrucosa is similar, but the clinical course is slower, the histology more granulomatous and the organism less common. In addition, the patient is not anergic. Chronic vegetating or blastomycotic pyoderma is almost identical, so exclusion of tuberculosis is always a must when considering the latter diagnosis. Halogenoderma may also appear similar. Verrucous carcinoma and squamous cell carcinoma can also have central clearing and serpiginous borders but the lesions are usually firm and the histology is different.

Therapy. Systemic multidrug regimens can be combined with surgical removal, if the lesion is small.

Cutaneous Tuberculosis in Patients with Normal Immunity

Cutaneous tuberculosis in a patient with intact cellular immunity always follows development of the primary complex and is thus a postprimary phenomenon. The lesions are characterized by distinct granulomas, few organisms and little risk of transmission. The patient's PPD test is always positive.

Tuberculosis Cutis Verrucosa
(RIEHL and PALTAUF 1886)

Synonyms. Butcher's wart, prosector's wart, warty tuberculosis

Definition. Inoculation tuberculosis in a patient with intact immunity and a healed primary complex.

Epidemiology. Most patients have some degree of occupational exposure to *M. tuberculosis* (physician, hospital worker, especially pathologists and dieners in autopsy suite) or *M. bovis* (farmer, veterinarian, slaughterhouse worker, butcher). The organism enters the skin through a tiny injury.

Etiology and Pathogenesis. Both bacteria elicit a local granulomatous response. Organisms are hard to find and patients are not likely to be contagious. The response to *M. bovis* tends to be more effective, so the infection is firmly localized, while with *M. tuberculosis* the lesions tend to be larger, ulcerated and the patient more likely to have associated lymphangitis.

Clinical Findings. The most common location for tuberculosis cutis verrucosa is the back of the hands, especially the fingers (Figs. 4.42, 4.43). Those in direct contact with animals may experience inoculation at other sites, such as the feet (through infectious particles falling into boots), beltline or chest (when grasping the animal). Multiple lesions can develop. The initial change is a small, firm, painless dusty red papule that slowly spreads over weeks and months and is surrounded by erythema. The overlying epidermis is often hyperkeratotic, resembling an inflamed wart. As the lesion spreads,

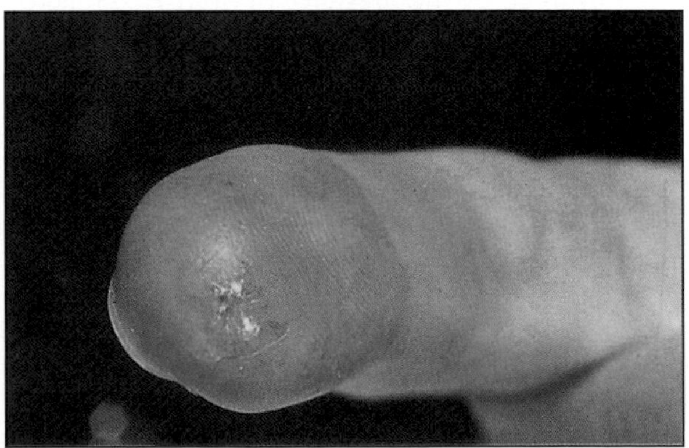

Fig. 4.42. Tuberculosis cutis verrucosa (prosector's wart)

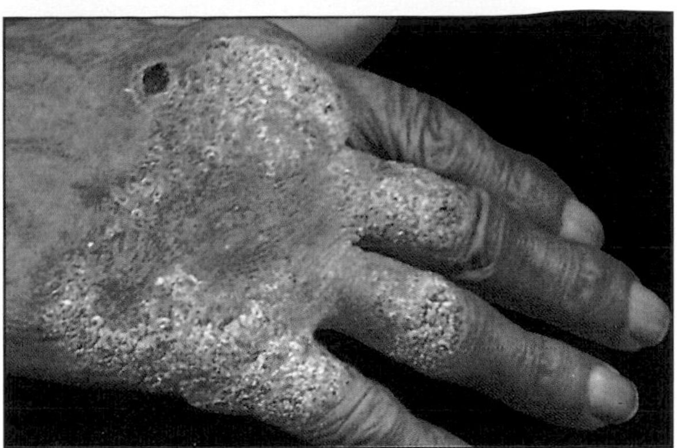

Fig. 4.43. Tuberculosis cutis verrucosa

there can be central healing with an atrophic scar, yielding annular and verruciform serpiginous lesions with an inflammatory base. When *M. tuberculosis* is responsible, the papules may become pustular, succulent and ulcerated. Then lymphangitis is not uncommon and lymphadenopathy may appear. Diascopy is negative.

Histopathology. The epidermis shows pseudoepitheliomatous hyperplasia. In the dermis numerous granulomas are present, but necrosis is uncommon. Ziehl-Neelsen staining is usually negative, although PCR can identify the mycobacterial DNA. Culture is positive.

Course and Prognosis. The outlook is good because of the patient's immune status and localized nature of the infection. If untreated, the changes are chronic with no spontaneous healing.

Differential Diagnosis. A swimming pool granuloma (*M. marinum*) is identical and can only be separated out by culture. Other infections introduced by inoculation such a sporotrichosis, nocardiosis, chromomycosis and deep fungi can also be similar. Ordinary warts may show central clearing and peripheral spread after cryotherapy but they are usually much less inflamed and more warty. Lupus vulgaris can have a verrucous form, but lupus nodules are always identifiable with diascopy, and after central clearing recurrences are not uncommon. Tertiary syphilis, halogenoderma, blastomycotic pyoderma, keratoacanthoma, squamous cell carcinoma and other tumors must be considered.

Therapy. This is one form of cutaneous tuberculosis in which monotherapy with isoniazid for 6 months is often successful, although some health groups recommend multidrug regimens. Local excision can speed the process. Radiation therapy 5 Gy weekly for 3 weeks is a useful adjunctive measure.

Public Health Measures. Most cases are work-related and should be so reported, in order to assure the patient of the benefits to which he is entitled.

Lupus Vulgaris

(WILLAN and BATEMAN)

Synonym. Tuberculosis cutis luposa

Definition. Most common post-primary highly destructive form of cutaneous tuberculosis in a patient with intact immunity. The Latin name lupus (= wolf)suggests that the disease is destructive.

Epidemiology. In the past lupus vulgaris had a prevalence of 4–6/100,000 in Germany. Today it has become quite uncommon, although it is still seen frequently in India and Asia. About 50,000 new cases appear yearly worldwide. Women are twice as likely to be affected as men. The social consequences are large because of the devastating cosmetic effects, just as with leprosy.

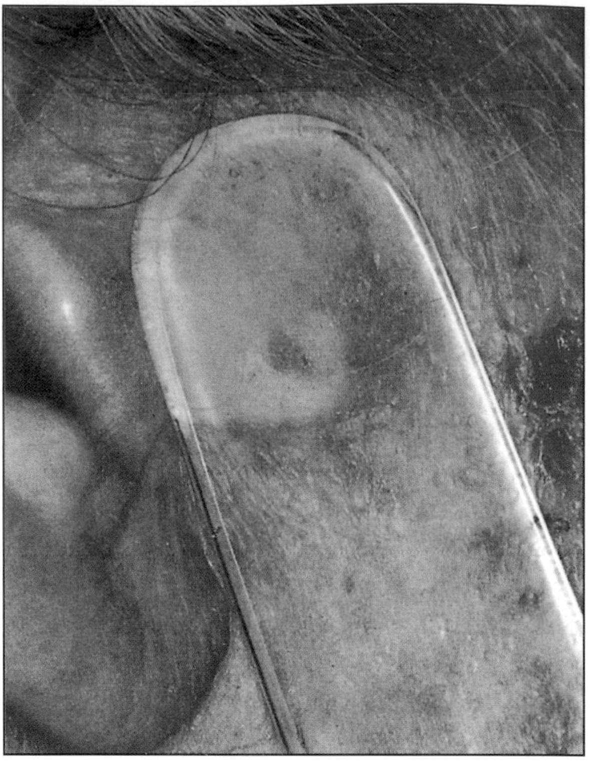

Fig. 4.44. Lupus vulgaris. Lupus nodule seen with diascopy

Etiology and Pathogenesis. Lupus vulgaris is a cutaneous form of postprimary or reactivation tuberculosis, usually associated with pulmonary disease. The patients all have a positive PPD test and about 50% have active involvement of another organ. *M. tuberculosis* can reach the skin endogenously or following inoculation. When tuberculosis cutis colliquativa breaks through the skin from the subcutaneous tissues, lupus vulgaris can develop. Gottron described this shift with the German term *Etagenwechsel*, changing stories or levels, as going from the basement to the attic. The terrain also plays an important role in lupus vulgaris. Acral areas are favored; reduced blood flow and cooling are probably the main determinants. The granulomas destroy the skin, subcutaneous tissue and even cartilage.

Clinical Findings. The acral areas, such as the nose, cheeks, rim of the ear, extensor surfaces of limbs, and the lateral surfaces of the buttocks and breasts, are favored. Usually the lesion is solitary and very slow-growing. It has been estimated that the diagnosis of lupus vulgaris is made about 5 years after the lesion first appears. Occasionally several lesions are seen and, in the rare setting of hematogenous spread of *M. tuberculosis* during an infection such as measles, multiple lesions can be found (lupus vulgaris postexanthematicus).

The primary lesion is the lupus nodule, a tiny 3–4-mm red-brown lesion. With diascopy, the findings become more characteristic (Fig. 4.44). A pin-head sized, apple jelly-colored or red-brown nodule is seen in the dermis, floating “like a piece of sago in tapioca pudding”. The nodules are surrounded by an thin, indistinct glassy rim. The color is determined by the presence of lipid-rich macrophages. Other granulomatous infiltrates can also have lupoid nodules; included in the group are sarcoidosis, rosacea, perioral dermatitis, lupus erythematosus and pseudolymphomas. In addition, Spitz nevi, because of their red-brown color and vascularity, can also occasionally show nodules on diascopy.

The second important clinical diagnostic technique is the use of a thin, blunt or rounded probe. When gentle pressure is applied to the center of the lesion, the probe penetrates the skin, and when it is withdrawn, often a drop of blood appears. The central epidermis is atrophic because of damage by the necrotizing dermal infiltrates. The other disorders with lupoid nodules have an intact epidermis and are not easily penetrated by a probe.

The progression of lupus vulgaris has been extensively subdivided, reflecting slightly varying clinical patterns as the red-brown papules slowly expand. The different names in themselves are not crucial, but together they reinforce the great variability of clinical presentation.

Lupus Spot. The initial lesion is of course small, easily overlooked and often confused with a hemangioma or Spitz nevus. Tiny lupus nodules can be identified by diascopy.

Lupus Vulgaris Planus. The lupus spot slowly grows. If it remains relatively flat and evolves into a patch, one speaks of lupus vulgaris planus. In this stage, there may rarely be spontaneous regression with an atrophic scar.

Lupus Vulgaris Exfoliativus. This form is characterized by extensive scale, as seen in psoriasis or Bowen disease (Fig. 4.45).

Lupus Vulgaris Verrucosus. Sometimes pseudoepitheliomatous hyperplasia dominates, so that warty lesions appear. They evolve much more slowly than warty tuberculosis, have a more red-brown color and show lupus nodules.

Lupus Vulgaris Tumidus (Hypertrophicus). If the infiltrate increases dramatically without marked regression, then larger nodules or plaques develop.

Lupus Vulgaris Ulcerosus. Usually necrosis of older parts of the lesion occurs, as the skin and associated structures are damaged by the granulomatous infiltrate. The result is the mutilation so intimately associated with lupus vulgaris.

Lupus Vulgaris Vegetans (Papillomatosus). Sometimes multiple papillomas develop at the edge of an erosion or ulcer, not dissimilar from the changes associated with a vegetative pyoderma or at the periphery of a venous leg ulcer.

Lupus Vulgaris Mutilans. The ears (Fig. 4.46) and nose (Fig. 4.47) can be destroyed. In contrast to tertiary syphilis, the bones of the nose are never attacked. Ectropion and distortion of the mouth are also possible. If the hands are involved, arthritic problems can develop. Neck involvement may restriction the range of motion.

Mucosal Lupus Vulgaris. The most common site of involvement is the nasal mucosa. Often the vestibule is affected; at other times the alae or the cartilaginous part of the septum. Thus the distal part of the nose can be extensively damaged. Oral lesions can occur. When the lacrimal gland is involved, the skin around the opening of the lacrimal duct can become infected. Usually the lupus nodules are more transparent, like frog eggs, but otherwise the process is similar.

Histopathology. The hallmark is caseating tuberculous granulomas. *M. tuberculosis* is present in very low numbers and never seen microscopically. The epidermis is usually atrophic although hyperkeratosis and occasionally pseudoepitheliomatous hyperplasia can occur. The microscopic tubercles are far smaller than the clinically visible lupus nodule, which consists of a conglomeration of tu-

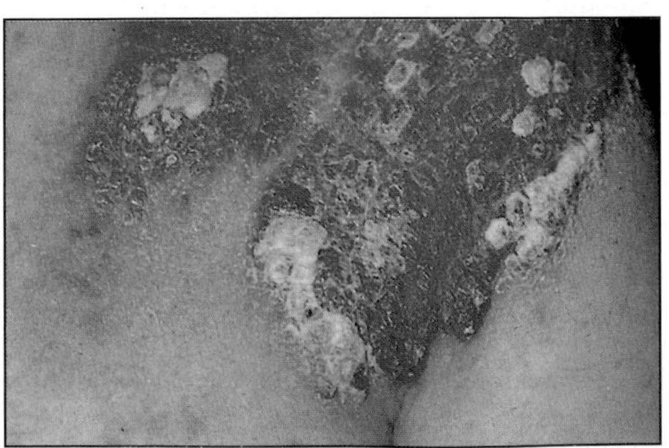

Fig. 4.45. Lupus vulgaris exfoliativus with psoriasiform lesion

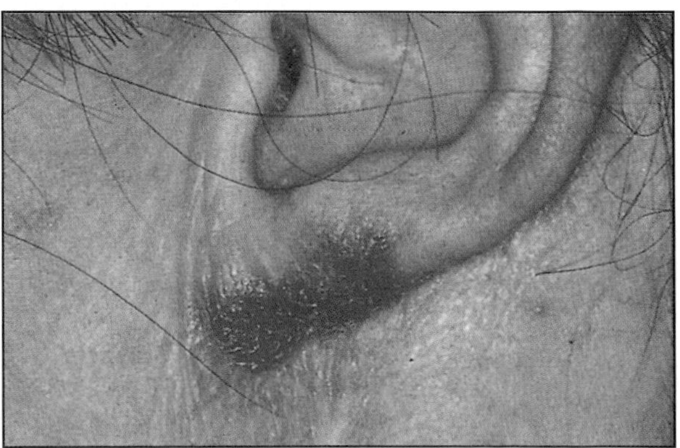

Fig. 4.46. Lupus vulgaris mutilans with destruction of ear lobe

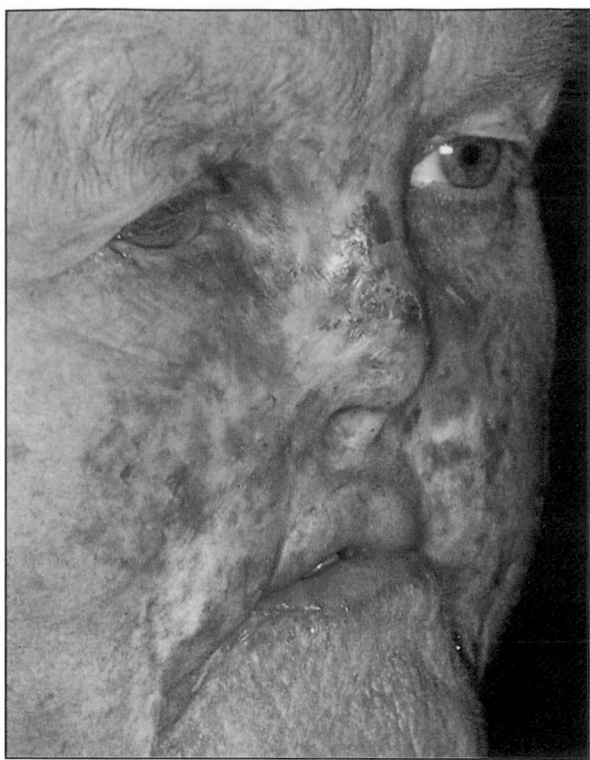

Fig. 4.47. Lupus vulgaris mutilans with nasal destruction

bercles. The histologic differential diagnosis includes rosacea, perioral dermatitis, sarcoidosis, tuberculoid leprosy and tertiary syphilis.

Laboratory Findings. The organisms can be identified via culture, animal inoculation or PCR.

Course and Prognosis. Lupus vulgaris is not contagious but very chronic, lasting months, years or even decades if untreated. Antituberculosis therapy leads to arrest of spread and then healing in a matter of months. While pulmonary changes are often present, active disease in the lungs or elsewhere is uncommon. Despite the often disabling clinical course when not treated, lupus vulgaris is a local phenomenon, with no severe systemic problems.

Over decades recurrences tend to develop in the scars; this is not seen with tertiary syphilis. Circular constricting scars on the limbs can produce distal elephantiasis. The main complication however is the develop of a squamous cell carcinoma, known as lupus carcinoma in German (Fig. 4.48). Thin hard scars are a greater risk than softer ones. The first change is the development of tiny hyperkeratotic papules, similar to actinic keratoses or radia-

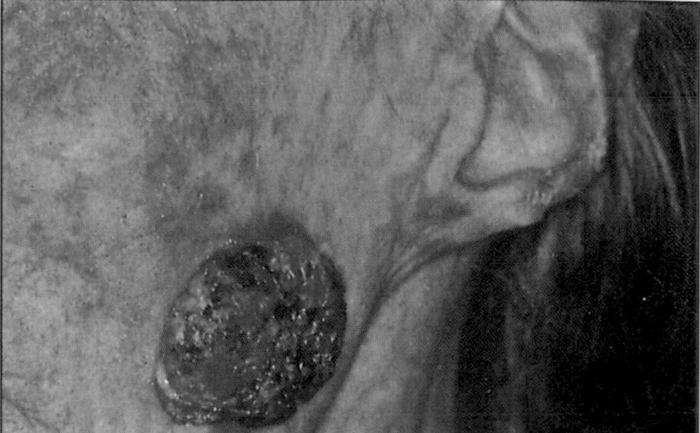

Fig. 4.48. Lupus vulgaris with squamous cell carcinoma

tion keratoses. Such lesions should be excised. When an invasive squamous cell carcinoma develops, it has the potential for metastasis and is considerably more dangerous than the same lesion evolving in an actinic keratosis. In the past, lupus vulgaris was treated with X-rays, which undoubtedly was a factor in the carcinogenesis.

Differential Diagnosis. The differential diagnosis is enormous and has been touched upon in both the clinical and histologic descriptions. In the past, the distinction between tuberoserpiginous syphilis and lupus vulgaris was difficult, but both have become rare. The syphilitic lesions develop far more rapidly, over weeks to a few months, never recur in the atrophic scar and respond promptly to supersaturated potassium iodide solution; today one relies primarily on the syphilis serology. In the case of sarcoidosis, the pulmonary picture is usually different, the hand changes have a distinctive radiological appearance and the granulomas usually are not necrotic.

Therapy

Systemic. Most patients today are treated with multidrug regimens. In this era of resistant organisms, it seems unwise to risk using a single agent. However, lupus vulgaris usually responds very well to isoniazid. The choice of agents should be based on regional resistance patterns and recommendations.

If isoniazid is used alone, the dosage is 5.0–6.0 mg/kg daily taken in a single dose before breakfast. Usually pyridoxine and vitamin B12 are administered simultaneously to avoid hematologic and neurologic problems. The main side effects are gastrointestinal complaints, hepatic toxicity, acral paresthesias and optic neuritis. The treatment must last many months; we usually treat for 6 months after complete resolution of the lesions. The cure rate is about 95%; if a cure is not achieved, then multidrug therapy must be used.

Other Measures. Small lesions can be excised, although antibacterial therapy should still be employed for 6 months. Sometimes phototherapy is used as an adjunct; it may help by increasing blood flow. Once the disease has been treated, plastic surgery procedures and the construction of facial prostheses are often needed.

Tuberculosis Cutis Colliquativa

Synonyms. Scrofuloderma, tuberculoid gumma

Definition. Chronic subcutaneous tuberculosis with sinus tracts draining to the skin.

Epidemiology. Scrofuloderma was formerly most common among children as a sequelae of *M. bovis* infection of the tonsils and cervical lymph nodes. It also occasionally appeared in the elderly as a sign of decreased immune response. Today it is rare.

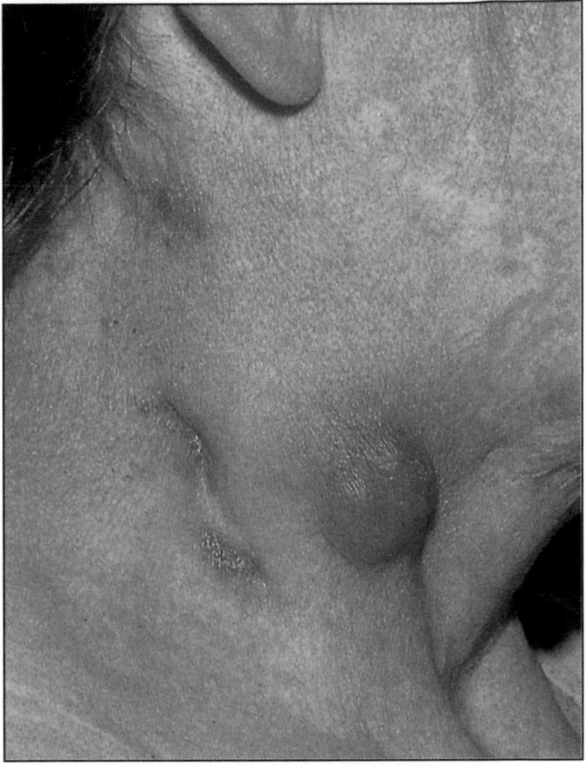

Fig. 4.49. Tuberculosis cutis colliquativa (scrofuloderma)

Etiology and Pathogenesis. Several different mechanisms are possible. The usual course is spread from involved lymph nodes, bones or other deeper structures. The bacteria may be introduced into the subcutaneous tissue by a contaminated needle, such as when doing a lumbar puncture for tuberculous meningitis. In the elderly, with decreased immunity, there may be hematogenous spread with seeding of subcutaneous fat.

Clinical Findings. The most common locations are over the lymph nodes of the neck, i.e., the submandibular, supraclavicular and lateral cervical areas (Fig. 4.49). When the spread is hematogenous, then multiple lesions, often on the trunk, are seen. Other sites may include the neck, groin and even tongue. If trauma is the cause, the site is obviously so localized.

The process is always the same. There are fluctuant, matted inflamed nodes which develop liquefaction necrosis and discharge through the overlying skin. Multiple sinus tracts form, associated with the appearance of new nodules and healing with scarring. A cheesy or pus-laden discharge is rich in organisms. The underlying structures become firmly adherent to the overlying skin, creating one large, thick draining mass. The end result is a complex scar with funnel-like channels, pieces of skin bridging two or more tracts, and an irregular surface. As discussed above, the adjacent dermis may become infected, so that the red-brown nodules of lupus vulgaris also appear.

Histopathology. The microscopic picture is usually one of massive necrosis. At the edge of the lesion, tuberculoid granulomas may be found. The organisms can usually be identified in the discharge and occasionally in the tissue sections.

Laboratory Findings. Cultures and animal inoculation are positive.

Course and Prognosis. In the past, scrofuloderma was a difficult problem because of the continued drainage and scarring. Today it is rare but easily treated.

Differential Diagnosis. Sporotrichosis, other deep fungi, lymphogranuloma venereum, actinomycosis and mixed bacterial infections, as well as acne inversa, can all appear similar. A syphilitic gumma is usually solitary and has less fistula formation. The cultures and serologic tests are diagnostic.

Therapy. Multidrug antibacterial therapy is required, usually for 9 months or longer. Surgical debridement will speed healing. In older individuals, the likelihood of involvement of other organs is high and should be sought.

Tuberculids
(Darier 1896)

Definition. Disseminated symmetric exanthems in patients with tuberculosis and hyperergic status.

Epidemiology. Tuberculids were always uncommon, and now that cutaneous tuberculosis is so rare, they have become even less common. In addition, many diseases which were formerly blamed on *M. tuberculosis*, such as rosacea-like tuberculid and lupus miliaris disseminatus faciei are now known to be unrelated.

Etiology and Pathogenesis. Id reactions are delayed allergic reactions to microbial antigens. They are described for bacteria (bacterid), fungi (mycid, fungal id) and viruses (virusid, viral id). In most cases, the organism cannot be proven to be present in the lesion. In some instances, microbial antigen-antibody complexes may be spread hematogenously, eliciting a distant vascular reaction. In other cases, the organisms or antigenic fragments of them are disseminated in small numbers and elicit an intense host allergic response. These two concepts obviously overlap. PCR and similar techniques have identified microbial DNA in lesions which were formerly held to be allergic and free of organisms.

Clinically tuberculids are symmetric and not associated with systemic signs or symptoms. The lesions are not contagious, because infectious intact bacteria are not present. The culture is always negative. PPD is always strongly positive. Mycobacteria are almost never identified by routine microscopy, culture or animal inoculation, but can be found on occasion with PCR. Tuberculids can also appear following BCG immunization, use of PPD skin testing and as part of a Jarisch-Herxheimer-like reaction at the start of antibacterial therapy. Microscopically all show tuberculoid granulomas, often centered around the dermal vessels. This suggests that mycobacterial antigens or immune complexes perhaps diffuse into the dermis from the vessels and elicit an inflammatory response.

Lichen Scrofulosorum
(Hebra 1860)

Synonym. Tuberculosis cutis lichenoides

Definition. Lichenoid cutaneous reaction in patient with active tuberculosis.

Etiology and Pathogenesis. Lichen scrofulosorum is seen most often in children with a primary complex. It can be seen in more disseminated disease, or following BCG or PPD usage.

Clinical Findings. The sites of predilection are the sides of the trunk. The primary lesion is a tiny peaked papule, usually with a keratotic cap, which may be follicular or perifollicular (Fig. 4.50). The color ranges between flesh tones and yellow-red-brown. The papules tend to arrange themselves in symmetric groups, often several centimeters in diameter, oval and organized along the skin lines. Such lesions are quite similar to those seen with the ointment version of the PPD test (Moro test). The eruption is asymptomatic and usually resolves spontaneously.

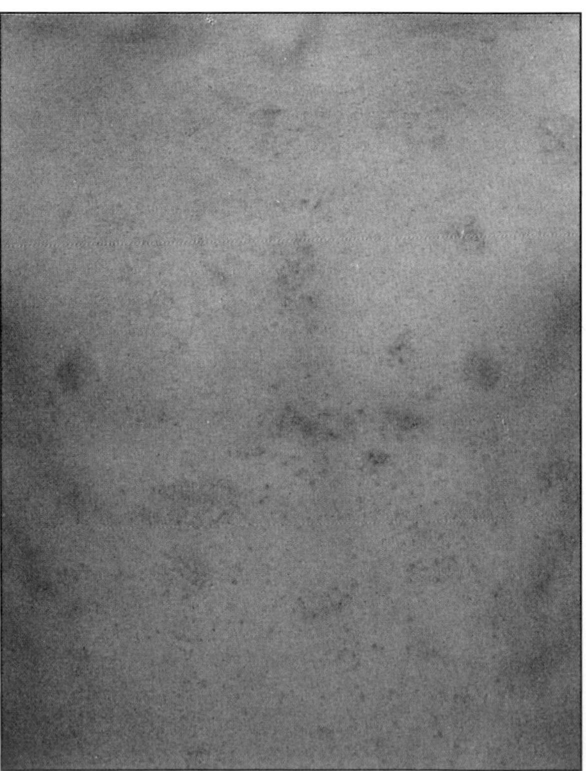

Fig. 4.50. Lichen scrofulosorum

Histopathology. Tiny tuberculoid structures are found in a perifollicular location. Tiny areas of necrosis can be seen. Occasionally there is a diffuse inflammatory infiltrate without tuberculoid structures. The eccrine ducts can also be involved by the process. No bacteria are seen in the Ziehl-Neelsen stain.

Laboratory Findings. Attempts to isolate organisms with culture or animal inoculation almost always fail. PCR is occasionally positive.

Differential Diagnosis. The presence of small, pointed hyperkeratotic papules is known as spinulosismus. Similar lesions can be seen as a syphilid (lichen syphiliticus in tertiary syphilis) or a fungal id (lichen trichophyticus with a inflammatory dermatophyte infection or following trichophytin injection). Similar lesions, but usually not grouped, can be seen with follicular lichen planus, lichenoid sarcoidosis or scurvy (lichen scorbuticus, usually with hemorrhage).

Therapy. If the lichen scrofulosorum is the result of BCG or PPD, no treatment is needed. Otherwise, a typical multidrug regimen should be implemented to treat the underlying tuberculosis.

Papulonecrotic Tuberculid

Synonym. Tuberculosis cutis papulonecrotica

Definition. Chronic, relapsing, hemorrhagic necrotic eruption with prominent vascular involvement in hyperergic patients.

Epidemiology. This eruption is extremely uncommon today; it was most often seen among girls and young women.

Etiology and Pathogenesis. Just as a PPD test can cause an intense local reaction and ulceration in hyperergic individuals, on rare occasion a hematogenous immunologic reaction directed against some tuberculous antigen can occur about the dermal vessels. Such rashes are bilateral and symmetric and patients always have a very strongly positive PPD test.

Clinical Findings. The typical locations are the extensor surfaces of the limbs, the lower aspects of the trunk and the buttocks. The eruption is more common in winter, improving in the summer. It is nonpruritic and painless. The lesions are scattered but generally symmetric and occasionally grouped. The primary lesion is a tiny red-brown papule that develops central necrosis with a pustule and later a crust. The lesions heal with hypo- or depigmented varioliform scars. Sometimes larger ulcers develop (ulcerated tuberculid).Typically scars are present along with fresh lesions. The lesions are usually asymptomatic. Occasionally there is an associated erythema induratum, and even less often there may be a transition to lupus vulgaris. In most cases there is a history of previous tuberculosis or radiologic evidence of lung or retroperitoneal involvement; active tuberculosis can be seen but is uncommon.

Histopathology. Papulonecrotic tuberculid is one of the lymphocytic vasculitides. It closely resembles pityriasis lichenoides et varioliformis acuta under the microscope. There is an intense lymphocytic perivascular infiltrate with occasional vessel destruction with fibrin deposition. In the adjacent dermis there may be necrosis and granulomatous inflammation, but classic tubercles are not found. The mycobacteria cannot be identified with Ziehl-Neelsen staining or culture, but sometimes their DNA is shown with PCR.

Course and Prognosis. The course is typically chronic over years with crops of new lesions and progressive scarring.

Differential Diagnosis. The main differential diagnostic point is pityriasis lichenoides et varioliformis acuta, but it has an acute course. Granulomatous changes are also uncommon in this disorder. Sometimes leukocytoclastic angiitis may be papulonecrotic, but neutrophils should predominate and no granulomatous changes are seen. When facial lesions are present, they closely resemble acne necrotica. The excoriations of prurigo simplex subacuta may appear similar but papulonecrotic tuberculid is not pruritic.

Therapy. A multidrug regimen should be employed. Under this antimycobacterial coverage, systemic corticosteroids may lead to more rapid healing.

Erythema Induratum

(Bazin 1861)

Synonyms. Tuberculosis cutis indurativa, nodose tuberculid

Definition. Panniculitis and vasculitis of the subcutaneous tissues of the legs in patients with hyperergic response. This disorder is both a panniculitis and a tuberculid; thus it is also considered in Chapter 21.

Epidemiology. Most cases occur in middle-aged women with evidence of impaired circulation in their legs, such as pernio, cutis marmorata or acrocyanosis.

Etiology and Pathogenesis. The mechanisms are the same as with the other tuberculids. Exposure to cold may also play a localizing role. As tuberculosis has become less common, more patients have been identified with nodular vasculitis, i.e., the same changes without tuberculosis. In our clinic we have used PCR to identify *M. tuberculosis* DNA in the tissue from a number of such patients, reconfirming our belief that this pattern is often related to tuberculosis, e.g., retroperitoneal tuberculosis or primary complex tuberculosis in the gastrointestinal tract. Ziehl-Neelsen stain, culture and animal inoculations are negative.

Clinical Findings. The lesions are usually multiple, symmetric and involve the calves. Firm subcutaneous nodules 1–2 cm in diameter arise with overlying erythema (Fig. 4.51). The lesions have sharp borders and evolve into thick plaques. They tend to resolve spontaneously, especially in the summer months, but can become quite thick, ulcerate, drain and heal with sunken scars. The ulcers are surprisingly painless. Other signs of a cold-sensitive peripheral vasculature such as acrocyanosis, cutis marmorata, hyperhidrosis, erythrocyanosis crurum puellarum and pernio follicularis are often present.

Histopathology. The key features are granulomatous inflammation about the vessels of the deep plexus, associated with a lobular panniculitis.

Course and Prognosis. The course is chronic over years. Worsening typically occurs in the winter. The persistent ulcerations and scarring are bothersome. The overall outlook is determined by the nature of the underlying tuberculosis.

Differential Diagnosis. The main differential is nodular vasculitis; thus PCR should be performed to identify the *M. tuberculosis*. The difference between nodular vasculitis and erythema induratum is almost philosophic. As the possibilities of identifying various microbial antigens increases, the existence of a truly idiopathic id-like panniculitis becomes less likely. Erythema nodosum is less nodular (despite the name), more painful, acute and bruise-like. It is found on the shins and never ulcerates. Polyarteritis nodosa can present with similar nodules, but the patient may be quite ill and the histology does not shown granulomas. Syphilitic gumma are also similar, but more likely to be asymmetric and disappear with supersaturated potassium iodide. Nodular pernio is even more seasonally related and does not ulcerate. The other forms of panniculitis discussed in Chapter 21 should be considered but erythema induratum has a distinctive picture.

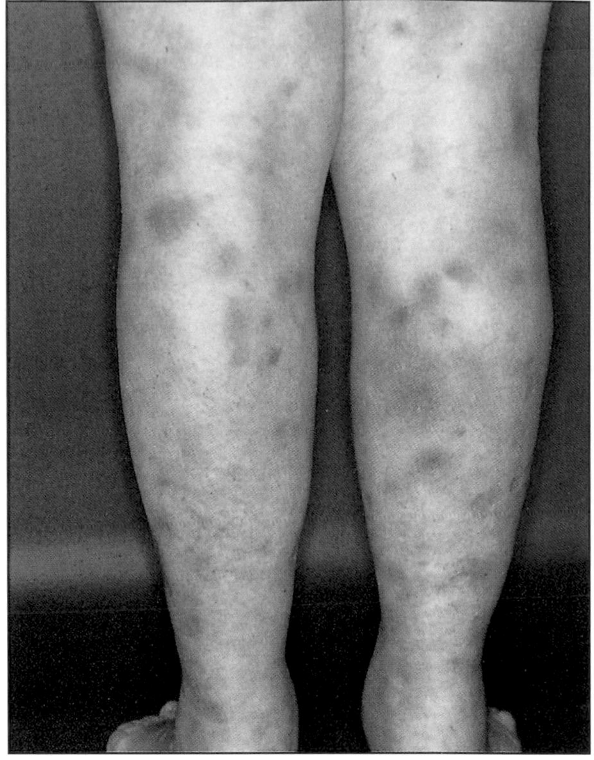

Fig. 4.51. Erythema induratum

Therapy. We have had good success using multidrug regimens to treat the tuberculosis. One must treat for 9–12 months. If no mycobacteria are identified, the risks of antituberculous therapy probably outweigh the benefits. One should also try to keep the legs warm, using compres-sion dressings, warm shoes, socks and pants (rather than skirts) and to keep rooms warmer than average in the winter. Warm baths may also help; in Germany nicotinic acid is added to baths and to creams to try to increase peripheral vasodilatation.

Pseudotuberculids

There are a number of diseases that were previously thought to be tuberculids, but today are not felt to be related to infection with *M. tuberculosis*. Their names frequently contain "lupus" or "tuberculosis," causing much confusion. The PPD test is usually negative; there is no evidence for present or past tuberculosis and neither *M. tuberculosis* nor its DNA is identified in the lesions.

Lupus Miliaris Disseminatus Faciei
(Fox 1878)

Definition. Symmetric, papulosquamous facial eruption with tuberculoid histology but no connection to tuberculosis. It may be part of the spectrum of rosacea or perioral dermatitis.

Etiology and Pathogenesis. This extremely rare disease is most common in young women although occasionally seen in men. Its cause is unknown.

Clinical Findings. As the name suggests, most lesions are facial. Occasionally the lateral aspects of the neck and even the trunk are affected. Small, soft, succulent blue-red or red-brown domed-shaped papules appear scattered about on otherwise normal skin (Fig. 4.52). They often develop a bit of scale and may shift towards being flat-topped. Tiny pustules also appear. The lesions are asymptomatic. There are no signs of rosacea such as erythema or telangiectases. Diascopy usually reveals some lupoid nodules but they are quite small and not aggregated. The probe test is negative. Cases have been described in association with erythema nodosum, occasionally triggered by *Yersinia.*

Histopathology. There are small tuberculoid granulomas with central necrosis and rims of epithelioid cells, giant cells and lymphocytes. The capillaries in the upper dermis are dilated.

Course and Prognosis. The course is usually chronic, lasting many months to a few years. The lesions do not ulcerate but sometimes heal with slightly atrophic flat scars.

Differential Diagnosis. The main differential diagnostic points are lupoid perioral dermatitis and small nodular sarcoidosis. Both may have a red-brown or lupoid appearance clinically and show granulomatous inflammation, although it is rarely as distinct as in lupus miliaris disseminatus faciei. Occasionally rosacea-like changes induced by topical corticosteroids acne may be quite similar. Sarcoidosis and lupoid syphilids are not usually confined to the face. Perioral dermatitis merges imperceptibly with lupus miliaris disseminatus faciei; they may be the same disorder in two different patient populations, as perioral dermatitis is almost never seen in men (Chap. 28).

Therapy
Systemic. Most patients do well with doxycycline or minocycline in routine acne dosages for several months. Isotretinoin is also effective. If the lesions are quite inflamed, a short course of mid-range systemic corticosteroids may produce improvement, but there is often a rebound flare. Finally, some clinicians endorse isoniazid as a monotherapy if all else fails.

Topical. Topical erythromycin or metronidazole creams, gels, or lotions are most useful and a sensible starting point. In severe cases, PUVA may also be helpful.

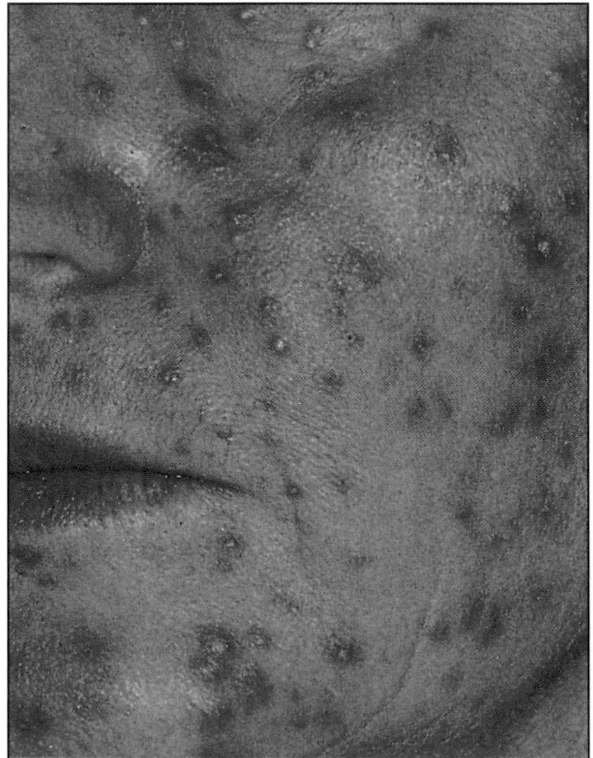

Fig. 4.52. Lupus miliaris disseminatus faciei

Rosacea-Like Tuberculid
(LEWANDOWSKY 1913)

No one is sure what LEWANDOWSKY was describing. Today one speaks of lupoid rosacea or lupoid perioral dermatitis.

Acneiform Tuberculid

Synonyms. Acnitis, folliclis, Barthélemy disease

These patients are similar to those with lupus miliaris disseminatus faciei but develop deeper small nodules. Today such cases are viewed as part of the spectrum of rosacea and perioral dermatitis.

Atypical Mycobacteria

There is nothing atypical about the other mycobacteria. They have the same characteristics in the laboratory as *M. tuberculosis*, but produce a different spectrum of diseases. The alternate term MOTT (mycobacteria other than tuberculosis) is not much better. The atypical mycobacteria tend to cause opportunistic infections and many members of the group are saprophytes. Infections are often associated with immunosuppression, minor injuries or associated organ damage.

Classification

One thing which is atypical about the group is the classification, which has perplexed physicians for many years. The Runyon groups refer to the growth properties. Table 4.12 lists just some of the members of this group. Most grow best at 37 °C but *M. ulcerans* and *M. marinum* grow at 32 °C. The photochromogens develop pigment in the presence of light, the scotochromogens do so in the absence of light and the nonchromogens never have pigmented colonies. The rapid growers develop colonies within 4 days while the others take many weeks. The final speciation of an atypical mycobacteria requires extensive laboratory efforts, considering growth rate and temperature and the presence of a battery of enzymes, as well as growth in NaCl and iron salts. A series of skin test antigens are also available; when used in patients with pulmonary disease, they help to speed the diagnosis, but are not helpful in diagnosing localized cutaneous disease.

Clinical Overview

Atypical mycobacteria are frequently found in water supplies or soil and transferred via droplets, dust or skin injuries. They most often cause pulmonary infection, similar to tuberculosis, or cervical lymphadenitis, especially in children. Table 4.13

Table 4.12. Atypical mycobacteria

Group	Name	Organism	Associated diseases
I	Photochromogens	*M. marinum*	Swimming pool granuloma
		M. kansasii	Pulmonary disease, lymphadenitis, sporotrichoid skin lesions
		M. simiae	Pulmonary disease in monkey handlers
II	Scotochromogens	*M. scrofulaceum*	Lymphadenitis
		M. szulgai	Pulmonary disease, lymphadenitis, skin lesions
		M. xenopi	Pulmonary disease; shares antigens with MAI
III	Nonchromogens	*M. avium-intracellulare*	Widespread disease in HIV/AIDS; pulmonary disease, lymphadenitis, rarely skin lesions
		M. ulcerans	Buruli ulcer
		M. haemophilum	Skin and soft tissue abscesses in immunosuppressed hosts
IV	Rapid growers	*M. chelonae*	Varied
		M. fortuitum	Varied
		M. smegmatis	Saprophyte

MAI *Mycobacterium avium-intracellulare*

Table 4.13. Cutaneous manifestations of atypical mycobacterial infections

Clinical pattern	Common causes	Less common
Swimming pool granuloma	*M. marinum*	–
Sporotrichoid nodules	*M. marinum*	*M. kansasii, M. chelonae, M. fortuitum*
Localized nodules, ulcers, sinus tracts	*M. chelonae, M. fortuitum*	*M. haemophilum*
Disseminated papules, nodules	*M. avian-intracellulare*	*M. kansasii*
Buruli ulcer	*M. ulcerans*	–
Erythema nodosum	*M. kansasii, M. avian-intracellulare*	–
Wound infections		Many (all rare)

Based on Table 3, page 1916 in Mandell et al. (1990).

lists some of the common skin findings which can be seen. The therapy is confusing and frequently changing. Multiple drug regimens are usually required and resistance is common. Most protocols include both antituberculosis drugs and other antibiotics. As discussed in Chapter 2, the usual regimens for *M. avian-intracellulare* include four to five antibiotics. We will now discuss the various skin diseases associated with atypical mycobacteria but leave the rest of the subject to infectious disease texts.

Swimming Pool Granuloma

Definition. Granulomatous infection following injury to skin with exposure to contaminated water.

Causative Organism. *Mycobacterium marinum.*

Epidemiology. Swimming pool granulomas develop following an injury such as an abrasion in water where *M. marinum* is present as a normal saprophyte. Lake Ponchartrain in New Orleans, Louisiana, is famous for the number of infections acquired by swimmers and waders. Small epidemics have been described from community swimming pools. It can also be isolated from fish. The other scenario is a minor injury to someone working with a heated aquarium.

Etiology and Pathogenesis. The organism is ubiquitous and grows best at 32 °C. It almost never causes systemic disease, just a cutaneous granulomatous response.

Clinical Findings. There is always some type of injury; *M. marinum* does not penetrate normal skin. After 2–4 weeks a single blue-red nodule begins to grow and often has a warty surface (Fig. 4.53). The lesion may reach a size of 1–2 cm and become ulcerated. The sites of predilection are the hands, feet, knees and elbows; in the case of aquarium injuries, only the hands are involved. In rare cases,

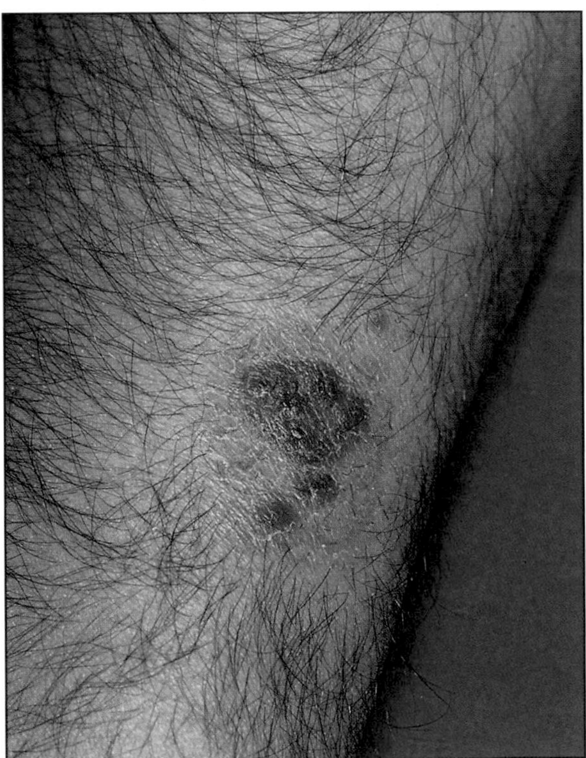

Fig. 4.53. Swimming pool granuloma

there may be ascending lymphatic spread with additional nodules in a sporotrichoid pattern or even lymphadenopathy.

Histopathology. The epidermis is usually hyperkeratotic and acanthotic. Tuberculoid granulomas are found in the dermis, often with central fibrinoid necrosis. The Ziehl-Neelsen stain is occasionally positive.

Laboratory Findings. The diagnosis must be confirmed by culture. The best plan is to do a skin biopsy and submit a piece of dermis to the laboratory with sufficient clinical information so that the appropriate tests for atypical mycobacteria are performed. Smears and scrapings are rarely helpful.

Differential Diagnosis. The diagnosis is usually clear. If the patient is in a risk group for inoculation tuberculosis, this must be considered and excluded by culture. All of the sporotrichoid lesions (Chap. 7) must be considered, but history and culture results are the answer.

Therapy. Small lesions should be excised or otherwise destroyed. Both cryotherapy and localized application of heat, such as with a Jon-E hand warmer, have also been recommended. For limited disease, single drug therapy with clarithromycin, trimethoprim-sulfamethoxazole, ciprofloxacin or doxycycline for 6 weeks is usually sufficient. If there is lymphatic disease, an antituberculosis regimen should be considered, based on in vitro sensitivity testing.

Buruli Ulcer

Synonyms. Bairnsdale or Searls ulcer (Australia), Kakerifu ulcer (Zaire), Kumusi ulcer (New Guinea)

Causative Organism. *Mycobacterium ulcerans*

Epidemiology. Buruli is a district in Uganda. Buruli ulcers have been described from wide areas of Africa, Australia, New Guinea, Southeast Asia and, rarely, from Mexico. The organisms has never been identified in the wild except in koalas but are be more common in moist or swampy areas. It is the most frequent cause of atypical mycobacterial skin disease worldwide

Etiology and Pathogenesis. The bacteria grows best at 32 °C and is thus confined to the skin, not tolerating higher internal temperatures. It produces a virulence factor, a polyketide known as mycolactone, which causes the skin damage. While this is the first polyketide to be isolated from mycobacteria, all mycobacterial genomes encode many similar products which may play a role in the pathogenesis of tuberculosis and leprosy. Most patients are children, so that perhaps some immunity to the toxin develops. BCG immunization also appears to provide protection.

Clinical Findings. Typically this is a minor injury, followed after several months by the appearance of a small papule or nodule which rapidly ulcerates. The most common sites are the legs, followed by the arms. There is the progressive striking destruction of the skin and subcutaneous tissue. Muscles, nerves and bones are exposed and occasionally damaged. The ulcer is surprisingly painless, but usually very rapid-growing, and ann entire limb may be involved. At some point, there is spontaneous resolution with severe scarring.

Histopathology. There is tremendous necrosis with little inflammation, as fits toxin-mediated damage. The organisms can be found at the edge of the ulcer.

Differential Diagnosis. The early lesions are nonspecific and all causes of infectious ulcers must be considered. As the changes become more dramatic, only pyoderma gangrenosum comes into question, but the clinical setting is quite different.

Therapy. Systemic antibacterial therapy has been disappointing. Excision is recommended whenever possible; grafting is usually required. Local heat therapy and hyperbaric oxygen have also been tried.

Mycobacterium avian-intracellulare Infections

Mycobacterium avian-intracellulare (MAI) has become commonplace and feared with the advent of HIV/AIDS (Chap. 2). Other immunosuppressed patients are also at risk. Formerly two mycobacteria were identified, *M. avian* and *M. intracellulare*, but they are so closely related that they are today grouped together. Most HIV/AIDS patients have MAI and require either prophylaxis or treatment. Any organ can be involved; the most common problems are chronic pulmonary disease, osteomyelitis and lymphadenopathy. Patients often present with night sweats or weight loss. Occasionally traumatic inoculation will produce localized skin lesions with ulcerations. When MAI is disseminated, multiple cutaneous papules and nodules can be seen.

Other Atypical Mycobacterial Infections

Mycobacterium kansasii is found in the midwestern and southcentral USA, California and Japan. It causes pulmonary changes resembling those found in tuberculosis, especially in patients with existing lung disease such as silicosis. Patients may develop hyperergic states, as in tuberculosis, leading to erythema nodosum or tuberculid-like reactions. Local lesions or sporotrichoid changes similar to those caused by *M. marinum* may occur; in immunosuppressed patients, more widespread disease can be seen.

Mycobacterium chelonae and *M. fortuitum* are widely distributed saprophytes in soil and water. They are often involved in wound infections and accidental inoculations; about two-thirds of all infections involve the skin. The two organisms are closely related but have different antibiotic sensitivities. *M. haemophilum* requires iron or blood to grow; it has caused subcutaneous abscesses in a small number of immunosuppressed patients and was first reported in Australia. For all these organisms, sensitivity testing should be used to determine the choice of antibiotics for long-term therapy. None of the infections are easy to treat.

Leprosy

Synonym. Hansen disease

Definition. Chronic minimally contagious infection with *M. leprae* involving primarily skin and nerves.

History. Leprosy has been a worldwide cause of disease since recorded history. The word leprosy comes from the Greek lepra (= scales) or the Indo-European lap (= peeling, removing scales). There is good evidence for the disease in ancient Egypt and China. Although leprosy is mentioned in the Bible as *Zaraath*, medical and biblical scholars are divided on if *M. leprae* infections are really being described. The next description of the leprosy we know comes during the time of Alexander the Great, around 330 B.C. The movements of the Roman troops and the Crusaders served to introduce leprosy to Europe. While it was common in Europe for a number of centuries, by the sixteenth century it was restricted to the Balkans, Scandinavia and the Mediterranean lands. Today leprosy is almost gone from Europe, reintroduced occasionally by the new surge of immigrants and the large numbers of tourists.

Many of the diseases called leprosy in the Middle Ages were clearly something else. Patients with syphilis, psoriasis, mycosis fungoides and pemphigus vulgaris were also deformed and probably labeled as lepers and banished from society. As late as the nineteenth century, Bateman, in London, wrote of and illustrated lepra graecorum, which was psoriasis. In many German cities, leprosaria and leper cemeteries existed until the eighteenth century. Some cities had rules requiring that lepers wear a special bell, so other people would be warned of their coming and could thus avoid them.

Causative Organism. *Mycobacterium leprae.* This acid-fast bacillus is 4–7 µm by 0.3–0.4 µm in size. It stains positively with a modified Ziehl-Neelsen stain; usually the Fite-Faraco modification is employed. The bacteria are often tightly packed together, like cigars in a box; these groups are called globi. *M. tuberculosis* stains with $AgNO_3$, while *M. leprae* does not. There is no culture medium for *M. leprae*; the organism can be grown in mouse foot pads or the nine-banded armadillo.

Epidemiology. Worldwide, the number of people infected with *M. leprae* is estimated at 2–3 million but dropping. The World Health Organization has as a goal the elimination of the organism in the next decade, although plenty of victims will still remain. The distribution today is in a belt around the world roughly bordered by 40° north and 40° south latitudes. The main foci of infection are the Indian subcontinent, Southeast Asia, Indonesia, the Philippines, tropical Africa and scattered areas in Latin America. In endemic areas, the prevalence is about 5/1000. In Germany, almost all cases are brought in by immigrants, although on rare occasion a tourist or, more likely, a foreign-aid worker (with a longer stay overseas) may be infected. In the USA, the vast bulk of cases are seen in immigrants from Southeast Asia and Latin America. Some cases have been seen in veterans of the Vietnam War and a few cases have been described in Louisiana and south Texas, primarily among individuals with intimate contact with armadillos (hunters, gourmets). There are no animal cases of leprosy. While the nine-banded armadillo is a carrier or vector, it does not suffer from this status.

Even though leprosy has always been feared as a contagious disease, it is hard to catch. Most patients are infected as children living in a household with an infected person. Children of both sexes are equally susceptible; among adults, men are at greater risk. When standards of hygiene are low, transmission is more probable. Only patients with lepromatous leprosy are likely to transmit the *M. leprae*.

Etiology and Pathogenesis. Even though leprosy is a very common infection, the exact mode of transmission is unclear. Droplet spread is the most likely explanation, as the nasal mucosa is frequently involved and patients with lepromatous leprosy release a large number of organisms. Open skin wounds may also seed the environment. Entry is probably through the upper respiratory tract and broken areas of skin. Insect vectors may mechanically transfer the bacteria, but they do not serve as a host or play a role in the life cycle. The sites of predilection of leprosy are the skin, mucosa, upper respiratory tract and peripheral nerves.

The incubation period for leprosy is very long. It has been estimated at 5 years for tuberculoid leprosy and twice that for lepromatous leprosy. Cases have developed 20 years after exposure, as in soldiers returning from the tropics. A small number of cases have been seen in children less than 3 years of age; in these cases placental transmission and maternal milk have been blamed.

There is probably no disease in which the interplay between the host immune response and the organism is more finely tuned than in leprosy. Despite extensive efforts, little is understood about individual susceptibility to *M. leprae*. There may be a genetic predisposition. In simplest terms, the initial exposure to the bacteria appears to induce tolerance with inadequate functioning of the clone of T helper cells that react to the agent. When this occurs, lepromatous leprosy results. If cellular immunity is adequate, tuberculoid leprosy is the clinical pattern. The tuberculoid patients have excellent immunity and few viable organisms, while those with lepromatous disease have a weak immune response against *M. leprae* and harbor many living organisms.

Several of the diagnostic tests actually fit well into a discussion of the pathogenesis. Often the organisms are stained in tissue sections. The bacterial index is the number of bacteria found in a skin smear or nasal smear; it ranges from 6^+, with many clumps of bacteria and over 1000 bacteria in an average field, to 1^+, with 1–10 bacilli in 100 fields. The morphologic index is the percentage of solid-staining bacteria, as these are the bacteria that are capable of reproduction and infection. In lepromatous leprosy, the morphologic index is typically about 20–25% prior to therapy but should drop to 0% over 6 months and is the usual way of monitoring therapy. The organism can also be identified with more modern techniques such as PCR. This is particularly valuable in unclear cases, as culture is still not possible for routine diagnosis. Mouse foot pad and armadillo inoculation are two research methods to cultivate *M. leprae*.

The lepromin test is used to determine the patient's immunity to *M. leprae* and offers prognostic help. It is not a diagnostic test, as many patients with tuberculosis will be positive. It tends to be positive in tuberculoid and borderline tuberculoid leprosy, but negative towards the lepromatous end of the spectrum. Several different antigens are available but none is available in Germany. They include:

- Standard lepromin antigen (Mitsuda-Hayasaki), made from macerated infected tissue from lepromatous leprosy patients
- Bacillus antigen (Dharmendra), which contains purified *M. leprae*
- Protein lepromin antigen (Olmos-Castro), which contains specific antigen components of *Mycobacterium leprae* wall

The most experience has been obtained with the standard test, which is read after 2 days (Fernandez reaction) and 3–4 weeks (Mitsuda reaction). The early reaction is usually a 2–5-mm erythematous papule that simply suggests prior exposure to mycobacteria. The later reaction is more nodular and if biopsied may show a granulomatous tissue response. It suggests the ability to mount a cell-mediated response to *M. leprae*. In screening surveys, children with positive lepromin tests almost never develop lepromatous leprosy.

In addition to the cellular immunity, there is also increased humoral immunity. Its beneficial role is hard to establish. The most common test searches for antibodies against the phenolic glycolipid lipid I (PGL I). Such antibodies are present in over 95% of lepromatous leprosy patients but in only 30–50% of tuberculoid leprosy patients. (In Germany, the tests are done at the Armaur-Hansen-Institute, Hermann-Schell-Str.7, D-97074 Würzburg,

Table 4.14. Ridley-Jopling classification of leprosy

Feature	TT	BT	BB	BL	LL
Infiltrated lesions	Defined plaques, central healing	Irregular plaques, partially raised edges, satellites	Variable lesions, often punched out centers	Papules, nodules	Nodules, diffuse thickening
Macular lesions	Single, small	Several, larger	Many, bizarre	–	Very many, confluent
Surface	Dry, scaly	Dry	Intermediate	Shiny	Shiny
Sensation	Usually absent	Diminished	Slightly diminished	Perhaps diminished	Intact
Hairs	Absent	Markedly decreased	Decreased	Slightly decreased	Normal
Mycobacteria	None	Rare	Moderate	Many	Very many
Lepromin test	+++	++/+	+/–	–	–

Tel.: +49-931-88 49 49). The antibodies play a major role in some of the leprosy reactions discussed below.

Clinical Findings. The clinical features will be described separately for the different types of leprosy even through there are frequent overlaps. The standard classification of Ridley and Jopling delineates five types ranging from lepromatous leprosy → borderline lepromatous → midborderline → borderline tuberculoid → tuberculoid leprosy. Some of the features are shown in Table 4.14 and Fig. 4.54; Table 4.15 compares the features of the two polar forms of leprosy. The dermatologist not experienced with leprosy should make it his goal not to miss a diagnosable case, and not worry about the exact classification or identification of indeterminate forms.

Table 4.15. Simplified comparison of tuberculoid and lepromatous leprosy

Feature	Tuberculoid	Lepromatous
Distribution of lesions	Few, asymmetrical	Many, asymmetrical
Margins	Sharp	Vague
Raised edge	No	Yes
Hypopigmentation	Marked	Mild
Surface	Dry, scaly	Smooth, shiny
Hair, sweat	Diminished	Less affected
Loss of sensation	Early, marked	Late, minimal
Nerve damage	Early, marked	Late, minimal
Bacterial index	Very low	High
Outcome	Healing	Progression

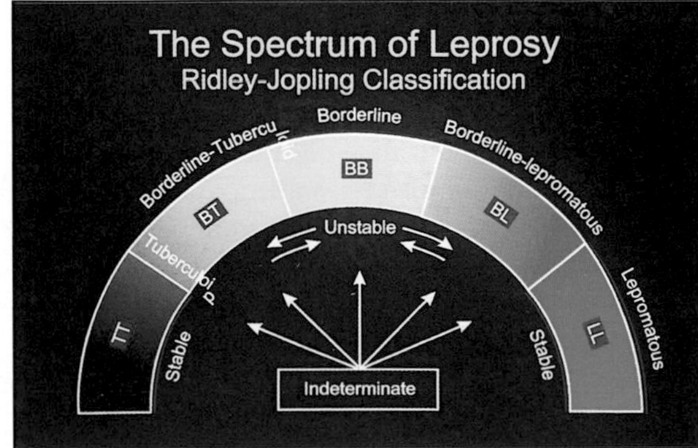

Fig. 4.54. Ridley-Jopling classification

Indeterminate Leprosy

Definition. Early, indistinct form of leprosy.

Early in its course, leprosy has few distinct features. Clinical changes are minor, confined to skin and nerves, few bacteria are present and the lepromin reaction may be weakly positive. Under the microscope the inflammatory changes are minimal and not typical.

Cutaneous Findings. There is usually a single, asymptomatic, hypopigmented ill-defined macule several centimeters in diameter. It is most common on the face, trunk or extensor surfaces of the limbs. If multiple lesions are present, they tend to be asymmetric. Cutaneous sensation may be slightly impaired but sweating is usually normal. Most patients are not seen by a physician at this stage.

Systemic Findings. There may also be involvement of nerves. A single thickened nerve may be present or a rare patient may present with an anesthetic patch.

Lepromatous Leprosy

Definition. Anergic progressive infection with *M. leprae* with many organisms and marked disfigurement.

Clinical Findings

Cutaneous Findings. The skin lesions are typically symmetric, small, shiny and usually confluent. The macules are round or oval and usually confined to covered body areas. The infiltrated plaques may arise from macules or independently; they have a distinct red-brown color, which of course varies greatly depending on the basic skin color of the patient. Such nodules are called lepromas. They have an indistinct border. The most striking involvement is facial, with infiltration of the forehead, chin, nose and ears, producing a leonine facies (Fig. 4.55). Skin folds are often spared, exaggerating the folded appearance. Infiltration of the ear lobes is very distinctive (Fig. 4.56). Another early sign is loss of the lateral aspects of the eyebrows. As the disease progresses, anhidrosis and anesthesia may develop. Certain areas are almost always spared in all types of cutaneous leprosy; they include the axillae, groin, perineum, scalp and midline of the back.

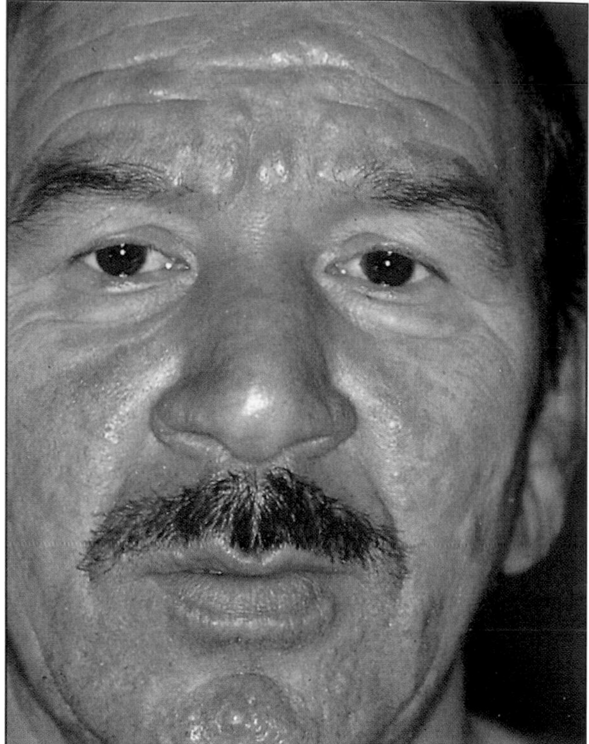

Fig. 4.55. Lepromatous leprosy

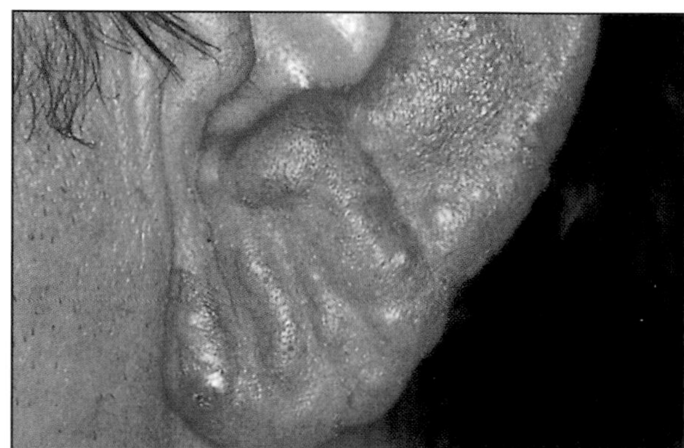

Fig. 4.56. Lepromatous leprosy

Mucosal Features. The nasal mucosa is almost always involved. Chronic nasal discharge, especially if hemorrhagic, should suggest leprosy in endemic areas. The proliferation may interfere with breathing and destroy the nasal septum with distal loss of substance (clover leaf nose of Gay-Prieto). Other mucosal surfaces, such as the lips, mouth and larynx, can also be infiltrated.

Systemic Findings. Peripheral nerve damage is slow to appear. Initially there is peripheral symmetric sensory loss, often temperature-dependent, and over the extensor surfaces of the extremities. The loss of sensation slowly spreads centrally. Pain is unusual. There may also be autonomic damage, as reflected by impaired sweating and vasomotor dysfunction. In lepromatous leprosy the involvement of major motor nerves occurs much later, as discussed under tuberculoid leprosy. In more advanced disease, the hands and feet become swollen and there is osteoporosis with osteolytic lesions and compression fractures. In addition, repeated often unnoticed trauma and secondary infections contribute greatly to the disability. Most patients have lymphadenopathy. Infiltrates may be found in the testes leading to sterility and gynecomastia.

Ocular Findings. The eye is affected in a number of ways in leprosy. Direct bacterial involvement occurs in lepromatous leprosy with infiltration of the conjunctiva, cornea and ciliary body. The eye is often involved in leprosy reactions, as considered below. In late lepromatous leprosy there may also be involvement of the facial nerve, as discussed under tuberculoid leprosy.

Lucio Leprosy. This rare severe form of lepromatous leprosy is seen primarily in Mexico. Most patients have both Spanish and Native American ancestry. The skin is diffusely infiltrated and shiny, so that the natural wrinkles are obliterated. Lucio leprosy has been designated as lepra bonita, or beautiful leprosy. The eyelids tend to thicken, the eyebrows are lost, and vocal cord involvement leads to hoarseness. The hands and feet swell such that the symptoms may be confused with those of myxedema. The feared Lucio reaction occurs in this subset.

Tuberculoid Leprosy

Definition. Noninfectious, form of leprosy with few organisms, good cellular immunity and few systemic problems other than nerve damage.

Clinical Findings

Cutaneous Findings. The lesions in tuberculoid leprosy are usually asymmetric, few in number and slow-growing. The initial lesions are small red or red-violet macules and papules which may be hyperesthetic. They slowly expand, have a sharply defined, often raised edge, may show central clearing and mild atrophy and are typically scaly and hypopigmented (Fig. 4.57). Some patients have a limited number of papules about body orifices; they tend to do very well. More typically the lesions are on the buttocks, trunk, face and extensor surfaces of the limbs. Loss of sensation, anhidrosis and hair loss occur.

Systemic Findings. Nerve damage is the major systemic finding in tuberculoid leprosy. Granulomatous inflammation damages the peripheral nerves, resulting in loss of function and in enlarged, firm palpable cords which can be clinically identified. The nerve involvement occurs earlier than in lepromatous leprosy and is more severe and asymmetric. Rather than early sensory changes, there may be paralysis and secondary muscle atrophy. The facial nerves are often involved; the rather blank expression which can result is named after St. Antonius. The vocal cords can also be paralyzed.

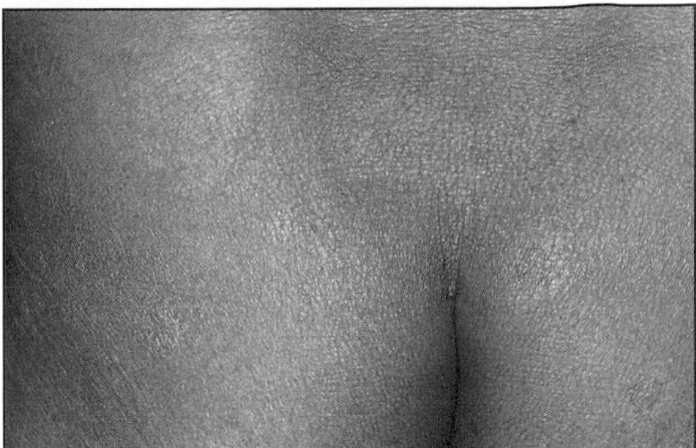

Fig. 4.57. Tuberculoid leprosy

The real problem in tuberculoid leprosy is extensive damage to the nerves and then the limbs. The nerves that are most likely to be affected are superficial, cooler (and thus more hospitable to *M. leprae*) and easily traumatized. There is early involvement of the ulnar and often the median nerves, producing lateral and medial claw-type changes of the hands. On the legs, the common peroneal nerve (causing foot drop) and posterior tibial nerve (producing anesthesia of the sole and wasting of intrinsic muscles) are most often affected. As a result of the dry, anesthetic skin, impaired healing and muscular paralysis, the skin is very sensitive to trauma. Minor injuries, inappropriate pressure from shoes, blisters and burns can all lead to extensive damage. Because of impaired proprioception, the foot may be unstable and repeatedly twisted or sprained. Scars complicate the picture.

Ocular Findings. The eyes are often affected in tuberculoid leprosy and in leprosy reactions. Most common is involvement of the facial nerve so that lagophthalmos develops, with incomplete blinking, dryness and corneal damage. If the first branch of the trigeminal nerve is affected, the eye can become anesthetic and even more easily damaged. Entropion is another cause of damage.

Borderline Leprosy

We will not go into detail on the three various stages of borderline leprosy but simply emphasize the main concepts. While tuberculoid and leproma-

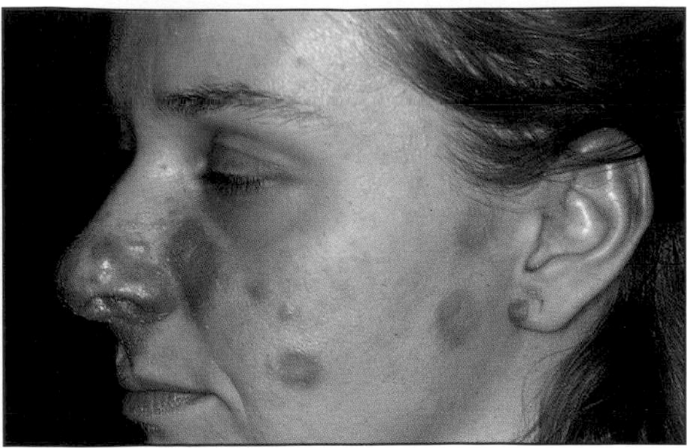

Fig. 4.58. Borderline leprosy

tous leprosy are relatively stable diseases, the borderline stages are often characterized by changes in immunity and so-called reactions, as considered below. Clinically there is an imperceptible swing from the features of one polar type towards the other. The borderline leprosy types tend to swing towards the tuberculoid pole with treatment, but spontaneously are more likely to go to the lepromatous end.

Midborderline (BB) leprosy is the most unstable form. There are many skin lesions, with some tendency to symmetry. These lesions may be shiny, as in lepromatous leprosy, but also have central dimpling or clearing and satellite lesions (Fig. 4.58). Nerve involvement is common and asymmetric. True borderline disease is less common than either borderline tuberculoid or borderline lepromatous disease.

In borderline tuberculoid (BT) leprosy, there is good immunity but nonetheless clinical evidence that everything is not as well-controlled as desired. The lesions may not have the perfect sharp border of tuberculoid leprosy, or may have a rim with occasional gaps. In other patients, there are simply too many lesions for ordinary tuberculoid leprosy. Nerve involvement is also more marked than in the polar form; while fewer nerves tend to be involved than in BB, the degree of damage is greater.

Pure neural leprosy is usually a form of borderline tuberculoid disease. It is most common in India. Most often only one nerve is involved, usually the ulnar. In rare cases, lepromatous leprosy or borderline forms may present with nerve damage only. The diagnosis is usually made on nerve biopsy.

In borderline lepromatous leprosy (BL), the skin lesions tend to have coalesced less than in the polar form. Papules and nodules still have borders, rather than fusing into diffuse infiltrates. Nasal, laryngeal and ocular involvement is much less common. Even though the patient is at risk of going on to develop lepromatous leprosy, the presence of borderline features is a better prognostic sign.

Histopathology. In indeterminate leprosy, the skin biopsy is rarely helpful; few organisms are identified. In more definite disease, the biopsy is usually quite helpful. In lepromatous leprosy, there are extensive infiltrates of foamy macrophages (Virchow cells) loaded with *M. leprae* which can be easily stained. As one moves towards the tuberculoid pole, the infiltration becomes more granulomatous with multinucleated giant cells and very few, if any, organisms.

Laboratory Findings. Many of the laboratory tests have already been mentioned. The lepromin test is primarily useful for following patients. In Western Europe, there are many false-positives from exposure to tuberculosis and BCG vaccine. Culture is difficult but PCR can be used to identify the organism in tissue. The presence of antibodies against various cell wall antigens of *M. leprae* is relatively specific and may speed the diagnosis in nonendemic populations.

The histamine test is similar to the control test in the ordinary prick testing for allergens. Patients with leprosy and impaired autonomic nervous function do not develop the triple response of Lewis but only a hive, with no peripheral erythema. A variety of sweat tests, using for example 0.1 ml of pilocarpine hydrochlorate 1:100 injected into a lesion, can be tried; the presence of sweating can be demonstrated with starch-iodide. Neither of these methods is very specific or sensitive.

Nontreponemal tests for syphilis are positive in about 30 % of patients, but the specific treponemal tests such as TPHA and FTA-ABS are negative. Other abnormal findings may include elevated cholesterol or triglycerides, cryoglobulinemia and hyperglobulinemia.

Diagnostic Criteria. The most important rule is never to overdiagnose leprosy. As many experienced leprologists warn, leprophobia is harder to treat than leprosy. In nonendemic areas, one must be careful to inquire about the patient's country of origin, foreign travel and prolonged living in endemic areas. The neurologic examination is crucial; in any patient suspected of leprosy, we do simple testing for sensation and motor function but also involve our neurology colleagues. In addition, the expertise of national leprosy or tropical disease centers should be sought.

Course and Prognosis. The biggest problem in leprosy is the presence of reactions. One speaks of downgrading when there is a loss of immunity and a shift towards the lepromatous pole, or of upgrading when immunity improves and tuberculoid features appear. Despite the sharp differences between these two concepts, reactions in both directions tend to be clinically similar. Three types of reactions are identified:

Type 1: This is the most common, reflecting a change in cellular immunity in borderline patients. Reversal is often associated with treatment, while downgrading only occurs in inadequately treated patients. In patients near the tuberculoid pole, skin lesions may become swollen and itchy but new lesions are uncommon. In contrast, in downgrading, as one moves towards the middle of the spectrum, new skin lesions often appear and tenosynovitis is common. Other systemic features are rare. While intuitively reactions moving towards the tuberculoid pole represent healing, they may be disastrous for the patient because of nerve damage, especially for those with BB or BT disease. Nerve involvement is rapid, with pain, swelling, tenderness and loss of function occurring.

The greatest risk is for patients with BB leprosy. They develop new skin lesions, as the old ones become swollen and painful. Many nerves may be involved and damage is extensive. The pain and weakness, coupled with malaise and diffuse edema, may incapacitate the patient. In patients nearer the lepromatous pole, the systemic effects are even more severe. The skin may become diffusely infiltrated. While many nerves are involved, damage tends to be mild. Orchitis may occur. These patients usually show upgrading reactions, often as treatment is starting; when they downgrade to lepromatous leprosy, the most frequent changes are more extensive mucosal disease. Microscopically, the diagnosis can often be made if a previous specimen is available for comparison. Reversal reactions tend to have more extensive giant cell formation and edema. In downgrading reactions, there is less cellular inflammation and fibrosis, associated with increased numbers of bacteria.

Type II: This reaction occurs only in BL and lepromatous leprosy patients, usually during treatment. About half of lepromatous leprosy patients experience this phenomenon. The high antibody levels are thought to lead to the presence of circulating immune complexes. There are similarities to a Jarisch-Herxheimer reaction, as bacterial killing is associated with increased risk. There is no reversal or downgrading. The most typical changes are deep, painful erythematous nodules, known as erythema nodosum leprosum. Unlike erythema nodosum, they are not limited to the shins but often involve the face or trunk. They may become pustular and drain, usually healing with brawny induration. The other main complications are marked iridocyclitis and neuritis. Under the microscope there is diffuse neutrophilic infiltration associated with foci of bacteria.

Lucio reaction: Patients with Lucio leprosy can develop an extensive severe vasculitis. It may appear prior to therapy, presenting as pink painful palpable nodules which can become hemorrhagic or necrotic. Larger lesions may develop bullae and heal with large eschars. Cryoglobulins are also present and abundant *M. leprae* can be found in the vessel walls.

Another even less common type of reaction is the development of histioid leprosy. Most patients have lepromatous leprosy or perhaps BL and have been on dapsone monotherapy. They develop numerous firm nodules which microscopically have marked fibrosis and may be mistaken for dermatofibromas; however, the nodules are very rich in organisms and their presence indicates resistance.

Patients with indeterminate leprosy may resolve spontaneously, but most enter the spectrum of determinate leprosy. Patients towards the tuberculoid pole may also spontaneously improve; their outlook is primarily determined by the degree of nerve and thus limb damage they have. Even after all signs of infection are gone, they may be severely disabled. Lepromatous leprosy is a polar disease which does not tend to improve or regress. The patients face a variety of serious problems including the obvious social implications of their facial deformities and limb defects. The ocular involvement may lead to blindness. Many male patients are sterile. Secondary amyloidosis can be seen and lead to chronic renal disease. Thus, the outlook is grimmer. If they are not adequately treated, their life expectancy is 10–15 years. The type I reactions in this group may also be life-threatening.

Differential Diagnosis. The differential diagnosis of cutaneous leprosy is endless. One should suspect leprosy in unexplained, hypopigmented scaly lesions, when other considerations include dermatophytosis, tinea versicolor, pityriasis alba, pityriasis rotunda and many others. Despite the popular impression, vitiligo is really not part of the differential diagnosis as leprosy almost never produces total depigmentation. In addition, infiltrated plaques or nodules suggest the entire differential diagnostic spectrum of cutaneous granulomatous infiltrates. Annular lesions with a raised border suggest granuloma annulare, granuloma multiforme, lupus erythematosus, sarcoidosis and tuberculosis. The facial nodules of lepromatous leprosy may be confused with leishmaniasis.

Therapy. The most important point is to emphasis to the patient that leprosy is eminently treatable today. There are effective antibacterial agents as well as many possibilities for reconstruction and rehabilitation. The therapy of leprosy is an uncomfortable problem for someone who is rarely confronted with the disease. The physician should check with an agency experienced in the problem and follow its guidelines exactly. If another physician is available with more experience, the case should be entrusted to his care. There are many schemes available for treating leprosy; they vary to some extent from region to region, reflecting the sensitivity of *M. leprae* to various antimicrobial agents.

Because of resistance, almost every patient today is treated with some type of combination therapy. The bacteriological and morphologic indexes are followed to assess the effectiveness of the regimen. The following minimum regimens are recommended by the World Health Organization.

- Lepromatous leprosy (as well as BB, BL): Dapsone 100 mg daily; rifampicin 600 mg once monthly; clofazimine 300 mg once monthly and 50 mg daily. The monthly doses are to be taken under observation. The treatment must be continued for 2 years after the skin or nasal smears have become negative.
- Tuberculoid leprosy (as well as BT): Dapsone 100 mg daily; rifampicin 600 mg once monthly under observation for 6 months.

Patients must be monitored carefully for the development of reactions. The main problem is in the BT-BB group with nerve damage. Some of the special features of these drugs are considered below.

Dapsone. Resistance is common, so that monotherapy is no longer acceptable. There is both primary resistance prior to therapy, which is as high as 50% in China, and secondary resistance following exposure to the drug, which approaches 100% in parts of Southeast Asia. Many groups recommend a lower dosage of dapsone in lepromatous leprosy, starting at 25 mg/week, working up over 6 months to the WHO recommendations to reduce the risk of reactions. In addition, DADPS (diacetyldiaminodiphenylsulfone; 225 mg) can be injected once monthly; it provides very low blood levels and probably helps select out resistant strains. Dapsone leads to invariable methemoglobinemia, and in individuals lacking glucose-6-phosphate-dehydrogenase (G6PD) there may be striking hemolysis. It may also cause peripheral neuropathies.

Rifampicin. This antibiotic produces the most rapid killing of *M. leprae*. After 1–2 weeks of therapy, there are no longer viable organisms found in the skin or nasal scrapings. Rifampicin inhibits bacterial RNA synthesis. Resistance is not a problem. While there may be transient elevations in liver enzymes, persistent rises mean the drug should be discontinued. There may also be CNS and bone marrow changes. Rifampicin interacts with a wide variety of medications, including oral contraceptives and coumarin. It should not be used in pregnancy.

Clofazimine. Another uncommon antimicrobial agent, clofazimine discolors urine, tears, sweat and skin, imparting a red-brown color. Resistance does not seem to be a problem. It is useful in treating erythema nodosum leprosum. The major side effects include gastrointestinal distress and impaired renal and hepatic function. The latter parameters should be monitored.

Alternate Drugs. Other antituberculosis drugs such as ethionamide and prothionamide may be used in special cases but are quite hepatotoxic. Streptomycin, thiosemicarbazone and second generation quinolones such as ciprofloxacin have also been employed. Many of these agents tend to be too expensive for the areas where leprosy is endemic.

Treatment of Reactions. Type 1 reactions are treated with systemic corticosteroids if there is evidence of nerve, eye or testicular involvement. Usually prednisone 40–80 mg daily is the starting dosage; this should be tapered over a period of weeks while continuing the antibacterial therapy. If the patient is on monotherapy, clofazimine is usually added. When the nerves are not involved, aspirin or chloroquine are most effective.

The treatment of choice for type 2 reactions is thalidomide. In the USA, until recently, it could only be used for this indication because of its known teratogenic effect. It is started at 400 mg daily and slowly tapered. In severe type 2 reactions, systemic corticosteroids may be needed. In addition, multidrug antibacterial therapy should be continued.

Lucio reaction is treated with systemic corticosteroids; thalidomide is not helpful. An aggressive antibacterial program featuring rifampicin is also required.

Surgical. Reconstructive surgery is the single most important contribution once the organism has been eradicated. Entire textbooks exist on the topic.

Prophylaxis. There are many efforts at developing a vaccine. Use of BCG has provided protection in some studies but not in others. Trials using BCG combined with killed *M. leprae* are under way. Dapsone can also be used for prophylaxis but the development of resistant strains is thereby encouraged.

Public Health Measures. Lepromatous leprosy is a reportable infection. Patients are infective, but this status is rapidly reversed with rifampicin. Thus, only a few need to be isolated for any length of time. Nonetheless, for social reasons, in many countries, lepromatous leprosy is still treated in leprosaria. Contacts of patients with lepromatous leprosy should be evaluated and followed for at least 5 years.

Primary Immunodeficiency Diseases

While secondary or acquired immunodeficiencies, especially HIV/AIDS, have occupied the center of attention in recent years, there are a number of rare genetic disorders in which individuals are born with defects in one or more facets of their immune response. In the past, many such patients died of infections in early life. Today the combination of earlier and more aggressive antibiotic therapy, more accurate identification of immune defects and, to some extent replacement or reconstitution of the immune response, have improved the outlook in this group. Almost all of these patients have cutaneous manifestations and bacterial infections. For these reasons, they are included in this chapter.

Epidemiology. All of these diseases are exceedingly rare. The overall incidence in the US is estimated at 1:10,000. All of the diseases are inherited, although the gene is not known in every case. Because several of the more common (or less rare) disorders are inherited in an X-linked recessive pattern, there is often a male predominance. Once a patient has been identified, the risk for siblings and children may be significant.

Clinical Findings. As Table 4.16 shows, one can suspect an immunodeficiency based both on the clinical disease pattern and the presence of various microorganisms. Many other organisms may be involved; those listed are commonly encountered. The key is to be suspicious when either uncommon organisms are found, infections involve unusual locations, recurrences are common or antibiotics fail to function as expected. A number of cutaneous signs and symptoms may also suggest primary immunodeficiency, as shown in Table 4.17. The most common dermatologic finding in addition to infections is dermatitis. There is often disagreement as to whether the patients have atopic dermatitis or a unique problem. This argument is philosophical today, although sophisticated analysis of the cells in individual inflammatory lesions may soon allow us to separate atopic dermatitis from clinically similar conditions. In the sections that follow, the wide range of immunodeficiency disorders will be discussed only briefly. Treatment in most cases is similar, consisting of prompt, directed antimicrobial therapy. Some attempts at immunologic reconstitution with bone marrow, stem cell transplants or gene therapy have been made.

Laboratory Findings

Humoral Immunity. The best test for humoral immunity is quantification of the major immunoglobulins. As a rough guideline, IgG < 200 mg/dl, IgA < 10 mg/dl and IgM < 10 mg/dl should raise the suspicion of a primary immunodeficiency. Serum protein electrophoresis is useful for detecting gammopathies but not reliable for identifying immunoglobulin deficits. One can also measure isohemagglutinins or immunoglobulins directed against specific common vaccines or infectious

Table 4.16. Features of primary immunodeficiency

Immune defect	Clinical findings	Prominent organisms
Humoral immunity	Recurrent infections Virulent infections with harmless bacteria Chronic sinus and airway infections Poor response to antibiotics Chronic diarrhea Failure to thrive	*Streptococcus pneumoniae* *Haemophilus influenzae*
Cell-mediated immunity	Severe viral infections Progressive disease after live virus vaccination Opportunistic infections Mucopurulent rhinitis Recurrent candidiasis Graft vs host disease Failure to thrive	*Candida albicans* Dermatophytes *Aspergillus, Fusarium* *Cryptococcus* *Nocardia* *Strongyloides* *Pneumocystis carinii* Mycobacteria *Listeria* *Legionella* Herpes viruses especially varicella-zoster and cytomegalovirus
Defects in granulocytes or phagocytes	Neutropenia Recurrent or progressive infections Infections with unusual, nonpathogenic organisms Infections in unusual locations Failure to respond to antibiotics	Aerobic gram-negative bacilli *Aspergillus, Fusarium* *Staphylococcus aureus* *Candida albicans*
Defects in complement	Seborrheic erythroderma Lupus-like syndromes Recurrent or severe *Neisseria* infections	*Neisseria gonorrhoeae* *Neisseria meningitidis*

Based on Tables 12-1 and 12-2 in Dahl (1996 pp. 148–149). with permission

Table 4.17. Differential diagnosis of skin findings in primary immunodeficiencies

Cutaneous findings	Likely associations
Severe dermatitis	Wiskott-Aldrich syndrome Hyper-IgE syndrome Ataxia telangiectasia
Recurrent boils, abscesses	Hyper-IgE syndrome Chronic granulomatous disease Chédiak-Higashi syndrome Leukocyte adherence defect syndrome Wiskott-Aldrich syndrome
Severe herpes infections	DiGeorge syndrome SCID
Marked verrucae	Selective IgM deficiency Hyper-IgM syndrome
Severe candidiasis	DiGeorge syndrome SCID Chronic mucocutaneous candidiasis

SCID; Severe combined immunodeficiency

Table 4.18. Types of primary immunodeficiencies

Primarily cellular immunodeficiency
X-linked recessive SCID
Adenosine deaminase (ADA) defect
Purine nucleoside phosphorylase (PNP) defect
Swiss-type autosomal recessive SCID
Bare lymphocyte syndrome (MHC defect)
Reticular dysgenesis
Absent $CD8^+$ T cells
Nezelof syndrome
Cartilage-hair hypoplasia
Primarily humoral immunodeficiency
X-linked agammaglobulinemia
Hyper-IgM syndrome
IgM deficiency
IgA deficiency
Transient hypogammaglobulinemia of infancy
Common variable immunodeficiency
Familial erythrophagocytic lymphohistiocytosis
Omenn syndrome
Immune defects with other abnormalities
DiGeorge syndrome
Hyper-IgE syndrome
Immunodeficiency with thymoma
Wiskott-Aldrich syndrome
Ataxia telangiectasia
Chronic mucocutaneous candidiasis
Phagocytic defects
Chronic granulomatous disease
Leukocyte adherence protein defect
Hereditary myeloperoxidase defect
Tuftsin defect
Lazy leukocyte syndrome
Onychotrichodysplasia and neutropenia
Cyclic neutropenia
Chédiak-Higashi syndrome
Complement defects
Isolated complement defects
Hereditary angioneurotic edema
Leiner syndrome

organisms. Tetanus vaccine is considered a safe test. Imaging of the pharynx to search for lymphoid tissues is also helpful. On a molecular level, B cells can be quantified and their surface antigens and degree of evolution analyzed.

Cellular Immunity. The best rough test is the number of circulating small lymphocytes, since most peripheral lymphocytes are T cells. Specific types of T cells, most often the absolute values and ratio of $CD4^+$ helper and $CD8^+$ cytotoxic cells, can also be measured. Functional tests of cellular immunity include a series of intradermal skin tests, usually tuberculin, candidin, trichophytin and tetanus toxoid. Challenge with a known sensitizer such as dinitrochlorobenzene (DNCB) can also be employed. Radiologic examination of the thorax can indicate the presence of a thymus. The ability of lymphocytes to react to antigens can be tested in vitro with either mitogen stimulation or antigen challenge.

Phagocyte Function. The number of neutrophils in the peripheral blood offers almost no insight into phagocyte function. A Rebuck window can be used to assess the migration of neutrophils into slightly damaged skin. Chemotaxis can be assessed by measuring the distance phagocytic cells migrate either randomly or in response to a challenge, either in agar or on filter paper. Adherence can be assessed by how well the cells stick to plastic laboratory dishes or by looking for adherence molecules. The nitroblue tetrazolium (NBT) test is a crude measure of oxidative function; normally about 10% of peripheral neutrophils will reduce NBT to a black dye.

Complement. The CH50 is the most widely used functional screening test. Individual components of complement can all be measured.

Other Tests. HIV infection should be excluded in both adults and infants with immunodeficiency.

Table 4.18 shows the different types of primary immunodeficiencies. Some are discussed in other chapters and thus are only referenced in the table.

Diseases with Impaired Cellular Immunity

Severe Combined Immunodeficiency

Etiology and Pathogenesis. Severe combined immunodeficiency (SCID) is not one disease but many. In almost all instances, the primary defect resides in T cells, with impaired activation of B cells by helper T cells. Qualitative and functional assessments show that both cellular and humoral immunity are impaired. There are many different forms.

- X-linked recessive SCID is characterized by a defect in the γ-chain of the interleukin (IL)-2 receptor; the gene is located at Xq13. This is the most common form, accounting for over 50% of cases.
- Adenosine deaminase (ADA) deficiency is inherited in an autosomal recessive fashion; it

accounts for another 25% of cases. When ADA is missing, the purine salvage cycle is interrupted and toxic materials accumulate, especially in immature lymphocytes. Defects in purine nucleoside phosphorylase (PNP) are less common, are also inherited in an autosomal recessive pattern and involve the same metabolic pathway.

- Swiss-type SCID was the first primary immunodeficiency to be described; it is inherited in an autosomal fashion and may in some cases include ADA or PNP defects.
- All other types of primary immunodeficiency are even more rare. They include the bare lymphocyte syndrome, with defects in MHC class II molecules; reticular dysgenesis, with a stem cell defect and absent $CD8^+$ suppressor-cytotoxic T cells. Both of these are also inherited in an autosomal recessive manner.

Clinical Findings. The major problems with infections become apparent as maternal immunoglobulins disappear from the infant. Typical skin findings are severe, chronic *Candida* infections and persistent viral infections, as well as pyodermas. Gastrointestinal, pulmonary and ear infections are also common. Use of live vaccines can be fatal. Patients usually have little evidence of lymphatic tissue. They are at risk for graft-vs-host reaction from maternal blood or transfusions.

Course and Prognosis. The infants usually die within the first year of life.

Therapy. Patients must be isolated in a germ-free (gnotobiotic) environment. Some are candidates for bone marrow transplantation. ADA deficiency was the first disease to be treated at the National Institutes of Health with somatic gene replacement and some of the other forms also appear to be good candidates for this approach.

Nezelof Syndrome
(NEZELOF 1964)

This is a milder form of combined immunodeficiency with thymic aplasia and dysfunctional immunoglobulins. Some of Nezelof's patients may have had a type of ADA or PNP deficiency. One importance difference from SCID is the lack of risk for graft-vs-host reaction.

Cartilage-Hair Hypoplasia
(MCKUSICK 1965)

Synonyms. Metaphyseal chondrodysplasia (McKusick type), short-limbed dwarfism with immunodeficiency

Etiology and Pathogenesis. Cartilage-hair hypoplasia is primarily limited to the Pennsylvania Amish, where it was identified by McKusick. The main immune defect is a lymphopenia leading to impaired cellular and humoral responses.

Clinical Findings. These patients are short-limbed dwarfs with excessive folds of skin, especially about the joints, which resemble cutis laxa but no elastic fiber defect is present. The joints may be hyperextensible. The hair is thin, pale and silky. Varicella infections are handled poorly. In addition, diarrhea and a variety of infections may be seen. Pyodermas and dermatitis are uncommon.

Immune Amnesia Syndrome

These patients have circulating lymphocytotoxic antibodies. Thus they suffer from episodic lymphocytopenia. During periods of immunodeficiency, they may have marked trouble with varicella. In addition, toxic epidermal necrolysis has been reported. There may be a persistent dermatitis, as well as recurrent infections.

Diseases with Impaired Humoral Immunity

X-Linked Agammaglobulinemia
(BRUTON 1952)

Synonym. Bruton syndrome

Etiology and Pathogenesis. The disease is inherited in an X-linked recessive pattern. The gene, located at Xq22, is known as *Btk* and codes for a cytoplasmic tyrosine kinase whose absence leads to blocked B cell differentiation.

Clinical Findings. Some patients have dermatitis but it is not common. Boils and abscesses are also unusual. A reactive dermatomyositis-like syndrome following enterovirus infections may occur. The main problem is recurrent or even continuous infections with encapsulated organisms such as

S. pneumoniae and *H. influenzae*. Conjunctivitis, bronchitis, pneumonia and otitis are common.

Hyper-IgM Syndrome

The disease is inherited in an X-linked recessive pattern with the mutation at Xq26. Affected boys have a defect in CD40, which interferes with interactions between T cells and B cells, especially the switch from IgM to IgG and IgA production. Patients may have recalcitrant warts, severe oral ulcerations and dermatitis. Respiratory tract infections are common, and hepatosplenomegaly, neutropenia and lymphadenopathy may develop.

Selective IgM Deficiency

Surprisingly, a deficiency in IgM alone is just as likely to lead to dermatitis. These patients do poorly with gram-negative organisms and *Neisseria meningitidis*; localized infections may rapidly lead to sepsis. Many individuals have no clinical problems.

Selective IgA Deficiency

This is the most common primary immunodeficiency, with an incidence of 1:600. There is a maturation defect in lymphocytes producing IgA. Most patients are asymptomatic. There are no specific skin findings, although a variety of diseases have been reported in association. Most common are persistent gastrointestinal or pulmonary infections, reflecting the repaired mucosal resistance. A variety of autoimmune disorders can be seen in adults with selective IgA deficiency including systemic lupus erythematosus, dermatomyositis and thyroiditis.

Transient Hypogammaglobulinemia of Infancy

These children fail to start producing IgG at the appropriate time. They are at risk for pyodermas and abscesses, as well as chronic diarrhea and recurrent respiratory infections. Most patients eventually begin to make IgG, but it may take several years. The defect appears to lie in the helper T cells; some patients are carriers for ADA deficiency.

Common Variable Immunodeficiency

This is not a single disease, but many different disorders involving the whole spectrum of T and B cell interactions and functions. It is also known as unclassifiable immunodeficiency, indicating the problems.

Immune Defects with Associated Abnormalities

DiGeorge Syndrome
(DiGeorge 1965)

This developmental abnormality has been associated with a wide variety of both gene and chromosomal defects, as well as diabetic, alcoholic and retinoid embryopathy. In its most limited form, involving the 3rd and 4th pharyngeal arches, there is absence or hypoplasia of the thymus and parathyroid glands, leading to defects in cell mediated immunity and tetany. In more severe variants, the changes extend to involve the heart and produce distinctive craniofacial abnormalities. There are no specific skin findings.

Hyper-IgE Syndrome

Synonyms. Job syndrome (et al. 1966), Buckley (1972) syndrome

Epidemiology. The incidence has been estimated at 1:500,000 in the USA.

Etiology and Pathogenesis. The disorder is inherited in an autosomal dominant pattern but the gene is unknown and the immunologic defect unclear. These patients have very high levels of IgE, often directed against staphylococci, as well as eosinophilia, elevated IgD levels and impaired neutrophilic chemotactic responses.

Clinical Findings. The classical triad is recurrent abscesses and pneumonia, associated with elevated IgE levels. These three findings are present in over 85% of patients. There may be recurrent cold abscesses – pyogenic infections of the skin and lungs, often without an appropriate inflammatory response or fever. The scalp is a particularly common site. In addition to infections with *H. influenzae* and *S. aureus*, pulmonary abscesses with *Aspergillus* are often described. Most patients also have a rather coarse facies with a broad nose (Fig. 4.59). Delayed eruption and shedding of teeth may occur. Often extraction of primary teeth is required. Other findings in adults include recurrent fractures, hyperextensible joints and scoliosis. A striking

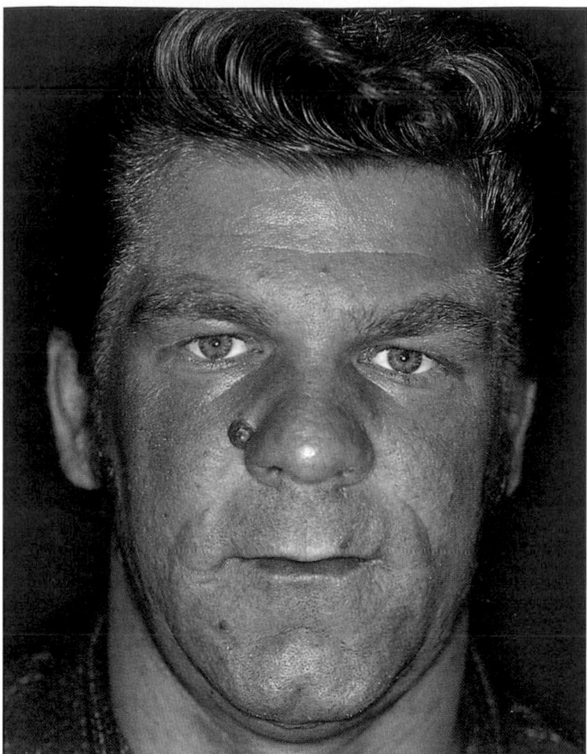

Fig. 4.59. Hyper-IgE syndrome

cutaneous finding is a severe chronic dermatitis, favoring the flexural areas and face. Sometimes the dermatitis may be papular or pustular. Dystrophic nails, often containing *C. albicans*, are also frequent. There is no sharp line of distinction either clinically or in the laboratory between these individuals and patients with atopic dermatitis, elevated IgE levels and recurrent staphylococcal infections.

Immunodeficiency with Thymoma

(Good 1954)

These patients have defects in both cellular and humoral immunity. The thymoma apparently interferes with B cell differentiation. When it is removed, reconstitution does not always occur. Patients often have recurrent skin infections, candidiasis and stomatitis, as well as a host of systemic infections.

Phagocytic Defects

Chronic Granulomatous Disease

Etiology and Pathogenesis. A wide variety of gene defects are responsible for the impaired phagocytic function in chronic granulomatous disease (CGD). Most if not all interfere with the function of cytochrome P558, which is essential for oxidation during phagocytosis. About 90% of cases are caused by a gene at Xp21.1, so most patients are males. Other autosomal genes may influence the same system.

Clinical Findings. Recurrent pyodermas, usually caused by *S. aureus* and often presenting as perianal or axillary abscesses, are common. Vesicular lesions have been described but their etiology is unclear. Scalp abscesses are also frequent. A persistent periorificial dermatitis may suggest the clinical diagnosis. Both stomatitis and gingivitis show that the normal oral bacteria are not managed well. Suppurative lymphadenopathy is often striking. Systemic findings are more pronounced and include osteomyelitis, pulmonary abscesses and granulomas and hepatosplenomegaly. Catalase-positive organisms such as *Serratia*, *Klebsiella* and *Aspergillus* are often responsible.

The mothers of affected boys with the most common gene often have Jessner lymphocytic infiltrate or discoid lupus erythematosus. In rare instances, systemic lupus erythematosus has been reported.

Laboratory Findings. The NBT reduction assay is usually negative. More sophisticated tests of oxidative metabolism are available.

Therapy. Long-term antibiotic therapy has been the mainstay. Some patients have been treated with interferon (INF)-γ and others with successful bone marrow transplantation.

Leukocyte Adhesion Deficiency

These children fail to produce lymphocyte function-associated antigen-1 (LFA-1). The defect is inherited in an autosomal recessive pattern and usually involves the β-chain (CD18). The antigen is required for many of the immune responses that require cell to-cell contact, so that chemotaxis, phagocytosis and natural killer (NK) cell function are impaired. Patients often present in the neonatal period with *P. aeruginosa* infections of the umbilicus, which may go on to produce extensive skin necrosis. Periodontal disease and delayed wound healing are also common. Some patients have been treated with bone marrow transplantation.

Myeloperoxidase Deficiency

The gene for myeloperoxidase is located at 17q22-q23; defects are inherited in an autosomal recessive pattern. Some patients with chronic mucocutaneous candidiasis have this defect. Both severe acne and pustular psoriasis have also been identified in such individuals, although most have minimal problems.

Tuftsin Deficiency

Tuftsin is a heavy chain molecule modified in the spleen to improve phagocytosis. Patients who have had a splenectomy are deficient in tuftsin and have problems with organisms which must be phagocytosed. There is a rare congenital tuftsin deficiency inherited in an autosomal dominant pattern.

Lazy Leukocyte Syndrome

The inheritance and cause of this disorder are poorly understood. Patients have normal bone marrow neutrophils but fail to mobilize the cells, leading to peripheral neutropenia. Both random migration and chemotaxis are impaired. Clinically patients usually present with recurrent stomatitis and gingivitis. Both systemic bacterial infections and dermatitis may also be seen.

Onychotrichodysplasia and Neutropenia

This rare disorder is inherited in an autosomal recessive pattern but the gene defect is unknown. Patients have sparse hairs, hypoplastic brittle nails and chronic neutropenia with counts around 1,000–2,000/ml. They frequently develop conjunctivitis, made wore by in-turning of their short eyelashes, as well as other bacterial infections.

Cyclic Neutropenia

These patients have precipitous drops in their neutrophil counts about every 3 weeks. The mechanism is poorly understood. At the time of the lower counts, they typically get a wide variety of bacterial infections, which may include pyodermas.

Complement Defects

The list of defects in complement factors is almost endless. Every factor has been described at least once as an isolated defect and almost all permutations have been seen. The most common cutaneous finding in this wildly heterogeneous group is lupus erythematosus-like illnesses, including Raynaud syndrome, vasculitis, photosensitivity, mucosal erosions and discoid skin lesions. Most of them are not characterized by positive antinuclear antibodies. Individuals with defects in the late components of the complement cascade have recurrent infections with *Neisseria meningitidis* and *N. gonorrhoeae*. Defects in C3 lead to a variety of infections, perhaps because of its central position in the cascade.

Miscellaneous Disorders

Many problems discussed elsewhere in this book may also occasionally be associated with immunodeficiency.

- Acrodermatitis enteropathica (Chap. 46): These patients have impaired chemotaxis which can be corrected by zinc. They also frequently have chronic candidiasis.
- Biotin-dependent carboxylase deficiency (Chap. 49): Patients with abnormalities in biotinidase and other carboxylases resemble those with acrodermatitis enteropathica. They often have candidiasis. The exact nature of the immune defect is unclear.
- Incontinentia pigmenti (Chap. 26): These rare patients have chemotactic and T cell defects.
- Darier syndrome (Chap. 17): The propensity of these patients to macerated infections of their damaged skin may be explained by chemotactic defects.

Bibliography

Flora of the Skin

Anthony RM, Noble WC, Pitcher DG (1992) Characterization of aerobic non-lipophilic coryneforms from human feet. Clin Exp Dermatol 17:102–105

Coyle MB, Lipsky BA (1990) Coryneform bacteria in infectious diseases: clinical and laboratory aspects. Clin Microbiol Rev 3:227–246

Hartmann AA (1990) The influence of various factors on the human resident skin flora. Semin Dermatol 9:305–308

Marcon MJ, Powell DA (1992) Human infections due to Malassezia spp. Clin Microbiol Rev 5:101–119

Schmidt A (1997) Malassezia furfur: a fungus belonging to the physiological skin flora and its relevance in skin disorders. Cutis 59:21–24

Williamson P, Kligman AM (1965) A new method for the quantitative Investigation of cutaneous bacteria. J Invest Dermatol 45:498–503

Clinical Aspects of Bacterial Skin Infections

Fite GL, Honolulu TH (1940) The fuchsin-formaldehyde method of staining acid-fast bacilli in paraffin section J Lab Clin Med 25:743–744

Gentry LO (1992) Therapy with newer oral beta-lactam and quinolone agents for infections of the skin and skin structures: a review. Clin Infect Dis 14:285–297

Koch R (1878) Untersuchungen über die Aetiologie der Wundinfektionskrankheit. Leipzig

Kutzner H, Argenyi ZB, Requena L et al. (1998) A new application of BCG antibody for rapid creening of various tissue microorganism. J Am Acad Dermatol 38: 56–60

Wiley EL, Beck B, Freeman RG (1991) Reactivity of fungal organisms in tissue sections using anti-mycobacteria antibodies. J Cutan Pathol 18:204–209

Toxin-Mediated Streptococcal and Staphylococcal Disease

Drage LA (1999) Life-threatening rashes: dermatologic signs of four infectious diseases. Mayo Clin Proc 74: 68–72

Jorup Ronstrom C, Hofling M, Lundberg C et al. (1996) Streptococcal toxic shock syndrome in a postpartum woman. Case report and review of the literature. Infection. 24:164–147

Manders SM, Heymann WR, Atillasoy E et al. (1996) Recurrent toxin-mediated perineal erythema. Arch Dermatol 132:57–60

Manders-SM (1998) Toxin-mediated streptococcal and staphylococcal disease. J Am Acad Dermatol 39:383–398

Margolis DJ, Horlick SE (1991) Group A streptococcus-induced bullous toxic shock-like syndrome. J Am Acad Dermatol 24:786–787

Resnick SD (1992) Staphylococcal toxin-mediated syndromes in childhood. Semin Dermatol 11:11–18

Stanford DG, Georgouras KE, Konya J et al. (1997) Toxic streptococcal syndrome. Aust J Dermatol 38:158–160

Veien NK (1998) The clinician's choice of antibiotics in the treatment of bacterial skin infection. Br J Dermatol 139 [Suppl 53]:30–36

Weiss KA, Laverdiere M (1997) Group A streptococcus invasive infections: a review. Can J Surg 40:18–25

Scarlet Fever

Altemeier WA III (1998) A pediatrician's view. A brief history of group A beta hemolytic strep. Pediatr Ann 27:264, 266–267

Aronson SM (1996) A rose by any other name. Med Health R 79:163–164

Barnett BO, Frieden IJ (1992) Streptococcal skin diseases in children. Semin Dermatol 11:3–10

Cherry JD (1993) Contemporary infectious exanthems. Clin Infect Dis 16:199–205

Cimolai N, Trombley C, Adderley RJ et al. (1992) Invasive Streptococcus pyogenes infections in children. Can J Public Health 83:230–233

Hsueh PR, Teng LJ, Lee PI et al. (1997) Outbreak of scarlet fever at a hospital day care centre: analysis of strain relatedness with phenotypic and genotypic characteristics. J Hosp Infect 36:191–200

Staphylococcal Scarlet Fever

Lina G, Gillet Y, Vandenesch F et al. (1997) Toxin involvement in staphylococcal scalded skin syndrome. Clin Infect Dis 25:1369–1373

Recalcitrant Erythematous Desquamating Disorder

Cone LA, Woodard DR, Byrd RG et al. (1992) A recalcitrant, erythematous, desquamating disorder associated with toxin producing staphylococci in patients with AIDS. J Infect Dis 165:638–643

Dondorp AM, Veenstra J, van der Poll T et al. (1994) Activation of the cytokine network in a patient with AIDS and the recalcitrant erythematous desquamating disorder Clin Infect Dis 18:942–945

Verbon A, Fisher CJ Jr (1998) Severe recalcitrant erythematous desquamating disorder associated with fatal recurrent toxic shock syndrome in a patient without AIDS. Clin Infect Dis 26:252–253

Neonatal Toxic Shock Syndrome-Like Exanthematous Disease

Takahashi N, Nishida H, Kato H et al. (1995) Exanthematous disease induced by toxic shock syndrome toxin 1 in the early neonatal period. Lancet 351:1614–1619

Takahashi N, Nishida H, Ino M et al. (1995) A new exanthematous disease in newborn infants. Acta Neonat Jpn 31:371–377

Recurrent Toxin-Mediated Erythema

Manders SM, Heymann WR, Atillasoy E et al. (1996) Recurrent toxin mediated perineal erythema. Arch Dermatol 132:1131–1132

Manders SM (1998) Toxin mediated streptococcal and staphylococcal disease. J Am Acad Dermatol 39:383–398

Kawasaki Disease

Akiyama T, Yashiro K (1993) Probable role of Streptococcus pyogenes in Kawasaki disease. Eur J Pediatr 152: 82–92

Ghazal SS, Alhowasi M, el Samady MM (1998) Kawasaki disease in a paediatric hospital in Riyadh. Ann Trop Paediatr 18:295–299

Smith PK, Goldwater PN (1993) Kawasaki disease in Adelaide: a review. J Paediatr Child Health 29:126–131

Pyoderma and Impetigo

Barnett BO, Frieden IJ (1992) Streptococcal skin diseases in children. Semin Dermatol 11:3–10

Brook I, Frazier EH, Yeager JK (1997) Microbiology of nonbullous impetigo. Pediatr Dermatol 14:192–195

Darmstadt GL, Lane AT (1994) Impetigo: an overview. Pediatr Dermatol 11:293–303

Noble WC (1998) Skin bacteriology and the role of Staphylococcus aureus in infection. Br J Dermatol 139 [Suppl 53]:9–12

Scales JW, Fleischer AB Jr, Krowchuk DP (1997) Bullous impetigo. Arch Pediatr Adolesc Med 151:1168–1169

Thestrup Pedersen K (1998) Bacteria and the skin: clinical practice and therapy update. Br J Dermatol 139 [Suppl 53]:1–3

Staphylococcal Scalded Skin Syndrome

Cribier B, Piemont Y, Grosshans E (1994) Staphylococcal scalded skin syndrome in adults. A clinical review illustrated with a new case. J Am Acad Dermatol 30: 319–324

Lyell A (1956) Toxic epidermal necrolysis: an eruption resembling scalding of the skin. Br J Dermatol 68:355–361

Lyell A (1979) Toxic epidermal necrolysis: (the scalded skin syndrome): a reappraisal. Br J Dermatol 100:69–86

Ritter von Rittershain G (1878) Die exfolative Dermatitis jüngerer Säuglinge. Zentralzeitung für Kinderheilkunde 2:3

Sheridan RL, Briggs SE, Remensnyder JP et al. (1995) The burn unit as a resource for the management of acute nonburn conditions in children. J Burn Care Rehabil 16:62–64

Nail Fold Infections

Chow E, Goh CL (1991) Epidemiology of chronic paronychia in a skin hospital in Singapore. Int J Dermatol 30:795–798

Weeks LE III, Scheker LR (1990) Upper extremity wound management. J Ky Med Assoc 88:337–341

Botryomycosis

Bonifaz A, Carrasco E (1996) Botryomycosis. Int J Dermatol 35:381–388

Defraigne JO, Demoulin JC, Pierard GE et al. (1997) Fatal mural endocarditis and cutaneous botryomycosis after heart transplantation. Am J Dermatopathol 19:602–605

Salvemini JN, Baldwin HE (1995) Botryomycosis in a patient with acquired immunodeficiency syndrome. Cutis 56: 158–160

Folliculitis

Annessi G (1998) Tufted folliculitis of the scalp: a distinctive clinicohistological variant of folliculitis decalvans. Br J Dermatol 138:799–805

Basarab T, Russell Jones R (1996) HIV-associated eosinophilic folliculitis: case report and review of the literature. Br J Dermatol 134:499–503

Baum J (1910) Ein Fall von sogenannter Acne urticata (Urticaria necroticans). In: Neisser A, Jacobi E (Hrsg) Ikonographia Dermatologica. Atlas seltener, neuer und diagnostisch unklarer Hautkrankheiten. Urban & Schwarzenberg, Berlin, pp 5–8

Berger RS, Seifert MR (1990) Whirlpool folliculitis: a review of its cause, treatment, and prevention. Cutis 45:97–98

Blume-Peytavi U, Chen W, Djemadji N et al. (1997) Eosinophilic pustular folliculitis (Ofuji's disease). J Am Acad Dermatol 37:259–262

Brenner S, Wolf R, Ophir J (1994) Eosinophilic pustular folliculitis: a sterile folliculitis of unknown cause? J Am Acad Dermatol 31:210–212

Buezo GF, Fraga J, Abajo P et al. (1998) HIV-Associated eosinophilic folliculitis and follicular mucinosis. Dermatology 197:178–180

Duarte AM, Kramer J, Yusk JW et al. (1993) Eosinophilic pustular folliculitis in infancy and childhood. Am J Dis Child 147:197–200

Dupond AS, Aubin F, Bourezane Y et al. (1995) Eosinophilic pustular folliculitis in infancy: report of two affected brothers. Br J Dermatol 132:296–299

Dyall-Smith D, Mason G (1995) Fungal eosinophilic pustular folliculitis. Aust J Dermatol 36:37–38

Faergemann J (1994) Pityrosporum infections. J Am Acad Dermatol 31:18–20

Fulton JE Jr, McGinley K, Leyden J et al. (1968) Gram-negative folliculitis in acne vulgaris. Arch Dermatol 98:349–353

Hoffmann E (1908) Perifolliculitis capitis abscedens et suffodiens: case presentation. Dermatol Z 15:122–123

Hoffmann E (1931) Zur Klassifizierung der atrophisierenden bzw. narbigen Alopecien und Folliculitiden. Arch Dermatol Syph 164:317–333

Jang KA, Chung ST, Choi JH et al. (1998) Eosinophilic pustular folliculitis (Ofuji's disease) in myelodysplastic syndrome. J Dermatol 25:742–746

Labandeira J, Suarez-Campos A, Toribio J (1998) Actinic superficial folliculitis. Br J Dermatol 138:1070–1074

Lazarov A, Wolach B, Cordoba M et al. (1996) Eosinophilic pustular folliculitis (Ofuji disease) in a child. Cutis 58: 135–138

Majors MJ, Berger TG, Blauvelt A et al. (1997) HIV-related eosinophilic folliculitis: a panel discussion. Semin Cutan Med Surg 16:219–223

McCausland WJ, Cox PJ (1975) Pseudomonas infection traced to motel whirlpool. J Environ Health 37:455–459

Mehregan AH, Coskey RJ (1968) Perforating folliculitis. Arch Dermatol 97:394–399

Misago N, Narisawa Y, Matsubara S et al. (1998) HIV-associated eosinophilic pustular folliculitis: successful treatment of a Japanese patient with UVB phototherapy. J Dermatol 25:178–184

Mizoguchi S, Setoyama M, Higashi Y et al. (1998) Eosinophilic pustular folliculitis induced by carbamazepine. J Am Acad Dermatol 38:641–643

Nieboer C (1985) Actinic superficial folliculitis, a new entity? Br J Dermatol 112:603–606

Noble WC (1998) Skin bacteriology and the role of Staphylococcus aureus in infection. Br J Dermatol 139 [Suppl 53]:9–12

Ofuji S, Ogino A, Horio T et al. (1970) Eosinophilic pustular folliculitis. Acta Dermatol Venereol [Stockh] 50:195–203

Plewig G, Jansen T (1998) Acneiform dermatoses. Dermatology 196:102–107

Ravikumar BC, Balachandran C, Shenoi SD et al. (1999) Disseminate and recurrent infundibulofolliculitis: response to psoralen plus UVA therapy. Int J Dermatol 38:75–76

Sahn EE (1994) Vesiculopustular diseases of neonates and infants. Curr Opin Pediatr 6:442–446

Steffen C (1985) Eosinophilic pustular folliculitis (Ofuji's disease) with response to dapsone therapy. Arch Dermatol 121:921–923

Teraki Y, Konohana I, Shiohara T et al. (1993) Eosinophilic pustular folliculitis (Ofuji's disease). Immunohistochemical analysis. Arch Dermatol 129:1015–1019

Vicente J, Espana A, Idoate M et al. (1996) Are eosinophilic pustular folliculitis of infancy and infantile acropustulosis the same entity? Br J Dermatol 35:807–809

Wagner A (1997) Distinguishing vesicular and pustular disorders in the neonate. Curr Opin Pediatr 9:396–405

Zirn JR, Scott RA, Hambrick GW (1996) Chronic acneiform eruption with crateriform scars. Acne necrotica (varioliformis) (necrotizing lymphocytic folliculitis). Arch Dermatol 132:1367, 1370

Furunculosis

Castanet J, Lacour JP, Perrin C et al. (1994) Juvenile pityriasis rubra pilaris associated with hypogammaglobulinaemia and furunculosis. Br J Dermatol 131:717–719

Eley CD, Gan VN (1997) Picture of the month. Folliculitis, furunculosis, and carbuncles. Arch Pediatr Adolesc Med 151:625–626

Golledge C (1994) Case of recurrent boils. Aust Fam Physician 23:2342

Tan HH, Tay YK, Goh CL (1998) Bacterial skin infections at a tertiary dermatological centre. Singapore Med J 39:353–356

Eyelid Infections

Black RL, Terry JE (1990) Treatment of chalazia with intralesional triamcinolone injection. J Am Optom Assoc 61:904–906

Donshik PC, Hoss DM, Ehlers WH (1992) Inflammatory and papulosquamous disorders of the skin and eye. Dermatol Clin 10:533–547

Olson MD (1991) The common stye. J Sch Health 61:138

Raskin EM, Speaker MG, Laibson PR (1992) Blepharitis. Infect Dis Clin North Am 6:777–787

Infections of Sweat Glands

Amren DP, Anderson As, Wanamaker LW (1966) Perianal cellulitis associated with group A streptococci. Am J Dis Child 112:546–552

Brehler R, Reimann S, Bonsmann G et al. (1997) Neutrophilic hidradenitis induced by chemotherapy involves eccrine and apocrine glands. Am J Dermatopathol 19: 73–78

Buezo GF, Requena L, Fraga Fernandez J et al. (1996) Idiopathic palmoplantar hidradenitis. Am J Dermatopathol 18:413–416

Landau M, Metzker A, Gat A et al. (1998) Palmoplantar eccrine hidradenitis: three new cases and review. Pediatr Dermatol 15:97–102

Sevila A, Morell A, Banuls J et al. (1996) Neutrophilic eccrine hidradenitis in an HIV-infected patient. Int J Dermatol 35:651–652

Shear NH, Knowles SR, Shapiro L et al. (1996) Dapsone in prevention of recurrent neutrophilic eccrine hidradenitis. J Am Acad Dermatol 35:819–822

Erysipelas

Bisno AL, Stevens DL (1996) Streptococcal infections of skin and soft tissues. N Engl J Med 334:240–245

Chartier C, Grosshans E (1996) Erysipelas: an update. Int J Dermatol 35:779–781

Eriksson B, Jorup Ronstrom C, Karkkonen K et al. (1996) Erysipelas: clinical and bacteriologic spectrum and serological aspects. Clin Infect Dis 23:1091–1098

Van der Meer JW, Drenth JP, Schellekens PT (1995) Recurrent erysipelas or erysipelas-like rash? Clin Infect Dis 22:881–882

Blistering Dactylitis

Woroszylski A, Duran C, Tamayo L et al. (1996) Staphylococcal blistering dactylitis: report of two patients. Pediatr Dermatol 13:292–293

Perianal Streptococcal Dermatitis

Bugatti L, Filosa G, Ciattaglia G (1998) Perianal dermatitis in a child. Perianal streptococcal dermatitis (PSD). Arch Dermatol 134:1147, 1150

Neri I, Bardazzi F, Marzaduri S et al. (1996) Perianal streptococcal dermatitis in adults. Br J Dermatol 135:796–798

Paradisi M, Cianchini G, Angelo C et al. (1993) Efficacy of topical erythromycin in treatment of perianal streptococcal dermatitis. Pediatr Dermatol 10:297–298

Skin Findings Associated with Streptococcal Infections

Cardullo AC, Silvers DN, Grossman ME (1990) Janeway lesions and Osler's nodes: a review of histopathologic findings. J Am Acad Dermatol 22:1088–1090

O'Dell ML (1998) Skin and wound infections: an overview. Am Fam Physician 57:2424–2432

Ecthyma

Duve S, Voack C, Rakoski J et al. (1996) Extensive inguinal lymphadenitis. Ecthyma with inguinal lymphadenitis. Arch Dermatol 132:823, 826

Cellulitis

Schwartz GR, Wright SW (1996) Changing bacteriology of periorbital cellulitis. Ann Emerg Med 28:617–620

Studer-Sachsenberg EM, Ruffieux P, Saurat JH (1997) Cellulitis after hip surgery: long-term follow-up of seven cases. Br J Dermatol 137:133–136

Necrotizing Fasciitis

Barton LL, Jeck DT, Vaidya VU (1996) Necrotizing fasciitis in children: report of two cases and review of the literature. Arch Pediatr Adolesc Med 150:105–108

Cha JY, Releford BJ Jr, Marcarelli P (1994) Necrotizing fasciitis: a classification of necrotizing soft tissue infections. J Foot Ankle Surg 33:148–155

Elliott DC, Kufera JA, Myers RA (1996) Necrotizing soft tissue infections. Risk factors for mortality and strategies for management. Ann Surg 224:672–683

Gamba MA, Martinelli M, Schaad HJ et al. (1997) Familial transmission of a serious disease-producing group A streptococcus clone: case reports and review. Clin Infect Dis 24:1118–1121

Jarrett P, Rademaker M, Duffill M (1997) The clinical spectrum of necrotising fasciitis. A review of 15 cases. Aust N Z J Med 27:29–34

Lewis RT (1998) Soft tissue infections. World J Surg 22:146–151

Weiss KA, Laverdiere M (1997) Group A Streptococcus invasive infections: a review. Can J Surg 40:18–25

Chronic Pyodermas

Al Rimawi HS, Hammad MM, Raweily EA et al. (1998) Pyostomatitis vegetans in childhood. Eur J Pediatr 157: 402–405

De Azua J, Sada y Pons C (1903) Pseudo-épithéliomas cutanés. Ann Derm Syph, Paris 4:745–746

Degos PR, Carteaud AL (1953) Pyodermite végétante d'hallopeau (forme en casque et en demi-cuirasse). Annales de Dermatologie 80:254–262

Holmes SC, Thomson J (1996) Recurrent chancriform pyoderma: report of a case with tongue lesions. Is Staphylococcus aureus implicated? Br J Dermatol 133:326–327

Nanta A, Bazex A (1937) Formes cliniques des pyodermites végétantes. Annales de Derm et de Syph 8:609–623

Rongioletti F, Semino M, Drago F et al. (1996) Blastomycosis-like pyoderma (Pyoderma vegetans) responding to antibiotics and topical disodium chromoglycate. Int J Dermatol 35:828–830

Erythrasma

Hartmann AA (1990) The influence of various factors on the human resident skin flora. Semin Dermatol 9:305–308

O'Dell ML (1998) Skin and wound infections: an overview. Am Fam Physician 57:2424–2432

Wharton JR, Wilson PL, Kincannon JM (1998) Erythrasma treated with single-dose clarithromycin. Arch Dermatol 134:671–672

Trichomycosis Axillaris

Hartmann AA (1990) The influence of various factors on the human resident skin flora. Semin Dermatol 9:305–308

Lestringant GG, Qayed KI, Fletcher S (1991) Is the incidence of trichomycosis of genital hair underestimated? J Am Acad Dermatol 24:297–298

Levit F (1990) Trichomycosis axillaris. J Am Acad Dermatol 22:858–859

Pitted Keratolysis

Omura EF, Rye B (1994) Dermatologic disorders of the foot. Clin Sports Med 13:825–841

Takama H, Tamada Y, Yano K et al. (1997) Pitted keratolysis: clinical manifestations in 53 cases. Br J Dermatol 137: 282–285

Vazquez-Lopez F, Perez-Oliva N (1996) Mupirocine ointment for symptomatic pitted keratolysis. Infection 24:55

Cutaneous Diphtheria

Coyle MB, Lipsky BA (1990) Coryneform bacteria in infectious diseases: clinical and laboratory aspects. Clin Microbiol Rev 3:227–246

Funke G, von Graevenitz A, Clarridge JE III et al. (1997) Clinical microbiology of coryneform bacteria. Clin Microbiol Rev 10:125–159

Gamlin C, Stewart GH (1994) Cutaneous diphtheria in Bristol. Commun Dis Rep CDR Rev 4:83–84

Hofler W (1991) Cutaneous diphtheria. Int J Dermatol 30: 845–847

Monsuez JJ, Mathieu D, Arnoult F et al. (1995) Cutaneous diphtheria in a homeless man. Lancet 346:649–650

Listeriosis

Horvat RT, Zahid MA (1994) Human listeriosis: case report and review. Kans Med 95:187–188, 192

Mylonakis E, Hohmann EL, Calderwood SB (1998) Central nervous system infection with Listeria monocytogenes. 33 years' experience at a general hospital and review of 776 episodes from the literature. Medicine (Baltimore) 77:313–336

Paul ML, Dwyer DE, Chow C et al. (1994) Listeriosis – a review of eighty-four cases. Med J Aust 160:489–493

Actinomycosis

Drancourt M, Oules O, Bouche V et al. (1993) Two cases of Actinomyces pyogenes infection in humans. Eur J Clin Microbiol Infect Dis 12:55–57

Sugano S, Matuda T, Suzuki T et al. (1997) Hepatic actinomycosis: case report and review of the literature in Japan. J Gastroenterol 32:672–676

Nagler R, Peled M, Laufer D (1997) Cervicofacial actinomycosis: a diagnostic challenge. Oral Surg Oral Med Oral Pathol Oral Radiol Endod 83:652–656

Nocardiosis

Freland C, Fur JL, Nemirovsky-Trebucq B et al. (1995) Primary cutaneous nocardiosis caused by Nocardia otitidiscaviarum: two cases and a review of the literature. J Trop Med Hyg 98:395–403

Kontoyiannis DP, Ruoff K, Hooper DC (1998) Nocardia bacteremia. Report of 4 cases and review of the literature. Medicine (Baltimore) 77:255–267

Schiff TA, Sanchez M, Moy J et al. (1993) Cutaneous nocardiosis caused by Nocardia nova occurring in an HIV-infected individual: a case report and review of the literature. J Acquir Immune Defic Syndr 6:849–851

Ye Z, Shimomura H, Kudo S et al. (1996) A case of lymphocutaneous nocardiosis with a review of lymphocutaneous nocardiosis reported in Japan. J Dermatol 23:120–124

Cat-Scratch Disease

Dunn MW, Berkowitz FE, Miller JJ et al. (1997) Hepatosplenic cat scratch disease and abdominal pain. Pediatr Infect Dis J 16:269–272

Jerris RC, Regnery RL (1996) Will the real agent of cat-scratch disease please stand up? Annu Rev Microbiol 50:707–725

Shinall EA (1990) Cat scratch disease: a review of the literature. Pediatr Dermatol 7:11–18

Bacillary Angiomatosis

Bastug DF, Ness DT, DeSantis JG (1996) Bacillary angiomatosis mimicking pyogenic granuloma in the hand: a case report. J Hand Surg Am 21:307–308

Fagan WA, DeCamp NC, Kraus EW et al. (1996) Widespread cutaneous bacillary angiomatosis and a large fungating mass in an HIV-positive man. J Am Acad Dermatol 35:285–287

Manders SM (1996) Bacillary angiomatosis. Clin Dermatol 14:295–299

Mohle-Boetani JC, Koehler JE, Berger TG et al. (1996) Bacillary angiomatosis and bacillary peliosis in patients infected with human immunodeficiency virus: clinical characteristics in a case-control study. Clin Infect Dis 22:794–800

Schlüpen EM, Schirren CG, Hoegl L et al. (1997) Molecular diagnosis of deep nodular bacillary angiomatosis and monitoring of therapeutic success. Br J Dermatol 136: 747–751

Stoler MH, Bonfiglio TA, Steigbigel RT et al. (1983) An atypical subcutaneous infection associated with acquired immune deficiency syndrome. Am J Clin Pathol 80:714–718

Trench Fever

Gluckman SJ (1996) Q fever and trench fever. Clin Dermatol 14:283–287

Tompkins LS (1996) Bartonella species infections, including cat-scratch disease, trench fever, and bacillary angiomatosis – what molecular techniques have revealed. West J Med 164:39–41

Bartonellosis

Alexander B (1995) A review of bartonellosis in Ecuador and Colombia. Am J Trop Med Hyg 52:354–359

Bass JW, Vincent JM, Person DA (1997) The expanding spectrum of Bartonella infections: I. Bartonellosis and trench fever. Pediatr Infect Dis J 16:2–10

Nosal JM (1997) Bacillary angiomatosis, cat-scratch disease, and bartonellosis: what's the connection? Int J Dermatol 36:405–411

Schwartzman W (1996) Bartonella (Rochalimaea) infections: beyond cat scratch. Annu Rev Med 47:355–364

Enterobacter Infections

Aliberti LC (1995) Enterococcal nosocomial infection: epidemiology and practice. Gastroenterol Nurs 18:177–181

Brook I (1998) Aerobic and anaerobic microbiology of infections after trauma in children. J Accid Emerg 15: 162–167

Klebsiella Group

Anderson MJ, Janoff EN (1998) Klebsiella endocarditis: report of two cases and review. Clin Infect Dis 26:468–474

Dennesen PJ, Bonten MJ, Weinstein RA (1998) Multiresistant bacteria as a hospital epidemic problem. Ann Med 30:176–185

Rhinoscleroma

Al-Serhani AM, Al-Qahtani AS, Arafa M (1998) Association of rhinoscleroma with rhinosporidiosis. Rhinology 36:43–45

Amoils CP, Shindo ML (1996) Laryngotracheal manifestations of rhinoscleroma. Ann Otol Rhinol Laryngol 105:336–340

Typhoid Fever

Lifshitz EI (1996) Travel trouble: typhoid fever – a case presentation and review. J Am Coll Health 45:99–105

Misra S, Diaz PS, Rowley AH (1997) Characteristics of typhoid fever in children and adolescents in a major metropolitan area in the United States. Clin Infect Dis 24:998–1000

Yersinosis

Giamarellou H, Antoniadou A, Kanavos K et al. (1995) Yersinia enterocolitica endocarditis: case report and literature review. Eur J Clin Microbiol Infect Dis 14:126–130

Taccetti G, Trapani S, Ermini M et al. (1994) Reactive arthritis triggered by Yersinia enterocolitica: a review of 18 pediatric cases. Clin Exp Rheumatol 12:681–684

Tripoli LC, Brouillette DE, Nicholas JJ et al. (1990) Disseminated Yersinia enterocolitica. Case report and review of the literature. J Clin Gastroenterol 12:85–89

Pneumococcal Infections

Campbell GD Jr, Silberman R (1998) Drug-resistant Streptococcus pneumoniae. Clin Infect Dis 26:1188–1195

Hill MD, Karsh J (1997) Invasive soft tissue infections with Streptococcus pneumoniae in patients with systemic lupus erythematosus: case report and review of the literature. Arthritis Rheum 40:1716–1719

Pastor P, Medley F, Murphy TV (1998) Invasive pneumococcal disease in Dallas County, Texas: results from population-based surveillance in 1995. Clin Infect Dis 26:590–595

Plouffe JF, Breiman RF, Facklam RR (1996) Bacteremia with Streptococcus pneumoniae. Implications for therapy and prevention. Franklin County Pneumonia Study Group. JAMA 275:194–198

Meningococcal Infections

Booy R, Kroll JS (1998) Bacterial meningitis and meningococcal infection. Curr Opin Pediatr 10:13–18

Corbett Feeney G (1996) A laboratory review of meningococcal infections in the west of Ireland. Ir J Med Sci 165:292–293

Ploysangam T, Sheth AP (1996) Chronic meningococcemia in childhood: case report and review of the literature. Pediatr Dermatol 13:483–487

Vibrio Infections

Kumamoto KS, Vukich DJ (1998) Clinical infections of Vibrio vulnificus: a case report and review of the literature. J Emerg Med 16:61–66

Mouzin E, Mascola L, Tormey MP et al. (1997) Prevention of Vibrio vulnificus infections. Assessment of regulatory educational strategies. JAMA 278:576–578

Helicobacter Infections

Veenendaal RA, Gotz JM, Lamers CB (1996) Mucosal inflammation and disease in Helicobacter pylori infection. Scand J Gastroenterol [Suppl] 218:86–91

Pseudomonas Infections

Chun WH, Kim YK, Kim LS et al. (1996) Ecthyma gangrenosum associated with aplastic anemia. J Korean Med Sci 11:64–67

Murphy O, Marsh PJ, Gray J et al. (1996) Ecthyma gangrenosum occurring at sites of iatrogenic trauma in pediatric oncology patients. Med Pediatr Oncol 27:62–63

Ng W, Tan CL, Yeow V et al. (1998) Ecthyma gangrenosum in a patient with hypogammaglobulinemia. J Infect 36:331–335

Paraskaki I, Lebessi E, Legakis NJ (1996) Epidemiology of community-acquired Pseudomonas aeruginosa infections in children. Eur J Clin Microbiol Infect Dis 15: 782–786

Actinetobacter, Moraxella and Branhamella Infections

Daoud A, Abuekteish F, Masaadeh H (1996) Neonatal meningitis due to Moraxella catarrhalis and review of the literature. Ann Trop Paediatr 16:199–201

Fish DN, Danziger LH (1993) Neglected pathogens: bacterial infections in persons with human immunodeficiency virus infection. A review of the literature (1). Pharmacotherapy 13:415–4139

Whipple Disease

Matsui T, Kayashima K, Kito M et al. (1996) Three cases of Pasteurella multocida skin infection from pet cats. J Dermatol 23:502–504

Koch CA, Mabee CL, Robyn JA et al. (1996) Exposure to domestic cats: risk factor for Pasteurella multocida peritonitis in liver cirrhosis? Am J Gastroenterol 91:1447–1449

Lyme Disease

Alonso-Llamazares J, Persing DH, Anda P et al. (1997) No evidence for Borrelia burgdorferi infection in lesions of morphea and lichen sclerosus et atrophicus in Spain. A prospective study and literature review. Acta Dermato Venereol (Stockh) 77:299–304

Bannwarth A (1941) Chronische lymphocytäre Meningitis, entzündliche Polyneuritis und "Rheumatismus." Ein Beitrag zum Problem Allergie und Nervensystem. Arch Psychiat Nervenkr 113:284–376

Berger BW (1997) Current aspects of Lyme disease and other Borrelia burgdorferi infections. Dermatol Clin 15: 247–255

Bergloff J, Gasser R, Feigl B (1994) Ophthalmic manifestations in Lyme borreliosis. A review. J Neuroophthalmol 14:15–20

Burmester GR (1993) Lessons from Lyme arthritis. Clin Exp Rheumatol [Suppl] 8:S23–27

Carlberg H, Naito S (1991) Lyme borreliosis – a review and present situation in Japan. J Dermatol 18:125–142

Coyle PK (1997) Borrelia burgdorferi infection: clinical diagnostic techniques. Immunol Invest 26:117–128

Horowitz HW, Sanghera K, Goldberg N et al. (1994) Dermatomyositis associated with Lyme disease: case report and review of Lyme myositis. Clin Infect Dis 18: 166–171

Jantausch BA (1994) Lyme disease, Rocky Mountain spotted fever, ehrlichiosis: emerging and established challenges for the clinician. Ann Allergy 73:4–11

Krbkova L, Stanek G (1996) Therapy of Lyme borreliosis in children. Infection 24:170–173

Leslie TA, Levell NJ, Cutler SJ et al. (1994) Acrodermatitis chronica atrophicans: a case report and review of the literature. Br J Dermatol 131:687–693

Malane MS, Grant Kels JM, Feder HM Jr et al. (1991) Diagnosis of Lyme disease based on dermatologic manifestations. Ann Intern Med 114:490–498

Nadelman RB, Wormser GP (1998) Lyme borreliosis. Lancet 352:557–565

Nagi KS, Joshi R, Thakur RK (1996) Cardiac manifestations of Lyme disease: a review. Can J Cardiol 12:503–506

O'Connell S (1993) Lyme disease: a review. Commun Dis Rep CDR Rev 3:R111–115

Oliver JH Jr (1996) Lyme borreliosis in the southern United States: a review. J Parasitol 82:926–935

Picken RN, Strle F, Ruzic-Sabljic E et al. (1997) Molecular subtyping of Borrelia burgdorferi sensu lato isolates from five patients with solitary lymphocytoma. J Invest Dermatol 108:92–97

Recommendation for the use of Lyme disease vaccine. Arch Dermatol 135:1425–1426. MMWR (1999) 48:11–13

Schmidt BL (1997) PCR in laboratory diagnosis of human Borrelia burgdorferi infections. Clin Microbiol Rev 10: 185–201

Seinost G, Golde WT, Berger BW et al. (1999) Infection with multiple strains of *Borrelia burgdorferi* sensu stricto in patients with Lyme disease. Arch Dermatol 135:1329–1333

Strle F, Maraspin V, Pleterski-Rigler D et al. (1996) Treatment of borrelial lymphocytoma. Infection 24:80–84

Strle F, Picken RN, Cheng Y et al. (1997) Clinical findings for patients with Lyme borreliosis caused by Borrelia burgdorferi sensu lato with genotypic and phenoty pic similarities to strain 25015. Clin Infect Dis 25:273–280

Weber K (1996) Treatment failure in erythema migrans – a review. Infection 24:73–75

Leptospirosis

Monno S, Mizushima Y (1993) Leptospirosis with acute acalculous cholecystitis and pancreatitis. J Clin Gastroenterol 16:52–54

Shaked Y, Shpilberg O, Samra D et al. (1993) Leptospirosis in pregnancy and its effect on the fetus: case report and review. Clin Infect Dis 17:241–243

Smythe L, Dohnt M, Norris M et al. (1996) Review of leptospirosis notifications in Queensland 1985 to 1996. Commun Dis Intell 21:17–20

Relapsing Fever

Cadavid D, Barbour AG (1998) Neuroborreliosis during relapsing fever: review of the clinical manifestations, pathology, and treatment of infections in humans and experimental animals. Clin Infect Dis 26:151–164

Myers SA, Sexton DJ (1994) Dermatologic manifestations of arthropod-borne diseases. Infect Dis Clin North Am 8:689–712

Clostridial Infections

Patel SB, Mahler R (1990) Clostridial pleuropulmonary infections: case report and review of the literature. J Infect 21:81–85

Present DA, Meislin R, Shaffer B (1990) Gas gangrene. A review. Orthop Rev 19:333–341

Schweitzer MA, Sweiss I, Silver DL et al. (1996) The clinical spectrum of Clostridium difficile colitis in immunocompromised patients. Am Surg 62:603–608

Settle CD, Wilcox MH (1996) Review article: antibiotic-induced Clostridium difficile infection. Aliment Pharmacol Ther 10:835–841

Zimmerman MJ, Bak A, Sutherland LR (1997) Review article: treatment of Clostridium difficile infection. Aliment Pharmacol Ther 11:1003–1012

Bites

Chidzonga MM (1998) Human bites of the face. A review of 22 cases. S Afr Med J 88:150–152

Garcia VF (1997) Animal bites and Pasturella infections. Pediatr Rev 18:127–130

Shewell PC, Nancarrow JD (1991) Dogs that bite. BMJ 303: 1512–1513

Vaughn JD (1996) Cat bites in primary care: a case report. Nebr Med J 81:163–165

Wiley JF Jr (1990) Mammalian bites. Review of evaluation and management. Clin Pediatr Phila 29:283–287

Young S (1997) Dog attacks. Aust Fam Physician 26:1375–1377

Zoonoses

General

Grisi L (1990) Parasitic zoonoses: selective review of some diseases in South America. Ann Parasitol Hum Comp 65 [Suppl 1]:79–82

Sanford JP (1990) Humans and animals: increasing contacts, increasing infections. Hosp Pract Off Ed 25:123–130, 133–134, 137–140

Erysipeloid

Connor MP, Green AD (1995) Erysipeloid infection in a sheep farmer with coexisting orf. J Infect 30:161–163

Razsi L, Sanchez MR (1994) Progressively enlarging painful annular plaque on the hand. Erysipeloid. Arch Dermatol 130:1311–1312, 1314–1315

Glanders

Al-Izzi SA, Al-Bassam LS (1989) In vitro susceptibility of Pseudomonas mallei to antimicrobial agents. Comp Immunol Microbiol Infect Dis 12:5–8

Smith AW, Vedros NA, Akers TG et al. (1978) Hazards of disease transfer from marine mammals to land mammals: review and recent findings. J Am Vet Med Assoc 173:1131–1133

Melioidosis

Dorman SE, Gill VJ, Gallin JI et al. (1998) Burkholderia pseudomallei infection in a Puerto Rican patient with chronic granulomatous disease: case report and review of occurrences in the Americas. Clin Infect Dis 26: 889–894

Golledge CL, Chin WS, Tribe AE et al. (1992) A case of human melioidosis originating in south-west Western Australia. Med J Aust 157:332–334

Lim MK, Tan EH, Soh CS et al. (1997) Burkholderia pseudomallei infection in the Singapore Armed Forces from 1987 to 1994 – an epidemiological review. Ann Acad Med Singapore 26:13–17

Anthrax

Doganay M, Aygen B (1997) Diagnosis: cutaneous anthrax. Clin Infect Dis 25:607, 725

Dragon DC, Rennie RP (1995) The ecology of anthrax spores: tough but not invincible. Can Vet J 36:295–301

Mallon E, McKee PH (1997) Extraordinary case report: cutaneous anthrax. Am J Dermatopathol 19:79–82

Shlyakhov E, Rubinstein E (1996) Evaluation of the anthraxin skin test for diagnosis of acute and past human anthrax. Eur J Clin Microbiol Infect Dis 15:242–245

Plague

Crook LD, Tempest B (1992) Plague. A clinical review of 27 cases. Arch Intern Med 152:1253–1256

Culliton BJ (1997) The microbial plague continues. Nat Med 3:1

Galimand M, Guiyoule A, Gerbaud G et al. (1997) Multidrug resistance in Yersinia pestis mediated by a transferable plasmid. N Engl J Med 337:677–680

Perry RD, Fetherston JD (1997) Yersinia pestis – etiologic agent of plague. Clin Microbiol Rev 10:35–66

Solomon T (1995) Alexandre Yersin and the plague bacillus. J Trop Med Hyg 98:209–212

Tularemia

Capellan J, Fong IW (1993) Tularemia from a cat bite: case report and review of feline-associated tularemia. Clin Infect Dis 16:472–475

Enderlin G, Morales L, Jacobs RF et al. (1994) Streptomycin and alternative agents for the treatment of tularemia: review of the literature. Clin Infect Dis 19:42–47

Kodama BF, Fitzpatrick JE, Gentry RH (1994) Tularemia. Cutis 54:279–280

Myers SA, Sexton DJ (1994) Dermatologic manifestations of arthropod borne diseases. Infect Dis Clin North Am 8:689–712

Risi GF, Pombo DJ (1995) Relapse of tularemia after aminoglycoside therapy: case report and discussion of therapeutic options. Clin Infect Dis 20:174–175

Brucellosis

Ablin J, Mevorach D, Eliakim R (1997) Brucellosis and the gastrointestinal tract. The odd couple. J Clin Gastroenterol 24:25–29

Corry JE, Hinton MH (1997) Zoonoses in the meat industry: a review. Acta Vet Hung 45:457–479

Habeeb YK, Al-Najdi AK, Sadek SA et al. (1998) Paediatric neurobrucellosis: case report and literature review. J Infect 37:59–62

Vallejo JG, Stevens AM, Dutton RV et al. (1996) Hepatosplenic abscesses due to Brucella melitensis: report of a case involving a child and review of the literature. Clin Infect Dis 22:485–489

Rat Bite Fever

Hagelskjaer L, Sorensen I, Randers E (1998) Streptobacillus moniliformis infection: 2 cases and a literature review. Scand J Infect Dis 30:309–311

Vasseur E, Joly P, Nouvellon M et al. (1993) Cutaneous abscess: a rare complication of Streptobacillus moniliformis infection. Br J Dermatol 129:95–96

Cunningham BB, Paller AS, Katz BZ (1998) Rat bite fever in a pet lover. J Am Acad Dermatol 38:330–332

Rat-bite fever – New Mexico (1996) MMWR 47:89–91

Wullenweber M (1995) Streptobacillus moniliformis – a zoonotic pathogen. Taxonomic considerations, host species, diagnosis, therapy, geographical distribution. Lab Anim 29:1–15

Other Zoonoses

Chang HJ, Miller HL, Watkins N et al. (1998) An epidemic of Malassezia pachydermatis in an intensive care nursery associated with colonization of health care workers' pet dogs. N Engl J Med 338:706–711

Groshek PM (1998) Malassezia pachydermatis. N Engl J Med 339:270–271

Lautenbach E, Nachamkin I, Schuster MG (1998) Malassezia pachydermatis. N Engl J Med 339:270–271

Tuberculosis

Bannon MJ (1999) BCG and tuberculosis. Arch Dis Child 80:80–83

DeRiemer K, Rudoy I, Schechter GF et al. (1999) The epidemiology of tuberculosis diagnosed after death in San Francisco, 1986–1995. Int J Tuberc Lung Dis 6:488–493

Eltringham IJ, Drobniewski F (1998) Multiple drug resistant tuberculosis: aetiology, diagnosis and outcome. Br Med Bull 54:569–578

Mault JR, Pomerantz M (1999) Mycobacterium tuberculosis and other mycobacteria. Chest Surg Clin North Am 9:227–238

WHO (1996) TB/HIV – a clinical manual. WHO, Geneva

Cutaneous Tuberculosis

Barbareschi M, Denti F, Bottelli S et al. (1999) Pulmonary tuberculosis revealed by lupus vulgaris in an immunocompetent patient. Eur J Dermatol 9:43–44

Boonchai W, Suthipinittharm P, Mahaisavariya P (1998) Panniculitis in tuberculosis: a clinicopathologic study of nodular panniculitis associated with tuberculosis. Int J Dermatol 37:361–363

Chong LY, Lo KK (1995) Cutaneous tuberculosis in Hong Kong: a 10 year retrospective study. Int J Dermatol 34: 26–29

Gooptu C, Marks N, Thomas J et al. (1998) Squamous cell carcinoma associated with lupus vulgaris. Clin Exp Dermatol 23:99–102

Kakakhel K (1998) Smultaneous occurrence of tuberculous gumma, tuberculosis verrucosis cutis, and lichen scrofulosorum. Int J Dermatol 37:867–869

Masellis P, Gasparini G, Caputo R et al. (1995) Tuberculosis verrucosa cutis which remained undiagnosed for forty three years. Dermatology 191:145–148

Moiin A, Downham TF Jr (1996) A slow growing lesion on the face. Lupus vulgaris. Arch Dermatol 132:83, 86

Nachbar F, Classen V, Nachbar T et al. (1996) Orificial tuberculosis: detection by polymerase chain reaction. Br J Dermatol 135:106–109

Pramatarov K, Balabanova M, Miteva L et al. (1993) Tuberculosis verrucosa cutis associated with lupus vulgaris. Int J Dermatol 32:815–817

Salazar JC, Bloom KE, Hostetter MK et al. (1996) Drug resistant tuberculosis verrucosa cutis in a Southeast Asian teenager. Pediatr Infect Dis J 15:834–836

Sehgal VN, Gupta R, Bose M et al. (1993) Immunohistopathological spectrum in cutaneous tuberculosis. Clin Exp Dermatol 18:309–313

Sutor GC, Ockenga J, Kirschner P et al. (1997) Tuberculosis cutis colliquativa during long term immunosuppressive therapy for rheumatoid arthritis. Arthritis Rheum 40: 188–190

Tur E, Brenner S, Meiron Y (1996) Scrofuloderma (tuberculosis colliquativa cutis). Br J Dermatol 134:350–352

Yates VM, Ormerod LP (1997) Cutaneous tuberculosis in Blackburn district (U.K.): a 15 year prospective series, 1981–1995. Br J Dermatol 136:483–489

Yerushalmi J, Grunwald MH, Halevy DH et al. (1998) Lupus vulgaris complicated by metastatic squamous cell carcinoma. Int J Dermatol 37:934–935

Tuberculids

Braun-Falco O, Thomas P (1995) Zum Tuberkulid-Begriff aus heutiger Sicht. Hautarzt 46:383–387

Degitz K, Steidl M, Thomas P et al. (1993) Aetiology of tuberculids. Lancet 341:239–240

Jordaan HF, Schneider JW, Schaaf HS et al. (1996) Papulonecrotic tuberculid in children. A report of eight patients. Am J Dermatopathol 18:172–185

Jordaan HF, Van Niekerk DJ, Louw M (1994) Papulonecrotic tuberculid. A clinical, histopathological, and immunohistochemical study of 15 patients. Am J Dermatopathol 16:474–485

Park YM, Hong JK, Cho SH (1998) Concomitant lichen scrofulosorum and erythema induratum. J Am Acad Dermatol 38:841–843

Ramdial PK, Mosam A, Mallett R (1998) Papulonecrotic tuberculid in a 2 year old girl: with emphasis on extent of disease and presence of leucocytoclastic vasculitis. Pediatr Dermatol 15:450–455

Roblin D, Kelly R, Wansbrough Jones M et al. (1994) Papulonecrotic tuberculide and erythema induratum as presenting manifestations of tuberculosis. J Infect 28:193–197

Schneider JW, Jordaan HF (1997) The histopathologic spectrum of erythema induratum of Bazin. Am J Dermatopathol 19:323–333

Vanhooteghem O, Doffiny Y (1996) Lichen scrofulosorum type tuberculids of the face. Dermatology 192:393–395

Pseudotuberculids

Hodak E, Trattner A, Feuerman H et al. (1997) Lupus miliaris disseminatus faciei – the DNA of Mycobacterium tuberculosis is not detectable in active lesions by polymerase chain reaction. Br J Dermatol 137:614–619

Swimming Pool Granuloma

Hoyen HA, Lacey SH, Graham TJ (1998) Atypical hand infections. Hand Clin 14:613–634

Lee MW, Brenan J (1998) Mycobacterium marinum: chronic and extensive infections of the lower limbs in south Pacific islanders. Aust J Dermatol 39:173–176

Posteraro B, Sanguinetti M, Garcovich A et al. (1998) Polymerase chain reaction-reverse cross-blot hybridization assay in the diagnosis of sporotrichoid Mycobacterium marinum infection. Br J Dermatol 139:872–876

Other Atypical Mycobacteria

Callahan EF, Licata AL, Madison JF (1997) Cutaneous Mycobacterium kansasii infection associated with a papulonecrotic tuberculid reaction. J Am Acad Dermatol 36: 497–499

Czelusta A, Moore AY (1999) Cutaneous Mycobacterium kansasii infection in a patient with systemic lupus erythematosus: case report and review. J Am Acad Dermatol 40:359–363

Griffith DE (1998) Mycobacteria as pathogens of respiratory infection. Infect Dis Clin North Am 12:593–611

Klein JL, Corbett EL, Slade PM (1998) Mycobacterium kansasii and human immunodeficiency virus co-infection in London. J Infect 37:252–259

Mandell GL, Douglas RG Jr, Bennett JE (eds) (1990) Principles and practice of infectious diseases, 3rd edn. Churchill Livingstone, New York

Ong EL (1999) Prophylaxis against disseminated Mycobacterium avium complex in AIDS. J Infect 38:6–8

Leprosy

Calderon P, Anzilotti M, Phelps R (1997) Thalidomide in dermatology. New indications for an old drug. Int J Dermatol 36:881–887

Choudhri SH, Magro CM, Crowson AN (1994) An Id reaction to Mycobacterium leprae: first documented case. Cutis 54:282–286

Nations SP, Katz JS, Lyde CB et al. (1998) Leprous neuropathy: an American perspective. Semin Neurol 18:113–124

Ramu G (1995) Clinical features and diagnosis of relapses in leprosy. Indian J Lepr 67:45–59

Sehgal VN (1994) Leprosy. Dermatol Clin 12:629–644

Style A (1995) Early diagnosis and treatment of leprosy in the United States. Am Fam Physician 52:172–178

Wathen PI (1996) Hansen's disease. South Med J 89:647–652

WHO Expert Committee on Leprosy (1998) World Health Organ Tech Rep Ser 874:1–43

Lepromatous Leprosy

Ajithkumar K (1998) Leprosy type 1 reaction as the first manifestation of borderline lepromatous leprosy. Br J Dermatol 139:922

Bainson KA, Van den Borne B (1998) Dimensions and process of stigmatization in leprosy. Lepr Rev 69:341–350

Barral-Netto M, Santos S, Santos I et al. (1999) Immunochemotherapy with interferon-gamma and multidrug therapy for multibacillary leprosy. Acta Trop 72:185–201

Cuevas-Santos J, Contreras F, McNutt NS (1998) Multibacillary leprosy: lesions with macrophages positive for S100 protein and dendritic cells positive for Factor 13a. J Cutan Pathol 25:530–537

Fajardo TT, Abalos RM, de la Cruz EC et al. (1999) Clofazimine therapy for lepromatous leprosy: a historical perspective. Int J Dermatol 38:70–74

Porche D (1999) Thalidomide: the past, present, and future. J Assoc Nurses AIDS Care 10:82–84

West BC (1998) Endemic lepromatous leprosy. Clin Infect Dis 27:1340–1341

Indeterminate Leprosy

Cossermelli-Messina W, Festa-Neto C, Cossermelli W (1998) Articular inflammatory manifestations in patients with different forms of leprosy. J Rheumatol 25:111–119

Jayakumar J, Aschhoff M, Job CK (1997) A case of morphoea with dermal neuritis as in indeterminate leprosy. Indian J Lepr 69:407–409

Saha K, Chattopadhya D, Kulpati DD (1998) Concomitant kala-azar, malaria, and progressive unstable indeterminate leprosy in an 8-year-old child. J Trop Pediatr 44:247–248

Sayal SK, Das AL, Gupta CM (1997) Concurrent leprosy and HIV infection: a report of three cases. Indian J Lepr 69:261–265

Tuberculoid Leprosy

Ng PP, Goh CL (1998) Sparing of tuberculoid leprosy patch in a patient with dapsone hypersensitivity syndrome. J Am Acad Dermatol 39:646–648

Pimentel MI, Sampaio EP, Nery JA et al. (1996) Borderline-tuberculoid leprosy: clinical and immunological heterogeneity. Lepr Rev 67:287–296

Ramesh V, Kulkarni SB, Misra RS et al. (1998) Sporotrichoid tuberculoid leprosy. Acta Derm Venereol 78:381

Borderline Leprosy

Croft R, Hossein D (1996) Case report: cutaneous lymphoma and borderline leprosy simulating lepromatous leprosy. Lepr Rev 67:145–147

Edward VK, Edward S, Shegaonkar S (1996) Dry skin lesions with marked hair loss in a case of BL leprosy. A case report. Lepr Rev 67:141–144

Zirn JR, Foitl DR, Shea CR (1996) Generalized rash in a Dominican immigrant. Borderline leprosy (Hansen's disease) with type 1 upgrading (ie, reversal) reaction. Arch Dermatol 132:82–83, 85–86

Primary Immunodeficiency Diseases

Bruton OC (1952) Agammaglobulinemia. Pediatrics 9:722–728

Dahl MV (1996) Clinical immunodermatology. Mosby, St. Louis

Buckley RH, Sampson HA (1981) The hyperimmunoglobulinemia E syndrom. In: Franklin EC (ed) Clincal immunology update. Churchill, Livingston, Edinburgh, pp 147–162

Davis SD, Schaller J, Wedgwood RJ (1966) Job's syndrome: recurrent "cold" staphylococcal abscesses. Lancet i:1013–1015

Di George AM (moderator) (1965) New concept of cellular basis of immunity. (Discussion of Cooper MD, Peterson RDA, Good RA). J Pediatr 67:907–908

Eley BS, Hughes J, Cooper M et al. (1997) Primary immunodeficiency diseases at Red Cross War Memorial Children's Hospital. S Afr Med J 87:1684–1688

Friedrich W (1996) Bone marrow transplantation in immunodeficiency diseases. Ann Med 28:115–119

Gribacher B, Holland SM, Gallin JI (1999) Hyper-IgE syndrome with recurrent infections – an autosomal dominant multisystem disorder. N Engl J Med 340:692–702

Knutsen AP, Wall D, Mueller KR (1996) Abnormal in vitro thymocyte differentiation in a patient with severe combined immunodeficiency-Nezelof's syndrome. J Clin Immunol 16:151–158

Makitie O, Kaitila I, Savilahti E (1998) Susceptibility to infections and in vitro immune functions in cartilage-hair hypoplasia. Eur J Pediatr 157:816–820

Markert ML, Hummell DS, Rosenblatt HM (1998) Complete DiGeorge syndrome: persistence of profound immunodeficiency. J Pediatr 132:15–21

McKusick VA, Eldridge R, Hastetler JA et al. (1965) Dwarfism in the Amish. II. Cartilage-hair Hypoplasia. Bull Johns Hopkins Hops 116:285–326

Nezelof C, Jammet ML, Lortholary P et al. (1964) L'hypoplasie héréditaire du thymus sa place et sa responsibilité dans une observation d'aplasie lymphocytare normoplasmacytaire et normoglbulininémique du nourissau. Arch Fr Pediatr 21:897–920

Ochs HD, Smith CI (1996) X-linked agammaglobulinemia. A clinical and molecular analysis. Medicine (Baltimore) 75:287–299

Uribe L, Weinberg KI (1998) X-linked SCID and other defects of cytokine pathways. Semin Hematol 35:299–309

CHAPTER 5

Sexually Transmitted Bacterial Diseases

Contents

Gonorrhea

Synonyms. GC, clap, drip

Definition. Infection primarily involving mucosal surfaces, producing prominent urethral discharge in men and capable of causing hematogenous infection.

Causative Organism. *Neisseria gonorrhoeae*, or the gonococcus, was identified by Albert NEISSER, the founder of the famous dermatology clinic in Breslau, Germany (now Wroclaw, Poland) in 1879. Another crucial member of the *Neisseriaceae* family is *N. meningitidis*, a common cause of meningitis. These two bacteria and a series of nonpathogenic relatives are all gram-negative aerobic diplococci (Fig. 5.1).

Epidemiology. Gonorrhea is one of the most common sexually transmitted diseases. WHO data suggests there are 25 million new cases yearly, ranking gonorrhea fourth among sexually transmitted diseases after trichomoniasis, chlamydial infections and genital warts. Humans are the only host for *N. gonorrhoeae* and transfer occurs only by direct mucosal contact, usually during sexual intercourse. The infection is often asymptomatic, making it difficult to track and control. The incubation period is highly variable, usually ranging between 1 and 6 days, but lasting up to 14 days.

Etiology and Pathogenesis. *Neisseria gonorrhoeae* prefers the columnar epithelium of the urethra, the cervical canal, the rectum and the conjunctiva. While the keratinizing epithelium of the adult vagina is quite resistant to *N. gonorrhoeae*, that

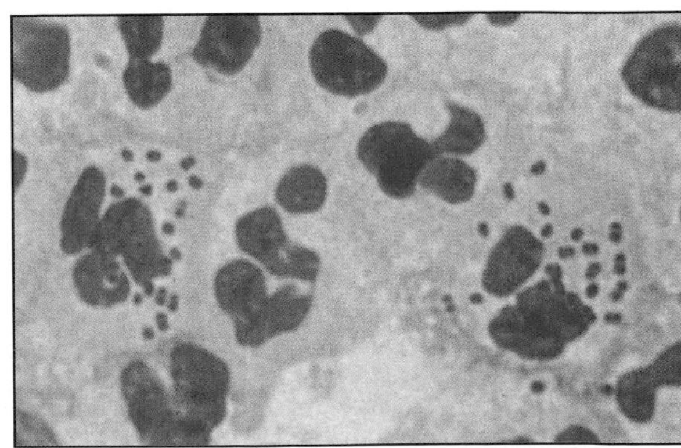

Fig. 5.1. *Neisseria gonorrhoeae*

of prepubertal girls, pregnant women and the elderly is more easily colonized. The false vagina constructed out of penile skin in some sex change operations may also be colonized. Surface adhesion molecules, such as the pilus and opaque proteins, help the bacteria to attach; then other membrane proteins attack the host epithelium and destroy surface IgA. Bacterial protein I is important in attachment, while bacterial protein II mediates endocytosis. The bacteria then cross the mucosal barrier and may be phagocytosed by circulating neutrophils, producing the marked pus that characterizes gonorrhea. Occasionally *N. gonorrhoeae* reaches the blood stream, causing sepsis. Certain types are more likely to spread systemically. No lasting immunity is achieved.

Clinical Findings. Infection with *N. gonorrhoeae* produces a broad spectrum of disease patterns. Crucial factors include the site of inoculation, the subtype of bacteria and the host's immune status. Asymptomatic infections are common. Most often, localized mucosal infections develop, but they may spread locally, ascending the genitourinary tract or evolve into sepsis. As part of the evaluation of any patient with suspected gonorrhea, the physician should do serologic testing for syphilis and be alert to the frequent presence of two or more sexually transmitted diseases simultaneously.

Gonococcal Urethritis in Men

This is the best known form of gonorrhea, known in slang as the clap or the drip because of the extensive, foul-smelling urethral discharge of pus. Most men are asymptomatic, developing both a discharge and dysuria 2–6 days after exposure. The urethral orifice is usually inflamed and there may be a balanitis because of the irritation from the discharge and secondary infection (Figs. 5.2, 5.3). A humorous but valuable question to ask a patient with urethral discharge is, "Is it so bad that you must throw away your underwear?" If the answer is positive, the diagnosis of *N. gonorrhoeae* infection is almost clinched. About 25% of patients have a

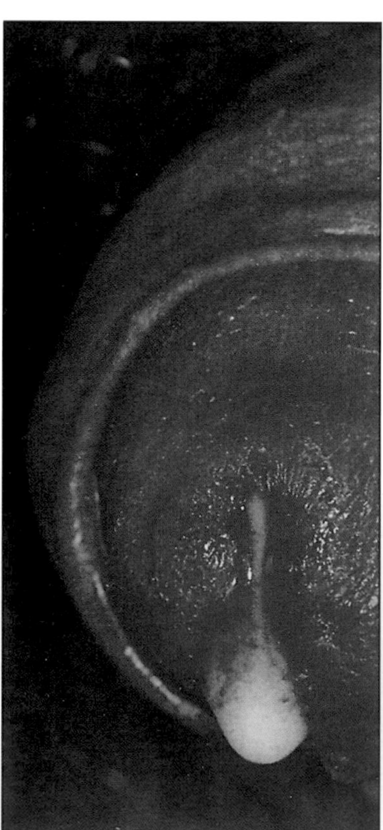

Fig. 5.2. Acute urethritis in gonorrhea

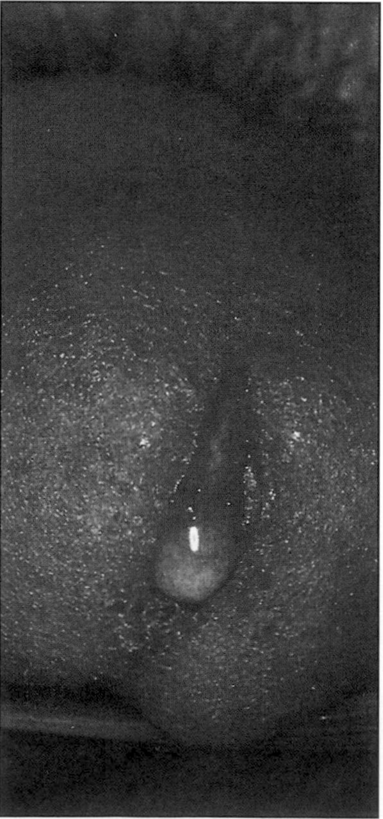

Fig. 5.3. Chronic urethritis in gonorrhea

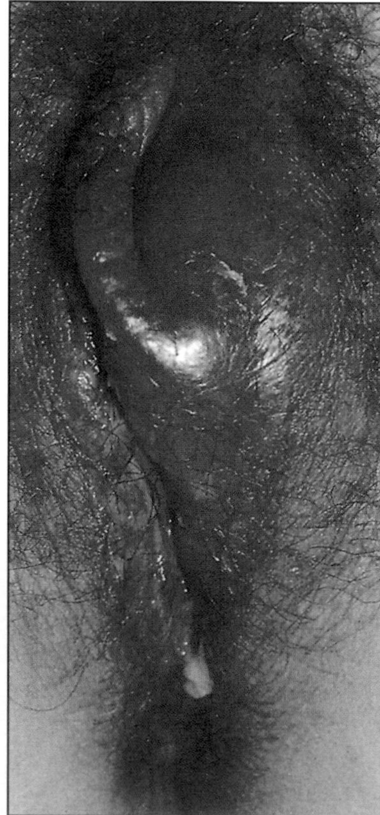

Fig. 5.4. Bartholin gland abscess in gonorrhea

scant discharge that cannot be distinguished from nongonococcal urethritis. Often they are asymptomatic during the day but have a drop of discharge in the morning (the so-called Bonjour drop or good morning sign). At least 10% are totally asymptomatic and identified only in epidemiological studies. The severe discharge clears after about 3 weeks and the entire process resolves over 6 months. No immunity is developed.

The evaluation of a patient suspected of having gonorrhea should include a search for lymphadenopathy and an evaluation of both the anal and the genital regions. The urethral smear is best obtained first thing in the morning, or in any event after the patient has not urinated for several hours. If the discharge is scant, material can be milked forward manually.

Local complications of urethral gonococcal infection were formerly feared but have today become quite uncommon. They include:

- Littré abscess involving periurethral glands
- Paraurethral abscesses
- Proximal urethral involvement with frequency and terminal hematuria
- Cowper gland abscess involving the bulbourethral glands, producing a swelling behind the base of the scrotum that can produce a proximal or Cowper stricture

In addition, occasionally solitary or multiple ulcers may be seen with gonorrhea. The lesions may involve genital skin and mucosa, typically have ragged edges and are covered with necrotic material. An accompanying urethritis or cervicitis may be absent. One should also always suspect a joint infection with *Treponema pallidum.*

Differential Diagnosis. If the discharge is scant or if the direct examination and culture are negative, one then must search for other forms of urethritis.

Ascending Gonorrhea in Men

Ascending infections of the male genital tract are very uncommon today. Prostatitis, seminal vesiculitis, and epididymitis are all possible; typically there is marked clinical overlap.

Only about 10% of all prostatitis is caused by *N. gonorrhoeae*. Acute prostatitis is characterized by fever, chills, inability to urinate and lower abdominal pain. On rectal examination, the prostate is swollen and tender. Culture of discharge or urine is the correct approach. Chronic prostatitis has less specific symptoms and a multifactorial basis. Prostate massage is often employed to produce a discharge that can be cultured to confirm the diagnosis.

Epididymitis is a feared complication of gonorrhea but in most cases is actually caused by other organisms; in only about 15% of cases is *N. gonorrhoeae* cultured. Usually there is the abrupt onset of unilateral scrotal pain and swelling. Examination initially reveals swelling at the base of the testis but soon the entire epididymis is swollen and the testis hard to localize. Ultrasound examination can help confirm the diagnosis. Often there is no urethral discharge. Obliteration of the vas deferens is a possible complication; thus ascending gonococcal infections can lead to sterility.

If ascending gonorrhea is suspected, additional culture material is needed. In acute prostatitis, a midstream urine suffices. In chronic prostatitis, often the four glass test is used: four specimens are cultured – initial urine, midstream urine, secretions after prostatic massage and final urine. If epididymitis is suspected, then a midstream urine and ejaculate should be cultured.

Differential Diagnosis. A long list of other bacteria can cause ascending infections; included are *Escheria coli*, a common cause in the insertive male homosexual, *Streptococcus faecalis, Staphylococcus aureus, Chlamydia trachomatis and Ureaplasma urealyticum.* The other organisms are usually transmitted nonsexually and follow genitourinary infections or surgery. *Mycobacterium tuberculosis* can cause both prostatitis and epididymitis, which is often bilateral. Other causes of acute unilateral scrotal pain include mumps, testicular torsion and testicular tumors.

Urogenital Gonorrhea in Women

The cervix and cervical canal are the most common site of infection in women. In about 75% of patients with gonococcal cervicitis, there is also an urethritis. In women who have had a hysterectomy, the urethra becomes the most common site. The most frequent complaint is discharge, often associated with burning on urination. With endometrial involvement, there may be vaginal bleeding. Over 50% of infected women are asymptomatic. This is a major factor in explaining the difficulties in controlling gonorrhea through public health measures.

On examination, one can identify the pus dis charge, as well as erythema and swelling of the cervix and easy bleeding on minimal contact. Sometimes pus can be expressed from the urethra. Local complications include infections of Skene's periurethral glands and Bartholin's labial glands (Fig. 5.4). In such cases there may be local swelling and pus visualized in the ostia of the ducts. Usually a Bartholin's gland abscess with *N. gonorrhoeae* is unilateral; all such abscesses should also be cultured for gonococci. Patients complain of pain when sitting or walking. In addition, there may be erythema and swelling of the labia, evolving into a vulvitis.

Obtaining material for culture is somewhat more complicated in women than in men. First the urethra should be examined and cultured. The Bartholin glands can be palpated and if any discharge is produced, it too is cultured. After this the speculum is inserted in the routine fashion, the cervix cleaned and then a culture taken from the cervical canal. In confusing cases multiple cultures may be needed; the yield is higher 2–3 days after menstruation. A rectal culture can also be taken, using a cotton-tipped applicator moistened in physiologic saline. At the same time, material should be obtained for routine bacterial, viral and candidal cultures, depending on the clinical situation.

Differential Diagnosis. Gonorrhea in women is often a culture diagnosis. Clinical signs and symptoms may be minimal and a wide variety of other organisms, including *C. trachomatis, Trichomonas vaginalis, Candida albicans,* herpes simplex virus and others can produce the same clinical picture. Mixed infections with two or more organisms are not uncommon.

Ascending Gonorrhea in Women

Neisseria gonorrhoeae may spread from the cervix to the endometrium, fallopian tubes, ovaries and then into the peritoneum. The exact degree of spread is often hard to determine, so one speaks of pelvic inflammatory disease (PID; Chap. 35). Menstruation, recent delivery and miscarriage all predispose a patient to ascending infections.

The endometrial involvement is typically minimal. There may be a bloody discharge or excessive menstrual blood flow. Usually the endometrium simply serves as a way station for the spread to the fallopian tubes. Salpingitis develops in 10–20% of cases of acute gonorrhea. The patients are often quite ill, with nausea, vomiting, abdominal pain and fever. Milder, more chronic cases may cause only vague abdominal complaints or dyspareunia. Physical examination reveals a cervical discharge, tenderness when the cervix is manipulated, guarding and rigidity of the abdominal wall and adnexal fullness and tenderness. The pain on examination may be so severe that the patient jumps in pain; this has been crudely designated the chandelier sign. In more chronic disease, thickened tubes and painful bilateral adnexal masses can be found. Fever, elevated neutrophil count and other laboratory signs of sepsis may be present. The chronic or late sequelae of ascending gonococcal infections include infertility, ectopic pregnancy and chronic abdominal pain, primarily from adhesions.

If the infection spreads further into abdomen, a perihepatic abscess may evolve. This unusual situation is known as the Fitzhugh-Curtis syndrome. Only about 10% of perihepatic abscesses are caused by *N. gonorrhoeae*; the most common causative organism is *C. trachomatis*. Often there is upper abdominal pain, radiating to the thorax and shoulders, as well as difficulty breathing. Signs of peritonitis may also be present. These symptoms may mask the genital tract findings. Abnormal liver function tests may be present. Laparoscopy shows characteristic violin string adhesions between the liver, peritoneum and other abdominal organs. These adhesions may later be responsible for chronic abdominal pain.

Women with ascending gonococcal infection will have a positive cervical smear in only about 50% of cases. Thus, culture of any discharge is essential. Gynecologic consultation, ultrasound examination and perhaps laparoscopy are essential. Appendicitis, ectopic pregnancy and strangulated ovarian tumor are other diagnostic considerations. Viral hepatitis can be excluded by liver function tests and sonography usually suffices to exclude cholecystitis.

Gonorrhea in Pregnancy

Gonorrhea's manifestation are very similar in the pregnant woman. Oropharyngeal gonorrhea may be more common. The key problem is the risk to the newborn infant; premature rupture of membranes, premature labor, chorioamnionitis and septic abortion are all potential complications. The infant may suffer from ophthalmia neonatorum or oropharyngeal gonorrhea. In many countries, cultures for *N. gonorrhoeae* are done routinely at the first pre-natal visit and repeated later if the mother is at risk for sexually transmitted diseases. All infants are treated prophylactically to avoid ophthalmologic disease.

Gonorrhea in Children

Gonorrhea in young girls is usually symptomatic. The prepubertal vaginal mucosa is readily infected by *N. gonorrhoeae*, producing a pus-laden discharge and local erythema and swelling. Pruritus and dysuria are also common complaints. The discharge may cause an irritant dermatitis of the upper thighs. When the labia are separated, the discharge is usually obvious.

The diagnosis is made on direct examination and culture. Any child with gonorrhea should be considered a victim of sexual abuse until proven otherwise. The unfortunate reality is that almost all such cases represent child abuse; fanciful stories of transmission from wash rags, bath water or toilet seats remain suspect. The help of pediatricians or social workers should be sought. Other sexually transmitted diseases should be excluded.

Differential Diagnosis. A vaginal foreign body, such as a small toy, bead, or even a piece of food, produces a severe and clinically similar vaginitis. Ultrasound can help exclude this possibility. Other infections caused by *T. vaginalis*, *C. albicans*, intestinal bacteria and even pin worms should be excluded by direct examination and culture.

Rectal Gonorrhea

Rectal gonorrhea is a problem in homosexuals and other practicing anal intercourse, but it also occurs in about 50 % of women with genital gonorrhea as a result of contamination. About 5 % of women and 40 % of homosexual men with gonorrhea present with rectal disease. The women are much more likely to be asymptomatic, while the men may complain of rectal discharge and pain. The perianal skin is usually normal, although it occasionally may be red and irritated by discharge.

Pharyngeal Gonorrhea

In about 5 % of patients the pharynx is the sole site of infection. About 25 % of women and homosexual men with urogenital infections also have pharyngeal involvement; in heterosexual men, the likelihood is about 5 %. The infection is the result of oral-genital sex, not kissing. Most patients are asymptomatic, emphasizing the need for routine pharyngeal cultures.

Ophthalmia Neonatorum

Neonatal ocular gonorrhea can be acquired via intrauterine infection or during passage through the vagina. Children infected in utero develop symptoms promptly after birth. A child born through an infected birth canal has a 30–50 % chance of getting infected. In this case a purulent conjunctivitis appears about 4–5 days after birth, although some cases are identified only on culture. The lids swell shut and the eyes are red and tender. If not treated promptly, the cornea may be eroded and perforated, leading to secondary glaucoma, conophthalmus and blindness. About 30 % of those with eye infections will also have oropharnyngeal gonorrhea.

For these reasons, prophylaxis is the best approach. The most effective method is to ensure that mothers do not have *N. gonorrhoeae*, but since this is not totally achievable, immediate instillation of an antibacterial agent into the eyes of every newborn is standard practice. Credé instituted silver nitrate prophylaxis in 1881; today silver nitrate 1 % aqueous solution is still appropriate, although both erythromycin 0.5 % and tetracycline 1.0 % ophthalmic ointments are also recommended. A single application suffices.

Differential Diagnosis. The silver nitrate prophylaxis can produce a chemical conjunctivitis, usually appearing 6–8 h after treatment and resolving over 24 h. The most common cause of neonatal conjunctivitis in most countries is *C. trachomatis*. The many other possible causes of conjunctivitis should be investigated with an ophthalmologist.

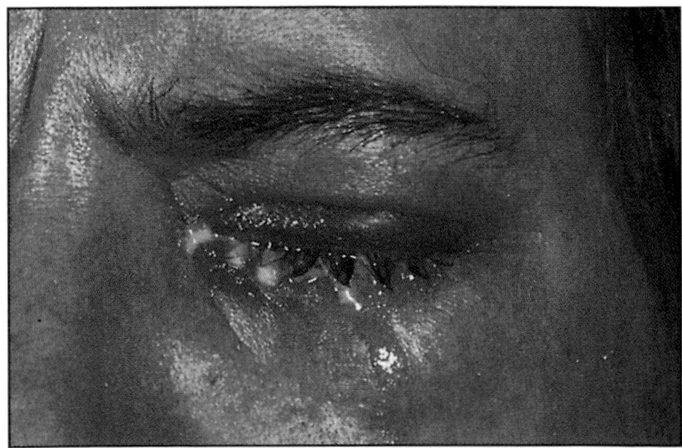

Fig. 5.5. Gonorrheal involvement of the eye in an adult

Gonococcal Conjunctivitis in Adults

Ocular infections in adults are even more aggressive, but fortunately they are rare (Fig. 5.5). Usually the mechanism is autoinoculation from an urogenital infection, so patients should be warned about this possibility. The early symptoms of tearing, burning and photophobia are easy to overlook; thus, one must always keep gonorrhea in mind as a cause of conjunctivitis.

Disseminated Gonococcal Infection

About 0.5–3.0% of patients with localized gonorrhea will develop disseminated infections. Women are far more often involved than men, comprising 60–97% of the patient population. Symptoms usually develop within 7 days of the menses or following a spontaneous abortion or delivery. Disseminated disease is usually caused by *N. gonorrhoeae* with the protein IA phenotype. This subtype causes few local problems and is very penicillin-sensitive. Since it is uncommon in homosexual populations, disseminated disease is equally unlikely. Perhaps 5–15% of patients with dissemination will have an inborn error in the late complement cascade involving C5–C9.

Disseminated gonococcal infections are characterized by episodic fever, polyarthritis and pustular skin lesions. The disease usually begins with arthralgias and tenosynovitis, but about 40% of patients have one or more acutely swollen effused joints. Typically, the wrists, fingers, ankles and knees are most often involved. In some patients a monoarthritis develops, either following more diffuse symptoms or as the presenting sign, usually several weeks after inoculation. Larger joints are almost always involved, especially the knees. The joint is red, swollen, fluctuant and has restricted motion. If not treated, a stiff joint may develop. The polyarthritis is probably caused by immune complex deposition, while the later monoarthritis is a result of true infection of the joint by the bacteria.

The skin lesions are usually acral or over the infected joint and appear as hemorrhagic papules and pustules that develop a crust and become necrotic (Fig. 5.6). Most patients have a small number of lesions, which can be mistaken for insect bites. Often they are painful, but in some patients they are ignored or escape notice. Histologically they are the prototype of an infectious or pustular leukocytoclastic vasculitis with fibrinoid vessel wall damage, small thrombi and exocytosis of erythrocytes. The organism is rarely cultured from the skin but can be identified in many cases with direct immunofluorescent techniques or electron microscopy.

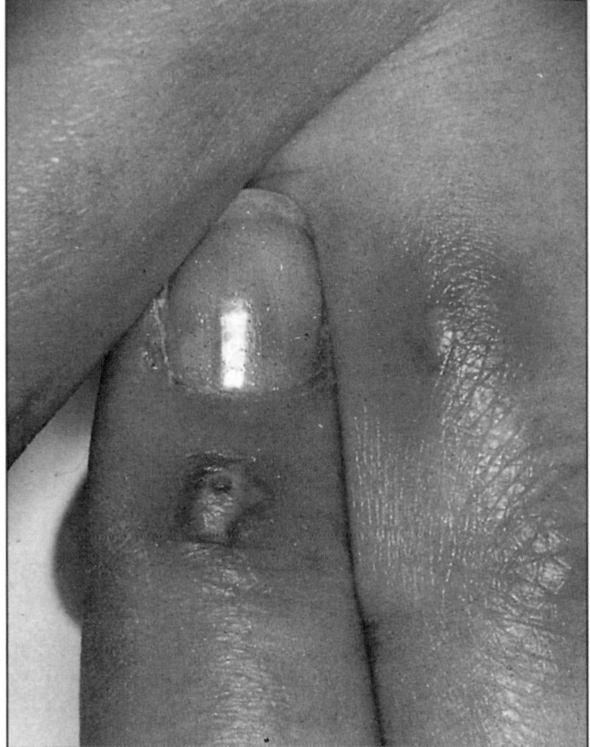

Fig. 5.6. Necrotic hemorrhagic pustules in disseminated gonococcal infection

There are many other possible sites of involvement. Hepatitis, endocarditis and meningitis are the most feared complications. Each may develop when the patient has no other typical signs or symptoms. A variety of reactive ocular problems, such scleritis, iritis and iridocyclitis also can be seen, as can osteomyelitis.

Differential Diagnosis. In full-blown cases, one must also consider chronic meningococcemia, other forms of sepsis, especially from gram-negative organisms, and leukocytoclastic vasculitis. When the joint changes dominate, Reiter syndrome is another possibility, along with reactive arthritis secondary to hepatitis B virus and rheumatoid arthritis.

Laboratory Findings

Direct Examination. The diagnosis of gonorrhea is based on microscopic identification of the organism and cultures. The secretions are spread on a glass slide, heat-fixed and stained with methylene blue or Gram stain. The *N. gonorrhoeae* are found with neutrophils as paired, bean-shaped cocci. They are blue on methylene blue staining but gram-negative. The methylene blue stain is only reliable for urethral discharge; in other sites, a Gram stain is needed. Extracellular or atypical organisms are usually nonpathogenic Neisseria; *N. meningitidis* is also found intracellularly and is identical. Direct identification has a specificity of almost 100% in the appropriate clinical setting, but is only highly sensitive when dealing with urethral discharge. Rectal and endocervical smears, as well as those from the urethra of asymptomatic men, have a sensitivity of 40–70% so they are rarely used.

Culture. Identification of the organism and determination of phenotype and antibiotic sensitivity are the standard for evaluation of gonorrhea. The organism is very sensitive to drying out, so a smear should be plated immediately or the material transported to the laboratory in an appropriate transport medium. Modified Thayer-Martin medium, which contains a variety of inhibitory antibiotics, is most often used. Sometimes it is wise to employ a second, less inhibitory medium to identify highly sensitive organisms. The cultures grow best at 36 °C in a CO_2-rich atmosphere. After 18–48 h, shiny gray colonies, variable in size, appear.

A variety of enzymatic tests and monoclonal antibody coagulation tests can be used to identify the two main serogroups. – protein IA (WI) and protein IB (WII/WIII). These steps allow one to exclude *N. meningitidis* and nonpathogenic Neisseria. Further serotyping can identify the serovars (serovariants) of *N. gonorrhoeae.*

Antibiotic Sensitivity. Neisseria gonorrhoeae was previously uniformly sensitive to penicillin. Over the past few decades resistance to antibiotics among *N. gonorrhoeae* has become a major public health problem. Both plasmid and chromosomal resistance may develop. Plasmid-mediated resistance involves the production of a penicillinase or β-lactamase. Penicillinase-producing *N. gonorrhoeae* have become common in the USA, especially in the coastal regions, and have been described throughout the world. Tetracycline resistance is also usually plasmid-mediated. The chromosomal resistance frequently affects multiple antibiotics; the most serious problem is presented by strains of spectinomycin-resistant organisms, initially reported in South Korea. In any event, the physician must be aware of antibiotic trends in his area and laboratory tests will usually determine sensitivity, even though treatment has been empirically undertaken.

Serology. No serologic testing for *N. gonorrhoeae* is available.

Other Methods. A variety of direct methods including DNA hybridization, direct immunofluorescent examination and ELISA are available but they have not as yet replaced culture and direct examination.

Diagnostic Criteria. The diagnostic approach to suspected gonorrhea varies greatly depending on the clinical setting. The following guidelines may be helpful.

- Heterosexual men: Direct examination of discharge and culture; urethral culture alone if asymptomatic
- Homosexual men: Urethral evaluation as above; rectal, pharyngeal culture
- Women: Urethral, rectal, cervical and pharyngeal cultures
- Children: The rectum, urethra, vagina and pharynx should be cultured and positive results identified by two independent methods
- Ocular: Cultures should be plated on both Thayer-Martin and nonselective media because *C. trachomatis* is quite likely
- Disseminated disease: Blood cultures are positive in far less than 50% of patients. Cultures from joints, CSF and skin, as well as direct identification in skin and fluids, still leave about half of patients with no direct proof of systemic infection. Thus it is crucial to culture the urogenital tract, rectum and pharynx, as up to 80% will be positive in one of these sites, even if asymptomatic. Finally, sexual partner(s) should also be cultured; this may also help confirm the diagnosis.

The skin biopsy may strongly suggest gonococcal vasculitis but should not be taken as confirmatory unless the organism is found. Many other bacteria also produce pustular vasculitis.

Therapy

The therapy of *N. gonorrhoeae* varies from region to region greatly and shifts often. We have cited the recommendations of the Centers for Disease Control in the USA, but each physician should follow the guidelines of the local health department. The mainstay of therapy is ceftriaxone, as resistance has not yet been observed and a single dose is curative in most cases. It may even treat an incubating syphilis infection. The oral cephalosporins and quinolones are also useful.

Uncomplicated Urogenital Gonorrhea. Cefixime 400 mg orally in a single dose, or ceftriaxone 125 mg IM in single dose, or ciprofloxacin 500 mg orally in a single dose, or ofloxacin 400 mg orally in a single dose are recommended.

A regimen effective against *C. trachomatis*, such as doxycycline 100 mg orally b.i.d. for 7 days, or azithromycin 1.0 g orally in a single dose is also effective against *N. gonorrhoeae*. Alternative regimens include other oral and intramuscular cephalosporins, other quinolones and spectinomycin 2.0 mg IM in a single dose (not effective for pharyngeal infections).

Uncomplicated Gonorrhea in Pregnancy. In pregnancy, cefixime, ceftriaxone or spectinomycin, in the above dosages, are recommended. Erythromycin or ampicillin should be used to cover against *C. trachomatis*.

Gonorrhea in Infants and Children. The mainstay is again ceftriaxone; the dosages are available in pediatric sources. It should also be used in asymptomatic infants born to mothers with gonorrhea. The dosages must be increased when there is evidence of disseminated disease.

Ocular Gonorrhea. A large dose of ceftriaxone is required; 1.0 g IM in a single dose is recommended. Infants should also receive ceftriaxone 25–50 mg/kg IV or IM in a single dose not to exceed 125 mg. Notice that the topical treatments are only for prophylaxis.

Pelvic Inflammatory Disease (Ascending Gonorrhea). Mixed infections are the rule so generally a complex in-hospital regimen is advised. The CDC recommends either cefoxitin or cefotetan plus doxycycline; both are administered intravenously. Once the patient has shown substantial improvement, after 24 h one may switch to oral doxycycline. Alternatively, IV clindamycin and gentamicin can be used, switching then to oral clindamycin or doxycycline. In Germany, cefoxitin, doxycycline and metronidazole are recommended. The goal is to cover against *C. trachomatis* and anaerobic bacteria as well as *N. gonorrhoeae*.

Disseminated Gonorrhea. Patients should be hospitalized. Initially they should receive ceftriaxone 1.0 g IM or IV every 24 h. Many alternatives are available. Once improvement is seen, after another 24–48 h they can be switched to cefixime 400 mg orally b.i.d. or ciprofloxacin 500 mg orally b.i.d. If meningitis or endocarditis is present, ceftriaxone 1–2 g IV every 12 h is needed; meningitis should be treated for 10–14 days and endocarditis for 4 weeks.

Other Considerations. A syphilis serology and HIV test should be performed. If the patient responds to a single dose regimen, no clinical follow-up is needed. HIV-positive patients can be treated in exactly the same way as outlined above. If symptoms recur, most often the explanation is a reinfection or a second untreated infection, but a resistant organism must be excluded. The patient's sexual partner(s) should be identified, examined and cultured. If the index case is symptomatic, then tracking should go back 30 days; if asymptomatic, 60 days. All sexual contacts during these periods should be treated. Sexual intercourse should be avoid until patient and partner are cured (therapy completed and no symptoms). In the case of gonorrhea in infants, the mother and her sex partner(s) should be evaluated, while in gonorrhea in children, all adolescents and adults with patient contact should be checked.

Public Health Measures. In most countries, infections with *N. gonorrhoeae* are reportable.

Other Forms of Urethritis

In some countries, dermatologists see most of the gonorrhea patients, so they must be familiar with the other causes of urethritis. In the past, when gonorrhea was more common and easier to diagnose, one spoke of nonspecific urethritis or nongonococcal urethritis. Today, in most cases, other infectious agents can be identified, although noninfectious urethritis also occurs. Simultaneous infection with two or more organisms is not uncommon but clinically confusing. One aspect has not changed: the other forms typically do not have the thick, pus-laden discharge associated with gonorrhea. In addition to examining a urethral smear and culture, a divided urine specimen may be helpful. More neutrophils in the first specimen than the second supports the diagnosis of urethritis.

Urethritis is traditionally viewed as a disease of men, as urethral infections of women are often asymptomatic. Nonetheless, the urethra in women may also be infected and should always be cultured. The same organisms that are associated with urethritis in men are linked with vaginitis in women (Chap. 35).

Chlamydia

Chlamydia cause more than half of all cases of urethritis. They are far more common than *N. gonorrhoeae* and are considered below. In the past, postgonococcal urethritis was a standard diagnosis, as patients developed urethritis after treatment for gonorrhea. Almost all cases represent a double infection with *N. gonorrhoeae* and *C. trachomatis*.

Mycoplasma

The mycoplasma are the smallest known free-living organisms; they have about half as much DNA as the smallest bacteria, lack a rigid cell wall and are immobile. But unlike viruses, they can grow on culture media. *Ureaplasma urealyticum* and *Mycoplasma hominis* are two mycoplasma that are part of the normal flora of the urethra, being found in up to 75% of sexually active individuals. While they have been blamed for a variety of infections, it appears that *U. urealyticum* is a true pathogen and responsible for about 25% of cases of urethritis. In contrast, *M. hominis* is more important in pelvic inflammatory disease. The urethritis is typically associated with a serous or white discharge, acid pH and sterile leukocytosis of the urine. The patient may complain of burning or itching. The diagnosis is one of exclusion, since so many patients are culture-positive. Not surprisingly, the mycoplasma cannot be seen on Gram stain or by other microscopic techniques. The only method of identification is culture on special media such as Shepherd's A7 medium with agar and serum. The colonies are so tiny they must be viewed with a microscope, but colony size and ability to split urea are used to separate the two main suspects.

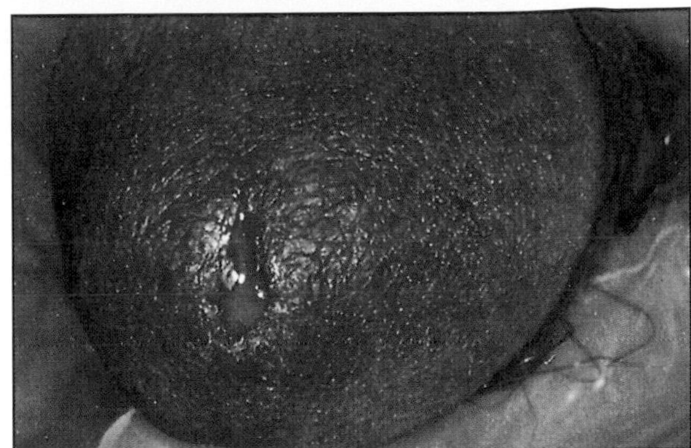

Fig. 5.7. Trichomonal urethritis

Therapy. Doxycycline 100 mg orally b.i.d. for 7 days is the standard. In case tetracyclines cannot be employed, azithromycin 1.0 g orally in a single dose, or erythromycin 500 mg orally q.i.d. for 7 days can be employed. Clindamycin 150 mg orally q.i.d. for 7 days is an alternative that is often used for the partner of a women with *M. hominis* pelvic disease.

Trichomoniasis

Trichomonas vaginalis is responsible for about 5% of cases of urethritis; it is covered in Chapter 6 but illustrated here as a contrast to gonococcal urethritis (Fig. 5.7).

Noninfectious Urethritis

Worry is an indirect cause of urethritis, although often not recognized as such. Some men, perhaps because of fear of an infection or guilt over a sexual practice, become fixated on their urethral function. They may also mechanically irritate their urethra by repeated milking or stripping. Examination shows only epithelial cells in the specimen and no inflammatory cells; culture may reveal *U. urealyticum*, the friendly traveler. Most patients are reassured by a careful examination and negative cultures. Other patients suffering from epididymitis erotica (minor pain and swelling secondary to sexual arousal but failure to ejaculate, commonly known in USA as "love nuts") may also have a trivial discharge. In some instances, the urethra has been mechanically damaged via the insertion of foreign objects. In such instances, the specimen is usually blood-tinged.

Other Bacteria

All the other causes of urethritis are uncommon. A variety of organisms have been blamed, but their exact roles are unclear. *Acinetobacter calcoaceticus* is a close relative of *N. gonorrhoeae* that can cause cystitis and prostatitis in patients with indwelling catheters; it may rarely produce urethritis, but is usually an innocent bystander. *Veillonella parvula* is a gram-negative anaerobic coccus that may be isolated but is rarely significant. *E. coli* causes epididymitis especially in homosexual men but rarely urethritis. Both staphylococci and streptococci can also on occasion be cultured. Treatment is directed by culture results. Finally any balanitis or balanoposthitis may secondarily cause irritation and urethral problems.

Yeasts

Candida albicans may involve the urethra, but usually presents as a balanitis or vaginitis with secondary urethritis. The presence of the yeast in a urethral or urine culture strongly suggest urethral involvement. Treatment can be with any of the imidazoles, such as itraconazole 100–200 mg daily for 7 days, or fluconazole 100 mg daily for 7 days.

Viruses

Herpes simplex virus (HSV) can cause a very painful urethritis, known as urethritis herpetica. In most cases, there is some sign of HSV infection of the genital mucosa. Rarely intraurethral HSV may occur and be extremely difficult to diagnose. Standard treatment with acyclovir 200 mg orally, five times daily for 5 days is effective. Other viruses such as cytomegalovirus, varicella zoster virus and measles virus may also produce urethral inflammation.

Reiter Syndrome

The combination of urethritis, arthritis and psoriasiform cutaneous changes should suggest Reiter syndrome (Chap. 14).

Chlamydial Infections

The chlamydiae occupy a special role between bacteria and viruses; they are obligate intracellular parasites, but still have many bacterial characteristics, such as both DNA and RNA, sensitivity to antibiotics, and the presence of a cell wall.

Causative Organisms

- *Chlamydia trachomatis* causes a wide spectrum of disorders, to be discussed below, as well as lymphogranuloma venereum, which is considered later in the chapter.
- *Chlamydia psittaci* is the causative agent of psittacosis or ornithosis, a infection transferred from birds (not just parrots) to humans, causing primarily pulmonary manifestations and fever.
- *Chlamydia pneumoniae* causes mild respiratory symptoms.

Epidemiology. *Chlamydia trachomatis* is the most common sexually transmitted infectious agent. It is two to four times more common than *N. gonorrhoeae*. In the USA, there are approximately 4 million new infections yearly. The organism causes so many different clinical problems that the epidemiologic features are impossible to summarize but will be alluded to below. It poses a threat not only to adults but also to neonates. In addition, the risk of sterility in both men and women is significant, producing obvious long-term effects.

Etiology and Pathogenesis. *Chlamydia trachomatis* has a number of serovars that have specific disease associations. The most common are shown in Table 5.1. *C. trachomatis* exists in two forms: the extracellular infectious elementary body and the intracellular replicative reticulate body. They attach

Table 5.1. Types of *Chlamydia trachomatis*

Serovariant	Disease	Transmission
A–C	Endemic trachoma	Hands, fomites, flies Perinatal
D–K	Pneumonia, inclusion conjunctivitis	
D–K	Urethritis, cervicitis, proctitis, many others (see text)	Sexual
L1, L2, L3	Lymphogranuloma venereum	Sexual

by a variety of mechanisms to the epithelial cells of the genitourinary tact, rectum and conjunctiva. The most favored host site is the cylindrical epithelial cell of the cervix. As the bacteria proliferate within the cell, they tend to effectively destroy their host. In other instances, chlamydiae may remain in host cells for long periods of time, providing a focus for recurrent disease. The inflammatory response against the necrotic host cells is usually rich in neutrophils and macrophages. *C. trachomatis* does not infect the vagina, causing vaginal symptoms only secondary to cervicitis. Ascending infections occur, just as with *N. gonorrhoeae* andare facilitated by the passage of sperm.

Clinical Findings. *Chlamydia trachomatis* causes a wide spectrum of genitourinary diseases, most of which are related and do not have significant skin findings. In many cases, the infections are asymptomatic, but when an incubation period can be determined, it is usually about 10–20 days. *C. trachomatis* also is responsible for considerable morbidity among infants and is a major cause of blindness.

Genitourinary Infections in Women

Cervicitis

The cervix is the main site of infection. Since only the cylinder cells are infected, the disease always presents as endocervicitis. Infections are more likely in women with an everted cervical os, since the susceptible cells are more exposed. Only about 50% of the patients are symptomatic, with a yellow-white slimy discharge that is often associated with pruritus and burning about the introitus. On physical examination, the cervix may show contact bleeding along with the discharge.

Pregnancy

The cervical infection makes transmission to newborns very likely, well over 50%. In addition, both premature rupture of membranes and thus preterm delivery are established complications. In pregnant patients, every effort should be made not to overlook *C. trachomatis.*

Endometritis

The endometrial epithelium is less hospitable than the cervical, but endometrial infections do occur. About half the patients with cervicitis also develop endometritis. Ovulation, muscular activity (such as with an orgasm) and intrauterine contraceptive devices also facilitate the upward spread, as do sperm. Clinically the patients have abdominal pain, increased menstruation and irregular bleeding, none of which are seen with simple cervicitis.

Pelvic Inflammatory Disease

Further ascending spread occurs in about 10% of patients. Clinically the patients have abdominal pain, tenderness and fever. Initially the tubes remain open, as the massive destruction of the ciliated epithelium seen with *N. gonorrhoeae* does not occur. Pyosalpingitis is very uncommon and suggests a mixed infection. Nonetheless the chronic inflammation and fibrosis of the tubes can lead to sterility. The chance is estimated as 20% for the first case of salpingitis and at 75% after three or more ascending infections. The risk of ectopic pregnancy also rises dramatically. The disease can spread further, causing an oophoritis, perioophoritis, peritonitis or even perihepatic abscess, in short, mimicking all the features of a *N. gonorrhoeae* infection. While one speaks of pelvic inflammatory disease, often ultrasound and laparoscopy allow one to more accurately localize the findings.

Bartholin Gland Infection

Chlamydia trachomatis is an uncommon cause of Bartholin gland infections. The problem is usually unilateral. The opening of the Bartholin duct onto the labia minora is often erythematous (Saenger point). The duct does not become closed, so an abscess, as seen with *N. gonorrhoeae*, usually does not develop.

Urinary Tract Infections

Urethritis occurs commonly, but only involving the proximal aspect of the urethra. Most patients are asymptomatic, but those who have symptoms complain of increased frequency and dysuria. About 70% of cases of urethritis in women are caused by *C. trachomatis.* The urethral meatus is erythematous and the smear shows neutrophils without any coliform bacteria. Hematuria or suprapubic pain suggest cystitis, which is not related to *C. trachomatis* infection.

Genitourinary Infections in Men

Urethritis

Chlamydia trachomatis is the most common cause of urethritis in men. It is responsible for over 50% of all cases and is far more common than gonorrhea. The condition was previously designated nonspecific urethritis, but this is inappropriate, as in most cases the causative organism can be found. Similarly postgonococcal urethritis is nothing more than a mixed infection with *N. gonorrhoeae* and *C. trachomatis*, in which the latter becomes apparent when the former is treated. For this reason, all therapy schemes for *N. gonorrhoeae* include appropriate treatment for *C. trachomatis*.

Clinically, the discharge is usually milder than in *N. gonorrhoeae*, but the two conditions cannot be separated with certainty and often coexist. Typical complaints are urethral discharge and dysuria. The urethral orifice may be erythematous. The discharge usually contains neutrophils.

Epididymitis

Chlamydia trachomatis can spread through the vas deferens to the epididymis. Usually the infection is acute and unilateral. The patient presents with pain, fever and chills, but in most cases is not as ill as with *N. gonorrhoeae* infection. The tenderness starts at the lower pole of the testis, but often spreads to the upper pole; the vas deferens may become thickened and indurated.

Proctitis

About 15% of proctitis in homosexual men is caused by *C. trachomatis*. In women, it may arise from autoinoculation from an infected cervical discharge. Clinical symptoms range from minor pain to prominent slimy, yellow discharge with associated anal dermatitis and pain on defecation.

Neonatal Infections

Newborns can be infected by passing through a cervix infected with *C. trachomatis*. The risk is about 60–70% that they will be infected. The two major problems are pneumonia, formerly known as pertussoid eosinophilic pneumonia, and a conjunctivitis that is not prevented by *N. gonorrhoeae* prophylaxis. The pneumonia is spread via aspiration. Many neonates have *C. trachomatis* in their pharynx, although they do not have pharyngitis. After a long incubation of 3–16 weeks, the infant may develop a crusted rhinitis, coughing and respiratory problems. Most cases resolve spontaneously without complications.

The eyes are infected by direct inoculation. Problems begin between days 5 and 12; by contrast, *N. gonorrhoeae* conjunctivitis usually appears before that. The conjunctivae are red, infiltrated and may develop lymphoid follicles. There is a pustular discharge. If not treated appropriately, the scarring and neovascularization can impair vision. Ulcerations do not occur. Venereal chlamydial conjunctivitis is a great problem in areas with a high incidence of cervical *C. trachomatis* infections. It far outweighs *N. gonorrhoeae* as a public health risk. There are overlaps between trachoma and inclusion conjunctivitis.

Other Ocular Infections

Trachoma

Endemic trachoma is one of or the major cause of blindness in the world. While eradication campaigns have reduced its prevalence, it still is a significant problem in parts of India, North Africa and the Middle East; it is also found among Native American in the desert Southwest of the USA. The reservoir is the eyes of infected individuals; the infection is spread by eye-hand-eye contact, fomites and perhaps even flies. Most children become chronically infected in the first few years of life; among adults, women have more acute disease, presumably because of more exposure to children. The combination of repeated infections, neovascularization of the cornea, proliferation of lymphoid follicles and conjunctival scarring leads to blindness; entropion is also a chronic problem.

Conjunctivitis of the Adult

Chlamydia trachomatis can also cause conjunctivitis in non-endemic areas. While it has been called swimming pool conjunctivitis, this is incorrect. In most cases, it is the result of self-inoculation from a genitourinary chlamydial infection with a discharge. Patients typically complain of tearing, a foreign body sensation and a pus-laden discharge. Usually the disease is self-limited.

Adult Pneumonia

Although the other chlamydiae are more common causes of pneumonia, *Chlamydia trachomatis* has been shown to produce pulmonary infections in immunosuppressed patients.

Laboratory Findings. In almost every case in which one considers *N. gonorrhoeae*, one must also consider *C. trachomatis*. The diagnosis is almost entirely dependent on direct identification, so obtaining appropriate material for the laboratory is the most important step in the evaluation. The specimen should be taken with a cotton applicator with a plastic or aluminum shaft; Dacron and wood both harm the organism. The appropriate transport medium should be used if the specimen is being sent away for diagnosis. *C. trachomatis* can be identified in a number of ways.

Direct Examination. Giemsa staining of ocular scrapings reveals intracellular inclusions of the organisms. When positive, this is very helpful, especially in trachoma surveys for which more sophisticated techniques are not available. Direct examination of cervical or urethral discharge may also, on rare occasions, show inclusions, but in most cases it serves only to exclude other causes.

Culture. Chlamydia trachomatis cannot be grown on culture media, only in cell cultures. While the lymphogranuloma venereum serovars are relatively easy to culture, the others are more fastidious. The most common cell line is a heteroploid mouse line known as McCoy cells. Culturing the organism is expensive, time-consuming and requires special laboratory facilities. It is usually reserved for research purposes.

Serology. Serologic evaluation plays a minor role, as there are many asymptomatic patients, and, in other cases, mucosal infections fail to elicit much of a systemic response. In patients with acute pelvic inflammatory disease, high IgA and IgG titers can be taken as a strong indication of infection.

Other Methods. The most useful technique is direct immunofluorescence examination of infected material with a monoclonal antibody directed against an antigen present in all serovars. Cervical or urethral scrapings have a higher yield than the purulent discharge. Kits are available so that the investigation be performed in 30 min in the office or clinic, with specificity and sensitivity greater than 90 %. Microimmunofluorescent serologic tests can also be used to identify the various serovars. Enzyme immunoassay and DNA hybridization tests are less accurate, especially where *C. trachomatis* is uncommon, but they allow more efficient screening programs.

Prognosis. The outlook for all chlamydial infections is good if they are promptly recognized and treated. If not, recurrent infections, scarring and neovascularization can lead to problems such as blindness and infertility.

Differential Diagnosis. The differential diagnosis in most cases include gonorrhea. In each organ system, a slightly different set of problems is likely. The differential diagnosis of urethritis has already been discussed earlier in this chapter while the approach to vaginal discharge is reviewed in Chap. 35.

Therapy. The tetracyclines are the mainstay of therapy. Doxycycline 100 mg orally b. i. d. for 7 days, or azithromycin 1.0 g orally in a single dose are recommended for uncomplicated genitourinary infections. Ofloxacin, erythromycin ethylsuccinate and erythromycin base are also effective; the latter is recommended for use during pregnancy.

In ascending or complicated infections, doxycycline should be continued for a longer period of time. Two weeks is usually suggested for epididymitis. In pelvic inflammatory disease, the regimen must also cover anaerobic organisms. Neonatal infections should be treated with systemic erythromycin. If topical erythromycin products are used, the eye problems may be controlled but the pharyngeal carriage can persist and lead to pneumonia or recurrent conjunctivitis.

Trachoma is generally treated with doxycycline 200 mg orally daily for 6 weeks.

Improved public health measures are likely more important than the choice of antibiotics.

Other Considerations. The sexual partners of patients with *C. trachomatis* infections should be examined, specimens obtained and if warranted treated. Routine gynecologic examinations should be accompanied by search for the organisms in patients at high risk, such as those with multiple partners, a new partner, or who failed to use condoms.

Public Health Measures. In most areas *C. trachomatis* infections are reportable.

Lymphogranuloma Venereum

(Hunter 1786; Durand-Favre 1913)

Synonyms. Lymphogranuloma inguinale (often confused with granuloma inguinale), lymphopathia venerea, climatic bubo, Durand-Nicolas-Favre disease

Definition. Sexually acquired chlamydial infection with small genital ulcerations and marked lymphadenopathy.

Causative Organism. *Chlamydia trachomatis* L1, L2, L3

Epidemiology. Lymphogranuloma venereum is most common in Asia, Africa and South America. In the USA, it is most prevalent in the Southeast, among homosexuals and among people returning from endemic areas, such as vacationers, soldiers and seamen. It is seen much more often in men.

Etiology and Pathogenesis. The lymphogranuloma venereum serovars are the only chlamydia capable of causing systemic infections and sepsis. They enter the body via the same mucosal attachment mechanisms, elicit a vigorous lymph node response and then cause systemic disease. They can be found in the blood, CSF and spleen. The pathology is different in men and women. In men, the main manifestations are inguinal buboes, reflecting drainage from the primary penile lesion to the regional lymph nodes. In women, the initial lesion is often more internal, the involved nodes are usually not palpable and often the disease presents at a more advanced stage. In homosexuals, rectal involvement is common. Theoretically at least, ocular inoculation is also possible, as one cause of the oculoglandular syndrome, along with cat-scratch fever and many other infections. The patient's immune response determines if an untreated infection will heal without sequelae or become chronic and more aggressive.

Clinical Findings. The clinical course is divided into three stages.

Primary Lesion (Stage I). The primary changes in lymphogranuloma venereum are nonspecific and subtle. The incubation period is at least 14 days, sometimes longer. The primary lesion is a small innocent papule, several millimeters in size, that evolves into a papulovesicle or papulopustule and then ulcerates. The flat small ulcer has a gray tone and a serous discharge. In men the primary lesion may be on the glans, in the coronal sulcus, or the prepuce or even the anterior part of the urethra. In contrast, in women, it often occurs on the cervix or in the vagina, and is thus not noticed; labial lesions do of course occur. Typically in either sex the primary lesion is ignored or diagnosed as trauma or HSV, or perhaps a syphilitic chancre or early chancroid lesion is considered. In some patients, especially from Africa, large, deep persistent ulcers have been identified, which may reflect a mixed infection. When the primary site of involvement is the rectum, diarrhea, a bloody discharge and multiple erosions may occur.

Bubo (Stage II). A bubo is an enlarged inguinal node, often associated with a sexually transmitted disease. After about 2 weeks, the infection spreads to the regional lymph nodes. In men, the buboes are usually unilateral and above the inguinal ligament, although sometimes they are found on both sides (Figs. 5.8, 5.9). They melt together in mats and may become as large a chicken egg or even a fist. While the overlying skin may become adherent, the lymph nodes usually are not fixed to deep structures. The painful masses are initially red, then blue-red and finally red-brown. Typically the lesion breaks down in the center, forming an abscess that drains to the skin surface through multiple sinus tracts. The discharge is purulent, gray-white or cream-like with chunks of necrotic tissue. Finally, the fistulae heal with cribiform scars.

In women and those with rectal disease, the perirectal and periaortic lymph nodes are most

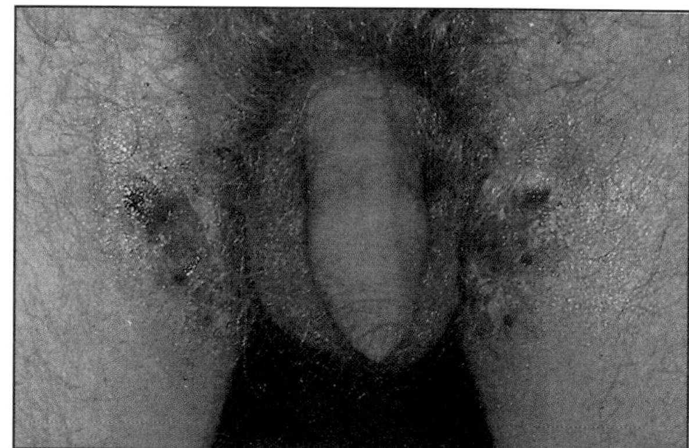

Fig. 5.8. Eroded lymphogranuloma venereum

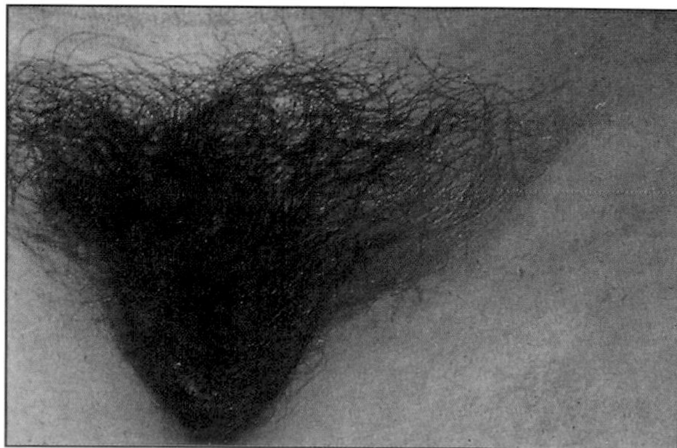

Fig. 5.9. Bubo in lymphogranuloma venereum

likely to be involved. Sometimes, if the inner aspect of the iliac crest is palpated in a relaxed patient, these intraabdominal buboes can be felt. The development of the buboes can be associated with a variety of systemic symptoms. Some patients never feel sick but most have at least some fever, chills and malaise. Initially there is a leukocytosis and then later a lymphocytosis. A variety of exanthems may be seen including erythema multiforme, erythema nodosum and transient, erythematous urticarial eruptions. Most common are arthritic complaints, such as arthralgias or even swollen joints. Meningeal signs (stiff neck, headache) are common and some patients develop meningitis or meningoencephalitis. Hepatitis and conjunctivitis are also seen.

Elephantiasis (Stage III). This stage was formerly felt to be a separate disease, known as esthiomène (Hugier 1849), èlèphantiasis de l'appareil gènital, anorectal symptom complex of Fournier and Jersild syndrome.

Much later in the disease course fibrosis and strictures can develop, compromising lymphatic return. Thus massive swelling and then fibrosis occurs, most typically involving the external genitalia of women. Sometimes the changes are highly localized, involving the clitoris or urethra (fish mouth urethra). In most cases one or both of the labia majora are involved, initially with a puffy swelling and later with either verrucous hyperplasia (as with other forms of lymphedema) or with keloidal tumors separated by deep folds. In addition to the elephantiasis, urethral strictures, urethral-vaginal fistulae, vaginal-anal fistulae and anal strictures may all develop. Esthiomène was long held to be a disease of women, but on rare occasion the penis or scrotum can be involved.

The other major problem is the anal-rectal symptom complex, which is almost limited to women and homosexuals. It can be the result of primary rectal or genital lymphogranuloma venereum infection. The perianal skin is typically involved; keloid-like swellings resembling hemorrhoids or condylomata acuminata may appear. They are known as "lymphorrhoids". The perianal lymph nodes (nodes of Gerota) are so enlarged and fibrosed that the rectum is compressed together over a length of 2–6 cm. The wall of the rectum is also infiltrated and thickened, so that passage of stool is painful and restricted. Rectal ulcers develop as do multiple cutaneous fistulae. After a period of time, the discharge through the fistulae ceases but they often fail to heal and are known as fistulae siccae.

Histopathology. Descriptions of the microscopic appearance of primary lesions can be found in dermatopathology texts, but in actuality a biopsy is a poor diagnostic approach and the findings are very nonspecific. The organisms cannot be identified, except by direct immunofluorescence staining; this method is more effective when examining the lymph nodes, which show stellate abscesses.

Laboratory Findings

Direct Examination. It is almost impossible to stain the organisms in direct preparations. Inclusion bodies are not seen.

Culture. The lymphogranuloma venereum serovars are easier to culture than the other chlamydiae, but still the procedure is delicate and expensive.

Frei Test. The Frei test was formerly considered specific for lymphogranuloma venereum but it is no longer employed. Frei (1930) used pus taken from buboes, but later the organism was cultured on chicken eggs. In either case, the material was injected in a patient to determine if previous exposure to *C. trachomatis* had occurred. The test antigen is no longer available or approved.

Serology. The complement fixation reaction is diagnostically useful. It becomes positive 2–4 weeks after the onset of the infection; fourfold titer rises are considered diagnostic, as is a single titer of >1:64. A negative titer rules out the diagnosis. Another serologic test is the micro-immunofluorescent test using a universal antigen for all *C. trachomatis* types. The titers in lymphogranuloma venereum are often >1:2000, far exceeding the levels reached in genitourinary infections.

Differential Diagnosis. The entire list of diseases with inguinal lymphadenopathy come into question, including HSV, syphilis, chancroid, granuloma inguinale, tuberculosis, Hodgkin disease and other lymphomas, plague and tularemia.

Therapy. The standard therapy is doxycycline 100 mg orally b.i.d. for 21 days. Erythromycin base 500 mg orally q.i.d. for 21 days is an acceptable alternative. The buboes should be drained by needle aspiration, entering through normal lateral skin. Incision of a bubo leads to many problems with healing.

Syphilis

Synonym. Lues

Definition. Worldwide infectious disease usually spread by sexual contact, involving multiple tissues including the skin, cardiac, skeletal and neurological systems.

Causative Organism. *Treponema pallidum.* Treponema means turning thread, referring to the dark field appearance, and pallidum means pale, for the organism is pale in the Giemsa stain (Fig. 5.10). *T. pallidum* is a spirochete; other pathogens in the family include the Borrelia and the Leptospira. There are also many nonpathogenic spirochetes; some are found in the mouth, making the diagnosis of oral syphilis slightly more difficult.

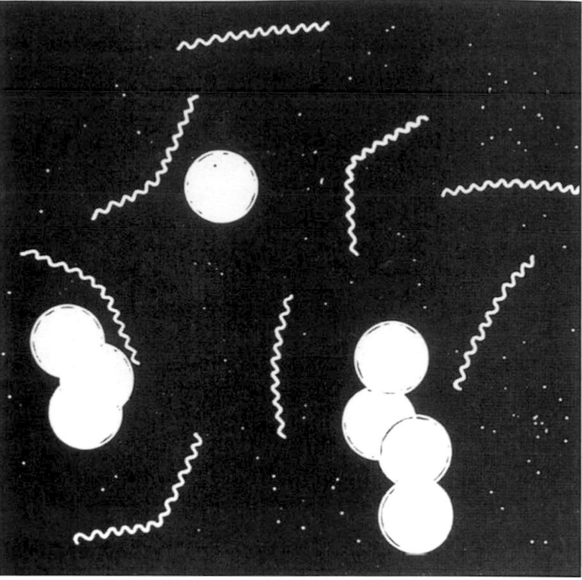

Fig. 5.10. Schematic drawing of *Treponema pallidum* in dark-field examination

Epidemiology

- Incidence: In the USA the incidence of syphilis has waxed and waned over the past 50 years but hovered around 10/100,000 per year. In the late 1970s – early 1980s, there was an upsurge in homosexual men, but this peak has declined. Similarly, there was a peak in syphilis, especially congenital syphilis, in the late 1980s in urban areas and the South, but it too has declined.
- Age: Most common in teenagers and young adults, ages 15–30.
- Sex: Equally common in both sexes in USA; in some societies, much more common in men, probably reflecting social patterns, not biological susceptibility.
- Race: Racial variations once again reflect social patterns.
- Occupation:. A major occupational hazard for prostitutes, otherwise none known.
- Other Risk Factors: Drug abuse, contraception, lack of circumcision.

Etiology and Pathogenesis. Syphilis has been a major public health problem for many years. While its exact origins are unclear, syphilis appears to have been introduced into Europe about the time of Christopher Columbus and then was spread by royal courts, marauding armies and the proverbial traveling salesman. It was the bane of many military campaigns. Until the twentieth century, there was no effective treatment for syphilis. The major cause of hospitalization in mental institutions was CNS syphilis, and the European tradition of large dermatology clinics began with the tremendous number of syphilitics requiring care. Table 5.2 shows some of the milestones in the understanding of syphilis. *History of Syphilis* (original French title *Le Mal de Naples: histoire de la syphilis*), by Claude Quétel (1990), is a fascinating social history of the disease.

T. pallidum is a tissue parasite, in contrast to the other spirochetes, which are primarily blood parasites. It is transferred by direct contact through tiny tissue injuries in the skin or mucosa just adjacent to the skin. The most common sites of entry are the genitalia and mouth. The organism then moves via the skin capillaries to the regional lymph nodes where it multiples in contact with tissues and lymphocytes until reaching high enough levels to cause clinical disease.

Most transfer from person to person occur through sexual contact; *T. pallidum* is so sensitive to drying out, temperature changes, pH changes and variation in O_2 levels that the fanciful "catching it from the toilet seat" is a good story, but little more. A patient with syphilis is only infectious for a limited period of time. In the absence of reinfection, 4 years can be taken as a maximum period of infectivity, with or without treatment. In early syphilis (defined below), the risk of infection ranges between 10% and 60%; in later stages, one must be very unlucky. Syphilis can of course also be transferred by blood, as seen in congenital syphilis and in transfusion-related transmission, which today is excluded by serologic testing of blood and

Table 5.2. Milestones in syphilis research

Researchers (year)	Accomplishment
METSCHNIKOW and ROUX (1903)	Transfer of syphilis to monkeys
SCHAUDINN and HOFFMANN (1905)	Discovery of *Treponema pallidum* Nobel Prize for Medicine 1906
WASSERMANN, NEISSER and BRUCK (1906)	Nontreponemal complement fixing reaction (Wassermann test)
EHRLICH and HATA (1910)	Salvarsan (preparation 606)
EHRLICH (1914)	Neosalvarsan (preparation 914)
MEINICKE and SACHS-GEORGI (1917)	Precipitation reaction; beginning of the so-called associated reactions
MAHONEY, ARNOLD and HARRIS (1943)	Penicillin for syphilis therapy
DEACON, FALCONE and HARRIS (1957)	FTA test
HUNTER, DEACON and MEYER (1964)	FTA-ABS test
RATHLEY, TOMIZAWA and KAMATSU (1965)	TPHA test
ATWOOD and MILLER (1969)	19S-IgM-FTA-ABS test

the inability of *T. pallidum* to survive usual blood storage procedures.

Experimental syphilis in laboratory animals has long played a crucial role. Transmissibility to monkeys was accomplished before the organism was identified. Most of the prepenicillin therapeutic measures were first tested in animals. The Nelson test, or *T. pallidum* immobilization test (TPI-test), was performed using patient serum and organisms cultured in rabbit testes.

Clinical Findings. In 1837 Ricord introduced the clinical division of syphilis into three stages – primary, secondary and tertiary. Primary syphilis is the stage of primary infection. Secondary syphilis is the phase during which *T. pallidum* has spread throughout the body, causing generalized changes. Both phases may overlap; after secondary syphilis heals, the patient enters a latency phase, in which he or she is seropositive and infective but lacks signs or symptoms. These phases are combined into early syphilis, as Table 5.3 shows. During the early latency period, the patient is at increasingly less risk of transferring the disease and suffering a relapse. In the infamous Oslo, Norway, and Tuskegee, Alabama, studies in which patients with syphilis were observed but not treated, 30–40% of patients developed signs of late syphilis, while the others, presumably with better immune responses healed spontaneously. The transition to late syphilis or from secondary to tertiary is fluid. Ricord was unaware that cardiovascular and neurosyphilis, including tabes dorsalis and general paresis of the insane, were actually syphilis; such information first became available with serologic and CSF testing.

Congenital syphilis is acquired by transplacental transfer of the organisms. Thus there is no primary lesion. When an infant is infected during birth, the process is closer to acquired syphilis. Syphilis associated with blood transfusions was known as "decapitated" syphilis, as the primary stage was skipped.

The incubation period of syphilis varies from stage to stage. The primary inoculation period or the time between inoculation and the appearance of the primary lesion is about 3 weeks. During this time, the patient has no signs or symptoms; positive laboratory tests first appear at about 2 weeks. If a sexual partner has documented early syphilis, the likelihood of transfer is high enough that most patients are treated prophylactically during this phase. The secondary incubation period is about 6 weeks, while the latency period between secondary and tertiary syphilis is highly variable.

Table 5.3. Stages of syphilis

Acquired syphilis	
Primary syphilis	Early syphilis
Secondary syphilis	Early syphilis
Early latent syphilis	Early syphilis
Late latent syphilis	Late syphilis
Tertiary syphilis	Late syphilis
Congenital Syphilis	

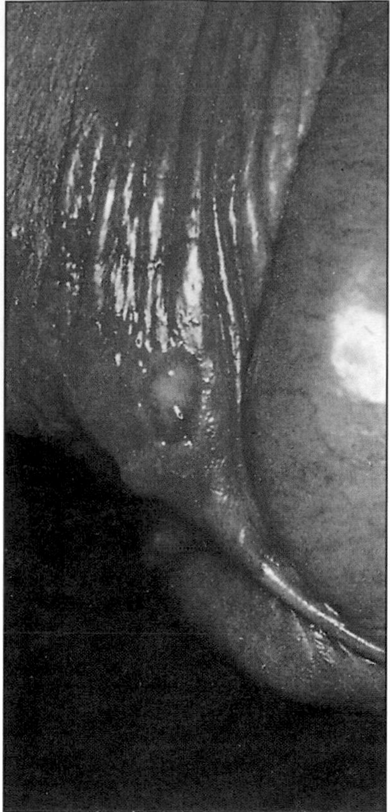

Fig. 5.11. Chancre: primary syphilis

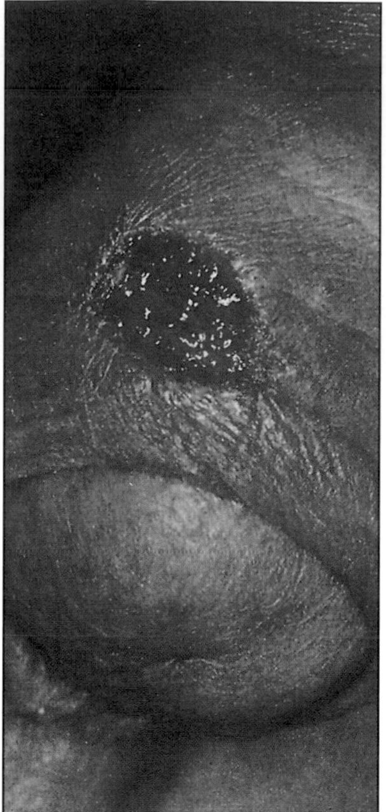

Fig. 5.12. Eroded chancre: primary syphilis

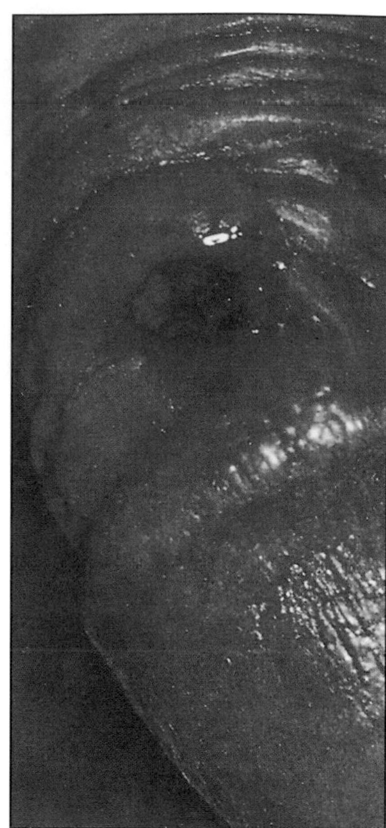

Fig. 5.13. Firm chancre: primary syphilis

Primary Syphilis

The primary lesion in syphilis is the chancre (HUNTER 1786; Figs. 5.11–5.18), which reflects the local proliferation of *T. pallidum* and is always full of organisms. After an incubation period of 3 weeks, the chancre appears along with regional lymphadenopathy. The presence of unilateral inguinal lymphadenopathy should always be followed by the search for a chancre and vice versa. The earliest lesion is a tiny papule which then expands. The most typical presentation is an erosion or minimal ulcer with a pink or ham color and a varnish-like shine. The usual size is 1–2 cm. The hard chancre (ulcus durum) has a firm, central punched-out defect with no undermining, in contrast to the soft chancre of chancroid. The periphery and base are indurated; the consistency has been likened to the firmness of a playing card. Occasionally marked necrosis may develop (ulcus phagedenicum gangrenosum). If the chancre is in an area where there is skin to skin contact, it is usually eroded. In other regions, it may be hyperkeratotic or crusted. Chancres typically yield a thin serous exudate when compressed or squeezed.

There are many clinical variations in chancres. While most lesions are solitary, multiple chancres can arise. There can be multiple inoculation sites, or kissing lesions can appear when a chancre is in contact with normal skin, as between the labia or between the glands and foreskin. The early papule is usually overlooked and, not infrequently, a small erosive chancre hidden under the foreskin or in a labial fold may also never be found. Edema indurativum is an unusual presentation, more common in women than men. There is massive induration and edema, usually involving the labia majora but also the foreskin and scrotum. The skin is firm swollen and has a copper-red color; usually a bubo is present. A chancre may be discovered in the urethra whose orifice is occluded by discharge. A final variant is reinduration. Here a primary lesion recurs as an indurated plaque following inadequate treatment. About 90 % of chancres are genital; extragenital lesions are more likely to be overlooked by the patient and physician.

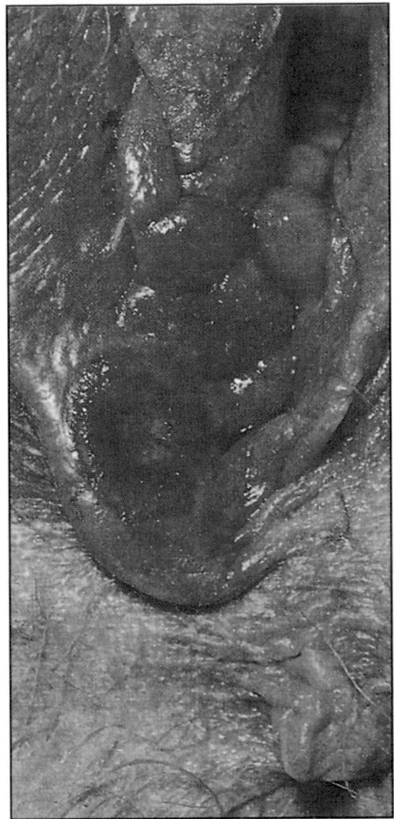

Fig. 5.14. Labial chancre: primary syphilis

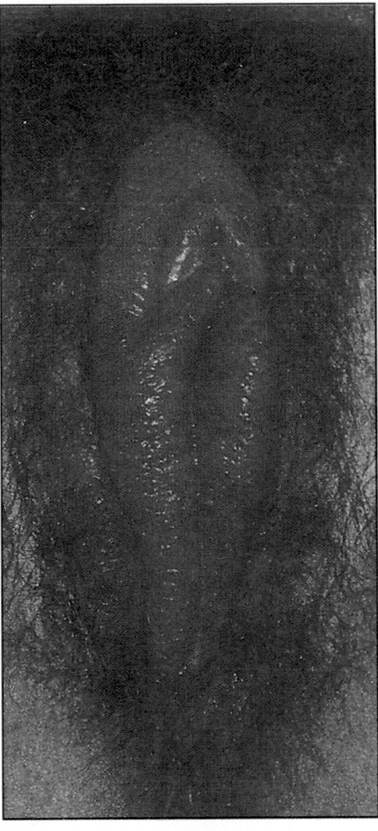

Fig. 5.15. Edema of labia with hidden chancre: primary syphilis

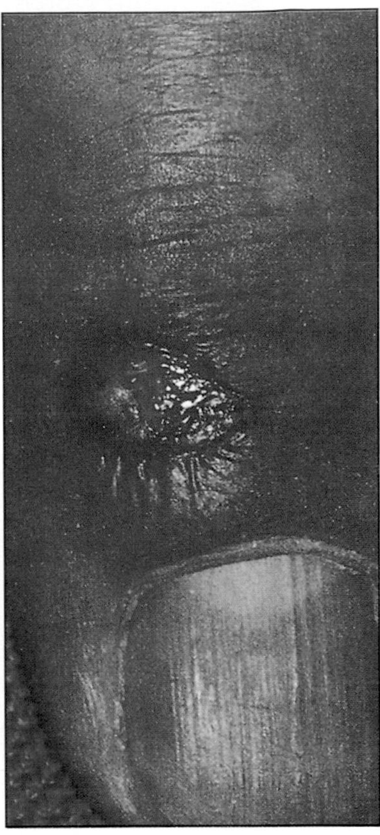

Fig. 5.16. Nongenital chancre: primary syphilis

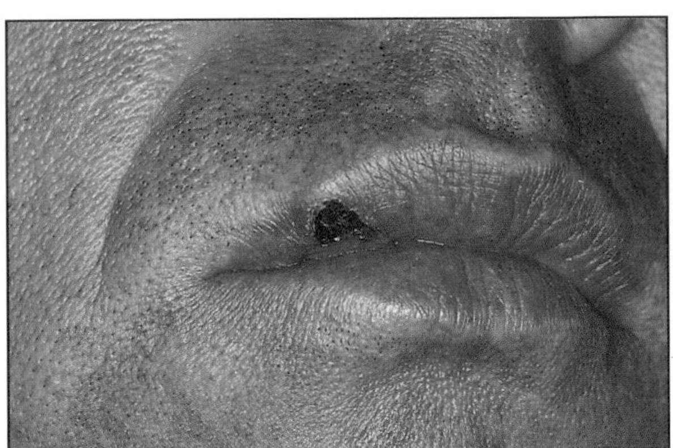

Fig. 5.17. Chancre of the lip: primary syphilis

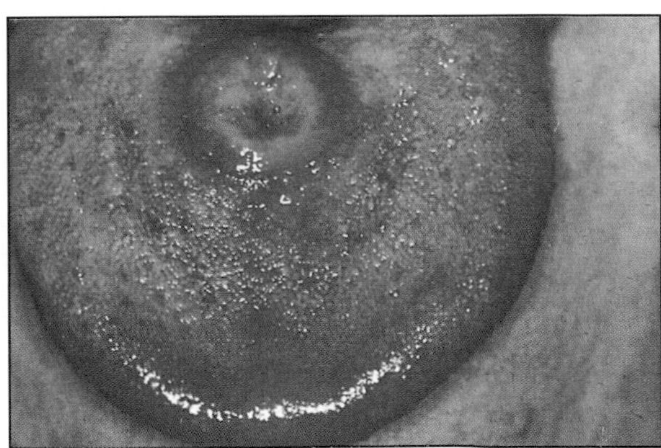

Fig. 5.18. Chancre of the tongue: primary syphilis

Genital Chancre. The most likely location in men is the glans and coronal sulcus. On the glans, a hard chancre is most frequently found while in the sulcus an erosive lesion is expected. Both types are equally common on the inner aspect of the foreskin. Periurethral lesions are unusual, and can be difficult to identify as they are associated with discharge and hard to palpate. Chancres on the shaft are also seen; those at the base of penis or adjacent abdominal skin are known as condom chancres. Other sites may include the perineum, scrotum and perianal region. In women most chancres are on the labia. The posterior commissure, the clitoris and the urethral orifice are also common

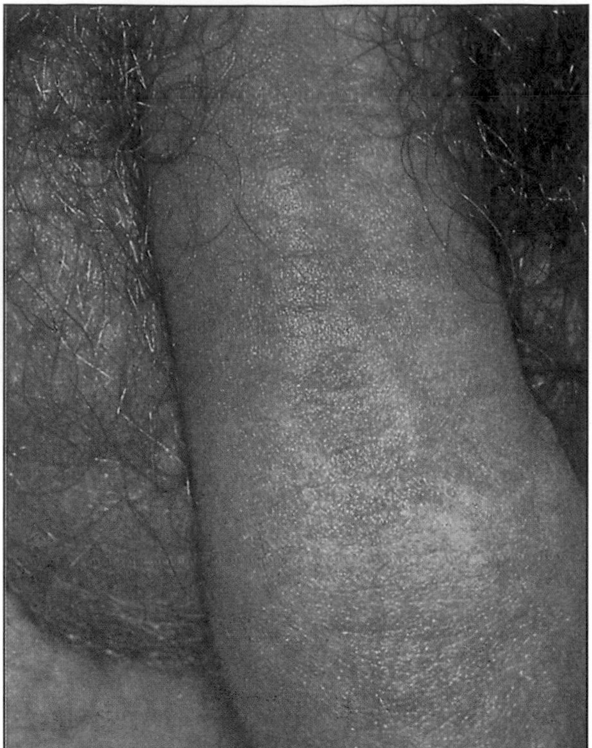

Fig. 5.19. Sclerosing lymphangitis: primary syphilis

sites. Vaginal and cervical lesions are uncommon and easy to overlook. In all locations erosive lesions are more common than firm deep ulcers.

Other primary genital presentations include an erosive balanitis from peri- or intraurethral lesions, focal edema and sclerosing lymphangitis of the dorsal vein of the penis (Fig. 5.19).

Extragenital Chancre. The location of extragenital lesions is only limited by the fantasy of the patient. The most common sites are the perianal and rectal region, as well as the mouth. The perianal region should be examined closely in women and male homosexuals; proctoscopic examination may be needed to identify rectal lesions. In the mouth, the lips are the most common site. Typically the chancre is on the inner side of the lip and easily overlooked; the tonsils are another common intraoral site. Other possibilities include the tongue, buccal mucosa and gingiva. The nipples, umbilicus, axillae, fingers and toes are also possible locations for chancres but no spot is impossible.

Regional Lymphadenopathy. Almost every chancre has associated lymphadenopathy. When the chancre is genital, the lesion is a bubo, usually unilateral. In every site, the regional nodes can be identified; only cervical chancres tend not to produce clinically apparent lymphadenopathy, because intraabdominal lymph nodes are involved. Even rectal chancres usually have inguinal as well as intraabdominal lymphadenopathy. The bubo is usually indolent and painless; ulcerations do not occur. The entire area may become hard and fuse together (syphilitic scleradenitis), but the overlying skin remains freely moveable. The area of the bubo is usually prominently involved in the lymphadenopathy of secondary syphilis.

Diagnostic Criteria

- Clinical suspicion based on history, primary lesion and regional lymphadenopathy.
- Identification of *T. pallidum* on dark-field examination: The dark-field examination is done using a special microscope in which only light that has been bent by the object in the field is seen through the objective. Thus the identified objects are white on a dark background. Clear fluid is squeezed from a moist lesion, placed on a slide with sterile saline and examined. Contamination with blood or other microorganisms makes the procedure very difficult. If a suspicious lesion has crusting or debris, it should be cleaned by using wet soaks prior to examination.
- Serologic reaction: The TPHA or VDRL tests are usually the first positive reactions, which typically appear 2–3 weeks after the chancre.

Differential Diagnosis. The hard chancre is usually fairly distinctive. Sometimes the soft chancre (ulcus molle) of chancroid may be similar, but in most parts of the world syphilis is much more common. Recent studies have shown that in chancroid-endemic regions, clinical diagnoses are often wrong and mixed infections common. An infected HSV infection or bacterial infection, perhaps following trauma, can also mimic a hard chancre, but more often are erosive. The entire differential of balanitis comes into question from eroded lesions of the glans. Firm persistent ulcers can represent carcinoma, so a biopsy may be needed. Primary lesions in other sites are most often mistakenly identified. For example, the syphilitic lesion of the finger formerly seen in physicians was usually diagnosed as a paronychium.

Secondary Syphilis

The secondary stage of syphilis starts at about the ninth week of the infection. The entire body is filled with *T. pallidum*, which have spread via the blood and lymphatics. The transition from primary to secondary syphilis is best viewed as an addition; in addition to the local spirochetosis there is now systemic spirochetosis. In early secondary syphilis the primary lesion is often still present. In other instances, it is already healed or was so small (microchancre) that it had been clinically overlooked. The lymphadenopathy usually persists into the secondary stage.

The spectrum of secondary syphilis is enormous. The most common sites of disease are the skin and mucous membranes, but the areas of localization are highly variable. The specific exanthems and enanthems are known as syphilids. The lesions are usually widespread, symmetrical and rich in *T. pallidum*, especially if weeping or involving mucosal surfaces. While almost everything is possible, the lesions of secondary syphilis are only very rarely pruritic, vesicular or bullous and they heal without scarring. Very late lesions in this phase may be asymmetric, localized and have so few organisms that they are hard to identify.

Diagnostic Criteria

We hesitate to give the diagnostic criteria before discussing the lesions but in the case of secondary syphilis an exception is warranted. Everything can be mistaken for secondary syphilis and vice versa. Fortunately most lesions, especially moist or mucosal lesions, are rich in *Treponema pallidum*, and serologic tests are invariably positive.

Clinical Findings

Macular Syphilid. The most subtle finding in secondary syphilis is the macular syphilid (Fig. 5.20). It was formerly designated as roseola, but that term today is usually reserved for measles. The picture is very monomorphic and always symmetrical. There are many small (2–4 mm) round or oval macules that tend to follow the skin lines. All degrees of severity can be seen from barely visible to as prominent as measles. The macules usually are indistinct, have little or no scale, and may sometimes be urticarial. The most common site is the trunk, especially the upper parts of the abdomen and flanks.

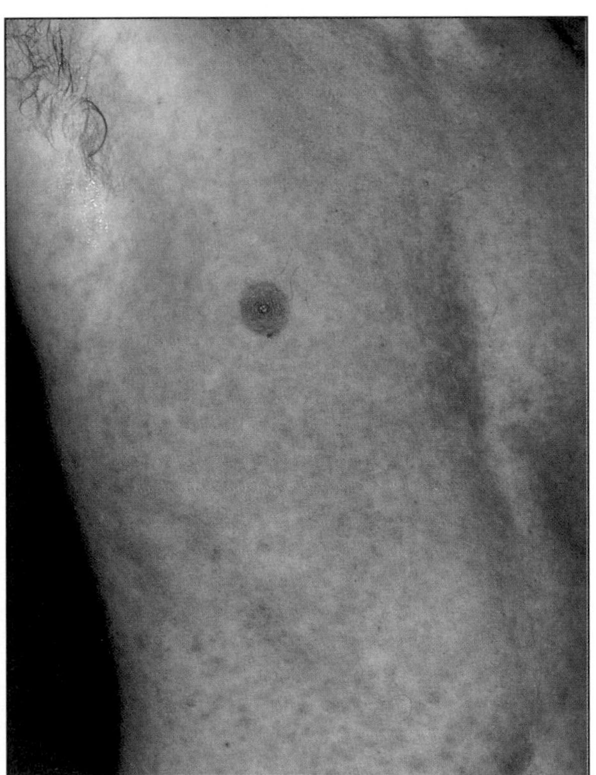

Fig. 5.20. Macular syphilid: secondary syphilis

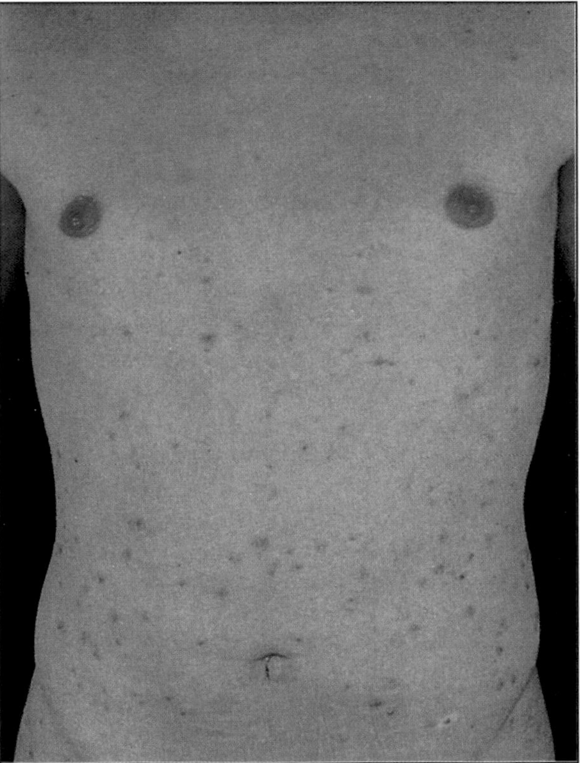

Fig. 5.21. Maculopapular syphilid: secondary syphilis

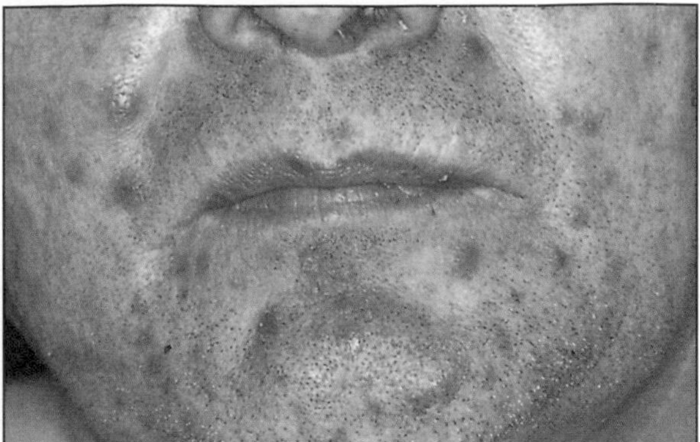

Fig. 5.22. Papular syphilid: secondary syphilis

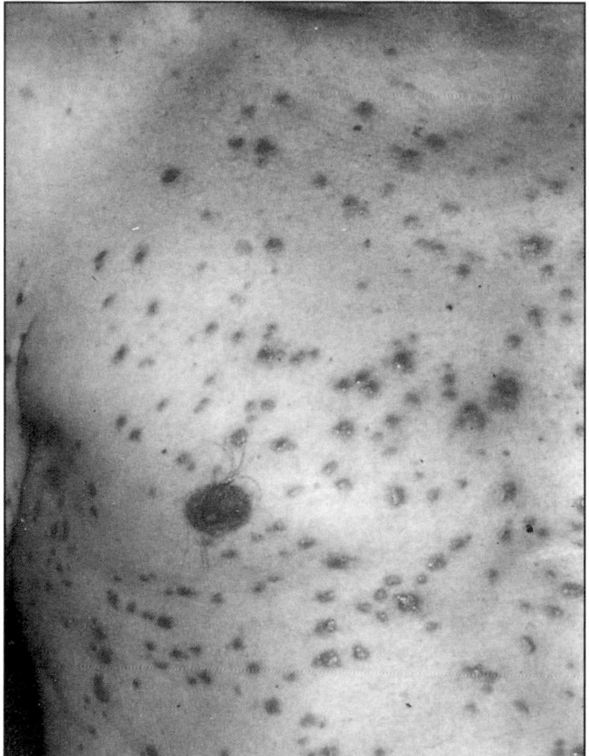

Fig. 5.23. Lichenoid papulonodular syphilid: secondary syphilis

The forehead is the most common facial location. When the extremities are involved, the flexural folds, palms and soles are most susceptible. The lesions tend to have few organisms.

Differential Diagnosis. In the past, the most common differential diagnosis was measles. In fact, the syphilitic exanthems were known as Kiel (a major German seaport) measles. The fever, Koplik spots, rhinitis and conjunctivitis of measles are all not seen. German measles typically has even smaller lesions and associated retroauricular lymphadenopathy. Any viral exanthem, including the primary rash of HIV, can mimic secondary syphilis. Scarlet fever may also be similar but usually has tongue changes. Drug eruptions usually involve the extremities, have larger lesions and heal with scaling.

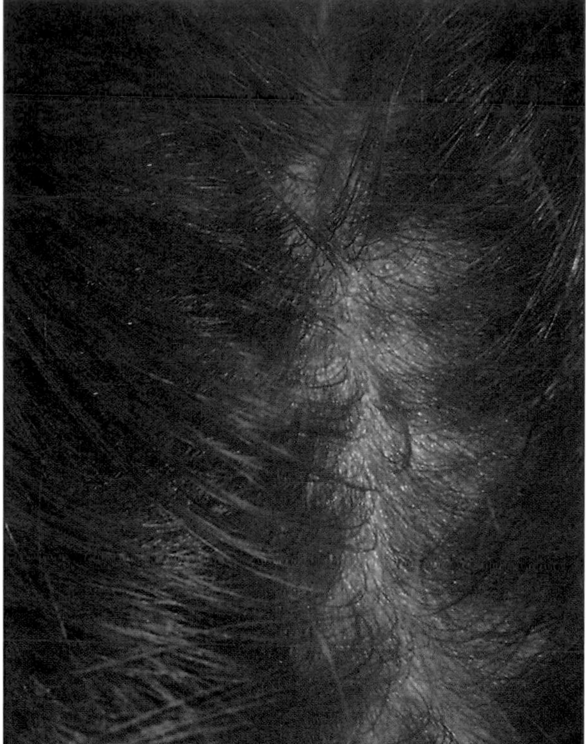

Fig. 5.24. Papular syphilid of the scalp: secondary syphilis

Papular and Papulosquamous Syphilid. This variant is about half as common as macular syphilid. There is a more intense inflammatory infiltrate producing papular lesions, sometimes in association with macules (Fig. 5.21). Later the papular lesions dominate; they tend to be firm, sharply circumscribed, flat-topped, often red-brown papules that may have a surface shine (Fig. 5.22). Thus they have been described as lenticular or lichenoid syphilids (Fig. 5.23). The papules tend to be painful when pressed with a probe. Most papular lesions are teeming with organisms. Their distribution is similar to the macular syphilid, concentrated on the trunk. On the forehead and scalp, the papules may be tender when the hair is combed or brushed (Fig. 5.24). When crusting occurs, they resemble impetigo and are known as impetiginous syphilid. As the papules evolve and age, many develop scale, often with a thin white collarette initially, known as Biett col-

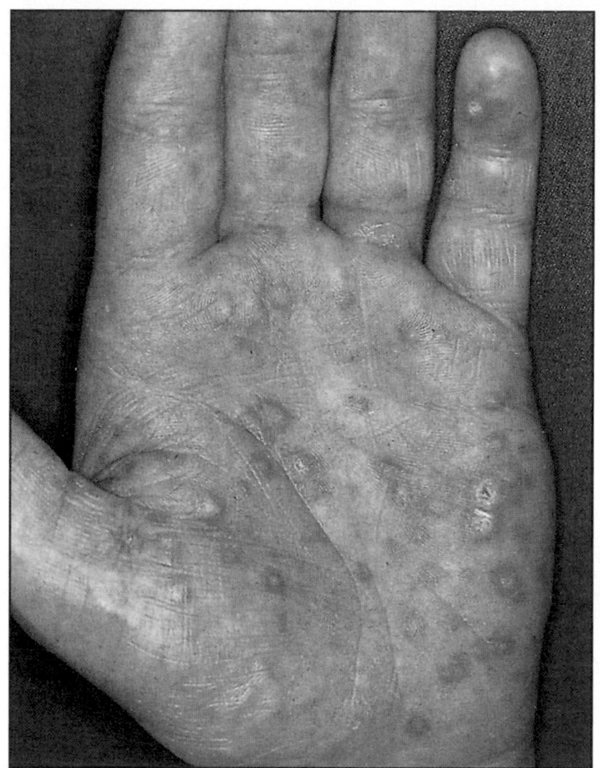

Fig. 5.25. Palmar syphilid: secondary syphilis

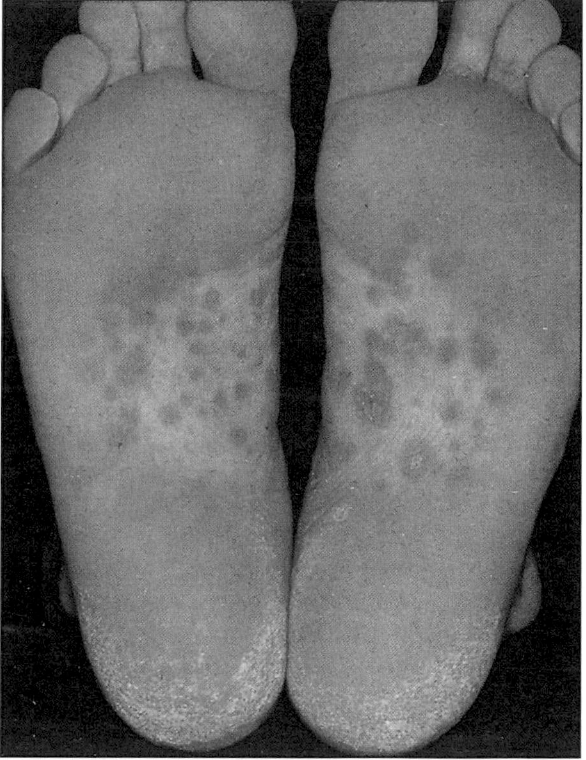

Fig. 5.26. Plantar syphilid: secondary syphilis

larette (1827). Later the scale may be more diffuse. When the palms and soles are involved, the lesions are usually hyperkeratotic and may resemble tinea pedis or even clavi or verruca. The palmar-plantar syphilids strongly suggest the correct diagnosis (Figs. 5.25, 5.26).

Differential Diagnosis. Lichen planus is usually quite pruritic. Pityriasis lichenoides chronica may appear similar but the collodium-like scale is not seen. Pityriasis rosea may also appear very similar but usually a herald patch is not present. Guttate psoriasis can appear identical and the red-brown color may suggest disseminated Kaposi sarcoma.

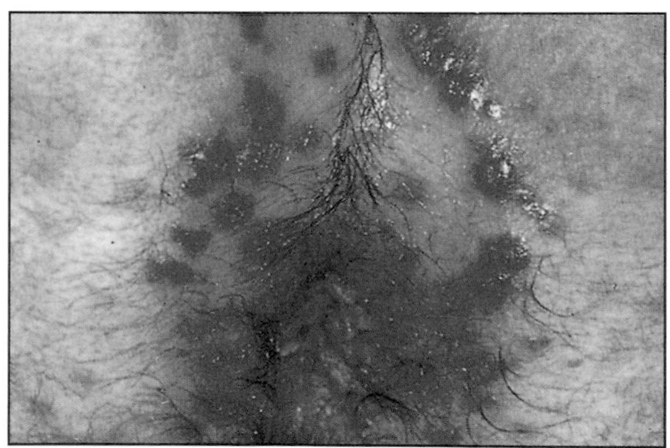

Fig. 5.27. Eroded weeping perianal papules: secondary syphilis

Other Papular Syphilids. Follicular involvement may occur, producing a pebbly surface with many ostial plugs. The crown of Venus refers to seborrheic dermatitis-like lesions along the hairline. Facial lesions often resemble impetigo, involve the nasolabial folds and are symmetrical. Papules at the corner of the mouth may resemble perlèche, but the latter rarely has such distinct papules. Interdigital papules can be seen on both the hands and feet, mistaken for warts, dermatophyte infections or dyshidrotic dermatitis. Papules along the nail fold can cause a paronychium that is usually not as acute as the primary lesion in the same site.

In blacks, annular syphilids are common. They have been called "nickel and dime" syphilids, because they resemble a scattering of coin-shaped lesions. The face and neck are the most common site.

Moist Papular Syphilids. Intertriginous papular lesions acquire a distinct appearance and are teeming with spirochetes (Fig. 5.27). They often have a

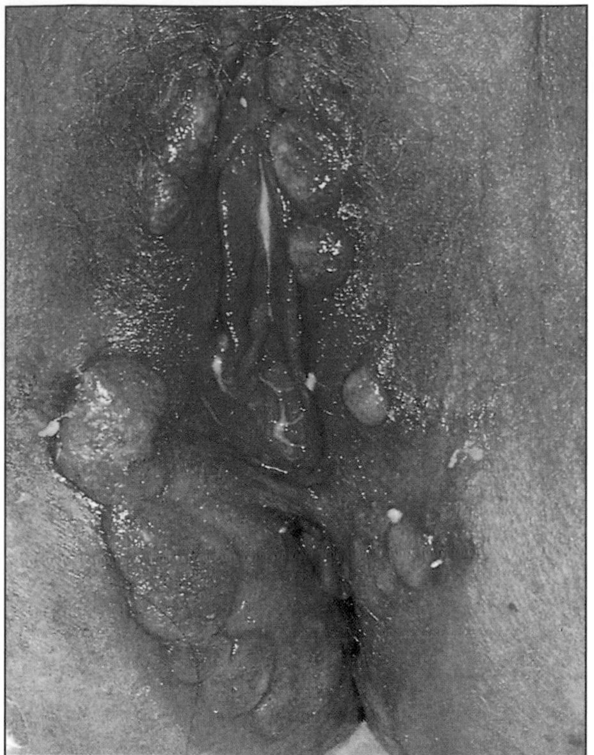

Fig. 5.28. Condylomata lata: secondary syphilis

sweet odor. When they occur in the genital or perianal region, they are known as condylomata lata. The most typical sites are the labia, anal rim and prepuce. Here they vary from broad-based minimally eroded plaques (Fig. 5.28) to vegetating papillomatous lesions to hypertrophic nodular or frambesiform (raspberry-like) proliferations. Other locations where erosive papules maybe seen include axillae, groin and umbilicus.

Differential Diagnosis. Condylomata acuminata is similar in appearance to the syphilids and the names of these two lesions are often confused. These human papilloma virus-induced lesions do not have a broad base, can be gently separated apart into individual papillomas even when massive and often have a cock's comb appearance when compressed between skin surfaces. The erosions of diaper dermatitis, especially when treated with corticosteroids (granuloma glutale infantum), may resemble syphilids. In the perianal region, sometimes hemorrhoids are incorrectly diagnosed.

Pustular Syphilid. All of the pustular forms are rare. They begin with a pustule and evolve rapidly, acquiring a crust and scale. They may range in size from tiny (miliary syphilid) to massive (obtuse syphilid) and are sometimes associated with follicles. The crust may become so massive that it is known as a carapace. In the past, pustular syphilis was confused with small pox, but that problem has disappeared.

Ulcerated Syphilid. Rarely, lesions may ulcerate and then heal with a scar. It is unclear why primary lesions so often ulcerate and secondary, so seldom. Presumably the initial injury facilitating entry is the explanation. Clearly ulcerated syphilid has many overlaps with the far more common erosive syphilid.

Malignant Syphilid

Synonyms. Lues maligna, rupial syphilis, pustulo-ulcerative syphilid

Malignant syphilid is an extreme and rare form, combining the ulcerative and pustular variants (Fig. 5.29). Papulopustular lesions become necrotic and form deep ulcers with thick dirty crusts. The walls of the ulcer are soft rather than indurated. There are usually relatively few lesions and the head and neck are favored. There may be associated oral mucosal changes. The patients are quite ill with fever, chills, weight loss and even hepatitis, but they do not have lymphadenopathy. Some may die if not treated promptly. Malignant syphilid appears more common in HIV- infected and other immunosuppressed patients, but usually there is no explanation. The patient simply never develops an appropriate immune response, while his or her sexual partner(s) handles the *T. pallidum* well. There is no proof that the organism is more virulent;

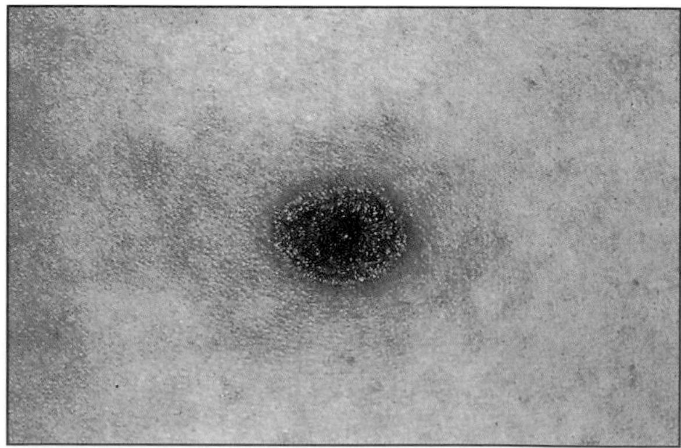

Fig. 5.29. Malignant syphilid: secondary syphilis

instead, the host defense is faulty. The serologic response is reduced and delayed, which may make the diagnosis difficult, but the organisms can be directly identified, for example with PCR.

Pigmentary Changes

The papulosquamous lesions of syphilis can heal with either hypo- or hyperpigmentation or both. The hypopigmentation is known as leucoderma specificum and is most common on the sides of the neck, spreading down to the anterior axillary folds. The many small 3–5-mm patches, irregular in shape and poorly circumscribed have been called the collar or necklace of Venus. They only slowly regiment and can be mistaken for early vitiligo, tinea versicolor, pityriasis lichenoides chronica, psoriatic leucoderma and psoriasis treated with anthralin (psoriatic pseudoleucoderma). Hyperpigmentation usually produces dark brown macules, known as pigmented syphilid, that resemble lichen planus or a resolving lichenoid drug eruption.

Alopecia

All types of hair loss are possible in secondary syphilis, ranging from localized patches to total alopecia. Hair loss occurs late in the secondary stage, about 8–12 weeks after the first secondary signs at a time when the serology is always positive. The hair loss may follow the distribution of the preceding exanthem. While patients may complain of diffuse hair loss, examination usually reveals focal yellow-red areas of alopecia that may coalesce in irregular patterns producing a moth-eaten appearance. The eyebrows and other hairy areas of the body may also be involved. Complete alopecia in a given patch, as seen in alopecia areata, is rare. In other instances there is diffuse loss and the entire scalp may have a light red-yellow color, suggesting diffuse inflammation.

Differential Diagnosis. The main question is usually alopecia areata. If multiple patches are present, if hair loss within the patch is incomplete, if explanation point hairs are missing or if lymphadenopathy is present, one should order a syphilis serology. In diffuse hair loss, if there any signs suggesting a systemic illness or fitting in with secondary syphilis, once again the serology is the answer.

Oral Mucosal Changes. About one-third of patients have oral mucosal changes. There may be erythematous macules and papules, but they soon become macerated and acquire a gray-white coating. The lesions are called mucous or opaline patches (Figs. 5.30, 5.31). On the dorsum of the tongue, the normal papillae seem to fuse together with the coalescent papules, producing smooth plaques or plaques lisses. When they thicken, then the tongue is described as a turtle-tongue, because of the fancied relationship between the dome-shaped nodules and a turtle's shell.

Differential Diagnosis. In their fully developed form, the oral lesions are fairy distinctive. Early on one may consider mucosal drug eruptions and viral exanthems, such as that caused by Epstein-Barr virus. Erosive lichen planus and lupus erythematosus produce broad flat erosions but these are much more chronic lesions.

Syphilitic Angina. Inflammation of the tonsils is typical for secondary syphilis. In German, it is known as specific angina, referring to the days when syphilis was specific and other diseases were

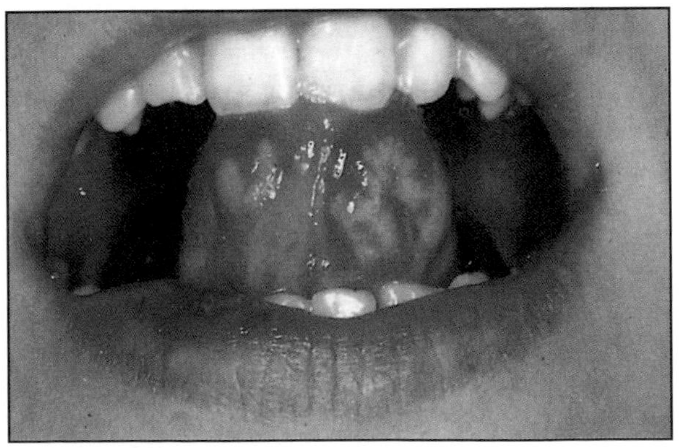

Fig. 5.30. Mucous patches: secondary syphilis

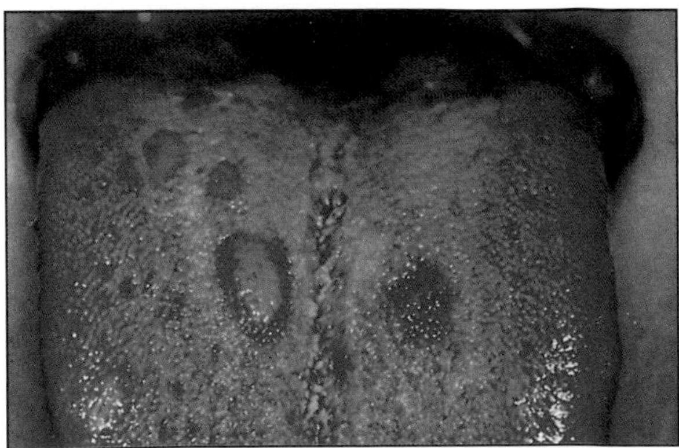

Fig. 5.31. Mucous patches: secondary syphilis

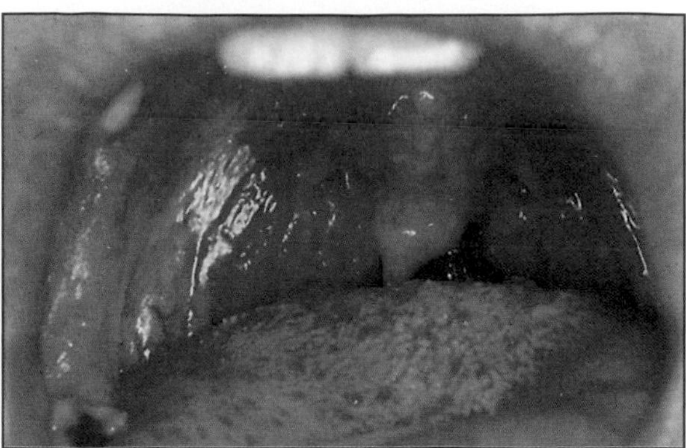

Fig. 5.32. Angina specifica: secondary syphilis

not. The tonsillitis reflects the underlying lymphadenopathy associated with the secondary stage. The tonsils are swollen, red and have a gray coating (Fig. 5.32). There may be a sweet smell and the patient often complains of pain on swallowing. Fever is usually absent. The primary tonsillar lesion is often unilateral and associated with unilateral cervical lymphadenopathy. Other bacterial and viral causes of tonsillitis should be excluded with the usual culture methods.

Lymphadenopathy. Every patient with secondary syphilis, except those with malignant syphilid, has diffuse lymphadenopathy, known as polyscleradenitis because of the multiplicity and firm nature of the nodes. The nodes are typically painless, not greatly enlarged, usually about 1–2 cm in size and freely movable. The overlying skin is not inflamed and the nodes never suppurate or ulcerate. The site of the primary bubo is almost invariably involved, but the cervical, axillary, antecubital, and inguinal nodes and many others may be affected. The famous syphilitic handshake involved glancing at the hand for a syphilid, and then reaching past the extended hand to attempt to palpate enlarged epitrochlear nodes about the elbow, a classic sign of secondary syphilis.

Systemic Manifestations. Most patients are surprisingly healthy, considering they have a widespread infection. Fever, loss of appetite and malaise are common. The major clinical problem involves the central nervous system, more specifically the meninges. About 40–50% of patients have some meningeal signs, such as a stiff neck or headaches, frequently occipital and at night. Many of these patients and some asymptomatic individuals have positive findings on CSF examination, including elevated protein, lymphocytosis and positive serologic tests. Aseptic meningitis develops in 1–2%. Since neurosyphilis is such a dreaded complication, the positive clinical findings and CSF are approached with caution. In the past, patients with meningeal signs were simply treated, and if any hints of persistent disease remained, then underwent CSF examination. Today, in light of problems with meningitis in HIV-positive patients treated with standard regimens, it is recommended that all such patients undergo CSF examination prior to therapy.

The other problems are less serious. Arthralgias are common and in some patients there is bone pain (dolores osteocopi) usually involving the long bones and perhaps reflecting subclinical periostitis. While most hepatitis in syphilis patients probably reflects a coincident viral infection, true syphilitic hepatitis does occur, usually in association with proctitis in homosexuals. An immune complex glomerulonephritis is also seen, as well as an uveitis. Many other rarer systemic problems can also occur, as discussed in specialized texts.

Latent Syphilis

The massive involvement with *T. pallidum* as seen in secondary syphilis is gradually brought under control by the immune response. The clinical features not only become less severe, but usually disappear entirely. In latent syphilis, the patient has no positive physical findings, in particular, no evidence of cardiovascular or neurological disease. Some criteria also require a negative CSF examination. Serologic examination is always positive; usually both nonspecific and specific treponemal tests are positive. Of untreated latent patients, two-thirds will remain latent or asymptomatic; one-third will develop tertiary syphilis. About half of this latter group will develop benign or gummatous tertiary syphilis, while the balance will manifest cardiovascular or CNS symptoms.

The distinctions between early latent syphilis and late latent syphilis are artificial. The biologic difference is crucial: early latent patients are infective; late latent patients can infect an infant transplacentally but are otherwise not contagious. Arbitrary cut-off points of 1, 2, or 4 years after the healing of secondary syphilis are used. When treatment is the issue, an untreated patient is regarded as having late latent syphilis after 1 year. Over 90% of relapses occur within 2 years. After 4 years, almost no patient is still infective. Patients who acquire transfusion-based syphilis are regarded as having late latent disease. The date of infection, the date of resolution and the serologic records are often unavailable. Some patients are serofast, even after treatment; others show seroreversal without treatment. In no case should seroreversal be equated with cure. Such patients may develop tertiary syphilis many years later. An untreated syphilis patient is always latent and almost always has positive, specific, treponemal serologic tests.

Recurrent Disease

During the early latency period recurrences are likely. They are best observed in the skin. The first recurrence is usually a recurrent macular syphilid, known as a recurrent roseola. Perhaps because all the areas where the skin was involved in the initial exanthem retain some immunity, recurrent syphilid seems to fill in the blanks. Thus the lesions are often annular, surrounding older lesions. Corymbiform lesions also usually represent a recurrence; a central papule or nodule is surrounded by many satellite lesions. Corymbiform means resembling the clusters of the ivy flower; a more dramatic term is bombshell lesions. A third typical form of skin recurrence is lichen syphiliticus. Multiple 2–3-mm papules, usually with a pointed surface and mild scale, are arranged about follicles and grouped in an area several centimeters in diameter. While there are many other causes of tiny follicular papules, none are typically so grouped.

Larger nodular lesions may also be seen and are often clinically misdiagnosed as malignant infiltrates. When seen on the legs, they resemble erythema nodosum but tend to ulcerate. After the first recurrence resolves, subsequent recurrences are much more widely spaced and most patients remain asymptomatic until tertiary syphilis starts. The skin lesions become less symptomatic, have many fewer organisms and are less symmetrical.

Similar signs of recurrence probably involve the same organs that are affected in secondary syphilis, but the nomenclature is not as well-established in the skin. Recurrent meningeal signs and symptoms are probably most common and certainly most crucial. In the past, recurrent disease was probably better identified. Today, one tends to make the diagnosis of tertiary disease without deliberating over the fine distinctions.

Tertiary Syphilis

The transition from early syphilis to late syphilis can last 10, 20 or even more years, or it can occur quite rapidly. The relationship between the patient's immune system and *T. pallidum* is decisive. The most typical response is a granulomatous one, reflecting a type IV immune reaction. The syphilitic gumma is the best known granulomatous lesion. In each organ, there is a balance between interstitial granulomatous inflammation, producing diffuse changes, and localized gummata, but the basic process is the same. Another key feature is the endarteritis that is seen in the skin but which plays a far more crucial role in the cardiovascular and central nervous systems. The final major mechanism is the relatively anergic state known as metasyphilis, in which there is parenchymal nervous tissue damage by the spirochetes and often a reversal of the serologic reactions, showing decreased immunity. The patients with a prominent granulomatous response and endarteritis are at less risk of developing parenchymal destruction.

If there is a typical case, then one could say that tertiary syphilis usually starts 3–5 years after secondary syphilis. The clinical lesions are asymmetric but usually grouped, show liquifactive necrosis and heal with atrophy or scarring. *T. pallidum* is almost impossible to find because of the excellent immunity of most patients. PCR has made it possible to identify the organisms in tissues. Certainly the patient is not infective. The lesions histologically show necrotic granulomas, known as syphilitic granulomas. About 70 % of gummata involve the skin, 10 %, the oral cavity, 10 % the bones and the balance are widely dispersed. In most instances there is peripheral spread of the destruction with associated central atrophy and scarring. In about 30 % of patients the nontreponemal serology is negative; almost all retain specific treponemal markers. One interesting aspect of tertiary syphilis is the use of potassium iodide as a therapeutic test; syphilitic gumma respond extremely rapidly to the administration of the salt. Administration of penicillin is an equally effective therapeutic test.

Clinical Findings. The skin findings can be divided into the tuberous or nodular cutaneous lesions and the subcutaneous gummata (singular gumma). These frequently overlap and should be viewed as the same response occurring at different tissue levels with different degrees of destruction. One

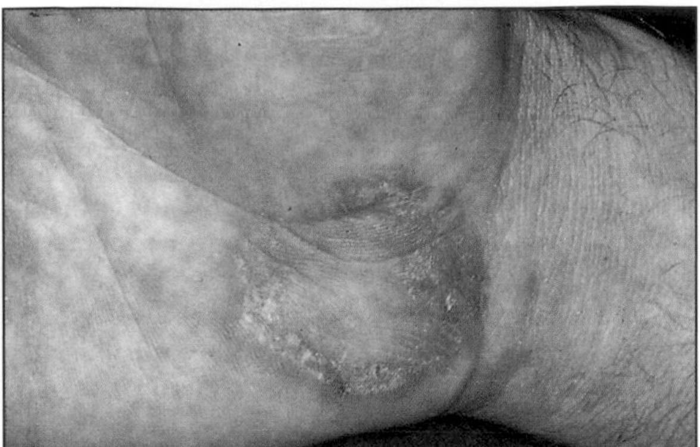

Fig. 5.33. Tuberous syphilid: tertiary syphilis

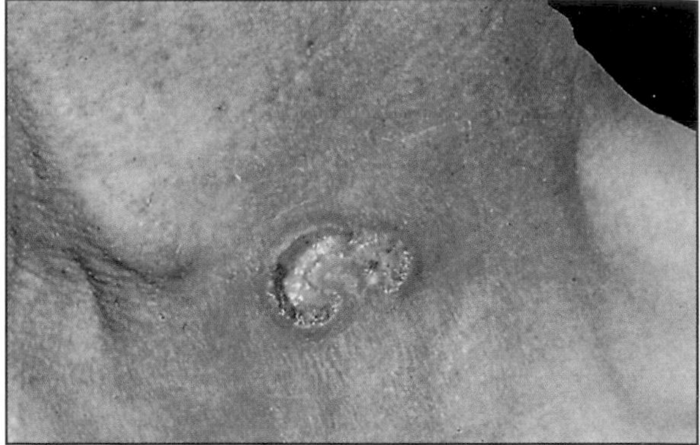

Fig. 5.34. Gumma: tertiary syphilis

can view a gumma as a superb host response to a local cluster of *T. pallidum* while the interstitial or parenchymal reactions are less severe but attack more widely dispersed organisms.

Tuberous Syphilid. The typical lesion consists of grouped papules that heal with atrophy. The most common sites are the face and scalp. The grouped lesions may intersect or overlap and may have an annular pattern (Fig. 5.33). The individual lesions are red-brown flat-topped papules with minimal scale. Lesions heal centrally with atrophy and either hyper- or hypopigmentation, as they progress peripherally. These wandering patterns have been called tubero-serpiginous syphilid.

When ulcers develop, they are similarly patterned, usually several millimeters in size and sharply punched out. The base of the ulcer is yellow and necrotic with oyster shell-like or rupial crusts. The ulcers heal centrally as they spread laterally. This pattern is known as tubero-ulcero-serpiginous syphilid.

Differential Diagnosis. The main differential diagnosis in the past was lupus vulgaris. While the syphilitic lesions appear similar, their speed of destruction is much greater. One says that what lupus vulgaris destroys in years, syphilis destroys in weeks to months. Diascopy does not reveal a lupoid infiltrate; recurrences within the scars rare unusual, while they are common in lupus vulgaris. Other considerations are cutaneous lymphomas, sarcoidosis (which rarely ulcerates) and deep fungal infections.

Gummata. The subcutaneous lesion of tertiary syphilis, the gumma, can appear anywhere on the skin. Features of all gumma are that they are surprisingly painless, not associated with lymphadenopathy and free of organisms. A subcutaneous nodule is the first change; it enlarges and becomes matted together with the underlying muscle and fascia as well as the overlying skin, which becomes livid red to brown, thickened and rubbery (hence, the name). Central necrosis occurs, producing first fluctuance and then a perforating, discharging ulcer (Fig. 5.34). The necrotic material is tenacious and can be drawn out into threads. The ulcers are often kidney-shaped. Gummata may become quite large, many centimeters in diameter, are tender to pressure but are not accompanied by lymphadenopathy. The lesions heal after weeks to months with a smooth white scar surrounded by a hyperpigmented band.

The depth and location of gummata are highly variable. They may involve any level from subcutaneous fat to periostium and bone. Massive destruction may occur, involving any of the intervening structures such as muscles, nerves and vessels. Common anatomic sites include the forehead, scalp, lips, neck, genitalia and tibia, but any site is possible. Most are solitary, but some patients develop multiple lesions. One special ulcer is the pseudochancre redux, a solitary penile gumma.

Differential Diagnosis. While tertiary syphilis is fairly unique and can be rapidly identified by serologic testing, one must think of other deep destructive processes such as tuberculosis (especially tuberculosis cutis colliquativa), actinomycosis (which also favors the neck), sporotrichosis, other deep fungi, lupus profundus (subcutaneous lupus erythematosus), lymphoma, ulcerated malignant tumors such as the rodent ulcer variant of basal cell carcinoma, ulcerated panniculitis or other granulomatous infections.

Oral Manifestations. The most notorious site for a gumma is the nasal septum, although such lesions have become rare. They may also involve the soft and hard palates, the sinuses and the tonsils. Bony or cartilaginous damage is the rule in the intraoral sites. Often, destruction of the nasal septum is followed by liquifactive necrosis of the floor of the nose (roof of the mouth) leading to palatal perforation. Soft palatal and tonsillar involvement leads to massive damage in the back of the mouth, with disappearance of the uvula and a resulting large V-shaped defect exposing the pharynx. The main differential diagnostic considerations include carcinomas, lymphomas, other malignant infiltrates and rarely tuberculosis.

Both tuberous syphilids and gumma may on rare occasion involve the inner aspect of the lips. Sometimes the upper lip is swollen (syphilitic macrocheilia) secondary to diffuse inflammation and sclerosis, mimicking Melkersson-Rosenthal syndrome or labial elephantiasis following recurrent HSV and erysipelas. On rare occasion diffuse ulcers occur, known as lues miliaris ulcerosa mucosa (Arndt 1926). They may be seen on the tonsils, gingiva or tongue as superficial bizarre erosions with a chewed border and small punched-out ulcers. The surface is covered with debris. While the term was suggested as a parallel to miliary tuberculosis, there is actually a significant contrast. In tuberculosis miliaris ulcerosa mucosa the ulcerations are rich in organisms, while in syphilis they are not.

The tongue may also be involved in several ways that have clinical and probably biologic overlaps. Tuberous lesions may develop. They tend to be small, but as they ulcerate and heal, they destroy the papillae, producing smooth, flat white scars. As such areas fuse, the dorsum of the tongue may become quite flat, sclerotic and even shiny. Another variant is interstitial glossitis, in which more diffuse changes occur. There is granulomatous inflammation involving the interstitial tissue of the tongue. If the inflammation is superficial, the surface may be focally attacked, producing flattening of the papillae. In the case of deeper interstitial involvement, the tongue initially may be swollen (syphilitic macroglossia) but later it becomes hardened and shrunken, although without ulceration. In contrast, gummata of the tongue are usually solitary, destroy the muscle fibers, ulcerate and heal with a deep pit or scar. The motility of the tongue is usually impaired.

All of the tongue changes provide a fertile ground for the development of carcinoma. Thus, in any case of squamous cell carcinoma of the tongue, one probably should order a syphilis serology. Conversely, the leukoplakia and atrophic changes seen on the tongue should be regularly monitored for changes suggesting malignancy. Other granulomatous disease, such as Melkersson-Rosenthal syndrome, and tumors, such as lymphomas and sarcomas, should also be excluded.

Other Internal Lesions. Bone involvement is the other common type of gumma. Bony lesions usually occur where the skin and bone are in close apposition, such as in the tibia, radius, clavicle, scapula, sternum and skull. Bone pains are typically worse in the evening. The classic lesion is osteomyelitis (or osteitis) of the medial end of the clavicle. Periostitis and sclerosing osteitis also occur, as well as juxtaarticular nodes, which are fibrous gummata, that is, they do not usually liquefy. Another joint change is gummatous involvement of the bursae, usually the olecranon, with rupture and discharge of gelatinous material; this is known as Verneuil's disease, a term which is also applied to acne inversa.

Gummata may also involve the liver, known as hepar lobatum, and are usually associated with parenchymal disease. They may also appear in the parotid gland, the stomach, the testes and almost every other organ.

Cardiovascular Syphilis. Many processes involve the cardiovascular system in tertiary syphilis. Men are more likely to be affected than women, and congenital syphilis does not cause cardiovascular problems. Before the days of antibiotics, about a third of cardiovascular disease in American blacks was caused by syphilis. About 10% of patients in the untreated series had aortic symptoms, but autopsies showed involvement in up to 80%. The main problems occur in the aorta. There is an infiltration of the media by spirochetes with resulting destruction leading to saccular aneurysms, mostly of the ascending aorta. These lesions do not dissect but about one-third rupture, while others damage the aortic valve and root. There is also a prominent endarteritis of the coronary vessels, often coupled with coronary artery ostial stenosis and leading to coronary artery disease, often at an early age without obvious risk factors. In addition, aortic regurgitation may develop. Finally, gummata may cause conduction defects or, rarely, destroy papillary muscles.

Today cardiovascular syphilis has become a rarity, but is nonetheless a fascinating problem. In the past, linear calcifications of the ascending aorta and eggshell calcifications of the descending aorta were considered classic signs of cardiovascular involvement. The treatment is surgical for the aortic problems, while penicillin therapy and standard medical management may help the coronary artery disease. The Jarisch-Herxheimer reaction, involving the massive kill-off of *T. pallidum* when penicillin therapy is started, may trigger cardiac symptoms and even immediate rupture of an aneurysm.

Neurosyphilis

All neurosyphilis is basically a meningitis, although in the tertiary stage one distinguishes between meningeal, vascular and parenchymal disease. The meningeal signs and rare aseptic meningitis seen in secondary syphilis do not necessarily correlate with later CNS involvement. Neurosyphilis is more common in patients affected at an early age, although it is not associated with congenital syphilis. Patients over the age of 40 are not at much risk, perhaps because they do not have time to develop neurologic signs and symptoms. Neurosyphilis has so many possible manifestations that it is a frustrating clinical diagnosis. There is one bright side; virtually every patient has positive serologic signs of syphilis and most have positive CSF findings, so if in doubt, search for syphilis.

It is important to recognize asymptomatic neurosyphilis. Some patients with late latent syphilis may have positive CSF findings or even subtle neurologic problems that are overlooked. Syphilis is usually curable at this stage, where more advanced neurologic disease is quite therapy-resistant. When untreated patients were followed, after 10 years about 20 % had abnormal CSF findings and of this group, one-third were symptomatic.

A wide variety of problems have been identified. Gummata may occur, destroying cranial nerves, causing local space occupying cortical lesions and meningeal irritation. They may present as a focal seizure disorder. The gummata are often difficult to distinguish from tumors and are therapy-resistant. Chronic meningitis may cause cerebral, cranial nerve or spinal symptoms. Cerebral endarteritis causes stroke-like problems at an early age as a result of thrombotic events; this is known as meningovascular neurosyphilis. Other problems include hemiparalysis and aphasia. In general, the meningovascular problems develop 5–10 years after secondary syphilis, while the more severe parenchymal problems appear even later.

The two most dreaded problems of neurosyphilis are general paresis of the insane and tabes dorsalis. Both involve invasion of neural tissue by *T. pallidum*, associated with reduced immunity. General paresis of the insane appears earlier, usually after 15–20 years; patients present with a combination of neurologic and psychiatric problems. Cerebral cortical destruction is the basic process. Patients with general paresis of the insane die a disturbing death, usually bed-ridden and thus succumbing to aspiration pneumonia or infection. Formerly such patients were the majority denizens of institutions for the mentally ill. Today the problems are usually recognized sooner and respond somewhat to treatment.

In tabes dorsalis, the key damage occurs in the posterior columns and the dorsal roots. There is progressive locomotor ataxia producing the foot slap walk, which generations of neurology professors could mimic so well during lectures. Romberg sign is positive, meaning that the patient cannot stand with the feet together and eyes closed. There are also shooting pains or lightening pains that appear suddenly, radiate and disappear. In addition, paresthesias are common. Deep tendon reflexes are absent. Frequently there are trophic ulcerations on the feet (mal perforans) and the joints may be damaged because of a lack of sensation. The reactive protective proliferative changes produce Charcot joints.

Several other special forms of neurosyphilis require mentioning. Cranial nerve involvement is common, but rarely isolated. The 7th and 8th nerves are most often involved, along with the nerves of ocular motility. Deafness is secondary to inner ear damage and is seen most often in congenital syphilis. However, it may also occur with tertiary syphilis, as may Menière disease. Even today a modest percentage of patients with sensorineural hearing loss or cochlear problems have an unexpected positive serologic test for syphilis.

The ocular manifestations of syphilis have filled entire books. Everything from keratitis, usually associated with congenital syphilis, to blindness can occur. The classic sign is the Argyll-Robertson pupil,a small irregular pupil that reacts to near vision but not to light or pain. Optic atrophy may also occur, usually with peripheral loss producing gun barrel vision and then blindness. On rare occasions, optic atrophy may be the first sign of tertiary syphilis. While optic atrophy usually reflects a neuritis, it may also be caused by gummata pressing on the nerve. Paralysis of the optic nerves and muscles may develop, caused by both gummata and inflammatory lesions. Finally, uveitis and chorioretinitis can also occur, as the ocular version of an overabundant inflammatory response. The eye findings are so diverse that they do not point to a single type or pattern of syphilis, but any patient with unexplained ocular problems deserves a serologic test for syphilis.

Congenital Syphilis

Synonyms. Connatal or prenatal syphilis is grammatically correct, but congenital syphilis is the standard term. Hereditary syphilis is incorrect and should not be used.

Definition. Syphilis caused by the transfer of *T. pallidum* from mother to infant during pregnancy.

Epidemiology. Congenital syphilis has become relatively uncommon because of the standard prenatal monitoring of syphilis serologies and the required testing of cord blood. There was an upsurge of congenital syphilis in the USA in the late 1980s; the risk factors are similar as for adult syphilis including AIDS, drugs abuse and prostitution. In addition, young mothers and mothers who first had intercourse at an early age are at greater risk.

Etiology and Pathogenesis. *Treponema pallidum* is usually transferred to the infant after the first trimester. During this early period the placenta is insufficiently developed and the risk of transfer is small, so if the mother acquires syphilis and is treated, no problems occur. If she is untreated, there are high blood levels of the organism and the placenta becomes infected. It is full of treponemes, enlarged and contains granulomas (Fränkel granulomas).

In the fourth to fifth month the fetus is overwhelmed by *T. pallidum* and the result is usually a spontaneous abortion. Over 80 % of children whose mothers had untreated syphilis early in pregnancy are stillborn. The organisms are found in the placenta, umbilical cord, amniotic fluid and fetus; in suspect cases, PCR can be employed. Maternal, fetal and amniotic fluid serologic tests are positive.

If the mother has late secondary syphilis, the numbers of organisms are smaller and, while the fetus is infected, it survives the intrauterine infection with stigmata. In late latent syphilis, the number of spirochetes is so small that some infants are infected, others not. Another scenario is when the mother acquires syphilis late in pregnancy. In this instance, blood levels may not suffice for infection, but there can be direct transfer during delivery. Technically the child has acquired syphilis. The most typical site for the chancre is the eyelid, except in breech deliveries.

The maternal antibodies are also transferred transplacentally, providing some protection and also confusing the interpretation of testing. As will be discussed in detail below, the IgM antibodies are not transferred transplacentally. If an infant is exposed in utero to *T. pallidum*, it will manufacture IgM antitreponemal antibodies. Thus a negative 19S IgM FTA-ABS test speaks against congenital syphilis, even when the mother is seropositive and the infant has other positive tests.

Clinical Findings. The clinical findings are all variations on the themes discussed under secondary syphilis. There is intense interstitial inflammation and frequently parenchymal invasion by *T. pallidum*. Because of the rapid metabolic processes in the skeleton during infancy, skeletal defects are far more prominent.

Early Congenital Syphilis

Synonym. Lues connata praecox

Clinical Findings

Cutaneous Findings. The changes are very similar to those of secondary syphilis. The papulosquamous lesions are most common on the face, trunk, palms, soles (Fig. 5.35) and especially diaper area,

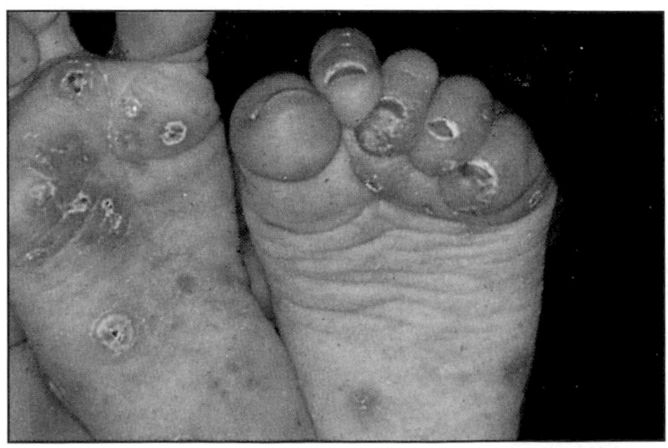

Fig. 5.35. Papular syphilid, early congenital syphilis

where they are frequently eroded. The lesions have a pink or red hint, but typically become red-brown. The end result may be hyper- or hypopigmented patches. The combination of anemia, jaundice and hyperpigmentation produces a café-au-lait tint. Other lesions may be crusted, resembling impetigo. The mucous patches are present in about one-third of infants; they are teeming with organisms and are highly infective, as are the condylomata lata, which may occur in the anogenital region and about other orifices.

There are other highly suggestive cutaneous changes. Because of nursing, the perioral area is subjected to considerable mechanical stress. Hochsinger infiltrates start as papules along the lips but then spread peripherally and coalesce. The indurated tissue tends to develop radial furrows and fissures that extend from the lips into the adjacent skin and are connected by transverse furrows. The changes, known as rhagades, are most prominent in the first months and heal with radial scars called Parrot furrows or Parrot lines.

In contrast to adult secondary syphilis, congenital syphilis may have vesicular or bullous lesions. These blisters are called pemphigus syphiliticus, but have nothing in common with pemphigus vulgaris. The subepidermal blisters reflect intense inflammation and are most often seen on the palms and soles but may extend onto the limbs. When they rupture, macerated plaques are left behind. At the same time, the palms and soles may be edematous and almost polished. Widespread desquamation may also occur.

Systemic Findings. Infants infected with syphilis may present with involvement of many organs, either at birth or in the first weeks of life. About a third have findings at birth; they are more likely to be premature, severely infected and, not surprisingly, do less well. The first sign is usually rhinitis or sniffles, secondary to the ulcerated nasal mucosa. The discharge is thick and often interferes with breathing and feeding. If not treated, the nasal bones may also be damaged producing the saddle nose deformity. An interstitial hepatitis with hepatosplenomegaly and fibrosis (Feuerstein (flint) liver) leads to jaundice in more than half the patients. There is marked lymphadenopathy – once again enlarged epitrochlear nodes are highly suggestive. Hemolytic anemia is also very common, sometimes associated with thrombocytopenia.

Over 90 % of infants have radiologic evidence of skeletal disease, although only a small percentage have clinical findings. The osteochondritis typically involves the long bones, with epiphyseal widening and damage and a moth-eaten appearance. Epiphyseal dislocation may occur; the classic location is the proximal end of the ulna producing a painful pseudoparalysis of the distal arm and hand known as Parrot pseudoparalysis. Other epiphyses can also be so affected. Later on, dactylitis is more common, as the osteochondritis involves the small bones of the digits.

Periostitis is also a later finding. It is more diffuse and appears radiologically as onion-skin calcification or multiple thin layers of calcification arranged outside the cortex of the affected bone. The two most common sites are the frontal bone of the skull, producing frontal bossing, and the tibia, producing bowed or saber shins (Fig. 5.37).

CSF examination is abnormal in about half the patients with increased protein, increased cells or positive serologic tests. While acute CNS disease is uncommon, residua often occur.

The pediatrician or pathologist may be able to make the diagnosis extremely early. The placenta is usually larger than expected, rich in granulomas and contains the organism. The umbilical cord has been described as the barber shop pole cord because there are red erythematous areas, blue cyanotic zones and chalky white necrotic areas within a smooth pale cord. These changes, known as necrotizing funisitis, are relatively diagnostic.

Prognosis. Infants who are treated promptly do well. The degree of permanent damage incurred prior to delivery is dependent on the timing of the infection of the fetus. Longer intrauterine infections are more likely to produce permanent damage.

Diagnostic Criteria. Children born to mothers with untreated or inadequately treated syphilis (such as those treated with erythromycin base during pregnancy), mothers treated in the last month of pregnancy and mothers in whom adequate serologic follow-up is not available should be evaluated for congenital syphilis. No infant should leave the hospital without the mother's serologic status having been evaluated at least once during pregnancy. In many populations, serologic testing is performed at delivery. Evaluation should include a nontreponemal test on the infant's sera, CSF analysis, bone survey, examination of placenta and umbilical cord, and, if all these are negative and suspicion remains, a 19S-IgM-FTA-ABS test.

Differential Diagnosis. The differential diagnosis of early congenital syphilis is usually that of the infant with sepsis and failure to thrive. In reality, most cases are diagnosed at latest on the cord blood results, but a mix-up is always possible and the clinician must keep the protean manifestations of congenital syphilis in mind.

Late Congenital Syphilis

Synonym. Lues connata tarda

Clinical Findings. In late congenital syphilis the changes or stigmata of congenital syphilis are discovered after 2 years of age, either because they were overlooked in the neonatal period, because the patient was relatively asymptomatic or because therapy was inadequate. One also uses the term late congenital syphilis to include the permanent sequelae of early congenital syphilis.

Definite Stigmata. These include the classic stigmata of congenital syphilis, known as the Hutchinson triad: Hutchinson incisors, interstitial keratitis and 8th nerve deafness. The deafness is so rare that the triad is more misleading than helpful. What is helpful is the lack of cardiovascular and CNS disease and the fact that all untreated patients are serologically positive. The other definite stigmata are listed below.

- Saddle nose: The sequelae of the sniffles and subsequent cartilage and bone damage in the nose produces a classic picture. The distal part of the nose is tilted back, as the bony part is absent or depressed (Fig. 5.36). In addition, there is too much skin because of the underlying damage, so that prominent radial folds are seen.
- Parrot lines: These are the radial deep furrows that are the result of the healed rhagades. They may also develop about the anus. What makes Parrot lines distinctive is that they extend through the vermilion and the skin.
- Interstitial keratitis: The ocular changes develop quite late, usually between age 6 and 20. The cloudy infiltrates begin at the limbus and gradually spread to involve the entire cornea. There may be an associated uveitis or chorioretinitis. Optic atrophy is also seen, but almost always associated with neurosyphilis.
- Dental changes:
  Hutchinson incisors. The permanent upper incisors are notched and taper from their base to the biting edge (Fig. 5.37). When the notching is minimal, one speaks of screwdriver incisors. Often a diastema is also present; that is, the teeth are set more widely apart than usual.
  Moon molars. Also known as mulberry molars, these are abnormal first molars in which the cusps are crowded together on the biting surface. They are subject to exaggerated caries and usually fall victim to the dentist.
- Gummata: These may arise just as in tertiary syphilis and tend to involve the bones of the skull

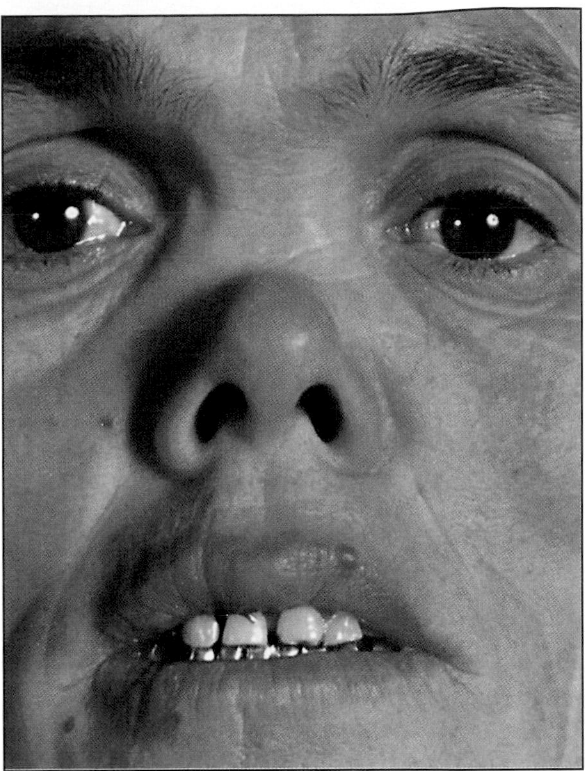

Fig. 5.36. Saddle nose and Parrot furrow, late congenital syphilis

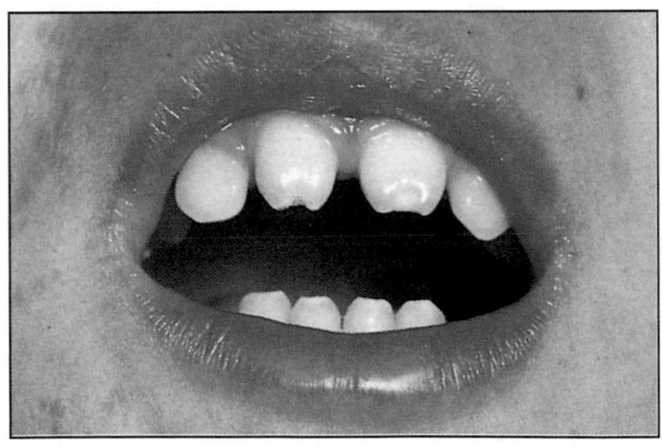

Fig. 5.37. Hutchinson incisors, late congenital syphilis

or tibia, but may erode through to the skin. The nasal septum is once again at risk, so a saddle nose can be acquired later in life.

Other Stigmata. There are a wide variety of bony changes that help support the clinical diagnosis. The classic changes are frontal bossing and saber shins (curved tibias; Fig. 5.38). The milder form of frontal bossing is known as caput natiforme or buttocks-like head, as both sides of the forehead are slightly enlarged and there is a prominent central cleft. The scapula and clavicle are also likely to be damaged; Higouménakis sign is a thickening of the medial aspect of the clavicle, but it may also occur secondary to a neonatal clavicular fracture, which is the most common bony injury during delivery. Dubois sign refers to a shortened fifth finger, in which the distal interphalangeal joint is proximal to the proximal interphalangeal joint of the fourth finger. A high arched or gothic palate is not specific but can be seen following bony destruction.

The articular involvement in congenital syphilis is somewhat different from that in tertiary syphilis. The larger joints, especially the knees, suffer from spontaneous effusions and are known as Clutton joints. These usually become apparent during adolescence, respond well to therapy, may resolve spontaneously and do not cause permanent joint damage. Finally, paroxysmal cold hemoglobinuria is highly suggestive of late congenital or untreated acquired syphilis. The patients typically have chills and void dark urine within 6 – 8 h of cold exposure, reflecting autohemolysis of erythrocytes.

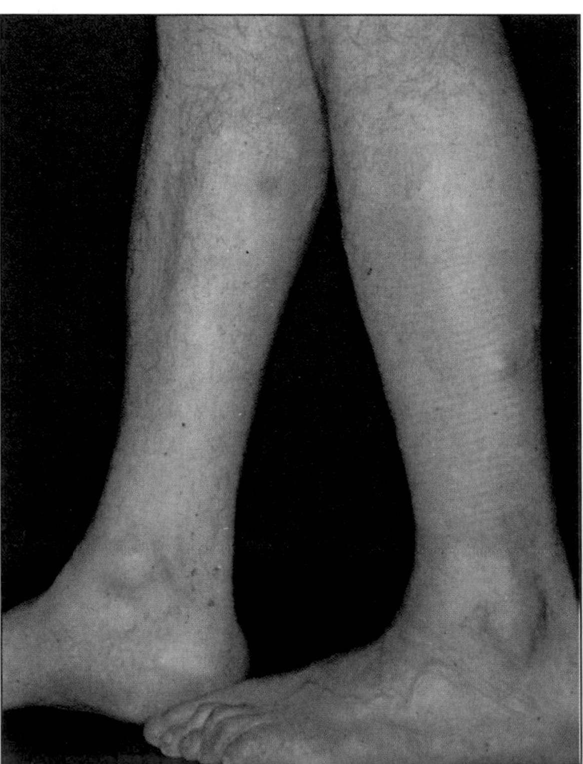

Fig. 5.38. Saber shins, late congenital syphilis

Histopathology. Histopathology does not play as much of a role in syphilis because of the focus on identification of the organism and serologic testing. Nonetheless, sometimes a lesion is biopsied when the clinician is not suspecting syphilis and does not mention it on the pathology slip. The dermatopathologist may still be able to suggest syphilis. The classic changes that suggest syphilis are plasma cell infiltrates, large, sausage-shaped granulomatous infiltrates and vascular changes, including endothelial swelling and true vasculitis.

Chancres are rarely biopsied but the organism can be identified with a Levaditi or Warthin-Starry stain. Depending on where the biopsy is taken, one may see an acanthotic, flat or ulcerated epidermis, as one moves centrally. At the base of the ulcer, there is a rich plasma cell infiltrate and prominent vessels.

In secondary syphilis, the histologic pattern varies as does the clinical one. There is a lymphocytic infiltrate, not as rich in plasma cells as in a chancre. There may be psoriasiform epidermal hyperplasia or lichenoid changes with atrophy. Often the perivascular infiltrates are prominent and bulbous or sausage-shaped. In later lesions, true granulomas are formed, once again distinguished by an admixture of plasma cells. In the eroded lesions of condylomata acuminata and mucous patches, the surface is teeming with organisms. As the granulomatous pattern appears, it becomes much harder to find spirochetes.

Gummata show marked necrosis with a mixed peripheral infiltrate, which once again usually includes plasma cells in addition to macrophages and giant cells. The peripheral vessels are also inflamed. The more superficial tuberous lesions may have tuberculoid granulomas without the extensive tissue damage of gummata. The organisms can be demonstrated in some instances with PCR but are not routinely found.

In congenital syphilis, the skin lesions are microscopically a variant of secondary syphilis. The bullous lesions show subepidermal blisters containing plasma cells and lymphocytes. The blister fluid and base are rich in spirochetes. Examination of the placenta and umbilicus may also give the first clues to syphilis, as granulomas, plasma cells and spirochetes can be found.

Laboratory Findings

Direct Examination. The ability to perform a dark-field examination is one of the almost holy skills of a dermatologist. The American Board of Dermatology still requires training in performing a dark-field test, but in many residency programs, the opportunities to learn the technique are few and far between. *T. pallidum* can be identified in tissue fluids because of its unique cork screw-like shape and motility. The organism is 5–15 μm long with very uniform, equal turns, spaced about as far apart as the width of the coil. In the center of the bacteria is a region that is less coiled. *T. pallidum* moves very slowly, turning about its long axis and folding or flexing in the central region. Other nonpathogenic spirochetes and *Spirillum minus* move more slowly and seem to purposefully move in a direction, while *T. pallidum* just bounces around, mimicking Brownian motion.

The way in which material is obtained for the dark-field examination is crucial. The crusted or eroded surface does not yield viable organisms. Instead the surface should be cleaned with a gauze pad dipped in sterile saline and then dried and lightly abraded with a second pad. Next, the deeper tissue fluid is expressed by massaging or milking the lesion, whether it be a chancre, condylomata lata, mucous patch or other lesion of secondary syphilis. The serum should be clear; it can be picked up with a platinum loop or touched to a glass slide. If it is cloudy, it is probably contaminated by erythrocytes and should be discarded. A good trick is to put a drop of sterile saline on the slide and then dip the loop in the solution, touch the lesion and so on several times. Finally the saline or serum is covered with a coverslip.

In dark-field microscopy, the spirochete is seen as a slowly moving spiral structure with a silver shine. The movements are slow, random and sometimes hard to find. One should search on low power and then confirm the presence of a *T. pallidum* with the 40x objective. As mentioned above, the nonpathogenic spirochetes are smaller, more hectic in their movement and less regularly coiled. Since there are a number of spirochetes in the oral mucosa, dark-field examination is most difficult there. Fortunately, mucous patches are usually teeming with organisms, but other oral lesions may be hard to evaluate. A good rule of thumb is that three separate dark-field examinations should be performed on a lesion before it is declared negative. A useful trick is to send the patient home and have them do several saline soaks to clean a lesion; then the dark-field examination can be repeated the next day with a better chance of success.

A lymph node puncture, as popularized by Hoffman, is often discussed but seldom done. If the cutaneous lesions are dark-field-negative, the lymph node can be aspirated and its contents examined by regular microscopy with special stains or PCR. Other fluids such as the blister fluid in the bullous lesions of congenital syphilis and the CSF may also be examined by the dark-field method.

Culture. Treponema pallidum cannot be cultured for routine purposes.

Other Methods. Monoclonal antibodies against various *T. pallidum* antigens and PCR can be employed to identify the organism in special settings.

Serology. The immunologic response to *T. pallidum* is a complex subject to which we have alluded frequently. The entire field was not designed to confuse dermatology residents but arose out of a necessity to have better tools to diagnose a major illness. One should never forget that tabes dorsalis and general paresis of the insane were not recognized as manifestations of syphilis until serologic tests were developed.

There are several basic rules to remember. First, despite the abundant number of antibodies that can be identified, there is little protective immunity against *T. pallidum*. Only during early untreated syphilis is the immunity high enough to prevent a superinfection. Thus reinfection can be taken as a sign that the prior syphilis was treated or had become latent. Second, the presence or absence of certain antibodies never should be taken as a sign of cure. That is, if a patient is untreated, even in the late latent phase when occasionally all serologic evidence disappears, the patient is still not cured. Third, there are two types of antibodies: (1) nonspecific or nontreponemal and (2) specific or treponemal. The former tend to diminish over time and with treatment; the latter are far more permanent. Figures 5.39 and 5.40 show the typical serologic course in untreated and treated syphilis.

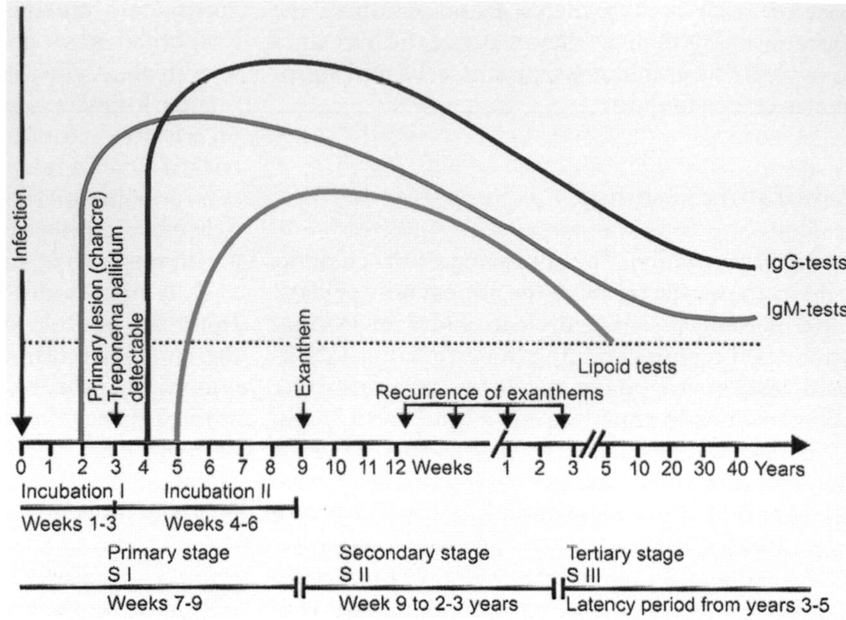

Fig. 5.39. Serologic pattern in untreated syphilis

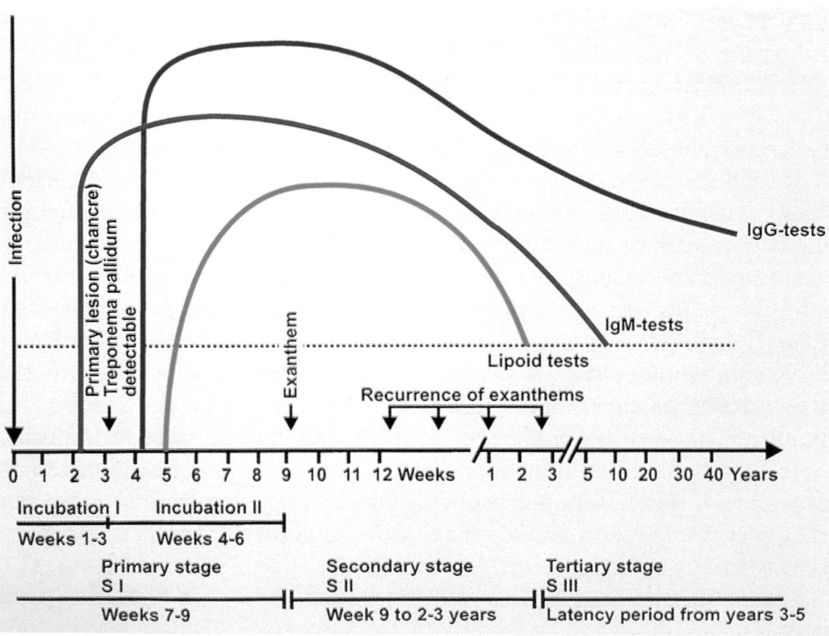

Fig. 5.40. Serologic pattern in treated syphilis

Over this century, a number of different tests have been developed. Many are no longer in use. The early tests were directed against phospholipids, primarily cardiolipin. The antigen in the VDRL (Venereal Disease Research Laboratory) test is a combination of cardiolipin, lecithin and cholesterol. Cardiolipin is a mitochondrial component that may be released by the tissue destruction associated with syphilis. The antibodies directed against cardiolipin are known as reagins. This is an unfortunate term, since it has nothing to do with the IgE reaginic antibodies found in atopic dermatitis. The specific tests against *T. pallidum* react in a variety of ways and with many different treponemal antigens. Most specific tests use extracts or homogenates of *T. pallidum*. Many cross-react with nonpathogenic treponemes and with the causative agents of the nonvenereal treponemal diseases.

The types of antibodies, their serum titers and their immunoglobulin classes vary as the body goes through the different stages of syphilis. The early response consists of IgM antibodies that are soon replaced by more specific IgG antibodies. This shift is seen in both specific and nonspecific antibodies. About 14 days after infection, antitreponemal IgM antibodies can be found, while antitreponemal IgG antibodies appear at about 21 days, roughly the time of the chancre. Nonspecific IgM appears at about 5 weeks, and IgG a week later. IgM requires continued stimulation of plasma cells by living *T. pallidum*, thus following treatment, IgM antibody titers drop the fastest. IgG is produced for many years in the absence of living organisms by memory-competent cells. In more than 90 % of patients, even after completely adequate treatment and a cure, the specific IgG antibodies persist forever. This state is known as serofast; in German one speaks of a *Seronarbe* or serum scar. In HIV patients with impaired immunity, the serofast state is less common; more than one-third of such patients with syphilis lose their specific antibodies. The nonspecific IgG antibody titers tend to drop gradually following treatment.

Nontreponemal Tests

Complement Fixation Reaction. Wassermann, Neisser and Bruck, in 1906, based their syphilis test on the complement fixation reaction described a few years earlier by Bordet and Gengou. They initially used an antigen extract from *T. pallidum*-infected fetal livers, but later switched to an extract from cow hearts known as cardiolipin. The Wassermann test is no longer employed.

Flocculation Reactions. Serum that contains reagins causes cardiolipin or other lipoid particles in a suspension to form a visible precipitate or flocculate. There are two main classes of flocculation tests.

- Rapid plasma reagin card (RPRC) test. The cardiolipin is attached to fine charcoal particles so that the reaction can be seen with the naked eye. Thus the test is also known as a macroflocculation test. Undiluted serum or plasma can be used. The test substrate is attached to a disposable card. After 30 min, one can assess if the charcoal particles have clumped together. Occasionally, with high titer serum, there may be a false-negative test, requiring dilution. The RPRC test is a rapid screening test, positive in early syphilis.
- Venereal Disease Research Laboratory (VDRL) test. This is the most widely used nontreponemal test; it is called the Harris test in some countries. The antigen is a mixture of cardiolipin, lecithin and cholesterol. Both serum and CSF can be studied by serial dilution techniques to provide titers of reactivity. The test is carried out on a slide with multiple wells, although today the procedure is usually automated. Once again, flocculation is observed, but since a microscopic is required, one speaks of a microflocculation test. The VDRL test is also suited to early diagnosis and, because the titers are easily obtained, their levels can be used to follow a response to therapy.

Treponemal Tests

All of the treponemal or specific tests are both more accurate and more permanent than the VDRL test. The treponemal tests are in general more expensive and more complicated, requiring specialized laboratories. The *T. pallidum* immobilization (TPI) test or Nelson test was quite specific, as it demonstrated immobilization of living organisms taken from rabbit testes, but it has been discontinued.

Fluorescent Treponema Antibody-Absorption (FTA-ABS) Test. Indirect immunofluorescence is used to identify antitreponemal antibodies. The antigen is a suspension of killed Nichols strain *T. pallidum* dried and fixed to a slide. The patient's serum is first reacted with fragmented nonpathogenic treponema to remove nonspecific antibodies developed against normal treponemes of the oral cavity. It is then allowed to react with the slide, where specific antibodies have been attached to the lyophilized spirochetes. A second reaction with fluorescently labeled antihuman immunoglobulins (or more specifically anti-IgG or anti-IgM; vide infra) allows identification of the reaction site. The FTA-ABS test is positive about 4 weeks after the infection starts and then remains positive for many years. It is used to confirm a positive nonspecific or screening test and is run at a standard dilution without titers. False-positive reactions may occur with lupus erythematosus and other diseases with anti-DNA antibodies or circulating immune complexes. The test is very time-consuming.

IgM-FTA-ABS and 19S-IgM-FTA-ABS Tests. This test is performed just as the FTA-ABS but with labeled anti-IgM antibodies in the second step. When both

IgG and IgM antibodies are present, the IgG may block attachment of the IgM, producing a false-positive test. For this reason, the 19S antibodies may be separated out first, so that one can test for IgM alone. IgM can be identified 14 days after infection, so this is the first test to turn positive with a new infection. Persistent IgM levels following treatment suggests persistent *T. pallidum* and a need for re-treatment. The IgM antibodies should disappear over about 24 months; an increase following therapy suggests reinfection. The presence of 19S-IgM antibodies in a newborn infant indicates a fetal response to *T. pallidum* rather than passive transfer from the mother.

T. pallidum Hemagglutination (TPHA) Test and Microhemagglutination-T. pallidum (MHA-TP) Test. In the TPHA test the antigen is a suspension of formalin-treated sheep erythrocytes coated with *T. pallidum* antigens. The patient's serum is purified of nonspecific heteroagglutins and then added to the suspension. Agglutination of the erythrocytes indicates the presence of specific antibodies. The entire test can be fully automated. The microhemagglutination version is quite similar, but is assessed microscopically.

A TPHA test is positive 3–4 weeks after infection and remains positive for many years. Occasionally, a patient with early syphilis who is promptly treated will lose his reactivity with the FTA-ABS test but will still be positive with the TPHA test. Thus, this test is totally unsuited for following disease course. Results can be obtained after about 4 h with the automated test. It is highly specific, relatively easy to do and quite reproducible. Thus it is the most important treponemal test in screening procedures. While the test lends itself to serial dilutions and thus titers, these values unfortunately do not correlate with the presence of live organisms and the need for therapy.

Use of Serologic Testing. There are several situations in which serologic testing can be employed: (1) as a screening test; (2) as a confirmatory test; (3) as a need for treatment test; (4) as a monitoring test; and (5) as a special test (especially for CNS disease).

Table 5.4 shows which test is best suited for each of these purposes, while Table 5.5 provides a simplified estimate of percent positive tests in various situations. Table 5.6 summarizes the status of the serologic tests for the various stages of syphilis.

Screening Test. This type of testing is used in epidemiologic studies, as part of routine evaluations, such as prenatal or pre-marital testing, and when there is a reason to suspect syphilis in a particular patient, such as the presence of other venereal diseases, HIV or a reasonable clinical or historical suspicion of infection. Usually the VDRL or RPRC is combined with the TPHA. The TPHA is positive earliest, in about 3–4 weeks, while the VDRL is most easily titrated and essential for following the disease course.

Confirmatory Test. On rare occasion, the TPHA will be positive and the FTA-ABS (or IgG-FTA-ABS) test negative. In this situation, the patient has had syphilis that was treated so early that the FTA-ABS did not remain positive. VDRL titers can also help

Table 5.4. Diagnostic use of serologic tests for syphilis

Purpose	Appropriate tests
Screening	TPHA VDRL or RPR
Confirmatory	VDRL titration IgG-FTA-ABS MHA-TP
Need for treatment	VDRL titration IgM-FTA-ABS 19S-IgM-FTA-ABS
Monitoring	VDRL titration 19S-IgM-FTA-ABS

Table 5.5. Percentage positive tests in various stages of syphilis

Test	Stage		
	Primary No Rx	Secondary No Rx	Late Post Rx
Nontreponemal			
VDRL	70	99	1
RPRC	80	99	0
Treponemal			
FTA-ABS	85	100	98
TPHA, MHA-TP	65	100	95

VDRL, Venereal Disease Research Laboratory; RPRC, rapid plasma reagin card; FTA-ABS, fluorescent treponema antibody-absorption; TPHA, MHA-TP, *T. pallidum* hemagglutination, microhemagglutination-*T. pallidum* (MHA-TP)

Table 5.6. Clinical stages of syphilis and serological results

Stage	Method			
	Nontreponemal	Treponemal		
		TPHA	IgG-FTA-ABS	19S-IgM-FTA-ABS
Untreated primary syphilis, seronegative	Nonreactive	Weakly reactive	Weakly reactive	Reactive
Untreated primary syphilis, seropositive	Reactive, rising	Reactive	Reactive	Reactive
Untreated secondary syphilis and reinfection	Reactive, high titer	Reactive	Reactive	Reactive
Untreated tertiary syphilis, neurosyphilis	Reactive (70%), nonreactive (30%) titers variable	Reactive	Reactive	Reactive (90%), nonreactive (10%)
Untreated congenital syphilis	Reactive with same or higher titer than mother	Reactive	Reactive	Reactive
Treated primary syphilis	Variable	Reactive	Reactive	Nonreactive (after 3–6 months)
Treated secondary syphilis	Variable	Reactive	Reactive	Nonreactive (after 6–18 months)
Treated tertiary syphilis	Variable	Reactive	Reactive	Nonreactive (after 12–24 months)
Treated neurosyphilis	Variable	Reactive	Reactive	Nonreactive
Exclusion in neonate with placentally transferred IgG antibodies	Reactive, same titer as mother but sinking	Reactive	Reactive	Nonreactive
Untreated reinfection	Reactive, rising titers	Reactive	Reactive	Reactive, rising titers

in this situation, but the TPHA is so accurate that in the routine setting no confirmation is needed.

Need for Treatment Test. Increased VDRL titers or the persistence or elevation of IgM titers suggests inadequate treatment and persistent stimulation by living *T. pallidum*.

Monitoring Tests. The VDRL titers should drop following treatment. This is the mainstay of long-term monitoring of the patient.

Special Tests. Evaluation of the CSF has taken on new importance with HIV/AIDS patients. A number of patients with HIV infections and secondary syphilis have developed neurosyphilis following what was thought to be adequate therapy. Thus, considerable attention must be paid to evaluating the CSF in such patients. The main indications are a patient with a positive serology and unclear neurologic problems, especially in whom there is an untreated or possibly inadequately treated secondary syphilis. This includes patients treated for secondary syphilis with benzathine penicillin, for as many as one in ten may require retreatment for possible neurosyphilis. Anyone with latent syphilis whose primary infection was more than 2 years in the past also needs CSF examination. The CSF usually shows signs of infection 3–5 years after the first infection. A negative CSF examination 5 years later means the chances of neurosyphilis are extremely small.

The same tests used in the serum can be used in the CSF. The standard tests are thus VDRL, TPHA and the 19S-IgM-FTA-ABS tests. In the VDRL test, the antigen amount is doubled. About 30–60% of patients with neurosyphilis have a negative CSF VDRL test, so it cannot be used alone; however, a positive CSF VDRL test does suggest CNS disease. TPHA activity in the CSF indicates a previous CNS infection. Titers higher than 1:10 are considered reactive. If the blood-brain barrier is not intact, false-positive test results can be obtained. The

FTA-ABS is similar but its titers are not helpful. If both FTA-ABS and TPHA tests are negative, a neurosyphilis is excluded. The IgM-FTA-ABS test can be used in untreated symptomatic neurosyphilis to demonstrate recent response to *T. pallidum*.

The CSF should be evaluated for cells, sugar, total protein, albumin and immunoglobulins. The correlation between serum and CSF levels of reactivity allows for closer assessment of the blood-brain barrier and the likelihood of active intrathecal infection. Either the TPHA-IgG index (normal 0.5–2.0, CNS infection > 3.0) or the TPHA index (CNS infection > 100) can be employed.

The CSF should be rechecked 1 and 2 years after treatment for neurosyphilis. The cell count drops first and the elevated protein more slowly. The VDRL titers drop and occasionally the antibodies disappear. If after 2 years the TPHA-IgG index is < 2.0 and/or the CSF TPHA titer has clearly dropped, then one can feel comfortable that treatment has been successful.

False-Positive Tests. One of the great problems with serologic testing for syphilis is the presence of false-positive tests. The early Wassermann test produced many false-positive reactions while the more purified VDRL test is much better. The following possibilities exist for false-positive tests: Technical mistakes may occur. In addition, there are rare individuals who have positive nonspecific tests, but no clinical findings and negative treponemal tests. All of the rest of the false-positive reactions are known as biologic false-positive reactions. A better term would be biologically nonspecific tests, since neither the test nor the result is false. Many infectious diseases cause a false-positive response to nontreponemal tests, presumably by tissue destruction and release or unmasking of mitochondrial antigens. These diseases are listed in Tables 5.7 and 5.8. There are several points worth emphasizing. Early HIV infection may produce a positive reaction, as may lymphogranuloma venereum and chancroid. Our list of infections does not pretend to be complete. Furthermore all the other spirochetal diseases produce positive nonspecific and specific tests; the glaring exception is *Borrelia burgdorferi*, which has a positive specific test, but a negative nonspecific test.

There are also a number of noninfectious diseases that may produce positive nonspecific tests. About 10% of patients over 70 years of age are reactive; the reasons are unclear. Both multiple transfusions and pregnancy also frequently produce positive reactions. Patients with the antiphospholipid (or lupus anticoagulant) syndrome are almost always positive (Chap. 18). Lupus erythematosus and the antiphospholipid syndrome patients may have positive specific tests; on occasion, the FTA-ABS will be positive and the VDRL negative. The fluorescent pattern is more beaded in lupus erythematosus but sometimes a TPI is needed. It is invariably negative. Finally, false-positive reactions in the CSF are mercifully extremely rare; CNS tumors may cause a positive CSF FTA-ABS test, but the serum test will be negative.

False-Negative Tests. These are a newer phenomenon. Patients with HIV break the rules. There

Table 5.7. False-positive serologic tests for syphilis

Disorder	Nontreponemal	Treponemal
Infectious diseases		
Lyme disease)	–	+
Relapsing fever	+	+
Yaws, pinta, bejel	+	+
Leptospirosis	+	+
Rat bite fever (*Spirillum minor*)	+	+
Other infections (see Table 5.8)	+	–
Noninfectious disorders		
Connective tissue disease	+	+/– (rare)
Rheumatic heart disease	+	–
Multiple transfusions	+	–
Drug addiction	+	–
Chronic liver disease	+	–
Pregnancy	+	–
Elderly	+	–

Table 5.8. Nonspirochetal infections with false-positive serologic reactions for syphilis

Bacteria	Tuberculosis; pneumococcal pneumonia; subacute bacterial endocarditis; leprosy; scarlet fever; mycoplasma
Viruses	Measles; varicella; hepatitis; Epstein-Barr virus infections; early HIV infection; vaccinia (vaccination)
Venereal diseases	Chancroid; lymphogranuloma venereum
Other	Malaria; trypanosomiasis

may be individuals with early syphilis but negative VDRL and IgM-FTA-ABS tests, or in a case of reinfection, the IgM may not rise. Similarly, patients with treated syphilis may lose their serofast state and not have positive TPHA tests.

Therapy

The treatment of syphilis can be summarized in one word: penicillin. Even after 50 years of use, there is no evidence of the resistance of *T. pallidum* to penicillin. How one treats syphilis is based on the absorption of the different penicillins, as well as on how well they cross the placenta and the blood-brain barrier. Studies have shown that long-term steady penicillin levels of about 0.03 IU/ml are needed for 7–10 days to adequate cure syphilis. *T. pallidum* divides every 33 h; thus if the inhibitory concentration sinks during this period, the organisms are able to overcome the antibiotic blockage of cell wall membrane synthesis and keep growing. The inhibition must be maintained for at least 7 days to obtain complete killing. In practice, one strives to maintain an optimal blood level for 2 weeks in early syphilis, 4 weeks in late syphilis and much longer in unusual variants such as syphilitic otitis.

Parenteral penicillin G is the treatment of choice. It can be used in its aqueous crystalline form intravenously, as aqueous procaine penicillin intramuscularly or as benzathine penicillin G as an intramuscular depot injection. The choice of regimen depends on the stage of the syphilis and the presence or absence of neurosyphilis. While benzathine penicillin G, 2.4 million units in a single dose, provides adequate levels of penicillin to treat ordinary early syphilis, it does not adequately penetrate the CSF, so that about one in ten patients may require retreatment. This problem was acceptable in the pre-HIV era, but serious neurosyphilis has occurred in appropriately treated patients, so that the current recommendations are in a state of flux.

Early Syphilis. Adults with primary, secondary or early latent syphilis should be given benzathine penicillin G, 2.4 million units IM in a single dose. Other, often more aggressive schemata involve procaine penicillin and probenecid, doxycycline, amoxicillin and probenecid or ceftriaxone. The recommended dosages are highly variable and should be obtained from local health authorities.

If the patient is allergic to penicillin, then tetracycline 500 mg orally q.i.d. for 2 weeks, or doxycycline 200 mg orally b.i.d. for 2 weeks is an acceptable alternative.

Children should be treated with similar regimens, modified for their weight. Sexual abuse must be excluded, as well as congenital syphilis.

Latent Syphilis. Early latent syphilis (present less than 1 year) is treated just like syphilis. Patients with latent syphilis present for more than 1 year should receive benzathine penicillin G, 2.4 million units IM weekly for a total of three doses.

Certainly these recommendations are conservative, and most clinicians would recommend a more aggressive approach. Alternate schedules involving doxycycline, amoxicillin and probenecid or ceftriaxone are available. In the case of penicillin allergy in latent syphilis, the official recommendation is doxycycline or tetracycline; if the infection is known to have been present less than 1 year, 2 weeks are recommended, otherwise 4 weeks.

Late Syphilis. Patients with cardiovascular disease or gummata but without evidence of neurosyphilis should receive benzathine penicillin G, 2.4 million units IM weekly for 3 weeks. Once again, many experts recommend more aggressive approaches. Patients with penicillin allergy can be treated with 4 weeks of doxycycline or tetracycline as outlined above. Some studies suggest that chloramphenicol, either IV or orally, for 30 days is more effective.

Neurosyphilis. The recommended therapy is aqueous crystalline penicillin G, 18–24 million units daily administered as 3–4 million units IV every 4 h for 10–14 days. An alternative is 10–14 days of procaine penicillin 2.4 million units IM daily plus probenecid 500 mg orally q.i.d.

No firm recommendations exist for treating neurosyphilis in penicillin-allergic patients. Desensitization appears the best approach. Some studies recommend doxycycline 100 mg IV b.i.d. for 30 days. When syphilitic otitis is present, the treatment should be prolonged to 6–12 weeks and prednisone 30–60 mg q.i.d. added. Similar recommendations have also been made for syphilitic uveitis and other situations in which the inflammatory response appears just as important as the infection.

Syphilis in Pregnancy. There is no proven effective alternative to penicillin, so wherever possible the mother should be desensitized and treated with penicillin. The tetracyclines stain the fetal teeth and bones, while the erythromycin base does not adequately treat the fetus. The other erythromycins cannot be used because of the risk of liver disease. Both azithromycin and ceftriaxone are under study in this difficult setting.

Early Congenital Syphilis. Patients should be treated with aqueous penicillin G, 100–150,000 units/kg per day IV (divided into two to three dosages) for 10 days, or procaine penicillin, 50,000 units/kg per day IM in a single dose for 10 days.

Modifications are detailed in specialized sources such as the CDC Guidelines or pediatric infectious disease texts, which should be consulted prior to embarking upon treatment.

Late Congenital Syphilis. Such patients should be treated just as those with late syphilis.

Syphilis in HIV/AIDS Patients. The occasional problems with loss of seroreactivity in HIV/AIDS, as well as the presence of false-positive reactions cause confusion. In general, HIV patients should always be treated with penicillin. In addition, the CSF must always be examined. The CDC recommends the same regimens as for non-HIV-infected individuals, but many other experts favor more aggressive schedules.

Jarisch-Herxheimer Reaction. The Jarisch-Herxheimer reaction occurs several hours after starting treatment for early syphilis, especially with penicillin. In those stages characterized by many viable *T. pallidum*, the rapid killing of the organism releases a heat-stable pyrogen and produces a general toxic reaction along with worsening of the syphilitic findings. It occurs in about 75% of patients with secondary syphilis, but can occur with any stage. The patient develops fever, chills, myalgias, headache, tachycardia, hyperventilation and often hypotension. The febrile reaction can be viewed as worthwhile, in that it may increase the killing of organisms just as in malaria therapy. Each patient should be warned about the possibility of such a reaction. Simultaneous administration of systemic or oral corticosteroids can ameliorate the attack, while the fever and other symptoms can be controlled with aspirin. In the case of cardiovascular disease and neurosyphilis, the Jarisch-Herxheimer can be catastrophic. For example, in severe aortitis, an aortic rupture can be precipitated. Similarly, the neurologic findings may become much more severe, especially in the parenchymal forms of neurosyphilis. Similar but not so dramatic signs and symptoms can be seen when other organisms are treated with antimicrobials; the reactions are also called Jarisch-Herxheimer reactions, although technically only the pyrogenic reaction in syphilis is so named.

Other Measures

Evaluation of partners. All at-risk partners should be evaluated. The time periods used to identify such individuals are 3 months for primary syphilis; 6 months for secondary syphilis and 1 year for early latent syphilis. Persons exposed to someone with early syphilis in the past 90 days should be treated prophylactically. Those exposed more than 90 days before can be treated presumptively if serologic tests are not immediately available and the chances of follow-up appear uncertain. If the duration of syphilis is unknown, VDRL titers >1:32 should be taken as a sign of early syphilis and infectivity. Long-term partners of patients with late syphilis should be checked.

Follow-up Evaluation. Every patient treated for syphilis should have a VDRL test after 3, 6 and 12 months and then yearly for 4 years. If penicillin alternatives are used, the evaluation may well include repeat CSF evaluation. The 19S-IgM-FTA-ABS test can be performed 1–2 years after the end of therapy to confirm the lack of living organisms.

In neurosyphilis, the control evaluations must be more frequent, perhaps every 3 months for 3 years and then every 6 months for a number of years. The CSF findings should also be followed every 6 months until the cells and protein have returned to normal.

Public Health Measures. Syphilis in all its forms is a reportable disease.

Nonvenereal Treponematoses

There are four diseases caused by treponemes that have many clinical and serologic similarities with syphilis, but they are not usually transmitted via sexual intercourse. The disorders and their causative agents are shown in Table 5.9. While we do not pretend to have more than a passing acquaintance with these diseases, they have such a fascinating history and reinforce so many aspects of the biology of syphilis that we will briefly review them.

Table 5.9. Other treponemal infections

Disease	Organism
Yaws	*Treponema pallidum* subspecies *pertenue*
Pinta	*Treponema carateum*
Endemic syphilis	*Treponema pallidum* subspecies *endemicum*

Yaws

Synonyms. Frambesia, pian, bouba, parru, parangi

Definition. Nonvenereal treponemal infection with early cutaneous lesions and late disabling musculoskeletal changes.

Causative Organism. *Treponema pallidum* subspecies *pertenue.* CASTELLANI identified *T. pertenue* in 1905 just after *T. pallidum* was discovered.

Epidemiology. Yaws covers wide areas of the earth between the Tropics of Cancer and Capricorn. It was previously prevalent in rural populations in Asia, Africa, Oceania, the Caribbean, and Central and South America. Heat and moisture favor the organism's spread. A common saying is "Yaws starts where the streets end". The slave trade may have been responsible for introducing it to the Americas. In the 1950 s, the infected population was estimated at between 50–100 million people. Today, the best guess is around 2 million, following an extensive eradication program with penicillin. Remaining foci are found in small areas of the northern coast of South America, with only hundreds of cases reported yearly. There has been a recent upsurge of new cases in West Africa, perhaps aided by the considerable political and social turmoil.

Etiology and Pathogenesis. The first infection with yaws usually occurs in childhood and is neither sexually nor connatally transmitted. The disease is spread by direct contact. Transmission by the fly *Hippelates pallipes* has been suggested but not proven. Patients with yaws have partial immunity against syphilis and vice versa, not surprising considering how closely the organisms are related. There are no cardiovascular or CNS problems in the tertiary stage.

Clinical Findings

Primary Yaws. After an incubation period of about 3 weeks, a primary lesion appears somewhere on the body. The most typical site is the leg below the knee. Mothers may infect their small children around the mouth. The primary lesion is known as a mother yaws. It consists of one or more grouped papules that become eroded, then ulcerated and then develop papillomatous granulation tissue. The proliferative stage resembles a raspberry, hence frambesia (French framboise = raspberry). The ulcer is soft and can become quite large. It is rich in spirochetes that can be easily seen in the secretions under dark-field examination. Most patients have regional lymphadenopathy and nonspecific findings such as fever, malaise and myalgias. The lesion heals after a few months, leaving behind an atrophic hypo- or hyperpigmented scar.

Secondary Yaws. Later, many smaller raspberry-like papules appear, usually starting 3–12 months after the first infection. They are spread symmetrically over the body, usually favoring the legs and trunk. The smaller lesions are less likely to ulcerate and heal spontaneously. They are rich in *T. pallidum* and known as daughter yaws, frambesiomas, or pianome. Several clinical variants have been identified, including a macropapular form, in which the secondary lesions resemble the mother yaws, and a micropapular form with smaller, more lichenoid papules that are less often ulcerated. In addition, macular and dyschromic hyperkeratotic lesions may also occur. The lesions heal spontaneously, usually with pigmentary changes but tend to recur. The most unusual clinical feature is the palmar-plantar changes, ranging from hyperkeratotic lesions to fissures to paronchyial changes. Since these lesions are quite painful, many patients, especially children, walk with a peculiar gait known as the crab yaws.

More problematic in the second stage is the bony involvement. Sometimes the primary lesion is overlooked and the children present with bone pain and a reluctance to use a limb. Just as in syphilis, they develop osteitis and periostitis. Mucosal changes are rare. Malaise, fever and diffuse lymphadenopathy are often present. Recurrences of the skin lesions are common and may come and go over a period of years.

Tertiary Yaws. The latent period usually lasts 5 or more years, so some children may show changes as early as age 5, but usually much later. Not all patients evolve into this stage, but exact numbers are lacking. There is no cardiovascular or CNS disease. The skin and skeletal system remain the two principle targets. In all situations, organisms are extremely rare. There are several clinical findings associated with this stage of disease.

- Nodular lesions. Most often a small number of verrucous nodules are found arranged in an annular pattern, sometimes coalescing to form a plaque. These lesions known as pianids.
- Gummata. The most common site is over the shins, where solitary painless deep-lying nodules develop and slowly ulcerate. Complications include bone destruction and joint ankylosis.
- Keratoderma. The hyperkeratotic changes become more severe and painful. There are usually poorly defined plaques along with punctate papules and crater-like pits.
- Bony changes. The long bones are most often involved; just as with congenital syphilis, saber shins are a common finding in children.
- Gangosa. Even though the oral mucosa is not usually involved, there may be massive midfacial destruction involving the nose and then indirectly the palate. Even though the tongue and larynx are not affected, the patient's voice is altered by the extensive destruction of skin, bone cartilage and mucosa. Gangosa means muffled voice in Spanish.
- Goundou. Once again the midface is involved but instead of destruction, there is reactive proliferation of the maxillae and nasal bone producing massive exostoses that may hamper sight.
- Juxtaarticular nodes. These fibrous subcutaneous nodules develop about the knees, elbows, hands and feet. Their etiology is poorly understood. In Brazil, even where yaws was common, the nodes were not seen, raising the question of their exact relationship to the infection.

Laboratory Findings. The organisms can be identified in most primary and secondary lesions either with dark-field examination or immunofluorescent staining. All of the techniques, including serology, discussed under syphilis are applicable here. If a patient has both yaws and syphilis, there is no way to determine the coinfection.

Differential Diagnosis. In the early stages, one must consider tropical ulcer, impetigo, impetiginized scabies, vegetating or blastomycotic-like pyoderma, tuberculosis, atypical mycobacteria, leishmaniasis, tungiasis and of course syphilis. Later on, syphilis, leprosy, tuberculosis, mucocutaneous leishmaniasis and pinta may appear similar. Any patient with skin and bone changes in an endemic area should be suspected of having yaws.

Therapy. Benzathine penicillin G, 1.2 million units in a single IM injection, is curative. Children can receive half the dose. All aspects except the hyperkeratotic lesions heal rapidly, resolving over weeks. The bony changes are arrested. Protocols for patients allergic to penicillin include tetracycline, doxycycline and chloramphenicol.

Widespread treatment of contacts or even entire villages is appropriate and has reduced the prevalence of yaws 50-fold in the past decades. The treatment is so simple that detailed public health investigations can be replaced by a request to bare one's buttocks or arm.

Pinta

Synonyms. Mal de pinto, carate

Definition. Nonvenereal treponemal infection that causes distinctive postinflammatory hypopigmentation.

Causative Organism. *Treponema carateum*

Epidemiology. Pinta is a very old disease, known to the advanced native civilizations of Mexico and Central America. Today is it uncommon, found only in remote areas of southern Mexico, Central America and northern South America. Several hundred cases are reported yearly, a marked reduction from two decades ago.

Etiology and Pathogenesis. Infection occurs through minor skin breaks. The treponemes then multiply locally and systemically just as with *T. pallidum.*

Clinical Findings. The inoculation period is about 21 days. The initial lesion is a smooth papule, usually on the extremities. Sometime several grouped papules appear and then coalesce into a large plaque, many centimeters in diameter, with a distinct raised border. While ulceration is uncommon, the primary lesion or lesions may persist for months to years before healing with a hypopigmented scar. The secondary lesions appear 3–12 months after

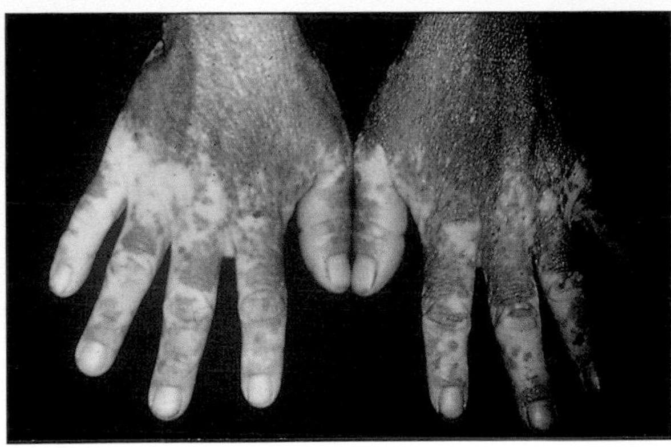

Fig. 5.41. Pinta with hypopigmentation. (Courtesy of Amado Saul, M.D., Mexico City, Mexico)

the appearance of the initial lesion; this means that, frequently, primary and secondary lesions are present simultaneously. The secondary lesions are small papules known as pintids, which heal slowly with dyschromic changes, producing white, gray, blue and brown flat macules. Pintids may continue to appear over many years. The primary and secondary lesions contain spirochetes. In the late stage, there are no destructive lesions but instead persistent hypo- or depigmentation, especially on the distal aspects of the arms and legs (Fig. 5.41). There are no skeletal, cardiovascular or CNS changes.

Histopathology. The early lesions are psoriasiform or, often, more lichenoid, with infiltrates impinging on the epidermal-dermal junction. Plasma cells are prominent, as is vascular involvement. Organisms can be identified with special stains. In the depigmented lesions, there is marked incontinence of pigment but residual melanocytes and occasional plasma cells, which may allow a distinction from vitiligo, in which melanocytes are lacking.

Laboratory Findings. Dark-field examinations are positive in the early stages. The serologic tests for syphilis become positive in the secondary stage and remain positive for life.

Prognosis. Since there are no systemic findings, pinta is less serious than the other treponemal diseases. Patients, however, find the pigmentary changes very distressing.

Differential Diagnosis. In the early stages, atopic dermatitis, dermatophyte infections, tinea versicolor and many other papulosquamous disorders can be considered. In the dyschromic stages, facial lesions are similar to melasma, which is also extremely common in the same populations. In the late stage, the main questions are vitiligo and leprosy, which also occurs in some of the same areas.

Therapy. A single IM injection of benzathine penicillin G, 1.2 million units, is curative. The early lesions clear in 4–6 months, while later lesions require longer and usually leave residual hypopigmentation. Totally depigmented lesions are not typically influenced by therapy. Once again, when a case is identified, mass inoculations of entire villages have been effective in reducing the impact of the disease.

Endemic Syphilis

Synonyms. Bejel (Syria, Iraq, other Arabic lands), sibbens (Scotland), radesyge (Norway), dichuchwa (South Africa), njovera (Rhodesia), sklerljevo (Balkans)

Definition. Endemic nonvenereal treponemal infection that has clinical overlaps with syphilis and yaws.

Causative Organism. *Treponema pallidum* subspecies *endemicum*.

Epidemiology. There are many focal areas of endemic or nonvenereal syphilis spread across the globe, concentrated in the Middle East and southern Caspian Sea area. Pockets also exist throughout Africa, Asia and Oceania. In the past, endemic syphilis was common in parts of Europe, but it is no longer found.

Etiology and Pathogenesis. Endemic syphilis is spread by direct contact or via common utensils. It has such a high penetrance in families that for years it was felt to be inherited. In actuality, the prevalence of the infection in the population and early acquisition of the disease make a systemic infection during pregnancy almost a biologic impossibility. Traditional drinking vessels were responsible for much of the transmission in the Balkans. In other societies, inoculation also appears to occur via the mouth.

Clinical Findings. The primary lesion is frequently lacking, supporting intraoral inoculation as a likely mode. The most common secondary lesions are also mucosal, including mucous patches, condylomata lata and lymphadenopathy. In addition, osteitis and periostitis occur. Late lesions include bony damage and gummata that may involve the skin. Gummata of the breast are described as common in nursing mothers; perhaps inoculation from an infected child triggers an exaggerated immune response. Cardiovascular and CNS problems can occur but they are extremely rare.

Laboratory Findings. The serologic tests are identical to those in syphilis.

Diagnostic Criteria. The only way to separate syphilis and endemic syphilis is via epidemiology – that is, investigating the community.

Therapy. The administration of 1.2 million units IM of benzathine penicillin G suffices. The mass treatment program in Bosnia in the 1960s, coupled with improved sanitation, led to virtual elimination of the disease, although some scattered reports suggest a recrudescence during the 1990s.

Chancroid

(Ducrey 1889)

Synonyms. Ulcus molle, soft chancre

Definition. Venereal infection characterized by large painful ulcers.

Causative Organism. *Haemophilus ducreyi* is a short gram-negative rod (1.25–1.40 × 0.55–0.60 μm) with rounded corners. The bacteria tend to form chains, often described as schools of fish (Fig. 5.42). Its more famous relative *H. influenzae* is a cause of cellulitis, especially in children (Chap. 4).

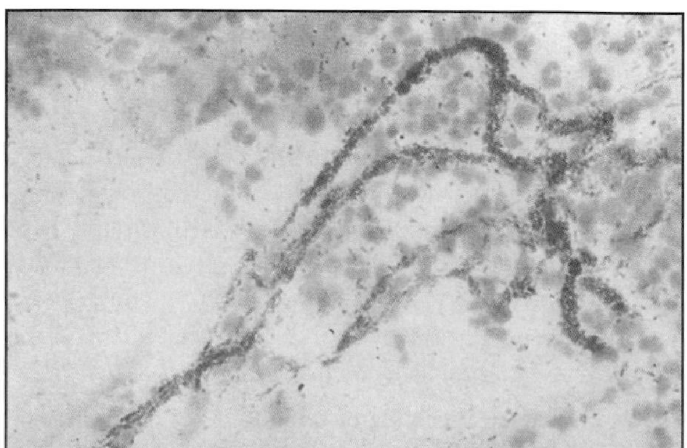

Fig. 5.42. *Haemophilus ducreyi*

History. Chancroid has been recognized as a separate disease, distinguishable from syphilis, since 1852. Ducrey, a Neapolitan bacteriologist, identified the causative agent in 1889, and Unna found the organisms in tissue sections 3 years later. Several groups cultured the bacteria at the turn of the century.

Epidemiology. Chancroid is a worldwide infection that is more common than syphilis. It is endemic in tropical Africa and southeast Asia, as well as India and parts of Central and South America. In Europe chancroid is relatively uncommon, although it continues to erupt in small pockets. In Germany, epidemics have occurred among Turkish immigrants in Berlin, Munich and other communities. In North America, there have been multiple outbreaks in urban centers in the past 15 years. The incidence has increased tenfold during this time. The disease is felt to be endemic now in New York City and south Florida.

Chancroid is most commonly diagnosed in black men who have visited prostitutes. It was much more common during the World Wars and ranked behind gonorrhea but ahead of syphilis among American soldiers in Korea. Chancroid was also a common problem during the Vietnam War. It now has renewed significance as its clinical lesion serves as an entry site for HIV in the same at-risk population. In Nairobi, detailed studies have shown a 2:1 male predominance without female carriers, as previously suspected. Other studies have shown a 10:1 male dominance, perhaps representing almost exclusive transmission by prostitutes with multiple partners. The presence of a foreskin is a risk factor, as chancroid is much less common among circumcised individuals.

Etiology and Pathogenesis. *Haemophilus ducreyi* enters the skin or mucosa through a minor break or tear. It is incapable of penetrating normal skin. The lipopolysaccharide composition of the cell wall appears to be an important virulence factor, dictating the degree of host inflammatory response, which contributes greatly to the tissue damage. Patients do not develop immunity.

Clinical Findings. The incubation period is usually 3–7 days, with maximum values of 2–10 days. The initial lesion is a small inconspicuous papule with peripheral erythema that rapidly develops into a pustule and then a soft painful ulcer. Typically the ulcer edge is somewhat raised and undermined (Fig. 5.43). One speaks of the "sign of the double border", as there is an advancing erythematous edge and then a thin, yellow necrotic zone. The ulcer is covered with yellow-gray necrotic material, beneath which is granulation tissue. The chancroid ulcer does not heal spontaneously, but becomes chronic and enlarges in the absence of therapy.

The most common location is the inner aspect of the foreskin; other sites in men include the frenulum and the coronal sulcus. In women the labia, urethral orifice and posterior commissure are most common; on occasion, the vagina or cervix can be involved. Anal lesions are common, both from anal intercourse and autoinoculation. Extragenital lesions may be found on the inner aspects of the thigh, the inguinal fold, about the mouth and on the breast, but they are quite rare.

Men typically have a single lesion, while women are more likely to have multiple lesions. The size is highly variable, ranging from dwarf chancroid (< 0.5 cm) to giant chancroid (2.0 cm). Many unusual variations have been described.

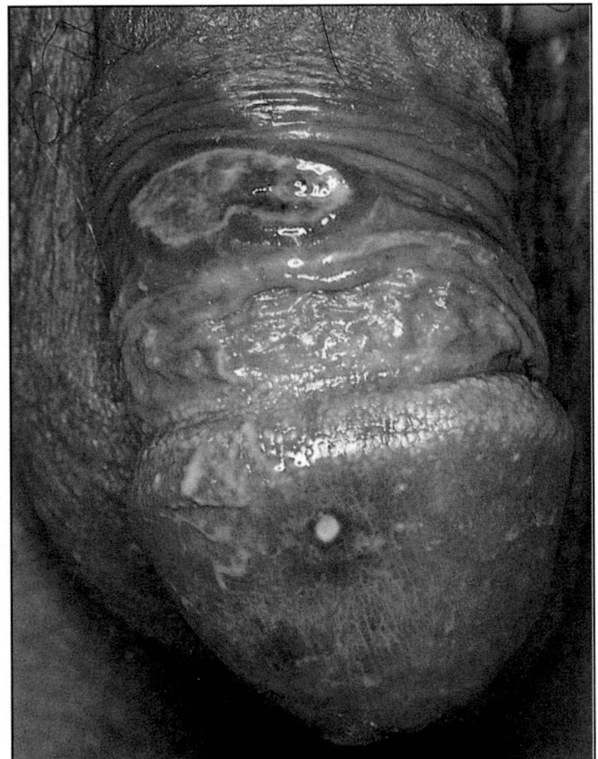

Fig. 5.43. Primary lesion in chancroid

- Follicular chancroid: The ulcer involves one or more follicles of the mons pubis.
- Papular chancroid: Granulation tissue rises from the base of the ulcer above the skin surface.
- Phagedenic chancroid: Mixed infection, usually with fusospirochetal organisms, produces massive ulcer and tissue destruction.
- Serpiginous chancroid: Progressive lesions extend towards the umbilicus or down the thighs; probably a variant of phagedenic chancroid.
- Transient chancroid: A tiny papule is overlooked but later lymphadenopathy appears.

About half the patients only have an ulcer; the rest develop lymphangitis or a bubo (Fig. 5.44). These patients are likely to feel ill and have fever or malaise. The lymphangitis is usually seen as a hardening of the dorsal penile vein; whenever such a change is found, the inner aspect of the foreskin should be examined for a possible clue to chancroid. At the base of the penis, a small abscess can develop, known as the bubo nucleus.

The bubo in chancroid is usually unilateral. It appears 1–2 weeks after exposure, so it may be present at the same time as the ulcer. The inguinal region is erythematous and swollen, and a group of lymph nodes become matted, painful and soon fluctuant. In about half the cases, the bubo ruptures, discharging a thick blood-tinged fluid. Fistulas develop and the skin at their openings becomes infected with *H. ducreyi*, producing more soft ulcers. Eventually the lesions heal with scarring but rarely become fibrotic.

Mixed ulcer. Simultaneous infection with *T. pallidum* and *H. ducreyi* is not unusual. Sexually transmitted diseases often occur together, but this specific combination is so common it has its own

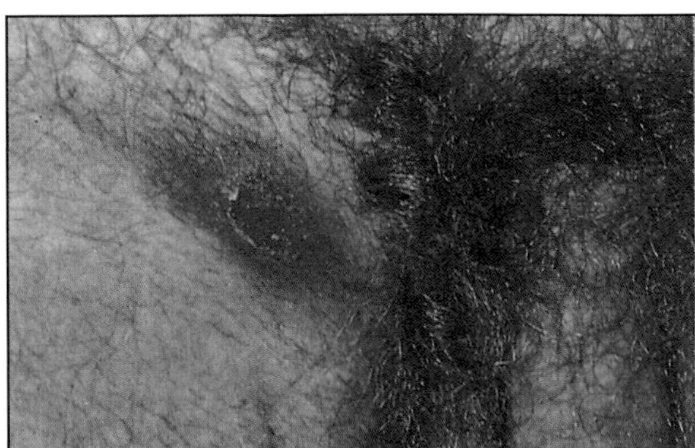

Fig. 5.44. Bubo in chancroid

name – mixed ulcer. The scenario is usually that the chancroid ulcer is present first and then the *T. pallidum* invade the damaged tissue, producing a hardening of the ulcer wall after another 2–3 weeks. Neither disease should be diagnosed without considering the other one.

Histopathology. The organisms can be seen in a biopsy from the base of the ulcer. Giemsa stain reveals them as both free and within macrophages in the granulation tissue. While the trizonal pattern of chancroid has been emphasized, it is neither common nor diagnostic. There is a superficial necrosis, mid-level granulation tissue and deeper inflammation.

Laboratory Findings

Direct Examination. Material taken from the ulcer or bubo can be spread on a slide and stained with methylene blue or Giemsa stain. The organisms' tendency to be arranged like "railroad tracks" or "a school of fish" provide many test questions, but in actuality these features are hard to identify. Direct examination is neither sensitive nor specific.

Culture. Identification via culture is the standard for *H. ducreyi*. All *Haemophilus* have complex culture requirements, which partially determine their speciation. An enriched blood-agar medium containing fetal calf serum, isovitalex and vancomycin grown in 5% CO_2 is preferred. The most standard medium in use today is the Nairobi medium, which contains two different enriched media in a biplate. Material is taken from the base of the ulcer or aspirated from the bubo. The sensitivity of the Nairobi medium in an endemic area is about 80%. The colonies are highly variable in size, giving the impression of a mixed culture, and can be slid about on the surface of the agar without disintegrating. A series of complex tests are needed to finally speciate the organisms.

Serology. Serologic evaluation plays no role in identifying *H. ducreyi*, but should be performed to exclude syphilis. An HIV test is also recommended. Both should be repeated after 6–12 weeks.

Other Methods. In experimental settings *H. ducreyi* can be identified with immunofluorescent examination, DNA blotting or PCR, but none of the techniques are used routinely. Formerly, the Ito-Reenstierna skin test was employed, in which *H. ducreyi* was injected into the skin and a delayed hypersensitivity reaction evaluated, but this test is no longer used and only employed to trick dermatology residents on examinations.

Prognosis. Chancroid does not resolve without treatment. Even without appropriate treatment, the buboes may proceed to rupture with the complications of scarring and tract formation. Phimosis, urethral fistulae, and deeper damage may also occur; human papilloma virus infections may develop in the healed ulcerations.

Diagnostic Criteria. The presence of a painful genital ulcer with negative dark-field examination and either appropriate clinical findings and/or negative Tzanck smear strongly suggests chancroid and can be taken as diagnostic for surveillance purposes. Multiple lesions and painful lymphadenopathy virtually clinch the diagnosis.

Differential Diagnosis. Table 5.10 shows the differential diagnosis between chancroid and a syphilitic chancre. A mixed ulcer should always be excluded. HSV infections can usually be separated by the presence of grouped smaller lesions and recurrence, but a primary HSV lesion in an immunosuppressed host can mimic chancroid. In endemic areas, one must also consider granuloma inguinale and the primary lesion of lymphogranuloma venereum. Nonvenereal ulcers must also be excluded, including mixed bacterial infections (chancriforme

Table 5.10. Differential diagnosis of chancroid and syphilis

	Chancroid	Chancre (syphilis)
Incubation period	3–7 days	3 weeks
Number	Usually multiple	Usually single
Consistency	Soft	Hard
Border	Undermined	Not undermined
Pain	Yes	No
Lymphadenopathy	Inflamed, soft, painful	Firm, hard

Table 5.11. Differential diagnosis of venereal buboes

	Syphilis	Chancroid	Lymphogranuloma venereum	Granuloma inguinale
Skin lesion	Present	Present	Often not seen	Extensive
Incubation period	3–12 weeks	1–2 weeks	2–12 weeks	1–2 months
Degree of lymphadeno-pathy	Bilateral, multiple	Unilateral, solitary node or fused mas	Usually unilateral and matted	Extensive
Nature of lymph nodes	Firm, rubbery	Soft	Multilocular with variable consistency and groove sign	Pseudobuboes (subcutaneous granulomas): lymph nodes only minimally affected
Pus	None	Thick, blood-tinged	Thick, creamy	Superficial pus from skin lesions
Overlying skin change	None	Bubo may rupture and heal with crater	Multiple sinus tracts	Primarily skin lesions
Pain	None	Marked	Marked	Somewhat
Spontaneous healing	Rapid	Usually fairly rapid without rupture	Slow (many months)	Very slow (months to years)

Based on Table 2 in Relman and Swartz (1995 p. 6).

pyoderma) sometimes following trauma, erythema multiforme, fixed drug reaction, aphthae and Behçet syndrome. Table 5.11 indicates the differential diagnosis of venereal buboes.

Therapy. Multiple effective regimens are available, including: azithromycin 1.0 g orally in a single dose, or ceftriaxone 250 mg IM in a single dose, or ciprofloxacin 500 mg orally b.i.d. for 3 days, or erythromycin base 500 mg orally q.i.d. for 1 week. Rare strains of the bacteria, especially in the Orient, have been resistant to erythromycin or ciprofloxacin.

In addition, disinfectant wet soaks or baths should be employed to debride the ulcer. The bubo should be aspirated; sometimes the procedure must be repeated. The lesion should not be incised.

Public Health Measures. Chancroid is a reportable disease.

Granuloma Inguinale

(McLeod 1888; Donovan 1905)

Synonyms. Granuloma venereum, donovanosis

Definition. Infection, usually sexually transmitted, characterized by extensive inguinal ulcerations.

Causative Organism. *Calymmatobacterium granulomatis* is small, poorly characterized gram-negative organism that grows intracellularly in macrophages.

Epidemiology. Granuloma inguinale is very uncommon in the USA and Europe, seen primarily in individuals returning from endemic areas. An epidemic was identified several years ago in Houston, Texas. The disease is most prevalent in New Guinea, India, the Caribbean and other subtropical regions. In New Guinea, as recently as 20 years ago, a quarter of patients attending sexually transmitted disease clinics had granuloma inguinale.

Etiology and Pathogenesis. The transmission of *C. granulomatis* is controversial. It is not an aggressive bacteria and sexual contact is not required. In children, there seems to be nonsexual spread, as they are infected by their parents during daily contact. In adults, there is sexual spread, but prolonged and multiple contacts are usually required. The organism is found in less than 50 % of steady partners of infected individuals. Rectal involvement is common in homosexuals.

Clinical Findings. The incubation period is poorly defined but ranges between 1 and 10 weeks. The initial lesions are small papules that erode and coalesce to produce beefy red ulcers. The most common sites are the foreskin and glans in men and the labia in women. About 80 % of patients have only genital lesions, while the rest have anal or inguinal involvement, most often in association with genital lesions. Facial lesions have on occasion been reported.

The lesions bleed easily on contact and are painful. They continue to expand, particularly into the perianal region by autoinoculation. Rarely, a true bubo develops, but most often there is no lymphadenopathy – instead subcutaneous granuloma formation in the inguinal region, known as a pseudobubo, is observed. Secondary infection with other bacteria often occurs. The ulcer border tends to become raised. Lymphedema is common as the fibrosis impairs lymphatic drainage. Systemic symptoms, including fever and weight loss, and distant spread involving bones, joints and liver have been described.

If the disease is not treated, it smolders along damaging tissue. On rare occasions, squamous cell carcinoma may develop in the ulcers or scars.

Histopathology. The ulcers are nonspecific and the bacteria hard to see with routine light microscopy. Using a Giemsa stain may help to find the parasitized macrophages (discussed below). Plastic embedding for thin sections also increases the yield.

Laboratory Findings. *Calymmatobacterium granulomatis* is very difficult to culture and no serologic testing is available.

Direct Examination. The only way to diagnose granuloma inguinale is via direct examination. Examining a crushed smear of granulation tissue spread over a glass slide, air-dried and stained with a Wright or Giemsa stain is standard. The organisms are identified as clusters of small dark bacteria within macrophages; they are known as Donovan bodies and may have a bipolar or safety pin staining pattern.

Differential Diagnosis. In endemic areas, all the other causes of genital ulcerations need to be considered, as discussed above. The ulcers of chancroid are most likely to resemble granuloma inguinale. In more advanced cases, the extensive fibrosis and destruction should suggest the answer.

Therapy. Trimethoprim-sulfamethoxazole, one double-strength tablet orally b.i.d. for at least 3 weeks, or doxycycline 100 mg orally b.i.d. for at least 3 weeks.

Therapy should be continued until the ulcerations have healed. Alternative regimens involve ciprofloxacin or erythromycin base. If no response is seen in the first few days of treatment, gentamicin 1 mg/kg IV every 8 h should be considered as an addition.

Public Health Measures. Granuloma inguinale is a reportable infection.

Bibliography

General

Brown TJ, Yen-Moore A, Tyring SK (1999) An overview of sexually transmitted diseases. Part I. J Am Acad Dermatol 41:511–529

Brown TJ, Yen-Moore A, Tyring S (1999) An overview of sexually transmitted diseases. Part II. J Am Acad Dermatol 41:661–680

Czelusta AJ, Yen-Moore A, Evans TY et al. (1999) Sexually transmitted diseases. J Am Acad Dermatol 41:614–623

Centers for Disease Control and Prevention (1997) 1998 Guidelines for treatment of sexually transmitted diseases. MMWR Morb Wkly Rep 47:1–116

Erbelding E, Quinn TC The impact of antimicrobial resistance on the treatment of sexually transmitted diseases (1997) Infect Dis Clin North Am 11:889–903

Evans BA, Kell PD, Bond RA et al. (1998) Racial origin, sexual lifestyle, and genital infection among women attending a genitourinary medicine clinic in London (1992). Sex Transm Infect 74:45–49

Harris JRW, Foster SM (1991) Recent advances in sexually transmitted diseases and AIDS. Churchill Livingstone, Edinburgh

Holmes KK, Sparling PF, Mårdh P et al. (1999) Sexually transmitted diseases. 3rd edn. McGraw-Hill, New York

Krowchuk DP (1998) Sexually transmitted diseases in adolescents: what's new? South Med J 91:124–131

McDonald LL, Stites PC, Buntin DM (1997) Sexually transmitted diseases update. Dermatol Clin 15:221–232

Gonorrhea

Biedenbach DJ, Jones RN (1996) Comparative assessment of Etest for testing susceptibilities of Neisseria gonorrhoeae to penicillin, tetracycline, ceftriaxone, cefotaxime, and ciprofloxacin: investigation using 510(k) review criteria, recommended by the Food and Drug Administration. J Clin Microbiol 34:3214–3217

Haugh PJ, Levy CS, Hoff Sullivan E et al. (1996) Polymyositis as the sole manifestation of disseminated gonococcal infection: case report and review. Clin Infect Dis 22: 861–863

Kirsch TD, Shesser R, Barron M (1998) Disease surveillance in the ER: factors leading to the underreporting of gonorrhea. Am J Emerg Med 16:137–140

Kissinger P, Clark R, Dumestre J et al. (1996) Incidence of three sexually transmitted diseases during a safer sex promotion program for HIV infected women. J Gen Intern Med 11:750–752

Lewis DA, Ison CA, Forster GE et al. (1996) Tetracycline resistant Neisseria gonorrhoeae. Characteristics of patients and isolates at a London genitourinary medicine clinic. Sex Transm Dis 23:378–383

Sherrard J, Barlow D (1996) Gonorrhoea in men: clinical and diagnostic aspects. Genitourin Med 72:422–426

Mycoplasma

Carlin EM, Barton SE (1996) Azithromycin as the first line treatment of non gonococcal urethritis (NGU): a study of follow up rates, contact attendance and patients' treatment preference. Int J STD AIDS 7:185–189

Janier M, Lassau F, Casin I (1997) Mycoplasma genitalium in male urethritis. Int J STD AIDS 8:534

Jensen JS, Hansen HT, Lind K (1996) Isolation of Mycoplasma genitalium strains from the male urethra. J Clin Microbiol 34:286–291

Koch A, Bilina A, Teodorowicz L, Stary A (1997) Mycoplasma hominis and Ureaplasma urealyticum in patients with sexually transmitted diseases. Wien Klin Wochenschr 109:584–589

Maeda S, Tamaki M, Nakano M et al. (1998) Detection of Mycoplasma genitalium in patients with urethritis. J Urol 159:405–407

Uno M, Deguchi T, Komeda H et al. (1996) Prevalence of Mycoplasma genitalium in men with gonococcal urethritis. Int J STD AIDS 7:443–444

Savio ML, Caruso A, Allegri R et al. (1996) Detection of Mycoplasma genitalium from urethral swabs of human immunodeficiency virus infected patients. New Microbiol 19:203–209

Taylor-Robinson D (1996) The history of nongonococcal urethritis. Sex Transm Dis 23:86–91

Taylor-Robinson D, Furr PM (1997) Genital mycoplasma infections. Wien Klin Wochenschr 109:578–583

Chlamydia

Busolo F, Camposampiero D, Bordignon G et al. (1997) Detection of Mycoplasma genitalium and Chlamydia trachomatis DNAs in male patients with urethritis using the polymerase chain reaction. New Microbiol 20:325–332

Jones RB (1991) New treatments for Chlamydia trachomatis. Amn J Obstet Gynecol 164:1789–1793

Meijer A, Kwakkel GJ, de Vries A et al. (1997) Species identification of Chlamydia isolates by analyzing restriction fragment length polymorphism of the 16 S 23 S rRNA spacer region. J Clin Microbiol 35:1179–1183

Ridgway GL (1992) Advances in the antimicrobial therapy of chlamydial genital infections. J Infect 25:51–59

Schwebke JR, Sadler R, Sutton JM et al. (1997) Positive screening tests for gonorrhea and chlamydial infection fail to lead consistently to treatment of patients attending a sexually transmitted disease clinic. Sex Transm Dis 24:181–184

Yealy DM, Greene TJ, Hobbs GD (1997) Underrecognition of cervical Neisseria gonorrhoeae and Chlamydia trachomatis infections in the emergency department. Acad Emerg Med 4:962–967

Lymphogranuloma Venereum

Davies N, Crown LA (1997) Lymphogranuloma venereum vs. incarcerated inguinal hernia: the Gordian knot unraveled. Tenn Med 90:278–279

Durand NJ, Favre (1913) Lymphogranulomatose inguinale subaigu d'origine génitale probable peut-être vénérienne. Buu Soc Med Hop Paris 35:274–288

Frei W (1925) Eine neue Hautreaktion bei Lymphogranuloma inguinale. Klin Wochenschr 1:2148–2149

Huguier PC (1849) Mémoire sur l'esthioméne ou dartre rongeante de la région vulvo-anale. Mem Acad Nat Méd 14:501–596

Papagrigoriadis S, Rennie JA (1998) Lymphogranuloma venereum as a cause of rectal strictures. Postgrad Med J 74:168–169

Kellock DJ, Barlow R, Suvarna SK et al. Lymphogranuloma venereum: biopsy, serology, and molecular biology (1997) Genitourin Med 73:399–401

Sevinsky LD, Lambierto A, Casco R et al. (1997) Lymphogranuloma venereum: tertiary stage. Int J Dermatol 36:47–49

Syphilis

History

Cates W Jr, Rothenberg RB, Blount JH (1996) Syphilis control. The historic context and epidemiologic basis for interrupting sexual transmission of Treponema pallidum. Sex Transm Dis 23:68–75

Fleming WL (1964) Syphilis through the ages. Med Clin North Am 48:587–612

Hudson MM, Morton RS (1996) Fracastoro and syphilis: 500 years on. Lancet 348:1495–1496

Luger A (1993) The origin of syphilis. Clinical and epidemiologic considerations on the Columbian theory. Sex Transm Dis 20:110–117

Quétel C (1990) History of Syphilis (original French title Le Mal de Naples: histoire de la syphilis). Polity, Cambridge, UK

Sartin JS, Perry HO (1995) From mercury to malaria to penicillin: the history of the treatment of syphilis at the Mayo Clinic – 1916–1955. J Am Acad Dermatol 32:255–261

Epidemiology and Biology

Felman YM (1993) Sexually transmitted diseases: selections from the literature since 1990. Syphilis: epidemiology. Cutis 52:72–74

Fraser CM, Norris SJ, Weinstock GM et al. (1998) Complete genome sequence of Treponema pallidum, the syphilis spirochete. Science 281:375–388

Magnusson HJ, Thomas EW, Olansky S (1956) Inoculation syphilis in human volunteers. Medicine 35:33–82

Miles TP, McBride D (1997) World War I origins of the syphilis epidemic among 20th century black Americans: a biohistorical analysis. Soc Sci Med 45:61–69

Nakashima AK, Rolfs RT, Flock ML et al. (1996) Epidemiology of syphilis in the United States, 1941–1993. Sex Transm Dis 23:16–23

Pennisi E (1998) Genome reveals wiles and weak points of syphilis. Science 281:324–325

St. Louis ME, Wasserheit JN (1998) Elimination of syphilis in the United States. Science 281:353–354

Wassermann, Neisser, Bruck, Schucht (1906) Weitere Mitteilungen über den Nachweiss spezifisch-luetischer Substanzen durch Komplementverankerung. Zeitschr Hyg Infektionskrnkh, vol. 55

Clinical Manifestations

Bernstein D, DeHertogh D (1992) Recently acquired syphilis in the elderly population. Arch Intern Med 152:330–332

Chapel TA (1978) The variability of syphilitic chancres. Sex Transm Dis 5:68–70

DiCarlo RP, Martin DH (1997) The clinical diagnosis of genital ulcer disease in men. Clin Infect Dis 25:292–298

Gjestland T (1955) The Oslo study of untreated syphilis: an epidemiologic investigation of natural course of syphilitic infection based upon restudy of Boeck-Bruusgaard material. Acta Derm Venereol (Stockh) 34:1–368

Hook EW, Marra CM (1992) Acquired syphilis in adults. N Engl J Med 326:1060–1069

Hunter J (1786) A treatise on the venereal disease. London

Rosen T, Brown TJ (1998) Cutaneous manifestations of sexually transmitted diseases. Med Clin North Am 82: 1081–1104

Talbot MD, Morton RS (1984) The Tuskegee study of untreated syphilis. Eur J STD 1:125–132

Congenital Syphilis

Bateman DA, Phibbs CS, Joyce T et al. (1997) The hospital cost of congenital syphilis. J Pediatr 130:752–758

Bennett ML, Lynn AW, Klein LE et al. (1997) Congenital syphilis: subtle presentation of fulminant disease. J Am Acad Dermatol 36:351–354

Blank S, McDonnell DD, Rubin SR et al. (1997) New approaches to syphilis control. Finding opportunities for syphilis treatment and congenital syphilis prevention in a women's correctional setting (see comments). Sex Transm Dis 24:218–226

Holder WR, Knox JM (1972) Syphilis in pregnancy. Med Clin North Am 56:1151–1160

Mascola L, Pelosi R, Blount JH (1985) Congenital syphilis revisited. Am J Dis Child 139:57–80

Nicoll A, Moisley C (1994) Ante-natal screening for syphilis. Br Med J 308:1253–1254

Sison CG, Ostrea EM Jr, Reyes MP et al. (1997) The resurgence of congenital syphilis: a cocaine-related problem. J Pediatr 130:289–292

Zenker PN, Berman SM (1991) Congenital syphilis: trends and recommendations for evaluation and management. Pediatr Infect Dis J 10:516–522

Neurosyphilis

de Souza MC, Nitrini R (1997) Effects of human immunodeficiency virus infection on the manifestations of neurosyphilis. Neurology 49:893–894

Flood JM, Weinstock HS, Guroy ME et al. (1998) Neurosyphilis during the AIDS epidemic, San Francisco, 1985–1992. J Infect Dis 177:931–940

Gordon SM, Eaton ME, George R et al. (1994) The response of symptomatic neurosyphilis to high-dose intravenous penicillin G in patients with human immunodeficiency virus infection. N Engl J Med 331:1469–1473

Luger A, Schmidt BL, Steyrer K et al. (1981) Diagnosis of neurosyphilis by examination of the cerebrospinal fluid. Br J Vener Dis 57:232–237

Malone JL, Wallace MR, Hendrick BB et al. (1995) Syphilis and neurosyphilis in a human immunodeficiency virus type-1 seropositive population: evidence for frequent serologic relapse after therapy. Am J Med 99:55–63

Marra CM, Gary DW, Kuypers J et al. (1996) Diagnosis of neurosyphilis in patients infected with human immunodeficiency virus type 1. J Infect Dis 174:219–221

Schoutens C, Boute V, Govaerts D et al. (1996) Late cutaneous syphilis and neurosyphilis. Dermatology 192: 403–405

Laboratory Tests

Bernard C, de Moerloose P, Tremblet C et al. (1998) Biological true and false serological tests for syphilis: their relationship with anticardiolipin antibodies. Dermatologica 180:151–153

Bromberg K, Rawstron S, Tannis G (1993) Diagnosis of congenital syphilis by combining Treponema pallidum-specific IgM detection with immunofluorescent antigen detection for T. pallidum. J Infect Dis 168:238–242

Clarkson KA (1956) Technique of darkfield examination. Med Tech Bull 7:199–207

Deacon WE, Lucas JB, Price EV (1998) Fluorescent treponemal antibody absorption (FTA/ABS) test for syphilis. JAMA 198:624–628

Huber TW, Storms S, Young P et al. (1993) Reactivity of microhemagglutinin, fluorescent treponemal antibody absorption, veneral disease research laboratory, and rapid plasma reagin card tests in primary syphilis. J Clin Microbiol 17:405–409

Keir G (1994) Cerebrospinal fluid proteins in neurosyphilis and HIV infection. Int J STD AIDS 5:310–317

Larsen SA, Steiner BM, Rudolph AH (1995) Laboratory diagnosis and interpretation of tests for syphilis. Clin Microbiol Rev 8:1–21

Lewis LL (1992) Congenital syphilis. Serologic diagnosis in the young infant. Infect Dis Clin North Am 6:31–39

Schultz DR (1997) Antiphospholipid antibodies: basic immunology and assays. Semin Arthritis Rheum 26: 724–739

Yinnon AM, Coury Doniger P, Polito R et al. (1996) Serologic response to treatment of syphilis in patients with HIV infection. Arch Intern Med 156:321–325

Young H, Moyes A, Seagar L et al. (1998) Novel recombinant-antigen enzyme immunoassay for serological diagnosis of syphilis. J Clin Microbiol 36:913–917

Zoechling N, Schluepen EM, Soyer HP et al. (1997) Molecular detection of Treponema pallidum in secondary and tertiary syphilis. Br J Dermatol 136:683–686

Treatment

1998 guidelines for treatment of sexually transmitted diseases. Centers for Disease Control and Prevention. MMWR Morb Mortal Wkly Rep 47:1–111

De Maria A, Solaro C, Abbruzzese M et al. (1997) Minocycline for symptomatic neurosyphilis in patients allergic to penicillin. N Engl J Med 337:1322–1323

Finelli L, Crayne EM, Spitalny KC (1998) Treatment of infants with reactive syphilis serology, New Jersey: 1992 to 1996. Pediatrics 102:127

Hook EW (1998) Is elimination of endemic syphilis transmission a realistic goal for the USA? Lancet 351 [Suppl 3]: 19–21

Levine WC, Berg AO, Johnson RE et al. (1994) Development of sexually transmitted diseases treatment guidelines, 1993. New methods, recommendations, and research priorities. STD Treatment Guidelines Project Team and Consultants. Sex Transm Dis 21:S96–101

Mashkilleyson AL, Gomberg MA, Mashkilleyson N et al. (1996) Treatment of syphilis with azithromycin. Int J STD AIDS 7 [Suppl 1]:13–15

Paryani SG, Vaughn AJ, Crosby M et al. (1994) Treatment of asymptomatic congenital syphilis: benzathine versus procaine penicillin G therapy. J Pediatr 125:471–475

Rolfs RT (1995) Treatment of syphilis, 1993. Clin Infect Dis 20 [Suppl 1]:23–38

Rolfs RT, Joesoef MR, Hendershot EF et al. (1997) A randomized trial of enhanced therapy for early syphilis in patients with and without human immunodeficiency virus infection. The Syphilis and HIV Study Group. N Engl J Med 337:307–314

Yaws

Backhouse JL, Hudson BJ, Hamilton PA et al. (1998) Failure of penicillin treatment of yaws on Karkar Island, Papua New Guinea. Am J Trop Med Hyg 59:388–392

Brown ST (1985) Therapy for nonvenereal treponematoses: review of the efficacy of penicillin and consideration of alternatives. Rev Infect Dis 7 [Suppl 2]:S318–326

Browne SG (1976) Treponemal depigmentation, with special reference to yaws. S Afr Med J 50:442–445

Engelkens HJ, Ginai AZ, Judanarso J et al. (1990) Radiological and dermatological findings in two patients suffering from early yaws in Indonesia. Genitourin Med 66: 259–263

Engelkens HJ, Judanarso J, Oranje AP et al. (1991) Endemic treponematoses. Part I. Yaws. Int J Dermatol 30:77–83

Engelkens HJ, Vuzevski VD, Judanarso J et al. (1990) Early yaws: a light microscopic study. Genitourin Med 66: 264–266

Garner MF, Backhouse JL, Daskalopoulos G et al. (1972) Treponema pallidum haemagglutination test for yaws. Comparison with the TPI and FTA-ABS tests. Br J Vener Dis 48:479–482

Koff AB, Rosen T (1993) Nonvenereal treponematoses: yaws, endemic syphilis, and pinta. J Am Acad Dermatol 29: 519–535

Noordhoek GT, Cockayne A, Schouls LM et al. (1990) A new attempt to distinguish serologically the subspecies of Treponema pallidum causing syphilis and yaws. J Clin Microbiol 28:1600–1607

Noordhoek GT, Engelkens HJ, Judanarso J et al. (1991) Yaws in West Sumatra, Indonesia: clinical manifestations, serological findings and characterisation of new Treponema isolates by DNA probes. Eur J Clin Microbiol Infect Dis 10:12–19

Noordhoek GT, Wieles B, van der Sluis JJ et al. (1990) Polymerase chain reaction and synthetic DNA probes: a means of distinguishing the causative agents of syphilis and yaws? Infect Immun 58:2011–2013

Rothschild BM, Rothschild C (1995) Treponemal disease revisited: skeletal discriminators for yaws, bejel, and venereal syphilis. Clin Infect Dis 20:1402–1408

Pinta

Engelkens HJ, Niemel PL, van der Sluis JJ et al. (1991) Endemic treponematoses. Part II. Pinta and endemic syphilis. Int J Dermatol 30:231–238

Fohn MJ, Wignall S, Baker Zander SA et al. (1988) Specificity of antibodies from patients with pinta for antigens of Treponema pallidum subspecies pallidum. J Infect Dis 157:32–37

Koff AB, Rosen T (1993) Nonvenereal treponematoses: yaws, endemic syphilis, and pinta. J Am Acad Dermatol 29: 519–535

Endemic Syphilis

Csonka G, Pace J (1985) Endemic nonvenereal treponematosis (bejel) in Saudi Arabia. Rev Infect Dis 7 [Suppl 2]: 260–265

Engelkens HJ, Niemel PL, van der Sluis JJ et al. (1991) Endemic treponematoses. Part II. Pinta and endemic syphilis. Int J Dermatol 30:231–238

Koff AB, Rosen T (1993) Nonvenereal treponematoses: yaws, endemic syphilis, and pinta. J Am Acad Dermatol 29: 519–535

Rothschild BM, Rothschild C (1995) Treponemal disease revisited: skeletal discriminators for yaws, bejel, and venereal syphilis. Clin Infect Dis 20:1402–1408

Sehgal VN (1990) Leg ulcers caused by yaws and endemic syphilis. Clin Dermatol 8:166–174

Tabbara KF (1990) Endemic syphilis (Bejel). Int Ophthalmol 14:379–381

Chancroid

D'Souza P, Pandhi RK, Khanna N et al. (1998) A comparative study of therapeutic response of patients with clinical chancroid to ciprofloxacin, erythromycin, and cotrimoxazole. Sex Transm Dis 25:293–295

Ducrey A (1889) Il virus dell'ulcera venerea. Gazz Internaz Med Chir 11:44

Eichmann A (1996) Chancroid. Curr Probl Dermatol 24: 20–24

Hammond GW (1996) A history of the detection of Haemophilus ducreyi, 1889–1979. Sex Transm Dis 23: 93–96

Jones CC, Rosen T (1991) Cultural diagnosis of chancroid. Arch Dermatol 127:1823–1827

Orle KA, Gates CA, Martin DH et al. (1996) Simultaneous PCR detection of Haemophilus ducreyi, Treponema pallidum, and herpes simplex virus types 1 and 2 from genital ulcers. J Clin Microbiol 34:49–54

Ortiz Zepeda C, Hernandez Perez E, Marroquin Burgos R (1994) Gross and microscopic features in chancroid: a study in 200 new culture-proven cases in San Salvador. Sex Transm Dis 21:112–117

Relman DA, Swartz MN (1995) Disease due to Chlamydia. In: Rubenstein E, Federman DD (eds) Scientific American Medicine first bound edition, vol 7. Scientific American, New York

Schmid GP, Sanders LL, Jr, Blount JH et al. (1987) Chancroid in the United States. Reestablishment of an old disease. JAMA 258:3265–3268

Schulte JM, Schmid GP (1995) Recommendations for treatment of chancroid, 1993. Clin Infect Dis 20 [Suppl 1]: 39–46

Trees DL, Morse SA (1995) Chancroid and Haemophilus ducreyi: an update. Clin Microbiol Rev 8:357–375

Granuloma Inguinale

Ahmed BA, Tang A (1996) Successful treatment of donovanosis with ciprofloxacin. Genitourin Med 72:73–74

Bassa AG, Hoosen AA, Moodley J et al. (1993) Granuloma inguinale (donovanosis) in women. An analysis of 61 cases from Durban, South Africa. Sex Transm Dis 20: 164–167

Hart G (1997) Donovanosis. Clin Infect Dis 25:24–30

Kharsany AB, Hoosen AA, Kiepiela P et al. (1997) Growth and cultural characteristics of Calymmatobacterium granulomatis – the aetiological agent of granuloma inguinale (Donovanosis). J Med Microbiol 46:579–585

Rosen T, Tschen JA, Ramsdell W et al. (1984) Granuloma inguinale. J Am Acad Dermatol 11:433–437

Sehgal VN, Sharma HK (1992) Donovanosis. J Dermatol 19:932–946

Protozoan Diseases

Contents

Introduction

Protozoa are single-cell eukaryotic organisms, classified on the basis of their morphology and means of locomotion. Many of them are familiar to high-school biology students who during their first encounters with a microscope may watch ciliated or flagellate organisms move about, or slower ameboid creatures gradually spread their pseudopodia. Table 6.1 shows just how ubiquitous protozoa are, how many serious diseases they cause and how many previously poorly understood or unknown organisms have acquired increased importance because of HIV/AIDS. Protozoa may have complex life-cycles, infections are typically difficult to treat and in most cases prophylactic immunization is ineffective. One redeeming feature is that the organisms are large enough to be seen in stool, other tissue fluids and histologic sections in many cases. We only consider a limited number of protozoan infections with cutaneous findings.

Leishmaniasis

Definition. Diverse protozoan infection found in most of the tropical world, featuring complex interplay between organism and host defense mechanisms with frequent cutaneous involvement.

Causative Organism. *Leishmania* species. Table 6.2 lists the various types of leishmaniasis and the associated organisms.

Epidemiology. Leishmaniasis is found in tropical and subtropical zones, except for Australia and Southeast Asia. Worldwide about 12 million people

Table 6.1. Common protozoan diseases

Organism	Disease	Distribution	Transmission
Leishmania	Leishmaniasis	Tropical and subtropical zones	Sandflies
Trichomonas vaginalis	Trichomonal vaginitis	Worldwide	Venereal
Entamoeba histolytica	Amebiasis	Worldwide	Water, food, fecal-oral
Trypanosoma brucei	Sleeping sickness	Africa	Tsetse fly
Trypanosoma cruzi	Chagas disease	South America	Reduviid bugs
Babesia	Babesiosis	North America, Europe	Ticks, transfusions
Toxoplasma gondii	Toxoplasmosis	Worldwide	Cats, transplacental
Plasmodium spp.	Malaria	Tropical and subtropical zones	Mosquitoes
Giardia lamblia	Giardiasis	Worldwide	Water, food, fecal-oral
Acanthamoeba spp.	Keratitis	Worldwide	Contact lenses
Pneumocystis carinii	Pneumonia in AIDS	Worldwide	Airborne
Cryptosporium spp.	Diarrhea in AIDS	Worldwide	Water, food, fecal-oral
Isospora spp.	Diarrhea in AIDS	Worldwide	Water, food, fecal-oral
Microsporidium spp.	Diarrhea in AIDS	Worldwide	Water, food, fecal-oral

Table 6.2. Classification of leishmaniasis

Clinical form	Species	Main distribution
Cutaneous leishmaniasis		
Solitary or limited cutaneous leishmaniasis		
Old World	*L. major*	Near and Middle East
	L. tropica	Near and Middle East, former USSR
	L. aethiopica	Ethiopia, Kenya
	L. infantum	Mediterranean countries
New World	*L. mexicana* complex	Mexico, Central America
	L. braziliensis complex	Central, South America
	L. mexicana amazonensis	Amazon basin
Diffuse anergic cutaneous leishmaniasis		
Old World	*L. aethiopica*	Ethiopia, Kenya
New World	*L. braziliensis* complex	South America
	L. mexicana amazonensis	South America
Chronic hypergic cutaneous leishmaniasis	*L. tropica*	Near and Middle East
Mucocutaneous leishmaniasis	*L. braziliensis* complex	South America, Panama
Visceral leishmaniasis		
Kala-azar	*L. donovani donovani*	India, East Africa
	L. infantum	Mediterranean countries
	L. chagasi	Central, South America
Post-kala-azar dermal leishmaniasis	*L. donovani donovani*	India

are infected and there are about 400,000 new infections yearly. In Europe the disease is found south of the 10°C yearly isotherm, roughly the area in which the olive tree grows. Tongue-like extensions go further north in the Balkans, Switzerland and Alsace. Individuals living in Central and Northern Europe frequently bring infections back from their travels, even though the protozoon has not established itself in the wild in these areas. In the New World, leishmaniasis is found from southern Mexico to Argentina. Around the world, the distribution is closely associated with the presence of sandflies of the *Phlebotomus* species.

Etiology and Pathogenesis. Leishmania are transmitted by sandflies which are small (1–2 mm), weak, low-flying insects living in stalls or primitive dwellings in which decaying vegetation can be found. They fly only at night. Vacationers living in upper stories are at little risk compared to those in nearby ground-level accommodation. In addition to sandfly bites, leishmaniasis can be transmitted by blood transfusions, and rarely transplacentally and even through intimate personal contact. Transmission usually involves an additional animal reservoir, usually a rodent or a dog, as well as the sandfly, which is usually of the species *Phlebotomus* but also *Lutzomyia* and *Psychodopygus*.

The protozoon has two basic forms: the amastigote and the promastigote. The amastigote is a 2–3 μm round or oval intracellular form (Fig. 6.1) found in humans and the mammalian reservoirs. It is transmitted to the insects where it develops into the 10–15 μm long and 2–3 μm wide flagellated promastigote which is then transmitted to the next potential host. Each species of leishmania has a favorite mammalian reservoir. Only *Leishmania donovani donovani* and *L. tropica* are primarily anthropomorphic.

Both forms have a nucleus and a small kinetoplast containing DNA. While the promastigotes from different species show minor differences, the

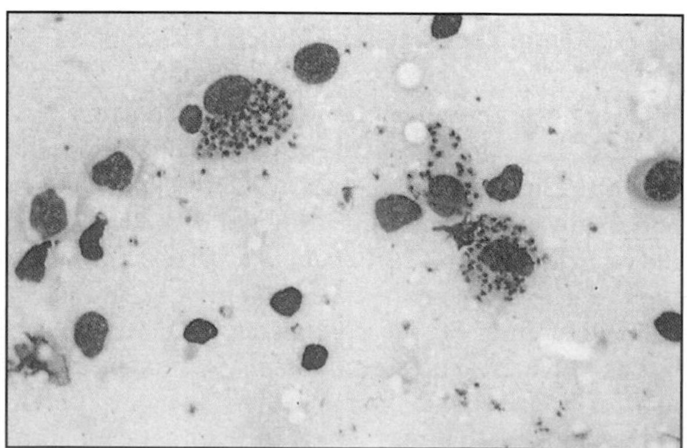

Fig. 6.1. Intracellular *Leishmania*

tissue forms or amastigotes are identical. In the past, the speciation was based on clinical features and geographic distribution. In recent years, leishmania have been subdivided based primarily on kinetoplast DNA studies, excretion products and isoenzyme studies. Monoclonal antibodies are available against many of the species surface antigens. Unfortunately, none of these methods is universally accepted as standard so confusion still exists.

The clinical spectrum of leishmaniasis can be best compared to that of leprosy. On one pole cutaneous leishmaniasis is found. The host develops a highly specific cell-mediated immunity which provides a life-long, parasite-specific immunity. The opposite pole is represented by visceral leishmaniasis, in which there is little evidence of an effective immune response. Intermediate forms include mucocutaneous leishmaniasis and disseminated cutaneous leishmaniasis in which there is an intense inflammatory reaction, but still local proliferation of the protozoa without systemic spread. In contrast to leprosy, the immune response in leishmaniasis is not only dependent on the host's immune status but also on the species of parasite. The combination of a given species and most likely geographic and climatic factors leads to biologically quite similar organisms producing radically different clinical pictures. While the clinical pattern often suggests the causative species or subspecies, the correlation is not perfect. On occasion, perhaps influenced by the host's status, organisms can act in unexpected ways. In other words, similar organisms can produce quite different pictures and almost all clinical patterns are produced by more than one organism.

There are few other infections in which the immune response and its role in controlling infection have been so intensively investigated. *Leishmania* species-specific immunoglobulins can be identified. The titers are especially high in patients with visceral leishmaniasis, where they appear to offer little protection. In contrast, macrophages and T cells appear to provide an important control in regulating the susceptibility of a host to the organism. Intracellular amastigotes are killed by the production of free oxygen radicals and hydrogen peroxide. This process is regulated by antigen-specific T cells. Those TH1 T cells that produce interferon (IFN)-γ and interleukin (IL)-12 are needed to efficiently eliminate intracellular parasites. The old Montenegro reaction, in which heat-treated leishmania are injected into the skin and the presence of a delayed or tuberculin-like reaction is observed, is mediated by the production of the above-mentioned cytokines, as in the clinical response in ordinary cutaneous leishmaniasis. Patients whose T cells are predominantly of the TH2 type which produce more IL-4 and less IL-12 and IFN-γ are more likely to develop disseminated cutaneous leishmaniasis or visceral leishmaniasis. In such patients, the Montenegro test is negative, but the immunoglobulin titers are elevated. The immunity conferred by the appropriate TH1 cells is life-long, but only for a single species of *Leishmania*. There is only one well-established exception: infection with *L. major* protects against a subsequent infection with *L. tropica*. If the immune system is weakened, such as in HIV/AIDS, there can be a loss of immunity, so that a clinical relapse may occur many years after the initial infection.

Cutaneous Leishmaniasis

Synonyms. There are many synonyms for the primary lesion in cutaneous leishmaniasis, reflecting the frequency of the disease in the Middle East. Names such as Baghdad boil, Delhi boil, Aleppo sore or Oriental sore are a few examples. They are all misleading because the distribution of the disease is far greater than the labeling suggests.

Epidemiology. Cutaneous leishmaniasis is restricted to warm countries where the appropriate sandflies are present. The entire Mediterranean basin is involved, including all of the islands. Dry sandy desert regions are the choice location. Thus the disease is found across the entire Near and Middle East, extending to the Indian subcontinent, the southern reaches of the former USSR and China. It is present in North Africa, but not in the tropical rain-forest regions. In the New World, there is an endemic focus in south-central Texas, but of greater importance is the widespread distribution of the disease throughout Mexico, especially the Yucatan, the Dominican Republic, and virtually all of Central and South America. Chile and Uruguay are generally held to be free of leishmania. While in general the vectors are found below 400 m above sea level, they extend to elevations of over 3000 m in the Ethiopian and Kenyan highlands and in the Andes. In the Old World, *L. major* is primarily a rural desert disease with gerbils as the main reservoir. In contrast *L. tropica* is a more urban disease with dogs as the reservoir. The hyrax or cony is the second host for the highland forms of *L. aethiopica*. In the New World, forest rodents are almost always the second host.

Clinical Findings. In endemic areas, the disease typically first appears in children. As mentioned already, the sandflies are tiny insects that fly weakly and close to the ground, only at night, and bite on exposed areas, such as the face and hands. The disease usually starts 2–4 weeks after the bite with a small erythematous papule which slowly grows over the next weeks to months. The border of the expanding papule or nodule is usually livid red while the central area may be ulcerated and covered with a crust (Fig. 6.2). Tiny satellite nodules may appear at the periphery or subcutaneous nodules may arise along the lymphatics in a sporotrichoid fashion. Aggressive local growth extending to the fat or muscle is rare. After 2–6 months, the growth stops, the nodule more extensively ulcerates (Fig. 6.3) and then heals with a characteristic cribriform scar. The lesions are usually asymptomatic, unless they cause ulcerations or more extreme tissue damage.

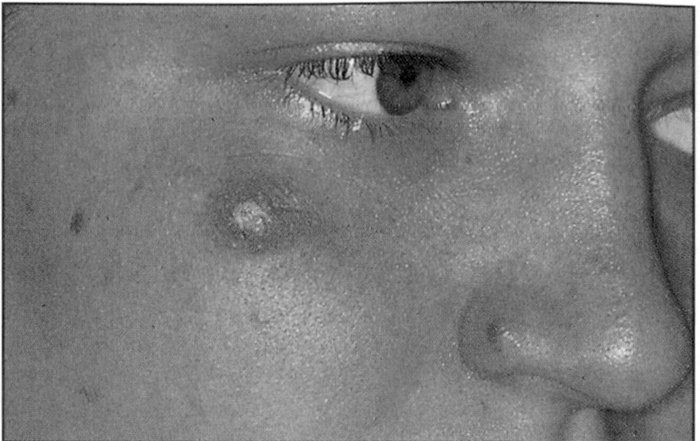

Fig. 6.2. Early lesion in Old World cutaneous leishmaniasis

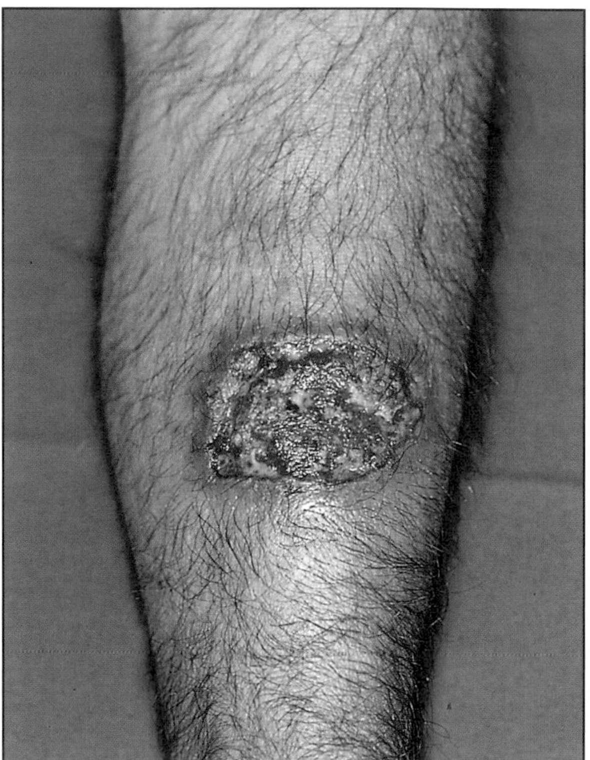

Fig. 6.3. More extensive ulceration in Old World cutaneous leishmaniasis

Solitary or Limited Cutaneous Leishmaniasis

Old World. There are many clinical variations determined to some extent by the species involved. In the Old World, the lesions tend to be self-healing and rarely a major health problem. *L. major* tends to cause multiple ulcerated lesions that resemble furuncles and are associated with lymphadenopathy. Sometimes the lesions resemble erysipelas, especially when the ear is involved. In contrast, *L. tropica* is more likely to cause a limited number of lesions, usually facial, without lymphadenopathy and with either an intact surface or superficial crusted ulcerations. The *L. major* form is known as wet leishmaniasis while that associated with *L. tropica* is described as dry. On rare occasions, the process remains active for more than 24 months; in such cases most often *L. major* is responsible. The multiple nonhealing lesions are called nonhealing chronic cutaneous leishmaniasis. In contrast, about 10% of patients with an *L. tropica* infection will develop a recurrence, often near the site of the original lesion. The lesions caused by *L. infantum* are similar to those caused by *L. major* but usually last for a shorter period of time; this form is especially common in the Mediterranean countries. With *L. aethiopica,* most patients have a typical locally limited self-healing lesion, but perhaps 20% go on to diffuse cutaneous leishmaniasis.

New World. In the New World, the clinical forms are somewhat different. In general, the disease is more variable and more aggressive. *L. mexicana* tends to cause a picture similar to *L. major* with multiple exudative lesions. One special feature is the frequency of ear involvement, especially in forest workers. When the cartilage is damaged by the ulcer, the healing is slow and the lesions painful. Such ear ulcerations are known as chiclero ulcers (a chiclero is a forest worker who harvests chicle from the sapodilla tree for chewing gum). Other regional names for typical cutaneous disease caused by *L. braziliensis* include uta in the Andean highlands and jungle yaws in the Amazon rain forests.

Diffuse Anergic Cutaneous Leishmaniasis

Both *L. aethiopica* and *L. braziliensis* can cause widespread cutaneous disease. About 20% of the patients in Ethiopia and Sudan have this form, as do many South Americans. In the latter case, an immunologically different variant of the *L. braziliensis* complex appears responsible. Usually multiple nonulcerated nodules appear, resembling lepromatous leprosy. Initially they may be arranged around the initial lesion, but later they are symmetrically distributed on the face and trunk. A keloidal variant is especially common in Honduras; it has also been called atypical cutaneous leishmaniasis. While there are high circulating antibody levels, the lesions are rich in parasites and there is no evidence of cell-mediated immunity, as demonstrated by a negative Montenegro test.

Chronic Hypergic Cutaneous Leishmaniasis

This form is subdivided into persistent and recurrent forms. Both are characterized by red-brown lupoid infiltrates that suggest sarcoidosis or cutaneous tuberculosis. Clinically the lesions are papules most often in the vicinity of a healed primary lesion. When the papules coalesce into a plaque, they resemble lupus vulgaris. Occasionally lesions may be keloidal.

Mucocutaneous Leishmaniasis

Leishmania braziliensis occasionally causes horrifying mucosal destruction, known as espundia (Fig. 6.4). The problem is more common in Brazil than in Central America. Occasionally *L. aethiopica* is responsible. Typically the primary ulcer heals and later a mutilating mucosal infection develops. Sometimes, the time interval may be as short as a few months, although the interval is usually months to a few years. In most cases, the involvement of the mucosa occurs via hematogenous or lymphatic spread, although in rare cases facial cutaneous leishmaniasis may be the cause.

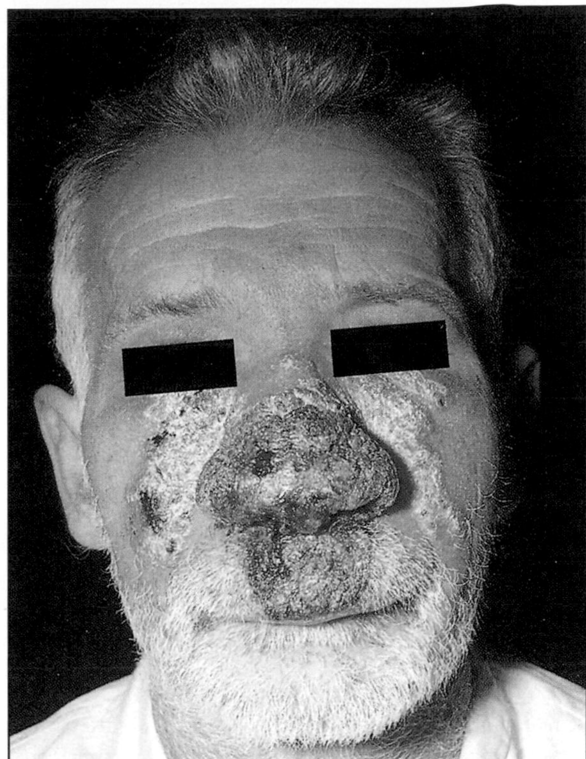

Fig. 6.4. New World mucocutaneous leishmaniasis

Most often the nasal septum is first involved. As it is damaged, the tip of the nose droops. This change combined with the swollen upper lip has led to the term tapir nose. The initial small submucosal lesion slow expands, ulcerates and causes tissue damage. Bacterial secondary infection with a wide variety of organisms occurs. In some cases, immunity develops and the disease is self-limited. Unfortunately, in others the destruction may be relentless affecting the oral cavity, the pharynx and even the trachea. Aspiration pneumonia secondary to inhalation of large clumps of necrotic parasite-laden tissue may cause death.

Histopathology. Just as with leprosy the histology varies with the immune status. When numerous organisms are present, such as in a young primary lesion or diffuse cutaneous leishmaniasis, they can be fairly easily found in histiocytes. In the typical primary lesion, there is a generous admixture of lymphocytes, plasma cells and histiocytes. Leishmaniasis may be misdiagnosed as B cell malignant lymphoma. Typically small 2–4 μm grouped intracellular organisms with a kinetoplast and no halo are found. Special stains are most helpful to exclude histoplasmosis which appears similar. Both PAS and Grocott silver stain are positive in histoplasmosis and negative in leishmaniasis. While the organisms are positive with the Giemsa stain, this feature is highly variable and not reliable. In later more granulomatous lesions, the number of organisms drops sharply and one only finds tuberculoid granulomatous inflammation. In mucocutaneous lesions, the secondary bacterial infection apparently helps destroy the organisms; in any event, they are very difficult to find.

Laboratory Findings

Direct Examination. Smears can also be examined. In this setting, Giemsa staining tissue may be more useful than it is on paraffin-fixed tissue. The leishmania stain basophilic but the kinetoplasts are eosinophilic and easily visualized. The organisms may be free or in histiocytes. The use of immunofluorescent antibodies directed against amastigotes (the tissue form) helps in the search.

Culture. The standard culture medium is Novy-McNeal-Nicolle medium, known as NNN medium. This and other modified blood agars yield the best results. The motile promastigotes proliferate. Aspirates or smears from lymph nodes or biopsies are most useful, as the surface contamination is avoided. Hamster inoculation can also be used. *L. mexicana* is easier to culture or transfer than *L. braziliensis.*

Serology. Antibodies are most prominent in the mucosal form and the diffuse cutaneous form. Either ELISA or indirect immunofluorescent studies may be done. The titers correlate to an extent with the disease course, but in endemic areas there is a high level of background positivity. In addition, the leishmanin or Montenegro test can be used to document cell-mediated immunity. The antigen is purified from promastigotes, so transmission of disease during testing is not a problem. The Montenegro test is negative in early or anergic cases and remains positive after a successfully healed primary infection, so its diagnostic usefulness is limited in endemic areas.

Other Methods. Speciation is accomplished via monoclonal antibodies, PCR analysis of DNA, isoenzyme measures, cultures in hamsters and ability to infect various sandflies

Differential Diagnosis. The differential diagnosis of leishmaniasis is lengthy. The nodular lesions are often confused with infectious processes such as furuncles, ecthyma or atypical mycobacteria infections, as well as tropical ulcers. The primary inoculation lesions of syphilis and tuberculosis may also be considered. Nodular lesions resemble malignant lymphoma, basal cell carcinoma or keratoacanthoma, while healing atrophic lesions resemble discoid lupus erythematosus. The diffuse forms resemble yaws or lepromatous leprosy. The hypergic lesions are similar to lupus vulgaris, sarcoidosis, sporotrichosis and other sporotrichoid infections. In the mouth and nose, one must consider malignant tumors, especially angiocentric lymphomas (formerly called lethal midline granuloma), pyoderma gangrenosum, treponematoses, deep fungal infections (primarily South American blastomycosis and histoplasmosis), nasal myiasis and noma.

Therapy. In all approaches to therapy of leishmaniasis it must be born in mind that many forms are self-limited, but that the potential exists for widespread disease. Most Old World leishmaniasis heals spontaneously and patients are not infectious, so little argument for toxic therapy can be made. Infections from Ethiopia, for example, have a significant risk of evolving into diffuse cutaneous leishmaniasis and should be treated, just as *L. braziliensis* infection can progress to destructive mucocutaneous disease and also warrants treatment.

Systemic. The primary systemic agents are the pentavalent antimony compounds, sodium stibogluconate (Pentostam) and meglumine antimonate (Glucantime). Pentostam is usually employed in the range of 10–20 mg/kg daily for 10–14 days. Higher dosages and longer therapy are needed for visceral, diffuse and resistant forms. Both antimony compounds must be administered intramuscularly and have a broad spectrum of side effects which are usually tolerated over the short term but which may cause problems if longer term therapy is needed. They include local pain and thromboses, as well as nausea, malaise, arthralgias and headaches. More serious are the anaphylactic reactions, cardiac arrhythmias, hemolytic anemia, renal and hepatic damage.

The official secondary choice is amphotericin B, used especially in mucocutaneous and diffuse forms in the same dosage ranges employed against deep fungi. Both itraconazole and ketoconazole are effective against some species of *Leishmania.* Because of their low toxicity and oral administration they are frequently employed but there exact role remains to be defined, especially since they have been most often used in self-limited forms of the disease. In some regimens, dapsone, rifampin, metronidazole, clofazimine and isoniazid are also used as alternates. Specialized sources that specifically address therapy of the species in question should be consulted for unusual or resistant cases. Allopurinol has recently been tried for cutaneous disease with some success.

Mucocutaneous disease has the highest relapse rate. In some studies, a recurrence rate of up to 50% has been found following antimonial treatment. Thus, amphotericin B should be considered for front-line treatment or used if a prompt response is not seen. Pentamidine isothionate is another possibility.

Topical. A myriad of topical approaches have been recommended for patients in whom the risk of mucocutaneous or disseminated disease is low. Both local heat (5 min at 55 °C) and cryosurgery can be tried. In addition, excision is often used. Finally topical or intralesional treatment with a variety of antimony compounds, as well as 15% paromomycin ointment in a vehicle with 10% urea or 15% methylbenzethonium chloride can be tried.

Other Measures. Immunotherapy with a variety of cytokines, usually combined with antimony compounds has been helpful in some cases where cell-mediated immunity was not present. Immunization with a mixed vaccine of live BCG and killed leishmania has also been studied in cutaneous leishmaniasis.

Prophylaxis. An effective vaccine for prophylaxis is not available. The best prophylaxis is control of the mammal vectors, selective spraying against sandflies, smaller mesh screens, sleeping at high levels of a home and similar simple avoidance measures.

Visceral Leishmaniasis

Kala-azar

Synonyms. Dumdum fever, Assam fever. In Hindi (*kala* = black, *azar* = fever)

Epidemiology. Visceral leishmaniasis is present in primarily rural areas with foci in India, Bangladesh, Pakistan, China, southern parts of the former USSR, sub-Saharan Africa, Turkey, the Mediterranean and parts of Mexico, Central and South America. In some regions, such as the Mediterranean, children are at particular risk and the disease is called infantile splenomegaly. The mammalian host varies widely from region to region. In India, humans appear to be the only hosts and the responsible sandfly feeds exclusively on humans.

Etiology and Pathogenesis. The main causative organisms are *L. donovani* in the Indian subcontinent and Africa, *L. infantum* in the Mediterranean basin and *L. chagasi* in South America. In rare cases, *L. tropica* appears responsible. Young and malnourished children are at the greatest risk. The ratio of disease to infections is about 1:5–10. The balance between the host immune status and the virulence of the organisms appears crucial. In general, cell-mediated immunity fails to develop appropriately. In rats, a single gene locus determining susceptibility to visceral leishmaniasis has been found, but in humans the situation appears more complex.

Clinical Findings. The initial inoculation lesion is a small papule or nodule that usually goes unnoticed. Only in rare cases does a distinctive ulcerated plaque appear. After a highly variable incubation period of 3–8 months, systemic symptoms appear. On rare occasions, the incubation period is as little as a few weeks or as long as many years. Visceral leishmaniasis is even more multifaceted than cutaneous leishmaniasis. The cutaneous findings are the least of the patients problems, and are considered below.

Systemic. The patient with visceral leishmaniasis is critically ill. Prior to the introduction of therapy, the disease was fatal in 75–95% of patients over 24 months. The most striking changes are hepatosplenomegaly, lymphadenopathy, bone marrow involvement with anemia, thrombocytopenia and leukopenia. The hematologic disorders are complex and probably reflect bone marrow involvement, hemolysis, hemodilution and splenic sequestration. The spleen and liver can become quite enormous, but jaundice is uncommon. Muscle pain may mimic dermatomyositis. The fever pattern may be characteristic with two daily peaks, but this cannot be relied upon. A variety of immunoglobulin abnormalities occur and there may be immune complex deposition in the kidneys, but renal failure is not a feature. Death may result from anemia, hemorrhage, concurrent infection or simply wasting and malnutrition. In HIV/AIDS patients, relapses have been described. Even if no documented history of visceral leishmaniasis is given, many patients in endemic areas have survived a subclinical infection.

Cutaneous Findings. Against this background the skin findings are insignificant. The main specific change is pigmented gray macules and patches, especially seen among light-skinned Indian patients; these gave rise to the name kala-azar. Most of the other changes are secondary to the severe disease. They include dry skin, hair loss, hemorrhages and oral mucositis. Post-kala-azar dermal leishmaniasis is considered below.

Histopathology. Dermatopathology is not helpful in diagnosing visceral leishmaniasis. If nodular lesions are present in the skin, a very rare event, then presumably organisms can be found, but this is not of much diagnostic benefit.

Laboratory Findings. The main diagnostic approaches are bone marrow aspiration and perhaps in early cases needle biopsy of the spleen. The organism can usually be identified directly or cultured on NNN medium. In massive infections, they can be found in the buffy coat of the blood. The presence of intercellular amastigotes or Leishman-Donovan bodies can be shown not only in the bone marrow, spleen and blood, but also in lymph node aspirates and liver biopsies. A rapid field test involving K39 antigen impregnated nitrocellulose strips has sensitivity and specificity over 98%. Polymerase chain reaction allows the detection of a single infected cell in 5–10 ml blood, and is the most sensitive technique. All the techniques discussed under cutaneous leishmaniasis can also be employed. Typically antibodies are present, but the Montenegro test is negative. Hamster inoculation leads to systemic disease, while when the leishmania involved in cutaneous disease are used, only a local response develops in the rodent.

Course and Prognosis. Without treatment, about 75–95% of patients with visceral leishmaniasis die within 2 years. The involvement of the liver, spleen, heart and bone marrow makes kala-azar a major public health problem. The good news is that about 95% of patients can be successfully treated.

Differential Diagnosis. The differential diagnosis of visceral leishmaniasis varies greatly from region to region and includes primarily nondermatologic infectious diseases such as malaria, typhoid fever, Chagas disease and many others. Leukemia and lymphoma must also be considered. The key to differential diagnosis is knowing where the patient has lived or traveled and ruling out leishmaniasis in patients with fever and organomegaly.

Therapy. The antimony compounds are the mainstays. Higher dosages and longer regimens are needed and should be sought in specialty sources. Pentamidine isothionate is effective against *L. donovani*, but usually reserved for treatment failures because of its toxicity. Amphotericin B, allopurinol and cytokines, such as IFN-γ are also employed. Amphotericin B in liposomal preparations seems especially promising. About 95% of patients can be cured. In immunocompetent hosts, relapses are rare and occur within the first 6 months after stopping therapy. If immunodeficiency, especially HIV/AIDS, appears then the risk or relapse is much greater.

Excellent supportive care, including hospitalization, supplemental nourishment and transfusions are valuable, but unfortunately often not obtainable. The same control measures discussed above are important.

Post-Kala-azar Dermal Leishmaniasis

Patients who survive visceral leishmaniasis are at risk of developing a chronic cutaneous form, usually called post-kala-azar dermal leishmaniasis. The classic triad for post-kala-azar dermal leishmaniasis is both hypopigmented and erythematous macules, as well as dermal nodules. About 5% of the East African patients show these changes during convalescence. Typically the papules appear on the face and extensor aspects of the extremities. On biopsy a tuberculoid infiltrate is found, and special stains may reveal a limited number of protozoa. Spontaneous resolution is the rule.

In Indian patients the situation is slightly different, as far more individuals, at least 20%, develop hypopigmented macules usually 1–2 years later. Linear urticarial lesions may appear. Over time, the hypopigmented macules may be decorated by numerous papules and nodules, with little tendency to spontaneous resolution. To the inexperienced, i.e., non-Indian observers, the clinical appearance is very similar to that of lepromatous leprosy.

The nodules show a dense lymphohistiocytic infiltrate, hyaline changes in the vessel walls and sclerosis of collagen. Organisms are sparse. They can be found only in nodular lesions, not in the hypopigmented macules and usually not in the bone marrow or other internal sites. In this setting, treatment is needed, using the same regimens as those available for kala-azar.

Trichomoniasis

(Donne 1836)

Definition. Common protozoan infection usually of female genital tract. This disease is illustrated in Chapter 5 and also discussed in Chapter 35.

Causative Organism. *Trichomonas vaginalis*

Epidemiology. Trichomoniasis is an extremely common infection, almost always transmitted via sexual or genital contact. The organisms can survive in a moist sponge for 90 min and in water at 36 °C for 24 h, so transmission by fomites is theoretically possible. Women are far more frequently involved and more likely to have symptoms. It is estimated that over 3 million women suffer an infection yearly in the USA. Worldwide the incidence is estimated at over 180 million cases yearly. Other studies suggest that 20% of women between 16 and 35 years of age have at least one infection. Of patients visiting a gynecologist, about 10–20% have *T. vaginalis*, while the proportion amongst prostitutes is around 50–75%. About 70% of women with gonorrhea also have trichomoniasis. Only about 5% of men visiting an STD clinic are positive, although 15% of those with a nongonorrheal urethritis have the organism. Men are more likely to be asymptomatic and serve as carriers. In addition, spontaneous resolution is often the case. In one study the prevalence of 70% in a group of symptomatic men dropped to 33% 2 weeks after the last sexual encounter. Coinfection with *Neisseria gonorrhoeae* is common; this should always be excluded.

Etiology and Pathogenesis. Three different trichomonads are potential human pathogens. The most common is *T. vaginalis*, but *T. tenax* is found in the mouth and may play a role in gingivitis and anaerobic oral infections as well as rarely causing pneumonia in predisposed patients, while *Pentatrichomonas hominis* is found in the colon and may be associated with bowel disease. All three protozoa are highly site-specific. The size of *T. vaginalis* varies from 4 to 45 µm in length and 2 to 14 µm in width. It has four smaller anterior flagella and a larger posterior flagellum embedded in the undulating membrane. The characteristic twitching motions allow one to spot the organism under the microscope. There are a variety of serologic subtypes which are not of clinical significance. *T. vaginalis* favors keratinizing mucosal surfaces, such as the urethra.

Clinical Findings. *T. vaginalis* does not grow on the skin, but favors the vagina, urethra, Skene glands and to a much lesser extent the cervix. Bladder and ureteral involvement is rare. In men, the urethra is the usual site; rarely the prostate, epididymis and prepuce are involved.

Women usually complain of a vaginal discharge, burning, dysuria or dyspareunia. An unpleasant odor may also be present, but should suggest *Gardnerella vaginalis*. The labia are often swollen. The cervix may have punctate hemorrhages producing a strawberry-like surface. This change is commonly seen with colposcopy, but is rarely identified with the naked eye. A white-yellow discharge and bubbles or froth strongly suggest *T. vaginalis*. Most men are asymptomatic. Some may have dysuria or a minimal urethral discharge; ascending involvement is very uncommon. The occasional case of balanoposthitis is probably secondary to the irritating discharge.

Laboratory Findings

Direct Examination. Evaluating material from the vaginal vault, cervix and urethra is the best diagnostic approach. The motile flagellates can be identified fairly readily. In women about 75% of infected individuals can be diagnosed with wet mount examinations. Slightly warming the slide and lowering the condenser on the microscope may increase the yield, but if available, either polarization or dark-field microscopy is more effective. The smear is usually rich in both neutrophils and mucosal epithelial cells, so that motion is the best way to find the organisms. Trichomonads are also often identified on Papanicolou smears. In men the yield is lower, so techniques such as collecting morning urine sediment, using a prostate massage or evaluating an ejaculate may be required.

Culture. A number of satisfactory culture media are available; all offer a sensitivity of about 95%. We use Bacto Kupferberg trichomonas medium. Simultaneously, a culture for gonorrhea should be performed.

Serology. The antibody response is variable and unreliable, so that no routine serologic testing is recommended.

Other Methods. Direct immunofluorescent, ELISA and latex agglutination tests are available. All are better than the wet mount but less sensitive than a culture.

Therapy

Systemic. Systemic therapy with metronidazole is the standard. Usually 1.5–2.0 g as a single dose or 500 mg twice daily for 5–7 days produces a 90–95% response rate. The single dose obviously has the best compliance and is usually preferred.The partner should be treated. In addition, asymptomatic patients identified via direct observation or culture should also be treated. Two newer closely related oral compounds, tinidazole and ornidazole, can also be used in a single-dose regimen.

While short-term therapy with metronidazole is simple and usually without problems, several aspects should be kept in mind. The biggest worry is that metronidazole is not approved in pregnancy; it cannot be used in the first trimester and is best avoided throughout. Unfortunately many pregnant women develop trichomoniasis. Some clinicians feel a single dose in the last two-thirds of pregnancy is safe. Others rely on time and ineffective topical measures. Both nausea and vomiting and secondary candidal infections are seen. The drug has a disulfuram-like action, so alcohol should be avoided. Long-term animal studies have suggested carcinogenicity, so repeated use should be avoided. The prothrombin time can be prolonged. Thus, one must be careful in patients with bleeding disorders or on anticoagulants. Metronidazole resistance can be seen. Often a higher dose for 5–7 days produces a cure. Determining sensitivity is complicated and not widely used.

Topical. There is no effective topical approach. In some countries, topical metronidazole is available. During pregnancy, topical imidazoles, such as clotrimazole vaginal tablets, can be tried.

Other Protozoan Infections

Most of the other organisms shown in Table 6.1 produce few cutaneous findings and rarely come to the attention of dermatologists. Others can occasionally produce skin findings which are briefly discussed below.

Amebiasis

(Losch 1875)

Synonyms. Amoebiasis, entamebiasis

Definition. Common protozoan bowel infection with rare cutaneous involvement.

Causative Organism. Entamoeba histolytica

Epidemiology. Amebiasis is primarily a tropical and subtropical disease, although the organism has been identified all over the world. In Central Europe, about 1% of individuals have an asymptomatic bowel infection; in homosexuals, the rate is about 20%. Many infections are brought from southern Europe. In tropical countries, the problem is much greater. About 50 million individuals yearly suffer from an infection and about 100,000 die. Serologic studies have shown positivity rates ranging from 80% in Calcutta to 6% in Mexico City.

Asymptomatic carriers are more likely to shed the cysts than are those with active disease. Inadequate personal hygiene, poorly protected sources of water, and the use of human excrement for fertilizer all contribute to the spread of the ameba. In western countries, direct spread is a more common pathway, especially among homosexuals. The cysts can be infectious for several months in cooler, moist areas; they are susceptible to heat and dryness.

Etiology and Pathogenesis. While there are a number of nonpathogenic ameba found in the colon, *E. histolytica* is the only major human pathogen. It can exist either as a dormant cyst or as an active motile trophozoite characterized by pseudopodia. Evaluation of the organism's isoenzymes and DNA has shown that two species occur; the pathogenic *E. histolytica* and the harmless *E. dispar* which causes intraluminal infections without invasion. Most asymptomatic cyst passers and many homosexuals carry *E. dispar*. When *E. histolytica* invades or penetrates the bowel wall, active infection occurs. The protozoon attaches to specific lectins and causes cytolysis by releasing a pore-forming enzyme. The invasion progresses, leading to ulcerations and eventually perforations. During this process, trophozoites can enter the bloodstream and migrate to the liver and occasionally other organs.

Clinical Findings

Systemic Findings. E. histolytica may cause an acute dysentery, a mild persistent infection or invasive disease. The acute amebic dysentery is characterized by blood and mucus in the stool. In later stages, fever, chills and headache may be found. In mild chronic amebiasis, the diagnosis is often irritable bowel syndrome or something equally nonspecific. When the trophozoites spread to the liver, a hepatic abscess may result.

Cutaneous Findings. In male homosexuals there may be direct inoculation of organisms into the penis or anal mucosa. In other patients, the skin of the perineum may be involved secondary to colonic disease or less commonly, the organism may move from a hepatic abscess to the skin. Clinically one finds purulent nodules, cysts and sinuses, usually with obvious underlying disease.

Histopathology. When an amebic cutaneous ulcer is biopsied, the trophozoite may be found in the dermis. It is usually 12–20 µm in diameter, has a clear cytoplasm, an eccentric nucleus and may contain erythrocytes. The overlying epidermis often shows pseudoepitheliomatous hyperplasia.

Laboratory Findings. Both cysts and trophozoites should be sought in the stool, scrapings and biopsy material. Trophozoites are taken as a sign of invasive disease. The diagnosis of amebiasis can be challenging, primarily because of the presence of similar or even identical (in the case of *E. dispar*) nonpathogenic organisms in the stool. In addition, patients with hepatic disease often do not shed cysts. Serologic tests, including direct immunofluorescence, ELISA and hemagglutination inhibition (HIA) are most useful when evaluating suspected amebic liver abscesses, which can often be identified with ultrasound or CAT scanning. The serologic tests are less useful in endemic areas, since chronic infections are common and the tests remain positive following therapy.

Differential Diagnosis. The differential diagnosis of amebic dysentery and liver disease is beyond the scope of this text. Amebiasis should be considered as a possible cause of cutaneous ulcers in the genital and perianal region in male homosexuals and in patients from endemic areas, especially those with gastrointestinal or hepatic complaints.

Therapy. Metronidazole is the mainstay of therapy, but many alternative agents are available and discussed in infectious disease texts. Surgery is often needed for amebic hepatic abscesses.

Trypanosomiasis

Sleeping sickness or African trypanosomiasis is a major health problem across vast areas of the African plains, causing considerable morbidity among cattle and their human associates. *Trypanosoma brucei* is inoculated by the bite of the tsetse fly. About 50% of patients develop a nodule at this site, followed weeks later by a more widespread papular eruption known as a trypanid. The neurologic symptoms predominate.

Chagas disease or American trypanosomiasis is seen through Central and South America. The causative organism is *T. cruzi*. Transmission occurs by the bite of a reduviid or kissing bug. The acute reaction at the bite site is known as a chagoma. The Romaña sign refers to bilateral orbital edema seen occasionally in the early stages. Chagas disease primarily involves the heart, intestines and CNS. Reactivation of cutaneous disease has been described following cardiac transplantation.

Babesiosis

(Smith 1893)

Synonym. Texas cattle fever

Babesia microti (in North America) and *B. divergens* in Europe are protozoan parasites of erythrocytes. While babesiosis has no cutaneous findings, it is of interest to dermatologists because it follows roughly the same pattern of distribution as *Borrelia burgdorferi* and is transmitted by the same ticks. When a patient with suspected borreliosis has high fever, chills, hemolytic anemia or fails to respond to standard therapy, babesiosis should be excluded by examination of a thick blood smear (just as with malaria). Patients with a splenectomy are at especially risk for infection. There is no standard therapy, although clindamycin and quinine in combination are usually recommended.

Toxoplasmosis

Definition. Widespread protozoan infection, usually associated with contact with house cats, and a major cause of CNS problems in HIV/AIDS patients, as well as congenital malformations and infections.

Causative Organism. *Toxoplasma gondii*

Epidemiology. Many humans have asymptomatic infections, acquired either by eating infected improperly cooked pork or because of contact with cat feces in kitty litter or sand boxes. About 10 % of individuals acquire the infection every decade, so that by age 70 years, up to 70 % of individuals show serologic signs of exposure, although most are asymptomatic. In France over 90 % of patients have positive serologic evaluations by 40 years of age.

Etiology and Pathogenesis. *T. gondii* is a protozoon which has a worldwide distribution and has become increasingly important during the HIV/AIDS epidemic as a cause of CNS disease and chorioretinitis. The definitive host for *T. gondii* are felines, primarily house cats. The organism takes three forms:

- Trophozoite: Circulating parasite which can enter almost every mammalian cell except for erythrocytes.
- Tissue cysts: When trophozoites settle in muscle or the CNS, they may divide, evolving into a pseudoencapsulated mass of organisms. When another animal eats such muscle, the disease can be transmitted.
- Oocysts: Only felines form oocysts, which are the sexual reproductive form of the protozoon, and are excreted in the feces.

Clinical Findings

Systemic Findings. The initial infection usually features lymphadenopathy, fever, headache and other symptoms resembling those seen in infectious mononucleosis. There may be a transient maculopapular rash during this stage. Patients with such symptoms and a negative test for mononucleosis should always be evaluated for toxoplasmosis. In most patients, the disease then becomes latent, but often cysts are formed in skeletal or cardiac muscle, the retina or the CNS. These cysts can be become reactivated during pregnancy, HIV/AIDS or other immunosuppression, often releasing viable protozoa and triggering new problems. Chronic persistent disease is most often in the form of chorioretinitis.

If a pregnant patient experiences an initial infection with *T. gondii*, the infant is at risk of intrauterine infection. Depending on the timing of the infection and the load of organisms transferred transplacentally, the results may range from a fetal death to marked fetal damage to less severe ocular or CNS disease manifested later in life. For this reason, pregnant women are usually checked for serologic signs of toxoplasmosis and if negative, advised to avoid cats or at least cat litter during their pregnancy. The main cutaneous finding in neonates is extramedullary hematopoiesis, producing red-blue nodules, known as the blueberry muffin syndrome.

In HIV/AIDS patients, toxoplasmosis is the most common cause of space-occupying CNS lesions. About 5–10 % of HIV/AIDS patients in the USA and a higher percentage in France develop CNS toxoplasmosis. In some it is the presenting sign of the disease.

Cutaneous Findings. Except for the extramedullary hematopoiesis, the cutaneous eruptions associated with toxoplasmosis are uncommon and poorly characterized. They are described as maculopapular, hemorrhagic or lichenoid.

Histopathology. Rarely the organism can be identified in a skin biopsy, occasionally even within the epidermis. Histologic evaluation of cysts leads to a rapid diagnosis as the protozoa can usually be readily identified.

Laboratory Findings. Serologic findings remain the mainstay of diagnosis. They are complicated by the high rate of positive reactions in many populations. The Sabin-Feldman dye test is standard, but complicated and often replaced by other tests. Rising IgG titers suggest active disease; in newborns, IgM titers are highly suggestive. Mouse inoculation tests or tissue culture inoculation are used to isolate the organism, especially in suspected congenital disease. More details on this complicated subject should be sought in specialized sources.

Differential Diagnosis. The differential diagnosis of toxoplasmosis is unlimited, depending on the clinical setting. In the newborn, the term TORCH syndrome is used as a mnemonic device to identify toxoplasmosis, other, rubella, cytomegalovirus and herpes simplex virus as causes of congenital infections with potential cutaneous hematopoiesis.

Therapy. Most patients require no treatment. Those with active chorioretinitis, myocarditis or CNS disease are usually treated with pyrimethamine, sulfadiazine and folic acid. The same regimen is used in HIV/AIDS. Sometime higher doses are suggested. Relapses and development of allergy to the sulfonamide are common. Clindamycin has also been employed, often used instead of sulfadiazine. Trimethoprim-sulfamethoxazole is another less-satisfactory possibility. During pregnancy, spiramycin is used, although it appears inferior to the standard combination.

Prophylaxis. Avoiding cat feces and improperly cooked meat is advisable for all, but crucial for pregnant patients. Serologic screening for toxoplasmosis during pregnancy appears cost effective. Screening is done early in pregnancy, and negative women are screened again at 20 weeks. If evidence of an early infection is found, either a termination or therapy can be considered. If still negative, the mother can be screened at term, to allow treatment of those with late and usually mild infections. The latter step has proven effective in reducing the number of patients with mental retardation and CNS disease.

Bibliography

Leishmaniasis

Ashford RW (1997) The leishmaniases as model zoonoses. Ann Trop Med Parasitol 91:693–701

Ashford RW (1999) Cutaneous leishmaniasis: strategies for prevention. Clin Dermatol 17:327–332

Ashford RW, Desjeux P, Raadt P de (1992) Estimation of population at risk of infection and number of cases of leishmaniasis. Parasitol Today 8:104–105

Azulay RD, Azulay DR Jr (1995) Immune-clinical-pathologic spectrum of leishmaniasis. Int J Dermatol 34:303–307

Berman JD (1997) Human leishmaniasis: clinical, diagnostic, and chemotherapeutic developments in the last 10 years. Clin Infect Dis 24:684–703

Canizares O, Haman RRM (eds) (1992) Clinical tropical dermatology, 2nd edn. Blackwell, Oxford

Davidson RN (1998) Practical guide for the treatment of leishmaniasis. Drugs 56:1009–1018

Dedet JP, Pratlong F, Lanotte G et al. (1999) Cutaneous leishmaniasis. The parasite. Clin Dermatol 17:261–268

Ghersetich I, Menchini G, Teofoli P et al. (1999) Immune response to Leishmania infection in human skin. Clin Dermatol 17:333–338

Grevelink SA, Lerner EA (1996) Leishmaniasis. J Am Acad Dermatol 34:257–272

Herwald BL (1999) Leishmaniasis. Lancet 354:1191–1199

Jha TK, Sundar S, Thakur CP et al. (1999) Miltefosine, an oral agent, for the treatment of indian visceral leishmaniasis. N Engl J Med 341:1795–1800

Koff AB, Rosen T (1994) Treatment of cutaneous leishmaniasis. J Am Acad Dermatol 31:693–708

Mehregan DR, Mehregan AH, Mehregan DA (1999) Histologic diagnosis of cutaneous leishmaniasis. Clin Dermatol 17:297–304

Moskowitz PF, Kurban AK (1999) Treatment of cutaneous leishmaniasis: retrospectives and advances for the 21st century. Clin Dermatol 17:305–315

Olliaro PL, Bryceson ADM, Uyemura K (1993) Practical progress and new drugs for changing patterns of leishmaniasis. Parasitol Today 9:323–328

Pearson RD, Sousa AQ (1996) Clinical spectrum of leishmaniasis. Clin Infect Dis 22:1–13

Postigo C, Llamas R, Zarco C et al. (1997) Cutaneous lesions in patients with viceral leishmaniasis and HIV infection. J Infect 35: 265–268

Salman SM, Rubeiz NG, Kibbi AG (1999) Cutaneous leishmaniasis: clinical features and diagnosis. Clin Dermatol 17:291–296

Samady JA, Schwartz RA (1997) Old World cutaneous leishmaniasis. Int J Dermatol 36:161–166

Samady JA, Janniger CK, Schwartz RA (1996) Cutaneous and mucocutaneous leishmaniasis. Cutis 57:13–20

Trichomoniasis

Gulmezoglu AM, Garner P (1998) Trichomoniasis treatment in women: a systematic review. Trop Med Int Health 3:553–558

Haefner HK (1999) Current evaluation and management of vulvovaginitis. Clin Obstet Gynecol 42:184–195

Hook EW III (1999) Trichomonas vaginalis – no longer a minor STD. Sex Transm Dis 26:388–389

Krieger JN (1995) Trichomoniasis in men: old issues and new data. Sex Transm Dis 22:83–96

Krieger JN, Verdon M, Siegel N et al. (1992) Risk assessment and laboratory diagnosis of trichomoniasis in men. J Infect Dis 166:1362–1366

Lewis DA, Habgood L, White R et al. (1997) Managing vaginal trichomoniasis resistant to high-dose metronidazole therapy. Int J STD AIDS 8:780–784

Nyirjesy P, Sobel JD, Weitz MV et al. (1998) Difficult-to-treat trichomoniasis: results with paromomycin cream. Clin Infect Dis 26:986–988

Paterson BA, Garland SM, Bowden FJ et al. (1999) The diagnosis of Trichomonas vaginalis: new advances. Int J STD AIDS 10:68–69

Pattman RS (1999) Recalcitrant vaginal trichomoniasis. Sex Transm Infect 75:127–128

Petrin D, Delgaty K, Bhatt R et al. (1998) Clinical and microbiological aspects of Trichomonas vaginalis. Clin Microbiol Rev 11:300–317

Sobel JD, Nagappan V, Nyirjesy P (1999) Metronidazole-resistant vaginal trichomoniasis – an emerging problem. N Engl J Med 341:292–293

Sorvillo F, Kerndt P (1998) Trichomonas vaginalis and amplification of HIV-1 transmission. Lancet 351:213–214

Thompson C, Malone JH (1998) Audit of diagnostic criteria for Trichomonas vaginalis in a genitourinary medicine clinic. Int J STD AIDS 9:364–365

Amebiasis

Anand AC, Puri P (1999) Amoebiasis revisited: pathogenesis, diagnosis and management. Trop Gastroenterol 20: 2–15

De Jonckheere JF, Brown S (1998) Non-Acanthamoeba amoebic infection. J Infect 36:349–350
Hashimoto K, Miner J (1996) Electron microscopy in AIDS-related infectious diseases. I. Acanthamoebiasis. J Dermatol 23:773–777
Helton J, Loveless M, White CR Jr (1993) Cutaneous acanthamoeba infection associated with leukocytoclastic vasculitis in an AIDS patient. Am J Dermatopathol 15: 146–149
Hunt SJ, Reed SL, Mathews WC et al. (1995) Cutaneous Acanthamoeba infection in the acquired immunodeficiency syndrome: response to multidrug therapy. Cutis 56:285–287
Katelaris PH, Farthing MJ (1995) Traveler's diarrhea: clinical presentation and prognosis. Chemotherapy 41 [Suppl 1]: 40–47
Loschiavo F, Guarneri B, Ventura-Spagnolo T et al. (1997) Cutaneous amebiasis in an Iranian immunodeficient alcoholic: immunochemical and histological study. Dermatology 194:370–371
Magana-Garcia M, Arista-Viveros A (1993) Cutaneous amebiasis in children. Pediatr Dermatol 10:352–355
May LP, Sidhu GS, Buchness MR (1992) Diagnosis of Acanthamoeba infection by cutaneous manifestations in a man seropositive to HIV. J Am Acad Dermatol 26: 352–355
Migueles S, Kumar P (1998) Primary cutaneous acanthamoeba infection in a patient with AIDS. Clin Infect Dis 27:1547–1548
Murakawa GJ, McCalmont T, Altman J et al. (1995) Disseminated acanthamebiasis in patients with AIDS. A report of five cases and a review of the literature. Arch Dermatol 131:1291–1296
Tai ES, Fong KY (1997) Fatal amoebic colitis in a patient with SLE: a case report and review of the literature. Lupus 6:610–612
Wortman PD (1996) Acanthamoeba infection. Int J Dermatol 35:48–51

Toxoplasmosis

Binazzi M (1986) Profile of cutaneous toxoplasmosis. Int J Dermatol 25:357–363
Dunn IJ, Palmer PE (1998) Toxoplasmosis. Semin Roentgenol 33:81–85
Fung HB, Kirschenbaum HL (1996) Treatment regimens for patients with toxoplasmic encephalitis. Clin Ther 18: 1037–1056
Lacroix C, Brun-Pascaud M, Maslo C et al. (1996) Co-infection of Toxoplasma gondii with other pathogens: pathogenicity and chemotherapy in animal models. Springer, Berlin Heidelberg New York, pp 223–233 (Current topics in microbiology and immunology, vol 219)
Pavesio CE, Lightman S (1996) Toxoplasma gondii and ocular toxoplasmosis: pathogenesis. Br J Ophthalmol 80: 1099–1107
Price RW (1996) Neurological complications of HIV infection. Lancet 348:445–452
Rabaud C, May T, Amiel C et al. (1994) Extracerebral toxoplasmosis in patients infected with HIV. A French National Survey. Medicine (Baltimore) 73:306–314
Rabaud C, May T, Lucet JC et al. (1996) Pulmonary toxoplasmosis in patients infected with human immunodeficiency virus: a French National Survey. Clin Infect Dis 23:1249–1254
Rodgers CA, Harris JR (1996) Ocular toxoplasmosis in HIV infection. Int J STD AIDS 7:307–309
Tomlinson DR, Fisher M, Coker RJ (1995) Management of protozoan infections in AIDS. The Jefferiss Wing Therapeutics and Protocols Group. Int J STD AIDS 6: 237–240

Fungal Diseases

Contents

Introduction

Fungi are aerobic organisms that form a cell wall and grow on or in organic material, forming a colony and reproducing either sexually or asexually. In contrast to plants, fungi do not manufacture chlorophyll. Without photosynthetic capabilities, they are dependent on other life forms. Such organisms are known as heterotrophs. Fungi are not in the plant kingdom, but form a kingdom of their own. Fungi differ from bacteria in that they have a true nucleus while most bacteria have a nuclear equivalent. The stable cell wall, primarily made of chitin, also distinguishes the fungi. Major components of the cell membrane are ergosterol and zymosterol, in contrast to the cholesterol found in mammalian cells. This offers a point of attack for many of the modern antifungal agents. While fungi can live as individual cells, often they are found in a community with various cell types acquiring specific functions, as in the case of larger fungi such as mushrooms.

A general botanical definition of fungus is: Any member of the kingdom of eukaryotic (having a true nucleus) saprophytic or parasitic organisms that lack chlorophyll, have a cell wall and have highly variable life cycles, reproducing sexually or asexually. For practical clinical purposes, fungi can be subdivided into dermatophytes, yeasts and molds.

Fungi are medically relevant for a number of reasons. They cause a variety of infections in humans, many of which have dramatic cutaneous manifestations. In addition, there are diseases where fungi appear to play a role, such as seborrheic dermatitis, where *Malassezia furfur* (*Pityrosporum ovale)* is often found. Furthermore, fungi are a significant cause of allergic disease, especially the spores of some molds. Other fungi produce toxins (such as aflatoxin from *Aspergillus flavus*, which can make various foods dangerous), hallucinogens or frank poisons. On the other hand, fungi are an essential part of the ecologic cycle and also of considerable benefit to man as a source of antibiotics, to say nothing of the yeasts using in baking and beer brewing.

Classification

The classification of fungi is complicated. The Deuteromycetes or fungi imperfecti are fungi awaiting classification. The true fungi or Eumycetes are capable of sexual reproduction. The manner of this reproduction helps determine the subclassification. The Zygomycetes form a zygote from the fusion of two identical spores. The more common Ascomycetes form spores in an internal sac or ascus, while Basidiomycetes form external spores. All these fungi also tend to reproduce asexually and are often identified in this form. In contrast, the Deuteromycetes have only been identified in an asexual form, but it is reasonable to assume they also have sexual forms. As Table 7.1 shows, some species of *Microsporum* and *Trichophyton* are Ascomycetes, while others are Deuteromycetes.

There are many ways of classifying fungi and their infections. In Germany, for instance, the DHS system is used – Dermatophytes, yeasts (*Hefe*) or molds (*Schimmelpilze*).

Dermatophytes live on keratin and infect the skin, hair and nails.

Yeasts are complicated; in some systems, they include only fungi that divide by simple budding, such as the Blastomycetes and the asexual form of *Cryptococcus neoformans*. Technically perfect yeasts are included under Ascomycetes as they are capable of forming mycelia under certain conditions. *Coccidioides immitis* and *Rhinosporidium seeberi* form large numerous internal spores; when the mother cell ruptures, the spores are released.

Molds are fungi that have a filamentous or mycelial component. In technical terms, a hypha (pl. hyphae) is a thread-like structure consisting of many oblong individual cells strung together. In contrast, a pseudohypha is a thread-like elongation from a single cell with constrictions or sphincters that mimic the cell walls in true hyphae. Many pathogens are present in the human at body temperature as yeasts but grow at room temperature with hyphae; included in this group are *Histoplasma capsulatum*, *Blastomyces dermatitidis*, *Sporothrix*

Table 7.1. Medically important fungi

Eumycetes – Fungi perfecti

Zygomycetes
- Mucorales
  - *Rhizopus* spp., *Mucor* spp. and many others
- Entomophthorales
  - *Conidiobolus* spp., *Basidiobolus* spp.

Ascomycetes
- *Geotrichum candidum*
- *Candida krusei*
- *Candida pseudotropicalis*
- *Piedraia hortae*
- *Aspergillus fumigatus*
- *Histoplasma capsulatum*
- *Blastomyces dermatitidis*
- *Trichophyton mentagrophytes*
- *Microsporum canis*
- *Microsporum gypseum*

Basidiomycetes
- *Cryptococcus neoformans*

Deuteromycetes – Fungi imperfecti

Blastomycetes – Yeasts
- *Candida albicans*
- *Candida tropicalis*
- *Malassezia furfur*
- *Trichosporon cutaneum (beigelii)*

Hyphomycetes – Molds
- *Aspergillus niger*
- *Aspergillus flavus*
- *Coccidioides immitis*
- *Hendersonula toruloidea*
- *Madurella mycetomatis*
- *Paracoccidioides brasiliensis*
- *Penicillium notatum*
- *Phaeoannellomyces (Exophilia or Cladosporium) wernickii*
- *Phialophora verrucosa*
- *Scopulariopsis brevicaulis*
- *Scytalidium hyalinum*
- *Sporothrix schenckii*

Dermatophytes
- *Epidermophyton floccosum*
- *Microsporum audouinii*
- *Trichophyton rubrum*
- *Trichophyton violaceum*
- *Trichophyton verrucosum*
- *Trichophyton tonsurans*
- *Trichophyton schoenleinii*
- *Trichophyton concentricum*

schenckii, Coccidioides immitis, Paracoccidioides brasiliensis and some of the agents of chromomycosis.

There are three types of mycelia or filamentous structures that serve different roles. The vegetative mycelia serve to anchor the fungal colony, while the submersed mycelia withdraw nutrients from the culture medium or host. The aerial mycelia are responsible for reproduction, releasing conidia (asexual spores) into the air. Mycelia are also divided into transparent and pigmented (dematiaceous). The nature of the conidia is used extensively to identify and classify fungi. One speaks of large, multicellular macroconidiae and small unicellular microconidiae. The three genera of dermatophytes are *Trichophyton, Microsporum* and *Epidermophyton.* The latter lack microconidiae, while all three genera can be differentiated on the basis not only of colony appearance and color but also of macroconidia shape.

Identification

Clinical Examination

In most instances, fungal infections can be diagnosed clinically. Skin lesions are typically slowly enlarging patches with scales and erythema more prominent at the periphery. In other instances, they may simply be hyperkeratotic. Hairs may be broken off, or there may be folliculitis or later alopecia. The nail changes are diverse but always have a degree of dystrophy and destruction. The clinical diagnosis of fungal infections is fraught with false-positive and false-negative assertions, so other diagnostic measures are usually employed to confirm the clinical suspicion.

Wood Light Examination

Fungi are diagnosed on the basis of both clinical and microbiologic criteria. Clinically, a Wood light examination will help identify some fluorescent species. *Microsporum audouinii, M. canis, M. distortum* and *M. ferrugineum* all fluoresce green, while *Trichophyton schoenleinii* shows a pale yellow fluorescence.

Obtaining Specimens

Material should be harvested carefully; this will increase the yield greatly. One should disinfect and then gently scrape scales from the skin surface with a sterile scalpel. If an intact blister or pustule is present, it can be disinfected and unroofed. The contents can be cultured and, in the case of dermatophytes, the roof examined for hyphae.

When nails are studied, one must obtain hyperkeratotic material from the nail bed and crumbly nail material. Once again, a small curette or scalpel is useful. One can also use a dermabrasion fraise to sand away infected nail for culture; here one must be careful not to release ground-up infectious nail material into the air. Potentially infected hairs can be plucked for examination and culture. In the oral cavity, either a platinum loop or sterile cotton-tipped applicators are needed. Another way to study the throat is to have the patient gargle a fixed amount of sterile water and then culture this. Finally, stool cultures can be done.

Microscopic Examination

The standard native examination or KOH examination is the quickest way to identify hyphae. The scales are placed on a glass slide, a drop or two of 15–20% KOH solution is added, and the slide is allowed to sit. In mycology laboratories the slides are kept in moist chamber for about 1 h, but clinicians tend to resort to gentle heating to speed the process. The KOH dissolves the keratin but leaves behind the hyphae. When 40% dimethylsulfoxide is added to the solution, the clearing is more immediate. If ink (Parker Blue-black Quink seems to work best) or other dyes (lactophenol cotton blue) are added, the hyphae are more easily identified. Optical whiteners can also be used, but then the specimen must be examined with an immunofluorescent microscope.

Hyphae, pseudohyphae, yeasts and spores can be seen. False-positive results occur when the normal keratinocyte cell walls are misinterpreted or when so-called mosaic fungi appear. The latter is an interaction between KOH and epidermal lipids that produces a network-like picture. No fungi are involved. This pattern disappears when the slide is allowed to cool, then reheated and reexamined. Hairs require special attention; one must ascertain whether the hyphae and spores are within the shaft (endothrix) or on the outside surface (ectothrix). Often the type of hair damage allows one to guess at the most likely agent. With nails, one must wait at least an hour and be aware that the yield is lower than with skin scales or hair. If looking for *Cryptococcus neoformans*, one should add ink to highlight the prominent capsule; this will only rarely apply to studies of skin specimens.

Histology

Another very useful technique is a skin biopsy. In the case of dermatophyte infections, some clinicians find a small punch biopsy more convenient than scraping; others do both. Another approach is to perform a tangential superficial excision of hyperkeratotic material. Nails are trimmed and the crumbly or altered material submitted, while plucked hairs can also be used. If a deep fungal infection is suspected, a biopsy is essential to obtain deep material not only for microscopic examination but also for culture. Specimens can be stained with either Gomori methenamine silver stain or periodic acid – Schiff (PAS) stain. The silver stain is more complicated but identifies fungal walls better. The PAS stain works well for dermatophytes in superficial scale, hairs or nails but is not as helpful when studying deep abscesses looking for a small yeast form. *Candida albicans* may be Gram positive. The capsule or clear space around *Cryptococcus neoformans* is also easily seen on histologic sections.

Culture

Culture is necessary to accurately identify a fungus. Usually Sabouraud medium is used. It consists of:

Glucose	20.0 or 40.0
Peptone	10.0
Agar-agar	15.0
Distilled water ad	1000

This produces either a 2% or a 4% agar, which is poured into glass tubes, where it is allowed to harden at an angle to increase surface area (slant tube), or into plastic Petri dishes. Often cycloheximide is added (400 mg/l) to inhibit contaminants, while different antibiotics are used to prevent bacterial growth (for example, penicillin and streptomycin). In the USA, Dermatologic Test Medium (DTM), as developed by Taplin in Miami, is popular. It contains a special color indicator, phenol red, which turns red after about 1 week if dermatophytes are present, as they raise the pH in the culture medium. DTM cultures cannot be used for speciation.

Ideally, dermatophyte cultures should be incubated at 25 °C. While laboratories have a special incubator, most dermatologists culture at room temperature. Yeasts and *Trichophyton verrucosum* require a temperature of 37 °C, so that if one is dealing with a yeast, especially a deep fungus with a yeast phase, then one should work with a suitably equipped laboratory. Yeasts and molds grow rapidly within a matter of days. Most dermatophytes require about 3 weeks to grow. The major problem with fungal cultures is contamination. Therefore, one should always disinfect the body surface before harvesting. If the patient is on systemic or topical antifungal therapy, false-negative results may be obtained. Many patients who present for the first time with a possible fungal infection have already been using over-the-counter imidazoles, so this problem has become more prevalent in recent years. One should stop all topical antifungal therapy for at least 1 week and then repeat the culture.

The exact diagnosis of a fungus begins with a detailed examination and description of the gross colony (Figs. 7.1, 7.2). While we have illustrated a few representative forms, the student or practitioner needs an atlas or slide set with pictures of the various colonies, or access to a mycology laboratory with a library of the regionally common cultures. One must evaluate the size of the colony, its surface (folded, smooth, furry, chunky and similar terms are used), its color, the nature of the underside and the periphery. To evaluate the macro- and microconidiae one uses lactophenol cotton blue and lifts off a bit of the colony either with a platinum loop or with transparent cellulose adhesive tape.

Other tests are more complicated and require some sort of specialized laboratory. *Malassezia furfur* does not grow on Sabouraud agar but can be grown on specialized media such as milk- or olive oil-based material incubated at 34 °C for at least 2 weeks. *Trichophyton mentagrophytes* and *Trichophyton rubrum* can be separated as follows: *Trichophyton rubrum* forms red pigment on potato agar and has a negative urease test. *Trichophyton mentagrophytes* can perforate hairs, while *Trichophyton rubrum* cannot. The L-histine test separates *Trichophyton rubrum*, which does not require the amino acid, from *Trichophyton megninii*, which does need it.

Identifying yeasts is more complicated. While *Candida albicans* is the most frequent pathogen presenting with small white smooth colonies, it can only be identified with certainty by means of the germ tube test. When yeasts are incubated in human serum for a few hours at 37 °C, only *Candida albicans* rapidly forms pseudomycelia. On rice agar, only *Candida albicans* and the almost identical *Candida stellatoidea* form thick-walled chla-

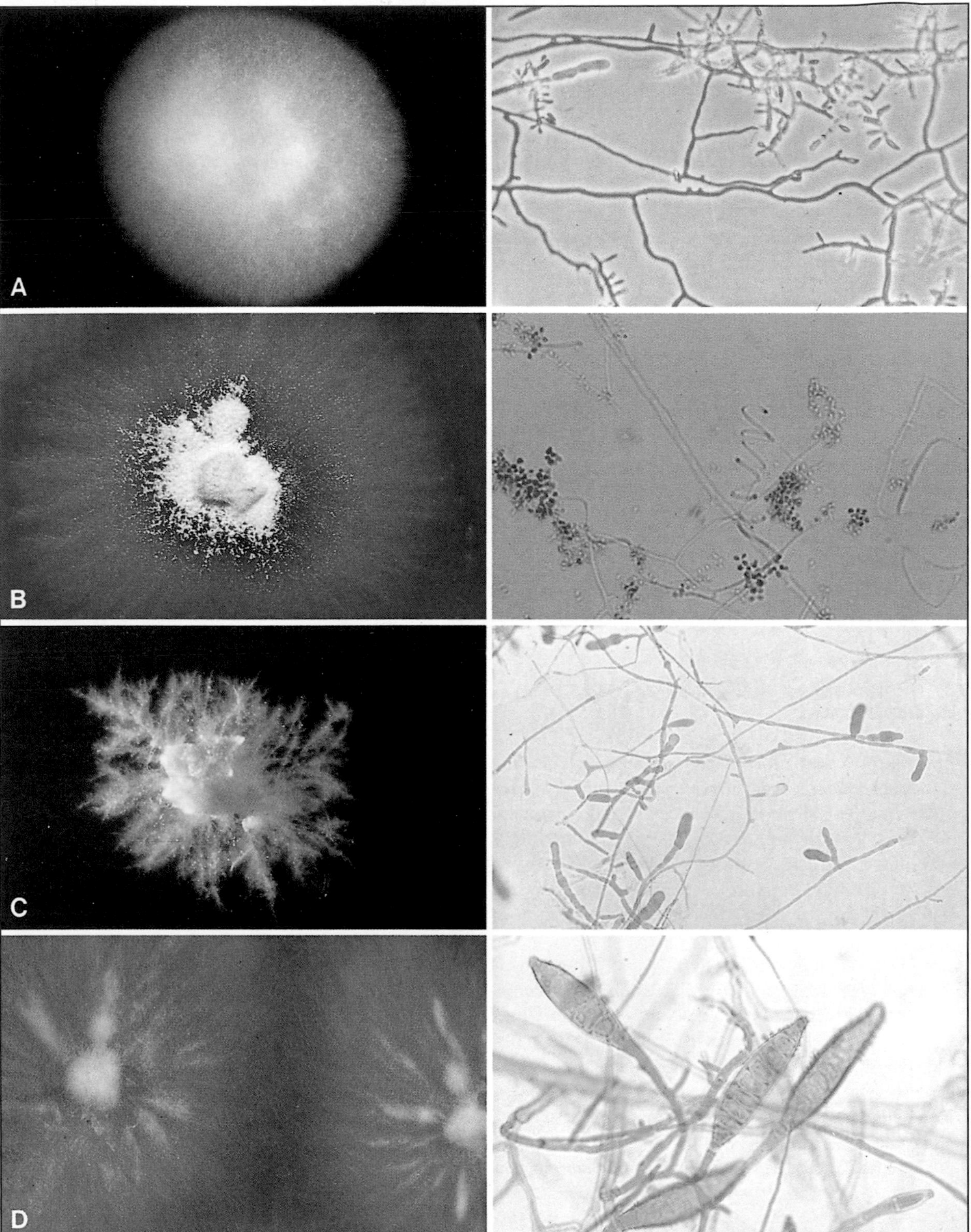

Fig. 7.1 A – D. Macroscopic and microscopic views of fungal cultures. **A** *Trichophyton rubrum*; **B** *Trichophyton mentagrophytes*; **C** *Epidermophyton floccosum*; **D** *Microsporum canis*

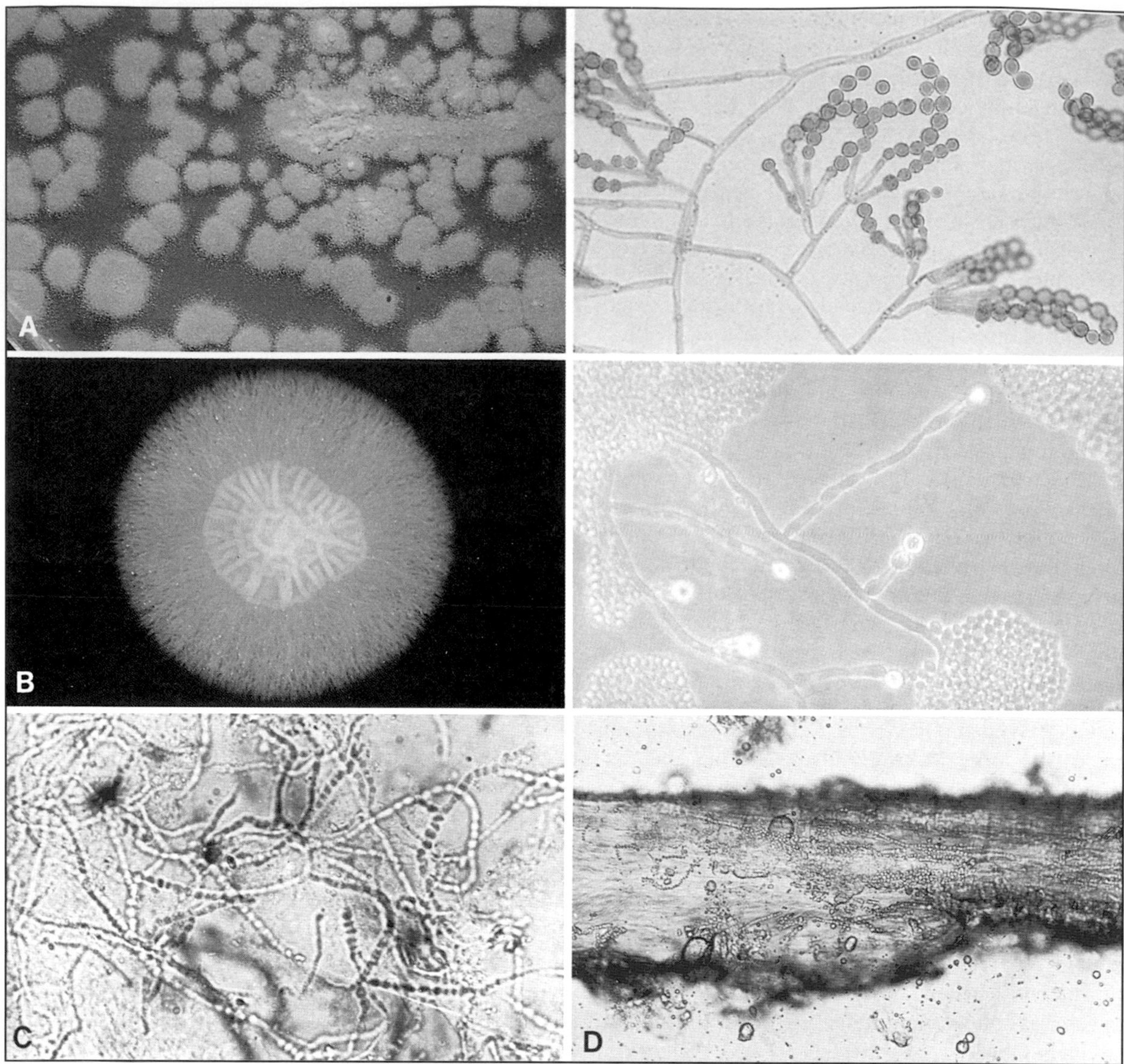

Fig. 7.2 A–D. Macroscopic and microscopic views of fungal cultures. **A** *Scopulariopsis brevicaulis* **B** *Candida albicans*. **C, D** Positive KOH examinations of scales (**C**) and hair (**D**)

mydospores. Further evaluations, including serotyping and subspeciation of *Candida albicans*, can help in epidemiologic studies.

Other Studies

Serologic studies play no role in studying dermatophytes but are needed for evaluating possible deep fungal infections including systemic candidiasis. Antifungal susceptibility can be tested just like antibiotic sensitivity. The standard disk test used for bacteria is only applicable when evaluating yeasts for flucytosine sensitivity. Otherwise more complicated procedures such as micro-dilution tests are needed. In HIV/AIDS patients or in patients who fail to respond to standard therapy, sensitivity studies are warranted. PCR studies are promising for the identification of dermatophytes. The „fingerprinting" DNA band detection method allows species and often subspecies to be characterized.

Clinical Classification

Another traditional classification of fungal infections is clinical. One can distinguish superficial, dermatophyte, yeast, subcutaneous and deep infections. There are clearly overlaps between these groups – for example, *Sporothrix schenckii* can cause both subcutaneous and deep infections – but we find them clinically useful.

Superficial Fungal Infections

The superficial infections are caused primarily by yeast forms.

Tinea Versicolor

(Eichstedt 1846)

Synonym. Pityriasis versicolor – we prefer this name since "tinea" should be reserved for dermatophyte infections.

Definition. Superficial scaly infection producing hypo- and hyperpigmentation.

Causative Organism. *Malassezia furfur*

Epidemiology. Tinea versicolor is more common in young adults than the elderly and is more often diagnosed in blacks. It is more common in tropical and humid climates, so that we see it more often in the summer months. Obesity, hyperhidrosis, occlusive clothing and inadequate hygiene also play a role.

Etiology and Pathogenesis. *Malassezia furfur* is a complicated organism. It is usually absent in newborns, but can be cultured from the nape or shoulders of a high proportion of asymptomatic individuals by 1 year of age. Exactly why it causes clinical disease in some is unclear. The organism requires lipids, just as for culture, so lipid-rich moist skin is one factor. The patient's immune status is another; in both renal transplant recipients and HIV/AIDS patients, tinea versicolor is very common.

The mechanisms of color change are also controversial. *Malassezia furfur* produces azelaic acid, which is capable of blocking melanin synthesis. Additionally, the increased thickness of the scale may have an umbrella-like effect, preventing tanning and making lesions more apparent. Darker lesions are accounted for by increased scale containing multiple organisms.

Adding to the confusion is the fact that *Malassezia furfur* and *Pityrosporum ovale* are the same organism. For historical reasons, when follicular involvement is present one uses the term pityrosporum folliculitis, but most biologists prefer the designation *Malassezia furfur*.

Clinical Findings. The sites of predilection are the nape, back and chest. The lesions spread to involve the lateral aspects of the trunk, occasionally reaching the umbilicus, thighs and upper inner aspects of the arms. Sharply bordered dirty yellow, red-brown or café-au-lait colored macules are first seen, usually only a few centimeters in diameter (Fig. 7.3). Later larger irregular patches may evolve. On other occasions, sharply defined hypopigmented macules and patches are seen (Fig. 7.4). The latter are more common in summer, supporting the concept that the surrounding skin is tanned, making them more apparent. Another explanation for the hypopigmentation is simply postinflammatory change as a lesion resolves. The term "versicolor" refers to the presence of both hyper- and hypopigmented

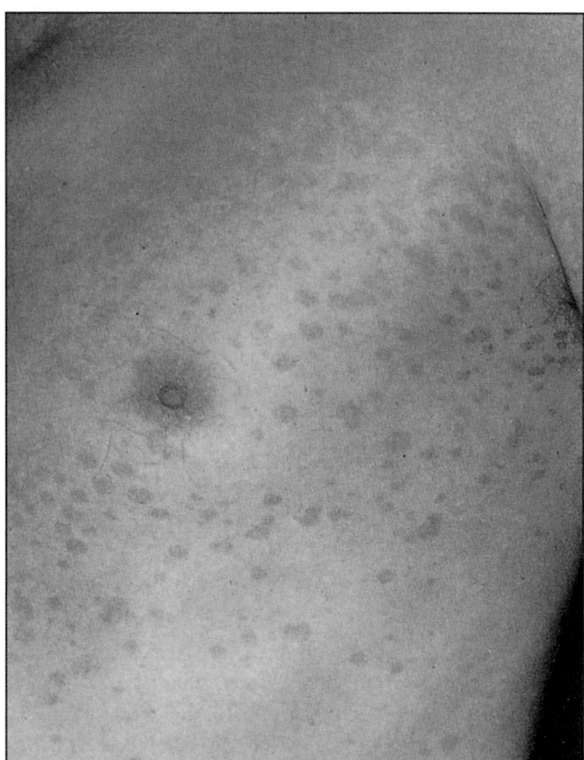

Fig. 7.3. Tinea versicolor with dark lesions

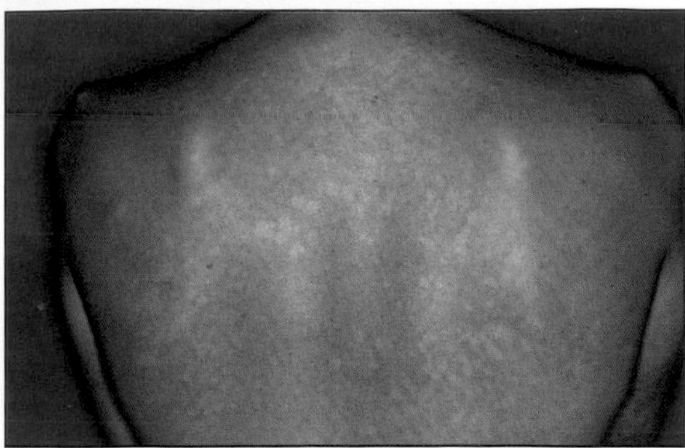

Fig. 7.4. Tinea versicolor with hypopigmented lesions

lesions. Wood light examination allows one to delineate the extent of the disease by highlighting the pigmentary changes; there is, in addition, a faint green-yellow fluorescence, but this is of little help.

Another crucial clinical feature is the presence of fine bran-like (pityriasiform) scale. If one scrapes the skin with a blade or tongue depressor, it is easy to produce the scales. This alone is almost diagnostic; other hypopigmented lesions, such as vitiligo, do not scale. The lesions are almost never pruritic and merely a cosmetic problem. Signs of inflammation are rarely seen. Patients frequently inquire whether the disease is contagious, since it is a fungal disorder. Almost everyone has *Malassezia furfur* as part of their normal flora; thus tinea versicolor is contagious only if the patient comes into contact with a rare uninfected individual.

The only situation where *Malassezia furfur* can be a true problem is in patients receiving hyperalimentation through tubes inserted in the chest region. Contamination of the lipid-containing medium either from the skin or other sources can lead to *Malassezia furfur* sepsis in immunocompromised hosts.

Histopathology. A biopsy from tinea versicolor is one of the invisible dermatoses. Usually one sees nothing, but with a fungal stain or careful study of the hematoxylin-eosin-stained stratum corneum, one can easily see multiple hyphae and spores.

Laboratory Findings. Usually the KOH is so strikingly positive that no other diagnostic investigations are carried out. Numerous short thick hyphae are seen admixed with grape-like clusters of spores. This picture, which has been described as "spaghetti and meatballs", is diagnostic for tinea versicolor. Cultures are difficult, and *Malassezia furfur* will not grow on routine Sabouraud agar.

Course and Prognosis. Recurrence is the rule. Patients should be counseled that since tinea versicolor results from the proliferation of otherwise normal flora, it is almost impossible to eradicate. Diligent personal hygiene will help keep the disease in check.

Differential Diagnosis. Postinflammatory hypopigmentation, such as pityriasis alba, and vitiligo can be excluded by the absence of scale. Hyperpigmented lesions may be confused with tinea corporis, seborrheic dermatitis and pityriasis rosea, but KOH examination usually answers the question. The most difficult diagnostic conundrum is when the patient has one or two small lesions with mild scale. Our rule is: if the lesions are on the trunk and scaly, think of tinea versicolor.

Therapy

Systemic. All of the oral imidazoles are effective. One can give itraconazole 200 mg daily for a week, or 400 mg daily for 2–3 days. We usually reserve oral therapy for cases that have failed topical therapy.

Topical. In Germany, most patients are treated with topical imidazoles, used both as a shampoo (ketoconazole or econazole) and as a body wash. It is reasonable to apply the material, work up a lather, let it sit for a few minutes and rinse. It is so difficult to be sure exactly where the disease ends that we have patients lather from their scalp to their groin. The patient should do this nightly for a week and then weekly for several weeks. Imidazole lotions such as Epi-Pevaryl PV are available in Europe; they are applied and left on overnight, then washed off in the morning. Solitary lesions are easily treated with any imidazole cream.

In the USA, shampoos containing selenium sulfide (Selsun and many others) or zinc pyrithionine (Head and Shoulders and others) are the most frequently used topical agents. They are lathered up on the involved areas, allowed to dry and then rinsed off. We follow the same regimen as with the imidazoles.

Prophylaxis. The risk of recurrence is so high that some patients prefer to simply use either an imidazole or selenium sulfide shampoo and treat their body every several weeks. Another approach is to prescribe itraconazole 200 mg to be taken every other week. In this low dose, there appear to be no side effects and recurrences are infrequent.

Pityrosporum Folliculitis

(POTTER et al. 1973)

Causative Organism. *Malassezia furfur*

Etiology and Pathogenesis. On rare occasions, especially in HIV/AIDS patients and other immunocompromised individuals, *Malassezia furfur* may infect hair follicles.

Clinical Findings. There is an acne-like eruption most often involving the back. The scattered monotonous lesions are tiny papules centered around follicles, occasionally evolving into pustules. As the lesions resolve, they heal with a brown, easily removed crust. In HIV/AIDS patients, the rash is usually very pruritic; in other patients it may be asymptomatic.

Histopathology. A biopsy reveals the diagnosis, as many *Malassezia furfur* organisms are found in an inflamed follicle or on a smear of debris.

Laboratory Findings. *Malassezia furfur* is difficult to culture under routine circumstances.

Differential Diagnosis. The differential diagnosis includes acne and acneiform lesions (Chap. 28) as well as all the forms of folliculitis (Chap. 4); the problem in HIV/AIDS patients is considered in Chapter 2.

Therapy. Topical azoles or selenium sulfide lotions or shampoos bring rapid relief. If pruritus is severe, several days of treatment with systemic azoles, such as discussed above, may bring more prompt healing. A 50 : 50 mixture of propylene glycol and water is an inexpensive maintenance therapy, applied twice weekly.

Neonatal Cephalic Pustulosis

(ARACTINGI et al. 1991)

Many babies with what has traditionally been identified as neonatal acne appear to have superficial infections with various *Malassezia* spp., most often *Malassezia sympodialis* but also *Malassezia furfur*. Onset is usually in the first few weeks of life, as colonization with *Malassezia* spp. occurs. Use of lipid-rich skin-care products may enhance the growth of these lipophilic agents. Typically a small number of pustules develop, usually on an erythematous base and not limited to follicular orifices. In rare cases there may be extensive erythema and many pustules. The predominant cell in the pustules is the neutrophil, but eosinophils are also found. Topical imidazoles bring prompt improvement.

Piedra

(BEIGEL 1865; HORTA 1911)

Synonyms. White piedra, black piedra, trichomycosis nodosa alba and nigra

Definition. Piedra is a superficial fungal infection of hairs that forms hard nodes on the hair shaft.

Causative Organisms. There are two types of piedra caused by totally unrelated organisms:

- White piedra: *Trichosporon cutaneum*, formerly *Trichosporon beigelii*
- Black piedra: *Piedraia hortae*

Trichosporon cutaneum is a yeast that forms a skin when cultured on a liquid. *Piedraia hortae* is a mold.

Epidemiology. White piedra is seen in the temperate regions of South America, Europe, Asia and the southern USA. It is relatively common in the area around Houston, Texas. Black piedra is more of a tropical disease, seen in South America, Asia and some Pacific islands.

Etiology and Pathogenesis. The mode of infection is unclear. There is probably person-to-person transmission, but also geophilic sources appear involved. In some societies, black piedra infection is allegedly encouraged.

Clinical Findings. Small firm nodules and concretions (*piedra* = stone) are attached to the hairs. In black piedra almost exclusively the scalp is involved, while in white piedra the pubic, axillary and beard hairs are more often affected. The hairs are more fragile, but there are no other symptoms. *Trichosporon cutaneum* can cause sepsis in immunosuppressed individuals; in these rare cases, there may be pustules and nodules in the skin.

Laboratory Findings. On microscopic examination, *Piedraia hortae* shows ascospores in a very organized (pseudoparenchymatous) fashion. *Trichosporon cutaneum* is softer and contains hyphae. Both fungi can be cultured on Sabouraud agar.

Differential Diagnosis. Nits, trichomycosis axillaris, hair casts, trichorrhexis nodosa and other hair shaft anomalies can all be easily excluded under the microscope.

Therapy. Shaving or cutting the hairs is probably sufficient. Some suggest treating the regrowing hairs with an imidazole lotion for several weeks.

Tinea Nigra

(Cerqueira 1891)

Definition. Superficial infection of palm or sole with dark pigmentation.

Causative Organism. *Phaeoannellomyces werneckii* (formerly *Exophiala werneckii* or *Cladosporium werneckii*)

Etiology and Pathogenesis. This mold is geophilic and dematiaceous; rarely, other fungi are involved. The infection is probably acquired from the environment, although person-to-person transmission is theoretically possible.

Clinical Findings. A sharply defined brown or black macule is found, usually on the sole but occasionally on the palm (Fig. 7.5). Scales are uncommon, and the lesion is asymptomatic; it resembles a silver nitrate stain.

Laboratory Findings. KOH examination reveals thick dark hyphae along with budding yeast cells.

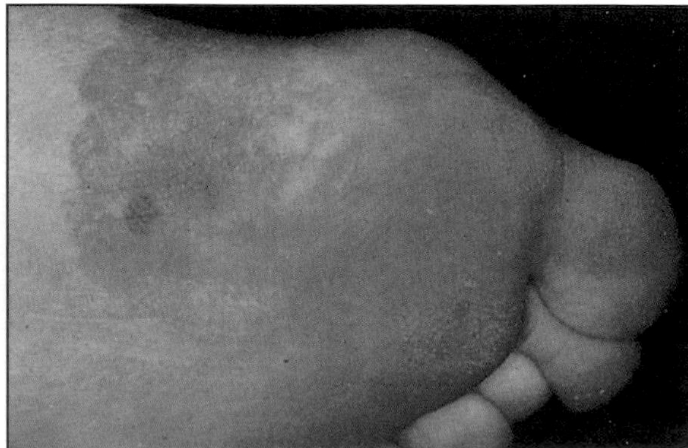

Fig. 7.5. Tinea nigra

In a biopsy specimen, the same structures are seen without special stains in the stratum corneum. They are demonstrated nicely with the methenamine silver stain.

Differential Diagnosis. The main differential diagnostic problem may be a melanocytic lesion; this is usually the reason for a biopsy.

Therapy. Topical keratolytics coupled with an imidazole and used for several weeks often bring a cure, although recurrence is not unusual. Benzimidazole has been reported as particularly effective, but few studies are available. Some recommend curettage prior to antifungal therapy.

Otomycosis

Otomycosis is a controversial condition. Many patients with seborrheic dermatitis or, less often, atopic dermatitis involving the outer ear may also have a variety of molds, usually from the genus *Aspergillus*. While otorhinolaryngologists firmly believe in primarily fungal infections of the external ear, many mycologists and dermatologists are skeptical. Even a response to imidazole creams is not convincing because they also help against seborrheic dermatitis. In the past, many patients with alleged otomycosis developed allergic contact dermatitis secondary to neomycin ear drops, but this problem has become less common.

Dermatophytoses

The dermatophyte infections can be considered either in a biologic way, considering the three genera and many species that infect humans, or in a clinical fashion. Dermatophytes also cause superficial fungal infections, but are traditionally separated. Each dermatophyte can produce a variety of clinical pictures. The English term tinea, with modifiers, is used to describe dermatophyte infections. The most common are:

- Tinea capitis (scalp)
- Tinea barbae (beard)
- Tinea faciei (face)
- Tinea corporis (trunk)
- Tinea inguinalis (groin)
- Tinea manus (hand), tinea manuum (hands)
- Tinea pedis (feet), tinea pedum (feet)
- Tinea unguis (nail), tinea unguium (nails)

Onychomycosis is a broader term than tinea unguis, as it include rare nail infections by yeasts and molds. There are several additional linguistic problems. Tinea inguinalis is often called tinea cruris but "crus" in Latin refers to the calf, not the groin. Tinea manus describes an infection of one hand; tinea manuum is correct when both hands are infected. For the feet the corresponding terms are tinea pedis and tinea pedum. For the nails, tinea unguis and tinea unguium are correct.

Epidemiology. There are about 40 species of dermatophytes, but only a few account for the vast bulk of human disease. Dermatophytes can also be classified based on their source. There are three groups:

- Anthropophilic Fungi. These fungi are acquired from other humans. They are generally well adopted to the human host and elicit little immune response. Thus, they are hard to eliminate. Examples are *Trichophyton rubrum*, *Trichophyton mentagrophytes* var. *interdigitale*, *Trichophyton schoenleinii* and *Microsporum audouinii.* (The term "var". is an abbreviation for "variety", indicating that this species has several varieties or subspecies).
- Zoophilic Fungi. These organisms are acquired from animals. Infections in a pet or farm animal are often mild or inapparent, so that the animal can be viewed as a carrier. When the fungus infects a human, it typically causes a marked inflammatory response. This intense reaction often leads to spontaneous healing. Some members of this group are *Microsporum canis*, *Trichophyton mentagrophytes* var. *mentagrophytes* and *Trichophyton verrucosum.*
- Geophilic Fungi. Much less common as causes of disease, these fungi are found in the soil or on vegetable matter. The best-known example is *Microsporum gypseum.*

Tinea pedis is probably the most common human infection, with its associated tinea inguinalis and tinea unguium. Men are far more often infected than women. Children are unlikely to get tinea pedis but most likely to have anthropophilic tinea capitis. Other species are limited to certain geographic areas, so they are relatively uncommon elsewhere, such as *Trichophyton concentricum* in the South Pacific, *Microsporum nanum* in Cuba or *Trichophyton megninii* in Sardinia and Portugal.

Etiology and Pathogenesis. Many factors determine the presence and clinical features of a fungal infection. The nature of the fungus plays a definite role. For example the *Trichophyton mentagrophytes* that caused such severe tinea pedis among US troops in Vietnam was an endemic strain, slightly different from those in the USA. In general, the more virulent a given dermatophyte, the less likely it is to have a sexual or perfect state.

The human host also plays a role – age, gender and race have been mentioned above. In addition, the immune status is important. Studies by the US Army during the Vietnam War showed a smaller fungal load was needed to establish an experimental dermatophyte infection in patients with atopic dermatitis. In addition, maceration, occlusion and minor skin trauma are also important factors in facilitating infection, as is a warm moist climate.

Once the inoculation is accomplished, the action appears to take place at the interface between the fungus and the exposed skin. The fungus must grow more rapidly than epidermal turnover rate. It also must produce a variety of enzymes capable of attacking and digesting keratin, although some studies suggest the organism prefers to spread between keratinocytes, not through them. The host response is reflected by the peripheral expanding band. Usually the growing organisms are slightly ahead of this scaly red area, where organisms are being shed and destroyed. Some patients may have dermatophytes without obvious signs of inflammation; this is known as noninflammatory tinea or tinea incognita. Prior treatment with topical antifungals or corticosteroids may also mask inflammation, producing a similar picture. While carriers are occasionally found, in most individuals there is some clinical sign of disease.

The host resistance to fungal infections is also crucial. Some aspects may be nonimmunologic. For example, changes in the free fatty acids of the scalp may cause relative resistance to *Microsporum audouinii* after puberty. Transferrin may also play a role by binding iron needed for fungal growth. The old serum inhibitory factor is probably transferrin; the relative paucity of tinea pedis in some tropical societies where people commonly go barefoot may be explained by the permanent iron-deficiency anemia introduced by parasites that produces high ferritin levels, as well as by the more important absence of occlusive shoes.

Both cellular and humoral immunity also play a role; the former is probably more important. When fungal antigens, such as trichophytin, are injected, both an acute (type I) and a late (type IV) reaction can be seen. Trichophytins are glycoproteins whose carbohydrates are responsible for the acute reaction and peptides for the delayed reaction. The trichophytin test is primarily used today to document intact cellular immunity. There is no evidence that it is associated with disease-protective immune functions. In experimental infections the trichophytin test becomes positive at about 30 days and second induced infections elicit a brisker defense response.

Laboratory Findings. The diagnostic approach will not be discussed for individual lesions. In all cases, KOH examination should be employed to rapidly identify a potential fungal infection and then culture used to accurately identify the species. If there is hair involvement, the hairs should be examined to see whether an ectothrix or endothrix infection is present. Often the yield on nails is so low with KOH examination that it helps to submit the trimmings and keratinous debris to a histology laboratory for PAS staining and tentative identification.

Tinea Capitis

Definition. Infection of the scalp by *Trichophyton* and *Microsporum* species.

There are several different types of tinea capitis, including infections acquired from other humans with a modest host response, those acquired from animals with a prominent host response, and favus, an especially chronic variant.

Epidemiology. Tinea capitis is more common in school-age children than adults. In epidemics with *Microsporum audouinii*, there are several striking features: male dominance, disappearance during puberty and, even in populations at risk, not much more than 20 % prevalence. Tinea capitis acquired from geophilic or zoophilic sources can occur in

Table 7.2. Common dermatophytes

Organism[a]	Ecology[b]	Common sites	Clinical features	Ecto/endo	Distribution
M. audouinii	A	Scalp	Noninflammatory	Ecto	Worldwide
M. canis	Z	Scalp	Inflammatory	Ecto	Worldwide
M. gypseum	G	Body	Rarely, favus		Worldwide
M. fulvum	G	Body			South America
M. ferrugineum	A	Scalp		Ecto	Africa, Asia, South America
M. nanum	Z	Body			Worldwide
T. mentagrophytes var. mentagrophytes	Z, A	Beard, feet	Inflammatory	Ecto	Worldwide
T. mentagrophytes var. *interdigitale*	A	Feet	Noninflammatory		Worldwide
T. rubrum	A	Feet, nails, groin, body	Both inflammatory and noninflammatory		Worldwide
T. verrucosum	Z	Body, beard	Inflammatory	Ecto	Worldwide
T. megninii	A	Body			Europe
T. tonsurans	A	Scalp	Black dot	Endo	Worldwide
T. violaceum	A	Scalp		Endo	Africa
T. soudanense	A	Scalp		Endo	Europe, Near East
T. schoenleinii	A	Scalp	Favus	Endo	
T. concentricum	A	Body			Pacific
E. floccosum	A	Feet, groin, axilla	Noninflammatory		Worldwide

[a] *M. Microsporum, T. Trichophyton, E. Epidermophyton*
[b] A anthropophilic, G geophilic, Z zoophilic

adult life, but is usually self-limited. In some series, blacks have been more commonly involved, especially with *Trichophyton tonsurans.*

Etiology and Pathogenesis. Virtually all *Microsporum* and *Trichophyton* spp. can cause tinea capitis, as Table 7.2 shows. *Microsporum* spp. always produce ectothrix infections, while *Trichophyton* spp. can cause both ecto- and endothrix. In an ectothrix infection, the fungi grow down along the follicle until they reach the zone of keratinization, known as the Adamson fringe. They do not invade nonkeratinized hairs. In an endothrix infection, they reproduce within the hair, weakening it so it often breaks off at the surface, sometimes producing a black dot.

Inflammatory Tinea Capitis

Inflammatory tinea capitis is usually caused by zoophilic and geophilic fungi, but sometimes there is an intense inflammatory response to an anthropophilic form. Typically there is an area of erythema and scale with local hair loss. (Fig. 7.6) Usually the border is sharply defined and inflamed. This an-nular shape with a sharp, often raised border probably led to the misleading name of "ringworm" for tinea capitis. Especially when zoophilic organisms are involved there may be pustules and deep induration, while in anthropophilic forms the inflammation tends to be less. Often there is massive destruction of the follicles, producing a boggy nodule with pustules, sinus tracts and drainage. This acute inflammatory nodule is known as a kerion (or kerion Celsi; *kerion* is the Greek word for honeycomb). It is often misdiagnosed as an acute staphylococcal infection and can be associated with lymphadenopathy. There is usually spontaneous resolution after a period of time, but often with scarring alopecia, which may also occur if treatment is not prompt.

Noninflammatory Tinea Capitis

Synonym. Epidemic tinea capitis

Both *M. audouinii* and *T. tonsurans* can appear in epidemics, spreading through schools, kindergartens and orphanages. In the epidemics in the USA in the 1950s, children were screened at school with a Wood light and parents worried about disinfecting procedures in barber shops or transmission via the seats in a bus or movie theater. In the past *M. audouinii* was the most common cause of epidemic tinea capitis in the USA. Today it is virtually extinct. *T. tonsurans* is the most common cause, while *M. canis* acquired from pets is also common. The most common source of *M. canis* is cats, not dogs.

Typically there are subtle small areas of fine scale with minimal hair loss. (Fig. 7.7) The lesions slowly expand, coalesce and cause wide areas of alopecia. Typically there are short stubby hairs amidst a scaly background with no inflammation. When *M. canis* is responsible, some erythema may be seen. As inflammation increases, there are transitions to inflammatory tinea capitis. One should search for black dots, as a clue to the presence of *T. tonsurans.*

Most *Microsporum* spp. show greenish fluorescence with a Wood light, so this examination is an effective way of screening for infection or determining whether the disease has spread away from the scalp. Individual hairs fluoresce; one must ignore the colors reflecting off the scales. A pet suspected of transmitting the disease can also be so inspected.

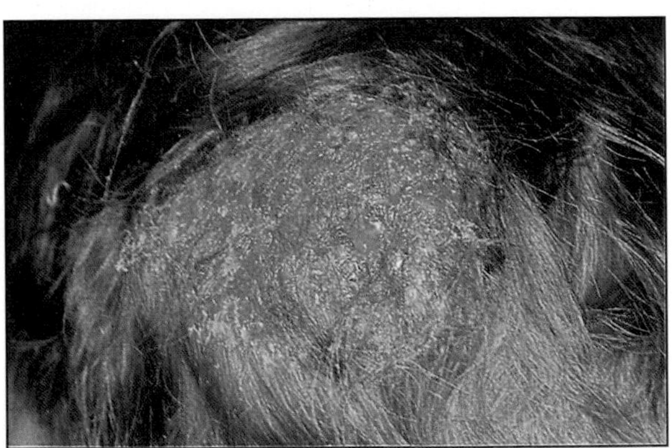

Fig. 7.6. Inflammatory tinea capitis

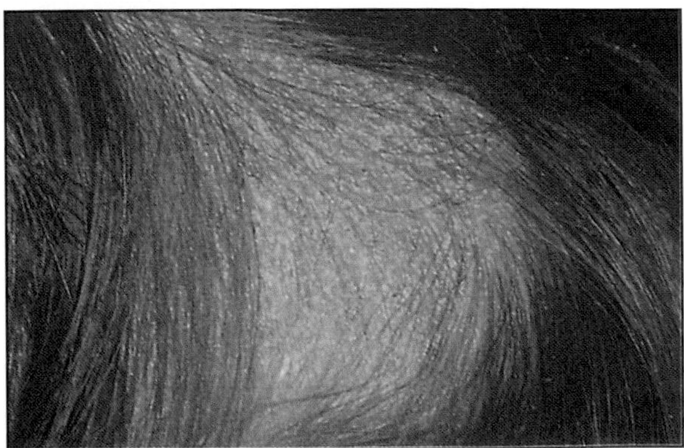

Fig. 7.7. Noninflammatory tinea capitis

Black-Dot Tinea Capitis

The main cause of black-dot tinea capitis is *T. tonsurans,* although any endothrix can produce the finding. The combination of relatively little inflammation, marked scaling (resembling seborrheic dermatitis) and multiple black dots strongly suggest *T. tonsurans* infection. The likelihood of scarring alopecia is greater than with other forms of noninflammatory tinea capitis but less than with inflammatory variants.

Favus
(Remak 1837)

Synonym. Tinea favosa

Definition. Chronic tinea capitis with large thick crusts and scarring alopecia.

Causative Organism. *Trichophyton schoenleinii*

Epidemiology. Favus is uncommon in Germany and USA. It is still endemic in parts of the Mediterranean Basin, Balkans and Near East, as well as Greenland.

Etiology and Pathogenesis. By definition favus is caused by *Trichophyton schoenleinii.* Rarely other dermatophytes will produce a similar clinical picture. Often almost all members of a family are infected. Early physicians suspected a genetic disorder. In some societies, ceremonial caps are responsible for transmission.

Clinical Findings. Children are most often affected. There is no tendency towards resolution during puberty; if untreated, the disease persists forever. Favus infections have been divided into three degrees of severity.

- In the mildest form, there is a loss of hair luster and a mild inflammation of the scalp, but no alopecia.
- In the next stage, there is more erythema and the typical scutula are present. They are small, compact, dish-like, sulfur-yellow scales and crusts; *scutulum* is Latin for little shield. The formation of each scutulum involves one or several hairs, which are then lost.
- In the most severe form, there is marked alopecia with central atrophic scarring and peripheral inflammation with scutula formation. The combination of the crusts, exudates and bacterial secondary infection produces an unpleasant odor that has been compared to the smell of mouse urine.

Occasionally, lesions on the nape and trunk are seen. Tinea unguium may be caused by *T. schoenleinii* but it is identical to that caused by other organisms.

Tinea Barbae

Causative Organisms. Zoophilic fungi, usually *T. verrucosum*

Epidemiology. Tinea barbae is a disease of males and almost always occurs in farmers, veterinarians and others with exposure to large animals. Rarely it may occur in a pet owner who sleeps with his face on an infected cat. In this latter case, the usual organism is *M. canis.* Tinea barbae caused by *T. verrucosum* is a reportable occupational dermatosis in Germany. Most cows have the fungus, so the question is simply when human contact occurs. Many young farm boys working for the first time with cattle get a scalp infection and kerion. Others have exposure later when they have terminal beard hairs.

Clinical Findings. This dermatophyte infection clinically presents as a severe deep folliculitis with erythema, nodular infiltrates, scales and pustules (Fig. 7.8). Shaving serves to spread the infection. Deep furunculoid nodules develop, still coated with pustules. The deep infectious lesions may coalesce, producing undermined confluent abscesses involving the entire anterior neck. The residual hairs are easily and painlessly plucked for diagnostic purposes. Marked regional lymphadenopathy is the

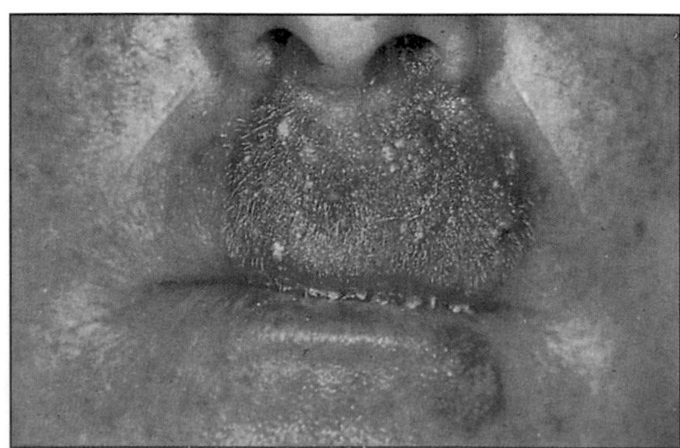

Fig. 7.8. Tinea barbae

rule. After 4–6 weeks, there is usually spontaneous resolution with a degree of immunity, as second bouts are unlikely. Scarring is much less severe than with inflammatory tinea capitis.

Differential Diagnosis. In the nineteenth century tinea barbae was known as sycosis parasitaria. "Sycosis" fancifully referred to a condition resembling figs, as the engorged grouped follicles reminded some of the inside of a fig. The hyphae of tinea barbae were easily recognized under the microscope, while the bacteria of staphylococcal folliculitis were not seen in the times before microscopic stains were available, so the latter condition was designated sycosis non parasitaria. Today the terminology is easier, but the differential diagnostic considerations the same. In addition, one must consider actinomycosis, tuberculosis (scrofuloderma), candidal folliculitis and other forms of folliculitis.

Tinea Faciei

Tinea faciei is probably the most often misdiagnosed form of tinea. The anatomy of the face occasionally prevents the development of annular or serpiginous lesions, although they are usually found (Figs. 7.9, 7.10). In addition, there are other scaly facial lesions, such as seborrheic dermatitis, atopic dermatitis, discoid lupus erythematosus and psoriasis, so that many clinicians occasionally fail to think of a dermatophyte infection when confronted with a facial rash. Tinea faciei is usually pruritic. The most striking cases of tinea faciei are produced by zoophilic fungi in patients, usually small children or women, who sleep in very close contact with their pets. In addition, tinea faciei is a typical postvacation disease in children who played with a stray cat while on holiday. While cats and dogs are the most common carriers, we have seen rashes caused by hamsters, rats and gerbils and have heard of more exotic species being responsible.

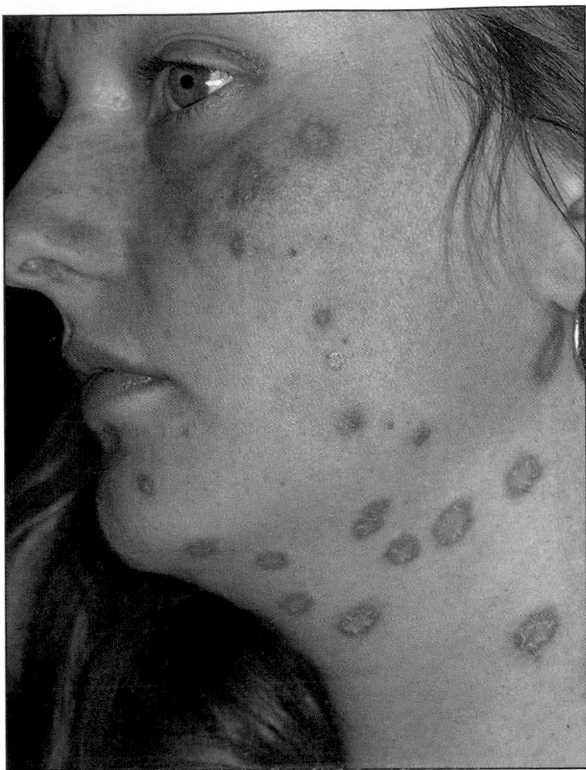

Fig. 7.9. Tinea faciei with annular lesions extending onto the neck

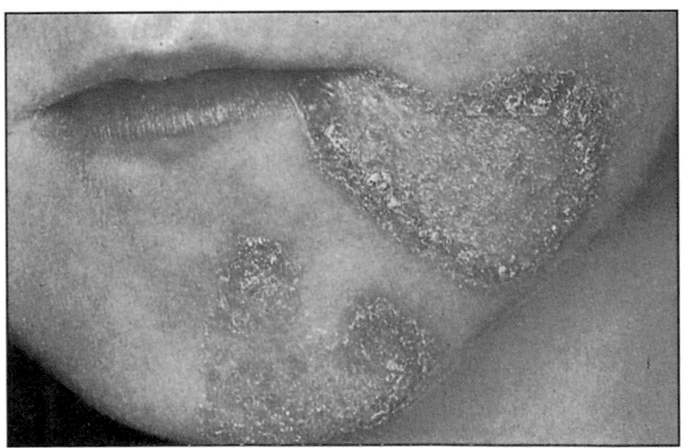

Fig. 7.10. Tinea faciei

Tinea Corporis

The classic dermatophyte infection or ringworm is tinea corporis. In most instances, the fungus is zoophilic or geophilic, acquired from pets or the soil. Anthropophilic fungi such as *T. rubrum* and *E. floccosum* can also be responsible. The typical lesion is a sharply bordered, peripherally spreading, slightly indurated patch or plaque. The border is often more red with prominent scale and pustules (Fig. 7.11). The scales are usually at the leading edge, pointing towards normal skin, whereas in pityriasis rosea they tend to point more towards the center of the lesion. In addition, the older central part of the lesion tends to resolve as the periphery advances. Pruritus is usually present. Sometimes one large lesion develops, but often there are multiple lesions that slowly spread and jump to uninvolved areas, so that with topical therapy one has

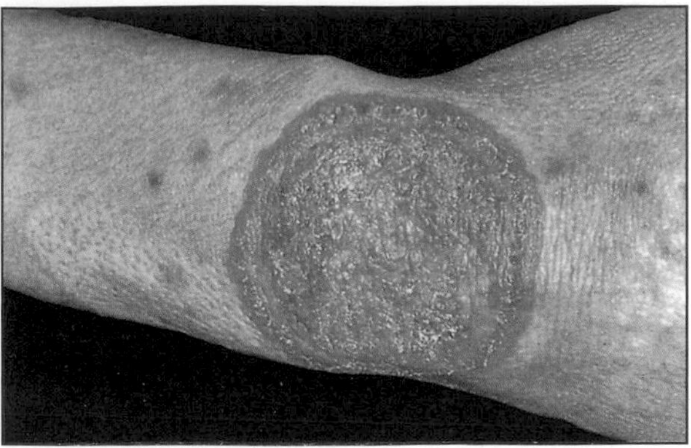

Fig. 7.11. Tinea corporis

the feeling of chasing lesions. In yet other patients, bizarre serpiginous, intersecting or confluent lesions develop, producing striking patterns.

Differential Diagnosis. The differential diagnosis of tinea corporis is endless. When a patient presents with just a target lesion of pityriasis rosea, often only the KOH examination can answer the question. If the patient reports the sudden appearance of many new lesions, the diagnosis is usually pityriasis rosea. Nummular dermatitis is also difficult to separate from tinea corporis. More chronic lesions can mimic psoriasis, seborrheic dermatitis and even mycosis fungoides. If a lesion has scales, a tinea should be excluded.

Tinea Inguinalis

Synonyms. Jock itch, eczema marginatum [Hebra]. Tinea cruris is often used but is incorrect.

Causative Organism. *Epidermophyton floccosum* most often occurs in the groin. On the other hand, if a patient has tinea pedis as well, the usual organism is *Trichophyton rubrum* or *Trichophyton mentagrophytes* var. *interdigitale.*

Epidemiology. Men are far more often affected than women, and tinea inguinalis is uncommon in children. Almost all patients have tinea pedis. The old advice "Always put your socks on before your underwear" is not a serious therapeutic recommendation but an easy way to remember the epidemiology. Thus one should check the feet of all patients with groin rashes. Person-to-person spread may occasionally occur but is much less likely than commonly thought. Finally, all the factors that lead to intertrigo, such as obesity, inadequate personal hygiene, hyperhidrosis, prolonged sitting on plastic or nonabsorbent surfaces, tight synthetic clothing and even diabetes mellitus, may play a role.

Clinical Findings. Slowly spreading erythematous patches with a scaly border are most often found on the upper inner aspects of the thighs, just where the scrotum usually touches the leg (Fig. 7.12). Scrotal involvement is relatively uncommon; occasionally the disease spreads to the perineum, perianal area and gluteal cleft. We have seen tinea inguinalis spreading out in such a perfect ring from the anus that it was diagnosed as allergic contact dermatitis to a toilet seat, although usually the eruption is asymmetric. In very rare cases other intertriginous areas, such as the axilla and submammary region, may be involved.

Differential Diagnosis. The main differential diagnostic considerations are simply intertrigo with no fungal infection, candidiasis, erythrasma, allergic contact dermatitis, inverse psoriasis and Hailey-Hailey disease. In addition, both atopic dermatitis and seborrheic dermatitis occasionally present in the groin.

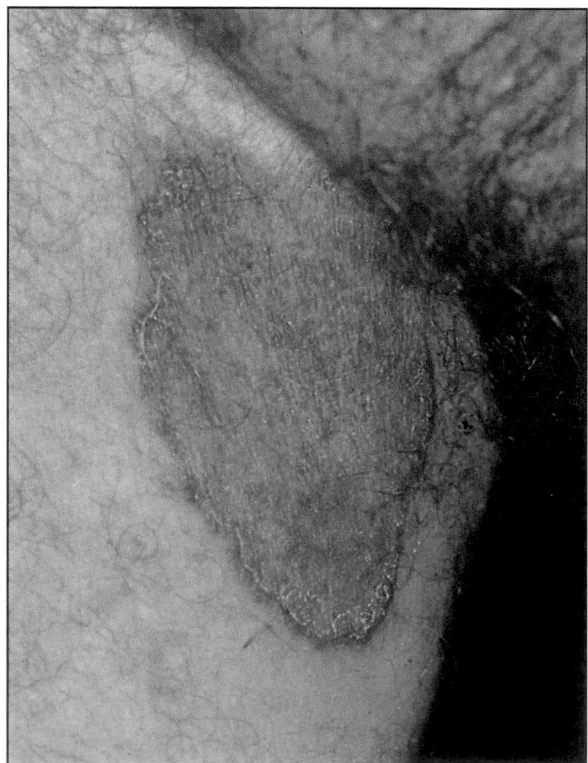

Fig. 7.12. Tinea inguinalis

Tinea Manus

Tinea manus is almost always secondary to tinea pedis. The most common organisms are *T. rubrum* and *T. mentagrophytes* var. *interdigitale*; less commonly, *E. floccosum* is found Very rarely, primary tinea manus may arise with occupational exposure to dermatophytes. Tinea manus may take many clinical forms, ranging from dyshidrotic to macerated, just as discussed under tinea pedis below. The most common variant is the hyperkeratotic form, characterized by fine, firmly adherent scale on an erythematous background, often with painful fissures (Fig. 7.13). Typically the fingertips and the metacarpal, thenar and hypothenar eminences are involved. The hands feel very dry and rough and the condition is often mistaken for a chronic wear-and-tear dermatitis. There is often nail involvement. One of the most dramatic variants of tinea manus is "one hand, two feet disease". Here patients have obvious diffuse tinea pedis, usually caused by *T. rubrum*, but with only one hand involved. The hand affected is often the dominant one, suggesting that direct inoculation is more likely onto the more active hand.

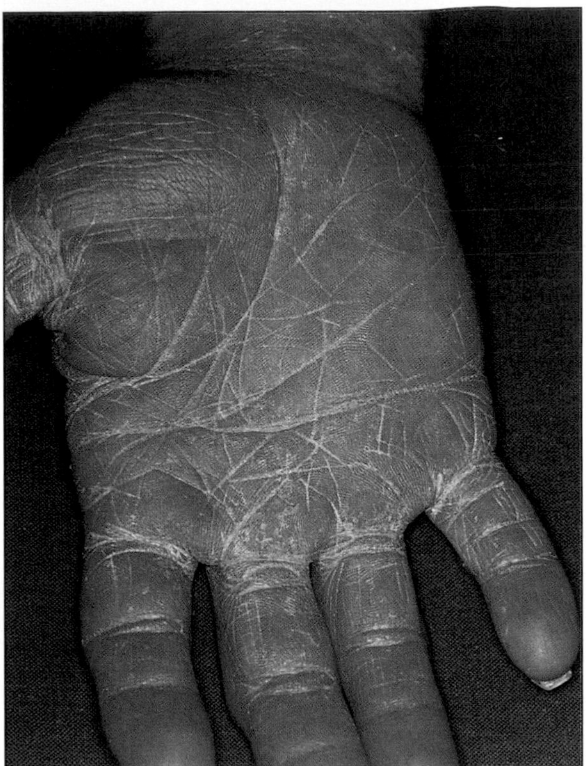

Fig. 7.13. Tinea manus

Differential Diagnosis. One must always check the feet and groin; sometimes the fungus is easier to identify there. In addition, psoriasis, dyshidrotic dermatitis, other forms of hand dermatitis and fungal id reaction should be considered. If the changes are symmetric, involving both hands, psoriasis or dermatitis is more likely, while asymmetric or unilateral changes suggest tinea. When the interdigital spaces or nail fold are involved, candidiasis is also a possibility but it does not cause hyperkeratotic lesions.

Tinea Pedis

Synonyms. Athlete's foot

Causative Organisms. The main causes are *T. rubrum, T. mentagrophytes* var. *interdigitale* and *E. floccosum*. To some extent, the fungal type correlates with the clinical forms discussed below.

Epidemiology. Tinea pedis is one of the most common diseases. In Germany, its prevalence is estimated at 15–30%. In the USA, studies in the South have shown a frequency of around 20%. Miners have shown a prevalence as high as 70%, and the problem is more common among athletes. It is also more common in warmer, moister climates.

Etiology and Pathogenesis. The spores of dermatophytes survive for months in shoes, carpets, bath mats, locker rooms and showers. The environs of hot tubs and thermal baths are often contaminated. The warm moist microenvironment in shoes, coupled with reduced hygiene, hyperhidrosis, increasing age and perhaps acrocyanosis, are predisposing factors. Using rubber sandals in community showers, carefully drying the feet, especially between the toes, and wearing clean shoes and socks are possible preventive measures. Because all the organisms are anthropophilic, once an individual contracts tinea pedis, he or she has it for a long time. Treatment brings remissions and periods when the organism cannot be cultured (called "cures" in drug studies) but eventual relapses are the rule.

Clinical Findings. Tinea pedis can present with a wide variety of clinical manifestations, which appear so dissimilar that they are often not recognized as the same disease. We identify the following types, hastening to add that overlaps are common.

- Chronic interdigital scaling
- Hyperkeratotic
- Dyshidrotic

In addition, nondermatophytes such as *Hendersonula toruloidea* and *Scytalidium hyalinum* as well as the mold *Scopulariopsis brevicaulis* may very rarely produce tinea pedis, although they more often cause onychomycosis.

Chronic Interdigital Scaling Type Tinea Pedis

Synonyms. Intertriginous type, macerated-erosive type

The most typical location is between the 3rd and 4th or the 4th and 5th toes, since these digits are usually more closely held together. Other interdigital spaces are not spared. When the toes are spread apart, one sees swollen, grayish-white skin, often with fissures (Fig. 7.14). When the area is scraped, as in doing a KOH examination, the scales come off easily, leaving behind erosions. The white scale and maceration can extend to the underside of the toes. Usually pruritus is minimal.

With marked hyperhidrosis, such as in the context of long hikes, lack of opportunity to change shoes or increased humidity, the maceration can cause marked flares with much pruritus. All of these conditions are present for infantry soldiers and for many other occupational groups. Among American troops in the Vietnam War, flares of tinea pedis were the second most common cause of disability, after actual wounds. Complicating the problem are two other factors: the ability of Gram-negative organisms to use the fungal infection as a portal and proliferate in the macerated spaces, producing a Gram-negative toe-web infection and the development of allergic contact dermatitis to traditional over-the-counter medications.

Hyperkeratotic Type Tinea Pedis

Synonym. Moccasin type

Patients with this type of tinea pedis are almost always infected with *T. rubrum* and usually have associated tinea unguium. They have dry, often thick scales typically covering the heels, the tips of the toes and the metacarpal pads (Fig. 7.15); once again, they are often unaware of a fungal infection and regard their problem as dry feet. On careful examination, as the scale turns the edge of the foot, erythema at the advancing border may be seen. Occasionally just one foot will be so extensively involved, in contrast to palmar-plantar keratoderma, which is bilateral and does not have nail involvement.

Dyshidrotic Type Tinea Pedis

Synonym. Recurrent blistering tinea pedis

In this variant, the patients are symptom free for long intervals and then experience the sudden eruption of pruritic grouped vesicles, usually on the instep (Fig. 7.16). The smaller vesicles are often cloudy or purulent and may coalesce, forming large fluid-filled blisters that eventually shed their roof, producing characteristic erosions with scale and erythema at the edge. The roof of such a blister is an

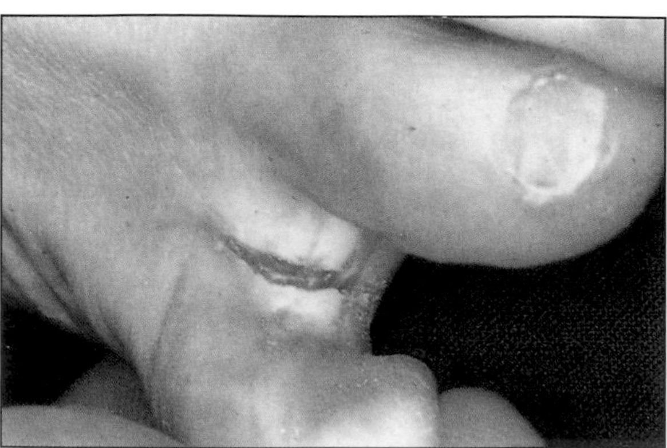

Fig. 7.14. Tinea pedis, chronic interdigital scaling type

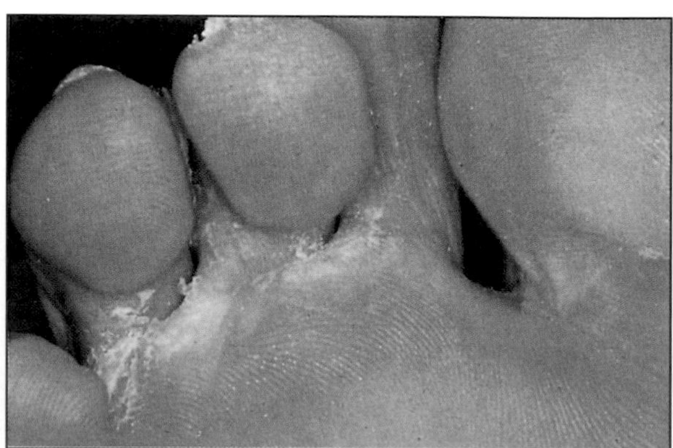

Fig. 7.15. Tinea pedis, hyperkeratotic type

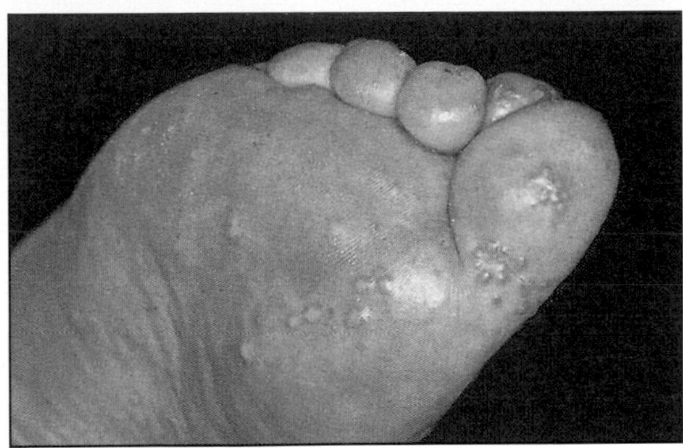

Fig. 7.16. Tinea pedis, dyshidrotic type

ideal specimen for a KOH examination. Typically recurrences come in the spring or summer, at least vaguely related to heat and humidity. In the USA this clinical pattern is almost invariably associated with *T. mentagrophytes* var. *interdigitale*.

Course and Prognosis. Tinea pedis is a chronic problem, no matter which clinical form is seen. The dyshidrotic form is recurrent, while the other two are persistent. There are several interesting variations. One hand, two foot disease is mentioned above. Another phenomenon involving the hands and less often the feet is the fungal id reaction, discussed below. Other complications include the Gram-negative toe-web infection and, more importantly, recurrent erysipelas, as the interdigital erosions serve as an entry site for bacteria. Post-bypass cellulitis, arising in the skin around a donor site for cardiac bypass surgery, is invariably associated with chronic tinea pedis.

Differential Diagnosis. The differential diagnosis varies with the clinical presentation. The interdigital type resembles simple intertrigo and occasionally candidiasis; gram-negative toe-web infection is usually a complication but can arise independently of tinea pedis. The hyperkeratotic type is usually confused with xerosis or palmar-plantar keratoderma when not inflamed; when the underlying skin is erythematous, then psoriasis, dermatitis, juvenile plantar dermatosis and lichen planus come into question. The dyshidrotic form must be distinguished from dyshidrotic dermatitis and pustular psoriasis of the palms and soles.

Tinea Unguium

Synonym. Onychomycosis (but this term also includes nondermatophyte fungal infections of the nails). We prefer the plural tinea unguium, as a single nail is rarely infected (tinea unguis).

Causative Organisms. *T. rubrum* is the most usual cause, but *T. mentagrophytes* var. *interdigitale* and *E. floccosum* are also common. Among the nondermatophytes, the yeasts *Candida albicans, Candida tropicalis, Hendersonula toruloidea* and *Scytalidium hyalinum*, as well as *Scopulariopsis brevicaulis, Onychocola canadenis* and other molds, may be responsible but usually represent contamination.

Epidemiology. Over 99% of onychomycoses are associated with a dermatophyte infection. Tinea unguium represents about 30% of all dermatophyte infections and accounts for 18–40% of all nail disorders.

Etiology and Pathogenesis. Initially there is tinea pedis, and perhaps tinea manus. The risk of tinea unguium is one reason to treat tinea pedis aggressively. The fungi grow under the nail plate, whether at the nail fold or distally, and eventually involve the nail bed. Impaired circulation, neuropathies, immune abnormalities and diabetes mellitus all predispose to tinea unguium. While it is rare to have involvement of the fingernails without the toenails, some occupational exposures may lead to this situation . For example, bakers often contract a candidal onychomycosis as the persistent exposure to water and sweet "nutrient" solutions facilitates infection, beginning as candidal paronychia but later involving the nail.

Clinical Findings. Toenails are far more likely to be involved than fingernails. When the hands are involved, always check the feet, for they too will almost certainly have fungus. Initially solitary nails are involved; later, many may be infected, but often one or more stay disease free. Traditionally several different types of tinea unguium are clinically identified.

Distal Subungual Onychomycosis. This is the most familiar and common form of tinea unguium. All of the organisms listed above can be responsible. The fungi reach the nail distally or laterally and slowly grow proximally to involve the nail bed and nail matrix. Initially there is a distal subungual proliferation that leads to nail-bed separation

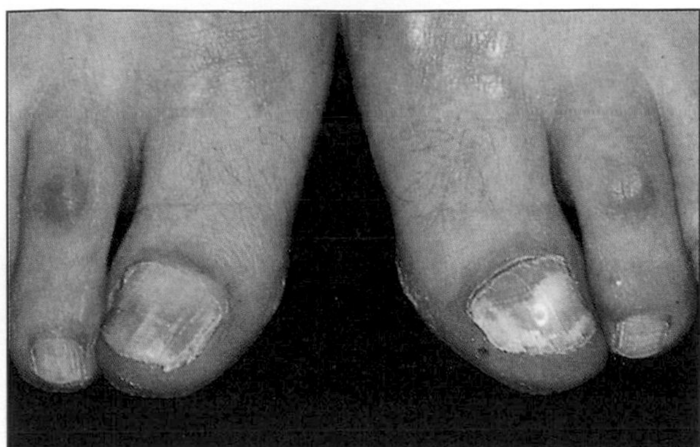

Fig. 7.17. Onychomycosis caused by *Trichophyton rubrum*

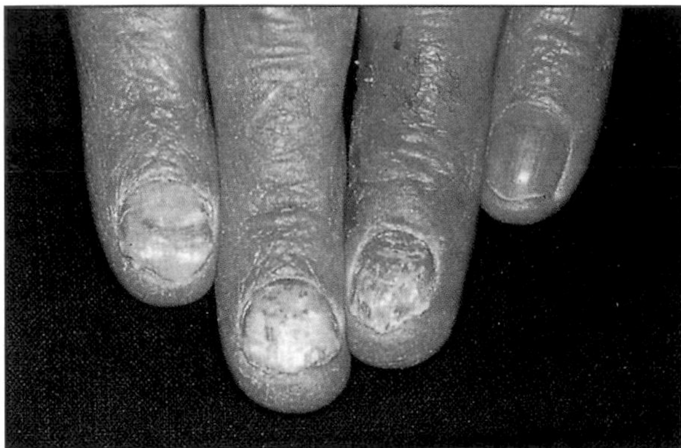

Fig. 7.18. Onychomycosis with marked dystrophy, caused by *Trichophyton rubrum*

(distal or semilunar onycholysis) and discoloration (Fig. 7.17). The fungi usually produce a dirty yellow color; when bacterial superinfection occurs, a dirty brown to green (*Pseudomonas aeruginosa*) color may develop. Nail dystrophy may also result (Fig. 7.18).

Proximal Subungual Onychomycosis. Only *Trichophyton* spp. have been proven to cause this variant. They penetrate the proximal nail fold and produce a white crumbly nail just at the nail fold. While this is the least common type of tinea unguium, it is much more frequent in HIV/AIDS patients. Initially the matrix is damaged so that nail growth is impaired. Later the nail is shed but regrowth is hampered.

White Superficial Onychomycosis. These changes are only seen on the toenails and usually caused by *T. mentagrophytes* var. *interdigitale* but also other *Trichophyton* spp. and some molds. There are small discrete white patches on the nail, easily overlooked, that are friable but can be scraped away, revealing a solid nail underneath. They may coalesce to form larger lesions.

Dystrophic Onychomycosis. In patients with chronic mucocutaneous candidiasis, there is often extensive nail destruction, producing thickened discolored crumbly nails. The entire nail is invaded by yeasts. *Candida albicans* is almost always responsible. A related problem is the presence of candidal paronychia with secondary nail unit damage. Once again, *Candida albicans* is the usual culprit but other *Candida* species, such as *C. tropicalis* and *C. parapsilosis*, have been identified. The lateral nail fold is usually swollen and red; often pus can be obtained by gentle squeezing and used for culture. When a paronychia is present, a dermatophyte infection alone is unlikely.

Dermatophytoma. Occasionally a ball of densely clumped hyphae may develop under the nail. Because it appears analogous to the balls of *Aspergillus* spp. that can arise in the lung, this change has been dubbed a dermatophytoma. A white, either linear or circular area is seen. When the nail is removed, the dense mass of organisms is found. Dermatophytomas may be responsible for some therapeutic failures, as the penetration of drugs into these masses appears inadequate for killing.

Unusual Causes of Onychomycosis. Several agents discussed later in this chapter occasionally cause nail disease. *Scopulariopsis brevicaulis* has been clearly shown to invade nail plate, often producing a cinnamon coloration. *Fusarium* spp. cause a superficial white onychomycosis. *Hendersonula toruloidea* and the perhaps related *Scytalidium hyalinum* cause dry or noninflammatory tinea pedis or manus, often with onychomycosis. None of these nondermatophytes respond to the imidazoles so they present treatment problems.

Differential Diagnosis. Someone once simplified this issue saying only three things can happen to a nail: "Trauma, psoriasis and fungal infection." While the true list is a little longer, including lichen planus, 20-nail dystrophy and perhaps nail damage secondary to other inflammatory dermatoses, one must exclude psoriasis and trauma. Neither is easy; psoriasis often co-exists with onychomycosis, that is, a psoriatic nail is easily infected with fungus, as is a damaged nail.

Granuloma Trichophyticum
(Majocchi 1883)

Synonym. Nodular granulomatous perifolliculitis of the legs, *Tinea der Unterschenkel* (German: tinea of the shins), Majocchi granuloma (incorrect, because Majocchi did not describe leg lesions).

Causative Organism. Usually *T. rubrum*

Etiology and Pathogenesis. When fungi are introduced into hair follicles, there may be a deep granulomatous inflammatory response to the infected structure. The fungi do not invade the dermis; they are confined to the keratin of the hairs in the lower two-thirds of the follicle. When the follicle ruptures, just as in any case of folliculitis, the follicular content released into the dermis triggers an immune response.

In Europe one distinguishes between the most common setting on the shins and appearance of the disease elsewhere as originally described by Majocchi. On the legs, the problem is much more common in women who have tinea pedis or tinea unguium and shave their legs, so shaving trauma has been blamed. In other sites, occlusion, topical corticosteroids, trauma and many other factors may play a role.

Clinical Findings. Red-brown papules and nodules are found, arranged in a follicular pattern and often penetrated by a hair. Sometimes the papules are grouped; in other instances, they coalesce into a plaque. Pustules are uncommon. At the edge of the lesion, scale can be seen. The most typical site is the shins in women who have follicular keratoses and acrocyanosis or even follicular pernio. Almost every patient has tinea pedis and tinea unguium. Lesions away from the shins are found more commonly in young adults who, once again, have a dermatophyte infection elsewhere. In the later setting, frequently a zoophilic fungus is involved, perhaps eliciting even more of an inflammatory response. The axillae, buttocks, groin and extremities are typical sites, suggesting that trauma and maceration play a role.

Histopathology. Often a biopsy is needed to confirm the diagnosis. Fungal elements are seen not only in the stratum corneum and hair shaft, but also in the granulomatous inflammatory response around the follicle. In the rare cases where the follicle is still intact, no hyphae are found in the dermis.

Laboratory Findings. One should attempt to grow the fungus from the hairs and scales, but because of the depth of the infection and the inflammatory response, sometimes results are negative.

Differential Diagnosis. All forms of persistent folliculitis should be considered. In addition, follicular dermatitis and follicular psoriasis may appear similar on the shins.

Fungal Id Reaction

A fungal id reaction is defined as a distant skin manifestation of an established fungal infection in which the lesions are "allergic", not infectious. The most typical setting is in association with tinea pedis. Sometimes when tinea pedis is flaring, the patient will simultaneously develop a dyshidrotic reaction with pruritic blisters on both the hands and feet. If KOH examination of the blister roof and culture are negative, then one can diagnose an id reaction. Both tinea pedis and dyshidrotic dermatitis are common, and they may occur simultaneously without a clear immunologic connetion.

The rarest fungal id reaction is lichen trichophyticus. Here one identifies small, pale red, pointed, grouped follicular papules on the trunk (Fig. 7.19). The differential diagnostic considerations include lichen planus, lichen syphiliticus and lichen scrofulosorum.

In all instances, the diagnosis of id reaction can be made only if there is a clear-cut fungal infection elsewhere, which is usually inflamed or flaring, suggesting a systemic immunologic antifungal reaction. Sometimes an id reaction develops when systemic antifungal therapy is initiated.

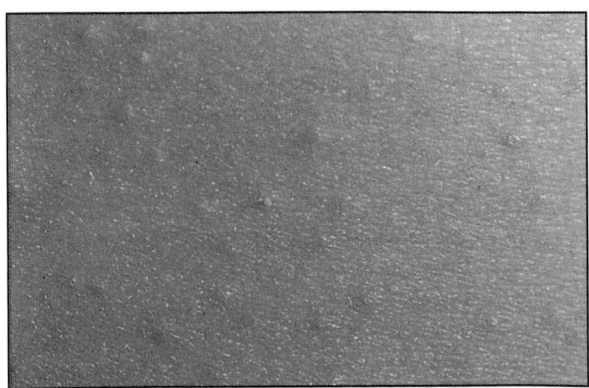

Fig. 7.19. Lichen trichophyticus

Tinea Imbricata

Synonym. Tokelau

Causative Organism. *Trichophyton concentricum*

Tinea imbricata is primarily limited to the islands of the Pacific Ocean, although the organism is also found in Malaysia, Ceylon, India, the Amazon Basin and elsewhere. Early explorers to the Pacific were fascinated by the presence of large concentric scaly rings that cover large areas of the body in decorative designs. Sometimes the scales are quite large; *imbricata* is Latin for tiled. The disease usually starts in childhood. The households are heavily contaminated by the organism, so that transmission mimics autosomal dominant inheritance. *T. concentricum* can also produce more ordinary dermatophyte lesions, but spares the hair and nails.

Therapy

Dermatophyte infections are so common and there are so many opportunities for therapy that this section contains more detail than most corresponding sections. Table 7.3 summarizes the many different antimycotic agents in use today. While often topical antifungal therapy is initiated as a therapeutic trial, at the latest before systemic therapy is started a culture-proven diagnosis should be available. If an apparent dermatophyte infection fails to response to antimycotic treatment, one should consider the remote possibility of a resistant strain or of a non-dermatophyte infection such as *Hendersonula toruloidea* or *Scytalidium hyalinum*. The usual explanation is a failure to follow the therapeutic regimen correctly. When treating zoophilic or geophilic fungal infections, one must bear in mind the likelihood of a spontaneous remission.

Systemic. A number of antifungal agents are available. The old standby griseofulvin has been supplanted in recent years first by ketoconazole, and then by fluconazole, itraconazole and terbinafine. Griseofulvin is effective only against dermatophytes, while the other agents have much broader spectra. The main indication for oral therapy is onychomycosis; other indications are widespread tinea corporis or tinea pedis where topical therapy has failed or is likely to fail. The official indications for the various agents cause a great deal of confusion, for different pharmaceutical firms have pursued different strategies in obtaining approval for their products. In general, griseofulvin is not

Table 7.3. Major antimycotic drugs

Class	Examples	Indications	Route	Form
Benzofuranes	Griseofulvin	Dermatophyte infections, especially in children; not onychomycosis	Oral	Tablet, suspension
Benzimidazoles	Ketoconazole	Tinea versicolor	Oral	Capsule
	Many others (Table 7.4)	All types of dermatophyte infections, tinea versicolor, candidiasis, seborrheic dermatitis,	Topical	Cream, solution, shampoo, vaginal tablet, troche, powder
Triazoles	Itraconazole	Onychomycosis, other dermatophyte infections	Oral	Capsule
	Fluconazole	Oral and vaginal candidiasis, dermatophyte infections	Oral	Capsule
Hydroxypyridones	Ciclopiroxol-amine	Dermatophyte infections	Topical	Cream, solution, powder
	Ciclopirox	Onychomycosis	Topical	Nail polish
Allylamines	Terbinafine	Dermatophyte infections Onychomycosis	Topical Oral	Cream Tablet
	Naftifine	Dermatophyte infections	Topical	Cream, gel
Morpholines	Amorolfine	Onychomycosis	Topical	Nail polish

as effective against tinea unguium as the newer agents, while ketoconazole has been widely replaced by equally effective agents with less hepatotoxicity. The other products are quite comparable and will be considered below.

The following rough guidelines can be used for duration of therapy and manner of administration, considering the three modern, almost equally effective agents: fluconazole, itraconazole and terbinafine. Tinea corporis and its variants require the shortest duration of therapy; 2–4 weeks of oral therapy usually suffices. When hairs are involved, a slightly longer period may be desirable, such as 4–6 weeks. When nails are infected, then longer-term therapy is needed. All three agents are stored to some extent in the growing nail, so daily usage for 3–6 months can be employed or interval therapy, where a higher dosage is taken at weekly intervals or for 1 week a month for 3–4 months. Significant differences between the various regimens are not generally recognized, so the physician's choice of agent should be based on compliance and cost. While griseofulvin is generally accepted as safe for children, the newer agents have obtained varying degrees of approval. Package inserts or other recent information should be consulted prior to prescribing systemic antifungals for children, and the parents should be carefully counseled.

An issue in treating dermatophyte infections is what defines a cure. The pharmaceutical companies and optimistic physicians define a cure as clinical improvement and a negative KOH and culture at a time 1–3 months after treatment. If one is dealing with an infection of the glabrous skin with no hair or nail involvement, this may be reasonable. Hair infections are somewhat more smoldering, but the real problem starts when talking about cures for tinea unguium. In our experience, if one waits a year after the patient has fulfilled the objective requirements for a cure, the chance of finding dermatophytes again is good. Companies may speak optimistically of 70–90% cure rates, when in reality the number is much lower, perhaps around 50%. In many instances it is difficult to decide in routine clinical practice whether one is confronted by recurrence or reinfection. Molecular biologic typing of dermatophytes may answer this important question. Retreatment is always possible and may sometimes involve a shorter course than the initial regimen.

Griseofulvin. The first oral antifungal agent, griseofulvin is derived from *Penicillium* molds. It inhibits fungal reproduction by blocking DNA synthesis, albeit in a poorly understood fashion. It is best absorbed with a fatty meal and at least partially reaches the skin through sweat – the "sprinkler effect". Griseofulvin is not stored in keratin, must be taken for long periods of time (up to 18 months for tinea unguium of the toenails) and is not very effective. For all these reasons, it has been replaced by newer medications. Some still recommend it for treating tinea capitis in children because of its excellent safety record in this setting and the lack of extensive data on use of the newer agents in children. It can also be used for tinea corporis and tinea pedis, but should not be used for tinea unguium.

In general, griseofulvin is a very safe drug. The main problems are hepatic toxicity, gastrointestinal bleeding, leukopenia and granulocytopenia. Thus hepatic and hematologic parameters should be monitored before and during treatment. Another concern is drug interactions. Griseofulvin blocks the effect of coumarin anticoagulants. In addition, it interferes with female hormone metabolism, leading to menstrual irregularities and perhaps even interfering with oral contraceptives. The latter is important because griseofulvin is not recommended in pregnancy. In addition, because it is metabolized in the liver, it should be avoided in patients with hepatic disease, especially acute intermittent porphyria and other hepatic porphyrias. It may cause flares of preexisting or subclinical lupus erythematosus, as well as photosensitivity, urticaria and other hypersensitivity reactions.

Griseofulvin is absorbed much better with high-fat meals. The ultramicrosize form, often on a polyethylene glycol matrix, is better absorbed. Initially patients may have gastrointestinal distress or headaches, but these tend to decrease in severity with continued use. The usual daily dosages are 500–1000 mg of the microsize form or 330–660 mg of the ultramicrosize form. There is a pediatric liquid microsize form; here the daily dosage is 10–15 mg/kg.

Ketoconazole. Ketoconazole is an imidazole that inhibits ergosterol synthesis in the fungal cell membrane. Fluconazole and itraconazole are in the same family. The target enzyme is a cytochrome P450-dependent 14-α-demethylase in the fungal microsomes. In high dosages it has an endocrinologic effect, as suggested by its use for advanced prostate cancer and Cushing syndrome. Ketoconazole is still recommended for some deep fungal infections, but is usually avoided for dermatophyte infections because of its side-effect profile.

The major risks are hepatotoxicity, hemolytic anemia, thrombocytopenia and leukopenia. About 1 in 10,000 users shows clinically apparent hepatitis. As with all the azoles, ketoconazole is not approved for use in pregnancy. Some patients may develop gynecomastia. Ketoconazole cannot be used with astemizole or terfenadine because of increased antihistamine levels and risk of cardiac arrhythmias. It increases the availability of coumarin, methylprednisolone, cyclosporine and several other agents. Since its uptake decreases when the gastric pH is increased, it is hampered by antacids and H2-blockers. Anyone prescribing ketoconazole should carefully check the entire list of cross-reactions and monitor the patient's hepatic and hematologic status. The usual dose for dermatophyte infections is 200 mg daily; for deep fungal infections, 400 mg is standard.

Itraconazole. Yet another inhibitor of ergosterol synthesis, itraconazole has a broad spectrum of action and a good safety profile. It is extensively used in deep fungal infections but is also approved for a variety of dermatophyte infections. While it causes the same problems as the other imidazoles, adverse events are extremely rare. It probably is the agent of choice for patients with hepatic problems who require systemic antifungal therapy. All the drug interactions discussed above for ketoconazole can occur with itraconazole and this is the main factor limiting the product's use. The drug is not recommended for use during pregnancy or in nursing mothers.

The usual dosage is 100 mg daily for 2–4 weeks for glabrous skin infections. For tinea unguium, the most extensive experience exists with a regimen involving 200 mg b.i.d. for 1 week, then a 3-week drug rest; three to four such cycles are recommended, depending on the clinical response. Involved toenails require longer-term therapy than fingernails.

Fluconazole. This agent works by the same mechanism as ketoconazole, inhibiting ergosterol synthesis in the cell membrane. It is not to be used in pregnancy and has the same list of side effects as ketoconazole but a much better safety record. Possible problems include hepatotoxicity, thrombocytopenia and leukocytopenia, as well as seizures. Drug interactions also occur but are more limited; coumarin's action is enhanced, as is that of tacrolimus and phenytoin.

Fluconazole has been used extensively for candidiasis, especially HIV/AIDS-related oropharyngitis and esophagitis, where it has been employed both for treatment and long-term prophylaxis. It is also available for one-shot therapy of vaginal candidiasis, as it is more effective and quicker than topical measures. It is used in bone marrow transplantation patients to prevent candidiasis. While the manufacturers first concentrated on obtaining approval for yeast infections, fluconazole is an effective antidermatophyte agent. It may be used in a daily dosage of 50–100 mg for 2–8 weeks, depending on the type of tinea, or in a once-weekly dosage of 150–300 mg for 3–4 months. In systemic candidiasis much higher dosages, up to 200–400 mg daily, are employed.

Terbinafine. A synthetic allylamine derivative, terbinafine causes the accumulation of squalene within cells, blocking sterol synthesis in a slightly different manner. Its spectrum is limited to dermatophytes and *Candida albicans*. Side effects are minimal; liver function should be monitored, and patients with preexisting liver disease should not be treated. Several instances of toxic epidermal necrolysis have been reported. Occasional patients report taste disturbances that are usually reversible. Flares of systemic lupus erythematosus have also been described after starting terbinafine. Drug interactions with rifampin, cimetidine and, to a lesser extent, with cytochrome P450-metabolized medications may occur. The drug probably can be used during pregnancy, but it is recommended to wait until the pregnancy is over before treating a dermatophyte infection or onychomycosis.

The usual dosage is 250 mg daily. Skin infections can be treated for 2–4 weeks. For nail infections, the usual recommendation is 250 mg daily for 6 weeks for fingernails, and 3–6 months (or longer) for toenails. Intermittent schemes are sometimes used, but are not officially endorsed.

Two other agents are not used for dermatophyte infections but for deep or systemic fungal infections. They are placed here for convenience and should not be confused with the above agents. Anyone using either of these toxic drugs should carefully acquaint themselves with the recommendations of the manufacturers and infectious disease experts.

Amphotericin B. This polyene damages sterols in the fungal cell membrane; a new form, amphotericin B lipid complex (ABLC), may have less nephrotoxicity. After administration of a test dose of 1 mg, therapy is usually started with 0.25 mg/kg daily administered over 6 h. The dosage is slowly increased in 0.25-mg increments to 1.0 mg/kg daily, occasionally going as high as 1.5 mg/kg. ABLC is given differently, 5.0 mg/kg over 2 h. Neither formulation penetrates the blood-brain barrier well; therefore, in many situations weekly intrathecal administration is needed. A variety of pretreatment medication schemes, including acetaminophen, antihistamines and antiemetics, should be considered. Major complications include the risk of permanent renal damage, especially if the total dose exceeds 5.0 g. Hematologic toxicity, cardiac arrhythmias and acute liver toxicity complete the list of major side effects.

Flucytosine. This fluorinated pyrimidine product interferes with the fungal DNA and RNA synthesis. It is recommended for systemic candidiasis, cryptococcosis and chromomycosis. It is rarely used as a single agent, but usually combined with amphotericin B. The oral dose is 50–150 mg/kg daily, depending on renal status. The toxicity is considerable, including renal failure, cardiac arrest, gastrointestinal hemorrhage and hematologic problems.

Topical. The number of topical agents is almost unlimited. In general topical therapy is sufficient for self-limited disease such as tinea corporis from a zoophilic species. It is unlikely to produce long-term cures in anthropophilic infections such as interdigital tinea pedis but often can effectively control the problem. Particular attention should be paid to the vehicle. Many products are available in several forms. Creams are usually most acceptable, but gels may perhaps allow better penetration and can be used if the skin is not broken. Solutions and pump sprays are more convenient for wider areas and interdigital use. When there is nail or hair involvement, topical therapy should be replaced, with rare exceptions, by systemic measures.

Older Products. All of these agents are available without a prescription in the USA.

- Whitfield Ointment. Before specific antifungal agents became available, keratolytics were used to remove the stratum corneum, in which the dermatophytes grow. The prototype of this family is Whitfield ointment, containing 12% benzoic acid and 6% salicylic acid. It is often irritating and the benzoic acid may cause allergic contact dermatitis. Nonetheless, Whitfield ointment is extremely inexpensive and an effective adjunct for hyperkeratotic infections. It may also be useful for superficial nondermatophyte onychomycosis.
- Undecylenic Acid. This fatty acid, as well as other fatty acids and their salts, is incorporated into a number of older over-the-counter preparations that are inexpensive and effective against simple infections of glabrous skin. The best-known such product in the USA is Desenex.
- Tolnaftate. Available widely as Tinactin and under other names, this is a modestly effective agent against dermatophytes only. It is also offered in combination with an absorbent powder.

These two compounds still require a prescription but are not widely used today.

- Amphotericin B. A major drug for systemic fungal infections, amphotericin B is effective topically against *Candida albicans* and dermatophyte infections.
- Haloprogin. This synthetic iodinated trichlorophenyl ether is effective against dermatophytes as well as *Candida albicans* and many bacteria. It is a good choice for toe-web infections.

Imidazoles. Table 7.4 shows the many different azoles available. All work in the same way by inhibiting ergosterol synthesis in the fungal cell wall. The main differences lie in the vehicles and costs. Many of the products are available over the counter in various countries. Some are approved for once-daily use, but it is unclear whether this is clinically relevant. Often it is cheaper to use a less expensive product twice daily.

Newer Agents

- Allylamines. Two members of this family, naftitine and terbinafine, are available for topical use. They have a narrower spectrum of action than

Table 7.4. Topical imidazole antifungal agents

Bifonazole	Miconazole
Clotrimazole	Omoconazole
Croconazole	Oxiconazole
Econazole	Sertaconazole
Fenticonazole	Sulconazole
Isoconazole	Tioconazole
Ketoconazole	

the imidazoles, reaching primarily dermatophytes. Topical terbinafine used once daily for a week to treat tinea pedis compares favorably with imidazoles.
- Hydroxypyridones. Ciclopiroxolamine 1% cream or solution is also effective against dermatophytes. In vitro it is also active against both gram-positive and gram-negative bacteria.
- Morpholines. Amorolfine has a spectrum similar to the imidazoles.

Special Products. Two nail polishes (or varnishes) containing 8% ciclopirox and 5% amorolfine respectively are available. These products are designed to be applied two to three times weekly. They may be effective for minor nail involvement, but in most cases serve to hold the infection in check rather than effecting a cure. Several combination products incorporating a corticosteroid and an effective antifungal agent are available in both Europe and the USA. These products are perhaps useful for the early treatment of an inflammatory exudative dermatophyte infection. After a week, one can use the antifungal alone. Unfortunately, such combination products are usually used in two other settings: diaper dermatitis, where the corticosteroid is often too strong, and situations were the clinician is not sure whether a dermatitis or a dermatophytosis is present, as in intertrigo. If we feel both antiinflammatory and antifungal actions are required, we tend to prescribe two separate products.

Other Measures. Surgical removal of infected nails was formerly quite popular. While patients still inquire about the procedure, it has fallen out of favor because of pain, likelihood of permanent matrix damage and resultant dystrophic nails and frequent reinfection. A less traumatic approach is the use of concentrated urea pastes. A 40% commercial product is available in Germany, or the following formula can be employed:

Urea nail paste

Urea	40.0
Thick liquid paraffin	15.0
White petrolatum	20.0
Bleached wax	5.0
Wool wax	20.0

Usually a quantity of 20–50 g is needed. The patient is instructed to protect the surrounding skin with zinc paste and the apply the urea paste under an occlusive dressing. We usually leave the dressing on for 48 h. The nail can then be cleaned, débrided and the process repeated. After 4–6 weeks, the diseased nail plate has been painlessly removed. In one formula, 1% bifonazole is added. While this approach may be preferable to surgery, it still is very laborious and time-consuming. Any attempt at removing a portion of the nail should be combined with systemic antifungal therapy if at all feasible. Nail removal is often the only treatment when the infection is caused by one of the unusual organisms not susceptible to imidazoles.

Yeasts

The main pathogenic yeast is *Candida albicans*. As mentioned above, several yeasts are traditionally grouped with the fungi causing superficial disease, namely *Malassezia furfur* and *Trichosporon cutaneum*. *Torulopsis* and *Rhodotorula* spp. are occasionally identified but rarely have clinical significance. The yeasts are sensitive to azoles and polyene antimycotic agents, such as amphotericin B and nystatin.

Candidiasis

Synonyms. Candidosis, moniliasis, thrush. Candidosis is actually the preferred term, as the ending "-iasis" has been designated for use with protozoan or helminthic infections. Nonetheless, candidiasis remains the most widely used term in the USA. Moniliasis, an ancient term, is totally incorrect, as *Monilia* is an entirely different fungus, used by Lederburg and Tatum in their Nobel prize studies because its linear arrangement of eight ascospores allows easy determination of recombination. It causes no human disease.

Definition. Infection with *Candida albicans*, usually involving moist areas with occlusion.

Causative Organism. *Candida albicans*

Epidemiology. *Candida albicans* is the most important member of its genus. Other species are discussed below. It is so common that epidemiology is a difficult topic. Little information is available. Virtually every individual in the world experiences at least one episode of clinically apparent candidal disease in his or her lifetime. Studies of females have shown this to be true with regard to candidal vaginitis.

Etiology and Pathogenesis. *Candida albicans* may be part of the normal flora of the oral cavity, gastrointestinal tract and external genitalia. Therefore it is often a problem to decide when it is a pathogen. Identification on culture in these sites does not suffice. Sometimes conversion to a pseudomycelial form is taken as suggestive. Thus, demonstration of pseudomycelia in a biopsy specimen obtained from the esophagus is as important as a positive culture. Quantifying the *Candida albicans* found in mouth washings, stool or other materials may also help. Finally, clinicopathologic correlation is essential; if erythema and other signs of inflammation are present, the organism is more likely to be playing a pathogenic role. Away from the mucosa and orifices, the identification of *Candida albicans* by culture strongly suggests an abnormal situation. The yeast's presence in the blood usually means sepsis.

Candidiasis has been described in German as an illness of the ill (*Krankheit der Kranken*). Those who are immunosuppressed, have diabetes mellitus, local factors that create a warm, moist milieu (obesity, diapers, incontinence, confinement to bed, drooling, poorly fitting dentures and many more) or even inherited inability to handle the yeast tend to suffer more. Oral contraceptives and pregnancy both are associated with greater susceptibility to candidiasis. Systemic antibiotics can lead to candidiasis by altering the fine system of checks and balances among the normal flora. Oral corticosteroids also predispose to candidal infections, perhaps by altering the glucose mechanism as well as inhibiting T cells. Virtually every HIV/AIDS patient has clinically significant oral or esophageal candidal infection at some point. Patients with a damaged epidermal barrier, such as those with atopic dermatitis, are at risk for colonization by *Candida albicans*, especially when treated with corticosteroids.

In both Germany and America, systemic candidiasis has become a fashionable diagnosis among those searching for an answer from practitioners of ecologic medicine. Individuals with depression, fatigue, palpitations and an endless list of complaints are told they have candidiasis and are given long and complicated treatment schemes. A patient who really has systemic candidiasis, i.e., candidal sepsis, is almost invariably immunosuppressed, extremely ill and will die if not treated. Patients who have positive yeast cultures from their mucosal surfaces, stool or other sources but are without appropriate symptoms or signs probably do not have significant disease.

Clinical Findings

Oral Candidiasis. As discussed in Chapter 33, *Candida albicans* is commonly found in the oropharynx. Everyone is familiar with the association of the yeast with white, cheesy easily removable plaques; this is known as thrush and is familiar to almost all lay people. One should bear in mind that candidal infections in the mouth can have many forms.

- Acute pseudomembranous candidiasis or thrush (Fig. 7.20).
- Chronic atrophic candidiasis, often under a denture.
- Chronic hyperplastic candidiasis with a single fixed plaque, falling into the clinical spectrum of leukoplakia.
- Acute atrophic candidiasis, including erosive candidiasis in immunosuppressed patients, some cases of gingivitis (especially in HIV/AIDS patients) and median rhomboid glossitis.
- Angular cheilitis or perlèche, common in children and those who drool, whether from a stroke or poorly fitting dentures. In children streptococcal infections may also cause perlèche.

Genital Candidiasis. Almost every women has at least one attack of vaginal candidiasis in her lifetime (Chap. 35). It is estimated that 30% of pregnancies feature candidiasis. In the case of recurrent infections, transfer from the perianal region may play a role. A diffuse scaling erythema may involve the external genitalia, spreading onto the inner aspects of the thighs. Men are less often affected (Chap. 34). In uncircumcised patients, especially older individuals, candidal balanitis is a frequent problem (Fig. 7.21), but more distant spread is uncommon.

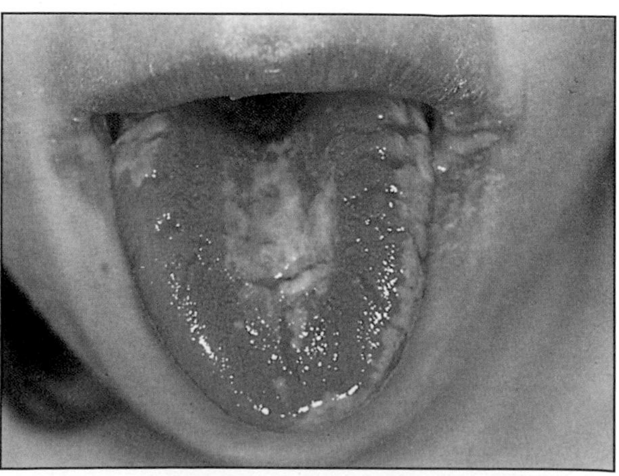

Fig. 7.20. Candidal glossitis and angular cheilitis

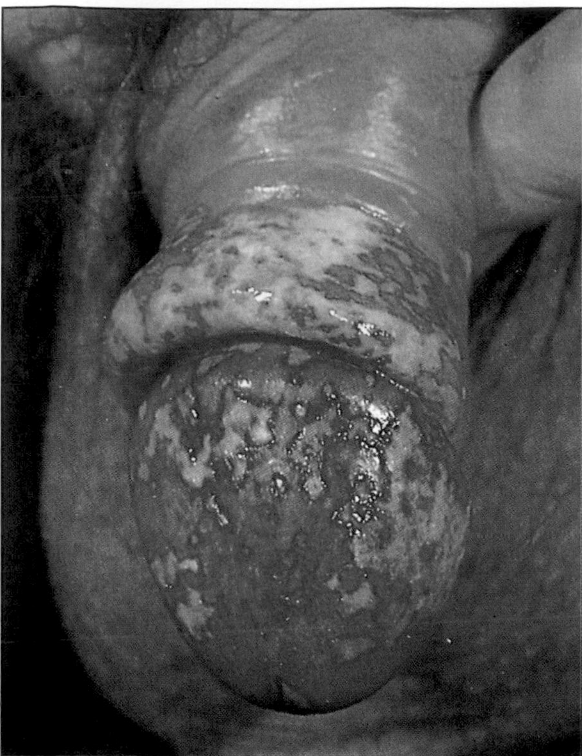

Fig. 7.21. Candidal balanitis

Interdigital Candidiasis. Also known as erosio interdigitalis blastomycetica, this uncommon type of candidal infection has a definite localization. It is almost always seen between the middle and ring fingers or the corresponding toes (Fig. 7.22). One explanation is that this web space is the least mobile in most patients, so that retention of sweat, soap and water leads to an irritation and then secondary infection with *Candida albicans*. Where the organism comes from is a mystery; one can suggest contact with the mouth or perianal region, but how does this explain the process on the feet? Typically there is an painful erosion surrounded by swollen macerated tissue.

Candidal Intertrigo. Intertriginous lesions are often secondarily infected by *Candida albicans* (Chap. 12). Typical sites include the groin, axillae and beneath the breasts (Fig. 7.23). A good clinical clue is the presence of satellite pustules at the periphery of the lesion, just beyond the typical erythema and light collarette scales.

Diaper Candidiasis. Many cases of diaper dermatitis (Chap. 12) are complicated by secondary infection with *Candida albicans* (Fig. 7.24). In infants, there is clearly transfer from the stools coupled with irritation and maceration. The same features are seen in incontinent elderly patients.

Candidal Paronychia. Candida albicans can cause painful, pus-laden infections of the nail fold and nail bed. An acute candidal paronychia is difficult to separate from a bacterial infection. Mixed infections involving *Candida albicans* and bacteria such as *Pseudomonas* spp. frequently occur. Often there is chronic damage to the cuticle, either through manipulation or persistent exposure to moisture. The periungual tissue is scaly, red, swollen and tender to pressure (Fig. 7.25). On manipulation, pus may ooze from the proximal or lateral nail fold. When *Candida albicans* causes onychomycosis, it is usually secondary to a chronic paronychia. More often there is a nail dystrophy, with transverse ridging, rather than nail invasion by the organisms. Occasional other candidal species may be identified.

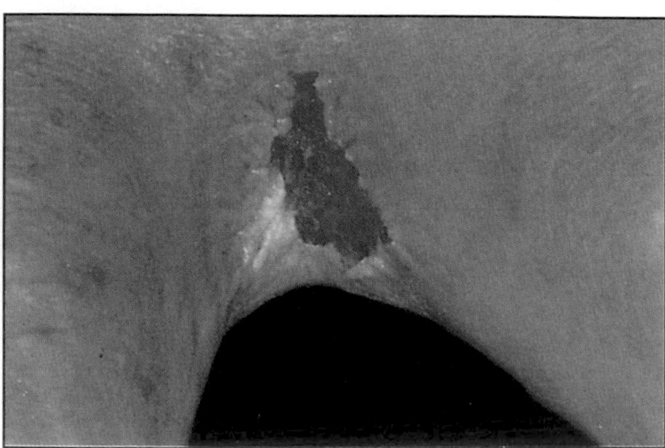

Fig. 7.22. Interdigital candidiasis

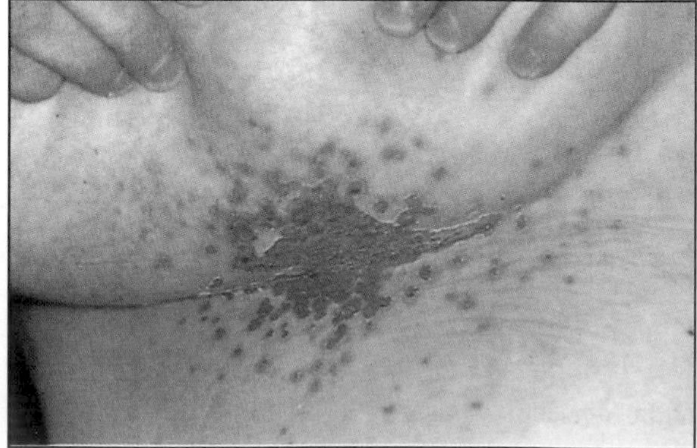

Fig. 7.23. Candidal intertrigo

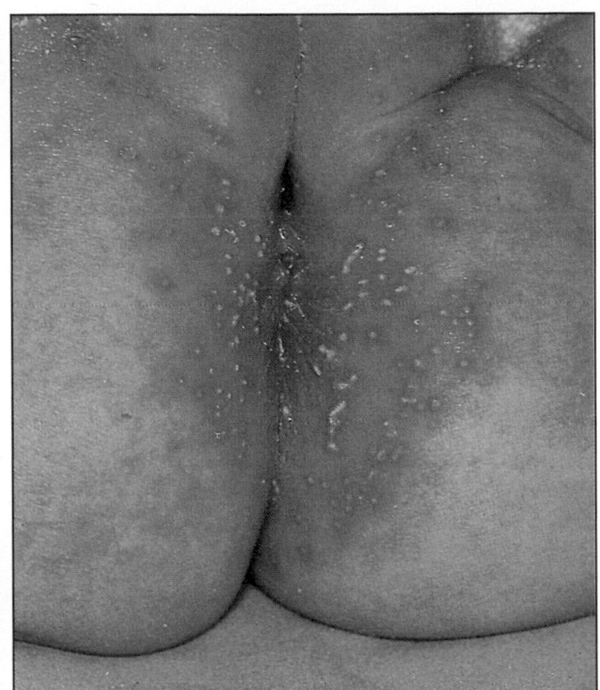

Fig. 7.24. Candidal diaper dermatitis in an infant

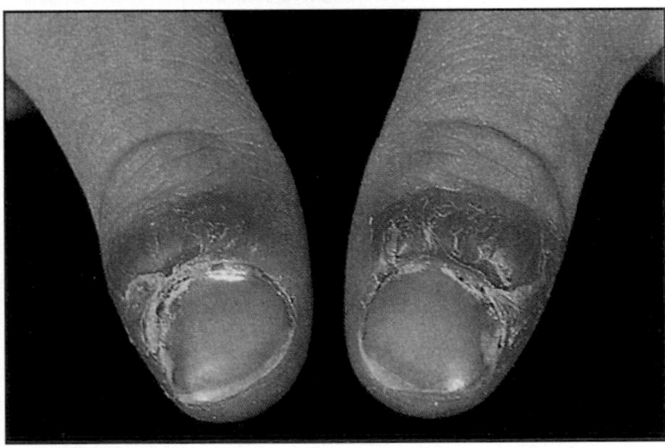

Fig. 7.25. Chronic candidal paronychia

Candidal Folliculitis. In rare circumstances, *Candida albicans* may cause folliculitis. The usual patient is an adult man with some degree of immunosuppression and involvement of the beard area. There may be pustules, crusts or deeper nodules around the hairs.

Candidal Esophagitis. This problem is almost entirely restricted to HIV/AIDS patients and is discussed in Chap. 2.

Neonatal Candidiasis. Several types of neonatal candidiasis may occur:

Congenital Candidiasis. This form occurs within a few hours of birth and represents intrauterine infection. The tiny patients have numerous small erythematous papules and pustules. In low-birth-weight infants, the risk of systemic disease is considerable, but most do well. Involvement of the palms and soles is typical, but the diaper area is usually spared. The evaluation of a newborn suspected of systemic disease is complex and should be carried out by specialists in neonatal infectious diseases. The differential diagnosis of the skin lesions includes all the other forms of neonatal pustular disease, including staphylococcal pustulosis, herpes simplex and syphilis but also the far less serious erythema toxicum and neonatal pustular melanosis.

Diffuse Neonatal Candidiasis. These patients develop papules, pustules and collarette scale several days after birth, representing a superficial infection acquired in the vaginal canal. They almost always do well.

Common Candidal Infections. Newborns may also have candidal infections of the mouth, usually thrush, or the diaper area.

Candidemia. Systemic candidiasis may develop in immunosuppressed patients, especially those with indwelling catheters, hyperalimentation and extensive antibiotic therapy. The patients present with sepsis but are hard to diagnose. Occasionally the skin may be the site of entry. In addition, tiny pink macules and papules, sometimes evolving into pustules, may be present. A biopsy specimen from such a lesion may reveal pseudomycelia, providing the most rapid diagnosis. More dramatic lesions may occur later in the disease course, including larger necrotic areas resembling ecthyma gangrenosum and even purpura fulminans. Systemic candidiasis should always be considered in the differential diagnosis of catheter-associated sepsis.

Histopathology. Biopsies are seldom done, but the presence of pseudomycelia in tissue suggests *Candida albicans* is pathogenic. The finding of a number of spores on an epithelial surface is less clear. An example of this is oral hairy leukoplakia, where candidal spores can be seen but the true pathogen is Epstein-Barr virus.

Laboratory Findings. *Candida albicans* can be readily identified on culture. One should use Sabouraud dextrose agar or a similar medium, incubate at 37 °C and check after 24–48 h. The smooth white colonies, usually less than 5 mm in diameter, are easily recognized. Microscopically, one sees blastospores, usually grouped in a cluster like grapes. If the blastospores become elongated and are arranged to resemble a chain, then one has a pseudomycelium. Chlamydospores are larger structures with a thicker wall that are almost specific for *Candida albicans*. Other candidal species are usually identified on the basis of fermentation tests.

Quantification of organisms in stool cultures can be helpful. In one system, 10^3 yeast cells per gram of stool is normal, 10^4–10^5 requires control and re-evaluation and 10^6 or more suggests significant infection.

Course and Prognosis. Most often candidal infections are chronic. One must pay particular attention to eliminating or ameliorating the predisposing factors.

Differential Diagnosis. The differential diagnosis varies with the location and is discussed in detail in other chapters.

Therapy. The mainstays of therapy are reducing moisture, where possible, and addressing predisposing factors.

Systemic. Fluconazole is the most widely used systemic anticandidal agent. It can be administered in a single dosage of 150 mg for vaginal candidiasis. It is also used in dosages of 50–100 mg daily for 7–14 days for oral candidiasis. Patients with nail bed involvement do better with oral therapy; if the nail itself is affected, they should be treated just like patients with tinea unguium. In addition, fluconazole is a mainstay of candidal prophylaxis in immunosuppressed patients and is often administered lifelong in HIV/AIDS patients to control candidal esophagitis. Other imidazoles can also be used, but fluconazole has the best safety record. Fluconazole resistance is a major concern in HIV/AIDS patients. If it is suspected, then antimycotic susceptibility testing should be performed.

Nystatin is an old polyene antimycotic agent. It is available as oral rinses, troches and pills. The medication is eliminated almost unchanged in the stool, so it cannot be used for internal treatment. It is often employed in dosages of 500,000–1,000,000 units t.i.d. for 7–10 days to treat apparent bowel infections. This is harmless and may be a way to help patients with positive stool cultures at significant levels with perianal or genital disease where contamination appears likely.

The agent of choice for candidemia is usually amphotericin B. In selected cases of catheter-related candidemia without evidence for severe disease, an imidazole may also be employed.

Topical. The azole creams, lotions and sprays discussed under dermatophytes are most widely used. Nystatin is effective topically and comes in a variety of forms including creams, ointments, pastes and powders. It is also combined with 1.0% hydrocortisone in some countries to treat diaper dermatitis. The various dyes, such as gentian violet, are less effective and if used at all should be prescribed at very low concentrations (0.1–0.5%) in an aqueous base. Otherwise there is a risk of cutaneous necrosis in intertriginous areas. Both azoles and nystatin are also available as troches and rinsing solutions for treating oral lesions.

Chronic Mucocutaneous Candidiasis

Definition. Persistent often granulomatous candidal infection of skin and mucosa in patients with immunodeficiency.

Epidemiology. Chronic mucocutaneous candidiasis is extremely rare. It is not one disease but several. In addition the clinical finding of persistent granulomatous candidal infections is seen in many other immunodeficiency states, such as selective immunoglobulin A (IgA) deficiency.

Etiology and Pathogenesis. There may be acquired or inherited defects in cellular or humoral immunity, occasionally associated with endocrine disease. While there is no standard classification of chronic mucocutaneous candidiasis, the following suffices.

- Chronic mucocutaneous candidiasis with endocrinopathy is inherited in an autosomal recessive pattern. Patients have early onset of chronic mucocutaneous candidiasis and may also have vitiligo and alopecia totalis. The cutaneous changes usually precede the endocrine diseases and run an independent course. The most common associated conditions are hypoparathyroidism and Addison disease.
- Chronic mucocutaneous candidiasis without endocrinopathy is another autosomal recessive disorder. The patients have mucocutaneous problems and may have low iron stores.

- Chronic mucocutaneous candidiasis with dermatophytosis may be the same as the above syndrome. Some patients have overlapping *Candida albicans* and, usually, *Trichophyton rubrum* infections.
- Chronic diffuse mucocutaneous candidiasis is a third distinct syndrome inherited in an autosomal recessive pattern. These patients are most likely to have chronic nail involvement and the serpiginous lesions described below. They also tend to have persistent mucosal granulomas and may have recurrent respiratory infections.
- Chronic localized mucocutaneous candidiasis is a sporadic disorder of childhood in which oral candidal granulomas and recurrent pulmonary infections are seen.
- Chronic mucocutaneous candidiasis with thymoma is the most common type of acquired disease in adults. Onset is usually in the third decade; mucocutaneous signs usually appear first. Associated problems may include myasthenia gravis, aplastic anemia and other hematologic disorders. In rare cases, systemic lupus erythematosus has been found.

Clinical Findings. Several clinical features should suggest chronic mucocutaneous candidiasis. Patients have therapy-resistant candidiasis in many sites. Probably oral thrush and vaginal candidiasis are most common. One clue is ocular involvement which is rare in all other forms of the disease. Typically there is a blepharitis (Fig. 7.26). Another feature is the presence of widespread erythematous inflammatory hyperkeratotic annular or serpiginous plaques of the skin, resembling a severe tinea corporis. *Candida albicans* infections are uncommon on glabrous skin in normal hosts.

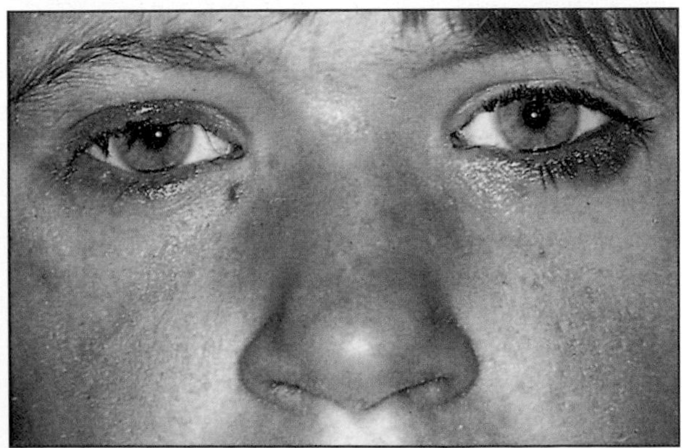

Fig. 7.26. Chronic mucocutaneous candidiasis with lid involvement

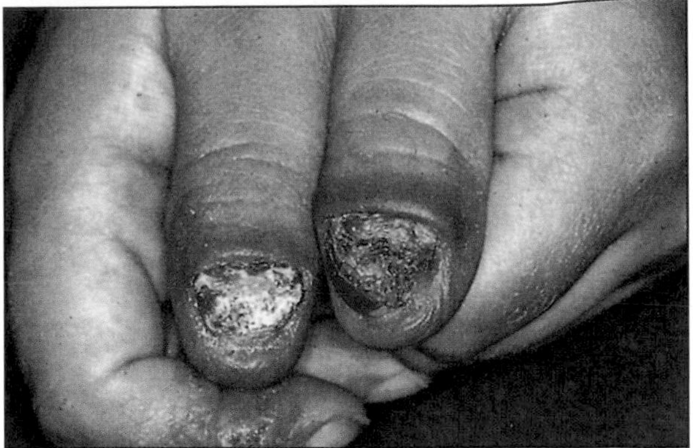

Fig. 7.27. Chronic mucocutaneous candidiasis with destructive paronychia

Typical sites in these immunosuppressed individuals are the flexural folds, face, scalp and hands. Nodular lesions may also develop; they have been called candidal granulomas. Finally, persistent paronychia and destructive nail lesions are seen (Fig. 7.27).

Histopathology. In the hyperkeratotic or psoriasiform lesions, hyphae and spores of *Candida albicans* are easily identified in the crusts and scales. A granulomatous response to *Candida albicans* is most unusual but may be seen in the nodular lesions. Often the organisms are sparse.

Laboratory Findings. Culture is useful for making the final diagnosis. There are no specific laboratory tests to confirm the diagnosis of the underlying disorder, but one should search for possible associated conditions.

Course and Prognosis. The course is chronic and sometimes fatal. It obviously depends on which subtype is present, the severity of the immunodeficiency and the nature of any associated disease.

Differential Diagnosis. In most instances, the diagnosis of chronic mucocutaneous candidiasis is straightforward, once it is considered. The hyperkeratotic lesions can often be mistaken for tinea corporis or psoriasis. The granulomatous nodules are puzzling but almost never present alone.

Therapy. The mainstay of therapy is long-term or even life-long oral treatment with an imidazole. While the most extensive experience has been accumulated with ketoconazole, there is no reason to think that the less toxic fluconazole is any less effective. In this special case, candidal susceptibility testing against the various imidazoles may be appropriate. As soon as therapy is stopped, the infections recur.

Other Yeast Infections

The other *Candida* species occasionally act as pathogens, as do other yeasts. Nonetheless, well over 90% of all candidal infections are caused by *Candida albicans*. Other members of the group can cause a variety of chronic cutaneous and systemic problems.

- *Candida tropicalis*. Systemic infections, especially in immunosuppressed patients, as well as nail disease and vaginitis.
- *Candida parapsilosis*. Nail disease, otitis externa and systemic infections.
- *Candida krusei*. Vaginitis, systemic infections.
- *Candida stellatoidea*. Vaginitis, systemic infections.
- *Candida glabrata (Torulopsis glabrata)*. Vaginitis, stomatitis, esophagitis, systemic infections, especially of the urinary tract.
- *Candida dubliniensis*. Stomatitis.
- *Rhodotorula rubra* and other species. Occasionally identified in catheter-associated infections, but their role as cutaneous pathogen remains unclear. Usually considered contaminants in cultures from skin and mucosal surfaces.

Subcutaneous Mycoses

Sporotrichosis

(Schenck 1898)

Definition. Infection usually following injury involving skin, subcutaneous tissues and often regional lymph nodes.

Causative Organism. *Sporothrix schenckii*. This dimorphous fungus exists in nature and in the laboratory at 22 °C in its mycelial variant and in tissues and at 37 °C as a yeast, the pathogenic form.

Epidemiology. *Sporothrix schenckii* is a relatively common pathogen. It is found on wood and other plant material, most often in tropical and subtropical regions, although it is common through most of the USA.

Etiology and Pathogenesis. There is almost always an injury, usually from a splinter or rose thorn. A famous epidemic occurred in a South African mine where the bracing timber was all contaminated. Sphagnum moss is often contaminated; here abrasions are more likely to produce localized skin disease. Rarely systemic disease may occur, following inhalation or ingestion. While animals may also be infected, transmission from animal to man or man to man has not be confirmed.

Clinical Findings. The classic form of sporotrichosis is the lymphocutaneous form. Here there is inoculation, usually on the hand. Typically several weeks after an often minor injury an inflamed papule or pustule appears. It may evolve into a deeper nodule or even an ulcer. The lesion is usually not diagnosed at this stage, and may heal spontaneously. But even as the primary site is improving, additional similar nodules appear in the lymphatic drainage of the site, each one typically more proximal than the last (Fig. 7.28). These deeper blue-red nodules may break through to the skin, producing a crusted ulcer; the more proximal lesions, i.e., those furthest away from the inoculation, tend not to ulcerate. Even though the course is chronic, the patient is not systemically ill.

There are several less common forms of sporotrichosis.

- Fixed cutaneous sporotrichosis may simply represent inoculation in a patient with previous exposure and good immunity or it may arise following more superficial injuries such as an abrasion. The lesions are typically crusted and verrucous and heal spontaneously with scarring

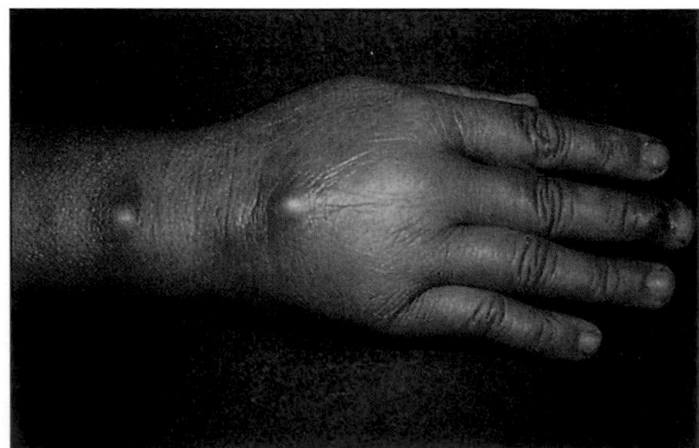

Fig. 7.28. Lymphocutaneous sporotrichosis

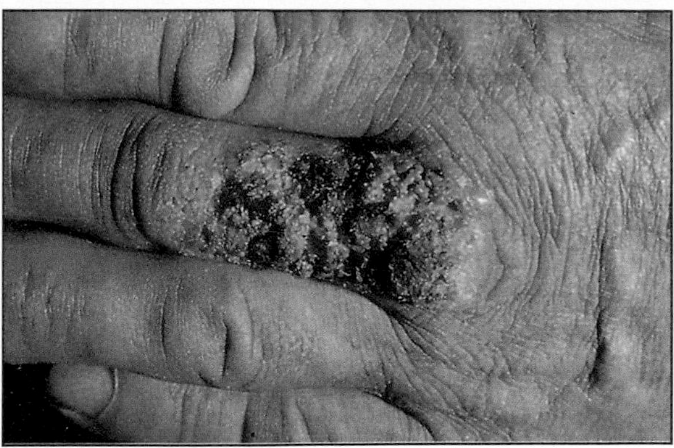

Fig. 7.29. Fixed cutaneous sporotrichosis

(Fig. 7.29). The most common sites are the face and trunk. We have seen large patches of sporotrichosis in gardeners who carry bundles of sphagnum moss held to their chest and abdomen.

- Mucocutaneous sporotrichosis may result from inoculation of the oral mucosa with a piece of wood or plant material, producing an ulcer. Since lymph node involvement also occurs, the mistaken diagnosis of an ulcerated squamous cell carcinoma is occasionally considered. Ocular inoculation may also occur.
- Disseminated cutaneous sporotrichosis is just what the name says – lesions like the lymphocutaneous form but scattered over the entire body, suggesting hematogenous spread. Such patients are often immunosuppressed.
- Primary pulmonary sporotrichosis results from inhalation. There are usually no cutaneous findings. Patients typically are older individuals who have other pulmonary disease and may develop infiltrates or cavitary disease.
- Systemic sporotrichosis is seen in immunosuppressed patients, especially those with HIV/AIDS. They may have disseminated cutaneous disease; bones, joints and muscles are most likely to be affected, but any organ can be involved. Pulmonary sporotrichosis may also disseminate.

Histopathology. *Sporothrix schenckii* can be difficult to find on biopsy specimens. There seem to be marked regional differences, as reports from Japan and Australia describe almost always finding fungal elements, while in other parts of the world, it appears more difficult. The localized hyperkeratotic lesions show pseudoepitheliomatous epidermal hyperplasia and granulomatous inflammation. In the lymphatic form, there is usually an abscess perhaps surrounded by granulomatous inflammation and a peripheral accumulation of lymphocytes and plasma cells. The yeasts are 4–6 µm in size, cigar-shaped and can be best seen with PAS or methenamine silver stains. Immunofluorescent stains may also help. The sporothrix asteroid body is a distinctive yeast form surrounded by an eosinophilic material with sunburst-like rays reaching a size of 25 µm. This feature is also known as the Splendore-Hoeppli phenomenon.

Laboratory Findings. The organism can be easily cultured on routine media growing within 3–5 days. The dimorphism is apparent, as the cultures held at room temperature are fluffy and white, later darkening, while those grown at 37 °C are cream-colored and smooth. Serologic tests may aid in evaluating systemic disease. The sporotrichin skin test is no longer employed.

Course and Prognosis. Most of the cutaneous lesions eventually heal, with scarring.

Differential Diagnosis. Table 7.5 shows the differential diagnosis for the lymphocutaneous form; such lesions are described as "sporotrichoid". Any inoculation of an organism can lead to ascending lymphatic spread nodules, but it is most common with atypical mycobacteria and *Nocardia brasiliensis.*

Therapy

Systemic. The standard of therapy for the cutaneous and lymphocutaneous forms is supersaturated potassium iodide. The usual dosage is 5 drops t.i.d., increasing gradually to 30–50 drops t.i.d. One should check thyroid function prior to the administration of so much iodide. Gastrointestinal tolerance is usually the limiting factor. It is convenient to give the solution mixed with orange juice. Therapy should be continued for 4–6 weeks past the resolution of lesions.

Table 7.5. Sporotrichoid lesions

Sporotrichosis
Nocardiosis
Tuberculosis
Atypical mycobacterial infection
Cat scratch disease
Anthrax
Tularemia

Amphotericin B is the traditional choice for systemic sporotrichosis and many other deep fungal infections, in the dosages discussed above. Itraconazole may be an acceptable safer alternative for cutaneous lesions and non-life-threatening systemic disease. Pulmonary lesions are usually treated with surgery and then amphotericin B. In HIV/AIDS patients, multi-drug regimens have had limited success.

Topical. No external therapy is worthwhile. Application of heat, e.g., with a hand warmer or heating pad, may speed resolution.

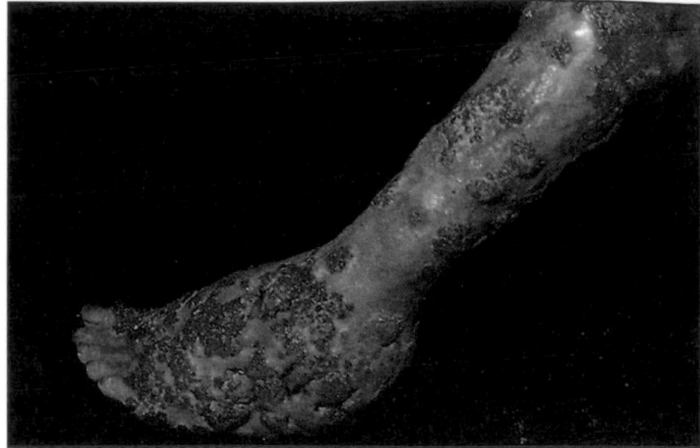

Fig. 7.30. Chromomycosis

Chromomycosis

(Lane and Medlar 1915)

Synonyms. Chromoblastomycosis, dermatitis verrucosa

Definition. Chronic spreading fungal infection, usually of the legs, with verrucous epidermal changes, typically caused by pigmented fungi.

Causative Organism. Many different agents can be responsible; almost all are pigmented or dematiaceous fungi found in soil and decaying vegetation. Five organisms are responsible for most cases: *Phialophora verrucosa, Fonsecaea (Phialophora) pedrosoi, Fonsecaea compacta, Cladosporium carrionii* and *Rhinocladiella aquaspersa.*

Epidemiology. Chromomycosis is most common in the tropics, typically occurring on the feet of those who go barefoot. Fungi present in the soil are inoculated into the skin via minor injuries.

Etiology and Pathogenesis. In contrast to mycetoma, the infection in chromomycosis remains localized to the skin, does not invade bone, produces exophytic changes and can be viewed as growing outward.

Clinical Findings. The feet are the most common site; occasionally trauma leads to inoculation on the hands or trunk. The initial lesion is a papule or pustule that slowly grows, producing widespread papillomas and hyperkeratotic or verrucous changes (Fig. 7.30). The foot is usually swollen and skip areas may occur. The process is painful. Secondary bacterial infection with lymphangitis and resulting lymphedema (elephantiasis chromomycetica) is not unusual. Ulceration may occur. In rare cases, systemic spread occurs. The course is chronic and progressive.

Histopathology. On biopsy the striking pseudoepitheliomatous epidermal hyperplasia is appreciated. In the dermis the dematiaceous fungi have a characteristic appearance. Brown fungal elements with a thick wall ranging in size from 5 to 12 µm are found; they are variously known as copper pennies, Medlar bodies or sclerotic bodies. They can also be found on KOH examination of discharge from the verrucous plaques.

Laboratory Findings. The organism should be cultured; usually Sabouraud medium with antibiotics is satisfactory. Some prefer to culture at 30 °C and growth is very slow, requiring 4–6 weeks. Because of these peculiarities, the laboratory should be consulted prior to culturing.

Differential Diagnosis. Once again, mycetoma has a different pattern, with downward growth, no verrucous changes and frequent bone involvement. Secondary verrucous changes with lymphedema of other causes may appear similar, but the history of an initial injury and local reaction is suggestive. Other infections, including leprosy, deep fungi, sporotrichosis and tuberculosis cutis verrucosa, may occasionally present with a similar picture, as may verrucous carcinoma.

Therapy. Local therapy is not effective. If a lesion is small, surgical excision, cryotherapy or local application of heat can be tried. Itraconazole is occasionally effective and can be tried; the recommended regimen is 200 mg daily for 6 months. If this fails or if the disease is rapidly progressive, a combination of flucytosine and amphotericin B is recommended.

Mycetoma

(VAN DYKE and CARTER 1860)

Synonyms. Eumycetoma, actinomycetoma, maduromycosis, Madura foot (if foot is involved).

Definition. Chronic invasive infection, usually of foot, with involvement of subcutaneous tissue and often bone, usually with draining sinus tracts often discharging grains.

Causative Organisms. Many different organisms can cause a mycetoma. When fungi are responsible one speaks of an eumycetoma. The responsible organisms are soil saprophytes, including *Madurella mycetomatis* and *Madurella grisea, Pseudallescheria boydii, Exophiala (Phialophora) jeanselmei* and many others that can be sought in specialized texts. When bacteria are responsible, sometimes the term actinomycetoma is applied. *Nocardia brasiliensis, Nocardia asteroides, Actinomadura madurae, Actinomadura pelletieri* and *Streptomyces somaliensis* are the most common causes of actinomycetoma. Note that *Actinomyces israeli*, the usual cause of actinomycosis (Chap. 4), does not cause actinomycetomas.

Epidemiology. Mycetomas occur most often in tropical areas but are also seen in temperate regions. Where individuals go barefoot, minor trauma can result in the inoculation of various soil saprophytes into the skin. There are marked regional variations; actinomycetoma is more common in Latin America, while eumycetoma predominates in Africa and Asia. The problem was apparently quite common in the Indian state of Madura. In Europe, most cases come from Romania and Bulgaria.

Etiology and Pathogenesis. The organism is inoculated into the skin. Little is known about the mechanism of infection. Host immunity presumably plays a role in localizing the disease. In contrast to chromomycosis, verrucous changes are unusual and the organisms tend to grow downward.

Clinical Findings. The three hallmarks are inflammatory swelling, sinus tracts and discharge of grains (Fig. 7.31). The grains are accumulations of the pathogens and may be white, yellow or black.

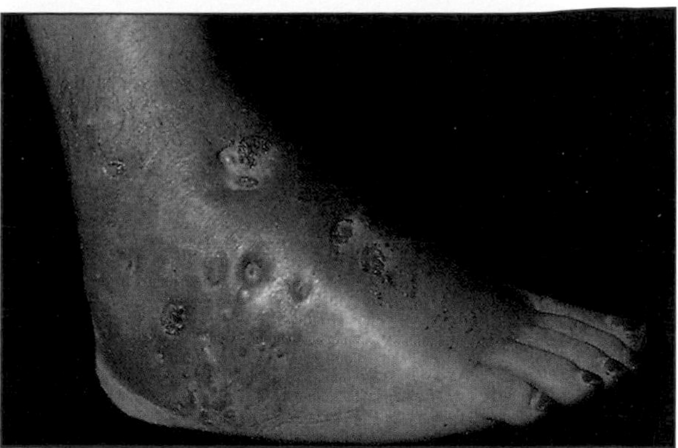

Fig. 7.31. Mycetoma

The initial lesion is a pustule or nodule that slowly expands and tends to grow downward. While the foot is the most common site, the hand may also be affected. The lesions are usually surprisingly painless but chronic, producing severe deformities.

Histopathology. The grains can be seen on biopsy, admixed with fibrosis and chronic inflammation. They can also be studied directly. Once again, the grains may be surrounded by eosinophilic clubs or spikes, another example of the Splendore-Hoeppli phenomenon. When Gram, PAS or silver staining is done, one can usually appreciate differences in thickness between the causative bacteria (1–2 μm) and fungi (4–6 μm). In addition, variations in staining quality occur between species, but the culture should be used for the final diagnosis.

Laboratory Findings. Black grains suggest an eumycetoma. Red grains indicate *Actinomadura pelletieri*, while white-to-yellow grains suggest an actinomycetoma. The grains can simply be crushed and plated on Sabouraud medium with and without antibiotics. The laboratory must be informed that one is searching for unusual organisms.

The limb should be studied with X-ray and other imaging techniques, searching for bone involvement.

Differential Diagnosis. In the head and neck region, actinomycosis can produce a woody inflammation with grains, but bone involvement does not occur. In addition, severe inflammatory tinea barbae, such as from *Trichophyton verrucosum*, can lead to deep-draining nodules. Osteomyelitis may drain towards the skin, producing a similar picture.

Therapy. There is no good therapy. Many patients require amputation or at least extensive surgical débridement. Small lesions should definitely be excised. In the case of eumycetoma, the results of using azoles, amphotericin B and flucytosine have all been disappointing. Nonetheless, it may be worth trying itraconazole, which seems to have the best record. When bacteria are identified, antimicrobial therapy should be tried. Recommended agents include trimethoprim-sulfamethoxazole, clindamycin, rifampin, streptomycin and dapsone. Infectious disease sources should be consulted for suggested dosages.

Systemic Fungal Infections

The systemic or deep mycoses are a group of infections somewhat on the border of dermatology. One must not make the mistake of considering them exotic diseases; rather, they are diseases with sharp regional variation. For example, if a German tourist spends 2 months in the San Joaquin Valley of California and returns home pregnant and with erythema nodosum, the German dermatologist must think of coccidioidomycosis. The systemic fungal infections can be divided in a number of ways. One can separate the obligate pathogens, which always cause disease, even if very subtle, from the facultative pathogens that are usually harmless but can cause trouble in an immunosuppressed host. All of the obligate pathogens are dimorphous fungi which in most cases enter the host via the respiratory route. In most instances, the initial pulmonary infection is mild or subclinical and heals spontaneously, so that therapy is not required. Perhaps 1 in 1000 healthy patients goes on to develop more widespread or persistent disease.

A number of patterns of skin involvement can be seen in the deep mycoses. Although they may vary in likelihood and detail among the different infections, in principle they are all similar.

Local Inoculation. If the patient has a good immune response, the organisms may be held in check at the site of entry in the skin, producing a lesion similar to inoculation tuberculosis. Many patients in endemic areas have good immunity since they have already had a subclinical infection.

Sporotrichoid Lesions. If the patient's immunity is less perfect, the deep fungi are all capable of lymphatic spread, as discussed under sporotrichosis.

Dissemination from the Skin. If the immunity is minimal, the skin may serve as a site of entry. This diagnosis should be made with reluctance. Most often, reactivation is the explanation for disseminated disease.

Dissemination to the Skin. Almost all the deep fungi can spread from internal organs to the skin, either via direct or hematogenous spread. These patterns vary and will be discussed under the individual causative organisms.

Hypersensitivity Reactions. Erythema nodosum and other immunologic reactions may reflect a deep fungal infection. They usually suggest a good prognosis.

Cryptococcosis

(Busse 1894; Buschke 1895)

Synonyms. Torula, Busse-Buschke disease, European blastomycosis

Causative Organism. *Cryptococcus neoformans.* There appear to be two major varieties: *Cryptococcus neoformans* var. *neoformans* and *Cryptococcus neoformans* var. *gatti.* The latter is limited almost exclusively to California, has an affinity for the bark of eucalyptus trees and may be more difficult to treat. Other cryptococci may cause disease in immunosuppressed hosts. The sexual forms of many have been identified. *Cryptococcus neoformans* exists in nature as a small budding yeast; when it grows in tissue, it usually develops a slimy or mucoid capsule that may block host defenses. It is a filamentous fungus at room temperature, but at 37 °C a yeast.

Epidemiology. *Cryptococcus neoformans* is found worldwide. It was first described in Berlin, but is present everywhere. The main source of infection appears to be the droppings of pigeons and other birds, although the birds themselves are not affected. The prevalence of cryptococcosis is unknown, as no good screening tests are available. Most patients with active disease are adults; the male: female ratio is 2:1. Children are rarely clinically involved. In the USA, about 10% of HIV/AIDS patients develop cryptococcosis.

Etiology and Pathogenesis. The initial infection almost always occurs via inhalation of the organisms. The mechanisms of spread are poorly understood. In most cases, the problem is with the host defense mechanisms, but the development of a capsule and perhaps direct inhibition of the host's cellular immunity may be contributions of the fungus.

Clinical Findings
Systemic Findings. The initial pulmonary infection is usually asymptomatic and limited. The most common site of spread is the CNS; cryptococcal meningitis is the usual presentation. In HIV/AIDS patients, the course may be surprisingly asymptomatic yet virulent. The prostate is often a hidden reservoir; renal and bone involvement is also common.

Cutaneous Findings. Primary inoculation cryptococcosis is thought to be extremely rare. Even if the skin is the only site involved, the answer is usually dissemination and the patient should be carefully evaluated and followed up. About 20% of patients with disseminated cryptococcosis have skin findings. The skin is the second most common site after the CNS. In HIV/AIDS patients, cutaneous disease is a definite sign of dissemination. The hematogenous spread produces a variety of cutaneous lesions, including papules, pustules, nodules, draining sinuses and ulcers. The most publicized change is the development of umbilicated nodules resembling molluscum contagiosum.

Histopathology. The fungi stain well with a PAS or methenamine silver stain. If they have their slimy capsule, they are unmistakable; the 2- to 4-µm yeast is surrounded by a wide clear capsule that stains with alcian blue or other mucin stains. If the capsule is not present, then the organisms can be found in giant cells, associated with granulomatous inflammation.

Laboratory Findings. The organisms can often be identified in the CNS or pus. When the fluid is stained with India ink, the capsule appears as a halo. The culture medium should not include cycloheximide. Tests for various fungal antigens in serum and CSF may be helpful.

Course and Prognosis. Most patients do not know that they have had cryptococcosis. Those who are immunosuppressed and then develop active disease require treatment. The prognosis is based on the speed with which therapy is instituted and the nature of the underlying disease.

Differential Diagnosis. The cutaneous lesions are usually not specific and if other findings are not present, they are first correctly diagnosed on biopsy.

Therapy. The standard therapy is a combination of flucytosine and amphotericin B. Fluconazole appears promising and is approved for cryptococcal meningitis. It can be given in dosages of 400 mg intravenously on the first day, then 200 mg orally for 10–12 weeks. The exact indications for choosing fluconazole remain disputed. Most agree that in HIV/AIDS, initial therapy should be with the older regimen, but that lifelong fluconazole prophylaxis (50–100 mg daily) is useful.

Blastomycosis
(Gilchrist 1894)

Synonyms. North American blastomycosis, Gilchrist disease

Causative Organism. *Blastomyces dermatitidis.* Another dimorphic fungus whose sexual form is known, this organism is filamentous at room temperature and a yeast at 37 °C.

Epidemiology. *Blastomyces dermatitidis* is primarily found in the Midwestern and South-Central parts of the USA. The hot spot is the area bordering the Ohio and Mississippi valleys. It is also occasionally found in Canada, Israel, Saudi Arabia and focally in Africa and India. It is a soil contaminant, usually found in moist or undisturbed areas.

Etiology and Pathogenesis. The organism is inhaled in spore form and begins its growth as a yeast in the lungs. Blastomycosis is not a problem among immunosuppressed patients, as the paucity of reports of its occurrence in HIV/AIDS patients dramatically underscores. It has a tendency to reactivate after many years.

Clinical Findings
Systemic Findings. The initial pulmonary infection is usually overlooked. Patients present with a cough and diffuse pulmonary infiltrates that resolve promptly. In some cases chronic pulmonary disease develops with cavitation. These patients are at risk for dissemination. About half the patients have bone involvement; the osteolytic lesions are usually asymptomatic. One quarter of male patients have prostate involvement. CNS disease is uncommon

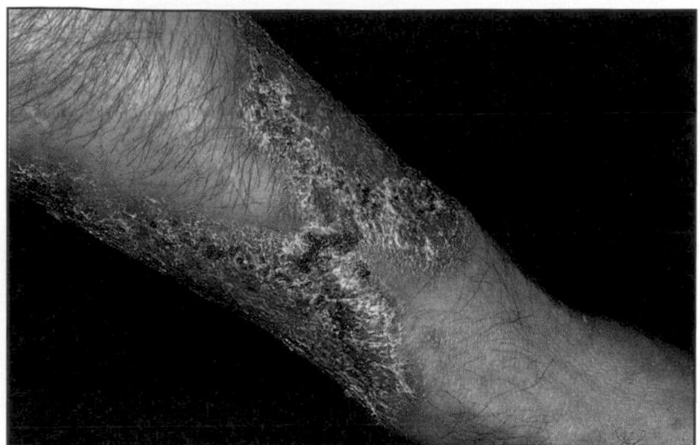

Fig. 7.32. Blastomycosis. (Courtesy of Robert H. Schosser, MD, Lexington, Kentucky)

but appears to be the one aspect of blastomycosis that is more severe in immunosuppressed paticnts.

Cutaneous Findings. About three-quarters of patients with extra-pulmonary disease have skin involvement. The most typical lesion is a verrucous nodule or plaque, usually on the face or extremities. It starts as a tiny papule and slowly advances with an active border, peripheral microabscesses and central healing (Fig. 7.32). Tiny occluded papillary vessels speckle the partially healed area, similar to the dots seen in a pared wart. Inoculation and sporotrichoid blastomycosis are uncommon but have been reported following contaminated wounds.

Histopathology. The epidermis shows pseudoepitheliomatous hyperplasia and intraepidermal microabscesses, reminiscent of pemphigus vegetans or iododerma. The organisms are quite large, 8–20 μm, with a refractile double wall and often a broad-based single bud. They stain well with PAS or methenamine silver stains.

Laboratory Findings. *Blastomyces dermatitidis* can be easily cultured. It produces a fluffy white colony at 30 °C. Serologic tests are not very helpful because they cross-react with histoplasmosis, but may be used to monitor disease.

Course and Prognosis. Most patients do well. Those with disseminated disease or cavitary pulmonary disease die if not treated appropriately.

Differential Diagnosis. The skin lesions resemble an ulcerated crusted tumor, such as a basal cell carcinoma or squamous cell carcinoma. Tuberculosis cutis verrucosa and other granulomatous infections may also be suggested, as well as halogenoderma.

Therapy. Limited pulmonary disease requires no treatment. For modest systemic disease without CNS involvement or other life-threatening problems, itraconazole or ketoconazole are the agents of choice. Both should be given at the upper range of tolerability for 6 months. In more severe cases, amphotericin B is required.

Histoplasmosis

(Darling 1906)

Synonyms. Histoplasmosis capsulati, American histoplasmosis, Darling disease

Causative Organism. *Histoplasma capsulatum* var. *capsulatum.* Another dimorphic fungus, it grows as a filamentous fungus in the soil and as a yeast in patients.

Epidemiology. Histoplasmosis is a disease of the Ohio and Mississippi valleys, overlapping greatly with blastomycosis in terms of home range. It is also found in localized areas of South America, Asia, Australia and even Africa. About 80% of the population in infected areas show evidence of past infection, although active disease is uncommon.

Etiology and Pathogenesis. The route of entry is once again the lungs. The primary infection usually occurs during childhood. The main source is soil contaminated by droppings of bats or of chickens or other birds. Plowing or otherwise working with contaminated soil is dangerous. Inoculation injuries can produce local disease.

Clinical Findings

Systemic Findings. The initial pulmonary infection is usually mild and overlooked. Occasionally there will be pneumonia associated with erythema nodosum, resolving with scattered lung calcifications. Chronic pulmonary histoplasmosis resembles chronic cavitary tuberculosis and represents reactivation in older men, often with a second lung disease such as emphysema.

The most serious form of histoplasmosis is the disseminated disease. In the acute form, there is lymphadenopathy, hepatosplenomegaly, bone marrow suppression, fever and weight loss, with a rapid downhill course. This frequently fatal form is most common in young children and in immunosuppressed individuals, especially those with HIV/AIDS. In chronic disseminated histoplasmosis, there are similarly widespread lesions, but a slower course. Meningitis and endocarditis are common features.

Cutaneous Findings. The acute infection may be associated with erythema nodosum or erythema multiforme, as an id reaction. Inoculation histoplasmosis is not uncommon. In the chronic disseminated disease, there may be ulcerations of the buccal and palatal mucosa, the tongue and the entire oropharynx and upper gastrointestinal tract. In HIV/AIDS patients, the incidence of skin involvement is less than 10%; in the general population it is even lower. Erythematous papules or nodules, ulcerations and even panniculitis may develop via hematogenous spread.

Histopathology. The dermis shows chronic granulomatous inflammation. The yeasts are very small, about 2–4 µm in diameter, and contained in macrophages. They too stain with both PAS and methenamine silver stains. While on routine sections there is often a clear space around each organism, there is no true capsule, despite the name.

Laboratory Findings. *Histoplasma capsulatum* grows very slowly. It can be cultured from the skin, mucosa or bone marrow. The culture is highly infectious, so the laboratory must be warned whenever there is the slightest suspicion of histoplasmosis. Fungal antigens can occasionally be detected in the serum, confirming the diagnosis. Paired serum specimens for complement-fixation testing are also helpful; a rise in titers usually represents acute infection. A histoplasmin test is available, but of limited utility in endemic areas. Its use may invalidate serologic testing.

Course and Prognosis. The outlook in the case of disseminated disease is grim, especially if the patient is immunosuppressed. The chronic pulmonary disease is disabling and also eventually fatal.

Differential Diagnosis. The skin lesions are not very diagnostic. Histoplasmosis should always be considered in the presence of oral ulcerations or otherwise unexplained cutaneous inflammatory lesions in individuals from endemic areas.

Therapy. If the patient is not immunosuppressed, both ketoconazole and itraconazole are approved as long as there is no evidence of CNS disease. In the acute disseminated form, or if there is CNS disease, then amphotericin B should be employed. In HIV/AIDS, following the use of amphotericin B, itraconazole is recommended for lifelong suppression.

African Histoplasmosis

Synonym. Histoplasmosis duboisii

Causative Organisms. *Histoplasma capsulatum* var. *duboisii.*

This dimorphic fungis is found in Africa and on the island of Madagascar. Despite the name, it is less common in Africa than ordinary *Histoplasma capsulatum.* Most infections are chronic soft tissue infections, although disseminated disease may occur. The organism is much larger in tissue than its close relative and has different culture characteristics. Treatment guidelines are unclear; most treat African histoplasmosis in the same way as histoplasmosis.

Coccidioidomycosis

(Wernicke 1892)

Synonyms. Valley fever, desert fever, San Joaquin fever

Causative Organism. *Coccidioides immitis*, another dimorphic soil fungus.

Epidemiology. The organism is limited to the Sonoran Desert of the Western USA and Mexico, as well as similar regions in Central and South America. It is a ubiquitous soil fungus, especially common around animal burrows. Infections are most common in summers following a rainy spring, when spores are blown around by dust storms and high winds.

Etiology and Pathogenesis. *Coccidioides immitis* is highly infective. Tourists, military personnel or migrant workers passing through the endemic zone can be infected with minimal exposure. Contaminated packing materials from the region have also transmitted the infection.

Clinical Findings

Systemic Findings. Once again, the initial infection is respiratory. About half of the patients are asymptomatic and the rest have mild symptoms. Some patients may have minor residual pulmonary disease, such as fibrosis or a small cavity. Sometimes there is a localized ball-like accumulation of the fungi, known as a coccidioidoma. Dissemination occurs in about 1:1000 patients, usually involving the CNS or bone. It is a major problem during pregnancy and in HIV/AIDS patients and is more common in black and Hispanic individuals.

Cutaneous Findings. Inoculation can produce a localized lesion. Erythema nodosum occurs in about one-quarter of diagnosed cases, most often in Caucasian women and rarely in black men. In the Sonoran Desert area, coccidioidomycosis is the most common cause of erythema nodosum. Other patients may have a diffuse maculopapular exanthem, resembling a viral exanthem, or erythema multiforme. In disseminated disease, papules and nodules favoring the face are the most common sign. Once again, they may mimic molluscum contagiosum, often favoring the nasolabial fold. More verrucous lesions, ulcers and deeper abscesses with draining sinus tracts may also occur.

Histopathology. The specimen shows chronic granulomatous inflammation but the organisms can usually be easily identified. The typical tissue form is a large spherule, 40–60 μm in diameter, loaded with endospores. They can usually be seen on routine staining but are enhanced by methenamine silver or PAS staining.

Laboratory Findings. The organism can be cultured, but once again, the plate is extremely infectious and must be handled under strict ventilation guidelines. The spherules can be readily identified in pus or CSF fluids because of their great size. The skin test becomes positive in the first days of the infection, so it is useful in nonendemic areas. Serologic testing is also helpful. The IgM precipitin antibodies appear in the first few weeks, while the IgG complement fixation antibodies occur later. A rising IgG titer points towards dissemination and, if positive in the CSF, suggests meningitis. Anergy is a poor prognostic sign, suggesting disseminated disease.

Course and Prognosis. The disseminated disease is potentially fatal if not recognized promptly. Patients from endemic areas tend to relapse if their immune status is altered. Erythema nodosum is usually associated with a good outcome; in some situations it can be viewed as protective. For example, among pregnant patients, almost none with erythema nodosum develop disseminated disease, while about one-third of those who fail to develop the skin findings evolve into widespread disease.

Differential Diagnosis. Infection with *Coccidioides immitis* must always be considered in patients who have lived or traveled in the endemic zone. The most distinctive finding is erythema nodosum early in the disease course; one should assume that coccidioidomycosis is the answer rather than reasoning in the other direction. In the case of cutaneous involvement in disseminated disease, the differential list is long but the biopsy findings highly specific.

Therapy. Fluconazole is the agent of choice for severe infections, even with meningeal involvement. Amphotericin B should be reserved for life-threatening situations or when there is no response or rising titers while on fluconazole. If the CNS is not affected, itraconazole and ketoconazole are also helpful.

Paracoccidioidomycosis

(Lutz 1908)

Synonyms. South American blastomycosis, Lutz-Splendore-Almeida disease.

Causative Organism. *Paracoccidioides brasiliensis*

Epidemiology. Paracoccidioidomycosis is limited to South and Central America. Its source in nature is poorly understood but is probably the soil, as it is typically a disease of men who work outdoors.

Etiology and Pathogenesis. The usual site of entry is the lungs. The organism has a propensity for dissemination. Even though the rate of infection is equal among sexes; the male:female ratio among patients with disseminated disease is about 15:1. Men as outdoor workers may receive a larger inoculum, or female hormones may somehow have an inhibitory action.

Clinical Findings

Systemic Findings. The acute pulmonary infection may be subclinical or resemble pneumonia. The chronic adult form features pulmonary destruction and invasion of the oral, nasal and intestinal mucosa. With dissemination, lymphadenopathy and adrenal involvement are common but any organ can be affected. In the juvenile or acute form, there is marked infection of the reticuloendothelial system with hepatosplenomegaly and bone marrow dysfunction, mimicking a hematologic malignancy.

Cutaneous Findings. The facial lesions are usually periorificial nodules that slowly expand and ulcerate. The crusted lesions may coalesce on the upper lip and around the nose (Fig. 7.33). At the same time there are usually painful mucosal ulcerations of the mouth and nose. The combination of lesions produces mid-facial disfigurement, resembling that of leishmaniasis, seen in the same parts of South America. Cervical lymphadenopathy is common and may create draining sinuses to the skin.

Histopathology. Biopsy shows pseudoepitheliomatous hyperplasia and granulomatous inflammation. The organisms are quite large, up to 60 µm. They have been described as having a steering-wheel appearance, because multiple, narrow-based buds radiate out from the central organism. The methenamine silver stain is the best way to identify them quickly.

Laboratory Findings. The organism can be cultured from the readily obtained pus. Serologic testing is also available. Titers can be helpful in following endemic cases, as well as in identifying the disease in a traveler.

Course and Prognosis. Untreated paracoccidioidomycosis can be a very aggressive disease. The juvenile form is frequently fatal, while the adult form is very destructive.

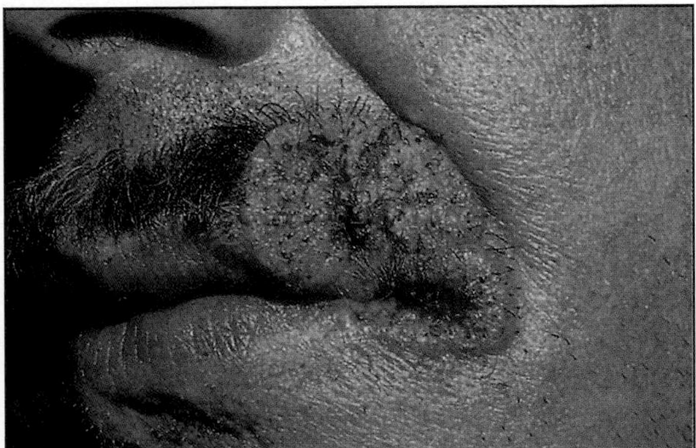

Fig. 7.33. Paracoccidioidomycosis

Differential Diagnosis. The differential diagnosis includes leishmaniasis, leprosy and other granulomatous infections.

Therapy. Itraconazole and ketoconazole have replaced amphotericin B except for the most ill patients, especially those with the juvenile form. Those who are treated with amphotericin B are then switched to an azole for completion of at least 6 months of therapy. Long-term sulfonamide therapy was formerly standard and may still be useful for maintenance.

Keloidal Blastomycosis

(Lôbo 1931)

Synonym. Lôbo disease

Causative Organism. *Loboa loboi*

This organism is classified as a deep fungus because it was considered related to paracoccidioidomycosis. Its life story is poorly understood, since it has not been successfully cultured. The endemic area is the northern part of South America and parts of Central America. It has also been described in dolphins in the Gulf of Mexico. The chronic infection is confined to the skin and subcutaneous tissue. Slowly growing, often annular or serpiginous nodules develop, with a smooth surface resembling a scar or keloid. In other instances, they may be more exophytic, creating cauliflower-like protuberances. Histologic examination reveals a distinct picture of highly refractile 6- to 12-µm fungal cells, many in large macrophages with a ground-glass cytoplasm. The only treatment is surgical; use of flucytosine and amphotericin B has been disappointing.

Opportunistic Fungi

Many of the organisms we have already discussed favor immunosuppressed hosts. Typical examples include *Candida albicans* and *Cryptococcus neoformans*. Candidemia or cryptococcal CNS disease are limited almost exclusively to the already ill. But there are other organisms, for the most part molds, that never cause disease in the healthy host. In this age of HIV/AIDS, transplantation of bone marrow and solid organs and aggressive chemotherapy, almost every organism known to microbiologists has caused at least one opportunistic infection. We will concentrate on the more common cutaneous invaders.

In any immunosuppressed patient with a papular, nodular or ulcerative skin lesion whose etiology is not absolutely clear, biopsy is recommended. At the same time, tissue should be submitted for culture, warning the laboratory of the problem, so that culture will be performed on appropriate media and the samples observed for a sufficient length of time.

Aspergillosis

Causative Organisms. *Aspergillus fumigatus, Aspergillus niger* and *Aspergillus flavus.* There are several other species, but these are the usual pathogens.

Etiology and Pathogenesis. All the molds are ubiquitous in nature, found on leaves and decaying vegetable matter, but also indoors, even in hospital air. *Aspergillus* is found in the lungs of many patients without causing disease. *Aspergillus flavus* produces aflatoxins that are highly carcinogenic in experimental animals but whose role in humans is unclear. In Africa and Southeast Asia, aflatoxins have been blamed for the high incidence of hepatocellular carcinoma.

Clinical Findings. *Aspergillus fumigatus* is involved in pulmonary disease in several ways. A fungal ball or aspergilloma may develop in a preexisting lung cavity, such as following tuberculosis. Some patients have an allergic reaction to *Aspergillus* with inflammation and swelling of the proximal bronchi, causing asthma. Other possible features are bronchial plugging, eosinophilia and a positive immediate prick test reaction. In yet other patients there may be invasive pulmonary disease secondary to immunosuppression.

The latter patients may have disseminated disease with cutaneous fungal emboli. *Aspergillus* tends to clog vessels, producing hemorrhage, infarcts and black eschars. A similar process may occur with local inoculation of the mold in a weakened host. This is known as primary cutaneous aspergillosis, and *Aspergillus flavus* is often found. Most patients have leukemia with markedly impaired immunity; the infections tend to occur at intravenous access sites or under dressings. In addition, burns and pyoderma gangrenosum may be secondarily infected with *Aspergillus.*

The same molds may cause disease in the ear and sinuses. *Aspergillus niger* is often identified in the external ear canal and is rarely a pathogen, although otomycosis is frequently diagnosed. In compromised hosts, it may behave aggressively. *Aspergillus flavus* may cause invasive sinusitis in the same settings.

Laboratory Findings. The hyphae of *Aspergillus* can be found in or adjacent to vessels. They are large structures that branch at sharp angles and are best seen with methenamine silver staining. The organisms can be cultured, but they are so ubiquitous that tissue demonstration is preferred.

Course and Prognosis. In compromised hosts, aspergillosis is rapidly fatal if not treated promptly.

Therapy. The usual therapy for disseminated aspergillosis is amphotericin B, but both ketoconazole and itraconazole are also effective against *Aspergillus* and can be employed if the situation is not life threatening, such as in a local infection around an access site.

Zygomycosis

Synonym. Phycomycosis

Causative Organisms. *Mucor, Rhizomucor, Rhizopus* and *Cunninghamella* species. Despite the old name of mucormycosis, *Mucor* is infrequently identified.

Etiology and Pathogenesis. These organisms, known collectively as bread molds, are very widespread and rarely cause disease.

Clinical Findings. The most common disease setting is nasal or sinus infection in patients with diabetes mellitus under poor control. Other immunosuppressed individuals are also at risk. Deferoxamine, a chelating agent used for iron overload in renal dialysis patients, also appears to favor these molds. The infection may spread rapidly, causing facial edema, bloody nasal discharge, orbital cellulitis, proptosis, cavernous sinus thrombosis and brain abscesses. In rare cases, there may be invasive pulmonary or gastrointestinal disease. Most patients succumb to this fulminant disease.

Local cutaneous disease may also occur. The most common scenario is secondary infection of a burn. Sometimes catheter-associated infections produce localized hemorrhagic dusky painful nodules and plaques. In other instances, in otherwise healthy trauma patients, the molds are introduced into the skin, perhaps under a cast, and produce pustules and plaques but little hemorrhage and have no tendency to invade vessels.

Histopathology. The large branching hyphae are not easily overlooked. They lack septa (coenocytic) and branch at right angles.

Laboratory Findings. The bread molds can be cultured, but a diagnosis must be based on immediate histologic study. Otherwise, the results of the culture can be incorporated into the autopsy report.

Therapy. Amphotericin B coupled with surgical débridement and control of the diabetes mellitus offer some hope.

Subcutaneous Phycomycosis

Synonym. Entomophthoramycosis

This tongue-twister is unlikely to be encountered by western dermatologists. It is included only for completeness. There are two principal forms of the disease, seen primarily in tropical Asia and Africa and caused by molds. *Basidiobolus ranarum* causes subcutaneous masses in children. *Conidiobolus coronatus* produces nasal and mid-facial swelling in adults, but not to the extremes discussed above. Both can be treated with supersaturated potassium iodide, or with amphotericin B if the former fails.

Hyalohyphomycosis and Phaeohyphomycosis

These terms support the fact that fungal terminology is confusing. They are used to describe infections by molds that are either glassy (hyalo-) or pigmented (phaeo-) and have septate hyphae. Many of the organisms causing chromomycosis also are included in this group when they cause other types of infections. Local inoculation can produce primary cutaneous disease or secondary infection of burns and damaged skin, but dissemination occurs only in immunosuppressed individuals.

The main pigmented or dematiaceous molds in the category are *Alternaria, Curvularia* and *Exophiala.* Among the hyaline molds, *Fusarium* and *Pseudallescheria boydii* are best known. While the latter is a common cause of mycetoma, it may also be found in the ear canal and cause skin or joint abscesses following penetrating trauma. *Fusarium* is another cause of hemorrhagic and necrotic skin lesions in compromised hosts, especially patients with severe burns or leukemia. In the Southwestern USA, these molds are the most common cause of mycotic keratitis.

All show hyphae on tissue examination and culture is needed for exact speciation.

They are all so uncommon that clear therapy guidelines do not exist. In life-threatening cases, amphotericin B is used; otherwise itraconazole and ketoconazole can be tried.

Other Rare Opportunistic Fungal Infections

Penicillium marneffei is the most common opportunistic fungal infection among HIV/AIDS patients in Southeast Asia. It has also been described in immunosuppressed patients who have visited that part of the world. The infection is typically disseminated with fever, anemia, weight loss and nodular or ulcerated skin lesions. The mortality rate is about 20%, even with aggressive treatment with amphotericin B for 2 weeks followed by 10 weeks of itraconazole 200 mg b.i.d. Secondary prophylaxis with itraconazole is recommended.

Paecilomyces lilacinus has been incriminated in endocarditis, eye infections and skin lesions in burn patients. A outbreak of multiple cutaneous infections with this unusual organism was reported among bone-marrow transplantation and other hematologic patients who received routine skin care with a hospital lotion infected with *Paecilomyces lilacinus.* Several developed systemic disease as well. No systemic antimycotic agents are effective against this otherwise harmless organism.

Presumed Fungal Infection

Rhinosporidiosis

Causative Organism. *Rhinosporidium seeberi*

This peculiar life form is found in South and Central America, India and Ceylon; occasional reports from the USA exist. It has never been cultured but is likely to be a fungus. It is found primarily on the nasal or ocular mucosa, where over years it produces a friable pedunculated mass. On rare occasions, the skin is affected. The striking feature is the presence of giant sporangia, 100–400 µm in diameter, containing thousands of apparent endospores. Treatment is surgical.

Algal Infections

Prototheca wickerhamii is a unicellular organism without chlorophyll that reproduces via endospores; it is ubiquitous in nature, not limited to water. It enters the skin via trauma or in wounds and produces localized inflammation with nodules, blisters and ulcers. Olecranon bursitis also occurs. Most affected individuals have been immunosuppressed. Dissemination has been described but is thought to be extremely uncommon; in animals, however, dissemination is the rule. The organisms are about 10 µm in size and contain internal septa with endospores. They stain with fungal stains and can be cultured on Sabouraud medium. Treatment is usually surgical; amphotericin B may also be effective.

Bibliography

General

Crissey JT, Lang H, Parish LC (1995) Manual of medical mycology. Blackwell Science, London

De Hoog GS, Guarro J (1995) Atlas of clinical fungi. Centralbureau voor Schimmelcultures. Baarn and Delft, Netherlands

Richardson MD, Warnock DW (1997) Fungal infection. Diagnosis and management. Blackwell Science, London

Superficial Mycoses

Aractingi S, Cadranel S, Reygagne P et al. (1991) Neonatal pustulosis induced by Malassezia furfur. Ann Dermatol 118:856–858

Assaf RR, Weil ML (1996) The superficial mycoses. Dermatol Clin 14:57–67

Bardazzi F, Patrizi A (1997) Transient cephalic neonatal pustulosis. Arch Dermatol 133:528–530

Faergemann J (1997) Pityrosporum yeasts – what's new? Mycoses 40:S29–S32

Figueras MJ, Guarro J, Zaror L (1996) New findings in black piedra infection. Br J Dermatol 135:157–158

Gueho E, Improvisi L, de Hoog GS et al. (1994) Trichosporon on humans: a practical account. Mycoses 37:3–10

Guidelines of care for superficial mycotic infections of the skin: Piedra (1996) J Am Acad Dermatol 34:122–124

Gupta G, Burden AD, Shankland GS et al. (1997) Tinea nigra secondary to *Exophialia werneckii* responding to itraconazole. Br J Dermatol 137:483–484

Gupta AK, Einarson TR, Summerbell RC et al. (1998) An overview of topical antifungal therapy in Dermatomycoses. A North American perspective. Drugs 55: 645–674

Hall J, Perry VE (1998) Tinea nigra palmaris: differentiation from malignant melanoma or junctional nevi. Cutis 62:45–46

Potter BS, Burgoon CF Jr, Johnson WC (1973) Pityrosporum folliculitis. Report of seven cases and areview of the Pityrosporum organism. relative to cutaneous diseases. Arch Dermatol 107:388–391

Rapelanoro R, Mortureux P, Couprie B et al. (1996) Neonatal *Malassezia furfur* pustulosis. Arch Dermatol 132:190–193

Reid BJ (1998) *Exophialia werneckii* causing tinea nigra in Scotland. Br J Dermatol 139:157–158

Sina B, Kauffman CL, Samorodin CS (1995) Intrafollicular mucin deposits in *Pityrosporum* folliculitis. J Am Acad Dermatol 32:807–809

Sunenshine PJ, Schwartz RA, Janniger CK (1998) Tinea versicolor: an update. Cutis: 65–68, 71–72

Dermatophytoses and Therapy

Abdel-Rahman SM, Powell DA, Nahata MC (1998) Efficacy of itraconazole in children with *Trichophyton tonsurans* tinea capitis. J Am Acad Dermatol 38:443–446

Bakos L, Bonamigo RR, Pisani AC et al. (1996) Scutular favus-like tinea cruris et pedis in a patient with AIDS. J Acad Dermatol 34:1086–1087

Budimulja U, Kuswadji K, Bramono S et al. (1994) A double-blind, randomized, stratified controlled study of the treatment of tinea imbricata with oral terbinafine or itraconazole. Br J Dermatol 130 43:29–31

Drake LA, Shear NH, Arlette JP et al. (1997) Oral terbinafine in the treatment of toenail onychomycosis: North American multicenter trial. J Am Acad Dermatol 37:740–745

Elewski BE (1998) Onychomycosis: pathogenesis, diagnosis, and management. Clin Microblol Rev 11:415–429

Evans EG (1998) Causative pathogens in onychomycosis and the possibility of treatment resistance: a review. J Am Acad Dermatol 38:32–56

Garcia-Sanchez MS, Pereiro M Jr, Pereiro MM, Toribio J (1997) Favus due to *Trichophyton mentagrophytes* var. *quinckeanum*. Dermatology 194:177–179

Graser Y, el Farl M, Presber W et al. (1998) Identification of common dermatophytes (*Trichophyton, Microsporum, Epidermophyton*) using polymerase chain reactions. Br J Dermatol 138:576–582

Hierholzer J, Hierholzer C, Hierholzer K (1994) Johann Lukas Schonlein and his contribution to nephrology and medicine. Am J Nephrol 14:467–442

Kick G, Korting HC (1998) Tinea barbae due to *Trichophyton mentagrophytes* related to persistent child infection. Mycoses 41:439–441

Korting HC, Klövekorn W, Klövekorn G (1997) Comparative efficacy and tolerability of econazole liposomal gel 1%, branded econazole conventional cream 1% and generic clotrimazole cream 1% in tinea pedis. Clin Drug Invest 14:286–293

Korting HC, Grundmann-Kollmann M (1997) The hydroxypyridones: a class of antimycotics of its own. Mycoses 40:243–247

Liu D, Coloe S, Baird R et al. (1997) PCR identification of *Trichophyton mentagrophytes* var. *interdigitale* and *T. mentagrophytes* var. *mentagrophytes* dermatophytes with a random primer. J Med Microbiol 46:1043–1046

Stevens DS (1995) Coccidioidomycosis. N Engl J Med 332:1077–1082

Tosti A, Piraccini BM, Stinchi C et al. (1998) Relapses of follow-up. Dermatology 197:162–166

Yeasts

Baran R (1997) Proximal subungual *Candida* onychomycosis. An unusual manifestation of chronic mucocutaneous candidosis. Br J Dermatol 137:286–288

Bjorses P, Aaltonen J, Horelli-Kuitunen N et al. (1998) Gene defect behind APECED: a new clue to autoimmunity. Hum Mol Genet 7:1547–1553

Guidelines/Outcome Committee (1996) Guidelines of care for superficial mycotic infections of the skin: mucocutaneous candidiasis. American Academy of Dermatology. J Am Acad Dermatol 34:110–115

Hoegl L, Thoma-Greber E, Röcken et al. (1998) HIV protease inhibitors influence the prevalence of oral candidosis in HIV-infected patients: a 2-year study. Mycoses 41:321–325

Hoegl L, Schönian G, Ollert M et al. (1998) *Candida sake*: a relevant species in the context of HIV-associated oropharyngeal candidosis? J Mol Med 76:70–73

Kick G, Korting HC (1998) Debilitating folliculitis barbae candidomycetica in a trumpeter: successful treatment with fluconazole. Mycoses 41:339–342

Kirkpatrick CH (1994) Chronic mucocutaneous candidiasis. J Am Acad Dermatol 31:14–17

Reich JD, Huddleston K, Jorgensen D et al. (1997) Neonatal *Torulopsis glabrata* fungemia. South Med J 90:246–248

Rello J, Esandi W, Diaz E et al. (1998) The role of *Candida* sp. isolated from bronchoscopic samples in nonneutropenic patients. Chest 114:146–149

Rosen RM (1996) Chronic mucocutaneous candidiasis with widespread dermatophyte infection: the trailing scale sign. Cutis 57:82–84

Safran DB, Dawson E (1997) The effect of empiric and prophylactic treatment with fluconazole on yeast isolates in a surgical trauma intensive care unit. Arch Surg 132:1184–1188; discussion 1188–1189

Samaranayake LP, Nair RG (1995) Oral *Candida* infections – a review. Indian J Dent Res 6:69–82

Tomsikova A (1998) Growing importance of non-*Candida* species as opportunistic pathogens. Cent Eur J Public Health 6:61–66

Tosti A, Piraccini BM, Vincenzi C et al. (1997) Itraconazole in the treatment of two young brothers with chronic mucocutaneous candidiasis. Pediatr Dermatol 14:146–148

Vincent JL, Anaissie E, Bruining H et al. (1998) Epidemiology, diagnosis and treatment of systemic *Candida* infection in surgical patients under intensive care. Intensive Care Med 24:201–216

Weers-Pothoff G, Havermans JF, Kamphuis J et al. (1997) *Candida tropicalis* arthritis in a patient with acute myeloid leukemia successfully treated with fluconazole: case report and review of the literature. Infection 25:109–111

Zaias-N (1997) *Candida*: a review of clinical experience with Lamisil. Dermatology 194:S10–S13

Sporotrichosis

Al-Tawfiq JA, Wools KK (1998) Disseminated sporotrichosis and *Sporothrix schenckii* fungemia as the initial presentation of human immunodeficiency virus infection. Clin Infect Dis 26:1403–1406

Karakayali G, Lenk N, Alli N et al. (1998) Itraconazole therapy in lymphocutaneous sporotrichosis: a case report and review of the literature. Cutis 61:106–107

Chromomycosis

Lee MW, Hsu S, Rosen T (1998) Spores and mycelia in cutaneous chromomycosis. J Am Acad Dermatol 39:850–852

Rivitti EA, Aoki V (1999) Deep fungal infections in tropical countries. Clin Dermatol 17:171–190

Silva JP, de Souza W, Rozental S (1999) Chromoblastomycosis: a retrospective study of 325 cases in Amazonic Region (Brazil). Mycopathologia 143:171–175

Mycetoma

Boiron P, Locci R, Goodfellow M et al. (1998) Nocardia, nocardiosis and mycetoma. Med Mycol 36:S26–S37

Davis JD, Stone PA, McGarry JJ (1999) Recurrent mycetoma of the foot. J Foot Ankle Surg 38:55–60

Mahaisavariya P, Chaiprasert A, Sivayathorn A et al. (1999) Deep fungal and higher bacterial skin infections in Thailand: clinical manifestations and treatment regimens. Int J Dermatol 38:279–284

Cryptococcosis

Aberg JA, Powderly WG (1997) Cryptococcosis. Adv Pharmacol 37:215–251

Hamilton AJ, Goodley J (1996) Virulence factors of *Cryptococcus neoformans*. Curr Top Med Mycol 7:19–42

Kauffman CA, Hedderwick S (1997) Opportunistic fungal infections: filamentous fungi and cryptococcosis. Geriatrics 52:40–42, 47–49

Korfel A, Menssen HD, Schwartz S et al. (1998) Cryptococcosis in Hodgkin's disease: description of two cases and review of the literature. Ann Hematol 76:283–286

Blastomycosis

Bradsher RW (1997) Therapy of blastomycosis. Semin Respir Infect 12:263–267

Chao D, Steler KJ, Gomila R (1997) Update and review of blastomycosis. J Am Osteopath Assoc 97:525–532

Vasquez JE, Mehta JB, Agrawal R et al. (1998) Blastomycosis in northeast Tennessee. Chest 114:436–443

Histoplasmosis

Akpuaka FC, Gugnani HC, Iregbulam LM (1998) African histoplasmosis: report of two patients treated with amphotericin B and ketoconazole. Mycoses 41:363–364

Butt AA, Carreon J (1997) *Histoplasma capsulatum* sinusitis. J Clin Microbiol 35:2649–2650

Gross ML, Millikan LE (1994) Deep fungal infections in the tropics. Dermatol Clin 12:695–700

Khalil MA, Hassan AW, Gugnani HC (1998) African histoplasmosis: report of four cases from north-eastern Nigeria. Mycoses 41:293–295

Onwuasoigwe O (1999) Fluconazole in the therapy of multiple osteomyelitis in African histoplasmosis. Int Orthop 23:82–84

Scheepers A, Lemmer J (1992) Disseminated histoplasmosis: aspects of oral diagnosis. J Dent Assoc S Afr 47: 441–443

Wheat J (1996) Histoplasmosis in the acquired immunodeficiency syndrome. Curr Top Med Mycol 7:7–18

Coccidioidomycosis

Galglani JN (1997) Coccidioidomycosis. Curr Clin Top Infect Dis 17:188–204

Herron LD, Kissel P, Smilovitz D (1997) Treatment of coccidioidal spinal infection: experience in 16 cases. J Spinal Disord 10:215–222

Myskowski PL, White NM, Ahkami R (1997) Fungal disease in the immunocompromised host. Dermatol Clin 15: 295–305

Paracoccidioidomycosis

Dos Santos JW, Michel GT, Londero AT (1997) Paracoccidioidoma: case record and review. Mycopathologia 137:83–85

Manns BJ, Baylis BW, Urbanski SJ et al. (1996) Paracoccidioidomycosis: case report and review. Clin Infect Dis 23:1026–1032

Lobomycosis

Brun AM (1999) Lobomycosis in three Venezuelan patients. Int J Dermatol 38:302–305

Elgart ML (1996) Unusual subcutaneous infections. Dermatol Clin 14:105–111

Restrepo A (1994) Treatment of tropical mycoses. J Am Acad Dermatol 31:S91–102

Rodriguez G, Barrera GP (1997) The asteroid body of lobomycosis. Mycopathologia 136:71–74

Taborda PR, Taborda VA, McGinnis MR (1999) *Lacazia loboi* gen. nov., comb. nov., the etiologic agent of lobomycosis. J Clin Microbiol 37:2031–2033

Aspergillosis

Latge JP (1999) *Aspergillus fumigatus* and aspergillosis. Clin Microbiol Rev 12:310–350

Paterson DL, Singh N (1999) Invasive aspergillosis in transplant recipients. Medicine 78:123–138

Van den Bergh MF, Verweij PE, Voss A (1999) Epidemiology of nosocomial fungal infections: invasive aspergillosis and the environment. Diagn Microbiol Infect Dis 34:221–227

Zygomycosis

Cuvelier I, Vogelaers D, Peleman R et al. (1998) Two cases of disseminated mucormycosis in patients with hematological malignancies and literature review. Eur J Clin Microbiol Infect Dis 17:859–863

Holland J (1997) Emerging zygomycoses of humans: *Saksenaea vasiformis* and *Apophysomyces elegans*. Curr Top Med Mycol 8:27–34

Lee FY, Mossad SB, Adal KA (1999) Pulmonary mucormycosis: the last 30 years. Arch Intern Med 159:1301–1309

Nenoff P, Kellermann S, Schober R et al. (1998) Rhinocerebral zygomycosis following bone marrow transplantation in chronic myelogenous leukaemia. Report of a case and review of the literature. Mycoses 41:365–372

Zavasky DM, Samowitz W, Loftus T et al. (1999) Gastrointestinal zygomycotic infection caused by *Basidiobolus ranarum*: case report and review. Clin Infect Dis 28: 1244–1248

Phycomycosis

Connolly JE Jr, McAdams HP, Erasmus JJ et al. (1999) Opportunistic fungal pneumonia. J Thorac Imaging 14:51–62

Linder N, Keller N, Huri C et al. (1998) Primary cutaneous mucormycosis in a premature infant: case report and review of the literature. Am J Perinatol 15:35–38

Mizutari K, Nishimoto K, Ono T (1999) Cutaneous mucormycosis. J Dermatol 26:174–177

Rhinosporidiosis

Shrestha SP, Hennig A, Parija SC (1998) Prevalence of rhinosporidiosis of the eye and its adnexa in Nepal. Am J Trop Med Hyg 59:231–234

Diseases Caused by Arthropods

Contents

This chapter is entitled Epizoonoses in the German edition. An epizoonosis is a disease caused by parasites living on the exterior surface of their host, for example on the skin. Because our scope is somewhat broader, including also arthropod bites by nonparasitic species and irritant contact dermatitis from simply touching other organisms, we have changed the title slightly. Two technical points must be made. First, it is incorrect to use to the term "insect bite" as both words are imprecise. Arthropods include insects, arachnids and many other animals. Insects have three body segments (head, thorax, and abdomen) and six legs, while arachnids, such as spiders, have two body segments (cephalothorax and abdomen) and eight legs. Centipedes and millipedes have bodies with many segments. Crustacea are another type of arthropod. Some *Cyclops* (water fleas) and crayfish are involved in the life-cycle of parasitic worms and are discussed in Chapter 9. In addition, some arthropods bite, that is inflict damage with their mouth parts, while others sting, using specially modified tail parts, such as bees and wasps. When a patient speaks of an insect bite, that is fine, but physicians should try to be more precise.

A number of factors determine the likelihood of arthropod assaults and their related diseases. They include both environmental and personal factors. At different times of the year in the same area, there may be marked differences. Mosquito bites are common in Alaska in summer but do not occur in winter. Even in tropical climates, there may be seasonal variation. In addition there are variants in microhabitat. Some arthropods favor fast-moving water; others, slow. Some fly only a few meters off the ground; others get much higher. A lack of personal hygiene or job and social requirements, such as walking many miles through water or washing clothes in a stream, may greatly increase the risk of exposure. The number of Europeans vacationing in tropical climates has greatly increased the number of previously uncommon epizootic diseases seen in more temperate countries.

Insects

Lice

Lice are insects with six legs, each equipped with strong claws. The females use an insoluble glue to glue their eggs, known as nits, to either hairs or clothing seams (Fig. 8.1). The larvae hatch in 8 days, go through three nymphal stages and are sexually mature after 2–3 weeks. They usually take a blood meal every few hours and cannot last more than a few days without blood. There are three major types of lice. A number of new names and subspecies have been described but they are of little clinical importance.

They are:

- *Pediculus humanus capitis*: head louse
- *Pediculus humanus corporis*: body louse
- *Phthirus pubis*: pubic louse

Pediculosis Capitis

Definition. Louse infestation of the scalp, frequently seen in school epidemics with no associated diseases.

Causative Organism. *Pediculus humanus capitis*, the head louse, has an elongated body and is 2–3.5 mm long.

Epidemiology. Children and individuals with long hair are more likely to be affected. The arthropods are transmitted from human to human, either via direct contact or by sharing combs, brushes and towels. Inadequate hygiene and close living conditions enhance their spread. Small epidemics are not uncommon in schools, much to the dismay of parents and teachers. Sharing of caps, combs and towels, as well as close contact during play, are held responsible.

Etiology and Pathogenesis. The louse lives on the scalp where it attaches its eggs or nits to the hair shaft. It feeds by taking a blood meal from the scalp. The bites tend to be pruritic and often become secondarily infected with bacteria following scratching. *Borrelia recurrentis*, the cause of louse-borne relapsing fever, can be transmitted by the head louse, but otherwise the insect is not a disease vector.

Clinical Findings. In general only the scalp is involved. Rarely eyebrows, eyelashes, pubic hairs or beard hairs may be affected. A favorite site is the area behind the ears (Fig. 8.2). Even though lice feed every few hours, it is usually a matter of days before symptoms appear. The bite produces an urticarial reaction. The delay suggests that at least part of the reaction is allergic. The intense itching and scratching often produce a dermatitis, called

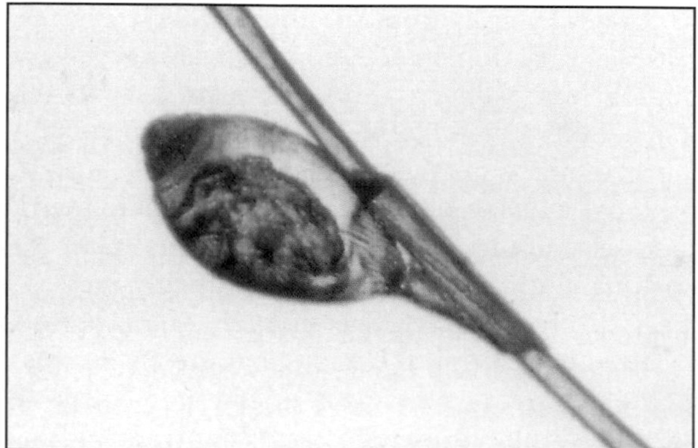

Fig. 8.1. Nit of *Pediculus humanus capitis* attached to scalp hair

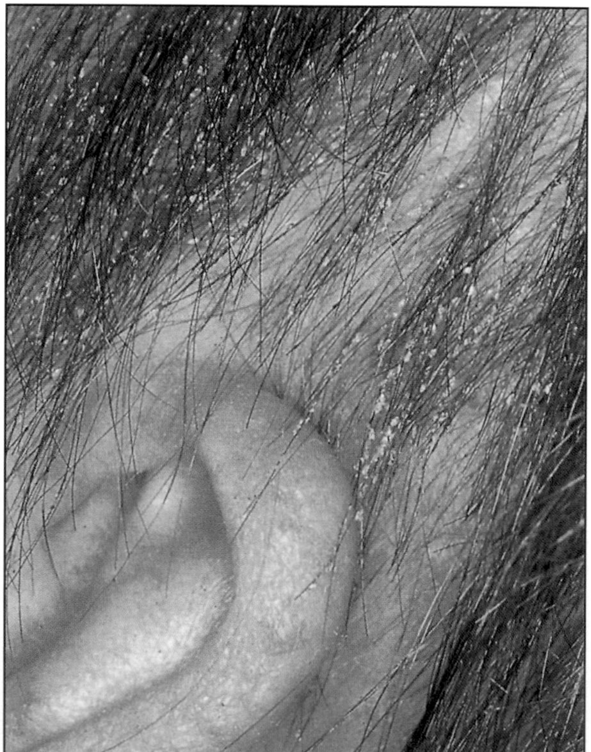

Fig. 8.2. Numerous nits and lice on scalp hair

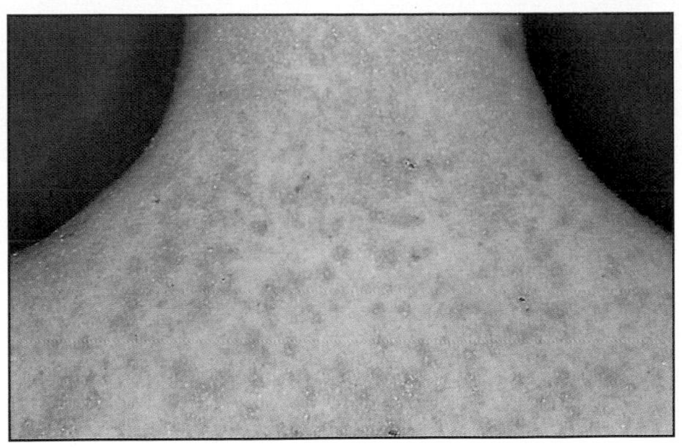

Fig. 8.3. Dermatitis on nape secondary to lice infestation of scalp

louse eczema in German (Fig. 8.3). Both the nits and the moving lice can be seen by the patients themselves or their carers, so usually the diagnosis is made for the physician. In more severe causes, there may be secondary bacterial infection and lymphadenopathy.

Laboratory Findings. One can examine either the louse or the nits under the microscope. The lice are straightforward. The nits are very firmly attached to the hairs and grow away from the scalp with the hairs. They resemble a bud branching away from the hair at an angle containing a 0.8-mm egg in a chitin hull. If the little cap, seen nicely in Fig. 8.1, is missing, then the egg has hatched. In patients with scalp pruritus and dermatitis, one should always search the hairs behind the ears carefully for nits.

Differential Diagnosis. Clinically, one must exclude atopic dermatitis, seborrheic dermatitis, impetigo, folliculitis and pityriasis amiantacea. Under the microscope, nits must be distinguished from hair casts, which are cylindrical and slide along the hair, and in the axilla from trichomycosis axillaris which is caused by clumping of bacteria.

Therapy. There are a number of possibilities. All balance minor degrees of toxicity against varying degrees of effectiveness.

Permethrin. This synthetic pyrethroid is probably the treatment of choice. Its method of action appears to be by altering the arthropod neural transmission, causing paralysis. It is available in the USA as Nix (1%) cream rinse. The product is applied for 10 min and rinsed off. There are no common side effects.

Pyrethrins. Chrysanthemums are the source of these agents which also interfere with nerve conduction. The pyrethrins are sold over-the-counter in the USA as RID and A-200, along with many other names. The major product in Germany is Goldgeist Forte (the strong golden ghost). Piperonyl butoxide is sometimes added to prolong their activity by blocking degradation. The pyrethrins are usually applied for 10 min and then rinsed off. Sometimes the procedure is repeated in 24–48 h. In Germany the same product is available as a spray; in this case one must be worried about terrarium and aquarium animals. In addition, this class should be avoided during pregnancy and in small infants.

Lindane or γ-Benzene Hexachloride. While used mainly for scabies, lindane is also effective against lice, but not as effective as the agents listed above. For head lice, it can be used as a shampoo or applied as a cream or gel. In Germany, the gel form is left on overnight, rinsed out, re-applied and then rinsed again after another 24 h. The procedure may be repeated in 1 week. In the USA, prolonged exposure to lindane has drawn undeserved criticism. Shampooing, leaving the lather on for 5–10 min, and then rinsing is recommended. Lindane should not be used in pregnancy or for small children.

Malathion. The most effective medication against head lice is this flammable organic insecticide, which kills a high percentage of arthropods very quickly. In a classic study, it achieved almost total lice kill within 5 min and a 95% ovicidal effect. It is no longer available in the USA, but is used in Germany and around the world.

No matter what the treatment, the ovicidal effect is not 100%. Some degree of resistance has been documented for each category of treatment. Since the nits take a week to hatch, the patient should be reexamined after that time and re-treated only if living lice are found. How to remove the nits is a problem that causes great concern. Some public health authorities refuse to recognize the over 90% ovicidal effect of most treatments and will not let appropriately treated children with nits back into school. While nit combs (very fine-toothed combs) or tweezers are helpful, and a rinse with one part kitchen vinegar to two parts water helps considerably to dissolve the nit glue, probably the best solution is a very short hair cut. At home, new combs and brushes should be purchased or the old ones disinfected in one of the antilouse preparations or in water at 60 °C for 5 min.

Public Health Measures. All contact individuals should be examined and treated as necessary.

Pediculosis Corporis

Synonyms. Pediculosis vestimentorum, vagabond's itch

Definition. Infestation associated with poor personal hygiene and the potential for disease transmission.

Causative Organism. *Pediculus humanus corporis*, the body louse, is very closely related to the head louse. There are subspecies that can cross-breed. For medical purposes, the two are separated on the basis of habitat, but entomologically, the issue is more complex (Fig. 8.4). Some entomologists distinguish among different subspecies infesting Orientals, Africans and Native Americans.

Epidemiology. Body lice are almost by definition associated with poor hygiene and unsanitary living conditions. For this reason, they are a disease of the homeless and common among both soldiers and civilians in war-torn areas. Simultaneous infestation with several louse types is not unusual.

Etiology and Pathogenesis. The body louse feeds on the body but lays its eggs on the clothes, especially favoring seams. The life-cycle is similar to that of the head louse. *P. humanus corporis* is a significant public health problem because it is capable of transferring several infectious diseases. It carries epidemic typhus (*Rickettsia prowazeki*), louse-borne relapsing fever (*Borrelia recurrentis*), and Wolhynia or trench fever (*Rochalimea quintana*). Students of history may know that all of these occurred as epidemics during both World War I and World War II.

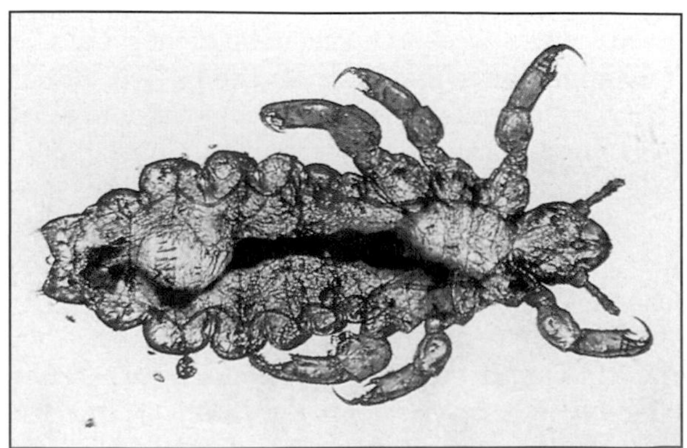

Fig. 8.4. *Pediculus humanus corporis*

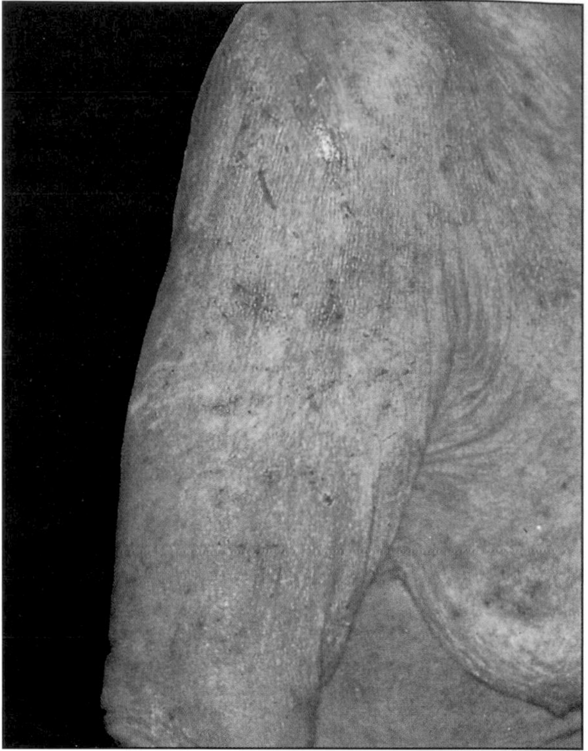

Fig. 8.5. Vagabond's skin

Clinical Findings. The saliva of the louse triggers erythema, urticarial lesions and intensely pruritic papules and nodules. Eventually the patient develops numerous excoriations, secondary infections and even lymphadenopathy. The combination of excoriations, hyperpigmentation, healed scars and secondary impetiginization is quite typical and is known as vagabond's skin or vagabond's itch (Fig. 8.5).

Laboratory Findings. The nits can be found in the clothing.

Differential Diagnosis. All pruritic dermatoses must be considered. In a homeless or unclean patient, it is easier to first exclude body lice by examining the seams than it is to worry about the entire differential diagnosis.

Therapy. The clothes must be disinfected. Washing and rinsing in hot water followed by ironing the seams usually suffices. Most patients will not do this, so it is simplest to turn them over to hospital social services who usually have a protocol involving new clothes or professional handling of the infested garments. The almost invariably present dermatitis should be treated with topical antipruritics or corticosteroids. In some settings a short course of oral antibiotics may be needed to treat the associated pyoderma.

Public Health Measures. Checking of contacts is ideal but rarely practical.

Pediculosis Pubis

Synonyms. Crabs, phthiriasis

Definition. Infestation usually involving the pubic hairs, although other hairy sites can be affected.

Causative Organism. *Phthirus pubis. Phthirus* is the correct spelling but the official nomenclature committee overlooked a misprint, so the form *Pthirus* may also be found.

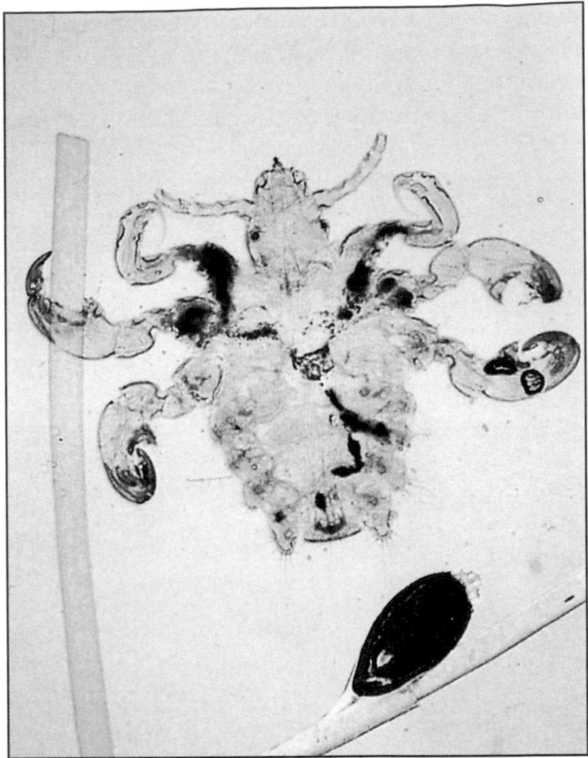

Fig. 8.6. Crab-shaped *Phthirus pubis* with nit

Epidemiology. Transmission in adults occurs most during sexual intercourse, although any intimate personal contact suffices. In children without pubic hairs, the scalp hairs and eyelashes are more often involved, although the infestation is uncommon in this age group. Shared wash cloths and underwear offer other possibilities for transmission.

Etiology and Pathogenesis. The pubic louse or crab is smaller than the head or body louse and has a broader, less-elongated body. Thus the resemblance to a crab is more than fanciful (Fig. 8.6). The second and third pairs of legs end in prominent claws that the louse uses to grasp hairs, usually close to their base. They breed slowly and attach their nits to the hairs, just as do head lice.

Clinical Findings. The preferred habitat for pubic lice is regions rich in apocrine glands. Thus they are most often found in the pubic and axillary hairs. Occasionally they may be found on abdominal or trunk hairs and on rare occasions they may be seen on the scalp, eyebrows and even eyelashes. Typically numerous lice and nits are seen by the patient, partner or parent (Fig. 8.7). Facial involvement is more common in children. The pruritus is modest so that excoriations are uncommon. A classic clinical finding is the maculae ceruleae (*tâches bleues*) – flat, indistinct blue-gray or slate-colored macules ranging in size from several millimeters to several centimeters. They result from the bite of the louse causing small intracutaneous hemorrhages involving blood whose hemoglobin has been altered by the saliva.

Laboratory Findings. The organisms can be easily found and identified under the microscope.

Therapy. All the treatments suggested for *P. humanus capitis* are effective. Often lindane lotion is left

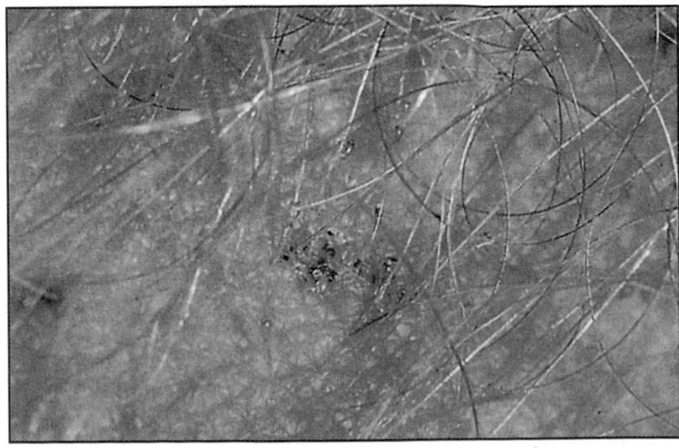

Fig. 8.7. *Phthirus pubis* adults and nits

on overnight and then rinsed out. In hairy individuals, the axillary and body hairs may also require treatment. Eyelash and eyebrow involvement is complicated; the safest treatment is simply repeated applications of petrolatum to suffocate the lice and then removal with tweezers. Physostigmine ophthalmic ointment 0.025% has been recommended on the basis that the medication paralyzes the lice, but it may just be an expensive way to apply petrolatum.

Public Health Measures. Contacts should be checked and treated.

True Bugs (Hemiptera)

Bedbugs

Causative Organism. *Cimex lectularius.* The bedbug is a member of the large family of biting bugs, known as *Wanzen* in German or Cimidae in entomologic terms.

Epidemiology. While other animals (such as swallows, chickens) also have Cimidae, their bugs cause only transient pruritic urticarial papules should they bite humans. The human bedbug *C. lectularius*, on the other hand, is a cause of significant human misery in temperate zones. Other species such as *C. hemipterus* and *C. rotundus* live in the tropics. Bedbugs are fond of darkness, so they spend their days in cracks along the floor boards, in furniture, behind pictures and in similar sites. In the past, it was very difficult to eradicate bedbugs from a room or house; modern insecticides have made the task somewhat easier.

Etiology and Pathogenesis. A female bedbug is 5 mm long and 3 mm wide; her mate is smaller. While the unfed bug is translucent, the sated version is enlarged and dark-red. Another feature is an unpleasant odor secreted by glands near the third pair of legs. The female bedbug lays two or three eggs daily. They develop over 1–2 months through several nymphal stages. The bedbug goes on the hunt for food in the night. It feeds about once weekly and can go for long periods of time without eating. It is probably attracted by the warmth and smell of its victim, either crawling to the bed or dropping down off the ceiling. In just a few minutes the blood meal is completed. The bedbug is not responsible for the transmission of diseases.

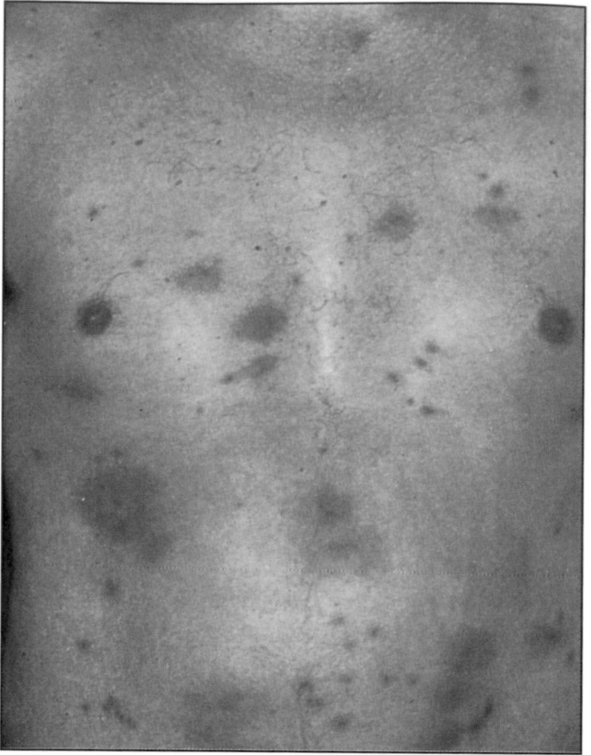

Fig. 8.8. Multiple bed bug bites

Clinical Findings. The typical clinical finding is several erythematous papules or urticarial lesions grouped together. Often three appear in a row (breakfast, lunch and dinner), but of course the bedbug does not keep count and both solitary bites and many lesions are common. The saliva causes urticaria and apparently an allergic reaction, as individuals with long exposure to bedbugs appear to react less (Figs. 8.8, 8.9). Diascopic examination reveals a hemorrhagic dot, the site of the bite, in the

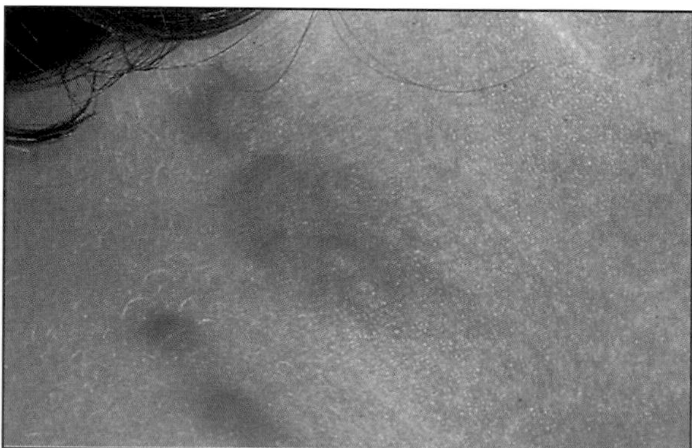

Fig. 8.9. Closer view of bed bug bites showing urticarial nature and linear arrangement

middle of many lesions. The most typical sites are arms, legs and face. On the face, lid edema may develop. The urticarial lesions evolve into firm papules that persist for several days and are typically pruritic and excoriated. Rarely blisters may appear, especially in areas with poor circulation. In patients with tolerance, the bites may produce no signs. Still, one may find spots of blood and bug feces on the sheets or bedclothes as a clue.

Laboratory Findings. Only rarely is a bug brought in by the patient. A biopsy of a lesion will show a typical arthropod bite reaction, but without any clue as to etiology.

Differential Diagnosis. Acute urticaria, other bites, papular urticaria or prurigo simplex acuta and erythema multiforme must all be considered. Since the diagnosis is clinical, often a definite answer is not available.

Therapy. Topical antipruritics or corticosteroids can be tried against the pruritus. In severe cases, systemic antihistamines can be used. Most important is having an exterminator inspect and treat the involved room.

Reduviid Bugs

Synonyms. Kissing bugs, conenose bugs, assassin bugs

The reduviid bugs are flying nocturnal insects capable of causing painful bites as well as transmitting *Trypanosoma cruzi*, the causative agent of Chagas disease. Several different species are involved in the transmission. The protozoa is found in the feces of the bug, so that fecal contamination of a bite is required. Should one encounter a kissing bug, it is wise to gently remove it, not slap or crush it. As far as biting goes, most of the bugs found in the USA are *Triatoma*. The kissing bugs typically bite around the mouth. Their painless bite can cause marked allergic reactions including giant urticaria, bullae and even anaphylaxis. Topical and systemic antipruritic measures usually suffice to treat the individual bite.

Beetles

Beetles (Coleoptera) are one of the largest families of insects. They range from the beloved lady bug to large beautiful scarabs to plant pests. The Meloidae and Oedemeridae beetles produce cantharidin, a blistering agent. The best known member of the family is *Lytta vesicata*, the Spanish fly. Most outbreaks of Meloidae blister beetle dermatosis occur in southern Europe in the summer months, although the beetles have a world-wide distribution. Oedemeridae are smaller beetles found in New Zealand and the Caribbean, especially the Florida Keys. Exposure to its blistering toxin can occur when the live beetle is handled, as it can exude from various joints. A crushed beetle is more likely to produce problems. Cantharidin is used to intentionally produce blistering in the treatment of warts and has alleged aphrodisiac properties because it causes bladder and urethral irritation when ingested.

A third group of blister beetles are those of the genus *Paederus* or rove beetles. These arthropods secrete paederin, a virulent blistering agent that elicits a prominent urticarial reaction as well as blisters.

Orthoptera

Grasshoppers, roaches and their relatives cause problems primarily by destroying crops. Even the fearsome praying mantis rarely bites humans. Cockroaches, more often the imported German cockroach, are an unfortunate reality of many dwellings, especially if unclean. Allergic reactions to their body parts and detritus are a major cofactor in causing asthma in inner city children.

Fleas

Fleas are among the most amazing athletes in the arthropod world. They cannot fly but can spring or jump great distances. They are highly specialized to a given host, but may leave this favored host to bite humans. Fleas are major vectors of human disease.

Human Fleas

Causative Organism. *Pulex irritans* is 2–4 mm long and can jump about 50 cm vertically and 60 cm sideways. An equally springy 6-foot human would have to achieve a high jump of 1000 feet and a long jump of 1200 feet.

Epidemiology. Fleas are a worldwide problem. They are disturbed by light and spend their time in tiny cracks and crevices, buried deep in carpet or in furniture. While they have become much less common with modern vacuum cleaners, they are still encountered. We also occasionally see patients with flea bites obtained in theaters or public transportation.

Etiology and Pathogenesis. Captive human fleas live about 18 months; other species have survived over 5 years in flea circuses. The female flea lays about 500 eggs which go through several larval forms over a 3–6-week period and then become an imago in a cocoon. In this form they can remain inactive for over 1 year. When the room shows signs of life, perhaps vibrations or localized warmth, the flea hatches and starts looking for a blood meal. A flea is a very flexible eater; it can feed several times daily or fast for weeks. The saliva contains anticoagulants, making feeding easier.

The human flea rarely transmits disease. In epidemics of plague, it is capable of transmitting *Yersinia pestis.*

Clinical Findings. Flea bites are typically multiple irregularly distributed wheals and papules on the covered body regions. The wheals are quite distinct because diascopic examination almost always identifies a central hemorrhagic bite site (Fig. 8.10). The hemorrhage is known as purpura pulicosa (flea purpura), and sometimes can be quite prominent (Fig. 8.11). Rarely individuals may react with large blisters. This is most common on the legs where large subepidermal blisters resembling bullous pemphigoid may arise. In children, sometimes there are a large number of bites producing papular urticaria. The presence of the hemorrhagic puncta helps one decide if all the lesions are bites or if some are allergic reactions to the bites (papular urticaria or strophulus).

Differential Diagnosis. Acute urticaria, papular urticaria, acute prurigo and other bites must be excluded. In the USA most flea bites are from dog or cat fleas. Rarely chicken pox may be confused with bites during the first few hours of its course.

Therapy. Topical and systemic antipruritic treatment suffices. The home should be evaluated by an exterminator. Because of the difficulty in distinguishing between the bites of *Pulex irritans* and those of dog and cat fleas, if pets are in the household they and their beds should be checked. Insect repellents are also useful.

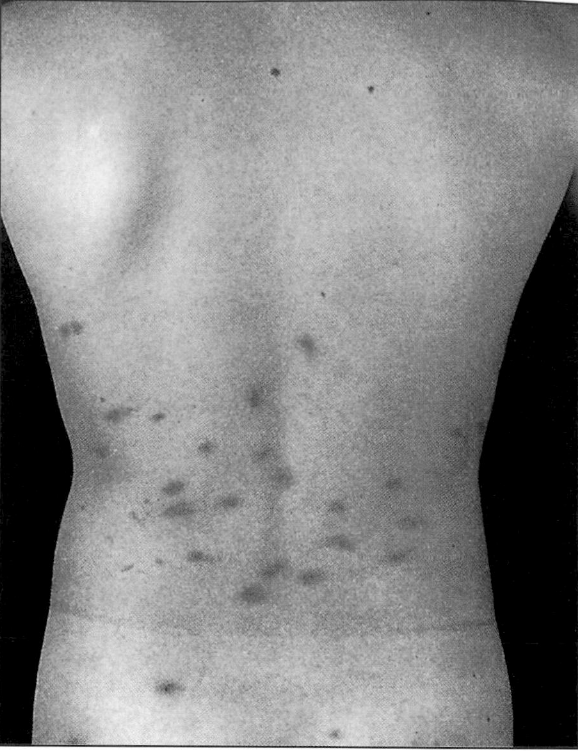

Fig. 8.10. Flea bites

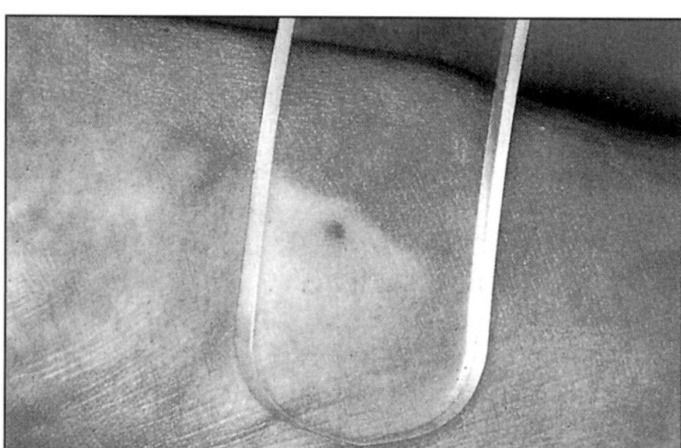

Fig. 8.11. Diascopy demonstrates the purpuric nature of a flea bite

Sand Fleas

Causative Organism. *Tunga penetrans*

Epidemiology. The sand flea is widespread in tropical America and Africa. It initially was native to the Americas, but was taken back to West Africa by slave traders on their return trips. It has since spread to the western coast of India as well. It lives in sandy soils, not necessarily beaches as often suggested.

Etiology and Pathogenesis. The pregnant 1.5-mm long female, also known as a chigoe or jigger, enters the skin of the feet of individuals visiting an infested beach. Over 1–2 weeks she achieves a size of about 1 cm. Her posterior with both the breathing apparatus and genitalia protrudes out of the skin. After laying about 300 eggs, the female dies.

Clinical Findings. The most typical sites for a sand flea attack are underneath the toenails and between the toes, but lesions can be found on the soles as well as about the genitalia. Initially there may be pruritus, erythema and pain, but soon it becomes clear that more than a bite has occurred as the body of the flea is observed. There is a marked foreign body reaction, resembling a furuncle with swelling, erythema and drainage of pus. Lymphangitis often occurs, and gas gangrene and tetanus have been described. In immunocompromised patients, there may often be a massive infestation.

Laboratory Findings. The worm can be identified if extracted. Alternatively, it can be found amidst marked inflammation in a biopsy specimen.

Differential Diagnosis. Often the lesion is mistaken for a subungual or plantar wart or a pyogenic granuloma.

Therapy. The worm must be mechanically removed or excised. Often a course of oral antibiotics is wise if secondary infection appears to be present. If patients have multiple lesions, a course of systemic thiabendazole (25–50 mg/kg daily for 2–4 days) or niridazole may be valuable. Using insecticides in shoes and socks when visiting tropical beaches may be useful prophylaxis.

Other Fleas

A variety of other fleas are responsible for both skin problems in humans and disease transmission. The cat flea (*Ctenocephalides felis*) and the dog flea (*C. canis*) are far more common than the human flea in the USA. Often the fleas only attack the pet owners when the pets are unavailable for a meal, such as away in a kennel. Then the fleas come out of hiding and avail themselves of the next best host. Children in close contact with pets are more likely to be bitten. Both multiple bites and papular urticaria may occur. The hemorrhagic puncta are not as often seen as with *Pulex irritans*. Rat fleas may transfer murine typhus and plague.

Hymenoptera

Hymenoptera are a large group, including bees, bumble bees, wasps, hornets and ants, all of which are capable of delivering painful stings that can lead to allergic reactions and even death.

Bees and Wasps

Etiology and Pathogenesis. Bees can only sting once. A bee's stinging apparatus has reverse barbs and is pulled out of the insect after its attack. In contrast, wasps and bumble bees can sting several times. Hymenoptera venoms are amazingly complex, leading to a variety of clinical symptoms and making desensitization a challenge. While native Northern European and North American bumble bees and honey bees are not aggressive, the African honey bees are quite aggressive and have been moving northward in the United States since coming from South America, where they were introduced from Africa. Wasps are typically encountered when eating outdoors in Europe. (In Bavaria many visitors to beer gardens place a special cover over their mug to keep wasps out.) Swallowing a drowning wasp can be life-threatening. Otherwise, wasps, hornets, and yellow-jackets are usually encountered only if one disturbs their nest.

Clinical Findings. The classic findings of bee sting are well known: pain, pruritus, erythema and swelling. Often the changes persist for several days. Periorbital bites are particularly likely to cause lid edema while those around the lips may produce a trunk-like swelling. The prominently decorated lips so fashionable today in the USA are called "bee sting lips". Occasionally the insects find their way into the mouth, where the risk of tongue and glottis edema with subsequent airway problems is great. Multiple stings can lead to widespread urticaria and to systemic toxicity, including cardiovascular problems. Repeat stings can produce a type I sensitivity against various components of the venom, placing the individual at risk of life-threatening anaphylaxis and laryngeal edema. On the other hand, there is some degree of hardening as bee keepers often scarcely notice bites and desensitization is possible in the clinic as well.

Therapy. The management of a bee or wasp sting is dependent on the presence or absence of sensitization. In a normal host, the stringer should be removed if still present. First-aid measures, such as applying ice to reduce spread of toxin, and use of topical antipruritic agents or corticosteroids suffice. If pruritus is intense, systemic antihistamines can be provided. If a more severe reaction begins to develop, then the patient must be handled just as in any other anaphylactic reaction.

Prophylaxis. Insect repellents may help somewhat, as well as not wearing colorful clothes, always wearing shoes and avoiding perfumes and other scented products. Patients with a previous history of allergic reaction should carry an emergency kit. Typically such kits contain injectable epinephrine, oral antihistamines a corticosteroid solution and a tourniquet. Corticosteroid and epinephrine inhalers may also be useful.

Immunotherapy or desensitization should be employed for anyone who has a systemic reaction to an insect sting. It can be considered in patients with a definite history of severe local reactions with positive RAST findings. Skin testing and immunization should be done in a setting where emergency care is available, since severe reactions to both prick testing and desensitization can occur. The risk of a severe reaction is reduced by about a factor of ten with adequate desensitization.

Ants

Most ants in both Europe and North America are harmless. In the southeastern United States, the imported red fire ant, *Solenopsis invicta*, and the black fire ant, *S. richteri*, are causing significant problems. While there are native species of *Solenopsis* capable of causing painful stings, they are not as aggressive as the imported species. The ants build large mounds, often in pastures but also along roadsides or in yards. If a human or animal ventures into this domicile, they are subjected to hundreds of painful stings. Their venom is highly toxic, containing primarily alkaloids of the piperidine family. The typical lesion is a tiny pustule with an erythematous, hemorrhagic halo, which can be reproduced by injecting the alkaloid. In many cases, the ants grab tightly with their jaws and then sting several times in a circular pattern as they swing around. Large urticarial lesions can arise, as well as systemic neurologic symptoms if many bites occur. In patients sensitized to the venom by previous exposure, anaphylaxis, shock and even death can occur. The bites can be treated with ice packs, oral antihistamines and topical antipruritics or corticosteroids. Secondary infection is so common that some prescribe oral antibiotics. If multiple bites are present, the patient should be monitored for more serious problems.

Diptera

Diptera include flies, mosquitoes and many related species. Their stings and bites cause local skin reactions, but in many cases they also transmit diseases. Furthermore, some fly larvae infest human skin while others ingest it. Their bites typically produce wheals that evolve into pruritic papules and nodules.

Mosquitoes

Etiology and Pathogenesis. Mosquitoes are the most significant arthropod disease vector. In many settings, there can be transovarian transmission, that is the offspring of an infected mosquito can be infective prior to even having a blood meal. Thus the arthropods serve as both reservoir and vector. The females take blood meals while the males drink plant products. There are thousands of different mosquitoes, only a few of which are adapted to transmit disease. The others are simply great pests, making large areas of the world uncomfortable for outdoor living over long periods of time. Mosquitoes require still water for breeding and development; thus, swamps, wetlands, and even puddles or old car tires are ideal habitats.

Mosquitoes can probably transmit any bloodborne disease. Among the diseases of which they are clearly vectors are some of mankind's greatest problems: malaria, filariasis, yellow fever, dengue and many types of encephalitis. It has been suggested that they may play a very small role in the spread of HIV/AIDS, but we suspect this is a theoretical concern.

Clinical Findings. The bites are usually multiple pruritic, often excoriated papules (Fig. 8.12). Secondary infection is common, especially in children. Bullous reactions are common; they are sometimes designated culicosis bullosa (Fig. 8.13). Just as with flea bites, occasionally mosquito bites on the shins or other sites may produce large blisters. These blisters are so dramatic and puzzling that they were formerly diagnosed as pemphigus hystericus (since the blister is subepidermal, pemphigoid hystericus would have been better). Such reactions are espe-

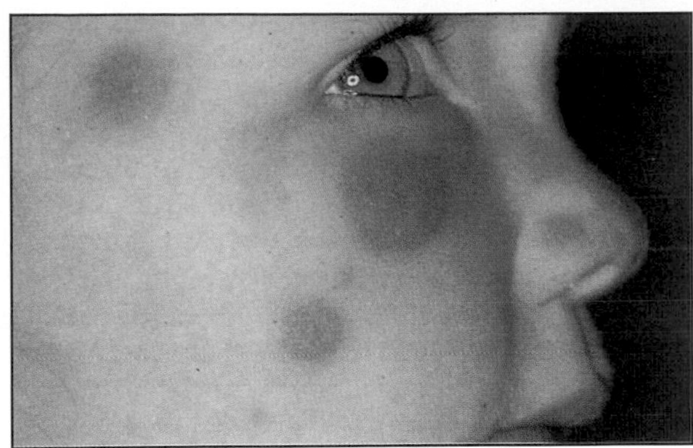

Fig. 8.12. Mosquito bites

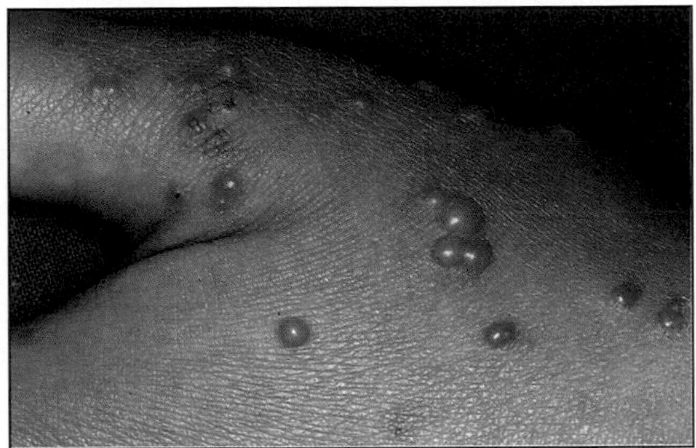

Fig. 8.13. Bullous reaction of mosquito bites

cially common in patients with chronic lymphocytic leukemia (Chap. 62). Systemic reactions to mosquito bites, even multiple ones, are uncommon but do occur in children.

Therapy. Antipruritic or corticosteroid creams or lotions are all that is usually needed. Occasionally oral antihistamines and/or antibiotics may be required.

Prophylaxis. Avoidance of mosquito bites is the wisest solution. Most insect repellents are also useful. In general they have earned their spurs against mosquitoes. Di-ethyltoluamide (deet) is most effective; one should seek the highest concentration in a suitable vehicle. In addition, protective clothing and mosquito netting are important. Studies have shown that in Africa, mosquito netting is about the most cost effective public health measure after sanitary drinking water. The mosquito habitat can also be attacked; there is no need for standing water around most homes. More large-scale attacks with insecticides, for example sprayed from airplanes, surely reduce the mosquito count, but their environmental risk:benefit ratio is controversial.

Flies

While most flies do not bite humans, those that do seem to make up for their comrades. In addition flies transfer a number of diseases. All flies are fairly well repulsed by insect repellents. The following is an incomplete list:

Deer and Horse Flies (Tabanidae)

These large flies are usually found in summer near water. They produce very painful urticarial lesions. In addition, deer flies transmit tularemia and loaiasis.

Stable Flies (*Stomoxys*)

Stable flies are known as *Wadenstecher* (calf biters) in German. They are found in the countryside. A typical scenario is a bite on the calf while pausing during a hike or bicycle ride. Large painful urticarial lesions evolve and heal very slowly.

House Flies (*Musca domestica*)

Bites are not the problems; they are rare and minor. Houseflies are responsible for transferring bacteria from spoiled food and excrement they favor to humans, usually via food. They carry no harmful organisms within their bodies, but serve as simple surface vectors.

Black Flies

Also known as buffalo gnats in the Northern USA and Canada, these flies bedevil canoeists as they live near fast flowing streams. They delight in biting about the face and crawling into the nares or ears. The nape is another favorite site. While the North American black flies *(Similium venustum)* do not transmit disease, their relatives in the genus *Similium* are the vectors of onchocerciasis in both Africa and Central and South America.

Sandflies

These flies are poor fliers, living and flying close to the ground. The major genera are *Phlebotomus* in Africa and *Lutzomyia* in the Americas. Their bites typically produce small urticarial papules, but the main problem is that they transmit leishmaniasis and bartonellosis, as well as Pappataci fever (sandfly fever) and several other viral febrile illnesses.

The sandflies in the USA (*Culicoides*), also known as no-see-ums, are small enough to easily pass through screening. They have extremely painful bites but transmit no diseases.

Tsetse Flies

These tiny creatures make vast areas of Africa almost uninhabitable as they are responsible for transmitting sleeping sickness or African trypanosomiasis.

Myiasis

Etiology and Pathogenesis. Myiasis is the presence of fly larvae in tissue (Fig. 8.14). There are two types of myiasis. Some larvae require the presence of living tissue. In most cases, animals are the intended host and humans accidental victims. This form is known as obligate or furuncular myiasis. In other situations, any fly can accidentally deposit its eggs in necrotic tissue, such as a wound or ulcer where the larvae may develop. A cofactor in such settings is usually a lack of cleanliness.

One major cause of human myiasis is the botfly (*Dermatobia hominis*) whose larvae are often transferred by mosquitoes. The usual host is cattle but humans can be involved. The range extends from the extreme southern USA into Mexico, and Central and South America. The rabbit botfly is the main endemic cause of myiasis in the USA. The screw-worm fly has been eradicated in the USA but causes major problems in cattle further south. The tumbu fly (*Cordylobia anthropophaga*) of tropical Africa lays its eggs on the ground or in clothing. The larvae usually grab a passing rat but may attach to humans, for example when lying on a beach that is contaminated. Other flies lay their eggs on mosquitoes, which may then transfer them to humans. Any fly can cause wound or accidental myiasis. Even the common house fly can invade wounds, although it never attacks the adjacent healthy tissue. Blow fly maggots were formerly sold for surgical wound debridement. In other species, the maggots move into normal tissue, increasing the amount of damage.

Clinical Findings. Furuncular myiasis not surprisingly mimics a furuncle (Fig. 8.15). The key feature is the presence of a tiny hole in the inflamed erythematous papule. With a loupe or dermatoscope, the spiracle or breathing tube of the warble or maggot can be seen. Sometimes multiple maggots are present and the lesion is fluctuant and hemorrhagic. A dead giveaway is a sensation of motion within a furuncle. In accidental myiasis, there is a pre-existing lesion, usually a leg ulcer, wound or ulcerated basal cell carcinoma. The bed of the wound is in motion as many tiny white "worms" move about.

Differential Diagnosis. One must consider furuncles, carbuncles and other deep infections.

Therapy. The maggot must be removed. The easiest technique is to anesthetize the area and extract the insect manually. Alternatively, the breathing hole can be occluded by petrolatum, chewing gum or household glue, eventually suffocating the maggot. Even more massive inflammation may occur after the animal's death. In some societies, a piece of fat meat is fastened over the hole. If one is lucky, the air-seeking maggot will migrate into the fat. When multiple maggots are present, surgical debridement is the best solution.

Larva Migrans

Rarely fly maggots, primarily from horse flies, can burrow under the skin, causing larva migrans. This

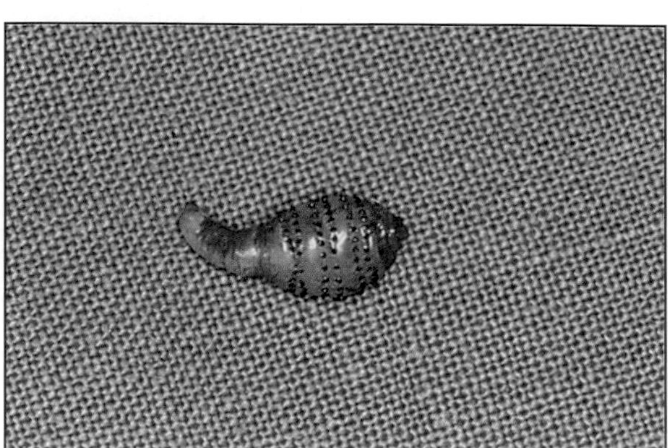

Fig. 8.14. Maggot or fly larva

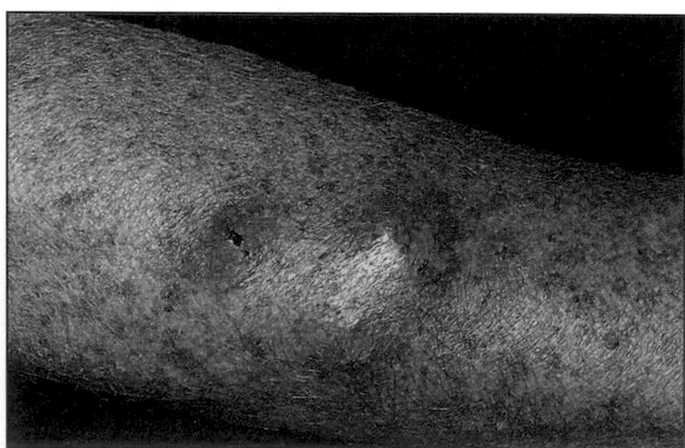

Fig. 8.15. Myiasis, resembling a furuncle

is discussed in Chapter 9, as larva migrans is usually caused by worms.

Butterflies and Moths

These lovely insects usually cause no damage themselves but their caterpillars have a variety of protective mechanisms, some of which can injure humans. Many caterpillars have fine hair-like spines that can introduce toxins into the skin. They may fall out of trees and land on victims, or even gain access through ventilation systems. Species often involved include larvae of the procession spinner (Thaumetopoeidae) and the bear spinner (Arctiidae) in Europe, as well as the gypsy moth (*Lymantria*), io moth (*Automeris io*) and several other species in the USA. The lesions are tiny urticarial papules, often in a linear arrangement, and often on the nape, face and arms. In the south of Germany, epidemics of gypsy moth caterpillar dermatitis have been seen in recent years.

Some adult moths may also cause pruritus and skin lesions. Best studied are those of the *Hylesia* genus. Major epidemics of brown tail moth (*H. alinda*) dermatitis have been reported from Cozumel, Mexico. In addition, Caripito itch has been described in the crew of a ship that stopped at Caripito, Venezuela. So many *Hylesia* were attracted to the ship's lights that 34 of 35 sailors developed a pruritic papulourticarial eruption, primarily on exposed skin surfaces.

Arachnids

Spiders

Spiders, along with scorpions, mites and ticks, are the medically important arachnids. Spiders are carnivores that live on other insects. Most pose no threat to humans other than a potentially painful bite. Even the large wolf, bird and tarantula spiders, despite their fearsome appearance, are generally harmless.

Black Widow Spider

Etiology and Pathogenesis. *Lactrodectus mactans* is a very widespread spider, missing only in the far north of the USA, middle Europe and the Far East. It is dark-gray to black. The female is 15 mm long, while the male is one-third as big. On the abdomen is a distinctive red hourglass marking. Black widows have earned their name because the female kills the male after mating, and becomes by her own action a widow. Black widows have a propensity for outhouses, but are also found in wood piles, barns, sheds and similar settings. Their main toxin is a neurotoxin, α-latrotoxin, which retards neuromuscular transmission.

Clinical Findings. The bite of the black widow is not a dermatologic problem, but an emergency medical one. When outhouses were more common, the penis was the most common site of the bite. Today hands and legs are favored locations. Often the bite is barely noticed and only tiny dots mark the site. Within a few minutes the patient experiences intense pain, associated with cramping, muscular rigidity and a variety of other symptoms including diaphoresis, nausea, vomiting, respiratory difficulty or even respiratory arrest. The grimacing facial expression has been called the lactrodectus facies. Several fatalities are reported yearly in the USA from black widow bites, usually in children and the elderly.

Differential Diagnosis. Most reported spider bites turn out to be bites of other insects. Either an accurate description or actually the spider itself are required for an accurate clinical diagnosis. If a bite is reported, and the patient has pain and cramping, then the likelihood is greater that a black widow was the perpetrator.

Therapy. Cooling the bite site with an ice cube, attempting to remove venom with suction and applying a tourniquet are all appropriate first-aid measures. Children, the elderly and patients with cardiovascular problems should be hospitalized. A horse serum antivenom is available. A 10% calcium gluconate solution (10 ml intravenously) appears to be the best approach for cramping; muscle relaxants and narcotics may also help.

Brown Recluse Spider

Etiology and Pathogenesis. Brown recluse spiders, *Loxoscleses reclusa* in the USA (and its close relatives *L. rufescens* in the Mediterranean and *L. laeta* in South America), are 8–15 mm long yellow-brown spiders with a typical fiddle marking on their thorax. In the USA, the central Mississippi and Missouri valleys are the hot-bed for brown recluse spiders. They live primarily in houses, especially closets, and sheds. Often individuals are bitten digging clothes out of a closet or putting on a garment. The spider's toxin contains a number of enzymes with necrolytic and hemolytic properties, but no single enzyme responsible for the massive tissue necrosis has been found.

Clinical Findings. The initial bite is not especially painful and may be overlooked. Within hours, erythema, swelling and pruritus develop. The rest of the course is highly variable. In some patients, nothing more happens. In others, a central bleb develops surrounded by ecchymoses. As the blister ruptures, a black eschar forms. When this is lost or removed, a deep ulcer often extending to muscle is seen. In yet others, the massive progressive tissue necrosis is associated with intravascular hemolysis, thrombocytopenia and even renal failure. Death is extremely rare.

Differential Diagnosis. The differential diagnosis of brown recluse spider bites is complex. Early on, they may be overlooked or ignored. Later, the entire range of large destructive ulcerations comes into question, including pyoderma gangrenosum, factitial lesions and infections, primarily mixed bacterial ones.

Therapy. The therapy is very controversial. Initial first-aid measures can include heat, elevation and rest. Three main recommendations have been made to treat early lesions before they become problematic:

- Surgical excision
- High-dose systemic corticosteroids
- Dapsone

No study has shown a clear advantage to one approach and the problems are obvious, as a large series of patients are needed because of the natural variability of the disease. We have the most experience with systemic corticosteroids, but respected colleagues endorse dapsone. Surgery is best avoided in our estimation. If the disease advances, standard supportive care for the hematologic problems is needed; an unfortunate few require renal dialysis.

Scorpions

Scorpions are widespread around the world, primarily in arid or semiarid climates. Scorpion bites are a major problem in Mexico, with an estimated 100,000 bites yearly and 800 fatalities. In North Africa, the magnitude of the problem is similar. Scorpions are large arachnids and most have pincers and a curved stinger arising from their segmented tail. They are capable of multiple stings. They live in dark spaces, are primarily nocturnal and sting only when disturbed. Typical scenarios include getting into a sleeping bag in the desert, putting on a shoe or garment, or reaching into a wood pile. Most scorpion bites are painful but not associated with local or systemic reactions. The most dangerous North American scorpions are the small bark scorpions, *Centruoides*. Their toxin causes a variety of sympathetic and parasympathetic problems, such as tachycardia, hypertension, salivation and lacrimation. In children there may be hyperactivity, while in adults the main neuromuscular effects involve the eyes. About 0.5% of scorpion bites wind up as fatalities.

The whip scorpion or vinegaroon is not a true scorpion. It has a thin whip tail, a painful bite and can squirt a painful liquid to defend itself. True scorpions bite and sting, but do not squirt.

Therapy. A number of antitoxins are available, varying from region to region. In addition, intensive supportive care is needed in some cases. The local wounds rarely cause problems.

Mites

Mites are small arachnids. They have eight legs, a small head and a large cephalothorax. Almost every species has its own mite, including humans. In addition, there are free-living mites, as well as those specialized for vegetable matter.

Scabies

(ARISTOTLE; HIPPOCRATES)

Synonyms. The itch, seven-year itch

Definition. Intensely pruritic infestation caused by human mite.

Causative Organism. *Sarcoptes scabiei* is a true human parasite. The female is 0.3–0.4 mm long; the male about half as big (Fig. 8.16).

Epidemiology. Transmission of scabies requires close personal contact, as Mellanby's elegant studies in World War II among conscientious objectors showed. While sexual intercourse is the usual

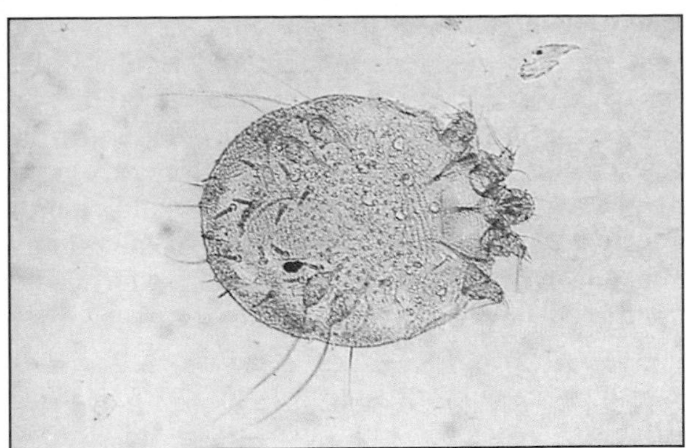

Fig. 8.16. *Sarcoptes scabiei*

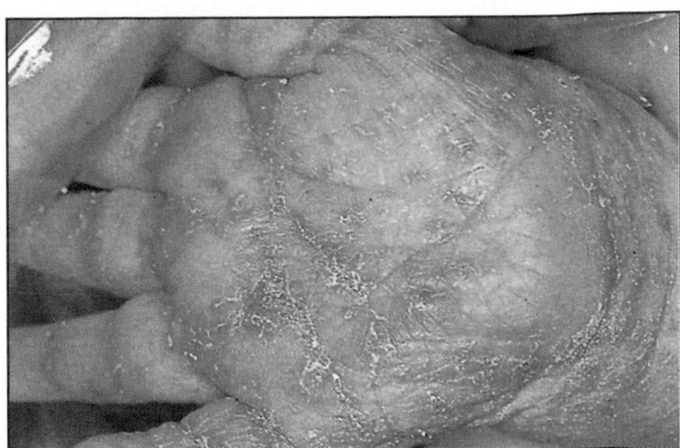

Fig. 8.17. Extensive scabies of palm with multiple burrows

method of spread among adults, sharing a bed or using the same underwear will also suffice. Scabies mites are easily spread among children and the degree of contact between parents and children is enough to spread the mites throughout a family. In addition, homeless individuals or others with inadequate hygiene, for example as a result of famine or war, are at risk. The mites can only live 2–3 days away from a human host. This means that airing clothes for 4 days, or leaving outdoors in freezing temperatures overnight, is sufficient to break the transmission cycle.

Etiology and Pathogenesis. After mating, the pregnant female crawls through the stratum corneum, tunneling her way with her strong mandibles. If a lesion is not excoriated one can see a tiny tunnel with a bump at the end where the female mite will be found. She lays two or three eggs daily, depositing them as well as feces (scybala) in the tunnel. After a matter of weeks, the adult dies. The eggs hatch in about 1 week and in about 3 weeks are mature adults. The larval and nymph forms, as well as the males, live on the skin surface. The male dies after mating.

When a human is infested for the first time, symptoms usually develop after 3–6 weeks, while after a reinfestation, they occur within 24 h. While the exact mechanisms are not understood, some degree of cellular immunity to mite proteins or byproducts must develop. The female produces a cement-like substance with which she stabilizes the tunnels; this may be the antigen.

Clinical Findings. The classic symptom is intense pruritus, especially at night in bed. There are two types of itch: the localized change associated with an individual lesion and the diffuse pruritus worse at night. The sites of predilection are the interdigital spaces, the anterior axillary folds, the umbilicus, the elbows and the genitalia, especially the gluteal cleft (Figs. 8.17, 8.18). In the most extensive studies of Mellanby (1972, 1973), the following distribution was seen: hands and wrists 63%, elbows 11%, feet 9%, genitalia 9%, buttocks 4%, axillae 2% and all the rest 2%.

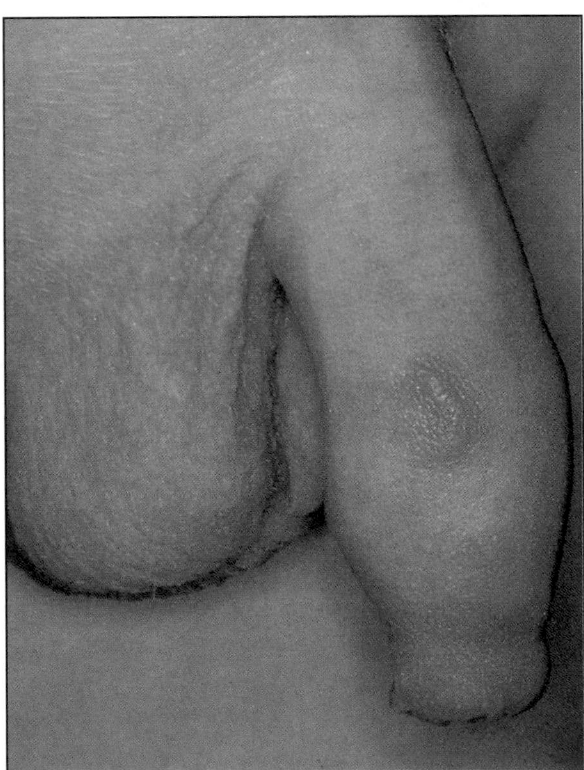

Fig. 8.18. Solitary burrow on shaft of penis with local inflammation

In two locations, involvement with scabies is almost clinically diagnostic. On the nipple and male genitalia (glans, shaft and scrotum) tiny scaly papules develop that are pathognomonic. In adults, the head and scalp are seldom involved; in infants on the other hand scalp involvement is typical. In addition, infants may have very extensive cutaneous disease with prominent nodular lesions on the trunk, palms and soles. The most diagnostic finding is an intact tunnel with a tiny dark dot, the mite at its end. More often one sees excoriations, impetiginization and crusting with a spectrum of secondary lesions.

The patient's general immune status and experience with *S. scabiei* play a role. In a normal host, the initial infection is asymptomatic for a period of time (usually about 6 weeks) during which time the individual is capable of transmitting the disease. For this reason, all family or living unit members must be treated, not just the itching ones.

In a patient who has previously had scabies, there is a more prompt pruritic allergic reaction. Erythematous papules develop at the tunnel entry sites and pruritic papules may appear as part of an urticarial reaction. That is, not every itching spot contains a mite. The intense pruritus leads to scratching and secondary infection. In children, the impetigo that arises may dominate the picture. Secondary allergic contact dermatitis may occur, as patients use a wide variety of antipruritics including the sensitizing topical antihistamines, as well as topical antibiotics. In endemic areas, older individuals may develop a degree of immunity. In a severely immune-deficient patient, as in HIV/AIDS, the mites may proliferate almost without resistance. Finally, in fastidious patients, the frequent washing and drying may remove many of the mites, so that the patient presents with few positive clinical findings but intense pruritus. This combination has been called scabies of the cleanly.

Histopathology. If one is lucky, the female mite may be identified within her tunnel in the stratum corneum. Otherwise, there is simply a lymphocytic perivascular infiltrate, often rich in eosinophils, and often associated with an excoriation. One must caution the laboratory to section carefully through all biopsies submitted from pruritic papules.

Laboratory Findings. If one is lucky enough to find an intact tunnel, then the diagnosis is easy. Dermatoscopic examination facilitates this search. Another trick is to apply fountain pen ink to the suspected area, leave for a while and wipe off. Sometimes tunnels are highlighted. The mite at the end of the tunnel can be removed with a needle or fine scalpel and viewed under the microscope. If one advances a relatively broad or blunt needle into the tunnel parallel to the skin surface and pushes until one reaches the dot at the end of the tunnel, then one can usually lift out the mite on the needle tip. Under the microscope, one can see the moving mite, the eggs or the red-brown scybala. Mineral oil is probably the best medium. Another trick if no clear tunnel is seen is to place a drop of mineral oil on the skin and gently scrape the surface with a scalpel; often one feels a pop as a mite is unroofed. Then the mineral oil is transferred to a slide for evaluation.

Differential Diagnosis. The differential diagnosis includes all pruritic skin disorders. In children, impetigo and atopic dermatitis are the most common problems. In adults, all forms of prurigo, dermatitis herpetiformis, folliculitis and all internal causes of pruritus have to be at least considered. The elderly are not spared from scabies but most often they have idiopathic pruritus. In rare patients, especially children, scabies will present as urticaria.

Diagnostic Criteria. If a mite is found, one needs no diagnostic criteria. But it is estimated that an adult has on average about 120 adult female mites on the body. Thus, finding a mite is equivalent to the needle in a haystack issue. Each clinician must determine which criteria suffice to institute presumptive treatment for scabies. In our experience, the typical lesions on the penis and nipple, the presence of a tunnel even without a mite and interdigital lesions are almost diagnostic. Severe pruritus, especially at night, of short onset or in multiple members of a living unit is also very suggestive.

Therapy. A number of effective treatments are available for scabies. The main rule is always to treat the entire family or all the contact individuals. Otherwise, a ping-pong effect develops, because individuals who are asymptomatic are infectious. This is impossible when hundreds of individuals are infected, as in some Third World villages or refugee settlements.

The following agents are appropriate.

Lindane (γ-Benzene Hexachloride). This is probably still the treatment of choice for adults. Applying lindane lotion twice is over 95% curative.

The problem is that lindane has neurotoxic effects when used on open skin, in infants or over long periods of time. This has produced much controversy about its use in pregnancy and infancy. While we are very cautious, in our experience, lindane used properly on intact skin is not dangerous. We recommend the following procedure which is also appropriate for the other agents discussed later.

- The patient and family members should be treated the same evening. All adults should apply lindane lotion from the head down, covering the entire body but paying special attention to between the fingers and toes, beneath the nails and in the genital region. Infants must also have their scalp treated as discussed below.
- The next morning everyone should bathe or shower, put on clean clothes and change their sheets. All clothes and bedding that can be washed should be washed. All other items should be either place outdoors in freezing temperatures overnight or hung up outdoors, or in a garage, attic or basement for 4 days. Dry-cleaning is also acceptable.
- Since lindane does not kill all the eggs, retreatment is needed. We treat two nights in a row and recommend retreatment 1 week later.
- Topical antipruritic or corticosteroid creams or ointments, or systemic antihistamines, may be prescribed for the itch. If impetigo is present, oral antibiotics are needed.
- Lindane should not be prescribed for pregnant or nursing women, or infants less than 1 year of age. It should not be used in patients with known neurologic problems to avoid potential medical-legal problems.
- While lindane resistance does not seem to be a problem in Europe or the USA, it is a factor in many other parts of the world.

Permethrin. Available as a 5% cream (Elimite), this newer antiscabetic medication is more effective than lindane, has fewer side effects and almost always suffices in a single overnight treatment. The only problem is that it is more expensive than lindane. Permethrin can be expected to work against lindane-resistant mites. Permethrin is the treatment of choice for infants, as well as pregnant and nursing women.

Benzyl Benzoate. This older product is rather irritating, especially in concentrations greater than 10%. It is still available in Germany but rarely used in the USA. If employed it must be used twice a day for 3 days.

Sulfur. Precipitated sulfur 5–10% in petrolatum is probably the safest treatment for scabies. If parents or their physician are worried about the dangers of insecticides, this product can be prescribed. A large prescription and lots of patience will be necessary, as the messy mixture must be applied twice daily for 7–10 days. Sulfur soaps, baths and dips are the mainstay of scabies treatment in endemic areas, such as poor villages in India.

Allethrin and Piperonyl Butoxide. This combination is available as an elegant spray (Spregal) in Germany. It is roughly as effective as lindane but has the same restrictions regarding pregnancy and infancy.

Crotamiton. Crotamiton (*N*-ethyl-*o*-crotonotoluide) 10% cream (Eurax) is an effective antipruritic, but not an especially effective antiscabetic preparation. It is usually applied 2 days in a row, and then washed off after a total of 48 h. It is nonirritating and is often suggested for use in pregnancy, but its toxicity has been poorly studied.

Ivermectin. The most recent development in the treatment of scabies is oral ivermectin. Approved only for onchocerciasis and other parasite infections, ivermectin is a macrolide that forms γ-aminobutyric acid that paralyses the parasites. Official approval is pending in both Germany and the USA. Ivermectin is usually given as a single 400-mg oral dose to adults. In crusted scabies (see below), retreatment after 1 week is recommended.

Infants less than 2 years of age require different treatment. Their scalp is more likely to be involved and must be more aggressively treated. The simplest approach is to apply permethrin cream from top to bottom in this group. If sulfur is used, one can still suggest lindane shampoo, not to be left on but just used twice to wash the scalp and then rinsed out. Otherwise the scalp must also be treated with sulfur soaps or shampoos.

Scabies Variants

Postscabetic Id

Our impression is that in individuals in whom the diagnosis has been missed, even after effective treatment, pruritus and allergic papules may persist for some time. This is such a common problem in children, especially in Asian infants brought to North America and Europe by adoption agencies, that it has acquired a special name. Most patients simply have pruritic papules in which no scabies mites can be found. Others have tiny pustules, specially on their hands and feet. Many have been treated several times for scabies. Topical antipruritics should be prescribed, unless one can document the presence of mites.

Postscabietic Pruritus

In some patients, the drying effects of the lindane lotion and the increased washing that often accompanies the treatment lead to extremely dry skin and associated pruritus. In addition, there may be a continuing allergic reaction to the mites with occasional tiny papules. In this setting, many patients demand retreatment. We make it a rule never to re-treat scabies without finding the organism. This sometimes angers or inconveniences the patient or parents, but there is the possibility of getting into the circle of repeated retreatment without a diagnosis. Topical antipruritic ointments usually suffice.

One should make a deliberate effort to spend some time with such patients, reassure them that a little itching is normal and search conscientiously for new lesions, while assuring them that permethrin or lindane have cure rates of more than 99% or 95%. If one fails to do this, some unfortunate patients drift into the realm of acarophobia or fear of scabies. They develop a monosymptomatic neurosis that can be totally disabling. They go from doctor to doctor, disappointed that no one can find their mites, often presenting envelopes or bottles filled with scrapings of skin scales and lint that they insist contain bugs. When reassurance and support fail to help these individuals, pimocide 2 mg daily may be helpful, ideally combined with psychiatric help.

Crusted Scabies

(Daniellsen and Boeck 1848)

Synonyms. Norwegian scabies, scabies crustosa

Daniellsen and Boeck described crusted or Norwegian scabies at about the same time they identified lepromatous leprosy, which was endemic in Norway in the middle of the last century. Presumably, many of the patients with crusted scabies had leprosy with impaired immunity.

In this vary uncommon variant of scabies, the patient fails to mount a resistance and the mites proliferate dramatically. In the past this was almost exclusively a disease of patients with Down syndrome, especially when institutionalized. Epidemics in nursing homes were not uncommon, as entire wards would be infested by one patient with "itchy psoriasis". Other institutionalized patients, and those with iatrogenic immunosuppression or intrinsic immunodeficiency were also at risk. Today these groups have been outnumbered by patients with HIV/AIDS.

The skin may be inhabited by thousands of mites per square millimeter. For unexplained reasons, there is a proliferative, hyperkeratotic response, so that clinically one sees thickened scales, mimicking psoriasis. The large adherent crusts are most often seen over the knees and elbows, as well as the hands and feet. In addition, the face and scalp are prominently involved. There may even be an erythroderma. Scrapings or a biopsy show many, many mites, so the diagnosis is easy. Treatment is difficult because the scales must also be removed. Traditionally lindane and keratolytic agents were combined. Today ivermectin seems ideal in such a setting, also combined with keratolytics.

Nodular Scabies

This is a persistent immunologic reaction to the allergic challenge of the mite. There are red-brown papules or nodules, usually several centimeters in diameter found in two clinical settings. In children they may occur anywhere on the body (Fig. 8.19), while in adults they are almost limited to the axilla and male genitalia. Microscopically there is a marked lymphocytic proliferation, as in a pseudolymphoma. The best treatment is topical or intralesional corticosteroids.

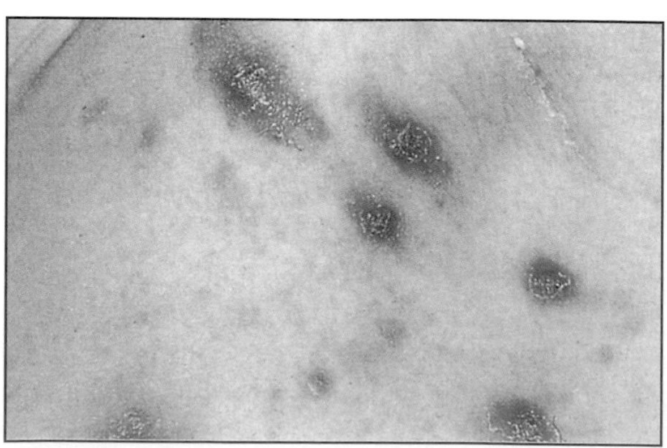

Fig. 8.19. Nodular scabies

Animal Scabies in Humans

Since almost every animal has its own *Sarcoptes* or closely related mite, it is not surprising that cats and dogs may have mites. The mites are specialized for just one host and cannot breed on other hosts. When they wind up on humans, they can cause itching and urticarial lesions that usually appear rapidly. There may be secondary infection and crusting, but the course is self-limited. The exception occurs when an individual sleeps with an untreated infested pet. Then the individual experiences continuous exposure and chronic problems. The distribution is different, in that the arms, chest and face are most often involved. In the animals, the mites cause pruritus, scaling, hair loss, crusting and often secondary infections. A good rule is that any patient with unclear pruritus and a pet with any skin symptoms or signs should take the pet to a veterinarian. In this case, the pet requires antimite treatment. The owner only needs antipruritic creams or oral antihistamines for a short time.

Cheyletiellosis

(Lomholdt 1917)

Synonyms. Walking dandruff, walking mange

There are a number of species of *Cheyletiella* infesting cats, dogs, rabbits and hares. They occur all around the world. On the animals, there tiny 0.5-mm mites live on the hairs, producing a flour-like fine scale, which on close examination moves. When the mites are transferred to humans, they may bite. They do not burrow either in humans or their animal hosts. Typically lesions are on the arms and abdomen. The eruption is quite variable with erythematous macules, papules and even vesicles. Pruritus is variable. If only one exposure occurs, such as when visiting a home with an infested pet, then the eruption is self-limited. If an animal keeper fails to diagnose their pet's infestation, then chronic problems arise. Just as with animal scabies, the human allergic response to *Cheyletiella* can be quite intense. In general, whether it be mites or fungi, humans react with a more excessive immunologic response to species that are usually present in animals. The animal needs to be treated, while in the human antipruritic measures suffice.

Environmental Mites

In the course of work and recreation, there are a number of chances for humans to come in contact with other mites. Usually an accurate history is the best way to sort out these confusing pruritic problems.

Dermanyssus gallinae seu avium, the chicken or bird mite, infests not only the birds but also their nests. In many parts of Europe, both pigeon mites and ticks are a problem in older dwellings. The mites live in nests or bird cages. When humans get in the way, such as by cleaning a bird cage or living in close proximity to birds, they become inadvertent hosts. Typically the skin reaction shows numerous small pruritic papules that are on occasion vesicular. They are often at the wrists or about the neck. Although the initial skin findings are irritant in nature, true allergies may develop, even associated with asthma. The latter diagnosis can be confirmed with prick testing and RAST.

Food mites are a slightly different story. *Tyroglyphi* are found in products such as flour, cheese, corn, tobacco leaves and dried fruits, such as copra (dried coconuts). Individuals involved in sorting and handling these products may develop an intense pruritus with multiple small papules on exposed surfaces. One slang expression for this problem is 'grocer's itch'. *Pediculoides ventricosus* is found on grain, beans and straw. It is a barely visible mite that parasitizes other pests. Individuals who sleep in straw, help with threshing, or pitch hay to store it in barns and silos are exposed to large numbers of grain mites. After a few hours, they have widespread pruritus, bright-red papules often with a central vesicle and urticarial lesions. The entire body can be covered and sometimes systemic symptoms develop. Those who carry bundles of hay or sacks of grain develop itchy papules on their shoulders, nape and arms. In all cases, topical and systemic antipruritic therapy is all that is needed.

House Dust Mites

The house dust mite, *Dermatophagoides pteronyssinus*, is commonly found in house dust, especially under conditions of high humidity. Many individuals become sensitized against the mites and their detritus, so that they experience type I allergic reactions, including rhinitis, conjunctivitis and asthma. It is unclear how much of a role house dust mites play in triggering atopic dermatitis but in at least some patients, patch testing with the mites induces a dermatitis-like reaction. RAST can also help confirm the diagnosis. Increased dust control, including special mattress and pillow covers, homes with leather furniture and wooden floors with few rugs and other such measures may help.

Hair Follicle Mites

(Henle 1841; Simon 1842)

Many animals have hair follicle mites, which in general are elongated worm-like organisms with eight small legs at their cephalic end. They are pathogens in some species, such as pigs where they produce terrible pustules and scarring about the eyes. In humans *Demodex folliculorum* is generally a harmless saprophyte. It may play a role in some types of folliculitis, especially in HIV/AIDS, as well as in severe pustular forms of rosacea. The load of *D. folliculorum* increases with age and is greatest in the facial (or acne-prone) sebaceous glands, as well as those of the eyelids, external ear and nipple. When a large number of mites are found, as in a very pustular rosacea, one can consider a trial of therapy. Sulfur, crotamiton and lindane all may be effective against *D. folliculorum*, although their actions are not clearly documented as regards either reducing the mite population or improving the clinical condition. Their presence may help explain why sulfur-containing compounds have traditionally enjoyed success against rosacea.

Trombidiosis

Synonyms. Harvest itch, chigger itch

In the Munich area, there is a nice tradition. Various communities describe the disorder as coming from the neighboring community. Two common terms in Munich are *Giesinger Beiß* and *Sendlinger Beiß*, but rest assured in Giesing and Sendling (two districts of Munich), the problem has a different name.

Causative Organism. Larval forms of *Trombicula*, a small plant mite. In Europe *Trombicula autumnalis*; in USA, *Eutrombicula alfreddugesi.*

Etiology and Pathogenesis. There are a wide variety of Trombiculidae that live on grasses, flowers, shrubs and vines. Their larvae cause intensely pruritic skin lesions. They attach to the human skin as the individual brushes past the plant. In Europe they are most common in late summer and fall. In the southeastern USA, they are present almost all

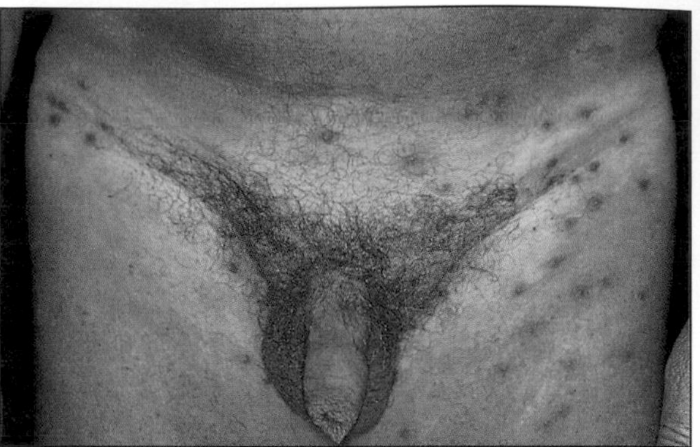

Fig. 8.20. Trombidiosis

year round. In order to get through the skin the tiny larva (< 0.1 mm) bores a shaft which it lines with an allergenic support substance. After feasting on blood, the larva drops off. The tiny adult mites in the USA are often red; thus, both the larval and adult forms are called red bugs, bête rouge, red mites, chiggers, jiggers or harvest mites. The term chigger is the most widely used one in the USA. It should not be confused with chigoe (or jigger), synonyms for *Tunga penetrans*. In Asia, harvest mites transmit scrub typhus.

Clinical Findings. The typical finding is several pruritic papules at an area of constriction of clothing, such as the sock line or belt line. Initially a small macule or wheal develops, but over 24–48 h it develops into a pruritic papule or papulovesicle, sometimes with hemorrhage (Fig. 8.20). The lesions are very persistent, lasting for several weeks, becoming excoriated and secondarily infected.

Differential Diagnosis. Other forms of arthropod bites are the only serious consideration. Early bites may be confused with urticarial lesions.

Therapy. Topical antipruritics or corticosteroids can be employed. Insect repellents are effective and should be applied about the clothing lines.

Ticks

Ticks are blood-sucking arachnids that cause a variety of problems in humans. There are two types of ticks: hard ticks (Ixodidae) (Fig. 8.21) and soft ticks without a chitinous dorsal plate (Argasidae). The two have slightly different life styles, for hard

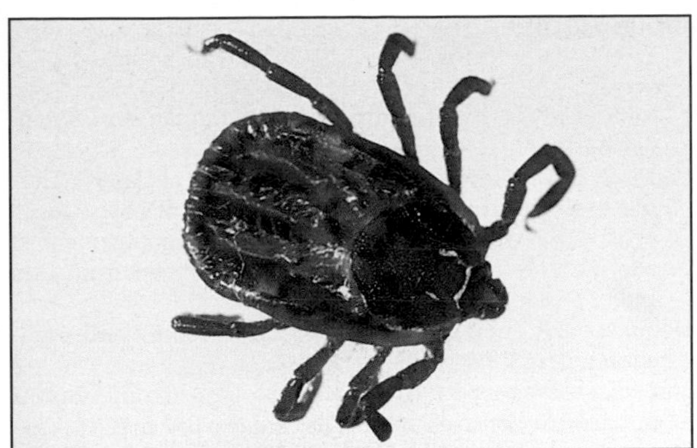

Fig. 8.21. *Ixodes ricinus*

ticks seek out passing animals moving great distances while soft ticks are primarily dwelling and nest parasites. Hard ticks feed once per stage, while soft ticks feed often.

Epidemiology. Ticks are very common and enjoy a world-wide distribution. They cause the most problems in situations where they or more often one of their vectors comes into close contact with humans. A good example for this is the spread of deer and their ticks carrying *Borrelia burgdorferi* into suburban areas of the East Coast of the USA, particularly the Lyme River Valley of Connecticut.

Etiology and Pathogenesis. The ticks and their larval stages attach to primarily mammalian hosts for their meals. In some species of ticks, each larval form has a preferred host and the life-cycle goes over several years with many complexities. For example *Ixodes ricinus* usually involves both a small rodent and a deer. Ticks typically insert their barbed mouthpiece (hypostom) into the host, releasing anesthetic and anticoagulant materials so that the bite is hardly noticed. The hard ticks feed for 3–12 days and then drop off; the soft ticks feed for only a short time. A number of bacteria, rickettsiae and viruses are transmitted by ticks. For each possible infectious agent, a certain amount of time is required before transmission can be accomplished. Because of the longer feeding time of hard ticks, they are most often the disease vectors. In addition, some ticks such as *I. holocyclus* in Australia and *Dermacentor andersoni* in the USA secrete neurotoxins that can cause life-threatening tick paralysis.

In Europe, *I. ricinus* transmits *B. burgdorferi* (Chap. 4) and tick-borne encephalitis, caused by a flavivirus. This type of encephalitis widespread in central Europe is known in Germany as FSME (*Frühsommer*, i.e. early summer, meningoencephalitis). It is most common in the forests of southern Germany and Austria. Active and passive immunization is available.

In North America, *I. dammini*, the deer tick, transmits *B. burgdorferi*, *Babesia microti* (a protozoon that causes Nantucket fever) and *Ehrlichia phagocytophilia* (a bacterium that causes human granulocytic ehrlichiosis). The Lone Star tick, *Amblyomma americanum*, transmits *E. chaffeensis* (a bacterium that causes human ehrlichiosis). The deer tick, the wood tick (*Dermacentor andersoni)* and the Lone Star tick are all responsible for transmitting Rocky Mountain spotted fever.

Ticks also transmit several other flavivirus diseases including various forms of encephalitis (Powassan fever in Canada, louping ill in the UK) and hemorrhagic fever (Omsk fever in Siberia). There are also three closely related tick-borne rickettsial diseases in Asia, Africa and Australia. Finally, some forms of *Borrelia recurrentis* (a spirochete that causes relapsing fever) are tick-borne; *Ornithodorus* in the southwestern USA and Mexico is often responsible. In Europe, relapsing fever is louse-borne but very uncommon.

Clinical Findings. Often the tick bite goes unnoticed. Many patients with borreliosis give no history of a tick bite. In other situations the patient may present to the doctor's office with an engorged tick firmly attached, but complaining of an irritated nevus or new growth (Fig. 8.22). In yet other situations, the tick bite is pruritic, presenting as a solitary red papule or nodule. When parts of the tick are left behind, a granulomatous reaction or pyoderma may develop. When *B. burgdorferi* has been transmitted, there may be an area of erythema

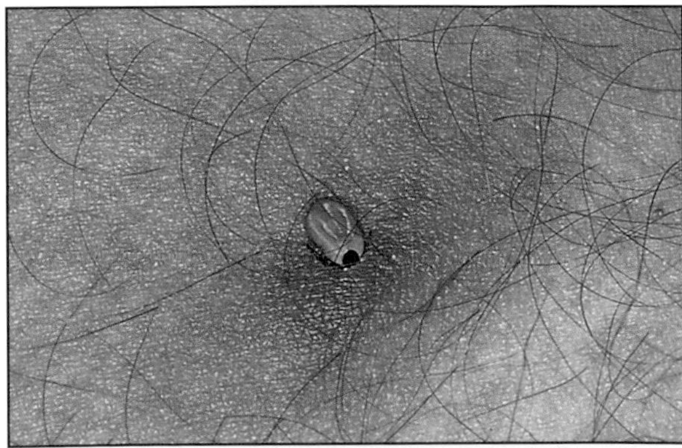

Fig. 8.22. Tick attached to patient with local inflammatory response

(erythema migrans) moving peripherally from the bite. Some ticks such as *Ornithodorus* in the southwestern USA and Mexico cause a more intense local reaction with vesiculation, eschar formation and then an ulcer.

Histopathology. Excisions of suspected tick bites are commonly submitted in Germany. The epidermis usually shows some damage while in the dermis there is an intense lymphocytic infiltrate admixed with eosinophils. With careful searching, one can often find some tick parts in the specimen.

Differential Diagnosis. The differential diagnosis of tick-borne diseases is endless. A solitary tick bite is usually fairly distinct, for most other bites are multiple. Occasionally a furuncle or infected cyst may initially appear similar. The possibility of lyme borreliosis should be serologically evaluated (Chap. 4).

Therapy. The main controversy in tick bites is how to remove the tick. One serious study showed that gentle twisting and extraction was as effective as any other method. Every society has a number of sure-fire methods, all of which often fail. If the tick is deeply embedded or if it has already been broken off, it is often simplest just to excise the lesion. A persistent inflammatory response can be treated with topical or intralesional corticosteroids.

Centipedes and Millipedes

Centipedes are long arthropods with one pair of legs per body segment. They have large pincer-like jaws with which they are capable of delivering a painful bite. Usually the jaws are large enough that two puncture wounds can be seen within a given bite site. House centipedes in general are helpful in pest control and rarely bothersome. Some of the larger centipedes, such as those found in desert regions are more dangerous. Millipedes, in contrast, have two pairs of legs per body segment, tend to coil up and do not bite.

Bibliography

General

Alexander J O'D (1984) Arthropods and human skin. Springer Berlin

Caumes E, Carriere J, Guermonprez G et al. (1995) Dermatoses associated with travel to tropical countries: a prospective study of the diagnosis and management of 269 patients presenting to a tropical disease unit. Clin Infect Dis 20:542–548

Hennessy DR (1997) Physiology, pharmacology and parasitology. Int J Parasitol 27:145–152

Mackey SL, Wagner KF (1994) Dermatologic manifestations of parasitic diseases. Infect Dis Clin North Am 8:713–743

Mehlhorn H (1988) Parasitology in focus. Springer, Berlin Heidelberg New York

Mumcuoglu Y, Rufli Th (1983) Dermatologische Entomologie. In: Metz J (Hrsg.) Beiträge zur Dermatologie, Bd. 9. Perimed Fachbuch, Erlangen

Pediculosis

Bainbridge CV, Klein GL, Neibart SI et al. (1998) Comparative study of the clinical effectiveness of a pyrethrin-based pediculicide with combing versus a permethrin-based pediculicide with combing. Clin Pediatr 37:17–22

Burkhart CG, Burkhart CN, Burkhart KM (1998) An assessment of topical and oral prescription and over the counter treatments for head lice. J Am Acad Dermatol 38: 979–982

Chouela E, Abeldano A, Cirigliano M et al. (1997) Head louse infestations: epidemiologic survey and treatment evaluation in Argentinian schoolchildren. Int J Dermatol 36: 819–825

Editorial (1998) Treating head louse infections. Drug Ther Bull 36:45–46

Eichenfield LF, Colon Fontanez F (1998) Treatment of head lice. Pediatr Infect Dis J 17:419–420

Hoehler F, Walicke PTI (1998) Comparative study of the clinical effectiveness of a pyrethrin based pediculicide with combing versus a permethrin based pediculicide with combing. Clin Pediatr (Phil) 37:17–22

Nguyen VX, Robert P (1996) Treatment of head lice. N Engl J Med 335:790

Bugs

Fletcher MG, Axtell RC (1993) Susceptibility of the bedbug, *Cimex lectularius*, to selected insecticides and various treated surfaces. Med Vet Entomol 7:69–72

Negromonte MR, Linardi PM, Nagem RL (1991) *Cimex lectularius* (Hemiptera, Cimicidae): sensitivity to commercial insecticides in labs. Mem Inst Oswaldo Cruz 86:491–492

Reduviid Bugs

Chimelli L, Scaravilli F (1997) Trypanosomiasis. Brain Pathol 7:599–611

Orthoptera

Schulaner FA (1997) Cockroach allergen and asthma. N Engl J Med 337:791

Tungiasis

Douglas Jones AG, Llewelyn MB, Mills CM (1995) Cutaneous infection with *Tunga penetrans*. Br J Dermatol 133: 125–127

Lowry MA, Ownbey JL, McEvoy PL (1996) A case of tungiasis. Mil Med 161:128–129

Sanusi ID, Brown EB, Shepard TG et al. (1989) Tungiasis: report of one case and review of the 14 reported cases in the United States. J Am Acad Dermatol 20:941–944

Wardhaugh AD, Norris JF (1994) A case of imported tungiasis in Scotland initially mimicking verrucae vulgaris. Scott Med J 39:146–X147

Hymenoptera

Glaspole L, Douglass J, Czarny D et al. (1997) Stinging insect allergies. Assessing and managing. Aust Fam Physician 26:1395–1399, 1401

Golden DB, Kwiterovich KA, Kagey-Sobotka A et al. (1998) Discontinuing venom immunotherapy: extended observations. J Allergy Clin Immunol 101:298–305

Muller UR (1998) Hymenoptera venom hypersensitivity: an update. Clin Exp Allergy 28:4–6

Wright DN, Lockey RF (1990) Local reactions to stinging insects (Hymenoptera). Allergy Proc 11:23–28

Myiasis

Davies HD, Sakuls P, Keystone JS (1993) Creeping eruption. A review of clinical presentation and management of 60 cases presenting to a tropical disease unit. Arch Dermatol 129:588–591

Jelinek T, Nothdurft HD, Rieder N et al. (1995) Cutaneous myiasis: review of 13 cases in travellers returning from tropical countries. Int J Dermatol 34:624–626

Kpea N, Zywocinski C (1995) "Flies in the flesh": a case report and review of cutaneous myiasis. Cutis 55:47–48

Lucchina LC, Wilson ME, Drake LA (1997) Dermatology and the recently returned traveller: infectious diseases with dermatologic manifestations. Int J Dermatol 36:167–181

Mattone Volpe F (1998) Cutaneous larva migrans infection in the pediatric foot. A review and two case reports. J Am Podiatr Med Assoc 88:228–231

Ng SO, Yates M (1997) Cutaneous myiasis in a traveller returning from Africa. Aust J Dermatol 38:38–39

Rao R, Nosanchuk JS, Mackenzie R (1997) Cutaneous myiasis acquired in New York State. Pediatrics 99: 601–602

Spiders

Anderson PC (1997) Spider bites in the United States. Dermatol Clin 15:307–311

Editorial (1996) Necrotic arachnidism Pacific Northwest, 1988–1996. MMWR Morb Mortal Wkly Rep 45:433–436

Smith DB, Ickstadt J, Kucera J (1997) Brown recluse spider bite: a case study. J Wound Ostomy Continence 24:137–143

Walker JS, Hogan DE (1995) Bite to the left leg. Necrotic ulcer from a brown recluse spider bite. Acad Emerg Med 2:223, 231, 234–237

Wilson DC, King LE Jr (1990) Spiders and spider bites. Dermatol Clin 8:277–286

Wright SW, Wrenn KD, Murray L et al. (1997) Clinical presentation and outcome of brown recluse spider bite. Ann Emerg Med 30:28–32

Yiannias JA, Winkelmann RK (1992) Persistent painful plaque due to a brown recluse spider bite. Cutis 50:273–275

Scorpions

Gateau T, Bloom M, Clark R (1994) Response to specific *Centruroides sculpturatus* antivenom in 151 cases of scorpion stings. J Toxicol Clin Toxicol 32:165–171

Zimmo S (1998) Desert dermatology. Clin Dermatol 16: 109–111

Scabies

Burkhart KM, Burkhart CN, Burkhart CG (1998) Our scabies treatment is archaic, but ivermectin has arrived. Int J Dermatol 37:76–77

Farrell AM, Ross JS, Bunker CB et al. (1998) Crusted scabies with scalp involvement in HIV 1 infection. Br J Dermatol 138:192–193

Huffam SE, Currie BJ (1998) Ivermectin for *Sarcoptes scabiei* hyperinfestation. Int J Infect Dis 2:152–154

Jaramillo Ayerbe F, Berrio Munoz J (1998) Ivermectin for crusted Norwegian scabies induced by use of topical steroids. Arch Dermatol 134:143–145

Lewis EJ, Connolly SB, Crutchfield CE III et al. (1998) Localized crusted scabies of the scalp and feet. Cutis 61:87–88

Mellanby K (1972) Scabies. EW Classey. Hampton, UK

Mellanby K (1973) Human guinea-pigs. Merlin, London

Cheyletiella

Scott DW (1998) Ivermectin usage for cheyletiellosis. J Am Acad Dermatol 38:1013

House Dust Mite

Ormstad H, Johansen BV, Gaarder Pl (1998) Airborne house dust particles and diesel exhaust particles as allergen carriers. Clin Exp Allergy 28:702–708

Simpson A, Hassall R, Custovic A et al. (1998) Variability of house-dust-mite allergen levels within carpets. Allergy 53:602–607

Spieksma FT (1997) Domestic mites from an acarologic perspective. Allergy 52:360–368

Demodicidosis

Barrio J, Lecona M, Hernanz JM et al. (1996) Rosacea like demodicosis in an HIV positive child. Dermatology 192:143–145

Castanet J, Monpoux F, Mariani R et al. (1997) Demodicidosis in an immunodeficient child. Pediatr Dermatol 14:219–220

Farina MC, Requena L, Sarasa JL et al. (1998) Spinulosis of the face as a manifestation of demodicidosis. Br J Dermatol 138:901–903

Forton F, Seys B, Marchal JL et al. (1998) *Demodex folliculorum* and topical treatment: acaricidal action evaluated by standardized skin surface biopsy. Br J Dermatol 138:461–466

Ticks

Falco RC, Fish D, D'Amico V (1998) Accuracy of tick identification in a Lyme disease endemic area. JAMA 280: 602–603

Ginsberg HS, Hyland DE, Hu R (1998) Tick population trends and forest type. Science 281:349–350

CHAPTER 9

Diseases Caused by Worms

Contents

Introduction

Climatic factors, limited hygiene, and a variety of daily activities including eating habits and obtaining water all contribute to a spectrum of infections caused by worms. All these infections are more common in subtropical and tropical regions and many have cutaneous features. While over 150 types of worms can infect humans, most are very rare or animal pathogens that reach humans only accidentally (Table 9.1). Some, however, cause major public health problems. Even though the variety of worm infections encountered in temperate lands is very limited, they are often overlooked, especially when imported by tourists or immigrants. There is no organ or organ system in which either worms or their larvae are not capable of establishing themselves.

Table 9.1. Major pathogenic worms

Scientific name	Common name
Nemathelminthes	Roundworms
Nematodes	Roundworms or thread worms
Enterobius vermicularis	Pinworm
Ascaris lumbricoides	Intestinal roundworm
Trichuris trichiura	Whipworm
Ancylostoma duodenale	Hookworm
Necator americanus	Hookworm
Ancylostoma braziliense, *A. caninum*	Dog and cat hookworm, cause cutaneous larva migrans
Strongyloides stercoralis	Dwarf round worm
Trichinella spiralis	
Wucheria bancrofti	
Brugia malayi	
Dirofilaria sp.	Zoonotic filaria
Toxocara canis, T. cati	Dog and cat roundworms
Gnathostoma spinigerum	
Loa loa	
Onchocerca volvulus	
Dracunculus medinensis	Guinea worm
Plathelminthes	Flat worms
Cestodes	Tapeworms
Taenia saginata	Cow tapeworm
Taenia solium	Pig tapeworm
Hymenolepsis nana	Dwarf tapeworms
Diphyllobothrium latum	Fish tapeworm
Echinococcus granulosus	Dog tapeworm
Echinococcus multilocularis	Fox tapeworm
Trematodes	Flukes
Schistosoma mansoni	
Schistosoma japonicum	
Schistosoma haematobium	
Trichobilharzia	Animal schistosomes
Clonorchis (Opisthorchis) sinensis	Chinese liver fluke
Opisthorchis felineus, *Opisthorchis viverrini*	Cat and dog liver flukes
Fasciolopsis buski	
Annelida	Segmented worms
Hirudinea	Leeches

Therefore, the manner of transmission, degree of involvement, and type of therapy all are complicated.

The mechanisms the body uses to protect against parasitic infections in general and worms in particular are poorly understood. Epidemiologic studies and experimental procedures have clearly shown that the immune status of the host is the most important factor in determining the course of the disease. When extracellular parasites, especially nematodes, are involved, IgE antibodies and T cell cytokines, primarily interleukin (IL)-4, appear to be most important. The strong activation of the immune system which occurs early in a parasitic infection and appears necessary to control it can also lead to inadvertent damage. The immediate hypersensitivity directed against the invaders produces a variety of allergic reactions while, in more severe and chronic worm infections, the later stages often resemble an autoimmune disease.

The skin can be involved either directly or indirectly. In some cases, it provides a barrier and even end-station for worm larvae unsuited for human hosts that have arrived accidentally. Two examples of this phenomenon are swimmers' itch and cutaneous larva migrans, as discussed below. Other worms can be viewed as dermatotropic, designed to spend long periods in the skin or subcutaneous tissue; the classic examples are guinea worm infection and onchocerciasis. Worms inhabiting the gut or other tissues may illicit allergic cutaneous reactions, especially if their larvae wander from one site in the body to another.

The diagnosis of parasitic infections requires the identification of the worm, its larvae, or its eggs. Traditionally, examining the stool for ova and parasites has been standard, but many infections never involve the gastrointestinal tract and even those that do may have only episodic shedding. In addition, there are nonpathogenic worms which may cause a great deal of confusion. Serologic examinations are often useful, especially in returning tourists who would not be expected to carry worms. Among natives, they are less helpful, as they may reflect prior exposure. In addition, polymerase chain reaction and other molecular biological techniques can be employed, but these are so sensitive that they may identify subclinical or coincidental infections.

Three main groups of worms assume medical importance:

- Nemathelminthes. The main class are the nematodes or roundworms. They are typically colorless, nonsegmented, circular in cross-section, and have a resistant cuticle and a hollow cavity containing digestive and sexual organs. Females and males are usually quite distinct.
- Plathelminthes. The flat worms contain two major classes:
  - Trematodes. The flukes are tongue- or lance-shaped and dorsoventrally flattened. All are hermaphroditic, except the schistosomes.
  - Cestodes. The tapeworms are band- or tape-like segmented worms, always hermaphroditic, which range in length from millimeters to several meters. When mature, they are found only in the gastrointestinal tract, but as larvae they can migrate. Each segment takes up nourishment directly from the bowel contents; the large members can steal enough nutrients to cause deficiency states in their hosts.
- Annelida. The segmented worms include ordinary earth worms, many marine and fresh water species, and leeches (*Hirudinea*). The last-named are the only medically important members of the group. Both marine and land forms exist who attach to their prey and remove blood. They are still prescribed medically to remove blood from extremities with delicate vascular supply, such as following a traumatic amputation, when arterial supply may overwhelm venous drainage. In addition, their saliva contains a family of anticoagulants which are being employed clinically. As a result, their bites tend to bleed for a period of time even after they detach or are removed. Occasionally, prurigo nodularis-like lesions develop. Otherwise, the annelids are harmless and not further discussed here.

Nematodes

Enterobiasis

Synonyms. Oxyuriasis, pinworm infection

Definition. Common intestinal parasitic infection often seen in temperate zones which usually presents with perianal signs and symptoms.

Causative Organism. *Enterobius vermicularis.* The females worms are 8–13 mm long, the males 2–5 mm.

Epidemiology. Enterobiasis is a worldwide problem affecting people of all social classes. About 400 million people are estimated to be infected. In the USA, it is most common in young school children; in some studies, a prevalence of 50 % has been found. In other parts of the world, the rates are even higher. Children tend to acquire the infection at their school or kindergarten and bring it home into their families.

The usual source of infection is fecal-oral spread, either as a source of reinfection or spread to others. Parents may be infected from their children. The eggs may remain viable outside the body for up to 20 days. If infected feces are used for fertilizer, the infection can be transferred by poorly washed vegetables such as lettuce. Once the infection is established, reinfection is the rule. If this is interrupted, the infection subsides after 4–8 weeks.

Etiology and Pathogenesis. The worms are found in the colon, cecum, and rectum. The females lay their eggs preferentially in the perianal region, perineum, and female genitalia, exiting the colon through the anus. The eggs may also be released within the colon and passed with bowel movements. The new eggs first hatch when they are ingested again. Thus the cycle is very simple, in contrast to that of certain other worms.

Clinical Findings. The patients are usually children in good health and many are asymptomatic. The main symptom is perianal pruritus, often worse at night. Some severe cases lead to loss of sleep. The inevitable scratching leads to transmission. Erosions and secondary infections may develop. Both molluscum contagiosum and human papilloma virus infections are common complications. In girls, a vulvovaginitis may occur from direct seeding of the genitalia by the worms. Occasionally, chronic urticaria is a symptom.

Laboratory Findings. The easiest way to find the eggs is to apply cellophane tape to the perianal skin early in the morning and attach it to a glass slide for microscopic evaluation. Sometimes, the worms themselves are found in the stool or on the skin or underwear. A stool examination will almost always reveal both.

Differential Diagnosis. Enterobiasis should be considered in the differential diagnosis of pruritus ani, especially in children. Any perianal dermatitis may be secondary to the itching induced by the worms.

Therapy

Systemic. Pyrantel pamoate (10 mg/kg; maximum 1 g), mebendazole (100 mg) or albendazole (400 mg) are used for a single treatment, which can be repeated in 2 weeks.

Topical. The perianal pruritus usually does not require treatment. Mild antipruritics such as polidocanol creams can be employed temporarily. If a secondary dermatitis develops, low potency corticosteroid creams may be useful. Warts or mollusca are treated in the standard fashion.

Other Measures. The fingernails should be kept short, the child encouraged to wash his hands after each bowel movement, and small children provided with tightly fitting underpants in the evening to reduce access.

Ascariasis

Synonyms. Ascaridiasis, roundworm infection

Definition. Common small intestinal worm infection whose cutaneous manifestations are usually allergic.

Causative Organism. *Ascaris lumbricoides.* The firm, elastic worms are about as thick as a pencil. The male is somewhat smaller than the female. They live primarily in the small intestine, which the female showers with 200,000 eggs daily.

Epidemiology. Ascariasis is the most common human worm infection, with about 1.25 billion individuals affected worldwide. Most infections are spread by the presence of eggs on poorly washed vegetables or from soil contaminated with feces and eggs. Direct spread from human to human is rare. The eggs become infective after several daysand remain so for many months.

Etiology and Pathogenesis. The freshly ingested eggs hatch in the small intestine and the larvae reach the lungs by passing through the wall and following the venous blood flow. In the lungs, they cause an eosinophilic inflammation known as Loeffler syndrome. Pulmonary symptoms are more common in reinfections; they include fever, wheezing, dyspnea, and infiltrates. After 9–10 days, the worms migrate up the trachea into the pharynx, where they are swallowed and land in the small intestine. Here they mature into adult worms and the cycle begins anew, usually lasting about 4 months. The adult worms can live for 1–2 years.

Clinical Findings. Most cases are asymptomatic. The worms are large enough to cause obstruction, volvulus, pain mimicking appendicitis, and even involve the biliary tree. The worms, their eggs, and their metabolic products lead to eosinophilia and allergic reactions such as urticaria in addition to the pulmonary problems. Thus, in patients with persistent eosinophilia and/or chronic urticaria, one should search for *Ascaris lumbricoides*.

Laboratory Findings. The stool should be examined for ova and parasites. Flotation and sedimentation methods are used to concentrate the eggs, facilitating identification. Occasionally, the worms are found in the stool or in vomitus. Elevated eosinophil counts and increased IgE levels are seen.

Therapy. The same agents recommended for *Enterobius vermicularis* can be used. Pyrantel pamoate can be given in a single dose (10 mg/kg; maximum 1 g). Mebendazole is given 100 mg b.i.d. for 3 days. Albendazole 400 mg in a single dose suffices.

Trichinosis

(von Zenker 1860)

Synonyms. Trichinellosis, trichiniasis

Definition. Infection by intestinal roundworms whose larvae migrate to muscles.

Causative Organism. *Trichinella spiralis*. The male worms are 1.4–2.0 mm long, the females 3.0–4.0 mm. There are other species of *Trichinella*, but most human infections are caused by *Trichinella spiralis*. In some classifications, the organism has been widely subdivided because of antigenic differences between worms from different parts of the globe.

Epidemiology. While trichinosis is thought of as a rare disease in the west, worldwide about 50 million people are infected. Surveys done at autopsy 50 years ago in the USA revealed a prevalence of over 15%, but today it is closer to 1% and diminishing. The most common source is pork that has been improperly cooked. The larvae are encysted in the muscle and released in the stomach following chewing and exposure to digestive enzymes. *Trichinella spiralis* is not often found in domestic animals in either Germany or the USA because of veterinary control of slaughtering facilities, which includes microscopic examination of muscle. In Germany, wild boars often carry the worm; many animals around the world, including polar bears, walruses, leopards, and hyenas, are often infected.

Etiology and Pathogenesis. The larvae mature rapidly in the small intestine. After 5–7 days, the female produces larvae which penetrate the bowel wall, enter lymphatics or veins, and are distributed throughout the body. They settle primarily in muscle.

Clinical Findings. The severity of the illness in humans is proportional to the number of larvae released. Many infections are subclinical. In typical infections, the first signs are acute muscle soreness and pain associated with periorbital edema. Usually there is marked eosinophilia. Fever, abdominal pain, and diarrhea may occur. The edema may also involve the palms and soles. Tiny hemorrhages can be seen beneath the nails as well as on the conjunctiva and retina. More severe complications include myocarditis with arrhythmias, bronchopneumonia, encephalitis, and even sepsis.

Laboratory Findings. The marked eosinophilia is usually the first clue. IgE levels will also be raised. Serologic studies such as enzyme-linked immunosorbent assay (ELISA) testing are also helpful, as is measurement of muscle enzymes. A muscle biopsy may be positive 10 days after infection, but the yield is much higher at 4 weeks.

Differential Diagnosis. In its early stages, trichinosis can be almost impossible to distinguish from acute dermatomyositis. The eosinophilia, muscle biopsy and clinical course usually provide the answer.

Therapy. Either mebendazole (200–400 mg t.i.d. for 3 days, then 400–500 mg t.i.d. for 10 days) or albendazole (400 mg b.i.d. for 6 days) are recommended. Thiabendazole has also been employed. In severe cases with cardiac or neurologic findings, systemic corticosteroids (20–60 mg prednisone daily for 10 days) can be used to reduce the allergic complications. In some instances, high dose intravenous corticosteroids are used at the beginning of therapy.

Prophylaxis. Detailed instructions are available for the cooking of potentially infected meat. In addition, prolonged holding in a deep-freeze unit can also deactivate the larva.

Public Health Measures. Trichinosis is a reportable disease in many localities.

Ancylostomiasis

Synonyms. Hookworm disease, uncinariasis, necatoriasis

Definition. Common chronic intestinal parasitic infection which usually manifests as iron deficiency anemia.

Causative Organisms. *Ancylostoma duodenale* and *Necator americanus.* In addition to these two human hookworms, on rare occasions animal hookworms can establish a life cycle in humans.

Epidemiology. Hookworm disease is the second most common worm infection, estimated to involve over 1 billion people worldwide. It was formerly very common in the USA, particularly the southeast, but increased hygiene has made it less of a problem. Transmission is from fecally contaminated soil. The eggs hatch into larvae which then can penetrate the skin, entering their new host. Thus, the problem is greatest in rural societies where people go barefoot and feces are either used for fertilizer or easily encountered about the home.

Etiology and Pathogenesis. The larvae penetrate the skin, typically on the feet. They reach the lungs via the lymphatics and veins, then pass up the airways, are swallowed, and settle in the small intestine. There they attach themselves, ingest blood, and reproduce with phenomenal numbers of eggs being passed in the stool.

Clinical Findings. The main findings are an eosinophilic pneumonitis as the larvae pass through the lungs and, later, iron deficiency anemia. Gastrointestinal symptoms are uncommon. As the larvae migrate through the skin, they elicit itching and localized urticarial lesions; this is known as ground itch, identical to that seen in cutaneous larva migrans. The eosinophilic stage may be associated with urticaria.

Laboratory Findings. Stool examination for ova and parasites suffices. The egg load may be light in early infections; on occasion, the worms lie dormant for a period of time.

Differential Diagnosis. Hookworm infection should be considered in all cases of iron deficiency anemia. The differential diagnosis of cutaneous larva migrans is considered below.

Therapy. Single dose therapy with mebendazole, albendazole or pyrantel pamoate is usually successful.

Cutaneous Larva Migrans

(Lee 1874)

Synonyms. Creeping eruption, creeping disease, plumber's itch

Definition. Infection of skin by various nematode larvae which migrate but never reach internal organs or complete their life cycle.

Causative Organisms. *Ancylostoma braziliense, Ancylostoma caninum, Ascaris suum, Bunostomum phlebotum*, and many others. Both *Ancylostoma duodenale* and *Necator americanus* cause similar findings, but because they progress to hookworm disease, their infections are not technically considered cutaneous larva migrans. In addition, *Dirofilaria, Gnathostoma spinigerum*, and *Strongyloides stercoralis* may also be responsible.

Epidemiology. The essence of the problem is penetration of the skin by mammalian hookworms or other larvae which are unable to mature there or pass on to another organ. Thus, exposure to soil contaminated by animal feces is essential. The soil may be contaminated by dog or cat hookworms as well as by those from humans. Another source is animals along a beach, where bathers may be infected. Miners, tunnel workers, plumbers crawling under homes, and those with similar occupations with exposure to moist, contaminated earth also are at risk.

Etiology and Pathogenesis. The worms elicit a host inflammatory response as they wander through the skin, but for unclear reasons they are unable to enter the blood stream and complete their life cycle.

Clinical Findings. Shortly after entering the skin, the larvae elicit intense pruritus with edema, tiny papules, and even papulovesicles. As the larvae begin to migrate, the classic wreath-like or winding road-like, minimally elevated, linear erythematous

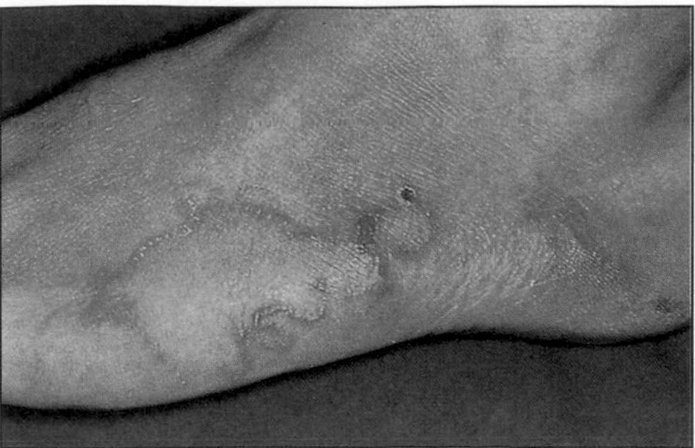

Fig. 9.1. Cutaneous larva migrans

tunnels become apparent (Fig. 9.1). The rate of migration varies with the species; *Strongyloides stercoralis* is the fastest. While the feet are most often involved, someone lying on a beach anywhere can the buttocks and shoulder blades where ground contact occurred (plumber's itch).

Because of pruritus, excoriations are common; the patient often scratches away the offending larvae. Secondary bacterial infections are common, including cellulitis.

Histopathology. With luck, one can find the larva with its chitinous coating within an intraepidermal tunnel. In most cases, the larvae never enter the dermis. There is an associated lymphocytic and eosinophilic infiltrate.

Laboratory Findings. Stool examination is worthless. Eosinophilia may be observed.

Differential Diagnosis. Myiasis, dirofilariasis, and strongyloidiasis can all appear similar. Identification of the organism is required.

Therapy

Systemic. Albendazole (400 mg daily for 2–3 days) is the therapy of choice. Thiabendazole also works but has considerably more side effects.

Topical. Topical thiabendazole can be effective, but it must be compounded. The oral suspension is frequently used topically but is less effective. We prefer 5–15% thiabendazole in hydrophilic ointment. This can be applied 2–3 times daily for 3–4 days, where possible with plastic wrap or tape occlusion. The cure rate in people with only a few lesions is close to 90%. While cryotherapy is also frequently recommended, we have had less success with it.

Dirofilariasis

Dirofilariasis, or zoonotic filariasis, results from the transmission of various animal filaria to humans via a mosquito bite. *Dirofilaria immitis*, the dog heartworm, can cause pulmonary symptoms in humans. A variety of other *Dirofilaria* from dogs, cats, raccoons, and even bears can cause cutaneous problems. The mosquito becomes infected when biting an infected animal and introduces larvae into the skin and subcutaneous tissues, so they are located deeper than typical cutaneous larva migrans.

The worms typically locate around the eyes, causing either periorbital edema or conjunctival infiltrates. They may also cause angioedema-like swellings elsewhere, especially on or near the genitalia. The infection is usually self-limited, so no therapy is needed.

Visceral Larva Migrans

There are other animal parasites that succeed in wandering about the body but never establish their life cycle within the human host. The two best known examples are toxocariasis and gnathostomiasis. *Toxocara canis* and *Toxocara cati* are ascaris-like worms infecting dogs and cats. When their eggs are ingested (or rarely when infected animals are eaten), the larvae hatch in the intestine and wander particularly to the lungs and eyes. In some parks in the USA, 30% of soil samples contain *Toxocara* eggs, so the possibility of infection is real, although transmission seldom occurs. *Gnathostoma spinigerum* is a nematode infecting dogs and cats in Southeast Asia; it has a complicated life cycle involving water fleas and fish. Human infection occurs from eating fermented or otherwise poorly cooked fish. The larvae may reach the CNS, causing eosinophilic cerebral abscesses. On rare occasions, cutaneous larva migrans has been described.

Strongyloidiasis

(Fülleborn 1926)

Synonyms. Larva currens, racing larva (Arthur and Shelley 1958)

Definition. Intestinal worm infection in which the larvae move rapidly through the skin and elicit intense itching.

Causative Organism. *Strongyloides stercoralis.* Rarely, *Strongyloides fülleborni* can be transferred from primates.

Epidemiology. *Strongyloides stercoralis* is a human parasite that can occasionally infect dogs, cats, and monkeys. It is distributed worldwide, primarily in tropical areas but occasionally seen in temperate zones. An estimated 80 million people worldwide are infected. Infection occurs when larvae hatch in fecally contaminated soil, enter the skin, pass to the lungs, ascend, are swallowed, and settle in the small intestine. Thus, the same risk factors discussed for hookworm and cutaneous larva migrans infections pertain.

Etiology and Pathogenesis. The parthenogenetic female attaches to the intestinal wall and lays eggs which develop into noninfectious rhabditiform larvae. These larvae usually pass with the stool and mature rapidly into infectious filariform larvae when deposited in the soil. Under appropriate oxygen conditions, filariform larvae may develop in the large intestine, penetrating the rectal mucosa or perianal skin and setting up a cycle of autoinoculation.

Clinical Findings. With the initial infection, there are changes identical to those with cutaneous larva migrans. *Strongyloides stercoralis* is famous for moving quickly, up to 5–15 cm/h, probably facilitated by the production of potent proteases. During the course of migration, there are allergic, primarily pulmonary symptoms associated with urticaria, which is often deep and persistent, lasting several days. The gut infection is often symptomatic, with diarrhea, pain, weight loss, and similar problems. The classic cutaneous change in strongyloidiasis is an intensely pruritic perianal rash with urticarial cords radiating out from the anus. In massive infections, especially in immunocompromised patients, *Strongyloides stercoralis* can be responsible for purpura, most often on the abdomen, and often associated with bacterial sepsis. Because of the autoinoculation, strongyloidiasis can last for many years.

Histopathology. The larvae can occasionally be found in a biopsy sample taken from the moving end of a lesion. When the purpuric lesions are biopsied, larvae may be found within small vessels.

Laboratory Findings. Examining stool for ova and parasites is the most reliable approach, but often must be repeated several times using enrichment techniques. If stool is maintained in the laboratory at the appropriate temperature and humidity, the larvae may hatch within 14 h. An ELISA test is also available. Eosinophilia is also usually present.

Differential Diagnosis. One must consider hookworm infections and cutaneous larva migrans, but the perianal problems usually point toward *Strongyloides stercoralis.*

Therapy. The treatment of choice is albendazole (400 mg daily for 3 days). Thiabendazole, mebendazole, and ivermectin are possible alternatives. Retreatment in 3 weeks is often recommended. Systemic corticosteroids should be avoided, as they seem to facilitate the infection.

Trichuriasis

Synonym. Whipworm infection

Causative Organism. *Trichuris trichiura.* The whipworm is another intestinal nematode spread by the fecal-oral route, usually via contaminated vegetables. It is a very common disorder, involving about 700 million people worldwide. The 3–5 cm adult worms are attached to the cecum or rectum, where they cause a variety of symptoms including bloody stools, abdominal pain, and even rectal prolapse, where they may be easily seen. In chronic childhood infections, severe anemia and even hypoproteinemia and growth retardation may also occur. Cutaneous findings are limited to an occasional urticarial reaction. Diagnosis is by examination of stool for ova and parasites. The treatment of choice is mebendazole.

Filariasis

(Bancroft 1880)

Synonyms. Bancroftian, Malayan, or Timorean filariasis

Definition. Tropical worm infection transmitted by mosquitoes in which the primary site of involvement is the lymphatic system.

Causative Organism. *Wucheria bancrofti*, *Brugia malayi*, and *Brugia timori*. The adult females are about 1 cm long, the males much smaller. The microfilariae are about 0.2 mm long.

Epidemiology. Filariasis is a worldwide tropical infection. *Wucheria bancrofti* is very widely spread, while *Brugia malayi* is more endemic to Asia and *Brugia timori* to a limited number of Indonesian islands. About 90 million people are infected. *Culex* mosquitoes, classic night biters, usually transfer the microfilariae, which also peak in the blood at night. In parts of Asia where *Aedes* mosquitoes, day feeders, are responsible, the microfilariae are present in the blood throughout the day, a remarkable adaptation. Thus, any conditions which favor breeding of mosquitoes or exposure to biting insects at night also facilitate filariasis. Humans are the only host for *Wucheria bancrofti*; for the *Brugia* species, cats, dogs, and monkeys are reservoirs of infection.

Etiology and Pathogenesis. The microfilariae pass to the regional lymph nodes, where they develop. The female releases new microfilariae into the blood stream, but they cannot develop within the host. Instead, they must be taken up by another mosquito, where they mature into an infectious form in the thoracic musculature. The adult worms continue to live in the lymph nodes, producing lymphatic obstruction and eventually edema.

Clinical Findings. There are some differences between *Wucheria bancrofti* and *Brugia malayi* infections, but the entire process is common to both. Many individuals are infected but asymptomatic. During World War II, USA troops demonstrated that the reverse is possible: several thousand soldiers developed symptoms, but microfilariae were found in only a handful of cases.

Signs and symptoms usually appear several months after the initial infection. Considering first infections with *Wucheria bancrofti*, the most typical symptoms are fever, chills, lymphangitis, and lymphadenopathy. The fever lasts for several daysand then disappears. In contrast to bacterial infections, the lymphangitis moves distally from infected lymph nodes. No microfilariae are found at this point. As the disease establishes itself, three major courses can be seen:

- Recurrent episodes of fever (acute recurrent filarial fever).
- Chronic pulmonary infections with asthma, eosinophilia, and tissue damage but without circulating microfilariae (tropical pulmonary eosinophilia syndrome).
- Progressive lymphedema leading to massive tissue thickening, especially of the legs and scrotum, and hydrocele and chyluria from obstruction. On rare occasions, the breasts and arms are involved. Such swollen limbs or scrotum are commonly called elephantiasis; the name is unfortunate but adequately describes the tragic cases of massively distorted limbs or a scrotum so large it must be carried in a wheelbarrow. The overlying skin becomes thickened and pebbly.

In *Brugia* infections, the recurrent fevers are more severe and the elephantiasis usually confined to the lower aspects of the legs, often unilateral.

Histopathology. Biopsy usually shows massively thickened skin with dilated lymphatics. One must be lucky to find organisms. Even in the lymph nodes, a granulomatous tissue response may often obscure the adult worms.

Laboratory Findings. The diagnosis is made by identifying the microfilariae in blood. They are motile and can be seen in a drop of fresh blood. The latent period during which none are found is 6–24 months for *Wucheria bancrofti* and 3–12 months for *Brugia malayi*. In addition, some patients have very low microfilariae loads and the daily variation must be taken into consideration. Special filters can be used to concentrate microfilariae, and acridine orange staining may aid identification. Serologic techniques are available but do not reflect the acuity of the disease, so they are of limited value in endemic areas.

Differential Diagnosis. Any patient with lymphangitis and/or lymphadenopathy arising after a tropical trip should be suspected of having filariasis. The fever and pulmonary syndrome can be caused by a variety of other worms and infections. In chronic cases, when only lymphedema is present, the history usually points one in the right direction.

Therapy

Systemic. Diethylcarbamazime is the treatment of choice. One recommended regimen involves gradually increasing doses, eventually using 3 mg/kg daily over 21 days. Initially, there may be a Jarisch-Herxheimer-like reaction, so most cases start with just 50 mg on day 1. Because diethylcarbamazine only kills microfilariae and not adults, yearly retreatment is recommended in endemic areas. Ivermectin (150 µg/kg twice yearly) represents a safer and easier approach and seems to be about as effective.

The allergic, febrile, and pulmonary symptoms are treated symptomatically.

Surgical. Surgery is the only hope for elephantiasis.

Prophylaxis. Insect repellents and mosquito netting are essential. In addition, either diethylcarbamazine or ivermectin can be taken every 2 weeks by travelers. In endemic areas, the addition of 0.1% diethylcarbamazine to salt has produced marked improvement. In a massive attack on filariasis, the pharmaceutical firm Smith Kline Beecham is donating enough albendazole to treat the 1.1 billion people at risk of acquiring the disease, in hopes of eliminating the problem by 2020.

Loiasis

(Gyout 1778; Cobbolt 1864; Argyll Robertson 1895)

Synonyms. Loa loa infection, Calabar swelling, Cameroon swelling, fugitive swelling, eyeworm disease of Africa, Loa loa filariasis

Definition. Infection with an African nematode that characteristically migrates through the skin and across the conjunctiva.

Causative Organism. *Loa loa.* The adult female worm is 5–7 cm long, the male about half as long.

Epidemiology. Loiasis is widely distributed in equatorial Africa, especially in the Congo River basin, where in some villages virtually all inhabitants are infected. About 30 million patients are estimated in Africa. The disease can not be acquired without visiting Africa. The disease is transmitted by the deerfly (*Chrysops*) which ingests microfilariae when feeding on a patient. The microfilariae mature in the deerfly and are then transferred to a new host. There is no known animal reservoir.

Etiology and Pathogenesis. The incubation period usually lasts several years but may be as short as a few months. The microfilariae mature in the connective tissue and then wander through the subcutaneous tissue as adult worms. The adult worm lives for over a decade. The wandering female worm, steadily shedding microfilariae, elicits a modest inflammatory reaction responsible for most of the signs and symptoms.

Clinical Findings. The initial complaint is usually pruritus, most commonly on the arms, chest, face, and scalp. The classic finding is a subcutaneous swelling containing the female worm; it is usually several centimeters in diameter and persists for a few days. At this time, eosinophilia may be extreme, up to 90%. Some patients may have severe allergic reactions with fever and giant urticaria. The most disturbing finding is the presence of the worm just beneath the conjunctiva, producing a migrating track associated with marked inflammation and irritation.

Histopathology. If a swelling is biopsied, the female worm may be found.

Laboratory Findings. The microfilariae can be identified in the blood. Eosinophilia is invariable.

Differential Diagnosis. One must initially consider other types of filariasis, especially *Wucheria bancrofti* and *Onchocerca volvulus. Mansonella streptocerca* is another nematode which can cause skin pruritus and swelling; it is found in the same part of Africa. Other *Mansonella* species cause only systemic disease, such as lung infections.

Therapy

Systemic. The same approach is used as for filariasis. Once again, Jarisch-Herxheimer reactions are common; often they must be blocked with antihistamines and corticosteroids. If the microfilariae load is high, there is a marked risk of allergic meningoencephalitis, so therapy should be left to experts.

Prophylaxis. Insect repellents and netting are even more important, as the deerfly is quite large and can be avoided. Extermination programs against the deerfly have failed. Either diethylcarbamazine or ivermectin can be used once weekly for prophylaxis.

Surgical. The worm is usually extracted from the eye and can be removed from a swelling.

Onchocerciasis

Synonym. River blindness

Definition. Common worm infection in tropical regions which frequently causes pruritus and blindness.

Causative Organism. *Onchocerca volvulus.* The female worms may be as long as 50 cm, while the males are about one-tenth as large.

Epidemiology. *Onchocerca volvulus* occur in equatorial Africa, Central and South America, and parts of Yemen and southwestern Saudi Arabia. Quite different clinical findings are seen in different lands – an unsolved puzzle. Even though extensive control programs have been instituted, especially in Africa, it is estimated that 50 million people worldwide are infected and about 3 million have been blinded. Some fertile river valleys have been deserted because of *Onchocerca volvulus* but are slowly being resettled today. The microfilariae are transmitted by female *Simulium*, tiny blackflies which breed along small, rapidly moving streams. They go through several development stages in these flies before being transferred to a new victim.

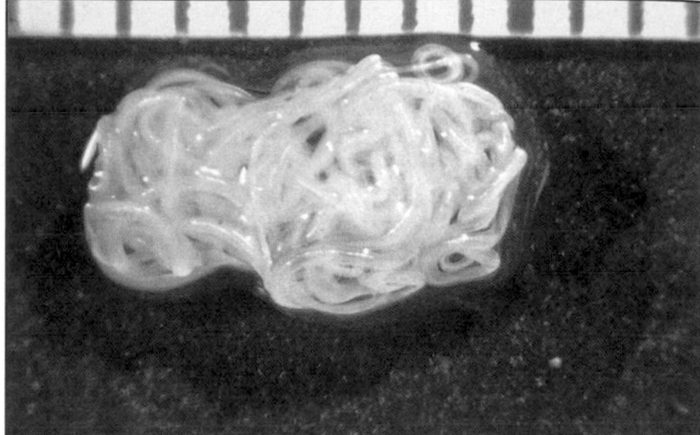

Fig. 9.2. Nodule of onchocerciasis

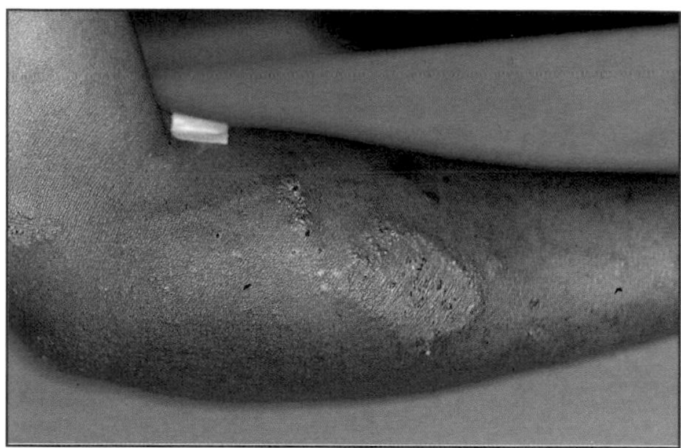

Fig. 9.3. Nodules and tracts of onchocerciasis secondary to migration of microfilariae

Etiology and Pathogenesis. The microfilariae move into the subcutaneous tissues of their new hosts and the large female and her tiny partner lie coiled together in fibrotic nodules, where they may live for many years. The female releases tiny, 0.3 mm microfilariae that wander through the host but show a special affinity for the skin and eyes. While they can be found in blood in heavy infections, their main activity is confined to tissue. Usually, 15–18 months pass after inoculation before microfilariae are present.

Clinical Findings. The clinical findings can be divided into several distinct groups:

- Subcutaneous Nodules or Onchocercoma. These nodules represent accumulations of paired worms, often with a host inflammatory and fibrous response (Fig. 9.2). Their distribution on the body varies in different parts of the world.
- Dermatitis. As the microfilariae begin to wander through the skin, they cause pruritus and urticaria. In addition, tiny papules known as craw-craw, not dissimilar to scabies, may appear. Over time, prurigo nodules and lichenification develop because of the intense scratching and secondary infection (Fig. 9.3).
- Depigmentation and Atrophy. On the legs, focal hypo- or depigmentation with retained pigment around the follicle gives a confetti-like picture. Since most patients are black, these changes are called leopard skin in some local tongues. The cause is felt to be postinflammatory hypopigmentation. In addition, a postinflammatory elastolysis develops, producing prematurely aged, thin skin. In the groin this is coupled with lymphadenopathy, producing loose hanging folds of skin (hanging groin sign).
- In later stages, the lymphadenopathy and lymphedema may predominate, just as with classic filariasis. Scrotal enlargement is more common than leg changes. Gynecomastia is also common in more advanced cases, but the cause is unclear.
- The eyes are another favorite site for the microfilariae. Most problems are caused by the inflammation which follows the destruction of micro-

filariae, with the release of various antigens which probably trigger a cross-reaction with ocular structures. The results are keratitis, chorioretinitis, iridocyclitis, lens opacity, and pannus formation. The pannus grows over the cornea, usually from the side or inferiorly, while in trachoma it usually grows from the superior pole downwards. The resulting loss of vision is known as river blindness. The classical picture is a young boy leading a chain of blind adults holding on to one another.

In Mexico, a slightly different picture may be seen, with an erysipelas-like infection of the cheeks, known as "erisipela de la costa" or coastal erysipelas. This is more common in younger patients, while older individuals develop purple or violet papules and plaques, designated "mal morado." Sometimes, in association with lymphadenopathy, one or both legs may become markedly hyperpigmented; this is known in Egypt and the Sudan as "sowda".

Histopathology. The nodules are often excised. This is one way to reduce the microfilariae. In such instances, the worms are readily identified. The microfilariae can also be spotted in biopsies from papules, but skin snips are more efficient.

Laboratory Findings. The microfilariae are identified by doing skin snips or tiny biopsies from papules. The tissue is placed in physiologic saline and after 30–60 min or, even better, after 1 day, examined with low power microscopy. Slit lamp microscopy can also be used to identify the microfilariae. Formerly, a low dose of diethylcarbamazine (25–50 mg) was administered; infected individuals have a Jarisch-Herxheimer reaction in this so-called Mazzotti test. When the microfilarial load is high, this approach is very dangerous and thus rarely used.

Differential Diagnosis. Clinically, onchocerciasis is fairly distinct when fully developed. When faced with someone who has pruritus and recently returned from the tropics, the idea is often considered, but usually another explanation such as scabies proves correct.

Therapy

Systemic. The same medications can be used as for filariasis. Ivermectin has proved especially effective for treating large populations. The manufacturer Merck has made it available gratis for control efforts in Africa. A dosage of 150 µg/kg is given once or twice yearly. This suffices to kill the microfilariae and reduce their release by the females. Diethylcarbamazine causes more of a Jarisch-Herxheimer reaction when treating full-blown infections. Either one is very effective against adult worms, whereas suramin kills the adults but with considerable side effects.

Surgical. Individual nodules can be excised.

Prophylaxis. There are attempts to kill the flies by making river beds unattractive for habitation. Recently, biodegradable insecticides have been applied with some success. Netting and repellents remain crucial. Today, whole populations are treated twice yearly with ivermectin; since the prevalence rates are over 90% in these areas, the difference between prophylaxis and treatment is a semantic one.

Dracunculiasis

Synonyms. Guinea worm infection, dracontiasis

Definition. Infection by a very long nematode which lives in the subcutaneous tissue and skin of the legs.

History. This is one of the oldest infections on record. Many feel that the serpent wrapped around the staff of Aesculapius, the god of healing, represents a guinea worm being extracted.

Causative Organism. *Dracunculus medinensis.* The female worm is up to 120 cm long, while the tiny male reaches only 2–4 cm.

Epidemiology. Guinea worm infection is found in Africa, India, and Yemen, but its range is shrinking. Recent estimates suggest that 100 million individuals are infected. In some localities, there is a high prevalence; in others, it remains an oddity. The only host is the human being. Larvae are released from the skin when the feet are immersed in fresh water ponds; tiny water crustaceans of the *Cyclops* family take up the larva. Reinfection occurs when the tiny crabs are ingested with drinking water. The trick is to avoid placing one's limbs in areas where drinking water is being obtained. In many areas, steps lead down to the water's edge to facilitate bathing, filling of water jugs, and washing clothes. Attempts to convert the inhabitants to using wells for drinking water has made major improvements.

Etiology and Pathogenesis. The swallowed crustaceans release the mature larvae in the intestine. They leave the intestine and migrate to the subcutaneous tissue, usually of the legs. Here, they slowly grow over a period of months; the male dies after 3–7 months, while the much larger female moves into the skin after 10–14 months. Here she produces an erythematous papule or blister which ruptures when the leg is placed in fresh water of the appropriate temperature. As the female's uterus prolapses, myriad larvae are released to be taken up again by *Cyclops.*

Clinical Findings. During the incubation period, most individuals are asymptomatic. As the female worm moves toward the skin, urticaria, eosinophilia, pulmonary problems, and other allergic manifestations may appear. Soon thereafter, the blister develops almost always over the ankle or knee, ulcerates, and then often becomes secondarily infected. These infections may extend into the deeper structures of the foot or knee, producing arthritis, ankylosis, and contractures.

Laboratory Findings. The female worm can often be seen. In addition, radiologic examination may show calcified subcutaneous worms. Both eosinophilia and elevated IgE levels are common.

Differential Diagnosis. While one can discuss the causes of foot ulcers at length, the presence of an ulcer with a long worm in it is specific.

Therapy. The traditional treatment is to extract the worm slowly by winding it about a match stick or twig, removing 3–5 cm daily. More dramatic attempts usually just break off the worm. Some suggest giving ivermectin or diethylcarbamazine simultaneously to facilitate removal. The medications do not kill the adult worms.

Prophylaxis. Eliminating step wells, filtering drinking water, and the use of biodegradable insecticides have put guinea worm infection on the verge of being eliminated.

Cestodes

Cestodes or tapeworms are responsible for a variety of illnesses but have few skin findings.

Taeniasis

Definition. Intestinal infection with either cattle or pig tapeworm.

Causative Organism. *Taenia saginata* or *Taenia solium*

Epidemiology. Taeniasis is a worldwide problem where meat is improperly cooked and cattle or pigs have access to human excrement. The names cattle tapeworm (*Taenia saginata*) and pig tapeworm (*Taenia solium*) are actually misnomers, as humans are the final host in both cases. The eggs are excreted in the stool, ingested by the intermediate host, and migrate through the body to encyst in the muscles. *Taenia solium* is more adaptable and can be spread by the fecal-oral route when there is close human contact and poor hygiene.

Etiology and Pathogenesis. If beef or pork is improperly cooked and the infected muscle ingested, the cyst opens and the immature worm attaches to the small intestine, where it matures. *Taenia saginata* may reach a length of 10 m while *Taenia solium* is only slightly smaller. These large worms absorb large amounts of nutrients, causing nutritional and obstructive problems.

Clinical Findings. Many patients are somewhat thin and surprised to discover at some point tapeworm segments in the stool or about their anus. Others are totally asymptomatic but have the tapeworm discovered at surgery for another problem. Yet others have abdominal pain, pancreatitis, anemia, hypoproteinemia, and similar problems. There are no skin findings.

Laboratory Findings. The diagnosis is based on stool examination for ova and parasites. Usually, only one worm is present, so after treatment the stool is examined to search for the scolex (head) of the worm.

Therapy. Niclosamide and praziquantel are currently recommended.

Cysticercosis

Definition. Human tissue infection by larvae of pig tapeworm.

Causative Organism. *Taenia solium*

Epidemiology. Only *Taenia solium* is capable of causing cysticercosis. There are several mechanisms; either the eggs of *Taenia solium* can be released in the upper intestine because of inadequate treatment or other triggers, or there can be fecal-oral spread with the ingestion of eggs from the patient or a close contact. The problem is most common in Central America and Eastern Europe.

Etiology and Pathogenesis. The eggs hatch and the larvae mature for 8–12 weeks, penetrate the intestine, and spread to the muscles and other human tissues rather than being confined to the bowel. While the larvae can invade any tissue, they typically cause problems in the CNS, eyes, and heart. Skin findings may call attention to the deeper problems.

Clinical Findings. The usual first finding is transient erythematous lesions, edema, and urticaria associated with eosinophilia. Later, the larvae may embed in muscles or subcutaneously, forming firm, permanent cysts called cysticerci cellulosae. When the cysts are formed in the heart, conduction disturbances are common, while in the eyes a variety of space-occupying problems occur. The most common severe complications involve the CNS with seizures, headaches, and pseudotumors. The combination of cutaneous swellings and seizures should always suggest cysticercosis.

Histopathology. If a nodule is excised, the larva can be found.

Laboratory Findings. Serologic tests are available. Often, the cysts are calcified and can thus be identified; both CAT scan and MRI have proven useful for evaluating CNS lesions.

Therapy. The treatment is very difficult, as the larvae are not as easily reached or as sensitive as the adults. Albendazole or praziquantel are recommended. The patient must be hospitalized because of the likelihood of severe CNS reactions when the organisms are killed. Often corticosteroids, antihistamines, and even antiepileptics are used to prepare the patient for this dramatic effect. Cysts in the skin and soft tissue can be removed; cardiac, ophthalmologic, or neurologic surgery may be required.

Other Tapeworms

Hymenolepsis nana Infection

The dwarf tapeworm is the most common tapeworm in the USA. It is only a few centimeters in length. Transmission is via the oral-fecal route or through fecally contaminated food. The symptoms are minor; only massive infections cause bowel problems such as pain and diarrhea. Epidemics may be seen in nursing homes and similar institutions. Treatment is with praziquantel or niclosamide. The closely related rat tapeworm *Hymenolepsis diminuta* can spread to humans if they ingest insects infected with the larvae; similarly, children may ingest the eggs of *Dipylidium caninum*, the dog and cat tapeworm.

Diphyllobothrium latum Infection

The fish tapeworm is found in lake regions in subarctic or temperate zones of Europe and North America. It has a complicated life cycle, as the eggs are excreted by the mammalian hosts and pass in *Cyclops* water fleas, where they mature. The invertebrates are eaten by fresh water fish; here the mobile larvae known as sparganum develop in the muscle. Humans and other fish-eating mammals are the final hosts. When they eat the fish, the sparganum is released and attaches to their intestinal wall. Most infections are asymptomatic; a classic finding is vitamin B12 deficiency. There are no skin findings. Treatment is with praziquantel or niclosamide.

Sparganosis

Sometimes the mobile sparganum of other *Diphyllobothrium* can penetrate the skin. The most common scenario is in Thailand, where frog flesh is used as an eye poultice. If the frog meat is infected with tapeworm larva, they may get under the conjunctiva, causing severe inflammation. Similarly, if fish or frogs infected with cat or dog tapeworms are eaten, the sparganum may migrate into the new, false host, producing subcutaneous nodules but never maturing. Rarely, CNS complications similar to cysticercosis may develop.

Echinococcosis

Synonym. Hydatidosis

Definition. Infection of humans by larvae of dog and fox tapeworms producing cysts in various organs. There are two rather different types of echinococcosis, caused by different species of the tapeworm.

Cystic Hydatid Disease

Synonyms. Unilocular echinococcosis, dog tapeworm disease

Causative Organism. *Echinococcus granulosus.* The dog tapeworm is 2–6 mm in length.

Epidemiology. The disease is most common where herds of herbivores are in close contact with dogs, in other words, mainly where sheep herding is common. *Echinococcus granulosus* is found in the sheep-raising regions of the western USA but has been almost eliminated in Australia and New Zealand. The sheep dogs are usually asymptomatic. The sheep are exposed to the dog droppings and the dogs are fed with infected sheep – a perfect cycle.

Etiology and Pathogenesis. *Echinococcus granulosus* has a simple life cycle. The eggs are passed by the dog or occasionally other canids and ingested by herbivores, where they mature in the liver and lungs, forming large cysts. The cycle is completed when the dog ingests a cyst containing the protoscolix (early head segment) of the tapeworm. It attaches to the intestinal wall to develop and breed. Humans are an accidental host and is infected when he ingests the eggs.

Clinical Findings. The most common site of involvement is the liver, which is affected in two-thirds of cases. In about 20 %, there is pulmonary disease. Other typical sites include the CNS, peritoneum, spleen, muscles, bones, skin, and subcutaneous tissues. *Echinococcus granulosus* typically forms solitary, usually unilocular cysts, ranging in size from several millimeters to more than 10 cm. If the cysts leak or are ruptured, anaphylactic reactions are common and larvae can be released to produce daughter cysts. Patients are asymptomatic for many years until either space-occupying lesions or impaired liver function appears. The subcutaneous cysts are fluctuant to firm, painless, fixed, noninflamed, and can be up to 10 cm in size. In contrast, cysticerci produce much smaller cysts. Large or dead cysts may calcify.

Laboratory Findings. If unilocular calcified cysts are identified, the diagnosis can be suggested by radiologic examination. Sonography, CAT scans, and MRI may also be used. The final diagnosis is usually made with laparoscopy to reduce leakage, anaphylaxis, and seeding. A wide variety of serologic tests are also available, including direct immunofluorescent testing with intact protoscolices and hemagglutination reactions with cystic fluid. ELISA and immunoblot testing is also available. Only about one-third of patients have eosinophilia.

Therapy. The ideal therapy is surgical excision of the cysts, which is usually attainable with *Echinococcus granulosus.* Both mebendazole (50 mg/kg daily) and albendazole (400 mg b.i.d.) are effective; either can be used in conjunction with surgery or tried as a primary treatment if the cysts are relatively small. Treatment should be continued for 3–6 months. If a cyst ruptures, praziquantel is the best "antiprotoscolicide."

Alveolar Hydatid Disease

Synonym. Multilocular echinococcosis

Causative Organism. *Echinococcus multilocularis.* The fox tapeworm is about the same size as the dog tapeworm.

Epidemiology. The cycle is quite different. The primary host is the fox, although occasionally other canids and even small cats can be infected. The intermediate hosts are usually rodents, especially mice, which eat the fox droppings, become infected, and are then eaten by a fox or other small mammal. Humans are infected by eating the eggs, which can be found on low-lying wild fruit or berries that are inadequately washed. In addition, cats and dogs may bring the infection into the home. Contact with their stools or bedding can also transfer the eggs to humans. The disease is most common in central Europe, Russia, Alaska, Canada, and occurs rarely in the north central USA.

Etiology and Pathogenesis. The ingested eggs hatch and the embryos are distributed to other organs, primarily the liver. The course is much more aggressive. *Echinococcus granulosus* cysts have a thick capsule and slowly expand. *Echinococcus multilocularis* cysts expand at their periphery with many small infiltrative nodules and blebs resembling a tumor growth. Daughter cysts with infective protoscolices are not found.

Clinical Findings. The disease is almost exclusively confined to the liver. Patients typically present with pain, a liver mass, or abnormal liver function. There may be seeding in other organs, including the subcutaneous tissue. When the cyst is cut into, the contents are gel-like. Leakage is less common, so allergic reactions are not as feared. Most patients are asymptomatic, but in some the cysts expand rapidly and do not respond to therapy, leading to death.

Laboratory Findings. The same diagnostic approach is used; often the irregular shape of the cyst allows a tentative diagnosis.

Therapy. Because the cysts are nonencapsulated and locally invasive, surgical removal is quite difficult. The same agents can be used as in *Echinococcus granulosus* infections but must be continued for at least 2 years. Often, lifelong treatment is required to prevent expansion.

Trematodes

The trematodes or flukes are flattened worms that attach to their hosts with two suction cup-like organs, the apical and ventral suckers. Most trematodes are hermaphroditic; an exception are the schistosomes. All trematodes have a complex life cycle involving a snail as intermediate host. Cercariae develop in the snail, are released, and then penetrate the skin or are swallowed with food or water. If the cercariae are intended for another species such as a duck, then they may irritate human skin but never mature, analogous to the failure of worm larvae to mature in cutaneous larva migrans.

Schistosomiasis

(Bilharz 1851)

Synonyms. Bilharziasis, snail fever

Definition. Common fluke infection that variably involves the liver and bladder as well as the skin and many other organs.

Causative Organism. *Schistosoma mansoni, S. haematobium*, and *S. japonicum*, as well as many other species. The worms are 5–25 mm long; the females are slightly larger than the males.

Epidemiology. Schistosomiasis is a very common and serious infection. It is estimated that there are over 200 million cases worldwide, including about 90 million in Africa. In general, *S. mansoni* is most common in Africa but has been introduced to South and Central America. *S. haematobium* is limited to Africa and the Middle East, while *S. japonicum* is found in China, Taiwan, and the Philippines (it has been extinct in Japan since 1978). Since infection occurs when the skin is penetrated by water-dwelling cercariae, the risk of infection increases as irrigation and agriculture expand. In addition, exposure is almost inevitable, as most bathing and drinking water sources are contaminated in endemic lands.

While there are distinct differences between the three main schistosomes, their life cycles are similar. There are also other schistosomes, but they are important only in very limited areas, as with *S. mekongi* in the Mekong delta. The eggs are passed in the urine (*S. haematobium*) or feces (*S. mansoni, S. japonicum*) into the body of water. They hatch into miracidia which enter the snail hosts, go through two generations, and leave the snail as fork-tailed cercariae which enter humans via the skin. The water must be about 25 °C and the snails usually prosper better at the edge of a lake or bank of a stream. *S. japonicum* may also infect domestic animals such as pigs and water buffalo, complicating control efforts.

Etiology and Pathogenesis. The cercariae go from the skin via the lymphatic system and veins to the splanchnic and urogenital venous plexi, where they mature into adult worms.

Clinical Findings. The cercariae cause a pruritic papular dermatitis. It is usually not as severe as that caused by nonhuman cercariae (swimmers' itch). Those with repeated infections and sensitization have more pruritus. The lesions are typically on the legs, when contact has been through step wells or working in irrigated fields; if bathing is the source, as with tourists, the lesions may be more widespread.

After a period of 3–10 weeks, an allergic febrile reaction occurs. Urticaria, edema, eosinophilia, arthritis, and fever may all accompany the establishment of the parasites in the internal organs. This acute reaction lasts a matter of days and then the slow chronic course of schistosomiasis begins.

The parasites breed in the venous plexi and cause marked obstruction. The eggs elicit a marked inflammatory and fibrous response, especially in the liver. *S. mansoni* primarily causes hepatosplenomegaly; in fact, schistosomiasis is known in some circles as Egyptian hepatosplenomegaly. Colonic pseudopolyps and pulmonary lesions are also relatively common. In contrast, *S. haematobium* primarily involves the bladder and may even lead to bladder cancer and renal failure. *S. japonicum* also primarily involves the liver, but its eggs are more likely to be found in ectopic sites such as the spinal cord and brain, where they may cause epilepsy.

The skin is another site for ectopic deposition of eggs. The ova elicit an intense inflammatory response, producing painless, verrucous papules and nodules primarily in the perineum and gluteal region (Fig. 9.4). Secondary infection, ulceration, and development of squamous cell carcinoma may all occur. Occasionally, such lesions are found on the trunk or about the umbilicus.

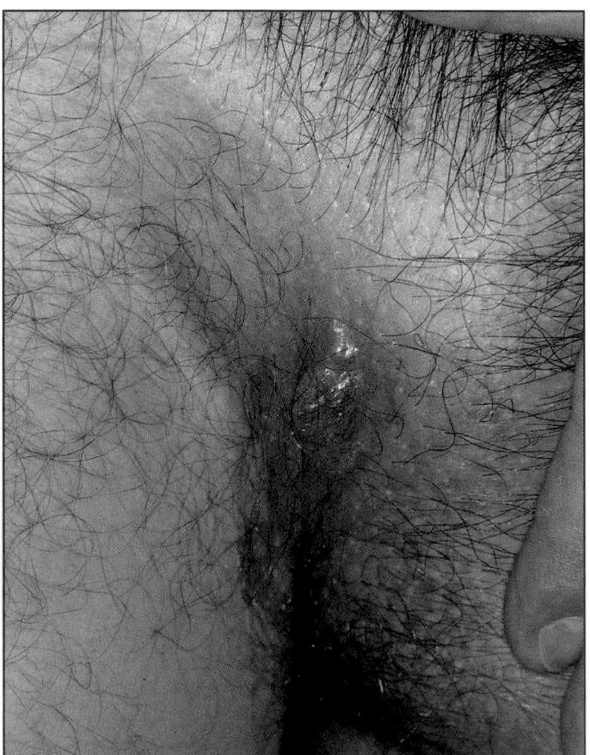

Fig. 9.4. Nodule of schistosomiasis

Histopathology. The cercarial papules show a modest eosinophilic infiltrate. It is difficult to find the cercariae in the skin. When the eggs are present in the chronic skin lesions, they can be identified associated with a dense eosinophilic and neutrophilic infiltrate.

Laboratory Findings. The eggs can be identified in the urine or stool as well as in the rectal mucosa, bladder wall, or liver. The shape of the egg can be used to determine the species of the infective organism. ELISA tests are most widely applied today, both to diagnose the infection accurately and to monitor therapy. In the past, anticercarial antibodies were used early in the disease course and, later, indirect immunofluorescent testing was used against the adult schistosomes.

Differential Diagnosis. The differential diagnosis includes most of gastroenterology and urology. As far as the skin lesions are concerned, the cercarial papules are usually too elusive to be diagnosed but can be confused with arthropod bites, early cutaneous larva migrans, other worm infections, and papular urticaria. The granulomas surrounding ectopic eggs are clinically confused with furuncles and ecthyma but often histologically straightforward.

Therapy. Praziquantel has revolutionized the approach to schistosomiasis. A total of 40–60 mg/kg divided into three doses over 1 day is the treatment of choice against all types of adult schistosomes. When CNS involvement is present, corticosteroids are often used to reduce the inflammatory edema associated with killing the flukes.

Prophylaxis. Eliminating the snails and reducing fecal contamination of bathing or agricultural water are helpful. If as a tourist one has a brief exposure to contaminated water, brisk rubbing of the skin, showering, and even massaging the skin with rubbing alcohol may help to prevent infection. Most recreational lakes in East Africa, long thought to be free of schistosomes, have been responsible for infections in recent years.

Swimmers' Itch

Synonym. Cercarial dermatitis

Definition. Infection of the skin by cercariae of nonhuman schistosomes.

Causative Organism. While many schistosomes can be responsible, most are members of the *Trichobilharzia* genus.

Epidemiology. Schistosomes that infect water fowl or small mammals also release the cercariae into water. The life cycle always involves a snail. Humans bathing in the water can easily be infected. This problem is common in the Great Lakes region, the inland lakes of Minnesota and Wisconsin, some coastal beaches in California, some of the alpine lakes around Munich, and many other locales. The snails tend to release the cercariae in the morning hours and especially when it is quite warm.

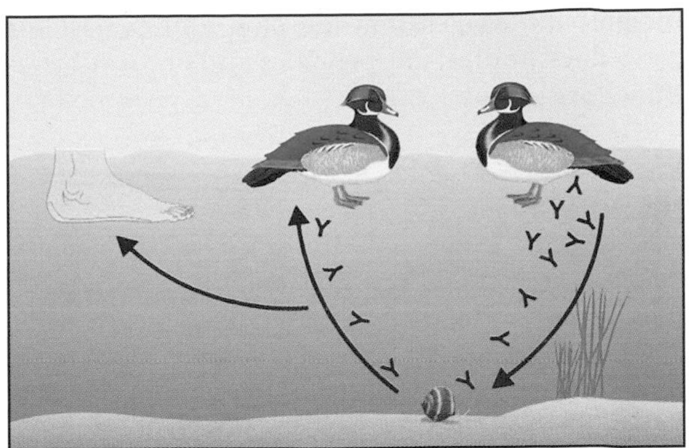

Fig. 9.5. Life cycle of swimmers' itch

Etiology and Pathogenesis. The cercariae cannot penetrate the human skin. They elicit an inflammatory response and die in a matter of days.

Clinical Findings. Swimmers' itch tells the story. Water exposure is required and an intensely pruritic macular eruption appears soon thereafter. In sensitized patients, the reaction is more severe, often urticarial, and occasionally accompanied by systemic symptoms. About 12 h later, pruritic papules begin to develop, surrounded by an erythematous base (Figs. 9.5, 9.6). The papules can coalesce and produce diffuse erythema and swelling. The cercariae die after 2–3 days and the rash disappears within a week. Some degree of sensitization is required. In the first infection, the cercariae last for about 2 weeks in the skin and the pruritic papules first develop after 5–14 days, so the course is slower and milder.

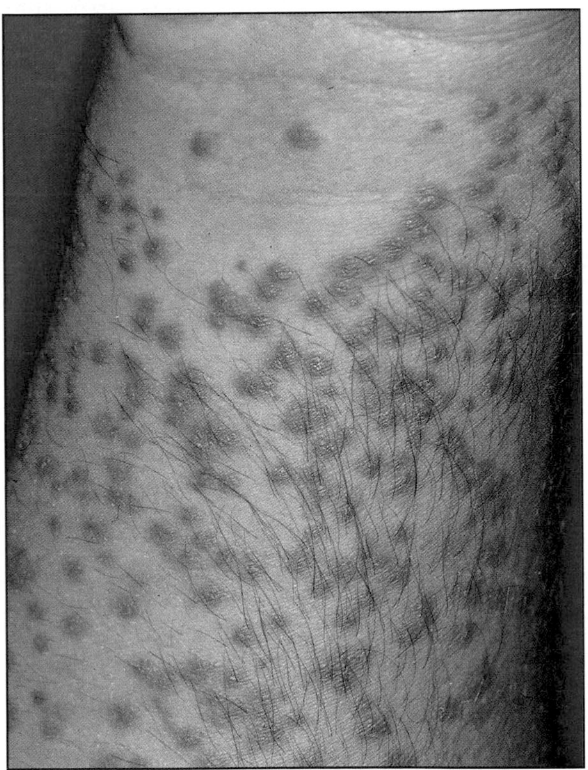

Fig. 9.6. Pruritic papules in swimmers' itch

Therapy. Topical antipruritics and oral antihistamines suffice. In severe cases, topical corticosteroids can be used; if systemic symptoms (other than pruritus) are present, oral corticosteroids may be needed.

Prophylaxis. The infection usually occurs in shallow water. Avoiding relatively still areas rich in vegetation and water fowl is wise, especially during the morning hours. Brisk toweling and use of rubbing alcohol may help.

Seabather's Eruption

Synonym. Marine dermatitis

Seabather's eruption is not a worm infection. It is often confused with swimmers' itch and is mentioned here for that reason. It is most common on the Florida coast and some Caribbean islands. The pruritic papular eruption occurs on skin covered by bathing suits, suggesting that something is trapped under the suit and held in contact with the skin. Possible causes include seaweed fragments, jellyfish larvae, crustacean larvae, and other small marine organisms. If the suit is removed promptly and a shower taken, no reaction occurs. Otherwise, over a period of time, pruritic erythematous papules may develop and persist for 7–10 days. Topical antipruritics and oral antihistamines are useful.

Clonorchiasis

Synonym. Oriental liver fluke disease

The Oriental liver fluke *Clonorchis sinensis* is found primarily in Asia, especially southeast China, Japan, Korea, Taiwan, and the Mekong Delta. It infects humans and fish-eating carnivores. The main problem is the use of fish ponds for the disposal of human excrement. The young worms enter the final host when an infected fish is eaten. They lodge in the biliary tree and cause obstruction and predispose to cholangiocarcinoma. Praziquantel is recommended.

Opisthorchiasis

The cat and dog flukes, *Opisthorchis felineus* and *Opisthorchis viverrini*, have a life cycle similar to that of *Clonorchis sinensis*. In parts of Thailand, up to 90% of villagers are infected, with a total of 10 million infected individuals. These flukes are the leading cause of cholangiocarcinoma worldwide. Once again, praziquantel is appropriate.

Fasciolopsiasis

Fasciolopsis buski, a large, up to 7 cm fluke, is common in Southeast Asia. The two main hosts are pigs and humans. While snails are intermediate hosts, the cercariae encyst on aquatic plants such as the water chestnut and bamboo. Eating the improperly prepared vegetables introduces the fluke into the intestine, where it causes inflammation and even obstruction. Massive allergic reactions may occur, complete with severe facial edema and eosinophilia. While avoidance is easy, praziquantel is the treatment of choice, should infection occur.

Bibliography

General

Crompton DW (1999) How much human helminthiasis is there in the world? J Parasitol 85:397–403

De Silva N, Guyatt H, Bundy D (1997) Anthelmintics. A comparative review of their clinical pharmacology. Drugs 53:769–788

Georgiev VS (1999) Parasitic infections. Treatment and developmental therapeutics. 1. Necatoriasis. Curr Pharm Des 5:545–554

Kaur V (1997) Tropical diseases and women. Clin Dermatol 15:171–178

Liu LX, Weller PF (1996) Antiparasitic drugs. N Engl J Med 334:1178–1784

Lucchina LC, Wilson ME, Drake LA (1997) Dermatology and the recently returned traveler: infectious diseases with dermatologic manifestations. Int J Dermatol 36: 167–181

Enterobiasis

Avolio L, Avoltini V, Ceffa F et al. (1998) Perianal granuloma caused by Enterobius vermicularis: report of a new observation and review of the literature. J Pediatr 132: 1055–1056

Hugot JP, Reinhard KJ, Gardner SL et al. (1999) Human enterobiasis in evolution: Origin, specificity, and transmission. Parasite 6:201–208

Villarreal O, Villarreal JJ, Domingo JA (1999) Progressive eosinophilia and elevated IgE in enterobiasis. Allergy 54:646–648

Ascariasis

De Almeida MM, Arede C, Marta CS et al. (1998) Atopy and enteroparasites. Allerg Immunol (Paris) 30:291–294

Dold S, Heinrich J, Wichmann HE et al. (1998) Ascaris-specific IgE and allergic sensitization in a cohort of school children in the former East Germany. J Allergy Clin Immunol 102:414–420

Sarinas PS, Chitkara RK (1997) Ascariasis and hookworm. Semin Respir Infect 12:130–137

Trichinosis

Clausen MR, Meyer CN, Krantz T et al. (1996) Trichinella infection and clinical disease. QJM 89:631–636

Ko RC (1997) A brief update on the diagnosis of trichinellosis. Southeast Asian J Trop Med Public Health 1:S91–S98

Ancylostomiasis

Grencis RK, Cooper ES (1996) Enterobius, trichuris, capillaria, and hookworm, including *Ancylostoma caninum*. Gastroenterol Clin North Am 25:579–597

Hotez PJ, Pritchard DI (1995) Hookworm infection. Sci Am 272:68–74

Prociv P, Croese J (1996) Human enteric infection with *Ancylostoma caninum*: Hookworms reappraised in the light of a "new" zoonosis. Acta Trop 62:23–44

Prociv P, Luke RA (1995) The changing epidemiology of human hookworm infection in Australia. Med J Aust 162: 150–154

Sarinas PS, Chitkara RK (1997) Ascariasis and hookworm. Semin Respir Infect 12:130–137

Cutaneous Larva Migrans

Albanese G, Di Cintio R, Beneggi M et al. (1993) Creeping eruption: a review of clinical presentation and management of 60 cases presenting to a tropical disease unit. Arch Dermatol 129:588–591

Elgart MLE (1998) Creeping eruption. Arch Dermatol 134: 619–620

Goto Y, Tamura A, Ishikawa O et al. (1998) Creeping eruption caused by a larva of the suborder *Spirurina* type X. Br J Dermatol 139:315–318

Lucchina LC, Wilson ME, Drake LA (1997) Dermatology and the recently returned traveler: infectious diseases with dermatologic manifestations. Int J Dermatol 36: 167–181

Sala G (1995) Larva migrans in Italy. Int J Dermatol 34: 464–465

Vaughan TK, English JC III (1998) Cutaneous larva migrans complicated by erythema multiforme. Cutis 62:33–35

Dirofilariasis

Degardin P, Simonart JM (1996) Dirofilariasis, a rare, usually imported dermatosis. Dermatology 192:398–399

Jelinek T, Schulte-Hillen J, Loscher T (1996) Human dirofilariasis. Int J Dermatol 35:872–875

Marty P (1997) Human dirofilariasis due to *Dirofilaria repens* in France. A review of reported cases. Parassitologia 39:383–386

Orihel TC, Helentjaris D, Alger J (1997) Subcutaneous dirofilariasis: single inoculum, multiple worms. Am J Trop Med Hyg 56:452–455

Pampiglione S, Gupta AP (1998) Presence of *Dirofilaria repens* and an insect immunocyte (plasmatocyte) in a human subcutaneous nodule, induced by a mosquito bite. Parassitologia 40:343–346

Santamaria B, Di Sacco B, Muro A et al. (1995) Serological diagnosis of subcutaneous dirofilariasis. Clin Exp Dermatol 20:19–21

Van den Ende J, Kumar V, van Gompel A et al. (1995) Subcutaneous dirofilariasis caused by *Dirofilaria (nochtiella) repens* in a Belgian patient. Int J Dermatol 34: 274–277

Visceral Larva Migrans

Chitkara RK, Sarinas PS (1997) Dirofilaria, visceral larva migrans, and tropical pulmonary eosinophilia. Semin Respir Infect 12:138–148

Kurokawa M, Ogata K, Sagawa S et al. (1998) Cutaneous and visceral larva migrans due to *Gnathostoma doloresi* infection via an unusual route. Arch Dermatol 134: 638–639

Tan JS (1997) Human zoonotic infections transmitted by dogs and cats. Arch Intern Med 22:1933–1943

Strongyloidiasis

Arthur RP, Shelley WB (1958) Larva currens: a distinctive variant of cutaneous larva migrans due to *Strongyloides stercoralis*. Arch Dermatol 78:186–190

Füllerborn F (1926) Hautguaddeln und "Autoinfektion" bei Strongyloidisträgern. Arch Schiffs Tropen-Hyg 30: 721–732

Jacob CI, Patten SF (1999) *Strongyloides stercoralis* infection presenting as generalized prurigo nodularis and lichen simplex chronicus. J Am Acad Dermatol 41:357–361

Kao D, Murakawa GJ, Kerschmann R et al. (1996) Disseminated strongyloidiasis in a patient with acquired immunodeficiency syndrome. Arch Dermatol 132:977–978

Mansfield LS, Niamatali S, Bhopale V et al. (1996) *Strongyloides stercoralis*: maintenance of exceedingly chronic infections. Am J Trop Med Hyg 55:617–624

Trichuriasis

Beach MJ, Addiss DG, Roberts JM et al. (1999a) Treatment of trichuris infection with albendazole. Lancet 16:237–238

Beach MJ, Streit TG, Addiss DG et al. (1999b) Assessment of combined ivermectin and albendazole for treatment of intestinal helminth and *Wuchereria bancrofti* infections in Haitian schoolchildren. Am J Trop Med Hyg 60:479–486

Lee WS, Boey CC (1999) Chronic diarrhoea in infants and young children: causes, clinical features, and outcome. J Paediatr Child Health 35:260–263

Filariasis

Chandrashekar R (1997) Recent advances in diagnosis of filarial infections. Indian J Exp Biol 35:18–26

Cunningham NM (1997) Lymphatic filariasis in immigrants from developing countries. Am Fam Physician 55:1199–1204

Meyrowitsch DW, Nguyen DT, Hoang TH et al. (1998) A review of the present status of lymphatic filariasis in Vietnam. Acta Trop 70:335–347

Orihel TC, Eberhard ML (1998) Zoonotic filariasis. Clin Microbiol Rev 11:366–381

Loiasis

Chandrashekar R (1997) Recent advances in diagnosis of filarial infections. Indian J Exp Biol 35:18–26

De Viragh PA, Guggisberg D, Derighetti M et al. (1998) Monosymptomatic Loa loa infection. Dermatology 197: 303–305

Onchocerciasis

Hagan M (1998) Onchocercal dermatitis: clinical impact. Ann Trop Med Parasitol 92:S85–S96

Kale OO (1998) Onchocerciasis: the burden of disease. Ann Trop Med Parasitol 92:S101–S115

Dracunculiasis

Hopkins DR, Ruiz-Tiben E, Ruebush T Jr et al. (1995) Dracunculiasis eradication: March 1994 update. Am J Trop Med Hyg 52:14–20

Hunter JM (1996) An introduction to guinea worm on the eve of its departure: dracunculiasis transmission, health effects, ecology, and control. Soc Sci Med 43:1399–1425

Kumate J (1997) Infectious diseases in the 21st century. Arch Med Res 28:155–161

Molyneux DH (1998) Vector-borne parasitic diseases – an overview of recent changes. Int J Parasitol 28:927–934

Taeniasis and Cysticercosis

Juckett G (1995) Common intestinal helminths. Am Fam Physician 52:2039–2048, 2051–2052

Kamal MM, Grover SV (1995) Cytomorphology of subcutaneous cysticercosis. A report of 10 cases. Acta Cytol 39:809–812

Matsushima H, Hatamochi A, Shinkai H et al. (1998) A case of subcutaneous cysticercosis. J Dermatol 25:438–442
Schmidt DK, Jordaan HF, Schneider JW et al. (1995) Cerebral and subcutaneous cysticercosis treated with albendazole. Int J Dermatol 34:574–579

Other Tapeworms

Griffin MP, Tompkins KJ, Ryan MT (1996) Cutaneous sparganosis. Am J Dermatopathol 18:70–72
Harris NR, Reifsnyder DN (1997) Subcutaneous living sparganum worms. Plast Reconstr Surg 99:2120–2121
Hutchinson JW, Bass JW, Demers DM, Myers GB (1997) Diphyllobothriasis after eating raw salmon. Hawaii Med J 56:176–177
Jeong SC, Bae JC, Hwang SH et al. (1998) Cerebral sparganosis with intracerebral hemorrhage: a case report. Neurology 50:503–506

Echinococcosis

Altintas N (1998) Cystic and alveolar echinococcosis in Turkey. Ann Trop Med Parasitol 92:637–642
Ambo M, Adachi K, Ohkawara A (1999) Postoperative alveolar hydatid disease with cutaneous-subcutaneous involvement. J Dermatol 26:343–347
Bhojraj SY, Shetty NR (1999) Primary hydatid disease of the spine: An unusual cause of progressive paraplegia. Case report and review of the literature. J Neurosurg 91:S216–S218
Bresson-Hadni S, Humbert P, Paintaud G et al. (1996) Skin localization of alveolar echinococcosis of the liver. J Am Acad Dermatol 34:873–877
Conchedda M, Palmas C, Bortoletti G, et al. (1997) Hydatidosis: a comprehensive view of the Sardinian case. Parassitologia 39:359–366
Erdener A, Sahin AH, Ozcan C (1999) Primary pancreatic hydatid disease in a child: case report and review of the literature. J Pediatr Surg 34:491–492
John M, Poole JE, Friedland IR (1995) Posterior neck mass in a 4-year-old boy. Pediatr Infect Dis J 14:1119, 1122–1124
Miguet JP (1996) Skin localization of alveolar echinococcosis of the liver. J Am Acad Dermatol 34:873–877
Vuitton DA (1997) The WHO Informal Working Group on Echinococcosis. Coordinating Board of the WHO-IWGE. Parassitologia 39:349–353

Schistosimiasis

Andrade Filho J de S, Lopes MS, Corgozinho Filho AA et al. (1998) Ectopic cutaneous schistosomiasis: report of two cases and a review of the literature. Rev Inst Med Trop Sao Paulo 40:253–257
Farrell AM, Woodrow D, Bryceson AD, et al. (1996) Ectopic cutaneous schistosomiasis: extragenital involvement with progressive upward spread. Br J Dermatol 135: 110–112
Kaur V (1997) Tropical diseases and women. Clin Dermatol 15:171–178
Lambertucci JR, Rayes AA, Serufo JC et al. (1998) Schistosomiasis and associated infections. Mem Inst Oswaldo Cruz 93:S135–S139
Mas-Coma MS, Esteban JG, Bargues MD (1999) Epidemiology of human fascioliasis: a review and proposed new classification. Bull World Health Organ 77:340–346
Rocha MO, Greco DB, Pedroso ER et al. (1995) Secondary cutaneous manifestations of acute schistosomiasis mansoni. Ann Trop Med Parasitol 89:425–430

Swimmers' Itch and Seabather's Eruption

Bastert J, Sing A, Wollenberg A et al. (1999) Aquarium dermatitis: Cercarial dermatitis in an aquarist. Dermatology 197:84–86
Chamot E, Toscani L, Rougemont A (1998) Public health importance and risk factors for cercarial dermatitis associated with swimming in Lake Leman at Geneva, Switzerland. Epidemiol Infect 120:305–314
Kumar S, Hlady WG, Malecki JM (1997) Risk factors for seabather's eruption: a prospective cohort study. Public Health Rep 112:59–62
Lindblade KA (1998) The epidemiology of cercarial dermatitis and its association with immunological characteristics of a northern Michigan lake. J Parasitol 84:19–23
MacSween RM, Williams HC (1996) Seabather's eruption – a case of Caribbean itch. BMJ 312:957–958
Segura Puertas L, Burnett JW, Heimer de la Cotera E (1999) The medusa stage of the coronate scyphomedusa *Linuche unguiculata* (thimble jellyfish) can cause seabather's eruption. Dermatology 198:171–172

Other Trematodes

Mirdha BR, Gulati S, Sarkar T, Samantray JC (1998) Acute clonorchiasis in a child. Indian J Gastroenterol 17:155
Shekhar KC (1995) Food-borne parasitoses in Malaysia. Epidemiological assessment and research needs. J R Soc Health 115:178–185
Shekhar KC, Nazarina AR, Lee SH et al. (1995) Clonorchiasis/opisthorchiasis in Malaysians. Case reports and review. Med J Malaysia 50:182–186
Woo PC, Lie AK, Yuen KY et al. (1998) Clonorchiasis in bone marrow transplant recipients. Clin Infect Dis 27:382–384

CHAPTER 10

Reactions to Medications

Contents

Introduction

Reactions to medications are an extremely common problem. In a general ambulatory practice, the likelihood of medication-related problems is about 5%. At least 20% of hospitalized patients experience an adverse drug reaction. The most common organ in which such reactions are apparent is the skin. About 0.1% of hospitalized patients will have a serious, potentially fatal cutaneous reaction.

While patients and physicians speak of allergic reactions and drug allergies, the immunology of drug eruptions is complex and poorly understood. All the basic types of immunologic reactions as outlined by Gell and Coombs can be seen. In addition, many medications have physiologic or toxic reactions which are dose-related. If the dose required for the adverse reaction far exceeds the usual dose, then the change is viewed as an adverse event. When the threshold for a reaction is close to the therapeutic level, as with many chemotherapy agents, then the reaction is accepted as a pharmacologic effect. Some medicines are capable of degranulating mast cells, for example aspirin and codeine, to produce a pseudoallergic reaction. Other medications cause problems in patients who lack a specific enzyme or other factor. For example, some patients slowly or poorly inactivate isoniazid. Biologic modifiers such as interferons are finding increasing usage. They cause reactions which are an exaggeration of their normal biologic role. Another variation, which is not discussed further in this chapter, is the complications of immunosuppression including viral infections and tumors. Finally, sometimes a reaction is very rare, occurs at low dosage, perhaps on the first exposure or without any evidence for immunologic changes; then one speaks of an idiosyncratic reaction. No matter what type of reaction is involved, once the offending agent is identified and stopped, improvement is usually prompt.

Drug reactions can resemble or even reproduce many of the diseases discussed throughout this text. In order to avoid repetition, we have discussed lichen planus-like (Chap. 14), bullous (Chap. 15), lupus erythematosus-like (Chap. 18) and acneiform (Chap. 28) reactions elsewhere and only mention them here.

The history is the key to intelligently evaluating patients with possible drug eruptions. First, one must be sure that the list of medications is complete. Patients tend to forget over-the-counter medications and even more often, products they have been taking for many years. In general, they are correct in assuming that a diuretic they have used for 10 years is not a likely cause of their rash, but sometimes it happens. One should be particularly suspicious of drugs taken in recent days, but there are cautions. If an allergic reaction is involved, then either prior exposure or a cross-reaction is required. Delayed reactions, such as serum sickness, occur 7–10 days after exposure, as the body mounts a response, as to an injection of horse-derived immunoglobulin. Idiosyncratic reactions can occur almost instantly, as can life-threatening anaphylactic reactions through an inadvertent rechallenge. Other medications, such as ampicillin, are notorious for causing late reactions. Finally, the medication may enter the body by unusual routes. Iodine toxicity has been described from usage of large amounts of Iodoform gauze to pack a wound. One must often repeat the history several times to get all the pertinent facts.

Cofactors may be involved. Considering ampicillin once again, the use of the antibiotic in a patient with infectious mononucleosis is very likely to cause a purpuric eruption. Erythema nodosum drug eruptions are much more common in women, suggesting a hormonal influence. The patient's HLA type may also play a role, as for example in drug-induced lupus erythematosus. Sunlight is another trigger; many drug reactions are either photoallergic or phototoxic.

Drug reactions are another great imitator. They can produce a wide spectrum of clinical pictures, ranging from lichen planus (gold salts) to pityriasis rosea (gold salts) to lupus erythematosus (hydralazine, for example). Some drug reactions occur in only one or two areas, and then mysteriously reoccur in these same sites on reexposure. Such a fixed drug reaction is commonly seen with tetracycline, phenolphthalein and phenobarbital. Nonetheless, the most common drug reaction is a diffuse macular exanthem or toxic erythema. The differential diagnostic question is usually drug reaction or viral exanthem. Sometimes, pruritus is the first or even only sign of a drug reaction. However, pruritus in the absence of any clinical lesions such as a macular exanthem or urticaria is uncommon, especially if cholestasis and other drug-induced liver malfunction is excluded. In other cases, paresthesias may be a clue, such as with isoniazid, griseofulvin or thalidomide.

To approach patients with potential drug eruptions, one needs a very current and handy source of information about the likelihood of different types of drug reactions with various medications. We recommend Bruinsma W, *A Guide to Drug Eruptions* as listed in general references.

Etiology and Pathogenesis

Even though cutaneous drug reactions cover a wide morphologic range and involve many different mechanisms, some immunologic and some toxic, we will try to discuss them simultaneously considering both the clinical appearance and the probable underlying disease mechanism. Table 10.1 summarizes most of these reactions.

Allergic Reactions

Allergic exanthems comprise the vast majority of all drug reactions. They develop when a medication is administered to which the patient has previously been exposed and against which he is capable of reacting. Two factors should be considered at this step. Medications usually are not a pure product containing just the active ingredient, but also have a vehicle consisting of allegedly inert ingredients. A patient may be allergic to a constituent of the vehicle, such as a dye or preservative. In addition, cross-reactions between chemically related pharmacologic agents occur. Both of these scenarios should be considered when a patient reacts to an agent to which he denies exposure, but the usual explanation is an inaccurate drug history.

Most drugs are relatively small molecules which function as incomplete antigens or haptens. They or their metabolites are bound in the body to various proteins, thus forming antigens which are recognized by the host as foreign triggering an immune response. The hapten determinants of most medications have not been determined. They are best identified for penicillin and some of the sulfonamides. The chemical structure of a product plays a considerable role in its antigenic or aller-

Table 10.1. Classification of drug reactions based on pathogenesis

Type of reactions	Examples
Allergic reactions	
Type I (reaginic)	Macular and urticarial exanthems
Type II (cytotoxic)	Thrombocytopenic purpura
Type III (immune complex)	Leukocytoclastic vasculitis Hemorrhagic and bullous exanthems Serum sickness
Type IV (delayed)	Diffuse exanthems (scarlatiniform, morbilliform, rubeoliform) Lichenoid reactions Fixed drug reactions Erythema multiforme Toxic epidermal necrolysis Chronic purpuric reactions Pseudolymphoma reactions
Toxic reactions	Embolization of medications Anagen and telogen effluvium Cutaneous necrosis (as from antimetabolite overdoses)
Pseudoallergic Reactions	
Intolerance reactions	Mast cell degranulation by codeine
Idiosyncratic reactions	Anaphylactoid reaction to ASA, radiocontrast material
Miscellaneous reactions	Jarisch-Herxheimer reaction
Provocation of preexisting or latent skin disease	Acne from hormones, psoriasis from β-blockers (Table 10.13)

genic properties. In the skin, allergic contact dermatitis against para compounds is common. Included in this group are a wide range of cyclic organic molecules substituted at the para position with reactive additions such as amino, hydroxy, nitro or halogen groups. Examples of para-substituted compounds, all of which may cross-react, include local anesthetics (procaine, benzocaine or tetracaine), antituberculous drugs (para-amino salicylic acid), oral antidiabetic agents and sulfonamides. Sensitization to a single chemical structure is described as monovalent sensitization. Group sensitization describes the situation with para compounds or similarly related structures. In polyvalent sensitization there is an allergy to a number of unrelated structures.

In many cases, the medication itself is not the sensitizer, but instead one of its metabolites. Often the metabolites are hard to identify. In addition, often a combination of events is required. For example, the patient may have an infection which predisposes him to react to an antibiotic; the classic example is the ampicillin rash in infectious mononucleosis. When the patient is rechallenged after being cured of the infection, he does not react to the medication.

It usually takes 8–12 days for the body to form antibodies and to be capable of reacting against a product. Many medications are used for short periods of time or are rapidly excreted from the body, so that the sensitized patient shows no reaction unless reexposure occurs. Other medications may still be present in the body so that a reaction is manifested during the first exposure. On reexposure, the reaction can proceed more rapidly. Antibody-mediated or humoral reactions may produce immediate reactions within minutes to hours, such as anaphylaxis or an Arthus reaction. Cell-mediated reactions require 24–48 h to develop and are alternatively referred to as delayed hypersensitivity, such as in allergic contact dermatitis or tuberculin testing. Observing the exact time sequence of a clinical allergic reaction is often helpful in providing a better understanding of the disease and identifying the causative agent.

Allergic drug reactions can be subdivided using the classification of immunologic reactions developed by Gell and Coombs (Chap. 1).

Type I or Anaphylactic Reactions

The responsible antigen is usually a relatively large protein molecule. Smaller molecules of medications most likely serve as haptens which are attached to a protein, in some instances after being metabolized, to form a complete antigen. Reactions to these structures are mediated by IgE antibodies, which do not fix complement. They develop following sensitization and may be reflected by an elevated serum IgE level. Various cytokines also play a role in regulating the production of IgE synthesis such as interleukin (IL)-4 which promotes synthesis and its antagonist interferon (IFN)-γ. Type II helper T cells (TH2) secrete IL-4 and thus help steer the process. The IgE molecules bind to cell-surface antigens, especially the high-affinity IgE receptors on the surface of tissue mast cells and circulating basophils. They also bind to eosinophils, monocytes and B cells, over both high- and low-affinity receptors. The linking of two IgE molecules by a molecule of antigen is known as cross-linking. It triggers a cascade of enzymatic reactions that lead to the release of mediators from the mast cells, basophils and other cells.
The mediators fall into three main groups.

- Lipid mediators: Leukotriene B_4, leukotriene C_4, platelet activating factor (PAF), and prostaglandin D_2
- Mediators of anaphylaxis: Histamine, serotonin, proteoglycans, serine protease
- Cytokines: IL-3, IL-4, IL-5, IL-6, tumor necrosis factor (TNF)-α

These substances cause dilatation and increased permeability of the vessels, chemotaxis of eosinophils and contraction of smooth muscles. The amunt of mediators released as well as the site of the reaction determine the clinical consequences. They include:

Anaphylactic Shock. Release of large amounts of histamine in the system suddenly produces bronchospasm, localized edema (especially laryngeal or glottic edema), diffuse vessel dilatation, hypotension and collapse. At the same time, there may be urticaria or angioedema.

Localized Reactions or "Shock Fragments". Sometimes the intense reaction is restricted to the tissue where the antigen-antibody reaction has occurred. Reactions such as acute blepharoconjunctivitis, rhinitis and asthma may be seen following exposure to pollen at the site of the antigen contact.

Cutaneous Reactions. When the antigen is transferred by the blood, reactions occur at those sites where it encounters mast cells bearing the IgE antibodies. A dermal reaction produces urticaria, while a deeper reaction leads to urticaria profunda or angioedema.

Type II Reaction or Cytotoxic Reaction

Such reactions are often triggered by medications. In this case the medication or antigen is bound to the cell surface where it reacts with IgG and IgM antibodies and fixes complement. Sometimes, the drug is a hapten and the complete antigen includes a cell membrane protein as well. The activation of the complement cascade leads to membrane destruction and cytolysis, often within hours. Typical clinical reactions include hemolytic anemia, allergic thrombocytopenia, allergic granulocytopenia and some forms of drug-induced agranulocytosis.

Type III Reactions or Immune Complex Reactions

There are two basic clinical types of immune complex reactions, the Arthus reaction and serum sickness. In the classical or experimental Arthus reaction, guinea pigs were sensitized to egg albumin by immunization. After a 2-week wait, the challenging antigen was injected intradermally. Initially immunoglobulins, usually IgG and IgM, form complexes which are found in the walls of small vessels. Complement activation occurs producing increased permeability. Neutrophils are called to the site where they release their lysosomal enzymes causing destructive inflammation with hemorrhage, leukocytoclasia and necrosis. The reaction begins within 4 h and may last up to 15 h.

Arthus-type reactions are characterized by an excess of soluble antigens, which leads to the formation of immune complexes. The clinical example closest to the experimental model is probably allergic or leukocytoclastic vasculitis. Sweet syndrome and erythema multiforme may also belong in this group. Triggers are usually medications or bacterial antigens. Sometimes local injections can also elicit an Arthus-like reaction; this is closer in form to the classic situation. In rare cases, the reaction can be confined to the injection site.

In serum sickness, the other main form of immune complex disease, the disease process is much slower. Serum sickness develops 4–14 days (most typically 9–10 days) after exposure to a new antigen. The trick here is that sufficient antigen with a long half-life is present to trigger an immune response with the production of antibodies and then the formation of immune complexes between the old antigen and the new antibodies. Foreign serum, such as that used in various vaccinations or the anti-T cell horse serum formerly used in transplantation, and a variety of medications, especially depot antibiotics or enzymes, are usually responsible. When a patient takes antibiotics for a number of days, the same process can occur towards the end of the course. Once again immune complexes are deposited in blood vessel walls and basement membranes of various organs.

The end effect is a disease known as serum sickness which is characterized by fever, urticarial lesions, lymphadenopathy, polyarthritis, neuritis, serositis and acute glomerulonephritis. Typical cutaneous findings include urticaria and purpura along the sides of the palms or soles, as well as erythema and swelling at an injection site, where the residual concentration of antigen is higher. Hemorrhagic lesions may also be seen. In milder cases, the only cutaneous sign may be urticaria. While most of the findings resolve over several days, the neurologic and joint manifestations may last longer.

If the patient is then reexposed to the triggering antigen, two types of reactions may be seen. If the time interval before reexposure is relatively long, perhaps a year or more, then a more rapid serum sickness develops within 2–7 days with a particularly intense local reaction at the site of injection. When reexposure occurs after a short period of time, the risk of anaphylaxis is considerable.

Type IV or Delayed Hypersensitivity Reactions

These reactions are also called cell-mediated reactions, since sensitized T cells are responsible and circulating antibodies are not found. In the initial sensitization reaction antigen-presenting cells interact with T cells with the help of a complex cytokine reaction to select a subset of T cells that are able to respond upon reexposure. Thus when an antigen is presented to a sensitized host, the appropriate T cells clonally expand and over a period of 24–48 h an immune response develops. Because of the time required for the cellular response, such reactions are known as delayed or late reactions.

The classic example of delayed hypersensitivity is the tuberculin reaction. When a sensitized host, already exposed to organism or to BCG immunization, is exposed to tuberculin antigen, the sensitized lymphocytes react with the antigen in the perivascular space. The cells recognize the antigen or fragments thereof via their T cell receptors. This releases a cascade of cytokines involving not only T cells but also macrophages and endothelial cells which produces inflammation. The best-established clinical equivalent of a delayed reaction is the typical drug-induced exanthem, which occurs as the body recognizes the antigen at many different cutaneous sites simultaneously. The pseudolymphoma-like drug reactions associated with phenytoin and other products may be an extreme variant, while a fixed drug eruption represents a localized pattern. Erythema multiforme and erythema nodosum may also belong in this category.

In an immunologically similar but clinically quite different pattern, a dermatitic reaction is seen. Here the process can be visualized as occurring with more epidermal participation. In allergic contact dermatitis, the antigen penetrates the stratum corneum and is taken up by Langerhans cells. At the same time, the adjacent keratinocytes are stimulated to produce a host of regulatory cytokines including granulocyte/macrophage colony-stimulating factor (GM-CSF), TNF-α and IL-1. The Langerhans cells move through the dermis to the regional lymph nodes where they interact with T cells to induce a subset of sensitized cells. When reexposure occurs, the sensitized T cells and antigen react in the skin, producing an intense local inflammatory reaction. The classic example of such a reaction is allergic contact dermatitis in which the reaction is usually confined to that area of the skin where an allergen is applied. But in more severe reactions, or if an allergen is initially applied topically and then later ingested (as often happens with antihistamines), a more widespread reaction known as hematogenous contact dermatitis may occur. Both of these problems are considered in greater detail in Chapter 12.

Toxic and Nonallergic Reactions

A number of drug reactions result from either toxic actions of the medication, exaggerated normal physiologic actions or poorly understood nonallergic mechanisms. Many of the reactions discussed above could also be included here; we have relied more on tradition than science in making this distinction.

Overdosage

The best example is perhaps the use of chemotherapy agents where the line between desired and undesired effects is very thin. Many patients experience hair loss or oral ulcerations even at doses which are appropriate for tumor control. Relative overdoses may occur in older patients with impaired renal function or infants with immature liver function. In the latter unmetabolized chloramphenicol can cause the gray baby syndrome. Finally, overdosage may lead to other side effects which then predispose to skin disease. A classic example is barbiturate coma in which the comatose patient develops pressure-induced ulcerations because he does not recognize impending pressure necrosis.

Cumulative Deposition

Some products slowly accumulate in the body because they are metabolized either very slowly or not at all. Hyperpigmentation following the long-term ingestion of clofazimine or phenothiazines is one example. Phenothiazines interact with melanosomes while clofazimine directly discolors the skin. Another example is argyria, where the patient slowly turns slate-gray as particles of silver accumulate in basement membranes especially around sweat glands. Other heavy metals may also be deposited, especially in the oral mucosa, such as bismuth and lead. Tetracycline and minocycline can discolor developing teeth, while minocycline can also cause diffuse hyperpigmentation as well as darkening of the gingiva, acne lesion and cutaneous osteomas. Arsenic causes a wide variety of changes decades after initially being used, including mottled hyperpigmentation (rain drops on a dusty road), palmaplantar keratoses and variety of cutaneous malignancies, especially Bowen carcinoma and superficial basal cell carcinoma.

Pharmacologic Reactions

Often to achieve a given effect, such as suppression of the immune reaction in pemphigus vulgaris with systemic corticosteroids, one must accept a series of expected pharmacologic reactions including osteoporosis, hypertension, steroid acne, hirsutism, skin fragility, i.e., Cushing syndrome. When systemic retinoids are used in therapeutic doses, they have the same spectrum of side effects as vitamin A.

Ecologic Changes

Antibiotics often predispose to candidiasis, as may cytostatic agents and corticosteroids. Similarly, other bacterial infections, particularly with resistant organisms, may be favored. Immunosuppression may also predispose to viral infections such as verrucae, herpes simplex or zoster.

Pseudoallergies

These are nonimmunologic hypersensitivity reactions that mimic an allergic reaction, especially anaphylaxis. Two types are described: intolerance reaction which is explained by the pharmacologic actions of the product and idiosyncratic reaction, which is not so explained.

Intolerance Reactions

Often patients are unable to metabolize a drug in the normal way because an enzyme is missing, so they react in an unexpected but pharmacologic manner. A classic example is the reduced level of glucose-6-phosphate dehydrogenase (G6PD) in many blacks and those of Mediterranean origin, which leads to methemoglobinemia and even hemolytic anemia when such individuals are given very low doses of dapsone. A person with normal G6PD levels experiences similar problems but at much higher doses. Another example is a patient with diffuse mastocytosis who cannot tolerate a mast cell degranulating agent such as codeine, which causes no problems for a normal individual. A final example is the use of coumarin in patients with an undiagnosed defect in protein C. Such individuals are at risk for coumarin necrosis early in the course of therapy.

Idiosyncratic Reactions

The concept of idiosyncrasy as a mysterious reaction is not acceptable. If one believes in the science of pharmacology, all reactions must have a pharmacologic basis. Nonetheless, some reactions resemble anaphylaxis but no IgE antibodies are found and in vitro mast cell degranulation does not occur. Examples of causative agents include contrast dyes, nonsteroidal antiinflammatory drugs, sulfites in wine or cheese, benzyl alcohol or dyes.

Jarisch-Herxheimer Reactions

A Jarisch-Herxheimer reaction may occur when a patient is given an effective antibacterial agent that kills so many organisms that the release of toxins causes a new set of symptoms. The classic Jarisch-Herxheimer reaction is seen when treating secondary syphilis, where fever, headache and a more intense syphlitic exanthem typically develop within hours of administration. Similar reactions have been seen when treating widespread often inflammatory dermatophyte infections with griseofulvin or imidazoles or when treating borreliosis with antibiotics.

Diagnostic Approach

The diagnosis of an allergic drug reaction has considerable significance for the patient who is then excluded from a presumably useful agent or family of agents and at the same time, in the case of an incorrect diagnosis, may be exposed to a potentially life-threatening agent needlessly. While it is easy to distinguish in theory between allergic and non-allergic reactions, it may often be quite hard in practice. In general, one attempts to document an allergic mechanism. If this cannot be shown, one assumes other factors are involved. The following diagnostic steps can be employed:

- Careful History. Normally the history is the most reliable clue to the diagnosis. Medications that have been taken in the past 14 days are particularly suspect. Agents that have been used for years are unlikely to be the cause of most reactions, whereas an agent never previously taken is unlikely to cause an allergic reaction for at least 7–10 days. If a patient has been sensitized to a structurally related compound, a cross-reaction can occur, so that there is a prompt clinical reaction to a newly introduced agent. One must always inquire about over-the-counter preparations which patients often ignore. In addition, sometimes the active ingredient is blamed when the vehicle, dyes or preservatives are responsible.

- Avoidance Test. One should stop as many medications as possible and see if the cutaneous reaction improves or resolves. This is not really a test, but the common-sense approach employed by almost all patients and physicians. We prefer to work closely with the patient's primary physician if confronted by an individual with a long list of necessary medications.

- Use Test. Rechallenge with a drug should be done only under carefully controlled conditions, usually in a hospital or outpatient area where emergency equipment is available. If a single drug is suspected, after the reaction has resolved, the patient can be cautiously rechallenged. If a drug reaction is suspected but no single agent stands out, one can discontinue as many drugs as possible and then gingerly reintroduce them. If the patient has experienced an anaphylactic reaction, toxic epidermal necrolysis or a similarly severe reaction, then rechallenge should be avoided or left for an expert working in a hospital setting.

- In Vivo Tests. A wide variety of tests can be employed including:

  Intracutaneous Tests. This approach is most useful when one suspects a type I reaction. Rub or scratch tests should be performed using dilute concentrations of the agent in question, before advancing to prick or intracutaneous injection. One starts with a very low antigen exposure, hoping to avoid anaphylaxis.

  Patch Tests. When a delayed or type IV reaction is suspected, patch testing is a useful tool. In special cases, the patch test can be applied to the healed site of a fixed drug reaction or to the leg, when trying to diagnosis fixed drug eruption or drug-induced pigmented purpura.

- In Vitro Tests. Unfortunately reliable in vitro tests are not available for most medications. The ideal situation would be to send the patient's blood to the laboratory where it would be tested against all the known medications, but the reality is different.

  RAST (Radioallergosorbent Test) or CAP (Carrier-Polymer) system. Here type I reactions are investigated to demonstrate an IgE in the patient's serum directed against a medication. At the present time, only the penicillin test is of practical use.

  Lymphocyte Transformation Tests. To identify type IV reactions, the patient's T cells are incubated with the suspected drug and then studied for lymphoblast-like transformation (increased nucleoprotein synthesis, morphologic changes). The procedure is not of great clinical importance. Frequently it is difficult to identify the exact antigen, for the medication itself may not stimulate the T cells, so one must use drug metabolites.

Clinical Manifestations

Exanthematous Reactions

Clinical Findings. Drug reactions are usually a difficult morphologic diagnosis. Most often they present as an exanthem and the differential diagnosis is "drug reaction versus viral exanthem." In Europe one speaks of morbilliform, rubeoliform and scarlatiniform eruptions, reflecting the resemblance to infectious exanthems (Figs. 10.1, 10.2). In elderly or hospitalized patients, drug reaction is often the answer, while in children, viral exanthems are more common. The reaction is usually type IV so that in a sensitized patient, the reaction occurs in 2–3 days, while in a nonsensitized patient, most reactions occur after 9–10 days. Ampicillin is notorious for causing reactions up to 2 weeks after initial exposure.

Despite frequent requests from our colleagues in other specialties, we find it most difficult to examine a patient and directly correlate a given clinical picture with a given drug. A disseminated drug exanthem may have a few accompanying clues: the extensor surfaces tend to be more prominently involved, there may be mucous membrane involvement (an enanthem), pruritus is more common than in viral exanthems and there may be peripheral blood eosinophilia, while a patient with an acute viral infection usually shows lymphopenia. While we think of drug reactions as only involving the skin, this attitude is almost 100% incorrect (with perhaps the exception of fixed drug reactions). Thus, a wide range of internal signs and symptoms may occur and should not be used as a reason to diagnose a viral exanthem instead of a drug reaction. Typical causative agents are shown in Table 10.2.

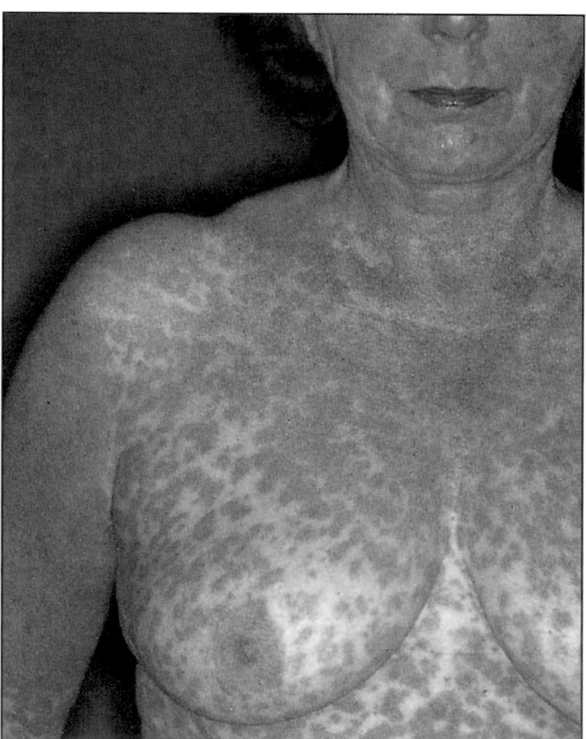

Fig. 10.1. Macular drug-induced exanthem

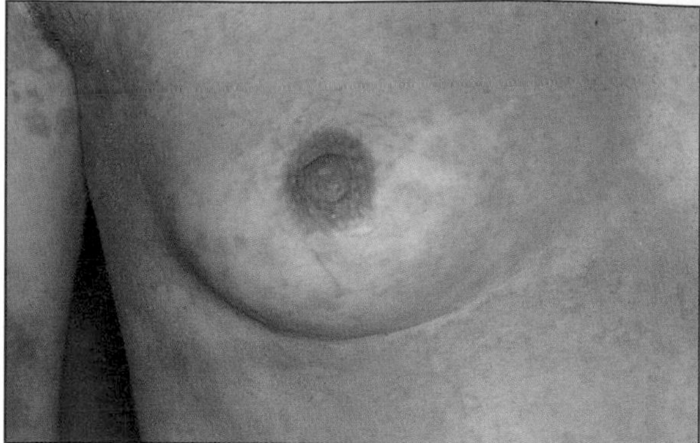

Fig. 10.2. Macular exanthem caused by ampicillin

It is most uncommon for a drug reaction to mimic acute dermatitis with erythema, weeping, scaling and crust. The most common scenario is a systemic reaction to an agent to which the patient has already been sensitized topically. This reaction is known as hematogenous contact dermatitis. Several patterns can occur: the eruption can be concentrated in the areas of previous allergic contact dermatitis, it can be widespread or it can mimic dyshidrotic dermatitis. In extreme cases, an erythroderma with dermatitis can develop virtually de novo. Perhaps the most striking example is the baboon syndrome, in which striking erythema develops in the flexural areas especially the buttocks (Fig. 10.3). The appearance of the buttocks has been compared to that of baboons and especially mandrills. There is no good explanation for the localization.

Macular exanthems may evolve to form vesicles, bullae or, if they become extreme, large eroded areas of erythroderma. In any case, the extensive damage at the epidermal-dermal junction produces epidermal instability and fragility. Such reactions are best viewed as an extreme version of a macular exanthem. The same drugs that cause ex-

Table 10.2. Drugs causing exanthematous drug reactions

Class	Examples	Frequency
Antibiotics	Penicillin, ampicillin Cephalosporins, tetracycline, streptomycin Erythromycin	High Medium Low
Sulfonamides	May cross-react with diuretics, antidiabetic agents	Medium
Nonsteroidal anti-inflammatory drugs	Phenacetin, aspirin indomethacin, phenylbutazone, oxyphenbutazone	Medium
Antiepilepsy drugs	Carbamazepine Phenytoin derivatives Barbiturates	High Medium Low
Psychotherapy drugs	Phenothiazines Benzodiazepines	Low Low
Miscellaneous drugs	Gold salts Allopurinol Isoniazid	High High Medium

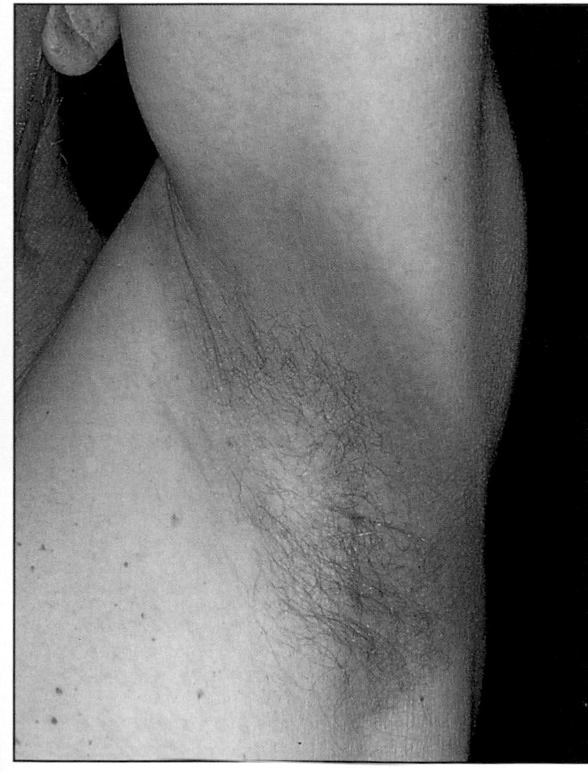

Fig. 10.3. Baboon syndrome

anthems, especially severe exanthems, cause vesicular eruptions.

Histopathology. Clinicians often request a skin biopsy to help rule in or rule out a drug eruption. Unfortunately, in most instances the microscopic appearance is not helpful. Typically one sees a sparse perivascular lymphocytic infiltrate, perhaps with a few eosinophils, and little more. More acute cases may have a more intense infiltrate with vessel wall swelling. In more advanced cases, there may be an interface dermatitis, regardless of whether the eruption clinically resembles lichen planus, erythema multiforme or lupus erythematosus. Some edema may be seen, reflecting the increased vessel permeability so often associated with drug reactions. Only a few special forms, such as some lichenoid reactions, fixed drug reactions, erythema multiforme and toxic epidermal necrolysis, have distinctive microscopic changes. These findings are discussed under the given disorders.

Therapy. The key to therapy is eliminating the causative agent. One must work with the patient's physician to make appropriate substitutions from chemically unrelated groups so that one does not create a new set of problems. For example, precipitating heart failure in a patient with pruritus by stopping all medications does not reflect a realistic assessment of risk-benefit.

Systemic. The standard of therapy is systemic corticosteroids, although it is unclear how much they actually help. Intuitively, clinicians feel that if they give corticosteroids early in the course of an immunologic action, they are bound to help. Another problem is that the differential diagnosis often includes viral and bacterial exanthems, where corticosteroids can be viewed as relatively contraindicated. If corticosteroids are given, then an adequate dosage should be employed; at least 60 mg prednisone daily, perhaps in two divided doses, should be prescribed. In addition, antihistamines are often helpful for relieving pruritus. When a type I reaction is suspected, it makes good sense to employ these agents.

Topical. Good topical nursing care can greatly speed the course of a drug reaction. The choice of an appropriate vehicle is probably most crucial, using a cream or ointment for dry lesions, and wet dressings with a lotion for weeping or eroded ones. Topical corticosteroids may be helpful for pruritic infiltrated lesions, such as lichenoid eruptions. As antipruritic agents they are expensive and ineffective and are not needed for a macular exanthem. If the main problem is pruritus, polidocanol added to an appropriate vehicle may offer relief.

Severe Skin Reactions

Definition. Acute life-threatening, usually drug-induced, disorders characterized by widespread loss of epidermis which prove fatal in about 20% of patients. Table 10.3 shows the classification of severe cutaneous reactions employed by the "*Dokumentationszentrum schwerer Hautreaktionen*" or "Center for Documenting Severe Skin Reactions", a study group based at the University of Freiburg in Germany. All of the data for which we do not provide other references reflect the experience of this group. The three diseases of most interest are Stevens-Johnson syndrome (SJS), toxic epidermal necrolysis (TEN) with maculae, and the SJS-TEN overlap. They represent a disease spectrum and will be referred to collectively as severe skin reactions.

Epidemiology. The German Center for Documenting Severe Skin Reactions has been collecting epidemiologic data since 1990 on hospitalized patients with severe skin reactions. The incidence is about two per million inhabitants. The reactions are slightly more common in women (a ratio of 55:45). Further details are shown in Table 10.4. The age distributions are also shown. Erythema multiforme majus is more common in individuals less than 40 years of age, while 75% of the patients with SJS/TEN overlap and TEN are older than 40 years. The severe skin reactions are associated with a mortality of about 18%.

The incidence of severe skin reactions in patients with HIV/AIDS is very high. It is estimated as at least 500-fold higher than in the general population. Patients with brain tumors or head injuries appear at greater risk, as do those with lupus erythematosus and bone marrow transplant recipients.

Etiology and Pathogenesis. Most severe skin reactions are caused by medications. The agents incriminated are shown in Table 10.5. The risk for

Table 10.3. Definitions of severe skin reactions

Type	Features
Erythema multiforme majus	Erosions or blisters involving less than 10% of the body surface Typical target lesions on the palms and soles Hemorrhagic-erosive lesions on at least one mucosal surface
Stevens-Johnson syndrome	Erosions or blisters involving less than 10% of the body surface Atypical target lesions and maculae primarily on the trunk Hemorrhagic-erosive lesions on at least one mucosal surface
Transition between Stevens-Johnson syndrome/toxic epidermal necrolysis	Erosions or blisters involving 10–30% of the body surface Widespread atypical target lesions and maculae Hemorrhagic-erosive lesions on at least one mucosal surface
Toxic epidermal necrolysis with maculae	Erosions or blisters involving more than 30% of the body surface Widespread target lesions and maculae Usually erosive mucosal lesions
Toxic epidermal necrolysis with diffuse erythema	Erosions or blisters involving more than 10% of the body surface No target lesions and maculae; noneroded skin erythematous or normal Usually erosive mucosal lesions

Table 10.4. Features of severe skin reactions

Reaction	Cause	Age <40 years (%)	Target lesions	Surface area involved (%)	Mortality (%)
Erythema multiforme majus	Herpes simplex	75	Typical, truncal	<10	1
SJS	Drugs	50	Atypical, truncal	<10	6
SJS/TEN	Drugs	25	Atypical, truncal	10–30	25
TEN	Drugs	25	Atypical, truncal	>30	40

Table 10.5. Medications causing severe drug reactions

Taken for short periods	Taken for long periods
Trimethoprim-sulfamethoxazole	Carbamazepine
Sulfonamides	Phenytoin
Aminopenicillins (ampicillin, amoxicillin)	Phenobarbital
Quinolones	Valproic acid
Cephalosporins	Lamotrigine
Corticosteroids	Oxicam types of NSAIDs
	Allopurinol

agents designated for long-term use, primarily the antiepileptics, seems greatest in the first 2 months of use. In one study where the relative risk of a severe skin reaction was calculated, patients taking corticosteroids also had an increased risk of a severe reaction, even when those with underlying collagen vascular diseases and CNS lesions were excluded. All of the drugs have a very low excess risk of severe skin reactions estimated at less than five cases per one million users per week. The mean interval between starting to take the medication and onset of skin symptoms is about 10 days. Any drug used in the past month should be considered as a possible trigger. Antipyretic and analgesic agents are particularly hard to study, as they may be taken for influenza-like symptoms that could represent an early severe skin reaction caused by some other agent. Sulfonamides appear to cause more problems in patients with diabetes mellitus. The three major antiepileptic agents, carbamazepine, phenytoin and phenobarbital, have a common metabolic pathway and may cross-react.

The pathogenesis of severe skin reactions is very poorly understood. In general, the reactions are held to be cell-mediated cytotoxic responses as the epidermis is infiltrated by activated lymphocytes. It is unclear whether the cytotoxic T cells directly damage the epidermis or release cytokines that stimulate apoptosis.

Clinical Findings. The severe skin reactions have a number of unifying features including target lesions, mucosal involvement and more than 10% of body surface area denuded. Target or iris lesions are a feature of erythema multiforme. In this disease the targets typically have a regular round form and three concentric rings: a purpuric, sometimes blistered center, a raised edematous pale intermediate ring and a sharp erythematous peripheral band. Atypical target lesions are seen in SJS and TEN. They are dark-red macules which have a central blister, may or may not be raised and have a poorly delineated border. The irregular target lesions tend to coalesce. The typical target lesions are usually acral, while the atypical target lesions are usually truncal.

About 90% of patients with severe skin reactions have mucosal involvement and almost as many have conjunctival disease. In the mouth one may see small aphthae, larger hemorrhagic erosions, and crusting of the lips (Fig. 10.4). There may be difficulty in eating and swallowing. Target-like lesions can be seen on the glans but are rare on the vaginal mucosa. Dysuria may result from urethral erosions. In the eyes, the initial change is usually conjunctival erythema, but there may be severe conjunctivitis and blepharitis. Healing tends to occur with strictures, stenoses and adhesions causing marked disability.

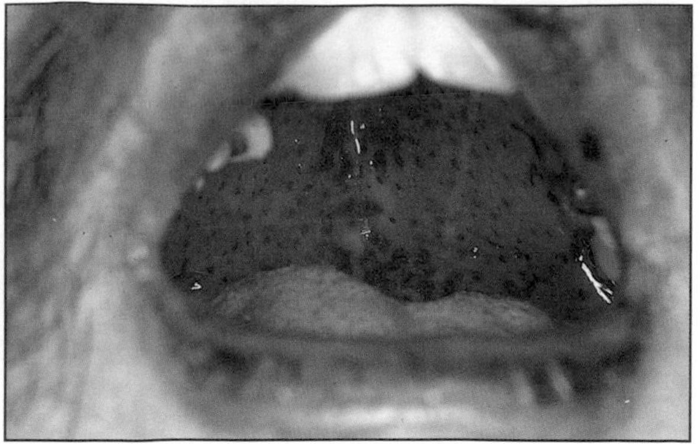

Fig. 10.4. Oral involvement in Stevens-Johnson syndrome

Erythema Multiforme

Erythema multiforme is discussed in detail in Chapter 14. It is traditionally divided into erythema multiforme minor and erythema multiforme majus or bullous erythema multiforme. The latter is included as a severe skin reaction but it is almost exclusively caused by herpes simplex. Other infections such as mycoplasma can also cause erythema multiforme majus but primarily in children and adolescents. Drugs are an uncommon source but often things are hard to sort out, because the patient has an underlying infection but has also received many medications.

Stevens-Johnson Syndrome

(Stevens and Johnson 1922)

Stevens and Johnson described two children with conjunctivitis, oral ulcerations and fever who had a disseminated primarily truncal eruption. They had dark-red erythematous macules some of which had a necrotic center. Because of imprecise descriptions, these lesions became known as target lesions and SJS was equated with erythema multiforme. As explained above this is incorrect; erythema multiforme majus and SJS are separate, but SJS overlaps with TEN. In children and adolescents, mycoplasma and other infections may be responsible for SJS; in adults it is almost always drug-related.

Stevens-Johnson Syndrome/Toxic Epidermal Necrolysis Overlap

These patients prove clinically the connection between these two disorders. They have severe SJS but do not fulfill the criteria for TEN and have a prognosis between the two extremes.

Toxic Epidermal Necrolysis

Synonyms. The nomenclature of toxic epidermal necrolysis is befuddling. It has also been called medication-related Lyell syndrome or scalded skin syndrome, but today the drug-related disorder is identified as toxic epidermal necrolysis and a somewhat similar clinical picture caused by staphylococcal toxins is known as staphylococcal scalded skin syndrome (SSSS). For clarity, we will only employ these two names.

Clinical Findings. Often a prodromal phase is described, but this very likely is related to an underlying viral or bacterial disease. In any event, patients may complain of fever, rhinitis, conjunctivitis or dysuria, suggesting that initial involvement often affects the mucous membranes. A diffuse macular exanthem appears on the trunk and face, which then spreads to involve the extensor surfaces of the limbs. The macular lesions rapidly coalesce and become bullous, forming large flaccid blisters (Fig. 10.5). Then large sheets of skin are shed, just as from a burn (Fig. 10.6). The shed skin has been described as laying on the dermis like a moist linen towel. The Nikolsky sign is strikingly positive:

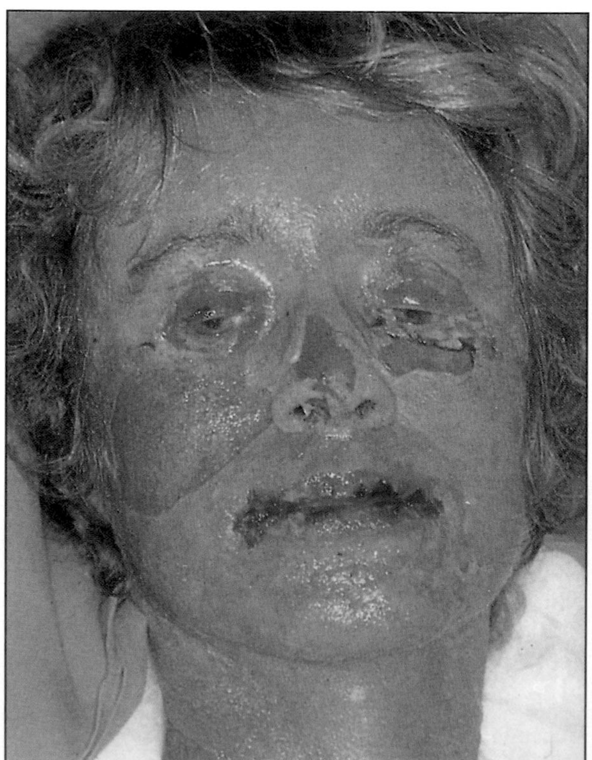

Fig. 10.5. Toxic epidermal necrolysis

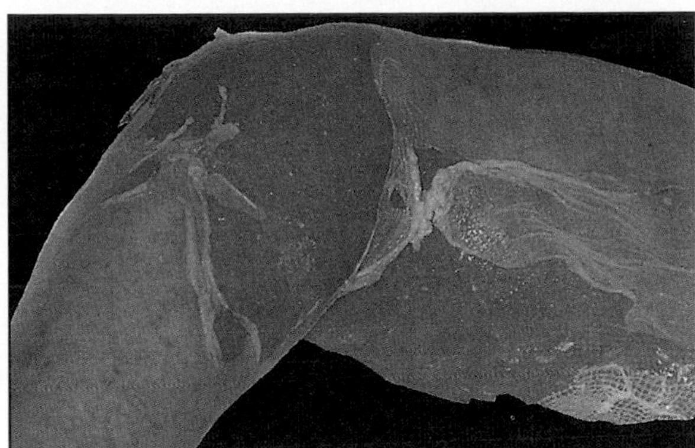

Fig. 10.6. Toxic epidermal necrolysis

when normal or erythematous skin is pressed from the side, it is easy to remove sheets of skin, as nursing personnel soon discover.

The nature of the macular lesions is used to define the two types of TEN. The most common variant is TEN with macules, in which atypical target lesions are seen on the trunk. They coalesce as they blister, causing widespread denudation. The other form of TEN is that associated with large areas of erythema which precede macules; this form is much less common.

The mucosal changes in TEN are identical to those in SJS and the overlap state, but may be more severe. The eyelids may often have hemorrhagic blisters while severe conjunctivitis may lead to scarring, symblepharon and even blindness. Immediate ophthalmologic consultation is imperative. The oral and genital mucosa may be similarly affected, interfering with feeding, urination and even defecation. In women genital adhesions between the labia minora are comparable to the ocular symblepharon.

The patients are also seriously ill. Typically fever persists and is accompanied by somnolence. The fluid loss is enormous with subsequent electrolyte abnormalities. In addition, glomerulonephritis, pneumonia and hepatitis may all develop, usually after the first week of illness. TEN is probably the most deadly skin disease; even with expert nursing care the fatality rate is about 40 %.

While the skin usually heals with little or no scarring, the hair and nails bear witness to the massive insult. Usually there is an anagen effluvium with marked hair loss, often coupled with telogen effluvium several months later. Some or all of the nails may be lost and those not lost typically show Beau lines. If nails are lost, pterygium-like scarring may develop so that either nail regrowth does not occur or is limited.

Histopathology. Microscopic evaluation provides a rapid way to identify TEN. A biopsy from an erythematous but not denuded area shows full-thickness epidermal necrosis with little if any lymphocytic infiltrate in the upper dermis. The dermis simply shows edema and vasodilatation – the so-called empty dermis. In contrast, in SSSS, the damage is subcorneal, so that the basal layer and lower spinous layer are virtually normal.

While frozen section evaluation of the blister roof reveals stratum corneum in SSSS and full-thickness epidermis in TEN, this technique is unfamiliar to most pathologists and more importantly to their technicians. We have seen a number of false interpretations. A punch biopsy is a minor insult in view of the gravity of the disease and is recommended. Immunohistochemical studies may identify CD8-positive cytotoxic lymphocytes along the epidermal-dermal junction and within the epidermis. The changes in the macular lesions of SJS and the overlap state are similar but usually not as severe.

Laboratory Findings. There are no specific findings that suggest TEN, but electrolytes and renal function should be monitored. Early in the disease the erythrocyte sedimentation rate may be elevated and the CBC may show an elevated hematocrit as a result of fluid loss.

Course and Prognosis. The mortality rates are shown in Table 10.4.

Differential Diagnosis. In a typical case, the differential diagnosis is simple. One must exclude SSSS, which usually affects children and younger adults and has a different microscopic picture.

While lengthy discussions concerning the separation of TEN from erythema multiforme and Stvens-Johnson syndrome have been written, they have little relevance in our opinion, as the disease processes overlap clinically and histologically. A somewhat different situation arises when patients are at risk for graft versus host disease. They often have had pretransplantation conditioning with radiation therapy and chemotherapy, which also influences their clinical appearance and biopsy results. In the transplantation unit, TEN is a very difficult diagnosis.

Other drug eruptions can appear similar. Patients with an extensive maculopapular drug eruption or erythroderma may have extensive desquamation which can be confused with TEN. Generalized bullous fixed drug eruption presents with well-defined oval plaques with a dusky violaceous color. While blisters occur, they involve less than 10% of the body surface. Fever, malaise and mucosal involvement are less common than in severe skin reactions. Finally, patients almost always give a history compatible with a previous more ordinary fixed drug eruption.

Extensive phototoxic reactions can also show widespread denudation. Inadvertent excessive radiation in PUVA therapy or use of too-concentrated solutions of topical psoralens are the usual causes. Acute generalized exanthematous pustulosis is a dramatic sudden pustular eruption (Chap. 16), usually caused by antibiotics. Patients have high fever and a diffuse edematous exanthem which is rapidly dotted by tiny pustules but no mucosal changes and heals rapidly.

In addition, both pemphigus vulgaris and bullous pemphigoid, when extensive enough, can appear similar. If any uncertainty exists, direct immunofluorescent examination should be performed to exclude this possibility. Some viral exanthems, particular in children, may have widespread cutaneous involvement and mucosal lesions very closely resembling those of SJS. We have seen this with Epstein-Barr virus infections.

Therapy. The therapy of TEN is best described as excellent burn care. It may be wise for both medical and medical-legal reasons to transfer all suspected or diagnosed TEN patients to the intensive care or burn unit. The principles of burn care include temperature control, regulation of fluid balance and avoidance or prompt treatment of secondary bacterial infections. In addition, the eyes and genital area should be given special attention, being regularly separated and treated with a neutral ointment to reduce the risk of adhesions. Each burn unit has its own approach to skin care which is best left in the hands of the experienced and dedicated nurses. The type of nursing care is the biggest determinant of survival. Fortunately, in TEN little dermal damage occurs and reepithelialization is usually prompt and the outlook better than the initial dismal clinical picture suggests.

The biggest controversy in treating TEN is the use of systemic corticosteroids. Many physicians feel that using high doses of corticosteroids early in the course of a reaction to a drug with a considerable risk for TEN, such as phenytoin, is intuitively wise and must help. No study has shown a clear benefit of systemic corticosteroids and several have shown detrimental effects, presumably because immunosuppression is not desirable in someone without an epidermis at risk for many infections. In the USA, the medical-legal situation has somewhat simplified the situation: there are enough experts who have stated that corticosteroids should not be used, so anyone doing the opposite is well-advised to carefully document their actions.

Pseudolymphoma Reactions

Synonym. Hypersensitivity syndrome. The term hypersensitivity syndrome is not ideal, as most drug reactions can be viewed as hypersensitivity reactions. But in this case it refers to a relatively specific mucocutaneous eruption with fever, lymphadenopathy, hepatitis and eosinophilia.

Etiology and Pathogenesis. The agents most often incriminated include the major antiepileptic drugs – carbamazepine, phenytoin and phenobarbital. Here the incidence is estimated at one reaction per 10,000 exposures. Sulfonamides, dapsone, allopurinol, minocycline and gold salts have also been incriminated. The mechanism seems to involve defects in normal enzymatic methods of detoxifying the medications. For the anticonvulsants, a defect in metabolizing arene oxide metabolites has been found in many patients. For sulfonamides, slow acetylator phenotype individuals are at greater risk.

Clinical Findings. The typical features are fever and rash, both present in over 80% of patients. The rash is usually morbilliform, but becomes confluent and edematous, with both purpura and blisters. Facial swelling is not uncommon. An equally high percentage of patients have lymphadenopathy. About 50% of patients have abnormal liver function tests, while a smaller number have eosinophilia and interstitial nephritis.

Histopathology. A well-developed lesion may show a cutaneous pseudolymphoma with a lymphocytic infiltrate, often with atypical cells and epidermotropism. Lymph node changes are reactive.

Laboratory Findings. Hepatic and renal function, as well as routine hematologic parameters, should be followed.

Course and Prognosis. The mortality associated with hypersensitivity reactions is about 8%. The usual cause of death is severe hepatitis, which can also persist as the rest of the findings begin to resolve. The lymphoid changes usually disappear, although lymphoma has been very rarely reported.

Differential Diagnosis. All the severe skin reactions can be considered. The liver disease, lymphadenopathy and striking eosinophilia tend to be unique. Denudation and mucosal changes are less prominent.

Therapy. There is no specific therapy other than withdrawal of the suspected medication and supportive care. One must remember that the three anticonvulsants cross-react, so all must be avoided in the future, a major problem for the neurologist responsible for seizure control.

Bullous Drug Reactions

A variety of medications may cause bullous disorders, including pemphigus vulgaris, bullous pemphigoid, linear IgA disease and even dermatitis herpetiformis. In the case of dermatitis herpetiformis, iodides and some other drugs may also exacerbate an existing disease. Bullous drug eruptions are considered in more detail in Chapter 15 along with the other blistering diseases. Drug-induced coma may produce bullous lesions via pressure necrosis perhaps combined with other toxic factors. PUVA therapy leads to blisters of the arms and legs in up to 10% of patients, while etretinate and acitretin tend to predispose the skin to forming friction blisters.

Serum Sickness Reactions

True serum sickness from serum administration is discussed above. In drug-induced serum sickness, often only an intense local reaction at the injection site and an urticarial exanthem develop. Foreign proteins such as immune serum, insulin, enzymes such as streptokinase, fresh cell suspensions and many others tend to be responsible. Probably the most common causes today are horse antithymocyte globulin and human diploid rabies cell vaccine. Antibiotics, especially depot forms for intramuscular use, may also cause serum sickness. Serum sickness reactions have also been described with minocycline, cephalosporins and propranolol. When patients develop serum sickness while taking a course of an antibiotic such as penicillin, the urticarial pattern usually predominates but often the predilection for the edges of the palms and soles provides a clue to the significant internal reaction.

Urticarial Reactions

There are frequently mixed reactions with both urticarial lesions and a macular exanthem. Patients may present with an exanthem but develop urticarial lesions. Yet other patients present only with urticaria, although here the history is usually very helpful as the hives are closely related temporally to an injection of contrast material, an injection of penicillin or a similar event. Urticarial reactions in general occur early in the course of therapy. Angioedema is not a common part of drug reactions, but an increasing number of angioedema reactions are caused by ACE inhibitors, and occasionally aspirin. Common causes are shown in Table 10.6. Pseudoallergic reactions are common, especially with aspirin and contrast media. Urticaria is discussed in greater detail in Chapter 11.

Vasculitic Reactions

Vasculitis is usually a type III reaction with immune complex deposition in vessel walls. Most leukocytoclastic angiitis (Chap. 22) is not drug-induced but one should be alert to the possibility. Perhaps 10% of cases of cutaneous vasculitis are caused by medications. Bacterial antigens are also an important trigger. A confusing situation arises when an infection is treated with antibiotics and then a vasculitis arises. When the patient is exposed to the drug after the infection has resolved, frequently no reaction occurs. Typical causative agents include ACE inhibitors, phenytoin and its derivatives, nonsteroidal antiinflammatory drugs, sulfonamides and thiouracils. The latter group, as well as levamisole, may cause earlobe vasculitis which has been mistaken for relapsing polychondritis. Amantadine can cause a livedo vasculitis when administered for prolonged periods. Hundreds of products have occasionally been implicated. As might be expected, there is overlap with the agents associated with purpura, as milder vessel wall damage will present as just purpura.

Table 10.6. Agents causing urticarial drug reactions

Agent	Frequency
Antibiotics (penicillin and related agents)	High
X-ray contrast media	High
Enzymes	High
Nonsteroidal antiinflammatory drugs	Medium
Aspirin	Low (also angioedema)
ACE inhibitors	Low (often angioedema)

Purpuric and Hemorrhagic Reactions

Most drug-induced purpura is toxic and expected, as antineoplastic agents kill megakaryocytes. In contrast, in rare instances type II reactions occur with direct cytotoxic damage to platelets and/or megakaryocytes. The platelet agglutination test can help identify allergic thrombocytopenia. The medication is mixed with the patient's platelets. When antibodies are present, platelet aggregation occurs. If complement is then added, lysis occurs. Other mechanisms of purpura include increased vessel fragility, as evaluated by the Rumpel-Leede test, and abnormalities of the clotting cascade. Some authorities divide drug-induced purpura into vascular purpura (vessel wall damage) and thrombocytopenic purpura, but many drugs cause both types of damage. Challenge tests to confirm a diagnosis of drug-induced purpura are potentially quite dangerous. If performed, they should be done in the hospital using very low levels of antigen challenge some weeks after the original eruption. Corticosteroid-induced purpura reflects decreased tensile strength of the perivascular collagen with shearing or tearing damage. Table 10.7 shows a selected list of such agents; much more information is available in Chapter 23 and in specialized texts.

When purpuric eruptions are severe, they may become hemorrhagic. This is most common in dependent areas such as the buttocks, thighs and scapula, or following trauma. Even subtle trauma such as that induced by electrocardiogram suction cups or blood pressure cuffs, can produce hemorrhage. Patients with underlying hematologic problems are also at greater risk. The same triggering agents are involved.

Table 10.7. Agents causing purpuric or hemorrhagic drug reactions

Quinine, quinidine
Thiazide diuretics
Sulfonamides
Pyrazolone derivatives
Phenothiazines
Furosemide
Gold salts
Indomethacin
Thiouracils

Another possible explanation for drug-induced purpura is an exacerbation of one of the pigmented purpuras. This group of disorders is characterized by lower extremity purpura, primarily reflecting chronic venous insufficiency. The defect appears to arise from a combination of increased local blood pressure and increased vessel wall fragility or permeability. Thus, any medication which influences these factors or clotting ability can worsen the problem. Sometimes patch tests performed on the back or especially on the legs may reproduce the problem. In most instances, pigmented purpura is idiopathic and has no relation to drugs. In the past carbamide, an old sleeping medication, was notorious for its ability to cause pigmented purpura. Today possible causes are meprobamate, carbamazepine, phenacetin and benzodiazepines.

Lichenoid Reactions

Many drug reactions resemble lichen planus either clinically or histologically (Chap. 14). This is not surprising because lichen planus appears to be a T cell mediated reaction against some epidermal antigens. In a lichenoid drug reaction, perhaps the medication is a hapten, combining with an epidermal structure to form an antigen. Lichenoid reactions usually occur after long periods of drug use, lending credence to their delayed nature. There may be subtle clinical differences between lichen planus and a lichenoid drug eruption. In the latter, the backs of the hands and feet are not so regularly involved and truncal lesions are common. Lichenoid drug eruptions are less monomorphic, often have

Table 10.8. Agents causing lichenoid drug reactions

Acyclovir
Antimalarials
Gold salts
Quinine, quinidine
Nonsteroidal antiinflammatory drugs
Penicillamine
Methyldopa
β-Blockers
Levamisole
Thiazides
Hepatitis B vaccine

scaling and crusting. Genital and mucosal involvement is less common in drug reactions. Microscopic examination may also give clues, as the prominent granular layer of lichen planus is less frequently seen, but often the histologic pictures are indistinguishable. Common causes are shown in Table 10.8.

Nodose Erythematous Reactions

Nodose reactions are deep-seated erythematous nodules, usually over the shins. They are also referred to as drug-induced erythema nodosum. Possible clues that erythema nodosum may be triggered by a drug include lack of bruising, multiple lesions and arm involvement. The reaction appears to most often be a type IV reaction, which can occasionally be confirmed by intradermal skin testing with the suspected cause. Since infection-related and idiopathic erythema nodosum are far more common, one should be reluctant to blame the reaction on medications. Possible causative agents include oral contraceptives, sulfonamides, aspirin, bromides, iodides and gold salts.

Fixed Drug Eruptions

Definition. Localized sharply circumscribed cutaneous drug reaction that recurs in exactly the same location on repeated exposure.

Etiology and Pathogenesis. A fixed drug eruption is one of the great immunologic puzzles. Some medications produce a sharply defined lichenoid drug reaction in the same location each time exposure occurs. Both the skin and mucous membranes may be involved. Exogenous agents are the only known cause of fixed drug eruption; it does not occur spontaneously or following infections. When the antigen is applied to or injected into the site after clinical healing has occurred, a reaction often occurs. In addition T cells can be isolated from active lesions and characterized; they are antigen-specific. Keratinocytes in the involved area express ICAM-1 and class II antigens and a lymphocyte chemotactic factor IP10 is present. This suggests a role for IFN-γ. Perhaps the tendency for the disease to recur in the same site is explained by the T cells being able to recognize altered antigens in the fomer lesion. The typical causative agents are shown in Table 10.9.

Table 10.9. Agents causing fixed drug eruptions

Most common	Others
Barbiturates	Penicillin
Paracetamol	Erythromycin
Phenolphthalein	Phenytoin
Pyrazolone derivatives	Halides
Sulfonamides	Antimalarials
Tetracyclines (often mucosal)	Quinine, quinidine and many more

Clinical Findings. Typically there are one or more sharply defined round, slightly edematous plaques, ranging in size from several millimeters to many centimeters. They have a characteristic dusky violet color and may become eroded. The most common sites are the distal aspects of the extremities (Fig. 10.7), palms and soles, glans penis (Fig. 10.8), scrotum and oral mucosa. The lesions may itch or burn. The lesions gradually fade over months, but typically leave behind subtle gray-brown postinflammatory hyperpigmentation. In darker skin, the hyperpigmentation may be very prominent and persistent.

When exposure to the medication occurs again, the reaction occurs at exactly the same site. If multiple attacks occur, the sites of action may eventually become quite dark. Typically the time interval between exposure and development of lesions shortens on repeated exposures. It usually occurs in days fitting with the apparent cellular mechanism. On the mucosa, broad erosions develop so that the disorder is often confused with herpes simplex infection, major aphthae or even pemphigus vulgaris.

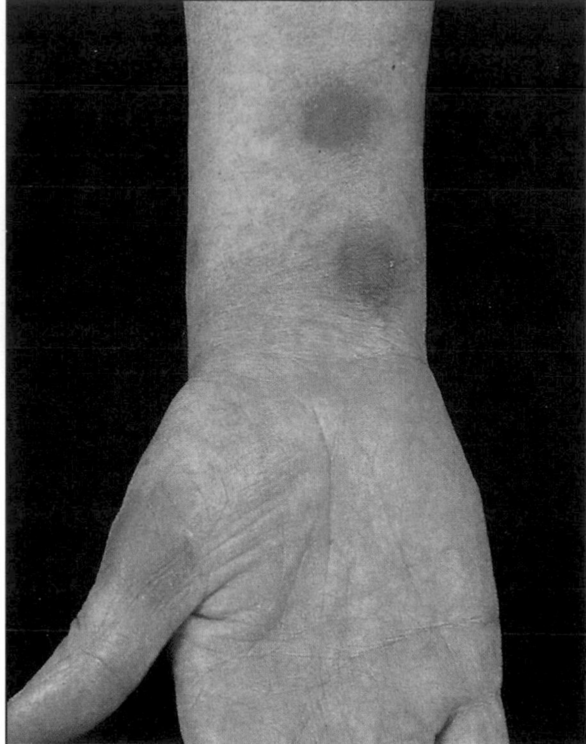

Fig. 10.7. Multifocal fixed drug reaction

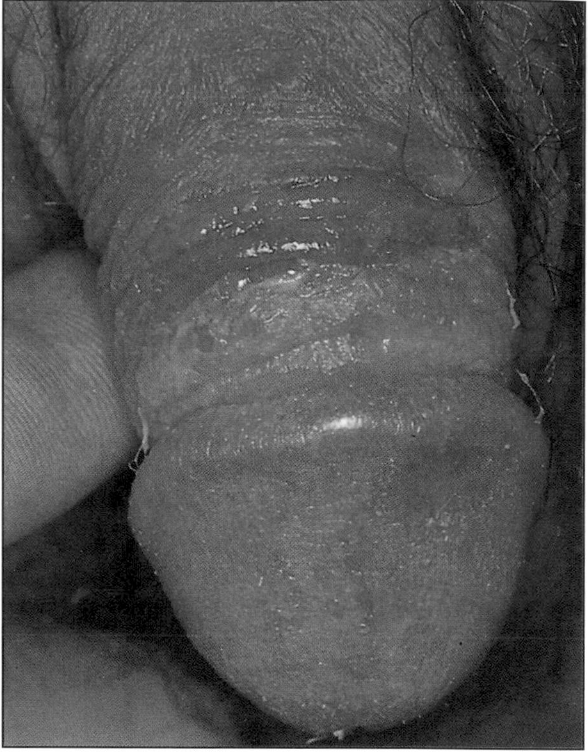

Fig. 10.8. Fixed drug reaction

The uncommon generalized bullous fixed drug eruption usually occurs in patients who previously have had ordinary fixed drug reactions. It may cover wide areas of the body, and have blisters and mucosal involvement, so it enters into the differential diagnosis of severe skin reactions.

Histopathology. A biopsy is often of great help. An acute lesion will show an intense lichenoid inflammation with an accumulation of lymphocytes at the epidermal-dermal junction. There is hydropic degeneration of the basal cells, often with necrosis and Civatte bodies. Edema is also common and there may be a subepidermal blister. In older or especially in recurrent lesions, melanophages rich in melanin are found in the superficial dermis.

Laboratory Findings. Patch testing may be useful. It should be performed on the quiescent lesional skin and on normal skin as a control. Only positive tests are helpful. If oral challenge is performed, one must be aware of occasional reports of generalized bullous fixed drug eruption following reexposure.

Differential Diagnosis. A fixed drug eruption is morphologically distinctive because of its unique color and tendency to recur in the same spot. Problems in diagnosis arise because many patients fail to associate the change with drug ingestion, considering it a bruise or arthropod bite reaction.

Therapy. The only therapy is avoidance. Topical corticosteroid creams can be used for relief of pruritus.

Acneiform Reactions

The main causes of acne-like eruptions are hormones and halogenated compounds. These problems are considered in more detail in Chapter 28. Corticosteroid-induced acne is probably the most common. It is seen in many adults taking systemic corticosteroids. The eruption tends to be widespread and consist primarily of plugged follicles. Both androgens and oral contraceptives may trigger or exacerbate acne. Halogen-induced lesions are more pustular without comedones. A wide variety of other drugs including phenytoin, isoniazid, cyclosporine, lithium and even tetracycline have been occasionally implicated. Acne is so common and flares so often that it is difficult to prove a relationship between a medication and the disease. A similar problem is flares of rosacea which have been described with acetazolamide, glymidine, nitrate compounds and psoralens.

Acute Generalized Exanthematous Pustulosis

Some patients taking antibiotics develop an acute widespread pustular eruption (Chap. 16). In some instances, bacterial infections are blamed, but these have usually been treated with antibiotics, confusing the issue. The eruption appears suddenly with a diffuse edematous erythematous exanthem which rapidly is covered by hundreds of tiny pustules with a red halo. The patient usually has fever and an elevated WBC count and may even have minimal mucosal disease. Healing is rapid and complete.

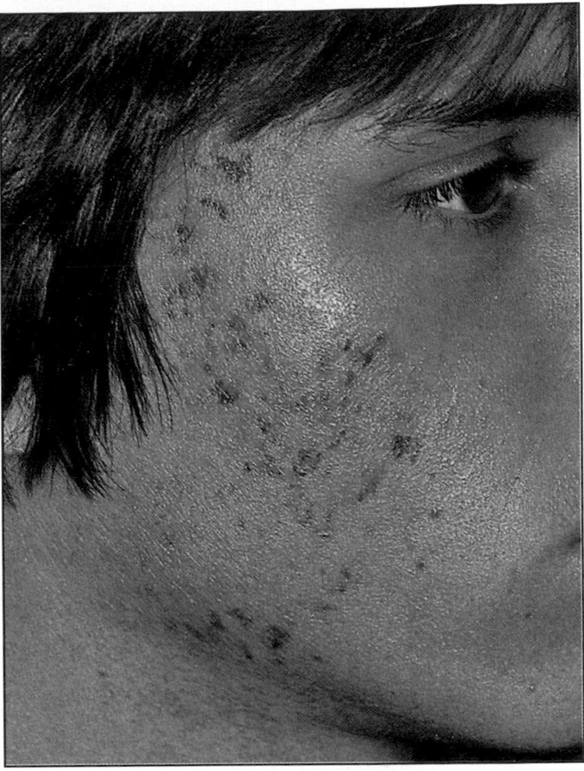

Fig. 10.9. Minocycline-induced hyperpigmentation

Lupus Erythematosus-Like Reactions

These reactions are considered in Chapter 18. The main drugs involved are hydralazine and procainamide although many others have been described. Skin involvement occurs in less than 25% of patients with drug-induced lupus erythematosus. In addition, most patients have antihistone antibodies.

Photosensitivity Reactions

Medications may either cause a toxic sunburn-like reaction by increasing the patient's sensitivity to light (phototoxic reaction) or may invoke immunologic mechanisms to produce a photoallergic reaction. Both types of problem are considered in Chapter 13.

Pigmentary Changes

The list of medications causing skin darkening is long. Often there is a complex interaction between the medication, its metabolites, melanin, iron and the dermal macrophages. Of special interest to dermatologists are the various disturbances associated with tetracyclines. In addition to the yellowish fluorescent staining of growing teeth and bones, tetracycline causes bluish discoloration of cutaneous osteomas. The mechanism is direct deposition of the drug. On the other hand, minocycline causes hyperpigmented scars by complexing with hemosiderin in the dermal melanophages, as well as causing a diffuse blue-gray hyperpigmentation more prominent in sunlight-exposed areas (Fig. 10.9).

Many cytostatic agents cause hyperpigmentation. Busulfan causes a diffuse darkening which resembles Addison disease. Others cause acral hyperpigmentation, especially adriamycin, bleomycin and cyclophosphamide, while yet others induce photosensitivity and darkening of sunlight-exposed areas. Phenytoin produces a brown hyperpigmentation in sunlight-exposed areas. Many hormonal products trigger melasma and localized hyperpigmentation of areas such as the nipples and genital mucosa. Corticosteroids may also cause hyperpigmentation. Antimalarials also cause a puzzling hyperpigmentation, usually over the shins, and with a peculiar blue-gray color. The mechanisms are unclear. Quinacrine can cause a yellow discoloration. Heavy metals also cause darkening of the skin, usually by direct deposition (Chap. 27).

Drug-induced hypopigmentation is rare. Often the hairs are lightened. Chloroquine may do this at the same time as causing darkening of the shins. A few other agents including etretinate have also been incriminated. Interleukin-2 may trigger vitiligo.

Granulomatous Reactions

These lesions are uncommon and may simply be a variant on the pseudolymphoma pattern, as similar agents are responsible and histologic patterns overlap. The lesions are usually erythematous often annular infiltrates involving the inner aspects of the arms and thighs. Clinically they resemble granuloma annulare, lupus erythematosus and erythema annulare centrifugum. On biopsy there is usually both a lichenoid epidermal pattern and a dermal picture resembling granuloma annulare. In some instances, atypical lymphocytes may be identified.

Sclerotic Reactions

Local sclerotic reactions have been reported with injections of vitamin K, pentazocine and heparin. Probably other agents such as insulin can also rarely trigger a fibrotic response with repeated use. Systemic medications felt to either trigger systemic sclerosis or cause a similar reaction in the skin include β-blockers, bromocriptine, carbidopa, tryptophan and valproic acid. In addition, as discussed in Chapter 18, a variety of toxic reactions, such as the toxic or Spanish oil reaction, industrial exposure to silica, silicones and other chemicals, may cause similar changes in the skin.

Hair Changes

Two types of toxic hair loss occur, depending on the medication, the dosage and many individual, poorly understood factors (Chap. 31). High dosages or acute toxicity leads to anagen effluvium (also known as immediate or dystrophic effluvium). The hairs come out rapidly over a period of days, are dystrophic anagen hairs under the microscope and produce the sudden alopecia so well known among chemotherapy patients.

In telogen effluvium the hair loss is more gradual and first begins several months after the insult. Microscopically the hairs are normal telogen structures and the loss is more diffuse, often not recognized by anyone but the patient and close associates. In addition there is pharmacologic androgenetic hair loss when susceptible patients, either men or women, are treated with hormones with androgenetic properties.

Typical causative agents include cytostatic agents, anticoagulants (both coumarin and heparin), oral contraceptives, other hormones (even the antiandrogen cyproterone acetate has been implicated), antithyroid drugs (both thiouracil and carbimazole derivatives), tamoxifen and clomifene. With many of the hormones, it is unclear whether the underlying endocrine disorder or the medication is the trigger.

Hypertrichosis is an uncommon problem, most often seen with cyclosporine and phenytoin, but also with a variety of other agents including systemic minoxidil. This property led to the eventual use of topical minoxidil as an approved treatment for some types of alopecia. All the drugs causing hirsutism are hormones with the possible exception of phenytoin which appears to cause both hypertrichosis and hirsutism.

Nail Changes

The effects of medications on nails are considered in Chapter 32. The most common change is nail dystrophy caused by toxic effects on the nail bed, usually from antimetabolites. The damage to the area of nail growth is reflected by transverse depressions (Beau's lines). Brittle nails may also result from such agents, as well as from retinoids. Most onycholysis is associated with light exposure, but sometimes the nail may be the only site of photosensitivity. A wide variety of pigmentary changes occur in the nail, producing both transverse and longitudinal pigmented streaks.

Toxic Reactions

While many of the above changes may be toxic reactions, in some instances there is no question. Such situations are considered below.

Necrosis Following Intramuscular Injections

(Freudenthal 1923; Nicolau 1925)

Synonyms. Embolia cutis medicamentosa, Nicolau syndrome

Definition. Following an intramuscular injection, hemorrhagic livid lesions develop and tend to progress to necrosis.

Table 10.10. Selected agents causing cutaneous necrosis

Class	Individual agents
Antibiotics	Penicillin, especially procaine and benzathine forms Streptomycin Sulfonamides Chlortetracycline
Antihistamines	Many, especially diphenhydramine
Rheumatologic agents	Phenylbutazone Acetaminophen
Miscellaneous	Local anesthetics (all) Corticosteroids, especially triamcinolone acetonide as depot form Vitamin B_{12}

Etiology and Pathogenesis. Livedo-like skin reactions were first described in the 1920s following the injection of bismuth salts for treating syphilis. They have been associated with a long list of intramuscular agents, reflecting primarily those medications which are frequently delivered via this route (Table 10.10). No matter how careful one is in administering an intramuscular injection, occasionally the medication enters an artery or its irritant action may cause arteriospasm, producing the same effect – distal ischemic necrosis. If an injection damages a nerve, it may cause not only pain but also vasoconstriction. Subsequent use of the agent typically does not produce a similar action, supporting the concept of direct toxic damage.

Clinical Findings. Within minutes to hours after an intramuscular injection, distal livid erythematous plaques develop, often with a livedo racemosa pattern, suggesting that an artery has been damaged (Fig. 10.10). The lesions are sharply demarcated, presumably confined to the area served by the vessel. Often the center of the area becomes more hemorrhagic and bullous, then later necrotic. The changes may extend into the deeper structures of the fat and muscle. Pain, nerve damage and decreased muscle function may occur. The deep wounds tend to heal with bizarre scars over many months.

Differential Diagnosis. Exactly the same pattern is seen after extravasation of chemotherapy agents. The two most notorious products are doxorubicin and daunorubicin, but many others have been implicated. Vasospasm caused by the intense irritation undoubtedly contributes to the direct toxicity.

Therapy. No good therapy exists. Attempts at reversing the vasospasm with a variety of vasodilators, including pentoxifylline, nicotinic acid and papaverine have proven relatively unsuccessful. Topical wound care is helpful in avoiding secondary infections, but the patient is still doomed to many months of a painful ulcer.

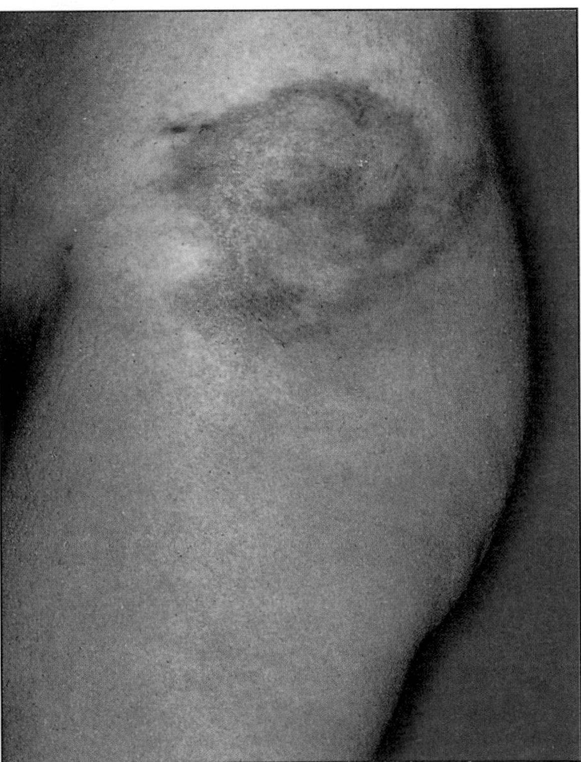

Fig. 10.10. Cutaneous necrosis following intramuscular injection of corticosteroid preparation

Anticoagulant Reactions

The coumarin derivatives are anticoagulants that inhibit the vitamin K-dependent blood clotting factors II, VII, IX and X that are manufactured in the liver. Balancing the dose of coumarin is a delicate matter and patients who are even slightly overtreated may have purpura or even hemorrhagic lesions. But sometimes there is a more dramatic reaction known as coumarin necrosis.

The typical patient is an older, often overweight, women who has just started treatment with the anticoagulant. She may develop hemorrhagic infarcts that spread rapidly and become necrotic. Typical sites of involvement are the breasts, abdomen and buttocks. The necrosis can be so extreme that a breast virtually undergoes autoamputation.

The mechanism appears to involve patients who are heterozygous for protein C, and unable to maintain an appropriate fibrinolytic response (Chap. 23). Those unfortunate individuals with a homozygous deficiency usually die in infancy of clotting problems, but the heterozygous patients have thromboembolic disease or escape detection. When coumarin is given, there is a brief window where the patient is in a hypercoagulable state as protein C levels are low but the other clotting factors have not yet been affected. This is explained by the very short half-life of protein C. Thus, during the induction phase of coumarin therapy, thromboses are even more likely and one of their clinical signs may be widespread skin necrosis. Paradoxically, coumarin should be continued but heparin added until the condition has stabilized.

One must also remember that a number of drugs besides vitamin K can antagonize coumarin. They include barbiturates, glutethimide, rifampin and cholestyramine. Hereditary resistance to coumarin is inherited in an autosomal dominant pattern. Patents who eat large amounts of vegetables such as broccoli which are rich in vitamin K are also somewhat resistant. Potentiating agents include anabolic steroids, phenylbutazone, clofibrate, aspirin, disulfuram, metronidazole, cimetidine, amiodarone, the imidazoles, third generation cephalosporins, tamoxifen, ciprofloxacin and related compounds.

Heparin necrosis has also been described, but it is much less common and has a totally different mechanism. Here heparin causes an immunologically mediated platelet adherence and consumption. Low molecular weight heparin may cause skin necrosis away from injection sites.

Coma Blisters

Etiology and Pathogenesis. Patients with a drug overdose, usually involving barbiturates, narcotics or other soporifics, may lie unconscious for many hours without moving a limb. The steady pressure induces tissue ischemia and necrosis, usually evolving into a blister. The process is similar to a decubitus ulcer but clinically moves at an accelerated pace. Similar changes are seen following carbon monoxide poisoning and in other coma patients, such as diabetic ketoacidosis. A final variable is the degree to which the offending drug accumulates in the eccrine glands, as accumulation appears to exaggerate the toxic effects.

Clinical Findings. Bullae, erosions and dusky hemorrhagic plaques develop on pressure points. The most common sites are the buttocks, scapulae and shoulders. Any dependent area can be damaged, simply depending on how the comatose individual is positioned. If carbon monoxide poisoning is involved, there may also be peripheral edema, as well as cherry-red skin discoloration because of the presence of carboxyhemoglobin.

Histopathology. The blisters are primarily subepidermal but can also be intraepidermal associated with spongiosis. Necrotic keratinocytes are present, and the eccrine glands may also show necrosis.

Therapy. Supportive care and attention to the underlying problem are foremost. Routine wound care is all that is required for the skin.

Carbon Monoxide Poisoning

This entity is not a drug reaction but is included here because it may have the same dermatologic changes as coma blisters.

Etiology and Pathogenesis. Carbon monoxide poisoning does not occur just from automobile exhausts in suicide attempts. It also results from faulty domestic gas appliances in inadequately ventilated rooms, most often affecting the poor but occasionally the wealthy, as the death of tennis star Vitas Gerulaitas in a Long Island guest quarters demonstrates. In addition, paint strippers containing methylene chloride are inhaled and converted to carbon monoxide in the body, and many other industrial exposures occur.

Clinical Findings. Any patient who is afebrile but complaining of nausea, vomiting, headache or other flu symptoms should be suspected of having carbon monoxide poisoning. Waiting for the classic cherry-red skin discoloration is futile. The level of carboxyhemoglobin in the skin is a very poor predictor. The bulk of the toxicity is caused by the ability of carbon monoxide to inhibit cytochrome oxidases. In addition to unconsciousness and cardiac problems, manifested best by ST segment depression on the EKG, there may be peripheral neuropathies, myolysis (leading to myoglobinuria and renal tubular necrosis) and hemolytic anemia.

While a dermatologist can expect to never diagnose a case of carbon monoxide poisoning, there are skin findings. In addition to the cherry-red discoloration, one may see facial and peripheral edema. In addition, if the patient becomes comatose, there may be pressure bullae in dependent areas.

Histopathology. The blisters are subepidermal and show epidermal necrosis. There may also be necrosis of the eccrine glands.

Differential Diagnosis. It is unclear whether there are significant differences between dependent blisters in coma patients when different processes are responsible. Barbiturate toxicity is quite similar as far as the skin findings are concerned. While there may be subtle histologic differences based on how much of the offending agent accumulates in the eccrine glands, they offer a poor way to discriminate between different etiologies. A history usually suffices.

Therapy. The most interesting approach is hyperbaric oxygen, which may be employed in patients who are unconscious, have cardiac problems or a carboxyhemoglobin level greater than 40 %. Otherwise, 100 % oxygen is administered by a tightly fitting facial mask or better an endotracheal tube, while at the same time electrolyte balance, particularly potassium levels, are monitored and manipulated carefully.

Reactions to Chemotherapeutic Agents

The cutaneous reactions seen in cancer chemotherapy patients are worthy of special consideration for several reasons. The first rule is that common things are common, even in this specialized setting. Toxic alopecia, horizontal nail ridging and mucosal erosions reflect the action of the drugs on rapidly growing tissues. In extreme cases, a toxic epidermal necrolysis-like reaction occurs or widespread cutaneous necrosis results from the same direct cellular toxicity. Exanthems and urticaria are the most common allergic reactions. Chemotherapy patients are almost invariably immunosuppressed, so concomitant infections should always be kept in mind. In most instances, cutaneous reactions are not reason enough to stop potentially life-saving treatment, so often one treats through reactions that would otherwise cause great alarm. Although chemotherapy is being done more often in community hospitals and even on an ambulatory basis, most of us see very few such reactions, for oncologists are familiar with those reactions associated with the regimens they use daily. We discuss a few special reactions and summarize others in Table 10.11.

Eccrine Reactions

Synonyms. Neutrophilic eccrine hidradenitis, eccrine syringomatous metaplasia

Many chemotherapy agents are concentrated and excreted in the eccrine sweat. This produces both irritation with the development of erythematous plaques and tiny pustules, known as neutrophilic eccrine hidradenitis. The same problem can be seen on the palms and soles of normal individuals, especially children, but on other body areas, it usually suggests some degree of toxic accumulation. Biopsy specimens show neutrophils infiltrating often necrotic eccrine ducts. In biopsy samples from some patients, there may be reactive proliferation of the ducts, known as eccrine syringomatous metaplasia. Finally, thiotepa accumulates in the sweat and causes hyperpigmentation in areas occluded, for example, with tape.

Acral Erythema

Several regimens employed primarily for hematologic malignancies or colon cancer are likely to induce erythema, swelling and pain of the digits. The infiltrated plaques resolve spontaneously with subsequent desquamation and postinflammatory hyperpigmentation. The effect is dose-related and tends to recur with each round of therapy but is harmless.

Table 10.11. Miscellaneous chemotherapy reactions

Drug	Reactions
Asparaginase	Urticaria, pseudocellulitis (marked swelling at injection site)
Bleomycin	Flagellate hyperpigmentation Nailfold and pressure hyperpigmentation Raynaud phenomenon Sclerotic reactions Eccrine reactions
Cytarabine	Acral erythema Eccrine reactions
Dactinomycin	Folliculitis (sterile)
Daunorubicin	Radiation enhancement Eccrine reactions Extravasation necrosis
Doxorubicin	Radiation enhancement Eccrine reactions Extravasation necrosis Acral erythema Changes in hair texture (straight to curly)
5-Fluorouracil	Flare of actinic keratoses Serpentine hyperpigmentation over veins Acral erythema Photosensitivity
Hydroxyurea	Lichen planus-like reaction Skin ulcers
Mechlorethamine	Contact dermatitis
Mitomycin	Facial flushing
Mitoxanthrone	Eccrine reactions
Thiotepa	Hyperpigmentation associated with sweat
Vinblastine	Extravasation necrosis
Vincristine	Extravasation necrosis

Pigmentary Changes

A wide variety of pigmentary changes may be seen. The most dramatic is the flagellate hyperpigmentation associated with bleomycin, in which dermal melanin deposition produces lesions that resemble the marks left by a large jellyfish (Fig. 10.11). Another puzzling reaction is the cutaneous hyperpigmentation overlying veins in patients treated with 5-fluorouracil. This change occurs in the absence of clinically apparent phlebitis. Some patients develop many new melanocytic nevi during treatment. Others may have multiple longitudinal pigmented nail stripes suggesting increased activity of nailfold melanocytes. The hair may lighten or darken. The flag sign of chemotherapy refers to the presence of dark bands in light hair of patients treated with methotrexate.

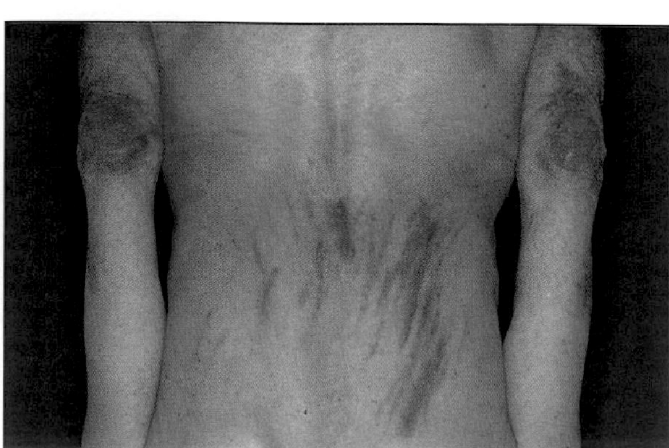

Fig. 10.11. Bleomycin-induced flagellate hyperpigmentation

Extravasation Reactions

Many agents are highly toxic and if they extravasate into the skin during intravenous infusions, marked damage may occur. The worst reactions are seen with doxorubicin and daunorubicin. If extravasation occurs, the physician and chemotherapy nurse should have a detailed plan of action. In some in-

Table 10.12. Provocation of latent or preexisting skin diseases by medications

Disease	Triggering medications
Acne	Hormones including oral contraceptives, corticosteroids, androgens and anabolic agents
Acne-like eruptions	Corticosteroids, lithium, tetracycline and many more (Chap. 28)
Allergic contact dermatitis	Many topical medications can cause allergic contact dermatitis. In rare instances, systemic use then leads to widespread disease (Chap. 12)
Bullous pemphigoid	Furosemide, sulfasalazine, phenacetin, penicillamine, nadolol
Dermatitis herpetiformis	Potassium iodide, other halogenated products, progesterone
Dyshidrosiform dermatitis	Penicillin, nickel
Lichen planus-like eruption	Gold salts, sulfonamides, *p*-amino salicylic acid, quinine, quinidine, arsenic, methyldopa, β-blockers, antimalarials
Lupus erythematosus	Hydralazine, procainamide, isoniazid, methyldopa, phenytoin, penicillamine, carbamazepine, primidone, thiouracil, and many more
Melasma	Phenytoin, estrogens, oral contraceptives
Pityriasis rosea	Gold salts, barbiturates, captopril, meprobamate, ketotifen, metronidazole
Pemphigus vulgaris	Penicillamine (especially in rheumatoid arthritis patients), ACE-inhibitors, some cephalosporins, clonidene, feprazone, glibenclamide, gold salts, nifedipine, penicillin, piroxicam, rifampicin, tiopronin
Porphyria cutanea tarda	Barbiturates, sulfonamides; also griseofulvin, phenytoin, sulfonylureas, estrogens, oral contraceptives, androgens and many others
Porphyria variegata	Chloroquine, hydroxychloroquine, oral contraceptives, griseofulvin, quinine, quinidine
Psoriasis	Lithium, gold salts, β-blockers, antimalarials
Pustular psoriasis	Same as above plus antibiotics, salicylates, opiates, withdrawal of corticosteroids, diltiazem. Anthralin in too-high concentrations

stances, local antidotes are recommended but in most cases supportive care is all that is available. In some centers, excision of damaged areas has been employed, but this approach is rarely recommended today. A minor variant of extravasation is toxic phlebitis which may present with erythematous cords or bands and overlying skin changes. In both instances, the recall phenomenon may be seen. When the agent is infused later, the previously damaged skin or vein may show erythema and swelling.

Radiation Reactions

Radiation recall is one of the most unusual chemotherapy reactions. A patient is treated initially with radiation therapy and then with chemotherapy. The drug therapy elicits a severe inflammatory response in the irradiated skin, often far exceeding the initial radiation dermatitis.

Irritation of Actinic Keratoses

Infusion of 5-fluorouracil may result in intense erythema of actinic keratoses. This phenomenon was the basis for the use of topical 5-fluorouracil in treating such lesions. In some instances, the actinic keratoses are relatively subtle, so that they are first noticed when they become red following treatment.

Provocation of Existing or Latent Skin Diseases

There is a long list of agents which may worsen an existing skin disease or trigger expression of a latent form of the disease; they are summarized in Table 10.12.

Bibliography

General References

Alanko K, Stubb S, Kauppinen K (1989) Cutaneous drug reactions: clinical types and causative agents: a five-year survey of inpatients (1981–1985). Acta Dermato Venereol (Stockh) 69:223–226

Arndt KA, Jick H (1976) Rates of cutaneous reactions to drugs. A report from the Boston Collaborative Drug Surveillance Program. JAMA 235:918–923

Bigby M, Jick S, Jick H et al. (1986) Drug-induced cutaneous reactions. A report from the Boston Collaborative Drug Surveillance Program on 15,438 consecutive inpatients, 1975 to 1982. JAMA 256:3358–3363

Bircher AJ (1996) Arzneimittelallergie und Haut. Georg Thieme Verlag, Stuttgart

Bork K (1988) Cutaneous side effects of drugs. Saunders, Philadelphia

Bork K (1999) Arzneimittelnebenwirkungen an der Haut, 2nd edn. Schattauer, Stuttgart

Bruinsma W (2000) Side effects in dermatology. Intermed Medical Publishers, Amsterdam

Chosidow O, Bourgault I, Roujeau JC (1994) Drug rashes: what are the targets of cell mediated cytotoxicity? Arch Dermatol 130:627–629

Cleach LL, Bocquet H, Roujeau JC (1998) Reactions and interactions of some commonly used systemic drugs in dermatology. Dermatol Clin 16:421–429

Coopman SA, Johnson RA, Platt R et al. (1993) Cutaneous disease and drug reactions in HIV infection. N Engl J Med 328:1670–1674

Fitzpatrick JE (1992) New histopathologic findings in drug eruptions. Dermatol Clin 10:19–36

Kramer MS, Leventhal JM, Hutchinson TA et al. (1979) An algorithm for the operational assessment of adverse drug reactions. I. Background, description, and instructions for use. JAMA 242:623–632

Litt JZ, Pawlak WA Jr (eds) (2000) Drug eruption reference manual. Partnenon, New York

Merk HF, Hertl M (1996) Immunologic mechanisms of cutaneous drug reactions. Semin Cutan Med Surg 15:228–235

Stubb S, Hekkila H, Kauppinen K (1994) Cutaneous reactions to drugs: a series of in-patients during a five-year period. Acta Dermato Venereol (Stockh) 74:289–291

Shapiro LE, Shear NH (1996) Mechanisms of drug reactions: the metabolic track. Semin Cutan Med Surg 15:217–227

Shear NH (1990) Diagnosing cutaneous adverse reactions to drugs. Arch Dermatol 126:94–97

Stern RS, Steinberg LA (1995) Epidemiology of adverse cutaneous reactions to drugs. Dermatol Clin 13:681–688

Vervloet D, Durham S (1998) Adverse reactions to drugs. BMJ 16(316/7143):1511–1514

Zürcher K, Krebs A (eds) (1992) Cutaneous drug reactions, 2nd edn. Karger, Basel

Exanthematous Reactions

Hasan T, Jansén DT (1983) Erythroderma: a follow-up of fifty cases. J Am Acad Dermatol 8:836–834

Sehgal VN, Srivastava G (1986) Exfoliative dermatitis. A prospective study of 80 patients. Dermatologica 173:278–284

Severe Skin Reactions

Assier H, Bastuji-Garin S, Revuz J et al. (1995) Erythema multiforme with mucous membrane involvement and Stevens-Johnson syndrome are clinically different disorders with distinct causes. Arch Dermatol 131:539–543

Bastuji-Garin S, Rzany B, Stern RS et al. (1993) Clinical classification of cases of toxic epidermal necrolysis, Stevens-Johnson syndrome, and erythema multiforme. Arch Dermatol 129:92–96

Becker DS (1998) Toxic epidermal necrolysis. Lancet 351:1417–1420

Braun-Falco O, Bandmann JH (1979) Das Lyell-Syndrom. Huber, Bern

Chan HL, Stern RS, Arndt KA et al. (1990) The incidence of erythema multiforme, Stevens-Johnson syndrome, and toxic epidermal necrolysis. A population-based study with particular reference to reactions caused by drugs among outpatients. Arch Dermatol 126: 43–47

Correia O, Chosidow O, Saiag P et al. (1993) Evolving pattern of drug-induced toxic epidermal necrolysis. Dermatology 186:32–37

Garcia-Doval I, LeCleach L, Bocquet H et al. (2000) Toxic epidermal necrolysis and Stevens-Johnson syndrome. Arch Dermatol 136:323–327

Mockenhaupt M, Schöpf E (1996) Epidemiology of drug-induced severe skin reactions. Semin Cutan Med Surg 15: 236–243

Roujeau JC (1997) Stevens-Johnson syndrome and toxic epidermal necrolysis are severity variants of the same disease which differs from erythema multiforme. J Dermatol 24:726–729

Roujeau JC, Stern RS (1994) Severe adverse cutaneous reactions to drugs. N Engl J Med 331:1272–1285

Roujeau JC, Kelly JP, Naldi L et al. (1995) Medication use and the risk of Stevens-Johnson syndrome or toxic epidermal necrolysis. N Engl J Med 333:1600–1607

Rzany B, Hering O, Mockenhaupt M et al. (1996) Histopathological and epidemiological characteristics of patients with erythema exudativum multiforme major, Stevens-Johnson syndrome and toxic epidermal necrolysis. Br J Dermatol 135:6–11

Rzany B, Correia O, Kelly JP et al. (1999) Risk of Stevens-Johnson syndrome and toxic epidermal necrolysis during first weeks of antiepileptic therapy: a case-control study. Study Group of the International Case Control Study on Severe Cutaneous Adverse Reactions. Lancet 353:2190–2194

Schöpf E, Stuhmer A, Rzany B et al. (1991) Toxic epidermal necrolysis and Stevens-Johnson syndrome. An epidemiologic study from West Germany. Arch Dermatol 127: 839–842

Stevens AM, Johnson FC (1992) A new eruptive fever associated with stomatitis and ophthalmia. Report of two cases in children. Am J Dis Child 24:526–533

Strom BL, Carson JL, Halpern AC et al. (1991) A population-based study of Stevens-Johnson syndrome. Incidence and antecedent drug exposures. Arch Dermatol 127: 831–838

Wolkenstein P, Revuz J (1995) Drug-induced severe skin reactions. Incidence, management and prevention. Drug Saf 13:56–68

Pseudolymphoma Reactions

Chopra S, Levell NJ, Cowley G et al. (1996) Systemic corticosteroids in the phenytoin hypersensitivity syndrome. Br J Dermatol 134:1109–1112

Conger LA Jr, Grabski WJ (1996) Dilantin hypersensitivity reaction. Cutis 57:223–226

De Vriese AS, Philippe J, Van Renterghem DM et al. (1995) Carbamazepine hypersensitivity syndrome: report of 4 cases and review of the literature. Medicine (Baltimore) 74: 144–151

Harris DW, Ostlere L, Buckley C et al. (1992) Phenytoin-induced pseudolymphoma. A report of case and review of the literature. Br J Dermatol 127:403–406

Morkunas AR, Miller MB (1997) Anticonvulsant hypersensitivity syndrome. Crit Care Clin 13:727–739

Vasculitic Reactions

Dubost JJ, Souteyrand P, Sauvezie B (1991) Drug-induced vasculitides. Baillieres Clin Rheumatol 5:119–138

Ekenstam EAF, Callen JP (1984) Cutaneous leukocytoclastic vasculitis. Clinical and laboratory features of 82 patients seen in private practice. Arch Dermatol 120:484–489

Lotti T, Ghersetich I, Comacchi C et al. (1998) Cutaneous small-vessel vasculitis. J Am Acad Dermatol 39: 667–687; quiz 688–690

Serum Sickness Reactions

Bielory L, Yancey KB, Young KB et al. (1985) Cutaneous manifestations of serum sickness in patients receiving antithymocyte globulin. J Am Acad Dermatol 13:411–417

Lawley TJ, Bielory L, Gascon P et al. (1984) A prospective clinical and immunologic analysis of patients with serum sickness. N Engl J Med 311:1407–1413

Lawley TJ, Bielory L, Gascon P et al. (1985) A study of human serum sickness. J Invest Dermatol 85:129–132

Lichenoid Reactions

Halevy S, Shai A (1993) Lichenoid drug eruptions. J Am Acad Dermatol 29:249–255

Fixed Drug Eruptions

Kanwar AJ, Bharija SC, Singh M et al. (1988) Ninety-eight fixed drug eruptions with provocation tests. Dermatologica 177:274–279

Kivity S (1991) Fixed drug eruption to multiple drugs: clinical and laboratory investigation. Int J Dermatol 30:149–151

Korkij W, Soltani K (1984) Fixed drug eruption. A brief review. Arch Dermatol 120:520–524

Mahboob A, Haroon TS (1998) Drugs causing fixed eruptions: a study of 450 cases. Int J Dermatol 37:833–838

Sowden JM, Smith AG (1990) Multifocal fixed drug eruption mimicking erythema multiforme. Clin Exp Dermatol 15(5):387–388

Acute Generalized Exanthematous Pustulosis

Moreau A, Dompmartin A, Castel B et al. (1995) Drug-induced acute generalized exanthematous pustulosis with positive patch tests. Int J Dermatol 34: 263–266

Roujeau JC (1991) Acute generalized exanthematous pustulosis. Analysis of 63 cases. Arch Dermatol 127:1333–1338

Spencer JM, Silvers DN, Grossman ME (1994) Pustular eruption after drug exposure: is it pustular psoriasis or a pustular drug eruption? Br J Dermatol 130:514–519

Drug-Induced Lupus Erythematosus-Like Reactions

Le Goff P, Saraux A (1999) Drug-induced lupus. Rev Rhum Engl Ed 66:40–45

Pramatarov KD (1998) Drug-induced lupus erythematosus. Clin Dermatol 16:367–377

Rubin RL (1999) Etiology and mechanisms of drug-induced lupus. Curr Opin Rheumatol 11:357–363

Granulomatous Reactions

Magro CM, Crowson AN, Schapiro BL (1998) The interstitial granulomatous drug reaction: a distinctive clinical and pathological entity. J Cutan Pathol 25(2):72–78

Hair Changes

Pillans PI, Woods DJ (1995) Drug-associated alopecia. Int J Dermatol 34:149–158

Tosti A, Misciali C, Piraccini BM et al. (1994) Drug-induced hair loss and hair growth. Incidence, management and avoidance. Drug Saf 10:310–317

Nail Changes

Piraccini BM, Tosti A (1999) Drug-induced nail disorders: incidence, management and prognosis. Drug Saf 21:187–201

Necrosis Following Intravascular Injections

Kohler LD, Schwedler S, Worret WI (1997) Embolia cutis medicamentosa. Int J Dermatol 36:197

Nagore E, Torrelo A, Gonzalez-Mediero I et al. (1997) Liveoid skin necrosis (Nicolau syndrome) due to triple vaccine (DTP) injection. Br J Dermatol 137:1030–1031

Ruffieux P, Salomon D, Saurat JH (1996) Livedo-like dermatitis (Nicolau's syndrome): a review of three cases. Dermatology 193:368–371

Anticoagulant Reactions

Comp PC (1993) Coumarin-induced skin necrosis. Incidence, mechanisms, management and avoidance. Drug Saf 8:128–135

Essex DW, Wynn SS, Jin DK (1998) Late-onset warfarin-induced skin necrosis: case report and review of the literature. Am J Hematol 57:233–237

Griffin JP (1994) Anticoagulants and skin necrosis. Adverse Drug React Toxicol Rev 13:157–167

Warkentin TE (1996) Heparin-induced skin lesions. Br J Haematol 92:494–497

Wutschert R, Piletta P, Bounameaux H (1999) Adverse skin reactions to low molecular weight heparins: frequency, management and prevention. Drug Saf 20:515–525

Coma Blisters and Carbon Monoxide Poisoning

Dunn C, Held JL, Spitz J et al. (1990) Coma blisters: report and review. Cutis 45:423–426

Kato N, Ueno H, Mimura M (1996) Histopathology of cutaneous changes in non-drug-induced coma. Am J Dermatopathol 18:344–350

Sanchez Yus E, Requena L, Simon P (1993) Histopathology of cutaneous changes in drug-induced coma. Am J Dermatopathol 15:208–216

Torne R, Soyer HP, Leb G et al. (1991) Skin lesions in carbon monoxide intoxication. Dermatologica 183:212–215

Reactions to Chemotherapeutic Agents

Baack BR, Burgdorf WH (1991) Chemotherapy-induced acral erythema. J Am Acad Dermatol 24:457–461

Bertelli G (1995) Prevention and management of extravasation of cytotoxic drugs. Drug Saf 12:245–255

Prussick R (1996) Adverse cutaneous reactions to chemotherapeutic agents and cytokine therapy. Semin Cutan Med Surg 15:267–276

San Angel F (1995) Current controversies in chemotherapy administration. J Intraven Nurs 18:16–23

Susser WS, Whitaker-Worth DL, Grant-Kels JM (1999) Mucocutaneous reactions to chemotherapy. J Am Acad Dermatol 40:367–398; quiz 399–400

Wenzel FG, Horn TD (1998) Nonneoplastic disorders of the eccrine glands. J Am Acad Dermatol 38:1–17; quiz 18–20

CHAPTER 11

Urticaria, Angioedema and Anaphylaxis

Contents

Urticaria

Definition. In English, "urticaria" refers to both a lesion and a disease. In Latin, things are clearer. The lesion, *urtica* or hive, is an erythematous, usually pruritic papule or plaque that appears and disappears over relatively short periods of times. The disorder, *urticaria*, features many hives; there are many different causes of urticaria and a wide variety of subtypes. The German name *Nesselfieber* refers to the typical skin reaction following contact with the stinging nettle (*Urtica dioica*), a common plant. While one distinguishes between acute and chronic urticaria, the individual lesions are almost always short-lived. Patients with chronic urticaria develop new lesions over many weeks, months or even years.

Epidemiology. Urticaria is one of the most common skin disorders. It appears that 20–30% of individuals have at least one attack of acute urticaria in their lifetime. Occasionally urticaria is combined with angioedema. About 3% of patients attending a German university dermatology clinic had urticaria. In adults there is about a 3:2 female:male ratio. The frequency of chronic urticaria is less clear. The prevalence has been estimated at 1–4%; rates of 6% have been reported from the Far East. In children acute urticaria is more common. There are also hereditary forms of urticaria, which also often first become apparent in childhood.

Etiology and Pathogenesis. A hive or urticarial lesion is the result of localized edema in the dermis following vasodilatation and increased vascular permeability with diffusion of serum and various mediators into the tissue. The typical urticarial reaction is similar to the triple response of Lewis seen when histamine is injected into the skin. There is initially erythema at the injection site secondary to vasodilatation; next the edema leads to a hive or edematous plaque; in the final stage there is an erythematous ring surrounding the hive as the axonal reflex produces more vascular changes.

The activation of cutaneous mast cells and their release of mediators is the unifying feature of most urticaria. Mast cells are found in the immediate vicinity of blood vessels; they release both preformed mediators (histamine, heparin, various enzymes) and newly manufactured ones (prostaglandins, leukotrienes). Histamine release is associated with mast cell degranulation, which can be seen with light or electron microscopy. This release is a metabolically active process; for a period of hours to days afterwards, the mast cells are refractory to stimulation as they manufacture new mediators. This explains the refractory phase between the disappearance of a hive and the appearance of new hive at a given site.

Many different stimuli can lead to release of mediators. The most common immunologic mechanism is immunoglobulin E (IgE)-mediated degranulation or a type I reaction of Gell and Coombs. Complement activation, other cytokines, nervous system stimulation, physical stimuli and various chemicals can also cause release. The classic IgE reaction develops when an allergen comes in contact with specific IgE on the mast cell surface and bridges between at least two IgE molecules, thus stimulating the mast cell membrane to trigger the cascade. The IgE is bound to the surface of the mast cells and basophils by a high-affinity, species-specific receptor. Thus for years it was only possible to demonstrate the presence of sensitizing antibodies via the Prausnitz-Küstner test, in which serum was transferred from a sensitive individual to another person who was then challenged with the allergen. Recent work has shown that eosinophils and also epidermal Langerhans cells also have the high-affinity IgE receptors.

There are direct interactions between mast cells and the nervous system. Electron microscopy has shown peripheral nerve fibers interacting with mast cells. Substance P is a direct liberator of histamine and probably involved in the axonal reflex. Conversely, histamine is a major cause of pruritus as it stimulates the peripheral sensory receptors. While most substances that cause pruritus work via histamine, there are other substances and pathways. The neural control of histamine release under normal conditions is unclear. Because the two systems are in such close contact, it appears likely that there may be continued interactions to modulate nerve reactivity and vessel tone. In some instances, such as cholinergic urticaria, the stimulus for urticaria appears almost entirely neural.

In many other urticarial disorders, such as familial cold urticaria, pressure urticaria and urticaria associated with pseudoallergy, other mediators such as serotonin, bradykinin, leukotrienes C_4, D_4 and E_4, prostaglandins and proteolytic enzymes appear important. This is of clinical relevance as such types of urticaria are far less responsive to antihistamines. Urticaria may also be associated with a variety of infectious disorders. Probably the two most common are infectious mononucleosis and hepatitis B, but many others have been described. Finally, there is contact urticaria, in which a material applied to the skin causes mast cell degranulation. Usually immunologic mechanisms are not involved; certain preservations in topical products such as sorbic acid are notorious for this effect. All of these mechanisms are discussed in more detail below.

Clinical Findings. The hive is a pruritic raised, often flat-topped lesion that is firm and has a sharp border (Fig. 11.1). When examined with diascopy, it may have a yellow tone, reflecting the serum in the skin. Sometimes the follicular openings will be prominent, especially if the lesion is compressed from the sides; this produces an orange skin appearance. Most hives are surrounded by a variably wide, patchy erythema.

Hives develop rapidly usually over minutes as preformed mediators are released. They show tremendous individual variation in color, size and shape. While most are red (urticaria rubra), if the edema is severe enough, the blood flow may be restricted, producing white tones (urticaria porcellanea). The size may range from a few millimeters in follicular urticaria to typical lesions several centimeters in diameter to enormous lesions covering whole body segments (urticaria gigantea). As the lesions spread peripherally, they may clear centrally (urticaria annularis) or intersect forming polycyclic or map-like patterns (urticaria circinata) (Fig. 11.2). When the swelling is in the deep dermis or subcutaneous tissue, then only a deep mass is seen or palpated (urticaria profunda); this is most common in angioedema, especially hereditary angioedema.

Rarely hives may become bullous (urticaria bullosa). This most commonly occurs on the shins following multiple insect bites with associated urticaria. In similar settings there may also be exocytosis of erythrocytes, producing hemorrhagic hives (urticaria hemorrhagica). While all other hives heal rapidly without leaving traces, hemorrhagic hives heal with hyperpigmentation, like any

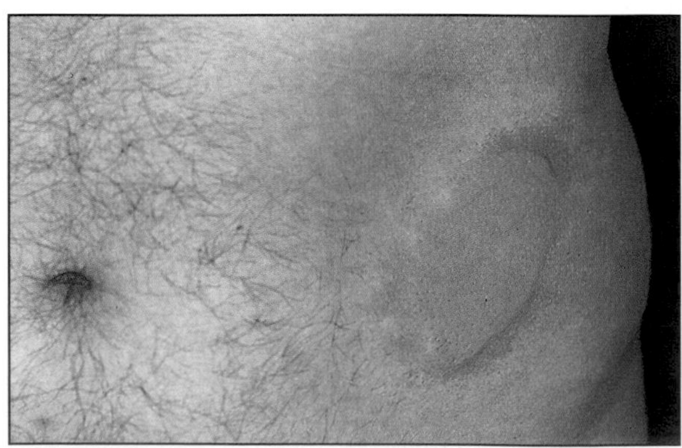

Fig. 11.1. Urticaria

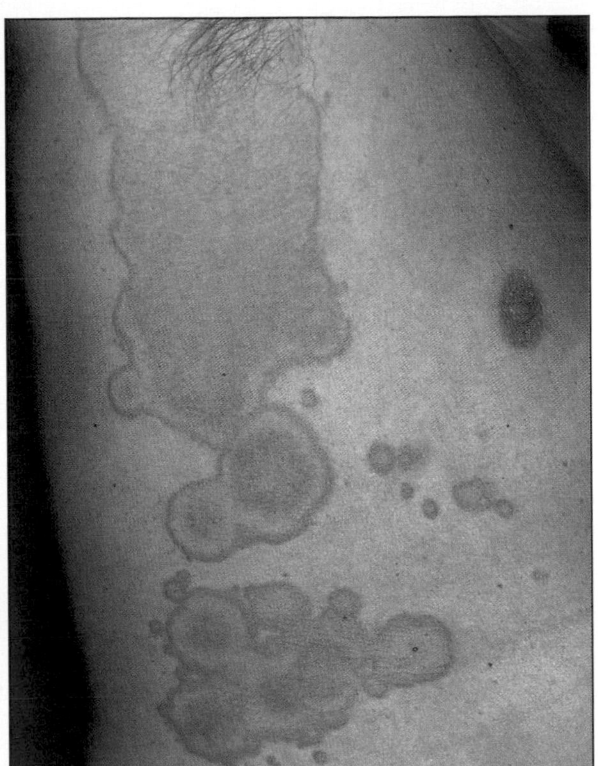

Fig. 11.2. Urticaria with wide variety of lesions in same patient

other hemorrhagic process. Finally, chronic hives may eventually lead to local hyperpigmentation secondary to melanocyte stimulation; this rare phenomenon, known as urticaria cum pigmentatione, has nothing to do with urticaria pigmentosa.

Hives develop rapidly and can disappear almost as fast. Sometimes the fluid is reabsorbed after 15–20 min. More often hives disappear over 3–8 h. If individual lesions of hives are present more than 24–48 h, then one should think of urticarial vasculitis or another urticarial variant in which histamine does not play a major role. One should even reconsider the diagnosis, for perhaps a cutaneous infiltrate is mimicking urticaria.

The pruritus associated with urticaria is usually extreme. Nonetheless, the lesions are almost invariably rubbed, not scratched. Excoriations following urticaria are extremely unusual. The itching is usually most severe as the hives develop; later it becomes more tolerable. As with so many other forms of pruritus, the problems become more severe in the evening, when the parasympathetic nervous system plays a more predominant role.

Another clinical variant is urticaria without hives. Many patients show a threshold for the development of hives when challenged by a stimulus. We have seen this most clearly in solar urticaria, where a low dose may cause pruritus; a modest dose, erythema; and a higher dose, urticaria. Thus some patients with chronic urticaria may present without hives and be misdiagnosed initially.

In most cases only the skin is involved in urticaria. In acute allergic reactions, such as to an antibiotic, there may be both urticaria and anaphylaxis-type problems. Here one may see laryngeal or glottic edema, as the patient suddenly becomes hoarse. Abdominal pain, diarrhea, bronchospasm and joint swelling are all rare. Occasionally there may be a fever with acute urticaria, as the German name *Nesselfieber* (hive fever) suggests. While the line between urticaria, angioedema and anaphylaxis is not sharply drawn, most patients with urticaria do not develop the deep or systemic problems and, conversely, most such patients do not have urticaria.

Histopathology. The histopathology of urticaria is not as spectacular as the clinical findings. There is edema in the papillary dermis. Often the superficial vessels are compressed while the deeper ones may be dilated. There is usually a sparse lymphocyte perivascular infiltrate. When neutrophils are prominent, one must consider urticarial vasculitis. Here one may also find leukocytoclasis and deposition of immunoglobulins and complement on direct immunofluorescence. In neutrophilic urticaria, there are dermal accumulations of neutrophils without vasculitis. Otherwise, histopathology plays little role in the diagnosis of urticaria and will not be mentioned in the sections to follow.

Course and Prognosis. The course of urticaria can be highly variable. In general, one distinguishes between acute and chronic urticaria. Acute urticaria usually resolves over 1–2 weeks. Contact urticaria disappears over hours. Different groups use different cut-off periods to identify chronic urticaria; we consider 6 weeks a reasonable break point. One can distinguish between chronic persistent urticaria, with hives almost every day, and chronic recurrent urticaria, in which there are disease-free intervals.

Therapy. The treatment of urticaria and related reactions is one of the most difficult aspects of dermatologic care. Patients are frequently frustrated, and doctors end up trying a long list of products that may or may not be helpful. The first step is clearly to try to remove the underlying cause, but often one cannot find the cause. The patient still requires treatment for a distressing problem. The approach to anaphylaxis is discussed separately below; patients with acute urticaria and systemic complaints may require some aspects of anaphylaxis treatment.

Antihistamines. Antihistamines are the mainstay of pharmacologic therapy. They are discussed in detail in Chapter 69 because they are employed so widely in dermatology. Some general tips for using antihistamines in urticaria patients include:

- Start out with the nonsedating products that can be given once daily. They are generally the simplest and most effective approach.
- If they fail, try several of the traditional agents; often it is wise to alternate them, using one at night and a different one during the day.
- The patient must be involved in planning the schedule. Just handing a patient a prescription for product X and saying "Take one twice a day" is silly. The patient must decide whether they are going to take the medication regularly to avoid attacks, or whether they are going to take the medication at the first sign of hives. In the latter case, the long- (and slow-) acting products are of little value. If the hives usually appear at night, a single evening dose may work. With cholinergic urticaria, the medication should be taken a few hours before exercise or other triggering activities.
- Counsel the patient carefully about side effects, as they may be taking the product for some time. Discuss drinking and driving precautions, as well as the many cross-reactions associated with some of the nonsedating agents that can cause cardiac rhythm disturbances. Terfenadine and astemizole should not be used with erythromycin or ketoconazole or in patients with a history of cardiac arrhythmias.

Other Systemic Agents. Even when antihistamines are used correctly and in maximum dosages, many patients fail to respond satisfactorily. A long list of alternative approaches have been endorsed over the years. None of them are clearly established, but many are well worth trying.

Corticosteroids. Systemic corticosteroids are part of the standard approach to anaphylaxis. Not surprisingly, they are also prescribed for acute urticaria, where their role is less clear. We do occasionally use short tapered courses of oral corticosteroids in acute urticaria. A typical regimen might start with 60 mg daily of prednisone and be tapered over 10–14 days. In chronic urticaria, a short burst of steroids may be useful to temporarily interrupt the disease process and give other therapies a chance to work. On very rare occasions, administration of low-dose corticosteroids on alternate days may be the only way to hold chronic urticaria in check, but we try hard to avoid this approach. Similarly, we do not use intramuscular triamcinolone acetonide for urticaria.

Psychotherapeutic Agents. We often choose doxepin in anxious or depressed patients, as it also has H1 and H2 action. Another possibility is to use phenothiazines such as promethazine or even other antidepressants or tranquilizers for urticaria. Opipramol is our favored agent in Germany. We suggest working with a psychiatrist who is experienced in the use of the products.

Other Medications. A number of other pharmacologic approaches have been recommended. One potentially useful group is the β-adrenergic agonists. Clearly parenteral epinephrine is effective in acute asthma. This property has inspired physicians to treat oral, more selective β-agonists in urticaria; anecdotal reports endorse albuterol, terbutaline and metaproterenol, but we view these drugs as primarily asthma medications. There are a host of other drugs, such as stanozolol, nifedipine and even more potent compounds such as methotrexate and cyclosporine, that occasionally help. Whether they are safer than low-dose corticosteroids on alternate days seems to be the key question, as they almost certainly are not as effective.

Mast Cell Stabilizers. A variety of substances can inhibit the release of mediators from mast cells, probably by blocking ion channels. Cromolyn sodium is the most widely used mast cell stabilizer but it is only effective topically and used in respiratory sprays, nose sprays or eye drops. While some individual physicians administer cromolyn systemically for chronic urticaria, it is hard to see how it reaches the skin. Ketotifen is the most effective mast stabilizer, but it is not available in the USA. Loratidine also inhibits mediator release.

Calcium. In Germany, the public and to some extent physicians place a great deal of faith in oral and even intravenous calcium to "seal" vessels and help against urticaria. Scientific support for this approach is lacking, and we do not employ calcium except for hypocalcemia, or as prophylaxis against corticosteroid-induced osteoporosis.

Blind Therapy. Shelley made popular the blind approach to chronic urticaria therapy in his marvelous little book "Consultations in Dermatology" over 25 years ago. He suggested treating the patients sequentially for a wide variety of possible underlying, missed infections. Possible approaches might include 1- to 2-week courses of:

- Antibiotics
- Anticandidal drugs
- Antifungal agents
- Antimalarial agents
- Deworming or amebicidal regimens in endemic areas
- Topical antiscabetic treatment

Such approaches are attractive, for the patient feels that something is being done. Unfortunately, they are expensive and potentially dangerous, without offering much evidence of efficacy. If there is reasonable suspicion of a particular underlying infectious trigger, such as tinea pedis or a history of sinusitis, then we too favor a trial of therapy. But blind trails are just that – blind!

Diet. Patients often ask about the relationship of their diet to their urticaria. Very little scientific information is available, but many anecdotes have been construed as evidence. On the other hand, urticaria following consumption of some foods (oysters and other shellfish, peanuts) has been reportedly repeatedly. For these reasons, we often employ a diet diary and a simple elimination diet.

Plasmapheresis. In severe unremitting urticaria, plasmapheresis has helped some patients. It may serve as a means of lowering levels of histamine-releasing autoantibodies.

Topical. The external treatment of urticaria is unrewarding. Topical distracters and antipruritic agents are the best bet. Lotions or cremes with polidocanol are most often used in Germany. Topical antihistamines have a local cooling and anesthetic effect but we avoid them as they are potent sensitizers. Once a patient is sensitized, they may be intolerant of certain systemic antihistamines. Topical corticosteroids are ineffective.

Hyposensitization. Hyposensitization or immunotherapy is discussed in connection with venom allergies, where it is an essential part of therapy. It is usually not indicated for chronic urticaria.

Types of Urticaria

There are many ways of classifying urticaria. The most common form is acute urticaria. In many cases, the patient never sees a physician as the process resolves rapidly. Histamine is the main mediator and often there is a history of an infection and ingestion of various medications, so that it is hard to decide which is the trigger. In chronic urticaria, about 15–20% of cases involve physical urticaria, 5–10% are allergic, 15–20% pseudoallergic and the rest remain unclear. The number of cases of idiopathic chronic urticaria that one diagnoses is a relative matter. Depending on how aggressively one searches and how willing one is to attribute the hives to a laboratory abnormality, one can identify an underlying disease as the cause in many or in very few cases. Table 11.1 shows the various types of urticaria.

Allergic Urticaria

Synonyms. Urticaria, hives, immunologic urticaria

Epidemiology. When patients speak of urticaria, this is the category to which they are usually referring. In most series allergic urticaria is common. This is usually a diagnosis of exclusion; in many instances, one simply concludes that the urticaria is or was allergic. If one were to define allergic urticaria as urticaria in which a relevant etiologic agent has been identified and avoidance has led to resolution of the skin findings, then the diagnosis would become less common. The onset is most often in young adult life, and women are more often affected than men. In the past, patients with atopic dermatitis were felt to have more allergic urticaria, but at least in the case of penicillin (the most common allergen), this is not true.

Etiology and Pathogenesis. The various triggers are considered below. A wide variety of immunologic reactions can be involved.

Immediate Urticarial Reaction. Type I reaction with IgE directed against allergen, usually with associated anaphylactic signs and symptoms.

Table 11.1. Types and causes of urticaria

Allergic
Foods
Medications
Aeroallergens
Other allergens
Contact urticaria (some)
Serum sickness
Toxic
Insects, Plants
Pseudoallergic (mast cell degranulators)
ASA, other analgesics, dyes, preservatives
Contact urticaria
Focus of infection
Parasites
Fungal infections
Bacterial, viral infections
Neoplasia
Physical
Mechanical (pressure, vibration, factitial)
Thermal (heat, cold)
Cholinergic (activity, stress)
Water
Light, other irradiation
Genetic
Muckle-Wells syndrome (amyloidosis, deafness & urticaria) (Chap. 41)
Enzyme defect
Angioneurotic edema
(C1 esterase inhibitor deficiency)
Inherited
Acquired (often with neoplasia)
Autoimmune disorders
Urticarial vasculitis
Systemic lupus erythematosus
Cryoglobulinemia
Paraproteinemia
Psychosocial conflicts
Stress
Depression
Many others
Endocrine disorders
Hyperthyroidism
Many others
Excessive mast cells (Chap. 63)
Mastocytoma
Urticaria pigmentosa
Telangiectasia macularis eruptiva perstans
Malignancies
Idiopathic

Delayed Urticarial Reaction. Once again, IgE is the mediator but the reaction appears 8–36 h after exposure to the allergen. An IgE-mediated reaction on the mast cell surface is involved but the mechanism for the delay is not clear. Perhaps the triggering allergen must be modified in vivo before it can cause trouble.

Serum Sickness. When a persistent antigen is introduced, such as horse serum or penicillin, especially in depot forms, then after 7–11 days a type III immune complex reaction may occur involving IgG antibodies and the foreign material. A typical clinical clue is the presence of urticarial lesions, initially along the sides of the hands and feet. IgE antibodies are also formed, probably explaining the frequent urticarial reactions. In drug-induced serum sickness, IgG antibodies play less of a role. The patient is also quite ill with a variety of systemic complaints, including arthritis, fever and lymphadenopathy.

Urticarial Vasculitis. In some instances, immune complexes are deposited in the dermal vessels, producing a leukocytoclastic vasculitis (Chap. 22). More often, the term urticarial vasculitis is used incorrectly to refer to urticaria in which the individual hives are long-lived, persisting more than 24 h.

Neutrophilic Urticaria (PETERS and WINKELMANN 1985). Neutrophilic urticaria is a histologic entity, not a clinical diagnosis. In some patients, or more likely in some urticarial lesions, there is an intense inflammatory infiltrate, probably secondary to up-regulation of mast cell cytokines. Neutrophils are found in the vessel wall and in the dermis, but there is no vasculitis.

Acute Urticaria

Definition. Urticaria of sudden onset lasting less than 6 weeks.

Etiology and Pathogenesis. Most cases of acute urticaria have a single exogenous trigger, although in most cases it is hard to define the cause with certainty. Possible causative factors are shown in Table 11.2.

Clinical Findings. Acute urticaria is the most common form of urticaria. Typically it occurs so rapidly that the patient is able to make a temporal association with a meal, medication or perhaps an arthropod sting. On occasion these associations are misleading, but most often they lead to the diagnosis. In addition, acute urticaria is sometimes associated with flushing, angioedema and anaphylaxis. In the delayed acute reaction, these valuable clues are much harder to find. Serum sickness is limited almost exclusively to exposure to foreign sera and penicillin. If the acute problems do not

Table 11.2. Causes of acute urticaria

Medications
Penicillins (most common, especially when parenteral)
ASA (also pseudoallergic), NSAIDs
Enzymes (such as pancreatic replacements)
Cephalosporins, sulfonamides
Paraminosalicylic acid
Isoniazid
Barbiturates
Meprobamate
Carbamazepine
Allergen extracts
Used for diagnosis or desensitization
Blood products
Hormones
Insulin
ACTH
Foreign proteins
Antisera
Fresh cell preparations
Vaccinations
Vitamins
Thiamine
Riboflavin
Inhalants (uncommon)
Pollens
Perfumes
Dust
Foods
Animals
Fish
Shellfish
Some meat (mutton)
Cheese (containing fungi)
Fruits
Strawberries
Walnuts
Gooseberries
Citrus fruits
Kiwi
Vegetables
Peanuts
Beans and peas
Tomatoes
Celery root
Dill
Miscellaneous
Cocoa
Chocolate
Quinine (tonic water)
Wine
Many spices
Insect antigens
Bee, wasp or hornet toxins following sensitization
Infections and infestations
Parasites (worms, scabies, others)
Infectious mononucleosis
Hepatitis B
Other acute infections

threaten the patient's life, then the course is usually uneventful with fairly rapid resolution.

Diagnostic Criteria. The diagnosis is usually based most heavily on history, although provocation tests, elimination diets, prick tests and RAST studies may be employed. Because there is a limited refractory period, prick tests are usually performed several weeks after resolution.

Urticaria in Children

Etiology and Pathogenesis. Urticaria in infants and children is almost always acute. It frequently has an infectious cause, or is secondary to medications used for infections, especially sulfonamides. Viral infections are far more commonly identified than bacterial ones. In western lands parasite infections play a minor role, but in less developed countries they are still important. We still see scabies presenting as urticaria. In children with atopic dermatitis, particular food items are an occasional cause of urticaria, usually early in life.

Clinical Findings. Clinically most children have ordinary hives, but there are several distinctive features. Lesions tend to be annular and often have punctate purpura. In acute annular urticaria, the lesions may spread to reach large sizes and persist for several days. Angioedema is present in over half the cases, a far higher proportion than seen in adults. Pruritus is often missing. While traditionally chronic urticaria has been thought to be rare, about 20 % of cases do last more than 6 weeks.

Differential Diagnosis. Urticarial lesions in small children are rarely biopsied, but we suspect there is an overlap with acute hemorrhagic edema of infancy (Chap. 22). Both are annular postviral eruptions.

Therapy. All the standard antihistamines can be used for short periods of time in children. The limiting factor is usually which products are available as elixirs or solutions.

Intermittent Urticaria

Definition. Hives that reappear at varying intervals over a period longer than 6 weeks.

Etiology and Pathogenesis. The cause is usually an allergic IgE reaction whose trigger has escaped the patient's attention, usually because of infrequent exposure or a low index of suspicion. The causative agents are the same as for acute urticaria but their patterns of exposure may be different. Medications and foods are the most likely causes.

Medications. Items that patients use infrequently are suspect, such as laxatives, headache products or pain medication taken primarily during menses. One should ask repeatedly about over-the-counter products, since many patients do not view these as medications. In addition, cross-reactions, such as those involving para-substituted benzole rings, may occur. In the later case, sulfonamides, sulfonylureas and "-caine" anesthetics may all cross-react.

Foods. Here only a food diary can help to find the elusive substance that is responsible for episodic attacks of hives. The many different possible causes have already been discussed.

Diagnostic Criteria. Once again, careful history and a diary are most helpful. Elimination diets and particular attention to medications, especially over-the-counter products, are crucial. Other tests can be employed just as for acute urticaria.

Course and Prognosis. Because chronic intermittent urticaria is so often caused by a food or medication allergy, one is more likely to detect the causative agent with a methodical approach and be able to eliminate the exposure.

Chronic Urticaria

Definition. Urticaria persisting for more than 6 weeks, either with the daily emergence of new wheals (chronic continuous) or with occasional hive-free periods (chronic recurrent).

Etiology and Pathogenesis. In most cases of chronic urticaria, the etiology is not found. Once pseudo-allergic reactions have been appropriately excluded and underlying diseases eliminated, the likelihood of finding a cause is low. One frequently reads of a given factor causing hives in a certain proportion of patients, but usually the causality is poorly established. Simply on a statistical basis, if one orders a large battery of tests, in each instance there is about a 5% chance of a false-positive result, because of the confidence intervals usually employed in laboratories. Thus if one orders 50 tests, the odds are overwhelming that a few will be abnormal. This cannot be equated with cost-effective evaluation of chronic urticaria, which most studies show does not exist. Unless there is clinical suspicion concerning a given organ system or triggering factor, blind searching rarely helps. First physical urticaria and pseudoallergic reactions, primarily idiosyncratic reactions to acetylsalicylic acid (ASA), should be excluded. Then the following possibilities should be explored.

Exogenous Factors

Medications. In contrast to acute urticaria, medications are rarely the cause of chronic urticaria. Once a drug allergy is developed, the reaction is usually so severe that all medications are stopped. Occasionally it is helpful to work with the attending physician to manipulate medications, especially if a patient is on multiple medications that may be interacting. In any event, the yield is low for chronic urticaria, even though it is high for acute urticaria.

Foods. Only products to which there is almost daily exposure, such as dairy products, eggs, grains, coffee and tea, are likely to cause chronic urticaria. Preservatives must also be considered; in this setting, tartrazine sensitivity, as a manifestation of ASA intolerance, should be ruled out.

Inhalation Allergies. Pollen sensitivity usually causes rhinitis, conjunctivitis or asthma. Urticaria is extremely unusual, except when associated with a severe variant of one of the mucosal reactions. Plant pollens are only present for limited seasons. Other aeroallergens, such as animal hairs and dander, house dust, house-dust mites, feathers and fibers (cotton, wool, kapok), are extremely rare causes of chronic urticaria.

Endogenous Factors

Infestations. Parasitic infestations are often overlooked, frequently cause urticaria, especially in children, and should be searched for diligently. A history of foreign travel should be obtained and the locally prevalent parasites, such as scabies and worms, excluded. Multiple stool evaluations for ova and parasites are mandatory.

Focus of Infection. In years past, endless searches for hidden infections were recommended, including evaluation of the sinuses, tonsils, teeth, gallbladder, fallopian tubes and prostate. Presumably the patient develops an allergic or mediator-driven-reaction to some bacterial product; perhaps toxic effects also play a role. While today foci of infection are viewed with more skepticism, if a patient has obvious dental problems or a history of sinusitis, chronic infections should be sought and treated.

Rheumatologic Disorders. Systemic lupus erythematosus may present with urticaria, but it is unusual for hives to be the only manifestation for any length of time. Nonetheless, an antinuclear antibody (ANA) assay is a reasonable part of any urticaria evaluation. In both rheumatoid arthritis and rheumatic fever, there are transient annular erythematous eruptions that may be confused with urticaria.

Autoimmune Urticaria (Graves et al. 1995). About 30% of patients with chronic urticaria have circulating autoantibodies. There are IgG antibodies directed against either IgE or, more often, the high-affinity IgE receptor FCεRI. These autoantibodies cause release of histamine from basophils. In some studies, the degree of urticaria correlated with the level of antibodies. The standard screening test for autoimmune urticaria is the injection of autologous serum, which induces a wheal and erythematous flare.

Underlying Malignancies. Virtually every malignancy has been reported at least once with urticaria. The relationship is made more secure when the chronic urticaria disappears when the tumor is treated and becomes even more certain if the urticaria reappears with a relapse. Certainly in elderly patients a tumor-directed history and reasonable screening procedures, such as fecal occult blood, chest X-ray, prostate and pelvic examination and Pap smear are appropriate. Further searches should probably be symptom-directed.

Gastrointestinal Disorders. Some believe that 60% of cases of chronic urticaria are caused by gastrointestinal problems, but the key word is "believe" as little information is available. Patients are eager to offer complaints such as bloating, constipation or even fatigue as signs of bowel involvement. In the past, both hypo- and hyperacidity were felt to be causes of urticaria, but this is no longer considered realistic. The theory is that various foods are improperly digested so that larger molecules are absorbed through the intestine and elicit an immunologic response.

A possible scientific explanation for the association of bowel complaints and urticaria has come to light in recent years. Some patients with chronic urticaria and *Helicobacter pylori* infections have had clearing of their skin lesions following appropriate antibiotic therapy. In addition, when collectives of chronic urticaria patients have been screened, there has been a higher incidence of asymptomatic *Helicobacter pylori* infection.

Another purported cause is intestinal candidiasis. Since 50% of normal individuals have *Candida albicans* in their stool at some time or other, it is easy to find the organism and then offer intestinal sterilization and recolonization with more attractive, safer species. There is certainly no harm in doing a stool culture and evaluating any reasonable bowel complaints, but the main goal probably should be to exclude silent bowel malignancies.

Endocrine Disorders. Urticaria associated with diabetes mellitus is usually caused by an insulin reaction. Hives can be seen with menses, pregnancy or climactericum, but a hormonal basis is poorly established, as oral contraceptives rarely cause hives. Hyperthyroidism may also be a trigger, but at least in some instances the flushing and warmth are confused with true urticaria. Hashimoto thyroiditis may also be found.

Other Systemic Disorders. Almost every disease has been associated with urticaria at least once. A skeptic might say, "There is no disease against which urticaria is protective." A wide variety of hematopoietic proliferative disorders are probably the most important for which to screen. In our experience, both Hodgkin disease and multiple myeloma occasionally have presented with chronic urticaria.

Emotional Factors. In truth, one is often faced with diagnosing idiopathic urticaria or saying, "It's your nerves" and diagnosing psychogenic chronic urticaria. There are no specific criteria for the latter diagnosis, although everyone agrees that the presence of recurrent disease with severe pruritus can certainly cause emotional distress and produce an anxious patient whose problem becomes that much more difficult to control.

Idiopathic Urticaria. Despite all the considerations already given and those to follow, there are large numbers of patients with acute, intermittent and especially chronic urticaria in whom no cause is found.

Clinical Findings. There are no specific clinical findings for chronic urticaria. One generalization is that persistent or chronic disease is less likely to be associated with angioedema and anaphylaxis. It is more likely to come on on in the evening or night, especially if idiopathic. Chronic urticaria may last for years; the longer it has been present, the less likely one is to find an explanation.

Diagnostic Approach. In our hands, a three-step approach to the diagnosis of chronic urticaria has proven most sensible and effective. Depending on the severity and chronicity of the patient's symptoms, one can alter the diagnostic measures.

Stage I: Basic Steps. A complete directed history, with attention paid to emotional factors, and a general physical examination, as suggested by the history, are essential. A questionnaire is often the most effective way to insure that a complete history is taken. It is also desirable to see the hives to be sure one is dealing with urticaria. If urticaria is present, then one can almost exclude hereditary and acquired angioneurotic edema. In addition, the family history will be helpful and levels of the C1 esterase inhibitor can be measured. Physical urticaria should be excluded by the history, the localization and the challenges with pressure, cold and exercise; cholinergic urticaria is a quick diagnosis if the distinctive lesions are reproduced. Flushing, scalp pruritus and lesions on the shoulders and face suggest idiosyncratic reactions to ASA.

Stage II: Intensive Evaluation. In this stage, one should repeat the history, often combined with a diary by the patient describing their diet and activities and the daily appearance of the hives. In addition, as suggested by the history, the triggering factors discussed in the previous section should be excluded as is deemed practical. Several studies have shown that almost no investigation is cost-effective in the absence of signs or symptoms. One should also consider changing or, if possible, discontinuing any systemic medications the patient is taking.

Prick testing (Chap. 12) may be useful in selected patients. Reactions to hazelnut, birch and mugwort (St. John's plant) may be positive in patients with food allergies because of cross-reactions; those with atopic dermatitis are most likely to so react. Prick testing and RAST with foods are often employed, but frequently yields false-positive and false-negative results. Intradermal injection of the patient's own serum is the best screening test for autoimmune chronic urticaria.

Stage III: Provocative Testing. Since so many cases of chronic intermittent urticaria are caused by foods and food additives, dietary manipulation can play a significant role. There are many ways to approach the problem, ranging from simple elimination diets that the patient does at home with the help of a dietitian to inpatient testing. At the extreme end of the spectrum are ecologic clinics where patients are maintained in allergen-free rooms for weeks and gradually reexposed to their "environment".

The simplest manipulation is avoidance, where the patient simply does not eat those items on which a degree of suspicion falls. Usually this approach does not achieve much, as it is hard to identify potential suspects. If one obvious item is responsible, the patient will find it. An elimination diet is the next step. Every country has its favorite elimination diet. One includes just potatoes and rice; another, a single meat, vegetable and fruit; another, tea and zwieback. In essence, a diet is chosen that is low in allergens and simple to control, although boring and often unpleasant for the patient. After 1 week, if no hives have occurred, foods or food groups are gradually added. Table 11.3 shows how the reexposure is managed at the University Dermatology Clinic in Munich. Each step or new addition can be performed after 1–2 days.

Another useful procedure is the oral provocation test for idiosyncratic reaction (OPTI), as shown in Table 11.4. It allows one to exclude pseudoallergies. The various food dyes listed are those tested for in Germany; in other countries, the list will undoubtedly be different. Such tests can only be done under medical supervision with emergency equipment available, as anaphylaxis is a possibility. Placebo tablets should be used, and ideally the physician evaluating the reaction should not know what the patient has received that day, i.e., the schedule should be varied. In addition to assessing the patient's symptoms and signs, one can also measure serum histamine levels following ingestion.

Table 11.3. Schedule for re-exposure to food groups following elimination diet

Step 1	Milk and milk products
Step 2	Carbohydrates and vegetables
Step 3	Meat
Step 4	Poultry and eggs
Step 5	Fish and seafood
Step 6	Mixed meals, including preservatives and dyes

Table 11.4. Oral provocation test for idiosyncratic reactions (OPTI)

Monday	Tartrazine 10–50 mg; parahydroxybenzoic acid ester 500 mg
Tuesday	Dye mixture I (5 mg each of chinolin yellow E104, yellow orange S 110, azorubin E122, amaranth E123 and cochinille red E124)
Wednesday	Dye mixture II (5 mg each of erythrosin D127, patent blue E131, indigotin E132, brilliant black E151 and iron oxide E172)
Thursday	Sodium benzoate 50–250–500 mg
Friday	Potassium disulfide 10–50–100 (300) mg
Monday	ASA 50–250–500 (1000) mg
Tuesday	Placebos, repeats, miscellaneous

Physical Urticaria

About 10–20% of cases of urticaria have a physical trigger. When one includes dermographism, the proportion is much higher. The mast cells are degranulated via some type of physical energy. The changes may be localized to the area of energy input or become widespread, with systemic symptoms. The cutaneous lesions may be classic hives or, more often, more fleeting urticarial erythematous reactions. In some cases, there is evidence for a type I reaction, while in others the trigger appears purely mechanical. Since the treatment for all the physical urticarias is similar, it will be covered once for pressure urticaria and then only additional therapeutic approaches will be mentioned for the other types. All of the challenges described to confirm the diagnosis of physical urticaria can potentially cause systemic symptoms of flushing, wheezing or anaphylaxis. Appropriate resuscitative equipment should be available during testing.

Dermographism

Dermographism is a common physical finding, present in 10–20% of individuals. It is not considered a disease per se. When the skin is manipulated by linear mobile pressure, such as from rubbing, scratching or moving a blunt object across the surface, several different reactions may occur.

Red Dermographism

Most commonly, after 15–20 s, the manipulated area become red through vasodilatation. Sometimes this erythema disappears and in other instances it spreads laterally with irregular borders. Because the mechanism is felt to be an axonal reflex following stimulation of the sensory nerves, this erythema has been called reflex erythema.

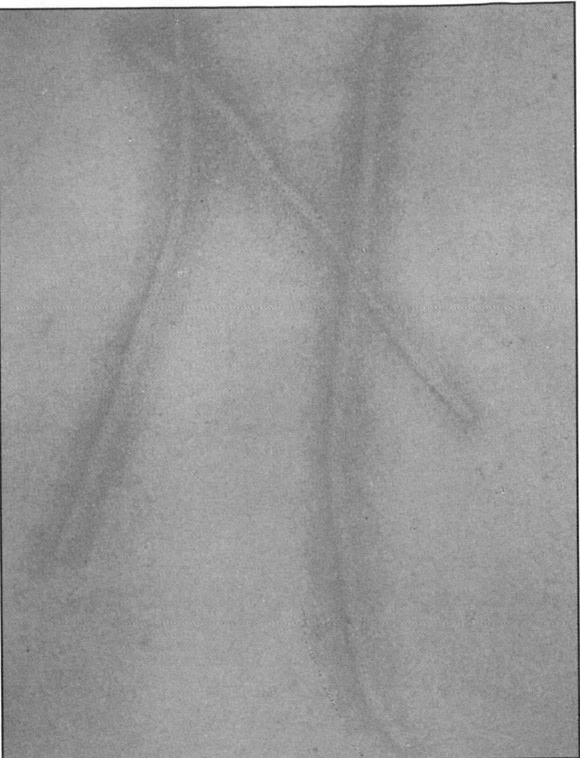

Fig. 11.3. Urticarial dermographism

Urticarial Dermographism

In some patients, after 3–5 min, a linear urticarial lesion develops in the traumatized area, presumably through the mechanical release of histamine and other mediators (Fig. 11.3). If one writes a word with a blunt object, then it will appear in raised red letters. The edema may last for 15–60 min and can be associated with itching. In the latent form of urticarial dermographism, the lesions appear after several hours and can last up to 24 h.

White Dermographism

In other instances, there is an anemic or white reaction. Both vasoconstriction and compression of vessels by tissue edema have been blamed for these changes. White dermographism is one of the minor criteria for the diagnosis of atopic dermatitis. Occasionally white dermographism may develop in patches of psoriasis, seborrheic dermatitis or other inflammatory disorders.

Symptomatic Immediate Dermographism

Synonyms. Urticaria factitia, dermographic urticaria

Etiology and Pathogenesis. Wheals appear within 10 min of applying a moderate stroking stimulus. The lesions can be induced by stroking the skin of the back with a spring-loaded stylus (dermographometer) so that a pressure of about 36 g/mm^2 can be applied. Stress appears to be an important co-factor in some patients.

Clinical Findings. In some instances, patients are so inclined towards dermographism that they develop linear urticarial reactions where there is pressure or rubbing from clothes, such as along the belt line, in the axilla, at the collar line and anywhere where elastic bands are used to hold garments in place. In addition, minor rubbing or scratching may produce urticarial lesions. A typical scenario is that the patients have severe pruritus, often in the morning or at night, rub or scratch themselves, induce urticarial lesions, which then trigger more pruritus, producing a vicious circle. This reaction seems particularly common in individuals under significant emotional stress.

There are two perhaps separate clinical variants:

Transient Urticaria Factitia. Some patients only have trouble with dermographism when taking medication, such as penicillin.

Urticaria Factitia Tarda. In this condition, the typical lesions of dermographism evolve into red streaks, without reflex erythema, which can last for hours to as much as several days. In other individuals, there may be delayed onset of the lesions.

Therapy

Systemic. Antihistamines form the basis of therapy. In all instances they work far better as potential prophylactic agents that they do to treat hives once present. A long-standing opinion holds that hydroxyzine is somewhat more effective in the various types of mechanical urticaria than its rivals, but there is individual variation and one must find the best product through a trial-and-error process. The long-acting and nonsedating antihistamines are generally more convenient for the patient. Sometimes more sedating products are best, especially in the evening. Minor tranquilizers may also be helpful.

Topical. External therapy with corticosteroids is not useful. Topical distracters or anesthetic agents (2–5% polidocanol) or cooling lotions may bring some relief. Topical antihistamines are often used for acute attacks, but their sensitizing potential makes them poor choices for chronic use in patients who are also likely to try many oral, possibly cross-reacting antihistamines.

Pressure Urticaria

Synonym. Delayed pressure urticaria

Etiology and Pathogenesis. Sustained physical pressure produces wheals. The pressure probably causes release of mast cell mediators, with the delay explained by recruitment of important mediators. Biopsies from later lesions show perivascular and interstitial mononuclear cells and eosinophils, suggesting some type of cellular response.

Clinical Findings. Persistent pressure may cause urticarial swelling. Usually several hours are required to produce a reaction, although sometimes a few minutes suffice. Typical scenarios include prolonged sitting (truck driver's urticaria) or persistent pressing such as during a dental procedure. Prolonged pressure from a belt or brassiere strap can be viewed as pressure or factitial urticaria, as both types are associated with dermographism (Fig. 11.4). While typical hives may develop, the swelling is usually deeper, although associated with an overlying erythema and thus often not correctly diagnosed. Patients may have systemic symptoms because of significant release of mediators. Prurigo dermatographica of Marcussen refers to prurigo (Chap. 25) following pressure urticaria.

Laboratory Findings. Weighted rods (1.5 cm diameter, weighing 2.5–4.5 kg) can be applied to the

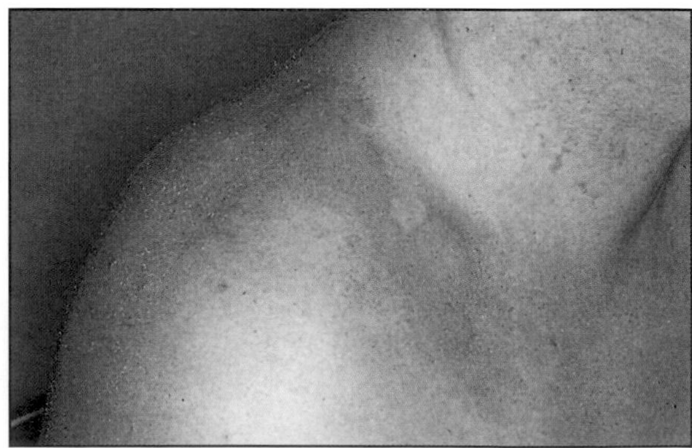

Fig. 11.4. Pressure urticaria

skin, or the dermographometer can be used at a pressure of 100 g/mm^2 for 70 s. Lesions may appear within 10–30 min (immediate pressure urticaria) or, most often, after 4–6 h (delayed pressure urticaria). Thus the site should be reobserved after a period of hours, or the patient asked to reobserve the site at home and report the next day. One should see a localized area of erythema and swelling, which may last 72 h.

Differential Diagnosis. Many patients with widespread hives develop lesions at pressure points, such as under a brassiere or on the belt line. Thus, one must always ask about and look for hives in other sites. If hives develop in nonpressure areas, then the diagnosis is simply urticaria, not pressure urticaria.

Therapy. Use of systemic antihistamines prior to exposure to pressure is the only choice, other than distracters to relieve pruritus.

Vibratory Angioedema

Synonym. Vibratory urticaria

Rare patients develop hives and deeper swelling within minutes of exposure to a vibratory stimulus. While rare familial cases have been described with autosomal dominant inheritance, most cases are acquired and sporadic. Probably the most common clinical presentation is swollen lips in a musician playing a wind or woodwind instrument. Use of massage vibrators and vibrating dildos has also triggered problems.

The standard test is the use of a vortex vibrator from a hematology laboratory; application to the forearm for 15 min usually evokes wheals and swelling.

Cold Urticaria

Synonyms. Urticaria e frigore

Epidemiology. Cold urticaria is one of the most common types of physical urticaria. It may be inherited in an autosomal dominant fashion, as familial cold urticaria or the much less common familial delayed cold urticaria. Most cases are acquired. Women are more often affected than men, and patients are typically middle aged.

Etiology and Pathogenesis. The two main forms of cold urticaria are:

- Acquired reflex cold urticaria in which exposure to cold ambient temperatures triggers a diffuse urticaria.
- Acquired contact cold urticaria in which direct contact with cold objects produces urticaria.

The various forms of cold urticaria have different pathologic mechanisms. In about half of the patients with acquired reflex cold urticaria, the Prausnitz-Küstner test is positive. This means that when serum from the patient is injected into a normal subject, that subject is made cold sensitive. In this age of HIV and other viral infections, such testing is no longer used. How an IgE mediates cold sensitivity has yet to be explained. The complement system does not appear involved.

A number of disorders have been associated with acquired cold urticaria. In some patients, the initial problem may be an infection, often upper respiratory tract or infectious mononucleosis. Ascariasis, syphilis and countless other focal infections and food allergies have also been implicated. Cold urticaria may be associated with cryoglobulins, cold agglutinins, cold hemolysins and cryofibrinogens, sometimes as a paraneoplastic marker for hematologic malignancies.

Clinical Findings

Acquired Reflex Cold Urticaria. In acquired reflex cold urticaria, the patients typically have symptoms after exposure to cold weather. Sudden changes in temperature, such as a cold wind, or exposure to cold water may also be triggers. The patient frequently reports chills or shivering prior to the hives (Fig. 11.5). The lesions tend to involve the trunk and proximal aspects of the extremities. The hives often disappear with exposure to warmth, such as taking a warm bath.

Acquired Contact Cold Urticaria. Acquired cold contact urticaria is different. Here the patient must directly handle something cold, such as frozen food or a chilled drink. The hives then develop on the hands. When such patients are exposed to cold temperatures, they may develop acral hives involving the ears, hands and perhaps feet.

These two groups have some common features. Both types of patients may experience dramatic symptoms after jumping into cold water, because of the massive release of histamine and other mediators. Ingestion of cold foods or liquids may produce local tingling around the mouth or, on rare occasions, systemic problems.

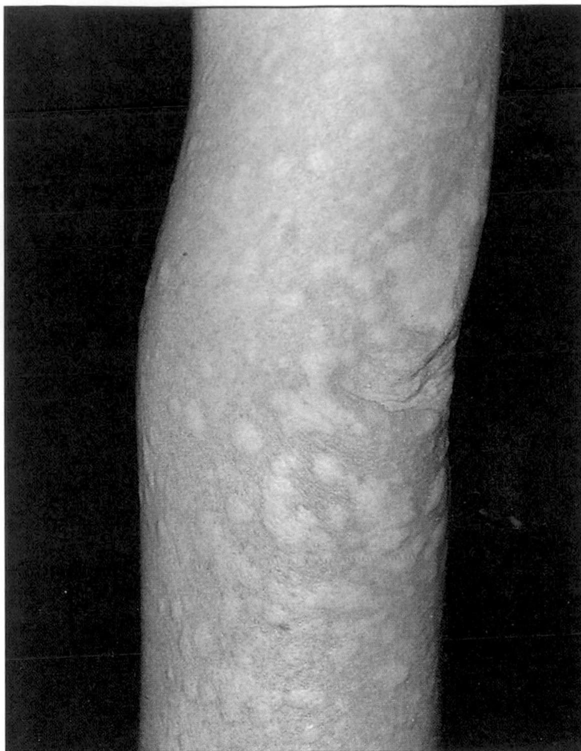

Fig. 11.5. Cold urticaria

Familial Cold Urticaria. In familial cold urticaria, there may be symptoms after cold exposure but prior to developing hives. Leukocytosis has been shown to precede attacks of urticaria, for example. In addition, arthritic changes, including swelling and pain of the distal joints, are often associated with attacks. Occasionally other symptoms such as fever, chills, headache and malaise may develop; all are uncommon in the acquired variant. The lesions may be erythematous, not urticarial, and on occasion are purpuric. They are more likely to involve nonexposed skin. In the delayed form of familial cold urticaria, the hives develop 9–18 h after cold exposure, so that the patient often overlooks the association at first.

Cold Erythema (Shelley and Caro 1962). Here the patients develop only erythema when challenged by cold.

Laboratory Findings. The ice-cube test is usually recommended, but actually a plastic bag filled with ice water is more appropriate, since it eliminates the possibility of aquagenic urticaria. The bag is applied to the skin for 20 min; upon removal and rewarming, the hives appear rapidly. If this test is negative and clinical suspicion is high, then an arm can be submerged in cold water at 5–10 °C for 10 min. To exclude acquired reflex cold urticaria, one must place the patient in a room at 4 °C for 30 min, but this is impossible to accomplish in our facilities; theoretically, the direct local challenge is almost always negative.

Therapy. Cyproheptadine, a serotonin inhibitor, has been recommended as slightly more effective in cold urticaria. Ketotifen and doxepin also have their supporters. In addition to the standard measures, treatment with intravenous penicillin has helped some patients with acquired cold urticaria; the mechanism is unknown. Usually 1 million units of benzylpenicillin are infused daily for 2–3 weeks.

Acquired Contact Heat Urticaria

Synonyms. Urticaria e calore

Etiology and Pathogenesis. In contrast to cold urticaria, heat urticaria is even more rare and even less well understood. Almost all cases are acquired and follow localized heat exposure. While the mast cells are presumably sensitive to increased temperatures, the mechanism is poorly understood. Familial delayed heat urticaria has been reported on occasion. Some view cholinergic urticaria as a form of heat urticaria.

Clinical Findings. Patients typically complain of swollen hands when handling hot vessels, washing dishes or similar tasks. Bath water appears rarely to be warm enough to cause problems for such individuals. Use of a hot-water bottle has also been implicated. The hives appear within minutes and are short-lived.

Laboratory Findings. The diagnosis can be confirmed by application of a warm vessel (38–50 °C) for 1–5 min to the inner aspect of the forearm. Wheals appear rapidly.

Rewarming Urticaria

Many individuals become flushed when coming from the cold into a warm room. Some may develop urticarial lesions. This reaction probably represents an over-enthusiastic vasodilatory response designed to rewarm the skin after cold exposure.

Solar Urticaria

Some individuals develop urticaria when exposed to solar irradiation. The problem of solar or light urticaria is discussed in Chap. 13.

Cholinergic Urticaria

Synonyms. Exercise urticaria, sweat urticaria, generalized heat urticaria

Definition. Development of tiny pruritic papules on an erythematous base following exercise or emotional stress.

Etiology and Pathogenesis. The etiology of cholinergic urticaria is not as clear as the name suggests. The intracutaneous injection of carbachol (1:4000) produces a hive with satellite lesions and erythematous fingers in about one-third of clinically clear cases. Probably many physiologic changes, induced by physical exercise or emotional stress, trigger these unusual hives. Histamine seems to be involved, as the blood histamine level rises. Passive transfer has been shown on rare occasions, but is usually negative.

Clinical Findings. Cholinergic urticaria is the hardest type to diagnose. The patient does not identify the lesions as hives because they are typically hundreds of very small (1–3 mm) papules usually with a yellow tint and a reflex erythema (Fig. 11.6). The lesions may coalesce, and occasionally larger hives may also be present. They typically last for less than 2 h. The trunk is the most common site. The patient usually describes pruritus following athletic activity, bathing, showering, eating or when under great emotional stress.

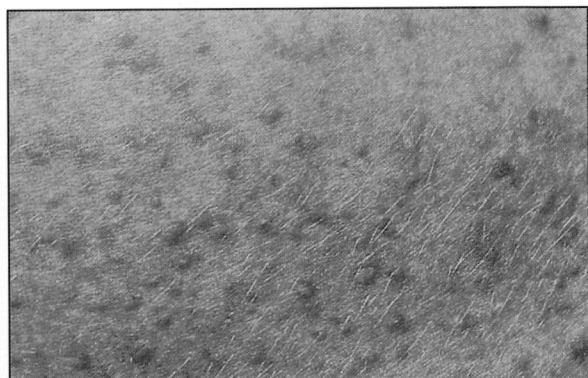

Fig. 11.6. Cholinergic urticaria

By far the most common trigger is exercise; some athletes suffer from this problem and with extreme activity also develop shock-associated signs and symptoms that are misdiagnosed. The problem tends to persist for months or years, but then disappears.

Laboratory Findings. The injection of pharmacologic mediators is not as important as a careful history and then an attempt to induce the eruption. The two standard tests are exercising to the point of sweating, often in an occlusive suit, or partial immersion in a warm bath (42 °C) for 10 min.

Therapy. Among the antihistamines, hydroxyzine appears to be most effective. Androgens such as danazol and stanozolol have been tried, but it is unclear whether the risk:benefit ratio is favorable. In addition, one should be cautious about prescribing such products for athletes. If emotional factors appear to be the trigger, tranquilizers may be of benefit.

Adrenergic Urticaria
(Shelley and Shelley 1985)

Synonym. Stress urticaria

Adrenergic urticaria is characterized by wheals surrounded by a white halo. It is very uncommon, but appears most often triggered by stress. The typical wheals can be reproduced with the intradermal injection of epinephrine or norepinephrine. This reaction can blocked by propranolol, which is also worth trying as a therapeutic agent in dosages of 25 mg b.i.d. or t.i.d.

Aquagenic Urticaria
(Shelley and Rawnsley 1964)

Etiology and Pathogenesis. Patients develop urticaria after contact with water at body temperature. This form of the disease challenges most of the rules of biology. How can one be allergic to water? The theory is that some water-soluble substance in the skin is released by water contact, enters the dermis and triggers mast cell degranulation.

Clinical Findings. The lesions are typically small intensely pruritic wheals, similar to cholinergic urticaria. which develop within minutes of contact with water and last for less than 2 h. Large hives do not appear.

Laboratory Findings. The standard challenge is a piece of gauze soaked in water at 37 °C and applied to the skin for 20 min. It should be kept warm with a heating pad at the same temperature. Testing must be done in an area where there is no breeze or draft to cause surface cooling. Alternatively, a bath at body temperature for 20 min can be used. Cold urticaria, localized heat urticaria and cholinergic urticaria should be excluded. Exclusion of the latter may be difficult because of its close clinical resemblance. Most cholinergic hives associated with swimming are cholinergic urticaria, not aquagenic or cold urticaria.

Differential Diagnosis. Aquagenic pruritus is the diagnosis when patients have pruritus following water exposure and develop no visible changes. Most probably have dry skin and are perhaps sensitive to chlorine and other chemicals in pool water. On rare occasions, aquagenic pruritus may be the presenting sign of hematologic malignancies.

Therapy. Since avoiding water is almost impossible, these patients usually require antihistamines.

Summation Urticaria

Many patients have two forms of mechanical urticaria simultaneously. The most typical combination is developing dermographism when cold, but many other combinations have been seen.

Contact Urticaria

Definition. Immediate local reaction of skin to allergen or irritant substance with initially localized erythema and edema appearing within 1 h and disappearing in a few hours.

Etiology and Pathogenesis. There are many clinical settings in which urticaria develops as a result of contact with an exogenous agent. In such instances, the urticaria is initially at least localized to the areas of contact and thus often asymmetric. There are two types of contact urticaria:

- Nonimmunologic contact urticaria is far more common and less severe, usually limited to the skin changes.
- Immunologic or allergic contact urticaria that is IgE mediated and may be associated with angioedema, asthma and anaphylaxis.

Nonimmunologic Contact Urticaria. Nonimmunologic contact urticaria can occur on first exposure to a given substance in the many individuals who come in contact with the material. It is generally limited to the skin and only rarely delayed. Typical causes include the following:

Plants. Many plants contains toxins in their leaves or other parts that are introduced into the skin via fine hairs and elicit wheals (Fig. 11.7). The classic example is the stinging nettle (*Urtica*).

Marine Animals. A variety of jellyfish and sea anemones cause urticaria as part of the direct action of their toxins.

Caterpillars. The toxic spines of a variety of caterpillars can cause urticarial reactions. The typical scenario is hundreds of caterpillars falling from trees and affecting a number of individuals with urticarial lesions on exposed surfaces. Even a shipboard epidemic of caterpillar urticaria has been described. The most commonly responsible moths in the USA are the hassock and gypsy moths. While in many instances histamine is released, there is also evidence for an IgE-mediated reaction. Patients may develop papular urticaria as allergic lesions apart from the direct contact.

Other Arthropods. Many different arthropods can induce urticarial reactions, usually around the site of their bites. Included as causative agents are bees, wasps, hornets, spiders, bed bugs, fleas, mosquitoes and ants. When the reaction is only toxic, it usually

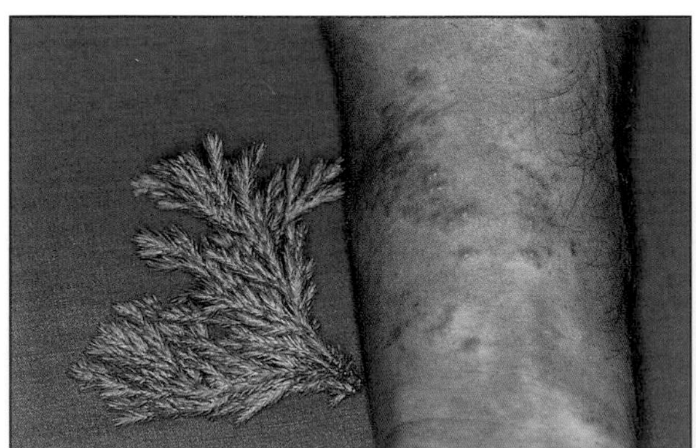

Fig. 11.7. Contact urticaria caused by *Thuja (Arbor vitae)*

resolves rapidly. Often there is an allergic aspect, manifested by evidence of IgE involvement, papular urticaria at distant sites and persistence of the reaction. Scabies can also present with urticaria, but in this case it usually represents sensitization.

Histamine Liberators. There are a number of substances not viewed as toxins that can directly cause release of histamine from mast cells. When they are applied topically, they produce localized urticaria. Included in this group are some fish, although almost all food reactions are allergic. Other selected examples are spices (mustard, cinnamon), fragrances (balsam of Peru, cinnamon aldehyde), medications (menthol, camphor, capsaicin, nicotinic acid esters, benzocaine, alcohol, bacitracin, polymyxin), metals (mainly cobalt salts), preservatives (benzoic acid, sorbic acid, formaldehyde) and many others.

Immunologic or Allergic Contact Urticaria. Allergic contact urticaria can be viewed as a rapid-acting relative of allergic contact dermatitis (Chap. 12). Patients are sensitized to a given compound and when it is applied to the skin, there is an IgE-mediated immediate urticarial reaction. Why some substances produce rapid urticarial reactions and others do not is unclear. Most materials that induce urticaria are proteins, but smaller molecules can act as haptens in producing an allergic contact urticaria. Associated systemic reactions are seen, so that the synonym "contact urticaria syndrome" has been proposed. In rare cases, the contact urticaria may have a delayed onset (4–6 h) or convert into a more typical allergic contact dermatitis. This form cannot develop on the first exposure, while a toxic reaction can occur with initial contact. Possible contact allergens include:

Animal Products. Hair, blood and other products may be responsible. Amniotic fluid is a major problem in veterinarians, who traditionally deliver baby animals without wearing gloves. Reactions to gelatin, wool and silk may fit into this category. As mentioned above, most of the insect toxins can sensitize individuals, later causing allergic reactions.

Plant Products. The most important vegetable agent today is latex. As the use of protective gloves has increased, the incidence of latex allergy in health care workers has risen dramatically and is probably over 10% in most societies. Patients with spina bifida are at particular risk. Those with latex allergy are also at risk of immediate reactions to various foods, such as bananas and tomatoes. Pollens and balsam of Peru may also be troublesome, as may a variety of woods, their oils and sawdust.

Foods. Almost every food has been described to produce immediate allergic reactions. Examples are citrus fruit peels, spices, potatoes, asparagus, tomatoes, onions, garlic, peanuts, dairy products, fish meal and honey. Protein contact dermatitis (Hjorth et al. 1976) is a type of immunologic contact urticaria seen almost exclusively in food handlers, who develop itching, erythema, urticaria and even dyshidrosiform changes within 30–60 min of handling certain fresh foods. Diagnosis can be very difficult in such patients, as some react to direct exposure with contact urticaria, others will have a positive patch or prick test, and yet others will only have a positive RAST.

Food allergens and plants may also elicit symptoms of the lips, tongue, oral mucosa and pharynx. Patients may complain of tingling, swelling or itching after eating a variety of foods, including apples, tomatoes and carrots. Often there is a cross-reaction with birch pollen, especially among patients with atopic dermatitis.

Medications. Topical antibiotics are frequent sensitizers. Penicillin is so allergenic that it is not used topically. Not only patients but also nurses and other health-care workers are at risk. Phenothiazines, pyrazolones, nitrogen mustard, benzocaine and even some corticosteroids have been responsible for acute allergic reactions.

Miscellaneous. A long list of other triggers includes ammonium persulfate (a bleach used by beauticians), epoxies, acrylics, some metal salts (primarily copper and nickel) and many preservatives.

Clinical Findings. The clinical findings have been discussed under the etiology. Not surprisingly, the main feature is urticaria at a site of contact with an allergen, arising immediately. Delayed onset, persistence and involvement of other organs, such as with asthma or even intestinal pain, suggests an immunologic mechanism.

Course and Prognosis. Most nonallergic reactions are a nuisance at worst, because large amounts of toxins are unlikely to be introduced. Unlucky exposure to a jellyfish is a possible exception. On the other hand, an allergic reaction is unpredictable. There are overlaps between localized allergic contact urticaria, allergic contact dermatitis, widespread urticaria and systemic symptoms, culminating for example in shock in a patient with latex allergy operated on by a surgeon wearing latex gloves.

Diagnostic Criteria. The diagnosis is usually suggested by the history. A modified patch test can be used to document suspected contact urticaria. The suspected allergen is occluded with a patch test for 20 min and then the reaction read after 30 min. In the case of food allergies, this is often inaccurate and further studies must be pursued.

Therapy. The main treatment is avoidance. Antihistamines are helpful in those cases that are histamine mediated, but usually pretreatment is required.

Pseudoallergic Urticaria

Synonym. Nonimmunologic urticaria

Definition. Urticaria produced by direct mast cell degranulation.

Etiology and Pathogenesis. A number of medications and diagnostic materials can produce urticaria by direct actions on mast cells, just as they can produce contact urticaria. The mechanisms are unclear, but when a mediator has been documented, it has usually been histamine. Some of the triggering agents are bases that may displace histamine, itself a base. Others may cause frank degranulation of the mast cell. By definition, IgE does not play a role, and other immunologic mechanisms have not been identified. In most instances the reaction is viewed as idiosyncratic, in that it is not dose related and shows no relationship to other expected toxic reactions. Pseudoallergic reactions are responsible for a fair number of cases of chronic urticaria in which an etiologic agent is identified.

Causative agents include the following:

Aspirin and Nonsteroidal Antiinflammatory Drugs. Aspirin causes both a type I allergic reaction and a pseudoallergic direct release of histamine from mast cells. About 1% of individuals taking ASA experience a reaction; how many are allergic is unclear. The same group of individuals may react to NSAIDs, as well as to azo dyes such as tartrazine and to benzoic acid complexes. There appears to be a familial tendency towards ASA pseudoallergy.

When one analyzes more limited groups, the prevalence of idiosyncratic ASA reactions becomes higher. It is estimated that 2–10% of patients with bronchial asthma are sensitive, while some groups have suggested that 25–50% of patients with chronic urticaria have such reactions. While the proportion is clearly significant, it is not that high in most series.

Other Medications. Opiates (morphine), pethidine, atropine and papaverine are notorious for producing flushing reactions and urticaria. A number of anesthetics, such as propanidid, thiopental, D-tubocurarine and succinylcholine, also cause histamine release. Occasionally, polymyxin and bacitracin may cause nonimmunologic urticaria. Sympathicomimetic agents, thiamine and iron salts have also been implicated.

Colloidal Volume Expanders. The mechanisms are confusing, but hydroxyethyl starches cause anaphylactic reactions in about 0.1% of cases, compared with 0.01% when human albumin is used. Direct mast cell effects as well as immune complex reactions are suspected.

Radiologic Contrast Material. At least 5% of patients who receive iodinated radiologic contrast material, usually using triiodinated benzoic acid, develop anaphylactic reactions. Iodine allergy is not a factor. Instead, mast cell degranulation, activation of the alternate complement pathway and release of serotonin from thrombocytes appear to be factors.

Food Additives. Benzoic acid, sorbic acid and tartrazine are often implicated. Tartrazine is not only an additive, but is also naturally present in a wide variety of yellow and green vegetables.

Clinical Findings. The acute pseudoallergic reaction is usually associated with at least some systemic symptoms. When patients with urticaria have conjunctival, nasal and respiratory symptoms, but no allergen is found, one should always consider a pseudoallergic reaction, especially triggered by ASA. Other clues include flushing, scalp pruritus and presence of a majority of the wheals on the upper part of the body. In patients with atopic dermatitis, the idiosyncratic reaction can combine with the underlying disorder to exaggerate the respiratory, nasal and ocular symptoms. Similarly, in a patient with chronic urticaria of a different cause, the presence of an idiosyncratic ASA reaction may worsen the symptoms.

Diagnostic Criteria. The diagnosis may be suggested by the history but can only be confirmed by an oral challenge or a provocation test. As shown in Table 11.4 and discussed above, gradually increasing dosages of the suspected agents are administered. A type I allergy must be excluded, usually via prick tests and in vitro identification of allergen-specific IgE.

Therapy. The same treatment recommended for acute urticaria is appropriate.

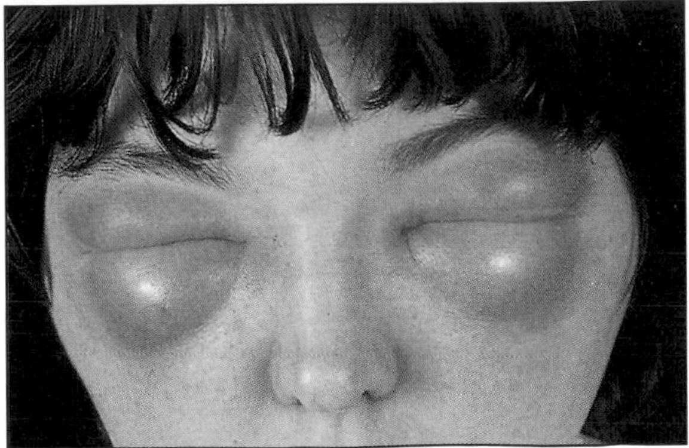

Fig. 11.8. Angioedema

Angioedema

(QUINCKE 1882)

Synonyms. Quincke edema, angioneurotic edema, urticaria profunda

Definition. Acute subcutaneous edema producing circumscribed irregular cutaneous swelling.

Etiology and Pathogenesis. Angioedema is in most cases a deeper expression of urticaria. It usually reflects a type I reaction, with the same possible triggers as suggested above. In hereditary, acquired and drug-related angioedema, elevated plasma bradykinin levels have been demonstrated, suggested it may be an important mediator. The most likely triggers for angioedema are bee and wasp stings, drug reactions, hyposensitization injections and certain foods, especially eggs, shellfish and nuts. Angiotensin-converting enzyme (ACE) inhibitors have been associated with life-threatening angioedema in several reports. Just as with urticaria, often one does not identify a cause.

Clinical Findings. Women are more often affected than men, and young adults are the typical target group. Ordinary angioedema is commonly clinically associated with urticaria. Sometimes there is a brief prodromal period, but usually the patient suddenly notices swelling of the skin and mucosa with little or no pruritus. Typical sites include the eyelids, lips, genitalia and distal parts of the extremities (Figs. 11.8, 11.9). The overlying skin is usually pale, occasionally slightly red. Usually there is one lesion or a small number. The swelling tends to reach its maximum size after several hours and then begins to recede. The entire process typically lasts 8–72 h.

The risk with angioedema is swelling of the tongue, larynx and/or pharynx, which can lead to airway obstruction and even death. On occasion, a tracheotomy is required. Other internal involvement rarely plays a clinical role except in hereditary angioedema where intestinal involvement is common and can be severe.

When angioedema recurs, it often involves the same site. Thus, over time the skin may be stretched

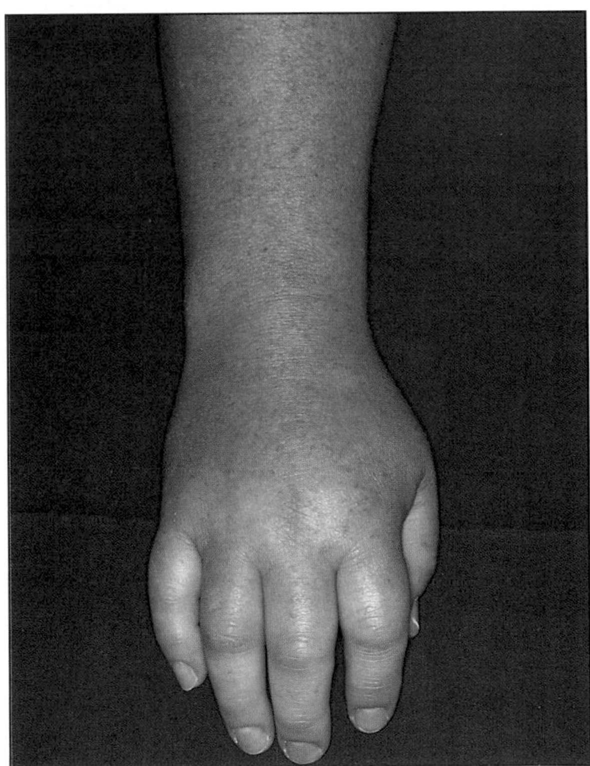

Fig. 11.9. Angioedema

and not regain its normal tone. This phenomenon is known as secondary dermatochalasis or secondary cutis laxa (Chap. 18).

Course and Prognosis. The outlook for any given attack is determined by the degree of airway involvement. Recurrent attacks without a known trigger are more dangerous than recurrent urticaria.

Diagnostic Criteria. The same approach discussed under acute urticaria is employed.

Differential Diagnosis. In contrast to urticaria, angioedema offers a number of differential diagnostic possibilities. First, one should consider the possibility of hereditary angioedema and the related acquired C1 esterase inhibitor (C1 INH) deficiency (Table 11.5). Hereditary angioedema almost never presents with urticaria, while in the acquired form hives may be found. Bowel symptoms are more common in hereditary angioedema. In any event, levels of C1 INH should be measured.

Episodic angioedema with urticaria and eosinophilia (GLEICH et al. 1984) is a very rare variant. It was initially felt to be part of the spectrum of hypereosinophilic syndrome, but is probably a separate, more benign disorder. The hives and swelling most often involve the head, neck and upper part of the trunk; the angioedema is relatively long-lived, persisting for a number of days. The edema is caused by eosinophil degranulation and release of major basic protein, which then triggers mast cell degranulation.

Acute allergic contact dermatitis can also present with marked swelling but there should be marked erythema, pruritus and often weeping or vesicles. Early attacks of zoster, especially involving the face, may present with massive swelling; they tend to be more erythematous and unilateral but can be quite hard to separate from angioedema. When the lips are involved, one should consider Melkersson-Rosenthal syndrome, but here the swelling is far more persistent. Erysipelas also begins with marked swelling, often around the lips, but the skin is erythematous, the lesions spread peripherally over time and the patient has fever and leukocytosis.

Hereditary Angioedema

Synonym. Hereditary angioneurotic edema (HANE)

Definition. Familial form of angioedema with defect in C1 INH and frequent bowel involvement.

Epidemiology. Hereditary angioedema is a rare disorder, found in less than 1% of patients with angioedema. The problems typically start in childhood or adolescence. Women are more often affected than men.

Etiology and Pathogenesis. The basic defect in hereditary angioedema is a defective C1 INH. The problem is inherited in an autosomal dominant pattern; that is, 50% levels of the C1 INH are sufficient to cause clinical problems. C1 INH is an

Table 11.5. Differential diagnosis of hereditary and ordinary angioedema

Features	Hereditary	Acquired
History	Onset in youth; often positive family history	Onset in adult life; no family history
Prodrome	Sometimes annular erythema	None
Trigger	Usually none (stress, trauma)	Usually none (medications, other allergens, pressure)
Symptoms		
Angioedema	Face, trunk, extremities	Face, mainly eyelids, mouth
Swelling	Diffuse often painful	None
Urticaria	None	Common
Abdominal colic	Present	Absent
Laboratory		
Plasma C1-INH activity	Reduced	Normal
Plasma C1-INH levels	Reduced or normal	Normal
Therapy	Danazol, C1 INH	Corticosteroids, antihistamines

α-globulin that not only modulates the complement cascade but also plays a role in kinin formation, blocking the activated Hagemann factor, kallikrein and plasmin. Most patients have reduced levels of the enzyme; some have a structurally abnormal and dysfunctional protein. Trauma, surgery, dental procedures, viral infections and perhaps emotional stress have been indicted as potential triggers.

Clinical Findings. The most reliable clinical finding is the presence of a family history of angioedema. Typically the patient experiences a prodromal period with malaise, headache or gastrointestinal symptoms, and then suffers acute angioedema. The lesions are painful, not pruritic, and urticaria is very uncommon. There is no typical site of predilection, but the likelihood of intestinal involvement is much higher than with ordinary angioedema. The acute edema of the intestinal wall may lead to transient obstruction and pain. Airway obstruction may also develop, just as with allergic angioedema. In some families, a significant number of members die before reaching middle age because of respiratory arrest following obstruction. The swelling usually lasts for 1–2 h and then spontaneously recedes. Recurrences are the rule.

Laboratory Findings. C4 levels should be reduced, giving the first clue. Today it is easier to measure C1 INH levels. In 85% of patients, these levels are reduced; in 15%, the enzyme is present in normal amounts, but dysfunctional. Repeated testing may be needed to identify the decreased enzyme levels.

Radiologic examination of the abdomen can demonstrate the bowel wall swelling but is not relied upon for diagnosis.

Differential Diagnosis. Acquired C1 INH deficiency should be considered, along with allergic angioedema and the other disorders considered under its differential diagnosis. Table 11.5 shows the differences between hereditary angioedema and ordinary angioedema.

Therapy. Treatment can be divided into several stages.

Acute Swelling. Management of the airway is the most important factor. Prior to effective pharmacologic management, many patients received permanent tracheotomies. The appropriate therapy is 1000–2000 IU of C1 INH concentrate; in severe cases this may have to be repeated. Relief is not immediate but takes place over hours. While the standard angioedema and anaphylaxis therapy, including epinephrine, corticosteroids and antihistamines, is often given, there is no proof that it is helpful.

Acute Prophylaxis. If a dental procedure or other operation involving the head and neck is planned, 500–1000 IU of C1 INH should be infused 30 min prior to the procedure. Some prefer to use danazol or ε-aminocaproic acid, but these agents are much slower to take effect.

Long-Term Prophylaxis. Prophylaxis is usually provided by the administration of an anabolic androgen, which stimulates liver synthesis of C1 INH and also increases C4 levels. Typically, danazol 50–600 mg daily is employed. Stanozolol 2–6 mg daily is also effective. Once control is achieved, one should reduce the dose as much as possible, especially in women to avoid masculinizing effects and hepatotoxicity. Finally, ε-aminocaproic acid or tranexamic acid, antifibrinolytic agents, may be employed, although androgens are usually more effective.

Acquired Angioedema with C1 INH Deficiency

When angioedema and C1 INH deficiency appear in adult life and there is no positive family history, two broad categories of disease are possible.

Caldwell Syndrome

(Caldwell et al. 1972)

Synonym. Type I acquired angioedema

Caldwell syndrome is the association of acquired angioedema with an underlying hematologic disorder. The most likely association is a monoclonal B cell proliferation, such as B cell lymphoma, chronic lymphocytic leukemia or multiple myeloma. Systemic lupus erythematosus has also be associated. Not all lymphoma or leukemia patients with low levels of C1 INH have angioedema. There is increased catabolism of C1 INH. One mechanism is apparently an antiidiotype antibody directed against the monoclonal immunoglobulin, with the resulting complex fixing C1 and consuming C1 INH. In contrast to hereditary angioedema, C1 levels are sharply reduced. The angioedema may precede other signs of disease by months or years. Treatment is directed against the underlying disorder; danazol is also effective.

Primary Acquired Angioedema

(Bork et al. 1987)

Synonym. Type II acquired angioedema

In this form, there are no associated disorders. Instead, the patient develops IgG or IgM antibodies directed against C1 INH. They block the binding of C1 and C1 INH, leading to increased levels of C1, which tends to create a vicious cycle further inactivating the enzyme. The most effective therapy for this form is ε-aminocaproic acid.

Table 11.6. Causes of anaphylaxis

Medications
Preservatives, dyes
Foods
Occupational exposure
Insect toxins
Aeroallergens
Seminal fluid
Echinococcal cysts
Cold, warmth, light
Contact urticaria
C1 INH deficiency
Systemic mastocytosis
Strenuous exercise/activity
Summation of above factors
Idiopathic

Anaphylaxis and Anaphylactoid Reactions

Etiology and Pathogenesis. Anaphylaxis is the maximal variant of the immediate IgE-mediated allergic reaction that affects the entire body. Usually the antigen is either injected or ingested and then spreads via the blood. On occasion, contact can be via the mucosal surfaces (aeroallergens) or even the skin (contact urticaria, even following severe patch test reaction). There is a massive release of mediators.

An anaphylactoid reaction refers to the same clinical reaction pattern, but in the absence of an acute type I reaction. Sometimes, an immune complex reaction such as serum sickness can also produce anaphylaxis. In other instances, no immunologic mechanism is discovered. The most common cause is the administration of intravenous contrast materials. Differentiation between anaphylaxis and an anaphylactoid reaction is a laboratory exercise; the acutely ill patient is treated in the same manner.

Table 11.6 lists some of the causes of anaphylaxis. The common triggers are medications, especially penicillin, hyposensitization injections, bee and wasp stings and food allergies, especially nuts, fish and shellfish. Sometimes the cause can be very subtle, such as the reaction to poppy seeds coating a roll. Latex is probably the most common cause of anaphylaxis following skin or mucosal contact; reports exist of anaphylaxis in latex-sensitive patients when a surgeon used latex gloves. While β-blockers rarely cause anaphylaxis, they can make it much worse. Summation anaphylaxis refers to the presence of several factors, each of which alone would probably not be sufficient to trigger anaphylaxis; for example, someone might exercise to excess after eating a food to which he or she is usually only minimally intolerant but then experience more dramatic symptoms.

Clinical Findings. The typical signs and symptoms are listed in Table 11.7. The skin is often but not always involved. In addition to the classic signs of acute urticaria and angioedema, an early clue may be tingling of the tongue, palms, soles and tip of the nose.

Differential Diagnosis. In a dermatologic practice, anaphylaxis is likely to occur only if hyposensitization is performed or, extremely rarely, following injections of medications. Thus the differential diagnostic considerations are limited. Most emergencies in dermatologic surgery suites are not anaphylaxis, but represent overdoses of local anesthetics, hyperventilation, syncope or exacerbation of an underlying cardiac or respiratory problem.

Therapy. Every physician must be prepared to treat anaphylaxis. Every practice should have an appropriately equipped emergency tray. Standards of care and recommended approaches vary from country to country; each individual must be sure he or she has access to the locally standard medications and equipment needed for resuscitation and that the office staff is trained in their use.

Exercise-Induced Anaphylaxis

Etiology and Pathogenesis. Exercise-induced anaphylaxis is one of the most dramatic types of anaphylaxis. It could be considered the anaphylactic

Table 11.7. Classification of anaphylactic reactions

Grade	Skin	Abdomen	Respiratory tract	Cardiovascular system
I	Pruritus, flushing, urticaria, angioedema	None	None	None
II	Pruritus, flushing, urticaria, angioedema	Nausea, cramps	Rhinorrhea, hoarseness, dyspnea	Tachycardia (Δ >20/min), hypotension (Δ >20 mmHg systolic), arrhythmias
III	Pruritus, flushing, urticaria, angioedema	Vomiting, defecation	Laryngeal edema, bronchospasm, cyanosis	Shock
IV	Pruritus, flushing, urticaria, angioedema	Vomiting, defecation	Respiratory arrest	Cardiac arrest

equivalent of physical urticaria. After vigorous exercise, patients may develop all the findings discussed above, and may progress to shock or even death. The same amount of exercise does not always produce the same results. The working hypothesis is that the release of endogenous opiates during exercise stimulates mast cell degranulation.

But the situation becomes more complex. In about one-third of the patients, food also plays a role. Both the amount of the allergen ingested and the interval between eating and exercise are crucial in determining whether anaphylaxis occurs or not. While the first patient had a shellfish allergy, many other foods, including hazelnuts, squid, and even wheat and chicken, have been incriminated. The foods are well tolerated when not associated with exercise.

Clinical Findings. Urticaria and angioedema may be seen, just as with ordinary anaphylaxis. The same signs and symptoms discussed above apply here.

Diagnostic Criteria. In many cases, prick tests and RAST are positive for the foodstuff in question. The final diagnosis sometimes must be made by challenge tests, varying the amount of food ingested, the delay before exercise and the amount of exercise.

Therapy. Antihistamines may have some prophylactic effect, but the patients should always exercise in the presence of another person and carry an epinephrine injector.

Hoigné Syndrome

(Hoigné and Schoch 1959)

Definition. Embolism and CNS symptoms following intramuscular injection of crystalline products.

Etiology and Pathogenesis. The pathogenesis of Hoigné syndrome is unclear. Presumably a subcutaneous or intramuscular injection is done improperly, resulting in an intravascular injection of a crystalline or particulate material, most often penicillin or corticosteroid. Hoigné syndrome is so rare that it is difficult to assess the risk realistically. In the case of corticosteroids, the particle size is now so small that untoward events are extremely unlikely. On the other hand, the dramatic clinical course makes it clear that one should do everything possible to avoid intravascular injections.

Clinical Findings. The most dangerous sites for injection are around the eyes and mouth. Some individuals avoid all injections from the corner of the mouth to the anterior hairline, but this is perhaps overcautious. Immediately following the injection, the patient develops anaphylaxis associated with severe neurologic manifestations, including agitation, confusion, visual and auditory hallucinations, panic reactions and even psychotic episodes. The patient may also have numbness and tingling, a peculiar taste in the mouth or cyanosis. In other instances, there may be loss of vision, sometimes permanent. Within minutes, the symptoms disappear, presumably as the embolic crystals dissolve.

Histopathology. The intravascular crystals have been demonstrated in a variety of organs.

Differential Diagnosis. The differential diagnosis is that of anaphylaxis. The Nicolau syndrome also follows the inadvertent intravascular injection of a medication, usually associated with an intramuscular injection in the buttocks, but leads to distal obstruction rather than the peculiar CNS findings seen here.

Therapy. The treatment is the same as for anaphylaxis; usually the patient suddenly improves as the resuscitative measures are in progress.

Bee, Wasp and Hornet Toxin Allergies

Epidemiology. About 4% of the population in Germany is allergic to stinging arthropods.

Etiology and Pathogenesis. Normally, when one is stung by a bee, wasp or hornet, the symptoms develop as a result of the toxin that is injected. After repeated exposures, an individual, such as a beekeeper or forest worker, may become allergic to the arthropod toxin. On subsequent exposure, a fulminant type I reaction may develop, as the effects of the toxins and the IgE-mediated reaction combine.

Clinical Findings. One should suspect that an allergy has developed when a bee or wasp sting causes severe local swelling, acute urticaria or angioedema. If anaphylaxis occurs, then one is past the point of suspicion.

Diagnostic Criteria. The diagnosis is suggested by history but should be confirmed by RAST and skin testing under close supervision, as the testing itself may also trigger anaphylaxis.

Therapy. Such patients should carry an allergy emergency kit. The contents of such a kit vary from country to country but usually include epinephrine in a preloaded syringe, antihistamines and oral corticosteroids. Patients should also wear an medical alert bracelet or necklace.

As a prophylactic measure, immunotherapy is most effective. The relevant allergen is administered in slowly increasing doses over a long period of time with the goal of improving or eliminating the patient's symptoms. Even though this procedure has been employed for almost a century, the mechanism of its action is unclear. IgG-blocking antibodies are the most attractive theory, but often they can not be demonstrated, so complex immunologic interactions are probably involved.

Hyposensitization is indicted for bee and wasp toxin allergies and should be considered for other clearly documented allergies, such as allergic rhinitis, conjunctivitis and asthma when the allergen can not be avoided, and the symptoms are difficult to control with ordinary therapeutic measures. In the case of bee and wasp toxins, hyposensitization is effective in reducing the risk of anaphylaxis in 80–90% of cases, as documented by sting provocation tests under controlled conditions. Pollen hyposensitization is usually carried out over a 3 year period; about 30% of patients become symptom free and 30% improve markedly; this leaves 40% disappointed. The role of hyposensitization in allergies to food, animal hair, house dust and house-dust mite is unclear. Patients with immune disorders, those who must take β-blockers and those who are noncompliant should not be desensitized.

The choice of allergen extracts is complicated and beyond the scope of this book. Individual firms offer a variety of different products that lend themselves to varying hyposensitization schemes. Bee and wasp toxin allergy is usually treated by an accelerated scheme on an inpatient basis. It is crucial to be certain that the RAST has confirmed the skin testing, that the identified allergens are clinically relevant and that standard treatment has not been successful. Patients often demand hyposensitization. One has to discuss in detail the slight but possible risk of death from anaphylaxis and the inherent failure rate, which for bee and wasp toxins is around 15%.

The administration of the allergen is usually subcutaneous. Intravascular injections can lead to anaphylaxis and intramuscular injections to severe pain. While the ordinary desensitization patient is observed for 30 min after the injection, those undergoing Hymenoptera desensitization are observed for 12 h. Individuals who are unwilling to wait should not be treated. Acute complications can include a severe local reaction with erythema and swelling, urticaria and anaphylaxis. With high doses of antigen, serum sickness can also develop. Late local reactions include a foreign body granuloma at the injection site. Sometimes the underlying disease can worsen. In general, appropriately administered hyposensitization provides a safe way to specifically alter the patient's immune response to selected allergens.

Bibliography

Urticaria, Angioedema and Anaphylaxis

General Aspects and Allergic Urticaria

Amin S, Lahti A, Maibach HI (eds) (1998) The contact urticaria syndrome. CRC Press, Boca Raton

Brostoff J, Challacombe SJ (eds) (1987) Food allergy and intolerance. Baillière Tindall, London

Champion RH, Greaves MW, Kobza-Black A et al. (1985) The urticarias. Churchill Livingstone, Edinburgh, pp 1–237

Charlesworth EN (1996) Urticaria and angioedema: a clinical spectrum. Ann Allergy Asthma Immunol 76:484–495

Greaves MW (1995) Chronic urticaria. N Engl J Med 332: 1767–1772
Haas N, Toppe E, Henz BM (1998) Microscopic morphology of different types of urticaria. Arch Dermatol 134:41–46
Henz BM, Zuberbier T, Grabbe J et al. (1998) Urticaria. Clinical, diagnosic and therapeutic aspects. Springer, Berlin
Heymann WR (1999) Chronic urticaria and angioedema associated with thyroid autoimmunity: review and therapeutic implications. J Am Acad Dermatol 40:229–232
Hide M, Francis DM, Grattan CE et al. (1993) Autoantibodies against the high-affinity IgE receptor as a cause of histamine release in chronic urticaria. N Engl J Med 328:1599–1604
Hide M, Francis DM, Grattan EH et al. (1994) The pathogenesis of chronic idiopathic urticaria: new evidence suggests an auto-immune basis and implications for treatment. Clin Exp Allergy 24:624–627
Jorizzo JL, Smith EB (1982) The physical urticarias: an update and review. Arch Dermatol 118:194–201
Juhlin L (1981) Modern approaches to treatment of chronic urticaria. In: Ring J, Burg G (eds) New trends in allergy. Springer, Berlin, pp 279–282
Juhlin L (1981) Recurrent urticaria: a clinical investigation of 330 patients. Br J Dermatol 104:369–381
Kanazawa K, Yaoita H, Tsuda F et al. (1996) Hepatitis C virus infection in patients with urticaria. J Am Acad Dermatol 35:195–198
Kozel MMA, Mekkes JR, Bossuyt PMM et al. (1998) The effectiveness of a history-based diagnostic approach in chronic urticaria and angioedema. Arch Dermatol 134:1575–1580
Leighton PM, MacSween HM (1990) Strongyloides stercoralis: the cause of an urticarial-like eruption of 65 years' duration. Arch Intern Med 150:1747–1748
Middleton E Jr, Reed CE, Ellis EF et al. (eds) (1998) Allergy: principles and practice. Mosby, St. Louis, 2 vols
Mittman RJ, Bernstein DI, Steinberd DR et al. (1989) Progesterone responsive urticaria and eosinophilia. J Allergy Clin Immunol 84:304–309
Monroe EW, Schul CI, Maize JC et al. (1981) Vasculitis in chronic urticaria: an immunopathologic study. J Invest Dermatol 76:103–107
Paul E, Greilich KD, Dominante G (1987) Epidemiology of urticaria. Monogr Allergy 21:87–115
Ring J, Brockow K, Ollert M et al. (1999) Antihistamines in urticaria. Clin Exp Allergy 29 [Suppl 1]:31–37
Sabroe RA, Francis DM, Barr RM et al. (1998) Anti-Fc-epsilon-RI auto antibodies and basophil histamine releasability in chronic idiopathic urticaria. J Allergy Clin Immunol 102:651–658
Sabroe RA, Greaves MW (1997) The pathogenesis of chronic idiopathic urticaria. Arch Dermatol 133:1003–1008
Settipane RA, Constantine HP, Settipane GA (1980) Aspirin intolerance and recurrent urticaria in normal adults and children. Epidemiology and review. Allergy 35:149–156
Sheehan-Dare RA, Henderson MJ, Cotteril JA (1990) Anxiety and depression in patients with chronic urticaria and generalized pruritus. Br J Dermatol 123:769–774
Stephens CJM, Black MM (1989) Perimenstrual eruptions: autoimmune progesterone dermatitis. Semin Dermatol 8:26–29
Wollenberg A, Hänel S, Spannagl M et al. (1997) Urticaria haemorrhagica profunda. Br J Dermatol 136:108–111

Physical Urticaria

Gorevic PD, Kaplan AP (1980) The physical urticarias. Int J Dermatol 19:419–435
Kaplan AP (1984) Unusual cold-induced disorders, cold-dependent dermographism and systemic cold urticaria. J Allergy Clin Immunol 73:453–456
Mayou SC, Kobza Black A, Eady RA et al. (1986) Cholinergic dermographism. Br J Dermatol 115:371–377
Winkelmann RK (1986) The histology and immunopathology of dermographism. J Cutan Pathol 12:486–492
Wong RC, Fairley JA, Ellis CN (1984) Dermographism: a review. J Am Acad Dermatol 11:643–652

Pressure Urticaria

Czarnetzki BM, Meentken J, Rosenbach T et al. (1984) Clinical, pharmacological and immunological aspects of delayed pressure urticaria. Br J Dermatol 111:315–323
Czarnetzki BM, Meentken J, Rosenbach T et al. (1985) Morphology of the cellular infiltrate in delayed pressure urticaria. J Am Acad Dermatol 12:253–259
Davis KC, Mekori YA, Kohler PF et al. (1986) Possible role of diet in delayed pressure urticaria – preliminary report. J Allergy Clin Immunol 77:566–569
Dover JSS, Kobza Black A, Ward AM et al. (1988) Delayed pressure urticaria. Clinical features, laboratory investigations, and response to therapy of 44 patients. J Am Acad Dermatol 18:1289–1298
Estes SA, Yung CW (1981) Delayed pressure urticaria. An investigation of some parameters of lesion induction. J Am Acad Dermatol 5:25–31
Winkelmann RK, Black AK, Dover J et al. (1986) Pressure urticaria: histopathological study. Clin Exp Dermatol 11:139–147

Cold Urticaria

Czarnetzki BM, Frosch PJ, Sprekeler R (1981) Localized cold reflex urticaria. Br J Dermatol 104:83–87
Grandel KE, Farr RS, Wanderer AA et al. (1985) Association of platelet-activating factor with primary acquired cold urticaria. N Engl J Med 313:405–409
Heavey DJ, Kobza-Black AK, Barrow SE et al. (1986) Prostaglandin D2 and histamine release in cold urticaria. J Allergy Clin Immunol 78:458–461
Neittaanmäki H (1985) Cold urticaria: clinical findings in 220 patients. J Am Acad Dermatol 13:636–644
Shelley WB, Caro WA (1962) Cold erythema: a new hypersensitivity syndrome. JAMA 180:639–642
Stafford CT, Jamieson DM (1986) Cold urticaria associated with C4 deficiency and elevated IgM. Ann Allergy 56:313–316

Cholinergic and Adrenergic Urticaria

Berth-Jones J, Grahham-Brown RAC (1989) Cholinergic pruritus, erythema and urticaria: a disease spectrum responding to danazol. Br J Dermatol 121:235–237
Czarnetzki BM, Galinski C, Meister R (1984) Cutaneous and pulmonary reactivity in cholinergic urticaria. Br J Dermatol 110:587–591
Hirschmann JV, Lawlor F, English JSC et al. (1987) Cholinergic urticaria. A clinical and histologic study. Arch Dermatol 123:462–467
Murphy GM, Greaves MW, Zollman PE et al. (1988) Cholinergic urticaria: passive transfer experiments from human to monkey. Dermatologica 177:338–340

Shelley WB, Shelley ED (1985) Adrenegic urticaria: a new form of stress-induced hives. Lancet ii:1031–1033

Aquagenic Urticaria and Pruritus

Bircher AJ (1990) Water-induced itching. Dermatologica 181:83–87

Czarnetzki BM, Breetholt KH, Traupe H (1986) Evidence that water acts as a carrier for an epidermal antigen in aquagenic urticaria. J Am Acad Dermatol 15:623–627

Lotti T, Teofoli P, Tsampau D (1994) Treatment of aquagenic pruritus with topical capsaicin cream. J Am Acad Dermatol 30:232–235

Newton JA, Singh AK, Greaves MW et al. (1990) Aquagenic pruritus associated with the idiopathic hypereosinophilic syndrome. Br J Dermatol 122:103–106

Shelley WB; Rawnsley HM (1964) Aquagenic urticaria: contact sensitivity reaction to water. JAMA 198:895–898

Steinmann HK, Greaves MW (1985) Aquagenic pruritus. J Am Acad Dermatol 13:91–96

Contact Urticaria

Accai MC, Brusi C, Francalanci S (1991) Skin tests with fresh foods. Contact Dermatitis 24:67–68

Kanerva L (1993) Contact urticaria. In: Burgdorf WHC, Katz SI (eds) Dermatology: progress and perspectives. Parthenon, New York, pp 745–749

Kligman A (1990) The spectrum of contact urticaria. Wheals, erythema and pruritus. Dermatol Clin 8:57–60

Lahti A (1980) Non-immunologic contact urticaria. Acta Derm Venereol (Stockh) 60 [Suppl 91]:3–43

Oranje AP, Aarsen RSR, Mulder PGH (1992) Food immediate-contact hypersensibility and elimination diet in young children with atopic dermatitis. Preliminary results in 107 children. Acta Derm Venereol (Stockh) 72 [Suppl 176]:41–44

von Krogh G, Maibach HI (1981) The contact urticaria syndrome – an updated review. J Am Acad Dermatol 5:328–342

von Krogh G, Maibach HI (1982) The contact urticaria syndrome. Semin Dermatol 1:59–66

Angioedema

Agostini A, Cicardi M (1992) Hereditary and acquired C1-inhibitor deficiency: biological and clinical characteristics in 235 patients. Medicine (Baltimore) 71:206–215

Alsenz J, Bork K, Loos M (1987) Autoantibody-mediated acquired deficiency of C1 inhibitor. N Engl J Med 316: 1360–1366

Bork K, Witzke G (1989) Long-term prophylaxis with C1-inhibitor (C1-INH) concentrate in patients with recurrent angioedema caused by hereditary and acquired C1-inhibitor deficiency. J Clin Immunol 83:677–682

Caldwell JR, Ruddy S, Schur PH et al. (1972) Acquired C1 inhibitor deficiency in lymphosarcoma. Clin Immunol Immunopathol 1:39–52

Chikama R, Hosokawa M, Miyazawa T et al. (1998) Nonepisodic angioedema associated with eosinophilia: report of 4 cases and review of 33 young female patients reported in Japan. Dermatology 197:321–325

Cicardi M, Bergamaschini L, Cugno M et al. (1991) Long-term treatment of hereditary angioedema with attenuated androgens: a survey of a 13-year experience. J Allergy Clin Immunol 87:768–773

Charlesworth EN (1996) Urticaria and angioedema: a clinical spectrum. Ann Allergy Asthma Immunol 76:484–495

Gleich GJ, Schroeter AL, Marcoux PL et al. (1984) Episodic angioedema associated with eosinophilia. New Engl J Med 310:1621–1626

Hakansson OM (1988) Menstruation-related angioedema treated with tranexamic acid. Acta Obstet Gynecol Scand 67:571–572

Helfman T, Falanga V (1995) Stanozolol as a novel therapeutic agent in dermatology. J Am Acad Dermatoi 32:254–258

Heymann WR (1997) Acquired angioedema. J Am Acad Dermatol 36:611–615

Heymann WR (1999) Chronic urticaria and angioedema associated with thyroid autoimmunity: review and therapeutic implications. J Am Acad Dermatol 40:229–232

Kozel MMA, Mekkes JR, Bossuyt PMM et al. (1998) The effectiveness of a history-based diagnostic approach in chronic urticaria and angioedema. Arch Dermatol 134: 1575–1580

Quincke HI (1882) Über akutes umbeschriebenes Hautödem. Monatshefte Prakt Dermatol 1:129–131

Sim TC, Grant A (1990) Hereditary angioedema: its diagnostic and management perspectives. Am J Med 88:656–664

Stoppa-Lyonnet D, Tosi M, Laurent J et al. (1987) Altered C1 inhibitor genes in type I hereditary angioedema. N Engl J Med 317:1–6

Tamayo-Sanchez L, Ruiz-Maldonado R, Laterza A (1997) Acute annular urticaria in infants and children. Pediatric Dermatol 14:231–234

Warin RP, Cunliffe WJ, Greaves M et al. (1986) Recurrent angioedema: familial and östrogen-induced. Br J Dermatol 115:731–734

Wollenberg A, Hänel S, Spannagl M et al. (1997) Urticaria haemorrhagica profunda. Br J Dermatol 136:108–111

Zurlo JJ, Frank M (1990) The long-term safety of danazol in woman with hereditary angioedema. Fertil Steril 53:64–72

Anaphylaxis

Brady WJ Jr, Luber S, Joyce TP (1997) Multiphasic anaphylaxis: report of a case with prehospital and emergency department considerations. J Emerg Med 15:477–481

Ewan PW (1998) Anaphylaxis. BMJ 316:1442–1445

Hoigné R, Schoch K (1959) Anaphylaktischer Schock und akute, nicht allergische Reaktionen nach Procain-Penicillin. Schweiz Med Wochenschr 89:1350–1356

Kagy L, Blaiss MS (1998) Anaphylaxis in children. Pediatr Ann 27:727–734

Muller U, Mosbech H, Blaauw P et al. (1991) Emergency treatment of allergic reactions to Hymenoptera stings. Clin Exp Allergy 21:281–288

Rueff F, Przybilla B, Müller U et al. (1996) The sting challenge test in Hymenoptera venom allergy. Position paper of the Subcommittee on Insect Venom Allergy of the European Academy of Allergology and Clinical Immunology. Allergy 51:216–225

Sampson HA (1998) Fatal food-induced anaphylaxis. Allergy 53:125–130

Schafer T, Przybilla B (1996) IgE antibodies to Hymenoptera venoms in the serum are common in the general population and are related to indications of atopy. Allergy 51: 372–377

van der Klauw MM, Wilson JH, Stricker BH (1996) Drug-associated anaphylaxis: 20 years of reporting in The Netherlands (1974–1994) and review of the literature. Clin Exp Allergy 26:1355–1363

Dermatitis

Contents

Introduction

A wide variety of unrelated diseases are included in this chapter. In the past, some have been called dermatitis and others, eczema. For the sake of uniformity we will only employ the term dermatitis; this is a radical change from the German version of this book in which dermatitis is used for acute disorders with a tendency toward spontaneous resolution and eczema for chronic diseases with little tendency to resolution. As a partial recognition of the European roots of this text, the term eczema is used in the synonyms. The derivations of the words do not help us much.

The word "dermatitis" is generally thought to be a translation of an ancient Greek word meaning inflammation of the skin (*derma-* + *-itis*), but it does not have such a distinguished etymology. According to Leider, it was coined later by analogy with other Greek words. "Dermatitis" is not really a noun but an adjective; just as "arthritis nosos" means disease of the joints, "dermatitis nosos" would mean disease of the skin. In both cases, the noun has been dropped and the adjective functions as a noun. In these structures, "-itis" does not mean inflammation.

The Greek roots of the word "eczema" are clear. Eczema is the "result of" (*-ma*) "boiling" (*-ze-*) "over" (*ec-*). Thus some would use it for more superficial reactions.

Even if one becomes frustrated with the terminology, one must pay careful attention to the problems. Probably between 15% and 25% of the workload of a typical dermatologic practice is devoted to the problems discussed in this chapter. Family practitioners and pediatricians are also concerned with many of these patients. The dermatitis family includes the noninfectious inflammatory disorders in which pathologic changes in the epidermis and upper dermis dominate the clinical picture. When acute, the main features are erythema, swelling, blisters, weeping and crusting, while more chronic lesions show reactive epidermal changes such as lichenification and scale. The diseases can be triggered by endogenous factors or by topical or systemic exposure to exogenous materials. Microscopically, acute dermatitis is characterized by spongiosis while chronic dermatitis features reactive epidermal changes; subacute falls in between the two poles.

Because the etiology of the dermatitis is for the most part unclear, any classification is fraught with problems. We will divide them as follows:

- Irritant contact dermatitis
- Allergic contact dermatitis
- Dyshidrotic dermatitis
- Seborrheic dermatitis
- Nummular dermatitis
- Atopic dermatitis
- Other forms of dermatitis

Irritant Contact Dermatitis

Irritant or toxic contact dermatitis results from the exposure of the skin to external agents that overwhelm the normal skin barrier function. This can result because the external agent is simply highly toxic (spilling hydrochloric acid on the skin), because of repeated exposures to agents of low toxicity (washing one's hands many times daily) or because of a variety of predisposing intrinsic factors, such as atopy.

Acute Irritant Contact Dermatitis

Synonyms. Acute nonallergic contact dermatitis, primary irritant dermatitis

Definition. Acute irritant contact dermatitis develops as a prompt inflammatory reaction when skin is exposed to an exogenous toxic agent.

Epidemiology. Acute irritant contact dermatitis is far more common than the better studied allergic contact dermatitis. While a number of factors moderate an individual's reaction to a toxic substance, anyone who has enough exposure will have trouble. Toxic substances are encountered in many work places, the home, the garden and in a variety of hobbies.

Etiology and Pathogenesis. There are many types of toxic reactions. Table 12.1 shows the basic differences between a toxic and an allergic reaction in the skin. The most dramatic example of a toxic reaction is tissue necrosis from a concentrated acid or base solution, which can produce its damaging effects in a matter of minutes. Less noxious agents require more time. The main protective barrier is the stratum corneum. Its thickness, the pattern of the corneocytes, the lipid layer and similar factors determine the skin's resistance. In general, the skin of the face, genitalia and intertriginous areas is more easily penetrated than other areas, while the palms and soles are relatively resistant. Hair follicles and sweat pores may allow shunting of material into the skin, but the discharge of sebum and sweat also has a protective action in coating and washing the stratum corneum.

The great range of skin irritability is partially explained by the factors shown in Table 12.2. For example, blacks not only have less sensitivity to UV radiation but they also have more resistance to irritation. In addition, individuals with type I skin not only are at risk for sunburn but also tend to have

Table 12.1. Major differences between toxic and allergic reactions

Parameter	Toxic	Allergic
Dose-dependent	Yes	Possible
Prior exposure required	No	Yes
Percentage exposed with reaction	High	Low
Immunity involved	No	Yes
Spread to non-exposed sites	No	Yes

Table 12.2. Exogenous and endogenous factors that influence toxic skin reactions

Exogenous
Type of irritant (chemical structure, pH)
Amount of irritant reaching skin (solubility, concentration, vehicle, duration and type of exposure)
Body region
Body temperature
Mechanical factors (pressure, rubbing, abrasion)
Climatic factors (temperature, humidity, wind)
Endogenous
Individual susceptibility towards given irritant
Sensitive skin in general
Atopy and especially atopic dermatitis
Lack of hardening
Racial factors
Sensitivity to UV radiation
Age

less resistance against toxic substances. The skin of older patients is more easily irritated. It is difficult to predict how one will react to a given toxic substance. But there are some people who simply have sensitive skin and find their skin continually irritated by otherwise relatively harmless substances.

The list of irritant or toxic substances is long but includes the following groups:

Physical Agents. UV radiation, X-rays, other ionizing radiation, laser rays, heat, cold and mechanical factors (Chap. 13).

Chemical Agents. Alkaline and acid solutions, organic solvents (xylol, toluene, benzene), fat solvents (acetone, carbon tetrachloride), detergents, croton oil, food stuffs (mustard, fruit acids), plants (Century plant, many others) and chemical warfare agents.

Phototoxic Agents. Chemicals that require exposure to UV radiation after being applied to skin (Chap. 13).

Airborne Irritants. Irritating dusts or fumes can cause marked facial irritation and swelling. Examples include various sawdusts and plastics, when they are cut, ground or heated.

The exact mechanisms of damage are highly variable. Free radicals may be formed which damage the keratinocytes. Various epidermal enzymes may be blocked. DNA synthesis and repair may be disturbed. Detergents damage first the epidermal lipid film and then the lipids in the cell membranes. Croton oil is a potent neutrophilic chemotactic agent. Organic solvents cause vasodilatation and intravascular thrombi. Dimethyl sulfoxide (DMSO) damages the lipid barrier and causes mast cell degranulation. Sodium lauryl sulfate is a surfactant found in some shampoos which is most often used as a standard irritant in product testing. Thus when one speaks of an irritant action, it may be far more complicated than the simple denaturation of proteins by an acid or a base.

Clinical Findings. Not surprisingly, the clinical spectrum is as variable as the possible etiologic agents. Typically there is some degree of erythema, ranging from pale pink to deep red, associated with hemorrhage, blisters, pustules, hives and epidermal changes such as crusts, scales and erosions. The skin damage is sharply localized to the areas of contact; distant spread does not occur (Fig. 12.1). Thus the lesions are usually asymmetric and sharply bordered. The history is often easy, as the cause-effect relationship is obvious to the patient. Sometimes the patient may hide this association.

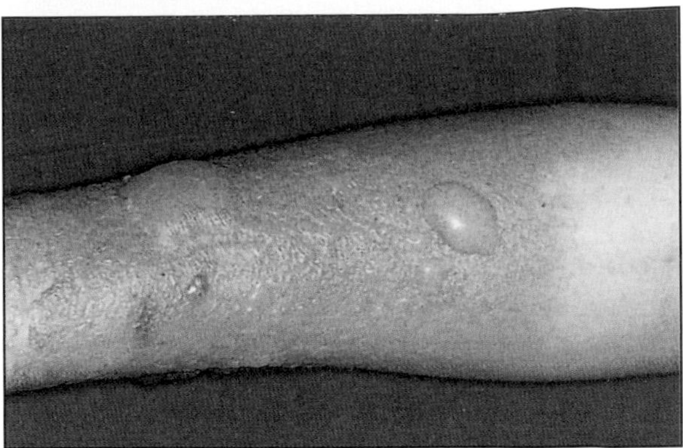

Fig. 12.1. Acute irritant contact dermatitis with bullae caused by an epoxy resin

Often there is a fairly logical pattern of lesion change over time. Hebra has shown this with croton oil, and any individual can notice it watching their own sunburn resolve. The stages have been somewhat artificially subdivided (Table 12.3). Not every individual goes through each stage; milder reactions do not necessarily blister and erode. Almost everyone has some degree of scaling (Fig. 12.2). The Latin terms are not crucial, but a nice tribute to the experimental work of Hebra. The symptoms are pruritus, burning or pain, depending on the severity of the reaction.

Histopathology. The epidermis shows spongiosis and intraepidermal vesicles or blisters. In more

Table 12.3. Stages of both irritant and allergic contact dermatitis

Stage	Clinical features
Erythematosum et oedematosum	Erythema, edema
Vesiculosum et bullosum	Blisters, bullae, usually superficial and rapidly becoming erosions
Madidans	Weeping erythematous erosions
Crustosum	Dried secretions, crusts
Squamosum	Shedding of crusts, scales; appearance of new epidermis beneath
Residual erythema	Skin appears normal except for erythema which fades over time

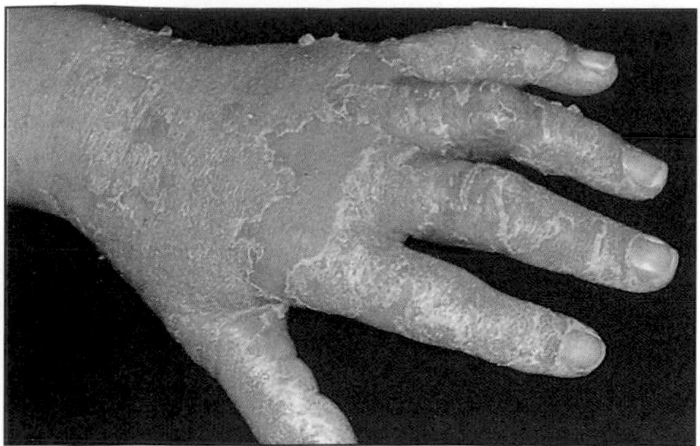

Fig. 12.2. Resolving irritant contact dermatitis with desquamation

extreme cases, there is epidermal necrosis or even no epidermis. In the dermis there is a perivascular infiltrate with exocytosis of neutrophils and lymphocytes, along with vasodilatation and edema. Acute irritant contact dermatitis is not often biopsied. In many cases the histologic picture is not specific, but the presence of more epidermal than dermal damage should suggest the possibility.

Course and Prognosis. The outlook is excellent as soon as the toxic agent is identified and removed. One possible sequel is development of an allergy against the toxic substance so that later allergic contact dermatitis occurs. A long-term sequela may be postinflammatory hypo- or hyperpigmentation following damage to the basal layer melanocytes.

Differential Diagnosis. The location of the irritant contact dermatitis determines the differential diagnostic considerations. While allergic contact dermatitis can usually be separated out, it remains a major consideration. Erysipelas is also erythematous, acute and painful. Usually a history of exposure is lacking and the patient is sick with fever, elevated white blood cell count and elevated erythrocyte sedimentation rate. Phototoxic reactions are similar, but limited to areas of UV radiation exposure and usually with a different history. Acute systemic lupus erythematosus and dermatomyositis may present with such intense facial erythema that they are mistaken for an airborne toxic reaction. The various forms of physical injury discussed in Chap. 13 must also be considered.

Therapy

Systemic. Usually none is needed. Systemic corticosteroids are not as helpful as in allergic contact dermatitis, but help reduce erythema and swelling. Often pain medication is needed.

Topical. The topical therapy of dermatitis is considered below.

Cumulative Irritant Contact Dermatitis

Synonyms. Nonallergic contact dermatitis, wear-and-tear dermatitis

Definition. Chronic dermatitis that develops following cumulative exposures to irritant substances; any single exposure would not be sufficient to produce clinical problems.

Epidemiology. Most industrial hand dermatitis falls into this category. Chronic exposure to irritating and drying substances such as water, cutting oils, chemicals, cement, tars and many others leads to a low-grade but troublesome dermatitis. Gloves are frequently used to protect the hands against environmental influences but they may contribute to the dermatitis through occlusion and abrasion. Most often the backs of hands and the forearms are involved. Housewives are also at risk; another synonym in the USA is "housewives' hands" or "housewives' dermatitis". In this case, repeated exposure to water, soaps, soiled diapers and the like is the problem. Individuals with the atopic diathesis are at greater risk. Finally, anyone required to wash their hands frequently such as health-care workers may also have trouble.

Etiology and Pathogenesis. As the many synonyms suggest, the crucial factor is repeated exposure to low-grade irritation. The skin has many defense mechanisms which must be broken down before the normally harmless irritation can produce clinical disease. In any group of people exposed to possibly irritating conditions, not all will develop a dermatitis. The variables include:

Buffering Capacity. The skin surface has a pH of about 5.7. Schade and Marchionini (1928) described this as the acid mantle. The skin is capable of buffering both acidic and basic solutions to a limited extent. When this capacity is exceeded, its deeper reaches are more easily damaged.

Water-Binding Capacity. The stratum corneum contains not only keratin but also water and fat-soluble substances that are released into the intercellular spaces by the keratinocyte as it evolves into a corneocyte. In addition, lipids reach the stratum corneum via the sebaceous glands. The water-binding substances are known as the natural moisturizing factors and consist of amino acids, sugars and lipids. If these substances are leached out of the stratum corneum, it can bind less water and becomes rougher and more likely to shed scales.

In the "bricks and mortar" model of the stratum corneum, the corneocytes are the bricks and the epidermal lipids are the mortar. A lack of epidermal lipids or quantitative variations, especially a loss of ceramide, lead to decreased water binding and drying out. In this way, the barrier function is damaged, transepidermal water loss increased, and it is easier for toxic substances to penetrate. Patients with atopy have a deficiency in ceramides which may in part explain their dry skin and sensitivity to irritants.

Skin Lipid Film. The skin lipid film is composed of the lipids contained in sebum as well as those contributed by the keratinocytes. The majority of the film is derived form sebum. The degree of sweating determines to what extent the film is diluted or altered by water. This lipid film also has antimicrobial properties. Repeated contact with soaps and detergents removes the lipid film faster than the body can restore it, resulting in drier skin.

Individual Factors. Not every person reacts in the same way to standardized irritant solutions, as a variety of test procedures with standardized panels of substances have shown. The main factor seems to be the dryness of the skin, so that patients with atopy or ichthyosis appear at particular risk.

Just as there is a long list of protective factors, there is an equally long list of agents ready to challenge the barriers. Table 12.4 shows some of the common irritants associated with various occupations. They include:

Chemicals. The number of irritating chemicals encountered primarily in the workplace as well as at home is too great to list. Alkali and acid solutions rapidly exhaust the skin's limited buffering capacity.

Detergents. Soaps, synthetic detergents (syndets), lipid solvents and other cleansing agents remove both the lipids and water-soluble substances. Repeated showering or bathing thus is drying, unless the skin is relubricated.

Organic Solvents. These agents also rapidly defat the skin. They include acetone, alcohols, benzene, benzol, carbon tetrachloride, toluene and many others.

Physical Agents. Contact with sand, dust, fabrics or even paper can be very drying. Wool is especially irritating to those with the atopic diathesis. In addition, UV radiation is drying, although it is at the same time immunosuppressive and stimulates epidermal thickening (*Lichtschwiele*) so its overall effects are hard to estimate.

Body Secretions. The irritating role of urine and stool is well known, but saliva and sweat can also be quite troublesome. Another source of trouble is the secretions that drain from a wound; a dermatitis surrounding an abrasion or injury is often not infectious but irritant.

Clinical Findings. Once the skin's defenses have been overcome via repeated exposure to the many different noxious agents which we encounter daily, a wide variety of clinical patterns may develop. In general, the chronic changes of lichenification, scaling and fissuring dominate, although more acute changes may also be seen, including erythema, swelling, blisters and crusts. Some of the clinical settings in which chronic irritation plays an important role are listed in Table 12.5. Many factors may be involved in each disorder. For example, dermatitis caused by plants may be irritant, allergic or photoallergic. In the sections to come, we consider in more detail the subgroups of chronic irritant contact dermatitis.

Chronic Irritant Hand Dermatitis

Etiology and Pathogenesis. This is the prototype of a chronic irritant contact dermatitis or cumulative toxic reaction. The cause is only rarely monofactorial; usually a number of factors combine to cause trouble. In housewives frequent exposure to water, detergents and other irritating substances is the main problem. Other groups at risk include hairdressers, nurses and other health-care workers. Among men, the main risk groups are those who work in the building trades with repeated exposure to cement and mortar, and machinists who are in constant contact with cutting oils and use harsh cleansers. Other at-risk groups include janitors and cleaners, printers, fishermen, butchers, barbers,

Table 12.4. Common irritants in various occupations

Occupation	Irritants
Bookbinder	Glue, solvents
Chemical and pharmaceutical industry	Detergents, soaps, solvents, wet conditions, numerous other irritants which t are dependen on exact tasks
Construction worker, tile layer, mason	Acids, cement, chalk, glues, paints, wet conditions, wood preservatives
Electrician, electrical industry worker	Metal cleaners, organic solvents, solder
Farmer	Animal products, cleaning supplies, diesel fuel, disinfectants, gasoline, oil, pesticides, plants, synthetic fertilizers
Food industry worker, baker, butcher, cook	Cleansers, crustaceans, detergents, fish, meat, pickling solutions, soaps, spices, vegetable and fruit juices, vinegar, wet conditions
Gardner, florist	Artificial fertilizers, compost, pesticides, plants and plant parts
Hairdresser	Hair dyes, shampoos, soaps, permanent wave solutions, wet conditions
Health personnel	Detergents, disinfectants, drugs, rubber gloves, soaps, solvents, wet conditions
Housewife	Cleaning supplies, detergents, foods polishes, soaps, wet conditions
Jeweler	Acids, bases, glues, polishes, rust remover, solder
Laundry worker, textile industry worker	Bleaches, depilatories, detergents, fibers, oxidizers and reducers, solvents, wet conditions
Metal worker, mechanic, molder, galvanizer	Antifreeze solutions, battery acids, cutting oils, defatting agents, detergents, greases, hand cleansers, soaps, solder, solvents
Miner	Cement, cleansing agents, dirt, oil, rock dust
Office worker	Carbonless copies, paper especially photocopy paper
Painter	Hand cleansers, paint removers, paints, solvents, thinners, wallpaper adhesives
Photographer	Bases, acids, oxidizers and reducers, solvents
Plastic industry worker	Acids, acryl monomers, diallylphthalates, diisocyanates, epoxy resins, oxidizers, solvents, styroles
Plumber	Hand cleansers, oils, solder, wet conditions
Printer	Acrylates, hand cleaners, lacquers, solvents
Rubber industry worker	Solvents, talc, zinc stearate
Shoe maker	Dyes, glues, polishes, solvents
Tanner	Acids, bases, oxidizers and reducers, proteolytic enzymes, solvents, wet work
Veterinarian	Animal byproducts, animal secretions, creosol, detergents, hypochlorite, soaps
Wood worker	Detergents, glues, polishes, solvents, wood preservatives

Table 12.5. Clinical diseases involving chronic irritant reactions

Chronic hand dermatitis	Stomal dermatitis
Juvenile plantar dermatosis	Airborne irritant dermatitis
Xerosis (asteatotic dermatitis)	Most dermatitis from wool and other textiles
Eyelid dermatitis	Many types of plant dermatitis
Lick cheilitis and dermatitis	Many reactions to topical medications
Diaper dermatitis	Many reactions to cosmetics
Perianal dermatitis	Adhesive tape reactions
Intertrigo	

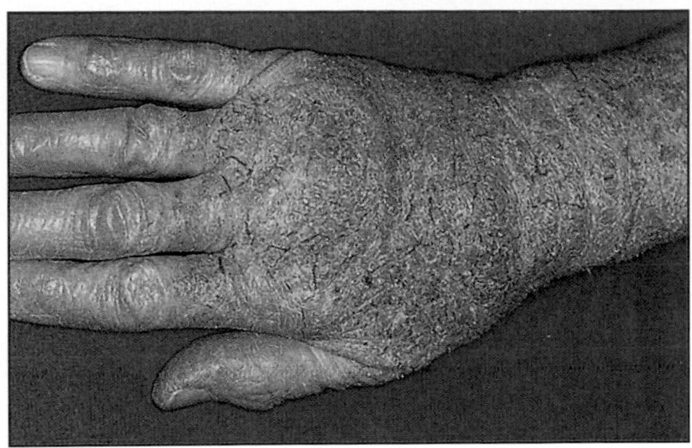

Fig. 12.3. Chronic irritant contact dermatitis

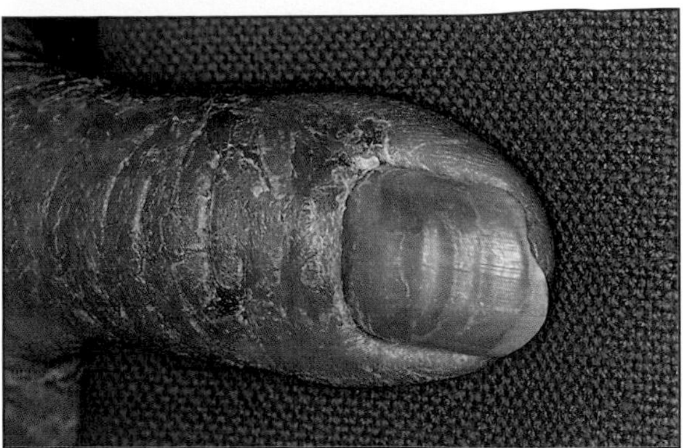

Fig. 12.4. Chronic irritant contact dermatitis of thumb with nail damage

gardeners, florists, automobile and truck mechanics, massage therapists, bakers, cooks and dental technicians. Clearly, both men and women can undertake any of these occupations in today's age of equal opportunities. Many patients have an underlying atopic diathesis and others go on to develop an additional allergic contact dermatitis.

Clinical Findings. The site of action is usually the back of the hands and the dorsal aspects of the forearms (Fig. 12.3). If the right hand is dominant, it is usually more severely affected. When hand dermatitis is more severe on the palms, dyshidrotic dermatitis and allergic contact dermatitis become more likely. Typically the dermatitis is inflammatory with simultaneous appearance of erythema, swelling and crusting. In contrast to acute irritant contact dermatitis, several stages appear at once.

Typically the lesions are asymmetric and diffuse or at least not sharply bordered. The skin is inflamed, perhaps slightly swollen and may show either acute changes such as blisters and crusts, or chronic changes such as lichenification and fissuring. Pruritus is common. Paronychia may develop and the resulting nailbed damage produces onychodystrophy (Fig. 12.4). In some cases, the lesions are limited to the fingers, especially when the irritating substances are contacted during fine work (dental plastics, glues) or when the contact is very local. Spread to skin which has not been in contact with the irritating substances does not occur, in contrast to allergic contact dermatitis where it is frequent.

Histopathology. Skin biopsy is rarely employed in this setting. The microscopic findings parallel the clinical ones ranging from acute to chronic inflammatory changes. In some cases, a biopsy is done to exclude psoriasis, but even this task is not easy. Modern immunohistochemical techniques still have not produced a foolproof way to separate allergic and toxic reactions.

Course and Prognosis. As the name suggests and even a minimum of clinical experience will reinforce, hand dermatitis tends to be recurrent and chronic. The typical patient has trouble for a while, experiences relative clearing and then relapses. Improvement is usually noted on weekends and during vacations. The unlucky one, especially when it is difficult to avoid exposure, has persistent disease. In addition, such patients use so many different products on the hands, partially under doctors' advice and partially out of frustration, that they are at risk of developing additional allergic contact dermatitis. A typical example is the construction worker who after a long battle with irritant contact dermatitis develops an allergy to chromate salts. The allergic contact dermatitis is usually more acute, wetter (more vesicles and blisters) and more likely to spread to nonexposed sites.

Diagnostic Criteria. The history, identification of risk factors (atopy, ichthyosis, dry skin of elderly) and physical examination usually suffice for the diagnosis. A particularly important question is how the hand dermatitis changes over weekends and during vacations, although a lack of improvement over weekends does not necessarily exclude occupational disease. In addition, patch testing should be performed to exclude allergic contact dermatitis. Since so many cases of chronic irritant contact dermatitis are work-related, there has been a long search for more definitive tests, but none has been found.

Buffering Capacity. Burckhardt (1957) developed tests to measure the ability of the skin to neutralize and resist basic solutions. These tests have been employed to test individuals prior to entering an at-risk occupation but they have shown little predictive value. In addition, they are not helpful in separating irritant contact dermatitis from allergic contact dermatitis.

Differential Diagnosis. The main differential diagnostic point is allergic contact dermatitis; the two conditions are not mutually exclusive. Clues suggesting psoriasis elsewhere should be sought. In addition, tinea manuum may be missed; this possibility should be excluded, especially in the presence of tinea pedis. Finally, other hybrid forms of hand dermatitis may exist, for example in the patient with atopic dermatitis who develops irritant contact dermatitis or dyshidrotic dermatitis. In most cases of hand dermatitis, it is reasonable to pursue the diagnosis of atopy a bit further, as discussed below.

Therapy. Avoidance, protective creams and gloves are the mainstays of prophylaxis. The selection of protective gloves depends on the penetration rate of the individual toxic substances or contact allergens through glove material. Gloves with lower sensitizing potential such as potassium dichromate-free leather gloves or thiuram-free rubber gloves are preferable. Topical corticosteroids are essential for more acute forms. The prophylactic measures first become valuable once the dermatitis has cleared. More detailed considerations are listed below under the different forms of irritant dermatitis.

Hyperkeratotic Palmoplantar Dermatitis

Synonyms. Hyperkeratotic rhagadiform palmoplantar dermatitis, tylotic dermatitis

Etiology and Pathogenesis. Why some patients develop a more hyperkeratotic hand dermatitis and why this particular form often also involves the feet is unclear. One possibility is that the patients have an ordinary dermatitis but an underlying tendency or genetic predisposition to keratinization abnormalities on the palms and soles. Another theory is that they often have atopy and over-respond to persistent palmoplantar inflammation. Allergic contact dermatitis and occupational exposure do not play prominent roles.

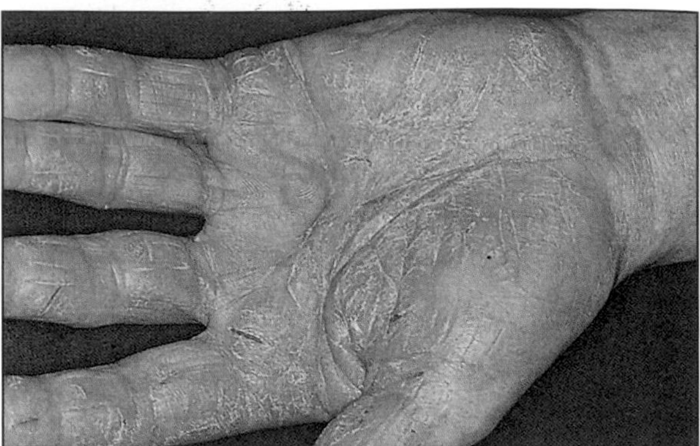

Fig. 12.5. Hyperkeratotic rhagadiform palmar dermatitis

Clinical Findings. The palms and soles are covered with a limited number of small, sharply bordered minimally inflamed plaques, covered with thickened yellow callus. A striking feature is the presence of deep cracks or rhagades (Fig. 12.5). The skin between the calluses may show fine scales. Small dyshidrosiform vesicles may be seen at the periphery. The hands and feet are not always simultaneously affected. The disorder is both very chronic and likely to recur.

Histopathology. A biopsy will usually just show marked hyperkeratosis and minimal inflammation, but it can be useful to exclude tinea manuum and help rule out other inflammatory disorders.

Differential Diagnosis. In contrast to chronic wear-and-tear hand dermatitis, this variant raises more differential diagnostic questions. The overlap with dyshidrotic dermatitis has already been mentioned. In addition, tinea manuum and pedis should be excluded. In rare cases, hypertrophic lichen planus and even discoid lupus erythematosus may present with hand dermatitis of this type.

Therapy. In addition to the standard therapies, several special approaches may be considered here.

Systemic. Low-dose oral retinoids (acitretin 10–20 mg daily) may be tried, even when psoriasis has not been proven.

Topical. Something must be done to loosen the scale. Traditionally salicylic acid is tried first; in Europe it is available combined with mid- to high-potency corticosteroids. Antipsoriasis therapy using anthralin or topical vitamin D derivatives (calcipotriol, tacalcitol) is another consideration. Hypertonic salt-water soaks, starting at 3% and working up to 10%, can be used. The hands and feet are soaked for about 10 min daily.

Other Measures. Hand and foot PUVA, or especially hand and foot PUVA bath therapy is another possibility.

Pityriasis Simplex

The term "pityriasis" was used by Galen to describe branny scaling. In general, it refers to slightly dry skin with fine scales. In Europe, pityriasis versicolor is used instead of tinea versicolor to describe the infection with *Malassezia furfur*. The other forms of pityriasis are less clear, but refer to dry scaly skin. Most patients have intrinsically dry skin such as elderly or prepubescent individuals or those with atopic diathesis. Other common factors include increased washing and reduced room humidity. In the USA the pityriasis family is considered a form of dry skin. Some of the subtypes of pityriasis identified include:

Pityriasis Simplex Capillitii. These patients have a dry scaly scalp, occasionally with pruritus, but without inflammation. In the USA they make the self-diagnosis of dandruff and rarely present to physicians. When there is little inflammation, then dandruff may be caused by excessive shampooing, whereas with seborrheic dermatitis, there is usually inflammation and frequent shampooing usually helps. In children, tinea capitis should be excluded. The possible role of *Pityrosporum ovale* is considered under seborrheic dermatitis. Treatment generally consists of decreasing shampooing, using a milder shampoo (not baby shampoo which is quite drying) and perhaps using a light oil such as a bath oil to lubricate the scalp.

Pityriasis Amiantacea. The nature of pityriasis amiantacea is a mystery. Amiantacea means asbestos-like referring to the thick adherent scales which pile up and resist removal (Fig. 12.6). Tinea is a misnomer; dermatophytes are not involved. Whether or not pityriasis amiantacea is an extreme form of pityriasis simplex is unclear. In any event, treatment is mechanical. We encourage patients to apply a lotion, oil or cream containing 3–5% salicylic acid, allow it to work for several hours, shampoo and then brush the scalp vigorously to remove scale. Other measures, such as tar shampoos and corticosteroids, can also be tried. Our last resort is to apply a corticosteroid cream followed by an oil with 3–5% salicylic acid; the scalp is occluded for several hours or overnight with a shower cap and then shampooed.

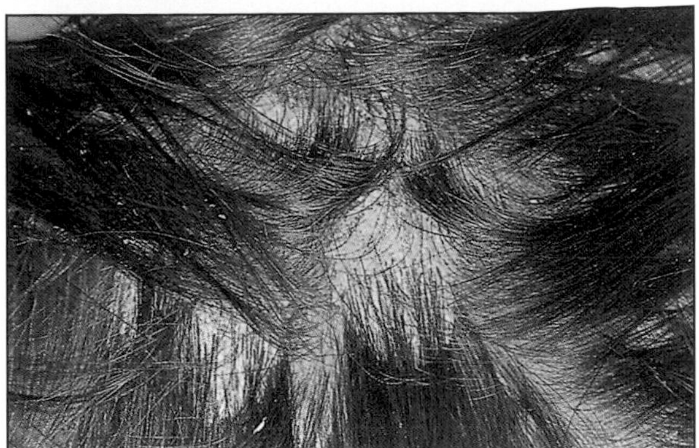

Fig. 12.6. Pityriasis amiantacea

Pityriasis Alba

Synonyms. Pityriasis simplex faciei, pseudoleukoderma

Small children, often those with atopic dermatitis, may present with circular fine scaly patches, most often on the cheeks. The condition is often misdiagnosed as tinea faciei, but this can be readily excluded with a KOH examination. Usually the problem is the result of too frequent or too aggressive cleansing. Common sense and a mild lubricant or a very low-potency corticosteroid cream or ointment suffice. The term pityriasis alba is employed because in darker skin individuals and in the summer, the patches appear lighter in color.

Asteatotic Dermatitis

Synonyms. Pityriasis simplex corporis, eczema hiemalis, dry skin eczema

Definition. The preferred German term, *Exsikkationsekzematid*, is difficult to define. Exsiccation or desiccation is the process of drying out. In English, the term eczematid is not used although it is common in German and French. Literally it simply means "eczema-like". In German, an eczematid is a predermatitic condition with scale, erythema, and very fine fissures.

Clinical Findings. The important fact is that skin can dry out in many ways. The beginner should not let the terms overwhelm him. The most typical

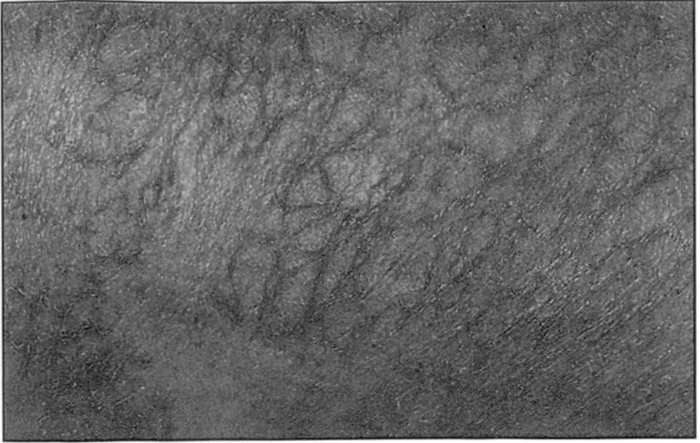

Fig. 12.7. Eczema craquelé

pattern is diffuse dryness with mild fine scaling and no erythema; this is xerosis. Localized disease, usually associated with at least mild inflammation has acquired different names.

- Localized dry areas are often called pityriasis simplex.
- Ichthyosis vulgaris-like pattern (Chap. 17).
- Asteatotic dermatitis. Some people dry out more intensely in localized areas. The favorite sites are the face and distal part of the extremities, where multiple 2–4-cm plaques may develop, usually with both prominent scale and erythema.
- Eczema craquelé. In this situation the skin dries out with larger scales separated by deep inflamed fissures resembling the *craquelé* work on glazed china (Fig. 12.7).
- Eczema cannelé. In this final variant, localized areas of dry skin are surrounded by a fissure, much as a moat surrounds a castle (Fig. 12.8). The base of the fissure is erythematous, as the dermal vessels can be seen. The term cannelé is from the adjectival form of the French *canneler*, to channel or groove.

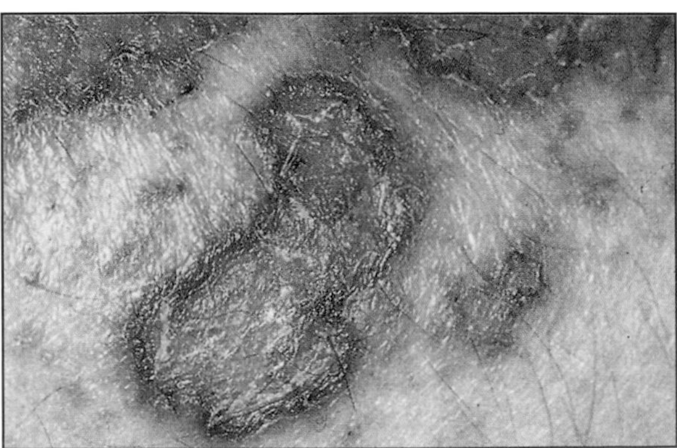

Fig. 12.8. Eczema cannelé

All these forms are typically pruritic. They tend to start in the fall when central heating is turned on and the environmental humidity is low.

Differential Diagnosis. Depending on the form, a variety of differential diagnostic questions arise. Localized lesions are often mistaken for dermatophyte infections, but the KOH examination quickly settles the issue. Inflamed lesions may resemble psoriasis. Pityriasis rosea and petaloid seborrheic dermatitis also appear similar, but close examination usually allows differentiation. More persistent lesions may suggest small-patch parapsoriasis.

Therapy. Limited bathing, avoidance of soaps and other cleansing agents and prompt relubrication usually work wonders.

Intertrigo

Definition. Intertrigo literally means rubbing between and refers to an acute superficial inflammatory process that arises where two pieces of skin rub together.

Etiology and Pathogenesis. The main risk factor for intertrigo is obesity. As an individual becomes fatter, there are more folds of skin which can come into contact, such as under the breasts, along the jowls and even where folds of abdominal skin pile up. There are also regions that come together regardless of obesity, such as the axillae, inguinal and genital regions, umbilicus, retroauricular region, between the digits, and in the uncircumcised, the prepuce. Anatomic peculiarities such as a funnel-shaped anus may be additional factors. Diabetes mellitus is usually listed as a risk factor, but it only plays a role in predisposing to overweight. When two pieces of skin are in contact, there is mechanical maceration coupled with reduced evaporation of sweat and increased growth of bacteria and fungi.

Clinical Findings. Acute intertrigo can arise if, for example, a person exercises heavily, perspires a great deal and sits in wet clothes for a while. An axillary or gluteal cleft intertrigo is not unusual but is self-limiting. Acute perianal or inguinal intertrigo is known in German as *Wolff*, an ancient German word. It is analogous to an acute irritant contact dermatitis. There is erythema, maceration, erosions and a weeping exudate with serous crusts.

Even more troublesome is chronic intertrigo, also called intertriginous dermatitis, and similar to chronic irritant contact dermatitis. Here the symmetric eruption is erythematous, scaly, pruritic and quite persistent. The most typical sites are under the breasts, in the anal region and between folds of abdominal fat. Fissures may develop in the depths of the folds. As one moves towards skin which does not fall into apposition, the changes disappear. The main complications are bacterial and candidal secondary infections, as the moist damaged skin is a fertile breeding ground. In addition, allergic contact dermatitis may occur, once again leading to lesions outside the area of contact.

Differential Diagnosis. Psoriasis may be most prominent in the intertriginous areas; one should search the scalp, nails and other predilection sites for clues. Seborrheic dermatitis may involve the axillae or inguinal regions, but usually there are clues on the scalp. Candidiasis should be excluded. Both Darier disease and Hailey-Hailey disease may present in intertriginous areas, as can pemphigus vegetans. When the latter disorders are suspected, a biopsy is helpful.

Therapy. The most important treatment is weight loss, but this is far easier to write than to achieve. In general, drying measures suffice. One can use a zinc oxide shake lotion. After bathing or showering, a blow dryer is a helpful tool to insure dryness without irritation. If corticosteroids are employed, a lotion or milk is the best form. Combinations of topical corticosteroids and imidazoles are often employed to reduce inflammation and simultaneously treat any possible candidal infection. Powders may help to lubricate the area but should first be employed when weeping has stopped, otherwise they will lead to clumping and worsen the problem.

Allergic Contact Dermatitis

Epidemiology. In our dermatology clinics, allergic contact dermatitis accounts for 5–15% of all inflammatory skin disease. The incidence of allergic contact dermatitis in the general population has been estimated to be between 1% and 10%. This means that in some populations as many as one person in ten has a clinically relevant contact allergy. The incidence of positive patch tests is somewhat higher. In more chronic cases, there may be a mixture of chronic irritant contact dermatitis and allergic contact dermatitis. Allergic contact dermatitis is equally common in men and women, although hand dermatitis appears more common in women.

Etiology and Pathogenesis. The patient becomes sensitized against one or more chemicals with which he comes into contact. The reaction is a classic Gell and Coombs type IV delayed hypersensitivity reaction (Chap. 1). The reaction may be acute or if less severe, exposure may persist over a longer period of time, often mixed with or masked by chronic irritant contact dermatitis. A number of factors play a role in the development of a topical allergy.

Ease of Sensitization. When a large number of people are exposed to a potential allergen, either in a test situation or in real life, only a small percentage develop allergic contact dermatitis. There are exceptions to this rule with allergens such as the *Rhus* allergen and deliberate sensitizers such as diphencyprone used in immunotherapy of alopecia areata. While there must be a genetic predisposition towards allergic contact dermatitis, HLA studies have not identified a clear risk group. Atopic patients are intrinsically less able to mount a normal immune response, so that in laboratory studies they are harder to sensitize. On the other hand, they have a less-effective skin barrier and are exposed to so many potential sensitizers that they wind up with more allergic contact dermatitis. Psoriasis patients also seem relatively resistant to allergic contact dermatitis. Clearly, impaired vascular or nervous supply to the skin, immune status and other underlying metabolic disorders may all play a role in determining how easy a particular individual is to sensitize. Unfortunately, the intricacies of such mechanisms remain a mystery.

Local Factors. Damaged skin is easier to sensitize. In simple terms, it is easier for the offending potential allergens to penetrate the stratum corneum. Thus damage to the stratum corneum from acids or alkalis, fissures or erosions, maceration and preexisting dermatitis of any type all predispose the patient to allergic contact dermatitis. The type of exposure also plays a role. For example, nickel-containing metals are more likely to sensitize when present in earrings used in pierced ears than when present in a ring.

The process of contact sensitization has been studied in considerable detail. It provides a clear immunologic model and has been used in many animal systems. Initially the allergen must be taken up and presented to the immune system where a specific reaction against it develops. This arm of the reaction is the induction phase or afferent limb. The immune response, causing the allergic contact dermatitis, is known as the elicitation phase or efferent limb.

Induction Phase. The concentration of the allergen, its chemical nature, the status of skin and the length of exposure all play a role in modulating induction. The chemical structure of the allergen allows only limited conclusions about the sensitizing potential to be drawn. The *para*-substituted benzene ring compounds, such as DNCB, are the most notorious sensitizers. About 90% of people are sensitized 5–7 days after a single exposure. Picryl chloride, thioglycolates and many plant proteins, such as those from *Rhus*, teak and primula, are also strong sensitizers. In contrast, nickel and dichromate ions are weak sensitizers, but nonetheless major causes of allergic contact dermatitis because so many individuals have repeated exposure to these substances. Both nickel jewelry allergy and dichromate hand dermatitis in masons often take many years to develop.

The sensitizing molecule is usually quite small. It is often a hapten which must be bound to a skin or serum protein to form a complete antigen. The antigen is then taken up by the antigen-processing cells which in the skin are the Langerhans cells. These bone marrow-derived macrophages account for 3–5% of the epidermal cells. With their dendrites they form a network of interacting cells able to identify bacteria, other organisms or foreign antigens. The characteristic ultrastructural marker of the Langerhans cell is the Birbeck granule which apparently is part of the phagocytic process. Langerhans cells are not only present in the epidermis but also in the dermis and lymph nodes. The new antigen is bound on their cell surface in association with the type II (HLA-DR) major histocompatibility complex antigen.

The next step is presentation of the antigen to the immune system, namely the T cells. Exactly where presentation occurs is unclear; it may occur in the epidermis or in the dermis or peripheral lymph nodes as the Langerhans cells migrate centrally. The primary T cell involved is the $CD4^+$ helper cell. The Langerhans cells present the antigen to the T cell receptor. CD4 interacts with the Type II MHC in a restricted fashion. While this interaction is known as the first signal, the second signal is provided by IL-1 which is secreted not only by Langerhans cells but also by keratinocytes to stimulate the T cells. The selection of antigen-specific memory T cells takes place in the paracortical zone of the regional lymph node. Both effector and suppressor T cells may be formed, modulating the immune reaction. Sensitized cells able to identify the allergen migrate back to the skin where they serve as forward observers for a potential re-exposure. Sensitization takes 5–7 days and may then persist for many years or forever.

Elicitation Phase. When the individual is reexposed to the antigen, even very small amounts are able to trigger a delayed immune response. Usually 24–48 h are required, although sometimes only 4–8 h are needed. The allergen, the degree of sensitization and the location of the exposure all help to determine how rapidly a response is mounted. The sensitized allergen-specific helper T cells identify the allergen via their receptors and become activated secreting a whole palette of cytokines (IL-2, IL-4, IL-6, IL-8, interferons). The cytokines call in the other cells needed for the inflammatory response, producing the allergic contact dermatitis. Contact dermatitis primarily involves the TH2 group of helper T cells. B cells may also play a role in the elicitation phase. While antibodies can occasionally be identified and immune complexes found during severe allergic contact dermatitis, the exact clinical significance is unclear.

The elicitation phase is often characterized by reactions outside the initial area of contact. This phenomenon helps clinically to separate allergic contact dermatitis from irritant contact dermatitis. The secretion of cytokines and the circulation of responsive lymphocytes throughout the body help explain the phenomenon. In addition, if a sensitized patient ingests an allergen or as is often the case a cross-reacting substance, there may be a wide spread allergic reaction, often referred to as hematogenous or systemic allergic contact dermatitis.

Resistance, Tolerance and Hardening. These immunologic terms are used loosely when discussing allergic contact dermatitis. Resistance or the fortunate inability to mount a delayed hypersensitivity response requires an impaired T cell system. In atopic dermatitis, psoriasis and HIV/AIDS there is experimental evidence of resistance, but its clinical significance is unclear.

Tolerance is a different matter. In this case, the immune system is manipulated so that an individual does not develop sensitivity to a given molecule. One of the best examples of tolerance is the Sulzberger-Chase phenomenon, described by the father of investigative dermatology in the USA, Marion B. Sulzberger (SULZBERGER 1929), and a famous immunologist, Jules Chase (CHASE 1946). They found that if an allergen is administered orally first, it is often difficult later to sensitize the patient. A more modern example from photoimmunodermatology is the ability to modulate allergic contact dermatitis by prior UV irradiation which reduces the number of Langerhans cells. Inducing tolerance after a patient is sensitized is a different problem; many efforts involving *Rhus* antigens have failed.

Hardening is purely a clinical phenomenon. It probably relates to the increased thickness of the epidermis and thus provides only local protection. Some patients despite clinically documented allergic contact dermatitis and positive patch tests show clinical improvement over weeks to months despite continuing exposure to the allergen. This phenomenon is both nonspecific and often not permanent. A hardened patient may experience a dramatic worsening. In addition, the positive patch test reaction does not change.

Contact Allergens. The number of known contact allergens is very large and continually growing. In addition, over the years the potentially important allergens change. For example, sunscreens, fragrances and corticosteroids were minor problems two decades ago; today they are responsible for many reactions.

Contact allergens which are potent sensitizers tend to cause fairly acute reactions. Probably the best example in North America is rhus dermatitis. In particular, rhus dermatitis from poison ivy is almost always vesicular or bullous. The *para*-substituted benzole products, caines and neomycin, also typically elicit a severe reaction. Other allergens such as nickel, chromate and thiurams in rubber more often cause a chronic problem, as manifested by ear-ring allergy from nickel, hand dermatitis in masons from chromates and rubber glove allergy in housewives.

History. Often a careful history can provide the diagnosis. The patient describes a localized reaction and can be helped to recall exactly what has been in contact with the involved area of the skin. One should always remember to ask what medications and over-the-counter products have been applied to the area, as patients generally do not suspect a medicine or a household remedy as the cause of a rash. An allergy to a hat band or adhesive tape may be very sharply localized. A reaction to neomycin or a topical anesthetic will also be localized, but less sharply bordered and with more of a tendency to spread (Fig. 12.9). Airborne contact dermatitis or that caused by volatile agents usually involves the face, nape, arms and hands (Fig. 12.10).

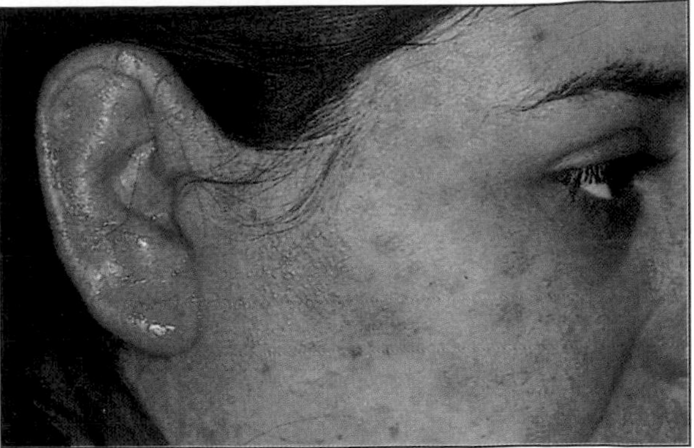

Fig. 12.9. Acute allergic contact dermatitis caused by neomycin ear drops

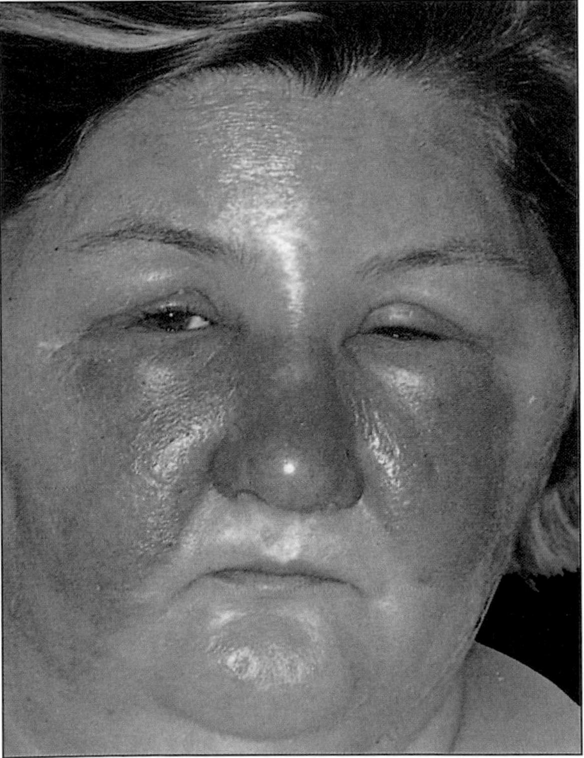

Fig. 12.10. Acute allergic contact dermatitis caused by turpentine vapors

Table 12.6. Common sources of allergens listed by body region

Region	Common allergen sources
Scalp	Cosmetics, barrettes
Forehead	Hat band, protective masks, airborne plant allergens, hair dyes
Eyelids	Cosmetics, ophthalmologic products, contact lens products, nail polish, airborne plant allergens
Ears	Hearing aids, eyeglass frames, jewelry, ear drops
Oral mucosa	Dentures, other dental materials, chewing gum, tooth paste, foods
Face	Cosmetics, hair dyes, toiletries, shampoos, sunscreens, protective masks, airborne plant allergens
Neck	Jewelry, cosmetics, clothing, hair dyes
Axilla	Deodorants and antiperspirants, other toiletries, clothing
Trunk	Clothing, metal zippers and buttons, cosmetics
Genitalia	Toiletries, condoms, spermicides, feminine hygiene products
Arms	Jewelry, cosmetics, clothing
Hands	Occupational exposure, gloves especially latex gloves, skin-protective creams, cosmetics, toiletries, jewelry
Legs	Toiletries, cosmetics, stockings, other clothes
Legs in stasis dermatitis	Topical antibiotics, other topical medications
Feet	Shoe material (chromates, rubber, glues), antifungals, dyes in socks and stockings
Perianal region	Hemorrhoid medications, disinfectants, other toiletries

Table 12.7. Common allergens in various occupations

Occupation	Allergens
Baker	Aromas and spices, lemon and almond oils, cinnamon, flour bleaches (ammonium persulphate), preservatives (benzoates), immediate-type allergy to proteins of eggs or flour
Electrician	Rubber and rubber-related products, metals, insulation material (colophony), resins (epoxy and formaldehyde)
Farmer	Pesticides, conservatives in greases, airborne plant fragments, feed additives (often photosensitizers), rubber
Gardner	Plant allergens (see text; think of airborne route), rubber, pesticides
Hairdresser	Permanent wave solutions (glycerol monothioglycollate, ammonium thioglycollate), fragrances, dyes (*para*-group, azo dyes), rubber, nickel (often present before entering profession)
Housewife	Foods, spices, rubber, soaps and cleansing supplies (fragrances, preservatives, turpentine), disinfectants, metals (chromates, nickel), cosmetics, immediate-type allergy to natural rubber latex
Health professionals	Rubber, fragrances, disinfectants (formaldehyde, glutaraldehyde, mercury salts), medications, immediate-type allergy to natural rubber latex
Mason and construction worker	Chromate and cobalt in cement, concrete hardeners, resins (epoxy and formaldehyde), insulation foam, rubber
Metal worker	Cutting oils, greases, soldering solutions, preservatives, fragrances, glues, rust preventatives, rubber, metals
Office worker	Copy paper, printer and copy inks, glues, rubber
Textile worker	Resins (formaldehyde), dyes, preservatives, stains, rubber

Table 12.6 shows common allergens or allergen sources which one should consider during evaluation of dermatitis in different body regions. When searching for a contact allergen, one must always remember that most products or workplaces contain a number of possible allergens. The suspected allergens must always be identified with patch testing.

In contrast, a chronic allergic contact dermatitis is often harder for the patient to identify. Often there is a preexisting irritant contact dermatitis. The most typical site is the back of the hands, although the face, neck, flexural aspects of the arms and scrotum are also common. Less frequent sites include the palms, soles, scalp and back. The location of the changes as well as a careful occupational and hobby history are mandatory. Table 12.7 identifies many of the risks associated with various professions and hobbies. In almost every case, one should also inquire about cleansers, protective creams and gloves. It is impossible to know every allergen in a given profession. The exposure will vary from company to company. Often a visit to the workplace by the physician will be required to piece things together. One must always remember that the vast bulk of job-related skin problems are irritant in nature, but never forget to search for the rare contact allergen and then be sure that it is relevant.

Contact Dermatitis from Plants. Another common source of allergens is plants. In North America, *Rhus* allergy is far and away the most common type of allergic contact dermatitis, recognized by every reasonably intelligent patient. It is the main cause of occupational disability for a variety of outdoor workers, especially telephone line repairmen, since the ground beneath a telephone line is heaven for a poison ivy plant. Poison oak and poison sumac have more limited geographic distributions but are equally allergenic. Patients allergic to *Rhus* react with a host of other plant substances including Japanese lacquer, true Indian laundry marking ink, mangoes, the husks of cashew nuts (not the nuts) and several others.

Florists and gardeners may develop allergies to the flowers, leaves, needles and even roots of a variety of plants. The best known allergy in Germany is to the *Primula* family, especially *Primula obconica*, usually called German primrose in other countries. The allergen is primin, a benzoquinone. While plant allergies usually involve the hands or arms, a patient sensitive to primrose may react with a diffuse facial eruption simply after being in a room with the offending plant. In such a situation, the physician may suspect a phototoxic or photoallergic reaction because of the distribution.

Another family of sensitizing plants is Compositae (or Asteraceae). The most notorious member of this family is ragweed, which is responsible for most of the late-summer/early-fall hay fever (allergic rhinitis) in the USA and is a common cause of airborne allergic contact dermatitis. The major allergens are sesquiterpene lactones. Marigold or *Calendula officinalis* is a problem in Germany, as many people use it for its curative properties; a number of first-aid ointments are sold with marigold extracts. Feverfew (a major problem introduced into India), daisies, asters and chrysanthemums also belong here. Liliaceae, including onions, garlic, hyacinths, and tulips cause problems with their bulbs. Tulip finger refers to the allergic contact dermatitis limited to the fingers that is associated with tulips. In contrast, narcissus usually causes an irritant reaction. In both cases, the finger tips are cracked and dry.

Table 12.8. Common allergens in topical medications

Category	Examples
Vehicle	Wool alcohols, cetyl alcohol
Preservative	Parabens, chloroacetamide, Euxyl K 400[a]
Active ingredients	Antibiotics, local anesthetics, antihistamines, sunscreens, corticosteroids, nonsteroidal anti-inflammatory drugs (bufexamac), older antifungals (not imidazoles)
Fragrances	Many

[a] Mix of phenoxyethanol and methyldibromoglutaronitrile

Another group of related products that cause a fair amount of allergic contact dermatitis is spices. Cinnamon, for example, is a common allergen in bakers, but must also occur in lovers of cinnamon buns. Other offenders include vanilla, chamomile, pepper, bay-leaf oil and nutmeg. Many tropical woods contain allergens; most often exposure is in the form of sawdust. Finally, plants provide a number of fragrances which also can sensitize.

Contact Dermatitis from Topical Medications. A crucial issue is the problem of a patient developing allergic contact dermatitis from a prescribed or over-the-counter topical product. Typically the underlying skin disorder is chronic, such as atopic dermatitis or a leg ulcer, and the patient has tried many different products and presents simply because of a worsening condition. Antibiotic ear drops are a common offender. Rarely are patients suspicious of a medication. Table 12.8 indicates some of the common problems.

Contact Dermatitis from Clothing. Formaldehyde is often found in wash-and-wear clothing; how often it causes a clinically significant reaction is unclear. Dark clothes, stockings and leather may be dyed with azoic or anthraquinone dyes while leather and green fabric may contain chromates (Fig. 12.11). Metal buttons, zippers and snap fasteners usually contain nickel, or perhaps cobalt. Sensitization from the exposed metal buttons in blue jeans is common and usually occurs in adolescents (Fig. 12.12). Rubber or elastic pieces may contain natural rubber latex, antioxidants, accelerators or dyes (Fig. 12.13).

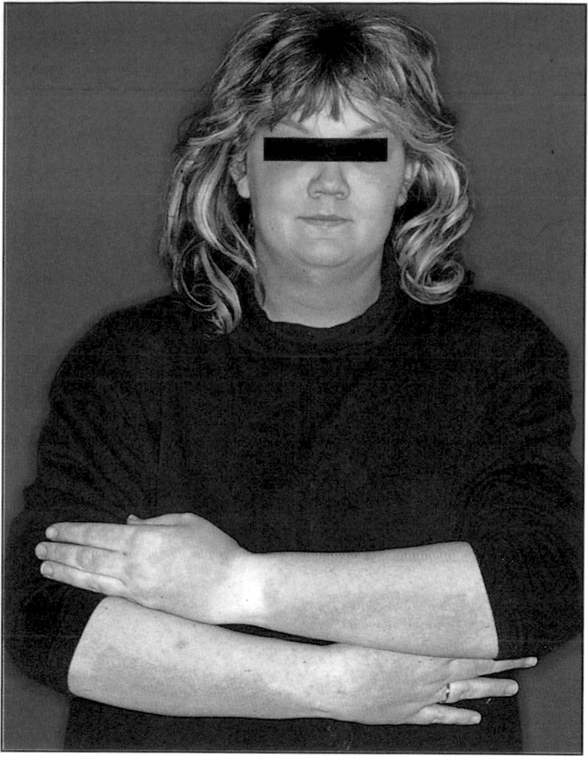

Fig. 12.11. Acute allergic contact dermatitis caused by black clothing dye. The area covered by wrist watch is spared

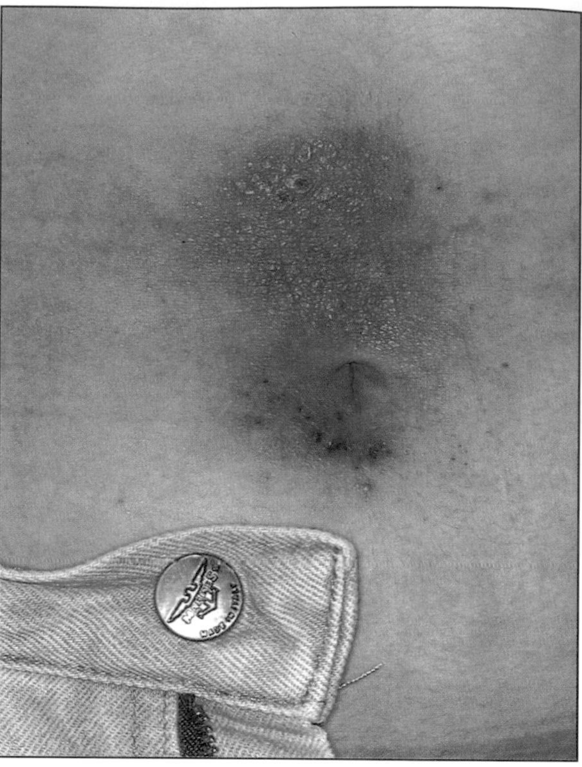

Fig. 12.12. Acute allergic contact dermatitis caused by nickel in button

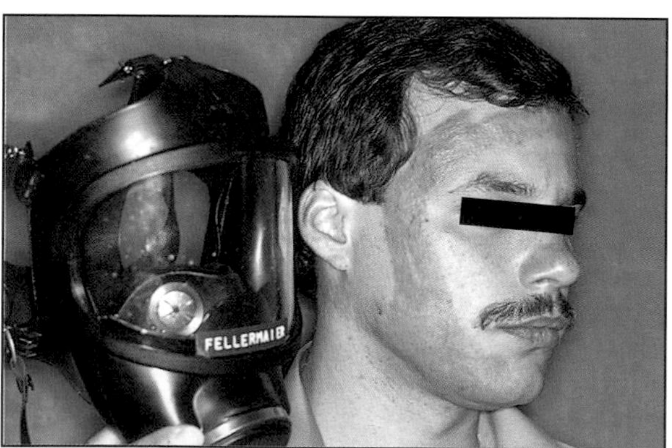

Fig. 12.13. Acute allergic contact dermatitis caused by rubber component in gas mask

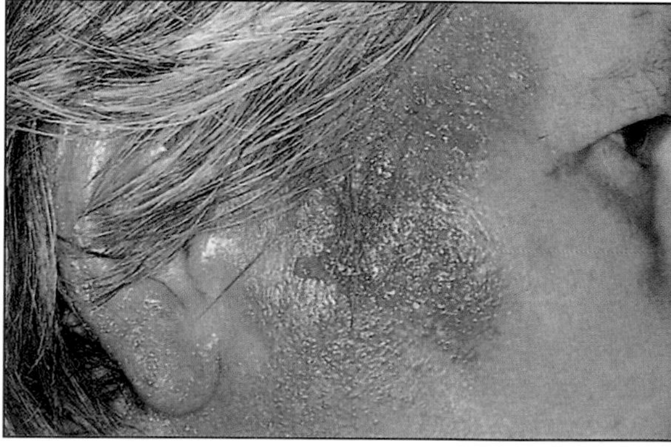

Fig. 12.14. Acute allergic contact dermatitis caused by hair dye

Contact Dermatitis from Jewelry. Nickel is the most common cause; in most cases, the individual already knows that they cannot wear costume jewelry. Some patients are so sensitive that they react with the small amounts of nickel found in gold or silver alloys. Others may react to cobalt or palladium. While reactions to gold salts are not rare, the metal itself is most infrequently an allergen.

Contact Dermatitis from Cosmetics. The most common offenders are fragrances and preservatives. The problems mentioned under medications in Table 12.8 also apply. In addition, one should consider formaldehyde and resins in nail polish and artificial nails, thioglycolates in permanent wave products and a wide variety of coloring agents (Fig. 12.14). In general, cosmetics are quite safe with a very low incidence of sensitization per use, but because they are so widely used on sensitive skin, an occasional case of allergic contact dermatitis is seen.

Clinical Findings. The clinical features of allergic contact dermatitis are as variable as the number of allergens, the sites to which they can be applied and the time-course of the reaction. In general, one should think of allergic contact dermatitis when a reaction is localized, has sharp or geometric borders and is not easily explained by any other form of dermatitis. In addition, the picture of acute allergic contact dermatitis is characterized by erythema, swelling and blisters while the more chronic reaction features epidermal reactive changes including lichenification, thick scale and fissuring. A wide range of pictures may evolve representing intermediates between these two poles. Each will be considered separately, but remember that overlaps are the rule.

Acute Allergic Contact Dermatitis

Clinical Findings. Acute allergic contact dermatitis develops after 24–48 h. The initial findings are limited to the area of contact, but dissemination may occur. Thus the early lesions are often asymmetric. Severe reactions often have swelling and blistering (Fig. 12.15). Just as with irritant contact dermatitis, there is a reasonably predictable series of events. The major clinical differences between irritant and allergic contact dermatitis are the more rapid onset of irritant contact dermatitis and the tendency of allergic contact dermatitis to disseminate. The widespread reaction is usually symmetric even though the primary reaction is not. In addition, a toxic reaction usually has sharper borders than an allergic one with a more uniform erythema.

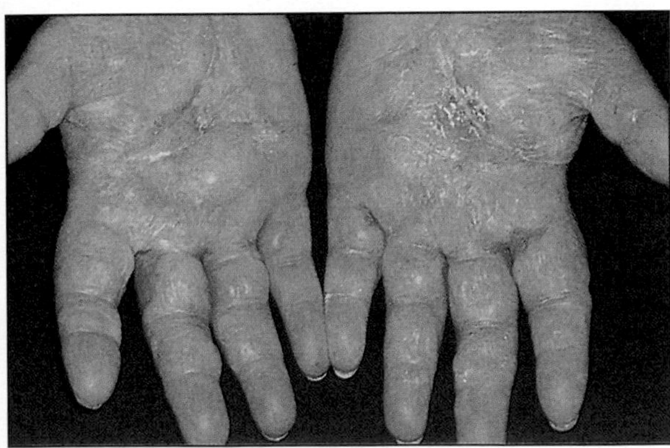

Fig. 12.15. Bullous acute allergic contact dermatitis caused by epoxy resin

Histopathology. The microscopic picture reveals a lymphocytic perivascular infiltrate, high dermal edema and spongiosis and exocytosis in the epidermis. As intuitively expected, the process here appears to be going from the dermal vessels to the epidermis, while in a toxic reaction the first step is epidermal damage. Nonetheless, the two pictures can overlap. Blisters arise as spongiotic vesicles fuse, and they may evolve into erosions and crusts.

Differential Diagnosis. The main differential diagnostic points are acute irritant contact dermatitis and those disorders listed under its differential diagnosis, such as erysipelas, acute systemic lupus erythematosus and dermatomyositis. When the eyelids are swollen, angioedema, early zoster and even exaggerated heliotrope eyelids of dermatomyositis may be considered.

Chronic Allergic Contact Dermatitis

Clinical Findings. Chronic allergic contact dermatitis can evolve from acute allergic contact dermatitis, creep up subtly with no acute phase or appear on top of chronic irritant contact dermatitis (Figs. 12.16, 12.17). Typical features include symmetric pattern, less sharp borders and distant spread. The distant lesions are typically papulovesicular and tend to lead both patient and doctor away from the correct diagnosis. As the name suggests, the problem is chronic with little tendency towards remission as the allergen is not identified and contact recurs. In addition, some allergens such as nickel, formaldehyde, fragrances and preservatives are so widespread that it is very difficult for a patient to truly avoid them, making the disease even more chronic.

The main feature of chronic allergic contact dermatitis is epidermal reaction. This layer is usually thickened and has increased scale (Fig. 12.18). Sometimes the scales are compact, producing a callus, and in other cases, they are mixed with secretions, yielding a crust. In contrast to acute allergic contact dermatitis, which tends to progress through stages, chronic allergic contact dermatitis shows a variety of lesions at the same time. Several relatively distinct clinical patterns are occasionally

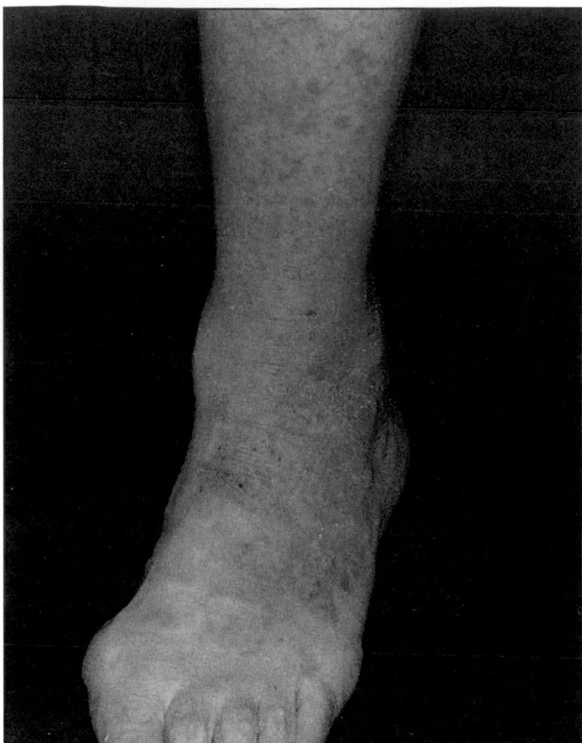

Fig. 12.16. Chronic allergic contact dermatitis caused by balsam of Peru

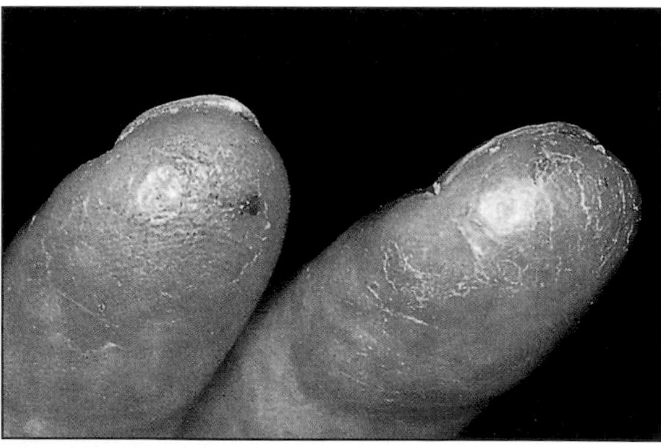

Fig. 12.17. Chronic allergic contact dermatitis in a dentist caused by local anesthetics

subdivided out of this complex picture. They include:

Lichenified Dermatitis. Sometimes intense pruritus leads to so much rubbing that the epidermis becomes thickened but smooth. This produces a superficial resemblance to lichen planus in that small smooth grouped papules can develop. In lichen planus, despite the intense pruritus, excoriations are almost never seen, while they are common here. Lichenification is also seen with lichen simplex chronicus and atopic dermatitis.

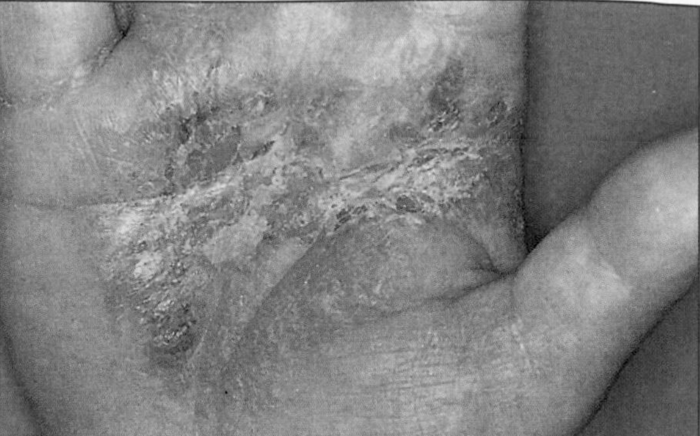

Fig. 12.18. Chronic allergic contact dermatitis with dyshidrotic features in a tailor caused by nickel in scissors

Dyshidrotic Dermatitis. This disorder is occasionally associated with allergic contact dermatitis, but most often it is idiopathic. It is discussed in detail below.

Histopathology. The epidermis shows some reactive changes (acanthosis, hyperkeratosis, parakeratosis). In the dermis there is a more intense, usually mixed inflammatory infiltrate. Spongiosis and exocytosis are less common. Sometimes the infiltrate is band-like or lichenoid, but this does not always correlate with the clinical picture of lichenification.

Differential Diagnosis. The differential diagnosis of chronic allergic contact dermatitis is so long that we have divided it into body regions.

Scalp. Psoriasis, atopic dermatitis, seborrheic dermatitis

External ear. Psoriasis, seborrheic dermatitis, chronic irritation (swimmer's ear from moisture)

Eyelid. Atopic dermatitis. If pustular or follicular, rosacea and *Demodex* infestations

Lips. The main consideration is lick cheilitis or lip chewing, especially in atopic dermatitis patients.

Hands. The palms are relatively protected by the thicker stratum corneum, so that the back of the hands are more prominently involved. Often the dominant hand is more severely involved. One must exclude chronic irritant contact dermatitis (far more common), atopic dermatitis, psoriasis and tinea manuum.

Fingertips. Atopic dermatitis and limited dyshidrotic dermatitis.

Nipples. Atopic dermatitis, scabies (usually smaller lesions and intense pruritus), if unilateral, Paget disease.

Leg. The most common cause is stasis dermatitis secondary to chronic venous insufficiency, but because so many medications are used, a secondary allergic contact dermatitis is not uncommon. Often the patient will have multiple positive patch tests and the challenge is to decide which are clinically important. Asteatotic dermatitis is also more common on the legs in the elderly. Sometimes the lesions will be psoriasiform; in this setting psoriasis should be excluded. While bacteria may be cultured from the lesions, their importance is unclear, as discussed under nummular dermatitis. When the dermatitis arises around a leg ulcer, the considerations are irritation from the wound secretions and contact dermatitis from a medication. In the case of a long-standing ulcer, especially with elevated margins, the rare presence of a squamous cell carcinoma or basal cell carcinoma should be excluded with a biopsy.

Genitalia. Chronic allergic contact dermatitis is rare on the genitalia, presumably because the acute reaction is so dramatic it is noticed. Atopic dermatitis and intertrigo are most common. One should exclude candidiasis. Very rarely, acquired zinc deficiency or glucagonoma syndrome may present with genital dermatitis.

Perianal Region (Chap. 67). Perianal dermatitis is often associated with psoriasis, seborrheic dermatitis or atopic dermatitis. Intertrigo, often associated with increased weight, decreased hygiene and anal discharge, is also common. While *Candida albicans* is often cultured, its role as a pathogen is unclear.

Mucosal Surfaces. Here swelling and erythema dominate, whether the eyelids, mouth or genitalia are involved. Allergic contact dermatitis is uncommon because of the relative resistance of the mucosal surfaces to sensitization. Table 12.9 lists the common allergens at various mucosal sites.

Table 12.9. Causes of mucosal type IV allergic reactions

Site	Allergens
Mouth	Toothpaste, mouthwash, dentures, denture adhesives, medications (rare, and then those designed to be sucked), chewing gum
Lips	Lipsticks, toothpastes, sunscreens, other lip balms
Conjunctiva	Eye drops, contact lens cleaners, eye cosmetics, sprays
Genitalia	Feminine hygiene products, spermicides, condoms, lubricants, disinfectants, topical medications

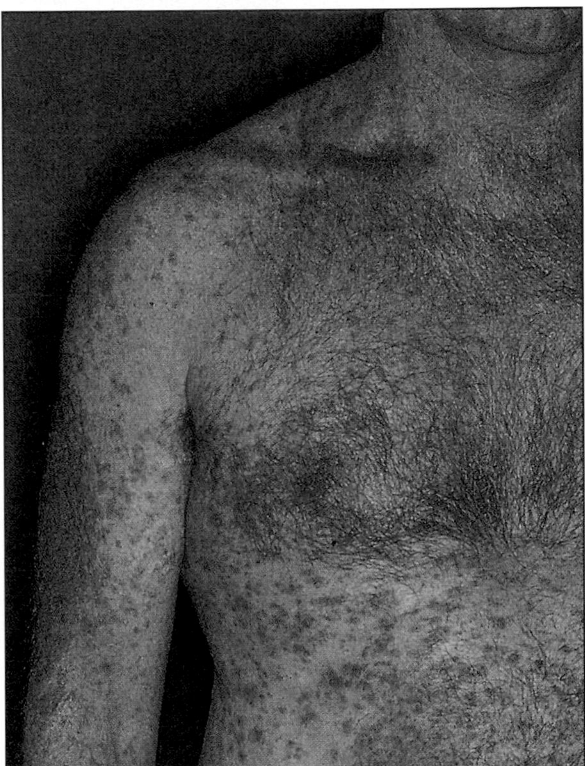

Fig. 12.19. Hematogenous allergic contact dermatitis

Hematogenous Allergic Contact Dermatitis

Once an individual has become sensitized to an allergen, then ingestion may also cause an allergic reaction. Several different clinical patterns can occur. The lesions are erythematous papules that are symmetrically distributed, occasionally follicular or vesicular, and evolve into crusted patches or plaques (Fig. 12.19). Occasionally dyshidrotic dermatitis may appear. In extreme cases, wide areas of skin can be involved approaching erythroderma. The baboon syndrome (Chap. 10) may be an extreme type of drug-related hematogenous allergic contact dermatitis. While this is similar to the distant spread seen in chronic allergic contact dermatitis, a focal site where the disease is concentrated is not found. Sometimes the site of the original allergic contact dermatitis or of a patch test may flare with systemic administration. Patients can become quite ill with elevated erythrocyte sedimentation rate, fever, lymphadenopathy, diarrhea and other problems.

A common scenario is sensitization to a topical agent when the same medication is also used systemically. For example, penicillin is such a good topical sensitizer that it should not be used topically, depriving many patients of a good medication. Thus most topical medications are ones that are rarely needed systemically. An exception is gentamicin, which we tend to avoid. Complicating the issue is the presence of cross-reactions, so that the patient is sensitized externally to one product and then receives a related product internally. An example which is discussed later is the cross-reaction between *p*-phenylenediamine and sulfonamides. Another problem group is the topical antihistamines. Diphenhydramine almost never causes allergies when administered systemically but is a potent topical sensitizer. Because it has mild anesthetic properties when used topically, diphenhydramine was a mainstay of Caldryl lotion (calamine lotion and diphenhydramine) as well as other topical poison ivy and sunburn medications. Patients who developed allergic contact dermatitis to the topical agent were at risk of having a severe reaction to the systemic agent received during subsequent medical care.

Diagnostic Criteria

Patch Testing. While a careful history, physical examination and a knowledge of likely allergens can lead to a guess about the etiology of a dermatitis, patch testing is required to confirm the diagnosis. The technique was developed by Jadassohn and Bloch (1895). Patch testing, or epicutaneous testing as it is called in Germany, is a provocation test. A known amount of allergen is applied to a small area of skin via a patch, which may be a piece of filter patch, an aluminum well or an impregnated gel. An allergic individual will react to the material, but a nonallergic person will not. The latter individual may very rarely develop an allergy via the testing. Thus we recommend patch testing only if there is clinical suspicion of contact allergy or if exclusion of contact sensitization is an essential part of the diagnosis of other dermatologic disorders. One should also avoid testing with materials with a high risk of sensitization.

Table 12.10. German standard patch test series

Material	Concentration (%)	Vehicle
Potassium dichromate	0.5	P
p-Phenylenediamine (free base)	1.0	P
Thiuram mix[a]	1.0	P
Neomycin	20.0	P
Cobalt chloride	1.0	P
Benzocaine	5.0	P
Nickel sulfate	5.0	P
Colophony	20	P
Isopropyl-*N*-phenyl-*p*-phenylene diamine	0.1	P
Wool wax alcohols	30	P
Mercapto mix[b]	2.0	P
Epoxy resin	1.0	P
Balsam of Peru	25.0	P
p-Tertiary butyl phenol formaldehyde resin	1.0	P
Formaldehyde	1.0	A
Fragrance mix[c]	8.0	P
Euxyl K 400[d]	1.0	P
Ammoniated mercury	1.0	P
Turpentine	10.0	P
Chloromethylisothiazolone	0.01	A
Paraben mix[e]	16.0	P
Cetostearyl alcohol	20.0	P
Thimerosal	0.05	P
Zinc diethyledithiocarbamate	1.0	P
Propolis	10.0	P
Bufexamac	5.0	P
Petrolatum	100.0	P

A, aqueous; P, petrolatum

[a] Thiuram mix 1.0%: tetraethylthiuram disulfide 0.25%, tetramethylthiuram disulfide 0.25%, tetraethylthiuram monosulfide 0.25%, dipentamethylene thiuram disulfide 0.25%

[b] Mercapto mix 2.0%: *n*-cyclohexyl benzothiazyl sulfenamide 0.5%, mercaptobenzothiazole 0.5%, dibenzothiazyl disulfide 0.5%, morpholinylmercaptobenzothiazole 0.5%

[c] Fragrance mix 8.0%: Cinnamic alcohol 1.0%, cinnamic aldehyde 1.0%, eugenol 1.0%, amyl cinnamic aldehyde 1.0%, hydroxycitronellel 1.0%, geraniol 1.0%, isoeugenol 1.0%, oak moss 1.0%

[d] Euxyl K 400 contains phenoxyethanol and methyldibromoglutaronitrile

[e] Paraben mix 12.0%: butyl-, ethyl-, methyl-, propyl-paraben, each 3.0%

Requirements for Testing. Patch testing must be carried out on normal skin. Ideally we wait at least 3 weeks after clearing of the skin lesions. Usually the back is used, but when a limited number of agents are tested, the upper, inner aspect of the arm can be used. The patient's dermatitis must be under control; if not, nonspecific reactions may occur at multiple test sites, known as the angry back syndrome. Severe stasis dermatitis on the legs is sufficient to trigger false-positive reactions; the back itself must not be involved. Conversely, UV radiation, topical or systemic corticosteroids and other antiinflammatory drugs may produce false-negative reactions.

Test Materials. Table 12.10 shows the materials tested for in the standard set used in Germany. For contrast, Table 12.11 compares this series to the standard test series used in Europe and the USA. Choosing what materials should be in a test series is a matter of checks and balances. Considering any one chemical, one must determine the concentration and vehicle that are most likely to a give an allergic reaction in a sensitive individual but unlikely to cause a toxic reaction in a nonsensitive person. Some substances such as neomycin must be tested in high concentrations, even though they are not used in such amounts in practice. Other substances are tested at far lower concentrations

Table 12.11. Comparison of the various standard patch test series

Material	German	European	USA	Major sources
Potassium dichromate	✓	✓	✓	Cement, many others
p-Phenylenediamine (free base)	✓	✓	✓	Dyes
Thiuram mix	✓	✓	✓	Rubber products
Neomycin	✓	✓	✓	Topical medications
Cobalt chloride	✓	✓		Metals
Benzocaine	✓	✓	✓	Local anesthetics
Nickel sulfate	✓	✓	✓	Metals, many others
Colophony	✓	✓	✓	Adhesives, waxes
n-Isopropyl-*n*-phenyl-*p*-phenylenediamine	✓	✓		Dyes
Wool wax alcohols	✓	✓	✓	Creams, ointments
Mercapto mix	✓	✓	✓	Rubber products
Epoxy resin	✓	✓	✓	Plastics, glues
Balsam of Peru	✓	✓	✓	Fragrances, flavorings
p-Tertiary butyl phenol formaldehyde, resin	✓	✓	✓	Glues
Formaldehyde	✓	✓	✓	Many sources
Fragrance mix	✓	✓		Fragrances
Euxyl K 400	✓			Preservative
Ammoniated mercury	✓			Indicator for inorganic mercury (amalgam)
Turpentine	✓			Paints
Chloromethylisothiazolone	✓	✓		Preservative
Paraben mix	✓	✓		Preservative
Cetostearyl alcohol	✓			Vehicle
Thimerosal	✓			Preservative
Zinc diethyledithiocarbamate	✓			Preservative
Propolis	✓			Vehicle
Bufexamac	✓			Topical antiinflammatory agent
Mercaptobenzothiazole		✓	✓	Rubber products
Imidazolidinyl urea (Germall 115)			✓	Preservative
Cinnamic aldehyde			✓	Fragrances, flavorings
Carba mix			✓	Rubber products
Ethylenediamine hydrochloride			✓	Stabilizer, antihistamine
Quaternium-15		✓	✓	Disinfectant
Black rubber mix 0.6%			✓	Rubber products
Clioquinol		✓		Topical antibacterial
Primin		✓		Plants
Petrolatum	✓			Control vehicle

than are commonly encounter. With nickel and potassium dichromate, the test concentration is very close to that used to produce an irritant reaction, so interpretation is difficult. Primarily we use standard patch test substances that are commercially available. Only if we cannot obtain a diagnosis using standard materials will we perform additional tests with suspicious products or components if available from the manufacturer. A patch test reaction to a nonstandardized material can only be considered as a true allergic reaction if ten healthy volunteers do not respond to the substance. If volunteer testing is considered unacceptable for whatever reason, then testing with nonstandardized materials should not be carried out. Only experienced clinicians should attempt to test nonstandardized materials.

The next question is the composition of the test panels. In the screening panel, the desire is to identify as many cases of clinically relevant allergic contact dermatitis without spending a lot of time and money. Most clinicians use a screening panel containing between 20 to 40 ingredients. The current recommended North America panel is twice as long as the FDA-approved panel. It includes sunscreens and topical corticosteroids, as well as other refinements. The FDA is beginning to realize that patch test materials are not medications and is relaxing its grip on their control, so patch testing should become easier for USA dermatologists.

To supplement the screening panel, a wide range of specialized test series are available. They are listed in Table 12.12. Some are obvious. For example, if a hairdresser comes to the office with a hand dermatitis, the hairdresser panel and the standard panel should be done, or if a patient with a leg ulcer secondary to chronic venous insufficiency reports pruritus and erythema at the periphery, the answer could be a medication, vehicle, fragrance or perhaps something else. Those individuals using large standard series will have less occasion to employ special panels.

Table 12.12. Available specialized patch test trays

Antioxidants/stabilizers	Medications
Fragrances	Antibiotics
Hairdressing products	Antimicrobials
Rubber-related chemicals	Corticosteroids
Preservatives	Miscellaneous
Cosmetics/household products	Ocular preparations
	Local anesthetics
Paints, plastics and glues	Sunscreens
Metal industry products, technical oils	Vehicles and emulsifiers
	Dental products
Plants	Amalgam, other fillings
Photography chemicals	Acrylates, related materials
Leather, textile dyes	
Disinfectants	
Photoallergens (for photopatch testing)	

Mechanics of Testing (Fig. 12.20). The test material is typically diluted in petrolatum or water. It is applied either to a piece of filter paper attached to an aluminum-backed paper (Al-test) or put into a small aluminum well attached to adhesive tape (Finn chamber). In the later case, aqueous solutions are placed on a filter paper that fits the well. Usually vertical rows of five to ten patches are applied. One can easily test numerous materials simultaneously. The trick is to carefully mark and record the materials so that the test results can be accurately interpreted. The patches are removed after 48 h. The different rows should be marked with a skin marker or fluorescent pen which is then reidentified under Wood's light, so that reexamination is accurate. The test sites are read after a 15–30 min and again at either 72 or 96 h. The second reading is mandatory, as delayed reactions are not unusual. The patient should also be told to return to the office if an even more delayed reaction arises, as may be the case with neomycin or *p*-phenylenediamine. Sometimes reactions first appear after 5–7 days.

Reading the Test. The standard scheme for reading patch tests is:

- – = No reaction
- ? = Doubtful reaction, only faint erythema
- +1 = Weak positive reaction with erythema, infiltration, possible papules
- +2 = Strong positive reaction with erythema, infiltration, papules, vesicles
- +3 = Extreme positive reaction with marked erythema, infiltration, confluent papules and vesicles
- IR = Irritant reaction

An allergic reaction extends beyond the borders of the patch and is irregular. An irritant reaction is confined to the shape of the patch. Another valuable clue is the course of the reaction after the patch is removed. A decrescendo reaction in which the inflammation decreases after 48 h, is typical for a toxic reaction, while a crescendo reaction with

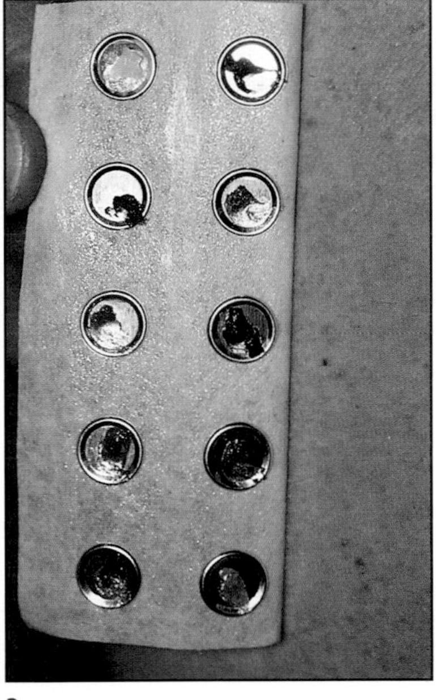
a

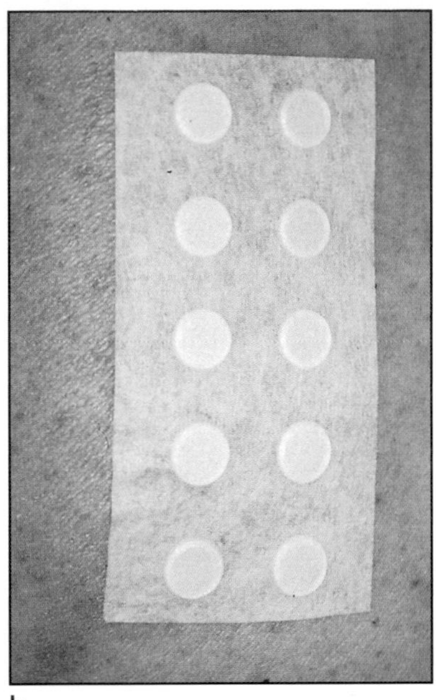
b

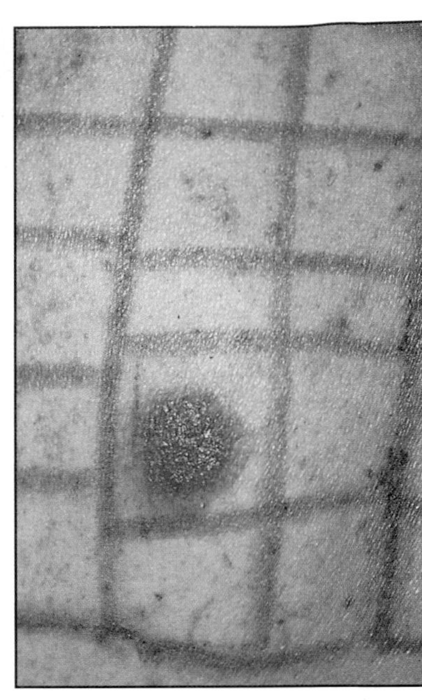
c

Fig. 12.20 a–c. Patch testing. **a** The test materials have been placed in Al-test wells. **b** The patch tests are firmly applied to the patient's back. **c** A positive patch test reaction is shown

more inflammation at 96 h indicates an allergic process. But it is far easier to distinguish irritant from allergic than it is to unequivocally interpret such patch tests. Considerable clinical expedience is required.

A positive reaction is present when at least a "+" reaction is present. If a "+" is present and the material is clinically relevant, the test can be repeated after several weeks. An old wisdom is that the interesting part of patch testing starts when the last patch has been read. False-positive reactions may occur because of the chosen concentration and vehicle. Such false-positive tests are frequently seen with fragrance mix, wool wax, cocamidopropyl betaine, metal salts and several other commercially available test substance. In addition, many patients have allergies that are not clinically relevant. The real challenge is to identify important relevant reactions. When one is evaluating an occupational problem, this becomes more difficult. The patient is convinced that any reaction means a problem and the insurance company and workman's compensation reviewers are skeptical of all results.

Interpreting the Results. In the most recent results from the North American Contact Dermatitis Group, 49 allergens were tested in over 3000 patients. Two-thirds of the patients had at least one positive allergic reaction and 57% had a reaction which was felt to be clinically relevant. About half the patients were identified with the standard 20-allergen kit and the rest were only identified because of the expanded array of test substances. This positivity rate is far higher than would be seen in daily practice, reflecting the specialized interests of the group members and referral patterns.

Table 12.13 shows the rate of sensitization to some common allergens in the USA and Germany. Several things jump out. One is the absence of lanolin. It has been argued that lanolin and wool wax alcohols are very weak sensitizers and that most reactions are part of the angry back syndrome. No one has succeeded in sensitizing animals or humans to lanolin under experimental conditions. Another is the presence of bacitracin and neomycin. These two rarely needed topical antibiotics are common allergens, reflecting poor prescribing practice by physicians. While sunscreens and corticosteroids are becoming more common allergens, they still have not caught up with the older sensitizers.

Monovalent Contact Allergy. When a patient reacts to a single substance, the question is: does it fit or not? A nurse with hand dermatitis reacting to rubber chemicals fits; the same person reacting to potassium dichromate is harder to explain. Some substances such as the chromates are so ubiquitous that they are hard to avoid; for example they may

Table 12.13. Sensitization rates (percent) to common contact allergens in USA and Germany

Allergen	USA (1994–1996)	Germany (1990–1995)
Nickel sulfate	14.3	15.7
Fragrance mix	NT	10.2
Neomycin	11.6	2.6
Balsam of Peru	10.4	6.5
Quaternium-15	9.2	NT
Formaldehyde	9.2	2.1
Thiuram mix	6.8	2.8
p-Phenylenediamine	6.8	5.0
Carba mix	5.7	NT
Thimerosal	NT	5.7
Cobalt chloride	NT	4.7
Wool wax alcohol	3.3	2.5
Ethylenediamine	2.9	NT
p-tert-butylphenol formaldehyde resin	2.7	0.9
Benzocaine	2.6	1.7
Colophony	2.6	3.4
Cinnamic aldehyde	2.4	NT
Potassium dichromate	2.0	4.6

NT, not tested with standard series

occur in cement, cement hardeners, impregnating materials, dyes, color film developers, leathers and tanning materials. Formaldehyde and nickel are other examples of widespread allergens. On the other hand, neomycin is easy to avoid by simply reading the label of all tubes of topical medicines.

Oligovalent Contact Allergy. When a patient reacts to several substances, there may be a connection. Sometimes the substances fit together chemically (group allergy) or arise from the same exposure (coupled allergy). In other instances, there is no connection and each must be interpreted separately.

Polyvalent Contact Allergy. When someone reacts to more than five substances, either they are very unlucky, or they have the angry back syndrome. Here patients with an existing dermatitis react in a nonspecific manner to many patches. Thus when multiple patches are positive, one should wait 3–4 weeks and then retest no more than 4–6 those substances which provoked a reaction at a time.

Group Allergy. Sometimes a patient will react to a series of chemically related compounds, after being exposed in nature to only one of them. A typical example is allergy to the *para*-amino compounds. A long list of substances have a benzene ring and *para*-substitution with NO_2, Cl, NH_2, OH and other molecules. A typical example is *p*-phenylenediamine as shown below:

Cross-reactions occur between these aniline dyes, sulfonamides, benzocaines and quinones. Other group allergies include the antibiotics neomycin, gentamicin, kanamycin, framycetin and paromomycin; phenothiazines; and triphenylmethane dyes such as gentian violet and brilliant green. Sometimes a substance may be metabolized in the body so that the altered structure may show an unexpected cross allergy.

Coupled Allergy. Here the materials are not chemically related but occur in the same setting. One example would be an allergy to nickel and rubber accelerators in a woman with a garter belt dermatitis or to chromate and cobalt in a cement worker with hand dermatitis.

Secondary Allergy. In this instance a patient might have a chromate-induced hand dermatitis which was treated with a corticosteroid-containing ointment. The allergy to the corticosteroid is truly secondary, as it would not have been employed were it not for the primary chromate problem.

Patient Counseling. The meaning of each positive patch test must be discussed with the patient. Printed material is no substitute for careful patient counseling. In the interests of time, most practitioners have prepared instruction sheets dealing with each allergen, pointing out where it is found, how it can be avoided and what are suitable substitutes. In some instances, the manufacturers of patch testing material provide such information in a form so that it can be inserted into an allergy pass which we give to all of our patients.

Additional Procedures. If patch testing is negative but a strong clinical suspicion exists, the suspicious substances should be retested. Similarly, borderline or clinically irrelevant positive tests can be repeated. False-positive reactions may result if patches are left on too long or are not properly applied, or if the test substance is present in the wrong concentration as a result of evaporation.

Use tests can also be employed, although they do not help to exclude an irritant reaction in most cases. Here the patient uses the suspected product ideally on just one side of the body and a neutral material such as petrolatum on the other side. After

2–3 weeks the sides are compared. If the usual site of use is quite resistant, such as the palms, the material can be tested on the antecubital fossa. Repeated open testing (ROAT) is also recommended when investigating the patient's tolerance of substances which have not been used. For example, even if a patient is sensitized to some fragrances, she may tolerate others.

Oral challenge tests are possible but best left in the hands of the experts. For example, a patient with hematogenous contact dermatitis and a positive nickel patch test, could be cautiously challenged with oral nickel to see if a reaction is elicited. Because of the risk of severe reactions, including anaphylaxis, this should be done in an inpatient or day-clinic setting.

In vitro testing of allergic contact dermatitis is possible in experimental settings but is not practical. In the lymphocyte transformation test, the suspected material is mixed with a culture of the patient's lymphocytes and DNA synthesis measured. In another test, the ability of the test chemical to inhibit the spontaneous migration of macrophages is measured.

Therapy

The treatment of acute and chronic allergic contact dermatitis and irritant contact dermatitis is a challenging problem. We have chosen to discuss it at length in one place, since there are few differences in the treatment of the acute and chronic phases of these intellectually quite different but clinically quite comparable disorders. In addition, the principles mentioned here are applicable to the treatment of most other forms of dermatitis.

Indifferent Therapy

Topical therapy requires a great deal of experience because it is crucial to adjust the vehicle to the stage of the disease. An experienced dermatologist can probably achieve more with carefully selected vehicles than a medical student with the most potent topical corticosteroid. For example, if one prescribes a solution for dry, cracking skin or an ointment for weeping lesions, then the active ingredient does not matter; the treatment will fail.

Indifferent therapy is a fancy way of saying: choose the right vehicle. One must consider the stage of the dermatitis, the region involved and the patient's skin type. In addition, one must try to avoid sensitizers and especially agents to which the patient is known to be sensitive. Below are some general suggestions for each stage of acute irritant contact dermatitis or allergic contact dermatitis.

Stage

Stadium Erythematosum et Oedematosum. This stage is often self-limited. Creams, lotions and shake lotions work best; ointments and pastes should be avoided.

Stadium Vesiculosum et Bullosum. Small vesicular lesions can still be treated with a shake lotion or lotion. When larger blisters are present, wet compresses are effective for cooling and debridement. They can then be followed by a cream or hydrophilic ointment. Widespread vesicles and blisters are best treated by baths.

Stadium Madidans et Crustosum. Once again wet compresses or baths can be used. They should not be used more than 2–3 days because they then become too drying. Following treatment, a hydrophilic cream is most appropriate.

Stadium Squamosum. In this late stage, a lipophilic cream or ointment is the best choice. Hydrophilic creams and lotions are too drying and disappear rapidly. If the skin is lichenified or hyperkeratotic, the ointment can be applied under occlusion using a household plastic wrap (such as Saran Wrap) to occlude the lesion. Occlusive corticosteroid-impregnated tapes are also available, but do not work as well as self-made occlusive dressings.

Localization

Intertriginous Regions. Occlusive materials and powders should be avoided. Lotions, creams and aqueous solutions are helpful. Powders are often prescribed but they tend to clump and make a mess. If no weeping is present, powders may lubricate the touching skin surfaces and thus help.

Palms. When the palms are quite hyperkeratotic, an ointment or paste should be used. Often mechanical debridement with a pumice stone or masonry-type sandpaper can be accomplished after soaking and prior to applying the medication. Localized hyperkeratotic areas can also be trimmed with a specialized blade. Adding salicylic acid (3–10%) to ointments may increase the keratolytic effect.

Scalp. Whatever one applies to the scalp must be easy to wash out. Thus hydrophilic creams and lotions are recommended. Solutions are easier to apply, but often too drying and irritating, especially if they contain alcohol. Some manufacturers produce ointments that have been chemically manipulated so they are easier to wash off.

Scrotum. The scrotum and eye lid are the thinnest skin on the body. The scrotum is easily dried out and shows maximum absorption. For example, 40 times as much hydrocortisone is absorbed on the scrotum as on the forearm. In addition, in the genital area, ointments are occlusive and poorly tolerated. Thus, although there is no ideal recommendation, a cream or cream-lotion is probably best. We often employ a zinc oil mixture. Shake lotions and tinctures are so irritating that the patient will not use them.

Skin Type

Patients with dry skin obviously need greasier treatment for any given stage than those with oily skin. Similarly, oily regions such as the forehead tolerate a much more drying approach than do intrinsically dry regions such as the shin.

Topical Therapy

The mainstay of topical dermatitis therapy is corticosteroids, but there are many tricks to using them and the search for alternatives continues. In the German-speaking countries of Europe many patients simply decline corticosteroids, so clinicians are being forced to find old and new substitutes.

Corticosteroids (Chap. 69). Corticosteroids are available in a wide range of strengths and in every conceivable vehicle. It is a rare day when one cannot find a corticosteroid suitable for a given condition. As already emphasized, the first step is to pick an appropriate vehicle. The next is to choose the correct strength. In general, it is simplest to use high potency corticosteroids initially and rapidly switch to less potent products as the disease improves. Finally, what is potent for the palm is too potent for the scrotum.

Usually once-daily or at maximum twice-daily therapy is sufficient for corticosteroids; they form a depot in the stratum corneum and are released from there. A well-known phenomenon is tachyphylaxis. If an individual uses the same corticosteroid for a long period of time, it looses effectiveness, so it makes sense to alternate products. In hyperkeratotic areas, corticosteroids can be used under occlusion, applied via an impregnated tape or even injected into stubborn plaques. Usually we inject 2–3 mg/ml triamcinolone acetonide into the dermis. Injecting into the subcutaneous fat simply increases systemic uptake and causes fat atrophy. When large areas, damaged skin or children are treated with higher potency topical corticosteroids, one must also remember that systemic absorption is occurring which can become clinically significant.

Alternatives to Corticosteroids. Both good medical practice and many patients' irrational fear of corticosteroids have pushed dermatologists into seeking steroid-sparing or alternative therapies for inflammatory dermatoses. Probably the best strategy is to use high-potency steroids and rapidly switch to either very low-potency agents or alternative agents. With this end in mind, many German pharmaceutical companies sell the vehicles in which their corticosteroids are mixed as a maintenance therapy. The active ingredient and vehicle can be alternated.

Nonsteroidal antiinflammatory drugs, primarily bufexamac, are used topically in Germany. They achieve at best the potency of 1% hydrocortisone and have a considerable risk of allergic contact sensitization. They are most popular among pediatricians. We do not employ them. In addition, some natural products, particularly those derived from the licorice plant, are sold as "natural corticosteroids"; their efficacy is minimal.

Tars and Tar-Like Substances. Probably the oldest alternative antiinflammatory therapy is tar and related products. Coal tar derivatives are available in elegant creams and bases, so that they no longer are so foul smelling or discoloring. In addition, shale oil (ichthammol or ichthyol) is available in a wide variety of formulations in Europe. While tars are most often used for psoriasis, they can also be employed for chronic, lichenified dermatitis. One must be cautious about both irritation and photosensitization when using coal tar.

Antimicrobial Agents. While dermatitis may appear infected and is often secondarily colonized by a variety of agents, antibacterial agents are not as efficacious as corticosteroids. Many dermatologists still add antibiotics to corticosteroid preparations, but this should be done in cooperation with a knowledgeable compounding pharmacist to avoid incompatibility. A variety of topical antimicrobials are available that lend themselves to treating dermatitis. Included are the iodophors such as povidone-iodine (Betadine), chlorhexidine (Hibiclens) and silver sulfadiazine (Silvadine). The first two are available in a variety of soaps, washes and cleansers, as well as ointments. In intertriginous areas, aqueous 0.1% gentian violet or brilliant green is still useful. We no longer prescribe these dyes because of recent European regulations, but instead only use them in the hospital for selected patients under direct supervision. Clioquinol (Vioform) is a modestly effective antibacterial and antifungal agent which is sold alone or mixed with a low-potency corticosteroid. It stains everything slightly yellow and is a rare cause of allergic contact dermatitis. If absorbed in sufficient amounts there is a theoretical risk of neurotoxicity, but we have never seen problems.

When employing topical antibiotics one must be aware of several factors in addition to their questionable efficacy. There is an increasing incidence of antibiotic resistance among many bacteria, so that common sense demands we limit the exposure of organisms to antibiotics. In addition, many antibiotics are potent topical sensitizers. They should therefore be used with caution so as not to deprive the patient of a potentially useful drug via the systemic route. The most widely prescribed topical antibiotics in the USA are neomycin and bacitracin, often in combination or with additional ingredients. Fusidic acid is widely used in Europe. Gentamicin should be avoided because it may be needed systemically. Mupirocin is highly effective against staphylococcal and streptococcal infections, but its cost usually prohibits its use for widespread disease. In general, antimicrobial agents including antibiotics are overused in this clinical setting and few studies have shown their efficacy.

Keratolytics. Hyperkeratotic and lichenified dermatitis can often be approached with something to loosen the scale, prior to or instead of corticosteroids. The most commonly prescribed agents are salicylic acid 5–10% in petrolatum, and urea 5–10% in a lipophilic cream or ointment. Urea is available mixed with corticosteroids; it increases the penetration and thus the potency of the corticosteroid. In Europe several high-potency corticosteroids are available with salicylic acid.

Systemic Therapy

Corticosteroids. Systemic corticosteroids are highly effective for acute allergic contact dermatitis, but rarely of value in irritant or chronic disorders. For example, in treating poison ivy allergic contact dermatitis, 40–60 mg prednisone daily tapered over 9–14 days is far safer, cheaper, and more effective than attempting to treat blisters and erosions with high-potency topical corticosteroids. Similar regimens are also useful for acute flares of dyshidrotic dermatitis, which is probably the most steroid-responsive type of "nonallergic" dermatitis. While chronic low-dose corticosteroids are effective for chronic hand dermatitis, they are difficult to justify medically.

Antibiotics. In general, if a dermatitis is secondarily infected, a short course of an oral antibiotic effective against *Staphylococcus aureus* and streptococci is simpler than topical therapy. Erythromycin has long been the favorite of dermatologists but the incidence of resistant strains is so high that other agents should be considered. Alternatives include cephalosporins and penicillinase-resistant penicillins, such as dicloxacillin.

Antihistamines. Despite the reputation of antihistamines as good antipruritic agents and "antiallergens", they are of only minimal value in allergic contact dermatitis and even less useful in irritant contact dermatitis. The ability of antihistamines to control all itch other than that mediated directly by histamine is related to their soporific action. Since histamine is not a major mediator in cell-mediated immunity, allergic contact dermatitis is not very amenable to such therapy.

Retinoids. As mentioned under hyperkeratotic hand dermatitis, it is sometimes worth a try to use a short course of systemic retinoids in carefully selected patients. We employ acitretin 10–20 mg daily for 1–4 weeks. It often enables one to turn the corner, without having to resort to long-term systemic corticosteroids.

Phototherapy

Ultraviolet radiation has long been used for dermatitis but the technique has been refined in recent years. Dyshidrotic dermatitis for example is fairly sensitive to UV radiation. Both UVB and PUVA can be employed. PUVA bath therapy, combined with special hand and foot sources, is a valuable new addition to the armamentarium. More widespread disease can also be treated. One must be very careful to avoid exceeding the minimum erythema dosage or minimum phototoxic dose, as erythema can trigger a dermatitic reaction.

In days gone by, soft X-rays and especially Grenz radiation were employed for severe or recalcitrant dermatitis, especially hand dermatitis. Typically 0.6–1.0 Gy were given every 8–10 days for a total of three exposures. If this approach is used, one should be careful not to use other irritating topical agents in combination. We no longer employ Grenz radiation in this setting.

Other Measures

Probably in no other area of dermatology are other measures such as protection, presentation, and maintenance care as important as in contact and irritant dermatitis. This can aptly be named corneotherapy, as it is intended to restore or maintain a well-functioning stratum corneum barrier. When one considers protection, most of the information applies best to hand dermatitis which is the major dermatologic cause of lost work days. Protective hand creams are available. Some are designed to protect against water-based irritants; others against oil-based materials. Studies have shown that such properties are not always true in the clinical setting. One must simply try different protective creams and see which one works best. In addition, one must be sure the patient has enough protective cream to cover the required areas; simply writing a prescription for one tube and saying good-by is a waste of time. Gloves are essential but often a mixed blessing. Patients who sweat a great deal may have even more trouble using gloves. In addition, sensitization to both natural rubber latex and other rubber components is possible. Finally, mild cleansing agents and good skin care are essential. In industrial settings, one must insist upon widely available mild cleansing products and hand creams which can be applied after cleansing.

In general soaps are quite drying and tend to worsen dermatitis. For this reason, in the past in German-speaking countries one used the terms *Waschverbot* or *Seifenverbot*, meaning that the patient should reduce washing to a minimum and only cleanse their skin with water. This is impractical in dirty industrial settings, but the modern synthetic detergents (syndets) have provided marked improvements. Soaps are usually alkaline and damage the epidermis by causing even more swelling. The syndets are neutral or even slightly acidic and much kinder to all skin, included damaged skin. Some patients are happy using a light oil as a cleansing agent.

When dermatitis is widespread and the patient's skin is dry, one can also use baths as a method of treatment, either adding oils or other active ingredients, as discussed under atopic dermatitis.

Avoiding the irritating substances is also a key feature. If an allergen is identified, sometimes it can be easily avoided, while in other instances it is so widespread (chromate, nickel, formaldehyde, fragrances, preservatives) that avoidance is difficult. In the USA, patients can be taught how to identify poison ivy and its relatives. If a given industrial product, for example a cutting oil or grease, is too irritating for a umber of workers, the firm can be persuaded to switch to a different product. Usually the workmen's compensation or similar insurance group can provide the physician with leverage when dealing with a reluctant employer.

Diet is often raised as an issue by the patient, but only rarely can one prove a definite association. Some exquisitely nickel-sensitive patients appear to develop a hand dermatitis upon exposure to nickel-rich foods. In addition, food may cause skin lesions to worsen in patients with contact sensitization to balsam of Peru, food dyes and preservatives and other orally ingested allergens. Dietary restriction is only recommended in the pre-phase of oral challenge tests or if a clear diagnosis of hematogenous allergic contact dermatitis has been made. Such a diagnosis can only be made in the inpatient setting with placebo-controlled double-blind challenge studies. In general, dietary manipulation plays little role in the treatment of dermatitis. If a patient thinks that some food, such as caffeine, nicotine, alcohol or chocolate (to pick a few items that are commonly incriminated), triggers a dermatitis, it is just common sense to avoid it, but even in such cases blinded challenges are usually negative.

Dyshidrotic Dermatitis

(Fox 1873)

Synonyms. Dyshidrosis, dyshidrotic eczema, pompholyx, cheiropompholyx, podopompholyx

Definition. Dermatitis of the palms and soles characterized by tiny water-filled vesicles which are usually quite pruritic. In Germany, distinctions are made among various types of dyshidrotic dermatitis based both on etiology and quality of the blisters, but in most other countries, the disorder is viewed as a single, poorly understood entity.

Epidemiology. Dyshidrotic dermatitis is one of the most common skin disorders. It has so many potential triggers that an epidemiologic picture is difficult to paint. One intriguing fact is its rarity among children and the elderly; most patients are young to middle-aged adults. In addition, dyshidrotic dermatitis is far less common in a very dry climate than it is in a temperate or humid climate.

Etiology and Pathogenesis. As the many names suggest, dyshidrotic dermatitis was long thought to be a disorder of the eccrine sweat glands. It consists of a vesicular dermatitis occurring on the thick skin of the palms and soles where it produces characteristic deep-seated vesicles. Careful histologic studies have shown that the vesicles do not reflect sweat duct occlusion. Nonetheless, many patients do have hyperhidrosis, confusing the issue somewhat. The eruption is somewhat more common during the summer, providing a weak but tantalizing link to sweating.

The number of possible causes or associated disorders is quite long and includes:

Manifestation of Atopic Diathesis. Many atopic patients have primarily dyshidrotic dermatitis in their adult life.

Id Reaction. Patients with tinea pedis may develop dyshidrotic dermatitis when the dermatophyte infection on their feet flares. The hands do not contain fungal elements. Id reactions are viewed as a distant allergic reactions to an infectious trigger. In the past, injection of trichophytin allergen produced a dyshidrotic flare on occasion.

Contact Allergy. In most cases, allergic contact dermatitis occurs on top of a dyshidrotic dermatitis, often caused by one of the many medications the patient has used. In rare cases, contact allergy may be the primary trigger of the vesicles, such as in allergic reactions to shoe inserts or sheepskin slippers. One should consider not only type IV allergy but also late-phase reactions to immediate-type allergens.

Systemic Allergic Reaction. Rarely patients with nickel sensitivity will develop dyshidrotic dermatitis when challenged inadvertently or intentionally with oral nickel. Cigarette smoking is also a known trigger of dyshidrotic reactions. The nickel in the cigarette smoke may be the explanation. Balsam of Peru and some dyes may also cause a similar reaction. In each case, the sensitization has probably occurred topically but systemic challenge produces the dyshidrotic reaction. One theory is that the materials selectively accumulate in eccrine sweat and then cause trouble on the palms and soles.

In addition, occasional drug reactions will be dyshidrosiform, but no medication is particularly known for causing this type of change. In Germany such reactions are also described as hematogenous allergic dyshidrotic dermatitis, in analogy to hematogenous allergic contact dermatitis.

Idiopathic. In the vast bulk of patients, no triggers or predisposing factors are found. Some physicians also list "psychogenic" as a cause, but we see no evidence that dyshidrotic dermatitis is more connected with stress or emotions than other types of dermatitis. Almost anyone whose hands are pruritic and difficult to use would become grouchy or upset.

Clinical Findings. The characteristic finding is pruritic, small symmetrically distributed relatively deep seated blisters on the palms and soles (Fig. 12.21). The most typical location is the sides of the second to the fifth fingers. The thumb is usually spared, and lesions on the sides of the digits are far more common than on the palmar or plantar surfaces. When the foot is involved, it is often the arch rather than the toes. Sometimes the blisters are very small and relatively asymptomatic. The lesions tend to come and go in crops. As they heal, erythematous scaly patches evolve (Fig. 12.22). If the right history is not obtained (asking about "water blisters"), the diagnosis may be missed.

There are several clinical variations on the theme of dyshidrotic dermatitis:

Pompholyx (Hutchinson 1876). This term is applied in Europe to the maximum variation of

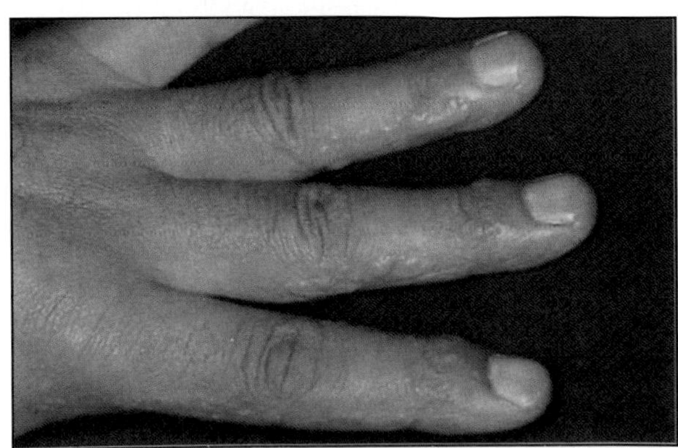

Fig. 12.21. Acute dyshidrotic dermatitis

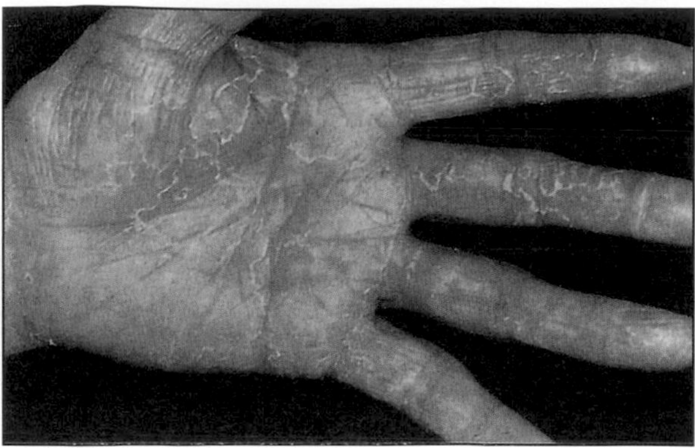

Fig. 12.22. Resolving dyshidrotic dermatitis with fine scaling

dyshidrotic dermatitis; that is, to the patients with large coalescing blisters. Such patients are at greater risk for secondary bacterial infections with lymphangitis. When large blisters are present and the plantar instep is prominently involved, the current diagnosis may be recurrent vesicular *Trichophyton mentagrophytes* infection of the feet and a fungal id reaction on the hands.

"Dyshidrotic Eczema." In German-speaking countries, this term is preferred to describe patients with underlying idiopathic dyshidrotic dermatitis (dyshidrosis) and secondary allergic contact dermatitis. There are clinical clues such as spreading of the erythema and vesicular reaction to the back of the hands or feet, as well as occasional distant reactions on nonacral sites. In some cases of chronic hand dermatitis, the erythema and epidermal reactive changes dominate and the blisters appear as a secondary phenomenon.

Dyshidrosis Lamellosa Sicca. Patients may overlook the blisters and present with fine collarette scales at the sites of the previous vesiculation. This is often a hint for the presence of the atopic diathesis, especially in summer time.

Histopathology. Dyshidrotic dermatitis is the prototype of acute spongiotic vesicular dermatitis. The typical hyperkeratosis of the palms and soles leads to more intact, better circumscribed blisters. In the upper dermis, edema and a lymphocytic perivascular infiltrate are found. Occasionally the blisters may sit in the acrosyringium.

Differential Diagnosis. How one approaches dyshidrotic dermatitis is a matter of controversy, but a few points are clear. One should always look at the feet and see if any vesicles or scaling are present. Foot involvement strongly suggest a dermatophyte infection, which can be easily confirmed or ruled out. Only in rare cases is localized tinea manuum vesicular. Second, if the disease has spread to the backs of the hands or feet, one should exclude allergic contact dermatitis by patch testing, perform prick tests and try to identify specific IgE antibodies in the serum eventually indicating immediate type allergy. When just small typical blisters, erythema and localized scales are found, one should inquire about the atopic diathesis.

The cause of dyshidrotic dermatitis is where the trouble starts. If one simply identifies a dermatophyte infection, atopic dermatitis or a positive patch test and then concludes that the etiology of dyshidrotic dermatitis is established, one is probably wrong. All four of these conditions (dyshidrotic dermatitis, atopic dermatitis, tinea pedis, a positive patch test) are extremely common, so the simultaneous appearance is not uncommon. To prove an association, the dyshidrotic dermatitis should flare with the fungal disease and disappear when the fungus is controlled. The same critical approach should be employed when considering the other disorders. In the vast majority of patients, dyshidrotic dermatitis remains a mystery with no clear triggering event.

Therapy

Systemic. Dyshidrotic dermatitis is a very difficult disease to treat. Fortunately it is often quite corticosteroid-responsive. Most patients do well with a short course of prednisone 40–60 mg daily tapered over 10–21 days. Bacterial secondary infections need to be treated with oral antibiotics. If a documented tinea pedis is present, it is worth trying a course of oral antifungal agents to see if the dyshidrotic dermatitis improves. There may be a Jarisch-Herxheimer-like reaction during the initial phase, with a worsening of the hand blisters. Some patients are so disabled by their dyshidrosis that they require a minor tranquilizer or mild soporific agent.

Topical. The simplest approach is ultra-high-potency topical corticosteroids for a period of 4–7 days, tapering rapidly to a milder agent and then skincare products. Some patients do better initially with a very drying form of corticosteroid such as a gel, solution or lotion. In any event, ointments and greasy creams should be avoided. Most find if they apply a corticosteroid to the early vesicles, they can reduce pruritus and prevent a severe attack.

If large blisters develop, then sometimes wet compresses, trimming of the blister roof, and use of antibacterial agents may be helpful. Tannic acid may be added to the compress water for its astringent effects, or an antibacterial agent (1% aluminum chloride or 1% silver nitrate) may be used.

Seborrheic Dermatitis

(Unna 1887)

Synonyms. Seborrheic eczema, dysseborrheic dermatitis, Unna disease

Definition. Chronic common dermatitis usually involving hair-bearing, intertriginous or sebum-rich areas.

Epidemiology. If one considers the entire spectrum of seborrheic dermatitis, including infantile, adult and elderly variants, then almost every individual at some time in their life has the disease. Many physicians and patients accept it as a normal variation rather than a disease. Probably 5% of the population has severe enough seborrheic dermatitis to seek medical attention. Men are more often affected than women.

Etiology and Pathogenesis. The cause of seborrheic dermatitis remains unclear but there are several not mutually exclusive suggestions.

Excessive Sebaceous Gland Activity. Traditionally one blamed the sebaceous glands. The excess secretion of sebum or seborrhea was felt to produce scales and irritation. This might help explain the presence of seborrheic dermatitis in infants whose sebaceous glands are quite active. The sebaceous theory would also explain the localization primarily on the scalp and face, but occasionally in other hairy areas. Most patients with seborrheic dermatitis have oily, sebum-rich skin. Clothing which is not absorbent may worsen the problem. In addition, patients with Parkinson disease have not only increased sebum flow but also increased frequency of seborrheic dermatitis. Qualitative changes in sebum have not been demonstrated.

Microbial Agents. Unna himself suggested that bacteria or *Pityrosporum ovale (Malassezia furfur)* might be responsible for seborrheic dermatitis. For many years, there has been controversy over the relative contributions of microbial organisms to the disease. Many physicians were skeptical, even though the lipophilic yeast *P. ovale* has long been accepted as part of the resident flora of the hairs and their lipid film. The observation in the early days of the AIDS epidemic that seborrheic dermatitis was more common in AIDS patients and responded to oral imidazole antifungal agents provided support for Unna's old hypothesis. Response to a therapeutic agent should not be taken as proof of causation. The oral and topical imidazoles have many other actions which could play a role in treating seborrheic dermatitis.

Immune System. As mentioned, severe seborrheic dermatitis is a possible sign of an early HIV infection. Nonetheless, it is a very common disease and most patients have no immune abnormalities.

Relationship to Psoriasis. Clinically severe seborrheic dermatitis and psoriasis of the scalp are very similar. Some clinicians use the term seborrhiasis or sebopsoriasis to describe this state. In addition, the onset of psoriasis or worsening of a preexisting psoriasis is also associated with HIV/AIDS. Histologically the two disorders also share some features.

Other Factors. The nervous system also appears to play a role. The most striking example is the severity of seborrheic dermatitis in Parkinson disease and its occurrence on only the involved side in stroke patients, or in the inappropriately innervated skin in syringomyelia. In many countries, the disease is more common in winter. Diet is frequently blamed for seborrheic dermatitis, both by patients and alternative medicine practitioners. A severe deficiency in many trace elements, such as zinc, free fatty acids and the B vitamins, can produce a seborrheic dermatitis-like rash. Normal seborrheic dermatitis does not respond to diets rich in these elements.

Clinical Findings. The prototypical lesions of seborrheic dermatitis are erythematous scaly patches, often pruritic. Typical locations include the scalp, hairline, eyebrows, glabella, sideburns, nasolabial folds, mustache region, behind the ears and within the ears (Fig. 12.23). Other sites may include the lateral neck, mid-chest, axillae, umbilicus and groin (Fig. 12.24). In rare instances the disease may spread to cover the entire body.

In the USA, the term dandruff is often equated with mild seborrheic dermatitis of the scalp. This is

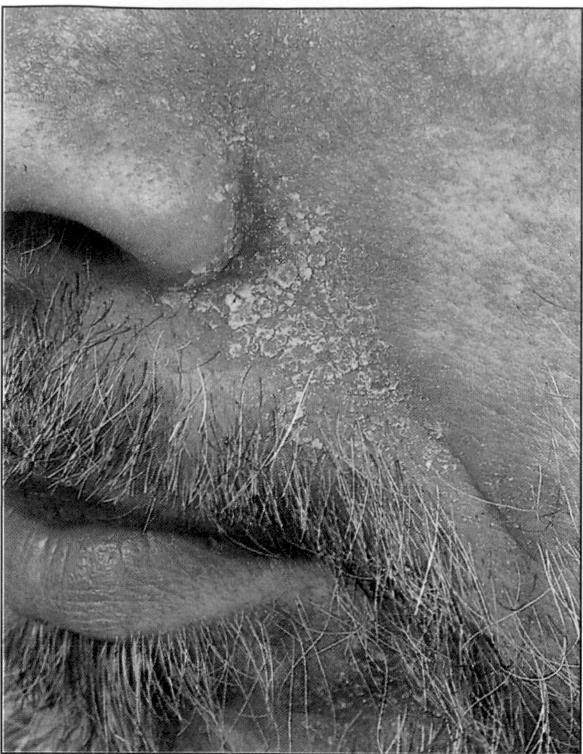

Fig. 12.23. Seborrheic dermatitis

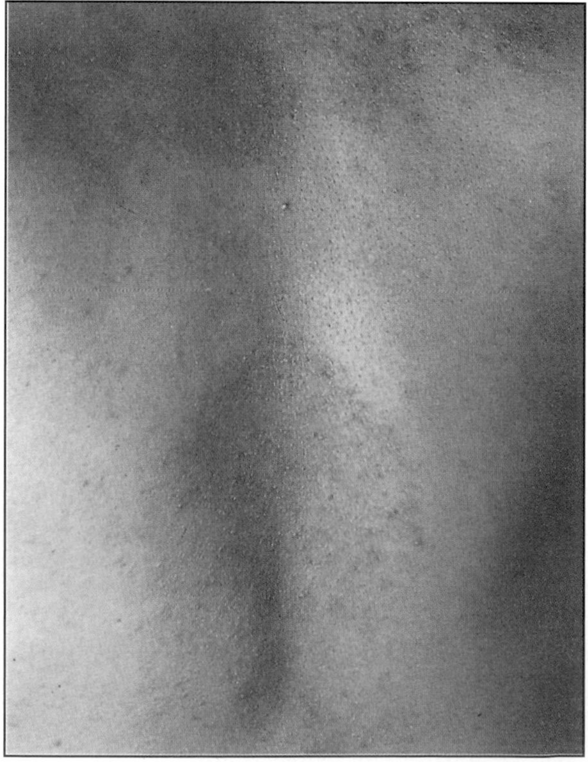

Fig. 12.24. Seborrheic dermatitis

not technically correct in our view, as seborrheic dermatitis (or any dermatitis) requires inflammation and thus erythema. Simply fine scaling of the scalp with no erythema is a variant of dry skin, best viewed as pityriasis simplex.

The mildest form of seborrheic dermatitis is known in German as seborrheic eczematid, suggesting a predermatitis or early condition. A greasy yellow branny scaling develops on irregular erythematous patches, especially about the eyebrows, nasolabial folds and ears. In some individuals, especially women, there is just paranasal erythema with scaling (erythema paranasale). Clinically this represents an overlap between seborrheic dermatitis and perioral dermatitis.

More severe seborrheic dermatitis appears slightly differently in various areas. The unifying feature is the presence of erythematous plaques with fine yellowish scale which develop in the typical sites mentioned above. On the scalp, usually the edge or hair line is favored, although occasionally there will be diffuse scalp erythema and scaling. Sometimes annular lesions are present, especially on the neck; they are termed petaloid (petal-like) seborrheic dermatitis and often mistaken for a dermatophyte infection. On the face, seborrheic dermatitis is occasionally light-provoked. Behind the ears, seborrheic dermatitis tends to fissure so that a secondary bacterial infection or irritant dermatitis may evolve. On the trunk, the most common site is the presternal region. Here, scale is less prominent, perhaps because it is rubbed away by the clothing and sweat; the French call this *eczéma flanellaire.* While seborrheic dermatitis is common in the axillae and groin, it is often misdiagnosed, described as a candidal infection, allergic contact dermatitis, intertrigo or something more esoteric.

Several special variants of seborrheic dermatitis have been described:

Disseminated Seborrheic Dermatitis. Occasionally seborrheic dermatitis may evolve into a more severe weeping eruption. Sometimes this occurs spontaneously and in other instances it is triggered by light or perhaps overly aggressive topical therapy. Immunosuppression may also play a role. In any event, the plaques become more pruritic, redder and tend to weep and crust. In addition to the typical sites, the nipples and flexural folds of the extremities may be involved, confusing the diagnosis.

Pityriasiform Seborrhoid. While this name is not well known in the USA, experienced colleagues will recognize the problem. This probably is best viewed as an acute severe form of petaloid seborrheic dermatitis. Most lesions are on the trunk, annular, scaly and follow the skin lesions, mimicking pityriasis rosea. No herald patch is present, the scale is not just collarette in form and the extremities and neck may be involved. The disease is stubborn but self-limited; stigmata of seborrheic dermatitis may remain. Perhaps this represents pityriasis rosea or inverse pityriasis rosea in a person who is susceptible to seborrheic dermatitis. We will have to learn the cause of either seborrheic dermatitis or pityriasis rosea to resolve this issue.

Seborrheic Erythroderma. Among elderly patients seborrheic dermatitis is probably the most common cause of erythroderma. Often either neglect or overly harsh treatment is the trigger. One must always exclude a drug-induced erythroderma and mycosis fungoides (Sézary syndrome). Lymphadenopathy is not associated with severe seborrheic dermatitis.

Seborrheic Blepharitis. Erythema, pruritus and mild scaling of the eye lids is a common problem. While it most often occurs in people with obvious seborrheic dermatitis elsewhere, when it is the only sign of the disorder, the diagnosis is puzzling.

Histopathology. The histology of seborrheic dermatitis is not very specific. The slightly acanthotic epidermis shows hyperkeratosis, parakeratosis and spongiosis. Accumulations of sebum in the stratum corneum represent the clinically obvious greasy scales. In the dermis there is edema and a lymphocytic perivascular infiltrate. Intraepidermal accumulations of neutrophils, elongation of the rete ridges and vessel tortuosity also suggest psoriasis. Munro microabscesses are not seen.

Course and Prognosis. Seborrheic dermatitis is a chronic condition. We tell every patient, "We can control your disease but not cure it." In addition, one should mention that there are overlaps with psoriasis. One school of thought is that seborrheic dermatitis triggers psoriasis via the Köbner phenomenon; we suspect the relation is a little closer. In at-risk individuals with sudden severe seborrheic dermatitis/psoriasis, one is obligated to rule out HIV/AIDS.

Differential Diagnosis. The differential diagnosis is lengthy but in practice, seborrheic dermatitis is a one-glance diagnosis (in German *Blick* diagnosis). In some countries, extensive patch testing to exclude allergic contact dermatitis and allergy work-ups to exclude atopic dermatitis are the standard, but the tendency towards saving money in health care means that this type of investigation will stop. A person with red scaly patches in the nasolabial folds and over the eyebrows has seborrheic dermatitis.

The biggest differential diagnostic question is psoriasis, and we have already acknowledged in several locations that often time will tell which disease is present. One should look for signs of psoriasis elsewhere and inquire about a family history. When the lesions are more inflamed or disseminated, the possibility of secondary bacterial or candidal infection should be entertained. Allergic contact dermatitis to the frames of eyeglasses may occasionally mimic seborrheic dermatitis behind the ears. Within the ears, the diagnosis of otomycosis is often made. Unfortunately, this is usually a mistake; true fungal infections of the external ear are uncommon. The fungi found in the ear are usually not pathogens. When the external ear shows erythema and scale, the answer is seborrheic dermatitis, allergic contact dermatitis to ear drops (often prescribed for the presumed fungal infection) or simple irritation, as in swimmer's ear when retained water causes trouble. In the nasolabial fold and occasionally in other sites, a more papular reaction should raise the question of perioral dermatitis, perhaps caused by too-potent topical corticosteroids prescribed for seborrheic dermatitis. When widespread lesions are present, one must consider pityriasis rosea. When faced with seborrheic erythroderma, one must exclude Sézary syndrome and a drug eruption.

Therapy. The main rule is "do no harm". As we have mentioned several times throughout this section, therapy is one of the triggers of worsening and spread. Almost all patients can be treated successfully with simple topical measures. The mainstays of therapy are shampoos, very low-potency topical corticosteroids and topical imidazoles.

Most patients with seborrheic dermatitis, even if they have only minimal scalp disease, do better with more frequent shampooing. The rare patient with very dry skin may worsen with increased use. The only truly medicated shampoo is ketoconazole shampoo which has been shown to reduce the numbers of *P. ovale* and produce more improvement in the erythema and scaling than the shampoo vehicle alone. Most patients do best when they use the ketoconazole shampoo every week or two. In between they should wash their scalp daily or every other day with either an ordinary cosmetically acceptable shampoo, a tar shampoo (tar shampoos are no longer available over-the-counter in Europe because of concerns about carcinogenicity, which we feel are exaggerated), a zinc pyrithione shampoo or a shampoo containing salicylic acid. Selenium sulfide shampoo is a favorite in the USA, but if used too frequently it causes a paradoxical scalp oiliness.

The other aspect of therapy is the use of either a topical corticosteroid or an imidazole cream. The corticosteroids work more quickly, but there is a natural reluctance to use them for a chronic disease on the face. If the patient has mild disease and can control the erythema and scale by using a low-potency corticosteroid on occasion, that is simplest. On the trunk, mid-potency corticosteroids can be employed, but they are rarely needed. If continuous treatment appears needed, it may be wiser to use any of the imidazole creams. In either case one daily application at night suffices. Clioquinol lotions or pastes are also very helpful and have no long-term side effects. Metronidazole creams, as used in rosacea, may also be helpful. Finally, there is a cream containing lithium salts available in Germany. This became available following the observation that some patients treated systemically with lithium for their manic-depressive disorder experienced improvement in their seborrheic dermatitis. In our experience, the order of efficacy is corticosteroids → imidazoles → others.

The scalp requires some therapeutic dexterity. If the scalp is severely involved, the patient is usually willing to use a corticosteroid cream or lotion at night and wash it out in the morning. Occlusion with a shower cap may also help. Very stubborn scalp lesions, can be treated with higher potency topical corticosteroids either as creams or gels. Tinctures containing either salicylic acid or a corticosteroid are often too drying. If very thick scales are present, they can be presoaked with baby oil, olive oil or 3–5% salicylic acid added to a water-miscible vehicle. After 1–2 h, or in rare instances overnight application, the scalp is washed removing most of the scale.

Seborrheic blepharitis is a special problem. One should work in conjunction with the ophthalmologist. Often low-potency corticosteroid creams are needed, but the risk of both glaucoma and periorbital steroid rosacea is considerable. Ophthalmologists tend to use antibiotic creams on the basis of the view that bacteria are a potential cause. A good compromise are the imidazole creams which are antibacterial and also help against seborrheic dermatitis. Washing the eyelids when shampooing may also be of benefit.

Systemic. While a number of systemic therapies are possible, they are rarely indicated for a chronic benign disease. In extremely severe cases, sometimes a short course of oral imidazoles (itraconazole or fluconazole) can be tried. Similarly, isotretinoin can be used to reduce sebum production, although the drying and erythema it produces may not be much better than the underlying disease. We employ very low dosages ranging from 10–20 mg daily to 10 mg three times weekly. Sometimes, if a patient has been mismanaged enough that they have disseminated disease, a short burst of oral corticosteroids may speed resolution. Finally, systemic antibiotics in acne-type regimens can be employed for refractory cases.

Infantile Seborrheic Dermatitis

Epidemiology. Almost every infant gets seborrheic dermatitis and usually grandmother knows how to treat it.

Etiology and Pathogenesis. The etiology of the disease in children is just as unclear as in adults. Seborrheic dermatitis may be more common in infants with atopy or a tendency towards psoriasis. Studies have shown that well over 50% of children with widespread seborrheic dermatitis have (or evolve into) atopic dermatitis. In this age group, *C. albicans* is identified in almost every case, both on the skin and in the stool. Perhaps in infants, *C. albicans* is another trigger, just as *P. ovale* may be in adults.

Clinical Findings. Seborrheic dermatitis is a little different in infants, who have more sebum and less hair. The onset is usually in the first 3 months but may occur later. The child has large greasy yellow scales which are often matted to the sparse scalp hairs (Fig. 12.25). We call the matted mass cradle cap. In German it is referred to as *Gneis*, which is also the word for a layered hard metamorphic rock. The word has been adopted by English-speaking geologists but not by dermatologists.

Typically there is little or no erythema. Occasionally erythematous plaques develop spontaneously;

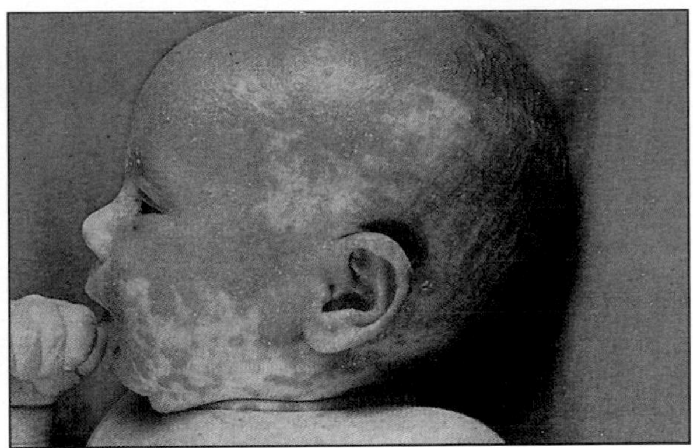

Fig. 12.25. Infantile seborrheic dermatitis

in other instances they are triggered by over-aggressive care. They are most often found in the axillae, umbilicus and diaper region, but sometimes the trunk is involved. The lesions may be eroded, raising the question of candidiasis, or become thickened and crusted. The British often call this condition napkin (diaper) psoriasis. It tends to resolve just as the milder forms do. Rare infants go on to develop severe erythrodermic seborrheic dermatitis.

Histopathology. Biopsy is often employed to exclude Langerhans cell histiocytosis. The features are similar to those in adults.

Differential Diagnosis. The absolute separation between seborrheic dermatitis and atopic dermatitis can be difficult. Seborrheic dermatitis starts earlier, does not itch, is less-often scratched and tends to have greasier scales. Atopic dermatitis starts later, is more pruritic and usually one parent or sibling has a positive history of atopy. Psoriasis should be diagnosed with caution; many cases resolve and probably represent severe seborrheic dermatitis. Scabies may present in infants with dermatitis, but the intense pruritus and excoriations lead one away from the diagnosis of seborrheic dermatitis. Persistent erythematous scaling, especially if hemorrhagic and therapy-resistant, or if in an infant who is doing poorly or has hepatosplenomegaly, deserves a biopsy to exclude Langerhans cell histiocytosis.

Therapy. Here the trick is to be gentle and mild. Encouraging the parent to frequently change diapers, use a mild cleanser and lubricate the skin after washing or bathing. The cradle cap can be treated by presoaking with baby oil or a hydrophilic cream or ointment, and then shampooing. While salicylic acid can be added to the pretreatment regimen, it is potentially toxic in infants and usually one can get by without it, relying on the mechanical properties of the oil.

The lesions in infants often tend to be moister, and thus drying approaches are often helpful. Aqueous 0.1% solutions of gentian violet may be applied to the intertriginous regions by the physician in selected cases; we no longer prescribe it for home use. An imidazole cream is also a good choice, covering against bacteria and *C. albicans*, as well as helping the inflammation. Clioguinol (0.5–1.0%) may also be useful. Low-potency corticosteroids can also be used when erythematous scaly patches are present, just as in adults. In the diaper area, with damaged barrier function, they are very well absorbed so additional caution is needed. In the past, creams containing 1% hydrocortisone and an anticandidal agent were available and often used, but today the combination agents typically contain stronger corticosteroids that are not appropriate for infants.

Leiner Syndrome

(Leiner 1908)

Everyone agrees Leiner syndrome is very rare. The real question is whether it exists or not. Patients have widespread seborrheic dermatitis evolving into exfoliative erythroderma, along with failure to thrive, lymphadenopathy, diarrhea and recurrent infections. A classic paper described Leiner syndrome as an autosomal dominant defect in C5 leading to defective opsonization. After a whole generation of young dermatologists had memorized this fact, but never seen a case, the trend switched. Today, one speaks of Leiner phenotype, as seen in a broad spectrum of immunodeficiency states in infants, including severe combined immunodeficiency, hypogammaglobulinemias, hyper-IgE syndrome and a variety of complement deficiencies (both C3 and C5), which can lead to impaired opsonization.

Nummular Dermatitis

(Devergie 1857)

Synonyms. Nummular eczema, microbial dermatitis, discoid dermatitis

Definition. Scattered, coin-shaped usually sharply bordered patches of dermatitis which typically show crusting and weeping.

Epidemiology. Nummular dermatitis is so poorly defined that epidemiologic data are difficult to acquire. Some authors feel it is a disease of the elderly; others state that it occurs primarily in children.

Etiology and Pathogenesis. The etiology is a mystery. In the past, nummular dermatitis was felt to be mediated by an allergy to bacterial antigens, hence the alternative names. The working theories included a reaction to bacterial antigens, similar to allergic contact dermatitis, and a cutaneous reaction to circulating factors from a focus of infection. Some patients even underwent cholecystectomy or extensive sinus surgery to remove such foci; in general, their nummular dermatitis remained. Secondary infection of the skin lesions with gram-positive bacteria is a common event, but it is generally agreed that nummular dermatitis is not primarily infectious. Bacterial contact allergies can be demonstrated in the laboratory, but whether or not they play a role in nature is unclear. Patients with atopic dermatitis often have nummular lesions. We separate out this group, but if one does not, then atopic dermatitis is the main "cause" of nummular dermatitis.

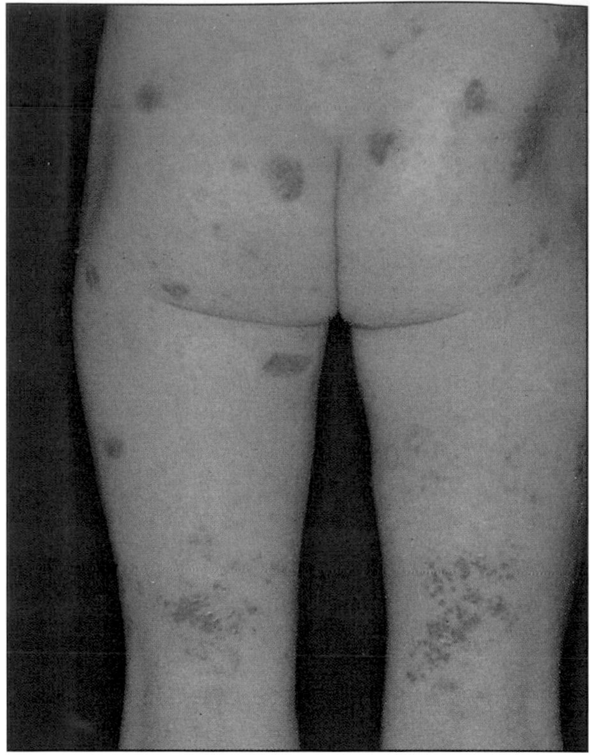

Fig. 12.26. Nummular dermatitis

Clinical Findings. The clinical features are what sets apart nummular dermatitis. The initial lesions are small (<1.0 cm) sharply bordered erythematous plaques which are often easier to palpate than to see. They may be edematous and have a few vesicles. As the acute inflammation leads to rupture of the vesicles, the larger expanding lesions tend to have yellow crust and scale (Figs. 12.26, 12.27). Pruritus is present and occasionally severe. Typical lesions are 5 cm or more in diameter and are usually round; nummular is derived from the Latin *nummulus* or "little coin". The nummular lesions are highly variable; most patients have just a couple of lesions but some may develop a widespread symmetric eruption. Typical locations include the legs and trunk, but peculiarly in younger patients involvement of the backs of the hands and feet is more common. Despite the thick crusted nature of the lesions, excoriations are not common and healing usually occurs without scarring other than mild pigmentary changes. There are no systemic problems and no mucosal involvement.

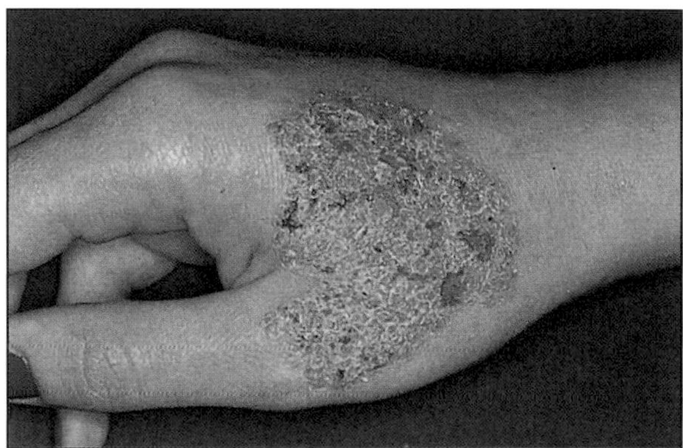

Fig. 12.27. Nummular dermatitis

Histopathology. The microscopic picture is not unique. The acanthotic epidermis shows spongiosis, blisters and serous crust, while the dermis features a perivascular lymphocytic infiltrate. In more severe cases, the epidermal reaction pattern may be psoriasiform, but microabscesses are absent.

Course and Prognosis. The course is chronic and frequently recurrent. Since the etiology is unknown, it is hard to do much more than treat lesions as they arise.

Differential Diagnosis. The differential diagnosis is quite lengthy. Solitary lesions are often confused with tinea corporis, but the KOH examination and culture can resolve the issue. In addition, the crusting and relatively adherent scale speak against a dermatophyte infection. Patches of psoriasis lack vesicles and crust. A single lesion can be confused with impetigo, especially since the culture is often positive.

When multiple lesions are present, the list of possibilities changes.

Nummular Atopic Dermatitis. Patients with the atopic diathesis may have nummular lesions; sometimes these are the only skin changes in a patient with unquestionable atopy. Typically the lesions are more acral, not so exudative or crusted and often more excoriated and lichenified. We believe these lesions are clinically distinct from classic nummular dermatitis in most cases.

Asteatotic Dermatitis. Elderly patients with dry skin often develop nummular patches, but dermatitis is usually absent. If erythema is present, it is minimal. Vesicles, crusting and scaling are absent. Simple lubrication produces improvement, which is not the case in nummular dermatitis.

Small-Patch Parapsoriasis. Typically patients with this disorder have more lesions, often prominently involving the trunk, although the extremities are not spared. The lesions are asymptomatic, never vesicular or crusted and very persistent. The biopsy in small-patch parapsoriasis is even less specific than that in nummular dermatitis.

Chronic Superficial Dermatitis. While this may be a variant of small-patch parapsoriasis, it is most common on the legs and inner aspects of arms of middle aged men. The lesions are sharply circumscribed, slightly red, oval or irregular plaques with fine scale.

Contact Dermatitis. In rare cases, allergic or irritant contact dermatitis can take a nummular form. This phenomenon has been reported with hematogenous contact dermatitis from nickel and chromate, and as a local reaction to medications. It is so rare that routine patch testing in nummular dermatitis is not needed.

Therapy

Topical. Nummular dermatitis is relatively corticosteroid-responsive, but also easy to exacerbate with overly enthusiastic approaches. We usually start with a high-potency corticosteroid cream or lotion in the exudative phase and switch to a weaker corticosteroid in a firmer vehicle as the lesions improve. When available, 0.1% gentian violet can be applied to weeping lesions prior to applying corticosteroids. Very stubborn, no longer exudative lesions can also be treated with corticosteroids under occlusion, Clioguinol is also very effective. Tars and ichthyol should be avoided in the acute phase, but may be quite helpful for more chronic lesions. After bathing, simply lubricating the patches is also wise, as they tend to otherwise dry out and persist even longer.

Systemic. While disseminated nummular dermatitis can be treated with a short burst of systemic corticosteroids, such an approach is almost never necessary. A short course of oral antibiotics, such as erythromycin, can also be helpful.

Distinctive Exudative Discoid and Lichenoid Chronic Dermatitis

(Sulzberger and Garbe 1937)

Synonyms. Sulzberger-Garbe disease, oid-oid disease

Sulzberger and Garbe described a form of dermatitis whose existence as a clinical entity has remained controversial for the past 50 years. One thing is for certain: the first word of their title, distinctive, was poorly chosen. They identified an intensely pruritic dermatitis which involved middle-aged and elderly men with a striking Jewish predilection (bearing in mind that many of their patients were Jewish). The key point in Sulzberger's eyes as he defended his disease many years later was the presence of both exudative discoid lesions and lichenification, involving resolving plaques and as discrete papules. The most typical sites are the penis and scrotum which are not favorite sites for nummular dermatitis. The neck, axillae and flexural surfaces of the arms are also often affected. Microscopic examination fails to reveal any specific clues, other than the presence of occasional eosinophils. Both a chronic course and recurrences are to be expected. This disorder tends to be resistant to the topical measures discussed for nummular dermatitis and often requires a short course of systemic corticosteroids to break the cycle.

Atopy

Definition. Coca and Cooke first used the term atopy in 1923; it is derived from the Greek *a-* (no),

-top- (place), *-y* (-ness). Just as utopia means the perfect place, atopy is the woeful state, as many patients with atopic diseases can testify. Atopy is a condition in which the individual is predisposed towards developing allergic asthma, allergic rhinitis, allergic conjunctivitis and atopic dermatitis. For the balance of this chapter we will use the terms rhinitis, conjunctivitis and asthma without the adjective allergic; in reference to atopy, they are assumed to be allergic. Atopy predisposes the individual to the production of IgE antibodies which are specific for common aeroallergens (grass or tree pollens, house-dust mite, cat dander). These allergens differ from very potent allergens such as insect venom or penicillin which may readily provoke sensitization in nonpredisposed individuals. In addition, continued exposure to less-potent allergens may sensitize all individuals, including those without atopy. Atopy does not have to lead to atopic diseases. In many individuals there are only clinical stigmata such as hyperlinearity of the palms and soles or white dermographism. On the other hand, atopy is generally first diagnosed when atopic diseases are present, making atopy somewhat of a circular definition, but nonetheless a useful clinical concept.

Epidemiology

- Prevalence. Atopy is becoming more common. It is estimated that up to 20% of people in industrialized countries will suffer from some aspect of atopic diseases during their life. This number is clearly increasing.
- Age. In general, atopic dermatitis is more prominent in infancy, rhinitis and conjunctivitis dominate in childhood and young adult life, and later on asthma and skin problems once again become common. The clinical course is quite variable; not all patients develop both atopic dermatitis and allergic asthma or rhinitis. The initial appearance of atopic dermatitis or inhalant disease can occur at any age. Nonetheless, 70% of patients have some symptoms during the first 2 years of life, usually involving the skin.
- Sex. Women are affected more often than men.
- Race. All races are affected, but the disease is more common and severe in whites.
- Genetics. No single gene has been identified. There is a gene on chromosome 6 which seems to control IgE response and is perhaps the best candidate. The appearance of atopic dermatitis in monozygotic twins is over 75%. If one parent has atopy, a child's risk is about 25%. If both parents are atopics, the risk increases to over 50%. These numbers support polygenic inheritance.
- Geography. Atopic diseases seem to be more common in industrialized countries and in the upper social levels, although asthma in the USA has shown an alarming increase in ghetto children, perhaps related to exposure to cockroach particles. Various features of modern life (heating, pets, indoor allergens, diet, hygiene and pollution) probably all play a role in the increase in atopic diseases.

Etiology and Pathogenesis. The immunologic reaction in atopy is a prototype for the type I reaction of Gell and Coombs. Specific IgE antibodies known as reagins or reaginic antibodies are formed against a wide variety of primarily environmental allergens (Table 12.14). These antibodies are bound to mast cells or basophils. There are several types of IgE-binding receptors. The major one on mast cells is the high-affinity IgE receptor $FC_{\varepsilon}R$ I. This receptor is identical to CD23 which regulates B cell differentiation. Two other receptors have been identified in a variety of cells including epidermal Langerhans cells. They are the low-affinity IgE receptor ($FC_{\varepsilon}R$ II) and IgE-binding protein (EBP). The specific IgE molecules bind to the mast cells via their Fc portion and the receptor; when they contact an allergen, adjacent molecules are connected or bridged, triggering a cascade of immunologic events.

Mast cells contain a long list of mediators, both preformed and nonstored. The preformed materials include inflammatory mediators such as histamine, heparin, tumor necrosis factor (TNF)-α, chemotactic agents such as eosinophil chemotactic factor, neutrophil chemotactic factor and many other enzymes. The mediators that are formed after stimulation include lipid-derived substances such as the prostaglandins, leukotrienes and platelet-activating factor, as well as a long list of cytokines such as interleukin (IL)-1, IL-3, IL-4, IL-5, IL-6 and

Table 12.14. Common allergens in atopy

Pollens (trees, grasses, weeds)
House dust mites
Animal dander or epithelial debris, especially from cats and dogs
Natural rubber latex
Weeping fig
Mold spores
Insect body parts, e.g., cockroaches

granulocyte/macrophage colony-stimulating factor (GM-CSF). As a result of this massive inflammatory cascade, inflammatory cells are recruited into the tissue, vascular permeability is increased and smooth muscle is constricted, along with many other effects.

The site of interaction of the allergen with mast cells determines the clinical problems. Allergic rhinitis (hay fever) and allergic conjunctivitis are prototypes of an immediate hypersensitivity, almost always allergen-related. Asthma may be predominantly allergic, but in the majority of patients, other factors also play a role. Unfortunately, the fourth member of the triad, atopic dermatitis, does not fit the picture so nicely. While the skin can react acutely with urticarial lesions following allergen exposure, most aspects of atopic dermatitis do not fit with immediate hypersensitivity.

Atopy tends to run in families and appears to be inherited in a polygenic fashion. In any event, up until now, no single locus for atopy has been identified. Certain HLA patterns have been identified, but the relative risk is not as striking as it is for dermatitis herpetiformis or similar disorders. In addition, environmental factors play a major role, as do stress and other emotional problems. One can best view a patient with atopy as a hyperreactor, perhaps because of a greater ability to release immunologic mediators (or a lesser ability to control their release). Many possible defects in the regulatory control have been investigated. For example, certain HLA class II molecules may preferentially bind various allergens, explaining the predisposition to reactivity. Another feature is alterations in the ratios and functions of the two main types of T helper cells, TH1 and TH2 cells. Under normal circumstances, TH1 cells produce IL-2, interferon (IFN)-γ and TNF-β, all of which support cell-mediated delayed hypersensitivity and are part of the usual response to intracellular pathogens and haptens. In contrast TH2 cells release IL-4, IL-5, IL-6, IL-9, IL-10, IL-13, all of which play a major role in B cell regulation and the response to extracellular pathogens such as parasites.

Many factors also point to a possible pathogenic role for IgE. Serum levels are usually raised and correlate with the severity and stage of the atopy. Nonaffected atopic skin has increased tissue IgE levels which are even higher in affected skin. The IgE molecules are specific for aeroallergens and bacterial superantigens in most cases. The role of eosinophils in the latter response is well known; IL-5 plays an important role in directing their trafficking. Patients with atopy have a relative predominance of TH2 cells, even in situations where TH1 would be more appropriate. For example, normal individuals usually do not mount an IgE response to aeroallergens, as do atopics. IL-4 appears potentially most important because of its autoregulatory role, as it further inhibits proliferation of $TH1_1$ cells. In addition, it increases IgE production, even converting IgM-producing cells to switch to IgE production. Not surprisingly, attempts to block IL-4 appear to be a promising early therapy for atopy.

Clinical Findings. Patients may present with any one of the four cardinal features of atopy, or with a variety of relatively specific stigmata. Often one family member may have one constellation (asthma and hay fever) while another has a different pattern (just atopic dermatitis). A child may have severe atopic dermatitis but as an adult only suffer from hay fever or have no atopic disease at all. Dermatologists in many countries do not treat pollen allergies and asthma, but it is essential to at least inquire about their presence.

Laboratory Findings. The diagnostic approach to atopy takes many forms. They include:

Skin Tests. In order to evaluate allergic causes of atopic diseases, a series of skin test procedures can be utilized. Standard series with common aeroallergen and food allergens are employed. If available, standardized commercial test solutions are the agents of choice for testing. Some institutions are very experienced in producing their own special safe standardized test solutions. Local regulatory guidelines should be observed when using self-made test materials in patients. We recommend skin prick tests with native material only if commercial test solutions are not available or if tests with these materials do not elicit positive test reactions in the patients despite clinical suspicion. If a nonstandardized material elicits a skin test reaction, we try to perform control tests in ten healthy volunteers. If more than two of the ten volunteers react in a similar way, the response can be regarded as nonspecific.

Patients with atopic diseases tend to exhibit sensitization to a broad array of aero- and food allergens. Not every skin reaction is clinically relevant, or it may help explain inhalant disease but be without significance for atopic dermatitis. On the other hand, patients with a clinical hypersensitivity reaction may not show sensitization to the causative allergen. The interpretation of such skin tests requires considerable medical skills. Besides skin testing and in vitro testing, a careful history, temporary avoidance of all allergens (for example via dietary restriction) and challenge tests are the mainstay of the allergy evaluation of affected patients.

Skin tests should be performed under precautionary conditions, including treatment of underlying asthma, discontinuation of β-blockers, threshold testing of suspected allergens and insertion of an intravenous line prior to testing allergens which are likely to cause anaphylactic reactions. Even with these measures, anaphylactic reactions may occur, so one should not undertake prick testing without being fully prepared to treat this medical emergency.

Skin tests are not reliable when the patient is taking corticosteroids or antihistamines which may block the reaction. Depending on the dose and duration of the corticosteroids, as well as the pharmacologic properties of the antihistamines, the patient should have discontinued these drugs for 1–6 weeks. Other systemic or topical medications may have similar effects. In addition, the skin lesions in patients with atopic dermatitis should be clear prior to skin testing. In patients who continue to require therapy, one can still attempt to do skin testing. If positive reactions occur, they may aid in making the diagnosis; if no reactions occurs, testing can be repeated later. Several different forms of skin testing can be used, varying the amount of exposure the patient receives.

Rub Test. In the case of potent, highly suspect allergens, the material (native substance or commercial test solution) can first be rubbed into the skin. A positive test occurs when urticarial lesions are found after 15–20 min, and application of an inert material does not elicit a similar reaction.

Prick Test. A drop of solution containing the allergen is placed on the skin and then a lancet is used to prick the epidermis, ideally without injury to dermal vessels (Fig. 12.28 a, b). Usually the forearm is the test site. Up to 40 substances can be tested on both arms. After 15–20 min, the test solutions are removed and the reactions are read. A positive reaction is a wheal with a diameter ≥2 mm and/or an erythema with a diameter ≥3 mm. We use histamine and physiologic saline as positive and negative controls. On occasion, late-phase reactions may occur 24–48 h after prick testing. Thus we ask the patient not to remove the skin test markings during this time period and to present again for a second reading if a late reaction does occur.

Scratch Test. In this variant, the skin is scratched, once again attempting not to cause bleeding, and then a drop of the test solution applied. The reading process is similar to a prick test, but nonspecific reactions may reduce the reliability of the scratch test. In addition, the risk of anaphylaxis is a little higher since more material is introduced. We do not recommend the scratch test.

Intradermal Test. In this form 0.03–0.05 ml of a sterile test solution are injected into the uppermost dermis (Fig. 12.28 c). Codeine and physiologic saline serve as control agents. Despite the dilution, the allergen concentration is 100–1000-fold higher than with prick testing and the risk of a systemic allergic reaction is greater. We recommend intradermal tests only if skin prick tests are negative.

Atopy Patch Test. Here aeroallergens are used for patch testing. A positive reaction site often resembles atopic dermatitis. The clinical relevance of this new approach is still being defined.

IgE Levels. Usually the PRIST (paper-radioimmunosorbent test) is used to determine the total serum IgE value. While an elevated serum IgE level cannot be used to diagnose atopic disease, it is frequently helpful. Normal levels vary with age but are usually less than 50 IU/ml; values >100 support the diagnosis of atopic disease, while those >1000 suggest the diagnosis. Patients with atopic dermatitis are more likely to have such levels than those with other forms of atopic disease.

In Vitro Testing. The basis of in vitro testing is the identification of specific IgE molecules directed against various allergens. The great advantage of in vitro testing is that it can be performed despite treatment with corticosteroids or antihistamines, or when the patient's skin condition or other medical problems point against skin testing. Interpretation of the test results must consider sensitization without clinical relevance (false-positive reaction) as well as clinically relevant allergy without sensitization (false-negative reaction) which may rarely occur in patients with atopic disease. False-negative tests are especially likely when IgG antibodies serve as blocking agents.

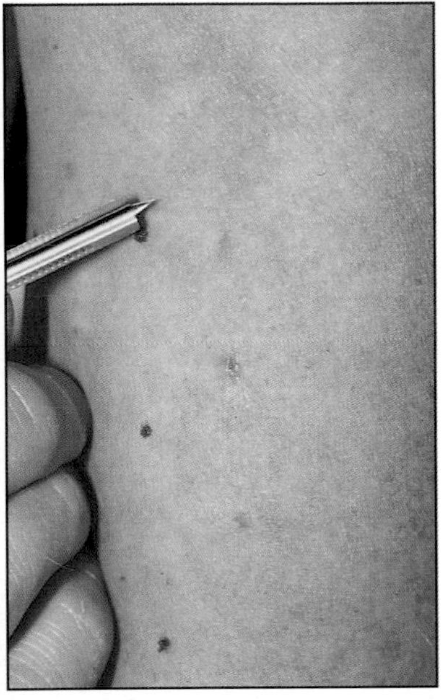
a

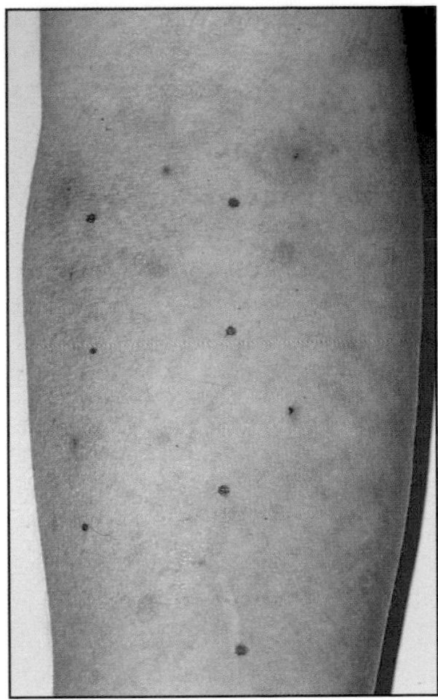
b

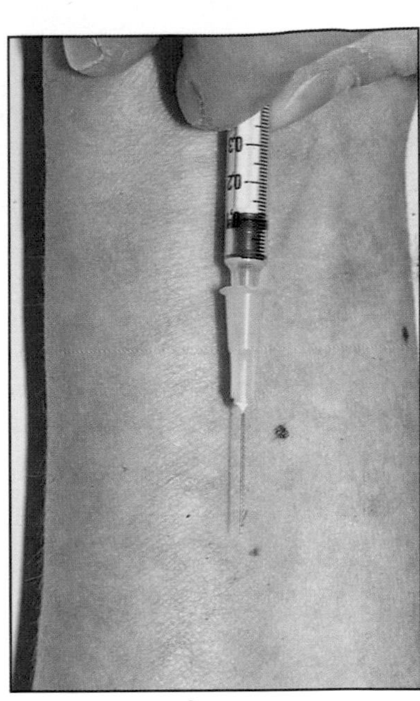
c

Fig. 12.28 a–c. Prick testing. **a** A lancet is used to prick the skin though the test material. **b** Several erythematous urticarial positive reactions are seen. **c** An intradermal test is demonstrated

ELISA. Various methods are available, either produced commercially or by experienced laboratories. All function on the same principle. Allergens are bound to paper discs or similar materials. The best known technique is RAST (radioallergosorbent test). When the patient's serum is added, allergen-specific IgE binds to the allergen epitopes. This bound antibody can be identified by a marker binding to the patient's IgE. Positive reactions can be quantified. Many different allergens are available, including pollens, house-dust mites, animal danders, natural rubber latex, weeping fig, molds, yeasts, insect toxins, penicillin and food allergens.

When a patient has high levels of IgE against specific allergens, these substances are likely to be provocative factors for atopic disease. In the situation where a major fraction of the total IgE is directed against a single allergen, this product is extremely likely to be clinically significant.

Other Tests. Research laboratories may study basophil release of histamine following allergen stimulation, immunoblotting to identify IgE binding to specific antigen epitopes, lymphocyte stimulation and many other procedures. All are of practical importance only if standardized and if the results are interpreted cautiously with respect to the patient's disease.

Provocation Tests. Allergens can be introduced in many ways. Tests should be done where emergency help is available. Food allergens can be tested by ingestion. Many studies have shown that double-blind, placebo-controlled studies are needed to reliably identify the rare patient with a true food allergy. Even in children where the parents and the physician are totally convinced that a food allergy is present, often a controlled study shows no reaction. The nasal mucosa can also be tested with allergens, as can the bronchi via an inhalation test. In the former case, mucosa swelling is measured, while in the latter various parameters of pulmonary function are studied.

Therapy. Therapy is discussed under the various disorders that make up atopy.

Inhalant Allergies

Synonyms. Rhinitis, conjunctivitis, asthma and related terms

Epidemiology. Inhalant allergies most commonly start in childhood or early adolescence. They are usually seasonal, occurring when a given tree, grass or weed is in action. For example, in the Midwest of the USA the biggest culprit is ragweed, blooming in late summer and causing misery up to the first frost. In Germany, the main allergens are hazelnut and alder in February and March, other trees including birch and poplar in April and the grasses in May and June. Typically the symptoms occur at about the same time each year, except when there has been a very mild or severe winter, altering nature's calendar. Some patients may suffer from allergy to various pollens, animal danders and house-dust mite and will develop symptoms throughout the entire year with seasonal peaks. Up to 25% of the patients with rhinitis or conjunctivitis will later develop asthma. In other patients remission of allergic symptoms occurs spontaneously.

Etiology and Pathogenesis. Very small amounts of allergen are sufficient to cause problems. For example, one study has suggested that 10–50 particles of pollen in 1 m^3 of air are sufficient. In most big cities, daily pollen counts are available. The nature of the immunologic reaction is considered under atopy.

Clinical Findings. The clinical findings vary with the site of action. They include:

Rhinitis or Hay Fever. Here the problems are sneezing, a marked increase in handkerchief use and impaired nasal breathing. Some patients present flu-like symptoms. Sometimes associated sinusitis develops.

Conjunctivitis. The eyes are red, swollen and intensely pruritic.

Pharyngitis. There may be a dry feeling in the back of mouth, sometimes associated with a disturbing itch and tiny hemorrhages. Postnasal drip from associated rhinitis complicates the problem.

Vulvitis. The vulval mucosa can also be exposed to pollens, such as when a small girl is playing in the fields and pollen finds its way into her underwear. One must be aware of the rare possibility in order to avoid suggesting child abuse.

Asthma. Attacks of asthma certainly can be triggered by allergens, although often there is no evidence of atopy, especially in those patients developing asthma for the first time in middle age or late adult life.

Food Allergy to Cross-reacting Allergens. Many food allergies in adults are acquired primarily by inhalant sensitization to aeroallergens. Allergic epitopes are located not only on pollen but also on fruit, nuts or vegetables. A botanical relationship between cross-reacting airborne and food allergens is not the rule. Ingestion of the respective food may cause a variety of symptoms including oral contact urticaria, rhinitis, conjunctivitis, asthma, abdominal complaints or even anaphylactic shock. Two typical examples seen in Germany are:

- Mugwort: celery
- Natural rubber latex: avocado, banana

Laboratory Findings. The dermatologist is Germany is often involved in the diagnosis of pollen allergy, performing prick tests and in vitro tests in an office laboratory.

Diagnostic Criteria. It is crucial to first take an accurate history and correlate the patient's problem with clinical findings and possible exposure to allergens. One should have a working diagnosis before starting prick testing. Most atopics react to a number of allergens and one must be a good detective to find out which one is relevant.

Differential Diagnosis. The differential diagnosis of these problem is beyond our scope. One must exclude infectious causes and medication-induced reactions, working along with an otorhinolaryngologist, ophthalmologist or pulmonary specialist.

Therapy. The mainstay of therapy is avoidance of allergens. Unfortunately this is usually quite difficult and only possible when dealing with indoor allergens. The most useful medications are systemic antihistamines, especially the nonsedating, once-daily varieties. Topical antihistamine eye and nose drops are also available. In addition topical mast cell-stabilizing agents such as the cromoglycates and corticosteroids are useful for rhinitis and conjunctivitis and via inhalers for asthma. A variety of leukotriene inhibitors are already in use for asthma. Patients have generally already tried the over-the-counter vasoconstrictor agents in the form of nose and eye drops.

Many dermatologists in Europe are involved in hyposensitization for inhalant allergies. In general, a patient should meet the following criteria:

- A well-defined allergy to one or a limited number of allergens
- Failure to achieve control with standard measures
- No contraindications

The patient must be aware that immunotherapy may not always cure symptoms completely and that additional symptomatic measures may be required. In addition to a clinical sense of improvement, patients may require fewer medications following desensitization or become less likely to develop asthma, even if their rhinitis or conjunctivitis does not entirely disappear. A very small number of patients experience severe anaphylactic attacks during hyposensitization and rarely a fatal reaction occurs.

Atopic Dermatitis

(WILLAN 1808)

Synonyms. Atopic eczema, endogenous eczema, eczema (in the USA, when a patient says eczema, they mean atopic dermatitis), neurodermatitis, neurodermitis (widely used in Europe), neurodermitis atopica. Suffice to say, we dermatologists will never agree on the best term for this disorder or on a suitable definition, as all these names make clear. Atopic dermatitis is that dermatitis associated with atopy; to go further requires a linguist.

Definition. Chronic usually pruritic and clinically variable skin disease associated with atopy.

Epidemiology. Atopic dermatitis and rhinitis are probably the two most common manifestations of atopy. The incidence of atopic dermatitis has increased dramatically in recent years. Prevalence rates of 1–30% have been found in a recent international study. In industrialized countries the rate is 5% (1–12%) in children. Over 50% have problems in the first year and over 90% before 5 years of age. In 60–70% of patients there is a positive family history of atopy. About 10–15% of the children have persistent problems after puberty and about the same percentage, but not the same individuals develop asthma.

Etiology and Pathogenesis. The overall immune mechanisms have been discussed above under atopy. The puzzle is why atopy – the prototypic immediate hypersensitivity disorder – is such a chronic disorder in the skin. Probably a number of exogenous and endogenous factors interact with the basic immunologic process to produce the final cutaneous disease (Fig. 12.29).

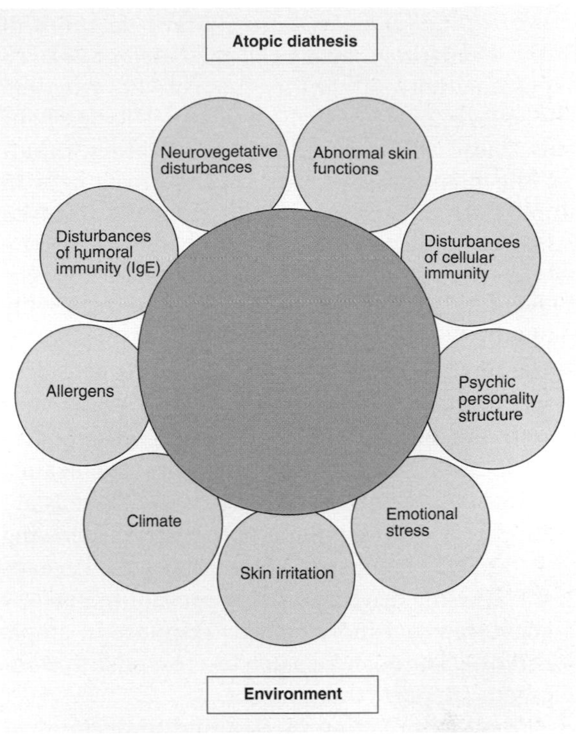

Fig. 12.29. Multifactorial pathogenesis of atopic dermatitis

Disturbed Humoral Immunity. As mentioned under atopy, there is a relative imbalance between $TH1_1$ and $TH21_2$ cells, leading to the overproduction of IL-4 which tends to favor immediate hypersensitivity. Early in life atopic patients develop immediate hypersensitivity to environmental materials which normally do not function as allergens. They have elevated levels of IgE directed against these specific allergens, and the excess IgE can be found in the skin. Sometimes the flares of atopic dermatitis correlate with other seasonal allergies, although more often they do not. Infants and children with atopic dermatitis may have food allergies, or at least positive prick or in vitro reactions against milk, eggs, fish, grains, and selected fruits and vegetables. Many mothers are relatively certain that their child's dermatitis worsens following a given food ingestion, even though this can be very hard to scientifically document. Studies have shown that among infants of atopic parents, fewer problems develop when the children are breast-fed for the first 6–9 months, supporting the role of cows' milk as an allergen. The aeroallergens can also play a role as surface allergens in airborne dermatitis caused by pollen or animal dander.

Disturbed Cellular Immunity. Many features of atopic dermatitis reflect a cell-mediated or delayed hypersensitivity, rather than an acute IgE reaction. The answer may lie in the epidermal Langerhans cells. These cells carry all the IgE receptors including the high affinity $FC_{\varepsilon}R$ I. Langerhans cells in atopic dermatitis, especially in clinically involved skin, have higher levels of $FC_{E}R$ I than normal skin; this feature can be used in the diagnosis. Thus the relevant IgE can bind to airborne or externally applied allergens, as well as to those present in the circulation. These antigen-presenting cells then move to the regional lymph nodes where they present the antigens. The Langerhans cells are able to induce $TH2_2$ cells which are directed against the stimulating antigen. More generic Th cells are usually TH1-type even in atopic patients, showing that the TH2 response is allergen-specific. Perhaps in this way, the drive towards IgE response in atopy is converted to a more cellular response in atopic dermatitis. The positive patch test response to aeroallergens supports this concept.

The overproduction of IL-4 and underproduction of IFN-γ also play a role here. IFN-γ is essential for the development of an appropriate cell-mediated response. Its underproduction may be critical. In addition, the $TH2_2$ cells secrete IL-5 which may help explain the elevated eosinophil levels and the presence of eosinophil basic protein in atopic skin, even when tissue eosinophilia is not marked.

Another possible mechanism would incorporate the clinical observation that breast-feeding reduces the incidence of atopic diseases. Atopic infants have a relative defect in secretory IgA which may favor the development of an IgE response, which then is not effectively controlled because of a lack of suppressor T cells. One example of this is the tendency of patients to develop more frequent and often more severe bacterial and viral infections. Many measures of delayed hypersensitivity are reduced, such as reduced T cell response to mitogens, reduced lymphocyte transformation test to viral antigens, reduced natural killer cell activity and a lower likelihood of developing allergic contact dermatitis in the experimental setting. In clinical practice, atopics often have more positive patch tests, but this presumably reflects their exposure to so many contact allergens through use of multiple topical agents.

Vascular Reactions. White dermographism is a hallmark of atopic dermatitis. When the skin is rubbed or scratched, vasoconstriction rather than vasodilatation occurs. Similarly, topical nicotinic acid esters when applied to normal skin produce erythema but they produce blanching in atopic dermatitis patients. Furthermore, injection of cholinergic agents such as acetylcholine produces blanching, not the normal erythema. Clinically these paradoxical responses may be manifest as lower digital temperatures or marked vasoconstriction when exposed to cold.

Szentivanyi (1968) proposed the β-adrenergic blockade theory of atopy. The blocked β receptors lead to increased α-adrenergic responsiveness, such as increased smooth muscle sensitivity. In addition, the increased sweat response of atopics to cholinergic agents would fit into this schema. Lichenification or epidermal response to trauma may also be enhanced by a reduced β-adrenergic response. Taking this theory further, perturbations in the balance between cAMP and cGMP have been postulated to explain the humoral perturbations seen in atopic dermatitis. cAMP does not rise in atopic leukocytes which are stimulated with histamine or prostaglandins, so perhaps these agents, once released by an IgE-mediated reaction, are not as well modulated in the atopic patient as in the normal individual.

Pruritus. Atopic dermatitis patients have one huge problem – pruritus. Some have even suggested that all the clinical features in the skin can be explained by the patients rubbing and scratching their skin in response to uncontrollable pruritus. The pruritus is more than a simple histamine-related phenomenon because antihistamines are relatively ineffective. Patients also have marked pruritus when exposed to wool. One idea is that atopics have a lowered pruritus threshold, but no one has figured out how to raise it. This fits in nicely with the alternative name of neurodermatitis.

Dry Skin. If one asks a group of adults about the need to frequently lubricate their skin, one can fairly reliably select out the atopics. They have very dry skin, often made worse by almost any cleansing agent or even just frequent exposure to water. Defects in the epidermal lipid film have been identified, especially in deficiencies in ceramides and a lack of δ-6-desaturase, thus causing epidermal barrier perturbation. The problem appears to be more than simply a mechanical defect in the film. One school of thought suggests that the defects in lipid synthesis lead to both altered prostaglandin, thromboxane and leukotriene synthesis as well as other immunologic abnormalities. Some patients respond to γ-linolenic acid which modulates the ω-6-fatty acid metabolism, offering some support for this hypothesis.

Abnormal Sweating. Almost every atopic dermatitis patient will complain that excessive sweating causes pruritus. Atopics sweat less than normal individuals and tend to avoid thermal stimuli such as a sauna. The mechanisms are unknown. One suggestion is that the abnormal stratum corneum inhibits the escape of sweat and that the retained sweat elicits an inflammatory response. Sweat also contains IgE and other mediators so it may cause urticarial lesions and erythema.

Bacterial Infections. It has long been known that atopic skin is more easily colonized by bacteria, usually *Staphylococcus aureus*. The bacterial super antigens are one trigger of the specific $TH2_2$ response discussed above. In addition, in some instances topical or systemic antibiotics produce a prompt improvement in atopic dermatitis.

Emotional Factors. There is no question that atopic dermatitis can appear or worsen when a patient is under emotional stress. Conversely, supportive psychological therapy can help many patients. But it is very difficult to explain the exact connections between CNS biochemical processes and the changes in the skin. An infant or child who is always itching and often sick may miss school or suffer from over-attentive parenting. Personality studies done later may reveal a variety of traits but it is not reasonable to say all of them are primary to the atopic patient; they may be epiphenomena.

Clinical Findings. Atopic dermatitis has a host of clinical features, varying greatly with the age of the patient. In young patients, the changes are quite acute, with erythema, blisters and crusts common. Later on, more chronic changes, include lichenification and prurigo papules, dominate the picture. The one constant appears to be pruritus with excoriations. Perhaps the acute reaction is more related to the initial IgE response while the later changes reflect the increasing dysfunction of cellular immunity.

Atopic Dermatitis in Infancy. As much as 80% of all dermatitis in infancy is an early manifestation of atopy. Problems usually start around the third month and male infants are more often affected than females, although later on, more women are involved. The early lesions usually are found on the lateral parts of cheeks and the scalp. Circumscribed erythematous patches, often evolving into papulovesicular plaques, are seen. They are intensely pruritic, soon damaged by excoriations, covered with crusts and often secondarily infected (Fig. 12.30). In German-speaking countries this exudative phase is known as *Milchschorf* (milk scale) because the rash is scaly, crusted and resembles burnt milk (Fig. 12.31). This extensive scalp crusting was formerly equated with seborrheic dermatitis but long-term studies have shown that far more infants with severe scalp dermatitis have atopic dermatitis.

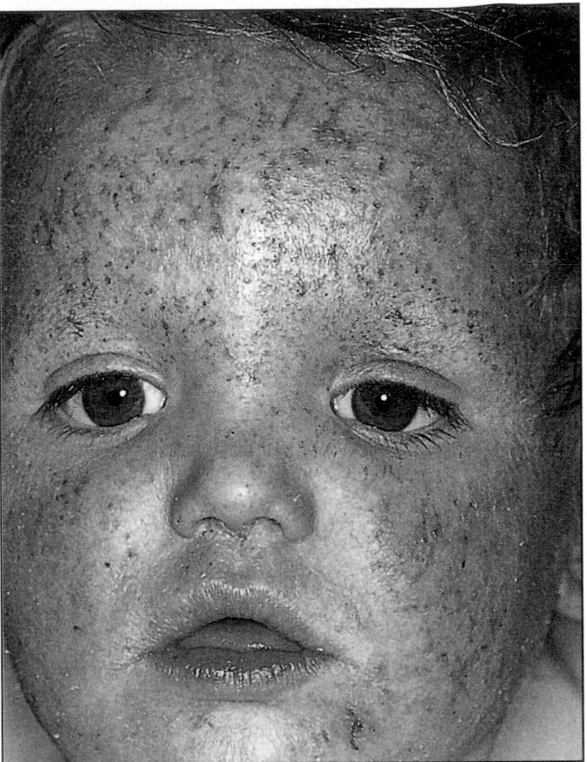

Fig. 12.30. Excoriated atopic dermatitis in an infant

The rash typically lasts for several months to years. The entire scalp and face may be covered and pruritic erythematous patches may develop on other areas. During the crawling stage the knees are at particular risk. Typically the extensor surfaces of the extremities are more involved than the flexor aspects, and often the diaper area is spared. The children often are whiners and have trouble sleeping because of the pruritus. About 50% clear by the end of 2 years.

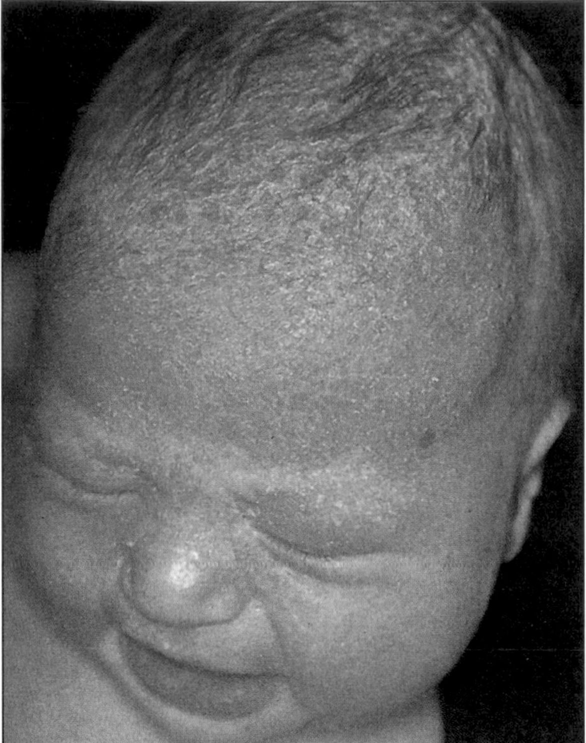

Fig. 12.31. Scalp scaling in infantile atopic dermatitis

Atopic Dermatitis in Childhood. Young children may develop these manifestations as sequelae to the exudative infantile form or de novo. Curiously, the skin tends to be dry rather than exudative and the predilection sites are the flexural areas – the antecubital and popliteal fossae and the dorsal aspects of the hands and feet (Fig. 12.32). A typical site is the skin on the dorsal aspect of the wrist. Other common areas of involvement include the nape, cheeks and eyelids. In German-speaking countries this stage was known as *Beugenekzem* or flexural eczema. The lesions are typically symmetric, irregularly bordered erythematous papules with excoriations, small crusts and then an inflammatory infiltrate and lichenification. The flexural areas almost always evolve into lichenoid papules, while the hands, for example, tend to be more exudative. Involvement of the nailfolds may produce an onychodystrophy. Localized moisture plays more of a role in this stage. Thumb-suckers often develop an exaggerated thumb dermatitis. Children playing in water in the summer often develop a one-hand dermatitis on their dominant hand. Atopic cheilitis secondary to lip licking is also common.

Atopic Dermatitis in Adolescents and Adults. In the older patients, the rash is once again symmetric but shifts its points of attack. The eyelids, forehead, perioral region, nape, neck, upper chest and shoulder girdle, flexural fossae and dorsal aspects hands are the classic sites (Fig. 12.33). The skin is diffusely dry. The mid-face is often pale, perhaps from vasoconstriction, just as the fingers occasionally are. On the face, the typical scenario is the sudden appearance of red patches, often following emotional stress, which do not usually lichenify. The skin acquires a gray-yellow color making the patient appear older and sadder. The most striking lichenification occurs in the flexural areas, backs of the hands and nape. The skin is diffusely red, thickened, with prominent skin markings and scales. The changes merge imperceptibly into the normal skin. While the argument has been made that lichenification is a direct result of rubbing and scratching, in some patients one can identify the pruritic lichenoid papules that also typify atopic dermatitis. On the trunk, larger patches evolve and often merge together.

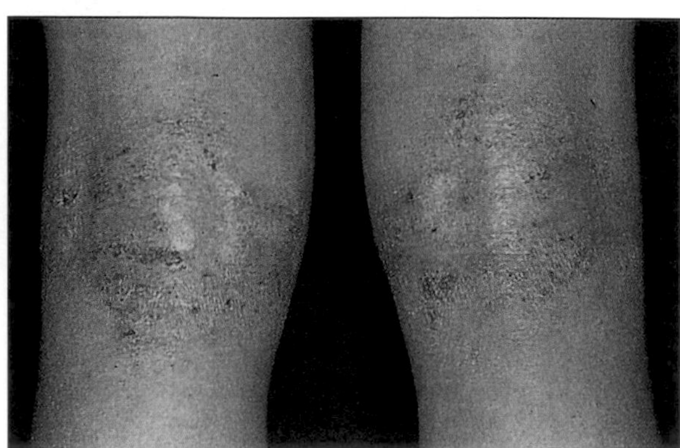

Fig. 12.32. Flexural involvement in atopic dermatitis

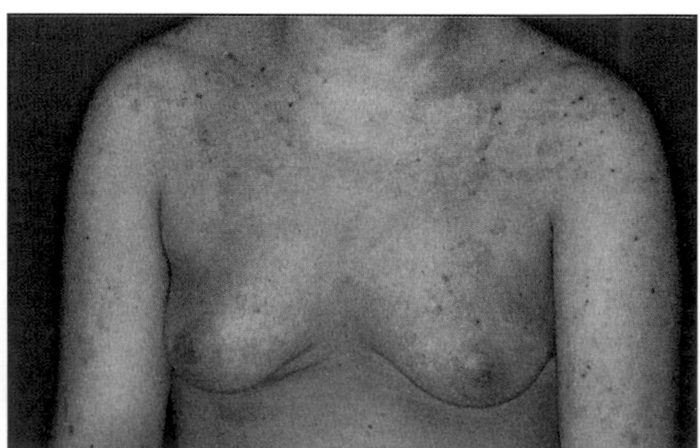

Fig. 12.33. Chronic atopic dermatitis in an adult

Postinflammatory hyperpigmentation is common. It is most frequently seen about the eyes (raccoon sign), often associated with increased skinfolds. On the sides of the neck, it may have a gray-brown reticular pattern (dirty neck sign). This may be a variant of macular amyloidosus, reflecting trauma and perhaps photodamage. In the late summer, when other areas are tanned, resolved patches of atopic dermatitis may be hypopigmented (pityriasis alba).

Pruritus is another unifying feature of adult atopic dermatitis. Patients often complain of being unable to sleep, relax or concentrate on work. Overwhelming attacks of pruritus may come on suddenly without warning, leading to incessant scratching. Patients' fingernails may be rubbed smooth (polished nail sign). Excoriations with hemorrhage and crusts are common.

When the disease is widespread and especially when bacterial secondary infections have been a problem, secondary or dermatopathic lymphadenopathy may develop. This can lead to diagnostic problems, as a common differential diagnostic challenge is distinguishing severe atopic dermatitis from Sézary syndrome.

Special Variants of Atopic Dermatitis. In adults there are many more subtle manifestations that often are not diagnosed as atopic dermatitis. The findings vary greatly from site to site and a given patient may only have one or two stigmata.

Scalp. Tiny hemorrhagic crusts associated with excoriations were formerly known as neurotic excoriations or acne necroticans miliaris capitis; they are simply scratched papules. The presence of pityriasiform scale and fine, thinned hair is also a possible clue. Often the hair line extends further down the forehead in atopic children. This change may represent a subtle form of traumatic hypertrichosis. In addition, there may be bilateral temporal thinning. Atopic scalp disease in the absence of clear cut signs of atopic dermatitis elsewhere is uncommon, so it can usually be easily separated from seborrheic dermatitis.

Eyelids. Many patients, usually women, present with recurrent eyelid dermatitis. Because the skin is so thin, swelling and lichenification occur relatively quickly. While some patients have allergic contact dermatitis, most are simply older atopics.

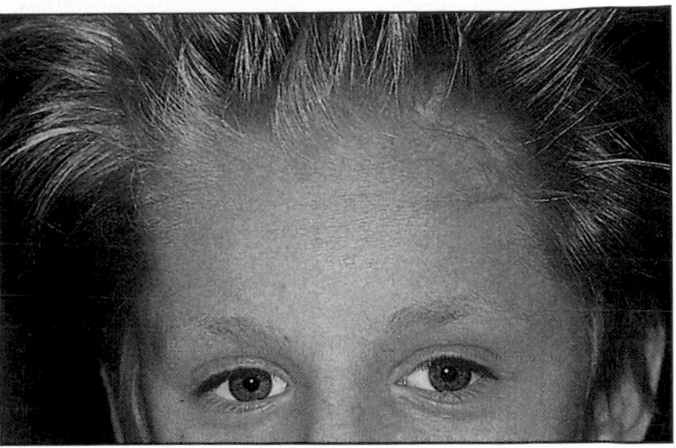

Fig. 12.34. Child with prominent Dennie-Morgan lines and Hertoghe sign

Periorbital Skin. A classic sign of atopic dermatitis is the exaggeration of the infraorbital folds or pleats (Dennie-Morgan sign in USA). Patients tend to have more than one fold, especially at an early age (Fig. 12.34). The sign is present in perhaps 70 % of atopic children, but is harder to use in adults and is present in a fair percentage of normal children, especially blacks. A related sign may be the nasal crease or saluter's sign. Some patients have a transverse fold on their nose, allegedly from repeatedly pushing their nose when rubbing and wiping during attacks of rhinitis. This must be separated from the congenital transverse nasal fold (Chap. 19). The lateral aspects of the eyebrows are often missing or sparse, perhaps from rubbing (Hertoghe sign).

Nape. Some patients clear everywhere else but have persistent nape lichenification. When it is localized, the diagnosis is lichen simplex chronicus but when it is more diffuse, the answer is usually atopic dermatitis. Some believe *Pityrosporum ovale (Malassezia furfur)* plays a role in atopic scalp and nape dermatitis. Imidazole creams and shampoos are often helpful, supporting this concept.

Earlobes. The lower attachment of the ear lobe to the neck may be inflamed and fissured. Sometimes crusting is present. In addition, there may be retroauricular erythema and crusting.

Lips. The lips give many clues to atopic dermatitis. Usually they are dry and scaly (cheilitis sicca), especially in the winter. Typical is a deep fissure in the center of the lower lip. The resulting lip licking leads to an inflammation of the adjacent skin. Infants and children may suck their lower lip,

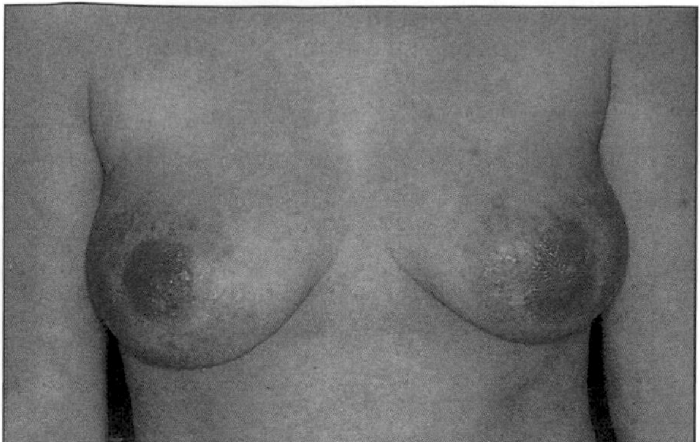

Fig. 12.35. Nipple dermatitis in atopic dermatitis

producing inflammation in a U-shaped pattern which is exactly covered by the upper anterior teeth when the patient is asked to bite their lower lip. Angular cheilitis or perlèche is also part of the clinical picture.

Nipples. Bilateral nipple dermatitis is usually atopic dermatitis. The lesions are usually fairly chronic (Fig. 12.35). Paget disease is almost never bilateral. The nipples are surprisingly resistant to allergic contact dermatitis.

Vulva. Lichenified atopic dermatitis of the vulva is very common in adult women. In our experience it is the most frequent form of vulvar dermatitis. The characteristic feature is marked lichenification leading to hypertrophy of the labia majora and extroversion of the labia minora, which tend to lose their mucosal characteristics (Fig. 12.36). Allergic contact dermatitis is a frequent sequel, as the desperate patients try many topical agents.

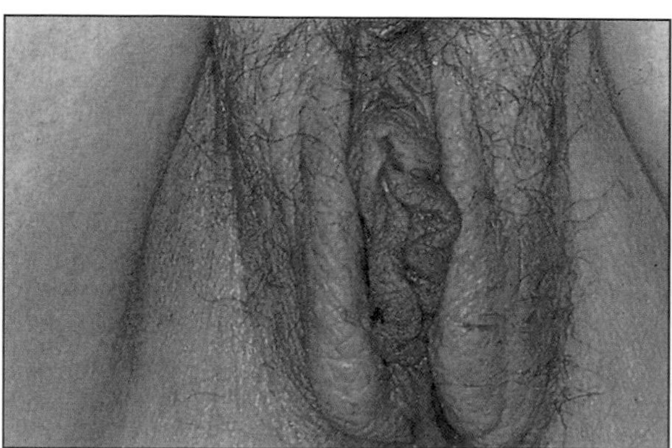

Fig. 12.36. Chronic lichenified vulvar dermatitis in atopic dermatitis

Hands. The hands pose a particular problem in atopic dermatitis. The classic picture is lichenification on the back of the wrists. Even well into adult life, this area may show flares of weeping and crusting. In other patients, the only stigma is localized often arcuate lichenified plaques with crusts, which clinically resemble nummular dermatitis. While it is a matter of terminology, we diagnose nummular atopic dermatitis if other stigmata of atopic dermatitis are presence and if the hands are favored. A bigger problem is the relationship of atopic dermatitis to chronic irritant hand dermatitis. It is estimated that 20–30% of hand dermatitis develops in atopic patients. Individuals who must frequently cleanse their hands are at greatest risk. The backs of the fingers and hands are usually red, crusted and fissured. Before one diagnoses chronic irritant hand dermatitis solely as an occupational disorder, one must pursue the possibility of atopic dermatitis, which in most cases would have existed prior to occupational problems. In addition, an allergic contact dermatitis must be excluded.

Palms. Hyperlinear palms or ichthyosis hands are present in a good percentage of atopic patients (Fig. 12.37). In addition these patients have dry skin. The

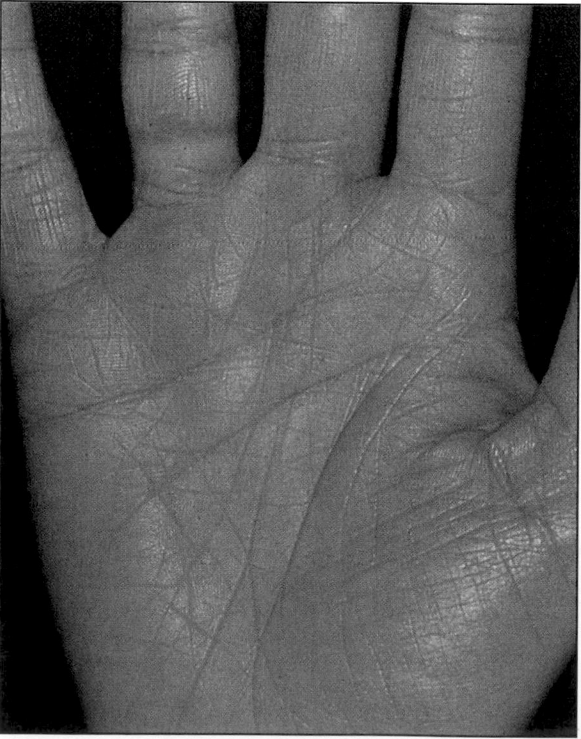

Fig. 12.37. Hyperlinear palms or ichthyosis hand in atopic dermatitis

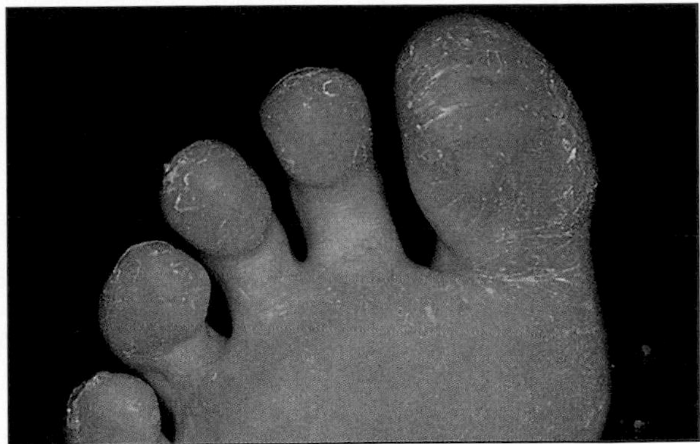

Fig. 12.38. Pulpitis sicca in atopic dermatitis

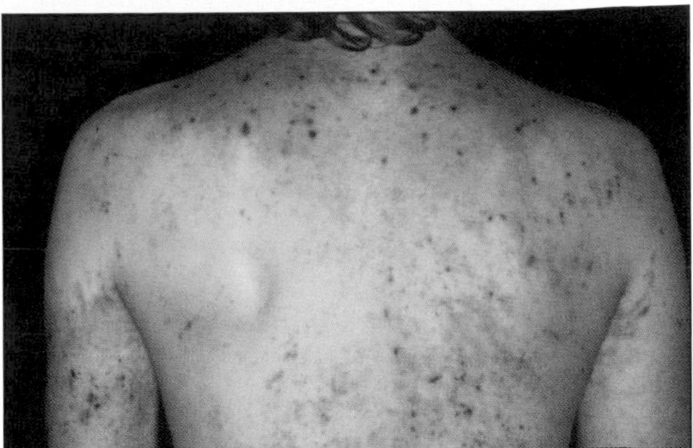

Fig. 12.39. Prurigo nodules in adult with atopic dermatitis

overlap between atopic dermatitis and ichthyosis vulgaris is discussed in Chap. 17. It has been suggested that 20–30% of atopic dermatitis patients have ichthyosis vulgaris; we are skeptical, and await with interest a specific genetic marker for ichthyosis vulgaris which could answer this question. We suspect that a high percentage of ichthyosis vulgaris patients may have atopy, but that a much lower percentage of atopy patients have true ichthyosis vulgaris. In both diseases the palms are similar with an increased number of creases and fine scale.

Fingers and Toes. The Latin term *pulpitis sicca* is not used much in English-speaking countries but it accurately describes the situation: dry skin over the tips (pulpa or ventral surface of the terminal phalanx) of the fingers and toes. Children are most often affected; they have erythematous digital tips, often with reduced skin markings and fine adherent scale (Fig. 12.38). Inexperienced observers often diagnose this as a dermatophyte infection, hence the term pseudomycosis. Onychodystrophy and secondary bacterial paronychiae may also be seen. In older patients, the relationship between atopic dermatitis and dyshidrotic dermatitis is often discussed. We view atopy as one of the predisposing factors to dyshidrotic dermatitis.

Prurigo. Adults with atopic dermatitis may develop small pruritic papules on the extensor surfaces of the extremities. Some may evolve into prurigo nodularis type lesions. Thus atopic dermatitis should be considered as one of the predisposing factors in the development of persistent pruritic excoriated papules (Fig. 12.39). In blacks, atopic dermatitis tends to be much more papular in nature and frequently has a follicular pattern. Periumbilical papules are common in children.

Pityriasis Alba. This feature is more common in young atopic patients. It features hypopigmentation and fine scaling, usually found on the cheeks or extremities. It is more often identified in black patients, who also tend to have even drier skin.

Lichen Spinulosus. Grouped hyperkeratotic follicular spines or plugs characterize this disorder. It is also more common in blacks, or once again perhaps more easily seen, since the plugs tend to be ivory white. The lesions are round, usually on the trunk and may be pruritic. They are far more discrete than the typical lichenified plaques and cannot result from just rubbing as the intrafollicular skin is normal.

Keratosis Pilaris. As keratosis pilaris is more common in individuals with dry skin, it is not surprising that many atopic children and young adults have it. The plugged follicles often associated with surrounding erythema are typically found on the extensor aspects of the thighs and outer upper aspects of the arms. Some atopic children may also develop follicular plugging on the cheeks, which can be mistaken for acne.

Light-Sensitive Atopic Dermatitis. A small percentage of patients, usually young women, experience seasonal flares. Typically the eruption is more exudative than that usually seen in adults, involving the dorsal aspects of the hands, the mid-face and the nape. A search for atopy is thus part of the evaluation of light-sensitive patients.

Cataracts. A small number of atopic dermatitis patients have cataracts. In our experience, it is less than 1%. Some careful studies have shown so few cases that no routine screening has been recommended. Others have estimated the incidence to be higher. Anterior subcapsular cataracts are most common; corticosteroid-induced cataracts are almost always posterior subcapsular. Cataracts were identified in atopic dermatitis patients long before corticosteroids were discovered. Nonetheless, lawyers have changed our approach to this problem. Any patient with atopic dermatitis for whom systemic corticosteroids are prescribed should have ophthalmologic evaluation. In addition, long-term topical corticosteroids about the eye can cause glaucoma, so they too should be considered a risk favor. Keratoconus and retinal abnormalities have also been described, but they are rare and not distinctive.

Histopathology. A biopsy is rarely used to diagnose atopic dermatitis, but occasionally performed to exclude other possibilities. Depending on the clinical stage of the disease, either an acute spongiotic dermatitis or a more chronic process with reactive epidermal changes may be found. While tissue eosinophilia is rare, eosinophilic basic protein is found in increased amounts in chronic lesions. In addition, mast cells are increased.

Laboratory Findings. Measuring the eosinophils and serum IgE may point one towards the diagnosis but neither is specific or sensitive enough to be taken as definite. Similarly, in vitro testing for allergen-specific IgE may offer clinical guidance but is also not specific. The presence of high levels of $FC_{\varepsilon}R$ I on Langerhans cell seems quite specific for atopic dermatitis but testing is not yet readily available.

Course and Prognosis. The prognosis for atopic dermatitis must be made very carefully. Formerly one told parents that in most cases their child would outgrow their atopic dermatitis. This is clearly bad advice; most atopics have some degree of skin involvement into adult life, even though the intensely pruritic exudative lesions do resolve. In addition, adults are likely to have rhinitis, conjunctivitis and asthma. Food allergies may occur at all stages of life. Finally there are a number of complications of atopic dermatitis, as listed below.

Complications. The major problem is the increased susceptibility to bacterial, viral and less-often fungal infections. Secondary staphylococcal infections are most common, producing impetiginous lesions which often lead to lymphadenopathy. Both the human papilloma virus and the molluscum contagiosum virus favor atopic children. A far more severe problem is the tendency of the herpes simplex virus to disseminate in such patients (Chap. 2). In the past, a major problem was the same tendency of the vaccinia virus, used for smallpox vaccinations, to disseminate causing a potentially fatal disease. Cowpox virus also seems to have a more aggressive course in atopic patients. Fungal infections are probably not intrinsically more common, but are often mistaken for an exacerbation of the dermatitis, treated with corticosteroids and thus become more severe. Patients with HIV/AIDS often experience a flare of their dermatitis, probably reflecting the even more dramatic immune alterations.

The main complications of atopic dermatitis are iatrogenic. For years, corticosteroids were viewed as a wonder drug in atopy and much of our knowledge of their topical side effects was derived from corticosteroid-treated atopic children. In infants there is sufficient absorption so that high to ultra-high-potency corticosteroids can cause measurable adrenal suppression, local skin damage (striae, steroid acne and others), growth suppression and even Cushing syndrome. Thus one must follow the guidelines for topical corticosteroids discussed under therapy. Growth retardation is another distressing problem. It is multifactorial in origin, perhaps reflecting protein loss secondary to severe skin disease (both via the skin and the bowel), chronic infections and inadequate nutrition.

Diagnostic Criteria. The diagnosis of atopic dermatitis is usually not difficult. The standard scheme of Hanifin and Rajka (1980) is now over two decades old. It is as follows:

- Definitive features present in all patients
  - Pruritus
  - Typical lesions, i.e. flexural lichenification in adults and facial involvement in children
  - Tendency towards chronic relapsing dermatitis
- Plus two or more of the following:
  - Personal or family history of atopy
  - Immediate prick test reactions
  - White dermographism
  - Anterior subcapsular cataracts
- Or four or more of the following:
  - Xerosis/ichthyosis/hyperlinear palms
  - Pityriasis alba
  - Keratosis pilaris
  - Facial pallor/infraorbital darkening

Dennie-Morgan infraorbital fold
Elevated serum IgE
Keratoconus
Tendency toward hand dermatitis
Tendency toward repeated cutaneous infections

Many of these features are difficult to reproduce among different observers or are very rare. For this reason many new schemes have been developed. We generally do not employ a scoring scheme but search for the following factors:

- Personal and family history of atopy
- History of food allergies
- Tendency to pruritus, especially after showers and baths, as well as in the winter
- Increased skin irritability, especially against wool and soaps
- Facial changes including Dennie-Morgan pleats, Hertoghe sign, lower frontal hairline (known as *Pelzmütze* in German, for fur cap) and dry lips
- Dry skin and scalp with fine scales
- Hyperlinear palms
- In adults, eyelid, nape, nipple and hand dermatitis
- Elevated IgE level
- Sensitization to common aeroallergens
- Functional skin changes such as white dermographism and reduced sweating

Differential Diagnosis. The differential diagnostic of atopic dermatitis includes most of the conditions listed in this chapter. But despite the long lists, in most cases the diagnostic is easy. In infants, problems include seborrheic dermatitis, which is usually less exudative and more likely to involve the diaper region, scabies, pyodermas and perhaps Langerhans cell histiocytosis, which has many clinical forms but usually a biopsy is specific. In adults, chronic irritant hand dermatitis is often associated with the atopic diathesis, even when other signs of atopic dermatitis are no longer present. Allergic contact dermatitis may appear to either mimic atopic dermatitis or be a complication of therapy. Acral nummular dermatitis and dyshidrotic dermatitis are both associated with atopy, so it is a semantic question whether they belong in the differential diagnosis.

A bigger problem in an intellectual sense but almost never a practical problem are the rare disorders in which atopic dermatitis has been described as a feature. In our experience, even though we hasten to add that none of us has had extensive dealings with these extremely rare problems, many patients have a dermatitis, but it rarely fulfils the criteria for atopic dermatitis. In addition, atopic dermatitis is present in around 5–10% of the population, so one could say that "having disease X fails to protect one from atopic dermatitis" rather than that "atopic dermatitis is a feature of disease X". Table 12.15 shows some of the disorders in which one can read of claims of associated atopic dermatitis. The disorders associated with elevated IgE all tend to overlap and have many features of atopic dermatitis. They may also be variations on the same theme with overproduction of IgE and relative inefficiency in handling intracellular infections. Wiskott-Aldrich syndrome patients have what is indistinguishable from atopic dermatitis and it resolves following bone marrow transplanta-

Table 12.15. Diseases allegedly associated with atopic dermatitis

Category of disorder	Disease	Chapter
Elevated IgE	Hyper-IgE syndrome	4
Immunodeficiency	Wiskott-Aldrich syndrome	23
	Ataxia-telangiectasia	13
	Bruton syndrome (X-linked hypogammaglobulinemia)	4
	Selective IgA deficiency	4
	Chronic granulomatous disease	4
Genodermatoses	Comèl-Netherton syndrome	17
	Phenylketonuria	39
	Hypohidrotic ectodermal dysplasia	30
	Biotin deficiency	49
	Hartnup disease	39
	Acrodermatitis enteropathica	46
	Langerhans cell histiocytosis	64

tion. The associations with the other immunodeficiencies are less clear. Among the miscellaneous disorders, ichthyosis vulgaris and Netherton syndrome are the most convincing; chronic granulomatous disease, for example, has exudative skin lesions but little else that reminds one of atopy (Chap. 4).

Therapy. The approach to atopic dermatitis varies with the age of the patient and the type of manifestations. Particularly when dealing with infants and children, it is important to win the parents to your side so that they are partners in a reasonable overall treatment scheme. If this means accepting a few things which the physician considers "unproved" such as avoiding certain foods (as long as the diet is sufficient), it probably is worth the sacrifice. We always tell the parents they are the most important member of the team, as they will have to make decisions on a daily basis that have a major impact on their child's current and future health. The physician can only be an advisor.

Systemic. Systemic corticosteroids are dramatically effective in atopic dermatitis, but should be avoided as much as possible. They work so well that the parents and patients often lose interest in the more time consuming, messier topical approach which is without question safer. When systemic corticosteroids are employed, they should be used over 1–2 weeks, and tapered rapidly. Systemic antibiotics are also helpful for acute flares or when secondary impetiginization has occurred. We use an effective antistaphylococcal agent, either a penicillinase-resistant penicillin or a cephalosporin. In addition, some patients improve dramatically when given a short course of itraconazole, suggesting that reducing the *Pityrosporum ovale* levels on the skin may also be useful. Oral antiherpetic drugs are required for eczema herpeticum.

Another issue is the use of antihistamines. In contrast to contact dermatitis, they theoretically should be helpful in atopic dermatitis. Several studies have shown that these drugs achieve most of their effectiveness via a sedating action, which can also be obtained with a mild benzodiazepine or hydroxyzine. Most parents and patients readily point out the limited effectiveness of antihistamines, but some patients respond so well that it is worth trying several of these agents.

A variety of more powerful and effective systemic agents seem effective, but their use is limited by cost and safety concerns. In most countries, they remain in the developmental stage. For example, cyclosporine and tacrolimus both are powerful antiatopy agents. In addition, IFN-γ, whose levels are reduced by the altered Th ratios, has shown promise in trials.

Topical. The goal of topical therapy is to control flares usually with corticosteroids and to design an effective system of maintenance care to reduce the number of flares as much as possible. Almost all the rules of using topical corticosteroids have been devised by trial and error in treating atopic patients. Careful attention must be paid to the vehicle; most atopics prefer a relatively lipophilic vehicle because of their underlying dry skin. It is better to use a relatively high-potency agent for a short time, but then rapidly back off to a weaker agent as soon as improvement is seen, usually after 4–7 days. After another 1–2 weeks, one should consider corticosteroid-free maintenance therapy. The side effects of corticosteroids used on young patients for a long time can be considerable. As an alternative over short periods of time, 0.3% tacrolimus ointment appears very promising but is not yet approved.

Topical antibiotics, usually fusidic acid ointment, can be helpful for early exudative lesions which are limited in number. Wet compresses can be used in the exudative stage to debride and cool the lesions before applying a corticosteroid. After applying the corticosteroid the patient may also wear moist pajamas; this "greasy-wet" approach is very effective. Oilated oatmeal baths may be used in the acute phases. For more chronic lesions, tars, ichthammol and corticosteroids under occlusion can be employed.

Maintenance therapy is crucial. Many manufacturers provide the vehicles for their corticosteroids in a relatively economic form to use once the active product is no longer needed. Otherwise various ointments and creams can be tried to find one or two that the patient likes. Most prefer something that is at least hydrophilic so that it can be applied to moist skin comfortably. Bath additives are also very popular and helpful. Two basic bath oils are available: those which stay on the surface of the water and those which are emulsified and disperse in the water. The former coat the patient on getting out of the tub and are less messy, but individual choice will determine which is used. The emulsified bath oils can also be applied directly to the skin after bathing. Bubble baths should be strongly discouraged; they are quite drying. Atopic patients should not use alkaline soaps; syndets are less irritating but still should only be used where the patient is truly dirty. Cleansing lotions or creams help cleanse and lubricate simultaneously.

Phototherapy. UV therapy has long been used in atopic dermatitis. In recent years, UVA1 therapy has been employed especially for acute flares. It is more effective than conventional UVA-UVB therapy and does not produce the heat and resultant sweating which makes so many atopic dermatitis patients uncomfortable. PUVA also brings a prompt improvement in severe atopic dermatitis. PUVA bath therapy avoids the complications of systemic PUVA and appears well-suited for this population.

Climatic Therapy. Some European countries including Germany have long been intrigued by the improvement many patients show when sent to spas either on the ocean or in the mountains at heights over 1500 m. Helgoland is a tiny island in the North Sea with the lowest pollen counts in Germany; similarly mountain resorts also have low pollen counts. House-dust mites are also absent at such heights. There are also considerable differences in the type of UV radiation the patient receives (less filtering in the mountains, more filtering at sea level) and clearly the changed environment and presumably pleasant surroundings also play a role.

Other Measures. The first question every patent of a child with atopic dermatitis asks is "What about diet?". Some have already manipulated the child's diet without success. If the parent notices that a particular product such as milk, eggs or citrus fruits seems to trigger flares in the dermatitis, then these suspected products can be evaluated via in vitro tests and controlled provocation trials. History is often misleading, so in patients with severe or recurrent skin lesions we recommend evaluation of food allergies even if the history fails to suggest any problems. Drastic elimination diets are to be avoided, as are "monodiets"; both often lead to caloric and vitamin deficiencies and growth difficulties. The data are quite good that breast-feeding is wise for at least the first 6 months; this is relevant if the mother, father or an older sibling has atopy. Some patients benefit from dietary supplements with γ-linolenic acid, usually in the form of evening primrose oil or borage oil.

The parents should be aware of the many possible irritating environmental factors and try to avoid them. The house or apartment should be kept relatively humid. Dust collectors should be avoided. While it sounds cruel, it is wise to have a pet-free household (no fur, no feathers). Exposure to cigarette smoke should also be eliminated. Patients should not try their luck with wool clothing or bed spreads; most simply do not tolerate it. As atopic patients get older, they should be encouraged to pursue a job or profession where they are not exposed to frequent skin irritation; that is, jobs such as auto mechanic, cook, baker and hairdresser should be discouraged. Patients should be aware of the risks involved with exposure to herpes simplex virus and should under no circumstances receive vaccinia.

Finally, what patients and their parents need most from their physician is a good friend, not a brilliant scientist. Most of the management of atopic dermatitis is common sense. An experienced mother who has raised one atopic child knows a great deal about treating the disease. The physician should be willing to work with the family, showing flexibility and understanding. Some personal and family situations are so complex that the ordinary office-based physician lacks the time and skills to intervene. In such instances, referral to those more experienced in social and psychiatric counseling is wise. In Europe there are some inpatient services devoted to the psychosomatic aspects of skin diseases, especially atopic dermatitis.

Dermatitis in Infants and Children

In German one speaks of *eczema infantum*. While there is no similar term in use in the USA, parents and physicians often simply say "eczema" and unwittingly group a number of only partially related disorders.

Atopic Dermatitis

Most childhood dermatitis is atopic dermatitis. The typical exudative form is rarely misdiagnosed, especially with a family history of atopy. Scalp involvement is typical; the lesions are usually inflamed. The diaper area is often spared. Onset is most often after 3 months or whenever breast-feeding is stopped.

Seborrheic Dermatitis

Infantile seborrheic dermatitis usually starts in the first 3 months, i.e. before atopic dermatitis, and almost always involves the diaper area and the scalp. The scalp lesions tend to be drier and less inflamed than in atopic dermatitis. A number of long-term studies have shown that the two disorders cannot be separated with certainty in infancy.

Lip Dermatitis

Probably a better name would be lick, chew and suck dermatitis. Patients both lick their lips and manipulate their lower lip. Atopic patients are most often involved as they tend to have dry lips and manipulate them (Fig. 12.40). The result is a chronic primary irritant dermatitis. Young infants who drool also develop a dermatitis about their lips, but it usually involves the corners of their mouths and is known as perlèche. In adults, lip dermatitis may represent allergic contact dermatitis but this is unlikely in children. The dermatitis can be complicated by herpes simplex virus and human papilloma virus infections, as well as by impetigo.

The most important therapy is to break the vicious cycle of dryness → licking → worse dryness. Usually a protective ointment or lipstick is most helpful. Low-potency corticosteroid ointments can be used for a few days. Zinc pastes are used for protection, especially at night.

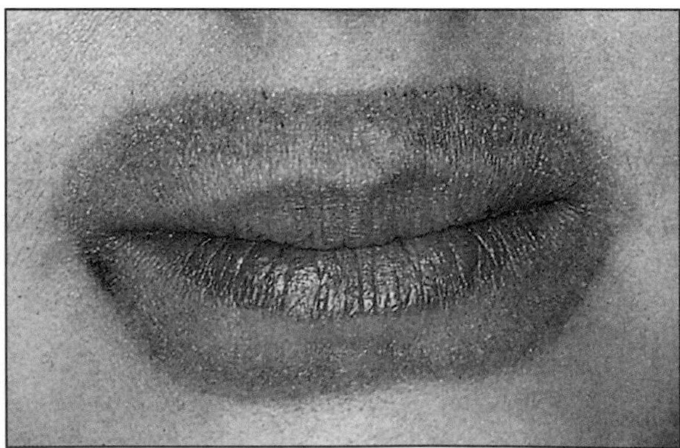

Fig. 12.40. Lip licker's dermatitis, usually associated with atopic dermatitis

Nummular Dermatitis

We feel most nummular dermatitis in children is atopic dermatitis. The lesions are more often acral and exudative, while in older children and adults they are truncal and drier.

Allergic Contact Dermatitis

Children develop less allergic contact dermatitis than adults. Perhaps it is just a matter of number of agents to which they are exposed and the duration of exposure. When allergic contact dermatitis develops, it is usually caused by a medication, often used for diaper dermatitis. Possibilities include neomycin, antihistamines, corticosteroids and local anesthetics. In addition, components of vehicles such as preservatives may be responsible.

Irritant Contact Dermatitis

This problem is much more common than allergic contact dermatitis, primarily because diaper dermatitis is an irritant contact dermatitis and almost every infant develops it. An often-discussed but uncommon irritant reaction is gentian violet necrosis. It is more common in Europe, perhaps because higher concentrations were used in the past. Because of the risk of an irritant reaction when applied to intertriginous or damaged skin, gentian violet should be compounded in a 0.1–0.25% aqueous solution and only used in the clinic or office, and not prescribed for home use.

Asteatotic Dermatitis

Children are not exposed to the occupational or housewive's wear-and-tear dermatitis but they subject their skin to enough challenges that a chronic irritant dermatitis can develop. Once again, children with dry skin, therefore primarily atopics, are at risk. Drying factors include too much bathing and swimming, excessive use of soaps, failure to lubricate the skin, wool clothes, crawling on rough surfaces and similar factors. Typical sites are the knees, elbows and in atopic patients, the cheeks and backs of the hands. The therapy is to avoid irritating factors and keep the skin lubricated. Very rarely low-potency topical corticosteroids can be employed for a short time. In older children, urea-containing creams are valuable, but the initial burning makes these products difficult to use in infants.

Diaper Dermatitis

(Jacquet 1905; Zahorsky 1915)

Synonyms. Diaper rash, dermatitis glutealis, dermatitis ammoniacalis

Epidemiology. Diaper dermatitis is the most common chronic irritant dermatitis of all. Our skin is simply not made to resist the repeated irritating action of urine and stool. In infants, it usually begins in the first months of life and lasts until toilet training is complete. The same problems trouble the elderly or infirm if they become incontinent. Usually a parent's care is better than that in a nursing home, so some of the worst diaper rashes are unfortunately in adults.

Etiology and Pathogenesis. The etiology of diaper dermatitis has been the subject of intense interest over the years and many theories have been advanced. In every case, the problem is multifactorial. The first step is the contact of the skin with irritating substances. Friction is the first problem, as the baby's skin rubs against the diapers, especially at the edges. Even with frequent diaper changes, the urine and stool are incubated against the skin with increasing warmth and humidity. The urine becomes more basic as ammonia is formed by bacterial enzymes especially from *Proteus* species. While ammonia was formerly considered a major role player, it is likely an innocent bystander responsible for little irritation. The stool often contains *Candida albicans* as well as various proteolytic enzymes. All these factors combine to break down the skin's resistance.

Clinical Findings. Diaper dermatitis obeys the rules for an irritant contact dermatitis. The reaction is initially erythematous and scaly. The sites of predilection are the convex curved areas, such as the upper parts of the thighs, buttocks, lower part of the abdomen and genitalia (Fig. 12.41). Typically the inguinal folds are spared as the diaper and irritating materials usually do not reach this area. As the inflammation becomes more severe, the erythema and swelling spreads. The infant becomes uncomfortable. The smell of ammonia is often prominent. Ordinary diaper dermatitis is often erosive. Inexperienced physicians sometimes equate erosions with infections or severe problems, but this is not the case. Crater-like erosions are called Jacquet dermatitis after the original describer (Jacquet 1905). Marked crusting suggests a secondary bacterial infection and peripheral pustules point to a candidal infection. Sometimes small papules develop when a diaper dermatitis is chronic; the term posterosive syphiloid refers to the similarity with a papular syphilid. Syphilis does not present with a diaper rash. A worrisome complication is an erosive meatal lesion, which may result in a few drops of blood on the diaper but is not a sign of ascending problems.

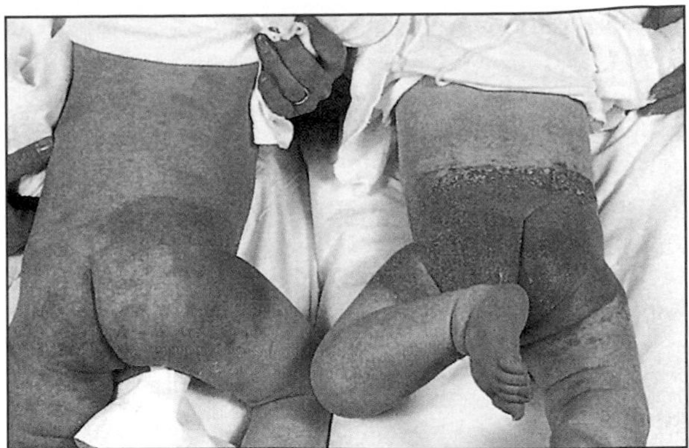

Fig. 12.41. Diaper dermatitis

Histopathology. Diaper rashes are not biopsied except to exclude Langerhans cell histiocytosis. Presumably they would show either acute or chronic dermatitis, perhaps with evidence of candidal secondary infection, i.e., pseudohyphae in the stratum corneum.

Course and Prognosis. Diaper dermatitis tends to be chronic, but shows improvement as the parents become more skilled in managing the problem. Allergic contact dermatitis may develop if sensitizing medications such as neomycin are used for long periods of time. The use of halogenated corticosteroids may produce a granulomatous response known as granuloma glutale infantum (Chap. 50).

Differential Diagnosis. The differential diagnosis is actually better stated as a search for underlying factors. A rash under the diapers is a diaper dermatitis. *Candida albicans* is often present in this region, even in asymptomatic patients, so that KOH and culture are not helpful in deciding when it is a pathogen. Even a positive stool culture for the yeast may not be clinically significant; some recommend quantitative stool cultures for this reason.

Several disorders predispose to diaper dermatitis. While the skin in atopic dermatitis is less resistant to irritation, diaper dermatitis is not as common or severe as expected. Another possibility is seborrheic dermatitis, which often involves the diaper area, more typically starting in the folds, which are involved late in a pure irritative reaction. Sometimes psoriasiform plaques develop. Only long-term studies can tell if such patients have or will have psoriasis. The British use the term napkin (diaper) psoriasis and estimate that about 20% of such patients will have psoriasis as adults. If the lesions are hemorrhagic, not present in the areas of irritation or become nodular, a biopsy should be done to exclude Langerhans cell histiocytosis. A painful perianal rash, especially with pain on defecation, suggest infectious streptococcal perianal disease which requires systemic antibiotics (Chap. 4).

Therapy

Other Measures. The most important measure is changing the diapers frequently. There are three possibilities: home-washed diapers, diaper services and disposable diapers. The super-high absorbency disposable diapers have reduced the incidence of diaper dermatitis simply by keeping the area dryer. The gels they contain take up a large amount of urine, thus keeping not only the skin but also the stools dry. Diaper services are more ecologically sound, as disposable diapers account for 2–5% of garbage in industrialized countries. Washing the diapers at home probably creates as much irritant contact dermatitis in the form of mother's hand dermatitis as it helps the infants. Occlusive rubber or plastic outer diapers should be eliminated.

Topical. Simple protective creams form the mainstay of care. Every culture has products which individuals, especially grandmothers, swear by. In addition, it is essential to clean the area with each diaper change and to change the diapers as frequently as possible, reducing skin-irritant contact. Water, baby oil and cleansing lotions are useful for cleaning. Packaged baby wipes are convenient but often irritating, as are soaps. Powders are acceptable. If the baby is relatively dry, a talcum powder will provide some lubrication. If the area is macerated, then perhaps a more absorbent powder is better. Corn starch powder, another of grandmother's favorites, is less desirable; when wet it often serves as a culture medium.

Anticandidal therapy often helps and carries little risk. If there are clinical signs of candidiasis, such as peripheral pustules, then an imidazole or nystatin paste should be used, either after each change or twice a day. Topical corticosteroids are often necessary to break the inflammatory cycle in a modest to severe diaper dermatitis. The combination of 1% hydrocortisone and nystatin in a paste or cream is a very useful product. Unfortunately, drug-regulatory agencies have insisted that combination products be clearly more effective than the initial product. This has forced pharmaceutical companies to add higher potency corticosteroids to the anticandidal agents making such combination products less suitable for infants.

Local bacterial infections can be tried with a topical antibacterial agent. We prefer clioquinol 0.5% in zinc oil or zinc paste. Neomycin is often used but in this setting of chronic applications may cause allergic contact dermatitis. Thus, bacitracin or bacitracin-polymyxin B ointments are most popular. If crusts are present, they can be loosened with moist compresses during the diaper change. When the eruption is exudative, one should switch to a lotion or cream, avoiding the usually occlusive pastes and ointments. A zinc shake lotion, perhaps with an oil added, is comforting and effective.

Systemic. Systemic therapy is rarely needed. If a candidal eruption is slow to respond, systemic nystatin is worth trying. Severe secondary bacterial infections can be treated with appropriate antibiotics, but often the resultant diarrhea makes the diaper dermatitis worse.

Intertrigo

While diaper dermatitis can be viewed as intertrigo, some infants develop intertrigo in other skin folds. Predisposing factors include being overweight, being clothed in nonabsorbent clothing, marked sweating because of excessive clothing or covers and lack of proper hygiene. Notice that all these factors are inflicted upon the infant by well-meaning parents.

The lesions are initially erythematous macules that are sharply bordered. They may develop vesicles and crusts. The typical locations are the nape, axillae and umbilicus, as well as the diaper area and perianal region. Involvement of the bases of folds or creases and the associated finding of miliaria lend credence to the diagnosis of intertrigo.

The differential diagnosis and therapy are identical to diaper dermatitis.

Pomade Crust

(Gartmann and Steigleder 1975)

If infants are treated with excessive amounts of ointments and pastes, thick adherent scales may develop. The typical sites are the inguinal and gluteal clefts, where large adherent gray-brown or yellow-brown polygonal scales are found. They are difficult to remove. Initially, it was assumed that they represented accumulated, improperly removed ointments, but instead, the scales appear to be part of a hyperplastic response of the epidermis to excessive occlusion. Long term use of ointments in adults, such as in treating stasis dermatitis, may produce a similar phenomenon. The scales can usually be removed by more aggressive soaks, use of light oils and discontinuance of the ointments or pastes.

Juvenile Plantar Dermatosis

Synonyms. Peridigital dermatosis, snowmobiler's feet, dermatitis hiemalis, atopic winter feet

Definition. Chronic irritant dermatitis of the feet almost exclusively limited to children.

Epidemiology. This disease appears more common in children with atopic dermatitis and is most uncommon in adults. The peak incidence is around 5 years of age, but problems may persist into adolescence. The reaction is definitely more common in the winter.

Etiology and Pathogenesis. Juvenile plantar dermatosis is a local chronic irritant reaction. Almost all patients have atopic dermatitis and dry skin. Major factors include occlusive shoes, nonabsorbent socks and the resultant excessive sweating. Clean socks and wool carpets serve as defatting agents. In the northern USA, it is more common in children wearing warm occlusive boots, i.e. snowmobile boots, in the cold months. Occasionally patients may develop changes on their fingertips. Here the use of wet gloves and mittens is suspected. A unifying theory of juvenile plantar dermatosis suggests that in patients with sensitive skin the alternate cycles of wetting and drying cause the irritant dermatitis.

Clinical Findings. The classic clinical finding is a almost perfectly symmetric plantar eruption involving the parts of the foot that are in contact with the shoe. Thus the instep is spared, while the pulps of the toes, the metatarsal heads and the heel are dry, erythematous and scaly (Fig. 12.42). The initial changes are often on the great toe. Occasionally the fingertips are also involved. The skin becomes thinned, easily fissured and scaly. The course is chronic, usually recurring in winter.

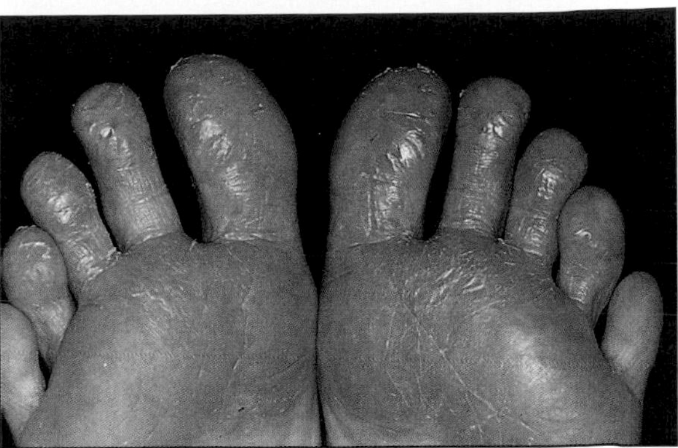

Fig. 12.42. Juvenile plantar dermatosis

Differential Diagnosis. Most often juvenile plantar dermatosis is misdiagnosed as tinea pedis. There is no reason for this; tinea pedis is never so symmetric and KOH and culture are negative in juvenile plantar dermatitis. An allergic contact dermatitis to shoe materials is the only serious possibility. This can be excluded by switching shoes or by patch testing.

Therapy. Most patients do better if greased. This means they should lubricate their feet before applying cotton socks. As unsanitary as it sounds, if the socks get a little greasy, it is probably helpful. When they come home from school, they should grease up again and not run around barefoot. Any ointment that feels good is fine. Hydrophilic ointments and urea-containing creams are usually well tolerated and helpful. The alternative approach – trying to keep the feet dry – is almost impossible because of the frequent winter temperature changes and occlusive shoes which induce sweating.

Dermatitis in the Elderly

As is so often the case, many of the forms of irritant dermatitis which are common in infants come to plague the elderly. Intrinsically dry skin, inappropriate or inadequate care, and incontinence all appear again as factors. While there is no dermatitis that only occurs in the elderly, the inflammatory dermatoses are usually less severe and allergic contact dermatitis is rare.

Asteatotic Dermatitis

Synonym. Xerosis of the elderly

Etiology and Pathogenesis. Dryness is the biggest factor in both dermatitis and pruritus in the elderly. Often habits that have been tolerated for 60 years, such as daily showers, using a antibacterial soap, not lubricating the skin, suddenly become too irritating and wreak havoc. Almost all elderly patients have low sebum production, especially on the extremities. Some have increased facial sebum production, especially those with CNS disease or Parkinson disease. The problem is usually worse in the winter and typically flares when central heating systems are turned on. A variety of internal problems, such as chronic renal disease, also cause dry skin, as may a variety of medicines, particularly the lipid-lowering agents.

Clinical Findings. Most patients complain of pruritus. It may be hard initially to appreciate that the skin is dry. Over a period of time the skin becomes rough, scaly and perhaps reddened. Eczema craquelé is particularly common in this group. The problem is chronic if the predisposing factors are not addressed.

Differential Diagnosis. The list of possible causes of dry skin and pruritus in the elderly is long. Drug reactions and underlying diseases, such as malignancies, renal and hepatic disease should be excluded. Some atopic patients will flare at this age, but the diagnosis is not critical, as the therapy is the same. Large-patch parapsoriasis and mycosis fungoides should be considered if localized therapy-resistant patches are present. Nummular lesions may be found, and in this age group, nummular dermatitis is usually an extreme variation of dryness and is not inflammatory. Dryness is so much more common than the other causes that it is simplest to first treat the dryness and if no improvement occurs, then investigate. Some elderly patients have unexplained pruritus without dry skin (Chap. 25).

Therapy. Patients or their carers must be convinced to correct the patterns of care that have triggered the problem. In addition, the skin must be lubricated. Bath or shower oils are useful, but because of the likelihood of elderly patients slipping in tubs, it is usually wiser to apply an oil or hydrophilic ointment after bathing. Low-potency topical corticosteroids can be used for short periods of time for particularly pruritic lesions. Lotions or creams containing polidocanol 2–5% are also effective.

Stomal Dermatitis

Epidemiology. Most colostomies and ileostomies are performed because of intestinal carcinomas. In such cases they are often temporary, or the patient has a relatively short life. In the case of inflammatory bowel disease, the procedures are likely to be performed in young individuals who will have to deal with the results for many years.

Etiology and Pathogenesis. Stomal dermatitis is a typical mixture of chronic irritant contact dermatitis and often secondary allergic contact dermatitis. A number of factors are important.

- Level of stoma. An ileostomy drains more irritating liquid material rich in enzymes and is more likely to cause trouble than a colostomy with its partially or fully formed stool.
- Quality of stoma. An ideal stoma is one that is supported by the abdominal muscles, properly placed on a relatively flat part of the abdomen and protrudes above the skin, emptying into the pouch.
- Nursing care. Most hospitals have enterostomy nurses who train patients to use a stoma and also serve as valuable resources for physicians.
- Preexisting disorder. Patients with inflammatory bowel disease are more likely to develop recurrences around a stoma than someone with a tumor resection.

Clinical Findings. The most common finding is erythema and weeping around the stoma. In most cases, the problem is irritation from the adhesive coupled with exposure to the body fluids. Secondary bacterial and candidal infections can occur but are uncommon, even though the organisms are easily cultured. Allergic contact dermatitis may develop to the stomal adhesive, plastic, deodorants or products used to protect, cleanse or treat the skin. Sometimes the Köbner phenomenon is seen, especially with psoriasis.

Therapy. A properly fitting stoma is essential. The stoma must fit as closely as possible into the opening of the bag. With time, the stoma may stretch or change so that revision is required. Protective creams around the stoma may help, but in our experience, they often interfere with adherence. The ideal situation is if a patient can train themselves to be continent, so that the skin about the stoma can have some time each day exposed to the air. When irritation develops, either a mild corticosteroid or a combination corticosteroid-imidazole or paste or cream is appropriate.

Occupational Dermatitis

Chronic irritant and/or allergic hand dermatitis is one of the most common occupational disabilities. After back injuries, it is the leading cause of disability in most industrialized nations. In Germany about 10% of all patients who receive compensation because they are unable to carry out their profession have hand dermatitis. Since occupational illnesses invariably lead to paperwork, our advice is to keep exceptionally good records on all working patients with hand dermatitis. Problems among those just learning a trade are even more important to recognize quickly. Hand dermatitis is a particular problem among, for example, apprentice hairdressers, veterinary students and fledgling auto mechanics.

Clues to an occupational cause or trigger include more trouble during the week, relative clearing on weekends, more dramatic clearing with vacations and more severe involvement of the dominant hand. Irritant dermatitis more often involves the dorsal aspects of the hands, as the palms intrinsically have more protection. Dyshidrosiform blisters may be present, but are less common. Secondary allergic contact dermatitis is always a possibility; sudden worsening, spread or blistering should suggest this consideration. Those in certain professions such mechanics, machinists, beauticians, bakers and butchers are at greater risk. Patients with atopic dermatitis are also more likely to have trouble, no matter what their line of work.

The approach to occupational dermatitis is determined by the laws in each country. We will cite the German rules, realizing they are not totally relevant in other countries but simply to show one system. All physicians must acquaint themselves with the correct approach in their own country.

Dermatologic Approach to Occupational Diseases

Work-related skin diseases are defined in Germany as "severe or recurrent skin diseases which have forced the individual to give up those occupational activities which are or could be responsible for the development, the worsening or recurrence of the disorder." In order to avoid patients being unable to work because of disease, and thus being entitled to workmen's compensation, family doctors and industrial physicians are encouraged to refer workers to dermatologists if there is any suspicion of occupational skin disease.

The dermatologist can then provide one of two documents:

- Dermatologist's Report. If the dermatologist feels the patient can keep working in the job, then he sends his treatment and prophylaxis recommendations to the patient's union which also serves as the patient's insurer for all occupational health problems. The union then interacts with the company physician or other company officials.
- Medical Notification of Occupational Disease. If the physician feels that the patient is no longer able to carry out his chosen profession, then a more complicated form is required. Three questions must be addressed:
  Is an occupational dermatitis present?
  Is it severe and/or frequently recurrent?
  Must the patient change his job?

All three questions must be answered "Yes" if the patient is to be declared disabled on dermatologic grounds. Once again the union must be informed. Often an independent dermatologist, either a public health physician or one employed by the union, then performs a detailed history, careful clinical evaluation, patch testing and other laboratory evaluation and comes up with a *Gutachten* or expert opinion.

The following points must be considered in the expert opinion.

Severity. An occupational dermatitis is severe when:

- Repeated dermatologic care has been needed
- The skin disease is widespread, painful, disabling, therapy-resistant and leaves residual damage
- Allergic contact dermatitis is documented, involving chemicals which cannot be avoided in the occupation

- The worker (patient) has been under continuous treatment for at least 6 months

If a patch test is positive, the clinical relevance is especially important. The degree of severity of the patch test, such as grade 3, has nothing to do with the severity of the disease. The patient's work records must document repeated exposure to the agent, usually in the background of irritant contact dermatitis. Simply stating that exposure at work was possible is not accepted as proof. In addition, there should be clinical clues that an allergic reaction is present, not just an irritant reaction.

Tendency to Recurrence. Repeated problems are defined as at least three episodes of illness, i.e. two recurrences. By definition, during the interval the patient must have been able to work and not receiving active treatment (skin maintenance and protective creams are excluded). If this is not the case, then the disease is viewed as continuous with waxing and waning, not as cured and relapsing.

Avoiding All Damaging Activities. In the past, only a fully trained worker was eligible for compensation. When the German work laws were revised, all workers who had to stop a given activity were included. This twist was designed to protect apprentices and people in training, as well as those performing general tasks, such as cleaning work, where no special training is involved. The tasks which cannot be tolerated may consume only part of the daily routine. For example, an experienced hairdresser who cannot do permanent waves or hair-dying jobs could still manage a shop, but a young worker with the same disability might have more trouble and would be eligible for retraining. If workers of their own accord stop a given task at work, without having failed aggressive treatment, their legal position is less secure.

Causal Relationship. A number of factors must be addressed. The relationship of the dermatitis to onset of work, weekends, vacations and daily variation in tasks should be documented. In most cases, the hands should be involved. A cement worker might get irritant contact dermatitis or even allergic contact dermatitis of the feet from cement powder and liquids accumulating in the boots.

Preexisting or Associated Disorders. Frequently patients with atopic dermatitis or psoriasis experience a worsening of their hand involvement at work. The first question the physician must answer is:

Is the occupational exposure responsible for 50% or more of the dermatitis, i.e., are exogenous causes greater than or equal to endogenous causes?

If yes, fine. If no, then:

Is the sequence of events such that the primarily endogenous problem has been made worse by work? For example, a young woman with clear atopic dermatitis but no major problems with her hands might develop severe hand dermatitis after 6 weeks in nursing school.

Correctly evaluating the causal relationship between work and hand dermatitis in patients with severe atopic dermatitis is challenging. More resources are available in Germany than in the USA. Nonetheless, no matter what the physician concludes, someone will be unhappy – the employer, the union, the insurance company or the patient. For each one, a fair amount of money is at stake. A detailed history and physical examination go without saying. Complete patch and prick testing, as well as other atopy-relevant tests, should be performed and evaluated in the background of previous results and the work exposure. The insurance company or union will usually pay for a visit to the workplace so the physician can see exactly how and why the patient is exposing or damaging their hands. Sometimes it is helpful to admit the patient for intensive hospital care. In Germany, patients are also sent to spas or rehabilitation clinics to recover completely; the insurance companies must approve this in advance.

When the doctor concludes that the work has been responsible for a worsening of the skin condition, then another set of legalistic phrases come into play.

- Was it a temporary worsening? Did the skin disease return to its previous, preoccupational damage status over a period of time, once work was stopped?

If yes, fine.

- If no, then there are two possibilities. The permanent worsening can either be unlimited or limited. When unlimited or dominating, the exogenous damage is felt to have triggered such a severe reaction, such as terrible hand psoriasis in a hairdresser, that while the future course is unpredictable, the occupational exposure has produced a new level of disease. In the permanent but limited worsening, the skin disease is worsened and unlikely to return to the previous healthier status, but also unlikely to flare or get a great deal worse.

Requirements for Legal Recognition. If all of the above conditions have been met, then the patient stands a good chance to receive compensation. He or she must give up all those activities that have led, or could have led, to the "development, worsening or recurrence of the disorder". For example, a mason or apprentice mason who is allergic to chromates cannot work any more. A mason cannot avoid cement in an effective way.

Degree of Disability. In Germany a system for assessing the degree of disability has been developed by occupational dermatologists cooperating with unions and insurance companies. The clinical findings, the degree of sensitization and how widespread are allergens are scored as 0 (none), 5 (minimal), 10 (moderate) and 15–20 (severe), and the degree of disability (which must be expressed as a percentage) is determined from the total score as shown in Table 12.16. Deviations from the numbers reached in the table are allowed. The skin findings should be described in terms of localization, severity and morphology (ulcers are worse than papules, for example). The presence of allergic contact dermatitis must be expanded by showing relevance and the number of cross-allergens. The degree of disability is not an assessment of the patient's inability to do the current job; it is an estimate of his reduced value on the total job market. For example, a chromate allergy has more far-reaching consequences than a neomycin allergy, for chromates are present in a long list of materials. If the patient is highly qualified, has many years experience and must give up a profitable profession, such as an orthopedic surgeon or dentist with a severe acrylate allergy, this should also be reflected in the report.

Table 12.16. Estimation of the degree of disability from dermatitis (Rudikoff 1998)

Total score	Degree of disability (%)
0–5	0
10–15	10
20–30	20
35–45	25
50–60	30
>60	>30

If the degree of disability is greater than 20%, the patient is also eligible to begin receiving a pension. The final pension must be determined 2 years after the onset of the case. The initial date of the case is usually the day that the third relapse is treated; in a severe unrelenting case, it is the date that the disorder was first treated. After this 2-year period, the degree of disability is relatively permanent. It is still subject to change, and any of the involved parties can request a reevaluation, but only if there is reason to think that the degree of disability has changed by more than 5%.

Role of Disability Insurance. By German law, the disability insurance company also is involved in occupational skin diseases. The accident or disability insurance company is required to do everything it can to prevent a permanent occupational disability. If a danger exists whereby the worker might develop an occupational hand dermatitis, the disability insurance company must provide him with protective equipment, encourage the employer to consider alternative techniques and similar tactics. If these dangers cannot be removed, then the disability insurance company also has responsibility for compensating the worker for lost income and paying for job retraining.

Bibliography

Irritant and Allergic Contact Dermatitis

Altekrueger I, Ackerman AB (1994) "Eczema" revisited. A status report based upon current textbooks of dermatology. Am J Dermatopathol 16:517–522

Benezra C, Ducombs G, Sell Y et al. (1985) Plant contact dermatitis. Mosby, St. Louis

Brasch J, Henseler T, Aberer W et al. (1994) Reproducibility of patch tests. J Am Acad Dermatol 31:584–591

Bruynzeel DP, Andersen KE, Camarasa JG et al. (1995) The European standard series. Contact Dermatitis 33:145–148

Bruze M, Emmet EA (1990) Occupational exposures to irritants. In: EM Jackson, R Goldner (eds) Irritant contact dermatitis. Dekker New York Basel, pp 81–106

Burckhardt W, Dorta T (1957) Die Alkaliresistenz bei Ekzemen verschiedener Genese und bei Neurodermitis. Dermatologica (Basel) 114:252–257

Chase MW (1946) Inhibition of experimental drug allergy by prior feeding of the sensitivity agent. Proc Soc Exp Biol Med 61:257–259

Coenraads PJ, Bleumink E, Nater JP (1975) Susceptibility to primary irritants. Age dependance and relation of contact allergic reactions. Contact Dermatitis 1:177–181

Cronin E (1980) Contact dermatitis. Churchill Livingstone, Edinburgh

Dooms-Goossens AE, Debusschere KM, Gevers DM et al. (1986) Contact dermatitis caused by airbone agents. J Am Acad Dermatol 15:1–10

Epstein E (1984) Hand dermatitis: practical management and current concepts. J Am Acad Dermatol 10:397–424
Gollhausen R, Przybilla B, Ring J (1989) Reproducibility of patch tests. J Am Acad Dermatol 21:1196–1202
Groot AC de (1994) Patch testing. Test concentrations and vehicles for 3700 chemicals, 2nd edn. Elsevier, Amsterdam
Guin JD (ed) (1995) Practical contact dermatitis. McGraw-Hill, New York
Hatch KL, Maibach HI (1995) Textile dye dermatitis. J Am Acad Dermatol 32:631–639
Hogan DJ, Dannaker CJ, Maibach HI (1990) The prognosis of contact dermatitis. J Am Acad Dermatol 23:300–307
Jackson EM, Goldner R (eds) (1990) Irritant contact dermatitis. Dekker, New York
Jadassohn J (1896) Zur Kenntnis der medicamentösen Dermatosen. Verhandlungen der Deutschen Dermatologischen Gesellschaft, 5. Congress, Wien 1895. Braunmüller, Vienna, pp 103–129
Lachapelle J-M, Ale SI, Freeman S et al. (1997) Proposal for a revised international standard series of patch tests. Contact Dermatitis 36:121–123
Liden S (1986) Contact dermatitis. Semin Dermatol 5:213–306
Lim KB, Tan T, Rajan VS (1986) Dermatitis palmaris sicca – distinctive pattern of hand dermatitis. J Clin Exp Dermatol 6:553–559
Lovell CR (1993) Plants and the skin. Blackwell Scientific Publ Oxford, London
Marks JG, Belsito DV, DeLeo VA et al. (1998) North American Contact Dermatitis Group patch test results for the detection of delayed-type hypersensitivity to topical allergens. J Am Acad Dermatol 38:911–918
Mathias CGT (1990) Prevention of occupational contact dermatitis. J Am Acad Dermatol 23:742–748
Memon AA, Friedmann PS (1996) "Angry back syndrome": a nonreproducible phenomenon. Br J Dermatol 135:924–930
Mennè T, Maibach HI (2000) Hand Eczema. CRC Press Boca Raton
Morren M-A, Janssens V, Dooms-Goossens A et al. (1993) α-Amylase, a flour additive: an important cause of protein contact dermatitis in bakers. J Am Acad Dermatol 29:723–728
Murray HE, Forsey RR (1975) Eczema craquelé. Arch Dermatol 111:1536
Rietschel RL (1997) Occupational contact dermatitis. Lancet 349:1093–1095
Rietschel RL, Fowler JF (1995) Fisher's contact dermatitis, 4th edn. Williams and Wilkins, Baltimore
Rycroft RJG, Frosch PJ (eds) (1994) Textbook of contact dermatitis. Springer, Berlin
Schade H, Marchionini A (1928) Zur physikalischen Chemie der Hautoberfläche. Arch Dermatol Syphil 154:690–716
Scheinman PL (1999) The foul side of fragrance-free products: What every clinician should know about managing patients with fragrance allergy. J Am Acad Dermatol 41:1020–1024
Schnuch A, Geier J, Uter W et al. (1997) National rates and regional differences in sensitization to allergens of the standard series. Contact Dermatitis 37:200–209
Sulzberger MB (1929) Hypersensitiveness to urophenamin in guinea pigs. I. Experiments in prevention and in desensitization. Arch Dermatol Syphilol 20:669–677
Thomson KF, Wilkinson SM (2000) Allergic contact dermatitis to plant extracts in patients with cosmetic dermatitis. Br J of Dermatol 142:84–88
Wilkinson SM, Burd R (1998) Latex – a cause of allergic contact eczema in users of natural rubber gloves. J Am Acad Dermatol 38:36–42

Dyshidrotic Dermatitis

Egan CA, Rallis TM, Meadows KP et al. (1999) Low-dose oral methotrexate treatment for realcitrant palmoplantar pompholyx. J Am Acad Dermatol 40:612–614
Kutzner H, Wurzel RM, Wolff HH (1986) Are acrosyringia involved in the pathogenesis of "dyshidrosis"? Am J Dermatopathol 8:109–116

Seborrheic Dermatitis

Bergbrant I-M (1991) Seborrhoeic dermatitis and Pityrosporum ovale: Cultural, immunological and clinical studies. Acta Derm Venereol (Stockh) 167:1–36
Braun-Falco O, Heiligemeier GP, Lincke-Plewig H (1979) Histologische Differentialdiagnose von Psoriasis vulgaris und seborrhoischem Ekzem des Kapillitiums. Hautarzt 30:478–483
Christensen OB, Möller H (1975) Nickel allergy and hand eczema. Contact Dermatitis 1:129–35
Cowley NC, Farr PM (1992) A dose-response study of irritant reactions to sodium lauryl sulphate in patients with seborrhoeic dermatitis and atopic eczema. Acta Derm Venereol (Stockh) 72:432–435
de Boer EM, Bruynzeel DP, Van Ketel WG (1988) Dyshidrotic eczema as an occupational dermatitis in metal workers. Contact Dermatitis 19:184–188
Devergie A (1857) Traité pratique des maladies de la peau. Librairie de Victor, Masson, Paris
Edman B (1988) Palmar eczema: a pathogenic role for acetylsalicylic acid, contraceptives and smoking? Acta Derm Venereol (Stockh) 68:402–407
Evans DIK, Holzel A, MacFarlane H (1977) Yeast opsonization defect and immunoglobulin deficiency in severe infantile dermatitis (Leiner's disease). Arch Dis Child 52:691–695
Goodyear HM, Harper JI (1989) Leiner's disease associated with metabolic acidosis. Clin Exp Dermatol 14:364–366
Green CA, Farr PM, Shuster S (1987) Treatment of seborrheic dermatitis with ketoconazole: II. Response of seborrheic dermatitis of the face, scalp and trunk to topical ketoconazole. Br J Dermatol 116:217–221
Leiner C (1908) Über Erythrodermia desquamativa, eine eigenartige universelle Hautdermatose der Brustkinder. Arch Dermatol Syph (Berlin) 89:65–76, 89:163–189
Lodi A, Betti R, Chianelli G et al. (1992) Epidemiological, clinical and allergological observations on pompholyx. Contact Dermatitis 26:17–21
Maietta G, Fornaro P, Rongioletti F et al. (1990) Patients with mood depression have a high prevalence of seborrhoeic dermatitis. Acta Dermato Venereol (Stockh) 70:432–434
Mathes KJ, Douglas MC (1985) Seborrhoeic dermatitis in patients with acquired immunodeficiency syndrome. J Am Acad Dermatol 13:947–951
McGinley KJ, Leyden JJ, Marples RR et al. (1975) Quantitative microbiology of the scalp in non-dandruff, dandruff, and seborrheic dermatitis. J Invest Dermatol 64:401–405

Meding B, Swanbeck G (1989) Epidemiology of different types of hand eczema in an industrial city. Acta Derm Venereol (Stockh) 69:227–233
Mennè T, Hjorth N (1983) Pompholyx-dyshidrotic eczema. Semin Dermatol 2:75–80
Pomodore P, Burrous D, Eedy DF et al. (1986) Seborrheic eczema – a disease entity or a clinical variant of atopic eczema. Br J Dermatol 115:341–350
Schechtman RC, Midgley G, Hay RJ (1995) HIV diseases and malassezia yeast: a quantitative study of patients presenting with seborrhoeic dermatitis. Br J Dermatol 133: 694–698
Tollesson A, Frithz A (1993) Essential fetty acids in infantile seborrhoic dermatitis. J Am Acad Dermatol 28:957–961
Unna PG (1921) Das seborrhoische Ekzem. Das Petaloid. Münch Med Wochenschr 18:547–548
Yates VM, Kerr REI, Frier K et al. (1983) Early diagnosis of infantile seborrheic dermatitis and atopic dermatitis – total and specific IgE levels. J Dermatol 108:639–645

Nummular Dermatitis

Abeck D, Strasser S, Braun-Falco O (1992) Exsudative diskoide lichenoide Dermatitis ("oid-oid-disease"). Akt Dermatol 18:280–282
Freeman K, Hewitt M, Warin AP (1984) Two cases of distinctive exsudative discoid and lichenoid chronic dermatosis of Sulzberger and Garbe responding to azathioprine. Br J Dermatol 111:215–220
Jansen T, Küppers Ü, Plewig G (1992) Exsudative diskoide und lichenoide chronische Dermatose Sulzberger-Garbe ("Oid-Oid-Disease")-Realität oder Fiktion. Hautarzt 43:426–431
Stevens DM, Ackerman AB (1984) On the concept of distinctive exsudative and lichenoid chronic dermatitis (Sulzberger-Garbe). Is it nummular dermatitis? Am J Dermatopathol 6:387–395
Sulzberger MB, Garbe W (1937) Nine cases of a discoid and lichenoid chronic dermatosis. Arch Dermatol Syphilol 36:247–278

Atopy

Abeck D, Mempel M (1998) *Staphylococcus aureus* colonization in atopic dermatitis and its therapeutic implications. Br J Dermatol 139:13–16
Alaiti S, Kang S, Fiedler VC et al. (1998) Tacrolimus (FK506) ointment for atopic dermatitis: a phase I study in adults and children. J Am Acad Dermatol 38:69–76
Atherton DJ (1988) Diet and atopic eczema. Clin Allergy 18:215–228
Bieber T, Salle H de la, Wollenberg A et al. (1992) Human epidermal Langerhans cells express the high affinity receptor for immunglobulin E (FcεRI). J Exp Med 175:1285–1290
Bousquet J, Lockey RF, Malling H-J (eds) (1998) WHO position paper allergen immunotherapy: therapeutic vaccines for allergic diseases. Allergy 53 [Suppl 44]:1–42
Butler M, Atherton D, Levinsky RJ (1982) Quantitative and functional deficit of suppressor T cells in children with atopic eczema. Clin Exp Immunol 50:92–98
Coleman R, Trembath RC, Harper JI (1997) Genetic studies of atopy and atopic dermatitis. Br J Dermatol 136:1–5
Cronin E, McFadden JP (1993) Patients with atopic eczema do become sensitized to contact allergens. Contact Dermatitis 28:225–228
Darsow U, Vieluf D, Ring J (1996) The atopy patch test: an increased rate of reactivity in patients who have an air-exposed pattern of atopic eczema. Br J Dermatol 135: 182–186
Der-Petrossian M, Seeber A, Hönigsmann H et al. (2000) Half-side comparison study on the efficacy of 8-methoxypsoralen bath-PUVA *versus* narrow-band ultraviolet B phototherapy in patients with severe chronic atopic dermatitis. Br J Dermatol 142:39–43
Di Nardo A, Wertz P, Gianetti A et al. (1998) Ceramide and cholesterol composition of the skin of patients with atopic dermatitis. Acta Derm Venereol (Stockh) 78: 27–30
Drake LA, Ceilly RI, Cornelison RL et al. (1992) Guidelines of care for atopic dermatitis. J Am Acad Dermatol 26: 485–488
Furue M (1994) Atopic dermatitis – immunological abnormality and its background. J Dermatol Sci 7:159–168
Hanifin JM (1997) Critical evaluation of food and mite allergy in the management of atopic dermatitis. J Dermatol 24:495–503
Hanifin JM, Chan S (1999) Biochemical and immunologic mechanisms in atopic dermatitis: New targets for emerging therapies. J Am Acad Dermatol 41:72–77
Hanifin JM, Rajka G (1980) Diagnostic features of atopic dermatitis. Acta Derm Venereol Suppl (Stockh) 92:44–47
Klein PA, Clark RAF (1999) An Evidence-Based Review of the Efficacy of Antihistamines in Relieving Pruritus in Atopic Dermatitis. Arch Dermatol 135:1522–1525
Krutmann J, Czech W, Diepgen T et al. (1992) Highdose UVA1 therapy in the treatment of patients with atopic dermatitis. J Am Acad Dermatol 26:225–230
Malling H-J (1993) Method of skin testing. Allergy 48 [Suppl 14]:55–56
Melnik BC, Plewig G (1989) Is the origin of atopy linked to deficient conversion of ω-6-fatty acids to prostaglandin E_1? J Am Acad Dermatol 21:557–563
Middleton E, Ellis EF, Yunginger JW et al. (eds) (1998) Allergy. Principles and practice, 5th edn. Mosby, St. Louis
Morren M-A, Przybilla B, Bamelis M et al. (1994) Atopic dermatitis: triggering factors. J Am Acad Dermatol 31: 467–473
Przybilla B, Eberlein-König B, Ruëff F (1994) Practical management of atopic eczema. Lancet 343:1342–1346
Przybilla B, Ring J (1990) Food allergy and atopic eczema. Semin Dermatol 9:220–225
Rajka G (ed) (1975) Atopic dermatitis. Major problems dermatol, vol 3. Saunders, London
Rajka G (1989) Essential aspects of atopic dermatitis. Springer, Berlin
Rencic A, Cohen BA (1999) Prominent pruritic periumbilical papules: a diagnostic sign in pediatric atopic dermatitis. Ped Dermatol 6:436–438
Rothe MJ, Grant-Kels JM (1996) Atopic dermatitis: an update. J Am Acad Dermatol 35:1–13
Rudikoff D, Lebwohl M (1998) Atopic dermatitis. Lancet 351:1715–1721
Ruzicka T, Ring J, Przybilla B (eds) (1991) Handbook of atopic eczema. Springer, Berlin
Rystedt I (1985) Prognostic factors in atopic dermatitis. Acta Dermato Venereol (Stockh) 65:206–213

Sampson HA (1988) The role of food allergy and mediator release in atopic dermatitis. J Allergy Clin Immunol 81: 635–645

Schultz Larsen F, Diepgen T, Svenson A (1996) The occurrence of atopic dermatitis in North Europe: an international questionnaire study. J Am Acad Dermatol 34: 760–764

Szentivanyi A (1968) The beta-adrenergic theory of the atopic abnormality in bronchial asthma. J Allergy 42:203

Werner Y, Lindberg M (1985) Transepidermal water loss in dry and clinically normal skin in patients with atopic dermatitis. Acta Derm Venereol (Stockh) 65:102–105

Zahorsky J (1915) The ammoniacal diaper in infants and young children. Am J Dis Child 10:436

Dermatitis in Infants and Children

Ashton RE, Russell-Jones R, Griffiths WAD (1985) Juvenile plantar dermatosis. Arch Dermatol 121:253–260

Gartmann H, Steigleder GK (1975) Inguinale „Pomaden“-Kruste der Säuglinge. Z Hautkr 50:667–669

Jones SK, English JSC, Forsyth A (1987) Juvenile plantar dermatosis – an 8-year follow-up of 102 patients. Clin Exp Dermatol 1:5–7

McKie RM (1982) Juvenile plantar dermatosis. Semin Dermatol 1:67–71

Patrizi A, DiLernia V, Ricci G et al. (1990) Atopic background of a recurrent papular eruption of childhood (frictional lichenoid eruption). Pediatric Dermatol 7:111–115

Patrizi A, Neri I, Marzaduri S et al. (1996) Pigmented and hyperkeratotic napkin dermatitis: a liquid detergent irritant dermatitis. Dermatology 193:36–40

Waisman M, Gables C, Sutton RL (1966) Frictional lichenoid eruption in children. Arch Dermatol 94:592–593

Weston WL, Lane AT, Weston JA et al. (1980) Diaper dermatitis: current concepts. Pediatrics 66:532–536

Wolff HH (1976) Windeldermatitis: Ein polyätiologisches Syndrom. In: Braun-Falco O, Marghescu S (Hrsg) Fortschritte der praktischen Dermatologie und Venerologie, Bd 8. Springer, Berlin S 9–17

Dermatitis in the Elderly

Newcomer VD, Young EM (1989) Geriatric Dermatology. Igaku-Shoin, New York, Tokyo

Thaipisuttikul Y (1998) Pruritic skin deseases in the elderly. J Dermatol 25(3):153–157

Beacham BE (1993) Common dermatoses in the elderly. Am Fam Physician 47(6):1445–1450

Beauregard S, Gilchrest BA (1987) A survey of skin problems and skin care regimes in the elderly. Arch Dermatol 123(12):1638–1643

Gupta G, Dawn G, Forsyth A (1999) The trend of allergic contact dermatitis in the elderly population over a 15 year period. Contact Dermatitis 41(1):48–50

Occupational Disease

Kanerva L, Elsner P, Wahlberg JE et al. (2000) Handbook of Occupational Dermatology. Springer, Berlin

Landrigan PJ, Baker DB (1991) The recognition and control of occupational disease. JAMA 266:676–680

CHAPTER 13

Diseases Caused by Environmental Exposure or Trauma

Contents

Mechanical Damage

The skin is exceptionally resistant to mechanical forces. Depending on the nature and duration of the mechanical stress, the skin response is quite variable. Acute pressure, such as the rubbing of a new pair of shoes, may produce separation within the epidermis or at the epidermal-dermal junction, creating a blister. Less severe chronic pressure produces a thickened epidermis with hyperkeratosis and acanthosis. A wide variety of clinical patterns may develop that are sometimes associated with hyperpigmentation.

Hyperpigmentation

Protracted rubbing or pressure from clothing, belts, suspenders, or prostheses may produce minimal skin thickening but pronounced hyperpigmentation, in which increased melanin production and incontinence of pigment both play a role. Such changes are far more common in overweight individuals, especially in intertriginous regions. A typical example is diffuse dark areas on the shoulders of heavy women secondary to the pressure from brassiere straps. There is no satisfactory treatment other than reducing the mechanical pressure. Bleaching creams bring little relief.

Blisters

Everyone has had a blister following marked physical activity. Common scenarios include rowing a boat for the first time, a session of hoeing in the garden, or a long hike (Fig. 13.1). Blisters can be disabling for soldiers or athletes, although they are generally only a nuisance. Patients with structural abnormalities at the epidermal-dermal junction, such as those with epidermolysis bullosa, tend to develop blisters when much smaller forces are applied. Some patients with mild variants of epidermolysis bullosa are first identified when forced to do heavy physical activity such as marching during initial military training.

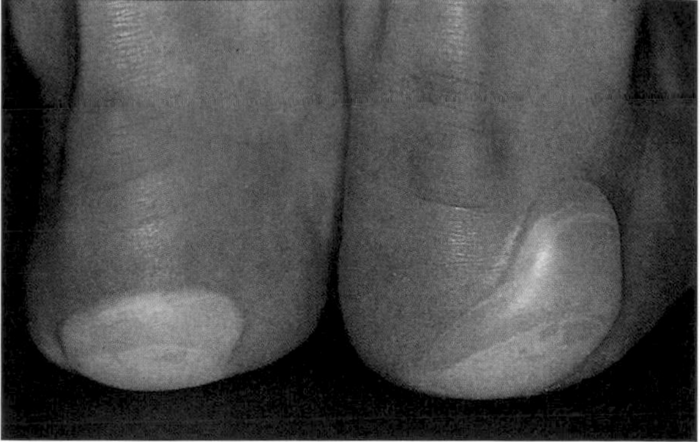

Fig. 13.1. Mechanical blisters

Therapy. Every culture has its own approach to blisters. In general, it is better to leave the blister roof intact, as it provides the best and most natural cover. When the blister is large and tense, a small drainage hole can be made. While the roof will not reattach, it can serve as a dressing until the new epidermis has a chance to develop. If the blister is denuded, then topical antimicrobials and protective dressing are appropriate. Systemic antibiotics are not needed unless there is evidence of a spreading infection.

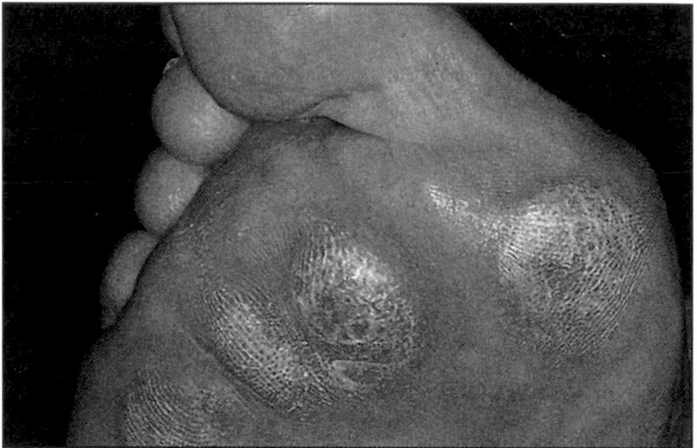

Fig. 13.2. Callus

Hyperkeratotic Changes

Reactive changes of acanthosis and hyperkeratosis produce a thickened epidermis that is then better able to resist mechanical forces. The thickened stratum corneum usually has a yellow tint. The various types of hyperkeratotic change are dependent on the localization and triggering factors.

Callus

Definition. Localized but not sharply bordered hyperkeratotic lesion that arises in response to chronic mechanical pressure.

Etiology and Pathogenesis. Any repetitive rubbing force can induce a callus. The same activities that acutely cause blistering lead to calluses as a protective reaction.

Clinical Findings. One need only to look at the hands of a competitive rower to see that symmetric calluses over the thenar and hypothenar eminences as well as the metacarpal heads and often the fingers provide the protection needed to withstand the great mechanical stresses involved. Other typical calluses are those just proximal to a ring or over the heel or metatarsal head when shoes do not fit properly (Fig. 13.2). The nature of the pressure and the presence of minor anatomic variations determine the location and form of the callus.

Sometimes calluses are an occupational marker. In the past, one spoke often of milkmaid's callus appearing typically on the dorsal surface of the thumb, which was flexed during milking. Guitar players often have calluses on their fingertips. Children who suck their thumbs or chew their fingers also develop typical lesions. Another interesting stigma is "prayer knees" – hyperkeratotic, often gray plaques over the tibial tuberosity in nuns and others who kneel for prolonged prayers. "Cleaning ladies' knees" are similar. In this location, a reactive hypertrichosis may also be present.

Clavus

Synonyms. Corn, soft corn

Definition. Small, sharply defined hyperkeratotic papule with a central plug or core.

Etiology and Pathogenesis. Corns typically develop in response to pressure from poorly fitting shoes or anatomic abnormalities, so that the most common location is the dorsolateral aspect of the fourth and fifth toes (Fig. 13.3). The central plug generally marks the underlying bony prominence, where the pressure is greatest. Corns are more common in women, because they tend to wear more tightly fitting shoes. A soft corn is a small hyperkeratotic papule usually between the fourth and fifth toes arising when the toes are squeezed too tightly together, such as in ballet dancers. In addition, soft corns often reflect an underlying bony spur, so that radiologic evaluation is appropriate.

Clinical Findings. The key finding for distinguishing a corn from a callus is the central plug or core. A typical corn is 5–8 mm in diameter, yellow, often dome-shaped, and usually sensitive to pressure. The central core or eye is generally the most sensitive region. There may be surrounding erythema; secondary infections may occur in patients with predisposing problems such as diabetes mellitus. Soft or interdigital corns are usually less sharply bordered and have a white, macerated surface. They are more likely to be overlooked or misdiagnosed.

Histopathology. The epidermis is hyperkeratotic, acanthotic, and does not contain koilocytes, although the granular layer may be prominent. A clavus will show the central plug if sectioned properly, while a callus will not. In the dermis, there is often edema, necrosis, and fibrosis, which can extend to the underlying joint capsule.

Differential Diagnosis. The most common clinical problem is to distinguish a plantar wart from a callus or clavus. Typically, there is callus formation around a plantar wart, making the problem more difficult. It is helpful to pare away the yellow, hyperkeratotic stratum corneum and look for the central plug of a clavus or the tiny punctate bleeding that suggests a verruca. If neither is found, a callus is usually the answer.

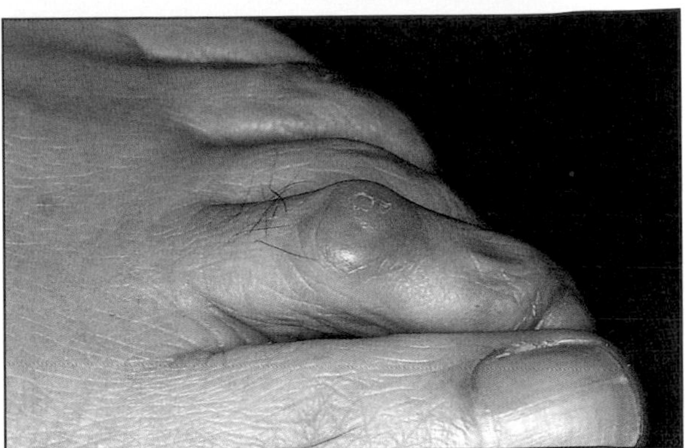

Fig. 13.3. Clavus

Therapy. Fortunately, all the therapies employed for treating verruca can be employed for other hyperkeratotic lesions. These include mechanical debridement, which may involve trimming with a special instrument or double-edged razor, sanding with a pumice stone or carborundum sandpaper, and salicylic acid plasters or solutions. Once the hyperkeratotic outer layer is removed, sometimes one can more accurately assess the underlying disorder. Pads, especially doughnut-shaped corn pads, are also popular. Annular pads may provide relief but can elevate the corn by causing pressure at its base.

Operative approaches to corns and calluses are best left to podiatrists or even orthopedic surgeons. They can most accurately assess whether an underlying bony defect requires correction, and they have more skill in operating in slow-healing areas. If fistulas develop, especially between the digits, surgery is often required. The surgical scars may serve as a nidus for renewed callus formation. The ideal solution is purchasing shoes that do not produce pressure and thus allow the problem to resolve slowly by itself. Once again, podiatrists can provide the best guidance and also recommend appropriate insets and pads.

Black Heel

(Crissey and Peachey 1961)

Synonyms. Pseudochromidrosis plantaris (Bazex et al. 1962), hyperkeratosis hemorrhagica (Rufli 1980)

Definition. Hemorrhage into stratum corneum caused by trauma.

Etiology and Pathogenesis. Sharp mechanical pressure applied to normally hyperkeratotic regions may produce hemorrhage into the stratum corneum. Basketball players are perhaps most prone, especially at the beginning of the playing season; but any activity associated with sudden stops and starts may be responsible. Dancers and individuals walking down mountains get similar lesions on their toes or beneath their toenails. Any mechanical pinching injury to the hands or feet may produce a similar change.

Clinical Findings. The patient usually presents concerned about a new melanocytic nevus on his foot and wants to be assured that it is not a malignant melanoma. Usually one can see linear or punctuate dark brown spots that represent hemorrhage in the stratum corneum (Fig. 13.4). Trimming may remove older lesions, as the hemosiderin migrates up with the scales. The changes are usually asymptomatic.

Histopathology. Even a tangential excision will show reddish brown pigment in the stratum corneum that is positive with an iron stain. If a malignant melanoma is a serious possibility, an biopsy should be done, as malignant melanoma also may bleed into the stratum corneum.

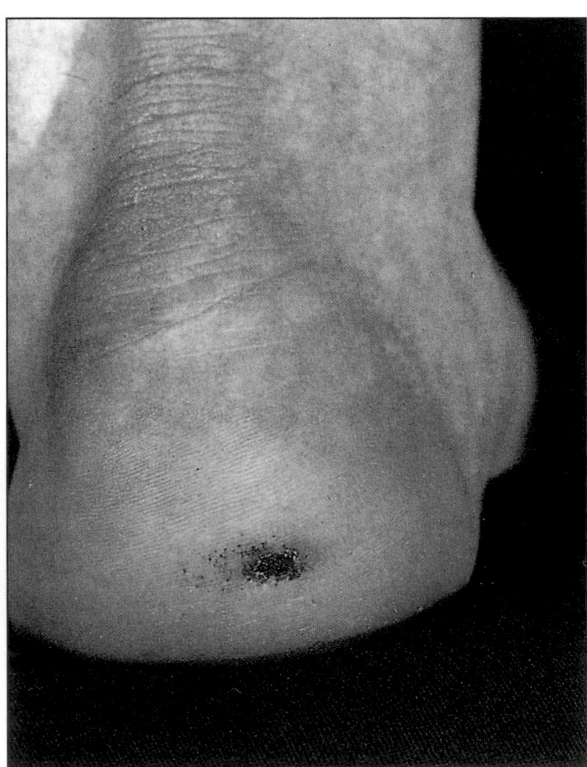

Fig. 13.4. Black heel

Differential Diagnosis. In addition to melanocytic lesions, traumatic tattoos may appear similar. If the history is inadequate, observation or biopsy usually answers the question.

Therapy. Once the diagnosis is clear, no therapy is required.

Acanthoma Fissuratum

(Epstein 1965)

Synonyms. Granuloma fissuratum, spectacle frame acanthoma.

Definition. Painful, callus-like lesion caused by eyeglass frames pressing on the ear or nose.

Etiology and Pathogenesis. The pressure from eyeglasses on the bridge of the nose, the junction of the ear with the scalp, or behind the ear may induce a special type of frictional lesion. There is typically an irregular hyperkeratotic lesion with a dermal granulomatous response.

Clinical Findings. Usually there is a unilateral skin-colored or inflamed flat nodule 0.5–1.0 cm in size, most often with a central dell or fissure. The lesion may be tender and occasionally discharges serous or pus-laden material. When one asks the patient to put on his glasses, the frame or earpiece typically hits the lesion dead center.

Histopathology. In addition to pseudoepitheliomatous hyperplasia and a central epithelial defect, the dermis shows granulomatous inflammation and fibrosis.

Differential Diagnosis. The differential diagnosis includes a basal cell carcinoma, especially when present on the nose. Behind the ear, one can also consider an inflamed epidermoid cyst and an inflammatory response to ingrown hairs.

Therapy. New glasses are a good start. If the lesion persists, intralesional or topical corticosteroids may be helpful. Excision may be required for large lesions but should always be combined with attention to the underlying problem. In our experience, opticians are surprisingly uninformed about this problem.

Decubitus Ulcer

Synonyms. Pressure sore, bedsore

Definition. Ulcer induced by prolonged pressure on the skin, leading to ischemic necrosis.

Etiology and Pathogenesis. A decubitus ulcer is the result of prolonged pressure that produces ischemic necrosis of the skin and even soft tissue. The best known decubitus are those over the ischial tuberosities in bedridden patients who are unable to move. While everyone is aware of the importance of turning and moving patients who are paralyzed or lack sensory input, often the sudden development of decubiti in injured patients, especially those in casts, comes as a surprise. Children may develop ulcers under a cast in a matter of days. Patients in poor general condition are more likely to develop decubiti, as are those individuals with peripheral vascular disease. The heels are another susceptible spot in such individuals.

Clinical Findings. Decubitus ulcers start as persistent, usually painless, livid edematous lesions directly over a bony prominence. They are often overlooked until the pressure produces necrosis with either blisters or a sharply demarcated dry lesion. As the skin integrity is progressively destroyed, the wound no longer remains dry but usually becomes infected and undermined and involves deeper structures such as fat, fascia, tendons, muscles, and even bones. If the patient has intact sensation, the lesions are painful. The long-term persistence of decubiti is one of the factors associated with amyloidosis.

Therapy. Prophylaxis is the best therapy. Skilled nursing is more important than fancy, expensive equipment. Turning immobile patients every 2–3 h, instructing their families in the appropriate procedures, being alert to problems under casts, and carefully inspecting skin at risk under good lighting are essential. Padding such as sheepskin mattress pads is helpful and not as expensive as later treatment of a decubitus ulcer. The role of special mattresses with alternating inflation patterns or that contain tiny plastic beads that are moved about is unclear. These are frequently used, both for prophylaxis and therapy; such beds are so expensive that they have a major impact on hospital budgets. One can say with certainty that they do not replace skilled nursing.

Once a decubitus ulcer has developed, the patient is in for a long haul. The lesions develop by definition in areas that are exposed to pressure and heal slowly. Topical and systemic antibiotics as well as a variety of protective dressings and creams play only a minor role. The main task is to avoid future pressure, which means even more intensive nursing procedures. Surgeons experienced in the management of decubiti should be consulted; both debridement and surgical coverage via a flap or graft are best instituted early but must be coupled with fastidious prophylaxis in the future.

Atypical Decubital Fibroplasia

(Montgomery et al. 1992)

Synonym. Ischemic fasciitis

The same patients who develop decubitus ulcers may also develop a subcutaneous mass over pressure points as a reactive response to prolonged ischemia. In most instances, the patients are elderly. The masses are clinically nondescript, but histologically there is a mixture of fibroblastic proliferation with atypical fibroblasts, necrosis, and new blood vessel formation. Such lesions can be simply excised; it is crucial not to misdiagnose them as sarcomas.

Disorders in Amputees

Definition. Primarily mechanically induced changes in the skin of an amputation stump.

Epidemiology. In the USA, there are an estimated 300,000 patients with leg amputations. In Germany, over 55,000 individuals are registered with amputations as a result of military duty. In younger adults, the main causes are trauma and military activities, while in older individuals peripheral vascular disease, especially associated with diabetes mellitus, is usually responsible.

Etiology and Pathogenesis. Arm amputations are associated with a variety of mechanical problems that arise in trying to couple the prosthesis to functional muscles. Leg amputations more often produce mechanical dermatoses. Walking is a complex task and new prostheses have complicated, often multiaxial knee joints, ankle joints, and flexible but not articulated feet. There are two basic systems:

- Conventional or exoskeleton prostheses, in which the entire prosthesis is functional and bears weight
- Modular or endoskeleton prostheses, in which a central tubular construction carries the weight but is covered by a primarily cosmetic surface

Wearing a prosthesis is anything but easy. The patient must initially overcome the emotional and physical shock of losing a limb, tolerate both actual and phantom pain, maintain good muscle tone and a constant body weight, and devote much time to getting used to the device and caring for both the stump and the prosthesis.

The amputation stump displays irregularities in temperature control. Typically, the skin covering the stump is cool and clammy but also tends to sweat more than the opposite, normal skin. Shear and rotation forces, pressure, rubbing, heat, and sweating affect the skin in combination. The prosthesis provides marked occlusion and often produces edema through suction as well as the lack of available muscle pumping. The end result is continuously traumatized, macerated skin.

Clinical Findings. In addition to examining the skin, one must learn to examine the prosthesis. Key factors include lack of contact at the distal end (producing edema), too much contact at the proximal sites (producing congestion), and local pressure points. One must work with the orthopedic surgeon to ensure that an optimal stump has been created, without bone spurs or sequestration.

Most of the problems seen on stump skin are familiar and not unique. The skin is macerated and may be secondarily infected. Any underlying dermatosis can become exacerbated by the prosthesis, including, for example, psoriasis or lichen planus. An underlying vasculitis may be more likely to ulcerate under the prosthesis. Edema secondary to cardiac disease may first become symptomatic in amputation sites.

Of particular interest are the dermatologic problems unique to prosthetic sites. They include:

- Infections. The stump skin has quantitatively more bacteria that tend to cause folliculitis and furuncles. When fungi are present, Majocchi granulomas may develop.
- Contact Dermatitis. Both irritant and allergic contact dermatitis are likely to develop. The increased sweating may help leach materials from the prosthesis. The main allergens include medications, especially topical antibiotics, as well as sensitizers found in leather, rubber, and plastics.
- Tumors. Keloids, traumatic neuromas, and true epidermal inclusion cysts are most common. Rare events include angiosarcomas in chronic lymphedemas and squamous cell carcinoma in chronic sinus tracts.

A variety of mechanical changes can also occur. The most common are calluses and clavi. Several unique findings may also appear:

- Stump Nodules. These tiny, true epidermoid cysts develop because of continuous follicular damage. Initially, hyperkeratotic follicular plugs appear. They enlarge, extend more deeply, and may evolve into cysts that can be painful and rupture. Shear pressure from skin folds rolling over the edge of the prosthesis appear to be the main cause.
- Stump Edema. The prosthesis is held in place with suction, but when distal or end contact is inadequate, the distal stump will swell as an extremely localized, severe variant of stasis dermatitis. The persistent edema can lead to exudates and ulcerations.
- Acroangiodermatitis (see Chap. 59). This is an extreme version of stasis dermatitis, producing small livid nodules that may be mistaken for tumors but are only proliferations of dilated vessels.
- Verrucous Hyperplasia. While verrucous changes can be seen in severe stasis dermatitis, they are more dramatic and more common in stumps. The combination of edema and friction produces a warty lesion which histologically shows papillomatosis, acanthosis and marked dermal fibrosis. Such lesions can be clinically confused with verrucous carcinomas, but malignant change is extremely rare. Improvement with conservative therapy is the rule.

Differential Diagnosis. The differential list is long and varied. In brief, one must exclude specific infectious processes such as bacterial folliculitis or warts, rule out allergic contact dermatitis, be alert to rare but potentially serious tumors, and remember that most stump dermatoses are caused by friction and other trauma.

Course and Prognosis. The patient will have a prosthesis for the rest of his life. With meticulous self-care and excellent professional attention, the prosthesis should be able to make his life more pleasant rather than create an additional burden.

Therapy. Prophylaxis is the best answer. The prosthesis must fit well and the patient be alert to local trauma, early signs of bacterial infection, and other such changes. Good local hygiene as well as antibacterial and drying measures are essential. Calluses and clavi can be treated with light sanding and mild keratolytics. Because of the need for lifelong therapy, potential sensitizing agents should be avoided. If edema develops, one must determine if it is a local phenomenon requiring prosthesis modification, local compression, and physical therapy or a systemic problem necessitating the intervention of an internist. The stump nodules can be injected with corticosteroids or excised, but recurrences are the rule. Verrucous hyperplasia is usually best managed by trying to reduce friction and edema.

Subcutaneous Emphysema

While few patients present to a dermatologist with subcutaneous emphysema, the clinical changes are in the skin and subcutaneous tissue.

Etiology and Pathogenesis. A number of disease processes can lead to the leakage of air into the skin. They include trauma, surgery, infection, perforation of a hollow internal organ, iatrogenic injuries, and self-inflicted damage. Free air spreads along deep fascial planes and through interstitial tissue following the path of least resistance. Probably the most common scenario is pneumothorax and pneumomediastinum, leading to swelling of the neck and even the face. Gas leaking from a ruptured bowel may reach the skin of the abdomen but also can ascend or descend. Facial fractures and extensive dental procedures have been associated with facial subcutaneous emphysema. Infections with gas-producing bacteria such as *Clostridium perfringens* are discussed in Chap. 4. In rare cases, patients may inject air into their skin.

Clinical Findings. In most instances, the underlying event will lead to obvious physical findings. The skin changes include swelling and, most strikingly, crepitation. When the skin is palpated, fine crackling sounds are heard as the air is moved about the subcutaneous compartment. There may be associated hemorrhage. The most typical changes are a swollen neck and puffy periorbital tissues when the thorax or head is involved. With abdominal leakage, there may also be genital swelling.

Differential Diagnosis. Edema, venous obstruction, and infiltrative processes may all appear similar, but none of these have crepitation.

Therapy. Treatment is directed at the underlying disease and closing whatever is leaking air, if technically possible. In anecdotal reports, inhaling 100% oxygen has seemed to promote resorption of the subcutaneous gas.

Thermal Injury

Most thermal injuries are burns. Other lesions such as erythema ab igne (Chap. 26) may result from prolonged exposure to lower temperatures.

Burns

Definition. Acute tissue damage caused by heat.

Etiology and Pathogenesis. The cause of burns is simple: excessive heat reaches the skin in the form of flames, fumes, hot liquids, or hot solids. But the number of ways in which burns can be acquired is limitless, including automobile accidents, industrial accidents, household mishaps, or simply the reckless use of fire. Small children are at special risk, from baths that are too warm to falling pots of hot water in the kitchen to playing with matches. Burns may also reflect abuse, especially in children and the elderly.

Clinical Findings. Burns are usually divided into three degrees of severity:

First Degree Burn (Superficial Burn). Only the outer layers of the epidermis are involved. The lesions are erythematous, perhaps swollen, invariably tender, and usually moist. They heal after several days with desquamation and perhaps hyperpigmentation.

Second Degree Burn (Partial Thickness Burn). Here the epidermis and perhaps uppermost aspects of the dermis are involved. The burns usually present with painful erythema and blisters that have a moist erythematous base and blanch with pressure (Fig. 13.5). The hairs may be singed, but their roots are intact. The area is not anesthetic. While healing is slower than with first degree burns and may be associated with secondary infection, the result is usually comparable, without scarring and perhaps with pigmentary changes.

Third Degree Burn (Full Thickness Burn). In this situation, there is major cutaneous damage involving the entire dermis and perhaps extending into the subcutaneous fat or even involving the underlying tendons, fascia, and bones (Fig. 13.6). The hairs can be easily epilated, as their roots are destroyed; the area tends to be pale, as the vascular supply is destroyed and anesthetic. If pale, the severity of the burn may be underestimated, but blanching is not present. If blood has coagulated in the dermal vessels, then the skin may be erythematous but, again, does not blanch. It is often difficult to distinguish between second and third degree burns in the first few days, so that one must wait until the depth of necrosis is more easily ascertained. The necrotic tissue forms a white or dark crust that is eventually shed, leaving behind a full thickness cutaneous defect that heals secondarily with a scar and lacks hairs and other adnexal structures.

The end result of a third degree burn is usually a difficult scar, both hyper- and hypotrophic with linear strands radiating in the lines of tension or pressure. Burns in flexural areas such as the antecubital or popliteal fossae are likely to scar, with restriction of motion and perhaps repeated ulceration or breakdown of tissue. Younger patients are more likely to get keloids. Burn scars are a potential precancerous lesion, as they may lead to squamous cell carcinomas after many years.

Systemic Findings. Depending on the type of burn, a variety of systemic problems may be anticipated. They include:

- Shock. The initial shock in a burn is identical to any other traumatic shock and can be treated with fluid replacement. Within a few days, burn-specific hypovolemic shock may develop secondary to fluid and protein loss from the denuded surfaces. This can be expected in adults with more than 20% surface area burns and children with more than 10%. The protein loss usually requires replacement with some type of colloid (albumin or plasma) to restore oncotic pressure.

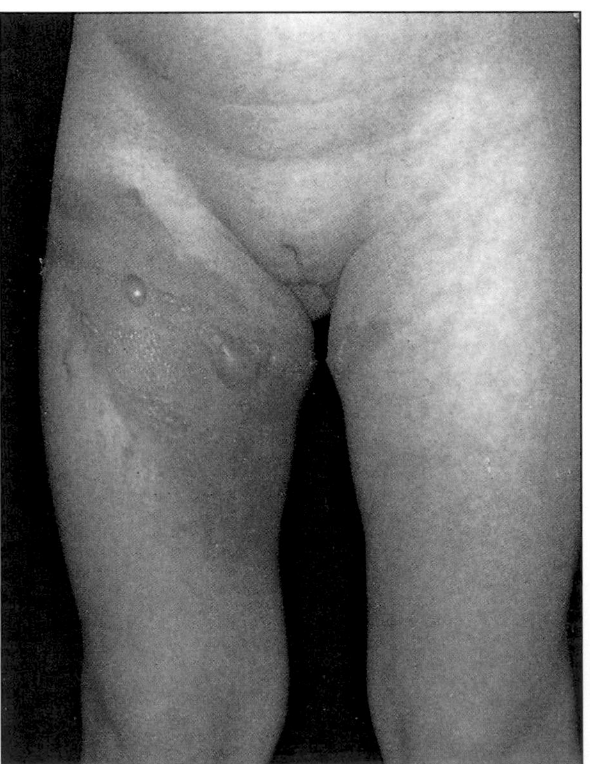

Fig. 13.5. Second degree burn

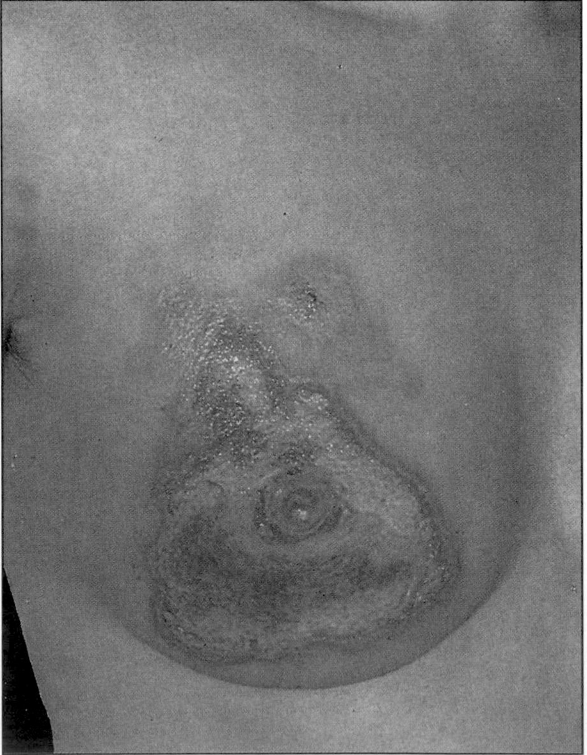

Fig. 13.6. Third degree burn

- Cardiac Disease. If electrical, the initial burn may be associated with cardiac rhythm disturbances. Later, hypovolemia, therapeutic fluid overload, and electrolyte disturbances threaten cardiac function.
- Pulmonary Disease. Inhalation of steam may directly damage the upper airway. In other cases, smoke inhalation causes primarily chemical irritation to the respiratory system and subsequent edema that may require intubation. Later, there may be fluid loss into the pulmonary bed.
- Renal Disease. Fluid and electrolyte imbalance, as well as hemoglobinuria and myoglobinuria, may lead to acute tubular necrosis.

Course and Prognosis. The rule of nines, developed by Wallace and shown in Table 13.1, is used to assess the degree of severity of a burn, usually expressed in percentage of body surface area involved. This value is crucial in planning the initial therapeutic approach. The standard rule of nines must be modified in infants and children because their skin surface area is relatively greater in comparison to their height and weight. The main predictors of death from a burn are extensive burn injury (> 40% of surface area), advanced age (> 60 years), and inhalation injury to the lungs. Patients with none of the risk factors have a < 1% fatality rate, with one factor 3%, with two factors 33% and, with all three factors, close to 90%.

Burns scars have a propensity to develop both basal cell and squamous cell carcinomas. All burn scars should be monitored for the life of the patient.

Table 13.1. The rule of nines, with modifications for infants and children

Body part	Newborn	Infant	Child	Adult
Head	21	19	15	9
Chest	16	16	16	18
Back	16	16	16	18
Arm	9.5	9.5	9.5	9
Leg	14	15	17	18
Genitalia	1	1	1	1

Therapy. In assessing burn patients, one usually moves rapidly from the clinical inspection to therapy. The differential diagnosis is usually nonexistent and laboratory evaluation is used to provide baseline values for monitoring electrolytes, hemoglobin, urine function and output and, often, blood gases. The therapy of burns is complicated and is best left in the hands of experts. If they are not extensive, more superficial burns can be handled on an outpatient basis, but it is prudent to let a burn center or burn management team decide which patients can be treated without admission.

Early management consists of extensive fluid replacement using a variety of formulas to infuse lactated Ringer solution or a similar product. In addition, a decision must be made about intubation and the cardiac condition assessed. Later on, the main challenges are avoiding fluid depletion or overload, maintaining appropriate electrolyte levels, monitoring renal function, and avoiding infection. In the early days of treatment, the most typical organisms encountered are gram-positive bacteria but, later, gram-negative bacteria, fungi, and viruses may play a role.

Topical. The topical therapy of minor burns can be accomplished by family physicians or dermatologists. First degree burns with an intact epidermis require only a bland dressing. Topical corticosteroids may help relieve inflammation. Neither topical nor systemic antibiotics are warranted for first degree burns.

Second degree burns should be cleaned and dressed. Following aspiration or drainage of fluid, intact blisters may be left for a day or two as a natural wound dressing. Broken blisters or other dead tissue should be removed. A dressing should consist of either a water-soluble ointment or ointment-impregnated gauze next to the skin, followed by gauze pads and some type of easily stretched dressing. Dressings can be left on several days unless there is marked weeping and drainage. Wound dressings such as colloid membranes, water-based gels, or other biosynthetic materials are also effective and may speed healing time while decreasing pain. Topical antibiotic dressings such as silver sulfadiazine cream or povidone-iodine products can be used if there is suspicion of infection.

Third degree burns are usually beyond the scope of the dermatologist. They require debridement and then some type of grafting, be it split thickness or meshed grafts, cultured keratinocytes, artificial skin, or other innovative coverings. Allografts or homografts (pigskin or preserved donor skin) may be used to provide temporary coverage when the skin loss is large. Keloid formation is a major problem that is best avoided by using pressure garments or dressings as soon as practicable.

Cold Injury

Cold injuries are invariably the result of man's inability to control his body temperature in the presence of environmental factors such as cold outdoor temperatures and wind. Generalized, diffuse or central cooling is known as hypothermia and is a major medical emergency associated with multiorgan damage. Cold water immersion and burial in snow (avalanche injuries) usually cause hypothermia. Exposure to cold air usually leads to localized injury unless escape and defense mechanisms are impaired or hindered. Localized cold injury in its most severe form is best designated as frostbite, while immersion foot, frostnip, and pernio are less severe variants. Cold-induced panniculitis is considered in Chapter 21.

Frostbite

Definition. Direct tissue injury that results when the skin temperature drops below 0 °C.

Epidemiology. Frostbite is a major military problem. Many armies, including those of Napoleon and Hitler, were stopped as much by frostbite as by enemy bullets. Aviators in World War II, especially the exposed gunners in large bombers, experienced high altitude frostbite. Baron de Larrey, Napoleon's surgeon, proposed guidelines that were still used for handling frostbite until the Korean War. During the 1950s, rapid rewarming at higher temperatures was introduced.

In addition to soldiers, outdoor workers and sportsmen are at the greatest risk. Properly dressed skiers may get frostbite of the cheeks, ears, or nose; those stranded in the cold are at risk of damage to their hands and feet, often requiring amputation. While hypothermia is a problem among the homeless and poor elderly, frostbite is seen less often, perhaps because these individuals are able to avoid freezing temperatures but still must endure long spells of weather just above freezing.

The intensity of the cold, humidity, wind, type of clothing, the presence of peripheral vascular abnormalities and other diseases, the use of alcohol, and the physical demands made on the individual all help determine the degree of cold injury.

Etiology and Pathogenesis. Frostbite is typically divided into four phases. The first signs of cooling are goose bumps (erection of the arrector pili muscles, which fluffs up the fur of other mammals but does little for humans) and shivering. Then the following phases evolve:

- Vasospastic (prefreeze) phase: Vasospasm, anesthesia, and plasma leakage are the hallmarks. Below 10 °C, sensation is markedly reduced, impairing the defensive mechanisms.
- Freeze-thaw phase: In this stage, ice crystals are formed in tissue, causing cellular damage and releasing a variety of mediators. Because of the warming effect of the circulation, skin must be cooled to at least −4 °C before it freezes. After that, the cooling and damage can proceed more rapidly. Nerves and vessels are more susceptible than muscles and bones.
- Vascular stasis phase: Blood flow is slowed, shunted, and halted as leakage, stasis, and edema may occur.
- Late ischemic phase: Thrombosis and other circulatory disruptions lead to tissue necrosis and gangrene.

Other classifications divide cold injury into direct cellular injury from cold and the secondary vascular changes associated with a variety of neurologic and chemical mediators.

Clinical Findings. The clinical findings in frostbite can be graded much as burns are:

First Degree Frostbite. This is a temporary and superficial freeze injury to the skin, presenting with a blanched anesthetic region that is rapidly rewarmed and becomes erythematous and painful but heals without sequelae.

Second Degree Frostbite. More severe or longer freezing that results in sufficient dermal damage to cause edema and superficial blister formation.

Third Degree Frostbite. Deep dermal damage occurs with vascular injury and hemorrhagic bullae and superficial necrosis.

Fourth Degree Frostbite. Tissue necrosis results as the entire skin is frozen and deeper layers are involved with either dry necrosis (mummification) or wet necrosis with infection (gangrene; Fig. 13.7). Totally frozen fingers or toes will evolve over a period of weeks into demarcated necrotic and damaged areas. Thus, amputations should be delayed if adequate nursing care is available.

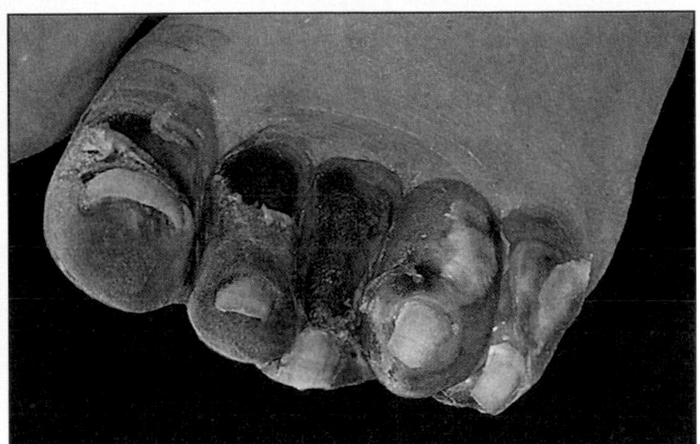

Fig. 13.7. Severe frostbite with necrosis

Course and Prognosis. Patients with superficial frostbite generally do well. Those with deeper lesions are at risk of losing digits or entire extremities. Even in the absence of such major loss, the extremities, especially the feet, may be hypersensitive to cold, experience pain, and show trophic changes such as lack of hairs and a tendency to ulcerate.

Therapy. In the field, no attempts at vigorous rewarming are recommended. Rubbing is particularly harmful and should be discouraged. Techniques of field rewarming such as placing patients next to space heaters or campfires are not wise, since freezing may occur during later transport. Once the patient is in a medical facility, the order of the day is rapid rewarming, usually via immersion in water heated to 40 °C. Hot tap water is too warm and causes burns. Systemic analgesics are usually required.

After rewarming, the skin care is identical to that of burn patients. As already mentioned, surgeons in civilian practice wait for natural delineation before amputating. In a military setting, cases of suspected fourth degree frostbite are often amputated to facilitate care; it is estimated that German military surgeons performed more than 15,000 amputations of limbs for frostbite in the winter of 1942–1943. If gangrene is severe and sepsis a problem, early amputation is sometimes endorsed.

Immersion Foot

Synonym. Trench foot

Definition. Cold damage caused by prolonged low temperature exposure without freezing.

Etiology and Pathogenesis. Immersion foot develops when the feet are exposed to low but not freezing temperatures over longer periods of time and is often associated with increased moisture. There is neurovascular damage but no ice crystal formation in the skin. The main risk group is probably members of the military, as the name trench foot suggests. Those engaging in outdoor activities are also at risk but usually have more opportunities for avoidance.

Clinical Findings. Initial symptoms include numbness and tingling. The skin may initially be erythematous but becomes pale and mottled as the extremity swells. Later, hyperemia develops associated with exquisite pain, ulcerations, and even gangrene. When the tissue damage resolves, the limb remains very sensitive to cold. Since immersion foot has a better prognosis than frostbite but may appear clinically quite similar, the history of exposure is crucial.

Therapy. Treatment is similar to that of frostbite, but one should be even more cautious regarding amputations.

Pernio

Synonym. Chilblains

Definition. Cold injury caused by modest cold exposure associated with peripheral vascular insufficiency of some kind.

Etiology and Pathogenesis. Pernio has many similarities to immersion foot since it too is associated with prolonged exposure to above-freezing temperatures. The major difference is the acral or other limited involvement and the lack of tissue loss. Affected individuals are most often women with impaired peripheral vasodilatory responses. Pernio develops most often in the changing fall and spring seasons and is more likely in those who are inadequately clothed for the rapidly changing temperatures. Tight shoes, thin socks, and tight gloves may all play a role. People who work in cold damp places such as butcher shops or meat packing plants are at special risk. Farmers who work their fields in the cold morning hours are also frequently affected.

Clinical Findings. Many patients may show other peripheral vegetative problems such as hyperhidrosis, acrocyanosis, or cutis marmorata. Pernio lesions are typically located on the dorsal aspects of the fingers and toes (Fig. 13.8), on the shins or inner

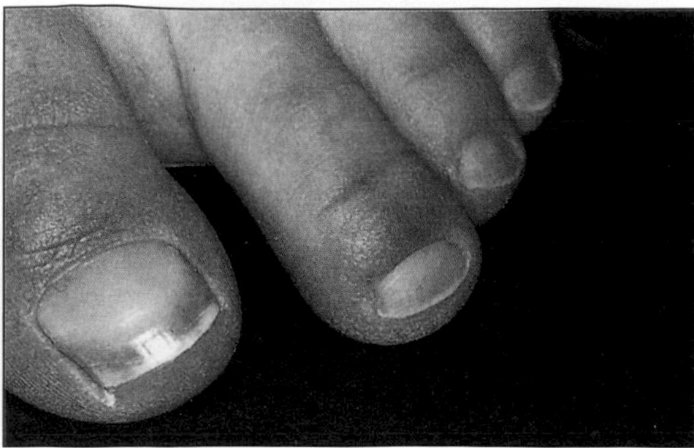

Fig. 13.8. Pernio

aspects of the knees and thighs, or occasionally on the breasts. They are blue-red, edematous, sharply bordered flat nodules that become pruritic, redder, and more painful when warmed. Pernio may present as very small perifollicular papules or large edematous vesicular lesions that may even ulcerate. The larger lesions overlap clinically with immersion foot.

Histopathology. The action is in the dermis, where there are edema, swollen vessels, and a lymphocytic infiltrate. Sometimes there may be vessel destruction, making pernio one of the few examples of a lymphocytic vasculitis. In more extreme cases, there may be subepidermal blisters or even epidermal damage.

Course and Prognosis. The outlook in pernio is good if one can avoid the triggering factors. If not, subsequent attacks tend to become more severe and the patient less tolerant of cold. Often, the tendency to develop pernio lessens with age.

Differential Diagnosis. Patients with lupus erythematosus may have similar lesions on their hands but do not usually have a typical history of exposure to cold (chilblain lupus). Erythema multiforme may also be suggested, but the seasonal pattern, the lack of herpes simplex virus infections, and the absence of target lesions suggest pernio. Larger lesions on the shins and thighs must be distinguished from erythema induratum, other forms of panniculitis, and sarcoidosis.

Therapy

Systemic. Vasodilator medications sound promising but rarely are helpful. Probably the safest approach is pentoxifylline 400 mg taken orally b.i.d. or t.i.d. Other vasodilator agents may shunt blood away from the acral regions.

Topical. Gradual rewarming is recommended. Both 10 % ichthyol in petrolatum and ointments containing nicotinic acid esters may be helpful.

Prophylaxis. Appropriate clothing is the answer. Electric or other hand warmers are a great aid.

Pernio Follicularis

Pernio follicularis lies somewhere between a normal variant and a disease. The relationship to cold exposure is less constant than in ordinary pernio and the lesions are more persistent. Typically, there are hundreds of livid-red follicular papules covering the shins, thighs, buttocks, or aspects of the arms (Fig. 13.9). There are often semi-permanent goose bumps (cutis anserina perpetua) as the arrector pili remain contracted. In addition, follicular keratoses may develop. This produces a rough feeling known as kitchen grater effect in German. While the lesions are most often simply a cosmetic problem, sometimes pruritus may be present. We suspect that most cases are never diagnosed but instead are lumped together with keratosis pilaris. There is no satisfactory treatment.

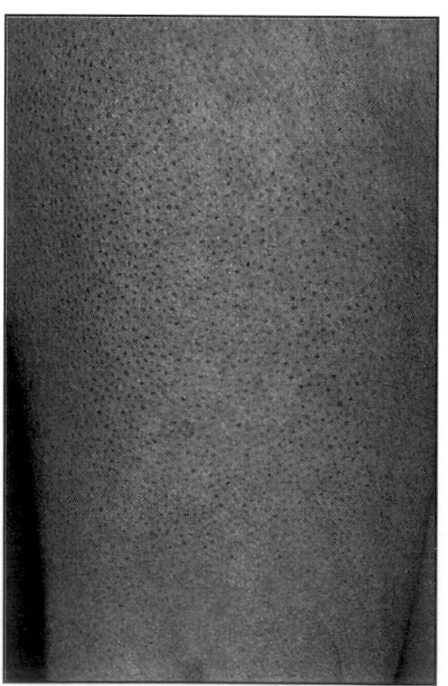

Fig. 13.9. Pernio follicularis

Acute Springtime Pernio
(KEINING 1940)

Clinical Findings. Egon Keining, the coauthor of the first two editions of this book, described young adults who developed pernio lesions on their cheeks, rims of their ears, and backs of their hands. The lesions tend to be edematous and are thus confused with erythema multiforme. Most today consider springtime pernio a variant of polymorphic light eruption.

Cryoproteinemias

The most common members of this rare group are the cryoglobulinemias (Chap. 40). Other, more rare hematologic disorders are discussed below. All of these disorders typically present as cold-induced purpura, usually on the legs and in a reticular pattern.

Cryofibrinogenemia
Cryofibrinogenemia is a very rare disorder in which fibrinogen and its related products precipitate in a reversible fashion in the cold. They are identified in anticoagulated blood, but heparin cannot be used for treatment, as it may produce false-positive precipitates. EDTA, citrate, or oxalate collecting tubes, all readily available, can be used. Cryofibrinogens can be found in healthy subjects during screening procedures. The disease is so rare that its pathophysiology is not understood. Cutaneous findings include purpura, hemorrhage, and ulceration. The search for an associated disease is mandatory; often a malignancy or thromboembolic disorder is found.

Cold Agglutinin Disease
Cold agglutinins appear in two clinical settings, but, in either case, they are IgM immunoglobulins that precipitate erythrocytes. In younger patients, they are polyclonal, triggered by infections such as infectious mononucleosis or *Mycoplasma*, short-lived, and harmless. In older individuals, they tend to be monoclonal and serve as a precursor or associated sign of B cell proliferation. Skin findings may include acrocyanosis, cold urticaria, and purpura, but the main clinical problem is hemolytic anemia, which may also be triggered by cold. The cold agglutinins usually react with the Ii system of erythrocyte antigens. On rare occasions, the monoclonal IgM may be present in large enough amounts to be seen on serum protein electrophoresis, but usually the hematology/immunology laboratory findings will make the diagnosis.

Paroxysmal Cold Hemoglobinuria
These patients have no skin findings, but their disorder is mentioned for completeness. In the past, paroxysmal cold hemoglobinuria was most often associated with syphilis, but today it is recognized to be triggered by a variety of infections. There is an IgG antibody directed against the P antigens of the erythrocytes. Patients have cold-induced hemolysis and dark urine.

Other Cold-Related Disorders

There is a wide variety of other disorders related to cold. For example, cold is one of the triggers of urticaria (Chap. 12). It also causes panniculitis (Chap. 21). Newborns placed on cold surfaces in the delivery room may develop subcutaneous fat necrosis, an extreme form of cold panniculitis. People holding cold Popsicles in the mouth can present with painful red plaques on their cheeks, once again representing panniculitis, despite the paucity of fat beneath the cheeks. Adiponecrosis e frigore describes the most common variant of cold panniculitis, involving overweight women, most often riders who are not dressed warmly enough. They get symmetric painful plaques on the inner aspects of their thighs or less often on their buttocks and breasts. The terms "rider's panniculitis" and "rider's pernio" are also used.

An iatrogenic form of cold injury is that caused by cryotherapy with liquid nitrogen. Usually, the procedure is uneventful, with localized erythema, swelling, and necrosis used to destroy verrucae or actinic keratoses. Sometimes, the necrosis far exceeds the intentions of the treating physician, either because of too long or too aggressive freezing, or because the patient has impaired peripheral circulation or an underlying cold sensitivity. While it is impractical to screen all patients for cryoglobulinemia prior to cryotherapy, one wishes that screening were careful. It is wise to at least ask adult patients whose extremities are to be frozen, such as young women with multiple verrucae of the legs, if they have problems with cold or to treat a few test lesions first.

Electrical Injury

Electrical current and lighting may also cause cutaneous injuries, although these patients usually present to the emergency department.

Electric Current

The burns caused by hot irons, heating coils on stoves, and exposed wires in a heating pad are no different from other burns. However, when electric current flows through the body following accidental exposure to high voltage, there is usually cutaneous damage. The victim tends to be "frozen" to the electrical circuit, so current surges through the body, causing massive internal damage. The muscle damage leads to myoglobinuria and may produce renal failure; compartment syndromes secondary to necrosis and swelling also occur. There is often an injury both where the current enters the body and where it leaves. Most often, the hand is the site of the entry injury (Fig. 13.10) and the foot usually represents the ground. There is often a sharply defined necrotic defect. Another feature is traces of metals underneath rings or other jewelry or associated with metallic prostheses, which may partially melt from the current. A special type of electrical burn is seen when small children chew on electrical cords. Typically, there is an ulcerated lip lesion which, in the absence of a history, may be mistaken for herpes simplex virus infection or impetigo. The underlying musculature tends to become necrotic and the labial artery may eventually be involved, leading to massive bleeding.

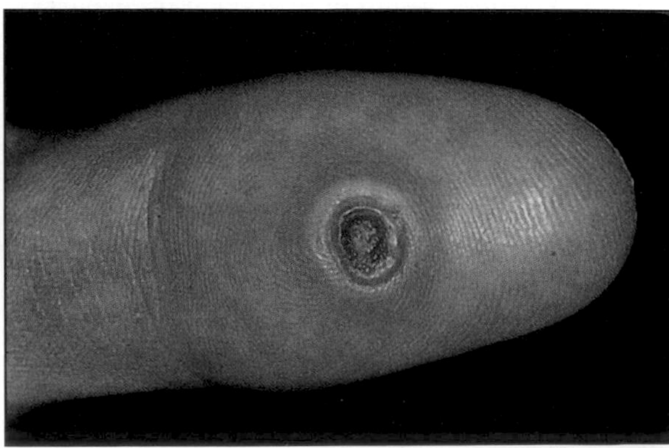

Fig. 13.10. Electrical burn, entry site

Lightening Injury

Etiology and Pathogenesis. Lightening develops when a flow of electric current is established between thunderclouds and the earth. Initially, the clouds are negatively charged and the earth positively. The initial leader stroke develops the connection between the clouds and the earth. Then the pilot stroke rises from the ground to meet the leader stroke and, finally, the return stroke strikes the ground. This cycle may be repeated several times with each lightning flash and is associated with thunder. Currents with more than 10,000 amperes and 100,000 volts arise briefly.

There are many types of lightning injury. The most feared is a direct hit, usually involving someone in an open area or in the mountains, perhaps carrying a conductor. Such individuals may be struck by the leader stroke, which, because of its lower energy levels, may paradoxically deliver more energy to the victim rather than skip over him. Splashing occurs when lightening hits a nearby structure and the energy jumps to the victim, while contact damage occurs when one is touching a struck object. Step voltage or ground current, which spreads through the earth or water following a strike, is less severe but may also cause problems. Finally, the same explosive and implosive forces that cause thunder may act upon a victim.

Clinical Findings. When lightening strikes, in most cases the voltage is so high and the duration so short that flashover occurs as the current envelops the body. Thus, focal entry and exit injuries are often lacking, but stories of victim's shoes or clothes being destroyed are true. The main problems associated with flashover are cardiac arrest and a wide variety of neurologic symptoms, but the massive muscle damage seen with electric current rarely occurs. Prolonged strikes are more likely to produce burns.

Lightening entry sites often show superficial streaking burns or peculiar fern-like figures, while the exit site may show anything from an erythematous macule to a necrotic charred defect. The lightening-damaged skin is usually not painful. The degree of damage is very difficult to assess early on, and almost trivial surface changes may wind up being associated with major deep destruction. Tympanic membrane rupture is frequent.

Histopathology. A biopsy from such lesions is an intellectual exercise and rarely needed. The same epidermal necrosis and elongation of the basal layer cells that is seen in biopsy specimens removed by electrocautery is also found here. The vessels are typically dilated and edema is present.

Course and Prognosis. The prognosis has little to do with the skin findings. Cardiac and neurologic damages are the most crucial in lightening strikes while, in electrical injuries, one must also worry about renal failure secondary to myoglobinuria.

Therapy. Routine burn therapy suffices for the skin.

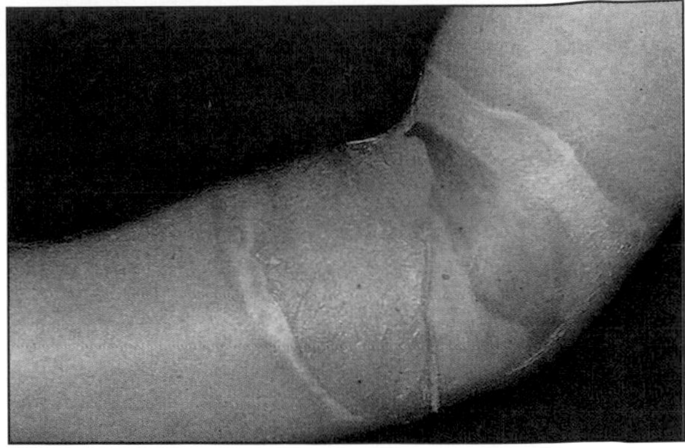

Fig. 13.11. Chemical burn from acetic acid

Chemical Injury

Etiology and Pathogenesis. Caustic or corrosive burns occur when a variety of strong acids or alkalis with tissue-destroying properties contact the skin. The nature of the injury and particularly the treatment are highly dependent on the exact nature of the chemical. Important factors include the composition of the chemical, its concentration, the duration of contact, and the type of skin damaged, i.e., the thickness of the stratum corneum. Most chemical injuries occur as accidents in the home or workplace. Another source of exposure is intentional chemical injury, such as throwing caustic substances onto a victim's face to cause scarring or blinding.

Acids usually denature proteins of the skin, which simultaneously neutralizes the acid. Thus, the lesions are relatively superficial and sharply bordered (Fig. 13.11). Various acids cause a rainbow of color changes in the necrotic skin. For example, sulfuric acid usually produces an immediate whitening followed by a dark crust. Nitric acid causes a yellow crust, while hydrofluoric acid is known for its initially innocent but later widely destructive lesions that may even extend to the bone. Hydrofluoric acid also easily penetrates small openings in otherwise satisfactory rubber gloves, causing digital burns and intense pain. Organic acids such as trichloroacetic acid are used to destroy superficial layers of the epidermis in skin peels and in higher concentrations to destroy verrucae and xanthelasmas. Hydroxyacids provide extremely superficial effects and are in vogue for reducing skin wrinkling. In high concentrations or with prolonged exposure, all of these less dangerous acids can produce significant damage.

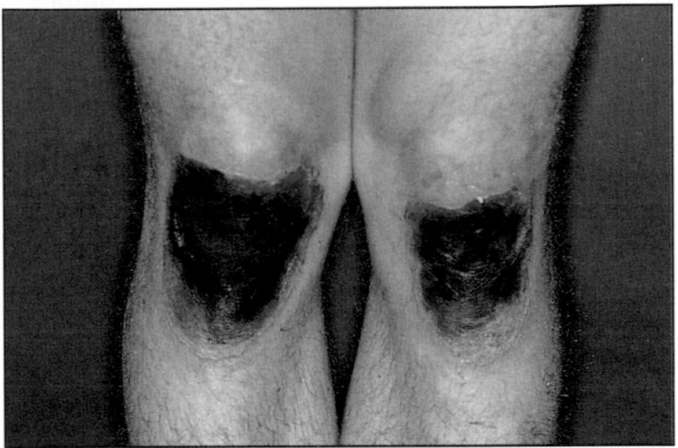

Fig. 13.12. Chemical burn from cement; the patient had worked on his knees in fresh cement

Alkalis or bases cause liquefactive necrosis, meaning that they dissolve the skin, making way for deeper and more severe penetration. The ulcer is often soft, swollen, and messy, not dry like an acid burn. In addition to the main lesion at the site of contact, there are almost always streaky lesions where the material has dripped or run. Sodium hydroxide is probably the most common destructive base, as it is present in many households for freeing up stopped toilets and drains, so it may inadvertently be spilled or even ingested. Ammonia, sodium carbonate, and especially cement are also common bases that may be quite damaging (Fig. 13.12). Potassium hydroxide (KOH) is used to dissolve skin and nails to make fungi easier to visualize.

Tar and asphalt burns are another special problem. The hot material not only causes a thermal burn but also may have chemical toxicity and, furthermore, sticks to the skin. While there is no good trick for removing these products, surface-active petroleum-based solvents are recommended. Standard organic solvents such as gasoline or kerosene may be absorbed and cause additional toxicity. Cement burns can sneak up on a patient, as he or she may work for hours in boots that are not tight or into which cement enters. At the end of the day, burns on the feet or hands under gloves are not uncommon. A final, unusual burn is that associated with ethylene oxide, which is used for cold sterilization in many operating suites and which may leave residues on surgical materials, leading to nurse, physician and, worst of all, patient burns.

Systemic effects should also be anticipated. For example, when using carbolic acid or phenol for deep peels, every physician is aware of the need for cardiac monitoring and the risk of renal damage. Hydrofluoric acid may cause hypocalcemia and tetany, while monochloroacetic acid can produce metabolic acidosis and CNS problems. Healing is usually uneventful, similar to that from a thermal burn, although keloids may be even more common with chemical burns.

Therapy. The treatment of chemical burns is not simple. The local poison control center should be contacted for information on antidotes. When in doubt, copious irrigation with water is usually correct, but wrong, for example, with phosphorus, where copper sulfate solution should be used. When hydrofluoric acid is involved, calcium gluconate gels or infusions should be employed, and it is usually wise to excise the damaged area. Afterwards, general burn care is appropriate.

Chemical Warfare Injuries

Mustard gas is a very damaging oily material. It was used extensively in World War I in France, and there are still areas where weekend hikers or farmers may stumble onto contaminated areas and receive burns. Technically, mustard gas is known as sulfur mustard or yperite after Ypres in Flanders; it is dichloroethyl sulfide. Mustard gas causes prompt blistering of the skin and prominent respiratory symptoms. The cutaneous lesions are slow to heal and scar badly. Chloramine is the military antidote, but it must be applied immediately. A similar chemical used in warfare is lewisite, which is slightly less toxic. The chelating agent dimercaprol or BAL (British antilewisite) has found other medical applications. Today, one speaks of using mustard gas medically; related compounds are used as alkylating agents in the treatment of some internal malignancies. Nitrogen mustard, N-methyl-2-2-dichloroethylamine, or mechlorethamine, is used as a very dilute topical solution to treat cutaneous T cell lymphomas.

Ionizing Radiation Injury

The major types of radiation in use today include standard X-rays or roentgen rays, Grenz rays, and γ-rays from radioactive cobalt or radium. The β-rays from strontium and α-rays from thorium X are hardly encountered anymore. Individuals are exposed to ionizing radiation either intentionally during radiation therapy, most often for systemic or cutaneous malignancies, through industrial exposure, or following a major accident such as at Chernobyl. In the past, hospital workers were at risk, as the dangers of ionizing radiation were not fully appreciated. Early dentists and dermatologists frequently developed radiation dermatitis of the digits or face. Workers painting clock dials with strontium were also exposed. Today, controls are so rigorous that, even in nuclear facilities or aboard nuclear-powered ships, workers have very little exposure.

Clinical Findings. Today, the term cutaneous radiation syndrome has been proposed to encompass the complex series of events that follow exposure to ionizing radiation. The following clinical stages have been identified.

Prodromal Stage. In this brief phase, lasting minutes to hours, there is erythema and pruritus, which resolves and is followed by a latent period.

Acute or Manifest Stage. This is equivalent to the old stage of acute radiation dermatitis and patients may have erythema, bulla, or ulcers, depending on the degree of exposure. Acute dermatitis may develop 6–12 days after exposure to radiation. A dose of more than 7 Gy is required for radiation erythema and subsequent dermatitis. Depending on the interval between exposures, smaller but repeated doses have a cumulative effect. In most instances today, radiation dermatitis is intentional, either because an area of skin is being treated or because the nature of the underlying lesion is such that the portals can not be arranged for sparing the skin. Radiation dermatitis can be graded, just as burns are, even though this subdivision is not included in the newer grading systems:

First Degree Radiation Dermatitis. The mildest form of radiation dermatitis consists of an erythema usually followed by patchy hyperpigmentation. Depending on the dose (about 4 Gy) and the half-value depth, there may be blocked sebum secretion and hair loss. Dryness and hair loss appear after about 3 weeks; regrowth usually starts after about 1–3 months. Today, the use of fluoroscopy to control various invasive radiologic procedures such as coronary reanastomoses has introduced a new source of acute radiation dermatitis: the overexposure to very small dose fluoroscopy levels. Ionizing radiation was used earlier to treat tinea capitis prior to the availability of systemic antifungal agents. Medical museums today contain the old helmets that were used to control the exposure of the various quadrants of the scalp via sliding panels. Similarly, radiation therapy was used for the treatment of acne because of its sebostatic effect, which was first matched by the oral retinoids. The use of ionizing radiation to treat benign disorders has fallen into disfavor.

Second Degree Radiation Dermatitis. Larger doses, in the range of 8–10 Gy, lead to more intense erythema, edema, blisters, and weeping wounds. Here, the loss of hair, sebaceous glands, sweat glands, and even nails may be permanent. The skin heals with telangiectases and pigmentary changes.

Third Degree Radiation Dermatitis. An acute radiation ulcer is typically painful, heals slowly, and always evolves into chronic radiation dermatitis. A radiation ulcer can be a disaster, especially over cartilage or bone. Today, severe damage usually reflects a mistake in dosimetry. Doses in the range of 12 Gy or higher are required.

Subacute Stage. In this phase, there may be persistent erythema and ulcerations.

Chronic Stage. Also known as chronic radiation dermatitis, this stage is the prototype of poikiloderma; there are telangiectases, hypo- and hyperpigmentation, and atrophy (Fig. 13.13). The skin may have a yellow hue (radiation elastosis) and is usually sclerotic. It is dry and appendages are lacking. While second degree acute changes heal with varying degrees of atrophy and pigmentary changes, third degree acute changes always lead to chronic radiation dermatitis. The effects of long-term exposure to much lower doses have been seen on the fingers of dentists who held film in patients' mouths, the hands of cardiologists who "played" with early fluoroscopy units, or even on the feet of salesmen who demonstrate fluoroscope units used to fit shoes.

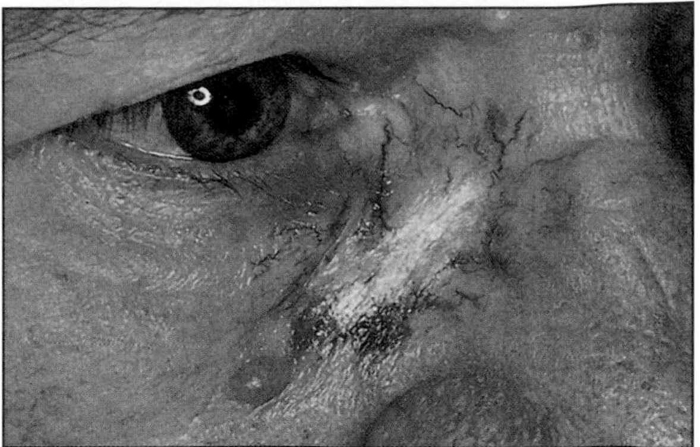

Fig. 13.13. Chronic radiation dermatitis following treatment of basal cell carcinoma; a recurrence is seen at the lower lateral border

The scars of chronic radiation dermatitis are famous for not improving with age, but worsening. The radiation dermatitis associated with Grenz rays as well as the obsolete α- and β-rays is more superficial and less likely to cause problems. Radiation delivered without medical supervision may also cause trouble. For example, in past, nonphysicians used it to perform epilation for women with facial hair; elderly female patients with poikiloderma of the upper lip and chin should always be thus questioned. Similarly, some patients with psoriasis, especially when localized to the nails, received excessive doses of radiation, either because their physicians were overenthusiastic or because they simply found a new physician when the old one said they had exceeded the safe level of 5–7 Gy. Radiation dermatitis is a fertile ground for the development of radiation ulcers, keratoses, and squamous cell carcinoma.

Radiation Fibrosis. Some patients who receive high dosages of radiation develop extensive cutaneous fibrosis, in contrast to the atrophy usually seen with lower dosages. This feature has been particularly noticed in victims of the Chernobyl accident, in whom low dose interferon α or γ seems to have ameliorated the problem.

Radiation Ulcer. Skin with chronic radiation damage lacks adequate vascularization and is easily injured, even by quite minor trauma. When ulcers develop in such areas, the lesions heal very poorly

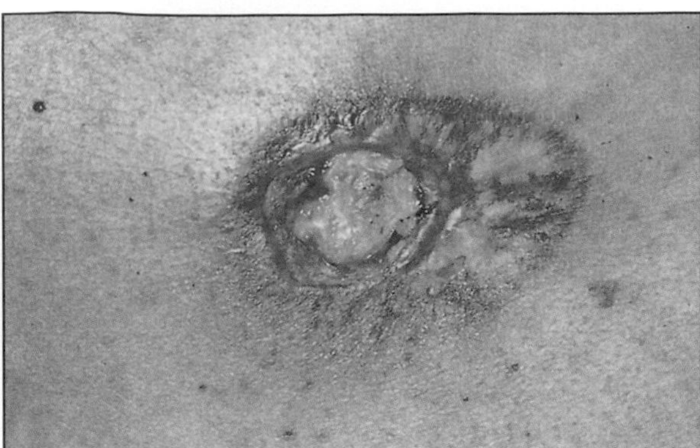

Fig. 13.14. Radiation ulcer

and rarely form sufficient granulation tissue. The ulcers are usually sharply bordered and have an adherent, fatty yellow base (Fig. 13.14). Except for very small lesions, the best approach is excision of the entire area and skin grafting, if needed.

Late Stage. In the late stage, all the features of chronic radiation damage may persist, but there is also the risk of cutaneous malignancies (Chap. 55). At a certain point, almost all chronic radiation dermatitis will develop into keratoses that are similar to actinic keratoses but which tend to be more hyperkeratotic and likely to evolve into squamous cell carcinoma. It is estimated that about 20% of patients with chronic radiation dermatitis develop squamous cell carcinomas. Basal cell carcinoma, malignant melanoma, and a variety of sarcomas have been described much less often.

Therapy. Acute radiation dermatitis is difficult to treat. There is no topical agent that has proven superior. Probably, petrolatum is as good as anything for erosive or crusted lesions. Some physicians suggest corticosteroid creams to reduce inflammation, but the effects are not dramatic. In severe cases, systemic corticosteroids are often administered.

Chronic radiation dermatitis requires tender, loving care. The patient must be aware that the affected piece of skin is fragile and must be guarded. Any minor ulceration should be viewed as a possible squamous cell carcinoma. Thus, small ulcers are best excised for histologic evaluation. When larger lesions are present, the answer is not as simple. Thickened areas should also be biopsied. If the sample shows no sign of malignancy and the patient does not want excision of the ulcer, wound dressings, especially hydrocolloid forms, are worth a try. IFN-γ may be helpful for treating radiation fibrosis; pentoxifylline, vitamin E, and superoxide dismutase have also been recommended.

Diseases Caused by Sunlight

Sunlight plays a major role in many dermatologic diseases. Photobiology is a well-defined scientific field, since the basic science aspects of sunlight, primarily its UV radiation, and its interactions with the skin, immune system, and even the psyche occupy the attention of a wide variety of physicians and scientists. Many dermatologists concern themselves primarily with phototherapy and the diagnosis of photodermatoses. The spectrum of skin disorders related to UV radiation ranges from acute sunburn, familiar to every individual, through the many forms of photoallergy to the diseases exacerbated by exposure, such as lupus erythematosus, and includes all of the aspects of skin with chronic UV radiation damage, including solar aging and most cutaneous malignancies.

Basic Science Aspects

Light refers to the entire spectrum of UV, visible, and infrared radiation. One feature of all light is that the radiation generally does not activate molecules producing ions, in contrast to the role of higher energy sources such as X-rays or γ-rays. Thus, one speaks of light as nonionizing radiation. The wave lengths of light range from 200 nm in short the UV to over 1 mm in the infrared.

Sunlight is ubiquitous and a rich source of light. About two-thirds of the sunlight's energy reaches the earth's surface. The balance is absorbed by ozone, water droplets, and particles of dust and dirt. Although there are marked variations depending on altitude, pollution, angle of the sun (season), and the ozone layer, the average dose reaching the earth's surface at noon is about 2–6 mW/cm^2. For the skin, UV radiation with wavelengths of 280–400 nm and visible light with wavelengths from 400 nm to 700 nm play the main roles. The wavelengths important for photobiology are shown in Table 13.2. The effects of UV radiation and visible light on the skin have been the best studied. Infrared radiation's biologic effects are less well-

Table 13.2. The electromagnetic spectrum

Type of radiation	Wavelength (nm)
Gamma rays	0.0001 – 0.14
X-rays	0.005 – 20
Ultraviolet radiation	
UVC	40 – 280
UVB	280 – 320
UVA	320 – 400
UVA2	320 – 340
UVA1	340 – 400
Visible light	400 – 800
Infrared radiation	800 – 10,000
Radio waves	$10^5 – 10^{15}$

understood but probably play a role both in chronic light damage and in heat transfer.

Ultraviolet Radiation

Ultraviolet radiation has been divided into three subtypes based on wavelength. The different photobiologic properties of the various types of UV radiation form the basis for the subclassification.

UVC Radiation (< 280 nm). The shortest wave UV radiation never reaches the earth's surface. It is screened out by the atmosphere, especially the ozone layer. Thus, with the shrinking ozone layer, there is concern that UVC may begin to play a biologic role. UVC is also blocked by window glass. Most experience with UVC has been acquired from artificial light sources such as xenon and mercury vapor lamps. Even from these sources, UVC is usually screened with a filter. UVC is toxic to cells and used for bactericidal purposes. Experimentally, UVC induces an erythema in the skin that becomes apparent about 6 h after exposure. Little browning occurs. UVC is especially irritating to the conjunctiva, so protective glasses should be worn when exposure to these wavelengths is possible.

UVB Radiation (280 – 320 nm). These wavelengths are responsible for sunburn. They reach the earth's surface, obtaining maximum intensity when the sun is directly overhead and filtering is thus minimal. Artificial light sources also contain UVB. Mercury vapor lamps emit at 297, 303, and 313 nm. UVB is somewhat less irritating to the conjunctiva than UVC. It, too, is blocked by window glass but penetrates quartz glass and water, explaining the risk of sunburn while swimming.

Sunburn or solar erythema usually develops 12 – 24 h after exposure to the sun. Erythema and inflammation are caused by the production and release of prostaglandins and related mediators from the damaged keratinocytes. There is also a delayed tanning as melanin production and transfer increase, occurring 48 – 72 h after exposure. In addition, 7-dehydrocholesterol undergoes photoisomerization on its way to forming biologically active vitamin D_3.

UVB exposure also leads to DNA, RNA, protein, and cell membrane damage, resulting in damage to the epidermis, connective tissue, and blood vessels. Along with photoimmunosuppression, mutations in the keratinocyte DNA are the main cause of solar carcinogenesis. That is, not only are cells damaged, but the body's ability to identify and destroy damaged cells is reduced.

UVB radiation also induces characteristic histologic changes. Erythematous skin shows dilated vessels with a lymphocytic perivascular infiltrate. The keratinocytes may show dyskeratotic changes representing early necrosis; these keratinocytes are known as sunburn or fried egg cells. There may be both intra- and intercellular edema in the epidermis, as well as dermal edema. The release of tumor necrosis factor-α from keratinocytes appears to play a major role in this reaction.

UVA Radiation (320 – 400 nm). Long considered less toxic than the shorter UV wavelengths, UVA is present in natural sunlight and reaches the earth's surface. The intensity of UVA in sunlight is 500 – 1000 times higher than UVB. Thus, during natural exposure, UVA causes both erythema and darkening. UVA erythema is immediate and does not involve toxic effects on keratinocytes. The UVA darkening is also rapid, arising via oxidation of melanin (the Meirowsky [1909] phenomenon) as well as stimulating melanin transfer and melanogenesis. But toxicity from UVA via sunlight is almost impossible, because sunburn or UVB toxicity is the limiting factor. That is, one cannot get a toxic dose of UVA in natural sunlight because by then one will already be "fried" by the UVB. The advent of artificial UVA sources as well as the availability of highly effective UVB sunscreens in the past two decades have made UVA far more important. UVA is divided into UVA1 (340 – 400 nm) and UVA2 (320 – 340 nm). The shorter UVA2 rays have some UVB-like effects, causing more erythema and producing DNA damage.

The biologic effects of UVA are quite different from those of UVB. UVA penetrates window glass, so photoreactions can occur in an automobile or indoors, despite adequate windows. Conjunctival irritation is minimal. Even in fairly large doses such as 100 J/cm^2 the epidermis shows no phototoxic changes. The dermal vessels may be dilated and surrounded by a mixed inflammatory infiltrate that may contain neutrophils and eosinophils in addition to lymphocytes. UVA is responsible for the vast majority of photoinduced drug reactions.

Visible Light and Infrared Radiation. The biologic effects of visible light on the skin are minimal. Patients with marked photosensitization, such as in cases of solar urticaria or some cases of chronic actinic dermatitis, may be sensitive to visible light. In higher doses, infrared radiation causes thermal damage, but it is unclear if it has other biologic roles. Animal studies have shown increased dermal damage when infrared radiation is added to UVB radiation. In addition, erythema ab igne (Chap. 26) is caused by infrared radiation.

Dosimetry

Clearly defined units are used to define light rays.

Watt = the power of the light source
Watt/s = joule = amount of energy released

Usually, the strength or power of a radiation source is give in watts (W) or milliwatts (mW), while the intensity is expressed as watts per unit area or W/cm^2. The dose is then expressed as J/cm^2.

$$\text{Dose} = \text{W/s/cm}^2 = \text{J/cm}^2$$

In the past, the amount of radiation given to a patient was often expressed or recorded simply in seconds or minutes. Modern machines are calibrated in J/cm^2 so that one can simply dial in the amount desired. The main variable is the age of the lightbulbs or tubes, which leads to considerable changes in energy released per second, the wavelength of the energy, and the radiation distribution pattern over the entire length of the light tube. Thus, calibration is still necessary. Devices with many light units for calibration are designed primarily for that unit and not very accurate when comparing several different units. Photobiologists have access to more expensive but more universal devices such as the Centra, made by Osram in Germany, which has special measuring heads for both UVA and UVB. Other devices such as a bolometer are used to assess monochromators, providing values in W or J/cm^2. In all cases, the distance of the patient from the light source must be considered, as the intensity of radiation quadruples if the distance from the source is halved. The role of time is linear; that is, for all practical purposes, 60 s exposure provides twice as many J/cm^2 as 30 s.

DNA Repair Mechanisms

There are three basic methods by which cells repair light-induced DNA damage:

- Excision Repair. The damaged DNA is excised and a correct replacement sequence is synthesized and inserted. Since radiation is not required, this mechanism is also known as dark repair; in genetic slang, it is described as cut and patch. Radioactive thymidine uptake can be demonstrated but at lower levels than during cell replication; thus, another synonym is unscheduled DNA synthesis. A series of enzymes are involved in the process of cutting out the defective piece and inserting a new one based on the intact paired DNA. The repair process is quite accurate. Patients with xeroderma pigmentosum have a variety of defects in excision repair.
- Postreplication Repair. In this situation, the damaged DNA is not directly repaired. Instead, it is ignored and then, during DNA replication, the errant segment replaced. This mechanism is fairly inaccurate, so it is likely to introduce mutations into the cell.
- Photoreactivation. One type of DNA damage is the formation of a cyclobutane ring. This ring can be split to restore the normal base pair sequence by an enzyme that is activated by visible radiation. Photoreactivation has best been shown in some marsupials. The presence of the photoreactivating enzyme in humans is disputed. The clinical importance of photoreactivation is clear; tests are underway involving the topical application of photoreactivating enzyme after sun exposure.

Skin Types

Fitzpatrick and coworkers developed the concept of skin types (Table 13.3) to categorize more quickly an individual's response to sunlight. The skin type is based on a person's reaction to 30 min of midday sunlight for the first time in the summer.

Table 13.3. Skin types (after FITZPATRICK 1988)

Skin type	Sunburn	Tan	Population
I	Always	Never	Celts
II	Always	Sometimes	
III	Sometimes	Always	
IV	Never	Always	
V	*	*	Dark-skinned persons (Native Americans, Mediterraneans, others)
VI	*	*	Blacks

* Such individuals may experience both tanning and sunburn under maximum sun exposure; they show no reactions after 30 min

All of the various reactions to light, be it sunlight or from artificial sources, show great individual variability, but the skin type is the quickest way to estimate roughly an individual's light susceptibility. Type I and II individuals are usually fair, may have blond or red hair, freckles, and blue eyes. However, one often encounters darker patients who easily burn or blue-eyed blondes who rarely burn. Persons with type I or II skin not only burn more easily but are at greater risk of chronic UV radiation damage, including basal cell carcinoma, squamous cell carcinoma and malignant melanoma, as shown by the Celtic population of Australia.

Pigmentation

Stimulation of the melanin system leads to tanning, darkening, or browning. Two types of pigmentation have been identified.

Immediate Pigmentation
(HAUSSER 1938)

Synonyms. Direct pigmentation, immediate pigmentation, Meirowsky phenomenon

Etiology and Pathogenesis. Melanin precursors are photooxidized to darker melanin. This occurs rapidly after exposure to UVA. The immediate pigmentation dose (IPD) is about 10–30 J/cm^2 at 330–400 nm. The pigment produced is ashy or grayish brown, as compared to the coffee brown color from UVB. Fewer joules are required if the skin is already tanned. Immediate pigmentation can be produced by an afternoon in natural sun, during psoralen plus ultraviolet A (PUVA) therapy, or by the UVA radiation used in tanning studios.

Late Pigmentation

Synonyms. Suntan, delayed pigmentation, melanogenesis, indirect pigmentation

Etiology and Pathogenesis. Late pigmentation appears 24–72 h after UV radiation exposure. While 297 nm wavelengths have the maximum effect on melanogenesis, the action spectrum extends from 250 nm to 400 nm. In the UVA region, the effect is 100–1000 times less than with UVB. The dosage required is known as the delayed pigmentation dose (DPD). Nonetheless, repeated UVA does lead to tanning, as experiments and the success of tanning studios show. In addition, there is about 1000 times as much UVA radiation in sunlight; so, despite its weaker activity, it does play a biologic role. The pigmentation remains for days or weeks.

Many factors determine how an individual tans. The amount and wavelength of UV radiation are crucial, but hormonal and genetic factors are also important. Under the influence of UV radiation, the basal layer melanocytes produce more melanin, which is packaged in melanosomes and transferred to keratinocytes via the dendrites. The production and transfer of melanin is considered in more detail in Chapter 26.

In some animals, the skin's response to radiation is controlled dramatically by melanocyte stimulating hormone (MSH). In humans, the role of MSH is confusing but clearly much less important. Little MSH is produced by the pituitary gland, and its role in pigmentation is unclear. Most MSH is derived from adrenocorticotrophic hormone (ACTH). The dark pigmentation in patients with Addison disease and excessive ACTH levels is the best evidence for at least some role for MSH. The role of estrogens is suggested both by pregnancy-induced darkening, such as of the nipples, and the interaction of hormones and light in melasma.

Lichtschwiele

(Miescher 1930)

The German term *Lichtschwiele* (light callus) describes the ability of the thickened stratum corneum to block the effects of light. The most practical example of this is the difference in tanning ability between the back, with 15–20 layers of stratum corneum, and the palms, with perhaps 200 layers. In addition, repeated UVB radiation produces thickening of the stratum corneum, while UVA radiation does not. This action of UVB radiation was one of the early justifications for phototherapy; today it appears that photoimmunologic factors better explain the benefits. In addition, the lack of a UVA lichtschwiele is another reason why a UVA tan does not protect as well as a UVB tan. The lichtschwiele persists for many weeks but disappears in the less sunny months.

Artificial Light Sources

A wide range of light sources are employed in dermatology, primarily for therapeutic purposes but also for diagnostic testing and research:

- Gas discharge lamps: The emission spectrum consists of characteristic bands (linear spectrum).
- Fluorescent lamps: These contain a variety of gases, often mercury, and are coated on the inside. The combination of the type of gas and the nature of the coating determines the emission spectrum. Both UVA and UVB fluorescent tubes are available. Some tubes also release UVC, which can be toxic, often causing keratoconjunctivitis. UVC lamps are used for sterilization.
- Low pressure mercury vapor lamps: These have a heavy band at 254 nm and are used primarily for sterilization.
- High pressure mercury vapor lamps: These are frequently small, home UV tanning lamps rich in UVB, known around the world as sunlamps. The UVC component is filtered out by the tube. The old Kromayer lamps also fell into this category.
- Super high pressure mercury lamps: These are the usual, monochromatic light sources used for diagnostic purposes and usually combined with a series of filters.
- High pressure mercury lamps with metal halide addition: The addition of various metal, e.g., iron, salts, can enrich selected parts of the spectrum, such as UVA. Many modern UVA lamps are of this type.
- Wood lamp: This special UVA lamp, usually a high pressure mercury lamp, has special filters to produce maximum radiation at about 365 nm. It is useful for diagnosing tinea versicolor, erythrasma, some forms of *Microsporum* infection, and for identifying depigmented areas (ash leaf macules in tuberous sclerosis, vitiligo) or hyperpigmented lesions (nevi, freckles) more clearly.
- Xenon arc lamp: Xenon lamps produce artificial light that most closely resembles sunlight. They form the mainstay of solar simulators, which are used to test photosensitivity or evaluate sunscreens, and are also found in many monochromators.

While many of the sources have a relatively wide spectrum, this can be reduced by selected filters which, unfortunately, at the same time reduce the intensity of the radiation. This is a particular problem with UVA. For example, to irradiate with 20–40 J/cm^2 using a conventional fluorescent source might require 20–60 min. Newer high intensity sources such as the metal halide ones can greatly reduce this time.

Monochromators (or monochromatic sources) are very useful in determining action spectra, such as for photosensitizing drugs or solar urticaria. They usually consist of a high pressure mercury or xenon light source and a prism or grid to produce a narrow wavelength of light. They are of low intensity, requiring a long time to deliver a given dosage, and also cover only small fields.

Photobiologic Testing Procedures

Table 13.4 shows the light sources used in our department for photobiologic testing.

Light Sensitivity

UVB Sensitivity. The minimal erythema dose (MED) is the smallest amount of radiation that will produce a sharply defined, uniform erythema after 24 h. The MED is used to assess reactions to UVB radiation using the *Lichttreppe* („steps of light“) technique of Wucherpfennig (1937). Defined areas of skin are exposed to increasing doses of radiation. Often, an opaque patch is used that has six to ten windows with opaque flaps which can

Table 13.4. Recommended light sources for photodiagnosis

Source	Wavelength (nm)	Main uses
UVB	280–320	Determination of MED Provocation of lupus erythematosus, polymorphic light eruption
UVA	320–400	Photopatch testing Determination of MPD
UVA1	340–400	Provocation of lupus erythematosus, polymorphic light eruption
Sun simulator	Mimics solar spectrum	Some sunscreen testing
Monochromator	Variable	Determination of action peak for solar urticaria; vary 10–25 nm/field

MED minimal erythema dose; MPD minimal phototoxic dose (DPD)

be closed at given time intervals. Usually, the difference in exposure between windows has a ratio of 1.25:1 or 1.4:1. One can use a solar simulator or lamp with a range of 280–350 nm to irradiate the areas. A typical sequence might go from 14 to 112 mJ/cm^2.

The areas are evaluated after 24 h and the area with the faintest hint of erythema is taken as the MED. There is some variation in MED, depending on the body region tested and the patient's skin type. The test site is usually on the buttocks. The MED also varies with wavelength (Table 13.5); if not otherwise specified, MED refers to UVB exposure. On a sunny, cloudless summer day spent outdoors, a fair individual can obtain up to 20 MED. Once the technique is standardized, the MED measurements can be used to assess a sunscreen by comparing the MED on treated and nontreated skin.

UVA Sensitivity. UVA sensitivity is somewhat more complicated. The ability of UVA to produce erythema is about 1/1000 that of UVB, so extremely long exposure would be required for a UVA MED. In addition, UVA erythema appears after 1–2 h, peaks after 12 h, and fades rapidly. A series of fields are exposed to about 5–40 J/cm^2 (note that the units are millijoules for UVB and joules for UVA) using a relatively intense source of UVA. The immediate pigmentation dose (IPD) is determined just after irradiation and the delayed pigmentation dose or minimal tanning dose (MTD) assessed after 24 h. One can use fluorescent UVA tubes or high pressure mercury lamps with metal halides. In patients with extreme photosensitivity, monochromators may be more appropriate.

Table 13.5. MED at various wavelengths

UV type	Wavelength (nm)	MED
UVB	300	0.038–0.053 J/cm^2
UVC	250	0.02 J/cm^2
UVA	360	20–50 J/cm^2

The minimal phototoxic dose (MPD) is the amount of UVA combined with a defined dosage of a photosensitizing agent, usually psoralen, that produces a similar erythema. The procedure is the same as with MED determination, but the reaction is read after 48 or 72 h. In some systems, the presence of tanning, instead of erythema, is used as the end point. The MPD can be determined prior to the institution of PUVA, just as the MED is determined prior to UVB therapy. The MPD for skin types I–III is usually around 0.2–2.0 J/cm^2.

Phototesting

Some dermatoses are elicited by radiation alone; examples are solar urticaria and polymorphic light eruption. In contrast, other disorders require a photosensitizing agent and radiation, as in the case of phototoxic and photoallergic dermatitis. Thus, the usual test procedure consists of exposing the skin to radiation both alone and in combination with suspected sensitizing agents. In every case, the goal of the test is reproduction of the clinical lesions suspected of being related to radiation. Most radiation reactions are mediated by UVA. As Table 13.6 shows, the amount of radiation required to produce a reaction varies greatly, from < 0.1 J/cm^2 in solar urticaria to > 40 J/cm^2 in polymorphic light eruption. Other than determining the MED, UVB testing hardly ever plays a role. Occasionally, UVB radiation is a factor in polymorphic light eruption.

Provocation Testing. It is often useful to attempt to reproduce a photosensitive dermatosis by repeated

Table 13.6. Average UVA dose to elicit reaction

Disease	Required UVA Dose J/cm^2
Solar urticaria	0.05–2.0
Photoallergic contact dermatitis	1–10
Phototoxic contact dermatitis	5–30
Hematogenous photoallergy	3–10
Persistent light reaction	0.5–5
Polymorphic light eruption	40–100
Hydroa vacciniformia	40–60

irradiation of a localized area. The procedure is most often used for polymorphic light eruption. The exact techniques are discussed with the descriptions of the respective diseases. Sometimes it is useful to perform a skin biopsy, as in the case of provoked lupus erythematosus. Provocation not only helps confirm the role of radiation in the disease and refine the diagnosis but, if sufficient testing is done, the wavelengths most responsible for the problem can be defined and the patient advised as to sunscreens and hardening measures.

Photopatch Testing. The suspected photoallergens are applied to the back as with ordinary patch testing but with two parallel sets. The most likely photoallergens are represented in standard test series such as the one developed by the German Photopatch Group (Table 13.7). After 24 h, one of the duplicate rows is exposed and irradiated with 5–10 J/cm^2 UVA. If deemed necessary, the irradiated sites can be covered again to avoid additional radiation through the clothing in sunny months. The reactions at both the irradiated and nonirradiated sites are read at 48, 72, and 96 h as well as days later in some cases. If an allergic reaction occurs only in the irradiated site and not in the corresponding nonirradiated site, one can diagnose a photoallergic reaction. A phototoxic reaction will also appear only in the irradiated area but will be strictly confined to the limits of the patch, just as with ordinary patch testing (Chap. 12). In addition, phototoxic reactions tend to be immediate, although delayed phototoxic reactions can be seen, as from psoralens.

Other Tests. Other types of phototesting are occasionally performed. All use UVA in the same range as photopatch testing:

- Systemic photoprovocation: The patient takes the suspected phototoxic or photoallergic medication and then is irradiated at the peak of the pharmacokinetic level, usually between 2 and 8 h.
- Prick or scratch phototesting: The suspected agent is introduced into the skin via a prick or scratch technique, just as with ordinary allergens (Chap. 12); then the site is irradiated.

Table 13.7. Recommended photopatch allergens

Agent	Concentration (%)
Tetrachlorsalicylanilide	0.1
5-bromo-4′-chlorsalicylanilide	1.0
Hexachlorophene	1.0
Bithionol	1.0
Sulfanilamide	5.0
Promethazine hydrochloride	0.1
Quinidine sulfate	1.0
Musk ambrette	5.0
Fragrance mix	8.0
4-amino benzoic acid	10.0
2-ethylhexyl-4-dimethyl-aminobenzoate	10.0
1-(4-isopropyl phenyl)-3-phenyl-1,3-propandione	10.0
4-tert-butyl-4′-methoxy-dibenzoylmethane	10.0
Isoamyl-4-methoxycinnamate	10.0
2-ethylhexyl-4-methoxycinnamate	10.0
3-(4-methylbenzylidene)-camphor	10.0
2-phenyl-5-benzimidazole sulfonic acid	10.0
Oxybenzone	10.0
Sulisobenzone	10.0

In both techniques the results are read immediately after irradiation and then 24–72 h later.

Radiation-Induced Skin Reactions

Three types of reaction occur: (1) reactions in normal skin as a result of too much radiation, be it acute (sunburn) or chronic (solar elastosis); (2) photodermatoses, in which the skin reacts to doses of radiation that would not cause trouble in a normal individual; (3) aggravation of existing dermatoses by radiation, such as a flare of lupus erythematosus induced by sunburn.

Photodermatoses are usually divided into primary disorders, in which the skin is sensitive to radiation but there is no underlying disorder identified, and secondary disorders, in which there is an established underlying problem such as a porphyria, lupus erythematosus, or xeroderma pigmentosum. Obviously, the latter separation is somewhat artificial, as the primary disorders also have an underlying etiology that has just not been discovered.

The wavelength of radiation that triggers a given reaction is known as the action spectrum. It is important to determine the action spectrum in order to be able to recommend the appropriate prophylactic and, to some extent, therapeutic measures. For example, sunburn is best avoided with UVB sunscreens, which, on the other hand, do little to protect against polymorphic light eruption, which is usually provoked by UVA radiation. In the latter case, a combined UVB and UVA sunscreen usually offers more help. Another example is erythropoietic protoporphyria, in which the action spectrum lies in the visible range at 400–410 nm (Soret band); in this case, an opaque or reflective screen is required.

Table 13.8. Sunlight-related changes in normal skin

Course	Features
Acute	Sunburn
	Suntan
	Immediate pigmentation
	Melanogenesis
	Lichtschwiele
	Immune suppression
Chronic	Photoaging
	Solar elastosis
	Telangiectases
	Carcinoma in situ
	Actinic keratoses
	Lentigo maligna
	Malignancies
	Basal cell carcinoma
	Squamous cell carcinoma
	Lentigo maligna melanoma
	(Probably other malignant melanomas)

Radiation Reactions in Normal Skin

The reaction of normal individuals to radiation is an attempt to protect against the acute and chronic effects of this energy. Unfortunately, often these protective mechanisms fail, producing sunburn instead of suntan and, more importantly, a wide range of chronic changes, as shown in Table 13.8. UV-induced erythema and pigmentation have already been discussed in this chapter, while malignant lesions are discussed in the relevant chapters dealing with tumors.

One very important aspect of photoinduced skin damage is UV-induced immunosuppression. A generation ago, it was believed that direct radiation damage to the DNA of the cells in the skin induced mutations that led to cancers. Today it is clear that the body has many mechanisms to repair such damage but that the immunosuppression induced by radiation facilitates the escape of such aberrant cells from the body's surveillance, increasing the risk of cancer formation. Today, photoimmunology is a new but well-established specialty of which photoimmunodermatology is a prominent subdiscipline. The most important milestone was the work of Kripke and her group on the antigenicity of UV-induced tumors: Using syngeneic mice, a range of tumors were induced using radiation. The tumors were transplanted to recipients; those which had been irradiated accepted the tumors, while nonirradiated animals rejected them. Thus, UV radiation induces a specific tolerance of UV-induced tumors.

Another major milestone was the discovery that it is much more difficult to induce allergic contact dermatitis in irradiated skin. When an antigen is applied to previously irradiated skin, a tolerance often develops. Langerhans cells, the epidermal antigen-presenting cells, present the antigen to the immune system. After UVB radiation or PUVA therapy, these cells are less adroit at presenting antigens, leading to a local immunosuppressive effect. They recover their effectiveness after 3–4 weeks.

The main effector cell in producing immune tolerance to both tumor-specific antigens and contact allergens is the suppressor T cell. Radiation can also lead to systemic tolerance towards both tumor antigens and allergens as well as reducing the reaction to organ transplants and some infectious agents. The mediators of systemic radiation-induced immunosuppression include urocainic acid, α-MSH, and a variety of cytokines. Urocanic acid develops in the stratum corneum through *cis-trans* photoisomerase formation. The other mediators are presumably released by keratinocytes following radiation exposure.

Sunburn

Etiology and Pathogenesis. Sunburn is a toxic reaction in the skin induced by the erythemogenic UVB wavelengths, mainly between 295 nm and 315 nm. It varies greatly from individual to individual, depending on skin type, degree of protection, season of the year, weather conditions, and duration of exposure. Sunburn is more likely when radiation is reflected from sand, water, or snow. In addition, at higher altitudes, the intensity of the radiation is stronger because there is less atmosphere to absorb the radiation, and the protective effects of moisture and dust droplets are reduced. The amount of previous exposure plays an important role, as both suntan and lichtschwiele are also protective. The immediate darkening is overwhelmed by the erythematous changes, so it has no importance.

Usually, multiple MEDs of exposure are required to produce sunburn. As a rule of thumb, an MED for noonday sun in the summer is about 20 min, so a day at the beach can produce up to 20 MED of exposure and sunburn. The main cause of the erythema is vasodilatation in the papillary dermis. The principle mediators in sunburn are prostaglandins; inhibitors such as indomethacin and aspirin can block the erythema by altering the degree of keratinocyte damage. As a result of keratinocyte damage, a variety of cytokines are released, including TNF-α and interleukin (IL)-6. The latter appears to trigger the appearance of acute phase proteins such as C-reactive protein, which is responsible for the systemic malaise associated with sunburn.

Clinical Findings. The clinical features of sunburn are known to everyone (Fig. 13.15). The erythema usually develops 4–6 h after exposure, peaks at 12–24 h and begins to fade by 72 h. When UV erythema is studied in the laboratory, the maximum erythema is interpreted at 24 h. The initial change is erythema associated with edema and a feeling of warmth and often malaise. Later, blistering and then peeling (desquamation) occur. In milder cases, the transition goes from erythema gradually to tanning or peeling. With more severe sunburn, the systemic symptoms become more problematic. Fever, nausea, vomiting, and headache may be seen; in extreme cases, circulatory collapse and heat stroke can be encountered. Ocular problems may also be encountered; UVC (only found in artificial sources) and short wavelength UVB radiation are especially irritating to the conjunctiva and may cause conjunctivitis, often known among skiers as snow blindness.

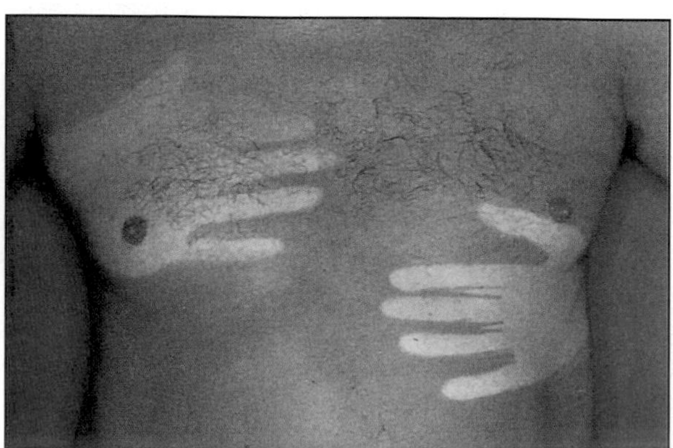

Fig. 13.15. Sunburn

Histopathology. The characteristic change is the development of dyskeratotic keratinocytes known as sunburn cells or fried egg cells. They are more common in the upper and middle stratum spinosum but can be found at all levels. As their name suggests, they are eosinophilic cells with a dark compact nucleus and pale cytoplasm. When damage is more severe, the individual cell necrosis can be replaced by frank epidermal necrosis and blisters. The superficial dermal vessels are dilated and may be surrounded by a mild lymphocytic infiltrate.

Differential Diagnosis. Phototoxic reactions induced by systemic medications such as doxycycline or the psoralens resemble an extreme sunburn. They are more likely to produce onycholysis than ordinary sunburn.

Therapy

Systemic. Aspirin or indomethacin can ameliorate a sunburn if taken promptly. Usually this is not possible, since the sunburn first becomes apparent hours after exposure and, by that point, these medications are not effective.

Topical. The treatment is that for a mild burn. Cool compresses, cooling lotions, and perhaps corticosteroid lotions or creams can be employed. In America, many over-the-counter sunburn remedies contain antihistamines or benzocaine anesthetics; both of these ingredients are likely to cause allergic contact dermatitis if repeatedly applied to damaged skin. We caution against their use.

Chronic Changes

Extrinsic photoaging describes the chronic changes induced by sunlight. It is to be distinguished from intrinsic or chronologic aging, which occurs in all skin but is often masked by photoaging. Comparing the skin of the face and axilla in an older patient rapidly demonstrates the differences. Photoaging is much more common in patients with skin types I and II and less prominent in blacks and other dark-skinned individuals.

Keratinocytes, melanocytes, and fibroblasts all are affected by endothelial cells, radiation. Damaged keratinocytes lead to actinic keratoses, which are irregular red to brown plaques, most often involving the face; histologically, they are in situ squamous cell carcinoma, so it should come as no surprise that they may evolve into invasive squamous cell carcinoma. Damage to melanocytes may produce changes ranging from patchy hyper- and hypopigmentation to malignant changes, as reflected by lentigo maligna and lentigo maligna melanoma. The role of sunlight in developing seborrheic keratoses is unclear, since many are found on the trunk; however, flat, tan-pigmented seborrheic keratoses are most common on the backs of the hands and face. They are usually called old age spots or liver spots by patients and lentigines by some physicians; we suspect that sunlight plays a role in their development.

The most obvious changes result from damage to the dermal fibroblasts. Solar elastosis refers to the combined damage to collagen, elastin, and ground substance, producing yellow papules or plaques which are represented microscopically by amorphous dermal deposits that readily stain with elastin stains. Many colorful terms have been applied to such skin, such as "sailors' skin" and "farmers' skin." Normal elastin comprises only a small percentage of the dermis, so it is surprising that it proliferates so much in response to chronic light exposure. UVB appears primarily responsible for solar elastosis, although UVA and even infrared light contribute. Damage to endothelial cells is reflected as telangiectases and purpura.

Variants on solar elastosis include the yellowish plaques of nodular elastosis usually seen on the temples as well as the heavily furrowed changes seen on the neck known as cutis rhomboidalis nuchae. Stellate pseudoscars are irregular white streaks, usually on the forearms, that reflect stretching of damaged collagen without known antecedent trauma. Senile purpura also occurs in the same region, probably because of both light- and age-induced vessel fragility. Erythromelanosis colli is the combination of telangiectasia and hypopigmentation usually prominent on the lateral aspects of the neck, with characteristic sparing of the submental region. All these changes show marked elastosis when examined histologically.

Table 13.9. Diseases often induced or worsened by sunlight or artificial radiation

Darier disease
Hailey-Hailey disease
Disseminated superficial actinic porokeratosis
Lichen planus
Herpes simplex
Lupus erythematosus
Lymphocytic infiltrate (especially Jessner-Kanof)
Seborrheic dermatitis
Dermatitis herpetiformis
Pemphigus foliaceus
Pemphigus erythematosus
Bullous pemphigoid
Psoriasis (uncommon)
Atopic dermatitis (uncommon)

Dermatoses Influenced by Ultraviolet Radiation

In contrast to the idiopathic or true photodermatoses, there is a long list of skin disorders (Table 13.9) characteristically induced or worsened by UV radiation. Probably the best example is lupus erythematosus, in which exposure to sunlight may not only induce cutaneous lesions but also cause a worsening of renal disease. The triggering role of UV radiation in herpes simplex virus infections, especially the labial lesions, is well known. In the case of lichen planus and psoriasis, there is often a local worsening in areas of sunburn, representing the Köbner phenomenon.

In contrast, some diseases are typically responsive to radiation and improve following a reasonable degree of exposure (Chap. 70). The classic example is psoriasis, in which phototherapy with a variety of sources is a mainstay. In other disorders such as acne, patients often describe an improvement in the summer; nonetheless, UV radiation is not used to treat acne as routinely today as it was in the past.

Primary Photodermatoses

The primary photodermatoses traditionally include not only the idiopathic forms of photosensitivity but also those reactions associated with a known toxic or allergic trigger as well as the entire spectrum of persistent light reactions, some idiopathic and some with a known trigger but a baf-

Table 13.10. Primary photodermatoses

Disease	Clinical picture	Frequency	Action spectrum
Idiopathic photodermatoses			
Solar urticaria	Urticaria	Very rare	UVA, UVB, UVC, visible light
Polymorphic light eruption	Monomorphous papules, vesicles, or plaques	Common	UVA, rarely UVB
Hydroa vacciniformia	Blisters, crusts, varioliform scars	Very rare	UVA
Actinic prurigo	Pruritic papules, plaques, lichenification	Very rare	UVA, UVB
Photodermatoses with known trigger			
Phototoxic reaction	Erythema, blisters (sunburn)	Fairly common	UVA
Photoallergic contact dermatitis	Dermatitis (localized)	Fairly common	UVA
Systemic photoallergic dermatitis	Dermatitis (disseminated, more papular)	Uncommon	UVA
Chronic actinic dermatitis			
Persistent light reaction	Lichenified dermatitis, often intensely pruritic	Uncommon	UVB, UVA visible light
Actinic reticuloid	Lichenified dermatitis, often intensely pruritic, atypical lymphocytic infiltrate microscopically	Uncommon	UVB, UVA visible light
Photosensitive eczema	Chronic dermatitis	Uncommon	UVB
Chronic photosensitive dermatitis	Chronic dermatitis	Uncommon	UVB, UVA
Photoaggravated atopic dermatitis	Chronic atopic dermatitis	Uncommon	UVB, UVA

flingly long course. Table 13.10 provides an overview of these disorders.

Solar Urticaria
(MERKLEN 1904)

Synonyms. Light urticaria, photoallergic urticaria

Definition. Urticaria induced by exposure to sunlight appearing within a few minutes of exposure.

Epidemiology. Solar urticaria is very rare and seen primarily in adults.

Etiology and Pathogenesis. The basic etiology of solar urticaria is simple; some patients develop urticaria almost immediately after light exposure. The rest of the explanation is baffling. A wide variety of wavelengths ranging from X-rays through UV radiation to include visible light and even infrared light may be responsible. In addition, passive transfer tests were positive in some patients; in this procedure, also known as the Prausnitz-Kuestner test, a patient's serum is injected into a normal host, who is then irradiated. For ethical reasons, this type of testing is no longer employed. Another test is to inject irradiated serum back into the patient's own skin and see if urticaria develops. In the past, solar urticaria patients were classified based on the action spectrum and the presence or absence of passive transfer. So many combinations were produced that one could best say that each solar urticaria patient had his own disease.

Today, the working concept is that the radiation is absorbed by a chromophore. This molecule is altered by the absorbed energy, forming the new photoallergen, which elicits a primarily IgE-mediated immune response. Antigen-specific IgE is bound to mast cells, so that subsequent exposures to the same radiation source may induce additional amounts of the photoallergen, which binds to the mast cells and produces urticaria in a typical type I Gell and Coombs reaction. Today, solar urticaria is divided into type I, in which the photoallergen is unique to the patient, and type II, in which the patient develops antibodies against a normal component of irradiated skin. The eliciting wavelength no longer serves for classification but only for more precise characterization.

Clinical Findings. Pruritus, erythema, and hives develop within minutes following exposure. Typically, there are lesions on nonirradiated as well as irradiated sites (Fig. 13.16). In extreme cases, the lesions can progress to giant hives or angioedema, especially when the unaware patient visits a tanning parlor for the first time. The course of the disease is usually chronic, persisting for many years, with little tendency to spontaneous cure.

Histopathology. The microscopic picture shows edema and a sparse lymphocytic perivascular infiltrate. In some cases, neutrophils and eosinophils may be found, with leukocytoclasis and evidence of degranulation along with deposits of complement factors.

Laboratory Findings. Upon phototesting, the hives develop within minutes after irradiation. The possible action spectrum is very broad, with individuals reported to react to UVA, UVB, UVC, and visible light. The action spectrum for a given patient can best be determined with a monochromator. The minimal urticaria dose (MUD) can also be assessed once the appropriate wavelength has been found. Use of a trial exposure to total body irradiation, as in a UV radiation source, is unwise because of the lack of specificity and risk of a severe reaction.

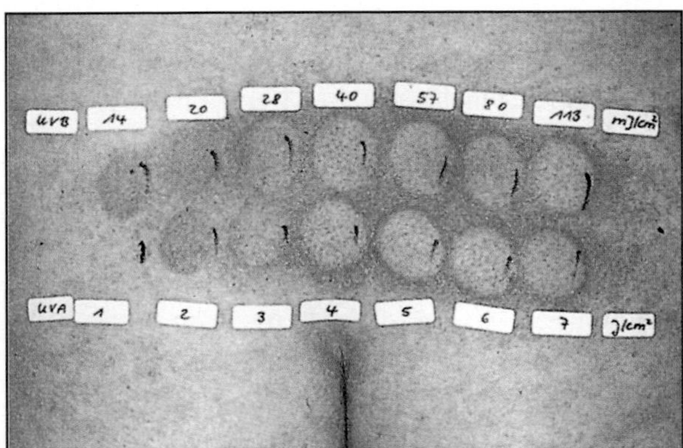

Fig. 13.16. Solar urticaria induced by phototesting

Differential Diagnosis. The main differential concern is erythropoietic protoporphyria, which is about as rare as solar urticaria. It should be excluded through appropriate hematologic testing (Chap. 44). In most instances, other forms of urticaria can be excluded by a careful history, while other radiation reactions usually have a much more delayed onset.

Therapy

Systemic. Despite the apparent role of histamine and other mast cell products in the pathogenesis, antihistamines are not a great relief for these unfortunate patients. Long-acting antihistamines can be tried, as they may occasionally help, but taking them after exposure is useless. Severely affected patients can be treated with azathioprine 50–100 mg daily.

Phototherapy. Following repeated UV radiation or visible light exposure, there is some hardening, presumably because the mast cells are exhausted and require time to resynthesize their mediators. This temporary clinical improvement lasts for only 2–3 days and thus provides little benefit. PUVA therapy is the treatment of choice. First, UV radiation or visible light in the appropriate action spectrum is used to provide temporary hardening. Then, during this lull, PUVA therapy is initiated, sometimes in association with systemic corticosteroid therapy, which can be tapered rapidly. It is usually necessary to continue PUVA therapy through the summer months, but many patients do not require it in the winter.

Other Measures. Plasmapheresis can also be employed in patients with a documented serum or plasma factor, but the cost:benefit ratios are usually not viewed as favorable.

Polymorphic Light Eruption

(RASCH 1900; HAUSMANN and HAXTHAUSEN 1929)

Synonyms. Polymorphous light eruption, summer prurigo (HUTCHINSON 1879), summer eruption, prurigo aestivalis, eczema solare

Definition. Common idiopathic photodermatosis that is always monomorphous in a given patient but shows a wide range of patterns between patients.

Epidemiology. Polymorphic light eruption (PMLE) is by far the most common form of idiopathic photodermatitis. It is estimated that at least 20% of individuals are affected. Most patients present in the spring or early summer, since some natural hardening occurs. Today, with the massive migration of tourists to sunny regions in the winter, PMLE has become a year-round disorder. In Europe, there is a strong female predominance, with estimates ranging as high as 9:1. In some reports from the USA, a 1:1 ratio is claimed but, in general, women appear to be at greater risk. Children may also be involved. While PMLE can occur in blacks, it is much less common and quite difficult to observe. The PMLE of Native Americans is described today as actinic prurigo, although it shares features with both PMLE and atopic dermatitis. Other patients with PMLE may also have stigmata of atopic dermatitis, and a positive family history is not uncommon.

Etiology and Pathogenesis. The cause of PMLE is unknown. The reaction is probably a type IV or delayed hypersensitivity reaction, based on the clinical course and histologic pattern. The responsible allergen has not been identified. Heat shock proteins may be involved as mediators. The patients show normal erythema and tanning responses. The action spectrum is usually in the UVA spectrum, but may fall into the UVB; some patients react to both wavelengths.

Clinical Findings. The key to PMLE is that, despite its name, it is an amazingly monomorphous eruption in any given patient. The variation from patient to patient may be enormous, as Table 13.11 demonstrates. The lesions develop hours to days after UV radiation and are limited to the irradiated areas. Initially, an irregular erythema is seen, usually accompanied by pruritus. Later, the individual lesions begin to develop and often coalesce.

Table 13.11. Morphologic variants of polymorphic light eruption

Papules
Hemorrhagic lesions
Plaques
Erythema multiforme-like lesions
Papulovesicles
Insect bite-like reaction
Vesiculobullous lesions

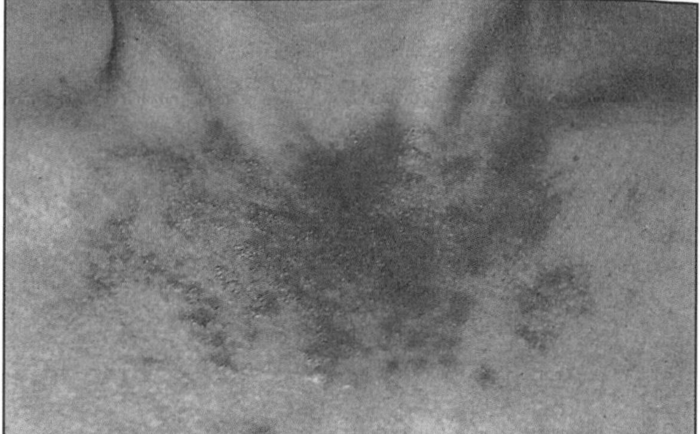

Fig. 13.17. Polymorphic light eruption

The most common variant is the papular or papulovesicular form, usually appearing in the décolletage and described by most women as sun poisoning or sun allergy. The side of the face (Fig. 13.17), the lateral part of the neck (Fig. 13.18), the upper lateral aspects of arms, and the backs of the hands are other common sites. A spread beyond irradiated areas is very uncommon. Dermatitis lesions with weeping, crusting, and scarring are not part of the clinical picture but may arise following excoriations or in patients with simultaneous

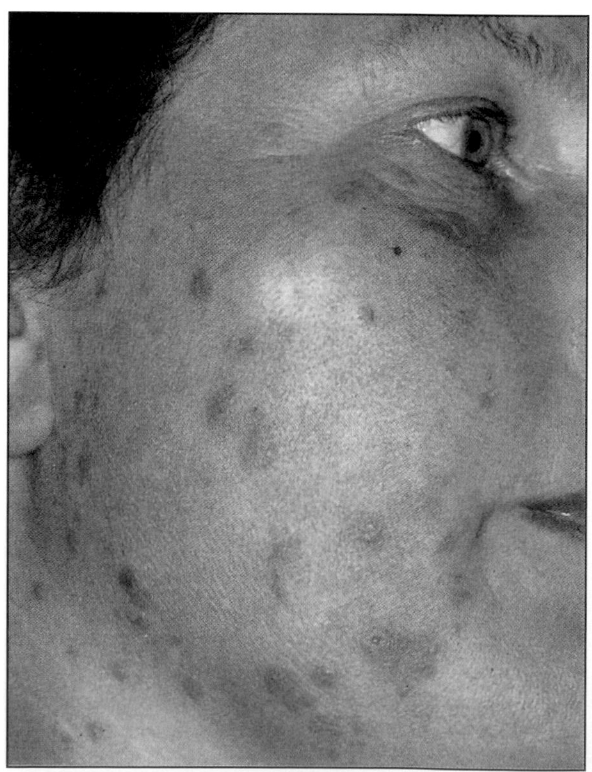

Fig. 13.18. Polymorphic light eruption

atopic dermatitis. The lesions resolve spontaneously over a period of days; in the presence of persistent sun exposure, there is usually hardening. However, the reaction is very likely to reoccur on re-exposure.

Juvenile spring eruption is a variant of PMLE affecting primarily boys or young men in the early spring. The most typical site is the helix of the ear, which is exposed to light, although other sites such as the hands or nose are sometimes involved. In several instances, outbreaks have been described in which a number of campers or soldiers developed this otherwise rare problem when exposed to a combination of sunlight and cold weather. Many equate this disorder with acute springtime pernio of Keining.

Histopathology. The histologic picture is not as varied as the clinical one. There is usually edema, a fairly intense lymphocytic perivascular infiltrate, and sometimes a minimal vacuolar change in the basal layer. Thus, lupus erythematosus may be closely mimicked. The mucin deposition of lupus erythematosus is not seen. There may be acanthosis.

Laboratory Findings. The lesions are fairly easily produced with phototesting. We prefer to irradiate relatively large fields (5x8 cm) at sites of predilection, such as forearms, with high doses of UVA (60–100 J/cm^2 daily), UVB (about 1.5 MED daily), and a combination of the two for 3 consecutive days. Most patients react to UVA or the combination; only a few react to UVB. Readings are done at 24, 48, and 72 h after irradiation. The induced lesions are compared clinically and histologically to the natural ones. The testing may induced disturbing, long lasting hyperpigmentation.

Course and Prognosis. This is a chronic disorder. In one study following patients over 30 years, about 25% were cleared, 50% had improved, and 25% were poorly or worse than at the onset of disease. The prevalence of thyroid disease was slightly increased in comparison to the normal population, but there was no increased risk of lupus erythematosus, confirming that the two disorders are separate.

Differential Diagnosis. The possibilities are limitless, based on the various morphologic patterns.

- Papulovesicular form: Atopic dermatitis, photoallergic dermatitis, prurigo simplex, and even hemorrhagic leukocytoclastic vasculitis
- Plaque form: Solar urticaria, erythropoietic protoporphyria, and erythema multiforme

Lupus erythematosus is also very similar, but the lesions usually require longer to develop and longer to resolve. The search for serologic evidence of lupus erythematosus and internal involvement may help clarify puzzling cases. Direct immunofluorescence examination of involved and uninvolved skin may also be needed. Experimental reproduction of the lesions with irradiation may also help; the lesions of PMLE develop in a few days, while those of lupus erythematosus take weeks.

Therapy. Topical antipruritic measures or corticosteroids bring some relief. The lesions usually resolve fairly promptly if light exposure is terminated.

Prophylaxis. Since no one traveling to an exotic location for a few weeks of winter sun is likely to avoid sun exposure, many other approaches to prophylaxis have been used. Sunscreens with good UVA coverage may be helpful. In addition, appropriate protective clothing and a more gradual exposure to the sun may bring benefits. A variety of systemic medications have been recommended, including β-carotene, chloroquine, nicotinamide, antihistamines, and calcium supplements. All show disappointing results, and we do not recommend them. Systemic corticosteroids, started in dosages ranging from 40–60 mg prednisone daily and tapering down over the course of the vacation can abort or ameliorate most cases, but the risk : benefit ratio is disputed.

The most effective prophylaxis is phototherapy. Prophylaxis must be started 4–6 weeks before exposure. Gradual exposure to either UVA or UVB, as required by the action spectrum, can induce hardening. If PMLE is induced, it can be treated as above. PUVA works even better for hardening and is probably the treatment of choice for severely affected patients. Extremely sensitive patients may require simultaneous use of systemic corticosteroids during PUVA.

Lupus Erythematosus

Lupus erythematosus is considered in detail in Chapter 18. Photosensitivity is a feature of most forms of lupus erythematosus. Repeated provocation similar to that for PMLE will produce skin lesions in photosensitive lupus erythematosus patients. We use the same large fields, but on the back, and the same dosages, again on 3 consecutive days. Changes first appear after 1–3 weeks and can be confirmed with biopsy. When lupus erythematosus patients are clearly photosensitive, then light avoidance is of great importance, as it may reduce the risk or severity of systemic complications.

Hydroa Vacciniformia

(BAZIN 1860)

Etiology and Pathogenesis. The cause of hydroa vacciniformia is unknown. It is an extremely rare type of photosensitivity, so that no large patient series have been compiled. In most patients, UVA appears responsible.

Clinical Findings. Hydroa vacciniformia usually starts in the first few years of life. Girls are more often affected than boys. The clinical picture is quite uniform. Skin findings are limited to sun-exposed areas. In the spring, erythematous papules and plaques develop on the nose, cheeks, tips of the ears, and backs of the hands. They evolve characteristically into blisters that are often hemorrhagic and acquire dark crusts. In the most severe cases, there may be accompanying systemic signs and symptoms. In addition, ocular involvement can occur, with both conjunctivitis and keratitis (Fig. 13.19).

These late, dark necrotic lesions tend to heal with depressed varioliform scars. In severe cases, the ears, nose, and distal parts of the fingers may be mutilated. In addition, postinflammatory hypo- and hyperpigmentation may occur. The corneal lesions may also scar, leading to visual damage. The attacks tend to occur each spring but often lessen as the patient reaches adolescence.

Histopathology. The epidermis shows far more necrosis than in other forms of photosensitivity. The typical changes of herpes simplex virus infection are not seen. In older lesions, the dermis shows perivascular inflammation and necrosis, often with the clinically apparent hemorrhage.

Laboratory Findings. Repeated provocation on the back with large doses of UVA, up to 30 J/cm^2 or more, may produce the typical hemorrhagic lesions.

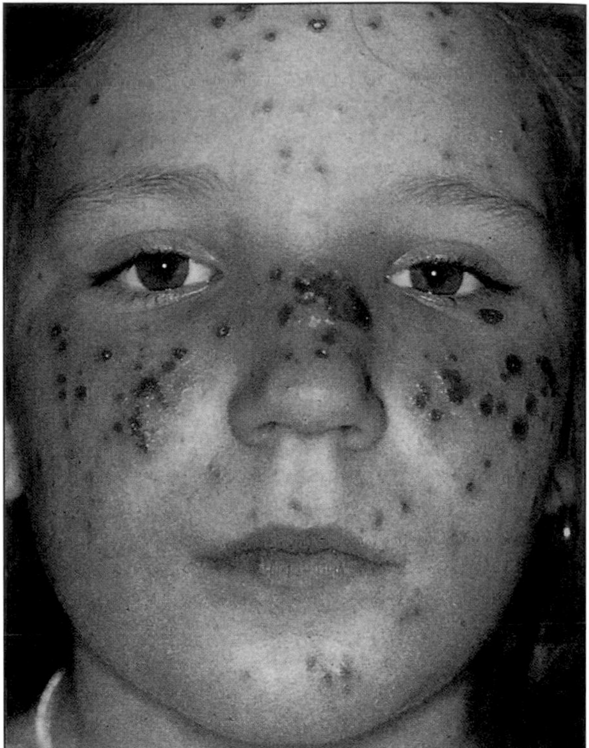

Fig. 13.19. Hydroa vacciniformia

Differential Diagnosis. The main problem is to exclude erythropoietic protoporphyria and congenital erythropoietic porphyria, both of which are characterized by early photosensitivity and scarring. In hydroa vacciniformia, porphyrin metabolism is normal.

Therapy. There is no good therapy except to avoid sunlight. Broad spectrum UVB and UVA sunscreens should be used in combination with chemical-free iron oxide or titanium dioxide blocking agents. Patients should also wear sunglasses with a high degree of UVA protection. If lesions develop, standard wound care is all that can be offered. If lesions continue to progress, systemic corticosteroids may also be employed.

Prophylaxis. Here, PUVA hardening can be tried, but patients are very sensitive and may not tolerate induction or may require systemic corticosteroids during induction. In contrast to erythropoietic protoporphyria, systemic protective agents such as β-carotene are not effective with hydroa vacciniformia.

Actinic Prurigo
(Lopez-Gonzáles 1961)

Epidemiology. Most patients have the onset of disease before they are 10 years of age. At least 50% show stigmata of atopic dermatitis. In Europe, most cases are sporadic and the disease is extremely uncommon. Among some Native Americans, including the Cree and Navajo, there is a strong family history. In the latter setting, the terms familial actinic prurigo or hereditary polymorphic light eruption are often used. In Central and South America, mestizos (individuals with mixed Spanish and Native American blood) are most often affected.

The classification of actinic prurigo is confusing, with some experienced observers not at all convinced that the disease in Native Americans is identical to the rare European entity and others unable to agree over the varying features seen in different racial groups of the Americas.

Etiology and Pathogenesis. The action spectrum for actinic prurigo lies primarily in UVA, although some patients are also responsive to the long end of the UVB spectrum. The mechanism of photosensitivity is unclear. Different HLA predilections have been shown in various tribes and in mestizos. Some patients show a paradoxical worsening of erythema when topical indomethacin is applied after exposure (recalling that indomethacin usually inhibits UVB erythema).

Clinical Findings. Clinically, actinic prurigo represents an overlap between atopic dermatitis and PMLE. Typical prurigo lesions are uncommon, which is why we are unhappy with the name. One very characteristic feature is the presence of an exudative cheilitis favoring the lower lip. Pruritus is prominent and the erythematous, edematous plaques that develop on the cheeks, neck, ears, arms, and hands soon tend to become excoriated and crusted. Initially, the findings are limited to skin exposed to sun. The course is very seasonal, with onset in spring and, occasionally, hardening in late summer (Fig. 13.20). Later on, there may be little sign of remission in the off-season, and involvement of nonexposed skin, such as on the back, is common. Actinic prurigo may improve in adolescence, but only a minority of patients, perhaps 25%, are fortunate enough to experience that. Others develop their disease in adult life.

Histopathology. The microscopic picture is not distinctive. There is a lymphocytic perivascular infiltrate, occasionally with eosinophils and accompanied by spongiosis and exocytosis. In older lesions, reactive epidermal changes such as acanthosis develop. Biopsy specimens from the lips often show a dense lymphoid infiltrate, sometimes with follicles. Thus, the term follicular cheilitis has been used, but it is an unfortunate choice, since confusion arises over the distinction between lymphoid follicle and hair follicle.

Differential Diagnosis. In the appropriate racial group, diagnosis is easy. Among Europeans, the dermatitic aspect of the eruption with the tendency to develop prurigo-like nodules and the cheilitis provide useful clues, but there are clearly many overlaps with light-sensitive atopic dermatitis and PMLE.

Therapy. The mainstay of therapy is topical and, in severe cases, consists of systemic corticosteroids. While β-carotene is not effective, thalidomide seems to offer promise under appropriate control.

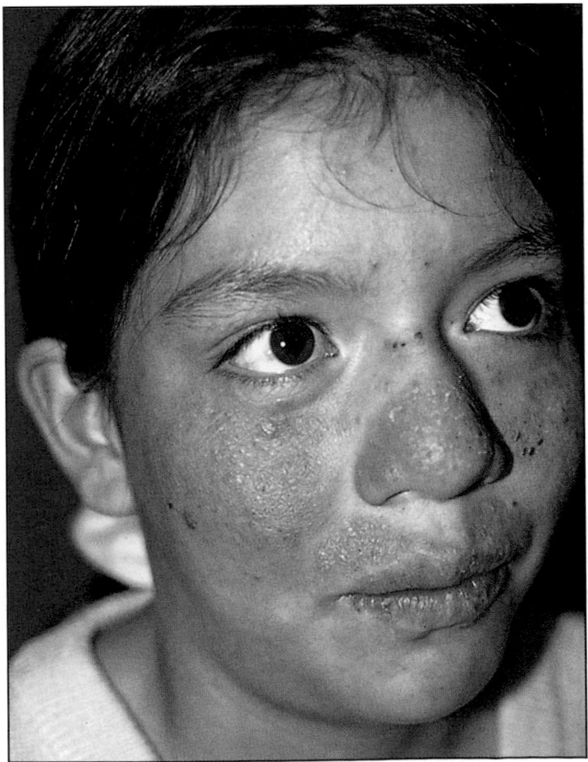

Fig. 13.20. Actinic prurigo. (Courtesy of Juan J. Ochoa, MD, Chihuahua, Mexico)

Because most patients in larger series live hundreds of miles from a medical center, experience with phototherapy is limited, but UVA or PUVA hardening appears worth trying, if technically possible.

Photodermatoses Caused by Exogenous Sensitizers

As Table 13.12 shows, such reactions can be best divided into phototoxic and photoallergic reactions. Table 13.13 further explains the differences between the two types of reactions.

Phototoxic Dermatitis

Definition. Photochemical reaction caused by direct interaction of radiation and photosensitizing substance, producing a sunburn-like reaction.

Epidemiology. Phototoxic reactions are quite common, because every person coming in contact with the suspected substance and sufficient sunlight experiences a reaction. Phototoxic substances can be ingested or applied topically. The most common situations are ingestion of phototoxic medications, sometimes intentionally, as in the case of PUVA therapy, and exposure to photosensitizing plants. Table 13.14 lists frequent topical phototoxic agents, while Table 13.15 shows the common phototoxic and photoallergic systemic medications.

Etiology and Pathogenesis. While sunburn and phototoxic reactions appear similar, the latter requires the presence of a chemical on or in the skin that magnifies the effect of the sunlight so that normally nonerythemogenic doses produce a sunburn-like picture. Photosensitizers can arise endogenously, as in the porphyrias or pellagra, but more often they reach the skin as a result of ingestion, topical application, or accidental contact. A major source of industrial exposure is the petroleum industry, as tars, oils, and a wide variety of other byproducts can be photosensitizers and much of the

Table 13.12. Pathogenesis of phototoxic and photoallergic skin reactions exposure to irradiation

Phototoxic reaction	Photoallergic reaction
↓	↓
Uptake of energy by reactive substance	Conversion of substance in (on) skin to a new hapten
↓	↓
Transfer of energy (free radicals, peroxides, heat)	Coupling with protein to form antigen
↓	↓
Toxic cell damage	Sensitization to new antigen
↓	↓
Acute phototoxic reaction	Re-exposure to light
	↓
	Immunologic reaction to new antigen
	↓
	Acute photoallergic reaction or chronic photoallergic dermatitis

Table 13.13. Clinical features of phototoxic and photoallergic reactions

Characteristic	Phototoxic	Photoallergic
Frequency	Common	Rare
Latency between first exposure and reaction	None	Always
Required light dosage	High	Low
Action spectrum	Narrow, usually long UVA	Wide, but also usually long UVA
Skin lesions	Sunburn-like; erythema, blisters	Dermatitis-like and polymorphic; papulovesicles, blisters, lichenification
Symptoms	Burning	Itching
Tendency to spread	None – only occurs in irradiated areas	Present – spreads to non-irradiated areas; old sites flare with re-exposure

Table 13.14. Topical phototoxic substances

Phototoxic Substance	Source
Acridine	Industrial exposure
Chlorpromazine	Swine food; reactions in farmers, veterinarians
Eosin	Histopathology laboratory, formerly lipstick
Furocoumarins	Many plants
Psoralens	Topical medications
Tars	Primarily industrial exposure, occasionally phototherapy

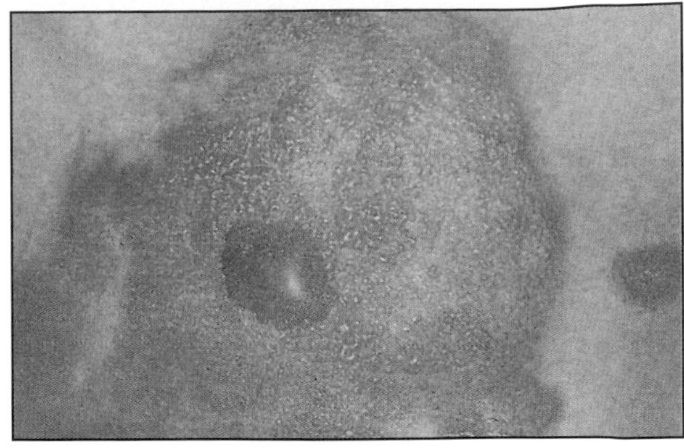

Fig. 13.21. Acute phototoxic contact dermatitis following topical psoralen use and irradiation

work with them is done in sunlight. The psoralens are modified furocoumarins that have been used topically and systemically, specifically because of their photosensitizing effects. Hematoporphyrins are used in combination with activating lasers for photodynamic therapy to destroy tumors. The main phototoxic medications include amiodarone, tetracyclines, nonsteroidal anti-inflammatory drugs, phenothiazines, and of course psoralens.

Phototoxic agents interact with radiation to produce free radicals, oxygen singlets, and peroxides. These reactive substances go on to damage keratinocytes. Both oxygen-dependent and oxygen-independent pathways for phototoxicity have been identified. The mediators of erythema are similar to those involved in sunburn.

Clinical Findings. The clinical findings are those of a sunburn, often severe and often unexpected. Spread to nonexposed areas is uncommn and always minimal (Fig. 13.21). Photoonycholysis and exaggerated postinflammatory hyperpigmentation are two features that may serve to distinguish phototoxic reactions from ordinary sunburn. When the photosensitizer is applied from the outside, as in the case of contact with a phototoxic plant such as giant hogweed, the typical pattern is one of streaked erythema and blisters.

Table 13.15. Phototoxic and photoallergic medications

Medication	Frequency	Phototoxic and/or photoallergic	Action spectrum (nm)
Amiodarone	High	Toxic	300–400
Chlorothiazides	Medium	Allergic	300–400
Fluoroquinolones	High	Toxic (mainly)	300–400
NSAIDs			
Piroxicam	Medium	Toxic	310–340
Carprofen	High	Both	310–400
Phenothiazines	Medium	Both	320–400
Psoralens	High	Toxic	320–380
Pyridoxine	Low	Allergic	320–400
Sulfonamides	Low	Allergic	315–400
Tetracyclines			
Base	Low	Toxic	320–400
Demeclocycline	High	Toxic	320–400
Doxycycline	Medium	Toxic	320–400
Minocycline	Low	Toxic	320–400

From Bruinsma (1995), with permission

Berloque Dermatitis

(Freund 1916; Rosenthal 1924)

Etiology and Pathogenesis. Berloque dermatitis is the result of the application of phototoxic oil of bergamot or related substances found in toilet water, perfume, aftershave lotion, and similar products. Limes are also very rich in oil of bergamot, so that individuals mixing gin-and-tonics in sunlight may develop erythema and hyperpigmentation on their fingers. The action spectrum is UVA. Traditionally, women were more likely to be affected than men. Very few phototoxic substances are still included in cosmetics.

Clinical Findings. The characteristic finding is erythema and even blisters following exposure to the sun but limited to a puzzling, often streaked pattern. The photosensitizing substance may drip or run downwards. The most common sites are the forehead, cheeks, neck, and perhaps upper parts of the chest (Fig. 13.22). Prominent postinflammatory hyperpigmentation is a typical characteristic. If the sun exposure is minimal, then the hyperpigmentation may appear with little or no erythema. This scenario often occurs on the neck, where a woman might place one or two drops of perfume and over months develop melasma-like hyperpigmentation. *Berloque* in French and *Berlocke* in German simply mean a pendant or trinket. Perhaps some early dermatologist felt the changes on the neck mimicked a piece of jewelry. Another typical feature is repigmentation in the following spring with UVA exposure.

Histopathology. Initially, there is toxic epidermal damage with necrotic keratinocytes. The basal layer melanin is increased and, in later stages, accumulates in the high dermal melanophages.

Differential Diagnosis. The streaking pattern usually gives the answer. If the erythematous phase is bypassed, melasma is the main problem, but this usually has a slightly different pattern. Often, both problems occur together.

Therapy. The main approach is to use an effective, fragrance-free UVA sunscreen and eliminate the phototoxic agent. A variety of agents can be applied for bleaching, including hydroquinone, azaleic acid, retinoids, and various combinations thereof. The trick is lots of patience and simultaneous use of UVA sunscreen.

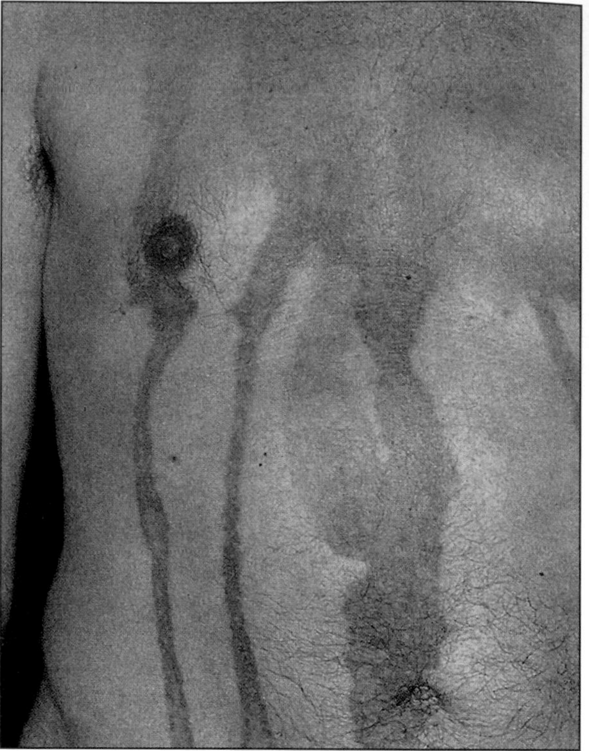

Fig. 13.22. Berloque dermatitis

Phytophotodermatitis

(Oppenheim 1917)

Synonyms. Dermatitis bullosa pratensis (Latin *Pratum*, or meadow) meadow grass dermatitis

Epidemiology. In the summer months, meadow grass dermatitis is especially common among sunbathers using grassy meadows. Children playing in such grass are also at risk. Patients using rotary string weedcutters while wearing short pants may get multiple tiny lesions on their legs where phototoxic weed fragments strike them. Individuals working at either harvesting or handling a wide range of vegetables may also have trouble, but in their cases the reaction is a painful hand dermatitis. Typical phototoxic plants include carrots, parsley, and celery, as well as many *Compositae* species including chrysanthemum, wormwood, thistles, and goldenrod. A major problem in many parts of Germany is the giant hogweed (*Heracleum* sp.), introduced from the Caucasus as a decorative, large (up to 3 m high) garden plant. It has spread rapidly to rights-of-way and along roads and railroad tracks. Contact with the juices of such a giant plant transfers large amounts of phototoxins that, in combination with sunlight, cause large blisters and burns.

Etiology and Pathogenesis. Many plants contain phototoxic substances. Most of these substances are furocoumarins, cyclic chemicals that react readily with light. The many sources of furocoumarins and related compounds were discussed above.

Clinical Findings. The typical patient has streaks of erythema and blisters following the pattern acquired by either lying upon or brushing against a phototoxic plant. Thus, exposed areas such as the face, arms, and legs are most often involved. The configuration tends to be quite bizarre, but spread to nonexposed areas does not occur (Fig. 13.23). Pruritus and even pain may be expected. Another classic feature is prominent hyperpigmentation as healing occurs. Once again, hyperpigmentation may reappear following marked sun exposure, as in the following spring.

Histopathology. Identical to other phototoxic dermatitis.

Differential Diagnosis. The main differential diagnosis is Rhus dermatitis (poison ivy and related disorders). One must simply know which plants are present in the local area. Rhus dermatitis is an allergic contact dermatitis (Chap. 12); light plays no role. In Munich, giant hogweed phototoxic dermatitis is the likely answer; the same patient in San Francisco probably has poison oak allergic contact dermatitis.

Therapy. It is often surprisingly difficult to convince patients of the etiology of their disorder. Until they are aware of the dangers of exposure to certain plants, avoidance is a problem. Topical corticosteroid lotions may help the early erythematous lesions. Once blisters are present, the lesions can be treated as a burn, using silver sulfadiazine cream or similar products.

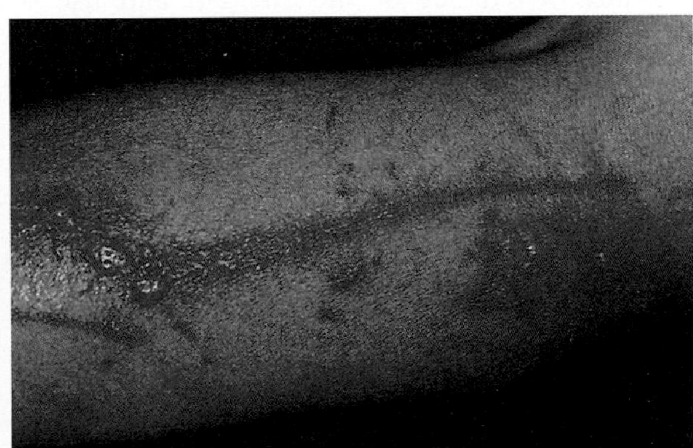

Fig. 13.23. Akute phytophototoxic contact dermatitis caused by contact with giant hogweed plant

Photoallergic Dermatitis

Definition. Cutaneous reaction involving a photoallergen and UVA radiation. Previous exposure to the allergen is required.

Etiology and Pathogenesis. Photoallergic dermatitis fulfills all the rules for allergic contact dermatitis. Prior exposure to an allergen is required and only a small percentage of those exposed develop an immune response and thus clinical symptoms. But, in this case, the presence of UV radiation is also required (Tab. 13.12). The photosensitizing substance can be applied topically or taken systemically. Once the patient is sensitized, then any method of exposure may lead to disease. Photoallergy is much less common than phototoxicity.

The interaction of the potential allergen, the skin, and UV radiation produces a modified substance, usually a hapten, that binds with normal skin proteins to form the true photoallergen. This new molecule triggers an immune response. When UV radiation and the allergen interact the next time in the skin, an allergic reaction occurs. It usually involves delayed hypersensitivity, as in allergic contact dermatitis, but may occasionally be IgE-mediated, producing photoallergic contact urticaria.

Two important wavelength spectra of the radiation can be studied. The first is that required to modify the allergen, known as the absorption spectrum. The second, is that required to trigger a clinical reaction, the action spectrum, suggesting that the modified allergen has a different chemical structure. While the absorption and action spectra can be identical, they are usually different. The action spectrum is usually UVA, although in rare cases, as with the sulfonamides and diphenhydramine, it lies within UVB. Many substances are capable of causing both phototoxic and photoallergic reactions, making testing very confusing. In addition, some substances can also cause ordinary allergic contact dermatitis. Photopatch testing is used to sort out the possibilities. Table 13.16 lists the common, topical photoallergic compounds.

Table 13.16. Topical photoallergic substances

Allergen	Comments
Halogenated salicylanilides (TCSA, TBSA)	Rarely found in soaps, disinfectants
Hexachlorophene	Disinfectant
Bithionol	Disinfectant
Musk ambrette	Fragrance in toiletries
PABA and related compounds	Sunscreen
Benzophenones	Sunscreen
Methoxycinnamates	Sunscreen
Parsol 1789	Sunscreen
Cyclohexanol	Sunscreen

A well-studied model for photoallergy was that caused by halogenated salicylanilides used in antibacterial soaps in the 1960s and early 1970s. They caused an epidemic of photoallergic dermatitis and also led to many cases of persistent or chronic light reactions. Fortunately, they have been removed from the market, and today the most common topical photosensitizers are sunscreens.

Clinical Findings. The clinical lesions of photoallergic contact dermatitis are pruritic, limited to sun-exposed skin where a photoallergen has been applied and thus sharply bordered. Erythema, papules, vesicles, and sometimes blisters may develop. Sometimes the exposure is more subtle. For example, many photosensitizers are present in animal feed products, so that a farmer may develop a reaction in exposed areas. In some instances, especially with the quinolones and related antimalarial compounds, a pattern may develop (Fig. 13.24). The triangle beneath the chin is typically spared and there is a sharp line across the upper arm at the sleeve level. In the winter months or with minimal sun exposure, the findings may be trivial and the patient simply complains of pruritus or minor erythema. If the diagnosis is not made and exposure to the allergen persists, a more chronic photoallergic dermatitis develops. In this form, lichenification is more likely and lesions may develop on nonirradiated areas.

Histopathology. Epidermal damage is uncommon. Spongiosis and lymphocytic perivascular infiltrates are seen early while, later on, epidermal reaction leads to acanthosis and parakeratosis.

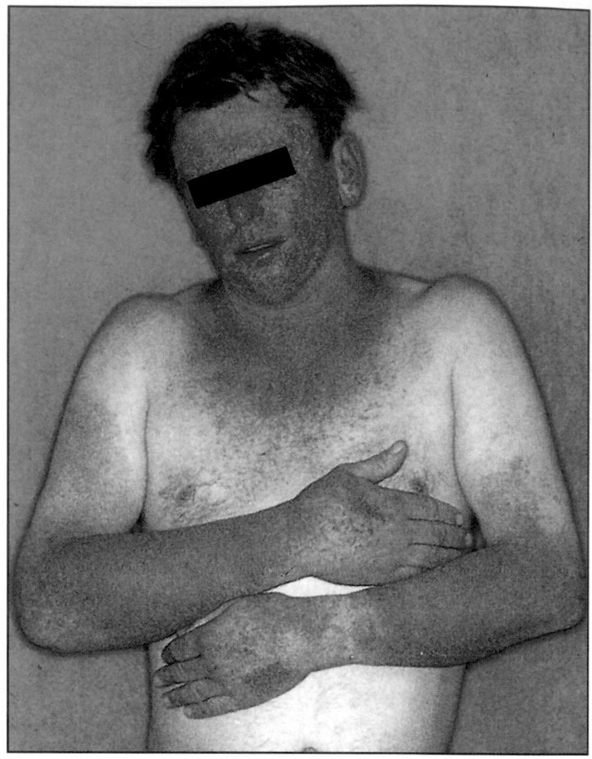

Fig. 13.24. Photoallergic contact dermatitis caused by chlorpromazine in animal feed

Differential Diagnosis. Sometimes, phototoxic and photoallergic reactions can be confused, but this is uncommon. The main differential diagnosis is systemic photoallergic reaction, which is more diffuse. Severe atopic dermatitis, especially if photoaggravated, may also be very similar. Photopatch testing is the proper way to identify photoallergic contact dermatitis.

Therapy. Avoidance of the allergen and use of UVA sunscreens and topical corticosteroids are the mainstays.

Systemic Photoallergic Dermatitis

When medications are taken that produce a photoallergy, then the reaction is systemic in nature. The typical causative drugs are shown in Table 13.15. The clinical reaction may be somewhat more diffuse and uniform in areas exposed to light since, when a topical agent is applied, areas are often missed or treated less or more intensely. Otherwise, the disorder is identical to photoallergic contact dermatitis.

Chronic Actinic Dermatitis

(Hawk and Magnus 1979)

Synonyms. Persistent light reaction, actinic reticuloid, chronic photosensitive dermatitis, photosensitive eczema

Definition. Pruritic dermatitis in areas exposed to sunlight that is triggered and maintained by sunlight alone, usually in relatively low doses, although there may be a past history of exposure to photosensitizing agents.

Epidemiology. All forms of chronic actinic dermatitis are rare. In general, they are problems of older men.

Etiology and Pathogenesis. Chronic actinic dermatitis is not a single disease, so not surprisingly it does not have a single, well-defined etiology. It encompasses a variety of different disorders defined briefly below and shown in Table 13.17.

Persistent Light Reaction (Wilkinson 1962). In the 1960s, individuals were identified with photoallergic dermatitis from halogenated salicylanilides who had persistent problems, even after exposure to the soaps was stopped and a reasonable amount of time had passed to assume safely that the disinfectants were no longer on or in the skin.

Table 13.17. Possible pathogenesis of chronic actinic dermatitis

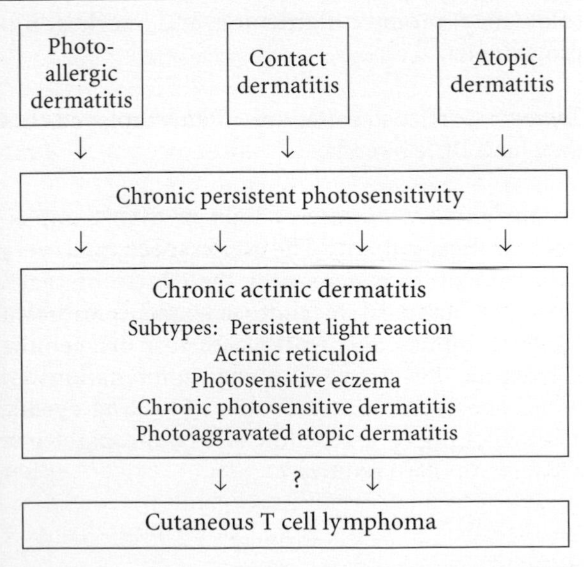

A peculiar change was noted in these patients: while UVA was required to trigger the initial photoallergic dermatitis, the persistent reaction was evoked by UVB. In addition, as the disease progressed, the action spectrum expanded even further in some cases, reincluding UVA and even encompassing visible light.

Actinic Reticuloid (Ive et al. 1969). Some patients with a clinical pattern identical to that of persistent light reactors show cytologicatypia of lymphocytes on skin biopsy. The infiltrate usually consists of atypical T cells resembling mycosis fungoides. The initial name reticuloid suggested that this was a pseudomalignancy but, in a few instances, the patients developed lymphomas. Sensitivity to both UVA and UVB as well as visible light has been described.

Photosensitive Eczema (Ramsay and Black 1973). These patients resemble the persistent light reactors but have no history of documented photoallergy. The action spectrum is as UVB. While photopatch testing is negative, some patients have positive routine patch tests, especially to chromates.

Chronic Photosensitive Dermatitis (Frain-Bell et al. 1974). In this group, action spectra in UVB and UVA were identified as well as a hodgepodge of positive patch and photopatch tests.

As one rereads the initial descriptions, the similarities between all these disorders far outweigh the differences. Thus, we endorse the concept of chronic actinic dermatitis. No matter what the predisposing event, the skin's photoimmune response is altered such that sunlight or artificial light alone is sufficient for perpetration of the dermatitis.

Clinical Findings. Patients are almost invariably elderly men with an intensely pruritic erythematous excoriated facial eruption. The forehead and nape are the most common sites, but the cheeks, ears, neck, and backs of the hands are also involved. The skin is thickened, furrowed, and often covered with scale (Fig. 13.25). Sometimes it may be very warm and weeping, even though no bacterial, fungal, or viral infection is identified. In some cases, a leonine facies evolves. The triangle under the chin and the retroauricular areas are often spared. There is frequently involvement of covered

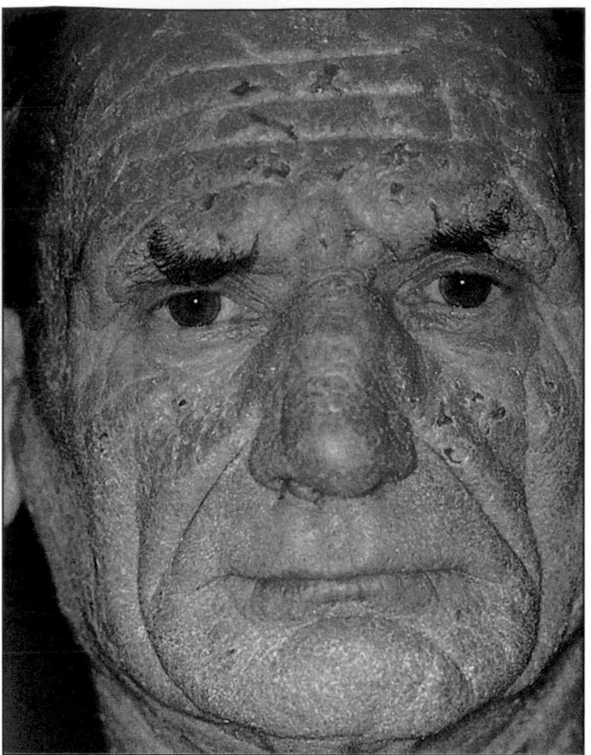

Fig. 13.25. Persistent light reaction

areas. The patients are so sensitive to light that the minimum amount of energy passing through their clothing may be enough to trigger a reaction. In addition, there may well be immunologic reactions spreading to truly nonexposed skin.

Histopathology. There is usually a chronic lichenified dermatitis with epidermal acanthosis, hyperkeratosis, and parakeratosis. The dermis shows a lymphocyte infiltrate that can be perivascular or lichenoid. Cytological atypia, a predominance of suppressor T cells, and epidermotropism all suggest actinic reticuloid.

Laboratory Findings. Low doses of UVB, UVA, and even visible light can elicit an erythematous reaction within 24 h. In addition, photopatch testing should be carried out using a dose of UVA below the erythema threshold.

Course and Prognosis. The outlook for these unfortunate older men is desperate. The dermatitis is so light-sensitive and pruritic that they frequently express suicidal thoughts. In addition, a given percentage of cases evolve into cutaneous T cell lymphoma.

Differential Diagnosis. We see little reason to distinguish between the various disorders listed under chronic actinic dermatitis. The action spectrum and results of patch and photopatch testing should be recorded, but which name is applied seems irrelevant. Serial biopsies should be performed to monitor the possible transition into cutaneous T cell lymphoma. The one disorder that may be slightly different is light-sensitive atopic dermatitis. If an individual has a clear history of atopic dermatitis but otherwise has disease that resembles chronic actinic dermatitis, we sometimes make this diagnosis.

In addition, one must be sure that no persistent photoallergic reaction is taking place. Sometimes, patients take medicines that only rarely are photosensitizing, so one should attempt photopatch testing with all possible offenders and inquire thoroughly about over-the-counter products. Finally, airborne contact dermatitis as caused by Rhus or *Compositae* may appear identical but is usually far more acute.

Therapy

Systemic. While there is no truly satisfactory approach, the use of azathioprine has proven to be relatively effective. Other immunosuppressive agents, including corticosteroids and cyclosporine, have also been employed.

Phototherapy. PUVA can be combined with corticosteroids to produce surprisingly good benefits. The initial dosage must be under the dermatitis threshold for the patient. A gradual increase in dosage coupled with reduction in corticosteroids may produce hardening and marked improvement.

Topical. Corticosteroids are often employed, but they have little benefit.

Prophylaxis. Avoidance of light is almost impossible for these patients. The action spectrum is very wide and often widens over the course of years. Even the standard incandescent and fluorescent lights in homes and workplaces may trigger the dermatitis. Protective clothing, combinations of broad spectrum sunscreens and blocking agents, and switching to a schedule with more nighttime activity are often required.

Secondary Photodermatoses

There are a number of disorders in which photosensitivity plays a major role in the clinical manifestations. Many have been covered in other chapters of this book and are listed in Table 13.18. Xeroderma pigmentosum, Bloom syndrome, and ataxia-telangiectasia, in which X-ray sensitivity is prominent, will be discussed here.

Table 13.18. Secondary photodermatoses

Cause	Disorder
Enzyme defects	Hartnup syndrome Phenylketonuria Xeroderma pigmentosum Cockayne syndrome Trichothiodystrophy
Loss of protection	Albinism Chediak-Higashi syndrome (pigment dilution) Vitiligo
Endogenous	Porphyrias
Photosensitive genodermatoses (various mechanisms)	Bloom syndrome Rothmund-Thompson syndrome
Increased X-ray sensitivity	Ataxia-telangiectasia Xeroderma pigmentosum

Xeroderma Pigmentosum

(Kaposi 1870)

Definition. Extremely uncommon genodermatosis with a variety of defects in DNA repair leading to photosensitivity, skin malignancies, and ocular and neurologic disease.

Epidemiology. Xeroderma pigmentosum is extremely rare. Less than 1000 patients have been identified worldwide. Most patients seen in Germany are from North Africa or Turkey. Consanguinity is often apparent in their family pedigrees.

Etiology and Pathogenesis. Patients with xeroderma pigmentosum are unable to repair radiation-induced DNA damage. The defects involve several enzymes needed to repair DNA; all are inherited in an autosomal recessive fashion. In 1968, Cleaver described the inability of some xeroderma pigmentosum patients to excise and replace UV radiation-induced thymidine dimers. While UVB appears most important, UVA and visible light also play a role.

A number of groups or types of xeroderma pigmentosum have been identified based on the ability of fused fibroblasts from two different patients to correct their corresponding deficiencies, as Table 13.19 shows. If both patients are in group A, then fused fibroblasts will still be unable to repair damage. If one patient is in group A and the other in group C, then the fused fibroblasts will have 50% levels of two different defects and be able to repair damage. The inability to repair DNA damage is felt to be responsible for the increased incidence of basal cell carcinoma, squamous cell carcinoma, malignant melanoma, and various soft tissue neoplasms. Patients with trichothiodystrophy and some types of Cockayne syndrome have similar DNA repair defects, but many lack skin cancers. Thus, the search continues for other abnormalities such as, perhaps, reduced immunologic surveillance, which could more fully explain the development of tumors in xeroderma pigmentosum.

The genetic defects in xeroderma pigmentosum are being gradually identified. Group A patients, which includes DeSanctis-Cacchione syn-

Table 13.19. Types of xeroderma pigmentosum

Group	Photosensitivity	Skin tumors	Neurologic disease	Comments
A	+++ (early)	SCC	++	Common in Japan, includes DS-C
B	+++		+	XP/CS
C	++/+++	SCC, BCC	–	
D	++	MM	–	XP/CS, TTD
E	+ (late)	BCC	–	
F	++		+	
G	++		+	XP/CS
Variant	+ (late)	BCC	–	

DS-C, DeSanctis-Cacchione syndrome; XP/CS, overlap of xeroderma pigmentosum and Cockayne syndrome; TTD, trichothiodystrophy; SCC, squamous cell carcinoma; BCC, basal cell carcinoma; MM, malignant melanoma.

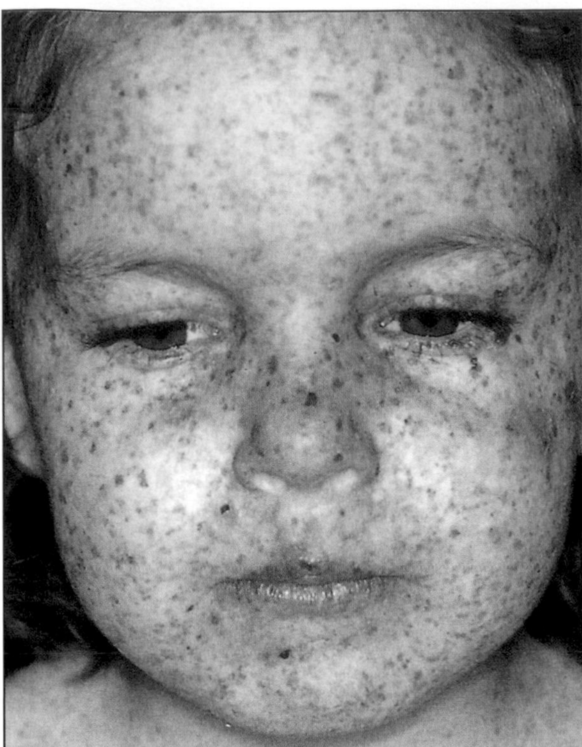

Fig. 13.26. Xeroderma pigmentosum in 3-year-old girl

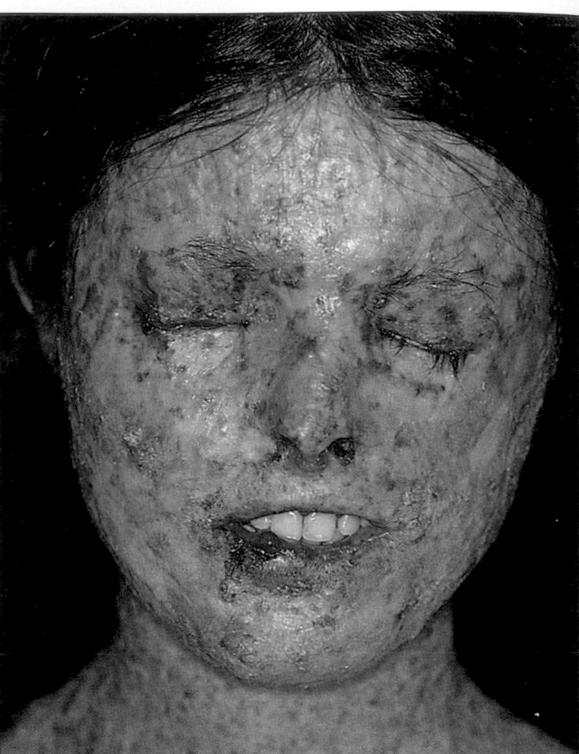

Fig. 13.27. Xeroderma pigmentosum in the same patient, now 15 years old, with far more extensive damage. The patient has had multiple cutaneous and soft tissue malignancies

drome patients with severe neurologic disease, have a mutation on chromosome 9 coding for a zinc finger protein, while group B patients have a mutation in a DNA helicase found on chromosome 2.

While the patients in groups A–I have defects in the early phases of excision repair, those of the variant group have a defect in postreplication repair. They were formerly identified as pigmented xerodermoid or caffeine-sensitive xeroderma pigmentosum (not because of a risk of drinking coffee but because in vitro caffeine corrects their repair defect to an extent). These patients develop skin changes in adult life that are considerably milder than those of the other xeroderma pigmentosum patients.

Clinical Findings. The initial clinical finding in xeroderma pigmentosum is extreme photosensitivity. Parents notice when their infant is first in sunlight that even minor exposure leads to crying and sunburn. The skin also tends to be dry and atrophic. It is essential to diagnose xeroderma pigmentosum at this stage; if one waits until the somewhat older child presents with the next stage of the disease – multiple cutaneous malignancies – then the battle is already partially lost. If unprotected, the skin develops a poikilodermatous appearance (hence, pigmentosum) with hyper- and hypopigmented areas, telangiectases, and varying degrees of erythema. Lentigenes and actinic keratoses appear in the first few years of life, while basal cell carcinomas, squamous cell carcinomas, and even malignant melanomas may be seen in childhood (Fig. 13.26). Typical in older patients is a significant degree of scarring and mutilation involving the nasal and orbital regions (Fig. 13.27). Different complementation groups show different tumors. Keratoacanthomas are also seen as well as soft tissue sarcomas, suggesting either deeper penetration of irradiation or other mechanisms.

Neurologic defects also occur; they, too, vary from group to group. The best defined is the DeSanctis-Cacchione syndrome, which is part of group A with severe mental retardation and dwarfism. In all, about 20–30% of xeroderma pigmentosum patients have neurologic findings. Deep tendon reflexes and audiometry are the most useful screening devices.

Ocular involvement is also common. About 40% of patients have photophobia, keratoconjunctivitis, and lid damage. The anterior part of the eye bears the brunt of the insult, as the retina is fairly well-protected. The same range of tumors seen on the skin also threatens the eye.

Histopathology. The individual tumors can be identified. There are no clues to xeroderma pigmentosum in nontumoral skin.

Laboratory Findings. The complementation group should be determined by turning to highly specialized laboratories. While waiting for the diagnosis, one should institute maximum light protection.

Course and Prognosis. The outlook is grim. The best hope for the patient is to be in a relatively mild complementation group and then to practice absolute avoidance of UV radiation. The risk of cutaneous malignancies is estimated as 2000 times greater than that of the general population, with a mean age of 8 years for the first tumor. The risk of internal malignancy is about 20-fold that of the general population.

Differential Diagnosis. In infants, congenital erythropoietic porphyria and erythropoietic protoporphyria, neonatal lupus erythematosus, and the other photosensitive genodermatoses should be considered. In a matter of months, the diagnosis of xeroderma pigmentosum becomes clear.

Therapy

Topical. Here, 5-fluorouracil can be tried in combination with topical retinoids. This type of approach may be useful if started early, when one is relatively certain of dealing only with actinic keratoses and lentigines. If an early basal cell carcinoma is treated, there is a risk of producing surface healing but allowing the tumor to grow deeply.

Systemic. Chemoprophylaxis with oral retinoids (usually isotretinoin) can be tried. The side effects are considerable, as relatively high doses (1.0–2.0 mg/kg daily) are needed and the therapy must be lifelong. Most studies have shown a reduction in the development of new tumors; little benefit is seen for existing lesions.

Surgical. The lesions can be treated by whatever surgical approach is felt most appropriate. Tumors develop rapidly, so patients should be checked every 2–3 months and sooner if a suspicious lesion is identified at home. Radiation therapy must be avoided. Dermabrasion of actinically damaged skin provides improvement for a fair period of time, as does superficial chemical peeling.

Prophylaxis. Absolute sunlight avoidance is the only approach. Sunscreens rarely suffice. Effective UV-absorbing sunglasses should also be prescribed. Acoma and Navajo Native American patients with xeroderma pigmentosum living at 1500 m above sea level with sunshine 360 days a year do terribly. The parents must reverse the child's diurnal rhythm to sleep in the day and activity at night. Not every family can comprehend or afford such steps.

Bloom Syndrome

(Bloom 1954)

Synonym. Congenital telangiectatic erythema

Definition. Congenital disorder with photosensitivity, dwarfism, and increased incidence of malignancies.

Epidemiology. Even though Bloom syndrome is inherited in an autosomal recessive pattern, about 75% of the patients are men. Over half the cases known have been reported in Ashkenazi Jews.

Etiology and Pathogenesis. Bloom syndrome is one of the chromosome instability syndromes. The responsible gene, BLM at 15q26.1, encodes a helicase; this group of enzymes helps separate and uncoil double-stranded DNA prior to replication. The cytogenetic hallmark of Bloom syndrome is increased numbers of sister chromatid exchanges. Other defects in DNA repair are also seen and the chromosomes are easily damaged in vitro by UV radiation.

Clinical Findings. The description photosensitive Jewish male dwarfs is a good summary. The patients are small at birth, usually under 2500 g, and remain small. They may have small genitalia but are able to reproduce. Their intelligence is normal. The face is distinctive, being narrow and pointed, with sunken cheeks. Other occasional findings include polydactyly, dental abnormalities, and a high or infantile voice. There is an increased incidence of diabetes mellitus.

The most obvious physical finding is the presence of matted telangiectases or telangiectatic erythema of the cheeks that appear very early in life, usually within the first month. The erythema spreads with exposure to sunlight to involve nose, eyelids, forehead and, later, the extensor surfaces of the arms. The combination of the essential telangiectasia and photosensitivity leads to a poikilodermatous picture. Often the patients blister easily with light exposure, especially on their lips. Multiple café au lait macules may be present. Despite the photosensitivity, cutaneous malignancies are relatively uncommon, perhaps because of the reduced life expectancy. Crusted scabies has also been described in such individuals.

Laboratory Findings. Typically, there are reduced levels of IgA and IgM.

Course and Prognosis. Two life-threatening problems can develop. Early in life, the reduced immunoglobulin levels predispose to recurrent pulmonary and gastrointestinal infections. Later, this problem tends to improve. Secondly, Bloom syndrome patients have an increased incidence of leukemia, lymphoma, Wilms tumor, and gastrointestinal carcinoma, so most who survive infancy die in the second or third decade from one of these malignancies.

Differential Diagnosis. While other photosensitive disorders, such as lupus erythematosus, should be considered, usually the very early onset of matted telangiectases prior to sun exposure associated with the small body size gives away the diagnosis.

Therapy. Avoidance of sunlight and regular evaluation to detect internal malignancies as soon as possible are both essential. The infections should be treated in the standard manner with antibiotics.

Ataxia-Telangiectasia

(Sillaba and Hanner 1926; Louis-Bar 1941)

Synonyms. Louis-Bar syndrome, cerebellar oculocutaneous telangiectasia syndrome

Definition. Rare disease with early onset of ataxia, telangiectases, immunologic defects, and an increased risk of malignancy.

Epidemiology. The incidence of this autosomal recessive inherited disorder is about 1:50,000–1:100,000. The sexes are equally affected.

Etiology and Pathogenesis. The defect is located on chromosome 11q22-q23. The gene, known as ATM, is a protein kinase responsible for signal transduction and meiotic recombination. The main problem is an inability to repair double-stranded DNA breaks. It appears that there are at least five complementation groups at this locus as well as an X-linked recessive type, in which the defect is in a DNA polymerase. Peculiarly, the risk in subsequent siblings is not 1:4 but closer to 1:8. In addition, characteristic changes occur on chromosomes 7 and 14 often involving lymphoma-associated oncogenes. The chromosomes are also sensitive to ionizing radiation and radiomimetic chemotherapy agents. While ataxia-telangiectasia patients may have increased spontaneous breakage, the most diagnostic feature is the in vitro sensitivity to ionizing radiation. Sister chromatid exchange rates are normal. Finally, heterozygotes for the ataxia-telangiectasia gene, while clinically normal, have a two- to six-fold relative risk of malignancy.

In the Nijmegen breakage syndrome, patients have craniofacial abnormalities, growth defects, infections, and early malignancies, but no ataxia or telangiectases. They have a defect in nibrin, a protein that interacts with the ATM gene.

Clinical Findings. The initial finding is usually ataxia presenting in the second or third year of life and becoming very apparent as the child either never walks or rapidly loses the ability to do so. Other typical finding include slurred speech, nystagmus, and oculomotor apraxia.

The telangiectases almost always appear first on the conjunctiva, usually after the onset of the ataxia. They spread to involve the ears, eyelids, cheeks and, rarely, the neck and flexural aspects of the arms and legs. Erythematous, reddish brown plaques may develop on the face and extremities. These have a raised border with central atrophy and even ulceration, resembling necrobiosis lipoidica diabeticorum (Chap. 50). Other cutaneous signs include café au lait macules, poliosis, hypertrichosis, and occasional diffuse hyperpigmentation which has been associated with a rapid downhill course.

The children suffer from frequent and severe sinopulmonary infections. They have defects in both cellular and humoral immunity. The latter is more obvious, as levels of IgA, IgE, and IgG may be reduced or even absent, but cellular parameters are also abnormal and the thymus is often small. There is a striking increase in lymphoreticular malignancies, often with typical cytogenetic translocations that activate oncogenes. Patients who survive these problems appear to be at risk for carcinomas as well.

Laboratory Findings. In addition to the immunoglobulin deficiencies, α-fetoprotein levels are low. This may also be useful in prenatal diagnosis. Both the cerebellar atrophy and the thymic hypo- or aplasia can be identified with imaging techniques.

Course and Prognosis. Those infants who survive their infections usually die in the second or third decade from malignant lymphoma or leukemia. Because of the ataxia, the patients are wheelchair-bound and usually have a poor quality of life.

Differential Diagnosis. Initially, the whole list of causes of childhood ataxia must be considered by the pediatrician or neurologist. Later, as the telangiectases become apparent, diagnosis is easier.

Therapy. Intravenous immunoglobulins are very helpful in reducing the frequency and severity of infections. Aggressive antibiotic treatment and pulmonary care may prolong life. In treating the tumors, one should avoid X-ray and radiomimetic medications.

Bibliography

Mechanical Skin Damage

Kligman AM, Klemme JC, Susten AS (eds) (1985) The chronic effects of repeated mechanical trauma to the skin. Liss, New York

Hyperpigmentation

Hata S, Tanigaki T, Misaki K et al. (1987) Incidence of friction melanosis in young Japanese women induced by using nylon towels and brushes. J Dermatol 14:437–439

Hidano A, Mizuguchi M, Higaki Y (1984) Friction melanosis. Ann Dermatol Venereol 111:1063–1071

Magana-Garcia M, Carrasco E, Herrera-Goepfert R et al. (1989) Hyperpigmentation of the clavicular zone: a variant of friction melanosis. Int J Dermatol 28:119–122

Blisters

Knapik JJ, Reynolds K, Barson J (1999) Risk factors for foot blisters during road marching: tobacco use, ethnicity, foot type, previous illness, and other factors. Mil Med 164:92–97

Naylor PF (1973) Cause of friction blisters. Lancet 1:495

Patterson HS, Woolley TW, Lednar WM (1994) Foot blister risk factors in an ROTC summer camp population. Mil Med 159:130–135

Peachey RD (1971) Factors affecting blister formation. Br J Dermatol 85:497

Hyperkeratotic Changes

Yoshii A, Ono T, Kayashima K et al. (1991) An unusual mechanical hyperkeratosis of the soles – health sandals keratosis. J Dermatol 18:291–294

Callus

Murray HJ, Young MJ, Hollis S et al. (1996) The association between callus formation, high pressures, and neuropathy in diabetic foot ulceration. Diabet Med 13:979–982

Pitei DL, Foster A, Edmonds M (1999) The effect of regular callus removal on foot pressures. J Foot Ankle Surg 38: 251–255

Clavus

Day RD, Reyzelman AM, Harkless LB (1996) Evaluation and management of the interdigital corn: a literature review. Clin Podiatr Med Surg 13:201–206

Richards RN (1991) Calluses, corns, and shoes. Semin Dermatol 10:112–114

Singh D, Bentley G, Trevino SG (1996) Callosities, corns, and calluses. Br Med J 312:1403–1406

Black Heel

Bazex A, Salvador R, Dupré A (1962) Chromidrose plantaire. Bull Soc Fr Dermatol Syphilgr 69:489–490

Crissey KT, Peachey JC (1961) Calcaneal petechiae. Arch Dermatol 83:501

Rufli T (1980) Hyperkeratosis haemorrhagica. Hautarzt 31: 606–609

Acanthoma Fissuratum

Benedetto AV, Bergfeld WF (1979) Acanthoma fissuratum. Histopathology and review of the literature. Cutis 24: 225–229

Betti R, Inselvini E, Pozzi G et al. (1994) Bilateral spectacle frame acanthoma. Clin Exp Dermatol 19:503–504

Dorn M, Plewig G (1981) Acanthoma fissuratum cutis. Hautarzt 32:145–148

Epstein E (1965) Granuloma fissuratum of the ears. Arch Dermatol 91:621–622

Thomas MR, Sadiq HA, Raweily EA (1991) Acanthoma fissuratum. J Laryngol Otol 105:301–303

Decubitus Ulcer

Allman RM, Laprade CA, Noel LB et al. (1986) Pressure sores among hospitalized patients. Ann Intern Med 105: 337–342

Diem E (1992) Decubitusprophylaxe und Therapie. Hautarzt 43:461–468

Hey S (1996) Pressure sore care and cure. Lancet 348:1511

Lydon P (1994) The local treatment of pressure sores. Ir Med J 87:72–73

Atypical Decubital Fibroplasia

Baldassano MF, Rosenberg AE, Flotte TJ (1998) Atypical decubital fibroplasia: a series of three cases. J Cutan Pathol 25:149–152

Montgomery EA, Meis JM, Mitchell MS et al. (1992) Atypical decubital fibroplasia. A distinctive fibroblastic pseudotumor occurring in debilitated patients. Am J Surg Pathol 16:708–715

Disorders in Amputees

Baptista A, Barros MA, Azenha A (1992) Allergic contact dermatitis on an amputation stump. Contact Dermatitis 26:140–141

Chalmers IM, Arneja AS (1994) Rheumatoid nodules on amputation stumps: Report of three cases. Arch Phys Med Rehabil 75:1151–1153

Gucluer H, Gurbuz O, Kotiloglu E (1999) Kaposi-like acroangiodermatitis in an amputee. Br J Dermatol 141: 380–381

Kohler P, Lindh L, Bjorklind A (1989) Bacteria on stumps of amputees and the effect of antiseptics. Prosthet Orthot Int 13:149–151

Levy SW (1995) Amputees: skin problems and prostheses. Cutis 55:297–301

Wlotzke U, Hohenleutner U, Landthaler M (1996) Dermatosen bei Bein-Amputierten. Hautarzt 47:493–501

Subcutaneous Emphysema

Doweiko JP, Alter C (1992) Subcutaneous emphysema: report of a case and review of the literature. Dermatology 184:62–64

Maggio KL, Maingi CP, Sau P (1998) Subcutaneous emphysema. Air as a cause of disease. Arch Dermatol 134:557–559

Samlaska CP, Maggio KL (1996) Subcutaneous emphysema. Adv Dermatol 11:117–151

Thermal Injuries

Kibbi AG, Tannous Z (1998) Skin diseases caused by heat and cold. Clin Dermatol 16:91–98

Kligman LH, Kligman AM (1984) Reflections on heat. Br J Dermatol 110:369–375

Burns

Andreassi L, Flori L (1991) Pharmacologic treatment of burns. Clin Dermatol 9:453–458

Baxter CR (1993) Management of burn wounds. Dermatol Clin 11:709–714

Bowden M, Grant S, Vogel B et al. (1988) The elderly, disabled and handicapped adult burned through abuse and neglect. Burns 14:447–450

Demling RH, LaLonde C (1989) Burn trauma. New York: Thieme Medical Publishers

Herndon DN (ed) (1996) Total burn care. London: WB Saunders

Lee RC, Astumian RD (1996) The physicochemical basis for thermal and non-thermal "burn" injuries. Burns 22:509–519

Miller JG, Carruthers HR, Burd DAR (1992) An algorithmic approach to the management of cutaneous burns. Burns 18:200–211

Renz BM, Sherman R (1992) Child abuse by scalding. J Med Assoc Georgia 81:574–578

Settle JAD (ed) (1996) Burns management. London: Churchill Livingstone

Cold Injury

Killian H (1981) Cold and frost injuries. Springer, Berlin

Frostbite

Bass M (1993) Treatment of frostbite. Alaska Med 35:141

Cattermole TJ (1999) The epidemiology of cold injury in Antarctica. Aviat Space Environ Med 70:135–140

Kanzenbach TL, Dexter WW (1999) Cold injuries. Protecting your patients from the dangers of hypothermia and frostbite. Postgrad Med 105:72–78

Lacour M, Le Coultre C (1991) Spray-induced frostbite in a child: a new hazard with novel aerosol propellants. Pediatr Dermatol 8:207–209

Immersion Foot

Irwin MS, Sanders R, Green CJ et al. (1997) Neuropathy in nonfreezing cold injury (trench foot). J R Soc Med 90:433–438

Mills WJ Jr, Mills WJ III (1993) Peripheral nonfreezing cold injury: immersion injury. Alaska Med 35:117–128

Pernio and Its Variants

Crowson AN, Magro CM (1997) Idiopathic perniosis and its mimics: a clinical and histological study of 38 cases. Hum Pathol 28:478–484

Goette DK (1990) Chilblains (perniosis). J Am Acad Dermatol 23:257–262

Keining E (1940) Die "Frühlingsperniosis" zum Unterschied von der Herbstperniosis. Dermatol Wochenschr 110:26

Spittell JA Jr, Spittell PC (1992) Chronic pernio: another cause of blue toes. Int Angiol 11:46–50

Skin Diseases Due to Electrical and Lightning Injuries

Ackerman AB, Goldfader GL (1971) Electrical burns of the mouth in children. Arch Dermatol 104:308–311

Armijo M, Naranjo R (1980) Electrical burns. J Dermatol Surg Oncol 6:843–845

Bartholomew CW, Jacoby WD, Ramchand SC (1975) Cutaneous manifestations of lightning injury. Arch Dermatol 111:1466–1468

Bingham H (1986) Electrical burns. Clin Plast Surg 13: 75–85

Hussman J, Kucan JO, Russell RC et al. (1995) Electrical injuries – morbidity, outcome and treatment rationale. Burns 21:530–535

Thomas SS (1996) Electrical burns of the mouth: still searching for an answer. Burns 22:137–140

Skin Damage Due to Chemicals

Barranco VP (1991) Mustard gas and the dermatologist. Int J Dermatol 30:684–686

McGovern TW, Christopher GW, Eitzen EM (1999) Cutaneous manifestations of biological warfare and related threat agents. Arch Dermatol 135:311–322

Momeni AZ, Enshaeih S, Meghdadi M et al. (1992) Skin manifestations of mustard gas. A clinical study of 535 patients exposed to mustard gas. Arch Dermatol 128:775–780

Sebastian G (1994) Praxisrelevante Therapieempfehlungen bei Flußsäureverätzungen. Hautarzt 45:453–459

Smith KJ, Smith WJ, Hamilton T et al. (1998) Histopathologic and immunohistochemical features in human skin after exposure to nitrogen and sulfur mustard. Am J Dermatopathol 20:22–28

Skin Disease Due to Ionizing Radiation

Kawakami T, Saito R, Miyazaki S (1999) Chronic radiodermatitis following repeated percutaneous transluminal coronary angioplasty. Br J Dermatol 141:150–153

Landthaler M, Hagspiel HJ, Braun-Falco O (1995) Late irradiation damage to the skin caused by soft x-ray radiation therapy of cutaneous tumors. Arch Dermatol 131: 182–186

Lichtenstein DA, Klapholz L, Vardy DA et al. (1996) Chronic radiodermatitis following cardiac catheterization. Arch Dermatol 132:663–667

Peter RU, Plewig G (eds) (1996) Strahlentherapie dermatologischer Erkrankungen. Blackwell, Berlin

Diseases Caused by Sunlight

Basic Science

Fitzpatrick TB (1988) The validity and practicability of sunreactive skin types I through VI. Arch Dermatol 124:869–871

Gilchrest BA, Park HY, Eller MS et al. (1996) Mechanisms of ultraviolet light-induced pigmentation. Photochem Photobiol 63:1–10

Harber LC, Bickers DR (1989) Photosensitivity diseases, 2nd edn. Decker, Philadelphia

Hausser I (1938) Über spezifische Wirkung des langwelligen ultravioletten Lichts auf die menschliche Haut. Strahlentherapie 62:315–322

Hözle E, Neumann N, Hausen B et al. (1991) Photopatch testing: the 5-year experience of the German, Austrian, and Swiss photopatch test group. J Am Acad Dermatol 25:59–68

Kim TA, Golden P, Ullrich SE et al. (1990) Immunosuppression by factors released from UV-irradiated epidermal cells: selective effects on the generation of contact and delayed hypersensitivity after exposure to UVA or UVB radiation. J Invest Dermatol 94:26–32

Kind P, Lehmann P, Plewig G (1993) Phototesting in lupus erythematosus. J Invest Dermatol 100:53–57

Krutmann J (1998) Therapeutic photoimmunology: photoimmunological mechanisms in photo(chemo)therapy. J Photochem Photobiol 44:159–164

Krutmann J (1995) Photoimmunology. Blackwell, Oxford

Lebwohl M, Hecker D, Martinez J et al. (1997) Interactions between calcipotriene and ultraviolet light. J Am Acad Dermatol 37:93–95

Lüftl M, Degitz K, Plewig G et al. (1997) Psoralen bath plus UV-A therapy. Possibilities and limitations. Arch Dermatol 133:1597–1603

Meirowsky E (1908) Über den Ursprung des melanotischen Pigments der Haut und des Auges. Bibliothek medizinischer Monographien; Bd. 4, Verlag von Dr. Werner Klinkhardt, Leipzig

Meirowsky E (1909) Über Pigmentbildung in vom Körper losgelöster Haut. Frankfurter Zeitschr der Path S 439–448

Miescher G (1930) Das Problem des Lichtschutzes und der Lichtgewöhnung. Strahlentherapie 35:403

Neumann NJ, Hölzle E, Lehmann P et al. (1994) Pattern analysis of photopatch test reactions. Photodermatology 10:65–73

Norris PG, British Dermatology Group (1994) British Photodermatology Group guidelines for PUVA. Br J Dermatol 130:246–255

Paul BS, Parrish JA (1982) The interaction of UVA and UVB in the production of threshold erythema. J Invest Dermatol 78:371–374

Scharffetter-Kochanek K, Wlaschek M, Brenneisen P et al. (1997) UV-induced reactive oxygen species in photocarcinogenesis and photoaging. Biol Chem 378:1247–1257

Vallat VP, Gilleaudeau P, Battat L et al. (1994) PUVA bath therapy strongly suppresses immunological and epidermal activation in psoriasis: a possible cellular basis for remittive therapy. J Exp Med 180:283–296

Walchner M, Messer G, Kind P (1997) Phototesting and photoprotection in LE. Lupus 6:167–174

Sunburn

Edwards EK Jr, Edwards EK Sr (1990) Sunburn and sunscreens: an update and review. Mil Med 155:381–383

Fitzpatrick TB (1975) Soleil et peau. J Med Esthet 2:33–34

Mallory SB (1990) Sunburn and sun reactions. Adolesc Med 1:375–384

Chronic Light-Induced Changes

Calderone DC, Fenske NA (1995) The clinical spectrum of actinic elastosis. J Am Acad Dermatol 32:1016–1024

Fisher GJ, Talwar HS, Lin J et al. (1999) Molecular mechanisms of photoaging in human skin in vivo and their prevention by all-trans retinoic acid. Photochem Photobiol 69:154–157

Kang S, Fisher GJ, Voorhees JJ (1997) Photoaging and topical tretinoin: therapy, pathogenesis, and prevention. Arch Dermatol 133:1280–1284

Scharffetter-Kochanek K (1997) Photoaging of the connective tissue of skin: its prevention and therapy. Adv Pharmacol 38:639–655

Solar Urticaria

Leenutaphong V, Hölzle E, Plewig G (1989) Pathogenesis and classification of solar urticaria: a new concept. J Am Acad Dermatol 21:237–240

Leenutaphong V, Hölzle E, Plewig G (1990) Solar urticaria: studies on mechanisms of tolerance. Br J Dermatol 122: 601–606

Roelandts R, Ryckaert S (1999) Solar urticaria: the annoying photodermatosis. Int J Dermatol 38:411–418

Uetsu N, Miyauchi-Hashimoto H, Okamoto H et al. (2000) The clinical and photobiological characteristics of solar urticaria in 40 patients. Br J Dermatol 142:32–38

Polymorphic Light Eruption

Elpern DJ, Morison WL, Hood AF (1985) Papulovesicular light eruption. A defined subset of polymorphous light eruption. Arch Dermatol 121:1286–1288

Hausmann W, Haxthausen H (1929) Die Lichterkrankungen der Haut. Strahlentherapie 11:62–71

Jansén CT, Karvonen J (1984) Polymorphous light eruption. A seven-year follow-up evaluation of 114 patients. Arch Dermatol 120:862–865

Lindmaier A, Neumann R (1991) Der PLD-Patient. Hauttyp, Hardening und andere Licht-assoziierte Merkmale. Hautarzt 42:430–433

Man I, Dawe RS, Ferguson J (1999) Artificial hardening for polymorphic light eruption: practical points from 10 years' experience. Photodermatol Photoimmunol Photomed 15:96–99

Norris PG, Hawk JLM (1990) Polymorphic light eruption. Photodermatology 7:186–191

Salomon N, Messer G, Dick D et al. (1997) Phototesting for polymorphic light eruption (PLE) with consecutive UVA1/UVB irradiation. Photodermatol Photobiol Photomed 13:72–74

Hydroa Vacciniforme

Bazin E (1862) Leçons thèoriques et cliniques sur les affections génériques de la peau. Delabrage 1, Paris, pp 132–134

Eramo LR, Garden JM, Esterly NB (1986) Hydroa vacciniforme. Diagnosis by repetitive ultraviolet-A phototesting. Arch Dermatol 122:1310–1313

Galosi A, Plewig G, Ring J et al. (1985) Experimentelle Auslösung von Hauterscheinungen bei Hydroa vacciniformia. Hautarzt 36:566–572

Gupta G, Mohamed M, Kemmett D (1999) Familial hydroa vacciniforme. Br J Dermatol 140:124–126

Hann SK, Im S, Park YK, Lee S (1991) Hydroa vacciniforme with unusually severe scar formation: diagnosis by repetitive UVA phototesting. J Am Acad Dermatol 25:401–403

Ketterer R, Morier P, Frank E (1994) Hydroa vacciniforme. Dermatology 189:428–429

Leroy D, Dompmartin A, Michel M et al. (1997) Factors influencing the photoreproduction of hydroa vacciniforme lesions. Photodermatol Photoimmunol Photomed 13:98–102

Sonncx TS, Hawk JL (1988) Hydroa vacciniforme: a review of ten cases. Br J Dermatol 118:101–108

Actinic Prurigo

Addo HA, Frain-Bell W (1984) Actinic prurigo – a specific photodermatosis? Photodermatol 1:119–128

Birt AR, Davis RA (1975) Hereditary polymorphous light eruption of American Indians. Int J Dermatol 14:105–111

Fusaro RM, Johnson JA (1980) Hereditary polymorphic light eruption in American Indians. Photoprotection and prevention of streptococcal pyoderma and glomerulonephritis. JAMA 244:1456–1459

Hölzle E, Rowold J, Plewig G (1992) Aktinische Prurigo. Hautarzt 43:278–282

Hojyo-Tomoka T, Granados J, Vargas-Alarcòn G et al. (1997) Further evidence of the role of HLA-DR4 in the genetic susceptibility to actinic prurigo. J Am Acad Dermatol 36:935–937

Lane PR, Sheridan DP, Hogan DJ et al. (1991) HLA typing in polymorphous light eruption. J Am Acad Dermatol 24:570–573

Lane PR (1997) Actinic prurigo. Photodermatol Photoimmunol Photomed 13:87–88

López-Gonzales G (1961) Prurigo solar. Arch Agent Dermatol 11:301–308

Magana M (1997) Actinic or solar prurigo. J Am Acad Dermatol 36:504–505

Photodermatoses Caused by Exogenous Sensitizers

Bowers AG (1999) Phytophotodermatitis. Am J Contact Dermat 10:89–93

Bruinsma W (1995) A guide to drug eruptions, 6th edn. File of Medicines, Oosthuizen, The Netherlands

Clark SM, Wilkinson SM (1998) Phototoxic contact dermatitis from 5-methoxypsoralen in aroma therapy oil. Contact Dermatitis 38:289–290

Fotiades J, Soter NA, Lim HW (1995) Results of evaluation of 203 patients for photosensitivity in a 7.3-year period. J Am Acad Dermatol 33:597–602

Gonzalez E, Gonzalez S (1996) Drug photosensitivity, idiopathic photodermatoses, and sunscreens. J Am Acad Dermatol 35:871–885

Gould JW, Mercurio MG, Elmets CA (1995) Cutaneous photosensitivity diseases induced by exogenous agents. J Am Acad Dermatol 33:551–573

Ibbotson SH, Farr PM, Beck MH et al. (1997) Photopatch testing – methods and indications. Br J Dermatol 136:371–376

Moore DE (1998) Mechanisms of photosensitization by phototoxic drugs. Mutat Res 422:165–173

Rünger TM, Lehmann P, Neumann NJ et al. (1995) Empfehlung einer Photopatch-Test Standardreihe durch die deutschsprachige Arbeitsgruppe "Photopatch-Test". Hautarzt 46:240–243

Chronic Actinic Dermatitis

Frain-Bell W, Lakshmipathi T, Rogers J et al. (1974) The syndrome of chronic photosensitivity dermatitis and actinic reticuloid. Br J Dermatol 91:617–634

Hawk JL, Magnus IA (1979) Chronic actinic dermatitis – an idiopathic photosensitivity syndrom including actinic reticuloid and photosensitive eczema. Br J Dermatol 101:24

Ive FA, Magnus IA, Warin RP et al. (1969) "Actinic reticuloid"; a chronic dermatosis associated with severe photosensitivity and the histological resemblance to lymphoma. Br J Dermatol 81:469–485

Lim HW, Cohen D, Soter NA (1998) Chronic actinic dermatitis: results of patch and photopatch tests with compositae, fragrances, and pesticides. J Am Acad Dermatol 38:108–111

Megahed M, Hölzle E, Plewig G (1991) Persistent light reaction associated with photoallergic contact dermatitis to musk ambrette and allergic contact dermatitis to fragrance mix. Dermatologica 182:199–202

Menage HD, Hawk JL (1993) The red face: chronic actinic dermatitis. Clin Dermatol 11:297–305

Murphy GM, Maurice PM, Norris PG et al. (1989) Azathioprine in the treatment of chronic actinic dermatitis: a double blind controlled trial with monitoring of exposure to ultraviolet radiation. Br J Dermatol 121:639–646

Norris PG, Camp RDR, Hawk JLM (1989) Actinic reticuloid: response to cyclosporin. J Am Acad Dermatol 21:307–309

Norris PG, Hawk JLM (1990) Chronic actinic dermatitis. A unifying concept. Arch Dermatol 126:376–378

Ramsay CA, Black AK (1973) Photosensitive eczema. Tran St Johns Hosp Dermatol Soc 59:152–158

Roelandts R (1993) Chronic actinic dermatitis. J Am Acad Dermatol 28:240–249

Wilkinson DS (1961) Photodermatitis due to tetrachlorsalicylanilide. Br J Dermatol 73:213–219

Zak-Prelich M, Schwartz RA (1999) Actinic reticuloid. Int J Dermatol 38:335–342

Xeroderma Pigmentosum

Auerbach AD, Verlander PC (1997) Disorders of DNA replication and repair. Curr Opin Pediatr 9(6):600–616

Chu G, Mayne L (1996) Xeroderma pigmentosum, Cockayne syndrome and trichothiodystrophy: do the genes explain the diseases? Trends Genet 12(5):187–192

Cleaver JE (1968) Defective repair replication of DNA in xeroderma pigmentosum. Nature 218:652–656

Copeland NE, Hanke CW, Michalak JA (1997) The molecular basis of xeroderma pigmentosum. Dermatol Surg 23(6): 447–455

Kraemer KH, Levy DD, Parris CN et al. (1994) Xeroderma pigmentosum and related disorders: examining the linkage between defective DNA repair and cancer. J Invest Dermatol 103:69–101

Lambert WC, Kuo HR, Lambert MW (1995) Xeroderma pigmentosum. Dermatol Clin 13:169–209

Van Steeg, Kraemer KH (1999) Xeroderma pigmentosum and the role of UV-induced DNA damage in skin cancer. Mol Med Today 5:86–94

Bloom Syndrome

Bloom D (1954) Congenital telangiectatic erythema resembling lupus erythematosus in dwarfs. Probably a syndrome entity. Am J Dis Child 88:754–758

Bloom D (1966) Congenital telangiectatic erythema syndrome and stunted growth. Arch Argent Dermatol 16:26–28

German J (1993) Bloom syndrome: a mendelian prototype of somatic mutational disease. Medicine Baltimore 72(6): 393–406

German J (1995) Bloom's syndrome. Dermatol Clin 13:7–18

German J (1997) Bloom's syndrome. XX. The first 100 cancers. Cancer Genet Cytogenet 93(1):100–106

Gretzula JC, Hevia O, Weber PJ (1987) Bloom's syndrome. J Am Acad Dermatol 17:479–488

Sirover MA, Vollberg TM, Seal G (1990) DNA repair and the molecular mechanisms of Bloom's syndrome. Crit Rev Oncog 2(1):19–33

Ataxia Teleangiectasia

Götz G, Eckert F, Landthaler M (1994) Ataxia-telangiectasia (Louis-Bar syndrome) associated with ulcerating necrobiosis lipoidica. J Am Acad Dermatol 31:124–126

Joshi RK, al Asiri RH, Haleem A et al. (1993) Cutaneous granuloma with ataxia telangiectasia – a case report and review of literature. Clin Exp Dermatol 18(5):458–461

Miller SJ (1965) The syndrome of Madame Louis-Bar. Trans Ophthalmol Soc U K 85:437–443

Savitsky K, Bar-Shira A, Gilad S et al. (1995) A single ataxia telangiectasia gene with a product similar to PI-3 kinase. Science 268:1749–1753

Swift M, Morrell D, Massey RB et al. (1991) Incidence of cancer in 161 families affected by ataxia-telangiectasia. N Engl J Med 26; 325(26):1831–1836

Erythemato-Papulo-Squamous Diseases

Contents

The diseases covered below all feature erythematous or papular lesions which often become covered with scale. The term papulosquamous is most often used in the USA but fails to correctly describe diseases such as pityriasis rosea which has erythematous macules and then scale, but never papules. Thus we prefer erythematosquamous, even though it is not widely used in English. Most of these diseases have an unclear etiology and their appearance in the same chapter should not be interpreted as evidence of any biologic relationship.

Erythemas

Flushing

Definition. Transitory facial reddening as a result of vasodilatation.

Etiology and Pathogenesis. Flushing is a common clinical phenomenon with many causes. Many pathogenic mechanisms come together to cause flushing, as shown in Table 14.1. In general, the vascular smooth muscles lose their tone as a result of decreased or altered neural stimuli. Coffee frequently causes flushing. For years, the caffeine was blamed for the problem, as a potent vasodilator. Instead, the temperature of the beverage is probably more important. Under laboratory conditions, warm water is more likely to produce flushing than cold coffee. The sudden reddening is probably con-

Table 14.1. Causes of flushing

Cause	Agent	Mediator
Emotions	CNS, peripheral nerves	Substance P
Physical factors	Heat	Multiple
Chemicals	Ethanol	Acetaldehyde
Medications	Nicotinic acid Disulfuram	Prostaglandins Acetaldehyde
Foods	Glutamates	Acetylcholine
Endocrine factors	Menopause Hyperendorphin syndrome	Gonadotropins Enkephalins
Tumors	Mastocytoma Carcinoid tumor Pancreatic carcinoma	Histamine, kinins Serotonin, prostaglandins Vasoactive intestinal protein (VIP)

trolled through the hypothalamic heat regulation center.

Alcohol consumption may create flushing in a variety of ways. Acetaldehyde, a metabolic product of ethanol, causes prompt flushing, especially in Asians who often lack the appropriate enzyme to metabolize the product. Alcohol dehydrogenase and β-hydroxylase may be blocked by medications enhancing alcohol-induced flushing. Disulfuram, chlorpropamide, griseofulvin, β-lactam antibiotics, metronidazole and phentolamine have been indicted. Sherry, other wines and some fish contain enough histamine to produce flushing, as do cheeses rich in tyramine. Monosodium glutamates also cause flushing, and because they are so often used in Chinese cooking, they are the usual cause of the Chinese restaurant syndrome.

In women with menopausal flushing, the serum estrogen and gonadotropin levels are usually only minimally altered as the problems begin, but in general estrogens can reduce the frequency of the flushing. They also can cause flushing by inhibiting tyrosine hydroxylase leading to increased CNS dopamine levels. Enkephalins have been proposed as mediators of the facial erythema in rosacea. Intravenous endorphins as well as idiopathic excess production of these CNS mediators (hyperendorphin syndrome) may also produce problems.

Clinical Findings. The patient complains of sudden facial erythema and warmth. Much less commonly, other body areas such as the neck or sternal region may be involved. Flushing during the menopause (hot flashes) is both common and notorious for its sudden onset and massive associated warmth. The flushing often spreads beyond the face. The skin temperature can be shown to be elevated and cardiac output increased because of the significant vasodilatation.

Differential Diagnosis. The differential diagnosis is discussed in the subsequent sections. The trick is to avoid overlooking flushing as a sign of underlying disease but at the same time avoid expensive and unrewarding testing in patients with an innocent history for idiopathic flushing.

Therapy. A variety of possible inhibitors can be tried. They block various aspects of flushing but none is reliably effective. Prostaglandins can be inhibited by some nonsteroidal antiinflammatory drugs and aspirin. Atropine blocks the glutamate-induced flush fairly well, but often with unacceptable side effects. Naloxone inhibits chlorpropamide-induced flushing and may ameliorate other CNS-mediated problems. Cyproheptadine hydrochloride is a serotonin inhibitor. Antihistamines can be used for histamine-mediated flush; they are covered under urticaria (Chap. 12).

Blushing

Definition. Emotionally induced, idiopathic flushing.

Etiology and Pathogenesis. In blushing, the vasodilatation appears to be regulated by emotional factors, but probably through many of the same pathways discussed above.

Clinical Findings. Blushing is clinically the same as flushing. Most patients are younger and are aware that stress or nervousness triggers their flushing. The erythema appears suddenly, may spread to the neck and upper anterior portion of the chest, and disappears rapidly. Such patients are often described as having psychovegatative dysregulation. This fancy term suggests that they tend to respond to emotional stress with more obvious physical findings. In addition to the flushing, hyperhidrosis and acrocyanosis may be seen.

Therapy. In general, no therapy is needed.

Persistent Facial Erythema

Clinical Findings. While this is rarely thought of as a disease, the finding of persistent mid-facial erythema is not uncommon. Familial cases have been described. Typical patients are young women, often with a short stocky build. They generally have pale or pasty skin color, but over their cheeks, nose and chin, there is persistent vasodilatation and even telangiectases. The perioral region is spared. The skin temperature is usually elevated in the involved area. The same patients may have ulerythema ophryogenes.

Therapy. Usually coverage with cosmetics is the simplest approach. Green make-up bases are most effective at masking erythema. Some patients respond to tetracycline, but often reject the needed long-term therapy.

Carcinoid Syndrome

Definition. Flushing associated with the presence of carcinoid tumor secreting vasoactive substances.

Etiology and Pathogenesis. The carcinoid syndrome is caused by a functioning paracrine tumor, usually arising in the small intestine and secreting serotonin and other vasoactive amines. Other tumor sites may include other parts of the gastrointestinal tract, ovaries, testes, pancreas or bronchi. In addition, other malignant tumors such as oat cell carcinoma of the lung, medullary carcinoma of the thyroid and islet cell tumor of the pancreas may also be responsible. Tumors of the gastrointestinal tract usually only cause symptoms when they have metastasized to the liver. The major active substance is serotonin which is metabolized in the liver by monoamine oxidase. Liver metastases can discharge serotonin directly into the circulation and tumors at other sites may also be able to bypass the liver.

Clinical Findings. The so-called serotonin flush typically appears and disappears rapidly, involves the face and neck and often has violet tones. It may spread to other parts of the body. Following repeated episodes, there may be a persistent erythema and then even a cyanosis if vessels remain dilated. The vasodilatation is usually caused more by histamines and other substances, while serotonin is responsible for the typical gastrointestinal symptoms of diarrhea, cramps and abdominal pain. Malabsorption and even pellagra (because too much tryptophan is converted to serotonin) may occur. Tachycardia is common. Right-sided endocardial fibrosis is a feared complication. The left side of the heart is usually spared because the active products are metabolized in the lungs. Some patients develop pulmonary stenosis, tricuspid regurgitation and right-sided heart failure; others have wheezing and shortness of breath.

Laboratory Findings. Serotonin is 5-hydroxytryptamine. It is metabolized to 5-hydroxyindolacetic acid (5-HIAA) and excreted in the urine. Normal urinary 5-HIAA excretion is <10 mg/day, whereas in carcinoid syndrome, excretion usually is >50 mg/day. A 24-h urine specimen must be analyzed after the patient has avoided foods rich in serotonin (bananas, avocados, walnuts and selected others) and medications such as phenothiazines which also interfere with the colorimetric test.

Diagnostic Criteria. Urinary 5-HIAA is the benchmark. Patients with mast cell disease typically have urticarial lesions, but may have similar clinical problems (Chap. 63). Patients with flushing and gastrointestinal, cardiac or pulmonary symptoms deserve an extensive work-up. Provocative tests are also described in the internal medicine literature but should be employed with care. Liver imaging studies are also required.

Therapy. The tumor is most often not resectable by the time it has been identified. There are many asymptomatic gastrointestinal carcinoids, such as in the appendix, but they are usually incidental findings. Occasionally pulmonary carcinoids can be resected. The metastatic tumors are hard to treat, but survival is usually quite long, up to 10–15 years. Streptozocin is the most-often employed agent, usually combined with 5-fluorouracil. Somatostatin usually blocks the flushing without altering 5-HIAA levels, which also speaks against the primary role of serotonin in the cutaneous problem. Cyproheptadine may also be useful, as well as phenothiazines, phentolamine (α-adrenergic blocker) and corticosteroids.

Familial Palmoplantar Erythema

(LANE 1929)

Synonyms. Erythema palmare et plantare hereditarium red palm syndrome, Lane syndrome

Clinical Findings. This uncommon disorder has its onset in early childhood. The mid-palm is spared, but the thenar and hypothenar eminences, distal part of the palm and fingertips are persistently red. The soles may be involved but to a lesser degree. The disorder appears to be inherited in an autosomal dominant pattern, but there is a male predominance.

Differential Diagnosis. Acquired palmoplantar erythema is the main differential question but a family history usually suffices. Erythema of acral regions (BRYAN and COSKEY 1967) is similar but the ears are also involved. There may be dental and skeletal abnormalities and the pattern of inheritance is autosomal recessive. Early or mild forms of palmoplantar keratoderma may also present with erythema; the clinical course should provide the answer.

Therapy. Nothing satisfactory has been found.

Acquired Palmoplantar Erythema

Synonyms. Erythema palmare et plantare symptomaticum, red liver palms

Clinical Findings. Acquired palmoplantar erythema is often a sign of chronic liver disease. Many patients develop a degree of palmoplantar erythema as a normal variant (Fig. 14.1). White or milk glass colored or banded nails should suggest the possibility of associated liver disease. The same changes may be seen in pregnancy, hyperthyroidism and a variety of other disorders. In addition, livid palms are often a marker of smoking and may also reflect an internal malignancy.

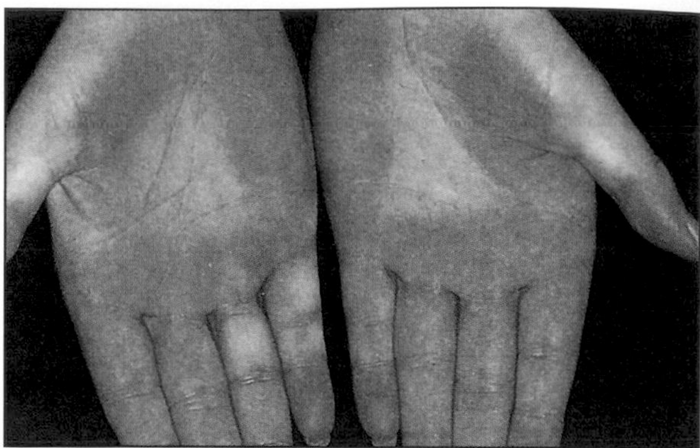

Fig. 14.1. Palmar erythema

Therapy. None available.

Other Erythemas

Several diseases are designated as erythemas but covered elsewhere in the text. They have other dominating features and do not enter into the differential diagnosis of an ordinary or figurate erythema. Examples include erythema toxicum neonatorum (Chap. 16) which usually has pustules, erythema elevatum diutinum (Chap. 22) which is a type of vasculitis, and erythema dyschromicum perstans (Chap. 26) which has a transient erythematous phase but usually presents with hyperpigmented lesions.

Figurate Erythemas

The figurate erythemas do not represent a group of related diseases, but instead refer to a series of unrelated entities that may present with annular or figurate red lesions which show peripheral spread. In addition to the entities discussed in this section, many other figurate erythemas exist. One should consider:

- Dermatophyte infections
- Urticarial reactions, including early urticarial stage of bullous pemphigoid
- Erythema multiforme
- Psoriasis

- Lupus erythematosus, especially subacute cutaneous lupus erythematosus and neonatal lupus erythematosus
- Sjögren syndrome especially in Asians

What appears to unify the figurate erythemas is that they represent a reaction against a given antigen, perhaps occurring near a vessel and then with peripheral diffusion into the adjacent skin. The differential diagnosis under each of the various disorders will not be repeated.

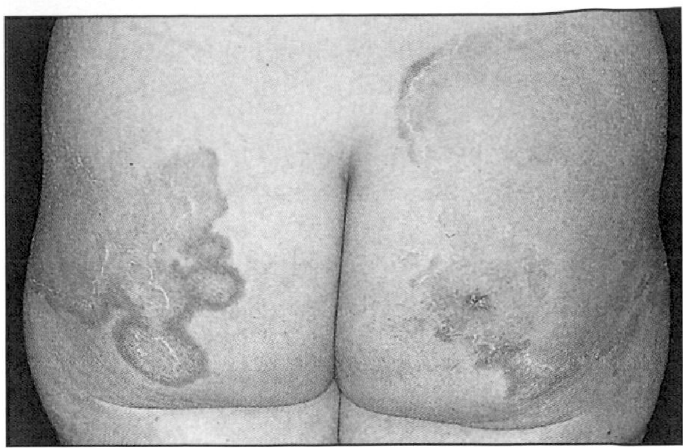

Fig. 14.2. Erythema annulare centrifugum

Erythema Annulare Centrifugum

[Darier 1916]

Epidemiology. This uncommon disorder occurs primarily in adults.

Etiology and Pathogenesis. Erythema annulare centrifugum represents a reaction to a wide variety of triggers. Commonly described associations include:

- Infections. Chronic dermatophyte infections are a fairly well established trigger. *Candida albicans* and a variety of bacterial infections have also been implicated.
- Tumors. Erythema annulare centrifugum can be considered an uncommon but genuine paraneoplastic sign. In a number of case reports, malignant tumors of the breast, gastrointestinal tract, lungs and other organs have been described with typical skin changes that disappear after excision of the tumor.
- Infestations. Intestinal worms, such as *Ascaris*, may be found.
- Food allergies to fish, cheese (especially blue cheese and other cheeses with active molds) and peanuts may be responsible.
- Drug reactions, such as to penicillin, have also been described, but probably fit better into the category of urticaria.

The problems with determining the cause of erythema annulare centrifugum are similar to those with urticaria. Many positive investigations have been reported, but it is often unclear if the etiologic factor is truly responsible for the skin finding or is simply a bystander. In most cases, no definite etiology is established.

Clinical Findings. The initial erythematous lesion resembles a hive does not resolve. Instead, its periphery slowly expands in an asymmetric fashion while central clearing occurs (Fig. 14.2). The result may be a series of intersecting circular and oval erythematous rings. Often there is fine collarette scale or punctate hemorrhage. The lesions spread over a period of days and resolve over weeks to months, as new lesions develop both in previously involved sites and in new regions. While any body part can be involved, the trunk is the most common site. The lesions are usually asymptomatic but may occasionally itch.

Histopathology. The hallmark is a prominent lymphocytic perivascular infiltrate in the dermis. If the infiltrate is relatively superficial, minimal epidermal changes (spongiosis, scale) may be found. When the infiltrate is deeper, the epidermis is spared. True vasculitis is not seen. Eosinophils may be present.

Therapy. The approach is the same as in chronic urticaria. If a possible etiologic agent is identified, the condition should be treated. Pruritic lesions can be treated with antihistamines or nonsteroidal antiinflammatory drugs.

Erythema Gyratum Repens

[Gammel 1952]

Etiology and Pathogenesis. Erythema gyratum repens is almost always a marker of internal malignancy. It has been associated with a long list of malignancies, involving the lungs, breasts, gastrointestinal tract and many other sites. It may occur in the absence of any tumor; we have seen it with tuberculosis.

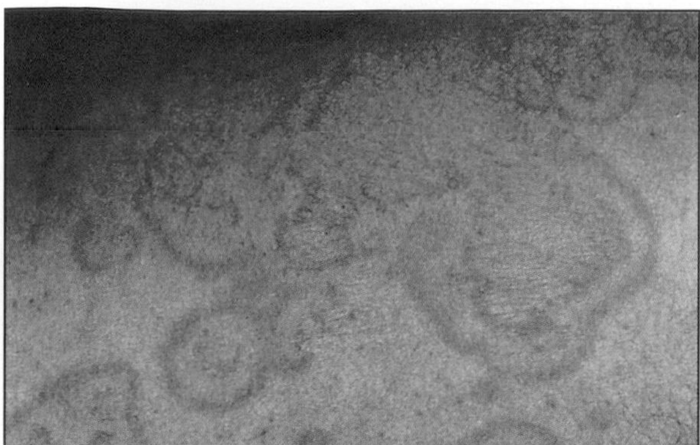

Fig. 14.3. Erythema gyratum repens

Clinical Findings. Because of its association with malignancy, erythema gyratum repens tends to occur in older patients. It is a rapidly spreading superficial erythematous eruption that produces bizarre intersecting wreaths and spirals (Fig. 14.3). The pattern has been compared to the grain of a sawn log, and since so many bands are present, the term zebra skin has been used. Once again the trunk is most often involved. Scale is characteristically present at the edge of the erythema. The eruption is often pruritic. The key feature is that erythema gyratum repens changes over minutes to hours, while erythema annulare centrifugum changes over days to weeks.

Histopathology. Once again there is a lymphocytic perivascular infiltrate, usually more intense in the upper dermis. Epidermal involvement is somewhat more likely, reflecting the almost invariable scale formation. Deposition of immunoglobulins in the basement membrane zone has been described, but does not help in the diagnosis.

Therapy. An extensive search for an underlying tumor is most important. Symptomatic treatment of the pruritus with antihistamines is appropriate.

Erythema Gyratum Perstans

(Colcott-Fox 1891)

Synonym. Familial annular erythema (Beare et al. 1966)

The clinical lesions are identical to those of erythema annulare centrifugum, but the disease is inherited in an autosomal dominant pattern. The lesions may begin shortly after birth or appear first in childhood. Most patients also have dermographism.

Annular Erythema of Infancy

In addition to erythema gyratum perstans, there are a number of other figurate erythemas described in infancy. Annular erythema of infancy typically features small papules that evolve into erythematous arches or rings without scale. Lesions last for several days and recur in cycles. Microscopic examination shows a perivascular lymphocytic infiltrate often with admixed eosinophils. This disease is probably closest to erythema annulare centrifugum.

There are also many peculiar variants of figurate erythemas in infants. In some instances, the lesions are scaly and may simply be unusual presentations of tinea versicolor so a KOH examination is always appropriate. In other instances, central atrophy develops; this is known as erythema gyratum repens atrophicans transiens (Gianotti and Ermacora 1975). In other cases, the histologic pattern shows neutrophilic perivascular deposits and nuclear dust with vessel destruction and the term neutrophilic figurate erythema of infancy has been suggested. The closest adult equivalent appears to be urticarial vasculitis. Finally, one must rule out neonatal lupus erythematosus (Chap. 18) which is often annular. In all cases except when *Malassezia furfur* is found, watching and waiting, rather than any specific treatment, is the only recommended course of action.

Erythema Marginatum

(Lehndorff and Leiner 1922)

Synonyms. Erythema circinatum, erythema annulare rheumaticum

Definition. Transient annular erythematous rash in children with rheumatic fever.

Etiology and Pathogenesis. The eruption is directly related to a streptococcal infection and probably represents an urticarial-type response to some streptococcal antigen.

Clinical Findings. About 20% of patients with acute rheumatic fever develop a transient erythematous rash. The most common site of involvement is the trunk. The initial lesions are pink macules that rapidly, over a period of minutes, spread to produce a polycyclic or serpiginous pattern. The bands of erythema are typically quite narrow, so the final pattern has been compared to chicken wire. Typically the cutaneous lesions appear along with a fever spike, often in the late afternoon. They usually disappear within hours to days, are asymptomatic and easily overlooked. Erythema marginatum is more common in patients with active carditis. It usually develops at about the same time as the typical joint and cardiac findings, but may appear weeks later.

Two other cutaneous manifestations of rheumatic fever are:

- Erythema Papulatum (Cockayne 1912). Tiny erythematous urticarial macules and papules appear on the knees and elbows. They do not evolve into annular lesions and resolve over a period of days to weeks. They clinically resemble granuloma annulare and are present in less than 5% of patients.
- Subcutaneous Nodules. Patients with more severe carditis may develop nodules over the extensor tendons of the extremities, the scalp and the spine. Histologically these nodules show extensive necrobiosis and are identical to granuloma annulare or rheumatoid nodules, but they tend to disappear in a matter of months.

Histopathology. There is a sparse perivascular infiltrate of neutrophils in the papillary dermis. This is a relatively uncommon finding that may help in a puzzling case.

Diagnostic Criteria. Both erythema marginatum and subcutaneous nodules are major criteria for the diagnosis of rheumatic fever. Evidence for a recent streptococcal infection should be sought, and cardiac and rheumatologic evaluations performed.

Differential Diagnosis. Patients with juvenile rheumatoid arthritis (Still disease) may also have a transient rash, similar to erythema marginatum. More often they have erythematous macules usually on the extremities which are relatively stable and not annular.

Therapy. The underlying rheumatic fever should be treated with antibiotics. The skin findings do not require any special therapy.

Erythema Scarlatiniforme Desquamativum Recidivans

(Féréol-Besnier 1878)

Definition. Typical localized or generalized erythema that resolves with desquamation similar to scarlet fever

Etiology and Pathogenesis. The etiology is unclear but some cases may represent staphylococcal scarlet fever (Chap. 4) and others, an unusual drug reaction. Implicated drugs include vitamin A, vitamin B_1 (thiamine), bismuth, gold, quinine, hydantoin, salicylates and diuretics. It has also been seen in cases of drug abuse.

Clinical Findings. The prodrome includes fever, chills and headache. Then a macular exanthem starts usually on the trunk and over days becomes generalized. The hands, feet and head are last to be involved. In the localized form, only the hands and feet are involved. As the erythema fades, there is characteristic desquamation, with the typical sock and glove shedding on the palms and soles, as well as larger scales on the trunk. While the skin findings resolve over a period of weeks, they may recur. A wide variety of other findings, such as gastrointestinal problems, arthritis and renal disease, have been described.

Histopathology. The epidermis shows focal parakeratosis with loss of the granular layer. In the dermis there is a mixed lymphohistiocytic perivascular infiltrate.

Differential Diagnosis. One must consider all scarlatiniform eruptions, including scarlet fever, tinea manuum and pedis, dyshidrotic dermatitis, pityriasis rubra pilaris and psoriasis.

Therapy. If an infectious disease is present, it should be treated with antibiotics. Otherwise topical antiinflammatory and keratolytic agents can be employed.

Necrolytic Migratory Erythema

[Becker et al. 1942]

Synonyms. Erythema necroticans migrans, glucagonoma syndrome

Definition. Paraneoplastic skin disorder associated with glucagon-secreting pancreatic islet cell tumor.

Epidemiology. This rare eruption is almost an obligate cancer marker. It is more commonly seen among postmenopausal women, with a 3:1 female to male ratio.

Etiology and Pathogenesis. Almost all patients have a glucagonoma. Most tumors are α-cell tumors; 80 % are malignant but usually slowly growing. Rare patients have been described without a tumor, some with underlying gastrointestinal disease (chronic pancreatitis, chronic hepatitis, carcinoma of the colon) and others in apparently good health (pseudoglucagonoma syndrome). While both glucagon itself and a variety of other metabolic products, such as amino acids, have been blamed for the eruption, its exact cause remains a mystery.

Clinical Findings. Fatigue and weight loss are usually the first symptoms. The rash most often begins in the perioral or inguinal region as red-brown macules that become superficially necrotic and then crusted (Fig. 14.4). Glossitis may also be present. This stage is often mistaken for *Candida albicans* infection. The erythematous macules may become vesicular, spread peripherally and form collarette scale. Once again, the peripheral spread produces unique, intersecting bands of erythema, most often with crusts and scales, in contrast to the other figurate erythemas.

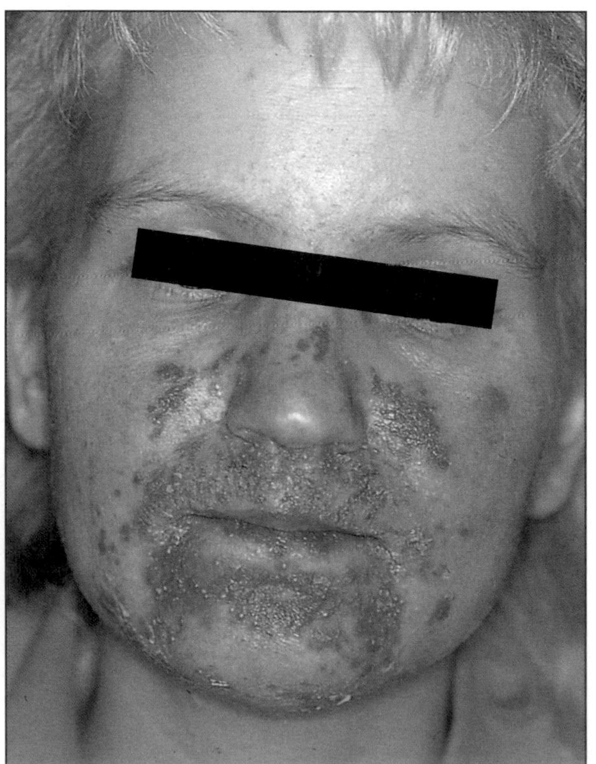

Fig. 14.4. Necrolytic migratory erythema

Histopathology. The epidermis is typically necrotic with reversal of staining (pale basal layer cells), dyskeratotic cells and acantholysis. Subcorneal pustule formation with neutrophils in the epidermis is identified. In older lesions, these changes are replaced by crust and scale. In the dermis there is a lymphohistiocytic perivascular infiltrate.

Laboratory Findings. The serum glucagon levels can be extremely high. Normal values are around 0.1 – 0.3 pg/ml, but patients have revealed values as high as 850 – 3000 pg/ml. In addition, the patients tend to have diabetes mellitus and anemia. An islet cell tumor can usually be identified by angiography, but clinical symptoms may appear while the tumor is still quite small and almost impossible to locate.

Differential Diagnosis. The combination of the rash and associated symptoms should suggest the diagnosis. The flexural involvement and crusting point away from the other figurate erythemas. Zinc deficiency may appear be quite similar, especially with inguinal and oral involvement. Hailey-Hailey disease also may have extensive groin erosions but the patients are in good health. Pustular psoriasis, subcorneal pustular dermatosis and pemphigus foliaceus should also be considered.

Course and Prognosis. Many patients can be cured by surgery. In those with inoperable or recurrent tumors, the disease progression is usually slow, so that 10 – 15-year survival is the rule. Following surgery, reappearance of the skin findings is a sensitive marker for tumor recurrence.

Therapy. If the tumor can be excised completely, then all symptoms including the necrolytic migratory erythema resolve. Those with multiple inoperable lesions are usually treated with streptozocin and sometimes 5-fluorouracil, which may decrease serum glucagon levels and produce improvement.

The cutaneous lesions are difficult to manage. Topical drying lotions, often with antibacterial substances added, seem to work best. Systemic corticosteroids have also been employed, but are difficult to use in patients with such abnormal glucose metabolism.

Multiforme and Nodose Erythemas

Erythema Multiforme

(HEBRA 1866)

Synonyms. Many complex names are no longer in use, but simply reflect the highly variable clinical nature of erythema multiforme; we will not inflict them upon the reader.

Definition. Acute heterogeneous allergic reaction with many possible triggering agents but characteristic symmetric target or iris lesions.

Etiology and Pathogenesis. There are many causes of erythema multiforme, but often one still fails to identify the specific trigger in a given patient. The most common causes are:

- Viral Infection. Oral herpes simplex virus often leads to erythema multiforme; genital herpes simplex virus is much less often associated. Typically the patient has had a cold sore on the lips 1–2 weeks before the erythema multiforme; the lip lesions may still be present. Recurrences are common. Other viruses have also been implicated but far less often. In the past, small pox vaccination was often involved.
- *Mycoplasma* Infection. Pulmonary mycoplasmal infections are more often associated with severe forms of erythema multiforme.
- Drugs. Common involved agents include sulfonamides, penicillins, tetracyclines, anticonvulsants (phenobarbital, phenytoin, carbamazepine), allopurinol, nonsteroidal antiinflammatory drugs and quinine derivatives.
- Streptococcal Infections. Occasionally erythema multiforme may appear several weeks after a streptococcal tonsillitis or pharyngitis.
- Miscellaneous. Other bacterial infections, deep fungal infections, malignant tumors and some autoimmune disorders (lupus erythematosus, Wegener granulomatosis, polyarteritis nodosa) also may be associated with erythema multiforme.

The pathogenesis of erythema multiforme has been best studied for the herpes simplex virus-associated form. Viral antigens and even DNA are present the dermis where they trigger a cell-mediated reaction. How this goes on to produce such symmetric lesions and also cause more widespread skin loss is unclear. In the case of the delayed appearance after streptococcal infection, a type IV reaction appears most likely. Others have suggested that the primary damage occurs in the epidermis and that the entire process is designed to eliminate epithelial antigens. Certain HLA associations have been described; they are not the ones typically associated with autoimmune diseases.

Clinical Findings. Erythema multiforme has been subdivided into several often overlapping forms. The key issues in classifying the disease are:

- Do different forms have different etiologies?
- Do different forms have better or worse outlooks?
- What is the significance of mucosal involvement?

While a number of groups have attempted to produce classification schemes, we have found the approaches of Revuz and his colleagues in Paris, as well as Schöpf and his colleagues in the German Center for Documenting Severe Skin Reactions, most useful. One can identify the following types of erythema multiforme and severe skin reactions (Table 14.2).

Minor Form. The minor, classic or Hebra form has symmetric target- or iris-shaped lesions almost invariably involving the hands, especially the dorsal aspects (Fig. 14.5). The typical lesion is initially an erythematous macule that enlarges and becomes annular. Within 1–2 days, the lesions are about 1 cm in size with a central area of hemorrhage, necrosis and blistering, surrounded by a pale cyanotic region and then enclosed by an erythematous peripheral band. This combination produces the classic, disease-defining target lesion. Lesions may coalesce, evolve into polycyclic patterns and show central healing. Sometimes the blisters dominate, so that erythema multiforme could also be considered under blistering diseases.

Mucosal involvement may occur but typically only the lips are involved. Often the patient has had a preceding herpes simplex virus infection so that the lip involvement is hard to assess. Trunk involvement is uncommon. The outlook in such cases is good. Healing is rapid but recurrences common.

Table 14.2. Classification of erythema multiforme and severe skin reactions

Type	Skin	Blisters (%)	Mucous membrane	Outlook	Recurrences	Cause
Minor	Acral target lesions	0	+/−	Excellent	Common	Herpes simplex virus
Major	Acral target lesions	<10	++	Good	Uncommon	Herpes simplex virus, mycoplasma
Stevens-Johnson syndrome (SJS)	Truncal erythematous macules	<10	++	Good	Uncommon	Drugs, herpes simplex virus, mycoplasma
SJS/TEN	Truncal erythematous macules	10–30	++	Fair	Rare	Drugs
Toxic epidermal necrolysis (TEN)	Truncal erythematous macules	>30	– (very rare)	Poor	Rare	Drugs

Most such cases are triggered by herpes simplex virus. A number of studies have identified herpes simplex virus markers in the skin in patients with idiopathic minor erythema multiforme and similarly antiviral therapy has ameliorated such problems, even in the absence of an obvious precursor lesion.

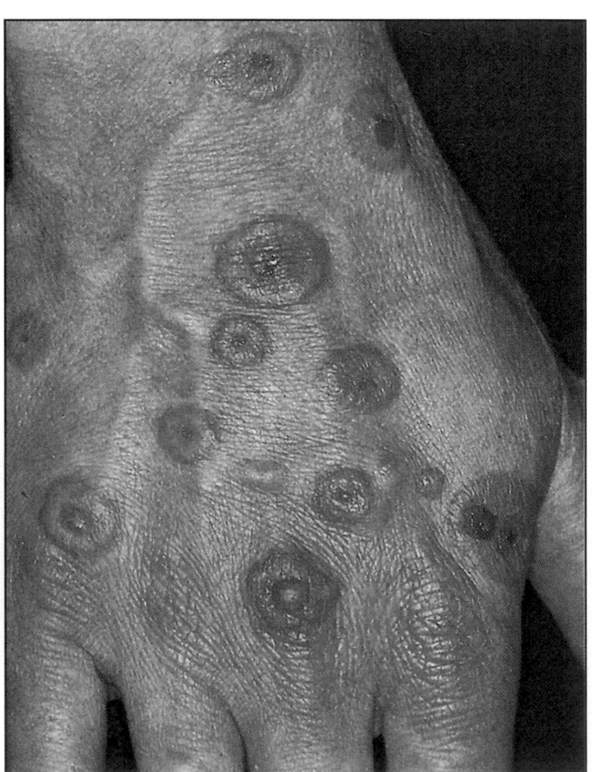

Fig. 14.5. Erythema multiforme

Major Form. Severe erythema multiforme is characterized by acral target lesions, but also by trunk involvement and blisters. The blisters are restricted to the center of target lesions and involve less than 10% of the body surface. All patients have mucosal involvement; the mouth, eyes and genital mucosa may be affected. Ocular involvement may produce scarring, while oral involvement can lead to nutritional difficulties. *Mycoplasma* and herpes simplex virus are the typical triggers. The prognosis is good and recurrences less common, since they are associated with herpes simplex virus.

Stevens-Johnson Syndrome. The skin lesions begin on the trunk as erythematous macules that coalesce. Target lesions may be seen but they are in the minority. Once again, blister formation does occur but is limited to less than 10% of the body surface. All patients have mucosal involvement. Drug reactions are the most likely trigger, but herpes simplex virus and *Mycoplasma* may rarely be involved, as well as other more uncommon infections.

Stevens-Johnson Syndrome/Toxic Epidermal Necrolysis Overlap. These patients typically have no target lesions, trunk involvement, involvement of 10–30% of the body surface with blisters and mucosal disease.

Toxic Epidermal Necrolysis. Such patients have greater than 30% body involvement with blisters, resulting in the loss of large sheets of skin which presents treatment problems identical to burn patients. They never start with target lesions, but

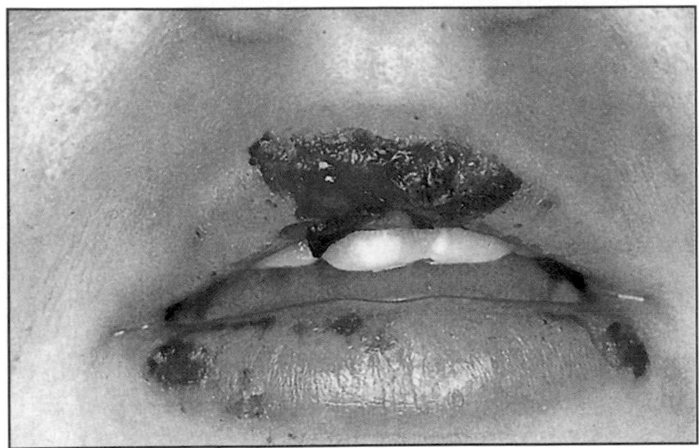

Fig. 14.6. Lip involvement in severe erythema multiforme

instead with erythematous macules on the trunk that rapidly spread and form blisters. Mucosal involvement is uncommon; when present, it is usually minimal. The risk of death is significant if the patients are not treated appropriately.

Toxic epidermal necrolysis and its overlap with Stevens-Johnson syndrome are discussed in more detail in Chapter 10.

The following additional clinical findings are also seen with erythema multiforme.

Mucosal Findings. Both severe erythema multiforme and Stevens-Johnson syndrome have mucosal involvement. The oral lesions most typically involve the lips, but may include the tongue, palate and buccal mucosa (Fig. 14.6). Typically large ulcers and erosions are seen, since the blisters are unstable. The lesions of intraoral herpes simplex virus are smaller and involve almost only the gingiva and lips. The ulcers may spread to the posterior oral cavity, pharynx, larynx and even lungs and esophagus. Genital involvement produces painful perianal, penile, scrotal and labial ulcers, while urethral involvement may lead to urinary retention.

Eye Findings. Many patients, perhaps as high as 90 %, have a mild conjunctivitis (Fig. 14.7). In some cases, it may be purulent. In the more severe forms, there are conjunctival blisters with symblepharon formation, corneal ulcers and iritis or uveitis. Permanent eye damage may result from the corneal lesions or the synechiae in about 10 % of patients with eye involvement. When patients have primarily oral and ocular involvement, the term Fuchs syndrome (Fuchs 1876) is employed. Such patients most often have herpes simplex virus as a trigger.

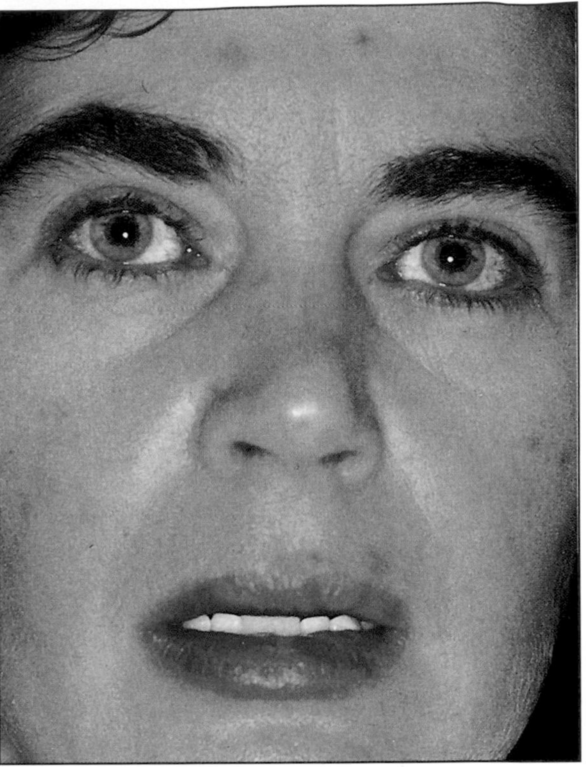

Fig. 14.7. Conjunctivitis with erythema multiforme (Fuchs syndrome)

Systemic Findings. Much has been made of the patient's general condition in classifying erythema multiforme. However, this aspect causes more confusion than clarity. There are several major variables. If infections are the suspected trigger, both the actions of the infectious agent and the antibiotics employed must be considered. If medications are suspected, both their profile and the complications of the underlying disease for which they were given confuse the picture. Patients with the minor form are generally well. All other patients tend to be ill with fever, arthralgias and myalgias. Those with oral involvement may have difficulty eating and drinking. The most feared complication is pulmonary disease, which can involve as many as 30 % of patients with major erythema multiforme and more advanced forms. Pneumonia commonly occurs and may lead to death. Other involvement, such as myocardial disease, renal failure, and gastrointestinal tract involvement is quite rare.

Histopathology. The histopathology provides one rationale for unifying such seemingly unrelated clinical findings. Initially there is a lymphocytic perivascular infiltrate with edema and mild exocytosis of red cells. Eosinophils are not preset. As the disease progresses, epidermal damage occurs. There is vacuolar degeneration of the basal layer and necrotic keratinocytes can be identified. In more severe cases, the entire epidermis may be necrotic. Subepidermal blisters result from the damage at the basement membrane zone. The presence of true vasculitis or neutrophils speaks against the diagnosis of erythema multiforme.

Immunofluorescent studies have not identified any disease-defining antibodies. C3 and IgM may be seen along the basement membrane zone and about the dermal vessels, but these findings are not specific.

Course and Prognosis. The outlook for minor or ordinary erythema multiforme is good. There is usually rapid resolution. In most instances herpes simplex is responsible and recurrences are likely. When other infections or drugs are responsible, the course is often stormier but the chance of recurrence far less.

Differential Diagnosis. The differential diagnosis is lengthy depending on the disease form. The approach to the more severe forms is explored in Chapter 10. The classic or minor form presents a wide differential diagnostic spectrum. Hand-foot-and-mouth disease typically has small oral ulcers without lip involvement and blisters on the hands, feet and buttocks that are not target-like. Leukocytoclastic vasculitis may present with acral erythematous lesions, but palpable purpura elsewhere and the lack of oral involvement help, as does a biopsy. Pemphigus vulgaris and bullous pemphigoid may both present with oral blisters and erythematous skin lesions. The clinical course and the histologic and immunofluorescent evaluation produce the answer. Dermatitis herpetiformis very rarely has acral and oral involvement.

Therapy

Systemic. The therapy of erythema multiforme depends heavily on the suspected trigger and the disease severity. No treatment is recommended after one episode. If the erythema multiforme is recurrent and extensive or persistent, herpes simplex is the usual trigger and treatment with acyclovir is an effective prophylaxis. One can either employ 200 mg five times daily for 5 days at the first sign of herpes simplex virus infection, or if this fails, use 200 mg twice or three times daily for long periods of time. One may treat for 1 year and see if recurrences have been aborted. The patient may wish to take a drug holiday after a year to see if the herpes simplex virus and erythema multiforme recur. If they do, the protocol appears safe for at least 5 years, if not longer. Patients with recurrent erythema multiforme without obvious signs of herpes simplex virus usually benefit as well from acyclovir prophylaxis, suggesting that they have subclinical herpes simplex virus triggering their erythema multiforme.

Once the erythema multiforme is in full swing, oral corticosteroids usually are effective in suppressing the disease manifestations. Doses of 60–100 mg prednisone daily tapered over a 3-week period are usually very helpful. However, there are some problems with corticosteroid use in erythema multiforme. They predispose the patient to additional infections and may lead to earlier recurrences of herpes simplex virus infections. The benefit of the agent in more severe disease forms, especially when administered later in the course, has not been documented and some studies have indicated a worsening. Many experts flatly state that systemic corticosteroids are inappropriate in toxic epidermal necrolysis. Ophthalmologists often recommend them to reduce ocular inflammation and retard scarring. Some prescribe systemic corticosteroids for severe drug reactions identified early in the disease course.

In contrast, everyone agrees that expert supportive care is the single most important factor in caring for the more severe forms. All the aspects of burn care, including infection prophylaxis, fluid restoration and wound care are essential. Consultation with ophthalmologists and internists is crucial towards obtaining the best outcome

Topical. Such measures are generally supportive and rarely dramatically effective. Early, noneroded target lesions can be treated with topical corticosteroid creams or lotions which seem to slow the disease progression. In most cases, erosions and crusts develop. They can be treated with wet soaks and then ointments, perhaps with antibacterial agents. In the flexural areas, drying measures are often helpful. Oral lesions may be treated with anesthetic gargles or rinses to make eating easier.

Acute Febrile Neutrophilic Dermatosis
(SWEET 1964)

Synonym. Sweet syndrome

Definition. Acute febrile illness with succulent erythematous lesions; often a marker for myeloproliferative disease.

Epidemiology. Most patients are middle-aged women with a 5:1 female to male ratio.

Etiology and Pathogenesis. Initially Sweet felt acute febrile neutrophilic dermatosis was an allergic reaction to an infectious agent. The disease may follow an acute respiratory infection, often with *Yersinia*. The histologic pattern is that of a vasculitis and immune complexes are occasionally identified. In the last decade it has become clear that many so-called idiopathic cases of Sweet syndrome represent early cases of leukemia.

Clinical Findings. The clinical findings are most impressive. The patient presents with fever, an elevated neutrophil count and succulent, tender dark red plaques and nodules (Fig. 14.8). The cutaneous findings can be somewhat variable ranging from the typical juicy plaques to erythematous patches to pustular lesions. Rarely bullous lesions are seen. The skin lesions usually heal uneventfully, but may last for many weeks if not treated.

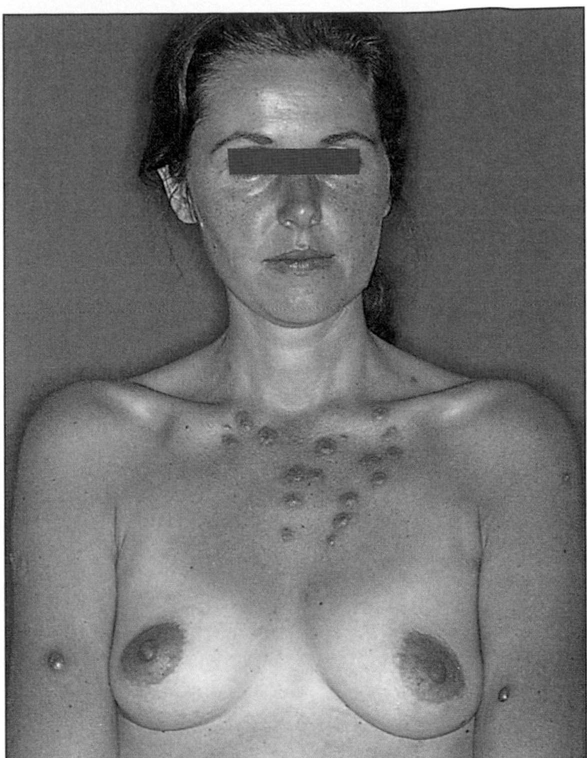

Fig. 14.8. Sweet syndrome

Histopathology. The chief finding is an intense dermal neutrophilic infiltrate, centered around vessels and often with nuclear dust. The upper dermis is edematous and the epidermis may show spongiosis and accumulations of neutrophils. Older lesions are dominated by lymphocytes. The vessel walls may be swollen, show fibrinoid degeneration reveal deposition of complement components and immunoglobulins with immunofluorescent staining.

Laboratory Findings. The erythrocyte sedimentation rate and the neutrophil count are elevated. The swing to the left may be dramatic with 70–90% neutrophils and a total leukocyte count of greater than 20,000/mm^3.

Differential Diagnosis. Erythema multiforme may appear similar, but typically has iris lesions and more acral involvement. In addition, the neutrophil count is not elevated and the biopsy lacks neutrophils. Erythema elevatum diutinum appears similar histologically but not clinically. Acute lupus erythematosus may present with infiltrated nodules; the serologic evaluation and histology should help differentiate. An overlap between Sweet syndrome and pyoderma gangrenosum is most often associated with myeloproliferative disorders, especially hairy cell leukemia. These patients have multiple superficial, often bullous lesions, and oral involvement may be seen, as well as neutrophilic infiltrates in internal organs. Finally, an evolving leukemia or malignant lymphoma may appear similar. Here the help of the hematopathologist is crucial.

Therapy

Systemic. The mainstay of therapy is systemic corticosteroids. One may start with 60 mg prednisone daily tapering over a 3-week period. Antipyretics should also be prescribed. Antibiotics are of no benefit. In nonresponsive or persistent cases, colchicine, dapsone or supersaturated potassium iodide can be tried.

Topical. Corticosteroid creams or lotions, as well as zinc shake lotions, can be tried for early lesions.

Erythematosquamous Diseases

Pityriasis Rosea
(Gibert 1860)

Definition. Acute, probably postinfectious dermatosis characterized by symmetric truncal lesions.

Epidemiology. Pityriasis rosea is a disease of adolescents and young adults. It tends to appear in cycles and is more common in the fall and winter months. It accounts for about 2% of dermatology outpatients. It is uncommon among siblings or other family members.

Etiology and Pathogenesis. Pityriasis rosea has long been assumed to represent a delayed reaction to a viral infection. The seasonal clustering and occasional occurrence among family members or classmates point in this direction. Clearly not all exposed individuals develop skin lesions. The most likely candidate at this writing is human herpes virus 7.

Clinical Findings. The clinical picture is quite distinct. Most patients can be diagnosed at a glance. The initial lesion, also known as the herald lesion or mother patch, is usually on the trunk. It is larger than the subsequent lesions, usually several centimeters in greatest diameter (Fig. 14.9). The lesion is initially red, but later pale pink with a collarette of scale that typically points centrally. The central part of the lesion is covered with fine scale and may appear atrophic or depressed. This initial lesion may be overlooked by the patient or diagnosed and treated as a dermatophyte infection.

Days to weeks later, the disease starts to spread, alarming the patient and usually prompting the first office visit. Many smaller oval scaly lesions are seen, often following the skin lines on the trunk, producing the so-called Christmas tree pattern. The trunk, abdomen and neck are the most frequent sites; the extremities and face are rarely involved. No mucosal lesions develop. The lesions typically do not itch or are only minimally symptomatic.

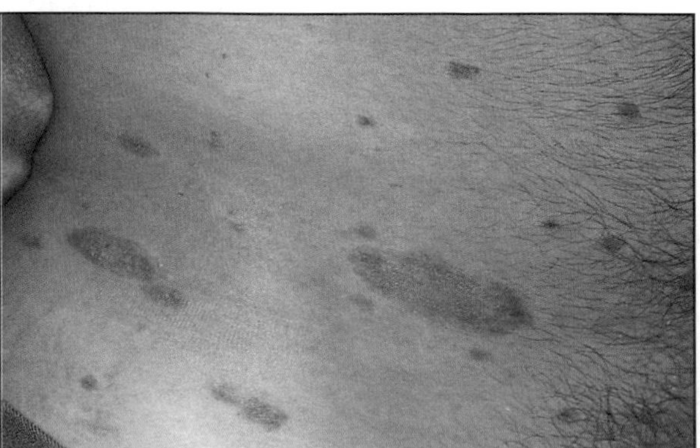

Fig. 14.9. Pityriasis rosea with large target lesion

The disease may take a slightly different course in black and Hispanic patients. Here the neck, face and distal aspects of the extremities are prominently involved; this pattern has been called inverse pityriasis rosea. The lesions tend to be much smaller, often appear to be follicular, typically are very pruritic and heal with significant postinflammatory hypopigmentation. In smaller children, lesions may have the same pattern but be more urticarial in nature. Other even less-common variants include hemorrhagic and vesicular forms.

Histopathology. The epidermis shows minimal, often focal, spongiosis and tiny parakeratotic accumulations or caps. In the dermis, there is a sparse perivascular infiltrate. Occasionally there is exocytosis of red cells.

Course and Prognosis. The disease persists for 3–6 weeks but may last for 3–4 months. Healing may occur with both postinflammatory hyperpigmentation and hypopigmentation. Recurrences are uncommon (approximately 1%).

Differential Diagnosis. Secondary syphilis can appear very similar; a serologic test for syphilis should be recommended to every pityriasis rosea patient. Tinea corporis can usually be excluded by the pattern, while the negative KOH examination is confirmatory. Early cases of psoriasis may appear similar, but should evolve differently. Petaloid seborrheic dermatitis has similar shaped scaly lesions, involving the neck, axillae and sternal region. Collarette scale is not seen. The disease is more chronic and usually there are other signs of seborrheic dermatitis present on the scalp or face. Drug eruptions may also mimic pityriasis rosea. The most classic agents are the gold salts, but captopril, isotretinoin, ketotifen and metronidazole have also been incriminated.

Therapy

Systemic. Antihistamines may be used for severe pruritus. Systemic corticosteroids are sometimes employed in black patients with severe disease and marked hypopigmentation, but their effect is minimal.

Topical. Patients should be encouraged not to wash frequently as this leads to dryness and secondary irritation. They should be encouraged to lubricate their skin well. A topical distracter may be added to whichever emollient cream or lotion the patient finds most acceptable. Topical corticosteroids are often prescribed. UVB radiation can be employed to help relieve pruritus.

One should be honest with the patient and explain that treatment will play little role in how rapidly their lesions disappear. Most patients are satisfied once they learn that the disease is harmless and self-limited, even though it looks so worrisome.

Pityriasis Rotunda

(Toyama 1906)

Pityriasis rotunda is an uncommon disorder in Western countries. Patients typically have multiple large scaly round or oval patches on their trunk or buttocks that become hyper- or hypopigmented. Most patients are Asian or black. In these groups, the lesions are usually less than 30 in number and generally hyperpigmented. There is no familial tendency and pityriasis rotunda may be a marker for an underlying malignancy or chronic illness. Occasionally it may evolve into mycosis fungoides. In whites, it is often familial, usually hypopigmented and not associated with underlying diseases. Familial cases have also been described in Asians. The microscopic picture is not helpful, usually showing modest hyperkeratosis and varying pigmentary changes. It seems that the familial cases may represent an uncommon form of congenital ichthyosis. In a parallel fashion, one could argue that the other form represents a variant of acquired ichthyosis which can also be a marker for systemic diseases. Early acquired cases must be separated from tinea corporis and large-patch parapsoriasis. Treatment is symptomatic with emollients. In some cases 10% urea creams used along with topical tretinoin have produced clearing.

Psoriasis

Definition. Inflammatory skin disease with increased epidermal proliferation usually characterized by erythematous lesions with silvery scale.

History. Psoriasis from the Greek word *psora* meaning scale has been known since antiquity. Robert Willan first described it more accurately at the beginning of the nineteenth century. He identified two separate types of psoriasis which von Hebra unified into a single disease.

Epidemiology. Psoriasis involves anywhere from 1–5% of the population, depending on what racial group is studied and how strict the diagnostic criteria are. In Western Europe psoriasis is about as common as diabetes mellitus. Psoriasis patients comprise about 6–8% of the patient load in a dermatology clinic. In the United States, it is striking how much less psoriasis, especially severe psoriasis, one sees in the southern part of the country as compared to the north, suggesting a possible role for light in controlling or suppressing the disease. Studies suggest that there is a hierarchy of susceptibility to psoriasis: white > Asian > black > Native American. We regard this finding skeptically. A classic paper states that Navajos do not get psoriasis, but one of us ran a clinic for Navajos for a decade and saw more than enough severe psoriasis, even in patients who were continually outdoors, such as shepherds.

Etiology and Pathogenesis. The cause of psoriasis remains elusive. But the search has yielded an enormous amount of information about cutaneous inflammation and epidermal cell kinetics, which has greatly expanded our knowledge of the skin and hopefully will pay rewards for the unfortunate patients with this disease. We will consider both the pathophysiologic basis of psoriasis and then the many predisposing factors.

A lesion of psoriasis is characterized by its sharp borders, erythema and increased scale. Thus the search for the etiology of psoriasis has concentrated on epidermal proliferation and differentiation, inflammatory changes and the dermal vasculature. Various research groups have claimed that each of these broad areas holds the answer, but at this time, there is no single concept that explains the many features of psoriasis. We will consider just some of the phenomena that have been explored, hoping to show both how complex psoriasis is and to perhaps give some clues as to the etiology.

Epidermal Turnover. The epidermis has a volume that is four to six times larger than normal skin from the same site. There are more keratinocytes and the individual cells are larger. Both DNA synthesis and mitotic rate are increased. The cell cycle is greatly speeded up. Basal cells in psoriasis turn

Table 14.3. Epidermal parameters in psoriasis

	Normal	Psoriasis
Mitoses	0.4%	2.5%
DNA synthesis	3–5%	20–25%
Cell cycle	457 h	37 h
Epidermal transit time	28 days	3–4 days
Cell metabolism	Normal	Markedly increased
Stratum corneum	Orthokeratotic	Hyperkeratotic, parakeratotic

over as fast as the rapidly growing cells of the small intestinal mucosa, dividing every 1.5 days. They also find their way to the stratum corneum more rapidly and are shed within 3–4 days (Table 14.3).

Epidermal Differentiation. The silvery scales are a quick indicator that the process of differentiation, which in the epidermis means formation of keratin, is disturbed. Histologically one sees an increased number of keratinocytes (hyperkeratosis) but with an abnormal stratum corneum containing cell nuclei (parakeratosis). The keratin proteins associated with differentiation (K5/14, K1/10) are reduced, while those associated with proliferation (K6/16) are increased. Electron microscopic evaluation shows reduced tonofilaments and abnormal desmosomes.

The cornified cell envelope also appears abnormal in psoriasis. This is an insoluble, very stable structure formed beneath the plasma membrane of differentiating keratinocytes. It consists of a variety of crosslinked proteins. Involucrin appears to be deposited first and then loricrin is attached. In psoriatic keratinocytes, the envelope is abnormal lacking the usual amounts of loricrin.

Initially abnormalities in cAMP/cGMP were held responsible for the increased turnover and decreased differentiation. In psoriatic keratinocytes cAMP is present in lower amounts, both because of reduced synthesis and increased degradation. This could explain the increased mitotic rate. Alterations in the arachidonic acid pathway have also intrigued investigators. Elevated levels of substances such as leukotriene (LT)B_4, 12-hydroxyeicosatetraenoic acid (HETE) or interleukin (IL)-8 could serve both as chemotactic agents for the invariably present inflammatory cells and as mitotic stimulators. Extracellular signals also play a major role, as keratinocytes in psoriatic skin express increased levels of epidermal growth factor (EGF) and transforming growth factor (TGF)-α. Unfortunately none of the epidermal changes is specific for psoriasis and it remains unclear what comes first.

Dermal Capillaries. The typical erythema and the punctate bleeding points of the Auspitz sign both indicate the presence of dilated vessels in psoriatic skin. The capillary loops are lengthened and more complex. In addition the capillaries and the postcapillary venules are more permeable, allowing leakage of cells and humoral factors into the dermis and eventually into the epidermis. Because of the elongated rete ridges and dermal papillae, the epidermis is far better served by vessels than that of normal skin. But there is little evidence that the capillary changes are the primary event.

Immunologic Effects. A variety of humoral changes have been demonstrated in psoriatic skin, although today more emphasis is placed on cellular changes. Psoriasis patients, especially those with severe and pustular disease, have elevated serum levels of IgA, and often IgG and even antinuclear antibodies. These antibodies can be shown in the stratum corneum, where they may stimulate complement and thus attract neutrophils.

Activated T cells in the psoriatic infiltrate emphasize the importance of cellular factors. The association with various HLA types, the effectiveness of cyclosporine and monoclonal CD4 antibodies that block T cells, and the ability of cytokines such as IL-2, interferon (IFN)-α and IFN-γ to induce psoriasis also support the role of T cells. T cell cytokines can also cause psoriatic-like changes in cultured keratinocytes.

An attractive theory to explain the triggering role of streptococcal infections in acute, eruptive or guttate psoriasis also involves T cells. Perhaps there are structural analogies between some streptococcal proteins and those expressed on keratinocytes. After a clone of T cells have been exposed to the correct streptococcal antigen, they may then be attracted to keratinocytes. This process could be HLA-limited, in that only certain HLA types are able to present the cross-reacting protein in such a way that it is recognized by the sensitized T cells. The T cell cytokines might then proceed to initiate the antiinflammatory response which is appropriately directed against bacteria, but becomes inappropriate when directed against keratinocytes.

Predisposing Factors. There are many factors that predispose a patient to psoriasis. Included are genetic factors, endogenous factors and a variety of exogenous triggers such as trauma, light and infections. The basic premises in explaining why some people get psoriasis are:

- There is a population of individuals who are genetically predisposed to psoriasis.
- Some or many of these individuals are exposed to the appropriate trigger and develop clinical psoriasis.

The two most promising lines of evidence for the genetic nature of psoriasis are family studies and HLA studies. The risk of psoriasis for a child with no family history of psoriasis is 1–2%. When one parent has psoriasis, the risk increases to 10–20%, while when both are affected, it is as high as 50%. Monozygotic twins show a 90% concordance for psoriasis. These numbers are typical for a polygenic or multifactorial pattern of inheritance. In addition, age at onset of disease appears to play an important role. Although no age group is spared from psoriasis, most cases begin either in adolescence or in the fifth decade. Siblings of patients with early onset psoriasis are at greater risk of developing the disease than siblings of those with later onset. There are conflicting data over severity of disease and age of onset; some studies suggest that early onset correlates with more severe disease.

The HLA picture in psoriasis is somewhat befuddling. Hundreds of HLA antigens have been studied in many psoriatic populations, producing a morass of data. In general, HLA-A2, -B13, -B17, -B27, -Bw57, -Cw2, -Cw6 and -DR7 have been most often identified as present in higher proportions in psoriasis patients. By combining age of onset and HLA pattern, one can identify two subtypes of common psoriasis.

- Type I: (early onset) <40 years of age; HLA-Cw6, -B57 and -DR7 over-represented; extended haplotypes EH57.1 and EH65.1 also increased; familial inheritance. Disease susceptibility genes appear present on chromosomes 4, q6p, 16, q17q and 20p; other linkage sites have also been suggested.
- Type II (late onset): >40 years of age; weaker HLA associations; no familial increased risk; greater likelihood of joint and nail involvement. The most common association is HLA-Cw2.

Other types of psoriasis may show other patterns. Psoriatic arthritis is associated with HLA-B27, along with Reiter syndrome and other seronegative arthropathies. Erythrodermic psoriasis is associated with B13 and B17, supporting the concept that it is a variant of ordinary psoriasis, not a separate disorder. Guttate psoriasis is most often associated with Cw6, while pustular psoriasis may be associated with B17 and B27 but is less-often familial. In addition, HLA types may help explain the geographic differences mentioned above. Many of the predisposing types are extremely uncommon in Native Americans or Eskimos. Cw6 conveys a higher risk in Asians, but the gene is less common. In Japanese, Cw7 and Cw11 are also increased in frequency. It has been suggested that Cw6 is the closest we have to a psoriasis gene and that many of the other associations can be explained by linkage to Cw6. In addition, Cw6 is more common in Northern Europeans than in blacks or Asians, following the trends for psoriasis.

A patient who is genetically predisposed to psoriasis may present in two ways:

- Genotypic or latent psoriasis: Normal skin and no way to diagnosis the disease in the laboratory
- Clinical psoriasis: Skin, nail or joint disease

Thus, treatment of psoriasis cannot provide a cure, in that the patient is returned to the latent or subclinical state.

Provocation Factors. Many different factors can trigger the eruption of psoriasis moving the patient in the wrong direction from latent to clinical disease (Fig. 14.10). These factors can be exogenous or endogenous. Trauma is probably the most important. It can be viewed as an intriguing experimental problem, a treatment method or a disturbing clinical phenomenon. Köbner described the latter. He noticed that trauma to normal skin in psoriasis patients often results days later in new psoriatic lesions. When the stratum corneum is removed from normal skin of a psoriasis patient, for example by tape stripping, about 10 days later typical psoriatic changes may occur (Fig. 14.11). It appears that epidermal damage and regeneration is the key; strictly dermal changes are not enough. It also appears that psoriasis patients go through cycles of increased and decreased susceptibility to the Köbner phenomenon. Reports in the literature describe surgical tangential excision of chronic stable psoriatic patches with good results.

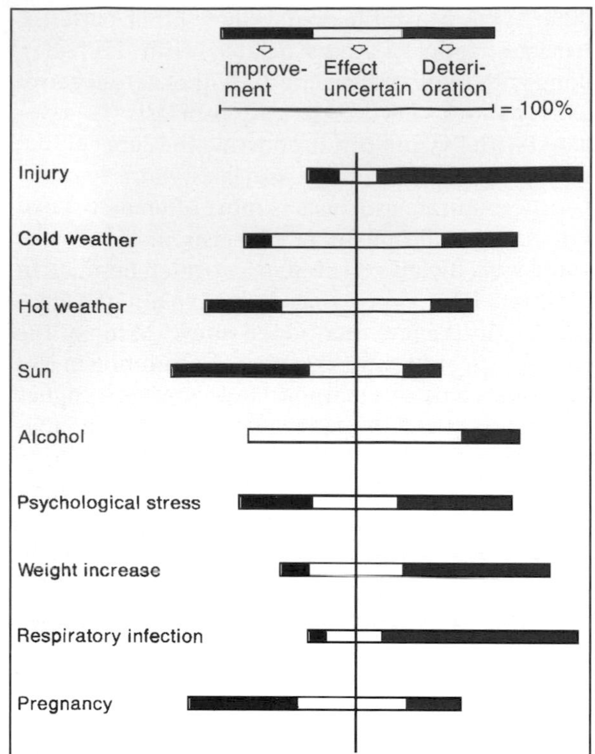

Fig. 14.10. Effects of endogenous and exogenous factors on psoriasis

Exogenous Provocation. There are many possible ways to trigger psoriasis. The risk depends on the stage of the patient's psoriasis. A patient with flaring disease is at far greater risk than a patient with stable disease and a few plaques on the knees and elbows. Factors include:

- Physical factors: Radiation (UV, X-ray), dermabrasion, other surgery, intradermal or subcutaneous injections, tattoos, vaccinations, insect bites, burns, scalds, abrasions, and even leech therapy or acupuncture
- Chemical factors: Chemical burns, other toxic exposures, chronic irritant dermatitis, even some topical psoriasis treatments
- Inflammatory dermatoses: Many other skin diseases, such as varicella zoster virus infections, pityriasis rosea, allergic contact dermatitis, or even positive prick, scratch or patch tests

One should thus be careful in treating acute psoriasis, perhaps using lower dosages of UV radiation and avoiding irritating chemicals. Similarly, when psoriasis flares in a localized region, such as the groin, one should search for a localized trigger such as a dermatophyte infection.

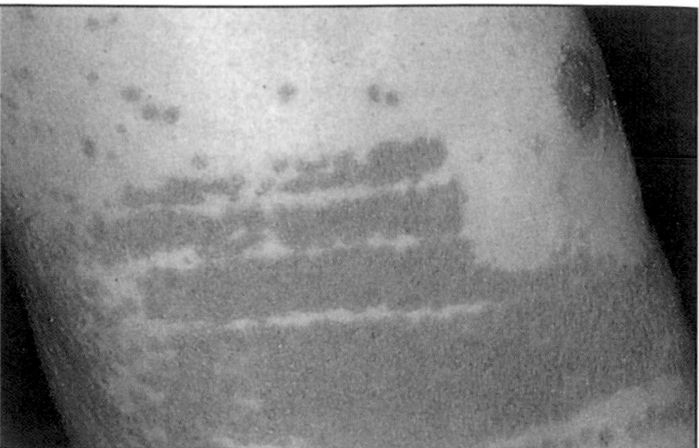

Fig. 14.11. Köbner phenomenon in psoriasis following removal of adhesive bandage

Endogenous Provocation. A number of endogenous factors also appear important:

- Infections. Most young patients with their first phenotypic expression of psoriasis experience an antecedent streptococcal throat infection. Often the initial clinical expression is guttate psoriasis. Later in life subsequent psoriatic flares are also often triggered by streptococcal pharyngitis.
  HIV/AIDS can lead to the onset or worsening of psoriasis. Roughly 5% of HIV/AIDS patients suffer from psoriasis. About one-third of HIV/AIDS patients with psoriasis experience a flare of existing disease and offer a family history of disease; the remainder develop psoriasis for the first time and often in atypical patterns or with arthritis. Typically these patients are affected after about 5 years as their cell-mediated immunity begins to drop, supporting the role of T cells in the disease process.
- Medications. Following reports of psoriatic flares during World War II when US troops in the Pacific were given antimalarials, the rule has been "No antimalarials for psoriasis or psoriatic arthritis". While later studies have shown that the risk is not great, we have seen severe reactions among vacationers. Beta-blockers, lithium, ACE-inhibitors, nonsteroidal antiinflammatory drugs and cimetidine have also been incriminated. In addition, a variety of biologic agents such as certain interferons, interleukins and GM-CSF often trigger psoriasis. Patients with psoriasis who are treated with systemic corticosteroids may flare when the medication is stopped. Pustular psoriasis may develop in this setting.
- Pregnancy and delivery
- Diet, alcohol and perhaps cigarette smoking

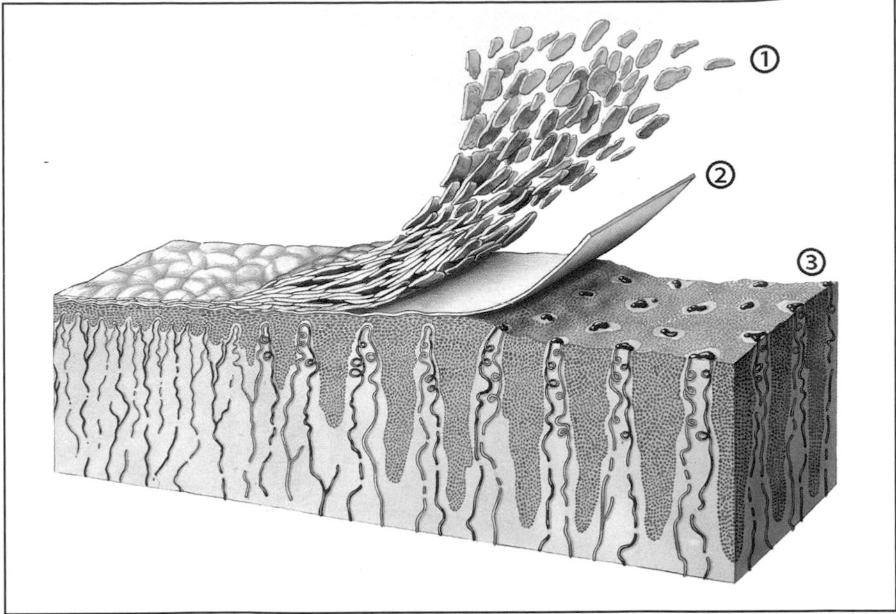

Fig. 14.12. Cross section of a lesion of psoriasis showing the clinical phenomenon of (1) candle sign, (2) last piece of skin and (3) Auspitz sign

- Hypocalcemia in renal dialysis patients or other settings
- Stress. Neural peptides and their receptors are elevated in psoriatic skin, supporting what patients have known for a long time – severe stress is a common trigger of psoriatic flares.

Clinical Findings. The clinical features of the individual lesion in psoriasis are monotonous. In contrast, the degree of involvement and localization vary greatly from patient to patient creating diagnostic difficulties. The primary lesion in psoriasis is erythematous and scaly. Initially a small red, inflamed sharply bordered macules appears, and is soon covered with silvery scale. Such lesions can appear anywhere. In more vascular areas, they can be more violet colored and be surrounded by a white area of vasoconstriction, known as a Woronoff ring. Three time-honored clinical features help confirm the diagnosis, but none is totally specific for psoriasis (Fig. 14.12). Before performing the tests, HIV/AIDS and syphilis should be excluded.

- Candle sign. When the scales are scratched away from the lesion, they fall off as tiny flakes that resemble scrapings from a candle.
- Sign of the Last *Häutchen* (last little piece of skin). If all the scale is removed, a moist, thin, translucent layer of skin covering the lesion is revealed. The lesion remains dry until this last level is reached.
- Auspitz Sign. If this last layer is removed, exposing the dermal papillae, punctate bleeding from the enlarged capillaries occurs (Fig. 14.13).

The clinical features of psoriasis varying greatly from patient to patient. The disease may explode suddenly in one patient, and remain fixed and chronic in the next. Signs of regression may be associated with the eruption of new areas. The eruptive lesions may be intensely pruritic, mildly so, or asymptomatic. The following factors help explain the different morphologic patterns.

Size of the Lesion. All lesions begin as small scaling macules but they may then take divergent paths as

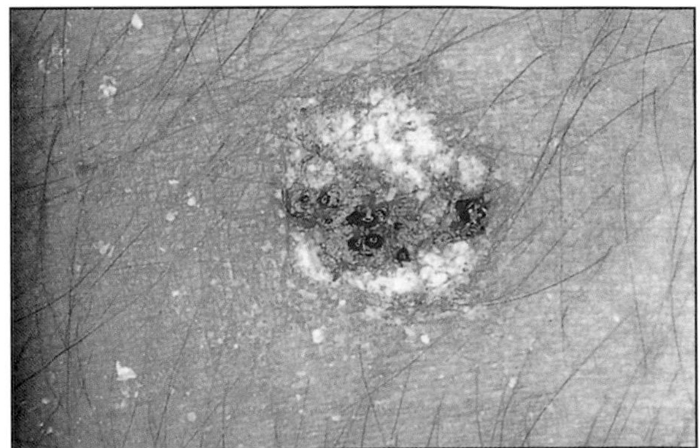

Fig. 14.13. Auspitz sign

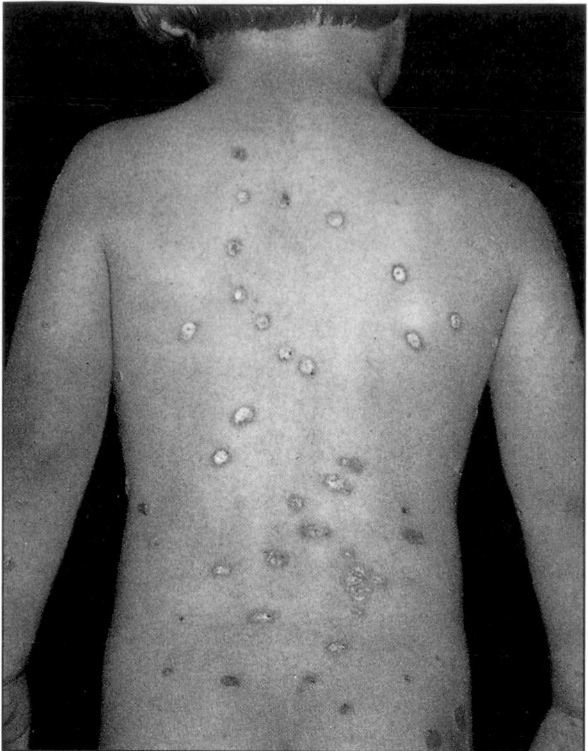

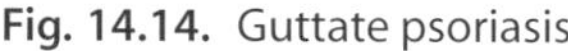

Fig. 14.14. Guttate psoriasis

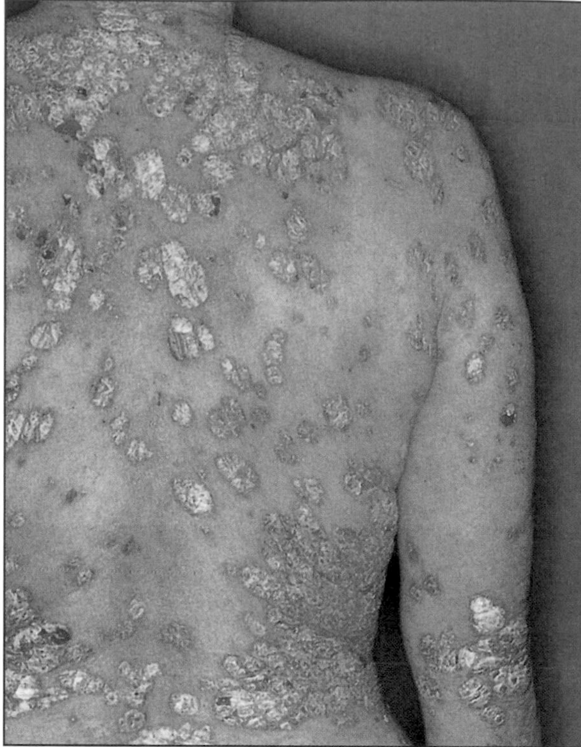

Fig. 14.15. Nummular psoriasis

they spread centrifugally. The following patterns are seen:

- Guttate Psoriasis. Lesions appear suddenly, are small or punctate, and have minimal scale. This variant is seen most often in children following streptococcal infections (Fig. 14.14), and may often heal with complete resolution after several months.
- Follicular Psoriasis. Uncommonly the punctate lesions are localized to the follicular orifices, especially on the trunk. The small often smooth lesions may mimic lichen planus (lichenoid psoriasis). When the lesion is scraped, its squamous nature is revealed.
- Nummular Psoriasis. In this most-common form, plaques several centimeters in diameter develop especially over the knees, elbows, buttocks, trunk and scalp (Fig. 14.15). Sometimes large plaques are seen simultaneously with new guttate lesions. (Fig. 14.16)
- Geographic Psoriasis. When many lesion coalesce, then very large plaques appear creating a pattern that fancifully resembles a map.
- Erythrodermic Psoriasis. Virtually the entire body is one large psoriatic patch. The patient has

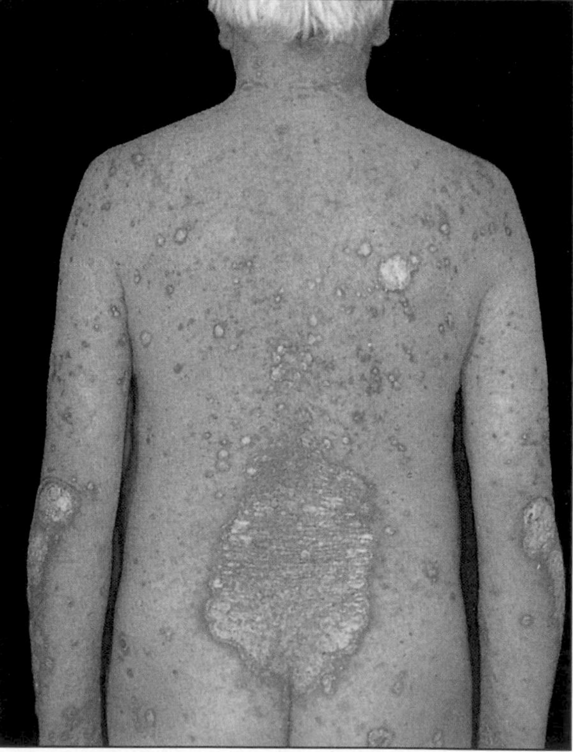

Fig. 14.16. Plaque psoriasis with scattered guttate lesions

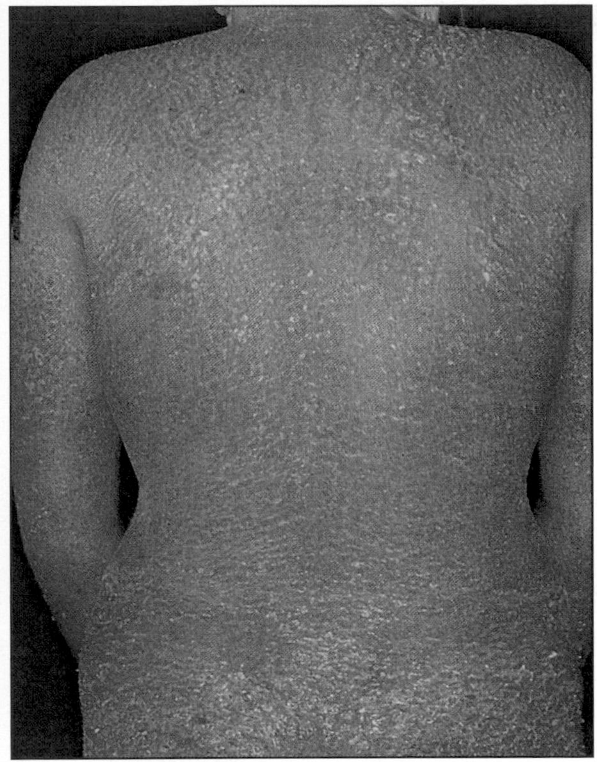

Fig. 14.17. Erythrodermic psoriasis

a dusky red color as the typical psoriatic scales give way to larger coherent sheets of stratum corneum or fine scale (Fig. 14.17).

Configuration. The combination of peripheral spread and central resolution produces complex patterns, such as:

- Annular Psoriasis. A peripheral ring of disease is present, surrounding an area of clearing.
- Gyrate Psoriasis. Intersecting annular lesions produce a more complex gyrate pattern (Fig. 14.18).
- Serpiginous Psoriasis. Occasionally long 1–2-cm wide curved plagues are left behind.

Sites of Predilection. Psoriasis has several favored locations. The classic sites of the knees and elbows are perhaps explained by trauma, as is nail disease (Fig. 14.19). The gluteal cleft disease may be triggered by sweating and sitting. The scalp is also a common location, although an easy explanation is not apparent. When obvious endogenous triggers are present, as in poststreptococcal guttate psoriasis, then the disease is disseminated. When the diagnosis of psoriasis is being considered, one should always examine the scalp, nails, knees, elbows and gluteal cleft.

Special Localization. Psoriasis may appear quite differently in different regions of the body.

- Scalp. This is an extremely common site for psoriasis. Typically the hair line (especially frontal) and the temporal regions are involved. The lesions usually spread to involve 1–2 cm of the adjacent skin (Fig. 14.20). If the patient has oily hair, the typical scale may be absent. If a patient has only scalp involvement, it is difficult both clinically and histologically to distinguish between psoriasis and seborrheic dermatitis. Hair loss is unusual in psoriasis. Patients with psoriatic erythroderma or severe pustular psoriasis may experience anagen effluvium, and any psoriasis patient may go through telogen effluvium following a flare of their disease. In rare cases, localized scalp involvement may be associated with hair loss, which in extremely rare cases has been documented as scarring alopecia.

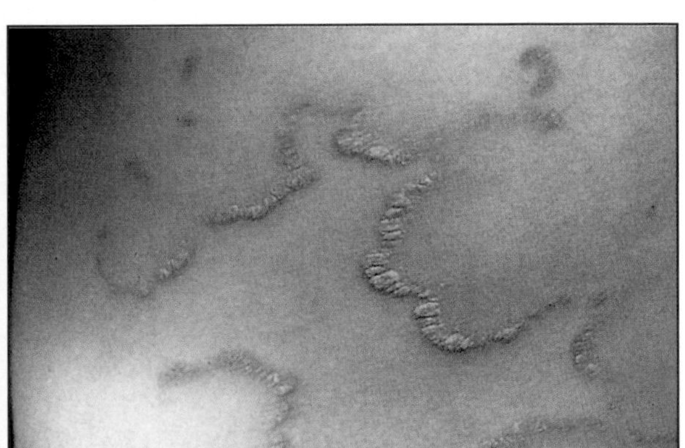

Fig. 14.18. Gyrate psoriasis

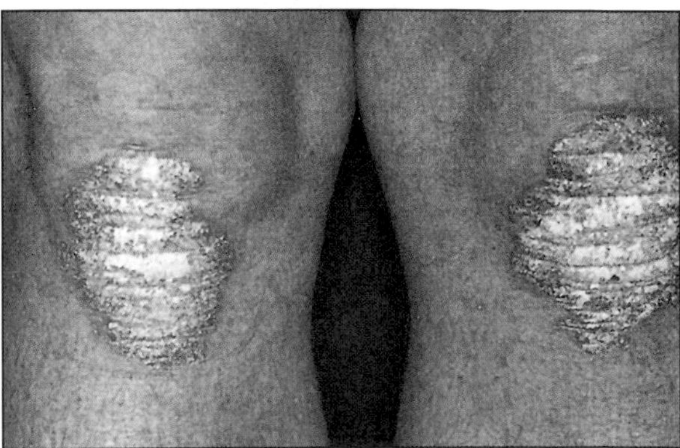

Fig. 14.19. Localized psoriasis

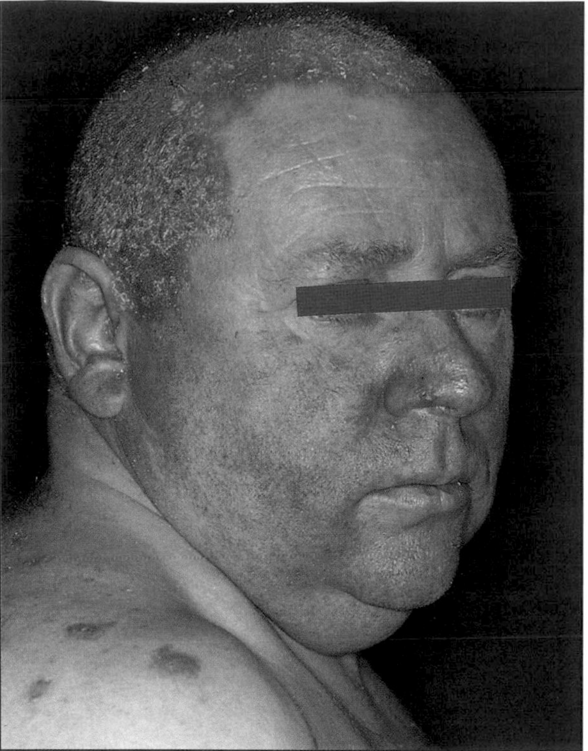

Fig. 14.20. Scalp psoriasis

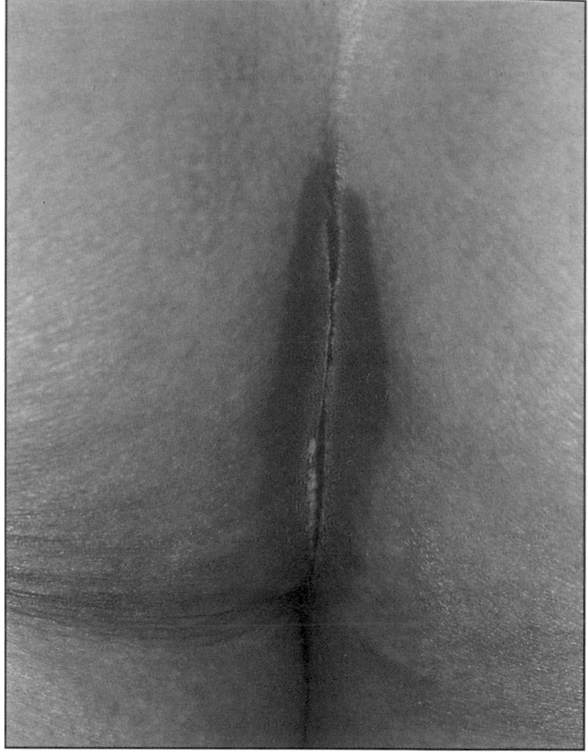

Fig. 14.21. Gluteal cleft erythema in psoriasis

- Intertriginous Regions. Psoriasis has a predilection for warm moist areas, such as the gluteal cleft, groin, axillae, umbilicus and beneath the breasts. The combination of the local traumatic factors, perhaps coupled with dermatophyte or *Candida albicans* infections, serves to trigger the psoriasis. In these areas, the scales are usually absent, so one sees an erythematous infiltrated plaque that is often pruritic. When only the flexural areas are involved, the term inverse psoriasis is employed. About 5% of patients have only inverse psoriasis, while perhaps 30% have involvement in this region as well as on other body parts. Behind the ears, psoriasis and seborrheic dermatitis are identical; often the patient suspects allergic contact dermatitis to eyeglass frames.
- Perianal Region. In the perianal area, psoriasis is usually pruritic. The lesions are typically sharply bordered, extend to the gluteal cleft and often have a midline fissure (Fig. 14.21). The sacral region is a another site of chronic stable psoriasis where it may be mistaken for chronic dermatitis, such as lichen simplex chronicus (Fig. 14.22). The lesions may occasionally be extremely thick (inveterate psoriasis) or warty (verrucous psoriasis).
- Penis. The penis may be the initial site of psoriasis in a fair percentage of young patients; in rare cases, it may be the only site. Penile psoriasis tends to be less scaly and present as a red infiltrated plaque with a varnished surface (Fig. 14.23). It must be distinguished from lichen planus, Zoon balanitis, Bowen disease, Bowenoid papulosis and candidiasis.
- Palms and Soles. At these sites psoriatic lesions are usually red, symmetric, sharply bordered

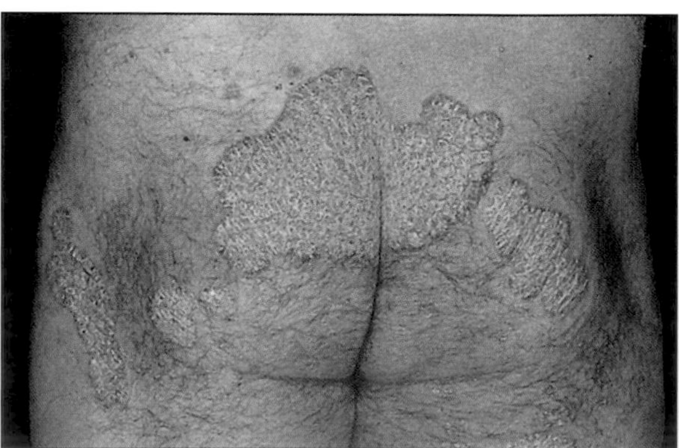

Fig. 14.22. Sacral plaque psoriasis

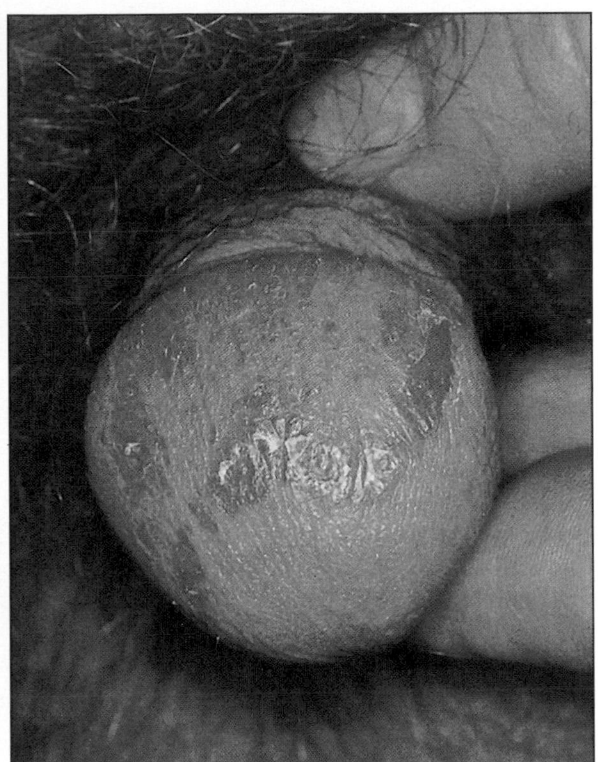

Fig. 14.23. Penile psoriasis

plaques with very adherent yellow scale and frequently with painful fissures (Fig. 14.24). Both chronic dermatophyte infections (such as *Trichophyton rubrum*) and chronic dermatitis appear similar. Occasionally psoriasis may be present between the toes (white psoriasis) where it is easily mistaken for tinea pedis; KOH examination is decisive. Reiter syndrome is very similar. Secondary syphilis and lichen planus should also be excluded.

Nail Involvement. About 30–50% of psoriasis patients have nail involvement; the numbers are even higher in those with psoriatic arthritis. Nail involvement is often an important diagnostic clue, usually involving multiple nails in a relatively symmetric fashion. All three anatomic parts of the nail unit, the matrix, nailbed and paronychium, may be affected.

When the matrix is involved, the most typical sign is pitting. Tiny areas of psoriasis in the matrix produce focal poorly compacted areas of parakeratosis in the nail. These concretions fall out, yielding a tiny pit. While most individuals occasionally have a nail pit, in psoriasis there may be large numbers involving many nails (Fig. 14.25). While alopecia areata patients may also have nail pits, the individual lesions are usually smaller and fewer in number. With more severe matrix disease, the nail may develop ridges and depressions.

The most reliable sign of nailbed disease is the oil spot, a small spot of psoriasis beneath the nail that shimmers through like a drop of oil with a yellow-brown color (Fig. 14.26). As the nail grows out, it is lifted away from the nailbed by the parakeratotic material, producing a white distal onycholysis. The crumbly material appears beneath the distal portion of the nail, where the patient typically scrapes it away with a nail file. The onycholysis can be quite severe, so that the nails are only loosely attached covering massive subungual debris.

In many patients there is involvement of both the matrix and nailbed, producing strikingly dystrophic crumbly nails (Fig. 14.27). The main differential diagnostic point is tinea unguium; the latter is asymetrical, involves fewer nails and may be associated with dermatophyte infections elsewhere. KOH examination and culture are needed to

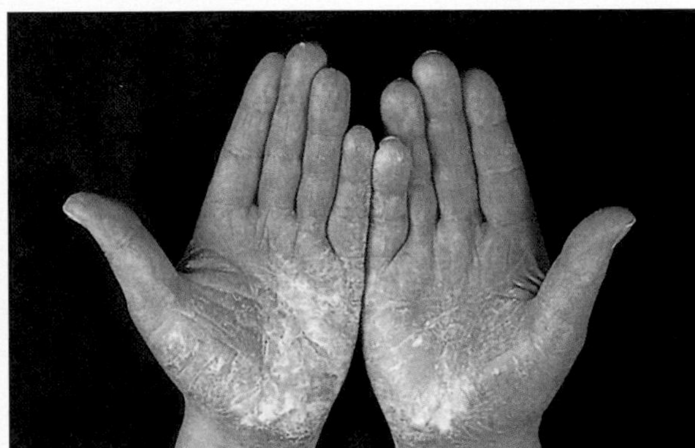

Fig. 14.24. Palmar psoriasis

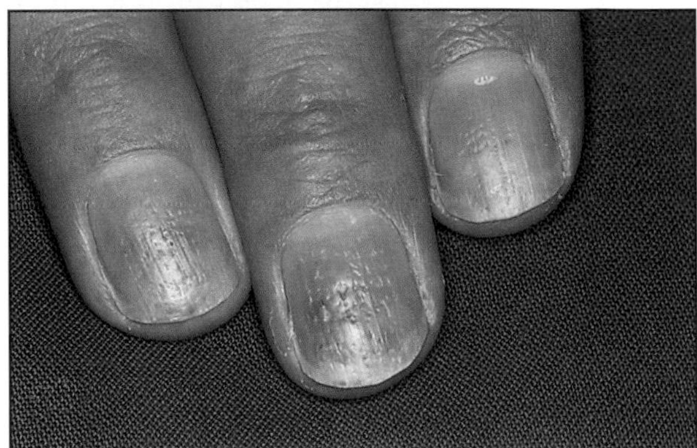

Fig. 14.25. Psoriatic nail involvement with pitting, onycholysis and oil spots

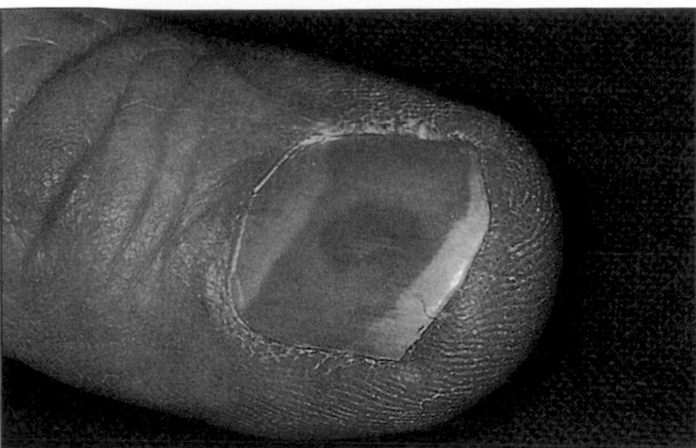

Fig. 14.26. Oil spot in psoriasis

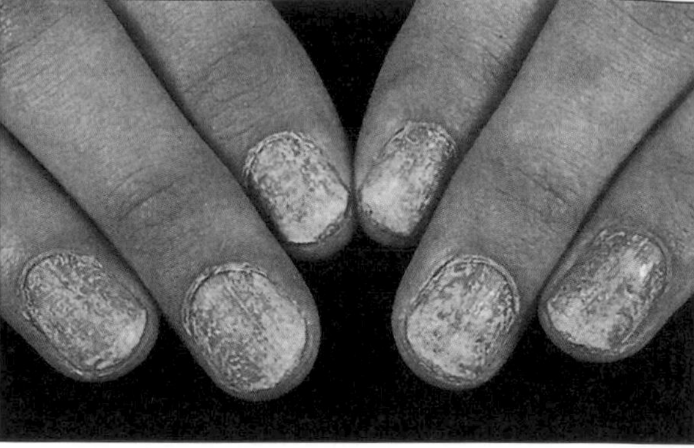

Fig. 14.27. Marked nail dystrophy in psoriasis

make the final diagnosis. Psoriasis and dermatophytes may occur simultaneously in the same nail.

Psoriasis also typically involves the tissues about the nail, producing quite striking paronychia. The cuticle is absent and there is swelling and erythema involving the entire nailfold and adjacent tissues (Fig. 14.28). Such changes are quite painful. They are almost always associated with significant nail dystrophy. The differential diagnosis includes bacterial and herpetic nailfold infections.

Mucosal Disease. Psoriatic disease in the mouth is most uncommon. Rare patients have pustular lesions on their lips, while still fewer with widespread, often pustular, psoriasis develop white, boggy, intraoral plaques with superficial pustules. Geographic tongue or benign migratory glossitis is a common condition that probably has no connection with psoriasis. The much rarer nontongue equivalent, known as migratory stomatitis, may represent intraoral psoriasis (Chap. 33).

Internal Manifestations. Except for psoriatic arthritis, which is discussed in detail below, psoriasis has surprisingly few internal manifestations. Despite the massive alterations in cutaneous status, there are no characteristic metabolic abnormalities. Uric acid levels may be elevated, but this is secondary to the rapid turnover of epidermal cells. In addition, very severe or erythrodermic psoriasis may be associated with an enteropathy, perhaps because of the massive protein loss. This phenomenon is not unique to psoriasis but is also seen with other types of widespread skin disease. The question of psoriasis and liver disease is frequently raised because of the hepatotoxic effects of methotrexate. While liver function test abnormalities may be more common in psoriasis, unfortunately so is alcohol abuse and that may be the explanation. Obesity appears to increase the likelihood of psoriasis manifesting itself. During World War I and World War II when there were multiple opportunities for under-nutrition and frank starvation in Europe, psoriasis became much less common. No characteristic lipoprotein abnormalities have been identified and low-fat diets have not proven their worth. Finally, psoriasis has been linked with diabetes mellitus, but both diseases are quite common and obesity may provide a link. Suffice it to say, “Psoriasis does not protect one from other common diseases.”

Symptoms. Psoriasis patients with any significant amount of involvement find their disease an emotional burden. Those of us without psoriasis are often cruel to its victims. A sense of repulsion as

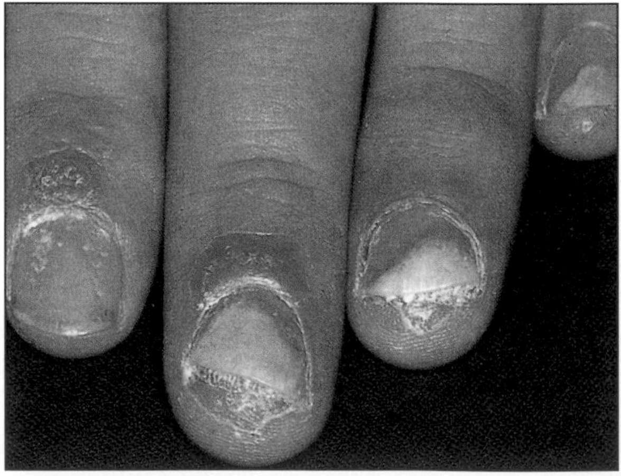

Fig. 14.28. Psoriatic nail involvement with onycholysis, crumbling and paronychia

someone sheds scales all over the floor or offers a hand with crumbly discolored nails is all too common. We tell our patients to seek sun and water, but they are turned away from swimming pools or spas and are too embarrassed to show themselves at the beach. Or we recommend applying an ointment to the entire body two or three times daily. Every young physician should be forced to undergo a topical psoriasis treatment regimen for a weekend to appreciate the practical difficulties. There is no wonder that patients are so eager for "clean" treatments such as methotrexate or PUVA, and so eager to flock where other psoriasis patients gather, such as at the Dead Sea.

Course. Psoriasis takes a highly variable course, depending on many factors such as age, localization and hopefully treatment. Sometimes individual lesions persist for years, in other cases new lesions replace older, regressing ones, and in rare cases, the patient remains clear for long periods of time. One can divide the natural history of psoriasis into three groups:

- Eruptive or Guttate Psoriasis. Patients are usually young, rapidly develop widespread disease, are pruritic and tend to display the Köbner phenomenon. The typical presentation is guttate psoriasis following streptococcal infection. On the positive side, the disease in these patients sometimes resolves entirely for many years. They should be treated with relatively mild measures because harsh treatments can elicit more psoriasis.
- Chronic, Stable Psoriasis. Here the typical scaly silvery plaques are found on the knees, elbows, gluteal cleft, trunk and scalp. Pruritus is uncommon and the Köbner phenomenon is rarely a problem. Individual lesions may resolve as new ones come. Such patients usually benefit from intensive local therapy.
- Unstable, Exudative Psoriasis. Such individuals tend to have more intense inflammation, less scale and more pruritus. While they may begin with typical small guttate lesions, they rapidly develop larger scales often with crusts. In a sense, they are a disaster waiting to happen, likely to evolve into psoriatic erythroderma or generalized pustular psoriasis. Of course, most patients during their lifetime fall into several of these categories, as switches frequently occur.

Clinical Scoring. Critical evaluation of therapeutic regimens requires a system of disease evaluation that is reproducible between different evaluators. We favor the Psoriasis Area and Severity Index (PASI). It allows a complex and detailed assessment that is particularly useful in inpatient settings and for pharmaceutical studies. The area of erythema, induration and desquamation is scored in four anatomic sites – head, arms, trunk and legs. The maximum score is 72 which represents severe, almost complete erythroderma.

Histopathology. Just as the clinical features are highly variable in psoriasis, so are the histologic findings. It is not surprising that a 3-mm red patch of guttate psoriasis has little in common with a thick plaque on the trunk present for years. The histologic changes help to explain the varying clinical picture. Any early macule has a modest lymphocytic perivascular infiltrate and more prominent vessels. Soon extravasation of erythrocytes occurs and mild epidermal hyperplasia is found. The scaly papules show mounds of parakeratosis, some epidermal hyperplasia, prominent mitoses in the lower levels of the epidermis, and the characteristic infiltration of neutrophils. Neutrophils typically wander through the epidermis to wind up in the stratum corneum. A small collection of neutrophils within this horny layer associated with parakeratosis is known as a Munro microabscess. When an accumulation of neutrophils is surrounded by a collar of necrotic epidermal cells whose cell walls are intact, thus resembling a sponge, one speaks of a spongiform pustule of Kogoj.

The fully developed scaly silvery plaque has the classic histologic features that are called psoriasiform, including uniform elongation of the rete ridges, a thinned suprapapillary plate, mounds of parakeratosis and more accumulations of neutrophils. There is exocytosis of erythrocytes and lymphocytes from the dilated and tortuous papillary vessels, producing the so-called squirting papillae. Resolving lesions begin to show fibrosis, fewer neutrophils, more compact parakeratosis and a gradual return of the normal epidermal architecture.

Differential Diagnosis. The differential diagnosis of typical psoriasis is limited. Usually a quick glance at the patient, often with a thorough examination of the typical predilection sites, provides the answer. Guttate psoriasis can be confused initially with pityriasis lichenoides et varioliformis acuta, pityriasis rosea and secondary syphilis. In addition, sometimes pityriasis rubra pilaris in its early stages can be hard to separate from psoriasis. In intertriginous areas, psoriasis must be distinguished from candidiasis, intertrigo and Hailey-Hailey disease. Scalp, face and chest involvement is similar to that in seborrheic dermatitis. Some view the two diseases as part of a spectrum, although we believe they are usually distinct. Chronic truncal lesions must be separated from nummular dermatitis, and small-plaque parapsoriasis, as well as tinea corporis. Nail psoriasis must be differentiated from tinea unguium. In almost all cases, examination of the classic predilection sites, as well as histopathologic evaluation, allow psoriasis to be diagnosed with certainty. The problem with psoriasis is rarely diagnosis or differential diagnosis; it is treatment.

Therapy

The treatment of psoriasis is both an art and a science. One has a variety of both topical and systemic measures available to remove scale, to reduce epidermal turnover and improve differentiation, to inhibit inflammation and to influence the complex immunologic reactions of psoriasis. While one can treat psoriasis, one cannot reverse the genetic predisposition to the disorder, so no patient is ever cured and relapses are the rule, not the exception. In addition, since the causes of psoriasis remain unclear, all therapy is empirical. Probably the most important aspect of psoriatic therapy is for the physician to enlist the aid of the patient and always be sensitive to the patient's needs. For example, it is much easier to ask a patient with a long history of psoriasis "Do you do better with a cream or ointment?" and then act accordingly, rather than to rely on one's extensive theoretical education to choose a product. But many doctors simply fail to take on the psoriasis patient as an equal partner in the treatment process.

Prophylaxis

Truly effective prophylaxis of psoriasis is not possible. Probably the best advice is to choose one's parents carefully. Patients with psoriasis would be well-advised to not marry partners with the disorder, for this greatly increases the risk for their children. However, often two psoriasis patients meet, perhaps visiting a psoriasis spa such as the Dead Sea, find that they finally have someone who understands their problem and wind up together. Genetic counseling for psoriasis is pretty much out of the question, because of the vast numbers of psoriasis patients and the few genetic counselors.

Another aspect of psoriasis is avoiding triggering factors. Patients with documented psoriasis or children of parent(s) with the disorder should have all possible streptococcal infections thoroughly investigated and aggressively treated. In addition, they should avoid medications known to trigger psoriasis, control their weight and avoid stress. Unfortunately the latter is easy to say and difficult to accomplish. Moderate exposure to sun and water appears helpful, while sunburn can elicit a flare. Specific topical prophylactic measures have not been proven effective.

Topical Therapy

Topical treatment of psoriasis is quick, safe and localized; it offers advantages over systemic therapy. One must pay careful attention to how reactive the patient is. A flaring patient must be treated relatively mildly, while a patient with stable disease can be approached more aggressively. The patient too must be aware that any topical treatment will require at least several weeks to show effects. Antipsoriatic medicines include a number of agents that are felt to be antiproliferative. Two of the agents, anthralin and tar, are messy, staining both patients and their environment. For this reason, they have traditionally been used for inpatient therapy regimens. As hospitalization becomes less financially acceptable, there has been a shift towards day care centers and also away from messy regimens. While corticosteroids and calcipotriol have thus won in favor, the real winners have been new forms of phototherapy, often combined with bath and/or psoralen therapy.

Keratolytics. Removal of scales is a key step in all topical psoriasis therapy, since the thick scales hamper the ability of all more active medications to reach metabolically active levels of the skin. The keratolytic mainstay is salicylic acid, which may be incorporated in creams or ointments in concentrations of 3–6% or used ready-mixed with propylene glycol in a 6% solution (Keralyt in the USA). Higher concentrations can be used on the palms and soles, while tinctures or more-readily washable mixtures are available for the scalp. Many medicated shampoos contain salicylic acid, but it is unclear how much effect it has during the brief exposure during washing. When the skin is damaged or wide areas are treated, especially in children, enough salicylic acid can be absorbed to cause salicylism.

Baths also play a role in removing psoriatic scale. Patients have traditionally soaked prior to receiving UV radiation therapy. Tar solutions may be added, as well as bath oils, but in recent years, salt solutions have become very popular in Germany. While ordinary industrial sodium chloride can be used at concentrations in the range 5–10%, companies have achieved financial and perhaps also medical success by reproducing the mineral content of Dead Sea water. Such high salt concentrations may damage tubs and plumbing, so the patient should be warned.

Anthralin. Known as both anthralin and dithranol, 1,8-dihydroxy-9-anthrone was introduced into dermatology in 1916 by Unna and Galewsky. Initially a closely related product, chrysarobin, from the bark of the South American araroba tree was employed, but the German drive to synthesize essential chemicals during World War I produced the synthetic replacement, which today is used almost exclusively. It has been shown to have a long list of possible actions, including interfering with DNA synthesis, creating free radicals in mitochondria, interfering with epidermal growth factor, and blocking prostaglandin activity. It is unclear which of these theoretical actions is clinically most important.

What is clear about anthralin is that it is capable of irritating the skin and staining the skin, clothes and sheets. When anthralin is ideally employed, it creates a mild erythema. In German, one says "The psoriasis is burned away in the fire of the anthralin". Great care should be taken to avoid too high a concentration or to treat a patient with flaring skin and produce irritation. Salicylic acid (0.5–1.0%) is added to anthralin as an antioxidant and preservative, but not for its keratolytic action. It is also a potential cause of irritation. If the skin does become too irritated, one must discontinue treatment for several days.

Anthralin was initially mixed in a paste formulation; today it is available in a variety of creams and ointments. In the US, Drithocream (0.1%, 0.25%, 0.5% and 1.0%, HP) as well as Dritho-Scalp (0.25%, 0.5%) are available. The ready-mixed products are much easier to use and stain less than the compounded formulations, which include anthralin 0.1–4.0% in petrolatum with 1% salicylic acid (Ingram) or anthralin 0.1–2.0% with 2% salicylic acid in zinc paste (Farber). Anthralin is also available in a micronized crystalline form, which is more stable and stainless.

The trick is to start with a low concentration and slowly work upwards, observing for mild erythema of adjoining skin and clinical effectiveness. While anthralin can be used alone for limited chronic disease, it is most often combined with baths and UV radiation. Typically, following a morning bath, the patient receives radiation (either UVB, selective UVB, or even combined UVB-UVA) and finally anthralin is applied. Today in North America, almost all anthralin therapy is the so-called minute therapy. The anthralin is applied in higher concentrations, working up to the 1.0% Drithrocream, which is comparable to a 3–4% mixed ointment, which is left on for periods of 30–60 min once or twice daily. It is then removed by bathing and the skin treated with an ointment or cream base. Minute therapy can also be easily combined with UV radiation. Another approach is to use topical corticosteroids during the day and anthralin overnight.

In acute or eruptive psoriasis, we may use anthralin pastes may be used, usually at a relatively low concentration, in combination with UV radiation. In more chronic disease, either pastes or ointments can be used and a higher concentration is tolerated. A patient with just a few stable plaques, such as on the knees and elbows, can use topical corticosteroids and anthralin at home effectively.

Tars. While tars formerly formed a major part of the topical therapeutic armamentarium of dermatologists, today they are much less popular. Concerns about carcinogenicity have led to the almost complete elimination of tars in Germany. Different federal agencies have taken different stances on this issue, so the availability and use of tar may vary geographically. In addition, many studies have shown that other methods of therapy are superior to tars in treating psoriasis.

Nonetheless tars are an integral part of dermatologic history and worthy of mention. Initially tars were obtained as a byproduct of petroleum distillation or from natural sources such as juniper, birch or pine trees. In his memoirs, Marion B. Sulzberger, MD, describes as a young resident fetching large barrels of tar from the city gas works in Zürich for use in Jadassohn's clinic. Tars contain aromatic polycyclic molecules, benzpyrenes, which are carcinogenic in laboratory animals. Ichthyol, a tar-like product from shale, has very few of these molecules. The carcinogenic activity of tar is difficult to assess. The first example of chemical carcinogenesis was the identification of scrotal cancers in chimney sweeps, as described by Sir Percival Pott. Patients with psoriasis have had the most extensive exposure to tars, but are also usually treated with UV radiation and other potential carcinogens.

Tars have been credited with many different mechanisms of action. While they sensitize the skin for phototherapy, as a monotherapy they do not show substantial benefits. Traditionally tars were used as a 1–5% mixture of crude coal tar in petrolatum or a 5–10% mixture of liquor carbonis detergens (LCD) in petrolatum. Later a number of more cosmetically acceptable products, including tar gels and creams, were developed. Tars are also available in a wide range of shampoos and bath oils; even these products now require a prescription in Germany although most feel that the short time of skin contact reduces any possible risk.

Almost all tars are used in combination therapy regimens. The classic Goeckerman regimen, developed at the Mayo Clinic over 70 years ago, included topical tars, baths and UV radiation. Today, highly modified regimens usually involve the same three components. Typically, the patient applies tar in the evening, removes it with mineral oil in the morning, bathes and then receives UV radiation. Following the treatment tar is once again applied. The Goeckerman regimen is no more effective than UV radiation alone, and we no longer employ it (Chap. 70).

Corticosteroids. Topical corticosteroids provide a rapid elegant way to control localized psoriasis. For this reason, they are loved by patients. The ultra-high-potency preparations, or mid- to high-potency products under occlusion, quickly reduce inflammation and induce regression of lesions. But the remissions induced by topical corticosteroids are typically shorter than those from anthralin or tar. In addition, lesions treated with corticosteroids are then less responsive to other methods. Finally, local side effects such as atrophy, striae, purpura, hypertrichosis, telangiectases and perioral dermatitis are possible, and less often with widespread disease sufficient absorption may occur to produce systemic effects. In addition, there may be a rebound flare or pustular reaction when corticosteroids are discontinued. While products with a better risk:benefit ratio continue to be developed, the side effects of corticosteroids will remain a part of long-term topical psoriasis therapy.

There are some body regions where corticosteroids remain the simplest approach. On the scalp, either corticosteroid lotions or tinctures are most cosmetically elegant. They can be combined with tar products for overnight use, or corticosteroid creams can be left on overnight and washed out in the morning. Another useful approach is to apply a keratolytic cream or lotion for several hours or overnight, wash the scalp, and then use a corticosteroid lotion. Facial lesions are best treated with low-potency corticosteroid creams. The dose must be kept as low as possible to avoid perioral dermatitis and other acneiform reactions. The newer products with a better safety profile such as mometasone or prednicarbate have proven especially useful in this setting. In intertriginous regions, either nonfluorinated products or low-potency fluorinated pastes are most effective.

Chronic lesions on the extremities or trunk can be treated with high-potency corticosteroids. Often they are combined with tar or anthralin, and in such combinations are applied overnight, often with plastic foil occlusion. In the morning the other product is used, followed where possible by phototherapy. In addition, tape impregnated with corticosteroid (Cordran tape in the USA) is helpful for solitary resistant lesions.

Corticosteroids are the mainstay of treating nail psoriasis. Ultra-high-potency products are applied under occlusion. In many cases, atrophy intervenes before a desired effect is achieved. Topical 5-fluorouracil cream can also be applied to the nailfold. Radiation therapy (3 × 1 Gy at weekly intervals) is extremely effective but fraught with problems. In the long term, controlling nail psoriasis is a matter of luck.

Vitamin D Analogues. Calcipotriol and tacalcitol are two vitamin D analogues that enhance the differentiation and reduce the proliferation of various cells including keratinocytes. They interact with keratinocyte vitamin D receptors like the natural product but have much less effect on renal and gut calcium metabolism. In addition, they appear to modulate lymphocyte function. They are roughly as effective as a mid- to high-potency corticosteroid in reducing erythema, scale and thickness of lesions. Ointments, creams and lotions are available but are very expensive, so they lend themselves only to treating small chronic lesions. Calcipotriol is used twice daily, while tacalcitol can be applied once daily. If less than 100 g are used weekly (a level few patients can afford to exceed), systemic effects are nonexistent. Early in the course of therapy, calcium levels can be checked, but it is not usually necessary. Topical irritation is the main side effect. Both can be combined effectively with phototherapy especially 311 nm UVB irradiation or other modalities, especially topical corticosteroids.

Retinoids. Tretinoin was initially tried in psoriasis because of its apparent peeling or keratolytic action in acne. The peeling is an irritant reaction not well suited to psoriasis patients. Since retinoids influence cell differentiation, a search for other agents effective in psoriasis was undertaken. Tazarotene, a third generation retinoid, available as a 0.01% gel, appears to be effective for mild to moderate psoriasis. Best results are seen when it is combined with UV radiation or topical corticosteroids.

Phototherapy

Most patients observe that their psoriasis improves during the summer with exposure to sunlight, often coupled with salt-water exposure at the seashore or perhaps less filtered light in the mountains. UV radiation appears to inhibit DNA synthesis, to influence the epidermal cytokine system and to modulate the antigen-processing cells. There are many ways today to obtain these benefits.

Natural Sunlight. Patients may travel to special clinics on the sea shore, such as the North and Baltic Seas in Germany or the Mediterranean beaches, where they can combine salt-water and sun exposure. Another possibility is to go to mountain resorts where more intense sun exposure is available. Finally, at the Dead Sea in Israel, not only is a very concentrated (28%) salt-water present, but also the level of UVA in the natural sunlight is much higher, because the site is over 390 m below sea level. The concentrated salt solutions seem to help loosen scale and may also deactivate epidermal cytokines. Some European patients spend 4–6 weeks at the Dead Sea and experience good results with relatively sustained remissions.

UVB Phototherapy. Of course, not every patient can travel to a spa for natural phototherapy, so many artificial units have been developed (Chaps. 13, 70). Psoriasis has been the stimulus for almost all of the advances in phototherapy, although a much larger spectrum of diseases is treated. Traditionally psoriasis was treated with UVB radiation, usually combined with tar (Goeckerman) or anthralin (Ingram). Today it can also be combined with retinoids or vitamin D analogues. Traditional UVB lamps cover the spectrum between 280 and 320 nm. Special lamps with both UVB and UVA peaking at 305 and 325 nm are widely used in Europe; they are known as SUP (selective ultraviolet phototherapy) lamps. The most effective part of the UVB spectrum against psoriasis is between 304 and 314 nm. A special narrow-spectrum light source with a maximum emission at 311 nm (Philips TL01) is even more effective. All three of these light sources are useful in treating psoriasis. The trick in each case is to identify the minimal erythema dosage, begin at or just below this level, and gradually increase exposure, avoiding sunburn.

Photochemotherapy (PUVA). While UVA light alone has little influence on psoriasis, it becomes a most effective treatment when combined with psoralens. The introduction of psoralens plus UVA (PUVA) in the mid 1970s represents one of the great advances in dermatologic therapy. Psoralens are furocoumarins, photosensitizers found in many plants. The ancient Egyptians recognized their photosensitizing properties and they were reintroduced into dermatology by el-Mofty in the 1950s for treating vitiligo. Psoralen molecules intercalate between strands of DNA, and when they are exposed to UVA, they form adducts with the DNA and thus interfere with cell proliferation. Initially it was felt they inhibited keratinocyte proliferation, but today PUVA therapy is viewed as more immunomodulatory.

Psoralens can be used systemically, topically or as bath therapy, in each instance combined with UVA. In the USA, two products are available. 8-methoxypsoralen (8-MOP, Oxsoralen) is used for psoriasis while trioxsalen (Trisoralen) is used primarily in vitiligo patients. Other psoralens such as 5-MOP are available in other parts of the world.

- Systemic PUVA. 8-MOP is taken internally prior to exposure to UVA. Both crystalline and liquid 8-MOP products are available in different countries. The usual dosage is 0.6–0.8 mg/kg. The liquid form is absorbed more rapidly and therefore taken 1.5 h before exposure, while the crystalline form is taken 2 h before exposure. Psoralen absorption is variable from patient to patient. The dosage range for the crystalline product is shown in Table 14.4.
  The advantages of oral psoralens include convenience. The patient is relieved of many of the messy topical treatments and baths, so the acceptance is high. In addition, PUVA is very effective and works rapidly. The disadvantages are considerable. The patient is made photosensitive and must avoid sun exposure for 24 h, use sunscreens and wear special sunglasses that screen UVA to reduce the risk of cataracts. Liver function tests should also be monitored. Failure to follow such instructions may lead to severe

Table 14.4. Dosage of 8-MOP in PUVA therapy

Body weight (kg)	8-MOP dose (mg)
<50	20
50–65	30
65–80	40
80–90	50
>90	60

phototoxic reactions, as may errors in either the radiation time or the dosage. Many patients also experience gastrointestinal distress or pruritus. Finally, some patients develop acral blisters. The mechanism is unknown but is invariably interpreted by the patient or lawyer as a phototoxic reaction.

There are also chronic side effects from PUVA. There is also an increased risk of squamous cell carcinoma, especially scrotal cancers, as well as increased skin aging and development of PUVA lentigenes. There may also be an increased risk of malignant melanoma. European studies show much less evidence of carcinogenesis than American studies, perhaps reflecting the high-dose short-term European approach as compared to the lower-dose long-term therapy popular in the USA. The risk of skin cancers is much higher in patients with a past history of treatment with arsenic, X-rays, methotrexate, cyclosporine or other immunosuppressive agents.

- PUVA Bath Therapy. This ingenious technique has all the advantages of topical therapy, but none of the disadvantages, since extremely low amounts of psoralens are applied via a bath prior to light therapy. Concentrations of 0.5–1.0 mg/l are used. A commercial solution (Meladinine) is available in Europe to serve as a stock solution. The patient bathes for 20 min in a 150-l bath at 37 °C and is then immediately irradiated. The photosensitivity resolves in about 20 min. Localized areas, such as the palms and soles, can also be treated by having the patient soak their extremities in the same fashion. Toxic reactions are most uncommon and results promising. In addition, PUVA bath therapy is also effective in many other disorders such as vitiligo, graft versus host disease, lichen planus and morphea.

Radiation Therapy

We no longer use this modality for psoriasis. X-rays work well for psoriasis. They were employed for nail disease as well as for chronic stable plaques on the knees and elbows. A typical regimen was 1.0–1.5 Gy weekly for 3 weeks. Unfortunately, patients tended to abuse the modality. After one physician had delivered the maximum total dose (perhaps 12 Gy or three or four rounds of therapy), the patient simply sought out another physician, denied having received radiation therapy and got additional treatment. Years later, many psoriasis patients apparently treated correctly with radiation therapy developed squamous cell carcinomas on their distal digits, knees or elbows.

Systemic Therapy

Systemic. Systemic treatment is very attractive to patients, just as radiation therapy is, because it avoids at least some of the messy topical regimens. A systemic therapy should not be considered efficacious unless more than 25% of patients benefit from it as monotherapy, for the spontaneous remission rate in psoriasis is relatively high, perhaps 15–25%.

Corticosteroids. While systemic corticosteroids work in psoriasis, they are rarely employed for skin disease alone. Occasionally they are the only modality capable of braking rampant psoriatic arthritis but usually alternatives exist. The problem with corticosteroids is twofold. There is a long list of systemic side effects, and since psoriasis is a chronic disease, all can be expected to occasionally appear. When systemic corticosteroids are discontinued, psoriasis almost always flares, sometimes with life-threatening pustular flares. Perhaps the best indication for systemic corticosteroids today is during the induction phase of PUVA in a patient with severe psoriasis, generalized pustular psoriasis or psoriatic erythroderma, and in this setting they may be combined with retinoids.

Cytostatic agents. A number of cytostatic agents have been tried in psoriasis, but methotrexate and to a lesser extent hydroxyurea are the only two still employed routinely. The initial idea was that cytostatic agents kill the rapidly dividing epidermal cells and shut off psoriasis. While their effects are dramatic, they probably modulate immune cells and thus cytokines far more than directly stopping epidermal cell growth. The main indication for cytostatic therapy is a patient with widespread or severe disease who has failed to respond to PUVA or cannot use PUVA (pruritus, lives too far from medical resources, must be outdoors). Severe disease includes psoriatic erythroderma, generalized or debilitating localized pustular psoriasis, psoriatic arthritis not responsive to conventional therapy, extensive large-plaque disease unresponsive to other measures and psoriasis that limits a patient's ability to earn a living. Sometimes too there are psychosocial reasons, as some patients simply demand a pill. It is good advice to force such patients to exhaust the safer treatment modalities at the risk of losing them to an unlucky colleague. The most important factor is to strive for marked improvement with a low dose, rather than total clearing with a higher, more dangerous dose.

- Methotrexate. The folic acid antagonist methotrexate is close to the ideal pill for psoriasis. It is relatively effective, helpful against psoriatic arthritis (approved in the USA for rheumatoid arthritis), can be used weekly, and is helpful in dosages with good safety profiles. On the other hand, one of the main causes for medical malpractice suits against dermatologists is adverse reactions to methotrexate, primarily hepatic. Thus one must carefully observe the contraindications as approved by the Food and Drug Administration and modified by Roenigk and colleagues; they are listed in Table 14.5.

  Methotrexate inhibits the enzyme dihydrofolate reductase. It has 10^5 times greater affinity for the enzyme than the natural substrate dihydrofolic acid. Thus the formation of tetrahydrofolic acid is blocked, leading to inhibition of purine synthesis. In addition, the further metabolism of tetrahydrofolic acid by thymidylate synthetase is partially inhibited. Leucovorin or citrovorum (N^5-formyl-tetrahydrofolic acid) or thymidine can reverse methotrexate toxicity by bypassing these blockage points. Methotrexate is usually administered orally and well absorbed, although it can be given intramuscularly or intravenously. It is excreted unchanged through the kidneys, but also metabolized in the liver to polyglutamated forms that are also potent.

  Methotrexate is rarely administered on a continuous basis. Instead it is given as pulse therapy. Some physicians place great faith in 25–50 mg (rarely 75 mg) intramuscularly or intravenously as a bolus, given every 10–14 days. Others give an oral dose of 15–25 mg in the same way. But probably 90% of physicians prefer the intermittent therapy, as popularized by Weinstein. In his regimen, methotrexate is given once weekly in three divided doses 12 h apart. This approach seems to maximize the antipsoriatic effect and reduce the side effects. Previously 20–50 mg in three divided dosages was used, pushing for total clearance, but almost always encountering hematologic and stomatologic problems. Today, following the plan of the rheumatologists, most dermatologists use 7.5–22.5 mg weekly, that is three doses of 2.5–7.5 mg every 12 h. Rheumatrex, the standard methotrexate package for rheumatoid arthritis in the USA, provides for weekly doses of from 5 to 15 mg. With lower dosages, one can achieve partial clearing, perhaps 75%, with almost no toxicity. The patient can then treat remaining lesions topically.

  The patient must be carefully monitored during therapy. While very complex recommendations are available, there are varying opinions. The one main rule is keep good records. The patient should sign an informed consent. We recommend devising a special methotrexate form that can be placed in a patient's records where the signed consent and also the results of laboratory evaluations can be tracked. Initially, the CBC and platelet count should be checked every 2 weeks, then later every 4 weeks. In addition, hepatic and renal function must be monitored. A baseline chest X-ray is needed, as well as repeat evaluation every 18–24 months because of the risk of pulmonary fibrosis.

  The real problem is how to follow hepatic disease. Methotrexate can induce hepatic fibrosis or even cirrhosis prior to causing diagnostic alter-

Table 14.5. Contraindications for methotrexate use in psoriasis

Childhood
Renal disease
Hepatic disease (including history thereof)
Pregnancy or nursing
Desire for children (contraception for both men and women during and for 3 months after therapy; many choose not to treat patients of child-bearing age)
HIV/AIDS or other immunodeficiency
Chronic infections
Gastric or duodenal ulcer
Anemia, thrombocytopenia or leukopenia
Drug or alcohol abuse or unwillingness to give up alcohol intake
Lack of cooperation from patient

ations in liver function tests. Thus, laboratory tests are not always sufficient, and unfortunately this is also the legal opinion in many jurisdictions. However, the exact protocol to follow is also unclear. Most agree that if the total dose of methotrexate does not exceed 1.5 g (that is, 15 mg/week for 2 years or 7.5 mg/week for 4 years) a liver biopsy is not needed. Once this level is reached, assuming the first biopsy is acceptable, it should be repeated each time the next 1.0–1.5 g has been administered. If the patient's history or initial laboratory evaluation suggests liver disease, then a pretreatment biopsy is appropriate. Serum levels of the amino-terminal propeptide of type III procollagen may be a sensitive way to monitor fibrosis. Various hepatic imaging techniques also show promise.

The acute side-effects of methotrexate are highly dose-dependent. Rapidly growing tissues, such as the oral mucosa (erosions), gastrointestinal tract (diarrhea, bleeding, ulcers), bone marrow (thrombocytopenia, leukopenia, anemia) and skin (anagen effluvium), are most often affected. With a marked overdose, the psoriatic plaques may become ulcerated. Often this toxic effect produces long-term improvement as a minor compensation. Occasionally, through medical or patient error, methotrexate overdosage occurs. In such instances, leucovorin can be administered, 20 mg intravenously immediately and then every 6 h as needed. In the rare cases of acute methotrexate renal toxicity, this approach is especially important to avoid or ameliorate renal failure. Chronic side effects are more subtle. In addition to the already discussed hepatotoxicity and pulmonary fibrosis, there may be chronic renal damage or inhibition of spermatogenesis.

- Hydroxyurea. Hydroxyurea blocks thymidine synthetase and thus interferes with DNA synthesis. It is most widely used today in treating sickle cell anemia and in thrombocythemia, as well as in a variety of solid tumor and leukemia protocols. While it is effective in psoriasis, it is not approved for this indication and is less effective and more toxic than methotrexate. The usual daily dosage is 500 mg twice or three times daily. Almost all patients develop a macrocytic anemia. The main toxic effects involve the kidneys and bone marrow, but hepatotoxicity does not occur. We see little reason to continue to employ hydroxyurea in psoriasis therapy.
- Other Cytotoxic Agents. A long list of other chemotherapy agents have been tried in psoriasis. Both 5-fluorouracil and azathioprine have their disciples but have won limited all-around acceptance and are not approved for psoriasis. 5-Fluorouracil must be administered intravenously, which makes it less attractive. However, many patients on regimens containing 5-fluorouracil for solid tumors, such as gastrointestinal carcinomas, find that their psoriasis improves. Azathioprine is occasionally employed as a second-line drug in psoriatic arthritis but it offers little for treating the skin lesions.

Cyclosporine. This medication, which has revolutionized organ transplantation, is derived from *Tolypocladium inflatum Gams*, a fungus discovered as a soil saprophyte in Hardanger Vidda, Norway, in 1970. It is a cyclic hydrophobic undecapeptide that inhibits the production by T cells of IL-2, a T cell growth factor, and thus shuts down the T cell activation and cytokine production cascade at an early point. Cyclosporine A is extremely effective in psoriasis. It has a rapid onset of action and is probably the treatment of choice for severe or explosive forms of both ordinary and pustular psoriasis. While it is also helpful for psoriatic arthritis, the onset of action is slower.

There are many contraindications to the use of cyclosporine for skin diseases listed in Table 14.6. While the only official contraindication is hypersensitivity to cyclosporine or to its vehicle castor oil (for intravenous use), this refers to patients having received an organ transplant. When dealing

Table 14.6. Contraindications for cyclosporine use in psoriasis

Pregnancy
Decreased renal function
Significant or difficult-to-control hypertension
Preexisting malignancy
HIV/AIDS or other chronic infections
Drug or alcohol abuse
Impairment of other major organs
Hyperuricemia or hyperkalemia
Use of medications that alter cyclosporine's bioavailability
Current UV radiation or PUVA therapy; significant previous phototherapy, X-ray radiotherapy or methotrexate

with a less serious disease, such as psoriasis, the contraindications are stricter, but because a much lower dose is used, the side effects are also far less.

The recommended initial dose is 2.5 mg/kg daily. If the patient shows the expected improvement after 1 month, this low level can be continued. If the improvement is not satisfactory, the dose can then be gradually increased to 5.0 mg/kg daily. In rare cases, such as life-threatening generalized pustular psoriasis, one may start with the higher dose. If after 6 weeks of 5.0 mg/kg daily, no improvement is seen, the patient has failed and therapy should be stopped. Similarly if patient compliance is not ideal, the treatment should be discontinued. If renal impairment or hypertension become problems, one can reduce the dosage gradually by 0.5–1.0 mg/kg and carefully monitor the problem.

No good guidelines exist for maintenance therapy with cyclosporine. Obviously the lowest possible dosage should be used and one should aim for improvement, not clearing. After six disease-free months, one should try to discontinue the medication. Unfortunately, relapses are to be expected. They usually occur within 10 weeks. While the patient is most often better off than before starting, occasional disastrous relapses, such as those seen with corticosteroids, may occur.

The main acute problem with cyclosporine is decreased renal function. The serum creatinine, potassium and uric acid may increase as the glomerular filtration rate decreases. As a rough guideline, if the serum creatinine increases over 30% of the baseline level, the dose should be reduced. While many of the changes are functional, renal vascular damage also occurs and is for the most part irreversible. About 10% of transplantation patients develop hypertension secondary to cyclosporine, but this is usually reversible with reduced dose and can be treated with antihypertensive agents. Additional side effects include tremors, gingival hyperplasia and hypertrichosis. The risk of developing internal malignancies is comparable to the risk with other immunosuppressive agents, so the patient should be evaluated prior to therapy and periodically thereafter with this risk in mind.

Laboratory monitoring should include three fasting creatinine levels prior to therapy. Then blood pressure, creatinine, electrolytes, uric acid and liver function tests should be checked every 2 weeks for the first 3 months and then every 4 weeks.

Retinoids. The aromatic retinoids, acitretin and etretinate, are a major option in treating severe psoriasis, including generalized pustular psoriasis and psoriatic erythroderma. Isotretinoin is not used in psoriasis. We only employ acitretin. Etretinate has a half-life over 120 days, while acitretin's value is about 50 h. Otherwise, the drugs are identical, for acitretin is the active form of etretinate. Both products have a significant effect on psoriasis, blocking epidermal proliferation, improving differentiation and modulating the inflammatory or immune response. As a monotherapy, they are not as effective as methotrexate, but they are often combined with other topical modalities or UV radiation.

The main contradiction to etretinate and acitretin is their use in a patient of child-bearing years. While both are teratogenic and should be used with considerable care in women of child-bearing potential, the margin of safety is better with acitretin. Nonetheless, paradoxically, a small amount of acitretin is metabolized back to etretinate, so that 2 years of contraception following cessation of drug therapy is recommended. The problem is not only a medical one, but also a medical-legal one, as has been seen with isotretinoin for acne. In general, there are few psoriasis patients who absolutely have to have a retinoid. If one initiates such therapy, then a lengthy consent form, pregnancy testing prior to starting therapy and contraception for 2 years after the end of treatment are strongly recommended.

Acitretin is prescribed in a single daily dose of 30–50 mg irrespective of the body weight for 2–4 weeks. As soon as improvement is seen, the dose should be reduced in an individualized way to the lowest possible level. After 8–12 weeks of therapy, about 70% of patients have a satisfactory response. With etretinate, one usually starts at 0.75–1.0 mg/kg daily for pustular psoriasis, but at the much lower level of 0.25 mg/kg daily for psoriatic erythroderma. The dose may have to be gradually increased. Within 2–4 weeks improvement should be seen and then one can taper, just as for acitretin.

Retinoids are typically combined with PUVA (Re-PUVA) or UVB (especially the 311 nm lamps). One tends to employ the retinoids first for 2–3 weeks. This flattens lesions and reduces scale, facilitating phototherapy. In all these situations the combination therapy is better than monotherapy and often excellent results are obtainable with a low retinoid dosage.

The side effects are similar to those of isotretinoin. They are dosage-related, mimic the effects of excessive vitamin A and almost all are reversible when the medication is stopped. Every patient experiences dryness of the lips, and often other areas of the skin, the eyes and nasal mucosa. Contact lens wearers may have to shift back to glasses. Diffuse hair loss may occur. Night vision is disturbed slightly. About 50% of patients develop elevated cholesterol and triglyceride levels, while 25% show abnormalities of liver function tests. The patients are almost always asymptomatic. More uncommon changes include bone and joint pain and pseudotumor cerebri, while there is a long list of extremely rare problems. In children, both products have skeletal side effects as they may produce premature closure of epiphyses. This is usually not a problem in psoriasis patients who receive such a short course.

Liver function tests, cholesterol and triglyceride levels must be checked prior to treatment, after 3–4 weeks and then every 3 months. If the patient is young or will be on long-term therapy, radiologic monitoring of the skeletal system is also wise.

Other Systemic Medications. There is a long list of preparations that have been employed in psoriasis. All are less effective than the standard approaches listed above but may have a use in severe or unusual situations.

- Fumaric Acid. Fumaric acid is a natural metabolite as part of the citric acid cycle. While the acid itself has no antipsoriatic activity, several of its esters do. A combination of fumaric acid monoethylester and similar esters (Fumaderm) is approved in Germany for severe psoriasis. Limited controlled studies evaluating the product point towards quite good results. While patients perceive fumaric acid esters to be safe because they are derived from a "natural product", the side effects are considerable, including flushing, gastrointestinal distress, fatigue and kidney disease. Plans are underway to produce and test a single fumaric acid ester. The efficacy of such a product will be easier to assess than the current product.
- Fish Oils. Since ω-3-fatty acids and other fish oils are theoretically capable of influencing the arachidonic acid cycle, they have been employed in a variety of inflammatory skin diseases, including psoriasis. The few clinical studies have shown little or no response.
- Antibiotics. Ampicillin was recommended three decades ago for pustular psoriasis, and subsequently, agents such as cephalosporins and penicillinase-resistant penicillins have been endorsed. In our hands, antibiotics are not beneficial in pustular psoriasis. Just because they are relatively harmless seems little reason to use them in a disease that is clearly not infectious. In guttate psoriasis, which is almost always triggered by streptococcal strains, it is reasonable to use antibiotics as part of the initial therapy if the throat culture is positive.
- Nonsteroidal Antiinflammatory Drugs. These products are often used in psoriatic arthritis. Since the role of prostaglandins and leukotrienes in psoriasis is well-established, it seems that manipulating this part of the inflammatory pathway would be a reasonable approach, but unfortunately numerous positive preliminary reports have failed to translate into any practical treatment breakthrough. In case reports, these agents have been blamed for triggering psoriasis.
- Colchicine. Usually employed for gout, colchicine influences neutrophils and has been recommended for pustular psoriasis, primarily the palmoplantar forms. Dosages are in the range 0.5–0.6 mg twice or three times daily. The initial reports were from Japan and subsequent American studies were not as glowing. Topical colchicine has also been employed with success for chronic stable plaques of psoriasis, but other approaches are easier.
- Gold. Gold salts, both intramuscular and oral, are not as effective in psoriatic arthritis as they are in rheumatoid arthritis. In some instances, the almost inevitable mucosal and cutaneous reaction to gold may trigger a flare of psoriasis, so one should be cautious.
- Oral Contraceptives. Some patients experience an improvement of their psoriasis during pregnancy. This phenomenon has led to therapeutic attempts with oral contraceptives, but both the presence of more effective agents and the increased medical-legal concerns about the risks of oral contraceptives have turned physicians away from this approach.

Diet

What a person eats surely plays some role in psoriasis but it is difficult to treat the disease by dietary manipulation. Reduced caloric intake usually helps psoriasis. As an extreme example, there are several reports documenting the reduced prevalence of psoriasis in times of war. Often patients report worsening of psoriasis coupled with gains in weight. The relationship of alcohol ingestion to psoriasis is difficult to document, but many clinicians suspect there is a negative association. Psoriasis in alcoholics is often therapy-resistant.

Many specific antipsoriatic diets have been proposed. Perhaps the change in diet, usually coupled with a reduction in calories and a generous placebo effect, explains the occasional efficacy of such measures.

Psoriatic Variants

Psoriatic Erythroderma

Psoriasis is one of the leading causes of erythroderma. About 1–2% of psoriasis patients experience erythroderma at some time in their life. Occasionally guttate or chronic stable psoriasis may flare, going on to cover the entire body. Patients with intense inflammatory lesions are more unstable and likely to show dissemination. But a far greater problem is erythroderma secondary to unsuccessful therapy. In the past, the major cause of both psoriatic erythroderma and generalized pustular psoriasis was the reduction or discontinuation of systemic corticosteroids; this is one reason such therapy is no longer considered acceptable. In addition, too aggressive topical therapy or UV radiation in an early eruptive stage of the disease may trigger erythroderma.

The patient is diffusely red with marked desquamation and often exudation. Usually clues as to the preexisting psoriasis are somewhere to be found, or at least the history helps. In very rare cases, a patient presents almost de novo with erythroderma and turns out to have psoriasis. The scales may be quite fine. Pruritus is usually present. The patient is often systemically ill with lymphadenopathy, fever, chills and fluid and protein loss. The acute respiratory distress syndrome is a another severe complication, also seen in patients with severe pustular psoriasis. The major problem, especially in the USA with its air-conditioned hospitals, is that it is often impossible in the summer to find a hospital room warm and humid enough for the shivering patient.

Differential Diagnosis. The differential diagnosis is discussed in greater detail under erythroderma. The main causes are drug eruptions, exacerbation of underlying skin diseases and lymphoma, especially mycosis fungoides. Depending on the special interests of the hospital, the proportion of each group may vary. But there is always an unfortunate group of erythrodermic patients in whom no explanation is found.

Pustular Psoriasis

Neutrophils in the epidermis are a classic feature of psoriasis. In this disease, pus does not equate with infection. In some forms of the disease, the collections of neutrophils are clinically obvious. Occasionally psoriasis patients treated under occlusion or with moist dressings may develop a secondary bacterial or candidal infection, which should be excluded, as the treatment is obviously different. The classification of pustular psoriasis is very confusing; we will present a scheme that has stood us in good stead, but acknowledge in advance that it is not universally accepted.

Generalized Pustular Psoriasis (von Zumbusch Type)

(von Zumbusch 1910)

Von Zumbusch was the founder of the Department of Dermatology at the Ludwig-Maximilian-University in Munich, Germany, where all four authors of this volume have spent varying amounts of their professional career. This form can be viewed as the maximum variant of acute, explosive psoriasis. Few clinical signs of classic psoriasis remain. The patient is acutely ill with fever, chills and often an elevated neutrophil count. Multiple erythematous patches and plaques dotted with pustules cover wide areas of the body (Figs. 14.29 and 14.30). The pustules may coalesce. Typically the palms and soles are involved. In addition, the oral mucosa, genital mucosa and even upper airways may show pustules. As the lesions dry out, they become scaly. Later in the course of the eruption, more typical psoriasis plaques may evolve.

Most often there is a trigger for von Zumbusch pustular psoriasis. In the past it was often the rapid

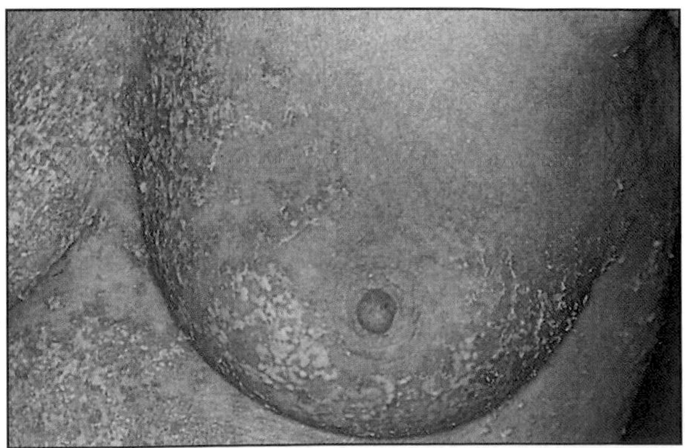

Fig. 14.29. General pustular psoriasis, von Zumbusch type

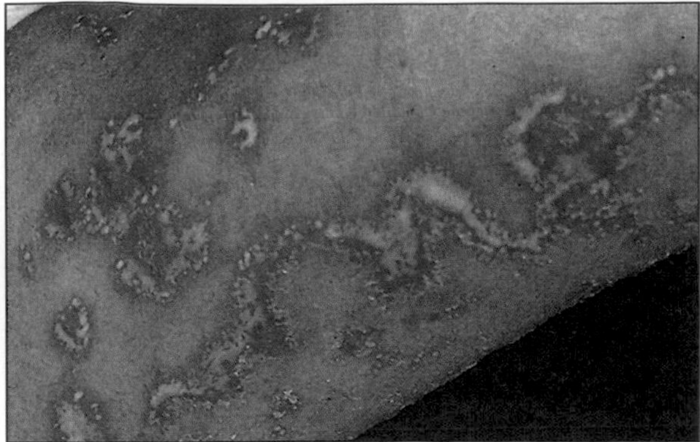

Fig. 14.30. Generalized pustular psoriasis, von Zumbusch type

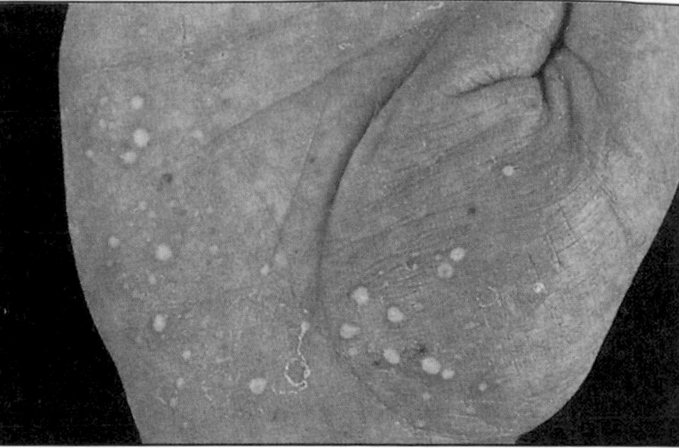

Fig. 14.31. Palmoplantar pustular psoriasis

reduction or termination of systemic corticosteroid therapy. Other medications such as β-blockers or antimalarial agents may also be responsible, as well as pregnancy or oral contraceptive use. The prognosis is serious; death may occur. The patients, despite having too many neutrophils, lack effective antibacterial activity and are at risk of life-threatening infections, especially pneumonia. In addition, the massive protein loss leads to an enteropathy and associated metabolic derangements. Unfortunately, such patients are at risk of recurrences, evenif they come through the first dramatic attack unscathed.

Psoriasis with Pustulation

Here a patient with chronic stable psoriasis develops weeping and pustules within individual lesions, triggered by the same factors discussed above or by aggressive topical therapy. The patient's general condition is usually unaffected.

Palmoplantar Pustular Psoriasis (Barber-Königsbeck Type)

(Barber-Königsbeck 1936)

In this relatively common variant, sharply defined erythematous plaques speckled with small pustules are limited to the palms and soles (Fig. 14.31). Daily new pustules appear and old ones dry up. On occasion the pustules develop on clinically normal skin or in association with the vesicles of dyshidrotic dermatitis. Large fissures eventually develop, which prove to be both painful and difficult to manage. The patients are not systemically ill.

The main differential diagnostic problem is palmoplantar pustulosis (Chap. 16) which is clinically similar to psoriasis. If the patient has no evidence of psoriasis elsewhere, and pustules on otherwise normal palmoplantar skin, then one can diagnosis palmoplantar pustulosis. The HLA associations are much less striking in such patients, speaking against the relationship with psoriasis. In some instances, there are histologic differences. Pustular psoriasis always starts with intraepidermal neutrophils and a unilocular pustule. Palmoplantar pustulosis may have a vesicle initially with associated spongiosis and only later show pustules.

Acrodermatitis Continua Suppurativa

While we consider acrodermatitis chronica suppurativa as a form of localized pustular psoriasis, we have for reasons of tradition covered it in Chapter 16 with other pustular diseases.

Impetigo Herpetiformis

This disorder of pregnancy, characterized by hypocalcemia, is best viewed as a variant of generalized pustular psoriasis (Chap. 16).

Erythema Annulare Centrifugum-Like Psoriasis (Annular Psoriasis)

This unusual variant features erythematous plaques especially on the extremities or trunk which show peripheral spread along with central healing, producing a figurate erythema. In many cases, tiny pustules can be discovered in the advancing border. A collarette scale develops pointing towards the center of the lesion rather than the periphery. The annular lesions change over days to weeks, but the disease process persists for years. Many patients also develop typical chronic psoriatic plaques. Histopathologic findings support the diagnosis of psoriasis.

Psoriatic Arthritis

Definition. Seronegative arthritis, often acral, which appears in association with psoriasis and has a relatively typical radiologic appearance.

Epidemiology. Psoriatic arthritis has a prevalence of 0.02–0.1%. About 5–7% of psoriasis patients have arthritis. Children are rarely affected. Over 70% of patients with psoriatic arthritis have preexisting psoriasis, while in about 10%, the two problems appear in the same time period. This leaves about 20% of patients who develop arthritis but lack any sign of psoriasis, although many later develop skin lesions.

Etiology and Pathogenesis. The connection between the skin and the joints in psoriasis remains somewhat a mystery. Certain HLA markers are more common and may have diagnostic and prognostic significance. They include A26, B17, B27, Cw6, DR3, DR4 and DR7. HLA-B27 is much more common in not only psoriatic arthritis, but also in ankylosing spondylitis and Reiter syndrome. Typically the serologic evaluation including both rheumatoid factor and ANA is negative. This led Moll and Wright (1973) to classify psoriatic arthritis as the prototype of the seronegative arthritides.

Clinical Findings. At least 70% of patients with psoriatic arthritis have nail changes (Fig. 14.32). It is most unusual to see an affected finger with swelling and destruction but without psoriatic nail lesions. Not only is the arthritis itself a problem, but such patients appear at greater risk for psoriatic erythroderma. Patients with fever and malaise at the onset of their joint problems are more likely to have a severe disease course. A number of types of psoriatic arthritis can be identified, incorporating clinical, serologic and radiologic parameters. Common features include digital involvement, sacroiliac disease and pain in areas of tendon insertions, such as the plantar fascia, known as esthesiopathy. In addition, the rheumatoid factor should be negative. However, striking differences in clinical pattern occur:

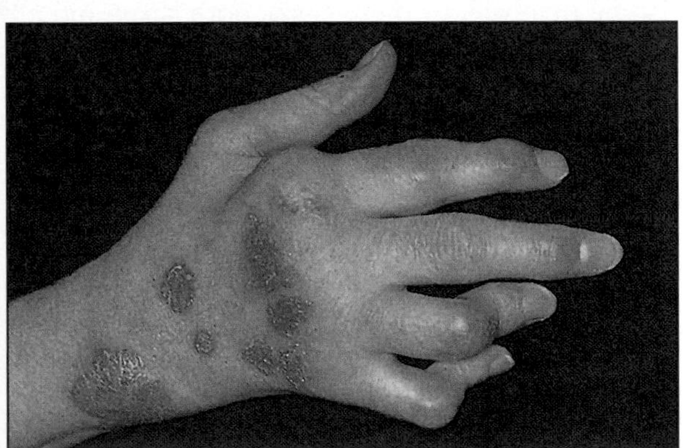

Fig. 14.32. Mutilating psoriatic arthritis with nummular psoriasis

Asymmetric Psoriatic Oligoarthritis. This is the most common form (>70%) and can appear as a monoarthritis. Typically distal digital joints are involved and progression to a more widespread form is rare. Usually synovitis and joint swelling is first identified. Later the digit typically is swollen, producing the so-called sausage finger.

Distal Interphalangeal Psoriatic Arthritis. Such patients have a maximal variant of the more common asymmetric form. Most or all of their distal interphalangeal joints are involved, so they have painful diffusely swollen fingers and toes. Men are more often involved than women. About 5–10% of psoriatic arthritis patients fall in this category.

Mutilating Psoriatic Arthritis. Fortunately this variant is also relatively uncommon, involving <5% of patients. They experience a widespread arthritis, with involvement not only of multiple digits, but also of the sacroiliac region and lower spine. The changes are thus similar to Reiter syndrome, but there is no sex predilection. The intense inflammation leads to bone and synovial damage, producing marked deformities, such as the classic collapsing or opera glass finger. Contractions also occur, culminating in a functionally impaired hand or foot.

Symmetric Psoriatic Arthritis. This variant most closely resembles rheumatoid arthritis; it accounts for about 15% of cases, strongly favoring women. The rheumatoid factor is negative and rheumatoid nodules are not found. Numerous small and large joints are involved. Typically the ulnar deviation is not as extreme as in rheumatoid arthritis, but the metacarpal joints are involved.

Psoriatic Spondyloarthritis. This uncommon variant (about 5%) is extremely similar to ankylosing spondylitis. Patients are usually men, HLA-B27^{+} and with severe psoriasis. While most often sacroiliac joint involvement is prominent, sometimes other parts of the spinal column are most affected.

Patients typically walk in a stiff manner and have characteristic restriction in their ability to bend and turn. There are minor radiologic differences between psoriatic spondyloarthritis and ankylosing spondylitis, but the two diseases form part of a spectrum.

Pustular Arthroosteitis [Sonozaki Syndrome (Sonozaki 1981)]. This rare disorder was first identified in Asians. Patients typically have palmoplantar pustular psoriasis associated with inflammation of the sternoclavicular joints or the other joints of the sternum. The sternal region is tender and the swollen joints show erosions on radiologic examination. Occasionally an osteomyelitis develops. Alkaline phosphatase levels may be elevated, along with the erythrocyte sedimentation rate and neutrophil count.

SAPHO [Syndrome, Acne Conglobata, Palmoplantar Pustulosis, Hyperostosis and Osteitis (Chamot et al. 1987)]. SAPHO also refers to patients with arthritis and palmoplantar dermatosis or pustular psoriasis. They also have severe acne and may have a slightly different spectrum of joint involvement than other patients in this group. There is a certain lack of logic since patients do not have both palmoplantar pustulosis and acne.

POPP (Psoriatic Onychopachydermoperiosteitis). POPP describes patients with nail onycholysis, painful soft tissue swelling of the digits and periosteal inflammation and thickening of bone (ivory fingers) without joint involvement.

The course in psoriatic arthritis is generally one of progressive disease. The rate of progression may vary greatly, and just as with rheumatoid arthritis, the disease may eventually burn out, but usually leaves a significantly disabled survivor.

Laboratory Findings. The single most important test in most settings is the rheumatoid factor, as patients with psoriatic arthritis are defined as rheumatoid factor negative. One must remember that there are a number of false-positive results with the examination for rheumatoid factor so occasionally one can encounter a patient with classic psoriatic arthritis and a positive test (Chap. 18).

Radiographic examination can help to confirm the diagnosis of psoriatic arthritis and more importantly to document disease progression. The changes vary as greatly as the various clinical forms and should be sought in a radiology text. In general, the fingers show narrowing of the joint space with marginal erosions and periarticular thinning; later there is ankylosis and osteolysis. Skeletal scintigraphy is a sensitive way to identify sites of involvement and monitor patients. Many other newer radiologic methods also lend themselves to the study of psoriatic arthritis.

Reiter Syndrome

(Stoll 1776; Brodie 1818; Fiessinger and Leroy 1916; Reiter 1916)

Synonyms. Sexually acquired reactive arthritis (SARA), Fiessinger-Leroy syndrome

Definition. Reiter syndrome is a chronic reactive disorder characterized by the triad of arthritis, urethritis and conjunctivitis which is triggered by a variety of infections.

Epidemiology. The incidence of Reiter syndrome is about 3/100,000. Most patients (70–90%) with Reiter syndrome are HLA-B27$^+$. The relative risk for such a patient is 37. Looking at it in the other direction, about 2% of patients with *Shigella* infections develop Reiter syndrome; if the patients are HLA-B27$^+$, the chance jumps to 20–25%.

There are two scenarios for Reiter syndrome. Endemic Reiter syndrome is associated with urethritis, in which case and almost exclusively young men are affected. While the triggering agent is not entirely clear, the best candidate is *Chlamydia trachomatis,* a common cause of urethritis. On the other hand, Reiter syndrome may also follow a gastrointestinal infection, usually *Shigella*, although *Salmonella*, *Yersinia* or *Campylobacter* may also be involved. In these cases, both sexes and all ages may be affected.

Etiology and Pathogenesis. While the exact mechanism remains unclear, it seems that bacterial antigens may mimic stretches of the HLA molecule and interfere with delicate immune control mechanisms. Patients who are HLA-B27$^-$ often have a cross-reacting, uncommon HLA type, but some lack any connection.

Clinical Findings. Reiter syndrome is one of the classic seronegative (rheumatoid factor-negative) spondylarthropathies. Others in the group include ankylosing spondylitis, psoriatic arthritis, and the arthritides associated with Crohn disease and ulcerative colitis and other reactive arthropathies.

Systemic Findings. Many organs can be involved but the most striking changes involve the musculoskeletal system.

- Arthritis. Most patients have rheumatologic manifestations. The most common changes are enthesopathies involving the tendons and ligaments, producing plantar fasciitis, achilles tendonitis, other types of tenosynovitis and occasionally true arthritis. Reiter syndrome is the most common cause of an oligoarthropathy in a young man. The weight-bearing joints of the legs and the sacroiliac joints are most often involved. Another typical finding is the swollen or sausage-shaped digits, also seen in psoriatic arthritis.
- Urethritis. The urethritis is often overlooked. When it is symptomatic, the patient usually has discharge with pus and/or blood as well as dysuria. More often there is only a serous discharge. The presence of circinate erythematous lesions with peripheral scale on the glans is known as circinate balanitis (balanitis erosiva circinata) and is a good clue to Reiter syndrome (Fig. 14.33). Chronic genitourinary problems may arise, most often chronic prostatitis, but they are uncommon.
- Ocular Disorders. Acute conjunctivitis is common. It is usually bilateral and mild, to the point of being overlooked. Some patients develop an iridocyclitis or uveitis which can be very persistent and disabling.
- Other Problems. A long list of other organs may rarely be involved. Conduction disturbances in the heart are probably the most worrisome and common of the rare findings. They may develop early in the disease course. Myocarditis and pericarditis have also been seen. Other uncommon problems include aortic insufficiency, optic neuritis, pleurisy, pulmonary infiltrates, thrombophlebitis and secondary amyloidosis. Despite the relationship to dysenteric bacteria, gastrointestinal symptoms are uncommon.
- HIV Infection. Reiter syndrome is both more common and more severe in HIV infected patients. As the immune status drops, the Reiter syndrome tends to be more severe, in contrast to rheumatoid arthritis which improves in the later stages of HIV/AIDS. The overlaps with psoriasis are even more frequent and puzzling in HIV-positive individuals. The same association with HLA-B27 is found. There is some suggestion that HIV alone may provoke a reactive arthritis, even in HLA-B27$^-$ patients. Occasionally Reiter syndrome is the first sign of HIV infection.

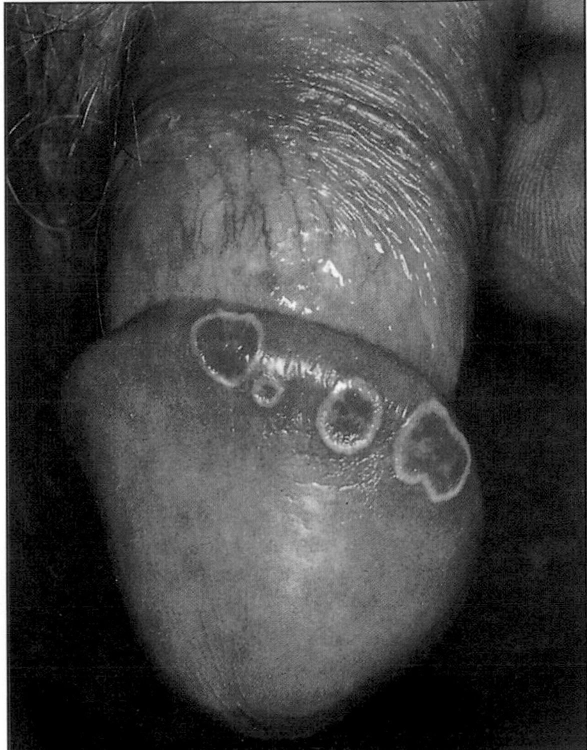

Fig. 14.33. Circinate balanitis in Reiter syndrome

Cutaneous Findings. The cutaneous spectrum of Reiter syndrome overlaps extensively with psoriasis. About 10% of patients have psoriasiform skin changes, which tend to be associated with the involved joints. The most characteristic change is hyperkeratotic lesions on the palms and soles. When they are callus-like, they are known as keratoderma blenorrhagicum (Fig. 14.34) but they are more often erythematous and pustular, just as in psoriasis. The fingers may be sausage-shaped and the nails can show psoriatic changes. Other common sites for the erythematous scaly patches include the umbilicus and scalp, although any place on the body may be affected.

In addition to the circinate balanitis, there may be oral mucosal lesions. Boggy red plaques may be found, usually on the buccal mucosa. They often develop a white keratotic surface. Rarely erosions and ulcerations are seen. Migratory glossitis (geographic tongue) may be present, and less commonly similar migratory lesions are seen on the buccal mucosa (migratory erythema).

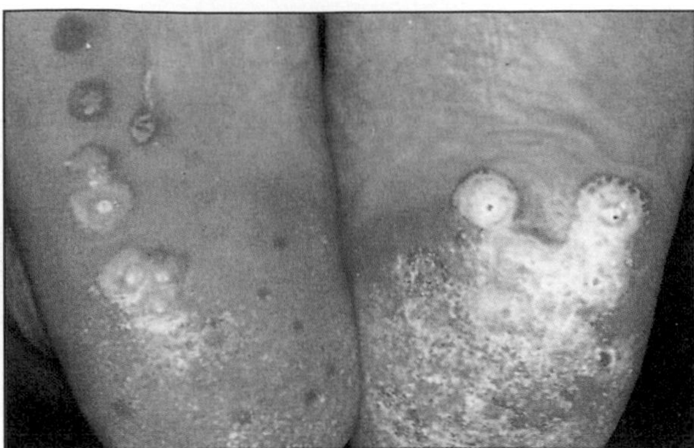

Fig. 14.34. Keratoderma blenorrhagicum in Reiter syndrome

Histopathology. The cutaneous lesions are identical to those of psoriasis.

Laboratory Findings. There are few specific findings for Reiter syndrome; it is a clinical diagnosis. HLA-B27 is useful but not diagnostic. The joint fluid usually has a high complement level rather than the low level present in rheumatoid arthritis. By definition, the rheumatoid factor is negative. Radiologic evaluation may be helpful in supporting the diagnosis.

Course and Prognosis. The outlook in Reiter syndrome is not as good as the term reactive arthritis suggests. The course of the arthritis may be progressive and disabling over years. After 5 years, 80% of patients still complain of musculoskeletal problems, which typically wax and wane. About 3% of patients have chronic cardiac or neurologic difficulties. Others lose vision from persistent uveitis. Chronic urethritis and strictures are rare, but chronic prostatitis appears more common. While the skin and mucosal problems may persist, they are rarely a major source of trouble.

Differential Diagnosis. When the classic findings are present, Reiter syndrome is an easy diagnosis. The hardest differential diagnosis is psoriatic arthritis, which typically has more skin involvement and more upper extremity arthritis. But overlaps are frequent. While the literature suggests a striking predominance in men, this is not entirely correct and leads to Reiter syndrome being overlooked in women with an incomplete presentation. When the uveitis dominates, Behçet syndrome is very hard to separate. The urethritis can be identified by a process of exclusion, as all cultures are negative, unless one is lucky and finds *Chlamydia trachomatis*.

Therapy

Systemic. If the disease presents with a urethritis or if *Chlamydia trachomatis* is cultured, then treatment with doxycycline 100 mg twice daily for 7–14 days is worth a try. Some groups recommend longer therapy to completely eradicate the organism but the benefits of such an approach are unclear. In the case of enteric or epidemic Reiter syndrome, if a known bacterial trigger is present in the community or cultured, then it too should be treated appropriately.

The arthritic symptoms are usually controllable with nonsteroidal antiinflammatory drugs. If not, methotrexate in low weekly dosages, as employed for rheumatoid arthritis, is probably the best alternative. The aromatic retinoids have also been employed, just as with psoriasis. Cyclosporine A is another possibility for severe and refractory cases. Systemic corticosteroids are also sometimes required.

HIV/AIDS patients should be treated cautiously. Immunosuppression can worsen both their Reiter syndrome and their HIV infection. Nonsteroidal antiinflammatory drugs and retinoids appear preferable to methotrexate and corticosteroids, and antiretroviral therapy helps some patients' arthritic problems.

Topical. The cutaneous lesions can be treated exactly as psoriasis.

Pityriasis Rubra Pilaris

(Devergie 1863)

Definition. Chronic hyperkeratotic erythematous dermatosis with a variety of clinical forms.

Epidemiology. Pityriasis rubra pilaris can appear in any age group, but follows a bimodal distribution, involving both children and adults.

Etiology and Pathogenesis. The cause of pityriasis rubra pilaris is totally unknown. Occasional familial cases have been described especially when onset is in childhood but most are sporadic. Several cases have been reported among HIV/AIDS patients, but pityriasis rubra pilaris is not usually associated with immunosuppression. In other instances, it may follow a severe infection. While pityriasis

Table 14.7. Classification of pityriasis rubra pilaris

Type	Prevalence (%)	Course	Clinical features
Adult			
Classic I	55	2–4 years	Abrupt onset, classic picture
Atypical II	5	Chronic	Slow onset, alopecia, localized lesions
Childhood			
Classic III	10	1–2 years	Same as classic adult
Circumscript IV	25	Chronic	Localized erythema and scale, often over joints
Atypical V	5	Chronic	Primarily palms and soles

After Griffiths WA, modified from COHEN and PRYSTOWSKY (1989)

rubra pilaris shares some features with psoriasis, it is a distinct disorder, probably more closely related to disorders of keratinization than to inflammatory processes.

Clinical Findings. Pityriasis rubra pilaris is characterized by follicular erythematous papules and more diffuse erythematous patches with pityriasiform scale. It has a variety of clinical forms (Table 14.7). The disease often smolders along in a relatively uncharacteristic form, causing patient distress and diagnostic confusion, before the patient develops classic findings and some observer makes the correct diagnosis. Often the disease process begins on the scalp with erythema and fine white scale. Facial patches may be deep red with thick crusts, especially in the nasolabial folds and eyebrows. On the body, pityriasis rubra pilaris starts as erythematous to salmon-colored patches that become papular and lichenified. Typically islands of normal skin are spared (Figs. 14.35, 14.36). Other common sites are the palms and soles, which are initially red

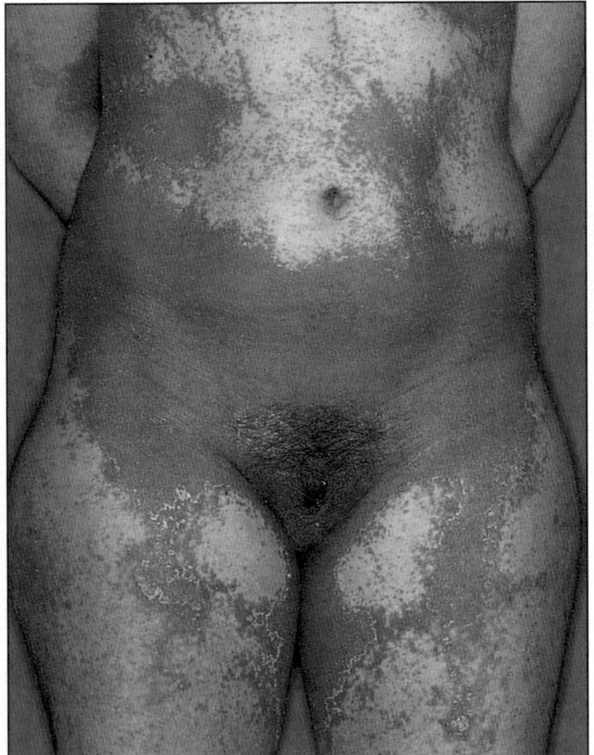

Fig. 14.35. Diffuse involvement with islands of sparing in pityriasis rubra pilaris

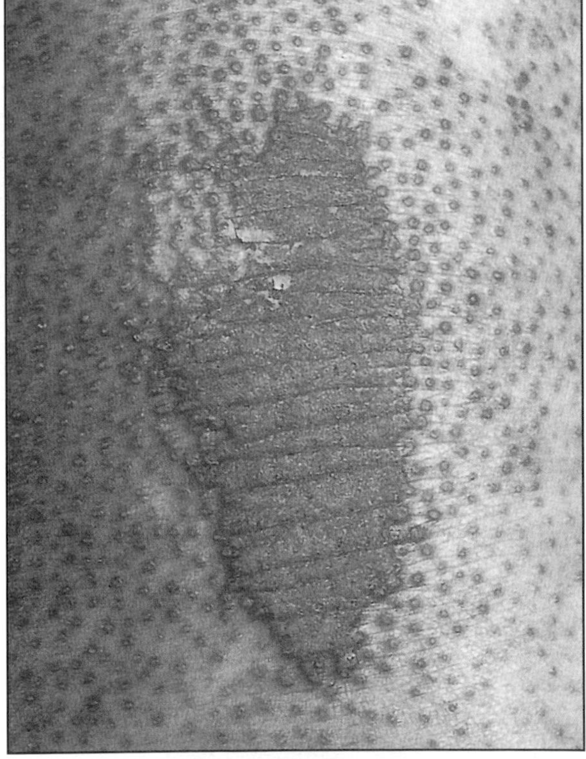

Fig. 14.36. Salmon-colored plaque with follicular involvement in pityriasis rubra pilaris

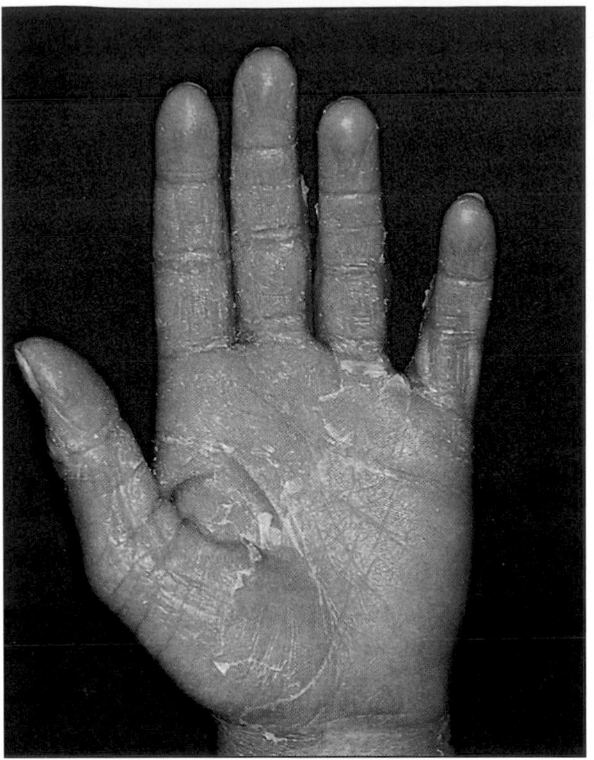

Fig. 14.37. Hyperkeratotic palm in pityriasis rubra pilaris

and then become hyperkeratotic and fissured, often with an orange hue (Fig. 14.37). The disorder is often pruritic.

When one looks closely, many of the individual lesions are small papules, usually centered about follicles. They are especially prominent on the fingers where they have been described as nutmeg-grater lesions. The papules are covered by a keratotic cap or dell and may contain a broken off hair. Sometimes the papules coalesce to produce a plaque, and conversely, sometimes they develop in erythematous areas. Nail changes may also be seen, including subungual hyperkeratoses, nailplate thickening and discoloration; pits, oil spots and other classic changes of psoriasis are not found. Oral lesions do not occur. Pityriasis rubra pilaris may rapidly evolve into an erythroderma. Usually at least a few islands of sparing are present and there are follicular papules and palmoplantar involvement pointing towards the correct diagnosis.

In children the disease usually starts slowly. About half the childhood patients have circumscribed pityriasis rubra pilaris with persistent papules and erythematous patches over the knees and elbows. These children are often misdiagnosed as psoriasis.

In the other variants, the classic features are present in limited or modified form. For example, the childhood atypical or type V variant has palms and soles that resemble classic pityriasis rubra pilaris. Whether there are any other unifying features awaits molecular biologic investigation of these rare problems.

Histopathology. Microscopic examination reveals acanthosis, a thickened granular layer and orthokeratosis alternating with parakeratosis both vertically and horizontally. Often parakeratotic shoulders are found at the openings of follicles, or actually plugging them. There may be spongiosis. In the dermis there is a lymphocytic perivascular infiltrate with few diagnostic features. The keratotic papules typically have lamellar follicular keratinization at the level of the sebaceous duct. A biopsy usually allows one to exclude psoriasis.

Course and Prognosis. The children with classic disease tend to clear rapidly, often within 1 year with treatment, while the adults usually respond over a period of several years.

Differential Diagnosis. The differential diagnosis has been discussed under the clinical features. In our experience, pityriasis rubra pilaris is frequently misdiagnosed. Early cases often resemble seborrheic dermatitis or psoriasis; the uncommon follicular variant of psoriasis is very similar. In addition, patients are seen with both pityriasis rubra pilaris and psoriasis. In children, the usual working diagnosis is atopic dermatitis. When the palm and sole involvement is prominent, one may consider palmoplantar keratoderma or another disorder of keratinization. The spiny keratotic papules may look lichenoid, but lack a violaceous color, and are not seen in the typical sites for lichen planus. If one keeps looking for islands of sparing, salmon color and palmoplantar disease, some puzzling papulosquamous disorders will eventually declare themselves as pityriasis rubra pilaris.

Therapy

Systemic. The retinoids have finally given us an effective agent in pityriasis rubra pilaris. Initially high-dose vitamin A was tried, but the retinoids have a better risk-benefit ratio. Both isotretinoin and the aromatic retinoids, acitretin and etretinate, are helpful. For isotretinoin and etretinate the dosage is between 0.5 and 1.0 mg/kg daily. Acitretin, which we prefer over etretinate, can be given at a dosage of 30–50 mg daily irrespective of weight. We have found it helpful to start at a low dosage and gradually increase. Contraception and all the other cautions discussed under both psoriasis and acne should be observed, anticipating that therapy for a longer time may be required. Thus skeletal monitoring is wise. If women of child-bearing age must be treated, isotretinoin is preferable.

Other systemic approaches include corticosteroids, methotrexate and even cyclosporine. While corticosteroids can reduce inflammation and may be helpful in the early part of the disease, they are required at levels that usually lead to side effects. Methotrexate has a similar track record. When it helps, it is often at high dosages. Pityriasis rubra pilaris is only minimally responsive to cyclosporine; this is yet another feature that sets it apart from psoriasis.

Topical. Topical corticosteroids, often under occlusion or combined with keratolytics such as urea, can effectively treat localized disease and reduce the need for systemic medications. Topical retinoids may also be employed, but one must remember that the skin is easily irritated in pityriasis rubra pilaris, leading to iatrogenic flares. For this reason, both phototherapy and photochemotherapy are usually not employed. Finding the best emollient for a given patient is very important in caring for this most stubborn disease.

Parapsoriasis

The German title of this section is "the so-called parapsoriasis group". This choice of words reflects the many uncertainties about the term parapsoriasis. Since Brocq first used the term in 1902 to describe a group of diseases of unknown etiology that he felt resembled psoriasis, the term parapsoriasis has led to primarily confusion and disagreement. While total agreement will never be achieved, we believe the following statements are reasonable:

- Parapsoriasis does not refer to a single disease or even to a group of related diseases but instead to several unrelated disorders.
- None of the diseases called parapsoriasis have anything in common with psoriasis, either on a clinical or histologic basis.

For these reasons we no longer use the term umbrella or group term parapsoriasis but instead refer to disorders that have evolved out of Brocq's initial befuddling scheme by their individual names. While we will give synonyms for completeness' sake, we warn the reader that the synonyms cause much confusion. Guttate parapsoriasis, for example, has been used for pityriasis lichenoides chronica, pityriasis lichenoides et varioliformis acuta and small-plaque parapsoriasis.

Pityriasis Lichenoides

Pityriasis lichenoides refers to two diseases that were for years felt to be separate but today are considered part of the same spectrum. They are pityriasis lichenoides et varioliformis acuta and pityriasis lichenoides chronica. While each will be considered separately, we feel they belong together as evidenced by clinical and histologic similarities and by overlap cases, which begin as pityriasis lichenoides et varioliformis acuta and wind up as pityriasis lichenoides chronica.

Pityriasis Lichenoides et Varioliformis Acuta

(MUCHA 1916; HABERMANN 1925)

Synonyms. Mucha-Habermann disease, PLEVA

Definition. Acute or subacute disease of unknown origin with hemorrhagic crusted lesions that heal with varioliform scars.

Epidemiology. Most patients are young adults and men are more commonly affected than women.

Etiology and Pathogenesis. While the cause of pityriasis lichenoides et varioliformis acuta is unknown, many physicians suspect an infectious etiology since the disease appears rapidly and favors adolescents and young adults. The target site is the superficial dermal vessels which are damaged by a true lymphocytic vasculitis. While occasional associated diseases have been described, they probably reflect coincidence, not etiology.

Clinical Findings. Pityriasis lichenoides et varioliformis acuta most often starts on the trunk with erythematous papules that continuously erupt over a period of weeks, developing scale and crust, and often ulcerating. The lesions may be hemorrhagic and vesicular (Fig. 14.38). They typically resolve with subtle scars. For all these reasons, the tongue twister of a name was coined: the lesions have scale

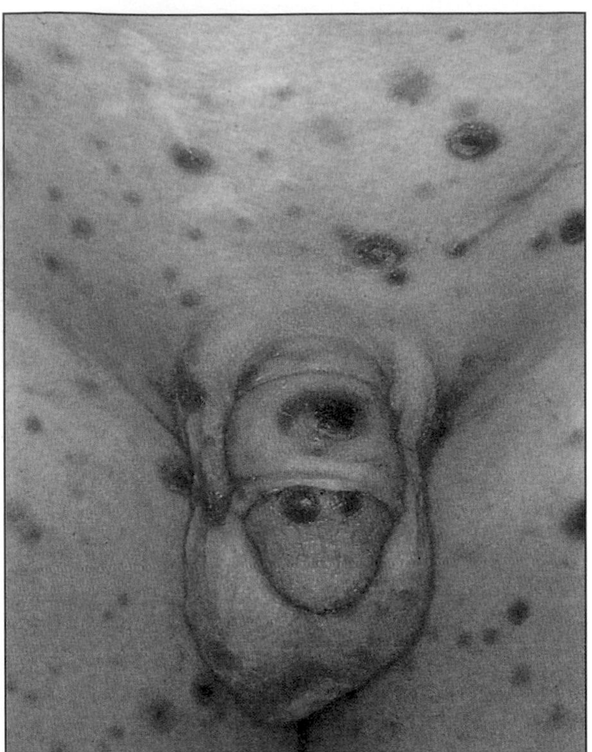

Fig. 14.38. Pityriasis lichenoides et varioliformis acuta

(pityriasis), may be papular (lichenoides) and erythematous, heal with scars (varioliformis) and appear suddenly (acuta). As a memory device, pityriasis lichenoides et varioliformis acuta has been described as looking like bad chronic chickenpox. Sometimes ulcerations dominate the picture; often they are associated with fever. Most patients are asymptomatic, often surprisingly since they look as though they should be sick. There is no mucosal involvement.

The disease resolves over weeks to months. The degree of scarring is dependent on how deep or ulcerated the lesions are. Some disease may not resolve in some patients but instead evolve into pityriasis lichenoides chronica, so the wise physician is cautious in counseling pityriasis lichenoides et varioliformis acuta patients. The time of transition to pityriasis lichenoides chronica is unclear. Some patients may have typical pityriasis lichenoides et varioliformis acuta for many months but always clinically acute, i.e. new lesions with hemorrhage, and others may develop a more chronic stable eruption.

Histopathology. Pityriasis lichenoides et varioliformis acuta is the prototypic disease featuring lymphocytic vasculitis. There is endothelial cell swelling and exocytosis of erythrocytes and lymphocytes, but few neutrophils and no nuclear dust. Fibrin deposition is not seen. Thus there are large accumulations of lymphocytes, primarily suppressor T cells, about the vessels. Some of the erythrocytes may reach the epidermis, where reticular degeneration and necrosis may also be seen. Immunofluorescent examination may reveal immunoglobulins (mainly IgM) and complement components in the basement membrane zone and about vessels.

Occasionally clinically typical cases of pityriasis lichenoides et varioliformis acuta may be found which on biopsy show striking atypia of the lymphocytes. Such cases overlap with lymphomatoid papulosis (Chap. 61).

Course and Prognosis. The course is difficult to predict. Most patients experience one or several flares of the disease and then heal spontaneously over weeks to months. Others continue to develop new lesions, but often of a milder form. The disease in yet others converts into pityriasis lichenoides chronica.

Differential Diagnosis. The differential diagnosis is limited. The lack of fever and oral involvement speak against varicella. In the early stages many other papulosquamous disorders can be considered such as guttate psoriasis and secondary syphilis but soon the hemorrhage and crusts make the diagnosis clearer and histology confirms the clinical impression.

Therapy

Systemic. Systemic antibiotic therapy is frequently recommended and reasonable to try. But many patients improve with no therapy and others continue to worsen under antibiotic treatment. Usually tetracycline (1.0–2.0 g daily), doxycycline (100–200 mg daily) or erythromycin (1.0 g daily) is recommended. In Germany sometimes penicillin is used. Whatever the choice, treatment should be carried out for 3–4 weeks.

Systemic corticosteroids can also produce prompt improvement, although when they are stopped, a relapse is the rule. One can view using corticosteroids as an attempt to interrupt the reactive process, hoping that the body will then revert to normal.

Very low-dose methotrexate therapy is amazingly effectively, but rarely used because of the self-limited nature of the disease and the age of the patients. Nonetheless, some feel that 2.5–10.0 mg weekly in a single dose is almost a therapeutic test for pityriasis lichenoides et varioliformis acuta. We caution against such diagnostic trials. Dapsone has also been endorsed, but we have no personal experience with it for this disease.

Topical. Topical therapy is strictly symptomatic and rarely useful. On the other hand, PUVA or PUVA bath therapy seem to work very well and should be considered as safe first-line choices. The disease tends to relapse when the PUVA treatment is stopped too early. We prefer PUVA bath therapy over all other approaches.

Pityriasis Lichenoides Chronica

(JADASSOHN 1894; JULIUSBERG 1899)

Synonyms. Parapsoriasis en gouttes, guttate parapsoriasis

Definition. Chronic papulosquamous eruption of unknown etiology with clinically distinctive lesions.

Epidemiology. Pityriasis lichenoides chronica is also a disease of young adults. About 20% of cases occur in children. It is more common than pityriasis lichenoides et varioliformis acuta.

Etiology and Pathogenesis. The etiology is unknown. While there is often a relationship to pityriasis lichenoides et varioliformis acuta, this advances our understanding little since the latter's etiology is also a mystery. Pityriasis lichenoides chronica is one of the many dermatologic diseases that have been linked with the concept of focus of infection. Other alleged associations include chronic urticaria, nummular dermatitis and palmoplantar pustulosis. While the theory is attractive, suggesting that chronic infections such as cholecystitis, tonsilitis, sinusitis, prostatitis or periodontitis may trigger skin disease, it is difficult to prove causality when the skin disease tends to resolve spontaneously.

Clinical Findings. The disease is almost always totally asymptomatic, so the patient usually presents with their rash in full bloom, wondering what is going on with their skin. The clinical picture is polymorphic for new lesions appear as old ones begin to fade (Fig. 14.39). The trunk and proximal parts of the extremities are the main sites of involvement. The initial lesions are 2–10-mm dome-

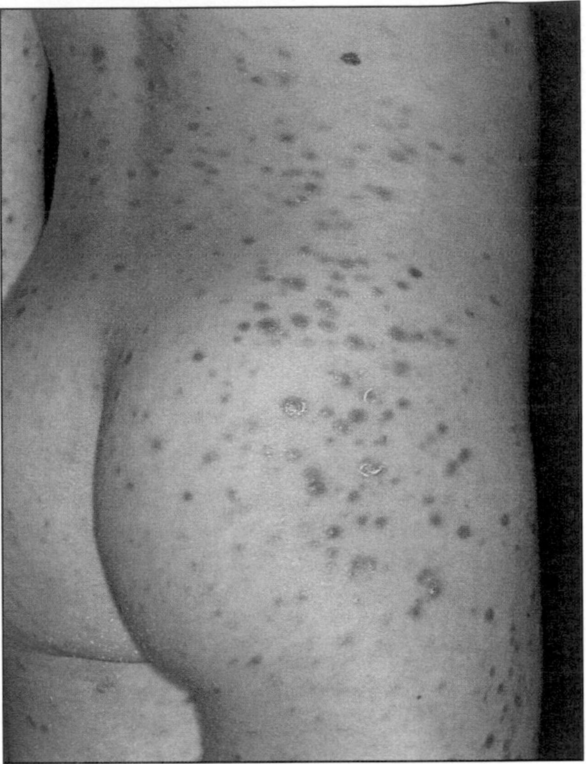

Fig. 14.39. Pityriasis lichenoides chronica

shaped red or red–brown papules, whose surface is either dull or has a slight shimmer. While there is a small amount of fine scale, it is only noticed when the lesion is scratched. Hemorrhagic lesions occur but are uncommon. The papules tend to expand as they become flatter and often either pale or more brown. They develop a more prominent compact scale that covers them.

After several more weeks, the lesion is entirely flat and has left behind the classic clinical sign of pityriasis lichenoides chronica – a thick, sharply defined single large scale. When this scale is peeled away, normal skin is revealed. The scale is described as *Oblaten*-like in German. *Oblaten* refers to the paper-thin wafers used in religious cermonies (Fig. 14.40). In America one speaks of the Scotch tape sign but the scale is opaque, not transparent. In darker individuals, pityriasis lichenoides chronica often heals with hypo- and hyperpigmentation.

The course may lasts months or even years. Even though the patient is asymptomatic, the chronic cosmetic problem is often quite distressing. Sometimes there may be a transition to pityriasis lichenoides et varioliformis acuta. This change has been more often observed following PUVA therapy. In

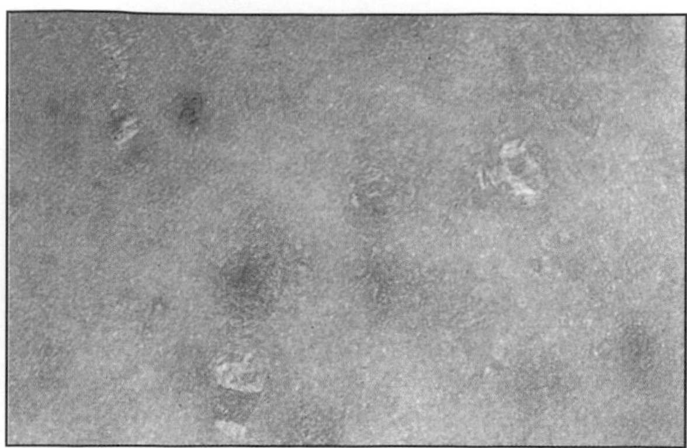

Fig. 14.40. *Oblaten* sign in pityriasis lichenoides chronica

other instances the conversion goes in the other direction, as pityriasis lichenoides et varioliformis acuta evolves into pityriasis lichenoides chronica.

Histopathology. The lymphocytic vasculitis seen in pityriasis lichenoides et varioliformis acuta may be present, but is much less prominent. Instead the perivascular lymphocytes also tend to form a lichenoid pattern along the epidermal-dermal junction. There may be spongiosis, minimal acanthosis and parakeratotic scale. Rarely accumulations of lymphocytes can be found in parakeratotic horny layer. Exocytosis of erythrocytes also occurs. In later lesions, the infiltrate is minimal and only the thick, compact scale seen. Immunofluorescent examination once again may reveal nonspecific deposition of immunoglobulins and complement components about the vessels and along the basement membrane zone.

Differential Diagnosis. While the initial lesions of pityriasis lichenoides chronica may resemble guttate psoriasis, the monomorphous nature of psoriasis usually allows a rapid distinction. Lichen planus is also a more uniform eruption and has far less scale, as well as frequent oral involvement. Secondary syphilis can also appear similar, but is more acute and monomorphous.

Therapy

Systemic. Just as in pityriasis lichenoides et varioliformis acuta, antibiotics, low-dose corticosteroids, methotrexate or dapsone can be tried. None are very effective and we tend to avoid them.

Topical. For many physicians, phototherapy is the treatment of choice. UVB, oral PUVA or PUVA bath therapy can all be tried. One must always discuss with the patient the possibility of triggering a disease flare with phototherapy. Climate therapy as discussed under psoriasis with sun exposure at the sea shore or higher elevations is also a possibility. In addition, topical corticosteroids are frequently recommended, but do little to influence the disease course.

Parapsoriasis en Plaques (Patch-Type Parapsoriasis)

After one has separated away pityriasis lichenoides et varioliformis acuta and pityriasis lichenoides chronica from the parapsoriasis group, one is still confronted with classification problems. Some physicians feel that all parapsoriasis en plaques is the same disease, a precursor of mycosis fungoides. Others feel confident in their ability to separate out two distinct diseases, only one of which is likely to evolve into mycosis fungoides. Further confusing the matter is that the French *en plaques* means patch, not plaque. We are splitters in this area, feeling that there are two separate diseases which rarely if ever overlap. Modern methods of molecular biology will certainly help to clarify this situation.

Small-Patch Parapsoriasis

Synonyms. Brocq disease (in Europe), chronic superficial dermatitis, digitate dermatitis, xanthoerythrodermia perstans

Definition. Persistent asymptomatic erythematosquamous eruption with very fine scales and with almost no risk of conversion to mycosis fungoides.

Epidemiology. The disorder is quite uncommon. Most patients are adult men.

Etiology and Pathogenesis. The etiology of small-patch parapsoriasis is unknown.

Clinical Findings. Most patients simply do not notice the onset of their disease. The lesions are subtle and asymptomatic, usually starting on the trunk or flexor surfaces of the extremities. Small slightly erythematous macules appear, usually covered with very fine scale. They slowly increase in number, usually reaching a size of less than five cm. Occasionally minimal pruritus is present. On the

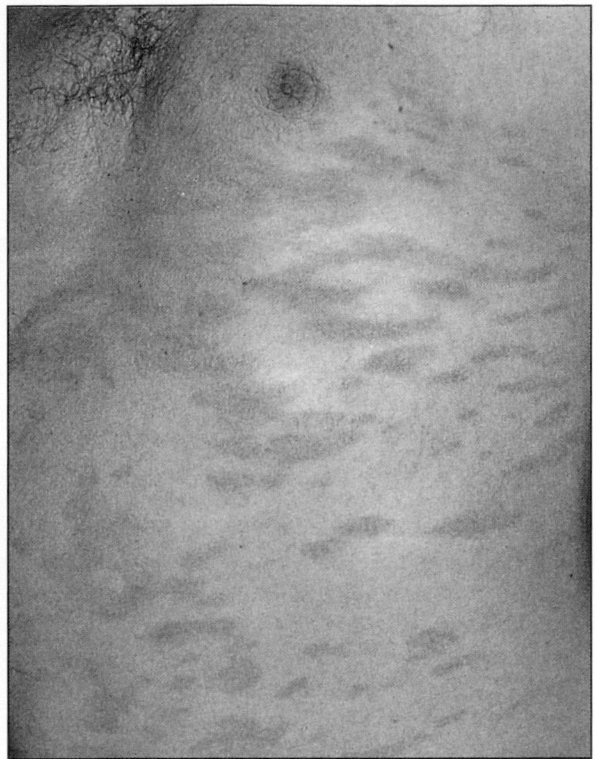

Fig. 14.41. Small-patch parapsoriasis

trunk they are often elongated and follow skin lines. Here they have been fancifully compared to the finger print marks that would be left behind after pressing one's hands on the skin (Fig. 14.41). Smaller lesions can coalesce or evolve into larger patches, so the name small-patch is relative. The scale is usually very fine and the lesions may have an indistinct border. Sometimes they have a yellow hue; then the term xanthoerythrodermia perstans is applied. Finally, some lesions have small surface tears in the stratum corneum that produce a coarse pattern which has been called pseudolichenification. When one looks closely, there is no sign of rubbing or scratching. There may be fine wrinkling which has been termed pseudoatrophy, as microscopically there is no thinning of the skin.

Histopathology. Microscopic examination reveals no diagnostic changes. The epidermis is virtually normal, although minimal spongiosis, parakeratosis or acanthosis may be seen. In the dermis there is a minimal lymphocytic perivascular infiltrate. Prominent exocytosis, vacuolar change in the basal layer and atypical lymphocytes are all not seen.

Course and Prognosis. The coarse of small-patch parapsoriasis is chronic. While the patients are not disturbed by their lesions, they are disturbed by the chronicity. Often the disease may wax and wane, improving in the summer, probably from natural sunlight. While long-term remissions are seen, they are the distinct exception. On the other hand, in our opinion, small-patch parapsoriasis is not a precursor of mycosis fungoides. Cases that are clinically typical and histologically bland do not convert and the patient can be reassured. Clinically or histologically atypical cases should be followed more closely.

Differential Diagnosis. The most common consideration is asteatotic dermatitis; small-patch parapsoriasis is more persistent. The most important differential diagnosis point is large-patch parapsoriasis, which can usually be distinguished by the clinical features discussed below, as well as the histology. Early cases may be confused with seborrheic dermatitis or nummular dermatitis, but these conditions are far more responsive to topical corticosteroids.

Therapy. There is no curative therapy. Topical corticosteroids bring temporary improvement; systemic corticosteroids are not warranted. We favor UVB radiation and short-term PUVA bath therapy; both produce improvement or clearing that lasts longer than that achieved with corticosteroids. In addition, many patients have dry skin and should be encouraged to use bath oils and lubricate their skin.

Large-Patch Parapsoriasis

Synonyms. Patch-stage mycosis fungoides, premalignant parapsoriasis

Definition. Early mycosis fungoides or cutaneous T cell lymphoma presenting with larger truncal patches, sometimes with pseudoatrophy and islands of normal skin.

Epidemiology. Most patients are middle-aged men. Once again, the disorder is uncommon.

Etiology and Pathogenesis. The etiology of mycosis fungoides is unknown. Various theories are discussed in Chap. 61.

Clinical Findings. The initial site is often the lower part of the trunk, buttocks, groin or axilla, although any body area can be involved. The breasts are a common site in females. At first only a small number of large irregular patches, often 8–10 cm in diameter, appear. They are erythematous, have a sharp border and may show pseudoatrophy (Fig. 14.42). When one carefully observes the lesions in appropriate light and manipulates the skin, a wrinkled skin surface is apparent suggesting atrophy, which cannot be substantiated by palpation or histologic examination. The patches are irregularly shaped and may have uninvolved areas inside their borders. They are erythematous, suggesting at least some infiltration by inflammatory cells. Lesions may slowly expand and new ones develop.

In most of those patients who live long enough, the disease evolves into frank mycosis fungoides. Danger signs include marked pruritus, palpable lesions (whether plaques or nodules, and whether within old lesions or appearing de novo) and lymphadenopathy. Rarely the lesions may show poikiloderma, which is also a sign of transition towards mycosis fungoides.

Histopathology. Early lesions may simply show minimal lymphocytic perivascular infiltrates without atypical lymphocytes or other characteristic changes. Often the first clue is subtle vacuolar change in the basal layer or modest epidermal atrophy. Later there may be a lichenoid pattern or exocytosis of lymphocytes. If Pautrier microabscesses or large cerebriform lymphocytes are found, the transition to mycosis fungoides has occurred. Often multiple biopsies over many years are needed to nail down the diagnosis. Modern molecular biologic investigations have generally identified clonality for the T cell receptor in the lymphocytes from large-patch parapsoriasis. Clonality alone cannot be taken as definitive proof of premalignancy or malignancy but it fits with the clinical course of this disease. Most cases of mycosis fungoides feature a helper T cell phenotype. Loss of pan-T cell markers usually occurs too late to be helpful.

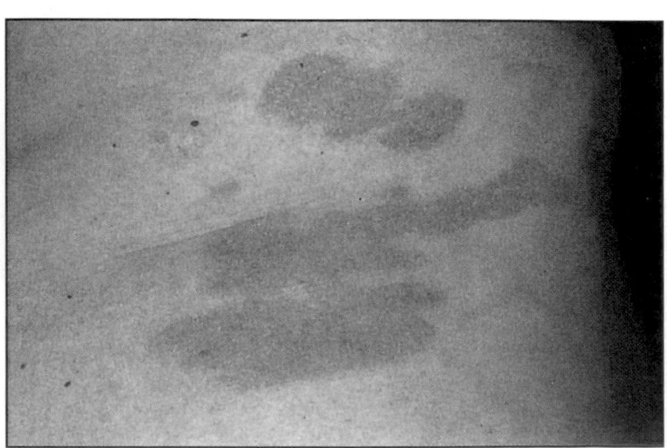

Fig. 14.42. Large-patch parapsoriasis

Laboratory Findings. The peripheral blood should be examined for Sézary cells. They are almost never present in the early stages of the disease but they should be periodically checked.

Course and Prognosis. The course of large-patch parapsoriasis is unpredictable. The disease in many patients evolves into mycosis fungoides, but the evolution can last 25 years. Recent studies have shown that carrying the diagnosis of large-patch parapsoriasis does not reduce one's life expectancy. Clinically most patients continue to develop new lesions but can be kept under fairly good control with a variety of therapeutic approaches. They require life-long surveillance.

Diagnostic Criteria. There is no sharp dividing line between large-patch parapsoriasis and mycosis fungoides. Most physicians are reluctant to unequivocally diagnosis mycosis fungoides, since it carries emotional and legal, i.e. insurance, implications for the patients, especially since there is little evidence that early recognition helps. Some use clinical criteria such as infiltration, nodules or poikiloderma; others wait until there is an unmistakable microscopic picture. Repeated clinical examinations and biopsies are the key to the correct diagnosis.

Differential Diagnosis. The main differential diagnostic point is small-patch parapsoriasis. The presence of infiltrates, larger lesions containing patches of normal skin, poikiloderma or typical histology leads one in the right direction. There are no other chronic diseases that resemble large-patch parapsoriasis, other than the variants discussed below.

Therapy. The most important question in large-patch parapsoriasis is: when do we treat the disease like a lymphoma? There are still two schools of thought:

- Treat aggressively at the first suspicion of mycosis fungoides, going for a total cure. Such physicians employ total body electron beam or X-ray radiation or chemotherapy early in the disease.
- Do no harm and treat conservatively for as long as possible, using topical corticosteroids or UV

radiation initially and then advancing to PUVA bath or PUVA therapy. Topical nitrogen mustard is another possibility.

We belong to the latter school, since so few patients who are aggressively treated enjoy long-term benefits. All of these possibilities are considered in greater detail in Chap. 61 where we deal with mycosis fungoides.

Poikilodermatous Large-Patch Parapsoriasis

Synonyms. Poikilodermia atrophicans vasculare (Jacobi 1906), prereticulotic parapsoriasis

Definition. Variant of large-patch parapsoriasis with clinical poikiloderma and a greater likelihood of malignant change.

Etiology and Pathogenesis. The etiology is unknown. We view this disease and the next closely related disorder, parakeratosis variegata, as variants of large-patch parapsoriasis and thus as initial mycosis fungoides.

Clinical Findings. Poikiloderma can best be remembered as a skin condition in which there is a rainbow of changes with hypo- and hyperpigmentation, telangiectases (or erythema) and atrophy. In this very uncommon variant, patients have large patches of poikiloderma, in the same distribution and with the same age and sex pattern as large-patch parapsoriasis. Often the initial lesion is simply erythematous but over a period of 1–2 years the poikilodermatous features evolve (Fig. 14.43). In contrast to connective tissue disorders, there is no sclerosis and no relation to areas of light exposure. The lesions are usually asymptomatic, but in a high percentage of cases, pruritus or infiltration augur the conversion to mycosis fungoides.

Histopathology. The changes and problems are the same as with large-patch parapsoriasis. Lesions usually show epidermal atrophy and telangiectases, but also vacuolar change in the basal layer.

Differential Diagnosis. Poikiloderma (Chap. 18) can be associated with a variety of congenital disorders, be a result of skin damage and healing or appear spontaneously in adult life associated with connective tissue disorders or mycosis fungoides.

Therapy. The approach is identical to that in large-patch parapsoriasis.

Parakeratosis Variegata

(Unna et al. 1890)

Synonyms. Parapsoriasis lichenoides (Brocq 1902), lichen variegatus (Radcliffe-Crocker 1900), retiform parapsoriasis

Definition. A persistent erythematosquamous disorder with lichenoid papules initially arranged in a linear pattern and evolving into a net-like pattern with associated atrophy, also viewed as a variant of large-patch parapsoriasis.

Epidemiology. This is a very rare variant of an already uncommon disorder.

Clinical Findings. While the distribution of parakeratosis variegata is identical to large-patch parapsoriasis, the individual lesions rarely show atrophy. Instead, they consist of numerous small smooth papules, are often arranged in linear, annular or net-like patterns. As they evolve they leave behind

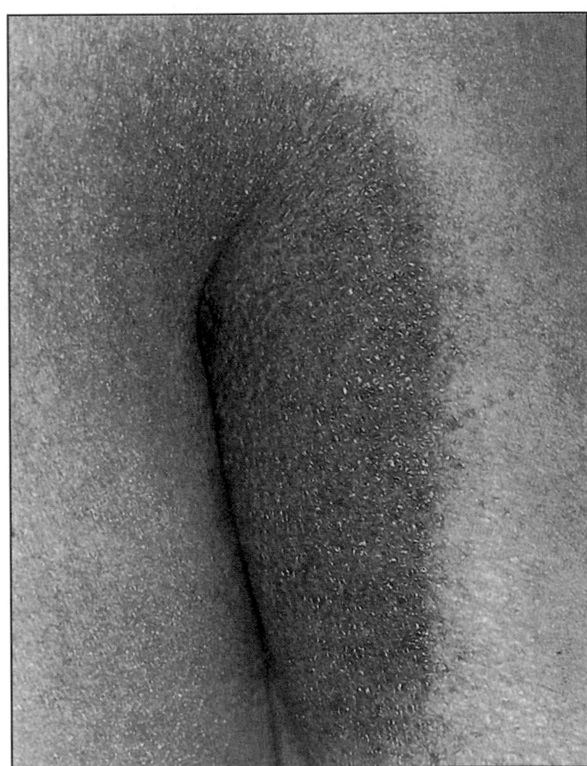

Fig. 14.43. Poikilodermatous large-patch parapsoriasis

a patterned hyperpigmentation. Telangiectases may also be seen, so the picture is one of poikiloderma but with papules and patterning. Between the papules and discoloration, small areas of normal skin remain. The eruption is usually asymptomatic. Alopecia may develop, both on the scalp and body.

Histopathology. The findings are very similar to those in large-patch parapsoriasis but the infiltrate not surprisingly tends to be more lichenoid and there is incontinence of pigment. In addition, dilated vessels may be seen in the papillary dermis. Once again, control biopsies are needed to exclude mycosis fungoides.

Course and Prognosis. The disease is very persistent, hard to treat and often evolves into mycosis fungoides.

Differential Diagnosis. The same problems as with large-patch parapsoriasis and its poikilodermatous variant exist here. In addition, lichen planus and erythema dyschromicum perstans must be considered in the early stages of the disease. Mucosal and nail involvement do not occur with parakeratosis variegata.

Therapy. PUVA bath and PUVA therapy seem to be most effective. Topical corticosteroids may bring temporary relief in the few cases that are symptomatic.

Papuloerythroderma

(Ofuji et al. 1984)

Papuloerythroderma is a rare disease of unknown etiology that may progress to a cutaneous malignant lymphoma. Its relationship to atopic dermatitis and psoriasis has been discussed but the clinical features are relatively distinct. Most patients are elderly men. It is characterized by intense pruritus and flat-topped red papules that characteristically spare the skin folds. The lesions have a cobblestone pattern, almost covering the skin, but not coalescing and leaving spared lines where folds occur. The histologic pattern is one of subacute dermatitis with dense lymphocytic perivascular infiltrates, often admixed with eosinophils, and usually favoring the papillary dermis. There may be associated eosinophilia and elevated IgE levels. The most effective treatment appears to be UV radiation or PUVA, perhaps combined with systemic corticosteroids when therapy is initiated. In the largest series of 17 patients, the disease in two patients evolved into definite mycosis fungoides, while two others had microscopic findings compatible with mycosis fungoides.

Erythroderma

(Baxter 1879; Montgomery 1933)

Synonym. Exfoliative dermatitis

Erythroderma refers to skin that is diffusely red and inflamed with varying degrees and types of scaling. There are many causes of erythroderma, but the most common are exacerbations of underlying skin diseases, drug reactions and underlying malignancies, primarily mycosis fungoides. Usually more than 90% of the skin is involved, but the residual islands of normal skin may be of great importance in the clinical diagnosis. For example, pityriasis rubra pilaris and mycosis fungoides are characterized by such spared areas. The scales may vary greatly, coming off in sheets in acute drug-induced erythroderma, but being smaller or finer in psoriasis or pityriasis rubra pilaris. Pruritus is common and often unbearable.

Unlike many other dermatologic disorders, erythroderma has profound effects on the entire body. The widespread inflammatory response, increased blood flow and marked desquamation all take their toll. The skin is usually infiltrated by a wide range of inflammatory cells that release a barrage of cytokines influencing virtually every organ. The vasodilatation and increased blood flow lead to chills and impaired temperature control. Hypothermia is a possible complication, especially when the patient lands in an air-conditioned hospital room. Increased evaporation, made possible by increased blood flow and damaged epidermal barriers, leads to dehydration and fluid problems. The basal metabolic rate is increased, often then calling into play secondary endocrine control mechanisms. Protein loss in the form of desquamation and exudation is significant, resulting in hypoproteinemia. Scales alone may account for up to 10 g/m^2 of protein loss daily. Typically there is hypoalbuminemia with a relative increase in immunoglobulins, especially γ-globulins. Protein-losing enteropathy may also lead to reduced levels of iron, folic acid and other vitamins, often producing a profound anemia. Cardiovascular, renal and hepatic complications are common. Both hair and nails are influenced by the increased demands; thus, telogen effluvium and transverse nail bands are expected. In more severe cases, anagen effluvium and even acute nail loss may occur.

If the erythroderma persists for any period of time, the patient's general condition will decline seriously. In the past, patients often died from erythroderma. Today far more advanced supportive care and to a lesser extent better diagnosis and care for the underlying skin condition have made this a rarity. A drug-induced erythroderma usually improves dramatically when the offending agent is identified and stopped. Occasionally it may evolve into toxic epidermal necrolysis, but even such patients do well with supportive care. Cases associated with malignancies tend to follow the underlying disease. Patients with erythroderma associated with a chronic skin disease such as psoriasis tend to be chronic. They improve but often relapse and often go for months or years on the verge of erythroderma. Clearly the prognosis too depends on the cause of the erythroderma.

Diagnostic Approach

The clinical diagnosis of erythroderma is usually straightforward. The issue is deciding what triggered or caused the problem. One can distinguish between primary and secondary erythroderma. In primary erythroderma, the condition arises on normal skin, usually as part of a drug reaction or as a marker for a malignancy, most often a malignant lymphoma. In secondary erythroderma, an underlying skin disease, e.g. psoriasis, atopic dermatitis or seborrheic dermatitis, flares, spreading to involve the entire skin. Finally, there are cases in which neither an underlying skin disease nor an exogenous trigger is identified.

In a study of about 200 erythrodermic patients, the distribution was as shown in Table 14.8. The following points should be considered in trying to narrow down the causes:

- History. The existence of a previous skin disease and how it was treated are crucial. In addition, a careful drug history and general history are needed. The age of the patient also plays a role: in infancy atopic dermatitis is common; in the elderly, one should think of seborrheic dermatitis. Table 14.9 indicates the different likely causes in different age groups.
- Clinical Features. One must search carefully for subtle signs of an underlying disease, such as gluteal cleft, nail or scalp involvement in psoriasis, various stigmata in atopic dermatitis, oral involvement in lichen planus or islands of sparing in pityriasis rubra pilaris. Many patients have lymphadenopathy which, while usually reactive or dermatopathic, may reflect an underlying lymphoma. If the diagnosis is unclear, a lymph node biopsy should be considered.
- Histopathology. One or even several skin biopsies should be done. While it sometimes dramatically solves the puzzle, it may be nondiagnostic. Usually the biopsy will allow one to rule out

Table 14.8. Causes of erythroderma

Type	Percent
Primary erythroderma	20
Secondary erythroderma	80
Psoriasis	25
Drug reaction	16
Atopic dermatitis	13
Allergic contact dermatitis	9
Seborrheic dermatitis	8
Internal malignancy	5
Others	4

Based on Thestrup-Pedersen K et al. 1988

Table 14.9. Likely causes of erythroderma in various age groups

Newborns	Ichthyosis (usually lamellar or bullous ichthyosiform erythroderma) Staphylococcal scalded skin syndrome Leiner disease Disseminated candidiasis Immunodeficiency disorders
Children	Atopic dermatitis Pityriasis rubra pilaris Psoriasis Staphylococcal scalded skin syndrome
Adults	Drug reactions Psoriasis Seborrheic dermatitis Atopic dermatitis Hematologic malignancies Pityriasis rubra pilaris Lichen planus Pemphigus foliaceus Crusted scabies

cutaneous T cell lymphoma. Epidermal necrosis should suggest early perhaps unexpected toxic epidermal necrolysis. Specific clues to psoriasis, atopic dermatitis or other dermatoses are usually blurred by the inflammation. One finds spongiosis, lymphocytic perivascular inflammation and edema. Later on parakeratosis or frank scale is found.

- General Evaluation. The patient should be carefully evaluated for underlying disease. Useful approaches include chest X-ray, computerized tomography of abdomen, pelvis and thorax, routine blood evaluation, iron and folic acid levels, immunoelectrophoresis, and perhaps bone marrow examination. The presence of a pre-existing dermatologic condition obviously narrows the search and allows one to avoid many steps in the diagnostic workup.

Types of Erythroderma

Drug-Induced Erythroderma

While many different agents can cause erythroderma, there are some notorious bad actors including phenytoin, carbamazepine, captopril, phenindione, cimetidine, diltiazem, nitrofurantoin, isoniazid, antimalarial agents, lithium salts and gold salts. Drug reactions usually appear first as macular exanthems that over time coalesce into erythroderma. They tend to improve promptly when the suspected agent is stopped, although they may still smolder for days to weeks. Sometimes they may present more rapidly with widespread erythema. Either type may develop blisters and even evolve into toxic epidermal necrolysis.

Another type of drug-induced erythroderma is allergic contact dermatitis. When the reaction is severe enough, the process may spread outside the areas where the offending agent was applied. This is referred to as hematogenous spread, which is not surprising since allergic contact dermatitis is mediated through circulating lymphocytes. Typical examples include poison ivy or a severe reaction to neomycin in a patient with a stasis ulcer who does not suspect a drug reaction and continues to apply the antibiotic as the allergic contact dermatitis blooms.

Erythroderma Caused by Underlying Dermatoses

About 60 % of erythroderma cases are caused by an exacerbation of an underlying dermatosis. In most instances, the characteristic signs of the skin disease are obscured by the intense inflammation, but often clues are to be found in the history or on the oral mucosa or nails. While all of the diseases that have been reported to cause erythroderma would form a long list, most cases in our experience come from one of the following disorders, all of which are covered in more detail elsewhere in the text.

- Atopic Dermatitis. In younger patients, this is the most likely cause of erythroderma. Usually a history of atopy is present. Pruritus is often extreme and associated secondary infections induced by scratching are common. Well-known atopic stigmata such as Dennie-Morgan lines, palmar hyperlinearity, or nail changes may help in the clinical diagnosis.
- Psoriasis. While generalized pustular psoriasis is the usual precursor of psoriatic erythroderma, ordinary psoriasis can also worsen and involve the entire body. Often too-aggressive therapy is responsible for the latter scenario, which develops more slowly than the pustular psoriasis outbreak. Psoriatic erythroderma with dwarfism is extremely uncommon.
- Pityriasis Rubra Pilaris. While this disease is uncommon in both children and adults, it accounts for a disproportionate share of the erythroderma cases. It seems as if almost every patient with classic pityriasis rubra pilaris experiences erythroderma at least once. The presence of islands of sparing with keratotic papules at their periphery and of thickened palms and soles are two good clinical clues.
- Seborrheic Dermatitis. When the elderly and infirm are either unable to care for their scalp and skin or are in a nursing home where such care is not adequate, their previously easily managed seborrheic dermatitis may flare dramatically. In this population, seborrheic dermatitis is one of the most common precursors of erythroderma, although one should always search carefully for an underlying malignancy and evaluate the drugs carefully, as often the history of seborrheic dermatitis leads one away from the correct diagnosis.
- Lichen Planus. The nails and oral mucosa are the best places to search for clues to lichen planus. The erythroderma is a very rare complication often reflecting over-aggressive treatment.
- Pemphigus Foliaceus. The face and upper part of the chest are most often involved. While pemphigus foliaceus is a blistering disorder, it may present primarily with erythroderma. Clues include moist

scaling, occasional circular areas of scaling that represent attempts at blister formation and generally a long history of some sort of facial rash.

- Crusted Scabies. Infections with *Sarcoptes scabiei* may lead to very widespread disease, particularly in elderly, handicapped or immunodeficient patients. Those with HIV/AIDS are also at risk. Not surprisingly, the pruritus is extreme. While one can speak of erythroderma, there is usually massive crusting, especially on the hands and feet. Often there is an eosinophilia. Often nursing personnel or acquaintances are also itching. Inappropriate care may also worsen the erythroderma. The *S. scabiei* are present in huge numbers and easily identified.

Erythroderma Associated with Hematologic Malignancies

Erythroderma from mycosis fungoides can be viewed as a flare of an underlying disease or as a sign of a T cell lymphoma. No matter what the perspective, classic large-patch parapsoriasis or early mycosis fungoides can evolve into widespread cutaneous disease with erythroderma. This conversion is a bad prognostic sign. Another similar problem is the Sézary syndrome, in which the patient is by definition erythrodermic, has circulating malignant T cells and lymphadenopathy. Biopsies of the skin and lymph nodes usually help establish the nature of the disease.

In contrast, erythroderma can also be a paraneoplastic marker for a wide range of hematologic malignancies, and even rarely for other tumors. In such cases, the onset is more rapid and there is no history of precursor lesions. The histologic examination of the lymph nodes or other tissue is crucial, because the skin changes are rarely caused by infiltrating tumor cells.

Idiopathic Erythroderma

This group is estimated as comprising between 10% and 20% of the total. In the past diagnoses such as Wilson-Brocq erythroderma or pityriasis rubra of Hebra were made. Today it is unclear if such terms make sense. In most cases of erythroderma, if one searches adequately and follows the patient long enough, a cause becomes evident. Occasionally it is tempting to say idiopathic but simply admitting one's own inability to solve the particular problem might be more appropriate. We rarely and reluctantly employ this diagnosis.

Therapy. The treatment of erythroderma is complicated. First, one must support the patient. This requires fluid restoration, often parenteral nutrition, vitamin supplements and careful monitoring at a minimum. If renal or cardiac failure occurs, it must be treated appropriately. If marked skin loss occurs, burn precautions should be instituted and the patient transferred to a burn unit. Second, if there is an underlying malignancy, then it must be found and treated. Finally, if an underlying skin disease is present, it should be treated indifferently at first and later in a more specific fashion. Remember that over-aggressive topical therapy is often the trigger for erythroderma.

Lichen Planus and Lichenoid Diseases

There is a long list of diseases that present with small papules, often pruritic. Since the prototype is lichen planus, they are called lichenoid. Some diseases are called lichenoid because they feature prominent skin markings as a result of prolonged rubbing, a picture known as lichenification. Yet other disorders are called lichenoid because of histologic similarities to lichen planus, that is the presence of a band-like lymphocytic infiltrate at the epidermal-dermal junction. Many of these only remotely related disorders are considered in this section.

Lichen Planus

(Wilson 1869)

Definition. Noninfectious, clinically and histologically typical, pruritic papular disease that often shows mucosal involvement and less frequently nail dystrophies or scarring alopecia.

Epidemiology. Lichen planus is a relatively common disease. In most clinics and practices, about 1% of the patients are affected. The prevalence in one study was around 0.5%. The average age of onset is about 40 years and there may be a slight female predominance.

Etiology and Pathogenesis. The etiology of lichen planus is a mystery. Two clues have emerged in recent years. First, lichen planus has striking clinical, histologic and immunologic similarities to graft versus host disease. In addition, a clear association between lichen planus and chronic hepatic disease has emerged, especially in Italy but also in studies from other countries including Germany. It is possible that altered hepatocytes express or mimic some basement membrane zone antigen inducing a cytotoxic T cell response against the region. Associations with HLA-B3 and -B5 have been suggested. Primary biliary cirrhosis, chronic active hepatitis and both hepatitis B and C have been associated with lichen planus.

In addition, some lichen planus is caused by medications. The classic example is gold salts; many other lichenoid drug eruptions are discussed in Chapter 10. Color film developing chemicals are also occasionally responsible. Finally, lichen planus is often blamed on emotional factors. However, patients with such an intensely pruritic rash are likely to be distraught and miserable, so the validity of such studies remains unclear.

Clinical Findings. Two hallmarks of lichen planus are intense pruritus and the presence of the Köbner phenomenon. Surprisingly, despite the pruritus, excoriations are rare, as the patients tend to rub, not scratch.

The typical lesion of lichen planus is a small smooth violaceous flat-topped papule (Fig. 14.44).

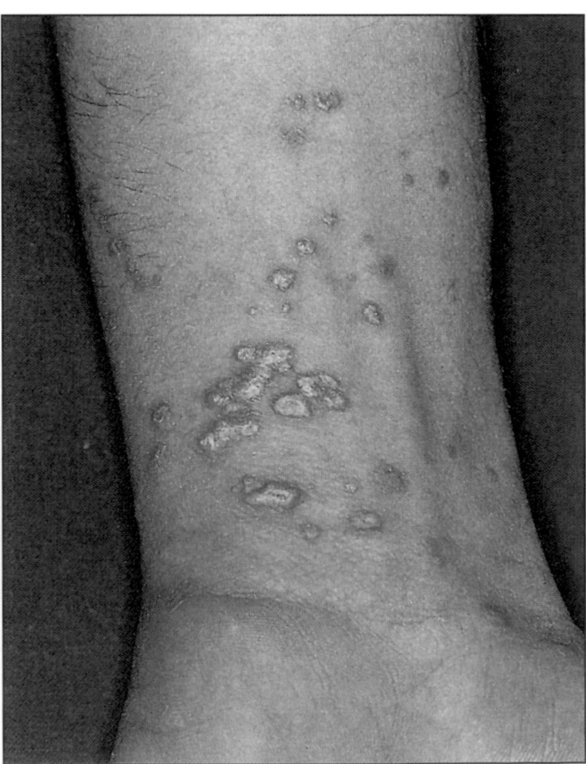

Fig. 14.44. Lichen planus

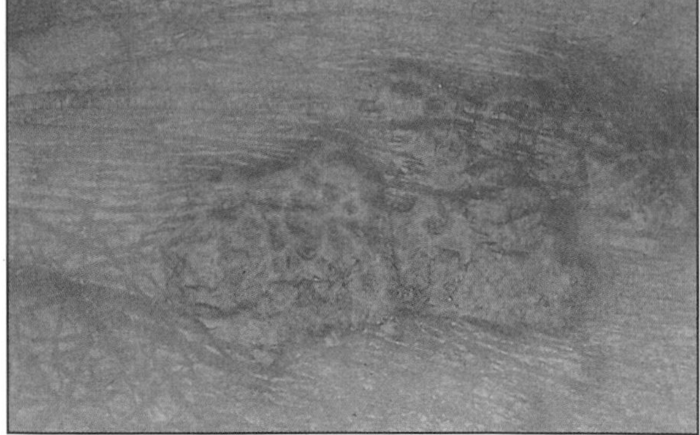

Fig. 14.45. Lichen planus with Wickham striae

The papules tend to coalesce producing patches, as the name lichen suggests; the grouped papules have some resemblance to growths on a tree or rock. Even the larger lesions are flat-topped, like a plateau in geologic terms. In addition, they are bordered by skin lines, so they have a polygonal shape. The surface often glistens. When one examines the surface carefully, the classic Wickham striae can be seen as a lacy network of fine white lines representing focal thickening of the granular layer (Fig. 14.45). While the color can be red, it is usually more red–blue or violet. Resolved lesions usually leave a brown postinflammatory hyperpigmentation. There are many clinical variants of lichen planus; these are summarized in Table 14.10 and discussed in the following paragraphs. Any one patient may have

Table 14.10. Clinical variants of lichen planus

Cutaneous lesions	Typical
	Elderly
	Localized
	Annular
	Linear
	Hypertrophic
	Nodular
	Atrophic
	Bullous
	Erosive
	Actinic
	Palmar-plantar
	Lupus erythematosus overlap
Appendageal	Nail
	Hair
	Lichen planopilaris (scalp)
	Follicular (elsewhere)
Mucosal	Oral
	Genital
	Anal

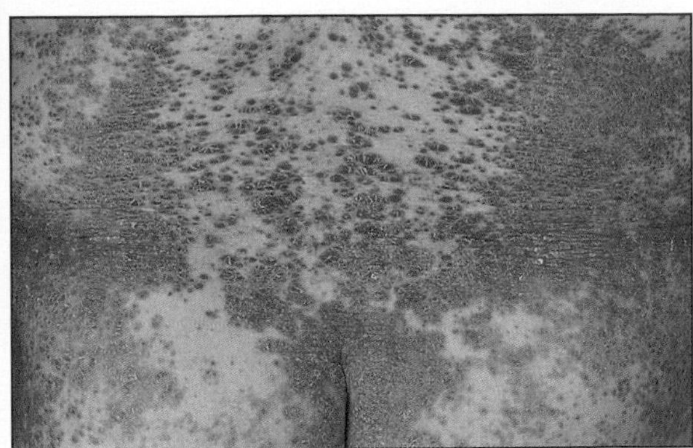

Fig. 14.46. Eruptive lichen planus

several forms, and many patients with skin disease have oral involvement, so the categories should in no way be taken as exclusive. They simplify the description of this protean disorder.

Eruptive Lichen Planus

In the typical patient, the individual lesions are for the most part distinct, although some may coalesce. The sites of predilection include the inner aspects of the wrists and the backs of the feet; other common sites include the neck, forearms, shins, genitalia and anal region. The trunk may also be involved, especially in those patients whose disease seems to run a more acute course and disseminates rapidly (Fig. 14.46). This form is also known as exanthematous lichen planus. In such patients the disease may rarely evolve into erythroderma. The face is almost never involved. One should always check for oral and nail disease as clues to the correct diagnosis. The course is usually self-limited, with perhaps 75% of patients clearing in 1 year and over 90% clearing in 2 years.

Localized Lichen Planus

Such patients have a limited number of larger plaques, often quite thick and infiltrated, with occasional typical papules at their periphery. The most common site is the shin, although the penis, neck and lower portion of the back are also common sites. The solitary lesions are more chronic and display prominent hyperpigmentation, but oral involvement is uncommon. On the shins, especially in Asians, one must consider lichen amyloidosus in the differential diagnosis.

Annular Lichen Planus

Lichen planus must be considered in the differential diagnosis of annular lesions. If one observed even a small papule, it may show a central dell, suggesting clearing. As larger plaques evolve, they too may be annular with central clearing, often with some hyperpigmentation.

Linear Lichen Planus

This very uncommon type of lichen planus presents with linear streaks of grouped papules, reaching for example from the axilla to the wrist or from the buttock down the leg. When the lesions follow Blaschko lines, the lichen planus is whorled or patterned. Presumably there is a somatic mutation in the involved regions. The differential diagnosis is extensive including ILVEN (inflammatory linear verrucous epidermal nevus), lichen striatus, linear psoriasis and lichen striatus. Histologic evaluation is usually necessary to decide the diagnosis, although clinical clues (nature of individual papules, mucosal or nail disease) may help.

Hypertrophic Lichen Planus

Hypertrophic or verrucous lichen planus is similar to the localized form. The most common site of involvement is the shin or dorsal aspect of the foot (Fig. 14.47). The lesions are intensely pruritic and this may be the type of lichen planus that is truly scratched, so that the prominent hyperkeratotic changes may be secondary. In any event, the thick lesions have marked scales that obliterate the fine markings so characteristic of the disorder. Sometimes the hyperkeratosis is more prominent around

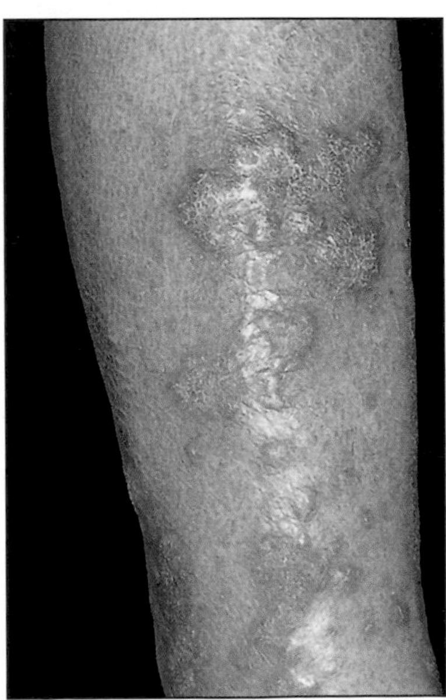

Fig. 14.47. Hypertrophic lichen planus

the follicles. Many patients have chronic venous insufficiency. If the lesions heal, they often do so with scarring. Malignant change has been described in hypertrophic lichen planus, just as it has in oral lichen planus. Both lichen simplex chronicus and a lichenified dermatitis must be excluded; usually the biopsy is distinctive.

Nodular Lichen Planus

Sometimes, the larger individual lesions may become nodular, so that one must think of prurigo nodularis. In the past, this form was called lichen planus obtusus, but the term has fallen into deserved ignominy.

Atrophic Lichen Planus

While lichen planus typically heals without any sequelae, except for postinflammatory hyperpigmentation, there is a significant dermal infiltrate so it is not surprising that occasionally atrophy develops. The lower aspects of the legs are the most common site. Typically small papules are replaced by tiny white depressed areas in which hairs and follicular openings are absent. Such lesions can coalesce or result from resolution of a larger plaque; then they mimic lichen sclerosus et atrophicus or even early disseminated morphea. Once again, a history of lichen planus elsewhere and the biopsy are decisive.

Bullous Lichen Planus

We distinguish between bullous lichen planus in which vesicles or bullae arise within the lesions of lichen planus and lichen planus pemphigoides in which the bullae arise in normal skin. Since there is an intense infiltrate at the epidermal-dermal junction, it is not surprising that separation may occur, producing a blister. Often when a biopsy specimen from lichen planus is processed, the epidermis and dermis become separated. On the oral mucosa, lichen planus is usually bullous, although most often only erosions are seen.

When lichen planus pemphigoides patients are evaluated, they appear to represent an overlap between bullous pemphigoid and lichen planus. Deposition of immunoglobulins and complement components at the basement membrane zone is found, but the circulating antibodies appear to react with a 200-kDa antigen along with the 180-kDa bullous pemphigoid II antigen.

Erosive Lichen Planus

In areas of trauma, such as on the plantar surface or between the toes, erosions may develop. They are very painful, chronic and heal poorly. When just ulcerations are present, the diagnosis of lichen planus is almost impossible; one must hope for clues elsewhere. Erosive lichen planus may be combined lichen planopilaris.

Actinic Lichen Planus

This variant is more common in tropical or subtropical areas, especially in the Middle East. It typically occurs on the sun-exposed areas of the face, neck and dorsal surfaces of the hands (Fig. 14.48). Most patients are children or young adults. Lesions may flare in the spring months in patients who live where the climate is seasonal. Similarly resolution may occur in the less sunny months. The facial lesions may resemble melasma. Whether this is best viewed as a lichenoid form of polymorphic light eruption or as a photosensitive variant of lichen planus is unclear. Summertime actinic lichenoid eruption features tiny papules and is discussed under lichen nitidus.

Palmoplantar Lichen Planus

This is one of the most disabling, painful and therapy-resistant variants of lichen planus. Verrucous or hyperkeratotic plaques are present on the palms

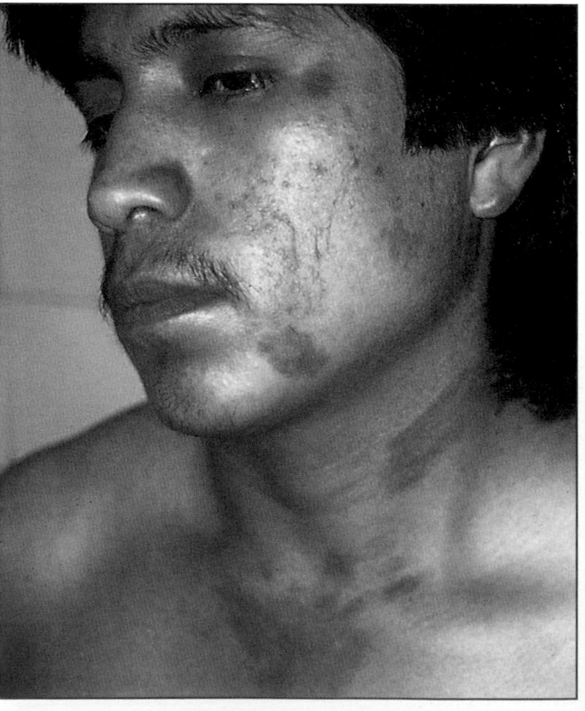

Fig. 14.48. Actinic lichen planus (courtesy of Juan J. Ochoa, MD, Chihuahua, Mexico)

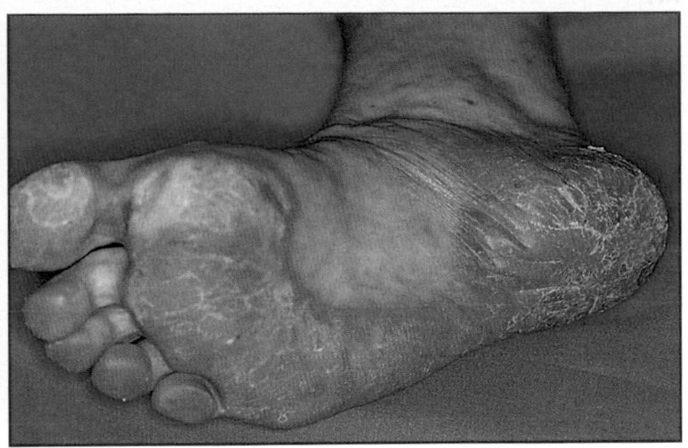

Fig. 14.49. Plantar hypertrophic lichen planus

and soles, often on the lateral borders but also on pressure points. The individual lesions simply appear hyperkeratotic, often with a yellow hue and often with little suggestion of lichen planus (Fig. 14.49). There may be associated ulcerations. The differential diagnostic list is long, including calluses, clavi, warts, hyperkeratotic palmoplantar dermatitis, porokeratosis, hyperkeratotic tinea pedis and even secondary syphilis.

Lichen Planus-Lupus Erythematosus Overlap

Both lichen planus and lupus erythematosus are relatively common disorders involving the epidermal-dermal junction. An overlap condition has been described, primarily in blacks. Whether it represents a variant of one of the two disorders (and if so, which one) or simply the unlucky coincidence of two similar disorders is unresolved.

Lichen Planus of the Nails

Nail involvement is often a valuable clinical clue in lichen planus. Not only do about 10% of patients have changes, but also on occasion the nail changes may be isolated. A wide variety of changes may be seen including longitudinal ridging, splitting, irregular pits, subungual hyperkeratoses and nail thinning. The end-stage of lichen planus of the nails is a pterygium. Often if the associated skin disease resolves, the nail damage may be arrested but often with irreversible scarring. Twenty-nail dystrophy may in some cases represent isolated nail lichen planus (Chap. 32).

Lichen Planopilaris

Scalp involvement with lichen planus leads to characteristic erythematous infiltrates around the follicular openings associated with scarring alopecia (Chap. 31). Some immunologic studies suggest differences between typical lichen planus and lichen planopilaris, but the presence of scalp disease in patients with ordinary lesions elsewhere suggests a unity. Sometimes only scalp disease is seen. Women seem to be more often affected. On the scalp, the main differential diagnostic question is lupus erythematosus. Often both routine histologic evaluation and immunofluorescent examination are required.

Follicular Lichen Planus

Follicular lichen planus presents with numerous red to red-brown hyperkeratotic papules each centered around a hair follicle. The lesions can coalesce into larger plaques. The term lichen planus acuminatus has also been used. While there is little clinical resemblance to ordinary lichen planus, typical lesions may be found elsewhere on the skin, scalp or mucosa and the histologic features are similar. The pebbly skin surface resembles a kitchen grater. Typical sites include the flexural surfaces of the extremities (inverse lichen planus), the neck, inner aspects of the thighs and sacral region. The association of follicular lesions, ordinary lichen planus and alopecia often with scarring is known as the Lasseur-Graham Little syndrome (LITTLE 1930). The differential diagnosis is once again different, including pityriasis rubra pilaris, follicular psoriasis, lichen trichophyticus, lichen syphiliticus and lichen scrophulosorum, but the biopsy is fairly distinct.

Oral Lichen Planus

While everyone agrees oral lichen planus is common, dermatologists and oral pathologists have different opinions. Most dermatologists suggest that about 50% of their patients have oral disease, but oral pathologists usually report that relatively few of their patients have cutaneous lesions. In addition, many patients have asymptomatic oral disease discovered by the dermatologist, while most dental patients have painful, ulcerative problems.

In the mouth, the typical papules of lichen planus are not seen. In addition, Wickham striae are larger, easily visible as lacy networks traversing primarily the buccal mucosa and vermilion but also seen on the gingiva and tongue (Fig. 14.50). The most common finding is painful erosions that may evolve into flat ulcerations. These lesions are difficult to treat, may heal with scarring in one area and then appear in another, and appear to be precancerous with a low but real risk of squamous cell carcinoma. Verrucous or fungating lesions may develop; they often represent a low-grade squamous cell carcinoma. Oral lupus erythematosus may appear quite similar, as may allergic contact stomatitis to dental materials.

Genital Lichen Planus

About 20% of male patients with lichen planus have genital lesions, with the glans the most common site. Both groups of small papules or a larger plaque may be seen. Annular lesions are also typically on the glans (Fig. 14.51). Typical papules may be seen on the shaft or scrotum; they clarify the diagnosis. Both psoriasis and lichen planus may present in young adults with no other cutaneous findings. Other possibilities include plasma cell balanitis of Zoon, erythroplasia of Queyrat and more acute problems such as candidiasis or secondary syphilis. Genital lichen planus in women tends to mimic oral disease, with lacy white streaks and erosions on the labia minora. Lichen planus is an uncommon cause of pruritus vulvae.

Anal Lichen Planus

In the perianal region lichen planus can be responsible for intense pruritus often with subtle physical findings. Papules are rare. Usually there is only a white shimmer to the skin or Wickham striae are seen. Uncovering inapparent lichen planus is perhaps one reason to do a biopsy in patients with pruritus ani.

Histopathology. Despite all of these quite different clinical variants, the histologic picture in lichen planus is relatively uniform. The key feature is a band-like infiltrate of T cells at the epidermal-dermal junction. The epidermis may be acanthotic with compact hyperkeratosis and focal wedge-shaped hyperplasia of the granular layer, which produces the Wickham striae. While most lesions show acanthosis, this will vary in hypertrophic or atrophic regions. The basal layer shows vacuolar change, along with colloid bodies, reflecting damaged often dyskeratotic keratinocytes. The rete ridges are often partially effaced by the infiltrate and the papillae somewhat widened, producing a classic saw-tooth pattern along the epidermal-dermal junction. In addition, the infiltrate may weaken the adhesion between the epidermis and dermis, producing small clefts. In older lesions, there is incontinence of pigment with melanin in dermal macrophages.

Biopsies from the scalp show a lymphocytic infiltrate extending into the dermis along the follicle, as well as follicular plugging and perifollicular fibrosis. In older lesions, only scarred tracts may be seen. Oral lesions typically lack most of the features of lichen planus. A nonulcerated white area should be sampled.

Immunofluorescent examination may reveal deposition of immunoglobulin and complement components at the epidermal-dermal junction. The PAS-positive colloid bodies also light up with this technique, but the changes are not specific enough to allow a definite diagnosis.

Course and Prognosis. The course of lichen planus is highly unpredictable. Eruptive lichen planus usually resolves in 6–12 months. Over 95% of patients are clear after 2 years and recurrences are uncommon. The most persistent forms of lichen planus are the hypertrophic and oral versions. In addition, lichen planopilaris usually leads to scarring alopecia and the nail damage is typically permanent.

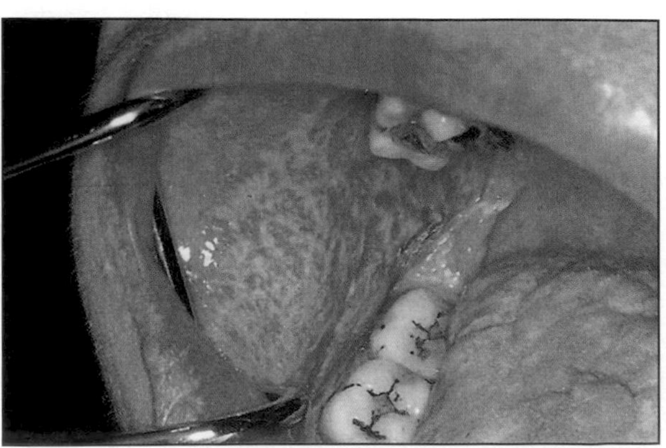

Fig. 14.50. Oral lichen planus

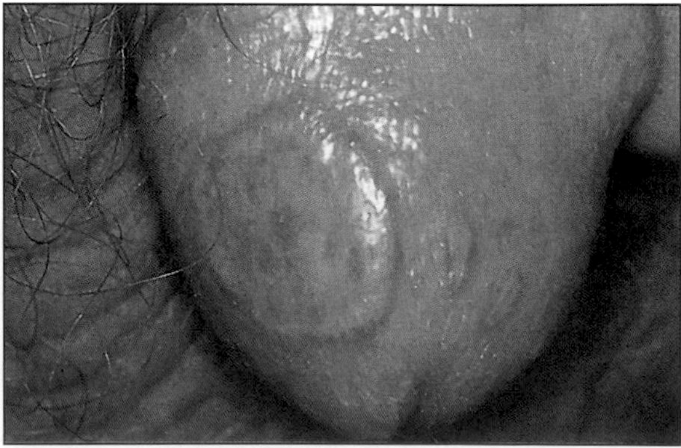

Fig. 14.51. Penile lichen planus

Differential Diagnosis. The differential diagnosis varies greatly depending on the type of lichen planus and has been discussed under the various variants. The histologic differential diagnosis is also challenging. Lichenoid drug eruptions usually contain some eosinophils and rarely reproduce perfectly classic lichen planus. They may have parakeratosis or lack the focal granular layer changes. However, in many instances, one must simply diagnose a lichenoid reaction pattern without being able to distinguish between lichen planus and a drug reaction.

Therapy. Lichen planus is a hard disease to treat. It is a persistent problem and most often the best one can achieve is an amelioration of symptoms until resolution occurs.

Systemic. The best-evaluated systemic therapy for cutaneous lichen planus is acitretin, although we suspect corticosteroids are most widely used. While the preferred approach is acitretin (25–50 mg daily), isotretinoin (0.3–0.5 mg/kg daily) can also be employed. We have found even lower doses of retinoids effective in oral disease.

Systemic corticosteroids do tend to suppress the inflammation and reduce pruritus. It is appropriate early in the disease course to use prednisone 20–40 mg daily for several weeks with reduction of dosage or switch to alternate-day therapy as soon as improvement is seen. Sometimes if one suppresses the disease early on, it will not recur as the corticosteroids are slowly tapered. In addition, topical therapy will be easier. Intramuscular triamcinolone acetonide 40 mg given once or twice at a 6-week interval is another approach. Often, lichen planus recurs as the corticosteroid effects wear off and one should not commit the patient to chronic therapy.

In oral disease and more severe cutaneous disease, a number of other agents have been employed with success including cyclosporine (2.5 mg/kg daily). While cyclosporine appears effective, the risk/benefit ratio and its suitability for chronic use must be weighed.

Many other systemic approaches have been recommended, including antimalarials, griseofulvin, antibiotics and isoniazid. It is unclear if any of these really bring any benefit or simply capitalize on the tendency of lichen planus to remit spontaneously. Antihistamines can be prescribed for the pruritus but they are often disappointing. Low molecular weight heparin has also be endorsed recently. Used as a monotherapy it relieved itch in many patients with lichen planus within 2 weeks.

Topical. Corticosteroids are the mainstay of topical therapy. One should employ high- to ultrahigh-potency forms, especially early in the disease to suppress inflammation. Lichen planus is one pruritic dermatosis where topical corticosteroids are effective in relieving itch. For isolated or hyperkeratotic lesions, corticosteroids under occlusion, corticosteroid-impregnated tapes or intralesional triamcinolone acetonide 2.5–5.0 mg/ml can be employed. As alternative approaches, one can try tars, anthralin or ichthammol but none compares to corticosteroids.

On the scalp, corticosteroid lotions and solutions are the best choice. In the mouth topical corticosteroids are the treatment of choice. Triamcinolone acetonide is available in adherent bases such as Orabase. The adherent bases are messy and patients dislike the glue-like texture. We tend to employ higher potency corticosteroid gels which are better tolerated. Lozenges containing corticosteroids are also available in some countries. As a final trick, a piece of gauze may be covered with a corticosteroid cream and placed against a lesion for 10 min several times daily. In addition, topical tretinoin in the gel form may be helpful, although it often burns. Topical cyclosporine also appears effective, but is very expensive. Finally, topical anesthetic mixtures may allow the patient to eat with more comfort.

PUVA and especially PUVA bath therapy seem effective for lichen planus and have become one of our first choices for extensive or highly pruritic cases. Extracorporeal photochemotherapy appears effective for erosive lichen planus of the mucosa.

Lichen Nitidus

(Pinkus 1907)

Definition. Dermatosis consisting of tiny papules that resemble lichen planus but histologically show tiny granulomas. This disorder is considered under granulomatous dermatoses in the German edition of the text but is placed here because of the clinical similarities to lichen planus.

Etiology and Pathogenesis. The etiology is unknown. The question remains – is lichen nitidus a disease on its own or a cousin of lichen planus? Clinically the two are very similar and some patients have both. However, histologically there are distinct differences, as lichen nitidus is granulomatous. At the next level, electron microscopy, there are once again similarities.

Clinical Findings. Hundreds of tiny white papules, usually 1–2 mm in size, are found. The most typical sites are the penis shaft and glans, the neck, flexural surfaces of the arms and less often the trunk (Fig. 14.52). The disease occurs more commonly in blacks and their lesions tend to be white. In light-skinned patients, the papules may be red or red–brown. The papules are polygonal and flat-tipped, just as in lichen planus, but they are much smaller, not inflamed and only rarely coalesce. The Köbner phenomenon may be seen. Occasionally secondary hemorrhage may occur. The lesions usually do not itch. The many clinical variants described with lichen planus are not seen.

Histopathology. Typically there is a focal granulomatous infiltrate in the papillary dermis, usually involving just two or three dermal papillae. On first glance the infiltrate appears lichenoid, but epidermal damage is rare. In addition, the infiltrate contains macrophages and usually a scattering of giant cells. The infiltrate is often enclosed by a collarette of elongated residual rete ridges at its periphery. Direct immunofluorescent examination is negative.

Course and Prognosis. The disorder is chronic and may heal with pigmentary changes.

Differential Diagnosis. The main differential diagnostic point is lichen planus; the biopsy is usually diagnostic. Other lichenoid disorders must also be considered, such as lichenoid forms of syphilis and tuberculosis, lichen spinulosus and many others.

Therapy. Usually no therapy is needed, for the problem is hidden and asymptomatic. Topical corticosteroids may produce some improvement. In difficult cases, systemic retinoids have been tried.

Actinic Lichen Nitidus

(Bedi 1978)

Synonym. Summertime actinic lichenoid eruption

Despite the name, this disease is not the same as actinic lichen planus. The patients have fine

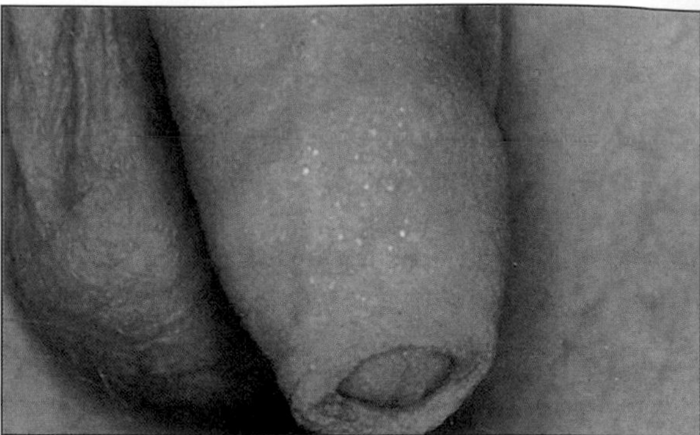

Fig. 14.52. Lichen nitidus

pinhead-sized papules that appear in sun-exposed areas. Some individuals also have other lesions more typical of lichen planus, just as is seen with lichen nitidus.

On biopsy the tiny papules are identical to lichen nitidus. Topical corticosteroid creams and sun protection are effective therapy.

Graft Versus Host Disease

Definition. Clinical syndrome in which immunocompetent leukocytes attack various tissues in an immunocompromised individual. Graft versus host disease refers to the entire disease picture, while graft versus host reaction refers to the expression of the disease in a single organ such as the skin.

Epidemiology. The most common setting for graft versus host disease is bone marrow transplantation, but it may develop in fetuses following maternal-fetal transfer of blood, following solid organ transplantation and after blood transfusions if the blood has not been irradiated or otherwise treated.

Etiology and Pathogenesis. The requirements for graft versus host disease include:

- Transfer of immunocompetent cells into an individual
- A relatively immunocompromised recipient
- Histoincompatibility between the host and the source of cells.

The immunology of graft versus host disease is complex. Functional lymphocytes must identify foreign antigens in their new host and then initiate a series of reactions that, while normally protective against invaders, in this setting attack the host. The major histocompatibility complex on human chromosome 6 consists of class I antigens (HLA-A, -B,-C) and class II antigens (HLA-D). Class I antigens are more widely expressed, are detected serologically and facilitate a suppressor and cytotoxic T cell response. Class II antigens have more limited expression, are more difficult to detect, and involve helper T cells. The class II antigens or immune response genes of animals modulate the cytotoxic action against class I antigens, so they appear to play a supervisory role. While both classes are important, there are other immune response genes or minor histocompatibility markers, so even perfect HLA matches among siblings may lead to graft versus host disease. In rare cases, graft versus host disease has been described following grafts between identical twins. The likelihood of graft versus host disease increases as the degree of HLA mismatch increases.

The initial reaction seems clearly to be initiated as host antigens are presented by antigen-processing cells to the donor T cells. These cells proliferate and then attack various host organs. Certain subpopulations of T cells are more responsible for the reaction and can be removed prior to transplantation. Natural killer cells are later recruited and may be responsible for some epidermal toxicity. In addition, various cytokines may also play a role in epidermal damage, as may reduced or altered functioning of Langerhans cells.

Clinical Findings. The clinical features are highly dependent on the type of transplantation that is performed. Graft versus host disease is most often associated with bone marrow transplantation, whereas in solid organ transplantation or blood transfusion, the risk is very low if all procedures are followed carefully. In the most common setting of bone marrow transplantation, the patient is treated with both chemotherapy (usually cyclophosphamide) and total body ionizing radiation prior to transplantation. These treatments are not needed in patients with severe intrinsic immunodeficiency, while in patients with leukemia more extensive pre-bone marrow transplantation chemotherapy is required. This pretreatment also profoundly affects the skin, reducing the number of Langerhans cells and disrupting the normal maturation of keratinocytes. In addition, the bone marrow may be treated with monoclonal antibodies to remove selected T cell subsets.

Immunosuppressive therapy is instituted at the time of transplantation. In bone marrow transplantation, the usual regimens contain cyclosporine and methotrexate, while in renal transplantation azathioprine usually replaces methotrexate and corticosteroids are added. Tacrolimus (FK-506) has replaced cyclosporine in many protocols. Mycophenolate is employed in some solid organ transplantation schemes. Antithymocyte or antilymphocyte globulin may be employed to control rejection reactions.

The main problems include infections, graft rejection and graft versus host disease. While the skin is an easy place to observe and help document the occurrence of graft versus host disease, it is not the crucial organ. Bowel disease and liver disease are the main serious risks and must be carefully monitored. Even with an HLA-matched sibling donor and appropriate immunosuppression, about two-thirds of all bone marrow transplantation patients develop graft versus host disease. Traditionally graft versus host disease is divided into acute and chronic forms.

Acute Graft Versus Host Disease

Clinical Findings. Acute graft versus host disease develops in the first few months after transplantation. Usually the reaction does not appear until 10–14 days, at which time the peripheral circulation has been repopulated with lymphocytes. Initial symptoms include diarrhea, fever, abdominal pain, jaundice, shortness of breath and often pruritus or painful skin. The initial sites of cutaneous disease often include the palms, soles and retroauricular region. Over a period of 1–2 days, a diffuse macular or papular exanthem appears, typically involving the axillae, lateral aspects of the trunk and extensor surfaces of the arms. At the same time there may be reddening of the nail folds or conjunctiva, as well as erosions of the oral and genital mucosa. Cutaneous graft versus host disease can be divided into four clinical categories based on the scheme from the University of Washington transplantation group:

Grade 1	Exanthem involving <25% of surface area
Grade 2	Exanthem involving >25% of surface area
Grade 3	Erythroderma
Grade 4	Blisters

Grade 3 and 4 skin disease may be life threatening by themselves, as all the problems of temperature control, fluid balance and infections are added to the already considerable difficulties of the patient. Milder disease tends to desquamate after a period of days, and then gradually fade away. Relapses may occur. The presence of acute graft versus host disease is not required for the eventual development of chronic graft versus host disease.

Histopathology. A similar grading scheme from the Washington group is available for the classification of histologic changes:

Grade 0	Normal skin or diseases unrelated to graft
Grade 1	Vacuolar change in basal layercells
Grade 2	Dyskeratotic cells in basal layer or follicle
Grade 3	Clefts and vesicles in basal layer
Grade 4	Separation of epidermis and dermis

Grade 4 disease is histologically as well as clinically almost identical to toxic epidermal necrolysis. A term often applied to graft versus host disease is satellite cell necrosis, which suggests that a single lymphocyte (the satellite cell) interacts with a keratinocyte to cause necrosis. The process is not this simple, although lymphocytes may be seen in close connection to keratinocytes. In addition, the finding is not specific.

When keratinocytes are stimulated by a variety of cytokines including IFN-γ they may express class II histocompatibility antigens. This feature may be found before other signs of the reaction. Langerhans cells trafficking, as host Langerhans cell are replaced by donor ones, and infiltration by natural killer cells can also be documented but their clinical significance is unclear.

Laboratory Findings. Liver function tests should be monitored. Many patients develop eosinophilia and thrombocytopenia. Stool output and bilirubin level are better predictors of the severity of graft versus host disease than skin findings.

Differential Diagnosis. The differential diagnosis is very difficult. Both viral exanthems and drug-induced exanthems can appear in the skin identical to grade 1 and 2 graft versus host disease. In addition, the pretransplantation regimens alter the skin, producing dyskeratotic cells similar to those associated with the reaction. More severe graft versus host disease is indistinguishable from toxic epidermal necrolysis. The rash of lymphocyte recovery occurs as the blood and skin are repopulated with lymphocytes; it too may be histologically identically to mild graft versus host disease. The presence of diarrhea and liver disease is probably the best clue to graft versus host disease.

Therapy

Systemic. The real issue is what type of treatment provides the best prophylaxis against graft versus host disease. With a prevalence of up to 70%, it is clear that the perfect approach has not been found. If the reaction does occur, the immunosuppressive regimen is manipulated in some way. If corticosteroids have not already been employed they may be added. Otherwise, the dose of cyclosporine or other agents may be increased, or newer modalities such as tacrolimus employed. In addition, thalidomide has been employed with good success. Recently anticytokine antibodies have been employed, but their exact role remains unclear. Another approach is the use of PUVA or PUVA bath therapy, which is better established in chronic disease.

Topical. Any mild emollient can be used during the desquamative phase. Patients with erythroderma or widespread skin loss require supportive care.

Chronic Graft versus Host Disease

Clinical Findings. Chronic graft versus host disease occurs more than 100 days after transplantation. It may overlap with a persistent acute graft versus host disease. One interesting risk factor is having a donor and recipient of opposite sexes; men who receive grafts from women are at special risk. Other risk factors include occurrence of acute graft versus host disease, advanced age and use of buffy coat cells to prevent rejection in aplastic anemia patients.

The clinical findings are quite variable and usually diagnosed in the skin. Initially there may be a papular eruption, thinning and splitting of the nails and oral erosions; the similarities to lichen planus are unmistakable. Later on, there may be sclerosis just as seen in morphea along with a sicca syndrome with dry mouth and eyes. The sclerotic skin may be dramatically hyperpigmented and tends to ulcerate, probably more readily than morphea (Fig. 14.53).

Systemic findings may include malabsorption, chronic liver disease, neuropathies, myositis, pulmonary fibrosis and an increased incidence of viral and bacterial infections.

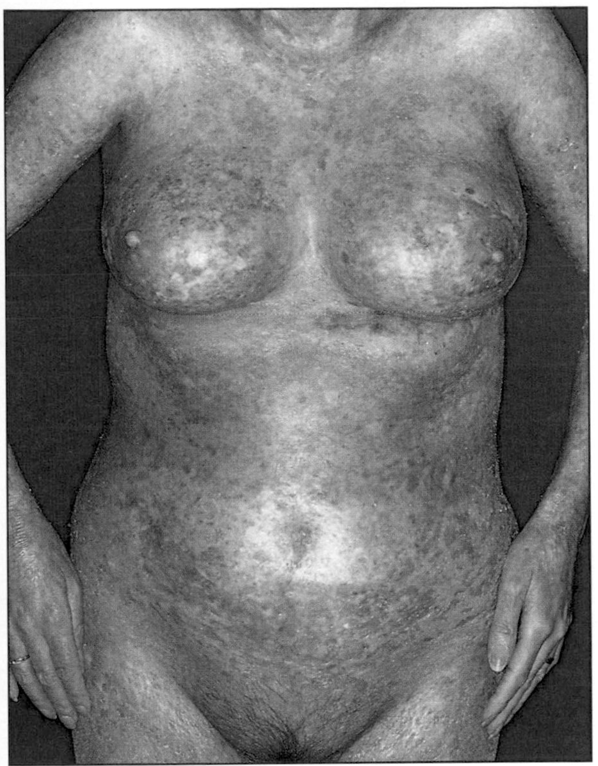

Fig. 14.53. Chronic graft versus host disease

Histopathology. The histologic features resemble those in lichen planus, morphea or Sjögren syndrome, depending on what type of lesion is biopsied. Sequential biopsies of the lip, assessing the degree of lymphocytic infiltrate about minor salivary glands, is an accepted way to monitor chronic graft versus host disease. The lichenoid papules tend to have less of a lymphocytic infiltrate than lichen planus and show more epidermal damage, while the sclerotic lesions are identical to those in morphea. The expression of class II antigens on keratinocytes may persist, and deposition of immunoglobulin and complement has been described at the epidermal-dermal junction.

Laboratory Findings. A number of autoantibodies can be identified, including antinuclear antibodies and antimitochondrial antibodies, as well as rheumatoid factor. Eosinophilia and hypergammaglobulinemia may also be present.

Differential Diagnosis. The differential diagnosis has already been discussed. It includes lichen planus, Sjögren syndrome and the whole spectrum of sclerotic skin disorders. Usually, the history of a recent bone marrow transplantation gives away the answer, so the problems are more theoretical, as compared to acute graft versus host disease, where it is often impossible to make a definite diagnosis with subsequent therapeutic implications.

Therapy. Manipulation of immunosuppression is the mainstay. Both PUVA and PUVA bath therapy have been amazingly effective in chronic graft versus host disease and may be the treatment of choice for the skin changes in this difficult problem.

Frictional Lichenoid Dermatitis

Synonyms. Juvenile papular dermatitis, recurrent summertime pityriasis of the knees and elbows (Sutton, Jr. 1956), frictional lichenoid eruption (Waisman and Sutton, Jr. 1966), sandbox dermatitis (Hjorth 1967), dermatitis du toboggan (Dupré et al. 1974)

Definition. Harmless lichenoid papular eruption of the knees and elbows in children.

Epidemiology. The disease is more often seen in boys, usually between the ages of 4 and 12 years and in the summer.

Etiology and Pathogenesis. The disease is more common in children with the atopic diathesis, but no other clues to its etiology exists. It probably does result at least in part from dry skin and friction, as all the colorful names imply.

Clinical Findings. Typically multiple grouped tiny papules appear on the knees, elbows, buttocks and backs of the hands (Fig. 14.54). The individual le-

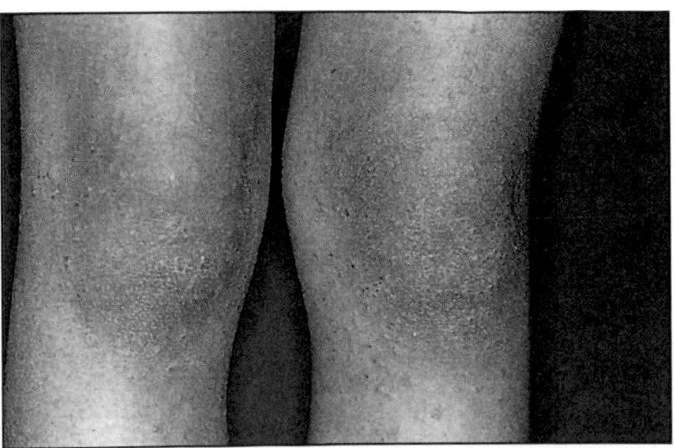

Fig. 14.54. Frictional lichenoid dermatitis

sions are 1–3 mm in diameter and have a pearly sheen. They may be slightly red or pale. Rarely mild scale or excoriations may be present, but most lesions are asymptomatic. The eruption usually resolves spontaneously, but may be expected to recur. Often the patients also have pityriasis alba, another sign of atopy.

Histopathology. Biopsies are not needed and rarely reported. A lymphocytic infiltrate in the superficial dermis is associated with mild epidermal reactive changes such as hyperkeratosis and acanthosis. The findings are by no means diagnostic.

Course and Prognosis. The disease frequently recurs in subsequent years. Sometimes it heals with hypopigmentation.

Differential Diagnosis. The main consideration is Gianotti-Crosti syndrome, which usually involves the face and distal parts of the extremities, and is self-limited. Lichen nitidus may occasionally appear similar but has a different histology.

Therapy. Any bland topical therapy suffices. Usually low-potency corticosteroids are employed, perhaps combined with urea. Emollients are also useful, especially after bathing.

Gianotti-Crosti Syndrome

Synonyms. Acrodermatitis papulosa eruptiva infantilis, papular acrodermatitis of children, papulovesicular acrolocalized syndrome

Definition. Papular lichenoid eruption in children, most often acrally located.

History. Gianotti described papular acrodermatitis of childhood in 1955, and Crosti and Gianotti published a longer paper in 1956. They later redefined it as associated with hepatitis B infections. Crosti and Gianotti in 1964 described papulovesicular acrolocalized syndrome, which was very similar but not associated with hepatitis B. After 30 years of wavering, it has generally become accepted that the two clinical pictures are identical and that many viruses can trigger the cutaneous reaction pattern. Some still reserve the diagnosis of Gianotti-Crosti syndrome for patients with documented hepatitis B virus infection.

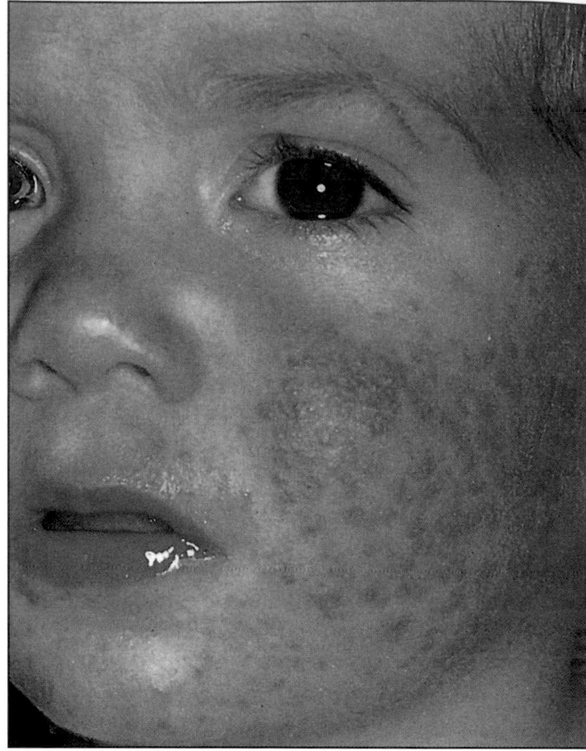

Fig. 14.55. Gianotti-Crosti syndrome

Epidemiology. Most patients are young children between 2 and 6 years of age.

Etiology and Pathogenesis. The trigger for Gianotti-Crosti syndrome is usually a viral infection, although most patients are asymptomatic. Even in countries such as Korea where hepatitis B virus is very common and responsible for almost all cases of Gianotti-Crosti syndrome, many of the children have no signs of liver disease. In addition to hepatitis B virus, many other viruses including Epstein-Barr virus, Coxsackie, ECHO, parainfluenza and even polio viruses have been identified, as well as streptococcal infections. Immunizations have also been blamed as triggers, as have medications.

Clinical Findings. In some cases there is a history of an antecedent illness but the vast majority of patients are healthy. The patient suddenly develops multiple succulent red papules typically involving the cheeks, buttocks, arms and legs but avoiding the flexural areas (Figs. 14.55, 14.56). In infants the lesions tend to be larger than in older children where the eruption has been described as micropapular. On the cheeks and buttocks confluent lesions are not unusual. Often the papules are lichenoid with a

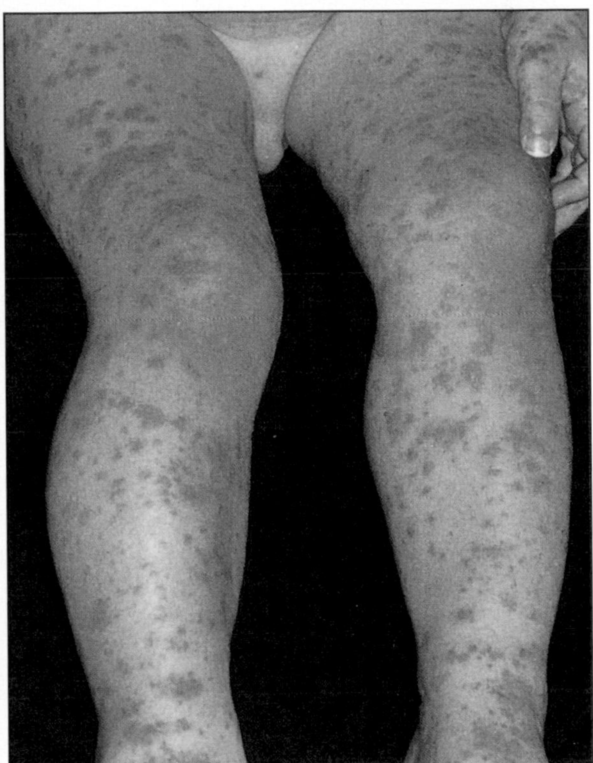

Fig. 14.56. Gianotti-Crosti syndrome

flat top and glistening surface; others may be hemorrhagic. Characteristically the lesions are not pruritic. They resolve over weeks and recurrences are uncommon. In patients with atopic dermatitis and in Down syndrome patients, the eruption may persist for a longer period of time.

Much has been written on the systemic findings in Gianotti-Crosti syndrome, but it is all misleading. The systemic findings occur only in those patients who have an active viral infection and then they reflect the underlying virus. Lymphadenopathy is more common in those children in whom hepatitis B virus is involved.

Histopathology. The epidermis shows spongiosis and mild acanthosis, as well as focal hyperkeratosis. The chief pathology is in the dermis where there is an intense lymphocytic perivascular infiltrate that may be associated with exocytosis of erythrocytes, vessel wall swelling and dilatation. There may also be papillary dermal edema. Despite the occasional lichenoid clinical appearance, a band-like infiltrate is not observed.

Laboratory Findings. In the absence of symptoms, knowing which virus is responsible is of little importance. We still check for hepatitis B virus because parents who read about the disease worry if their child has hepatitis. Usually the surface antigen (HB_s-AG) is most reliable. Other laboratory investigations should be directed towards the patient's symptoms or recent exposures.

Differential Diagnosis. Frictional lichenoid dermatitis may appear similar but is more localized and not inflamed. Occasionally Langerhans cell histiocytosis may present with small papules in a minimally ill child; the biopsy should exclude this diagnosis. While widespread lichen planus is an uncommon childhood disease, it should be considered.

Therapy. Indifferent topical care is all that is needed. Zinc shake lotion is often helpful. Many feel that topical corticosteroids worsen Gianotti-Crosti syndrome. We occasionally employ low-potency corticosteroid creams early in the disease if the lesions are pruritic.

Lichen Simplex Chronicus

(Vidal 1886)

Synonyms. Circumscribed neurodermatitis, lichen Vidal

Definition. Common pruritic skin disorder, usually sharply localized and characterized by skin thickening and prominent skin markings.

Epidemiology. Lichen simplex chronicus is a very common disease. It appears to be more common among women than men.

Etiology and Pathogenesis. Lichenification is a common phenomenon. It describes the response of the skin to repetitive irritation with thickening and more prominent skin markings. For example, lichenification is common in atopic dermatitis, usually in the flexural areas and on the nape. Lichen simplex chronicus features lichenification, but it is sharply localized and often there is no clear history of a preexisting dermatitis. Nonetheless, it is generally agreed that lichen simplex chronicus is caused by rubbing and scratching the skin. Why it so often involves such a limited area and why there are such common sites of predilection remains unclear. Many patients have atopic dermatitis and some have defined lichen simplex chronicus as part of

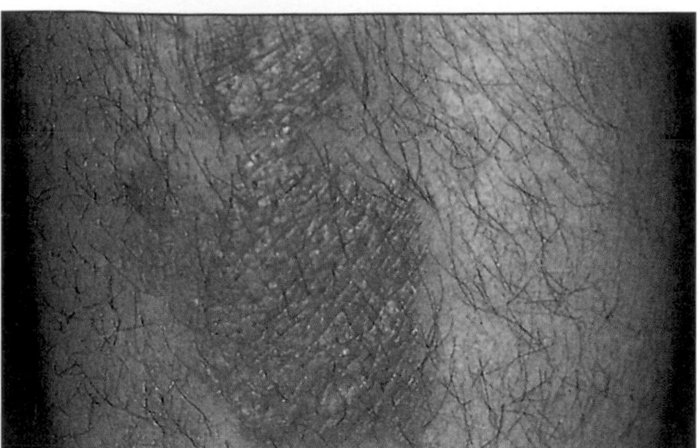

Fig. 14.57. Lichen simplex chronicus

the atopic diathesis. Others have blamed a variety of internal disorders, none of which is regularly involved. Many patients do show other signs of emotional stress such as nail chewing, compulsive smoking or similar behavior.

Clinical Findings. Following rubbing or scratching, sharply circumscribed areas of thickened skin with prominent markings develop. The most typical sites are the nape (lichen nuchae) and distal extremities (Fig. 14.57). The genitalia and upper eyelids are also common sites, perhaps because the skin is so thin in those regions. The typical patient has a single lesion, although occasionally several are present. Both patients and physicians sometimes refer to the lesion as a "worry spot" or "worry patch". While the primary lesion is a papule, when one carefully looks at the lesion one can identify three zones:

- In the middle a thickened plaque with prominent skin lines.
- Surrounding it are multiple small papules, usually skin colored or pale red.
- At the periphery postinflammatory hyperpigmentation extends in an irregular fashion several centimeters into the adjacent skin.

While most lesions are pink or red, some may lose color centrally, especially on the face and in darker skinned individuals. The lesions tend to be round or oval, but can be linear or assume other bizarre shapes. The disease is chronic; even when therapy produces temporary improvement, relapses are likely.

There are also several clinical variants of lichen simplex chronicus.

Lichénification Géante

(Brocq and Pautrier 1936)

Synonym. Lichen giganteus

In the genital region, lichen simplex chronicus may be more papillomatous and at the same time show maceration and crusting. Typically the scrotum or labia majora are involved showing red juicy plaques that are intensely pruritic. Recurrent bacterial infections may complicate the picture leading to elephantiasis-like changes. A biopsy should be performed to exclude pemphigus vegetans and Hailey-Hailey disease.

Verrucous Lichen Simplex Chronicus

Patients with chronic venous insufficiency may develop markedly verrucous plaques on the distal aspects of the shins or the dorsal surface of the foot. The central usually smooth zone is covered by thick compact scales. The pruritus is once again intense. The main differential diagnosis is hypertrophic lichen planus, although lichen amyloidosus and lipoid proteinosis can also show such changes. A biopsy is decisive. Such patients should additionally be treated with compression wraps, stockings or Unna boots.

Histopathology. The epidermis shows hyperkeratosis, parakeratosis and acanthosis with characteristic elongation and thickening of the rete ridges that may join together at their bases. The capillaries in the papillary dermis are dilated and surrounded by a primarily lymphocytic infiltrate.

Course and Prognosis. The course is usually protracted. If a lesion is treated early in the disease course, the response is rewarding. If the patient suffers from psychological problems, the lesions are more likely to be persistent.

Differential Diagnosis. If the patient has many lesions, one should look for other signs of atopic dermatitis. The standard differential question includes localized lichen planus and lichenified dermatitis. Histologically one can readily rule out lichen planus, while the concept of lichenified dermatitis is a more philosophical one, since many believe that lichen simplex chronicus also fits into this category. When the three zones are not seen, when signs of acute inflammation such as weeping or crusts are found or when marked spongiosis and exocytosis are present on microscopic study, one leans towards the diagnosis of dermatitis. Many other disorders can present as a single pruritic patch, so that a biopsy is always reasonable to exclude problems such as mycosis fungoides, sarcoidosis or lichen amyloidosus.

In addition, there are other problems with localized pruritus that show some overlaps. The lesions of prurigo nodularis are multiple, smaller and dome shaped. Notalgia paresthetica typically involves the scapular area but otherwise may be similar to lichen simplex chronicus (Chap. 25).

Therapy

Systemic. Both antihistamines and minor tranquilizers may be of help in relieving the pruritus and helping patients modify their behavior. In some instances, psychological counseling is helpful.

Topical. The best approach is topical corticosteroids either under plastic foil occlusion via impregnated tape.

Often wrapping the lesion with an Unna boot for a week will produce marked improvement by hindering access. Another useful agent, if available, is tar which produces surprisingly good results. One can use 2–5% liquor carbonis detergens in zinc paste or a commercially available tar cream.

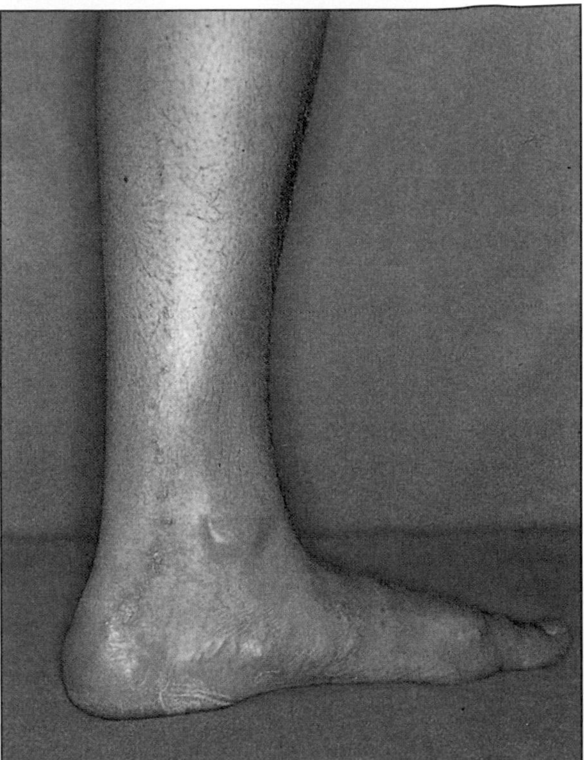

Fig. 14.58. Lichen striatus

Lichen Striatus

Definition. Subacute linear inflammatory dermatitis of unknown etiology.

Epidemiology. Most patients are children or adolescents, and women are more often affected.

Etiology and Pathogenesis. The etiology is unknown. Often the lesions follow Blaschko lines with typical whorls. Lichen striatus is probably the best example of blaschkitis (Chap. 1). Somatic mosaicism presumably creates regions of skin that are more susceptible to inflammatory stimuli. Others feel that the distribution is dermatomal and that perhaps neural factors are involved. Patients with the atopic diathesis may be more frequently affected.

Clinical Findings. The initial lesions are small red papules without Wickham striae or central dells that combine to form a 2–20-mm wide band usually running along a limb (Fig. 14.58). The evolution of the lesion may last 3–5 weeks. Sometimes the entire limb may be involved, although short segments are usual. There may be skip areas. Psoriasiform scaling may develop. Pruritus is rarely seen, as far example when the diaper region is involved in infants. Nail lesions have occasionally been reported, such as splitting and onycholysis. Multiple lesions are most uncommon. The disease is self-limited and usually resolves in months but may persist several years.

Histopathology. The key feature is the presence of scattered dyskeratotic cells in the upper layers of the epidermis, which separates lichen striatus from clinically similar disorders. The epidermis also shows acanthosis and hyperkeratosis with minimal spongiosis. There is a lymphocytic perivascular infiltrate with is usually limited to the upper dermis but occasionally involves deeper vessels. Sometimes edema and exocytosis occur.

Differential Diagnosis. The possibilities include many of the variants of linear epidermal nevus, including inflammatory linear verrucous epidermal nevus (ILVEN). These lesions are usually identified at birth and persist indefinitely. Often, a linear epidermal nevus is overlooked in early infancy when it is relatively flat and then first noticed when it becomes hyperkeratotic or inflamed. If the epidermal changes are not prominent histologically, often one cannot separate the two possibilities. Linear psoriasis, linear lichen planus and linear porokeratosis can be excluded with a biopsy.

Therapy. None is needed, which is just as well since none is available. The rare lesions that itch can be treated with antipruritic agents such as polidocanol creams or topical corticosteroids.

Bibliography

Erythemas

Flushing

Wilkin JK (1993) The red face: flushing disorders. Clin Dermatol 11:211–223

Blushing

Drott C, Claes G, Olsson R (1998) Successful treatment of facial blushing by endoscopic transthoracic sympathicotomy. Br J Dermatol 138:639–643

Flushing in Carcinoid Syndrome

Roberts JL, Marney SR, Oates JA (1979) Blockage of the flush associated with metastatic gastric carcinoid by combined H1 and H2 receptor antagonists. Evidence for an important role of H2 receptors in human vasculature. N Engl J Med 300:236–238

Smith AG, Greaves MW (1974) Blood prostaglandin activity associated with noradrenaline-provoked flush in the carcinoid syndrome. Br J Dermatol 90:547–551

Familial Palmoplantar Erythema

Lane JE (1929) Erythema pamare hereditarium. Arch Dermatol Syphilol 20:445–448

Bryan HG, Coskey RJ (1967) Familial erythema of acral regions. Arch Dermatol 95:483–486

Figurate Erythemas

Hurley H, Hurley JP (1984) The gyrate erythemas. Semin Dermatol 3:327–336

Saurat JH, Janin-Mercier A (1984) Infantile epidermodysplastic erythema gyratum responsive to imidazoles. A new entity? Arch Dermatol 1320:1601–1603

Summerly R (1964) The figurative erythemas and neoplasia. Br J Dermatol 76:370–373

Erythema Annulare Centrifugum

Bressler GS, Jones RE Jr (1981) Erythema annulare centrifugum. J Am Acad Dermatol 4:597–602

Darier J (1916) De l'érythème annulaire centrifuge (érythème papulocirciné migrateur et chronique) et de quelques éruptions analogues. Ann Dermatol Syph 7:57–76

Jilson D (1954) Allergic confirmation that some cases of erythema annulare centrifugum are dermatophytids. Arch Dermatol Syphilol 70:355–359

Mahboob A, Haroon TS (1998) Drugs causing fixed eruptions: a study of 450 cases. Int J Dermatol 37:833–838

Mahood JM (1983) Erythema annulare centrifugum. A review of 24 cases with special reference to its association with underlying disease. Clin Exp Dermatol 8:383–387

Reichel M, Wheeland RG (1991) Inflammatory carcinoma masquerading as erythema annulare centrifugum. Acta Derm Venereol (Stockh) 73:138–140

Shelley WB (1965) Erythema annulare centrifugum due to Candida albicans. Br J Dermatol 77:383–384

Trying SK (1993) Reactive erythemas: erythema annulare centrifugum and erythema gyratum repens. Clin Dermatol 11:135–139

Erythema Gyratum Repens

Albers SE, Fenske NA, Glass LF (1993) Erythema gyratum repens: direct immunofluorescence findings. J Am Acad Dermatol 29:493–494

Barber PV, Doyle L, Vickers KM, et al. (1978) Erythema gyratum repens with pulmonary tuberculosis. Br J Dermatol 98:465–468

Boyd AS, Neldner KH, Menter A (1992) Erythema gyratum repens: a paraneoplastic eruption. J Am Acad Dermatol 26:757–762

Gammel JA (1952) Erythema gyratum repens – skin manifestations in a patient with carcinoma of breast. Arch Dermatol Syphilol 66:494–505

Garret SJ, Roenigk HH Jr (1998) Erythema gyratum repens in a healthy woman. J Am Acad Dermatol 26:121–122

Kawakami T, Saito R (1995) Erythema gyratum repens unassociated with underlying malignancy. J Dermatol 22:587–589

Kurzrock R, Cohen PR (1995) Erythema gyratum repens. JAMA 273:594

Annular Erythema of Infancy

Gianotti F, Ermacora E (1975) Erythema gyratum atrophicans transiens neonatale. Arch Dermatol 111:615–616

Erythema Gyratum Perstans

Beare JM, Frogatt P, Jones JH (1966) Familial annular erythema. An apparently new dominant mutation. Br J Dermatol 78:59–68

Friedman SJ, Winkelmann RK (1987) Familial granuloma annulare. Report of two cases and review of the literature. J Am Acad Dermatol 16:600–605

Erythema Marginatum

Burke JB (1993) Erythema marginatum. Arch Dis Child 30:359–365

Gadrat J (1983) Sur les érythèmes rhumatismaux. Ann Dermatol Syph 9:1045–1051

Green ST, Harnlet NW, Willocks L (1990) Psittacosis presenting with erythema-marginatum-like lesions – a case report and a historical review. Clin Exp Dermatol 15:225–227

Erythema Scarlatiniforme Desquamativum Recidivans

Lausecker H (1954) Das Erythema scarlatiniforme desquamativum recidivans. Arch Dermatol Syphilol 198:529–548

Landthaler M, Michalopoulos M, Schwab U et al. (1985) Erythema scarlatiniforme desquamativum recidivans localisatum. Hautarzt 36:581–585

Necrolytic Migratory Erythema

Becker SW, Kahn D, Rothman S (1942) Cutaneous manifestations of internal malignant tumors. Arch Dermatol Syphilol 45:1069–1080

Burton JL (1993) Zinc and essential fatty acid therapy for necrolytic migratory erythema. Arch Dermatol 129:246

Doyle JA, Schroeter AL, Rogers RS III (1979) Hyperglucagonemia and necrolytic migratory erythema in cirrhosis – possible pseudoglucagonoma syndrome. Br J Dermatol 101:581–587

Kheir SM, Omura EF, Grizzle WE et al. (1986) Histologic variation in the skin lesions of the glucagonoma syndrome. Am J Surg Pathol 10:445–453

Marinkovich MP, Botella R, Datloff J et al. (1995) Necrolytic migratory erythema without glucagonoma in patients with liver disease. J Am Acad Dermatol 32:604–609

Sheperd ME, Raimer SS, Tyring SK et al. (1991) Treatment of necrolytic migratory erythema in glucagonoma syndrome. J Am Acad Dermatol 25:925–928

Sinclair SA, Reynolds NJ (1997) Necrolytic migratory erythema and zinc deficiency. Br J Dermatol 136:783–785

Vandersteen PR, Scheithauer BW (1985) Glucagonoma syndrome. A clinicopathologic, immunocytochemical and ultrastructural study. J Am Acad Dermatol 12:1032–1039

Multiforme and Nodose Erythemas

Erythema Multiforme

Aslanzadeh J, Helm KF, Espy JM et al. (1992) Detection of HSV-specific DNA in biopsy tissue of patients with erythema multiforme by polymerase chain reaction. Br J Dermatol 126:19–23

Aurelian L, Kokuba H, Burnett JW (1998) Understanding the pathogenesis of HSV-associated erythema multiforme. Dermatology 197:219–222

Bedi TR, Pinkus H (1976) Histopathological spectrum of erythema multiforme. Br J Dermatol 95:243–250

Choy AC, Yarnold PR, Brown JE et al. (1995) Virus induced erythema multiforme and Stevens-Johnson syndrome. Allergy Proc 16:157–161

Drago F, Parodi A, Rebora A (1995) Persistent erythema multiforme: report of two new cases and review of literature. J Am Acad Dermatol33:366–369

Duvic M, Reisner EG, Dawson DV et al. (1983) HLA-B15 association with erythema multiforme. J Am Acad Dermatol 8:493–496

Fabbri P, Panconseni E (1993) Erythema multiforme ("minus" and "maius") and drug intake. Clin Dermatol 11:479–489

Foedinger D, Anhalt GJ, Boecskoer B et al. (1995) Autoantibodies to desmoplakin I and II in patients with erythema multiforme. J Exp Med 181:169–179

Hewitt J, Ormerod AD (1992) Toxic epidermal necrolysis treated with cyclosporine. Clin Exp Dermatol 17:264–265

Huff JC (1988) Therapy and prevention of erythema multiforme with acyclovir. Semin Dermatol 7:212–217

Huff JC, Weston WL, Tonnesen MG (1983) Erythema multiforme: a critical review of characteristics, diagnostic criteria and causes. J Am Acad Dermatol 8:763–775

Lemak MA, Davis M, Bean SF (1986) Oral acyclovir for the prevention of herpes-associated erythema multiforme. J Am Acad Dermatol 15:50–54

Lewis DA, Brook MG (1992) Erythema multiforme as a presentation of human immunodeficiency virus seroconversion illness. Int J STD AIDS 3:56–57

Lyell A (1979) Toxic epidermal necrolysis (the scalded skin syndrome): a reappraisal. Br J Dermatol 100:69–86

Lyell A, Gordon AM, Dick HM (1967) Mycoplasmas and erythema multiforme. Lancet ii:1116–1118

Miura S, Smith CC, Burnett JW et al. (1992) Detection of viral DNA within skin of healed recurrent herpes simplex infection and erythema multiforme lesions. J Invest Dermatol 98:68–72

Rzany B, Hering O, Mockenhaupt M et al. (1996) Histopathological and epidemiological characteristics of patients with erythema exudativum multiforme major, Stevens-Johnson syndrome and toxic epidermal necrolysis. Br J Dermatol 135:6–11

Shelley WB (1967) Herpes simplex virus as a cause of erythema multiforme. JAMA 201:153–156

Todd P, Halpern S, Munro DD (1995) Oral terbinafine and erythema multiforme. Clin Exp Dermatol 20:247–248

Wuepper KD, Watson PA, Katzmierowski JA (1980) Immune complexes in erythema multiforme and the Stevens-Johnson syndrome. J Invest Dermatol 74:368–371

Acute Febrile Neutrophilic Dermatosis

Cohen PR (1993) Pregnancy-associated Sweet's syndrome: world literature review. Obstet Gynecol Surv 48:584–587

Cohen PR, Kurzrock R (1987) Sweet's syndrome and malignancy. Am J Med 82:1220–1226

Cohen PR, Holder WR, Tucker SB et al. (1993) Sweet syndrome in patients with solid tumors. Cancer 72:2723–2731

Driesch P van den (1994) Sweet's syndrome: acute febrile neutrophilic dermatosis. J Am Acad Dermatol 31:535–556

Hofmann C, Braun-Falco O, Petzoldt D (1976) Akute febrile neutrophile Dermatose (Sweet-Syndrom). Dtsch Med Wochenschr 101:1113–1118

Jeanfils S, Joly P, Young P (1997) Indomethacin treatment of eighteen patients with Sweet's syndrome. J Am Acad Dermatol 36:436–439

Kemmett D, Hunter JAA, Berth-Jones J et al. (1989) Sweet's syndrome and malignancy: a case associated with multiple myeloma and review of the literature. Br J Dermatol 121:123–128

Kemmett D, Hunter JAA, Berth-Jones J et al. (1989) Sweet's syndrome: a clinicopathologic review of twenty nine cases. J Am Acad Dermatol 23:503–507

Storer JS, Nesbitt LT, Galen WK et al. (1983) Sweet's syndrome: a review. Int J Dermatol 22:8–12

Sweet RD (1964) An acute febrile neutrophilic dermatosis. Br J Dermatol 76:349–356

Sweet RD (1979) Acute febrile neutrophilic dermatosis – 1978. Br J Dermatol 100:93–99

Tikjob G, Kassis V, Klem-Thomsen H et al. (1985) Acute febrile neutrophilic dermatosis and abnormal bone marrow chromosomes as a marker for preleukemia. Acta Derm Venereol (Stockh) 65:177–179

Walker DC, Cohen PR (1996) Trimethoprim-sulfamethoxazole-associated acute febrile neutrophilic dermatosis: case report and review of drug-induced Sweet's syndrome. J Am Acad Dermatol 34:918–923

Pityriasis Rosea

Aiba S, Tagami H (1985) Immunohistologic studies in pityriasis rosea. Arch Dermatol 121:761–765

Aoshima T, Komura J, Ofiji S (1981) Virus-like particles in the herald patch of pityriasis rosea. Dermatologica 162: 64–65

Arndt KA, Paul BS, Stern RS et al. (1983) Treatment of pityriasis rosea with UV radiation. Arch Dermatol 119:381–382

Björnberg A, Hellgren L (1962) Pityriasis rosea: a statistical, clinical and laboratory investigation of 826 patients and matched healthy controls. Acta Derm Venereol (Stockh) 42 [Suppl 50]:1–68

Drago F, Ranieri E, Malaguti F et al. (1997) Human herpesvirus 7 in pityriasis rosea. Lancet 349:1367–1368

Gibert GM (1860) Traité pratique des maladies de la peau et de la syphilis, 3rd edn. Plon, Paris, p 402

Leenutaphong V, Jiamtom S (1995) UVB phototherapy for pityriasis rosea. A bilateral comparison study. J Am Acad Dermatol 33:996–999

Marcus-Faber BS, Bergman R, Ben-Porath E et al. (1997) Serum antibodies to parvovirus B19 in patients with pityriasis rosea. Dermatology 194:371

Messenger AG, Knox EG, Summerly R et al. (1982) Case clustering in pityriasis rosea: support for role of an infective agent. Br Med J 284:371–373

Panizzon R, Bloch PH (1982) Histopathology of pityriasis rosea Gibert. Qualitative and quantitative lightmicroscopic study of 62 biopsies of 40 patients. Dermatologica 165:551–558

Parsons JM (1986) Pityriasis rosea update:1986. J Am Acad Dermatol 15:159–167

Pierson JC, Dijkstra JW, Elston DM (1993) Purpuric pityriasis rosea. J Am Acad Dermatol 28:1021

Pityriasis Rotunda

Aste N, Pau M, Biggio P (1997) Pityriasis rotunda: a survey of 42 cases observed in Sardinia, Italy. Dermatology 194: 32–35

Grimalt R, Gelmetti C, Brusasco A et al. (1994) Pityriasis rotunda: report of a familial occurrence and review of the literature. J Am Acad Dermatol 31:866–871

Psoriasis

General

Abel EA, DiCicco LM, Orenberg EK et al. (1986) Drugs in exacerbation of psoriasis. J Am Acad Dermatol 15:1007–1022

Ashcroft DM, Li Wan A, Williams HC et al. (1999) Clinical measures of disease severity and outcome in psoriasis: a critical appraisal of their quality. Br J Dermatol 141: 185–191

Baker BS, Fry L (1992) The immunology of psoriasis. Br J Dermatol 126:1–9

Beutner EH (ed) (1984) Autoimmunity in psoriasis. CRC, Boca Raton

Bos JD (1988) The pathomechanism of psoriasis; the skin immune system and cyclosporine. Br J Dermatol 118: 141–155

Eedy DJ, Burrows D, Bridges JM et al. (1990) Clearance of severe psoriasis after allogenic bone marrow transplantation. BMJ 300:908

Gottlieb SL, Gilleaudeau P, Johnson R et al. (1995) Response of psoriasis to a lymphocyte-selective toxin ($DAB_{389}IL$-2) suggests a primary immune, but not keratinocyte, pathogenic basis. Nat Med 1:442–447

Kulick KB, Mogavero H Jr, Provost TT et al. (1983) Serologic studies in patients with lupus erythematosus and psoriasis. J Am Acad Dermatol 8:631–634

Menssen A, Trommler P, Vollmer S et al. (1995) Evidence for an antigen-specific cellular immune response in skin lesions of patients with psoriasis vulgaris. J Immunol 155:4078–4083

Naldi L, Peli L, Parazzini F (1999) Association of early-stage psoriasis with smoking and male alcohol consumption. Arch Dermatol 135:1479–1484

Obuch ML, Maurer TA, Becker B et al. (1992) Psoriasis and human immunodeficiency virus infection. J Am Acad Dermatol 27:667–673

Poikolainen K, Karvonen J, Pukkala E (1999) Excess mortality related to alcohol and smoking among hospital-treated patients with psoriasis. Arch Dermatol 135: 1490–1493

Prinz JC, Gross B, Vollmer S et al. (1994) T cell clones from psoriasis skin lesions can promote keratinocyte proliferation in vitro. Eur J Immunol 24:593–598

Roenigk HH, Maibach HI (eds) (1998) Psoriasis, 3rd edn. Dekker, New York

Valdimarson H, Baker BS, Jonsdottir I et al. (1986) Psoriasis: a disease of abnormal keratinocyte proliferation induced by T lymphocytes. Immunol Today 7:256–259

Valdimarsson H, Sigmundsdottir H, Jonsdottir I (1997) Is psoriasis induced by streptococcal superantigens and maintained by M-protein-specific T cells that cross-react with keratin? Clin Exp Immunol 107 [Suppl 1]: 21–24

Vollmer S, Menssen A, Trommler P et al. (1994) T lymphocytes derived from skin lesions of patients with psoriasis vulgaris express a novel cytokine pattern that is distinct from that of T helper type 1 and T helper type 2 cells. Eur J Immunol 24:2377–2382

Wrone Smith T, Nickoloff BJ (1996) Dermal injection of immunocytes induces psoriasis. J Clin Invest 98:1878–1887

Genetics

Christophers E, Henseler T (1992) Psoriasis type I and II as subtypes of nonpustular psoriasis. Semin Dermatol 11:261–266

Elder JT, Henseler T, Christophers E et al. (1994) Of genes and antigens: the inheritance of psoriasis. J Invest Dermatol 103:150S–153S

Farber EM, Nall ML, Watson W (1974) Natural history of psoriasis in 61 twin pairs. Arch Dermatol 109:207–210

Henseler T (1998) Genetics of psoriasis. Arch Dermatol Res 290:463–476

Henseler T, Christophers E (1985) Psoriasis of early and late onset: characterization of two types of psoriasis vulgaris. J Am Acad Dermatol 13:450–456

Jenisch S, Henseler T, Nair RP et al. (1998) Linkage analysis of human leukocyte antigen (HLA) markers in familial psoriasis: strong disequilibrium effects provide evidence for a major determinant in the HLA-B/-C region. Am J Hum Genet 63:191–199

Karvonen J (1975) HL-A antigens in psoriasis with special reference to the clinical type, age of onset, exacerbation after respiratory infections an occurrence of arthritis. Ann Clin Res 7:301–311

Karvonen J, Tiilikainen A, Lassus A (1975) HL-A antigen in patients with persistent palmoplantar pustulosis and pustular psoriasis. Ann Clin Res 7:112–115

Lerner MR, Lerner AB (1972) Congenital psoriasis. Arch Dermatol 105:598–602

Lomholt G (1963) Psoriasis: prevalence, spontaneous course and genetics. A census study on the prevalence of skin diseases on the Faroe Islands. G.E.C. GAD, Copenhagen

Matthews D, Fry L, Powles A et al. (1996) Evidence that a locus for familial psoriasis maps to chromosome 4q. Nat Genet 14:231–233

Nair RP, Guo SW, Jenisch S et al. (1995) Scanning chromosome 17 for psoriasis susceptibility: lack of evidence for a distal 17q locus. Hum Hered 45:219–230

Nair RP, Henseler T, Jenisch S et al. (1997) Evidence for two psoriasis susceptibility loci (HLA and 17q) and two novel candidate regions (16q and 20p) by genome-wide scan. Hum Mol Genet 6:1349–1356

Russell TJ, Schultes LM, Kuban DJ (1972) Histocompatibility (HL-A) antigens associated with psoriasis. N Engl J Med 287:738–740

Tomfohrde J, Silverman A, Barnes R et al. (1994) Gene for familial psoriasis susceptibility mapped to the distal end of human chromosome 17q. Science 264:1141–1145

Trembath RC, Clough RL, Rosbotham JL et al. (1997) Identification of a major susceptibility locus on chromosome 6p and evidence for further disease loci revealed by a two stage genome-wide search in psoriasis. Hum Mol Genet 6:813–820

Clinical Features

Braun-Falco O (1963) Zur Morphogenese der psoriatischen Hautreaktion. Eine morphologisch-histochemische Studie. Arch Klin Exp Dermatol 216:130–154

Braun-Falco O, Christophers E (1974) Structural aspects of initial psoriatic lesions. Arch Dermatol Forsch 251:95–110

Braun-Falco O, Schmoeckel C (1977) The dermal inflammatory reaction in initial psoriatic lesions. Arch Dermatol Res 258:9–16

Christophers E, Parzefall R, Braun-Falco O (1973) Initial events in psoriasis: quantitative assessment. Br J Dermatol 89:327–334

Farber EM, Nall L (1992) Nail psoriasis. Cutis 50:174–178

Farber EM, Nall L (1992) Nonpustular palmoplantar psoriasis. Cutis 50:407–410

Farber EM, Nall L (1993) Psoriasis associated with human immunodeficiency virus/acquired immunodeficiency syndrome. Cutis 52:29–35

Lazar AP, Roenigk HH (1987) Aids and psoriasis. Cutis 39:347–351

Nickoloff BJ (1987) Interferons and psoriasis – 1987 perspective. Dermatologica 175:1–4

Ragaz A, Ackerman AB (1979) Evolution, maturation and regression of lesions of psoriasis. Am J Dermatopathol 1:199–214

Therapy

Abel EA, DiCicco LM, Orenberg EK et al. (1986) Drugs in exacerbation of psoriasis. J Am Acad Dermatol 15:1007–1022

Abels DJ, Kattan-Byron J (1985) Psoriasis treatment at the Dead Sea: a natural selective ultraviolet phototherapy. J Am Acad Dermatol 12:639–643

Altmeyer PJ, Matthes U, Pawlak F et al. (1994) Antipsoriatic effect of fumaric acid derivatives. Results of a multicenter double-blind study in 100 patients. J Am Acad Dermatol 30:977–981

Berth-Jones J, Hutchinson PE (1992) Vitamin D analogues and psoriasis. Br J Dermatol 127:71–78

Berth Jones J, Voorhees JJ (1996) Consensus conference on cyclosporine microemulsion for psoriasis, June 1996. Br J Dermatol 135:775–777

Bos JD, Meinardi MM, Van Joost T et al. (1989) Use of cyclosporine in psoriasis. Lancet 2:1500–1502

Calzavara Pinton PG, Ortel B, Carlino et al. (1993) Phototesting and phototoxic side effects in bath PUVA. J Am Acad Dermatol 28:657–659

Collins P, Rogers S (1992) The efficacy of methotrexate in psoriasis – a review of 40 cases. Clin Exp Dermatol 17:257–260

Ellis CN, Voorhees JJ (1987) Etretinate therapy. J Am Acad Dermatol 16:267–291

Ellis CN, Gorsulowsky DC, Hamilton TA et al. (1986) Cyclosporine improves psoriasis in a double-blind study. JAMA 256:3110–3116

Ellis CN, Fradin MS, Hamilton TA et al. (1995) Duration of remission during maintenance cyclosporine therapy for psoriasis. Relationship to maintenance dose and degree of improvement during initial therapy. Arch Dermatol 131:791–795

Esgleyes Ribot T, Chandraratna RA, Lew Kaya DA et al. (1994) Response of psoriasis to a new topical retinoid, AGN 190168. J Am Acad Dermatol 30:581–590

Farber EM, Nall L, Morhenn V et al. (1987) Psoriasis. Proceedings of the Fourth International Symposium. Elsevier, New York Amsterdam London

Farber EM (1992) History of the treatment of psoriasis. J Am Acad Dermatol 27:640–645

Farber EM, Harris DR (1970) Hospital treatment of psoriasis. A modified anthralin program. Arch Dermatol 101:381–389

Gollnick H, Bauer R, Brindley C et al. (1988) Acitretin versus etretinate in psoriasis. Clinical and pharmacological results of a German multicenter study. J Am Acad Dermatol 19:458–469

Gollnick HP (1996) Oral retinoids – efficacy and toxicity in psoriasis. Br J Dermatol 135 [Suppl 49]:6–17

Greaves MW, Weinstein GD (1995) Treatment of psoriasis. New Engl J Med 332:581–588

Heidbreder G, Christophers E (1979) Therapy of psoriasis with retinoid plus PUVA: clinical and histological data. Arch Dermatol 264:331–337

Henseler T, Christophers E, Hönigsmann H (1987) Skin tumors in the European PUVA Study. Eight year follow-up of 1643 patients treated with PUVA for psoriasis. J Am Acad Dermatol 16:108–116

Ingram JT (1954) The approach to psoriasis. Brit Med J ii:591–594

Jekler J, Swanbeck G (1992) One-minute dithranol therapy in psoriasis: a placebo-controlled paired comparative study. Acta Dermato Venereol (Stockh) 72:449–450

Kerkhof PC van de (1998) An update on vitamin D3 analogues in the treatment of psoriasis. Skin Pharmacol Appl Skin Physiol 11:2–10

Kerscher M, Volkenandt M, Plewig G et al. (1993) Combination phototherapy of psoriasis with calcipotriol and narrow-band UVB. Lancet 342:923

Koo JY (1998) Tazarotene in combination with phototherapy. J Am Acad Dermatol 39: S144–S148

Koo J, Lebwohl M (1999) Duration of remission of psoriasis therapies. J Am Acad Dermatol 41:51–59

Kragballe K, Dam TN, Hansen ER et al. (1994) Efficacy and safety of the 20-epi-vitamin D3 analogue KH 1060 in the topical therapy of psoriasis: results of a dose-ranging study. Acta Derm Venereol 74:398–402

Lebwohl M, Ellis C, Gottlieb A et al. (1998) Cyclosporine consensus conference: with emphasis on the treatment of psoriasis. J Am Acad Dermatol 39:464–475

Lebwohl M, Poulin Y (1998) Tazarotene in combination with topical corticosteroids. J Am Acad Dermatol 39:S139–S143

Lowe NJ, Wortzman MS, Breeding J et al. (1983) Coal tar phototherapy for psoriasis reevaluated: erythemogenic versus suberythemogenic ultraviolet with a tar extract in oil and crude coal tar. J Am Acad Dermatol 8:781–789

Marks JM (1986) Cyclosporin A treatment of severe psoriasis. Br J Dermatol 115:745–746

Menne T, Larsen K (1992) Psoriasis treatment with vitamin D derivatives. Semin Dermatol 11:278–183

Menter A, Cram DL (1983) The Goeckerman regimen in two psoriasis day care centers. J Am Acad Dermatol 9: 59–65

Michel G, Kemeny L, Homey B et al. (1996) FK506 in the treatment of inflammatory skin disease: promises and perspectives. Immunol Today 17:106–108

Morel P, Revillard JP, Nicolas JF et al. (1992) Anti-CD4 monoclonal antibody therapy in severe psoriasis. J Autoimmun 5:465–477

Mrowietz U, Christophers E, Altmeyer P (1999) Treatment of severe psoriasis with fumaric acid esters: scientific background and guidelines for therapeutic use. Br J Dermatol 141:424–429

Ortel B, Perl S, Kinaciyan T et al. (1993) Comparison of narrow-band (311 nm) UVB and broad-band UVA after oral or bath-water 8-methoxypsoralen in the treatment of psoriasis. J Am Acad Dermatol 29:736–740

Peter RU, Ruzicka T (1992) Cyclosporin A in der Therapie entzündlicher Dermatosen. Hautarzt 43:687–694

Powles AV, Cook T, Hulme B et al. (1993) Renal function and biopsy findings after 5 years' treatment with low-dose cyclosporine for psoriasis. Br J Dermatol 128:159–165

Powles AV, Hardman CM, Porter WM et al. (1998) Renal function after 10 years' treatment with cyclosporine for psoriasis. Br J Dermatol 138:443–449

Prinz JC, Braun-Falco O, Meurer M et al. (1991) Chimeric CD4 monoclonal antibody in treatment of generalized pustular psoriasis. Lancet 338:320–321

Roenigk HH Jr, Auerbach R, Maibach H et al. (1998) Methotrexate in psoriasis: consensus conference. J Am Acad Dermatol 38:478–485

Runne U, Kunze JJ (1982) Short-duration ("minutes") therapy with dithranol for psoriasis: a new out-patient regimen. Br J Dermatol 106:135–139

Shroot B (1986) Anthralin. Dermatologica 173:261–263

Speight EL, Farr PM (1994) Calcipotriol improves the response of psoriasis to PUVA. Br J Dermatol 130:79–82

Steigleder GK, Orfanos CE, Pullmann H (1979) Retinoid-SUP-Therapie der Psoriasis. Z Hautkr 54:19–23

Stern RS (1997) Psoriasis. Lancet 350:349–353

Stern RS, Nichols KT, Vakeva LH (1997) Malignant melanoma in patients treated for psoriasis with methoxsalen (psoralen) and ultraviolet A radiation (PUVA). N Engl J Med 336:1041–1045.

Stern RS, Lange R, Members of the Photochemotherapy Follow-up Study (1988) Non-melanoma skin cancer occurring in patients treated with PUVA five to ten years after treatment. J Invest Dermatol 91:120–124

Streit V, Wiedow O, Christophers E (1994) Innovative Balneotherapie mit reduzierten Badevolumina: Folienbäder. Hautarzt 45:140–144

Studniberg HM, Weller P (1993) PUVA, UVB, psoriasis, and nonmelanoma skin cancer. J Am Acad Dermatol 29:1013–1022

Tanew A, Ortel B, Rappersberger K et al. (1988) 5-methoxypsoralen (Bergapten) for photochemotherapy. Bioavailability, phototoxicity, and clinical efficacy in psoriasis of a new drug preparation. J Am Acad Dermatol 18:333–338

Vallat VP, Gilleaudeau P, Battat L et al. (1994) PUVA bath therapy strongly suppresses immunological and epidermal activation in psoriasis: a possible cellular basis for remittive therapy. J Exp Med 180:283–296

Walters IB, Burack LH, Coven TR et al. (1999) Suberythemogenic narrow-band UVB is markedly more effective than conventional UVB in treatment of psoriasis vulgaris. J Am Acad Dermatol 40:893–900

Wang JTC, Krazmien RJ, Dahlheim CR (1986) Anthralin stain removal. J Am Acad Dermatol 15:951–955

Weinstein GD (1996) Safety, efficacy and duration of therapeutic effect of tazarotene used in the treatment of plaque psoriasis. Br J Dermatol 135 [Suppl 49]:32–36

Zachariae H, Abrams B, Bleehen SS et al. (1998) Conversion of psoriasis patients from the conventional formulation of cyclosporin to a new microemulsion formulation: a randomized, open, multicentre assessment of safety and tolerability. Dermatology 196:231–236

Zachariae H (2000) Liver biopsies and methotrexate: A time for recondsideration? J Am Acad Dermatol 42:531–534

Zaun H (1985) Orale Glukokortikosteroidtherapie bei Psoriasis vulgaris: Pro und Contra. Hautarzt 36:13–15

Pustular Psoriasis

Baker H, Ryan TJ (1968) Generalized pustular psoriasis. A clinical and epidemiological study of 104 cases. Br J Dermatol 8:771–793

Barber HW (1936) Pustular psoriasis of the extremities. Guy Hosp Rep 86:108

Braun-Falco O, Weidner F (1968) Psoriasis vom Typ des Erythema anulare centrifigum mit Pustulation. Hautarzt 19:109–115

Braun-Falco O, Berthold D, Ruzicka T (1987) Psoriasis pustulosa generalisata – Klassifikation, Klinik und Therapie. Übersicht und Erfahrungen an 18 Patienten. Hautarzt 38:509–520

Khan SA, Peterkin GA, Mitchell PC (1972) Juvenile generalized pustular psoriasis. A report of five cases and a review of the literature. Arch Dermatol 105:67–72

Pearson LH, Allen BS, Smith JG Jr (1984) Acrodermatitis continua of Hallopeau: treatment with etretinate and review of relapsing pustular eruptions of the hands and feet. J Am Acad Dermatol 11:755–762

Peter RU, Ruzicka T, Donhauser G et al. (1990) Acrodermatitis continua-type of pustular psoriasis responds to low-dose cyclosporine. J Am Acad Dermatol 23: 515–516

Shelnitz LS, Esterly NB, Honig PJ (1987) Etretinate therapy for generalized pustular psoriasis in children. Arch Dermatol 123:230–233

Zelickson BD, Muller SA (1991) Generalized pustular psoriasis. A review of 63 cases. Arch Dermatol 127:1339–1345

Zumbusch LR von (1909–1910) Psoriasis und pustulöses Exanthem. Arch Dermatol Syph 99:335

Psoriatic Arthritis

Braun-Falco O, Ruzicka T (1994) Psoriatic arthritis. Int J Dermatol 33:320–322

Carette S, Calin A, McCafferty JP et al. (1989) A double-blind placebo-controlled study of auranofin in patients with psoriatic arthritis. Arthritis Rheum 32:158–165

Chamot AM, Benhamou CL, Kahn MF et al. (1987) Acne-pustulosis-hyperostosis-osteitis syndrome. Results of a national survey Rev Rheum Mal Osteoartic 54:187–196

Farr M, Kitas GD, Waterhouse L et al. (1988) Treatment of psoriatic arthritis with sulphasalazine: a one year open study. Clin Rheumatol 7:372–377

Feldges DH, Barnes CG (1974) Treatment of psoriatic arthropathy with either azathioprine or methotrexate. Rheumatol Rehabil 13:120–124

Gupta AK, Matteson EL, Ellis CN et al. (1989) Cyclosporine in the treatment of psoriatic arthritis. Arch Dermatol 125:507–510

Moll JMH (1986) Psoriatic arthropathy. In: Mier PD, Kerkhof PCM van de (eds) Textbook of psoriasis. Churchill Livingstone, Edinburgh, pp 55–83

Olsen TG (1981) Chloroquine and psoriasis. Ann Intern Med 94:546–549

Ruzicka T (1996) Psoriatic arthritis. New types, new treatments. Arch Dermatol 132:215–219

Salvarani C, Zizzi F, Macchioni P et al. (1989) Clinical response to auranofin in patients with psoriatic arthritis. Clin Rheumatol 8:54–57

Seideman P, Fjellner B, Johannesson A (1987) Psoriatic arthritis treated with oral colchicine. J Rheumatol 14: 777–779

Sonozaki H, Mitusi H, Miyanaga Y et al. (1981) Clinical features of 53 cases with pustulotic arthro-osteitis. Ann Rheum Dis 40:547–553

Watts RA, Crisp AJ, Hazleman BL et al. (1993) Arthroosteitis: a clinical spectrum. Br J Rheumatol 32:403–407

Reiter Syndrome

Aho K, Ahvonen P, Lassus A et al. (1974) HL-A 27 in reactive arthritis. A study of Yersinia arthritis and Reiter's disease. Arthritis Rheum 17:521–526

Barron KS, Reveille JD, Carrington M et al. (1995) Susceptibility to Reiter's syndrome is associated with alleles of TAP genes. Arthritis Rheum 38:684–689

Brewerton DA, Caffrey M, Nicholls A et al. (1973) Acute anterior uveitis and HL-A 27. Lancet 2:994–996

Butler MJ, Russell AS, Percy JS et al. (1979) A follow-up study of 48 patients with Reiter's syndrome. Am J Med 67:808–810

Fiessinger N, Leroy E (1916) Contribution à l'étude d'une épidémie de dysenterie dans la Somme (juliett-octobre 1916) Bull Soc Med Hôp 40:2030–2069

Hughes RA, Keat AC (1994) Reiter's syndrome and reactive arthritis: a current view. Semin Arthritis Rheum 24: 190–210

Marks JS, Holt PJ (1986) The natural history of Reiter's disease – 21 years of observations. Q J Med 60:685–697

Reiter H (1916) Ueber eine bisher unbekannte Spirochaeteninfektion (Spirochaetosis arthitica). Dtsch Med Wochenschr 42:1535–1536

Willkens RF, Arnett FC, Bitter T et al. (1981) Reiter's syndrome. Evaluation of preliminary criteria for definite disease. Arthritis Rheum 24:844–849

Yli Kerttula UI (1984) Clinical characteristics in male and female uro-arthritis or Reiter's syndrome. Clin Rheumatol 3:351–360

Pityriasis Rubra Pilaris

Braun-Falco O, Ryckmanns F, Schmoeckel C et al. (1983) Pityriasis rubra pilaris: a clinico-pathological and therapeutic study with special reference to histochemistry, autoradiography, and electron microscopy. Arch Dermatol Res 275:287–295

Cohen PR, Prystowsky JH (1989) Pityriasis rubra pilaris: a review of diagnosis and treatment. J Am Acad Dermatol 20:801–807

Davidson CL, Winkelmann RK, Kierland RR (1969) Pityriasis rubra pilaris – follow up study of 57 patients. Arch Dermatol 100:175–183

Devergie A (1857) Pityriasis pilaris. In: Traité practique des maladies de la peau, 2nd edn. Martinet, Paris pp 454–464

Dicken CH (1994) Treatment of classic pityriasis rubra pilaris. J Am Acad Dermatol 31:997–999

Fleissner J, Happle R (1981) Etretinate in the treatment of juvenile pityriasis rubra pilaris. Arch Dermatol 117:749–750

Goldsmith LA, Weinrich AE, Shupack J (1982) Pityriasis rubra pilaris response to 13-cis-retinoic acid. J Am Acad Dermatol 6:1710–1715

Grimnalt R, Gelmetti C, Brusasco A et al. (1994) Pityriasis rotunda: report of a familial ocurrence and review of the literature. J Am Acad Dermatol 31:866–871

Martin AG, Weaver CC, Cockerell CJ et al. (1992) Pityriasis rubra pilaris in the setting of HIV infection: clinical behaviour and association with explosive cystic acne. Br J Dermatol 126:617–620

Meyer P, Voorst PC van (1989) Lack of effect of cyclosporine in pityriasis rubra pilaris. Acta Derm Venereol 69:272

Pavlidakey GP, Hashimoto K, Savoy LB et al. (1985) Stanazolol in the treatment of pityriasis rubra pilaris. Arch Dermatol 121:546–548

Piamphongsant T, Akaraphant R (1994) Pityriasis rubra pilaris: a new proposed classification. Clin Exp Dermatol 19:134–138

Soeprono FF (1986) Histologic criteria for the diagnosis of pityriasis rubra pilaris. Am J Dermatopathol 8:277–283

Vanderhooft SL, Francis JS, Holbrook KA et al. (1995) Familial pityriasis rubra pilaris. Arch Dermatol 131:448–453

Parapsoriasis

Altmann J (1984) Parapsoriasis: a histopathological review and classification. Semin Dermatol 3:14.21
Brocq L (1902) Les parapsoriasis. Ann Dermatol 3:433–468
Burg G, Dummer R (1995) Small plaque (digitate) parapsoriasis is an abortive cutaneous T cell lymphoma and is not mycosis fungoides. Arch Dermatol 131:336–338
Burg G, Hoffmann-Fezer G, Nikolowski J et al. (1981) Lymphomatoid papulosis. Acta Derm Venereol (Stockh) 61:491–496
Cliff S, Cook MG, Ostlere LS et al. (1996) Segmental pityriasis lichenoides chronica. Clin Exp Dermatol 21:464–465
English JC, Collins M, Bryant-Bruce C (1995) Pityriasis lichenoides et varioliformis acuta and group-A beta hemolytic streptococcal infection. Int J Dermatol 34:642–644
Fink-Puches R, Soyer HP, Kerl H (1994) Febrile ulceronecrotic pityriasis lichenoides et varioliformis acuta. J Am Acad Dermatol 30:261–263
Gelmetti C, Rigoni C, Alessi et al. (1990) Pityriasis lichenoides in children: a long term follow-up eighty-nine cases. J Am Acad Dermatol 23:473–478
Habermann R (1925) Über die akut verlaufende, nekrotisiernde Unterart der Pityriasis lichenoides (pityriasis lichenoides et varioliformis acuta). Dermatol Z 45:42–48
Hood AF, Mark EJ (1982) Histopathologic diagnosis of PLEVA and its clinical correlation. Arch Dermatol 118:478–482
Hu CH, Winkelmann RK (1973) Digitate dermatosis. A new look at symmetrical small plaque parapsoriasis. Arch Dermatol 107:65–69
Jacobi E (1906) Fall zur Diagnose. (Poikilodemia vascularis atrophicans). Verh Deut Dermatol Ges, 9th Congress, pp 321–323
Jadassohn J (1894) Über ein eigenartiges psoriasiformes und lichenoides Exanthem. In: Verhandlung Deut Dermatol Ges, 4th Congress Breslau, p 524
Juliusberg F (1899) Über die Pityriasis lichenoides chronica (psoriasiform-lichenoides Exanthem). Arch Dermatol Syph 50:359–374
Kikuchi A, Naka W, Harada T et al. (1993) Parapsoriasis en plaques: its potential for progression to malignant lymphoma. J Am Acad Dermatol 29:419–422
Lambert WB, Everett MA (1981) The nosology of parapsoriasis. J Am Acad Dermatol 5:373–395
Le Vine MJ (1983) Phototherapy for pityriasis lichenoides. Arch Dermatol 119:378–380
Longley J, Demar L, Feinstein RP et al. (1987) Clinical and histological features of pityriasis lichenoides et varioliformis acuta in children. Arch Dermatol 123:1335–1339
Maekawa Y, Nakamura T, Nogami R (1994) Febrile ulceronecrotic Mucha-Habermann`s disease. J Dermatol 21:46–49
Mucha V (1916) Über einen der Parakeratosis variegata (Unna) bzw. Pityriasis lichenoides chronica (Neisser-Juliusberg) nahestehenden eigentümlichen Fall. Arch Dermatol Syphilol 123:586–592
Muhlbauer JE, Bhan AK (1984) Immunopathology of PLEVA. J Am Acad Dermatol 10:783–795
Panizzon RG, Speich R, Dazzi H (1992) Atypical manifestations of pityriasis lichenoides chronica: development into paraneoplasia and non-Hodgkin lymphomas of the skin. Dermatology 184:65–69
Radcliffe-Crocker H (1905) Xanthoerythroderma perstans. Br J Dermatol 17:119–134
Rogers M (1992) Pityriasis lichenoides and lymphomatoid papulosis. Semin Dermatol 11:73–79
Rongioletti F, Rivara G, Rebora A (1987) Pityriasis lichenoides et varioliformis acuta and acquired toxoplasmosis. Dermatologica 175:41–44
Ross S, Sanchez JL (1990) Parapsoriasis. A century later. Int J Dermatol 29:329–330
Suarez J, Lopez B, Vilalba R et al. (1996) Febrile ulceronecrotic Mucha-Habermann disease: a case report and review of the literature. Dermatology 192:277–279
Takahashi K, Atsumi M (1993) Pityriasis lichenoides chronica resolving after tonsillectomy. Br J Dermatol 129:353–354
Truhan AP, Hebert AA, Esterly NB (1986) Pityriasis lichenoides in children: therapeutic response to erythromycin. J Am Acad Dermatol 15:66–70
Unna PG, Santi DR, Pollitzer S (1890) Über die Parakeratosen im Allgemeinen und eine neue Form derselben (Parakeratosis variegata). Monatsch Prakt Dermatol 10:404–412, 444–459
Vella Briffa D, Warin AP, Calnon CD (1979) Parakeratosis variegata: a report of two cases and their treatment with PUVA. Clin Exp Dermatol 4:537–541

Papuloerythroderma

Depaire F, Dereure O, Guilhou J (1996) Ofuji's papuloerythroderma: report of a new case responding to PUVA. Acta Derm Venereol (Stockh) 76:93–94
Dwyer CM, Chapman RS, Smith GD (1994) Papuloerythroderma and cutaneous T cell lymphoma. Dermatology 188:326–328
Garcia-Patos V, Repiso T, Rodriguez-Cano L et al. (1996) Ofuji papuloerythroderma in a patient with the acquired immunodeficiency syndrome. Dermatology 192:164–166
Harris DW, Spencer MJ, Tidman MJ (1990) Papuloerythroderma – clinical and ultrastructural features. Clin Exp Dermatol 15:105–106
Ofuji S, Furukawa F, Miyachi Y et al. (1984) Dermatologica 169:125–130
Tay YK, Tan KC, Wong WK et al. (1994) Papuloerythroderma of Ofuji: a report of three cases and review of the literature. Br J Dermatol 130:773–776

Erythroderma

Abel EA, Lindae ML, Hoppe TR et al. (1988) Benign and malignant forms of cutaneous erythroderma: cutaneous immunophenotypic characteristics. J Am Acad Dermatol 19:1089–1095
Boyd AS, Menter A (1989) Erythrodermic psoriasis. J Am Acad Dermatol 21:985–991
Hasan T, Jansen CT (1983) Erythroderma. A follow-up of fifty cases. J Am Acad Dermatol 8:836–840
Krook G (1960) Hypothermia in patients with exfoliative dermatitis. Acta Derm Venereol 40:142–160
Montgomery H (1933) Exfoliative dermatosis and malignant erythroderma: the value and limitations of histopathologic studies. Arch Dermat Syphil 27:253

Nicolis GD, Hewig EB (1973) Exfoliative dermatitis. A clinicopathologic study of 135 cases. Arch Dermatol 108:788–797
Pal S, Haroon TS (1998) Erythroderma: a clinico-etiologic study of 90 cases. Int J Dermatol 37:104–107
Rubins AY, Hartmane IV, Lielbriedis YM et al. (1992) Therapeutic options for erythroderma. Cutis 49:424–426
Sentis HJ, Willemze R, Scheffer E (1986) Histopathologic studies of Sézary syndrome and erythrodermic mycosis fungoides: a comparison with benign forms of erythroderma. J Am Acad Dermatol 15:1217–1226
Shuster S, Wilkinson P (1963) Protein metabolism in exfoliative dermatitis and erythroderma. Br J Dermatol 75:344–353
Sigurdsson V, Toonstra J, Vloten WA van (1997) Idiopathic erythroderma: a follow-up study of 28 patients. Dermatology 194:98–101
Thestrup-Pedersen K, Halkier-Sørensen L, Søgaard H et al. (1988) The red man syndrome. J Am Acad Dermatol 18:1307–1312
Walsh NM, Prokopetz R, Tron VA et al. (1994) Histopathology in erythroderma: review of a series of cases by multiple observers. J Cutan Pathol 21:419–423
Winkelmann RK, Buechner SA, Diaz-Perez JL (1984) Pre-Sézary syndrome. J Am Acad Dermatol 10:992–999
Worm AM, Taaning E, Rossing N (1981) Distribution and degradation of albumin in extensive skin disease. Br J Dermatol 104:389–396

Lichen Planus

Acactingi S, Chosidow O (1998) Cutaneous graft-versus-host disease. Arch Dermatol 134:602–612
Annessi G, Signoretti S, Angelo C et al. (1997) Neutrophilic figurate erythema of infancy. Am J Dermatopathol 19:403–406
Bellman B, Reddy RK, Falanga V (1995) Lichen planus associated with hepatitis C. Lancet 346:1234
Black MM (1977) What is going on in lichen planus. Clin Exp Dermatol 2:303–310
Camisa C, Hamaty FG, Gay JD (1998) Squamous cell carcinoma of the tongue arising in lichen planus: a case report and review of the literature. Cutis 62:175–178
Cram DL, Kierland RR, Winkelmann RK (1966) Ulcerative lichen planus of the feet. Arch Dermatol 93:692–701
Cribier B, Frances C, Chosidow O (1998) Treatment of lichen planus. An evidence-based medicine analysis of efficacy. Arch Dermatol 134:1521–1530
Crotty CP, Su WPD, Winkelmann RK (1980) Ulcerative lichen planus. Follow-up of surgical excision and grafting. Arch Dermatol 116:1252–1256
Ellgehausen P, Elsner P, Burg G (1998) Drug-induced lichen planus. Clin Dermatol 16:325–332
Fellner MJ (1980) Lichen planus. Int J Dermatol 19:71–75
Hintner H, Tappeiner G, Hönigsmann H et al. (1979) Lichen planus and bullous pemphigoid. Acta Dermato Venereol (Stockh) 59 [Suppl 85]:71–76
Katzenellenbogen I (1962) Lichen planus actinicus (lichen planus in subtropical countries). Dermatologica 124:10–20
Kronenberg K, Fretzing D, Potter B (1971) Malignant degeneration of lichen planus. Arch Dermatol 104:304–307
Oliver GF, Winkelmann RK (1993) Treatment of lichen planus. Drugs 45:56–65
Plotnick H, Burnham TK (1986) Lichen planus and coexisting lupus erythematosus versus lichen planus-like lupus erythematosus. Clinical, histologic, and immunopathologic considerations. J Am Acad Dermatol 14:931–938
Powell FC, Rogers RS, Dickson ER et al. (1986) An association between HLA DR1 and lichen planus. Int J Dermatol 114:473–478
Ragaz A, Ackerman B (1981) Evolution, maturation and regression of lesions of lichen planus. New observations and correlation of clinical and histologic findings. Am J Dermatopathol 3:5–25
Sehgal VN, Abraham GIS, Malik GB (1972) Griseofulvin therapy in lichen planus: a double-blind controlled trial. Brit J Dermatol 87:383–385
Shklar P (1968) Erosive and bullous oral lesions of lichen planus. Arch Dermatol 97:411–416
Tosti A, Peluso AM, Fanti PA et al. (1993) Nail lichen planus: clinical and pathologic study of twenty-four patients. J Am Acad Dermatol 28:724–730
Wilson E (1869) On leichen planus. J Cutan Med Dis Skin 3:117–132
Woo TY (1985) Systemic isotretinoin treatment of oral and cutaneous lichen planus. Cutis 35:385–393

Lichen Nitidus

Chen W, Schramm M, Zouboulis CC (1997) Generalized lichen nitidus. J Am Acad Dermatol 36:630–631
Mihara M, Nakayama H, Shimao S (1991) Lichen nitidus: a histologic and electron microscopic study. J Dermatol 18:475–480
Pinkus F (1907) Über eine neue knochenformige Hauteruption: Lichen nitidus. Arch Dermatol Syph 85:11–36
Smoller BR, Flynn TC (1992) Immunohistochemical examination of lichen nitidus suggests that it is not a localized papular variant of lichen planus. J Am Acad Dermatol 27:232–236

Actinic Lichen Nitidus

Bedi TR (1978) Summertime actinic lichenoid eruption. Dermatologica 157:115–125
Hussain K (1998) Summertime actinic lichenoid eruption, a distinct entity, should be termed actinic lichen nitidus. Arch Dermatol 134:1302–1303

Graft Versus Host Disease

Aractingi S, Chosidow O (1998) Cutaneous graft-versus-host disease. Arch Dermatol 134:602–612
Atkinson K, Horowitz MM, Biggs JC (1988) The clinical diagnosis of acute graft-versus-host disease: a diversity of views amongst marrow transplant centers. Bone Marrow Transplant 3:5–10
Chosidow O, Bagot M, Vernant JP et al. (1992) Sclerodermatous chronic graft-versus-host discase. Analysis of seven cases. J Am Acad Dermatol 26:49–55
Darmstadt GL, Donnenberg AD, Vogelsang GB (1992) Clinical, laboratory, and histopathologic indications of the development of progressive acute graft-versus-host disease. J Invest Dermatol 99:397–402
Ferrara JL, Deeg HJ (1991) Graft-versus-host disease. N Engl J Med 324:667–664
Gale RP, Horowitz MM, Butturini A et al. (1992) What determines who develops graft-versus-host disease: the graft or the host (or both)? Bone Marrow Transplant 10:99–102

Greinix HAT, Volc-Platzer B, Rabitsch W et al. (1998) Successful use of extracorporeal photochemotherapy in the treatment of severe acute and chronic graft-versus-host disease. Blood 92:3098–3104

Kelemen E, Szebeni J, Petranyi GG (1993) Graft-versus-host disease in bone marrow transplantation: experimental, laboratory, and clinical contributions of the last few years. Int Arch Allergy Immunol 102:309–320

Loughran TP Jr, Sullivan K, Morton T et al. (1990) Value of day 100 screening studies for predicting the development of chronic graft-versus-host disease after allogeneic bone marrow transplantation. Blood 76:228–234

Rowe JM, Ciobanu N, Ascensao J et al. (1994) Recommended guidelines for the management of autologous and allogeneic bone marrow transplantation. A report from the Eastern Cooperative Oncology Group (ECOG). Ann Intern Med 120:143–158

Saurat JH (1981) Cutaneous manifestations of graft-versus-host disease. Int J Dermatol 20:249–256

Saurat JH, Gluckman E, Bussel A et al. (1975) The lichen planus-like eruption after bone marrow transplantation. Br J Dermatol 93:675–681

Schiller G, Gale RP (1993) Is there an effective therapy for chronic graft-versus-host disease? Bone Marrow Transplant 11:189–192

Siadak MF, Kopecky K, Sullivan KM (1994) Reduction in transplant-related complications in patients given intravenous immuno globulin after allogeneic marrow transplantation. Clin Exp Immunol 97 [Suppl 1]: 53–57

Tanaka K, Sullivan KM, Shulman HM (1991) A clinical review: cutaneous manifestations of acute and chronic graft-versus-host disease following bone marrow transplantation. J Dermatol 18:11–17

Volc-Platzer B, Hönigsmann H, Hinterberger W (1990) Photochemotherapy improves chronic cutaneous graft-versus-host disease. J Am Acad Dermatol 23:220–228

Frictional Lichenoid Dermatitis

Asthon RE, Russel-Jones R, Griffiths WAD (1985) Juvenile plantar dermatosis. Arch Dermatol 121:253–260

Jones SK, English JSC, Forsyth A (1987) Juvenile plantar dermatosis – an 8-year follow-up of 102 patients. Clin Exp Dermatol 1:5–7

McKie RM (1982) Juvenile plantar dermatosis. Semin Dermatol 1:67–71

McKie RM, Husain SL (1976) Juvenile plantar dermatosis. A new entity? Clin Exp Dermatol 1:253–260

Moller H (1972) Atopic winter feet in children. Acta Dermato Venereol (Stockh) 52:401–405

Sutton RL, Jr (1956) Diseases of the skin, 11th edn. Mosby, St. Louis, p 898

Waisman M, Sutton RL (1966) Frictional lichenoid eruption in children. Arch Dermatol 94:592–593

Gianotti-Crosti Syndrome

Baldari U, Monti A, Righini MG (1994) An epidemic of infantile papular acrodermatitis (Gianotti-Crosti syndrome) due to Epstein-Barr virus. Dermatology 188: 203–204

Braun-Falco O, Rupec M (1964) Über das Gianotti-Crosti-Syndrom (Acrodermatitis papulosa eruptiva infantilis). Med Klin 52:210–214

Caputo R, Gelmetti C, Ermacora E (1992) Gianotti-Crosti syndrome: a retrospective analysis of 308 cases. J Am Acad Dermatol 26:207–210

Carrascosa JM, Just M, Ribera M (1998) Papular acrodermatitis of childhood related to poxvirus and parvovirus B19 infection. Cutis 61:265–267

Crosti A, Gianotti F (1956) Dermatosi infantile eruttiva acroesposta di probabile orgine virosica. Minerva Dermatol 31 (Suppl 12):483

Crosti A, Gianotti F (1964) Ulteriore contributo alla conoscenza dell'acrodermatite papulosa infantile. G Ital Derm 105:477

Gianotti F (1955) Rilievi di una particolare casisistica tossinfettiva caratterizzata da eruzione eritemato-infiltrativa desquamativa a focolai lenticolari, a sede elettiva acroesposta. G Ital Derm Sif 96:678–697

Gianotti F (1973) Papular acrodermatitis of childhood. Arch Dis Child 43:794–799

Gianotti F (1979) Papular acrodermatitis of childhood and other papulovesicular acro-located syndromes. Br J Dermatol 100:49–59

James WD, Odom RB, Hatch MH (1982) Gianotti-Crosti-like eruption associated with Coxsackie A-16 infection. J Am Acad Dermatol 6:862–866

Lowe L, Hebert AA, Duvic M (1989) Gianotti-Crosti syndrome associated with Epstein-Barr virus infection. J Am Acad Dermatol 20:336–338

Ramelet A-A (1984) Mononucléose infectieuse avec manifestations cutanées à type d'acrosyndrome de Gianotti-Crosti. Dermatologica 168:19–24

Sagi EF, Linden N, Shonval D (1985) Papular acrodermatitis of childhood associated with hepatitis A virus infection. Pediatr Dermatol 3:31–33

Spear KL, Winkelmann RK (1984) Gianotti-Crosti syndrome. Arch Dermatol 120:891–896

Taieb A, Plantin P, du Pasquier P et al. (1986) Gianotti-Crosti syndrome: a study of 26 cases. Br J Dermatol 115:49–59

Lichen Simplex Chronicus

Berlin C (1939) Lichenification gigantea (Lichenification géante of Brocq and Pautrier). Arch Dermatol 39:1012–1020

Brocq, Pautrier (1910) Über einige abnormale Formen von Lichenifikation. Arch Dermatol Syph 99:421

Kantor GR, Resnik KS (1996) Treatment of lichen simplex chronicus with topical capsaicin cream. Acta Derm Venereol 76:161

Kinsella LJ, Carney-Godley K, Feldmann E (1992) Lichen simplex chronicus as the initial manifestation of intramedullary neoplasm and syringomyelia. Neurosurgery 30:418–421

Robertson IM, Jordan JM, Withlock FA (1975) Emotions and skin (III) – the conditioning of scratch responses in cases of lichen simplex. Br J Dermatol 92:407–412

Singh G (1973) Atopy in lichen simplex (neurodermatitis circumscripta). Br J Dermatol 88:625–627

Vidal E (1886) Du lichen (lichen, prurigo, strophulus) Ann Derm Syph 7:133–154

Lichen Striatus

Gianotti R, Restano L, Grimalt R (1995) Lichen striatus – a chameleon: an histopathological and immunohistological study of forty-one cases. J Cutan Pathol 22:18–22

Grosshans E, Margot L (1990) Blaschkite de l'adulte. Ann Dermatol Venereol 117:9–15

Herd RM, McLaren KM, Aldrige RD (1993) Linear lichen planus and lichen striatus – opposite ends of a spectrum. Clin Exp Dermatol 19:335–337

Karp DL, Cohen BA (1993) Onychodystrophy in lichen striatus. Pediatr Dermatol 10:359–361

Kaufman J (1974) Lichen striatus with nail involvement. Cutis 14:232–234

Taieb A, El-Youbi A, Grosshans E et al. (1991) Lichen striatus: a Blaschko linear acquired inflammatory skin eruption. J Am Acad Dermatol 25:637–642

Toda K, Okamoto H, Horio T (1986) Lichen striatus. Int J Dermatol 25:584–585

Tosti A, Peluso AM, Misciali C (1997) Nail lichen striatus: clinical features and long-term follow-up of five patients. J Am Acad Dermatol 36:908–913

Blistering Diseases

Contents

This group of primarily chronic diseases have blisters as their primary clinical feature. The site of action may be within the epidermis, at the epidermal-dermal junction or in the very uppermost dermis. In some instances, the disorders are congenital with abnormal structural proteins. In other instances, they are acquired and described as autoimmune because they feature antibodies against structural components of the epidermis and epidermal-dermal junction. Still other blistering diseases have other mechanisms, such as the porphyrias (Chap. 44), or are entirely mysterious as is the case for bullous disease of diabetes (Chap. 48).

Basic Science Aspects

In order to understand why cells fall apart, one must at least have an overview of what keeps them together. Figures 15.1 and 15.2 show the major structures involved in the process of holding epidermal cells together and attaching them to the dermis at the epidermal-dermal junction. The cells of the mid-epidermis have long been called the spinous layer. This refers to how they stay together, that is via connecting structures known as desmosomes which are thickenings in the cell membrane which temporarily hold two keratinocytes together. Thus, when the cells retract during fixation, they remain attached by molecules designated as integrins, leading to elongations or spines which terminate at the desmosomes. As the cells move from the basal layer to the stratum corneum, they continuously form and break attachments. Desmosomes can best be viewed by electron microscopy. They show both intracellular and intercellular components, making a large sandwich which consists of several layers: cytoplasmic plaque–cell membrane–intercellular attachments–cell membrane–cytoplasmic plaque.

At a higher magnification, within the keratinocyte, the keratin intermediate filaments can be seen to connect to the plakin proteins which are found just beneath the cell membrane. The main constituents of the plakin cytoplasmic plaque or mat are desmoplakin I and II, as well as desmocollin, envoplakin, periplakin and plakoglobin. Also attached to this mat or plaque are the transmembrane components, desmogleins and desmocollins, members of the cadherin family. The extracellular domain of the cadherin binds to a homologous sequence on a cadherin from another cell, completing the bridge. The glycocalyx or intercellular cement is a gel rich

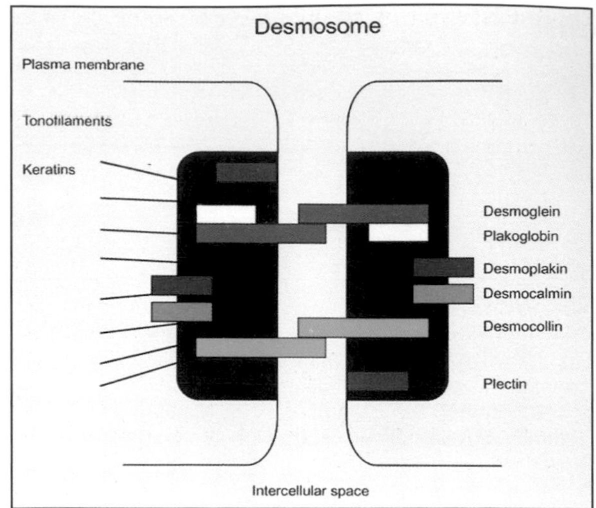

Fig. 15.1. Diagram of desmosome

in glycoproteins which provides some adherence, but allows diffusion and gradual motion. While a number of autoantibodies are directed against desmosomal elements, surprisingly few inherited defects have been described. A mutation in plakophilin 1 has been associated with increased skin fragility and a variety of epidermal defects.

Desmosomes are a specific characteristic of epithelial cells. In the past electron microscopy was used extensively to characterize tumors. Finding desmosomes in a cutaneous tumor meant one was dealing with a squamous cell carcinoma. There are other types of epidermal attachment bodies, including hemidesmosomes which attach to a basement membrane. In addition there are focal adherens plaques made up of integrins, adherens junctions formed by cadherins and gap junctions which allow the passage of ions and small molecules facilitating

Fig. 15.2. Diagram of epidermal-dermal junction

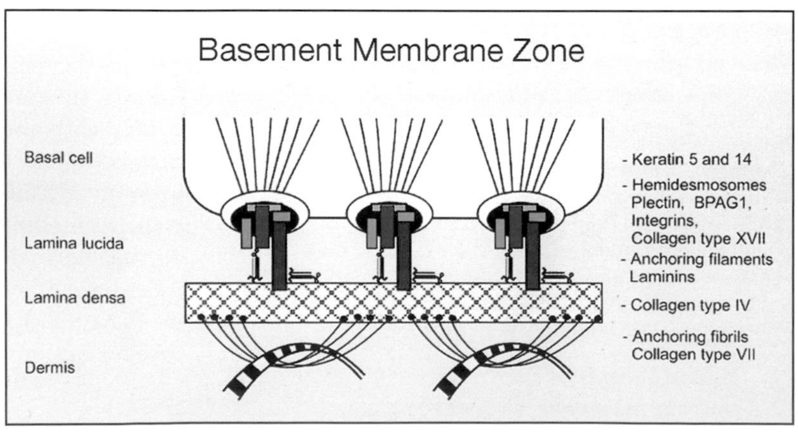

communication by soluble factors. Some of these other attachments are not restricted to epithelial cells.

As one views the epidermal-dermal junction at progressively higher magnifications, the complexity of its organization becomes obvious. By light microscopy the epidermal-dermal junction is barely visible, although it can be better appreciated with PAS stain. In lupus erythematosus, it appears thickened. On ultrastructural examination, more complexity becomes apparent. The basilar keratinocytes are attached to the basement membrane by hemidesmosomes, localized thickenings of the inferior pole. Underneath the hemidesmosomes is an electron-lucid area (the lamina lucida), an electron-dense area (the lamina densa), and finally the anchoring filaments and other fibrous elements of the upper dermis (sublamina densa zone). All these elements interact to form a firmly adherent but flexible junction between the epidermis and dermis.

Many of the molecules which participate in this process have been identified. The keratin intermediate filaments, primarily those of keratins 5 and 14, attach to the hemidesmosomes, which contain plectin and bullous pemphigoid antigen 1 (BPAG1), a 230-kDa protein with homologies to desmoplakin. Plectin is involved in anchoring the intermediate filaments to the plasma membrane. The integrin $\alpha 6\beta 4$ extends from the hemidesmosome into the lamina lucida, while BPAG2 also known as type XVII collagen, extends through the lamina lucida, connecting hemidesmosomes to the lamina densa. Since the anchoring filaments are found in the same area, it may be that BPAG2 as well as laminin 6 form these structures. Other antigens associated with the anchoring filaments include the antigen recognized by 19-DEJ-1 and uncein; both are poorly characterized. Laminin 5 was formerly held to be the major component of the lamina lucida, but recent studies indicate it is concentrated in the lamina densa and may extend to the hemidesmosomes. Nidogen helps attach laminin 1 to the lamina densa, which is comprised primarily of type IV collagen and perlecan. The anchoring fibrils composed of type VII collagen anchor the lamina densa to the dermis. They originate and terminate in the lamina densa, forming semicircular loops.

Study of this region has undergone a number of changes as new techniques have become available. Light microscopy alone seldom allows a specific diagnosis. Even when a blister is identified, its exact level and associated disease are difficult to determine. Both Achilles Civatte and Walter Lever used light microscopy to separate pemphigus from dermatitis herpetiformis and bullous pemphigoid because of acantholysis in the former. In the mid-1960s Beutner, Jordon and colleagues introduced immunofluorescent examination, both direct and indirect, to more accurately define diseases such as pemphigus vulgaris and bullous pemphigoid. Immunoelectron microscopy made it possible to more accurately identify the site of deposition of immunoreactants. Several modifications of the above techniques have proven highly useful. When normal human epidermis is exposed to a 1 M NaCl solution, separation occurs within the lamina lucida and various antigens of the basement membrane zone are made more easily accessible for specific antibodies. Thus, indirect immunofluorescent examination using salt-split skin allows one to map the epidermolysis bullosa acquisita antigen (type VII collagen) to the base of the separation and the BPAGs to the top. The same technique can be used for direct immunofluorescent testing, as the patient's tissue is incubated in the salt solution. Immunomapping is another valuable tool as shown in Table 15.1. If a panel of antibodies are used, such as antibodies to BPAG2, laminins, and type IV collagen, the level of separation can be mapped. This simplified scheme is rarely used today; instead more sophisticated mapping using the antigens listed in Table 15.2 and others is employed.

In the past few years, the use of a wide variety of molecular genetic techniques, including immunoblotting, gene sequencing, protein analysis, generation of transgenic animals, creation of partial anti-

Table 15.1. Simplified immunofluorescent mapping of epidermolysis bullosa blisters

Type of blister	Bullous pemphigoid antigens	Laminins	Type IV collagen
Epidermal (simplex)	Base	Base	Base
Junctional	Roof	Base	Base
Dermal (dystrophic)	Roof	Roof	Roof

Table 15.2. Acquired and inherited diseases associated with various components of the epidermal basement membrane zone

Antigen	Level	Inherited defects	Autoantibodies
Keratins 5, 14	Basal cell	EB simplex	
Plectin	Lamina lucida (hemidesmosome)	EB with muscular dystrophy	
BPAG1	Lamina lucida (hemidesmosome)		Bullous pemphigoid, herpes gestationis
BPAG2	Lamina lucida	Generalized atrophic benign (junctional) EB	Bullous pemphigoid, herpes gestationis, cicatricial pemphigoid, linear IgA disease
Integrin α6 β4	Lamina lucida	Junctional EB with pyloric atresia	
Laminin 5	Lamina lucida	Junctional EB Herlitz type and others	Cicatricial pemphigoid
Type VII collagen	Dermis	Dystrophic EB	Epidermolysis bullosa acquisita, bullous eruption of systemic lupus erythematosus, porphyria cutanea tarda

EB, epidermolysis bullosa

genic epitopes, transfection of cells with target antigens and many other approaches have allowed an even more accurate understanding of the dermal-epidermal junction and its associated diseases. Structures that are targets in acquired blistering diseases have also been shown to be the site of mutations in inherited blistering disorders such as epidermolysis bullosa. For example, patients with one type of cicatricial pemphigoid have autoantibodies against laminin 5 or 6, while mutations in the same molecules cause the Herlitz or letalis form of junctional epidermolysis bullosa.

In the past a great deal of emphasis was placed on the frequency with which immunofluorescent examinations were positive. Today for most diseases one can say that direct immunofluorescent examination is positive in almost all cases, depending on the degree of sophistication of the laboratory, and that circulating antibodies for indirect immunofluorescent examination are present in slightly fewer cases. Salt-split human skin has greatly increased the yield for most diseases involving the basement membrane zone, as have the more sophisticated techniques such as immunoblotting and ELISA. Today none of the autoimmune blistering diseases is diagnosed without at least one positive test identifying the presence of autoantibodies.

The pathogenesis of the blistering diseases has remained difficult to elucidate. Even though intuitively one assumes that the specific antibodies are causing disease, they could just as easily reflect another process. For example, inflammation, such as a viral infection, or trauma, such as a burn, could expose or alter normal proteins, making them more antigenic. Similarly genetic variation in structural proteins or molecules involved in specific immune reactions or loss of self-tolerance (via the HLA antigens) could trigger autoimmune processes. While there are some structural proteins that lead to inherited disorders when altered by a mutation and also serve as targets of autoantibodies, there are others that tend to present either as mutations or as antibody targets. In some instances injecting the autoantibodies into an experimental animal does not reproduce disease because of interspecies differences in epitopes. A wide variety of tricks have been employed to create disease models, such as producing antibodies in one species of laboratory animal and transferring them to another, or immunizing an animal with an epitope of a suspected antigen.

A complex issue is the relationship between medications and the autoimmune blistering disorders. Most textbooks contain long lists of drugs that may cause pemphigus vulgaris, bullous pemphigoid and other disorders. Both ionizing and ultraviolet radiation have also been incriminated. There are many problems inherent in such analyses. First, many of the lists were compiled using diagnoses which were not made using the current standard techniques. Next, most patients with bullous pemphigoid are elderly and may be taking several medications. In addition, the blistering disorders especially pemphigus vulgaris are severe enough that repeat challenges are usually not undertaken. Furthermore, one can always argue that the medication or irradiation triggered or revealed an already present disorder, perhaps by altering the immune status. While we have discussed the incriminated agents under the various diseases, we are skeptical that medications are a major cause of autoimmune blistering diseases and suggest they are more likely to expose or make more prominent an already-existing perhaps subclinical disorder. Nonetheless, if a possible offending agent is identified, it is well worth eliminating the medication and observing the patient's course.

Epidermolysis Bullosa

Epidermolysis bullosa refers to a group of hereditary diseases all of which present at birth or early in life with blisters of the skin or mucosa. Inheritance occurs in both autosomal dominant and autosomal recessive patterns. The blisters can arise spontaneously but are most often associated with minor trauma. For this reason, the group is also known as the mechanobullous disorders. The diseases have traditionally been grouped according to the level of separation – within the epidermis, at the epidermal-dermal junction or in the upper dermis. The variants with deeper involvement are those that most often scar. The main clinical problem is secondarily infected erosions that heal poorly. Often other epithelial structures, such as hair, nails, teeth and oral mucosa are involved. These features are also helpful in subdividing this befuddling list. New mutations leading to new subtypes of epidermolysis bullosa are described regularly, but Table 15.3 gives an overview of the major types. We suspect that within a matter of years, this classification will be regarded as a dinosaur. As more and more gene defects are identified, undoubtedly some clinical forms of epidermolysis bullosa will be unified, i. e., one gene may be responsible for several clinical types. In addition, others will become more complex as mutations in several genes will be shown to produce similar clinical changes.

Prenatal diagnosis is possible in many cases. In those instances where the genetic defect is known, gene analysis can be used. In suspected junctional epidermolysis bullosa, a fetal skin biopsy can be used to assess the possible reduction in hemidesmosomes, while in dystrophic epidermolysis bullosa, the same procedure may allow one to analyze type VII collagen. Most often, immunomapping is done on fetal skin biopsies, if a specific defect is suspected.

The differential diagnosis of epidermolysis bullosa is primarily the other forms of epidermolysis bullosa, so we will not repeatedly discuss it but emphasize difficulties. One area of confusion is epidermolysis bullosa acquisita. Although the name is similar and epidermolysis bullosa acquisita can occasionally be seen in children, the two disorders have little in common clinically. Epidermolysis bullosa acquisita resembles bullous pemphigoid, cicatricial pemphigoid or porphyria cutanea tarda. Therapy for epidermolysis bullosa is discussed at the end of the section, as it is similar for all variants.

Epidermolysis Bullosa Simplex

Synonym. Epidermolytic epidermolysis bullosa

The diseases in this group are primarily inherited in an autosomal dominant pattern and tend to form mechanical blisters that heal without scarring. They usually are confined to the skin although some are associated with systemic disorders. The genetics of the three main variants, the Köbner, Weber-Cockayne and Dowling-Meara types, have been greatly clarified by transgenic mice studies. The mutations lie in the genes for keratins 5 (chromosome 12q) and 14 (chromosome 17q), the main keratins of the basal layer keratinocytes. The Dowling-Meara patients have the most severe clumping of keratin filaments. The location of the mutation in the keratin gene determines how it affects the keratin arrangement and this correlates well with the clinical severity. The principle histologic change in almost all forms of epidermolysis bullosa simplex is basal layer clefting and cytolysis, known as epidermolytic blistering. Inflammatory cells are sparse. Immunofluorescent mapping with bullous pemphigoid antisera can be used to

Table 15.3. The types of epidermolysis bullosa

Major category	Disease	Inheritance
Epidermal EB (EB Simplex (EBS))		
Localized	EBS of hands and feet (Weber-Cockayne)	AD
	EBS with anodontia/hypodontia (Kallin)	AR
Generalized	EBS, Köbner variant	AD
	EBS herpetiformis (Dowling-Meara)	AD
	EBS with mottled hyperpigmentation	AD
	EBS, Ogna variant	AD
	EBS superficialis	AD
	EBS with muscular dystrophy	AR
	EBS, Mendes da Costa variant	XLR
Junctional EB (JEB)		
Localized	JEB inversa	AR
	JEB, acral variant	AR
	JEB, progressiva variant	AR
Generalized	JEB, gravis variant (Herlitz)	AR
	JEB with pyloric stenosis	AR
	JEB, mitis variant (generalized atrophic benign EB)	AR
	Cicatricial JEB	AR
Dystrophic (DEB)		
Localized	RDEB, inversa variant	AR
	DDEB, acral variant	AD
	DDEB, pretibial variant	AD
	RDEB, centripetal variant	AR
Generalized	DDEB, Cockayne-Touraine variant	AD
	DDEB, Pasini variant (albopapuloid variant)	AD
	RDEB, gravis variant (Hallopeau-Siemens)	AR
	RDEB, mitis variant	AR
Miscellaneous	Congenital localized absence of skin (Bart)	AD
	Kindler syndrome	AR?
	Transient bullous dermolysis of the newborn	AD/AR

AD, autosomal dominant; AR, autosomal recessive; DDEB, dominant dystrophic epidermolysis bullosa; DEB, dystrophic epidermolysis bullosa; EB, epidermolysis bullosa; EBS, epidermolysis bullosa simplex; JEB, junctional epidermolysis bullosa; RDEB, recessive dystrophic epidermolysis bullosa; XLR, X-linked recessive; see text for other terms

show that the cleavage is within the basal layer. Electron microscopy can also be used to confirm the diagnosis.

This description is not repeated for each disorder, although exceptions are noted.

Epidermolysis Bullosa Simplex, Köbner Variant

(Köbner 1896)

Synonym. Epidermolysis bullosa simplex generalisata

Epidemiology. This is the most common member of the group with an incidence of 1:50,000 births, showing just how rare the rest of the group is. The disease is more common in men than in women.

Etiology and Pathogenesis. The disease is inherited in an autosomal dominant pattern. Mutations arise in the genes encoding both keratins 5 and 14. While a variety of abnormal catabolic enzymes have been identified, they presumably arise secondarily to extensive mechanical epidermal damage.

Clinical Findings. Some patients are affected at birth and the rest tend to develop problems as they begin to crawl. While areas of mechanical stress cause the worst problems, the entire body tends to have fragile skin. The typical infantile pressure points of heels, buttocks, elbows, shoulders and occiput may be the first areas to be involved (Fig. 15.3, 15.4). A child hospitalized for early orthopedic surgery may develop widespread erosions. Oral lesions and nail dystrophies are uncommon. Transient milia may arise. Palmoplantar keratoderma and hyperhidrosis are common. The lesions heal without scarring. While there are no systemic problems, the continuous burden of trying to avoid or treat blisters places considerable stress on the patient and parents. Overlaps between this variant and the Weber-Cockayne variant occur, often within a family, which is not surprising since both involve mutations in the same molecules.

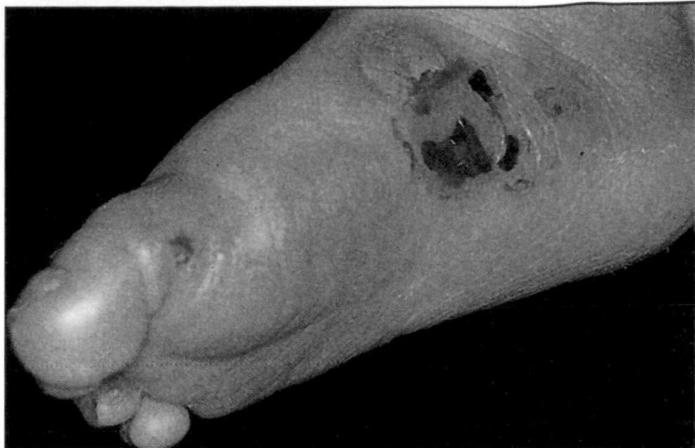

Fig. 15.3. Epidermolysis bullosa simplex of the hands and feet (Köbner variant)

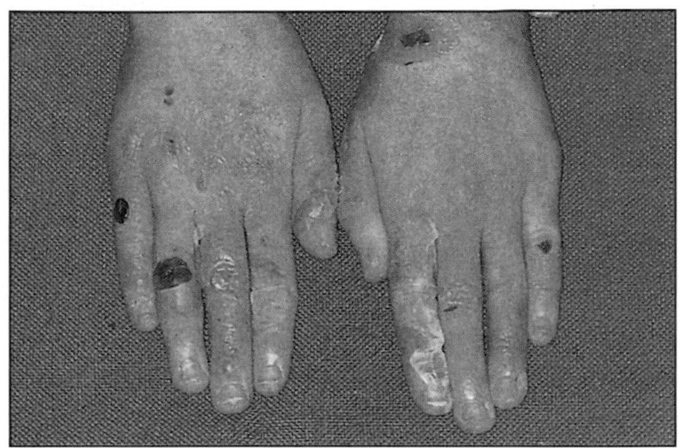

Fig. 15.4. Epidermolysis bullosa simplex feet (Köbner variant)

Course and Prognosis. Patients may improve during puberty, but the tendency to form blisters easily remains. Most have more trouble in warm weather.

Epidermolysis Bullosa Simplex of the Hands and Feet

(Weber 1926; Cockayne 1938)

Synonyms. Epidermolysis bullosa simplex localisata, Weber-Cockayne syndrome, epidermolysis bullosa manuum et pedum aestivalis, recurrent bullous eruption of the hands and feet

Etiology and Pathogenesis. Mutations are found in the genes for keratins 5 and 14 in this autosomal dominant inherited disease. Trauma and heat are key factors. The many synonyms almost tell the story: increased friction, sweating and heat lead to blisters on the hands and feet.

Clinical Findings. Some patients develop blisters during infancy. About one-third have intraoral blisters from sucking on a bottle. Other extracutaneous changes are not found. The nails are normal. Most patients will remain free of symptoms until they become teenagers or young adults. They may develop blisters and erosions on their hands and feet when starting competitive sports, hard manual labor or the military. Long summer time marches in the military frequently produce such severe blisters that an unexpected case is unearthed. Poorly fitting shoes, ski boots and more recently in-line skates may also play a role. The history will reveal a discrepancy between the degree of mechanical stress and the development of blisters. The patients do better in cooler weather. The erosions heal without scarring. An association with macular amyloidosis has been reported, probably reflecting dropping of keratin into the upper dermis. There are no systemic problems.

Epidermolysis Bullosa Simplex with Anodontia/Hypodontia

(Nielsen and Sjölund 1985)

Synonym. Kallin syndrome. Kallin was the family name of the first patients.

Patients typically develop localized acral blisters not at birth, but in infancy. They have missing or absent teeth, oral erosions, nail dystrophies and sparse hair which may normalize in adult life. The disorder is extremely rare and inherited in an autosomal recessive pattern. The basic defect is unknown.

Epidermolysis Bullosa Simplex Herpetiformis
(Dowling and Meara 1954)

Synonyms. Epidermolysis bullosa simplex, Dowling-Meara type

Etiology and Pathogenesis. While mutations of the same keratin 5 and 14 genes are involved in this autosomal dominant inherited disease, they seem to occur at a more crucial location for the function of the keratin molecule leading to early clumping of tonofilaments in basal layer keratinocytes.

Clinical Findings. As the name suggests, the blisters are often grouped in a herpetiform manner and sometimes have an erythematous base. They are present either at birth or shortly thereafter; at this age, they may be large, confluent and life-threatening. They often are serous or hemorrhagic. Later they become more localized and herpetiform. The blisters appear more inflamed than in the other variants. Patients typically have palmoplantar keratoderma and thickened nails. Patients may also have natal teeth or lack teeth. While the lesions heal without scarring, milia occur as does postinflammatory hypo- and hyperpigmentation. Later in life patients tend to improve.

Histopathology. The basal layer damage may be so severe that the blister is mistaken for a subepidermal blister. Abundant eosinophils and even neutrophils may also be found. Another distinctive feature is the presence of dyskeratotic cells, perhaps reflecting the keratin clumping which is best seen with electron microscopy.

Epidermolysis Bullosa Simplex with Mottled Hyperpigmentation
(Fischer and Gedde-Dahl 1979)

This very uncommon condition resembles both localized and generalized epidermolysis bullosa simplex but the patients also have mottled hypo- and hyperpigmentation on the trunk. It is unclear if the changes are truly postinflammatory, i. e., if they directly follow blisters. Some have palmoplantar keratoderma, and nail and oral lesions may occur. The disorder is inherited in an autosomal dominant pattern.

Epidermolysis Bullosa Simplex, Ogna Variant
(Gedde-Dahl 1971)

This extremely rare disorder was first described in the Ogna region of southwest Norway. The disease is inherited in an autosomal dominant pattern. While the whole skin can be affected, acral blisters are most troublesome. They tend to appear in childhood and are worse in the summer. The blisters are often hemorrhagic. Nail dystrophies are common.

Epidermolysis Bullosa Simplex Superficialis
(Fine et al. 1989)

This extremely rare autosomal dominant disorder is the exception among the epidermolysis bullosa simplex family. Clinically it is not unique, featuring diffuse blisters, milia, oral lesions and nail dystrophies early in life. But the level of separation is in the upper cells of the epidermis, usually subcorneal. While the biopsy findings are identical to those in peeling skin syndrome, the latter does not show blisters and has a more steady pattern of shedding.

Epidermolysis Bullosa Simplex with Muscular Dystrophy
(Salih et al. 1985)

Synonym. Epidermolysis bullosa simplex letalis

Clinically this form of epidermolysis bullosa simplex is characterized by widespread blistering at birth often associated with muscular dystrophy or other neuromuscular problems. Scarring is common, in contrast to the other forms of epidermolysis bullosa simplex. Hair, nail, tooth and oral mucosal disease is often seen. Many of these patients die early, often without a clear explanation; hence the term letalis. A defect in plectin appears to be the cause, as anchoring of the cytoskeleton to the plasma membrane is defective in both the skin and muscles. The split occurs just above the basal keratinocyte plasma membrane. Thus, this is the one type of epidermolysis bullosa simplex which does not involve keratin mutations.

Epidermolysis Bullosa Simplex, Mendes da Costa Variant
(Mendes da Costa 1908)

Synonyms. Epidermolysis bullosa simplex, macular dystrophic type; epidermolysis bullosa hereditaria, typus maculatus; epidermolysis bullosa simplex, Amsterdam type; X-linked epidermolysis bullosa simplex

This very rare form of epidermolysis bullosa simplex has been described primarily in Dutch patients. It is inherited in an X-linked recessive pattern, so that only males are involved. Infants develop widespread blisters which heal with both reticulated hyper- and hypopigmentation and macular atrophy. A wide variety of other defects including acrocyanosis, alopecia, nail anomalies, corneal dystrophies and more importantly microcephaly have been identified. The life expectancy is considerably shortened.

Junctional Epidermolysis Bullosa

The separation in junctional epidermolysis bullosa occurs in the lamina lucida zone of the basement membrane. All forms are inherited in an autosomal recessive fashion, suggesting that in most instances, a 50% decrease in a component of the lamina lucida is not enough to cause obvious disease. Many of the structures of the lamina lucida have been found to be missing in various forms of junctional epidermolysis bullosa, such as BPAG2 in generalized atrophic benign epidermolysis bullosa, several components of laminin 5 in the Herlitz or lethal form, and integrin $\alpha6\beta4$ in junctional epidermolysis bullosa with pyloric atresia. In the past, all forms of junctional epidermolysis bullosa were feared as fatal, but as the subclassification of epidermolysis bullosa has improved, many relatively harmless junctional variants, some localized with mosaic patterns, have been described.

Once again, routine histology is not very helpful. If an intact blister is obtained, the separation appears to be subepidermal, since the defect is located within the epidermal-dermal junction itself. Immunomapping localizes the defect to the appropriate level but does not suffice for the diagnosis which is usually made with monoclonal antibodies directed against the various components of the lamina lucida and lamina densa.

Junctional Epidermolysis Bullosa, Gravis Variant
(Herlitz 1935)

Synonyms. Epidermolysis bullosa letalis, Herlitz syndrome, junctional epidermolysis bullosa of Herlitz

Etiology and Pathogenesis. Inherited in an autosomal dominant pattern, this form appears to be caused by defects in laminin 5, a key component of the lamina lucida. Laminin 5 is composed of three subunits, α-3, β-3 and γ-2, each encoded by a separate gene on two different chromosomes. All three are candidate genes for junctional epidermolysis bullosa, gravis variant.

Clinical Findings. In most cases there are widespread hemorrhagic blisters present at birth. They lead to massive denudation and fluid loss, so that many patients in the past succumbed during early life. Sepsis and protein loss are the two main causes of death, but today the disease is by no means uniformly fatal and the name letalis should not be used. The ruptured blisters evolve into chronic granulation tissue, especially about the mouth and nail folds, leading to paronychia. The oral mucosa is regularly involved with blisters and erosions extending into the respiratory and gastrointestinal tracts. Pyloric stenosis has been described. Urologic complications including hydronephrosis and urethral scarring have also been identified. Some patients are born lacking areas of skin (see Bart syndrome below).

Histopathology. The blister in Herlitz disease is the best studied of this group because of its relatively greater frequency. It is the prototype for a junctional blister. By light microscopy, the blister appears to be subepidermal, but electron microscopy demonstrates the split in the lamina lucida, often with reduced hemidesmosomes. Antigen mapping shows BPAG2 in the blister roof, laminin on the floor and roof and type IV collagen on the floor.

Junctional Epidermolysis Bullosa with Pyloric Stenosis
(El Shafie et al. 1979)

The association of epidermolysis bullosa and pyloric stenosis is confusing. Recent studies have shown that in at least some patients the integrin $\alpha6\beta4$ is missing in the lamina lucida. In the past it was felt that most patients described as having epidermolysis bullosa with pyloric atresia had

Herlitz disease, although pyloric atresia has been described in other forms of the disease. Whether clinical features or the missing integrin will prove to be the best way of separating this category awaits the test of time.

Generalized Atrophic Benign Epidermolysis Bullosa
(Hashimoto et al. 1976)

Synonyms. Junctional epidermolysis bullosa, mitis variant; nonlethal junctional epidermolysis bullosa; junctional epidermolysis bullosa, non-Herlitz variant; epidermolysis bullosa atrophicans generalisata mitis, type Disentis

Etiology and Pathogenesis. This tongue twister of a name, usually abbreviated to GABEB, indicates one of the newest but best-established forms of epidermolysis bullosa. The defect in this autosomal recessive inherited variant is primarily in the BPAG2. Some feel that the case from Disentis, Switzerland, is a late onset variant of the Herlitz form but most include it here. One pedigree shows a defect in the laminin β-3 chain, supporting the overlap between junctional epidermolysis bullosa, Herlitz type, and generalized atrophic benign epidermolysis bullosa.

Clinical Findings. This disorder is similar to the Herlitz variant with the patients showing widespread spontaneous or mechanically induced blistering at birth. The massive granulation tissue is not seen; instead the lesions heal with widespread atrophic patches. The backs of the hands are typically involved. The nails are usually destroyed. Milia are not present. Alopecia is common but oral involvement mild, although dental anomalies are seen. The children improve with time.

Cicatricial Junctional Epidermolysis Bullosa
(Haber et al. 1985)

In the past, all forms of epidermolysis bullosa with severe scarring were considered to be dystrophic. This rare form, also inherited in an autosomal recessive pattern, is the exception that proves the rule. There is widespread disease at birth, with blistering extending into the upper respiratory and gastrointestinal tracts. The mitten deformities discussed under dystrophic epidermolysis bullosa appear and the anterior nares is often stenotic. The other blisters heal with atrophic scars. Scarring alopecia and dental abnormalities have also been reported.

Junctional Epidermolysis Bullosa, Progressiva Variant
(Gedde-Dahl 1971)

Synonyms. Junctional epidermolysis bullosa neurotropica, epidermolysis bullosa progressiva

In contrast to most other forms of epidermolysis bullosa, this variant worsens with age and is thus called progressive. The disorder is inherited in an autosomal dominant pattern. Blisters typically start in late childhood or adolescence and are primarily acral and oral. As they heal, the renewed skin lacks markings; this is especially true on the fingertips where the fingerprint pattern is erased. Palmoplantar keratoderma and nail dystrophies are usually present. There is progressive hearing loss.

Junctional Epidermolysis Bullosa Inversa
(Ridley 1977)

Synonym. Epidermolysis bullosa atrophicans inversa

This extremely uncommon disorder is inherited in an autosomal recessive pattern and presents with neonatal blistering. Later the blistering is milder and confined to the body folds, hence inversa. The lesions typically heal with atrophic white streaks, also called albostriate lesions. Nail, dental and oral mucosal lesions have been reported.

Dystrophic Epidermolysis Bullosa

In this most severe form of epidermolysis bullosa, the separation occurs in the upper part of the papillary dermis, involving the network of type VII collagen and the rest of the anchoring apparatus. The scarring is most extreme, milia formation is very common, the nails are usually damaged and in some forms, mitten deformities of the hands and feet cause significant problems. In addition, the scars of dystrophic epidermolysis bullosa are premalignant; patients who live long enough develop a variety of squamous cell carcinomas. This category is particularly confusing as it is divided into both localized and systemic forms, as well as split into dominantly inherited and recessively inherited types. Microscopically, the split appears as a relatively uninflamed subepidermal or dermolytic blister. Electron microscopy shows a sparse or damaged anchoring fiber network while immunomapping shows a blister with BPAG2, laminin and type IV collagen in its roof.

Recessive Dystrophic Epidermolysis Bullosa, Gravis Variant

(Hallopeau 1896; Siemens 1925)

Synonyms. Epidermolysis bullosa dystrophica of Hallopeau and Siemens, epidermolysis bullosa dystrophica generalisata mutilans

Epidemiology. This is the most common of the dystrophic forms of epidermolysis bullosa but is still rare. There are about 10,000 patients in the USA.

Etiology and Pathogenesis. It is inherited in an autosomal recessive pattern. There is a mutation in the gene for type VII collagen located on chromosome 3p21. The anchoring fibrils are either severely damaged or missing, also in nonaffected skin. Elevated levels of collagenase have been measured, suggesting excessive catabolism of the damaged fibrils.

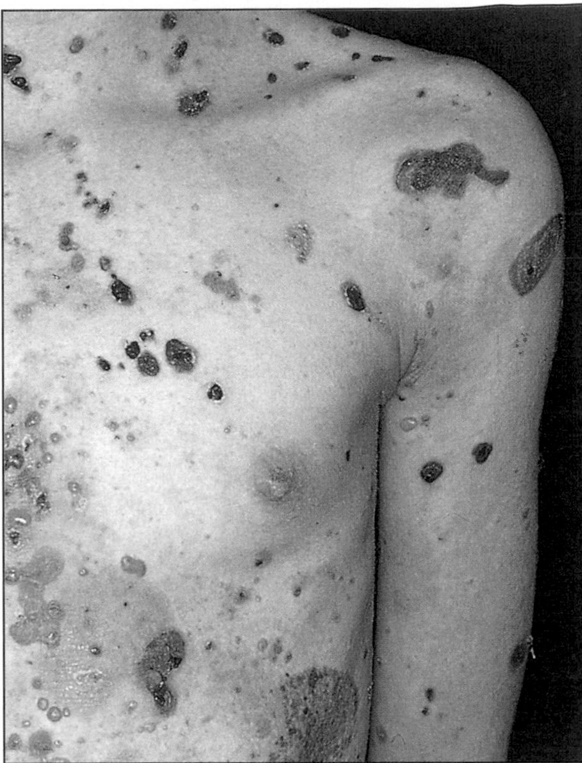

Fig. 15.5. Recessive dystrophic epidermolysis bullosa, gravis variant, with widespread blisters

Clinical Findings. Problems usually start at birth or shortly thereafter. Congenital absence of skin may be found. The skin is extremely fragile, forming large flaccid hemorrhagic blisters, both spontaneously and secondary to trauma (Fig. 15.5). The blisters are most typically acral or on the buttocks (Fig. 15.6). The skin heals with atrophy and both hypo- and hyperpigmentation. The fingertips lose their dermatoglyphic pattern. Milia are very common, especially on the ears and backs of the hands. Acrocyanosis and hyperhidrosis of the palms and soles may be present; the rest of the skin is typically dry. The nails may be absent or dystrophic. The hair is typically sparse and pseudopelade-like areas can be found (Fig. 15.7).

The most devastating problem is the extreme scarring of the hands and feet leading to the mitten deformities (Fig. 15.8). Initially, there are adhesions between the digits, but insidiously over time the individual digits become indistinct as the hand or foot fuses into a scarred mass. The patients are at considerable risk of developing squamous cell carcinoma both on their mitten hands and less often feet, suggesting a secondary role for sunlight. Contractures involving other joints may also develop.

The oral mucosa is often involved so that feeding may be hampered and the tongue or lips fused to the gingival mucosa. Other mucosal sites including the genital, anal and ocular areas may also be affected with scarring. Intraoral and esophageal squamous cell carcinomas have also been reported, as well as secondary amyloidosis. Dental abnormalities are common, including missing or deformed teeth and severe caries. Because of the feeding problems and widespread denudation leading to

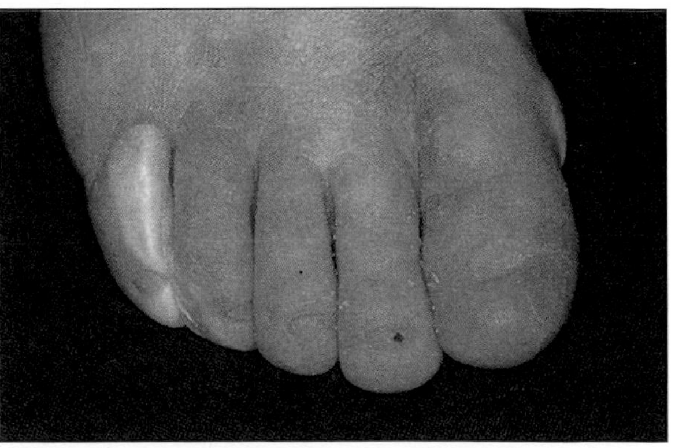

Fig. 15.6. Recessive dystrophic epidermolysis bullosa, gravis variant, with loss of toenails and fresh blister

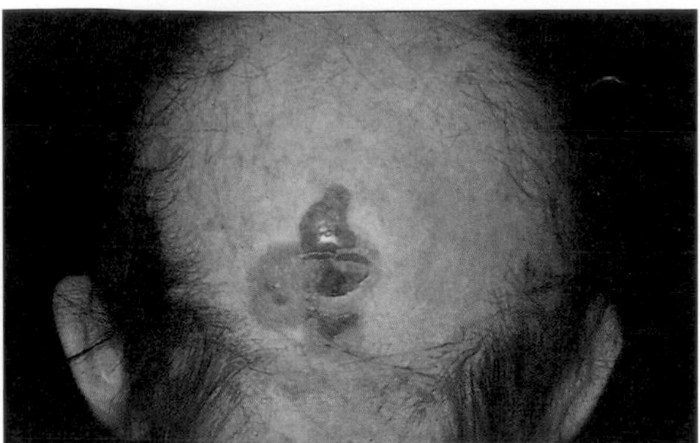

Fig. 15.7. Recessive dystrophic epidermolysis bullosa, gravis variant, with blister, ulceration and alopecia of pseudopelade type

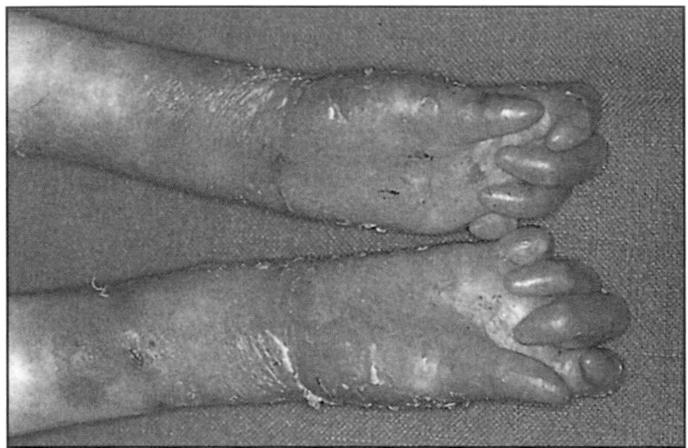

Fig. 15.8. Recessive dystrophic epidermolysis bullosa, gravis variant, with skeletal deformities and early mitten formation

fluid loss, electrolyte imbalances and malnutrition are other worrisome complications.

Histopathology. Routine histology is rarely helpful as the blisters are seldom preserved. Blistering occurs in the upper dermis beneath the lamina densa. With antigen mapping, all of the usual components, such as BPAG2, laminin and type IV collagen are found in the blister roof. The anchoring fibrils are missing or damaged on electron microscopy and staining with antibodies directed against them is accordingly reduced.

Course and Prognosis. The course is usually quite difficult for the patient and parents. Intensive nursing care is required to avoid and treat blisters and secondary infections. The risk of deformities and carcinomas is high. Conservation of the teeth is a great challenge.

Differential Diagnosis. It can be very difficult to separate the recessive and dominant forms of dystrophic epidermolysis bullosa, which can have disastrous consequences for genetic counseling. Electron microscopy was for decades the standard, but mistaken diagnoses were made. Both diseases involve mutations in type VII collagen. In many instances a specific mutation can be identified and used for exact diagnosis, i. e., present on one or two alleles. In other families, linkage analysis may be helpful.

Recessive Dystrophic Epidermolysis Bullosa, Mitis Variant

This disorder more closely resembles dominant dystrophic epidermolysis bullosa but the pattern of inheritance is recessive. Such rare pedigrees document the frustration in sorting out the type of epidermolysis bullosa in a single patient.

Dominant Dystrophic Epidermolysis Bullosa, Cockayne-Touraine Variant

(Cockayne 1933; Touraine 1943)

Synonyms. Epidermolysis bullosa dystrophica hyperplastica, epidermolysis bullosa dystrophica localisata (but today considered a generalized form)

Epidemiology. This is the only other relatively common form of dystrophic epidermolysis bullosa. It is about half as common as the more severe recessive form.

Etiology and Pathogenesis. This type is inherited in an autosomal dominant pattern with a mutation in the gene for type VII collagen on chromosome 3p21. The anchoring fibrils are decreased to absent in the areas predisposed to blistering, such as the extremities. They may be normal in nonaffected areas, but this is not a reliable way to separate the dominant and recessive forms of dystrophic epidermolysis bullosa.

Clinical Findings. The blisters appear at birth or early infancy and favor the extremities but can be widespread. The buttocks and shins are sites of predilection. While most blisters heal with milia and atrophic scars, some evolve into keloidal tumors, as suggested by the name hyperplastica. Some patients are born with localized absence of skin. The ocular mucosa is often involved. The upper respiratory and gastrointestinal tracts are rarely affected. While the hair and teeth are normal, the nails are often involved, either being absent or markedly dystrophic. Squamous cell carcinomas may develop in the scarred skin, but their appearance is much less common than in the recessive forms of dystrophic epidermolysis bullosa.

Dominant Dystrophic Epidermolysis Bullosa, Pasini Variant

(Pasini 1928)

Synonyms. Epidermolysis bullosa albopapuloidea, albopapuloid dominant dystrophic epidermolysis bullosa, Pasini syndrome

Etiology and Pathogenesis. This form is an allelic variant of the more common Cockayne-Touraine form, as there are mutations in type VII collagen.

Clinical Findings. As the name suggests, the hallmark clinical feature is the presence of albopapuloid lesions, white perifollicular papules that appear on the trunk in puberty. While some may be scars, others seem to arise in normal skin. The most common site is the lumbosacral region. The lesions slowly enlarge, reaching about 1.5 cm. Otherwise, the Pasini variant is very similar to the Cockayne-Touraine variant.

Recessive Dystrophic Epidermolysis Bullosa, Inversa Variant

(Gedde-Dahl 1971)

Synonyms. Epidermolysis bullosa dystrophica inversa of Gedde-Dahl, dermolytic dystrophic epidermolysis bullosa inversa

This form of epidermolysis bullosa presents with widespread blisters but later in life they are predominantly confined to the intertriginous regions. The oral and esophageal problems are severe, quite similar to those in the noninverse form discussed below. While scarring develops, milia are uncommon and no mitten deformities develop. The nails and teeth are usually damaged, and corneal erosions may be a problem.

Diagnostic Criteria. The diagnosis of the various types of epidermolysis bullosa is an immense challenge when one is confronted with a newborn with the first case of epidermolysis bullosa in the family. Around the world there are expert referral centers which can help in analyzing a biopsy to identify both the level of split and in many cases the exact nature of the defect. The parents should be carefully examined and questioned to pursue the possibility of autosomal dominant transmission but epidermolysis bullosa is not often overlooked. If autosomal dominant epidermolysis bullosa is the answer, the proband usually carries a mutation. Consanguinity suggests that the disorder is inherited in an autosomal recessive pattern.

Prenatal diagnosis is possible in many situations. Usually a fetal skin biopsy is needed. It can be analyzed in much the same way as an adult biopsy with light microscopy, electron microscopy, antigen mapping and staining with a battery of monoclonal antibodies to identify the missing or damaged components. In those types where the gene defect has been identified, DNA analysis may be helpful. Prenatal diagnosis will be of most use to families with one child having autosomal recessive dystrophic epidermolysis bullosa.

Therapy. In contrast to the diagnostic advances, the therapy of epidermolysis bullosa remains frustrating. The most important factors are expert nursing which can only be achieved by having skilled nurses and ideally parents of other epidermolysis bullosa children coach and teach the new parents. The self-help groups for patients and their parents have made a great difference. In addition, parents should be encouraged to experiment since each case is slightly different. The treatment of epidermolysis bullosa is also associated with many checkered, unproved therapies, not surprising when one considers the magnitude of the defect and how desperate the parents become.

Systemic. The ultimate systemic therapy will be gene therapy. Ideally patients' stem cells of keratinocytes can be transfected with the missing genes and then reapplied in the form of a skin graft. While this has not yet been achieved, it is not science fiction.

Phenytoin inhibits collagenase so it has been tried for patients with recessive dystrophic epidermolysis bullosa, who usually have elevated levels of the enzyme. Some patients with junctional epidermolysis bullosa have also improved. While some argue for trying phenytoin in these settings, one must remember that in larger placebo-controlled double-blind studies, no significant improvement has been seen. The same must be said for systemic corticosteroids, vitamin E, antimalarials and a long list of other agents tried with enthusiasm in the past.

The most important oral therapy is judicious supplementation of vitamins and minerals, because of the loss through denuded skin. There is no evidence that excessive administration is helpful. The other essential is culture-directed carefully chosen systemic antibiotics for cutaneous and soft tissue infections. Because the patient faces a lifetime of encounters with bacteria via denuded skin, one must continuously worry about resistant strains.

Topical. The mainstays of therapy are biologic dressings, nonadherent gauze, nonsensitizing topical antibiotics and fluff wraps. When one considers how often dressings must be changed, the costs are significant and one must be prepared to deal with insurance companies and social agencies.

A wide variety of biologic or artificial wound dressings have made the life of the epidermolysis bullosa patient a little bit easier in the past decade. Dressings that do not have an adhesive component are preferred, otherwise when they are removed, a second blister may be induced. Old reliables such as petrolatum-impregnated gauze are still useful and cost effective. Depending on the type of lesion (dry, crusted versus weeping, exudative) one may have to use several different dressings simultaneously in the same patient. In those patients who tend towards mitten formation, primarily recessive dystrophic epidermolysis bullosa, dressings should routinely be used between the fingers. Thicker dressings are often needed on the feet to combine protection with padding. In addition, custom-made shoes can go along way towards reducing plantar blisters. One rule is almost inviolable: no tape. Conforming or self-adhering elasticized gauze is much better.

One must resist the temptation to treat every weeping erosion as an infection. Open skin is routinely colonized by a variety of gram-positive bacteria, but one must develop the skill to only treat the clinically relevant, severe infections. The second problem is topical sensitization because of life-long use and open skin. Mupirocin is a useful agent, but its cost limits its usefulness. Silver sulfadiazine is not advised in infants but can be employed later. Bacitracin, fusidic acid and povidone-iodine products are also effective. Any topical antibiotic must be used gingerly in patients with widespread blistering because of systemic absorption.

Surgical. Surgery is often needed in the more severe forms of epidermolysis bullosa. The mitten deformities can be repaired and squamous cell carcinomas should be excised totally as soon as possible, because the risk of metastasis is considerable. Routine skin grafting is quite complicated, but the use of cultured keratinocytes has been possible in some cases to provide temporary covering.

Other Measures. Depending on the type of involvement, a dentist, ophthalmologist and gastroenterologist should be involved in the continuing care of patients. The pediatrician should help with diet recommendations and general monitoring.

Miscellaneous Blistering Diseases of Infancy

Congenital Localized Absence of Skin

(Bart et al. 1966)

Synonym. Bart syndrome

Etiology and Pathogenesis. Bart syndrome is probably not a single entity. As mentioned above, localized absence of skin has been reported with several types of junctional and dystrophic epidermolysis bullosa. The basic question is: are the denuded areas simply deep in utero blisters or do they reflect areas where no skin was ever present such as in aplasia cutis congenita? Bart's original patients showed autosomal dominant inheritance and probably represented a variant of dominant dystrophic epidermolysis bullosa.

Clinical Findings. At birth, denuded areas of subcutaneous tissue are exposed. This occurs most frequently on the legs and buttocks. In addition, blisters are present at birth, involving the skin and oral mucosa; they heal with scarring. The tendency to blistering lessens with time. Most patients have nail dystrophy

Kindler Syndrome

Kindler syndrome features both blisters and poikiloderma. It is discussed in Chap. 18. The blistering defect has not been clearly defined.

Transient Bullous Dermolysis of the Newborn

(Hashimoto et al. 1985)

Synonyms. Congenital self-healing mechanobullous dermatosis

Several different patients have been described with generalized blistering of the skin and mucous membranes present at birth or infancy but resolving over the first year of life. Residua include milia and minimal atrophic scarring. Both autosomal dominant and autosomal recessive inheritance has been suggested. The blisters are below the lamina densa. The defect appears to lie in the packaging or secretion of type VII collagen by the basilar keratinocytes.

Congenital Erosive and Vesicular Dermatitis
(Cohen et al. 1985)

Synonym. Congenital erosive and vesicular dermatitis with reticulated scarring

This rare disorder presents at birth with vesicles, diffuse erosions, deeper ulcerations and crusts. The disorder appears to be sporadic and perhaps follows an untoward intrauterine event. Most patients have been premature and had a variety of CNS defects. Wide areas are affected with up to 75% of the skin denuded. The face, palms and soles are spared. Peculiarly the lesions heal within the first month of life with a characteristic reticulated scarring. The skin has a cobblestone-like texture, often following Blaschko lines. The raised areas are normal or hypopigmented while the depressed areas are typically hyperpigmented. Scarring alopecia and absent or dystrophic nails may result. The histopathologic features have not been well established.

The differential diagnosis is extensive including aplasia cutis congenita (usually less widespread with deeper defects), focal dermal hypoplasia (linear outpouching of thinned skin and fat). Bart syndrome (skin loss usually limited to legs with continued blistering) and congenital infections (more extensive associated abnormalities). While the scarring resembles poikiloderma, the latter entity is rarely present at birth. In the early stages, treatment is that of epidermolysis bullosa. Later one must pay particular attention to heat intolerance, since the scarred areas lack adequate eccrine glands.

Intrauterine Epidermal Necrosis
(Ruiz-Maldonado et al. 1998)

This very rare disorder is lethal, occurring in very ill premature infants. The children are born with extensive areas of skin loss, but without blisters. The head, knees, elbows, hands and feet are spared. A wide variety of grave systemic findings have also been reported. Two patients were twin girls, suggesting inheritance in an autosomal recessive or X-linked recessive pattern. In the few studied cases, biopsy has shown epidermal debris with some regeneration, dermal inflammation and calcification of hair follicles. The epidermis adjacent to the denuded areas showed features of apoptosis including individual cell necrosis, vacuolar changes and Civatte bodies.

Pemphigus Diseases

The pemphigus family includes a number of diseases which feature intraepidermal blisters with acantholysis. Adhesions between epidermal cells are dissolved, most often by autoimmune mechanisms. Mucosal surfaces may also be involved. The Tzanck smear, today used primarily to diagnose herpes simplex virus infections, was developed to diagnose pemphigus vulgaris by the identification of free floating acantholytic keratinocytes (pemphigus cells) in the blister fluid. Both direct immunofluorescent examination of perilesional skin and indirect immunofluorescent examination of the patient's serum can reveal the presence of antibodies directed against various epidermal adhesion components.

The pemphigus family is often divided into pemphigus vulgaris and pemphigus vegetans, which involve the entire epidermis, and the more superficial forms of pemphigus, including pemphigus foliaceus, pemphigus erythematosus and endemic Brazilian pemphigus (fogo selvagem), as well as IgA pemphigus and paraneoplastic pemphigus. All of these disorders have an immunologic basis. Table 15.4 summarizes the target antigens for the major forms of pemphigus.

Hailey-Hailey disease or familial chronic benign pemphigus is a disorder of epidermal differentia-

Table 15.4. Antigens in pemphigus disorders

Disease	Antigens
Pemphigus vulgaris	Desmoglein 3
Pemphigus foliaceus	Desmoglein 1
Paraneoplastic pemphigus	Desmoglein 3, desmoglein 1, plakin proteins and others

tion and shows no evidence of autoimmune phenomena; it is covered in Chapter 17. Histologically it features marked acantholysis, but otherwise is unlikely to be confused with any of the autoimmune blistering diseases.

Pemphigus Vulgaris

Definition. Pemphigus vulgaris is an acquired chronic disease in which blisters develop on normal-appearing skin and mucous membranes. In the past, when untreated or poorly treated, it was often fatal. Because of the presence of pathogenic antibodies, it is one of the prototypes of an autoimmune skin disease.

Epidemiology. Pemphigus vulgaris is a rare disease of adult life, equally uncommon in men and women, with peak onset between 30 and 60 years of age. It can be seen transiently in infants of affected mothers, rarely occurs in children and may involve the very elderly. In Jewish populations, in which the disease is more common, there is a strong HLA association with DR4/DRw6. In Jerusalem, the incidence is around 1.5/100,000, in New York around 0.5/100,000, and in Finland, < 1/1,000,000. In areas where the incidence is higher because of the presence of many Jews, pemphigus vulgaris is far more common than pemphigus foliaceus. In other countries, the two are about equally common.

Etiology and Pathogenesis. The site of action in pemphigus vulgaris is the desmogleins, the cadherins that extend from the desmosomal plaque into the intercellular space where they join desmogleins from adjacent keratinocytes. Desmoglein 1 is expressed primarily in the upper levels of the epidermis and weakly in mucosa while desmoglein 3 is expressed through the epidermis and strongly in mucosa. Damage or absence of desmoglein 1 does not lead to mucosal lesions, as desmoglein 3 alone is sufficient to keep mucosal surfaces intact.

The pemphigus antibodies attach to the extracellular domain of desmoglein and interfere with its attachment to similar domains on other cells, reducing cell-cell adherence. At the same time they may activate a signaling pathway to increase proteinase production, aiding acantholysis. Some patients have antibodies that activate cholinergic receptors which also appear to play a role in cell adhesion. Complement factors, plasminogen activator and other inflammatory mediators may also play a part in propagating the reaction. The pemphigus antibody is a pathogenic antibody, not an epiphenomenon. In most patients, the antibody titers and immunoglobulin subclasses correlate to the disease status and can be useful in predicting the course. Infants born to mothers with pemphigus vulgaris receive IgG pemphigus antibodies which can cause transient acantholytic skin lesions. Similar antibodies can cause acantholysis in vitro when complement and other mediators are blocked. Finally, when IgG pemphigus antibodies are purified and injected into newborn mice, a blistering dermatitis with typical pemphigus vulgaris histology is produced.

Occasionally medications may cause pemphigus vulgaris. The two drugs which appear to be most reliably involved are penicillamine and captopril. Both contain sulfhydryl groups which may interact with the sulfhydryl groups in desmoglein 1 or desmoglein 3. The prevalence of pemphigus in patients taking long-term penicillamine for rheumatoid arthritis or Wilson disease is over 5%. There is a marked predominance of pemphigus foliaceus. The findings of both direct and indirect immunofluorescent examinations are similar to those in the naturally occurring disease, with antibodies against the appropriate desmogleins. Other drugs with sulfhydryl groups, and even food with similar configurations such as garlic, have also been incriminated. In addition, some cytokines have been associated with pemphigus, as have physical damage including ionizing radiation and PUVA.

Clinical Findings. The onset of pemphigus vulgaris is often insidious. A small flaccid clear blister may develop, often in the umbilicus. It ruptures and evolves into an inflamed erosion. Centrally crusts may form as the blisters spread peripherally (Fig. 15.9). New blisters can develop on top of the old one. Hemorrhagic blisters are uncommon. In at least half the cases, the process begins in the mouth. Here the blisters are rarely found intact, but break rapidly so that the patient presents with painful erosions which are often misdiagnosed (Fig. 15.10). In rare cases, the ocular mucosa may be involved first, so that the patient presents with a chronic conjunctivitis or blepharitis.

As the disease progresses, the intertriginous areas (axilla, beneath the breasts, groin) are often next to be involved. Presumably the rubbing in this area separates already weakened intercellular adhesions. Gradually blisters of variable size appear over the entire body surface. They are typically flaccid

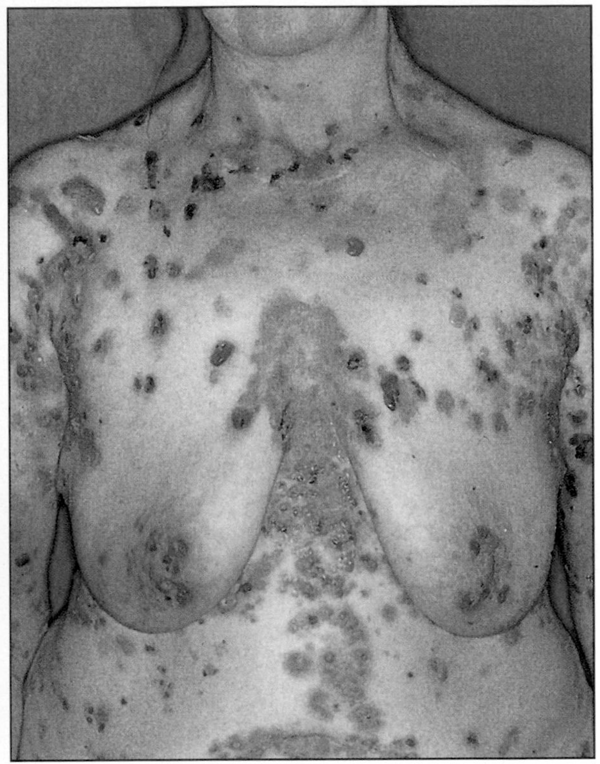

Fig. 15.9. Pemphigus vulgaris

and clear or have cloudy white contents with a peripheral erythematous band. The thin blister roofs break easily, leaving behind eroded patches which dominate the clinical picture. The erosions continue to spread and crust, as new blisters continue to develop.

If one pushes clinically normal skin in the vicinity of a blister to the side, one can push the upper layers of the epidermis away. This is known as the Nikolsky sign (NIKOLSKY 1896). A second, known as the Asboe-Hansen sign (ASBOE-HANSEN 1970) or the Nikolsky II sign, is the spreading of an intact blister laterally when gentle pressure is applied. Both signs demonstrate the fragility of the clinically normal skin. In periods of remission, they may both be negative.

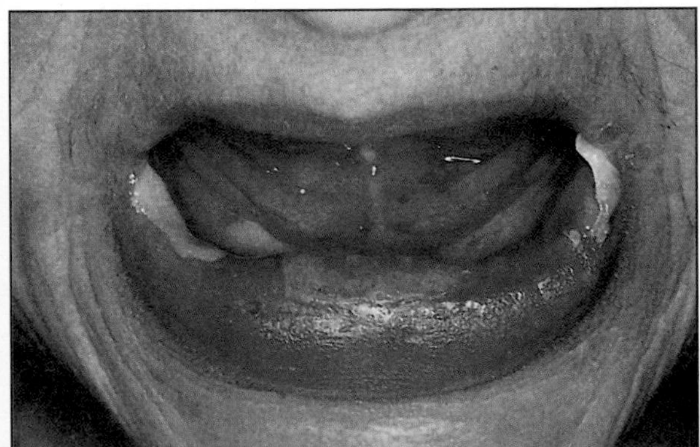

Fig. 15.10. Oral blisters and erosions in pemphigus vulgaris

The patients are usually surprisingly asymptomatic at first. Pruritus is not a common feature. Instead, they complain initially of pain, especially when the mouth is involved. Systemic involvement is possible in all sites where the epithelia react with the autoantibodies. For example, Papanicolau smears may remove large numbers of cervical epithelial cells which can confuse the pathologist. Esophageal involvement, usually proximal, can produce symptoms such as severe heartburn. Rectal and urethral inflammation may present with blood in the stool or urine.

Histopathology. When an early blister or better the edge of blister is biopsied, one typically sees acantholysis. Often the basal layer remains attached, producing the so-called tombstone effect. The blister usually contains serum in addition to the acantholytic keratinocytes. Later lesions may show inflammatory infiltrates, necrotic keratinocytes and crusting, but at this stage, the biopsy is only rarely diagnostic.

The blisters can also be analyzed via cytology smears. TZANCK (1947) identified the acantholytic cells in smears taken from the base of freshly opened blisters. Once the slide has been stained with a routine cytology stain, one sees loosely arranged epidermal cell complexes, sometimes with a hint of intercellular adhesions. The keratinocytes typically have a perinuclear clear zone about a single dark nucleus, so that a pemphigus blister can usually be separated with certainty from one caused by herpes simplex virus or bullous pemphigoid. Nonetheless, the Tzanck smear is only a rapid screening test which cannot be used for a final diagnosis.

Immunofluorescent Examination. Direct immunofluorescent examination of perilesional skin shows the deposition of immunoglobulins and complement components (C1q, C3, C4) between the epidermal cells (Fig. 15.11). No matter what the level of the blister is, most epidermal cells are coated by immunoglobulin. The dominant immunoglobulin in pemphigus is IgG, especially IgG_4. Occasionally in biopsies from the oral mucosa and even the skin, IgA may also be seen. Today the presence of only

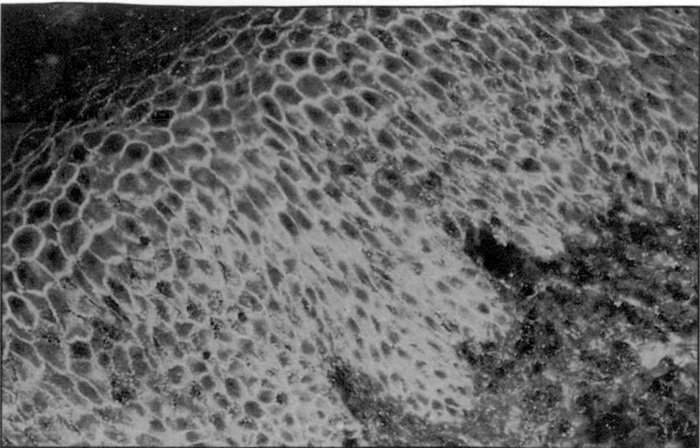

Fig. 15.11. Direct immunofluorescent examination in pemphigus vulgaris

IgA in an intercellular pattern associated with blisters and acantholysis leads to the diagnosis of IgA pemphigus, as discussed below. In patients with only oral mucosal involvement, direct immunofluorescent examination of uninvolved skin, such as from the buttocks, may be positive allowing an earlier diagnosis.

The presence of circulating antibodies can be demonstrated in virtually every patient via indirect immunofluorescent examination. The usual substrate is monkey esophagus on which the characteristic net-like intercellular staining pattern is seen. The titers measured with indirect immunofluorescent examination often correlate with the disease course, dropping during remissions and rising during flares. Some studies have shown the titers may rise before the clinical flare, offering predictive value. The autoantibodies in drug-induced pemphigus vulgaris react in the same way in the immunofluorescent studies as those from the spontaneous disease.

False-positive pemphigus antibodies can also be seen in a variety of totally unrelated clinical settings, including toxic epidermal necrolysis and burn patients where the mechanical dissolution of the epidermal cells may expose altered antigens which elicit a clinically irrelevant immune response. Furthermore, relatives of patients with pemphigus vulgaris may have circulating antibodies without clinical evidence of disease. In the case of myasthenia gravis, the pemphigus antibodies are undoubtedly of immunologic significance, but only rare patients have both neurologic problems and skin disease. Acetylcholine receptor autoantibodies interfere with neurotransmission explaining most of the neurologic problems.

Laboratory Findings. The desmoglein ELISA as developed by Amagai and his group represents a major advance in the diagnosis of pemphigus disorders. Desmogleins 1 and 3 are expressed in a baculovirus system in which the proteins are present in their important conformational epitopes. The desmoglein ELISA is commercially available, can be done in most experienced laboratories, is quantitative, correlates well with previous immunofluorescent examinations and has become a valuable tool. If a serum sample is positive against desmoglein 3, the diagnosis is pemphigus vulgaris, regardless of reactivity against desmoglein 1. Conversely, if a specimen is positive against desmoglein 1 and negative against desmoglein 3, the diagnosis is pemphigus foliaceus. Patients with mucosal dominant pemphigus vulgaris usually have only antibodies against desmoglein 3, while those with mucocutaneous diseases often have antibodies against both desmogleins.

Routine laboratory evaluations are helpful to document the presence of secondary infections, electrolyte imbalance or malnutrition.

Course and Prognosis. The course of pemphigus vulgaris is unpredictable. Prior to the use of systemic corticosteroids, the disease was usually fatal over a 1–3-year period. The major causes of death were infections, fluid loss (as in a burn patient) and malnutrition. Oral involvement often made eating and drinking extremely painful, so that weight loss was common. The erosions and crusts involving the eyes, nose, urethra, genitalia and anus also contributed to the general sense of misery. Today, the outlook is brighter with a variety of therapeutic approaches possible. The main cause of death is now long-term complications of immunosuppressive therapy.

Differential Diagnosis. The main differential diagnostic consideration is other forms of pemphigus. The desmoglein ELISA has facilitated the distinction between pemphigus vulgaris and pemphigus foliaceus. The other major consideration is bullous pemphigoid. While it is easy to list criteria to separate these two disorders (Table 15.5), one must remember that it was not until the 1940s that Civatte and later Lever called our attention to these differences. Prior to that, it was simply realized that older patents with alleged "pemphigus" did better. Occasionally linear IgA disease may present with widespread erosions, but the immunofluorescent examination will clarify the diagnosis. In addition

Table 15.5. Major differences between pemphigus vulgaris and bullous pemphigoid

Feature	Pemphigus vulgaris	Bullous pemphigoid
Age	Middle aged	Elderly
Clinical pattern	Monomorphous	Polymorphous
Blister	Easily broken, flaccid	Stable, tense
Blister fluid	Clear to white	Often hemorrhagic
Oral involvement	Common	Less common
Nikolsky sign	Positive	Negative
Tzanck smear	Acantholysis	No acantholysis
Immunofluorescent examination	Intercellular deposits	Basement membrane zone deposits
Major antigens	Desmogleins 3 and 1	BPAG2 (type XVII collagen)

these patients have intense pruritus. Bullous drug reactions and erythema multiforme may also appear similar in the beginning of the disease course. One should not forget about drug-triggered pemphigus and fail to discontinue an agent such as captopril while treating pemphigus vulgaris. When only oral lesions are present, one may initially think of severe aphthae. Both lupus erythematosus and lichen planus can also appear similar in the mouth. Today the answer in all cases is immunofluorescent examination and the ELISA testing to identify specific antidesmoglein antibodies.

Therapy

Systemic. The mainstay of systemic therapy is corticosteroids, which have changed the entire picture for pemphigus patients. There are two major issues: what dose is needed to get the patient under control and how can we avoid long-term side effects. We start with 1.0 mg/kg daily of oral prednisone and occasionally go up to 1.5 or 2.0 mg/kg. But we rapidly employ steroid-sparing agents and try not exceed the magic level of 1.0 mg/kg. At this dose acute problems with corticosteroids including aberrant sugar metabolism and electrolyte imbalance occur infrequently, and the long-term morbidity is reduced.

There are many ways in which corticosteroids can be manipulated. One approach is to administer intravenous pulse corticosteroid therapy. When we use pulse therapy, the typical dosage is methylprednisolone 500 mg i.v. on three consecutive days once monthly; this usually allows reduced maintenance levels of oral corticosteroids.

Once blistering has stopped and a remission has been achieved, usually over 4–6 weeks, one can taper to a daily maintenance dose, ideally in the range of 5–15 mg prednisone. At this stage alternate day regimens, such as 20–40 mg prednisone q.o.d. are helpful. When corticosteroids are administered every other morning, the pituitary-adrenal axis functions on the off day. Unfortunately, the immunosuppression also suffers on the off day. Many patients with pemphigus vulgaris respond well to alternate day therapy so we almost always try this approach.

The long-term side effects of systemic corticosteroids are multiple, affecting almost every organ. Even in one's haste to get pemphigus vulgaris under control, one should not forget the prophylactic measures discussed in Chapter 69. Because of all these problems, the push is to avoid administering systemic corticosteroids over long periods of time. A number of corticosteroid-sparing agents have been employed. They include:

- Azathioprine has been used the most. It can be started relatively early in the disease course while the patient is still on high doses of corticosteroids. The dosage ranges between 50 and 200 mg daily. The onset of action of azathioprine is usually estimated at 4–6 weeks, so it is just becoming effective as one is forced to taper the corticosteroids.
- Cyclophosphamide 50–200 mg daily is probably the most effective agent in this group, but is more toxic than azathioprine. It appears to have more selectivity for plasma cells. Major side effects include cystitis, neutropenia, sterility and a 5–10% life-time risk of tumors, including lymphomas, leukemias and solid neoplasms. Monthly cyclophosphamide pulse therapy (0.5–1.0 g intravenously) as used in lupus nephritis is another approach.
- Methotrexate 15–30 mg orally or intravenously once weekly can also be used. If administered orally it can be used in divided doses, as discussed under psoriasis.
- Mycophenolate mofetil 1.0 g b.i.d. appears promising but we have not had extensive experi-

ence. In many centers, it has become the first line steroid-sparing agent in bullous diseases.

- Chlorambucil 4–8 mg daily, or cyclosporine 2.5–5.0 mg daily are more rapid acting and are usually introduced as the corticosteroids are being tapered.
- Gold salts enjoyed a period of popularity, but their side effect profile sets them apart even from the toxic agents above; we do not use them. Gold sodium thiomalate and aurothioglucose must be given intramuscularly; oral gold or auranofin is less toxic but also appears to be less effective.

As one introduces steroid-sparing agents, one introduces another long list of possible side effects, such as hemorrhagic cystitis from cyclophosphamide, hypertension and decreasing renal function from cyclosporine or hematologic problems from azathioprine. In addition immunosuppression increases the risk of bacterial or fungal infections, reactivation of tuberculosis and long-term tumor development.

There are two other drastic measures which we occasionally employ.

- High-dose intravenous immunoglobulin G (IVIG). Infusions of 0.25–0.5 g/kg daily of IVIG have a rapid anti-inflammatory effect and a down regulating potential on the autoantibodies. Treatment can be provided for several (2–5) days and then repeated every 4 weeks. Rapid clinical responses and a decrease in the CD4/CD8 T cell ratio are discussed in case reports and open trials. IVIG should be used to supplement systemic corticosteroids or steroid-sparing agents, not as a monotherapy.
- Plasmapheresis offers an effective but expensive way to reduce antibody levels. It is usually performed in three day cycles every 4–8 weeks. Just as with IVIG, it supplements more standard treatment.

Topical. The external treatment goes a long way towards determining how comfortable the patient is. Mild cases or early noneroded lesions may respond transiently to topical corticosteroids, but usually these agents are not helpful. Routine care as for burns is most important, with attention to secondary infections. Both 0.1–0.5% aqueous gentian violet and silver sulfadiazine can be useful. Antibacterial agents can also be added to baths, but one should be alert to the possibility of massive absorption. The oral lesions require special care, using topical anesthetic agents for comfort. Many patients will require help in cleaning their mouth.

Pemphigus Herpetiformis

(Jablonska et al. 1975)

Synonym. Dermatitis herpetiformis with acantholysis (Floden and Gentele 1955)

Etiology and Pathogenesis. The differences between pemphigus herpetiformis and pemphigus vulgaris are not totally clear. In most patients desmoglein 1 is the target antigen, but in some patients desmoglein 3 appears more important. The antibodies in pemphigus herpetiformis may be directed against different epitopes on the desmoglein molecules leading to acantholysis via other complement-independent mechanisms.

Clinical Findings. Pemphigus herpetiformis combines the clinical features of dermatitis herpetiformis with microscopic and immunopathologic features of pemphigus vulgaris. Patients have intense pruritus and small grouped vesicles on an erythematous base which may occur in the predilection sites for dermatitis herpetiformis (Fig. 15.12). Oral involvement is relatively uncommon.

Histopathology. The biopsy findings can be quite variable, changing with the age of the lesion, and often do not point to the correct diagnosis. In some instances acantholytic blisters containing eosinophils or neutrophils may be seen. Other lesions have only eosinophilic spongiosis, the accumulation of eosinophils in the epidermis seen in a variety of blistering disorders. Yet other patients may have intraepidermal pustules filled with neutrophils or eosinophils. The typical papillary dermal abscesses of dermatitis herpetiformis are not seen.

Immunofluorescent Examination. The immunofluorescent examination offers the best chance of making the diagnosis of pemphigus herpetiformis. Both direct and indirect immunofluorescent examination reveals fluorescence about epidermal cell surfaces, usually heaviest in the upper aspects of the epidermis.

Course and Prognosis. Pemphigus herpetiformis has a milder course than pemphigus vulgaris or pemphigus foliaceus. The disorder in some patients may evolve into one of these forms.

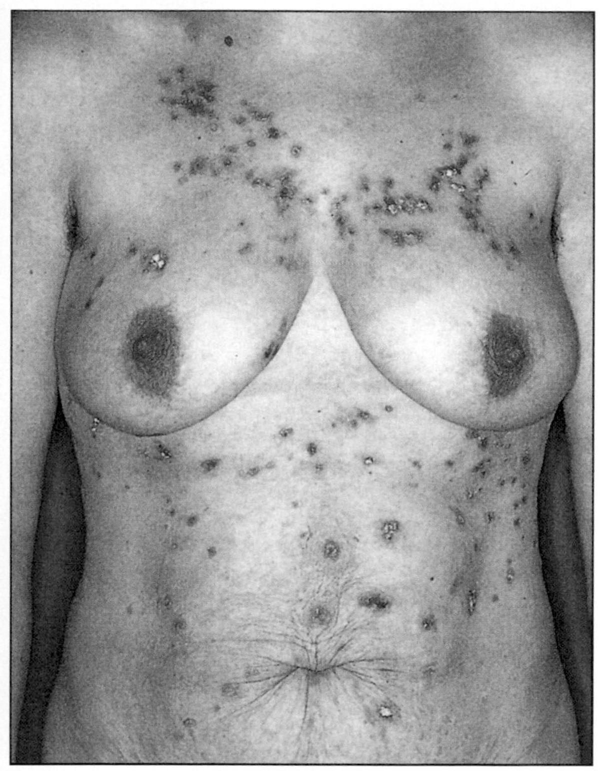

Fig. 15.12. Pemphigus herpetiformis

Differential Diagnosis. The disorder is often misdiagnosed as dermatitis herpetiformis, linear IgA disease or bullous pemphigoid. Pemphigus vulgaris and pemphigus foliaceus are separated on clinical and histologic features, since they have identical immunologic pictures.

Therapy. Dapsone is the initial treatment of choice, usually at a dose of 100–300 mg daily. To avoid dapsone toxicity, it may be wise to supplement a lower dapsone dose with systemic corticosteroids. In addition, azathioprine and cyclophosphamide have been employed with success.

Overlap Between Pemphigus Vulgaris and Bullous Pemphigoid

Very rare patients may have acantholytic blisters but circulating autoantibodies against both the intercellular attachments (as in pemphigus vulgaris) and the basement membrane zone (as in bullous pemphigoid). Some patients may just be unlucky and actually have both diseases. In other patients, one set of antibodies may represent an epiphenomenon. One should also think of paraneoplastic pemphigus. This disorder is often associated with a malignant lymphoma or thymoma and has a confusing array of autoantibodies.

Pemphigus Vegetans

Definition. Variant of pemphigus in which there is a localized vegetating papillomatous response. Two subtypes have been traditionally described.

Etiology and Pathogenesis. The target antigens and immunopathology of pemphigus vegetans are unclear. Both desmoglein 1 and 3 have been described. Some patients with IgA pemphigus also have vegetating lesions. We suspect that any relatively smoldering acantholytic process will allow bacterial overgrowth, as the skin is not shed so rapidly. The response to such chronic infection may be the vegetating lesions.

Pemphigus Vegetans, Neumann Type
(Neumann 1876)

The Neumann type of pemphigus vegetans develops as part of ordinary pemphigus vulgaris. In this sense, it is an exaggeration of the normal intertriginous pattern. Sometimes, the vegetating phase first begins with corticosteroid therapy. The eroded patches do not heal but develop papillomatous growths or vegetations. Typical intertriginous locations include the axilla, groin, perianal region (Fig. 15.13), and female genitalia, but also the nasolabial folds and corners of the mouth. The granulation tissue can dry out and then produce a warty surface with painful fissures. The biopsy reflects the clinical picture. Acanthosis and papillomatosis dominate, but intraepidermal eosinophils are a clue. Occasionally suprabasilar acantholysis and acantholytic cells can be found. The immunofluorescent examination confirms the diagnosis of pemphigus vegetans. Often the differential diagnosis is more difficult. Condylomata acuminata and condylomata lata must both be excluded in the perianal and genital regions. Halogenodermas are also a consideration, as are blastomycosis, blastomycotic pyoderma and the even rarer vegetating form of bullous pemphigoid. The therapy and prognosis are those for pemphigus vulgaris, although the vegetating lesions tend to be more therapy-resistant. Additional helpful tools include intralesional corticosteroids, soft x-rays and surgical debridement of vegetations in refractory cases.

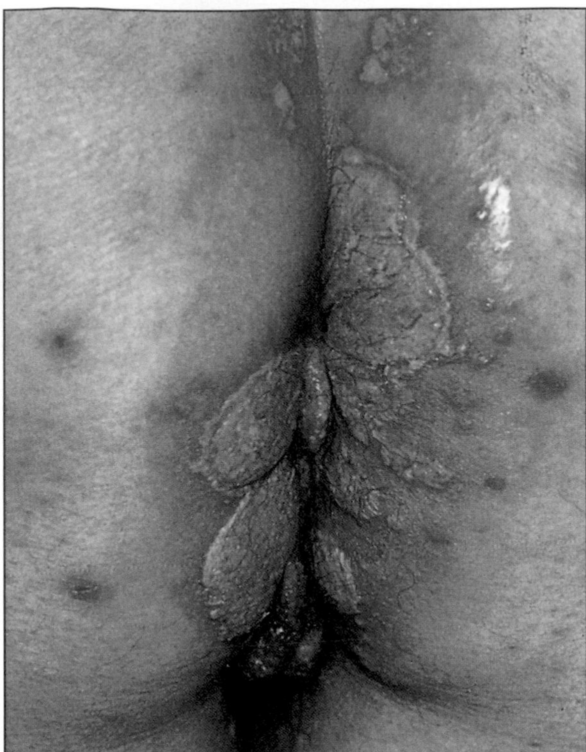

Fig. 15.13. Pemphigus vegetans, Neumann type

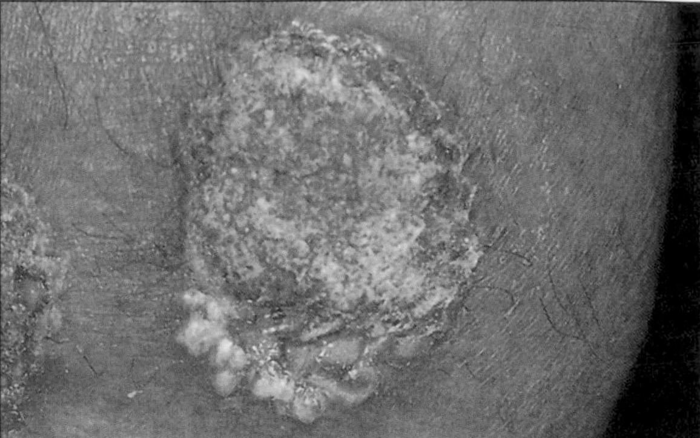

Fig. 15.14. Pemphigus vegetans, Hallopeau type

Pemphigus Vegetans, Hallopeau Type
(Hallopeau 1898)

The Hallopeau type presents as a disease sui generis without any obvious lesions of pemphigus vulgaris. The primary lesion is more likely to be a pustule which ruptures and then develops both papillomatous hyperplasia, granulation tissue and new pustules at the periphery (Fig. 15.14). The typical locations are once again the flexural areas, although lesions can be seen on the scalp and other areas. The lesions tend to be painful, foul smelling and often secondarily infected. The histologic features are identical to those of the Neumann type. On occasions, the Hallopeau type may also evolve into pemphigus vulgaris. In general, the Hallopeau type is more corticosteroid-responsive. Surgical debridement, intralesional corticosteroids or antibiotic therapy may be tried to control the local vegetating growths.

Pemphigus Foliaceus
(Cazenave 1850)

Definition. Type of pemphigus with very superficial acantholysis producing more erosions than blisters.

Epidemiology. Pemphigus foliaceus is also a very uncommon disorder, perhaps even less frequent than pemphigus vulgaris. While most patients are adults, pemphigus foliaceus is the most common type of pemphigus in children.

Etiology and Pathogenesis. The major antigen in pemphigus foliaceus is desmoglein 1. The antibodies to desmoglein 1 are pathogenic in neonatal mice. While desmoglein 1 is expressed on mucosal surfaces, it is not necessary to maintain mucosal integrity. Most cases of drug-induced pemphigus are clinically pemphigus foliaceus.

Clinical Findings. Pemphigus foliaceus typically starts on the scalp, face, sternum or lateral aspects of the chest and thorax. The initial lesions are broad flat blisters, often never appreciated as such by the patient, which easily rupture and evolve into fine wet sheets of scales (Fig. 15.15). The scales have been compared to puff pastry. The upper layer of the epidermis is actually floating on a bed of serum, so weeping and crusting are inevitable. Bacterial colonization may lead to a foul smell.

As the eruption spreads, it may come to resemble an erythroderma, with widespread areas of red moist patches, decked with crust and scale. Just as with pemphigus vulgaris, the intertriginous lesions evolve slightly differently without scaling. Lesions below the knees or elbows are unusual. Older lesions

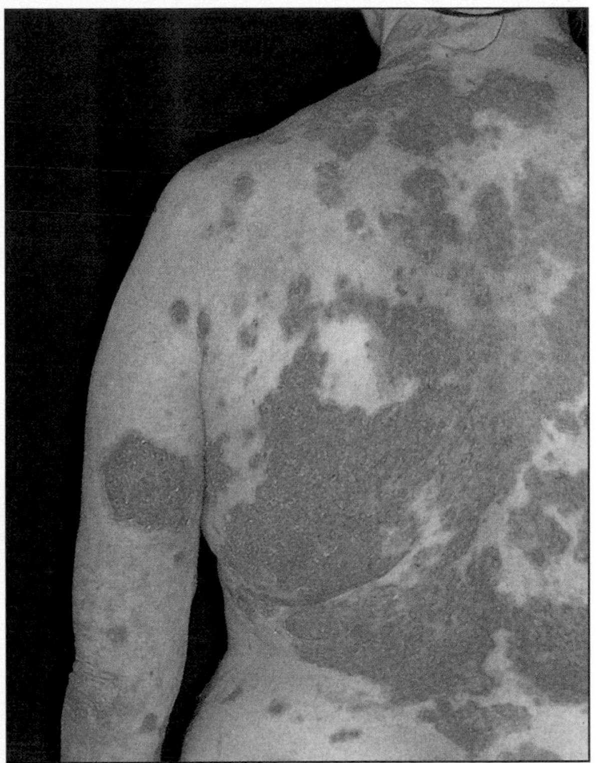

Fig. 15.15. Pemphigus foliaceus

on the trunk may become quite thickened. Oral and ocular lesions are almost unheard of. The Nikolsky sign is usually positive.

Histopathology. The lower and mid reaches of the epidermis are normal or spongiotic. The acantholysis is found in the upper stratum spinosum or stratum corneum. Dyskeratotic cells as well as reactive epidermal changes such as acanthosis and papillomatosis may be seen. The dermis often shows perivascular or diffuse inflammatory infiltrates, sometimes rich in eosinophils. The Tzanck smear is once again positive. Because of the more superficial location of the acantholysis, some of the free keratinocytes are dyskeratotic.

Immunofluorescent Examination. Routine direct and indirect immunofluorescent examinations cannot always separate pemphigus vulgaris and pemphigus foliaceus. In both situations, the entire epidermis can be stained in a net-like pattern, but in most cases of pemphigus foliaceus, autoantibodies are confined to the upper aspects of the epidermis. To separate pemphigus vulgaris and pemphigus foliaceus the desmoglein ELISA is most efficient. Patients with pemphigus foliaceus have antibodies against desmoglein 1 but not against desmoglein 3.

Course and Prognosis. The course of pemphigus foliaceus is quite chronic in adults. The prognosis is about as dismal in untreated patients as that of pemphigus vulgaris. In adults, the pattern is often one of waves. Some patients flare in the summer, supporting the photosensitive nature of the disease. In children spontaneous healing may occur after a number of years.

Differential Diagnosis. Initially the clinical diagnosis may be seborrheic dermatitis or impetigo but the course and a biopsy rapidly exclude those considerations. Lupus erythematosus is another possibility, as discussed below.

Therapy. The approach is just as with pemphigus vulgaris, but usually lower doses of systemic corticosteroids suffice. Early or mild cases may also respond to dapsone, which is worth a try because of its better safety profile. Antimalarials are occasionally helpful. Topical corticosteroids may be sufficient to control some lesions. With widespread erosions, disinfectant ($KMnO_4$ or clioquinol) or astringent (tannic acid) baths may be helpful.

Brazilian Pemphigus

(Vieira 1940)

Synonyms. Fogo selvagem, endemic pemphigus

Definition. Endemic South American illness, perhaps infectious in origin, that resembles pemphigus foliaceus.

Epidemiology. Brazilian pemphigus occurs not surprisingly in Brazil but also in parts of Argentina, Paraguay, Bolivia, Peru and Venezuela. The disease occurs primarily at the interface between civilization and tropical nature. For example, special pemphigus hospitals built on the periphery of Sao Paulo three decades ago are today surrounded by the megalopolis and far away from the source of their patients. Men are far more often affected, usually outdoor workers. Patients treated in urban areas frequently flare when returning to rural areas. Most patients live within 10 km of rivers or lakes. The general distribution follows the same pattern as that of the black fly *Simulum prinosum*, and the number of cases peaks as the fly population does. Finally, transmission has not been described via patient contact or blood products.

Etiology and Pathogenesis. All of the above epidemiologic data strongly suggest that an infectious agent, probably transmitted by the black fly is the trigger. HLA alleles may also play a role, as some families are affected and others are spared. In general, genetically related family members are more often affected than unrelated, i.e., two siblings or parent-child involvement is more common than spouse-spouse or spouse-parent-in-law. Some HLA haplotypes appear to confer protection and others, susceptibility.

Clinical Findings. The patient usually complains of burning and pain. The Portuguese term *fogo selvagem* means wild fire. The superficial blisters are once again primarily on the face and scalp but also involve the trunk. They quickly evolve into weeping, crusted erosions. Oral involvement does not occur. The Nikolsky sign is positive.

Histopathology. The histology and immunofluorescent examinations are very similar to those in pemphigus foliaceus. The indirect immunofluorescence titers tend to be very high and correlate with the disease status.

Course and Prognosis. Prior to the introduction of systemic corticosteroids, the disease had a poor prognosis. Today some patients are cured while others must be maintained on long-term therapy. The mortality is estimated at 5%.

Therapy. The same approaches as discussed under pemphigus vulgaris and pemphigus foliaceus are employed. Usually lower dosages of prednisone can be employed and the maintenance levels are reached more easily. In Brazil, the usual duration of therapy is 2–4 years.

Pemphigus Erythematosus

(Senear and Usher 1926)

Synonyms. Pemphigus seborrheicus, Senear-Usher disease

Definition. Variant of pemphigus foliaceus which overlaps with lupus erythematosus.

Etiology and Pathogenesis. While pemphigus foliaceus often clinically resembles lupus erythematosus, a small subgroup of patients have immunologic markers for both diseases. This variant is even more likely than pemphigus foliaceus to be triggered by light or drugs. The antigens involved have not been characterized.

Clinical Findings. Just as with pemphigus foliaceus, the eruption begins with erythematous patches on the sun-exposed areas, primarily the face, scalp and décolletage. Sometimes small symmetric patches are present, rather than more diffuse disease. The facial lesions strongly resemble those of lupus erythematosus or even seborrheic dermatitis, while those on the trunk tend to be more eroded and crusted, suggesting the correct diagnosis. The oral mucosa is not involved. The patients are usually relatively symptom-free.

Histopathology. The superficial acantholysis of pemphigus foliaceus is once again found. In addition, there may be basal layer vacuolar degeneration and a lymphocytic perivascular infiltrate which impinges on the thickened basement membrane zone. The Tzanck smear shows acantholytic and dyskeratotic keratinocytes but also many leukocytes.

Immunofluorescent Examination. Direct immunofluorescent staining identifies IgG antibodies against the intercellular adhesion molecules in the same diffuse pattern as in pemphigus foliaceus. Between 50% and 70% of the patients have a positive LE band test in more chronic lesions. A small number may also have antinuclear antibodies directed against the keratinocyte nuclei, but in about 80% the antinuclear antibodies are identified in the serum. Highly specific lupus erythematosus antibodies such anti-DNA, -Sm or -Ro are not found. If the clinical suspicion of pemphigus erythematosus is high, the immunologic tests should be repeated at 2–4-week intervals.

Course and Prognosis. In most cases, the disease persists. Sometimes the blistering may become more severe, so that one speaks of a transition to pemphigus foliaceus, although this is admittedly more a semantic than a medical issue. Other rare patients may develop signs of systemic lupus erythematosus, such a lupus nephritis. Finally, thymomas and myasthenia gravis can occur.

Differential Diagnosis. The main considerations are seborrheic dermatitis and lupus erythematosus.

Therapy. When systemic therapy is used, moderate dosages of systemic corticosteroids usually suffice. As alternative agents, antimalarials and dapsone are both occasionally successful. Patients with few lesions can often be treated exclusively with topical corticosteroids, perhaps under occlusion or using a corticosteroid-impregnated tape. Even cryotherapy is helpful for early lesions. Sun protection is essential.

IgA Pemphigus

Synonym. Intercellular IgA vesiculopustular dermatosis

Two similar diseases have been described under the rubric of IgA pemphigus. One is termed subcorneal pustular dermatosis and may have flaccid pustules, while the other is usually less distinct clinically and was originally identified histologically. Both types have been described in patients with HIV/AIDS.

IgA Pemphigus, Subcorneal Pustular Dermatosis Type

(Wallach et al. 1982)

Patients with subcorneal pustular dermatosis (Chap. 16) have flaccid pustules (Fig. 15.16), no sign of systemic disease, subcorneal neutrophilic pustules and tend to respond to dapsone. In most cases, both direct and indirect immunofluorescent examination is negative, but in some instances, deposition of IgA is identified in the upper one-third of the epidermis in the pattern of pemphigus foliaceus. Often repeated direct immunofluorescent examinations are required. Several days of systemic corticosteroid therapy is sufficient to block IgA production making testing negative. The autoantigen is desmocollin 1, another desmosomal cadherin, as best shown by reacting serum from such patients with cells constructed to express only this desmocollin in vitro.

An additional feature of subcorneal pustular dermatosis is an association with IgA gammopathy. In most instances, patients have either epidermal deposition of IgA or an IgA gammopathy, but not both. While several cases of IgA pemphigus have been reported in which such a gammopathy was present, the patients had both IgA and IgG autoantibodies, making their classification problematic.

This variant tends to have a relatively benign course and often responds to dapsone. It is unclear if there are two diseases – IgA pemphigus resembling subcorneal pustular dermatosis and classic Sneddon-Wilkinson subcorneal pustular dermatosis, or if there is only one disorder and one must search long and hard for the IgA markers. Patients classically described with subcorneal pustular dermatosis appear most likely to have widespread cutaneous disease and pemphigus vegetans-like involvement of the flexures, but a clinical separation is impossible.

Intraepidermal Neutrophilic IgA Dermatosis

(Huff et al. 1985; Wallach 1986)

Epidemiology. Most common in elderly patients, but so rare that other features have not been identified.

Etiology and Pathogenesis. The etiology is unknown. One case was described in a child with homozygous α_1-antitrypsin deficiency and liver transplantation, requiring prednisone and cyclosporine. Another was seen in a patient with HIV/AIDS. The target for the IgA is unclear; in one case, it was desmoglein 3.

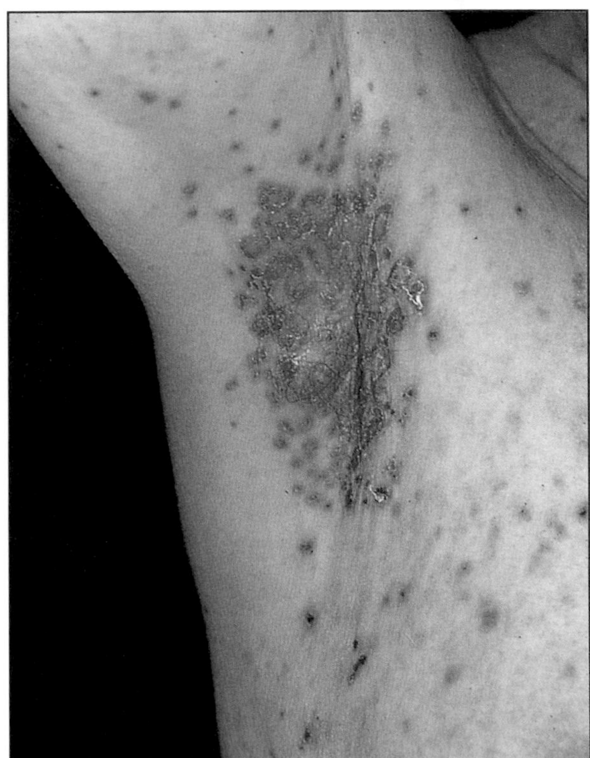

Fig. 15.16. IgA pemphigus

Clinical Findings. The patients typically present with fragile pustules, small blisters and superficial erosions. The most common site is the trunk; intertriginous regions are also commonly involved. Pruritus may be a problem. Oral lesions are very rare.

Histopathology. There are subcorneal and intraepidermal pustules filled with neutrophils, occasional eosinophils and occasional acantholytic cells. In the dermis is a predominantly neutrophilic infiltrate.

Immunofluorescent Examination. Direct immunofluorescent examination reveals IgA deposited in a pattern resembling that seen in pemphigus vulgaris. Rare patients also have IgG antibodies; their classification is problematic. The indirect immunofluorescent examination is positive in about half of cases.

Course and Prognosis. The disorder is chronic over many years, with little tendency to remission. On the other hand, the patients tend to do better than with other forms of pemphigus vulgaris and require less-aggressive therapy.

Differential Diagnosis. Impetigo can be separated by bacterial cultures and direct immunofluorescent examination, although it is identical microscopically. Other forms of pemphigus, linear IgA disease and dermatitis herpetiformis should also be considered, as well as necrolytic migratory erythema.

Therapy. Dapsone is often effective, and should probably be tried before systemic corticosteroids. Topical corticosteroids should be tried on new lesions. Pustules can be opened and treated with topical antiseptics.

Paraneoplastic Pemphigus

(Anhalt et al. 1990)

Definition. Polymorphic eruption with mucosal involvement in which patients have acantholytic blisters and pemphigus-like antibodies, as well as underlying neoplasms.

Epidemiology. Paraneoplastic pemphigus is an uncommon disorder which has been described under a number of misleading names such as tumor-associated pemphigus vulgaris and tumor-associated lichen planus.

Etiology and Pathogenesis. The hallmark is an association with an underlying neoplasm. The most common tumors are hematologic neoplasms such as non-Hodgkin lymphoma and chronic lymphocytic leukemia. Other hematologic disorders which may be found include Castleman disease or giant follicular hyperplasia (a benign B cell proliferation) and Waldenström macroglobulinemia. In addition both thymomas and myasthenia gravis can be present. Sarcomas and carcinomas have only rarely been indicted.

The mechanisms of cutaneous disease remain unclear. Somehow the tumor induces synthesis of autoantibodies that react with a variety of epithelial structures. This may be accomplished by the tumor expressing epithelial adhesion antigens, so that the autoimmune response is actually a misled anti-tumor response. Cell-mediated cytotoxicity may also play a role, suggesting that the immune pathways are quite complex.

Antibodies are directed against many different components of hemidesmosomes and keratinocytes. If one or two of these antibodies are missing, one should not exclude the diagnosis of paraneoplastic pemphigus. Almost all patients have antibodies against desmoglein 3 and about two-thirds react against desmoglein 1. Other antigens include the plakin proteins (desmoplakin I and II, envoplakin, periplakin and plakoglobin) and BPAG1 which seems analogous to desmoplakin I in the hemidesmosome. Finally antibodies are also found directed against plectin and a 170-kDa protein whose identity is unknown. Desmogleins are transmembrane proteins and more likely to play an initial role. Anti-desmoglein 3 antibodies have been identified using a desmoglein ELISA and seem to cause bronchial epithelial involvement.

Clinical Findings. The most important clinical finding is the presence of severe, often hemorrhagic, painful oral erosions (Fig. 15.17). The lips are typically involved with thick crusted erosions, and the intraoral disease extends throughout the oropharynx. The conjunctiva, genitalia, perianal region and even nailfolds may also develop painful erosions. The palms and soles, upper aspects of the trunk and the extremities are sites of predilection. The cutaneous lesions are quite polymorphic, causing considerable diagnostic confusion. Sometimes intact blisters are seen, as in bullous pemphigoid or erythema multiforme. The Nikolsky sign may be positive. In other instances, the prominent rosette formation associated with linear IgA

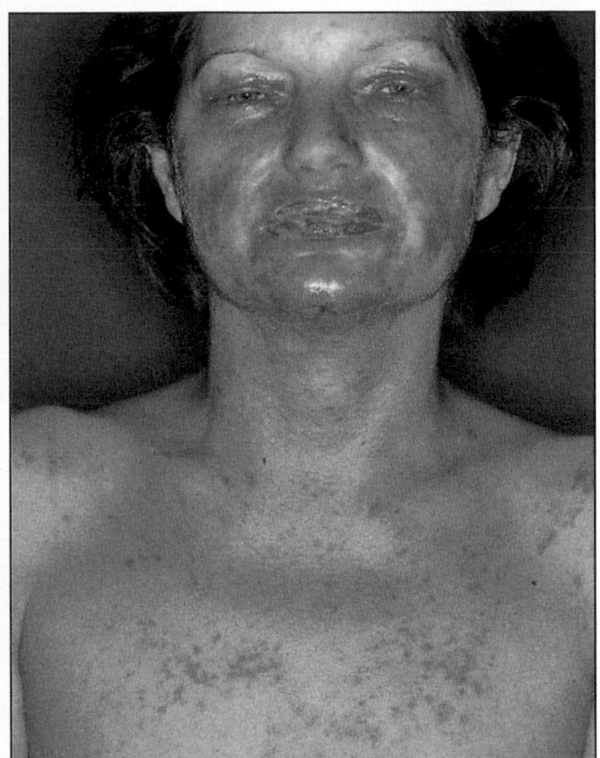

Fig. 15.17. Paraneoplastic pemphigus

dermatosis is found. Finally, infiltrated violaceous papules, resembling lichen planus, may develop either de novo or more often as secondary changes in eroded lesions.

Histopathology. The pathology varies greatly depending on the type of lesion. The blisters tend to show suprabasilar acantholysis, even though the diseases they resemble most closely are nonacantholytic subepidermal blistering disorders. In addition, there may be vacuolar basal layer damage associated with a lichenoid dermal lymphocytic infiltrate. In papulosquamous lesions, the acantholysis may be absent. Multiple biopsies are frequently required to make the diagnosis.

Immunofluorescent Examination. Direct immunofluorescent examination shows deposition of IgG antibodies directed against the epithelial cell surfaces. False-negative tests are common so multiple biopsies may be needed. Occasionally direct immunofluorescence will also show basement membrane zone deposition of immunoglobulin and complement. Indirect immunofluorescent examination reveals circulating pemphigus-like antibodies. To separate paraneoplastic pemphigus from pemphigus vulgaris, one can employ two indirect immunofluorescence substrates: monkey esophagus and rodent bladder epithelium. Serum from patients with paraneoplastic pemphigus will react with both substrates. In addition special laboratories can identify the serum antibodies via immunoprecipitation studies.

Laboratory Findings. Routine investigations should be pursued until an underlying tumor is identified.

Course and Prognosis. The outlook depends on that of the underlying tumor. If the tumor is benign, some patients show dramatic improvement once it is removed. Malignant tumors not only have their associated morbidity, but the blistering disorder tends to be more severe and hard to treat. About 90% of the first 33 patients died of the disease or complications of its (not the tumor's) treatment. A peculiar respiratory failure syndrome mediated by autoantibodies responds poorly to treatment. Thus pulmonary physicians should be involved in the disease management as soon as any lung involvement is suspected and should perform bronchoscopy to obtain tissue for direct immunofluorescence.

Differential Diagnosis. The list is very long. All the blistering disorders mentioned in this chapter can be mimicked. In addition, lichen planus and erythema multiforme may be considered initially.

Therapy. Treatment is difficult. The oral lesions are extremely refractory to all approaches and interfere greatly with eating. The same immunosuppressive agents used for pemphigus vulgaris can be tried, but all are less effective. Recent use of adjuvant IVIG in the same dosages outlined above appears promising.

Pemphigoid Diseases

The pemphigoid group includes a series of chronic diseases in which blisters form within the lamina lucida of the basement membrane. The blister roof is thus the entire epidermis so it is more stable. Frequently the blisters are hemorrhagic, fluid-filled and tense. No acantholysis occurs, so the Tzanck test is negative. Antibodies are directed against various components of the basement membrane zone. Once again they can be identified

Table 15.6. Antigens in the pemphigoid group

Disorder	Antigens
Bullous pemphigoid	BPAG2, BPAG1, laminin 5, 105-kDa antigen, 200-kDa antigen
Herpes gestationis	BPAG2, (?)BPAG1
Cicatricial pemphigoid	BPAG2, laminin 5, laminin 6, integrins
Linear IgA dermatosis	BPAG2 and fragments thereof, laminin, integrins, type VII collagen, (?)BPAG1
Epidermolysis bullosa acquisita	Type VII collagen
Dermatitis herpetiformis	Unknown, perhaps tissue transglutaminase

by both direct and indirect immunofluorescent examination. The study of the pemphigoid group has cast considerable light on the structure of the basement membrane zone. Table 15.6 summarizes the target antigens in the subepidermal blistering disorders.

Bullous Pemphigoid

(Lever 1953)

Definition. Relatively common chronic blistering disease that features tense blisters on an erythematous base.

Epidemiology. Bullous pemphigoid is primarily a disease of the elderly. The mean age of onset is 76 years with a 1.8:1 male to female ratio among German patients. Patients with HLA- DQB1*0301 appear predisposed. Childhood cases have also been classified as chronic bullous disease of childhood, confusing the epidemiology.

Etiology and Pathogenesis. Two target antigens have been identified in the hemidesmosomes. The split occurs predominantly in the upper part of the lamina lucida, just beneath of the basal layer keratinocytes, where these proteins are found. The serum of patients with bullous pemphigoid has been used to identify these antigens in normal skin, so in this case, the disease has helped to define the normal anatomy. The antigens are:

- BPAG2 or type XVII collagen is a 180-kDa transmembrane component of hemidesmosomes that spans the lamina lucida and reaches the lamina densa with its carboxy terminal portion. Another important region is the noncollagenous domain 16A (NC16A) which is just beneath the hemidesmosome.
- BPAG1 is a 230-kDa protein associated with inner plaques of hemidesmosomes. It is thought to interface with the keratin intermediate filament cytoskeleton of basal keratinocytes.

More than 95% of bullous pemphigoid patients have antibodies against BPAG2 or BPAG1. BPAG2 is much more important since it is extracellular and more likely to be a site for the initiation of the disease. BPAG1 may be exposed after the disease is in full swing and then involved as a second antigen. The binding of autoantibodies against BPAG2 can be analyzed in detail by antigen mapping. Binding to the NC16A domain in the vicinity of the keratinocyte membrane is more likely to be associated with bullous pemphigoid or herpes gestationis, while in cicatricial pemphigoid, the C-terminal region may more often be the target. In addition to these well established antigens, several other target antigens are rarely found in patients who clinically appear to have bullous pemphigoid. Included in this group are laminin 5 and the 105-kDa and 200-kDa antigens which have not been fully characterized.

The binding of IgG autoantibodies can activate the complement cascade, triggering the clinically apparent inflammatory reaction involving neutrophils and eosinophils which results in a subepidermal blister. While it has been difficult to show a pathogenic role for these antibodies in experimental settings, very complicated approaches, such as immunizing animals against various epitopes of BPAGs, have succeeded in producing the disease. The problem seems to be the lack of interspecies homology between the relevant epitopes of BPAG2.

Bullous pemphigoid may also be a paraneoplastic marker. It is well-agreed that a percentage of the primarily elderly patients have an associated tumor. The number has been estimated at 15–20%.

The question is: is this number higher than in the general age-matched population? Most studies have shown that it is not, but it is still appropriate to at least screen for an underlying malignancy in a bullous pemphigoid patient.

Medications may also cause bullous pemphigoid, but even less often than pemphigus vulgaris. The only large study identified patients with bullous pemphigoid as being more likely to be taking antihypertensive agents and diuretics, the two medications which many elderly patients take regardless of their skin status. If antibasement membrane zone antibodies are present, they are usually of a very low titer and may be accompanied by other autoantibodies directed against other components of the epidermis. In some patients, the disease resolves promptly when the medication is stopped; in other mostly younger individuals, it behaves like the idiopathic version. The classic drug incriminated in bullous pemphigoid is furosemide, although many other agents are mentioned occasionally. Perhaps the mechanism is that any medication which induces a bullous drug reaction by whatever means can expose the BPAGs or alter the inflammatory response to them. In addition UV radiation, PUVA therapy and x-rays have been reported to trigger bullous pemphigoid. Perhaps such reactions are analogous to the Köbner reaction in a susceptible individual.

Bullous pemphigoid has been reported in coexistence with a wide variety of other diseases, some of which may also have an autoimmune basis. Included in the list are dermato- or polymyositis, pemphigus vulgaris, pemphigus foliaceus, dermatitis herpetiformis, systemic lupus erythematosus, ulcerative colitis, various forms of nephritis, rheumatoid arthritis, lichen planus and psoriasis.

Clinical Findings. The initial lesions are often urticarial and the patient may smolder along for weeks or even months with what are mistaken as hives. Just as with ordinary urticaria, the lesions are intensely pruritic. At some point the blistering begins. Sites of predilection include the side of the neck, axilla, groin, upper inner aspects of the thighs and the abdomen. Large tense often irregular blisters develop either within the urticarial plaques or on normal skin (Fig. 15.18). The early blisters may resemble those of erythema multiforme. They may reach many centimeters in size, have bizarre configurations and typically contain blood and serum. Some blisters are frankly hemorrhagic; this strongly suggests the diagnosis.

The blisters are fairly resistant to breakage. When they do rupture, erosions appear, usually with blister formation at their periphery, resulting in rosettes of blisters, a typical feature of all subepidermal blistering diseases (Fig. 15.19). The erosions typically have bloody crusts, as the superficial dermal vessels are exposed. In the intertriginous areas, the lesions rupture sooner, so patients are more likely to present with erosions. In rare cases the scalp can be involved. The Asboe-Hansen sign is

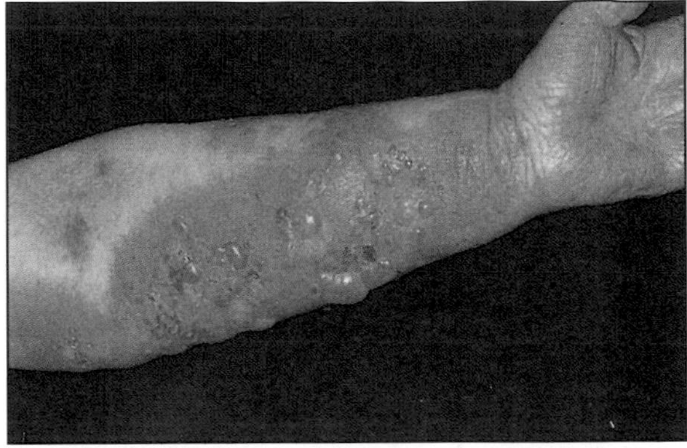

Fig. 15.18. Bullous pemphigoid with tense blisters on erythematous base

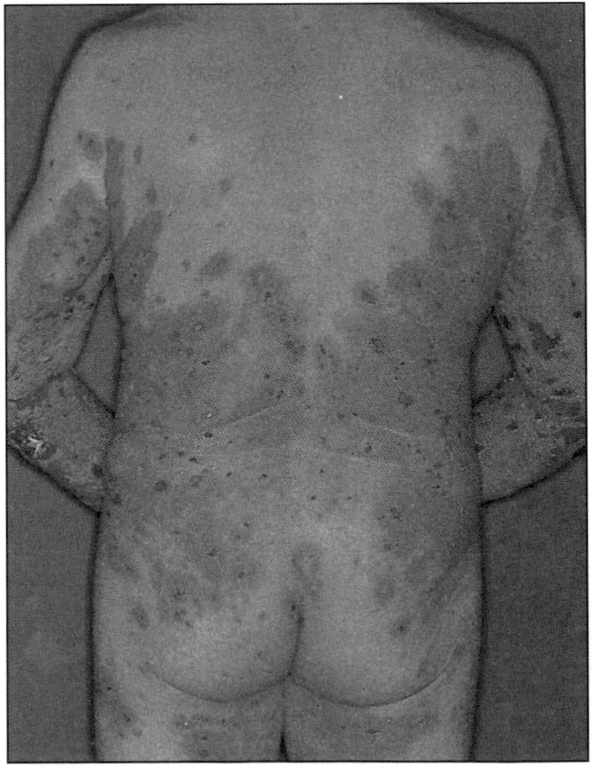

Fig. 15.19. Bullous pemphigoid

usually positive, and on occasion the Nikolsky sign is positive at the edge of blisters.

Mucosal lesions are less common than in pemphigus vulgaris. Very few patients present with only oral lesions, but 20–30 % have either tiny blisters or painful sharply bordered erosions in the mouth. The other mucosal surfaces are almost always spared, so that if for example ocular involvement is present, one should think of an alternative diagnosis.

Many different clinical variants of bullous pemphigoid have been described. In some instances, typical bullae are not appreciated and the diagnosis is first made by immunofluorescent examination. These forms are discussed below.

Histopathology. The hallmark is a subepidermal blister. The blister roof is the entire epidermis which often appears entirely normal. Early lesions may show tiny subepidermal microvesicles, which are also seen at the edge of more developed blisters. The blister fluid usually contains fibrin and eosinophils but not acantholytic cells. Both cell-poor and cell-rich variants of bullous pemphigoid can be found. In the former, there is almost a naked blister with a sparse lymphocytic perivascular infiltrate, perhaps admixed with a few eosinophils. In contrast, the cell-rich or inflammatory variant shows an intense perivascular infiltrate containing lymphocytes, neutrophils and eosinophils. There may be a true vasculitis with endothelial swelling and nuclear dust.

Immunofluorescent Examination. When the perilesional skin is examined by direct immunofluorescence, almost every patient has deposition of C3 and most have IgG, usually IgG_4. In addition IgG_2, IgG_3 (the main complement activator), IgM and even IgA can be found. Sometimes early in the disease only C3 will be present. The line of deposition is a thick, sharply defined band just beneath the basal keratinocytes within the basement membrane zone (Fig. 15.20).

Indirect immunofluorescent examination produces similar results with a sharp band of IgG deposits seen in more than 80 % of patients. The preferred substrate is normal human skin or patient skin which has been separated in the lamina lucida via incubation in 1.0 M NaCl solution. The antibodies attach in most cases just to the upper side of the split; when both sides are labeled, the upper is always more intense. While staining on the epidermal side is highly specific for bullous pemphigoid, dermal staining can be seen with epidermolysis bullosa acquisita and cicatricial pemphigoid. While the autoantibody titers in indirect immunofluorescent examination have traditionally been thought not to correlate with the disease course, recent studies with larger numbers of patients have shown that there is a significant correlation.

Course and Prognosis. The outlook for bullous pemphigoid is probably most determined by the nondermatologic status of the patient. While bullous pemphigoid is a chronic disease, it usually can be controlled by systemic corticosteroids. Unfortunately, many older patients develop abundant complications from the corticosteroids and have an increased risk of infections. In addition, the burden of a chronic widespread disease may lead to loss of appetite, weight loss and depression complicating their management. In the days before corticosteroids, the mortality was estimated at 40 %, compared to greater than 95 % in pemphigus vulgaris. In addition, the disease tends to relent or even remit after a period of years.

Diagnostic Criteria. For classic bullous pemphigoid, a large study with multivariate analysis has suggested that the most important diagnostic associations are absence of atrophic scars, absence of head and neck involvement, absence of mucosal involvement and age greater than 70 years. When three of these four criteria are present in a patient with a subepidermal blistering disease, the disease is extremely likely to be bullous pemphigoid. Nonetheless, the diagnosis should be confirmed by immunologic methods.

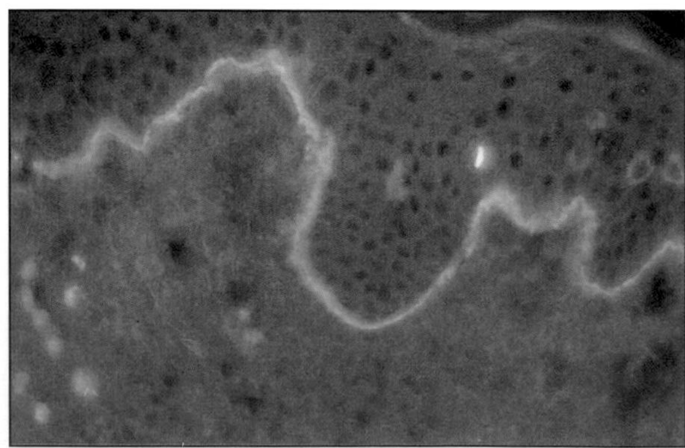

Fig. 15.20. Direct immunofluorescent examination in bullous pemphigoid

Differential Diagnosis. The other blistering diseases form the main differential diagnostic considerations. Once again, it seems easy to separate bullous pemphigoid and pemphigus vulgaris but our forebears had much difficulty until immunofluorescent examination became routine. When dermatitis herpetiformis, linear IgA dermatosis or epidermolysis bullosa acquisita presents with large tense blisters, it is easy to go wrong. The variants discussed below are almost always misdiagnosed at first. Early lesions mimic either urticaria or erythema multiforme, but the disease course is totally different. Large blisters on the legs may be confused with bullous arthropod bite reactions, which are especially common in patients with chronic lymphocytic leukemia (Chap. 62), and bullous disease of diabetes mellitus.

Therapy

Systemic. One must remember that the main cause of death today in patients with bullous pemphigoid is side effects of therapy. Corticosteroids are the mainstay. Because one is dealing with an elderly population, all the cautions discussed under pemphigus vulgaris are even more important. Fortunately, lower dosages are usually required, in the range of 30–60 mg daily of prednisone. Often one can even start with alternate-day therapy or switch rapidly to it. The same steroid-sparing agents can be employed; azathioprine and chlorambucil are probably most often used. We use azathioprine 100–150 mg initially but then taper to 50 mg daily. Chlorambucil 4–6 mg daily is the usual dose. Mycophenolate mofetil has been shown to be effective in recent studies and may even become the steroid-sparing agent of choice if larger studies support its efficacy. Methotrexate once weekly in the usual psoriasis or rheumatoid arthritis dosages (5–15 mg, either oral or intravenous) is also effective.

Even more harmless agents can also be tried in combination; dapsone is occasionally effective. In addition, some patients respond to antibiotics, either macrolides or tetracyclines in the usual dosages, sometimes combined with nicotinamide. Plasmapheresis can reduce the antibody titer and produce clinical improvement.

Topical. One must not forget topical corticosteroids, as they are the safest for these patients. Often high-potency agents applied to the early erythematous lesions can limit or stop the development of blisters. Once erosions are present, the same topical care recommended for epidermolysis bullosa and pemphigus vulgaris is appropriate.

Variants of Bullous Pemphigoid

There are a number of variants of bullous pemphigoid. Some are readily recognized as belonging to the family, but have peculiar or limited clinical features. Others are first identified on immunofluorescent studies. All are treated as outlined above.

Urticarial Bullous Pemphigoid

This form is in most cases not a variant, but simply the early stage of bullous pemphigoid. The urticarial lesions in some patients may persist for months to years and may evolve into modest blisters resembling erythema multiforme. While the direct immunofluorescent examination from perilesional skin is usually positive, multiple biopsies may be required. Indirect immunofluorescence is positive in at most 30 % of cases.

Vesicular Bullous Pemphigoid

(Bean et al. 1976)

Synonyms. Polymorphic bullous pemphigoid, herpetiform bullous pemphigoid

This disorder clinically resembles dermatitis herpetiformis, with multiple, intensely pruritic or burning tiny vesicles. Large tense blisters never develop. Histologically, the lesions also resemble those of dermatitis herpetiformis but the immunofluorescent examination findings are typical for bullous pemphigoid, as is the response to therapy. Systemic corticosteroids are effective, while dapsone and sulfapyridine are not.

Dyshidrosiform Bullous Pemphigoid

(Levine et al. 1979)

Some patients have tense small blisters confined to the palms and soles. Inevitably they are diagnosed as dyshidrotic dermatitis and treated with topical corticosteroids, which often help. A second differential diagnostic possibility is a dyshidrotic tinea pedis. If lesions compatible with bullous pemphigoid are found elsewhere on the body, the diagnosis may come sooner. Otherwise, it is often delayed. Modest dosages of corticosteroids are effective, so treatment for dyshidrotic dermatitis may further mask the issue.

Seborrheic Bullous Pemphigoid

(Schnyder 1969)

This peculiar disorder resembles lupus erythematosus or pemphigus erythematosus. Most patients are elderly women. Histologically the blister is subepidermal. Both direct and indirect immunofluorescent examination supports the diagnosis of pemphigoid, but the circulating IgG titers are usually very low. Relatively low dosages of systemic corticosteroids are effective.

Vegetating Bullous Pemphigoid

(Winkelmann and Su 1979)

Synonym. Pemphigoid vegetans

This disorder is analogous to pemphigus vegetans. While the groin and axilla are typical sites for erosions in pemphigoid, in rare instances there may be a granulomatous or vegetating response. The face and scalp may also be involved. The light microscopic picture is dominated by the reactive epidermal changes, but the immunofluorescent examination confirms the diagnosis of pemphigoid. In the differential diagnosis one must also consider halogenodermas, blastomycotic pyoderma and blastomycosis.

Localized Bullous Pemphigoid

(Eberhartinger and Niebauer 1961; Person et al. 1976]

Some patients have only a limited number of blisters localized to a given region. Most patients are elderly and the shins and scalp are the most common sites. Confusion may arise in the summer with bullous arthropod bite reactions which are also common over the shins. In women, localized vulvar pemphigoid is occasionally seen. The lesions in adults must be distinguished from localized cicatricial pemphigoid (Brunsting-Perry disease) which tends to be located on the head and neck and is scarring, as well as from localized epidermolysis bullosa acquisita. Patients with localized bullous pemphigoid may occasionally develop generalized lesions after a period of time. The local lesions can be controlled with topical corticosteroids.

Prurigo Nodularis-like Bullous Pemphigoid

(Yung et al. 1981)

Synonym. Pemphigoid nodularis

In this very uncommon disorder patients have localized disease with a hypertrophic local response. Thus the healing lesions resemble those of prurigo nodularis, just as is the case in some forms of pemphigus foliaceus. Once again, bullae may be found in association or there may be a history of previous blistering.

Herpes Gestationis

(Bunes 1811; Milton 1872)

Synonyms. Pemphigoid gestationis, dermatitis multiformis gestationis

Definition. Uncommon blistering disease associated with pregnancy, but otherwise similar to bullous pemphigoid.

Epidemiology. Herpes gestationis is almost exclusively limited to pregnancy. It may persist in the postpartum period (rarely starting during this time) and can also be triggered by oral contraceptives. The incidence is estimated at 1 : 50,000.

Etiology and Pathogenesis. The target antigen in herpes gestationis is BPAG2. Somehow antigen processing and presentation is altered in the placenta so that normally innocuous epitopes become antigenic. While almost all cases of herpes gestationis appear during pregnancy, the disease can also be seen in association with hydatidiform moles and choriocarcinomas. The former contain placental tissue; the latter, fetal.

The majority of patients have circulating antibodies against BPAG2, mainly directed at the NC16A domain. Some also have antibodies against BPAG1. The IgG antibodies are pathogenic. In addition to the skin, they attach to the basal membrane of the amnion, where they form immune complexes with complement activation. Decades ago, these IgG complement-fixing antibodies were known as the herpes gestationis factor. The antibodies also cross the placenta where they cause self-limited disease in infants.

There are also definite HLA associations. About 75% express HLA-DR3; 50% HLA-DR4 and 35–40% both. About 50% of fathers have HLA-DR2.

HLA-DR4 is very uncommon in blacks and this may explain the even greater rarity of herpes gestationis in this group.

Clinical Findings. Herpes gestationis is an intensely pruritic eruption that starts in the second or third trimester. The initial lesions are most often urticarial and confined to the abdomen (Fig. 15.21). Over a period of days, the eruption can generalize usually sparing the face and mucous membranes. In at least half the cases, the palms and soles are covered with deep tense painful blisters. The individual lesions are identical to those of bullous pemphigoid, except perhaps more pruritic. Large tense, often hemorrhagic blisters, small herpetiform vesicles and urticarial plaques are admixed. There is often a flare at the time of delivery and then gradual resolution, sometimes associated with menstrual flares. About 5% of infants born to mothers with herpes gestationis have blisters and are diagnosed readily as having neonatal herpes gestationis. Another 10% have erythematous macules or papules which to a trained eye suggest the disease. The skin changes in these infants resolve spontaneously within weeks.

When the disease starts in the postpartum period, it occurs within the first few days. About 25% of patients experience a flare if given oral contraceptives. The disease often recurs in subsequent pregnancies. The chance of a skipped pregnancy, i.e., a successful subsequent pregnancy with no herpes gestationis, has been estimated at about 5% although our patients have not been this unlucky. Patients with herpes gestationis are at risk for a variety of other autoimmune diseases. The most common association is with Graves disease. Although the two rarely occur at the same time, at least 10% of herpes gestationis patients develop hyperthyroidism. Hashimoto thyroiditis and pernicious anemia have also been described.

Histopathology. The blisters in herpes gestationis are somewhat more inflammatory than in even cell-rich bullous pemphigoid. Eosinophils may dominate. In addition, the complement-mediated reaction at the epidermal-dermal junction may produce basal layer necrosis. There may be intraepidermal vesicles, foci of eosinophils (eosinophilic spongiosis) and the so-called inverted teardrop sign, where the upper aspect of the dermal papillae is widened, prior to coalescing with adjacent papillae to form the blister.

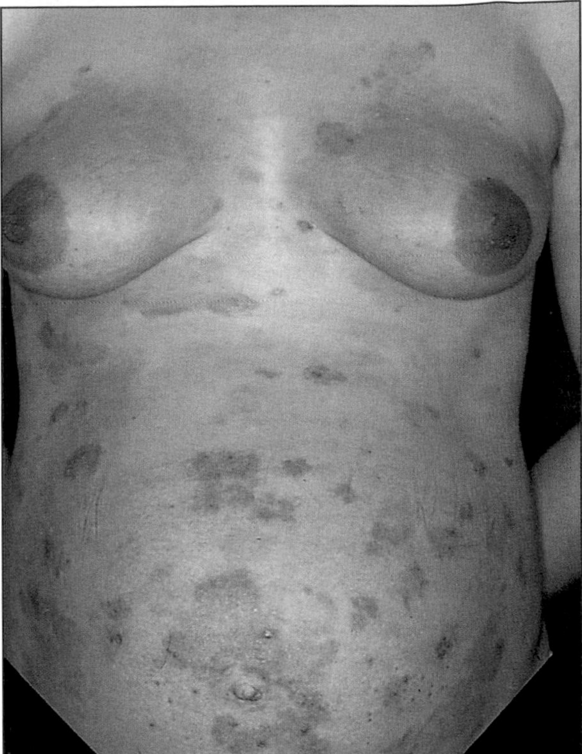

Fig. 15.21. Herpes gestationis

Immunofluorescent Examination. Direct immunofluorescence always shows C3 in the basement membrane zone. In about 50% of patients, IgG (usually IgG_1 and IgG_3) and even IgA may be found. The placental basement membrane shows similar changes. When indirect immunofluorescence is performed, IgG_1-labeled antibodies should be used; then the test is usually positive. In addition, these antibodies can be identified through their ability to fix complement. Salt-split skin can be used for mapping; then the C3 is found on the epidermal roof of the blister.

Laboratory Findings. There may be peripheral eosinophilia. Patients with herpes gestationis should have regular thyroid function tests.

Course and Prognosis. The individual eruption will clear, usually after a few menstrual flares, if pregnancy and oral contraceptives are avoided. The greatest question has been what the risk is to the mother and especially the child. In the past, one read about a high risk of spontaneous abortions and stillborn infants. This is incorrect. Several recent careful studies have shown that there is a tendency for prematurity and small for gestational age births, because of relative placental insufficiency. None of the recent studies has identified increased numbers of spontaneous abortions or stillborn infants.

Differential Diagnosis. Bullous pemphigoid, dermatitis herpetiformis and systemic lupus erythematosus may all flare in pregnancy. Urticaria, erythema multiforme, bullous Sweet syndrome and drug reactions are also important considerations. Initially one may also think of scabies because of the extreme pruritus. The urticarial lesions may be confused with pruritic urticarial papules and plaques of pregnancy but herpes gestationis soon becomes vesicular. The final answer is usually provided by immunofluorescent examination.

Therapy

Systemic. Sometimes one can avoid systemic therapy; this is usually the wish of the mother. If needed, systemic corticosteroids can be used safely in the later stages of pregnancy. They appear to be safe for the infant, as assessed by birth weights, lack of malformations and subsequent course. The dosage required is usually less than that for bullous pemphigoid: perhaps 20–40 mg prednisone daily. In addition, one can usually begin to reduce the dose once the pregnancy is over. The many steroid-sparing agents recommended anecdotally have an even less reassuring safety profile in pregnancy; we prefer to avoid them. Pyridoxine 400–900 mg daily is harmless, and some women do well with dapsone which is safe in pregnancy, as proven by its use in leprosy. Diphenhydramine also has an acceptable safety profile in pregnancy and can be used against pruritus. The patient should later be encouraged to use nonhormonal contraception.

Topical. Corticosteroid creams may alleviate the symptoms somewhat and help reduce or postpone the need for systemic agents. Topical anesthetics such as polidocanol can also be tried. Zinc oxide shake lotions are useful for drying out the lesions.

Cicatricial Pemphigoid

(Lever 1942)

Synonyms. Benign mucous membrane pemphigoid, scarring pemphigoid

Definition. Chronic blistering disease which favors mucosal surfaces, especially the conjunctiva, but also involves the skin and typically scars.

Epidemiology. Cicatricial pemphigoid is primarily a disease of the elderly and is far more common in women.

Etiology and Pathogenesis. Recent studies have shown that cicatricial pemphigoid is not one entity but several. Some patients have IgG antibodies against BPAG2, located on the epidermal side of salt-split skin. Usually the carboxy terminal domains are recognized by autoantibodies, but the NC16A domain closer to the keratinocyte membrane can also be the target. Others have the same class of antibodies but directed against laminin 5, an adhesion molecule at the interface between the lamina lucida and lamina densa, thus on the dermal side of salt-split skin. Yet other patients have antibodies directed against hemidesmosomal integrins $\alpha6$ and $\beta4$, as well as against other molecules. In some studies ocular medications, especially those used for glaucoma, have been incriminated as a cause of cicatricial pemphigoid. When the disease is limited to the eyes and associated with topical medications, the term pseudo-ocular cicatricial pemphigoid is employed. We are skeptical that there is a difference, as many patients with cicatricial pemphigoid have only ocular involvement and maybe the glaucoma is a reflection of early ocular disease. Immunologic and immunogenetic findings are similar in the two groups.

Clinical Findings. Cicatricial pemphigoid can present in a variety of ways, most often not involving the skin. Only 25% of patients have cutaneous lesions, more than 90% have oral lesions and an estimated 60–70% have ocular lesions. The skin lesions cannot be distinguished from those of bullous pemphigoid, herpes gestationis or epidermolysis bullosa acquisita except for their tendency to scar. They may evolve into hyperpigmented atrophic patches, but never scar to the degree seen on the mucosa. On the scalp, the blisters may lead to pseudopelade. On rare occasion, widespread blisters develop mimicking bullous pemphigoid.

Ocular Lesions. Cicatricial pemphigoid may exclusively affect the eyes (ocular cicatricial pemphigoid). Typical clinical features include a chronic scarring conjunctivitis with progressive subconjunctival fibrosis, fornix foreshortening and synechia formation between the bulbar and palpebral conjunctiva (Fig. 15.22). The disease may initially involve only one eye, often remaining so localized for up to 1–2 years. Conjunctival blisters are rarely

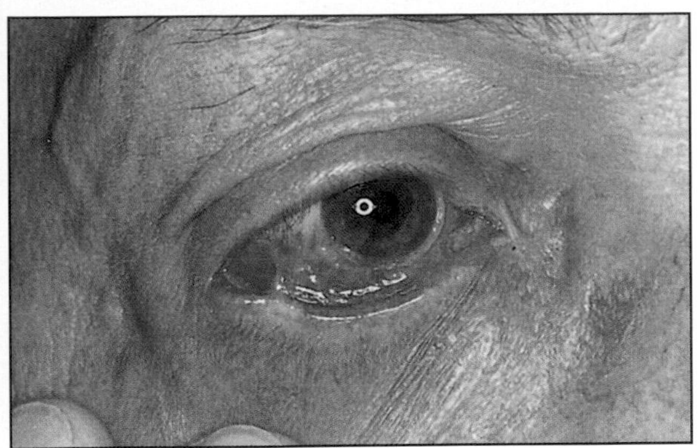

Fig. 15.22. Cicatricial pemphigoid

observed. Unfortunately, most patients are diagnosed in the later stages when scarring has occurred. Complications associated with scarring include lid entropion with trichiasis, corneal vascularization, keratitis and even blindness. Lacrimal duct and Meibomian duct obstruction as well as loss of goblet cells are all responsible for the development of a dry eye through reduction in the tear film. Glaucoma exists or develops in up to 25% of patients.

Oral Lesions. In the mouth, blisters are once again rare. Most patients present with scattered painful erosions or with desquamative gingivitis with smooth erosions along the fixed gingiva. Sometimes the mucosa can be peeled away, a useful but disturbing clinical sign comparable to the Nikolsky sign. Scars are once again a problem. The tongue may be truly tied if the frenulum is involved. If the buccal mucosa is scarred, there may be difficulty chewing and swallowing. Labial and very rarely laryngeal mucosal changes may interfere with speech. In general the oral scarring is less significant than the ocular. Both localized and vegetating lesions have also been described in the mouth.

Other Mucosal Surfaces. The larynx, esophagus and genitalia are potential sites. On other mucosal surfaces, adhesions and strictures are also a problem. Vulvar cicatricial pemphigoid is extremely difficult to separate from localized bullous pemphigoid.

Histopathology. If an intact blister is found, it shows a subepidermal separation similar to that found in a bullous pemphigoid blister. Mucosal biopsies typically show marked inflammation with a mixture of inflammatory cells. Later there is fibrosis and vascular proliferation, as expected in a scar.

Immunofluorescent Examination. Direct immunofluorescent examination is positive in 50–60% of cases, showing IgG, C3 and occasionally IgA in the basement membrane zone. The ideal site for a biopsy is the perilesional erythematous zone. Often repeated biopsies are required to obtain a positive result. Routine indirect immunofluorescence is only positive in fewer than 50% of cases. More sophisticated studies can usually show antibodies against either BPAG2 or laminin 5. Salt-split skin exposes both of these antigens better and should be used.

Course and Prognosis. Ocular cicatricial pemphigoid is a distressing chronic disease. Treatment is often difficult and blindness a feared complication, occurring in 20–60% of cases. The oral lesions are usually a great nuisance, being painful and interfering with eating and drinking. Stenosis of the larynx or pharynx can lead to life-threatening complications. Rarely squamous cell carcinoma may develop in mucosal scarring. The skin lesions are troublesome but not as significant as the ocular or oral changes.

Differential Diagnosis. The differential diagnosis varies with the site. In the skin, the other autoimmune blistering diseases should be considered. The ocular lesions must be distinguished from scarring after chemical burns or trauma. In the mouth, ulcerative lichen planus and ulcerative lupus erythematosus appear very similar. Both linear IgA dermatosis and epidermolysis bullosa acquisita may also present with desquamative gingivitis.

Therapy

Systemic. Standard treatment with systemic corticosteroids is more successful for the cutaneous lesions but usually does not help the ocular and oral lesions. Cyclophosphamide is felt to be the most effective systemic immunosuppressive agent. Azathioprine may also be used, usually in combination with corticosteroids. Dapsone may be successful for oral lesions and mild ocular disease, usually in doses of 50–150 mg daily. Both isotretinoin and acitretin may also help, even though they dry out an already dry mucosal and corneal surface. Cyclosporine (2.5–5.0 mg/kg daily) has also been reported to be helpful, but appears not to help the ocular disease much.

Topical. Corticosteroids can be used topically, usually in special adhesive pastes for the mouth. Stubborn oral erosions lend themselves well to intralesional triamcinolone acetonide. Topical cyclosporine may also help oral lesions. The ocular lesions are best left to an ophthalmologist.

Surgical. Surgery should only be attempted after systemic antiinflammatory agents have been given a chance to work. Lysis or removal of skin adhesions and correction of scars brings a great deal of relief. Surgery can also be combined with intralesional or topical corticosteroids. Localized lesions that ulcerate and do not heal, whether in the mouth or on the skin, can be excised and covered with a graft, which generally takes well in medically controlled disease. Correction of the entropion and trichiasis by the ophthalmologist may prevent further scarring and damage but the conjunctiva should not be traumatized.

Localized Cicatricial Pemphigoid

(Brunsting and Perry 1957)

Synonym. Brunsting-Perry disease

Clinically these patients are fairly distinct. They are elderly men with scarring blisters on the scalp, forehead and nape. They do not have oral or ocular lesions. Light exposure may play a role. The lesions fulfill the immunologic criteria for cicatricial pemphigoid. Both bullous pemphigoid (usually localized elsewhere) and epidermolysis bullosa acquisita may appear similar. Treatment is the same as for cicatricial pemphigoid, but occasionally one can get by with topical or intralesional corticosteroids.

Disseminated Cicatricial Pemphigoid

(Provost et al. 1979)

This very rare disorder is defined almost entirely by immunofluorescent testing. The patients have no oral or ocular lesions, but develop widespread pruritic erythematous blisters that are often hemorrhagic. The trunk and extremities are involved. The lesions are often misdiagnosed as artifacts. They crust readily and heal with atrophic white scars. New blisters may form on the scars, creating a distinctive clinical picture. Except for the scarring, they cannot be separated clinically from bullous pemphigoid. Histologically there is a subepidermal blister identical to blisters of bullous pemphigoid, but in later lesions there may be fibrosis and new blood vessels, as evidence of the scarring. Some cases represent epidermolysis bullosa acquisita, but others show antibodies against one of the many cicatricial pemphigoid antigens. Serologic search for antibodies is usually not successful. Treatment is as discussed under cicatricial pemphigoid. Because only the skin is involved, the response is often somewhat better.

Linear IgA Dermatosis

(Chorzelski and Jablonska 1979)

Synonyms. IgA pemphigoid, polymorphic pemphigoid

Definition. Linear IgA disease is not a single clinical disease; it is an immunopathologic finding – the presence of a linear band of IgA at the epidermal-dermal junction.

Etiology and Pathogenesis. Many target antigens have been described for linear IgA disease. The main antigen appears to be BPAG2 and more often proteolytic fragments of this, especially the 120-kDa fragment. Integrin $\alpha6\beta4$, laminin and type VII collagen are also targets, as well as BPAG1. Reactions may occur on a mucosal surface, since this is where IgA production predominates. There may be overlaps with bullous pemphigoid. Similar clinical features are seen especially in children and cases have been described with both IgA and IgG antibodies. The latter are usually directed against BPAG1. Vancomycin and several cytokines have been reported as possible causative agents.

Clinical Findings. Two main groups comprise the rainbow spectrum of linear IgA dermatosis. About 10% of patients with clinically typical dermatitis herpetiformis have a linear deposition of IgA rather than the typical granular pattern. They also lack the HLA pattern and gluten-sensitive enteropathy of dermatitis herpetiformis. They are also more likely to have oral erosions, which are not seen in classic dermatitis herpetiformis. The second main group are patients with chronic bullous disease of childhood, who typically have large blisters with a rosette pattern. Still other patients have large blisters on an urticarial base, as in bullous pemphigoid. Finally, the smallest group have mucous membrane erosions as in cicatricial pemphigoid.

Histopathology. The microscopic picture matches whatever clinical disease is mimicked.

Immunofluorescent Examination. Direct immunofluorescent examination shows a linear band of IgA, usually IgA_1, rarely IgA_2 or IgA dimers, deposited at the basement membrane zone. When other immunoglobulins, especially IgG are present, it is more logical to diagnose bullous pemphigoid. In about 60 % of patients, the indirect immunofluorescent examination is also positive. The best substrates are salt-split human skin and monkey esophagus. The IgA antibodies react with a wide spectrum of antigens. IgA directed against reticulin, endomysium and gliadin are not seen; they are only found in classic dermatitis herpetiformis.

Immunoelectron microscopy reveals IgA deposited at several levels. One site is the upper lamina lucida, just as in bullous pemphigoid, where the candidate antigens are 97-kDa and 120-kDa molecules which seem to be proteolytic fragments of BPAG2. Other possible targets include laminin and various integrins. In yet other cases, the split occurs in the sublamina densa region where type VII collagen may be the target.

Differential Diagnosis. The differential diagnosis includes the entire spectrum of subepidermal blistering disorders. The relationship to chronic bullous disease of childhood is most confusing, as suggested below.

Therapy. In general, patients whose condition resembles bullous pemphigoid respond better to corticosteroids, while those with a dermatitis herpetiformis-like clinical picture tend to be sulfone- or sulfapyridine-responsive, although not as exquisitely so as dermatitis herpetiformis.

Epidermolysis Bullosa Acquisita

(Roenigk et al. 1971)

Definition. Epidermolysis bullosa acquisita is a chronic scarring bullous disease with antibodies against type VII collagen in the basement membrane zone.

Epidemiology. Epidermolysis bullosa acquisita is a very uncommon disease which typically presents in adult life and is slightly more common in women. Childhood cases, even in infants, have been reported. It may be more prevalent in blacks.

Etiology and Pathogenesis. The unifying feature in epidermolysis bullosa acquisita is the presence of antibodies against type VII collagen. When proteins from the human basement membrane are immunoblotted with epidermolysis bullosa acquisita serum, both 320-kDa and 145-kDa molecules are found. The larger molecule is intact type VII collagen while the two smaller ones are its components: a rod-like 145-kDa collagenous domain which extends into the sublamina densa as a component of the anchoring fibrils, and a globular 145-kDa noncollagenous domain which attaches to the lamina densa. Most of the antibodies attack the globular region.

There is an increased frequency of HLA-DR2 in epidermolysis bullosa acquisita patients. In addition, epidermolysis bullosa acquisita has been associated with a long list of other diseases, including diabetes mellitus, Crohn disease, systemic lupus erythematosus and many others. As better criteria have been defined for the diagnosis, the apparent disease associations have become less common.

Clinical Findings. Epidermolysis bullosa acquisita can present in a variety of ways. Patients may shift from one form to the other. In general early in the disease course, lesions tend to be more inflammatory, while later on the skin fragility and scarring dominate.

Noninflammatory Type. About 50 % of patients present with the clinical picture of porphyria cutanea tarda but with negative serum and urine porphyrin levels. Most often the sun-exposed areas are involved with fragile skin which forms blisters and heals with milia (Fig. 15.23). In contrast to porphyria cutanea tarda, blisters may also be found on non-sun-exposed skin, a good clinical clue. This

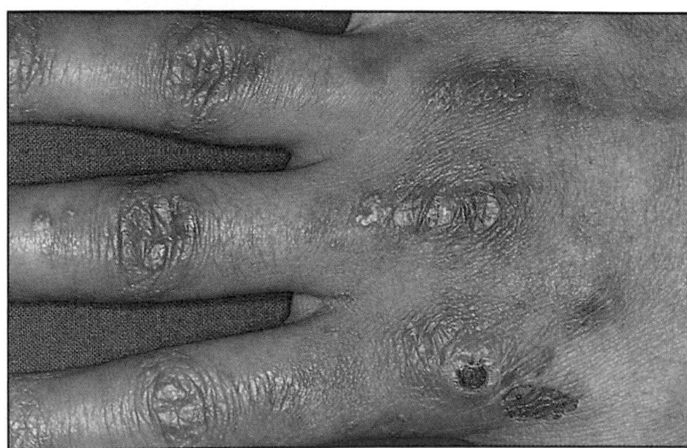

Fig. 15.23. Epidermolysis bullosa acquisita

variant may also present with blisters on pressure points, such as the knees and elbows, alopecia or mutilating nail dystrophies.

Inflammatory Type. Some patients have urticarial lesions, large tense blisters and pruritus. Their lesions tend to heal with less scarring. Typical sites are the trunk and flexural aspects of the extremities. About 5% of patients with classic bullous pemphigoid, proven with routine immunofluorescent studies, actually have antibodies against type VII collagen. One should suspect epidermolysis bullosa acquisita in bullous pemphigoid patients who are therapy-resistant and in whom the diagnosis has been made without using salt-split skin or antigen mapping.

Mucosal Type. The third major group resemble cicatricial pemphigoid with scarring erosions primarily in the mouth, but also involving other mucosal surfaces.

Histopathology. When an intact blister is obtained, it is clearly subepidermal. The degree of inflammation reflects the clinical situation so that one can see intensely inflamed lesions rich in neutrophils or even eosinophils or almost naked blisters. Recurrent lesions may show dermal fibrosis, but the thickening of the basement membranes seen in porphyria cutanea tarda is not present.

Immunofluorescent Examination. Direct immunofluorescent examination shows C3, IgG and occasionally IgA and IgM at the basement membrane zone in perilesional skin. C3 and other complement components are never seen alone; if this is the case the diagnosis is bullous pemphigoid. Routine indirect immunofluorescent examination is positive in fewer than 50% of patients and gives a similar pattern. Immunoelectron microscopy shows the deposits both in the lamina densa and the anchoring fibrils. In more chronic lesions, the deposits tend to be more dermal.

While clues can be obtained from the direct immunofluorescent examination, more detailed studies must be done to confirm the diagnosis. Salt-split skin is the most efficient way to diagnose epidermolysis bullosa acquisita. If the patient has circulating antibodies, salt-split normal skin can be used. Epidermolysis bullosa acquisita serum marks the floor of the blister which is at the level of the lamina lucida, while bullous pemphigoid antibodies mark the epidermal roof. If the patient has no circulating antibodies, then a biopsy of perilesional skin can be salt-split and direct immunofluorescent examination performed with similar results. Almost all dermal labeling with salt-split skin represents either epidermolysis bullosa acquisita or bullous systemic lupus erythematosus.

Course and Prognosis. Epidermolysis bullosa acquisita is a very chronic disease. It can be very difficult to treat and seldom remits.

Differential Diagnosis. The clinical differential diagnosis depends on the clinical subtype of the disease. The inflammatory lesions resemble bullous pemphigoid, linear IgA dermatosis, cicatricial pemphigoid and even pemphigus vulgaris. The mucosal lesions are identical to those of cicatricial pemphigoid. Finally, the scarring lesions suggest hereditary epidermolysis bullosa, but this can be excluded by history. There may also be superficial similarities to porphyria cutanea tarda and bullous amyloidosis.

Further confusing the issue is the fact that several other disorders involve type VII collagen. The dystrophic forms of epidermolysis bullosa have mutations in the collagen molecule. In porphyria cutanea tarda and the bullous eruption of lupus erythematosus the separation is also in the sub-lamina densa zone, but each disease has other specific markers (urine porphyrins and antinuclear antibodies, respectively).

Therapy. The treatment of epidermolysis bullosa acquisita is difficult. Many patients are first identified as having epidermolysis bullosa acquisita when their bullous pemphigoid proves therapy-resistant. If the disease is inflammatory, it still makes sense to try prednisone at doses of 1.0 mg/kg daily. If this is ineffective, cyclosporine has been touted as the most effective alternative agent, although we have had little success with it. The usual starting dose is 5 mg/kg daily until blistering is controlled followed by a somewhat reduced dose. Dapsone may also be helpful, especially in the mucosal variants. Recently IVIG has given promising results in some patients. Colchicine 500 mg twice to three times daily, vitamin E 600–1200 mg daily and plasmapheresis have also been successful on occasion.

Dermatitis Herpetiformis

(Duhring 1884)

Synonyms. Duhring disease, Duhring-Brocq disease, dermatite polymorphe douloureuse

Definition. Dermatitis herpetiformis is a chronic intensely pruritic clinically polymorphic dermatitis with characteristic granular IgA deposition in the dermal papillae.

Epidemiology. Dermatitis herpetiformis is relatively common in comparison to the other rare diseases discussed in this chapter. It has a prevalence of 1:5,000–10,000 in Northern European populations and is even more uncommon in blacks. The onset of the disease is usually in adolescence or young adulthood. The male to female ratio is 3:2.

Etiology and Pathogenesis. Dermatitis herpetiformis shows a very strong HLA predisposition. The classic pattern is HLA-A1 (75%), -B8 (88%), -DR3 (DRB1*0301) (95%) and -DQA1*0501/DQB1*0201 (>95%). The relative risk ratio for dermatitis herpetiformis is 15–20:1. The same HLA profile predisposes to celiac disease and many patients with dermatitis herpetiformis have gluten-sensitive enteropathy. Although perhaps only 10% have gastrointestinal symptoms, if one investigates further, about 25% show evidence of malabsorption and 60–70% show villous atrophy and lymphocytic infiltrates when a small-bowel biopsy is taken. In addition, patients may note worsening of their disease when eating a gluten-rich diet and many benefit from a gluten-free diet, just as in celiac disease.

The bulk of the antibodies in dermatitis herpetiformis are IgA in type. They are directed against a number of target antigens. One target antigen is tissue transglutaminase. There are also autoantibodies against gliadin and reticulin. The latter cross-react with the smooth muscle endomysium and jejunal submucosal connective tissue. Transglutaminase appears to be a major autoantigen of endomysium. Circulating immune complexes of IgA and perhaps dietary elements might settle in the sublamina densa region where they could trigger an inflammatory response leading to blisters.

Many other autoimmune diseases are also associated with dermatitis herpetiformis. About 40% of patients have thyroid antimicrosomal antibodies and a wide range of thyroid disease are seen, including both hyper- and hypothyroidism as well as thyroid malignancies. Over half have gastric parietal cell antibodies, and both gastric atrophy and hypochlorhydria are common. An increased prevalence of *Helicobacter pylori* infection has also been found. Other associations with Sjögren syndrome, systemic lupus erythematosus, rheumatoid arthritis, dermatomyositis and myasthenia gravis are blamed on the HLA predilection. Finally, patients with dermatitis herpetiformis have a significant lifetime risk of gastrointestinal lymphoma, perhaps from the persistent immunostimulation in the gut.

Another oddity in dermatitis herpetiformis is the exquisite sensitivity to halogen salts, especially potassium iodide. Dietary excesses in iodine, such as shellfish, can trigger a flare of disease, as can ingestion of supersaturated potassium iodide or even use of topical iodine products. Some expectorants contain iodides. Even iodinated salt may cause problems in some patients, so it is best avoided.

Clinical Findings. While the clinical manifestations of dermatitis herpetiformis can be highly variable, as the French name suggests, the unifying problem is intense itching or even pain. The disease may start slowly or explode over a short time. Typically pruritic erythematous macules and papules develop over the knees, elbows, shoulder girdle, scalp and buttocks. The Cottini variant (Cottini 1955) is limited to the knees and elbows, probably the most classic sites.

The lesions are quite polymorphous; some may be urticarial, others vesicular. When small grouped (herpetiform) blisters on an erythematous base are present in a classic site in a young adult, the diagnosis is easy (Fig. 15.24). Unfortunately, sometimes the tiny vesicles are hard to see and can be best

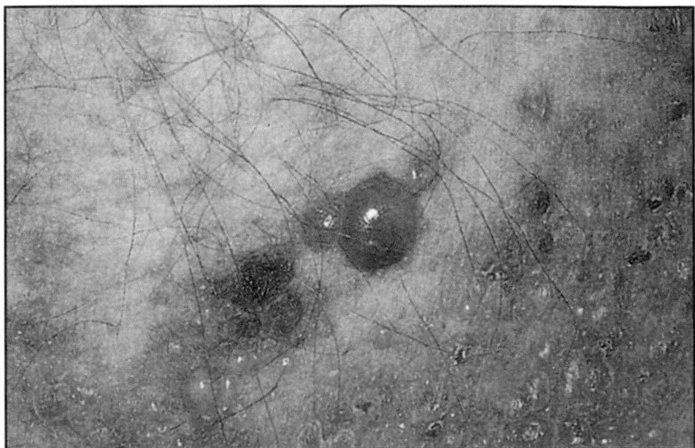

Fig. 15.24. Dermatitis herpetiformis with grouped blisters

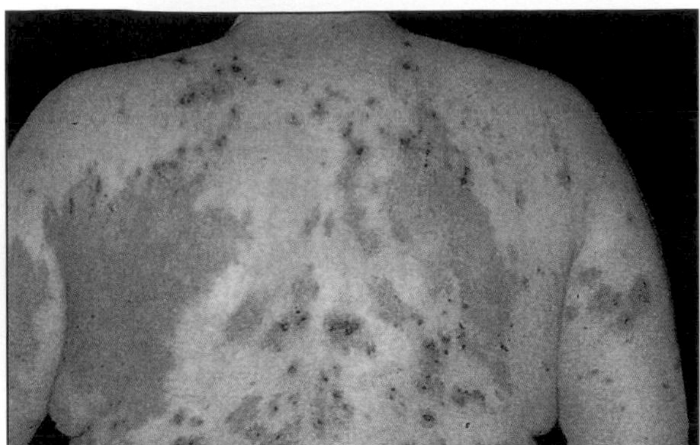

Fig. 15.25. Dermatitis herpetiformis

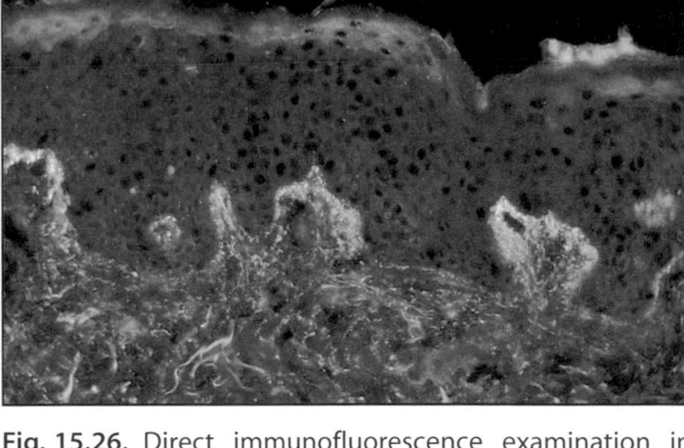

Fig. 15.26. Direct immunofluorescence examination in dermatitis herpetiformis

palpated. Even though they are relatively resistant to trauma, the vesicles are scratched intensely so that often one only sees excoriations (Fig. 15.25). A good trick is to ask a patient to cover a new lesion with a dressing rather than scratching it and to come to the office the next day. Such a lesion both clinically and histologically may pave the way to the correct diagnosis.

Occasionally large blisters form. This phenomenon is most common in children, in elderly patients, when therapy is suddenly stopped and when linear IgA dermatosis is present. Secondary hyperpigmentation is very common. Some patients present with prurigo nodularis-like lesions or secondarily infected excoriations. Yet others have circinate bizarre patterned vesicles and pustules at the periphery of an erythematous often crusted patch. Oral mucosal involvement is extremely rare.

Despite the role of gastrointestinal findings in the disease's pathophysiology and even treatment, few dermatitis herpetiformis patients present with intestinal complaints. Most are surprised when the physician recommends an investigation of that area.

Histopathology. The classic feature in dermatitis herpetiformis is the presence of subepidermal blisters which have papillary microabscesses at their periphery. The fusion and expansion of these papillary accumulations leads to blisters. The predominant inflammatory cell is the neutrophil, although occasionally eosinophils will be observed. While the microabscesses suggest dermatitis herpetiformis, they can be seen in other subepidermal blistering diseases. Electron microscopy has shown that the action appears to start in the upper dermis with edema, inflammation and damage to fine collagen fibers. The level of separation is often within or just below the lamina lucida, perhaps because it is the weakest link.

Immunofluorescent Examination. About 90% of dermatitis herpetiformis patients have granular deposits of IgA in the dermal papillae on direct immunofluorescent examination (Fig. 15.26). The antibodies are usually IgA_1. These deposits are present throughout the skin, although they are more common and intense in predilection sites. The biopsy should be taken from perilesional skin or from the buttock if no active lesions are present. The antibody deposits tend to be fairly permanent, even after successful treatment, but can wane with long-term gluten-free diets or over time. Indirect immunofluorescent examination is not positive for the skin antibodies.

Antibodies to tissue transglutaminase, reticulin and smooth muscle endomysium can be identified and their titers measured. They are positive in the 70–80% of patients who have some evidence of gastrointestinal disease. Probably all three systems measure the same antibodies, just using different substrates. The antigliadin antibodies are different, showing no cross-reactions.

The other 10% of clinically typical dermatitis herpetiformis patients have linear deposition of IgA.

Course and Prognosis. The course of dermatitis herpetiformis is chronic. The patients are at risk for intestinal lymphoma and a variety of autoimmune diseases, so they should be monitored. This is easy to overlook when a person has been receiving dapsone for 30 years and simply calls for refills. Typically the disease waxes and wanes, and most patients adjust their diet and therapy to their disease state.

Differential Diagnosis. The patients with linear IgA disease cannot be sorted out clinically, although they are more likely to have large blisters, lack the specific HLA associations, do not have gluten-sensitive enteropathy, intestinal lymphoma or autoimmune disease and do not have autoantibodies against transglutaminase, smooth muscle endomysium or reticulin.

The other differential diagnostic possibilities in dermatitis herpetiformis are numerous. When blisters are present, the possibilities are those discussed in this chapter. Occasionally an acute eruptive case or a flare will resemble erythema multiforme. More nodular lesions may suggest Sweet syndrome, while the circinate lesions closely resemble those of subcorneal pustular dermatosis.

More often the intense burning or pruritus drives the differential diagnostic considerations, so that patients with scabies, excoriations, papular urticaria and even Grover disease, and the elderly with pruritus, are biopsied to exclude dermatitis herpetiformis. Dermatitis herpetiformis simply does not start in the elderly, although it can be misdiagnosed or overlooked and thus first diagnosed in an older individual. When crusted excoriated papules and nodules are present, one must consider the many types of prurigo, as well as atopic dermatitis.

Therapy. The therapy of dermatitis herpetiformis is so specific that one can actually speak of a diagnostic trial of therapy. The pruritus responds almost overnight to dapsone. Because dapsone is so effective, both patients and physicians tend to get sloppy in using it. The effective dosage is highly variable and the patient should be encouraged to find the lowest dose for symptom control. While the average range is 50–150 mg daily, many get by on 50 mg every other day.

Dapsone requires hematologic monitoring during the induction phase. A deficiency in glucose-6-phosphate dehydrogenase (G6PD) should be excluded prior to institution of therapy. Baseline hepatic and renal function tests should also be performed. Then the expected methemoglobinemia and hemolysis must be monitored until the changes are stable. In addition, a wide variety of idiosyncratic reactions can be seen including peripheral neuropathies, usually motor, leukopenia and agranulocytosis (independent of the expected hematologic effects), hepatitis, cholestatic jaundice and renal damage. The mechanism of action of dapsone is unknown. It clearly is a drug with many functions, as manifested by its use in leprosy, *Pneumocystis carinii* infections and toxoplasmosis. In dermatitis herpetiformis dapsone produces dramatic improvement in the skin without affecting the gut changes at all.

When dapsone is not tolerated, sulfapyridine is the usual alternative. The dosage required is 500–2000 mg daily. Sulfapyridine causes similar hematologic problems, although less often, as well as renal stones when used in higher dosages, and has a significant risk of cutaneous reactions. Only those few patients who cannot tolerate dapsone and who can be controlled on lower doses are good candidates for sulfapyridine. In the USA it has become an orphan drug and is difficult to obtain; it is not available in Germany.

A gluten-free diet is clearly beneficial, if the patient can be motivated to stick to it. We refer our patients to a dietitian experienced in treating celiac disease for counseling. Oats seem to be better tolerated than wheat, rye or barley. The gluten-free diet does many things. It reduces the need for dapsone and helps the skin problems, but it also improves the more serious gastrointestinal changes and may reduce the risk of small-bowel lymphoma. This advantage has not been shown in dermatitis herpetiformis but in isolated gluten-sensitive enteropathy.

Topical. Both topical corticosteroids and antipruritic agents can be used, but usually dapsone is so effective that the patient has little desire to spend time on such measures.

Lichen Planus Pemphigoides

(Schreiner 1930)

Lichen planus is discussed in detail in Chapter 14. Lichen planus pemphigoides is characterized by blisters arising in patients with lichen planus, both in lesional skin and on normal skin. Bullous lichen planus or lichen planus vesiculosus refers to bullae arising only in lesions of lichen planus as a result of weakening of the epidermal-dermal junction through the intense inflammatory infiltrate.

In contrast, in lichen planus pemphigoides, blisters can arise independently of infiltrate, and immunofluorescent examination reveals distinct subepidermal deposits of immunoglobulin and complement. There are conflicting studies as to the nature of the target antigen. In the most recent studies, the NC16A domain of BPAG2 appears to be the most common target. There is an epitope in this domain with which serum from most lichen planus pemphigoides patients reacts and with which serum from bullous pemphigoid patients does not react. Other patients in the past who were studied with cruder methods had antibodies against structures in the lamina densa or upper dermis. Most patients require systemic corticosteroids, but many respond very rapidly and may not need long-term therapy.

Bullous Diseases in Childhood

All of the blistering diseases discussed in this chapter can occur in childhood, although they are quite rare and may be clinically different. Even herpes gestationis can produce a transient erythematous vesicular eruption in the newborn. Not only are the diseases rare but the terminology is confusing. Nonetheless, today exactly the same diagnostic criteria are applied as in adults and we will simply summarize briefly some of the unique features.

Chronic Bullous Disease of Childhood

(Bean et al. 1970)

Synonym. Linear IgA dermatosis

Etiology and Pathogenesis. Bean and others initially defined chronic bullous disease of childhood on clinical grounds, describing infants with multiple grouped blisters, often arranged around an initial lesion in a rosette fashion. Later it became obvious that many subepidermal blistering disorders, especially in childhood, could have rosettes. While the vast bulk of such patients have linear IgA dermatosis, some have IgG antibodies and thus childhood bullous pemphigoid.

Clinical Findings. The onset is usually between 2 and 5 years of age. Typically there are large, often pruritic blisters arranged in a rosette fashion (Fig. 15.27). The usual sites are the perioral region, genitalia and upper inner thighs. The blisters are often misdiagnosed as bullous impetigo, but fortunately almost as often respond to antibiotics, just as bullous pemphigoid occasionally does. Oral lesions are common, present in 60–70% of patients.

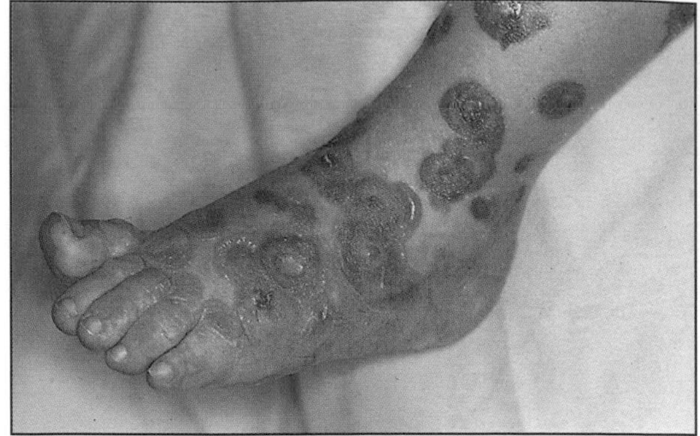

Fig. 15.27. Linear IgA disease in a child with clinical rosette pattern

Histopathology. A subepidermal blister is seen, just as in the adult forms.

Immunofluorescent Examination. About 50–70% of patients have linear deposition of IgA which tends to be in the lamina lucida. Antigen mapping shows type IV collagen on the blister base. Others have a picture identical to bullous pemphigoid.

Course and Prognosis. The disease is chronic from the perspective of a parent and child but tends to resolve after a few years or at puberty.

Therapy. Linear IgA in childhood is corticosteroid-responsive. Both dapsone (2 mg/kg daily) and sulfapyridine (100 mg/kg daily) may also be effective. Both may induce remissions, usually with 6–12 months of therapy. Patients may still develop occasional blisters, but relapses are uncommon.

Dermatitis Herpetiformis

When young children develop dermatitis herpetiformis, they are often homozygous for HLA-A1, -B8, -DR3(DRB1*0301), -DQA1*0501/DQB1*0201, meaning that both their parents have one such haplotype. Otherwise, the disease is identical to the adult form. Adolescents often develop dermatitis herpetiformis, so after puberty it should not be considered unusual. In some younger patients, the disease resolves, but it is likely to recur in adolescence. While dermatitis herpetiformis does not usually have large blisters, it too can present with rosettes. Involvement of the palms and soles may also occur, perhaps because this skin is softer and thinner in children. Triggering by iodine seems more common than in adults, so that any child with a blistering eruption should be investigated for exposure to iodine. In addition, adenovirus 12 has been suggested as a possible etiologic factor in children.

Differential Diagnosis. Scabies can be bullous in children, especially young infants, so the differential diagnosis is harder. In addition, bullous arthropod bite reactions can be seen, often on the legs with large blisters even with rosettes.

Bullous Pemphigoid

(BEAN et al. 1970)

Clinical Findings. Two clinical subtypes of juvenile bullous pemphigoid are seen. One is the central type, with either facial or genital involvement. While boys are more often affected, in young girls, bullous pemphigoid may be limited to the vulva. The second form is acral involving the hands and feet. In the latter form, rosettes are somewhat more common. Otherwise the lesions are typical for bullous pemphigoid with urticarial lesions and tense blisters. Oral involvement is rare. The distinctions between chronic bullous disease of childhood and juvenile bullous pemphigoid are a matter of definition and by no means agreed upon.

Therapy. Systemic corticosteroids are the treatment of choice. Often therapy for several months suffices, in sharp contrast to the adult disease. Dapsone, sulfapyridine, antibiotics and nicotinamide may also be effective.

Cicatricial Pemphigoid

Except for a rare patient with linear IgA dermatosis confined to the mouth, scarring mucosal disease seems not to occur in children.

Epidermolysis Bullosa Acquisita

Epidermolysis bullosa acquisita can occur in childhood or infancy, even rarely being confused with epidermolysis bullosa. In children, it usually resembles chronic bullous disease of childhood but often has severe mucosal involvement. It can only be defined with immunologic studies. The disorder in some patients appears to remit spontaneously and in others is usually responsive to prednisone and dapsone.

Pemphigus Vulgaris

Childhood pemphigus vulgaris appears most likely to present with oral involvement. Over 90% of children have mucosal involvement, so that aphthae or other forms of stomatitis are often diagnosed. The cutaneous lesions favor the seborrheic areas, so clinical separation from pemphigus foliaceus is difficult. The treatment is identical to that in adults. Once again, remissions occasionally occur. Neonatal pemphigus vulgaris may be seen in infants born to mothers with active pemphigusvulgaris; it is usually mild and always self-limited.

Pemphigus Foliaceus

Pemphigus foliaceus appears more common than pemphigus vulgaris in childhood. The erythematous crusting lesions favor the seborrheic areas and the disorder is often misdiagnosed as seborrheic dermatitis or impetigo. Systemic corticosteroids are usually quite effective. Sometimes one can get by with a potent topical corticosteroid, especially in patients with a limited number of lesions. While therapy for several years may be required, the disease remits eventually in most patients remit .

Brazilian Pemphigus

Brazilian pemphigus is likely to be the most common blistering disease of childhood, as it is estimated that 15–20% of patients are children. The disease tends to be more disabling in childhood, especially in those areas where treatment and monitoring are not readily available. The skin may be excoriated and secondarily infected. Children are described with bone and muscle wasting, as they become inactive because of the intense burning and pain from their disease.

Bibliography

Basic Science Aspects

Aumailley M, Krieg T (1996) Laminins: a family of diverse multifunctional molecules of basement membranes. J Invest Dermatol 106:209–214

Christiano AM, Uitto J (1996) Molecular complexity of the cutaneous basement membrane zone. Exp Dermatol 5: 1–11

McGrath JA (1999) Hereditary diseases of the desmosomes. J Dermatol Sci 20:85–91

McGrath JA, McMillan JR, Shemanko CS et al. (1997) Mutations in the plakophilin 1 gene result in ectodermal dysplasia/skin fragility syndrome. Nat Genet 17:240–244

Shimizu H (1998) New insights into the immunoultrastructural organization of cutaneous basement membrane zone molecules. Exp Dermatol 7:303–313

Uitto J (1997) Clinical implications of basic research on heritable skin diseases. J Dermatol 24:690–700

Epidermolysis Bullosa

Anton-Lamprecht I, Schnyder UW (1984) Prenatal diagnosis of epidermolysis bullosa hereditaria: a review. Semin Dermatol 3:229–240

Bart BJ, Gorlin RJ, Anderson VE et al. (1966) Congenital localized absence of skin and associated abnormalities resembling epidermolysis bullosa. A new syndrome. Arch Derm 93:296–304

Bruckner-Tuderman L, Mitsuhashi Y, Schnyder UW et al. (1989) Anchoring fibrils and type VII collagen are absent from skin in severe recessive dystrophic epidermolysis bullosa. J Invest Dermatol 93:3–9

Cockayne EA (1947) Recurrent bullous eruption of the feet. Br J Dermatol 59:109–112

Cohen BA, Esterly NB, Nelson PF (1985) Congenital erosive and vesicular dermatosis healing with reticulated supple scarring. Arch Dermatol 121:361–367

Christiano AM, Bart BJ, Epstein EH Jr et al. (1996) Genetic basis of Bart's syndrome: a glycine substitution mutation in type VII collagen gene. J Invest Dermatol 106:1340–1342

Christiano AM, Fine J-D, Uitto J (1997) Genetic basis of dominantly inherited transient bullous dermolysis of the newborn: a splice site mutation in the type VII collagen gene. J Invest Dermatol 109:811–814

Dowling GB, Meara RH (1954) Epidermolysis bullosa resembling juvenile dermatitis herpetiformis. Br J Dermatol 66:139–143

El Shafie M, Stidham GL, Klippel CH et al. (1979) Pyloric atresia and epidermolysis bullosa letalis: a lethal combination in two premature newborn siblings. J Pediatr Surg 14:446–449

Fine J-D, Johnson L, Wright T (1989) Epidermolysis bullosa simplex superficialis. A new variant of epidermolysis bullosa characterized by subcorneal skin cleavage mimicking peeling skin syndrome. Arch Dermatol 125: 633–638

Fine J-D, Bauer EA, Briggaman RA et al. (1991) Revised clinical and laboratory criteria for subtypes of inherited epidermolysis bullosa. J Am Acad Dermatol 24:119–135

Fischer T, Gedde-Dahl T (1979) Epidermolysis bullosa simplex and mottled skin pigmentation. Clin Genet 15: 228–238

Gedde-Dahl T (1971) Epidermolysis bullosa: a clinical genetic and epidemiological study. John Hopkins Press, Baltimore, pp 1–180

Haber RM, Wedad H, Ramsay CA et al. (1985) Cicatricial junctional epidermolysis bullosa. J Am Acad Dermatol 12:836–844

Hashimoto K, Schnyder UW, Anton-Lamprecht I (1976) Epidermolysis bullosa hereditaria with junctional blistering in an adult. Dermatologica 152:72–86

Hashimoto K, Matsumoto M, Iacobelli D (1985) Transient bullous dermolysis of the newborn. Arch Dermatol 121: 1429–1438

Hintner H, Wolff K (1982) Generalised atrophic benign epidermolysis bullosa. Arch Dermatol 118:375–384

Hovnanian A, Christiano AM, Uitto J (1993) The molecular genetics of dystrophic epidermolysis bullosa. Arch Dermatol 129:1566–1570

Ishida-Yamamoto A, McGrath JA, Chapman SJ et al. (1991) Epidermolysis bullosa simplex (Dowling-Meara type) is a genetic disease characterized by an abnormal keratin-filament network involving keratins K5 and K14. J Invest Dermatol 97:959–968

Jonkman MF, Jong MCJM de, Heeres K et al. (1996) Generalized atrophic benign epidermolysis bullosa. Arch Dermatol 132:145–150

Kon A, Nomura K, Pulkkinen L et al. (1997) Novel glycine substitution mutations in COL7A1 reveal that the Pasini and Cockayne-Touraine variants of dominant dystrophic epidermolysis bullosa are allelic. J Invest Dermatol 109:684–687

Lin AN, Carter DM (1992) Epidermolysis bullosa: basic and clinical aspects. Springer, Berlin

Nielsen PG, Sjuland E (1985) Epidermolysis bullosa simplex localisata associated with anodontia, hair and nail disorders. Acta Derm Venereol (Stockh) 65:526–530

Olaisen B, Gedde-Dahl T (1973) GPT-epidermolysis bullosa simplex (EBS Ogna) linkage in man. Hum Hered 23: 189–196

Pasini A (1928) Dystrophie cutanée bulleuse atrophiante et al. bo-papuloide. Ann Dermatol Syph (Paris) 9:1044–1066

Reed WB, College J, Francis MJO et al. (1974) Epidermolysis bullosa dystrophica with epidermal neoplasms. Arch Dermatol 110:894–902

Ridley CM (1977) Epidermolysis bullosa with unusual features: inversa type. Pro R Soc Med 70:576–577

Ruiz-Maldonado R, Duran-McKinster C, Carrasco-Daza D et al. (1998) Intrauterine epidermal necrosis: report of three cases. J Am Acad Dermatol 38:712–715

Salih MA, Lake BD, el Hag MA et al. (1985) Lethal epidermolytic epidermolysis bullosa: a new autosomal recessive type of epidermolysis bullosa. Br J Dermatol 113:135–143

Shaw DW, Fine J-D, Piacquadio DJ et al. (1997) Gastric outlet obstruction and epidermolysis bullosa. J Am Acad Dermatol 36:304–310

Vailly J, Gagnoux-Palacios L, Dell'Ambra E et al. (1998) Corrective gene transfer of keratinocytes from patients with junctional epidermolysis bullosa restores assembly of hemidesmosomes in reconstructed epithelia. Gene Ther 5: 1322–1332

Wakasugi S, Mizutari K, Ono T (1998) Clinical phenotype of Bart's syndrome seen in a family with dominant dystrophic epidermolysis bullosa. J Dermatol 25: 517–522

Pemphigus Vulgaris and Pemphigus Variants

Aberer W, Wolff-Schreiner EC, Stingl G et al. (1987) Azathioprine in the treatment of pemphigus vulgaris. A long-term follow-up. J Am Acad Dermatol 16:527–533

Ahmed RA, Blose DA (1984) Pemphigus vegetans. Neumann type and Hallopeau type. Int J Dermatol 23:135–141

Amagai M (1996) Pemphigus: autoimmunity to epidermal cell adhesion molecules. Adv Dermatol 11:319–352

Amagai M, Klaus-Kovtun V, Stanley JR (1991) Autoantibodies against a novel epithelial cadherin in pemphigus vulgaris, a disease of cell adhesion. Cell 67:869–877

Anhalt GJ, Kim SC, Stanley JR et al. (1990) Paraneoplastic pemphigus. An autoimmune mucocutaneous disease associated with neoplasia. N Engl J Med 323: 1729–1735

Asboe-Hansen G (1970) Diagnosis of pemphigus. Br J Dermatol 83: 81–92

Basset N, Guilot B, Michel B et al. (1987) Dapsone as initial treatment in superficial pemphigus. Report of nine cases. Arch Dermatol 123:783–785

Braun-Falco O, Abeck D, Meurer M (1991) Isolierter Pemphigus vulgaris der Mundschleimhaut – Pemphigustest: Diagnosesicherung mittels direkter Immunfluoreszenzuntersuchung an unbefallener Körperhaut. Hautarzt 42:623–626

Brown MV (1954) Fogo selvagem (pemphigus foliaceus). Review of the Brazilian literature. Arch Dermatol 69: 589–599

Bystryn JC, Steinman NM (1996) The adjuvant therapy of pemphigus. An update. Arch Dermatol 132:203–212

Bystryn JC, Abel E, DeFeo C (1974) Pemphigus foliaceus. Subcorneal intercellular antibodies of unique specificity. Arch Dermatol 110:857–861

Diaz LA, Sampaio SAP, Rivitti EA et al. (1989) Endemic pemphigus foliaceus (Fogo Selvagem): II. Current and historic epidemiologic studies. J Invest Dermatol 92:4–12

Fine J-D (1995) Management of acquired bullous skin diseases. N Engl J Med 333:1475–1484

Grundmann-Kollmann M, Korting HC, Behrens S et al. (1999) Mycophenolate mofetil: a new therapeutic option in the treatment of blistering autoimmune diseases. J Am Acad Dermatol 40:957–960

Harman KE, Black MM (1999) High-dose intravenous immune globulin for the treatment of autoimmune blistering diseases: an evaluation of its use in 14 cases. Br J Dermatol 140:865–874

Hashimoto T, Kiyokawa C, Mori O et al. (1997) Human desmocollin (Dsc1) is an autoantigen for the subcorneal pustular dermatosis type of IgA pemphigus. J Invest Dermatol 109:127–131

Hodak E, David M, Ingber A et al. (1990) The clinical and histopathological spectrum of IgA-pemphigus – report of two cases. Clin Exp Dermatol 15:433–437

Huff JC, Golitz LE, Kunke KS (1985) Intraepidermal neutrophilic IgA dermatosis. N Engl J Med 313:1643–1645

Ishii K, Amagai M, Komai A et al. (1999) Desmoglein 1 and desmoglein 3 are the target autoantigens in herpetiform pemphigus. Arch Dermatol 135:943–947

Jablonska S, Chorzelski T, Beutner EH et al. (1975) Herpetiform pemphigus, a variable pattern of pemphigus. Int J Dermatol 14:353–359

Jansen T, Plewig G, Anhalt GJ (1995) Paraneoplastic pemphigus with clinical features of erosive lichen planus associated with Castleman's tumor. Dermatology 190:245–250

Korman NJ (1990) Pemphigus. Dermatol Clin 8:689–700

Lever WF (1953) Pemphigus. Medicine 32:1–123

Lever WF (1979) Pemphigus and pemphigoid. J Am Acad Dermatol 1: 2–31

Lever WF, Schaumburg-Lever G (1984) Treatment of pemphigus vulgaris. Results obtained in 84 patients between 1961 and 1982. Arch Dermatol 120:44–47

Messer G, Sizmann N, Feucht H et al. (1995) High-dose intravenous immunoglobulins for immediate control of severe pemphigus patients. Br J Dermatol 133:1014–1016

Nishikawa T (1999) Desmoglein ELISAs. Arch Dermatol 135: 195–196

Nousari HC, Detering R, Wojtczack H et al. (1999) The mechanism of respiratory failure in paraneoplastic pemphigus. N Engl J Med 340:1406–1410

Ongenae KC, Temmermann LJ, Vermander F et al. (1999) Intercellular IgA dermatosis. Eur J Dermatol 9: 85–94

Robinson ND, Hashimoto T, Amagai M et al. (1999) The new pemphigus variants. J Am Acad Dermatol 40: 649–671

Senear FE, Usher B (1926) An unusual type of pemphigus combining features of lupus erythematosus. Arch Dermatol Syph 13:761–781

Stanley JR (1989) Pemphigus and pemphigoid as paradigms of organ-specific, autoantibody-mediated diseases. J Clin Invest 83:1443–1448

Stanley JR (1999) Therapy of pemphigus vulgaris. Arch Dermatol 135:76–78

Vieiera JP (1940) Nova contribucões ao estudo de pênfigo foliáceo (fogo-selvagem) no Estado de São Paulo. Emprésa Gráfica da „Revistas dos Tribunais

Wallach D (1986) Intraepidermal neutrophilic IgA dermatosis. N Engl J Med 315:66–67

Wallach D, Foldes C, Cotenot F (1982) Pustulose souscornée, acantholyse superficielle et IgA monoclonale. Ann Dermatol Venereol (Paris) 109: 959–963

Wolff H, Kunte C, Messer G et al. (1999) Paraneoplastic pemphigus with fatal pulmonary involvement in a woman with a mesenteric Castleman tumour. Br J Dermatol 140: 313–316

Bullous Pemphigoid

Ahmed AR, Maize JC, Provost TT (1977) Bullous pemphigoid. Clinical and immunologic follow-up after successful therapy. Arch Dermatol 113:1043–1046

Bean SF, Michel B, Furey N et al. (1976) Vesicular pemphigoid. Arch Dermatol 113:1402–1404

Chan LS, Fine J-D, Briggaman RA et al. (1993) Identification and partial characterization of a novel 105-kD lower lamina lucida autoantigen associated with a novel immune-mediated subepidermal blistering disease. J Invest Dermatol 101:262–267

Eberhartinger C, Niebauer G (1961) Zur prognose und Therapie des Pemphis vulgaris und ähnlicher Erkrankungen. Hautarzt 12:503–508

Fox B, Odems RB, Findlay RF (1982) Erythromycin therapy in bullous pemphigoid: possible anti-inflammatory effects. J Am Acad Dermatol 7:504–510

Gohestani RF, Nicolas JF, Rousselle P et al. (1997) Diagnostic value of indirect immunofluorescence on sodium chloride-split skin in differential diagnosis of subepidermal autoimmune bullous dermatoses. Arch Dermatol 133:1102–1107

Jablonska S, Chorzelski TP, Blasczyk M et al. (1984) Bullous diseases and malignancy. Semin Dermatol 3:316–326

Jung M, Kippes W, Messer G et al. (1999) Increased risk of bullous pemphigoid in male and very old patients: a population-based study on incidence. J Am Acad Dermatol 41:266–268

Korman NJ (1998) Bullous pemphigoid. The latest in diagnosis, prognosis, and therapy. Arch Dermatol 134:1137–1141

Lever WF (1979) Pemphigus and pemphigoid. J Am Acad Dermatol 1:2–31

Levine N, Freilich A, Barland P (1979) Localized pemphigoid simulating dyshidrosiform dermatitis. Arch Dermatol 115:320–321

Liu HN-H, Su DWP, Rogers RS III (1986) Clinical variants of pemphigoid. Int J Dermatol 25:17–27

Nunzi E, Rongioletti F, Parodi A et al. (1988) Dyshidrosiform pemphigoid. J Am Acad Dermatol 19:568–569

Person JR, Rogers RS III (1977) Bullous pemphigoid responding to sulfapyridine and the sulfones. Arch Dermatol 113: 610–615

Person JR, Rogers RS III, Perry HO (1976) Localized pemphigoid. Br J Dermatol 95:531–534

Provost TT, Maize JC, Ahmed AR et al. (1979) Unusual subepidermal bullous disease with immunologic features of bullous pemphigoid. Arch Dermatol 115:156–160

Sato M, Shimizu H, Ishiko A et al. (1998) Precise ultrastructural localization of in vivo deposited IgG antibodies in fresh perilesional skin of patients with bullous pemphigoid. Br J Dermatol 138:593–601

Schmidt E, Obek K, Bröcker E-B et al. (2000) Serum levels of autoantibodies to BP180 correlate with disease activity in patients with bullous pemphigoid. Arch Dermatol 136:174–178

Schnyder MMU (1969) Pemphigoide séborrhéique. Entité nosologique nouvelle? Bull Soc Fr Dermatol Syphiligr 76:320

Stone SP, Schroeter AL (1975) Bullous pemphigoid and associated malignant neoplasms. Arch Dermatol 111:991–994

Winkelmann RK, Su WPD (1979) Pemphigoid vegetans. Arch Dermatol 115:446–448

Yung CW, Soltani K, Lorincz AL (1981) Pemphigoid nodularis. J Am Acad Dermatol 5:54–60

Zillikens D, Kawahara Y, Ishiko A et al. (1996) A novel subepidermal blistering disease with autoantibodies against a 200-kDa antigen of the basement membrane zone. J Invest Dermatol 106: 465–470

Zillikens D, Mascaro JM, Rose PA et al. (1997) A highly sensitive enzyme-linked immunosorbent assay for the detection of circulating anti-BP180 autoantibodies in patients with bullous pemphigoid. J Invest Dermatol 109: 679–683

Herpes Gestationis

Chimanovitch I, Schmidt E, Messer G et al. (1999) IgG_1 and IgG_3 are the major immunoglobulin subclasses targeting epitopes within the NC16 A domain of BP180 in pemphigoid gestationis. J Invest Dermatol 113:140–142

Holmes RC, Black MM, Jurecka W et al. (1983) Clues to the aetiology and pathogenesis of herpes gestationis. Br J Dermatol 109:131–139

Jenkins RE, Hern S, Black MM (1999) Clinical features and management of 87 patients with pemphigoid gestationis. Clin Exp Dermatol 24:255–259

Morrison LH, Labib RS, Zone JJ et al. (1988) Herpes gestationis autoantibodies recognize a 180-kD human epidermal antigen. J Clin Invest 81:2023–2026

Shornick JK, Black MM (1992) Fetal risks in herpes gestationis. J Am Acad Dermatol 26:63–68

Shornick JK, Bangert JL, Freeman RG et al. (1983) Herpes gestationis: clinical and histological features of 28 cases. J Am Acad Dermatol 8:214–224

Vaughan Jones SA, Black MM (1999) Pregnancy dermatoses. J Am Acad Dermatol 40:233–241

Cicatricial Pemphigoid

Ahmed AR, Kurgis BS, Rogers RS III (1991) Cicatricial pemphigoid. J Am Acad Dermatol 24:987–1001

Balding SD, Prost C, Diaz LA et al. (1996) Cicatricial pemphigoid autoantibodies react with multiple sites on the BP180 extracellular domain. J Invest Dermatol 106: 141–146

Brunsting LA, Perry HO (1957) Benign pemphigoid? A report of seven cases with chronic, scarring herpetiform plaques about the head and neck. Arch Dermatol 75: 489–501

Chan LS, Majmudar AA, Tran HH et al. (1997) Laminin-6 and Laminin-5 are recognized by autoantibodies in a subset of cicatricial pemphigoid. J Invest Dermatol 108:848–853

Kirtschig G, Caux F, McMillan JR et al. (1998) Acquired junctional epidermolysis bullosa associated with IgG autoantibodies to the α subunit of laminin-5. Br J Dermatol 138: 125–130

Lever WF (1942) Pemphigus conjunctivae with scarring of the skin. Arch Dermatol Syph 46:875–880

Michel B, Bean SF, Chorzelski T et al. (1977) Cicatricial pemphigoid of Brunsting-Perry. Arch Dermatol 113: 1403–1405

Pandya AG, Warren KJ, Bergstresser PR (1997) Cicatricial pemphigoid successfully treated with pulse intravenous cyclophosphamide. Arch Dermatol 133:245–247

Rogers RS III, Seehafer JR, Perry HO (1982) Treatment of cicatricial (benign mucous membrane) pemphigoid with dapsone. J Am Acad Dermatol 6:215–223

Wolff K, Rappersberger K, Steiner A et al. (1987) Vegetating cicatricial pemphigoid. A new subset of the cicatricial pemphigoid spectrum. Arch Dermatol Res 279S: 20–37

Linear IgA Dermatosis

Bhogal B, Wjnarowska F, Marsden RA et al. (1987) Linear IgA bullous dermatosis of adults and children: an immunoelectron microscopic study. Br J Dermatol 117: 289–296

Chorzelski TP, Jablonska S (1979) IgA linear dermatosis of childhood (chronic bullous disease of childhood). Br J Dermatol 101:535–542

Collier P, Wojnarowska F, Allen J et al. (1994) Molecular overlap of the IgA target antigens in the subepidermal blistering diseases. Dermatology 189S:105–107

Kárpáti S, Stolz W, Meurer M et al. (1992) Ultrastructural immunogold studies in two cases of linear IgA dermatosis. Are there two distinct types of this disease? Br J Dermatol 127:112–118

Mobacken H, Kastrup W, Ljunghall K et al. (1983) Linear IgA dermatosis. A study of ten adult patients. Acta Derm Venereol (Stockh) 63:123–128

Pas HH, Kloosterhuis GJ, Heeren K et al. (1997) Bullous pemphigoid and linear IgA dermatosis sera recognize a similar 120-kDa keratinocyte collagenous glycoprotein with antigenic cross-reactivity to BP180. J Invest Dermatol 108:423–429

Pulimood S, Ajithkumar K, Jacob M et al. (1997) Linear IgA bullous dermatosis of childhood: treatment with dapsone and co-trimoxazole. Clin Exp Dermatol 22:90–91

Zambruno G, Manca V, Kanitakis J et al. (1994) Linear IgA bullous dermatosis with autoantibodies to a 290 kd antigen of anchoring fibrils. J Am Acad Dermatol 31:884–888

Epidermolysis Bullosa Acquisita

Callot-Mellot C, Bodemer C, Caux F et al. (1997) Epidermolysis bullosa acquisita in childhood. Arch Dermatol 133:1122–1126

Gammon WR, Briggaman RA, Woodley DT et al. (1984) Epidermolysis bullosa acquisita – a pemphigoid-like disease. J Am Acad Dermatol 11:820–832

Kofler H, Wambacher-Gasser B, Topar G et al. (1996) Intravenous immunoglobulin treatment in therapy-resistant epidermolysis bullosa acquisita. J Am Acad Dermatol 34: 331–334

Kurzhals G, Stolz W, Meurer M et al. (1991) Acquired epidermolysis bullosa with the clinical feature of Brunsting-Perry cicatricial bullous pemphigoid. Arch Dermatol 127: 391–395

Megahed M, Scharffetter-Kochanek K (1993) Epidermolysis bullosa acquisita – successful treatment with colchicine. Arch Dermatol Res 286:35–40

Roenigk HH Jr, Ryan JG, Bergfeld WF (1971) Epidermolysis bullosa acquisita. Report of three cases and review of all published cases. Arch Dermatol 103:1–10

Zhu XJ, Niimi Y, Bystryn JC (1990) Epidermolysis bullosa acquisita. Incidence in patients with basement membrane zone antibodies. Arch Dermatol 126:171–174

Dermatitis Herpetiformis

Cottini GB (1955) Dermatite herpétiforme de Duhring symétrique et localisée aux genoux et aux coudes. Ann Dermatol Syph 82:285–286

Crabtree JE, O'Mahony S, Wyatt JI et al. (1992) *Helicobacter pylori* serology in patients with coeliac disease and dermatitis herpetiformis. J Clin Pathol 45:597–600

Dieterich W, Laag E, Bruckner-Tuderman L et al. (1999) Antibodies to tissue transglutaminase as serologic markers in patients with dermatitis herpetiformis. J Invest Dermatol 113:133–136

Duhring LA (1884) Dermatitis herpetiformis. JAMA 3:225–229

Ermacora E, Prampolini L, Tribbia G (1986) Long-term follow-up of dermatitis herpetiformis in children. J Am Acad Dermatol 15:24–29

Floden CH, Gentele H (1955) A case of clinically typical dermatitis herpetiformis presenting acantholysis. Acta Derm Venereol 35:128–131

Hardman CM, Garioch JJ, Leonard JN et al. (1997) Absence of toxicity of oats in patients with dermatitis herpetiformis. N Engl J Med 337:1884–1887

Katz SI, Strober W (1978) The pathogenesis of dermatitis herpetiformis. J Invest Dermatol 70:63–75

Rhodes LE, Tingle MD, Park BK et al. (1995) Cimetidine improves the therapeutic/toxic ratio of dapsone in patients on chronic dapsone therapy. Br J Dermatol 132: 257–262

Lichen Planus Pemphigoides

Bouloc A, Vignon-Pennamen MD, Caux F et al. (1998) Lichen planus pemphigoides is a heterogeneous disease: a report of five cases studied by immunoelectron microscopy. Br J Dermatol 138:972–980

Schreiner K (1930) Lichen ruber pemphigoides und lichen ruber vesiculosus. Arch Dermatol Syph 161:647–657

Zillikens D, Caux F, Mascaro JM et al. (1999) Autoantibodies in lichen planus pemphigoides react with a novel epitope within the C-terminal NC16 A domain of BP180. J Invest Dermatol 113:117–121

Bullous Diseases in Childhood

Bean SF, Good RA, Windhorst DB (1970) Bullous pemphigoid in an 11-year-old boy. Arch Dermatol 102: 205–208

Bhogal B, Wojnarowska F, Marsden RA et al. (1987) Linear IgA bullous dermatosis of adults and children. Br J Dermatol 117:289–296

Chorzelski TP, Jablonska S (1979) IgA linear dermatosis of childhood (chronic bullous disease of childhood). Br J Dermatol 101:535–542

Faber WR, Joost TH van (1973) Juvenile pemphigoid. Br J Dermatol 89:519–522

Gianotti F, Ermacora E, Prampolini L et al. (1986) Dermatitis herpetiformis in childhood. Long-term follow-up of dermatitis herpetiformis in children. J Am Acad Dermatol 15:24–30

Marsden RA (1982) The treatment of benign chronic bullous dermatosis of childhood, and dermatitis herpetiformis and bullous pemphigoid beginning in childhood. Clin Exp Dermatol 7:653–663

Marsden RA, McKee PH, Bhogal B et al. (1980) A study of benign chronic bullous dermatosis of childhood and comparison with dermatitis herpetiformis and bullous pemphigoid. Clin Exp Dermatol 5:159–176

Nemeth AJ, Klein AD, Gould EW et al. (1991) Childhood bullous pemphigoid. Clinical and immunologic features, treatment, and prognosis. Arch Dermatol 127: 378–386

Rosenbaum MM, Esterly NB, Greenwald MJ et al. (1984) Cicatricial pemphigoid in a 6-year-old child: report of a case and review of the literature. Pediatr Dermatol 2: 13–22

Schiffner JH (1982) Therapy of childhood linear IgA dermatitis herpetiformis. J Am Acad Dermatol 6:403–404

Surbrugg SK, Weston WL (1985) The course of chronic bullous disease of childhood. Pediatr Dermatol 2:213–215

Trueb RM, Didierjean L, Fellas A et al. (1999) Childhood bullous pemphigoid: report of a case with characterization of the targeted antigens. J Am Acad Dermatol 40:338–344

Wojnarowska F, Marsden RA, Bhogal B et al. (1988) Chronic bullous disease of childhood, childhood cicatricial pemphigoid, and linear IgA disease of adults. J Am Acad Dermatol 19:792–805

Pustular Diseases

Contents

One unusual feature of the skin is its tendency to form sterile pustules. Nondermatologists have often been taught to equate pus with infection and find the nonchalance of dermatologists' approach to pus puzzling. While many bacterial, viral, and fungal infections in the skin are indeed pustular, there are also many patients who present with sterile pustules. The prototypical pustular disease is psoriasis. Presumably, a number of noninfectious triggers can also produce the appropriate cytokines for eliciting a pustular response in the skin. In this chapter, we will discuss the idiopathic pustular diseases, dividing them as shown in Table 16.1 into acral and generalized conditions while also distinguishing between the childhood and adult forms.

Table 16.1. Idiopathic pustular diseases

Localized acral pustules	
Children	Infantile acropustulosis
	Parakeratosis pustulosa
Adults	Acrodermatitis continua suppurativa
	Palmoplantar pustulosis
	Acute acropustulosis
	Erosive pustular dermatosis of the scalp
Generalized pustules	
Children	Erythema toxicum neonatorum
	Transient neonatal pustular melanosis
	Incontinentia pigmenti
Adults	IgA pemphigus foliaceus
	Subcorneal pustular dermatosis
	Impetigo herpetiformis
	Acute generalized exanthematous pustulosis
	Eosinophilic pustular folliculitis

Acral Pustular Diseases

Childhood Acropustulosis

Infantile Acral Pustulosis
(Kahn and Rwylin 1979)

Synonym. Acropustulosis infantilis

Definition. Disease of infants with pruritic pustules primarily on the palms and soles.

Epidemiology. While there are about 50 cases reported in the literature, we suspect this disorder is somewhat more common. It has been described more often among black male children, but that may simply reflect where the first authors happened to describe the disease. Recent reports have represented all races and show equal sex distribution. The disease can be present at birth and usually begins in the first 4 months of life, although it can appear in older infants.

Etiology and Pathogenesis. The cause is unknown. The main question is always scabies. Some children, especially Asian orphans brought to the USA and northern Europe, may have a prolonged pustular response after being appropriately treated for long-standing scabies. This is known as the postscabetic id reaction. While some cases of infantile acropustulosis clearly are postscabetic, many offer no such history. The problem may be more common in children with atopic dermatitis.

Clinical Findings. The changes are primarily limited to the hands and feet and are intensely pruritic. Other body regions such as the trunk and scalp may also show an occasional pustule. The primary lesion is a 1–2 mm vesicle that arises on an erythematous base and develops within 24 h into a pustule. Later, it develops a collarette scale with crust. Some patients may have stigmata of atopic dermatitis. In addition, peripheral blood eosinophilia and IgE level may be elevated.

Histopathology. Biopsy shows an intraepidermal, unilocular vesicle or pustule with minimal spongiosis at the periphery. The initial changes start apparently in or just above the basal layer. The contents include neutrophils, eosinophils, other inflammatory cells, and keratinocytes, all of which can be seen in a blister smear. Immunofluorescent studies are negative.

Course and Prognosis. The course is chronic and frustrating. While the disease eventually resolves, it may wax and wane for 2–3 years. Typically, flares come every several weeks over a period of years.

Differential Diagnosis. In newborns, erythema toxicum neonatorum and transient neonatal melanosis are both more common. Only the acral distribution helps, but the chronic course provides the diagnosis. The relationship to scabies has been discussed above. Typical vesiculopustular infections in infants, such as herpes simplex virus, *Candida albicans*, and even impetigo are rarely acral. Dyshidrotic dermatitis and pustular psoriasis do not occur in infants, but infantile acropustulosis may well be immunologically related to one of them. If the lesions are around the nail folds and mouth, acrodermatitis enteropathica should be considered.

Therapy. Initial reports enthusiastically described the use of dapsone and sulfapyridine. Both these medications cause more hematologic problems in children than adults and we have not been impressed by their effectiveness. Oral erythromycin has also been endorsed but shows little effect. Corticosteroids bring little response, used either systemically or topically. Probably the best approach is to use topical antipruritic agents, such as polidocanol, or distracters such as a menthol or calamine shake lotion.

Parakeratosis Pustulosa
(SABOURAUD 1931)

Etiology and Pathogenesis. This disorder is probably not as rare as the limited number of case reports suggests. It is unclear whether parakeratosis pustulosa is a specific entity or simply a manifestation of acral dermatitis of many types. Patients are usually children, often with atopic diathesis or psoriasis. They develop periungual erythema with fine scaling that usually precedes the nail changes. In some cases, there are distal subungual pustules evolving into hyperkeratotic changes, nail dystrophies, and onycholysis. Often only one finger, usually the index finger, is affected. Resolution is usually spontaneous. While a dermatophyte infection should be excluded, fingernail involvement in children is an uncommon fungal manifestation. Treatment with topical corticosteroids may speed resolution. Recurrences are common.

Adult Acropustulosis

Acrodermatitis Continua Suppurativa
(HALLOPEAU 1890)

Synonyms. Dermatitis repens (CROCKER 1888), acrodermatitis perstans

Definition. Pustular eruption concentrated on the tips of the digits with nail damage that usually represents localized psoriasis.

Epidemiology. This uncommon disorder is perhaps more common among women.

Etiology and Pathogenesis. While the cause of acrodermatitis continua suppurativa is a mystery, the clinical resemblance to psoriasis is so striking that we view this as localized psoriasis. Similar changes can be seen in patients with a flare of psoriasis or with widespread pustular psoriasis. A association with HLA-B27 has been reported, as have flares triggered by trauma or infections.

Clinical Findings. The classic finding is sterile pustules on erythematous skin at the tips of the fingers and toes, often leading to nail loss and nail bed scarring (Figs. 16.1, 16.2). Often there is a history of trauma (crush injury, thorn, insect bite) or infection (paronychia). In the latter case, we suspect the initial diagnosis of infection is often

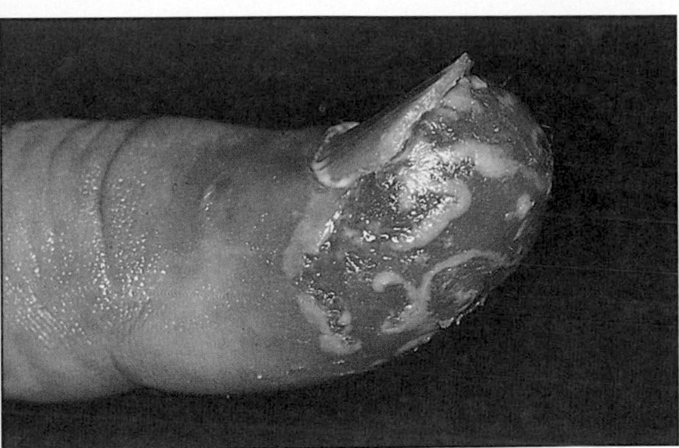

Fig. 16.1. Acrodermatitis continua suppurativa with pustules, acute stage

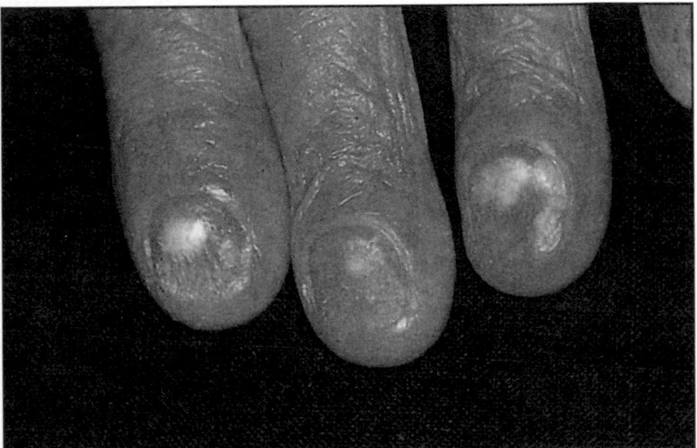

Fig. 16.2. Acrodermatitis continua suppurativa with nail damage, chronic stage

simply wrong. Usually the problem does start with a single digit, in contrast to the multiple-digit involvement of generalized pustular psoriasis. When the disease remains limited to one digit, some prefer the term dermatitis repens, even during recurrences.

Initially there are painful, sharply bordered erythematous plaques in the vicinity of the nail. They rapidly develop pustules and fuse together, forming bizarre lakes of pus. In other instances, the pustules remain discrete small lesions. As they age, they dry, forming a honey-colored crust with layers of peripheral scale. New lesions advance proximally, moreso on the ventral than the dorsal sides of the digits. The episodes of erythema, pus, and scaling recur and spread relentlessly. The border to the normal skin is always sharp and sometimes slightly elevated. There may be pruritus, but more often the patient complains of pain and impaired use of the involved digits. When the hands are involved, as is usually the case, the cosmetic impairment is also considerable.

In later lesions, the nail is almost invariably damaged. Often it is lost and scarring occurs in the nail fold, so that the new nails are dystrophic. The digital tips may become puffy and swollen, almost clubbed. While the distal skin appears atrophic, it usually can regenerate normally if the inflammatory process is halted. In addition, the distal phalanxes may show osteoporosis or even loss of bony structures on X-ray examination.

Histopathology. Microscopic examination confirms the relationship to psoriasis. The unilocular pustule contains primarily neutrophils that seep through the epidermis covering the lesion, producing a spongiform pustule of Kogoj. The epidermal cells show a sponge-like necrosis. In the papillary dermis, the vessels are elongated and tortuous, while there is mixed inflammatory infiltrate.

Course and Prognosis. The course is usually one of recurrences and gradual spread. The risk of a generalized pustular psoriasis makes predicting the course difficult. Spontaneous regressions can occur, but no prudent physician would claim to have a cure.

Differential Diagnosis. When the lesions first appear, the main differential diagnoses are a paronychium and herpetic whitlow. Thus, bacterial and viral cultures and a Tzanck test are appropriate. When more chronic, almost granulomatous changes are present, one must consider disorders such as mucocutaneous candidiasis and acrodermatitis enteropathica, which may feature pustular acral lesions with nail destruction but usually offer countless other clues. Chronic tinea ungium should be excluded but is rarely pustular.

Therapy

Systemic. A wide variety of potent drugs are used for this problem, because topical therapy brings so little and the process can be so disabling. The use of aromatic retinoids such as acitretin, initially 30–75 mg daily with lower maintenance doses, is probably most effective. Systemic corticosteroids, usually prednisone 40–60 mg daily with tapering, usually suppress the disease but flares often occur when they are stopped. On rare occasions, widespread flares have been reported in this setting, producing very unhappy patients. Because of the relationship to psoriasis, methotrexate has also been used, most often 15–25 mg orally weekly. Cyclosporine 2.5–5.0 mg daily also seems effective, as does fumaric A acid in routine dosages. Each of these medications deserves careful monitoring. Isolated reports describe colchicine (500 mg orally b.i.d.), especially in Japanese patients, and dapsone (50–150 mg orally daily) as being helpful. While we have had little success with these agents, they may be worth trying because of their better safety profile. One additional possibility is clofazimine, an agent used to treat leprosy which apparently has immunostimulatory effects and is occasionally effective in pustular psoriasis. The usual dose is 200–300 mg daily; the main side effect is a pinkish red discoloration of the skin and urine.

Phototherapy. Hand and foot or bath psoralen plus ultraviolet A (PUVA) therapy is probably the best approach. Either can be combined with acitretin. Radiation therapy (soft X-rays 1–2 Gy once weekly for 3 weeks) is very effective, but its use for benign conditions has wrongly fallen into disrepute.

Topical. If topical corticosteroids are to be tried, then one should start with very high potency agents. It is usually possible to occlude them for a few hours with plastic household wraps or the tips of plastic gloves. Intralesional triamcinolone acetonide (2.5–5.0 mg/ml diluted with an anesthetic) is useful for limited lesions but painful and very likely to produce permanent atrophy. Both anthralin and tars can be used just as in psoriasis therapy; we have had more luck with short contact anthralin therapy in combination with corticosteroids. Vitamin D_3 analogues are also effective and deserve a trial.

Palmoplantar Pustulosis

(Andrews et al. 1934)

Synonyms. Pustulosis palmaris et plantaris, pustular bacterid (of Andrews)

Definition. Idiopathic chronic pustular eruption concentrated on the palms and soles.

Epidemiology. Palmoplantar pustulosis is relatively common, seen more often in women (3:1 ratio) and usually starting between 20 and 60 years of age.

Etiology and Pathogenesis. The principle difference between palmoplantar pustulosis and acrodermatitis continua suppurativa is the clinical distribution. Many cases represent a variant of pustular psoriasis. Andrews felt, as the name suggests, that palmoplantar pustulosis was a bacterid or response to a focal, overlooked bacterial infection. In the heyday of "pustular bacterid mania", general surgeons loved the dermatologists, because patients were referred for cholecystectomy, tonsillectomy, or sinus surgery in hopes of curing palmoplantar pustulosis. The chance of success was no better than random chance. Several interesting factors remain unexplained:

- Palmoplantar pustulosis is much more common in smokers.
- Patients often have an exaggerated reaction to intradermal injections of streptococcal or staphylococcal antigens.
- Individuals with atopy appear at greater risk.

No relationship to HLA-B27 has been found; an increased frequency of HLA-B8, -Cw6, and -DR3 was reported. While pustular drug eruptions mimicking pustular psoriasis occur with systemic antibiotics, they appear rarely to be limited to the extremities.

Clinical Findings. Most often, there is a symmetric distribution of pustules involving the palms and soles (Fig. 16.3). The pads of the fingertips are the most common site. The lesions may begin in an asymmetric pattern, but with time they become

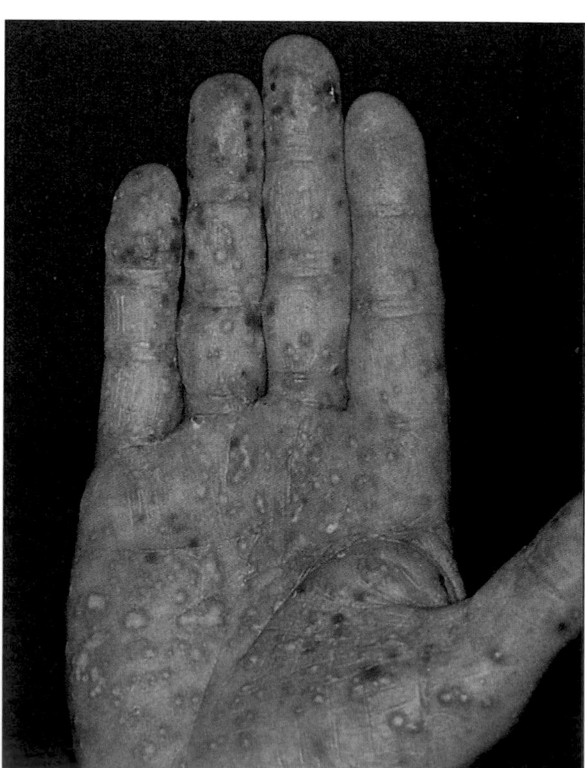

Fig. 16.3. Palmoplantar pustulosis

more uniform. On the hands, the thenar and hypothenar eminences are most reliably affected, but on the feet the instep or arch is more likely to be involved. The interdigital spaces are spared, as are the nails and dorsal aspects of the digits in most cases. Typically there are lesions in many stages of evolution adjacent to each other. One sees 1–5 mm intact fresh pustules, dry yellowish brown lesions, small accumulations of crust and scale, and the residual collarette scale. There may also be a diffuse irregular erythema of the palms and soles.

In other words, palmoplantar pustulosis seems to stop where acrodermatitis continua suppurativa starts. Another difference is that the pustules of palmoplantar pustulosis arise in relatively normal skin without much erythema. The process is usually relatively asymptomatic or somewhat pruritic. A number of associated diseases have been described. To some extent, the literature is befuddled because some groups still believe in the bacterid theory and others do not. The best association is with arthritis of the sternocostoclavicular joints (Sonozaki syndrome). The joints are swollen, tender, and contain a sterile neutrophilic infiltrate; there are similarities to the SAPHO syndrome (Chap. 28). Another association with both hyper- and hypoparathyroidism has been described.

Histopathology. The initial lesion is a vesicle arising in the basal layer and slowly shed at the same time that neutrophils migrate in, producing the pustule. Thus evolves the classic picture of a unilocular neutrophilic pustule. The dermis shows relatively little inflammation.

Course and Prognosis. The course tends to be chronic. In most cases, widespread disease does not develop.

Differential Diagnosis. Since palmoplantar pustulosis is probably a variant of pustular psoriasis, the two cannot be separated with certainty. Other clues for psoriasis should be sought, such as nail pitting or oil spots, scalp involvement, gluteal cleft redness, and the like. Both dyshidrotic dermatitis and inflammatory tinea manuum and pedum should be excluded. A biopsy will show fungal hyphae in the later case and there is more likely to be interdigital changes. In the chase of dyshidrotic dermatitis, the lesions usually start on the sides of the digits. A biopsy from a fresh lesion of dyshidrotic dermatitis is less likely to contain neutrophils and more likely to have intense spongiosis. Acrodermatitis continua suppurativa is more acral, more erythematous, and more likely to damage nails.

Therapy. The same principles discussed for acrodermatitis continua suppurativa above apply here.

Acute Acropustulosis

Occasionally, acute generalized exanthematous pustulosis is limited to the palms and soles (vide infra).

Erosive Pustular Dermatitis of the Scalp

(Pye et al. 1979)

Synonym. Pustular ulcerative dermatosis of the scalp

Definition. Chronic pustular, erosive, scarring scalp inflammation that leads to scarring alopecia.

Epidemiology. This uncommon disorder has been described primarily among elderly women with age of onset between 60 and 90 years. Similar problems have been reported in African men. It may follow trauma and zoster involving the first branch of the trigeminal nerve.

Etiology and Pathogenesis. The etiology is unknown. In most cases, the pustules are sterile but, once they break, a wide spectrum of bacteria and fungi can be cultured. The relationship to trauma, the presence of leukocytoclastic vasculitis, and the rapidly spreading ulcerations have tempted some to classify this as pyoderma gangrenosum of the scalp.

Clinical Findings. The lesions on the scalp show a chronic course with frequent flares. Flat pustules, erosions, and crusts evolve, usually associated with pruritus (Fig. 16.4). The pustules are not localized

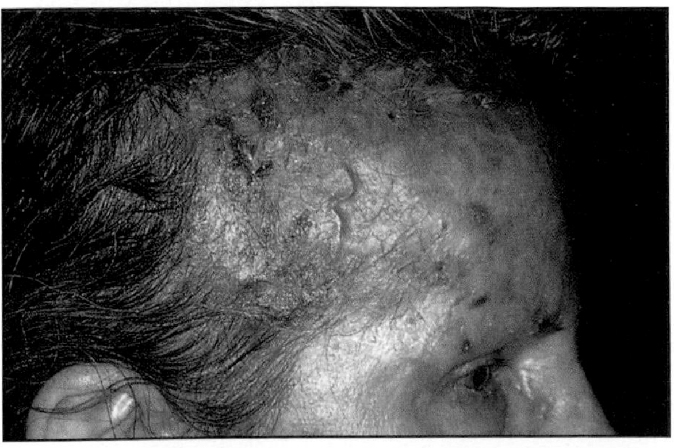

Fig. 16.4. Erosive pustular dermatitis of the scalp

specifically to the hair follicles, so this disorder is slightly different from other forms of scarring folliculitis. Over time, focal areas of scarring resembling pseudopelade develop.

Histopathology. Biopsy does not help understand the disease. The pustules are usually subcorneal, perhaps suggesting a relationship to subcorneal pustular dermatosis. Occasionally, hints of leukocytoclastic vasculitis are seen, but this not unusual at the periphery of ulcerations of any type. Plasma cells may be numerous. Immunofluorescent examination is negative.

Course and Prognosis. The course is chronic. The hairs tend to be glued together by the dried exudates, which is painful and cosmetically disturbing. In several patients, squamous cell carcinoma developed in the areas of scarring.

Differential Diagnosis. Probably the most common differential diagnostic point is a secondarily infected scalp dermatitis. Chronic pyodermas with a vegetative response may appear similar but lack the pustular stage. Primary bacterial folliculitis can be excluded by repeated cultures, and primary fungal infections of the scalp are rare in adults. One must also consider subcorneal pustular dermatosis, pustular psoriasis, and all the forms of pustular and scarring folliculitis that can be excluded by careful observation and biopsy. Eosinophilic pustular folliculitis may also involve the scalp. As mentioned above, there may be overlaps with pyoderma gangrenosum.

Therapy

Systemic. There is no good therapy. Systemic antibiotics rarely bring any persistent improvement. Oral isotretinoin has been helpful in some cases, as has zinc supplementation. The combination of erythromycin and zink may be helpful in some cases. Systemic corticosteroids bring prompt temporary improvement, but as soon as they are tapered, a flare can be anticipated.

Topical. Some patients respond at least temporarily to high potency topical corticosteroid lotions or gels. Ointments should be avoided. Topical antibiotics usually fail. Topical disinfectants are probably the wisest choice.

Generalized Pustular Diseases

Generalized Pustular Diseases in Children

In newborns and infants, there are a number of benign pustular disorders that must be distinguished from a series of potentially life-threatening problems. One must exclude staphylococcal pustulosis (a variant of bullous impetigo), disseminated herpes simplex virus infection, and diffuse candidiasis. In slightly older infants, after 1–2 months of age, neonatal scabies is often pustular. In addition, incontinentia pigmenti may feature pustules, as may Langerhans' cell histiocytosis. But the following two benign disorders are far more common and should be considered first.

Erythema Toxicum Neonatorum

(Leiner 1912)

Synonyms. Erythema neonatorum, erythema toxicum, toxic erythema of the newborn

Definition. Harmless, common, short-lived erythematous eruption of newborns. The word "toxicum" is misleading and has been dropped in Germany.

Epidemiology. Between 30 % and 50 % of newborns develop erythema toxicum neonatorum. It is so common that dermatologists rarely get a chance to see it unless they make a habit of visiting the newborn nursery and simply looking at all the patients. No racial or sexual predilection has been shown. Subtle erythemas are undoubtedly overlooked in black infants, but most cases are identified. The disorder is more common in full-term infants than premature ones.

Etiology and Pathogenesis. The etiology is unknown. Even though eosinophils are a key feature, there is no evidence for an allergic reaction. Most have concluded that erythema toxicum neonatorum represents part of the normal transition from the watery womb to the dry external environment.

Clinical Findings. Erythema toxicum neonatorum appears most often in the first 2 days of life. It may occasionally be present at birth and even less often during the first 2 weeks. The primary lesions are widespread erythematous macules, usually most prevalent on the trunk and proximal parts of the extremities. They often coalesce, become elevated and urticarial, or develop into pustules. The most typical lesion is an erythematous macule with a central, firm yellow papule; Hurwitz called this the "flea-bitten rash of the newborn." The palms and soles are usually spared; on the scalp, the lesions look more like folliculitis. The infant is otherwise healthy.

Histopathology. The pustule is either subcorneal or intraepidermal. It may be associated with a follicle. The most striking feature is the overwhelming predominance of eosinophils, which may also be seen on a smear of the pustule contents. In the dermis, there is a perivascular infiltrate consisting of both neutrophils and eosinophils.

Course and Prognosis. The typical rash lasts 2 days. Healing is spontaneous, but occasionally one must wait 7–14 days. The lesions heal without scarring or hyperpigmentation.

Differential Diagnosis. The differential diagnosis is mentioned above. The most difficult question is excluding miliaria crystallina or miliaria rubra, which usually are found on the buttocks, lower part of the back, or intertriginous regions. Miliaria is almost as common, usually starts later in life, and has more discrete lesions that are either tiny noninflamed vesicles or more deeply seated erythematous papules. One subtle difference is that erythema toxicum neonatorum usually starts as a flat macule, while miliaria begin as tiny papules involving sweat ducts. In sum, the two are almost indistinguishable clinically. The blister smear in miliaria does not contain eosinophils.

Therapy. No therapy is needed. If something is desired, a zinc oxide shake lotion can be offered.

Transient Neonatal Pustular Melanosis

(Ramamurthy et al. 1976)

Synonym. Transient neonatal pustulosis

Definition. Transient, self-limited pustular eruption in newborns, almost limited to blacks.

Epidemiology. Seen in up to 4% of American black infants, transient neonatal pustular melanosis may also be seen in other infants, where its frequency is estimated at 0.1%.

Etiology and Pathogenesis. The cause is unknown. It has been suggested that transient neonatal pustular melanosis is simply erythema toxicum neonatorum in blacks, but neither the clinical course nor the lack of eosinophils fit in with this explanation.

Clinical Findings. The skin lesions are always present at birth. Very superficial vesicles and pustules as well as hyperpigmented macules with a fine collarette scale are seen. The latter are the result of intrauterine rupture of pustules. As more fragile pustules break and dry out, more macules evolve. The most common sites are the nape and neck. Other locations include the buttocks, lower aspects of the back, and forehead. Erythematous macules or firm yellow pustules on an erythematous base are not seen. The child is otherwise healthy.

Histopathology. The pustular lesions are similar to erythema toxicum neonatorum except that neutrophils dominate, although eosinophils can be present. The same findings are seen on a smear from a pustule. These hyperpigmented lesions have not been extensively studied but appear to have increased basal layer pigmentation and not postinflammatory dermal hyperpigmentation.

Course and Prognosis. The pustules cease forming after a few days. The hyperpigmented lesions resolve over a period of months.

Differential Diagnosis. The differential diagnosis is mentioned in the introduction above.

Therapy. No therapy is needed; again, a drying lotion can be prescribed.

Transient Cephalic Neonatal Pustulosis

(Aractingi et al. 1991)

Synonym. Neonatal *Malassezia furfur* pustulosis

Etiology and Pathogenesis. This uncommon disease features pustules of the face in neonates ranging from several days to 1 month in age. The disorder has been blamed on *Malassezia furfur*, but in other cases no organism is found. Since *Malassezia furfur* is present in normal infants and not detected in ordinary cultures, its pathogenic role is difficult to prove. The most common sites are the forehead, chin, neck, and scalp; the pustules tend to have an erythematous halo. The main differential point is neonatal acne, but there are no comedones and the pustules can coalesce, a feature not often seen in acne. The eruption is self-limited, although topical imidazoles can be employed.

Generalized Pustular Disorders in Adults

Subcorneal Pustular Dermatosis
(SNEDDON and WILKINSON 1956)

Synonyms. Subcorneal pustulosis, Sneddon-Wilkinson disease

Definition. Chronic, noninfectious pustular dermatosis occasionally associated with a gammopathy.

Epidemiology. This uncommon disorder predominantly affects adult women (4 : 1 ratio) but has been described in children. When associated with an IgA gammopathy, it overlaps with pyoderma gangrenosum, Sweet syndrome, and inflammatory bowel disease.

Etiology and Pathogenesis. The cause is a mystery. The blisters are sterile. The main question is the relationship to IgA pemphigus foliaceus (Chap. 15). Evidence is accumulating that these two disorders are either identical or closely related.

Clinical Findings. Flaccid fragile blisters form on the trunk, proximal part of the extremities, and intertriginous region (Fig. 16.5). The head, palms, soles, and oral mucosa are almost always spared. The primary lesion is a small, firm pustule that only becomes flaccid as it expands. Its contents are either cloudy or purulent; a sheet of neutrophils may accumulate at the base of the blister much like a hypopyon in the anterior chamber of the eye. The periphery is usually erythematous. The patients are generally asymptomatic.

The most typical clinical picture develops as the lesions enlarge and their fragile roofs break. Circinate, sometimes polycyclic, crusted erosions with peripheral collarette scales and tiny new pustules form an almost unmistakable picture. In addition, the lesions heal with a livid tone that shifts to a mild hyperpigmentation.

In the gammopathy-associated cases, there may be ulcerations with necrotic undermined borders or more nodular erythematous infiltrates, supporting the overlap in this setting with pyoderma gangrenosum or Sweet syndrome.

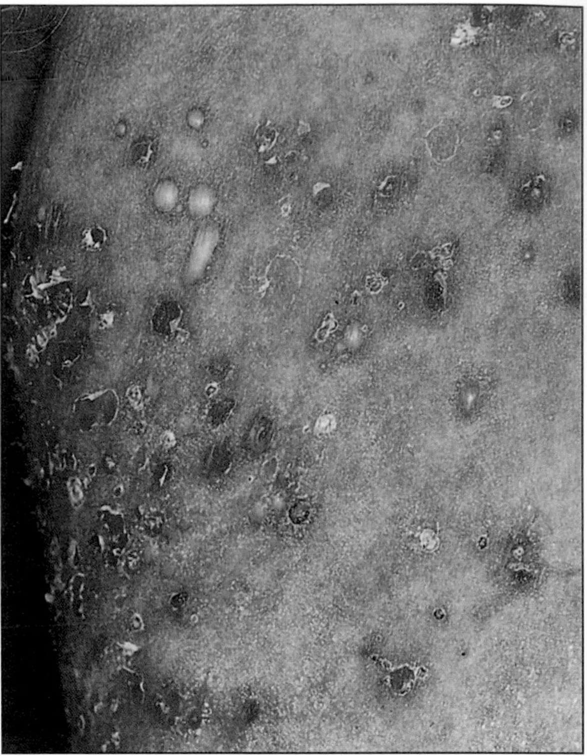

Fig. 16.5. Subcorneal pustular dermatosis

Histopathology. The pathology is not diagnostic. There is a subcorneal pustule filled with neutrophils that are also seen on a smear from the pustule. Bacteria are not seen in the pustule or on the smear, helping to separate it from impetigo. The action is only in the upper layer of the epidermis; the granular layer is usually intact. While spongiosis may be present, acantholysis is not seen. In the dermis there is a mixed perivascular inflammatory infiltrate.

Course and Prognosis. The disease is chronic. Older patients should be monitored periodically to exclude the presence of an IgA gammopathy.

Differential Diagnosis. The main initial differential diagnostic point is impetigo, which is excluded by bacterial culture and the chronic course. The relationship to pustular psoriasis has long been disputed, but patients with subcorneal pustular dermatosis lack scalp and nail involvement and are no more likely to have psoriatic lesions elsewhere than the general population. In addition, when von Zumbusch type pustular psoriasis is as widespread as the subcorneal pustular dermatosis, the patients are very ill with fever and an elevated neutrophil count. Acute generalized exanthematous pustulosis is a pustular drug reaction that may be similar but resolves rapidly. Pemphigus foliaceus and especially IgA pemphigus foliaceus (intraepidermal neutrophilic IgA dermatosis) are similar but diagnosed with direct immunofluorescent examination. The classic erosions with peripheral scale and pustules suggest necrolytic migratory erythema and the erythema annulare centrifugum variant of psoriasis; the former can be excluded with glucagon levels, the latter on the basis of associated features.

Therapy

Systemic. Dapsone is generally effective in dosages ranging from 50 mg to 150 mg daily. When remissions occur, a lower dose can be used or the drug stopped, as the waxing and waning is relatively independent of therapy. Corticosteroids are disappointing. Probably the best approach in dapsone-resistant cases is an oral retinoid, either acitretin or isotretinoin.

Phototherapy. PUVA, either alone or combined with retinoids, is effective. PUVA bath therapy also appears to be a reasonable approach.

Topical. External therapy is frustrating. Early lesions can be treated with high potency corticosteroid lotions; ointments should be avoided. Later on, the pustules can be opened and the erosions treated like any other open wound.

Impetigo Herpetiformis

(Hebra 1872; Kaposi 1887)

Definition. An uncommon disease with widespread erythema and pustules, usually presenting in pregnancy and leading to critical if not fatal problems.

Epidemiology. Some define impetigo herpetiformis as associated with pregnancy and others associate it with hypocalcemia; these definitions alter the epidemiology. But, in general, it occurs in the second half of pregnancy and is likely to recur in subsequent pregnancies. It may also develop in the postpartum period and is rarely seen in men and nonpregnant women. Finally, it has been described after thyroid surgery, presumably because of the well known problem of inadvertent parathyroidectomy.

Etiology and Pathogenesis. We view impetigo herpetiformis as a unique variant of generalized pustular psoriasis, triggered either by pregnancy or abnormal calcium metabolism or perhaps both. The mechanisms of the disease interactions are unknown.

Clinical Findings. The clinical features are alarming. The patients are sick with fever, chills, and headache. There may be signs of hypoparathyroidism (low calcium, positive Chvostek and Trosseau signs, tetany). Abdominal complaints such as nausea, vomiting, diarrhea, and even peritonitis, as well as renal failure and peripheral neuropathies may develop. In addition, the skin changes are striking. The initial lesions are infiltrated erythematous patches, primarily in the intertriginous regions, then the trunk and proximal aspects of the extremities. Small pustules develop on this inflamed background, enlarge, and coalesce. The lakes of pus dry out centrally and develop a collarette scale that points centrally, not peripherally (trailing collarette scale, also seen in erythema annulare centrifugum). The patches can fuse into circinate or serpiginous figures. In extreme cases, the patient develops a pustular erythroderma. The tongue may have tiny pustules as well as glassy punctae or gyrate lesions similar to those from candidiasis.

Histopathology. The microscopic picture is identical to pustular psoriasis, with large spongiform pustules of Kogoj. Occasionally, acantholytic cells and eosinophils may be seen.

Laboratory Findings. The erythrocyte sedimentation rate and neutrophil count are elevated. There is often proteinuria and hypoalbuminemia. Iron deficiency followed by anemia may develop. In addition, calcium levels may be lowered. Renal function should finally be monitored.

Course and Prognosis. There is general agreement that both the mother and infant are threatened. Maternal deaths are seen from hypocalcemia, hyperthermia, and cardiac or renal failure. Arguments can be made to terminate the pregnancy for the sake of the mother. In addition, stillbirths, premature abortions, and low weight for gestation infants may result.

Differential Diagnosis. In a pregnant woman with diffuse pustules who is sick, diagnosis is straightforward. In other settings, the distinction from pustular psoriasis is semantic. Subcorneal pustular dermatosis may also appear similar, but the patients are never as ill.

Therapy. The first and most difficult consideration concerns the further management or termination of the pregnancy.

Systemic. Managing the electrolyte and protein loss, and the probable hypoparathyroidism, and monitoring the renal and cardiac functions are best left in the hands of an internist working with the obstetrician. The mainstay of dermatologic management is systemic corticosteroids, which pose less of a threat to mother and child than the disease does. Usually 60–80 mg prednisone daily is sufficient to bring the eruption under control. It should be tapered very slowly to avoid flares, which can be devastating, and continued at least until the pregnancy is over. If the patient is not pregnant, then all the measures discussed under pustular psoriasis can be employed.

Topical. The eruption is so severe that topical measures are largely futile. Topical corticosteroid lotions may bring some relief. To reduce the likelihood of secondary infections, the erosions should be managed as any other open lesion with topical antibacterial measures.

Acute Generalized Exanthematous Pustulosis

(MacMillan 1973; Tan 1974)

Synonyms. Pustulosis acuta generalisata, acute generalized pustulosis, acute generalized exanthematous bacterid

Definition. Acute generalized pustular exanthem that resolves over a matter of weeks.

Epidemiology. This form is very uncommon; no statistics are available.

Etiology and Pathogenesis. Most eruptions appear 7–10 days after antibiotic use. Since antibiotics are used to treat infections, the possibility also exists that the underlying infection is the trigger, in the sense of a bacterid. β-Hemolytic streptococcal infections are most often incriminated, usually as bronchitis or pharyngitis. In children, acute viral illnesses may also be pustular. Another possible explanation is the triggering of pustular psoriasis in susceptible patients, but the benign course speaks against this possibility. Another consideration is immune complex disease, since in some cases leukocytoclastic vasculitis is identified on biopsy. Finally, in rare cases, no cause is even suggested.

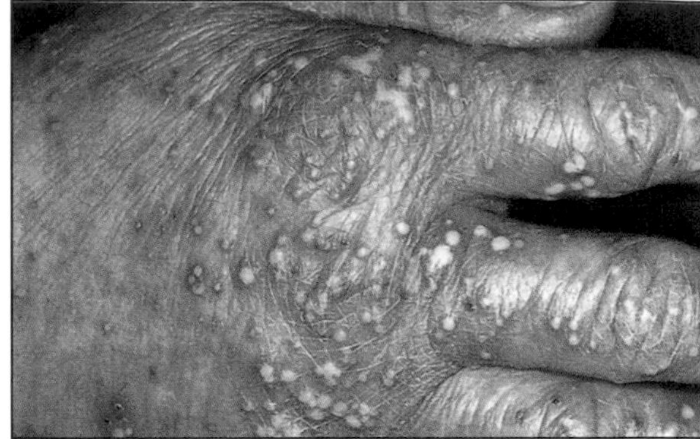

Fig. 16.6. Acute generalized exanthematous pustulosis

When drugs are involved, the most common agents are β-lactam antibiotics, macrolides, tetracyclines, other antibiotics, carbamazepine, nystatin, isoniazid, furosemide, diltiazem, and some nonsteroidal antiinflammatory drugs. Dactinomycin causes a pustular folliculitis that is probably closely related.

Clinical Findings. The pustules appear suddenly simultaneously with widespread distribution. They are several millimeters in size, with a narrow erythematous halo. On the backs of hands and feet as well as on wrists and ankles, they tend to be closely grouped (Fig. 16.6), whereas on the trunk, scalp, and distal portions of the extremities, they are more diffuse. The oral mucosa, palms, and soles are usually spared. The yellow pustules rupture, develop erosions with brown crusts, peripheral scale, and then heal, often with hyperpigmentation.

In some cases, only the hands and feet are involved; this variant is known as acute acropustulosis.

There may be systemic symptoms, but they probably depend more on the underlying disorder than the reaction. Elevated erythrocyte sedimentation rate and elevated neutrophil count, occasionally with eosinophilia and fever, are most common. Hematuria is rarely seen. When vasculitis is present, circulating immune complexes may be identified.

Histopathology. Biopsy simply shows an intraepidermal unilocular pustule. The pustule is sterile and the predominant cells are neutrophils, which can also be demonstrated on a smear. Occasionally, acantholytic cells are present, as well as minimal spongiosis. In the dermis there is a mixed perivascular infiltrate, sometimes with minimal leukocytoclastic vasculitis. Immunofluorescent studies are not specific.

Course and Prognosis. The disease resolves spontaneously, usually after 10–28 days.

Differential Diagnosis. The differential diagnosis is extensive. Pustular psoriasis usually involves sicker patients and a more chronic course. Injections of granulocyte-macrophage (GM)-CSF may induce a Sweet syndrome-like picture but also pustular lesions at the injection site and erythroderma. In addition, pustular lesions and folliculitis are part of the phenytoin hypersensitivity reaction, which also involves fever and lymphadenopathy, usually appearing a few weeks after starting therapy.

Therapy. Usually, a topical, drying shake lotion or corticosteroid lotion suffices. Systemic corticosteroids have been employed in severe cases, usually starting with 60 mg prednisone daily and tapering rapidly.

Bibliography

Infantile Acropustulosis

Dromy R, Raz A, Metzker A (1991) Infantile acropustulosis. Pediatr Dermatol 8:284–287

Kahn G, Rywlin AM (1979) Acropustulosis of infancy. Arch Dermatol 115:831–833

Mancini AJ, Frieden IJ, Paller AS (1998) Infantile acropustulosis revisited: history of scabies and response to topical corticosteroids. Pediatr Dermatol 15:337–341

Newton JA, Salisbury J, Mardsen A et al. (1986) Acropustulosis of infancy. Br J Dermatol 115:735–739

Van Praag MC, Van Rooij RW, Folkers E et al. (1997) Diagnosis and treatment of pustular disorders in the neonate. Pediatr Dermatol 14:131–143

Vignon-Pennamen MD, Wallach D (1986) Infantile acropustulosis. A clinicopathologic study of six cases. Arch Dermatol 122:1155–1160

Parakeratosis Pustulosa

Hjorth N, Thomsen K (1967) Parakeratosis pustulosa. Br J Dermatol 79:527–532

Sabouraud R (1931) Les parakératoses microbiènnes du bouts des doigts. Ann Dermatol Syphil 11:206

Tosti A, Peluso AM, Zucchelli V et al. (1998) Clinical findings and long-term follow-up of 20 cases of parakeratosis pustulosa. Pediatr Dermatol 15:259–263

Acrodermatitis Continua Suppurativa

Behrens S, von Kobyletzki G, Hoffmann K et al. (1997) PUVA-Bad-Photochemotherapie bei Acrodermatitis continua suppurativa Hallopeau. Hautarzt 48:824–827

Hallopeau M (1890) Sur une asphyxie locale des extremities avec polydactylite suppurative chronique et pouseés epheméres dermatitae pustuleuse disséminée et symetrique. Bull Soc Fr Dermatol Syph 1:39–45

Kuijpers AL, van Dooren-Grebe RJ, van de Kerkhof PC (1996) Acrodermatitis continua of Hallopeau: response to combined treatment with acitretin and calcipotriol ointment. Dermatology 192:357–359

Pearson LH, Allen BS, Smith JG Jr (1984) Acrodermatitis continua of Hallopeau: treatment with etretinate and review of relapsing pustular eruptions of the hands and feet. J Am Acad Dermatol 11:755–762

Piraccini BM, Fanti PA, Morelli R et al. (1994) Hallopeau's acrodermatitis continua of the nail apparatus: a clinical and pathological study of 20 patients. Acta Derm Venereol (Stockh) 74:65–67

Palmoplantar Pustulosis

Andrews GC, Birkman FW, Kelly RJ (1934) Recalcitrant pustular eruptions of the palms and soles. Arch Dermatol Syphil 29:548–563

Burge SM, Ryan TJ (1985) Acute palmoplantar pustulosis. Br J Dermatol 113:77–83

Eriksson MO, Hagforsen E, Lundin IP et al. (1998) Palmoplantar pustulosis: a clinical and immunohistological study. Br J Dermatol 138:390–398

Lindelöf B, Beitner H (1990) The effect of grenzray therapy on pustulosis palmoplantaris. Acta Dermatol Venereol (Stockh) 70:529–531

Stevens DM, Ackerman BA (1984) On the concept of bacterids (pustular bacterid, Andrews). Am J Dermatopathol 6:281–286

Erosive Pustular Dermatosis of the Scalp

Bieber T, Ruzicka T, Burg G (1987) Erosive pustulöse Dermatitis des Kapillitiums. Hautarzt 38:687–689

Caputo R, Veraldi S (1993) Erosive pustular dermatosis of the scalp. J Am Acad Dermatol 28:96–98

Jacyk WK (1988) Pustular ulcerative dermatosis of the scalp. Br J Dermatol 118:441–444

Pye RJ, Peachey RDG, Burton JL (1979) Erosive pustular dermatosis of the scalp. Br J Dermatol 100:559–566

Watanabe S, Takizawa K, Hashimoto N et al. (1989) Pustular dermatosis of the scalp associated with autoimmune diseases. J Dermatol 16:383–387

Erythema Toxicum Neonatorum

Ferrandiz C, Coroleu W, Ribera M et al. (1992) Sterile transient neonatal pustulosis is a precocious form of erythema toxicum neonatorum. Dermatology 185:18–22

Schwartz RA, Janniger CK (1996) Erythema toxicum neonatorum. Cutis 58:153–155

Transient Neonatal Pustular Melanosis

Hansen LP, Brandrup F, Zori R (1985) Erythema toxicum neonatorum mit Pustulation versus transitonische neonatale pustulöse Melanose. Hautarzt 36:475–477

Ramamurthy RS, Reveri M, Esterly NB et al. (1976) Transient neonatal pustular melanosis. J Pediatr 88:831–835

Wyre HW, Murphy MO (1979) Transient neonatal pustular melanosis. Arch Dermatol 115:458

Transient Cephalic Neonatal Pustulosis

Aractingi S, Cadranel S, Reygagne P et al. (1991) Neonatal pustulosis induced by Malassezia furfur. Ann Dermatol Venereol 118:856–858

Bardazzi F, Patrizi A (1997) Transient cephalic neonatal pustulosis. Arch Dermatol 133:528–530

Niamba P, Weill FX, Sarlangue J (1998) Is common neonatal cephalic pustulosis (neonatal acne) triggered by Malassezia sympodialis? Arch Dermatol 134:995–998

Subcorneal Pustular Dermatosis

Bauwens M, De Conick A, Roseeuw D (1999) Subcorneal pustular dermatosis treated with PUVA therapy. A case report and review of the literature. Dermatology 203–205

Chimenti S, Ackerman AB (1981) Is subcorneal pustular dermatosis of Sneddon and Wilkinson an entity sui generis? Am J Dermatopathol 3:363–376

Ise S, Ofuji S (1965) Subcorneal pustular dermatosis. A follicular variant? Arch Dermatol 92:169–171

Kasha EE, Epinette WW (1988) Subcorneal pustular dermatosis (Sneddon-Wilkinson disease) in association with a monoclonal IgA-gammopathy: A report and review of the literature. J Am Acad Dermatol 19:854–858

Lutz ME, Daoud MS, McEvoy MT et al. (1998) Subcorneal pustular dermatosis: a clinical study of ten patients. Cutis 61:203–208

Sneddon IB, Wilkinson DD (1956) Subcorneal pustular dermatosis. Br J Dermatol 68:385–394

Sneddon IB, Wilkinson DS (1979) Subcorneal pustular dermatosis. Br J Dermatol 100:61–68

Stolz W, Bieber T, Meurer M (1989) Its the atypical neutrophilic dermatosis with subcorneal IgA deposits a variant of pemphigus foliaceus? Br J Dermatol 120:276–279

Impetigo Herpetiformis

Breier-Maly J, Ortel B, Breier F et al. (1999) Generalized pustular psoriasis of pregnancy (impetigo herpetiformis) Dermatology 198:61–64

Hebra F (1872) Über einzelne während der Schwangerschaft, dem Wochenbette, und bei Uterinalkrankheiten der Frauen zu beobachtende Hautkrankheiten. Wien Med Wochenschr 48:1197–1202

Kaposi M (1887) Impetigo herpetiformis. Arch Dermatol Syph 19:273–296

Moynihan GD, Ruppe JP (1985) Impetigo herpetiformis and hypoparathyroidism. Arch Dermatol 121:1330–1331

Acute Generalized Pustulosis

Beylot C, Doutre MS, Beylot-Barry M (1996) Acute generalized exanthematous pustulosis. Semin Cut Med Surg 15:244–249

Braun-Falco O, Luderschmidt C, Maciejewski W et al. (1978) Pustulosis acuta generalisata. Eine ungewöhnliche Erscheinungsform von leukozytoklastischer Vaskulitis. Hautarzt 29:371–377

MacMillan AL (1973) Generalized pustular drug rash. Dermatologica 146:285–291

Roujeau JC, Bioulac-Sage P, Bourseau C et al. (1991) Acute generalized exanthematous pustulosis. Analysis of 60 cases. Arch Dermatol 127:1333–1338

Tan RSH (1974) Acute generalized pustular bacterid. An unusual manifestation of leukocytoclastic vasculitis. Br J Dermatol 91:209–215

Zelickson BD, Muller SA (1991) Generalized pustular psoriasis. A review of 63 cases. Arch Dermatol 127:1339–1345

CHAPTER 17

Disorders of Keratinization

Contents

Basic Science Aspects

The disorders of keratinization can be best understood within the framework of normal epidermal differentiation. The outermost layer of the epidermis, the stratum corneum, provides the interface between man and his external world. The epidermis is a multiple layered keratinizing squamous epithelium. Besides keratinocytes, there are three other important cell populations in the epidermis: melanocytes, Langerhans cells or epidermal antigen-processing cells and Merkel cells which appear to function as mechanoreceptors interacting with peripheral nerves. On ultrastructural examination, the melanosomes are characterized by immature melanosomes (stage I–II), the Langerhans cells by Birbeck granules, the Merkel cells by dense core granules, and the keratinocytes by tonofilaments and desmosomes.

The rete pegs form a three-dimensional jigsaw puzzle-like mesh with the dermal papillae providing epidermal-dermal cohesion. On a finer level, the hemidesmosomes and basement membrane zone complete the attachment. Mechanical trauma, proteolytic enzymes, 1.0 M salt solutions and heat can all destroy the attachment, producing epidermal-dermal separation.

The basic scaffolding of the epidermis is provided by the meshwork of tonofibrils, which are fine bundles of the keratin intermediate filaments. They attach to the desmosomes and the hemidesmosomes, as well as form a network around the nucleus. The intermediate filaments or 10-nm filaments are so named because they are larger than the actin microfilaments but smaller than the myosin and tubulin filaments. The various intermediate filaments help distinguish types of epithelial cells, and monoclonal antibodies against them are used in pathology to determine the differentiation of many epithelial tumors. The desmosomes are continually being opened and closed as the keratinocytes migrate upwards. They can almost be viewed as magnetic junctions. The autoantibodies in several variants of pemphigus are directed against proteins of the desmosome.

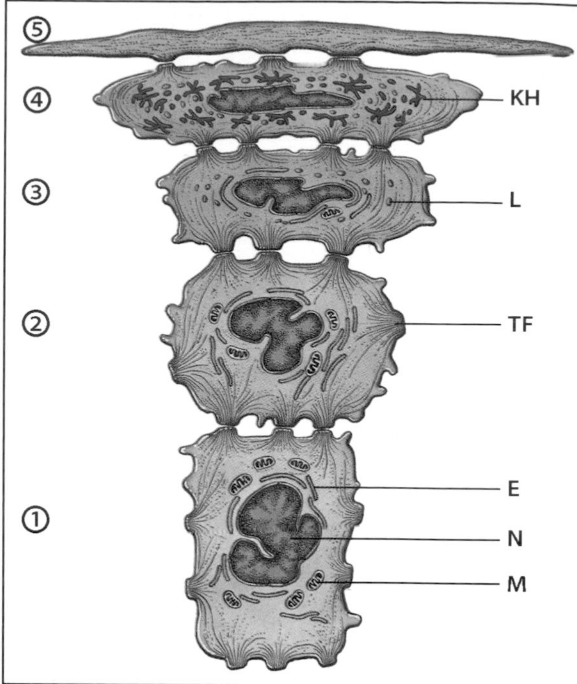

Fig. 17.1. Schematic view of keratinization. *1* Stratum basale; *2, 3* Stratum spinosum; *4* Stratum granulosum; *5* Stratum corneum. *M* Mitochondrion, *N* nucleus, *E* endoplasmic reticulum, *TF* tonofilament bundle, *L* lamellar body, *KH* keratohyaline granule

Types of Keratinocytes

The different layers of the epidermis can be readily distinguished and have different functions. As Fig. 17.1 shows, the cell morphology changes from a columnar vertical orientation to a flattened horizontal appearance in the course of differentiation towards the surface. Throughout the book we use the Latin and English names for these layers interchangeably.

- Stratum Basale (Basal Layer). The cells are vertically oriented, and about 5% show mitoses. The keratin intermediate filaments or tonofilaments (8–10 nm) can be seen as they aggregate into tonofibrils (25 nm). This is the beginning of the process of keratinization. The basal layer keratinocytes are also able to synthesize some of the components of the basement membrane zone including bullous pemphigoid antigen 1, type IV collagen, some of the laminins and fibronectin. This capacity has been best studied in wound healing. In addition, on their surface they display a number of integrins which bind to basement membrane and extracellular matrix protein ligands.
- Stratum Spinosum (Spinous Layer). These rhomboidal cells have an extensive intermediate filament network. The desmosome attachments are firm enough that when the epidermis is fixed for routine histology, shrinkage occurs between the desmosomes so the cells appear to be held together by spiny processes. The cells are more rounded or polygonal. Lamellar bodies (membrane-coating granules, Odland bodies, keratinosomes) also appear in the upper stratum spinosum. They are found near the external surface of the cells and eventually discharge their lipid contents to form the epidermal lipid barrier.
- Stratum Granulosum (Granular Layer). This layer is normally only two or three cells thick; it may be absent in pathological conditions such as porokeratosis, psoriasis and ichthyosis vulgaris and is much thicker on the palms and soles. The flat cells have a horizontal orientation. The keratohyaline granules contain profilaggrin,

which is converted to filaggrin as the conversion to stratum corneum occurs. Filaggrin binds keratin together in the lower layers of the stratum corneum, but is then degraded.

- Stratum Lucidum. Found only on the palms and soles, this opaque layer consists of densely packed markedly elongated but still nucleated keratinocytes in which the intermediate filaments and filaggrin are already combined.
- Stratum Corneum (Cornified or Horny Layer). The keratinocyte (also called a corneocyte) is no longer nucleated; it is a dry shadow of its former self. Many enzymes appear during the transition to this stage. They are needed for destroying the nucleus and other organelles, opening the lamellar bodies, converting profilaggrin to filaggrin and forming the cornified envelope. The latter develops just beneath the plasma membrane of the keratinocyte; precursor molecules include involucrin, loricrin and many others; These are linked together by transglutaminases, which are classic marker enzymes for this region. The best known so-called late markers of differentiation are filaggrin, involucrin and loricrin. Involucrin is a very primitive α-helical flexible protein that contains a regular number of glutamic acids in positions favorable to forming cross-linkages with lysyl groups. Involucrin expression is abnormal in psoriasis. Loricrin is contained in L-granules, is extremely insoluble, rich in glycine and serine, and helps to glue materials together in the cornified envelope once it is released.
The residual filaggrin in the corneocytes is degraded into free amino acids and other compounds which can bind water. These substances are known as the natural moisturizing factor (NMF); they are also described as the non-keratin part of the corneocyte or as natural humectants. Right at the transition from the stratum granulosum to the stratum corneum there is also an extracellular accumulation of lipids and polysaccharides that provides a coating for the corneocytes and resistance against water. Loss of these lipids and the NMF leads to drying out of the skin.
Electron microscopic observation shows that the corneocytes contain a thick accumulation of relatively contrast-poor intermediate filaments embedded in a homogeneous matrix mainly comprising filaggrin. The cell membrane is also much thicker because of the addition of the cornified envelope; it is about 15 nm thick and attached to the protein envelope by a layer of ω-hydroxyceramides. The corneocyte continues to lose water and flatten until it is shed. This loss is not noticed and is thus described as insensible desquamation. If more scales are shed, this is known as dander in animals or dandruff in humans. On X-ray diffraction, the epithelial keratins are primarily arranged in the α or coiled pattern, as compared to the β-pleated sheet of amyloid. A variety of chemical bonds hold the keratins in this secondary structure; disulfide bonds appear particularly important.

Types of Keratins

The process of keratinization is very complex. Approximately 30 epithelial cytokeratins have been recognized. We will refer to these substances as keratins. They are subdivided first into acidic and basic keratins and then divided on the basis of their molecular weight. Almost all keratins are only expressed in fixed pairs, one basic and one acidic. In the human epidermis, types 5 and 14 are expressed in the basal layer, while types 1 and 10 are seen in the higher layers. Mutations in type 5 or 14 lead to the changes of epidermolysis bullosa simplex, while mutations in type 1 or 10 cause disturbances in differentiation discussed in this chapter. Abnormalities in the matrix protein filaggrin or the cornified envelope proteins involucrin and loricrin also lead to an abnormal final structure. The major components of the desmosomes, such as plakoglobin and the cadherins desmoplakin and desmocollin can be altered by mutations, leading to inherited disorders of keratinization and adherence, or can be the target of antibodies leading to autoimmune blistering disorders.

Epidermal Lipids

The epidermal lipids have been the focus of much exciting work in recent years. The model of the epidermis as brick and mortar is perhaps simplistic but has contributed to our understanding of many diseases. In the simplest terms, the keratins and other proteins provide the bricks and the epidermal lipids are the major component of the mortar. For the most part, mutations in structural proteins are inherited in an autosomal dominant pattern, while mutations in enzymes which lead to lipid disturbances are inherited in an autosomal recessive pattern. The main neutral lipids are glycerolphosphatides, triglycerides, free fatty acids, free and esterified sterols, and saturated aliphatic carbohydrates. In addition, complex sphingolipids such as ceramides and glycosylceramides are found in the skin and nervous system, helping explain why there are inherited disorders affecting both systems.

The lipid patterns change during the process of keratinization and appear to play an active role in guiding the process. In the basal cells, the most prominent lipids are the phospholipids as the primary components of the plasma membrane. As keratinization progresses, the neutral lipids and sphingolipids become more prominent eventually forming the lipid lamellae of the stratum corneum. Abnormalities in the lipids can lead to abnormal barrier function, lack of cohesion and abnormal desquamation. Often the normal shedding is delayed, leading to retention hyperkeratosis.

Epidermal Turnover

The major protective barrier interacting with the outer world is provided by the shedding scales of the stratum corneum. Other species have a thick, almost inert cuticle, a coating of slimy protein or very thick hard scales. In humans the stratum corneum must be constantly renewed. One can divide the epidermis into two compartments:

- Proliferative compartment: Stratum basale and perhaps lower part of stratum spinosum, especially in acanthotic areas.
- Differentiating compartment: The bulk of the stratum spinosum, as well as the stratum granulosum and stratum corneum.

Under normal conditions, mitoses are only found in the basal layer. There is about one mitosis per 400 basal cells when one studies sections of fixed tissue. Studies with [^{3}H]thymidine show that at any given time, about 5% of basal cells are synthesizing DNA (S_1 phase). The stem cells divide to produce another stem cell and a basal cell with limited life expectancy which divides a number of times. The basal cells then slowly migrate to the stratum granulosum, forming and reforming desmosomes and undergoing differentiation. It is estimated that the passage from the basal layer to the stratum granulosum takes 14 days, and the interval between the stratum granulosum and final desquamation is another 14 days, for a total epidermal turnover time of above 28 days.

When the turnover is accelerated as in psoriasis, pityriasis rubra pilaris and some forms of ichthyosis, the total time may be as short as 8–10 days. The stratum corneum may still show normal orthokeratotic keratinization or it may have marked parakeratosis, suggesting impaired cornification. The proliferation and differentiation phases are not automatically coupled.

The intrinsic control of the epidermal cell cycle rate is one of the persistent mysteries of dermatology. Many theories have been advanced but few have stood the test of time. The response of the keratinocytes to injury, UV radiation and other stimulatory factors is slightly better understood. The keratinocytes are far more active cells than initially thought. When stimulated, they secrete a vast array of cytokines, may express more basement membrane zone antigens and frequently express a pair of keratins, 6 and 16, not seen in normal skin. Epidermal growth factor (EGF) and its receptor form one mechanism of control. When EGF binds to the EGF receptor, the latter dimerizes and via tyrosine kinase initiates a series of phosphorylation events that eventually influence the nucleus, guiding differentiation and activation. For example, EGF is capable of turning on keratins 6 and 16. Intracellular interleukin (IL)-1 may also play a role, as when it is released from an injured cell, it is first able to bind to its receptors on the neighboring cells triggering activation.

A number of other factors also help control epidermal differentiation. Most work through nuclear receptors and several have therapeutic implications. Nuclear receptors are proteins that bind firmly to their trigger or stimulatory molecule and also interact with the DNA to modulate the transcription of various genes. The retinoid receptors are best understood. There are two major groups known as RAR and RXR. The former bind most tightly to retinoic acid, while the latter interact with 9-*cis*-retinoic acid. The complex interaction of the different retinoids and the their receptors helps explain the role of these agents in disorders of epidermal differentiation. The retinoids in general downregulate expression of differentiation markers such as keratins 1 and 10 and filaggrin. While we are most interested in their epidermal effects, retinoids may also cause some leukemic cells to differentiate more normally. Vitamin D also plays an important role in epidermal differentiation, acting to promote or upregulate the process. There are also specific nuclear receptors for vitamin D which is also converted to its most active metabolite, vitamin D_3 or 1,25-dihydroxycholecalciferol, in keratinocytes. Keratinocytes also have receptors for thyroid hormones and steroid hormones, but the details of the interactions are less clear.

Epidermal Function

The intact stratum corneum is responsible for limiting water loss and thus evaporative heat loss. When it is damaged, as in psoriasis, both fluid loss and hypothermia may develop. The sebum from the sebaceous glands forms a fine outer film over the stratum corneum, supplementing the role of the epidermal lipids in protecting against water-soluble substances as well as providing a smoother surface. The NMF bind water and thus make a major contribution to smoothness. The epidermis has a pH of 5.7; thus the outer layer has been referred to as the "acid mantle" of the skin. Syndets have been designed with a pH of about 5.7 so that they will not challenge the limited buffer capacity of the epidermis as alkaline soaps do. The epidermis also thickens with repetitive trauma (lichenification) or UV radiation (the *Lichtschwiele*). All of these features are explored in more detail elsewhere in this volume.

Clinico-pathological Correlations

The disorders covered in this chapter all have some defect in keratinization. Some show rapid epidermal turnover (proliferation hyperkeratosis); others, delayed desquamation (retention hyperkeratosis). The end result is similar: the accumulation of thick, clinically obvious scale. These scales may be present at birth or appear later, either widely distributed, arranged about follicles or as focal lesions. In most cases the lesions are identified clinically.

Microscopically one can see a number of changes including a thickened stratum corneum; increased number of mitoses, even in higher levels of the epidermis; and changes in thickness. While acanthosis is most common, ocessionally atropy occurs. The granular layer is thicker in proliferative hyperkeratosis, but normal inretention hyperkeratosis. Nuclei may be retained in the stratum corneum (parakeratosis). Unusual changes include acanthokeratolysis or epidermolytic hyperkeratosis in which there is clumping of keratin and separation of cells in the upper layers of the epidermis, and cornoid lamella, when parakeratotic columns form, as in porokeratosis.

We have divided the disorders of keratinization into seven major groups:

- Ichthyoses: Diffuse hyperkeratotic disorders which in most cases reflect an underlying genetic defect in either keratins or lipids (bricks or mortar) and appear either at birth or in infancy; in rare cases, they can be acquired, caused by underlying tumors, medications or other triggers
- Palmoplantar keratodermas: Thickening alterations confined to the palms and soles, usually because of mutations in keratins which are only expressed in these regions
- Erythrokeratodermias: Rare group of disorders with both erythema and increased scaling
- Follicular keratoses: Diseases in which the hyperkeratotic changes are for the most part confined to hair follicles
- Dykeratotic-acantholytic disorders: Diffuse or localized keratoses which have a distinctive microscopic picture
- Porokeratoses: Diseases with a cornoid lamella
- Other disorders

These divisions are not mutually exclusive or sharply defined. In addition, Darier disease usually has lesions arranged in a follicular pattern but can involve hairless areas and even mucosal surfaces.

Happle has demonstrated that the same mutations which result in widespread disorders of keratinization when inherited from one's parent(s) and expressed in all cells, can cause localized areas of change when the mutation develops in a somatic cell on its way to forming part of the epidermis. Such lesions usually follow Blaschko lines. A corollary of Happle's thesis is that if the somatic mutation also involves gonadal tissue, i.e., if it occurs early in embryonic life, then a person with a localized mutation could transmit the widespread disease to his offspring. This feature was first convincingly shown in patients with epidermolytic epidermal nevi (Chaps. 19, 52) whose children had widespread epidermolytic hyperkeratosis, also known as congenital bullous ichthyosiform erythroderma.

Ichthyoses

The ichthyoses are a large heterogeneous group of disorders, typically involving most of the body and usually present at birth or shortly thereafter. Traupe, whose monograph on this subject *The Ichthyoses* is very informative, has divided them into four workable categories, as shown in Table 17.1.

Another useful listing is that of Williams, who has attached DOC (disorders of cornification) numbers to each entity; these are given under the synonyms. The therapy of all these disorders is similar, so it is discussed at length under the most common form, ichthyosis vulgaris, and then only briefly mentioned for the rest if additional approaches are available.

Ichthyosis Vulgaris

Synonyms. Autosomal dominant ichthyosis vulgaris, ichthyosis simplex, DOC 1

Definition. Most common disorder of keratinization with diffuse scaling and highly variable degree of involvement.

Epidemiology. The most common ichthyosis, with estimates of prevalence ranging from 1:250 to 1:500. The highly variable expression means that many patients are not diagnosed as having ichthyosis but as having dry skin. This is particularly true in blacks. There is a clear association with atopic dermatitis.

Etiology and Pathogenesis. The defect in ichthyosis vulgaris appears to lie in the profilaggrin molecule, which is missing in severe forms and reduced in milder forms. The exact genetic defect for this disorder which is inherited in an autosomal dominant pattern has not been determined but it is likely to be a structural defect in filaggrin. The epidermal turnover is very slow, so ichthyosis vulgaris is the prototype of a retention hyperkeratosis.

Clinical Findings. The scaly lesions are not present at birth but usually appear in the first few months. In rare cases, the problems first become apparent later. The sites of predilection are the extensor surfaces of the extremities and the trunk. The symmetrically distributed light-gray scales vary in quality from thick adherent shiny plates to simply dusty accumulations which when scratched leave a mark just as when one touches a dusty surface. The truncal lesions tend to be thicker, and those on the face and scalp thinner. The rims of the ears are often scaly. The antecubital and popliteal fossae are typically spared, as are the inguinal and axillary regions (Fig. 17.2). Almost all patients have hyperlinear palms and soles, known in German as ichthyosis hand. In addition many have keratosis pilaris or follicular keratosis. The eyelids are unaffected. There is no mucosal involvement.

About 25–33% of patients have atopic dermatitis. Looking at the problem backwards, about 2–4% of randomly chosen atopic dermatitis patients have histologic evidence of ichthyosis vulgaris. Once the gene for ichthyosis vulgaris is identified, the latter number can be accurately refined. When an ichthyosis vulgaris patient has severe pruritus or flexural involvement, the answer is usually atopic dermatitis. Many atopic dermatitis

Table 17.1. Types of ichthyosis

Noncongenital (vulgar) ichthyoses		Congenital ichthyoses	
Skin only	**Skin and associated manifestations**	**Skin only**	**Skin and associated manifestations**
Ichthyosis vulgaris	Associated steroid sulfatase deficiency	Lamellar ichthyoses (including collodion baby)	Sjögren-Larsson syndrome
XLR ichthyosis	Multiple sulfatase deficiency	Harlequin ichthyosis	Trichothiodystrophy syndromes
	Refsum syndrome	Epidermolytic ichthyoses	Comèl-Netherton syndrome
		Ichthyosis hystrix Curth-Macklin	Dorfman-Chanarin syndrome
		Peeling skin syndrome A	XLD chondrodysplasia punctata
		Peeling skin syndrome B	Ichthyosis hystrix Rheydt (HID) Ichthyosis follicularis with atrichia and photophobia

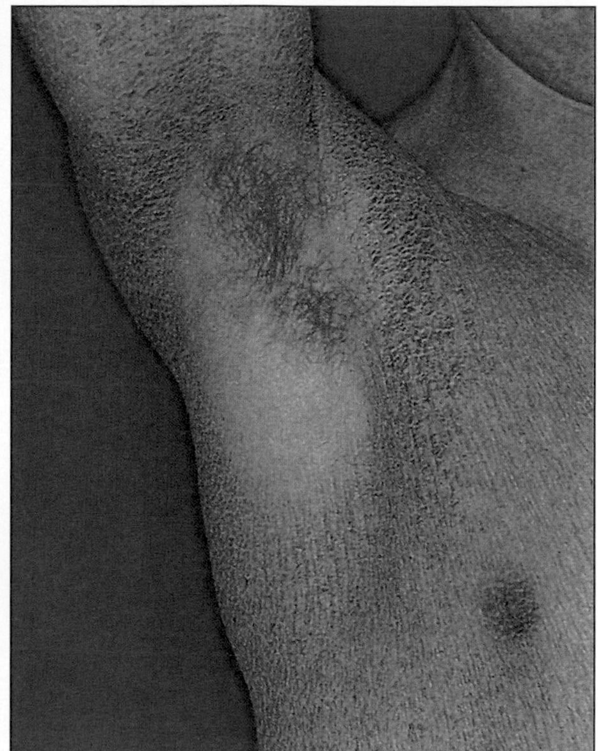

Fig. 17.2. Ichthyosis vulgaris

patients also have hyperlinear palms, so here the relationship is not quite as clear. Ichthyosis vulgaris patients do not have CNS or other associated defects to a greater extent than the general population.

Histopathology. The classic finding is the presence of minimal compact orthokeratosis associated with an absent granular layer. Follicles often are plugged. The dermis is normal; inflammation is either secondary to treatment, infection or atopic dermatitis. Electron microscopy reveals abnormal keratohyaline granules, a finding which supports the role of filaggrin in the pathogenesis. The distinction between dry skin and mild ichthyosis vulgaris remains unclear. The best test is a skin biopsy searching for a reduced granular layer. Since this distinction is rarely of clinical importance, the biopsy is usually not done.

Course and Prognosis. The disease tends to wax and wane. Most patients are better in the summer. In addition, there is usually improvement at puberty so that the patient's impression is often that of only dry skin. The patients should avoid drying soaps, not use sensitizing topical agents because their period of exposure is likely to be long, and receive the same job counseling as atopic dermatitis patients.

Differential Diagnosis. Ichthyosis vulgaris is the mildest of the ichthyoses. One should search for flexural sparing and hyperlinear palms. X-linked recessive ichthyosis is the closest form clinically.

Therapy

Systemic. In contrast to some of the other ichthyoses, for ichthyosis vulgaris the use of systemic retinoids is rarely indicated and not very helpful. In those patients whose "severity" is actually a manifestation of atopic dermatitis, retinoids may produce worsening.

Topical. The mainstays of topical therapy are avoiding drying measures and proper lubrication. During the first few years of life, bath or shower oils and bland ointments suffice. Later on, one may employ creams or lotions containing urea, lactic acid or table salt as humectants; these products cause too much pruritus in infants.

Genetic Counseling. While the risk of transmission to offspring is 50%, the disease is mild enough that few patients desire to alter their family planning.

X-Linked Recessive Ichthyosis

(Wells and Kerr 1965)

Synonyms. X-linked ichthyosis, DOC 2

Definition. Uncommon ichthyosis with dirty brown scales which is seen only in men.

Epidemiology. The incidence has been estimated at between 1:2000 and 1:6000 male births.

Etiology and Pathogenesis. The gene involved in X-linked recessive ichthyosis is the steroid sulfatase gene located at Xp22.3, an unusual part of the X chromosome which does not always undergo inactivation under the terms of the Lyon hypothesis. This means that even in individuals "normal" at this locus, there is a different gene dosage in men and women. In the skin, steroid sulfatase functions in the stratum granulosum to convert cholesterol sulfate to cholesterol. When this process is deranged, the lamellar lipid film is more adhesive, leading to less shedding of scale and retention hyperkeratosis. The defective gene can be identified, but there are other laboratory tools for the diagnosis.

Clinical Findings. There may be fine scales present in the first weeks of life. But the characteristic dark brown rhomboid scales first appear at age 3–4 months. The nape is almost always involved, producing the poorly named dirty neck sign. Old reports spoke of ichthyosis nigricans, but this has caused confusion. At least 25% of patients have fine light scales as in ichthyosis vulgaris, so false diagnoses were made. The trunk and extensor aspects of the extremities are once again the major sites, but flexural sparing, hyperlinear palms and keratosis pilaris are all unlikely to be seen.

X-linked recessive ichthyosis is associated with several problems. Depending on the pedigree, the incidence of corneal opacities involving Descemet membrane has been estimated as high as 50% but is much lower in our experience. In addition, female carriers may have both mild ichthyosis, especially on the nape and extremities, and allegedly also ocular findings, but this is not a reliable screening test. A more important problem for both the mother and affected son is the steroid sulfatase deficiency in the placenta which may lead to inadequate cervical dilatation and problems with labor. At least 20% of the boys have cryptorchism which in some cases leads to hypogonadism.

Histopathology. The biopsy shows a thickened stratum corneum, a normal granular layer and perhaps even mild epidermal atrophy. In some pedigrees, the granular layer has been reduced. There are no diagnostic ultrastructural features.

Laboratory Findings. Steroid sulfatase levels can be measured, both to detect patients and carriers. Unfortunately, this test is available in only a few laboratories in the world. The simplest test is to order a routine lipoprotein electrophoresis; the increased cholesterol sulfate and reduced cholesterol leads to an increased rate of migration for the β-lipoproteins. The laboratory must know what the physician is seeking, otherwise this feature will be overlooked. In addition, cholesterol sulfate (and aryl sulfatase C, an isoenzyme) levels in corneocytes, red blood cell membranes and serum can be measured in specialized centers.

Course and Prognosis. The disease tends to smolder along, without the improvement seen in ichthyosis vulgaris. While the severity of the skin disease varies from pedigree to pedigree greatly, in any given family the features tend to be relatively consistent and permanent.

Differential Diagnosis. The main issue is separating ichthyosis vulgaris and X-linked recessive ichthyosis.

Therapy. In severe cases, systemic retinoid therapy has proven effective, probably by altering the lipids of the stratum corneum. It can be used to produce a temporary remission which can then hopefully be prolonged with adequate topical care.

Genetic Counseling. The mother and other appropriate female relatives should be aware they are carriers, not so much because of the severity of the skin problems but so they can alert their obstetrician to possible difficulties in subsequent pregnancies. In addition, the patient with X-linked recessive ichthyosis must tell his daughters they are obligate carriers.

Associated Steroid Sulfatase Deficiency

A number of other important genes are located close to the steroid sulfatase gene. If a deletion is larger, it may include some of these genes, producing a contiguous gene syndrome. Two closely linked genes are those for Kallman syndrome (hypogonadotrophic hypogonadism and anosmia) and X-linked recessive chondrodysplasia punctata. Possible linkage to a gene for hypertrophic pyloric stenosis has also been described. Thus patients may present with the skin changes of X-linked recessive ichthyosis but with a whole spectrum of other problems.

Multiple Sulfatase Deficiency

Synonyms. Sulfatidosis, DOC 13

Multiple sulfatase deficiency is a severe neuropediatric disorder inherited in an autosomal recessive pattern. Patients develop normally for the first several years and then begin to show striking losses in mental capacity and motor abilities. The ichthyosis is usually mild and the least of their problems. There is no successful therapy; prenatal diagnosis is possible.

Refsum Syndrome

(REFSUM 1945)

Synonyms. Heredopathica atactica polyneuritiformis, DOC 11

Definition. Extremely rare ichthyosis associated with lipid abnormalities and neurologic problems.

Epidemiology. Refsum was a Norwegian neurologist who identified the first cases in his native land. Fewer than 100 cases have been reported in the intervening half century.

Etiology and Pathogenesis. Refsum syndrome belongs to the general family of peroxisome abnormalities. Peroxisomes perform a wide variety of tasks including bile acid and cholesterol biosynthesis. They are often associated with dysmorphic features, neurological problems and hepatic abnormalities. In classical Refsum syndrome, the patients have ichthyosis and a defect in the α-oxidation of phytanic acid. In at least some individuals the error is in the peroxisomal enzyme phytanoyl-CoA hydroxylase; in other cases, it may be in phytanic acid α-oxidase. Both defects are inherited in an autosomal recessive pattern. Phytanic acid is a byproduct of chlorophyll metabolism that accumulates. The elevated phytanic acid levels may lower the free cholesterol levels by esterification and subsequent storage, thus mimicking X-linked recessive ichthyosis or it may interfere with free fatty acid metabolism.

Clinical Findings. The ichthyosis usually begins to appear gradually, often in childhood or around the time of puberty. The skin changes are similar to those in ichthyosis vulgaris; hyperlinear palms may be seen. A peculiar finding is the presence of yellow melanocytic nevi because of lipid storage. More severe problems include loss of vision from retinitis pigmentosa, cardiac arrhythmias and a whole spectrum of neurological problems including bilateral sensorineural deafness, cerebellar ataxia and peripheral polyneuropathies.

Histopathology. On routine light microscopy, the skin appears identical to that in ichthyosis vulgaris. When a biopsy is fixed in alcohol and a Sudan stain done, lipid droplets are found in the keratinocytes. The same inclusions can be shown with ultrastructural examination.

Laboratory Findings. Specialized laboratories can measure the elevated phytanic acid.

Differential Diagnosis. One must consider both ichthyosis vulgaris and X-linked recessive ichthyosis. In some cases, the retinitis pigmentosa or deafness is the first sign, shifting the differential diagnosis in those directions.

Therapy. Dietary restriction of phytanic acid can lead to marked improvement. The patient must restrict intake of green vegetables and milk products. The diet must be introduced slowly or the disease can temporarily worsen. In such flares, plasmapheresis has been employed. The skin is treated with routine topical care.

Genetic Counseling. The problem with Refsum syndrome is that the diagnosis is usually delayed until well into adult life. Thus, the parents are likely to have had more children before discovering their problem. Prenatal diagnosis and heterozygote testing, searching for the missing or reduced enzyme, is possible.

Lamellar Ichthyosis

(RIECKE 1900)

Synonym. Ichthyosis congenita

There are three types of lamellar ichthyosis which are clinically quite similar and account for most cases of congenital ichthyosis. In addition, most collodion babies evolve into this category. The two most common forms are inherited in an autosomal recessive pattern but have biochemical differences while there is a much rarer autosomal dominant form. As a group their incidence is less than 1:10,000 births.

Lamellar Ichthyosis with Transglutaminase Deficiency

Synonyms. Nonerythrodermic lamellar ichthyosis (NELI), classic lamellar ichthyosis, DOC 4

Etiology and Pathogenesis. The disease is inherited in an autosomal recessive pattern; the defective gene is located on chromosome 14 and codes for transglutaminase-1. This defect can be identified in cultured keratinocytes or identified histochemically in frozen skin sections.

Clinical Findings. The various forms of lamellar ichthyosis show striking overlaps and it is only in recent years that they have been separated out. In this type, the clinical findings will gradually be refined now that a definite biochemical marker is available. Many patients are born as a collodion baby with a thick membrane which splits and is then shed. They develop thick dark scales which are polygonal and separated by fissures (Fig. 17.3). Despite the name, there is also an associated erythema. The palms and soles may be macerated are not as hyperkeratotic as other variants. The face may be distorted as ectropion of the lower lid, eclabion (distorted widely opened lips, unfortunately called fish mouth) and adherence of the external ears to the scalp may be seen (Fig. 17.4). The hair may be sparse and nail dystrophies occur.

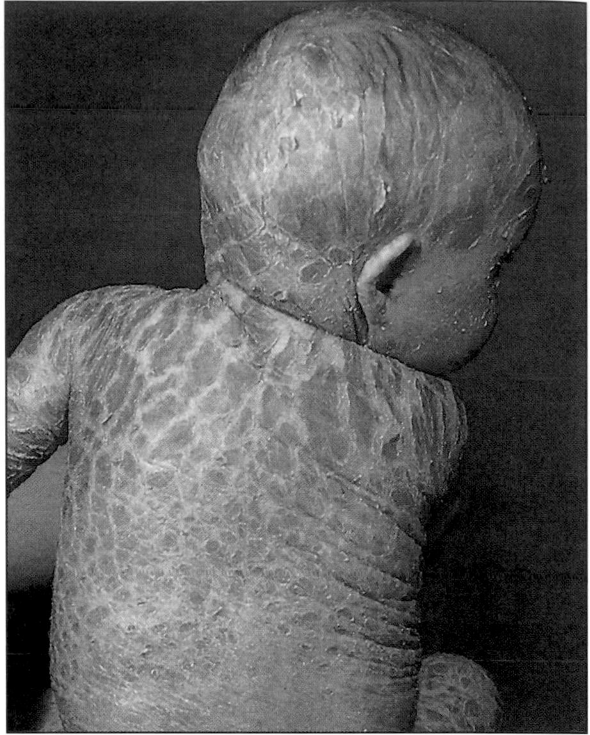

Fig. 17.3. Lamellar ichthyosis with transglutaminase deficiency

Histopathology. The epidermis shows orthokeratosis with a prominent granular layer. This is an example of a proliferative hyperkeratosis. Increased mitoses can be found, and the epidermal turnover is reduced. A wide range of ultrastructural findings have been reported in lamellar ichthyosis, but unfortunately they correlate poorly with the clinical pattern and can only be applied by those few centers with extensive experience.

Course and Prognosis. The disease persists throughout life. Both the skin and ocular problems are quite disabling. Patients may have temperature intolerance because of plugged eccrine ducts.

Differential Diagnosis. The main differential diagnostic considerations are the other forms of lamellar ichthyosis. In adults, severe X-linked recessive ichthyosis can appear similarly.

Therapy

Systemic. Both of the autosomal recessive forms of lamellar ichthyosis are severe enough that systemic retinoids are often used. Even in infants where the risks of growth retardation are significant, the choice is still often to use the retinoids. Generally acitretin 0.3–0.5 mg/kg is employed. Prior to treatment there should be baseline radiologic examination of the spine and large joints, but yearly re-examinations are no longer recommended. Only in the presence of symptoms or a marked dropping off from the normal growth curve are re-examinations needed. Interval therapy is encouraged. Hepatic function, as well as cholesterol and triglyceride levels, should be checked periodically.

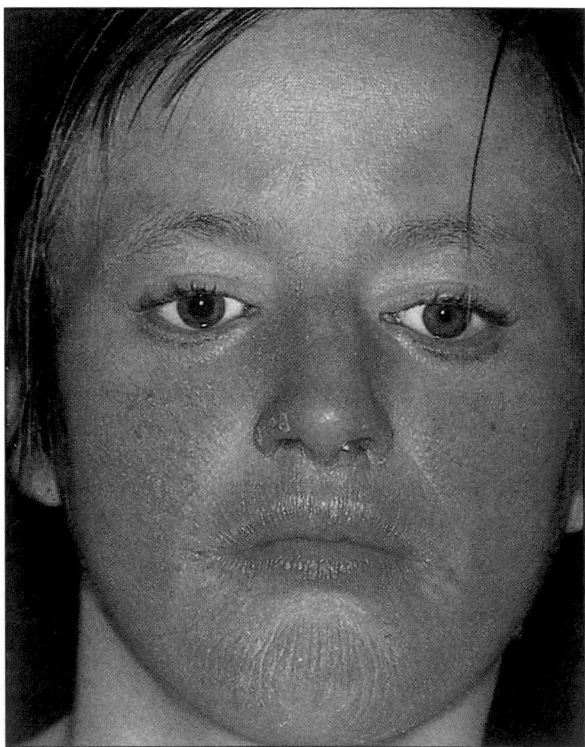

Fig. 17.4. Lamellar ichthyosis with transglutaminase deficiency

Topical. Lactic acid, especially in the form of buffered ammonium lactate is an effective topical agent. A combination of urea 10% and lactic acid 5% in a bland vehicle seems helpful. Topical retinoids help. We have found mixing either the gel or cream forms designed for acne with an emollient vehicle in a ratio of 1:2 to 1:4 helpful.

Genetic Counseling. Fetal skin biopsy has been employed for the diagnosis but one is on the border because the characteristic changes occur after 20 weeks.

Nonbullous Congenital Ichthyosiform Erythroderma

Synonyms. Autosomal recessive lamellar ichthyosis with normal transglutaminase levels, erythrodermic lamellar ichthyosis (ELI), DOC 5

Etiology and Pathogenesis. The etiology is not known. We suspect because of the wide variety of ultrastructural features described that this group contains more than one basic defect. In several families, a mutation has been mapped to chromosome 2q33–35, but the gene function is unknown.

Clinical Findings. These patients present at birth with erythroderma and sometimes with a collodion membrane. The erythroderma tends to fade and they develop somewhat finer, gray-white scales which are diffusely distributed (Fig. 17.5). Palmoplantar keratoderma, nail dystrophies and alopecia may also be seen. Ectropion is less likely.

Histopathology. There may be more parakeratosis and less hyperkeratosis than in the transglutaminase deficiency form, but this is a poor way to tell the two apart.

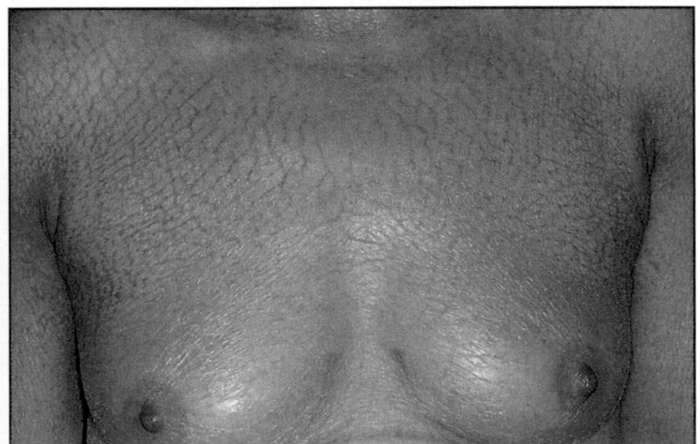

Fig. 17.5. Non-bullous congenital ichthyosiform erythroderma

Course and Prognosis. The disease is quite persistent and relentless.

Differential Diagnosis. Once again, the other forms of lamellar ichthyosis must be excluded. In older patients, there may be clinical overlaps with ichthyosis vulgaris.

Therapy. The same approaches as discussed for the non-inflammatory form apply here.

Autosomal Dominant Lamellar Ichthyosis
(Traupe et al. 1984)

Synonym. DOC 6

Etiology and Pathogenesis. The gene has not been identified.

Clinical Findings. Patients may present as a collodion baby. They later are covered by diffuse dark-gray scales that involve all areas of the body but are prominent on the extensor surfaces where they become lichenified. There may be massive palmar hyperkeratosis with thick yellow scales that occasionally even reach the dorsal aspect of the foot. The palms are usually only minimally involved. Pruritus may be present. The penetrance of the disease is poor with skipped generations and the expressivity is variable.

Histopathology. The stratum corneum may have parakeratosis. On ultrastructural examination, the zone of transition between the stratum granulosum and stratum corneum is often widened.

Course and Prognosis. The course is relatively benign but the pruritus may be troublesome.

Differential Diagnosis. One must consider X-linked recessive ichthyosis and the others forms of lamellar ichthyosis.

Therapy. Usually mild topical measures suffice. Oral retinoids are also effective and can be used if needed.

Collodion Baby

Collodion baby is a clinical description not a disease. All three forms of lamellar ichthyosis as well as other forms of ichthyosis can present with collodium-like sheets of scale covering the body like a membrane. The sheets have usually begun to split at birth and then slowly are shed. The newborns are at great risk for fluid loss, electrolyte imbalance and infections. They require intensive care, usually in a moist chamber with a neutral emollient lotion. Perhaps 10% of collodion babies evolve over a period of months to have normal skin, and this condition has been called self-healing collodion baby or lamellar ichthyosis of the infant, a misleading name. The basis defect is unclear, but the disorder appears to be inherited in an autosomal recessive pattern. Ultrastructural studies have been used to predict which type of ichthyosis will evolve, but it is probably most practical to measure the transglutaminase-1 levels, enquire about affected parents and advise watching and waiting.

Harlequin Ichthyosis

Synonyms. Ichthyosis congenita gravis, harlequin fetus, keratoma malignum, DOC 7

Definition. Most extreme form of congenital ichthyosis with striking keratotic plates separated by deep fissures.

Etiology and Pathogenesis. The gene has not been located. It is likely that several different defects may cause this alarming clinical picture. In most cases, autosomal recessive inheritance seems likely.

Clinical Findings. The newborn infants are covered with thick, armor-like scales, divided by erythematous fissures. Ectropion and eclabion are often present; digits may be mummified or distorted. The appearance is justly described as grotesque. Many infants are stillborn and others die during the first days because their respiratory motions are limited by their shell. The condition in those who survive this period evolves into a severe variant of lamellar ichthyosis.

Histopathology. The stratum corneum is massively thickened, while the stratum granulosum and balance of the epidermis are normal to thinned. On electron microscopic examination, the lamellar bodies have been reduced to absent in some cases.

Course and Prognosis. In the past, the name harlequin fetus was used. But enough children have survived that this additional stress should be spared the parents. The surviving patients do about as well as those with severe lamellar ichthyosis.

Differential Diagnosis. At birth there is no differential diagnosis. Later on other severe forms of ichthyosis could be suggested but the history answers the question.

Therapy. At birth moisturizing measures, temperature control, artificial ventilation and nasogastric feeding are required. Oral retinoids are helpful, although we are skeptical if they are responsible for the survival of patients, since they do not work rapidly enough. They certainly make the first few years of life more tolerable and should be employed. Surgery can help the ocular, labial and digital problems.

Genetic Counseling. The changes are so dramatic that a fetal skin biopsy can be used for diagnosis.

Epidermolytic Ichthyoses

There are several unrelated diseases whose unifying feature is the histologic picture of epidermolytic hyperkeratosis. Because this change involves keratins which are first expressed in the upper part of the stratum spinosum, superficial blisters and erosions are often a clinical feature. All of the disorders are inherited in an autosomal dominant pattern. The group has a frequency estimated at 1:100,000 or less; bullous ichthyosiform erythroderma is the most common.

Bullous Congenital Ichthyosiform Erythroderma

(Brocq 1902)

Synonyms. Epidermolytic hyperkeratosis, bullous ichthyosis, DOC 3

Etiology and Pathogenesis. Mutations in either the keratin 1 or 10 gene are responsible for this ichthyosis. These keratins are expressed as part of terminal differentiation so the changes appear in the upper parts of the epidermis. The disease is inherited in an autosomal dominant pattern. Patients with epidermolytic epidermal nevus may have a mosaic mutation in one of these genes and have parented children with the full-blown disorder.

Clinical Findings. At birth the infants are erythrodermic, have diffuse blistering and almost appear

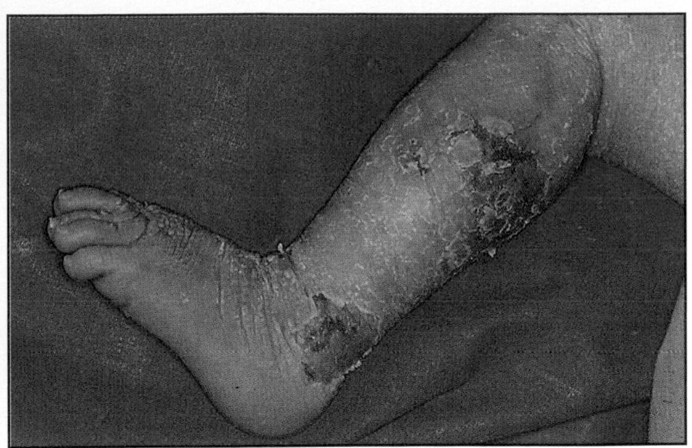

Fig. 17.6. Bullous congenital ichthyosiform erythroderma

burned. Nonetheless focal hyperkeratotic areas may be seen presaging things to come. During the first year, the blistering and erythema gradually resolve and thick dark warty spines or plates evolve (Fig. 17.6). The nape, axilla, groin and flexural folds are sites of predilection; the skin may appear corrugated and is foul smelling. Occasional blisters still arise, often at sites of pressure. Those patients with keratin 1 mutations tend to have palmoplantar keratoderma; those with keratin 10 mutations do not.

Histopathology. The biopsy findings are so striking that bullous ichthyosiform erythroderma was the first disease to be diagnosed microscopically following prenatal skin biopsy. The abnormal keratin 1 or 10 leads to acanthokeratolysis. As the name suggests, this is the combination of epidermal thickening and dishesion. The keratin tonofilaments can be seen as dark clumps on light microscopy; ultrastructural examination reveals them arranged about the nucleus in a shell-like pattern.

Course and Prognosis. The patient can expect occasional bullous flares. Some patients end up with relatively localized disease after puberty.

Differential Diagnosis. Early on the main differential diagnostic question is the neonatal blistering disorders. The clinical features and microscopic pattern provide a definite answer.

Therapy

Systemic. The mainstay of therapy is oral retinoids. One must titer the dose carefully. The lowest level which controls the hyperkeratotic changes is preferred. When this dose is increased, the tendency to blistering may be exacerbated. Short courses of acitretin should be employed for flares. In addition, antibiotics should be employed for suspected pyodermas.

Topical. In contrast to other forms of ichthyosis, these patients tend to get superficial infections. They may benefit from antibacterial soaps routinely. The skin is quite sensitive, so only mild keratolytics should be employed.

Annular Epidermolytic Ichthyosis

Synonym. Autosomal dominant ichthyosis exfoliativa

One pedigree has shown a focal dinucleotide mutation in keratin 10, and perhaps the relatively mild clinical features are explained by the tiny defect. Inheritance is autosomal dominant. In many ways, this is a mild localized variant of bullous ichthyosiform erythroderma. Patients may have mild erythroderma and blisters at birth, but the characteristic feature is the presence of many annular gray hyperkeratotic plaques with a peripheral erythematous border. The skin retains its tendency to blister and becomes easily infected. The histology is that of epidermolytic hyperkeratosis, but with less clumping of keratohyaline. Treatment is similar to that recommended for bullous ichthyosiform erythroderma.

Ichthyosis Bullosa of Siemens

(Siemens 1937)

This rare disorder, also inherited in an autosomal dominant pattern, is caused by a mutation in keratin 2e, an unusual nonpaired keratin expressed only in the stratum granulosum. The patients have a tendency to very superficial blisters that heal without scarring, as well as hyperkeratotic plaques, especially on the extremities and about the umbilicus. No erythroderma is present. The biopsy shows relatively superficial mild epidermolytic hyperkeratosis. Topical therapy usually suffices, but oral retinoids in low dosages may be tried.

Ichthyosis Hystrix

Ichthyosis hystrix is not a single disease but a group of very rare unrelated disorders. The term hystrix is Greek for porcupine. All the patients have very dark thick, often spiny scales.

Ichthyosis Hystrix Curth-Macklin
(OLLENDORFF-CURTH and MACKLIN 1954)

Synonym. DOC 8

While this variant is inherited in an autosomal dominant pattern, no mutation in a keratin gene has been found. The patients have diffuse verrucous plaques, involving the entire trunk, the flexural surfaces of the extremities and the palms and soles. Blisters are not found. While light microscopy shows epidermolytic hyperkeratosis, ultrastructural examination reveals relatively normal tonofilaments with concentric shells around the nucleus. Many keratinocytes are binucleate. Oral retinoids can be employed.

Ichthyosis Hystrix Lambert

This famous but rare disease has become extinct. The Lamberts were a family of porcupine men who became famous at side shows in England in the eighteenth century. The spines covered their entire body, sparing the genitalia, face, palms and soles. The pedigree has apparently died out.

Ichthyosis Hystrix Rheydt
(ANTON-LAMPRECHT 1976, SCHNYDER 1977)

Synonyms. Hystrix-like ichthyosis with deafness (HID)

Rheydt is the name of a German town where one of the first pedigrees was identified. These rare patients have erythroderma during early life which then evolves into a widespread hystrix-like hyperkeratosis. Clinically the disease resembles the Curth-Macklin type but all patients have sensorineural deafness. They also are very susceptible to bacterial and fungal infections, and may have scarring alopecia. The histologic picture shows papillomatosis, acanthosis and vacuolated "bird's eye" keratinocytes in the granular layer. Electron microscopy reveals a distinct picture which was the initial basis for separating out this syndrome. The keratinocytes are swollen and the intracellular matrix contains a granular mucinous material. The disease is very responsive to retinoids. The main differential diagnostic considerations are ichthyosis hystrix Curth-Macklin where deafness is uncommon and KID syndrome which has localized hyperkeratotic patches, not true ichthyosis.

Peeling Skin Syndrome
(FOX 1921; WILE 1924)

Synonyms. Familial continual skin peeling, keratolysis exfoliativa congenita, DOC 21

Traupe has pointed out that there are actually two peeling skin syndromes, as described by Fox and Wile. Both are very rare and inherited in an autosomal recessive pattern.

Peeling Skin Syndrome A (Fox). There is a generalized continued shedding or peeling of the entire skin, including the face. This has been compared to the shedding of skin by a reptile. The split occurs in the lower part of the stratum corneum, apparently through still intact keratinocytes rather than between cells. The peeling is asymptomatic and simply a great annoyance. There are no associated disorders, except for tiger-tail hairs, typical for trichothiodystrophy, seen in one case.

Peeling Skin Syndrome B (Wile). These patients may present with an erythroderma at birth and have associated findings such as growth retardation, aminoaciduria and increased skin infections. They have isolated erythematous lesions which then peel, leaving superficially denuded red patches with a peripheral collarette which can be further peeled. The epidermis is psoriasiform with an absent or reduced granular layer and marked parakeratosis. The split occurs at the level of the granular layer. Traupe has suggested an association with Comèl-Netherton syndrome.

Sjögren-Larsson Syndrome
(SJÖGREN and LARSSON 1957)

Synonym. DOC 10

This rare disorder is inherited in an autosomal recessive pattern. The initial cases and most large pedigrees have come from Sweden but it is seen around the world. There is a defect in the gene for the fatty aldehyde component of fatty alcohol oxidoreductase.

At birth, the infants are usually erythrodermic with diffuse scaling, often lamellar. Later they develop darker more spiny or corrugated scales which typically spare the face. Larger sheets of scale may also be found. As is the case with many disorders of fat metabolism, the other major system involved is the CNS with mental retardation and paraplegia, often with a scissors gait. The retina shows glistening dots, punctate areas of glial degeneration; this reliable finding is present in all patients after age 1–2 years. The biopsy shows uniform papillomatosis and acanthosis. The main differential diagnostic considerations are bullous ichthyosiform erythroderma, mild forms of lamellar ichthyosis and trichothiodystrophy. Dietary manipulation can be attempted and retinoids are helpful for the skin problems. Many patients are wheelchair-bound and little concerned about their skin; others are greatly bother by pruritus. The enzyme defect can be identified in fibroblast assays and thus also used for prenatal diagnosis; fetal skin biopsies have also been employed.

Trichothiodystrophy Syndromes

This confusing group of disorders is further discussed in Chapter 31. The unifying feature is the presence of trichothiodystrophy – brittle hair with longitudinal splitting which under polarizing light shows alternating dark and light bands. Because of these bands, the hair has been called tiger-tail hair or zebra hair. While such hairs can also be found in otherwise normal individuals, they are seen in a number of related disorders burdened by a baffling array of acronyms (Table 17.2). All are inherited in an autosomal recessive pattern. The nature of the mutation is unclear, as PIBIDS patients have a DNA repair gene mutation identical to group D xeroderma pigmentosum patients. Tay syndrome patients may have a defect in a closely linked gene. Patients with BIDS syndrome have no skin changes and will not be considered further. The important message is to examine the hair in patients with congenital ichthyosis, especially those with associated dysmorphic and CNS features.

Table 17.2. The trichothiodystrophies

Disorder	BIDS	IBIDS (Tay)	PIBIDS
Photosensitivity			x
Ichthyosis		x	x
Brittle hair	x	x	x
Impaired intelligence	x	x	x
Decreased fertility	x	x	x
Short stature	x	x	x

Tay Syndrome

(Tay 1971)

Synonyms. IBIDS, DOC 14

The patient may be born as a collodion baby, but later evolve to have diffuse fine scales and erythema. Often palmoplantar keratoderma is present, as well as nail dystrophies. Increased bacterial infections may be seen. Systemic findings include mental retardation, ataxia, hypogonadism and short stature, often with a progeria-like face.

PIBIDS. This disorder represents the combination of photosensitivity and Tay syndrome. Despite having the same mutation as xeroderma pigmentosum patients, PIBIDS patients do not develop increased numbers of skin cancers. Nonetheless, they should use adequate sunscreens. The DNA repair defect can be identified via prenatal diagnosis.

Comél-Netherton Syndrome

(Comél 1949; Netherton 1958)

Synonyms. Ichthyosis linearis circumflexa, DOC 9

Definition. This very uncommon syndrome is inherited in an autosomal recessive pattern. It has three cardinal features: ichthyosis, hair shaft abnormalities and atopic dermatitis.

Clinical Findings. At birth almost all patients have an erythroderma. Some soon develop ichthyosis linearis circumflexa which features distinctive hyperkeratotic erythematous migratory plaques with circinate, polycyclic or serpiginous patterns. The clinical hallmark is the presence of two parallel lines or bands of scale at the periphery; for unclear semantic reasons, this is called double-edged scale. If one wishes to use the analogy of razor blades, then it is a twin-edged scale. Other patients have a congenital ichthyosiform erythroderma pattern but this may later evolve into ichthyosis linearis circumflexa. The more severely involved patients are more likely to have hypotrichosis, but almost all show trichorrhexis invaginata or other structural hair abnormalities. The hair condition can improve with time.

The patients with widespread disease show a range of other problems. They have massively elevated IgE, other immune defects and a tendency towards infections. *Pseudomonas* infections are a common cause of death during infancy. In addition, they tend to develop hypernatremia as a result of dehydration and perhaps other factors. There is also growth retardation. Many patients have typical features of atopic dermatitis, which is coupled with an increased incidence of food allergies, frequent asthma and the high IgE.

Histopathology. The microscopic picture is psoriasiform with parakeratosis, acanthosis and a peculiar eosinophilic material just below the stratum corneum. The two parallel bands of scale can be seen if the sections are aligned properly. Microscopic examination of the hairs usually leads to a rapid diagnosis, although sometimes one must search repeatedly to find the typical structural changes.

Differential Diagnosis. In the severe cases at birth, ichthyosis is often not considered. The differential diagnosis includes severe seborrheic dermatitis, including Leiner syndrome, severe atopic dermatitis and immune deficiency states. Later one must remember that there are patients with ichthyosis linearis circumflexa alone.

Therapy. In the first year, skilled pediatric care is probably the answer for the severe cases. There is no special treatment for ichthyosis linearis circumflexa; keratolytics can be tried but may irritate the atopic skin. This is one form of ichthyosis where one may consider low potency topical corticosteroids. Retinoids have been described as effective for the ichthyotic component but will worsen the atopic aspects.

Dorfman-Chanarin Syndrome

(Dorfman et al. 1974; Chanarin et al. 1975)

Synonyms. Neutral lipid storage disease, ichthyosis and neutral lipid storage disease, DOC 12

This very rare autosomal recessive inherited disorder involves abnormal lipid metabolism but the responsible gene has not been identified. Most German patients are of Mediterranean background. The skin findings resemble congenital ichthyosiform erythroderma. There may be CNS, musculoskeletal and ocular changes. Intracellular lipid vacuoles can be present in circulating neutrophils, as well as in a variety of other cells including keratinocytes. Thus a skin biopsy fixed in alcohol may be useful. Lipid vacuoles may also be found in the obligate carrier parents. Refsum syndrome patients also have epidermal lipid vacuoles, but in Dorfman-Chanarin syndrome patients, the phytanic acid levels are normal.

X-Linked Dominant Chondrodysplasia Punctata

(Conradi 1914; Hünermann 1931)

Synonyms. Conradi-Hünermann syndrome, X-linked dominant ichthyosis, DOC 17

Etiology and Pathogenesis. Chondrodysplasia punctata refers to stippled calcifications of the epiphyses. Confusion can result when a physical or laboratory finding is equated with a disease. Conradi and Hünermann described patients with severe skeletal defects who also had cutaneous changes. While they and many others were confident they were describing an autosomal dominant disorder, Happle convincingly showed that the classic Conradi-Hünermann syndrome is inherited in an X-linked dominant fashion. Only girls are involved. Presumably male infants carrying just the one abnormal gene do not survive. At least one case has been described in a Klinefelter syndrome patient, a man with two X chromosomes. But the X chromosome has been almost completely analyzed and the gene for this disorder remains elusive. Peroxisome function may also be abnormal.

Clinical Findings. At birth, the young girls have widespread erythema with whorled scaling following Blaschko lines. While the erythema clears, the focal scaly areas may persist. In addition, follicular atrophoderma develops, as well as patchy alopecia. The face is typically flattened, over half the patients have cataracts, often congenital, and there is a wide range of severe skeletal defects. Intelligence is normal.

Histopathology. A skin biopsy or examination of scale shed in the nursery may be helpful, revealing calcium deposits in the keratinocytes especially in follicular epithelium. Later on these changes are difficult to find, but ultrastructural examination may reveal electron-dense calcium crystals in the same cells.

Therapy. Usually mild therapy suffices. The most important aspect for the patient is skilled orthopedic and ophthalmologic care.

CHILD Syndrome
(Happle et al. 1980)

Synonym. DOC 16

Definition. CHILD syndrome features congenital hemidysplasia, unilateral ichthyosiform erythroderma and limb defects.

Etiology and Pathogenesis. Inheritance is also in an X-linked dominant pattern with female predominance and chondrodysplasia punctata may be seen on radiologic examination. It is caused by heterozygous mutations in the gene NSDHL (NAD(P)H steroid dehydrogenase-like protein), which maps to Xp28 and encodes an enzyme, which controls a step in the cholesterol biosynthetic pathway. While CHILD syndrome is a variant of the epidermal nevus syndrome, the cutaneous lesions are so similar to those of other types of ichthyosiform erythroderma that we include the disorder here.

Clinical Findings. The cutaneous changes are usually unilateral, show a sharp demarcation on the anterior and posterior midline of the trunk and predilection for the body folds (ptychotropism; Fig. 17.7). The lesions are typically erythematous, have yellow hyperkeratotic scales and may have spines. The nails on the involved side may be thickened. The sharp demarcation and relative permanency of the lesions fits better with an epidermal nevus, but bilateral lesions may be seen and some individual lesions may wax and wane. The skeletal defects are usually on the same side of the body as the predominant cutaneous changes, usually featuring hypoplasia or aplasia of various limb bones. Cardiac, renal and other internal abnormalities are also occasionally seen.

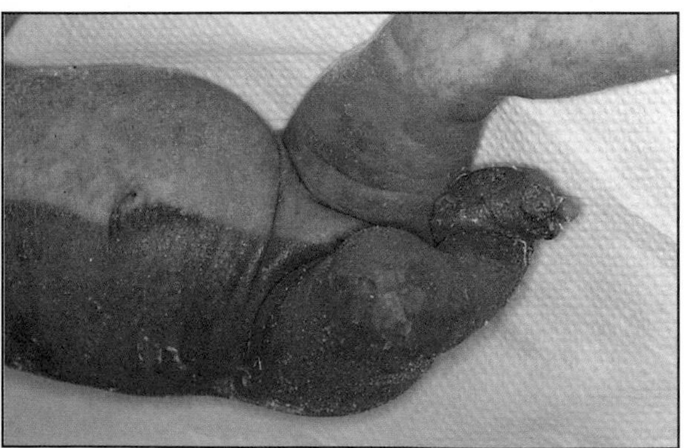

Fig. 17.7. CHILD syndrome

Histopathology. The epidermis shows psoriasiform hyperplasia with a pale-staining stratum corneum. On ultrastructural examination, lamellar bodies may be defective.

Laboratory Findings. Radiological evaluation may be diagnostic; the combination of limb defects and chondrodysplasia punctata is pathognomonic.

Differential Diagnosis. The cutaneous findings are so striking that there is usually no differential diagnosis.

Therapy. Treatment is difficult. The inflammation is persistent, the skin barrier often inadequate and secondary infections tend to occur. Routine keratolytic and antiinflammatory measures can be tried. Low dose oral retinoids may help.

Ichthyosis Follicularis with Atrichia and Photophobia

The inheritance of this uncommon form of ichthyosis is unclear. Boys seem to be more often affected than girls. The classic clinical findings are striking follicular keratoses and congenital atrichia, along with a mild ichthyosis in the intervening skin. The patients also have striking photophobia but no other ocular abnormalities. The biopsy supports the presence of follicular plugging. The differential diagnosis includes other forms of atrichia, keratosis follicularis spinulosa decalvans and perhaps mild ichthyosis vulgaris. Topical therapy usually suffices.

Acquired Ichthyosis-Like Conditions

There are a number of disorders in which the patients develop diffuse ichthyosis-like scaling. Acquired ichthyosis is not a syndrome but a clinical description which should prompt the search for an underlying disorder. Table 17.3 shows the disorders most often associated with an adult-onset ichthyosis-like scaling. The two most common are not mentioned because they are normal variants. Many individuals with dry skin, especially blacks, develop lamellar scales on their legs and occasionally trunk. Similarly, elderly patients with dry skin may also acquire thicker distinct scales. Reduced bathing and increased lubrication are what these two groups require.

Table 17.3. Disorders associated with acquired ichthyosis-like scaling

Category	Diseases
Paraneoplastic	Hodgkin disease malignant lymphomas Carcinomas (rarely)
Infections	Leprosy Tuberculosis HIV/AIDS Acute infections (rare and self-limited)
Nutritional deficiencies	Pellagra Vitamin A deficiency (and excess) Kava consumption
Medications	Nicotinic acid Other lipid lowering agents Allopurinol Cimetidine Lithium Retinoids
Miscellaneous	Sarcoidosis Inflammatory bowel disease Hypothyroidism Down syndrome

Palmoplantar Keratodermas

The palmoplantar keratodermas (PPK) are another befuddling area. It is now apparent that many involve mutations in specific keratins that are only expressed on the palms and soles. For example, keratins 6 and 16 are found in palmar and plantar skin, but also in mucosal, and hair- and nail-associated tissue, always in a suprabasal position. In contrast, keratin 9 is only found in the skin of the palms and soles. Other PPK are caused by mutations not related to keratin but to other structural proteins. PPK fall into the ectodermal dysplasia spectrum. Many have abnormalities of hair or nails; teeth are less often involved. Table 17.4 shows those forms of palmoplantar keratoderma covered elsewhere in the text or considered too rare for more detailed discussion.

Another important consideration is acquired versus inherited variants. The spectrum of acquired PPK is considered as a single category at the end of this section. A final consideration is the relationship of PPK to malignancy. Several forms of acquired PPK are paraneoplastic markers, while in

Table 17.4. Other types of palmoplantar keratoderma

Disease	Inheritance	Main features	Chapter
Tyrosinemia II (Richner-Hanhart)	AR	PPK, corneal dystrophy	39
Acrokeratoelastoidosis	AD	Polygonal papules along sides of hands and feet	18
Pachyonychia congenita	AD	Several types, all with focal PPK and specific keratin defects	32
Punctate keratoderma with hyperpigmentation (Cole syndrome)	AD	Punctate PPK and diffuse hyperpigmented macules	
Punctate keratoderma of the palmar creases	Acq	Acquired PPK with warty lesions limited to the palmar (and to lesser extent plantar) creases; quite common in blacks	
Olmsted syndrome	Acq	Severe PPK, flexion deformities and auto-amputation of digits, periorificial hyperkeratotic plaques	
PPK with sclerodactyly (Huriez)	AD	Sclerodactyly with atrophy, diffuse PPK, squamous cell carcinoma in atrophic areas, also gastrointestinal tumors	
Hidrotic ectodermal dysplasia (Clouston)	AD	Diffuse PPK, alopecia, nail changes, mental retardation, skeletal defects, deafness	
Congenital poikiloderma with blisters	AD	Punctate and linear PPK, reticulate hyperpigmentation, lack of dermatoglyphics, nail, hair, teeth defects, hypohidrosis	15, 18
PPK with deafness (Bart-Pumphrey)	AD	Extensive focal PPK, sensorineural deafness, leukonychia	

Acq, Acquired; AD, autosomal dominant; AR, autosomal recessive; PPK, palmoplantar keratoderma

a few of the inherited forms there are associated malignancies. In addition, both malignant melanoma and squamous cell carcinoma have been rarely described in the abnormal acral skin in various types of PPK.

The differential diagnosis in each case includes the other morphologically similar disorders. For the most part, treatment is mechanical with removal of scale using a pumice stone, sharp blade or even masonry-type sandpaper. Keratolytic agents may soften the thickened scale somewhat, but rarely suffice alone. Systemic retinoids may be helpful in severe cases, but most patients get by without them.

Diffuse Palmoplantar Keratodermas

Epidermolytic Palmoplantar Keratoderma

(Thost 1880; Unna 1883; Vörner 1901)

Synonyms. Keratosis palmoplantaris diffusa Vörner-Unna-Thost, Unna-Thost disease, Vörner disease

Epidemiology. This is the most common form of PPK but it took over a century to recognize this fact. For many years, Unna-Thost disease was defined as the common PPK while Vörner disease, the epidermolytic variant of PPK, was felt to be rare. Most patients with classic PPK have the epidermolytic variant, including descendants of some of the original pedigrees. Estimates of frequency are as high as 1:200 in Northern Sweden, but 1:10,000–1:20,000 is probably more reasonable.

Etiology and Pathogenesis. The genetic defect is a mutation in keratin 9 on chromosome 17q.

Clinical Findings. The findings are fairly distinct clinically, with diffuse bilateral symmetric yellow waxy plaques covering the palms and soles. Onset of problems is usually during childhood. Fissures are common. The periphery of the lesions is distinctive with an erythematous border, which may blister. The thickened skin typically just turns the corner working its way onto the lateral aspects of the hands and feet; this is known as transgredience (Fig. 17.8). Dermatophyte infections are uncommon. Knuckle pads and clubbed digits have been described. Patients often complain of hyperhidrosis.

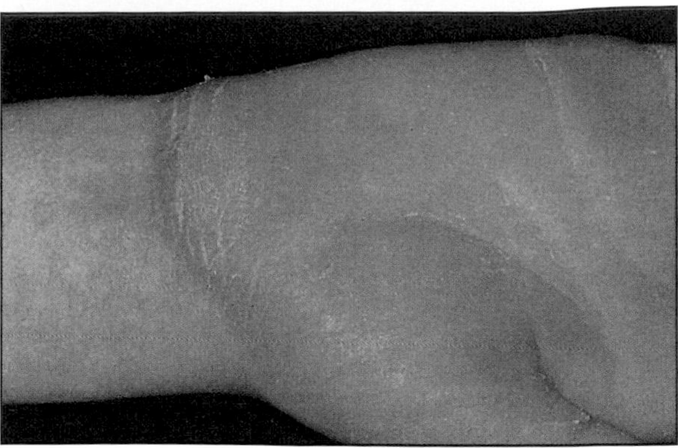

Fig. 17.8. Palmoplantar keratoderma, Vörner type

Histopathology. There is massive compact hyperkeratosis with epidermolytic hyperkeratosis in the upper stratum spinosum and stratum granulosum. Electron microscopic examination shows cytoplasmic vacuoles and clumped perinuclear tonofilaments.

Differential Diagnosis. The nonepidermolytic autosomal dominant PPK has been shown to be very uncommon in recent years. Occasional pedigrees are identified with appropriate histology in which there have been linkages to keratin genes. A 100-year history of mistaken diagnoses supports the fact that the different types cannot be separated clinically.

Mal de Meleda

(Stulli 1826)

Synonyms. Keratosis palmoplantaris transgrediens et progrediens Mljet (Meleda), mutilating palmoplantar keratoderma type Gamborg-Nielsen

Epidemiology. Meleda or Mljet is a small island in the Adriatic Sea just off the coast of Dalmatia. This unique form of PPK was reported here many years ago. It is inherited in an autosomal recessive pattern and its prevalence reflects the consanguinity found on the small island. The gene defect has not been found. Even today, many patients around the world have Adriatic roots.

Clinical Findings. The problem begins with palmoplantar erythema in the first weeks of life and evolves to look similar to epidermolytic PPK but the keratosis is transgredient, i.e. it progresses onto the dorsal aspects of the fingers and toes. There may be sufficient keratoderma to cause secondary finger contractures especially of the fifth finger which may even be shortened. Other lesions may involve the knees or elbows, and sometimes the perioral region. Nail dystrophies are common. Oral leukokeratosis has been reported in some pedigrees. Biopsy shows diffuse hyperkeratosis without epidermolytic changes. Retinoids appear to be helpful, but the problem is life-long.

Progressive Palmoplantar Keratoderma
(Greither 1952)

Synonyms. Greither syndrome, keratosis palmoplantaris diffusa transgrediens et progrediens

Etiology and Pathogenesis. Progressive PPK is inherited in an autosomal dominant pattern, closely related to erythrokeratodermia variabilis. Both are linked to the Rhesus blood group on chromosome 1p36. The diseases can clinically overlap, so perhaps contiguous gene deletions are involved.

Clinical Findings. In the first years of life, patients develop a diffuse symmetric PPK with small pits and hyperhidrosis. Later the disease creeps centrally to involve the backs of the hands and feet, the ankles, knees and elbows (Fig. 17.9). The progress is slowly progressive until adult life and then stabilizes. The biopsy findings simply show marked hyperkeratosis. Mechanical treatment measures usually suffice.

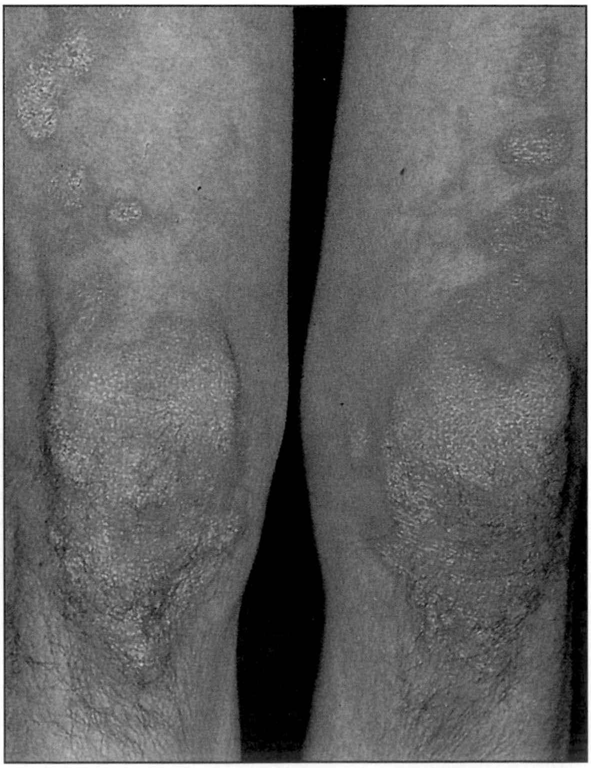

Fig. 17.9. Progressive palmoplantar keratoderma

Papillon-Lefèvre Syndrome
(Papillon and Lefèvre 1924)

Synonyms. Keratosis palmoplantaris diffusa with periodontopathia, palmoplantar keratoderma with periodontal disease

Papillon-Lefèvre syndrome is a rare autosomal recessive syndrome whose genetic defect is not known. Patients have diffuse PPK with a modest tendency towards progression, developing plaques on the dorsal aspects of the hands and feet, as well as the knees and elbows (Fig. 17.10). They have marked hyperhidrosis, a foul odor and tend to develop pyodermas. Some patients have phagocytic defects. The major clinical problem is severe periodontal disease which destroys both sets of teeth (Fig. 17.11). The early loss of the primary teeth

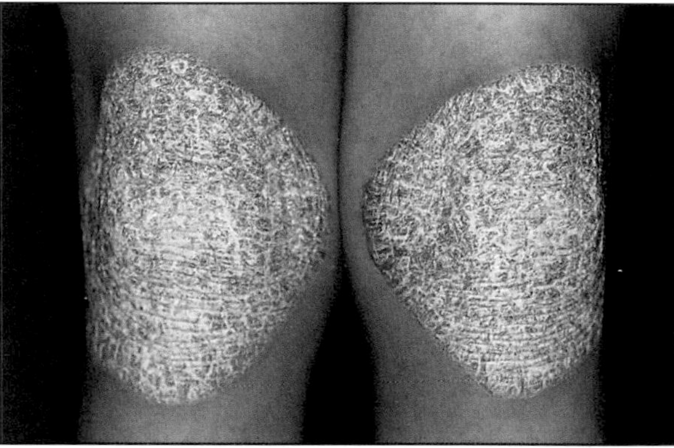

Fig. 17.10. Papillon-Lefèvre syndrome

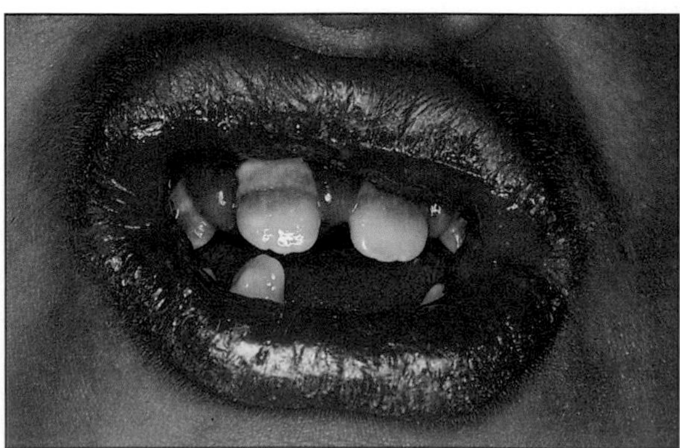

Fig. 17.11. Papillon-Lefèvre syndrome

may lead to undergrowth of the maxilla and mandible. Retinoids seem to help not only the skin but also the dental problems. One must work closely with a dentist to insure maximal prophylactic care.

Vohwinkel Syndrome

(Vohwinkel 1929)

Synonyms. Keratosis palmoplantaris mutilans, keratoma hereditaria mutilans, mutilating palmoplantar keratoderma

Etiology and Pathogenesis. This autosomal dominant disorder appears to involve a mutation in involucrin on chromosome 1q21.

Clinical Findings. The clinical features are characteristic: there is diffuse PPK with hyperhidrosis, a yellow tone and distinctive pits producing the so-called honeycomb pattern. Hyperkeratotic lesions may spread to the usual sites of the dorsal hands and feet as well as knees and elbows. Here they form linear or starfish-like hyperkeratoses. Finally, there may be pseudo-ainhum or auto-amputation of digits as deep constricting creases form. The nails are often clubbed. Finally, most patients have sensorineural deafness.

Histopathology. The biopsy is nonspecific, showing a papillomatous, acanthotic pattern with prominent hyperkeratosis, focal parakeratosis and thickened stratum granulosum.

Therapy. Oral retinoids usually help reduce the keratoderma and arrest the auto-amputation process. Plastic surgery may be required for more advanced lesions to release contractures or constricting bands.

Howel-Evans Syndrome

(Howel-Evans et al. 1958)

This very rare autosomal dominant cancer-associated genodermatosis was first described in a pedigree from the Liverpool area. Only a limited number of involved families have been identified since. The patients have mutations in the keratin gene clustered on chromosome 17q. They develop diffuse PPK in childhood, usually worse on the feet. During puberty, they typically acquire leukokeratosis. Over 90% of those in the family with PPK develop carcinoma of the esophagus by age 60 years.

Schöpf Syndrome

(Schöpf et al. 1971)

Synonyms. Palmoplantar keratoderma with lid cysts, Schöpf-Schulz-Passarge syndrome

This syndrome is inherited in an autosomal recessive pattern; the defect is unknown. The patients have a relatively mild, diffuse erythematous keratoderma association with hypodontia, hypotrichosis, nail dystrophies and eyelid cysts. The latter are apocrine hidrocystomas which tend to appear late in life. In addition, multiple eccrine syringofibroadenomas (Mascaro tumor) and squamous cell carcinomas have been described on the acral surfaces in older patients.

Punctate Palmoplantar Keratoderma

(Buschke and Fischer 1910; Brauer 1913)

Synonyms. Keratosis palmoplantaris papulosa, papular palmoplantar keratoderma, keratosis papulosa, papulotranslucent acrokeratoderma, Davis-Colley syndrome

Etiology and Pathogenesis. The genetic defect is unknown. The disorder is inherited in an autosomal dominant pattern and may be linked to the cancer family syndrome.

Clinical Findings. The many synonyms describe the clinical picture well. Small hyperkeratotic papules, usually several millimeters to 1 cm in size, appear in young adult life (Fig. 17.12). They may have a central dell or a plug which when removed leaves behind a small crater with a keratotic wall, resembling a volcano. The lesions tend to coalesce into larger plaques over the pressure points. Nail

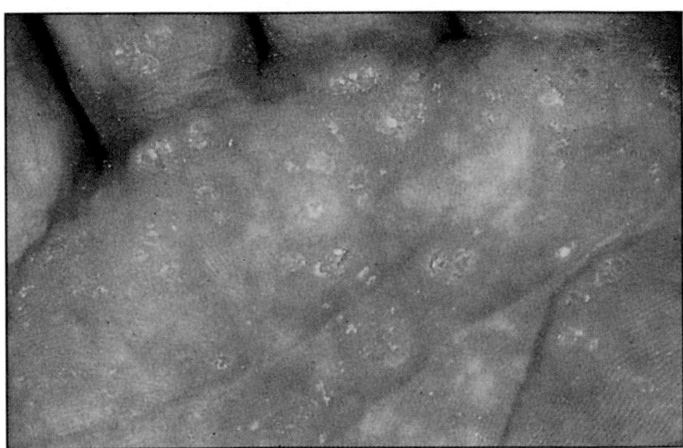

Fig. 17.12. Punctate palmoplantar keratoderma

dystrophies may occur. There is considerable variation between pedigrees.

Histopathology. Light microscopy shows marked hyperkeratosis with focal parakeratosis especially at the openings of the sweat ducts. Ultrastructural studies show clumping of the tonofilaments and desmosomal abnormalities suggesting a defect in cell adhesion rather than a keratin defect.

Differential Diagnosis. In the differential diagnosis for punctate keratodermas, one must exclude old warts, calluses, Darier disease, arsenical keratoses and the many forms of acquired punctate keratoderma. Another common form of punctate palmoplantar keratoderma is punctate porokeratosis.

Therapy. Rare patients respond to oral retinoids.

Striate Palmoplantar Keratoderma

(Brünauer 1923; Fuhs 1924; Siemens 1929)

Synonyms. Keratosis palmoplantaris areata, keratosis palmoplantaris varians, Brünauer-Fuhs-Siemens syndrome, palmoplantar keratoderma of Wachter

Etiology and Pathogenesis. The defect in this autosomal dominant disorder has been mapped to a cluster of genes on chromosome 18q12 coding for the adherins desmoglein and desmocollin.

Clinical Findings. The initial lesions usually are plantar and start in childhood. Round or oval hyperkeratotic papules, often yellow-brown and inflamed, appear first. They tend initially to be grouped into small clusters but evolve into linear lesions often running from the palm or sole onto the digits (Fig. 17.13). The lesions both interfere with motion and tend to be sensitive to pressure. Extensive walking or manual labor is both painful and results in the development of more lesions.

Histopathology. Light microscopy is not helpful. Electron microscopy shows abnormalities of the tonofilaments, fitting together with the genetic findings.

Therapy. Oral retinoids may rarely be helpful.

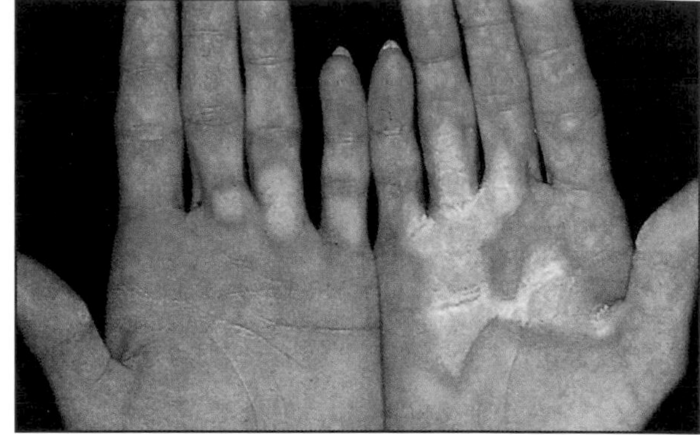

Fig. 17.13. Striate palmoplantar keratoderma

Acquired Palmoplantar Keratoderma

Acquired PPK should only be diagnosed after a detailed family history. Many hereditary forms of PPK have a late onset. Acquired diffuse PPK has been described as a tumor marker in several individual patients. Acquired punctate PPK formerly was most often associated with inorganic arsenic exposure; patients also have the typical pigmentary changes and an increased incidence of skin and internal malignancies. Rarely patients with nonarsenic-related acquired punctate keratoderma may also have underlying malignancies. Acquired filiform porokeratosis also frequently heralds an underlying malignancy. Another type of keratoderma that is today uncommon is the hyperkeratotic lesions seen in late or recurrent secondary syphilis. These copper brown often painful lesions are known as clavi syphilitici. They can be viewed as a hyperkeratotic form of the usual scaly lesions of the palms and soles in late secondary syphilis.

Erythrokeratodermias

Several rare disorders are technically best grouped as erythrokeratodermias. Ichthyosis by definition involves the entire integument, whereas in contrast these disorders show local erythema and hyperkeratosis.

Keratosis-Ichthyosis-Deafness Syndrome

(Burns 1915)

Synonyms. Erythrokeratodermia progressiva, KID syndrome, Senter syndrome, DOC 15. Because the skin lesions are not truly ichthyotic, Traupe has

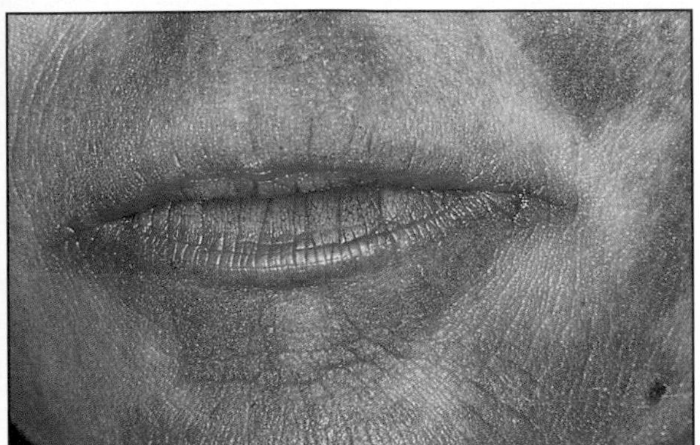

Fig. 17.14. Keratosis-ichthyosis-deafness syndrome

suggested renaming KID syndrome as keratitis-ichthyosis-like hyperkeratosis-deafness syndrome.

While KID syndrome may well be inherited in an autosomal dominant pattern, most cases have been sporadic and the genetic defect unclear. The characteristic lesions are symmetric, sharply circumscribed dirty brown verrucous plaques on an erythematous base (Fig. 17.14). They appear during the first year of life and slowly progress. Sites of predilection include the cheeks, chin, nose, ears, knees, elbows and dorsal aspects of hands and feet. Patients also have a leathery fine palmoplantar keratoderma. The trunk is usually spared or may show a fine scale. Associated defects include sensorineural deafness, a keratitis with prominent neovascularization and scarring alopecia. KID syndrome is a precancerous condition as squamous cell carcinomas have developed in both the skin lesions and on the oral mucosa. The microscopic picture is nonspecific. Differential diagnostic considerations include ichthyosis hystrix Rheydt, ichthyosis bullosa Siemens and other forms of erythrokeratodermia. Oral retinoids may be helpful; in addition, they should theoretically reduce the risk of tumor formation.

Erythrokeratodermia Variabilis

(Mendes da Costa 1925)

Synonyms. Erythrokeratodermia figurata variabilis, Mendes da Costa syndrome, keratosis rubra figurata, DOC 18

Etiology and Pathogenesis. The gene for erythrokeratodermia variabilis localizes to the Rh locus on chromosome 1p36 just as that for progressive PPK; both are inherited in an autosomal dominant pattern.

Clinical Findings. Classically erythrokeratodermia variabilis has two different skin findings. There is a migratory erythema which may start during infancy or childhood. The lesions appear over a matter of hours and may last for a week or two. Sometimes patients complain of burning. The red patches are often polycyclic or map-like. They seem to be influenced by weather, stress and hormonal changes. In addition, there are more persistent, hyperkeratotic plaques which favor the extremities and buttocks, and may show a stocking and glove pattern. The distal lesions may resemble chronic psoriasis. Some patients have a progressive palmoplantar keratoderma, fitting with the genetic overlap.

Histopathology. The epidermis shows papillomatosis, acanthosis, orthohyperkeratosis and focal parakeratosis.

Differential Diagnosis. Psoriasis and other erythrokeratodermias are the main considerations.

Therapy. Oral retinoids, primarily acitretin, appear to be the treatment of choice. An interval therapy combined with topical keratolytics is most acceptable. PUVA therapy has also produced favorable results.

Symmetrical Progressive Erythrokeratodermia

(Darier 1911; Gottron 1922)

Synonyms. Gottron syndrome, DOC 20

This autosomal dominant genodermatosis features symmetric, well-circumscribed hyperkeratotic red-brown plaques with an erythematous base on the extremities. The lesions start in early childhood and are slowly progressive. There may be prominent PPK and rare facial involvement, but the trunk is always spared. The plaques continue to spread until puberty but afterwards may show some regression. The microscopic picture is dominated by parakeratosis. Oral retinoids appear effective for the keratotic component, while PUVA therapy leads to a reduction in the erythema.

Other Forms of Erythrokeratodermia

There are several other disorders which best fit into this category. They are shown in Table 17.5.

Table 17.5. Other forms of erythrokeratodermia

Disorder	Inheritance	Features
EKD with ataxia (Giroux-Barbeau, DOC 23)	AD	Acral plaques in infancy which improve, ataxia and other CNS problems
CHIME syndrome	AR ?	Colobomata, heart defects, ichthyosiform dermatosis (i.e. EKD), mental retardation, ear defects
EKD en cocardes (Degos)	AD	Migratory annular EKD
Erythrokeratolysis hiemalis (Oudtshoorn skin, DOC 19)	AD	Erythematous plaques on palms and soles, trunk and extremities symmetric erythematous figurate lesions which peel periodically especially in winter. Almost limited to South African Boers

AD, autosomal dominant; AR, autosomal recessive; DOC, disorder of cornification (Williams); EKD, erythrokeratodermia

Follicular Keratoses

In a number of conditions, the hyperkeratosis is limited or most prominent in the hair follicle, forming clinically apparent plugs. Follicular ichthyosis is discussed above under the ichthyoses.

Keratosis Pilaris

Synonyms. Keratosis follicularis, lichen pilaris (both used in Germany, but beware – in English keratosis follicularis is Darier disease and lichen pilaris is a variant of lichen planus), keratosis suprafollicularis

Epidemiology. Keratosis pilaris is a very common disorder, seen far more often in young women. In some studies, almost 50 % of young women have at least a trace of keratosis pilaris, raising the question as to whether it is really a disease. It is associated with a long list of other diseases including atopic dermatitis and ichthyosis vulgaris. In addition, all the follicular atrophodermas are preceded by a keratosis pilaris-like lesions.

Clinical Findings. Far and away the most common location is the upper outer aspect of the arm. Other sites include the buttocks and lateral aspects of the thighs and calves. When one runs a hand over the skin surface, there is a grater effect. Many tiny keratotic plugs fill the follicular orifices (Fig. 17.15). When a plug is removed, sometimes a curled up hair may be found. Sometimes the plug may resemble tiny spines. Often there is marked livid erythema about the follicles. In Germany this is known as pernio follicularis. It is not true pernio but a combination of acrocyanosis and keratosis pilaris. The surrounding skin shows variable degrees of erythema and dryness.

Histopathology. While a biopsy is not needed, it shows a patulous follicle filled with keratin. There is no evidence for epithelial abnormalities, suggesting that the resulting scales are somehow more adherent to one another. There are no signs of inflammation.

Differential Diagnosis. Keratosis pilaris lesions on other body sites should raise the question of an associated disorder. One should consider ichthyosis vulgaris, other forms of ichthyosis and atopic der-

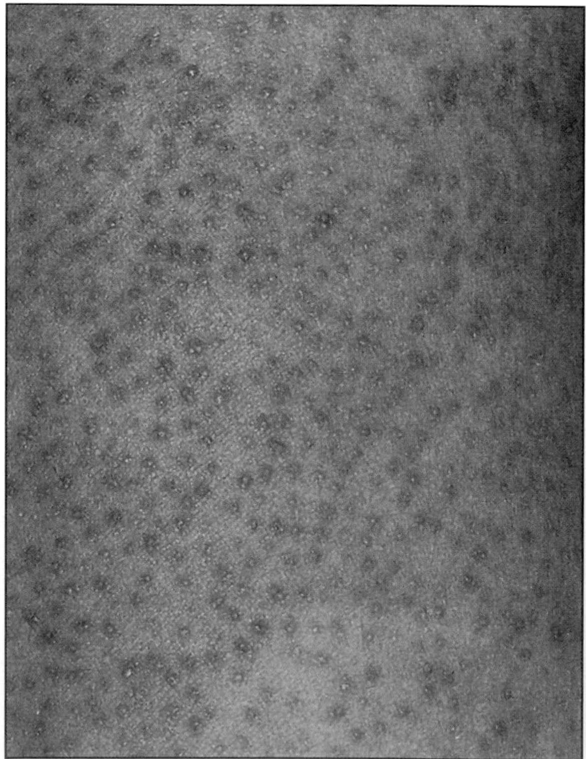

Fig. 17.15. Keratosis pilaris

matitis. Rare cases of follicular lichen planus may mimic keratosis pilaris, but usually lichen planus is more pruritic and erythematous.

Therapy. Keratosis pilaris is difficult to treat. Keratolytics including lactic acid, urea, salicylic acid and table salt are often effective. Topical retinoids are not as effective as one might suspect; the plugged follicles in keratosis pilaris are quite different from comedones. Mechanical removal of scale with a coarse sponge or similar product is also helpful.

Ulerythema Ophryogenes

(Unna and Raenzer 1889)

Synonym. Keratosis pilaris rubra atrophicans faciei (Gans 1925)

This uncommon disorder may be inherited in an autosomal dominant pattern but is usually sporadic. It affects children and young adults, involving the cheeks and lateral aspects of the eyebrows (Fig. 17.16). There is usually an associated erythema and the lesions may heal with scarring, leading to loss of the lateral aspects of the eyebrows. The areas are rough on palpation. The same patients often have keratosis pilaris. The disease tends to improve over time and can be treated just as keratosis pilaris. In rare cases with marked erythema, low-potency topical corticosteroids can be tried for short periods of time.

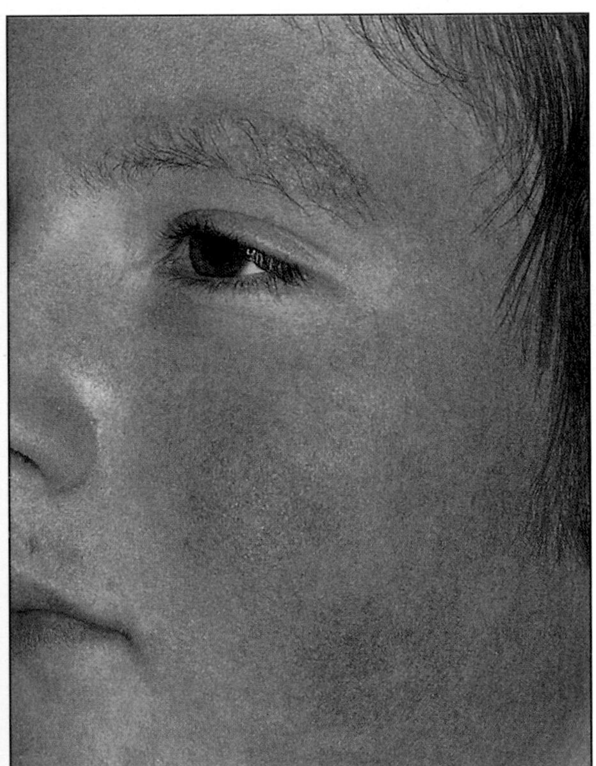

Fig. 17.16. Ulerythema ophryogenes

Keratosis Follicularis Spinulosa Decalvans

(Lameris 1905; Siemens 1926)

Synonyms. Siemens syndrome, DOC 24

The genetics of this rare syndrome are unresolved; both X-linked recessive and X-linked dominant inheritance have been suggested. At least one responsible gene has been mapped to Xp21.1–p22.2. Boys are more often and more severely affected than girls. There are plugged follicles apparent early in life usually involving the face, neck and extremities. They resolve with hyperpigmentation, milia and follicular atrophoderma. There is usually photophobia associated with conjunctivitis and corneal trauma, perhaps from the hyperkeratotic lesions on the eyelids. In addition, scarring alopecia of the scalp and eyebrows appears, probably also related to plugged follicles and inflammation. Palmoplantar keratoderma may also be seen. The differential diagnosis includes ichthyosis follicularis with atrichia and photophobia.

Lichen Spinulosus

Synonym. Spinulosismus

The nature of lichen spinulosus is unclear. Some define it as round to oval patches of grouped follicular plugs; others as a spiny variant of keratosis pilaris. It has been described several times in HIV/AIDS patients, showing a possible overlap in this group with pityriasis rubra pilaris. A number of other disorders may also show grouped tiny follicular plugs including the rare lichenoid fungal id reaction (lichen trichophyticus), lichen scrofulosorum, punctate porokeratosis and the other spiny keratoses mentioned below.

Hyperkeratosis Follicularis et Parafollicularis in Cutem Penetrans

(Kyrle 1916)

Synonyms. Kyrle disease, perforating disorder of renal disease

This rare disease is considered in Chapter 25 along with prurigo nodularis. It does not appear to be a primary disorder of keratinization.

Follicular Hyperkeratotic Spicules
(Heidenström and Tottie 1944)

Patients with multiple myeloma may rarely develop hyperkeratotic spicules on the face, especially the nose. Recent studies have shown that these follicular plugs are cryoglobulins. Presumably the nose is a favored site because it is acral and cooler, but also has large easily plugged follicles. Occasional cases have been described in association with other diseases, such as HIV/AIDS, Crohn disease, renal failure and vitamin A deficiency, as well as in normal individuals. In such cases, the follicular spicule consist of keratin.

Dyskeratotic-Acantholytic Disorders

Darier Disease
(Darier 1889; White 1889)

Synonyms. Dyskeratosis follicularis, keratosis follicularis, Darier-White disease

Definition. Common genodermatosis with widespread distinct dyskeratotic changes.

Epidemiology. Darier disease is one of the most common genodermatoses. The incidence is estimated at 1:50,000 births, but the patients have a normal life expectancy and frequently large pedigrees are encountered. Men appear either more often or more severely affected than women.

Etiology and Pathogenesis. While the gene has been located on chromosome 12q23–24, the mechanism of abnormal keratinization is unclear. Electron microscopic studies show abnormal tonofilament-desmosome complexes; the dyskeratotic cells do not arise from the acantholytic cells. UV radiation is a well-established trigger.

Clinical Findings. The clinical features of Darier disease involve not only the skin but also the oral mucosa and nails, demonstrating how false the name dyskeratosis follicularis is. The disease usually begins in adolescence or early adult life. The typical lesions are tiny keratotic papules; they are usually several millimeters in diameter, have a firmly adherent gray–brown keratin cap and are most often found in the seborrheic areas, such as the neck (the nape is often the first site of involvement), mid-chest, axillae, groin, and later scalp and extremities (Fig. 17.17). When the caps are scratched away, a tiny dell is left behind; sometimes it is follicular but often it is not. The initial lesions are very subtle and usually either overlooked or misdiagnosed for many years.

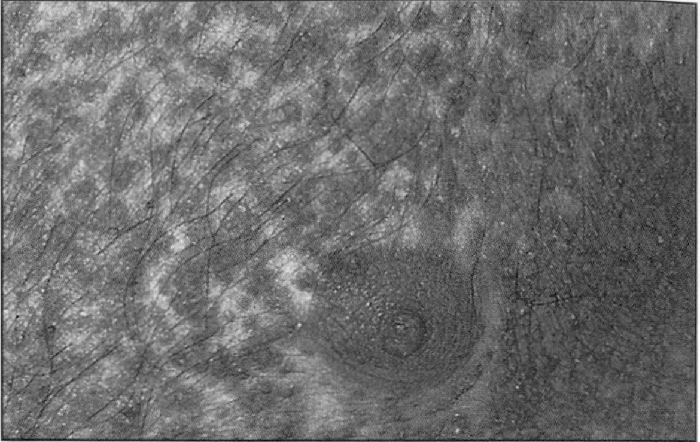

Fig. 17.17. Darier disease

Over time the lesions coalesce, become thicker and more distinctive with a dirty appearance. The large plaques may weep or have a greasy crust (Fig. 17.18). In the intertriginous areas, the lesions become macerated, malodorous and often secondarily infected. Several studies have shown chemotactic defects, perhaps explaining the tendency to infection. Nodular lesions and blisters are most uncommon. Pruritus may be a problem, especially with widespread or inflamed lesions.

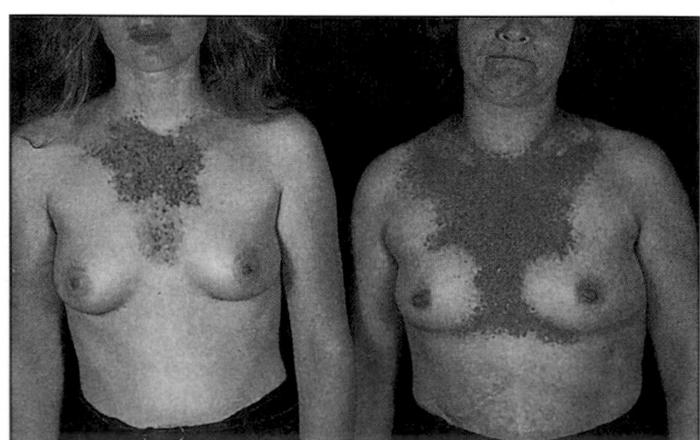

Fig. 17.18. Darier disease in a mother and daughter

Head. On the face one usually thinks of severe seborrheic dermatitis. The scalp, when involved, may present with massive crusts, suggesting pityriasis amiantacea or favus. Hair loss is usually minimal despite the severe inflammation.

Palms and Soles. Tiny pits develop, sometimes with little keratotic plugs. Minute disturbances in dermatoglyphics can be used for the early diagnosis of Darier disease. A very rare variant of Darier disease has extraordinary disabling palmoplantar keratoderma. Surprisingly these patients can be helped by excision and split-thickness skin grafting.

Hands. The classic lesions on the dorsal and lateral aspects of the hands are tiny flat-topped verrucous excrescences, known as acrokeratosis verruciformis of Hopf. These lesions are discussed in more detail below.

Nails. The nails often show distal notches, subungual hyperkeratosis and red and white longitudinal bands (Fig. 17.19). Marked nail dystrophies may evolve over time.

Linear Lesions. Some patients may present with a focal, often linear eruption following Blaschko's lines. This disorder has been called linear Darier disease or zosteriform Darier disease. It probably represents a focal, genetically limited form of the disorder (Chap. 19).

Nipples. Sometimes just the nipples are extremely hyperkeratotic. Dermabrasion or shave excision of the keratotic mass is most effective.

Oral Mucosa. White grouped papules are found, initially on the palate or buccal mucosa but they may become very widespread. The pattern is often described as cobblestone (Fig. 17.20). Similar lesions are seen on the genital mucosa but Papanicolau smears are usually not influenced.

Histopathology. The microscopic features of Darier disease are quite distinct. Both dyskeratosis and acantholysis are seen. Individual cell keratinization leads to a variety of abnormal keratinocytes in the upper epidermis: corps ronds are the round eosinophilic cells in the stratum spinosum, while the smaller nuclear remnants in the stratum granulosum are known as grains. In addition, there is separation of the suprabasilar keratinocytes. Often the basal layer is retained, producing the tombstone pattern seen so often in pemphigus vulgaris. The dermis often shows considerable inflammation. Sometimes the changes are very focal, so one must search carefully through the biopsy to find them.

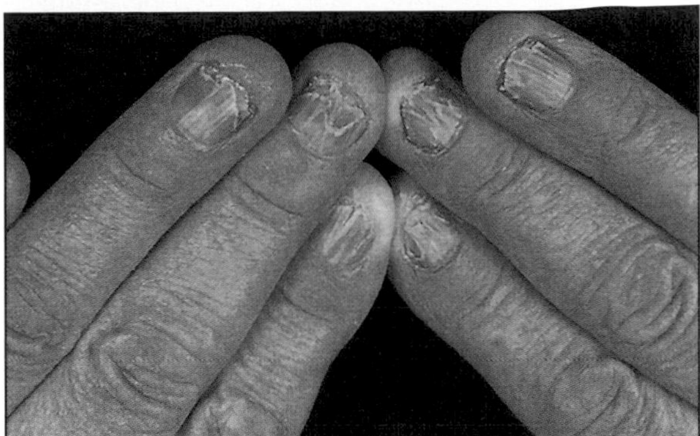

Fig. 17.19. Nail involvement in Darier disease

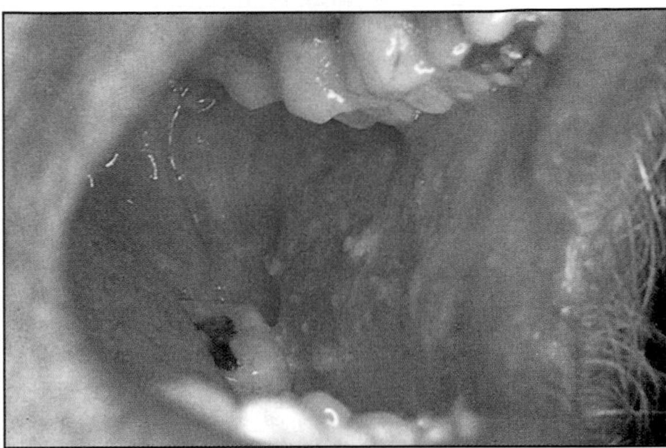

Fig. 17.20. Mucosal involvement in Darier disease

The changes of Darier disease, generally described as focal acantholytic dyskeratosis, are also seen in linear epidermal nevus, Grover disease, warty dyskeratoma, rare cases of punctate palmoplantar keratoderma, familial dyskeratotic comedones, acantholytic actinic keratosis, focal and multiple acantholytic dyskeratomas and as an incidental finding.

Course and Prognosis. In most patients, the disease worsens during the first years of its appearance and is then relatively stable. The two most dramatic triggers are sunburn and herpes simplex virus infections. Patients with Darier disease who are susceptible to recurrent herpes simplex virus infections should be given suppressive antiviral therapy. Otherwise the risk of a widespread flare, sometimes with systemic involvement, remains high. Any patient with a sudden worsening of

Darier disease and no sunburn should be suspected of having herpes simplex virus infection. Bacterial infections and vegetating lesions may become a problem in eroded intertriginous areas.

Differential Diagnosis. The clinical differential diagnosis includes seborrheic dermatitis, Hailey-Hailey disease, and Grover disease. When the intertriginous involvement is severe, one may think of pemphigus vegetans or acanthosis nigricans. The scalp disease can suggest favus or pityriasis amiantacea. The similarities between a zosteriform variant of Darier disease and a linear epidermal nevus with focal acantholytic dyskeratosis are puzzling; the former should wax and wane while the latter should be permanent. Otherwise, they appear identical.

Therapy

Systemic. Oral retinoids have made life easier for patients with severe Darier disease, but many do not require such aggressive therapy. Acitretin appears more effective than isotretinoin. Interval therapy should be used, but the disease recurs shortly after cessation. Systemic antibiotics and anti-herpes simplex therapy are also very useful.

Topical. Topical corticosteroids may reduce inflammation, topical antimicrobials may help control infection and topical retinoids may slightly decrease scaling, but none is extremely successful. If the patient can tolerate the retinoids over a period of time, they offer the most hope.

Surgical. Excision of difficult areas, such as the soles, scalp or axillae followed by split-thickness grafting is often amazingly successful.

Grover Disease

(Grover 1970)

Synonym. Transitory acantholytic dermatosis (TAD)

Definition. Acquired highly pruritic dermatosis with dyskeratosis and acantholysis.

Epidemiology. Grover disease is a disease of older men; it is very uncommon in woman or young adults. Most have dry skin and typically flare in the winter as central heating is turned on and the skin begins to dry out. Other patients have more trouble in the summer as their problems appear to be triggered by sunlight.

Etiology and Pathogenesis. The etiology is unknown.

Clinical Findings. The cardinal finding is pruritus. The site of action is the trunk, where one sees or can palpate many tiny discrete succulent or keratotic papules (Fig. 17.21). Sometimes tiny vesicles are appreciated; other lesions have a frank crust. Sometimes the lesions are grouped together.

Histopathology. There are usually small areas of acantholytic dyskeratosis as in Darier disease. Sometimes several biopsies are needed to find them. The histologic pattern can also more closely resemble Hailey-Hailey disease or pemphigus. Sometimes there is spongiosis in addition to acantholysis. That is, there are varying degrees of dyskeratosis, acantholysis and inflammation, features which can vary from biopsy to biopsy in the same patient. Immunofluorescent examination is negative. Occasionally a Tzanck smear is positive, showing acantholytic cells.

Course and Prognosis. The name is a misnomer. Grover originally stated that most cases cleared up after 2 months. When the patients lubricate their

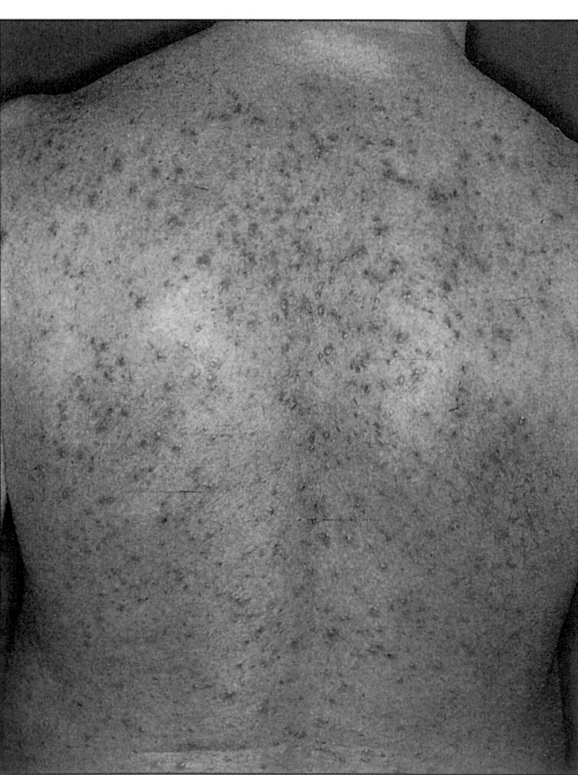

Fig. 17.21. Grover disease

skin, many resolve more quickly, but most relapse the next winter. In addition, some patients are very therapy-resistant and have trouble with Grover disease for many years.

Differential Diagnosis. The lesions look like a mild folliculitis or follicular dermatitis. One must also consider scabies, miliaria (in the summer cases), acneiform drug eruptions and dermatitis herpetiformis, as well as other causes of pruritus.

Therapy

Systemic. Oral retinoids bring a prompt resolution, but in this age group there are often reasons not to use them. Similarly, systemic corticosteroids have been employed to control the pruritus until topical therapy starts to work. Antihistamines especially at bedtime may bring relief.

Topical. Many patients do well with intensive lubrication and use of topical anesthetics such as polidocanol.

Phototherapy. UV radiation is helpful except for those rare patients in whom light is a trigger. PUVA bath therapy seems to be the treatment of choice, as many of these patients do not tolerate oral PUVA therapy.

Hailey-Hailey Disease

(Hailey and Hailey 1939)

Synonym. Familial benign chronic pemphigus

Definition. Acantholytic genodermatosis with no connection to the pemphigus family of autoimmune blistering disorders.

Epidemiology. Hailey-Hailey disease is a relatively common disease with the same order of incidence as Darier disease. The principle trigger factors are heat, sweating and friction. Some patients also flare with sunlight and superficial bacterial, viral or candidal infections.

Etiology and Pathogenesis. The disorder is inherited in an autosomal dominant pattern. The gene is located on chromosome 3q21–24 but its function is not known. Because of the many similarities to Darier disease, including ultrastructural evidence of abnormal tonofilament-desmosome complexes, the assumption is that there is a mutation in a structural gene needed in epidermal adherence and differentiation.

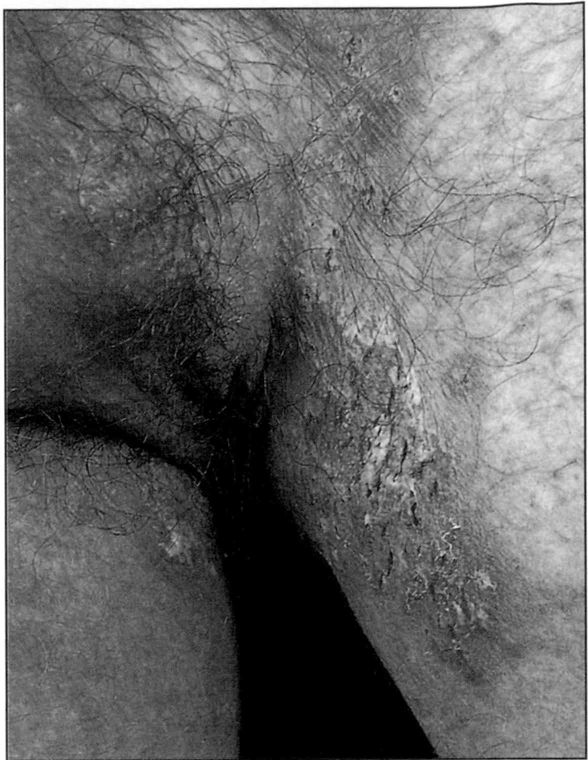

Fig. 17.22. Hailey-Hailey disease

Clinical Findings. The onset of the disease is usually in young adult life. The patches of Hailey-Hailey disease have been described in America as a dirt road drying out after a rain storm (Fig. 17.22). For readers in Lapland this will say very little, but it captures the image. The sites of predilection are areas of maceration and friction – the axilla, groin, perianal region and lateral aspects of the neck. While the initial lesion is an erythematous broad flaccid blister, it is often destroyed and overlooked (Fig. 17.23). The ruptured blisters evolve into dermatitis plaques with crust and multiple fissures. The lesions are usually symmetric and round, oval or circinate. The intertriginous lesions may weep, become foul smelling and develop papillomatous vegetations. When one looks carefully at the edge of lesions, small blisters can often be found. Pruritus is not as common or severe as in Darier disease, but can be quite troublesome. Occasionally a punctate palmoplanter keratoderma may be present, as well as longitudinal nail stripes, but both of these findings are much more common in Darier disease. Oral lesions do not occur.

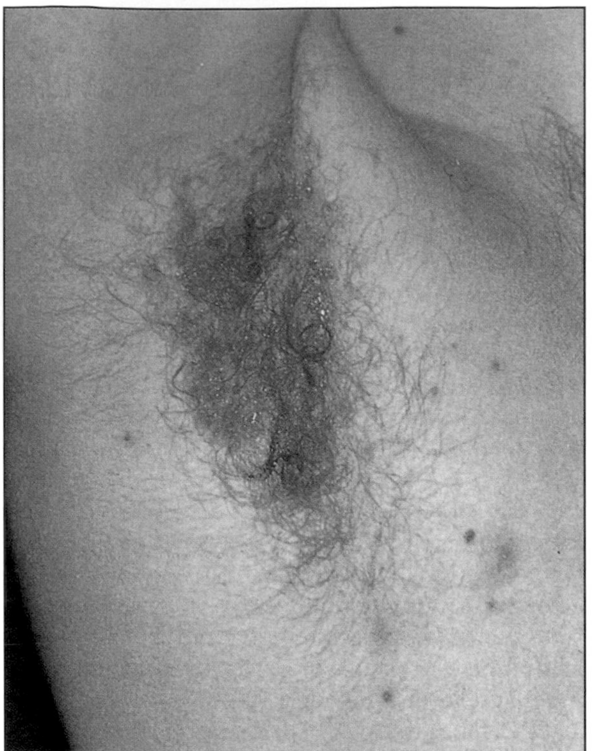

Fig. 17.23. Hailey-Hailey disease

Histopathology. The acantholysis in Hailey-Hailey disease has been compared to a dilapidated brick wall. There is diffuse acantholysis as the epidermis appears to collapse. Dyskeratotic cells are uncommon. The epidermis is often acanthotic with villous projections. Blisters are only seen when a biopsy is taken from the edge of a lesion. In the dermis there is often a fair amount of inflammation. Immunofluorescent examinations are negative.

Course and Prognosis. The disease waxes and wanes. Particularly disturbing to the patient are the flares which are often associated with bacterial, viral or candidal infections. Huge erosive weeping plaques in the groin are a difficult home nursing problem.

Differential Diagnosis. Hailey-Hailey disease is easy to misdiagnose. Many cases are missed at first as intertrigo or candidiasis. If only the groin or axilla is involved, Darier disease can be hard to exclude, especially since the nail and palmar changes, as well as the histologic findings, may be identical. In general, the pattern of distribution is different and Darier disease shows far more dyskeratosis. Later on the groin lesions can be mistaken for pemphigus vegetans. Here the lack of eosinophils and the negative direct immunofluorescence are decisive in favor of Hailey-Hailey disease.

Therapy

Systemic. Oral antibiotics are quite useful during flares. Oral corticosteroids will reduce inflammation, but predispose to more trouble with infections. Oral retinoids are also worth a try but they are not as reliably effective as in Darier disease.

Topical. Disinfectant measures such as gentian violet 0.1–0.5% aqueous solution, clioguinol or antibacterial cleansing solutions may reduce the flares. Some patients find topical corticosteroids helpful. Mixtures which also include antibacterial or antifungal agents are useful. Ointments should be avoided. Topical retinoids, either in their most dilute form or mixed with an appropriate vehicle to reduce their concentration, can be helpful but most often are too irritating.

Surgical. Dermabrasion, CO_2 laser destruction or excision followed by split-thickness skin grafting are all surprisingly effective to treat localized disease such as in the groin or axillae. Often the donor dominance lasts for many years.

Acrokeratosis Verruciformis

(Hopf 1931)

These patients have multiple flat-topped verrucous papules on the dorsal aspects of the hands and feet (Fig. 17.24). The lesions often have a polygonal pattern, mimicking lichen planus or plane warts. They may fuse together into larger plaques. In almost all cases, acrokeratosis verruciformis is associated

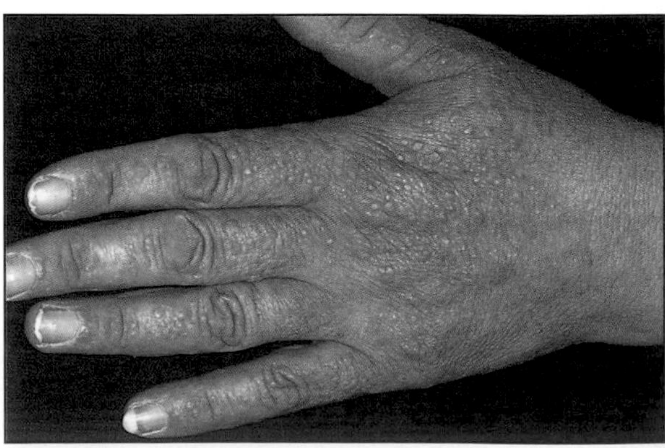

Fig. 17.24. Acrokeratosis verruciformis

with Darier disease, but in rare cases it may appear spontaneously or be inherited in an autosomal dominant pattern. In such cases it may represent partial expression of the gene for Darier disease. If the patient has any other even minor clues, such as dermatoglyphics, suggesting Darier disease, we prefer that diagnosis. If a specimen is carefully sectioned, usually focal dyskeratotic and acantholytic changes can be found. The differential diagnosis includes flat warts, epidermodysplasia verruciformis and acrokeratoelastoidosis and its variants. Individual lesions can be excised, curetted or destroyed with cryotherapy or a suitable laser.

Focal and Disseminated Acantholytic Acanthomas

Some patients have solitary or multiple papules dominated by acantholysis and dyskeratosis. Depending on whether acantholysis or dyskeratosis dominates, the lesions are designated acantholytic acanthoma or dyskeratotic acanthoma (papular acantholytic dyskeratosis). They differ from Grover disease because the lesions are nonpruritic, fewer in number, larger and more likely to be permanent. The genitalia in women are the most common sites for this disorder which in that setting should not be confused with localized pemphigus vulgaris.

Warty Dyskeratoma

This benign tumor is often clinically warty and microscopically shows Darier-like changes. It is discussed in Chapter 54.

Familial Dyskeratotic Comedones

(Carneiro et al. 1972)

This autosomal dominant disorder is characterized by hundreds or thousands of comedones, often appearing during puberty along with ordinary acne vulgaris. But these lesions are unusual on several counts. They can involve most of the body, sparing only the mucous membranes, scalp, palms and soles. Microscopically, they are more rectangular or patulous than an acne comedo and contain dyskeratotic and acantholytic cells in their plug. They do not always involve a hair follicle and, may not be true comedones, but instead keratotic invaginations. This further separates them from nevus comedonicus. Finally, the comedones are very difficult to treat, although topical retinoids are recommended. Laser destruction is also useful.

Porokeratoses

This family also shows the problems of naming a disease after a histologic finding. Porokeratosis is defined by the presence of a cornoid lamella in a keratotic lesion. The cornoid lamella is a column of parakeratotic cells arising from a focus in the epidermis where the stratum granulosum is either reduced or abnormal. Despite the name, there is little evidence that the defect is associated with the eccrine pore.

Porokeratosis of Mibelli

(Mibelli 1893)

Synonyms. Parakeratosis centrifugata atrophicans, parakeratosis Mibelli

Epidemiology. Porokeratosis of Mibelli is usually an acquired lesion, although occasional reports of autosomal dominant inheritance are found. Men are more often involved (2 : 1).

Etiology and Pathogenesis. Porokeratosis may represent a clonal expansion of a keratinocyte defect. Porokeratosis frequently seems to be associated with immunosuppression; it is more common in renal transplant patients, for example.

Clinical Findings. The lesions may appear at any age and are often multiple. The extremities are the favored sites, although the trunk, face and even glans have been involved. The initial lesion is a small red papule with a central keratotic spine. The lesion spreads peripherally with a distinctive white "ditch" surrounding it (Fig. 17.25). Set in the depression is a sheet of scale – the microscopic cornoid lamella. The central part of the lesion is often clinically atrophic. The periphery may have a wreath-like or circinate pattern. The lesions may reach a size of several centimeters, but usually are asymptomatic.

Two variants are:

- Linear porokeratosis: Some linear epidermal nevi following the lines of Blaschko show multiple cornoid lamella; in other cases, the lesions develop and grow later in life. Then one must

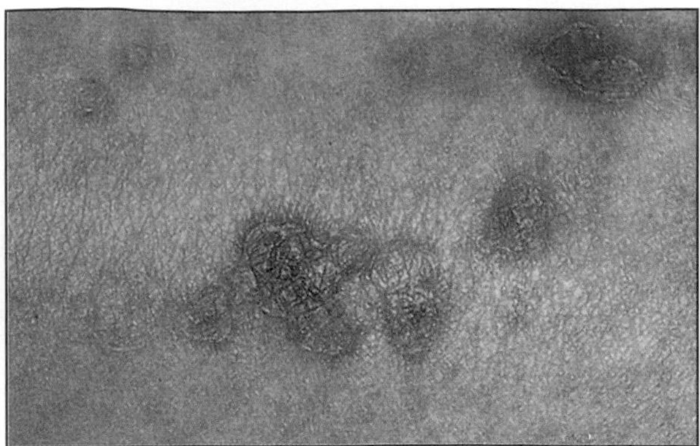

Fig. 17.25. Porokeratosis of Mibelli

view them as a linear variant of porokeratosis of Mibelli.
- Giant porokeratosis: Occasional lesions may reach a size of 10–20 cm with a thick wall, central scarring and a risk of malignant change.

Histopathology. It is often difficult to identify a cornoid lamella. Ideally one should take a small thin ellipse perpendicular to the border and have it cut along its long axis. Then the search is simpler. The epidermis is atrophic. There is no relationship between the cornoid lamellae and sweat pores. The dermis typically shows a sparse nonspecific lymphohistiocytic infiltrate. Sometimes the damage under the cornoid lamella is more severe and dermal collagen appears to be being extruded; this rare finding is known as perforating porokeratosis. Ultrastructural examination shows irregular basal cells, vacuolar degeneration in the granular layer and tonofilament clumping.

Course and Prognosis. Porokeratosis of Mibelli on rare occasions shows conversion to malignancy. While squamous cell carcinoma in situ (Bowen disease), frank squamous cell carcinoma with fatal metastases and basal cell carcinoma have been identified, this phenomenon is very rare in our experience.

Differential Diagnosis. Sometimes the lesions lack a distinctive border, perhaps because of keratolytic or emollient therapy. Then they may resemble a patch of dermatitis, Bowen disease, or an actinic keratosis, depending on the location.

Therapy. In general, all therapeutic measures are disappointing. Any destructive treatment is worth trying. Excision is most definitive, but often the problems with excising a 2–3-cm lesion around the ankle lead to alternative approaches. Cryotherapy may be helpful, as may other destructive measures. Occasionally topical retinoids or 5-fluorouracil over a long period of time may be helpful.

Disseminated Superficial Actinic Porokeratosis

(Chernosky and Freeman 1967)

Synonym. DSAP

Disseminated superficial actinic porokeratosis is a far more widespread variant of porokeratosis. Women are more often affected than men. While autosomal dominant inheritance has been described, most cases are sporadic. Sunlight appears to play a role. Patients develop many flat annular lesions on the backs of the hands, the dorsal aspects of the forearms and over the shins (Fig. 17.26). The lesions often have a less distinctive border than those in porokeratosis of Mibelli and may be more inflamed. The same patients usually have multiple actinic keratoses. On biopsy, the cornoid lamella requires even more searching, but the atrophy is often suggestive of the correct diagnosis. While the

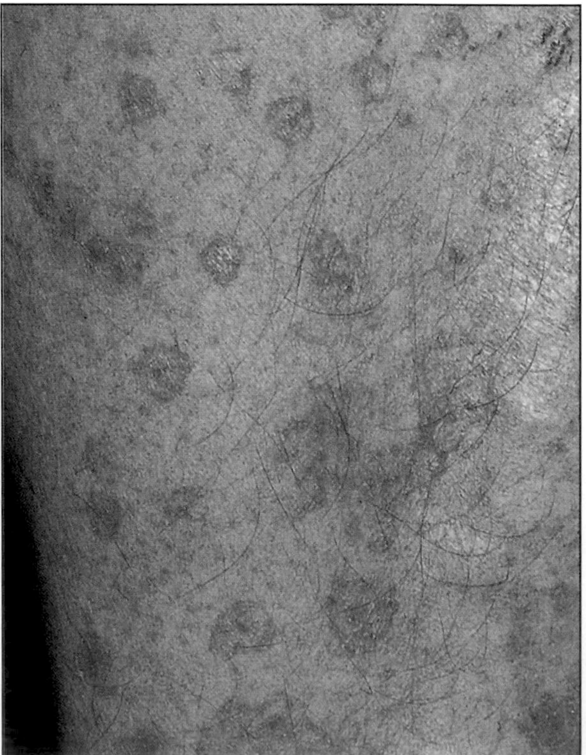

Fig. 17.26. Disseminated superficial actinic porokeratosis

risk of malignant change for any one lesion is small, monitoring is required because so many lesions are present. Sunscreens should be encouraged. Superficial destruction with cryotherapy, lasers or topical 5-fluorouracil can be tried.

Punctate Palmoplantar Porokeratosis

Synonyms. Punctate porokeratosis, spiny keratoderma

This autosomal dominant disorder typically begins in adolescence. Patients develop tiny spines on the palms and soles mimicking the spines on a music box drum. The lesions show no tendency to peripheral spread and remain small. Microscopically there is columnar parakeratosis and granular layer changes. Some argue that the typical ultrastructural changes of porokeratosis of Mibelli are not present. The differential diagnosis includes the other forms of punctate keratoderma. Mechanical abrading and keratolytics are usually helpful.

Porokeratosis Palmoplantaris Punctata et Disseminata

(Guss et al. 1971)

Some patients with punctate porokeratosis may also develop lesions away from the palms and soles, just as with almost all other forms of palmoplantar keratoderma. In contrast to disseminated superficial actinic porokeratosis, non-light-exposed areas are involved and the lesions are usually more papular, resembling warts or arsenical keratoses. Malignant degeneration has been described, but must be much less common than in the other forms.

Filiform Porokeratotic Palmoplantar Keratoderma

Several groups have described the relatively sudden eruption of multiple filiform spines on the palms and soles as an acquired marker of internal malignancy.

Porokeratosis Plantaris Discreta

Podiatrists frequently encounter solitary, endophytic keratotic lesions that may represent old plantar warts or clavi. Even though the lesions have a distinct parakeratotic column, it is not a true cornoid lamella. We view such parakeratosis as a feature of thick, traumatized skin of the feet and do not include such lesions with the rest of the porokeratosis family.

Other Keratotic Disorders

Hyperkeratosis Lenticularis Perstans

(Flegel 1958)

This very rare disorder, inherited in an autosomal dominant pattern, is more common in women and usually presents in adult life as hyperkeratotic papules on the lower aspects of the legs and dorsal surface of the feet. Rarely other parts of the body including the oral mucosa may be affected. The lesions are 2–4-mm red-brown keratotic papules that are usually asymptomatic. Biopsy shows a keratotic cap over an atrophic epidermis with an underlying focal lichenoid dermal infiltrate; a very distinctive picture indeed. There is no follicular involvement. Some ultrastructural studies have shown missing or defective lamellar bodies. Treatment is very difficult. Topical therapy does little, and the disease is usually not severe enough to justify extensive surgery, oral retinoids or corticosteroids. Sometimes PUVA therapy, especially PUVA bath therapy, or topical 5-fluorouracil may prove helpful.

Keratosis Lichenoides Chronica

(Kaposi 1896; Nékam 1938)

Synonyms. Lichenoid trikeratosis, Nékam disease

Clinical Findings. This rare chronic dermatosis is grouped as a variant of lichen planus by some individuals but has enough unique features to be mentioned on its own. Most patients are older men, although some patients first present in childhood or young adult life. The classical findings are hyperkeratotic lichenoid papules, striate or plaque-like keratoses and psoriasiform scaly patches (Fig. 17.27). The lesions usually start with lichenoid papules on the trunk or over the knees or elbows. Occasionally there is facial erythema and scale, suggesting seborrheic dermatitis or lupus erythematosus. Mucosal lesions, involving both the eyes and mouth, are rare but can be very disturbing. Even blindness has been reported as a late sequel.

Histopathology. The various lesions have quite different pictures. The papules closely resemble those

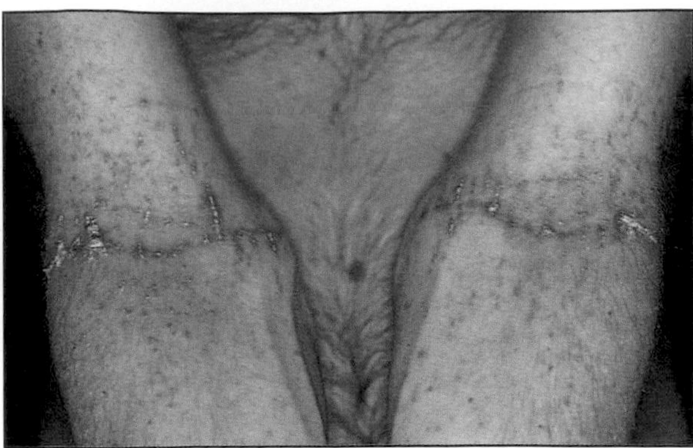

Fig. 17.27. Keratosis lichenoides chronica

of lichen planus. The more keratotic plaques may even show follicular plugging with an associated dermal inflammatory response. Sometimes microabscesses are seen, strongly suggesting psoriasis. Without a history, diagnosing keratosis lichenoides chronica from a single biopsy would be almost impossible. One should biopsy several different lesions if suspicious.

Differential Diagnosis. The differential diagnosis includes a long list, such as lichen planus, psoriasis, Reiter disease, Darier disease, pityriasis rubra pilaris and even lupus erythematosus. Usually the answer is found histologically with much diligence.

Therapy. No good therapy exists. Topical corticosteroids may reduce inflammation but the keratotic areas remain. Topical or even oral retinoids are worth considering. Both oral and bath PUVA have also been helpful.

Nipple Hyperkeratosis

Synonyms. Keratosis areolae mammae naeviformis (Otto), hyperkeratosis areolae mammae naeviformis

Some women have hyperkeratotic excrescences on their nipples. In some cases, they reflect an epidermal nevus, as Otto described, but these should become apparent at the latest during puberty. Lesions with a later onset are harder to explain. There may be hormonal influences or the keratoses may represent a reaction to a nipple dermatitis or trauma. Localized Darier disease can also present on the nipples. Dermabrasion or tangential excision is the best therapeutic approach in any event.

Multiple Minute Digitate Hyperkeratoses

Some patients have hundreds or thousands of asymptomatic nonfollicular tiny papules, most commonly on their trunk. The onset is in adult life. It has been suggested that the lesions are inherited in an autosomal dominant fashion.

Acanthosis Nigricans

(Pollitzer 1891)

Definition. Multiple small gray-brown verruciform papules most often in flexural areas which may be associated with a variety of underlying disorders.

Etiology and Pathogenesis. Acanthosis nigricans results from stimulation of epidermal growth in predisposed areas by either excessive levels of insulin, insulin-like growth factor, other epidermal growth factors, medications or tumor-related factors. The exact mechanism of these relationships are unclear, as the wide range of associated disorders discussed in the classification demonstrates. Ollendorff-Curth published the traditional classification of acanthosis nigricans almost 50 years ago. We have modified it somewhat (Table 17.6) but as the discussion makes clear, there are still problems.

Benign Acanthosis Nigricans. This is an extremely uncommon group of disorders with autosomal dominant inheritance. Typically the skin lesions develop in childhood and improve in adolescence. Women are more often affected than men. There is an overlap with pseudoacanthosis nigricans since obesity also tends to run in families.

Syndrome-Associated Acanthosis Nigricans. A long list of syndromes have been associated with acanthosis nigricans. The most fascinating are those with insulin resistance and high circulating insulin levels. Gorlin has subdivided this category into several more workable groups. All patients have peripheral resistance to insulin and varying degrees of diabetes mellitus.

- Defect in Insulin Receptor (Type A of Kahn). The HAIR-AN syndrome (hyperandrogenism, insulin resistance and acanthosis nigricans) is most common in adolescent women who may also have polycystic ovaries. The insulin receptor on the cell surface is defective so enormous circulating levels of insulin are produced. Leprechaunism, generalized lipodystrophy and Rabson-

Table 17.6. Classification of acanthosis nigricans

Feature	Benign forms					Malignant (paraneoplastic) AN
	Benign AN	AN associated with various syndromes	AN associated with endocrine disease	Pseudo-AN	Drug-induced AN	
Inheritance	AD	As the syndrome	Sporadic	Sporadic	Sporadic	Sporadic
Sex	F ≫ M	M = F	M = F	F ≫ M	M = F	M = F
Onset	Childhood	Childhood	Variable	Adolescence	Adult	Adult
Clinical features	Moderate involvement of flexural areas, may improve after puberty	Highly variable; in insulin resistance syndromes may be severe	Varies with endocrine disorder	More common in darker individuals and those who are over weight; associated with skin tags	Moderate	Severe, often with involvement of extremities and oral mucosa; associated with skin tags; Leser-Trélat sign; may be pruritic
Associated findings	None	Varies with syndrome; often high insulin levels	Acromegaly; pituitary tumors; Cushing syndrome; others	Obesity	History of medication use (nicotinic acid, corticosteroids, estrogens)	Underlying tumor, most often gastrointestinal adenocarcinoma

AN = acanthosis nigricans

Mendenhall syndrome also have defective insulin receptors.

- Presence of Autoantibodies (Type B of Kahn). Older patients with autoantibodies against the insulin receptor and usually multiple other autoantibodies and autoimmune disease, such as Sjögren, systemic lupus erythematosus, vitiligo and alopecia areata.
- Postreceptor Abnormalities (Type C of Kahn). Patients are similar to those of type A but have normal receptors.
- Obesity. Typically young female patients often with hyperandrogenism develop acanthosis nigricans but have normal receptors and no autoantibodies. Thus a postreceptor mechanism has been postulated (here is an obvious overlap with pseudoacanthosis nigricans). One can reasonably argue that acanthosis nigricans associated with obesity reflects some disturbance in the insulin receptor pathway which cannot be found in pseudoacanthosis nigricans.
- Generalized Lipodystrophy (Chap. 21). These patients have profound insulin resistance and diabetes mellitus with loss of fat, massive acanthosis nigricans and hirsutism, inherited in an autosomal recessive pattern.
- Prader-Willi Syndrome (Pollitzer 1891). The result of a deletion of parental 15q11–13, this usually sporadic disorder features obesity, hypogonadism, failure to thrive, and hypertonia. Patients have reduced skin pain sensitivity and almost always have open picked sores and multiple scars from such lesions, as well as acanthosis nigricans. Many have diabetes mellitus.
- Leprechaunism. Inherited in an autosomal dominant pattern, this disorder features failure to thrive, unusual facies, retarded bone age and sexual precocity along with acanthosis nigricans and diabetes mellitus. The problem seems to be with that part of the insulin receptor that binds both insulin and insulin-like growth factor. Unfortunately patients with several different disorders have been fancifully compared to the Irish leprechauns or little people.
- Rabson-Mendenhall Syndrome. Another insulin receptor disorder, probably inherited in an autosomal recessive pattern, in which patients have multiple dental anomalies, macroglossia, en-

larged genitalia, pineal gland hyperplasia, and acanthosis nigricans.

In addition to this long and by no means complete list there are yet other syndromes that may have acanthosis nigricans. All of the inherited disorders that result in elevated levels of corticosteroids, estrogens, progesterones, pituitary hormones and other growth-controlling hormones can produce acanthosis nigricans. In addition, there are some syndromes without obvious endocrine features in which acanthosis nigricans is nonetheless common. They include:

- Bloom Syndrome. Photosensitive, often Jewish, dwarfs with facial telangiectases and increased chromosome fragility and elevated sister chromatid exchange rates; autosomal recessive inheritance (Chap. 22).
- Crouzon Syndrome. Craniofacial dysostosis, increased fingerprint markings, hypoplastic maxilla producing pseudo-prognathism, exophthalmos, beaked nose, and acanthosis nigricans. Inherited in an autosomal dominant pattern.
- Beare-Stevenson Syndrome. Cutis verticis gyrata, acanthosis nigricans, craniosynostosis, cleft palate and hypodontia.

Acanthosis Nigricans Associated with Endocrine Disease. Just as many inherited endocrine disorders feature acanthosis nigricans, the same effects on the skin can be created by a range of acquired endocrine diseases. Acromegaly is most common, but pituitary tumors including Cushing syndrome, Addison disease, polycystic ovary disease, juvenile, insulin-dependent diabetes mellitus and many other underlying diagnoses are possible.

Pseudoacanthosis Nigricans. Many reject the concept of pseudoacanthosis nigricans, and we use the term only because it is so widely accepted. Studies have shown that acanthosis nigricans is relatively common in overweight dark-skinned adolescents, especially women. These individuals often have elevated insulin levels or some degree of insulin resistance. Their acanthosis nigricans may improve if they lose weight.

Drug-induced Acanthosis Nigricans. Many hormones such as corticosteroids and estrogens can under rare circumstances produce acanthosis nigricans. Agents used to interfere with lipid metabolism such as nicotinic acid and tripanarol also cause acanthosis nigricans, while rarely an acanthosis nigricans-like eruption has been associated with phenytoin.

Malignant (Paraneoplastic) Acanthosis Nigricans. This is the most important form of acanthosis nigricans and one of the most intriguing cutaneous markers of internal malignancies. Unfortunately it is also almost a death notice, for few patients whose tumor has advanced far enough to create acanthosis nigricans survive. Almost all tumors are carcinomas. About 60% arise in the stomach, 30% in other gastrointestinal organs and 10% elsewhere. In roughly 20% of cases, the skin changes appear first, and these patients have the best chance. In another 60% the two problems appear at about the same time while in the remaining 20% the tumor is well established before skin signs appear. When the tumor is excised, the acanthosis nigricans may disappear, but on the gloomy side, its reappearance usually heralds metastatic disease.

Clinical Findings. All the various forms of acanthosis nigricans appear clinically similar. The most widespread and severe disease is found in malignant acanthosis nigricans. The findings are symmetrical, typically involving the axillae and lateral aspect of the neck, as well as the groin, flexural areas of the limbs, umbilicus and nipples. The findings are symmetrical, typically involving the axillae sites (Figs. 17.28 and 17.29). More widespread disease, especially with oral, orbital or nostril findings, should suggest an underlying tumor. Most lesions are totally asymptomatic. If maceration occurs, there may be some pruritus. Tripe palms and soles probably represent acanthosis nigricans of these areas. Associated findings may include multiple skin tags and eruptive seborrheic keratoses (Leser-Trélat sign; Chap. 65).

The individual lesions are tiny, closely grouped, velvety papules. As they are brushed, normal skin can be seen at the base of the villous projections. Initial lesions may have a dirty yellow or gray color, but more advanced lesions are brown or black. In the inguinal area, accumulations resembling a cock's comb may appear. This may be a result of the frequent maceration. Often the middle part of a region will be hyperkeratotic while at the periphery the papules are smaller and there is a poorly defined transition to simple hyperpigmentation. On the palms and soles, there are exaggerated skin markings and velvety overgrowth, resembling the lining of the intestine and leading to the term tripe palms. In the mouth, the most common change is

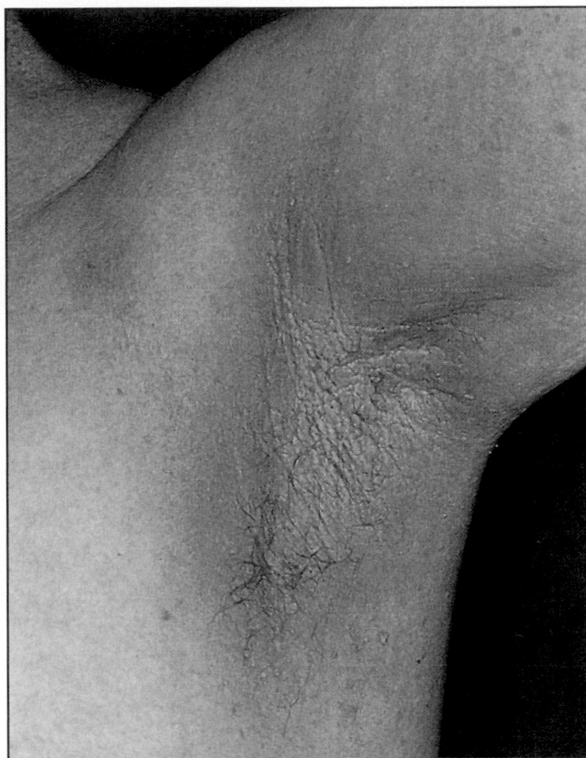

Fig. 17.28. Acanthosis nigricans

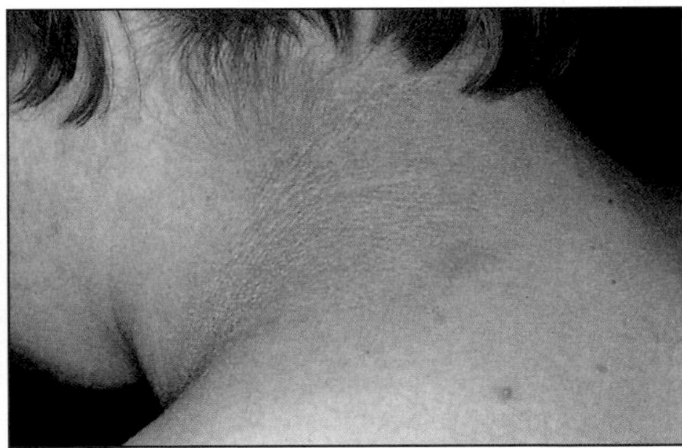

Fig. 17.29. Acanthosis nigricans

plaques on the tongue, although tiny papules can also appear on the lips and in extreme cases form warty excrescences.

Histopathology. Acanthosis nigricans is a histologic misnomer; there is no acanthosis and little hyperpigmentation. Instead, there is papillomatosis (church spires) and hyperkeratosis. When increased melanin is found, it is located in the basal layer. Despite the dramatic clinical picture, the microscopic findings are not remarkable and are identical to those in an acrochordon, small seborrheic keratosis or epidermal nevus.

Differential Diagnosis. Sorting out which type of acanthosis nigricans is present is enough of a challenge. Fortunately, there are not any serious differential diagnostic considerations. Multiple skin tags in an obese person appear similar but are probably a variation on the same biologic theme. Some forms of ichthyosis may appear very similar on the neck, but usually there are other more hyperkeratotic changes elsewhere. Occasionally Hailey-Hailey disease or pemphigus vegetans may be considered if the lesions are macerated. Confluent and reticulated papillomatosis is histologically similar but clinically quite different.

Therapy

Systemic. Oral retinoids, either isotretinoin or acitretin, bring transient improvement, but the disease relapses as soon as the medications are stopped. Thus, they are hardly ever employed. Overweight patients may dramatically improve if they lose weight.

Topical. There is no good topical therapy. Retinoids are probably the best approach; the patient must try to balance improvement against irritation. Other keratolytics such as salicylic acid or urea are only helpful in mild cases. The patient should be encouraged to use antibacterial syndets and to dry the area carefully, perhaps with a hair dryer. Secondary maceration can be treated with topical antibacterial or antifungal agents as appropriate.

Confluent and Reticulated Papillomatosis

(Gougerot and Carteaud 1927)

Synonym. Gougerot-Carteaud syndrome

Definition. Uncommon dermatosis consisting of multiple small flat papules arranged in a net-like pattern

Etiology and Pathogenesis. There are two completely different interpretations of the cause of confluent and reticulated papillomatosis. In some patients especially infants and children, *Malassezia furfur* has been identified, suggesting that confluent and reticulated papillomatosis is nothing more than a clinical variant of tinea versicolor. In others the same risk factors, darker skin and obesity, are present as in pseudoacanthosis nigricans and the disorder is considered a close relative of acanthosis nigricans. In the same light, it has occasionally been described in families. In our experience, *M. furfur* cannot be identified in every case, but this may reflect technical problems since the yeast is usually identified on microscopic examination, and difficult to culture.

Clinical Findings. The individual lesions are small papules, similar to plane warts or seborrheic keratoses. They are less than 5 mm in diameter and have a gray-brown color. The unique feature is that they are arranged in lacy or net-like patterns and may also coalesce into larger patches. The most common sites are the mid-chest, nape and back. On the neck, the lesions are very similar to those of acanthosis nigricans. In the initial description, Gougerot and Carteaud described three variants – pigmented verruciform, coalescing reticular and confluent nummular – reflecting the patterns described above. The lesions are asymptomatic, but tend to persist and are cosmetically annoying.

Histopathology. Histopathologic findings include papillomatosis and hyperkeratosis. Thus confluent and reticulated papillomatosis is another disease with church spires, so the histologic differential is that discussed under acanthosis nigricans. A Kolt examination or PAS stain is recommended to exclude *M. furfur*.

Differential Diagnosis. The main differential diagnosis is acanthosis nigricans; often the two blend together.

Therapy. It is probably worth trying topical antimycotic agents, even if KOH examination is negative. The easiest method is to use imidazole shampoos and have the patient employ them as a liquid soap. Other possibilities include topical retinoids. When the disease is localized, gentle curettage is a time-consuming but effective approach. Anecdotal reports endorse the use of oral minocycline or doxycycline for 3 – 6 weeks, an unusually long period to treat a superficial infection. In rare cases, systemic retinoids can be considered.

Granular Parakeratosis

(Northcutt et al. 1991)

Granular parakeratosis typically involves the axilla, but may effect other flexural areas. It presents with erythematous keratotic papules and plaques. The most unique feature is the striking parakeratosis seen microscopically. This change appears to reflect a derangement in the processing of profilaggrin to filaggrin. The differential diagnosis includes allergic and irritant contact dermatitis as well as Hailey-Hailey disease. Treatment is difficult but topical corticosteroid lotions appear most reasonable. Topical isotretinoin may also be helpful.

Dermatosis Papulosa Nigra

This disorder is almost entirely limited to blacks, and is covered in Chapter 72. The individual lesions are tiny papules on the cheeks which resemble small seborrheic keratoses or plane warts, so they fall into the same general class as acanthosis nigricans and confluent and reticulated papillomatosis.

Bibliography

Reviews

Ammirati CT, Mallory SB (1998) The major inherited disorders of cornification. New advances in pathogenesis. Dermatol Clin 16:497 – 508

Bale SJ, DiGiovanna JJ (1997) Genetic approaches to understanding the keratinopathies. Adv Dermatol 12:99 – 113

Elias PM (1983) Epidermal lipids, barrier function, and desquamation. J Invest Dermatol 80:44s – 49s

Happle R, Kerkhof PCM van de, Traupe H (1987) Retinoids in disorders of keratinization: their use in adults. Dermatologica 175 [Suppl 1]: 107 – 124

Irvine AD, McLean WH (1999) Human keratin diseases: the increasing spectrum of disease and subtlety of the phenotype-genotype correlation. Br J Dermatol 140: 815 – 828

Ishida-Yamamota A, Tanaka H, Nakane H et al. (1998) Inherited disorders of epidermal keratinization. J Dermatol Sci 18:139 – 154

Leigh IM, Lane EB, Watt FM (1994) The keratinocyte handbook. Cambridge University Press, Cambridge

Moss C, Savin J (1995) Dermatology and the new genetics. Blackwell Scientific Publications, Oxford

Novice FM, Collison DW, Burgdorf WHC et al. (1994) Handbook of genetic skin disorders. Saunders, Philadelphia

Traupe H (1989) The ichthyoses. A guide to clinical diagnosis, genetic counseling, and therapy. Springer, Berlin

Williams ML, Elias PM (1987) Genetically transmitted, generalized disorders of cornification. The ichthyoses. Dermatol Clin 5:155 – 178

Williams ML, Elias PM (1993) From basket weave to barrier. Unifying concepts for the pathogenesis of the disorders of cornification. Arch Dermatol 129:626 – 629

The Ichthyoses

Aras N, Sutman K, Tastan HB et al. (1994) Peeling skin syndrome. J Am Acad Dermatol 30:135 – 136

Bäfverstedt B (1941) Fall von genereller, naevusartiger Hyperkeratose, Imbecillität, Epilepsie. Acta Dermato Venereol (Stockh) 22:207 – 212

Bale SJ, Compton JG, DiGiovanna JJ (1993) Epidermolytic Hyperkeratosis. Semin Dermatol 12:202–209

Basarab T, Smith FJ, Jolliffe VM et al. (1999) Ichthyosis bullosa of Siemens: report of a family with evidence of a keratin 2e mutation, and a review of the literature. Br J Dermatol 140:689–695

Bichakjian CK, Nair RP, Wu WW et al. (1998) Prenatal exclusion of lamellar ichthyosis based on identification of two new mutations in the transglutaminase 1 gene. J Invest Dermatol 110:179–182

Brocq L (1902) Erythrodermie congénitale ichthyosiforme avec hyperépidermotrophie. Ann Dermatol Syph Ser 4:1–31

Brusasco A, Cavalli R, Cambiaghi S et al. (1994) Ichthyosis Curth-Macklin: a new sporadic case with immunohistochemical study of keratin expression (letter). Arch Dermatol 130:1077–1079

Brusasco A, Veraldi S, Tadini G et al. (1998) Localized peeling skin syndrome: case report with ultrastructural study. Br J Dermatol 139:492–495

Castano Suarez E, Segurado Rodriguez A, Guerra Tapia A et al. (1997) Ichthyosis: the skin manifestation of multiple sulfatase deficiency. Pediatr Dermatol 14:369–372

Chanarin I, Patel A, Slavin G et al. (1975) Neutral lipid storage disease: a new disorder of lipid metabolism. Br Med J 1:553–555

Choate KA, Williams ML, Elias PM et al. (1998) Transglutaminase 1 expression in a patient with features of harlequin ichthyosis: case report. J Am Acad Dermatol 38: 325–329

Comél M (1949) Ichthyosis linearis circumflexa. Dermatologica 98:133–136

Conradi E (1914) Vorzeitiges Auftreten von Knochen und eigenartigen Verkalkungskernen bei Chondrodystrophia foetalis hypoplastica. Jahrb Kinderh 80:86–97

Curth H, Macklin MT (1954) The genetic basis of various types of ichthyosis in a family group. Am J Hum Genet 6:371–382

Dale BA, Kam E (1993) Harlequin ichthyosis. Variability in expression and hypothesis for disease mechanism. Arch Dermatol 129:1471–1477

Dorfman ML, Hershko C, Eisenberg S et al. (1974) Ichthyosiform dermatosis with systemic lipidosis. Arch Dermatol 110:261–266

Fartasch M, Williams ML, Elias PM (1999) Altered lamellar body secretion and stratum corneum membrane structure in netherton syndrome. Arch Dermatol 135:823–832

Fox H (1921) Skin shedding (keratolysis exfoliativa congenita). Report of a case. Ann Dermatol Syphilol 3:202

Haftek M, Cambazard F, Dhouailly D et al. (1996) A longitudinal study of a harlequin infant presenting clinically as non-bullous congenital ichthyosiform erythroderma. Br J Dermatol 135:448–453

Happle R (1979) X-linked dominant chondrodysplasia punctata. Review of literature and report of a case. Hum Genet 53:65–73

Happle R, Koch H, Lenz W (1980) The CHILD syndrome. Congenital hemidysplasia with ichthyosiform erythroderma and limb defects. Eur J Pediatr 134:27–33

Happle R, Traupe H, Grobe H et al. (1984) The Tay syndrome (congenital ichthyosis with trichothiodystrophy). Eur J Pediatr 141:147–152

Hennies HC, Kuster W, Wiebe V et al. (1998) Genotype/-phenotype correlation in autosomal recessive lamellar ichthyosis. Am J Hum Genet 62:1052–1061

Huber M, Rettler I, Bernasconi K et al. (1995) Mutations of keratinocyte transglutaminase in lamellar ichthyosis. Science 267:525–528

Hünermann C (1931) Chondrodystrophia calcificans congenita alos abortive Form der Chondrodystrophie. Zschr Kinderh 51:1–19

Ishida-Yamamoto A, McGrath JA, Judge MR et al. (1992) Selective involvement of keratins K1 and K10 in the cytoskeletal abnormality of epidermolytic hyperkeratosis (bullous congenital ichthyosiform erythroderma). J Invest Dermatol 99:19–26

Jeon S, Djian P, Green H (1998) Inability of keratinocytes lacking their specific transglutaminase to form cross-linked envelopes: absence of envelopes as a simple diagnostic test for lamellar ichthyosis. Proc Natl Acad Sci USA 95:687–690

Kolde G, Happle R, Traupe H (1985) Autosomal-dominant lamellar ichthyosis: ultrastructural characteristics of a new type of congenital ichthyosis. Arch Dermatol Res 278:1–5

Korge BP, Krieg T (1996) The molecular basis for inherited bullous diseases. J Mol Med 74:59–70

McGrath J, Cerio R, Wilson-Jones E (1991) The phenotypic heterogenicity of bullous ichthyosis – a case report of three family members. Clin Exp Dermatol 16:25–27

Melnik B, Kuster W, Hollmann J et al. (1989) Autosomal dominant lamellar ichthyosis exhibits an abnormal scale lipid pattern. Clin Genet 35:152–156

Nanda A, Sharma R, Kanwar AJ et al. (1990) Dorfman-Chanarin syndrome. Int J Dermatol 29:349–351

Netherton EW (1958) A unique case of trichorrhexis nodosa – "bamboo hairs". Arch Dermatol 778:483–487

Norton SA, Ruze P (1994) Kava dermopathy. J Am Acad Dermatol 31:89–97

Ollendorff-Curth H, Macklin MT (1954) The genetic basis of various types of ichthyosis in a family group. Am J Hum Genet 6:371–382

Paige DG, Emilion GG, Bouloux PM et al. (1994) A clinical and genetic study of X-linked recessive ichthyosis and contiguous gene defects. Br J Dermatol 131:622–629

Powell J, Dawber RPR, Ferguson DJP et al. (1999) Netherton's syndrome: increased likelihood of diagnosis by examining eyebrow hairs. Br J Dermatol 141:544–546

Refsum S (1945) Heredoataxia hemerolopica polyneuritiformis et tidligere ikke beskrevet familial syndrome? En forelobig modelelse. Nord Med 28:2682–2685

Riecke E (1900) Über Ichthyosis congenita. Arch Dermatol Syph (Wien) 54:289–340

Rizzo WB (1993) Sjögren-Larsson syndrome. Semin Dermatol 12:210–218

Rizzo WB (1998) Inherited disorders of fatty alcohol metabolism. Mol Genet Metab 65:63–73

Saeki H, Kuwata S, Nakagawa H et al. (1998) Deletion pattern of the steroid sulphatase gene in Japanese patients with X-linked ichthyosis. Br J Dermatol 139:96–98

Sahn EE, Weimer CE Jr, Garen PD (1992) Annular epidermolytic ichthyosis: a unique phenotype. J Am Acad Dermatol 27:348–355

Sato-Matsumura KC, Matsumura T, Kumakiri M et al. (2000) Ichthyosis follicularis with alopecia and photophobia in a mother and daughter. Br J Dermatol 142:157–162

Schnyder UW (1977) Ichthyosis hystrix typus Reydt (ichthyosis hystrix gravior mit praktischer Taubheit). Z Hautkr 52:763–766

Siemens W (1937) Dichtung und Wahrheit über die "Ichthyosis bullosa", mit Bemerkungen zur Systematik der Epidermolysen. Arch Dermatol Syph (Berlin) 175:590–608

Sjögren T, Larsson T (1957) Oligophrenia in combination with congenital ichthyosis and spastic disorders. A clinical and genetic study. Acta Psychiatr Scand 32 [Suppl 113]: 1–108

Smith DL, Smith JG, Wong SW et al. (1995) Netherton's syndrome: a syndrome of elevated IgE and characteristic skin and hair findings. J Allergy Clin Immunol 95:116–123

Srebrnik A, Brenner S, Ilie B et al. (1998) Dorfman-Chanarin syndrome: morphologic studies and presentation of new cases. Am J Dermatopathol 20:79–85

Steijlen PM, Perret CM, Schuurmans Stekhoven JH et al. (1990) Ichthyosis bullosa of Siemens: further delineation of the phenotype. Arch Dermatol Res 282:1–5

Tay CH (1971) Ichthyosiform erythroderma, hair shaft abnormalities, and mental and growth retardation. A new recessive disorder. Arch Dermatol 104:4–13

Traupe H, Kolde G, Happle R (1984) Autosomal dominant lamellar ichthyosis: a new skin disorder. Clin Genet 26:457–461

Traupe H, Kolde G, Hamm H et al. (1986) Ichthyosis bullosa of Siemens: a unique type of epidermolytic hyperkeratosis. J Am Acad Dermatol 14:1000–1005

Van Neste D, Caulier B, Thomas P et al. (1985) PIBIDS: Tay's syndrome and xeroderma pigmentosum. J Am Acad Dermatol 12:372–373

Wells RS, Kerr CB (1965) Genetic classification of ichthyosis. Arch Dermatol 92:1–6

Wile UJ (1924) Familial study of three unusual cases of congenital ichthyosiform erythroderma. Arch Dermatol Syph 4:487–498

Williams ML (1992) Ichthyosis: mechanisms of disease. Pediatr Dermatol 9:365–368

Williams ML, Feingold KR, Grubauer G et al. (1987) Ichthyosis induced by cholesterol-lowering drugs. Implications for epidermal cholesterol homeostasis. Arch Dermatol 123:1535–1538

Wöhrle D, Barbi G, Schulz W et al. (1990) Heterozygous expression of X-linked chondrodysplasia punctata. Complex chromosome aberration including deletion of MIC2 and STS. Hum Genet 86:215–218

Palmoplantar Keratodermas

Bart RS, Pumphrey RE (1967) Knuckle pads, leukonychia and deafness. A dominantly inherited syndrome. N Eng J Med 276:202–207

Brauer A (1913) Über eine besondere Form des hereditären Keratoms (Keratoma dissipatum hereditarium palmare et plantare). Arch Dermatol 114:211–236

Brünauer SR (1923) Zur Vererbung des Keratoma hereditarium palmare et plantare. Acta Derm Venereol (Stockh) 4:489–503

Buschke A, Fischer W (1910) Keratodermia maculosa disseminata symmetrica palmaris et plantaris. In: Neisser A, Jacobi E (eds) Ikonographia dermatologica, vol 1. Urban and Schwarzenberg, Berlin, pp 183–192

Camisa C (1986) Keratoderma hereditaria mutilans or Vohwinkel's syndrome. J Am Acad Dermatol 14:512–514

Christiano AM (1997) Frontiers in keratodermas: pushing the envelope. Trends Genet 13:227–233

Clarke CA, Howel-Evans AW, McConnell RB (1957) Carcinoma of oesophagus associated with tylosis. BMJ 1:945

Cole LA (1976) Hypopigmentation with punctate keratosis of the palms and soles. Arch Dermatol 112:998–1000

Covello SP, Irvine AD, McKenna KE et al. (1998) Mutations in keratin K9 in kindreds with epidermolytic palmoplantar keratoderma and epidemiology in Northern Ireland. J Invest Dermatol 111:1207–1209

Fluckiger R, Itin PH (1993) Keratosis extremitatum (Greither's disease): clinical features, histology, ultrastructure. Dermatology 187:309–311

Frias-Iniesta J, Sanchez-Pedreño P, Martinez-Escribano JA et al. (1997) Br J Dermatol 136:935–938

Fuhs H (1924) Zur Kenntnis der herdweisen Keratosen an Händen und Füßen. Acta Derm Venereol (Stockh) 5:11–58

Greither A (1952) Keratosis extremitatum hereditaria progrediens mit dominantem Erbgang. Hautarzt 3:198–203

Hanhart E (1947) Neue Sonderformen von Keratosis palmoplantaris. Dermatologica 94:286–308

Helm T, Spigel GT, McMahon J et al. (1998) Striate palmoplantar keratoderma: a clinical and ultrastructural study. Cutis 61:18–20

Howel-Evans W et al. (1958) Carcinoma of the esophagus with keratosis palmaris et plantaris (tylosis): a study in two families. Q J Med 27:413

Huriez C, Deminati M, Agache P et al. (1969) Génodermatose scléro-atrophiante et kératodermique des extrémités. Ann Dermatol Syphilgr 96:135–146

Irvine AD, McLean WH (199) Human keratin diseases: the increasing spectrum of disease and subtlety of the phenotype-genotype correlation. Br J Dermatol 140: 815–828

Itin PH, Lautenschlager S (1995) Palmoplantar keratoderma and associated syndromes. Semin Dermatol 14:152–161

Kellum RE (1989) Papillon-Lefevre syndrome in four siblings treated with etretinate. A nine-year evaluation. Int J Dermatol 28:605–608

Kogoj F (1934) Die Krankheit von Mljet („Mal de Meleda"). Acta Derm Venereol (Stockh) 15:264–299

Küster W, Becker A (1992) Indication for the identity of palmoplantar keratoderma type Unna-Thost with type Vörner. Thost's family revisited 110 years later. Acta Derm Venereol (Stockh) 72:120–122

Lestringant GG, Frossard PM, Adeghate E et al. (1997) Mal de Meleda: a report of four cases from the United Arab Emirates. Pediatr Dermatol 14:186–191

Maestrini E, Monaco AP, McGrath JA et al. (1996) A molecular defect in loricrin, the major component of the cornified cell envelope, underlies Vohwinkel's syndrome. Nat Genet 13:70–77

Magro CM, Baden LA, Crowson AN et al. (1997) A novel nonepidermolytic palmoplantar keratoderma: a clinical and histopathologic study of six cases. J Am Acad Dermatol 37:27–33

Nazarro V, Blanchet-Bardon C, Mimoz C et al. (1988) Papillon-Lefèvre syndrome. Ultrastructural study and successful treatment with acitretin. Arch Dermatol 124: 533–539

Olmstead HC (1927) Keratodermia palmaris et plantaris congenitalis: report of a case showing associated lesions of unusual location. Am J Dis Child 33:757–764

Paoli S, Mastrolorenzo A (1999) Keratosis palmoplantaris varians of Wachters. J Eur Acad Dermatol Venereol 12: 33–37

Papillon MM, Lefèvre P (1924) Deux cas de kératodermie palmaire et plantaire symétrique familiale (maladie de Meleda) chez le frère et la soeur. Coexistence dans les deux cas d'altérations dentaires graves. Bull Soc Fr Dermatol Venereol 31:82–87

Patrizi A, DiLernia V, Patrone P (1992) Palmoplantar keratoderma with sclerodactyly (Huriez syndrome). J Am Acad Dermatol 26:855–857

Ratnavel RC, Griffiths WA (1997) The inherited palmoplantar keratodermas. Br J Dermatol 137:485–490

Schöpf E, Schulz HJ, Passarge E (1971) Syndrome of cystic eyelids, palmo-plantar keratosis, hypodontia and hypotrichosis as a possible autosomal recessive trait. Birth Defects Orig Art Ser 7(8):219–221

Siemens HW (1929) Keratosis palmaris-plantaris striata. Arch Dermatol 157:392–408

Stevens HP, Kelsell DP, Bryant SP et al. (1996) Linkage of an American pedigree with palmoplantar keratoderma and malignancy (palmoplantar ektodermal dysplasia Type III) to 17q24. Literature survey and proposed updated classification of keratodermas. Arch Dermatol 132:640–651

Stevens HP, Kelsell DP, Leigh IM et al. (1996) Punctate palmoplantar keratoderma and malignancy in a four-generation family. Br J Dermatol 134:720–726

Thost A (1880) Über erbliche Ichtyosis palmaris et plantaris cornea. Inaugural Dissertation, University of Heidelberg

Unna PG (1883) Über das Keratoma palmare et plantare hereditarium. Vierteljahresschr Dermatol Syph 15:231–270

Verplancke P, Driessen L, Wynants P et al. (1998) The Schopf-Schulz-Passarge syndrome. Dermatology 196: 463–466

Vohwinkel KH (1929) Keratoma hereditarium mutilans. Arch Dermatol Syph 158:354–364

Vörner H (1901) Zur Kenntnisse des Keratoma hereditarium palmare et plantare. Arch Dermatol Syph (Berlin) 56: 3–31

Erythrokeratodermias

Baden HP, Bronstein BR (1988) Ichthyosiform dermatosis and deafness. Report of a case and review of the literature. Arch Dermatol 124:102–106

Burns FS (1915) A case of generalized congenital keratoderma. J Cutan Dis Dermatol 33:255–260

Darier MJ (1911) Erythro-kératodermie verruqueuse en nappes, symétrique et progressive. Bull Soc Fr Dermatol Syph 2:252–264

Degos R, Delzant O, Morival H (1947) Erytheme desquamatif en plaques, congenital et familial (genodermatose nouvelle?) Bull Fr Soc Dermatol Syph 54:442

Findlay GH, Nurse GT, Heyl T et al. (1977) Keratolytic winter erythema or "oudtshoorn skin": a newly recognized inherited dermatosis prevalent in South Africa. S Afr Med 52:871–874

Giroux JM, Barbeau A (1972) Erythrokeratodermia with ataxia. Arch Dermatol 106:183–188

Gottron H (1922) Congenital angelegte symmetrische progressive Erythrokeratodermie. Zentralbl Haut Geschl Krankh 4:493–494

Gray LC, Davis LS, Guill MA (1996) Progressive symmetric erythrokeratodermia. J Am Acad Dermatol 34:858–859

Mendes da Costa S (1925) Erythro- et keratodermia variabilis in a mother and a daughter. Acta Derm Venereol (Stockh) 6:255–261

Papadavid E, Koumantaki E, Dawber RP (1998) Erythrokeratoderma variabilis: case report and review of the literature. J Eur Acad Dermatol Venereol 11:180–183

Rajagopaalan B, Pulimood S, George S et al. (1999) Erythrokeratoderma en cocardes. Clin Exp Dermatol 24:173–174

Follicular Keratoses

Barron DR, Hirsch AL, Buchbinder L et al. (1987) Folliculitis ulerythematosus reticulata: a report of four cases and brief review of the literature. Pediatr Dermatol 4:85–89

Friedman SJ (1990) Lichen spinulosus. Clinicopathologic review of thirty-five cases. J Am Acad Dermatol 22:261–264

Heidenström N, Tottie M (1944) Haut- und Gelenkveränderungen bei multiplem Myelom. Acta Dermatol Venereol 2:192–199

Kim TY, Park YM, Jang IG et al. (1997) Idiopathic follicular hyperkeratotic spicules. J Am Acad Dermatol 36:476–477

Kunte C, Loeser C, Wolff H (1998) Folliculitis spinulosa decalvans: successful therapy with dapsone. J Am Acad Dermatol 39:891–893

Poskitt L, Wilkinson JD (1994) Natural history of keratosis pilaris. Br J Dermatol 130:711–713

Rand R, Baden HP (1983) Keratosis follicularis spinulosa decalvans. Arch Dermatol 119:22–26

Siemens HW (1926) Keratosis follicularis spinulosa decalvans. Arch Dermatol 151:384–386

Dyskeratotic-Acantholytic Disorders

Antley CM, Carrington PR, Mrak RE et al. (1998) Grover's disease (transient acantholytic dermatosis): relationship of acantholysis to acrosyringia. J Cutan Pathol 25:545–549

Beier C, Kaufmann R (1999) Efficacy of erbium: YAG laser ablation in Darier disease and Hailey-Hailey disease. Arch Dermatol 135:423–427

Burge SM, Wilkinson JD (1992) Darier-White disease: a review of the clinical features in 163 patients. J Am Acad Dermatol 27:40–50

Burkhart CG, Burkhart CN (1998) Tazarotene gel for Darier's disease. J Am Acad Dermatol 38:1001–1002

Carneiro SJC, Dickson JE, Knox JM (1972) Familial dyskeratotic comedones. Arch Dermatol 105:249–251

Casanova JM, Pujol RM, Taberner R et al. (1999) Grover's disease in patients with chronic renal failure receiving hemodialysis: Clinicopathologic review of 4 cases. J Am Acad Dermatol 41:1029–1033

Chapman-Rolle L, DePadova-Elder SM, Ryan E et al. (1994) Persistent flat-topped papules on the extremities. Acrokeratosis verruciformis (AKV) of Hopf. Arch Dermatol 130:508–509

Darier J (1889) Psorospermose folliculaire végétante. Ann Derm Venereol 3(10):597–612

Davis MD, Dinneen AM, Landa N et al. (1999) Grover's disease: clinicopathologic review of 72 cases. Mayo Clin Proc 74:229–234

Grover RW (1970) Transient acantholytic dermatosis. Arch Derm 101:426–434

Hailey H, Hailey H (1939) Familial benign chronic pemphigus. Arch Dermatol 39:679–685

Hopf G (1931) Über eine bisher nicht beschriebene disseminierte Keratose (Akrokeratosis verruciformis). Dermatol Z 60:227–250

Metze D, Hamm H, Schorat A et al. (1996) Involvement of the adherens junction-actin filament system in acantholytic dyskeratosis of Hailey-Hailey disease. A histological, ultrastructural, and histochemical study of lesional and non-lesional skin. J Cutan Pathol 23:211–222

O'Malley MP, Haake A, Goldsmith L et al. (1997) Localized Darier disease. Implications for genetic studies. Arch Dermatol 133:1134–1138

Parsons JM (1996) Transient acantholytic dermatosis (Grover's disease): a global perspective. J Am Acad Dermatol 35:653–666

Price M, Russel Jones R (1985) Familial dyskeratotic comedones. Clin Exp Derm 10:147–153

Sakuntabhai A, Ruiz-Perez V, Carter S et al. (1999) Mutations in ATP2A2, encoding a Ca^{2+} pump, cause Darier disease. Nat Genet 21:271–277

Sánchez-Carpintero I, España A, Idoate MA (1999) Disseminated epidermolytic acanthoma probably related to trauma. Br J Dermatol 141:728–730

Tada J, Hashimoto K (1998) Ultrastructural localization of cell junctional components (desmoglein, plakoglobin, E-cadherin, and beta-catenin) in Hailey-Hailey disease, Darier's disease, and pemphigus vulgaris. J Cutan Pathol 25:106–115

Van Geel NA, Kockaert M, Neumann HA (1999) Familial dyskeratotic comedones. Br J Dermatol 140:956–959

White JC (1889) A case of keratosis (ichthyosis) follicularis. J Cutan Dis 7:201–209

Wolff HH, Chalet MD, Ackermann AB (1977) Transitorische akantholytische Dermatose (Grover). Hautarzt 28:78–82

Zarour H, Grob JJ, Andrac L et al. (1992) Palmoplantar orthokeratotic filiform hyperkeratosis in a patient with associated Darier's disease. Classification of filiform hyperkeratosis. Dermatology 185:205–209

Porokeratoses and Other Disorders

Alpsoy E, Yilmaz E, Aykol A (1997) Hyperkeratosis of the nipple: report of two cases. J Dermatol 24:43–45

Balus L, Donati P, Amantea A et al. (1988) Multiple minute digitate hyperkeratosis. J Am Acad Dermatol 18:431–436

Bohm M, Luger TA, Bonsmann G (1999) Disseminated superficial actinic porokeratosis: treatment with topical tacalcitol. J Am Acad Dermatol 40:479–480

Braun-Falco O, Bieber T, Heider L (1989) Keratosis lichenoides chronica – Krankheitsvariante oder Krankheitsentität? Hautarzt 40:614–622

Chernosky ME, Freeman RG (1967) Disseminated superficial actinic porokeratosis (DSAP). Arch Dermatol 96: 611–624

Fimiani M, Rubegni P, Andreassi L (1996) Linear palmo-plantar porokeratotic hamartoma. Br J Dermatol 135: 492–494

Fisher CA, LeBoit PE, Frieden IJ (1995) Linear porokeratosis presenting as erosions in the newborn period. Pediatr Dermatol 12:318–322

Flegel H (1958) Hyperkeratosis lenticularis perstans. Hautarzt 9:362–364

Friedman SJ, Herman PS, Pittelkow MR et al. (1988) Punctuate porokeratotic keratoderma. Arch Dermatol 124: 1678–1682

Gougerot H, Carteaud A (1927) Papilomatose pigmentée inominée. Cas pour diagnostic. Bull Soc Fr Derm Syph 34:719–721

Gus SB, Osbourn RA, Lutzner MA (1971) Porokeratosis plantaris, palmaris et disseminata. A third type of porokeratosis. Arch Dermatol 104:366–373

Herranz P, Pizarro A, De Lucas R et al. (1997) High incidence of porokeratosis in renal transplant recipients. Br J Dermatol 136:176–179

Ito M, Fujiwara H, Maruyama T et al. (1991) Morphogenesis of the cornoid lamella: histochemical, immunohistochemical, and ultrastructural study of porokeratosis. J Cutan Pathol 18:247–256

Jurecka W, Neumann RA, Knobler RM (1991) Porokeratoses: immunohistochemical, light and electron microscopic evaluation. J Am Acad Dermatol 24:96–101

Kaposi M (1886) Lichen ruber moniliformis – Korallenschnurartiger Lichen ruber. Arch Derm Syph 1:1–32

Konstantinov KN, Sondergaard J, Izuno G et al. (1998) Keratosis lichenoides chronica. J Am Acad Dermatol 1998 38:306–309

Li TH, Hsu CK, Chiu HC et al. (1997) Multiple asymptomatic hyperkeratotic papules on the lower part of the legs. Hyperkeratosis lenticularis perstans (HLP) (Flegel disease). Arch Dermatol 133:910–914

Mehregan DA, Vandersteen P, Sikorski L et al. (1995) Axillary granular parakeratosis. J Am Acad Dermatol 33(2 Pt 2):373–375

Metze D, Rütten A (1999) Granular parakeratosis – a unique acquired disorder of keratinization. J Cutan Pathol 26: 339–352

Mibelli V (1893) Contributo allo studio della ipercheratose dei canali sudoriferi (porokeratosi). G Ital Mal Ven 28: 313–355

Nékam L (1938) Sur la question du lichen moniliformis. Presse Med 46:100

Northcutt AD, Nelson DM, Tschen JA (1991) Axillary granular parakeratosis. J Am Acad Dermatol 24(4):541–544

Pollitzer S (1891) Acanthosis nigricans. In: Unna PG, Morris M, Besnier E, et al. (eds) International atlas of rare skin diseases. HK Lewis, London, pp 1–3

Sasson M, Abigal DK (1996) Porokeratosis and cutaneous malignancy. A review. Dermatol Surg 22:339–342

Sawai T, Hayakawa H, Danno K et al. (1996) Squamous cell carcinoma arising from giant porokeratosis: a case with extensive metastasis and hypercalcemia. J Am Acad Dermatol 34:507–509

Schaller M, Korting HC, Kollmann M et al. (1996) The hyperkeratotic variant of porokeratosis Mibelli is a distinct entity: clinical and ultrastructural evidence. Dermatology 192:255–258

Schamroth JM, Zlotogorski A, Gilead L (1997) Porokeratosis of Mibelli. Overview and review of the literature. Acta Derm Venereol (Stockh) 77:207–213

Webster CG, Resnik KS, Webster GF (1997) Axillary granular parakeratosis: response to isotretinoin. J Am Acad Dermatol 37(5 Pt 1):789–790

Yanklowitz B, Harkless L (1990) Porokeratosis plantaris discreta. A misnomer. J Am Podiatr Med Assoc 80:381–384

CHAPTER 18

Diseases of Connective Tissue

Contents

A wide variety of quite different diseases are discussed in this chapter. Their one unifying feature is abnormalities of the dermis, both quantitative, such as atrophy or hypertrophy, and qualitative with abnormal collagen, elastin, fibroblasts and ground substance. At the same time such disorders typically also affect the adnexal structures, nerves and vessels all of which are in intimate relation with the connective tissue. The heterogeneity of these disorders is underscored by the various etiologic factors: inherited disorders, infections, autoimmune diseases and inflammatory processes whose causes are poorly understood. There are many overlaps with other chapters. Blistering diseases, some of which involve constituents of the very uppermost layers of the dermis, are covered in Chapter 15. Connective tissue nevi are dealt with in Chapter 52, while scars, keloids and tumor-like proliferations are considered in Chapter 59.

Basic Science Aspects

The most important components of the connective tissue (Fig. 18.1) include:

- Cells: fibroblasts
- Fibers: collagen, elastic, reticulin
- Ground substance: proteoglycans, salts, water

Fibroblasts

Fibroblasts are a heterogeneous group of mesenchymal cells with various types of differentiation. They produce all the fibers and most of the components of the ground substance or extracellular matrix.

Collagen

Collagen has long been a subject of research because of its commercial importance in the leather and gelatin industries, just as the wool industry was the first to concern itself with hair. Collagen is not one protein but instead comprises a large family of different molecules, as shown in Table 18.1, which does not pretend to be complete, only representative. About 30 different collagen genes, encoding the various chains designated in column two of Table 18.1, have been identified. Many different chromosomes are involved; that is, few clusters of collagen genes exist.

Several different types of collagen have been described based on their structure and function:

- Interstitial collagens (types I, II, III, V, XI) form fibrils and account for most of the body's collagen. They are the major structural proteins whose molecular characteristics are discussed below.
- Basement membrane collagens (types IV, VII) are found in the lamina densa and anchoring fibrils (Chap. 15).
- Microfibrils (type VI) form networks and help to bind larger fibrils together.
- FACIT (fibril-associated collagen with interrupted triple helices) (types IX, XII, XIV) have large globular domains and help type I or II collagen organize.
- Vascular collagen (type VIII) is secreted by endothelial cells.
- Type X collagen is a globular protein regulated by processes that involve cartilage growth and bone formation.
- Transmembrane collagen (type XVII) is the bullous pemphigoid antigen 2, an essential component of the basement membrane zone (Chap. 15).

The mechanical stability of collagen derives from its special structural features. The interstitial collagens are all about 300 nm long and have a diameter of 1.4 nm. The polypeptide chains, each about 1000 amino acids long, are arranged in a triple helix. The secondary structure of the coiling is such that every third amino acid is glycine and every fifth proline or hydroxyproline. The fibrillar collagens have long

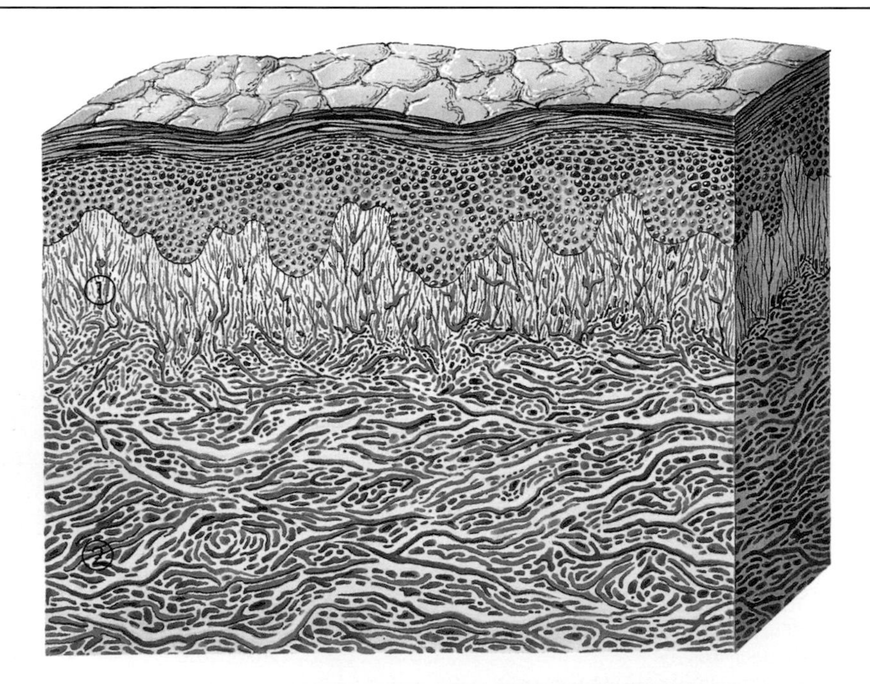

Fig. 18.1. Overview of the dermis with fine elastic fibers in the papillary dermis ① and thicker ones in the reticular dermis ②

Table 18.1. The collagen family

Type	Chains	Structure	Location
I	α1(I), α2 (I)	Large fibrils	Skin, tendon, ligament, bone, cornea
II	α1(II)	Fibrils	Cartilage, vitreous, cornea, vertebral disc
III	α1 (III)	Fibrils	Fetal skin, skin, vessels, GI tract
IV	α1(IV), α2 (IV), others	Meshwork	Basement membrane
V	α1(V), α2(V), α3(V)	Fine fibrils	Widespread
VI	α1(VI), α2(VI), α3(VI)	Microfibrils	Widespread
VII	α1(VII)	Anchoring fibrils	Skin, oral mucosa
VIII	α1(VIII), α2(VIII)	Lattice	Vessels especially embryonic, Descemet membrane
IX	α1(IX)	FACIT (see text)	Associated with type II
X	α1(X)	Lattice	Hypertrophic, mineralizing cartilage
XI	α1(XI), α2(XI), α3(XI)	Fibrils	Cartilage
XII	α1(XII)	FACIT	Associated with type I
XIV	α1(XIV)	FACIT	Associated with type I
XVII	α1(XVII)	Transmembrane	Keratinocytes and BMZ; also known as BPAG 2

helical domains and smaller globular domains. Some of the collagens, designed more for linking and binding, have primarily globular domains. Type I collagen consists of two molecules of α1(I) and one molecule of α2(I). Many of the other collagens are trimers of three identical chains; some are more complicated. For example, the basement membrane collagen type IV is composed of various arrangements of five different chains.

Several other proteins, such as pulmonary surfactant and the complement factor C1q have collagenous sequences and structures but play no role in the extracellular matrix.

The manufacture of collagen is a complicated process. While it is not as orderly as shown, for didactic purposes the following scheme may be helpful:

- Synthesis of pre-pro-α chains on ribosomes.
- Excision of signal peptide to form pro-α chains.
- Modification of procollagen chains including:
  - Hydroxylation of proline to hydroxyproline involving two prolyl hydroxylases and hydroxylation of lysine to hydroxylysine via lysyl hydroxylase. These enzymes require ascorbic acid, Fe^{2+} and O_2; they are inhibited by β-lactam antibiotics, minoxidil and a variety of other agents.
  - Glycosylation of hydroxylysine
- Organization into procollagen triple helix in the endoplasmic reticulum with disulfide bonds linking the strands.
- Secretion of the soluble procollagen into the extracellular matrix.
- Cleavage of the N-terminal and C-terminal propeptides by procollagen N and procollagen C proteinases, which can be inhibited by metal chelators and synthetic peptides.
- Assembly of fibrils. The triple helical structure left when the proteases are finished is the collagen fibril. In type I collagen, the 300-nm fibrils, also known as tropocollagen, are arranged in a quarter stagger or quarter overlapping pattern, so that on electron microscopy a banded pattern with dense stripes every 70 nm is seen.
- Cross-linking of chains via lysyl oxidase which requires copper and can be inhibited by β-aminopropionitrile, a chemical derived from the sweet pea (*Lathyrus odoratus*) and responsible for lathyrism.

The above describes the process for the interstitial or fibrillar collagens. The other types are manipulated somewhat differently at the end. The FACIT collagens are arranged onto the surface of fibrils. Type IV forms a meshwork for the basement membrane zone. Type VI consists of tetramers associated end to end to form thin microfibrils. Type VII consists of dimers formed by overlapping C terminal regions. Types VIII and X form hexagonal networks more fixed than type IV.

In routine hematoxylin-eosin sections, the collagen fibers are pink, stained with eosin. They are also weakly PAS-positive. In general, it is very difficult to discern individual bundles or to comment on the nature of the collagen on light microscopy. Electron microscopy can be used to achieve better resolution. Monoclonal antibody stains are available for several of the molecules; those directed against type IV and type VII collagen are especially used in studying the epidermal-dermal junction.

Elastic Fibers

The elastic fibers are dwarfed in number or mass by the collagen fibers and ground substance. They represent only a few percent of the dermal fibers, but are responsible for many important mechanical properties including distensibility and elasticity. A network of elastic fibers is seen running parallel to the epidermis amidst the collagen fibers of the reticular dermis. In the papillary dermis a much finer network is seen consisting of the horizontal oxytalan fibers and the vertical elaunin fibers which extend almost to the lamina densa.

Elastic fibers have two main components, as demonstrated at the electron microscopic level:

- Elastin: the central amorphous core of the fiber consists of this protein with relative molecular mass of 72 kDa which is organized as a cross-linked polymer. It accounts for about 95% of the elastic fiber.
- Fibrillins: two different electron-dense glycoproteins, known as fibrillin-1 and fibrillin-2, surround the elastin core and are also the main components of elaunin and oxytalan.

The production of elastin is not as complex as that of collagen but involves similar steps. The gene for elastin is located on chromosome 7, containing a number of different exons with the possibility for alternative splicing to create a wide variety of elastin molecules. While most collagen is made by fibroblasts, elastin can be manufactured not only by fibroblasts but also by smooth muscle cells.

- Synthesis of tropoelastin chains on ribosomes
- Excision of signal peptide to form 72-kDa tropoelastin
- Modification of tropoelastin by hydroxylation of proline to hydroxyproline
- Secretion of the soluble tropoelastin into the extracellular matrix
- Cross-linking of chains via lysyl oxidase

The elastin molecule is a far more variable molecule than collagen. It consists primarily of nonpolar amino acids. The arrangement of the glycine molecules is not as regular. The main attachments between tropoelastin molecules are the lysine linkages which can form quite complex bonds involving a group of cyclic structures known as desmosines and isodesmosines. Thus the lysine content of elastin is about one-sixth of that in tropoelastin. The lack of copper and the presence of β-aminoproprionitrile can inhibit cross-linking via lysine and produce striking defects in elastin.

The arrangement of the elastin molecules is quite random and no specific coiling or pattern is identified. The fibrillin fibers appear to serve as a framework for the elastin polypeptides. They are 350-kDa cysteine-rich fibers which are also very stable. Fibrillin-1 is found in the skin, periosteum and lens. Defects in fibrillin-1 lead to Marfan syndrome which not surprisingly shows skin, bone and lens abnormalities. Fibrillin-2 is more of a regulatory protein, sharing the same distribution as elastin. It is defective in congenital contractural arachnodactyly, a marfanoid syndrome.

Elastic fibers are very resistant to both acids and bases. Initially elastin was defined as what was left over after boiling skin at 100 °C in dilute NaOH for 45 min. Elastin consists of alternating hydrophobic regions and hydrophilic regions rich in cross-linkages. In the crudest terms, elastin can be viewed as a coiled mass of fibers attached along the fibrillin network. When tension is applied, the fibers are straightened out, perhaps exposing the small hydrophobic areas to the watery environment. Refolding to once again hide the hydrophobic areas may be what gives elastin its ability to snap back.

A number of special stains are available to visualize elastic fibers in tissue. The orcein (Pinkus), resorcin-fuchsin (Weigert), aldehyde fuchsin and Verhoeff-van Gieson stains (hematoxylin-ferric chloride) are among the standard techniques. Each laboratory seems to have a favorite stain. Elastic fiber stains are essential for identifying many of the diseases discussed in this chapter. Often it is wise to biopsy a similar area of normal skin so that the dermatopathologist has a control for comparison.

Reticulin Fibers

The reticulin fibers (also called reticulum fibers) are fine fibers seen along the basement membrane zone and around hair follicles and sweat glands. They are visualized best with a silver stain. Their molecular basis remains unclear.

Ground Substance

The amorphous material in which the connective tissue fibers are embedded is known as ground substance. Its biomechanical-functional role in the skin is often underestimated. The main constituents of the ground substance are neutral and acid mucopolysaccharides such as hyaluronic acid, dermatan sulfate and chondroitin sulfate which are coupled with proteins and known as proteoglycans. Water, salts, glycoproteins and other proteins are also part of the mixture. The regulation of the qualitative and quantitative composition of the ground substance and the interactions between the individual components are poorly understood.

Hereditary Disorders of Connective Tissue

Ehlers-Danlos Syndrome

(van Meekeren 1682; Tschernogubow 1891; Ehlers 1901; Danlos 1908)

Ehlers-Danlos syndrome is not a single disease but instead is a number of only partially related syndromes. They are presented in detail in Table 18.2 and the text only expands upon the table.

Table 18.2. Syndromes associated with Ehlers-Danlos syndrome

Type	Name	Inheritance	Frequency	Skin	Other organs	Defect
I, II	Classical	AD	80%	Hyperextensibility	Joint laxity, mitral valve prolapse, hernias, premature rupture of membranes	Perhaps type V collagen
III	Benign hypermobile	AD	10%	Minimal hyperextensibility	Severe joint laxity, mitral valve prolapse	Perhaps type V collagen
IV	Vascular (Sack-Barabas)	AD (AR?)	5%	Thin, inelastic skin with prominent vessels	Acral joint laxity, rupture of vessels, bowel, uterus, acrogeria	Mutations in type III collagen at 2q31
V	XLR	XLR	Very rare	Hyperextensibility, hemorrhage	Modest joint laxity	Lysyl oxidase (?)
VI	Kyphoscoliosis	AR	Rare	Hyperextensibility, hemorrhage	Scoliosis, ocular disasters, neonatal hypotonia	Lysyl hydroxylase deficiency at 1p36
VII	Arthrochalasis	AD/AR	Rare	Minimal changes	Small stature, marked joint laxity, multiple dislocations,	Defect in procollagen protease(s) AR 7q22; defect in pro-α2(I) or pro-α1(I) AD
VIII	Periodontitis	AD	Rare	Hyperextensibility, hemorrhage, pretibial scars	Severe periodontal disease	Decreased type III
IX	Occipital horn	XLR	Rare	Mild hyperextensibility	Occipital exostoses, hernias, joint laxity	Lysyl oxidase deficiency due to copper transport defect
X	Fibronectin	AR	Very rare	Mild hyperextensibility, petechiae	Mild joint laxity	Mutation in fibronectin
XI	Large joint hyper motility	AD	Rare	Minimal changes	Laxity and dislocations of large joints	Unknown

AD, autosomal dominant; AR, autosomal recessive; XLR X-linked recessive

Epidemiology. Types I and II are far and away the most common. Type III accounts for about 10% of cases and type IV for about 5%. All the rest are rare, while types V and X are so rare that their existence has been questioned.

Etiology and Pathogenesis. The etiology of the most common types (types I, II and III) remains unclear. The latest evidence suggests defects in type V collagen with mutations in several different chains. Type IV Ehlers-Danlos is caused by mutations in type III collagen, a major component of vessel walls. Defects in the procollagen α1(III) gene as well as processing defects have been identified. Some studies have shown that mutations earlier on the gene produce more profoundly defective collagen which correlates with more severe disease, but this finding awaits confirmation. In type VI, there is a defect in lysyl hydroxylase, leading to reduced cross-linking of collagen. Two causes of type VII Ehlers-Danlos have been described. The autosomal dominant form is caused by a structural mutation in procollagen α2(I) in the N-terminal propeptide. In the autosomal recessive form, the collagen is normal but the enzyme procollagen N-protease is defective. Type IX Ehlers-Danlos is a puzzler. Both Menkes syndrome and this form of Ehlers-Danlos have defects in the same gene, a copper transport gene, but the clinical findings are quite different.

Clinical Findings. We briefly review the clinical features of the more common or interesting types.

Types I and II. The classic patients with Ehlers-Danlos fall in this group. Type I patients have hyperextensible skin; it can be stretched and snaps back (Fig. 18.2). But this skin is easily damaged and tends to heal with peculiar scars. They may resemble cigarette paper, simply gape or be molluscoid with herniation of dermis and fat into the protuberant scar (Fig. 18.3). Surgical scars may also heal poorly. The dermal vessels are easily damaged, leading to hemorrhages and ecchymoses.

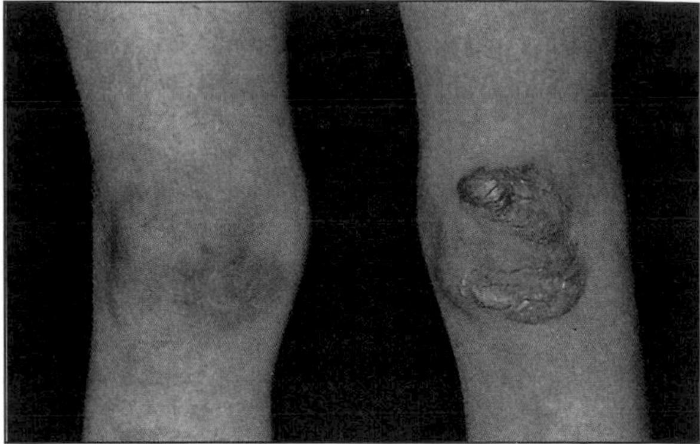

Fig. 18.3. Type I Ehlers-Danlos syndrome; molluscoid scars

The patients have varying degrees of joint hyperextensibility (Fig. 18.4). They were formerly described as elastic men or found employment as contortionists in circuses and side shows. Some ballet dancers appear to have Ehlers-Danlos syndrome. Older patients often have degenerative arthritis. Synovial cysts may develop and extend into the skin following joint trauma. Many can touch their nose with their tongue; this is known as the Gorlin sign (one of many Gorlin signs). About 50% of these patients will have mitral valve prolapse. Hernias are another common problem. Type I Ehlers-Danlos is also characterized by premature rupture of membranes in labor; this is probably the most reliable way to separate type I and type II.

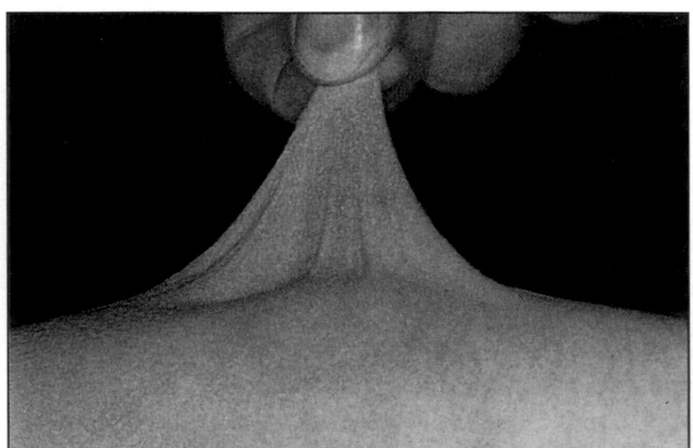

Fig. 18.2. Type I Ehlers-Danlos syndrome; hyperelastic skin

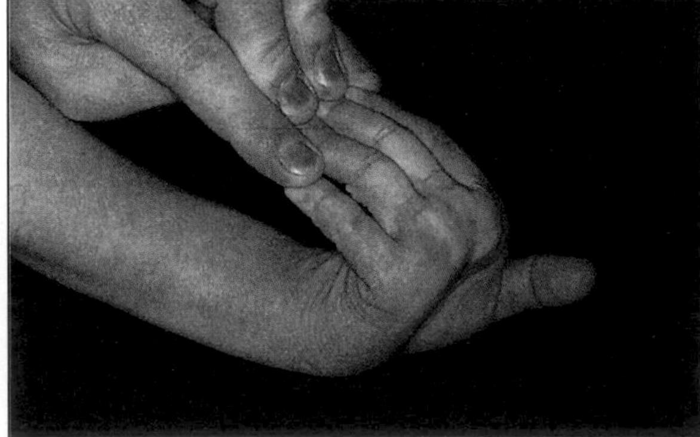

Fig. 18.4. Type I Ehlers-Danlos syndrome; joint hyperextensibility

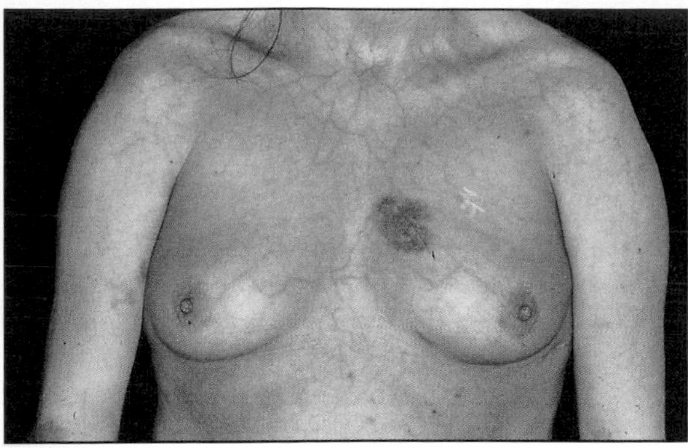

Fig. 18.5. Type IV Ehlers-Danlos syndrome; prominent veins and bruises

Type III. These individuals have striking hypermobility of their large and small joints but minimal skin changes and lack molluscoid pseudotumors. They typically have leg pains, degenerative arthritis and are at risk for mitral valve prolapse. Premature labor and congenital hip dislocations are not increased as compared to the general population.

Type IV. The skin is inelastic and so translucent that the vessels are easily seen. The major risk is that of rupture of the aorta, as well as of other viscera. Many patients have an acrogeric facies. In other patients a bleeding tendency because of vessel fragility is the dominant problem (Fig. 18.5). Yet other patients give a family history of sudden death following arterial bleeds, bowel rupture or uterine rupture during pregnancy. Type IV patients rarely survive into the fifth decade.

Type VI. These scoliotic patients with marked joint problems are at risk for both ocular rupture and retinal detachment. Their skin is the least of their problems. They may present as floppy newborns. If they are lucky enough to be diagnosed at this stage, ascorbic acid can be quite helpful.

Type VII. These small patients with scoliosis suffer from recurrent dislocations. They have few skin problems except for fragility. Typically they have marked joint laxity and hip dislocations at birth.

Type IX. The occipital horns are exostoses on the occiput that can be palpated and seen on X-rays. The patients have extensible skin which tends to droop as in cutis laxa, hernias and bladder diverticulae. This disease was formerly known as X-linked recessive cutis laxa.

Histopathology. The skin biopsy is a great disappointment in studying Ehlers-Danlos. It can be used as a source of fibroblasts to culture for genetic studies.

Laboratory Findings. In addition to the genetic tests already mentioned, one can do serum copper and ceruloplasmin levels which are decreased in type IX. In many instances, prenatal diagnosis is possible.

Course and Prognosis. The prognosis depends completely on the type of Ehlers-Danlos.

Differential Diagnosis. In some cases early on, cutis laxa may come into the question. Type IV enters into the differential diagnosis of premature aging syndromes. Occasionally Marfan syndrome may superficially resemble Ehlers-Danlos but the two can usually be separated clinically.

Therapy. There is no good therapy other than caution, with one dramatic exception. The very rare but disabling type VI responds to ascorbic acid. Otherwise, one can only practice damage management. The type IV patients should have baseline echocardiographic evaluation and be followed by a skilled cardiologist.

Restrictive Dermopathy

(Antoine 1929; Witt et al. 1986)

Synonym. Late fetal epidermal dysplasia

Etiology and Pathogenesis. Fewer than 50 patients with this disorder have been reported. It appears to be inherited in an autosomal recessive pattern. While it has been grouped with both disorders of keratinization and aplasia cutis congenita, it appears to be distinct. The defect appears to be either exaggerated fetal keratinization or abnormal fetal fibroblasts with aberrant integrin expression. Neither hypothesis has been well proven.

Clinical Findings. Almost all patients are premature. They have a fixed facial expression, an open mouth with everted lips ("o" position), small chin and often ectropion. Their skin is either firm, thickened and scaly or atrophic and thinned; usually both types of skin are present. The limbs are flexed, almost as if the patient were trapped within tightened skin. The contractures and immobilization at such an early age produce a whole spectrum of bony deformities. The lungs are also underexpanded. In some pedigrees pyloric stenosis is found. Other internal organs are usually not affected.

Histopathology. The epidermis is atrophic. The dermis is thin, lacks appendages and usually has collagen bundles arranged parallel to the skin surface.

Course and Prognosis. The outlook is poor.

Stiff Skin Syndrome

(ESTERLY and MCKUSICK 1971)

Synonyms. Esterly syndrome, congenital fascial dystrophy

The stiff skin syndrome sounds similar to restrictive dermopathy but is entirely different. Patients are born with or soon develop stone-hard areas of skin bound to the underlying tissues, most commonly over the thighs and buttocks. Microscopic study of the skin shows increases in both fibrous tissue and in some instances in mucins. There appear to be two forms of the disease. In the autosomal dominant version, the patients have joint contractures but few other associated findings and do relatively well. The autosomal recessive form is known as Parana syndrome (CAT et al. 1974). These patients have more widespread hardening of the skin, almost becoming entrapped inside their integument and have hyperpigmentation and hypertrichosis, as well as a variety of systemic problems.

Osteogenesis Imperfecta

(EKMAN 1788; SARTORIUS 1826; VROLIK 1849)

Epidemiology. There are four major types of osteogenesis imperfecta, all of which have been subdivided. Many osteogenesis imperfecta syndromes have also been described. The most common is the mildest or type I. The incidence is estimate at 1:20,000 births.

Etiology and Pathogenesis. A wide variety of mutations have been described in both collagen $\alpha 1$ (I) on chromosome 17q22 and collagen $\alpha 2$(I) on chromosome 7q22. Types I and IV are inherited in an autosomal dominant pattern, while types II and III are more heterogeneous and show both autosomal dominant and recessive inheritance.

Clinical Findings. These patients are unlikely to come to a dermatologist for help with their underlying disease.

Type I. These minimally affected patients have thin skin with easy bruising and distinctive blue sclerae. The major problem is multiple fractures of the long bones and scoliosis. With puberty, the fracture risk tends to stabilize. They also tend to develop hearing loss from otosclerosis and sensorineural changes. A classic finding is dentinogenesis imperfecta or faulty development of dentin. The teeth are an unusual translucent brown color; the enamel is normal but fractures away because of the poor dentin. Most patients wind up with complete crowns. The radiographs of the mouth are characteristic because the dental pulps opacify.

Type II. The fractures occur in utero, so most patients are stillborn or die in the neonatal period. Limbs may be avulsed during delivery.

Type III. These infants have multiple fractures in utero, but tend to survive and somewhat stabilize. They are usually markedly deformed with progressive scoliosis, which often leads to cardiorespiratory problems.

Type IV. In this group, the sclerae are not blue. They, too have thin, easily bruised skin and fractures at birth and in childhood which tend to stabilize.

Therapy. Nothing effective is available, other than good specialist care and caution.

Prenatal Diagnosis. Gene defects can be identified and abnormalities in type I collagen synthesis or interaction identified in cultured fibroblasts.

Cutis Laxa

(ALIBERT 1855)

Synonyms. Dermatochalasis, generalized elastolysis, loose skin syndrome

Cutis laxa refers to several inherited disorders of elastin in which the skin lacks elasticity and thus becomes droopy or pendulous.

Epidemiology. All forms of cutis laxa are extremely rare; the autosomal recessive form is most common.

Etiology and Pathogenesis. The genetic defects in cutis laxa have not been well defined. In the autosomal dominant forms, there is presumably a structural defect in elastin, while in the autosomal recessive forms, there may be reduced production of tropoelastin mRNA reflecting an enzymatic or control defect. The X-linked recessive variant of cutis laxa is now classified as Ehlers-Danlos syndrome type IX.

Clinical Findings. In the autosomal recessive form, there are typical skin and also extensive systemic findings, while the autosomal dominant form is mostly limited to the skin. The skin is very slack, so that even young infants have the "hush puppy" or "basset hound" look with prominent jowls and eyelids (Figs. 18.6, 18.7). Parents with the disease can often identify it in their newborn children by the loose perioral structures. The skin can be stretched a long distance but then returns very slowly. The patients soon look much older than their age. A classic picture shows an affected child looking much older than his parents. The systemic problems include emphysema, intestinal and bladder diverticulae, hernias and occasionally joint laxity.

Histopathology. Skin biopsy reveals reduced and fragmented elastic fibers.

Course and Prognosis. Those patients with only skin involvement do well. In those with systemic disease, the lung involvement is crucial. Neonates can die from hypoplastic lungs, while emphysema with all its sequelae influences adult life.

Differential Diagnosis. There are many associated syndromes with cutis laxa. Some are listed below. Occasionally in early stages of the disease, the clinical symptoms overlap with Ehlers-Danlos syndrome, especially type IX.

Therapy. No therapy is available other than surgical correction of the functional and cosmetic defects.

Conditions Related to Cutis Laxa

There are a number of other conditions, both inherited and acquired, which have similarities to cutis laxa and must be considered in the differential diagnosis.

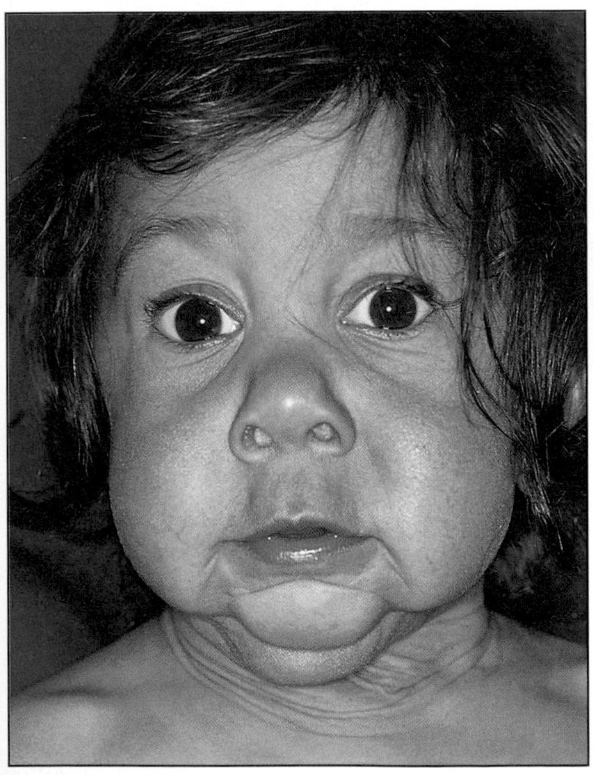

Fig. 18.6. Cutis laxa; patient at 1 year of age

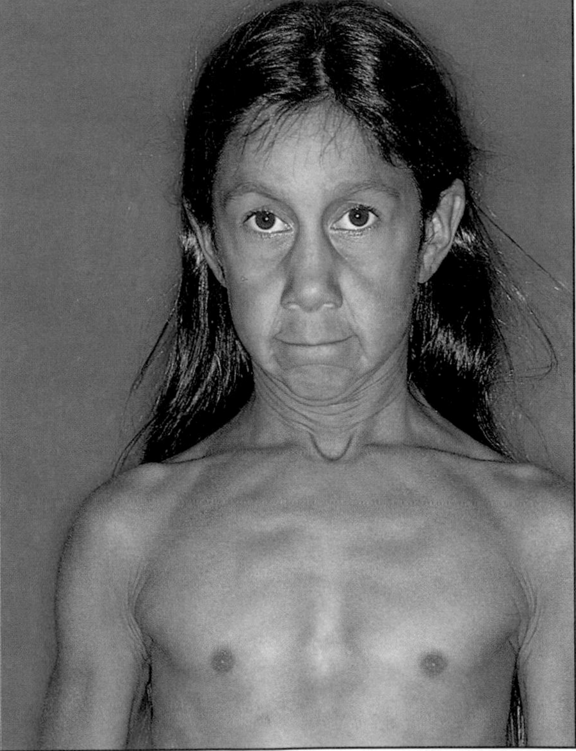

Fig. 18.7. Cutis laxa; same patient 6 years later

Acquired Cutis Laxa

As rare as cutis laxa is, acquired cutis laxa is even rarer. In this condition patients develop normally to a point and then following some inflammatory skin disorder, begin to show the same cutaneous changes as cutis laxa. Triggers may include urticarial eruptions, dermatitis herpetiformis-like disease, infections and many other poorly characterized conditions. The best-studied connection between infection and elastic fiber damage is acrodermatitis chronica atrophicans, not usually included in this group.

Ascher Syndrome

(Laffer 1909; Ascher 1920)

Etiology and Pathogenesis. While most cases are sporadic, autosomal dominant inheritance has been suggested. The genetic defect is not known but is assumed to involve elastic fibers.

Clinical Findings. Ascher syndrome is the combination of premature blepharochalasis, a double lip and occasional thyroid enlargement. The eyelids may initially show angioneurotic edema-like swelling, but usually show redundant tissue in childhood or young adult life, interfering with vision. The involved lip is usually the upper lip, with a horizontal fold of excess tissue seen at the junction of its cutaneous and mucosal parts. The redundancy is often not seen when the mouth is closed, but as the patient opens his or her mouth, the fold becomes apparent. In some patients thyroid enlargement is present but thyroid disease is unusual.

Histopathology. Surprisingly, there is little evidence of elastic tissue damage. When blepharoplasty is performed, the excised tissue is primarily herniated fat, while the excessive labial tissue is fairly normal.

Course and Prognosis. The outlook is good; severe systemic problems do not occur.

Differential Diagnosis. Both premature blepharochalasis and double lip may occur sporadically as isolated findings. The Mounier-Kuhn syndrome is the association of the Ascher syndrome with tracheal and bronchial diverticulae. Melkersson-Rosenthal syndrome and isolated granulomatous cheilitis may appear similar, but eyelid involvement is uncommon and the biopsy shows granulomatous inflammation. The Hughes syndrome of acromegaloid features, thickened oral mucosa, bulbous nose and joint laxity can begin with lip changes.

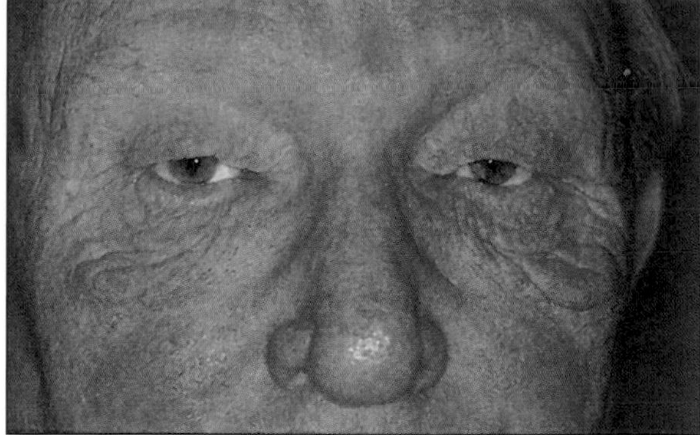

Fig. 18.8. Blepharochalasis

Therapy. Surgical correction of both the eyelid and lip defects is possible.

Blepharochalasis

Almost every older person gets some degree of sagging of the skin beneath the eyes and of drooping of the upper lid (Fig. 18.8). This is a normal part of aging, perhaps accelerated by recurrent infections and swelling in the periorbital area, as well as by genetic factors and cigarette smoking. The surgical correction of blepharochalasis is known as a blepharoplasty; it is a common procedure.

Prune Belly Syndrome

These rare patients have features of cutis laxa, but the most striking changes are a wrinkled lax abdominal wall since the abdominal muscles are lacking. They have renal and intestinal abnormalities as well as hip dysplasias. A defect in elastic fibers has not been documented.

Pseudoxanthoma Elasticum

(Darier 1896)

Synonyms. Grönbald-Strandberg syndrome, elastorrhexis generalisata et systemica (Touraine)

Epidemiology. The prevalence of pseudoxanthoma elasticum has been estimated at around 1/100,000.

There is a consistent 2:1 female predominance, even though there is no evidence for X-linked recessive inheritance. The South African patients tend to have less cardiovascular and more severe ophthalmologic disease.

Etiology and Pathogenesis. Pseudoxanthoma elasticum is inherited in both autosomal recessive and autosomal dominant patterns. Most large series of patients suggest that about 90% of the cases are inherited in an autosomal recessive pattern. Two decades ago Pope proposed a complicated classification scheme with four types of pseudoxanthoma elasticum with different clinical manifestations; later workers have not been able to duplicate this scheme. One gene for pseudoxanthoma elasticum has been localized to chromosome 16p13.1, but the gene itself and the function of its protein remain a mystery. Prenatal diagnosis is not available.

While the key abnormalities in pseudoxanthoma elasticum are fragmented elastic fibers that are calcified, the mechanism is not known. There is both increased production of elastin and of glycosaminoglycans, but how one or both of these structures lead to calcification is unclear. Calcium and phosphorus metabolism is generally normal, but in rare patients with other causes of hypercalcemia or hypervitaminosis D, the pseudoxanthoma elasticum can take a more rapid course.

Clinical Findings

Cutaneous Findings. The cutaneous lesions usually begin during adolescence and are typically the first manifestation. Numerous round, oval or even linear, slightly elevated papules and patches are found, favoring the flexural areas, such as the neck, axillae, umbilicus, groin, antecubital and popliteal fossae (Fig. 18.9). The lesions are initially yellow-violet but soon loose their inflammatory component and become yellow-white, which perhaps prompted Darier to suggest the term pseudoxanthoma. As the lesions develop, the skin acquires a rough bumpy thickened texture which has been compared to chicken skin. The areas of involvement tend to slowly expand peripherally. The skin loses its elasticity and secondary cutis laxa-like changes may develop.

About 5% of patients develop small annular lesions consisting of crusted papules. They are either elastosis perforans serpiginosa or very closely related. Because the abnormal elastic fibers in sporadic elastosis perforans serpiginosa and that associated with other disorders are not usually calcified, some refer to the elastosis perforans serpiginosa-like lesions in pseudoxanthoma elasticum as perforating pseudoxanthoma elasticum.

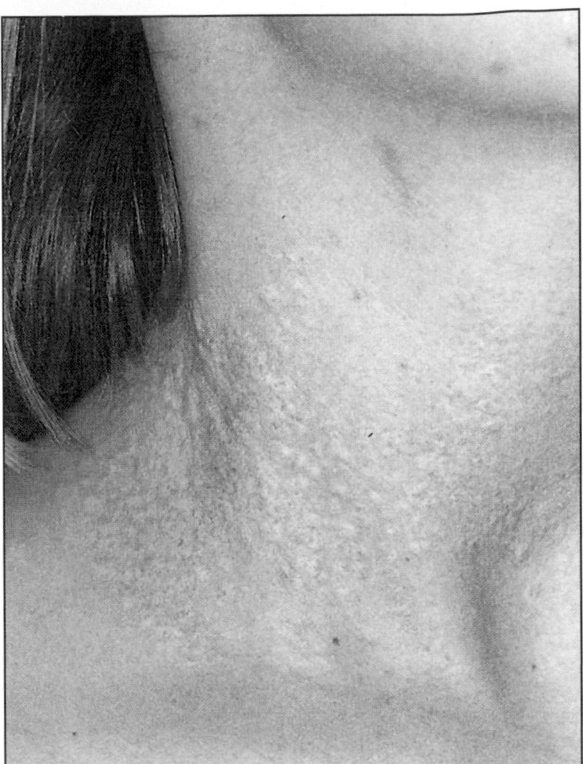

Fig. 18.9. Pseudoxanthoma elasticum

Systemic Findings. The major systemic findings are confined to the eyes and cardiovascular system. About two-thirds of patients have visual problems by 40 years of age. Often they first present to the ophthalmologist, even though the skin lesions are already present. The first ophthalmologic finding is usually mottled retinal pigmentation which appears about the time of the skin findings. The classic clinical feature is angioid streaks or ruptures in the Bruch membrane, which are also seen in many other disorders including Marfan syndrome, Ehlers-Danlos syndrome, sickle cell anemia and Paget disease of bone. The Bruch membrane is a thin elastic layer in the retina. As it calcifies and hardens, it splits, often with radiating rays or spokes. Retinal neovascularization (nets) and then retinal hemorrhage lead to loss of central vision, although blindness is rare.

The peripheral arteries are most severely affected by the calcification of the elastic media. The first symptom is often intermittent claudication in young adult life. Another suggestive finding is gastric artery hemorrhage. Coronary artery disease and strokes can occur, but are rare. Some patients present with premature cardiovascular disease and are found to have pseudoxanthoma elasticum on skin biopsy even though they do not have typical cutaneous lesions.

Histopathology. The skin biopsy is highly characteristic. The elastic fibers are swollen and fragmented; these changes are called elastorrhexis. Sometimes they are clumped into little balls – the so-called clumps of wool. While the changes can be easily seen on hematoxylin-eosin sections, a von Kossa stain for calcium demonstrates them dramatically. In addition, the Hale stain is positive as increased glycosaminoglycans are present. Ultrastructural studies show that the calcium deposition begins on the elastin, not the fibrillin, and slowly proceeds. It can be found in clinically normal skin. Other sophisticated studies have shown that in older lesions there is also an increased production of elastin, perhaps as a response to the damage. If a patient is at risk for pseudoxanthoma elasticum because of family history, a biopsy of a traumatic scar or even normal skin may show the confirmatory histologic changes before cutaneous or ocular examination is positive.

Laboratory Findings. The calcium and phosphate levels are always normal and there is no need to do more than screen them for the rare presence of an unrelated calcium disorder. More important is to monitor the cholesterol and triglycerides as is discussed under therapy.

Course and Prognosis. The outlook is better than most suggest. Central vision loss is the biggest problem. Most patients do not have early cardiovascular mishaps.

Differential Diagnosis. The early cutaneous lesions can be mistaken for the thin skin of Ehlers-Danlos syndrome with prominent follicles. Later on, the picture is quite specific. When rheumatoid arthritis patients are treated with penicillamine, they may develop pseudoxanthoma elasticum-like lesions.

Therapy. Pseudoxanthoma elasticum is a good example of a genetic disease for which many treatment possibilities exist. Moderate dietary calcium restriction appears helpful; daily intake should be restricted to 600–800 mg. No more than the minimum daily requirement of vitamin D should be taken. Close ophthalmologic follow-up is most important. Noncontact sports should be recommended, as strenuous exercise and heavy lifting are common triggers of retinal hemorrhage. The presence of elevated cholesterol or triglycerides can accelerate the cardiovascular disease, so dietary or medical management is essential. Early attention to exercise should help develop peripheral collateral circulation. Since platelet counts are often down in pseudoxanthoma elasticum, patients should avoid aspirin and similar compounds. Turning to the skin, once the lesions are stable, excision is a possibility. Surgery seems to work best on the neck, which is fortunate since this is the most visible region likely to develop cutis laxa-like changes.

Acquired Pseudoxanthoma Elasticum

There are a number of conditions which may mimic pseudoxanthoma elasticum either clinically or histologically. In general, ulcerations, keratotic lesions and discharge of necrotic calcified material (perforating pseudoxanthoma elasticum) are more common in the acquired forms. They include:

Saltpeter-Induced Pseudoxanthoma Elasticum (Christensen 1978). A number of Scandinavian farmers were identified with pseudoxanthoma elasticum-like changes, primarily in their antecubital fossae. They had only cutaneous changes without ocular or cardiovascular problems. All had been in contact with fertilizer containing saltpeter which had caused skin irritation and erosions. While the lesions looked like typical pseudoxanthoma elasticum, they tended to ulcerate more easily. Sophisticated studies showed specific apatite crystals in the dermis. Other occupational exposure to calcium salts, as in mine workers, has induced similar changes.

"Ordinary" Acquired Pseudoxanthoma Elasticum. In the USA, the most common scenario is plaques on the breasts and around the umbilicus of black, obese, multiparous women. The patients usually have no other stigmata of pseudoxanthoma elasticum and develop their cutaneous lesions later in life. Clinically, the lesions are more papular and keratotic than the usual "chicken skin".

Penicillamine. Treatment of rheumatoid arthritis patients with penicillamine also produces pseudoxanthoma elasticum-like lesions. The elastic fibers in penicillamine-related pseudoxanthoma elasticum have a thickened bramble bush or "lumpy-bumpy" pattern on electron microscopy.

Papillary Dermal Elastolysis. This is probably a fancy name for sunlight-damaged skin, but on rare occasions solar elastosis may mimic pseudoxanthoma elasticum.

Marfan Syndrome

(Marfan 1896)

Epidemiology. The incidence of Marfan syndrome is about 1:10,000. Many mild cases are not identified. About 30% of cases represent new mutations; advanced paternal age has been identified in this group.

Etiology and Pathogenesis. The affected protein in this autosomal dominant inherited disorder is fibrillin-1, coded on chromosome 15. The fibrillin molecule is quite large (350 kDa) and a wide variety of mutations have been found leading to the abnormal synthesis, secretion and matrix formation of the protein. Many families with Marfan syndrome have their own mutation, making diagnosis and prenatal diagnosis difficult.

Clinical Findings. The skin findings in Marfan syndrome are rarely of clinical significance. Patients may develop prominent or early striae distensae, and some have elastosis perforans serpiginosa. The facies is distinctive with a long head (dolichocephaly), high arched palate and prominent lips. The internal problems are most obvious in three organ systems:

- Skeletal. Patients are tall. The ratio of the upper body segment to the lower body segment is reduced (i.e. legs longer than trunk) and their wingspread is often greater than their height (>1.03; 1 is abnormal). The hands are long and thin (arachnodactyly) and a number of measurements, such as the metacarpal index, can also aid in the diagnosis. Joint laxity is also present, but usually not to the same extent as in Ehlers-Danlos syndrome. The Steinberg thumb sign (thumb when extended across palm reaches ulnar border) and the Walker-Murdoch wrist sign (when grasping the wrist with the opposite hand, the thumb and little finger touch) are not specific, but may suggest the diagnosis. Pectus excavatum or carinatum and pes planus are also often seen. In more severely affected patients, there may be scoliosis and joint problems.
- Cardiovascular. While the diagnosis is usually made on skeletal findings, the problem is with the cardiovascular system. Patients often have mitral valve prolapse, but the real danger is a gradual dilatation of the ascending aorta with the risk of rupture or dissection. About 70% of young adults have a dilated aortic root. The carotid arteries may also be weakened.
- Ophthalmic. About two-thirds of patients have ectopia lentis (dislocated lens) because fibrillin-1 is essential to the lens support structures. The dislocation is most often upwards. Most patients are myopic.
- Miscellaneous. Bilateral inguinal hernias, lung cysts, spontaneous pneumothorax and chronic emphysema are also common.

This general description fits a number of professional basketball players and every so often a sudden death in a tall athlete leads to the diagnosis of Marfan syndrome. In the tall Nilotic blacks, the same decreased upper segment: lower segment ratio is present without any evidence for Marfan syndrome.

Course and Prognosis. The prognosis is almost entirely dependent on the cardiac status.

Differential Diagnosis. There is a long list of disorders which occasionally resemble Marfan syndrome, usually because of a similar facies. Several of interest to dermatologists include:

- Congenital contractural arachnodactyly or Beals-Hecht syndrome. In this related disorder, there is a defect in fibrillin-2. The changes are more acral and contractures tend to develop, but cardiac problems are not seen.
- Homocystinuria. These patients appear similar but the defect is inherited in an autosomal recessive pattern. They have frequent thrombotic episodes and do not have the aortic problems. While they also have ectopia lentis, the dislocation is usually downward. All patients suspected of Marfan syndrome without a positive family history should be screened for homocystinuria.
- Multiple endocrine neoplasia type 2B (Chap. 65). Multiple endocrine abnormalities, mucosal neuromas and a lack of cardiac findings distinguish these patients. The disorder is inherited in an autosomal dominant pattern with mutations in tyrosine kinase receptor. The patients are at risk for medullary carcinoma of the thyroid.

Therapy. The cardiac problems are life-threatening and require a referral to a cardiac surgeon with experience in Marfan syndrome who can do baseline studies and help decide when to prophylactically replace the ascending aorta with a graft. Cardiac β-blockers may delay the need for the operation.

Premature Aging Syndromes

In addition to cutis laxa, there are a number of other disorders in which the patients appear older than their stated age and are at risk for a variety of systemic problems. Their skin is typically atrophic, wrinkled, sclerotic or poikilodermatous. Subcutaneous fat may be scant, the hair prematurely gray, and the cutaneous vessels prominent. One old review lists over 150 premature aging syndromes. We have chosen to discuss only the most common of these rare disorders, realizing that few will wind up in dermatologic practices.

Progeria

(Hutchinson 1886; Gilford 1904)

Synonyms. Progeria infantilis, Hutchinson-Gilford syndrome

Epidemiology. Just to show how rare progeria is, the incidence has been estimated at 1/10,000,000. Since the lifespan is about a decade, the prevalence is extremely low.

Etiology and Pathogenesis. The etiology is unknown. Familial cases are poorly documented and no patient has ever reproduced. Despite the severity of the disease, there are no useful biochemical or genetic markers.

Clinical Findings. Typically the patients are normal at birth but grow slowly and become clinically obvious before 2 years of age. Their appearance has been liked to a "plucked bird" which a large skull, frontal bossing, bulging eyes, beaked nose, small chin and no scalp, eyelid or eyebrow hairs. The acral skin is usually tight and shiny. Nail dystrophies are usual. The sunlight-exposed areas may develop hypo- and hyperpigmentation. The subcutaneous fat is markedly reduced.

The systemic symptoms are multiple. Osteoporosis and secondary fractures cause considerable disability. The patients are usually of normal intelligence, although obviously socially compromised by their tragic course. They show no signs of sexual maturation and do not develop cataracts.

Histopathology. Skin biopsy reveals epidermal atrophy with increased collagen and/or elastin in the dermis. The adnexal structures and subcutaneous fat are reduced.

Course and Prognosis. The outlook is grim. The patients usually die in the second decade of life of widespread arteriosclerosis, leading to coronary artery disease or strokes.

Differential Diagnosis. All the diseases discussed in this section should be considered.

Therapy. Standard therapy of the cardiovascular problems should be attempted. Hormonal replacement has proven disappointing.

Acrogeria

(Gottron 1941)

Synonym. Gottron syndrome

Etiology and Pathogenesis. This very rare disorder is inherited in an autosomal recessive pattern. Many cases are type IV Ehlers-Danlos syndrome. Patients without skin hyperextensibility, joint hyperflexibility and cardiac findings are more likely not to have Ehlers-Danlos syndrome.

Clinical Findings. The cutaneous changes appear at birth or early in life. The skin of the hands and feet becomes atrophic and tight. Often there is a short erythematous stage first, similar to acrodermatit is chronica atrophicans. The subcutaneous fat is reduced. The face also appears aged, especially as the chin is often small and the nose beaked (Fig. 18.10). Some patients develop elastosis perforans serpiginosa. Nail dystrophies, prominent vessels and poorly healed scars may also be seen, as well as a gradual overlap with the cutaneous findings of type IV Ehlers-Danlos syndrome. The hair is normal. The patients are usually of small stature but have normal sexual development and no cataracts.

Course and Prognosis. The outlook is reasonable, perhaps better than the more typical type IV Ehlers-Danlos syndrome patients. Nonetheless, the risk of a vascular catastrophe is present. Clearly

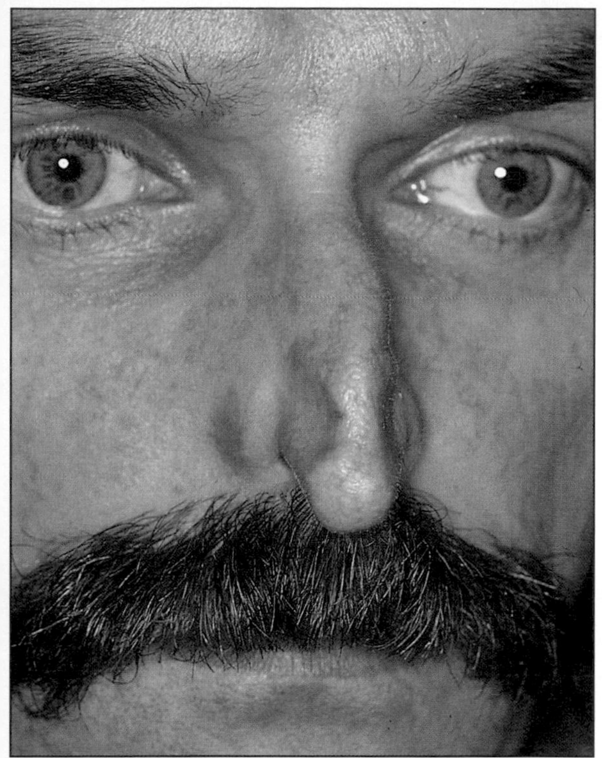

Fig. 18.10. Acrogeria

those acrogeric patients with normal type III collagen have a better outlook.

Therapy. No effective treatment is available.

Werner Syndrome

(Werner 1904)

Synonyms. Progeria adultorum, pangeria

Epidemiology. Werner syndrome is the most common of the premature aging disorders with an estimated incidence of 1/1,000,000. Large pedigrees have been found in Japan and Sardinia.

Etiology and Pathogenesis. Werner syndrome is inherited in an autosomal recessive pattern. The gene is located at 8p12-p11 and is a DNA helicase of the RecQ family which helps to unwind nucleic acids prior to cell duplication.

Clinical Findings. The hallmark of Werner syndrome is normal development for the first decade of life. Then the trouble starts with growth arrest and acceleration of many aging-associated problems. While the onset of the disease is usually in the mid-teens, it may be delayed until as late as 30 years of age. The skin changes usually begin on the shins and feet, with loss of subcutaneous fat, and tight atrophic, often poikilodermatous features. Hyperkeratoses appear over bony prominences, such as on the sole and over the knees and ankles. Large slow-to-heal ulcers develop, both within these calluses and secondary to vascular problems. Soft tissue calcifications may also be present.

A typical clinical picture evolves. The patients are quite small, usually less than 1.60 m. They have tiny hands and feet and spindly limbs. The face is also characteristic. The nose is beaked or pinched and the cheeks sunken because of fat loss, producing the bird-faced appearance. There is early balding and gray hair. Cataracts are common; they are usually posterior, subcapsular. The eyes are prominent and ears often tight and fixed. The facial expression is restricted and the voice is typically high-pitched.

Of greater concern are the development of diabetes mellitus and severe arteriosclerotic vascular disease, and an increased risk of many different tumors, including hematologic malignancies, sarcomas, meningiomas and carcinomas, as well as a variety of cutaneous malignancies. The ankle and heel ulcers may evolve into squamous cell carcinoma. There is also hypogonadism and premature menopause.

Laboratory Findings. Urinary hyaluronic acid may be elevated. The glucose metabolism is usually abnormal.

Course and Prognosis. Death is usually in the fourth or fifth decade from cardiovascular disease.

Therapy. Conventional therapy should be tried, such as insulin and cardiovascular drugs. Careful monitoring can reduce the risk of tumors.

Metageria

(Gilkes et al. 1974)

Metageria is the rarest of the premature aging syndromes. Skeptics doubt its existence because described patients have all appeared to have overlap features of several different premature aging syndromes. The pattern of inheritance is not established, but may be autosomal recessive. Patients are generally tall with a tight, bird-like face and resultant pseudoexophthalmos. They have a gradual loss of subcutaneous fat, starting in infancy, and typically have digital ulcerations secondary to arterial compromise. They have fine scalp hair and develop little pubic or axillary hair. Starting in puberty poikilodermatous changes appear on the neck and trunk. Both diabetes mellitus and arteriosclerosis appear to be more common. While life expectancy is reduced, the outlook is better than for similar syndromes.

Cockayne Syndrome

(Cockayne 1936)

Epidemiology. Cockayne syndrome is about as rare as progeria.

Etiology and Pathogenesis. Cockayne syndrome is inherited in an autosomal recessive pattern. Several families have been identified with Cockayne syndrome and the same DNA repair defect as that seen in xeroderma pigmentosum groups B and D. In addition, two different genes have been tentatively identified in other Cockayne syndrome patients, known as Cockayne syndrome A and B. The Cockayne syndrome genes appear to be transcription coupling or regulating genes. The DNA repair genes in xeroderma pigmentosum also play a role in regulating transcription.

Clinical Findings. The onset of problems is at birth or early in life. The cutaneous hallmark of Cockayne syndrome is severe photosensitivity. Typically there are poikilodermatous changes over the face, neck and backs of the hands. Despite the relationship to xeroderma pigmentosum, there is not an increased incidence of skin cancers. Some patients have a prominent butterfly rash, mimicking lupus erythematosus. The subcutaneous fat is also scant.

The patients are small with microcephaly, sunken eyes, a thin nose and large ears. The hands and feet may also be disproportionately large. There are diffuse myelin defects with progressive neurologic deterioration and mental retardation. Cataracts, specked retinal pigment, sensorineural deafness and severe caries also occur.

Course and Prognosis. Death usually occurs in the second or third decade. The neurologic changes are most devastating.

Differential Diagnosis. The differential diagnosis initially is primarily of those photosensitive disorders presenting in childhood, such as xeroderma pigmentosum, Bloom syndrome, Hartnup syndrome and the other forms of poikiloderma. Initially progeria may be similar, but the facial rash does not develop and premature aging is more accelerated.

Therapy. Sunscreens should be provided, but the more significant problems are not treatable.

Myotonic Dystrophy

(Curschmann and Steinert 1909)

Synonyms. Dystrophia myotonica, Curschmann-Steinert syndrome, Steinert syndrome

Epidemiology. The incidence of myotonic dystrophy is reported as 1/10–20,000, but is probably much higher. The onset is usually delayed and mild cases are often overlooked.

Etiology and Pathogenesis. The disorder is inherited in an autosomal dominant pattern, but with considerable variability in expressivity and penetrance. The gene, known as DMPK (dystrophia myotonica protein kinase), is located on chromosome 19 and has a unique mechanism. The likelihood of clinical disease depends on the number of trinucleotide CTG repeats within the gene, just as in Huntington chorea. How this phenomenon leads to disease awaits unraveling. A second locus may exist on chromosome 3q.

Clinical Findings. The onset of signs and symptoms in myotonic dystrophy is usually young adult life. Some patients have already started a family before discovering they carry an inheritable illness. The striking finding is the myotonia. It can be demonstrated by asking the patient to tightly grasp your finger; when you rapidly extract your finger, the patient cannot relax the grip and experiences painful "cramps" or muscle spasms. Most patients come to fear this simple test. They may also have muscle atrophy, loss of fat, cardiac conduction defects, cataracts, premature baldness and graying, thus conveying an impression of premature aging which is never as severe as the other disorders mentioned above. Infants may have hypotonia and die in utero or in the neonatal period. Such a scenario is most common if the mother has myotonic dystrophy, even if she had the typical late onset.

Such patients are likely to come to the attention of the dermatologist because they have multiple pilomatricomas. The tumors are typically on the scalp, but can be anywhere. They are often quite large and can be painful, in contrast to solitary pilomatricomas (Chap. 57).

Differential Diagnosis. These patients do not have poikiloderma and their disease should not be confused with other premature aging syndromes. Often the only finding in this direction is frontal balding. The neurologic findings lead to the diagnosis.

Congenital Poikilodermas

Poikiloderma is defined as the combination of cutaneous atrophy, hypo- and hyperpigmentation, often reticulated, and telangiectases. Many disorders have only part of this triad. Often skin atrophy is lacking. Examples include Bloom syndrome and ataxia-telangiectasia (Chap. 13). Another group of disorders often called poikilodermatous are those with mottled or speckled hyper- and hypopigmentation (Chap. 26).

The prototype of poikiloderma is radiation dermatitis. Chronic sunlight-damaged skin may also become poikilodermatous. Many of the connective tissue disorders, cutaneous lymphomas and a host of other disorders are considered examples of acquired poikiloderma. Poikiloderma atrophicans vasculare (Jacobi 1906) is not a disease entity but is one pattern associated with mycosis fungoides. Most of the disorders with premature aging have poikilodermatous features. Based primarily on tradition, a number of disorders are viewed as congenital poikilodermas. We review only the most common members of this family. Table 18.3 shows some of the disorders.

Rothmund-Thomson Syndrome
(von Rothmund 1868; Thomson 1923)

Synonym. Poikiloderma congenitale. In the USA, one usually speaks of Rothmund-Thomson syndrome. In Europe, one separates the two, Rothmund syndrome is associated with cataracts, while Thomson is not.

Epidemiology. Rothmund-Thomson syndrome is quite rare. There is a female predominance. The considerable variance among cases suggests that several disorders over the years have been lumped together.

Etiology and Pathogenesis. Rothmund-Thomson syndrome is inherited in an autosomal recessive pattern. In many patients, consanguinity is found. The locus appears to be on chromosome 8, causing genomic instability, acquired somatic mosaicism and trisomy of the chromosome. The gene appears to be another RNA helicase. Patients both with and without cataracts have displayed mutations at the same site.

Clinical Findings. The initial clinical finding is erythematous cheeks, which soon develop a characteristic reticulate pattern with generally a coarse livedo-like network (Fig. 18.11). These changes begin during the first year of life. They soon spread to involve the ears, chin, forehead and later the extremities and buttocks. The trunk is typically spared.

The patients may also have photosensitivity and some develop acral keratoses, which can evolve into squamous cell carcinoma. The hairs, sebaceous and sweat glands may be reduced or absent (Fig. 18.12). All have a small stature. About 50% have cataracts with onset in early childhood. Other

Table 18.3. Types of poikiloderma

Syndrome	Inheritance	Cataracts	Leukoplakia	Blisters	Keratoses	Sclerosis
Rothmund-Thomson	AR	+/–	–	–	+/–	–
Dyskeratosis congenita	XLR	–	+	–	–	–
Kindler	?AR	–	–	+	–	–
Poikiloderma with blisters	?AR	–	–	+	+	+/–
Hereditary acrokeratotic poikiloderma	AD	–	–	+/–	+	–
Hereditary sclerosing poikiloderma	AD	–	–	–	–	+

AD, autosomal dominant; AR, autosomal recessive; XLR, X-linked recessive

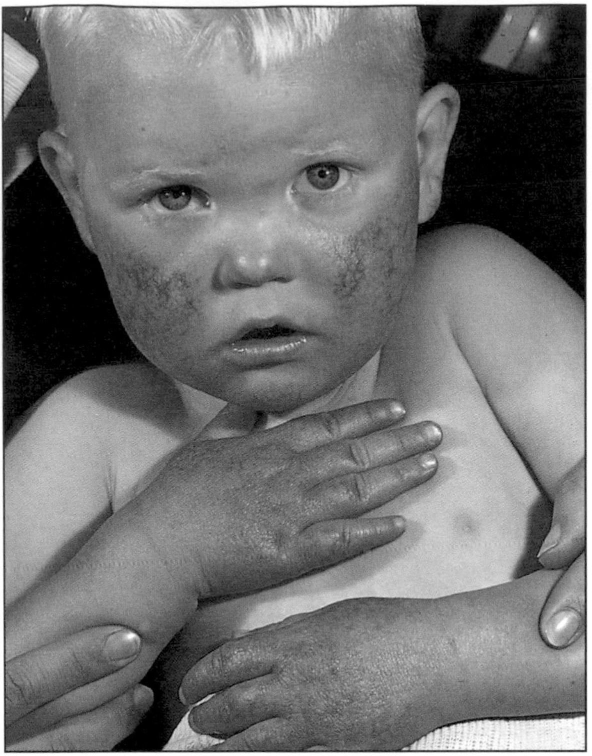

Fig. 18.11. Rothmund-Thomson syndrome with prominent poikiloderma

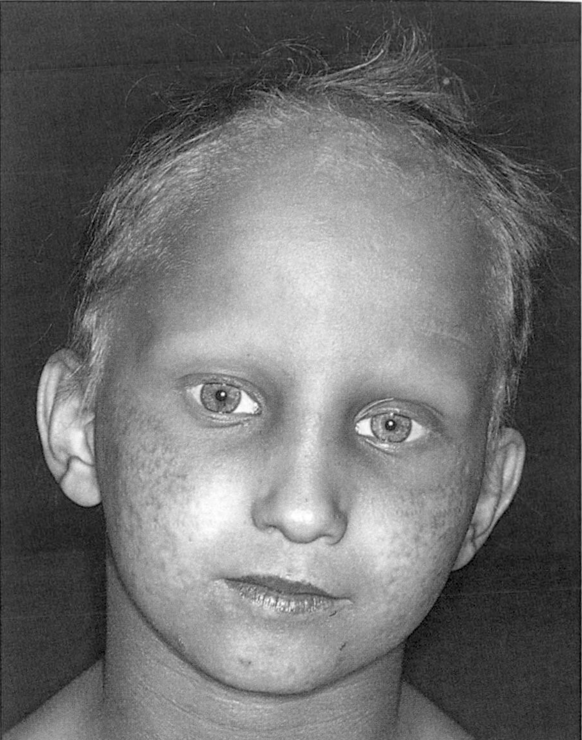

Fig. 18.12. Rothmund-Thomson syndrome with less poikiloderma but hair loss in a patient with cataracts

features include hypogonadism, skeletal abnormalities such as bowing of the tibia, small hands and feet, hypoplastic thumbs and dental abnormalities. The intelligence is normal. There is a risk of osteosarcoma.

Course and Prognosis. The life expectancy is normal if no malignancy intervcnes.

Therapy. Sunscreens are essential and careful monitoring is needed.

Dyskeratosis Congenita

(Zinsser 1910; Engman 1926; Cole et al. 1930)

Synonym. Zinsser-Cole-Engman syndrome

Etiology and Pathogenesis. This X-linked recessive inherited disorder is caused by the DKC1 gene located at Xq28 wich encodes dyskerin, a nucleolar protein. Rare cases with apparent autosomal dominant and autosomal recessive inheritance have been described; they await further study now that a putative gene has been found. Dyskeratosis congenita is one of the chromosome breakage syndromes and also can show an elevated sister chromatid exchange rate.

Clinical Findings. Most of the findings are confined to the skin and mucous membranes. Almost all patients have a reticulated dusky brown gray hyperpigmentation with atrophy and telangiectases. This usually starts during childhood. The face, trunk and thighs are the most common sites. Chronic tearing with conjunctivitis and blepharitis is common. Often the lacrimal duct is hypoplastic. The nails are atrophic or absent. Pterygium of the nails is common, as well as thin or sparse hair. Mild palmoplantar keratoderma may be present. Axillary hyperhidrosis is frequently described, perhaps as a compensatory change, for the rest of the skin is usually quite dry.

The most significant change is seen on the mucous membranes where there are diffuse hyperkeratotic patches, not only involving the mouth but also the genital and anal mucosa (Fig. 18.13). Malignant degeneration is almost expected with conversion to squamous cell carcinoma occurring in young adult life. Dental abnormalities are common. In addition, about half the patients develop Fanconi-type pancytopenia with its sequelae.

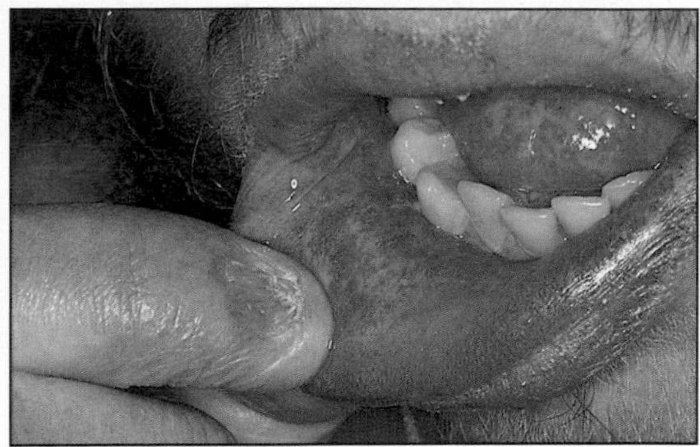

Fig. 18.13. Dyskeratosis congenita with dystrophic nails and verrucous mucosal changes

Course and Prognosis. The outlook is poor both because of the mucosal squamous cell carcinomas and because of the risk of bone marrow failure. Some patients have been treated with bone marrow transplantation. A puzzling twist is the resemblance of their normal skin to that associated with graft-versus-host disease.

Differential Diagnosis. The most challenging differential diagnostic consideration is Fanconi anemia.

Fanconi Anemia

(FANCONI 1927)

Synonyms. Fanconi aplastic anemia, Ehrlich-Fanconi syndrome, congenital pancytopenia. There are many Fanconi syndromes, so it is best not to employ that term.

Etiology and Pathogenesis. Patients with Fanconi anemia have a high incidence of spontaneous chromosome breaks and often reveal tri- or quadriradial figures. The sister chromatid exchange rate is normal. In vitro and in vivo their cells are extremely sensitive to clastogens (chemicals causing chromosome breakage) such as mitomycin C. There are five complementation groups and the genes have been identified in several instances, but their exact function is unclear. The sensitivity to clastogens can be used for prenatal diagnosis with cultured fetal cells.

Clinical Findings. Patients have pancytopenia, skeletal abnormalities (especially involving the thumb and radius), renal anomalies, mental retardation and small size, along with a host of other problems. Their skin shows mottling with diffuse hyperpigmentation, as well as focal hypopigmentation and café au lait macules. The darkening may be very prominent in the skin folds. The outlook is poor because of the high incidence of leukemias and later solid tumors.

Therapy. Once again, bone marrow transplantation is the only real therapy. The skin problems require no treatment.

Kindler Syndrome

(KINDLER 1954)

Synonyms. Kindler-Weary syndrome is probably incorrect, as most feel that Weary described a slightly different disorder, hereditary acrokeratotic poikiloderma.

Etiology and Pathogenesis. This rare, probably autosomally recessively inherited, disorder combines features of a mild epidermolysis bullosa with poikiloderma. The exact nature of Kindler syndrome awaits defining. Pathologic studies have identified blisters in several different layers, no gene defect has been found and no clear explanation for the photosensitivity is available. The poikiloderma appears to be more than a postinflammatory phenomenon; otherwise it would be seen more often in other forms of epidermolysis bullosa.

Clinical Findings. Infants have acral blistering which improves with time but may produce proximal webbing of digits and prominent cutaneous atrophy. In some pedigrees, there are also acral keratoses. The skin is atrophic, telangiectatic and wrinkled, out of proportion to the amount of clinical scarring. Some patients have reduced dermatoglyphics. Others appear to have impaired sweating, presumably because of the damage to sweat ducts during blister formation and scarring. The poikiloderma starts in areas of sunlight exposure as the patients have moderate photosensitivity, but later may appear on non-light-exposed sites. Nail dystrophies and oral, esophageal and genital mucosal lesions also have been reported in some pedigrees.

Poikiloderma with Blisters

(BRAIN 1952; MARGHESCU and BRAUN-FALCO 1965)

Synonyms. Brain syndrome, Marghescu-Braun-Falco syndrome

Etiology and Pathogenesis. This very rare disorder appears to be inherited in an autosomal recessive pattern. Patients are more likely to be women. The gene or genes have not been identified.

Clinical Findings. Blisters appear at birth or early in life. They are often acral, posttraumatic and usually subepidermal. As the tendency to blistering resolves, the patients develop extensive poikiloderma primarily on the face and neck but also on the extensor surfaces of the forearms and shins. There are verrucous palmoplantar lesions which may interfere with motion, along with sclerotic atrophic fingers. Milia were common in Brain's patients but not present in those of Marghescu and Braun-Falco. Hair, nail and tooth anomalies have also been described. Some of the patients have had small stature but normal mental status and no cataracts.

Hereditary Acrokeratotic Poikiloderma

(Dowling 1936; Greither 1958; Weary 1971)

Synonyms. Poikiloderma with keratoses, Dowling syndrome, Greither syndrome, Weary syndrome

This disease, or more likely group of diseases, is inherited in an autosomal dominant pattern. There is frequently an inflammatory early stage with initial acral erythema and blisters and later flexural involvement. The acral skin is often atrophic and develops numerous warty papules which persist. They may also involve the knees and elbows. In some pedigrees, the poikilodermatous changes are described as primarily facial, in others, as flexural, raising the question once again of heterogeneity. The patients are otherwise normal without cataracts, mental retardation or hypogonadism.

Hereditary Sclerosing Poikiloderma

(Weary et al. 1969)

Synonym. Weary syndrome

In another autosomal dominant inherited disorder, the key findings are acral sclerosis and atrophy associated with diffuse hypo- and hyperpigmentation. Telangiectases are not seen. The onset of the skin changes is in childhood. The skin resembles xeroderma pigmentosum or arsenical changes, but there is no increase in malignancies. There may be hyperkeratotic or sclerotic bands in the flexural areas. Some of these patients have mandibuloacral dysplasia with mandibular hypoplasia, dysplastic clavicles, failure of cranial suture closure, shortened phalanges and atrophic acral skin, as well as poikiloderma.

Acquired Cutaneous Atrophy

The very general heading applies to a wide variety of disorders all of which are acquired and show varying degrees of thinning of the skin. The atrophy may involve the dermis or less often the subcutaneous fat. It may be focal or diffuse. Epidermal atrophy alone is rarely appreciated clinically.

Aging Skin

Epidemiology. The changes that occur in skin as we age are well known. One must distinguish between intrinsic aging and extrinsic or solar aging. The onset and degree of solar aging depends on the skin type and degree of exposure. Patients who are fair, have worked outdoors and have lived in the tropics are more likely to show early signs of change. The cutaneous signs of extrinsic aging involve both the epidermis and dermis. The epidermal changes include actinic keratoses and cutaneous malignancies, while the dermis features alterations in the elastic fibers and wrinkling. The signs of intrinsic aging appear later and can only be appreciated in skin which has not had much sunlight exposure. They include dryness, fine wrinkling and atrophy.

Etiology and Pathogenesis. The mechanisms of skin aging are poorly understood and complex. The intrinsic clock ticks steadily, but can be influenced by such factors as nutrition and exercise.

A number of changes can be documented in intrinsically aged skin. The epidermis is thinned and the epidermal-dermal junction is smoother or less interdigitated. Thus the epidermis is more easily separated from the dermis. The epidermal turnover rate is slowed. Both melanocytes and Langerhans cells are decreased in number. The amount of vitamin D synthesis per unit area per joule of UV radiation drops. Because the skin is dry, hydrophilic substances are less-well absorbed. The dermis is more clearly thinned, has reduced fibroblast function, has fewer mast cells and is less vascular. Functional studies show that it is less elastic and less resistant to trauma.

The mechanisms of solar aging are also barely understood. The action spectrum for aging has not been identified, although it is generally estimated that the UVB spectrum is responsible for more epidermal damage and UVA for primarily dermal changes. There is cumulative damage to the epidermis and dermis which exceeds the reparative abilities of the keratinocytes and fibroblasts. While there are probably individual differences in repair of solar damage, we are only able to measure them in extreme cases, such as in xeroderma pigmentosum. The inhibition of Langerhans cells function by UV radiation is well studied. At the same time in intrinsically aged skin, the number of Langerhans cells decreases, showing the interplay between the two not-so-independent processes. In general, solar aging in many ways appears to represent an acceleration of the intrinsic aging process.

Clinical Findings. Intrinsic aging can best be observed on the buttocks of an older individual. The skin is finely wrinkled, often drier and perhaps thinner. The decreased function of the sebaceous and sweat glands makes the skin more susceptible to xerosis when exposed to frequent washings or too much soap and detergent. Except for these minor changes, intrinsically aged skin appears relatively normal.

Sunlight-damaged skin varies considerably from location to location on the body and has thus acquired many different names. The unifying feature is poikiloderma with atrophic skin, hypo- and hyperpigmentation and telangiectases.

Arms and Backs of Hands. Here the skin is thin and easily injured, presumably because of loss of dermis and fat (Fig. 18.14). Typical findings include:

- Senile purpura (Bateman 1815): The support for the dermal vessels is also reduced. Minor damage can produce large hemorrhagic lesions which are almost exclusively limited to this region, although rarely much smaller purpuric macules can be seen on the face (Chap. 23).
- Stellate pseudoscars: These white atrophic starlike or bizarre patterned lesions are true scars but follow such minor damage that the patients do not recall the event or consider the lesion a scar (Fig. 18.15).
- "Age spots" or "liver spots:" The dark sharply bordered uniformly colored patches on the backs of the hands usually represent flat seborrheic keratoses, although occasionally they may be melanocytic in nature or a pigmented actinic keratosis.
- Hypertrophic actinic keratoses: While actinic keratoses are more common on the face, those on the backs of the hands are often hyperkeratotic or even dome-shaped. They resemble a keratoacanthoma but do not arise suddenly. The risk of conversion to squamous cell carcinoma is less for these lesions than for facial actinic keratoses.

Face. The amount of atrophy on the face is less, but the number of actinic keratoses, basal cell carcinomas and squamous cell carcinomas greater. The solar elastosis is more common, seen in virtually every biopsy taken from older facial skin. A number of different types of solar elastosis are discussed below. Other changes more common on the face include:

- Wrinkles: Many different types of wrinkles are seen. The most prominent are the deep furrows that arise perpendicularly to the muscles of facial expression, called both worry lines and smile

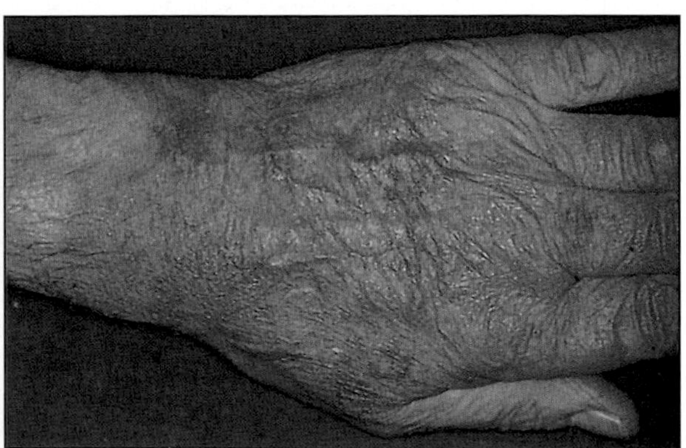

Fig. 18.14. Atrophic skin on the back of the hand with foci of senile purpura

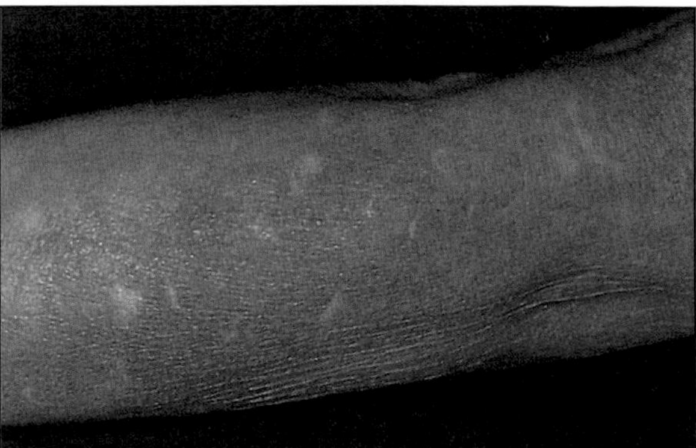

Fig. 18.15. Stellate pseudoscars

lines. They are also useful in cutaneous surgery since they can be used to hide an excisional scar. Smaller periorificial radiating lines, known as crows' feet at the corner of the eyes, but also seen about the mouth are a minor version of the same phenomenon. Injection of botulinum toxin may relieve these wrinkles. Other wrinkle lines result from the sagging of the facial skin, such as those just anterior to the ears and below the jaw line; they represent loss of elasticity. Finally, fine wrinkles are also seen as a combination of solar and intrinsic aging.

- Pigmented lesions: A wide variety of flat pigmented lesions can be seen, including flat seborrheic keratoses, pigmented actinic keratoses and solar or senile lentigines. All can be flat, slowly growing, range in color from tan to dark-brown and often can only be separated with certainty via a skin biopsy. They are discussed in Chapter 58.
- Erythrosis interfollicularis colli: The combination of speckled follicular hypopigmentation and erythema on the lateral neck is well known. When tan hyperpigmentation is also present, one can speak of erythromelanosis (Chap. 26).

Histopathology. The epidermis is thinned and the epidermal-dermal junction flatter. There may be focal atypia even in skin not clinically suggestive of actinic keratosis. In the dermis, the thinning is hard to appreciate but varying degrees of elastosis are found.

Differential Diagnosis. The diagnosis of aged skin is obvious. The problem is to identify the actinic keratoses and possible carcinomas as well as separate out the various flat pigmented lesions.

Therapy. Sunscreens or sunlight avoidance are the obvious answers to avoid damage. Intensive efforts to develop agents which reverse the cutaneous aging process have once again come into vogue. In the USA 0.025% tretinoin has been approved in a cream vehicle (Renova) for the treatment of photodamaged skin. Hydroxy acids and a variety of topical peeling agents are also used, while chemical peeling and laser skin resurfacing are also available. Studies showing increases in epidermal thickness and production of more collagen and ground substance following treatment form the basis for optimism about at least partially reversing age-related changes in the skin.

Atrophy of Chronic Disease

Many chronically ill patients or starved patients develop pale, thin skin that lacks tone and fails to return to its normal position when pinched or lifted up. The principal causes are loss of subcutaneous fat from reduced nutrition, loss of turgor from dehydration and undoubtedly loss of vitamins and other essential nutritional ingredients. There is often an associated diffuse anagen alopecia. Patients with eating disorders may present with a milder version of such atrophy, while terminally ill patients and starved patients are the best examples of advanced cases.

Neurogenic Atrophy

If the regional innervation of the skin is damaged, there are many trophic changes. The term "glossy skin and fingers" has been applied, as the skin becomes thin, smooth and either red or cyanotic, but usually paradoxically moist from hyperhidrosis. Mechanical blisters, hyperkeratotic lesions, nail dystrophies and dysesthesias also occur. Similar changes are seen in reflex sympathetic dystrophy. Depending on the degree and level of nerve damage, there may also be changes in the underlying fat, muscle and even bone.

Pressure Atrophy

Constant pressure can also damage the skin. If the pressure exceeds the ability of the vascular system to supply nutrients, then a pressure ulcer develops (Chap. 13). If the pressure is either less constant or less severe, other changes can be seen. If the mechanical forces are applied for a long enough period of time, the changes can be permanent. One good example of trivial pressure atrophy can be seen under a ring which is slightly too tight and worn for years. Fat is particularly prone to pressure atrophy, so seemingly minor injuries to the fat, especially of the thighs, may produce long-term atrophy. The hair follicles are also sensitive to pressure, such as that from tight ponytails or "corn rows" leading to traction alopecia or that from carrying loads on the head leading to hair loss, for example, in women carrying baskets or water containers long distances in various African and Asian cultures.

Moulin Syndrome

(Moulin 1992)

Synonym. Acquired pigmented atrophic band-like dermatosis following Blaschko lines

Clinical Findings. This rare disorder has only recently been identified. Patients present with unilateral hyperpigmented, atrophic plaques on the trunk in a linear pattern following Blaschko lines. Similar lesions may be seen on the ipsilateral limbs. The age of onset is not at birth, but usually in childhood or adolescence. The plaques are soft, not sclerotic. They remain relatively stable over many years.

Histopathology. The epidermis shows basal layer hyperpigmentation while the dermis is of normal thickness and composition. Presumably the clinical atrophy reflects changes in the subcutaneous fat although this has not been confirmed.

Differential Diagnosis. Linear scleroderma is usually suggested but the skin is not sclerotic. Atrophoderma of Pasini and Pierini may appear similar, but has not been described as linear and usually has some dermal atrophy. The pattern resembles linear and whorled nevoid hypomelanosis, but the latter is not atrophic and is usually present at birth.

Therapy. Moulin syndrome is a cosmetic disturbance usually requiring no therapy.

Progressive Hemifacial Atrophy

(Parry 1825; Romberg 1846)

Synonyms. Hemiatrophia faciei progressiva, Romberg syndrome, Parry-Romberg syndrome

Epidemiology. Hemifacial atrophy is uncommon and equally distributed among men and women. Most cases are sporadic.

Etiology and Pathogenesis. The cause is unknown. In some cases underlying neurologic disease is present. In others, there is a history of previous trauma. Rarely there is a positive family history, suggesting autosomal dominant inheritance.

Clinical Findings. The onset of the problem is in the first two decades of life. There is usually unilateral facial pain in the distribution of the trigeminal nerve associated with a disfiguring scarring involving the skin, subcutaneous fat and bone (Fig. 18.16). The involved facial half appears smaller; the eye appears to lie deep, and the opening of the mouth is narrowed. The orbital ridge may be notched and the process typically extends onto the scalp, with loss of eyelashes, eyebrows and scalp hair. Poliosis may also occur. The tongue and larynx can also show unilateral involvement. Rarely the shoulder region or the contralateral side may be affected. The skin is tight, thin, and occasionally shows hypo- or hyperpigmentation, as well as hypohidrosis. There may be contralateral focal or Jacksonian epilepsy.

Histopathology. Surgical specimens show dermal sclerosis, atrophy of the fat and normal but distorted bone. Even in the early stages, the inflammatory changes of scleroderma are not present.

Course and Prognosis. The disease usually burns out after a period of years. Then the changes are permanent, unless corrective surgery is performed.

Differential Diagnosis. The age-old argument is the relationship between progressive hemifacial atrophy and linear scleroderma. In general, scleroder-

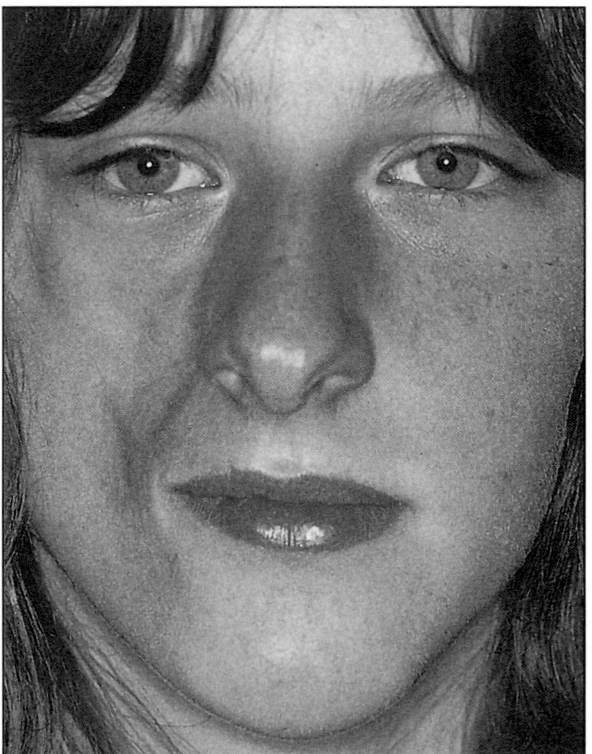

Fig. 18.16. Hemifacial atrophy

ma does not involve the bone, has an inflammatory phase, and is not associated with neurologic problems. But one can argue equally convincingly that progressive hemifacial atrophy is simply severe localized scleroderma triggered by a neurologic event. Progressive facial lipodystrophy is a similar process, equally difficult to separate out.

Therapy. Lesions are probably best treated just as morphea. UVA-1 and bath PUVA both appear worth a try. Later, plastic surgery is the most reasonable approach. Injection of the patient's own fat or artificial collagen products may be beneficial, but the defects are often too large for this approach.

Atrophoderma

Atrophoderma or atrophodermia is not a helpful term. It has been applied to a variety of unrelated disorders and says nothing that atrophy does not say. Generalized atrophoderma (Pasini-Pierini disease) is discussed later in this chapter as we view it as a variant of scleroderma. The other major category is follicular atrophoderma which we will consider here.

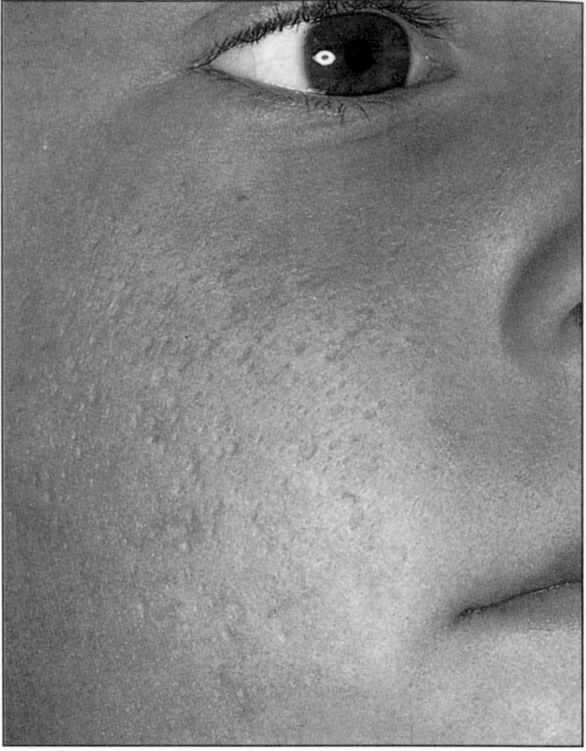

Fig. 18.17. Atrophodermia vermiculata

Etiology and Pathogenesis. In some cases, such as acne, there is a history of follicular inflammation and the follicular atrophoderma is simply a localized atrophic scar. The term perifollicular elastolysis was suggested to describe these lesions because of the tentative identification of elastases in various bacteria found in acne lesions but not in *Propionibacterium acnes.* In atrophoderma vermiculatum, there is often a history of preexisting follicular plugging. In other cases, there is no explanation.

Clinical Findings. The typical lesion is a small pit or dell around a hair follicle, or more often distributed in the pattern of hair follicles, but with no hairs left because of scarring.

The major clinical variants are:

Atrophodermia Vermiculata (Darier 1920) or Atrophoderma Vermiculatum. The whole topic of follicular keratoses is explored in Chapter 17. Children with follicular plugging of the cheeks often develop sharply defined pits or even worm-like scars on the cheeks (Fig. 18.17).

Perifollicular Elastolysis. Many acne patients develop white scars in a follicular pattern typically on the chest, back or lateral part of the neck. The lesions may be slightly herniated or depressed. In rare other cases, for example associated with mid-dermal elastolysis, similar scars may be seen.

Chondrodysplasia Punctata, CHILD Syndrome, and Other X-linked Dominant Disorders. These may have follicular atrophoderma as a minor feature.

Bazex Syndrome. In this autosomal dominant inherited disorder, follicular atrophoderma is associated with multiple basal cell carcinomas, hypohidrosis and hypotrichosis.

Rombo Syndrome. The main features of this autosomal dominant inherited syndrome are facial milia, atrophodermia vermiculata, acral cyanosis, alopecia and multiple trichoepitheliomas and basal cell carcinomas in adult life.

Nicolau-Balus Syndrome. These patients have prominent atrophodermia vermiculata associated with multiple milia and syringomas. The disorder is inherited in an autosomal dominant pattern.

Histopathology. In follicular atrophoderma a large dilated pore or follicle is seen. Special stains may show reduction in peripheral elastic fibers. This supports the concept of perifollicular elastolysis. Rarely scarring adjacent to the atrophic area is seen. In contrast to an acne comedo, the patulous follicle is empty and lacks inflammation.

Therapy. The lesions improve with age but can be treated with punch excision and closure or dermabrasion if needed.

Disorders of Elastic Fibers

In addition to the inherited defects in elastic fibers discussed above, there are acquired changes. Elastolysis refers to a diffuse or localized loss of elastic fibers, while elastosis indicates an increase. The only common elastosis is that seen in skin with actric damage. Some congenital mesenchymal malformations are dominated by elastic fibers. These lesions, known as congenital elastomas or elastoses, are one variant of connective tissue nevus (Chap. 52).

Anetoderma

Synonyms. Macular atrophy, localized elastolysis

Definition. Anetoderma is the localized loss or decrease in elastic fibers.

Epidemiology. Several pedigrees have been reported in which multiple family members had anetoderma but no clear pattern of inheritance has been established.

Etiology and Pathogenesis. The etiology of anetoderma is known in some cases. Two generations ago, it was often associated with healed syphilis. *Borrelia burgdorferi* infections may play a role. Often a healed varicella or herpes zoster will produce anetoderma rather than typical scars, perhaps suggesting a deeper inflammatory process. Sometimes the lesions of lupus erythematosus, mycosis fungoides or mast cell disease resolve with focal defects. In recent years anetoderma has been described in association with HIV/AIDS and the whole spectrum of the antiphospholipid syndrome. True scars and large plaques of atrophy by definition are not anetoderma. There must be some inflammatory damage to the elastic fibers or the induction of an elastase enzyme, but the mechanisms remain fuzzy.

Clinical Findings. The characteristic change in anetoderma is a round or more often oval, sharply bordered area of thinned skin several millimeters is size. The lesions may be solitary, widely scattered or often grouped. The trunk and upper aspects of the thighs are the most likely locations (Fig. 18.18). The skin may clinically appear thinned, described as cigarette paper skin with fine wrinkling and visible vessels (Fig. 18.19). In other cases, the dermal fat may herniate out through the defect. Even if the latter is not the case, one can often palpate the tiny herniation, as the digit drops into the subcutaneous fat.

Traditionally anetoderma has been subdivided into a number of groups, based on the presence or absence of precursor lesions. These precursor lesions are somewhat mysterious, since if a known clinically identified precursor such as varicella causes anetoderma, most people speak of secondary anetoderma or anetoderma-like changes. We suspect that there is idiopathic anetoderma in which we simply have no knowledge of the initial

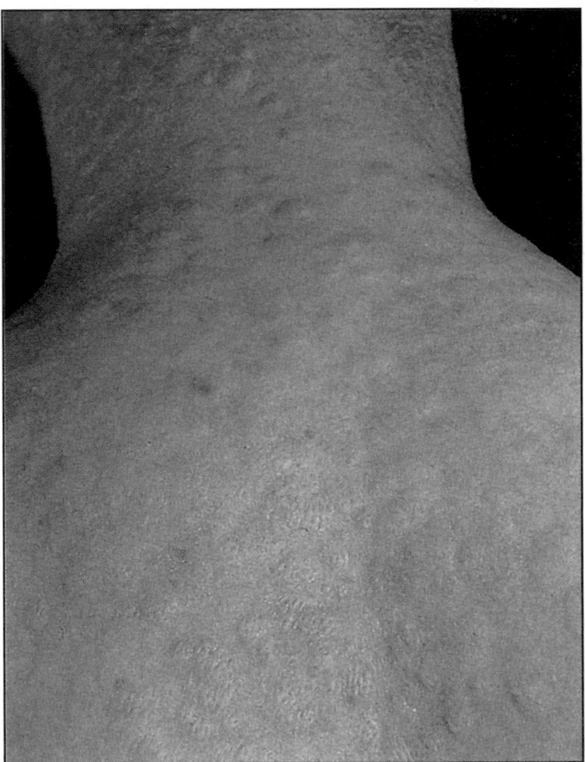

Fig. 18.18. Anetoderma

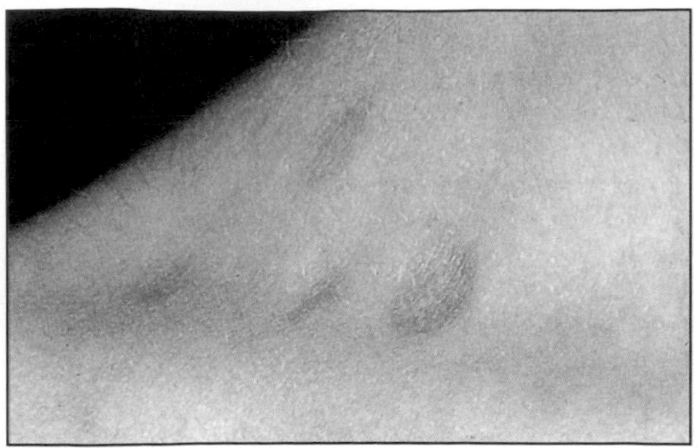

Fig. 18.19. Anetoderma; closer view of depressed lesions covered by thin skin

insult and that these various phases have a similar pathogenesis. Nonetheless, we have listed them separately.

Jadassohn type (Jadassohn 1892). In this type, there is an inflammatory stage with focal erythema and swelling evolving into anetoderma.

Pellizari type (Pellizari 1884). Here the precursor lesions are allegedly urticarial in nature but often persistent over a period of weeks. In extreme cases, bullae can be seen (Alexander type; Alexander 1904). The biopsy shows more edema and less inflammation. Often these two types are combined as Jadassohn-Pellizari anetoderma.

Schwenninger-Buzzi type (Schwenninger and Buzzi 1889–1899). In this variant, the inflammatory stage is not present or is better said to be subclinical. The patient and physician first notice the atrophic lesions, most commonly on the trunk.

Histopathology. The histology of established anetoderma is clear. There is a focal decrease or even absence of elastic fibers. To identify this chance with certainty, it is advantageous for the dermatopathologist to receive normal skin for comparison. One can either do an excision biopsy which includes both normal and diseased skin, or submit two biopsies – one from a lesion and one from a corresponding area of normal skin.

The pathology of the inflammatory stage is by definition unclear. If one knew what the inflammatory stage was, then the process would not be so mysterious. Edema and varying degrees of lymphohistiocytic perivascular and periadnexal inflammation have been described.

Differential Diagnosis. True secondary causes of anetoderma can usually be excluded by the history and examination. The biopsy rarely provides clues in this direction. Early lichen sclerosus et atrophicus or morphea can appear similar, but usually become sclerotic at some point. The lesions in focal dermal hypoplasia are anetodermic, as is nevus lipomatosus, but these disorders traditionally are not grouped here.

Course and Prognosis. Since the development of anetoderma is so poorly understood, the likelihood of a patient developing new lesions is hard to predict. The lesions are stable and unlikely to change.

Therapy. Antibiotic therapy has been recommended in the acute stage. Later on lesions can be excised, but the cosmetic results are not very satisfying.

Striae Distensae

Synonyms. Striae, stretch marks

Epidemiology. Striae are among the most common cutaneous findings. During puberty 70% of girls and 40% of boys, and during pregnancy 90% of women develop them.

Etiology and Pathogenesis. The main risk factor in striae is sudden weight gain, as the skin appears to be simply stretched. Striae typically develop perpendicularly to the direction of stretch. In experimental settings, stretching the skin alone does not appear to induce striae. The weight gain may be a baby, a tumor, additional fat or muscle mass. Hormones also play a role. Striae are a known complication of both Cushing disease and syndrome and can result from the local use of high-potency corticosteroids. This is more likely in children and in areas of the body predisposed to striae formation. There are also individuals who develop striae, especially during puberty, without significant weight gain or body-building activity. In such a case, one should consider connective tissue disorders such as Marfan syndrome.

Clinical Findings. Early striae are usually erythematous or blue-red elevated lesions (striae rubrae) (Fig. 18.20). Typically there are multiple firm linear parallel bands of varying widths and lengths. Later they gradually become white and deposed or atrophic (striae albae). The minimally sunken skin is

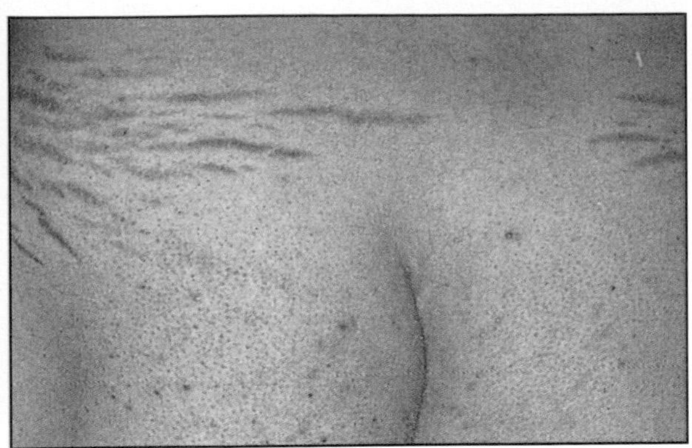

Fig. 18.20. Striae distensae

finely wrinkled and occasionally tiny herniations of fat can be appreciated. The sites of predilection are the buttocks and upper parts of the thighs. During pregnancy, the abdomen is the favorite site, usually more laterally, as well as the breasts. In weight lifters, the shoulder girdle is a common location. In Cushing disease, the axillae are a common site.

Several variations on striae have been described.

Stria Migrans (Shelley and Cohen 1964). These authors described a single stria running along the thigh of a teenager and increasing in longitudinal length, rather than stretching in size. We have seen the same phenomenon following topical corticosteroid use, but it is quite rare.

Transverse Striae (Burket et al. 1989). These striae are found on the lower part of the back, not a fatty or stretched area, and are horizontally arranged. In some cases they show increased elastin and have also been described as linear focal elastosis.

Histopathology. Microscopic studies have confused the study of striae, perhaps because they have been for the most part random biopsies, not carefully timed to follow the course of the disease. Equally convincing reports describe increased and decreased amounts of elastic fibers. If striae are analogous to other scars, then initially the dermis should be rarefied so both elastic fibers and collagen are decreased. Later perhaps there is a disproportionate increase in elastic fibers in abnormally staining collagen. Clumped and distorted elastic fibers can be found at the edge of a lesion.

Course and Prognosis. The striae gradually improve with time as they become more skin-colored, but never resolve.

Differential Diagnosis. The lesions themselves are distinctive and well known. The trick is not to overlook a treatable underlying or predisposing condition.

Therapy. Avoiding weight gain and a bit of luck are the only treatments. The preventive creams sold to pregnant women in many countries have never been proven effective. Exercise programs are admirable but probably do not directly influence striae. There is some evidence that topical tretinoin may reduce the severity of striae, but both its efficacy and particularly its safety in pregnancy have been questioned.

Mid-dermal Elastolysis

(Shelley and Wood 1977)

Synonym: Elastolysis mediodermalis

Epidemiology. Mid-dermal elastolysis is not as uncommon as the few reports would suggest. It appears to be a disease of middle-aged women.

Etiology and Pathogenesis. There is no explanation for the loss of elastic fibers in the mid-part of the dermis.

Clinical Findings. The abdomen, flanks and upper aspects of the thighs are the sites of predilection. Often it is difficult to see the very fine wrinkling that the patient has usually noticed under close observation. While some patients describe initial erythema, it is rarely observed. Large patches evolve and often fuse together. The main finding is the diffuse wrinkling which disappears when one stretches the skin. In addition, tiny white papules, called perifollicular protrusions, 3–5 mm in diameter, may be seen; they allegedly merge into the wrinkles.

Histopathology. The hematoxylin-eosin stain is normal. With elastic stains, amazingly the mid-dermal elastic fibers are absent, even though those in the papillary and deeper dermis are totally normal. Occasionally a scant, but not diagnostic, perivascular lymphohistiocytic infiltrate is seen.

Course and Prognosis. The lesions remain subtle but permanent.

Differential Diagnosis. Early lesions raise the question of acquired cutis laxa, but never become so severe. Similarly pseudoxanthoma elasticum and perifollicular elastolysis should be considered.

Actinic Elastosis

Synonyms. Solar elastosis, senile elastosis

Definition. Alterations in the dermis of sunlight-exposed skin which may be detected clinically, while histologically showing increased amounts of material that stains positively with elastic stains.

Epidemiology. Solar elastosis occurs in every white adult who has had any degree of sunlight exposure. It is more common in type I-II skin, in outdoor workers and in those living in the tropics. It typically begins in the fourth to fifth decade, but may be seen sooner in special risk groups. It is almost never seen clinically in black skin.

Etiology and Pathogenesis. The effective wavelengths for solar damage are not known. Because UVA penetrates more deeply than UVB, it is assumed that it plays a role in solar elastosis. Infrared can also cause elastosis, as seen in erythema ab igne. The exact mechanism remains a mystery, but there is so little turnover in dermal collagen and so much more collagen than elastin that it is hard to explain how the dermis in sunlight-exposed skin acquires so much material which stains positively for elastic fibers. There is a shift towards the production of more elastic fibers with increased levels of elastin and fibrillin mRNA, but in addition, sunlight-damaged collagen appears to express elastin-like surface fibers.

Clinical Findings. Any sunlight-exposed skin may show elastosis histologically. Often there are no distinct clues, but in other cases there may be a yellowish tint. The distinct clinical entities associated with solar elastosis are considered separately below.

Histopathology. The epidermis is usually atrophic and may show atypia of basal cells, even when no actinic keratosis is present. In the dermis are varying amounts of elastosis. The new material has a blue-gray tint on routine microscopy and can be seen approaching the epidermal-dermal junction but there is always a Grenz zone of normal pink dermis just under the basement membrane zone. This upper area may contain newly synthesized collagen. Sometimes the damaged material shows thick coils or fibers, but often these can first be seen with an elastic fiber stain. When one stains a specimen from the face of an older adult with an elastic fiber stain, one is often amazed at just how extensive the solar elastosis is.

Course and Prognosis. The solar elastosis continues to progress. While it is a marker for other solar damage and thus for the risk of actinic keratoses and squamous cell carcinomas, in itself, elastosis carries no malignant risk.

Therapy. In general, sunscreens are the answer, but by the time elastosis has developed, it is really too late. More superficial and milder forms of elastosis respond to topical retinoids; one can demonstrate reversal of the elastic fiber staining and increased synthesis of ground substance. Topical 5-fluorouracil does not appear to greatly influence the dermal fibers. Dermabrasion and superficial laser removal have also be used. The regenerating fibroblasts appear to manufacture more normal collagen and elastin.

Cutis Rhomboidalis Nuchae
(Jadassohn 1925)

The clinical picture of deep furrows in rhomboid pattern on the nape associated with thickened skin and yellow plaques is known as farmer's neck or sailor's neck (Fig. 18.21). It can also be seen in photosensitive patients such as those with porphyria. It is uncommon in women, because of the usual protection of the nape by the hair. Sometimes comedones are also seen and they may contain multiple small hairs (trichostasis spinulosa). Microscopically, the deposits of elastic-staining material are massive.

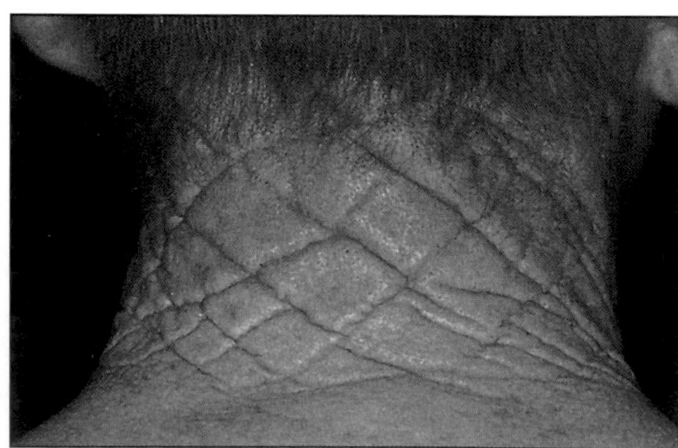

Fig. 18.21. Cutis rhomboidalis nuchae

Elastoma Diffusum
(Dubreuilh 1892)

While this term is rarely applied in the USA, the condition is quite common. Patients may present with widespread, sharply bordered plaques, usually on the forehead, cheeks or lateral portion of the neck. Frequently comedones are seen, overlapping with Favre-Racouchot disease. Sometimes a single plaque or nodule may be seen. Such nodular lesions are often mistaken for a basal cell carcinoma and biopsied or excised. Microscopically one sees massive elastosis without any tumor cells. Another confusing clinical situation is hemorrhage into a plaque of elastosis. This is analogous to the hemorrhage seen in amyloidosis, but the cause is lack of vessel support from elastosis without any underlying systemic disease.

Lemon Skin
(Milian 1921)

Synonym. Peau citréine

This is a variant of elastoma diffusum but clinically unique. It is almost always limited to the lateral forehead, where patients have patches or plaques with atrophy, prominent pale papules which represent residual hair follicles, and often yellow deposits of elastotic material.

Favre-Racouchot Disease
(Favre and Racouchot 1951)

Synonym. Nodular elastosis with cysts and comedones

The synonym says it all. The typical patient is an older man who begins to develop comedones. The most common site is the malar ridge, but the lateral aspects of the cheeks, the inferior periorbital region, the temples and less often the nose and ears may be involved. Often yellow nodules or plaques of elastosis are also seen, as well as numerous tiny cysts, some of which may become several centimeters in size (Fig. 18.22). Microscopic examination reveals marked elastosis admixed with tiny cysts and comedones which are usually rectangular in shape with a wide opening (in contrast to more spherical acne comedones with a relatively narrow opening). Topical retinoids are not as helpful as might be expected but they should be tried. Individual lesions can be expressed. Low-dose oral isotretinoin

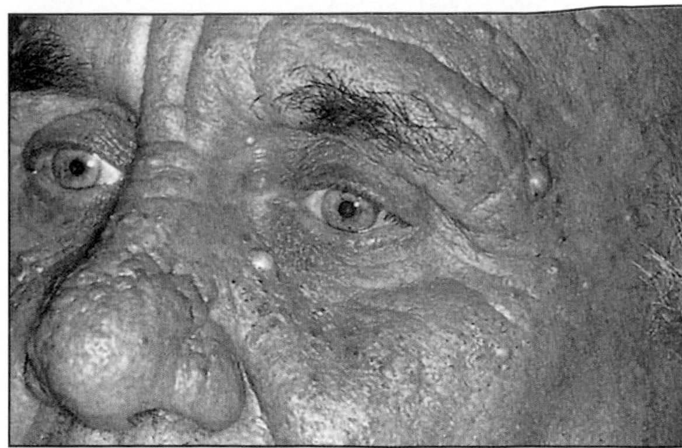

Fig. 18.22. Favre-Racouchot disease

0.1–0.2 mg/kg for a few months usually produces improvement which may last for some time. Dermabrasion may also be useful.

Elastotic Ear Papules
(Carter et al. 1969)

Occasionally yellow papules, usually multiple, develop on the antihelix in patients with other signs of chronic sunlight exposure. They are usually small, not painful and not crusted or ulcerated. The differential diagnosis includes basal cell carcinoma, gouty tophus and chondrodermatitis nodularis helicis. If the clinical clues do not allow distinction, a biopsy will settle the issue, as it shows diffuse elastosis.

Other Forms of Elastosis

Smokers' Elastosis. Heavy smokers tend to have ash gray-yellow discoloration of their facial skin with marked drooping. It is difficult to totally separate this feature from solar elastosis, but many of the individuals have no other stigmata of solar damage. In a large retrospective study of premature wrinkling, sunlight exposure and smoking history appeared to be independent risk factors. Histologic studies have also shown increased and fragmented elastic fibers in smokers' skin as compared to site-matched skin from nonsmokers.

Radiation Elastosis. Radiation dermatitis also shows elastotic changes. Sometimes yellow plaques or nodules can be found in association with more typical poikilodermatous changes.

Uremic Elastosis. Uremic patients also can develop elastotic changes in the skin. This change has become quite uncommon because of the more prompt treatment of renal failure with dialysis and transplantation.

Acrokeratoelastoidosis

There are a number of different disorders which are clinically so similar that we suspect they are related. All feature papules, plaques and nodules located almost exclusively at the junction between the palmar and dorsal skin of the hands or feet (the line of transgredience) along the thenar and hypothenar eminences. Nonetheless they have been subdivided based primarily on histologic appearance. All represent some form of dermal degenerative change. There is no satisfactory form of treatment.

Acrokeratoelastoidosis Verruciformis
(Costa 1953)

This disorder is the best described of the group. It was originally reported from South America and is still most often found there. In some instances, autosomal dominant inheritance has been described. The patients are usually outdoor workers and it is likely that sunlight, trauma and a genetic predisposition combine forces. In addition to the plaques along the sides of the hands, similar changes have been described on the feet and occasionally on the dorsal surfaces. Tightly aggregated, often umbilicated yellow papules are seen. Diascopic examination makes the deposits more dramatic. They often have a rhomboidal shape, and sometimes a hyperkeratotic surface (Fig. 18.23). The key microscopic finding is the presence of massive elastosis along with regionally typical changes in the epidermis.

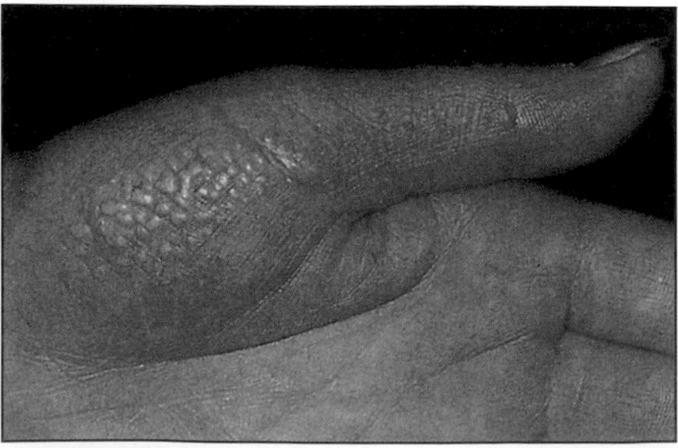

Fig. 18.23. Acrokeratoelastoidalis

Keratoelastoidosis Marginalis

Synonyms. Degenerative collagenous plaques, digital papular calcific elastosis

This lesion is confined to the line of transgredience in the notch between the thumb and index finger. Most cases have been described from South Africa. The lesions are large plaques which tend to calcify more often than the other lesions, but also show striking elastosis and are probably the same as the South American variant.

Focal Acral Hyperkeratosis

This disorder is clinically identical to acrokeratoelastoidosis and may also be autosomally dominantly inherited or occur sporadically. Microscopic evaluation shows focal orthohyperkeratosis often with some epidermal atrophy in a clavus or corn pattern. No elastic fiber changes are present.

White Fibrous Papulosis
(Shimizu et al. 1989)

Synonyms. Fibroelastolytic papulosis, pseudoxanthoma elasticum-like papillary dermal elastolysis

While this disease was first described only in Japanese, it has been seen in a number of racial groups. The cause is unknown but it probably represents an aging response. Patients are typically adults who have many small white papules on their nape. In other instances, the lesions coalesce, forming plaques, and may have a yellowish hue. Lesions may extend into the hairline or even involve the axillae and supraclavicular fossa. Under the microscope, there is fibrosis and homogenization of the papillary dermis coupled with loss of fine elastic fibers in this area, as well as clumping of thickened elastic fibers in the reticular dermis. There is no connection with pseudoxanthoma elasticum, either clinically or histologically. While the problem is harmless, individual lesions can be excised.

Colloid Milium
(Wagner 1863)

Synonyms. Elastosis colloidalis conglomerata, colloid degeneration of the skin

Etiology and Pathogenesis. While colloid milia appear to be a type of nodular solar damage, they do not show elastotic change microscopically. Ultrastructural studies show an amorphous substance with fine 2-nm filaments that may represent elastic fiber or fibrillin degeneration. Others speculate that a new fibrous protein is secreted by the sunlight-influenced fibroblasts.

Clinical Findings. Several types of colloid milium have been identified. The classic lesions are waxy papules in sunlight-damaged skin, usually on the back of the hands, cheeks, nape or ears. Less often other sunlight-exposed areas are involved. Usually multiple yellow, glassy translucent soft papules are present. They may range in size from 0.2 cm to 2.0 cm. If one makes a tiny incision, the gelatinous material can often be expressed; this is not possible with nodular elastosis or amyloidosis. Sometimes the lesions appear vesicular. In yet other instances, multiple confluent papules form a plaque (en plaque colloid degeneration). Sometimes the adjacent skin also is yellow or papular, reflecting the associated solar elastosis. In the rarest variant, the lesions may be pigmented.

Histopathology. The overall pattern is dome-shaped. The epidermis is usually thinned, but the striking change is large amorphous dermal deposits with clefts. Solar elastosis is always seen. The nature of the colloid is difficult to determine. It is most easily distinguished from amyloid based on the size of the deposits, but this does not work when contrasting nodular amyloidosis and nodular colloid degeneration. Colloid is usually negative with amyloid stains but occasionally may be weakly positive. Electron microscopy is the most reliable way to separate the two as the amyloid fibers are much thicker.

Course and Prognosis. The lesions are stable and have no malignant potential.

Differential Diagnosis. The main clinical question is nodular solar elastosis, as well as basal cell carcinoma, adnexal tumors and nodular amyloidosis. On the hands, the whole spectrum of acrokerato-elastoidosis may come into question. A pigmented lesion can be confused with a malignant melanoma.

Therapy. Any destructive therapy, such as excision, curettage, laser destruction or dermabrasion can be employed.

Juvenile Colloid Milium

(Wooldridge and Frerichs 1960)

This extremely rare disorder, perhaps inherited in an autosomal recessive pattern, shares only its name with the far more common adult colloid milium. Children develop translucent yellow brown papules on the nose, upper lip and upper aspects of the cheeks. Occasionally the nape and hands may be involved. They arise before sunlight damage can be a factor. While juvenile colloid milium appears identical by light microscopy and with special stains, it contains densely packed 8–10-nm filaments believed to represent degenerating keratin filaments, suggesting an epidermal origin similar to amyloidosis.

Perforating Dermatoses

There are a number of unrelated dermatoses in which perforation or transepidermal elimination seems to occur. The classic perforating disorders are shown in Table 18.4. Both elastosis perforans serpiginosa and reactive perforating collagenosis seem to reflect the elimination of damaged dermal materials through epidermal channels or defects. All forms of suppurative folliculitis (Chap. 4) eventually show perforation as the inflammatory infiltrate within the follicle damages the wall of the follicle and eventually reaches the dermis. Note that in this case, the direction of perforation is from outside into the dermis, underscoring the lack of unity of this concept. Kyrle disease is classified as a dyskeratotic condition. Kyrle's original cases are difficult to interpret, but we suspect he was describing a chronic suppurative folliculitis with marked pruritus and resultant prurigo nodularis changes secondary to manipulation. Most likely Kyrle disease and perforating disorder of renal disease are very similar (Chap. 25).

In addition, granuloma annulare (Chap. 50) often shows discharge of necrobiotic collagen through epidermal defects, as do larger rheumatoid nodules. Finally, periumbilical perforating pseudoxanthoma elasticum often has hyperkeratotic papules with transepidermal elimination of calcified elastic fibers. In rare instances, these patients have other stigmata of pseudoxanthoma elasticum, but usually they do not.

Table 18.4. Perforating dermatoses

Disease	Clinical features	Microscopic features	Chapter
Elastosis perforans serpiginosa	Annular grouped papules, often on nape keratotic	Abnormal elastic fibers within intraepidermal channels	18
Reactive perforating collagenosis	Crusted excoriated papules and nodules; often Köbner phenomenon	Cup-shaped channel filled with abnormal collagen and topped by crust	18
Perforating folliculitis	Hyperkeratotic follicular plugs, associated with inflammation	Follicular plug with lateral destruction of wall, often retained hairs	4
Kyrle disease (perforating disorder of renal disease)	Multiple pruritic hyperkeratotic nodules, often associated with renal disease, diabetes mellitus	In most instances overlap features of perforating folliculitis and prurigo nodularis; sometimes no follicular structures are identified	17

Elastosis Perforans Serpiginosa

(LUTZ 1953; MIESCHER 1955)

Synonyms. Elastoma intrapapillare perforans verruciforme (Miescher), keratosis follicularis serpiginosa (Lutz)

Epidemiology. Most cases of elastosis perforans serpiginosa are seen in patients with underlying connective tissue diseases or other problems, but it is occasionally seen sporadically. Associated disorders include Wilson disease, Ehlers-Danlos syndrome, pseudoxanthoma elasticum, osteogenesis imperfecta, Marfan syndrome, Down syndrome and perhaps some of the premature aging syndromes and congenital poikilodermas. It is a disease of children and young adults, and more common in men.

Etiology and Pathogenesis. The etiology is unknown in most cases. The best-established cause is in patients with Wilson disease taking penicillamine. Some patients with Wilson disease develop elastosis perforans serpiginosa without exposure to the medication. Elastic fibers in the papillary dermis become thickened and are eliminated through the epidermis.

Clinical Findings. The sites of predilection are the nape, neck, cheeks and extremities. Numerous small erythematous keratotic or verruciform papules are arranged closely together forming annular, circinate or serpiginous plaques (Fig. 18.24). Typically there is central clearing and peripheral spread. Most patients have just one or two lesions which are asymptomatic.

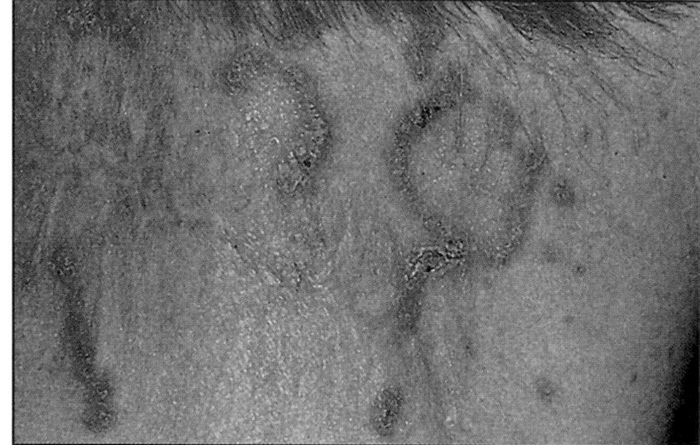

Fig. 18.24. Elastosis perforans serpiginosa

Histopathology. The epidermis is hyperkeratotic and acanthotic. There is an accumulation of altered elastic fibers in the papillary dermis which tend to stain basophilic with hematoxylin-eosin as well as positively with routine elastic fiber stains. This material is eliminated through the epidermis (transepidermal elimination) via channels which often have a corkscrew pattern on sectioning. Associated with the abnormal elastic fibers are usually neutrophils and sometimes nuclear debris. The exact nature of the channels is unclear. In some instances their lining resembles the hair follicle or eccrine duct, but in other cases, it is difficult to determine the nature of the channel.

Course and Prognosis. The prognosis is that of the underlying condition. The lesions of elastosis perforans serpiginosa are chronic and a cosmetic annoyance.

Differential Diagnosis. Clinically, porokeratosis of Mibelli often is suggested, especially in early lesions. Occasionally reactive perforating collagenosis or perforating granuloma annulare may be similar, but the biopsy is decisive.

Therapy. Lesions can be excised, curetted or treated with cryotherapy. Laser destruction is also reasonable. The sites of elastosis perforans serpiginosa tend to form keloids easily. Occasionally intralesional steroids are helpful and avoid the scarring problems.

Reactive Perforating Collagenosis

(Woringer and Laugier 1963; Mehregan et al. 1967)

Synonym. Collagenoma perforans verruciforme (for the solitary lesion)

Epidemiology. This is a very rare disorder which takes two forms. Children typically have multiple lesions and there may be a positive family history although the inheritance is unclear. In those with adult onset, there is usually a solitary lesion, called collagenoma perforans verruciforme.

Etiology and Pathogenesis. The etiology of both types is unknown. Some have dismissed reactive perforating collagenosis as a disease sui generis suggesting that in all cases, it is simply a response to trauma. Others claim that the trauma required for induction of the lesion is often trivial and that those rare children with the disease get many lesions.

Clinical Findings. Pruritic papules develop in response to trauma, most often on the arms, legs and other accessible sites. The Köbner phenomenon is frequently seen, with papules arranged along a scratch line. They soon become umbilicated with a central adherent keratotic plug and heal with scarring over 2–6 weeks. In adults, the disorder is usually secondary to pruritic dermatoses and clinically identical to prurigo nodularis. Rarely a solitary hyperkeratotic crusted lesion which is not clinically distinct may appear.

Histopathology. The epidermis is damaged and perhaps replaced by a crust. The collagen in the upper dermis is no longer eosinophilic but instead basophilic and necrotic. Bundles of this damaged collagen are found at the interface between the dermis and crust and often tunneling through the crust.

Differential Diagnosis. The main differential diagnostic considerations are lichen simplex chronicus and prurigo nodularis.

Therapy. Individual lesions can be excised. Intralesional corticosteroids may also be helpful.

Lichen Sclerosus et Atrophicus

(Hallopeau 1887; Darier 1892)

Synonyms. Lichen sclerosus, lichen albus, white spot disease (Johnson and Sherwell 1903), balanitis xerotica obliterans (on male genitalia)

Epidemiology. Lichen sclerosus et atrophicus (LSA) is more common among females with two distinct peaks: in the fifth to sixth decade and prior to puberty. The disease appears less common in blacks. Familial cases have been described but there is no suggestion of an inheritance pattern.

Etiology and Pathogenesis. The etiology is unknown. The female predominance suggests hormonal factors. LSA is occasionally associated with autoimmune disorders, but no clear defect has been found. There are many similarities with morphea and on occasion the same patient may have LSA and morphea or lichen planus.

Clinical Findings. On the skin, LSA can start as a single patch or as diffuse macules. Sites of predilection include the side of the neck, the clavicular region, the shoulders, the area between and beneath the breasts and the flexural surfaces of the forearms. Early lesions in the form of lichenoid papules are only rarely seen. Most common are porcelain or perhaps blue-white, flat or minimally elevated, round or oval plaques, usually less than 1 cm in diameter. They often have a pink-red inflammatory border and typically slowly expand and coalesce, forming irregular larger lesions (Fig. 18.25). Older lesions appear more atrophic with a parchment texture to the epidermis and frequent comedo-like follicular hyperkeratoses. There may be blisters formed by separation at the epidermal-

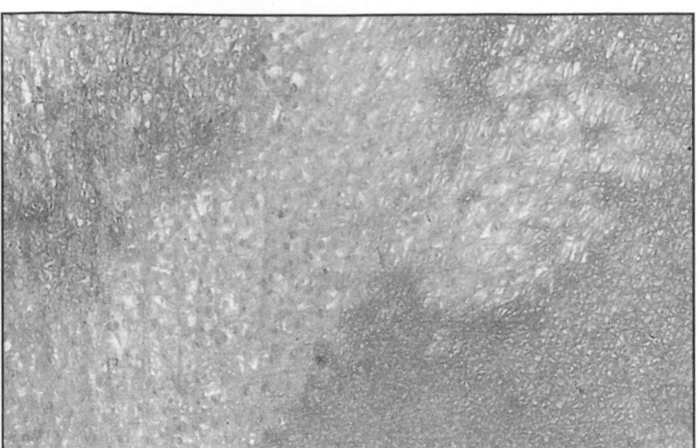

Fig. 18.25. Lichen sclerosus et atrophicus with follicular keratoses

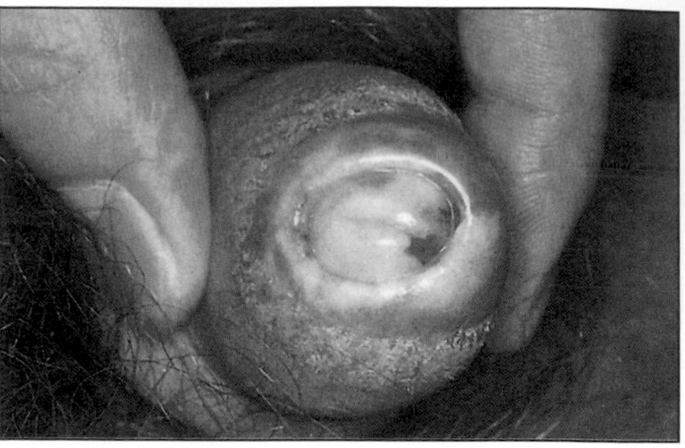

Fig. 18.26. Lichen sclerosus et atrophicus with phimosis (also known as balanitis xerotica obliterans)

dermal junction, and these are frequently filled with fluid which acquires a gelatinous consistency.

On the genitalia, the vulva, perineum and perianal region are the most common sites of involvement in women; the glans and prepuce in men (Fig. 18.26). Other genital lesions are illustrated in Chaps. 34 and 35. Here the tendency to scarring or contractures is more prominent, and hemorrhagic blisters are common. The genital lesions, especially in women, are characteristically very pruritic. The combination of mild scarring and hemorrhage in small children often raises the specter of child abuse. Infantile perianal pyramidal protrusion arises on the perianal medium raphe in young girls. It is a soft asymptomatic red or skin-colored swelling which in at least some cases is early lichen sclerosus et atrophicus. The same changes on the glans, prepuce and urethral meatus lead to synechia, phimosis and difficulty in urinating. While the penile involvement was described as a separate illness, balanitis xerotica obliterans, it is LSA (Chap. 34). Older scarred or contracted lesions have been designated kraurosis vulvae or kraurosis penis, but neither term is employed today. Very rarely, oral mucosal lesions are seen; they are white plaques, typically on the buccal mucosa or under the tongue.

Histopathology. LSA has a distinctive histologic pattern. The epidermis is atrophic and may show follicular plugging. The upper dermis is pale staining, containing edematous, swollen collagen. Special stains show that this area has few if any elastic fibers. Blisters arise just below the epidermal-dermal junction, presumably because of the edema, and are frequently filled with blood-tinged fluid. Widely dilated vessels and lymphatics are found. Beneath the altered dermis is a band-like lymphocytic infiltrate. While a variety of positive immunofluorescent findings have been reported, none is specific.

Course and Prognosis. The course of LSA is definitely chronic in adults, and more chronic than previously thought in children. While spontaneous remissions do occur, there is usually residual atrophy and the disease sometimes starts again later in life. In adults, genital LSA is a potential premalignant condition. In both women and less often men squamous cell carcinomas may arise in typical lesions of LSA. Usually the tumor develops in a longstanding hyperkeratotic papule or plaque, often described as leukoplakia. Occasionally, a persistent erosion turns out to be a tumor. Thus both hyperkeratotic and eroded areas deserve special attention.

Several disease associations have been described with LSA. There may be a connection between widespread LSA and diabetes mellitus in adults, so it is reasonable to check for this. In other cases, LSA has been associated with lichen planus, lupus erythematosus and vitiligo. In some cases one disease or the other was likely misdiagnosed, or histologic confirmation was not obtained.

Differential Diagnosis. Well-developed LSA is unmistakable. The early multiple white macules and papules are clinically identical to vitiligo and the confetti-stage of systemic sclerosis. Histologically, both the sclerosis of systemic sclerosis and the hyalinization and loss of elastic fibers of LSA may take some time to become apparent. Similarly, if a patient has a single plaque on the shoulder with a violaceous border, clinically both morphea and LSA are possibilities. Some have suggested that LSA is morphea confined to the upper part of the dermis with epidermal changes; we believe the two entities can usually be separated.

Therapy

Systemic. Systemic corticosteroids are not helpful. Oral retinoids may produce improvement, but require careful monitoring in the predominantly female patient group and further study. Antimalarials are also recommended, but we have had little success.

Topical. Intralesional corticosteroids (2.5–5.0 mg/ml of triamcinolone acetonide) are extremely effective and we consider them the treatment of choice. Numerous studies have shown that high-potency corticosteroids are more effective than topical estrogen, progesterone or testosterone preparations. In young boys with phimosis secondary to LSA, corticosteroids often provide marked relief. Both UVA-1 and bath PUVA therapy appear promising alternatives.

Surgical. The blisters often heal better if unroofed with a tangential excision. The phimosis and meatal problems should be treated by a urologist. Any persistent ulcer or nodule should be biopsied and then managed appropriately. In generations past, LSA (under the name kraurosis) was taken as an indication for vulvectomy; this was incorrect.

Scleroderma

The sclerodermas are a group of disorders in which after an initial inflammatory change, the skin becomes sclerotic, that is, the dermis becomes thickened and hardened. Scleroderma can be localized or widespread in the skin and associated with internal organ involvement. Despite clinical similarities and an identical histologic pattern, it is reasonable to separate the localized form and the widespread form because of their strikingly different course and prognosis. Systemic forms can be life-threatening, while the localized forms can be distressing or disfiguring but never fatal. Pseudoscleroderma or scleroderma-like disorders are those in which the skin resembles scleroderma but there is an underlying cause or trigger known, such as porphyria cutanea tarda or chemical exposure. The term sclerodermiform is used to describe sclerotic lesions, such as a sclerodermiform or sclerosing basal cell carcinoma, which has a sclerotic stroma but would never be mistaken for scleroderma.

Morphea

Synonyms. Sclerodermia circumscripta, localized scleroderma

Epidemiology. Morphea is an uncommon disorder. It is more frequent in women by a 2–3:1 ratio. Young adults (20–40 years of age) are most often affected, but about 15% of patients are children less than 10 years of age. The disease is rare in blacks.

Etiology and Pathogenesis. In most instances, the etiology is unknown. In some individuals, trauma appears to be a trigger. *Borrelia burgdorferi* is not the cause of morphea, but may produce focal sclerotic lesions in acrodermatitis chronica atrophicans. The response of occasional cases of morphea to high-dose penicillin therapy was known long before *Borrelia burgdorferi* was identified. The active agent may be a metabolite of penicillin such as penicillamine.

Clinical Findings. Morphea begins with a patchy, peripherally expanding erythema. As the erythema disappears centrally, a slowly spreading yellow-white lesion evolves (Fig. 18.27). It consists of a firm plate-like plaque, which is fixed to the underlying tissue but over which the epidermis can be easily moved. The ivory-colored hardened area is bordered by a blue-pink or violet ring of erythema – the lilac ring. While the sclerotic areas are usually permanent, over many years they can become atrophic, with loss of hairs and sweat glands, as well as hypo- and hyperpigmentation (Fig. 18.28). A number of clinical variants of morphea exist, including:

Plaque-Like Morphea. One or more 1–10-cm plaques develop, usually on the trunk.

Guttate Morphea. In this variant many small sclerotic macules cover the trunk. This form, as well as the previous one, are often confused with LSA, but in most instances, the histology is helpful.

Disseminated Morphea. Some patients have many lesions of morphea. At times the entire body appears to be involved and one speaks of generalized morphea. The disease in such patients may

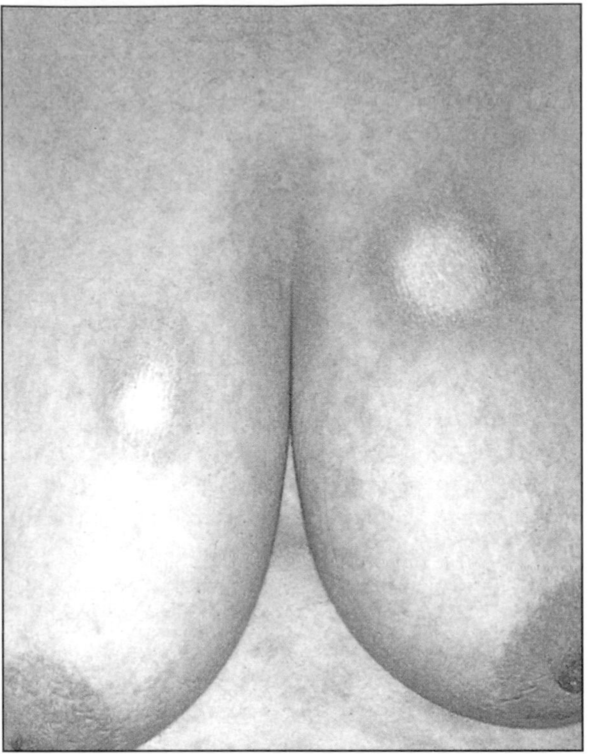

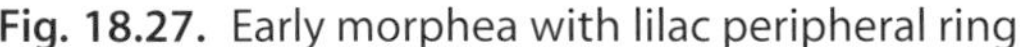

Fig. 18.27. Early morphea with lilac peripheral ring

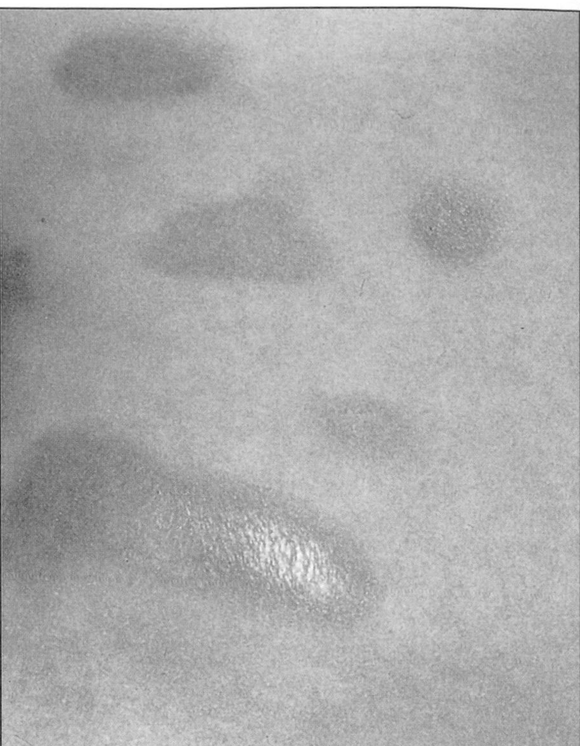

Fig. 18.28. More advanced and disseminated morphea

evolve into or be mistaken for systemic sclerosis, so close monitoring is appropriate. Positive antinuclear antibodies (ANA) values may be seen, as discussed under systemic sclerosis.

Linear Morphea. There are two quite distinct variants of this type. Both are also often called linear scleroderma.

- En Coup de Sabre. The band-like lesion typically extends vertically in a paramedian position from the eyebrows to the scalp, causing scarring alopecia. Occasionally underlying bone damage or abnormal neurologic findings may be seen. This suggests an overlap with progressive hemifacial atrophy (Fig. 18.29).
- Linear Morphea of the Limbs. The typical patient is young with a sclerotic band extending down one limb, usually a leg (Fig. 18.30). The sclerosis may interfere with joint motion and limb growth. Such patients often have positive ANA findings, in contrast to most other forms of morphea. Radiologic and electromyographic investigations may be abnormal.

Atrophoderma of Pasini and Pierini (Pasini 1923; Pierini and Vivoli 1936). This uncommon form is

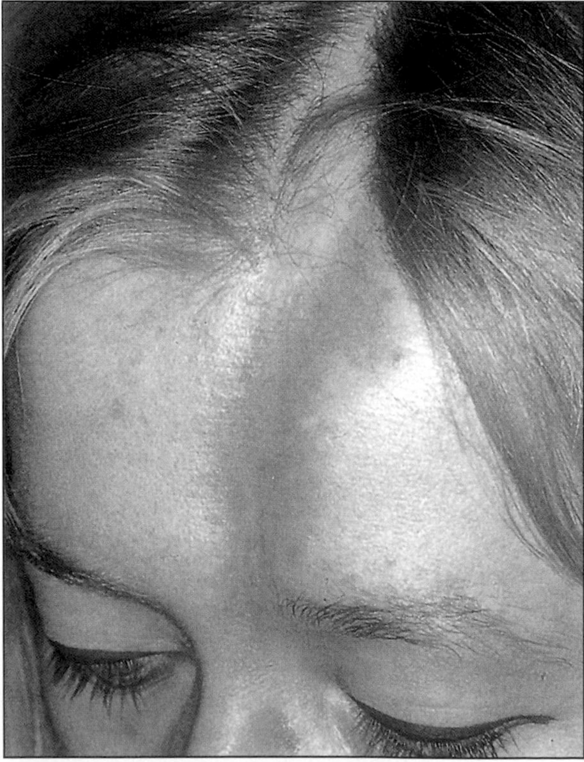

Fig. 18.29. Linear morphea; en Coup de Sabre

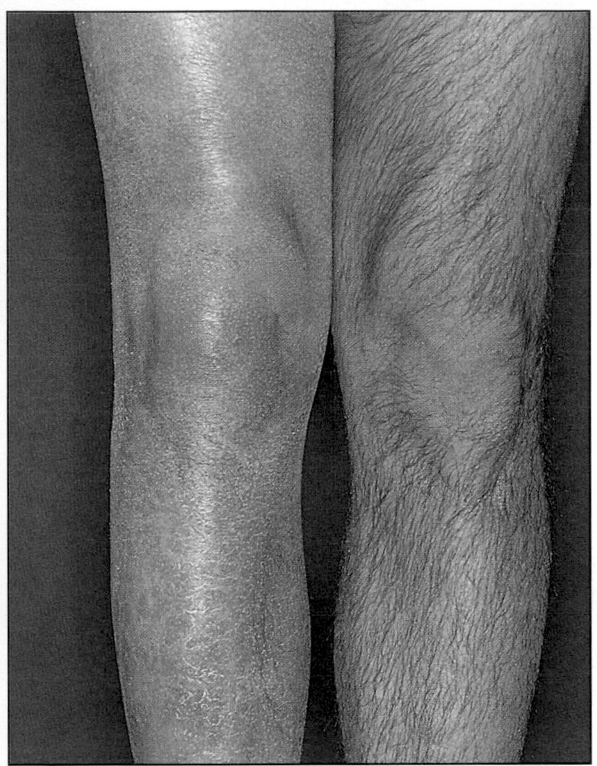

Fig. 18.30. Linear morphea of one limb

also known as erythematous localized morphea. The site of predilection is the trunk, especially the lower part of the back and buttocks. One or more round or oval plaques develop with a diffuse lilac color (*forme lilacée* of Gougerot). Rather than becoming sclerotic, the lesion becomes atrophic and depressed with a characteristic sharp drop-off at the edge. Histologic studies of the depressed area fail to show sclerosis, but the patients typically develop morphea at other sites, or an individual lesion may evolve into morphea. While we have no quarrel with those who prefer to classify atrophoderma of Pasini and Pierini as an idiopathic atrophy, our experience strongly suggests a relationship to morphea.

Nodular Morphea. Rarcly morphea will be nodular mimicking a keloid. Helpful for the diagnosis are the presence of more typical lesions elsewhere and the normal elastic fiber stain, as contrasted to the diminished pattern in a keloid.

Bullous Morphea. Subepidermal blisters may form as the sclerotic dermis is pulled away from the epidermis. The bullae usually appear in a well-established plaque of morphea and are more a curiosity.

Morphea Profunda. This form features sclerosis in the connective tissue septae of the subcutaneous fat and in the underlying muscle fascia. Thus, no inflammatory changes are seen on the skin. Instead, the skin is bound to the deeper structures and typically has a bumpy or depressed surface.

Fascial Morphea. In this most uncommon form, the sclerosis develops in the muscle fascia, usually the flexural tendons on the forearm. Typical manifestations are pain and contractures, mimicking a carpal tunnel syndrome. If the problem progresses, the joint motion may be restricted and the muscles damaged. While the diagnosis is difficult if no cutaneous involvement is present, it should be suspected in a patient with morphea and arm or wrist problems.

Disabling Pansclerotic Morphea of Children (Diaz-Perez et al. 1980). This tragic variant occurs in children and destroys their life. The involvement by morphea is so widespread and severe that multiple joint contractures and other mutilating changes develop. Later the trunk and face maybe affected (Fig. 18.31). The children often cannot feed themselves and frequently fall victim to the vicissitudes of chronic disease, including malnutrition and chronic infections.

Histopathology. As highly varied as the above clinical descriptions are, the microscopic picture in each case is about the same. Early on there is a dense primarily lymphocytic inflammatory infiltrate around the superficial and deep vascular plexi. Eosinophils are usually present, and may sometimes be quite prominent. Very typical is the inflam-

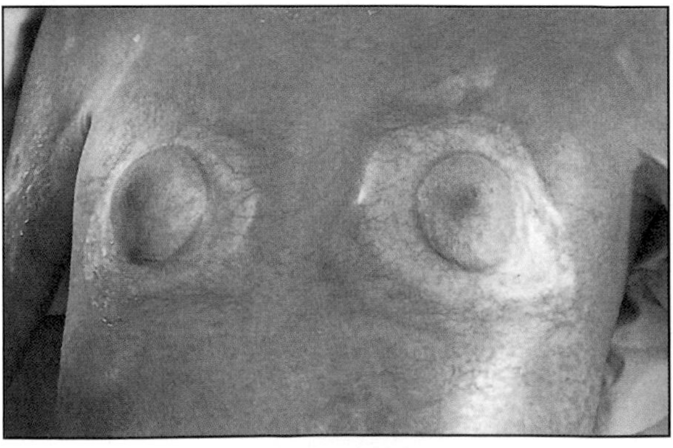

Fig. 18.31. Disabling pansclerotic morphea; the preservation of the nipple and a small amount of breast tissue is common in morphea and scleroderma

mation at the junction between the dermis and the subcutaneous fat which may evolve into a panniculitis. If the dermis is changed, there is simply mild edema. Sometimes individual bundles of collagen are swollen or separated.

Later on, the sclerotic changes dominate. The dermal connective tissue proliferates, usually at the expense of the subcutaneous fat. The inflammatory cells disappear and few fibroblasts are found in the collagen fibers which are thickened and arranged parallel to the epidermal surface. Involvement of the papillary dermis is common. The adnexal structures are frequently reduced in numbers; often only the arrector pili muscles survive to represent the hair follicle. The eccrine sweat glands are found at a much higher level. While they are described as entrapped, actually there is new collagen beneath them. Vessels often appear compressed or slit-shaped. Despite all these alterations, the elastic fiber network is almost unchanged, a valuable clue in separating morphea from both scars and perhaps LSA.

In morphea profunda and disabling pansclerotic morphea, fibrosis and inflammation are much deeper involving the fat septae and muscle fascia. During the inflammatory phase lymphoid follicles are common especially in the fat septae. Eosinophils may be prominent, but their absence does not preclude the diagnosis. Eosinophilic fasciitis, a related disorder, is considered separately below.

Ultrastructural studies show a localized increase in collagen fibrils but with a reduced diameter and much more internal variability than seen in normal skin. In addition, the vessels may have a thickened endothelial lining with more prominent fenestrations and a thickened basement membrane.

Laboratory Findings. The routine evaluation is usually normal. Occasionally circulating eosinophilia is seen. ANA studies done using HEp-2 cells as substrate may be positive in patients with linear morphea and disseminated morphea.

Course and Prognosis. While morphea is a persistent and unpredictable disease, it is usually not a permanent one. At some point, the inflammatory process diminishes, and even the sclerosis can lessen. Typical plaques of morphea are present on average for 1.5–4 years, while the linear forms last longer. The secondary changes, such as pigmentary changes, muscle atrophy and contractures, as well as the facial deformity in en coup de sabre, are more permanent. Occasionally ulcerations may develop in old lesions of morphea. These commonly occur on the legs and are slow to heal and hard to treat. Calcification is uncommon in morphea, but it too is a long-term problem.

Therapy. There is no uniformly successful therapy. Most patients can be treated topically and expectantly, but occasionally systemic therapy is needed for the progressive and destructive variants.

Systemic. A wide variety of systemic therapies have been recommended. Penicillin and other antibiotics are often given but there is no controlled study establishing their efficacy. Phenytoin has been recommended for linear morphea of the limbs but it has been disappointing in our hands. The Mayo Clinic experience with antimalarials, either chloroquine or hydroxychloroquine one tablet daily, is good. They may be the treatment of choice with appropriate cautions and controls. If antimalarials fail to work after a period of 3–6 months or the disease is progressive and destructive, systemic corticosteroids should be employed. If this fails acitretin, cyclosporine, penicillamine and cyclophosphamide can be considered. We are reluctant to give dosages as no regimen is well-established as safe and effective.

Topical. Many patients do well with simple emollients. In the inflammatory stage, it is well worth trying a mid- to high-potency corticosteroid; often the results are good. Intralesional corticosteroids may also be effective and are convenient if only a small number of lesions are present. In addition, vitamin D analogs may be helpful.

Phototherapy. Bath PUVA therapy is extremely effective for many forms of morphea and we currently consider it the treatment of choice, finding it safer and more effective than the systemic therapies discussed above. Treatment with UVA1 radiation in dosages ranging from 10 to 50 J/cm^2 also seems to work well. It has been shown to activate interstitial collagenase, a metalloprotein essential for collagen remodeling.

Other Measures. If there is restriction of joint motion, physical therapy is essential. The patients should avoid strenuous activity during the acute phase of their disease but should always strive to retain their range of motion.

Systemic Sclerosis

Synonyms. Scleroderma, systemic scleroderma, progressive systemic sclerosis (PSS). We prefer the term scleroderma and have retained it when describing the skin. But we have yielded to international convention and used systemic sclerosis throughout the text.

Epidemiology. The illness is uncommon. In the USA the prevalence is estimated at 105/1,000,000. There are between about 3 and 12 new cases per 1,000,000 yearly with a mortality of 2–4/1,000,000. Women are far more often affected than men; the ratio ranges between 3:1 and 5:1. Marked geographic or racial variations are not seen. The disease is very rare in children; it appears to be more severe in older patients. About 80% of patients first seek medical attention in the third to seventh decade. Almost all have cutaneous involvement.

Etiology and Pathogenesis. The cause of systemic sclerosis is unknown. Speculation centers on several areas: genetic factors, microchimerism, autoimmune processes, abnormally reactive vessels, inappropriate regulation of collagen synthesis and environmental factors. One can view the pathophysiology of systemic sclerosis as a spectrum

inflammation ↔ sclerosis ↔ vascular disease.

Genetic Factors. In some patients with systemic sclerosis and their families, increased numbers of chromosome breaks and sister chromatid exchanges have been identified. A factor in the serum of these individuals increases chromosome breaks in vitro in normal individuals. Various HLA associations have also been found: HLA-B8 seems to be associated with a more severe course, while HLA-DR5 and DR12 are associated with a milder course and anticentromere antibodies. Various genetic markers seem more common in different subtypes.

Microchimerism. Several studies have shown persistence of fetal stem cells in women with systemic sclerosis, suggesting that these cells could induce a chronic graft-versus-host reaction in the women.

Autoimmune Factors. A wide variety of ANA have been shown, to some extent correlating with certain forms of the disease. Cellular immune factors have been identified. There is a relative decrease in T cells with increased in vitro reactivity of T cell subsets against both skin and muscle.

Vascular Changes. A number of organs show primarily vascular changes in systemic sclerosis, such as the kidney and lungs. In addition, Raynaud phenomenon is one of the cardinal cutaneous signs. Both hyperactive vessels and vessel obstruction because of medial sclerosis and endothelial proliferation appear to be relevant.

Collagen Synthesis. Fibroblasts from systemic sclerosis patients have been shown to produce much more collagen in culture than those from control individuals. Furthermore there is a shift towards type V collagen.

Environmental Factors. A number of clear environmental associations with scleroderma diseases have been established. The most recent example is the eosinophilia-myalgia syndrome associated with impure tryptophan; this is discussed below. Another scenario was the Spanish toxic oil story in the early 1980s. Contaminated rapeseed oil produced an acute illness followed by chronic neurologic problems and sclerodermatous skin changes. The work of groups in Pittsburgh and Leipzig has shown a possible role for silica. The potential role of silicone, as in breast implants, remains a major controversy. Radiation therapy may also cause scleroderma, but the relationship between radiation-induced sclerosis and scleroderma is unclear. Perhaps mutations and cell damage trigger autoimmune processes.

Clinical Findings. Systemic sclerosis is a polymorphic disorder. Two major forms (Table 18.5) are distinguished:

- Limited systemic sclerosis with a slow course, primarily acral skin changes and modest systemic disease, usually associated with anticentromere antibodies
- Diffuse systemic sclerosis with a potentially aggressive course, truncal skin involvement and multiorgan disease, often associated with anti Scl-70 antibodies

There are also several more unique forms that do not fit easily into the major categories. Included in this group are:

- CREST syndrome. Synonyms: Thibièrge-Weissenbach syndrome (Thibièrge-Weissenbach 1911), Winterbauer syndrome (Winterbauer 1964)
  - Calcinosis
  - Raynaud syndrome

Table 18.5. Classification of systemic sclerosis

Limited form	Diffuse form
Long prodrome with Raynaud phenomenon	Short interval (<1 year) between onset of Raynaud phenomenon and development of skin changes
Limited peripheral skin disease (acrosclerosis; changes restricted to below the elbows)	Skin changes on trunk and extremities
Calcinosis, telangiectases	Tendon rubs
Later, pulmonary hypertension and renal involvement	Pulmonary fibrosis, gastrointestinal, myocardial
Capillary telangiectases in nailfold	Capillary drop out in nailfold
Anticentromere (CENP) antibodies	Scl-70 (topoisomerase I) antibodies but no anticentromere antibodies

  - Esophageal disease
  - Sclerodactyly
  - Telangiectases
  - (Anticentromere antibodies)
- CREST syndrome with severe pulmonary disease; these patients usually have antifibrillarin (U_3-RNP) antibodies.
- Dermatomyositis-systemic sclerosis overlap in which patients can have PM-Scl (PM-1) antibodies.

We will now consider the multiple aspects of systemic sclerosis separately, but emphasizing that the disease is an active flowing process with many overlaps.

Prodrome. The early complaints are usually nonspecific; fatigue, headaches, depressive and low-grade fevers may all be seen and overlooked. Vasomotor disturbances in the extremities may also be present. Patients may show acrocyanosis or cutis marmorata with cold sensitivity and perhaps paresthesias but without the classic clinical signs of Raynaud syndrome. At this stage, the autoantibodies can sometimes be detected, greatly aiding in the diagnosis.

Raynaud Phenomenon. Raynaud phenomenon refers to cold-induced vascular spasms, particularly on the hands, that go through three phases: painful ischemia (white skin), local cyanosis (blue skin) and erythema on revascularization (red skin). Raynaud phenomenon is seen in 60–90% of systemic sclerosis patients and is a hallmark of the limited form (Chap. 22).

Limited Systemic Sclerosis (Acrosclerosis and Sclerodactyly). This form is the most common cutaneous variant of systemic sclerosis, far more often seen in women. It begins on the fingers with doughy edematous only minimally red swelling, which extends to the hands and occasionally the wrists (Fig. 18.32). Involvement of the feet is possible. As the process progresses, the skin becomes tight, waxy and cannot be picked up or squeezed into folds. The skin changes lead to reduced joint mobility (dermatogenous contractures). The fingers are typically folded slightly into the position of function (unfortunately described as claw-like) and eventually become fixed (Fig. 18.33). The fingertips show tiny necrotic ulcerations, the so-called rat-bite ulcers – a term which we avoid. The soft tissue, muscles and bones may also show pressure atrophy. The finger pads are often flattened so the digits appear pointed (Madonna fingers)

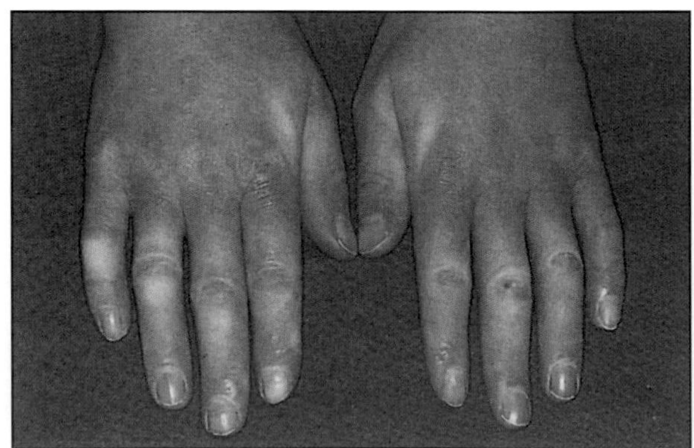

Fig. 18.32. Systemic sclerosis with swollen erythematous hands and ulcerations

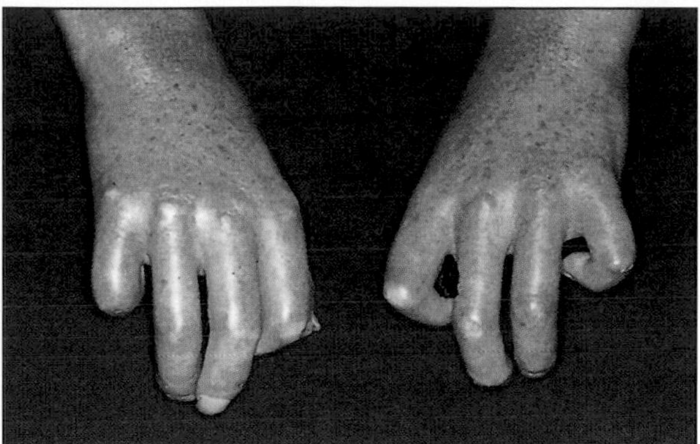

Fig. 18.33. Systemic sclerosis with contractural deformity of the hands

and may be mutilated by the destructive changes. The nailfolds show tiny hemorrhages and subungual keratoses, while a variety of nail dystrophies arise from the vascular and traumatic changes.

A second common site of involvement in the acral form is the face. There is a loss of expression, sometimes called the scleroderma mask or amimia. The face appears smaller because the skin is tight and the subcutaneous tissues reduced. The nose is often beaked, the cheeks and forehead without folds and the lips thin (Fig. 18.34). The mouth gradually evolves into a tight small oval orifice that is difficult to move (microstomia); patients look as if they want to whistle but cannot. The hard skin usually has a white-yellow tone.

Diffuse Systemic Sclerosis. These patients usually start with edema and tightness of the trunk which then spreads peripherally to involve the extremities. Men are as often affected as women. Raynaud phenomenon usually appears later as the hands become involved, rather than as a presenting sign. Early in the disease, involvement of muscles, joints and internal organs is common (Table 18.6). A variety of positive antinuclear antibodies are present, as well as elevated erythrocyte sedimentation rate and elevated immunoglobulins. This form is sometimes described as the febrile arthritic variant. Use of the limbs is made difficult by the contractures and when the trunk is involved, even respiratory motions are impaired. Overlaps with dermatomyositis or even systemic lupus erythematosus may occur. Diffuse systemic sclerosis has an unfavorable prognosis. Death can occur

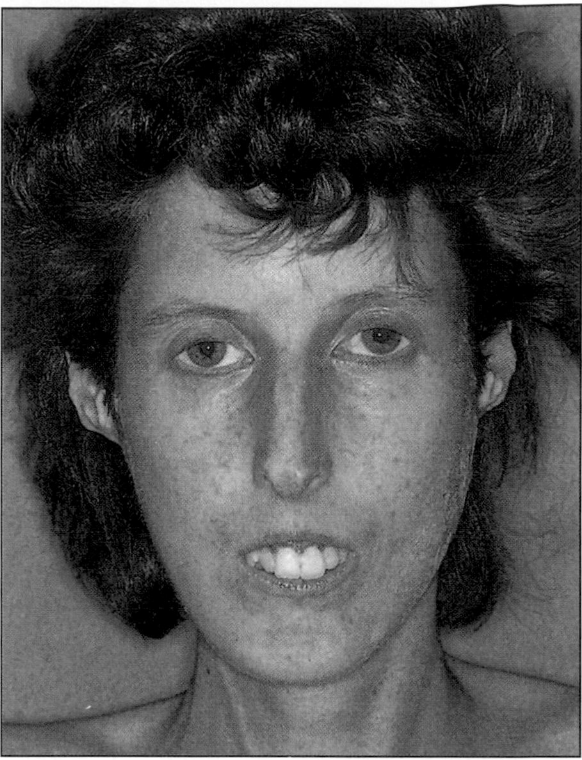

Fig. 18.34. Systemic sclerosis with typical facial appearance

Table 18.6. Systemic manifestations in systemic sclerosis

Organ or disease	Percentage of patients with involvement
Skin	90-95
Raynaud phenomenon	60-90
GI tract	90
Esophagus	45-75
Stomach	6-25
Intestine	10-57
Lungs	40-60
Heart	50-90
Pericardium	11
Kidneys	35-70
Hypertension	21
Anemia	27
Joints	25-50
Tendons, tendon sheaths	25
Skeletal muscles	20

The great variability in our numbers reflects the many different sources and the variety of methods used to make a diagnosis

within 3–5 years, while in the acute malignant form, death occurs within months.

Other Skin Changes. Telangiectases are commonly seen on the digits and face. They are frequently described as matted, as several small vessels appear to have coalesced. Early cases, especially in blacks, may show a perifollicular speckled hypo- to depigmentation that can be confused with vitiligo. Sometimes, the combination of pigmentary changes, atrophy and telangiectases produces a poikilodermatous picture. A scarring or sclerodermatous alopecia may be seen, as well as loss of eccrine and sebaceous glands producing a dry skin. The tiny digital ulcers are most common, but larger ulcers on the legs may also be seen.

Calcinosis. Subcutaneous calcification occurs in all the CREST patients and about 25% of the total group, usually on the digits with focal dermal or subcutaneous masses that are discharged via painful ulcerations. Women are far more often affected than men (10:1). Larger deeper deposits are seen less often about the hips, spinal column, knees and elbows, also contributing to loss of motion.

Mucosal Involvement. The lips are thin and the mouth hard to open. Oral hygiene and routine dental care become difficult. The salivary gland ducts are often sclerotic leading to reduced saliva flows. The esophageal involvement with decreased peristalsis may lead to retained or regurgitated food. All these factors lead to a marked increase in caries. The oral mucosa may develop sclerotic and atrophic areas. The tongue becomes smooth and firm, while its motion is restricted. The frenulum may be thickened (Fig. 18.35).

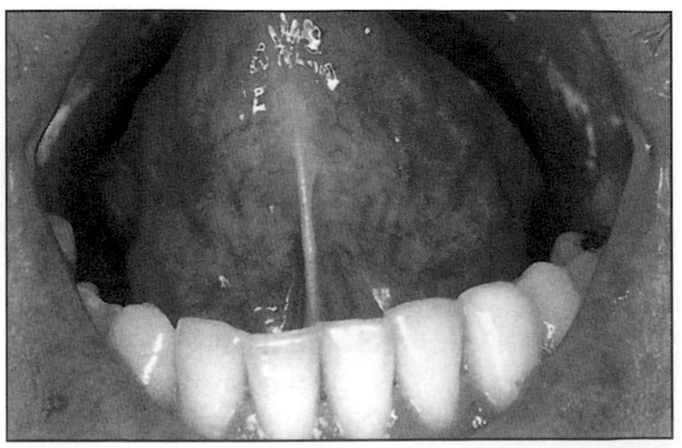

Fig. 18.35. Systemic sclerosis with involvement of frenulum

There are also diagnostic periodontal changes which also contribute to loss of teeth. The periodontal ligaments become widened, so that systemic sclerosis may have a classic radiologic appearance. Local microvascular changes are probably responsible. In addition, there is resorption of bone, probably secondary to pressure and disuse.

Gastrointestinal Tract. Almost 90% of patients have some form of gastrointestinal involvement. The most common site is the esophagus with symptoms of reflux and dysphagia. Radiologic examination shows reduced peristalsis, atonic dilatation, mucosal atrophy, ulcerations, Barrett esophagus and stenosis of the lower segment. Manometric studies show a lack of relaxation during swallowing, while contrast studies demonstrate delayed emptying. The stomach is least-often involved, showing atrophy, esophageal reflux because of lost sphincter tone and occasionally ulcerations. The small and large intestine often have reduced motility leading to constipation, large bowel diverticulae, gas dissecting into the intestinal wall and even obstruction or paralytic ileus. Conversely, diarrhea may occur secondary to bacterial overgrowth and fat malabsorption.

Lungs. The principal change is fibrosis, detected in about 40% of patients by chest radiography but in a higher number by pulmonary function tests and an even higher number at autopsy. The two main changes are pulmonary hypertension and diffuse interstitial fibrosis, often culminating in pulmonary insufficiency or cor pulmonale. The pulmonary hypertension is particularly likely to flare after pregnancy. The fibrosis predisposes the patients to alveolar cell carcinoma. A final problem is aspiration pneumonia because of the esophageal problems.

Larynx. Involvement of the vocal cords may lead to hoarseness and a rough or deep voice.

Heart. The most typical cardiac change is diffuse interstitial myocardial fibrosis. The individual muscle fibers are compressed by a fibrotic sheath, leading to arrhythmias, conduction defects and heart failure. A second problem is myocardial Raynaud phenomenon. Patients with systemic sclerosis often have exercise-induced perfusion defects with normal coronary angiograms. Pericardial fibrosis leads to a further restriction in cardiac function, while pericardial effusions present an acute problem. In addition there are cardiac stresses caused by the pulmonary hypertension, arterial hypertension and renal disease.

Kidneys. Significant renal involvement occurs in about 25 % of patients with systemic sclerosis. The classic change is nephrosclerosis in which there is onion-skin thickening of the vessel walls secondary to intimal proliferation, just as seen in severe hypertension. Initially renal problems are generally mild with minimal proteinuria, reduced creatinine clearance and mild hypertension. Malignant hypertension can evolve as the end stage of nephrosclerosis with renal infarcts, tubular atrophy and a shrunken kidney. In turn, oliguria and then renal failure evolve. It is estimated that 40 % of the fatalities associated with systemic sclerosis are related to the kidneys.

Eyes. Dry eyes are a problem especially in those patients who overlap with Sjögren syndrome. In addition, cataracts may occur at an earlier age than expected.

Musculoskeletal System. The main changes are the contractures secondary to both skin involvement and fibrosis of the tendons and their sheaths. Crepitance or tendon sheath rubs are a classic clinical finding. There may be a mild inflammatory arthritis. Juxtarticular bone erosions can occur, particularly on the distal digits, where acral osteolysis or absorption is also a possibility. This process occurs independently of infection or ulceration and may be caused by microvascular changes. Cystic and sclerotic changes in the digits may also be appreciated radiologically.

The muscles may show a myopathy that mimics polymyositis with proximal group weakness. Such patients often have a systemic sclerosis-dermatomyositis overlap, also known as sclerodermatomyositis. In other instances, muscle atrophy arises from disuse secondary to contractures and tightened skin.

Histopathology. The cutaneous histopathology of systemic sclerosis is similar to that of morphea. The papillary dermis is usually spared and inflammatory changes are minimal. The involvement in the other organs is beyond the scope of this book, although diagnostic changes can often be seen in renal or lung biopsies.

Laboratory Findings. A variety of abnormal results reflect the underlying inflammation, including elevated erythrocyte sedimentation rate, elevated neutrophil count, increased C-reactive protein and immunoglobulin perturbations. Anemia is frequently seen, probably reflecting chronic disease more than any one specific cause. Other tests are useful in documenting the degree of organ malfunction, such as renal function tests or muscle enzymes. About 5 % of patients have a biologic false-positive syphilis serology, while up to 25 % may show cold agglutinins, but only rarely cryoglobulins.

In contrast, the search for antinuclear antibodies using a sensitive substrate such as HEp-2 can be helpful in both diagnosing and subdividing systemic sclerosis, thus offering prognostic help. Table 18.7 indicates some of the available tests. ANA tests are positive in over 90 % of diffuse disease and 50 % of those with the limited form.

Table 18.7. Antibody tests in scleroderma

Immunofluorescent pattern	Antigens	Cutaneous features	Frequency (%)	Specificity
Nucleolar	Nucleolar ribonucleoproteins (nRNP)	Diffuse or limited scleroderma	50	Fair
	RNA polymerases	Diffuse scleroderma	25	High
	Nuclear proteins PM-1 (PM-Scl), Ku	Scleroderma-polymyositis overlap	<5	Very high
Centromere (large speckles)	Centromere proteins (CENP)	Limited scleroderma CREST syndrome	50	High
Diffuse (fine speckles)	Scl-70 (Topoisomerase I)	Diffuse scleroderma	25	High
Homogeneous	Histones	Localized scleroderma	50%	Average

Rheumatoid factor is positive in about 30 %. Scl-70 topoisomerase I antibodies are a poor prognostic sign; they are best determined by doing an immunodiffusion test with extracted nuclear antigens and by ELISA. Direct immunofluorescent examination of the skin may reveal immunoglobulins and complement about the vessels in a nondiagnostic pattern.

Course and Prognosis. The course and prognosis are highly dependent on the clinical pattern and correlate somewhat with the ANA pattern. In general the limited form does much better than the severe form and women, although far more often affected, have a better outlook than men. The main causes of death are cardiovascular, renal and pulmonary disease. Spontaneous remissions or reversals are very unlikely; a relentless course is the rule – the only question is how widespread and severe the disease will become.

Differential Diagnosis. In fully developed cases, there is no differential diagnosis except for pseudoscleroderma. In early stages, both systemic lupus erythematosus and dermatomyositis must be considered. Often the disease course first allows a definite diagnosis. There are several overlap syndromes such as the PM-Scl-positive polymyositis-scleroderma overlap, mixed connective tissue disease, Sjögren syndrome-scleroderma overlap and others, which confuse the issue.

Therapy. The lack of understanding of the etiology coupled with the variable course of the disease make identifying and evaluating therapeutic efforts very difficult. For example, skin tightness or degree of skin involvement are often used as parameters, but they are notoriously difficult to quantify. Tests such as pulmonary function tests are more reproducible, but then less-often influenced by therapy.

Therapeutic efforts can be directed against the three major pathophysiologic factors:

- Inflammation: Corticosteroids, cyclophosphamide other immunosuppressive agents
- Sclerosis: UVA-1, bath PUVA, penicillamine, extracorporeal photopheresis, interferon (IFN)-γ
- Vascular disease: Vasodilators, other rheologic agents, physical therapy

Systemic. Corticosteroids may be helpful in the acute inflammatory stage. The myositis of the overlap disease responds very well to corticosteroids, but otherwise there is disagreement on their efficacy. Some reports suggest that corticosteroids worsen renal disease. For pulmonary involvement cyclophosphamide pulse therapy is given. Cyclosporine clearly can worsen the renal status and has not been dramatically effective.

Three treatments which are aimed at reducing collagen synthesis are penicillamine, extracorporeal photopheresis and IFN-γ. Penicillamine is used at relatively low dosages of 250–1500 mg daily for many years with careful monitoring renal function and other well-known side effects. Some groups in Germany prefer to use intravenous penicillin G 10 million IU units daily for 3 weeks, with the rationale that penicillamine is one of the metabolic products. The initial excitement over extracorporeal photopheresis has not held up and we do not employ it for systemic sclerosis. In a preliminary study, 20 patients were treated with IFN-γ 50 μg subcutaneously three times weekly for 1 year. Their skin score stabilized and there was no sign of increased visceral problems. IFN-γ inhibits collagen production by fibroblasts and is not overcome by TGF-β, which induces fibroblast function and has been found to be elevated in lesional skin of some systemic sclerosis patients.

The vascular problems are relatively amenable to management. Raynaud phenomenon is best managed by avoidance measures, such as avoidance of cold, stopping smoking and use of vasodilating agents. Calcium channel antagonists are probably the best choice, but orthostatic hypotension often arises. Vasodilators only work as long as the vessels are not embedded in such sclerotic connective tissue that they cannot respond. Reflux esophagitis should be treated by small meals, raising the head of the bed and H2 antagonists. Antibiotics may help the bacterial overgrowth and malabsorption. Strict control of blood pressure is the best approach to the renal disease. Angiotensin-converting enzyme inhibitors appear to retard the development of uremia. Standard therapeutic approaches are recommended for the cardiac and pulmonary problems, as well as the other assorted disorders that arise.

Topical. The ulcers are most difficult to treat. Nitroglycerin ointment has helped some patients and is worth trying in addition to standard approaches.

Phototherapy. Oral PUVA has been successfully used in many cases. It appears to modulate the immune response and also to affect collagen synthesis. In recent years, bath PUVA has shown similarly beneficial results. Bath PUVA can be limited to the hands and feet. Medium- to high-dose UVA1 radiation alone can also be employed. We favor the use of the various phototherapy regimens in systemic sclerosis because of their efficacy and safety.

Other Measures. Physical therapy is absolutely essential to help the patient retain as much motion as possible. In addition, emotional support should be provided, by the physician, his or her own staff and often by the local scleroderma support group.

Pseudoscleroderma

Pseudoscleroderma refers to diseases with clinical changes resembling diffuse scleroderma but which have other causes. Table 18.8 lists the main causes of pseudoscleroderma. Several of special interest are discussed below while others can be found elsewhere in the text.

Eosinophilic Fasciitis
(SHULMAN 1974)

Synonyms. Diffuse fasciitis with eosinophilia, Shulman syndrome

Epidemiology. This rare disease is seen more often in men.

Etiology and Pathogenesis. Whether eosinophilic fasciitis is a separate disease or a variant of localized scleroderma remains unanswered. We view it as a separate disease. Often it appears to be triggered by strenuous physical activity.

Clinical Findings. The disorder typically arises in young adult life. Patients suddenly develop scleroderma-like skin changes without associated Raynaud syndrome. Involvement is usually symmetric and most often affects the arms. The skin is initially doughy, but then becomes hard and firmly bound to the underlying structures so that contractures can develop rapidly (Fig. 18.36). The lesions may be acutely painful. Systemic

Table 18.8. Types of pseudoscleroderma

Category	Examples	Chapter (if not 18)
Congenital disorders	Werner syndrome	
	Other premature aging syndromes	
Deposition disorders	Scleredema adultorum	43
	Scleromyxedema	43
	Amyloidosis (usually acral)	41
Metabolic conditions	Porphyria cutanea tarda	44
	Phenylketonuria	39
	Glycogen storage diseases	43
	Diabetic stiff hand syndrome	48
Chronic venous insufficiency	Dermatosclerosis of the lower leg	22
Connective tissue disorders	Systemic lupus erythematosus	
	Dermatomyositis	
	Eosinophilic fasciitis	
	Overlap syndromes	
Paraneoplastic syndromes	Carcinoid syndrome (especially metastatic)	14
	Multiple myeloma (scleromyxedema, POEMS syndrome)	40
Chronic graft-versus-host disease		14
Exogenous factors	Eosinophilia-myalgia syndrome (contaminated L-tryptophan)	
	Vinyl chloride	
	Trichlorethylene	
	Toxic oil syndrome	
	Silica	
	Silicone (disputed)	

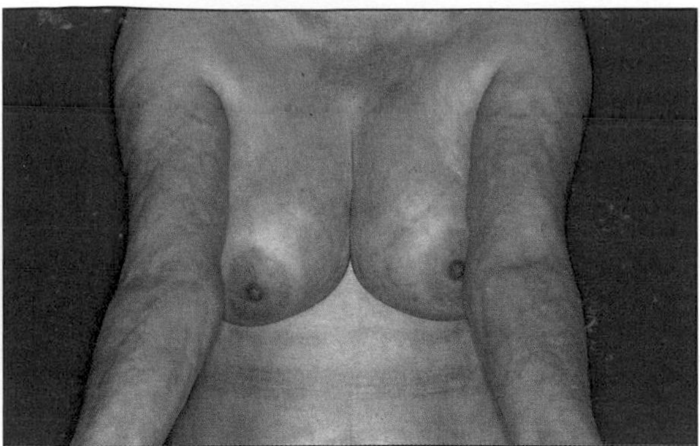

Fig. 18.36. Shulman syndrome with puffy involvement of both arms

manifestations are uncommon, suggesting an overlap disorder.

Histopathology. The biopsy may show typical cutaneous changes of scleroderma but with a generous admixture of eosinophils. In other instances, the dermis is relatively normal. The key pathology is in the fascia. This layer is usually two to three cells thick, but in eosinophilic fasciitis it may be as thick as the overlying skin. It is impossible to adequately sample the fascia with a punch biopsy. A long thin ellipse should be excised down to the muscle and carefully fixed in a stretched position, i.e., not allowed to curl up. The fascia will not only be thickened but also be infiltrated by many eosinophils. The direct immunofluorescence (DIF) examination may show immunoglobulins at the epidermal-dermal junction, about vessels or diffusely scattered through the dermis.

Laboratory Findings. Typically there is marked blood eosinophilia, often as high as 50%, coupled with elevated immunoglobulins and an elevated erythrocyte sedimentation rate. ANA testing is usually negative. Bone marrow examination will also show increased eosinophils and plasma cells.

Differential Diagnosis. Scleroderma adultorum may also appear rapidly.

Course and Prognosis. The disease is so rare that the course is hard to predict. In some patients total resolution has occurred, while others have gone on to develop systemic sclerosis or overlap disorders.

Therapy. In contrast to systemic sclerosis, systemic corticosteroids appear highly effective. One can start with prednisone 60 mg daily and slowly taper the medication. At the same time, physical therapy is essential to avoid disabilities.

Eosinophilia-Myalgia Syndrome

Epidemiology. In the late 1980s a syndrome involving myalgias, peripheral blood eosinophilia and a variety of systemic manifestations was identified in patients taking L-tryptophan. Elegant detective work traced the involved amino acid supplements to a limited number of manufacturers, primarily Japanese, and identified several contaminants in the manufacturing process which appeared responsible for the disorder. While new cases have ceased to appear since the FDA banned the sale of L-tryptophan as a dietary supplement, many patients still suffer from this problem. Most patients are women, as the supplements were often self-prescribed for premenstrual symptoms.

Etiology and Pathogenesis. A contaminant in the L-tryptophan is felt to be responsible, but some patients may have simply taken too much of the noncontaminated product.

Clinical Findings. The skin changes are similar to those in scleroderma. Initially there is an erythematous papular rash and then edema; later the skin becomes indurated and thicker. The dominant changes are muscle weakness and an overwhelming sense of fatigue. While systemic changes other than muscle involvement are uncommon, pulmonary and hepatic disease has been described.

Histopathology. The skin biopsy often shows mucin during the early or papular stage. Later biopsies show similar changes to those in scleroderma but have far more eosinophils.

Laboratory Findings. The eosinophil count is dramatically raised, often >30,000/mm^3, although only 1000 cells are required for the CDC working definition.

Course and Prognosis. Some patients have had long protracted courses, but most have improved, even if they have not totally recovered.

Differential Diagnosis. Trichinosis, periarteritis nodosa, polymyositis, eosinophilic fasciitis, eosinophilic myositis and fulminant forms of systemic sclerosis must be excluded.

Therapy. Stopping L-tryptophan is the answer. Many other approaches, including systemic corticosteroids, have been tried but it is impossible to evaluate their effectiveness.

Toxic Oil Syndrome

Contaminated rapeseed oil was distributed in the Madrid region in 1981. The patients developed severe myalgias, eosinophilia and scleroderma, as well as neurologic, pulmonary and hepatic abnormalities. More than 20,000 individuals were affected and almost 500 died. During the acute stage, the main problems were pneumonitis (which caused most of the deaths) myalgias and eosinophilia. Acutely, erythematous papules and exanthems were seen. On biopsy, many of the papules represented papular mucinosis. Later on, the major problems were peripheral neuropathies and scleroderma especially involving the legs. The condition in some patients evolved into systemic sclerosis. Large amounts of unsaturated fatty acid anilides, mostly derived from oleic and linoleic acid, were identified in culprit oil samples and are believed to be responsible for the disease.

Scleredema and Scleromyxedema

Scleredema and scleromyxedema (Chap. 43) are two unrelated diseases in which deposits of mucinous material are present in the dermis producing sclerotic skin. Scleredema usually involves the back and is unlikely to be confused with scleroderma. Scleromyxedema may have acral sclerotic changes which are quite similar to those in systemic sclerosis.

Sclerema Neonatorum

While sclerema neonatorum was erroneously called neonatal scleroderma in the past, it is not related to scleroderma. It is primarily a disease of the fat (Chap. 21).

Lupus Erythematosus

(Cazenave and Schedel 1838; Kaposi 1872; Osler 1895)

Under the term lupus erythematosus (LE) one finds a spectrum of disease with variation in course and prognosis. Overlapping clinical, histologic and laboratory findings which may change during the course of the disease make the distinctions difficult. The three major forms of LE are:

- Discoid lupus erythematosus (DLE) or chronic cutaneous lupus erythematosus
- Subacute cutaneous lupus erythematosus (SCLE)
- Systemic lupus erythematosus (SLE)

Discoid Lupus Erythematosus

Synonyms. Lupus erythematodes chronicus, chronic cutaneous lupus erythematosus

DLE is a poor term, because it is used both to describe a type of chronic hypertrophic scarring skin lesion and to describe a disease, i. e., the chronic primarily cutaneous form of LE. Nonetheless, it is so well accepted that we reluctantly employ it.

Epidemiology. DLE is the most common form of cutaneous lupus. It is more common in women than men with the ratio ranging from 2:1 to 4:1. Its incidence is estimated at more than 1:200 in black women. About 5% of patients first diagnosed with DLE later show systemic involvement and are diagnosed as having SLE. The disease typically affects young patients, with onset between 20 and 40 years of age. In children, even if the skin lesions are typical for DLE, one should suspect SLE. Familial cases have been described, probably reflecting HLA patterns.

Etiology and Pathogenesis. The underlying cause of DLE is unknown. One working hypothesis is that it is an autoimmune disease in which genetically predisposed individuals are stimulated by a variety of factors including UV radiation, usually UVA but occasionally UVB or both, but also stress, infections and even temperature changes. These exogenous forces lead to epidermal cell death and the exposure or revealing of normally intracellular antigens, such as the nucleoproteins Ro, La, snRNP and double-stranded DNA, which then trigger an autoimmune response characterized in the laboratory by the presence of ANA. The increased formation of these antigens, and many others, on the cell surface can lead to an aberrant cellular and humoral immune response. In DLE, the damage appears to be primarily restricted to skin.

Clinical Findings. The lesions of DLE are most commonly found on the face. Typical sites are the forehead, nose and cheeks. When both cheeks are

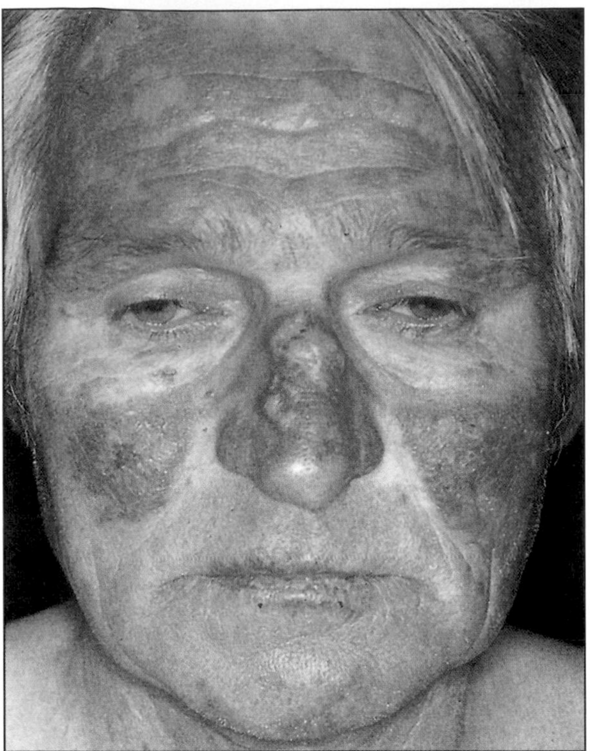

Fig. 18.37. Discoid lupus erythematosus

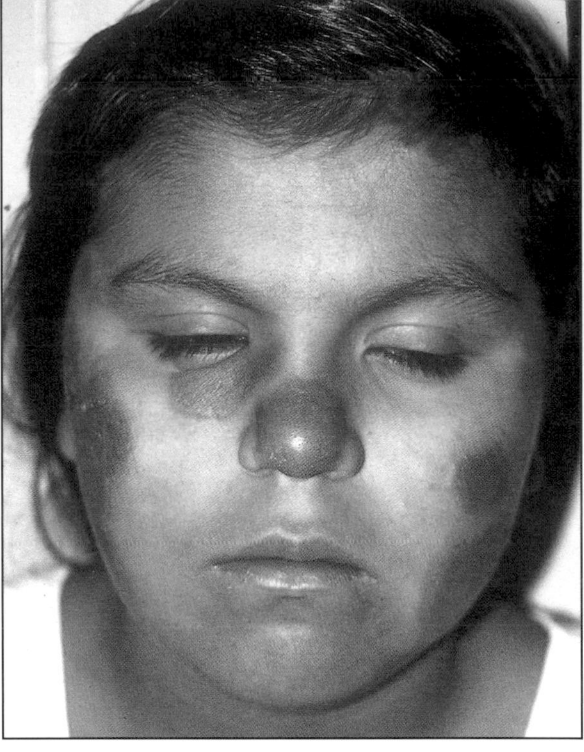

Fig. 18.38. Discoid lupus erythematosus; hyperpigmentation in a Hispanic patient. (Courtesy of Juan J. Ochoa, MD, Chihuahua, Mexico)

involved, one speaks of a butterfly rash. Other sites include the eyelids, the ears including the ear canal where sunlight normally does not reach, the scalp and the décolleté area (Figs. 18.37, 18.38). Much less often the disease is more disseminated, involving the trunk and extremities; in such cases, the likelihood of SCLE and SLE is greater. The lesions can be provoked by sunlight or experimentally induced with ultraviolet irradiation (Fig. 18.39).

Each lesion is characterized by erythema, hyperkeratosis and atrophy. The lesions start with persistent, often bilateral, indurated erythematous papules and plaques. The plaques slowly grow peripherally, becoming more plate-like or discoid and often coalescing (Fig. 18.40). Centrally they are covered by firmly adherent white-yellow scale, which is usually painful when removed. When one peels off a piece of scale with a tweezers and observes the undersurface with a loupe, one sees hyperkeratotic spicules which represent follicular plugs. This is known as the carpet tack sign. Another finding is hyperesthesia which is noticed when one rubs across a plaque with a fingernail or instrument. Sometimes only the follicular plugs are seen.

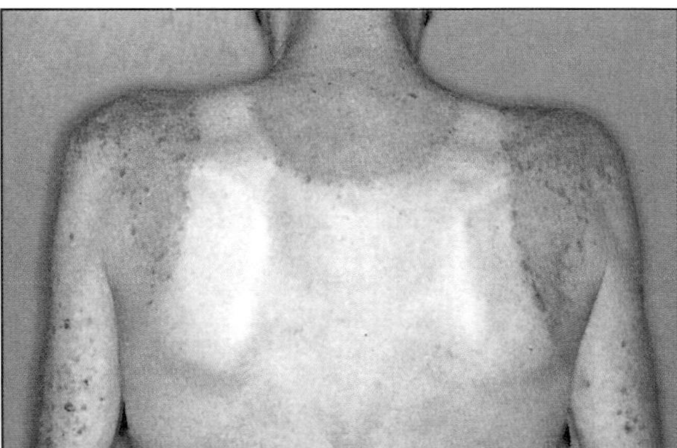

Fig. 18.39. Discoid lupus erythematosus; lesions induced by sunlight exposure

The lesions continue to evolve. The periphery is typically raised and erythematous while the center gradually becomes pale and depressed, reflecting atrophy. The keratotic plugs and follicular openings disappear as scarring progresses. Pigmentary changes are expected. Black skin almost always becomes hypo- or depigmented, while white skin may show hyperpigmentation and frequent telangiectases. Sometimes the border is quite sharp and the center

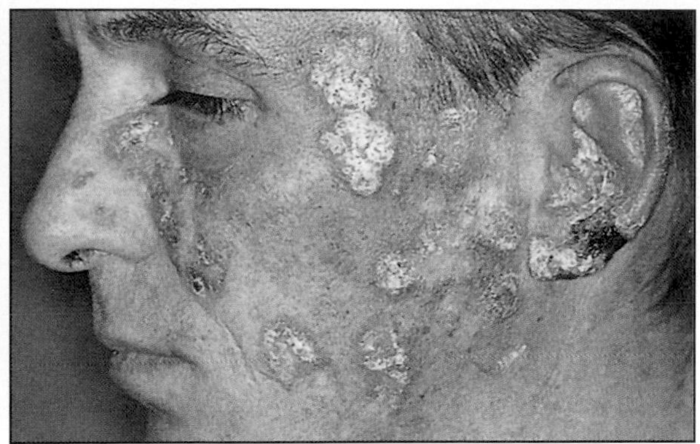

Fig. 18.40. Discoid lupus erythematosus; hyperkeratotic lesions, hypopigmentation and mutilation

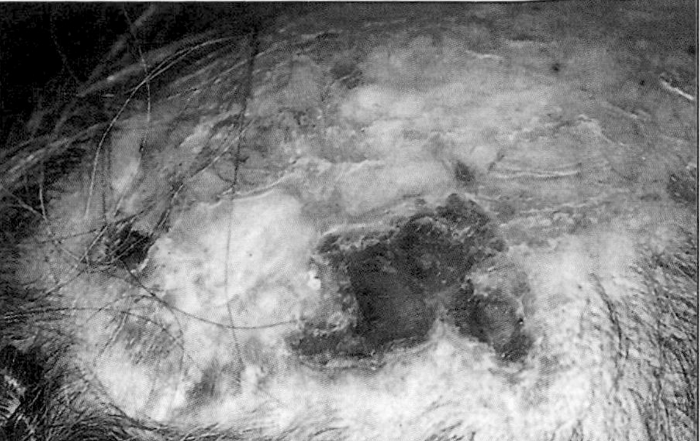

Fig. 18.41. Discoid lupus erythematosus; scarring alopecia and ulcerations

definitely depressed. Such lesions are most common on the nose and ear, are often mistaken for a basal cell carcinoma and can be quite destructive.

There are a number of clinical variants of cutaneous LE:

Scarring Alopecia. DLE often involves the scalp, especially in black women. Sometimes there will be only scalp involvement, first revealed when the patient removes a wig. While erythema, atrophy and depigmentation are seen, the most striking feature is the hair loss, as the follicles are scarred beyond repair producing pseudopelade status (Fig. 18.41).

Lupus Tumidus. Some patients develop extensive lymphocytic infiltrates leading to elevated nodular lesions, rather than depressed atrophic ones. The most common sites are the face and trunk.

Hypertrophic Lupus Erythematosus. The lesions of hypertrophic LE typically involve the forearms or the face. They are domed nodules with a thick scale that resemble a keratoacanthoma or hypertrophic actinic keratosis. In our experience, the reports of multiple keratoacanthoma in LE reflect this feature. Hypertrophic LE is notoriously hard to treat.

Lupus Profundus (HEBRA and KAPOSI 1875; IRGANG 1954). The subcutaneous fat may be involved in lupus erythematosus, either alone or in association with overlying or separate skin lesions. Typically there are deep painful nodules with an erythematous surface, most often on the shoulders, thighs, buttocks or breasts (Fig. 18.42). The lesions can ulcerate or heal with deeply depressed scars. Histologically, there is a lymphocytic panniculitis, often with lymphoid follicles.

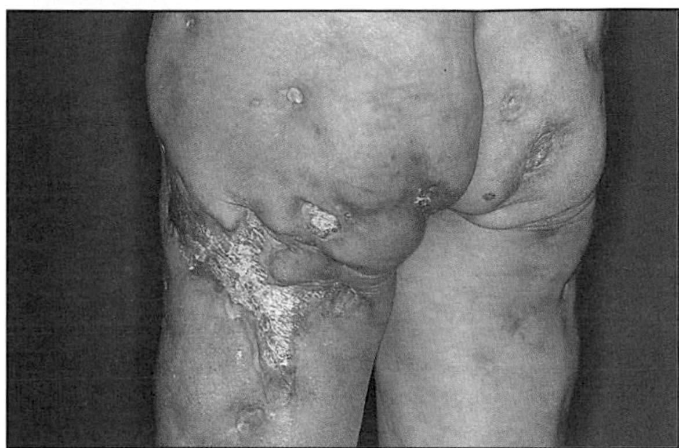

Fig. 18.42. Lupus profundus

Lupus Erythematosus Hypertrophicus et Profundus (BEHÇET 1942). While this term is rarely used, the clinical situation it describes is real. Some patients present with hypertrophic tumoral lesions, often as facial plaques, which extend deeply and involve the fat, and heal with irregular scars.

Chilblain Lupus. Some patients develop acral lesions which are typically associated with acrocyanosis, often as the first sign of SLE (Fig. 18.43). There are large, well circumscribed blue-red flat nodules with tiny keratotic plugs and hyperesthesia. The sites of predilection are the dorsal and lateral aspects of the fingers, although the toes, nose, and ears can also be affected. The tendency towards central atrophy and scarring is minimal.

Bullous Lupus Erythematosus. While DLE often shows signs of epidermal-dermal junction separation histologically, bullous lesions are unusual clinically but can be seen. The bullous eruption of SLE

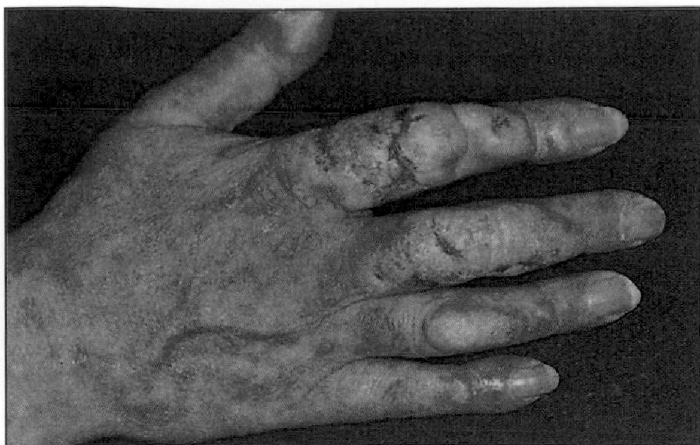

Fig. 18.43. Chilblain lupus

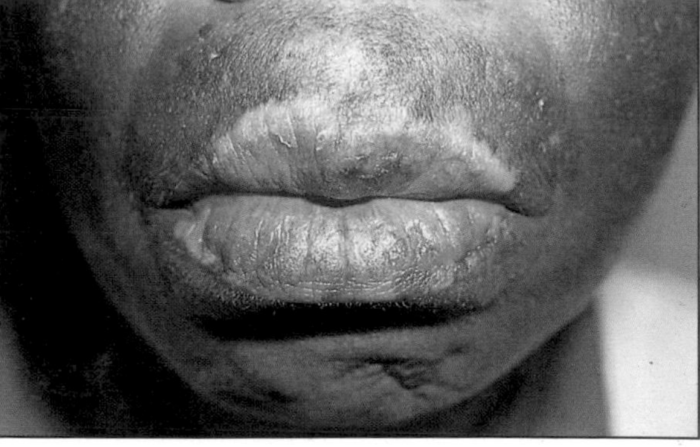

Fig. 18.45. Lip involvement in discoid lupus erythematosus; patient later developed systemic lupus erythematosus. (Courtesy of Robert Swerlick, MD, Atlanta, Georgia)

resembles that seen in dermatitis herpetiformis or linear IgA disease and is discussed below.

Mucinous Lupus Erythematosus. Once again, many lesions of LE show mucin microscopically, but some patients present with lesions mimicking papular mucinosis. Most typically they have small papules on acral sites or the back but sometimes larger plaques, such as in lupus profundus, are found. In yet other instances they may have scalp involvement, as seen in follicular mucinosis (Chap. 43).

Mucosal Changes. The buccal or palatal mucosa is often involved in DLE. Typically there are erythematous patches, often with a white hyperkeratotic veil, which can be eroded (Fig. 18.44). In contrast to oral lichen planus, the lesions are usually relatively asymptomatic and Wickham striae are absent. Lip lesions can also be seen; the lower lip is more likely to be affected (Fig. 18.45). Erythema, swelling, crusts

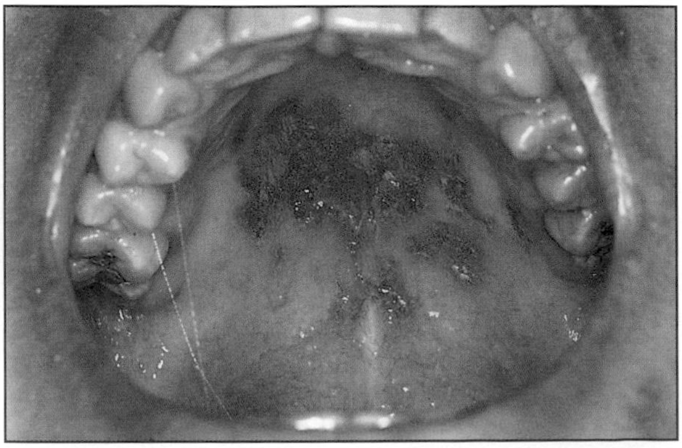

Fig. 18.44. Oral involvement in discoid lupus erythematosus

and erosions may be present. Similar lesions can be seen on the genital and anal mucosa, as well as on the conjunctiva.

Histopathology. The histology of DLE is fascinating because it exactly reflects the clinical picture. The epidermis is usually atrophic with plugged follicles. The basilar keratinocytes show vacuolar degeneration, while the microscopic (or PAS-positive) basement membrane zone is more prominent and thickened. In the dermis there are lymphocytic infiltrates about the vessels and adnexal structures, and scattered diffusely. Perifollicular infiltrates are especially common. In addition, mucin is common, as are telangiectases. Both collagen and elastic fibers are damaged. The infiltrate can extend to the subcutaneous fat, where typically there is both lobar and septal involvement with lymphoid follicles.

Immunofluorescent Examination. About 90% of biopsies of lesions which have been present for more than 6 months show deposition of IgG and C3, and to a lesser extent IgM and IgA, in a diffuse irregular band at the epidermal-dermal junction (Fig. 18.46). The antigens responsible for the reaction are not known, except in the case of bullous LE. It has been suggested that the basement membrane zone simply serves as a trap for a variety of circulating immunoglobulins but we suspect the answer is even more complex. In early lesions or those treated with topical corticosteroids for a number of weeks, the DIF may show fine granular deposits of IgM or be negative. In patients with rosacea, multiple telangiectases and perhaps sunlight damage, there may be similar results, most often IgM.

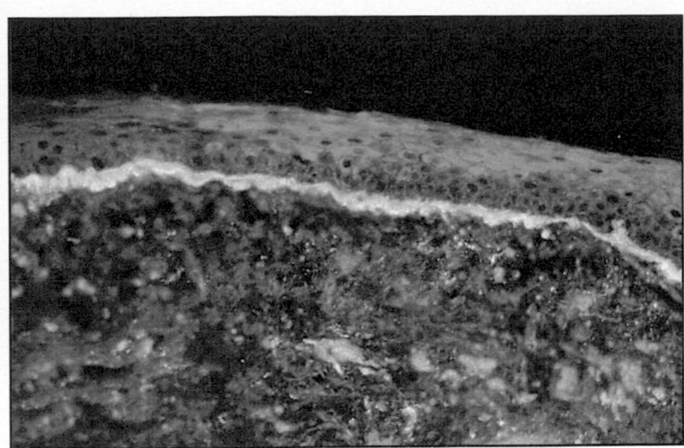

Fig. 18.46. Direct immunofluorescent examination in discoid lupus erythematosus; typical shaggy band of IgM at the epidermal-dermal junction

A positive DIF test in normal skin is a criterion for SLE, it does not occur in DLE.

Laboratory Findings. Formerly a positive ANA meant a patient had SLE and not DLE. With more sensitive substrates, about 25% of DLE (and perhaps 50% of disseminated DLE) patients have positive ANA. Occasionally antibodies against Ro or U_1-RNP will be found, but dsDNA, La or Sm antibodies suggest systemic disease.

Course and Prognosis. The course of DLE is difficult to predict. Each patient with newly diagnosed DLE should be evaluated for signs of SLE, including complete physical examination, routine screening blood tests, ANA on a sensitive substrate and perhaps histologic and immunofluorescent examination of lesional, sunlight-exposed and nonexposed skin. If all these tests are negative, then one can diagnose DLE as LE limited to the skin. About 5% of these patients over the years will develop symptoms of SLE. Another scenario is the presence of cutaneous LE in a patient with SCLE or SLE. This is much more common; perhaps 20% of SLE patients have discoid lesions. These patients often have arthritis and Raynaud phenomenon and are less likely to have renal disease.

DLE should also be viewed as a precancerous condition. It is unclear if the photosensitivity, immune defects, DNA repair defects or even loss of pigment are pathophysiologically relevant. In any event, squamous cell carcinoma may develop in chronic lesions of DLE. Sometimes mutilation can occur (the term lupus refers to a wolf or a progressive destructive lesion). Such changes are more typically seen on the nose and ears. The scarring alopecia is permanent and often of great concern to the patient.

Differential Diagnosis. The differential diagnosis is lengthy and has been alluded to under the clinical variants discussed above. Occasionally lupus vulgaris and LE can be hard to tell apart, especially if LE has a lupoid infiltrate on diascopy or if lupus vulgaris is erythematous and keratotic. The biopsy settles the issue. In the case of polymorphic light eruption, nodular lesions of LE can be very difficult to separate out. LE is more likely to have mucin, while polymorphic light eruption usually has more edema microscopically. Phototesting (Chap. 13) can also help separate the two. Eventually LE will develop either clinical atrophy or histologic epidermal damage. Rosacea, when plaque-like, can be confusing but is never atrophic. The hematoxylin-eosin biopsy is always distinct although false-positive DIF examinations can occur. In early stages, one can also think of seborrheic dermatitis, psoriasis, tinea faciei and corporis, and when only a few lesions are present, actinic keratoses. There are also actinic keratoses that resemble LE microscopically, so on rare occasion, one must simply await the course.

The special forms of LE raise different differential diagnostic questions:

Scarring Alopecia. The usual causes of scarring alopecia, including lichen planus, chronic folliculitis, sarcoidosis and pseudopelade should be considered.

Lupus Tumidus. Such lesions are histologically difficult to distinguish from a polymorphic light eruption or lymphocytic infiltration of Jessner-Kanof, both clinically and histologically. Malignant lymphoma can also be similar. Granuloma faciale is also similar, but has a different histology.

Hypertrophic Lupus Erythematosus. Hypertrophic actinic keratosis and keratoacanthoma should be excluded.

Lupus Profundus. One must consider the other forms of panniculitis and especially subcutaneous malignant lymphomas.

Chilblain Lupus. The differential diagnosis includes dermatomyositis, pernio and sarcoidosis.

Oral Mucosal Changes. The lip lesions closely resemble those in actinic keratoses. The intraoral lesions suggest lichen planus, autoimmune blistering diseases or other forms of leukoplakia.

Therapy

Systemic. The standard systemic therapy is antimalarials, usually hydroxychloroquine 200 mg or chloroquine 250 mg daily. We use almost exclusively hydroxychloroquine which appears to be a safer choice. The usual starting dose is one tablet twice daily for 10–14 days, followed by a reduction to a single tablet daily. The major concern with the antimalarials is retinal toxicity. While both cumulative dosage and high daily dose have been indicted, the latter seems to be more critical. For chloroquine a dose of 4 mg/kg daily should not be exceeded, and for hydroxychloroquine, a dose of 6.5 mg/kg daily. In addition, a baseline ophthalmologic examination should be obtained and the patients should be asked about photophobia and visual problems, as well as checked every 3–6 months.

There are several other precautions with antimalarials. They should not be used in patients with G6PD deficiency, pregnancy or liver disease. Hematologic parameters should be monitored because of the risks of thrombocytopenia and neutropenia. In addition, some patients with psoriasis may flare on antimalarials but this risk is much lower than previously estimated. Very few psoriatic flares were seen among US soldiers in Vietnam, but the dose of antimalarial agents they took for prophylaxis was much lower. Other less-common complications include mucosal and cutaneous hyperpigmentation, lightening of the hairs, toxic exanthems, muscle weakness and psychiatric disease.

About 75% of patients show improvement. Usually one should wait 3 months before deciding that the antimalarials are not helping. If they help but have toxic side effects, quinacrine 100–200 mg daily can be used; it causes skin yellowing but has no eye toxicity. Other alternatives include acitretin 10–50 mg daily or isotretinoin 0.2–0.5 mg/kg daily, as well as dapsone 50–150 mg daily, all of which are used primarily in disseminated DLE and SCLE. The role of systemic corticosteroids is controversial. In general, they are not indicated for cutaneous LE, although sometimes a short burst can help control a severe flare. Low-dose methotrexate 10–15 mg weekly is another possible option. Azathioprine (50–150 mg daily) and cyclophosphamide (50–200 mg daily) are used primarily for renal disease in SLE, but may play a role in selected severe cases, as may high-dose intravenous immunoglobulin G (IVIG) and experimental immunologic regimens. Thalidomide seems particularly useful for mucosal ulcers and scalp involvement, but there are concerns about its use, such as the teratogenicity in a young female population, as well as the development of polyneuropathy.

Topical. Topical or intralesional corticosteroids are usually effective for early lesions before scarring has developed. High-potency corticosteroids, perhaps under occlusion, or using a tape impregnated with the corticosteroid, are needed. DLE is one strong exception to the rule of no high-potency corticosteroids on the face.

Surgical. Cryotherapy is effective especially for hyperkeratotic lesions. Hair transplantation can be used for the alopecia if enough donor hair is available and the disease is no longer active.

Prophylaxis. Sunscreens with high UVA and UVB protection factors must be used religiously. Products which combine sunscreens and physical blocking agents are even better. Makeup with additional sunscreens is effective for many patients, offering coverage and protection simultaneously. Routine monitoring for possible signs of SLE should be performed.

Subacute Cutaneous Lupus Erythematosus

(Sontheimer et al. 1979)

Synonyms. Lupus erythematodes superficialis, superficial disseminated lupus erythematosus

Epidemiology. SCLE is less common than DLE or SLE. The extreme female predominance of SLE does not hold. Onset is usually between 30 and 40 years of age. Drug-induced and photosensitive forms may also appear later in life.

Etiology and Pathogenesis. The etiology is as unclear as for DLE. Sunlight is a very reliable trigger. Some cases appear to be drug-induced, such as from thiazide diuretics, perhaps by altering UV sensitivity. SCLE has the most uniform immunogenetic profile of all forms of LE. Over 70% of the patients with annular lesions and 25% of those with papulosquamous changes are HLA-B8, DR3, DQw2 and DRw52. They have high titers of antibodies against Ro (SSA) and often La (SSB) and show signs of polyclonal B cell activation.

Clinical Findings. The classic features of SCLE are marked UV sensitivity, widespread lesions that heal without scarring (Fig. 18.47). The sites of predilection are the shoulder, chest, back and extensor surfaces of the arms; facial involvement is uncommon. In the papulosquamous or psoriasiform variant, there are numerous oval or round plaques ranging in size from 0.5 to 3.0 cm that frequently have psoriasiform scale at their periphery. The scale is less well developed and less oriented towards follicles so the carpet tack sign is usually negative. When depressed scars are uncommon, lesions frequently resolve with hypopigmentation and a fine wrinkled surface, mimicking vitiligo. In the annular form, there are larger flatter lesions with a prominent raised scaly periphery and central clearing. Sometimes the border is vesicular or weeping, resembling erythema multiforme. This subtype has been called the Rowell syndrome (ROWELL 1963). Facial and periungual telangiectases, alopecia and mucosal involvement are all more common than in DLE.

In contrast to the findings in DLE, there are often signs of systemic involvement, although rarely as dramatic as in SLE. Fatigue, weakness and low-grade fevers are nonspecific findings. Myalgias, arthralgias, sicca syndrome and leukocytoclastic vasculitis may occur; CNS and renal disease are uncommon.

Histopathology. The changes are less dramatic than in DLE. The epidermis may show minor atrophy and vacuolar change while the dermal lymphocytic infiltrate is usually sparse.

Immunofluorescent Examination. The LE band test is positive in only 50–60% of lesions. In contrast to the findings in DLE, an IgG band may be found in 40–50% of biopsies from sunlight-exposed normal skin and in 20–30% from sunlight-protected skin.

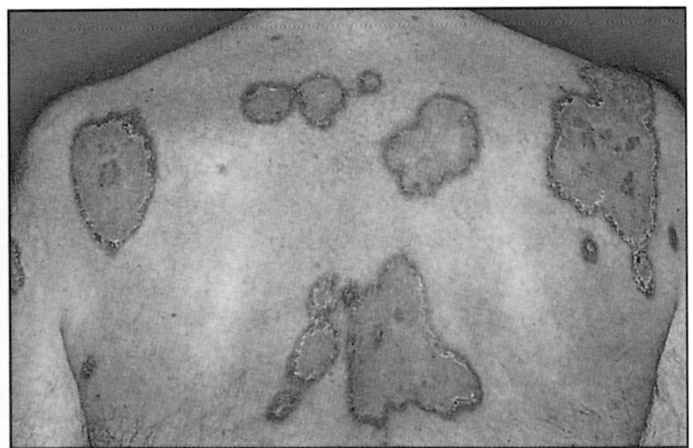

Fig. 18.47. Subacute cutaneous lupus erythematosus

Laboratory Findings. Two decades ago SCLE was described as ANA-negative LE. With better substrates, over 90% of patients are now found to have a positive ANA. Characteristic antibodies are those directed against Ro, present in 20–35% of cases, often simultaneously with anti-La. About 30–40% have antibodies against dsDNA but usually in low titer. The rheumatoid factor is positive in 20%.

Course and Prognosis. The course of SCLE is persistent with flares and periods of improvement. About 50% eventually fulfill the criteria for SLE, but then have a milder disease course than those who begin with SLE. Since neonatal LE is associated with Ro and La, these patients' infants are at risk.

Differential Diagnosis. Psoriasis, tinea corporis and seborrheic dermatitis are frequently confused. All forms of photosensitivity must also be considered.

Therapy. The approaches are similar to the approaches to DLE. Antimalarials are somewhat less effective, dapsone is often helpful and thalidomide is very effective. Systemic corticosteroids may be used for flares, especially with systemic manifestations such as vasculitis. Long-term corticosteroid therapy is not needed. Topical corticosteroids alone are rarely sufficient. Sunscreens are essential.

Systemic Lupus Erythematosus

Epidemiology. SLE is a disease of women; the ratio is about 10:1. The age of onset is usually in young adult life. Blacks and Asians appear to be more often affected. There are familial cases and an increased concordance in monozygotic twins.

Etiology and Pathogenesis. The etiology is unknown, just as with DLE. In the white population SLE is associated with both HLA-B7, DR2 and HLA-B8, DR3; the latter is linked to the complement gene null allele mutation C4A*Q0. Other genetic factors appear to play a role, as there is a clear association with certain alleles of the tumor necrosis factor genes and with complement deficiencies, of both the activation pathway and the membrane attack complex. While every single complement factor has been associated with SLE, the most common are deficiencies of C2 and C4. In general, C2 deficiency patients tend to have more severe cutaneous findings, less severe systemic problems and are often Ro-positive. C4 involves two pairs of alleles, 4A and 4B. Inheritance of the single null allele C4A*Q0 (an allele that makes no protein) is probably the most common complement defect in LE. These patients have normal levels of C4. To become deficient, multiple alleles must be missing; this is uncommon.

The possible role of viruses has been debated for years. There are LE-like diseases in laboratory animals that are viral in nature. Either the viral infection could expose usually protected antigens to the immune system or the infection could alter the immune response. More recently endogenous retroviral sequences have been suggested as a cause of systemic autoimmune diseases, especially SLE. The ability of retroviruses to alter immunity is most dramatically seen in HIV/AIDS, but a number of autoimmune diseases in laboratory animals appear to also be retroviral in nature. Female hormones, both endogenous and exogenous, are possible triggers, as is UV radiation (UVB or UVB + UVA, rarely UVA alone). UV radiation can trigger systemic flares, such as worsening of renal disease, as well as the expected cutaneous changes. The role of other medications is discussed below.

The spectrum of immune defects identified in SLE is large. Both cellular and humoral immunity is altered, involving T cells, B cells, granulocytes, monocytes and macrophages. Characteristic are polyclonal B cell stimulation with increased immunoglobulin secretion, primarily IgG, as well as lymphocytopenia. The latter primarily involves T cells and may be mediated by antilymphocyte antibodies. The cellular immunity appears intact, but evaluation of acute severely ill patients may reveal functional abnormalities. Lymphocytes and macrophages tend to have altered cytokine secretion patterns, while erythrocytes show a reduced number of complement receptors, leading to reduced removal of circulating immune complexes. A wide spectrum of autoantibodies are present and relied upon for diagnosis. The pathogenicity of many of these antibodies is still unclear, although it appears that immune complexes involving anti-dsDNA antibodies may be responsible for vasculitis in the kidneys, CNS, serosal surfaces and skin. Antibodies against T cells, B cells, natural killer (NK) cells, granulocytes, monocytes and erythrocytes can all play a clinically significant role, by destroying or incapacitating the cells.

Clinical Findings. The diagnostic criteria of the American College of Rheumatology (ACR), formerly called the American Rheumatism Association (ARA), are shown in Table 18.9. If the patient has four of the criteria, then the diagnosis of SLE is made. One can see that the criteria were not formulated with careful dermatologic input. For example, a patient with a malar rash, discoid rash, photosensitivity and oral ulcerations, in other words, a typical if severe DLE patient, technically has SLE. There

Table 18.9. American Rheumatism Association (ARA) criteria for the diagnosis of systemic lupus erythematosus (from 1971, revised 1982, annotated 1997)

Clinical features		
1	Malar rash	
2	Discoid rash	
3	Photosensitivity	
4	Oral ulcers	
5	Arthritis	
6	Serositis	Pleuritis or pericarditis
7	Renal disorder	Proteinuria >0.5 g daily or cellular casts
8	CNS disorder	Seizures or psychotic reaction
Laboratory features		
9	Hematologic disorder	Hemolytic anemia or leukopenia or lymphopenia or thrombocytopenia
10	Immunologic disorder	Antibodies against Sm or dsDNA; biological false-positive syphilis serology
11	Positive ANA	

is a specificity of 96% (4% false positives) and a sensitivity of 90% (10% false negatives).

Cutaneous Findings. Only 80% of SLE patients have cutaneous findings; as a dermatologist, one often guesses that almost all do. The four most specific lesions, malar rash, discoid lesions, photosensitivity and oral ulcerations, have already been discussed under DLE. The face can be quite severely involved and acutely inflamed (Fig. 18.48). Sometimes there is a persistent facial erythema (erythema perstans) which can involve the entire face with poorly circumscribed irregular scaly patches. In other instances, there are papulovesicular lesions which can evolve into pityriasiform or atrophic macules. The lesions on the trunk are similar to those in DLE and SCLE; one potential difference is the greater likelihood of hemorrhagic areas.

Acral lesions are probably more common in SLE. Persistent patchy erythematous macules may be present on the palms, soles, digital tips and nail folds (Fig. 18.49). These often reflect vasculitis and may ulcerate or become hyperkeratotic and painful. Subungual hemorrhages are often seen, as well as digital and nailfold telangiectases (Fig. 18.50).

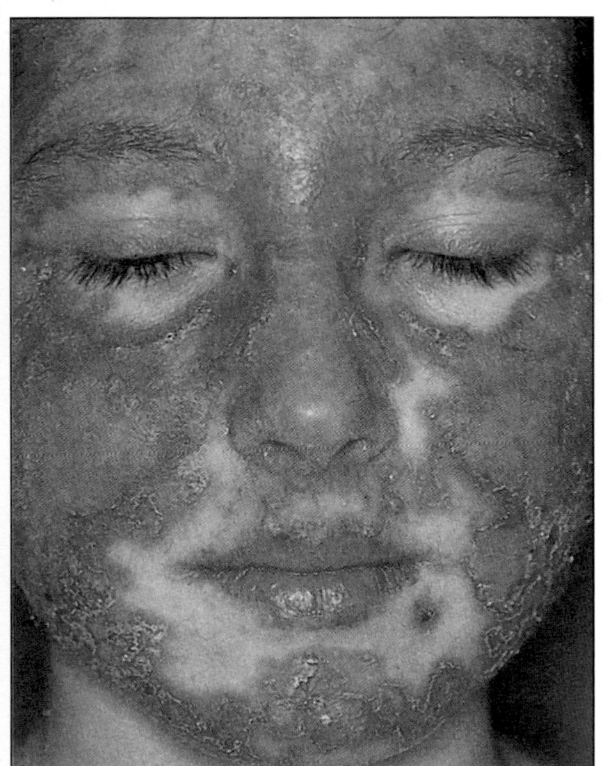

Fig. 18.48. Systemic lupus erythematosus; photosensitivity leading to severe facial erythema and scaling

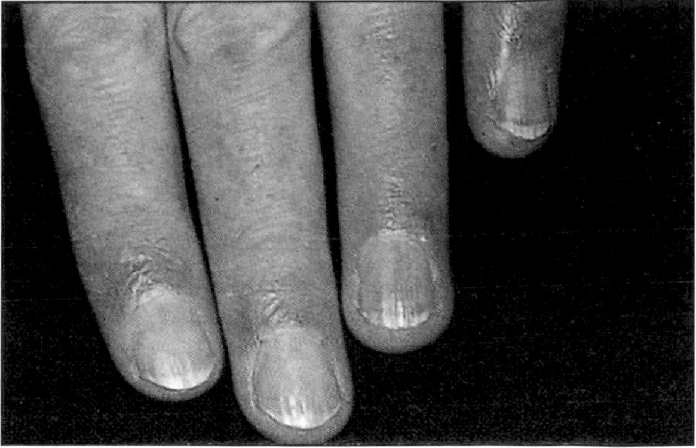

Fig. 18.49. Systemic lupus erythematosus; periungual erythema

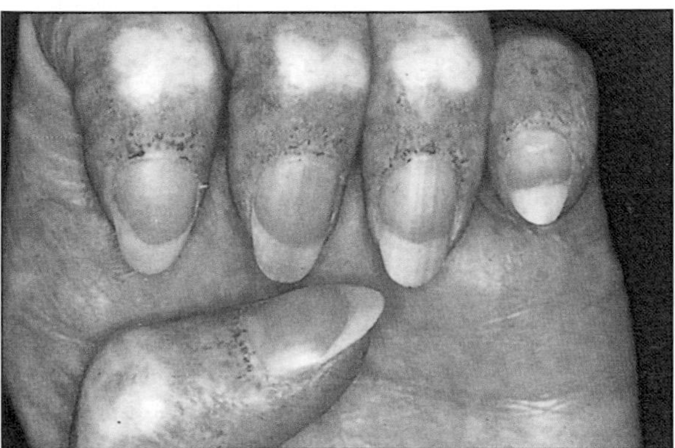

Fig. 18.50. Systemic lupus erythematosus; nailfold telangiectases and loss of finger tip substance

The knees and elbows may have reticular erythematous patches with special tendency to superficial ulcerations and atrophy.

Vasculitis is a general feature of SLE, taking many forms. Classic leukocytoclastic angiitis appears in about 20% of patients. The presence of persistent urticarial lesions, which on biopsy show true vasculitis and are associated with hypocomplementemia is known as urticarial vasculitis. Livedo racemosa is present in another 10–15% of patients, often as a marker for the antiphospholipid antibody syndrome. Such patients are more likely to develop thrombotic problems, widespread ulcerations and even gangrenous changes. In livedo racemosa, the vasculitis is accompanied by marked fibrin deposition in the dermal vessels. The fingertip lesions may represent a proliferative endothelial process with vascular occlusion (as seen in rheumatoid arthritis), part of the spectrum of acrocyanosis and Raynaud phenomenon (present in perhaps 25% of SLE patients) or cold-triggered lupus pernio.

Necrobiotic lesions can be seen. Fairly typical rheumatoid nodules are found in a small percentage of SLE patients. In addition, smaller papules may be seen on the hands and feet that histologically reveal both vasculitis and necrobiosis. They have been called rheumatoid papules or palisaded neutrophilic and granulomatous dermatitis of collagen vascular disease. All are more typical in patients with rheumatoid arthritis.

Bullous lesions may also occur in SLE. When one speaks of the bullous eruption of SLE, one is referring to a subepidermal blistering eruption which resembles dermatitis herpetiformis, features antibodies against type VII collagen or other proteins of the basement membrane zone and responds well to dapsone. This is typically seen in young blacks with severe SLE, high ANA titers and most often facial lesions. In addition, patients with severe flares of SLE, such as those induced by a sunburn, may have vesicles or blisters within their established lesions. Finally, SLE may appear in association with other blistering disorders, the most distinctive of which is pemphigus erythematosus (Chap. 15).

Patients with SLE may have a severe diffuse alopecia which often worsens as the disease flares. It is best viewed as a nonscarring telogen effluvium. The tiny broken off hairs along the frontal scalp line are known as lupus hairs but are not specific. Scarring discoid lesions of the scalp may also develop. In contrast to systemic sclerosis and dermatomyositis, calcification is very uncommon in all forms of LE. The same oral mucosal changes described under DLE also occur in SLE, but only rarely do they represent the first sign of the disorder.

The overall picture is that about 60 % of patients have an acute rash (malar, photosensitive or vasculitic). Another 20 % have lesions of DLE or SLE. Of the remaining 20 %, even though their skin is free, one should look for nailfold changes, diffuse hair loss or oral mucosal lesions. The course of the skin changes is unpredictable. Generally, skin flares run along with systemic flares. Sometimes even erythroderma develops. Lesions may heal with fine wrinkling and atrophy, only to recur, while others may persist for months or years.

Systemic Findings. The spectrum of systemic findings in SLE is lengthy, as almost any organ can be affected. We only cover the most common and important ones superficially, considering first those mentioned in the ARA criteria. Patients often complain of fever, malaise or fatigue. The causes of their feeling unwell are protean.

Arthritis. Almost all patients suffer from arthralgias, usually distal and very painful or even disabling. Most often there is pain without swelling, but acute polyarthritis can also occur. It primarily involves the proximal interphalangeal and metacarpal-phalangeal joints, and can cause destructive changes, although they are uncommon. Similarly, probably 50 % of patients have myalgias, but frank myositis is uncommon. Avascular necrosis of the femoral heads is another skeletal complication. In most cases, the patient has received high doses of systemic corticosteroids but the necrosis appears to be intrinsically associated with SLE.

Serositis. About 50 % of patients have serosal problems. A young women with sterile pericarditis, pleuritis or especially both should always be suspected of having SLE. Sterile peritonitis can also occur. The most typical scenario is the suspicion of a pulmonary embolus because of pain, but no radiologic confirmation.

Renal Disease. About 50 % of patients also have renal lesions. The spectrum of renal disease is dependent on how hard one looks for problems. Almost all patients may have mild proteinuria or hematuria. If renal biopsies are done routinely, mesangial lupus nephritis can be identified. This disorder is relatively harmless and usually not treated, other than by routine monitoring of proteinuria and renal function, as well as attention to possible hypertension. Elevated titers of antibodies against dsDNA and decreased complement levels may also reflect renal disease.

Other histologic patterns include focal proliferative glomerulonephritis, which also tends to resolve and then membranous glomerulonephritis often associated with the nephrotic syndrome or diffuse proliferative glomerulonephritis leading to renal failure and hypertension. The exact classification of renal SLE is complex, highly dependent on morphologic studies and of limited prognostic use because the morphologic diagnosis may change with time.

CNS Disease. The CNS manifestations are protean. The psychotic processes in SLE can be devilishly hard to separate from those associated with high-dose corticosteroid therapy and opportunistic CNS infections. Epilepsy, transient ischemic episodes and strokes may occur, but the problems may also be as minor as a headache or attention disorder. Peripheral neuropathies, especially cranial nerve palsies, may also be seen. A variety of techniques have been tried to increase the ability to diagnose CNS lupus. EEG and contrast magnetic resonance imaging appear most useful.

Hematologic Disorders. A variety of autoantibodies lead to autoimmune cytopenias, which serve as diagnostic clues. About 50% of patients are anemic, although it is usually an anemia of chronic disease. Hemolytic anemia is uncommon. Leukocytopenia is very common; the white cell count usually ranges between 2000 and 4000/mm^3. Lymphocyte counts may also be low. Less than 1500/mm^3 is considered suggestive of LE. Finally, thrombocytopenia is often present. Counts less than 100,000/mm^3 are suggested by the criteria, but symptoms are rarely present until much lower levels are reached or if there is an associated anticoagulant or inhibitor. The most serious hematologic problems are associated with antiphospholipid (APL) antibodies and are discussed below.

Cardiac Involvement. While 30–50% of patients have cardiac problems, most have pericarditis. Myocarditis with associated arrhythmias and cardiac failure may also be seen. The well-known Libman-Sacks endocarditis with verrucous vegetations on the valves and endocardium is quite rare.

Other Organs. In addition to the pleurisy, there may be pneumonia, loss of lung volume, adult respiratory distress syndrome and even intraalveolar hemorrhage. While 25% of patients may have hepatosplenomegaly, lupoid hepatitis is much more uncommon. Gastrointestinal problems including nausea, vomiting, diarrhea and bleeding may occur. Perhaps 20% of patients have esophagitis, gastritis or bowel involvement. Ocular findings include retinal hemorrhages with cotton-wool exudates, as well as uveitis, episcleritis and optic neuritis. Perhaps 15–20% of patients have overlapping Sjögren syndrome with dry eyes or other features.

Histopathology. The microscopic changes in SLE are frequently less dramatic than those in DLE. There may be modest vacuolar change and a sparse lymphocytic infiltrate with dermal edema and mucin. When dealing with SLE, one must search hard for vasculitis, either leukocytoclastic or fibrinoid, since this is clinically important and helps set SLE apart from DLE.

Immunofluorescent Examination. The LE band test has been discussed under DLE. Table 18.10 summarizes its use in diagnosing SLE. Another use if trying to make the diagnosis of SLE in a puzzling case is to biopsy sunlight-exposed normal skin. Such skin shows less specificity than nonexposed skin but the sensitivity is greater. If possible, the biopsies for the LE band test should be taken before systemic (or even local) corticosteroid use.

Laboratory Findings. One can order an endless number of laboratory tests in SLE. They fall into a number of categories.

General Tests. The erythrocyte sedimentation rate is almost always elevated and to some extent can be used to follow the disease course. The dsDNA titer and various complement levels are also used in this regard, but are far more costly. Elevated levels of acute phase reactants (C-reactive protein, β2-microglobulin) can be found. The urine should be checked for hematuria and casts, and renal function monitored.

Hematologic Tests. A positive Coombs tests or signs of cytopenia are part of the diagnostic workup, as

Table 18.10. Clinical use of the lupus erythematosus band test

Clinical diagnosis	Site of biopsy	Positive tests (%)
DLE	Diseased skin	90
	Light-exposed skin	–
	Protected skin	–
SCLE	Diseased skin	90
	Light-exposed skin	20
	Protected skin	–
SLE	Diseased skin	90
	Light-exposed skin	>50
	Protected skin	>50

indicated in the criteria and discussed above under hematologic disorders.

Immunologic Tests. Increased immunoglobulins (usually polyclonal IgG), sometimes cryoglobulins and rheumatoid factor, can all be found. Some patients, especially with CNS or renal disease, have evidence of circulating immune complexes. Such patients often have low complement levels. Antibodies against parietal, thyroid, muscle and nerve cells may also be found, but are rarely of clinical significance.

Antinuclear Antibodies. Over 90% of patients have positive ANA identified with indirect immunofluorescent examination. The principle of the test consists of using a substrate such as HEp-2 cultured epithelial carcinoma cells which have a high nuclear to cytoplasmic ratio. The cells and the patient's serum, diluted to standard concentration, are placed on slides. After various incubation steps, fluorescently labeled antihuman immunoglobulin is added to identify sites in the nucleus or cytoplasm where the patient's serum has attached.

The pattern of immunofluorescent staining can be identified, as homogeneous, membranous, speckled, nuclear or centromere as shown in Table 18.11. Different laboratories have varying degrees of skill and interest in fine-tuning the fluorescent pattern. Today the exact identification of protein targets has made the pattern more of a screening procedure.

If a positive ANA is found, then the serum is diluted to a series of standard titers to quantify the amount of antibodies present. While such titers are often used as crude markers of disease activity, they are seldom helpful. In contrast, titers of anti-dsDNA and antihistone antibodies appear useful, especially in following the reduction in the amount of systemic immune activation, renal disease and the resolution of drug-induced LE, respectively. In addition, further confirmatory tests such as immunodiffusion, ELISA or immunoprecipitation are employed to exactly identify the antigen specificity. Native or dsDNA can be identified using single-cell flagellates of the *Crithidia* genus as a substrate for indirect immunofluorescent examination because dsDNA is found in their flagellar apparatus.

The various antigens are shown in Table 18.12 and their disease associations in Table 18.13. Anti-native dsDNA antibodies are quite specific for SLE, being present in 40–90% of patients. The titers appear clinically relevant in many cases. Antibodies against single-stranded DNA are nonspecific. Anti-Sm is also seen in 10–30% of LE patients and is often associated with severe renal or CNS disease. Anti-Sm along with U_1-RNP is part of the extractable nuclear antigen (ENA), a mixture of ribonucleoproteins and other nuclear proteins essential for protein synthesis. Anti-U_1-RNP is a marker for mixed connective tissue disease.

Ro and La are proteins of both nuclear and cytoplasmic origin that can be expressed on the cell surface. Anti-Ro and anti-La are seen in 40–60% of patients, usually in those with SCLE or with milder SLE without renal or CNS problems. Anti-Ro or anti-La combined with anti-dsDNA or anti-Sm is associated with severe disease, so the combination of antibodies must be considered. The role of anti-Ro, anti-La and U_1-RNP in pregnancy is discussed under neonatal LE. They can also be found in

Table 18.11. Patterns of immunofluorescence in antinuclear antibody (ANA) testing

Pattern	Antigens	Antibodies	Disease(s)
Homogeneous	Chromatin	dsDNA, histone	SLE, drug-induced LE
Rim or peripheral	Chromatin, nuclear membrane	dsDNA	SLE
Fine speckled	Nuclear RNP	Sm	SLE (nephritis)
		Ro	SLE, Sjögren
		La	SLE
		U_1-RNP	SLE, MCTD
	Chromatin	Ku	SLE, scleroderma, myositis
		Topoisomerase I (Scl-70)	Scleroderma
Discrete speckled	Centromere	Centromere	CREST
Nucleolar	Nucleolar RNP	U3-RNP	Scleroderma
	Other nucleolar proteins	RNA polymerase I (PM-Scl)	Scleroderma

Table 18.12. Antinuclear antibodies (ANA) in systemic lupus erythematosus

Antigen	Frequency (%)
Native double-stranded DNA (dsDNA)	40–90
U_1-RNP (nuclear)	40–60
Sm (part of ENA)	10–30
rRNP (ribosomal)	10
Ro (SSA)	40–60
La (SSB)	20–30
Ku (part of ENA)	10
Histones	70

Table 18.13. Diagnostic and prognostic meaning of various antinuclear antibodies in systemic lupus erythematosus

Clinical association	Antinuclear antibodies
Severe SLE with multiple organ involvement	dsDNA (high titer), Sm; also Ro but not alone
SLE with CNS disease	dsDNA, rRNP
Less severe SLE, SCLE, neonatal LE, MCTD	Ro, La, U_1-RNP
SLE with polymyositis	Ku
SLE with antiphospholipid syndrome	dsDNA and antiphospholipid antibodies
Drug-induced SLE	Histones

Sjögren syndrome, systemic sclerosis and polymyositis.

Many other antigens also play a role. While about 70% of SLE patients have antibodies against histones, almost all patients with drug-induced SLE do, and they rarely have other antibodies. Anti-Ku suggests the overlap of SLE and polymyositis, while anti-rRNP is associated with CNS disease. Antiphospholipid antibodies are found in 30–40% of SLE patients.

Course and Prognosis. The course of SLE is very difficult to predict, even though the pattern of ANA gives one a start. The typical course waxes and wanes. Probably the crucial factors are the degree of renal involvement and the avoidance of infections. The use of systemic corticosteroids has altered the previous dismal outlook with death in weeks to months. Today, the 5-year survival following diagnosis of SLE is well over 90%. Even those with diffuse proliferative glomerulonephritis have an 80% 5-year survival. Other factors that play a role in determining the course include:

- Age of onset: Children and young adults do worse than those with onset later than 50 years of age. This is in contrast to the reverse pattern in systemic sclerosis and dermatomyositis.
- Gender: Men do worse than women.
- Pregnancy: While in the past it was often suggested that LE was likely to flare during pregnancy, controlled studies have not supported this. Nonetheless, if there is a severe flare of SLE in a pregnant woman, both the mother and child may be at risk. The biggest problems are pregnancy-induced hypertension and an associated antiphospholipid syndrome with thrombotic events. Anti-Ro antibodies can cause neonatal LE but do not appear to jeopardize the pregnancy.
- Other triggers: Sunlight, medications and perhaps viral infections are other possible provoking factors for SLE.

Differential Diagnosis. The differential diagnostic considerations in SLE are broad. If there are no typical cutaneous signs, often the possibility is overlooked. For example, fever and malaise, polyarthritis with leukopenia or purpura, therapy-resistant polyarthritis, "idiopathic" thrombocytopenic purpura in an adult, mild glomerulonephritis without hypertension, unexplained pleurisy or pericarditis and myocardial or endocardial changes in a young women are all scenarios in which we have seen SLE overlooked.

Important considerations usually include the other connective tissue disorders. Usually repeated ANA tests and careful clinical observation allow a distinction. Drug-induced SLE should always be kept in mind. Acute cases of SLE may be confused with bacterial endocarditis, meningococcemia, disseminated gonococcal disease, rheumatic fever, other types of glomerulonephritis, vasculitis and serum sickness, to name but a few possibilities. The cutaneous changes may suggest seborrheic dermatitis, polymorphic light eruption, drug eruptions and erythema multiforme. The CNS changes are very difficult to identify; they resemble multiple sclerosis and may be mimicked by corticosteroid-induced psychotic changes.

Therapy. Good common sense is probably the least controversial aspect of SLE therapy. Avoidance of sunlight, physical and emotional stress, as well as bed rest during times of flare are essential. Monitoring of renal, CNS and hematologic status is also needed. The most useful tests are urine protein, creatinine clearance, erythrocyte sedimentation rate, CBC and titer of anti-dsDNA.

Systemic. While many patients with SLE are treated almost exclusively with systemic corticosteroids, this is not necessarily wise. They are unquestionably effective over the short term, but their long-term effects on survival are poorly documented, while their side effects are numerous. Patients with polyarthritis, serosal syndromes, skin disease and other non-life-threatening manifestations can often be managed with antimalarials and nonsteroidal antiinflammatory drugs.

The major indications for systemic corticosteroids are renal and CNS disease. Thus there is rarely a need for a dermatologist alone to administer systemic corticosteroids. Usually one starts with relatively high doses of prednisone (1–2 mg/kg daily) but then carefully works down to a level which controls the disease but has as few side effects as possible. Because many SLE patients will be on some dosage of corticosteroids for their entire life, the cautions discussed in Chapter 70 are crucial. Alternate-day regimens should be tried but often fail to control the disease adequately. Pulse therapy (methylprednisolone 0.5–1.0 g IV daily for 3 days, repeated every 4–6 weeks) may be used for severe vasculitis or renal disease. In therapy-resistant cases, a wide range of other options have been tried. They include total lymphoid irradiation, plasmapheresis, extracorporeal photopheresis and IVIG.

The role of cyclosporine in SLE renal disease remains unclear. Steroid-sparing agents such as azathioprine (50–150 mg daily) or cyclophosphamide (50–150 mg daily) can be considered. The latter is often given as pulse therapy monthly to reduce the effects of the hemorrhagic cystitis, combined with low-dose corticosteroid therapy. This seems the best approach for most patients with lupus nephritis. End-stage renal disease is managed by dialysis and transplantation, just as in patients with other causes. Interestingly, recurrent LE nephritis in a transplanted kidney is rare.

Topical. The cutaneous lesions are treated just as under DLE, usually with topical corticosteroids. Sunscreens with good protection against both UVA and UVB are mandatory.

Neonatal Lupus Erythematosus

(McCuistion and Schoch 1954)

Etiology and Pathogenesis. Neonatal lupus erythematosus (NLE) occurs in infants whose mothers almost always have anti-Ro antibodies, but may occasionally have anti-La or anti-U_1-RNP antibodies. Only about 5% of the children born to such women develop neonatal NLE, although the repeat risk is about 25%. Many of the mothers may be asymptomatic when their child presents with NLE. The antibodies are transferred across the placenta and react with fetal skin and cardiac muscle.

Clinical Findings. The skin lesions are erythematous patches, usually annular or circinate, most often on the face and trunk. They spread peripherally and have a scaly border. The lesions are present at birth or appear soon thereafter. The other organ that is regularly involved is the heart. About 75% of patients with NLE develop a congenital atrioventricular heart block. Antigens on the conducting fibers in the heart are also attacked by the anti-Ro antibodies. Many patients with congenital heart block and anti-Ro antibodies have no cutaneous changes. The skin changes resolve spontaneously, usually in the first months. The heart block may be critical after birth, requiring a pacemaker.

Histopathology. The microscopic picture is identical to that of SCLE.

Laboratory Findings. Almost all NLE is associated with anti-Ro antibodies in the mother and usually the child. Anti-La antibodies may also be found but usually not alone. Very rarely U_1-RNP appears responsible. The antibodies disappear by 6–9 months of age.

Course and Prognosis. The extent and severity of the heart block determines the course in the child. The mother has the same outlook as any other mother with SLE or SCLE. Subsequent children are at risk, as discussed above.

Differential Diagnosis. The differential diagnosis in the mother is that of SCLE. In the child, one must consider other causes of neonatal annular eruptions. Most are idiopathic; some may be familial or associated with *Malassezia furfur* infection.

Therapy. The skin findings in the child require no therapy. The cardiac problems may require a pacemaker. Series looking at the use of prednisone during pregnancy in mothers with a variety of LE-associated antibodies have shown little benefit.

Drug-Induced Systemic Lupus Erythematosus

Synonym. Pseudo-SLE

Epidemiology. The concept of drug-induced SLE is a confusing one. Most patients with frank drug-induced SLE are adult men usually taking cardiac medications. There are a number of variables. Some patients are probably destined to develop SLE and the drugs they are taking at the time play no role. In other instances, the medications may cause photosensitivity which may then trigger the LE. Drug-hypersensitivity reactions, when severe, may include fever, lymphadenopathy, serositis and similar findings, thus mimicking SLE. Many medications cause positive ANA titers without producing SLE. Finally, some authors have tried to distinguish between drug-induced SLE and drug-induced SCLE.

Etiology and Pathogenesis. There are a number of agents which clearly produce an SLE-like disorder in a reproducible fashion. The most reliable causes are shown in Table 18.14, but at least 50 other drugs have been implicated. Of patients taking procainamide, 90% develop positive ANA titers within 1 year, but only 30% have signs and symptoms of SLE. With hydralazine, about 40% have positive ANA titers and 6% have clinical features of SLE. None of the other drugs have numbers anywhere near this high. Other drugs implicated include thiazide diuretics, usually associated with SCLE and photosensitivity, as well as estrogens which typically cause flares of existing SLE.

The mechanisms of action are unclear, although genetic predisposition may well play a role. In some instances, the medications may simply be unmasking a preexisting LE. In other cases, the combination of the medication and a normal structure may create a significant autoantigen as a hapten or the metabolism of a drug may be abnormal, producing immunologically active byproducts.

Table 18.14. Major causes of drug-induced systemic lupus erythematosus

Hydralazine
Procainamide
Isoniazid
Methyldopa
Chlorpromazine
Hydantoin derivatives
Penicillamine
Carbamazepine
Primidone
Thiouracils

The most common agents are listed first

Clinical Findings. Cutaneous findings as well as renal and CNS disease are rare. The typical manifestations of drug-induced SLE include fever, arthralgias and serositis. Transient and nonscarring skin lesions, usually in light-exposed areas, occur in fewer than 25% of patients, perhaps because the offending drug is usually stopped before the skin changes can properly develop.

Histopathology. The skin biopsy is not helpful in sorting out the problem. Usually the changes are minimal.

Laboratory Findings. The classic feature is the presence of antibodies against ssDNA without antibodies against dsDNA. By exclusion this suggests the presence of antihistone antibodies, as the histones are better exposed in the single-stranded substrate. One can also identify antihistone antibodies directly by ELISA. Antihistone antibodies are usually absent in drug-induced SCLE. No laboratory test unequivocally separates spontaneous SLE from drug-induced SLE.

Course and Prognosis. In most instances, once the drug is stopped, the disease slowly disappears and eventually the antibodies also fade away. Patients are at risk to react to other drugs associated with LE. If a patient fails to improve, then one concludes that he has SLE which was unmasked by the medication.

Differential Diagnosis. True SLE along with other photosensitivity and hypersensitivity reactions come into question. Serial serologies and clinical observation usually answer the question.

Therapy. No therapy is required, but symptomatic treatment of the arthralgias may be useful. In some cases, short courses of systemic corticosteroids may be employed. Skin changes can be encouraged to fade more rapidly with topical corticosteroids.

Antiphospholipid Syndrome

(Harris et al. 1983)

Synonyms. Lupus anticoagulant syndrome, anticardiolipin syndrome, Hughes syndrome

Epidemiology. The antiphospholipid syndrome (APS) is an uncommon disorder seen more often in young women. About 2% of normal people have APL antibodies, as do about 30% of SLE patients, but most do not have the characteristic clinical features.

Table 18.15. Features of antiphospholipid syndrome

Arterial and venous thromboses
Fetal wastage
Livedo racemosa
Leg ulcerations without other risk factors
Raynaud phenomenon
Peripheral gangrene
Purpura and ecchymoses
Subungual splinter hemorrhages
Widespread skin necrosis

Etiology and Pathogenesis. The hallmark of the antiphospholipid syndrome is the presence of either APL antibodies or anticardiolipin antibodies (ACA). The major APL antibodies are the lupus anticoagulant antibodies (LAC). Thus the major group of the antiphospholipid syndrome can be subdivided into the LAC syndrome and the ACA syndrome. In addition, it is separated into the primary form and the secondary form when another disorder such as SLE is present.

LAC is a misnomer for many reasons. Most patients do not have LE and the in vivo effect of the antibody is a procoagulant. In vitro there is a prolonged whole blood clotting time and prothrombin time. The LAC antibodies are immunoglobulins, usually IgG, that block various phospholipid surface structures. The ACA is also usually IgG, although IgM and IgA may also be represented. ACA can be associated with autoimmune diseases or infection. Biologic false-positive tests for syphilis are common. Many patients have both LAC and ACA specificities. Both classes of antibodies appear not to be just epiphenomena, but to play a direct role in causing thromboses.

Clinical Findings

Systemic Findings. The clinical features of the antiphospholipid syndrome are shown in Table 18.15. There are some differences between patients with predominantly ACA or LAC antibodies. The ACA are more common and associated with arterial and venous thromboses, while the LAC are usually seen with just venous thromboses. The most common venous event is deep vein thromboses of the legs, while the most common arterial event is cerebral thromboses with transient ischemic attacks and strokes. Other possibilities include pulmonary embolus, hepatic, renal, retinal and adrenal vein thromboses, as well as myocardial, mesenteric, hepatic and renal infarctions and peripheral ischemia and gangrene. When multiple thromboses and infarctions occur simultaneously, the outlook is grim, as disseminated intravascular coagulation or thrombotic thrombocytopenic purpura is mimicked. High-titer ACA are most often associated with fetal loss, but LAC antibodies alone may be found. Once loss has occurred, subsequent pregnancies are also at risk.

Associated disorders in secondary antiphospholipid syndrome include autoimmune diseases, especially SLE and systemic sclerosis, vasculitis disorders, infections, hematologic disorders including leukemias, malignant lymphomas and paraproteinemias, thrombotic thrombocytopenic purpura, polycythemia vera, renal failure with dialysis and a variety of medications, showing considerable overlap with drug-induced LE. The biggest risk is that associated with SLE. About 10–25% of SLE patients develop secondary antiphospholipid syndrome. The risk of fetal loss for such patients is at least 50%.

Cutaneous Findings. Most of the cutaneous findings are also explained by vascular occlusion. About half of the patients present with skin findings, while the rest develop systemic problems or experience fetal loss first. Livedo racemosa is the most common change. About half the patients with livedo racemosa have APL antibodies, and many have SLE. Typically they have livedo racemosa associated with ulcerations and even gangrene. The Sneddon syndrome is the combination of livedo racemosa and cerebrovascular accidents. While most patients have either ACA or LAC antibodies, some do not.

Although in most cases of antiphospholipid syndrome there is no vessel wall inflammation but just occlusion, vasculitis can be seen (Chap. 22). Livedo vasculitis refers to the association of livedo racemosa with cutaneous ulcerations, atrophie blanche and segmental hyalinization of vessels. Some of these patients have antiphospholipid syndrome, suggesting another overlap. These patients are more likely to have their ulcerations in the spring and summer. True necrotizing vasculitis usually means the patient has an underlying SLE with secondary antiphospholipid syndrome. In either case, leg ulcers are common, usually about the ankles. When patients with SLE develop leg ulcers, one should always suspect the antiphospholipid syndrome. The ulcers can go on to resemble pyoderma gangrenosum, widespread necrosis or digital gangrene. Other patients may have painful nodules, reflecting microthrombi in vessels, or larger more obvious superficial thrombophlebitis.

A number of other disorders have been associated with the antiphospholipid syndrome but the relationships remain unclear. The lesions can heal to resemble those of Degos syndrome, and in rare cases, antibodies have been found in patients with Degos syndrome. Similarly, the presence of LAC antibodies may predispose patients to develop anetoderma secondary to dermal ischemia. ACA have also been identified in a significant number of patients with systemic sclerosis, not surprisingly those with vasculitic problems and clinical overlap with SLE. While APL antibodies are most often associated with SLE, they may also rarely be seen in DLE. The association of cutaneous T cell lymphoma and antiphospholipid syndrome probably reflects the stimulation of B cells by the neoplastic T cells and thus aberrant antibody production, including LAC and ACA antibodies.

Histopathology. While the skin findings are not specific, the presence of noninflammatory small vessel thrombosis should raise the question of antiphospholipid syndrome. The thrombi may be seen when one biopsies painful nodules, thromboses, or the edges of ulcers or other necrotic processes. In addition, changes usually seen with stasis dermatitis, such as hemosiderin deposition, multiple small thick-walled vessels in the papillary dermis and fibrosis may be seen, both away from the legs and without other signs of chronic venous insufficiency. Segmental or hyalinizing vasculitis is less common, but may be present; it is more often found in Sneddon syndrome and livedo vasculitis. Noninflammatory thrombi also suggest sickle cell anemia, coumarin necrosis, cryoglobulinemia, protein S and C abnormalities including purpura fulminans, thrombocythemia and some cutaneous emboli.

Laboratory Findings. High-titer IgM and IgG ACA, especially when persistent, strongly suggest antiphospholipid syndrome. The presence of the LAC antibodies can be documented by an abnormal activated thromboplastin time, kaolin clotting time or dilute Russell viper venom time. Most patients with SLE and antiphospholipid syndrome have anti-dsDNA antibodies. Biologic false-positive syphilis serology, thrombocytopenia and a positive Coombs test may also be found, as well as clues to secondary causes of the antiphospholipid syndrome.

Course and Prognosis. The outlook is not good, but varies depending on the associated disorders. The severe multiorgan vascular involvement has the worst prognosis, but obviously multiple cerebral or coronary insults are not conducive to long-term enjoyment of life. In addition, the threat to each pregnancy is potentially a major family disaster.

Differential Diagnosis. The differential diagnosis is lengthy, including all the types of vasculitis and disorders of coagulation, as well as the many causes of fetal loss and the other numerous secondary or associated disorders.

Therapy. The therapeutic approach takes several forms. Prophylaxis of thrombosis in patients identified by chance or via skin findings, but without a previous thrombosis has not been proven effective. Nonetheless, they tend to receive prophylaxis when faced with major surgery or immobilization or if they have associated risk factors. If thromboses occur, both heparin and coumarin have their supporters but long-term studies with clear guidelines are sparse. The need for long-term prophylaxis following a thrombosis seems clear. The best suggestion is probably life-long coumarin anticoagulation, perhaps coupled with low-dose aspirin. Low molecular weight heparin may be useful for acute attacks. The best approach to fetal loss is also confusing. Studies have looked at both prednisone and a combination of aspirin and heparin. The latter is probably preferable. Coumarin is not appropriate during pregnancy and must be stopped.

Dermatomyositis

(Wagner 1863; Unverricht 1887)

Synonyms. Dermatomyositis sine myositis, amyopathic dermatomyositis (when there is only skin involvement), lilac disease (childhood form). Polymyositis is a closely related idiopathic inflammatory myopathy without skin involvement.

Epidemiology. Dermatomyositis is an uncommon disorder. The incidence is estimated at 5–10/1,000,000 in adults and 1–3/1,000,000 in children. While the adult form usually begins between 40 and 60 years of age, the juvenile form has a peak onset at 8–10 years of age. While women are two to three times more affected than men, among children there is a slight male predominance. When there are overlap features present, women are almost exclusively involved. Blacks are far more often affected; the incidence may be as high as 30/1,000,000 in black women. In adults, polymyositis is more common, while children almost always have dermatomyositis.

The standard classification of Bohan and Peter (1975) is often used and is still helpful, although there are outrider cases. Table 18.16 presents a modified version.

Etiology and Pathogenesis. The etiology is unknown. An autoimmune process is likely involved with the presence of both humoral and cell-mediated responses directed against muscle components. Viral infections are suspected to be triggering agents, perhaps by damaging muscle fibers and revealing new or altered antigens to the immune system. Most attention has been directed against Coxsackie B viruses, as some studies have shown an increased incidence of antibodies to this group in dermatomyositis. In addition, there appears to be molecular mimicry between some picornavirus RNA and histidyl-tRNA synthetase. Marked physical stress may also play a role via the same mechanisms, especially in individuals of selected HLA types.

Even though some clinical features of dermatomyositis and polymyositis are similar, the nature of muscle damage appears different. In polymyositis, the cell-mediated response appears more important, with cytotoxic T cells directed against components of the muscle fibers. In contrast, in dermatomyositis the changes appear to be more humoral in nature, with a B cell infiltrate and antibodies directed against the muscular microvasculature with evidence of complement-mediated damage.

A number of autoantibodies have been identified, although the system has not been as thoroughly explored as in LE. Most patients have at least one ANA and about one-third have myositis-specific antibodies.

Finally, there has long been interest in the possible association between polymyositis and dermatomyositis and internal malignancies. The risk estimates have varied from negligible to more than 50%. Our clinical impression is that there is an increased risk, especially among patients over 45 years of age. A Swedish study (Sigurgeirsson 1992) has shown a relative risk of 3.4 for men and 2.4 for women with dermatomyositis. Other studies have shown an internal malignancy to be present in about 15–25% of patients with dermatomyositis and 3–10% of those with polymyositis. The skin and muscle changes may precede the clinical identification of the tumor, may appear simultaneously or later. Further proof of the association is the resolution of the polymyositis or dermatomyositis following resection of the tumor and a recurrence during tumor relapse. The associated tumors follow the distribution in the general population: among men, lung and gastrointestinal tumors are most common; among women, breast and ovarian cancers.

Table 18.16. Classification of polymyositis/dermatomyositis (after Bohan and Peter 1975)

Category	Frequency (%)
Polymyositis	35
Dermatomyositis	30
Malignancy-associated polymyositis and dermatomyositis	10
Childhood polymyositis or dermatomyositis	5
Overlap syndromes and inclusion body myositis	20

Clinical Findings. The classic target organs are the skin and skeletal muscle. Patients may present with muscle disease first, have only muscle disease, start with cutaneous manifestations or in rare cases never develop muscle problems. About 20% of patients followed in a large university dermatology clinic over a 10-year period had no muscle changes.

Cutaneous Findings. While there are several cutaneous changes that are highly suggestive of dermatomyositis, often the skin findings are nonspecific, as the name suggests. Many patients have a photo-

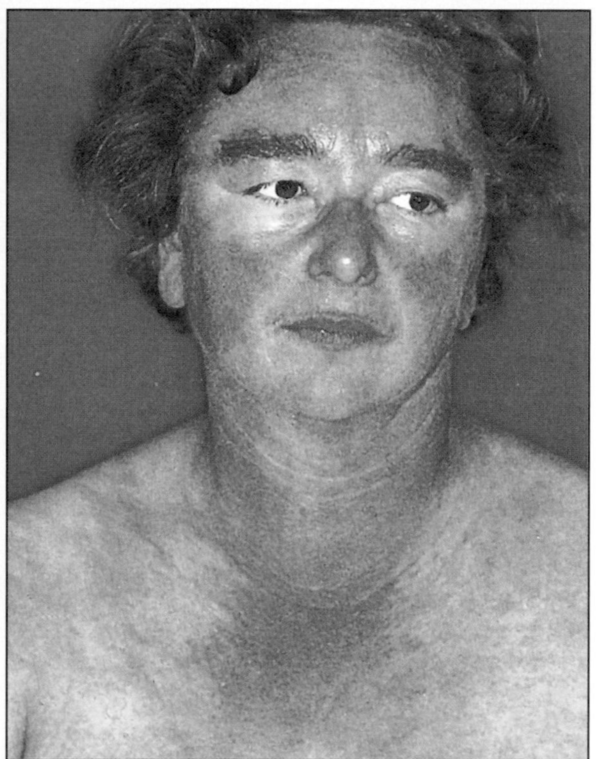

Fig. 18.51. Dermatomyositis

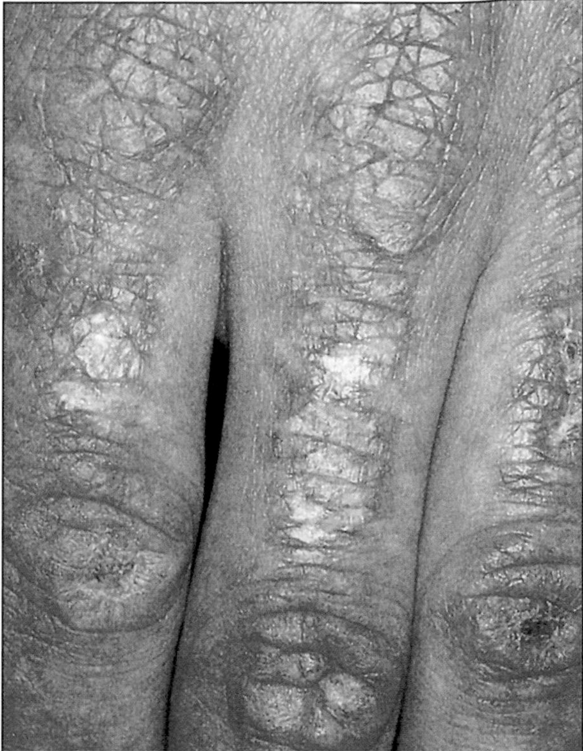

Fig. 18.52. Dermatomyositis; Gottron papules

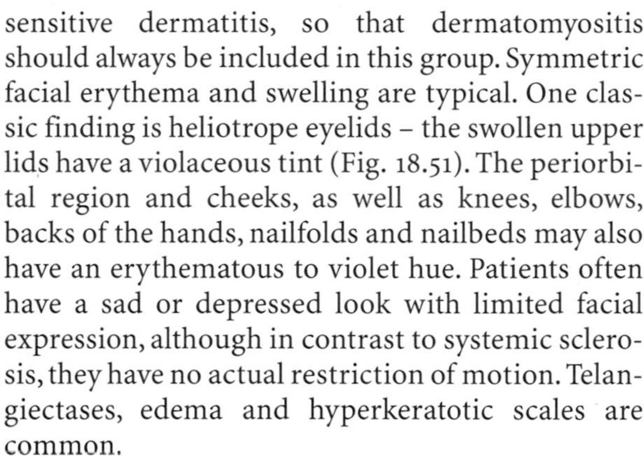

sensitive dermatitis, so that dermatomyositis should always be included in this group. Symmetric facial erythema and swelling are typical. One classic finding is heliotrope eyelids – the swollen upper lids have a violaceous tint (Fig. 18.51). The periorbital region and cheeks, as well as knees, elbows, backs of the hands, nailfolds and nailbeds may also have an erythematous to violet hue. Patients often have a sad or depressed look with limited facial expression, although in contrast to systemic sclerosis, they have no actual restriction of motion. Telangiectases, edema and hyperkeratotic scales are common.

Later characteristic changes may be found on the backs of the digits, as there are violaceous flat-topped papules and plaques over the knuckles and interphalangeal joints, known as Gottron papules (Gottron 1954; Fig. 18.52). These lesions may resolve with atrophy and a parchment-like texture. The cuticles are often tender or painful to touch – the Keining sign (Keining 1939) – and feature linear telangiectases. Similar telangiectases are seen on the gingival mucosa. More diffuse poikilodermatous changes are found in the light-exposed areas. In other instances, the skin lesions may mimic pityriasis rubra pilaris with palmoplantar keratoderma and erythematous hyperkeratotic papules. Rarely lichenoid papules, blisters and necrotic areas can be seen. Both diffuse alopecia and localized hypertrichosis may occur.

In children, the cutaneous features are a bit different. The face is often lilac-colored or violaceous (lilac disease); eyelid involvement may be striking. Soft tissue calcification is frequent, causing confusion with CREST syndrome. Typical sites include the digits, elbows and buttocks. Ulcerations and discharge of chalky material are common. Because of fat involvement, there may be atrophy and bound-down areas, once again suggesting sclerosis.

Systemic Findings. The onset of systemic problems is usually insidious, beginning with fever, malaise and diffuse weakness. The proximal muscles of the extremities are first involved. Typical problems include inability to comb the hair, or to rise from a sitting or kneeling position, or to climb stairs. When the neck muscles are affected, the patient's head may unwillingly droop. Involvement of the appropriate muscles can lead to dysphagia, dyspnea or dysphonia. Reflexes are usually present but reduced; sensory disturbances do not occur. In fulminant cases, such as in tumor-associated dermatomyositis in adults, the patient may wind up virtually helpless. In children, such dramatic courses are uncommon. There can be relentless sclerosis and calcification of the muscles, tendons and ligaments leading to massive disability.

While arthritis or Raynaud phenomenon suggest an overlap syndrome, arthralgias and morning stiffness are often present. Arthritis may also be associated with pulmonary fibrosis and anti-Jo1 antibodies. In children, pulmonary involvement is uncommon. Cardiac changes are more frequent in dermatomyositis than polymyositis. They include myocarditis, cardiomyopathies, arrhythmias and even cor pulmonale. Marked muscle destruction can lead to myoglobinuria and acute renal failure. Dysphagia can complicate the pulmonary picture by causing aspiration pneumonia. In children, acute gastrointestinal problems may develop secondary to a necrotizing arteritis with ulcerations and infarctions. Other difficulties include ocular muscle weakness, carpal tunnel syndrome and osteoporosis secondary to systemic corticosteroids.

Histopathology. The biopsy picture of dermatomyositis is best described as being almost LE. When one sees epidermal atrophy, vacuolar changes, telangiectases, mucin deposition or lymphocytic infiltrates, but one is not convinced that LE is present, then one should consider dermatomyositis as a second possibility. When calcification is present in older lesions, dermatomyositis becomes a very good guess. While DIF examination may show immunoglobulins, predominantly IgM, about the vessels and even at the junction, a classic LE band is not found.

In contrast, the muscle biopsy may show specific changes. One should biopsy a clinically involved, tender muscle; often the deltoid is used. Electromyography may be useful to identify the most involved muscles increasing the yield. The muscle biopsy should be generous and the muscle bundle mounted in an appropriate clamp for transport to a specialized laboratory. The pattern of involvement is patchy. Often badly damaged muscles are adjacent to normal tissue. The inflammation is concentrated around vessels and the perimysium. The muscle fibers are initially edematous, but later they lose their transverse bands and become vacuolated or homogenized, and indeed almost empty sarcolemmal tubes may be found. The perifasicular infiltrates are rich in lymphocytes, plasma cells and histiocytes. Inclusion body myositis is characterized by distinctive granular vacuoles in the muscle fibers.

Laboratory Findings. A variety of nonspecific findings may be present. The erythrocyte sedimentation rate is usually elevated. There may be a leukocytosis with lymphopenia and eosinophilia. The rheumatoid factor is positive in 10–20% of patients. Most important is the documentation of muscle damage. The most helpful enzyme is creatine phosphokinase. The transaminases, aldolase and LDH may also be raised. Creatine phosphokinase is raised in about 90% of patients, but there are individuals with active muscle disease and normal enzyme levels, mandating further searches. It may be helpful to measure the creatine kinase isotypes, because CK3 is most associated with skeletal muscle damage. The 24-h urinary *creatine* levels may be elevated as the first sign of the disease. To avoid misunderstanding, one should be sure the laboratory is aware of the purpose of the test, otherwise a standard 24-h urinary creatinine may be done.

Table 18.17 identifies the positive autoantibodies found in dermatomyositis and polymyositis. About 50% of patients have ANA; the number is much lower among children. No antibodies correlate with cancer risk. Anti-Mi-2 antibodies are specific for dermatomyositis but are only present in 10–30%

Table 18.17. Autoantibodies in dermatomyositis and polymyositis

Antibody	Frequency (%)	Antigen	Clinical association
Anti-Mi-2	10–30	Nucleoproteins (30–240 kDa)	DM
Anti-Jo-1	15–40	Histidyl-tRNA synthetase	PM > DM, often pulmonary fibrosis
Anti-SRP	5–10	Signal recognition protein	PM > DM
Anti-PM-Scl	5–10	Nucleolar proteins (20–110 kDa)	PM > DM, often with systemic sclerosis overlap
Anti-U1-RNP	10–20	Ribonucleoproteins (22, 33, 68 kDa)	Mixed connective tissue disease
Anti-Ku	<5	Nucleoproteins (70, 86 kDa)	PM and SLE

of patients. The antisynthetase antibodies are more common in polymyositis than in dermatomyositis; the best known member of the group is anti-Jo-1 which is present in 15–40% of patients. The combination of myositis, pulmonary fibrosis, Raynaud syndrome and arthritis is often known as the antisynthetase syndrome. Other antisynthetase antibodies are less common in dermatomyositis (<5%) but associated with similar changes. Anti-signal recognition protein (anti-SRP) antibodies are associated with severe polymyositis and dermatomyositis in which case pulmonary fibrosis is not present. Anti-PM-Scl suggests the dermatomyositis/systemic sclerosis overlap syndrome, while anti-Ku is seen in LE/polymyositis overlaps and anti-U_1-RNP points to mixed connective tissue disease.

Another useful test is electromyography, which is not only helpful to find appropriate muscles for biopsy, but may also reveal the so-called myopathy pattern. This consists of a triad of small polyphasic potentials during contraction, fibrillation with positive sharp potentials and increased irritability during the insertion of probes and bizarre high-frequency discharges during mechanical stimulation. Often it is wise to biopsy the muscle opposite the one studied by electromyography to avoid artifacts. Magnetic resonance imaging can be used to confirm muscle damage and loss of mass, but does not provide exact diagnostic information.

Course and Prognosis. The prognosis in dermatomyositis and polymyositis of adults is dependent on the presence or absence of an underlying tumor. While some patients experience a very rapid downhill course, in most the story is one of waxing and waning with a long period of disability. In some lucky individuals, the disease may permanently remit. The mortality in adults is estimated at 10–20%; in children, 5–15%. Major life-threatening events include respiratory failure, aspiration pneumonia and renal failure secondary to myoglobinuria. The complications of therapy are also disturbing. Corticosteroids are invariably employed as first-line therapy and may rarely lead to corticosteroid myopathy and rapid worsening. In children, even when the disease burns out, there may be major problems with calcifications and contractures, but no increased cancer risk.

Diagnostic Criteria. The major diagnostic criteria used for dermatomyositis and polymyositis are progressive symmetric proximal muscle weakness, muscle biopsy with myositis and necrosis, elevated serum muscle enzymes, especially creatine kinase, characteristic autoantibodies, typical electromyographic changes and distinctive cutaneous changes.

Differential Diagnosis. The main differential diagnostic considerations are other connective tissue disorders and overlap states, when cutaneous involvement is present. The final diagnosis is usually based on the clinical course and serologic findings. In children, dermatomyositis may be easily confused with systemic sclerosis; one should lean towards dermatomyositis since it is so much more common.

While the list of muscle diseases which resemble polymyositis is long, one which should be considered is trichinosis. The roundworm *Trichinella spiralis* is ingested by eating raw or inadequately cooked pork (or rarely bear). The encysted larvae are liberated in the stomach, where they embed themselves in the intestinal mucosa, mate and then the female releases myriad new larvae which are carried around the body. They land in skeletal muscle tissues, causing tenderness and damage, as well as blocking the facial lymphatics, which yields periorbital edema. There is usually eosinophilia. The diagnosis can be made on muscle biopsy or more often with serologic testing.

Therapy

Systemic. The mainstay of treatment is immediate relatively high-dosage systemic corticosteroids. Usually prednisone 1–2 mg/kg is employed. Triamcinolone and dexamethasone are usually avoided because they cause more myopathy than prednisone. Once the prompt antiinflammatory effect has been achieved, the corticosteroids can be slowly tapered, usually following the serum muscle enzyme levels as a guide. Often therapy over years is required.

Probably two-thirds of patients have an inadequate response or require such high doses of prednisone that additional therapy is needed. The most popular steroid-sparing agent is methotrexate, usually given intravenously in dosages of 15–45 mg weekly. Both azathioprine and cyclophosphamide can also be employed in the usual dosage ranges. Various combinations of prednisone and cytotoxic agents appear to be more helpful than prednisone alone, although clear studies are lacking. Cyclosporine appears of limited effectiveness. Plasmapheresis has been disappointing. Long-term, medium to high-dose IVIG has become established as an effective adjunctive therapy in both children and adults.

The skin lesions can be treated with hydroxychloroquine, as discussed under discoid LE.

Topical. The skin lesions can be treated with low- to mid-potency corticosteroids. Sunscreens should be employed. There is no good treatment for the calcification. Standard ulcer care can be employed.

Other Measures. Bed rest during the acute phase is important but as soon as the inflammation subsides, activity is equally valuable. Physical therapy not only contributes to the patient's general well-being but also reduces the problems associated with calcification and contractures.

Mixed Connective Tissue Disease

(Sharp et al. 1972)

Synonym. Sharp syndrome

Definition. While there are many overlap syndromes, Sharp described a relatively specific disorder defined by a specific ANA pattern.

Epidemiology. Most patients are women (4:1) and the disease begins in the fourth to fifth decade.

Etiology and Pathogenesis. The cause of the disease is not known.

Clinical Findings. Mixed connective tissue disease (MCTD) usually begins like systemic sclerosis with Raynaud phenomenon and edematous fingers and hands which later become indurated. About 60% of patients have arthralgias. While arthritis may develop, deformities are rare. Other patients may have myalgias and even myositis. Esophageal disorders and pulmonary fibrosis suggest an overlap with systemic sclerosis, while serositis and CNS disease confirm the relationship to LE. Vasculitis, renal disease and Sjögren syndrome are rather uncommon.

The cutaneous findings are often not dramatic. The most common are DLE lesions. Other changes include sclerodactyly, diffuse alopecia, facial erythema and periungual telangiectases and erythema. In children, both the cutaneous and systemic findings can be more severe.

Histopathology. The skin lesions have no unique features on routine light microscopy.

Immunofluorescent Examination. DIF reveals positively staining nuclei in the diseased or normal epidermis. While this change can be seen in any disorder with high ANA titers, it is most common in MCTD. The LE band test may also be positive.

Laboratory Findings. General laboratory evaluations will confirm the wide spectrum of clinical involvement, such as elevated muscle enzymes if myositis is present. The diagnosis is based on specific ANA findings. The hallmark is the presence of antibodies against U_1-RNP, one of the many antibodies directed against small ribonucleoproteins with HEp-2 cells, there is a characteristic speckled pattern. More sophisticated analysis identifies the target protein as the 68–70 kDa U_1-RNP complex which is part of a splicing enzyme. The presence of anti-U_1-RNP antibodies alone strongly suggests MCTD. Patients with SLE with anti-Sm antibodies almost always have anti-U_1-RNP antibodies as well. Rarely patients with MCTD will have antibodies against dsDNA, Ro or La, while on occasion patients with systemic sclerosis or cutaneous LE may have anti-U_1-RNP antibodies.

Course and Prognosis. The outlook is generally better than in LE, systemic sclerosis or dermatomyositis.

Differential Diagnosis. The differential diagnosis includes the other forms of connective tissue disease discussed above.

Therapy. Systemic corticosteroids are usually effective. Rarely steroid-sparing agents may be needed. In some cases, nonsteroidal antiinflammatory drugs are sufficient to control the arthralgias. If cutaneous LE is present, topical corticosteroids can be used.

Rheumatoid Arthritis

Definition. Severe symmetric inflammatory polyarthritis of unknown etiology which is chronic, progressive and destructive.

Epidemiology. Rheumatoid arthritis is one of the most common chronic diseases. It has a prevalence of about 1% with a 3:1 female to male ratio. The typical age of onset is between 25 and 50 years. The prevalence increases with age so that by 70 years of age, about 5% of women are affected. The disease is also more common in blacks and Asians; it is especially prevalent in Pima Indians. There is an increased incidence in first-degree relatives.

Etiology and Pathogenesis. The cause of rheumatoid arthritis is unknown. The trigger of the destructive immune response is unclear, but infectious agents are most often postulated. About 70% of Europeans with rheumatoid arthritis are HLA-DR4-positive, as compared to 15% in the general population, yielding a relative risk ratio of 4.5:1. Certain polymorphisms in HLA-DR4 are especially likely to be present. Shared epitopes between these self-proteins and various infectious agents may be recognized.

Antigenic peptides are presented bound to HLA-DR4 and -DR1 molecules, triggering an inflammatory response which involves the synovium and endothelium as well as many other sites. The synovial lining develops villous folds, thickens and is rich in plasma cells and lymphocytes. The hyperplastic synovial tissue is known as pannus. It may damage articular structures and interfere with motion.

Rheumatoid factor is an IgM or IgG antibody which reacts with selected regions of the Fc fragment of autologous IgG. It is present in the serum where it may be diagnostically useful but is also deposited in tissues, often as immune complexes, and is capable of activating complement. Thus it is likely to play a pathogenic role in promoting the inflammatory process. Many other autoantibodies are also present. Most of the cutaneous findings are related either to vasculitis or to necrobiosis which itself may be associated with vessel disease.

Clinical Findings. While patients with rheumatoid arthritis often have skin problems, dermatologists are only rarely involved in the diagnosis and management of this disease so the systemic problems will only be reviewed briefly.

Systemic Findings. The disease can present rapidly but usually evolves slowly. The arthritis is symmetric and often involves the small joints of the hands and wrists. Other common sites are the shoulders, cervical spine, knees and feet. Typical symptoms include stiffness in the morning or following activity, pain, tenderness, warmth and swelling. On physical examination, fluid or soft tissue swelling can be seen in the involved joints. A wide variety of characteristic hand deformities develop, the most obvious of which is ulnar deviation of the fingers. The proximal interphalangeal and metacarpophalangeal joints are more often involved; the distal interphalangeal joints are usually spared. Subluxation of the vertebrae of the upper cervical spine, especially of the atlantoaxial joint, can cause cervical cord compression or even transection. Other musculoskeletal problems include bursitis, muscle weakness, popliteal (Baker) cysts and carpal tunnel syndrome.

Other systemic findings include vasculitis which may produce a peripheral neuropathy, as well as bowel, cerebral or myocardial infarctions. Peripheral nerves may also be compressed. Ocular symptoms are because of associated Sjögren syndrome, present in 10–15% of patients. Peripheral ulcerative keratitis may also develop and appears to be a marker for high rheumatoid factor titers. Scleritis occasionally leads to perforation (scleromalacia perforans). Pericarditis, pleuritis and pulmonary fibrosis are also seen.

Cutaneous Findings. The skin changes in rheumatoid arthritis are numerous. While none is pathognomonic, many strongly suggest the diagnosis.

Rheumatoid Nodules. About 20% of patients have such nodules, usually present over pressure points, especially the elbows (Fig. 18.53). In some instances, the patients may have minimal articular problems. Nodules may also involve internal organs. Larger or traumatized lesions may become ulcerated. The major histologic feature is necrobiosis (Chap. 50).

Interstitial Granulomatous Dermatitis. Linear subcutaneous bands, most typically involving the axillae and trunk, are rare but very suggestive of rheumatoid arthritis. Clinically they are unique. Histo-

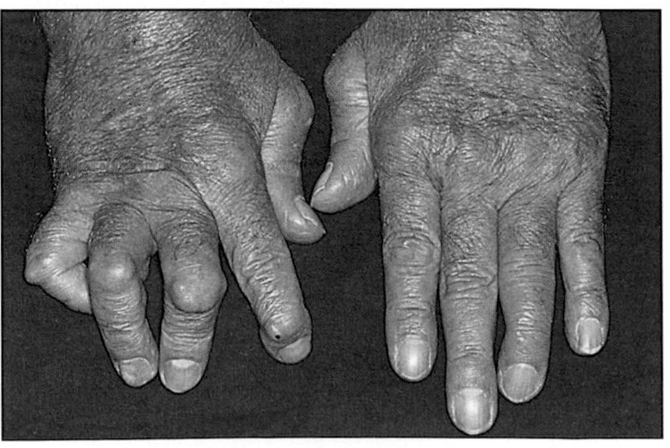

Fig. 18.53. Rheumatoid nodules in patient with severe rheumatoid arthritis

logically, there are areas of necrobiosis, usually in the lower half of the dermis, associated neutrophils and eosinophils but no mucin. While there are microscopic similarities to granuloma annulare and rheumatoid nodule, we consider this process distinct.

Rheumatoid Neutrophilic Dermatitis. Most patients with this uncommon disease have severe rheumatoid arthritis and develop tiny papules and nodules usually over the knees and elbows. On biopsy a dense dermal infiltrate comprised primarily of neutrophils is found. Vasculitis is not present. The differential diagnosis includes rheumatoid nodules, erythema elevatum diutinum and Sweet syndrome. Only the latter is likely to be confused histologically, but typically the lesions are larger boggy plaques.

Vascular Reaction Patterns. Palmar erythema, most prominent on the thenar and hypothenar eminences, is common, just as it is in liver disease and pregnancy. Raynaud phenomenon is very uncommon. Livedo reticularis may be present, but livedo racemosa is more ominous.

Vasculitis. Blood vessel damage in rheumatoid arthritis takes many forms. Tiny digital infarcts are most common. They appear about the nails and the tips of the fingers. Here small digital arteries are involved. Because these tiny ulcerations are relatively painless, they can be easily overlooked. They may cause a small pit or depressed scar, or a groove in the nail. Microscopic examination usually shows intimal proliferation and occlusion, resembling the layers of a cut onion.

Leukocytoclastic angiitis may also occur usually presenting with purpura, palpable lesions and ulcerations. Most lesions involve the extremities. More extensive vascular disease may also occur, with ecchymoses, necrosis and ulcerations. Livedo racemosa may be present. Accelerated rheumatoid vasculitis describes patients with fever, malaise and massive tissue infarction, including cardiovascular damage. It is very similar to polyarteritis nodosa.

Leg Ulcers. There are many types of leg ulcers in rheumatoid arthritis. Most common are stasis ulcers as the underlying disease often interferes with activity. On occasion arterial ulcers may develop. Of the chronic diseases seen in association with pyoderma gangrenosum, rheumatoid arthritis is probably most common. Cryoglobulinemia may also lead to multiple relatively superficial ulcerations. While rheumatoid ulcers are often blamed on corticosteroids, this association appears poorly documented. In immunosuppressed patients, a variety of infections can present as ulcerations so any puzzling ulcer should be examined for bacteria and deep fungi.

Fistulous Tracts. Draining sinus tracts are common in rheumatoid arthritis and have many causes. Most common is a deep rheumatoid nodule which ulcerates and drains. Periarticular cysts may also drain, especially if they become infected. Vasculitis of the subcutaneous structures or even deeper viscera may cause necrosis and subsequent drainage. Finally, soft tissue infections are more likely in this population. Thus any draining sinus tract should be investigated promptly.

Nail Changes. Nailbed infarcts may be seen. Red lunulae have also been described. In addition, rheumatoid arthritis may be associated with the yellow nail syndrome (Chap. 33).

Other Cutaneous Findings. Genital and perianal aphthoid ulcerations may be seen, suggesting either Behçet syndrome or inflammatory bowel disease. Neutrophilic panniculitis has been reported in rare instances. Sclerotic changes may involve the hands. Cold flexed fingers describes such patients who may represent an overlap between rheumatoid arthritis and systemic sclerosis. Some patients develop transparent skin, especially on the backs of their hands. Secondary or wear-and-tear amyloidosis (Chap. 41) is also seen. Finally, many of the cutaneous side effects of long-term systemic corticosteroid therapy are common in rheumatoid arthritis patients.

Histopathology. Some of the histopathologic features have been alluded to above. In a patient with connective tissue disease, the presence of necrobiosis, granulomatous inflammation, neutrophilic infiltrates or vasculitis in the skin should suggest the possibility of rheumatoid arthritis.

Laboratory Findings. No one single test is diagnostic. Rheumatoid factor is present in about 75% of patients. Over 25% will have positive ANA, while p-ANCA is positive in about the same number. Anti-MPO antibody is uncommon and thus helpful in this situation. Many patients are anemic and may have elevated platelet counts. Synovial fluid examination and radiologic examination are helpful in assessing the joints but only rarely lead to the primary diagnosis.

Diagnostic Criteria. Specific diagnostic criteria from the American College of Rheumatology are available in internal medicine and rheumatology texts.

Course and Prognosis. The course of rheumatoid arthritis is highly variable. Some patients have repeated brief attacks (palindromic or recurrent rheumatoid arthritis). Others resolve entirely, but most experience either episodic attacks with residual damage or slowly progressive disease. Rare individuals will have severe rapidly progressive disease which is often therapy-resistant.

Differential Diagnosis. The differential diagnosis of rheumatoid arthritis is beyond our scope. It is more important for a dermatologist to consider the possibility of rheumatoid arthritis when encountering any of the skin manifestations that are occasionally associated with the disease.

Therapy. Treatment of rheumatoid arthritis is a multidisciplinary task. Some patients can be treated with analgesics or nonsteroidal antiinflammatory drugs, but most require some type of immunosuppressive or disease-modifying therapy. Usually sulfasalazine, gold salts, methotrexate, penicillamine or antimalarial agents are employed first. Corticosteroids, azathioprine and cyclophosphamide are typically reserved for treatment failures, although the exact choice of agents is complex and controversial. Orthopedic surgery is also extremely helpful, either to stabilize joints or increasingly to insert artificial joints. Physical therapy is also essential to insure that muscle strength is retained and contractures do not become a problem. Bed rest should be avoided.

In many instances cutaneous problems respond to the systemic agents. Rheumatoid nodules can be excised if troublesome or infected, and multiple nodules have been reported to improve with penicillamine. Severe rheumatoid vasculitis is often treated with systemic corticosteroids, even if the rest of the clinical picture would not warrant this intervention. Similarly, plasmapheresis and high-dose IVIG have been employed when there is vasculitis with high titers of circulating rheumatoid factor or immune complexes.

Variants of Rheumatoid Arthritis

A number of different diseases are generally considered forms of rheumatoid arthritis although evidence for similar etiology is often lacking.

Felty Syndrome

(Felty 1924)

Felty syndrome is the association of rheumatoid arthritis, splenomegaly and leukopenia. Patients are particularly likely to have extensive leg ulcers, as well as perianal and genital ulcerations. Rheumatoid vasculitis is both common and frequently severe. Some individuals have multiple rheumatoid nodules. The patients are often bed-ridden, emaciated and depressed, presenting a tremendous therapeutic challenge.

Juvenile Rheumatoid Arthritis

Synonyms. Juvenile chronic arthritis. Still disease is often used as a synonym but this is not correct.

Juvenile rheumatoid arthritis is a chronic polyarthritis with onset in childhood. It is usually divided into several groups based on the disease pattern at onset.

- Typical adult-type rheumatoid arthritis occurs in older children who have a poor outlook.
- Still disease with systemic involvement at onset. These patients have a distinctive rash, fever (often spiking in the afternoon), minimal arthritis, organomegaly, lymphadenopathy, pleurisy and pericarditis. Rheumatoid factor is often negative.
- Polyarticular disease tends to affect young girls and has only minimal systemic findings.
- Pauciarticular disease often affects teenage boys who have sacroiliac involvement. Thus it is equivalent to juvenile ankylosing spondylitis.

Cutaneous Findings. The classic rash of Still disease is present in only about 25% of juvenile rheumatoid arthritis patients but in a much higher percentage of those with Still disease. It consists of evanescent small salmon-pink macules and papules usually on the trunk, the limbs or occasionally the face, which are more common in the afternoon with the fever spike, and often have a peripheral pallor. The Köbner phenomenon may occur. The lesions do not spread and should not be confused with erythema marginatum of rheumatic fever (Chap. 4). The microscopic picture is not specific and no skin treatment is required.

Adult Still Disease

Rarely adults may also have Still disease. The rash is also usually present, and may precede other findings, or persist for many years. Since the arthritis is often minimal and the rheumatoid factor frequently negative, the diagnosis may be overlooked. Many patients present with a fever of unknown origin.

Miscellaneous Connective Tissues Disorders

We describe some reactive and proliferative fibrotic processes here. Many other related disorders are discussed in Chapter 59 under fibrous tumors and fibromatoses. There is no clear line of distinction.

Knuckle Pads

Synonym. Tylositates articuli

Epidemiology. Most cases are sporadic although familial associations exist. The onset is usually in childhood or adolescence. There is a strong association with other fibromatoses, such as Dupuytren contracture.

Etiology and Pathogenesis. The etiology is poorly understood. In some families, the disorder appears to be inherited in an autosomal dominant pattern. In these patients the onset is usually in childhood, gradual and symmetric. In the Bart-Pumphrey syndrome, there is autosomal dominant inheritance of knuckle pads, leukonychia, palmoplantar hyperkeratosis and deafness. The genes have not been identified. We suspect that trauma plays a crucial role in all cases, even when there is a genetic predisposition. Minor vascular damage has also been postulated to be a factor.

Clinical Findings. Knuckle pads are symmetric, sharply defined cushion-like pads that are located over the proximal and distal interphalangeal joints of the hands. They rarely involve the thumb or tips of the digits, and typically are located on the lateral aspect of the joint, not directly over it. They are usually less than 1 cm in diameter, have a smooth surface and a hyperpigmented periphery. They are permanent.

Histopathology. The epidermis shows typical changes for the digits. The chief pathology is in the dermis where there is a marked thickening of the collagen bundles. Electron microscopy shows increased numbers of myofibroblasts.

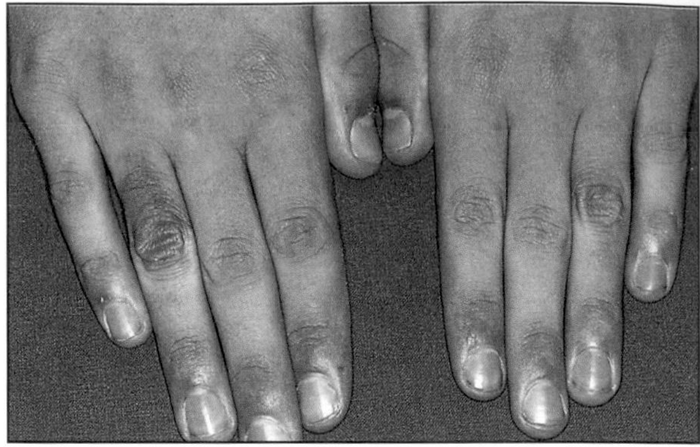

Fig. 18.54. Mechanically induced knuckle pads (false knuckle pads)

Differential Diagnosis. The main differential diagnostic consideration is false knuckle pads or calluses, which are clearly related to trauma, are asymmetric, poorly circumscribed and arise later in life (Fig. 18.54). Other disorders discussed below should also be considered.

Therapy. No successful therapy exists.

Kauschwielen

(Garrod 1893; Meigel and Plewig 1976)

Synonyms. Chew pads, reactive knuckle pads

Etiology and Pathogenesis. There is no widely accepted English name for this disorder. The German term *Kauschwiele* means literally chew-callus. This concisely summarizes the etiology. Patients suck, chew and otherwise manipulate their digits with their mouths producing a characteristic reaction.

Clinical Findings. The lesions are usually asymptomatic, develop slowly and initially fail to bother the patients or their parents. Typically the radial aspects of the second to fifth fingers are involved, as these are the easiest to chew. Usually the eruption is symmetric (Fig. 18.55). The skin may be raw and appears to be pressed or stamped out. The thickening is greater between the joints and the skin may be folded along the long axis of the finger. If the patient stops chewing, the disorder improves.

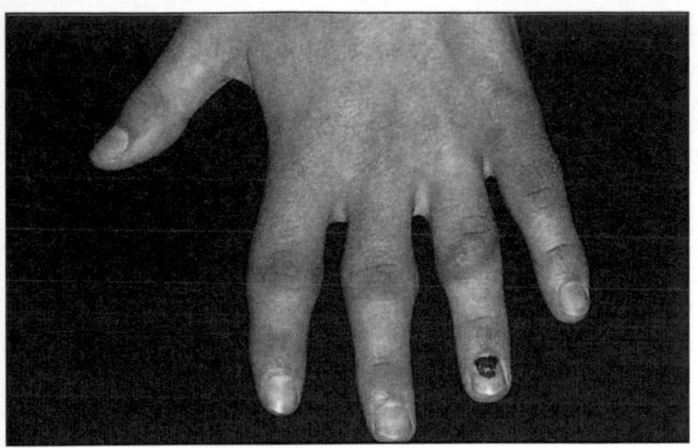

Fig. 18.55. Kauschwielen

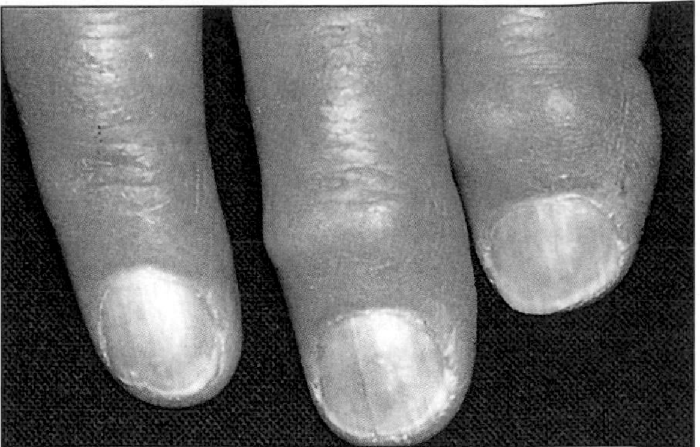

Fig. 18.56. Heberden nodes

Histopathology. The biopsy simply shows reactive epidermal changes (acanthosis, papillomatosis) and dermal fibrosis.

Differential Diagnosis. True knuckle pads are more circumscribed and over the knuckles. Digital calluses from work are also usually over the knuckles but more diffuse. Other digital fibrous tumors, gouty tophi and tuberous xanthomas may appear similar but are readily distinguished by history and biopsy.

Therapy. The best therapy is to stop chewing and manipulating the digits. Healing may be hastened with topical corticosteroids, applied under occlusion at night. Emotional support or even psychologic guidance may also be beneficial.

Pachydermodactyly

(Verbov 1975)

These patients, usually young men, have symmetric thickening and swelling of the proximal phalanges. Usually the second to fourth fingers are involved. If the patients are carefully observed, almost all of them as a matter of habit interlock their fingers and then apply pressure. It is conceivable that the repeated episodes of minor trauma play a role in predisposed individuals. Some patients also have carpal tunnel syndrome, supporting the idea of an underlying tendency towards fibrosis. While the lesions are rarely biopsied, they show mild dermal fibrosis. Patients with pachydermoperiostosis have thickened digits but also many other distinguishing features. No good therapy exists.

Heberden Nodes

(Heberden 1802)

Patients with chronic degenerative arthritis (osteoarthritis) typically develop hard nodules on the dorsal or lateral aspects of their digits about the joints (Fig. 18.56). The lesions are very common, present in over half of women more than 60 years old and to a lesser extent in men. There appears to be a familial tendency to develop the nodules. The typical sites are the distal interphalangeal joints of the second, third and fifth fingers. When the proximal interphalangeal joints are affected, one speaks of Bouchard nodes. The lesions develop in association with exostoses and cartilaginous proliferations. The nodules are somewhat movable. They may become quite large and interfere with function. Occasionally gelatinous cysts develop and may rupture. Typically there may also be lateral deviation of the terminal phalanx.

Gouty tophi, rheumatoid nodules, tuberous xanthomas and digital fibromas may appear similar. Heberden nodes have a distinctive radiologic appearance, and the others can to some extent be sorted out with a biopsy. Often Heberden nodes are present simultaneously with tophi. A biopsy should be performed only if serious clinical questions exist, as healing is slow and a disabling digital ulcer may develop. No therapy other than treating the pain is available.

Dupuytren Contracture

(Dupuytren 1831)

Synonyms. Fibromatosis palmaris, palmar fibromatosis

Epidemiology. Dupuytren contracture is primarily a disease of older men. About 2–6% of the population are affected. In older age groups, up to 20% of men are affected to some degree. In women, the disease appears later. There appears to be autosomal dominant inheritance, with an association with knuckle pads and other fibromatoses, such as Ledderhose disease, Peyronie disease and even fibrosis of the male breast. In such cases, one speaks of polyfibromatosis. Alleged associations with liver cirrhosis, diabetes mellitus, alcoholism and even AIDS are difficult to sort out because of the commonness of all the disorders.

Etiology and Pathogenesis. The etiology remains unclear. Genetic predisposition, trauma and perhaps vascular ischemia stimulate the fibroblastic proliferation and the transition to myofibroblasts which then furthers the contractures.

Clinical Findings. Dupuytren contracture is slowly progressive and often bilateral. It is divided into four grades:

- Grade I. Circumscribed palpable nodules on the palmar aponeuroses, most often involving the fourth digit
- Grade II. Minimal contractures with slightly restricted metacarpal-phalangeal joint motion
- Grade III. Restriction of proximal interphalangeal joints or proximal thumb joint
- Grade IV. In addition, restriction of distal interphalangeal joints

Initially the patient simply notices a thickening in the palm, which moves with digital motion. If the disease progresses, there is inevitable restriction of motion and occasionally pain. The overlying skin becomes attached to the fibrous proliferation. As the patient attempts to straighten the digits, the aponeurotic bands, which become more prominent, can be palpated (Fig. 18.57).

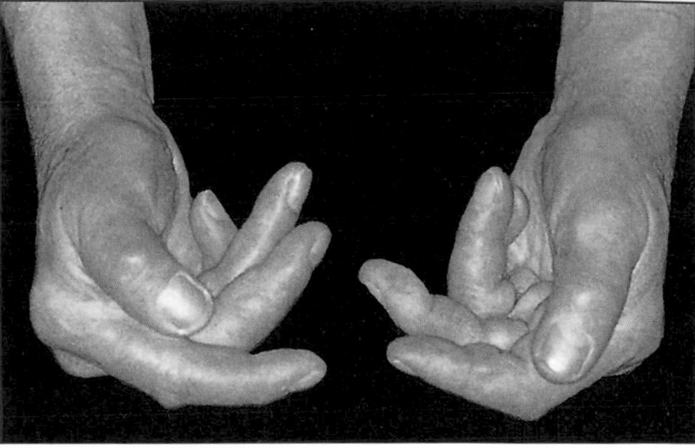

Fig. 18.57. Dupuytren contracture

Histopathology. The initial nodules are rich in fibroblasts and can be mistaken for a tumor. Later the proliferation is quite cell-poor, resembling a tendon. Electron microscopy reveals myofibroblasts.

Course and Prognosis. In severe cases, the hand is permanently held as a fist, predisposing to intertrigo and candidiasis in the permanent creases.

Differential Diagnosis. There is no true differential diagnosis. Calcifying aponeurotic fibroma can be similar but appears in children (Chap. 59). Campodactyly refers to a hereditary or acquired flexion contracture of the proximal interphalangeal joint of the fifth finger. The condition is painless and usually starts in childhood.

Therapy. In general, the best treatment is surgical excision which is usually highly successful. In early stages, intralesional corticosteroid injections and even soft X-ray therapy (4 Gy daily for 2 days, then 2-month pause, repeated for a total dose of 24 Gy) are employed. Radiation therapy may make subsequent surgery more difficult. No topical therapy is effective.

Ledderhose Disease

(LEDDERHOSE 1895)

Synonyms. Fibromatosis plantans, plantar fibromatosis

Ledderhose disease is similar to Dupuytren contracture but involves the plantar surface (Fig. 18.58). It is much less common than Dupuytren contracture. In addition, restriction of joint motion

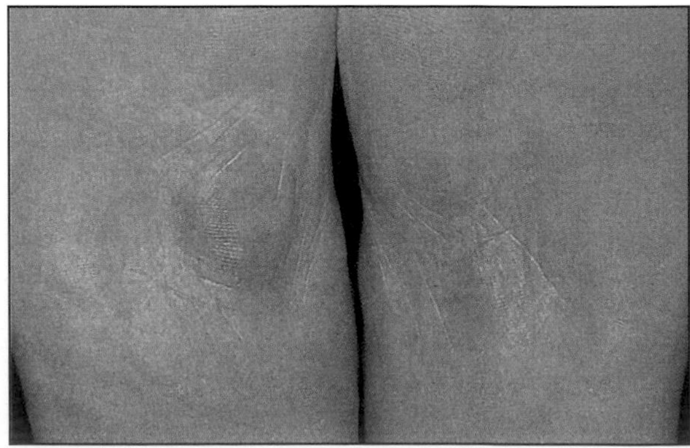

Fig. 18.58. Ledderhose diseas

through contractures occurs infrequently. The great toe is most often involved. Treatment is similar.

Peyronie Disease

(DE LA PEYRONIE 1743)

Synonyms. Induratio penis plastica, fibromatosis penis, deviated penis

History. François de la Peyronie was the personal physician of King Louis XIV of France; the disease appears to have royal origins.

Epidemiology. Uncommon disorder; usually first noticed after 40 years of age.

Etiology and Pathogenesis. The etiology is unknown. The association with other fibromatoses is well documented; 10% of patients also have Dupuytren contracture.

Clinical Findings. The initial finding is usually a focal area of hardening just behind the glans on the dorsal aspect of the penis. The fibrosis involves the tunica albuginea with localized or diffuse changes which typically spread proximally. One can palpate plate-like, ring-like or pencil-like areas of hardening. The penile septum and corpora cavernosa may also be affected. Rarely there is ventral, even periurethral hardening. Urination is normal.

When the penis is flaccid, the hardened areas are scarcely noticed. The erect penis tends to deviate to one side or upwards, producing the most puzzling manifestation of Peyronie disease. The overlying skin is always freely movable, in contrast to Dupuytren contracture. Problems can include pain on intercourse, and even secondary impotence with its associated emotional problems.

Histopathology. The tunica albuginea shows initially cell-rich inflammatory and then later cell-poor nodules and masses of myofibroblastic proliferation. There may be secondary calcification and even dysplastic formation of cartilage and bone. While the term penile bone is sometimes used, it is incorrect. True penile bone can rarely be seen in humans and is an embryologic relic of the common penile bones of several other species of mammals.

Laboratory Findings. Both ultrasound and magnetic resonance imaging can be used to further document the changes. Calcified or ossified areas can be seen on routine radiographs.

Course and Prognosis. The pain tends to decrease after a period of months. In some patients, the fibrosis regresses, while in others, it progresses so that striking deviation of the penis occurs. Malignant change is not seen.

Differential Diagnosis. Once again, the clinical picture is so classic that the diagnosis is usually easy. In early cases, the clinical findings may be subtle unless the erect penis is seen. In unusual cases (such as early age, ulceration or the like) one may wish to do a biopsy to exclude a soft tissue tumor.

Therapy. Treatment is difficult. Early lesions can be treated with intralesional corticosteroids or radiation therapy, just as Dupuytren contracture. Irradiation is helpful in 30–50% of patients, especially relieving pain. Other techniques such as telecesium radiation and electron beam (6–9 meV electrons) therapy have also been helpful in specialized centers. Surgery is a final resort, but less successful than with the other fibromatoses, with postoperative impotence a potential problem.

Bibliography

General

Kühn K, Krieg T (eds) (1986) Connective tissue: biological and clinical aspects. Karger, Basel

Mutasim DF, Adams BB (2000) A practical guide for serologic evaluation of autoimmune connective tissue diseases. J Am Acad Dermatol 42:159–174

Prockop DJ, Kivirikko KI (1995) Collagens: molecular biology, diseases, and potentials for therapy. Annu Rev Biochem 64:403–434

Royce PM, Steinman B (eds) (1993) Connective tissue and its heritable disorders. Wiley-Liss, New York

Schumacher HR Jr (ed) (1993) Primer on the rheumatic diseases. Arthritis Foundation, Atlanta

Hereditary Disorders of Connective Tissue

Aoyama T, Francke U, Gasner C et al. (1995) Fibrillin abnormalities and prognosis in Marfan syndrome and related disorders. Am J Med Genet 58:169–176

Ascher KW (1920) Blepharochalasis mit Struma und Doppellippe. Mbl Augenhk 65:86–97

Beighton P, De Paepe A, Steinmann B et al. (1998) Ehlers-Danlos syndrome: revised nosology, Villefranche, 1997. Ehlers-Danlos National Foundation (USA) and Ehlers-Danlos Support Group (UK). Am J Med Genet 28:31–37

Burrows NP, Nicholls AC, Yates JRW et al. (1996) The gene encoding collagen αa_1 (V) (COL5A1) is linked to mixed Ehlers-Danlos syndrome type I/II. J Invest Dermatol 106:1273–1276

Cat I, Magdalena NI, Marinoni LP et al. (1974) Letter: Parana hard-skin syndrome: study of seven families. Lancet 1:215–216

Christensen OB (1978) An exogenous variety of pseudoxanthoma elasticum in old farmers. Acta Derm Venereol (Stockh) 58:319–321

Colige A, Sieron AL, Li SW et al. (1999) Human Ehlers-Danlos syndrome type VII C and bovine dermatosparaxis are caused by mutations in the procollagen I N-proteinase gene. Am J Hum Genet 65:308–317

Danielsen L (1979) Morphological changes in pseudoxanthoma elasticum and senile skin. Acta Derm Venereol (Stockh) 59 [Suppl 83]:1–79

Danlos H (1908) Un cas de cutis laxa avec tumeurs por contusion chronique de coudes et des genoux (xanthoma juvenile pseudo-diabetique de MM. Hallopeau et Mace de Lepinay. Bull Soc Fr Derm Syph 19:70–72

Darier J (1896) Pseudoxanthoma elasticum. Monatsschr Prakt Dermatol 23:609–616

Dembure PP, Janko AR, Priest JH et al. (1987) Ascorbate regulation of collagen biosynthesis in Ehlers-Danlos syndrome, type VI. Metabolism 36:687–691

Ehlers E (1901) Neigung zu Hämorrhagen in der Haut, Lockerung mehrerer Artikulationen. Dermatol Zschr 8: 173–174

Esterly NB, McKusick VA (1971) Stiff skin syndrome. Pediatrics 47:360–369

Foster K, Ferrel R, King-Underwood L et al. (1993) Description of a dinucleotide repeat polymorphism in the human elastin gene and its use to confirm assignment of the gene to chromosome 7. Ann Hum Genet 57:87–96

Grönblad E (1933) Pseudoxanthoma elasticum and changes in the eye. Acta Derm Venereol (Stockh) 13:417–422

Happle R, Stekhoven JH, Hamel BC et al. (1992) Restrictive dermopathy in two brothers. Arch Dermatol 128:232–235

Kuivaniemi H, Peltonen L, Kivirikko KI (1985) Type IX Ehlers-Danlos syndrome and Menkes syndrome: the decrease in lysyl oxidase activity is associated with a corresponding deficiency in the enzyme protein. Am J Hum Genet 37:798–808

Laffer WB (1909) Blepharochalasis. Report of a case of this trophoneurosis involving also the upper lip. Cleveland Med J 8:131–135

Marfan AB (1896) Un cas de deformation congénitale des quatre membre, plus prononcées aux extrémités, caractérisée par l'allongement des os avec un certain degré d'aminicissement. Bull Soc Méd Hop 13:220–226

Mau U, Kendziorra H, Kaiser P et al. (1997) Restrictive dermopathy: report and review. Am J Med Genet 71: 179–185

Nielsen AO, Christensen OB, Hentzer B et al. (1978) Salpeter-induced dermal changes electron-microscopically indistinguishable from pseudoxanthoma elasticum. Acta Derm Venereol (Stockh) 58:323–327

Nuytinck L, Sayli BS, Karen W et al. (1999) Prenatal diagnosis of osteogenesis imperfecta type I by COL1A1 null-allele testing. Prenat Diagn 19:873–875

Paige DG, Lake BD, Bailey AJ et al. (1992) Restrictive dermopathy: a disorder of fibroblasts. Br J Dermatol 127: 630–634

Pepin M, Schwarze U, Superti-Furga A et al. (2000) Clinical and genetic features of Ehlers-Danlos syndrome type IV, the vascular type. N Engl J Med 342:673

Pope FM (1974) Two types of autosomal recessive pseudoxanthoma elasticum. Arch Dermatol 110:209–212

Pope FM (1975) Historical evidence for the genetic heterogeneity of pseudoxanthoma elasticum. Br J Dermatol 92:493–509

Ramirez F, Gayraud B, Pereira L (1999) Marfan syndrome: new clues to genotype-phenotype correlations. Ann Med 31:202–207

Richard MA, Grob JJ, Philip N et al. (1998) Physiopathogenic investigations in a case of familial stiff-skin syndrome. Dermatology 197:127–131

Sanchez MR, Lee M, Moy JA et al. (1993) Ascher syndrome: a mimicker of acquired angioedema. J Am Acad Dermatol 29:650–651

Sherer DW, Sapadin AN, Lebwohl MG (1999) Pseudoxanthoma elasticum: an update. Dermatology 199:3–7

Sillevis Smitt JH, van Asperen CJ, Niessen CM et al. (1998) Restrictive dermopathy. Report of 12 cases. Dutch Task Force on Genodermatology. Arch Dermatol 134:577–579

Sorokin Y, Johnson MP, Rogowski N et al. (1994) Obstetric and gynecologic dysfunction in the Ehlers-Danlos syndrome. J Reprod Med 39:281–284

Strandberg J (1929) Pseudoxanthoma elasticum. Zentralbl Hautkr 31:689

Tschernogubow AN (1892) Über einen Fall von Cutis Laxa. Mtschr Prakt Dermatol 14:76

Van Meekeren JA (1682) De dilatabilitate extraordinaria cutis. Obersavtiones Medichochirugicae, Chap. 32, Amsterdam

Witt DR, Hayden MR, Holbrook KA et al. (1986) Restrictive dermopathy: a newly recognized autosomal skin dysplasia. Am J Med Genet 24:631–648

Wooldridge WE, Frerichs JB (1960) Amyloidosis: a new clinical type. Arch Dermatol 82:230–234

Premature Aging Syndromes

Blaszczyk M, Depaepe A, Nuytincle L et al. (2000) Acrogeria of the Gottron type in a mother and son. Eur J Dermatol 10:36–40

Cleaver JE, Thompson LH, Richardson AS et al. (1999) A summary of mutations in the UV-sensitive disorders: xeroderma pigmentosum, Cockayne syndrome, and trichothiodystrophy. Hum Mutat 14:9–22

Cockayne EA (1936) Dwarfism with retinal atrophy and deafness. Arch Dis Child 11:1–8

Curshmann J (1912) Über familiäre atrophische Myotonie. Deut Zschr Nervenheilk 45:161–202

Eriksson M, Ansved T, Edstrom L et al. (1999) Simultaneous analysis of expression of the three myotonic dystrophy locus genes in adult skeletal muscle samples: the CTG expansion correlates inversely with DMPK and 59 expression levels, but not DMAHP levels. Hum Mol Genet 8:1053–1060

Fleischmajer R, Nedwich A (1973) Progeria (Hutchinson-Gilford). Arch Dermatol 107:253–258

Gilford H (1904) Progeria: a form of senilism. Practitioner 73:188–217

Gilkes JJ, Sharvill DE, Wells RS (1974) The premature ageing syndromes. Report of eight cases and description of a new entity named metageria. Br J Dermatol 91:243–262

Gottron H (1941) Familiäre Akrogerie. Arch Dermatol 181:571–583

Gray MD, Shen JC, Kamath-Loeb AS et al. (1997) The Werner syndrome protein is a DNA helicase. Nat Genet 17: 100–103

Hutchinson J (1886) Case of congenital absence of hair with atrophic condition of the skin and its appendages. Lancet I:923
Pesce K, Rothe MJ (1996) The premature aging syndromes. Clin Dermatol 14:161–170
Steinert H (1909) Myopathologische Beitrage. I. Über das klinische und anatomische Bild des Muskelschwunds der Myotoniker. Deutsch Zschr Nervenheilk 37:58–104
Venencie PY, Powell FC, Winkelmann RK (1984) Acrogeria with perforating elastoma and bony abnormalities. Acta Derm Venereol (Stockh) 64:348–351
Werner O (1904) Über Katarakt in Verbindung mit Sklerodermie. Dissertation, University of Kiel
Wiedemann HR (1948) Über Greisenhaftigkeit im Kindesalter, insbesondere die Gilfordsche Progerie. Z Kinderheilkd 65:670–697

Congenital Poikilodermas

Brain RT (1952) Poikiloderma congenitale (Thomson). Proceedings of the 10th international congress on dermatology, London. pp 531–533
Burgdorf W, Kurvink K, Cervenka J (1977) Sister chromatid exchange in dyskeratosis congenita lymphocytes. J Med Genet 14:256–257
Cole HN, Rauschkolb JE, Toomey J (1930) Dyskeratosis congenita with pigmentation, dystrophia unguis and leukokeratosis oris. Arch Dermatol Syphilol 21:71
Engman M (1926) A unique case of reticular pigmentations of the skin with atrophy. Arch Dermatol Syphilol 13: 685–686
Fanconi G (1927) Familiäre, infantile, perniciosaähnliche Anämie. (Pernizioses Blutbild und Konstitution). Jahrb Kinder 117:257–280
Hassock S, Vetrie D, Giannelli F (1999) Mapping and characterization of the X-linked dyskeratosis congenita (DKC) gene. Genomics 55:21–27
Kindler T (1954) Congenital poikiloderma with traumatic bulba formation and progressive cutaneous atrophy. Br J Derm 66:104–111
Kitao S, Lindor NM, Shiratori M et al. (1999) Rothmund-Thomson syndrome responsible gene, RECQL4: genomic structure and products. Genomics 61:268–276
Marghescu S, Braun-Falco O (1965) Über die kongenitalen Poikilodermien: ein analytischer Versuch. Dermatol Wochenschr 15:9–19
Rothmund A von (1868) Über Cataracte in Verbindung mit einer eigentümlichen Hautdegeneration. Arch Ophthalmol 14:159–182
Thomson MS (1923) A hitherto undescribed familial disease. Br J Dermatol Syph 35:455
Weary PE, Hsu YT, Richardson DR et al. (1969) Hereditary sclerosing poikiloderma. Report of two families with an unusual and distinctive genodermatosis. Arch Dermatol 100:413–422
Weary PE, Manley WF Jr, Graham GF (1971) Hereditary acrokeratotic poikiloderma. Arch Dermatol 103:409–422
Zinsser F (1910) Atrophia cutis reticularis cum pigmentatione, dystrophia unguium et leukoplakia oris. In: Nesser AQ, Jacobi E (eds) Ikonographia dermatologica. Urban and Schwarzenberg, Berlin, pp 219–223

Acquired Cutaneous Atrophy

Darier J (1920) Atrophodermie vermiculée des joues avec kératoses folliculaires. Bull Soc Fr Dermatol Syphil 27:345
Jadassohn J (1892) Über eine eigenartige Form von "Atrophia maculosa cutis". Arch Dermatol Syph [Suppl] 1:342–358
Kligman AM (1969) Early destructive effect of sunlight on human skin. JAMA 210:2377–2380
Moulin G, Hill MP, Guliiaud VP et al. (1992) Acquired atrophic pigmented band-like lesions following Blaschko's lines [in French]. Ann Dermatol Venereol 119:729–736
Romberg MH von (1846) Trophoneurosen. In: Klinische Ergebnisse. Berlin, pp 75–81
Shelley WB, Cohen W (1964) Striae migrans. Arch Dermatol 90:193–194
Singh M, Bharija SC, Belhaj MS et al. (1985) Romberg's syndrome: a case report. Dermatologica 170:145–156
Uitto J (1986) Connective tissue biochemistry of the aging dermis. Age-related alterations in collagen and elastin. Dermatol Clin 4:433–446
Winer LH (1936) Atrophodermia reticulatum. Arch Dermatol Syphil 34:980
Wollenberg A, Baumann L, Plewig G (1996) Linear atrophoderma of Moulin: a disease which follows Blaschko's lines. Br J Dermatol 135:277–279
Zheng P, Lavker RM, Kligman AM (1985) Anatomy of striae. Br J Dermatol 112:185–193

Disorders of Elastic Fibers

Balus L, Amantea A, Donati P et al. (1997) Fibroelastolytic papulosis of the neck: a report of 20 cases. Br J Dermatol 137:461–466
Burket JM, Zelickson AS, Padilla RS (1989) Linear focal elastosis (elastotic striae). J Am Acad Dermatol 20: 633–636
Carter VH, Constantine VS, Poole WL (1969) Elastotic nodules of the antihelix. Arch Dermatol 100:282–285
Costa OG (1953) Acrokeratoelastoidosis: a hitherto undescribed skin disease. Dermatologica 107:164–167
Ebner H, Gebhard W (1977) Colloid milium: light and electron microscopic investigations. Clin Exp Dermatol 2:217–226
English DT, Martin GC, Reisner JE (1971) Dermabrasion for nodular cutaneous elastosis with cysts and comedones. Favre-Racouchot syndrome. Arch Dermatol 104:92–93
Favre M, Racouchot J (1951) L'élastéidose cutanée nodulaire à kystes et à comédones. Ann Dermatol Syphil 78: 681–702
Graham JH, Marques AS (1967) Colloid milium: a histochemical study. J Invest Dermatol 49:497–507
Hashimoto K, Katzman RL, Kang AH et al. (1957) Electron microscopical and biochemical analysis of colloid milium. Arch Dermatol 111:49–59
Hashimoto K, Miller F, Bereston AS (1972) Colloid milium. Arch Dermatol 105:684–694
Jordaan HF, Rossouw DF (1990) Digital papular calcific elastosis: a histopathological, histochemical and ultrastructural study of 20 patients. J Cutan Pathol 17(6):358–370
Jung EG, Beil EV, Anton-Lamprecht J et al. (1974) Akrokeratoelastoidosis. Hautarzt 25:127–133
Miller WM, Ruggles CW, Rist TE (1979) Anetoderma. Int J Dermatol 18:43–45
Oikarinen AI, Palatsi R, Adomian GE et al. (1984) Anetoderma: biochemical and ultrastructural demonstration of

elastin defect in the skin of three patients. J Am Acad Dermatol 11:64–72
Pellizzari C (1884) Eritema orticato atrofizzante: atrofia parziale idiopatica della pelle. G Ital Mal Ven 19:230–243
Plewig G, Braun-Falco O (1971) Behandlung von Comedonen bei Morbus Favre-Racouchot und Acne venenata mit Vitamin A-Säure. Hautarzt 22:341–345
Schwenninger E, Buzzi F (1889–1899) Multiple benign tumour-like new growths of the skin. In: Unna PG, Morris M, Besner E et al. (eds) International atlas of rare skin diseases, vol 5, part 1, chap 15. Voss, Hamburg, pp 4–5
Shelley WB, Wood MG (1977) Wrinkles due to idiopathic loss of mid-dermal elastic tissue. Br J Dermatol 97:441–445
Shimizu H, Kimura S, Harada T et al. (1989) White fibrous papulosis of the neck: a new clinicopathologic entity? J Am Acad Dermatol 20:1073–1077
Shuster S (1979) The cause of striae distensae. Acta Derm Venereol (Stockh) 59 [Suppl 85]:105–108
Venencie PY, Winkelmann RK (1984) Histopathologic findings in anetoderma. Arch Dermatol 120:1040–1044
Venencie PY, Winkelmann RK, Burton AM (1984) Anetoderma. Arch Dermatol 120:1032–1039

Perforating Disorders

Bong JL, Fleming CJ, Kemmett D (2000) Reactive perforating collagenosis associated with underlying malignancy. Br J Dermatol 42:390–391
Fretzin DF, Beal DW, Jao W (1980) Light and ultrastructural study of reactive perforating collagenosis. Arch Dermatol 116:1054–1058
Hill VA, Seymour CA, Mortimer PS (2000) Pencillamine-induced elastosis perforans serpiginosa and cutis laxa in Wilson disease. Br J Dermatol 142:560–561
Kirsch N, Hukill PB (1977) Elastosis perforans serpiginosa induced by penicillamine. Arch Dermatol 113:630–635
Kumar V, Mehndiratta V, Sharma RC et al. (1998) Familial reactive perforating collagenosis: a case report. J Dermatol 25:54–56
Laugier P, Woringer F (1963) Refléxions au sujet d'un collagénome perforant verucciforme. Ann Dermatol Syph 90:29–36
Lutz W (1953) Keratosis follicularis serpiginosa. Dermatologica 106:318–320
Mehregan AH (1968) Elastosis perforans serpiginosa. A review of the literature and report of 11 cases. Arch Dermatol 97:381–393
Mehregan AH (1977) Perforating dermatoses: a clinicopathologic review. Int J Dermatol 16:19–27
Mehregan AH, Schwartz OD, Livingood CS (1967) Reactive perforating collagenosis. Arch Dermatol 96:277–282
Miescher G (1955) Elastoma intrapapillare perforans verruciforme. Dermatologica 110:254–266
Patterson JW (1984) The perforating disorders. J Am Acad Dermatol 10:561–581
Patterson JW (1989) Progress in the perforating disorders. Arch Dermatol 125:1121–1123

Lichen Sclerosis et Atrophicus

García-Bravo B, Sánchez-Pedreno P, Rodríguez-Pichardo A et al. (1988) Lichen sclerosus et atrophicus. A study of 76 cases and their relation to diabetes. J Am Acad Dermatol 19:482–485
Hart WR, Norris JH, Helwig EB (1975) Relation of lichen sclerosus et atrophicus of the vulva to development of carcinoma. Obstet Gynecol 45:369–377
Kint A, Geerts ML (1975) Lichen sclerosus et atrophicus. J Cutan Pathol 2:30–34
Meffert JJ, Davis BM, Grimwood RE (1995) Lichen sclerosus. J Am Acad Dermatol 32:393–416
Mihara Y, Mihara M, Hagari Y et al. (1994) Lichen sclerosus et atrophicus. A histological, immunohistochemical and electron microscopic study. Arch Dermatol Res 286:434–442
Powell JJ, Wojnarowska F (1999) Lichen sclerosus. Lancet 353:1777–1783
Wallace HJ (1971) Lichen sclerosus et atrophicus. Trans St John's Hosp Dermatol Soc 57:9–30

Scleroderma

Barnes L, Roduan GP, Medsger TA et al. (1979) Eosinophilic fasciitis – a pathologic study of twenty cases. Am J Pathol 96:493–518
Bell SA (1996) The toxic oil syndrome: an example of an exogenously induced autoimmune reaction. Mol Biol Rep 23:261–262
Bell SA, Hobbs MV, Rubin RL (1992) Isotype-restricted hyperimmunity in a murine model of the toxic oil syndrome. J Immunol 148:3369–3376
Coyle HE, Chapman RS (1980) Eosinophilic fasciitis (Shulman syndrome) in association with morphea and systemic sclerosis. Acta Derm Venereol (Stockh) 60:181–182
Diaz-Perez JL, Connolly SM, Winkelmann RK (1980) Disabling pansclerotic morphea of children. Arch Dermatol 116:169–173
Doyle JA, Conolly SM, Winkelmann RK (1982) Cutaneous and subcutaneous inflammatory sclerosis syndromes. Arch Dermatol 118:886–890
Eidson M, Philen RM, Sewell CM et al. (1990) L-tryptophan and eosinophilia-myalgia syndrome in New Mexico. Lancet 335:645–648
Fleischmajer R (1979) The pathophysiology of scleroderma. Int J Dermatol 16:310–318
Golitz LE (1980) Fasciitis with eosinophilia: the Shulman syndrome. Int J Dermatol 19:552–555
Hein R, Behr J, Hundgen M et al. (1992) Treatment of systemic sclerosis with gamma-interferon. Br J Dermatol 126:496–501
Jabłońska S (ed) (1975) Scleroderma and pseudoscleroderma. Polish Medical Publishers, Warsaw
Krausner RE, Tuthill RJ (1977) Eosinophilic fasciitis. Arch Dermatol 113:1092–1093
Krieg T, Meurer M (1988) Systemic scleroderma. Clinical and pathophysiologic aspects. J Am Acad Dermatol 18:457–481
Krieg T, Perlish JS, Mauch C et al. (1985) Collagen synthesis by scleroderma fibroblasts. Ann N Y Acad Sci 460: 375–386
Lüftl M, Degitz K, Plewig G et al. (1997) Psoralen bath plus UV-A therapy. Possibilities and limitations. Arch Dermatol 133:1597–1603
Michet CJ Jr, Dogle JA, Ginsburg WW (1981) Eosinophilic fasciitis: report of 15 cases. Mayo Clin Proc 56:27–34
Nelson JL (1998) Microchimerism and the pathogenesis of systemic sclerosis. Curr Opin Rheumatol 10:564–571
Pasini A (1923) Atrofodermia idiopatica progressiva. (Studio clinico ed istologico). Gior Ital Mal Vener 64:785–809

Pierini LE, Vivoli D (1936) Atrofodermia idiopatica progressiva (Pasini). Gior Ital Derm 77:403–409

Sackner MA (1962) The visceral manifestations of scleroderma. Arthritis Rheum 5:184–196

Shulman LE (1974) Diffuse fasciitis with hypergammaglobulinemia and eosinophilia: a new syndrome? J Rheumatol [Suppl] 1:46

Silman AJ (1997) Scleroderma – demographics and survival. J Rheumatol 48S:58–61

Subcommitee for Scleroderma Criteria of the American Rheumatism Association (1980) Preliminary criteria for the classification of systemic sclerosis (scleroderma). Arthritis Rheum 23:581–590

Tan FK, Arnett FC, Antohi S et al. (1999) Autoantibodies to the extracellular matrix microfibrillar protein, fibrillin-1, in patients with scleroderma and other connective tissue diseases. J Immunol 163:1066–1072

Thibiérge G, Weissenbach RJ (1911) Concrétions calcaires sous cutanées et sclérodermia. Ann Dermatol Syph 2: 129–155

Varga J, Uitto J, Jimenez SA (1992) The cause and pathogenesis of the eosinophilia-myalgia syndrome. Ann Intern Med 116(2):140–147

Winterbauer RH (1964) Multiple telangiectasia, Raynaud's phenomenon, sclerodactyly, and subcautaneous calcinosis. Bull Johns Hopkins Hosp 114:361–383

Lupus Erythematosus

Bettinotti MP, Hartung K, Deicher H et al. (1993) Polymorphism of the tumor necrosis factor-beta gene in systemic lupus erythematosus: TNFB-MHC haplotypes. Immunogenetics 37:449–454

Burlingame RW (1997) The clinical utility of antihistone antibodies. Autoantibodies reactive with chromatin in systemic lupus erythematosus and drug-induced lupus. Clin Lab Med 17:367–378

Burlingame RW, Boey ML, Starkebaum G et al. (1994) The central role of chromatin in autoimmune responses to histones and DNA in systemic lupus erythematosus. J Clin Invest 94:184–192

Callen JP (1982) Chronic cutaneous lupus erythematosus. Arch Dermatol 118:412–416

Callen JP (1985) Systemic lupus erythematosus in patients with chronic cutaneous (discoid) lupus erythematosus. Clinical and laboratory findings in seventeen patients. J Am Acad Dermatol 12:278–288

Casciola-Rosen LA, Anhalt G, Rosen A (1994) Autoantigens targeted in systemic lupus erythematosus are clustered in two populations of surface structures on apoptotic keratinocytes. J Exp Med 179:1317–1330

Chan LS, Lapiere J-C, Chen M et al. (1999) Bullous systemic lupus erythematosus with autoantibodies recognizing multiple skin basement membrane components, bullous pemphigoid antigen 1, laminin-5, laminin-6, and type VII collagen. Arch Dermatol 135:569–573

Davies EJ, Snowden N, Hillarby MC et al. (1995) Mannose-binding protein gene polymorphism in systemic lupus erythematosus. Arthritis Rheum 38:110–114

Davis BM, Gilliam JN (1984) Prognostic significance of subepidermal immune deposits in uninvolved skin of patients with systemic lupus erythematosus: a 10-year longitudinal study. J Invest Dermatol 83:242–247

Dekle CL, Mannes KD, Davis LS et al. (1999) Lupus tumidus. J Am Acad Dermatol 41:250–253

Deng JS, Sontheimer RD, Gilliam JN (1984) Relationships between antinuclear and anti-Ro SS-A antibodies in subacute cutaneous lupus erythematosus. J Am Acad Dermatol 11:494–499

Fischer GF, Pickl WF, Fae I et al. (1994) Association between chronic cutaneous lupus erythematosus and HLA class II alleles. Hum Immunol 41:280–284

Franco HL, Weston WL, Plebes C et al. (1981) Autoantibodies directed against sicca syndrome antigens in the neonatal lupus syndrome. J Am Acad Dermatol 4: 67–72

Fritzler MJ (1994) Drugs recently associated with lupus syndromes. Lupus 3:455–459

Gaffney PM, Kearns GM, Shark KB et al. (1998) A genome-wide search for susceptibility genes in human systemic lupus erythematosus sib-pair families. Proc Natl Acad Sci USA 95:14875–14879

Gilliam JN, Sontheimer RD (1981) Distinctive cutaneous subsets in the spectrum of lupus erythematosus. J Am Acad Dermatol 4:471–475

Guenther LC (1983) Inherited disorders of complement. J Am Acad Dermatol 9:815–839

Hahn BH (1998) Antibodies to DNA. N Engl J Med 338: 1359–1368

Hartung K, Baur MP, Coldewey R et al. (1992) Major histocompatibility complex haplotypes and complement C4 alleles in systemic lupus erythematosus. Results of a multicenter study. J Clin Invest 90:1346–1351

Hebra F, Kaposi M (1875) On disease of the skin, including exanthemata. New Sydenahm Society 4:1–247

Hochberg MC (1997) Updating the American College of Rheumatology revised criteria for the classification of systemic lupus erythematosus. Arthritis Rheum 40: 1725–1734

Ioannides D, Golden BD, Buyon JP et al. (2000) Expression of SS-A/Ro and SS-B/La antigens in skin biopsy specimens of patients with photosensitive forms of lupus erythematosus. Arch Dermatol 136:340–346

Irgang S (1954) Apropos du lupus erythemateux profond. Ann Derm Syph 81:246–249

Kephart DC, Hood AF, Provost TT (1981) Neonatal lupus erythematosus: new serologic findings. J Invest Dermatol 77:331–333

Klinenberg, Wallace DJ, Quismorio FP et al. (1990) DuBois' lupus erythematosus, 5th edn. Williams and Wilkins, Philadelphia

Lahita RG (ed) (1998) Systemic lupus erythematosus. Academic Press, New York

McCuistion CH, Schoch EP Jr (1954) Possible discoid lupus erythematosus in newborn infant: report of a case with subsequent development of acute systemic lupus erythematosus in mother. Arch Dermatol 70: 782–785

Milliard LG, Rowell NR (1978) Chilblain lupus erythematosus (Hutchinson). Br J Dermatol 98:497–506

Olansky AJ (1982) Bullous systemic lupus erythematosus. J Am Acad Dermatol 7:511–516

Peter JB, Shoenfeld Y (1996) Autoantibodies. Elsevier, Amsterdam

Provost TT (1979) Subsets in systemic lupus erythematosus. J Invest Dermatol 72:110–113

Provost TT, Watson R, Gammon WR et al. (1987) The neonatal lupus syndrome associated with U_1-RNP (nRNP) antibodies. N Engl J Med 316:1135–1138

Prystowsky SD, Gilliam JN (1975) Discoid lupus erythematosus as part of a larger disease spectrum. Arch Dermatol 111:1448–1452

Rowell NR et al. (1963) Lupus erythematosus and erythema multiforme-like lesions. A syndrome with characteristicimmunological abnormalities. Arch Dermatol 88:176–180

Rupec RA, Petropoulou T, Walchner M et al. (2000) Lupus erythematosus tumidus and chronic discoid lupus erythematosus in carriers of X-linked chronic granulomatous disease. Report of two cases and review of the literature. Eur J Dermatol 10:184–189

Ruzicka T, Goerz G (1981) Dapsone in the treatment of lupus erythematosus. Br J Dermatol 104:53–56

Ruzicka T, Meurer M, Bieber T (1988) Efficiency of acitretin in the treatment of cutaneous lupus erythematosus. Arch Dermatol 124:897–902

Salmon JE, Millard S, Schachter JA et al. (1996) FcγRIIA alleles are heritable risk factors for lupus nephritis in African Americans. J Clin Invest 97:1348–1354

Sanchez NP, Peters MS, Winkelmann RK (1981) The histopathology of lupus erythematosus panniculitis. J Am Acad Dermatol 5:673–680

Shen GQ, Shoenfeld Y, Peter JB (1998) Anti-DNA, antihistone, and antinucleosome antibodies in systemic lupus erythematosus and drug-induced lupus. Clin Rev Allergy Immunol 16:321–334

Sheth AP, Esterly NB, Ratoosh SL et al. (1995) U_1RNP positive neonatal lupus erythematosus: association with anti-La antibodies. Br J Dermatol 132:520–526

Sontheimer RD, Thomas JR, Gilliam JN (1979) Subacute cutaneous lupus erythematosus. A cutaneous marker for a distinct lupus erythematosus subset. Arch Dermatol 115:1409–1415

Stein LF, Saed GM, Fivenson DP (1997) T cell cytokine network in cutaneous lupus erythematosus. J Am Acad Dermatol 36:191–196

Tan EM (1982) Special antibodies for the study of systemic lupus erythematosus. An analysis. Arthritis Rheum 25:753–756

Tan EM, Cohen AS, Fries JF et al. (1982) The 1982 revised criteria for the classification of systemic lupus erythematosus. Arthritis Rheum 25:1271–1277

Tani M, Shimizu R, Ban M et al. (1984) Systemic lupus erythematosus with vesiculobullous lesions. Arch Dermatol 120:1497–1501

Tappeiner G (1983) Disease states in genetic complement deficiencies. Int J Dermatol 21:175–191

Walchner M, Messer G, Kind P (1996) Phototesting and photoprotection in LE. Lupus 6:167–174

Walchner M, Leib-Mösch C, Messer G et al. (1997) Endogenous retroviral sequences in the pathogenesis of systemic autoimmune disease. Arch Dermatol 133:767–771

Walchner M, Meurer M, Plewig G et al. (2000) Clinical and immunological parameters during thalidomide treatment of lupus erythematosus. Int J Dermatol 39:1–6

Watson R, Kang E, May M et al. (1988) Thrombocytopenia in the neonatal lupus syndrome. Arch Dermatol 124:560–563

Antiphospholipid Syndrome

Conley CL, Hartmann RC (1952) A hemorrhagic disorder caused by circulating anticoagulant in patients with disseminated lupus erythematosus. J Clin Invest 31:621–622

Douketis JD, Crowther MA, Julian JA et al. (1999) The effects of low-intensity warfarin on coagulation activation in patients with antiphospholipid antibodies and systemic lupus erythematosus. Thromb Haemost 82:1028–1032

Gibson GE, Gibson LE, Drage LA et al. (1997) Skin necrosis secondary to low-molecular weight heparin in a patient with antiphospholipid antibody syndrome. J Am Acad Dermatol 37:855–859

Gibson GE, Su WP, Pittelkow MR (1997) Antiphospholipid syndrome and the skin. J Am Acad Dermatol 36:970–982

Greaves M (1999) Antiphospholipid antibodies and thrombosis. Lancet 353:1348–1353

Harris EN, Boey ML, Mackworth-Young CG et al. (1983) Anticardiolipin antibodies: detection by radioimmunoassay and association with thrombosis in systemic lupus erythematosus. Lancet 26:1211–1214

Hughes GRV (1993) The antiphospholipid syndrome: ten years on. Lancet 342:341–344

Johansson EA, Niemi KM, Mustakallio KK (1977) A peripheral vascular syndrome overlapping with systemic lupus erythematosus. Dermatologica 155:257–267

McNeil HP, Chesterman CN, Krilis SA (1991) Immunology and clinical importance of antiphospholipid antibodies. Adv Immunol 49:193–279

Moore JE, Mohr CF (1952) Biologically false-positive serologic tests for syphilis: type, incidence and cause. JAMA 150:467–473

Munther AK, Cuadrado MJ, Mujic F et al. (1995) The management of thrombosis in the antiphospholipid-antibody syndrome. N Engl J Med 332:993–997

Nahass GT (1997) Antiphospholipid antibodies and the antiphospholipid antibody syndrome. J Am Acad Dermatol 36:149–168

Nilsson IM, Astedt B, Hedber V et al. (1975) Intrauterine death and circulating anticoagulant (antithromboplastin). Acta Med Scand 197:153–159

Out JH, Bruinse HW, Derksen RHWM (1991) Anti-phospholipid antibodies and pregnancy loss. Hum Reprod 6: 889–897

Stephens CJM (1991) The antiphospholipid syndrome. Clinical correlations, cutaneous features, mechanism of thrombosis and treatment of patients with the lupus anticoagulant and anticardiolipin antibodies. Br J Dermatol 125:199–210

Dermatomyositis

Al-Janadi M, Smith CD, Karsh J (1989) Cyclophosphamide treatment of interstitial pulmonary fibrosis in polymyositis dermatomyositis. J Rheumatol 16:1592–1596

Basta M, Dalakas MC (1994) High-dose intravenous immunoglobulin exerts its beneficial effect in patients with dermatomyositis by blocking endomysial deposition of activated complement fragments. J Clin Invest 94: 1729–1742

Bernstein RM, Morgan SH, Chapman J et al. (1984) Anti-Jo-1 antibody: a marker for myositis with interstitial lung disease. BMJ 289:151–152

Bohan A, Peter JB (1975) Polymyositis and dermatomyositis. N Engl J Med 292:344–347, 403–407

Bohan A, Peter JB, Bowman RL et al. (1977) Computer-assisted analysis of 153 patients with polymyositis and dermatomyositis. Medicine 56:255–286

Bonnetblanc JM, Bernard P, Fayol J (1990) Dermatomyositis and malignancy. A multicenter cooperative study. Dermatologica 180:212–216

Bowles NE, Sewry CA, Dubowitz V et al. (1987) Dermatomyositis, polymyositis, and Coxsackie-B-virus infection. Lancet1:1004–1007

Callen J (2000) Dermatomyositis. Lancet 355:53–57

Cosnes A, Amaudric F, Gherardi R et al. (1995) Dermatomyositis without muscle weakness: long-term follow-up of 12 patients without systemic corticosteroids. Arch Dermatol 131:1381–1385

Dalakas MC, Illa I, Dambrosia JM et al. (1993) A controlled trial of high-dose intravenous immune globulin infusions as treatment for dermatomyositis. N Engl J Med 329:1993–2000

Drake LA, Dinehart SM, Farmer ER et al. (1996) Guidelines in care for dermatomyositis. J Am Acad Dermatol 34:824–829

Esteve E, Cambie MP, Serpier H et al. (1994) Paraneoplastic dermatomyositis: efficacy of intravenous gammaglobulin. Br J Dermatol 131:917–918

Euwer R, Sontheimer RD (1991) Amyopathic dermatomyositis. J Am Acad Dermatol 24:959–966

Ghali FE, Stein LD, Fine J-D et al. (1999) Gingival telangiectases. Arch Dermatol 135:1370–1374

Ghate J, Katsambas A, Augerinou G et al. (2000) A therapeutic update on dermatomyositis/polymyositis. Int J Dermatol 39:81–87

Gianini M, Callen JP (1979) Treatment of dermatomyositis with methotrexate and prednisone. Arch Dermatol 115:1251–1252

Gottron HA (1954) Zur Dermatomyositis nebst Bemerkungen zur Poikilodermatomyositis. Dermatol Wochenschr 130:923–930

Hiketa T, Matsumoto Y, Ohashi M et al. (1992) Juvenile dermatomyositis: a statistical study of 114 patients with dermatomyositis. J Dermatol 19:470–476

Janis J, Winkelmann RK (1986) Histopathology of the skin in dermatomyositis. Arch Dermatol 97:640–648

Kasteler JS, Callen JP (1997) Low-dose methotrexate administered weekly is an effective corticoid-sparing agent for the treatment of the cutaneous manifestations of dermatomyositis. J Am Acad Dermatol 36:67–71

Keining E (1939) Versammlung Casus 3 und 4. Dermatol Wochenschr 109:1198–1199

Kovacs SO, Kovacs SC (1998) Dermatomyositis. J Am Acad Dermatol 39:899–920

Lister RK, Cooper ES, Paige DG (2000) Papules and pustules of the elbows and knees: an uncommon clinical sign of dermatomyositis in oriental children. Ped Dermatol 17:37–40

Metzger AL, Bohan A, Goldberg LS et al. (1974) Polymyositis and Dermatomyositis; combined methotrexate and corticosteroid therapy. Ann Intern Med 81:182–189

Sansone A, Dubowitz V (1995) Intravenous immunoglobulin in juvenile dermatomyositis – four year review of nine cases. Arch Dis Child 72:29–32

Sigurgeirsson B (1992) Skin disease and malignancy. An epidemiological study. Acta Derm Venereol (Stockh) Suppl 178:1–110

Sigurgeirsson B, Lindelöf B, Edhag O et al. (1992) Risk of cancer in patients with dermatomyositis or polymyositis. A population-based study. N Engl J Med 326:363–367

Targoff IN, Johnson AE, Miller FW (1990) Antibody to signal recognition particle in polymyositis. Arthritis Rheum 33:1361–1370

Unverricht H (1887) Über eine eigentümliche Form von akuter Muskelentzündung mit einem der Trichinose ähnelnden Krankheitsbilde. Münch Med Wochenschr 34:488–492

Wagner E (1863) Fall einer seltenen Muskelkrankheit. Arch Heilkd 4:282–283

Woo TY, Callen JP, Voorhees JJ et al. (1984) Cutaneous lesions of dermatomyositis are improved by hydroxychloroquine. J Am Acad Dermatol 10:592–600

Mixed Connective Tissue Disease

Black C (1981) Mixed connective tissue disease. Br J Dermatol 104:713–719

Chubik A, Gilliam JN (1978) A review of mixed connective tissue disease. Int J Dermatol 17:123–133

Guldner HH, Netter HJ, Szostecki C et al. (1988) Epitope mapping with recombinant human 68 kDa (U1) ribonucleoprotein antigen reveals heterogeneous autoantibody profiles in human autoimmune sera. J Immunol 141:469–475

Matsuoka Y, Miyajima S, Okada N (1998) A case of calcinosis universalis successfully treated with low-dose warfarin. J Dermatol 25:716–720

Reimer G, Huschka W, Keller J et al. (1983) Immunofluorescence studies in progressive systemic sclerosis (scleroderma) and mixed connective tissue disease. Br J Dermatol 109:27–36

Sharp GC, Irvin WS, Tan EM et al. (1972) Mixed connective tissue disease: an apparently distinct rheumatic disease syndrome associated with a specific antibody to an extractable nuclear antigen (ENA). Am J Med 52:138–159

Rheumatoid Arthritis

Ginsberg MH, Genant HK, Yu TF et al. (1963) Rheumatoid nadulosis: an unusual variant of rheumatoid disease. Arthritis Rheum 18:49–58

Gordon DA, Stein JL, Broder I (1973) The extra-articular features of rheumatoid arthritis. Am J Med 54:445–452

Ichikawa MM, Murata Y, Higaki Y et al. (1998) Rheumatoid neutrophilic dermatitis. Eur J Dermatol 8(5):347–349

Isdale IC, Bywaters EGL (1956) The rash of rheumatoid arthritis and Still's disease. Q J Med 49:377–387

Jorizzo JL, Daniels JC (1983) Dermatologic conditions reported in patients with rheumatoid arthritis. J Am Acad Dermatol 8:439–457

Kaminski MJ (1996) Skin disorders associated with rheumatic disease. Clin Podiatr Med Surg 13:139–153

Mashek HA, Pham CT, Helm TN et al. (1997) Rheumatoid neutrophilic dermatitis. Arch Dermatol 133:757–760

Pun YLW, Barraclough DRE, Muirden KD (1990) Leg ulcers in rheumatoid arthritis. Med J Aust 153:585–587

Still GF (1896) On a form of chronic joint disease in children. Med Chir Trans 80:47. Reprinted in: Am J Dis Child 1978; 132:192–200

Miscellaneous Diseases

Allison JR Jr, Allison JR Sr (1966) Knuckle pads. Arch Dermatol 93:311–316

Bart RS, Pumphrey RG (1967) Knuckle pads, leukonychia and deafness. A dominantly inherited syndrome. N Engl J Med 276:202–207

Connelly TJ (1999) Development of Peyronie's and Dupuytren's diseases in an individual after single episodes of trauma: a case report and review of the literature. J Am Acad Dermatol 41:106–108

Evans RA (1986) The aetiology of Dupuytren's disease. Br J Hosp Med 35:198–199

Fitzgerald AM, Kirkpatrick JJ, Naylor IL (1999) Dupuytren's disease. The way forward? J Hand Surg 24:395–399

Guberman D, Lichtenstein DA, Vardy DA (1996) Knuckle pads – a forgotten skin condition: report of a case and review of the literature. Cutis 57:241–242

Kelâmi A, Pryor JP (eds) (1982) Peyronie's disease (induration penis plastica). Progress in reproductive biology and medicine, vol 9. Karger, Basel

Kodama BF, Gentry RH, Fitzpatrick JE (1993) Papules and plaques over the joint spaces. Knuckle pads (heloderma). Arch Dermatol 1239:1044–1045, 1047

Kopera D, Soyer HP, Kerl H (1995) An update on pachydermodactyly and a report of three additional cases. Br J Dermatol 133:433–437

Landthaler M, Kodalle W, Braun-Falco O (1983) Röntgenweichstrahlentherapie der Induratio penis plastica. Hautarzt 34:171–174

Ledderhose G (1895) Ledderhose syndrome. Plantar aponeurositis and fibrous nodules of the flexor tendons resulting in clawfoot. Über Zerresungen der Plantarfascie. Langenbeck Arch Klin Chri 48:853–856

Meigel WN, Plewig G (1976) Kauschwielen, eine Variante der Fingerknöchelpolster. Hautarzt 27:391–395

Nesbit RM (1965) Congenital curvature of the phallus. Report of 3 cases with description of corrective operation. J Urol 93:230

Peyronie F de la (1743) Sur quelques obstactles, qui s'opposent à l'éjaculation naturelle de la semence. Mém Acad Chir, Paris 1:425

Ramer JC, Vasily DB, Ladda RL (1994) Familial leukonychia, knuckle pads, hearing loss, and palmoplantar hyperkeratosis: an additional family with Bart-Pumphrey syndrome. J Med Genet 31:68–71

Verbov J (1975) Pachydermodactyly: a variant of the true knuckle pads. Arch Dermatol 111:524

Warthan TL, Rudolph RI, Gross PR (1973) Isolated plantar fibromatosis. Arch Dermatol 108:823–825

Williams JL, Thomas GG (1970) The natural history of Peyronie's disease. J Urol 103:75–76

Young ID, Fortt RW (1981) Familial fibromatosis. Clin Genet 20:211–216

CHAPTER 19

Malformations and Genetic Disorders

Contents

The principles of genetic disorders are considered in Chapter 1. In this chapter we will discuss a variety of malformations, as well as some of the major genodermatoses.

Malformations

Aplasia Cutis Congenita

(CORDON 1767)

Synonym. Aplasia cutis circumscripta

Definition. Congenital circumscribed skin defect which heals with scarring.

Epidemiology. Aplasia cutis congenita occurs in about 1:3000 births; almost all cases are solitary.

Etiology and Pathogenesis. The cause of aplasia cutis congenita is unknown. In most instances, it is believed to represent a sporadic intrauterine event. While it has been associated with maternal use of methimazole, intrauterine herpes virus infections, and amniotic defects, in most cases no etiology is found. Complicating the matter is the association of aplasia cutis congenita with a variety of genodermatoses such as focal dermal hypoplasia and epidermolysis bullosa, and chromosomal disorders, primarily trisomy 13. Finally, a number of syndromes include aplasia cutis congenita as a regular feature. Even the ordinary solitary scalp defect may be inherited in an autosomal dominant pattern.

In many instances, failure of embryonic tissue lines to fuse may be the explanation. On the scalp, the lesions usually are over suture lines. On the face, there are three main regions in which closure does not occur:

- Lateral temple where frontal facial and maxillary lines meet, as seen in facial focal dermal hypoplasia and Setleis syndrome
- Nasolabial fold area as in MIDAS syndrome
- Preauricular region where the maxillary and mandibular processes fuse

Clinical Findings. The most common finding is a localized oval scalp defect, usually posterior of the midline and of varying depth (Fig. 19.1). The lesions may include dermal defects with a mem-

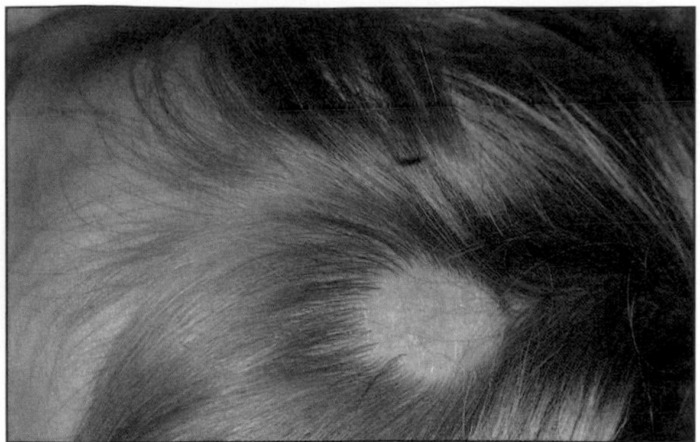

Fig. 19.1. Aplasia cutis congenita

branous cover to epidermal erosions, full-thickness skin loss, or defects in the underlying muscles, bones, and even meninges. About two-thirds of all lesions are solitary and not associated with underlying defects. In other cases there may be multiple lesions and involvement of other parts of the body.

A search should be made for associated defects. The following groups are usually recognized (Table 19.1). A few points in the table deserve further consideration:

- Group 1. The most common form of aplasia cutis congenita.
- Group 2. Probably the best-established association of aplasia cutis congenita with limb defects is the Adams-Oliver (1945) syndrome, which is inherited in an autosomal dominant pattern and also features extensive cutis marmorata. There are distal limb defects often associated with constricting bands and terminal swelling. Other reported associations include cardiovascular anomalies, spina bifida, and auricular malformations.
- Group 3. Fetus papyraceous is a mummified fetus. One of a pair of twins dies and is compressed and mummified by the living partner. The partner may develop aplasia cutis congenita; in this instance the evidence is best for the vascular or thrombotic etiology. Amniotic bands are also more common in this group, as are ischemic contractures.
- Group 5. The aplasia cutis congenita seen in epidermolysis bullosa is very likely more than just a deep mechanical erosion. An intrauterine blister at the appropriate time could interfere with the epithelial-mesenchymal interaction and lead to a permanent defect. Experts argue whether aplasia cutis congenita with pyloric atresia is part of epidermolysis bullosa (Chap. 15).
- Group 6. Aplasia cutis congenita is regularly seen in trisomy 13 (Patau [1960] syndrome) and 4p deletion. It is also part of focal dermal hypoplasia, MIDAS syndrome, and oculocerebrocutaneous syndrome, all discussed below. The Johanson-Blizzard (1971) syndrome is inherited in an autosomal recessive pattern; it features aplasia cutis congenita of scalp, sparse hair, hypoplastic nasal alae, pancreatic insufficiency, and a variety of other defects.

Table 19.1. Classification of aplasia cutis congenita (ACC)

Group	Inheritance	Type of ACC	Other features
Isolated ACC	AD; sporadic	Usually single, on scalp	None
ACC with limb defects	AD	Variety of syndromes, almost all AD	Limb reduction usually involving legs, other malformations
ACC on trunk +/– other defects	Sporadic	Associated with fetus papyraceous – see text	Placental infarcts, limb defects, fibrous constriction bands
ACC with preauricular skin defects	Uncertain	Bilateral oval patches in preauricular region	None
ACC with EB	Varies with type of EB	Typically on limbs, may be extensive	Occasionally pyloric atresia
ACC with other syndromes	Varies	Highly variable	Varies with disorder
ACC with teratogen exposure	Sporadic	Highly variable, often on trunk and extensive	Methimazole may also cause imperforate anus

AD, autosomal dominant; EB, epidermalysis bullosa

Histopathology. Most studies are not very satisfactory, as biopsy of an absent structure is impossible. Once the lesion has healed, the biopsy shows an atrophic scar. Histopathology is not needed to diagnose aplasia cutis congenita. Immunomapping of perilesional skin may help to exclude epidermolysis bullosa.

Laboratory Findings. Other tests are needed only if one is trying to identify one of the associated syndromes.

Differential Diagnosis. The differential diagnosis is really aimed at classifying the type of aplasia cutis congenita. Nevus sebaceous appears as a bald spot at birth but without a defect. A biopsy will help here. Ectopic neural tissue involves a skull defect, so imaging studies should be done if any question exists. Our advice is that if a single midline posterior lesion is present, a family history should be taken and the parents and siblings examined for a typical scar. If this is negative, no further evaluation is needed. If the lesions are not on the scalp, then a search of associated problems is mandatory.

Therapy. No therapy is needed. The defects usually heal spontaneously. If deep structures are exposed, the defect can be covered with a flap or graft.

Pseudoainhum

(Portal 1685; Streeter 1930)

Synonyms. Amniotic band syndrome, early amnion rupture sequence, congenital constriction band syndrome, Streeter bands

Definition. Congenital fibrous bands usually involving a limb.

Epidemiology. The incidence has been estimated at 1:5000.

Etiology and Pathogenesis. The theory is that early rupture of the amnion leads to the formation of bands which apparently can attach to the fetus and cause developmental abnormalities by constriction. Bands are seen fairly frequently on routine ultrasound examinations but they rarely restrict fetal motion or cause problems. The best support for this hypothesis is provided by studies in rodents where the amnions were ruptured intentionally. In almost all cases, the event appears sporadic; family reports are rare and not convincing.

Clinical Findings. Tight constriction bands are found, producing indentations in the soft tissue and occasionally leading to amputation of a digit or even a limb. There is usually distal swelling because of impaired venous or lymphatic return. Deep ankle grooves are most common. While only the limbs are typically involved, occasionally there may be trunk defects. Cleft lip and palate and CNS defects have also been described.

Histopathology. In most cases, dermal fibrosis representing a thickened fibrous band have been described, usually on operative material. Some have identified possible amniotic residua in the bands, but this seems far-fetched.

Differential Diagnosis. The differential diagnosis is quite diverse:

- Adams-Oliver syndrome combines constricting bands and aplasia cutis congenita.
- Ainhum is a disease limited almost exclusively to blacks, regularly involving the fifth toes and probably secondary to trauma. It is acquired, not congenital.
- Michelin tire syndrome babies have deep, symmetric circumferential grooves but no limb defects.
- Constricting bands also may be seen in Vohwinkel syndrome (mutilating palmoplantar keratoderma), mal de Meleda, and hereditary sclerosing poikiloderma.
- Yaws, leprosy, and even dermatophyte infections may lead to autoamputation.
- In adults, linear scleroderma may produce constricting bands.

Therapy. The constricting bands can usually be released by surgical procedures.

Cutis Verticis Gyrata

(Jadassohn 1906)

Synonyms. Pachydermia verticis gyrata, cutis verticis plicata, bulldog scalp

Definition. Congenital or acquired folding of excessive scalp skin to produce thick, corrugated folds.

Epidemiology. Cutis verticis gyrata is uncommon. It can be present at birth, either alone or as part of

Table 19.2. Classification of cutis verticis gyrata

True cutis verticis gyrata
Idiopathic (not associated with syndrome in otherwise healthy individual)
Endocrine
Acromegaly
Myxedema
Congenital myxedema (cretinism)
Associated with syndromes
Pachydermoperiostosis
Beare-Stevenson syndrome: widespread cutis verticis gyrata, acanthosis nigricans, craniofacial dysostosis
Turner syndrome
Pseudo cutis verticis gyrata
Cerebriform dermal nevus (Orkin sign)
Focal mucinosis
Nevus lipomatosus
Connective tissue nevus
Neurofibroma
Leukemia cutis with extensive infiltrates

a variety of syndromes, or become apparent in adult life.

Etiology and Pathogenesis. The cause of cutis verticis gyrata is unknown. In Turner syndrome, where edema of the scalp is common, cutis verticis gyrata may be seen. Because the same changes are always seen in bulldogs and basset hounds, it seems reasonable to assume that the human condition can be genetically determined in an analogous way. We designate the folded skin over a defined dermal process such as a dermal nevus or mucin deposition as pseudocutis verticis gyrata. Table 19.2 shows the various disorders associated with this finding.

Clinical Findings. Most commonly, the scalp is involved. There appears to be simply too much skin, so it is folded up (Fig. 19.2). Skin color is usually unchanged. The hairs over the folds or gyri are usually reduced, but normal in the sulci. When palpated, the folds are soft and spongy. The folds may be as thick as an adult's finger. The lesions usually progress.

If cutis verticis gyrata is present elsewhere on the body, one should be very suspicious of an associated syndrome or underlying dermal tumor or deposit. In our experience, an underlying dermal nevus is the most common cause in infants. It tends to be sharply bordered and may be somewhat darker. In the idiopathic form, men appear to be affected more often, although it may just be easier to see small patches with them. Onset is generally in adolescence. Often a barber notices the changes first. In other instances, the patient complains of the maceration and foul odor caused by secondary infections.

The cutis verticis gyrata mental deficiency syndrome is characterized by an association between the cutaneous findings with mental retardation and therapy-resistant epilepsy.

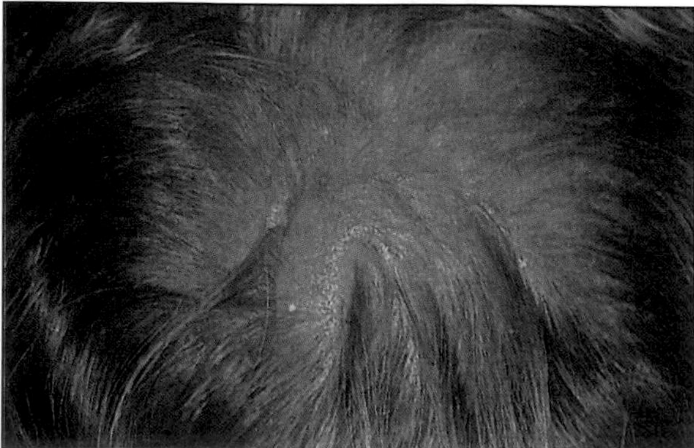

Fig. 19.2. Cutis verticis gyrata

Histopathology. The macroscopic pictures shows the prominent folds. If a dermal tumor or deposit is present, as in pseudocutis verticis gyrata, it can be identified. Otherwise the skin is normal.

Differential Diagnosis. The differential diagnostic considerations are shown in Table 19.2. The question is one of identifying associated disorders; the clinical finding is quite specific.

Therapy. Surgical excision, if desired.

Pachydermoperiostosis

(Friedrich 1868; Touraine et al. 1935)

Synonyms. Touraine-Solente-Golé syndrome, idiopathic hypertrophic osteoarthropathy

Etiology and Pathogenesis. This rare genodermatosis is usually sporadic but may be inherited in an autosomal dominant or, less often, autosomal recessive fashion. There is a 9 : 1 male : female ratio.

Clinical Findings. The hallmarks of pachydermoperiostosis are cutis verticis gyrata, thickened and coarse facial skin with increased sebaceous glands, periostosis, and clubbing of the fingers and toes. Patients may suffer from hyperhidrosis and often have oily skin because of the increased sebaceous glands. The eyelids may be thickened, giving the patient a worried look.

Periostosis refers to a thickening of the periosteum with formation of new bone by the osteoblasts of this outer membrane. Trauma and infection are the typical causes of periosteal reaction, but in pachydermoperiostosis the process is idiopathic. The bones, especially of the digits, are deformed; this, coupled with soft tissue swelling, produces clubbed digits and spade-like hands and feet. The cylindrical thickening of the limb bones may be painful. Magnetic resonance imaging of the long bones of the extremities and scalp can help to identify minor or early lesions. While the problems are annoying, the outlook is good.

Histopathology. The epidermis is normal while the dermal layer is greatly thickened, mimicking scleroderma. The presence of prominent sebaceous glands may be a clue to the correct diagnosis.

Differential Diagnosis. The differential diagnosis of clubbing is covered in Chapter 33. Acquired pachydermoperiostosis, also called hypertrophic pulmonary osteoarthropathy, is a paraneoplastic phenomenon associated with small-cell lung carcinoma. Acromegaly should be excluded as it, too, shows thickened hands and clubbing (Chap. 48). Thyroid acropachy (EMO syndrome; Chap. 43) is also similar. Acro-osteolysis refers to the dissolution of the terminal phalanxes on radiologic examination; the digits are often spade-shaped. It is associated with a long list of inherited disorders, including KID syndrome and Papillon-Lefèvre syndrome. It may also present associated with chronic inflammation and neurologic deficits, as in syphilis, leprosy, psoriasis, and systemic sclerosis. Finally, exposure to polyvinyl chloride causes similar findings.

Polydactyly

Synonym. Supernumerary digit

Polydactyly, or an excess number of digits, is seen in a long list of syndromes. Of interest to dermatologists are oral-facial-digital syndrome type 1 and Ellis-van Creveld (1940) syndrome. Polydactyly is usually ulnar and ranges from a fully formed sixth (or higher) digit to part of a digit. Autoamputation of such digits may occur in utero, leaving a small dermal papule on the lateral aspect of the fifth digit known as rudimentary polydactyly. If a bony center is identified on histologic or radiologic examination or if a joint is present, the diagnosis is clear. In other instances, only residual dermal nerves are found, resembling an amputation neuroma.

Developmental Cysts, Sinuses, and Rests

The head and neck region has a complex embryology, as the pharyngeal pouches and clefts interact to form the various structures of the face and neck. Many development cysts and sinuses are formed; all are discussed in Chapter 53. Fistulas of the lips as well as dental sinus tracts are covered in Chapter 33.

Accessory Tragus

(Meckel 1826)

Synonyms. Choristoma, congenital cartilaginous rest of the neck

Etiology and Pathogenesis. This relatively common malformation results from the incomplete migration and closure of the first branchial arch to form the tragus so that cartilage rests are left behind in the skin. They are found in 1–2% of all otorhinolaryngology patients. Much less common are similar lesions along the anterior border of the sternocleidomastoid muscle, representing defects in the closure of other arches.

Clinical Findings. A tiny papule or nodule is found anterior to the ear (Fig. 19.3). Often, the central cartilaginous core can be palpated. The preauricular lesions usually have abundant vellus hairs. Associated findings may include preauricular pits and sinuses, which are usually absent for the neck

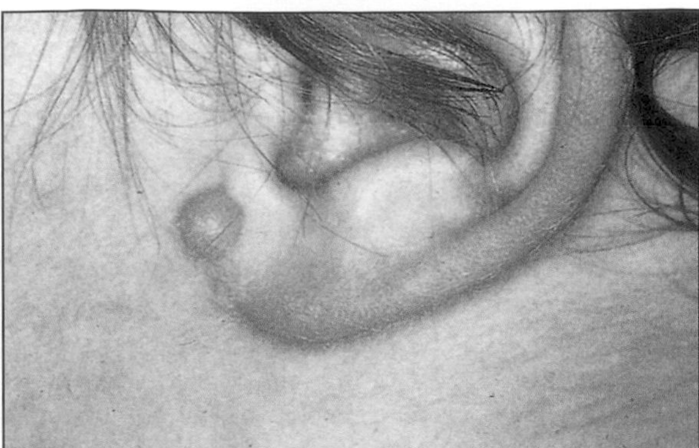

Fig. 19.3. Accessory tragus

lesions. In addition, accessory tragi may be associated with deafness in a wide variety of syndromes.

Histopathology. The biopsy shows normal skin covering a small piece of normal cartilage. Most nonacral chondromas are actually just such cartilaginous rests. The accessory tragus has many tiny vellus hair follicles; when no cartilage is found, the diagnosis of hair follicle nevus is often made. We consider the anatomic location of an accessory tragus diagnostic and reserve the term hair follicle nevus for the rare epidermal nevus with hair follicle differentiation.

Differential Diagnosis. While the diagnosis is usually clear because the cartilage can be felt, the only other likely consideration is a melanocytic nevus.

Therapy. Surgical excision is appropriate. If there is any suggestion of a cyst, sinus, or ear problem, consultation should be sought.

Accessory Nipple

Synonym. Polythelia

Etiology and Pathogenesis. Accessory nipples fall along the milk line running from the axilla to the groin. They are viewed as embryologic remnants. Sometimes associated breast tissue is present; this condition is called polymastia.

Clinical Findings. The most common location for an accessory nipple is on the milk line just below the breast (Fig. 19.4). Accessory breast tissue is more common in the other direction in the axilla. Typically, there is a papillomatous, reddish brown papule or nodule with a central dell and radial folds. It may be erectile, show a few coarse hairs, change with periods, or even leak milk during nursing, depending on the degree of associated breast tissue. Smaller lesions are often confused with nevi, neurofibromas, or dermatofibromas. Occasionally, lesions are found away from the milk line, such as on the back or even the legs. Polythelia maybe associated with renal malformations, but this connection is disputed.

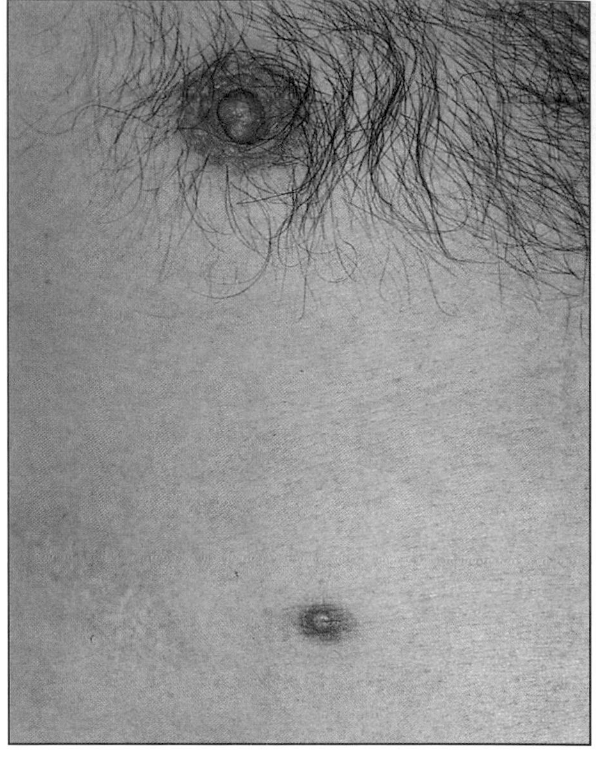

Fig. 19.4. Accessory nipple

Histopathology. Microscopically, there is a proliferation of smooth muscle associated with ductal epithelium. Often there is hyperpigmentation of the basal layer, reflecting the clinically darker tones of the nipple.

Therapy. The decision for surgery is made if differential questions exist or the lesion is troublesome.

Painful Piezogenic Papules

(Shelley and Rawnsley 1968)

Synonym. Multiple fat herniations

Definition. Herniation of fat along the edge of the heel or, less often, the thenar eminence.

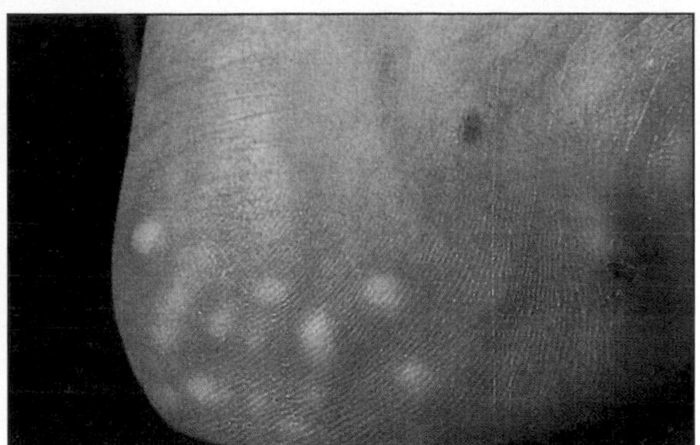

Fig. 19.5. Painful piezogenic papules

Epidemiology. Over 20 % of individuals have piezogenic papules, which only rarely are painful.

Etiology and Pathogenesis. Fat extrudes up into the dermis and even between bundles of collagen. Presumably, weight-bearing and sudden pressure, as in sports, are the triggers. Fat is usually contained by multiple fibrous septae which are perhaps reduced in number or strength.

Clinical Findings. Small, reducible, protruding nodules are seen along the border of one or both heels and along the line of transgredience (Fig. 19.5). They are more easily seen when a patient stands on one leg. Multiple lesions are often present; more than 20 are not unusual. The nodules are either skin-colored or yellow. They are somewhat firm when palpated but tend to disappear when the patient is horizontal. A hernia-like defect is usually not observed. On rare occasions, individuals will complain that one or more of the lesions are intensely painful.

Histopathology. Fat is seen compressing or extending into the dermal collagen.

Differential Diagnosis. Neural or eccrine tumors are considered most often when the lesions are painful. When multiple lesions are present and become more prominent with standing, the diagnosis is clear.

Therapy. Usually no therapy is needed. Excision with subcutaneous closure can be employed for painful lesions.

Transverse Nasal Line
(Cornbleet 1951)

Synonym. Stria nasi transversa

The transverse nasal line is a common malformation located at the upper border of the tip of the nose. It may simply be a pink line, which becomes more obvious with vasodilatation, or actually a tiny groove. In blacks, it is often hyperpigmented. Embryologically, it lies over the junction between the lesser and greater alar cartilage. Its location at a line of fusion may explain why it is a predilection site for comedones and milia. The transverse nasal line may be confused with the allergic salute (Myers 1960), which is a series of small transverse furrows in wrinkles of patients with allergic rhinitis who repeatedly rub and twitch their noses.

Dorsal-Ventral Transposition

In embryogenesis, a variety of genes are responsible for cell positioning, including those which determine dorsal-ventral, left-right, anterior-posterior, and proximal-distal relationships. The function of such genes is essential for limb development and the appropriate location of cutaneous structures in laboratory animals and presumably in humans. An interesting example was that of a young black child with a patch of more darkly pigmented, normal nonplantar skin with hairs running along the sole of his foot. The changes were not dissimilar from those observed in mice with defects in various dorsalizing and ventralizing genes.

Neural Heterotopias

Synonyms. Nasal glioma, rudimentary meningocele, primary cutaneous meningioma, meningeal hamartoma

Etiology and Pathogenesis. Neural heterotopias or ectopic neural tissue arises when neural elements fall outside their usual locations during embryogenesis. The most common such tumor is a nasal glioma, in which glial tissue is found at the root of the nose. Ectopic meningeal tissue is usually found on the scalp.

Clinical Findings. Nasal glioma typically presents as a congenital, smooth, reddish gray nodule up to 3 cm in diameter. Often the nose is flattened and hypertelorism develops. Lesions may be surrounded by a ring of dark hair (hair collar sign). While about 60% of lesions are cutaneous, the balance may be intranasal. Rudimentary meningoceles are similar nodules or plaques found on the scalp, in most cases along suture lines. In about 20% of cases there is a connection with the brain, usually through a bony defect with a dumbbell pattern on imaging studies.

Histopathology. A nasal glioma consists primarily of astrocytes and glial tissue, but neurons are uncommon. The rudimentary meningocele may be cystic and contains meningothelial cells in a collagenous matrix.

Differential Diagnosis. Nasal gliomas can be mistaken for dermoid cysts or hemangiomas, as they often have the same reddish gray sheen. Gliomas are present at birth, do not grow, and have a smooth surface. Another major differential diagnostic point is an encephalocele, in which case a fluid-filled connection with the ventricular system is present.

Therapy. In case of any suspected nasal glioma or heterotopic neural tissue, neurosurgical consultation and imaging advice is mandatory. When a dermatologist attempts to excise a tumor with CNS connections, problems are not far away. Once the diagnosis and extent of the lesion are clear, a neurosurgeon or pediatric surgeon should remove the lesion.

Phakomatoses

Phakomatosis is an awkward term from the Greek words "phak" (lens), "oma" (tumor), and "osis" (condition) used to described syndromes with cutaneous, neurological, and ocular manifestations. We are not trying to make the word popular again but simply use it as an umbrella term for a group of disorders widely scattered throughout the German version of this text. For example, neurofibromatosis could be discussed under both pigmentary lesions and mesenchymal tumors, but we have placed it here.

Neurofibromatosis

Neurofibromatosis is not one disease but a group of clinically related disorders. The Riccardi classification is unnecessarily complex and being continuously refined by newer genetic studies.

Neurofibromatosis Type 1

(VON RECKLINGHAUSEN 1882)

Synonyms. Von Recklinghausen disease, NF-1

Definition. Common neurocutaneous disorder featuring cutaneous neurofibromas and café-au-lait macules as well as a variety of systemic problems.

Epidemiology. Neurofibromatosis is one of the most common genodermatoses. It has an incidence of 1:3000–5000 and is seen among all racial groups.

Etiology and Pathogenesis. This disease is inherited in an autosomal dominant pattern. The gene, neurofibromin, is a very large gene with many exons located on chromosome 17q11.2. About 50% of patients represent new mutations. One function

Table 19.3. Diagnostic criteria for neurofibromatosis type 1

The patient must have two or more of the following criteria:
Six or more café-au-lait macules Children: the lesions must be >5 mm in diameter Adults: the lesions must be >15 mm in diameter
Two neurofibromas or one plexiform neurofibroma
Axillary or inguinal freckling
Optic nerve glioma
Two or more Lisch nodules
Distinctive bony lesion (sphenoid dysplasia or thinning of long bone cortex with or without pseudoarthrosis)
First degree relative with neurofibromatosis type 1

of neurofibromin is to provide negative feedback control of the ras growth factor or oncogene by stimulating its inactivation. In the absence of neurofibromin, there are disturbances in growth control and development of tumors. The exact pathogenesis of the highly variable features is not understood. In the skin, the presence of numerous mast cells may play a role.

Clinical Findings. The features of neurofibromatosis can vary greatly from patient to patient within a pedigree, evoking the genetic arguments of variable expressivity and incomplete penetrance. The diagnostic criteria developed at a National Institutes of Health consensus conference are given first because they outline the clinical features so nicely. Two of the following seven criteria shown in Table 19.3 establish the clinical diagnosis of NF-1.

Cutaneous Findings. There are many distinctive skin findings in NF-1.

Café-au-Lait Macules. These flat, tan macules are usually the first sign of NF-1 (Fig. 19.6; Chap. 26). While most lesions are present in early life, some may appear later. Others may disappear in adulthood. While about 85% of patients have multiple café-au-lait macules, there is no correlation between the number of lesions and the severity of the syndrome. The palms, soles, and genitalia are usually spared. Darker skinned individuals tend to have more café-au-lait macules and the diagnostic criteria may be less useful with them.

Axillary Freckling. Also known as Crowe sign (Crowe and Schull 1953), axillary freckles are tiny café-au-lait macules. They are most common in the groin and axillae, tend to develop in puberty, and are present in about 70% of patients.

Neurofibroma. Almost every patient has at least a few neurofibromas (Chap. 59). Some may be disfigured by hundreds of the tumors. The lesions are soft flesh-colored to red brown papules and nodules, often pedunculated (Fig. 19.7). They appear as herniations which can be pushed back into the dermis. Neurofibromas of the nipple are extremely suggestive of NF-1.

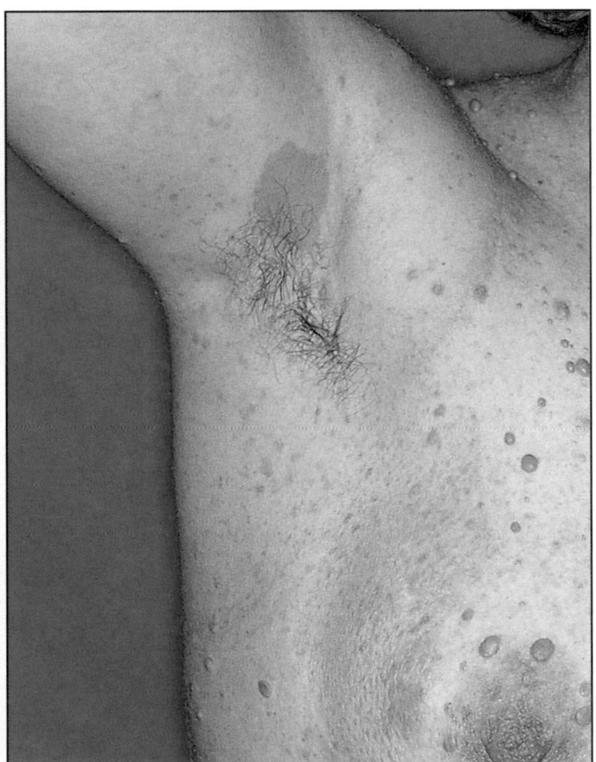

Fig. 19.6. Neurofibromatosis 1 with café-au-lait macule, axillary freckling, and neurofibromas

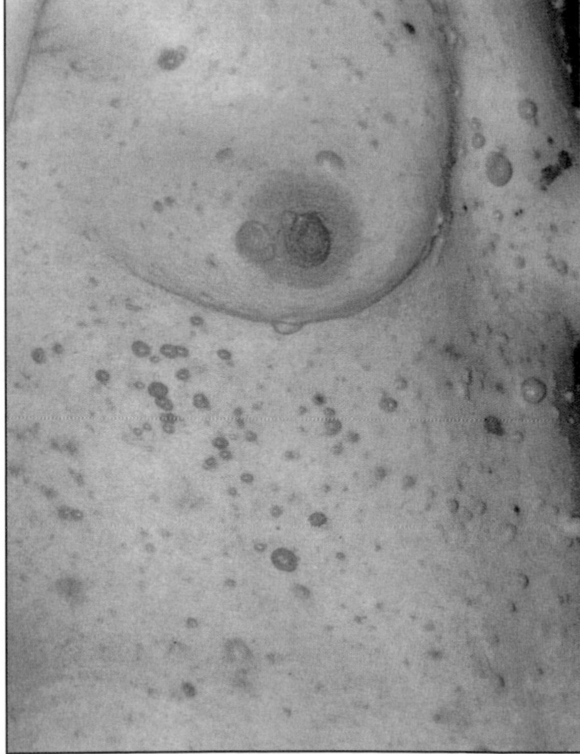

Fig. 19.7. Multiple neurofibromas, including highly significant nipple lesion

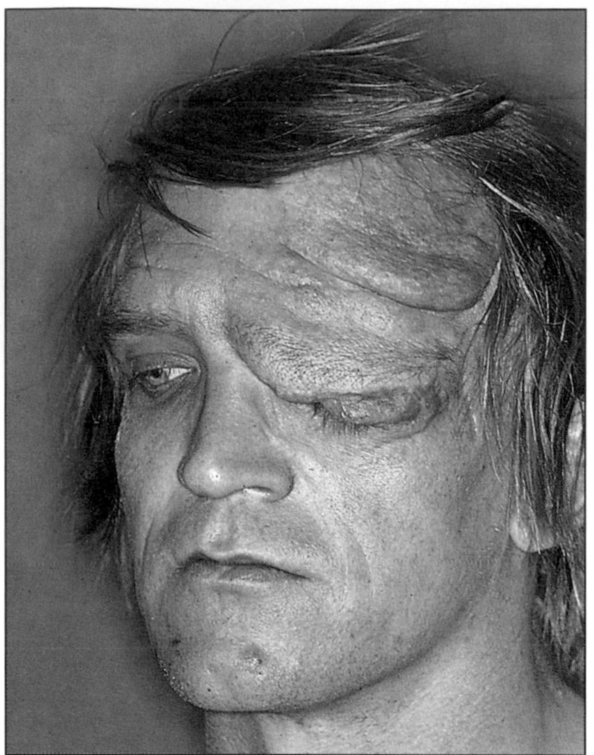

Fig. 19.8. Plexiform neurofibroma

Plexiform Neurofibroma. Most plexiform neurofibromas are deeper subcutaneous tumors. More superficial lesions can be palpated; they are often described as a "bag of worms" (Fig. 19.8). The epidermis may be darker, have excess hairs, or even be atrophic. Larger tumors may be associated with excessive folds of overlying skin resembling localized cutis laxa.

Pruritus. Intense pruritus can be a severe problem for some patients. In our experience, it usually affects individuals with hundreds of neurofibromas, suggesting that mast cell degranulation could play a role.

Pigmentation. Pale olive green or yellow pigmentation of the entire skin.

Juvenile Xanthogranulomas. The presence of multiple juvenile xanthogranulomas and neurofibromatosis is a paraneoplastic marker of juvenile chronic myelogenous leukemia.

Systemic Findings. The number of internal organs involved is quite long; we will only mention the more common problems.

CNS. The most common tumor is optic glioma, which may cause blindness. While 15% of patients may have optic gliomas, less than 5% have signs or symptoms from the tumor. Other CNS tumors also occur, including meningiomas and astrocytomas. About 5–10% of patients are mentally retarded, while learning disorders and other minor problems are more common.

Eye. Lisch (1937) nodules are hamartomas of the iris not dissimilar to dermal melanocytic nevi. They are present in over 90% of adults but not useful for early diagnosis. They are difficult to see with the naked eye and best visualized in slit lamp examination. The nodules are asymptomatic.

Ear. While acoustic neuromas are described occasionally, they should immediately suggest central neurofibromatosis, NF-2.

Musculoskeletal. Over half the patients have scoliosis and in 5% it is a significant disability. Pseudoarthrosis or bowing of the long bones usually involves the tibia and is seen early in life, making this change diagnostically useful. Winging or sphenoid dysplasia is seen radiologically, not clinically.

Endocrine. Both precocious and delayed puberty can be seen. Premature onset is usually associated with a functioning endocrine tumor, often a pituitary adenoma. About 1% of patients have pheochromocytoma.

Vascular. Renovascular hypertension may occur; cerebral and gastrointestinal vessels may also be abnormal. Blood pressure should be monitored in all patients; hypertension may not be idiopathic but is secondary to renal artery stenosis or pheochromocytoma.

Malignancies. The two most common malignancies are juvenile chronic myelogenous leukemia and malignant schwannoma. Most malignant peripheral nerve sheath tumors arise in the deep plexiform neurofibromas of NF-1; they are confusingly designated both as neurofibrosarcoma and malignant schwannoma. Rhabdomyosarcoma and Wilms tumor may also occur.

Histopathology. The microscopic skin lesion patterns are not unique. The café-au-lait macules show increased basal layer pigmentation without an increase in melanocytes. They may contain melanin macroglobules, but this is not unique to NF-1 lesions. In similar fashion, solitary and syndrome-associated neurofibroma are microscopically identical.

Laboratory Findings. There are no specific laboratory tests. The gene is very large and many different mutations are responsible for NF-1, making molecular diagnosis difficult.

Course and Prognosis. The psychosocial burden for patients with full-blown NF-1 is immense. A prognosis is difficult to offer. The neurofibromas continue to develop. If a malignancy develops, the outlook is obviously worse. Other life-threatening complications may include vascular disease, especially in the CNS, and space-occupying or functional benign tumors.

Differential Diagnosis. The differential diagnosis of NF-1 is complicated. Firstly, the diagnosis cannot be made on the clinical or histologic features of either café-au-lait macules or neurofibromas. Multiple café-au-lait macules are seen in many diseases; the list is so long that it is easier just to remember that they are not specific. The only real clinical issue is in patients who present only with café-au-lait macules. In a child with one or two café-au-lait macules, no other features, and no family history, it is simply not possible to determine whether NF-1 is present. On the other hand, multiple neurofibromas strongly suggest the diagnosis, as do axillary freckling and Lisch nodules.

In addition to the other types of neurofibromatosis, there are a number of diseases which can be confused with NF-1:

- WATSON (1967) syndrome: Apparently allelic to NF-1, Watson syndrome also features pulmonic stenosis, short stature, and mental retardation.
- Neurofibromatosis-Noonan syndrome overlap: Some patients have features of both NF-1 and Noonan syndrome, including short stature and a webbed neck.
- LEOPARD syndrome (Chap. 58): Multiple lentigines and a host of systemic problems characterize this rare disorder which is clinically completely different from NF-1. Multiple café-au-lait macules may be present, but so are thousands of lentigines.
- Carney syndrome (Chap. 58): This also features multiple lentigines with a variety of cardiac and cutaneous myxomas and a range of unusual endocrine tumors.
- McCune-Albright syndrome (Chap. 58): The café-au-lait macules tend to be larger and usually does not cross the midline. The main feature is bony defects which can be seen radiologically.
- WESTERHOF syndrome (1978): This is extremely rare but features both café-au-lait macules and hypopigmented macules along with mental retardation.

Therapy. Individual neurofibromas which are large or painful can be excised. Café-au-lait macules can be destroyed with lasers or cryotherapy, but most are on the trunk and do not bother the patient. Ketotifen has been recommended for the intense pruritus; in our experience, it is better than other antihistamines. Some feel that one may modify the disease course by inhibiting mast cells over a long period of time.

Prenatal Diagnosis. The large size of the gene makes prenatal diagnosis a challenge. In a family with a number of affected individuals, linkage markers are usually employed for molecular diagnosis, be it prenatal or in a patient at risk. Such studies are primarily helpful for either a family in which one parent has NF-1 or for counseling an individual from an NF-1 pedigree who has no clinical findings. Genetic studies are seldom helpful in studying a child with a single café-au-lait macule to confirm the presence of NF-1 as a sporadic event because of the multiplicity of possible mutations. This makes genetic counseling in neurofibromatosis even more challenging. Because neurofibromatosis is so common, dermatologists are occasionally tempted to do genetic counseling themselves. As mentioned in Chapter 1, there are many reasons for leaving this in the hands of experts.

Other Types of Neurofibromatosis

Central Neurofibromatosis

Synonyms. Acoustic neurofibromatosis, NF-2

Epidemiology. The incidence is about 1:40,000; thus, NF-2 is much rarer than NF-1.

Etiology and Pathogenesis. This syndrome is also inherited in an autosomal dominant pattern. The gene is located on chromosome 22q and codes for a protein known as schwannomin or merlin. The protein is intimately involved in growth signaling

Table 19.4. Diagnostic criteria for neurofibromatosis type 2

The patient must satisfy either the first or second set of criteria:
Bilateral acoustic neuromas (eighth cranial nerve tumors)
or
A first degree relative with neurofibromatosis type 2 and either:
A unilateral acoustic neuroma
or
Two of the following:
Neurofibroma
Meningioma
Glioma
Schwannoma
Juvenile posterior subcapsular lenticular opacity

pathways and linking the cytoskeleton to the plasma membrane. Once again, about half of the patients represent spontaneous mutations. Variable expressivity is much less common than in NF-1, so the pedigree often gives the diagnosis.

Clinical Findings. The clinical diagnostic criteria are shown in Table 19.4. The most consistent clinical feature is acoustic neuromas, which are bilateral in over 90% of patients and often lead to deafness. They tend to appear during puberty or young adulthood. About 30% of patients have café-au-lait macules, but as many as six lesions is uncommon. Around 60% have neural tumors; most of these are schwannomas, although neurofibromas and overlap tumors can be identified. Deeper or plexiform neural tumors are proportionally more common; the overlying skin can be hyperpigmented and hairy. Axillary freckles are not seen and Lisch nodules are rare. Juvenile xanthogranulomas have been described but not in association with leukemia, as is seen in NF-1. Juvenile posterior subcapsular cataracts are also relatively common. A variety of other neural tumors can also be found, including other schwannomas (an acoustic neuroma is a type of Schwann cell tumor), meningiomas, and spinal gliomas.

Course and Prognosis. The outlook is not good because of the likelihood of hearing and sight loss. The most common cause of death is CNS tumors, usually in adults.

Differential Diagnosis. Until acoustic neuromas are found, the cutaneous lesions can be mistaken for NF-1.

Another rare syndrome is neurilemmomatosis or schwannomatosis. Patients have multiple cutaneous neurilemmomas as well as a range of CNS tumors. They do not regularly have neurofibromas or acoustic neuromas but usually represent a variant of NF-2 with the same gene defect.

Therapy. The acoustic neuromas can be identified with a variety of imaging techniques and then surgically removed. Radiation therapy also appears to be an alternative.

Segmental Neurofibromatosis

Segmental neurofibromatosis (NF-5) features neurofibromas and café-au-lait macules confined to one body segment. It probably represents a somatic mutation; as with other such disorders, the risk of a germline mutation cannot be excluded, so these patients should be regarded as capable of having children with true NF-1. Occasionally, patients with segmental neurofibromatosis will be found within pedigrees of NF-1, or patients with typical NF-1 will have a segment following Blaschko lines in which they have many more neurofibromas.

Neurofibromatosis with Only Café-au-Lait Macules

There are some families in which multiple café-au-lait macules are present and no other features of NF-1 are seen. Linkage studies suggest that this very rare disorder is not linked to the neurofibromin gene. An alternative explanation would be that only a small part of the gene is mutated, i.e., that part responsible for café-au-lait macules. If an individual presents with only café-au-lait macules, he should be followed, because the most likely diagnosis is NF-1. If no other features appear by puberty, then this diagnosis should be entertained.

Tuberous Sclerosis

(Balzer and Grandhomme 1886; Pringle 1890; Bourneville 1890)

Synonyms. Pringle disease, Bourneville disease. Epiloia (epilepsy, low intelligence, adenoma sebaceum) is a term we prefer not to use.

Definition. Neurocutaneous syndrome with a variety of skin lesions as well as a range of systemic problems, including CNS lesions and seizures.

Epidemiology. Tuberous sclerosis is less common than NF-1; it has an incidence of about 1:10,000. About 75% of patients represent new mutations. The lower incidence of familial cases reflects the impaired reproductive capacity of patients with tuberous sclerosis.

Etiology and Pathogenesis. Tuberous sclerosis is an interesting disease to geneticists. For years, there were arguments about whether the disease tracked to chromosome 9q34 or 16p13. The answer is that two unrelated genes cause tuberous sclerosis. They are known as TSC1 (9q34) and TSC2 (16p13); the gene product of TSC2 is tuberin. The TSC2 mutation is more common, accounting for perhaps two-thirds of all cases. Presumably, both gene products are growth control genes acting in subsequent or very closely connected steps in a common pathway. In a given family, only one gene defect is found. Based on clinical features, it is impossible to guess which mutation is present.

Clinical Findings

Cutaneous Findings. The cutaneous findings are clearly not the most important problem for the patient, but they often lead to diagnosis.

Adenoma Sebaceum. While histologic studies have shown that these lesions are misnamed, as they are not adenomas of sebaceous gland origin, we will retain the clinical term. Initially there are pinhead-sized, skin-colored, red or yellow papules favoring the nasolabial folds and chin. The lesions increase in size and number, may become confluent, and have fine telangiectases (Fig. 19.9). They may remain relatively subtle, even in adult life, or become disfiguring. While the prevalence of adenoma sebaceum is often listed at around 50% in tuberous sclerosis patients, we suspect that it is much higher but that there is marked variation in expressivity.

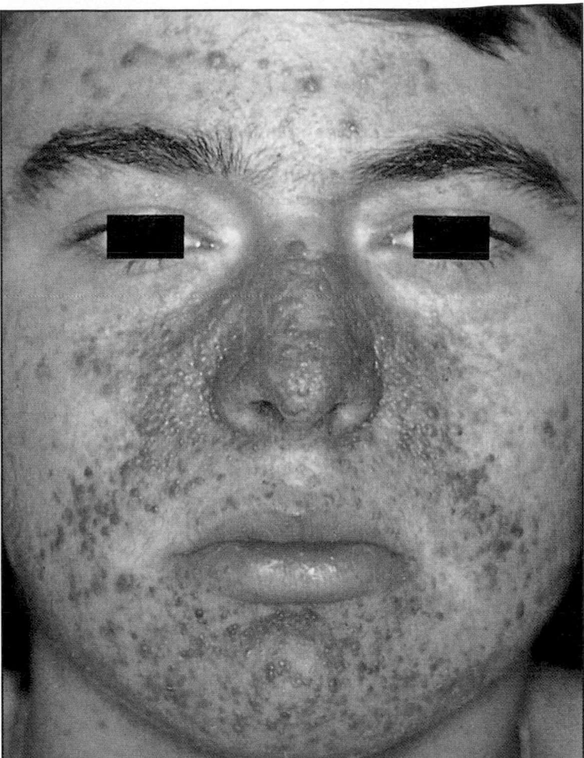

Fig. 19.9. Adenoma sebaceum in tuberous sclerosis

Ash Leaf Macule. Often the first sign of tuberous sclerosis is scattered hypopigmented macules, most commonly found on the trunk. While the classic lesion is an oval or elliptical lesion on the back resembling an ash leaf, more irregular macules or confetti-like lesions may be found. The latter are more common on the shins. About 90% of patients have some hypopigmented lesions when examined closely. They can be more easily identified with Wood light examination, which is recommended for all infants with unexplained seizures and for screening first degree relatives of tuberous sclerosis patients.

Connective Tissue Nevus. Also known as a shagreen patch, this lesion is usually in the lumbosacral region. It has a convoluted surface often described as cobblestone-like (Fig. 19.10). Shagreen originally referred to the rough skin of a shark or a ray but later came to be used for any hide tanned with a rough surface pattern. In any event, the connective tissue nevus consists of grouped firm papules and nodules. It is present in perhaps 25% of patients. In our judgment, the closely related fibrous plaque of the face is a variant of connective tissue nevus.

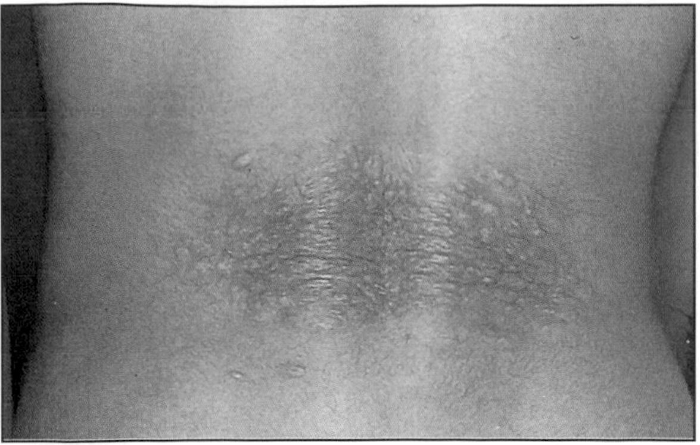

Fig. 19.10. Connective tissue nevus in tuberous sclerosis

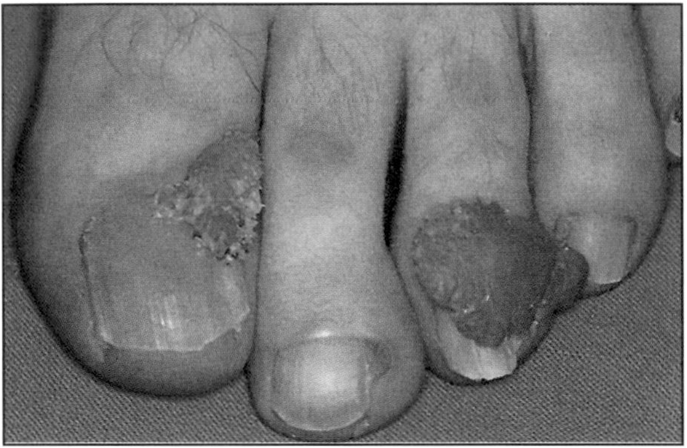

Fig. 19.11. Koenen tumor in tuberous sclerosis

Koenen (1932) Tumor. The Koenen tumor is a sub- or periungual fibroma. When small, it may be easily overlooked. Larger lesions are distinctive and tend to destroy part of the nail (Fig. 19.11).

Café-au-Lait Macules. Tuberous sclerosis patients frequently have one or more café-au-lait macules but never have axillary freckling or neurofibromas.

Oral Lesions. Gingival fibromas, tiny fibrous papules of the oral mucosa, and enamel pits are all relatively common (Fig. 19.12).

Systemic Findings. The list of systemic problems is long and we mention only the most common here.

CNS. The pathologic CNS defect is the presence of tubers, which are hamartomas consisting of astrocytes. They almost always cause seizures. Over 80 % of tuberous sclerosis patients suffer from epilepsy, which is often the presenting complaint in infancy. The other major problem is mental retardation, which affects about 50 % of patients to varying degrees. Depending on the society studied, a significant percentage of patients permanently hospitalized because of mental retardation have tuberous sclerosis. In some studies, this number has been as high as 5 %. In addition, calcified subependymal gliomas are often found and are fairly specific.

Heart. Rhabdomyomas are common, benign cardiac tumors that may be detected on prenatal ultrasound studies. They may cause conduction defects and interfere with appropriate muscular and valvular function.

Kidney. Renal angiomyolipomas are also almost specific for tuberous sclerosis. They are present in about 20 % of patients and can cause pain or hemorrhage. Renal cysts are also common; the TSC2 gene is very close to one of the adult-onset polycystic kidney genes, so this may be one clinical sign for differentiating the two gene effects. Renal failure may result and is the leading cause of death. Renal cell carcinoma may also occur.

Eyes. Retinal hamartomas, also known as phakomas, are often found but rarely cause visual problems. Larger lesions may have a mulberry pattern.

Lungs. Large cysts may produce a honeycomb pattern and pneumothorax and lead to respiratory failure.

Skeleton. Periosteal bone formation and phalangeal pseudocysts can sometimes be identified on radiologic studies.

Malignancies. Malignant tumors are rare in tuberous sclerosis. Occasionally, renal cell carcinoma or aggressive astrocytomas are described.

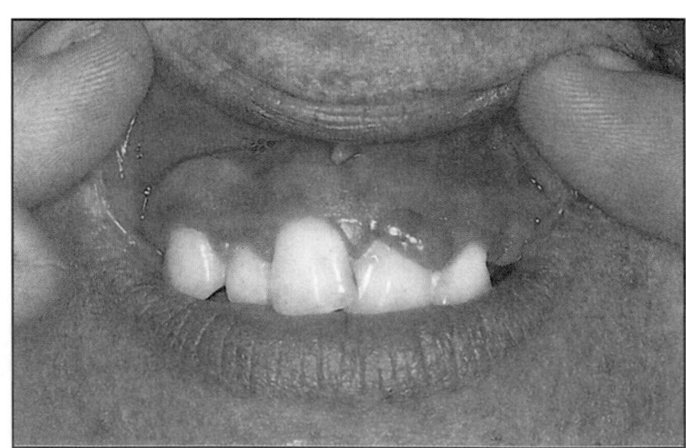

Fig. 19.12. Oral fibromas in tuberous sclerosis

Histopathology. Sebacious adenomas are angiofibromas (Chap. 59). They may contain sebaceous glands simply because they are so common in the sites of predilection. Some argue that the more yellow lesions are true sebaceous lesions, while the redder nodules are typical angiofibromas. Koenen tumors are also angiofibromas. The connective tissue nevi are indistinguishable from sporadic versions of the same lesion (Chap. 52). The hypopigmented macules contain melanocytes, in contrast to vitiligo. Apparently, there is impaired transfer of melanin from the melanocytes to keratinocytes, although detailed studies are lacking.

Laboratory Findings. Magnetic resonance imaging is the best way to identify the tubers and confirm the diagnosis. Other imaging procedures such as computerized tomography can also be employed but involve radiation on a small patient. Ultrasound is useful to check for cardiac rhabdomyomas, renal tumors, and cysts. EKG or echo electrocardiogram will elucidate the nature of the conduction defects.

Course and Prognosis. Patients without mental retardation have relatively normal life expectancies. Most require seizure medication. Cardiac and renal problems also contribute to morbidity and mortality.

Differential Diagnosis. Early facial adenoma sebaceum can be confused with acne. Later, the differential diagnosis includes nevoid basal cell carcinoma syndrome (Chap. 56), multiple trichoepitheliomas (Chap. 57), and other syndromes with multiple adnexal tumors. Koenen tumors are confused with verruca or other digital fibrous tumors. The connective tissue nevi may resemble nevus lipomatosis.

In rare instances, individuals and even families present with adenoma sebaceum or Koenen tumors but no other stigmata of tuberous sclerosis. Only molecular genetic studies can clarify the relationships of such patients to tuberous sclerosis. Connective tissue nevi are somewhat more common. They are usually sporadic but may be familial and are also seen in Buschke-Ollendorff syndrome (Chap. 52).

Therapy. The facial lesions can be destroyed with lasers, dermabrasion, electrosurgery, or tangential excision. All methods bring improvement for some time, but recurrences are the rule. Other cosmetically disturbing lesions can be excised. Both the cardiac and renal problems require expert internal medicine management. Renal transplantation has been required for some patients.

Prenatal Diagnosis. Either linkage studies or mutation detection can be performed. In addition, the cardiac rhabdomyomas can be recognized on ultrasound.

Von Hippel-Lindau Syndrome

(Jackson 1872; von Hippel 1895; Lindau 1926)

While von Hippel-Lindau syndrome is classically viewed as a phakomatosis, cutaneous involvement is infrequent. This rare disease with an incidence of 1:40,000 is inherited in an autosomal dominant pattern. The gene, known as VHL, inhibits a transcription control protein known as elongin. Patients have cerebellar and retinal angiomas as well as occasionally cutaneous vascular malformations. Facial port wine stains have been described. In our experience, such patients almost never present to dermatologists. It is not necessary to search for VHL mutations in patients with congenital vascular malformations unless the family history points toward von Hippel-Lindau syndrome. About 50% of patients develop renal cell tumors, usually bilaterally and at an earlier age than sporadic tumors. Pheochromocytomas are also seen. Of special interest is the presence of VHL gene mutations in about 80% of sporadic renal cell carcinomas.

Other Genodermatoses

Focal Dermal Hypoplasia

(Jessner 1921; Goltz et al. 1962; Gorlin et al. 1963)

Synonyms. Goltz syndrome, Goltz-Gorlin syndrome, congenital ectodermal and mesodermal dysplasia, osteooculodermal dysplasia

Epidemiology. Focal dermal hypoplasia is a rare disorder, with about 250 patients described. The male:female ratio is about 1:10.

Etiology and Pathogenesis. Focal dermal hypoplasia is an X-linked dominant disorder. While the gene has been reported on Xp22.31, such cases were actually occurrences of MIDAS syndrome. In any event, the basic gene defect is unknown.

Clinical Findings. Focal dermal hypoplasia involves so many organs in so many ways that it is hard to find a proper niche for it. The multiple findings are all present at birth.

Cutaneous Findings. The skin typically has linear atrophic telangiectatic areas following the Blaschko lines. The skin is so thin that the terms "cigarette paper atrophy" or "scarring" have been used (Fig. 19.13). There may be herniations or bulges of fat producing soft nodules in the same pattern. There are often tiny papillomas around the mouth and anus, sometimes with a verrucous surface. In some cases, areas will be ulcerated at birth and heal with deeper scarring. Nail dystrophies and scarring alopecia both can develop. Apocrine nevi are very rare (Chap. 52), but when they do occur, it is usually in association with focal dermal hypoplasia.

Systemic Findings. At birth, the most dramatic findings are often skeletal; there may be claw hands or feet (Fig. 19.14), simple syndactyly, scoliosis, or major limb defects. Ocular abnormalities include coloboma, microphthalmia, and decreased visual acuity. Dental abnormalities are common. Many other structural abnormalities can be seen, especially on the face. Perhaps a quarter of the patients have mild to moderate mental retardation.

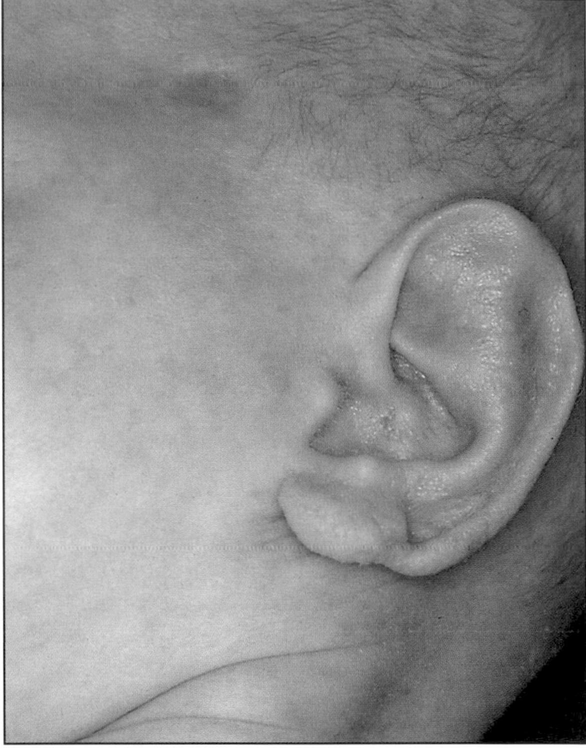

Fig. 19.13. Focal atrophic lesion on temple in focal dermal hypoplasia

Histopathology. Skin biopsy can be very helpful. If an atrophic lesion is biopsied, the subcutaneous fat may be found in virtual opposition to the epidermis, with no more than wisps of fibrous dermis. The papillomas have a different configuration but are otherwise similar.

Laboratory Findings. Most patients in infancy have osteopathia striata or linear striations in the epiphyses of long bones. This can be readily appreciated on routine X-ray and greatly aid the clinical diagnosis of infants with multiple anomalies.

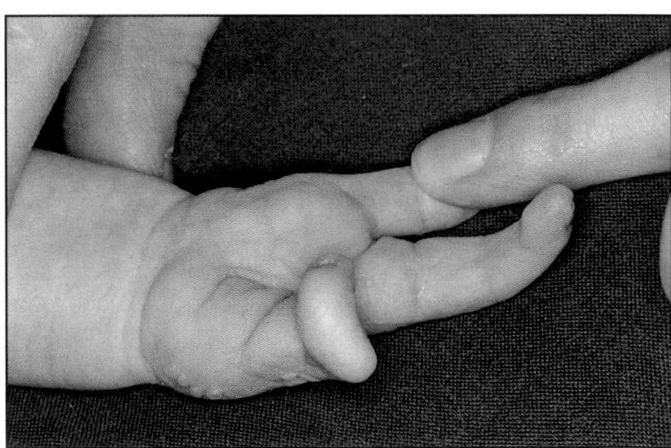

Fig. 19.14. Malformed hand in focal dermal hypoplasia

Course and Prognosis. The patients are generally severely handicapped by their orthopedic and ocular problems.

Differential Diagnosis. The rare mild patients may present with one or two fatty herniations, which are identical to nevus lipomatosus, or with multiple papillomas, which are confused with warts. The differential diagnosis also includes the rare syndromes listed below.

Therapy. Surgery can usually reduce the skeletal problems and may improve the visual difficulties. Large herniated tumors which are painful or disturbing can be excised, as can the papillomas.

Variants of Focal Dermal Hypoplasia

MIDAS Syndrome

(Happle et al. 1993)

MIDAS is an acronym for microophthalmia, dermal aplasia, and sclerocornea. Dermal aplasia is probably closer to scars of aplasia cutis congenita, since herniation of fat is not seen. None of the other changes of focal dermal hypoplasia is found. This disorder has been mapped to X22.1–22.3 and is inherited in an X-linked dominant pattern.

Focal Facial Dermal Hypoplasia

(Brauer 1928; McGeoch and Reed 1973)

Synonyms. Brauer syndrome, nevus aplasticus

Brauer described almost 40 patients with tiny, atrophic pseudoscars on the temples in a large pedigree showing inheritance in an autosomal dominant pattern and no associated features. In a large Australian family, there was a possible association with gastrointestinal carcinomas.

Setleis Syndrome

(Setleis 1963)

Synonym. Bitemporal aplasia cutis congenita

Most patients are reported in isolated clusters in Puerto Rico, suggesting autosomal recessive inheritance. There are bilateral temporal focal dermal hypoplasia, upward-slanting eyebrows, a flattened nose, lowered hairline, and often a cleft chin. Many patients are initially diagnosed as showing obstetric forceps injury. These patients do not have aplasia cutis congenita, but the differences are slight, as the atrophic skin may be eroded.

Oculocerebrocutaneous Syndrome

(Delleman and Oorthuys 1981)

Synonym. Delleman-Oorthuys syndrome

In this rare sporadic syndrome, patients have focal areas of missing or atrophic skin, called both aplasia cutis congenita and focal dermal hypoplasia. The most common site is the face. They also have orbital cysts and multiple periorbital skin tags, some of which contain striated muscle and can show independent motion. They also have cerebral malformations. It has been suggested that oculocerebrocutaneous syndrome is an example of an autosomal, dominant, lethal mutation surviving only in the mosaic state.

Oral-Facial-Digital Syndrome Type I

Synonym. Papillon-Léage and Psaume (1954) syndrome, OFD I

There are several oral-facial-digital syndromes which are poorly defined but apparently unrelated. The most common is OFD I, but it is still quite rare. It is inherited in an X-linked dominant pattern. The principal cutaneous finding is of multiple milia that evolve into pitted scarring known as follicular atrophoderma (Chap. 18). The tongue is often lobulated and the lips fail to juxtapose, leaving a small central hole (drinking straw sign). Finally, there is polydactyly. In OFD II syndrome (Mohr 1941), milia are absent but the thumbs are typically duplicated, rather than other digits.

Proteus Syndrome

(Cohen and Hayden 1979; Wiedemann et al. 1983)

Etiology and Pathogenesis. Proteus syndrome is one of the epidermal nevus syndromes (Chap. 52). It is believed to represent a somatic mutation to a lethal autosomal dominant gene, but this gene has not been identified. All cases have been sporadic.

History. Proteus was a Greek god who was polymorphous and could change his shape at will. Wiedemann chose this name to indicate dramatically how variable the clinical appearance of the syndrome can be. Joseph Merrick, the Elephant Man made famous by a stage play and movie of the same name, almost certainly had Proteus syndrome and not neurofibromatosis, as has often been suggested. Castings of his soles show the typical cerebriform changes.

Clinical Findings

Cutaneous Findings. The most striking cutaneous findings are hyperkeratotic epidermal nevi and palmoplantar connective tissue nevi that produce cerebriform changes on the hands and feet. A variety of mesenchyme malformations are also seen, including nevus flammeus, hemangiomas, lymphangiomas, and lipomas.

Systemic Findings. The underlying theme is asymmetric growth which may result in macrocephaly, unequal limbs, enlarged or distorted hands and feet, and a variety of other malformations. Ocular defects are common and highly variable. Moderate mental retardation is present in about 50% of patients. Despite the hamartomatous nature of the disorder, malignant degeneration appears rare.

Differential Diagnosis. The presence of an enlarged limb (hemihypertrophy) may suggest a variety of systemic disorders with dermatologic features:

- Encephalocraniocutaneous lipomatosis (Chap. 59) is probably a variant of Proteus syndrome.
- Mafucci syndrome (Chap. 59) features hemangiomas and endochondromas. There are probably overlaps between it and Proteus syndrome.
- Klippel-Trénaunay-Weber syndrome (Chap. 52) usually involves only one limb.
- Neurofibromatosis should not be confused with Proteus syndrome. The deformities induced by large plexiform neurofibromas with overlying loose skin only remotely resemble the lesions in Proteus syndrome, although both are very disfiguring.
- Tumors such as rhabdomyosarcoma, Wilms tumor, hepatoblastoma, and neuroblastoma also produce isolated limb enlargement.

Therapy. Dermatologic management has little to offer. Skilled orthopedic care can correct some of the skeletal defects. In other cases, amputation is the only answer.

Chromosomal Syndromes

Since skin problems are usually only a minor part of these patients' problems, we will review the cutaneous findings only briefly.

Turner Syndrome

(Ullrich 1930; Bonnevie 1934; Turner 1938)

Synonyms. Ullrich-Turner syndrome, Bonnevie-Ullrich syndrome, XO syndrome

Epidemiology. Turner syndrome affects about one in 10,000 female births, but over 95% of XO fetuses are lost in the first trimester. Turner syndrome accounts for 20% of spontaneous abortions.

Etiology and Pathogenesis. The karyotype in Turner syndrome is 45,XO, i.e., one X chromosome is missing. An error in gamete formation is the usual explanation. In most cases, only the maternal X chromosome is present. Partial loss of an X chromosome and mosaicism can also play a role. Maternal age has no role.

Clinical Findings. As a rule of thumb, about one-third of Turner syndrome patients are diagnosed at birth, one-third in childhood, and one-third at adolescence. If the malformations are severe enough, the diagnosis at birth is easy, but often the patients are simply viewed as small girls for a number of years before an investigation is undertaken.

Cutaneous Findings. At birth, a webbed neck and lymphedema of the limbs may be discerned in an infant who later remains small for its age. The webbed neck is a residual result of bilateral fetal cystic hygromas, which are widely dilated, malformed lymphatics. The peripheral lymphedema also usually resolves. Later, the patients have multiple melanocytic nevi and tend to develop keloids easily.

Systemic Findings. In childhood, coarctation of the aorta usually leads to the diagnosis, as every pediatric cardiologist seeing a small girl with this problem orders a karyotype. In other cases, primary amenorrhea brings the girl to a doctor's attention, as the patients have streak gonads. The face is usually somewhat triangular, the chest broadened (shield chest) with wide-set nipples, and the posterior hairline is low. The fourth and fifth fingers tend to be shortened and a variety of nail anomalies can be seen. In addition to the cardiac changes, renal malformations such as horseshoe kidneys can occur. The patients are intellectually normal but have impaired spatial orientation.

Laboratory Findings. Buccal smears reveal a lack of Barr bodies. The diagnosis is confirmed with a karyotype, as complex chromosomal rearrangements or losses may on occasion be found.

Differential Diagnosis. The main differential diagnostic consideration is Noonan (Noonan and Ehmke 1963) syndrome, which is inherited in an autosomal dominant pattern with highly variable expressivity. Patients can appear very similar to cases of Turner syndrome, with small stature, webbed neck, lymphedema, and multiple melanocytic nevi. They, too, have cardiac defects, most often atrial septal defects, and pulmonic stenosis. Noonan syndrome is about as common as Turner syndrome but is underdiagnosed. There is also a Noonan-neurofibromatosis overlap syndrome.

Therapy. If required, the webbed neck, coarctation, and other malformations can be surgically repaired. Estrogen replacement therapy, usually combined with growth hormone, increases the growth rate and induces secondary sexual characteristics. Women thus treated can carry a fertilized donated egg to full term.

Prenatal Diagnosis. While the risk of a second child with Turner syndrome is no greater than with the general population, most families want to be sure. In addition, the risk does increase along with other, more complex chromosomal changes. In additional to karyotype analysis, ultrasound for measuring nuchal skin thickness is helpful.

Klinefelter Syndrome

(Klinefelter et al. 1942)

Epidemiology. The frequency is about 1:500 male births. The risk increases with advanced maternal age.

Etiology and Pathogenesis. These patients are usually 47, XXY. In some instances they may have even more additional X chromosomes.

Clinical Findings. Klinefelter syndrome is discussed in Chapter 67 because the diagnosis is often made when a man presents for an infertility workup. The patients tend to be tall, with relatively long legs and truncal obesity. They are sterile, with small genitalia, gynecomastia, and sparse axillary and pubic hair. They also have prominent varicose veins and, as a result, often stasis dermatitis and leg ulcerations. Mild mental retardation and antisocial behavior appear common.

Laboratory Findings. Buccal scrapings reveal the presence of Barr bodies, not otherwise seen in males. Karyotyping confirms the diagnosis.

Differential Diagnosis. Although the patients are not truly marfanoid, the differential diagnosis listed in Chapter 18 should be considered.

Therapy. Hormone replacement allows development of secondary sexual characteristics. Most patients benefit from treatment of their varicosities. Psychological and educational counseling is probably the most important consideration if the patients are identified in childhood.

Prenatal Diagnosis. Karyotype analysis can be easily done, as is standard for older mothers or in families where one child has already been identified.

Down Syndrome

(Séguin 1846; Down 1866)

Synonym. Trisomy 21. Unfortunately, Down used the term Mongolian idiocy, which insults the patients and does an injustice to Asians.

Epidemiology. The incidence of Down syndrome is about 1:700 live births but increases profoundly with maternal age. Once again, over two-thirds of trisomy 21 conceptions end in spontaneous abortion. About 15% of individuals institutionalized for mental retardation have this disorder.

Etiology and Pathogenesis. In most cases there is nondisjunction of the maternal chromosome 21 during meiosis. Rarely, the paternal chromosome may be duplicated and in a small percentage of families the syndrome is the result of a translocation. They have brain deposits of β-amyloid protein, as do patients with Alzheimer's disease; the gene for this protein is located on chromosome 21.

Clinical Findings

Cutaneous Findings. The number of skin changes in Down syndrome is lengthy, but none of the problems is severe. Infants tend to have cystic hygromas and nuchal thickening. The most annoying problem is severe xerosis, often associated with erythema and lichenification. In addition, syringomas, elastosis perforans serpiginosa, and alopecia areata all appear more common. The single palmar crease is probably the best known characteristic but it is not specific.

Systemic Findings. Details should be sought in the pediatric or medicine literature. Patients are often identified because of an enlarged furrowed tongue, flat face, dysplastic ears, and epicanthic folds. They have a variety of skeletal defects. The main problems include mental retardation, cardiac anomalies, increased incidence of leukemia, and a host of other changes. The life expectancy is around 40 years.

Laboratory Findings. Karyotype analysis answers the question.

Differential Diagnosis. There is no serious differential diagnosis; at birth, cretinism may come into question.

Therapy. Standard therapy should be offered. Aggressive early repair of cardiac anomalies has advanced the survival age. Many patients do well in sheltered work programs and most societies are trying to keep Down syndrome individuals in their homes as long as feasible.

Prenatal Diagnosis. This syndrome is the main reason for checking the fetal karyotype whenever the mother is older than 35 (or even 30) years. Women who already have a child with Down syndrome or are aware of a translocation are also screened. Many new methods of diagnosis exist, including measurement of α-fetoprotein, ultrasound assessment of nuchal skin thickness and, most recently, identifying trisomic fetal cells in the maternal blood.

Bibliography

Aplasia Cutis Congenita

Adams FH, Oliver CP (1945) Hereditary deformities in man due to arrested development. J Hered 36:3–7

Bart BJ, Gorlin RJ, Andersen VE et al. (1966) Congenital localized absence of skin and associated abnormalities resembling epidermolysis bullosa. Arch Dermatol 93: 296–304

Frieden IJ (1986) Aplasia cutis congenita: a clinical review and proposal for classification. J Am Acad Dermatol 14: 646–660

Johanson A, Blizzard R (1971) A syndrome of congenital aplasia of the alae nasi, deafness, hypothyroidism, dwarfism, absent permanent teeth, and malabsorption. J Pediatr 79:982–987

Kruk-Jeromin J, Janik J, Rykala J (1998) Aplasia cutis congenita of the scalp. Report of 16 cases. Dermatol Surg 24:549–553

Küster W, Traupe H (1988) Klinik und Genetik angeborener Hautdefekte. Hautarzt 39:553–563

Küster W, Lenz W, Kääriänen H et al. (1988) Congenital scalp defects with distal limb abnormalities (Adams-Oliver-syndrome): report of ten cases and review of the literature. Am J Med Genet 31:99–115

Leaute-Labreze C, Depaire-Duclos F, Sarlangue J et al. (1998) Congenital cutaneous defects as complications in surviving cotwins. Aplasia cutis congenita and neonatal Volkmann ischemic contracture of the arm. Arch Dermatol 134:1121–1124

Patau K et al. (1960) Multiple congenital anomaly caused by an extra autosome. Lancet i:790–793

Zvulunov A, Kachko L, Manor E et al. (1998) Reticulolineal aplasia cutis congenita of the face and neck: a distinctive cutaneous manifestation in several syndromes linked to Xp22. Br J Dermatol 138:1046–1052

Pseudoainhum

Krunic AL, Ljiljana M, Novak A et al. (1997) Hereditary bullous acrokeratotic poikiloderma of Weary-Kindler associated with pseudoainhum and sclerotic bands. Int J Dermatol 36:529–533

Peterska ES, Karom IM (1964) Congenital pseudo-ainhum of the finger. Arch Dermatol 90:12–14

Raque CJ, Stein KM, Lane JM (1972) Pseudo-ainhum constricting bands of the extremities. Arch Dermatol 105: 434–438

Rushton DI (1938) Amniotic band syndrome. Br Med J 286:919–920

Takahashi H, Ishida-Yamamoto A, Kishi A et al. (1999) Loricrin gene mutation in a Japanese patient of Vohwinkel's syndrome. J Dermatol Sci 19:44–47

Cutis Verticis Gyrata

Farah S, Farag T, Sabry MA et al. (1998) Cutis verticis gyrata-mental deficiency syndrome: report of a case with unusual neuroradiological findings. Clin Dysmorphol 7:131–134

Fesel R, Plewig G, Lentrodt J (1990) Cutis verticis gyrata. Hautarzt 41:502–505

Kolawole TM, Al-Orainy IA, Patel PJ et al. (1998) Cutis verticis gyrata: its computed tomographic demonstration in acromegaly. Eur J Radiol 27:145–148

Schepis C, Palazzo R, Cannavo SP et al. (1990) Prevalence of primary cutis verticis gyrata in a psychiatric population: association with chromosomal fragile sites. Acta Derm Venereol (Stockh) 70:483–486

Unna PG (1907) Cutis verticis gyrata. Monatsschr Prakt 45: 227–233

Pachydermoperiostosis

Demirpolat G, Sener RN, Stun EE (1999) MR imaging of pachydermoperiostosis. J Neuroradiol 26:61–63

Lindmaier A, Raff M, Seidl G et al. (1989) Pachydermoperiostose. Klinik, Klassifikation, und Pathogenese. Hautarzt 40:752–757

Sinha GP, Curtis P, Haigh D et al. (1997) Pachydermoperiostosis in childhood. Br J Rheumatol 36:1224–1227

Touraine A, Solente G, Golé L (1935) Un syndrome ostéodermopathique: la pachydermie plicaturée avec pachypériostose des extrémités. Presse Med 43:1820–1824

Polydactyly

Ellis RW, van Creveld S (1940) A syndrome characterized by ectodermal dysplasia, polydactyly, chondrodysplasia and congenital morbus cordis. Report of three cases. Arch Dis Child 15:65–84

Shapiro L, Juhlin EA, Brownstein MH (1973) Rudimentary polydactyly. An amputation neuroma. Arch Dermatol 108:223–225

Suzuki H, Matsuoka S (1981) Rudimentary polydactyly (cutaneous neuroma) case report with ultrastructural study. J Cutan Pathol 8:299–307

Acessory Tragus

Brownstein MH, Wanger N, Helwig EB (1971) Accessory tragi. Arch Dermatol 104:625–631

Cohen PR, Gilbert BE (1993) Pathological cases of the month. Acessory tragus. Am J Dis Child 147:1123–1124

Acessory Nipple

Leung AKC, Robson WLM (1989) Polythelia. Int J Dermatol 28:429–433

Toumbis-Joannou E, Cohen PR (1994) Familial polythelia. J Am Acad Dermatol 30:667–668

Weinberg SK, Motulsky AG (1976) Aberrant axillary breast tissue: a report of a family with six affected women in two generations. Clin Genet 10:325–328

Painful Piezogenic Papules

Laing VB, Fleischer AB (1991) Piezogenic wrist papules. A common and asymptomatic finding. J Am Acad Dermatol 24:415–417

Plewig G, Braun-Falco O (1973) Piezogene Knötchen. Druckbedingte Fersen- und Handkantenknötchen. Hautarzt 24:114–118

Shelley WB, Rawnsley HM (1968) Painful feet due to herniation of fat. JAMA 205:308–309

Transverse Nasal Line

Cornbleet T (1951) Transverse nasal stripe of puberty (stria nasi transversa). Arch Dermatol 63:70–72

Myers WA (1960) The nasal crease. JAMA 174:1204–1206

Okinduro OM, Burge SM (1994) Congenital milia in the nasal groove. Br J Dermatol 130:800

Piqué E, Olivares M, Farina MC et al. (1996) Congenital nasal comedones – report of three cases. Clin Exp Dermatol 21:220–221

Shelley WB, Shelley ED, Pansky B (1997) The transverse nasal line: an embryonic fault line. Br J Dermatol 137:963–965

Dorsal-Ventral Transposition

Dragan L, Lorincz AL, Medenica MM et al. (1999) Graft-like plantar lesion secondary to possible dorsal-to ventral cutaneous transposition. J Am Acad Dermatol 40:769–771

Nasal Glioma

Argenyi ZB (1996) Cutaneous neural heterotopias and related tumors relevant for the dermatopathologist. Semin Diagn Pathol 13:60–71

Sanjuan-Rodriguez S, Diaz-Pino P, Ortiz-Barquero MC et al. (1998) Frontal extranasal glioma. Cir Pediatr 11:81–83

Neurofibromatosis

Atit RP, Crowe MJ, Greenhalgh DG et al. (1999) The NF1 tumor suppressor regulates mouse skin wound healing, fibroblast proliferation, and collagen deposited by fibroblasts. J Invest Dermatol 112:835–842

Crowe FW, Schull WJ (1953) Diagnostic importance of café au lait spot in neurofibromatosis. Arch Intern Med 91: 758–766

Johnson NS, Saal HM, Lovell AM et al. (1999) Social and emotional problems in children with neurofibromatosis type 1: evidence and proposed interventions. J Pediatr 134:767–772

Karnes PS (1998) Neurofibromatosis: a common neurocutaneous disorder. Mayo Clin Proc 73:1071–1076

Klose A, Peters H, Hoffmeyer S et al. (1999) Two independent mutations in a family with neurofibromatosis type 1 (NF1). Am J Med Genet 83:6–12

Landau M, Krafchik BR (1999) The diagnostic value of café-au-lait macules. J Am Acad Dermatol 6:877–890

Lisch K (1937) Über Beteiligung der Augen, insbesondere das Vorkommen von Irisknötchen bei der Neurofibromatose (Recklinghausen). Z Augenheilk 93:137–143

Mautner VF, Lindenau M, Baser ME et al. (1997) Skin abnormalities in neurofibromatosis 2. Arch Dermatol 133: 1539–1543

von Recklinghausen FD (1882) Über die multiplen Fibrome der Haut und ihre Beziehungen zu den Neuromen. Festschrift für R. Virchow. Hirschwald, Berlin, p 138

Riccardi VM (1999) Neurofibromatosis: phenotype, natural history, and pathogenesis, 3rd edn. Baltimore. The Johns Hopkins University Press

Watson GH (1967) Pulmonary stenosis, café-au-lait spots, and dull intelligence. Arch Dis Child 42:303–307

Westerhof W et al. (1978) Hereditary congenital hypopigmented and hyperpigmented macules. Arch Derm 114:931–936

Wolkenstein P, Frèche B, Zeller J et al. (1996) Usefulness of screening investigations in neurofibromatosis type 1: a study of 152 patients. Arch Dermatol 132:1333–1336

Tuberous Sclerosis

Arslan A, Ciftci E, Cetin A et al. (1998) Tuberous sclerosis: Ultrasound, CT, and MRI features of two cases with multiple organ involvement. Aust Radiol 42:379–382

Borelli S (1999) Koenen, Kothe und die periunfualen Fibrome bei tuberöser Sklerose. Hautarzt 50:368–369

Bourneville DM (1880) Sclérose tubéreuse des circonvolutions cérébrales, idiotie, et épilepsie hémiplégique. Arch Neurol (Paris) I:81–89

Jozwiak S, Schwartz RA, Janniger CK et al. (1998) Skin lesions in children with tuberous sclerosis complex: their prevalence, natural course, and diagnostic significance. Int J Dermatol 37:911–917

Koenen J (1932) Eine familiäre hereditäre Form von tuberöser Sklerose. Acta Psychiat (Kbh) 1:813–821

Kothe R (1903) Zur Lehre von den Talgdrüsengeschwülsten. Arch Dermatol Syph 68:33–54

Pringle JJ (1890) A case of congenital adenoma sebaceum. Br J Dermatol 2:1–14

Sampson JR, Whittemore VH (eds) (1999) Tuberous sclerosis complex, 3rd edn. Oxford University Press

Young J, Povey S (1998) The genetic basis of tuberous sclerosis. Mol Med Today 4:313–319

Von Hippel-Lindau Syndrome

von Hippel E (1895) Vorstellung eines Patienten mit einem sehr ungewöhnlichen Aderhautleiden. Bericht 24. Versammlung der Ophth Ges, p. 169

Lamiell JM, Salazar FG, Hsia YE (1989) Von Hippel-Lindau disease affecting 43 members of a single kindred. Medicine 68:1–29

Lindau A (1926) Studien über Kleinhirnzysten. Bau, Pathogenese und Beziehungen zur Angiomatosis retinae. Acta Path Microb Scand 3:1–28

Maher ER, Bentley E, Yates JRW et al. (1991) Mapping of the von Hippel-Lindau disease locus to a small region of chromosome 3p by genetic linkage analysis. Genomics 10:957–960

Focal Dermal Hypoplasia

Barre V, Drouin-Garraud V, Marret S et al. (1998) Focal dermal hypoplasia: description of three cases. Arch Dermatol 5:513–516

Boothroyd AE, Hall CM (1988) The radiological features of Goltz syndrome: focal dermal hypoplasia. A report of two cases. Skeletal Radiol 17:505–508
Goltz RW (1992) Focal demal hypoplasia syndrome. An update. Arch Dermatol 128:1108–1111
Goltz RW, Peterson WC, Gorlin RJ et al. (1962) Focal dermal hypoplasia. Arch Dermatol 86:708–717
Gorlin RJ, Meskin LH, Peterson WC et al. (1963) Focal dermal hypoplasia syndrome. Acta Derm 43:421–440
Happle R, Daniels O, Koopman RJ (1993) MIDAS syndrome (microphthalmia, dermal aplasia, and sclerocornea): an X-linked phenotype distinct from Goltz syndrome. Am J Med Genet 47:710–713
Jessner M (1921) Breslauer dermatologische Vereinigung. Arch Dermatol Syph 133:48
Larregue M, Duterque M (1975) Striated osteopathy in focal dermal hypoplasia. Arch Dermatol 1311–1315
McGeoch AH, Reed WB (1973) Familial focal facial dermal dysplasia. Arch Dermatol 107:591–595

Setleis Syndrome

Setleis H et al. (1963) Congenital ectodermal dysplasia of the face. Pediatrics 32:540–548

Oculocerebrocutaneous Syndrome

Delleman JW, Oorthuys JW (1981) Orbital cyst in addition to congenital cerebral and focal dermal malformations: a new entity? Clin Genet 19:191–198
Loggers HE, Oosterwijk JC, Overweg-Plandosen WCG (1992) Encephalocraniocutaneous lipomatosis and oculocerebrocutaneous syndrome. Ophthalmic Paediatr Genet 13:171–177
Moog U, de Die-Smulders C, Systermans JMJ et al. (1997) Oculocerebrocutaneous syndrome: Report of three additional cases and aetiological considerations. Clin Genet 52:219–225

Oral-Facial-Digital Syndrome

Mohr OL (1941) A hereditary sublethal syndrome in man. Skr Norske Vidensk Akad 14:1–18
Papillon-Léage E, Psaume J (1954) Une nouvelle malformation héreditaire de la muquese buccale. Brides et freins amormaus. Rev Stomat 55:209–227

Proteus Syndrome

Cohen MM, Hayden PW (1979) A newly recognized hamartomatous syndrome. Birth Defects 15:291–296
Rizzo R, Pavone L, Micale G (1993) Encephalocraniocutaneous lipomatosis, Proteus syndrome, and somatic mosaicism. Am J Med Genet 47:653–655
Sigaudy S, Freouille C, Gambarelli D et al. (1998) Prenatal ultrasonographic findings in Proteus syndrome. Prenat Diagn 18:1091–1094
Wiedemann HR, Burgio GR, Aldenhoff P et al. (1983) The proteus syndrome. Partial gigantism of the hands and/or feet, nevi, hemihypertrophy, subcutaneous tumors, macrocephaly or other skull anomalies and possible accelerated growth and visceral affections. Eur J Pediatr 140:5–12

Turner Syndrome

Bonnevie K (1934) Embryological analysis of gene manifestation in Little and Bogg's abnormal mouse tribe. J Exp Zool 67:443–520
Haeusler G (1998) Growth hormone therapy in patients with Turner syndrome. Horm Res 49:62–66
Hall JG, Gilchrist DM (1990) Turner syndrome and its variants. Pediatr Clin North Am 37:1421–1440
Turner HH (1938) A syndrome of infantilism, congenital webbed neck, and cubitus valgus. Endocrinology 23: 566–574
Ullrich O (1930) Über typische Kombinationsbilder multiper Abortungen. Zeitschr Kinderh 49:271–276
Zinn AR, Tonk VS, Chen Z et al. (1998) Evidence for a Turner syndrome locus or loci at Xp11.2-p22.1. Am J Hum Genet 63:1757–1766

Noonan Syndrome

Char F, Rodriguez-Fernandez HL, Scott CI et al. (1972) The Noonan syndrome – a clinical study of 45 cases. Birth Defects Orig Art Ser 8:110–118
George CD, Patton MA, el Sawi M et al. (1993) Abdominal ultrasound in Noonan syndrome: a study of 44 patients. Pediatr Radiol 23:316–318
Noonan JA, Ehmke DA (1963) Associated noncardiac malformations in children with congenital heart disease. J Pediatr 63:468–470

Klinefelter Syndrome

Klinefelter HF Jr, Reifenstein EC Jr, Albright F (1942) Syndrome characterized by gynecomastia, aspermatogenesis without A-leydigism, and increased excretion of follicle-stimulating hormone. J Clin Endocr 2:615–627
Mandoki MW, Sumner GS (1991) Klinefelter syndrome: the need for early identification and treatment. Clin Pediatr 30:161–164
Mark HF, Alter D, Mousseau P (1999) Klinefelter syndrome. Arch Pathol Lab Med 123:261
Meschede D, Louwen F, Nippert I et al. (1998) Low rates of pregnancy termination for prenatally diagnosed Klinefelter syndrome and other sex chromosome polysomies. Am J Med Genet 80:330–334

Down Syndrome

Down JL (1866) Observations on an ethnic classification of idiots. London Hosp Clin Lect Rep 3:259–262
Scherbenske JM, Benson PM, Rotchford JP, James WD (1990) Cutaneous and ocular manifestations of Down syndrome. J Am Acad Dermatol 22:933–938

Inflammatory Diseases of Cartilage

Contents

Inflammatory diseases of cartilage are relatively uncommon but are occasionally encountered by dermatologists. There is often a traumatic component, whether dramatic as in a cauliflower ear or subtle as in chondrodermatitis nodularis helicis. The ears are exposed and very susceptible to cold injury. In addition, sometimes cutaneous vasculitis involves the ears, especially drug-induced vasculitis. Because of the poor vascular supply of the cartilage, any damage tends to be chronic and difficult to treat.

Chondrodermatitis Nodularis Helicis

(Winkler 1915)

Synonyms. Chondrodermatitis nodularis chronica helicis, sleeper's ear, painful ear nodule

Definition. Painful inflammatory nodule on the upper aspect of the helix.

Epidemiology. This relatively common problem is seen more often in men than women, usually occurs in late adult life and more often affects the right ear.

Etiology and Pathogenesis. The cause of chondrodermatitis nodularis helicis is unclear. It may be a response to persistent minor trauma, such as might be induced during sleeping. Nuns have a similar change where their stiff head covering presses on their ears. More striking trauma or cold injury usually induces more diffuse change. Some histologic studies have indicated involvement of hair follicles in the process, but we are sceptical and suspect secondary involvement as the ear is rich in hairs.

Clinical Findings. The typical lesion is a round or oval nodule, perhaps 4 mm in diameter, located on the border of the helix, most often on the superior or posterior aspect (Fig. 20.1). The nodule is usually firmly bound to the underlying cartilage. It is usually skin-colored or even pearly, but can be slightly red; the adjacent skin may also show inflammation. There is often a central scale or crust, which when removed reveals a tiny ulceration. Removing the accumulation is usually painful. A key clinical feature is pain or at least tenderness to touch. Many patients complain of having to sleep on the other ear or not being able to hold a telephone to their ear.

Histopathology. The histologic features are fairly distinct. The central crust or scale is reflected as a small dell in the epidermis or even as an ulcer. The dermis and perichondrium show chronic granulomatous inflammation and even necrosis. There may be deposits or fibrin and transepidermal elimination of damaged elastin and collagen. An interesting feature is the occasional presence of small glomus-like arteriovenous anastomoses, which may account for some of the painful features. In addition, there is usually solar elastosis. The underlying cartilage may be normal or show some damage, but should not show distinct infiltration by inflammatory cells; the latter is far more suggestive of relapsing polychondritis.

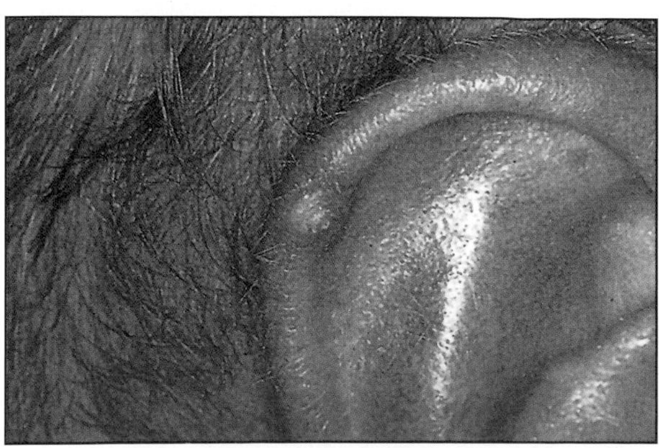

Fig. 20.1. Chondrodermatitis nodularis helicis

Course and Prognosis. If not treated, chondrodermatitis nodularis helicis is a persistent disorder that tends to worsen. Multiple lesions may develop, sometimes following excision.

Differential Diagnosis. A number of different lesions may develop on the helix. Chondrodermatitis nodularis helicis tends to be exactly on the edge of the helix and painful. Weathering nodules tend to be multiple, small and nonpainful white nodules on the free margin of the helix. On biopsy they may show elastosis, calcification or both. Thus, they have also been referred to as elastotic or calcified ear nodules. A small basal cell carcinoma or squamous cell carcinoma may be quite similar, but usually is located a little bit more posteriorly, that is, away from the edge of the helix. Darwin ear, or an auricular tubercle, is a protuberance on the posterior aspect of the ear, arising from the superior aspect of the helix; it is an embryologic abnormality of no consequence that has been taken to be an atavistic trait, hence the name Darwin. In younger patients, granuloma annulare may appear quite similar. Finally, a gouty tophus must also be considered.

Therapy. In most cases surgery is needed. Very small lesions can sometimes be treated by injection of intralesional triamcinolone acetonide 2.5–5.0 mg/ml in an anesthetic solution. Cryotherapy or tangential excision may help in early cases. Laser excision or destruction is another possibility.

There are several ways to approach the problem surgically. One can perform a wedge-shaped excision to include the damaged cartilage, but this may be excessive. Alternatively one can also lift up a flap of the damaged skin, smooth down the easily exposed cartilage and then reattach the skin. In the absence of the irritating protruding cartilage, the skin usually heals.

Relapsing Polychondritis

(von Jaksch-Wartenhorst 1923)

Synonyms. Polychondritis recidivans et atrophicans, polychondritis, polychondropathia

Definition. Idiopathic, probably autoimmune damage to articular and nonarticular cartilage causing arthritis, ear pain and occasionally respiratory problems.

Epidemiology. Fewer than 400 patients have been reported with relapsing polychondritis; most have been from Europe or North America. Neither sex is favored. Most patients are middle-aged adults. In a large study the average age was 51 years with a range of 13–84 years. No racial or genetic predilection has been described.

Etiology and Pathogenesis. Relapsing polychondritis is an autoimmune disorder involving immunity to type II collagen, which is the major component of both articular and nonarticular cartilage. It has been associated with psoriasis, rheumatoid arthritis, systemic lupus erythematosus, Behçet disease, a variety of systemic vasculitides, ulcerative colitis, Crohn disease, Sjögren syndrome, thymoma, myasthenia gravis and others.

Antibodies have been identified to type II collagen, as well as to a variety of other collagen molecules. While the antibodies may represent an epiphenomenon following damage to cartilage and unmasking of various epitopes, many factors suggest they are pathogenic. Rats injected with native type II collagen develop inflamed ears. The antibodies are most often directed against native undamaged collagen and are more likely to appear, or develop higher titers, during disease flares. While antibodies against type II collagen can be found in rheumatoid arthritis patients or normal individuals, they are much more common in relapsing polychondritis. Finally, immunoglobulin and complement may be found in the damaged cartilage, suggesting that immune-mediated cartilage damage occurs.

Clinical Findings. In about 90% of cases the key clinical feature is chronic painful inflammation of ears (Fig. 20.2). There is typically swelling and erythema with pain; often the ear lobe is somewhat spared. The process may be bilateral, unilateral or shift from side to side. Individual attacks usually last 1–2 weeks, while the interval between attacks is highly variable. Eventually, floppy or cauliflower ears may develop. The nasal cartilage is also often involved (in perhaps 50–70% of cases). Here the features are similar, but the end effect is a saddle or depressed nose.

The other major feature is arthritis, which involves up to 80% of patients. Both large and small joints may be involved and the process may be widespread or monoarticular. The changes may be migratory and effusions are common. Relapsing

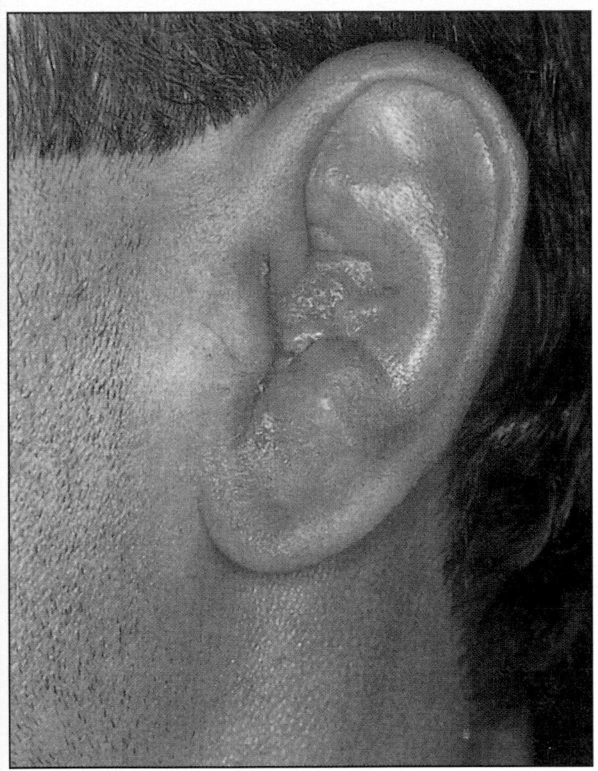

Fig. 20.2. Relapsing polychondritis

polychondritis is difficult to diagnose precisely on the joint findings alone.

Other signs and symptoms are protean but fortunately rare. Involvement of the respiratory cartilage can lead to dyspnea as the bronchi collapse. Ocular changes are multiple but include conjunctivitis, iritis, episcleritis and keratitis. Inner ear involvement may cause tinnitus or vertigo, as well as hearing problems. Involvement of the renal arteries may cause renal disease, while damage to the aortic elastic fibers can produce aneurysms. Yet other patients may present with fever of unknown origin.

Histopathology. Biopsy of the ear is often the easiest way to diagnose the disease. The cartilage is pale and infiltrated by both lymphocytes and neutrophils. In later stages it may be fragmented or fibrosed. Immunofluorescent examination may show deposition of immunoglobulins and complement.

Laboratory Findings. There is no specific laboratory test. The erythrocyte sedimentation rate is usually elevated, and up to 50% of patients may have circulating antibodies against type II collagen. Less specific findings include an elevated WBC, anemia, proteinuria and increased urinary acid mucopolysaccharides.

Course and Prognosis. Patients with primarily ear, nose and joint involvement are greatly inconvenienced but do acceptably well. About one-third of patients die from their disease. The main causes of death are pulmonary failure, ruptured aneurysms, systemic vasculitis, renal failure and infections. A large Mayo Clinic study showed 5- and 10-year survival rates of 74% and 55%.

Differential Diagnosis. The systemic disease must be separated from rheumatoid arthritis, Wegener granulomatosis, Reiter syndrome and other forms of acute arthritis and vasculitis. The differential of the ear changes includes cold injury, other types of vasculitis, gout, granuloma annulare and trauma, but the relapsing nature soon suggests the correct answer. Drug-induced vasculitis secondary to thiouracil use often involves the ears, resembling relapsing polychondritis. The association of relapsing polychondritis with aspects of Behçet syndrome is known as the MAGIC syndrome (mouth and genital ulcers with inflamed cartilage).

Therapy. The mainstay of therapy for those patients with severe arthritis or internal involvement is systemic corticosteroids. Initially relatively high doses of prednisone are required, such as 40–60 mg daily; a typical maintenance dose is perhaps 20 mg daily. In patients with a less than satisfactory response, additional immunosuppressive therapy can also be considered. The arthritis may often be managed with nonsteroidal antiinflammatory drugs. Colchicine 500 mg twice daily may also be tried. While dapsone has been proposed as an effective agent, our experience has been disappointing. If it has any role, it may be to ameliorate the acute inflammation in patients with primarily ear involvement. All such therapy is hard to evaluate because of the relapsing nature of the disease.

Cauliflower Ear

Synonyms. Wrestler's ear, boxer's ear, auricular pseudocyst

Definition. Traumatic damage to ear resulting in hemorrhage, fibrosis and deformity.

Epidemiology. Almost all patients give a history of boxing or wrestling; occasionally other trauma is involved. Thus, except for the newly liberated female boxers, almost all patients are men.

Etiology and Pathogenesis. Trauma is the problem. Bleeding occurs between the cartilage and perichondrium, producing a blood- or fluid-filled space known as an auricular pseudocyst. In other cases, the cartilage itself splits with intracartilage hemorrhage. The hemorrhage eventually forms a thrombus, may resolve, but often calcifies. Later there is a proliferative response by the damaged cartilage.

Clinical Findings. Initially, a cystic lesion may be found, usually over the flat cartilage forming the plate of the ear (Fig. 20.3). An anterior location is more common than a posterior position, i.e., behind the ear. Later the hemorrhage may evolve into a firm, perhaps calcified nodule. Even later, the irregular bumpy nodules so well known as cauliflower ear predominate.

Differential Diagnosis. The history of trauma is usually obvious. Some try to distinguish between hemorrhage beneath the perichondrium and within the cartilage, but we suspect many individuals have both types of changes as they are exposed to repeated trauma.

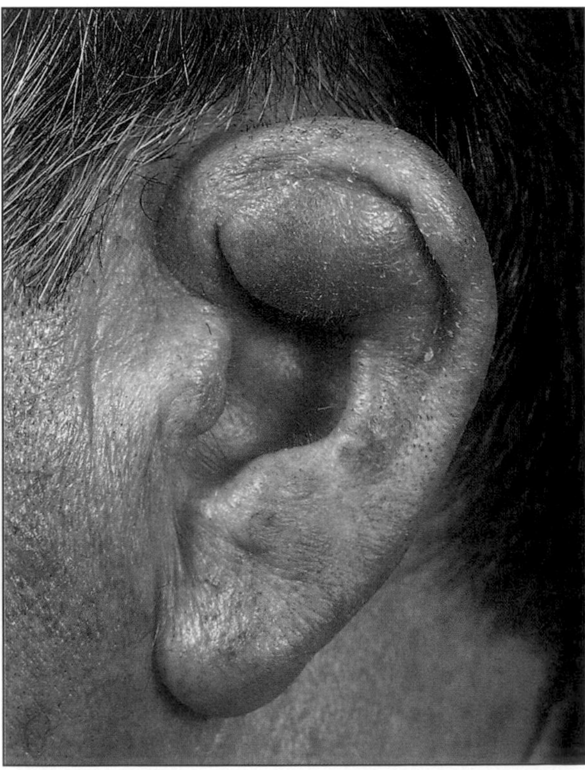

Fig. 20.3. Cauliflower ear

Therapy. Avoidance is the best therapy. Protective headgear has been proven to help, but as wrestlers and boxers advance in their career, they are inclined to discard the headgear. Fresh cystic lesions are best drained. The old proliferative or calcified nodules must be excised, once the patient has concluded his or her combative career.

Bibliography

Chondrodermatits Nodularis Helicis

Bottomley WW, Goodfield MD (1994) Chondrodermatitis nodularis helicis occurring with systemic sclerosis – an under-reported association? Clin Exp Dermatol 19: 219–220

Goettle DK (1980) Chondrodermatitis nodularis chronica helicis: a perforating necrobiotic granuloma. J Am Acad Dermatol 2:148–154

Long D, Maloney ME (1996) Surgical pearl: surgical planing in the treatment of chondrodermatitis nodularis chronica helicis of the antihelix. J Am Acad Dermatol 35: 761–762

Munnoch DA, Herbert KJ, Morris AM (1996) Chondrodermatitis nodularis chronica helicis et antihelicis. Br J Plast Surg 49:473–476

Santa Cruz DJ (1980) Chondrodermatitis nodularis chronica helicis. Arch Dermatol 68:241–255

Taylor MB (1991) Chondrodermatitis nodularis chronica helicis – successful treatment with carbon dioxide laser. J Dermatol Surg Oncol 17:862–864

Winkler M (1915) Knötchenförmige Erkrankung am Helix (Chondrodermatitis nodularis chronica helicis). Arch Dermatol Syph 121:278–285

Relapsing Polychondritis

Askari AD (1984) Colchicine for treatment of relapsing polychondritis. J Am Acad Dermatol 10:507–510

Barranco VP, Minor DB, Solonom H (1976) Treatment of polychondritis with dapsone. Arch Dermatol 112:1286–1288

Firestein GS, Gruber HE, Weisman MH et al. (1985) Mouth and genital ulcers with inflamed cartilage: MAGIC syndrome. Am J Med 79:69–72

Fujimoto N, Tajima S, Ishibashi A et al. (1998) Acute febrile neutrophilic dermatosis (Sweet's syndrome) in a patient with relapsing polychondritis. Br J Dermatol 139:930–931

Jaksch-Wartenhorst R von (1923) Polychondropathia. Wien Arch Inn Med 6:93–100

Labarthe MP, Bayle-Lebey P, Bazex J (1997) Cutaneous manifestations of relapsing polychondritis in a patient receiving goserelin for carcinoma of the prostate. Dermatology 195:391–394

McAdam LP, O'Hanlan NA, Bluestone R et al. (1976) Relapsing polychondritis: prospective study of 23 patients and a review of the literature. Medicine (Baltimore) 55: 193–215

Miyasaka LS, de Andrade Junior A, Bueno CE et al. (1998) Relapsing polychondritis. Rev Paul Med 116:1637–1642

Orme RL, Nordlund JJ, Barich L et al. (1990) The MAGIC syndrome (mouth and genital ulcers with inflamed cartilage). Arch Dermatol 126:940–944

Shah RP, Shah VR, Reichmuth DA et al. (1999) Man with inflamed ears. Hosp Pract 34:35–38

Weinberger A, Myers AR (1979) Relapsing polychondritis associated with cutaneous vasculitis. Arch Dermatol 115: 980–981

Yang CL, Brinckman J, Rui HF et al. (1993) Autoantibodies to cartilage collagens in relapsing polychondritis. Arch Dermatol Res 285:245–249

Cauliflower Ear

Vogelin E, Grobbelaar AO, Chana JS et al. (1998) Surgical correction of the cauliflower ear. Br J Plast Surg 51:359–362

Khalak R, Roberts JK (1996) Images in clinical medicine. Cauliflower ear. N Engl J Med 335:399

Diseases of the Subcutaneous Fat

Contents

The subcutaneous fat serves as a source of insulation, padding or protection and as an energy storage center. The thickness of the fat varies greatly from person to person and from region to region. No fat is found on the eyelids and male genitalia, but elsewhere metabolic, hormonal and genetic factors interact to determine the amount of fat accumulated. The fat lies between the dermis and the fascia of the muscles, tendons and ligaments. It is divided by fibrous septa, bands of connective tissue that connect the dermis to the fascia (Fig. 21.1). The true functional unit of fat is the microlobule, a small collection of fat cells serviced by a single vessel; the microlobule has no distinct, easily discerned boundaries, but the larger lobule is encased by fibrous septa. The septa carry the vessels, arteries, veins and lymphatics to the fat and also serve as pathways to the dermis and epidermis.

Panniculitis

Inflammation of the subcutaneous fat is called panniculitis. There are many possible etiologies, including trauma, infection, connective tissue disease and vasculitis (Table 21.1). Unfortunately, almost all types of panniculitis look clinically similar. They present as indurated red to red-brown nodules on the legs. Some heal with hyperpigmentation; others ulcerate and scar. In rare cases, they discharge an oily liquid; liquefying panniculitis is not associated with erythema nodosum but is otherwise not very specific. In our experience, it is probably most often seen with α1-antitrypsin deficiency. Histologists divide panniculitis into septal and lobular types. The prototype of septal panniculitis is erythema nodosum, while most of the other forms are predominantly located in the lobules. There are many overlaps and the histologic picture often does not correlate with clinical findings. In general, inflammatory disease of the dermis does not involve the fat, but when there is vasculitis involving the deep dermal vessels, then the fatty tissue is at least at risk. Similarly, when the fat is inflamed, the lowest aspects of the dermis may be secondarily involved.

While there are many elegant and often confusing classifications of panniculitis, the clinical approach can be simplified. The first question is

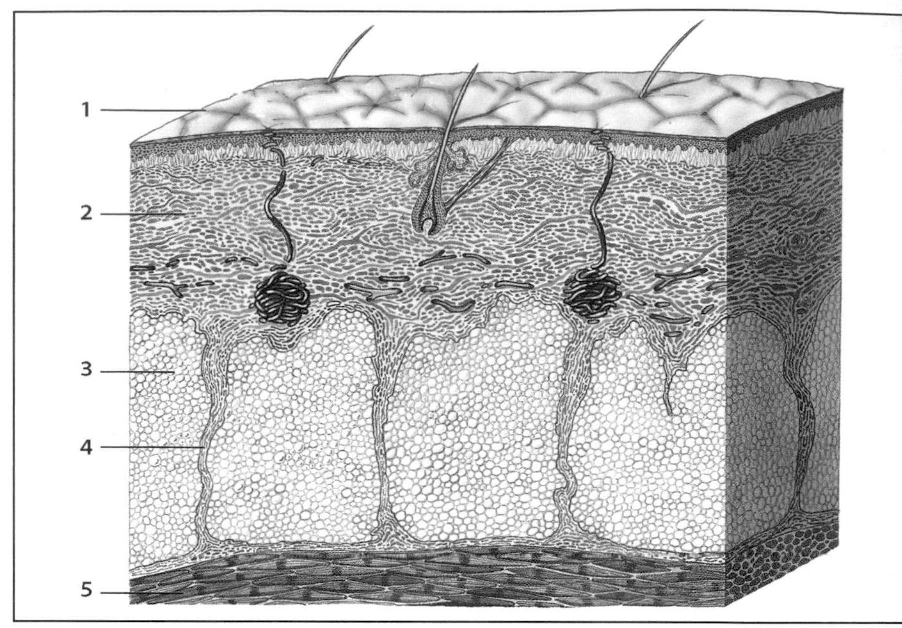

Fig. 21.1.
Diagram of fat layer
1 epidermis
2 dermis
3 fat lobule
4 fat septum
5 fascia

Table 21.1. Types of panniculitis

Types of panniculitis
Erythema nodosum
Vasculitis
Nodular vasculitis
Secondary to other types of vasculitis
Connective tissue disease
Lupus erythematosus
Systemic sclerosis
Infections
Tuberculosis (erythema induratum)
Many others
Physical
Cold
Trauma
Injections
Artifact
Metabolic
Pancreatic disease
α1-Antitrypsin deficiency
Sclerema neonatorum
Neonatal fat necrosis
Gout
Calciphylaxis
Proliferative disorders
Lymphomas and leukemias
(Cytophagic histiocytic panniculitis)
Metastases and direct extension of tumors
Miscellaneous
Lipodermatosclerosis (chronic venous insufficiency)
Subcutaneous granulomas
Medication induced
Eosinophilic panniculitis
Weber-Christian disease
Lipogranulomatosis subcutanea

simple: Is it erythema nodosum or not? Erythema nodosum is far more common than all the other forms of panniculitis together and can often be identified clinically as discussed below. If the answer is not erythema nodosum, a biopsy should be performed to determine whether septal or lobular involvement predominates. At the same time, one must search for vasculitis and other clues to associated diseases, such as lupus erythematosus. Foreign bodies, cold damage, artifactual injury and sometimes even pancreatic disease also leave histologic evidence. In addition, one must often perform extensive laboratory testing to exclude the various underlying causes of panniculitis. Both the inflamed fat and other tissues should be studied to exclude an infectious etiology, especially if the onset of the lesions is sudden. The differential diagnosis is shortened or even eliminated for most of the disorders in this chapter, as all of the various types of panniculitis form the differential considerations for each other.

Erythema Nodosum

(Hebra 1860)

Synonym. Erythema contusiforme

Definition. Common panniculitis, usually involving shins, often presenting with erythematous or bruised nodular lesions.

Epidemiology. Erythema nodosum is far more common in women than in men (6:1 ratio) and appears primarily in young adults.

Etiology and Pathogenesis. The pathogenesis of erythema nodosum is unclear, but it represents some form of allergic reaction to an almost endless list of triggers. One need only compare a German and an American dermatology text to see how one must adjust the search for associated diseases depending on where one lives. In the southwestern USA coccidioidomycosis is a common cause, while in Scandinavia one must think of sarcoidosis and *Yersinia* infections. A specific cause for erythema nodosum is found in about half the cases. Possible causes include the following:

Infections. In Europe, *Yersinia* infection with diarrhea and then later typical leg lesions is a common scenario. Streptococcal throat infections in children may trigger erythema nodosum; often at the same time they produce rheumatic fever. Erythema nodosum may represent part of the primary host response to tuberculosis, cat-scratch fever, psittacosis, lymphogranuloma venereum, toxoplasmosis or a deep fungal infection such as coccidioidomycosis or histoplasmosis.

Sarcoidosis. Erythema nodosum may be associated with sarcoidosis in both early and late stages of the disease. Löfgren syndrome (1946) refers to the association of erythema nodosum with bilateral hilar lymphadenopathy, fever, cough and arthralgias; it is a variant of sarcoidosis.

Inflammatory Bowel Disease. Both Crohn disease and ulcerative colitis may be associated with erythema nodosum. About 10% of patients with either disease may have panniculitis; on occasion the cutaneous changes precede the diagnosis of bowel disease, but only rarely do they precede gastrointestinal symptoms.

Blind Loop Syndrome. Patients with intestinal bypass surgery or gastrointestinal motility problems may develop a blind loop of bowel with bacterial overgrowth. Combining characteristics of infection and immune reaction, the blind loop syndrome usually features cutaneous pustular vasculitis, but can also cause panniculitis, which generally resembles erythema nodosum. Sometimes vasculitis is present, suggesting nodular vasculitis or erythema induratum.

Medications. Oral contraceptives and estrogens are a common trigger, but the figures may be distorted since erythema nodosum is most common among young women, many of whom are likely to be taking the medications. Antibiotics, especially sulfonamides, salicylates, halogen salts and gold salts have also been incriminated. In general drugs play a minor role in erythema nodosum.

Clinical Findings. Depending on the cause there may be a prodromal stage, usually reflecting the initial infection with a microbial trigger. Patients with idiopathic and drug-induced erythema nodosum usually lack systemic complaints. One should inquire about diarrhea, sore throat, foreign travel, exposure to ill individuals and bowel symptoms.

The patient suddenly develops several poorly defined, tender red subcutaneous nodules over the tibial surfaces (Fig. 21.2). While erythema nodosum can appear above the knees and even on the arms, such a pattern should raise the question of other types of panniculitis. The lesions are painful on palpation and typically go through a color progression, beginning bright red, becoming red-brown and then, as healing occurs, taking on the typical yellow-green color of a bruise (hence the

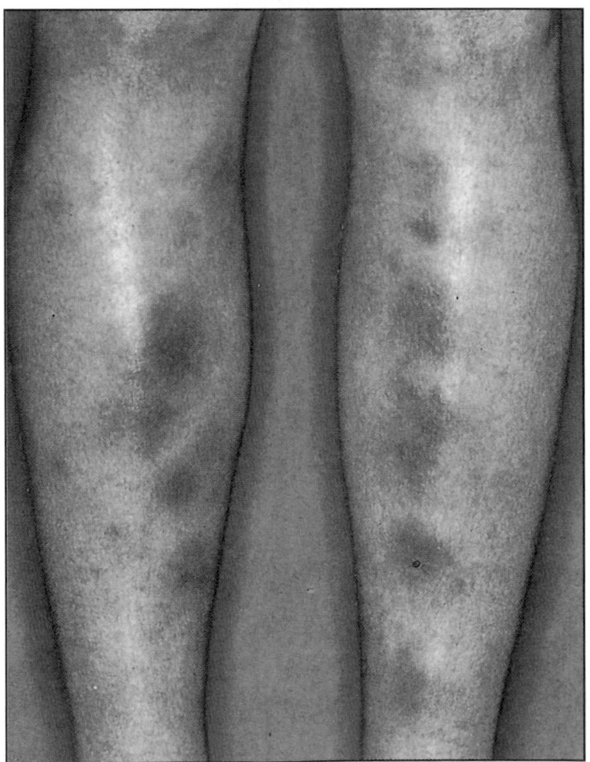

Fig. 21.2. Erythema nodosum

name erythema contusiforme). Individual lesions may slowly enlarge and new lesions appear. The lesions never ulcerate and always heal without scarring; there may be postinflammatory hyperpigmentation. The disease course lasts 3–6 weeks; recurrences are not unusual, especially in the idiopathic form.

We use erythema nodosum to describe this typical disease course and nodose erythema to describe the reaction pattern.

Variants. Erythema nodosum migrans (BÄFVERSTEDT 1954) is a variant of erythema nodosum. Subacute nodular migratory panniculitis of VILANOVA and PIÑOL-AGUADÉ (1956) is probably the same disease. Almost all patients are female and some are pregnant. Often there is antecedent pharyngitis. The lesions are confined to one leg, starting on the lower anterolateral aspect and slowly spreading over the shin. A complex polycyclic lesion may be produced, showing central healing with yellow sclerotic areas at the same time as the active erythematous border spreads.

Histopathology. Proper biopsy is essential. Erythema nodosum is the prototype of a septal panniculitis, meaning that the main inflammation is in the fat septa. Since the septa may be as much as a centimeter apart, a long, deep biopsy is required. Punch biopsies often fail to reach fat or, if they are deep enough, fail to sample a septum. The most effective biopsy specimen is a very narrow ellipse, perhaps 3–4 cm in length and 5 mm in width extending to the fascia.

Histopathologic findings include a normal epidermis and upper dermis. There is a nonspecific perivascular infiltrate in the deep dermis, but the main pathology is a mixed infiltrate in the fat septa, spilling over into the lobules. The early infiltrate contains lymphocytes, eosinophils and neutrophils. Sometimes small granulomas may be found, especially in older lesions or in patients with granulomatous diseases such as sarcoidosis. No vasculitis is present.

Laboratory Findings. An endless number of laboratory tests can be ordered, but blind tests rarely yield any worthwhile information. The erythrocyte sedimentation rate is usually elevated and can be used to follow the disease, although clinical signs suffice. Depending on the part of the world where the patient is seen, a detailed history should be taken and appropriate laboratory tests performed. For example, if a young pregnant patient on the East Coast of the USA develops her problem a few weeks after visiting Arizona, one must exclude coccidioidomycosis, which can be a devastating illness in pregnancy. On the other hand, an otherwise healthy young women who has no risk factors and a few typical lesions does not require an expensive laboratory workup.

Differential Diagnosis. The main differential diagnostic point is the other forms of panniculitis discussed in this chapter. Erythema nodosum is the most common and most clinically typical. Lesions that are persistent, ulcerated, do not involve the shins or occur in men should raise the question of another diagnosis. The biopsy can help, distinguishing between septal and lobular panniculitis, but often the final diagnosis is achieved by clinical means. The only other likely diagnosis is vasculitis, but patients with deep periarteritis nodosa are usually more ill and the lesions are often ulcerated. Factitial lesions should always be kept in mind; the thighs are easier to inject or damage than the area below the knee.

Therapy

Systemic. Aspirin or nonsteroidal antiinflammatory drugs are usually sufficient for pain relief. Bed rest and compression stockings or band ages should be employed. Supersaturated potassium iodide (SSKI) 5–10 drops t.i.d. can also be tried, especially in more chronic or granulomatous forms. Thyroid status should be monitored in such cases. Systemic corticosteroids, usually 40 mg prednisone daily tapered rapidly to alternate-day therapy, is usually helpful but should be reserved for refractory cases. Obviously, the most important therapy is that directed against any underlying triggering disease.

Topical. External therapy has little to offer. Some mild cases may be helped by topical corticosteroids, perhaps under occlusion.

Nodular Vasculitis

(BAZIN 1861)

Synonyms. Erythema induratum. The terms erythema induratum of Bazin and erythema induratum of WHITFIELD (1901) have been used to separate two clinically similar disorders; the former associated with tuberculosis and the latter considered idiopathic. MONTGOMERY's (1945) term of nodular vasculitis has been used both as an umbrella term for both disorders and as a synonym for erythema induratum of Whitfield.

Definition. Nodular more persistent panniculitis usually on posterior aspect of calf and often associated with tuberculosis.

Epidemiology. Nodular vasculitis is a chronic disease of middle-aged women. It is more likely to affect patients with poor circulation in their legs, as manifested by erythrocyanosis, cold pasty skin, livedo reticularis, perifollicular erythema or pernio. Perhaps 5–10% of cases are described in men; these patients are probably more likely to have evidence of tuberculosis.

Etiology and Pathogenesis. Work in our Munich clinic and other centers has identified *Mycobacterium tuberculosis* in many of these lesions using polymerase chain reaction (PCR) techniques (Chap. 4). In other patients, there is clear evidence of tuberculosis elsewhere, reinforcing the concept of a tuberculid. Thus, we prefer to think of erythema induratum as tuberculosis-related panniculitis and nodular vasculitis as a clinically similar but uncommon problem in which there is no evidence of association with the tubercle bacillus. If tuberculosis is not identified, in most instances no etiology is found.

Clinical Findings. Nodular vasculitis usually presents as red-brown nodules on the calves, rather than over the shins as is the case with erythema nodosum. The nodules may enlarge into plaques; they are painful, may liquefy, often ulcerate and heal very slowly. New lesions tend to appear as older ones heal. The disease often flares with the onset of cold weather. Lesions can occur anywhere on the body and may be unilateral.

Histopathology. The microscopic picture adds further confusion to the problem. The usual histologic picture is focal lobular panniculitis There may be fat necrosis, perhaps secondary to vascular change. Within the septa there is some degree of vasculitis, usually with both vessel wall destruction and granuloma formation. In other cases, there is more diffuse lobular panniculitis with neutrophilic vasculitis of small and large dermal vessels. Perhaps immune complexes containing organisms or other triggering agents are deposited in the vessels, leading to both vessel inflammation and fatty damage. The inflammatory infiltrate is mixed. As with other forms of panniculitis, later lesions can be more granulomatous and foamy.

While nodular vasculitis and erythema induratum cannot always be separated microscopically, the latter may have more fat necrosis and larger granulomas involving the dermis. If tiny tuberculoid granulomas are seen scattered throughout the lower dermis and the septa, erythema induratum becomes a better choice.

Laboratory Findings. Tuberculosis should be sought. Specimens can be evaluated with PCR to identify the DNA of the organisms.

Differential Diagnosis. Cutaneous periarteritis nodosa may appear quite similar. Patients may have livedo racemosa. In the biopsy specimen, a larger vessel, usually in the deep dermis, is involved with secondary fatty damage. Often the distinction is not as clear as this; it may be hard to tell whether the fat or the vessel is the primary target. One should sample as fresh a lesion as possible.

In rare cases, other forms of vasculitis such as leukocytoclastic vasculitis and even superficial thrombophlebitis may cause septal panniculitis. Behçet syndrome may feature vasculitis extending into panniculitis. Pernio may reveal a lobular panniculitis histologically, but the cutaneous lesions are usually acral or on the ears and not clinically suggestive of panniculitis.

Connective Tissue Panniculitis

Not surprisingly, disorders that involve the dermal connective tissue may also involve the fat and frequently have a septal component. Panniculitis is most common in lupus erythematosus and systemic sclerosis, but has also been described with dermatomyositis and Sjögren syndrome.

Lupus Erythematosus Profundus

(KAPOSI 1875; IRGANG 1954)

Synonym. Lupus panniculitis

Clinical Findings. Lupus erythematosus profundus is lupus erythematosus involving the subcutaneous

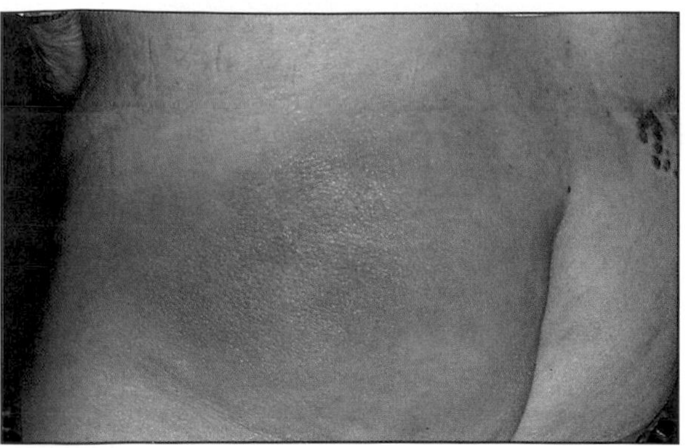

Fig. 21.3. Lupus erythematosus profundus

fat (Chap. 18). In general, the lesions do not overlap with typical lower extremity panniculitis. They are larger, less nodular, more plaque-like or indurated and often involve the cheeks, shoulder girdle, hips, thighs or breasts (Fig. 21.3). Liquefaction is a frequent change. The lesions tend to heal with a sunken scar. The overlying skin may show hyperpigmentation or depigmentation, or even typical changes of discoid lupus erythematosus.

Histopathology. The septa show nodular infiltrates containing lymphocytes, plasma cells and histiocytes, sometimes around vessels. In addition, there is lobular panniculitis, often with fat cell necrosis and mucin deposition. In the later stages, fibrosis occurs. It is critical to examine the overlying dermoepidermal junction; there may be features of lupus erythematosus there, such as vacuolar change, atrophy or follicular plugging, even in the absence of clinical changes. In addition, the dermis often contains mucin. PAS staining may reveal a thickened basement membrane zone.

Immunofluorescent Examination. A lupus erythematosus band may be identified, clinching the diagnosis.

Therapy. Antimalarial agents appear to be the best therapy for lupus erythematosus profundus.

Scleroderma Panniculitis

Almost all types of systemic sclerosis may have associated panniculitis. The primarily lymphocytic perivascular dermal infiltrate extends into the thickened septa and reaches the periphery of the fat lobules, which are eventually replaced by extensively fibrosed, enlarged septa. The end result is a thickened skin, rather than the typical red nodules of panniculitis. In a reverse variant, the same fibrotic process may extend upward from the fascia in eosinophilic fasciitis. Clinically there are large, flat, deep indurated areas, usually on the extremities. A useful phlebologic sign is the so-called negative vein sign; when the leg is returned to the horizontal position from an elevated position, the veins tend to remain collapsed. Systemic corticosteroids remain the treatment of choice for eosinophilic fasciitis.

Infectious Panniculitis

There are two basic mechanisms by which infectious organisms can cause panniculitis: direct infection of the fat and an immunologic reaction, with perhaps immune complexes deposited in the small vessels of the septa and even in the microlobules. There are also two points of attack; directly through the skin or via the blood. Inoculation of organisms via either a bite or trauma can elicit an intense local reaction involving the fat, while a disseminated reaction is more likely to be bloodborne, representing either sepsis or an immunologic reaction. Immunosuppressed patients appear to be at far greater risk.

The number of organisms that can cause panniculitis is almost endless. Deep fungi can be involved either via direct inoculation or as a cause of erythema nodosum. Actinomycosis, nocardiosis, chromomycosis and sporotrichosis are also potential causes. The other mycobacteria also may be involved; in leprosy one speaks of erythema nodosum leprosum. Ordinary bacterial infections appear rarely to cause direct infection of the fat, but some, such as *Yersinia*, trigger erythema nodosum. In a more distant sense, a brown recluse spider bite can even be viewed as panniculitis when it reaches the fat, as it almost always does. Finally some parasitic infections feature worms or other forms wandering through the fat, where they too cause inflammation.

If the cause of panniculitis is unclear, tissue should be submitted for culture to identify both anaerobic and aerobic bacteria, fungi and atypical mycobacteria. It is difficult if not impossible to accomplish this with a swab or needle aspirate. Positive culture results for bacteria should be viewed skeptically; often the organisms are only secondarily present. Treatment should be guided by culture and histologic identification of the infective organism, as well as by a consideration of whether a direct infection or an immunologic response is involved.

Physical Panniculitis

Many different types of injury to the fat can produce inflammation. Once the fat is injured it is slow to heal, so that persistent inflammation and atrophy often occur. There is an overlap between traumatic panniculitis and lipoatrophy or lipodystrophy.

Cold Panniculitis

Infants and children are especially susceptible to cold panniculitis. Neonatal fat necrosis may represent subtle cold injury. In infants, the cheeks and chin are usually involved, as these are the only areas exposed during a normal baby-buggy ride during cold weather. In children and occasionally in adults cold panniculitis has occurred on the cheeks after holding a popsicle or similar cold treat in the mouth, rather than licking it. Among adults, overweight women are at greatest risk. Skiing, motorcycling and especially horse riding are likely causes; in German one speaks of rider's thighs or rider's panniculitis, typically involving the thighs or buttocks.

Clinically all the lesions appear the same, as diffuse livid areas that are initially cold to the touch and when palpated reveal subcutaneous nodules or plaques (Fig. 21.4). The lesions resolve over a number of weeks, often healing with a depression. There is no effective therapy, so warm clothing and appropriate exposure times are most important.

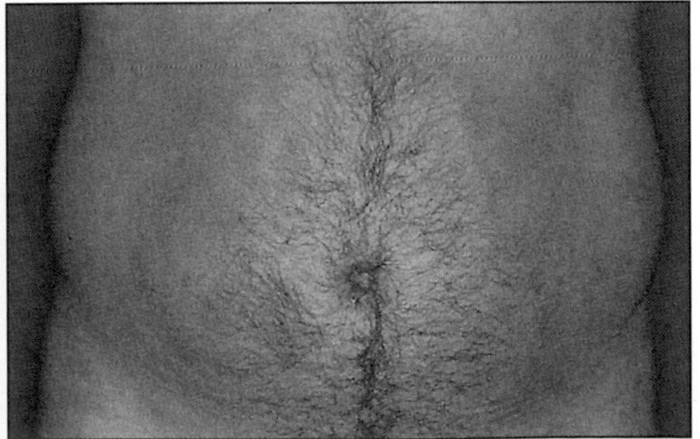

Fig. 21.4. Cold panniculitis in worker who was not clothed warmly enough; symmetry suggests an exogenous cause

Traumatic Panniculitis

Clinical Findings. Any type of blunt trauma can lead to fat damage. Once again, women seem more susceptible. The damaged fat yields lipids, which are broken down to fatty acids that are then irritating, aggravating the initial injury. The breasts, thighs, shins, arms and buttocks are the most likely sites. A distinct type of fat trauma is the injury to the thighs that inexperienced water skiers suffer from the tow rope and handle; such injuries produce semicircular depressions on the thighs known as semicircular lipoatrophy. The initial lesion is usually a bruise with the typical color spectrum of such an injury. However, on deeper palpation there are irregular painful nodules or more plate-like induration that heals with a depression. On the breasts, the depressed scars frequently raise the question of carcinoma if there is no clear history of trauma.

One special type of posttraumatic panniculitis is self-healing panniculitis of young women. Some patients appear to develop inflammatory nodules over their shins far out of proportion to the actual trauma. The lesions may heal with liquefaction and drainage. In another special variant, the trauma may be very localized and heal with a distinct moveable nodule. This change has been called encapsulated nodulocystic fat necrosis.

Histopathology. The chain of events in traumatic fat necrosis is similar to that in other forms of panniculitis. Initially necrosis may predominate, along with an intense neutrophilic infiltrate. Both are good clues to a traumatic etiology. Later the infiltrate is more likely to be lymphohistiocytic, and in the end stage there is a combination of foamy histiocytes and multinucleated giant cells, some containing lipid vacuoles. The term lipogranuloma has been applied here, but it is very nonspecific. In the end, fibrosis dominates.

The lesions of encapsulated fat necrosis contain lobules of honeycombed necrotic fat surrounded by a fibrous capsule. The pseudocysts can be lined by a crenellated cuticle-like ceroid-rich membrane, leading to the alternate histologic term of membranous fat necrosis or membranous lipodystrophy. The latter change can be seen in the late stages of many forms of panniculitis in which there is sufficient necrosis.

Therapy. There is no good therapy. The smaller lesions are sometimes excised, more for diagnostic certainty than as a true therapeutic intervention.

Postinjection Panniculitis

Synonyms. Paraffinoma, silicone granuloma, oil granuloma, sclerosing lipogranuloma

Etiology and Pathogenesis. In certain clinical settings, silicone, paraffin (mineral oil in American terms) and similar viscous fluids have been injected by physicians or, more often, by patients. Liquid silicone was used for breast enlargements in the USA and still is employed around the world; this is in contrast to the use of silicone-filled bags used for augmentation or reconstruction of the breast. Everyone agrees that silicone injected directly or leaking from an implant can induce a foreign body response. The breast implant issue centers around whether small amount of silicone can trigger autoimmune disease.

In addition, patients have been known to inject various oils into their genitalia, particularly the penis, presumably for purposes of enlargement and increased sexual satisfaction. Transvestites unable to obtain medical aid have also used such injections to alter their body contours.

Clinical Findings. The surprising finding is that the injection works, at least for some time. Eventually, sometimes after a large number of years, pain, erythema and induration develop, followed by ulcers, sometimes with discharge of oily material. The viscous fluids are able to wander somewhat through the body, so the reactions may not be at the exact injection site. For example, patients with breast injections have developed inflammation of their hands. When multiple sinus tracts develop with discharge of material, especially on the penis, one speaks of sclerosing lipogranuloma.

Histopathology. Microscopic evaluation reveals a classic Swiss-cheese pattern with large holes or vacuoles in the fibrosed fatty tissue. Abundant macrophages are present. Spectroscopy has been used to identify the chemical nature of the injected material.

Therapy. Smaller lesions can be easily excised. Larger ones may require grafting, but it is wise to remove as much of the lesion as possible. Malignant degeneration has been described with the development of a variety of sarcomas.

Factitial Panniculitis

Synonyms. Artifactual panniculitis, psychogenic panniculitis

Etiology and Pathogenesis. There is little difference between factitial panniculitis and the injection of oily liquids by the patient. In this setting, one usually thinks of the injection of either abused medicines (especially pentazocine, but also morphine, pethidine and others) or an incredible range of substances designed to produce an acute reaction. The patients' imaginations really know no limit; we have encountered injections of milk, blood, urine, stool, bacterial cultures, paint thinner, turpentine, hair spray and many others. All elicit a classic foreign body reaction, often associated with toxic damage to the fat.

Clinical Findings. The major risk group is drug abusers. Apart from them, women are more likely to have factitial panniculitis than men, and medical personnel are a second significant risk group. The lesions are in sites that one can reach, often on the left side of the body in a right-handed individual, usually on the extensor surfaces and frequently grouped. Typical lesions are inflamed nodules often with ulcerations. Pentazocine causes massive woody induration over a wide area. The patient may have fever and other signs of infection. Any of the panniculitis types mentioned above can be mimicked.

The possibility of a factitial panniculitis or any factitial dermatitis must always be borne in mind. Lesions that fail to respond to treatment or recur despite appropriate measures should arouse suspicion. Often one can occlude an involved area for a week with an Unna bandage to see whether there is improvement, although some patients inject through their protective wrapping. Many of the patients are already under psychiatric care. Their self-injection can be viewed as a cry for help. Often they wander from one care faculty to another, seeking new doctors as their secret is diagnosed.

Histopathology. The biopsy shows acute neutrophilic inflammation and fat necrosis. Material should be submitted for culture. Polarization microscopy should be performed on all types of panniculitis but is especially valuable in revealing foreign materials. Laser-assisted high-pressure liquid chromatography has been employed to identify minute amounts of foreign materials in this clinical setting.

Therapy. The acute situation should be treated with antibiotics to cover a mixed range of organisms, pending culture results. The longer-term approach is less satisfactory. Most patients appear to need this abnormality, and when discovered they move on. Nonetheless, social and psychiatric care should be offered.

Metabolic Panniculitis

A number of underlying diseases may present with or, more often, be associated with panniculitis.

Pancreatic Panniculitis

Both carcinoma of the pancreas and acute or chronic pancreatitis can lead to panniculitis. The suspected cause is the release of lipases by the damaged organ or tumor; these enzymes are assumed to act upon the fat to produce painful subcutaneous nodules. In contrast to most of the other forms of panniculitis, any area of the body can be involved. Patients may have fever, malaise and a variety of other symptoms. The biopsy shows ghost cells, or poorly outlined necrotic fat cells produced by enzymatic degradation. These zones are typically surrounded by neutrophils with nuclear dust. When such changes are seen one should suggest pancreatic panniculitis, although the picture is not totally specific. Later on calcification frequently occurs, lending the necrotic lipocytes a basophilic appearance. Serum amylase and lipase should be measured and the pancreas imaged. Research studies have demonstrated elevated enzyme levels in the nodules.

α1-Antitrypsin Deficiency

(WARTER et al. 1972)

Etiology and Pathogenesis. α1-Antitrypsin deficiency is a genetically determined defect. There are many alleles of the α1-antitrypsin gene. The PiZZ homozygous genotype is usually found; only rarely are heterozygotes involved. α1-Antitrypsin is the major serum protease inhibitor (Pi). Initially α1-antitrypsin deficiency was described as a cause of emphysema in children and young adults. The enzyme is easily inhibited by cigarette smoke. Other manifestations include neonatal hepatitis and panniculitis.

Clinical Findings. The panniculitis in α1-antitrypsin deficiency is often a draining or liquefying variant, frequently associated with minor trauma. Initially painful nodules arise, not necessarily limited to the legs. Patients often describe the drainage of an oily material, which may also be encountered when attempting a biopsy. Thus ulcers often result. These may be progressive, associated with fever and other systemic symptoms, and occasionally the outcome is fatal. Surprisingly, the pulmonary and hepatic findings rarely occur in the same patients as the panniculitis.

Histopathology. The biopsy results are similar to other forms of lobular panniculitis. Initially there is necrosis, often associated with large numbers of neutrophils which leak into the dermis. Later foamy and then fibrotic stages are seen.

Laboratory Findings. Levels of α1-antitrypsin can be measured in the serum as a screening measure. The exact genotype is determined via polyacrylamide gel analysis. All cases of liquefactive panniculitis and all cases in which panniculitis has been recorded in another member of the family should be so analyzed.

Therapy. Acute attacks can be aborted by infusion of α1-antitrypsin. The enzyme has a short half-life and infusions must be frequently repeated. Genetically modified forms of the enzyme that are more resistant to degradation offer advantages. Dapsone is frequently employed to, presumably, inhibit the neutrophilic response; some patients require only dapsone, others can reduce their need for enzyme replacement. Colchicine has been used in a similar way. Danazol appears to raise the level of α1-antitrypsin and may also be tried.

Neonatal Fat Necrosis

(CAUSE 1879)

Synonyms. Adiponecrosis subcutanea neonatorum, subcutaneous fat necrosis of the newborn

Epidemiology. Neonatal fat necrosis affects healthy new born infants; it has no predilection for premature or sickly newborns.

Etiology and Pathogenesis. The exact cause is unknown, but the major factors appear to be trauma (usually in the form of pressure, such as during a difficult birth), anoxia, cold and perhaps hypercalcemia. There may be an association with maternal diabetes mellitus. The relative deficiency of oleic acid and the higher percentage of saturated fatty acids in the newborn fat may also play a role.

Clinical Findings. The hallmark of neonatal fat necrosis is hard, deep, often symmetric plaques, typically over pressure points such as the buttocks, scapulae and thighs as well as on the arms and cheeks. The overlying skin is violaceous and stony hard, while the periphery is sharply delineated. The lesions are usually asymptomatic but sometimes painful. They typically develop in the first days or weeks of life. Some lesions may liquefy, drain and calcify, but most resolve spontaneously without scarring over a period of weeks.

Histopathology. The microscopic picture may be distinctive, especially if a frozen section is studied. Fine crystals of fat, actually triglycerides, are preserved extending from the walls of the lipocytes. The same crystals can be found in giant cells. In addition, there is a mixed inflammatory infiltrate and fat necrosis.

Differential Diagnosis. The main differential diagnostic consideration is sclerema neonatorum.

Therapy. No therapy is required.

Sclerema Neonatorum
(Usenberg 1718; Soltmann 1899)

Synonyms. Sclerema adiposum neonatorum, Soltmann syndrome, fat sclerosis of the newborn

Epidemiology. This extremely rare disorder occurs in premature or otherwise weakened infants during the first weeks of life. It is usually associated with a serious underlying disorder such as congenital heart disease, sepsis or respiratory distress. In the past it was more often seen with congenital syphilis.

Etiology and Pathogenesis. The cause is a total mystery; hypothermia, maternal illness and disorders of fatty acid metabolism have been postulated.

Clinical Findings. The onset is usually between days 2 and 4 of life. There is a sudden diffuse induration that typically climbs the body, starting on the shins and then spreading to involve the entire skin surface, sparing the palms, soles and genitalia. The skin is initially doughy but then becomes very firm. Its color swings between yellow-white and mottled and has been compared to cadaver skin. The infant often ceases to move its limbs, perhaps because of the induration, and may have difficulty with respiration. Many other reported systemic findings are probably related to the underlying problems.

Histopathology. The classic histologic findings are dermal edema and crystallization of the fat cells. There may be mucin in the dermis, but the changes in the fat are more important for the diagnosis. On gross examination of the biopsy specimen, the fat appears as a white uniform mass. The septa are widened by edema. The fat cells contain abundant crystals with little inflammation, in contrast to neonatal fat necrosis with abundant inflammation and few crystals. Often the crystals are arranged in a starburst pattern. Necrosis and calcification are not seen.

Course and Prognosis. The already weakened infant is at grave risk; the mortality rate is estimated at 50–75% but is undoubtedly greatly influenced by the underlying risk factors. In those who survive, the skin heals spontaneously and completely.

Differential Diagnosis. The main issue is neonatal fat necrosis, which occurs in healthy infants in limited areas, such as over pressure points or with cold exposure, and shows more inflammation on biopsy.

Therapy. Optimal supportive care and treatment of the underlying problems is crucial. Both high-dose systemic corticosteroids and antibiotics are usually tried, in view of the gloomy outlook. Recent or controlled studies are not available, and no one has extensive clinical experience.

Other Forms

Both gouty tophi (Chap. 47) and calciphylaxis (Chap. 45) can present with inflamed nodules in the subcutaneous fat.

Proliferative Disorders

Cytophagic Histiocytic Panniculitis
(Winkelmann and Bowie 1980)

Winkelmann and colleagues identified a group of patients with panniculitis who did very poorly, often with hemorrhagic disorders, infections and multisystemic disease.

Today this term is rarely used, since more sophisticated markers have made it clear that most cases represent a subcutaneous T cell lymphoma. Some patients with marked erythrophagocytosis and a chronic course have an Epstein-Barr virus infection. The patients have widely distributed red-brown nodules, often ulcerated. Microscopically there is panniculitis involving both lobules and septa. The key histologic feature is phagocytosis of erythrocytes and lymphocytes by histiocytes that are still functional and not obviously malignant. These laden histiocytes have been called bean-bag cells. Even in Winkelmann's series the patients did so poorly that many observers were skeptical of the reactive nature of the disease. Today lymphoma appears to be the answer in most instances; lymphoma experts consider subcutaneous T cell lymphoma a relatively specific entity (Chap. 62).

Other Malignant Processes

A variety of other lymphomas and leukemias can have fat involvement. The accumulations of malignant cells in the fat produce red-brown, often ulcerated nodules that can appear anywhere on the body. On biopsy, the malignant cells may not be recognized amidst the necrotic fat and marked granulomatous inflammatory response. Angiocentric immunoproliferative lesions such as lymphomatoid granulomatosis are also likely to have panniculitis. Moreover, all the tumors that can metastasize to the skin may also land in the subcutaneous fat, where they can mimic panniculitis. Furthermore, primary fatty tumors, although usually involving deeper sites, can present in the subcutaneous location. All these possibilities emphasize the need for biopsy in all but the most clear-cut cases of panniculitis.

Miscellaneous Types of Panniculitis

Lipodermatosclerosis

Synonyms. Sclerosing panniculitis, hypodermitis sclerodermiformis

Etiology and Pathogenesis. Most patients are middle-aged or older women with some degree of chronic venous insufficiency. Occasionally arterial disease, previous thrombophlebitis or chronic lymphedema may be a factor. Some patients, however, have no sign of underlying vascular disease.

Clinical Findings. The early stage of lipodermatosclerosis is often confused with cellulitis, as it has diffuse erythema and warmth. In other instances, the changes are more nodular, or linear, following a vein. The most typical site is the medial aspect of the calf just above the ankle. Gradually the process becomes sclerotic, often cuff-like and slowly expanding. There may be faint erythema at the periphery of the plaque, just as in scleroderma. The skin become indurated, firm and depressed. Pain is a typical feature, at all stages. Ulcerations are characteristically very slow to heal. Because of this pattern, panniculitis often not considered. We suspect this is the most underdiagnosed or misdiagnosed form of panniculitis.

Histopathology. Early lesions show a septal and lobular panniculitis, sometimes with fat necrosis or infarction. The septa may have prominent vessels. As the process progresses, the dermis becomes thickened and sclerotic, blending with thickened septa. Sometimes a superficial biopsy will show only dermal thickening and the fatty changes will be missed.

In the lobules, fatty microcysts are formed. The cyst wall is lined by an eosinophilic membranous material. This has produced a befuddling list of names, confusing clinical features with histologic findings. The histologic changes have been called membranous lipodystrophy or membranocystic change; they are probably most often seen in traumatic fat necrosis and lipodermatosclerosis, but can be seen in many other situations.

Differential Diagnosis. The list here is somewhat different than for the more typical nodular forms of panniculitis. One must exclude scleroderma, morphea, borreliosis, lupus profundus and post-traumatic and postinfectious scarring.

Therapy. There is no good therapy. Adequate compression stockings and similar support may help early in the disease, but later on no measures are dramatically successful. Stanazolol is the latest drug to be recommended, but the sclerosis is hard to influence.

Subcutaneous Granulomas

Granuloma annulare, necrobiosis lipoidica diabeticorum and sarcoidosis can all wind up one layer deeper than normal and produce panniculitis rather than a dermal nodule. They typically extend down the septa but then involve and even replace the fat lobules. The diagnosis is histologic, and the treatment is usually either excision or intralesional corticosteroids.

Medication-Induced Panniculitis

Nodose erythemas are occasionally related to medications; the main agents are oral contraceptives, sulfonamides, salicylates, phenytoin and gold salts. The artificial sweetener aspartame has also been indicted. Iodide or bromide salts cause nodular lesions that can be viewed as a type of panniculitis. More remotely, radiation therapy may produce what has been described as pseudosclerodermatous panniculitis, a mixture of sclerosis and fatty inflammation.

Probably the most interesting drug-induced panniculitis is postcorticosteroid panniculitis. This rare reaction occurs primarily in children, usually several days after abruptly stopping a relatively high dose of systemic corticosteroids. Multiple subcutaneous nodules develop, which microscopically show the same crystal needles in giant cells often seen in neonatal fat necrosis. Resolution is spontaneous.

Weber-Christian Syndrome

(Pfeifer 1892; Weber 1925; Christian 1928)

Synonyms. Panniculitis nodularis nonsuppurativa febrilis et recidivans, Pfeifer-Weber-Christian syndrome, (Pfeifer)-Weber-Christian disease, recurrent febrile nodular panniculitis

Etiology and Pathogenesis. The etiology of Weber-Christian syndrome is unknown. As the abundance of synonyms makes clear, it is a poorly understood disorder. Some major groups feel Weber-Christian syndrome does not exist; others use the term for all panniculitis with systemic involvement, and yet others consider it a rare but specific type of panniculitis. Patients with pancreatic panniculitis and subcutaneous T cell lymphoma fit Weber-Christian syndrome quite well. One can imagine that derangements involving other cells, organisms or enzymes, might produce a similar picture. We always try to detect an underlying cause for an ill patient with panniculitis; if we find no explanation after repeating searching, we reluctantly and tentatively diagnose Weber-Christian syndrome. Winkelmann has also reached this conclusion; he recently reviewed 30 cases previously diagnosed as Weber-Christian syndrome and was able to make a more specific diagnosis in each case.

Clinical Findings. The Latin name for Weber-Christian syndrome, panniculitis nodularis nonsuppurativa febrilis et recidivans, describes the problem well. Patients develop subcutaneous masses associated with episodes of fever; the lesions heal with prominent atrophy and tend to recur (Fig. 21.5). The disease appears in adult life, and women appear to be more often affected. Typically the onset of the disease is acute, with fever, malaise, gastrointestinal complaints and even arthritis; the sudden onset suggests an infectious trigger. Soon numerous subcutaneous masses appear, often distributed in a symmetric fashion and typically tender. While the legs are the most common site, any part of the body can be involved except for the face. The lesions may liquefy, ulcerate and discharge

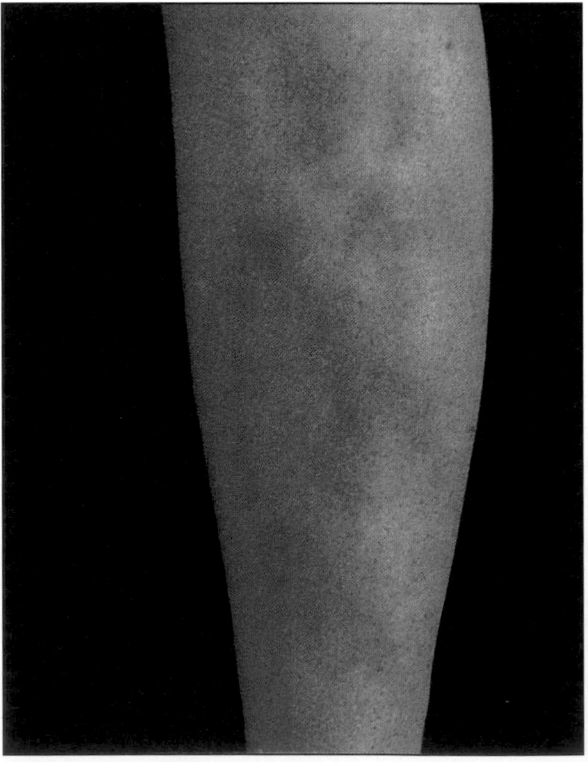

Fig. 21.5. Liquefying panniculitis, initially classified as Weber-Christian disease but in retrospect likely to represent α1-antitrypsin deficiency

a serous or oily material, but this is uncommon. In some patients, fever is not prominent and liquefaction more common; while this has been called afebrile nodular (or liquefactive) panniculitis, it usually represent $\alpha 1$-antitrypsin deficiency. In some cases involvement of the intraperitoneal or abdominal fatty tissue has been shown.

Histopathology. The microscopic picture is not specific but shows a changing pattern. Early lesions show lobular panniculitis with marked infiltration of neutrophils. Later on, there is a prominent granulomatous response with foamy histiocytes. The late lesions simply show fibrosis.

Laboratory Findings. There is no specific laboratory test. Nonetheless, extensive investigations are required to exclude the other systemic causes of panniculitis. For us, Weber-Christian syndrome is a diagnosis of exclusion.

Course and Prognosis. The course tends to be chronic with relapses. The outlook depends on the degree of systemic problems. In some cases, the disease is fatal and even on autopsy no other explanation (such as a minute pancreatic tumor) is found.

Differential Diagnosis. The main differential points are infectious panniculitis and that associated with pancreatic disease.

Therapy. Usually high-dose corticosteroids are employed; often we use 60–80 mg prednisone daily for 7–10 days followed by careful reduction. A variety of steroid-sparing agents have been tried, but none has shown itself to be especially effective. If an infectious trigger is suspected, antibiotic therapy may be tried.

Rothmann-Makai Syndrome

(Rothmann 1894; Makai 1928)

Synonyms. Lipogranulomatosis subcutanea, oleogranuloma, spontaneous panniculitis, spontaneous lipogranulomatosis

Etiology and Pathogenesis. Unknown. The very existence of Rothmann-Makai syndrome is disputed.

Clinical Findings. Adolescents and middle-aged women appear to be most often involved. Subcutaneous nodules develop suddenly and without associated systemic findings. While they are most common on the legs, they may appear anywhere on the body, including the face. They are tender during their early stage, and usually slide freely between the skin and fascia. Larger lesions may appear plate-like. The overlying skin is usually normal.

Histopathology. There is a lobular panniculitis that often has a granulomatous component. One allegedly common feature is the presence of tiny accumulations of liquefied fat (oil cysts), associated with foamy histiocytes. Thus, the microscopic picture is similar to Weber-Christian syndrome and traumatic panniculitis.

Differential Diagnosis. The most common differential point is erythema induratum or nodular vasculitis. Larger lesions may resemble a syphilitic gumma.

Therapy. Nonsteroidal antiinflammatory drugs or systemic corticosteroids seem the most reasonable approach, once an infectious etiology has been excluded. Compression stockings or bandages should also be used.

Lipoatrophy and Lipodystrophy

The distinction between lipoatrophy (thinning or disappearance of the fat) and lipodystrophy (abnormal growth of the fat) has not been observed by our forefathers, so this next section is confusing and complicated beyond all reason. Adding insult to injury is the concept of *Wucheratrophie*, anglicized as wucher atrophy. This almost metaphysical concept suggests that fat grows (the German verb *wuchern* means to grow profusely or proliferate) as it becomes atrophic; even enthusiasts have trouble selling this idea. Lipoatrophy can be divided into localized and systemic forms, some of which are congenital, others acquired. In the localized lesions, trauma probably plays a frequent role. In more diffuse lesions, especially congenital ones, the endocrine control of fat metabolism is probably altered, often with abnormal insulin or insulin-like growth factor receptors responsible. Other types of fat proliferation have traditionally been viewed as lipomas (Chap. 59). For practical purposes, one can treat fat atrophy and fat dystrophy as synonyms.

Localized Lipoatrophy

The fat may disappear following a clinically recognized inflammatory process or trauma, or just mysteriously. Typically one finds one or more flat or depressed areas on the extremity. The presence of clinical erythema and of inflammation on biopsy suggest that the inflammatory process is still active and the atrophy may expand.

Corticosteroid Lipoatrophy

Injections of corticosteroids may cause both dermal and fat atrophy. The latter usually results when an intramuscular injection is delivered too superficially or when a joint is missed. In contrast, intradermal injection of corticosteroids is usually intentional, to treat a keloid or provide local anti-inflammatory action, but nonetheless dermal thinning may occur, just as with high-potency topical steroids. Dermal thinning alone is usually clinically subtle.

The most typical lesion is a nonerythematous depression, usually several centimeters in diameter, over the triceps or buttocks (Fig. 21.6). The skin may be slightly pale and have telangiectases. In blacks, the depigmentation may be more striking than the depression. Such lesions are often clinically diagnosed as atrophoderma, but on repeated questioning the patient or parent usually admits that a shot of corticosteroid has been administered, often for arthritis, asthma, allergic rhinitis or similar problems. Usually the lesions develop over a period of weeks to months and resolve slowly over years. Sometimes the atrophy is permanent. Microscopically the collagen appears pale and thin; there may a mild granulomatous response to the corticosteroid, especially if it contains sizable crystals.

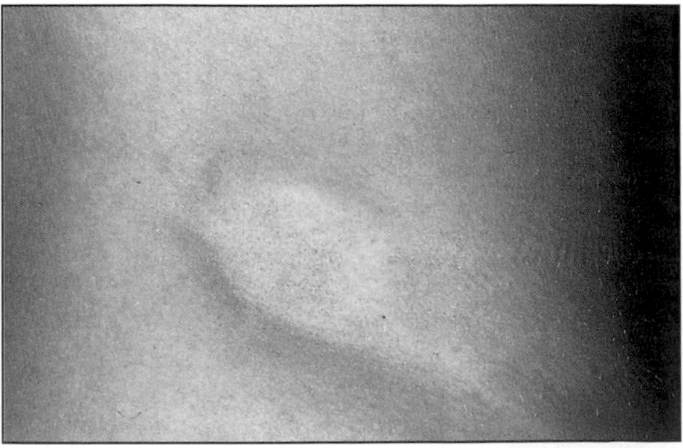

Fig. 21.6. Atrophy and hypopigmentation following corticosteroid injection

Insulin Lipodystrophy

Repeated injections of insulin, as required in diabetes mellitus, may lead to fat atrophy. On rare occasions, there may be fat hypertrophy, lending some justification to the term dystrophy. Women and children are at greater risk. Acidic insulins cause more problems; the newer highly purified and often synthetic insulins are least troublesome. The atrophy has no obvious clinical connection to urticaria and other local allergic reactions. It may even occur away from the sites of injection, although this is uncommon. The change usually starts within the first two years of using insulin. In some patients, granulomatous hypertrophic nodular reactions occur along with fat atrophy, suggesting a foreign body type reaction. In others, immunofluorescent examination suggest immune complex deposition. The only treatment is to religiously vary injection sites and experiment with different types of insulin. The addition of dexamethasone or another corticosteroid to the injection has been suggested, but this complicates the entire procedure greatly, increasing the risk of infections (from multiple mixing procedures) and of corticosteroid side effects.

Annular Lipoatrophy and Semicircular Lipoatrophy

(Ferreira-Marques 1953 [annular]; Gschwandtner and Münzberger 1974 [semicircular])

Synonyms. Lipoatrophia anularis, lipoatrophia semicircularis

As with so many of the disorders of fat, this process almost exclusively involves women. It presents as a depressed semicircular or annular band around the thigh, often bilateral. Lesions can also be seen on biceps region. The initial but incorrect explanation was the wearing of tight jeans that pressed into the fat of the thighs when the wearer was seated (Fig. 21.7). Similar lesions have been described on the shoulders of large-breasted women, where the pressure from bra straps seems causative. Another almost distinct variant involves the ankles, described as annular atrophy of the ankles (Shelley and Izumi 1970). We have seen similar changes in

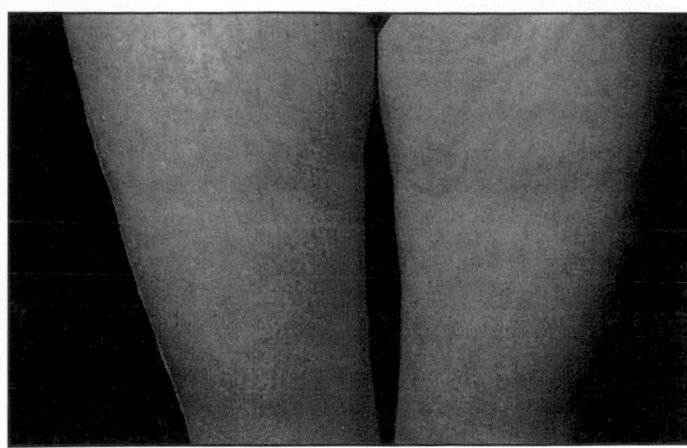

Fig. 21.7. Semicircular lipoatrophy

female water skiers, where they are clearly post-traumatic. In some patients, one can not elicit any history of trauma. While there is no satisfactory therapy, often spontaneous resolution occurs. In others, the process is painful, progressive and may hamper use of a limb. In our experience, the more distal lesions are more permanent and troublesome.

Lipodystrophia Centrifugalis Abdominalis Infantilis

(IMAMURA et al. 1971)

Epidemiology. This tongue twister is primarily a disease of young Japanese children with a 2:1 female predominance. Over 80% of cases appear before the age of 5 years. The cause is unknown.

Clinical Findings. The skin changes usually begin in the axilla or groin. As a result of the disappearance of fat, deep depressions appear and spread centrifugally to involve large parts of the abdominal or thoracic skin. Typically the area has an erythematous tint or often a distinct erythematous border with scale. The regional lymph nodes are often enlarged. The lesions usually improve spontaneously, and sometimes complete resolution occurs.

Histopathology. The periphery shows a mixed inflammatory infiltrate, while centrally the fatty layer is diminished or absent. Occasionally the fat may show liquefaction.

Differential Diagnosis. Both morphea and its variant atrophoderma of Pasini and Pierini, as well as borreliosis, appear similar. Progressive lipodystrophy is more extreme and more permanent.

Therapy. No therapy is well established. Both systemic and topical corticosteroids are usually recommended.

Local Inflammatory Lipoatrophy

(PETERS and WINKELMANN 1980; BILLINGS et al. 1987)

Synonyms. Localized lipoatrophy, atrophic connective tissue panniculitis, lipoatrophic panniculitis

Etiology and Pathogenesis. In our view, this is an unfortunate term for with panniculitis who evolve into prominent lipoatrophy. Autoimmune panniculitis might be a better term, as associations have been suggested with Hashimoto thyroiditis, juvenile rheumatoid arthritis and juvenile diabetes mellitus.

Clinical Findings. Most patients are children with involvement of the extremities and occasionally the buttocks. During the acute phase, they have typical red-brown nodules of panniculitis; often, however, these are quite large, ranging up to 20 cm in diameter. As such plaques coalesce and resolve, there is marked loss of fat, often associated with cutis laxa-like changes of the overlying skin.

Histopathology. The histology initially shows lobular panniculitis and later granulomatous inflammation with loss of fat.

Differential Diagnosis. All the forms of panniculitis discussed earlier in this chapter should be considered. In addition, underlying diseases should be aggressively ruled out, as panniculitis is an uncommon problem in children.

Partial and Generalized Lipoatrophy

A number of different syndromes are included here. All are rare and are summarized briefly. Even at major teaching centers, such patients are a once a decade event.

Partial Progressive Lipodystrophy

(BARRAQUER 1906; HOLLÄNDER 1910; SIMONS 1911)

Synonyms. Barraquer-Simons syndrome, Holländer-Simons syndrome, partial lipodystrophy, progressive lipodystrophy, Weir-Mitchell syndrome, cephalothoracic lipodystrophy

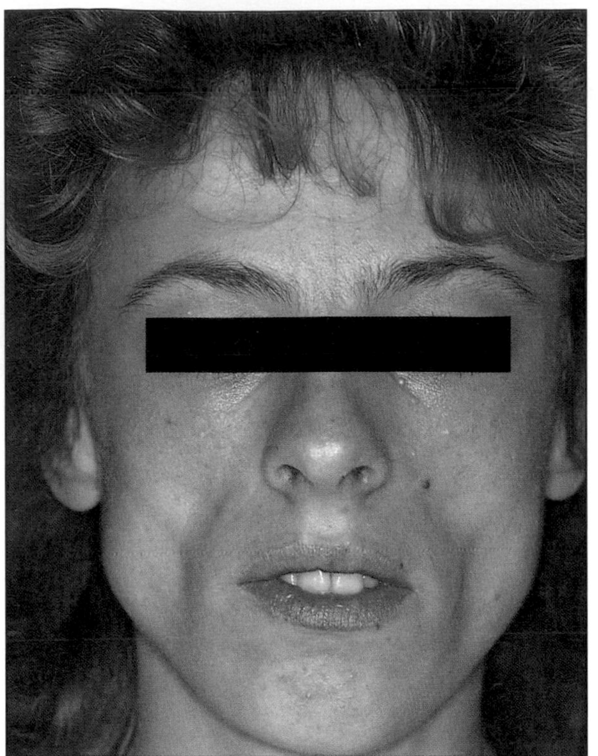

Fig. 21.8. Partial progressive lipodystrophy

Etiology and Pathogenesis. The cause is unknown. As the list of synonyms suggests, this is probably not a single disorder. There may be a genetic component, although most cases appear acquired, often following a febrile illness or associated with another major medical problem. The female to male ratio is 4:1. Many patients have a glomerulonephritis whose etiology is somewhat better understood. The C3 nephritic factor is an IgG antibody directed against the C3 complex.

Clinical Findings. Typically there is loss of fat involving the face, trunk and arms, producing a cachectic look (Fig. 21.8). Usually the buttocks and legs are normal or even carry extra fat. Many other clinical variants have been described with other patterns of involvement. The associated renal disease is present in 50% of patients; it may precede the fat changes. Despite the disturbing appearance and the renal disease, the patients do relatively well.

Differential Diagnosis. All the other types of lipoatrophy should be considered. Until more definitive tests are available, this disease category will remain almost impossible to sort out. Table 21.2 shows the major subtypes.

Therapy. Transplantation of fat via liposuction and reinjection may improve the facial appearance, but does not provide permanent relief.

Partial Lipodystrophy, Dunnigan and Köbberling Types

(Dunnigan et al. 1974; Köbberling et al. 1975)

Synonyms. Partial face-sparing lipodystrophy, reverse partial lipodystrophy, Dunnigan-Köbberling syndrome

Face-sparing lipodystrophy adequately describes these rare disorders, which for unclear reasons only affect women. One gene has been identified at 1q21–q24, so the female dominance remains a mystery. In the Dunnigan variant, the loss of fat involves the trunk and extremities, while in the Köbberling type, only the extremities are involved. In both cases the musculature and veins appear prominent. A number of associated symptoms have

Table 21.2. Types of lipodystrophy

	Generalized		Partial		
	Berardinelli-Seip	**Lawrence**	**Dunnigan**	**Köbberling**	**Barraquer-Simons**
Inheritance	AR	Sporadic	? XLD	? XLD	Sporadic
M:F	Equal	Women > men	Only females	Only females	Women > men
Localization	Face, trunk, extremities	Face, trunk, extremities	Trunk, extremities	Extremities	Face, chest, arms
Onset	Birth, infancy	Childhood, puberty	Puberty, young adulthood	Puberty, young adulthood	Childhood, puberty

been reported, including acanthosis nigricans, hirsutism, diabetes mellitus and lipid abnormalities; in the Dunnigan type, the labia may appear enlarged because of the loss of fat around them. Often there is resistance to insulin or insulin-like growth factor. The only treatment is management of the associated diabetes mellitus, which is often very difficult because of the lack of effect of insulin.

Congenital Generalized Lipoatrophy
(BERADINELLI 1954; SEIP 1959)

Synonyms. Beradinelli-Seip syndrome, lipoatrophic diabetes

Etiology and Pathogenesis. This very rare disease appears to be inherited in an autosomal recessive pattern. The hallmark is marked insulin resistance; patients may have blood insulin levels, as high as 5000 units/ml. The basic defect is unclear but appears to involve either abnormalities of the diencephalon-hypophyseal axis or membrane insulin receptors.

Clinical Findings. Either at birth or early in life, the patients lose their buccal fat, producing a characteristic facies with gaunt cheeks, large ears and hypertelorism. Initially they appear very muscular, as their fat is so scant. Skeletal growth is accelerated during the first years of life, so that in their early school years, these children are often mistakenly thought to be extremely athletic, when in fact they are just the opposite. Other cutaneous findings include hirsutism and acanthosis nigricans, both of which may be extreme. Some patients may have xanthomas. The systemic findings are more troublesome. In addition to severe insulin-resistant diabetes mellitus, there is usually hepatomegaly caused by lipid deposits, true genital hypertrophy, masculinization of the girls and in about 50% of cases, mental retardation.

There is no good treatment.

Acquired Generalized Lipoatrophy
(LAWRENCE 1946)

The acquired form of generalized lipoatrophy is quite similar to the congenital form. It is sporadic, usually involves women, and often follows an infection or other serious illness. Because of the later onset, the sexual precocity and skeletal changes are not seen, but the fat atrophy, other skin changes and diabetes mellitus are similar.

Other Diseases of Fat

Lipedema
(ALLEN and HINES 1940)

Synonyms. Painful fat syndrome, painful lipedema of the legs

Clinical Findings. This disease, although described by vascular physicians at the Mayo Clinic, has never really caught on in America and is diagnosed far more often in Europe. The patients are almost all older women with swollen legs, usually with sparing of the feet; inelegantly called piano legs. The swelling is symmetrical, quite firm and very painful, especially around the knees. The swelling increases when the patient stands a great deal, and only slowly recedes when the legs are elevated. Some patients have had lipid abnormalities, and in others unclear abnormalities in the fat composition of the legs have been reported. The course is progressive and painful.

Differential Diagnosis. The main question is whether lipedema exists. If it does, then it is very similar to lymphedema. In Dercum disease (Chap.

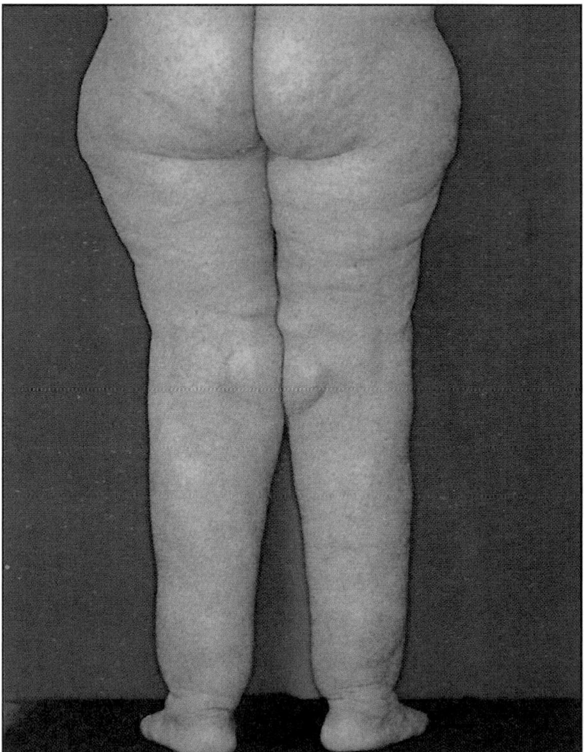

Fig. 21.9. Lipedema

59), painful lipomas are present but the disease is not as diffuse. In lipodermatosclerosis, the legs are painful but the changes more localized.

Therapy. Compression bandages or stockings should be tried.

Cellulite

Cellulite is not a disease but an almost normal finding. Young women may complain of changes of the skin and fat of their thighs and buttocks. When the skin is pushed together, an orange-peel appearance becomes more prominent. The alignment of the fat septa in these areas in women is such that when there is an increase in fat, the skin puckers a bit. Some patients may complain of minor pain or other vague symptoms. Some women simply easily add fat in these regions; the problem becomes more severe with weight gain and age. There is no good treatment other than weight loss and exercise. In recent studies, both massage and ultrasound have proven disappointing.

Bibliography

Panniculitis

Patterson JW (1991) Differential diagnosis of panniculitis. Adv Dermatol 6:309–329; discussion 330

Peters MS, Su WP (1992) Panniculitis. Dermatol Clin 10: 37–57

White WL, Wieselthier JS, Hitchcock MG (1996) Panniculitis: recent developments and observations. Semin Cutan Med Surg 15:278–299

Erythema Nodosum

Bäfverstedt BO (1954) Erythema nodosum migrans. Acta Derm Venereol (Stockh) 48:381–384

Cribier B, Caille A, Heid E et al. (1998) Erythema nodosum and associated diseases. A study of 129 cases. Int J Dermatol 37:667–672

Vilanova X, Pinol Aguadè J (1959) Subacute nodular migratory panniculitis. Br J Dermatol

Waltz KM, Long D, Marks JG Jr et al. (1999) Sweet's syndrome and erythema nodosum: the simultaneous occurrence of 2 reactive dermatoses. Arch Dermatol 135: 62–66

Nodular Vasculitis

Cho KH, Kim YG, Yang SG et al. (1997) Inflammatory nodules of the lower legs: a clinical and histological analysis of 134 cases in Korea. J Dermatol 24:522–529

Montgomery H, O'Leary PA, Barker NW (1945) Nodular vascular disease of the legs. JAMA 128:335–341

Naschitz JE, Boss JH, Misselevich I et al. (1996) The fasciitis-panniculitis syndromes. Clinical and pathologic features. Medicine (Baltimore) 75:6–16

Schneider JW, Jordaan HF (1997) The histopathologic spectrum of erythema induratum of Bazin. Am J Dermatopathol 19:323–333

Yus ES, Simon P (1999) About the histopathology of erythema induratum–nodular vasculitis. Am J Dermatopathol 21: 301–306

Lupus Erythematosus Profundus

Hebra F, Kaposi M (1875) On disease of the skin, including exanthemata. New Sydenham Society, London

Holland NW, McKnight K, Challa VR et al. (1995) Lupus panniculitis (profundus) involving the breast: report of 2 cases and review of the literature. J Rheumatol 22:344–346

Irgang S (1954) Apropos du lupus erythemateux profond. Ann Dermatol Syph 81:246–249

Kundig TM, Trueb RM, Krasovec M (1997) Lupus profundus/panniculitis. Dermatology 195:99–101

Martens PB, Moder KG, Ahmed I (1999) Lupus panniculitis: clinical perspectives from a case series. J Rheumatol 26: 68–72

Infectious Panniculitis

Aleman CT, Wallace ML, Blaylock WK et al. (1999) Subcutaneous nodules caused by *Pseudomonas aeruginosa* without sepsis. Cutis 63:161–163

Callahan TE, Schecter WP, Horn JK (1998) Necrotizing soft tissue infection masquerading as cutaneous abcess following illicit drug injection. Arch Surg 133:812–817; discussion 817–819

De Argila D, Rodriguez-Peralto JL, Ortiz-Frutos J (1996) Septal panniculitis associated with infectious mononucleosis. Dermatology 192:291

Patterson JW, Brown PC, Broecker AH (1989) Infection-induced panniculitis. J Cutan Pathol 16:183–193

Cold Panniculitis

Aroni K, Aivaliotis M, Tsele E et al. (1998) An unusual panniculitis appearing in the winter with good response to tetracycline. J Dermatol 25:677–681

Ben-Amitai D, Metzker A (1996) Cold panniculitis in a neonate. J Am Acad Dermatol 35:651–652

Ter Poorten JC, Hebert AA, Ilkiw R (1995) Cold panniculitis in a neonate. J Am Acad Dermatol 33:383–385

Traumatic Panniculitis

De Groot AC (1994) Is lipoatrophia semicircularis induced by pressure? Br J Dermatol 131:887–890

Nagore E, Sanchez-Motilla JM, Rodriguez-Serna M et al. (1998) Lipoatrophia semicircularis – a traumatic panniculitis: report of seven cases and review of the literature. J Am Acad Dermatol 39:879–881

Winkelmann RK, Barker SM (1985) Factitial traumatic panniculitis. J Am Acad Dermatol 13:988–994

Postinjection Panniculitis and Factitial Panniculitis

Drago F, Rongioletti F, Battifoglio ML et al. (1996) Localised lipoatrophy after acupuncture. Lancet 347:1484

Lee JS, Ahn SK, Lee SH (1995) Factitial panniculitis induced by cupping and acupuncture. Cutis 55:217–218

Pancreatic Panniculitis

Bem J, Bradley EL III (1998) Subcutaneous manifestations of severe acute pancreatitis. Pancreas 16:551–555

Dahl PR, Su WP, Cullimore KC, Dicken CH (1995) Pancreatic panniculitis. J Am Acad Dermatol 33:413–417

Durden FM, Variyam E, Chren MM (1996) Fat necrosis with features of erythema nodosum in a patient with metastatic pancreatic carcinoma. Int J Dermatol 35:39–41

α1-Antitrypsin Deficiency

Edmonds BK, Hodge JA, Rietschel RL (1991) Alpha 1-antitrypsin deficiency-associated panniculitis: case report and review of the literature. Pediatr Dermatol 8:296–299

Eriksson S (1996) A 30-year perspective on alpha 1-antitrypsin deficiency. Chest 110:237S–242S

Linares-Barrios M, Conejo-Mir IS, Artola Igarza JL et al. (1998) Panniculitis due to alpha 1-antitrypsin deficiency induced by cryosurgery. Br J Dermatol 138:552–553

Warter J, Storck D, Grosshans E et al. (1972) Syndrome de Weber-Christiane associé à un déficit en alpha1-antitrypsine: Enquète familiale. Ann Med Interne (Paris) 123:877–882

Neonatal Fat Necrosis

Balazs M (1987) Subcutaneous fat necrosis of the newborn with emphasis on ultrastructural studies. Int J Dermatol 26:227–230

Hernandez-Martin A, de Unamuno P, Fernandez-Lopez E (1998) Congenital ulcerated subcutaneous fat necrosis of the newborn. Dermatology 197:261–263

Liu FT, Dobry MM, Shames BS et al. (1993) Subcutaneous nodules and hypercalcemia in an infant. Subcutaneous fat necrosis of the newborn. Arch Dermatol 129: 898–902

Mather MK, Sperling LC, Sau P (1997) Subcutaneous fat necrosis of the newborn. Int J Dermatol 36:450–452

Sclerema Neonatorum

de Silva U, Parish LC (1994) Historical approach to scleroderma. Clin Dermatol 12:201–205

Jardine D, Atherton DJ, Trompeter RS (1990) Sclerema neonatorum and subcutaneous fat necrosis of the newborn in the same infant. Eur J Pediatr 150:125–126

Cytophagic Histiocytic Panniculitis

Craig AJ, Cualing H, Thomas G et al. (1998) Cytophagic histiocytic panniculitis – a syndrome associated with benign and malignant panniculitis: case comparison and review of the literature. J Am Acad Dermatol 39: 721–736

Okamura T, Niho Y (1999) Cytophagic histiocytic panniculitis – what is the best therapy? Intern Med 38:224–225

Ostrov BE, Athreya BH, Eichenfield AH et al. (1996) Successful treatment of severe cytophagic histiocytic panniculitis with cyclosporine. Semin Arthritis Rheum 25: 404–413

Winkelmann RK, Bowie EJ (1980) Hemorrhagic diathesis associated with benign histiocytic, cytophagic panniculitis and systemic histiocytosis. Arch Intern Med 140: 1460–1463

Lipodermatosclerosis

Herouy Y, May AE, Pornschlegel G et al. (1998) Lipodermatosclerosis is characterized by elevated expression and activation of matrix metalloproteinases: implications for venous ulcer formation. J Invest Dermatol 111: 822–827

Sheth R, Poonevala V (1997) Lipodermatosclerosis: a postphlebitic syndrome. Int J Dermatol 36:931–932

Vowden K (1998) Lipodermatosclerosis and atrophie blanche. J Wound Care 7:441–443

Medication-Induced Panniculitis

McCauliffe DP, Poitras K (1991) Aspartame-induced lobular panniculitis. J Am Acad Dermatol 24:298–300

Weber-Christian Syndrome

Christian HA (1928) Relapsing febrile nodular nonsuppurative panniculitis. Arch Intern Med 42:338–351

Pfeiffer V (1892) Über einen Fall von herdweiser Atrophie des subcutanen Fettgewebes. Dtsch Arch Klin Med 50: 438–449

Weber FP (1925) A case of relapsing nonsuppurative nodular panniculitis, showing phagocytosis of subcutaneous fat cells by macrophages. Brit J Dermatol S 37:301–311

White JW Jr, Winkelmann RK (1998) Weber-Christian panniculitis: a review of 30 cases with this diagnosis. J Am Acad Dermatol 39:56–62

Rothmann-Makai Syndrome

Chan HL (1975) Panniculitis (Rothmann-Makai), with good response to tetracycline. Br J Dermatol 92:351–354

Makai E (1928) Über Lipogranulomatosis subcutanea. Klin Wochenschr 7:2343–2346

Rothmann M (1894) Über Entzündung und Atrophie des subcutanen Fettgewebes. Virchows Arch Pathol Anat 136:159–169

Insulin Lipoatrophy

Asherov J, Mimouni M, Laron Z (1979) Successful treatment of insulin lipoatrophy. A case report. Diabete Metab 5: 1–3

Murao S, Hirata K, Ishida T, Takahara J (1998) Lipoatrophy induced by recombinant human insulin injection. Intern Med 37:1031–1033

Involutional Lipoatrophy

Dahl PR, Zalla MJ, Winkelmann RK (1996) Localized involutional lipoatrophy: a clinicopathologic study of 16 patients. J Am Acad Dermatol 35:523–528

Peters MS, Winkelmann RK (1986) The histopathology of localized lipoatrophy. Br J Dermatol 114:27–36

Annular Lipoatrophy and Semicircular Lipoatrophy

Ferreira-Marques J (1953) Lipoatrophia anularis. Ein Fall einer bisher nicht beschriebenen Krankheit der Haut (des Pannikulus adiposus). Arch Dermatol Syph 195: 479–491

Gschwandtner WR, Münzberger H (1974) Lipoatrophia semicircularis. Hautarzt 25:222–227

Shelley WB, Izumi AK (1970) Annular atrophy of the ankles: a case of partial lipodystrophy. Arch Dermatol 102: 326–329

Lipodystrophia Centrifugalis Abdominalis Infantilis

Imamura S, Yamada M, Ikeda T (1971) Lipodystrophia centrifugalis abdominalis infantilis. Arch Dermatol 104: 291–298

Local Inflammatory Lipoatrophy

Billings JK, Milgraum SS, Gupta AK et al. (1987) Lipoatrophic panniculitis: a possible autoimmune inflammatory disease of fat. Report of three cases. Arch Dermatol 123:1662–1666

Peters MS, Winkelmann RK (1980) Localized lipoatrophy (atrophic connective tissue disease panniculitis). Arch Dermatol 116:1363–1368

Partial and Generalized Lipoatrophy

Barraquer R (1906) Histoire clinique d'un cas d'atrophie du tissue cellulo-adipeux. Barcelona

Berardinelli W (1954) An undiagnosed endocrinometabolic syndrome: report of 2 cases. J Clin Endocr Metab 14: 193–204

Cronin CC, Higgins T, Molloy M (1995) Lupus, C3 nephritic factor and partial lipodystrophy. Q J Med 88:298–299

Dunnigan MG, Cochrane MA, Kelly A et al. (1974) Familial lipoatrophic diabetes with dominant transmission. A new syndrome. Q J Med 43:33–48

Gedde-Dahl T Jr, Trygstad O, Van Maldergem L et al. (1996) Genetics of the Berardinelli-Seip syndrome (congenital generalized lipodystrophy) in Norway: epidemiology and gene mapping. Berardinelli-Seip Study Group. Acta Paediatr [Suppl] 413:52–58

Griebel M, Mallory SB (1988) Generalized weight loss in a child. Arch Dermatol 124:571–576

Holländer E (1910) Über einen Fall von fortschreitendem Schwund des Fettgewebes und seinem kosmetischen Ersatz durch Menschenfett. Münch Med Wochenschr 57: 1794–1795

Köbberling J, Willms B, Kattermann R et al. (1975) Lipodystrophy of the extremities. A dominantly inherited syndrome associated with lipatrophic diabetes. Humangenetik 29:111–120

Lawrence RD (1946) Lipodystrophy and hepatomegaly with diabetes, lipaemia, and other metabolic disturbances. A case throwing new light on the action of insulin. Lancet 1:724–731, 773–775

Mamalaki E, Katsantonis J, Papavasiliou S et al. (1995) A case of partial face-sparing lipodystrophy combining features of generalized lipodystrophy. J Am Acad Dermatol 32: 130–133

Seip M (1959) Lipodystrophy and gigantismus with associated endocrine manifestations: a new diencephalic syndrom? Acta Paediatr 48:555–574

Seip M, Trygstad O (1996) Generalized lipodystrophy, congenital and acquired (lipoatrophy). Acta Paediatr [Suppl] 413:2–28

Senior B, Gellis SS (1964) The syndromes of total lipodystrophy and of partial lipodystrophy. Pediatrics 33: 593–612

Simons A (1911) Eine seltene Trophoneurose („Lipodystrophia progressiva"). Z Neurol 5:29–38

Lipedema

Bilancini S, Lucchi M, Tucci S et al. (1995) Functional lymphatic alterations in patients suffering from lipedema. Angiology 46:333–339

Dimakakos PB, Stefanopoulos T, Antoniades P et al. (1997) MRI and ultrasonographic findings in the investigation of lymphedema and lipedema. Int Surg 82:411–416

Rudkin GH, Miller TA (1994) Lipedema: a clinical entity distinct from lymphedema. Plast Reconstr Surg 94: 841–847; discussion 848–849

Cellulite

Draelos ZD, Marenus KD (1997) Cellulite. Etiology and purported treatment. Dermatol Surg 23:1177–1181

Kligman AM (1997) Cellulite: facts and fiction. J Geriatr Dermatol 5:136–139

Piérard GE, Nizet JL, Piérard-Franchimont C (2000) Cellulite. From standing fat herniation to hypodermal stretch marks. J Am Dermatopath 22:34–37

Rosenbaum M, Prieto V, Hellmer J et al. (1998) An exploratory investigation of the morphology and biochemistry of cellulite. Plast Reconstr Surg 101:1934–1939

Scherwitz C, Braun Falco O (1978) So called cellulite. J Dermatol Surg Oncol 4:230–234

Diseases of the Blood Vessels

Contents

In this chapter we will consider diseases in which malformations, functional abnormalities or inflammation of the arteries, arterioles, capillaries, venules and veins play a major role. A certain amount of overlap with other chapters is unavoidable. Some vascular malformations are considered under nevi (Chap. 52), while the role of the vessels is also emphasized in allergic reactions (Chap. 11).

Basic Science Aspects

The three-dimensional network of the cutaneous vasculature is shown in Figure 22.1. The two dermal networks run parallel to the skin surface and are connected by vertically oriented vessels. The deep dermal plexus is at the level of the dermal-subcutaneous junction. From it arise vessels serving the adnexal structures as well as connecting to the superficial dermal plexus in the subpapillary dermis. From this plexus, individual capillary loops serve the dermal papillae. The venous system is similarly arranged. In addition to supplying nutrients, the cutaneous vessels are active in temperature control. This explains their relatively large size in comparison to other organs. The width of the lumen of the arteries and arterioles is regulated by neural pathways controlling the smooth muscles of the media. The acral arteriovenous anastomoses control the distal blood flow, shunting blood away from the capillary system when they are open. Increased arterial blood flow produces erythema, while a restricted or overextended venous supply leads to cyanosis.

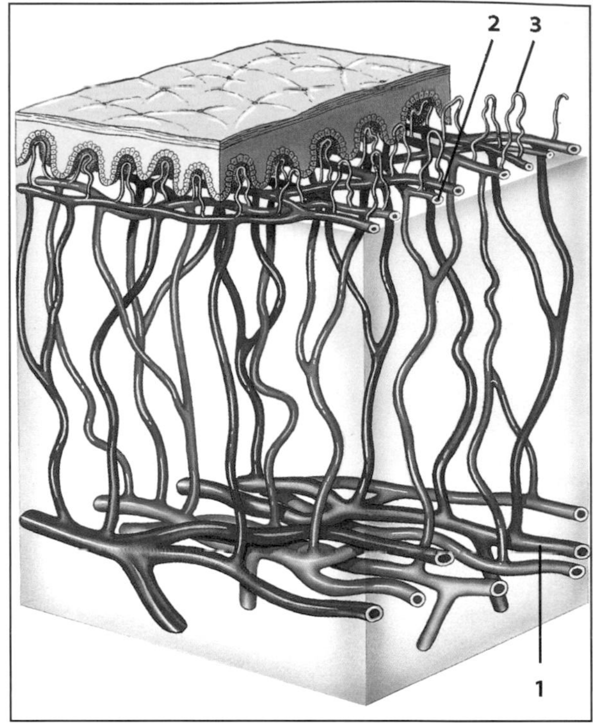

Fig. 22.1. Vascular network of the skin: *1* deep plexus, *2* superficial plexus, *3* capillary loops

While it is difficult to identify the type of vessel with routine methods, ultrastructural and histochemical studies have shown that they are usually capillaries or postcapillary venules.

Telangiectasia

Definition. Telangiectasia is the permanent dilation of preexisting small vessels (arterioles, capillaries, venules) that are blood-red in color and shine through the skin (Fig. 22.2). A single lesion is a telangiectasis, but usually multiple lesions (telangiectases) are present.

Telangiectases can be so numerous in a given area that they produce an erythema, known as telangiectatic erythema. When such a lesion of matted small vessels is examined closely, the individual lesions can be seen. When diascopy is performed, the vessels fade. Microscopic examination reveals small dilated vessels in the dermal papillae.

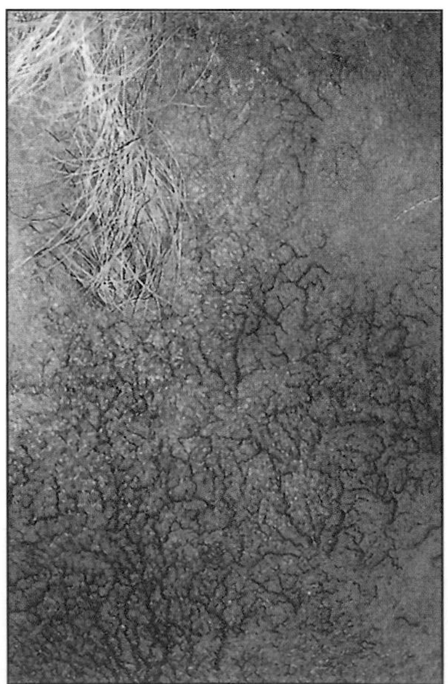

Fig. 22.2. Telangiectases

All telangiectases can be treated with electrosurgical devices, usually using a fine cat's whisker needle at a low setting. In addition, a variety of lasers are very effective. Oral tetracycline has been recommended for diffuse conditions but rarely produces lasting betterment. Often, the telangiectases are the least of the patient's problems and require no treatment.

Clinically, one can distinguish between primary and secondary telangiectasia. Poikiloderma refers to the association of telangiectases, atrophy, and hypo- or hyperpigmentation. Thus, all patients with poikiloderma have telangiectases. This family of disorders is considered in Chapter 18.

Primary Telangiectasia

Hereditary Hemorrhagic Telangiectasia

(Babington 1865; Rendu 1896; Osler 1907)

Synonym. Osler-Weber-Rendu syndrome

Definition. Widespread disorder with cutaneous telangiectases and frequent arteriovenous malformations.

Epidemiology. Hereditary hemorrhagic telangiectasia has a prevalence ranging from 1:3000 to 1:40,000, depending on the ethnic group studied.

Etiology and Pathogenesis. The disease is inherited in an autosomal dominant pattern, but 20% of patients do not have a positive family history. The basic defect is unknown, but most patients show inheritance at 9q33. Others have a defect localized on chromosome 12q. Abnormalities in both transforming growth factor-β receptor (endoglin) and activin receptor-like kinase have been identified, so it is likely that hereditary hemorrhagic telangiectasia is not one disease but several.

Clinical Findings. Almost every patient has telangiectases, but the more systemic arteriovenous malformations are less constant. Patients tend to present with bleeding problems, most often persistent nosebleeds. Gastrointestinal bleeding and hematuria are other signs. About 10% of individuals never report bleeding. The cutaneous lesions appear later in life, but by 40 years of age, almost every patient has telangiectases, particularly on the lips, ears, oral mucosa, and conjunctiva (Fig. 22.3, 22.4). Acral lesions are also common, including subungual ectatic vessels. Spider angiomas and larger malformations are uncommon. Bleeding from cutaneous lesions is very rare.

The same dilated vessels are found throughout the body, especially in the nasal mucosa, gastrointestinal tract, lungs, and genitourinary system, producing a wide range of symptoms in addition to bleeding. Some patients may present with anemia. CNS involvement may lead to focal neurologic signs and symptoms. Pulmonary and hepatic arteriovenous malformations pose the second greatest threat after bleeding. The pulmonary lesions may produce chronic pulmonary insufficiency with dyspnea, cyanosis, and clubbing of the fingers. They may also release septic emboli that can lead to brain abscesses. In the liver, cirrhosis may develop and worsen after the transfusions necessary to treat episodes of internal bleeding. Despite all these problems, the life expectancy is relatively good.

Histopathology. The upper dermis shows enlarged and ectatic capillaries, while in the deeper dermis aberrant, larger, thick-walled vessels are found.

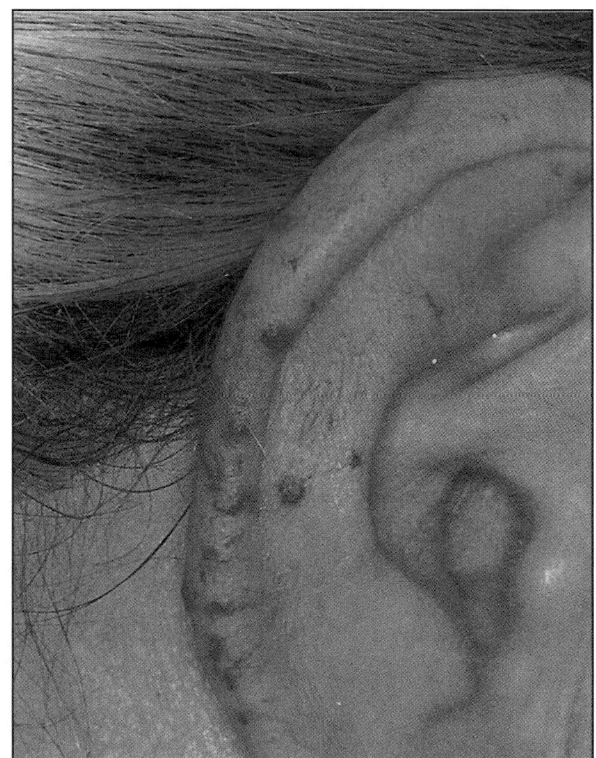

Fig. 22.3. Hereditary hemorrhagic telangiectasia

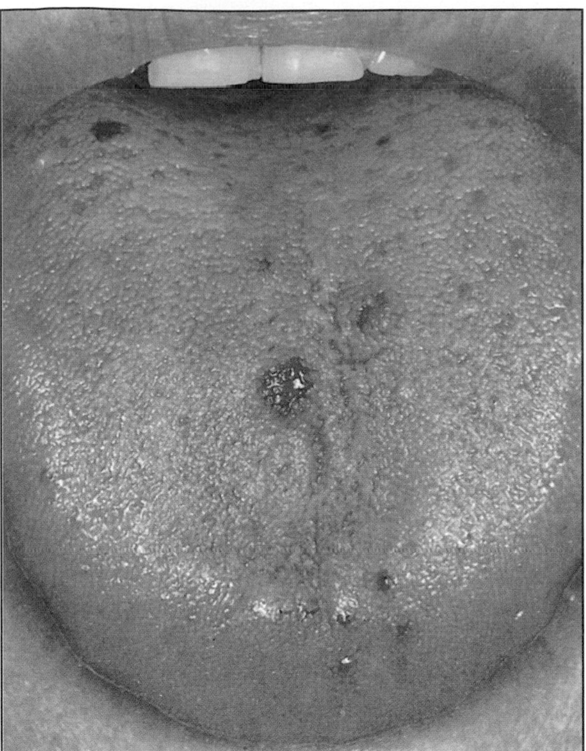

Fig. 22.4. Hereditary hemorrhagic telangiectasia

Differential Diagnosis. In patients with a positive family history and associated bleeding problems, the diagnosis is easy. In other cases, multiple spider nevi, multiple cherry angiomas, and the diseases associated with multiple angiokeratomas all come into question.

Therapy. The cutaneous lesions usually require no therapy, although they can be destroyed with electrosurgery or lasers. Acute nosebleeds usually require packing, while patients with chronic problems may benefit from a ligation of the major septal vessels. The almost inevitable anemia from gastrointestinal bleeding can usually be treated with iron. If endoscopic examination reveals especially large malformations, they too can be coagulated with a laser. The pulmonary arteriovenous shunts can be treated surgically or blocked with intravascular catheterization techniques. Aminocaproic acid has been effective in some patients with recurrent severe bleeding. The usual dosage is 1.0–1.5 g daily. Both pulmonary and hepatic function should be monitored. Acute neurologic problems should be aggressively investigated, as they may represent a cerebral embolus or abscess.

Hereditary Benign Telangiectasia

This very uncommon disorder must be distinguished from hereditary hemorrhagic telangiectasia. It too is inherited in an autosomal dominant pattern. The lesions are not present at birth but develop during childhood. As with all the generalized telangiectasias, the individual lesions are highly variable, ranging from small, pinhead-sized macules to mats or complex intertwining vascular aggregations. The sites of predilection are the face, neck, and upper part of the trunk; the vermilion border may be involved. In contrast to hereditary hemorrhagic telangiectasia, there is no mucosal involvement and no bleeding. In addition, in the latter disorder, the telangiectases usually appear much later.

Generalized Essential Telangiectasia

This uncommon disorder is probably not a single entity. Patients are typically girls who begin developing telangiectases in late childhood or early adult life. The lesions initially appear on the upper parts of the legs and slowly progress to involve the abdomen, trunk, and rarely the neck, face, or legs. The telangiectases are varied in appearance, ranging from solitary macules to retiform lesions to coalesced sheets (Fig. 22.5). Lesions of the conjunctiva and other mucosal surfaces are common. Associated findings are rare, but gastrointestinal bleeding has been described. The main task is to exclude any underlying disorder, such as a connective tissue disease. Individual lesions can be destroyed, but camouflage is wiser.

Unilateral Nevoid Telangiectasia

Synonym. Unilateral dermatomal superficial telangiectasia

Two separate problems are collected under this rubric. Congenital unilateral nevoid telangiectasia is far more common in boys (in contrast to the other forms of generalized telangiectasia) and develops in childhood. The typical assortment of telangiectatic lesions is present but in localized distribution. Despite the name, the pattern follows Blaschko lines, not dermatomes, typically involving the face, chest, or an arm. There are no associated findings. In some patients with acquired telangiectases, either during pregnancy or in association with liver disease, the distribution may also be seg-

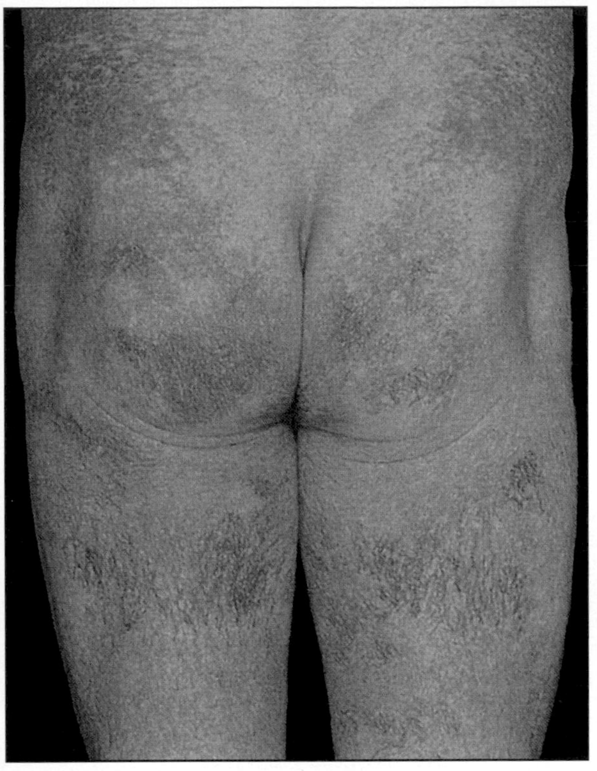

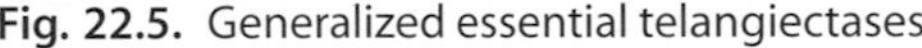

Fig. 22.5. Generalized essential telangiectases

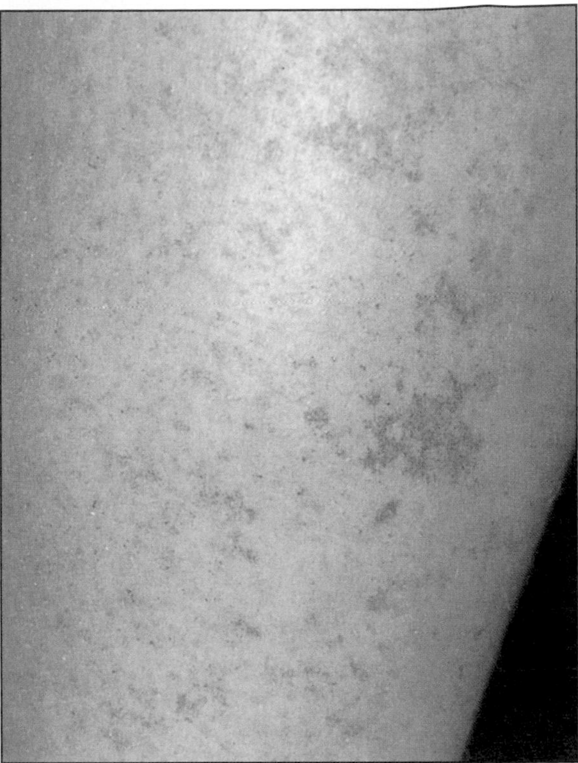

Fig. 22.6. Angioma serpiginosum

mental. The congenital lesions tend to be permanent; those that are acquired may improve spontaneously.

Angioma Serpiginosum

(Hutchinson 1889; Crocker 1899)

Definition. Uncommon vascular manifestation consisting of telangiectases that appear after infancy but may be interpreted as nevus.

Clinical Findings. Angioma serpiginosum is an uncommon and peculiar disorder. It appears almost exclusively in women, usually on the buttocks, thighs or arms. The initial lesion consists of several grouped, punctate ectatic capillaries that become apparent during puberty. It may slowly enlarge as new puncta arise peripherally, producing an annular or serpiginous pattern (Fig. 22.6). If central regression occurs, the entire area acquires a red hue. The ectatic vessels are difficult to compress with a glass spatula. The lesions may continue to grow slowly for years.

Histopathology. Dilated small vessels are seen in the superficial dermis. There is no incontinence of pigment or inflammation.

Differential Diagnosis. Both Osler-Weber-Rendu syndrome and Fabry syndrome (as well as the other, even rarer diseases with angiokeratomas) should be considered, but the distribution is wrong for the former, and the latter usually has systemic findings by the time skin lesions appear. The most common differential diagnostic point is a pigmented purpura, but there is no hemosiderin deposition here, and the lesions are usually not located on the legs.

Therapy. Either no therapy or treatment with a tunable dye or copper laser is appropriate.

Secondary Telangiectasia

Sometimes telangiectases arise as a result of exposure to exogenous factors or in association with other diseases.

Exogenous Causes

Chronic exposure to sunlight is probably the most common cause. Most individuals develop a few telangiectases on their cheeks and nose over the years in association with solar damage. In some individuals, the telangiectases dominate over the other changes. Chronic radiation dermatitis is rich in telangiectases, while long-term use of topical corticosteroids can produce similar effects, usually associated with atrophy. Systemic corticosteroids or estrogens also tend to cause telangiectases. Chronic cold exposure can lead to telangiectatic changes, especially on the calves of women.

Erythromelanosis Interfollicularis Colli
(Leder 1944)

Synonym. Erythrosis interfollicularis colli

This tongue twister is a clinically specific form of sun-induced skin damage that involves the side of the neck and occasionally the décolletage area (Fig. 22.7). The changes always have sharp borders, and the shaded areas underneath the chin and behind the ear are spared. Numerous telangiectases coalesce, producing an erythema interrupted by the pale perifollicular areas. In addition, there may be some incontinence of pigment, probably analogous to melasma. The changes are generally permanent, so the best approach is avoidance of light or the use of sun screens. In some patients, topical retinoids produce an improvement.

Endogenous Causes

As mentioned above, hormones and chronic liver disease are the two main factors. In many instances, the two triggers are intertwined. Many connective tissue diseases feature multiple telangiectases; included in the list are systemic sclerosis, lupus erythematosus, dermatomyositis, and acrodermatitis chronica atrophicans. In systemic sclerosis, the telangiectases may be very prominent, as in CREST syndrome where the T stands for telangiectases.

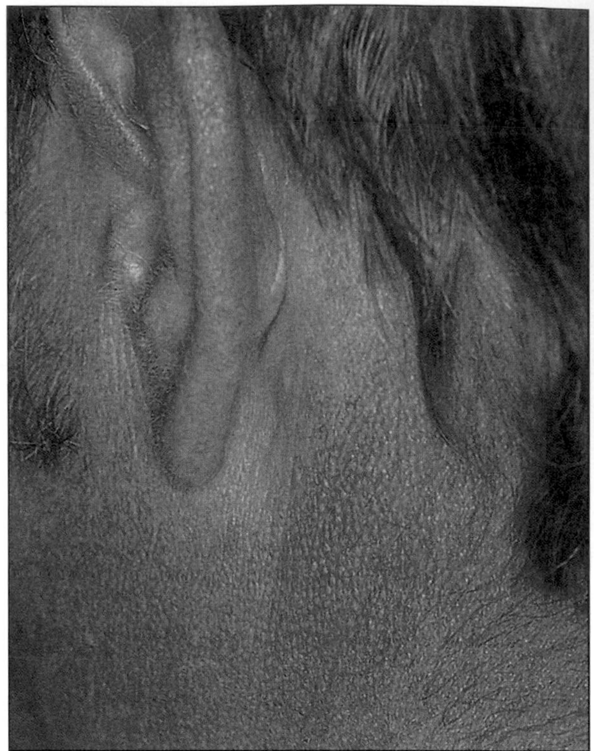

Fig. 22.7. Erythromelanosis interfollicularis colli

Dilated Vessels

Nevus Araneus

Synonym. Spider nevus

Definition. Acquired vascular lesion with small vessels radiating from a central source.

Etiology and Pathogenesis. Spider nevi are not present at birth and are not true nevi. They are usually classified under telangiectases but appear to involve a larger central vessel.

Clinical Findings. Spider nevi are most common on the face of girls and young women. Centrally, one sees a small, pinhead-sized vessel which may pulsate (Fig. 22.8). Radiating out from it are a series of small capillaries, producing the spider image. Occasionally, multiple spider nevi may erupt during pregnancy. They are also more common in patients with chronic liver disease, where they may become quite large and the central vessel may resemble a hemangioma. In addition, patients with connective tissue disease, especially CREST syndrome, may have many spider nevi. In patients with liver dis-

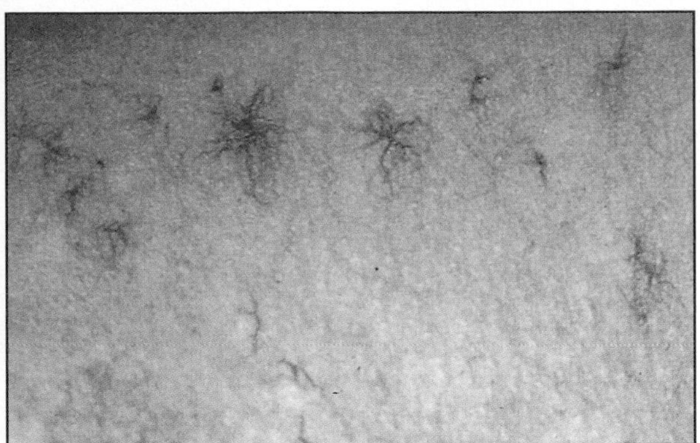

Fig. 22.8. Spider nevi

ease, the trunk is often involved, while those with CREST may have facial, truncal, and especially acral lesions.

Histopathology. If the biopsy is serendipitously sectioned along the right planes, one can see an enlarged central vessel with radiating branches.

Therapy. Either electrocautery with a very fine needle (cat's whisker needle) at a very low setting or a laser can be used. Larger or recurrent lesions can be excised.

Venous Ectasias

Synonyms. Venectasia, phlebectasia

Venous ectasias are easy to separate from telangiectases, as they tend to be blue or violet, have a larger diameter, are often several centimeters long, and have an irregular course. Sometimes they have a starburst pattern around a central, even larger vessel. In German these lesions are known as *Besenreiser* varicosities, referring to the branched twigs formerly used to make brooms. In English, the lesions are called spider, starburst, or sky rocket veins (Fig. 22.9). Similar accumulations of dilated veins may be seen over the rib cage (cougher's crown in German) in patients with chronic pulmonary diseases and along the sides of the feet in early chronic venous insufficiency (corona phlebectatica). Because these vessels are somewhat larger, they can be treated with sclerotherapy, as discussed below, as well as with some lasers.

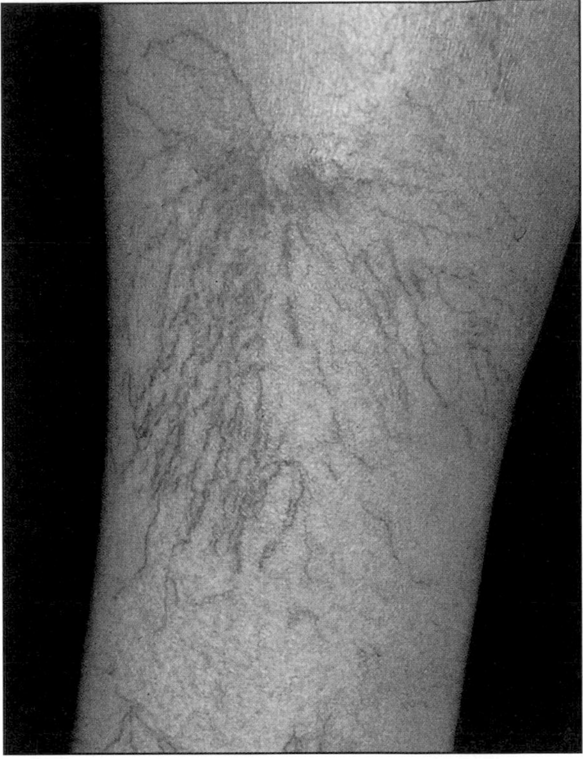

Fig. 22.9. Starburst veins

Functional Angiopathies

Chronic functional disturbances involving the arterioles, capillaries, and venules lead to a variety of clinical pictures, all of which have reduced cold tolerance as a feature. In general, the vascular musculature regulates blood flow away from the skin at inappropriate times. While the changes are a nuisance and can occasionally lead to serious problems, they are in general much less troublesome than disorders in which the vessels are structurally damaged.

Acrocyanosis

Synonym. Acroasphyxia

Definition. Acral cyanosis associated with reduced skin temperature and often hyperhidrosis or boggy swelling.

Epidemiology. Acrocyanosis is a disease primarily of women. The problems usually begin in puberty and generally disappear in the fourth or fifth decade. The problems are worse in cold damp climates or when one must work in such an environment, such as in a butcher shop handling cold meat.

Etiology and Pathogenesis. The exact cause is not known; many factors probably interact. A dysregulation of the peripheral circulation is the problem. In some instances, acrocyanosis appears to be familial, and many patients express emotional instability. More precise neurologic explanations have been suggested such as a defect in the diencephalonic-hypophyseal axis, spinal reflexes, or temperature sensitivity of the vascular smooth muscle. In any event, the oxygen-depleted blood remains in the dilated postcapillary venules while the arterioles show increased muscle tone and reduced flow. Acrocyanosis may also be associated with myeloproliferative disorders. It has been reported in HIV/AIDS patients following amyl and butyl nitrate abuse.

Clinic Findings. The most typical areas of involvement are the hands and feet, but the nose, cheeks, ears, buttocks, lateral inferior aspects of the breasts, arms, and legs may also be affected. The blue-red areas are cold to the touch, while the palms and soles are moist. The hands often evidence a cushion-like, doughy swelling. Some patients complain not only of cold hands but of a numb feeling (acrocyanosis chronica anesthetica). While patients experience increased problems with cold exposure, the problem is present to some extent over longer periods of time, rather than occurring suddenly and then disappearing.

The iris shutter sign is a helpful diagnostic test. When one presses on the bluish skin with a finger, a pale area is produced (Fig. 22.10). It gradually disappears as the circle closes from the periphery moving centrally. In normal skin, the color returns almost simultaneously in all areas from the base. Furthermore, there is a temporary hyperemia, producing a brighter red spot (known in German as the cinnabar spot, because of the red color of this mercury salt). Soon the cyanosis returns.

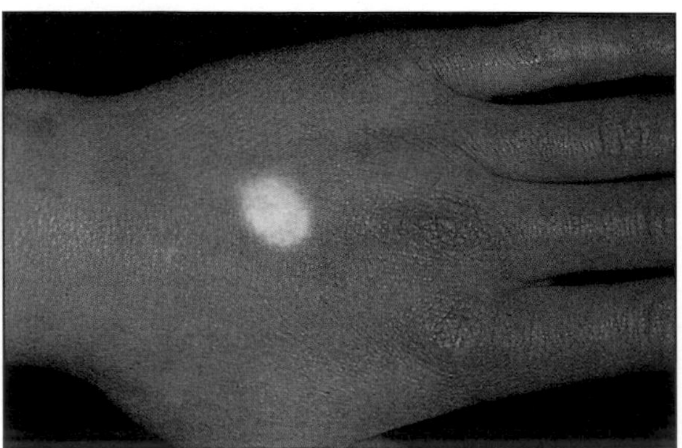

Fig. 22.10. Acrocyanosis with the iris shutter sign

Course and Prognosis. Patients tend to have less trouble with acrocyanosis as they get older. The acrocyanotic skin seems to be a fertile ground for other skin disorders. Probably the best established association is with lupus vulgaris. In addition, pernio and the pernio variants of both lupus erythematosus and sarcoidosis are more common in acral, cold areas. Bacterial infections are slower to heal, and there may be an increased incidence of fungal and candidal infections, as well as of human papilloma virus infections.

Differential Diagnosis. Acrocyanosis may be associated with chronic cardiac and pulmonary disease because of impaired circulation. In some neurologic disorders, there may be abnormal peripheral blood flow. In both cryoglobulinemia and cold agglutinin disease, acrocyanosis may be severe, although it is usually somewhat episodic. In acrodermatitis chronica atrophicans, the skin is atrophic, there is no cold intolerance, and the serologic tests for *Borrelia burgdorferi* are positive. Raynaud syndrome and disease feature more episodic problems with a distinctive clinical cycle of blanching and rewarming.

Therapy. There is no satisfactory therapy. Protection from cold with appropriate clothing and a wise choice of activities are essential. Exercise, massages, and exposure to warmth, as in saunas and baths, may play a beneficial role. A variety of irritating substances such as salicylic acid and nicotinic acid derivatives appear to stimulate peripheral blood flow and can be tried as topical treatments, although their value is often challenged.

Livedo Reticularis

Synonym. Cutis marmorata

Definition. Harmless physiologic condition in which vascular constriction produces white patches in often acrocyanotic skin associated with prominent veins, yielding a marble-like pattern. We will use cutis marmorata and livedo reticularis interchangeably for this disorder, and reserve the term livedo racemosa for the more serious marbled condition associated with vessel wall damage or intravascular obstruction. This is in keeping with European usage and in direct contrast to American terminology, in which livedo reticularis is used for both conditions.

Epidemiology. Up to 50% of young women are affected; the problem is uncommon in men. Most patients also have acrocyanosis.

Etiology and Pathogenesis. The mechanisms are probably the same as in acrocyanosis, but the vessels of the deep dermal plexus are involved, producing the characteristic marbled pattern. The veins are dilated and the arteries constricted. Livedo reticularis is a normal response in infants and in anyone exposed to cold.

Clinical Findings. Often the same individual with acrocyanosis will show a transition to a large net-like pattern of livedo reticularis on the calves or forearms (Fig. 22.11). The same pattern can be seen on the thighs, upper aspects of the arms, buttocks, and trunk. Typically, the pattern shifts over time and disappears following warming or rubbing of the skin. Sometimes macular exanthems are difficult to recognize against the marbled background. There are no symptoms.

Course and Prognosis. Just as with acrocyanosis, livedo reticularis tends to disappear with increasing age.

Differential Diagnosis. The main consideration is livedo racemosa, as discussed below.

Therapy. The same considerations discussed under acrocyanosis apply here. Most patients require no therapy.

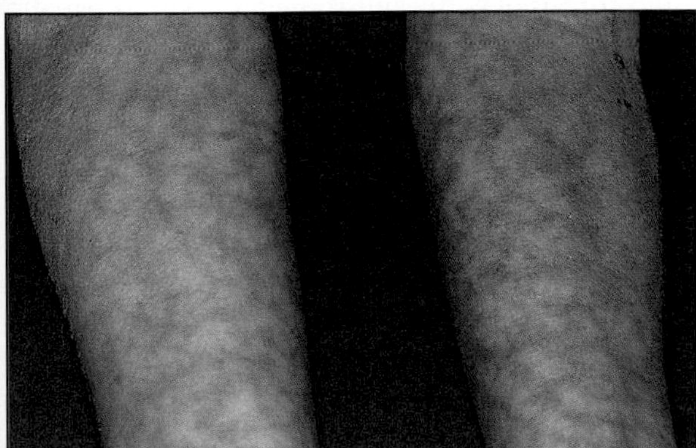

Fig. 22.11. Livedo reticularis

Pseudoleukoderma Angiospasticum

This variant of livedo reticularis presents with a white checkered pattern of the palms, soles, flexural aspects of the forearms, and buttocks. Some people tend to react to emotional stress by developing this pattern, which is also more common in cigarette smokers. Once again, there is central arteriolar spasm with peripheral vasodilation producing pale areas. Diascopy produces uniform blanching, confirming that there is no true hypopigmentation.

Erythrocyanosis Crurum Puellarum

(Klingmüller 1925)

Definition. Variant of acrocyanosis with cyanosis and puffy swelling caused by chronic cold exposure.

Epidemiology. Once again, this variant is more common in young women, especially among chubby young girls. Wearing short skirts or thin stockings may be other predisposing factors.

Etiology and Pathogenesis. The well-developed fatty layer not only protects the deeper structures from cold, but leaves the skin isolated and more susceptible to cold and reduced circulation. Thus, these patients with acrocyanosis have severer changes.

Clinical Findings. Patients have acrocyanosis and often either keratosis pilaris or its variant perniosis follicularis, in which the plugged follicles have a livid border. The erythrocyanosis usually involves the inner aspects of the thighs and can extend down to the calves. There are blue patches admixed with light red areas. The iris shutter effect is positive. When the cyanotic areas are rubbed or pressed, they develop arterial hyperemia, producing dark red blotches, the cinnabar spots. Vessel leakage causes edema and a puffy or doughy skin. Pernio-like nodules may develop. Here the physiologic changes are somewhat more persistent than in ordinary acrocyanosis. Even though some improvement occurs with rewarming, there may be residual changes.

Course and Prognosis. The changes improve over time and also with loss of weight. The same disorders associated with acrocyanosis are more common.

Differential Diagnosis. Pernio and panniculitis should be considered.

Therapy. The same approaches discussed under acrocyanosis are appropriate.

Erythema Ab Igne

Erythema ab igne is a reaction to chronic heat that features both reticulated erythema and hyperpigmentation. It is discussed in more detail in Chapter 26.

Erythromelalgia

(Mitchell 1872; Gerhardt 1892)

Synonyms. Erythralgia, erythermalgia. These three terms describe overlapping diseases. Some clinicians distinguish between erythermalgia or erythralgia as a primary disorder and erythromelalgia as secondary to hematologic diseases.

Definition. Episodic attacks of diffuse erythema of an extremity associated with marked skin warming and pain.

Epidemiology. Most patients with idiopathic or primary erythromelalgia are young or middle-aged adults, usually women. In Norway, the incidence is around 3 per million. Familial cases with onset in childhood are also seen. The pattern in those with the secondary forms follows the distribution of the underlying disease.

Etiology and Pathogenesis. Three rather separate clinical settings can be identified.

- Primary Form (Erythermalgia). Patients with erythermalgia experience problems when exposed to heat, physical activity, or emotional stress. They seem to have a critical temperature, ranging between 32 °C and 37 °C, but usually just below normal body temperature, above which problems occur. Studies have shown that heat is responsible for the pain, not the increased blood flow. The defect seems to be one of vasomotor control.
- Secondary to Hematologic Disease (Erythromelalgia). Any disease with elevated platelet counts, such as idiopathic thrombocythemia or polycythemia vera, can lead to erythromelalgia. Platelet-mediated thrombosis seems to be coupled to stimulation of vascular wall smooth muscle development by platelet-derived growth factor (PDGF).
- Secondary to Vascular or Neurologic Diseases. Vessel wall damage (arteriosclerosis, peripheral occlusive disease, diabetes mellitus, hypertension, pernio) or neurologic disorders can also lead to reduced flow and platelet activation. In addition, medications that interfere with vasomotor control or platelet function can trigger attacks.

Clinical Findings. Patients with idiopathic disease typically have a sudden onset of bilateral erythema, swelling, and warmth in their hands. Often there is also hyperhidrosis and tenderness to touch. The feet, lower aspects of the legs, and occasionally forearms can be involved. Additional exposure to heat causes great pain, while cooling, as with cold water or ice cubes, brings relief. Attacks may last minutes to over an hour. Recurrences are the rule, but often there is a period of days of relative tolerance following an episode. The secondary forms tend to be less symmetric, more often involve the feet, and can progress to peripheral gangrene. There may be associated paresthesias.

Histopathology. While biopsy is very rarely needed, with luck one can separate the primary and secondary forms. In primary erythromelalgia, there are no vessel changes, while in the secondary forms, one may find thrombi in the vessels.

Laboratory Findings. Any patient with erythromelalgia should have a hematologic evaluation.

Course and Prognosis. The outlook for the primary form is one of chronic annoying problems, while in the secondary form, the underlying disease determines the prognosis.

Differential Diagnosis. Raynaud syndrome is often confused with erythromelalgia, but is usually triggered by cold and has a cyclic progression with initial vasospasm. Burning feet syndrome has similar symptoms but different physical findings. Reflex sympathetic dystrophy occurs under different circumstances and is more permanent.

Therapy. The best treatment is cold, e.g., immersion in cold water. Some patients grasp a cold drink or hold ice cubes in their hands. Others keep a cold pack usually used for treating aches and pains in their freezer ready for action. Some patients do well with desensitization, using hand and foot baths with gradually increasing temperatures. This may provide relief for days to a week.

The role of aspirin is confusing. The erythromelalgia associated with thrombocythemia is very responsive to low dosages of aspirin, ranging from 80 to 325 mg daily. Idiopathic erythromelalgia may respond to higher dosages. Serotonin reuptake inhibitors also appear to be useful and may be worth trying in severe or refractory cases.

Burning Feet Syndrome

(Stannus 1912)

Definition. Painful burning of the feet, usually associated with internal or neurologic disorders, or vitamin deficiency.

Etiology and Pathogenesis. A wide variety of disorders causes burning feet syndrome. Many different peripheral neuropathies, including those associated with polyarteritis nodosa, diabetes mellitus, alcoholism, tumors, and space-occupying spinal cord lesions, can be responsible. In addition, vitamin B deficiencies often associated with malabsorption may be a factor. Thalidomide and isoniazid may also be responsible. In recent years, burning feet syndrome has been described in HIV/AIDS patients. The mechanisms are unclear.

Clinical Findings. Painful tingling and burning of the feet most often appear at night, perhaps triggered by the warmth of the bedding. In other individuals, the problem begins during the day, often upon activity. The changes usually start over the first metatarsal head where one may also note hyperhidrosis and muscle spasms. If the patient pulls the covers away or hangs his feet over the end of the bed, relief is obtained. Immersing the feet in cold water also helps.

Differential Diagnosis. Patients who suffer frostbite often have persistent paresthesias of their extremities. This has been shown to be particularly common in soldiers who have experienced frostbite; perhaps compensation issues also play a role here. There are many other neurologic disorders with painful paresthesias of the extremities. A neurologist should be involved in evaluating such cases. Often no cause is found.

Therapy. Treating the underlying disease is most important. Foot baths with increasing temperatures may produce improvement, as may avoidance of warmth such as by wearing light clothing and footwear. The role of aspirin is debated; low dosages are worth trying. While vitamins are often recommended, they are only helpful in those rare cases in which a deficiency is documented.

Restless Legs Syndrome

(Wittmack 1861; Ekbom 1945)

Synonyms. Anxietas tibiarum, Wittmack-Ekbom syndrome

This problem is mentioned primarily because it is often confused with burning feet syndrome. Patients develop pain and paresthesias at night that force them into a relentless, restless movement of their legs. Often lying face down in bed helps. Many alleged triggers have been suggested, including pregnancy, anemia, cold, uremia, hyperinsulinemia, and malabsorption. Vasomotor disturbances have also been suggested, but acrocyanosis or mottling is not seen. In rare instances, familial cases with presumed autosomal dominant inheritance have been described. In other instances, emotional factors clearly play a role. The wide diversity of this list suggests immediately that the syndrome is heterogeneous and poorly understood. There is no satisfactory treatment.

Reflex Sympathetic Dystrophy

(Mitchell 1872)

Synonyms. Sudeck atrophy (Sudeck 1900), causalgia, posttraumatic neuralgia

Definition. Reflex sympathetic dystrophy is a so-called deafferentation syndrome. An extremity becomes painful and even swollen following an injury to its afferent nerve pathway.

Epidemiology. Reflex sympathetic dystrophy is usually a disease of older adults. It occurs in over 10% of patients with myocardial infarctions, where it is usually called the shoulder-hand syndrome. It also develops in 5–10% of patients with nerve injuries to their limbs.

Etiology and Pathogenesis. The mechanisms are poorly understood. Many types of injuries including fractures, surgical procedures, blunt trauma, and even prolonged immobilization have been implicated. The generally accepted theory is that the altered afferent fibers erroneously overstimulate central sympathetic pathways. The result is increased sympathetic tone in the limb.

Clinical Findings. A variety of signs and symptoms may occur. There is usually severe unrelenting pain and increased sensitivity of a limb. Patients may describe hyperpathia (exaggerated pain response) or allodynia (perverted pain response, such as sharp deep pains following tickling). Typically, the patient resists movement of the affected limb, often wears a sling, and avoids examination. Some complain of hyper- or hypohidrosis, others of either very warm or very cold limbs. Often there is a diffuse swelling of the limb; in chronic cases, atrophy may be seen. Vasospastic attacks may occur, mimicking Raynaud syndrome.

Laboratory Findings. The bone may show patchy demineralization, known as Sudeck atrophy. In other patients, there is increased radionuclide uptake in the involved limb.

Course and Prognosis. If the diagnosis is made promptly and therapy instituted, the outlook is good. If the problem is ignored, the patient is usually doomed to years of suffering.

Differential Diagnosis. All the entities considered above must be ruled out. Usually the history of injury or myocardial infarction, the varying sympathetic signs and symptoms, and the guarding of the limb by the patient suggest the diagnosis.

Therapy. Aggressive physical therapy is the most important approach. If improvement is not prompt, chemical, surgical, or pharmacologic sympathetic nerve blockade should be undertaken. Vasodilator drugs may also be helpful, as well as other treatments discussed below for Raynaud syndrome.

Raynaud Syndrome and Raynaud Disease

(RAYNAUD 1862)

Definition. The terminology of Raynaud phenomenon, syndrome, and disease is confusing. We will use the following terms:

- Raynaud phenomenon: Clinically characteristic vasospastic changes involving the hands and feet, usually in a symmetric fashion.
- Raynaud syndrome: Recurrent episodes of Raynaud phenomenon, associated with the diseases shown in Table 22.1.

Table 22.1. Causes of Raynaud syndrome

Types of problem	Examples
Structural changes	Thoracic outlet obstruction (cervical rib syndrome, scalenus anticus syndrome) Carpal tunnel syndrome
Trauma	Following injuries or operations Reflex sympathetic dystrophy Vibratory tools (jackhammer operator) Repetitive tasks (piano player, typist) Hypothenar hammer syndrome (mechanics, butchers using hand as hammer)
Vascular diseases	Arteriosclerosis Thromboangiitis obliterans Polyarteritis nodosa Other forms of vasculitis Emboli, thrombi Arteriovenous fistulas
Connective tissue diseases	Systemic sclerosis Lupus erythematosus Dermatomyositis Rheumatoid arthritis Sjögren syndrome
Neurologic diseases	Peripheral neuropathies Syringomyelia Multiple sclerosis Herniated disc
Hematologic diseases	Cold agglutinins Cold hemolysins Cryoglobulinemia Macroglobulinemia (Waldenström) Paroxysmal hemoglobinuria Polycythemia vera
Intoxication	Ergotismus Heavy metals Cyanide salts in alcohol Some mushroom toxins Vinyl chloride derivatives Trichloroethylene
Medications	Intraarterial injections Bleomycin Methysergide Ergot preparations Clonidine Bromocriptine β-adrenergic blockers
Miscellaneous	Neoplasms Hypothyroidism

- Raynaud disease: If no underlying cause is found for Raynaud syndrome, we diagnose Raynaud disease.

Epidemiology. Raynaud disease is most common among women (5:1) and usually appears in young adult life. Raynaud syndrome follows the distribution of the underlying disorders.

Etiology and Pathogenesis. The exact mechanism is unknown. Abnormalities of the sympathetic innervation, increased cold sensitivity of the vascular smooth muscle, increased blood viscosity, and changes in the hypothalamic temperature control center have all been identified. Probably multiple factors interact.

Clinical Findings. The episodic development of symmetric painful vasospasm involving the peripheral vessels is typical. The sudden ischemia involves one or more fingers, the toes, and even the nose, ears, and tongue (Fig. 22.12). There are three classic phases that distinguish Raynaud syndrome from other types of vasospasm.

- Arterial Spasm. The involved fingers are white and stiff.
- Cyanosis. The fingers become dark blue or violet.
- Arterial Hyperemia. As part of a compensatory mechanism, the arterial blood flow increases, producing bright red fingers.

The frequency and duration of the attacks vary greatly from individual to individual. Usually the hyperemic phase is the most painful, much as frostbite is first painful after thawing and revascularization begins. While many attacks are triggered by cold, on occasion there is no obvious cause. Emotional factors can also trigger attacks. With repeated episodes, more permanent changes develop. The fingers and toe remain somewhat swollen, and because of damage to the distal vessels, thinning and atrophy of the distal parts of the digits appear. Tiny ulcerations may be seen; they are ungraciously described as rat bite necroses and heal with small, pitted scars. The nails may become dystrophic. On radiologic examination, resorption of the distal phalanx can be documented.

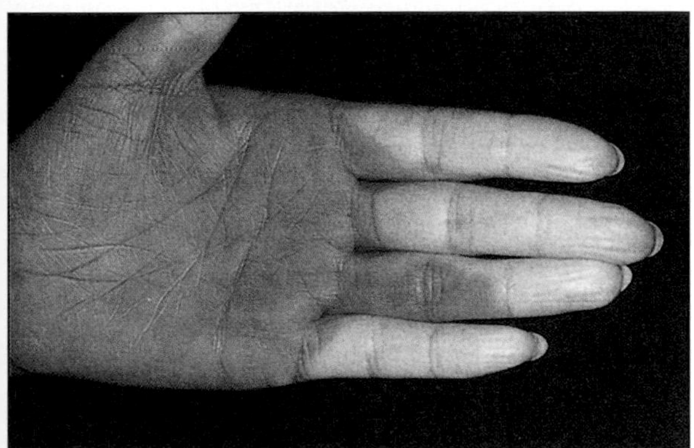

Fig. 22.12. Raynaud phenomenon

Diagnostic Criteria. The clinical features of Raynaud syndrome are so typical that usually a careful history leads to the diagnosis. Often an attack can be provoked by immersing the hands in cold water for 10–15 s. All of the disorders shown in Table 22.1 should be excluded. If organic vascular disease is suspected, angiography is recommended.

Patients with systemic sclerosis, especially its acral form, often present with Raynaud syndrome. In addition, digital atrophy, scarring, and tightening suggest systemic sclerosis. If over a 2-year period the changes are stable, then that diagnosis becomes less likely. Any patient with Raynaud syndrome should undergo repeated serologic evaluation to search for the anti-centromere antibodies typical of CREST syndrome (Chap. 18).

Course and Prognosis. In Raynaud disease, the outlook is good, though the problem remains annoying. Patients may have to avoid cold climates or jobs with cold exposure, but with care, they do well. If they have an associated underlying disease, then they can expect another range of problems.

Differential Diagnosis. The differential diagnosis is limited if careful attention is paid to the three-phase process. Other forms of peripheral vasospasm discussed above lack this pattern.

Therapy. There is no single satisfactory therapy. Avoidance of cold is far and way the most important action to undertake. Moving to a warmer climate is estimated to help 50% of patients. Any underlying problem should be treated as aggressively as possible. Smoking should be avoided because of the peripheral vasoconstrictive action of nicotine. Physical measures such as warm baths, underwater massage, and hand exercises are helpful. Warm oil (called hot paraffin in Europe) hand baths seem to produce more lasting vasodilation.

Windmilling of the arms at the beginning of an attack may help minimize it. Biofeedback techniques have also proven helpful.

Surgical techniques may be useful for thoracic outlet obstruction or carpal tunnel syndrome, as well as in a well-defined reflex sympathetic dystrophy, but routine partial or total sympathectomies are no longer performed because of the disappointing results.

Topical treatments are usually not helpful. Nitroglycerine ointment or paste, designed for treatment of angina, may be helpful, especially in healing ulcerations more rapidly. It has little effect during an acute attack.

Systemic therapy is only used for patients with frequent, severe attacks. There is no agent which works rapidly enough to be taken just when the attacks occur. Nifedipine is probably the most widely used agent, diltiazem is also effective, but verapamil less so. Ketanserin also appears promising.

Digitus Mortuus

Synonyms. Dead finger, corpse finger

This common but rarely reported problem may represent an incomplete form of Raynaud syndrome. Most patients are women who suddenly develop a white painless digit following exposure to cold, usually the ring or middle finger. The problem resolves rapidly and often disappears entirely. A small percentage of the patients go on to develop Raynaud syndrome, often with an underlying cause. Cold avoidance is usually the only therapy needed.

Cutaneous Emboli

While emboli to cerebral and pulmonary vessels are much better known because of their far-reaching consequences, a number of different types of cutaneous emboli create relatively distinctive clinical findings.

Bacterial Emboli

When bacterial colonies grow on heart valves or within the great vessels, clumps can be dislodged and settle in the skin. These deposits are also known as septic metastases. The bacterial masses block vessels, often towards the end of the arterial circulation. As a result, the patients with sepsis develop hemorrhagic, painful, flat-topped nodules. These are most common on the fingertips or tips of the toes, but can also be seen on the nose. When associated with subacute bacterial endocarditis, these lesions are known as Osler nodes (Chap. 2). Microscopically, at first glance one sees a small vessel vasculitis, but Giemsa staining usually allows one to identify clumps of bacteria.

Fat Emboli

Fat emboli develop following a major trauma, such as a fractured femur, when pieces of fat from the bone marrow get into the circulation. This can also happen following trauma to fatty tissue, operations, and even liposuction. Petechial lesions are found, most often in the axillae, but also on the neck and conjunctivae. Patients often have multiple internal emboli, and thus may present with fever, confusion, or cardiorespiratory problems. On biopsy, one can find intra- and extravascular accumulations of fat along with collections of erythrocytes. Electron microscopic studies have shown fatty deposits in tears of the vessel wall. The serum lipase levels are often elevated and the platelet count reduced. Commonly, patients are treated with heparin, dextran and occasionally systemic corticosteroids.

Cholesterol Emboli

Patients who have large, fragile, cholesterol-rich atheromas of the aorta or great vessels can develop emboli. The intestine is most commonly involved but the skin can also be affected. Usually, there is no apparent cause, although anticoagulation, arterial catheterization, and trauma may all be responsible. Small pieces of the atheromatous material lodge in distal vessels, once again most often involving the fingers or toes. Sometimes a pattern of livedo racemosa is produced. Cholesterol crystals can be seen in the vessels; this should always be sought for in skin biopsies for peripheral occlusive disease. There is no specific treatment.

Myxoid Emboli

Atrial myxomas can release fragments of tumor tissue. Smaller pieces can end up in the skin, often producing livedo racemosa changes on the legs along with small nodules. On biopsy, the myxoid material is seen in and around the vessels. Most atrial myxomas are sporadic, but some may be associated with Carney syndrome (Chap. 58).

Emboli from Other Tumors

Rarely, a solid tumor may erode into a vessel, and fragments may be transported to distal sites, so that the metastases present as arterial occlusive disease. In other instances, rare intravascular tumors, such as chemodectomas of the aorta, behave in the same way. There is also an intravascular, large B cell lymphoma (Chap. 61). When such lesions are biopsied, abundant tumor cells are seen in the vessel.

Vasculitis

Cutaneous vasculitis is a common, important disease complex that is subject to a multiplicity of classification schemes. The most recent, widely accepted Chapel Hill classification was published in 1994 and is shown in Table 22.2. Even for small vessel vasculitis, refinements are possible, as cutaneous leukocytoclastic angiitis involves venules, while Henoch-Schönlein purpura may also involve capillaries. Some problems from the dermatologic point of view are immediately obvious. The lesions of Henoch-Schönlein purpura and cutaneous leukocytoclastic angiitis are clinically identical in the skin.

Infections may cause vasculitis by direct involvement of the vessel wall, as in Rocky Mountain spotted fever or gonorrhea, or by inducing immune complexes. Drugs rarely cause vasculitis but when they do, it may involve several immune mechanisms.

Table 22.2. Chapel Hill classification of vasculitis

Large vessel vasculitis
Giant cell arteritis
Takayasu arteritis
Medium-sized vessel vasculitis
Polyarteritis nodosa
Kawasaki disease
Small vessel vasculitis
ANCA-positive
Wegener granulomatosis
Churg-Strauss syndrome
Microscopic polyangiitis
Immune complex
Henoch-Schönlein purpura
Cutaneous leukocytoclastic angiitis

Modified from Jennette et al. 1994

Table 22.3. Vasculitis classified by inflammatory infiltrate

Histologic pattern	Examples
Leukocytoclastic	Henoch-Schönlein purpura Leukocytoclastic angiitis
Lymphocytic	Connective tissue vasculitis Drug-induced vasculitis
Granulomatous	Wegener granulomatosis Churg-Strauss syndrome Microscopic polyangiitis
Giant cell	Giant cell (temporal)arteritis Polymyalgia rheumatica Takayasu arteritis
Not classifiable/ relationship to vasculitis uncertain	Degos syndrome Pyoderma gangrenosum Thromboangiitis obliterans

Many other classifications are equally helpful in understanding the process. In Germany, vasculitis is often identified as primary (no known trigger, initially involving a vessel) and secondary (associated with an underlying disease). Classic examples of each type are Takayasu arteritis and gonococcal vasculitis, respectively. Unfortunately, in many cases there is considerable overlap; for example, cutaneous leukocytoclastic angiitis is idiopathic in about 50% of cases and associated with an underlying disorder in the rest. Table 22.3 lists the various types of vasculitis in the skin based on the nature of the histologic pattern or inflammatory infiltrate. Finally, there is a long list of diseases in which the action is clearly in the cutaneous vessels, such as erythema multiforme, Behçet disease, Sweet syndrome, pityriasis lichenoides et varioliformis acuta, and pernio, which for a variety of reasons are not described as vasculitis.

Etiology and Pathogenesis. Many different disease processes can lead to cutaneous vasculitis. The structure of the terminal arterioles, capillaries, and venules, the hydrostatic pressure and temperature determine which section of the vascular tree and which body regions are involved. In general, the favored site for most cutaneous vasculitis is the legs. The trigger and the pathogenic mechanism determine the nature of the infiltrate, depending on whether lymphocytes, neutrophils, eosinophils, or platelets are primarily activated. The release of inflammatory mediators and enzymes, especially from mast cells, plays a major role in determining the course of the disease. The formation of immune complexes triggered by infections, drugs, tumors or other antigens, as well as the activation of the complement cascade, are also important. The clinical course is dependent on how fast corrective factors can begin working. If the vessel wall is sufficiently damaged, then exocytosis, leukocytoclasia, fibrin deposition, and necrosis may result. In even more chronic processes, a histiocytic or giant cell response may lead to granuloma formation.

Diagnostic Criteria. Approaching the diagnosis of a vasculitis with cutaneous manifestations is like opening Pandora's box. One never knows how many organ systems will need to be explored or how many other specialists called in for help. Nevertheless, the most common cutaneous vasculitis is leukocytoclastic angiitis, which is confined to the skin. The typical lesion is palpable purpura; many other hemorrhagic, purpuric and necrotic changes can be seen. It is essential to biopsy a fresh lesion, and ideally one above the knees, as the lower aspects of the legs often show vessel changes caused by chronic venous insufficiency, which may confuse the histologic picture. In addition, it is usually wise to do an excisional biopsy down to the fat; a punch biopsy may miss the site of activity, especially in livedo vasculitis.

The history should address all the triggers, while the general examination and laboratory investigations are designed to exclude those associated conditions that could reasonably be expected to play a role. In this day of cost containment, one cannot simply order all known tests related to vasculitis, but must rely on the history and clinical presentation to help choose the appropriate tests. A patient with obvious clues indicating internal involvement, such as CNS symptoms, peripheral neuropathy, hematuria, or respiratory symptoms, requires a more detailed investigation.

A reasonable baseline series might include a complete CBC, erythrocyte sedimentation rate, C-reactive protein, platelet count, clotting status, liver enzymes, and renal function parameters. Serum electrophoresis, a search for cryoglobulins, rheumatoid factor, and antinuclear antibodies, and screening complement levels are also needed. Antineutrophil cytoplasmic antibodies (ANCA) are very valuable in assessing necrotizing and granulomatous vasculitis. Cytoplasmic or cANCA are directed against proteinase 3 and are present in 90% of patients with Wegener granulomatosis, but almost never in other individuals. In contrast, perinuclear or pANCA are directed against myeloperoxidase and are less specific; they are seen in Churg-Strauss syndrome and microscopic angiitis.

No matter what schemes one employs, and how much testing one does, there will always be unclear cases of vasculitis. The main efforts of the dermatologist should be directed toward not missing serious, treatable systemic diseases that present with cutaneous vasculitis.

Large Vessel Vasculitis

Giant Cell Arteritis

(Hutchinson 1889; Horton et al. 1932)

Synonyms. Temporal arteritis, cranial arteritis, Horton syndrome

Definition. Granulomatous vasculitis predominately involving vessels of the head and neck.

Epidemiology. Giant cell arteritis is a disease of the elderly. The peak incidence occurs at 70 years of age. Women are slightly more often involved than men. The prevalence has been estimated at about 0.5%.

Etiology and Pathogenesis. It is unclear why selected vessels are so preferentially involved and why the elderly are at such risk. A cellular immune reaction against the internal elastic lamina or smooth muscle cells has been postulated but not substantiated. Giant cell arteritis is related to polymyalgia rheumatica, as discussed below.

Clinical Findings. The cranial arteries are most often involved. After a brief prodrome, patients typically complain of headache or visual disturbances. The headaches may be unilateral or bilateral, but usually occur over the temple. The temporal artery is swollen, tender, and often covered by erythematous swollen skin (Fig. 22.13). As the disease progresses, the temporal pulse may be reduced or absent. Purpura, blisters, and necrosis, as well as hair loss, may occur in this region. Not all patients will have temporal artery involvement. The second most common site is the occipital arteries. Another interesting feature is claudication upon chewing because of involvement of the ar-

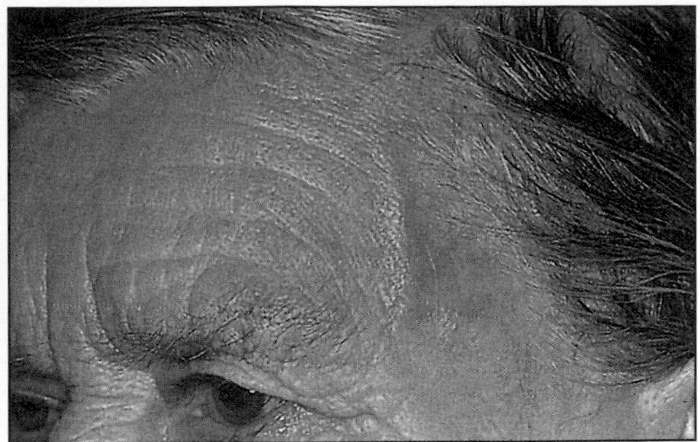

Fig. 22.13. Temporal arteritis

teries to the masseter muscles, or even tongue claudication.

Over half the patients have ocular symptoms. Transitory visual problems, known as amaurosis fugax, appear first because of inadequate vascular supply to the optic nerve. Later, ptosis, diplopia, and blindness may develop. About 40% of patients suffer visual loss, and in this group three-quarters have bilateral problems. Other vessels that may be involved include the coronary arteries and the aortic arch.

Histopathology. Biopsy of an involved temporal artery shows a neutrophilic infiltrate of the vessel wall with intimal proliferation, fragmentation of the internal elastic lamina, and, later, a lymphohistiocytic infiltrate with numerous giant cells and fibrosis. Because the histologic changes are segmental, with normal areas intervening, a generous segment of artery must be obtained and carefully sectioned. Doppler ultrasonography or angiography may help select the appropriate site for a biopsy.

Laboratory Findings. The erythrocyte sedimentation rate is usually strikingly elevated, often to greater than 100 mm/h. Values above 40 mm are suspicious. Acute phase proteins are raised, and there may be leukocytosis. Muscle enzymes are negative, as is electromyography. On rare occasions, pANCA is positive.

Course and Prognosis. The main risk is blindness. Otherwise the disease tends to run an episodic course and resolves completely in 4–24 months.

Differential Diagnosis. The differential diagnostic considerations of headache in the elderly are numerous, but if the temporal artery is tender, and visual complaints or other signs of polymyalgia rheumatica are present, the diagnosis should be suggested.

Therapy. The key is prompt institution of systemic corticosteroids, which can prevent blindness. Usually 60–80 mg of prednisone daily, or occasionally even higher levels, often in divided doses at first, is required. Once remission is obtained, the dosage can be reduced to 7.5–20 mg daily, but the therapy should continue for at least 1 year. Others recommend longer periods, as recurrences may be seen when the medication is discontinued. The erythrocyte sedimentation rate may be useful to monitor the disease course.

Polymyalgia Rheumatica

There are few cutaneous manifestations of polymyalgia rheumatica. It is closely related to giant cell arteritis, but occurs in a younger age group and favors women by a 2:1 ratio. It is about as common as rheumatoid arthritis. Patients present with severe pain and weakness in the proximal muscle groups without arthritis. About 25% also have giant cell arteritis. Morning stiffness is a common problem, and there may be associated anemia, fever, and malaise. Rheumatoid arthritis can be excluded by the lack of distal involvement and the negative rheumatoid factor, while polymyositis can be excluded because of the negative results for muscle enzymes, muscle biopsy, and electromyography. In some instances, even without temporal artery symptoms, a biopsy of the artery may show giant cell changes and confirm the diagnosis. Once again, corticosteroids are the answer, but lower dosages, such as prednisone 30–40 mg daily suffice if there are no ocular or cranial findings. The dose can be tapered to 5–10 mg daily, but this therapy may be required for many years.

Takayasu Arteritis

(Adams 1827; Takayasu 1908)

Synonyms. Pulseless disease, young Oriental female disease

Definition. Arteritis of the aorta and its main branches.

Epidemiology. This unusual form of giant cell arteritis is most common in the Orient and primarily affects young women between 15 and 30 years of age.

Etiology and Pathogenesis. The cause is unknown. A variety of experimental approaches suggest an autoimmune basis. Both antinuclear antibodies and clinical lupus erythematosus have been seen in association with Takayasu arteritis.

Clinical Findings. The most typical findings arise from the obliteration of the brachiocephalic, carotid and subclavian arteries, producing the pulseless state suggested by the name. Patients usually present with fever, malaise, and weight loss. Occasionally, there is an iritis. Cerebrovascular insufficiency and claudication of the arms are the main results of the obliteration. Fainting while turning the head is a typical sign, and the same sort of visual problems seen in giant cell arteritis may occur. Takayasu described perimacular arteriovenous fistulas. In addition, aneurysms may form and more peripheral thrombi may develop. Many patients have hypertension.

Cutaneous findings are limited. Occasionally, ulcerations and necrosis of regions of the face and scalp may develop, but this is surprisingly rare considering the degree of occlusion. Raynaud syndrome is relatively common. Erythema nodosum-like lesions may be seen; it is unclear whether these reflect peripheral arteritis or are a manifestation of tuberculosis, which is often seen in these patients. Digital papules may develop with a granulomatous histology but no clear vasculitis.

Histopathology. Biopsy of a vessel shows far more intense intimal proliferation and damage than seen in giant cell arteritis. Later, patchy destruction of the media with mixed infiltrates, fibrosis, and occasional giant cells may also be seen, predisposing to aneurysm formation and thrombi.

Laboratory Findings. The erythrocyte sedimentation rate is elevated but not as high as in giant cell arteritis. Once again, the acute phase proteins and the neutrophil count are also increased. ANCA is almost always negative; occasionally, ANA may be positive.

Course and Prognosis. The outlook is poor. About 25% of patients die in the first 2 years, and the average survival is about 5 years.

Differential Diagnosis. There are many other diseases that can present with occluded branches of the aorta. The most common one is severe arteriosclerosis, while in younger patients, congenital abnormalities may be responsible. With the proper demographic features, one should always consider Takayasu arteritis.

Therapy. Corticosteroids are the mainstay of therapy. Usually, dosages in the range of 30 mg of prednisone daily are recommended. Controlling the blood pressure and blocking platelet aggregation are also essential.

Medium-Sized Vessel Vasculitis

Polyarteritis Nodosa

(Rokitansky 1852; Kussmaul and Maier 1866)

Synonyms. Periarteritis nodosa, panarteritis nodosa, Kussmaul-Maier syndrome

Definition. Necrotizing vasculitis of medium-sized or small arteries, especially at bifurcations.

Epidemiology. Polyarteritis nodosa is more common in men (3:1) than women and usually involves middle-aged adults. The prevalence in western populations has been estimated at 5:100,000.

Etiology and Pathogenesis. In most cases no cause is identified. Hepatitis B and C virus antigenemias seem to be major triggers in some populations. Other possible causes include streptococcal antigens, serum sickness, cryoglobulinemia, other autoimmune diseases, amphetamine abuse, and rarely other drugs or toxins. In recent years, HIV/AIDS has become a common cofactor in polyarteritis nodosa. While familial Mediterranean fever is rare, patients with this disease are also likely to develop polyarteritis nodosa.

Clinical Findings

Systemic Findings. There is often a long prodromal period with fever, malaise, weight loss, arthralgias, and other nonspecific complaints. The type and localization of inflamed arteries determine the rest of the problems. The kidneys are involved in over 70% of patients. There is usually a necrotizing glomerulitis or damage to the renal arteries, producing parenchymal damage and eventually uremia. The peripheral nervous system is involved in 50%

of cases; the central, in 25%. Cerebrovascular damage can lead to strokes, paralysis, or blindness, while peripheral neuropathies are common. Abdominal vessel damage may present with a wide variety of acute abdominal signs secondary to infarction. Cardiac disease is uncommon but usually manifests as coronary artery damage or conduction defects.

Cutaneous Findings. About one-third of patients has involvement of cutaneous vessels, but the clinical findings are highly variable. Most commonly, livedo racemosa-like changes, often with ulcerations, are seen (Fig. 22.14). This is the usual presentation in HIV/AIDS patients. Urticaria-like nodules may develop, but are longer lived than urticaria because of the vessel damage. Small aneurysms and nodular scarring may produce palpable changes along subcutaneous or muscular arteries. Panniculitis and purpura or ecchymoses may also be seen.

Histopathology. Often a skin biopsy can help in the diagnosis, if a nodular lesion is adequately sampled. There is inflammation of the arteries of the deep dermal plexus, initially with fibrinoid necrosis, and then later with dense neutrophilic and eosinophilic infiltrates and thrombosis. In the late stages, both granulation tissue and fibrosis may be seen.

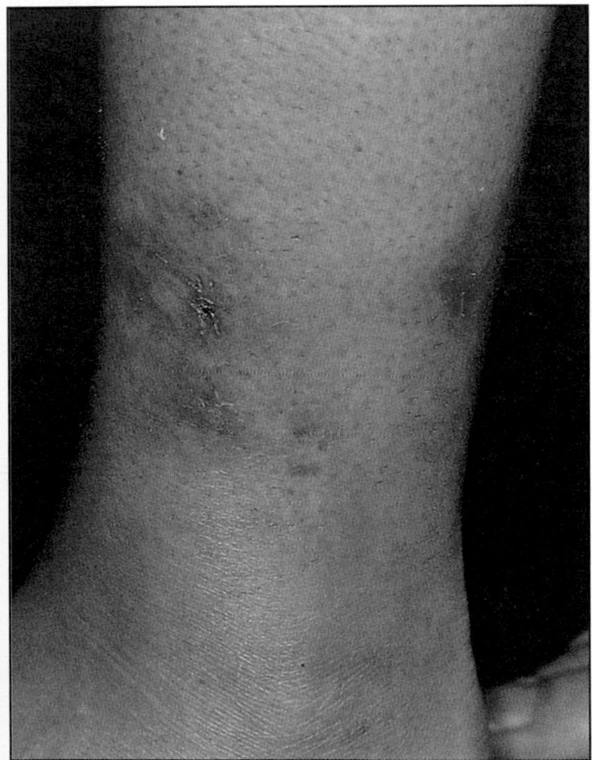

Fig. 22.14. Polyarteritis nodosa

Laboratory Findings. The diagnosis is primarily based on histologic evidence of vasculitis. Imaging studies may help to find involved vessels for use in directing the biopsy. Abdominal or renal angiography may reveal typical changes at vessel bifurcations. Muscle biopsies may also be useful if no obvious site for a histologic study suggests itself. The erythrocyte sedimentation rate is usually elevated, and both leukocytosis and eosinophilia are often present. ANCA is usually negative.

Course and Prognosis. The outlook depends on the pattern of organ involvement. On average, 60% of patients survive 5 years with modern treatment. Two decades ago, the 5-year survival rate was under 20%. Cutaneous involvement is said to be a marker of a better prognosis.

Differential Diagnosis. The list is endless, depending on which organ is involved.

Therapy. Most patients are treated initially with prednisone 1 mg/kg daily. If this fails to arrest the disease, the Fauci regimen is employed: prednisone 1 mg/kg daily combined with cyclophosphamide 1–2 mg/kg daily. The cyclophosphamide is given as a single morning dose. Adequate hydration, monitoring of urine output, and cystitis prophylaxis with mesna are all important. In addition, neutrophil count and renal function should be monitored and contraception practiced. As improvement is seen, the prednisone dose should first be reduced. When a remission is obtained, usually after 3–6 months, the therapy can be switched to a monthly bolus with cyclophosphamide (15–20 mg every 3–4 weeks). Both azathioprine and methotrexate have also been used to sustain remissions. In patients with chronic hepatitis B and C infections, interferon-α (and perhaps ribavirin) can also be considered.

Cutaneous Polyarteritis Nodosa

(Lindberg 1931; Fisher and Orkin 1964)

Synonyms. Polyarteritis nodosa cutanea

Clinical Findings. This entity is disputed. There is no question that some patients have polyarteritis nodosa limited to their skin and do better; the argument concerns whether they have a different disease or just have polyarteritis nodosa with a favorable pattern of involvement. Again, livedo racemosa-like changes on the legs are the most typical finding. Nodose lesions, ulcerations, and extreme tenderness of the arch of the foot are also seen. The cutaneous disease continues along for years but is not threatening to the patient, who should be evaluated periodically for signs of systemic involvement.

Therapy. Topical corticosteroids can be tried, but most patients, at least on occasion, require the systemic version. The Fauci regimen is not recommended if the disease is limited to the skin. We have used azathioprine successfully in patients with therapy-resistant ulcers.

Kawasaki Disease

(Kawasaki et al. 1967)

Synonyms. Mucocutaneous lymph node syndrome (MLNS), acute febrile mucocutaneous lymph node syndrome

Definition. Acute febrile disorder of unknown etiology with characteristic mucocutaneous lesions and medium-sized vessel vasculitis, especially involving the coronary arteries.

Epidemiology. Kawasaki disease has been known for many years in Japan, where over 30,000 cases have been registered. It was initially described in the USA, in Hawaii, but is seen in all parts of the world, although not as commonly as in Japan. Most patients are under 5 years of age, and half the cases involve infants less than 3 years old.

Etiology and Pathogenesis. The etiology of Kawasaki disease remains a mystery. The sudden onset and fever point towards an infection, but the agent has not been identified. The most likely suspects are staphylococcal or streptococcal toxins (Chap. 4). In any event, there is an intense immunologic reaction with vasculitis, circulating immune complexes, and other aberrations. Some epidemics have been associated with carpet cleaning, leading to the suggesting that a toxic reaction to a cleaning chemical or an allergic reaction to the housedust mite might be the trigger.

Clinical Findings. Kawasaki disease can be viewed as triphasic. In the initial or febrile phase, the patient has a high fever, associated with conjunctival injection, dry red lips, stomatitis, a variety of cutaneous findings, and lymphadenopathy. This period lasts until about day 12 of the disease. During the subacute phase, lasting until day 30, the patient is at greatest risk of death from coronary thrombosis and may develop arthritis and arthralgias. The fever and skin findings resolve. In the final or convalescent phase, which lasts weeks to months, the patient gradually recovers, although a small number may die in this stage, also from cardiac disease.

Cutaneous Findings. Over 90 % of patients develop a widespread rash, usually on day 3–5 of their illness. Typically, the first sign is reddening of the palms and soles; the rash then spreads to involve the trunk and extremities over a period of days. Individual lesions are usually red macules that may coalesce. In many instances, the rash is pruritic. It may remain maculopapular or evolve into urticarial plaques, scarlatiniform macules with prominent flexural involvement, or truncal target lesions clinically identical to erythema multiforme. The most common pattern is symmetric urticarial lesions, while the most distinctive change is the desquamative scarlatiniform perianal rash. Blister formation and crusts are not seen. The lesions are not purpuric but blanch with pressure.

The palms and soles are almost invariably reddened, and most patients have firm edema of the extremities. The skin appears stretched over the dorsal hands and feet, and the digits swollen. After 2–3 weeks, the classic acral desquamation occurs, as large sheets of skin are shed, usually beginning just beneath the tips of the nails. Almost all patients develop Beau's lines or horizontal nail furrows, reflecting nail matrix damage.

The most typical oral finding is lip changes, which may including erythema, cracking, and crusting. Almost as common is the strawberry tongue, produced by erythema and mild desquamation, making the papillae prominent.

Systemic Findings. Kawasaki disease has a broad pattern of internal involvement but the most important changes involve the heart.

- Coronary Artery Disease. About 20 % of patients have clinical cardiac disease, although much higher percentages have ECG or coronary angiography abnormalities. Towards the end of the acute phase, serious cardiac problems become apparent, including rhythm disturbances, heart failure, valvular disease, and sudden death from coronary artery occlusion and related damage.

- Ocular Disease. The conjunctival vessels are simply dilated, producing injection without inflammation or true conjunctivitis. Ocular damage does not occur. The changes persist for several weeks.
- Lymphadenopathy. Despite Kawasaki's original emphasis, this is a relatively nonspecific finding. About half the patients have cervical lymphadenopathy, often unilateral and involving a single node.
- Arthritis. Many patients complain of joint pain but about a quarter will have swellings and effusions of large joints. The problem is self-limited.
- CNS. About 25 % of patients have aseptic meningitis, while almost all show lethargy, irritability, or other neurologic signs.
- Other Organs. Gastrointestinal problems include diarrhea, hepatitis, and abdominal pain. Pyuria is common, but renal disease rare. Apparently, urethral inflammation is responsible.

Histopathology. The skin lesions lack a characteristic microscopic picture. There is a lymphocytic perivascular infiltrate associated with dilated vessels. Occasionally, one is able to identify a small artery with true vasculitis, but this characteristic histologic feature is far more often found in autopsy studies of the coronary vessels.

Laboratory Findings. The most significant finding is thrombocytosis, which appears to correlate with the highest risk of coronary disease. Values during the second phase may exceed 1.0 – 1.5 million/mm^3. The neutrophil count is also elevated, and many other nonspecific signs of inflammation may be found. The erythrocyte sedimentation rate is useful in following the disease course.

Course and Prognosis. The rate of death is less than 1 % in Japan, involving primarily male infants and occurring during the first month of the disease. Later, cardiac problems do occur, including second infarctions.

Diagnostic Criteria. Table 22.4 shows the diagnostic criteria. When coronary ultrasound or coronary angiography shows coronary vessel disease in a young infant with a febrile mucocutaneous illness, then the other criteria are usually relaxed.

Table 22.4. Diagnostic criteria for Kawasaki disease

Fever for at least 5 days
Four of the following five changes:
Edema of the hands and feet followed by desquamation
Exanthem
Conjunctival injection
Oral changes (cracked lips, strawberry tongue)
Cervical lymphadenopathy

Differential Diagnosis. The differential diagnosis is extensive, involving many febrile illnesses. However, the criteria generally allow a definitive diagnosis. The skin findings alone are rarely diagnostic; the perianal desquamation appears most specific, along with the digital desquamation. Infantile periarteritis nodosa is probably a variant or close relative of Kawasaki disease; it has a higher mortality rate and lacks the mucocutaneous findings but also selectively involves the coronary vessels.

One serious differential diagnostic problem is distinguishing early Kawasaki disease from Rocky Mountain spotted fever, which may also present with palmar erythema and high fever. Fortunately, the two diseases have different endemic areas; when any doubt exists, specific immunofluorescent tests for *Rickettsia* can be performed and the patient treated with the presumptive diagnosis of Rocky Mountain spotted fever.

Therapy. The therapy of Kawasaki disease is out of the hands of the dermatologist. The skin findings can be treated symptomatically but this is not where the problem lies. All patients should be treated with intravenous γ-globulin and aspirin. While the risk of Reye syndrome as a complication of aspirin therapy is real, the risk of coronary artery disease is greater. If the patient develops varicella or influenza during the convalescent phase, aspirin should be stopped.

ANCA-Positive Small Vessel Vasculitis

While there are many overlaps between Wegener granulomatosis, Churg-Strauss syndrome and microscopic polyangiitis, it is usually possible to separate them using both clinical and laboratory criteria. While all three may show involvement of arteries, in most instances the action centers around arterioles, capillaries, and venules.

Initially, microscopic polyangiitis was considered a variant of polyarteritis nodosa involving smaller vessels, but today clinical features and ANCA results strongly place it with its granulomatous cousins, Wegener granulomatosis and Churg-Strauss syndrome.

Wegener Granulomatosis

(KLINGER 1932; WEGENER 1936)

Definition. Granulomatous necrotizing vasculitis with preferential involvement of the upper airways, lungs, kidneys, and skin.

Epidemiology. Wegener granulomatosis is primarily a disease of middle-aged men. It is relatively uncommon.

Etiology and Pathogenesis. The etiology is unknown. While the presence of cANCA is quite specific, their role in the pathogenesis remains to be shown. It has been speculated that an infectious agent triggers the immune response against proteinase 3, but how this translates into the clinical features is unclear.

Clinical Findings

Systemic Findings. The course of Wegener granulomatosis is usually biphasic. The early phase generally features localized inflammation of the sinuses or upper airway and is often misdiagnosed. Over two-thirds of patients have sinusitis or pulmonary infiltrates at presentation. Later, the patient has all the features of systemic vasculitis with fever, malaise, weight loss, and multiorgan disease. Sometimes the acronym ELK disease is used, to suggest the frequent involvement of the *e*ars, nose, and throat-*l*ungs-*k*idneys. There may be sinus pain and a purulent hemorrhagic rhinitis that is treated with antibiotics until a biopsy shows vasculitis and granuloma formation. There may be destruction of the nasal bones causing a saddle nose or ulcerative defect, as well as pulmonary damage with hemoptysis, and necrotizing glomerulonephritis leading to renal failure. Ocular involvement is also common, with conjunctivitis, episcleritis, and dacrocystitis. Arthritis, peripheral neuropathies, and rarely CNS disease with cerebellar and cranial nerve damage can also occur.

Cutaneous Findings. About half the patients have cutaneous findings, but they are often not specific. Urticarial and maculopapular exanthems are most common; they may ulcerate (Fig. 22.15). Other findings including purpura, subcutaneous nodules, and panniculitis. Oral mucosal ulcerations, especially of the hard palate (Fig. 22.16), and friable gingival hyperplasia are other features.

Histopathology. Cutaneous biopsies rarely show granulomatous vasculitis. Often there is only a necrotizing vasculitis with neutrophils. Similarly, in

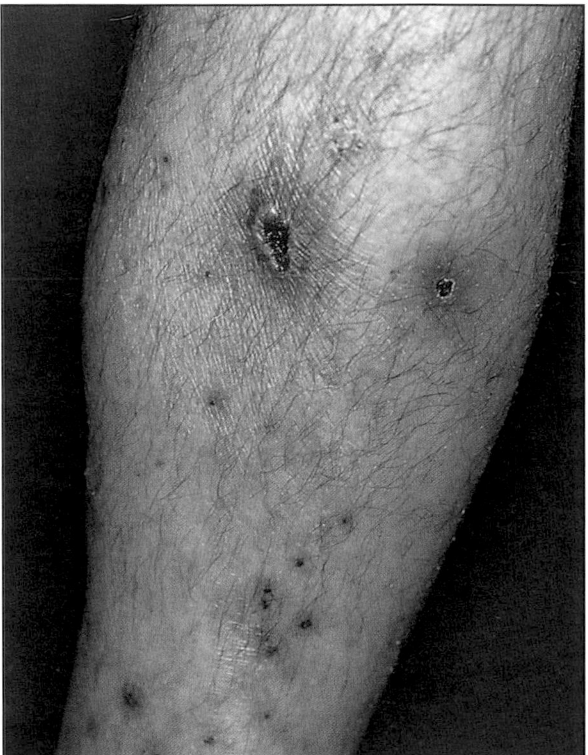

Fig. 22.15. Wegener granulomatosis; cutaneous ulcerations

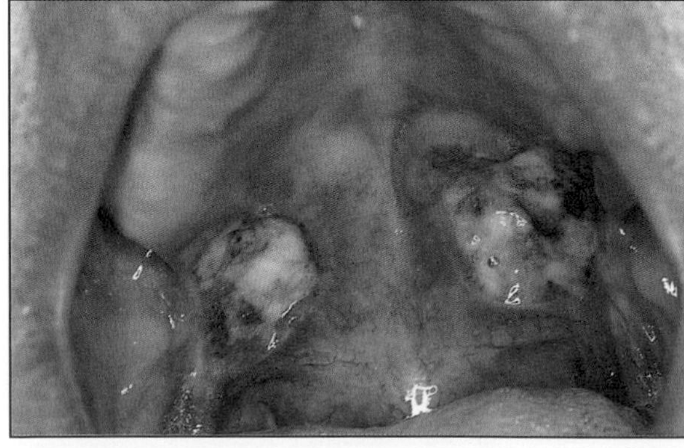

Fig. 22.16. Wegener granulomatosis; destructive oral ulcerations

the kidney, granulomatous changes are uncommon. Biopsies from the lungs and upper airways are more likely to provide evidence of diagnostic granulomatous vascular changes. Direct immunofluorescent examination is negative.

Laboratory Findings. The expected changes in acute phase proteins and erythrocyte sedimentation rate are found in the acute stage, along with thrombocytosis and leukocytosis. The most important test is for cANCA, which is not only specific (>95%) but also sensitive (50–80%, depending on stage of the disease). In addition, the cANCA titers can be used to monitor the disease status.

Course and Prognosis. Prior to the use of cytostatic drugs, about 90% of patents with multisystemic disease died within 2 years. Today about 90% survive. Patients with more limited disease do much better. Massive pulmonary damage and renal failure are the main causes of death.

Differential Diagnosis. The other necrotizing vasculitides can have overlapping features. Polyarteritis nodosa rarely has pulmonary and upper airway changes. A wide variety of pulmonary diseases, including tuberculosis, sarcoidosis and systemic mycoses, should be considered. Upper airway destruction may suggest syphilis or malignant lymphoma. Lymphomatoid granulomatosis occupies a position between Wegener granulomatosis and malignant lymphoma, although most classify it today with the latter. Severe skin ulcerations may suggest pyoderma gangrenosum.

Therapy. Once again, the Fauci regimen discussed under polyarteritis nodosa is usually employed with the same precautions. In contrast to polyarteritis nodosa, cyclophosphamide is more effective and can be used as a monotherapy. Pulse therapy with cyclophosphamide is another possibility. In all cases, the dose should be calibrated against the total leukocyte count. In early cases, especially those with relatively mild organ damage, trimethoprim-sulfamethoxazole may be helpful. This antimicrobial agent is also useful in preventing relapses. Cyclosporine, intravenous immunoglobulins, and methotrexate all are promising but await further confirmation.

Churg-Strauss Syndrome

(Churg and Strauss 1951)

Synonyms. Churg-Strauss granulomatosis, allergic granulomatosis, allergic angiitis and granulomatosis

Definition. Granulomatous necrotizing vasculitis primarily involving the respiratory tract and associated with asthma and eosinophilia.

Epidemiology. Churg-Strauss syndrome is more common in women and usually starts during middle age.

Etiology and Pathogenesis. The cause of this extremely rare disorder has not been elucidated. Recently, several cases have been associated with the use of zafirlukast, a leukotriene receptor antagonist. Because zafirlukast is used almost exclusively in patients with preexisting pulmonary disease, this relationship remains unclear but nonetheless a tantalizing clue.

Clinical Findings. Patients usually present with asthma or rhinitis. They may develop fulminant pulmonary disease with eosinophilic infiltrates that also may involve the gastrointestinal tract. Later the patients enter the vasculitis phase; the two major tract organs are the heart (coronary arteries and myocardium) and nervous system; renal disease is less common and milder. The most specific skin finding is painful nodules often on the scalp or distal extremities and typically symmetric. Purpuric papules and ulcerations are also common, as a reflection of vasculitis. About 40% of patients have cutaneous involvement; less than 10% present with skin findings.

Histopathology. The nodules demonstrate what are now called Churg-Strauss granulomas (Chap. 50): palisading granulomas with central basophilic necrosis, giant cells, neutrophils, and eosinophils. Leukocytoclasia is usually present. The purpuric lesions are more likely to reveal necrotizing vasculitis with eosinophils but without the granulomatous reaction.

Laboratory Findings. The eosinophilia is usually striking and may be associated with increased IgE levels. Eosinophilia may also be seen in the bronchial lavage. The erythrocyte sedimentation rate and acute phase proteins are elevated. pANCA is positive in about 70% of cases.

Course and Prognosis. Cardiac disease accounts for about 50% of the mortality, with pulmonary damage being the second major factor. Most patients do well with therapy.

Differential Diagnosis. Most often the differential diagnosis initially centers around asthma and other respiratory problems. Later, Churg-Strauss syndrome must be separated from other forms of necrotizing vasculitis.

Therapy. Most patients respond well to prednisone 60 mg daily with tapering as clinical improvement appears. Both daily and pulse cyclophosphamide treatment can be employed for refractory cases.

Microscopic Polyangiitis

(Zeek et al. 1948; Davson et al. 1948)

Synonyms. Microscopic polyarteritis, hypersensitivity angiitis

Definition. Necrotizing vasculitis with few or no immune deposits affecting small vessels.

Etiology and Pathogenesis. Microscopic polyangiitis is considered part of the spectrum of polyarteritis nodosa by some. Strictly by definition, it refers to those cases of small vessel disease involving the arterioles, capillaries, and venules. Some patients may have involvement of arteries such as in muscle or peripheral nerves, but many do not. The reverse is not true; a patient with polyarteritis nodosa cannot have involvement of the small vessels. Hepatitis B and C viruses do not play a role in microscopic polyangiitis.

Clinical Findings. Microscopic polyangiitis affects the kidneys in 90% of cases; musculoskeletal, gastrointestinal, and pulmonary involvement are also found in more than half of patients. The most dangerous problem is alveolar capillaritis with hemorrhage, which can be rapidly fatal. About 40% of patients have cutaneous findings, either purpura, urticaria-like nodules, or ulcerations, but dermatologists seldom think of this diagnosis.

Histopathology. Biopsy reveals fibrin necrosis of small vessels without granulomatous change. Direct immunofluorescent examination does not reveal a typical pattern, although rarely, small amounts of immune reactants may be identified.

Laboratory Findings. The most helpful test is for pANCA, which is positive in around 80% of patients. Standard signs of inflammation such as erythrocyte sedimentation rate, acute phase reactants, and leukocyte count are also elevated. A renal biopsy is usually undertaken and shows glomerulonephritis.

Course and Prognosis. The outlook is generally good with aggressive systemic therapy; in the past, most patients died of renal or pulmonary disease.

Differential Diagnosis. The differential diagnosis shows the frustrations of dealing with vasculitis. A patient with purpura, abdominal pain, and nephritis may have microscopic polyangiitis with a grave outlook or Henoch-Schönlein purpura with a good outlook. Exact classification of the level and type of vessel damage as well as immunofluorescent studies are required to provide a diagnosis.

Therapy. The same therapeutic approach discussed under Wegener granulomatosis is appropriate here. Thus, it is not crucial to distinguish with final certainty between these two possibilities before starting therapy for life-threatening renal or pulmonary disease. The Fauci regimen induces remission of the glomerulonephritis in about 80% of patients and is equally effective in relapses.

Lymphomatoid Granulomatosis

(Liebow et al. 1972)

Initially, patients were described with granulomatous vasculitis of the lungs, kidney, CNS, and skin. The cutaneous lesions were ulcerated plaques or nodules. The infiltrates were unusual because they showed cytologic atypia. Today it is clear that most if not all of these cases are angiocentric lymphomas (Chap. 61).

Immune Complex Vasculitis

Leukocytoclastic Angiitis

(Gougerot 1932; Ruiter and Brandsma 1948)

Synonyms. Vasculitis allergica, leukocytoclastic vasculitis, cutaneous necrotizing venulitis, hypersensitivity angiitis, anaphylactoid purpura, immune complex vasculitis, Henoch-Schönlein purpura (as a special variant)

Definition. Symmetric purpuric exanthem caused by immune complex vasculitis of the cutaneous capillaries and venules.

The Chapel Hill classification uses the terms cutaneous leukocytoclastic angiitis and Henoch-Schönlein purpura as two separate categories. We view Henoch-Schönlein purpura as a form of leukocytoclastic angiitis. Although the term leukocytoclastic angiitis may seem foreign to dermatologists, it is preferred to leukocytoclastic vasculitis because of the involvement of the capillaries and venules, not the arteries.

Epidemiology. Leukocytoclastic angiitis is relatively common. There are no age or sex predilections.

Etiology and Pathogenesis. The key event is the deposition of immune complexes in the walls of the capillaries and venules (Fig. 22.17). This event can be documented by immunofluorescent or electron microscopic studies. The deposits are primarily subendothelial. They represent the beginning of a complex chain reaction involving complement activation, leukocyte chemotaxis, release of cytokines and lysosomal enzymes, and vessel wall destruction. The final results are exocytosis of erythrocytes and necrosis. Mast cell activation is important, as often the injection of histamine can produce a similar lesion. Despite the name leukocytoclastic, lymphocytes also play a major role. They are especially prominent in vasculitis associated with autoimmune diseases and in drug-induced forms (Chap. 10). In most cases, the process is a type III reaction of Gell and Coombs, closely related to the Arthus reaction or serum sickness. Table 22.5 shows some of the antigens that have been implicated in leukocytoclastic angiitis.

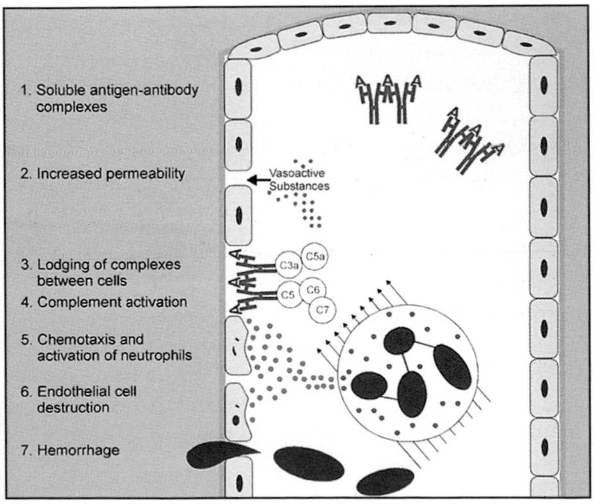

Fig. 22.17. Pathogenesis of leukocytoclastic angiitis

Clinical Findings. The cutaneous features of leukocytoclastic angiitis are highly variable and may change rapidly. Almost all eruptions are symmetric, and the legs are most heavily involved. There is often swelling and pain. Hemorrhage is always present, although it may vary depending on the vessel's location and size. Diascopy fails to blanch the lesions. The Rumpel-Leede test is often positive.

Table 22.5. Typical triggers of cutaneous vasculitis

Type of trigger	Examples
Infections	
Viral	Hepatitis B Hepatitis C Herpes simplex Dengue Cytomegalovirus Coxsackie
Bacterial	Streptococci *Treponema pallidum* *Borrelia burgdorferi* *Mycobacterium tuberculosis* *Mycobacterium leprae*
Fungi	*Candida albicans* Dermatophytes (id reaction?)
Protozoa	Trypanonsomes *Falciparum* (malaria)
Worms	*Ascaris lumbricoides* *Onchocerca volvulus* Schistosomes
Tumors	Lymphomas, leukemias Gammopathies Cryoglobulinemia Many solid tumors
Autoimmune diseases	Lupus erythematosus Rheumatoid arthritis Systemic sclerosis Dermatomyositis Inflammatory bowel disease
Medications	Nonsteroidal antiinflammatory drugs Antibiotics, mainly sulfonamides Phenytoin derivatives ACE inhibitors Thiouracils
Foods	Dyes Preservatives Natural salicylates

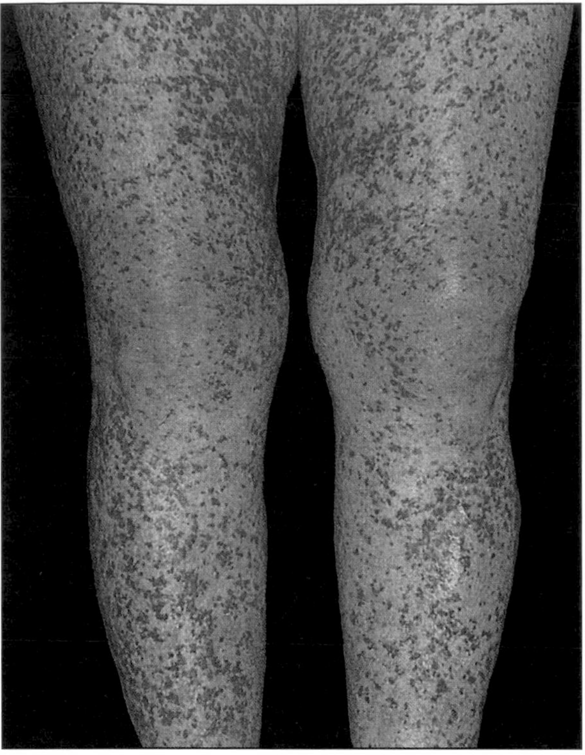

Fig. 22.18. Leukocytoclastic angiitis with purpura

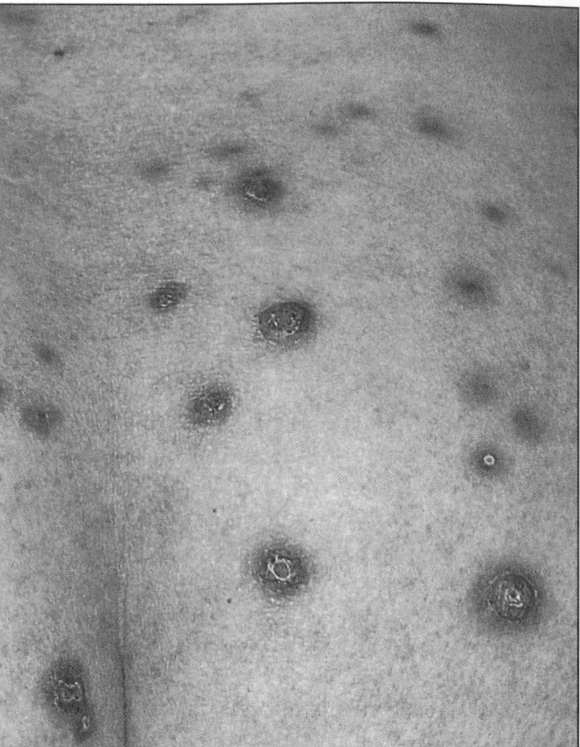

Fig. 22.20. Leukocytoclastic angiitis; papulonecrotic form

Mucosal surfaces are spared. The following clinical patterns can be seen, with wide degrees of overlap:

- Hemorrhagic Type. This is the classic picture of palpable purpura. Early lesions are tiny purpuric macules that may enlarge to reach a size of several centimeters (Fig. 22.18). The lesions do not disappear with diascopy (Fig. 22.19). Some of the larger lesions are usually palpable, separating leukocytoclastic angiitis from other types of purpura (Chap. 23). As the disease progresses, new lesions may appear as the older ones begin to regress with the typical color changes of a resolving bruise.
- Hemorrhagic-Necrotic Type. Larger lesions may evolve into flat red-black areas of necrosis.
- Papulonecrotic Type. The hemorrhagic papules can develop central ulcerations and crust, healing with varioliform scars. This form is more common over the extensor surfaces, especially the knees and elbows (Fig. 22.20).
- Polymorphous-Nodular Type. Hemorrhagic macules, papules, urticarial lesions, and nodules appear admixed. Tiny blisters and larger bullae may also develop, as a reflection of edema and necrosis (Fig. 22.21). Gougerot described this form as maladie trisymptomatique – or even pentasymptomatique depending on the variety of lesions present.
- Annular Type. Some individuals may present with annular purpuric lesions. While this is common in acute hemorrhagic edema of infancy, it is decidedly rare in older children and adults.
- Pustular Type. Sometimes accumulations of neutrophils are so pronounced that pustules form and then rapidly crust.

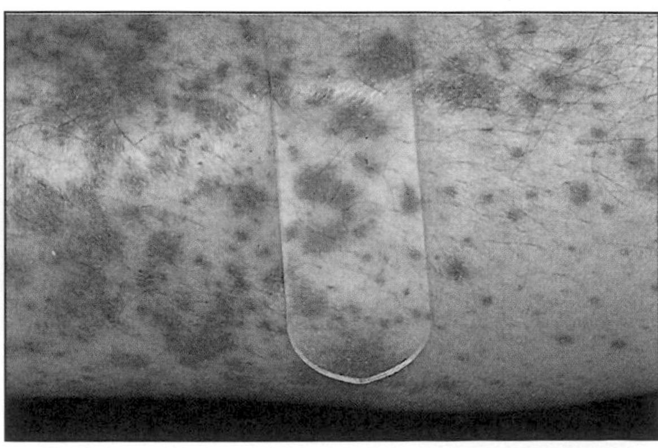

Fig. 22.19. Leukocytoclastic angiitis with lack of blanching on diascopy

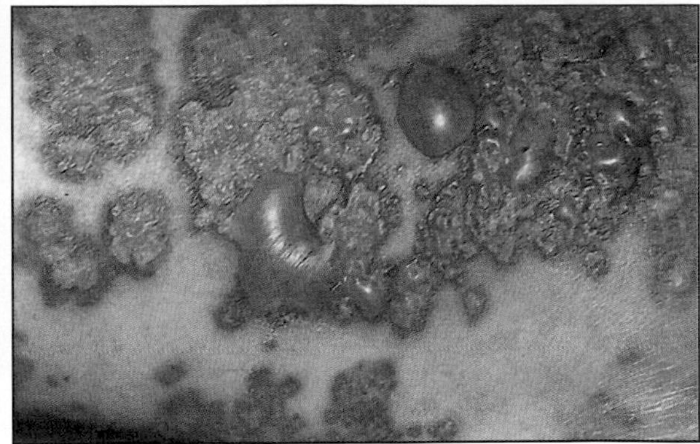

Fig. 22.21. Leukocytoclastic angiitis; bullous-necrotic form

- Urticarial Vasculitis. Sometimes only urticarial lesions are present. This has been documented best in patients with hypocomplementemia and arthritis, as discussed below.

Involvement of Internal Organs. Many patients with leukocytoclastic angiitis have varying degrees of arthralgias. As discussed above, except with Henoch-Schönlein purpura, significant internal organ involvement is uncommon with leukocytoclastic angiitis and, if present, should suggest microscopic polyangiitis. Despite the problems induced by attempts at classification, all patients with cutaneous leukocytoclastic angiitis should be evaluated for renal and gastrointestinal involvement, as these are most common. Other organ systems should be investigated if there are signs or symptoms.

Histopathology. The classic picture is one of damage to the small vessels of the papillary dermis. There is exocytosis of erythrocytes, accumulations of neutrophils with nuclear dust or debris (leukocytoclasia), fibrin deposition in the vessel wall, and focal necrosis of the dermis. Early lesions may be dominated by lymphocytes and have little vessel destruction; late lesions may show primarily necrosis.

Immunofluorescent Examination. Early lesions almost always have intra- and perivascular deposition of C3, IgG, and IgM. In Henoch-Schönlein purpura, by definition, IgA is found.

Laboratory Findings. In order to exclude other causes of purpura, the clotting parameters and platelet numbers should be assessed. In experimental situations, evidence for circulating immune complexes can be sought. Otherwise, the laboratory should be employed judiciously to identify suspected associated disorders.

Course and Prognosis. The outlook varies with the presence of associated disorders or known triggers. Leukocytoclastic angiitis associated with medications, foods, or infections resolves rapidly when the responsible agent is removed. If patients have an underlying chronic disease, such as rheumatoid arthritis, then they are likely to have long-term difficulties with their vasculitis, with waxing and waning of problems. In patients with idiopathic leukocytoclastic angiitis confined to the skin, the course is subacute to chronic. The proportion of patients with underlying disease varies greatly depending on the nature of the reporting institution.

Diagnostic Criteria. The approach to a patient with suspected leukocytoclastic angiitis should include:

- Documenting the diagnosis with histologic evaluation
- Searching for trigger factors
- Excluding involvement of internal organs

Differential Diagnosis. The differential diagnosis varies with the type of lesion. When only purpura is present, one must consider all the conditions discussed in Chap. 23. In very early cases, only a biopsy can distinguish between the onset of leukocytoclastic angiitis and pigmented purpura. The papulonecrotic type resembles pityriasis lichenoides et varioliformis acuta and papulonecrotic tuberculid. When pustules or dusky necrotic lesions are present, septic vasculitis associated with gonococcemia or meningiococcemia (as well as many other bacteria, rarely) must be excluded. In these instances, the lesions are usually fewer in number, but it is essential not to miss the diagnosis because of the need for antibiotic therapy. Embolic disease must be suspected when scattered painful nodules are present, especially acrally. The polymorphous form is similar to erythema multiforme; biopsy is decisive here as erythema multiforme is never associated with vasculitis.

Therapy. The most important factors are to remove possible triggers and to treat any underlying disorder. Patients generally do better with bed rest, elevation of the legs, and compression bandaging of the lower aspects of the legs.

Topical. High potency corticosteroid creams under occlusion may help in treating early lesions.

Systemic. Systemic corticosteroids are the most effective treatment, starting in dosages of 60 mg of prednisone daily and tapering over several weeks, but they are suppressive, not curative, so recurrences are expected. In addition, they may mask or interfere with the treatment of underlying disorders. The range of additional possibilities is almost as confusing as the classification. Some authors endorse starting with antihistamines, but we have had little success with these agents. For relief of pain, the nonsteroidal antiinflammatory drugs are often helpful, although one must remember that they are also a likely trigger. Colchicine 0.5 mg b.i.d.or t.i.d. or dapsone 50–150 mg daily may also be effectivc. In scvere cases, azathioprine and other cytostatic agents as well as plasmapheresis can be employed.

Henoch-Schönlein Purpura

(Schönlein 1832; Henoch 1868)

Synonyms. Purpura rheumatica, as well as all the synonyms for leukocytoclastic angiitis. The European designation of Schönlein-Henoch purpura is historically more correct.

Definition. IgA-dominant immune complex vasculitis frequently involving the skin, gut, and kidneys, and often associated with arthralgias.

Epidemiology. Henoch-Schönlein purpura is a disease of children primarily between the ages of 4 and 11 ycars. The peak is 5 years of age. There is a 2:1 male predominance in children, but among adults this is reversed. Often, there are disease peaks in the spring and fall.

Etiology and Pathogenesis. In about 60% of patients, an infectious trigger can be found. Often there is a history of a preceding upper respiratory infection, such as streptococcal tonsillitis. A wide variety of both bacteria and viruses has been implicated. In other instances, antibiotics (used to treat the respiratory infection), other medications, foods, and immunizations may be responsible. The role of IgA suggests that the challenge may often be mucosal. In most cases, IgA can be identified with immunofluorescent examination of the skin (and kidneys when necessary). Other immunoglobulins and C3 may also be deposited. Some patients with typical Henoch-Schönlein purpura have no IgA deposits. Conversely, patients with Berger disease (a different entity than thromboangiitis obliterans or Buerger disease) develop hematuria often following upper respiratory infections and have IgA nephropathy. When their normal skin is biopsied, IgA is often found.

Clinical Findings. Usually, the purpuric skin lesions follow the respiratory infection by 2–3 weeks. The exanthem usually lasts 10–14 days. In severe cases, the whole range of vasculitic lesions, including urticarial nodules, blisters, and hemorrhagic necrosis, can be seen. In contrast to cutaneous leukocytoclastic angiitis, a wide range of systemic problems is anticipated.

- Arthralgias. About 60% of patients have arthralgias, complaining of pain when they move their knees, ankles, elbows, and hands. Periarticular edema is felt to be the cause of the problems. Inflammation and joint effusions are very rare.
- Abdominal Complaints. As described by Henoch, over half the patients have abdominal problems. Typical complaints include nausea, vomiting, cramping, hematemesis, and melana. The problems result from bowel wall edema and focal vasculitis. Many children are in such distress that they are hospitalized for suspected appendicitis, but are usually rescued by identification of the cutaneous lesions.
- Renal Disease. About half the patients have hematuria or proteinuria, but a much smaller percentage has impaired renal function. The glomerulonephritis is associated with IgA deposits. Microscopically, one can distinguish between focal intracapillary and diffuse proliferative glomerulonephritis. In about 5% of patients, the diffuse glomerulonephritis progresses to endstage renal disease.
- Other. Both CNS and pulmonary involvement is uncommon. Scrotal and testicular hemorrhage has been reported in up to 20% of boys, causing intense pain.

Histopathology. The microscopic picture is identical to that discussed above under leukocytoclastic angiitis.

Laboratory Findings. The renal status must be monitored carefully. If decreasing renal function or marked hematuria is identified, a renal biopsy is indicated. Antistreptolysin titers are raised in about

30% of patients. Otherwise, the same approach suggested for leukocytoclastic angiitis should be followed.

Course and Prognosis. Henoch-Schönlein purpura is generally benign and self-limited. In most cases, resolution occurs over 4–6 weeks. The unlucky patients with severe renal involvement may face a long-term (even life-long) struggle.

Differential Diagnosis. A distinction must be made between microscopic polyangiitis, which may also present with purpura, abdominal pain, and renal disease, and Henoch-Schönlein purpura. In the former, far more aggressive treatment is required. In most instances, the presence of IgA in the skin or kidney offers reassurance. In other instances, fine microscopic differences in the renal involvement may help distinguish between the two.

Therapy. Most patients with Henoch-Schönlein purpura heal spontaneously with bed rest and supportive care. Underlying infections should be treated. If progressive renal disease is identified, the treatment is controversial. The most recent studies suggest that combined treatment with systemic corticosteroids and azathioprine gives the best results. Anticoagulant therapy has also been suggested. Plasmapheresis may be employed. Infusions of factor XIII (which is often reduced) have helped relieve the abdominal pain.

Acute Hemorrhagic Edema

(Snow 1913; Finkelstein 1938; Seidlmayer 1940)

Synonyms. Acute hemorrhagic edema of infancy, acute hemorrhagic vasculitis, Finkelstein disease, Seidlmayer postinfectious cockade purpura

Acute hemorrhagic edema is a striking form of cutaneous vasculitis usually seen in infants less than 24 months of age. We have also seen it in older children (Fig. 22.22). It may well be triggered by infectious agents, although no definite associations have been made. We suspect it is simply a variant of leukocytoclastic angiitis, perhaps associated with angioedema. Cases have been described in which an older sibling has Henoch-Schönlein purpura and the younger sibling, acute hemorrhagic edema.

Infants present with fever, edema of the limbs, and a striking polymorphous exanthem, often identified as erythema multiforme. For this reason, early reports described erythema multiforme as

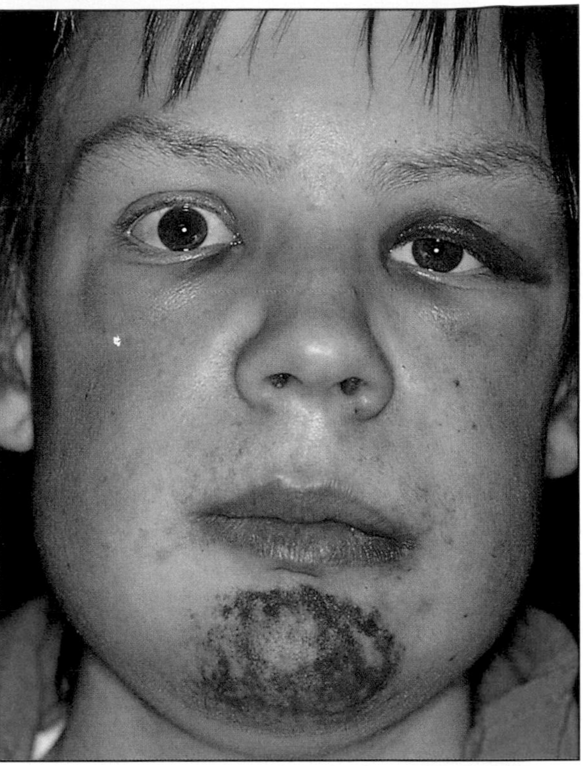

Fig. 22.22. Acute hemorrhagic edema in an older child

showing vasculitis in infants but not adults. The lesions frequently have a target or rosette pattern and often appear on the face and the extremities. They resolve rapidly over days without blister formation or necrosis. There are no systemic manifestations. No therapy is required, unless there is clear evidence for an untreated underlying infection.

Urticarial Vasculitis

(McDuffie et al. 1973)

Synonyms. Hypocomplementemic vasculitis, hypocomplementemia-urticaria-vasculitis syndrome

Definition. Urticarial vasculitis can be defined in several ways. We prefer the most strict or restrictive definition, meaning the conjunction of leukocytoclastic vasculitis, urticaria, and a variety of systemic problems, most often associated with hypocomplementemia. Some clinicians define urticarial vasculitis as urticaria with persistent individual lesions lasting more than 24 h that on biopsy show leukocytoclastic vasculitis, regardless of systemic findings.

Etiology and Pathogenesis. The causes of urticarial vasculitis are as protean as those of urticaria and of vasculitis. The pathophysiology is that of vasculitis, as the urticarial lesions and the occasional angioedema simply reflect leakage through a damaged vessel. The list of associated disorders is long and includes systemic lupus erythematosus, Sjögren syndrome, and serum sickness; most cases are idiopathic. Those patients with hypocomplementemia are more likely to have systemic lupus erythematosus.

Clinical Findings. Most patients are adult women. The urticarial lesions usually appear first. The hives are sharply circumscribed, erythematous, blanch upon diascopy, and may have tiny purpuric areas. While most lesions disappear within 24 h, some last up to 3–5 days and may heal with hyperpigmentation, reflecting leakage of erythrocytes. Systemic symptoms typically include fever, malaise, and myalgias with arthritis and arthralgias. Virtually every other organ system can be involved; other features may include lymphadenopathy, paraproteinemia, hepatosplenomegaly, abdominal pain, glomerulonephritis, headache, renal disease, gastrointestinal distress, ocular inflammation, and acute and chronic respiratory problems.

Histopathology. The histopathology defines the disease. There should be unequivocal leukocytoclastic vasculitis on biopsy. A lymphocytic infiltrate does not suffice.

Laboratory Findings. About 50% of patients show hypocomplementemia. The erythrocyte sedimentation rate is usually elevated. One should search for signs of other organ dysfunction and associated diseases. There may be an elevated leukocyte count and eosinophilia.

Course and Prognosis. The course is chronic. Patients with hypocomplementemia tend to have associated disorders and do less well.

Differential Diagnosis. The differential diagnosis includes all types of urticaria (Chap. 11) and leukocytoclastic angiitis, so it is extensive.

Therapy. The treatment of urticarial vasculitis is different from other forms of urticaria. Antihistamines may be used but are often ineffective. NSAIDs may help the skin and joint findings. When systemic involvement is present, systemic corticosteroids are usually prescribed. If they fail, various steroid-sparing agents, including azathioprine, 6-mercaptopurine, and cyclosporine, can be tried.

Schnitzler Syndrome

(Schnitzler et al. 1974)

This is an association of urticarial vasculitis with a monoclonal macroglobulinemia and with hyperfibrinogenemia. Severe headaches are a typical feature. Both the hives and the underlying hematologic disorder are difficult to treat. We view Schnitzler syndrome as a variant of urticarial vasculitis.

Serum Sickness

Serum sickness is the prototype of an immune complex vasculitis and has many similarities with the experimental Arthus reaction. It is discussed in Chap. 11.

Miscellaneous Forms of Vasculitis

Vasculitis with Autoimmune Diseases

Fairly distinct forms of leukocytoclastic angiitis are seen in lupus erythematosus, rheumatoid arthritis, and Sjögren syndrome. All are discussed in Chapter 18. It is debated whether the vasculitis takes a different form because of the underlying disease or whether there are pathologic differences. In all three diseases, the vasculitis is likely to be dominated by lymphocytes with less leukocytoclasia.

Vasculitis is a constant feature of rheumatoid arthritis, but usually only involves the synovial vessels. In more advanced cases, especially those with high titers of rheumatoid factor, more widespread vasculitis is seen. Presumably, the rheumatoid factor, other immunoglobulins, and complement form immune complexes. Polyneuropathy is probably the most common manifestation; bowel perforations, myocardial infarctions, and CNS damage also occur. In the skin, purpura, ulcerations, and infarctions may be seen, as well as subcutaneous nodules. Tiny infarcts about the nailfolds and on the pulp of the digits occur in about 25% of patients. They are usually painless, last for a few days, and fade with a brown hue. Painful papules can occur in the digit pulp; they are often confused with emboli but result from a characteristic onion-skin-like intimal proliferation and occlusion, rather than true inflammation.

Just as with rheumatoid arthritis, many of the extraglandular features of Sjögren syndrome are explained by vasculitis. In the skin, the whole spectrum of leukocytoclastic angiitis is seen. Urticarial vasculitis is particularly common, and both Waldenström hypergammaglobulinemic purpura and cryoglobulinemia may occur.

In systemic lupus erythematosus, ordinary leukocytoclastic angiitis is the most common form. Urticarial vasculitis may also be seen. The main concern in lupus erythematosus with vasculitis is the possibility of underlying CNS or renal vascular damage. In addition, livedo vasculitis (see below) is present in some lupus erythematosus patients. Patients with a genetic deficiency in C2, who often have systemic lupus erythematosus, tend to have cutaneous vasculitis, usually a severe form.

Hypergammaglobulinemic Purpura

(WALDENSTRÖM 1943)

Some authors consider this a form of vasculitis. The histologic picture is variable, only occasionally showing vessel damage. We consider it in Chapter 40.

Cryoglobulinemia

Deposition of cryoglobulins in a vessel triggers the vasculitic process. In other words, cryoglobulinemia combines occlusion and inflammation. This disorder, which primarily affects the skin and kidneys, is considered in more detail in Chapter 40.

Tumor-Associated Vasculitis

Many different myelo- and lymphoproliferative diseases cause vasculitis by a wide variety of mechanisms. These include monoclonal gammopathies, abnormal cytokine responses, deposition of malignant cells in vessels (angiocentric and angiotropic lymphomas). Solid tumors may also cause vasculitis; in most causes an immune complex mechanism is suspected although rarely proven.

Nodular Vasculitis

Inflammation of the deep dermal vessels is often associated with panniculitis. Erythema induratum of Bazin and nodular vasculitis are similar, but PCR techniques have identified *Mycobacterium tuberculosis* DNA in some erythema induratum lesions. The clinical picture is indurated nodules on the legs, and the vasculitis is usually in the larger vessels of the deep dermal plexus, so the disease is closer to cutaneous polyarteritis nodosa than leukocytoclastic angiitis, although many texts include it here.

Inflammatory Bowel Disease

Both ulcerative colitis and Crohn disease may be associated with leukocytoclastic angiitis. Often the lesions are pustular, and the histologic pattern may be granulomatous. Just as with nodular vasculitis, the larger vessels of the deep plexus are frequently involved, although in some instances a clinically typical palpable purpura appears.

Erythema Elevatum Diutinum

(RADCLIFFE-CROCKER and WILLIAMS 1894)

Definition. Form of chronic vasculitis usually presenting with symmetric papules, plaques and nodules on the extremities.

Epidemiology. This rare disorder more often affects women than men.

Etiology and Pathogenesis. The cause of erythema elevatum diutinum is unknown. It may represent a type of leukocytoclastic vasculitis reflecting an immunologic response against streptococcal or other bacterial antigens. It has been described in association with Crohn disease, another inflammatory disorder of unclear but perhaps infectious origin.

Clinical Findings. The most common sites are the extremities, especially the knees, elbows, and backs of the hands and feet (Fig. 22.23). Multiple papules

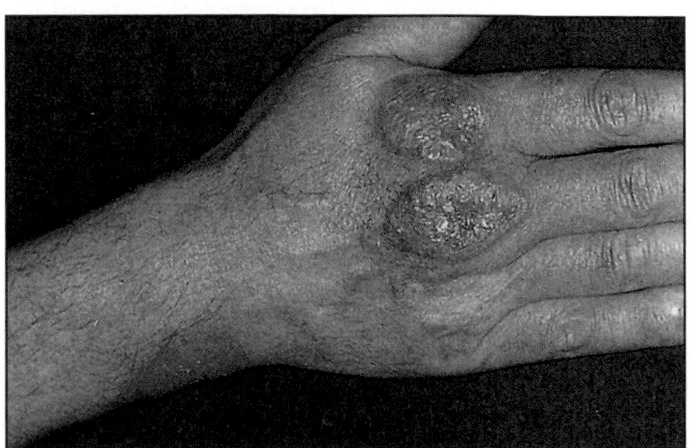

Fig. 22.23. Erythema elevatum diutinum

and nodules are present in a symmetric fashion. Occasionally, larger plaques develop with a central depression. They may be annular. While early lesions tend to be red, later on they acquire reddish brown tones. Hemorrhage and ulceration are extremely uncommon. The lesions are often painful and heal with hyperpigmentation.

Many patients have arthralgias, and peripheral ulcerative keratitis has been reported, but other internal problems are rare. Vasculitis in other organs does not seem to occur. An association with gout has been reported. The disease course is chronic, over years; individual lesions may disappear as new ones develop.

Histopathology. Microscopic examination reveals a diffuse dermal infiltration of neutrophils and eosinophils despite the chronic nature of the lesions. The dermal blood vessels are damaged with fibrin deposits, leukocytoclasia, and nuclear dust. Older lesions may be more granulomatous or even fibrotic. Necrobiosis is not seen.

A histologic variant is extracellular cholesterolosis (Urbach et al. 1932), in which there are cholesterol clefts and a granulomatous response. Despite these findings, an abnormal lipid metabolism has not been identified.

Laboratory Findings. In some instances, rheumatoid factor titers may be elevated in the absence of other signs of rheumatoid arthritis. Rare patients may have a paraproteinemia, perhaps associated with a plasmacytoma; anti-thrombin III deficiency has also been seen.

Course and Prognosis. The disease persists over years. Individuals lesions wax and wane, or disappear entirely.

Differential Diagnosis. Lesions are often identified clinically as granuloma annulare, but the individual lesions are much more succulent and red brown; in addition, no necrobiosis is present.

Therapy. Dapsone is the single most effective agent, in doses of 50–150 mg daily. Trimethoprim-sulfamethoxazole may also be helpful, as are systemic corticosteroids. Often antibiotic therapy is tried because of the possibility of bacterial triggering, but it usually offers little improvement. Intralesional corticosteroids are helpful for treating individual painful lesions.

Pyoderma Gangrenosum

(Brunsting et al. 1930)

Synonym. Dermatitis ulcerosa

Definition. Chronic progressive cutaneous necrosis of unknown etiology, often associated with underlying diseases.

Epidemiology. Little is available on the frequency of pyoderma gangrenosum. The disease is rare but often occurs in patients under the care of other specialists.

Etiology and Pathogenesis. The cause of pyoderma gangrenosum is unknown. Many factors point towards it being a type of vascular disease. It is associated with diseases that often have vasculitis, such as gammopathies and inflammatory bowel disease. It is very difficult to prove a vascular origin, and a wide range of immunologic defects have been identified, suggesting that many are epiphenomena. The clinical presence of pathergy or the development of a lesion at a site of minor trauma suggests an overenthusiastic immunologic reaction.

Table 22.6 shows some of the diseases associated with pyoderma gangrenosum. In the case of rheumatoid arthritis and inflammatory bowel disease, the underlying disease is almost always well-established and flaring at the time pyoderma gangrenosum appears. With IgA gammopathies, the opposite is true; pyoderma gangrenosum is quite often the first sign of the underlying disease. Most series suggest that, in about 50% of patients, an underlying disease will be found, while in the others, the reluctant diagnosis of idiopathic pyoderma gangrenosum is made.

Clinical Findings. The clinical examination is everything in pyoderma gangrenosum. There is probably no other such serious dermatologic disease that is diagnosed almost entirely on clinical features. While any part of the skin can be involved, most lesions are on the legs. The initial lesion is an inflamed, red, often pustular papule or nodule that is frequently mistaken for a furuncle or insect bite reaction. Often there is a history of previous, usually minor, trauma. The lesion ulcerates and rapidly expands laterally, producing a large, relatively flat ulcer with a swollen necrotic base and a raised, dusky erythematous border (Fig. 22.24). The border is usually undermined and may have tiny pieces of

Table 22.6. Diseases associated with pyoderma gangrenosum

Category	Examples
Inflammatory bowel disease	Ulcerative colitis * Crohn disease *
Other gastrointestinal disorders	Carcinoid syndrome Gastric and duodenal ulcers Diverticulitis
Arthritis	Rheumatoid arthritis * Seronegative arthritis (+/– inflammatory bowel disease) * Chronic recurrent multifocal osteomyelitis
Hematologic disease	Monoclonal gammopathy (usually IgA) * Multiple myeloma Polycythemia vera Paroxysmal nocturnal hemoglobinuria Malignant lymphoma Myelocytic leukemias * Other myeloproliferative disorders * Hairy cell leukemia * Congenital deficiency of leukocyte adhesion proteins
Hepatic disease	Hepatitis C Chronic active hepatitis Primary biliary cirrhosis
Immunologic disease	Systemic lupus erythematosus Complement deficiencies
Miscellaneous	Post-operative, post-traumatic Sarcoidosis HIV/AIDS Solid tumors Acne conglobata Acne inversa Behçet disease

* The most significant disorders

necrotic epidermis still attached. Multiple lesions may fuse together. The ulcers are invariably painful. The course may be explosive and, if untreated, expose muscles, nerves, vessels, fascia, and even bones. Many patients have associated fever, malaise, and arthralgias. In other individuals, the expansion is slower and dominated by a raised, exudative granulomatous response. When the lesions heal, the scarring is described as cribiform or sieve-like, with many little burrows and indentations.

A major feature of pyoderma gangrenosum is pathergy, but it is often overemphasized. Pathergy describes the induction of a lesion by trauma, often quite minor, such as a needle stick for blood drawing. Some use pathergy as part of the diagnostic criteria for pyoderma gangrenosum, even trying to induce it. Those patients with pathergy are at special risk, as, should they require surgery, they may have devastating problems; however, only about 25% of patients have this feature. Behçet disease is another disorder in which pathergy is frequently seen.

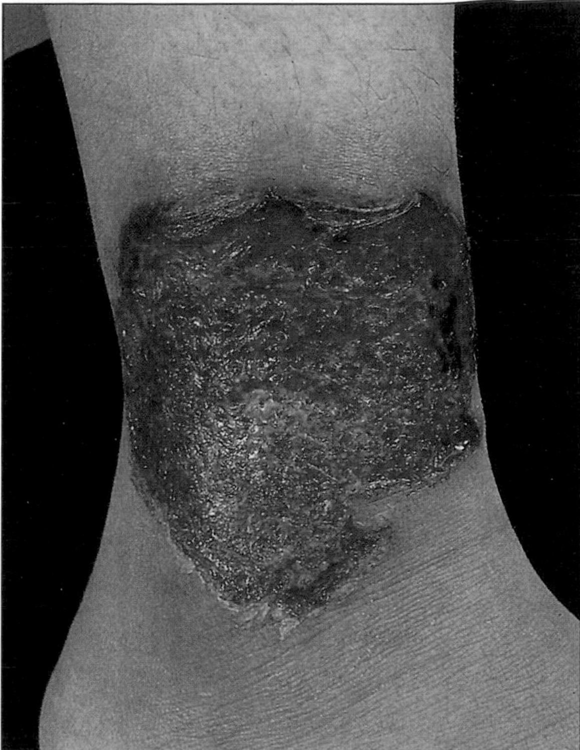

Fig. 22.24. Pyoderma gangrenosum

Many clinical variants of pyoderma gangrenosum have been described.

- Bullous Pyoderma Gangrenosum. This variant is clinically important as it is more likely to be associated with hematologic malignancies, such as hairy cell leukemia, myelogenous leukemia, and other myelodysplastic conditions. The lesions are more superficial and frequently either start with bullae or have bullae at their borders. Bullous Sweet syndrome is associated with the same group of disorders but usually does not have such prominent ulcerations. Clearly, the two disorders are connected somehow, as some patients have both disorders.
- Malignant Pyoderma (Perry et al. 1968). Initially this condition was considered to be separate

from pyoderma gangrenosum because it was on the head and neck, was rarely associated with underlying diseases, and lacked the erythematous border. Today, it is considered to be a variant of pyoderma gangrenosum.

- Pyostomatitis Vegetans. This pustular vegetative disease of the oral mucosa is also associated with inflammatory bowel disease and may be oral pyoderma gangrenosum (Chap. 33).
- Peristomal Pyoderma Gangrenosum. Patients with inflammatory bowel disease may develop extensive ulcerations about their stoma site or in their wound. In addition, the pustular eruption of ulcerative colitis is probably also pyoderma gangrenosum.
- Postoperative Cutaneous Gangrene (Cullen 1924). Other patients may also develop pyoderma gangrenosum-like changes following surgery. Usually, a bacterial wound infection is suspected, but the rapid course and failure to respond to antibiotics suggest a different answer.
- Genital Pyoderma Gangrenosum. Vulvar, penile, and scrotal pyoderma gangrenosum have all been identified. Often the differential diagnosis of Behçet syndrome is suggested, but the ulcers are too large. Once again, mixed synergistic bacterial infections must be excluded
- Superficial Granulomatous Pyoderma. These patients have a more superficial, slowly spreading ulcer, usually on the trunk, with a heaped up border and draining sinuses. Microscopically, there is granulomatous inflammation in the dermis, which does not fit with pyoderma gangrenosum. This may be a variant of pyoderma gangrenosum triggered by an infectious agent, similar to blastomycotic-like pyoderma but not as deep. It is unclear to us how to interpret this rare phenomenon.
- Subcutaneous Pyoderma Gangrenosum. The disease process may start in the fat, causing massive destruction and then breaking through to the skin. There is usually a massive purulent discharge and, not surprisingly, far deeper destruction.
- Extracutaneous Pyoderma Gangrenosum. Sterile neutrophilic deposits have been described in the heart, lungs, gastrointestinal tract, and CNS. Often they are first identified at autopsy.

Histopathology. A biopsy of the advancing edge of a lesion may, if one is lucky enough, reveal neutrophils and fibrin in the superficial vessels. In one large series, about 40% of patients had histologic evidence of vasculitis. Thrombosis of small vessels may also be seen. Later on, massive tissue destruction is noted with massive neutrophilic infiltrates accompanied by lymphocytes, plasma cells, histiocytes, and even giant cells.

Immunofluorescent Examination. Most groups have found immunoglobulins and complement in the vessel walls at the edge of lesions, but others have been unable to repeat this. Immune complexes have not been demonstrated.

Laboratory Findings. The laboratory is only useful to search for possible underlying disorders. Bacterial and deep fungal infections should be excluded, but confusion is very rare.

Course and Prognosis. If the underlying disease is treatable, the outlook is good; if not, the patient is in trouble from both directions. In patients with idiopathic pyoderma gangrenosum, the usual story is waxing and waning over many years.

Differential Diagnosis. True bacterial and deep fungal infections, factitial disease, and panniculitis are the main problems to be excluded. The main infectious cause of such extensive destruction is synergistic bacterial infections, such as noma and related disorders (Chap. 4).

Therapy. The most important treatment is that of the underlying disease. For some inflammatory bowel disease patients, this may be carried as far as resection of the involved bowel.

Systemic. Many patients have already been treated with antibiotics before the diagnosis is made, but they usually have no effect. The mainstay of therapy is systemic corticosteroids, usually starting with prednisone 60–80 mg daily. If this does not promptly arrest the spread of the disease, higher dosages (up to 120 mg daily) or intravenous methylprednisolone pulse therapy should be considered. Most patients with severe pyoderma gangrenosum develop corticosteroid-related problems. For this reason, many steroid-sparing agents have been employed. In our experience, dapsone is helpful in less severe cases and for maintenance, usually in dosages of 50–150 mg daily. Sulfasalazine has been endorsed, even for patients without inflammatory bowel disease. Clofazimine 100–300 mg daily has also helped some patients. Cyclosporine in doses of up to 8 mg/kg daily is often dramatically effective, and similar results have been reported for tacrolimus. Finally, many immunosuppressive drugs have been employed; in recent years mycophenolate mofetil has shown special promise, but controlled studies are lacking. Intravenous human immunoglobulin has also been effective; typical regimens include 1.0 g/kg daily for 2 days, repeated monthly for four to six courses.

Topical. Patients require gentle wound care, limb elevation, and bed rest. One should keep the surgeons away from the wound, as both debridement and grafting are frequently tried without success. Very early lesions can be treated with intralesional or very potent topical corticosteroids to try and abort their spread. Both topical cyclosporine and tacrolimus have been helpful in selected cases.

Livedo Racemosa

(Ehrmann 1907)

Synonym. Vasculitis racemosa

Definition. Livedo racemosa is a net-like or lacy, often bizarre, generally permanent pattern of livid skin changes which reflects underlying vessel damage, be it due to occlusion or inflammation. We distinguish it from the transient changes of livedo reticularis discussed earlier.

Epidemiology. Livedo racemosa is an uncommon disorder, but probably underdiagnosed as many patients present with nondermatologic problems.

Etiology and Pathogenesis. There are many different underlying causes of livedo racemosa (Table 22.7). The diagnosis of idiopathic livedo racemosa is a diagnosis of exclusion, and such patients should be regularly reevaluated. The mechanisms of the disease are highly variable. The major vessels in the deep dermal plexus become partially or totally occluded, producing the unusual distribution of blood.

Clinical Findings. Typical findings include blanchable, irregularly formed, blue-red vascular markings that have been compared to lightning bolts, stripes, or irregular nets (Fig. 22.25). The larger areas have tiny finger-like projections extending into the adjacent skin. The overall pattern resembles a garden plant with runners or tendrils. The buttocks, lower part of the back, upper aspects of the arms, and the lower parts of the legs, especially

Table 22.7. Causes of livedo racemosa

Inflammatory vascular diseases
Polyarteritis nodosa
Cutaneous polyarteritis nodosa
Lupus erythematosus
Anticardiolipin syndrome
Sneddon syndrome
Dermatomyositis
Arteriosclerosis
Thromboangiitis obliterans
Pancreatitis
Bacterial endocarditis
Rheumatic fever
HIV/AIDS
Syphilis
Tuberculosis
Drugs (oral contraceptives?, nicotine?, quinidine?)
Occlusive vascular diseases
Arterial emboli
Thrombocythemia
Cryoglobulinemia
Gammopathy
Coagulopathies
Intraarterial injections
Decompression illness (bends) in divers

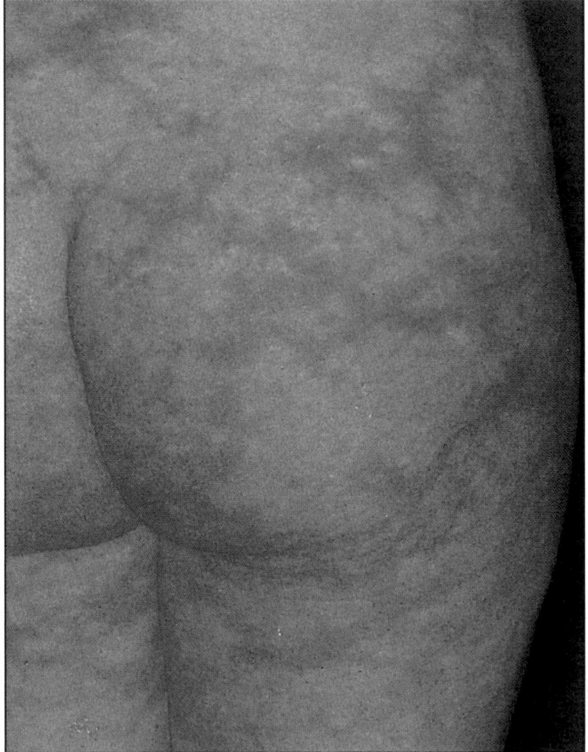

Fig. 22.25. Livedo racemosa

the plantar instep, are the most characteristic sites. Nodular lesions and ulcerations are uncommon, but suggest an active underlying disease. There may be intense pain, especially with plantar involvement.

Histopathology. The site of the biopsy is crucial. Often the abnormal vessels are found in the paler, apparently normal skin, rather than in the livid area. Thus, a generous biopsy extending into the subcutaneous fat, coupled with multiple sections, is often required to identify either occlusion or inflammation. When vasculitis is present, it is usually segmental, and the wall is thickened with amorphous or hyaline material.

Laboratory Findings. There are no specific laboratory findings. Appropriate tests should be ordered as directed by the history to identify or exclude underlying disease.

Therapy. The only satisfactory therapy is to treat the underlying disease. Anticoagulation or at least platelet inhibition, as well as rheologic agents (pentoxifylline, for example), are worth trying. Sometimes nonspecific antiinflammatory agents such as NSAIDs (also with antiplatelet activity), corticosteroids, colchicine, dapsone, or azathioprine are tried in the standard dosages. Our advice is to continue looking for the cause and only treat the symptoms, such as pain or ulcerations.

Anticardiolipin Syndrome

This syndrome, often associated with systemic lupus erythematosus, is probably the best understood underlying cause of livedo racemosa. It is considered in greater detail in Chapter 18.

Sneddon Syndrome

(Sneddon 1965)

The cutaneous changes of livedo racemosa may be combined with systemic artenal disease in Sneddon syndrome, which may be a variant of antiphospholipid syndrome. Cerebral, coronary, renal and peripheral arteries may become occluded. Any patient, especially a younger individual, with a stroke should be searched for evidence of livedo racemosa. The patients may present with paralysis, seizures, visual disturbances, or vague symptoms that are mistaken for psychosomatic problems. Many of the patients are smokers, and among women, the use of oral contraceptives also appears to be a risk factor. Histologically there is endarteritis obliterans.

Livedo Vasculitis

(Feldaker et al. 1955)

Synonyms. Livedo reticularis with summer ulcerations, livedoid vasculitis. This disease is incorrectly called livedo reticularis, but the patients actually have livedo racemosa.

Definition. Livedo racemosa on the lower parts of the legs combined with therapy-resistant ulcerations.

Etiology and Pathogenesis. This rare disorder is probably not a single disease, but is most often associated with systemic lupus erythematosus and antiphospholipid syndrome.

Clinical Findings. Whenever livedo racemosa involves the foot and ankle region, it tends to be painful. Some patients develop ulcerations about their ankles, more often in warm weather than in cold (Fig. 22.26). The ulcers tend to heal with white

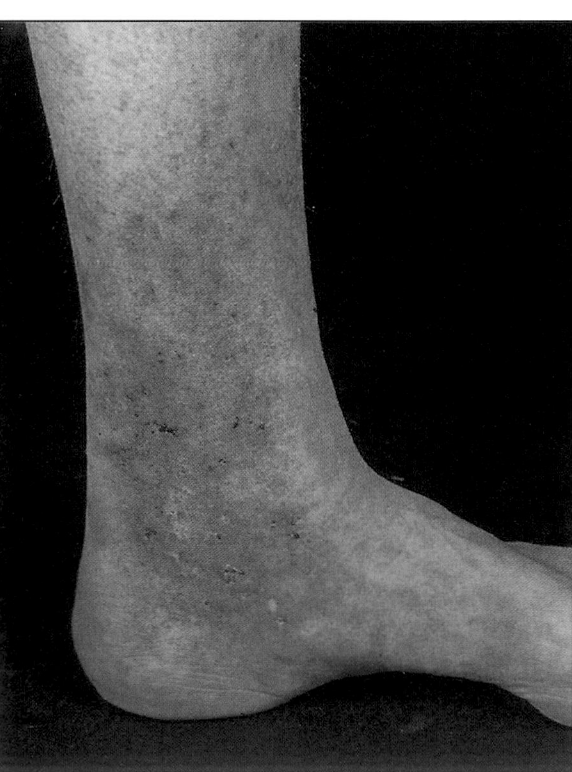

Fig. 22.26. Livedo racemosa with ulcerations

telangiectatic scars, leading to the diagnosis of atrophie blanche.

Histopathology. Segmental hyaline vasculitis is present. There may also be dermal fibrosis, hemosiderin, and other changes appropriate to chronic vascular leakage about the ankle. Direct immunofluorescent examination often reveals deposition of IgG and C3 in the vessel walls.

Laboratory Findings. Anticardiolipin and lupus anticoagulant antibodies should be sought.

Therapy. Standard ulcer care is needed. The same therapeutic approach discussed above, using anticoagulants, platelet activation inhibitors, pentoxifylline, or immunosuppressive agents, can be tried, but there is no single uniformly effective agent.

Cutis Marmorata Telangiectatica Congenita
(VAN LOHUIZEN 1922)

Synonyms. Nevus vascularis reticularis, congenital livedo reticularis, congenital generalized phlebectasia

Definition. Congenital persistent mottling of the skin associated with a variety of other defects.

Etiology and Pathogenesis. This rare disorder probably represents an inherited defect in the ability of the vessels to respond to cold, but the genetics have not been clarified. Occasionally, segmental lesions are seen, suggesting mosaicism. In some families, paradominant inheritance appears to be involved. Such patients tend to have atrophy and scarring.

Clinical Findings. The changes are usually present at birth and expand over a period of months. There is mottled erythema that is more permanent than the physiologic livedo reticularis of infants, and thus closer to livedo racemosa (Fig. 22.27). In addition, there are telangiectases and permanently dilated larger vessels. Cutaneous ulcerations and atrophy, including limb atrophy, may occur. Other patients have a more telangiectatic pattern that may overlap with Klippel-Trénaunay-Weber syndrome, as this group tends to develop limb hypertrophy.

A long list of associated findings have been described. It has been suggested that 25–50% of patients with cutis marmorata telangiectatica congenita have other congenital anomalies, but we suspect that patients without other changes are under-reported. The defects are too numerous to list but include other vascular changes, especially involving the heart, great vessels, and CNS, skeletal changes, glaucoma, and embryologic defects in the urogenital tract.

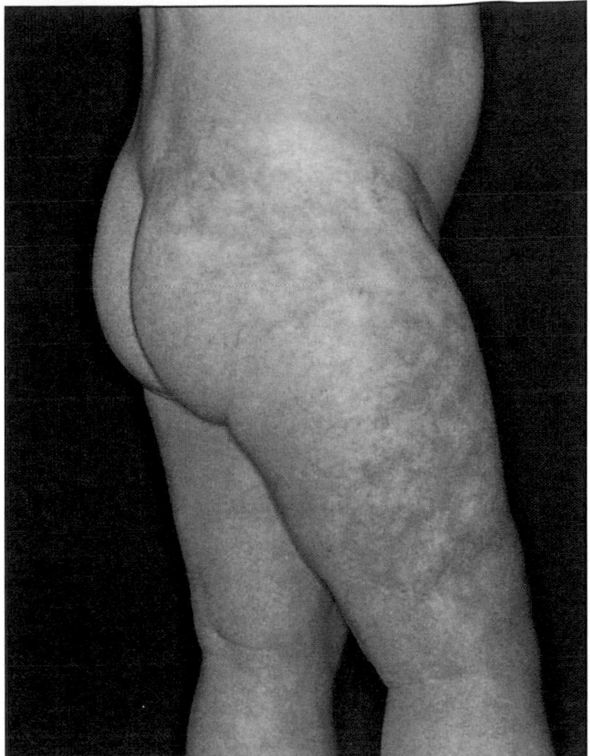

Fig. 22.27. Cutis marmorata telangiectatica congenita

Histopathology. A wide range of enlarged vessels may be seen, but in other instances, the defect appears to be primarily physiologic and the vasculature is microscopically normal.

Course and Prognosis. The course is dependent on the associated findings. In patients with only skin changes, the outlook is good. The mottling improves during childhood, but the excessive vessels, such as the telangiectases, remain. Minor amounts of scarring and ulceration persist, as do limb changes.

Differential Diagnosis. Neonatal lupus erythematosus may have mottled skin but the lesions improve rapidly. Vascular malformations are more sharply localized and not so temperature sensitive.

Therapy. Avoidance of cold is the only helpful approach.

Malignant Atrophic Papulosis

(Köhlmeier 1941; Degos et al. 1942)

Synonyms. Papulosis maligna atrophicans, Köhlmeier-Degos syndrome, Degos syndrome, thromboangiitis cutaneointestinalis disseminata, lethal intestinocutaneous syndrome

Definition. Idiopathic vascular occlusive disease with papules that evolve into atrophic white scars and frequent gastrointestinal vascular problems.

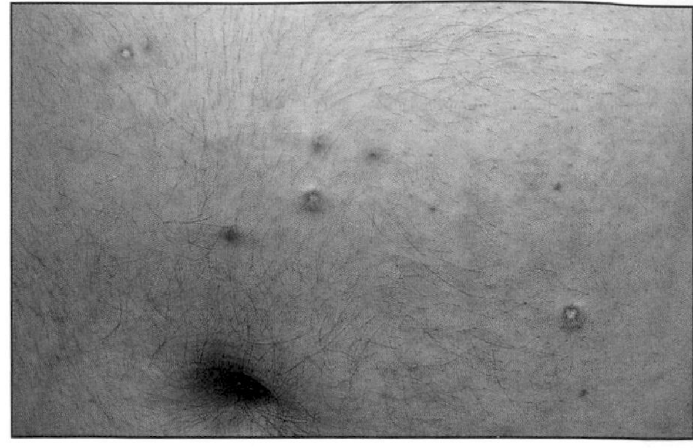

Fig. 22.28. Malignant atrophic papulosis

Epidemiology. The disorder is very rare, usually appears in young and middle-aged adults, and was initially felt to show a male predominance. Recent reports suggest the sex ratio is about equal.

Etiology and Pathogenesis. The etiology is unknown. Köhlmeier thought this was a variant of thromboangiitis obliterans, but was incorrect. There is still no consensus about whether the precipitating event is a vasculitis or a hypercoagulable state, perhaps in association with the antiphospholipid syndrome. Malignant atrophic papulosis has recently been described in a patient with HIV/AIDS.

Clinical Findings

Systemic Findings. Infarcts in the small bowel and CNS are the most common changes. The systemic difficulties generally follow the cutaneous ones. Patients may present with fever, abdominal pain, cramping, hematemesis, and bloody stools. Others may have intestinal infarcts discovered first on endoscopic examination or at autopsy. The most frequent cause of death is intestinal perforation and peritonitis. For this reason, the disease was described as "malignant." The CNS may also be involved, producing a variety of problems depending on the site and size of the infarct. Rarely, ocular and renal vascular disease have been reported. Some patients have no systemic abnormalities.

Cutaneous Findings. The trunk and abdomen are the most common sites of involvement. Disseminated, 3–5 mm, pale red papules appear in small crops. They are usually asymptomatic. After several days, their central portion becomes porcelain-white (Fig. 22.28). Other lesions develop further necrosis and ulcerations, healing with white atrophic scars, often with peripheral hyperpigmentation.

Histopathology. The microscopic picture in a well-developed lesion is classic. There is vessel destruction of arterioles in the deep dermis producing a wedge-shaped infarct that heals with sclerosis and mucin deposition. Lymphocytes may be seen along the junction between the scar and normal dermis, as well as about the vessels, which tend to show intimal thickening. In biopsy samples from early lesions, a lymphocytic vasculitis can be identified. Direct immunofluorescent examination is usually negative.

Laboratory Findings. Systemic lupus erythematosus should be excluded.

Course and Prognosis. The term malignant is inappropriate. Atrophic papulosis would be preferable. Patients with only cutaneous involvement tend to do relatively well. While the life expectancy of patients with gastrointestinal involvement was formerly estimated as 5 years, better supportive care has extended this limit.

Differential Diagnosis. All the diseases associated with livedo racemosa should be considered. Even though malignant atrophic papulosis does not usually have a livedo pattern, it has the same characteristic white scars seen so often in the latter setting. Some patients with systemic lupus erythematosus also develop atrophic white scars, so this more common diagnosis must be ruled out.

Therapy. This disease is too rare for any controlled studies. Anticoagulants, corticosteroids, and surgical intervention have shown little benefit. Today, most patients are treated with inhibitors of platelet aggregation, such as low-dose aspirin, occasionally combined with dipyramidole.

Peripheral Occlusive Arterial Disease

When peripheral arteries are either narrowed (stenotic) or occluded, the end organ is underperfused. For the dermatologist, the most common consequences are pain and necrosis of the extremities, but one must always keep in mind that internal organs (CNS, heart, kidneys, etc.) may also be involved. The most important causes of peripheral occlusive disease are arteriosclerosis, diabetic angiopathy, thromboangiitis obliterans, thromboses, and emboli. The latter are often responsible for acute complete arterial occlusion as they seed peripherally and may block either a healthy artery or one damaged by another process.

Clinical Stages

Peripheral occlusive disease, especially of the legs, is divided into four stages as originally proposed by Fontaine (Table 22.8).

- Stage I: symptom-free. Even though studies may demonstrate narrowing or occlusion of a vessel, there is adequate collateral circulation so that, even with activity, the individual is asymptomatic.
- Stage II: pain with activity. The most typical symptom is intermittent claudication; pain forces the patient to cease walking or some other activity. Stage II can be divided into IIa (able to walk more than 50 m without pain) and IIb (pain before reaching 50 m).
- Stage III: pain on resting. The patient has pain in his legs even when resting in the horizontal position.
- Stage IV: necrosis. Localized (IVa) or more diffuse (IVb) areas of necrosis result from decreased perfusion.

One should consider how well the functional and clinical stages correlate. For example, there are patients with pain on rest and necrosis, but others who have only very mild claudication and nonetheless recalcitrant ulcers.

Diagnostic Procedures

While many elegant tools are available to study the peripheral circulation, one should not overlook the simple nontechnical aspects of the evaluation.

Inspection

The skin color should be compared between sides after the patient has had time to adapt to the room temperature. With chronic arterial disease, the skin is often pale, especially when the legs are raised above the level of the heart. With acute occlusion, the paleness is more pronounced (*Leichenblässe*, or pale as a cadaver in German) and coupled with intense pain. Erythema can be a sign of inflammation or reactive hyperemia. Both dilatation of the venules and reduced hemoglobin levels contribute to the cyanosis. One should compare the filling of the veins between the two legs, as well as search for edema, necroses, ulcerations, and scars. The diameter of the legs should be measured at

Table 22.8. Classification of peripheral occlusive arterial disease

Stage	Compensation	Vessel changes	Blood supply	Symptoms
I	Complete	Narrowing or extensive collaterals	Only minimally reduced	None
IIa	Partial	Marked stenosis or complete closure with adequate collaterals	At rest, adequate; with activity, incompetent	Claudication after > 50 m
IIb	Partial	As IIa	As IIa	Claudication at <50 m
III	Poor	Occlusion with few collaterals	Inadequate at rest	Claudication, pain at rest, often at night or with legs levated
IV	Absent	Occlusion of one or more vessels without collaterals	Ischemia at rest	Necrosis, gangrene

standard reference points. Dry skin, inadequate wound healing, nail dystrophies, and dermatophytosis are also associated with inadequate circulation.

Palpation

The radial and ulnar arteries should be checked on both arms. If any pulses are missing, then the brachial, axillary, and subclavian arteries should be investigated. On the legs, the most important pulses are the dorsalis pedis artery on the back of the foot, the posterior tibial artery just behind the medial malleolus, the popliteal artery (best identified with the knee slightly flexed), and the common femoral and external iliac arteries in the groin. Palpation usually allows one to recognize an arterial occlusion and estimate its level. The following subtypes of occlusion were proposed by Ratschow:

Arms
- Shoulder girdle type: Occlusion of subclavian artery
- Upper arm type: Occlusion of brachial artery
- Peripheral type: Occlusion distal to elbow

Legs
- Pelvic type: Occlusion proximal to groin, with failing inguinal pulses
- Thigh type: Occlusion of femoral artery with palpable pulse in groin but not in popliteal space
- Calf type: Occlusion distal to knee with palpable popliteal pulse but one or more distal pulses absent

In addition, palpation can identify nodules in an artery in polyarteritis nodosa, changes in caliber from an aneurysm, thrills from an arteriovenous fistula, and variations in skin temperature.

Auscultation

Stenoses and arteriovenous fistulas cause thrills or flow disturbances that can be heard well before they can be palpated. If there is no auditory clue to blood flow, this means either unrestricted normal flow or complete occlusion.

General Examination

In all patients with peripheral occlusive disease, one should search for hypertension, diabetes mellitus, hyperlipidemia, and gout. In addition, evidence of arterial functional problems in the heart, kidneys, and brain should be sought.

Functional Testing

Ratschow Test. This procedure is valuable for assessing peripheral occlusive disease of the legs. The patient lies on his back and holds his legs in an upright or vertical position. He may support his thighs, or the examiner may offer support at the heels. The foot should be flexed and extended 20–50 times over about 2 min. In the normal individual, there is no change in the skin color of the foot. In those with impaired circulation, patchy pale areas appear, most often on the sole and usually associated with pain.

Next, the patient sits up and lets his legs hang over the side of the examining table. In normal subjects, a reactive hyperemia appears in 3–5 s, followed by complete vein filling in 5–12 s, rarely requiring 20 s. In those with peripheral arterial disease, the hyperemia first appears after 20–60 s, often with cyanosis. Vein filling may require 20–180 s. False-positive results may be obtained when the patient has cold feet or marked vasoconstriction, as from nicotine. If the venous valves are incompetent, the venous refilling cannot be evaluated. False-negative results may occur with very well-compensated occlusion, such as with superb collateral vessels, and following sympathectomy. When edema or inflammation is present, the test is difficult to interpret. The same test can be done on the arms, which are held upright while the patient makes a fist many times. Later, the arms are allowed to hang at the sides.

Walking Test. The patient is asked to walk on a level surface, such as a long corridor, going 120 steps/min or one double step per second, using a metronome if needed. A treadmill can be used if available. The patient walks until pain forces him to stop. More than 200 m is normal; less than 50 m shows impaired circulation. If the walking tests are frequently repeated, as when assessing a therapy, the patient's condition may improve, producing a false-positive increase in distance that does not reflect improved perfusion.

Diagnostic Equipment

While many apparatuses are available to assess arterial flow, we mention only a few that are especially useful.

- Blood Pressure Cuff. Blood pressure can be compared between sides both on the arms and legs. If performing this test frequently, a larger cuff for use on the thigh should be obtained to minimize errors.
- Doppler Ultrasound Test. This technique allows an objective and very sensitive measurement of flow speed in the vessels. It is especially useful for identifying markedly stenosed vessels that cannot be found with palpation. Once such vessels have been located, the blood pressure over them can be measured with a cuff.
- B-Scan Ultrasound. Using this modification, one can obtain images, either cross-sectional or longitudinal, of the vessels near the skin surface. Stenoses, aneurysms, and shunts can be easily identified. When a Doppler duplex scanner is incorporated, then the direction and speed of the blood flow are presented on the monitor in a color-coded pattern.
- Oscillography. With this device one can identify the pulse curve of large and small vessels. The shape of the curve gives clues to stenoses and sclerotic changes in the vessel wall.
- Plethysmography. With this flow volume technique, one determines the blood pressure-dependent variation in volume of the body region under study. The value is given in ml/100 ml of tissue per minute. One can measure the reactive hyperemia by measuring not only the maximum volume but also the time course during refilling after an arterial block is removed.
- Thermography. The use of infrared-responsive sensors allows one to measure the surface temperature of various regions. The devices are sophisticated enough that the course of an artery can be followed simply by the slightly increased temperature in the overlying skin.
- Partial Oxygen Tension. The partial oxygen tension can be measured on the surface or in deeper tissues using a microprobe. Thus, one can document the reduced oxygen tension in the vicinity of an ulcer.
- Angiography. Visualizing the vessels following injection of contrast medium is often the definitive procedure, especially if vascular surgery is planned. With digital subtraction angiography, the contrast of the images is improved, allowing a more exact interpretation.

Arteriosclerosis

Synonym. Atherosclerosis

Definition. Arteriosclerosis or hardening of the arteries results from medial thickening secondary to smooth muscle hyperplasia as well as from intimal thickening. Usually, there is associated atherosclerosis with intimal damage and focal deposits of lipids and calcium salts.

Epidemiology. Arteriosclerosis is an inevitable consequence of aging. It is the most common cause of peripheral occlusive disease. Typically, problems begin around the age of 50 years in men and somewhat later in women. Men are affected more often, but the male predominance has decreased in recent years. Some of the risk factors include genetic predisposition, improper diet, obesity, lack of activity, stress, smoking, hypertension, diabetes mellitus, hyperlipoproteinemia (Chap. 37), and gout. Most often, several of these risk factors are present in an affected individual.

Etiology and Pathogenesis. Arteriosclerosis represents a combination of inflammatory and degenerative processes. The medial thickening is probably safely viewed as reactive. The key issue is whether elevated blood lipids can cause disease or whether there must first be another form of intimal damage. In any event, the intima suffers minor damage, and then deposition of lipids begins, forming initially fatty streaks and then plaques. Mucopolysaccharides and proteins are also deposited, eventually producing a small microthrombus on the vessel wall. This in turn may further stimulate fibrosis of the vessel wall, with subsequent calcification and blockage of the lumen. Finally, the risk of more extensive thrombosis and embolization increases.

Clinical Findings. Peripheral arteriosclerosis shows all the symptoms of increasing arterial occlusion. In the legs, the pelvic and thigh types of occlusion are more common than more distal changes. The degree of occlusion should be graded. The necrosis and gangrene in stage IV disease usually begins with marked pain in the calf or toes (Fig. 22.29). The skin is cold and either livid or very pale. Within hours to days, sharply bordered necrosis appears in a pattern determined by the distribution of the blocked vessel and its branches. If the dead tissue remains dry or mummified (dry

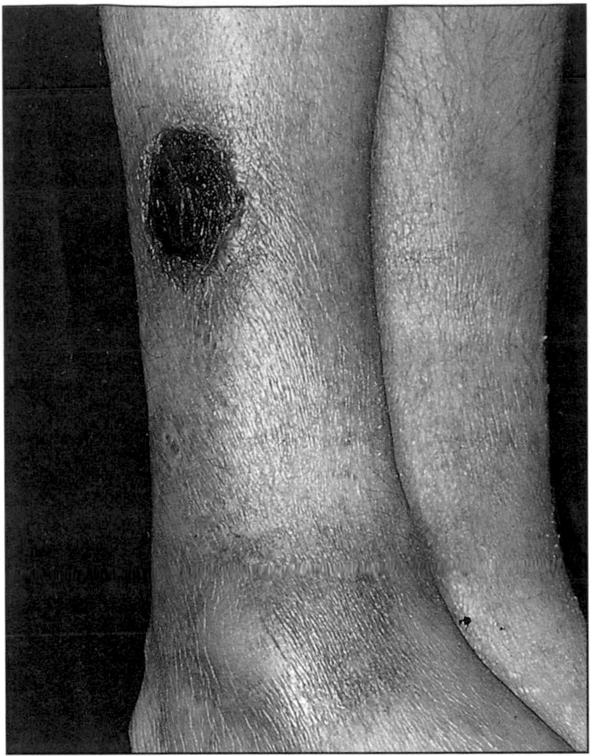

Fig. 22.29. Lividity and gangrene associated with arteriosclerotic vascular disease

gangrene), the patient is at little additional risk. If the necrosis area becomes moist (wet gangrene), this suggests secondary infection. One should search for other signs of diabetes mellitus or hyperlipidemia (xanthelasmas, xanthomas, arcus lipoides).

Histopathology. While biopsies are not done for the diagnosis, sometimes a damaged artery is found as part of a wound debridement or amputation. The arterial lumen is reduced by the lipid-rich plaques with foam cells and fibrosis. The internal elastic lamina is usually damaged, and the media is often calcified.

Laboratory Findings. The list of desired tests is long, but all of the risk factors listed above should be investigated. The blood lipid status requires special attention.

Course and Prognosis. The course is chronic and progressive, but there is considerable individual variation, depending both on therapy and success in modifying risk factors. The real prognosis is usually based on the degree of involvement of other arteries, e.g., in the heart, kidney, and CNS, rather than the severity of the skin disease, which can be viewed as a warning sign.

Differential Diagnosis. The differential diagnosis is usually limited. Thromboangiitis obliterans should be excluded, as should more disease-specific angiopathies such as those associated with diabetes mellitus and syphilis.

Therapy. The most important measure is to attempt to alleviate the various risk factors, by dietary management, increased physical activity, stopping smoking, and appropriate treatment of the underlying disease. Dermatologists must work closely with internists and vascular surgeons to assure that no important approach is overlooked. Table 22.9 summarizes our therapeutic approach.

Systemic. Depending on the stage of the disease, platelet aggregation inhibitors, vasodilators, and anticoagulants are the main options. In stage II disease, exercise may be helpful to increase the patient's physical reserve. In all stages, the patient should be encouraged to lose weight as well as engage in modest physical activity, which promotes the development of collateral vessels. The main thrust in recent years has been re-opening the occluded vessels in stages II–IV. Percutaneous transluminal angioplasty is very popular; usually a balloon is used to dilate an occluded segment and sometimes a stent is placed. Intravascular lasers can destroy the occlusion and make a new patent channel. In both cases, both aspirin and anticoagulation are used. Fibrinolytic therapy with streptokinase, urokinase, or plasminogen activator can also be employed, as is more commonly done for coronary artery disease. Elaborate stents are available for treating the larger vessels of the legs, and even the aortic bifurcation. Finally, damaged vessels can either be replaced with grafts or bypassed.

Topical. Meticulous skin care and treatment of interdigital tinea pedis are important prophylactic measures. There is no sensible way to increase arterial blood flow through application of cutaneous irritants or the like. The cutaneous vessels are usually already maximally vasodilated, and additional flow might steal blood from more vital, deeper structures.

The main goal in treating the necrosis and eventual gangrene that may result is to avoid infection by using antiseptic or antibiotic agents. The necro-

Table 22.9. Treatment of peripheral occlusive disease

Major feature Stage	Asymptomatic I	Claudication II	Pain at rest III	Necrosis IV
Treat risk factors	+	+	+	+
Treat myocardial insufficiency	+	+	+	+
Platelet aggregation inhibition (aspirin)	+	+	+	+
Increase physical activity	+	+		
Vasodilators		+		
Rheologic measures		+	+	+
Lumen-opening measures (PTA, fibrinolysis, surgery)		+	+	+
Anticoagulation (especially after PTA, surgery)	+	+	+	+
Antibiotics if suspicious of infection				+

PTA, percutaneous transluminal angioplasty

tic tissue should otherwise be left alone until the extent of damage delineates itself. The adjacent skin can be protected with a zinc oxide paste. Appropriate nursing measures help avoid development of pressure sores on already compromised skin. If erysipelas or cellulitis is suspected, cultures and systemic antibiotics should be used. Once the extent of necrosis is clear, surgical debridement or even amputation may be necessary.

Superficial Migratory Gangrene

Occasionally, a unique clinical picture develops of superficial spreading ulcerations with little tendency towards healing. The mechanism is obliteration of a cutaneous arteriole with a resultant infarct. The problem is rare, but most common in elderly women, where it occurs on the back of the foot and the shin. Exact angiologic evaluation is required to make the diagnosis. In the differential diagnosis, one must consider pyoderma gangrenosum and artifactual damage. The treatment is the same as for arteriosclerosis.

Diabetic Angiopathy

A number of vascular problems are associated with diabetes mellitus. One distinguishes between macro- and microangiopathy. The macroangiopathy is virtually the same as arteriosclerosis, but is about 10–20 times more common in diabetic patients and appears 10–20 years earlier. It usually begins peripherally and is more rapidly progressive, more widespread, and more likely to involve the arms. Medial calcification is very common. Both internal complications such as coronary artery disease and cutaneous ones such as gangrene are found more often (Fig. 22.30). Diabetic microangiopathy on the other hand features massive hyaline thickening of the basal membrane of arterioles, capillaries, and venules with endothelial cell proliferation and lumen occlusion. Because of the frequent simultaneous presence of diabetic neuropathy, the reflex control of the vascular flow is frequently impaired.

The macroangiopathy is responsible for diabetic gangrene, while the microangiopathy may be responsible for smaller acral ulcerations. Diabetic brown spots or shin spots and perhaps necrobiosis lipoidica diabeticorum may also be related

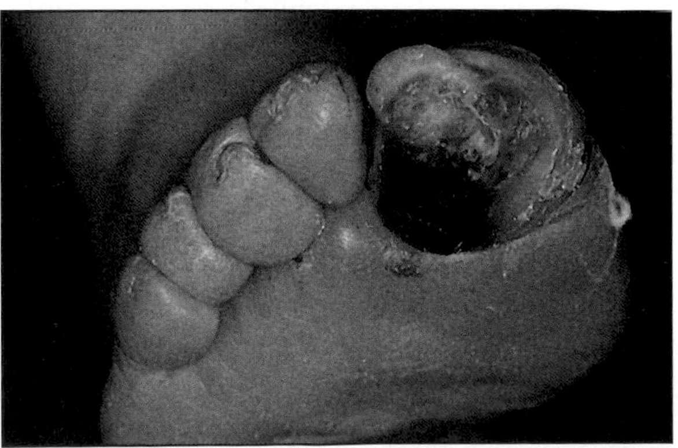

Fig. 22.30. Diabetic gangrene

to the microangiopathy. In addition, the increased incidence of bacterial and candidal infections in diabetes mellitus may be associated with the impaired vascular supply. The therapeutic approach is the same as for arteriosclerosis, combined with the need for excellent diabetic control.

Thromboangiitis Obliterans

(Friedländer 1876; von Winiwarter 1879; Buerger 1908)

Synonyms. Endangiitis obliterans, endarteritis, Buerger disease, Winiwarter-Buerger disease

Definition. Inflammatory arterial occlusive disease especially in the legs of younger men who smoke.

Epidemiology. Most patients are men between 25 and 45 years of age. Smoking is a major risk factor.

The disease is more common in Israel, eastern Europe, and the Orient.

Etiology and Pathogenesis. It is controversial whether thromboangiitis obliterans is an inflammatory or an occlusive disease, as it combines features of both. The etiology is unknown; infections, hormonal influence, cold, and genetic predisposition have all been blamed. An inflammatory endothelial lesion appears to be the trigger for the endothelial proliferation, thrombosis, and later arteriosclerosis.

Clinical Findings. The initial findings most often appear on just one leg, although later the opposite limb is usually also affected. An early sign may be superficial thrombophlebitis; in about one-third of patients erythematous macules and indurated nodules appear. These are painful, either to pressure or spontaneously, and resolve over 1–2 weeks with hyperpigmentation, while new lesions often develop simultaneously.

The first sign of beginning arterial occlusion is usually a sense of fatigue or heaviness in the leg, often combined with paresthesias or a cold feeling. Sometimes the foot appears very pale. As the degree of occlusion increases and the supply of oxygen decreases, there are a variety of symptoms, once again divided into stages I–IV and classified according to the level of occlusion. In stage III disease, in addition to pain at rest, there may be bizarre, painful erythematous lesions as well as petechiae. In stage IV disease, there are typically necrotic ulcers on the tips of the toes. The necrotic lesions can also involve the bottom of the toes, metatarsal heads, heels, back of the foot, and even calves. The necrosis can be quite extreme, so that one or more digits are lost. In more advanced disease, the arms and hands are involved in a similar fashion (Fig. 22.31). The pain is frequently very severe and relentless. In addition, sympathetic nerve activity is increased, with hyperhidrosis, coolness, and cyanosis. There may be increases in the number of dermatophyte and bacterial infections. Involvement of coronary, mesentery, and CNS arteries is extremely rare.

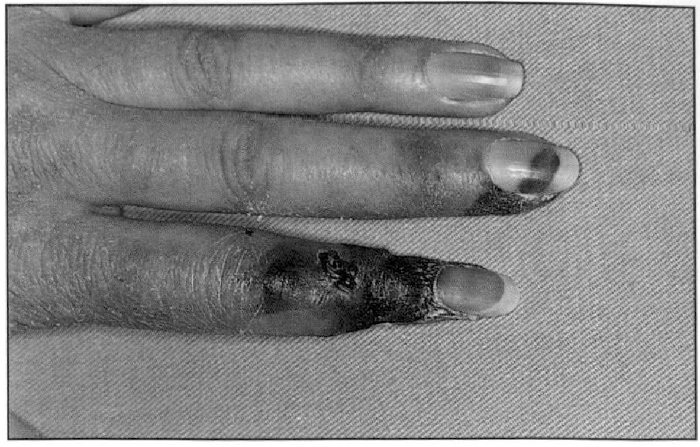

Fig. 22.31. Thromboangiitis obliterans

Histopathology. Early lesions usually show neutrophilic infiltration of an edematous arterial wall, supporting the importance of inflammation in the pathogenesis. Later there is occlusion with a mixed infiltrate, endothelial cell proliferation, thrombosis with tiny channels of recanalization, and a striking folding of the internal elastic membrane.

Laboratory Findings. No specific laboratory test is available. All of the procedures discussed above can be used to identify impaired flow, with absent pulses, pallor, decreased blood flow, and segmental occlusions. On angiography, the collateral vessels are often very tortuous or corkscrew-like, just as with diabetic collateral vessels.

Course and Prognosis. The prognosis is better than in arteriosclerosis because of the lack of cardiac and CNS involvement. Many patients lose digits and eventually require amputation of one or both legs.

Diagnostic Criteria. Since thromboangiitis obliterans is a clinical diagnosis, the following features are helpful:

- Onset before age 40 years
- Male patient
- Smoker
- Associated superficial, often migratory, thrombophlebitis

Differential Diagnosis. Arteriosclerosis is similar, but more likely to involve larger vessels and have associated internal disease. In addition, it usually becomes apparent at a later age. In Raynaud syndrome, digital ulcers may be seen, but usually the damage is less extensive. The anoretic agents fenfluramine and dexfenfluramine increase serotonin levels and may lead to pronounced digital arterial spasm and necrosis.

Therapy. The first, second, and third most important factors are stopping smoking. If the patient continues to smoke, amputations are inevitable. Avoidance of cold and minor trauma is crucial. Sympathectomy may help alleviate the residual arterial insufficiency once the patient has stopped smoking. Vasodilator therapy is unrewarding. The necrotic areas are treated by standard ulcer therapy.

Hypertensive Ulcer

(MARTORELL 1945)

Synonym. Arterial ulcer, Martorell ulcer

Etiology and Pathogenesis. This quite rare problem arises from a combination of hypertension and vessel changes. The arterioles appear to become stenotic, presumably because of the intraluminal pressure. The muscle layer becomes thicker, and there are hyaline deposits in the media. Minor trauma may play a role in initiating the ulceration.

Clinical Findings. Most patients are women, usually middle-aged. The typical location is just above the lateral malleolus, in contrast to the medial malleolus as occurs with stasis ulcers. The ulcers are usually sharply punched out and often quite large and painful. Furthermore, they are very therapy-resistant.

Differential Diagnosis. The differential diagnosis of leg ulcers is shown in Table 22.14 and discussed below, as 95% are venous ulcers.

Therapy. The main task is to control the hypertension. Standard ulcer care is adequate, once this has been accomplished. Compression therapy is not wise because of the arterial nature of the problem. Usually, nonsteroidal antiinflammatory drugs are sufficient to control the pain.

Diseases of the Veins

Diseases of the veins are a very common problem in western countries. For dermatologists, venous diseases of the legs are most important. In Germany, for example, with a population of 80 million people, about 12 million suffer from varicose veins, and about 1 million have leg ulcers as a result of this chronic venous insufficiency. Venous diseases place significant demands on workmen's compensation and the health insurance system. In the USA, chronic venous insufficiency is awkward to treat, as family physicians, internists, dermatologists, and surgeons do not have extensive training in all aspects of the problem. In Germany, chronic venous insufficiency has traditionally been a disease diagnosed and treated by specially trained dermatologists.

Basic Science Aspects

Anatomy

In the legs, the blood is returned to the heart via superficial (epifascial) and deep (subfascial) veins. The two systems are connected by perforating (transfascial) veins. The most important superficial veins are the greater and lesser saphenous veins. The greater saphenous vein drains the medial part of the dorsal venous plexus and then runs along the medial aspect of the leg from just anterior to the medial malleolus, curving gently posteriorly about the knee and then to the groin, where it penetrates the deep fascia at the saphenous opening and joins the femoral vein. In the groin, a number of veins enter the greater saphenous, forming the venous cross or star. Included in this group are the superficial epigastric vein, the superficial circumflex iliac vein, and the superficial external pudendal vein. The lesser saphenous vein drains the lateral part of the dorsal venous plexus, runs behind the lateral malleolus and then subfascially below the popliteal fossa, where it enters the popliteal vein at varying locations. The greater and lesser saphenous veins are connected by the dorsal venous plexus on the back of the foot and by a variety of connecting

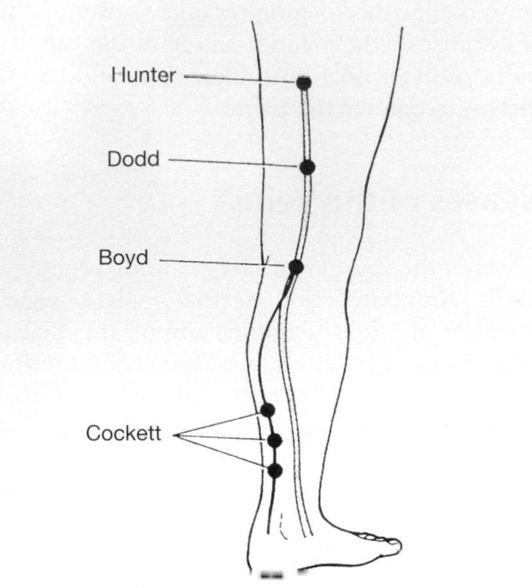

Fig. 22.32. Important perforating veins

veins. In addition, both have numerous perforating veins to the deep system.

The distal representatives of the deep system are the paired anterior and poster tibial veins and the fibular veins, which join the popliteal and the superficial femoral veins, then later the deep femoral vein. These deep veins are intramuscular and run parallel to arteries of the same name. On the calf, the most important intramuscular veins are the gastrocnemii and solei veins. All these veins along with their surrounding musculature are supported by the fascia lata or fascia cruris.

Some of the perforating veins are of such clinical importance that they have specific names (Fig. 22.32). The Cockett veins connect the posterior arcuate vein (a branch of the greater saphenous vein) with the posterior tibial vein. The Boyd, Dodd, and Hunter veins connect the greater saphenous vein with the deep veins.

Physiology

The veins are part of a low pressure system. Their main role is to return blood to the heart. In addition, the venous tone or volume helps modulate the functional blood volume. There are a number of forces driving the blood back to the heart. When contraction occurs, a suction pressure is applied to the venous system. In addition, the movement of the diaphragm produces a two-phase pump mechanism. Both of these systems are only effective in the thorax and possibly, to a limited extent, in the abdomen.

In the legs, the veins have a pressure of 15 mm Hg when the patient is prone and 90 mm Hg when upright. This pressure gradient is overcome by the muscle-joint pumping system. The contraction of the leg muscles squeezes the inter- and intramuscular deep veins and the perforating veins. If the venous valves are intact, this creates a unidirectional flow in the direction of the heart. When the muscle relaxes, the vein is opened and exerts a distal suction effect. As one walks, this combination of squeezing and sucking advances the blood centrally.

Around the joints, the effects are more complex. The veins are connected to the adjacent tendons and fascia so that when the joint bends, the vein is opened up, increasing its cross-sectional area and once again exerting a suction action. This typing of pumping plays a key role in the dorsal venous plexus and the small saphenous vein. The great saphenous vein has few fascial connections and is drained primarily through perforating veins. While all the muscles work together, the main pumping action comes from the contraction of the calf muscles and the movement of the ankle joint.

Diagnostic Procedures

History

The following points are important in the patient's history: other family members with venous disease, pregnancies, use of oral contraceptives, occupation (prolonged standing), previous thromboses, operations, prolonged immobilization, and anticoagulant therapy. With regard to the current problem, one should inquire about symptoms (tightness, fullness, cramps, restless legs, pain), increasing difficulties with warm weather, with prolonged standing or sitting, and with menses, and if the feet become more swollen toward evening.

Inspection

The nature of existing varicosities, the presence of trophic skin changes (loss of hair, smooth or dry skin), pigmentary changes, and ulcerations should be documented. It is easiest to assess the veins when the patient is standing on a small platform. The presence of stasis dermatitis, hyperpigmentation (usually red-brown from pigmented purpura), dermatosclerosis, atrophie blanche, ulcers, and scars all suggest chronic venous insufficiency. Thus, these features usually reflect valvular insufficiency in either the superficial, deep, or perforating systems. Unilateral changes such as increased circumference, increased venous markings, increased warmth, or suprapubic varicosities all suggest a thrombosis or postthrombotic state. One should also pay attention to skeletal deformities and impaired motion or use of joints.

Palpation

By touching the skin, one can estimate the skin temperature, assess the presence and degree of edema, and identify fascial holes when the perforating veins are incompetent. Firm, painful cords or bands suggest thrombophlebitis, while tender pressure points hint at phlebothrombosis. In addition, the induration of dermatosclerosis may be a sign of chronic venous insufficiency.

Functional Testing

The century-old classic tests of Trendelenburg to identify reflux in the great saphenous vein or its perforating veins and of Perthes to assess the patency of the deep veins are not reliable enough to be used primarily. They offer a quick orientation but must be confirmed with the various techniques discussed below.

Diagnostic Equipment

Doppler Ultrasound

Doppler ultrasound is a rapid, reliable, noninvasive method of evaluating veins. A pencil-thick sound head sends out continuous sound waves at 4 or 8 MHz. These waves cannot be heard by the human ear. By using a contact gel, the sound head can be placed on the skin, and the waves pass through the skin into the blood vessels where they are reflected by erythrocytes. The reflection leads to a change in frequency (Doppler principle); the reflected waves are taken up by the receiver in the sound head and then presented either as audible sound waves or in a graphic display. The frequency of the sound tone correlates with the speed of blood flow in the vessel. The venous Doppler signal is low frequency and varies with respiration, while the arterial signal is high frequency. Some devices only measure the speed of flow (unilateral Doppler); others are also able to indicate the direction (bidirectional Doppler). A-mode ultrasound presents the echo signals as waves of varying amplitude, much like an ECG or oscilloscope picture. By contrast, B (brightness)-mode ultrasound produces images.

Doppler ultrasound can be used to evaluate the following:

- Valve function in the superficial, deep, or perforating veins.
- Start- and end-point of the pathologic venous reflux.
- Presence of thigh or pelvic thrombosis when a larger vein is involved; smaller thrombi are difficult to find.

Diagnosis of Superficial Venous Reflux

Greater Saphenous Vein. The sound head is placed over the saphenous opening where the multiple veins enter, and the standing patient is asked to perform a Valsalva maneuver. In a healthy person, there is no sound, as the flow stops. In someone with valve insufficiency, there is a retrograde noise. The sound head is then moved distally to determine the extent of the venous insufficiency.

Lesser Saphenous Vein. The head is placed over the vein in its epifascial location in the popliteal region or on the outer posterior aspect of the calf. Then the Valsalva maneuver is induced, or compression is applied to the inferior aspect of the popliteal space or the calf muscles. Loud retrograde signals indicate insufficient valves.

Perforating Veins. The head is placed over the fascial gap, which has been identified by palpation. The veins above and below are compressed with tourniquets or the periphery is compressed with a rubber ring. When the patient moves his foot, or when the distal muscles are compressed, a sound is heard as regurgitation from the deep to superficial veins occurs because of incompetent valves.

Diagnosis of Deep Venous Reflux. Insufficiency of the deep accompanying veins in the calf can be identified by compressing the adjacent muscles. If one presses proximally, nothing should be heard, while on relaxation there is a normal tone as physiologic drainage occurs. If compression is applied distally, the normal flow tones are increased; when compression ceases, the sounds should also cease. If regurgitation is heard, the valves are defective.

The paired posterior tibial calf veins are found about the medial aspect of the ankle adjacent to the comparable artery. When the calf is compressed, reflux can be heard as a marker for incompetent valves. In the popliteal space, the vein is lateral to the artery. Either compression of the thigh or decompression of the calf can elicit the sound of reflux. The superficial femoral vein can be found in the area of the adductor canal, while the common femoral vein lies in the inguinal fold. Either the Valsalva maneuver or compression of the distal third of the thigh can be used to test valve patency.

Diagnosis of Thrombosis. In the case of pelvic vein thrombosis, the flow signals in the inguinal region are no longer discontinuous, i.e., they no longer vary with respiration. As an expression of the increased venous pressure distal to the thrombosis, they have a higher frequency and are continuous. The Valsalva maneuver produces no stoppage. When the thrombosis is in the thigh, then similar changes in the flow signal can be heard over the popliteal fossa.

Collateral veins may offer spontaneous sounds, often called S-sounds, which are not increased by the compression of distal veins. If the thrombosis lies between the site of compression and the sound head, then the compression will also not produce any increase in flow sounds (A-sounds). Doppler ultrasound is not very effective in evaluating the calf. The presence of three veins with frequent opportunities for connections leads to weak sounds that are difficult to evaluate. While Doppler ultrasound is very specific in diagnosing reflux, it is only suggestive in the case of thrombosis. This diagnosis should be confirmed by duplex sonography or phlebography.

Light Reflection Rheography

This noninvasive electronic-optical technique is also known as photoplethysmography. Infrared radiation is directed into the skin and its reflection measured. Since filled vessels reflect less radiation than empty ones, the brightness of the measuring field decreases as the vessel fills.

The usual place for measurement is just above the medial malleolus. The seated patient flexes and extends the foot ten times; this empties not only the deep and superficial veins but also the venous plexus of the skin, which connects with the deep veins via subcutaneous collecting veins and perforating veins. A reduction in venous pressure correlates in an almost linear fashion with the reduction in volume and reduced vessel surface area. Using a computer program, the light reflection rheographic curve can be analyzed to show the maximum reflection difference as a measure of venous drainage and the venous filling time. This is the time needed to refill the plexus after the exercise is stopped. In healthy patients, this is achieved via the arteries, capillaries, and venules, while in patients with incompetent venous valves, retrograde filling occurs. In healthy individuals, the filling time is greater than 25 s; the shorter it is, the greater the venous insufficiency. This technique has also become standard and widely employed. In contrast to Doppler ultrasound, it provides information about the global function of the venous system, rather than about one vein.

Phlebodynamometry

In this procedure, the venous pressure is directly measured. A vein is punctured on the dorsal surface of the foot. A pressure sensor then measures the true venous pressure during a prescribed set of motions (knee bends, standing on tiptoes). The loss in pressure with activity in healthy patients is about 60 mmHg; this parameter as well as the refill time provide insight into the effectiveness of the muscle-joint pump. While this is the most exact procedure, it is painful and has several complications (such as hematoma and phlebitis), so it is not routinely employed.

Impedance Plethysmography

A tourniquet is applied to the thigh to produce venous blockage. An expandable measurement band on the calf is used to measure the increase in volume (in ml/100 ml tissue) and, once the obstruction is removed, the loss of the volume (in ml/100 ml tissue per min). This procedure is not very reproducible but gives information about the venous capacity of the lower part of the leg, venous back flow, venous elasticity, and the capillary filtration rate.

Phlebography

In addition to all these functional tests, morphologic information such as provided by phlebography is also very important. Such studies are indicated prior to surgery when an exact diagnosis cannot be made with the other techniques, for example, when dealing with venous malformations, arteriovenous fistulas, and the postthrombotic syndrome. Furthermore, phlebography is, together with Duplex sonography, the standard method for diagnosing deep vein thrombosis. In ascending phlebography, the contrast medium is injected into a dorsal foot vein after compression above the ankle has insured that superficial epifascial drainage is blocked. When the patient performs a Valsalva maneuver, the contrast medium will be forced back into the superficial system at the major junction in the groin, in the popliteal fossa, or via perforating veins if there is valve insufficiency. In this way, both the functional dynamics and morphology can be studied.

Contraindications to phlebography include contrast medium allergy, major illnesses especially involving the thyroid and kidneys, severe lymphedema, and advanced peripheral arteriosclerosis. Pregnancy is a relative contraindication. In addition, the study should not be performed unless the results promise to offer therapeutic direction or are required for medical-legal reasons. The main complications are allergic and toxic reactions to the contrast medium, as well as thrombophlebitis.

Duplex Sonography

Here an image-forming system using B-mode ultrasound in real time technique is combined with simultaneous Doppler evaluation and usually enhanced with color coding. In a noninvasive manner, flow direction, volume, and speed can be determined, while the vein volume, wall, valves, and surrounding tissue are visualized. In many instances, there is no longer a need for phlebography. Despite the high cost of the equipment, duplex sonography has won wide acceptance in recent years.

Varicosities

Synonym. Varicose veins

Definition. Veins, most often in the legs, that are widened either in a hose-like or more focal pattern and also elongated so that they run in a convoluted pattern.

Epidemiology. Varicose veins are especially common in industrialized countries. In a study in Basel, Switzerland, 9% of adults had medically relevant varicosities, while 3–4% had conditions requiring treatment. The prevalence of varicosities increased linearly with age; in 70-year-old individuals, they were ten times more common than in 35-year-olds. Other studies have shown even higher figures. A study in Tübingen, Germany, found that 15% of individuals have clinically relevant varicosities, while another university dermatology clinic series identified problems in 50% of a group of randomly chosen patients. Their problems were classified as 25% mild, 10% moderate, and 15% severe. Women are twice as likely as men to have varicosities of the legs.

Etiology and Pathogenesis

Primary Varicosities. Age, familial predisposition, and hormonal factors (female, multiple pregnancies, oral contraceptives) play a major role. Alterations in the vessel wall lead to a loss of contractile elements and an increase in connective tissue, so that the veins are dilated, and the valves become incompetent. Primary varicosities usually appear around age 20 years and in the area of the great saphenous vein. The visually thickened, snake-like or coiled veins usually appear before valvular defects do in the proximal termination of the vein. Later the valvular problems spread distally. Increased intraabdominal pressure generates retrograde pressure pulses that hasten the process.

Varicosities in Pregnancy. About one-third of women develop varicosities during their first pregnancy; with multiple pregnancies, the number increases to about two-thirds. In addition to the typical lesions on the legs, vulvar, suprapubic, and even vaginal varicosities may appear. The main factors appear to be genetic predisposition and the increased intraabdominal pressure with blocked venous return. Many of the enlarged veins improve following delivery.

Secondary Varicosities. Vascular malformations such as absent or inadequate valves, arteriovenous fistulas, or more massive changes such as seen in Klippel-Trénaunay-Weber syndrome can also lead to varicosities. The most common cause of secondary varicosities is deep vein thrombosis. They can also develop following acute venous obstruction, e.g., from extravascular compression, or as part of the postthrombotic syndrome. Here, there is recanalization of veins, but the valve function is impaired. The muscle pump thus forces blood in both directions, raising pressure in the deep system, so that the blood is forced through the perforating veins into the superficial system. The superficial veins are dilated and then also develop valvular problems. Patients with primary varicosities are more likely to develop thrombophlebitis or phlebothrombosis, so combinations are likely.

Clinical Findings. The individual veins are both dilated and elongated. They are most apparent in the superficial cutaneous branches of the leg, but any vein can be involved (Fig. 22.33). Table 22.10 shows the most commonly affected leg veins. Varicosities of the superficial and perforating veins can be diagnosed by inspection and palpation, while the deeper veins must be assessed with Doppler ultrasound and other techniques. The degree of insufficiency can be estimated as shown in Table 22.11. Initially, varicosities are a cosmetic problem but asymptomatic. Some patients develop a heavy or tense feeling in their legs and may have edema in the evening. Spider veins are nearly always asymptomatic.

Course and Prognosis. Varicosities continue to worsen as one ages. Most patients wind up with chronic venous insufficiency. Thus, early treatment to control the proximal insufficiency before distal damage occurs is wise. Similarly, sections of the venous system that are no longer functional can often be removed.

Following often minor trauma, there may be extensive bleeding from a damaged superficial varicosity. In patients whose judgment is impaired, such as someone who is drunk and stumbles, fatal bleeds have been reported. The extremity should be elevated and a pressure dressing applied. In some instances, it is necessary to tie off a vein under local anesthesia. Once the acute event is resolved, the problem should be addressed with sclerotherapy or surgery.

Therapy. Compression stockings or dressings can be employed in very early cases. Class I compression stockings should be worn by all pregnant

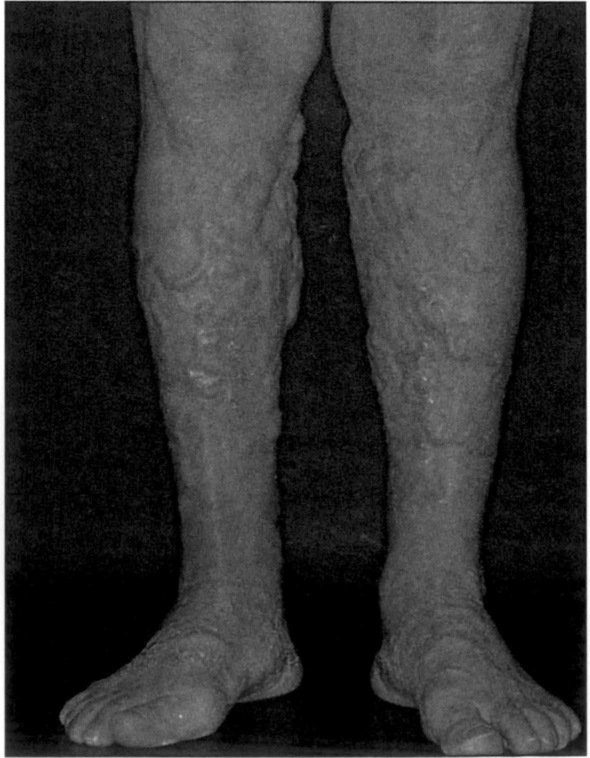

Fig. 22.33. Multiple varicose veins

Table 22.10. Varicosities of the legs

Superficial system

Subcutaneous

Major trunks – greater saphenous vein, lesser saphenous vein

Branches – medial and lateral accessory veins, anterior and posterior arcuate veins

Reticular varicosities – net-like venous proliferations without connections to major veins

Intradermal

Spider veins – enlarged small veins usually on thigh and side of the foot

Perforating system

The perforating veins mentioned under anatomic considerations are those most likely to be affected.

Deep system

Dilated deep veins not clinically apparent but can be detected with various noninvasive techniques

Table 22.11. Insufficiency of major superficial veins (Hach classification)

Greater saphenous vein	
Stage I	Insufficiency in inguinal region
Stage II	Reflux to above the knee
Stage III	Reflux past the knee
Stage IV	Reflux to medial malleolus
Lesser saphenous vein	
Stage I	Insufficiency at junction with popliteal vein
Stage II	Reflux to mid-calf
Stage III	Reflux to lateral malleolus

women. Those with vein problems or symptoms should use class II stockings. In general, invasive approaches are more appropriate in young patients to avoid chronic venous insufficiency. The preoperative evaluation, as discussed under the various techniques, is crucial to determine patency of the deep system and identify incompetent superficial segments and perforating veins. Some patients with early varicosities have no abnormalities of the collecting system. Treatment is discussed in more detail later in the chapter, but sclerotherapy or operations such as vein stripping, tying off perforating veins and ligating the saphenous vein at the saphenous opening are all useful.

Thrombophlebitis

Superficial Thrombophlebitis

Definition. Acute focal inflammation of the vein wall (phlebitis) and adjacent tissue (periphlebitis) often with thrombus formation and partial or complete occlusion. When the process occurs in a varicosity, one speaks of varicophlebitis. In German, the term phlebothrombosis is used in place of deep vein thrombosis. One avoids the argument about which came first – the inflammation (thrombophlebitis) or the clot (phlebothrombosis).

Epidemiology. The incidence of thrombophlebitis is around 1%. While only 2% of 20-year-old individuals have suffered thrombophlebitis, about 25% of 70-year-old persons have.

Etiology and Pathogenesis. The Virchow triad of vessel wall damage, reduced flow rate, and increased likelihood of clotting still summarizes the risk factors well. In addition, local factors such as trauma, arthropod bite reaction, injection of irritant medications, or incorrect injection of almost anything, infiltration of an intravenous line or catheter, and any localized intense inflammation can play a role. There are other risk factors such as prolonged immobilization, underlying malignancies, pancreatic disease, and immunologic diseases.

Clinical Findings. One can identify a painful, localized, often linear erythema and swelling about a vein. In some instances, the vessel feels like a tender cord (Fig. 22.34). Apart from pain, there are few systemic findings. In rare instances, in patients with particularly severe disease or secondary infection, there may be fever, elevated erythrocyte sedimentation rate, and leukocytosis. After the acute changes resolve, the skin may remain hyperpigmented over an indurated, scarred, often occluded or incompetent vein (phlebosclerosis).

Histopathology. The vein wall is loaded with inflammatory cells, while the lumen shows a thrombus. In later stages, the thrombus may show varying degrees of canalization, fibrosis, and calcification.

Course and Prognosis. The outlook is generally good, especially with appropriate therapy. Usually, resolution occurs over days to weeks. In rare cases, the area can ulcerate; around the ankle, there is a sudden or postphlebitis ulcer. Occasionally, there is bacterial secondary infection and then sepsis. Only under extremely rare circumstances, as when the thrombus involves the greater saphenous vein just before it joins the femoral vein, is there any risk of embolization.

Therapy

Systemic. Low-dose heparin is often employed, primarily to reduce the risk of spread to deep veins.

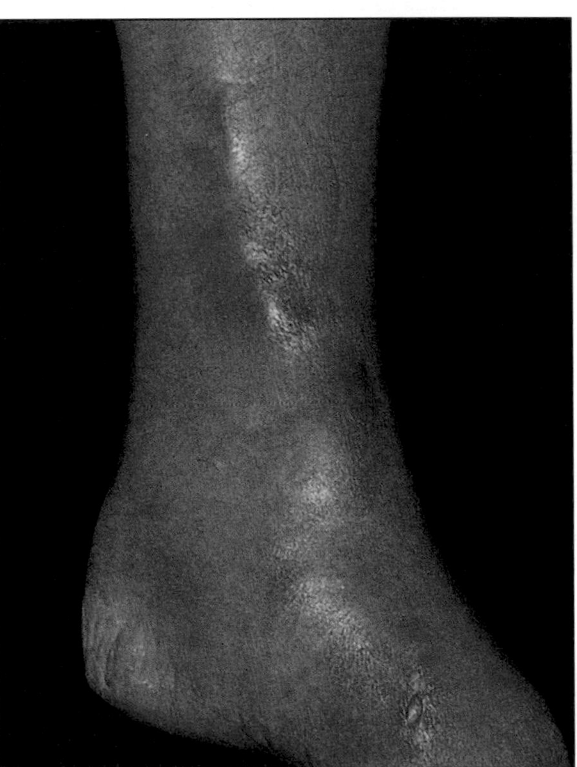

Fig. 22.34. Superficial thrombophlebitis

When the thrombus is located in the greater saphenous vein in the groin, some surgeons prefer to excise the thrombus, while others recommend higher doses of heparin. Aspirin or nonsteroidal antiinflammatory drugs can be given for pain relief. Antibiotics are only prescribed if an infection has been documented.

Topical. The most important measures are a firm compression bandage and mobilization. The bandage fixes the thrombus, while the physical activity increases the muscle-joint pump action and speeds up blood flow. When such patients are kept in bed, the tiny risk of more extensive thrombus formation and embolization is increased. Sometimes the clot can be expressed from the vein via a small incision; this often brings quicker relief. Cold packs may also bring relief. In Europe, topical heparin creams and gels are sometimes employed; data supporting their effectiveness are minimal.

Superficial Migratory Thrombophlebitis

Synonyms. Thrombophlebitis migrans, thrombophlebitis saltans

Definition. Recurrent thrombophlebitis at different locations often as a sign of underlying disease.

Epidemiology. Men are more often affected than women; most patients are young or middle-aged adults.

Etiology and Pathogenesis. The etiology is unknown. Sometimes there is an association with thromboangiitis obliterans or the diseases usually associated with deep vein thrombosis. In other instances, there may be an underlying malignancy, such as carcinoma (most often pancreas, lung, prostate), lymphoma or leukemia, or systemic diseases such as Behçet syndrome.

Clinical Findings. The most common location is the extensor surface of the legs. The typical inflamed, cord-like lesions appear over a long period of time in various, sometimes interconnected, veins. The patient is symptom-free except for pain and occasional fever. Although the individual lesions heal over 2–3 weeks, the course is chronic. Sometimes there may be spontaneous remission, while in other cases the thrombophlebitis follows the course of the underlying disease.

Differential Diagnosis. Because of the frequent localization on the legs, both erythema nodosum and panniculitis come into consideration. Histology is definitive.

Therapy. The main goal is to find or exclude underlying disorders. Treatment is the same as for ordinary thrombophlebitis.

Superficial Sclerosing Phlebitis
(Favre 1929; Mondor 1939)

Synonyms. Mondor disease, phlébite en fil de fer

Definition. Superficial phlebitis that produces a firm cord with relatively little secondary change.

Etiology and Pathogenesis. This uncommon disorder remains a mystery. Trauma, surgery, ionizing radiation, adjacent infections, and many other factors have been considered.

Clinical Findings. The most common variant is Mondor disease, which is more common in women (3:1) than men and involves the lateral thoracic vein. There is a firm linear subcutaneous cord, often as thick as a knitting needle or pencil, that runs along the edge of the ribs. The overlying skin is normal. If the patient raises his arms, the changes are easier to see. Rarely, there may be multiple or bilateral lesions, involvement of the thoracogastric or superficial epigastric veins, or involvement of smaller branches of the main vein. There is often a sharp localized pain that can be mistaken initially for cardiac or intraabdominal disease. Resolution is spontaneous in a matter of weeks; sometimes the skin may become puckered for a short time, causing concern when the breast is involved. Other locations are less common, but any superficial vein can be affected. Sclerosing phlebitis of the penis (Chap. 34) is another variant. The arms, legs, and neck veins may show similar changes.

Therapy. If pain is significant, nonsteroidal antiinflammatory drugs can be used. Topical therapy is not needed.

Deep Vein Thrombosis

Synonyms. Deep thrombophlebitis, thrombophlebitis profunda, phlebothrombosis, venous thrombosis

Table 22.12. Risk factors for venous thrombosis

Bed rest for more than several days
Major surgery within past 4 weeks, especially of the femur, prostate, abdomen
Paralysis or immobilization of a leg or foot
Pregnancy
Oral contraceptives
Advanced age
Active cancer
Trauma to leg
Heart failure
Autoimmune diseases
Family history of deep vein thrombosis
Hypercoagulability disorders

Definition. Thrombosis of deep veins, often of the pelvic region or legs, with risk of pulmonary embolism.

Epidemiology. Deep vein thrombosis is a common disorder that is a major cause of morbidity and death in hospitalized patients. The major risk factors are shown in Table 22.12. These risk factors should not provide false reassurance. In most cases, deep vein thrombosis is unexplained or associated with generally harmless activities such as prolonged sitting in an airplane (economy class syndrome) or even strenuous physical activity. A recent study confirmed the increased incidence of deep vein thrombosis in cancer patients, but did not find that blind searching for internal malignancies in patients with an individual thrombus was fruitful. Patients with varicosities and superficial thrombophlebitis are also at greater risk. Studies have shown thrombi in the legs of about 50 % of patients following hip or prostate surgery; most remain subclinical, but this value indicates the magnitude of the problem. Sometimes the deep vein thrombosis is first suggested by a pulmonary embolism.

Etiology and Pathogenesis. Once again the Virchow triad – vessel wall damage, reduced flow, and abnormal clotting – is important. In the case of deep vein thrombosis, the presence of the hypercoagulable state assumes even greater importance (Table 22.13). When deep vein thrombosis occurs in a young individual, is recurrent or associated with a positive family history, then the presence of one of these defects becomes more likely.

Trousseau sign refers to the association between deep vein thrombosis and an underlying malignancy. Many mechanisms are possible, including invasion of the vessel wall by tumor cells, compression of a vessel, and the hypercoagulable state. Almost all tumor patients have some evidence of activation of their coagulation system, even though only a few have problems. A recent Danish study showed that deep vein thrombosis may precede clinical diagnosis of the cancer but did not endorse blind screening, simply a careful history and clinical examination. Often there are complex interactions. For example, following surgery both platelets and prothrombin levels are elevated; during pregnancy, factor V, prothrombin, and fibrinogen may be elevated; and infections and myocardial infarcts are associated with raised fibrinogen levels.

Clinical Findings. There are few serious disorders whose clinical diagnosis is so inexact. In recent years, a variety of objective diagnostic measures have become routine and must be employed because of the dangers involved when a deep vein thrombosis is overlooked. In active patients, there may be sudden clinical findings that suggest the diagnosis. The typical triad is pain, cyanosis, and edema, but sometimes there are no clinical signs. In incapacitated, bed-ridden individuals, the changes are often minimal or overlooked, so that the diagnosis is first made when pulmonary embolism develops. Early signs may include pain in the calf or sole or a heavy sensation in the leg. The leg pain is usually worse when the leg is dependent, when walking or even when coughing. Dilated superficial veins may be present (Pratt warning veins). On palpation, the involved leg is thicker, may have pitting edema, and occasionally tenderness can be identified over the affected deep vein. The thighs and calves should be measured. A 3 cm difference in circumference, measured 10 cm below the tibial tuberosity, suggests a deep vein thrombosis on the larger side. Assessment of the thighs is not as

Table 22.13. Major causes of hypercoagulability

Protein S and protein C deficiencies
Factor V mutation (Leiden)
Antithrombin III deficiency
Prothrombin mutation
Increased factor VIII levels
Structural defects in fibrinogen, plasminogen
Antiphospholipid syndrome (lupus anticoagulant, anticardiolipin antibody)
Homocystinuria
Malignancy (Trousseau sign)
Medications (especially oral contraceptives)

standardized. In more advanced lesions, there may be fever, chills, and tachycardia.

A number of pain provocation tests are routinely employed, but are fraught with false-positive and false-negative results.

- Payr sign: Marked tenderness of the sole.
- Homan sign: Dorsal flexion of the foot causes pain in the calf.
- Sigg sign: Hyperextension of the knee causes pain in the popliteal fossa.
- Lowenberg test. A blood pressure cuff is applied to each calf and inflated until painful. A difference of 20 mmHg between the two sides suggests a deep vein thrombosis.

The most feared complication is a pulmonary embolism. Most pulmonary emboli arise from thromboses in the iliofemoral or pelvic veins. Their clinical features are very nonspecific; in extreme cases, patients may be asymptomatic or die suddenly. Common symptoms include restlessness, anxiety, fever, shortness of breath, cough, chest pain, and impaired respiratory motion. Signs may include tachycardia, tachypnea, and inspiratory rales. One cannot separate pulmonary embolism and the underlying deep vein thrombosis; they should be approached as a diagnostic unit.

There are also a number of late complications, often grouped together as the postthrombotic syndrome. They include secondary varicosities, chronic venous insufficiency, stasis ulcers, and other problems discussed below.

Diagnostic Criteria. The clinical diagnosis of both deep vein thrombosis and pulmonary embolism is usually incorrect. Continuous wave (CW)-Doppler and compression duplex sonography of the femoral and popliteal veins form the most effective approach, being highly sensitive (>90%) in diagnosing the more dangerous popliteal or femoral vein problems. These methods are less sensitive for calf vein thrombosis. Other diagnostic tools include impedance plethysmography and other objective noninvasive tests as well as measurement of plasma D-dimer (a fibrin-specific substance) levels. Phlebography may be needed if the clinical findings and noninvasive tests are contradictory. If a pulmonary embolism is suspected, the standard approaches include ventilation-perfusion lung scans and then pulmonary angiography if questions still exist.

Differential Diagnosis. Other causes of edema, lymphatic problems, lipedema, erysipelas, cellulitis, and muscle injuries should all be considered.

Therapy. Such patients are usually treated by internists. In some situations, the patient may be hospitalized on a dermatology service so that the treatment is provided in consultation.

The mainstay is anticoagulation, initially with heparin and then with coumarin. In Germany, low-molecular-weight heparin has all but replaced unfractionated heparin. It is easier to use, safer, and just as efficacious in treating deep vein thrombosis. In pregnancy, coumarin cannot be used. Other contraindications for anticoagulation are relative but include advanced age, hypertension with systolic levels above 200 mm Hg, bleeding disorders, and gastrointestinal ulcers. Administration in the immediate postoperative period is a very difficult decision, to be made in consultation with the surgeon.

When extensive proximal vein thrombosis or pulmonary embolism is identified, thrombolytic therapy with streptokinase or urokinase may be considered. If the patient has active bleeding, a high risk of bleeding or cannot receive heparin, then an inferior vena cava filter of some type is usually inserted. On some occasions, the thrombus can be removed surgically with a catheter; this is especially helpful for fresh iliofemoral thrombi.

Calf vein thromboses present a difficult management decision. In most cases, they are small, self-limited and resolve spontaneously. Many protocols recommend following patients with suspected deep vein thrombosis of the calf for several weeks with repeat ultrasound to identify the 15–20% in whom the thromboses extend into the proximal veins. Others feel that anticoagulation is the better approach.

The duration of anticoagulant therapy is also confusing. In a patient with no risk factors, 3 months is recommended. A recent large study showed that patients treated for 1 year or longer had fewer recurrences. If a correctable risk factor is present, treatment should be continued until the risk is resolved. In pregnancy, heparin is used until delivery and then coumarin is administered for 4–6 weeks postpartum. Patients with a malignancy, an underlying defect, or recurrent disease require long-term therapy; some clinicians suggest treating for 1 year and then observing; others recommend life-long treatment because of the mortality associated with pulmonary embolism. In addition, treatment may reduce the risk of the post-thrombotic syndrome.

Complications of therapy include bleeding, lack of effectiveness, heparin-induced thrombocytopenia, heparin-induced osteoporosis (especially in pregnancy), and both coumarin- and, rarely, heparin-induced skin necrosis (Chap. 10).

Prophylaxis. Clearly, avoidance is the best approach. For this reason, patients are encouraged to ambulate as soon as possible following operations and wear compression stockings. When ambulation is impossible, physical therapy exercise programs in bed can be arranged. High-risk patients, such as those undergoing hip surgery, are usually anticoagulated prophylactically, most often with low-molecular-weight heparin.

Diseases Associated with Hypercoagulability

There are a number of diseases associated with increased coagulability. They are of importance not just in thromboses but also in disseminated intravascular coagulation (Chap. 23) and its related disorders. There is a striking vascular bed variation in the type of thromboses associated with different defects. Apparently, vessels in various locations release different signaling patterns, so that one defect may cause leg vein thromboses and the other, cerebral thromboses. All may also cause adverse outcomes of pregnancy, such as preeclampsia, abruptio placentae, severe growth retardation, or intrauterine fetal death.

Antiphospholipid Syndrome

This syndrome is often associated with lupus erythematosus and is discussed in Chapter 18. Briefly, antiphospholipid antibodies are anticoagulants in vitro, prolonging several hemostatic parameters but clinically leading to thromboses. The cause of the hypercoagulability is unclear.

Antithrombin III Deficiency

This essential modulator of hemostasis inactivates thrombin and activated procoagulant factors. Its deficiency may be hereditary or acquired. Most patients are heterozygous for the genetic defect but have only modest reductions in antithrombin III. They typically present with mesenteric vein thrombosis in adult life and have more trouble during pregnancy and when taking oral contraceptives. Most affected adults are asymptomatic but may have trouble if they undergo abdominal surgery. Patients who are homozygous are more likely to have arterial thromboses. Acquired antithrombin III deficiency may result from heparin usage, in disseminated intravascular coagulation, and in a variety of other settings. Prophylactic treatment is with coumarin, while acute thromboses are treated with heparin and replacement of antithrombin III.

Protein C and Protein S Deficiency

Protein S and protein C combine forces to maintain adequate fibrinolysis. Homozygous protein C deficiency causes fatal purpura fulminans in infancy (Chap. 23). Heterozygotes are relatively common, with a prevalence of about 1:300 in western populations. Some are asymptomatic but others have an increased number of deep vein thromboses, often appearing at an early age without clear triggers. Cutaneous necrosis with coumarin therapy is also related to protein C. Coumarin inhibits protein C production much more rapidly than the hepatic coagulation factors, so a period of hypercoagulability occurs. Protein S deficiency is also usually inherited in an autosomal dominant pattern, and patients are at risk for deep vein thrombosis. Rare patients with two abnormal protein S genes probably have a course similar to homozygous protein C deficiency.

Factor V Mutation

Mutations in factor V may lead to a resistance to inactivation by proteins C and S and subsequent hypercoagulability. The most common mutation is known as the Leiden mutation (G1691A) and is a significant factor in western European populations. Here, too, increased arterial and venous thromboses are common, including cerebral and coronary thromboses.

Prothrombin Gene Mutation

A very specific mutation (G20210A) in the 3′ untranslated region of the prothrombin (factor II) gene is the second most common genetic determinant of deep vein thrombosis of the legs, ranking only behind factor V mutation. Prothrombin is converted to thrombin by factor X and then converts fibrinogen to fibrin. The mutation leads to higher plasma concentrations of prothrombin, presumably because of reduced breakdown. The defect is inherited in an autosomal dominant pattern and leads to increased arterial and venous thromboses, including coronary and cerebral thromboses.

Homocystinuria

Patients with homocystinuria (Chap. 39) have long been known to have an increased incidence of thromboses. The mechanisms involve vascular wall damage and impaired protein C activation. While the homozygous disease is uncommon, many individuals, perhaps up to 1–2% of the general population, have only one defective gene. Although they are referred to in formal genetics as carriers, these persons have an increased risk of thromboembolic disease.

Chronic Venous Insufficiency

Definition. Skin changes on the legs that appear secondary to impaired venous flow. In the USA, stasis is used as an imprecise equivalent term.

Epidemiology. In Germany, chronic venous insufficiency is very common, affecting more than 5 million individuals (7–10% of the total population). Over 1 million have a stasis ulcer. The problem is more common in women, presumably because of pregnancies and oral contraceptives.

Etiology and Pathogenesis. Chronic venous insufficiency can develop from incompetent superficial, deep, or perforating veins. It may be associated with primary or secondary varicosities. The postthrombotic syndrome is also associated with this problem.

The incompetent veins lead to pathologic reflux, with increased blood volume and pressure in the veins of the calves. Capillary dilation results, with leakage between the endothelial cells, which are forced apart. Fluids, erythrocytes, and protein are all deposited in the interstitial tissue. The leakage causes edema, and the erythrocytes lead to a variety of color changes. The foreign substances trigger the fibroblasts towards increased collagen synthesis, producing dermatosclerosis (also known as dermatoliposclerosis). In these sclerotic areas, the microcirculation is impaired, with tortuous vessels and occlusion producing atrophie blanche. The leakage of fibrinogen coupled with disturbed fibrinolysis results in pericapillary fibrin cuffs. Both the sclerosis and the fibrin cuffs impede the diffusion of oxygen into the tissue. The resulting hypoxia predisposes patients to ulcerations and impaired wound healing. In addition, leukocytes aree trapped in the area and may release their destructive enzymes, compounding the problem.

Clinical Findings. Three grades (WIDMER) of chronic venous insufficiency are identified:

- Grade I: Edema, corona phlebectatica paraplantaris
- Grade II: Trophic or degenerative skin changes (edema, dermatitis, hyperpigmentation, hypodermitis, dermatosclerosis, atrophie blanche)
- Grade III: Stasis ulcer or scars from healed ulcer

Corona Phlebectatica Paraplantaris. Here, tiny spider veins appear about the ankle and on the skin just above the instep. They are always asymptomatic (Fig. 22.35).

Edema. The lymphatic system is no longer able to handle the increased interstitial fluid, so edema develops. It is worse following prolonged standing or in the evening, and disappears overnight because of the patient's horizontal position. Often the

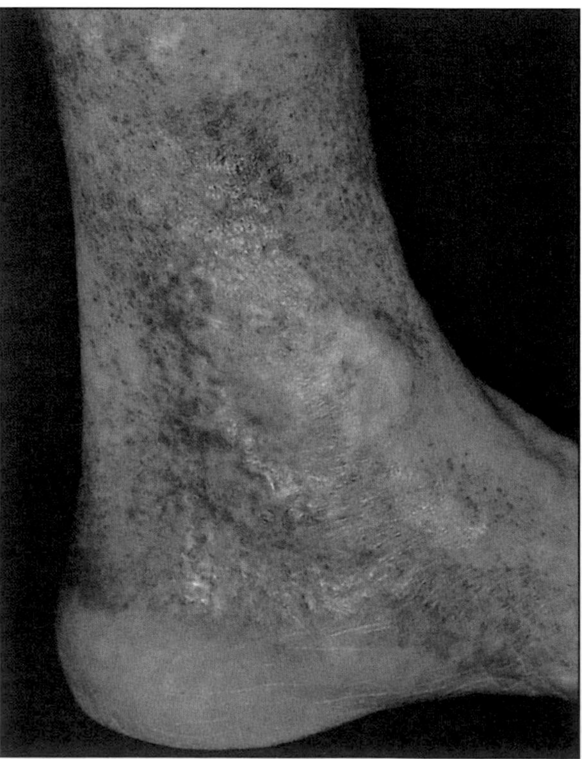

Fig. 22.35. Chronic venous insufficiency with pigmentary changes and corona phlebectatica

first location for edema is the area between the medial or lateral malleolus and the Achilles tendon; this is known as the Bisgaard space.

Stasis Dermatitis. The initial inflammation involves the perivascular aspects of the dermis, but soon the epidermis is affected. There is usually erythema coupled with weeping, scales, and crusts. Pruritus may be severe, so that excoriations are common. Often the changes begin over perforating veins or over varicosities on the distal aspects of the leg. Stasis dermatitis is not a single entity. The skin of the legs is drier than most other body sites, and often nummular dermatitis appears in this location. In addition, a wide variety of topical agents are used, often over many years, so the risk of irritant or allergic contact dermatitis is significant. Patch testing belongs to the evaluation of suspected stasis dermatitis. Sometimes the allergic contact dermatitis will show hematogenous spread with distant lesions developing. This same phenomenon, imprecisely called an id reaction, can also occur with severe stasis dermatitis, often with ulceration; a more generalized dermatitis can develop, almost as a sympathy reaction.

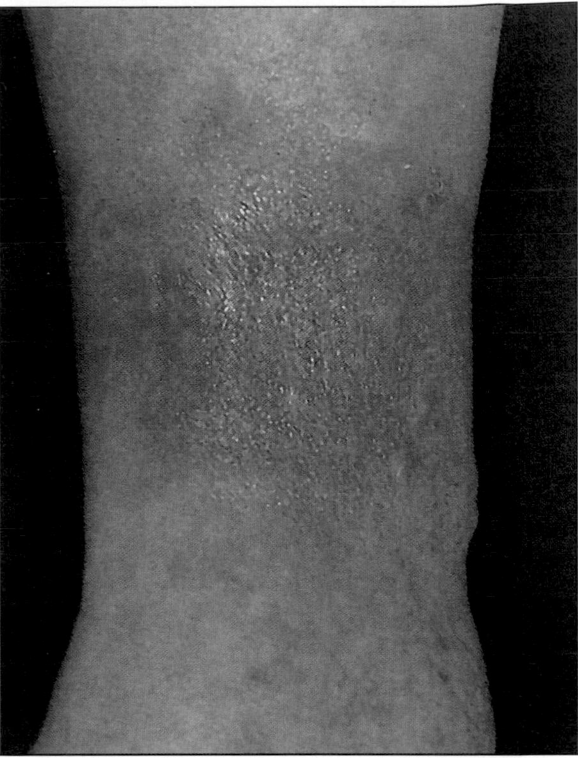

Fig. 22.36. Chronic venous insufficiency with hypodermitis

Hyperpigmentation. The extracellular erythrocytes pose a problem; they are irritating, and the body lacks a method of easily recirculating its hemoglobin. Thus, hemosiderin deposits begin to accumulate. Initially, one sees only purpura with small red macules that resist diascopy. Soon these areas become yellow brown (purpura jaune d'ocre). Larger patches also develop, but typically a speckled pattern is retained. The most common site is about the malleoli, especially medially, but the changes are often seen over incompetent perforating veins. Occasionally, the pigmentation may diminish over time (months) with adequate compression therapy, but it is relatively persistent. Sometimes there is associated postinflammatory hyperpigmentation involving melanin which is even more permanent.

Hypodermitis. A tense, sometimes tender, erythematous infiltrate may involve the distal aspects of the leg. The leaked irritating substances cause a noninfectious inflammation and edema that have also been called pseudoerysipelas (Fig. 22.36). Histologically, the main findings are edema, vessel wall thickening, and lymphohistiocytic infiltrates. In contrast to erysipelas, the patient is well. Most view this as the first stage of dermatosclerosis.

Dermatosclerosis (Dermatoliposclerosis). The same process of leakage and deposition of irritating substances stimulates the fibroblasts to produce more collagen. At the same time, pericapillary fibrin cuffs develop. The combination of impaired vascular permeability and a more resistant dermis leads to decreased diffusion of oxygen and nutrients. Clinically, dermatosclerosis is typically hyperpigmented and circumferential, wrapping about the leg just above the ankle. The skin is bound down firmly to the underlying fat and resists pinching or folding. Often the follicle openings are difficult to identify. Later, there may be striking edema above the constrictive band. Many colorful terms have been applied such as spats-like sclerosis, armored stenosis, and the inverted champagne bottle sign. The sclerotic changes limit joint motion and reduce the effectiveness of the muscle pump, creating a vicious circle. Both systemic sclerosis and panniculitis are frequently considered in the differential diagnosis, especially in the USA where dermatologists tend to be less familiar with chronic venous insufficiency.

Pachydermy. As a reaction to marked and persistent edema, in some instances the skin responds not only with thickening but also with papillomatous and verrucous changes. In the USA, sometimes the term verrucous lymphedema is employed. An associated problem may be recurrent erysipelas, often involving toe web infections, and leading to elephantiasis nostras with more lymphatic impairment.

Histopathology. Biopsies are a poor way to diagnose chronic venous insufficiency. Some of the features have been alluded to above, but in most cases, there are no specific changes, and one can only exclude other possibilities.

Laboratory Findings. No specific tests need be ordered.

Differential Diagnosis. The differential diagnosis is endless, because of the protean clinical features of chronic venous insufficiency. It is probably easier to first consider chronic venous insufficiency when trying to make a diagnosis around the ankle or lower shin than to worry about the many possibilities.

Therapy. We will consider the treatment of varicosities and chronic venous insufficiency together, since they are similar. The goal is to increase or restore venous return. The muscle-joint pump should be activated, usually by increased physical activity or through physical therapy. Incompetent veins should be removed or hemodynamically closed off via sclerotherapy.

Topical. The mainstay of treating stasis dermatitis is "do not harm." The incidence of allergic contact dermatitis is very high in this population, and most of the offending agents are part of the prescriptions. In general, bland protective creams and low- to mid-potency corticosteroid creams and ointments suffice. If a weeping dermatitis develops, wet-to-dry dressings and antiseptic dyes, as discussed under leg ulcers below, may be useful.

Systemic. In patients with severe stasis dermatitis and an id reaction, a short burst of systemic corticosteroids is very effective. We use prednisone 60 mg daily tapered over 9–14 days. There is no effective systemic therapy for chronic venous insufficiency. In the USA, many physicians employ diuretics. They are relatively ineffective against the localized mechanical edema of chronic venous insufficiency and often display their side effects before any antiedema effect is seen. In Germany, a number of drugs are viewed as protecting against edema; one natural product from horse chestnuts known as aescin has shown efficacy comparable to mild compression therapy. Other bioflavinoids, Hamamelis (witch hazel), and rutinoids are also employed. In our opinion, if they are effective, their role is minimal. Rheologic agents, such as pentoxifylline, are also endorsed, although controlled studies are lacking.

Compression

Compression Bandages. These bandages allow one to apply a titered pressure to the tissues and veins. The increased pressure works against the hydrostatic and hemodynamic forces producing edema and also reduces the venous volume, which corrects some valve insufficiency. The muscle pumping is made more effective, so the blood volume in the legs is reduced and the blood velocity increased. In addition, tissue fibrinolysis appears improved, so the fibrin cuffs may be lysed.

Compression bandages are chosen when the leg is edematous or when significant dermatitis or an ulcer is present. All of these effects are only possible when the correct bandage is chosen, and the patient collaborates by activating the muscle-joint pump system. Contradictions to compression dressings include arterial disease of the legs, especially if the pressure at the ankle is less than 60 mmHg. Patients with heart failure may also not tolerate the shifts in fluid volume and should be approached carefully.

Types of Dressings. Usually, elastic bandages are used. Once patients have received proper instructions, they can remove their bandages in the evening and reapply them in the morning. Correct application is essential, and an experienced nurse or physical therapist should work with the patient and his family until the techniques have been learned. Incorrectly applied bandages, especially when the proximal ones exert more pressure than the distal, cause more harm than good. Each reader has probably seen a well meaning patient with elastic bandages almost pathetically draped around the leg, providing no support or pressure.

Many different types of bandages are available, in various widths and with various degrees of tension. We favor firm, hard-to-stretch bandages as they achieve a higher pressure. They are available in a self-adhering form that is more convenient for many patients. On the feet and about the ankles, a narrower (6–8 cm) bandage should be used than for the calf (10–12 cm). The bandage should be applied with the foot in dorsal extension, the pressure points padded with cotton, and the depressions filled with foam rubber or a similar product. The wrapping must be uniform with no slits or spaces, which will only fill up with edema. The tension or degree of compression must decrease as one moves proximally. In almost all cases, below-the-knee wrapping suffices.

Sometimes Unna boot or zinc paste bandages are used. These are firmer and more permanent, designed to be left on for several days. They are applied in the clinic by an experienced nurse or physician. Because they are not elastic, they exert deeper pressure and are preferred by some when wrapping a calf thrombosis. Over time they become loose, so they must be frequently checked and replaced. The Brann bandage combines inner elastic and outer inelastic components.

Compression Stockings. Compression stockings can be used when the edema has been reduced and when the skin is relatively free of acute problems. They are also recommended for thrombosis prophylaxis, such as during pregnancy or following surgery. Ready-made and custom compression stockings are available. They are available in four classes in Germany.

- Class I (~20 mmHg): Mild varicosities, pregnancy, heavy feeling in legs
- Class II. (~30 mmHg): More advanced varicosities, following vein surgery, thrombophlebitis and with healed stasis ulcers
- Class III. (~40 mmHg): Severe chronic venous insufficiency, postthrombotic syndrome, patients who are very active
- Class IV (~60 mmHg): Marked lymphedema, elephantiasis

The antithrombosis stockings [often known as TEDS (thromboembolic devices) in the USA] have a pressure of about 15 mmHg and are only useful to patients during bed rest. All ambulatory patients have pressures higher than this and thus do not benefit. Patients often assume that what they received in the hospital must be good and therefore use these stockings.

Compression stockings can be ordered in varying lengths (calf, knee, mid-thigh, and entire leg) depending on the location of the incompetent veins and the proximal insufficiency point. They should be replaced about every 6 months, as they wear out from both use and laundering. The patient should always have two acceptable pairs to alternate. They are usually not worn when a weeping dermatitis or a florid ulcer is present and are contraindicated in arterial disease. Young patients often reject them for cosmetic reasons, and older patients often have great trouble getting into them.

Intermittent Compression. These devices are flexible plastic boots, resembling the inflatable casts used by emergency medical teams. They extend from the foot to the thigh and are connected to a compressor. In regular cycles, they are inflated from distal to proximal and subsequently deflated, providing physiologic draining. They are very good for patients who cannot employ their muscle-joint pump. They are often employed prophylactically following high-risk surgery, and offer help in severe lymphedema. Contraindications include active infection in the leg, thrombophlebitis, peripheral arterial disease, especially stages III and IV, and heart failure.

Sclerotherapy

Principle. The intravascular injection of an irritating substance induces an iatrogenic thrombophlebitis that leads to vessel lumen obliteration. The two main sclerosing materials are polidocanol (ethoxysclerol 0.5–4.0%) and sodium iodide (4–8%). The endothelium of the widened damaged vein is somewhat more sensitive to the irritating substance than the normal vein wall. A thrombus forms, fills the vessel within 24 h, and is organized over 1–3 weeks. Recanalization may occur, just as with natural thrombi. The larger the vein, the more likely this event.

Indications. The main indications are spider veins, reticular varicosities, and small to mid-sized tortuous nodose varicosities, as well as small branches of larger superficial veins without incompetent transfascial communication.

Contraindications. There are many contradictions, including allergies to the sclerosing material, arterial occlusive disease, cardiac, renal, and hepatic diseases, malignancies, wasting, and nonambulatory status. Relative contraindications include deep vein thrombosis in the past year, acute or recurrent superficial thrombophlebitis, any inflammatory or febrile illness, allergic diseases, or plans for marked physical activity or a dramatic climate change. Weeping stasis dermatitis or an infected stasis ulcer are also reasons not to perform sclerotherapy; in contrast, a clean ulcer will often heal better if the nearby varicosities are sclerosed.

Most authors recommend not performing sclerotherapy in the first 3 months or the last 6 weeks of pregnancy. During the remainder of pregnancy, sclerotherapy can be performed as long as minor procedures are done that require no bed rest. The varicosities that first appear during pregnancy should be observed following delivery, because many disappear or improve and require no treatment. Menstruation and use of oral contraceptives present no problems as far as sclerotherapy is concerned.

Technique

Plan. The sclerotherapy should begin at the proximal insufficiency point. Once this is closed, often the more distal lesions improve spontaneously. In addition, the incompetent perforating veins should be treated. After that one can attack large superficial veins, their branches, and solitary, reticular, and spider varicosities. It may be wise to treat the perforating veins and other varicosities about an ulcer first.

Injection Method. The skin is disinfected. The patient either stands or lets his legs hang over the edge of the table. Thick short needles are inserted into the filled veins; no tourniquet is used. The dripping of venous blood into a basin confirms the correct placement of the needle. The patient now lies down, and the leg is raised slightly above the horizontal. This is more convenient when using a special phlebology tilt table. The sclerosing material is slowly injected, trying to maximize contact with the damaged wall segment.

Amount of Sclerosing Material. We usually use polidocanol. At first, only 0.5 ml of the lowest (0.5%) concentration is injected, to see how the patient tolerates the procedure. Then higher doses are used, ranging from 0.5 ml to 2.0 ml of 1–3% solution. One or two large varicosities or many smaller ones can be treated in one sitting. Spider veins are routinely treated with a very fine needle and 0.5% solutions; one attempts to inject just enough to blanch the lesion.

Postoperative Care. After the injection, the site is compressed with gauze, and then a generous compression bandage is applied to the limb. After treatment and bandaging, the patient must walk for 30 min. Even if he has problems with pain, he must leave the bandages on and keep walking. He must be aware that the desired thrombophlebitis will cause stinging and other discomforts. The dressings are removed several days after the procedure. At the same time, other veins can now be treated. We usually wait 1 week between injections. After the first treatment, the patient wears compression bandages or preferably stockings for 2–4 weeks.

Complications

Immediate Complications. Rarely, urticarial reactions or anaphylactic shock may occur. Sclerotherapy should only be done in rooms in which resuscitation equipment and easy access are available. Sometimes anxious patients may faint prior to or at the beginning of the procedure; this should not be confused with anaphylaxis and can be treated by simply having the patient lie down with the legs elevated, easily accomplished in a phlebology suite.

If the sclerosing material winds up adjacent to the vessel, the area should be infiltrated with physiologic saline to dilute the material. Other clinicians inject hyaluronidase, corticosteroids, or lidocaine without epinephrine. Intraarterial injection should be impossible if the procedure is done appropriately. Nonetheless, it does occur occasionally in the groin, popliteal fossa, behind the medial malleolus, and on the back of the foot. Heparin should be immediately injected, and the patient transferred to an intensive care unit, where he must be evaluated by vascular surgeons; most patients receive fibrinolytic therapy as a prophylaxis.

Later Complications. When the inflammation is excessive, stronger compression and more extensive walking are recommended. If the pain is severe, nonsteroidal antiinflammatory drugs can be prescribed. Sometimes intravascular clots develop; they can be expressed through a tiny incision. If necrosis is severe, debridement may be necessary. Deep vein thromboses and emboli are feared, but with proper technique and postoperative care, they are extremely rare. Often there is postinflammatory hyperpigmentation over the sclerotherapy site.

Surgery

Vein Stripping. The procedure is only done following appropriate studies to determine the proximal and distal points of insufficiency. Doppler ultrasound, duplex sonography, or phlebography may be employed. The expected result can be estimated using light reflex rheography with compression of the proximal point. The standard procedure is the Babcock approach, in which the branches of the venous star or cross that meet the greater saphenous vein are first tied off in the groin, and then the vein is removed. This approach reduces recurrences. The high ligation-avulsion can be done as an isolated procedure for varicosities of the proximal part of the thigh and inguinal region, but is usually combined with removal of the greater saphenous vein to the distal insufficiency point. The lesser saphenous vein is stripped after a similar ligation-avulsion procedure in the popliteal space. As the vein is removed, major branches and perforators are tied off.

Perforating Veins. Incompetent perforating veins, especially in the Cockett group, are often better handled surgically than with sclerotherapy. They must be individually identified and then tied off and removed. Both epifascial and subfascial procedures can be performed. Endoscopic approaches are also possible.

Congenital Absence of Venous Valves

This rare disorder is inherited in an autosomal dominant pattern, so that men and women are equally involved. Lower extremity edema begins around puberty and typically improves at night or with elevation. Most patients develop varicosities, stasis dermatitis and leg ulcers, all of which are uncommon in lymphedema. Imaging studies show total or partial absence of valves in the superficial and deep veins, but intact lymphatics.

Stasis Ulcer

Synonyms. Ulcus cruris venosum, venous ulcer

Definition. Ulcer of the distal part of the shin or ankle region secondary to chronic venous insufficiency, with loss of skin and subcutaneous tissue damaged by inadequate perfusion and nutrition.

Epidemiology. Stasis ulcers are a major cause of morbidity. As mentioned above, about 1 million Germans have stasis ulcers. They cause a great deal of lost time from work, consume a number of in-hospital days, and place demands on home nursing care and family members.

Etiology and Pathogenesis. The pathogenesis of stasis ulcers has been discussed under chronic venous insufficiency. Ulcers represent one end-point as the inadequately supplied sclerotic tissue breaks down, and healing is impaired to a great extent. Sometimes minor trauma is responsible, but in other cases the ulceration is spontaneous. Blow-out ulcers arise directly over a perforating vein. Sometimes a superficial thrombophlebitis will ulcerate. In addition, both bacterial infections and severe allergic contact dermatitis can evolve into ulcers.

Clinical Findings. The most common site of stasis ulcers is the medial aspect of the leg around and above the ankle (Fig. 22.37). Their form is variable, sometimes oval, sometimes serpiginous, sometimes quite bizarre. Often multiple ulcers develop and fuse together (Fig. 22.38). Large ulcers can envelop the entire limb; they are known as spat ulcers in Germany because they resemble this piece of apparel (Fig. 22.39). In other instances, the ulcers may be located directly over thrombosed veins (Fig. 22.40). The ulcers have varying degrees of depth, sometimes exposing underlying structures. They tend to contain necrotic debris and pus, with varying amounts of granulation tissue. Usually, the edges are sharply punched out. The degree of pain is unpredictable. Small ulcers, especially in atrophie blanche, can be exquisitely painful, while some enormous ulcers are relatively asymptomatic.

A number of complications can arise. Secondary bacterial, and occasionally fungal, infections are

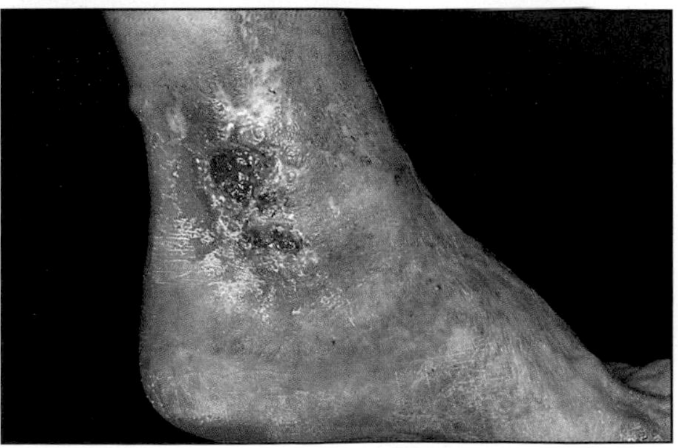

Fig. 22.37. Stasis ulcer

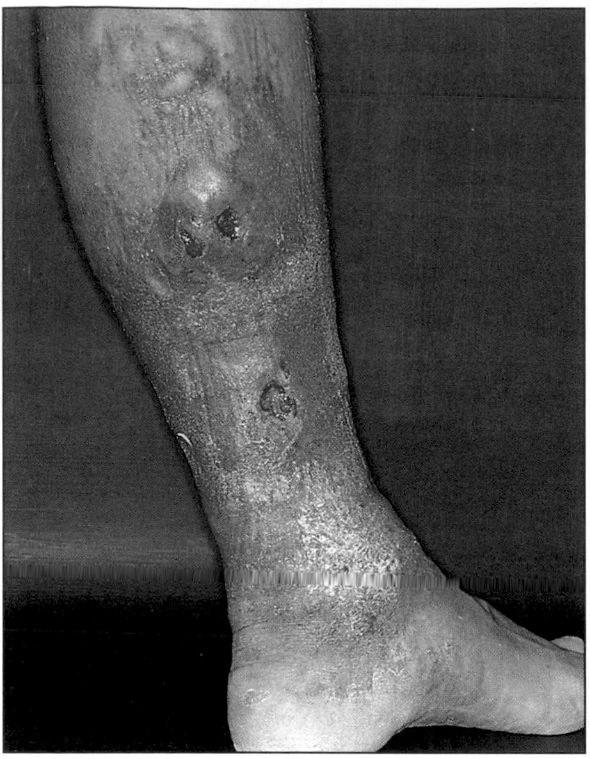

Fig. 22.38. Multiple stasis ulcers as well as dermatosclerosis

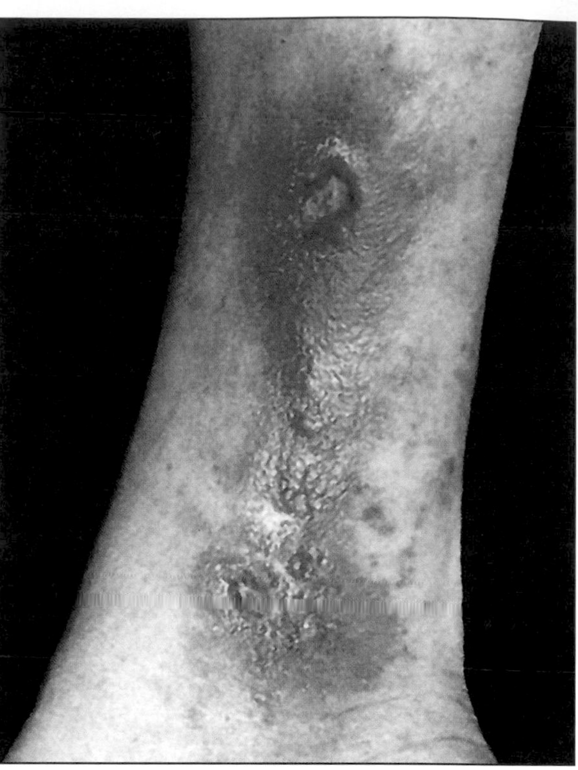

Fig. 22.40. Ulcerations over sites of thrombophlebitis

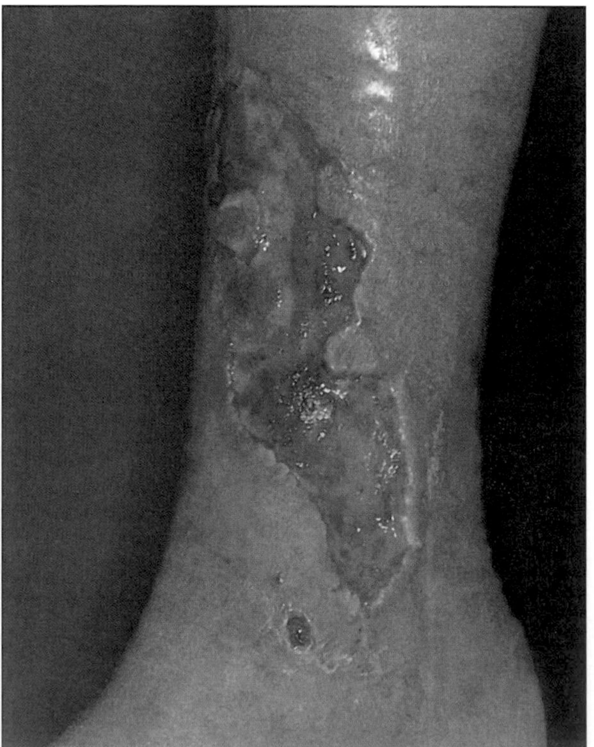

Fig. 22.39. Large stasis ulcer; also known as "spat" ulcer

the rule in dirty necrotic areas. The clinical challenge is to decide when the bacteria are responsible for the problem so that the appropriate therapy can be administered. The ulcer secretions often cause an erosive dermatitis, which may spread rapidly and even ulcerate itself. This change must be distinguished from allergic contact dermatitis. Patients with a stasis ulcer are exposed to an amazing list of topical preparations, both from physicians and through their own selection. The prevalence of allergic contact dermatitis in such patients approaches 80%. Patch testing is always worthwhile. Common sensitizers include antibiotics (neomycin), balsam of Peru, local anesthetics (benzocaine family), fragrances, preservatives, antiseptics (clioquinol), and vehicles (wool wax alcohols, lanolin, lanette). Very rarely, a squamous cell carcinoma may develop in the ulcer wall; this is known as a Marjolin ulcer.

Histopathology. Biopsy is primarily useful to exclude an ulcerated tumor. When searching for vasculitis, the edge of an ulcer is an unsatisfactory location. Many vessels in this site show a chronic inflammatory infiltrate.

Course and Prognosis. Stasis ulcers are usually very chronic; they may persist for years or even decades. Even if healing is achieved through intensive treatment, recurrences are the rule, unless the underlying defects can be corrected.

Differential Diagnosis. Table 22.14 lists the major causes of leg ulcers. Despite the many possible etiologic factors, in an ordinary medical or dermatologic practice, the vast majority (well over 90%) of leg ulcers will be stasis ulcers. The problem is not to overlook another cause. One should remember that often two factors are involved, such as an arterial and venous ulcer, or a stasis ulcer with secondary allergic contact dermatitis.

Therapy. The mainstay of treatment is that of the underlying varicosities and chronic venous insufficiency. If one can improve the venous return, the ulcer will heal with little or no other attention.

Topical. Local therapy is only an adjutant to phlebologic measures. It may speed up the wound healing.

Cleansing. If large amounts of necrotic tissue are present, mechanical debridement with curettage is the simplest approach. We have found EMLA an effective anesthetic in this setting. A variety of proteolytic enzymatic creams and ointments are also available; they contain collagenases, elastases, fibrinases, or other bacterial enzymes. These can be applied once or twice daily to the wound, with careful cleansing after each application. We rarely use these products for more than 1 week.

Disinfection. In Europe, painting the ulcers with colored disinfectant solutions is often beloved. Every clinic has its favorite solution, including silver nitrate (2–5% in water), gentian violet (0.1–0.5% in water), and brilliant green (1% in water). Wet-to-dry soaks using tap water and clean (not sterile) cotton rags provides cooling and debridement; this can be modified by adding clioquinol (1:1000), potassium permanganate (1:1000–1:5000), or silver nitrate (1:1000) to the solution. The dyes stain, so the patient must be warned. An advantage of wet-to-dry soaks is that they can be performed with the legs elevated. Patients can also soak their feet and ankles in a foot bath.

Table 22.14. Causes of leg ulcers

General category	Examples
Chronic venous insufficiency	Posttraumatic Postthrombophlebitis Postthrombotic syndrome, including familial disorders of coagluation (protein C, protein S, antithrombin III, factor V and others)
Arterial disease	Arteriosclerosis Thromboangiitis obliterans Small vessel vasculitis Polyarteritis nodosa Diabetic angiopathy Hypertension Arteriovenous fistulas Aneurysms
Trauma	Primary trauma (mechanical, thermal, chemical) Scars (burns, postoperative, others) Artifact
Infections	Ecthyma (deep pyoderma) Deep mycoses Gumma (tertiary syphilis) Leprosy (combined with neurologic damage) Lupus vulgaris Leishmaniasis Diphtheria
Dermatoses	Pyoderma gangrenosum Erythema induratum Pernio Systemic sclerosis Systemic lupus erythematosus (especially lupus profundus) Necrobiosis lipoidica diabeticorum
Neurologic	Any type of paralysis Peripheral nerve lesions
Neoplastic[a]	Basal cell carcinoma Squamous cell carcinoma (especially in scar) Verrucous carcinoma (epithelioma cuniculatum) Lymphoma Kaposi sarcoma Malignant melanoma (rare, usually amelanotic)
Genetic defects	Sickle cell disease Hypercoagulability disorders Prolidase deficiency Klinefelter syndrome Familial leg ulcers (in absence of defect in coagulation or any of above disorders) Medications Hydroxyurea

[a] The tumors become ulcerated and mimic an ulcer; most often residual tumor is seen.

Stimulating Granulation. Silver nitrate ointment ($AgNO_3$ 1.0; white petrolatum ad 100.0) is an old favorite. Polysaccharide granules can also be used; either Debrisan or Duoderm are satisfactory. The Duoderm granules can then be combined later with the Duoderm colloid dressing or any similar product. The granules tend to dry out an ulcer and are only used for a few days.

Stimulating Epithelialization. If the ulcer basis is clean and granulation tissue covers the base, then epithelialization is not a problem. Sometimes the edges are scraped or slit to speed up the process.

Wound Dressings. The vast array of new wound dressings have contributed to ulcer care. The most useful are the hydrocolloid dressings, which can be left on for 2–7 days depending on how much exudate accumulates and how well the adjacent skin tolerates the adhesive. Hydrogels are useful for shorter periods of application, while films may be useful for very small or superficial lesions. In the case of very recalcitrant ulcers, some of the newer, more complex, and extremely expensive artificial skins can be considered.

Surgical Approaches. A clean ulcer can often be treated with skin grafting to speed healing. Mesh grafting is usually preferred, although pinch grafting can also be employed. Shave excision of the ulcer and the surrounding dermatosclerosis followed by coverage with a mesh graft produces surprisingly good healing. A paratibial fasciotomy has also won acceptance in recent years, especially when an ulcer is associated with marked dermatosclerosis or the postthrombotic syndrome. The fascia is split on the medial side. An incision is made on the calf and the excision extended subcutaneously through the fascial plane to the region of the medial malleolus. At the same time, perforating veins are tied off. The splitting of the fascia reduces the pressure in the deep compartment and allows communication between the sub- and epifascial regions. In ideal cases, new capillaries extend from the muscles to the subcutaneous tissues, improving the microcirculation and assisting in ulcer healing. Usually, the ulcer is covered with skin grafts at the same time.

Treating the Adjacent Skin. The skin around an ulcer is always at risk of maceration, allergic contact dermatitis, or further ulceration. It must be protected, even if clinically normal, during ulcer therapy. We prefer a zinc oxide paste. If the adjacent skin is erythematous and scaling, i.e., shows signs of stasis dermatitis, low to mid-potency topical corticosteroids can be employed.

Atrophie Blanche

(Milian 1929)

Synonym. Capillaritis alba

Definition. Area of white atrophic scarring usually with telangiectases in a bizarre pattern.

Etiology and Pathogenesis. The nature of atrophie blanche has long been discussed. Some groups speak of primary atrophie blanche when describing the scars in the antiphospholipid syndrome and livedo vasculitis, and consider the same clinical lesions in chronic venous insufficiency as secondary. To us, atrophie blanche is a type of scarring associated with many vascular disorders. It may be more dependent on small artery occlusion in combination with inadequate perfusion and venous stasis.

Clinical Findings. One or more patches several centimeters in size are found about the ankle. In their early phase, they may be livid red and inflamed, but soon they become depressed, turn white, and often contain small vessels. The white areas may have a hyperpigmented periphery. The most important clinical feature is the tendency of atrophie blanche to develop small painful ulcerations – regardless of the underlying or associated disease (Fig. 22.41). The ulcers can coalesce and are notoriously therapy-resistant.

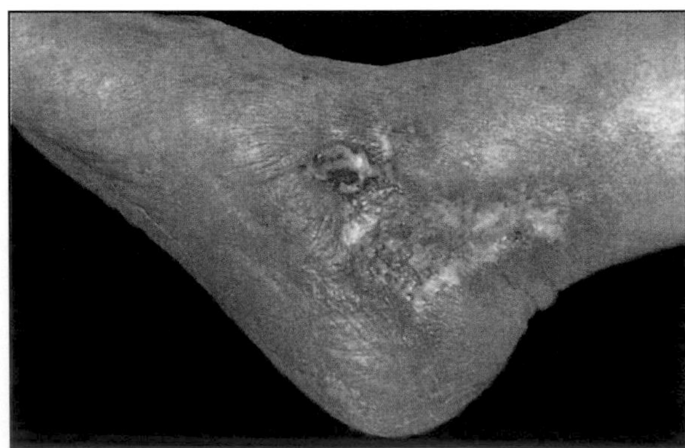

Fig. 22.41. Atrophie blanche with ulceration

Histopathology. Microscopic examination is not a good way to make the diagnosis. The biopsy site will almost certainly ulcerate. Since both chronic venous insufficiency and antiphospholipid syndrome are characterized by fibrin deposits around vessels, often the distinction cannot be made. If intravascular fibrin thrombi are found, chronic venous insufficiency is unlikely. In addition, the expected epidermal atrophy and dermal sclerosis are seen.

Differential Diagnosis. The differential diagnosis includes all forms of vasculitis that can occasionally heal with such changes, the antiphospholipid syndrome and its related disorders, and other types of leg ulcers. Usually, the history and the changes in the adjacent skin are more helpful than examining the atrophie blanche.

Therapy. If the primary cause is chronic venous insufficiency, then aggressive compression is required. Often "finger pointing" varicosities can be found at the periphery; they should be sclerosed or ligated. Paratibial fasciotomy may also be useful. Aspirin or other inhibitors of platelet aggregation can be beneficial, as can heparin for short periods of time. Some studies have shown benefits from pentoxifylline, but we have not been impressed with the results. Topical treatment is rarely helpful. Very early cases may be helped by topical corticosteroids. If an ulcer develops, standard care is appropriate.

Acroangiodermatitis

(Mali et al. 1965; Chaix 1926; Favre 1941)

Synonym. Pseudo-Kaposi sarcoma

Definition. Prominent reactive change with vessel proliferation and fibrosis, associated with chronic venous insufficiency and vascular malformations.

Etiology and Pathogenesis. Increased venous pressure may lead to proliferation and dilation of veins of the superficial plexus. The most common cause is chronic venous insufficiency, but similar changes have been described in vascular malformations, congenital or acquired arteriovenous fistulas, paralyzed legs, and even amputation stumps. There is no association with human herpes virus 8, as seen in Kaposi sarcoma.

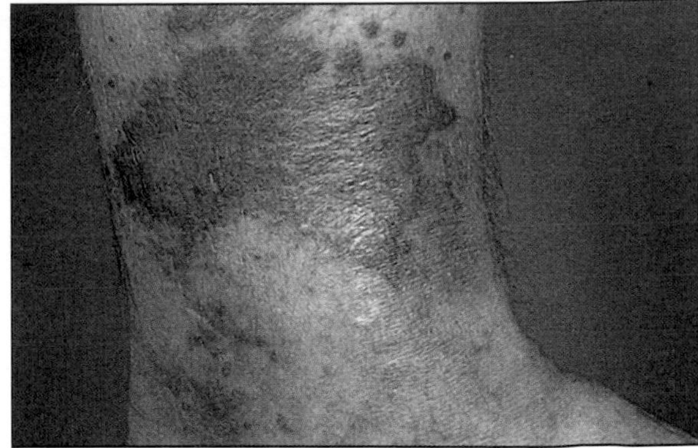

Fig. 22.42. Acroangiodermatitis

Clinical Findings. Multiple papules, nodules, and plaques may develop, sometimes in band-like or bizarre configurations (Fig. 22.42). In the center, the sharply defined lesions are usually bright red, while at their periphery they are more red-brown. The most common location is the dorsal aspect of the foot, with lesions involving the base of the great and second toes, but the ankle and lower aspect of the shin can also be affected. There is usually associated edema. In the case of chronic venous insufficiency, the lesions are often bilateral. In the other scenarios, the underlying clinical defect is obvious, as the patient has signs of a vascular or neurologic problem. Here the lesions tend to be unilateral.

Histopathology. The findings are those of stasis dermatitis. There are dilated vessels, mild edema, hemosiderin deposition, fibrosis and patchy lymphohistiocytic infiltrates. The vessels are round and lack atypia.

Differential Diagnosis. While clinically the lesions may mimic Kaposi sarcoma, there is no question histologically. In addition, the associated clinical findings of chronic venous insufficiency or a vascular or neurologic problem usually point one in the right direction.

Therapy. The underlying disease should be treated. If the cause is chronic venous insufficiency, compression and sclerotherapy usually bring improvement. Early flat lesions sometimes improve with topical corticosteroids.

Postthrombotic Syndrome

Definition. Chronic venous insufficiency following deep vein thrombosis.

Etiology and Pathogenesis. Following a resolved deep vein thrombosis, there is usually some degree of lumen occlusion and valve insufficiency. Although there are usually adequate collaterals, if adequate compression therapy is not pursued, eventually complications develop.

Clinical Findings. Any of the features of chronic venous insufficiency can develop, but most often the sequence involves edema, secondary varicosities, and ulceration.

Diagnostic Criteria. If the patient does not give a clear history of a deep vein thrombosis, then the diagnosis can be difficult. The various objective methods including light reflection rheography, phlebodynamometry, and impedance plethysmography can document the deep vein impairment.

Therapy. The most important step is compulsive compression therapy immediately following the treatment of a deep vein thrombosis, as well as prophylactic anticoagulation. The patient should be encouraged to avoid a job or hobby with prolonged standing. Physical therapy, maintenance of ideal weight, and regular walking are also essential.

Stasis-Arthritis Syndrome

Definition. Musculoskeletal disorder secondary to a tendency towards persistent plantar flexion associated with chronic venous insufficiency.

Etiology and Pathogenesis. In some instances, dermatosclerosis may be extensive and involve the fascia of the ankle joint and the tissue about the Achilles tendon. The pressure and pain forces the patient to walk in a position of plantar flexion, e.g., on tip-toes. If this is not corrected promptly, the patient experiences atrophy of the dorsiflexor muscles, atrophy of the Achilles tendon, and a worsening of the chronic venous insufficiency as the muscle-joint pump does not operate. Finally, the joints become stiffened; in the worst case, the foot winds up in a permanent tip-toe position. It is truly a vicious circle.

Clinical Findings. Most patients are older women with marked dermatosclerosis and refractory or recurrent stasis ulcers. In any case, all the stigmata of chronic venous insufficiency are likely to be present.

Differential Diagnosis. Other neurologic and orthopedic causes of persistent plantar flexion of the foot should be sought. All of them can also lead to a worsening of chronic venous insufficiency.

Therapy. Aggressive compression therapy should be combined with skilled physical therapy. The goal is to mobilize the joint. Often exercise bicycles and even more ergometric devices are helpful. In some instances, the dermatosclerosis must be approached surgically.

Bibliography

Hereditary Hemorrhagic Telangiectasia

Babington BG (1865) Hereditary epistaxis 2:362–363

Guttmacher AE, Marchuk DA, White RI Jr (1995) Hereditary hemorrhagic telangiectasia. N Engl J Med 333(14): 918–924

Haitjema T, Westermann CJ, Overtoom TT et al. (1996) Hereditary hemorrhagic telangiectasia (Osler-Weber-Rendu disease): new insights in pathogenesis, complications, and treatment. Arch Intern Med 156(7):714–719

Harries PG, Brockbank MJ, Shakespeare PG et al. (1997) Treatment of hereditary haemorrhagic telangiectasia by the pulsed dye laser. J Laryngol Otol 111:1038–1041

Osler W (1907) On multiple hereditary telangiectases with recurrent hemorrhage. Q J Med 1:53–58

Rendu H (1896) Epistaxis répetées chez un sujet porteur de petits angiomes cutanés et muqueux. Bull Soc Méd Hôp, Paris 13:731–733

Rius C, Smith JD, Almendro N et al. (1998) Cloning of the promotor region of human endoglin, the target gene for hereditary hemorrhagic telangiectasia type 1. Blood 92: 4677–4690

Shovlin CL (1997) Molecular defects in rare bleeding disorders: hereditary haemorrhagic telangiectasia. Thromb Haemost 78:145–150

Weber FP (1907) Multiple hereditary development angiomata (telangiectases) of the skin and mucous membranes associated with recurring haemorrhages. Lancet ii:160–162

Hereditary Benign Telangiectasia

Gold MH, Eramo L, Prendiville JS (1989) Hereditary benign telangiectasia. Pediatr Dermatol 6:194–197

Puppin D, Rybojad M, Morel P (1992) Hereditary benign telangiectasia: two case reports. J Dermatol 19:384–386

Ryan TJ, Wells RS (1971) Hereditary benign telangiectasia. Trans St John's Hosp Dermatol Soc 57:148–156

Zahorcsek Z, Schneider I (1994) Hereditary benign telangiectasia. Dermatology 189:286–288

Generalized Essential Telangiectasia

Checketts SR, Burton PS, Bjorkman DJ et al. (1997) Generalized essential teleangiectasia in the presence of gastrointestinal bleeding. J Am Acad Dermatol 37:321–325

Driban NE (1982) Progressive essentielle Teleangiektasien. Hautarzt 35:500–501

McGrae JD Jr, Winkelmann RK (1963) Generalized essential teleangiectasiae. JAMA 185:909–913

Shelley WB (1971) Essential progressive teleangiectasia: successfull treatment with tetracycline. JAMA 216:1343–1344

Unilateral Nevoid Telangiectasia

Hynes LR, Shenefelt PD (1997) Unilateral nevoid telangiectasia: occurence in two patients with hepatitis C. J Am Acad Dermatol 36:819–822

Taskapan O, Harmanyeri Y (1998) Acquired unilateral nevoid telangiectasia syndrome. J Am Acad Dermatol 39:138–139

Tok J, Berberian BJ, Sulica VI (1994) Unilateral nevoid telangiectasia syndrome. Cutis 53:53–54

Angioma Serpiginosum

Cox NH, Paterson WD (1991) Angioma serpiginosum: a simulator of purpura. Postgrad Med J 67:1065–1066

Gerbig AW, Zala L, Hunziker T (1995) Angioma serpiginosum, eine Hautveränderung entlang den Blaschko-Linien? Hautarzt 46:847–849

Long CC, Lanigan SW (1997) Treatment of angioma serpiginosum using a pulsed tunable dye laser. Br J Dermatol 136:631–632

Erythromelanosis Colli

Hellwig S, Schonermark M, Raulin C (1995) Treatment of vascular malformations and pigment disorders of the face and neck by pulsed dye laser, Photoderm VL and Q-switched ruby laser. Laryngorhinootologie 74:635–641

Schroeter CA, Neumann HA (1998) An intense light source. The photoderm VL-flashlamp as a new treatment possibility for vascular skin lesions. Dermatol Surg 24:743–748

Nevus Araneus

Enta T (1994) Dermacase. Nevus araneus (spider telangiectasia). Can Fam Physician 40:1105–1112

Venous Ectasias

Wiek K, Vanscheidt W, Ishkanian S et al. (1996) Selektive Photothermolyse von Besenreiservarizen und Teleangiektasien der unteren Extremität. Hautarzt 47:258–263

Functional Angiopathies

Acrocyanosis

Davis E (1992) Oscillometry of radial artery in acrocyanosis and cold sensitivity. J Mal Vasc 17:214–217

Hoegl L, Thoma-Greber E, Poppinger J et al. (1999) Butyl nitrite-induced acrocyanosis in an HIV-infected patient. Arch Dermatol 135:90–91

Mangiafico RA, Malatino LS, Santonocito M et al. (1996) Plasma endothelin-1 concentrations during cold exposure in essential acrocyanosis. Angiology 47:1033–1038

Livedo Reticularis

Choi HJ, Hann SK (1999) Livedo reticularis and livedoid vasculitis responding to PUVA therapy. J Am Acad Dermatol 40:204–207

Gould JW, Helms SE, Schulz SM et al. (1998) Relapsing livedo reticularis in the setting of chronic pancreatitis. J Am Acad Dermatol 39:1035–1036

Morell A, Botella R, Silvestre JF et al. (1996) Livedo reticularis and thrombotic purpura related to the use of diphenhydramine associated with pyrithyldione. Dermatology 193:50–51

Nonaka Y, Sibue K, Shimizu A et al. (1997) Lipo-prostaglandin E1 therapy for livedo reticularis with ulceration. Acta Derm Venereol (Stockh) 77:246–247

Erythromelalgia

Davis MDP, O'Fallon WM, Rogers RS et al. (2000) Natural history of erythromelalgia. Arch Dermatol 136:330–336

Drenth JP, Michiels JJ (1992) Clinical characteristics and pathophysiology of erythromelalgia and erythermalgia. Am J Med 93:111–114

Kalgaard OM, Seem E, Kvernebo K (1997) Erythromelalgia: a clinical study of 87 cases. J Intern Med 242:191–197

Michiels JJ, Drenth JP, Van Genderen PJ (1995) Classification and diagnosis of erythromelagia and erythermalgia. Int J Dermatol 34:97–100

Mørk C, Kvernebo K (2000) Eryhtromelalgia – a mysterious condition? Arch Dermatol 136:406–409

Rudikoff D, Jaffe IA (1997) Erythromelalgia: response to serotonin reuptake inhibitors. J Am Acad Dermatol 37:281–283

Burning Feet Syndrome

Galer BS, Lipton RB, Kaplan R et al. (1991) Bilateral burning foot pain: monitoring of pain, sensation, and autonomic function during successful treatment with sympathetic blockade. J Pain Symptom Manage 6:92–97

Stogbauer F, Young P, Kuhlenbaumer G et al. (1999) Autosomal dominant burning feet syndrome. J Neurol Neurosurg Psychiatry 67:78–81

Restless Legs Syndrome

Ekbom KA (1945) Restless legs. A clinical study of a hitherto overlooked disease in the legs characterized by peculiar paresthesia ("anxietas tibarum"), pain and weakness and occurring in two main forms, asthenia crurum parasthetica and asthenia crurum dolorosa. A short review of parasthesias in general. Acta Med Scand [Suppl] 158:1–123

Metcalfe RA, MacDermott N, Chalmers RJ (1986) Restless red legs: an association of the restless legs syndrome with arborizing telangiectasia of the lower limbs. J Neurol Neurosurg Psychiatry 49 (7):820–823

Reflex Sympathetic Dystrophy

Faria SH, Flannary JC (1998) Reflex sympathetic dystrophy syndrome: an update. J Vasc Nurs 16:25–30

Kurvers HA (1998) Reflex sympathetic dystrophy: facts and hypothesis. Vasc Med 3:207–214

Nath RK, Mackinnon SE, Stelnicki E (1996) Reflex sympathetic dystrophy. The controversy continues. Clin Plast Surg 23:435–446

Sudeck P (1900) Über die akute entzündliche Knochenatrophie. Arch Klin Chir 62:147–156

Raynaud Syndrome and Raynaud Disease

Creutzig A, Caspary L, Freund M (1996) The Raynaud phenomenon and interferon therapy. Ann Intern Med 125:423

Gasbarrini A, Serricchio M, Tondi P et al. (1996) Association of Helicobacter pylori infection with primary Raynaud phenomenon. Lancet 348:966–967

Maricq HR, Valter I, Maricq JG (1998) An objective method to estimate the severity of Raynaud phenomenon: digital blood pressure response to cooling. Vasc Med 3:109–113

Raynaud AG (1862) De l'asphyxie locale et la gangrene symetrique des extremites. Paris (Thesis)

Spencer-Green G (1998) Outcomes in primary Raynaud phenomenon: a meta-analysis of the frequency, rates, and predictors of transition to secondary diseases. Arch Intern Med 158:595–600

Vergon JM, Barthelemy JC, Riffat J et al. (1992) Raynaud's phenomenon of the lung. A reality both in primary and secondary Raynaud syndrome. Chest 101:1312–1317

Cutaneous Emboli

Watsky KL (1995) Sporotrichoid nodules in an immunocompromised host. Cutaneous emboli of Fusarium. Arch Dermatol 131:1329–1330

Watsky KL, Eisen RN, Bolognia JL (1990) Unilateral cutaneous emboli of Aspergillus. Arch Dermatol 126:1214–1217

Fat Emboli

Richards RR (1997) Fat embolism syndrome. Can J Surg 40:334–339

Vedrinne JM, Guillaume C, Gagnieu MC (1991) Diagnosis of fat emboli. Ann Intern Med 114:339

Cholesterol Emboli

Becker KA, Schwartz RA, Rothenberg J (1997) Leg ulceration and the cholesterol embolus. J Med 28:387–392

Bell SP, Frankel A, Brown EA (1997) Cholesterol emboli syndrome – uncommon or unrecognized? J R Soc Med 90:543–546

Peat DS, Mathieson PW (1996) Cholesterol emboli may mimic vasculitis. BMJ 313:546–547

Rumpf KW, Schult S, Mueller GA (1998) Simvastin treatment in cholesterol emboli syndrome. Lancet 352:321–322

Vasculitis

Bacon PA (1993) Systemic vasculitic syndromes. Curr Opin Rheumatol 5:5–10

Jennette JC, Falk RJ, Andrassy K et al. (1994) Nomenclature of systemic vasculitides. Proposal of an international consensus conference. Arthritis Rheum 37:187–192

Jennette JC, Falk RJ (1997) Small-vessel vasculitis. N Engl J Med 337:1512–1523

Jorizzo JL (1993) Classification of vasculitis. J Invest Dermatol 100:106S–110S

Schellong MS, Niedermeyer J, Bernhards J et al. (1993) Problems of classification in necrotizing vasculitis. Adv Exp Med Biol 336:345–348

Large Vessel Vasculitis

Giant Cell Arteritis

Dummer W, Zillikens D, Schulz A et al. (1996) Scalp necrosis in temporal (giant cell) arteritis: implications for the dermatologic surgeon. Clin Exp Dermatol 21:154–158

Horton BT, Magath TB, Brown GE (1932) An undescribed form of arteritis of the temporal vessels. Proc Staff Meet Mayo Clin 7:700–701

Karanjia ND, Cawthorn SJ, Giddings AE (1993) The diagnosis and management of arteriitis. J R Soc Med 86:267–270

Polymyalgia Rheumatica

Salvarani C, Macchioni P, Boiardi L (1997) Polymyalgia rheumatica. Lancet 350:43–47

Swannel AJ (1997) Polymyalgia rheumatica and temporal arteritis: diagnosis and management. Br Med J 314:1329–1332

Takayasu Arteritis

Hall S, Barr W, Lie JT (1985) Takayasu arteritis. A study of 32 North American patients. Medicine 64:89–99

Procter CD, Hollier LH (1992) Takayasu's arteritis and temporal arteritis. Ann Vasc Surg 6:195–198

Schwarz-Eywill M, Breitbart A, Csernok E et al. (1993) Treatment modalities and ANCA in Takayasu's arteritis. Adv Exp Med Biol 336:497–501

Takayasu M (1908) A case of strange anastomosis of the central vessels of the retina. J Jpn Ophthalmol Soc 12:554

Medium-Sized Vessel Vasculitis

Polyarteritis Nodosa and Cutaneous Polyarteritis Nodosa

Callen JP (1993) Cutaneous vasculitis and other neutrophilic dermatoses. Curr Opin Rheumatol 5:33–40

Daoud MS, Hutton, KP, Gibson LE (1997) Cutaneous periarteritis nodosa: a clinicopathological study of 79 cases. Br J Dermatol 136:706–713

Fisher I, Orkin M (1964) Cutaneous form of periarteritis nodosa – an entity? Arch Dermatol 89:180–189

Fortin PR, Larson MG, Watters AK et al. (1995) Prognostic factors in systemic necrotizing vasculitis of the polyarteritis nodosa group – a review of 45 cases. J Rheumatol 22:78–84

Guillevin L, Lothe F (1998) Treatment of polyarteritis nodosa and microscopic polyangiitis. Arthritis Rheum 41:2100–2105

Guillevin L, Lhote F, Amouroux J et al. (1996) Antineutrophil cytoplasmic antibodies, abnormal angiograms and pathological findings in polyarteritis nodosa and Churg-Strauss syndrome: indications for the classification of vasculitides of the polyarteritis nodosa group. Br J Rheumatol 35:958–964

Kussmaul A, Maier R (1866) Über eine bisher nicht beschriebene eigentümliche Arterienerkrankung (Perarteriitis nodosa), die mit Morbus Brightii und rapid fortschreitender allgemeiner Muskellähmung einhergeht. Deut Arch Klin Med 1:484–518

Langford CA, Sneller MC (1997) New developments in the treatment of Wegener's granulomatosis, polyarteritis nodosa, microscopic polyangitis, and Churg-Strauss syndrome. Curr Opin 9:26–30

Lindberg K (1931) Ein Beitrag zur Kenntnis der Periarteriitis nodosa. Acta Med Scand 76:183

Moreland LW, Ball GV (1990) Cutaneous polyarteriitis nodosa. Am J Med 88:426–430

Sheth AP, Olson JC, Esterly NB (1994) Cutaneous polyarteritis nodosa of childhood. J Am Acad Dermatol 31:561–566

Kawasaki Disease

Barron KS, Shulman ST, Rowley A et al. (1999) Report of the National Institutes of Health Workshop on Kawasaki Disease. J Rheumatol 26:170–190

Chung CJ, Stein L (1998) Kawasaki disease: a review. Radiology 208:25–33

Hall M, Hoyt L, Ferrieri P et al. (1999) Kawasaki syndrome-like illness associated with infection caused by enterotoxin B-secreting Staphylococcus aureus. Clin Infect Dis 29:386–389

Kawasaki T (1967) Acute febrile mucocutaneous syndrome with lymphoid involvement with specific desquamation of the fingers and toes in children. [in Japanese] Arerugi 16:178–222

Leung DY, Meissner C, Fulton D et al. (1995) The potential role of bacterial superantigens in the pathogenesis of Kawasaki syndrome. J Clin Immunol 15(6):11–17

ANCA-Positive Small Vessel Vasculitis

Hagen EC, Ballieux BE, van Es LA et al. (1993) Antineutrophil cytoplasmatic autoantibodies; a review of the antigens involved, the assays, and the clinical and possible pathogenetic consequences. Blood 81:1996–2002

Niles JL (1996) Antineutrophil cytoplasmic antibodies in the classification of vasculitis. Annu Rev Med 47:303–313

Wegener Granulomatosis

Duna GF, Galperin C, Hoffman GS (1995) Wegener's granulomatosis. Rheum Dis Clin North Am 21:949–986

Hoffman GS (1993) Wegener's granulomatosis. Curr Opin Rheumatol 5:11–17

Jennings CR, Jones NS, Dugar J et al. (1998) Wegener's granulomatosis – a review of diagnosis and treatment in 53 subjects. Rhinology 36:188–191

Klinger H (1931) Grenzformen der Periarteriitis nodosa. Frankf Zschr Pathol 42:455–480

Knight JM, Hayduk MJ, Summerlin D-J et al. (2000) "Strawberry" gingival hyperplasia. Arch Dermatol 136:171–173

Lynch JP, Hoffman GS (1998) Wegener's granulomatosis: controversies and current concepts. Comp Ther 24:421–440

Reinhold-Keller E, Kekow J, Schnabel A et al. (1994) Influence of disease manifestation and antineutrophil cytoplasmic antibody titer on the response to pulse cyclophophamide therapy in patients with Wegener's granulomatosis. Arthritis Rheum 37:919–924

Wegener F (1939) Über eine eigenartige rhinogene Granulomatose mit besonderer Beteiligung des Arteriensystems und der Nieren. Beitr Path Anat 102:36–68

Churg-Strauss Syndrome

Bottero P, Venegoni E, Riccio G et al. (1990) Churg-Strauss syndrome. J R Soc Med 83:651–652

Behrens R, Holzhausen HJ, von Poblozki A et al. (1998) Eosinophil cationic protein in a 39-year-old patient with Churg-Strauss syndrome. Dtsch Med Wochenschr 123:6–11

Churg J, Strauss L (1951) Allergic granulomatosus, allergic angiitis, and periarteritis nodosa. Am J Pathol 27:277–294

Davis NDP, Dauod MS, McEvoy MT et al. (1997) Cutaneous manifestations of Churg-Strauss syndrome: a clinicopathologic correlation. J Am Acad Dermatol 37:199–203

Masi AT, Hunder GG, Lie JT et al. (1990) The American College of Rheumatology 1990 criteria for the classification of Churg-Strauss syndrome (allergic granulomatosis and angiitis). Arthritis Rheum 33:1094–1101

Vogel PS, Nemer J, Sau P (1992) Churg-Strauss syndrome. J Am Acad Dermatol 27:821–824

Microscopic Polyangiitis

Davson J, Ball J, Platt R (1948) The kidney in periarteritis nodosa. QJ Med 17:175–202

Guillevin L, Durand-Gasselin B, Cevallos R et al. (1999) Microscopic polyangiitis: clinical and laboratory findings in eighty-five patients. Arthritis Rheum 42:421–430

Irvine AD, Bruce IN, Walsh MY et al. (1997) Microscopic polyangiitis. Delineation of a cutaneous-limited variant associated with antimyeloperoxidase autoantibody. Arch Dermatol 133:474–477

Penas PF, Porras JI, Fraga J et al. (1996) Microscopic polyangiitis. A systemic vasculitis with a positive P-ANCA. Br J Dermatol 134:542–547

Zeek PM (1948) Studies on periarteritis nodosa. III. The differential between the vascular lesions of periarteritis nodosa and of hypersensitivity. Am J Pathol 24:889–917

Lymphomatoid Granulomatosis

Bekassy AN, Cameron R, Garwicz S et al. (1990) Lymphomatoid granulomatosis in children. J Rheumatol 17:571–572

Liebow AA, Carrington CR, Friedman PJ (1972) Lymphomatoid granulomatosis. Hum Pathol 3:457–558

Magro CM, Tawfik NH, Crowson AN (1994) Lymphomatoid granulomatosis. Int J Dermatol 33:157–160

Tong MM, Cooke B, Barnetson RStC (1992) Lymphomatoid granulomatosis. J Am Acad Dermatol 27:872–876

Leukocytoclastic Angiitis

Abe Y, Tanaka Y, Takenaka M et al. (1997) Leucocytoclastic vasculitis associated with mixed cryoglobulinaemia and hepatitis C virus infection. Br J Dermatol 136:272–274

Claudy A (1998) Pathogenesis of leukocytoclastic vasculitis. Eur J Dermatol 8:75–79

Gougerot H (1932) Septicémie chronique indéterminée caractériseé par de petits nodules dermique ("dermatitis nodularis non necroticans"), éléments érythémo-papuleux, purpura. Bull Soc Fr Dermatol Syph 39:1192–1194

Jennette JC, Tuttle R, Falk RJ (1993) The clinical, serologic, and immunopathologic heterogeneitiy of cutaneous leukocytoclastic angiitis. Adv Exp Med Biol 336:323–326

Papi M, De Pita O, Frezzolini A et al. (1999) Prognostic factors in leukocytoclastic vasculitis: what is the role of antineutrophil cytoplasmic antibody? Arch Dermatol 135:714–715

Ruiter M, Brandsma CH (1948) Arteriolitis allergica. Dermatologica 97:265–271

Sais G, Vidaller A, Jucgla A et al. (1997) Adhesion molecule expression and endothelial cell activation in cutaneous leukocytoclastic vasculitis. An immunohistologic and clinical study in 42 patients. Arch Dermatol 133:443–450

Henoch-Schönlein Purpura

Baselga E, Drolet BA, Esterly NB (1997) Purpura in infants and children. J Am Acad Dermatol 37:673–705

Henoch H (1868) Über den Zusammenhang von Purpura und Intestinalstörungen. Berlin Klin Wochenschr 5:517–519

Kraft DM, McKee D, Scott C (1998) Henoch-Schönlein purpura: a review. Am Fam Physician 58:405–408

Lanzkowsky S, Lanzkowsky L, Lanzkowsky P (1992) Henoch-Schönlein purpura. Pediatr Rev 13:130–137

Schönlein JL (1832) Allgemeine und spezielle Pathologie und Therapie. Etinger, Würzburg

Acute Hemorrhagic Edema

Finkelstein H (1938) Lehrbuch der Säuglings Krankheiten, 4th edn. Auff, Amsterdam, pp 814–830

Ince E, Mumcu Y, Suskan E et al. (1995) Infantile acute hemorrhagic edema: a variant of leucocytoclastic vasculitis. Pediatr Dermatol 12:224–227

Long D, Helm KL (1998) Acute hemorrhagic edema of infancy: Finkelstein's disease. Cutis 61:283–284

Seidlmayer H (1940) Die früchtinfantile, postinfektiose Kokarden-Purpura. Zschr Kinderheilk 61:217–255

Serna MJ, Leache A, Sola MA (1994) Targetlike lesions in an infant. Infantile acut hemorrhagic edema (AHE). Arch Dermatol 130:1055–1059

Snow IM (1913) Purpura, urticaria and angioneurotic edema of the hands and feet in a nursing baby. JAMA 61:18–19

Urticarial Vasculitis

Black AK, Lawlor F, Greaves MW (1996) Consensus meeting on the definition of physical urticarias and urticarial vasculitis. Clin Exp Dermatol 21:424–426

Eads TJ, Fretzin S, Lewis C (1998) Pruritic, painful eruption. Urticarial vasculitis. Arch Dermatol 134:231–234

Hamid S, Cruz PD Jr, Lee WM (1998) Urticarial vasculitis caused by hepatitis C virus infection: response to interferon alpha therapy. J Am Acad Dermatol 39:278–280

McDuffie FC, Sams WM Jr, Maldonado JF (1973) Hypocomplimentemia with cutaneous vasculitis and arthritis. Possible immune complex syndrome. Mayo Clin Proc 48:340–348

Mehregan DR, Gibson LE (1998) Pathophysiology of urticarial vasculitis. Arch Dermatol 134:88–89

Papadavid E, Yu RC, Tay A et al. (1996) Urticarial vasculitis induced by centrally acting appetite suppressants. Br J Dermatol 134:990–991

Schnitzler Syndrome

de Kleijn EM, Telgt D, Laan R (1997) Schnitzler's syndrome presenting as fever of unknown origin (FUO). The role of cytokines in its systemic features. Nether J Med 51:140–142

Puddu P, Cianchini G, Girardelli CR et al. (1997) Schnitzler's syndrome: report of a new case and review of the literature. Clin Exp Rheumatol 15:91–95

Schnitzler L, Schubert B, Boasson J et al. (1974) Urticaire chronique, lésions osseuses, macroglobulinémie IgM: maladie de Waldenström? Bull Soc Dermatol Syphil 81:363

Tomkova H, Shirafuji Y, Arata J (1998) Schnitzler's syndrome versus adult onset Still's disease. Eur J Dermatol 8:118–121

Hypergammaglobulinemic Purpura (Waldenström)

Finder KA, McCollough ML, Dixon SL et al. (1990) Hypergammaglobulinemic purpura of Waldenström. J Am Acad Dermatol 23:669–676

Katayama J (1995) Clinical analysis of recurrent hypergammaglobulinemic purpura associated with Sjogren syndrome. J Dermatol 22:186–190

Senecal JL, Chartier S, Rothfield N (1995) Hypergammaglobulinemic purpura in systemic autoimmune rheumatic diseases: predictive value of anti-Ro(SSA) and anti-La(SSB) antibodies and treatment with indometacin and hydroxychloroquine. J Rheumatol 22:868–875

Waldenström J (1943) Zwei interessante Fälle mit Hyperglobulinämie. Schweiz Med Wochenschr 78:927

Yamamoto T, Yokohama A (1997) Hypergammaglobulinemic purpura associated with Sjogren's syndrome and chronic C type hepatitis. J Dermatol 24:7–11

Tumor-Associated Vasculitis

Carson's S (1997) The association of malignancy with rheumatic and connective tissue diseases. Semin Oncol 24:360–372

Kurzrock R, Cohen PR (1993) Vasculitis and cancer. Clin Dermatol 11:175–187

Maestri A, Malacarne P, Santini A (1995) Henoch-Schönlein syndrome associated with breast cancer. A case report. Angiology 46:625–627

Nashitz JE, Yeshurun D, Eldar S et al. (1996) Diagnosis of cancer-associated vascular disorders. Cancer 77:1759–1767

Stashower ME, Rennie TA, Turiansky GW et al. (1999) Ovarian cancer presenting as leukocytoclastic vasculitis. J Am Acad Dermatol 40:287–289

Nodular Vasculitis

Cho KH, Lee DY, Kim CW (1996) Erythema induratum of Bazin. Int J Dermatol 35:802–808

Degitz K, Messer G, Schirren H et al. (1993) Successful treatment of erythema induratum of bazin following rapid detection of mycobacterial DNA by polymerase chain reaction. Arch Dermatol 129:1619–1620

Ollert MW, Thomas P, Korting HC et al. (1993) Erythema induratum of Bazin. Evidence of T-lymphocyte hyperresponsiveness to purified protein derivative of tuberculin: report of two cases and treatment. Arch Dermatol 129:469–473

Sanz-Vico MD, De Diego V, Sanchez Yus E (1993) Erythema nodosum versus nodular vasculitis. Int J Dermatol 32:108–112

Inflammatory Bowel Disease – Associated Vasculitis

Magro CM, Crowson AN (1999) A clinical and histologic study of 37 cases of immunoglobulin A-associated vasculitis. Am J Dermatopathol 21:234–240

Salmi M, Jalkanen S (1998) Endothelial ligands and homing of mucosal leukocytes in extraintestinal manifestations of inflammatory bowel disease. Inflamm Bowel Dis 4:149–156

Erythema Elevatum Diutinum

Bachmeyer C, Aractingi S (1996) Erythema elevatum diutinum with HIV-2 infection. Lancet 347:1041–1042

LeBoit PE, Cockerell CJ (1993) Nodular lesions of erythema elevatum diutinum in patients infected with the human immunodeficiency virus. J Am Acad Dermatol 28:919–922

Orteu CH, McGregor JM, Whittaker SJ et al. (1996) Erythema elevatum diutinum and Crohn disease: a common pathogenic role for measles virus? Arch Dermatol 132: 1523–1525

Radcliffe-Crocker H, Williams C (1894) Erythema elevatum diutinum. Brit J Dermatol 6:1–9

Sangueza OP, Pilcher B, Martin-Sangueza J (1997) Erythema elevatum diutinum: a clinicopathological study of eight cases. Am J Dermatopathol 19:214–222

Urbach E, Epstein E, Lorenz K (1932) Extrzelluläre Cholesterinose. Arch Dermatol Syph 166:243–272

Yiannis JA, El-Azhary RA, Gibson LE (1992) Erythema elevatum diutinum: a clinical and histopathologic study of 13 patients. J Am Acad Dermatol 26:38–44

Pyoderma Gangrenosum

Brunsting LA, Goeckerman WH, O'Leary PA (1930) Pyoderma (ecthyma) gangrenosum. clinical and experimental observations in five cases occurring in adults. Arch Dermatol 22:655–680

Callen JP (1998) Pyoderma gangrenosum. Lancet 351:581–585

Chow RK, Ho VC (1996) Treatment of pyoderma gangrenosum. J Am Acad Dermatol 34:1047–1060

Dourmishev AL, Miteva I, Schwartz RA (1996) Pyoderma gangrenosum in childhood. Cutis 58:257–262

Ko CB, Walton S, Wyatt EH (1992) Pyoderma gangrenosum: associations revisited. Int J Dermatol 31:574–577

Long CC, Jessop J, Young M et al. (1992) Minimizing the risk of postoperative pyoderma gangrenosum. Br J Dermatol 127:45–48

Perry HO, Winkelmann RK, Muller SA et al. (1968) Malignant pyodermas. Arch Dermatol 98:561–576

Powell FC, Su WP, Perry HO (1996) Pyoderma gangrenosum: classification and management. J Am Acad Dermatol 34:395–409

Livedo Racemosa

Asherson RA, Cervera R (1993) Antiphospholipid syndrome. J Invest Dermatol 100:21S–27S

Zala L, Braathen LR (1994) Livedo racemosa: a report of five cases. Dermatology 189:421–424

Sneddon Syndrome

Alegre VA, Winkelmann RK, Gastineau DA (1990) Cutaneous thrombosis, cerebrovascular thrombosis, and lupus anticoagulant – the Sneddon syndrome. Report of 10 cases. Int J Dermatol 29:45–49

Daoud MS, Wilmoth GJ, Su WP et al. (1995) Sneddon syndrome. Semin Dermatol 14:166–172

Schellong SM, Weissenborn K, Niedermeyer J et al. (1997) Classification of Sneddon's syndrome. Vasa 26:215–221

Sneddon IB (1965) Cerebrovascular lesions and livedo reticularis. Brit J Derm 77:80–85

Zelger B, Sepp N, Stockhammer G et al. (1993) Sneddon's syndrome. A long-term follow-up of 21 patients. Arch Dermatol 129:437–447

Livedo Vasculitis

Feldaker M, Hines EA Jr, Kierland RR (1955) Livedo reticularis with summer ulcerations. Arch Dermatol 72:31–42

Cutis Marmorata Telangiectatica Congenita

Baxter P, Gardner-Medwin D, Green SH et al. (1993) Congenital livedo reticularis and recurrent stroke-like episodes. Dev Med Child Neurol 35:917–921

Lohuizen CH, van (1922) Über eine seltene angeborene Hautanomalie (Cutis marmorata Telangiectactica). Acta Derm Venereol (Stockh) 3:202–211

Picascia DD, Esterly NB (1989) Cutis marmorata teleangiectatica congenita: report of 22 cases. J Am Acad Dermatol 20:1098–1104

Rupprecht R, Hundeiker M (1997) Cutis marmorata teleangiectatica congenita. Hautarzt 48:21–25

Wheeler PG, Medina S, Dusik A et al. (1998) Livedo reticularis, developmental delay and stroke-like episode in a 7-year-old male. Clin Dysmorphol 7:69–74

Malignant Atrophic Papulosis

Assier H, Chosidow O, Piette JC et al. (1995) Absence of antiphospholipid and anti-endothelial cell antibodies in malignant atrophic papulosis: a study of 15 cases. J Am Acad Dermatol 33:831–833

Degos R, Delort J, Tricot R (1942) Dermatite papulosquameuse atrophiante. Ann Dermatol Syph 21:148–150

Katz SK, Mudd LJ, Roenigk HH (1997) Malignant atrophic papulosis (Dego's disease) involving three generations of a family. J Am Acad Dermatol 37:480–484

Köhlmeier W (1940) Multiple Hautnekrosen bei Thromboangiitis obliterans. Arch Dermatol 181:783–792

Snow JL, Muller SA (1995) Degos syndrome: malignant atrophic papulosis. Semin Dermatol 14:99–105

Yag-Howard C, Shenefelt PD (1998) Multiple pink papules with white, depressed centers. Malignant atrophic papulosis (Degos disease). Arch Dermatol 134:233–236

Peripheral Occlusive Arterial Disease

Altstaedt HO, Berzewski B, Taschke (1993) Treatment of patients with peripheral arterial occlusive disease Fontaine stage IV with intravenous iloprost and PGE 1: a randomized open controlled study. Prostaglandins Leukot Essent Fatty Acids 49:573–578

Horsch S, Claeys L (1994) Epidural spinal cord stimulation in the treatment of severe peripheral arterial occlusive disease. Ann Vasc Surg 8:468–474

LoGerfo FW (1992) Peripheral arterial occlusive disease and the diabetic: current clinical management. Heart Dis Stroke 1:395–397

McCulloch JM, Kemper CC (1993) Vacuum-compression therapy for the treatment of an ischemic ulcer. Phys Ther 73:165–169

Pemberton M, London NJ (1997) Colour flow duplex imaging of occlusive arterial disease of the lower limb. Br J Surg 84:912–919

Diabetic Angiopathy

Bierhaus A, Ziegler R, Nawroth PP (1998) Molecular mechanisms of diabetic angiopathy – clues for innovative therapeutic interventions. Horm Res 50:1–5

Stehouer CD, Lambert J, Donker AJ et al. (1997) Endothelial dysfunction and pathogenesis of diabetic angiopathy. Cardiovasc Res 34:55–68
Tooke JE, Shore AC, Cohen RA et al. (1996) Diabetic angiopathy: tracking down the culprits. J Diabetes Complications 10:173–181

Thrombangiitis Obliterans
Buerger L (1908) Thromangiitis obliterans: a study of the vascular lesions leading to presenile spontaneous gangrene. Am J Med 136:567–580
Mishima Y (1996) Thromangiitis obliterans (Buerger's disease). Int J Cardiol 54:S185–187
Suzuki S, Yamada I, Himeno Y (1996) Angiographic findings in Buerger disease. Int J Cardiol 54: S189–195
Zellerman GL, Lin MT, Rosen T (1998) Chronic ulcerations in the upper and lower extremities. Thrombangiitis obliterans (Buerger disease). Arch Dermatol 134:1019–1023

Hypertensive Ulcer
Henderson CA, Highet AS, Lane SA et al. (1995) Arterial hypertension causing leg ulcers. Clin Exp Dermatol 20: 107–114
Martorell F (1945) Las úlceras supramaleolares por arteriolitis de los grandes hipertensos. Actas Inst Policlinico (Barcelona) 1:6–9
Nikolova K (1995) Treatment of hypertensive venous leg ulcers with nifedipine. Methods Find Exp Clin Pharmacol 17:545–549

Diseases of the Veins
Kappert A (1998) Lehrbuch und Atlas der Angiologie, 13th edn. Huber, Bern
Rabe E (1994) Grundlagen der Phlebologie. Kagerer Kommunikation, Bonn
Ramelet AA, Monti M (1999) Phlebology. Elsevier, Amsterdam
Ruckley CV, Fowkes FGR, Bradbury AW (eds) (1999) Venous disease, epidemiology, management and delivery of care. Springer, London
Tibbs DJ, Sabiston DC, Davies MG et al. (eds) (1997) Varicose veins, venous disorders, and lymphatic problems in the lower limbs. Oxford University Press, Oxford
Wienert V (1993) Beinveneninsuffizienz, 2nd edn. Schattauer, Stuttgart

Varicosities
De Roos KP, Neumann HA (1998) Muller's ambulatory phlebectomy for varicose veins of the foot. Dermatol Surg 24:465–470
Evans CJ, Fowkes FG, Hajivassiliou CA et al. (1994) Epidemiology of varicose veins. A review. Int Angiol 13: 263–270
Goldman MP, Weiss RA, Bergan JJ (1994) Diagnosis and treatment of varicose veins: a review. J Am Acad Dermatol 31:393–413
Goldman MP, Sadick NS, Weiss RA (1995) Cutaneous necrosis, teleangiectatic matting, and hyperpigmentation following sclerotherapy. Etiology, prevention, and treatment. Dermatol Surg 21:19–29
Morrow PL, Hardin NJ, Karn CM et al. (1994) Fatal hemorrhage by varicose veins. Am J Forensic Med Pathol 15: 100–104
Palfreyman SJ, Lochiel R, Michaels JA (1998) A systemic review of compression therapy for venous leg ulcers. Vasc Med 3:301–313
Smith SR, Goldman MP (1998) Tumescent anesthesia in ambulatory phlebectomy. Dermatol Surg 24:453–456

Thrombophlebitis
Bergqvist D, Jaroszewski H (1986) Deep vein thrombosis in patients with superficial thrombophlebitis of the leg. Br Med J 292:658–659
Campbell B (1996) Thrombitis, phlebitis, and varicose veins. Br Med J 312:198
Guex JJ (1996) Thrombotic complications of varicose veins. A literature review of the role of superficial venous thrombosis. Dermatol Surg 22:378–382

Superficial Migratory Thrombophlebitis
Fiehn C, Pezzuto A, Hunstein W (1994) Superficial migratory thrombophlebitis in a patient with reversible protein C deficiency and anticardiolipin antibodies. Ann Rheum Dis 53:843–844
Vaughan MM, Thomas WE (1995) Thrombophlebitis migrans in association with acute relapsing pancreatitis. Br J Surg 82:674
Walsh-McMonagle D, Green D (1997) Low-molecular-weight heparin in the management of Trousseau's syndrome. Cancer 80:649–655

Superficial Sclerosing Phlebitis
Chiedozi LC, Aghahowa JA (1988) Mondor's disease associated with breast cancer. Surgery 103:438–439
Cox EM, Siegel DM (1997) Mondor disease: an unusual consideration in a young woman with a breast mass. J Adolesc Health 21:183–185
Favre JP, Becker F, Lorcerie B et al. (1992) Vascular manifestations in homocystinuria. Ann Vasc Surg 6:294–297
Diamantopoulos EJ, Yfanti G, Andreadis E (1999) Giant-cell arteritis presenting as Mondor disease. Ann Intern Med 130:78–79
Mondor H (1939) Tronculite souscutanée de la paroi thoracique antéro-laterale. Mem Acad Chir 65:1271–1278

Deep Vein Thrombosis
Bounameaux H, de Moerloose P, Perrier A et al. (1994) Plasma measurement of D-Dimer as a diagnostic aid in suspected venous thromboembolism: an overview. Thromb Haemost 71:1–6
Brandjes DPM, Büller H, Hejboer H et al. (1997) Incidence of the postthrombotic syndrome and the effects of compression stockings in patients with proximal venous thrombosis. Lancet 349:759–762
Cogo A, Lensing AWA, Koopman MMW et al. (1998) Compression ultrasonography for diagnostic management of patients with clinically suspected deep vein thrombosis: prospective cohort study. Br Med J 316:17–20
Ginsberg JS (1996) Management of venous thromboembolism. N Engl J Med 335:1816–1828
Hirsh J, Weitz JI (1999) New antithrombotic agents. Lancet 353:1431–1436
Lensing AWA, Prandoni P, Prins MH et al. (1999) Deep vein thrombosis. Lancet 353:479–485

Martineau P, Tawil N (1998) Low-molecular-weight heparins in the treatment of deep-vein thrombosis. Ann Pharmacother 32:588–598
Nordström M, Lindblad B, Anderson H et al. (1994) Deep venous thrombosis and occult malignancy: an epidemiological study. Br Med J 308:891–894
Partsch H, Kechavarz B, Köhn H et al. (1996) The effect of mobilisation of patients during treatment of thromboembolic disorders with low-molecular-weight heparin. Int Angiol 16:189–192
Rosendaal FR (1999) Venous thrombosis: a multicausal disease. Lancet 353:1167–1173
Schulman S, Granqvist St, Holmström M et al. (1997) The duration of oral anticoagulant therapy after a second episode of venous thromboembolism. N Engl J Med 336:393–398
Wheeler HB, Hirsch J, Wells P et al. (1994) Diagnostic tests for deep vein thrombosis. Arch Intern Med 154: 1921–1928

Diseases Associated with Hypercoagulability

Brigden ML (1997) The hypercoagulable state. Who, how, and when to test and treat. Postgrad Med 101:249–262
Girolami A, Simioni P, Scarano L et al. (1997) Venous and arterial thrombophilia. Haematologica 82:96–100
Milian G (1929) Les atrophies cutanées syphilitiques. Bull Soc Fr Dermatol 36:865–871
Nachman RL, Silverstein R (1993) Hypercoagulable states. Ann Intern Med 119:819–827
Rao AK, Sheth S, Kaplan R (1997) Inherited hypercoagulable states. Vasc Med 2:313–320
Rosenberg RD, Aird WC (1999) Vascular-bed-specific hemostasis and hypercoagulable states. N Engl J Med 340:1555–1564
van den Belt AG, Sanson BJ, Simioni P et al. (1997) Recurrence of venous thromboembolism in patients with familial thrombophilia. Arch Intern Med 157:2227–2232
Zoller B, Garcia de Frutos P, Hillarp A et al. (1999) Thrombophilia as a multigenic disease. Haematologica 84:59–70

Antithrombin III Deficiency

Demers C, Ginsberg JS, Hirsh J et al. (1992) Thrombosis in antithrombin-III-deficient persons. Report of a large kindred and literature review. Ann Intern Med 116: 754–761
Rosendaal FR, Heijboer H (1991) Mortality related to thrombosis in congenital antithrombin III deficiency. Lancet 337:1545
Seguin J, Weatherstone K, Nankervis C (1994) Inherited antithrombin III deficiency in the neonate. Arch Pediatr Adolesc Med 148:389–393

Protein C and Protein S Deficiency

Aiach M, Gandrille S, Emmerich J (1995) A review of mutations causing deficiencies of antithrombin, protein C and protein S. Thromb Haemost 74:81–89
Allaart CF, Poort SR, Rosendaal FR et al. (1993) Increased risk of venous thrombosis in carriers of hereditary protein C deficiency defect. Lancet 341:134–138
Amster MS, Conway J, Zeid M et al. (1993) Cutaneous necrosis resulting from protein S deficiency and increased antiphospholipid antibody in a patient with systemic lupus erythematosus. J Am Acad Dermatol 29:853–857
Baccard M, Vignon-Pennamen MD, Janier M et al. (1992) Livedo vasculitis with protein C system deficiency. Arch Dermatol 128:1410–1411
Falanga V, Bontempo FA, Eaglstein WH (1990) Protein C and protein S plasma levels in patients with lipodermatosclerosis and venous ulceration. Arch Dermatol 126: 1195–1197
Libow LF, DiPreta EA, Dyksterhouse DL (1997) Cutaneous heparin necrosis in a patient with heterozygous protein S deficiency. Cutis 59:242–244
Phillips WG, Marsden JR, Hill FG (1992) Purpura fulminans due to protein S deficiency following chickenpox. Br J Dermatol 127:30–32
Schramm W, Spannagl M, Bauer KA et al. (1993) Treatment of coumarin-induced skin necrosis with a monoclonal antibody purified protein C concentrate. Arch Dermatol 129:753–756
Weir Nu, Snowden JA, Greaves M et al. (1995) Livedo reticularis associated with hereditary protein C deficiency and recurrent thromboembolism. Br J Dermatol 132:283–285

Factor V Mutation

Bertina RM, Koeleman BPC, Koster T et al. (1994) Mutation in blood coagulation factor V associated with resistance to activated protein C. Nature 369:64–67
Dahlbäck B, Carlsson M, Svensson PJ (1993) Familial thrombophilia due to previously unrecognized mechanism characterized by poor anticoagulant response to activated protein C: prediction of a cofactor to activated protein C. Proc Natl Acad Sci USA 90:1004–1008
Desmarais S, de Moerloose P, Reber G et al. (1996) Resistance to activated Protein C in an unselected population of patients with pulmonary embolism. Lancet 347:1374–1375
Hoerl HD, Tabares A, Kottke-Marchant K (1996) The diagnosis and clinical manifestations of activated protein C resistance: a case report and review of the literature. Vasc Med 1:275–280
Munkvard S, Jorgensen M (1996) Resistance to activated protein C. A common anticoagulant deficiency in patients with venous leg ulceration. Br J Dermatol 134:296–298
Peus D, von Schmiedeberg S, Pier A et al. (1996) Coagulation factor V gene mutation associated with activated protein C resistance leading to recurrent thrombosis, leg ulcers, and lymphedema: successful treatment with intermittent compression. J Am Acad Dermatol 25:306–309
Zöller B, Dahlbäck B (1994) Linkage between inherited resistance to activated protein C and factor V gene mutation in venous thrombosis. Lancet 343:1536–1538

Prothrombin Gene Mutation

De Stefano V, Martinelli I, Mannucci PM et al. (1999) The risk of recurrent deep venous thrombosis among heterozygous carriers of both factor V Leiden and the G2021A prothrombin mutation. N Engl J Med 341:801–806
Martinelli I, Sacchi E, Landi G et al. (1998) High risk of cerebral-vein thrombosis in carriers of a prothrombin-gene mutation and in users of oral contraceptives. N Engl J Med 338:1793–1797
Poort SR, Rosendaal FR, Reitsma PH et al. (1996) A common genetic variation in the 3′-untranslated region of the prothrombin gene is associated with elevated plasma prothrombin levels and an increase in venous thrombosis. Blood 88:3698–3703

Homocystinuria

den Heijer M, Koster T, Blom HJ et al. (1996) Hyperhomocystinemia as a risk factor for deep vein thrombosis. N Engl J Med 334:759–762

Favre JP, Becker F, Lorcerie B et al. (1992) Vascular manifestations in homocystinuria. Ann Vase Surg 6:294–297

Makris M (1998) Hyperhomocystinemia is a risk factor for venous and arterial thrombosis. Br J Haematol 101:18–20

Mandel H, Brenner B, Beranet M et al. (1996) Coexistence of hereditary homocystinuria and factor V Leiden – effect on thrombosis. N Engl J Med 334:763–768

Chronic Venous Insufficiency

Anderson JH, Geraghty JG, Wilson YT et al. (1990) Paroven and graduated compression hosiery for superficial venous insufficiency. Phlebology 5:271–276

Cheatle TR, Scurr JH, Coleridge Smith PD (1991) Drug treatment of chronic venous insufficiency and venous ulceration: a review. J R Soc Med 84:354–358

Dunn JM, Cosford EJ, Kernick VFM et al. (1995) Surgical treatment for venous ulcers: is it worthwhile? Ann R Coll Surg Engl 77:421–424

Goren G (1991) Injection sclerotherapy for varicose veins: history and effectiveness. Phlebology 6:7–11

Groen G, Yellin AE (1995) Minimally invasive surgery for primary varicose veins: limited invaginated axial stripping and tributary (hook) stab avulsion. Ann Vasc Surg 9:401–414

Kistner RL (1997) Classification of chronic venous disease. Vasc Surg 3:217–218

Leu HJ (1993) Morphological findings in chronic venous insufficiency. Phlebology 8:48–49

Leu AJ, Leu HJ, Franzeck UK et al. (1995) Microvascular changes in chronic venous insufficiency – a review. 3:237–245

Lynch TG, Dalsing MC, Ouriel K et al. (1999) Developments in diagnosis and classification of venous disorders: non-invasive diagnosis. Cardiovasc Surg 7:160–178

Motykie GD, Caprini JA, Arcelus JI et al. (1999) Evaluation of therapeutic compression stockings in the treatment of chronic venous insufficiency. Dermatol Surg 25:116–120

Oesch A (1993) 'Pin-stripping': a novel method of atraumatic stripping. Phlebology 8:171–173

Piller MH, Ernst E (1998) Horse-chestnut seed extract for chronic venous insufficiency. A criteria based systematic review. Arch Dermatol 134:1356–1360

Porter JM, Moneta GL (1995) International Consensus Committee on Chronic Venous Disease. Reporting standards in venous disease: an update. J Vasc Surg 21:635–645

Widmer LK, Kamber V, Leu HJ (1978) Dokumentation und Einteilung. In: Widmer LK (ed) Venenkrankheiten: Häufigkeit und sozialmedizinische Bedeutung. Hans Huber Verlag, Bern, pp 17–32

Stasis Ulcer

Black SB (1995) Venous stasis ulcers: a review. Ostomy Wound Manage 41:20–30

Gosain A, Sanger JR, Yousif NJ et al. (1991) Basal cell carcinoma of the lower leg occuring in association with chronic venous stasis. Ann Plast Surg 26:279–283

Gourdin FW, Smith JG (1993) Etiology of venous ulceration. South Med J 86:1142–1146

Padberg FT (1999) Surgical intervention in venous ulceration. Cardiovasc Surg 7:83–90

Schmeller W, Gaber Y, Gehl H-B (1998) Shave therapy is a simple, effective treatment of persistent venous leg ulcers. J Am Acad Dermatol 39:232–238

Other Diseases Associated with Chronic Venous Deficiency
Atrophie Blanche

Bisalbutra P, Kullavanijaya P (1993) Sulfasalazine in atrophie blanche. J Am Acad Dermatol 28:275–276

Cooper DL, Bolognia JL, Lin JT (1991) Atrophie blanche in a patient with gamma-heavy-chain disease. Arch Dermatol 127:272–273

Suarez SM, Paller AS (1993) Atrophie blanche with onset in childhood. J Pediatr 123:753–755

Acroangiodermatitis

Chaix A (1926) La dermite pigmentée et purpurique des membres inférieurs. Lésions pré-erosive des ulcéres dits variqueux. Lyon (Thesis)

Favre M (1941) Nouvelle pratique dermatologique. Paris, p. 413

Landthaler M, Stolz W, Eckert F et al. (1989) Pseudo-Kaposi's sarcoma occurring after placement of arteriovenous shunt. J Am Acad Dermatol 21:499–505

Mali JWH, Kuiper JP, Hamers AA (1965) Acroangiodermatitis of the foot. Arch Dermatol 92:515

Rao B, Unis M, Poulos E (1994) Acroangiodermatitis: a study of ten cases. Int J Dermatol 33:179–183

Yi JU, Lee CW (1990) Acroangiodermatitis. A clinical variant of stasis dermatitis. Int J Dermatol 29:515–516

Postthrombotic Syndrome

Biguzzi E, Mozzi, Alatri A et al. (1998) The post-thrombotic syndrome in young women: retrospective evaluation of prognostic factors. Thromb Haemost 80:575–577

Ernst E (1992) Rheology of the post-thrombotic syndrome. J Mal Vasc 17:93–96

Leizorovicz A (1998) Long-term consequences of deep vein thrombosis. Haemostasis 28:1–7

Prandoni P, Lensing AW, Cogo A et al. (1996) The long-term clinical course of acute deep venous thrombosis. Ann Intern Med 125:1–7

Rutherford RB (1996) Pathogenesis and pathophysiology of the post-thrombotic syndrome: clinical implications. Semin Vasc Surg 9:21–25

CHAPTER 23

Disorders of Hemostasis

Contents

Introduction

Hemostasis is a complex problem. Endothelial cells, megakaryocytes and platelets, clotting factors, fibrinolysis components and their inhibitors are all intertwined in a system designed to rapidly seal off vessel damage without producing extensive clotting or occlusion. Normally, there is a delicate balance between the factors favoring hemostasis and those opposing it. If the hemostatic system is inappropriately activated, a thrombosis results. If on the other hand the system fails to function effectively, hemorrhage occurs. Since the skin is often the first site where hemorrhage is seen, dermatologists must have a basic understanding of hemostasis. We have deliberately simplified this chapter, leaving out rare disorders and only touching on the basic scientific aspects of platelet function, the coagulation cascade, and fibrinolysis. A number of different disturbances can lead to hemorrhage:

- Platelet Defects. Both quantitative and qualitative platelet defects can produce bleeding problems.
- Coagulation Defects. Quantitative or qualitative defects in components of the coagulation cascade can lead to inadequate hemostasis. Many of these problems are inherited.
- Fibrinolysis. Fibrin may either be present in insufficient amounts or broken down too rapidly.
- Vascular Defects. Sometimes capillaries leak because of increased pressure as in chronic venous insufficiency (Chap. 22). In other instances, there is vessel wall damage from trauma or inflammation. In idiopathic purpura, it is assumed that the vessel wall permeability is the main factor, since platelet function, coagulation, and fibrinolysis can be much more exactly studied.

Diagnostic Approach

History. Often the history gives the first clues. One should inquire about the following:

- Hemostatic problems in other family members; if so, what pattern of inheritance, what diagnoses have been made

- Nature of bleeding: spontaneous, posttraumatic, frequency, duration
- Underlying diseases: hematologic malignancies, other tumors, chronic renal disease, chronic hepatic disease
- Recent problems: infections, transfusions, immunizations
- Medications: pay special attention to aspirin, anticoagulants, immunosuppressive or chemotherapy agents

Clinical Findings. One should observe the type of bleeding, which may range from tiny petechiae to huge hematomas.

- Petechiae. These small (1–5 mm) areas of leakage usually represent defects in the platelet system or vascular wall abnormalities. They occur spontaneously and are discrete but may coalesce. The most typical locations for petechiae are sites of increased intravascular or mechanical pressure. Thus, they are more common on the feet and distal aspects of the legs, for example. Blanching does not occur with pressure, allowing one to rule out telangiectases. There is no edema or erythema, as would be seen with vasculitis. Purpura refers to the exanthem produced by petechiae; the Latin root simply means purple. Some use purpura to define small areas of bleeding that are nevertheless larger than petechiae.
- Ecchymoses. Ecchymosis comes from the Greek for a pouring out of blood and refers to a large flat extravasation. Suggillation is a wonderful word derived from the Latin term to beat someone up and refers to bruises or black and blue marks. Hematoma indicates a deep bleeding with swelling. All these lesions are usually sharply bordered, often asymmetrical, and go through characteristic color changes from purple to blue to green-yellow.

The type of cutaneous hemorrhage gives clues as to the underlying hematologic defect:

- Patients with thrombocytopenia tend to have petechiae; even with marked platelet defects, large areas of bleeding are relatively uncommon. Petechiae can also involve mucosal surfaces. Typical sites include the conjunctiva, nasal and oral mucosa. In the mouth, larger lesions are more common. Other organs which may show petechial-like bleeding include the retina, intestine, kidneys, and CNS. Increased menstrual bleeding may also occur.
- Ecchymoses and hematomas suggest a coagulation defect, as classically seen in hemophilia. There is often associated hemorrhage in the soft tissues and joints, which is not seen with platelet defects.
- In individuals with vasculitis, there is usually a mixture of petechiae and palpable lesions, sometimes associated with erythema and edema. This combination, known as palpable purpura, is discussed in Chapter 22.
- In complex hemostatic problems, such as disseminated intravascular coagulation (DIC), there is often a combination of ecchymoses and petechiae. The underlying large bleeding problem produces a consumptive coagulopathy, leading to decreased platelets and secondary petechiae.

Laboratory Findings. The laboratory evaluation of hemostasis is complex; the number of tests which can be ordered is almost inconceivably large, and the selection should be left to specialists. Nonetheless, a logical approach to screening tests should form part of the dermatologist's knowledge base, as shown in Table 23.1. For example, the classic Rumpel-Leede test in which a tourniquet is applied to the biceps area for 10 min and the distal skin observed for petechiae is a good test for vascular wall integrity.

Platelet-Related Hemostatic Diseases

A reduced number of platelets is known as thrombocytopenia; the normal range is 140,000–400,000/µl. When the platelet count drops below 30,000–40,000/µl, bleeding may result. In addition, functional defects in platelets (thrombocytopathia)

Table 23.1. Stepwise approach to hemostatic diagnosis

Component	Useful screening tests
Platelets	Platelet count Bleeding time Platelet morphology
Coagulation	Prothrombin time (Quick test) Activated partial thromboplastin time (aPTT) Thrombin time
Fibrinolysis	Reptilase time Fibrinogen Fibrin split products
Vessel wall	Rumpel-Leede test

may occur; there may be inherited problems, such as abnormal membrane proteins, or acquired defects, often induced by medications.

Thrombocytopenia

Definition. Thrombocytopenia is defined as peripheral platelet counts of less than 140,000/µl.

Etiology and Pathogenesis. Congenital thrombocytopenia is most uncommon; we will only discuss the Wiskott-Aldrich syndrome. There are several mechanisms of acquired thrombocytopenia (Table 23.2). Most important are impaired production or increased destruction. Splenic sequestration and dilution are other possibilities.

Clinical Findings. Petechiae represent the main symptom of thrombocytopenia. They typically occur on the distal aspects of the legs or at sites of pressure. If other factors come into play, such as vessel wall changes or altered coagulability, then they may appear with higher platelet counts. Minor injuries can lead to ecchymoses. One should look for conjunctival hemorrhages and ask about epistaxis and bleeding gums, as well as searching for hematuria and melena. Retinal hemorrhages are not only dangerous in themselves but may suggest underlying CNS bleeding.

Many other clues can be found on physical examination. Fever should suggest infection, systemic lupus erythematosus, or thrombotic thrombocytopenic purpura, but is usually not present in idiopathic thrombocytopenic purpura or drug-induced thrombocytopenia. Splenomegaly suggests sequestration or a malignant lymphoma. Jaundice and palmar erythema indicate chronic liver disease.

Table 23.2. Causes of thrombocytopenia

Production defects
- ***Reduced numbers of megakaryocytes***
  - Bone marrow aplasia or hypoplasia
  - Aplastic anemia
  - Megakaryocyte aplasia
  - Ionizing radiation
  - Myelosuppressive medications
  - Bone marrow infiltration or replacement: Leukemia, lymphoma, metastatic carcinoma; osteomyelofibrosis, storage diseases
  - Impaired platelet production: Drugs (Table 23.4); viral infections, especially rubella
- ***Ineffective development of megakaryocytes***
  - Nutritional defects (folic acid, Vitamin B_{12})
  - Alcohol
  - Myeloproliferative diseases
- ***Unknown or mixed causes***
  - Chronic renal disease

Increased removal
- ***Nonimmunologic***
  - Disseminated intravascular coagulation (early)
  - Thrombotic thrombocytopenic purpura and related disorders
  - Vasculitis
  - Preeclampsia and eclampsia
  - Kasabach-Merritt syndrome
  - Adult respiratory distress syndrome
  - Hemodialysis
  - Heart-lung machine
- ***Immunologic***
  - *Primary:* idiopathic thrombocytopenic purpura
  - *Secondary:* autoimmune diseases, especially systemic lupus erythematosus; hematologic malignancies; HIV/AIDS; drugs (quinine, quinidine, many others; Table 23.4, heparin); alloantibodies (posttransfusion purpura)

Sequestration
- Hypersplenism

Dilution
- Massive transfusions
- Massive bleeding

Laboratory Findings. The platelet count and bleeding time are the most important parameters. Occasionally, automated counting machines will give a falsely low value, as platelets aggregate in the anticoagulated blood specimen. One must always correlate platelet count with platelet number and morphology on a blood smear. The peripheral blood smear is also needed to identify associated erythrocyte damage in thrombotic thrombocytopenic purpura or leukocyte abnormalities in leukemias or anemias. The bleeding time will be prolonged in any platelet deficiency; if the bleeding time is prolonged although the platelet count is above 440,000/µl, a functional defect involving the platelets is likely. Bone marrow examination is also required. Coagulation studies are normal.

Hereditary Thrombocytopenia

Wiskott-Aldrich Syndrome

(Wiskott 1937; Aldrich et al. 1954)

Definition. Familial thrombocytopenia with impaired immunity, increased risk of infections, and dermatitis.

Epidemiology. This very rare disorder has an incidence of about 1:500,000. It is inherited in a X-linked recessive pattern.

Etiology and Pathogenesis. The genetic defect is located on the X chromosome at Xp11.3–11.2, so almost all affected patients are male. Female carriers are asymptomatic since the X chromosome carrying the defective gene appears to be selectively inactivated. The gene is known as WASP, and the defective product may be sialophorin, a surface glycoprotein on neutrophils, lymphocytes, and platelets. The patients have diffuse immune defects involving both their cell-mediated and humoral limbs. Both helper and suppressor T cell function is abnormal. Typically, IgM is markedly reduced while the other immunoglobulins are elevated. The platelets are small and lack organelles, but are also destroyed by phagocytes in the bone marrow; thus, despite the presence of normal megakaryocytes, platelet function is impaired. The platelet half-life is only 2–3 days, compared with the normal range of 4–5 days.

Clinical Findings. The clinical features are protean. The platelet defects lead to petechiae which can be present at birth, associated with umbilical stump or circumcision bleeding. Internal organ bleeding is common. The chronic dermatitis is clinically indistinguishable from atopic dermatitis and tends to improve with age. One clinical difference may be the presence of hemorrhage in the dermatitic lesions (Fig. 23.1). The immune deficiency presents the major problem early in life, as bacterial infections such as pneumonia and meningitis are both common and severe, encapsulated organisms causing the most trouble. Later, pyodermas, otitis media, human papilloma virus and molluscum contagiosum infections occur commonly. Herpes simplex, varicella, and cytomegalovirus infection can take a fulminant and fatal course.

Laboratory Findings. The reduced number of small platelets, decreased IgM level, and lowered T cell counts all point towards the diagnosis. The genetic defect can be identified for confirmation, carrier identification, and prenatal diagnosis.

Course and Prognosis. The outlook is poor. Those patients who do not succumb to infections or bleeding problems are at great risk for leukemias, lymphomas, and even solid tumors.

Differential Diagnosis. All the different immunodeficiency syndromes (Chap. 4) must be considered. While atopic dermatitis is a clinical consideration, almost at first glance one notices that the patient has other problems.

Therapy. The only satisfactory treatment is bone marrow transplantation, assuming an appropriate donor can be found. Appropriate antibiotic and antiviral therapy, immunoglobulin replacement, platelet transfusions, and other supportive measures are warranted. Splenectomy may help

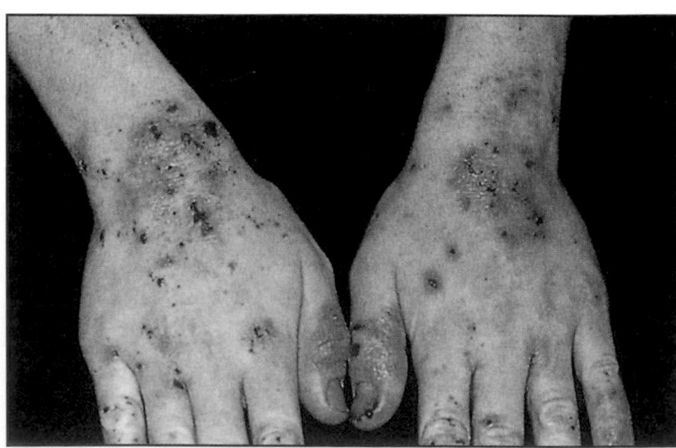

Fig. 23.1. Dermatitis in Wiskott-Aldrich syndrome

the platelet problem but increases the infectious risk.

Acquired Thrombocytopenia

Thrombocytopenia Secondary to Impaired Platelet Production

Etiology and Pathogenesis. Many different mechanisms are involved in this type of thrombocytopenia.

Bone Marrow Damage. Both radiation therapy and cytotoxic drugs may damage or ablate the bone marrow, leading to decreased platelets along with pancytopenia.

Bone Marrow Infiltration. The bone marrow may be replaced by metastatic tumors, lymphoproliferative disorders, or fibrosis.

Impaired Platelet Production. Some medications, especially thiazide diuretics, can selectively impair platelet production. Childhood rubella and cytomegalovirus infections may also lead to thrombocytopenia. In this setting there are decreased numbers of normal megakaryocytes.

Impaired Megakaryopoesis. Vitamin B_{12} and folic acid deficiency lead to defective megakaryocytes, as well as anemia. Alcohol also exerts many effects, including a toxic effect on megakaryocyte precursors as well as arrested maturation; typically micromegakaryocytes are found in the bone marrow. In many myeloproliferative diseases, structurally abnormal megakaryocytes are seen.

The mechanisms behind the reduced platelet count seen in 15–50% of patients with chronic renal failure are poorly understood.

Clinical Findings. Once again, the dermatologic features include purpura and occasionally ecchymosis. The underlying disturbance determines the overall clinical pattern and the appropriate therapeutic approach.

Thrombocytopenia Secondary to Increased Platelet Destruction

Etiology and Pathogenesis. In this scenario, the peripheral platelet consumption cannot be matched by increased bone marrow production. The platelet half-life is reduced to several hours and the turnover increased by up to five-fold. The number of megakaryocytes in the marrow is normal or raised, and the platelet volume is increased as larger, more immature cells are released.

On a pathogenic basis, this group of disorders is somewhat artificially divided into nonimmunologic and immunologic forms, depending on whether antiplatelet antibodies are present. Regarding both drug reactions and infections, there appears to be considerable overlap.

Thrombotic Thrombocytopenic Purpura
(Moschcowitz 1924)

Synonyms. Moschcowitz syndrome, thrombotic microangiopathy

Definition. Thrombotic thrombocytopenic purpura (TTP) is characterized by the pentad of thrombocytopenia, hemolytic anemia with fragmented erythrocytes, neurologic deficits, fever, and impaired renal function.

Epidemiology. TTP is very uncommon, with a incidence of 1:50,000. There is a slight female predominance, and most patients are between 20 and 50 years of age.

Etiology and Pathogenesis. The term TTP does not refer to a single disease or to a single pathogenic process. The best defined mechanism is the failure of a metalloprotease to degrade large polymers of von Willebrand factor in patients with recurrent TTP. In those with acute episodes, there appears to be inhibition of the metalloprotease by an IgG autoantibody whose trigger awaits elucidation. In all cases, fibrin is deposited in small vessels, trapping and damaging platelets and erythrocytes, microthrombi develop and occlude small vessels.

The most common form is primary or idiopathic TTP, although in some cases the cause can be identified. The best established one is the relationship with hemorrhagic colitis and Shiga toxin from *Escherichia coli* 0157 and *Shigella dysenteriae.* The antiplatelet drug ticlopidine very rarely causes TTP, but the affected patients tend to have a rocky course; oral contraceptives, penicillin, chemotherapy agents, and cyclosporine have also been implicated, as have pregnancy and metastatic carcinoma.

Clinical Findings. Usually, TTP is an acute fulminant disease, but it can take an intermittent or chronic course. The clinical picture varies tremendously from patient to patient depending on the site of the microthrombi. The main cutaneous signs are petechiae and ecchymosis. Many patients are jaundiced as they have profound hemolytic anemia. Most have fever and neurologic problems including paresthesias, paralysis, seizures, and a disturbed level of consciousness. Renal disease is common but typically mild, with proteinuria and mild elevations in creatinine. Abdominal symptoms, cardiac conduction abnormalities, acute pulmonary failure, and retinal hemorrhages or detachment are less common features. About 25% of patients have hepatosplenomegaly.

Histopathology. Occasionally, platelet-rich thrombi can be seen in the small vessels of the superficial plexus. No vasculitis is present. The same thrombi can be seen on bone marrow and gingival biopsies.

Laboratory Findings. The peripheral blood shows thrombocytopenia, leukocytosis, anemia, reticulocytosis, and marked erythrocyte damage (fragmented cells known as schistocytes). LDH is clearly elevated, bilirubin somewhat raised, and haptoglobin either very low or absent. Typical platelet counts are 10,000–50,000/μl. Bone marrow examination shows increased production of leukocytes, erythrocytes, and megakaryocytes. Mild or moderate hematuria and proteinuria are found. The coagulation studies are normal, although fibrin split products may be augmented as a sign of increased fibrinogen turnover. The direct Coombs test is negative. During the acute phase, serum levels of platelet-specific proteins such as β-thromboglobulin and platelet factor 4 are raised.

Course and Prognosis. In the past, the mortality was over 90%. Most patients died within the first 10 days of their disease. Today it is around 10–15%.

Differential Diagnosis. Adult hemolytic uremic syndrome (HUS) is very closely related to TTP. There are differences only in the distribution of organ involvement; HUS patients have more severe renal disease and fewer CNS problems. Other differential diagnostic possibilities include systemic lupus erythematosus and Evans syndrome.

Therapy. TTP is an acute medical emergency not likely to be treated by dermatologists. Details should be sought in an internal medicine text.

Hemolytic-Uremic Syndrome

(Gasser et al. 1955)

The hemolytic-uremic syndrome (HUS) is a variant of TTP most commonly found in children. It often occurs in epidemics, suggesting an infectious trigger. Often *Escherichia coli* 0157 or *Shigella dysenteriae* is identified in the stool; the bacteria secrete a verotoxin which is held responsible for the platelet aggregation. The renal disease is usually pronounced, and commonly the platelet-rich thrombi are identified on renal biopsy. The other manifestations, including petechiae and ecchymoses, are similar to TTP. Most cases resolve spontaneously, but some require renal dialysis.

Immune-Mediated Acquired Thrombocytopenia

Immune-mediated platelet destruction is common and takes many forms. Both idiopathic thrombocytopenic purpura and autoimmune thrombocytopenia associated with other autoimmune diseases are seen by dermatologists from time to time. Most thrombocytopenia are associated with medication or infections and immunizations. Even when antiplatelet antibodies are not identified, platelet destruction may result from circulating immune complexes and activation of the complement cascade.

Immune Thrombocytopenic Purpura

(Werlhof 1735)

Synonyms. Morbus haemorrhagicus maculosus, immune thrombocytopenic purpura, Werlhof disease

Definition. Autoimmune disorder with antiplatelet antibodies and marked thrombocytopenia.

Epidemiology. Immune thrombocytopenic purpura (ITP) is typically divided into two forms. Acute ITP is a disease of children; in 80% of cases it develops following a viral infection. The incidence is about 6/1000 yearly, involving boys and girls. The age peak is 1–6 years. The chronic form involves adults beginning between 20 and 40 years of age. There formerly was a 4:1 female predominance, and only rarely is a predisposing infection implicated. HIV/AIDS infection has changed this aspect; in many communities, it is now the most common cause of ITP, so that the risk group matches that of HIV infection, producing a male shift.

Etiology and Pathogenesis. In the acute form, the most likely explanation is that there is a cross-reaction between antiviral antibodies and platelet antibodies. The destruction of platelets in the spleen is so marked that the bone marrow cannot compensate. The trigger for the chronic form is unknown, but the immunology is better studied. Over 90% of patients have platelet-associated immunoglobulin, usually IgG (PA-IgG). The immunoglobulins are directed against a platelet glycoprotein receptor, and the main problem is increased splenic destruction of PA-IgG-labeled platelets. The platelet half-life correlates with the platelet count and is reduced to a matter of hours. The bone marrow production is increased two- to five-fold, but cannot effectively compensate.

The relationship between ITP and systemic lupus erythematosus is complex. Purpura may be an early manifestation of systemic lupus erythematosus in as many as 10% of patients, and present without characteristic immunologic parameters. The old fear that splenectomy might accelerate systemic lupus erythematosus in these underdiagnosed patients has not been substantiated. Thyroid disease is present in about 10% of ITP patients. Thus, one should search for systemic lupus erythematosus and check thyroid function in all apparent ITP patients; how one then classifies the individuals is unclear.

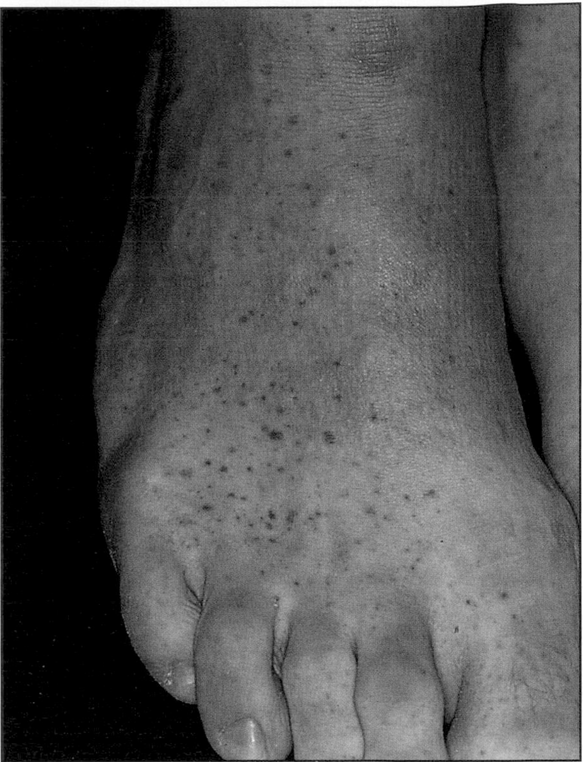

Fig. 23.2. Immune thrombocytopenic purpura

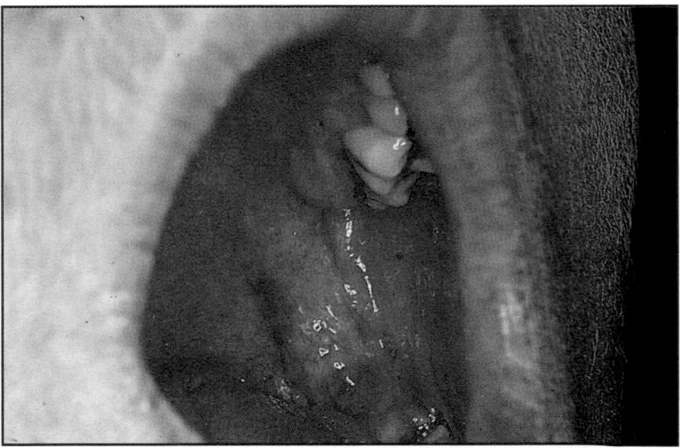

Fig. 23.3. Oral lesions in idiopathic thrombocytopenic purpura

Clinical Findings. Once again, petechiae and ecchymosis are seen (Fig. 23.2). Usually, the hair follicles are spared, and there are no epidermal changes such as scaling. Both lymphadenopathy and splenomegaly are uncommon. Even though typical platelet counts are below 20,000/µl, the degree of purpura is mild. Uterine bleeding may be a problem in adults. Some divide ITP patients into those with just purpura and those with mucosal bleeding (wet purpura) who are at greater risk for severe problems (Fig. 23.3). In children with acute ITP, about 5% have evidence of internal bleeding from retinal, gastrointestinal, or urogenital sites; the incidence of CNS bleeds is less than 1%. Some children may have splenomegaly.

Laboratory Findings. The platelet count is usually <20,000/µl, while a peripheral smear is otherwise normal. PA-IgG and other autoantibodies are identifiable in about 90% of cases. Bone marrow examination usually reveals an increased megakaryocytic response, with giant and immature forms.

Course and Prognosis. In children, spontaneous remission is the rule. This usually occurs after 2–6 weeks, and recurrences are uncommon. In adults, the disease is chronic. The mortality rate is about 1–5%, most often from CNS bleeds. There may be short remissions with increased platelet counts, but the counts soon drop. Bacterial or viral infections may trigger profound drops. As the patients age, the risk of intracranial bleed increases; for example, a 60-year-old patient has about a 20-fold risk compared with a 30-year-old with the same platelet count.

Differential Diagnosis. Evans syndrome represents the association of ITP with Coombs-positive hemolytic anemia. Secondary forms of immune-mediated thrombocytopenia are clinically identical, but have a different history or background.

Therapy. In children, therapy is usually not needed. In adults, unless the platelet level drops below 30,000/μl, treatment can also be withheld. Common sense advice includes avoiding strenuous physical activity, sports in which trauma is common, and medications which have any influence on platelet function(especially aspirin and nonsteroidal anti-inflammatory drugs). The patients should use a soft toothbrush and an electric razor. Intramuscular injections should be avoided, and pressure should be applied to venipuncture sites for about 10 min.

Therapy is guided by the bleeding problems and not by the platelet count. It is best left to the hematologist. The mainstay of therapy is systemic corticosteroids, usually in dosages of around 1 mg/kg daily. Splenectomy is usually the next step in patients who do not respond to or tolerate corticosteroids. Intravenous immune globulin 1.0 g/kg daily produces a prompt but temporary increase in platelets and can be used prior to surgical procedures or during severe acute hemorrhages. Patients who respond well to immune globulin are more likely to do well with splenectomy. In refractory patients, azathioprine 2 mg/kg daily appears to be the best option. Pulse corticosteroid therapy, danazol, and vincristine have also been recommended.

Secondary Immune-Mediated Thrombocytopenia

The thrombocytopenia associated with systemic lupus erythematosus, rheumatoid arthritis, Hodgkin disease, malignant lymphoma, and chronic lymphocytic leukemia is very similar to ITP. Autoimmune thyroid diseases such as Hashimoto disease and Grves disease should be excluded, as they require quite different therapy. Other associated diseases may include myasthenia gravis and systemic sclerosis. The situation is often complicated by aspects of the underlying disease, such as bone marrow infiltration, splenic sequestration, or other autoimmune phenomena. In addition, treatment of the underlying malignancy may further compromise the megakaryocytes. If feasible, the same approaches discussed under ITP are applied here.

HIV-Associated Immune Thrombocytopenia

Epidemiology. About 3–9% of HIV-infected patients have thrombocytopenia. As their disease progresses, the prevalence increases to over 50%.

Etiology and Pathogenesis. The similarities between ITP and HIV/AIDS thrombocytopenia far outweigh the differences. In HIV/AIDS, circulating immune complexes are extremely common, and the autoantibodies have slightly different targets. Direct damage to megakaryocytes can be seen. Furthermore, HIV/AIDS patients are exposed to a variety of drugs which show bone marrow toxicity and further reduce the platelet count.

Clinical Findings. About one-third of patients with HIV-associated thrombocytopenia have clinical bleeding problems. CNS bleeding is a major risk in hemophiliacs with HIV infection but less common in other risk groups. Purpura can be seen in patients with asymptomatic HIV infection as well as in AIDS patients. In the former group, it usually cannot be distinguished from ITP. There may be a slightly higher incidence of mucosal bleeding among HIV/AIDS patients.

Therapy. Usually, antiviral therapy results in an increased platelet count. Systemic corticosteroids are the next choice. The role of a splenectomy is unclear in this patient group. Other approaches discussed under ITP may be appropriate.

Infection-Related Thrombocytopenia

Etiology and Pathogenesis. Usually, infection-related thrombocytopenia has a mixed pathogenesis. Typical infections include malaria, gram-negative sepsis, varicella, and infectious mononucleosis. There is increased peripheral consumption of platelets, but occasionally, direct megakaryocyte toxicity is also implicated. The mechanisms of peripheral destruction include platelet aggregation and consumption, direct microbial damage to platelets, platelet adherence to altered vessel walls, and immune complex-mediated damage. In most of these infections, there are varying degrees of evidence for immune damage, including anti-platelet antibodies.

Clinical Findings. The clinical features can range from petechiae to marked ecchymoses and internal bleeding. The prognosis and treatment are based on the underlying disease.

Medication-Related Immune Thrombocytopenia

Epidemiology. This problem is more common in the elderly, probably because they are exposed to more medication. There appears to be a female predilection.

Etiology and Pathogenesis. Most medication-related thrombocytopenia results from the induction of autoantibodies that contribute to platelet destruction. The medication may bind to the platelet surface, creating a new antigen which triggers an immune response. In some instances, the resultant autoantibodies can react with platelets in the absence of the medication, so they are indistinguishable from those seen in ITP. In other cases, both the antibody and the medication must be present to trigger platelet damage; this is the situation with quinine and quinidine. In other situations, such as with gold, the platelet membrane is altered so that it becomes antigenic, but the medication itself does not serve as a hapten. The list of drugs occasionally associated with thrombocytopenia is long and should be sought in the sources listed in Chapter 10.

Clinical Findings. Probably, most drug-induced thrombocytopenia is overlooked. Usually, the first manifestations are mild with petechiae on the legs. Upon re-exposure to the mediation, the bleeding may become more severe and be associated with fever and chills.

Laboratory Findings. The diagnosis is very difficult; usually the history is the most important aspect. Two in vitro tests have been developed – inhibition of clot retraction and platelet agglutination – but neither is very reliable. Identifying the circulating antibodies is a task for specialized laboratories.

Therapy. If a drug-induced thrombocytopenia is suspected, the medication must be avoided, as subsequent attacks tend to be more severe. Usually stopping the offending agent suffices. If there is severe bleeding, either corticosteroids or intravenous immunoglobulins can be used, as discussed under ITP.

Heparin-Associated Thrombocytopenia

The action of heparin on platelets is complex but common. Two different processes are involved in heparin-induced thrombocytopenia (HIT). In type I HIT there is a mild, always reversible decline in platelet count just after starting treatment. In contrast, type II HIT starts 6–14 days after onset of therapy and causes marked thrombocytopenia not associated with bleeding but instead with life-threatening venous and arterial thromboembolic events.

Epidemiology. HIT is probably the most common medication-induced platelet problem. Type I disease occurs in over 10 % of patients, while type II is less common, but presents in up to 5 % of patients treated with unfractionated heparin. The incidence is significantly reduced when low molecular weight heparin is employed. The mortality of type II HIT has been estimated as 20–50 %.

Etiology and Pathogenesis. The type of heparin, the route of administration, and the dose hardly affect the outcome. Even the use of a heparin-coated catheter may cause type I disease, where platelet aggregation is stimulated, mildly reducing the count. In type II disease, there is an IgG antibody directed against platelet factor 4/heparin complexes which causes platelet aggregation, endothelial wall damage, and thrombosis.

Clinical Findings. Type I HIT is rarely noticed. Mild purpura may be seen. In type II disease, the patient may be critically ill with multiple thromboses and even pulmonary and cerebral emboli. The risk of thromboembolic problems rises as the platelet count drops; it is usually less than 50,000/µl and may fall below 10,000/µl. The cutaneous disease can be extensive, but it is secondary and the least of the patient's problems.

Laboratory Findings. The presence of the antibodies in type II HIT can be shown in vitro using platelet aggregation and secretion tests in the presence of various levels of heparin. ELISA methods can be used to identify the antibodies.

Therapy. In type I, heparin therapy can be continued, while in type II, it must be stopped. Because of the risk of type II HIT, many clinicians start coumarin at the same time as instituting heparin therapy. Coumarin should be continued as heparin is stopped if thrombocytopenia develops. If HIT is probable or diagnosed, low-molecular-weight heparin should not be used. Direct thrombin inhibitors such as hirudin (derived from leeches) and related compounds appear promising in this setting.

Alloantibody Immune-Mediated Thrombocytopenia

Allo- (or iso)antibodies are exogenous antibodies which are important in several types of thrombocytopenia. Examples include neonatal purpura with maternal antibodies damaging fetal platelets and posttransfusion purpura in which the recipient has antibodies against platelet antigens from the donor. Patients who require multiple platelet transfusions, such as those with acute leukemia or severe forms of thrombocytopenia with frequent bleeds, are at risk to develop antibodies against any number of platelet antigens. In such a case, they become refractory to the benefits of a platelet transfusion. Sometimes using single donor transfusions helps in this setting.

Thrombocytopenia Through Sequestration

In a normal human, about 30 % of the entire platelet mass is stored in the spleen, from whence the platelets move rapidly in and out. In a variety of forms of hypersplenism, the sequestration of the platelets can increase in a linear fashion with the spleen size, so that up to 80 % are hidden here. Platelet counts under 50,000/µl are unusual, because of bone marrow compensation. The platelet half-life may be somewhat reduced. Bleeding problems, including purpura, are uncommon. If the splenomegaly is associated with chronic hepatic disease and impaired coagulation, then bleeding problems are far more likely.

Thrombocytopenia Through Dilution

Ordinary stored blood contains nonviable platelets, so after 6–10 units have been replaced, the patient has few functioning platelets. In addition, there is no immediate bone marrow reserve. Patients with bleeding and volume replacement with expanders or similar agents also develop thrombocytopenia. Depending on clinical indications, platelet transfusions may be needed.

Thrombocythemia

Peripheral platelet counts greater than 400,000/µl are considered abnormal. The cause is always increased marrow production of megakaryocytes, either as a primary disease or secondary to a variety of stimuli. The main problem seems to be an overproduction of ineffective platelets, as patients have trouble with bleeding as well as with thrombosis, so antiplatelet agents should be considered carefully.

Primary Thrombocythemia

Myeloproliferative disorders, polycythemia vera, chronic myelogenous leukemia, osteomyelofibrosis, and primary or essential thrombocythemia all represent clonal proliferations of hematopoietic stem cells. Thus, a pure idiopathic proliferation of megakaryocytes and platelets is rare; usually, there is an associated increase in erythrocytes or leukocytes. The most common association is between polycythemia vera and thrombocythemia. Individuals with these conditions are likely to suffer erythromelalgia (Chap. 22). Patients with polycythemia vera tend to have thromboses, whereas those with isolated thrombocythemia are more likely to have bleeding problems. Leg ulcers may also develop. The platelet counts are usually higher; the polycythemia vera study group has suggested 800,000/µl and exclusion of any other bone marrow disorder as the criteria for essential thrombocythemia. Patients often have counts over 800,000/µl with isolated reports as high as 15,000,000/µl. There is a very poor correlation between the platelet count and the clinical problems. Treatment is complex because of the frequent presence of underlying disease and the problems of balancing bleeding versus thrombosis. The usual approach is oral hydroxyurea, which itself appears to trigger leg ulcers in this unique patient group. Interferon-α is effective in lowering the platelet count, while anagrelide, an imidazo-quinazoline compound, also appears effective.

Secondary Thrombocythemia

The list of diseases associated with elevated platelet counts is long. It includes chronic infections and inflammatory diseases (tuberculosis, sarcoidosis, rheumatoid arthritis, polyarteritis nodosa, osteomyelitis, Crohn disease, and ulcerative colitis), tumors (Hodgkin disease, malignant lymphomas, and some carcinomas), iron deficiency, stress, trauma, surgery, alcohol withdrawal, correction of B_{12} deficiency, and following splenectomy. Of particular interest is that many of these problems are also associated with thrombocytopenia, showing how fragile the balance is. The treatment is that of the underlying disorder.

Functional Abnormalities of Platelets

Functional platelet disorders are diagnosed by clinical problems with hemostasis, a prolonged bleeding time, and a platelet count usually greater than 100,000/μl. In contrast to those individuals with thrombocytopenia, such patients tend to have more ecchymoses and less often petechiae. The main clinical problem is drug-induced dysfunction; the hereditary disorders are only likely to be encountered on tests, not in daily practice.

Hermansky-Pudlak Syndrome

This pigmentary disorder is discussed in Chap. 26. Patients have platelets which lack dense bodies and are unable to store all the necessary mediators. They fail to aggregate irreversibly, leading to bleeding problems. The biggest problems arise with aspirin use; fatal bleeding accidents have been described.

Pseudo-von Willebrand Syndrome

Von Willebrand factor (vWF) is the only member of the clotting cascade synthesized and stored in platelets and endothelial cells, rather than in the liver. Thus, disorders involving it can be viewed as platelet or coagulation problems. It is the carrier molecule for Factor VIII, but also has binding sites for platelet glycoproteins I b and II b – III a, heparin, and collagen. The Ib site is most important for adhesion, while the II b – III a site is responsible for aggregation (and is blocked by the new monoclonal antibodies and peptides which prevent thrombosis). Large multimers of vWF are stored in the Weibel-Palade bodies of endothelial cells, as well as being released to the circulation. In pseudo-von Willebrand syndrome, the platelet glycoprotein IIb binds excessively well to vWF, causing platelet aggregation and depletion of vWF multimers. Agglutination in the presence of ristocetin is markedly increased. Desmopressin is contradicted here.

Membrane Disorders

Platelets adhere to damaged endothelium through a variety of membrane receptors. Patients with Bernard-Soulier syndrome lack the platelet glycoprotein I b – IX, the factor on the activated platelet that binds to vWF. They have impaired platelet adhesion to wound surfaces. Those with Glanzmann thrombasthenia lack the II b – III a complex which binds to fibrinogen, causing platelet aggregation. They may have severe mucosal bleeding.

Acquired Defects in Platelet Function

The diseases listed in Table 23.3 often lead to defects in platelet function. Usually the changes are subclinical, but if the patient is challenged with medications or has concomitant hematologic problems, hemorrhage may result.

Drug-Induced Platelet Dysfunction

Drug-induced platelet dysfunction is common, but usually not of clinical importance. In most instances, there is abnormal platelet aggregation and a prolonged bleeding time (Table 23.4).

Aspirin is the most commonly used antiplatelet agent. Within an hour of ingesting aspirin, the patient's platelets are profoundly altered for the duration of their lifetime, which is 7 – 12 days. Aspirin irreversibly inhibits cyclooxygenase blocking both platelet secretion and aggregation. A usual dose of 500 – 600 mg prolongs the bleeding time by several minutes in a normal individual. While most individuals do not experience bleeding problems when taking aspirin, they may have problems during surgical or dental procedures. The effects of aspirin last for 5 – 7 days after it is discontinued. If the patient has other problems, such as uremia or alcoholism, the effect of aspirin is severer. Other nonsteroidal antiinflammatory drugs have less severe and shorter term effects on the platelets.

Ticlopidine is a potent antiplatelet agent used in patients who are intolerant of aspirin which inhibits

Table 23.3. Disorders of platelet function (thrombocytopathies)

Hereditary disorders
Granule abnormalities
Hermansky-Pudlak syndrome
Factor abnormality
Pseudo-von Willebrand disease
Membrane abnormalities
Bernard-Soulier syndrome: Ib-IX absent
Glanzmann thrombasthenia: IIb-IIIa absent
Acquired disorders
Production of abnormal platelets
Hematologic diseases (polycythemia vera, myelogenous leukemia, essential thrombocythemia)
Alteration of normal platelet function
Medications
Chronic renal disease
Antiplatelet antibodies
Extracorporeal circulation
Chronic liver disease

Table 23.4. Medication-related platelet changes

Medication-related platelet changes
Production defects
Bone marrow toxicity
Most chemotherapy regimens
Impaired platelet production
Thiazides, amrinone, ethanol, estrogen, trimethoprim-sulfamethoxazole
Increased destruction
Heparin
Quinine, quinidine
Gold salts, rifampin, sulfonamides, oral hypoglycemic agents, valproic acid
Altered function
Inhibitors of cyclooxygenase
Aspirin
Nonsteroidal antiinflammatory drugs
Miconazole
Inhibitors of platelet-fibrinogen binding and platelet aggregation
Ticlopidine
Membrane changes
β-Lactam antibiotics (with other mechanisms)
Volume expanders (dextran, hydroxyethyl starch)

platelet-fibrinogen interactions. Many β-lactam antibiotics are also guilty of altering platelet function, making their use in septic patients at risk for bleeding a therapeutic challenge.

Disorders of Coagulation

The coagulation and fibrinolysis cascades are even more complex than the platelet system. Quantitative or qualitative defects in the coagulation proteins lead to perturbations of coagulation and fibrinolysis. There are both hereditary deficiencies in coagulation factors, such as hemophilia, and acquired deficiencies. Factors II, VII, IX, and X are vitamin K dependent, as are proteins S and C. In the case of fibrinolysis, most problems are acquired. Defects in coagulation lead to continued bleeding and are considered in this chapter. There are also a number of hypercoagulable states, many of which are associated with thromboses and are discussed in Chapter 22.

Hereditary Coagulopathies

For almost all the clotting factors, congenital deficiencies have been identified. Most are inherited in an autosomal recessive pattern, although in many cases the heterozygotes may also have mild bleeding tendencies. Homozygous patients tend to have ecchymoses and hematomas, not purpura.

Hemophilia

Definition. Bleeding disorder associated with deficiency in Factor VIII or IX.

Epidemiology. Hemophilia A (Factor VIII deficiency) and hemophilia B (Factor IX deficiency, Christmas disease) are both inherited in an X-linked recessive pattern. The genes have been identified at Xq28 and Xq27. Hemophilia A is about five times as common as hemophilia B; together they have a incidence of about 1:10,000 in German men. The history of hemophilia is fascinating to students of European history, as Queen Victoria was a carrier, and her male descendants in the royal houses of Europe were frequently affected, including the last crown prince of Russia.

Etiology and Pathogenesis. The Factor VIII gene is enormous, encoding a protein with a molecular weight of 330 kDa. Defects may lead to a lack of production of the protein Factor VIII:C (coagulant activity) or to abnormal proteins with varying degrees of dysfunction. Factor VIII:C is bound to vWF and combines with Factor IX:C at the end of the intrinsic pathway to cleave Factor X, starting the conversion of prothrombin to thrombin. Defects in either factor lead to impaired thrombin generation and poor clotting.

Clinical Findings. The main features are bleeding into joints, soft tissue, and internal organs. Ecchymoses and hematomas are common in the skin, as well as prolonged bleeding from even minor trauma or dental procedures.

Laboratory Findings. The activated partial thromboplastin time (aPTT) is prolonged, while the prothrombin time, thrombin time, and bleeding time are normal. Specific assays identify a deficiency in either Factor VIII:C or IX:C and quantify the defect.

Course and Prognosis. The coagulation factor activity is the main determinant of the prognosis.

- Less than 1% activity: Trouble in infancy, bleed at circumcision, spontaneous hemarthroses
- 1–5% activity: Onset in childhood; usually posttraumatic bleeding, rare hemarthroses
- 5–20% activity: Tend to have trouble after surgery, dental extraction, trauma
- 20–50% activity: Little trouble, may reach adult life and then have initial problems following major trauma or surgery

In recent years, infection with HIV/AIDS has radically altered the prognosis. Today the risk of infection during therapy has almost been eliminated by the use of careful donor selection and sophisticated virus inactivation procedures.

Differential Diagnosis. The main differential diagnostic consideration is von Willebrand disease. Inhibitory autoantibodies against Factor VIII:C can be seen in a wide variety of autoimmune diseases such as rheumatoid arthritis, systemic lupus erythematosus, dermatitis herpetiformis, and ulcerative colitis, as well as in association with gammopathies, pregnancy, and penicillin therapy.

Therapy. The mainstay is replacement therapy with Factor VIII concentrate. Today the risk of transmission of HIV, hepatitis B, and hepatitis C is almost zero. Recombinant Factor VIII is available but expensive. In addition to maintenance replacement, special approaches are needed for preoperative priming and managing acute bleeds. Desmopressin is useful for managing minor bleeds in modestly affected patients. Aspirin should never be administered. Some patients develop antibodies to Factor VIII and require concentrates with activated factor VIIIa. Factor IX concentrate is also available and is equally safe.

von Willebrand Disease

(von Willebrand 1926)

Definition. Group of disorders with quantitative or qualitative defects in von Willebrand factor (vWF).

Epidemiology. There are about ten different types of von Willebrand disease, but we shall discuss only the classic type I form. This is the most common bleeding disorder, with a frequency of around 0.5–1.0% in Europe.

Etiology and Pathogenesis. The gene for vWF is located on chromosome 12. The disease is inherited in an autosomal dominant pattern. The 270-kDa molecule is manufactured in endothelial cells and platelets and serves not only as a carrier for Factor VIII, but is also the main ligand in platelet adherence and aggregation.

Clinical Findings. The most common problem is mucosal bleeding, but there is tremendous variability. Some patients first discover they have a problem as adults when they experience bleeding following trauma or major surgery. Women may have increased menstrual bleeding as the first clue.

Laboratory Findings. The sorting out of the many subgroups of von Willebrand disease is beyond our scope. One can assess both vWF levels and function. The aPTT can be slightly prolonged because vWF is required for Factor VIII function. The bleeding time can be prolonged depending on the sensitivity of the method used; the platelet count is normal.

Therapy. Depending on the type, the two mainstays of therapy are desmopressin for patients with a reduced level of functionally normal vWF and replacement therapy with Factor VIII concentrates rich in vWF for those in whom the molecule is absent or dysfunctional.

Acquired Coagulopathies

The main categories of acquired coagulopathies are shown in Table 23.5.

Table 23.5. Major types of acquired coagulopathy

Defects in hepatic production of clotting factors
Vitamin K deficiency
Medications (coumarin, heparin, thrombolytics)
Acquired anticoagulants
Gammopathies
Marked blood loss and transfusions with dilution effect
Impaired fibrinolysis
Consumption coagulopathies, especially disseminated intravascular coagulation

Hepatic Defects

Etiology and Pathogenesis. Parenchymal liver damage leads to either reduced manufacture of clotting factors (II, V, VII, IX, X), inhibitors (proteins C and S, antithrombin III) or inadequate clearance of activated factors. The prothrombin time is the best measure of hepatic synthesis, as long as there is no vitamin K deficiency. There may be associated splenomegaly with platelet sequestration, as well as other platelet defects, such as those associated with alcohol. In addition, there may be consumption of fibrinogen and plasminogen, along with increased fibrinolysis. Thus, bleeding in severe hepatic disease is quite complex. The inability to clar activated factors also predisposes to DIC.

Clinical Findings. Cutaneous findings are rare, but both petechiae and ecchymoses are seen. Bleeding from esophageal varices and gastric or duodenal ulcers poses a far greater threat.

Laboratory Findings. The mainstays are the prothrombin time, aPTT, fibrinogen level, platelet count and bleeding time. Individual liver-dependent factors can also be assayed to evaluate the severity of the defect and to monitor substitution therapy.

Therapy. The therapy is difficult. Fresh-frozen plasma is usually required. Vitamin K should be given. If the platelet count is reduced, platelet transfusions may help.

Vitamin K Deficiency

Vitamin K is a fat-soluble vitamin required for the synthesis of Factors II, VII, IX, and X as well as proteins S and C. When it is lacking, both cutaneous and systemic bleeding can occur. Vitamin K deficiency is further discussed in Chapter 49.

Drug-Induced Hemorrhage

The drug-induced causes of hemorrhage are fairly predictable; the main offenders are coumarin, heparin, and thrombolytic therapy. Coumarin antagonizes vitamin K. The cause of bleeding can either be an overdose of coumarin or the administration of another drug which increases its action. The number of interactions with coumarin are numerous and complex; many drugs used by dermatologists prolong the prothrombin time by a variety of mechanisms. Included in the latter group are, for example, erythromycin, trimethoprim-sulfamethoxazole, metronidazole, and several of the imidazoles. On the other hand, rifampicin and griseofulvin reduce the prothrombin time by increasing the metabolic clearance of coumarin. The main clinical problems are ecchymoses, mucosal bleeding, and occasionally gastrointestinal bleeding. Usually decreasing the coumarin dosage, avoiding the interaction, and administering vitamin K suffice for treatment. If marked bleeding is present, various concentrates such as PPSB in Germany which contain Factors II, VII, IX, and X can be administered. Coumarin-induced skin necrosis is a dramatic event covered in Chapter 10.

Heparin causes bleeding through several mechanisms, but its main role is the potentiation of antithrombin III, as well as the platelet problems discussed above. The main clinical problems in the case of overdosage are hematomas and ecchymoses. The prothrombin time, thrombin time, and aPTT are all prolonged, but the reptilase time is normal. Normally stopping the infusion of heparin is adequate, because of its short half-life (30 min); in addition, reversal is possible with protamine sulfate. All forms of thrombolytic therapy have hemorrhage as their main complication, but most often the problem is oozing at vascular entry sites. CNS bleeds present the main serious complication.

Acquired Anticoagulants

Some patients have circulating proteins, usually antibodies, that inhibit coagulation factors. The main underlying diseases are collagen vascular disorders and lymphoproliferative diseases, or this can occur during pregnancy. Some medications, such as penicillin, sulfonamides, and phenytoin, may also act as antigens. The most common target antigens are Factors VIII and IX, although others have been described. The best clinical clue is the failure of the addition of normal plasma to correct a prolonged prothrombin time or aPTT. Lupus anticoagulants have to be differentiated because they interfere in vitro with coagulation assays but clinically cause thrombosis. The treatment is the same as for the factor deficiency; immunosuppressive therapy may also be tried to inhibit antibody production.

Gammopathies

The abnormal immunoglobulins associated with multiple myeloma and other gammopathies can block platelet function and interfere with coagulation. For example, IgA myeloma is associated with Factor V deficiency, while both IgA and IgM proliferations can reduce Factor VII deficiency. Plasmapheresis rapidly corrects the bleeding defect, but treatment must be directed at the underlying disease.

Gammopathies can cause purpura in many others ways, including vasculitis, such as that associated with cryoglobulinemia. Waldenström macroglobulinemia is a monoclonal IgM gammopathy which causes purpura through hyperviscosity, but usually larger areas of necrosis are also present. In the similarly named, totally unrelated, and extremely uncommon Waldenström purpura, there is a polyclonal gammopathy with poorly explained petechiae. The key clinical point is to check elderly patients with unexplained purpura for a gammopathy.

Fibrinolysis

Primary defects in fibrinolysis are rare. Most often fibrinolysis is associated with DIC. The fibrin D dimer test identifies the degradation products found in DIC. The two main causes of primary fibrinolysis are prostate surgery, through the release of large amounts of endogenous urokinase, and the bite of the Western diamondback rattlesnake, which directly introduces plasminogen activator and causes fibrinolysis. Other poisonous snake bites cause massive tissue destruction and then DIC.

Disseminated Intravascular Coagulation

(BARRAUD 1904)

Synonym. Consumption coagulopathy

Definition. Disseminated intravascular coagulation (DIC) is a complex hemostatic disturbance with many causes which lead to increased fibrin formation, thromboses, and bleeding.

Etiology and Pathogenesis. The various causes of DIC are listed in Table 23.6. The most common one is gram-negative sepsis, while massive trauma, burns, and metastatic tumors are other common causes. DIC is not a disease but a symptom of many different diseases, all of which reach a similar catastrophic end-point by slightly different pathways.

Four overlapping phases can be identified, as hemostatic mechanisms overwhelm their inhibitors.

- Hypercoagulability. The triggering event is usually uncontrolled hemostasis in which thrombin causes massive platelet activation and conversion of fibrinogen to fibrin to produce platelet-fibrin clots, especially in small vessels.
- Fibrinolysis. The expected control processes lead to the destruction of fibrin clots but overshoot, starting the vicious circle which characterizes the process.
- Plasminemia. Fibrin deposition triggers the unbridled production of plasmin, which further interferes with clotting and degrades fibrinogen and fibrin.
- Decompensatory Phase. The thrombin activation overwhelms the protein C, protein S, and antithrombin III control cycles, resulting in thromboses in arteries and veins. The resultant occlusion and tissue necrosis further drives the reaction. Since both thrombin and plasmin attack fibrinogen, soluble fibrin and fibrin split products (D dimers) are indicators of DIC.

Table 23.6. Causes of disseminated intravascular coagulation

Infections
Gram-negative sepsis, meningococcemia, Rocky Mountain spotted fever, some viral infections
Malignancies
Leukemia, especially acute promyelocytic leukemia
Carcinomas, more likely when metastatic
Obstetric problems
Preeclampsia and eclampsia
Amniotic fluid embolus
Abruptio placentae
Retained placental products
Trauma
Massive trauma especially crush injuries
Burns
Extensive surgery
Heatstroke
Abnormal or artificial vascular surfaces
Kasabach-Merritt syndrome
Use of heart-lung machine
Immunologic reactions
Incompatible blood transfusions (usually ABO)
Anaphylaxis
Immune complexes (such as post-varicella)
Bites
Some snake bites
Brown recluse spider bites

Clinical Findings. If the course of DIC is relatively slow or compensated, the thrombotic events tend to dominate, while in fulminant cases, the hemorrhagic events are key. While the skin is not the main site of activity, over 70% of patients have skin lesions. Bleeding problems such as purpura, ecchymoses, and hemorrhagic bullae as well as thromboses with occlusion and necrosis can be seen. The microvascular thrombi often cause a microangiopathic hemolytic anemia, as the tiny fibrin nets can be viewed as damaging the erythrocytes. The main cause of death is shock, resulting from tissue necrosis and massive fluid leakage, as well as many other, poorly understood factors. The thrombotic events tend to involve the heart, lungs, liver, and kidneys, causing a wide range of problems. Hemorrhages usually manifest as hematomas, internal bleeding, or leakage from vascular access sites.

Histopathology. The skin biopsy may show fibrin thrombi in small vessels. Later necrosis dominates the picture.

Laboratory Findings. The laboratory diagnosis of DIC is complex, as so many crucial factors are changing simultaneously. Typical findings include damaged erythrocytes on a peripheral smear and progressive thrombocytopenia despite normal marrow megakaryocytes. All coagulant assays tend to be abnormal. Fibrinogen is reduced, while fibrin monomer and fibrin split products are raised. Sequential monitoring of these parameters may be needed to confirm the diagnosis.

Course and Prognosis. The outlook for DIC is determined by how effectively the underlying disorder can be controlled. Mortality rates are very high.

Therapy. The most important factor is to treat the underlying or triggering disease, while also trying to correct hemodynamic imbalance, i. e., shock and hypoxemia. Heparin is occasionally tried in low dosages to antagonize thrombin by interacting with antithrombin III. The evidence is best for heparin use in acute promyelogenous leukemia; in other circumstances, it takes considerable courage to give heparin to an oozing, bleeding patient. Platelet transfusion and fresh-frozen plasma may be used when bleeding is the paramount symptom. The problem is that any interruption of the vicious circle may cause as much harm as good.

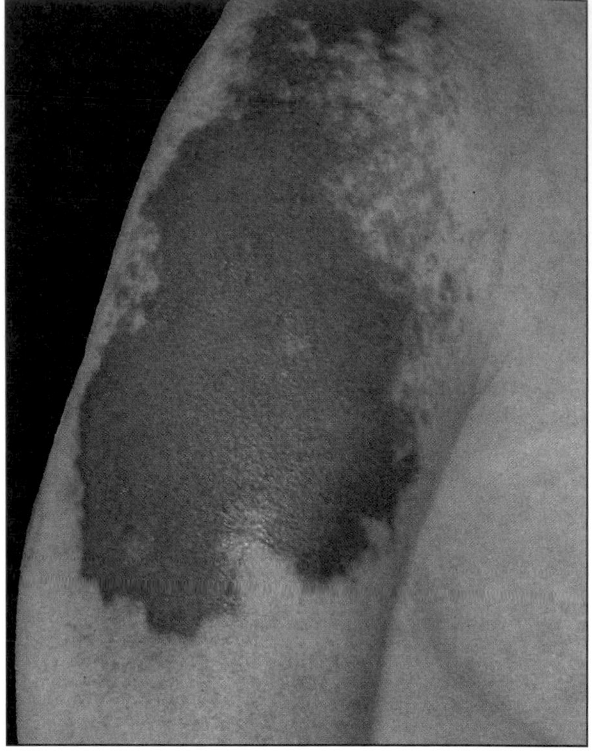

Fig. 23.4. Purpura fulminans

Purpura Fulminans

Definition. A form of DIC usually seen in children and usually associated with either a bacterial infection or markedly disturbed protein S and protein C metabolism.

Etiology and Pathogenesis. The main causes of purpura fulminans are gram-negative sepsis, meningococcemia, varicella, and Rocky Mountain spotted fever. Originally, purpura fulminans was described in children as an idiopathic reaction occurring in the recovery period following a banal infection, usually varicella, streptococcus, or other febrile exanthems. In addition, infants with homozygous defects in proteins S or C may present with severe purpura fulminans as well as internal vascular catastrophes. Sometimes no triggering event is identified, but increasingly transient defects in proteins C or S are found in such cases. The thromboses in purpura fulminans seem to involve primarily the venous side of the vascular tree.

Clinical Findings. The early lesions may be petechial, but soon ecchymoses develop (Fig. 23.4). Symmetric lesions, usually on the limbs, are typical. They are tender, expand rapidly, become bullous or necrotic, and coalesce to produce extensive skin loss. At the same time, there are usually systemic signs of DIC.

Therapy. The approach to the patient is that discussed under DIC. If a triggering infection is documented, it must be treated aggressively. Often the DIC occurs as the infection is resolving; this is particularly true of purpura fulminans associated with varicella. The patients with disorders of proteins S and C are usually treated with coumarin, but the results are disappointing. The use of protein C concentrates appears to be a promising option.

Waterhouse-Friderichsen Syndrome

(Waterhouse 1911; Friderichsen 1918)

Synonym. Meningococcal sepsis

Definition. Acute meningococcal sepsis with DIC and hemorrhagic adrenal necrosis.

Epidemiology. Infections with *Neisseria meningitidis* are discussed in Chapter 4. Most involve infants or children less than 4 years of age. About

5–10% of these individuals develop a fulminant disease with meningitis, sepsis, and DIC. Other gram-negative infections can also cause DIC, but the term Waterhouse-Friderichsen syndrome is usually reserved for meningococcal disease.

Etiology and Pathogenesis. The scenario discussed under DIC develops along with acute, bilateral adrenal hemorrhage, leading to adrenal insufficiency.

Clinical Findings. The cutaneous lesions are of diagnostic and prognostic value. Any patient with purpura and fever, especially an infant, should be suspected of having meningococcal disease. The early petechiae may be subtle, but later there are often ecchymoses. Lesions greater than 1 cm in size or confluent are associated with a severer disease course. Marked necrosis and gangrene, even to the point of necessitating amputations, are seen in extreme cases.

Histopathology. In addition to the fibrin thrombi of DIC, one may find leukocytoclastic vasculitis with abundant nuclear debris. Numerous gram-positive organisms can be found in the vessel wall. Even scrapings from petechiae may reveal bacteria.

Laboratory Findings. *Neisseria meningitidis* can be cultured from the CSF or peripheral blood. Both peripheral leukocytosis and CSF leukocytosis with elevated protein and decreased sugar can be found. All of the parameters discussed under DIC are implicated in more advanced cases.

Course and Prognosis. In full-blown Waterhouse-Friderichsen syndrome, the mortality rate is about 70%. The necrotic skin lesions heal with scarring.

Differential Diagnosis. Early on, this includes other febrile illnesses associated with purpura, such as Rocky Mountain spotted fever, enteroviral infections, *Haemophilus influenzae* infections, and endocarditis. Later, the extensive purpura in an infant makes the diagnosis clearer.

Therapy. Penicillin G, 300,000 units/kg daily (maximum of 24 million units) intravenously every 2 h is the initial treatment. Usually treatment for 7–10 days suffices. In addition, the supportive measures discussed under DIC apply. Contacts of the patient should be considered for antibiotic prophylaxis, usually with rifampin.

Kasabach-Merritt Syndrome

(Kasabach and Merritt 1940)

Synonyms. Giant hemangioma syndrome, hemangioma-thrombocytopenia syndrome

Definition. Association of hemangioma with thrombocytopenia and DIC.

Etiology and Pathogenesis. The Kasabach-Merritt syndrome is a disease of infants usually less than 3 months of age who have a congenital hemangioma or vascular malformation. Even though the term giant hemangioma syndrome has been used, it is misleading because the underlying lesion is almost always a tufted angioma or a Kaposiform hemangioendothelioma (Chap. 59). The reduced blood flow velocity is felt to increase platelet attachment to convoluted vessels, perhaps with abnormal endothelial cells. The platelet aggregation triggers DIC.

Clinical Findings. The patients have a vascular lesion which may be large, rapidly increasing in size, or show signs of thrombosis. Occasionally, it will be found in the liver or spleen, rather than the skin. Usually, the first sign is the development of petechiae. Later, more extensive purpura or ecchymoses are seen, along with hemolytic anemia, bleeding, and rarely the other problems associated with DIC.

Laboratory Findings. The first sign is thrombocytopenia, which is a warning. If one waits until hemolytic anemia, increased fibrin split products, or other signs of DIC are present, one has missed a window of opportunity.

Therapy. The main task is to remove the vascular malformation or hemangioma. If the problem is identified early, the bleeding defect can be controlled with fresh-frozen whole blood while surgical removal of the hemangioma is attempted. Alternatively, laser destruction can be tried. Often high-dose corticosteroids are employed because they too cause regression of hemangiomas (Chap. 59). If full-blown DIC develops, then the treatment approach may include heparin or inhibitors of platelet aggregation such as aspirin and dipyridamole.

Vessel-Related Hemorrhage

Into this group fall those diseases in which purpura is present but neither platelet function nor coagulation is deranged. Instead, the hemorrhage occurs through damaged or incompetent vessel walls. Petechiae are most commonly seen with capillary leakage, but if larger vessels are damaged, ecchymoses can also be seen.

Many different factors can damage the vessels. Vasculitis (Chap. 22) leads to purpura via vessel wall destruction. Leukocytoclastic angiitis, the most common from of vasculitis, is known as palpable purpura. In addition, elevated venous pressure can lead to leakage. In scurvy, vitamin C deficiency leads to vessel leakage, although vitamin C ingestion does not help prevent leakage in healthy individuals. Many infections cause transient purpura, probably through vessel wall damage as well as by influencing the hemostatic system. Hereditary vascular diseases such as hereditary hemorrhagic telangiectasia (Chap. 22) or connective tissue diseases such as Marfan syndrome or Ehlers Danlos syndrome (Chap. 18) may involve weakened vessels.

Acquired Vascular Purpura

Senile Purpura
(BATEMAN 1815)

Synonym. Purpura senilis

Definition. Common purpura in older individuals practically limited to the extensor surfaces of the arms.

Epidemiology. Extremely common, especially in individuals who have had extensive sun exposure or used corticosteroids.

Etiology and Pathogenesis. Chronic solar radiation is felt to be the main predisposing factor. The vessel walls appear to be more fragile. Mechanical trauma is the immediate cause of the purpura. Similar changes can be seen after prolonged systemic or topical use of corticosteroids (steroid purpura); the medication appears to inhibit collagen synthesis in the same, already damaged skin areas.

Clinical Findings. The most common site is the backs of the hands and the extensor surfaces of the forearms. Up to 5 cm in size, sharply bordered, red or blue-red, hemorrhagic patches with bizarre shapes appear relatively suddenly (Fig. 23.5). While there is only rarely a clear history, trauma is the cause. The lesions slowly evolve into brown patches as hemosiderin is deposited. The adjacent skin is thin and often shows white stellate scars, often caled pseudo-scars because a history of trauma is lacking. Sometimes the lesional skin can be documented to be stretching over a period of days. Rarely, lesions are seen on the legs, feet or face.

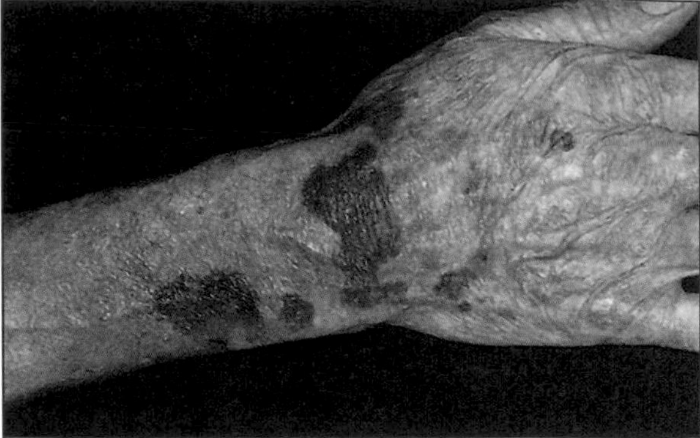

Fig. 23.5. Senile purpura

Therapy. There is no therapy other than attention to the predisposing factors and avoidance of trauma.

Orthostatic Purpura
(SCHULTZ 1918)

Synonyms. Purpura orthostatica, purpura jaune d'ocre

Definition. Petechiae on dependent surfaces which usually evolve into brown macules.

Epidemiology. Extremely common in elderly patients.

Etiology and Pathogenesis. Increased hydrostatic pressure in the capillaries of the legs leads to leakage of erythrocytes, causing petechiae. Thus, these changes are very commonly seen in chronic venous insufficiency. The deposited red cells are not easily scavenged, so hemosiderin deposition and hyperpigmentation occur. Often there is a secondary increase in melanin as well.

Clinical Findings. The most typical location is the distal third of the shins and the area around the ankle, as well as the dorsal surface of the feet. Occasionally, the forearms or hands may be affected. Tiny petechiae appear and undergo the typical color change from red to yellow to ochre, and occasionally to deep brown or black. The macules may coalesce. The dyschromia is usually permanent.

Therapy. Treatment of the chronic venous insufficiency is all that can be done. Medications alleged to inhibit capillary leakage are usually ineffective.

Mechanical Purpura

Many different activities can induce petechiae. Annular petechiae following the use of suction EKG electrodes is well-known. Another very common type of mechanical purpura is a hickey or medallion d'amour, usually seen on the neck following the combined application of kissing and suction. Tiny petechiae on the anterior axillary folds, hips, and dorsal surfaces of the feet, especially in women, reflect pressure from wearing apparel. Petechiae on the upper part of the trunk may be seen following the Valsalva maneuver, heavy coughing, blowing hard on a musical instrument, glass blowing, and similar activities. Often there is a minor predisposing factor such as aspirin use. While systemic amyloidosis is rare (Chap. 41), it often presents with traumatic purpura or ecchymoses, so if any clinical question remains, a biopsy is warranted.

Factitial Purpura

Synonym. Purpura factitia

Purpura may occur as a result of mechanical damage to the skin. Changes can be as innocent as bleeding into areas which have been intensively scratched or into lines of dermographism. In other instances, the patient may have manipulated their skin, such as by repeated pinching. Often localization is the clue; factitial purpura involves easily reched sites and often the same site repeatedly. In other instances, patients may be taking coumarin surreptitiously. Often such patients work in health-related professions. Hematologic studies should give a clue to this problem, which should be left to the care of psychologists or psychiatrists.

Paroxysmal Finger Hematoma
(Achenbach 1957)

Synonyms. Achenbach syndrome, finger apoplexy

Definition. Painful spontaneous hematoma of the fingers.

Etiology and Pathogenesis. This phenomenon is relatively uncommon but surely under-reported. The etiology is unknown, but there seems to be localized vessel fragility or ectatic vessels. In some cases, there is a history of minor trauma. Most patients are women.

Clinical Findings. Suddenly, a painful hematoma appears either in the hollow of the palm or the palmar aspect of the base of the finger. There may be swelling into the interdigital space. The sites typically exposed to trauma, such as fingertips or the thenar or hypothenar eminences, are rarely implicated. The lesion resolves spontaneously, but recurrences can be seen. In the interval, one may be able to identify ectatic veins at the site of prior injury.

Laboratory Findings. All hematologic parameters are normal.

Therapy. None required. Patients should try to avoid mechanical trauma, but this is easier said than done.

Metabolic Causes of Vessel-Related Purpura

Vitamin C Deficiency

Synonyms. Scurvy (adults), Moeller-Barlow disease (children)

In the past, scurvy was a major problem among salors and buccaneers, as dramatically expressed in the literature of seafaring nations. One of the hallmark features of scurvy is perifollicular petechiae, especially on the legs and associated with corkscrew hairs (Chap. 49). Gingival bleeding as well as deeper muscle and joint hematomas also occur. Vitamin C appears essential for the integrity of the collagen in the vessel wall. If vitamin C is the cause of hemorrhage, 300–500 mg daily rapidly reverses the problem. The use of vitamin C in other types of vessel-related purpura is often recommended but unsupported.

Diabetes Mellitus

Vessel damage is common in diabetes mellitus. The best known site is the retina, but Binkley spots on the legs represent tiny petechiae. The under-lying problem appears to be nonglycosylated proteins which accumulate in the walls of small vessels.

Corticosteroids

Both Cushing disease and syndrome, as well as the chronic or excessive use of topical or systemic corticosteroids, can lead to vessel fragility and purpura. Often there are overlaps with senile purpura. Despite the often extensive purpura, the hemostatic parameters are normal.

Pigmented Purpuric Dermatoses

Several, probably related disorders are usually grouped together in this category. In most instances, the changes are chronic and unlikely to improve. Histology does not help much to separate the different clinical variants. Pigmented purpuric dermatoses are common and the standard explanation for purpura in older individuals. The therapy is identical for all variants.

Etiology and Pathogenesis. Since the etiology is unknown, it is difficult to say exactly how closely related or distantly separated these entities are. All these disorders have a sparse, pericapillary, lymphocytic infiltrate. Other typical histologic features include thick-walled vessels with a proliferation of new tiny vessels, as well as the deposition of hemosiderin in macrophages and free in the upper dermis. The vessel changes probably reflect their location on the lower legs. There may also be epidermal dermatitic changes and pruritus. One comprehensive scenario might be:

inflammation → vessel wall damage → leakage → purpura → hemosiderin deposition.

There are other possible contributing factors. Occasionally, a mild hemorrhagic pigmented dermatosis may be associated with a viral infection or even food intolerance; such cases may resolve promptly. Drugs are often blamed and undoubtedly play a role in some cases. The old soporific carbromal was frequently incriminated; in some instances patch testing showed a delayed hypersensitivity to the agent. The patch testing appears more sensitive if performed on the shins or on a site where the stratum corneum has been tape-stripped. In some instances, there appears to be a narrowing of the small arteries in the superficial plexus, followed by dilatation of the capillaries and leakage. Such assessments are difficult to make in vivo, but it is easy to imagine that the vascular tone plays a role in leakage, as does the hydrostatic pressure.

Progressive Pigmented Purpura
(Schamberg 1901)

Synonyms. Dermatosis pigmentaria progressiva, Schamberg disease

Epidemiology. This is the most common of the hemorrhagic pigmented dermatoses and probably the most common purpura. Most patients are adults. It is similar to orthostatic purpure but occurs without evidence of chronic venous insufficiency.

Clinical Findings. The purpura usually begins symmetrically on the shins and occasionally may spread to the thighs, arms, or trunk. Initially, there are irregularly shaped, red-brown macules and patches of varying sizes (Fig. 23.6). The classic feature is the presence of tiny petechiae at their periphery, producing a speckled pattern. This distinctive appearance has been called Cayenne pepper spots. Cayenne is an island off the coast of South America famous for its peppers, but the description is fanciful. It has also been applied to multiple tiny telangiectases. The color later turns yellow brown, and there may be atrophy. New lesions continue to appear so that a kaleidoscopic pattern is

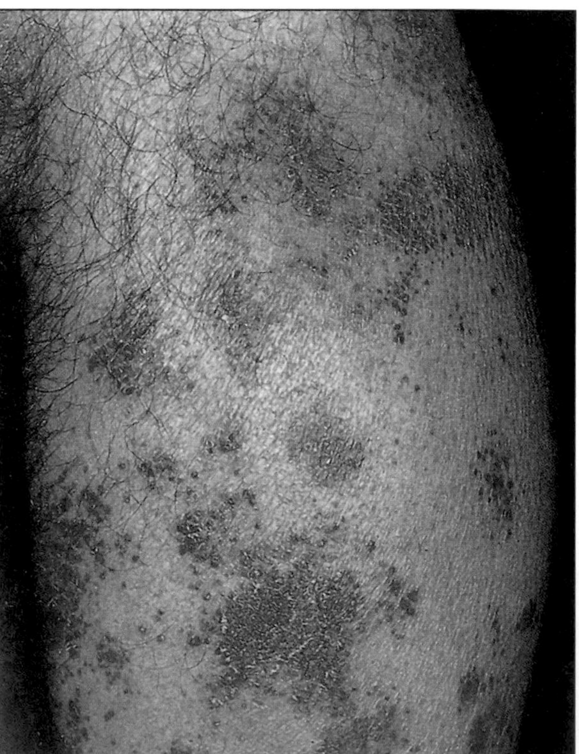

Fig. 23.6. Progressive pigmented purpura

formed. In severe cases, the shins become almost uniformly hyperpigmented.

Histopathology. There is a perivascular lymphocytic infiltrate associated with hemorrhage; later, the appearance of hemosiderin correlates with the shift from red to yellow-brown. Iron can be demonstrated in macrophages using a variety of special stains.

Therapy. There is no satisfactory treatment. In some cases, topical emollients or corticosteroids produce relief from pruritus and short-term improvement. PUVA and even PUVA bath therapy may be useful in severe cases. Measures to improve chronic venous insufficiency and the resultant decrease in hydrostatic pressure are also beneficial, primarily by reducing disease progression.

Purpura Annularis Teleangiectoides
(Majocchi 1896)

Synonym. Majocchi purpura

Epidemiology. Very uncommon and usually seen in middle-aged men.

Etiology and Pathogenesis. The telangiectases seen in this disorder support the observation that sometimes there is narrowing of small arterioles followed by dilation of capillaries and leakage.

Clinical Findings. The early purpuric lesions are seen on the legs, sometimes associated with telangiectases. They assume an annular or serpiginous pattern. The arms and trunk can also be involved. The initial color is dark red but later becomes rust brown and then yellow brown. The punctate lesions may coalesce, the telangiectases often disappear, and there may even be a hint of atrophy in the center of the lesion. The course is chronic.

Therapy. See Progressive Pigmented Purpura above.

Lichenoid Purpuric Dermatitis
(Gougerot and Blum 1925)

Synonyms. Gougerot-Blum disease, purpuric pigmented lichenoid dermatitis

Clinical Findings. The lesions resemble those of progressive pigmented purpura, but within the hemorrhagic patches one finds grouped polygonal papules resembling lichen planus (Fig. 23.7). The papules are initially red but later acquire a blue-red or brown sheen; Wickham striae are absent. In some instances, the lichenoid papules develop away from obvious purpuric areas.

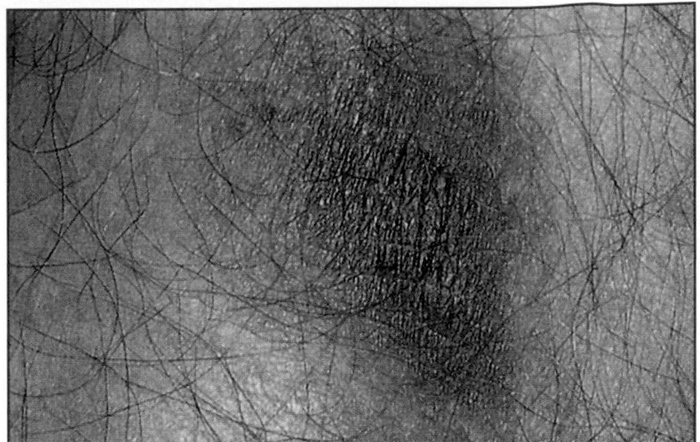

Fig. 23.7. Lichenoid purpuric dermatitis

Histopathology. There is epidermal thickening and a band-like dermal infiltrate, associated with vascular proliferation and hemorrhage. The classic changes of lichen planus are not seen. The infiltrate seems to lie at the same level as lichen planus but does not attack the epidermis.

Therapy. See Progressive Pigmented Purpura above.

Eczematid-Like Purpura
(Doucas and Kapetanakis 1953)

Synonyms. Doucas-Kapetanakis disease, itching purpura (Loewenthal 1954)

Etiology and Pathogenesis. This form has more epidermal involvement. Thus, contact dermatitis and mechanical irritation have been suspected as possible triggers.

Clinical Findings. In this variant, the trunk is likely to be involved along with the legs. Most patients are older men. The few purpuric patches usually have pityriasiform scale or even crust. Tiny petechiae are once again found at the periphery. Pruritus is common, and excoriations may be seen.

Histopathology. The epidermis shows spongiosis, scale, and crusting, while in the upper dermis, the inflammatory infiltrate is more prominent than in ordinary progressive pigmented purpura.

Therapy. In this form, topical corticosteroids often help resolve the inflammatory component.

Lichen Aureus

(Martin 1958)

Synonym. Lichen purpuricus

Etiology and Pathogenesis. The cause of lichen aureus may be different than those of the other pigmented purpuras. The petechiae and subsequent pigmentary changes can be confined to a small area over an incompetent perforating vein.

Clinical Findings. Two characteristics are used loosely to define lichen aureus: localized nature and yellow tone. Most lesions are circular patches with tiny lichenoid papules associated with purpura or even bruise-like changes in the background skin. The usual site is the distal aspect of the legs (Fig. 23.8) or the abdomen. In some instances, the purpura may follow a segmental distribution. The lichenoid papules may have a yellow border, and the entire patch varies from reddish brown to yellow-brown.

Histopathology. There may be a band-like dermal infiltrate of lymphocytes, but it usually is not confused with lichen planus. Often there is even a Grenz zone of normal papillary dermis. Hemosiderin deposits are prominent, and there may be mild signs of epidermal reaction.

Therapy. See progressive pigmented purpura above. If an incompetent perforating vein is identified, it can be tied off or sclerosed.

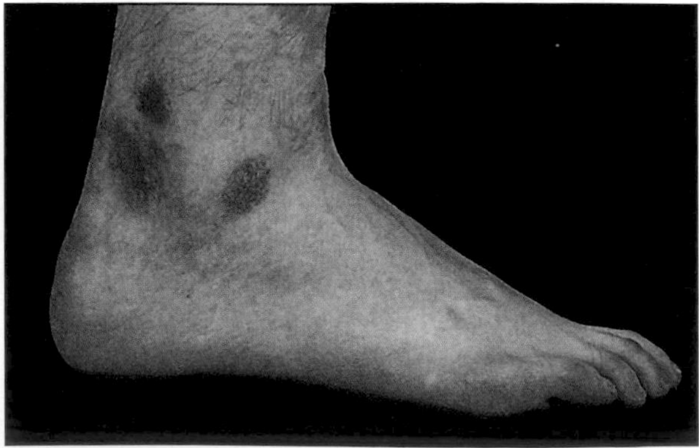

Fig. 23.8. Lichen aureus

Other Forms of Purpura

Langerhans Cell Histiocytosis

Tiny purpuric lesions, especially associated with scaling and crusting in seborrheic areas should suggest Langerhans cell histiocytosis. A good rule in infants is to biopsy a purpuric diaper rash or scalp dermatitis (Chap. 64).

Embolic Purpura

Just as emboli can cause thrombosis, they may produce sufficient vessel damage and changes in pressure in the capillary bed to produce acute purpura. The typical embolic purpuric lesions involve the fingertips; when they are associated with subacute bacterial endocarditis, they are known as Janeway spots, but they can also be caused by atrial myxomas, infected artificial heart valves, cholesterol particles, metastatic carcinomas, and leukemia. Sometimes a biopsy will identify not only purpura but also an embolus in a small vessel. Emboli are discussed in Chapter 22.

Gardner-Diamond Syndrome

(Gardner and Diamond 1955)

Synonyms. Painful bruising syndrome, autoerythrocyte sensitization syndrome, DNA sensitization syndrome, psychogenic purpura

Definition. Spontaneously appearing, painful nodules that evolve over 24 h into ecchymoses.

Epidemiology. Gardner-Diamond syndrome is either incredibly rare or does not exist, depending on one's view. Almost all patients are women, most of whom are involved in the health-care professions.

Etiology and Pathogenesis. The working hypothesis is that some patients become sensitized to part of the red blood cell membrane, perhaps phosphatidyl serine. Then even minor leakage can trigger a prompt allergic response (whose details remain unclear), vascular damage, further leakage, and ecchymosis. Some of these patients respond to an intradermal injection of erythrocytes, leukocytes, or even purified DNA with a hemorrhagic lesion. Many of the patients have marked emotional problems and have access to needles and syringes; the suspicion of a factitial purpura always haunts them and their physicians.

Clinical Findings. There is a prodrome of pruritus and burning, followed by the sudden appearance of an erythematous, indurated, often subcutaneous nodule. The most typical sites are the arms and legs, but the trunk and face can also be involved. Over days, an ecchymosis develops and heals without scarring. Occasionally, mild hyperpigmentation may remain. Some patients have associated symptoms and signs such as fever, cramps, nausea, or vomiting, but subjective indicators of underlying disease are absent.

Histopathology. The microscopic findings have been poorly described. Apparently, there is hemorrhage associated with edema and almost no inflammation.

Laboratory Findings. The intracutaneous injection of erythrocytes, leukocytes, or DNA is the standard approach. One should inject at a site the patient cannot reach, inject a control substance (physiologic saline), and perform the same test on enough volunteers to be sure that one can interpret a significant reaction.

Differential Diagnosis. The main consideration is artifactual purpura.

Therapy. There is no adequate therapy. Some patients benefit from psychotherapy, but the disease is too rare for any controlled studies.

Bibliography

General

Baselga E, Drolet BA, Esterly NB (1997) Purpura in infants and children. J Am Acad Dermatol 37:673–705

Hirsh J, Weitz JI (1999) New antithrombotic agents. Lancet 353:1431–1436

Kottke Marchant K (1994) Laboratory diagnosis of hemorrhagic and thrombotic disorders. Hematol Oncol Clin North Am 8:809–853

Manco-Johnson MJ (1997) Disorders of hemostasis in childhood: risk factors for venous thromboembolism. Thromb Haemost 78:710–714

Piette WW (1994) The differential diagnosis of purpura from morphlogic perspective. Adv Dermatol 9:3–9

Shopnick RI, Brettler DB (1996) Hemostasis: a practical review of conservative and operative care. Clin Orthop 328:34–38

Platelet-Related Hemostatic Diseases

Blanchette VS, Rand ML (1997) Platelet disorders in newborn infants: diagnosis and management. Semin Perinatol 21:53–62

Rodgers GM (1999) Overview of platelet physiology and laboratory evaluation of platelet function. Clin Obstet Gynecol 42:349–359

Wiskott-Aldrich Syndrome

Aldrich RA, Steinberg AG, Campbell DC (1954) Pedigree demonstrating a sex-linked recessive condition characterized by draining ears, eczematoid dermatitis and bloody diarrhea. Pediatrics 13:133–139

Haddad E, Cramer E, Riviere C et al. (1999) The thrombocytopenia of Wiskott Aldrich syndrome is not related to a defect in proplatelet formation. Blood 94:508–518

Kuska B (1996) Wiskott-Aldrich syndrome is a "wonderful mystery". J Natl Cancer Inst 88:1258–1261

Ochs HD (1998) The Wiskott-Aldrich syndrome. Semin Hematol 35:332–345

Wiskott A (1937) Familiärer angeborener Morbus Werlhoffi? Mschr Kinderh 68:212–216

Thrombotic Thrombocytopenic Purpura

Chen DK, Kim JS, Sutton DM (1999) Thrombotic thrombocytopenic purpura associated with ticlopidine use: a report of 3 cases and review of the literature. Arch Intern Med 159:311–314

George JN, Gilcher RO, Smith JW et al. (1998) Thrombotic thrombocytopenic purpura-hemolytic uremic syndrome: diagnosis and management. J Clin Apheresis 13:120–125

Hayward CP, Sutton DM, Carter WH et al. (1994) Treatment outcomes in patients with adult thrombotic thrombocytopenic purpura-hemolytic uremic syndrome. Arch Intern Med 154:982–987

Moake J (1998) Moschcowitz, multimers and metalloprotease. N Engl J Med 339:1629–1631

Musio F, Bohen EM, Yuan CM et al. (1998) Review of thrombotic thrombocytopenic purpura in the setting of systemic lupus erythematosus. Semin Arthritis Rheum 28:1–19

Hemolytic-Uremic Syndrome

Gasser C et al. (1955) Hämolytisch-üramische Syndrome: Bilaterale Nierenrindennekrosen bein akuten erworbenen hämolytischen Anämien. Schweiz Med Wschr 85:905–909

Siegler RL (1995) Hemolytic uremic syndrome in children. Curr Opin Pediatr 7:159–163

Stewart CL, Tina LU (1993) Hemolytic uremic syndrome. Pediatr Rev 14:218–224

Immune-Mediated Acquired Thrombocytopenia

Johnson JR, Samuels P (1999) Review of autoimmune thrombocytopenia: pathogenesis, diagnosis, and management in pregnancy. Clin Obstet Gynecol 42:317–326

Kiefel V, Freitag E, Kroll H et al. (1996) Platelet autoantibodies (IgG, IgM, IgA) against glycoproteins IIb/IIa and Ib/IX in patients with thrombocytopenia. Ann Hematol 72:280–285

Pulkrabek SM (1996) Platelet antibodies. Clin Lab Med 16:817–835

Idiopathic Thrombocytopenic Purpura

George JN, Woolf SH, Raskob GE (1998) Idiopathic thrombocytopenic purpura: a guideline for diagnosis and management of children and adults. American Society of Hematology. Ann Med 30:38–44

Karpatkin S (1997) Autoimmune (idiopathic) thrombocytopenic purpura. Lancet 349:1531–1536

Law C, Marcaccio M, Tam P et al. (1997) High-dose intravenous immune globulin and the response to splenectomy in patients with idiopathic thrombocytopenic purpura. N Engl J Med 336:1494–1498

Secondary Immune-Mediated Thrombocytopenia

Blanco R, Martinez-Taboada VM, Rodriguez-Valverde V et al. (1997) Successful therapy with danazol in refractory autoimmune thrombocytopenia associated with rheumatic diseases. Br J Rheumatol 36:1095–1099

Boumpas DT, Austin HA, Fessler BJ et al. (1995) Systemic lupus erythematosus: emerging concepts, part 1: renal, neuropsychiatric, cardiovascular, pulmonary, and hematologic disease. Ann Intern Med 122:940–950

Diehl LF, Ketchum LH (1998) Autoimmune disease and chronic lymphocytic leukemia: autoimmune hemolytic anemia, pure red cell aplasia, and autoimmune thrombocytopenia. Semin Oncol 25:80–97

Yashiro M, Nagoshi H, Kasuga Y et al. (1996) Evans syndrome associated with Graves' disease. Intern Med 35:987–990

HIV-Associated Immune Thrombocytopenia

Fabris F, Sgarabotto D, Zanon E et al. (1993) The effect of a single course of alpha-2B-interferon in patients with HIV-related and chronic idiopathic immune thrombocytopenia. Autoimmunity 14:175–179

Lord RV, Coleman MJ, Milliken ST (1998) Splenectomy for HIV-related immune thrombocytopenia: comparison with results of splenectomy for non-HIV immune thrombocytopenic purpura. Arch Surg 133:205–210

Louache F, Vainchenker W (1994) Thrombocytopenia in HIV infection. Curr Opin Hematol 1:369–372

Infection-Related Thrombocytopenia

Al-Majed SA, al-Momen AK, al-Kassimi FA et al. (1995) Tuberculosis presenting as immune thrombocytopenic purpura. Acta Haematol 94:135–138

Lotric-Furlan S, Strle F (1995) Thrombocytopenia – a common finding in the initial phase of tick-borne encephalitis. Infection 23:203–206

Mayer JL, Beardsley DS (1996) Varicella-associated thrombocytopenia: autoantibodies against platelet surface glycoprotein V. Pediatr Res 40:615–619

Yamaguchi S, Kubota T, Yamagishi T et al. (1997) Severe thrombocytopenia suggesting immunological mechanisms in two cases of vivax malaria. Am J Hematol 56:183–186

Medication-Related Immune Thrombocytopenia

Aster RH (1999) Drug-induced immune thrombocytopenia: an overview of pathogenesis. Semin Hematol 36:2–6

Kelton JG (1998) Dealing with drug-induced thrombocytopenia. Hosp Pract Off Ed 15:37–48

Heparin-Associated Thrombocytopenia

Demasi R, Bode AP, Knupp C et al. (1994) Heparin-induced thrombocytopenia. Am Surg 60:26–29

Gross AS, Thompson FL, Arzubiaga MC et al. (1993) Heparin-associated thrombocytopenia and thrombosis (HATT) presenting with livedo reticularis. Int J Dermatol 32:276–279

Walenga JM, Bick RL (1998) Heparin-induced thrombocytopenia, paradoxical thromboembolism, and other side effects of heparin therapy. Med Clin North Am 82:635–658

Warkenin TE, Levine MN, Hirsh J et al. (1995) Heparin-induced thrombocytopenia in patients treated with low-molecular-weight heparin of unfractionated heparin. N Engl J Med 332:1330–1335

Thrombocythemia

Barbui T, Finazzi G (1999) Clinical parameters for determining when and when not to treat essential thrombocythemia. Semin Hematol 36:14–18

Griesshammer M, Bangerter M, Sauer T et al. (1999) Aetiology and clinical significance of thrombocytosis: analysis of 732 patients with an elevated platelet count. J Intern Med 245:295–300

Kutti J, Wadenvik H (1996) Diagnostic and differential criteria of essential thrombocythemia and reactive thrombocytosis. Leuk Lymph 22:41–45

Murphy S, Peterson P, Iland H et al. (1997) Experience of the Polycythemia Vera Study Group with essential thrombocythemia: a final report on diagnostic criteria, survival, and leukemia transition by treatment. Semin Hematol 34:29–39

Tefferi A, Hoagland HC (1994) Issues in the diagnosis and management of essential thrombocythemia. Mayo Clin Proc 69:651–655

Vora AJ, Lilleyman JS (1993) Secondary thrombocytosis. Arch Dis Child 68:88–90

Yohannan MD, Higgy KE, al Mashhadani SA et al. (1994) Thrombocytosis. Etiologic analysis of 663 patients. Clin Pediatr Phila 33:340–343

Pseudo-von Willebrand Syndrome

Kunishima S, Heaton DC, Naoe T (1997) De novo mutation of the platelet glycoprotein Ib alpha gene in a patient with pseudo-von Willebrand disease. Blood Coagul Fibrinolysis 8:311–315

Marchese P, Saldivar E, Ware J et al. (1999) Adhesive properties of the isolated amino-terminal domain of platelet glycoprotein Ib alpha in a flow field. Proc Natl Acad Sci USA 96:7837–7842

Disorders of Coagulation

Lusher JM (1996) Screening and diagnosis of coagulation disorders. Am J Obstet Gynecol 175:778–783

Rao AK, Sheth S, Kaplan R (1997) Inherited hypercoagulable states. Vasc Med 2:313–320

Hemophilia

Antonarakis SE (1995) Molecular genetics of coagulation factor VIII gene and hemophilia A. Throm Haemost 74:322–328

Kay MA, High K (1999) Gene therapy for the hemophilias. Proc Natl Acad Sci USA 96:9973–9975

Lillicrap D (1998) The molecular basis of haemophilia B. Haemophilia 4:350–357

Von Willebrand Disease

Lethagen SR (1995) Pathogenesis, clinical picture and treatment of von Willebrand's disease. Ann Med 27:641–651

Rinder MR, Richard RE, Rinder HM (1997) Acquired von Willebrand's disease: a concise review. Am J Hematol 54:139–145

Hepatic Defects

Mammen EF (1994) Coagulation defects in liver disease. Med Clin North Am 78:545–554

Rereira SP, Langley PG, Williams R (1996) The management of abnormalities of hemostasis in acute liver failure. Semin Liver Dis 16:403–414

Vitamin K Deficiency

Shearer MJ (1995) Vitamin K. Lancet 345:229–234

Sutor AH (1995) Vitamin K deficiency bleeding in infants and children. Semin Thromb Hemost 21:317–329

Thorp JA, Gaston L, Caspers DR et al. (1995) Current concepts and controversies in the use of vitamin K. Drugs 49:376–387

Gammopathies

Appenzeller P, Leith CP, Foucar K et al. (1999) Cutaneous Waldenström macroglobulinemia in transformation. Am J Dermatopathol 21:151–155

Finder KA, McCollough ML, Dixon SL et al. (1990) Hypergammaglobulinemic purpura of Waldenström. J Am Acad Dermatol 23:669–676

Kaneko Y, Murakami H, Matsushima T et al. (1993) Idiopathic thrombocytopenic purpura and monoclonal gammopathy of undetermined significance accompanied by urinary bladder carcinoma. Clin Exp Rheumatol 11:217

Keren DF (1993) Coagulation disorders in patients with monoclonal gammopathies. Hematol Oncol Clin North Am 7:1153–1159

Miyagawa S, Fukumoto T, Kanauchi M et al. (1996) Hypergammaglobuliaemic purpura of Waldenström and Ro/SSA autoantibodies. Br J Dermatol 134:919–923

Robert F, Mignucci M, McCurdy SA et al. (1993) Hemostatic abnormalities associated with monoclonal gammopathies. Am J Med Sci 306:359–366

Torok L, Borka I, Szabo G (1993) Waldenström's macroglobulinaemia presenting with cold urticaria and cold purpura. Clin Exp Dermatol 18:277–279

Disseminated Intravascular Coagulation

Baglin T (1996) Disseminated intravascular coagulation: diagnosis and treatment. BMJ 312:683–687

Barraud S (1904) Über extremitätengangrän im jugendlichen Alter nach Infektionskrankheiten. Deut Zschr Chir 74:237–297

Bick RL (1994) Disseminated intravascular coagulation. Objective laboratory diagnostic criteria and guidelines for management. Clin Lab Med 14:729–768

Hardaway RM, Williams CH (1996) Disseminated intravascular coagulation: an update. Compr Ther 22:737–743

Levi M, Ten-Cate H (1999) Disseminated intravascular coagulation. N Engl J Med 341:586–592

Purpura Fulminans

Bergmann F, Hoyer PF, D'Angelo SV et al. (1995) Severe autoimmune protein S deficiency in a boy with idiopathic purpura fulminans. Br J Haematol 89:610–614

Darmstadt GL (1998) Acute infectious purpura fulminans: pathogenesis and medical management. Pediatr Dermatol 15:169–183

Kreuz W, Veldman A, Escuriola-Ettinghausen C et al. (1998) Protein C concentrate for meningococcal purpura fulminans. Lancet 351:986–987

Smith OP, White B (1999) Infectious purpura fulminans: diagnosis and treatment. Br J Haematol 104:202–207

Waterhouse-Friderichsen Syndrome

Locker GJ, Wagner A, Peter A et al. (1995) Lethal Waterhouse-Friderichsen syndrome in posttraumatic asplenia. J Trauma 39:784–786

Ryan CA, Wenman W, Henningsen C et al. (1993) Fatal childhood Waterhouse-Friderichsen syndrome. Pediatr Infect Dis J 12:250–251

Varon J, Chen K, Sternbach GL (1998) Rupert Waterhouse and Carl Friderichsen: adrenal apoplexy. J Emerg Med 16:643–647

Kasabach-Merritt Syndrome

Enjolras O, Wassef M, Mazoyer E et al. (1997) Infants with Kasabach-Merritt syndrome do not have "true" hemangiomas. J Pediatr 130:631–640

Ettlinger JJ, Fleming PJ, Joffe HS et al. (1996) Cavernous haemangioma with Kasabach-Merritt syndrome: treatment with alpha-interferon. J R Soc Med 89:55–56

Schulz AS, Urban J, Gessler P et al. (1999) Anaemia, thrombocytopenia and coagulopathy due to occult diffuse infantile haemangiomtosis of spleen and pancreas. Eur J Pediatr 158:379–383

Velin P, Dupont D, Golkar A et al. (1998) Neonatal Kasabach-Merritt syndrome healed by complete surgical excision of the angioma. Arch Pediatr 5:295–297

Senile Purpura

Lewis AB, Gendler EC (1996) Resurfacing with topical agents. Semin Cutan Med Surg 15:139–144

Factitial Purpura

Shelley ED, Shelley WB, Talanin NY (1997) The mysterious case of the premenstrual purple chin. Cutis 60:147–149

Paroxysmal Finger Hematoma

Achenbach W (1957) Ematomi parossistici della mano. Athena, Rome. 23:187–189

Layton AM, Cotterill JA (1993) A case of Achenbach's syndrome. Clin Exp Dermatol 18:60–61

Parslew R, Verbov JL (1995) Achenbach syndrome. Br J Dermatol 132:319

Pigmented Purpuric Dermatoses

Ratnam KV, Su WP, Peters MS (1991) Purpura simplex (inflammatory purpura without vasculitis): a clinicopathologic study of 174 cases. J Am Acad Dermatol 25:642–647

Smoller BR, Kamel OW (1991) Pigmented purpuric eruptions: immunopathologic studies supportive of a common immunophenotype. J Cutan Pathol 18:423–427

Progressive Pigmented Purpura

Ghersetich I, Lotti T, Bacci S et al. (1995) Cell infiltrate in progressive pigmented purpura (Schamberg's disease): immunophenotype, adhesion receptors, and intercellular relationships. Int J Dermatol 34:846–850

Kano Y, Hirayama K, Orihari M et al. (1997) Successful treatment of Schamberg's disease with pentoxifylline. J Am Acad Dermatol 36:827–830

Nagata K, Danno K, Tanaka S (1999) Unilateral Schamberg disease in a 14-year-old Japanese boy. J Dermatol 26:348–351

Reinhold U, Seiter S, Ugurel S et al. (1999) Treatment of progressive pigmented purpura with oral bioflavonoids and ascorbic acid: an open pilot study in 3 patients. J Am Acad Dermatol 41:207–208

Purpura Annularis Teleangiectoides

Honda M, Saijo S, Tagami H (1997) Majocchi's disease in a newborn baby: a familial case. Br J Dermatol 137:655–666

Kim HJ, Skidmore RA, Woosley JT (1998) Pigmented purpura over the lower extremities. Purpura annularis telangiectoides of Majocchi. Arch Dermatol 134:1477–1480

Lichenoid Purpuric Dermatitis

Krizsa J, Hunyadi J, Dobozy A (1992) PUVA treatment of pigmented purpuric lichenoid dermatitis (Gougerot-Blum). J Am Acad Dermatol 27:778–780

Lotti T, Ghersetich I, Panconesi E (1994) Why should we use PUVA treatment in pigmented purpuric lichenoid dermatitis. J Am Acad Dermatol 30:145

Eczematid-Like Purpura

Doucas G, Kapetanakis J (1953) Eczematid-like purpura. Dermatologica 106:86–95

Lowenthal LJ (1954) Itching purpura. Brit J Derm 66:95–103

Lichen Aureus

Dippel E, Schröder K, Goerdt S (1998) Zosteriformer Lichen aureus. Hautarzt 49:135–138

Marten R (1958) Case for diagnosis. Trans St Johns Hosp Dermatol Soc 40:93

Rubio FA, Robayana G, Herranz P et al. (1997) Abdominal lichen aureus in a child. Pediatr Dermatol 14:411

Gardner-Diamond Syndrome

Anderson JE, DeGoff W, McNamara M (1999) Autoerythrocyte sensitization (psychogenic purpura): a case report and review of the literature. Pediatr Emerg Care 15:47–48

Berman DA, Roenigk HH, Green D (1992) Autoerythrocyte sensitization syndrome (psychogenic purpura). J Am Acad Dermatol 27:829–832

Gardner FH, Diamond LK (1955) Autoerythrocyte sensitization. A form of purpura producing painful bruising following autosensitization to red blood cells in certain women. Blood 10:675–690

Gomi H, Miura T (1994) Autoerythrocyte sensitization syndrome with thrombocytosis. Dermatology 188:160–162

Moll S (1997) Psychogenic purpura. Am J Hematol 55:146–147

Diseases of the Lymphatics

Contents

The diseases of the lymphatics appear almost exclusively on the legs. Only occasionally are the arms, trunk and even head involved. The visual evidence of lymphatic disease is lymphedema, an edema or swelling that is the result of impaired lymphatic return. The protein-rich lymph accumulates in tissue when reabsorption is hindered or when the lymphatics are absent (congenital absence or surgical removal) or blocked. One speaks of two types of lymphedema.

- Primary Lymphedema. These patients usually lack lymphatics. In some cases there may be agenesis or fibrosis of the lymph nodes. Difficulties become apparent early in life, at the latest during adolescence. The problem can be unilateral or bilateral and may be familial or sporadic.
- Secondary Lymphedema. This disease usually appears in older individuals. It, too, can be either uni- or bilateral. Principal causes include damage to the lymphatics through trauma, surgery or radiation, external compression by tumors or obliteration by metastatic tumor cells or inflammatory processes. Typical infections that lead to lymphatic damage include filariasis, erysipelas and other deep streptococcal infections and herpes simplex. The latter two often interact to produce lymphedema.

Clinical Findings. The clinical features of all types of lymphedema are similar. The affected limb has an increased circumference, feels heavy and has a restricted range of motion. The skin and subcutaneous tissue eventually become thickened; this is known as pachyderma. Stemmer sign refers to the fact that, with lymphedema, the skin over the metatarsal-phalangeal joint cannot be pinched up into a fold. If the lymphedema persists, the thickened skin may develop verruciform changes (mossy foot) and hyperpigmentation. Nail changes such as onychodystrophy and onychogryposis may develop, along with discoloration and slowed growth. Lymphadenopathy is not usually a feature of lymphedema but may be seen with recurrent erysipelas and metastatic tumors.

Therapy. The treatment of all forms of lymphedema is similar and will only be discussed once. In Germany one speaks of "complex physical antiedema therapy." This form of treatment includes manual physical therapy in the form of lymphatic drainage – a type of massage designed to aid lymph flow. It must be coupled with compression dressings or stockings, usually class III or IV (Chap. 22), appropriate physical activity and meticulous skin care. While it is difficult to convince small children to wear compression devices and it is expensive to replace the garments as the child grows or as the devices wear out, all the trouble is well worthwhile. After fibrosis has occurred, treatment is very difficult.

Medical therapy of lymphedema is disappointing. Diuretics are often described but generally produce little benefit and often have a variety of side effects as they must be employed for many decades. In more acute tumor-associated lymphedema, sometimes diuretics make the patient more comfortable. The single most important medical measurement is prompt treatment of erysipelas (Chap. 4) to avoid recurrences and postinfectious lymphedema. Tinea pedis should be aggressively treated, as it often predisposes to erysipelas.

Surgical measures are in their infancy. Previously, large excisions were performed, removing skin, subcutaneous tissue and fat; these "clean-up" operations provided little benefit. Today, a variety of microvascular procedures are available to perform autologous lymphatic transplantation to circumvent local areas of obstruction or defective drainage. The main indications are localized congenital absence of lymphatics or lymph nodes, secondary lymphedema following lymph node resection or radiation and to repair traumatic damage.

Primary Lymphedema

Hereditary Primary Lymphedema

Hereditary Congenital Lymphedema Type I

(Nonne 1892; Milroy 1928)

Synonyms. Nonne-Milroy disease, congenital trophedema

Definition. Congenital lymphedema of early onset involving the legs.

Etiology and Pathogenesis. This very rare disorder presumably reflects a dysplasia or hypoplasia of the lymphatics. Inheritance appears to be autosomal dominant, but girls are affected far more often than boys.

Clinical Findings. The onset of problems is in childhood. Initially there is painless pitting edema of the lower parts of the legs and the feet that is produced by the persistent edema. A typical clinical finding is puffy, almost pillow-like, pads on the backs of the feet (Fig. 24.1). Later, fibrosis develops, the edema is no longer easily compressible and the skin becomes bound to the underlying subcutaneous tissue. The skin surface usually remains unremarkable. The swelling may extend to the inguinal fold, but never beyond. The hands and forearms are involved only in exceptional cases. The lymphedema is cosmetically very disturbing, interferes with the choice of shoes and restricts athletic activity.

Histopathology. Microscopic examination yields little. Even when lymphedema is prominent, on routine sections lymphatics are hard to identify and rarely described as increased. In later stages, dermal and subcutaneous fibrosis becomes apparent.

Course and Prognosis. Although the onset is in early life, there may be worsening with puberty. Frequent streptococcal infections exacerbate the problem. Eventually the patient is at risk for lymphangiosarcoma, as well as significant restriction of activities.

Therapy. Early and consequent treatment is required. It is hard to convince the parents to start treatment in infancy, but that is the wisest decision.

Hereditary Congenital Lymphedema Type II

(Meige 1889)

Synonyms. Meige disease, late-onset lymphedema, late-onset trophedema

Definition. Lymphedema that usually appears around puberty and involving the legs.

Etiology and Pathogenesis. This disease is probably similar in nature to type I disease but starts around puberty. Why the lymphatics suddenly cease

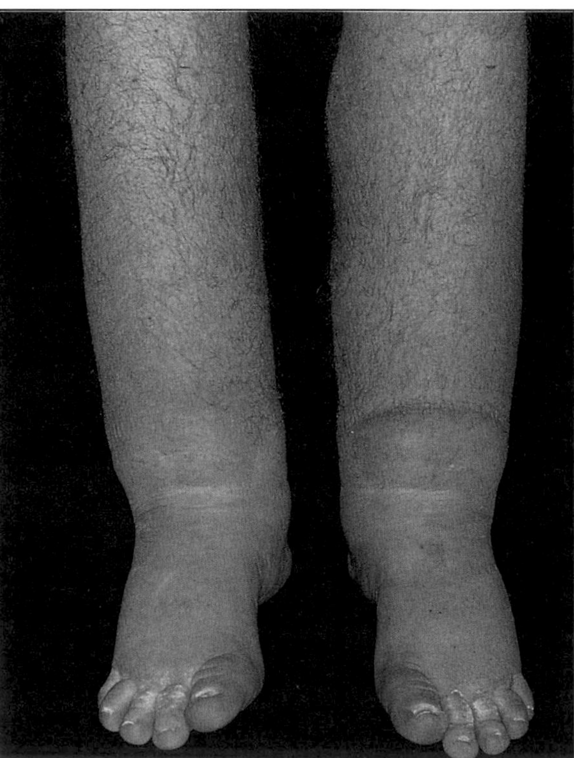

Fig. 24.1. Bilateral primary lymphedema

to function properly is not understood. Once again, girls are affected more often than boys and a variety of patterns of inheritance have been discussed.

Clinical Findings. The lymphedema is very similar to that of type I disease but appears later in life. When examining a 25 year old woman with lymphedema, it is impossible to determine which form she has without asking questions. The course and prognosis are identical.

Therapy. As above

Turner Syndrome

Turner syndrome appears in about 1:2500 female births. It is caused by the loss of an X chromosome in a gamete or early embryo, producing a 45 XO genotype and an abnormal female phenotype. Lymphatic problems include cystic hydroma, chylothorax and hydrops fetalis, as well as lymphedema of the hands and feet. The latter tends to improve with time. Prenatal ultrasound can often be used to make the diagnosis, along with chromosome analysis. The differential diagnosis includes Noonan syndrome, in which the lymphedema is more persistent and cardiac problems are common (Chap. 19).

Other Associated Disorders

Many different problems have been described associated with congenital lymphedema. In most instances, these diseases are exceedingly rare and poorly understood.

- Yellow nail syndrome (Chap. 32): In addition to the yellow nails and pleural effusions, there may be lymphedema of the extremities or even the face.
- Distichiasis-lymphedema syndrome: Patients have late-onset lymphedema along with a double row of eyelashes.
- Hennekam syndrome: Described in an isolated population on the Zuider Zee, these Dutch patients show autosomal recessive inheritance. They have widespread congenital lymphedema, most severe on the legs and genitalia, periorbital edema, dental anomalies, intestinal lymphangiectases and mild mental retardation. Mücke syndrome is very similar.
- Figueroa syndrome: Cleft lip and cleft palate associated with late-onset lymphedema, probably inherited in an autosomal dominant pattern.
- Lymphedema with recurrent cholestasis: Patients have cholestasis, intense pruritus and dental enamel defects.
- Lymphedema with intestinal lymphangiectases

Nonhereditary Primary Lymphedema

The distinction between hereditary and nonhereditary primary lymphedema is not sharp. Since the pattern of inheritance is often unclear and the responsible genes remain unknown, it is difficult to decide if a given case is truly sporadic or the start of a pedigree. Nonetheless, most authors attempt the separation.

Essential Congenital Lymphedema

The onset is at birth or in early life and the course identical to that of type I lymphedema, discussed above. The family history is negative.

Essential Lymphedema

Synonyms. Lymphedema praecox, lymphedema tardum

Definition. All primary lymphedema that is noncongenital and nonfamilial.

Epidemiology. This is the most common form of lymphedema. In 65% of patients the disease appears between the ages of 10 and 24 years; this is known as lymphedema praecox. Later onset is called lymphedema tardum. Women are far more often affected.

Etiology and Pathogenesis. The cause is unknown. Lymphangiography shows aplasia of the larger lymphatic vessels but it is unclear why the system functions for years and then fails.

Clinical Findings. Initially the patient may notice swelling of the feet or ankles, often in summer and often associated with menses. Differentiation from venous edema is difficult. Initially the fluid drains when the legs are elevated. Later the edema progresses proximally and becomes more permanent. The course and prognosis are those of the congenital variant.

Secondary Lymphedema

Acute Lymphangitis

Acute ascending lymphatic infection is a common sequel of a bacterial infection of the extremities. The patient notices a red, often tender streak or stripe running in a vertical fashion over the involved lymphatic (Fig. 24.2). In the days prior to antibiotic therapy, this was a dangerous sign and most patients still associate it wisely with a spreading infection. The associated lymphedema and lymphadenopathy is usually not a major problem. Once the bacterial infection is treated, the problems generally resolve. Streptococcal infections are notorious for causing lymphangitis but also for damaging the lymphatics so that subsequent infections and eventually persistent lymphedema can develop.

Elephantiasis

Definition. Deformity of body part because of persistent lymphedema, destruction of lymphatics, fibrosis and reactive cutaneous changes.

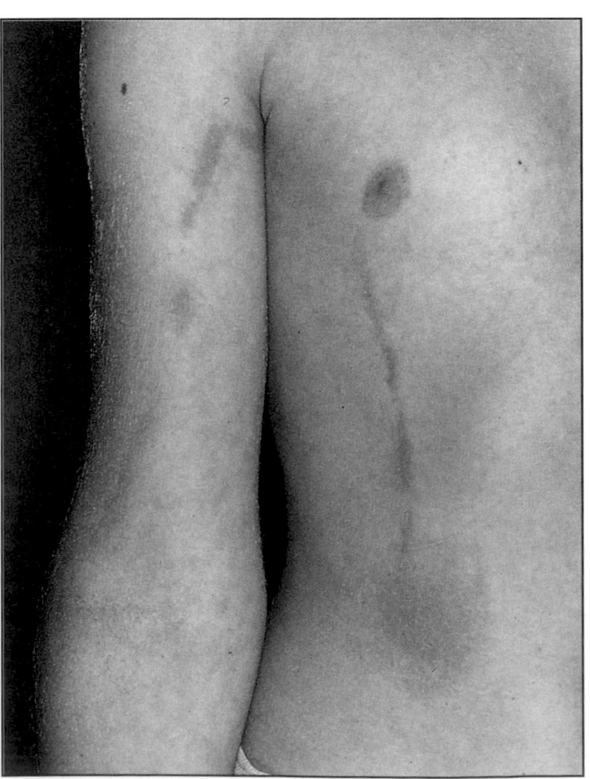

Fig. 24.2. Lymphangitis associated with insect bite reaction

Epidemiology. In some settings, such as those parts of the world with endemic filariasis, elephantiasis is common. In western countries, it is often seen in association with surgery or radiation, so that one can describe it as common in selected clinical settings.

Etiology and Pathogenesis. There are many different causes of elephantiasis, as shown in Table 24.1. The following three terms are typically applied.

Elephantiasis Tropica. This disease is caused by filiaria (Chap. 9). There is typically scrotal enlargement, which may become grotesque.

Elephantiasis Chromomycetica. Chromoblastomycosis (Chap. 7) may produce a swollen limb with focal scarring.

Elephantiasis Nostras. Nostras is Latin for "our", suggesting that this type of elephantiasis is not exotic or tropical but seen in our countries. The main causes include:

- Chronic or Recurrent Erysipelas. In this most common scenario, tinea pedis or gram-negative toe web infections produce tiny portals of entry for streptococci, which tend produce erysipelas and also cause lymphatic damage. As the foot remains more swollen, minor injuries are more likely and penetration by streptococci is facilitated, setting up a vicious cycle.
- Recurrent Herpes Simplex Infection. Herpes simplex infections often predispose to streptococcal infections by damaging the epidermis, creating an entry site. Recurrent fever blisters associated with recurrent erysipelas is the most common cause of persistent swelling of the upper lip, often called the tapir sign. The virus can produce similar changes in the penis, scrotum, labia or other body parts, either alone or with secondary bacterial infections (Fig. 24.3).
- Chronic Inflammatory Diseases. Patients with both severe acne and rosacea can develop persistent lymphedema, especially about the glabella, eyelids and bridge of the nose (Chap. 28).
- Granuloma Inguinale (Chap. 5). Marked genital elephantiasis (esthiomène) is a classic feature of infection with *Calymmatobacterium granulomatis.*
- Thrombophlebitis. Marked inflammation of the vein and especially the tissue around the vein can lead to lymphatic destruction and secondary lymphedema. It is often hard to separate the ede-

Table 24.1. Differential diagnosis of secondary lymphedema

Mainly unilateral	Mainly bilateral
Venous	Functional
Thrombosis (leg or iliac vein)	Stasis edema (prolonged standing)
Iliac vein blockage, as from bony spur	Premenstrual edema
Postthrombotic syndrome	Edema of pregnancy
Malignant tumors	Nutritional
Uterus and ovaries	Chronic malnutrition
Prostate	Protein deficiency
Breast	Protein-losing enteropathy
Lymphoma	Internal diseases
Various sarcomas	Cardiac failure
Fungus	Renal failure
Chromoblastomycosis	Chronic hepatic disease
Virus	Cutaneous diseases
Recurrent herpes simplex	Generalized pustular psoriasis
Bacteria	Medications
Streptococci (recurrent erysipelas)	Oral contraceptives
Postcellulitis	Psoralens
Syphilis (edema indurativum)	Corticosteroids
Granuloma inguinale	Antihypertensives, diuretics
Worms	
Filariasis	
Mechanical	
Surgery	
Radiation	
Trauma	
Inflammation	
Angioedema	
Hereditary angioneurotic edema	
Acne and rosacea	
Reflex sympathetic dystrophy	

ma of venous stasis from lymphatic obstruction in this clinical setting.

- Tumors. A variety of carcinomas, sarcomas and even malignant melanoma can cause lymphedema by two mechanisms – external compression of lymphatics or occlusion via metastatic spread within the vascular spaces.
- Surgery or Radiation. When the lymphatics are destroyed, such as in a radical procedure or lymph node dissection, or when they are irradiated, secondary obstruction often develops (Fig. 24.4).

Clinical Findings. The initial finding is just as with primary lymphedema, that is, there is innocent puffy swelling. The major difference is that the chances are more likely that the lymphedema is unilateral and often involves body regions other than the legs. If the underlying factors cannot be controlled, the swelling increases, becomes more permanent and fibrosis results. Often, the function of a limb, such as walking, is disturbed. The overlying skin is initially smooth and white-yellow. Later it becomes blue-red and then dirty brown. Simultaneously, it thickens, developing verruciform hyperplasia (Fig. 24.5). As the disease further progresses, the excrescences of the skin are cauliflower-like, easily macerated and routinely secondarily infected with bacteria and fungi, producing a foul-smelling, virtually untreatable picture known as mossy foot.

Histopathology. Usually the changes are so extreme in the late stages of elephantiasis that the dilated lymphatics, dermal fibrosis and reactive epidermal changes can be seen. The unwary may confuse the histological picture of elephantiasis with a lymphangioma (Chap. 59).

Laboratory Findings. Laboratory tests are useful primarily for excluding underlying diseases. Vascular imaging studies such as lymphangiography

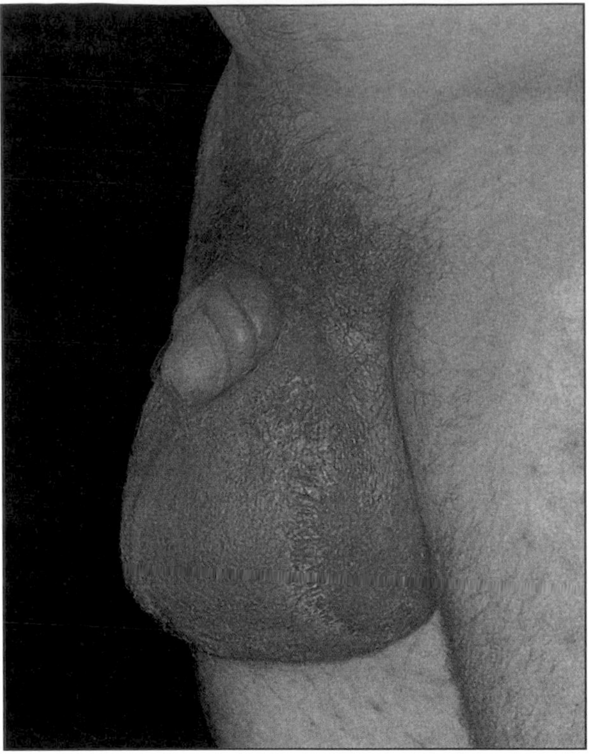

Fig. 24.3. Scrotal elephantiasis following recurrent erysipelas

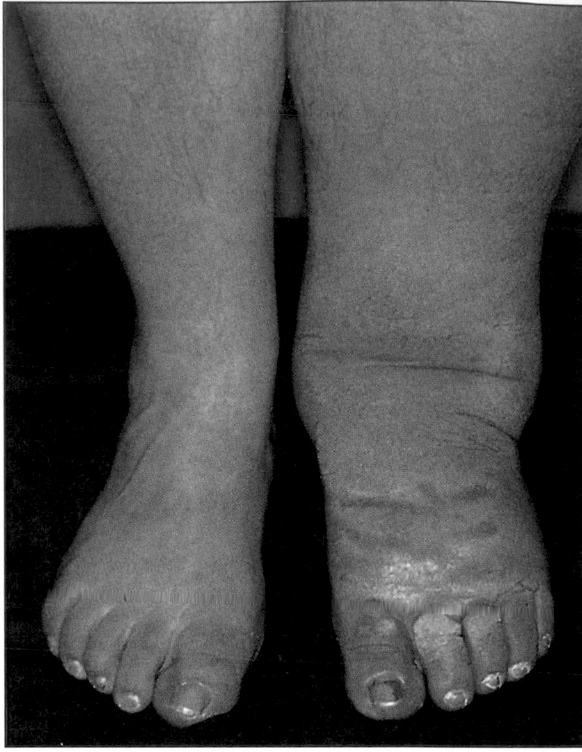

Fig. 24.5. Chronic lymphedema with verrucous changes following recurrent erysipelas

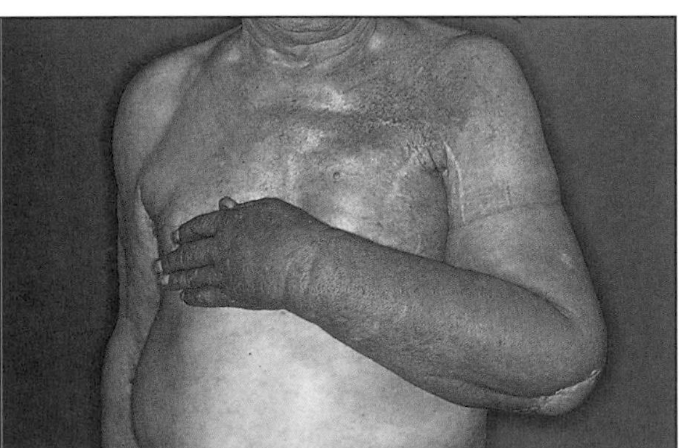

Fig. 24.4. Edematous lymph following radical mastectomy and radiation therapy

and the other studies mentioned in Chapter 22 can be used to separate lymphatic disease from that also involving the arteries and veins.

Course and Prognosis. The course is usually progressive and hard to interrupt. In the case of erysipelas, recurrent infections often run a milder course with less fever and a lower erythrocyte sedimentation rate. Nonetheless the lymphatic damage continues. A very rare but feared complication is the development of a lymphangiosarcoma in the area of chronic lymphedema. This change is most common in a swollen arm following radical mastectomy, where the term Stewart-Treves syndrome (Chap. 59) is applied. It can occur in all types of chronic lymphedema.

Differential Diagnosis. The diagnosis of elephantiasis – swelling secondary to lymphatic disease – is usually easy. The differential diagnosis is also usually straight-forward and includes the various causes discussed under etiology.

Therapy. The underlying disease must be treated. Early in the course, compression stockings are helpful, but once fibrosis is prominent they bring little relief. Careful foot care is essential and specially fitted shoes are often required. Later, one must try to prevent secondary bacterial and fungal infections. Topical antifungal products can be used routinely; most also have an antibacterial action. Monthly injections of depot penicillin may reduce the incidence of erysipelas. Both corticosteroids and oral retinoids have been employed in severe cases with variable results. Plastic surgical efforts can reduce the mass of the lymphedema but are reserved for desperate cases because of the risks of scarring, infection and tissue breakdown.

Cutaneous Chylous Reflux

(Kinmouth and Taylor 1964)

Etiology and Pathogenesis. If lymphatic flow is obstructed, there may be leakage of lymphatic fluid and chyle in a retrograde fashion into the skin. Chyle is lymphatic fluid draining the bowel where it has picked up lipids and is thus milky or cloudy, while other lymphatic fluid is generally clear. Two types of primary cutaneous chylous reflux have been described: type I, associated with dilated lymph vessels, and type II, associated with diminished lymph vessels. In addition, all the causes of lymphedema already discussed can also lead to this problem.

Clinical Findings. Most patients have lymphedema, either primary or secondary, with obvious cutaneous involvement. In some of the congenital cases, there has been an associated vascular malformation. On rare occasions, there may be intestinal or other internal lymphatic defects without limb lymphedema.

The clinical findings are striking. Tiny drops of white milky or clear fluid are found, most often on the upper thigh or in the genital region. Sometimes the drops may be arranged about pubic hairs. In other cases, they mimic vesicles. The involved skin is usually erythematous and may be swollen.

Histopathology. Microscopic examination reveals dilated lymph vessels filled with proteinaceous material.

Course and Prognosis. The problem is chronic, but usually the lymphedema can be improved.

Differential Diagnosis. The differential diagnosis includes milia, lymphangioma circumscriptum (Chap. 59), and herpetic lesions.

Therapy. There is no satisfactory treatment.

Artifactual Lymphedema

Synonym. Secrétan syndrome

Rarely patients may induce lymphedema by repeated self-induced trauma (Chap. 25).

Congenital Absence of Venous Valves

This rare disorder is usually mistaken for lymphedema. It is inherited in an autosomal dominant pattern, so that men and women are equally involved. Lower extremity edema begins around puberty and typically improves at night or with elevation. Most patients develop varicosities, stasis dermatitis and leg ulcers, all of which are uncommon in lymphedema. Imaging studies show total or partial absence of valves in the superficial and deep veins, but intact lymphatics.

Bibliography

Andersson HC, Parry DM, Mulvihill JJ (1995) Lymphangiosarcoma in late-onset hereditary lymphedema: case report and nosological implications. Am J Med Genet 56:72–75

Campisi C (1999) Lymphoedema: modern diagnostic and therapeutic aspects. Int Angiol 18:14–24

Casley-Smith JR (1999) Benzo-pyrones in the treatment of lymphoedema. Int Angiol 18:31–41

Cerri A, Gianni C, Corbellino M et al. (1998) Lymphangiosarcoma of the pubic region: a rare complication arising in congenital non-hereditary lymphedema. Eur J Dermatol 8:511–514

Chern LC, Lin CS, Wong CK (1989) Cutaneous chylous reflux. Br J Dermatol 120:695–700

Evans AL, Brice G, Sotirova V et al. (1999) Mapping of primary congenital lymphedema to the 5q35.3 region. Am J Hum Genet 64:547–555

Ferrell RE, Levinson KL, Esman JH et al. (1998) Hereditary lymphedema: evidence for linkage and genetic heterogeneity. Hum Mol Genet 7:2073–2078

Foldi E (1998) The treatment of lymphedema. Cancer 83:2833–2834

Hershko A, Hirshberg B, Nahir M et al. (1997) Yellow nail syndrome. Postgrad Med J 73:466–468

Larralde M, Gardner SS, Torrado MV et al. (1998) Lymphedema as a postulated cause of cutis verticis gyrata in Turner syndrome. Pediatr Dermatol 15:18–22

Mangion J, Rahman N, Mansour S et al. (1999) A gene for lymphedema-distichiasis maps to 16q24.3. Am J Hum Genet 65:427–432

Marcks P (1997) Lymphedema. Pathogenesis, prevention, and treatment. Cancer Pract 5:32–38

Meige H (1899) Le trophoedème héréditaire. Nouv Icon Salpetriere 12:453–480

Milroy WF (1892) An undescribed variety of hereditary edema. NY Med J 56:505–508

Mortimer PS (1998) The pathophysiology of lymphedema. Cancer 83:2798–2802

Nonne M (1891) Vier Fälle von Elphantiasis congenita hereditaria. Arch Path Anat 125:189–196

Partsch H (1995) Assessment of abnormal lymph drainage for the diagnosis of lymphedema by isotopic lymphangiography and by indirect lymphography. Clin Dermatol 13:445–450

Rajan TV, Gundlapalli AV (1997) Lymphatic filariasis. Chem Immunol 66:125–158

Rockson SG (1998) Precipitating factors in lymphedema: myths and realities. Cancer 83:2814–2816

Routh HB, Bhowmik KR (1994) Filariasis. Dermatol Clin 12: 719–727

Szuba A, Rockson SG (1997) Lymphedema: anatomy, physiology and pathogenesis. Vasc Med 2:321–326

Szuba A, Rockson SG (1998) Lymphedema: classification, diagnosis and therapy. Vasc Med 3:145–156

Thiadens SR (1998) Current status of education and treatment resources for lymphedema. Cancer 83:2864–2868

Tunkel RS, Lachmann E (1998) Lymphedema of the limb. An overview of treatment options. Postgrad Med 104: 131–134

Pruritus, Prurigo, Self-Induced Disease, Psychiatric Disease and Neurologic Disease

Contents

Pruritus

Definition. Pruritus is the Latin word for itching.

Basic Science Aspects

Pruritus is classified along with pain as a nociceptive response. Nociceptors are located primarily in the skin and abdominal viscera. They respond to both external and internal conditions, such as physical and chemical stimuli. The stimulus is found unpleasant by the host. The afferent sensation of pruritus is closely linked to the efferent motor response of scratching as a spinal reflex, which can be controlled by higher centers. Pruritus develops exclusively in the skin, in contrast to pain, which can arise in many organs. The tickle sensation is closely related to pruritus, but usually not as unpleasant. Tickling induces a similar motor response but the victim does not actually scratch the skin, spontaneously interrupting the reaction. In addition, tickling is usually associated with laughter while pruritus is not. Another difference is that tickling usually diminishes with repeated stimulation while pruritus shows no adaptation.

Pruritus can best be understood by reviewing the cutaneous innervation. The skin is a richly innervated structure, containing sensory and motor fibers. Some areas are much richer in nerves than others; one need only compare two-point discrimination on different parts of one's own body, for instance the fingertips versus the back or thigh. The major cutaneous sensations are pain, pruritus, touch, pressure and temperature. The autonomic nerves, both sympathetic and parasympathetic, are the main efferent or motor nerves, controlling adnexal smooth muscle contraction and thus regulating sweating, cutaneous vascular supply and even temperature control, by contracting the arrector pili muscles to fluff up the body hair.

The cutaneous nerves are divided into A or myelinated and C or nonmyelinated fibers. The A fibers serve mechanical nociceptors, specific structures that respond to a variety of stimuli. The C fibers, on the other hand, are known as polymodal fibers and they connect primarily to the rich plexus of free nerve endings. Pruritus is transmitted to the CNS via C fibers.

The main specific receptors in the skin are primarily tactile and include the following:

- Free nerve endings are the major source of information. They are distributed in dense interconnecting networks and are responsible for the fine perception associated with an individual hair being moved, as well as for two-point discrimination. They also are primarily responsible for heat and pain sensation.
- Meissner corpuscles are most common on the palms and soles, nipples and genitalia. They consist of coils of axons and Schwann cells, are located high in the dermis just below the epidermal-dermal junction and serve as mechanoreceptors.
- Pacini (or Vater-Pacini) corpuscles are located deep in the dermis and resemble an onion under the microscope, consisting of a central nerve and many layers of flattened Schwann cells. They sense deep pressure.
- Golgi-Mazzoni corpuscles are similar in function to Pacini corpuscles, also found in the fingertips, but involve a larger nerve with more branching and fewer lamellae.
- Ruffini corpuscles consist of a dense branching network of nerves in the deep dermis without the concentric arrangement of Pacini corpuscles. They sense continuous pressure and are also known as slowly adapting cylindrical receptors.
- Merkel cells lie in the basal layer of epidermis and connect with free nerve endings. C fibers develop a terminal bulb that touches the Merkel cell; this is as close as nerves usually get to the epidermis, although fetal skin sometimes shows intraepidermal nerve fibers. Merkel cells are presumed to be touch receptors.
- The *Haarscheibe* or hair disc is a highly sensitive touch receptor, best developed in the area around the vibrissae (whiskers) of cats, rabbits and similar animals. The epidermis is thickened, contains an increased number of Merkel cells and is served by a rich network of nerves. While humans have hair discs, their physiologic role is probably minor.
- Krause end bulb or mucocutaneous receptors are located near the epidermal-dermal junction and function as cold or rapidly adapting receptors.

The nerve receptors in the skin form a complicated transmission network that has a resting potential of 60–80 mV. This potential is produced by increased intracellular K^+ and increased extracellular Na^+ and Cl^- concentrations, producing a transmembrane imbalance. Upon electrical or chemical stimulation, the K^+ ions leave the cell, triggering a wave-like depolarization impulse that extends via the spinal chord to the brain. After discharge there is an influx of Na^+ ions that must be pumped out via ATP-dependent processes to set up the conditions for firing again. This refractory period varies in length depending on the type of nerve. Depolarization is connected with the release of many mediators, including neuropeptides, especially substance P, as well as more standard neurotransmitters such as norepinephrine and acetylcholine. Free nerve endings often interact with mast cells.

The neurologic mechanisms of pruritus are complex and not well understood. A number of theories have been proposed and probably all have an element of truth. They include:

- Specificity theory: certain fibers transmit itch
- Intensity theory: low-intensity stimuli cause itch; higher-intensity stimuli, pain
- Selectivity theory: some of the peripheral receptors have specific central connections that enable them to transmit itch messages
- Pattern theory: itch is transmitted as a complex pattern of individual nerve firings

The nature of the mediators involved in pruritus is equally unclear. While one often thinks of antihistamines as the answer for itch, histamine is by no means the best-established mediator, and not surprisingly many forms of pruritus do not respond well to non-sedating levels of antihistamines. Potential mediators include histamine, kinins, prostaglandins, peptidases, opioids and neuropeptides. The role of central opioids in pruritus awaits clarification. Depletion of substance P by repeated application of capsaicin ameliorates some cutaneous pain (such as postherpetic neuralgia) as well as itching. Substances such as bile salts may directly stimulate nerve endings or mast cells to cause pruritus.

Clinical Aspects

Pruritus is the most common unpleasant experience involving the skin. At a low level it is merely annoying, but it may actually torture the patient, interfere with sleep and lead to inability to complete tasks at work and at home. Children with pruritus, primarily those with atopic dermatitis, are often less effective in school. Patients have even committed suicide because of uncontrollable pruritus. Thus, it is no wonder that the itching patient seeks medical aid and is demanding of the physician's time and skills. With the exception of the very common dry skin pruritus, especially of the elderly, the complaint of pruritus requires a detailed history, careful examination and usually at least screening laboratory testing.

The history should establish the nature of the pruritus. In some cases itching remains localized; a given area itches and is scratched, without significant spread. In other instances, localized itching and scratching trigger a more diffuse crescendo reaction. It is very rare for the itch to be incessant. One should inquire about triggers such as temperature changes (warm baths, cold showers, coming inside, going outside). In other situations, especially with scabies, pruritus is worse at night. If a patient claims to itch all the time with unvarying severity, there is invariably a marked emotional overlay to the complaints. Sometimes a given skin lesion, such as in prurigo simplex subacuta, may itch until it is scratched sufficiently to cause bleeding and a erosion; then the itching stops. In many settings, once pain occurs, pruritus is somehow blocked out.

On physical examination, it is important to separate the secondary excoriations from a primary skin disorder. Excoriations are typically linear and occur where the patient can reach with his hands. Thus the arms, chest, thighs and shoulders are probably the most common sites. The middle of the back is typically spared, although with a back scratcher, this rule loses value. This pattern of sparing has been called the reverse butterfly sign; the Greek word for the area that cannot be reached is acnestis. Few people scratch with just one finger; most use their entire hand so parallel linear lesions are seen. Often one such line is more prominent than the others. The scratch is usually erythematous, with many tiny erosions scattered along it; fresh ones are usually weeping or bloody, while older ones are crusted. Secondary infections are common, and once a bacterial infection is established, it can be spread by scratching. In both scabies of the cleanly and dermatitis herpetiformis, it is very difficult to find primary lesions. One can instruct the patient to cover their next primary lesion with an adhesive bandage, make a concerted effort to scratch elsewhere and present to the office as soon as possible for evaluation. In addition to excoriations, some patients may have smooth, almost shiny fingernails. These have been described as the polished nails of chronic pruritus.

Pruritus Secondary to Skin Disorders

Synonym. Pruritus cum materia

Dermatoses

In some situations, the cause of the pruritus is obvious. Patients with atopic dermatitis typically have marked pruritus; they have other stigmata of their disease, so diagnosis is usually easy. Similarly, lichen planus, psoriasis, insect bites and drug eruptions are usually easy to identify. Patients with urticaria have marked pruritus but may not have lesions when examined; they rub and do not scratch, so they do not have excoriations. One must specifically ask about hives or wheals. In the case of mast cell disease, sometimes distinct lesions are present; in other cases, the involvement is subtle and diffuse. In dermatitis herpetiformis, excoriations are often the only findings; in young adults with itching elbows, knees, scalp and genitalia, this diagnosis should be considered. Except for the scalp, scabies has a similar distribution and is far more common. Sometimes folliculitis is pruritic, especially in HIV/AIDS patients.

Subtle Skin Disturbances

In German, one speaks of minimal dermatoses. The message is the same; in some patients, the underlying skin disorder is quite subtle. For example, in the winter months, the combination of frequent bathing and central heating dries out many individuals' skin, leading to mild scaling and pruritus. This problem is more common in patients with atopic diathesis. Sometimes, it can be more severe, associated with obvious scaling and erythema. Older individuals are more often affected, and parts of the body without much sebum, such as the upper arms and thighs, dry out first.

Urticarial dermographism is equally subtle. While about 20% of the population has dermographism, it causes pruritus in only a small proportion. Itching is most common in the evening. In atopic patients wool clothing is often the trigger. Urticaria can be almost invisible. Sometimes heat, cold and even water may trigger urticarial lesions that are transient but intensely pruritic.

Aquagenic pruritus is fascinating, for it is hard to imagine an allergic or toxic reaction to water, but it does occur. By definition, water of any temperature causes pruritus within a matter of minutes when applied to the skin, presumably by activating either mast cells or mediators. Furthermore, this form of pruritus may be associated with underlying systemic diseases such as hypereosinophilic syndrome, polycythemia rubra vera or other hematologic disorders.

Infestations

Any patient who complains of pruritus should be examined with the possibility of scabies in mind. If other family members have pruritus or severe itching at night, the level of suspicion is raised. One should also examine the nape for *Pediculus humanus capitis*, the pubic hairs for *Phthirus pubis* and the clothing seams for *Pediculus humanus corporis*.

Pruritus Secondary to Systemic Disease

Synonyms. Pruritus sine materia, pruritus without skin disease

The list of systemic diseases associated with pruritus is lengthy. Table 25.1 shows just a sampling of the more common problems. One should search for obvious clues in the history or physical examination, such as jaundice, uremic frost, lymphadenopathy and the like. The usual situation is that there is no obvious explanation for the itching and one must carefully weigh the costs of extensive testing against the likely yield. Internal medicine and neurologic consultation may on occasion be helpful. In our experience, pruritus secondary to medications is often overlooked. While most pruritic drug reactions are associated with an exanthem, Table 25.2 shows those that may present with just pruritus. In addition, PUVA therapy may produce severe itching. Hydroxyethyl starches [poly(O-2-hydroxyethyl) starch] are used as volume expanders and infused to treat tinnitus; they often produce long-term pruritus. The starch particles can sometimes be identified in the skin with electron microscopy.

Table 25.1. Systemic diseases associated with pruritus

CNS disorders
Multiple sclerosis
Tumors
Tabes dorsalis, general paresis
Liver disorders
Cholestasis
Primary biliary cirrhosis
Extra hepatic biliary obstruction
Acute hepatitis
Renal disorders
Chronic renal failure, even with dialysis
Endocrine disorders
Hypo- and hyperthyroidism
Secondary hyperparathyroidism (renal failure)
Hypoparathyroidism
Diabetes mellitus
Hematologic disorders
Polycythemia rubra vera
Multiple myeloma
Iron deficiency anemia
Systemic mastocytosis
Hypereosinophilic syndrome
Malignancies
Any carcinoma, especially if metastatic
Carcinoid syndrome
Malignant lymphomas, especially Hodgkin disease
Leukemias
Pregnancy
Pruritus of pregnancy
Infestations
Ascariasis
Onchocerciasis
Oxyuriasis
Trichinosis
Ancylostomiasis
Schistosomiasis
Filariasis
Psychological diseases
Anxiety
Obsessive compulsive disorders
Monosymptomatic psychoses (delusions of parasitosis, others)
Psychogenic pruritus
HIV/AIDS

Table 25.2. Medications associated with pruritus

Histamine liberators
Opioids
CNS stimulants
Belladonna alkaloids
Barbiturates
Oral contraceptives
Hepatotoxic drugs
Biologic response mediators (interferons, interleukins, others)

Idiopathic Pruritus

Synonym. Pruritus simplex

If neither a cutaneous nor a systemic explanation for the pruritus can be found, one is faced with the diagnosis of idiopathic pruritus. This diagnosis is very unsatisfactory, leaving the patient unhappy and the doctor puzzled. In the elderly, mild pruritus is often almost normal, so that in an older patient with dry skin, one can make the working diagnosis of idio-

Table 25.3. Systemic therapy of pruritus

Agent	Comments
Antihistamines; H1 and H2 blockers	Sedating classes more useful; trial and error; combine different classes, H1 and H2
Antiinflammatory	
Nonsteroidal antiinflammatory drugs, aspirin	Both may occasionally help by blocking prostaglandins, but may also cause pruritus
Mast cell stabilizers	
Cromoglycate	Helps in mastocytosis; perhaps for aquagenic pruritus; not useful in other situations
Ketotifen	Mast cell stabilizer and antihistamine; helps for neurofibromatosis itching, aquagenic pruritus
CNS Agents	
Doxepin	Antihistamine plus tranquilizer
Other tricyclic antidepressants	Often helpful in low doses for depressed itchy individuals
Opiate antagonists (naloxone, others)	Helpful in primary biliary cirrhosis, under study for other forms
Sedatives, tranquilizers	Mild sedation takes the edge off itch
Ion exchange	
Cholestyramine	Helpful for a variety of conditions but hard to use
Activated charcoal	Best established in pruritus of renal failure; large amounts required
Placebo	In desperate cases, worth a try

pathic pruritus and initiate therapy. Otherwise, we are reluctant to make the diagnosis. Sometimes, psychological or psychiatric consultation can be of assistance, as the pruritus may be a call for help.

Therapy. Obvious the first goal is to treat the underlying disease. If nothing is found, or if treating the underlying disorder does not relieve the pruritus, then symptomatic therapy is needed.

Systemic. Table 25.3 shows some of the approaches available. One general caution is that ordinary antihistamines are not as helpful as often expected. For many pruritic conditions, they only help when they produce minor sedation. This has been shown nicely in atopic dermatitis and is probably true in many other instances. Systemic corticosteroids are often employed for pruritus, but in the absence of an antiinflammatory disorder, their use appears unwise.

Topical. Unfortunately, the topical approach to pruritus is often underestimated. Many patients have dry skin, so the first step should be lubrication with bland ointments or bath oils. One can add a variety of distracters, such as menthol, or topical anesthetics, such as polidocanol, to provide cost-effective relief. Some of the other topical measures are shown in Table 25.4. Topical capsaicin deserves a special word. It depletes substance P and presumably reduces itching in this way. Although initially approved for postherpetic neuralgia, it has also been used for fibromyalgia with painful trigger points and localized pruritus, such as notalgia paresthetica. The cream must be applied at least 4 times daily; it may cause pruritus initially and should not be used on larger areas.

Table 25.4. Topical therapy of pruritus

Agent	Comments
Antihistamines	Helpful in short term (insect bites, etc.) but high potential for allergic contact dermatitis; recently seen with topical doxepin
Corticosteroids	Expensive and disappointing in the absence of inflammatory skin disease
Tars	Small subset of patients respond well to tars or tar baths
Crotamiton	Expensive, perhaps helpful for localized lesions
Anesthetics	Most penetrate stratum corneum poorly, more useful on mucosal surfaces; polidocanol, pramoxine effective on skin
EMLA	Useful for very localized lesions, such as prurigo nodularis
Capsaicin	Helpful for localized itch or pain

Other Measures. UV radiation is probably the most useful adjunct. Even sunbathing must help, since pruritus tends to be less severe in sunny months. UVB is the best therapy for uremic pruritus; some dialysis centers have sun beds. UVB 311-nm lamps appear to work best. In some instances UVA and UVA 1 are also effective. Both PUVA and PUVA bath therapy have been employed for a variety of puzzling pruritic conditions with success.

Prophylaxis. Most pruritus can be greatly helped by simply having the patients bathe less often, use a mild soap or syndet, only wash where they are dirty (face, hands, feet, groin, axillae), pat rather than rub their skin dry and immediately lubricate the affected areas.

Prurigo

Definition. In Latin prurigo simply means the itch. It has two separate meanings in dermatology: a group of itchy diseases, and a special type of lesion. As a collective term, prurigo refers to a group of unrelated itchy disorders that in most cases are scratched or excoriated. The primary lesion is usually a tiny urticaria-like seropapule, known as a prurigo papule. The lesions are small, erythematous and edematous, occasionally with a tiny serum-filled blister, but unlike true urticaria they do not disappear over a period of hours without leaving a trace. Most often they evolve, with the help of scratching, into a hyperpigmented nodule with scale. Prurigo may also be used to describe papules or nodule secondary to manipulation of other itching disorders; prurigo nodules with atopic dermatitis are common, no matter what name one applies to them.

Prurigo is not a common concept in American dermatology. Except for prurigo nodularis and actinic prurigo, it is scarcely mentioned in American textbooks. Indeed, there is no other group of diseases with so many synonyms and so much confusion over the classification and meaning of the individual disorders. Nonetheless, we have retained the term and will discuss the various entities, as the concept has stood us in good stead. Table 25.5 shows the main features of the major subtypes of prurigo.

Prurigo Simplex Acuta

(Brocq)

Synonyms. Prurigo simplex acuta infantum, acute prurigo, strophulus infantum

Definition. Recurrent pruritic allergic reaction, primarily in children, generally secondary to arthropod bites or stings.

Epidemiology. Prurigo simplex acuta is most common in children 2–8 years of age, especially in the summer and early fall.

Table 25.5. Types of prurigo

Disease	Primary lesion	Secondary lesion	Residual lesion	Pruritus
Prurigo simplex acuta	Urticarial seropapule, often with red border	Dome-shaped, crusted, varicelliform papule	Hyper- or hypo-pigmented patch	Intense; scratching and rubbing
Prurigo simplex subacuta	Small mosquito bite-like urticarial (sero)papule	Scratched, crusted hemorrhagic papule	Usually central depigmented patch with peripheral hyperpigmentation	Intense; lesion usually scratched until open, bleeding; then pruritus less. No scratch marks on noninvolved skin
Prurigo simplex chronica	Small mosquito bite-like urticarial (sero)papule	Keratotic dome-shaped nodule with peripheral hyperpigmentation	No regression	Intense and long-lasting; nodules continuously manipulated
Prurigo nodularis	None (see text)	Hyperkeratotic dome-shaped nodule with peripheral hyperpigmentation	No regression	Intense and permanent; rubbing more common than scratching

The overlaps between prurigo simplex chronica and prurigo nodularis are discussed in the text

Etiology and Pathogenesis. This disorder most closely resembles urticaria. In our opinion it is generally the result of an arthropod bite or sting; we say this because it is more common in rural areas, in the summer months, and generally resolves when the patient is hospitalized. In addition, patients with prurigo simplex acuta are more likely to have positive prick-test reactions to arthropod antigens. We suspect it is a combined type I and type IV reaction.

Other causes have been suggested – dietary intolerance, especially in overweight children eating sweets or not totally ripe fruit, or the eruption of teeth (tooth pox) – but we find these concepts hard to accept.

Clinical Findings. A totally healthy child suddenly presents with intensely pruritic seropapules with a pale red elevated border (Fig. 25.1). The lesions are usually widely scattered but may be grouped. The trunk and extremities are most often involved. The very first lesion is a tiny soft urticarial papule whose center shows a yellow color on diascopy, representing the initial exudation of serum. Sometimes a tiny, barely visible vesicle develops, while in other instances it becomes larger and clinically apparent (strophulus bullosus).

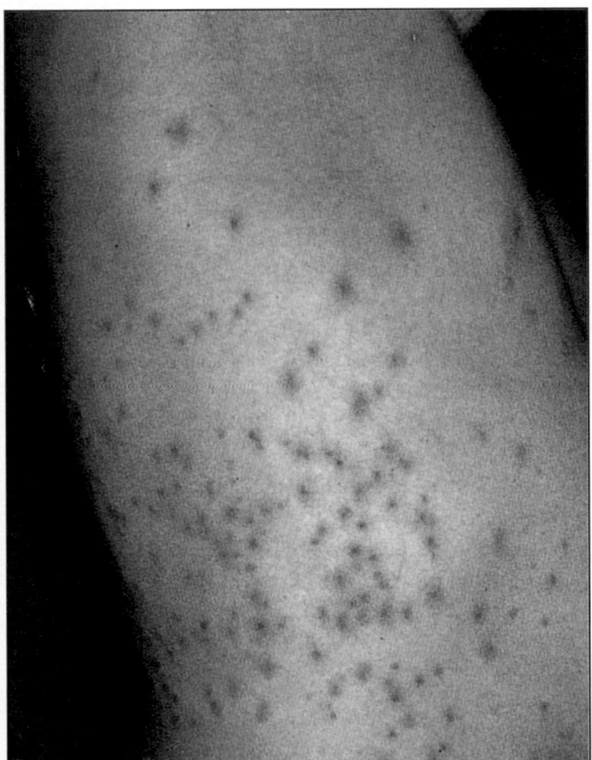

Fig. 25.1. Prurigo simplex acuta

Usually the seropapule evolves rapidly into a firm hard papule, losing its erythematous border. This is the most intensely pruritic stage, so that the lesion is almost invariably scratched and often denuded, producing a crust. Secondary impetiginization is common. Healing usually occurs without scarring, but sometimes with hyper- or hypopigmentation. Lesions in various degrees of evolution are frequently seen together, so that a varicelliform pattern develops. Mucosal involvement is not seen.

Histopathology. A fresh seropapule shows intraepidermal, often subcorneal, blister with edema and a mild lymphocytic perivascular infiltrate, often admixed with eosinophils. After excoriation, the lesion shows either an erosion or crust and has a more intense infiltrate.

Course and Prognosis. Lesions in various stages of evolution may be mixed together, producing a varicelliform picture. Secondary impetiginization occasionally occurs. Typical is that a miserable child is hospitalized and clears dramatically even before treatment has a chance to be effective.

Differential Diagnosis. The main problem is distinguishing prurigo simplex acuta from multiple insect bites. Some physicians feel that all prurigo simplex acuta lesions are bites, but we feel that more often there are some bites and then an allergic reaction. Severe cases can mimic varicella, but oral involvement is lacking, the scalp is free and the child is not febrile. The blister fluid contains no viral elements. Scabies and trombidiosis may be considered but can usually be excluded by their clinical features. Scabies involves the genitalia, groin and axillae and itches more severely at night, while chigger bites are usually fewer in number and confined to the legs or present at sites where clothing causes an impasse.

Therapy. Oral antihistamines and topical antipruritic agents, such as lotions containing polidocanol or menthol, are most useful. Sometimes a drying lotion suffices.

Prurigo Simplex Subacuta

(Brocq)

Synonyms. Urticaria papulosa chronica, subacute prurigo, strophulus adultorum, lichen urticatus

Definition. Subacute or chronic inflammatory dermatosis with typical clinical picture and history of pruritus.

Epidemiology. About two-thirds of patients are women, mostly in their 20s or after menopause. Men are usually older than 50 years when affected. Arthropod reactions play no role, i.e., there are no seasonal or regional differences in distribution. Most patients have at least neurotic behavior patterns and may overreact to the pruritus. Some have an underlying atopic diathesis.

Etiology and Pathogenesis. The true etiology is unknown. Probably a wide variety of factors can elicit pruritus and then in a small subset of individuals distinctive papular lesions arise and are excoriated. Some have suggested a follicular location for the lesions, but this is not always the case. Many subcategories of prurigo simplex subacuta have been defined, more likely reflecting the pruritic background rather than any other connection.

They include some of the entities listed in Table 25.6. In addition, a variety of hormonal, gastrointestinal and gynecologic causes have been postulated, as well as the presence of focal infections. In the vast majority of cases, no cause is identified. The mechanism appears to involve an initial type I reaction coupled with a later type IV reaction with a prominent cellular infiltrate.

Clinical Findings. The most striking feature is the intense pruritus, which is relieved when the patient scratches the lesion until it bleeds. Excoriations almost never extend to the adjacent normal skin; this clinical feature helps distinguish prurigo simplex subacuta from other pruritic dermatoses (Fig. 25.2). The primary lesion is a pink seropapule with a central vesicle that can be palpated as a tiny grain. The lesion is so pruritic that it is immediately attacked and rarely seen by the physician. The typical sites are the shoulder girdle and the lateral aspects of the thighs. The same lesions on the face are called acne urticata.

The secondary lesions are what the physician must recognize. There are crusted excoriations and even excavations, which are sharply bordered. The crust usually has at least some blood in it. The size is highly variable. The intervening skin is normal. In contrast to

Table 25.6. Variants of prurigo

Name	Description
Actinic prurigo	Type of photosensitivity, most often seen in Native Americans
Prurigo aestivalis or Hutchinson prurigo	Type of photosensitivity, variant of polymorphic light eruption
Prurigo Besnier	Nodular prurigo reaction in patients with atopic dermatitis
Prurigo diabetica	Prurigo in patients with diabetes mellitus
Prurigo dermatographica of Marcussen	Prurigo following pressure urticaria
Prurigo dysmenorrhoica	Prurigo prior to menses; perhaps autoimmune progesterone dermatitis
Prurigo gestationis or prurigo gravidarum	Old term that is hard to incorporate into modern terminology (Chap. 36)
Prurigo hepatica	Prurigo secondary to hepatic disease
Prurigo lymphatica	Prurigo in patients with malignant lymphoma or leukemia
Prurigo lymphogranulomatotica	Prurigo in patients with Hodgkin disease
Prurigo leukodystrophica	Postinflammatory hypopigmentation associated with prurigo, usually in patients with atopic dermatitis
Prurigo melanotica (Pierini-Borda)	Postinflammatory hyperpigmentation associated with prurigo, usually in dark-skinned individuals
Prurigo paraneoplastica	Prurigo secondary to underlying malignancy
Prurigo pigmentosa	Primarily seen in Oriental patients; prurigo associated with reticulate hyperpigmentation
Prurigo uremica	Prurigo secondary to chronic renal disease

Included in this table are true variants of prurigo as discussed in this chapter, as well as diseases that have been named prurigo

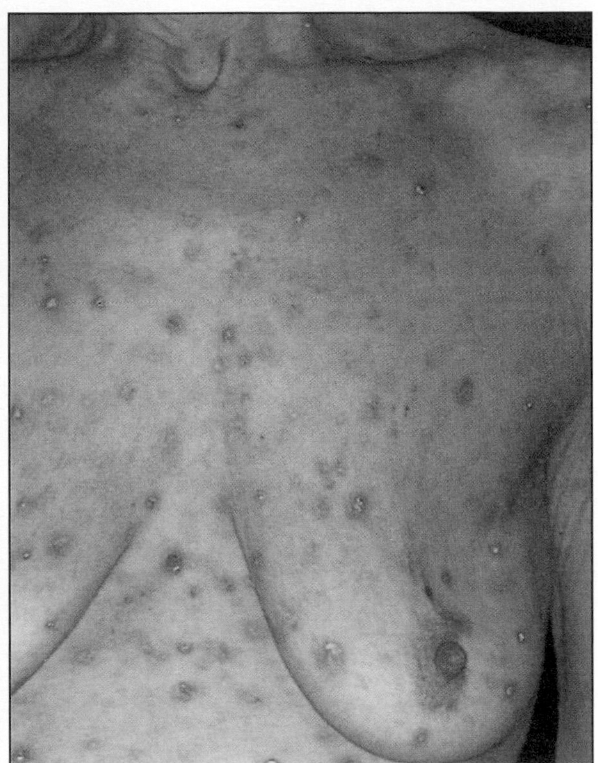

Fig. 25.2. Prurigo simplex subacuta

prurigo simplex acuta, hypopigmented, often atrophic scars with a hyperpigmented periphery are common. Thus a dimorphous picture develops with crusted lesions and scars, but only rarely with primary lesions. Lichenified lesions, seen so often in other itchy dermatoses, do not develop. The palms, soles and mucosa are spared.

Histopathology. The microscopic features reflect the clinical stages. The acute stage is identical to prurigo simplex acuta; in some reports, the early edema is within the follicular epithelium. Later the epidermis is acanthotic and may contain lymphocytes and eosinophils, often located within an intraepidermal or subcorneal blister. The excoriation comes to dominate the picture, while the dermal infiltrate is more mixed. As epidermal regeneration occurs, dermal fibrosis and new vessels with thickened walls can be found.

Laboratory Findings. If the history points towards disease in a given organ system, it should be investigated. Blind screening is rarely helpful.

Course and Prognosis. The prognosis is unsatisfactory. If the underlying condition improves (or, in the case of pregnancy, resolves), improvement can be expected.

Differential Diagnosis. The distinction between prurigo simplex subacuta and neurotic excoriations can be difficult. A history of intensely pruritic red bumps is needed to diagnosis prurigo simplex subacuta, even if one does not clinically see a primary lesion. Patients with atopic dermatitis may develop similar lesions, but they have other stigmata of their underlying disease. Occasionally, nodular lesions may develop in dermatitis herpetiformis, but they are uncommon. Nodular scabies has fewer larger lesions that are not so pruritic. Prurigo aestivalis (summer prurigo) is a form of photosensitivity; the lesions are confirmed to the face and arms.

Therapy

Systemic. Antihistamines, usually with soporific action, or minor tranquilizers are generally the mainstay of therapy. Some feel that hydroxyzine is more effective than other antihistamines. Systemic corticosteroids usually produce little effect and the disease recurs rapidly. If internal disease is identified, such as diabetes mellitus, it should be treated. The question here, as with urticaria, reads: Is blind treatment of possible internal diseases, such as arbitrary use of antibiotics, antifungal agents or similar drugs, justified? We tend to employ such agents only in desperate cases. Antimalarial agents and oral contraceptives have been used in the same manner.

Topical. Both topical distracters and anesthetics such as polidocanol lotion or pramoxine can be tried. High-potency corticosteroids can also be employed. The itching is so focal that some patients can be taught to use an antipruritic medication rather than destroying the lesion.

Other Measures. Just as for ordinary pruritus, radiation with UVB, UVA and PUVA, as well as PUVA bath therapy, can be considered.

Acne Urticata

(Kaposi 1893)

Acne urticata is prurigo simplex subacuta confined exclusively to the face (Fig. 25.3). Almost all patients are young women with emotional problems. Premenstrual flares may be seen. Other underlying causes are not usually found. The lesions are identical to those discussed above, with, once again, intensive pruritus. The differential diagnosis includes a number of acneiform lesions. Acne vulgaris does not itch. In acne excoriée, definite acne lesions are manipulated

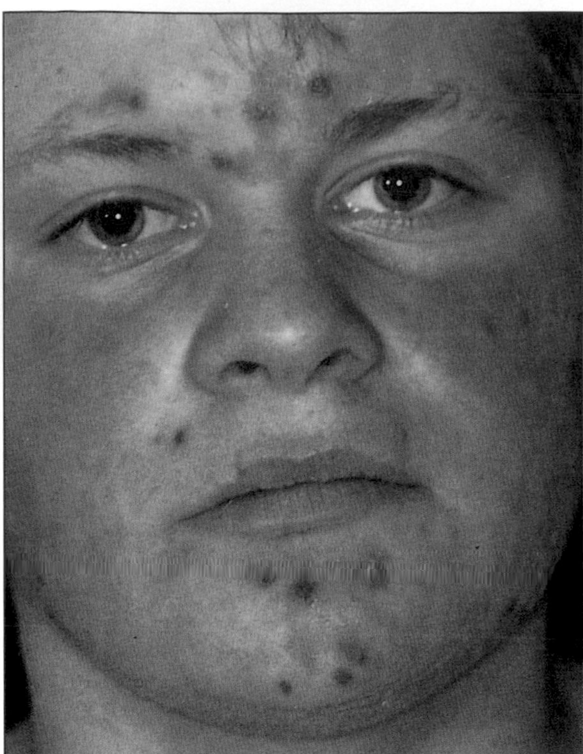

Fig. 25.3. Acne urticata

and excoriated. In acne necrotica, the changes are primarily pustules that involve the hairline; they too are scratched away, healing with varicelliform scars. The therapy is just as unrewarding as for the nonfacial form.

Prurigo Simplex Chronica

Synonyms. Chronic prurigo, urticaria perstans

Prurigo simplex chronica is closely related to prurigo nodularis; we view the latter as the maximal variant of the former. The causes are the same as prurigo simplex subacuta, but the lesions tend to persist as hyperpigmented dome-shaped nodules, usually 0.4–1.0 cm in diameter with a hyperkeratotic surface. While theoretically a primary seropapule can be seen, practically this is a very rare occasion. The histopathology is identical to that discussed below under prurigo nodularis. If both typical bloody crusted excoriations of prurigo simplex subacuta and hyperkeratotic nodules are present, one can consider this diagnosis. We view it as a stage between prurigo simplex subacuta and prurigo nodularis, not as a sharply defined disease. A nodular variant of bullous pemphigoid has been described, so if there is a history of bullae or oral lesions, it may be wise to perform an immunofluorescent examination to rule out this possibility.

Therapy. The therapy is the same as for prurigo nodularis with a few alterations. Intralesional corticosteroids are the best treatment for the nodules; an alternative is high-potency corticosteroid creams or ointments under occlusion. Cryotherapy and even laser destruction have also been employed.

Prurigo Nodularis

(Hyde and Montgomery 1909)

Definition. Very pruritic dermatosis characterized by persistent nodules.

Epidemiology. Thirty years ago prurigo nodularis was considered by some as almost pathognomonic for uremia. With the advent of dialysis and renal transplantation, it has become less common. Probably the biggest group are patients with severe atopic dermatitis or at least an atopic diathesis. The same underlying emotional risk factors discussed for other prurigo forms, such as depression and psychosocial problems, apply here.

Etiology and Pathogenesis. The French term *lichénifications circonscrits nodulaires chroniques* reflects the close overlap between lichen simplex chronicus and prurigo nodularis. Some feel that the prurigo nodule is simply the result of persistent rubbing and lichenification, perhaps at the site of a previous bite, folliculitis or prurigo lesion. The role of the dermal nerves in prurigo nodularis has long been debated. They are more prominent but it is unclear whether they are reactive or play a role in triggering the pruritus. In addition, a potential role for proteinases and other constituents of eosinophilic granules has been suggested. Elevated serum immunoglobulin E (IgE) and increased incidence of immediate reactions to pollens, dust and house dust mites support the role of underlying atopy.

Clinical Findings. Once again, the key feature is pruritus. The lesions are almost limited to the distal aspects of the extremities, in contrast to prurigo simplex subacuta. The face and trunk are spared. There is usually a modest number of symmetrically distributed, isolated firm nodules with a size ranging from 0.5 to 3.0 cm (Fig. 25.4). The intervening skin is normal or occasionally hyperpigmented. Early lesions

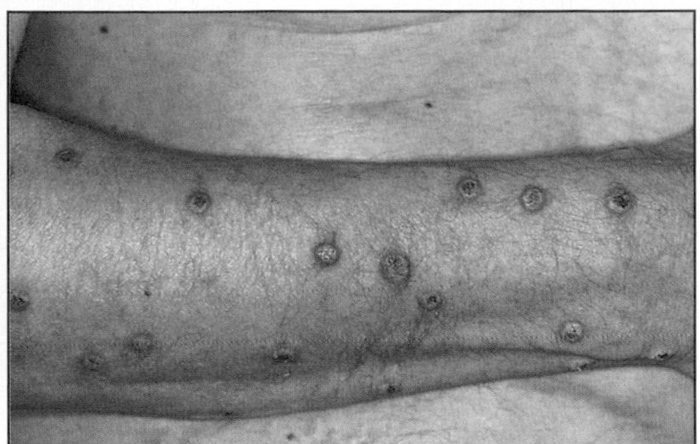

Fig. 25.4. Prurigo nodularis

may have an erythematous tone; later the color is red-gray or more of a dirty gray; with side lighting, the surface is dull, not shiny. Because the nodules continue to itch, they are often excoriated or crusted, sometimes with bloody debris.

Histopathology. The epidermis shows acanthosis and hyperkeratosis, while in the upper dermis is a mixed inflammatory infiltrate. The only difference from lichen simplex chronicus is the dome-shaped profile on low-power visualization of an entire lesion. Mast cells and eosinophils may be increased. As mentioned above, thickened dermal nerves and prominent Schwann cells may be seen; occasionally tiny neuromas are formed (Pautrier neuroma).

Course and Prognosis. The course is chronic and the patient miserable. Suicidal ideation is not uncommon.

Differential Diagnosis. On the legs, verrucous lichen planus must be considered; the lesions are sometimes quite similar even on biopsy. One should look for more typical lichen planus elsewhere, especially on mucosal surfaces that are unaffected by prurigo. When multiple smaller nodules are present, along with crusted excoriations, one can entertain the diagnosis of prurigo simplex chronica. The prurigo nodules in atopic dermatitis are accompanied by other disease manifestations and the intervening skin is usually not normal. Even today, it may be wise to exclude underlying renal disease in severe cases.

Therapy

Systemic. The ordinary measures of antihistamines and even corticosteroids usually fail. Thalidomide 100–200 mg daily has often been effective; it is probably worth a try in severe cases, as long as pregnancy can be excluded and neurologic complications are monitored. Pimocide and other psychopharmaceutic agents can be tried, perhaps in cooperation with a psychiatrist. Dapsone and clofazimine have been proposed, but since the process is not primarily inflammatory, it is not surprising that they often fail to help. In some cases azathioprene 50–150 mg daily is effective.

Topical. Simple topical therapy is doomed to failure. As a minimum, corticosteroids under occlusion or intralesionally are needed. We usually use triamcinolone acetonide 5–10 mg/ml, employing a topical anesthetic for dilution. Cryotherapy, laser destruction and even excision of especially annoying lesions may be contemplated.

Other Measures. Once again, UVB, UVA and PUVA are often helped. PUVA bath therapy seems a good way to treat localized lesions.

Hyperkeratosis Follicularis et Parafollicularis in Cutem Penetrans

(Kyrle 1916)

Synonyms. Kyrle disease, perforating disorder of renal dialysis

Etiology and Pathogenesis. Following Kyrle's original description, this poorly understood disorder was classified as a disorder of keratinization, as Kyrle believed he could identify both follicular and parafollicular hyperkeratotic lesions. Later Mehregan and Coskey (1968) described perforating folliculitis, with plugged inflamed follicles on the legs and damage to the follicle wall. These two descriptions, Kyrle's "in cutem penetrans" and Mehregan and Coskey's "perforating folliculitis", led to the concept of perforating dermatoses, also discussed in Chapter 18.

As patients with chronic renal disease began to be routinely treated with dialysis, the disorder was rediscovered. In addition to their well-known pruritus, some of these individuals developed prurigo nodularis-like lesions. The problem appears particularly common in those individuals with diabetic renal disease. We believe that Kyrle disease, perforating folliculitis and perforating disorder of renal disease all represent the combination of chronic folliculitis and prurigo nodularis. Familial cases have been described but are poorly documented; they probably represent unrelated disorders of keratinization.

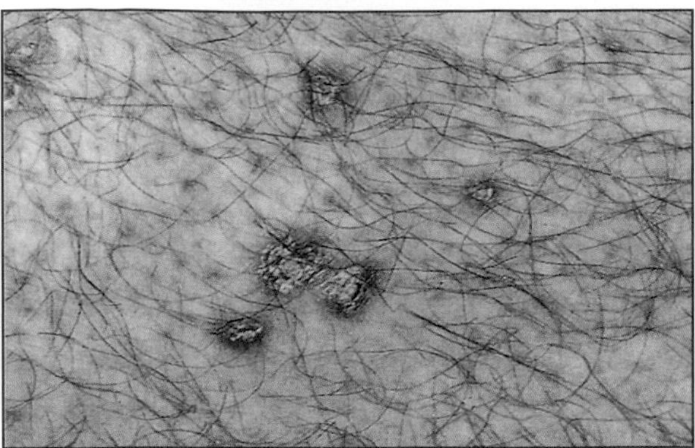

Fig. 25.5. Hyperkeratosis follicularis et parafollicularis in cutem penetrans

Clinical Findings. There are hyperkeratotic papules and plaques, some with crust and some domed-shaped with a central plug (Fig. 25.5). They range in size from 2–3 mm to 1–2 cm. Excoriations are also present in most cases. Often there is a linear pattern to the lesions suggesting the Köbner phenomenon. The legs are most often involved, especially the shins, but the arms and trunk may also be affected.

Histopathology. The microscopic findings have led to most of the confusion in describing this disease complex. The key feature is the presence of cornified plugs of keratin in a follicular or epidermal invagination. Because of the chronic changes, a well-developed follicle is not seen. Kyrle believed most lesions were not follicular and this concept is repeated in many modern texts. The so-called epidermal invaginations (parafollicularis) are old distorted follicles. In addition, there may be focal dyskeratosis, reactive epithelial hyperplasia and chronic dermal inflammation, which is occasionally suppurative. The keratotic plugs are described as penetrating the epidermis, but this is so illogical that it hardly deserves comment. The concept of plugged, chronically manipulated follicles with prurigo nodularis changes seems not only more reasonable but also biologically feasible.

Differential Diagnosis. The major differential diagnostic point is prurigo nodularis. Hyperkeratosis lenticularis perstans (Flegel disease) (Chap. 17) has acral keratoses which are usually smaller and not pruritic. The other perforating disorders, such as elastosis perforans serpiginosa, are completely distinct.

Therapy. Treatment is most difficult, as almost all patients today have complex medical histories. UVB phototherapy is probably the most effective approach; systemic retinoids help but are often not acceptable or tolerated.

Prurigo Pigmentosa

(NAGASHIMA et al. 1971)

Definition. Uncommon papular pruritic disease that heals with reticulate hyperpigmentation.

Epidemiology. Prurigo pigmentosa has been reported primarily in Japan but is occasionally seen in other parts of the world. Most patients are young women, who are usually affected in the spring and summer months.

Etiology and Pathogenesis. The etiology is unknown.

Clinical Findings. The initial lesions are pruritic erythematous papules. They occur most often on the trunk and nape. Involvement of the intrascapular and sternal areas is especially common. The primary lesions often coalesce, forming urticarial plaques. Scale may be seen. After a period of days to weeks, the lesions disappear, leaving behind reticulated hyperpigmented patches that persist for months to years. New pruritic lesions may arise on the background of pigmentary changes, as they continue to develop over a period of 6–12 months. While other sites may be involved, the mucous membranes are spared. There are no associated systemic findings.

Histopathology. The microscopic findings are not specific. There is a lichenoid dermatitis following by postinflammatory hyperpigmentation with melanophages.

Differential Diagnosis. The differential diagnostic considerations include all the lichenoid dermatoses, especially lichen planus. The question here is similar to that regarding erythema dyschromicum perstans – Is this dermatosis unique, or is it a variant of lichen planus? When erythematous plaques are found between the breasts of a young woman, one must also consider reticulated erythematous mucinosis, but the histology is definitive. The hyperpigmented lesions resemble macular amyloidosis.

Therapy. The literature suggests that dapsone 50–100 mg daily or minocycline 100–200 mg daily for several weeks both ameliorates the pruritus and reduces the pigmentation.

Self-Induced Skin Diseases

There are many situations in which a dermatologist may encounter patients who have created their skin symptoms or lesions. We divide self-induced skin disease into several categories (Table 25.7). We will first briefly discuss these different variants and then review the skin findings of the most common forms in more detail. Several of the problems are considered below under "Psychiatric Disorders".

Simulated Diseases

In all these situations, the patient is deliberately creating the impression that he has a disease in order to achieve some benefit. The term "malingering" is often applied in the USA. Probably the most common examples are workmen's compensation problems and "whiplash" injuries, in which the financial advantages of disease are obvious. It is estimated that about 0.5% or less of patients in a general medical practice have such simulated symptoms or signs, while more than 2% of those presenting for dermatologic evaluation of work-related conditions fall into this category.

False Symptoms

In this setting, the patient claims to have problems that he does not have. Dermatologists are rarely involved. One could imagine a patient complaining of extreme pruritus or cutaneous pain, but fortunately for our specialty these patients usually choose headaches, visual disturbances, tinnitus, chest pain or musculoskeletal pain as their problem.

Table 25.7. Types of self-induced skin disease

Types of self-induced skin disease
Patient is conscious of manipulation
Patient admits manipulation
Simulated disease
False symptoms
Artifacts
Pathomimicry
Induced disease
Obsessive-compulsive disorders
Patient unable to admit manipulation
Münchhausen syndrome
Münchhausen by proxy syndrome
Patient is not conscious of manipulation
True dermatitis artifacta
Delusions of parasitosis and related disorders

Artifacts

Here the patient creates objective signs of disease, such as simulating fever by heating a thermometer, drinking blood to suggest gastrointestinal bleeding, injecting blood in the bladder or adding it to urine to suggest hematuria, and many others. Because the skin is so accessible, it is a common site for artificial changes. The various ways in which dermatitis artifacta can appear are discussed below. Other scenarios include manipulating patch test results or deliberately interfering with wound healing in order to suggest inadequate surgical results. One should be suspicious of such artifacts if the following factors are present:

- The patient stands to gain from a disease
- The history does not fit with the physical findings and frequently changes
- The clinical findings do not fit with any well-established dermatologic condition

Pathomimicry

These patients have a disease but they are able to induce its appearance through the normal pathogenic mechanisms. It is almost impossible for a physician to spot, much less prove, such manipulations. Examples include a patient with pemphigus vulgaris or bullous pemphigoid who stops his immunosuppressive therapy and allows disease to flare, or someone with a known drug allergy who surreptitiously ingests the medication. An equally puzzling problem is a nonresolving allergic contact dermatitis. A patient may know what substance is responsible for the allergic contact dermatitis and continue to apply it, producing a therapeutic dilemma. This situation has been called dermatitis autogenica. In other instances, patients with atopic dermatitis may apply irritating or drying substances, such as alcohol or urine, to their already damaged skin, exaggerating the process.

Induced Disease

The most interesting of these patients have infectious diseases that they have created by inoculating themselves with microbes. A classic report describes young men in a Russian village deliberately infecting each other with *Trichophyton schoenleinii* to cause favus and perhaps avoid military duty. Others deliberately damage their skin in a fashion similar to dermatitis artifacta patients, but they do so to obtain an advantage and they usually do not take much risk.

Therapy. Such patients should be confronted. If the physician has evidence that manipulation has occurred, then the situation should be discussed with the patient, mentioning both the medical and legal consequences of such behavior.

Dermatitis Artifacta

Epidemiology. These patients damage their skin in the same way as simulant patients, but they cannot admit to the manipulation. They also are not malingering, as they have no obvious gain from their disorder. Women are more commonly involved than men. Most patients are young adults, but the entire age spectrum can be represented. A disproportionate number of patients have been treated for psychiatric disease. Many are involved in health care, e.g., nurses or social workers; physicians are rarely affected.

Etiology and Pathogenesis. A respected colleague, when lecturing about dermatitis artifacta, always tells his students, "You can ask me anything you want but why." Indeed, it is extremely difficult to comprehend why individuals intentionally inflict damage on themselves. The skin is the favorite site, being easily accessible and often presented in an ostentatious manner. Most individuals would be reluctant to drip acid on their liver or inject milk into their heart, but with the skin they find it easier.

The major underlying theme is an attempt to alter or escape from an unsatisfactory situation, by calling attention to oneself as a patient, victim or bearer of a mysterious problem. The patients have a severe psychiatric problem but are otherwise cooperative, allowing multiple diagnostic or therapeutic measures. They often have other psychosomatic or psychiatric problems. In a review of 15,000 psychiatric consultations, 93 patients had artifactual disease. Of this group, 21 had skin damage.

Clinical Findings. One must have a high degree of clinical suspicion to diagnose dermatitis artifacta. There is no one clinical picture that fits. Instead, one should consider dermatitis artifacta whenever a clinical picture does not fit into a logical diagnostic pattern. The lesions are usually found on the extremities, chest or face, i.e., the areas that can be conveniently reached.

Ordinary manipulation with the fingers can produce hemorrhagic, ulcerated or swollen areas (Fig. 25.6). Usually exogenous materials are used to facilitate damage, often leaving telltale signs. When a sharp object is used, linear streaks and lines, finer and deeper than a scratch from a fingernail, may be seen (Fig. 25.7). Often several tentative cuts are seen, just as on the wrists of those who attempt suicide by slashing an artery. When cigarettes are used to burn the skin, multiple circles of uniform size are seen. If caustic material is applied, there is often streaking or dripping, producing suggestive markings. Injections of urine or feces often induce cellulitis and fever; typical is the presence of multiple unusual organisms on culture. Injections of foreign material may cause a factitial panniculitis; the male genitalia are often involved. The creativity of such patients should never be underestimated.

Diagnostic Criteria. The best diagnostic method is to occlude the lesion and observe the tendency for healing. Confronting the patient with the working diagnosis of dermatitis artifacta can be very dangerous, driving them to suicide or at the very least to another physician. The damage done by a false diagnosis is potentially enormous. If a patient has a true skin disease and is diagnosed as dermatitis artifacta, not only is appropriate treatment delayed but marked hostility may arise.

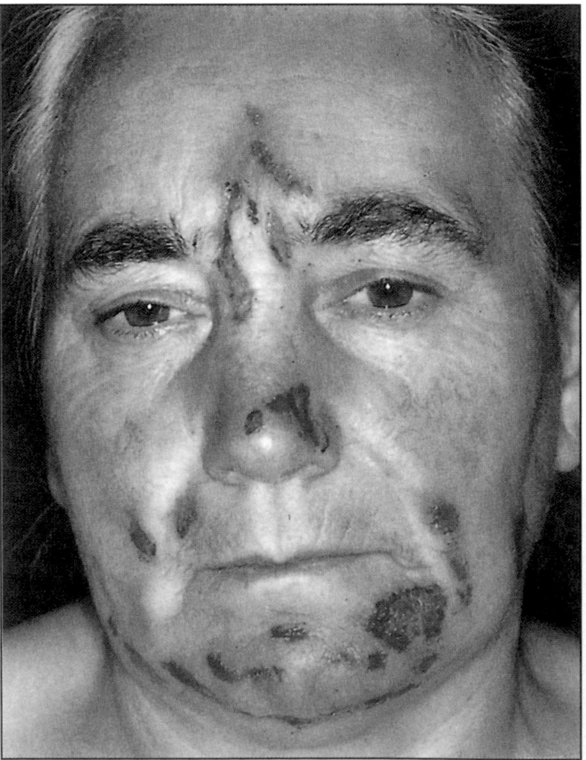

Fig. 25.6. Dermatitis artifacta caused by manipulation with the fingers

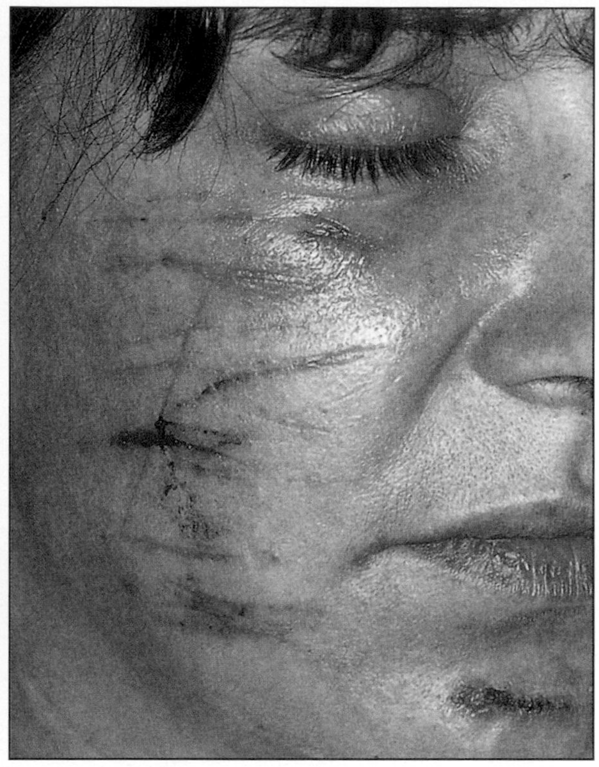

Fig. 25.7. Dermatitis artifacta caused by a sharp object

Course and Prognosis. It is important not to forget that dermatitis artifacta can be coupled with true skin problems, most often cellulitis and sepsis. Since the manipulation is often performed under insanitary conditions, or involves the introduction of contaminated material into the skin and subcutaneous tissues, infections may result, typically involving multiple organisms, some of which are not usual skin pathogens. Until the patient's underlying emotional problem is resolved, the situation is likely to continue. If one approach is blocked, e.g., by removing access to needles, usually another avenue will be opened, perhaps one more dangerous to the patient.

Differential Diagnosis. The usual differential diagnosis involves a wide variety of infectious and inflammatory diseases, including pyoderma gangrenosum, vasculitis and panniculitis. It is perhaps most important to exclude neurologic, vascular and infectious causes of ulcerations.

Cultural barriers may interfere with an accurate diagnosis; in many societies, including Russia and Vietnam, healers perform cupping, applying heated small glasses to the skin. As the air in the glass cools, a vacuum is created and the suction produces circular hemorrhagic patches. Some include extreme forms of piercing and implantation of objects in the skin of the genitalia as self-mutilation, but the diagnosis is at least obvious. In some Oriental societies, glass or metal beads are implanted subcutaneously on the penis or on other parts of the genitalia to increase sexual satisfaction.

Another related differential diagnosis category involves drug abusers, who create a broad spectrum of skin lesions, ranging from superficial ulcerations from skin popping to track marks from recurrent superficial phlebitis and thrombosis, nasal septal perforations from cocaine sniffing, and cellulitis and sepsis from introduced infections, often with unusual organisms.

Therapy. The individual lesions usually heal under occlusion. Topical or systemic antibiotics are needed to treat secondary infections. Confrontation brings little benefit when dealing with these patients. They often become aggressive and usually seek other sources of care. It is very difficult for a dermatologist to work with such patients. They strictly refuse to see a psychiatrist, the only specialist who might be helpful. In addition, there is an ethical and legal dilemma for the dermatologist, as it is probably inappropriate to try and trick the patient by searching for evidence to support the induction of lesions, by using laboratory tests to uncover artifactual disease or by providing psychiatric consultation under the guise of "having another doctor interested in your problem visit with you."

Münchhausen Syndrome and Related Disorders

A final scenario, more the problem of psychiatrists and administrators, is Münchhausen syndrome (Asher 1951), named after a German folklore character who told fantastic stories, such as tying his horse to a post during a snowstorm and waking to find the horse hanging from the church steeple. Patients with Münchhausen syndrome create a complex disease picture, usually with a lengthy history and multiple bizarre symptoms, and visit many hospitals, seeking help but often leaving suddenly and with anger. They may undergo multiple dangerous operations for uncontrollable pain or similar problems. In some instances, they may use dermatitis artifacta as part of their complex illness. In Münchhausen syndrome by proxy, a parent or spouse may induce a severe injury or disease and create a bizarre story around their child or mate. In children, the risk of underlying damage is so great that a skull X-ray and skeletal survey are appropriate. Particularly in the case of children, where the mother is the usual perpetrator, the physician's duty to protect the child overweighs any other considerations regarding medical privacy. In another example a husband may inject material into his wife's breast and then bring her to the doctor for care. In most instances, it is felt appropriate to report adults with Münchhausen syndrome to medical societies, social services or hospitals in order to prevent the patient from undergoing unneeded testing or procedures.

Factitial Lymphedema

(SECRÉTAN 1901)

Synonym. Secrétan syndrome

Repeated relatively mild trauma may produce swelling and erythema of the skin with hemorrhage. The German term for this is *Klopfartefakt* (pounding artifact). Some patients are simulants, seeking exterior gain, while other cases are similar to dermatitis artifacta. Secrétan was a Swiss insurance agent who unravelled such a case. The usual site is the dorsal surface of the nondominant hand, although the shin may also be involved. The end result is fibrosis and a persistent localized lymphedema. There may be other signs of artifactual skin damage, but no suggestion of underlying lymphatic disease. Attempts at treatment are just as frustrating as for other artifactual disease.

Psychiatric Disorders

The importance of psychiatry in dermatologic disease is unquestioned. Many major dermatology clinics in Germany, including ours in Munich, have doctors specialized in both psychosocial medicine and dermatology. One should always remember that for many patients a visit to the doctor, no matter what the specialty, is a plea for help, often unrelated to the specific complaint, be it cutaneous, gastrointestinal or musculoskeletal. Thus, by taking at least a partial history and attempting to get to know one's patients, one can often sense or identify an underlying problem. Unfortunately, the nature of reimbursement schedules in most countries keeps dermatologic doctor-patient interactions brief. One good time to expand this relationship is during minor surgical procedures, once the patient is relaxed, anesthetized and pain-free.

Psychiatric referrals are often tricky. Most patients have deliberately chosen a nonpsychiatrist, even if they suspect they may need psychiatric help. To simply say "I can't help your itching; you must see a psychiatrist" is inevitably a failure. One can hope that the patient will sense the need for further help; often asking "What other specialists do you think we should ask for help?" will get the patient to mention the dreaded word first. Another approach is to suggest consultation with a doctor who has experience with difficult problems like the current one. This is much easier in a clinic than when the patient must go to a different office where "Psychiatry" is boldly stated on the door.

Therapy. Many dermatologists with sufficient training and experience in internal medicine or psychiatry feel comfortable prescribing psychiatric drugs. We generally prefer to do this in connection with a psychiatrist. A number of different agents can be useful. Anyone employing them should be well aware of the potential side effects and especially the numerous drug interactions. Agents potentially useful in dermatologic patients include:

- Antidepressants. Doxepin is an excellent antihistamine in dosage levels of 10–25 mg daily. In much higher dosages (75–200 mg daily) it is a safe antidepressant. For patients with obsessive-compulsive disorders, the tricyclic inhibitor of serotonin uptake, clomipramine is approved by the FDA. The usual starting dose is 25 mg daily, increased every week by 25 mg until the therapeutic effect is achieved. While the maximum recommended dose is 250 mg daily, we encourage dermatologists to stop much sooner, perhaps at 100 mg. Fluoxetine, a nontricyclic serotonin uptake inhibitor can also be used; the dose ranges between 20–60 mg daily.
- Tranquilizers. Almost all tranquilizers are benzodiazepines. In a dermatologic practice, they should only be used for short periods, such as when situational anxiety makes an atopic dermatitis flare dramatically. In addition, the most common kinds of "anxiety", stage fright or related disorders, are best treated with β-blockers.
- Antipsychotic medications. Pimocide in a dosage range of 1–6 mg daily is usually the best treatment for monosymptomatic psychoses. In Europe, a closely related compound, fluspirilen, is also employed. Some psychiatrists prefer more traditional medications such as haloperidol, but we have had good results with pimocide.

Many skin diseases have frequent and obvious emotional components. Atopic dermatitis and psoriasis may flare with stress and make their victims as miserable emotionally as physically. In other situations, such as with dermatitis artifacta, one senses an underlying psychological problem, but it is often vague. In contrast, there are two categories of disease where dermatology and psychiatry clearly interact.

Delusions of Parasitosis

(Thibierge 1894, Ekbom 1938)

Synonyms. Acarophobia, parasitophobia, Ekbom disease

Definition. Monosymptomatic psychosis in which patients are certain they have parasites, even though they do not.

Epidemiology. Most patients are women of middle age or older, often with fastidious habits in earlier years.

Etiology and Pathogenesis. The true monosymptomatic psychosis is characterized by hallucinatory phenomena, delusions and a convincing history of being able to see and describe the bugs. Some patients may have suffered from a documented scabies as the trigger; others never have had a true infestation.

Clinical Findings. Patients present with varying degrees of excoriations, as they attempt to remove or destroy the imagined parasites, which may be mites, worms or other life forms. They may use tweezers, knives or even ice picks to attack the invaders, producing significant wounds that heal with scarring. The usual sites are once again those that are accessible – arms, thighs, breasts and face. Typically they bring a small bottle or envelope full of "animals". Microscopic examination reveals the content to be scales, lint and dirt, but there is no use trying to convince the patient of this fact. A patient so informed will simply never return to the physician again.

Differential Diagnosis. When a patient complains of bugs, mites or parasites, there are several possibilities. First and foremost, one must exclude a true but subtle infestation. There may be a history of excessive use of lindane or other antiscabetic medications, so that neurologic effects of such medications should be considered. Second, patients with organic brain disease, toxic psychosis (drugs or medications, such as corticosteroids) or underlying medical disorder associated with pruritus (such as renal failure) may complain of bugs. In addition, some patients are obsessed with having parasites, but when confronted, know they do not. Finally, others have a phobia of contact with other individuals or animals to avoid infestation.

Therapy. Topical antipruritics can be prescribed but achieve little. The answer is pimocide. The challenge is to convince the patient to take the medicine.

Other Monosymptomatic Psychoses

Several other disorders are similar to delusions of parasitosis. They include delusions of facial asymmetry, other physical malformations, marked halitosis or bromhidrosis (unpleasant body odors). Psychologists tell us that no one has a truly symmetric face; if individuals are shown pictures purporting to portray their whole face, but actually constructed from either the left or right side and its mirror image, most will be somewhat perplexed and uncomfortable.

Another closely related group is delusions of venereal diseases, "AIDS phobia" and cancerophobia. Patients present with minimal changes on their genital skin, such as normal pearly penile papules or ectopic sebaceous glands, or with a minor traumatic erosion. Some can be reassured, but others demand repeated testing for syphilis or AIDS and never really accept their lack of disease. Others may be convinced that they have a cancer, often in the mouth, and demand repeated biopsies or other tests. Such patients should be treated with pimocide or fluspirilen; most wind up in the care of psychiatrists.

Obsessive-Compulsive Disorders

Definition. Personality traits where the individual performs conscious, repetitive damaging actions may result in distinctive patterns of self-mutilation.

Epidemiology. In general, there is a striking female predominance. The age of onset varies somewhat with the manifestation; trichotillomania or lip licking occur earlier than neurotic excoriations.

Etiology and Pathogenesis. Patients have a rigid personality; they are afraid of making mistakes and thus indecisive. They may admit to their habits, unable to understand why they are so driven, or may blatantly deny any self-manipulation. Some habits, such as continuous hand washing or repetitive rearrangement of a desk or an entire household, are also related. This tendency seems to be intimately connected with serotonin transmission, as the agents that produce the most improvement all interfere with CNS serotonin uptake.

Clinical Findings. The spectrum of findings is broad; some patients may pick at their skin or hairs when nervous or upset, while others are totally unable to function because of their preoccupation with certain physical tasks, which are often self-destructive. To some extent, disorders such as lichen simplex chronicus and prurigo nodularis may be considered manifestations of a obsessive-compulsive disorder, as they result from repetitive manipulation. More classical examples include neurotic excoriations, trichotillomania, trichotemnomania (obsessive cutting of the hair), onychotillomania and lip licking.

Neurotic excoriations are often confused with dermatitis artifacta and there are overlaps. Patients often have a ritualized approach to picking, scratching or otherwise damaging their skin. The sites of involvement are the arms, thighs, breasts and upper outer aspects of the back. Some patients claim to identify primary fleeting pruritic lesions; others admit to damaging virgin skin. In contrast to dermatitis artifacta, instruments are almost never used, just the fingernails. Sometimes the complaints are unusual; one patient described enjoying hearing the sound of scratching. Depressed patients may also present with neurotic excoriations; they are less likely to admit to manipulating. Typically, fresh crusted lesions and scars in varying degrees of healing are seen.

Trichotillomania is common in infants and small children, where it may simply be a sign of boredom. In older children, adolescents and young women it is always associated with psychiatric disease. Typically the patient is a young woman who has a conflict with her mother; the father is not interested or involved. Invariably, the physician is confronted by a girl and an angry mother who wants to help. The clinical aspects of trichotillomania are discussed in Chap. 31. Onychotillomania is more than nail biting; patients usually use tweezers, scissors or even larger tools to pick and destroy their nails, complaining that something is under their nails. Thumb or finger sucking beyond infancy may also fit into this general category. Young lip lickers often have the atopic diathesis and sensitive perioral skin; later, they invariably bite and chew their lips, producing a dermatitis in the skin within reach.

Ordinary nail chewing and thumb sucking probably should be excluded from this category. They are quite common and usually not associated with apparent psychiatric disease. Many individuals outgrow these traits, and others use them as a harmless nervous outlet; some may chew their nails while others smoke a cigarette or pace restlessly.

Differential Diagnosis. The differential diagnosis is discussed in the various chapters dealing with these diseases. One's obligation is to exclude any primary skin disease.

Therapy. As mentioned above, various inhibitors of serotonin uptake, such as clomipramine and fluoxetine, are usually most effective. If depression is the apparent diagnosis, doxepin should be considered.

Neurologic Disorders

Any disease in which cutaneous sensation is altered may lead to inadvertent skin damage and delayed healing. Probably worldwide the best example is leprosy. We will consider just a sample of neurologic diseases with cutaneous findings.

Neurotrophic Ulcerations

Synonyms. Malum perforans, *mal perforant* (French), anesthetic ulcer, Morvan ulcer. A common but incorrect term is mal perforans, mixing the French and Latin terms.

Definition. Chronic painless ulceration that develops at a pressure point in association with neurologic disease.

Etiology and Pathogenesis. The chronic ulceration develops in skin which lacks sensation and probably other vegetative functions. Many neurologic problems can lead to sensory disturbances, including syringomyelia, congenital absence of pain, tabes dorsalis, a variety of peripheral neuropathies including those associated with leprosy, diabetes mellitus and alcoholism, peripheral nerve injuries and spinal or central defects.

Clinical Findings. Neurotrophic ulcers have certain sites of predilection. Most commonly they arise on the soles, especially over the first and fifth metatarsal heads, as well as the heel. The initial finding is usually a callus, which develops as a protective response to the inappropriate, often too steady pressure. The callused area may be relatively anhidrotic as well. As a result of the continuing pressure or even a minor injury, a thin fissure or crack appears within the callus. It enlarges, often becomes infected, undermines the callus, and develops central necrosis and then an ulcer. Thus, the ulcer is typically surrounded by callus and is painless. At the base of the ulcer, there is usually no granulation tissue and no other signs of healing. The underlying bone is at risk of osteomyelitis; osteoporosis may also be present because of the lack of appropriate pressure and use.

Differential Diagnosis. It is important to rule out vascular insufficiency and a primary ulcerated skin tumor, such as a verrucous carcinoma (carcinoma cuniculatum) or malignant melanoma, which on the sole can be amelanotic and ulcerated. The neurologic diagnosis is best left in the hands of a neurologist. One should inquire about alcohol consumption, diabetes mellitus, syphilis and neurologic problems.

Therapy. Taking weight off the ulcer is most important. In the short term, bed rest with aggressive wound care is needed. Necrotic tissue should be debrided. One should work with orthopedic surgeons to obtain special shoes that redistribute the weight to less damaged parts of the foot. Routine foot care is essential, both to monitor healing of the ulcer and later to keep the calluses trimmed to reduce the risk of recurrence. If there is no underlying vascular disease, such ulcers usually heal with this approach.

Trigeminal Neurotrophic Ulcer

Synonym. Trigeminal trophic syndrome

Definition. Neurotrophic ulceration usually involving the ala nasi secondary to anesthesia caused by trigeminal damage.

Etiology and Pathogenesis. This rare problem is usually the result of iatrogenic damage to the gasserian ganglion, as when alcohol is injected because of severe trigeminal neuralgia. Occasionally it may be associated with more peripheral damage to the trigeminal nerve, cerebral vascular disease or with neurologic diseases such as syringomyelia. Typically there is anesthesia or paresthesia in the second branch of the trigeminal nerve and the patient proceeds to create a sharply circumscribed ulcer (Fig. 25.8). Why damage in this area is so likely to cause an ulcer is unclear. Some patients have associated psychological problems.

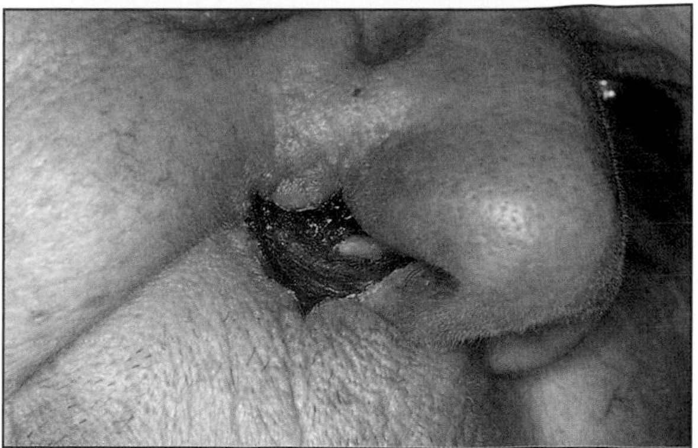

Fig. 25.8. Trigeminal neurotrophic ulcer

Clinical Findings. The German term *Nasenflügelgeschwür* (ulcer of the nasal ala) nicely describes the clinical situation. A long time may elapse between the damage to the nerve and the eventual ulceration. The patient usually admits to being disturbed by the dysesthesia or altered sensation on the cheek and nose and to manipulating the area. The ala nasi is typically erythematous, crusted and eroded. As manipulation continues, ulceration or even a full-thickness defect involving the cartilage may develop. Even with almost grotesque changes, the patient has no pain and is surprisingly tolerant of the defect. Secondary infection may occur, complicating the problem.

Differential Diagnosis. The main differential diagnosis is ulcerated destructive basal cell carcinoma or other tumor. Thus a biopsy is wise.

Therapy. If the patient has insight into their disease, convincing them to stop manipulating the area and then applying an occlusive dressing until healing has occurred is ideal. Then a plastic surgeon can usually reconstruct the ala. Some patients continue to manipulate the area, producing a chronic problem. Transcutaneous electrostimulation of the nerve has sometimes proven helpful.

Acroosteopathia Ulceromutilans Familiaris

(Thévenard 1942)

Synonyms. Hereditary sensory neuropathy type I, hereditary sensory radicular neuropathy, Thévenard syndrome

Definition. Combination of plantar neurotrophic ulcerations, acroosteolysis and sensory neuropathy, inherited in an autosomal dominant pattern.

This rare disorder is inherited in an autosomal dominant fashion but the gene defect is not known. There are defects in both the sensory and autonomic nerves. The first symptoms occur in adolescence and usually involve the hands and feet; hypohidrosis, reduced sensation, acrocyanosis and swelling of digits may be seen. Sensations of temperature, pain and light touch may all be distorted. Occasionally pyramidal tract signs such as hyperreflexia or a positive Babinski sign may be found. Neurotrophic ulcers typically develop in young adult life and remain a difficult problem. Attention to foot care is essential and special shoes must be worn. There is frequently peroneal muscle atrophy. The bones, especially those of the digits, develop osteoporosis and osteolysis, as seen on radiologic examination. Other causes of neurotrophic ulcers, as well as the entire list of hereditary sensory neuropathies, must be excluded.

The much rarer type II hereditary sensory neuropathy is inherited in an autosomal recessive pattern and begins earlier in childhood.

Acroosteopathia Ulceromutilans Nonfamiliaris

(Bureau and Barrière 1955)

Synonyms. Bureau-Barrière syndrome, neuropathic acrodystrophy

Definition. Acquired chronic polyneuropathy with neurotrophic ulcerations and acroosteolysis.

Epidemiology. Almost all patients are men who develop a peripheral stockings-and-gloves neuropathy, usually between 40 and 60 years of age.

Etiology and Pathogenesis. The key predisposing factors appear to be chronic alcoholism and diabetes mellitus. Patients are often outdoor workers, such as construction workers or vintners, who spend long hours wearing rubber boots and exposed to cold. Homeless individuals are also at risk. The best guess is that this is a peripheral neuropathy with multiple etiologic factors, including toxic damage from alcohol, vitamin deficiency and cold injury.

Clinical Findings. The clinical features include:

- Neurologic Changes. These are constant and include dysesthesia and loss of temperature sensation, usually extending to the mid-shin coupled with hyperhidrosis (in contrast to the hypohidrosis of the hereditary disorder). Both temperature changes and emotional stimuli can trigger the sweating. The Achilles and patellar reflexes are reduced to absent. Later there may be muscular atrophy associated with cramping or severe leg pain.
- Neurotrophic Ulcerations. These are identical to the changes described above (Fig. 25.9).
- Tissue Hypertrophy. The feet develop lymphedema and later elephantiasis-like changes. Secondarily there can be verrucous hyperplasia or pachyderma. Such feet are at particular risk for recurrent erysipelas with further lymphatic damage and more swelling.
- Bony Changes. The distal bones initially show osteoporosis and eventually osteolysis. The phalanges and even the distal metatarsal heads can appear as if chewed away. Spontaneous fractures and subluxations are complications. The vascular supply is normal.
- Liver. Almost all patients have alcoholic liver disease.

Differential Diagnosis. The history usually allows one to exclude hereditary sensory neuropathies, while the multiplicity of signs and symptoms separa-

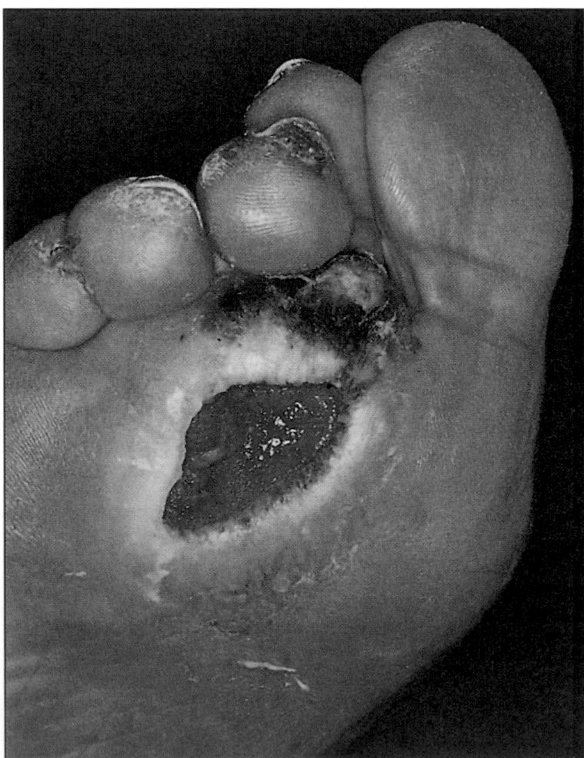

Fig. 25.9. Neurotrophic ulcer in acroosteopathia ulceromutilans nonfamiliaris

tes these cases from ordinary neurotrophic ulcers, although they may represent an extreme form of this problem.

Therapy. The approaches discussed above are important. Stopping alcohol intake, eating an adequate diet and taking vitamin supplements are all wise, but hard to accomplish. Special shoes, careful foot care and often reconstructive surgery are needed. In Germany α-liponic acid is recommended for the polyneuropathy, while quinine can be tried for the leg cramps. Both orthopedic surgeons and neurologists are usually involved in the care of such patients.

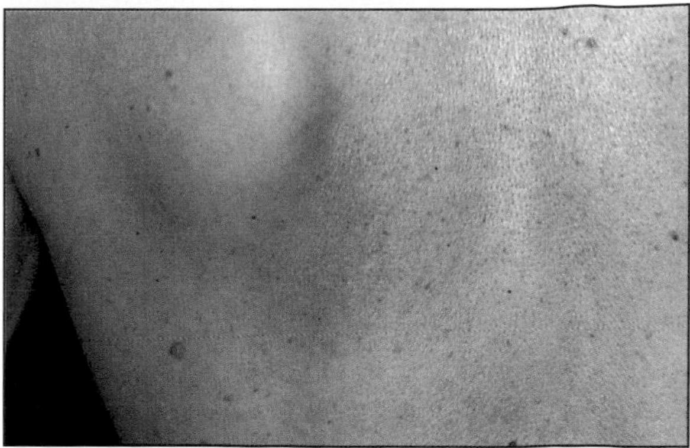

Fig. 25.10. Notalgia paresthetica

Notalgia Paresthetica

(Astwazaturow 1934)

Definition. Isolated neuropathy involving the skin over or near the scapula.

Etiology and Pathogenesis. The cause of notalgia paresthetica is unknown. There appears to be some sort of damage to thoracic nerves T2–T6 involving the posterior rami. On rare occasion, imaging studies may show impingement or other such changes, but in most cases such searches reveal nothing.

Clinical Findings. Patients usually present with a localized patch of altered sensation overlying the scapula. The problem is almost always unilateral and the patient outlines an oval area. While pruritus is the most common complaint, others may describe burning, tingling or even reduced sensation. Yet others may present not because of the neurologic findings but because of a hyperpigmented patch in the same area (Fig. 25.10). The area usually has somewhat reduced sensation when tested.

The course is unpredictable. In some patients there is spontaneous resolution; in others, the dysesthesia persists; and in a third group papular changes develop, resembling mild lichen simplex chronicus.

Histopathology. Biopsy has cast some new ideas on the nature of notalgia paresthetica. Biopsy specimens are usually obtained only when there are pigmentary changes; one sees reactive epidermal changes and incontinence of pigment. As the lesions become more thickened, amorphous deposits of macular amyloid may be seen as a secondary change. The early work on macular amyloid emphasized its frequent location near the scapula, and we suspect the two processes overlap. The amyloid is a marker for keratin and is derived from damaged keratinocytes; there is no connection with systemic amyloidosis.

Differential Diagnosis. Except for the processes already discussed, there is really no differential diagnosis.

Therapy. Topical capsaicin appears to represent a significant improvement for this problem. The commercially available 0.025 Zostrix cream can be applied four to six times daily over a period of months. Initially there is burning and even worsening, but usually improvement is seen after a week or two. Topical anesthetics, antipruritics and corticosteroids can also be tried.

Meralgia Paresthetica

Synonym. Roth (1895) – Bernhardt (1895) syndrome

The only other common local paresthesia involves the skin of the outer upper thigh. Patients usually complain of numbness or pain, and do not have skin changes. The neurology is better understood, as the lateral femoral cutaneous nerve is entrapped in the inguinal ligament. Sometimes obesity or excessively tight clothing is responsible. If not, surgical freeing of the nerve may be necessary.

Pants Paresthesia Syndrome

(Fisher 1995)

This puzzling syndrome affects primarily middle-aged men who complain of intense itching and burning when they wear certain pants. We have seen several patients; all were successful businessmen who realized the complaint sounded implausible, but were still distressed. Neurologic examination is negative. In some cases there may be an irritant or allergic contact dermatitis caused by dyes or formaldehyde, while in other instances the fabric may be mechanically irritating. In yet other cases, no logical explanation is found. Experimenting with different fabrics seems helpful, and usually a topical anesthetic cream is beneficial.

Cluster Headaches

(Bing 1930; Horton 1941)

Synonyms. Erythroprosopalgia (red facial pain), Bing-Horton syndrome

Cluster headaches are well known. They tend to come in groups, so that a patient may have a burst of five to ten headaches over a period of weeks and then be symptom free for years. Patients develop unilateral facial pain, always involving the same side, with tearing, conjunctival erythema and even rhinorrhea. They may develop redness and swelling of the eyelids and even the forehead, which can then be mistaken for erysipelas or angioedema. Treatment is best left to a nondermatologist; ergot derivatives, nonsteroidal antiinflammatory drugs, systemic high-dose corticosteroids and supplemental oxygen therapy all have their adherents. The skin findings require no attention, but the patient deserves a correct diagnosis.

Bibliography

Basic Science Aspects

Birder LA, Perl ER (1994) Cutaneous sensory receptors. J Clin Neurophysiol 11:534–552

Nakamura A, Shiomi H (1999) Recent advances in neuropharmacology of cutaneous nociceptors. Jpn J Pharmacol 79:427–431

Pruritus

Bernhard JD (ed) (1994) Itch: mechanism and mangement of pruritus. McGraw-Hill, New York

Greaves MW, Wall PD (1996) Pathophysiology of itching. Lancet 348:938–940

Hautkappe M, Roizen MF, Toledano A et al. (1998) Review of the effectiveness of capsaicin for painful cutaneous disorders and neural dysfunction. Clin J Pain 14:97–106

Jones EA, Bergasa NV (1999) The pruritus of cholestasis. Hepatology 29:1003–1006

Kam PC, Tan KH (1996) Pruritus – itching for a cause and relief? Anaesthesia 51:1133–1138

Kantor GR, Bernhard JD (1995) Investigation of the pruritic patient in daily practice. Semin Dermatol 14:290–296

Leung AK, Wong BE, Chan PY et al. (1998) Pruritus in children. J R Soc Health 118:280–286

Teofoli P, Procacci P, Maresca M et al. (1996) Itch and pain. Int J Dermatol 35:159–166

Prurigo Simplex Acuta, Prurigo Simplex Subacuta and Acne Urticata

Braun-Falco O (1961) Zur Kenntnis der Urticaria papulosa chronica. Med Welt 12:1371–1374

Clark AR, Jorizzo JL, Fleischer AB (1998) Papular dermatitis (subacute prurigo, "itchy red bump" disease): pilot study of phototherapy. J Am Acad Dermatol 38:929–933

Howard R, Frieden IJ (1996) Papular urticaria in children. Pediatr Dermatol 13:246–249

Jordaan HF, Schneider JW (1997) Papular urticaria: a histopathologic study of 30 patients. Am J Dermatopathol 19:119–126

Jorizzo J, Gatti S, Smith EB (1981) Prurigo: A clinical review. J Am Acad Dermatol 4:723–728

Kaposi M (1893) Pathologie und Therapie der Hautkrankheiten. Urban & Schwarzenberg, Wien, p 530

Salfeld K (1957) Zur Frage der Abgrenzung von Acne urticaria (Kaposi), acne excoriée des jeunes filles (Brocq) und "neurotic excoriations". Hautarzt 8:546–549

Shelnitz LS, Paller AS (1990) Hodgkin's disease manifesting as prurigo nodularis. Pediatr Dermatol 7:136–139

Streit V, Thiede R, Wiedow O et al. (1996) Foil bath PUVA in the treatment of prurigo simplex subacuta. Acta Derm Venereol 76:319–320

Prurigo Nodularis

Braun-Falco O, Marghescu S (1967) Prurigo nodularis Hyde-artige Reaktion durch Blutegelbiß. Hautarzt 18:112–115

Hann SK, Cho MY, Park Y-K (1990) UV treatment of generalized prurigo nodularis. Int J Dermatol 298:436–437

Hyde JN, Montgomery FH (1909) A practical treatise on diseases of the skin for the use of students and practioners, 8th edn. Lea and Febiger, Philadelphia, pp 174–175

Lindley RP, Rowland Payne CME (1989) Neural hyperplasia is not a diagnostic prerequisite in nodular prurigo. J Cutan Pathol 16:14–18

Mattila JO, Vornanen M, Katila ML (1997) Histopathological and bacteriological findings in prurigo nodularis. Acta Derm Venereol (Stockh) 77:49–51

Nahass GT, Penneys NS (1994) Merkel cells and prurigo nodularis. J Am Acad Dermatol 31:86–88

Rowland Payne CME, Wilkinson JD, McKee PH et al. (1985) Nodular prurigo – a clinico-pathological study of 46 patients. Br J Dermatol 113:431–439

Sheskin J (1975) Zur Therapie der Prurigo nodularis Hyde mit Thalidomid. Hautarzt 26:215

Winkelmann RK (1984) Thalidomide treatment of prurigo nodularis. Acta Derm Venereol (Stockh) 64:412–417

Zelickson BD, McEvoy MT, Fransway AF (1989) Patch testing in prurigo nodularis. Contact Dermatitis 20:321–325

Hyperkeratosis Follicularis

Harman M, Aytekin S, Akdeniz S et al. (1998) Kyrle's disease in diabetes mellitus and chronic renal failure. J Eur Acad Dermatol Venereol 11:87–88

Igarashi A, Ishibashi Y, Otsuka F et al. (1991) Disease associated with sarcoidosis and renal failure. Int J Dermatol 30:211–212
Kyrle J (1916) Über einen ungewöhnlichen Fall von universeller follikulärer und parafollikulärer Hyperkeratose (Hyperkeratosis follicullaris et parafollicularis in cutem penetrans). Arch Dermatol Syph 123:466–493
Mehegan AH, Coskey RJ (1968) Perforating folliculitis. Arch Dermatol 97:394–399

Prurigo Pigmentosa

Kobayashi T, Kawada A, Hiruma M et al. (1996) Prurigo pigmentosa, ketonemia and diabetes mellitus. Dermatology 192:78–80
Liu MT, Wong CK (1994) Prurigo pigmentosa. Dermatology 188:219–221
Nagashima M, Oshiro A, Shimizu N (1971) A peculiar pruriginous dermatosis with gross reticular pigmentation. Jap J Dermatol 81:38–39
Schepis C, Siragusa M, Palazzo R et al. (1996) V Prurigo pigmentosa treated with minocycline. Br J Dermatol 135: 158–159

Self-Induced Skin Diseases, Artifacts, Münchhausen

Antony SJ, Mannion SM (1995) Dermatitis artefacta revisited. Cutis 55:362–364
Asher (1951) Münchhausen' Syndrom. Lancet 1:339–341
Joe EK, Li VW, Magro CM et al. (1999) Diagnostic clues to dermatitis artefacta. Cutis 63:209–214
Koblenzer CS (1996) Neurotic excoriations and dermatitis artefacta. Dermatol Clin 14:447–455
Secrétan H (1901) Oédeme dur et hyperplasie traumatique du métacarpe dorsal. Rev Med Suisse Romande 21: 409–416

Psychiatric Disorders

Ekbbom K (1938) Praeseniler Dermat-zooenwahn. Acta Psychiat Scand 13:227–259
Jones MK, Whitmont S, Menzies RG (1996) Danger expectancies and insight in spider phobia. Anxiety 2:179–185
Logsdail S, Lovell K, Warwick H et al. (1991) Behavioural treatment of AIDS-focused illness phobia. Br J Psychiatry 159:422–425
Allan SJ, Doherty VR (1995) "Naevophobia". Clin Exp Dermatol 20:499–501

Acroosteopathia Ulceromutilans Familiaris and Nonfamiliaris

Bureau Y, Barrière H (1955) Acropathies pseudosyringomyeliques des membres inferieur. Sem Hôp (Paris) 31: 1419–1429
Thévenard A (1942) L' arcopathie ulcero-mutilante familaris. Rev Neurol (Paris) 74:193–212
Vanhooteghem O, Lateur N, Hautecoeur P et al. (1999) Acropathia ulcero-mutilans acquisita of the upper limbs. Br J Dermatol 140:334–337

Notalgia Paresthetica

Astwazaturow M (1934) Über parästhetische Neuralgien und eine besondere Form der selben – Notalgia paresthetica. Dtsch Z Nervenheilkd 133:188–196 (in German)
Eisenberg E, Barmeir E, Bergman R (1997) Notalgia paresthetica associated with nerve root impingement. J Am Acad Dermatol 37:998–1000
Goulden V, Toomey PJ, Highet AS (1998) Successful treatment of notalgia paresthetica with a paravertebral local anesthetic block. J Am Acad Dermatol 38(1):114–116
Massey EW (1998) Sensory mononeuropathies. Semin Neurol 18:177–183
Wallengren J, Klinker M (1995) Successful treatment of notalgia paresthetica with topical capsaicin: vehicle-controlled, double-blind, crossover study. J Am Acad Dermatol 32:287–289

Meralgia Paresthetica

Bernhardt M (1895) Über isoliert im Gebiete des N. cutaneus femoris externus vorkommende Paresthesien. Neurol Zbl 14:242–244
Roth WK (1895) Meralgia paresthetica. Karger, Berlin
Shelley WB, Shelley ED (1998) Aquadynia: noradrenergic pain induced by bathing and responsive to clonidine. J Am Acad Dermatol 38:357–358
Wiezer MJ, Franssen H, Rinkel GJ et al. (1996) Meralgia paraesthetica: differential diagnosis and follow-up. Muscle Nerve 19:522–524
Williams PH, Trzil KP (1991) Management of meralgia paresthetica. J Neurosurg 74:76–80

Pants Paresthesia Syndrome

Allen DI (1994) Tight pants syndrome. JAMA 271:1628
Fisher AA (1995) Contactants that produce pruritus and paresthesia with invisible reactions. Cutis 55:269
Fisher AA (1996) The pants paresthesia syndrome: a ten-year follow-up. Cutis 58:199–200
Giele HP (1995) The wonderbra syndrome. Plast Reconstr Surg 96:503

Cluster Headaches

Bing R (1930) Über Erythromelalgie und Erythroprosopalgie. Nervenarzt 3:506–512
Horton BT (1941) The use of histamine in the treatment of specific types of headaches. JAMA 116:377–383
Manzoni GC (1999) Cluster headache and lifestyle: remarks on a population of 374 male patients. Cephalalgia 19: 88–94
Mathew NT (1997) Cluster headache. Semin Neurol 17:313–323

CHAPTER 26

Disorders of Melanin Pigmentation

Contents

Basic Science Aspects

Melanin is the most important determinant of skin color. The type of melanin and how it is packaged in melanosomes and transferred to keratinocytes determines one's skin color. Other factors influencing skin color include the relative amounts of oxidized and reduced hemoglobin and the presence of carotenoids. Melanin provides the main protection against ultraviolet radiation. Thus, individuals with defects in melanin production, such as albinos, are at risk for marked sun-induced skin damage and tumor induction, especially if they live in countries with long hours of sunlight. In contrast, dark skin is relatively resistant to damage by chronic sunlight exposure. The only obvious disadvantage that such individuals have is impaired vitamin D synthesis when light levels are low. Evolutionists have argued for generations whether dark skin evolved as an advantage for those in the tropics or whether lighter skin evolved as an advantage for those further north who otherwise would have been ravaged by rickets. Another possible advantage of melanin is its effectiveness as a free-radical scavenger, perhaps helping protect against cell damage in a second way in addition to blocking light.

Melanocytes

Melanocytes are the cells in the epidermis that manufacture melanin. They are spaced between the basal keratinocytes; in routine sections about every tenth basal cell is a melanocyte (Fig. 26.1). The melanocyte is a clear dendritic cell, transferring packaged melanin in melanosomes to adjacent keratinocytes (Fig. 26.2). It has been estimated that every melanocyte is connected with about 36 keratinocytes, forming the epidermal melanin unit. Melanocytes are clear in routine sections because their cytoplasm shrinks.

The cutaneous melanocytes arise from the embryologic neural tube. As the neural tube closes, a group of cells migrate dorsolaterally, forming the neural crest. They are the precursors of many tissue elements, including peripheral neurons, Schwann cells, glial cells, a variety of skeletal and connective tissue components and the melanocytes of the skin, uveal tract, inner ear and leptomeninges. The melanocytes of the retina evolve from an outpouching of the primitive forebrain known as the neural endoderm. These primitive melanocytes are known as melanoblasts. The control of melanocyte migration is poorly understood, but one important signaling pathway involves the c-*kit* protooncogene, a tyrosine kinase receptor that binds to a hematopoetic growth factor. All melanocytes have tyrosinase and manufacture melanin, but only the cutaneous melanocytes are normally capable of transferring melanin to other cells; Masson called them "secretory melanocytes" for this reason. They reach the skin and hair follicle in about the third fetal month. While the basal layer melanocytes are a relatively stable population normally, the hair follicle melanocytes have a cyclic profile, increasing in number and activity as new anagen hairs are induced by the interaction between the hair matrix and the dermal papillae. Many pigmentary disorders involve both skin and hair melanocytes, but in some situations only one population is affected.

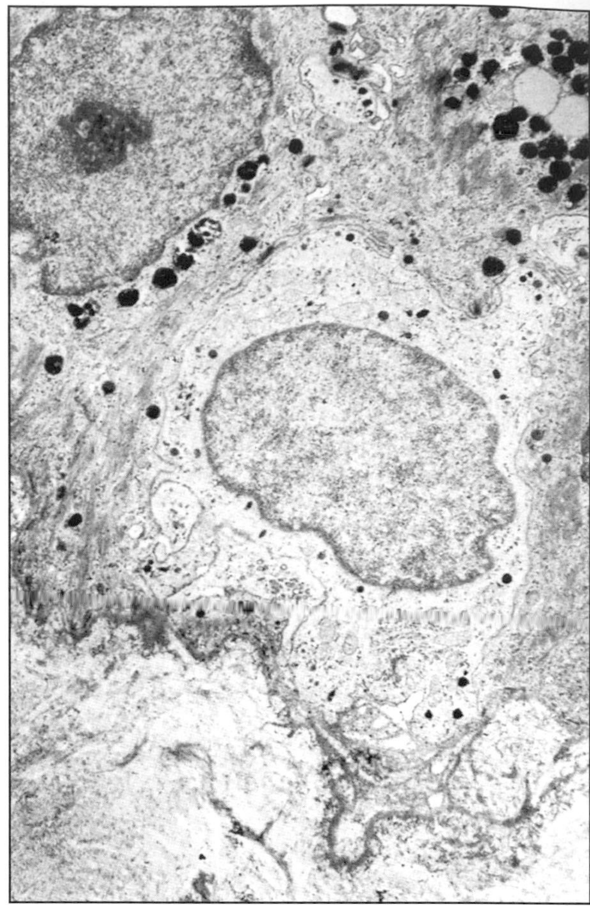

Fig. 26.2. Electron microscopy showing a melanocyte between two keratinocytes. The dense bodies in the keratinocytes are melanosomes that have been transferred (× 8200)

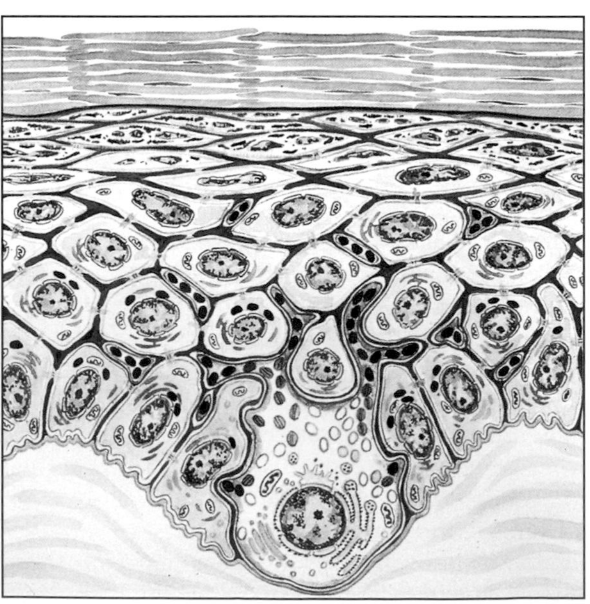

Fig. 26.1. Central clear dendritic melanocytic in close proximity to many keratinocytes with transfer of melanosomes

There are surprisingly few racial or sexual differences in distribution of melanocytes. The activity of the melanocytes, the nature of the melanosomes and the efficiency of the transfer determine the color differences. The number of melanocytes per square millimeter of skin varies greatly from site to site. The face and genital region have the highest numbers, estimated at around 1100–1300 melanocytes/mm^2. The number of melanocytes increases in chronically light exposed skin but decreases with age.

Melanocytes are highly dendritic cells, although this is hard to appreciate in ordinary sections. Occasionally the section will by chance show a pigmented dendrite or two. When the epidermis is separated from the dermis and then stained with the DOPA method developed by Bloch in the 1920s, the true dendritic nature of the melanocyte is better appreciated. The melanocyte can be viewed as a unicellular gland, since its purpose in life is the manufacture and secretion of melanin.

Electron microscopy reveals a large clear cell without tonofilaments and without desmosomal contacts to adjacent cells. There are, however, structures resembling the hemidesmosomes of keratinocytes by which they are attached to the lamina densa. As with all secretory cells, there is a prominent endoplasmic reticulum and Golgi apparatus. Tyrosinase and other enzymes are formed in the rough endoplasmic reticulum and transferred to tiny vesicles, known as melanosomes. These organelles are divided into four stages, as shown in Table 26.1 Thus stage I and II melanosomes are found only in melanocytes, while stage III and IV can be found in a variety of cells, but mainly keratinocytes. The melanosomes migrate to the ends of the dendrites, which are motile because of 100-Å cytofilaments. These fine pigment-laden cell extensions insinuate between keratinocytes, where they are clipped off by the keratinocytes transferring the pigment.

Table 26.1. Types of melanosomes

Stage	Features
I	Spherical, tyrosinase positive, but no melanin
II	Oval, containing filaments with 7 mm periodicity
III	Contain melanin but internal structure still visible
IV	Full of melanin, electron-dense or opaque

Melanin Production

The biochemistry of melanin production is centered around the enzyme tyrosinase, but is extremely complex and not well understood. The key amino acid in melanin production is tyrosine or hydroxyphenylalanine. In melanosomes tyrosine is converted to DOPA (dihydroxyphenylalanine) and then oxidized to DOPA-quinone. Bloch's reaction adds DOPA to sheets of skin where rapid oxidation produces brown DOPA-quinone, an unequivocal way to identify melanocytes and their dendrites. Tyrosinase, a copper-containing enzyme encoded on chromosome 11q14–21, is required for these first two steps but also apparently plays a regulatory role for the rest of the process, along with other enzymes and a variety of cofactors such as metal ions. Levels of tyrosinase mRNA and enzyme are about the same in black and white skin.

The pathway for the final production of melanin is known as the Raper-Mason pathway, but it is considerably more complex than originally suggested by these scientists. At the level of DOPA-quinone, the process diverges. Several enzymes form a series of bicyclic products including leukoDOPAchrome (cycloDOPA); DOPAchrome; 5,6-dihydroxyindole; and indole-5,6-quinone. A tautomerase reaction produces similar molecules but with carboxylic acid attached. These products polymerize to form eumelanins. The pheomelanins and trichromes are formed by adding glutathione or cysteine to DOPA-quinone through a variety of polymerization steps. Thus there are three types of melanin in human skin:

- Eumelanins: dark brown or black, cyclic, insoluble.
- Pheomelanins: red, yellow, contain sulfur, not cyclic, soluble in alkali solutions.
- Trichromes: intensive red, rich in sulfur, otherwise similar to pheomelanin.

The eumelanins are responsible for dark-colored hair, while pheomelanins are found in blond and red hair, where trichromes are also prominent. In the skin, there is usually a mixture but clearly darker skinned individuals have predominantly eumelanin.

Melanosomes and Skin Color

The arrangement of melanosomes within the keratinocytes is different in black and white skin. A keratinocyte in a black may contain 400 melanosomes, while that in a white might have only 100. In whites, Orientals and American Indians, the melanosomes are about 0.6 × 0.3 µm in size and often complexed together. In blacks and Australian Aborigines, they are much larger, about 1.2 × 0.6 µm, and lie singly rather than in complexes. In whites the melanosomes already begin to undergo degradation in the lower layers of the epidermis, while in blacks melanosomes are found in all epidermal layers, including the stratum corneum. The melanosomes in hairs are generally much larger than in the skin.

Regulation of Pigmentation

Both the basic skin and hair colors and the tendency to tan or darken with light exposure are inherited characteristics. The skin or hair color is determined primarily by the color, size, quantity and distribution of the melanosomes. The major factor changing one's basic color is sun exposure. Two types of darkening occur:

- Immediate pigmentation. Exposure to UVA produces darkening over a matter of minutes to hours as immature forms of melanin are oxidized, becoming darker, and melanosomes are moved rapidly to the ends of the dendrites for transfer (Meirowsky phenomenon).
- Late pigmentation. UVB light produces elevated tyrosinase levels, increased number of melanosomes containing more melanin and increased transfer to keratinocytes. This takes days to weeks. In addition, there is also an increase in the number of functioning melanocytes when sunlight or UV radiation exposure is more chronic.

The degree to which an individual responds to light with tanning has been subdivided into the six skin types as popularized by Fitzpatrick (1975). This entire topic is explored further in Chapter 13.

There are other factors that also control pigment. Lerner, a dermatologist, and Takahashi (1956) discovered melanocyte-stimulating hormone (MSH), a pituitary hormone which, in a variety of vertebrate models, plays a key role in regulating melanin production (Chap. 48). Both α- and β-MSH have been identified; neither is produced in humans in quantities sufficient to play a significant role. ACTH and β-lipotropin are other pituitary hormones that also potentially can influence pigmentation. There are structural similarities between MSH and ACTH, so that the hyperpigmentation seen in Addison's disease may be secondary to excessive MSH or MSH-like activity. In tissue culture experiments, human melanocytes become more dendritic and darker under the stimulation of MSH. The placenta and fetal pituitary also secrete MSH, which certainly plays a role in the development of the pigmentary system and may be responsible for some of the pigmentary changes seen in pregnancy such as melasma and darkening of melanocytic nevi. Estrogens also appear to be significant, as melasma is almost limited to women, but also requires sun exposure and often elevated hormonal levels. The areolae, the linea alba and genitalia may darken in pregnancy (Chap. 36).

Pigmentation is stimulated by various growth factors secreted by keratinocytes in response to UV radiation damage. Examples include GM-CSF, nitric oxide and many others. Another strong stimulus is the presence of small DNA fragments, especially thymidine dinucleotides, which are released during the DNA repair process.

Finally melatonin, a pineal gland hormone that is active in regulating skin color in many lower vertebrates, probably plays no role in human pigmentation. Currently it is widely used in attempts to regulate the sleep cycle in international travelers.

Clinical Correlations

As this all too brief overview makes clear, there are many places where things can go wrong in the pigmentation process. One can divide the disorders of melanin pigmentation in a number of ways:

- Increased or decreased pigment. When the skin is darker, one speaks of hyperpigmentation. Lighter patches reflect hypopigmentation, while totally white patches with no melanin at all represent amelanosis (melanin was never present) or depigmentation (melanin has been destroyed).
- Localized or diffuse changes. Many of the localized forms of hyperpigmentation are considered in Chapter 58, since they enter into the differential diagnosis of melanocytic nevi. They involve a focal increase in melanocytes or focal overproduction of melanin. Diffuse changes reflect systemic processes and are considered below.
- Congenital or acquired disorders. Pigmentary changes caused by enzymatic defects are almost invariably genetic in nature, while other forms of both hypo- and hyperpigmentation may be congenital. Other processes, such as melasma, are almost always acquired.

Localized Hyperpigmentation

Melasma

Synonyms. Chloasma, mask of pregnancy

Definition. Localized facial hyperpigmentation seen primarily in women, triggered by sunlight and hormonal changes.

Epidemiology. Melasma is a very common problem, especially among native populations in Latin America living at high altitudes. In some villages in Guatemala, the prevalence has been estimated at over 80 % in adult women.

Etiology and Pathogenesis. The three main factors in the development of melasma are female hormones, sunlight and genetic predisposition. Melasma is one of the physiologic forms of hyperpigmentation in pregnancy; while it usually resolves to some extent after delivery, some traces remain. Similarly, about 10–20 % of women taking oral contraceptives develop melasma, which may also be a marker for other causes of elevated estrogen levels such as secreting tumors.

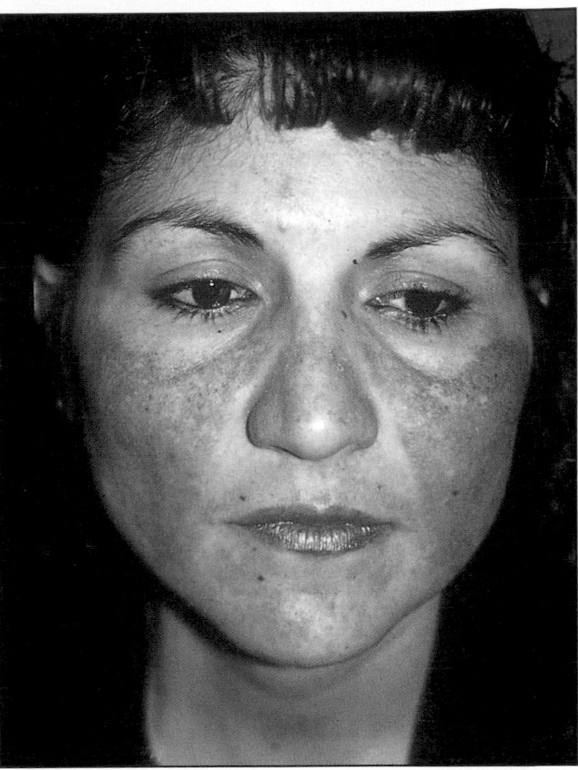

Fig. 26.3. Melasma in a Hispanic patient (courtesy of Juan J. Ochoa, MD, Chihuahua, Mexico)

Clinical Findings. Melasma is an irregular hyperpigmentation mostly confined to the face or neck of women (Fig. 26.3). The typical locations are the forehead, temples, cheeks and upper lip. The color ranges from yellow-tan to brown but may occasionally have a bluish hue. Initially small bizarre patches are present but they tend to darken, enlarge and blend together with time. This produces a mask-like effect. The lesions increase in size and number and darken with sun exposure.

Histopathology. Biopsy is not needed for the diagnosis, but examination of the specimen shows increased melanin in the basal layer keratinocytes and incontinence of pigment. The presence of increased melanin in the epidermis provides a rationale for treatment with bleaching agents.

Differential Diagnosis. Melasma-like hyperpigmentation may be produced by a chronic phototoxic reaction to cosmetics. This blends into the picture of melanosis perioralis et peribuccalis of Brocq. Men may also be affected; phototoxic reactions to after-shave lotions are usually responsible. Some systemic medications, most notably phenytoin and chlorpromazine, may produce photosensitivity and later facial hyperpigmentation that mimics melasma. Finally, some terminally ill patients with cachexia develop unexplained facial darkening.

Therapy. The best treatment is avoidance of further sun exposure and use of sun-blocking agents. This usually allows the melasma to regress somewhat, as it typically does over the winter in northern areas. The only effective bleach is hydroquinone, which is available in 2 % formulations over the counter in the USA and as 3–4 % preparations on prescription. It can be combined with a sunscreen (for example, the Solaquin products in the USA). The Kligman formula, containing hydroquinone, tretinoin and a low-potency corticosteroid, can be mixed or obtained commercially in some countries. It is available as Pigmanorm from Widmer in Europe. One word of caution: Even higher concentrations of hydroquinone creams are available in other countries, ranging up to 8–10 %. These creams are designed to bleach normal black skin and are too strong. They may lead to exogenous ochronosis. In addition, both tretinoin and azelaic acid have bleaching action and can also be tried as single agents. Finally, camouflage cosmetics are often the best solution, simply disguising the darkened areas.

Secondary Hyperpigmentation

Definition. Hyperpigmentation following the action of exogenous factors on the skin.

Etiology and Pathogenesis. Secondary hyperpigmentation is the result of two main mechanisms. It may be caused by an increased number of melanocytes and/or increased production of melanin with increased transfer to keratinocytes. This produces a brown hyperpigmentation, which is more likely to be spontaneously reversible and also more easily bleached. The second pathway is the deposition of melanin in the dermal melanophages. This produces a blue-gray color and is more permanent. As many of the examples below show, both types of hyperpigmentation may develop with the same stimulus.

Clinical Findings. There are many different types of secondary hyperpigmentation, which are clinically best divided on the basis of the triggering mechanism.

- Mechanical Hyperpigmentation. Chronic mechanical irritation produces darkening of the skin in many settings. Both overproduction of melanin by irritated melanocytes and incontinence of pigment secondary to trauma are factors. For example, hyperpigmentation may be seen at the belt line, under brassiere straps, suspenders or knapsack (backpack) straps. In addition, the groin, axilla and neck may be hyperpigmented in overweight individuals, presumably from the chronic rubbing of skin against skin, as well as from garments. Finally, pruritic dermatoses often lead to scratching, damage to the epidermal-dermal junction and then patchy postinflammatory hyperpigmentation.
- Thermal Hyperpigmentation. Infrared irradiation and exposure to heat may cause erythema and then hyperpigmentation. Erythema ab igne is discussed in more detail below.
- Actinic Hyperpigmentation. Tanning is the result of solar stimulation of melanin production and transfer; it is well known and totally reversible. In addition, ionizing radiation may also stimulate increased melanin production. Chronic actinic hyperpigmentation is most common on the sides of the neck. The correct term for this change is erythrosis interfollicularis colli or erythromelanosis colli, although in America it is often erroneously called poikiloderma of Civatte. Typically there are white macules around the follicles while the skin in between is hyperpigmented and telangiectatic. The changes are prominent on the lateral aspect of the neck and spare the submental region.
- Chemical Hyperpigmentation. Toxic chemical agents that damage the epidermis may produce hyperpigmented residual lesions. The best example is contact with the World War I chemical agents, sulfur mustard and nitrogen mustard. Soldiers who were sprayed with the chemical or contacted it on the ground developed massive edema and blisters that healed with hyperpigmentation. Today nitrogen mustard is a chemotherapeutic agent; both patients and nurses may develop irritation and later hyperpigmentation if they handle the drug. Phototoxic reactions involving the furocoumarins also producing darkening. The classic example is the use of psoralens for a more rapid tan, as they stimulate melanogenesis. Similar, in PUVA therapy, the patient always becomes tanned. Topical use of furocoumarins can also produce a tan, or, if it elicits a more intense inflammatory response, then incontinence of pigment. Two diseases caused by topical exposure to furocoumarins are meadow dermatitis (in German, *Wiesengräserdermatitis*) as natural meadows contain a variety of photosensitizing grasses, and berloque dermatitis, when photosensitizing furocoumarins are employed in cosmetics.
- Postinflammatory Hyperpigmentation. This is the waste basket, suggesting that any process that causes inflammation at the epidermal-dermal junction can lead to hyperpigmentation. Many different dermatoses can be involved. Typical examples include lichen planus, psoriasis, lupus erythematosus, atopic dermatitis, lichen simplex chronicus and some forms of urticaria. In such situations the inflammation may stimulate melanin production. In other instances, the source of the hyperpigmentation is clearly incontinence of pigment. For example, the scars of zoster are often darker. An even better example is the fixed drug reaction, which is recognized by its gray-brown or gray-blue color and by the microscopic presence of dermal melanophages.

Histopathology. Biopsy sections usually show deposition of melanin in dermal macrophages (melanophages). In some cases, there may be increased melanin in the basal layer keratinocytes.

Differential Diagnosis. The different causes discussed above must be considered. There is a long list of unusual forms of localized hyperpigmentation, considered below.

Therapy. To whatever extent the hyperpigmentation is epidermal, bleaching agents may bc tried, as discussed under melasma. Dermal hypopigmentation improves with time if the triggering agents are removed, but bleaching agents are usually futile.

Erythema ab Igne

Synonym. Livedo reticularis e calore

Definition. Chronic reticulated erythema caused by exposure to infrared radiation.

Etiology and Pathogenesis. There are many different causes of erythema ab igne. Classically it was described on the shins and inner aspects of the thighs of women who sat in front of open fires or room stoves. Chronic use of a hot water bottle or electric heating pad produces the same changes; erythema ab igne of the abdomen has been touted as a sign of chronic pancreatitis for this reason, but it is not specific. Some occupations with marked heat exposure, such as bakers, foundry workers, and blacksmiths are also predisposed to the condition. In the Orient, erythema ab igne has been described in Chinese sleeping on beds of hot bricks, Indians holding pots of hot coals on the skin and Japanese who used pocket heaters (similar to the old Jon-E hand warmer in the USA).

Clinical Findings. The most striking change is a reticulate erythema which evolves into a reticulate hyperpigmentation (Fig. 26.4). When the hyperpigmentation predominates, one speaks in Europe of heat melanosis. The changes are relatively permanent. The patients do not have a history of cold intolerance.

Histopathology. The microscopic changes include epidermal atrophy, incontinence of pigment, and an lichenoid dermal infiltrate. Thus the lesion may be confused with lupus erythematosus. There is usually marked dermal elastosis and there may be a variety of changes in the keratinocytes ranging from mild atypia to squamous cell carcinoma.

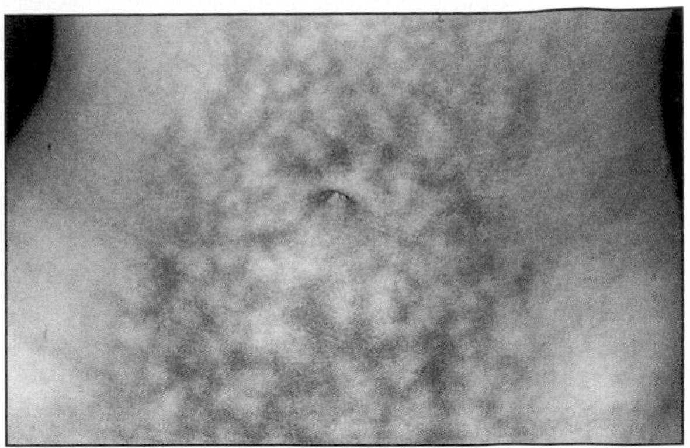

Fig. 26.4. Erythema ab igne from an electric heating pad

Course and Prognosis. Erythema ab igne is a precancerous condition. In India, the ulcers developing within the reticulated erythema are known as kangri sores or kangri ulcers and represent squamous cell carcinoma. Isolated reports of such changes in Western patients also exist.

Differential Diagnosis. The main consideration is livedo reticularis which is transitory and lacks pigmentary changes.

Therapy. No therapy is available. By stopping the heat exposure, progression can be halted. The area should be monitored for the rare development of a squamous cell carcinoma.

Localized Hyperpigmentation of the Face and Neck

There are a series of closely related facial dermatoses that we consider equivalent. All are phototoxic reactions to cosmetics, soaps, other skin care products or industrial chemicals such as tars and oils. We will describe them as separate disorders primarily for historical interest. All enter into the differential diagnosis of melasma.

Periocular Hyperpigmentation

Brunettes are particularly likely to develop brown to brown-black periorbital hyperpigmentation. Brocq described this as *masque biliaire*, suggesting incorrectly that it was a marker for biliary disease. Sometimes patients are described as having "raccoon eyes". They complain of continually being told that they look tired or unhealthy. Occasionally families are identified with this problem. When the hyperpigmentation is most prominent in the medial corner of the eye and the medial aspects of the lids, one should think of Jellinek sign for hyperthyroidism and run the appropriate tests. There is no effective treatment.

Riehl Melanosis

(Riehl 1917)

Riehl described a facial hyperpigmentation in Vienna during World War I and attributed it to improper nutrition. This explanation was clearly incorrect; today Riehl melanosis is either ignored as a disease or lumped together with melanodermitis toxica as a pigmented photocontact dermatitis. We have chosen the latter course.

Melanodermitis Toxica

(Hoffmann and Habermann 1918)

Definition. Postinflammatory hyperpigmentation caused by the topical application of photosensitizing agents and subsequent light exposure.

Etiology and Pathogenesis. Patients who use cosmetics with photosensitizing ingredients, such as members of the coumarin family, develop inflammation and then hyperpigmentation. Similarly, tar products have been incriminated, as has carbolated petrolatum. In addition, industrial exposure to cutting oils that splatter or are rubbed on the face may also produce hyperpigmentation.

Clinical Findings. The cheeks, chin, side of the neck and sometimes the V of the chest are initially inflamed, but this erythema is usually subtle and not even noticed. The postinflammatory reaction is far out of proportion to the insult, yielding diffuse brown-violet patches. The hyperpigmentation is relatively permanent.

Histopathology. The main sign is pronounced incontinence of pigment, with melanin both free and in melanophages in the upper dermis. There may be minimal signs of inflammation such as lymphohistiocytic perivascular infiltrates or minimal spongiosis.

Therapy. Avoidance of the causative agents is the best approach. While bleaching can be tried, as in melasma, it is less effective because the pigment is deeper and epidermal melanin is not increased.

Poikilodermie Réticulée Pigmentaire du Visage et du Cou

(Civatte 1923)

Civatte described an unusual reaction that he felt was caused by a photocontact reaction (melanodermitis toxica) or hormones (melasma). He attached the tongue-twister of a name given above – reticulated pigmented poikiloderma of the face and neck. The key word is "reticulated". Most often the reticulated pattern reflects photodamage, although rarely both photocontact dermatitis and melasma may show such features. Today the diagnosis is no longer made.

Melanosis Perioralis et Peribuccalis

(Brocq 1923)

Synonyms. Peribuccal pigmentation of Brocq, erythrose péribuccale pigmentaire Brocq

Etiology and Pathogenesis. Once again, most patients probably have a photocontact dermatitis. In others, the disorder resembles perioral dermatitis and may reflect a postinflammatory stage of this disorder.

Clinical Findings. Most patients are middle-aged women, although occasionally men are involved. Initially red-brown patches appear around the mouth and spread irregularly in a peripheral fashion, involving the chin and upper lip (Fig. 26.5). Sometimes initially tiny papules are present, and the typical white perioral sparing of perioral der-

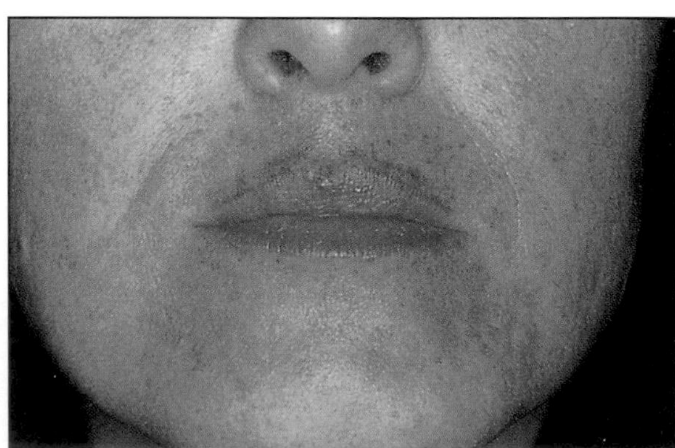

Fig. 26.5. Melanosis perioralis

matitis may be seen. The cheeks and even temples can be involved. Later the lesions usually acquire gray-black tones. The hyperpigmentation is relatively permanent.

Histopathology. Usually just postinflammatory hyperpigmentation is present. On occasion, granulomatous inflammation may be seen.

Therapy. Bleaching regimens are doomed to failure, given that these patients are very sensitive to irritation. In early cases, particularly if there is a hint of perioral dermatitis, it is worth employing the antibiotic therapy so effective in this disorder.

Incontinentia Pigmenti

(BLOCH 1926; SULZBERGER 1928)

Synonym. Bloch-Sulzberger syndrome

Definition. Uncommon genodermatosis with prominent skin involvement but also typically ocular, skeletal and CNS defects.

Epidemiology. Incontinentia pigmenti is a very rare disorder. Over 97 % of the reported cases of involve girls and women. Men with the disease may have Klinefelter syndrome or may be mosaics.

Etiology and Pathogenesis. This X-linked dominant disorder is caused by a mutation on chromosome Xp11.21, but the gene's function is unknown. X-linked dominant disorders are usually fatal in males, so primarily females are affected.

Clinical Findings

Cutaneous Findings. The skin findings in incontinentia pigmenti are traditionally divided into three phases, although there are actually four stages that overlap.

Vesicular Stage. In utero or in the first weeks of life, inflammatory lesions are present. The hallmark is vesicles and bullae arranged in a linear fashion following the lines of Blaschko; on biopsy, the blisters are rich in eosinophils. The lesions may appear pustular. Erythematous macules may also be present. The inflammatory lesions are usually short-lived and resolve spontaneously (Fig. 26.6).

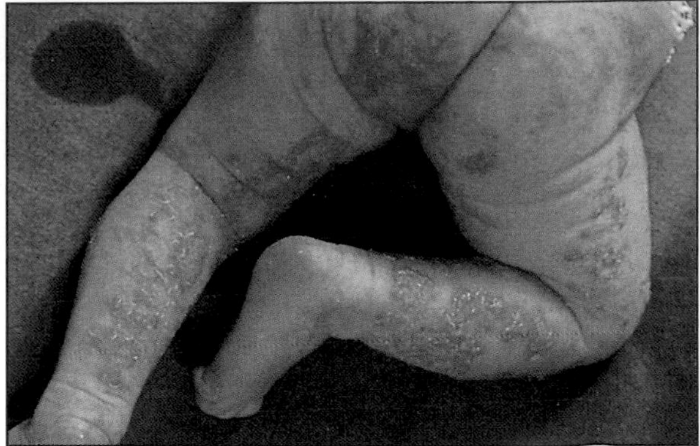

Fig. 26.6. Incontinentia pigmenti, bullous stage

Verrucous Stage. These same lesions tend to evolve into linear hyperkeratotic papules and nodules resembling verrucae. The extremities are most often involved. A particularly typical sign is an elongated "wart" running the length of the palm or sole. At the same time, lichenoid papules may be present. These lesions typically appear between the 2nd and 6th weeks of life and last for a period of weeks or months.

Hyperpigmented Stage. While lesions in the verrucous stage seem to evolve from inflammatory lesions, the classic hyperpigmented lesions are most common on the trunk and usually have no clear precursors. Presumably the intense inflammation in the early stages leads to postinflammatory hyperpigmentation, even in areas where the inflammation has not been clinically prominent. The blue-gray lesions are marbled, showing whorls and swirls once again along lines of Blaschko. They have been compared to Chinese letters (Fig. 26.7). This hyperpigmentation is relatively permanent.

Hypopigmented Scarring Stage. Many adult patients with incontinentia pigmenti have hypopigmented scars, especially on the legs. Typically they do not sweat in these regions, and they may have noticed this themselves. On occasion, this will be the only stigma in a mother of a child with obvious incontinentia pigmenti. Related findings include scarring alopecia and nail dystrophies. Sweat testing with starch-iodide or other methods is an elegant way to demonstrate this defect.

Systemic Findings. At least 50 % of the patients have abnormalities in other organ systems. Most common is dental involvement, with conical or peg teeth or absence of some adult teeth. A wide variety

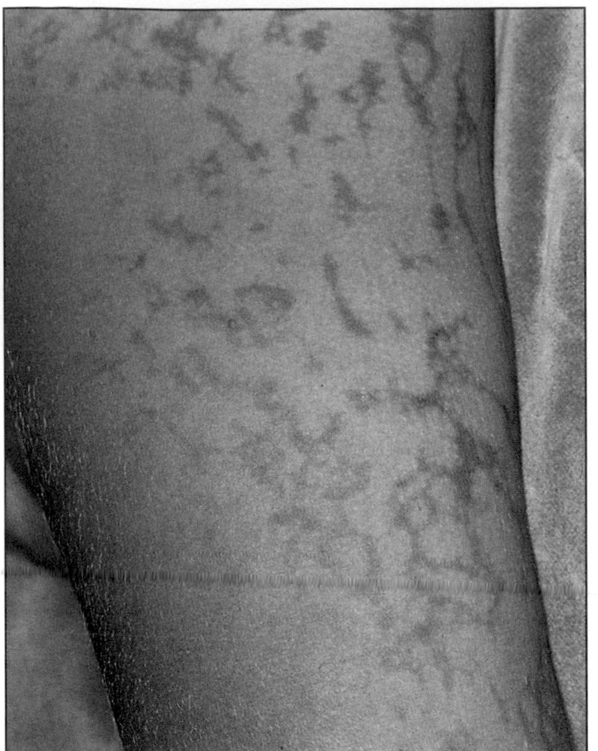

Fig. 26.7. Incontinentia pigmenti, hyperpigmentation

of ocular (optic atrophy, uveitis, strabismus, cataracts, retrolental masses such as pseudogliomas, retinal vascular disease) and CNS (mental retardation, seizures, spastic paralysis) problems may occur. The skeletal abnormalities so common in other X-linked dominant disorders are uncommon, as are congenital cardiac defects.

Histopathology. Skin biopsy may be very effective in aiding the diagnosis. The inflammatory lesions show either an eosinophil-rich dermatitis or a spongiotic blister laden with eosinophils. Dyskeratotic cells may be present, but they are more common in the hyperkeratotic stage. The hyperpigmented lesions show melanin and melanophages in the papillary dermis; the melanocytes are normal. The hypopigmented lesions are typical scars with dermal fibrosis and reduced to absent adnexal structures.

Laboratory Findings. Infants may have peripheral eosinophilia; values as high as 50 % of the total neutrophil count have been described.

Course and Prognosis. The key factors are the ocular and CNS problems. Most older children and adults are not troubled by their skin changes.

Differential Diagnosis. Not surprisingly, the differential diagnosis varies with the stage. The infants evoke the entire spectrum of neonatal blistering and pustular disorders, including congenital infections (TORCH), neonatal herpes simplex virus infections, staphylococcal infections and some of the variants of epidermolysis bullosa, as well as epidermolytic hyperkeratosis. The childhood blistering diseases, such as linear IgA disease, are not typically present at birth. Scabies in infants may have eosinophilic blisters and nodular lesions, but once again is uncommon in the first month of life. The hyperpigmented lesions are relatively specific, especially when coupled with a history of the pre-existing lesions. Surprisingly, incontinentia pigmenti achromians (hypomelanosis of Ito) sometimes enters the picture, as it is difficult, particularly in dark-skinned patients, to decide what is abnormal – the light or the dark areas.

Therapy. The inflammatory lesions, particular if denuded, should be treated with standard wound care to avoid secondary infections. There is no effective treatment for the other stages. Genetic counseling should be offered, although in our experience few women decide not to have children because of their disease.

Erythema Dyschromicum Perstans

(Ramirez 1957; Convit et al. 1961)

Synonyms. Ashy dermatosis, *los cenicientos*

Definition. Uncommon disorder with hyperpigmented blue-gray patches, usually on the back; almost exclusively limited to Hispanics.

Epidemiology. Erythema dyschromicum perstans is very uncommon. Even in Mexico, there is marked regional variation, as it is uncommon in the northern part of the country.

Etiology and Pathogenesis. The cause of erythema dyschromicum perstans is unknown. It occurs almost exclusively among Latin Americans, and debate has continued for 40 years whether it is a primary inflammatory dermatosis with a distinctive postinflammatory stage or whether it represents the end stage of a variety of diseases, including lichen planus pigmentosus.

Clinical Findings. In its early stages, erythema dyschromicum perstans is characterized by blue-

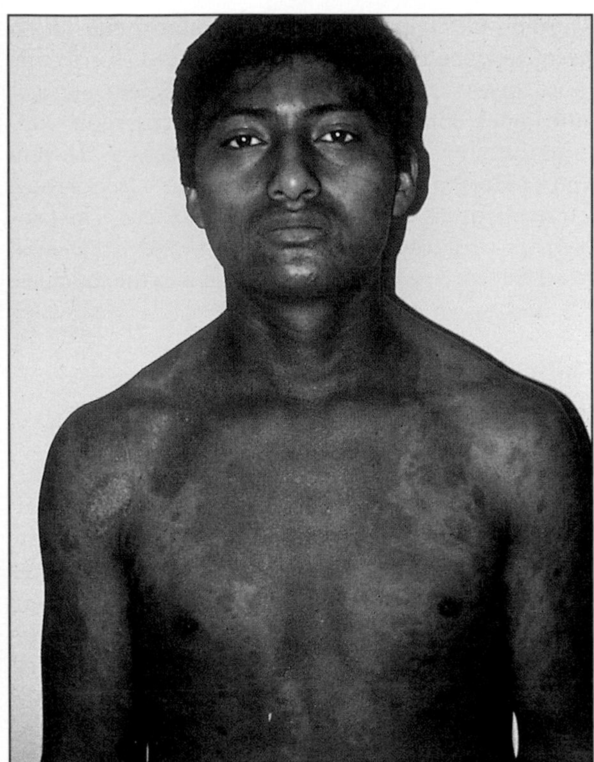

Fig. 26.8. Erythema dyschromicum perstans (courtesy of Juan J. Ochoa, MD, Chihuahua, Mexico)

gray macules and patches with an erythematous border. Papules, so common in lichen planus, are not seen. The back is the most common site of involvement, although the face, neck, chest and even arms may also be affected. Since the lesions are asymptomatic, few patients consult a physician in this alleged acute stage. Later on the lesions are flat, blue-gray or ashy patches with indistinct borders (Fig. 26.8). The lesions are relatively permanent, although new ones may develop over the years.

Histopathology. When the border of an active lesion is biopsied, there is an interface dermatitis with vacuolar change in the basal layer keratinocytes and necrosis. In the upper dermis a lymphocytic perivascular infiltrate is present; the lichenoid band of lichen planus is uncommon. Later lesions are dominated by incontinence of pigment with prominent melanophages.

Course and Prognosis. The hyperpigmentation is persistent.

Differential Diagnosis. All the causes of localized hyperpigmentation must be considered. Individual lesions most closely resemble the terminal stages of a fixed drug eruption. Whether late pigmented lichen planus is different or not is a question of definition.

Therapy. Because the pigment is in the dermis, bleaching is futile.

Pigmentatio Maculosa Eruptiva Idiopathica

(Degos and Ossipowski 1954)

Synonyms. Pigmentatio idiopathicamaculosa acquisita (Sakae 1941), melanosis lenticularis generalisata (Gottron 1943), *kleinfleckige Pigmentdermatose* (Rupec and Vakilzadeh 1971).

Etiology and Pathogenesis. The etiology and even the existence of this disorder is unclear. Perhaps it is best viewed as the Central European equivalent of erythema dyschromicum perstans, a mysterious postinflammatory disorder where the inflammatory stage is poorly documented. We suspect that in some cases it represents the end stage of lichen planus.

Clinical Findings. The typical lesions are small red-brown or brown macules, ranging in size from 0.5 to 2.5 cm and sharply bordered. The most common site is the side of the neck, although the trunk and extremities are also involved. The mucosal surfaces are spared. Most patients are children and adolescents. The lesions are relatively stable but may regress over a period of months or years.

Histopathology. In the early phase, there is basal cell liquefaction. Later, both increased basal layer pigmentation and incontinence of pigment are found, resembling melasma. Lymphohistiocytic perivascular infiltrates are also described, but they are hardly specific.

Differential Diagnosis. Postinflammatory hyperpigmentation following viral exanthems or drug eruptions are the most likely considerations. In the USA such lesions are seen as a sequel of inverse pityriasis rosea, a common variant among blacks.

Therapy. There is no satisfactory treatment, but some spontaneous improvement can be expected.

Reticulate Hyperpigmentation

Reticulate or mottled hyperpigmentation results from the presence of hyperpigmented macules aggregated in a reticulate or net-like pattern. The individual macules are typically ephelis-like, i.e., they have varying degrees of pigment and indistinct borders. The neck, axilla and groin appear particularly predisposed to this type of pigmentary change. Many of the poikilodermas (Chap. 18) such as dyskeratosis congenita or poikiloderma with blisters have a mottled pattern. Often the presence of telangiectases and especially atrophy is difficult to determine. Many of the secondary forms of hyperpigmentation, such as erythema ab igne, also tend to have lacy networks of hyperpigmentation. In addition, there are a number of rare disorders in which this pattern is featured; some are discussed below. There is no effective treatment for any of them, although individual pigmented lesions can be destroyed with a variety of lasers. Table 26.2 lists just a few examples of diseases associated with this type of pigmentary change.

Dowling-Degos Disease

(Degos and Ossipowski 1954; Smith et al. 1971)

Synonym. Reticulated pigmented anomaly of the flexures

The characteristic finding is small brown macules distributed symmetrically in the axillae and groin, occasionally involving the flexural surfaces. The macules fuse together to form a reticulated pattern, and later other areas of the body may be involved. Pigmented pits in the perioral and palmar regions have been described. Onset is usually in adult life. While most cases are sporadic, some pedigrees suggest autosomal dominant inheritance. Microscopic examination shows increased melanin in the basal layers and epidermal hyperplasia similar to a seborrheic keratosis, often with a lacy adenoid pattern. The problem is progressive, hard to treat, and occasional basal cell carcinomas have developed in the macules.

Table 26.2. Other examples of reticulate hyperpigmentation

Disease	Chapter
Dyskeratosis congenita	18
Kindler syndrome	18
Poikiloderma with blisters	18
Rothmund-Thomson syndrome	18
Epidermolysis bullosa simplex with mottled hyperpigmentation	15
Pachyonychia congenita with amyloidosis	17
Macular amyloidosis	41
KID syndrome	17

Haber Syndrome

(Sanderson and Wilson 1965)

This disorder is most likely inherited in an autosomal dominant pattern. Patients have a persistent rosacea-like dermatitis and multiple small pigmented seborrheic keratoses, which are particularly common in the axillae and groin. Thus the clinical appearance is often reticulate as the lesions merge together. There is an increased incidence of basal cell carcinoma, but most lesions arise on the face in association with the persistent erythematous nodules.

Reticulate Acropigmentation of Kitamura

(Kitamura 1953)

These patients initially have pigmented macules on the backs of their hands and feet, sometimes associated with palmar pits. The dermatoglyphic pattern shows characteristic disruptions in the ridges. Most affected individuals have been Orientals. Onset is usually in childhood and the hyperpigmentation slowly creeps proximally. There is also epidermal atrophy and, in some instances, not only increased melanin but also increased melanocytes, as in a lentigo. Some authors have suggested that Dowling-Degos disease and reticulate acropigmentation of Kitamura are either identical or closely related.

Symmetric Acropigmentation of Dohi

(Dohi 1924)

Synonym. Dyschromatosis symmetrica hereditaria.

This disorder is also primarily limited to Orientals. It features acral hyper- and hypopigmentation, producing a poikiloderma-like picture. Neither atrophy nor palmar pitting is seen. The pigmented areas show increased melanin with incontinence of pigment, while the pale areas lack melanocytes.

Dermatopathia Pigmentosa Reticularis
(Komaya 1924)

Synonym. Oberste-Lehn-Hauss Syndrome

In contrast to the other reticulate disorders, these patients develop pigmented macules on their trunk, nape, shoulders and hips during childhood. The macules blend together to form a net-like pattern. Associated alopecia and onychodystrophy have been reported, as well as some instances of autosomal dominant inheritance.

Naegeli-Franceschetti-Jadassohn Syndrome
(Naegeli 1927; Franceschetti and Jadassohn 1954)

Synonyms. Naegeli syndrome, chromatophore nevus syndrome

This rare syndrome has been primarily studied in large Swiss pedigrees. It is inherited in an autosomal dominant pattern and features reticulate hyperpigmentation, palmoplantar keratoderma, hypohidrosis and dental defects. The pigment is often blue-gray, suggesting deposition of melanin in dermal melanophages as well as in keratinocytes. It appears in infancy, favors the trunk and flexural areas, and tends to fade in adulthood.

Diffuse Hyperpigmentation

Diffuse hyperpigmentation has many different causes. Wide areas of the body are darkened, sometimes in a speckled pattern but in other cases without a hint of individual lesions.

Endocrine Hyperpigmentation

The endocrine disorders are considered in more detail in Chap. 48. While hyperpigmentation can be a feature of several endocrine problems, it is rarely the sole manifestation.

Addison Disease
(Addison 1855)

The hyperpigmentation is most prominent in light-exposed areas and in areas that tend to be darker in normal individuals, such as the knees, elbows and knuckles. The nipples and palmar creases also darken. There also may be prominent involvement of the oral, genital and rectal mucosa. Both freckling and vitiligo may be present. Since the adrenal gland is damaged or not responsive to ACTH, the feedback loop is interrupted and high levels of ACTH and MSH are present and probably cause the pigmentary change. Ectopic hormone-producing tumors, such as small-cell carcinoma of the lung, can also secrete ACTH or MSH and produce pigmentary changes.

Cushing Disease
(Cushing 1912)

When the cause of hyperadrenalism is an ACTH-secreting pituitary adenoma, there is often hyperpigmentation. There may be simultaneous secretion of MSH or the previously discussed homologies between the two molecules may be responsible for the activity. Ectopic hormone-secreting tumors, such as small-cell carcinoma of the lung, may also be responsible. Mucosal involvement is uncommon. In iatrogenic Cushing disease, hyperpigmentation is uncommon, confirming the possible importance of ACTH rather than corticosteroids.

Acromegaly

Pituitary adenomas may also produce growth hormone, as may occasionally ectopic tumors. Diffuse darkening may result, presumably once again because of overlaps with MSH.

Hyperthyroidism

About 10% of patients with hyperthyroidism have diffuse hyperpigmentation, similar to Addison disease. The mucosal surfaces and pressure points are not prominently involved. Some of these patients may have pituitary tumors that secrete thyroid-stimulating hormone and perhaps MSH analogs, but in others the mechanism is unclear.

Pregnancy

While pregnancy is hardly an illness, the pigmentary changes are striking (Chap. 36). The nipples, genital mucosa and linea alba darken, and melasma commonly develops. While the exact mechanisms are unclear, elevated MSH values have been measured in pregnancy and placental production of the protein has been postulated.

Hyperpigmentation Secondary to Other Systemic Disorders

Hemochromatosis (Chap. 46), also known as bronze diabetes, is one of the most common genetic disorders. Cirrhosis, cardiac failure, arthritis and diabetes mellitus are the main features. The skin has a metallic-gray sheen. Even though there is marked iron deposition in the skin, the pigmentation is caused by incontinence of pigment. Patients with vitiligo and hemochromatosis have depigmented patches, which on biopsy are laden with iron but lack melanin.

A wide variety of other disorders are occasionally associated with diffuse hyperpigmentation but the mechanisms are unclear. In many cases, a distorted pituitary gland function and increased MSH-like activity is blamed. Chronic infections, malnutrition, Hodgkin disease, chronic renal disease, other forms of cirrhosis and porphyria cutanea tarda have all been incriminated, but lucid descriptions are lacking.

Hyperpigmentation Secondary to Cutaneous Disorders

Sometimes, patients with systemic sclerosis, lupus erythematosus and dermatomyositis have diffuse darkening. In the past, ACTH therapy may have been the trigger and occasionally anti-malarial agents are incriminated. In other patients there is no apparent explanation. Any erythroderma can heal with diffuse hyperpigmentation, secondary to widespread incontinence of pigment. Finally, in metastatic malignant melanoma, if the tumor load is great enough, there may be circulating levels of melanin and its products in the blood. They are deposited in the dermis, both free and in melanophages, producing a blue-gray color.

Hyperpigmentation Caused by Medications

A variety of medications interact with the melanin system. The most obvious one is ACTH, which has an MSH-like action. Oral contraceptives play a role in melasma; drug-induced melasma is far less reversible than that associated with pregnancy. Psoralens combined with sunlight or UVA cause exaggerated tanning. Phenytoin and related compounds induce melasma-like changes in about 10 % of patients, mainly females. In addition to the facial involvement, the neck and arms may be affected. There is increased basal layer melanin and incontinence of pigment.

In other situations, a medication, the melanin system, light, and sometimes even lipofuscin and hemosiderin all combine to produce shades of brown, gray and blue. The phenothiazines cause a blue-gray hyperpigmentation, more pronounced in sun-exposed areas. Physical complexes between the medication and melanosomes are found. Antimalarial agents also interact with melanocytes to cause hyperpigmentation, most typically in sun-exposed areas. However, two other common sites are the shins and the oral mucosa, so chloroquine at least must have intrinsic hyperpigmenting qualities in addition to its interaction with the melanin system. The tetracyclines, especially minocycline, cause a variety of changes, including pigmented cutaneous osteomas, blue-gray pigmentation in acne scars, gray hyperpigmentation in sun-exposed areas and, least often, a diffuse muddy-brown hyperpigmentation involving the entire body. In most cases, the pigment seems to result from chelation of the tetracycline with heme products. The list of cancer chemotherapy agents that cause hyperpigmentation is long; they may produce localized lesions as well as more diffuse changes. Bisulfan causes diffuse hyperpigmentation with prominent nipple darkening mimicking Addison's disease. 5-Fluorouracil causes a variety of photo-related and postinflammatory pigmentary changes. A wide variety of poorly understood mechanisms are involved.

Melanosis Diffusa Congenita

(van Bogaert 1948)

Synonyms. Dyschromatosis universalis hereditaria, diffuse neurocutaneous melanosis

Definition. Diffuse hyperpigmentation present at birth without other signs or symptoms.

Etiology and Pathogenesis. Unknown. Usually sporadic, but cases in siblings have been reported.

Clinical Findings. The infant is born with diffuse dirty gray-brown hyperpigmentation involving the entire body (Fig. 26.9). In some cases, the color has been extremely dark. The axilla, groins, palms and soles are less dark. In some patients, thin hair, nail changes and keratosis pilaris have also been seen. There may be some lightening over time.

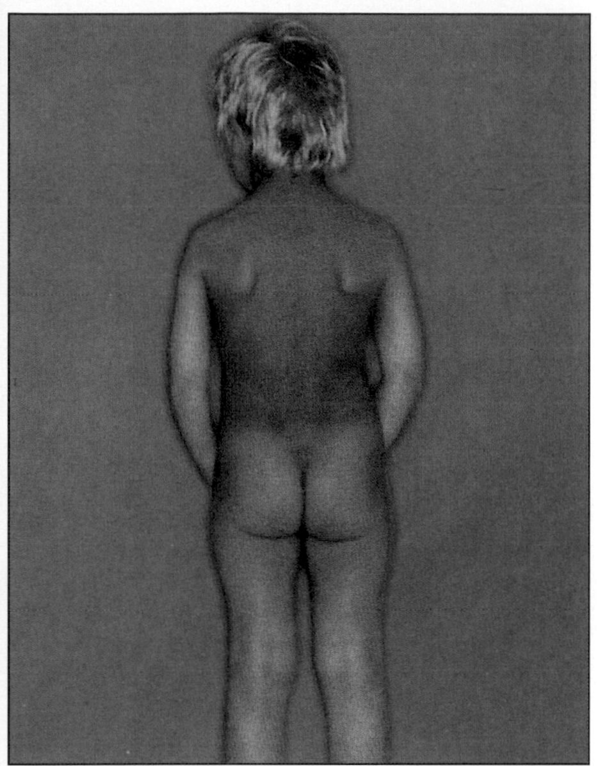

Fig. 26.9. Melanosis diffusa congenita

Histopathology. The excess pigment is melanin. There is incontinence of pigment but the main change is marked increased in melanin in the keratinocytes. There seems to be decreased destruction of melanosomes in the epidermis, as pigment is seen at high levels. In addition, complex melanosomes are uncommon.

Differential Diagnosis. There is really no differential diagnosis for this rare disorder. Most often the first reaction is a question about the true parenthood. In the even rarer universal acquired melanosis or carbon baby syndrome (Ruiz-Maldonado et al. 1978), the infants are apparently normal at birth but soon become very dark.

Therapy. None

Amelanosis and Hypomelanosis

There are several mechanisms for hypopigmentation as shown in Table 26.3. The changes may be diffuse or localized. Acquired hypopigmentation is usually postinflammatory in nature.

Table 26.3. Types of hypopigmentation

Defect	Example
No melanocytes	Vitiligo
Absent signaling molecule (c-*kit*)	Piebaldism
Diminished tyrosine	Phenylketonuria
Diminished/absent tyrosinase	Albinism

Phenylketonuria

Patients with phenylketonuria lack tyrosine so they are diffusely pale. This disorder is discussed in Chapter 39.

Albinism

Definition. Absence of melanin in the skin, hair and eyes because of congenital defects in melanin production and transfer. There are many different types of albinism. The dermatologist encounters them infrequently.

Epidemiology. The most common form of albinism is the tyrosinase-positive variant, which has an incidence of around 1:15,000 in blacks and perhaps half that much in whites. All other forms are much rarer. There are isolated populations, such as in Biafra or on the coastal islands of the southeastern USA where albinism is more prevalent. Many forms of albinism are more common in blacks.

Etiology and Pathogenesis. Melanin is absent in the skin, hairs and eyes to varying degrees in the different types of albinism. Almost all forms of albinism are inherited in an autosomal recessive pattern, as befits enzymatic disorders. The most obvious defect in albinism is the absence of tyrosinase. Patients lacking tyrosinase are not surprisingly known as tyrosinase-negative albinos and they represent the most severe form of the disease. The many other variants all have defects in later stages of melanin synthesis, packaging and transfer. Tyrosinase-positive albinism is more common than the classic tyrosinase-negative disease.

The two main organs affected in albinos are the skin and the eyes. The separation into ocular and oculocutaneous albinism is somewhat artificial. Patients with so-called ocular albinism may have skin defects and even be diagnosed on this basis.

Table 26.4. The major types of albinism

Type	Inheritance	Skin	Hair	Red eye reflex	Vision	Skin cancers	Tyrosinase in hair bulb	Melanosomes
Tyrosinase negative	Autosomal recessive	White	White	++++	----	++++	-	I–II
Tyrosinase positive	Autosomal recessive	Cream	Yellow	++	---	+++	++++	I–III
Hermansky-Pudlak	Autosomal recessive	Cream-gray	Tan	++	--	+++	+	I–III, large
Chédiak-Higashi	Autosomal recessive	Pink	Gray	++	–/+	++	++++	IV, very large

For example, X-linked ocular albinism patients, as well as female carriers, regularly have melanin macroglobules in their normal skin. Patients with cutaneous stigmata of albinism almost always have ocular findings. The ocular problems are not only caused by the obvious lack of ocular protection, with the iris and retinal pigment abnormalities and the prominent red reflex. Melanin plays a key role in the "wiring" of the optic pathways and other neural circuits in the brain, so that absence or shortage of melanin causes nerve-pathway-based visual defects, such as nystagmus.

Clinical Findings. The clinical findings are listed in Table 26.4. This list does not pretend to be exhaustive.

Tyrosinase-Negative Albinism

A wide variety of point mutations in the tyrosinase gene on chromosome 11q14–21 have been identified. These individuals are totally white with white-blond hair and blue eyes. They never tan and while they may have melanocytic nevi, the lesions are pale or red colored. Their ocular problems are severe, with visual acuity ranging from 20/200 to 20/400. Since they have no melanin in their retinas, they have the most prominent red reflex of all albinos. Because they have absolutely no photoprotection, they are at risk for the development of actinic keratoses, basal cell carcinomas and malignant melanomas, which by definition are amelanotic.

The yellow and platinum forms are considered variants of tyrosinase-negative albinism in which there is enough enzymatic activity to produce some hair color and slightly pigmented freckles and nevi. Yellow mutant albinism is most common among the Pennsylvania Amish.

Tyrosinase-Positive Albinism

This is the most common type of albinism, especially among blacks. It was first described among the Zuni Indians of New Mexico. Affected individuals have a defect on chromosome 15q11, but its exact role is unclear. While the skin is white at birth, it may acquire a pink to cream hue, especially in blacks. The patients usually have yellow-brown hair, blue to yellow-brown irides and pigmented freckles and melanocytic nevi. Malignant melanomas are not such a problem as in tyrosinase-negative albinos. The ocular problems are not as severe.

Minimal Pigment Albinism

This variant is very similar to the platinum form of tyrosinase-negative albinism. It awaits further classification.

Brown and Rufous Albinism

These variants are present in Africa and New Guinea. Patients are light brown in color and do not tan. Some have rufous hair. They have about the same risk of skin cancers as their white neighbors in Africa and only minimal visual problems. Inheritance is in an autosomal recessive pattern. Mutations in the TYRP1 gene, which encodes a melanosomal glycoprotein, have been found in these patients.

Hermansky-Pudlak Syndrome

(Hermansky and Pudlak 1959)

This autosomal recessive disorder has a fascinating history. It is found primarily in Puerto Rico but also in the Netherlands, Switzerland, India (Madras), and

Japan (Nagasaki); isolated cases are identified around the world. The gene, known as *HPS*, is on chromosome 10q23. While the gene product is unknown, it appears to function in lysosomes and melanosomes. The Puerto Rican patients have a specific 16-base pair duplication in exon 15 of the gene.

The patients have tyrosinase-positive albinism with cream to light-brown hair, freckles and pigmented melanocytic nevi, together with ocular problems (Fig. 26.10). Of greater interest are the hematologic disturbances, with abnormal platelets, so that patients may present with bleeding problems, including petechiae and ecchymoses. The platelets have ultrastructural abnormalities, described as storage pool abnormalities. They fail to store various essential mediators and do not aggregate normally. The bleeding is worsened by aspirin, which should therefore be avoided. Cells of the monocyte-macrophage lineage contain lipofuscin or ceroid inclusions, which may be found in the lungs (pulmonary fibrosis), gastrointestinal tract (granulomatous colitis) and heart (cardiac myopathy).

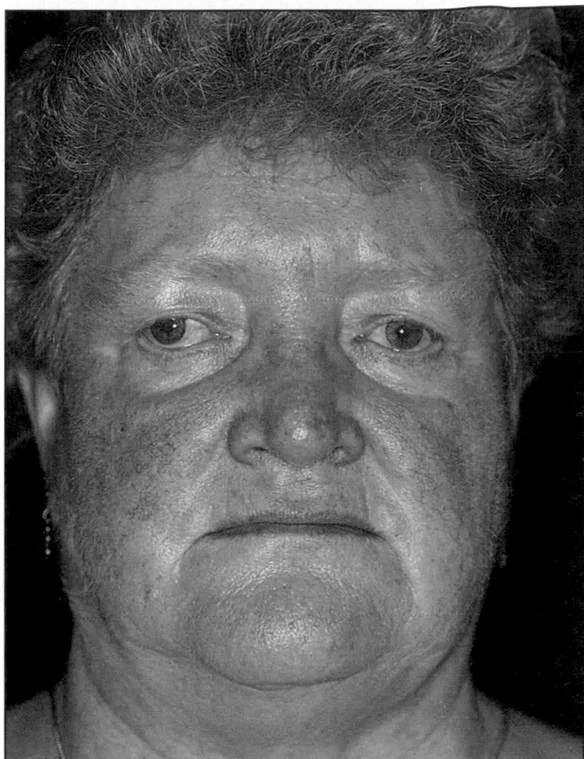

Fig. 26.10. Hermansky-Pudlak syndrome

Chédiak-Higashi Syndrome

(Beguez Cesar 1943; Steinbrinck 1948; Chédiak 1952; Higashi 1954)

Synonym. Bequez Cesar-Steinbrinck-Higashi syndrome

The Chédiak-Higashi syndrome is also inherited in an autosomal recessive pattern. These patients appear to have a defect in a gene encoding for a lysosomal protein. Patients are best described as having pigmentary dilution. Thus, Caucasian patients may appear almost totally white, like tyrosinase-negative albinos, while darker-skinned patients may have a grayish tinge. The hair has a metallic color. More severe manifestations include failure to thrive and chronic recurrent infection. The skin is frequently involved, with pyodermas and deep abscesses. Oral ulcerations and periodontal disease also occur. Respiratory tract infections pose a more significant problem. The most troublesome aspect of Chédiak-Higashi syndrome is the so-called accelerated phase or accelerated reaction, a lymphohistiocytic lymphoma-like proliferation that occurs in over 80% of patients. It involves the liver, spleen and lymph nodes and is associated with anemia, bleeding episodes and overwhelming infections leading to death.

Chédiak-Higashi syndrome is best diagnosed by examination of a peripheral blood smear, which will show large granules in neutrophils. A skin biopsy specimen usually appears entirely normal but may show melanin macroglobules and perhaps sparse dermal melanin. However, ultrastructural examination reveals large abnormal type IV melanosomes that are transferred to keratinocytes with difficulty and degraded more rapidly.

Griscelli Syndrome

Synonym. PAID (partial albinism, immunodeficiency) syndrome

This syndrome resembles Chédiak-Higashi syndrome; the patients have silver-gray hair and pale skin with focal depigmentation. There appears to be a mutation in the myosin 5 gene. There are large melanosome inclusions, as in Chédiak-Higashi syndrome, but no neutrophil inclusions. These patients, too, suffer from multiple immunodeficiencies, have a broad range of pyogenic infections, develop hepatosplenomegaly and also demyelinating CNS disease.

Autosomal-Dominant Albinism

Synonyms. Cutaneous albinism, cutaneous albinoidism

This disorder is inherited in an autosomal-dominant pattern and features minimal eye findings, so that many prefer not to classify it as a form of albinism. The patients have pink skin, pale hair and there is about the same risk of actinic damage as in the other tyrosinase-positive forms.

Cross-McKusick-Breen Syndrome

Synonyms. Cross syndrome, oculocerebral syndrome with hypopigmentation

This extremely rare disorder has been identified in Amish populations and is inherited in an autosomal recessive pattern. Patients have hypopigmented skin and hair but may have a few dark hairs or pigmented nevi. The basic defect may involve the melanocytes, which have been reported as decreased; the patients are tyrosinase positive.

Histopathology. Routine light-microscopic evaluation is often requested by the uninitiated but is of little value. DOPA incubation may or may not result in melanin production, depending on the nature of the enzyme defect. Ultrastructural examination reveals reduced to absent melanin in stage I–II melanosomes, while stage III–IV melanosomes are not seen and the silver stain is usually negative.

Laboratory Findings. When plucked hairs are incubated in tyrosine, those from tyrosine-negative albinos cannot manufacture melanin. Hairs from other albinos can produce pigment to varying degrees. Today most studies involve identifying the specific mutations involved in the various defects. In both Hermansky-Pudlak and Chédiak-Higashi syndrome, hematologic studies are very helpful.

Course and Prognosis. As far as the skin findings go, the main issue is sun avoidance. In African albinos, both malignant melanoma and squamous cell carcinoma are frequent causes of death. In the USA, the ocular problems are the main factor in limiting quality of life.

Differential Diagnosis. The differential diagnosis includes all the forms of albinism discussed above, as well as the other forms of diffuse hypopigmentation described below. All are very rare.

Therapy. There is no effective treatment except prophylaxis, such as sun avoidance or high-potency sunscreens.

Other Types of Congenital Hypomelanosis

A long list of disorders are often confused with albinism. Technically, they involve an abnormality of melanocytes, rather than of melanin production. Sometimes they have been called albinoidism, but this simply adds to the confusion. Two such conditions, autosomal-dominant albinism and the Cross-Breen-McKusick syndrome, are usually discussed under albinism. In addition, Chédiak-Higashi syndrome is not strictly albinism, as it involves a defect in the transfer of melanosomes.

Piebaldism

(Morgan 1786)

Synonyms. Partial albinism, congenital white patches, white forelock syndrome

Definition. Fixed localized depigmentation, usually involving the face, caused by congenital absence of melanocytes.

Epidemiology. Piebaldism is a rare disorder, with an incidence of less than 1:20,000.

Etiology and Pathogenesis. Piebaldism is a disorder of autosomal-dominant inheritance involving a mutation of the c-*kit* protooncogene on chromosome 4q12. This gene is important for melanocyte trafficking in the embryologic period, and as a result of its dysfunction certain areas of the body lack melanocytes.

Clinical Findings. Piebaldism has often been mistaken for albinism or vitiligo. However, several clinical features allow a ready distinction. First, the areas of pigment loss are circumscribed and fixed at birth. Second, there are always areas of normal pigmentation. Typically the depigmentation is most prominent in the midline, involving the forehead, producing the white forelock (circumscript or localized poliosis), midface, sternum and parts of the upper abdomen, as well as knees and elbows. The totally white areas are usually surrounded by a hyperpigmented ring and have islands of pigmented skin within them.

Histopathology. Biopsy shows a total lack of melanocytes. Light microscopy is not sufficient, since Langerhans cells may occupy the basal layer sites not filled by melanocytes. Electron-microscopic examination shows a clear picture – no melanocytes, no melanosomes and no melanin.

Differential Diagnosis. Vitiligo is also often considered. However, vitiligo is rarely present at birth, is often acral and most importantly increases with time, something which is never seen in piebaldism. The main differential diagnosis point is nevus depigmentosus, which may actually represent a very localized form of piebaldism. Further genetic studies are needed to clarify this issue. Waardenburg syndrome must also be excluded.

Therapy. There is no good therapy, although melanocyte transplant procedures seem more appropriate here than in vitiligo, for once the defect is repaired, it should stay repaired. The current mainstay is cosmetic coverage.

Waardenburg Syndrome

(Klein 1950; Waardenburg 1951)

Synonym. Klein-Waardenburg syndrome

Definition. Waardenburg syndrome is an inherited disease characterized by piebald-like lesions of the skin and hair. Additional manifestations include heterochromia iridis, dystopia canthorum and deafness.

Etiology and Pathogenesis. Waardenburg syndrome is heterogeneous. While it is often simply defined as piebaldism and deafness, genetic studies have shown this is incorrect. Mutations in the transcription factor PAX3 on chromosome 2q35 are responsible for classic Waardenburg syndrome (WS1) and a variant with musculoskeletal involvement (WS2). A mutation in the microphthalmia gene, which codes another transcription factor, causes a phenotype without dystopia canthorum (WS3). All three of these forms are inherited in an autosomal-dominant pattern. A fourth variant, WS4, is inherited in an autosomal-recessive pattern and associated with Hirschsprung disease.

Clinical Findings. The key cutaneous findings in Waardenburg syndrome are a white forelock and depigmented patches with hyperpigmented islands, much in the distribution of piebaldism. Some patients may have white eyelashes and eyebrows. The key clinical findings are sensorineural deafness, which is present in about 25% of patients, and Hirschsprung disease, involving 5%. Other findings on physical examination include dystopia canthorum or lateral displacement of the inner canthi with normal interpupillary distance, heterochromia iridis (also common in the Dalmatian dog, the canine equivalent of piebaldism), synophrys (eyebrows growing together at the midline) and a broad nasal root. Despite the rarity of Waardenburg syndrome, it accounts for about 2% of all cases of congenital deafness in children.

Histopathology. Biopsy is not needed but once again reveals missing melanocytes.

Therapy. The cutaneous lesions defy therapy. Of great importance is not to overlook the cutaneous and dysmorphologic clues that point towards deafness or gastrointestinal disease.

Congenital Poliosis

Some patients are born with just white forelocks and no other defects. Once again, this may be a variant of piebaldism. The genetic defect has not been identified, but its presence in several generations suggests inheritance in an autosomal-dominant pattern.

Black Locks, Albinism and Deafness Syndrome

Synonyms. BAD syndrome

These patients have a dramatic appearance with snow-white hair but focal black locks. In addition, they have diffuse hypopigmentation except for occasional tan macules. They suffer from both deafness and visual defects. On biopsy, no melanocytes are present in the white areas, while there are normal melanocytes and melanosomes in the dark areas. The basic defect is unknown.

Tietz Syndrome

(Tietz 1963)

This poorly documented syndrome consists of hypopigmentation of the skin and hair combined with severe deafness. The eyes are not involved except for hypoplasia of the brows. Inheritance is autosomal dominant.

Woolf Syndrome

(Woolf et al. 1965)

Synonym. Woolf-Dolowitz-Aldous syndrome

This is another form of piebaldism associated with deafness and heterochromia iridis. It was described in the Hopi Indians as albinism, but was later clearly shown to be piebaldism, once the patients were undressed and fully examined. It is transmitted in an X-linked recessive pattern.

Ziprkowski-Margolis Syndrome

(Margolis 1962; Ziprkowski 1962)

Another of the confusing litany of piebaldism-like disorders associated with deafness, the Ziprkowski-Margolis syndrome appears to be inherited in an X-linked recessive pattern. It has also been described as albinism; in some reports, melanocytes have been identified. Some equate it to Woolf syndrome.

There is one clear message from all of these syndromes: Until the genetic defects are clarified, it is impossible to discuss them in detail. However, the role of melanocytes in the neural pathways of hearing may be just as crucial as in vision.

Incontinentia Pigmenti Achromians

(Ito 1952)

Synonym. Hypomelanosis of Ito

Definition. Localized swirled hypopigmentation following lines of Blaschko, usually present at birth.

Epidemiology. While incontinentia pigmenti achromians is rare, it may overlap with nevus depigmentosus and linear and whorled nevoid hypomelanosis, which are somewhat more common.

Etiology and Pathogenesis. Incontinentia pigmenti achromians is not an inherited disorder but represents mosaicism for a number of different chromosomal segments carrying many unrelated genes. It is often difficult to determine whether the light or the dark segments of skin are normal. There is sufficient clinical variability to suggest that incontinentia pigmenti achromians may well embrace several disorders.

Clinical Findings. The cutaneous manifestation of incontinentia pigmenti achromians has incorrectly been described as the reverse of incontinentia pigmenti. Here the defect is one of hypopigmentation and patients have swirls and whorls of lighter-colored skin, usually following Blaschko lines. The term "chocolate marble cake hypopigmentation" has been employed. The lesions are usually present at birth, but may become more prominent in the first year of life. They may progress or regress minimally but are most often stable. Wood light examination delineates the hypopigmentation more sharply. The inflammatory precursor lesions so typical of incontinentia pigmenti do not occur. The exact nature of the pigmentary defect remains unclear.

There is a high incidence of systemic findings, including seizures, mental retardation, strabismus, dental anomalies and skeletal problems.

Histopathology. Electron-microscopic evaluation reveals a decreased number of melanocytes, with defective function. Melanogenesis is reduced, and transfer of melanosomes to keratinocytes is impaired. The suggestion is that there are two types of melanocytes in the skin, one of which does not produce or transfer melanin well.

Differential Diagnosis. Both nevus depigmentosus and linear and whorled nevoid hypermelanosis can be similar and may represent part of the same mosaic disease process following the lines of Blaschko. If this is the case, nevus depigmentosus or nevus achromicus is the least extreme variant, as a congenital hypopigmented area, present at birth, usually segmental and stable. Linear and whorled nevoid hypermelanosis involves similar or larger focal hyperpigmented lesions, also present at birth but with increased basal layer melanin. There are considerable clinical and laboratory overlaps between these disorders and incontinentia pigmenti achromians.

Hypopigmented Macules in Tuberous Sclerosis

Infants with tuberous sclerosis (Chap. 19) may have localized depigmented areas present at birth. These have been described as ash-leaf macules, although they can have a variety of shapes. Wood light examination makes them more prominent and should be performed in all infants with seizures, since these macules are often the first and only sign of tuberous sclerosis. Electron-microscopic findings suggest a defect in the transfer of melanosomes to keratinocytes.

Depigmentation

Depigmentation refers to the loss of normal pigmentation. By definition, it is not present at birth. Depigmentation may occur without any obvious cause, may have a triggering reaction or may be secondary to inflammatory dermatoses during the healing phase. The latter phenomenon is also known as leukoderma, such as in psoriatic or syphilitic leukoderma.

Vitiligo

Definition. Acquired loss of melanocytes leading to areas of depigmentation and sometimes associated with uveitis and other autoimmune phenomena.

Epidemiology

- Prevalence. 1–2% among whites, higher among blacks
- Age. Usually starts in childhood or young adult life
- Sex. No gender predilection
- Race. Far more of a problem in darker-skinned individuals
- Occupation. Chemically induced depigmentation seen in janitorial workers who are in contact with para-phenolic compounds or hydroquinones mimics vitiligo, but is considered a different disorder.
- Genetics. Often familial, but exact inheritance unclear. Up to four different genes have been discussed.

Etiology and Pathogenesis. The bottom line is that the cause of vitiligo is unknown. There are three major theories; probably each of these mechanisms plays a role in selected patients. Each hypothesis has convincing scientific arguments both for and against:

- Autoimmune Hypothesis. An autoimmune reaction could develop against melanocytes during the process of their normal turnover in the basal layer. Cytotoxic antigens could be developed against the melanocytes and destroy them. Many autoantibodies can be demonstrated in vitiligo patients, but those against melanocytes are among the hardest to find. In addition, the inflammatory reaction at the active edge of a vitiligo patch usually shows lymphocytes.
- Neural Hypothesis. Vitiligo lesions often follow a dermatomal pattern, so it has been suggested that a neurochemical mediator is responsible for destroying the melanocytes.
- Self-Destruction Hypothesis. A toxic intermediary of melanin synthesis destroys the melanocytes.

Initially the melanocytes produce less melanin. Presumably in this early phase, the destructive process is reversible, explaining the better treatment responses when lesions are treated promptly. Later, the melanocytes are destroyed. Sometimes the deeper hair follicle melanocytes are also destroyed, but often they remain relatively unaffected and a potential source for repopulating the skin with pigment-producing cells.

In any event, a wide variety of illnesses may be associated with vitiligo. Some of them may also give a clue to the etiology of the disorder. Thyroid disorders are the most common associated factor, being found in as many as 30% of the patients. Both hyperthyroidism, including Graves disease, and hypothyroidism, along with Hashimoto thyroiditis, may be found. Other possibly related endocrinologic disorders include Addison disease and both insulin-dependent and adult-onset diabetes mellitus. A wide range of other autoimmune disorders are also associated with vitiligo. They include pernicious anemia, lupus erythematosus, systemic sclerosis, myasthenia gravis, Crohn disease, primary biliary cirrhosis, Sjögren syndrome and alopecia areata. Patients with systemic sclerosis often have a confetti-like pattern of hypopigmentation. Finally, vitiligo can be seen in patients with malignant melanoma, usually as a good prognostic sign since it suggests an effective immune reaction against the tumor cells. Halo nevi may also be seen in patients with vitiligo.

In addition, a wide variety of autoantibodies can be identified in vitiligo patients. Commonly found are antithyroid antibodies, antigastric parietal cell antibodies and antiadrenal cortical cell antibodies. Unfortunately these antibodies often have little clinicopathologic correlation. While it is surely worth looking for an associated disease in vitiligo, usually it is just that – an interesting association and not a cause. Even when the associated disorder is treated, the vitiligo is unlikely to respond.

Trigger factors for vitiligo abound, but once again they are not usually clinically applicable. The Köbner phenomenon can be very dramatic in vitiligo. When patients are in an active phase, developing new lesions, minor skin trauma can lead to depigmentation. Marked sunburn is also an interesting trigger. Here one can speculate that melanocytes have been damaged, perhaps "over-exerted" themselves to produce more pigment, and have released products that then trigger the autoimmune response. Other triggering events such as emotional stress and severe systemic illnesses (ignoring the associated endocrine and autoimmune disorders) are difficult to analyze.

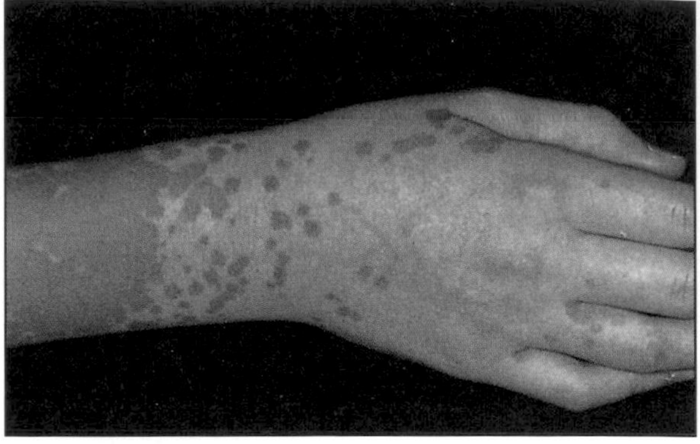

Fig. 26.12. Vitiligo

Clinical Findings. The key clinical finding in vitiligo is the acquired onset of an increasing number of initially hypopigmented and then depigmented macules, patches and later even broad sheets of skin (Figs. 26.11, 26.12). While vitiligo can appear at any age, it usually starts in individuals between the ages of 10 and 30 years. Over 50% of the patients report having their vitiligo by 20 years of age. Initially, small pale or white patches appear; they are easier to see when the adjacent skin is either dark or tanned. Wood light examination is very helpful, especially when examining pale individuals. At first there are usually a small number of patches, ranging in size from less than 1 cm to several centimeters. Their border is very sharp and they may be surrounded by hyperpigmented skin. As the patches increase in number they fuse, creating bizarre intersecting lesions. Patients occasionally complain of itching, but inflammation is almost never seen clinically. Sometimes the lesions become red and painful when sunburn is incurred.

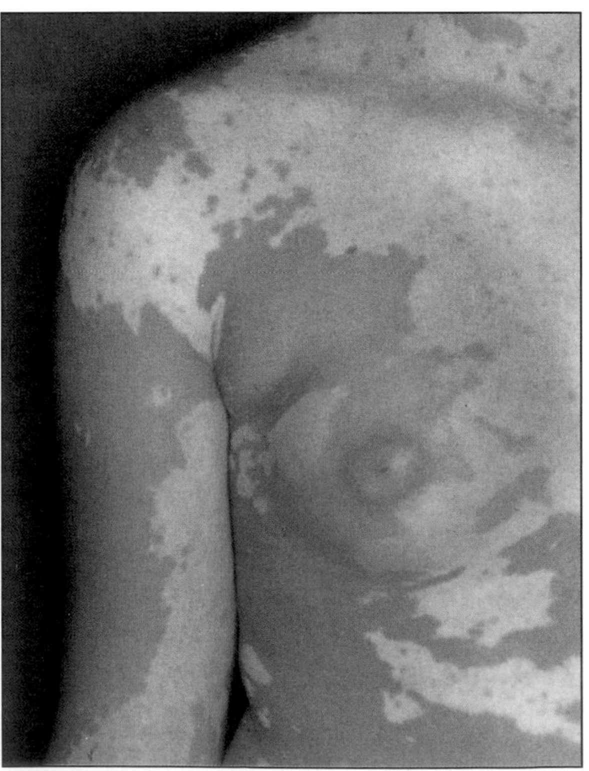

Fig. 26.11. Vitiligo

The sites of predilection are the somewhat more pigmented skin regions, such as the backs of the hands and feet, genitalia, head, neck, axillae and nipples. The early lesions are often periorificial. The hairs may depigment (acquired poliosis) or they may retain their natural color, even if the scalp is white. In the early phases, especially in blacks and other dark-skinned individuals, one may see trichrome vitiligo – the three colors are the white patch, the normal skin color and the hypopigmented brown or tan areas between normal and diseased skin. The mucosal surfaces are normal.

Just as with albinism, the interplay between the melanocytes of the eyes, ears and skin is apparent in vitiligo. The prototype is Vogt-Koyanagi-Harada syndrome, but patients with ordinary vitiligo may also develop uveitis. Thus, any ocular signs or symptoms merit prompt referral. In addition, in admittedly skewed series, about 40% of vitiligo patients had pigmentary retinal defects (almost always asymptomatic) and 15% had hints of deafness.

The clinical features are used to classify vitiligo. We employ the scheme shown in Table 26.5.

Histopathology. Biopsy of a lesion should reveal an absence of melanocytes and no basal layer melanin. However, we mention this only to condemn routine biopsy as a useful diagnostic tool in vitiligo. Some

Table 26.5. Types of vitiligo

Localized vitiligo
Focal: one or more patches, not segmental
Segmental: one or more patches, following a dermatomal pattern
Generalized vitiligo
Acrofacial: multiple lesions involving face and hands
Common: irregularly but widely distributed patches
Universal vitiligo
Virtually the entire body is depigmented. Usually some patches of normal skin remain
Mixed vitiligo
Combination of two or more of the above patterns

patients still have clear cells in the basal layer, as Langerhans cell slide into the lower layers, and thus vitiligo can only be diagnosed with certainty by means of electron-microscopic procedures or DOPA incubation, if the physician does not trust his clinical judgment. If the edge of a lesion is biopsied, one can find a T cell infiltrate, often somewhat lichenoid in nature. Biopsy may be appropriate to rule out some of the differential diagnostic considerations listed below.

Laboratory Findings. If clinical findings suggest associated disease, appropriate tests should be ordered. Thyroid status should be assessed. Other routine screening is not cost effective.

Course and Prognosis. Vitiligo is a frustrating disease. Many patients are shunned by their acquaintances so that emotional problems are not uncommon. In some societies, vitiligo is confused with leprosy, probably more on a cultural than a scientific basis, and the patients are truly outcasts. In widespread vitiligo, there is a risk of severe actinic damage in the unprotected areas. In occasional patients ocular problems may worsen the quality of life.

If the disease has been present for many years or is predominantly acral, neither spontaneous resolution nor a response to therapy is likely. In our experience, patients with atopic dermatitis have more persistent and severe vitiligo. While complete clearing is unlikely, many patients improve during the summer months. Often the repigmentation comes from the hair follicles, just as it does in a variety of therapeutic settings.

Differential Diagnosis. While the differences between vitiligo, piebaldism and nevus depigmentosus are often discussed, this question is usually easily settled. Vitiligo is almost never present at birth and generally expands, while the other two are present at birth and stable. The main differential point clinically is postinflammatory hypopigmentation, which should not reach depigmentation and should improve with time. For example, depigmented atopic dermatitis of the cheeks or lateral aspects of the arms, known as pityriasis alba, is often diagnosed as vitiligo in black children. Another pitfall is tinea versicolor; any pale or white lesion should be scraped and examined for hyphae and spores. Tinea versicolor may be present as a solitary hypopigmented lesion. In addition, early lesions of systemic sclerosis are vitiligo-like, but usually with many smaller confetti-like lesions, often centered around follicles. Similarly, the first clinical sign of lichen sclerosus et atrophicus may be hypopigmented patches. If there is a history of another dermatitis, or lesions are still present, then leukoderma is a good possibility, such as in some healing psoriatic and syphilitic lesions. Hypopigmented lesions may be seen in leprosy; one should test for sensation and palpate the appropriate peripheral nerves. Finally, an occupational history is needed to exclude exposure to depigmenting agents, and one should inquire about the use of hydroquinone bleaching agents, especially if they are available over the counter.

Therapy. The long list of suggested therapies for vitiligo simply confirms that we have no good approach. The cornerstone of therapy is a long discussion with the patient, explaining the disadvantages of all the different treatments. Nonetheless, patients are often so distressed and desperate that it is a rare physician who can get away without at least trying several different treatment modalities. None of the partially effective treatments are appropriate for children. Before starting treatment, it is probably worthwhile to document any associated abnormalities. As mentioned above, this will play little role in treating the skin, but it is better, for instance, to document a primary biliary cirrhosis before therapy than to be blamed for it later.

Systemic

PUVA. The mainstay of systemic therapy is the psoralens, combined either with natural light or UVA radiation sources in the office. PUVA can be delivered either topically or orally. In our practice in Germany, we only treat patients in the office, but we realize that financial aspects and great distances make this impossible in other lands. The following guidelines are offered.

- Oral PUVA Therapy
  A quantity of 0.3 mg/kg of 8-methoxypsoralen (Oxsoralen-Ultra) 90 min before exposure (if not tolerated, 0.6 mg/kg of trimethylpsoralen can be taken 2 h before exposure).
  Initial dose of 1–2 J/cm², increasing by 1 J each treatment.
  Two treatments weekly, often up to 100–300 in total.
- PUVA-Sol Therapy (Psoralen-Sun Therapy)
  0.6 mg/kg of trimethylpsoralen taken 2 h before exposure is employed; sometimes a lower dose is recommended.
  Patients are instructed to start with 5 min of midday sun (between 10 a.m. and 3 p.m.) and work up to 30 min in 5 min portions. They must always go out at the same time of day and should treat themselves no more than three times weekly.
  All the routine precautions (protective glasses, sunscreens, liver function testing) discussed under PUVA for psoriasis apply here.
- PUVA Bath Therapy
  8-Methoxypsoralen is added to bath water to a final concentration of 0.5 mg/l. Patients soak for 20 min.
  Initial dose of 0.1–0.2 J/cm².
  This technique is also discussed in more detail in Chapter 14.

Regardless of which type of PUVA is chosen, lesions of the face and neck respond in over 60% of cases; the rate on the hands and feet is much lower. We currently favor the PUVA bath technique because it has fewer side effects. Patients with skin types IV–VI do much better than those with paler skin. In any given case, no promises can be made, except that a relatively high UVA dose may be needed, so the patient must be careful to use sunscreens and be aware of the risk of solar elastosis, actinic keratosis and carcinoma in years to come. PUVA is usually not used in children.

PAUVA, KUVA. These two unfamiliar acronyms refer to combining UVA irradiation with phenylalanine or khellin. Neither has associated phototoxicity, but the effectiveness remains disputed. Neither product is approved for this use in USA or Germany.

Beta-carotene. Beta-carotene can produce an orange-yellow skin color by deposition of the vitamin in the stratum corneum. The dosage is 25–30 mg three to six times daily. The patient can adjust the dose to that necessary to discolor the skin. While the carotenes are usually harmless, liver function should be checked prior to treatment and after several months. Most vitiligo patients are not very gratified to have yellow spots instead of white spots. The medication is senseless in dark-skinned patients.

Topical

Corticosteroids. Treatment of a limited number of early lesions has been reported to result in repigmentation in 10–80% of patients. Our results unfortunately approach the lower end of the scale. Nonetheless, one can use low- to mid-potency corticosteroids applied once or twice daily. This offers almost the only way to treat children. If steroid acne develops, one should stop the treatment to avoid more permanent changes.

Psoralens. The use of topical psoralens and either UVA irradiation or sunlight is very difficult to titrate. There have been so many toxic reactions in the USA that the product 1% Oxsoralen Lotion is no longer available. In any event, the concentration is too high. If one is determined to try topical therapy, a maximum concentration of 0.1% can be used in the office or 0.001% for use at home. The lotion is painted on and followed by the exposure as outlined above under PUVA and PUVA-Sol. Just as with PUVA bath therapy, one does not have to worry about systemic effects, just about increased local photosensitivity.

UV Radiation. Narrow-band 311-nm UV-B radiation is favored by some. It can be given in suberythemal doses several times weekly for up to several hundred treatments.

Sunscreens. Even though patients hardly think of sunscreen application as therapy, it is essential for two reasons. One, while vitiligo skin is not at as much risk of skin cancer development as albino skin, the problem is still real. In addition, by using a sunscreen, the normal skin does not tan as much, so the contrasts are less apparent.

Camouflage. A number of excellent cover-up cosmetics are available in most countries. In the USA the best-known is Covermark but there are many worthy competitors. In addition, a variety of stains are available, utilizing natural dyes (such as walnut dye) and dihydroxyacetone (Man-Tan-like products).

Total Depigmentation. In desperate cases, with widespread disease and unsatisfactory results, one can attempt to bleach the remaining normal skin, producing uniformly depigmented skin. In our opinion, one should always make the patient mull this approach over for several months before embarking upon it, as many dissatisfied customers are produced. The standard product is 20% monobenzylether of hydroquinone (Benoquin Creme in the USA). It should be applied daily or every other day to the normal skin. The melanocytes are destroyed by a toxic reaction involving the tyrosinase pathway. The major side effect is an irritant or occasionally allergic contact dermatitis. Over many months, at great expense, it is possible to produce diffuse vitiligo. Two cautions: 20% monobenzylether of hydroquinone produces depigmentation at distant sites so it should never be used for depigmenting stubborn local hyperpigmentation. In addition, acquired ochronosis is a considerable risk and may produce an even worse cosmetic problem.

Surgical. The surgical approach to vitiligo is the newest and most creative. When pigmented skin is grafted onto vitiligo patches, often the transferred melanocytes repigment the pale area. Obviously surgical repigmentation makes the most sense in patients with stable vitiligo. The various techniques are beyond our scope but possible approaches include suction blister grafts, mini-punch grafts and transfer of either pure melanocyte cultures or mixed epidermal cultures to a prepared site.

Vogt-Koyanagi-Harada Syndrome

(Vogt 1906; Harada 1926; Koyanagi 1929)

The Vogt-Koyanagi-Harada syndrome is an acquired disorder, usually manifest in the third to fifth decade. The etiology is unknown. It appears much more common among Orientals. Initially there is an acute febrile process, often with neurologic signs, suggesting a viral infection. The next step is the development of bilateral uveitis with the threat of retinal detachment and blindness. At the same time, there is disturbed hearing or even deafness. The cutaneous findings appear much later and are less crucial but include vitiligo, alopecia areata and poliosis of scalp hair, eyebrows and eyelashes (Fig. 26.13). Because they occur last, these interesting cutaneous changes rarely help in making the initial, key diagnosis. The ocular and auditory inflammatory lesions respond to high dose systemic corticosteroids and other immunosuppressive regimens. Cycloplegics are used to reduce the risk of retinal detachment.

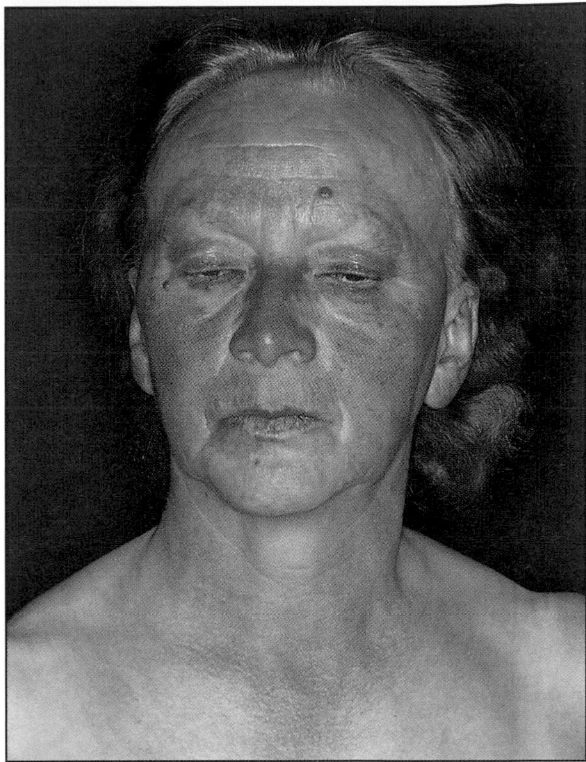

Fig. 26.13. Vogt-Koyanagi-Harada syndrome

A useful mnemonic device is "too bad for PUVAD" (P = poliosis, U = uveitis, V = vitiligo, A = alopecia, D = deafness).

Allezandrini Syndrome

The Allezandrini syndrome is an uncommon variant of vitiligo, featuring unilateral retinal degeneration, ipsilateral facial vitiligo, poliosis, most often of eyebrows and eyelashes, and deafness. Its etiology is unclear.

Idiopathic Guttate Hypomelanosis

(Costa 1951; Cummings and Cottel 1966)

Synonyms. Hypomelanosis guttata idiopathica, leucoderma lenticulare disseminatum (Argüelles-Casals and Gonzalez 1969)

Definition. Common disorder with multiple tiny confetti-like hypopigmented macules, usually on extremities of adults.

Epidemiology. While rarely discussed, this is probably the most common acquired hypopigmentation. Many individuals have at least a few lesions.

Etiology and Pathogenesis. The cause remains a mystery.

Clinical Findings. Typically hundreds of maculae measuring 2–5 mm are found on calves and shins, as well as the forearms. The lesions are scattered like confetti and are totally asymptomatic, but also totally permanent. (Fig. 26.14) They are best seen on Wood light examination or in the summer when individuals are more tanned.

Histopathology. Melanocytes are present in the lesions, but the number of melanosomes is reduced and transfer perhaps hindered.

Differential Diagnosis. Occasionally systemic sclerosis can present in an identical fashion, so one should at least take a history and inquire about symptoms. On rare occasions, lichen sclerosus et atrophicus may also have a confetti-like phase.

Therapy. None

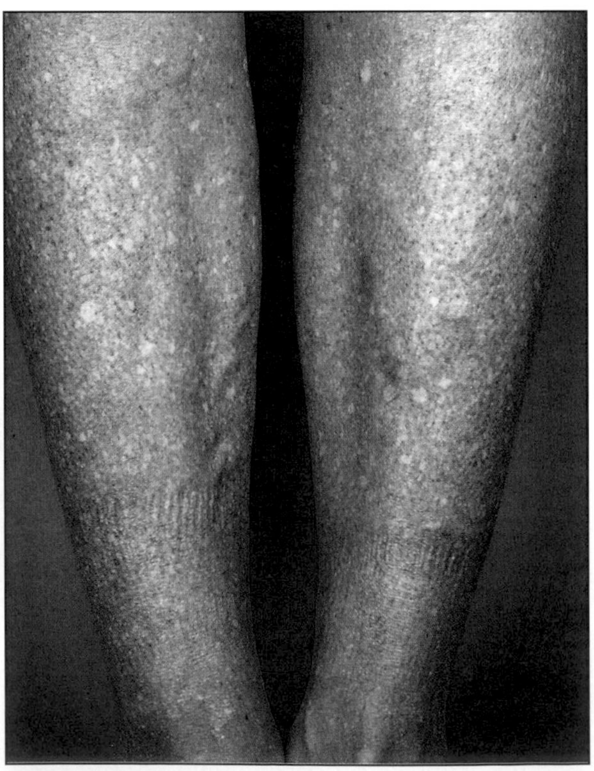

Fig. 26.14. Idiopathic guttate hypomelanosis

Chemical Leukoderma

Several occupational exposures can produce vitiligo-like lesions. The hands are most commonly involved, just as in ordinary vitiligo, but usually there is a history of preceding dermatitis. When melanogenesis is blocked, these changes may be reversible. Often, however, the melanocytes are destroyed, and then the damage is permanent.

The best-known example is exposure to hydroquinone, the same product use to bleach darkened skin in melasma and to complete depigmentation in vitiligo. It has been used as an anti-oxidant in both the leather and rubber industries. Typically there are irregular patches on the hands; the problem is far more common – or perhaps just more easily noticed – in blacks. Sometimes the lesions are confetti-like. Initially the changes may be reversible, but hydroquinone eventually destroys melanocytes. In extremely sensitive individuals, depigmentation has been seen following use of an adhesive plaster containing hydroquinone products.

The second most common industrial source is disinfectants containing para-tertiary butylphenols or amylphenols. Such products are often used in hospitals and clinics. These chemicals competitively compete with tyrosine and probably damage melanocytes in other ways. They produce a clinical picture similar to that seen with hydroquinone but are also absorbed, so that there may be cutaneous lesions at distant sites. More disturbingly, there is a tendency for associated hepatosplenomegaly and thyroiditis, the latter confirming the intriguing if poorly understood connection between the thyroid gland and vitiligo. If the insult is noticed early enough and exposure stopped, some natural repigmentation may occur and enough melanocytes may remain to make some type of PUVA therapy reasonable.

Medication-Induced Hypopigmentation

A variety of medications may cause hypopigmentation. Both the various topical retinoids and azelaic acid as used in treating acne may produce lightening of skin color. Benzoyl peroxide is well known as a hair-bleaching agent, but it also may cause some irregular lightening of dark skin. Intralesional corticosteroids, or even corticosteroids used for rheumatologic or orthopedic purposes, may cause localized depigmentation. A common scenario is depigmentation of the anatomic snuff box following injection for Quervain tenosynovitis with ascending color changes proximally up the arm. Similarly, atrophic lesions following corticosteroid injections in the deltoid or buttocks may also be depigmented. These changes are almost exclusively limited to black patients. Chloroquine also causes hypopigmentation of the hair; this phenomenon starts 2–3 months after therapy. Initially the root of the hair changes color and then of course the entire hair becomes pale as it grows out. The reaction is primarily seen in patients with light-colored hair. Para-aminobenzoic acid and interleukin-2 have been described to cause vitiligo or vitiligo-like changes, while etretinate and vitamin E may also cause lightening of hair color.

Depigmentation Secondary to Cutaneous Disorders

Permanent Depigmentation

Permanent depigmentation is no more than a scar involving the melanocytes. In some cases, e.g., following trauma, surgery or burn, there is an obvious scar. In other cases the scenario is more subtle, such as hypopigmentation following radiation exposure. In addition, any disease with inflammation at the epidermal-dermal junction can produce hypopigmentation, as seen in lichen sclerosus et atrophicus, lupus erythematosus and systemic sclerosis, especially in blacks. Severe drug reactions such as toxic epidermal necrolysis may also produce pseudo-albinism.

Temporary Depigmentation

Temporary or postinflammatory hypopigmentation or leukoderma follows many inflammatory dermatoses. Usually the damage is minimal and the process is spontaneously reversible. Several mechanisms are possible: inhibition of melanogenesis, blockage of transfer, or an "umbrella effect" limiting the amount of sunlight that reaches diseased skin. In hyperproliferative dermatoses, such as psoriatic leukoderma, perhaps the transfer cannot be completed because the keratinocytes are turning over so rapidly. In syphilitic leukoderma, the spirochetes are alleged to damage the melanocytes directly, but the hypopigmentation may simply be postinflammatory. The hypopigmentation in leprosy also involves chronic damage at the epidermal-dermal junction and is associated with anesthetic and hypohidrotic changes. In tinea versicolor the argument goes on whether the umbrella effect is responsible or whether the azelaic acid made by the organism interferes with melanogenesis, or whether both occur.

Pseudoleukoderma

In some situations, what appears to be a lightening of the skin color actually represents a contrast phenomenon. For example, there are two types of psoriatic pseudoleukoderma. In one, treatment with anthralin products that are oxidized in the skin produces a brown hyperpigmentation of the adjacent normal skin. Similarly, with PUVA therapy for psoriasis, the adjacent normal skin is excessively tanned. In either case, the psoriatic lesions appear hypopigmented. In general this is a positive finding, suggesting that the psoriasis is resolving.

Pityriasis alba or atopic pseudoleukoderma is also quite common, especially on the cheeks of children with dry skin or atopic dermatitis. It is also seen on the extremities. Apparently the hyperkeratotic scale blocks the effects of UV irradiation so that the area remains lighter in summer. There may also be some interference with melanogenesis, for lesions can develop in the winter, perhaps secondary to dryness and mild inflammation. Pityriasis alba is more easily identified in dark-skinned children; whether it is more common in this group remains unclear.

Angiospastic pseudoleukoderma is a common finding, although the term is rarely employed. Many patients, especially teenage girls, have white areas on the distal parts of their extremities as a result of localized anemia secondary to vasospasm of superficial cutaneous vessels. It may become more prominent following cold exposure or emotional disturbances. The same phenomenon is also seen on the buttocks; in German it is called *Weissfleckung* (condition of white spots), but it has not acquired a name in English.

Leukomelanoderma

In several disorders hypo- and hyperpigmentation appear together. A prime example is the "raindrops on a dusty road" of chronic arsenic poisoning (Chap. 55). Similarly, in systemic sclerosis the confetti-like or vitiligo-like hypopigmentation may be accompanied by dark areas. Mycosis fungoides is also characterized by hypo- and hyperpigmented lesions; they tend to be larger patches. In addition, there is often an element of pseudoleukoderma, as many patients are treated with PUVA. Erythroderma caused by drugs [antimalarials, sulfonamides, penicillin, phenytoin, barbiturates and others, especially those containing heavy metals (mercury or gold)] may heal with a leukomelanoderma. This can also be seen after the regression of generalized lichen planus and the exanthem of syphilis (Chap. 5).

Bibliography

General

Eller M, Ostrom K, Gilchrest B (1996) DNA damage enhances melanogenesis. Proc Natl Acad Sci USA 93:1087–1092

Fitzpatrick TB (1975) Soleil et peau. J Med Esthet 2:33–34

Gilchrest B, Park H, Eller M et al. (1996) Mechanisms of ultraviolet light-induced pigmentation. Photochem Photobiol 63:1–10

Lerner AB, Takahashi Y (1956) Hormonal control of melanin pigmentaton. Recent Progr Hormone Res 12:303

Mishima Y (1994) Molecular and biologic control of melanogenesis through tyrosinase genes and intrinsic and extrinsic regulatory factors. Pigment Cell Res 7:376–387

Circumscribed Hyperpigmentation

Brocq L (1923) L'erythrose pigmentée péri-buccale. Presse Med 31:727–728

Civatte A (1923) Poikilodermie réticulée pigmentaire du visage et du cou. Ann Dermatol Syphil 6:605–620

Danese P, Zanca A, Bertazzoni M (1997) Familial reticulate acropigmentation of Dohi. J Am Acad Dermatol 37: 884–886

Degos R, Ossipowski B (1954) Dermatose pigmentaire réticulées des plis. Ann Dermatol Syphil 81:147–151

Grimes P (1995) Melasma. Etiologic and therapeutic considerations. Arch Dermatol 131:1453–1457

Kitumara K, Akamatsu S, Hirokawa K (1953) Eine besondere Form der Akropigmentation: Akropigmentic reticularis. Hautarzt 4:152–156

Komaya G (1924) Symmetrische Pigmentanomalie der Extremitäten. Arch Dermatol Syphil 147:389–393

Riehl G (1917) Über eine eigenartige Melanose. Wien Klin Wochenschr 30:780–781

Sanderson K, Wilson H (1965) Haber's syndrom: familial rosacea-like eruption with intra-epithelioma. Br J Dermatol 77:1–8

Schnur R, Heymann W (1997) Reticulate hyperpigmentation. Semin Cutan Med Surg 16:72–80

Smith E, Dowling G, Wilson Jones E (1971) Acquired axillary and inguinal pigmentation: An epidermal naevoid abnormality not to be confused with acanthosis nigricans. Br J Dermatol 85:295–296

Sulzberger MB (1928) Über eine bisher nicht beschriebene congenitale Pigmentanomalie (Incontinentia pigmenti). Arch Dermatol Syph 154:19–32

Incontinentia pigmenti

Bloch B (1926) Eigentümliche, bisher nicht beschriebene Pigmentaffektion (Incontinentia pigmenti). Schweiz Med Wochenschr 56:404–405

Francis J, Sybert V (1997) Incontinentia pigmenti. Semin Cutan Med Surg 16:54–60

Gorski J, Burright E (1993) The molecular genetics of incontinentia pigmenti. Semin Dermatol 12:255–265

Happle R (1985) Lyonization and the lines of Blaschko. Hum Genet 70:200–206

Mevorah B, Politi Y (1997) Genodermatoses in women. Clin Dermatol 15:17–29

O'Brien J, Feingold M (1985) Incontinentia pigmenti. A longitudinal study. Am J Dis Child 139:711–712

Secondary Hyperpigmentation

Baranda L, Torres-Avarez B, Cortes-Franco R et al. (1997) Involvement of cell adhesion and activation molecules in the pathogenesis of erythema dyschromicum perstans. Arch Dermatol 133:325–329

Berger R, Hayes J, Dixon S (1989) Erythema dyschromicum perstans and lichen planus: are they related? J Am Acad Dermatol 21:438–442

Convit J, Kerdel-Vegas F, Rodriguez G (1961) Erythemia dyscromia perstans: hitherto undescribed skin diseases. J Invest Derm 36:457–462

Cox N, Long E (1991) Dowling-Degos disease and Kitamura's reticulate acropigmentation: support for a concept of a single disease. Br J Dermatol 125:169–171

Finlayson RG, Sams MJ, Smith JG (1966) Erythema ab igne. A histopathological study. J Invest Dermatol 46:104–108

Foerster H, Schwartz L (1939) Industrial dermatitis and melanosis due to photosensitization. Arch Dermatol 39:55–68

Ing E, Buncic J, Weiser B et al. (1992) Periorital hyperpigmentation and erythema dyschromicum perstans. Can J Ophthalmol 27:353–355

Knox J, Dodge B, Freeman R (1986) Erythema dyschromicum perstans. Arch Dermatol 97:262–272

Ramirez C (1967) The ashy dermatosis (erythema dyschromicum perstans). Epidemiological study and report of 139 cases. Cutis 3:244–247

Sharad P, Marks R (1977) The wages of warmth: changes in erythema ab igne. Br J Dermatol 97:179–186

Diffuse Hyperpigmentation

Addison T (1855) On the constitutional and local effects of the suprarenal capsula. Samuel Highley, London

Cushing H (1912) The pituitary body and its disorders. Lippincott, Philadelphia

Franceschetti A, Jadassohn W (1954) A propos de "l'incontinenti pigmenti" dlimitation de deux syndromes diffrents figurant sous le meme terme. Dermatologica 108:1–28

Naegaeli O (1927) Familiärer Chromatophorennaevus. Schweiz Med Wochensch 57:48

Ruiz-Maldonado R, Tamayo L, F Ruiz-Maldonado Fernández-Diez J (1978) Universal acquired melanosis. Arch Dermatol 114:775–778

Stefanato C, Bhawan J (1997) Diffuse hyperpigmentation of the skin: a clinicopathologic approach to diagnosis. Semin Cutan Med Surg 16:61–63

van Bogaert L (1948) La mlanose neuro-cutane diffuse hrdo-familiale. Bull Acad Roy Med Belg 13:307

Depigmentation and Hypopigmentation

Beguez Cesar A (1943) Neutropenia cronica maligna familial con granulaciones atipicas de los leucocitos. Bol Soc Cubana Pediat 15:900–922

Boersma B, Bos J, Westerhof W (1995) Repigmentation in vitiligo vulgaris by autologous minigrafting: results in nineteen patients. J Am Acad Dermatol 33:990–995

Boissy R, Zhao H, Oetting W et al. (1996) Mutation in and lack of expression of tyrosinase-related protein-1 (TRP-1) in melanocytes from an individual with brown oculocutaneous albinism – a new subtype of albinism classified as oca3. Am J Hum Genet 58: 1145–1156

Boissy R, Nordlund J (1997) Molecular basis of congenital hypopigmentory disorders in humans: a review. Pigment Cell Res 10:10–24

Bologna J, Pawelek J (1988) Biology of hypopigmentation. J Am Acad Dermatol 19:217–255

Chédiak M (1952) Nouvelle anomalie leucocytaire de charactère constitutionnel et familial. Rev Hematol (Paris) 7:362–367

Cowan C, Halder R, Grimes P et al. (1986) Ocular disturbances in vitiligo. J Am Acad Dermatol 15:17–24

Cummings K, Cottel W (1966) Idiopathic guttate hypomelanosis. Arch Dermatol 93:184–186

Fleisher L, Zeligman I (1960) Cutaneous finding in phenylketonuria. Arch Dermatol 81:898–903

Giebel L, Spritz R (1991) Mutations of the KIT (mast/stem cell growth factor receptor) protooncogene in human piebaldism. Proc Natl Acad Sci USA 88:8696–8699

Hermansky F, Pudlak P (1959) Albinism associated with hemorrhagic diasthesis and unusual pigmented reticular cells in the bone marrow: report of two cases withhistochemical studies. Blood 14:162–169

Higashi O (1954) Congenital gigantism of peroxidase granules. Tohoku J Exp Med 59:315–322

Ito M (1952) Studies on melanin. XI. Incontinentia pigmenti achromians. A singular case of nevus depigmentosus systematic N.S. bilateralis. Tohoku J Exp Med Suppl 55: 57–59

Jimbow K (1997) Tuberous sclerosis and guttate leukodermas. Semin Cut Med Surg 16:30–35

Kahn G (1970) Depigmentation caused by phenolic detergent germicides. Arch Dermatol 102:177–187

Klein D (1950) Albinisme partiel (leucisme) avec surdi-mutit, blpharophimosis et dysplasie myo-osto-articulaire. Helvet Paediat Acta 5:38–58

King RA, Hearing VJ, Creel DJ et al. (1995) In: Scriver CR, Beaudet AL, Sly WS, Valle D (eds) The metabolic and molecular bases of inherited disease, 7th edn. McGraw-Hill, New York, pp 4353–4392

Koyanagi Y (1929) Dysakusis, Alopecie und Pollinosis bei schwerer Uveitis nicht traumatischen Ursprungs. Klin Monatsbl Augenheilkd 82:194–211

LePoole I, van den Wijngaard R, Westerhof W et al. (1993) Presence or absence of melanocytes in vitiligo lesions: an immunohistochemical investigation. J Invest Dermatol 100:816–822

LePoole C, Boissy R (1997) Vitiligo. Semin Cutan Med Surg 16:3–14

Loomis C (1997) Linear hypopigmentation and hyperpigmentation, including mosaicism. Semin Cutan Med Surg 16:44–53

Margolis E (1962) A new hereditary syndrome sex-linked deaf mutism associated with total albinism. Acta Genet Statist Med 12:12–19

Morgan J (1786) Some account of a motley coloured or pye Negro girl and mulatto boy. Trans Amer Philos Soc 2:392–395

Nagle D, Karim M, Woolf E et al. (1996) Identification and mutation analysis of the complete gene for Chediak-Higashi syndrome. Nat Genet 14:307–311

Nekal K, PeBenito R, Orlow S (1996) Analysis of 54 cases of hypopigmentation and hyperpigmentation along the lines of Blaschko. Arch Dermatol 132:1167–1170

Njoo MD, Westerhof W, Bos JD et al. (1999) The development of guidelines for the treatment of vitiligo. Arch Dermatol 135:1514–1521

Oh J, Bailin T, Fukai K et al. (1996) Positional cloning of a gene for Hermansky-Pudlak syndrome, a disorder of cytoplasmatic organelles. Nat Genet 14:300–306

Oliver E, Schwarz L, Warren LH (1939) Occupational leukoderma. JAMA 113:927–928

Orlow S (1997) Albinism: an update. Semin Cutan Med Surg 16:24–29

Park S, Albert D, Bolognia J (1992) Ocular manifestations of pigmentary disorders. Dermatol Clin 10:609–622

Pastural E, Barrat J, Dufourcq-Lagelouse R et al. (1997) Griscelli disease maps to chromosome 15q21 and is associated with mutations in the Myosin Va gene. Nat Genet 16:289–292

Rinchik E, Bultman S, Horsthemke B et al. (1993) A gene for the mouse pink-eyed dilution locus and for human type II oculocutaneous albinism. Nature 361:71–76

Ruiz-Maldonado R, de la Luz Orozco-Covarrubias M (1997) Postinflammatory hypopimentation and hyerpigmentation. Semin Cutan Med Surg 16:36–43

Schallreuter K, Lemke R, Brandt O et al. (1994) Vitiligo and other diseases: coexistence or true association? Hamburg study on 321 patients. Dematology 188:269–275

Schiaffino M, Ballabio A, De Luca M et al. (1996) The ocular albinism type 1 gene product is a membrane glycoprotein localized to melanosomes. Proc Natl Acad Sci USA 93: 9055–9060

Spritz R (1997) Piebaldism, Waardenburg syndrome, and related disorders of melanocyte development. Semin Cutan Med Surg 16:15–23

Steinbrinck E (1948) Über eine neue Granulationanomalie der Leukocyten. Deut Arch Klin Med 193:577–581

Sybert V (1994) Hypomelanosis of Ito: a description, not a diagnosis. J Invest Dermatol 103 [Suppl]:141S–143S

Tezcan I, Demir E, Asan E et al. (1997) A new case of oculocerebral hypopigmentation syndrome (Cross syndrome) with additional findings. Clin Genet 51:118–121

Tietz W (1963) A syndrome of deaf-mutism associated with albinisms showing dominant autosomal inheritance. Am J Hum Genet 15:259–264

Toro J, Turner M, Gahl W (1999) Dermatologic manifestations of Hermansky-Pudlak syndrome in patients with and without a 16-base pair duplication in the *HPS1* gene. Arch Dermatol 135:774–780

Tourian A, Sidbury J (1983) Phenylketonuria and hyperphenylalaninemia. In: Stanbury J, Wyngaarden J, Fredrickson D et al. (eds) The metabolic basis of inherited disease, 5th edn. McGraw-Hill, New York, pp 270–286

Urabe K, Hori Y (1997) Dyschromatosis. Semin Cut Med Surg 16:81–85

Waardenburg P (1951) A new syndrome combining developmental anomalies of the eyelids, eyebrows, and nose root with pigmentary defects of the iris and head with congenital deafness. Am J Hum Genet 3:195–253

Webb D, Clarke A, Fryer A et al. (1996) The cutaneous features of tuberous sclerosis: a population study. Br J Dermatol 135:1–5

Westerhof M, Nieuweboer-Krobotova L (1997) Treatment of vitiligo with UV-B radiation vs topical psoralen plus UV-A. Arch Dermatol 133:1525–1528

Woolf C, Dolowitz D, Aldous H (1965) Congenital deafness associated with piebaldness. Arch Otolaryngol 82:244–250

Ziprowski L et al. (1962) Partial albinism and deaf-mutism due to a recessive sex-linked gene. Arch Dermatol 86: 530–539

Dyschromias

Contents

Dyschromias result when endogenous or exogenous pigments are deposited in the skin. Melanin pigmentation is considered separately (Chap. 27). The pigmentary changes may be diffuse or localized, usually depending on the source and route of exposure to the pigment.

Endogenous Dyschromias

Hemosiderosis

In most instances, the iron-rich pigment hemosiderin is deposited in the skin following degradation of erythrocytes. A number of scenarios may occur. The first is subtle leakage such as in stasis dermatitis and the progressive pigmented purpuras. Here the pigment may range in color from red-orange (purpura jaune d'ocre) to red-brown to brown. Ecchymoses following mechanical trauma, such as deep bruises or the well-known black eye or shiner go through predictable color changes from red-orange to red-blue or even deeper blue (the shiner), then red-yellow and finally pale yellow-tan. Permanent pigmentary changes are uncommon. It is unclear why microleakage often produces permanent discoloration and major leakage usually does not.

In sickle cell anemia, hemolysis of erythrocytes may occur, followed by leakage of hemosiderin and related products into the skin, producing more diffuse color changes. Traumatic hemorrhage into the stratum corneum produces a deep-blue or black color, which may be mistaken for a melanocytic lesion. The most typical site for the trauma is the heel, so the term "black heel" is often heard, but the tips of the toes or the toenails are most often involved. Often physical activity to which the patient is unaccustomed is responsible, such as at the beginning of a basketball season, when "black heel" is common, or a long night of vigorous dancing or walking down a steep trail, both of which typically produce "black toe".

In hemochromatosis (Chap. 26), although iron is deposited in the skin, the bronze color is the result of melanin. In less dramatic situations, the initial deposition of iron may also stimulate melanogenesis, so that for example in dermatofibromas, there is often not only iron but also melanin found. Finally, exogenous iron may also be deposited in the skin. When particles containing iron are driven into the skin, such as in a machine shop accident, they may eventually rust. Another scenario is the superficial injection of iron-containing medications.

Bile Pigments

Jaundice is well known to all physicians. It results from the deposition of bilirubin in the skin in hepatic disease, especially acute hepatitis. The skin acquires a yellowish hue, as do the sclerae. Experienced clinicians can reasonably estimate the bilirubin level by examining the sclerae. There is a fair amount of racial variation, as many dark-skinned individuals normally have somewhat discolored sclerae. When biliverdin, a precursor of bilirubin, is deposited in the skin, the tint is more yellow-green. This may be a clue to primary biliary cirrhosis or carcinoma of the gall bladder. The bile salts seem to stain the elastic fibers in the skin particularly well.

The main differential diagnostic consideration is carotenemia where the sclerae are normal (see below). Other causes of xanthoderma (yellow skin) include medications, such as quinacrine, that can also rarely discolor the sclerae.

Bronze Baby Syndrome

[Rubaltelli et al. 1983]

This peculiar situation develops when newborns are treated with phototherapy for hyperbilirubinemia. After 1–3 days they may develop a generalized bronze to gray discoloration of the skin, serum and urine. Apparently the newborn liver lacks sufficient biliverdin reductase to metabolize and excrete all the accumulating pigments. Thus a nontoxic photooxidation product of bilirubin or of the copper-porphyrin metabolism accumulates and discolors the skin. When phototherapy is stopped, the discoloration resolves over a few weeks. No treatment is needed.

Carotenemia

[von Baelz 1896]

Synonyms. Carotinosis, aurantiasis cutis

Carotenoids are yellow pigments that contribute to the normal skin color. They are maximally stored in hyperkeratotic skin, such as the palms and soles. When serum carotenoid levels are elevated, deposition may occur in these areas and also peculiarly on the tip of the nose. Infants are often affected, as they seem not to metabolize carotene well and are often fed excessive amounts of carrots and other yellow vegetables, usually as juices. In tomatoes and some berries, the main carotenoid is lycopene, which produces similar skin changes. The yellow color in oranges, a form of tartrazine yellow, may also cause pigmentary changes. Adults may also develop carotenemia, either from dietary excesses or from taking beta carotene for intentional pseudotanning (yellowing), for sun protection in erythropoietic protoporphyria and other light dermatoses, or as part of a vitamin regimen (Fig. 27.1). In these cases, changing the dietary habits produces improvement.

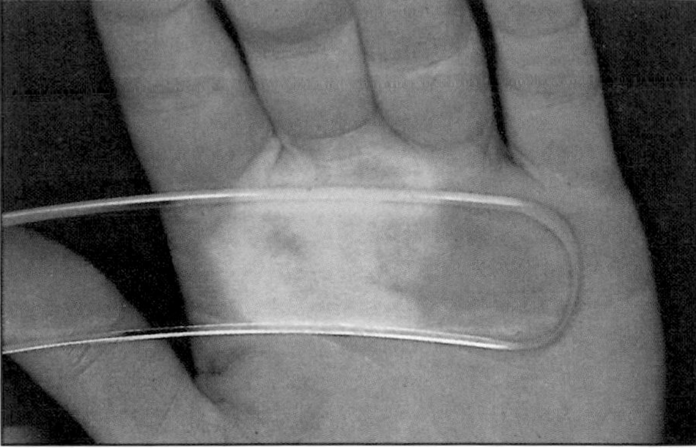

Fig. 27.1. Carotenemia

A far more difficult problem involves those patients who develop carotenemia because they are unable to convert carotene into vitamin A. The discoloration can be a valuable clue to hypothyroidism, nephrotic syndrome, other types of nephritis and some forms of hyperlipoproteinemia. In all instances, the sclerae are free, there is no pruritus and the bilirubin level is normal, so jaundice can be quickly excluded.

High doses of vitamin A usually lead to toxic side effects, such as desquamation and dry skin, as well as elevated liver enzymes, before any yellow color occurs. In fact, a yellow discoloration from vitamin A is more likely to be drug-induced jaundice than carotenemia.

Ochronosis

Ochronosis is caused by the deposition of homogentisic acid in the skin, cartilage and other tissues in the rare metabolic disease, alkaptonuria (Chap. 39). The missing enzyme in this autosomal recessive inherited disease is homogentisic acid oxidase, essential in the tyrosine pathway. The dark-brown pigment is deposited in the skin, where it produces a brown sheen. Color changes are most obvious in areas overlying cartilage, such as the ears and nose, because this tissue is also deeply discolored. The conjunctivae are also darkened. More important are the deposits in cartilage, tendons and ligaments, which produce a severe arthritis. In addition, cardiac accumulations may cause arrhythmias and other dysfunction. No satisfactory treatment exists.

Exogenous Dyschromias

The exogenous dyschromias can be caused by the ingestion, topical application or injection of a variety of materials. Many are caused by medications so that there is considerable overlap with the problems discussed in Chapter 10. The pigmentary changes induced by heavy metal salts are particularly important for they bind to a variety of dermal structures and are relatively permanent. While it is sometimes difficult to identify the salts in the skin with routine measures, a wide variety of modern analytic methods have virtually solved this problem.

Argyria

Argyria results from the deposition of fine particles of silver in the skin and mucosal surface. These particles produce a gray to gray-black discoloration that is darker in sun-exposed areas. The nail beds may also be affected. Microscopically the silver particles are bound primarily to basement membranes especially about the eccrine sweat glands and also to elastic fibers. They can be seen by ordinary light microscopy or with dark-field microscopy. Electron microscopy reveals the electron-dense particles very well and shows their distribution to be more widespread, as they are also taken up in macrophages.

Exposure to silver takes many forms. Topical discoloration may occur on the ocular, nasal or oral mucosa following prolonged use of silver nitrate solutions. If this practice is carried to extremes, systemic absorption may occur, so that the entire body is discolored. Silver sulfadiazine is a popular topical antimicrobial cream, used extensively in burn centers (it is often called "burn butter"). When used to excess, it too may produce argyria. Prolonged usage of silver salts as bleaching agents may cause discoloration (Fig. 27.2). In addition, silver salts were previously used systemically in the treatment of gastric ulcers and other gastrointestinal problems. Finally, workers in a variety of industries can be exposed to silver dust that is then inhaled and later distributed throughout the body. In systemic absorption, the gingiva and nail beds may also be discolored, along with the skin. There is no effective treatment.

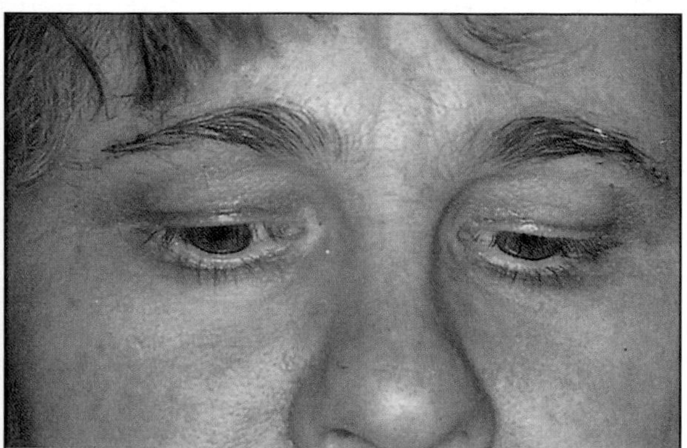

Fig. 27.2. Argyria

Chrysiasis

Gold salts cause a blue-gray, occasionally reticular, pigmentation in the skin and sclerae. Once again, the discoloration is more prominent in sun-exposed areas, emphasizing the interaction between exogenous pigments, sunlight and the melanin system. Gold salts are used in both oral and injectable forms in the treatment of rheumatoid arthritis and other autoimmune disorders. The injectable forms are far more likely to cause discoloration. While chrysiasis is relatively unlikely, it may appear fairly soon in the therapeutic regimen or after a long latency period. Once again, the particles are permanently bound to the dermal fibers and stored in macrophages, so that no treatment is available. When examined with the electron microscope, the particles are much coarser and more irregular than with silver. Patients treated with gold salts should be instructed to always use sunscreens and avoid excessive sun exposure.

Bismuth

The use of bismuth salts has taken an upsurge with their demonstrated effectiveness in the treatment of *Helicobacter pylori* infections. However, Pepto-Bismol and related products do not cause discoloration in all but the most unusual circumstances. In the past, bismuth salts were injected in the treatment of syphilis and occasionally lichen planus. The bismuth sulfide salts typically caused oral ulcerations and a distinctive gray-black pigmentation of the marginal gingivae (the bismuth line). There may also be cutaneous discoloration similar to those seen in argyria. Bismuth salts can have considerable renal toxicity, which was a limiting factor in their use for syphilis.

Mercury Pigmentation

Synonym. Hydrargyrosis

Mercury poisoning is also quite a fashionable topic today with all the interest in amalgam reactions (Chap. 33). In the past mercury salts were one of the mainstays of topical therapy, also used as bleaching creams and in a variety of ophthalmologic preparations. When used for long periods of time, they caused a local gray-brown discoloration, especially on the eyelids and in the skin creases. In addition, a variety of systemic medications including mercury diuretics and calomel were formerly prescribed and could produce diffuse pigmentary changes, although other toxic reactions usually came first. Industrial exposure to mercury vapors can cause a severe pneumonitis. Finally, the two sources most patients worry about – broken mercury thermometers and merthiolate – are relatively unimportant. Once again, the particles are found in the dermis about basement membranes, along elastic fibers and in macrophages.

Chronic mercury toxicity, especially in children, is most likely to cause acrodynia or pink disease. Affected individuals have cool digits because of arterial constriction but an overlying pink or red tone through compensatory vasodilatation. There may also be hyperhidrosis, tachycardia and CNS signs of irritability. If levels are high enough, mercury salts can be identified in the urine. Penicillamine can be used to increase the elimination of mercury.

Other Metal Salts

Chronic ingestion of bromides, such as in some over-the-counter tranquilizers, may produce a macular brown pigmentation primarily in the sun-exposed areas. Usually mental changes and bromoderma precede the pigmentary changes. Lead poisoning produces gingival discoloration similar to that from bismuth.

Exogenous Ochronosis

Secondary or exogenous ochronosis is far more common than the rare alkaptonuria. Here only cutaneous changes are present, with no joint or eye changes. The discoloration is secondary to misuse of hydroquinone. Just as many pale individuals avidly seek to become darker through tanning, many dark-skinned people avidly use bleaches to lighten their skin tone. The ordinary 2–4% cremes and gels can cause the problem in rare cases, but in countries where higher concentrations, ranging up to 8–12%, are readily available, the incidence is much higher. The hydroquinone blocks homogentisic acid oxidase and the acid accumulates in the skin. Typically the face is involved, as it is most often bleached. The cheeks are mottled and blue-brown. Caviar-like dark papules may develop, known as ochronotic or pigmented colloid milium.

The skin biopsy specimen is identical in both types of ochronosis. Large irregular collagen bundles are seen. With hematoxylin-eosin staining they appear yellow-brown but are enhanced and blackened by crystal violet or methylene blue stain. The papules contain damaged collagen and coarse pigment granules.

Black Dermographism

Some patients complain of black pigmentation under jewelry objects. The explanation is usually that various skin-care products such as powders with zinc oxide, titanium dioxide or talcum have abraded infinitesimal amounts of the silver or other metal away and deposited it in the skin. Sometimes the problem is exacerbated in patients with hyperhidrosis.

Other Local Dyschromias

In European dermatology clinics where a wide variety of medicinal dyes are used for their antiseptic and drying qualities, an array of discolorations are seen. Painting a wound with silver nitrate, potassium permanganate, gentian violet, brilliant green, Castellani's paint, Arning's solution or other examples can produce relatively long-lasting discoloration. Usually the pigment is confined to the stratum corneum, but when the nails are discolored, they can retain pigment for a long time. Sometimes when open wounds are treated, the pigment reaches the dermis, where it may persist for long periods of time. This problem often occurs with Monsel solution (ferric subsulphate) when it is used for hemostasis following tangential excisions or curettage procedures. Iron salts are responsible for the discoloration. In our clinic we no longer employ

Monsel solution. Henna is widely used as a natural hair dye and as a semipermanent decorative body paint, producing "disappearing" tattoos. In some Middle Eastern cultures, it is employed to dye the nails, palms and soles. The main active ingredient is 2-hydroxy-1,4-naphthoquinone, which has features of a bleaching and an oxidizing agent.

Medication-induced Pigmentary Changes

Here we include only a small sample of the pigmentary changes that can be induced by medications. They are also discussed in Chapters 10 and 26.

- Quinacrine causes a yellow discoloration of the skin. It is no longer used in malaria, but is occasionally employed in connective tissue diseases when ocular problems prevent the use of chloroquine and hydroxychloroquine.
- Amiodarone is a potent antiarrhythmic agent that causes photosensitivity in a considerable number of patients and a blue-gray discoloration in a small number who are forced to take it over long periods of time. The cheeks and forehead are most commonly involved. The pigment is a lipofuscin that is deposited in dermal macrophages.
- Clofazimine is a leprosy medication causing red urine and a pink to red-brown skin color. A ceroid-like pigment has been identified in the dermal macrophages.
- Minocycline, when used for long periods of time in acne therapy or for pulmonary disorders, causes a variety of pigmentary changes including blue-gray deposits on the face, shins and oral mucosa. Cutaneous osteomas may also be discolored. The pigment is rich in iron and may represent minocycline-iron complexes.

Tattoos

Definition. A tattoo is a permanent change in skin color produced by introducing a pigmented particle into the skin.

Decorative Tattoos

Decorative tattoos are a part of many cultures. In Western countries, they have traditionally been associated with soldiers and sailors, but today have acquired a widespread popularity. Psychologists divide patients with tattoos into three main groups: those with one or few decorative tattoos; those with ritual tribal or gang-related tattoos; and those with multiple tattoos often covering most of the body. Patients in the first two categories have no more psychologic disease than the general population, while those in the last group frequently have other problems.

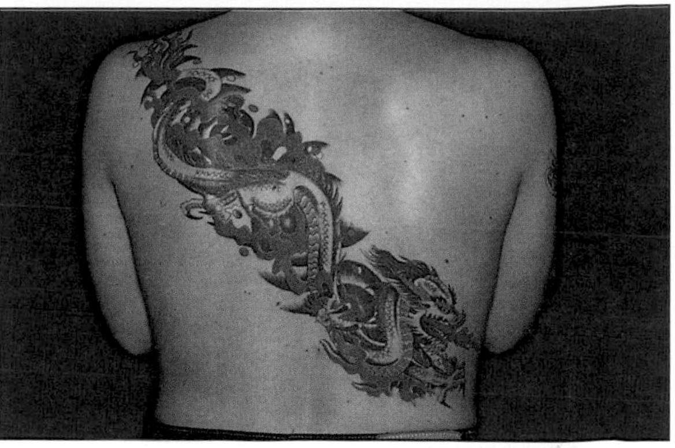

Fig. 27.3. Professional multicolored tattoo

Tattoos may be done professionally where sterile pigment is injected with specialized needles to a standard depth in the dermis (Fig. 27.3), or they may be done in an amateur fashion where a variety of pigments, such as ink, ashes and the like, are introduced into the dermis by repeated sticks with an ordinary needle. When black pigments, such as India ink, are used, the Tyndall effect produces the familiar blue-black tone. Red is usually obtained with cinnabar (mercuric sulfide), while cadmium salts provide yellow hues and chromium salts produce the green tones. Cobalt aluminate salts yield a light-blue color and various iron salts yield brown tones. In addition, many other salts, a variety of natural dyes and today, many synthetic dyes are used.

The main acute risk with tattooing is the transfer of infectious agents. If a tattoo parlor is properly run, this risk should be small. Bacterial (pyoderma, syphilis, tuberculosis) and viral (hepatitis B and C, HIV, HPV) infections can be acquired during tattooing. Later, allergic reactions to the metal salts may develop. Typically the reaction is localized, so that an animal with red eyes will appear to be crying as severe allergic contact dermatitis is caused by the mercury salts used for the red colors (Fig. 27.4). Less often there may be more widespread allergic reactions. It has been postulated that an allergic contact dermatitis to mercury salts in a tattoo may make a patient intolerant of dental amalgam, but this remains controversial. Cadmium

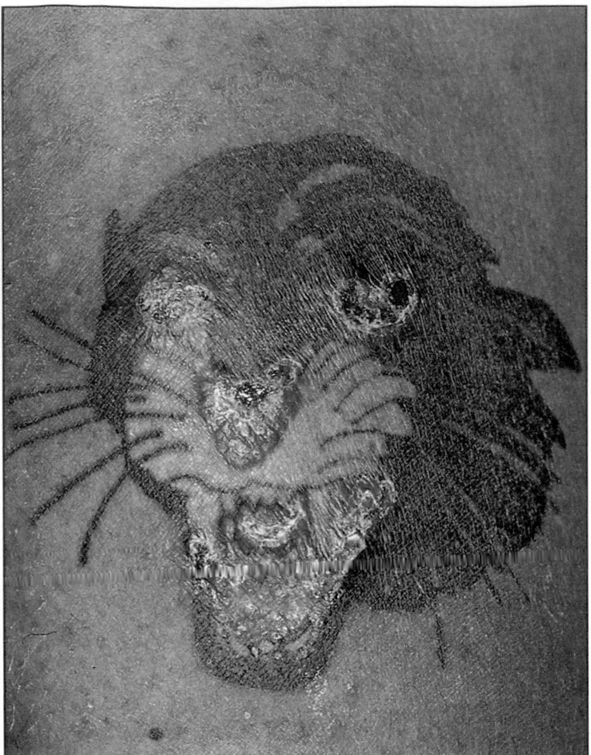

Fig. 27.4. Professional tattoo with allergic contact dermatitis to red ingredients

salts may cause a phototoxic reaction. A variety of foreign body reactions may also occur. Most often there is a foreign body granuloma, more common when nonprofessional dyes are used. Sometimes there is a sarcoidal reaction to the salts, clinically presenting as a nodule that histologically reveals naked granulomas. Such patients may have sarcoidosis. In other instances, the microscopic picture is one of a pseudolymphoma. Finally the Köbner phenomenon may occur, so that psoriasis or lichen planus appears in a tattoo. In reverse, the cutaneous exanthems of syphilis may spare red tattoos as the mercury salts have an inhibitory or toxic action against the spirochetes.

Therapy. Many patients request removal of tattoos. Sometimes their taste has changed, in other instances, they are now carrying the name of the wrong woman or man, or in a new profession or life style, the tattoos are a considerable stigma. The removal of decorative tattoos is difficult, especially amateur ones, which tend to be deeper and have larger pigment particles. Today the use of a variety of pulsed lasers (Chap. 70), which literally explode or micronize (break into tiny pieces) the tattoo pigment, is the best treatment. Older methods including excision, dermabrasion and salabrasion are less effective and far more likely to produce scars. In this field, the laser has truly proven itself superior.

Accidental Tattoos

There are a wide variety of settings in which particles may be accidentally introduced into the skin. They include:

- Coal dust tattoos. Coal miners may rub particles of coal into their skin during their work. The typical coal miner's stripes are blue-gray stripes on the shoulders and upper back, the result of repeated episodes of bumping the back against tunnel walls and roofs.
- Powder tattoos. The most common cause today is an accident with a firecracker. Misfires of guns, especially the black powder weapons enjoying a revival in the USA, produce a similar effect. Most often the face is involved and thousands of tiny particles of powder and packaging material are driven into the skin (Fig. 27.5). The eyes are also typically damaged, so that all such patients should be seen by an ophthalmologist.
- Dirt tattoos. Following car or bicycle accidents or sport injuries, particles of dirt from the ground may be implanted in deep abrasions. Often silica products are implanted, which later may elicit a foreign body granuloma. A sarcoidal granuloma following a road accident tattoo is far more likely in patients with sarcoidosis; it can be viewed as a variant of scar sarcoidosis.
- Amalgam tattoos. This most common tattoo occurs when a dentist introduces a piece of amalgam during a filling procedure. There is then a blue-gray macule on the buccal or gingival mucosa, very near an amalgam filling. Often a blue nevus or malignant melanoma is considered clinically, but they are rare and amalgam tattoos, very common. Histologically mercury particles are seen along the basement membranes and elastic fibers. If the diagnosis is clear, no therapy is needed.
- Hemosiderosis. When iron particles are introduced into the skin, they may rust and later acquire a red-brown color. Iron products that are injected superficially may discolor the skin. Rusty acupuncture needles have been blamed for tiny rust spots.
- Other accidents. Trivial accidents, such as being stabbed or stabbing oneself with a fountain or

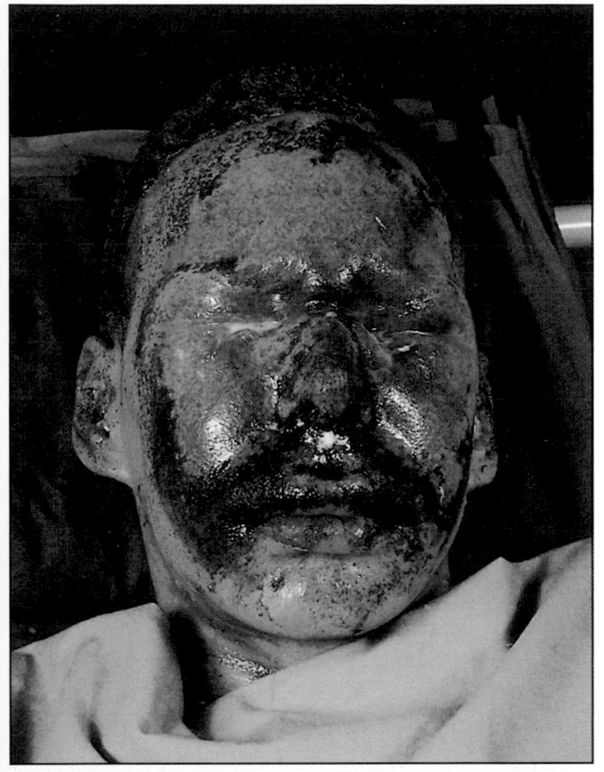

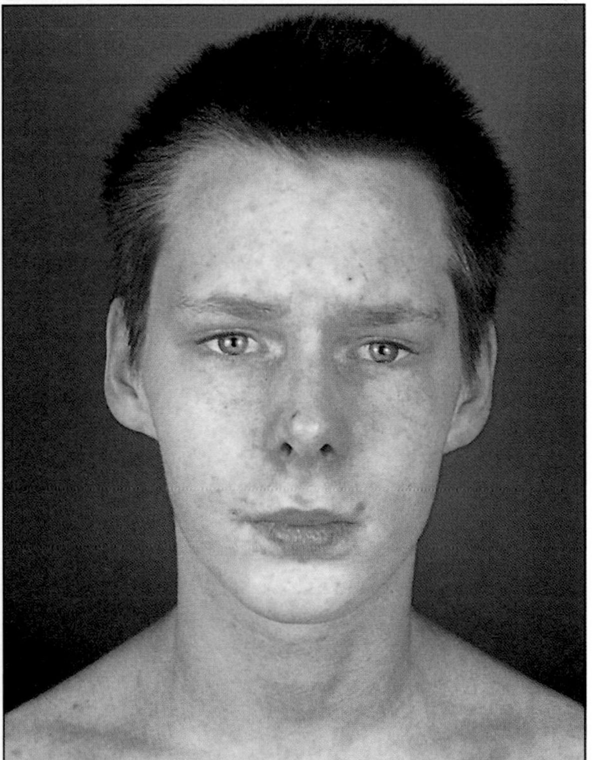

Fig. 27.5. Traumatic powder tattoo before (a) and after (b) treatment

ballpoint pen or lead pencil, or injuring oneself with a dirty tool, may produce a discolored macule that years later is mistaken for a melanocytic process.

Therapy. If the traumatic induction of pigment is obvious, as following an accident, the best plan is immediate removal. In the case of powder tattoos, all particles should be removed from the eyes by an ophthalmologist. If general anesthesia is required for this, then the dermatologic treatment can be performed simultaneously. Otherwise, local anesthesia usually suffices for the skin therapy. Physiologic saline is used, along with sterile hand and tooth brushes to debride the wounds deeply enough to remove all particles. Single deep particles can be removed with a needle, fine tweezers or a biopsy punch. If removal is done in the first few days, the results are usually excellent. Road and sport accidents can be treated similarly. Residual lesions can be excised later, as needed.

Bibliography

General

Fulk CS (1984) Primary disorders of hyperpigmentation. J Am Acad Dermatol 10:1–16

Endogenous Dyschromias

Ashley JR, Littler CM, Burgdorf WHC. Bronze baby syndrome: report of a case. J Am Acad Dermatol 1985; 12:325–8

Bilimoria S, Keczkes K, Williamson D. Hypercarotenaemia in weight watchers. Clin Exp Dermatol 1979; 4:331–5

Kopelman A, Brown R, Odell G. The bronze baby syndrome: a complication of phototherapy. J Pediatr 1972; 81: 466–72

Micali G, Di Stefano AG, Nasca MR et al. (1998) A 46-year-old man with a 4-year history of diffuse brownish black pigmentation. Endogenous ochronosis (alkaptonuria). Arch Dermatol 134:98–101

Monk BE, Metabolic carotenemia. Br J Dermatol 1982; 106: 485–7

Purcell SM, Wians FH, Ackermann AB et al. Hyperbilirubinemia in bronze baby syndrome. J Am Acad Dermatol 1987; 16:172–7

Purcell SM, Wians FH Jr, Ackerman NB Jr et al. (1987) Hyperbiliverdinemia in the bronze baby syndrome. J Am Acad Dermatol 16:172–177

Rubaltelli FF, Jori G, Reddi E (1983) Bronze baby syndrome: a new porphyrin-related disorder. Pediatr Res 17:317–330

Exogenous Dyschromias

Altmeyer P, Hufnagel D (1975) Chrysiasis. Nebenwirkung einer intramuskulären Goldtherapie. Hautarzt 26: 330–333

Basler RSW. Minocycline-related hyperpigmentation. Arch Dermatol 1985; 121:606–8

Bleehen SS, Gould DJ, Harrington CI et al. Occupational argyria; light and electron microscopic studies and X-ray microanalysis. Br J Dermatol 1981; 104:19–26

Bruce S, Tschen JA, Chow D (1986) Exogenous ochronosis resulting from quinine injections. J Am Acad Dermatol 15:357–361

Buckley WR, Terhaar CJ. The skin as an excretory organ in argyria. Trans St John's Hosp Dermatol Soc Lond 1973: 59:39–44

Burge KM, Winkelmann RK. Mercury pigmentation. Arch Dermatol 1970; 102:51–61

Connor T, Braunstein B (1987) Hyperpigmentation following the use of bleaching creams. Arch Dermatol 123:105–110

Gordon G, Sparano BM, Iatropoulos MJ. Hyperpigmentation of the skin associated with minocycline therapy. Arch Dermatol 1985; 121:618–23

Granstein RD, Sober AJ (1981) Drug- and heavy metal-induced hyperpigmentation. J Am Acad Dermatol 5:1–18

Kennedy C, Molland EA, Henderson WJ et al. Mercury pigmentation from industrial exposure. Br J Dermatol 1977; 96:367–74

Lawrence N, Bligard CA, Reed R et al. (1988) Exogenous ochronosis in the United States. J Am Acad Dermatol 18:1207–1211

Le Cleach L, Chosidow O, Peytavin G et al. Blue-black pigmentation of the legs associated with pefloxacin therapy. Arch Dermatol 1995; 131:856–7

Sakurai I, Skinsnes OK, Histochemistry of B 663 pigmentation: ceroid-like pigmentation in macrophages. Int J Lepr 1977; 45:343–54

Shelley WB, Shelley ED, Burmeister V (1987) Argyria: the intradermal "photograph", a manifestation of passive photosensitivity. J Am Acad Dermatol 16:211–217

Smith RW, Leppard B, Barnett NL et al. Chrysiasis revistied: a clinical and pathological study. Br J Dermatol 1995; 133:671–8

Waitzer S, Butany J, From L et al. (1987) Cutaneous ultrastructural changes and photosensitivity associated with amiodarone. J Am Acad Dermatol 16:779–787

Tattoos

Alster TS. Q-switched alexandrite laser treatment (755 nm) of professional and amateur tattoos. J Am Acad Dermatol 1995; 33:477–9

Björnberg A. Allergic reactions to chrome in green tattoo markings. Acta Derm Venereol (Stockh) 1959; 39: 23–9

Björnberg A. Allergic reactions to cobalt in light blue tattoo markings. Acta Derm Venereol (Stockh) 1961; 41: 259–63

Karge HJ (1978) Bürstenbehandlung von Schmutztätowierungen. Hautarzt 29:281–282

Michel S, Hohenleutner U, Bäumler W et al. (1997) Der gütegeschaltete Rubinlaser in der Dermatotherapie. Hautarzt 48:462–470

Schwartz RA, Mathias CA, Muller CH et al. Granulomatous reaction to purble tattoo pigment. Contact Dermatitis 1987; 16:198–202

Shelley WB, Shelley ED, Burmeister V (1986) Tattoos from insulin needles. Ann Intern Med 105:549–550

Soroush V, Gurevitch AW, Peng SK (1997) Malignant melanoma in a tattoo: case report and review of the literature. Cutis 59:163–166

Sowden JM, Byme JPH, Smith AH et al. Red tattoo reactions: X-ray microanalysis and path test studies. Br J Dermatol 1991; 124:576–80

Symposium on tattoos. J Dermatol Surg 1979; 5:14–70.

Taaffe A, Knight A, Marks R. Lichenoid tattoo hypersensitivity. Br Med J 1978; i:616–18

Taylor AJW. Tattooing among male and female offenders of different ages in different types of institutions. Genet Psychol Monogr 1970; 81:81–119

Tope WD, Arbiser JL, Duncan LM. Black tattoo reaction: the peacock's tale. J Am Acad Dermatol 1996; 35:477–9

CHAPTER 28

Diseases of the Sebaceous Glands

Contents

Basic Science Aspects

The distribution of the sebaceous glands in the skin is highly variable. Sebaceous glands are almost always associated with a hair follicle; the most common exception are the ectopic or free sebaceous glands of the lips and other mucosal surfaces known as Fordyce glands. There are three types of hair follicles with differing types of sebaceous glands:

- Terminal hair follicle (for example, scalp hairs): a large thick hair is associated with large sebaceous glands
- Vellus hair follicle (for example, fine facial hair in women): a thin hair and small sebaceous glands are seen
- Sebaceous follicle: a midsized hair is combined with large sebaceous glands; such an arrangement is seen only in humans, especially on the face, the upper parts of the chest and the back, the sites of predilection for acne vulgaris.

A sebaceous follicle has four parts: the keratinized follicular infundibulum, the hair, the sebaceous gland and the sebaceous duct, which connects the gland to the infundibulum. The large, cauliflower-like, convoluted sebaceous glands secrete sebum, which passes through the duct, into the follicle and then to the skin surface. Sebum is a light yellow viscous fluid whose approximate composition is: glycerides and free fatty acids 57%, squalenes 12%, wax and sterol esters 29%, free sterols 2%. The bacterial lipases, especially those of *Propionibacterium* spp., split the free fatty acids away from the di- and triglycerides; these fatty acids have a chain length between C_6 and C_{22}.

The amount of sebum varies from individual to individual, and possibly among races; the composition, however, is relatively uniform. Diet has relatively little influence; only when the patient is fasting or starving does sebum production decline. Treatment with retinoids, estrogens, antiandrogens and some antimetabolites may reduce sebum production.

Secretion of sebum is holocrine; this means that the cells of the sebaceous gland disintegrate as they migrate towards the gland center and release their sebum. The turnover time is about 14 days. The flow of sebum is relatively continuous. The fluid remains relatively thin and flows freely as it moves through the duct and then the follicle to the skin surface. The infundibulum is divided into two parts. The distal portion, or acroinfundibulum, is very similar to the adjacent epidermis. It displays keratinization with a granular layer and corneocytes which are shed into the lumen. The lower part, or infra-infundibulum, is quite different. It shows a distinct pattern of keratinization, often called trichilemmal keratinization, where there is no granular layer and the keratinocytes do not flatten out as much as they break off. The stratum corneum provides a poor barrier function. The shed corneocytes are transported to the surface by the flow of sebum and perhaps the hair growth.

Sebaceous follicles are most common in the face, behind the ears, on the upper parts of the chest and back and, to a certain extent, on the upper outer aspects of the arms. These are the areas in which acne vulgaris is found. Clinically these areas tend to be somewhat oilier than the rest of the body. As one moves distally and acrally, the number of sebaceous glands declines. None are found on the palms and soles. In areas rich in sebaceous glands, such as the face, the skin surface lipids predominantly come from the sebum; the epidermal lipids from keratinocytes make only a small contribution. In areas with few sebaceous glands, the contribution of the epidermal lipids is greater.

Sebum production is relatively high at birth, but soon declines and remains low until puberty, when it increases. The production of androgens seems to be the main factor controlling the development of the glands and production of sebum. The level of sebum production at the end of puberty is the adult baseline level, which then stays constant through most of adult life. The beginning of sebum production, or sebarche, precedes menarche by about a year.

Sebum production can be quantitatively measured. The techniques include washing the skin with an organic solvent and then determining the amount of lipids in a gravimetric fashion; blotting the skin with cigarette or filter paper; and absorbing the lipids onto clay and then weighing. Photoelectric crystals can be applied to the skin surface to measure lipids, or pieces of impregnated cellophane-tape material can be applied to the skin; they undergo colorimetric changes based on the amount of sebum available. Normal patients studied with the cigarette paper technique on the forehead produce around 1 mg of sebum/10 cm^2 every 3 h; less than 0.5 mg suggests sebostasis or dry skin, and more than 1.5 – 4.0 mg is considered excessive, as in seborrhea.

Sebostasis and Xerosis

Everyone is familiar with patients with dry skin, who are often referred to as having sebostasis. They are typically individuals with the atopic diathesis who not only have dry skin but also dry hair; often they also suffer from hypohidrosis, or reduced sweating. These patients also have defects in the epidermal lipid layer primarily involving ceramides; technically this is known as asteatosis or atopic xerosis and is slightly different from sebostasis. Nonetheless, the two overlap and the patients experience similar problems.

Both inappropriate bathing measures and decreased humidity in the winter because of central heating tend to exacerbate dry skin. This may be manifested in a number of ways:

- Fine (pityriasiform) scales, often involving the scalp as well as the body
- Larger thicker scales, as in ichthyosis vulgaris
- Eczema craquelé, which looks like a dried-out film of mud with erythematous skin between the patches
- Asteatotic dermatitis, in which the skin dries out in small patches, perhaps similar to nummular dermatitis

Perhaps as a result of immunologic defects, patients with atopic dermatitis are quite likely to have bacterial colonization, especially with *Staphylococcus aureus*. Atopic dermatitis patients with acne vulgaris often represent a difficult management problem, as their skin does not tolerate topical retinoids, benzoyl peroxide and peeling agents well.

Therapy. The simplest step is to restrict the amount and length of bathing, to reduce the water temperature somewhat and to encourage minimal use of a mild soap. Harsher soaps, bubble baths and similar products should be discouraged. The skin must be lubricated repeatedly, but especially during or after bathing. A bath oil can be added directly to the tub, but this is messy and causes slippery tubs. Shower gels or oils are useful or one can apply a bath oil to the skin after bathing or showering, rinsing and patting the skin dry. Vigorous drying with a coarse towel is also best avoided. In addition, a wide range of lubricating creams can be used after bathing, either for the entire body or, more often, for stubborn or especially troublesome spots. Ointments that are water miscible, such as Aquaphor and Eucerin, are especially helpful, as are lotions containing either lactic acid or urea.

Seborrhea

Seborrhea or oily skin is a common phenomenon, but an uncommon diagnosis; it is perhaps better considered a normal variation. The skin in areas rich in sebaceous glands acquires a sheen. When one touches the nasolabial folds, the forehead or behind the ear, the skin feels greasy or oily. Patients especially women, may complain about their appearance. In addition, the hair is often greasy, difficult to manage and the scalp tends to develop scales. Eyeglasses may appear smeared because surface lipids are so easily transferred to the lens surface. The combination of excessive sebum and infrequent bathing often leads to an unpleasant, almost rancid body odor.

The patient's genetic predisposition is the most important factor in determining the degree of seborrhea; hormones play a secondary role. In elderly patients seborrhea tends to remit somewhat but otherwise it remains a lifelong problem. Androgens stimulate sebum production and estrogens block it indirectly via the pituitary axis. Antiandrogens block the role of hormones at the glandular level by inhibiting the attachment or activation of androgens to the sebaceous glands. The most effective inhibitor of sebum production is the retinoid isotretinoin, 13-*cis*-retinoic acid.

In summer and in warm climates seborrhea tends to be more of a problem. It is often accompanied by increased sweating; in fact, it is sometimes difficult to determine whether sebum or sweat is mainly responsible for the skin's condition. In the winter months or in dry climates, the problem is less severe, supporting the idea that sweating is at least a cofactor. Emotional factors may also play a role; seborrhea is clearly more severe in both Parkinson disease and encephalitis lethargica. In addition, seborrhea is a predisposing factor for a long list of dermatoses, such as acne vulgaris, gram-negative folliculitis, seborrheic dermatitis and rosacea.

Therapy
Systemic. Both estrogens and isotretinoin may provide improvement, but they are rarely prescribed for seborrhea alone because of an unacceptable risk-benefit ratio. If isotretinoin is employed, 2.5–5.0 mg daily is often sufficient to produce dramatic improvement. We may prescribe 10 mg every other or every 3rd day. This is a far lower dosage than needed for acne vulgaris.

Topical. Patients usually resort to repeated cleansing or washing but with little benefit. Often the measures simple produce an irritated, still oily skin. Cleansing the skin with an alcohol solution or simply using tissue paper several times a day is probably as efficient as other, more complicated approaches.

Acne

Acne Vulgaris

Acne vulgaris (hereafter referred to as acne) is one of the most common skin diseases. Almost every individual has some degree of acne during puberty, with spontaneous resolution occurring in early adult life. Occasionally the disease persists into the fourth decade or even remains a lifelong problem. In general, the earlier acne begins, the more likely it is to be severe and persistent. While both sexes are equally frequently involved, the more severe forms occur more often in men, probably because of hormonal influences. Because of the involvement of the face with considerable cosmetic problems, acne is a major psychosocial problem for many teenagers and young adults. For this reason, acne should always be taken seriously by the treating physician; nothing is more discouraging to the distressed young patient than to hear, "Oh, it's just acne."

Definition. Disease that arises in areas rich in sebaceous glands and characterized by seborrhea, comedo formation, inflammatory pustules and papules, and scars.

Epidemiology. The epidemiology of acne is hard to document. Almost every individual has acne at some point in their life and most teenagers benefit from at least topical treatment.

Etiology and Pathogenesis. Many factors interact to produce acne in a given patient. They include genetic factors, sebum production, hormones, bacteria, and properties of the sebaceous follicle. Immunologic factors probably play a secondary role.

Genetics. The tendency to acne is clearly inherited, but an exact pattern has not been identified. This suggests multifactorial inheritance. The child of parents who both had acne has a greater than 50% chance of being affected.

Sebaceous Glands and Sebum. Almost all acne patients have increased sebum production. Eunuchs, who lack male hormones and have very dry skin, do not get acne. Acne patients have larger sebaceous glands and produce more sebum than patients with normal skin. Nonetheless, increased sebum is not both necessary and sufficient; patients with Parkinson disease, who have extremely high sebum levels, do not get acne. Agents that block sebum production lead to an improvement in acne.

Sebum in the sebaceous glands and ducts is sterile and contains no free fatty acids. The true sebaceous cysts of steatocystoma multiplex also contain sebum with triglycerides and no free fatty acids; they rarely become inflamed. The microenvironment of the infundibulum favors the growth of *Propionibacterium acnes* and *Staphylococcus epidermidis.* Both of these bacteria are part of the normal flora of the facial skin, but if they proliferate, they contribute to the development of acne. Their lipases split di- and triglycerides, producing free fatty acids. The free fatty acids comprise about 20 % of the skin surface lipids in acne patients. They are comedogenic, by altering the pattern of keratinization in the infundibulum. In addition, they are chemotactic, attracting neutrophils to the follicle, producing pustules and papules. The combination of the damaged follicular wall from the free fatty acids and the increased intrafollicular pressure secondary to the inflammation leads to ruptured follicles, nodules, abscesses, and scars.

Microorganisms. Every sebaceous follicle is rich in bacteria and fungi. They are part of the normal flora but may be quantitatively increased. Acne is not an infectious disease, and the acne pustules are not pyodermas. The main fungus is *Malassezia furfur* (also known in the past as *Pityrosporum ovale*). This dimorphous agent is found in the acroinfundibulum between the most superficial keratin scales but is not felt to play a role in acne. In the midinfundibulum *Staphylococcus epidermidis* and other micrococci are found. As one moves deeper into the follicle, the microaerobic propionibacteria predominate. There are three types of *Propionibacterium*: *Propionibacterium acnes* (type I), *Propionibacterium granulosum* (type II) and the most uncommon *Propionibacterium parvum* (type III). Since propionibacteria produce porphyrins, sebaceous follicles rich in these bacteria tend to fluoresce coral red under Wood light. *Propionibacterium acnes* produces lipases that play a major role in acne, as discussed above. *Demodex folliculorum*, the hair follicle mite, is not involved in acne. It is uncommon in young adults but seen more often in older patients.

Hormones. Prior to puberty, the sebaceous follicles are small and not capable of developing into acne lesions. In puberty androgenic stimulation, primarily from testosterone but also from other ovarian and adrenal hormones, stimulates the growth of the sebaceous glands and thus the production of sebum. The adrenal glands produce a variety of androgens, including androstenedione and dehydroepiandrosterone sulfate. The increased adrenal production prior to menarche may explain why sebarche so often precedes menarche.

Sebaceous glands have androgen receptors on their cell surface. Testosterone itself is inactive and must be converted to 5 α-dihydrotestosterone (DHT) by the enzyme 5α-reductase. DHT then enters the cell, is carried to the nucleus attached to cytoplasmic receptors and then, via the complex messenger system, influences nuclear mechanisms. In both sexes, the physiologic levels of androgens are high enough to ensure almost maximal sebaceous gland activity. In men, most DHT comes from testosterone, while in women androstenedione is the main precursor. The conversion of testosterone to DHT is 30 times greater in acne skin than in normal skin. Anabolic steroids with androgenic effects increase the sebum production; even in men who already have seborrhea, a 10–20 % increase is possible, which may lead to an severe exacerbation of acne (bodybuilder's acne). Estrogens, either as contraceptives or naturally produced during pregnancy, reduce sebum production by inhibiting the production of androgens via the pituitary axis. The exact role of natural progesterones is unclear, but many synthetic progesterones have an androgenic action. Antiandrogens may either block attachment of testosterone to the cell receptors or inhibit 5 α-reductase. Cyproterone acetate and chlormadinone acetate both block attachment; the former is available in Europe combined with an estrogen (Diane-35, Dianette) and used to treat acne in women.

Abnormal Keratinization. The first detectable sign of acne is the increased production and accumulation of corneocytes in the acroinfundibulum. The keratinized cells are not shed but clump together forming a microcomedo. Comedones are thus a result of follicular proliferation and retention hyperkeratosis. The initial pathogenic event is unclear. The flow of sebum is not blocked; the sebaceous glands appear normal, although later they may become smaller. However, the increased sebum flow may still be responsible for the formation of comedones. The process of keratinization, be it in the skin or in a hair follicle, is complex, depending on dissolution of desmosomes and formation of a lipid-rich intracellular cement from both the keratinosomes (Odland bodies) and other cell lipids. Perhaps the rapid flow of sebum dilutes the lipid coat in the follicle, reducing the levels of cholesterol, ceramides and linoleic acid, which then leads to disordered keratinization. In addition, disordered follicular keratinization leads to an increased permeability of the follicle wall, allowing fluids and inflammatory cells to pass more easily and allowing *Propionibacterium acnes* to proliferate more readily. Whatever the mechanism, hundreds of corneocytes are pressed on top of another, much like the layers of an onion, and saturated with lipids; this produces the comedo, the primary lesion of acne.

Follicular Reactivity. The infrainfundibulum of acne patients responds to a variety of physiologic and exogenous stimuli more readily than that of patients without acne. The reasons for this increased follicular reactivity are unknown. However, comedogenic agents such as halogenated cyclic hydrocarbons, as well as petrolatum, tar products and some cosmetics, cause more problems (chloracne, cutting oil acne, cosmetic acne) in acne patients. In addition, agents such as corticosteroids, isoniazid and potassium iodide are more likely to cause a pustular follicular response in acne patients. In this case, the inflammatory response comes first, followed by comedones.

Immunology. Immunologic evaluation reveals no primary immunologic problem in acne patients. Instead, their intact immune system leads to the secondary inflammatory response. Patients show increased reactivity to *Propionibacterium acnes*, as manifested by elevated antibody levels and a more pronounced prick-test reaction. The significance of secretory IgA in the sebum is unclear. Patients with more severe acne, such as acne conglobata, show reduced delayed hypersensitivity to the standard test agents. Because of chronic inflammation, patients with severe acne inversa are at risk for secondary amyloidosis, which is nonetheless a rare event.

Clinical Findings

Acne lesions can be divided into primary, noninflamed lesions; secondary, inflamed lesions; and postinflammatory scars. Even though the acne cysts, fistulated comedones and scars no longer appear inflamed clinically, histologic evaluation reveals the signs of chronic inflammation.

Primary Noninflammatory Lesions

Follicular Cast or Filament

Many follicles, especially those of the lateral part of the nose, are filled with pasty plugs or casts. Gentle pressure allows the patient or physician to extrude this material. While patients think of this normal variation as a comedo, it is not one. Instead, a cluster of corneocytes is loosely clumped around a vellus hair but a channel is present, allowing for the flow of sebum and often containing *Propionibacterium acnes* and other bacteria. Rarely, true comedones may develop from follicular casts. Patients often attempt to treat the nasal lesions with topical retinoic acid and are disappointed to observe that the casts do not respond nearly as well as comedones elsewhere on their face.

Microcomedo

The first detectable change in a sebaceous follicle is the microcomedo; it can only be identified microscopically as an early plug in the infrainfundibulum. The proliferation and retention hyperkeratosis leads to a tightly compressed layer of corneocytes that blocks the follicle so that the distal part expands much like a balloon.

Closed Comedo (Whitehead)

As the corneocytes accumulate, the plug becomes more complete. The infrainfundibulum is filled with whitish material, while the acroinfundibulum remains tightly closed. When the skin is stretched, skin-colored or whitish papules are seen; occasionally the central pore or follicular opening is visible. When squeezed, the whitehead can be emptied through the pore, producing a white, pasty mass on the skin surface.

Open Comedo (Blackhead)

The open comedo usually develops from a closed comedo, but it can arise directly from a microcomedo. Here the acroinfundibulum is also dilated by the larger, more compacted plug. The comedo plug consists of densely compacted corneocytes, bacteria (*Propionibacterium acnes*, *Staphylococcus epidermidis*), distally *Pityrosporum ovale* and sebum. Channels in the plug allow sebum to course through. The vellus hair at the base of the follicle continues to grow but does not reach the surface; it is trapped in the plug. Thus a long-standing comedo may contain 10–15 hairs. From the number of hairs and the length of the hair cycle, one can estimate the age of a comedo. If the hairs are extruded through the follicle wall into the dermis, they elicit a foreign body reaction.

As the closed comedo develops, the sebaceous glands become smaller. In older lesions, they are often reduced in size. In some inflammatory acne lesions, sebaceous glands can no longer be identified. Thus it seems unlikely that sebum is a significant factor in the inflammatory component of acne. The dark distal part of the open comedo is black because of the presence of melanin; blacks have darker blackheads, while albinos have white ones. The dark color does not come from oxidation of lipids, from exogenous material or from lack of cleanliness.

Secondary Inflammatory Lesions

Any primary lesion can become inflamed. At this point, immunologic mechanisms appear to become more important. Some patients, such as those with acne conglobata, are so reactive that massive inflammation occurs as a result of microcomedones, so that closed and open comedones are rarely seen. In acne mechanica, mechanical or irritant factors are responsible for producing inflammation of preexisting comedones.

Papule and Pustule

The follicular epithelium becomes damaged, with spongiosis, and accumulation of initially neutrophils and then lymphocytes. Eventually, the epithelium ruptures; the comedo contents elicit an intense inflammatory reaction in the dermis. This entire process leads to both papules, when the inflammation is relatively deep, and pustules, when the process is more superficial.

Indurated Nodule

These persistent deep lesions are the result of a long-lasting dermal inflammatory stimulus, often from hair fragments. Such lesions clinically resemble an inflamed epidermoid cysts and are often called acne cysts, although they have no cystic structure unlike true acne cysts. They may wax and wane over weeks to months.

Abscess

Sometimes a group of papules and pustules will coalesce; this is particularly likely in acne conglobata. Indurated erythematous nodules develop which tend to drain an mixture of blood, pus and sebum. They then persist as weeping, crusted, painful lesions that heal with widespread scars.

Draining Sinus

These complex lesions are typical of severe acne conglobata and acne fulminans. They typically occur in the nasolabial region, the bridge of the nose, the mandibular region and the neck. Linear fluctuant abscesses develop; they may be up to 10 cm in length and contain numerous sinus tracts or fistulas connecting them to the skin surface. When manipulated, they often yield foul-smelling secretions at several sites. They tend to heal slowly over a period of months to years but then to relapse during new inflammatory attacks. Often surgical treatment is required.

Postinflammatory Lesions and Scars

These lesions are the result of severe acne that has healed to an extent.

Fistulated Comedones

Two or more comedones are joined by scar tissue and sinus tracts. Such lesions evolve as abscesses containing multiple follicles or comedones heal with scaring. Most common are the double comedones, which are usually found on the neck or back. Typically one can pass a probe from one opening to the next.

Cyst

True epidermoid cysts develop often in acne patients, presumably from repeated insults to the follicular epithelium. Common sites are behind the ears and along the eyebrows. Lesions tend to be 1–5 cm in size, elevated and with a prominent central pore. Perhaps because of their location, they are more likely to rupture than ordinary cysts. They can be shelled out easily through a small incision.

Scar

The variety of scars in acne is rich. Scarring is generally the main concern of the patient. Typical scars include tiny ice-pick or punched lesions, nodular scarring around a follicle mimicking a milium or closed comedo, small nodules, larger keloidal scars, especially on the chest and back, and large cigarette-paper-thin scars as a result of healed abscesses and pigmentary changes.

There are striking differences in the clinical expression of acne that should be reflected in the therapeutic plan. Acne patients range from individuals with several closed comedones, visible only on close examination, to systemically ill patients with large abscesses, ulcerations and, rarely, even bone involvement in acne fulminans. Acne vulgaris can be divided into three stages: comedonal acne, papulopustular acne and acne conglobata. In addition, there are a number of special variants of acne that are considered after the discussion of acne vulgaris.

Comedonal Acne. Open and closed comedones predominate; they are seen primarily on the face (Fig. 28.1). Only rarely are inflamed lesions present. The lesions tend to appear early in puberty, starting around the nose and midface, as well as on the forehead. Most patients have seborrhea. Mild cases with only a few lesions are usually easy to treat; patients with more severe forms, such as with hundreds of closed comedones, are difficult to manage.

Papulopustular Acne. In these patients, the inflammatory process predominates so that one sees both papules and pustules. Not only the face but also the chest and back may be involved. In addition to the inflamed erythematous lesions, comedones are also present, although sometimes few in number. In patients with a rapid clinical course, sometimes comedones are not clinically visible because microcomedones become inflamed so early in the disease course. Indurated or deeper lesions may also be present. Once again, almost all patients have seborrhea. Scarring usually occurs.

Acne Conglobata. This is the most severe form of acne vulgaris and affects men more often than women. In addition to the above-mentioned lesions, patients tend to have abscesses, draining sinuses, fistulated comedones and scars, often both keloidal and atrophic (Figs. 28.2, 28.3). The chest and back are usually just as prominently involved as the face; the disease may be even more widespread reaching the arms, abdomen, buttocks and even scalp. The fistulated or duplex comedones are especially typical (Fig. 28.4). Cysts also tend to be a problem; they may become repeatedly inflamed, rupture and drain foul-smelling material.

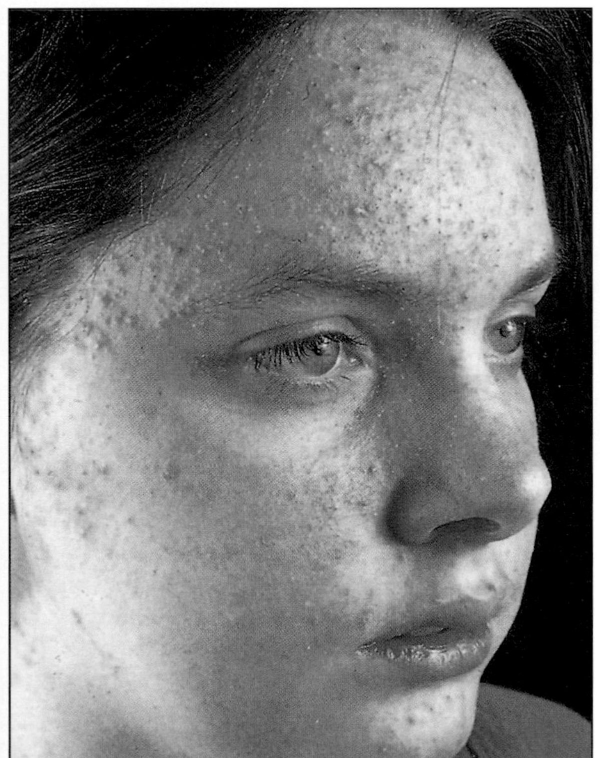

Fig. 28.1. Comedonal acne

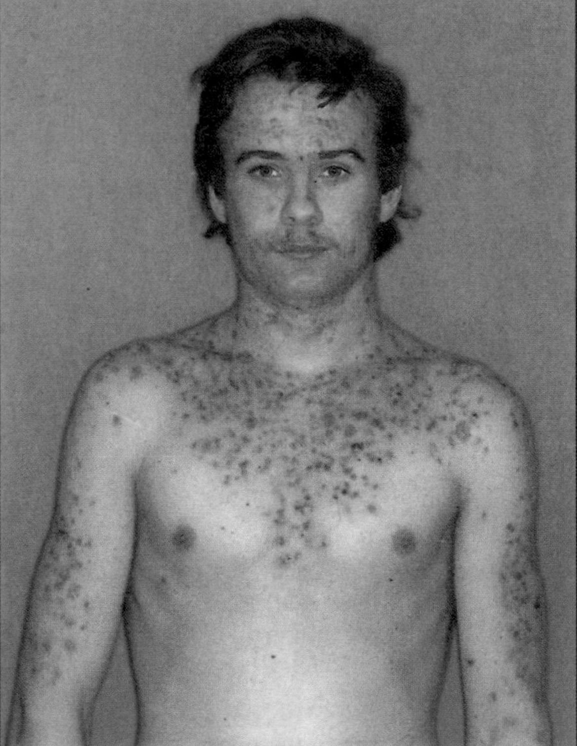

Fig. 28.2. Acne conglobata

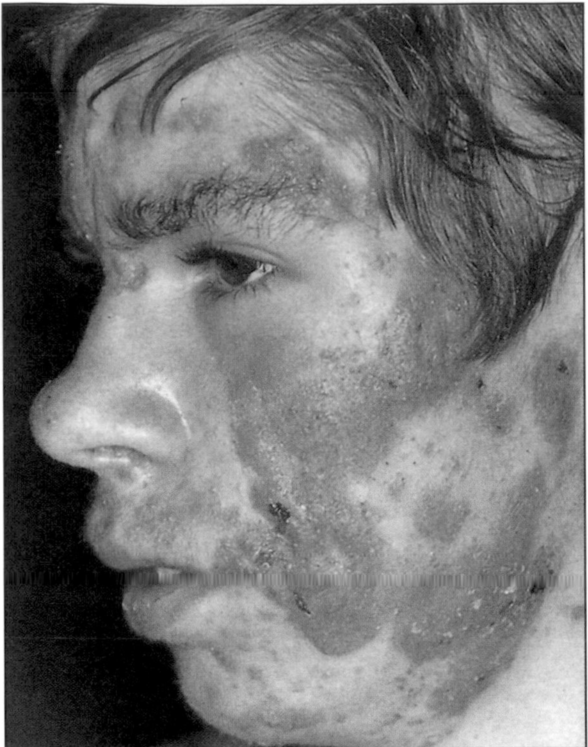

Fig. 28.3. Acne conglobata

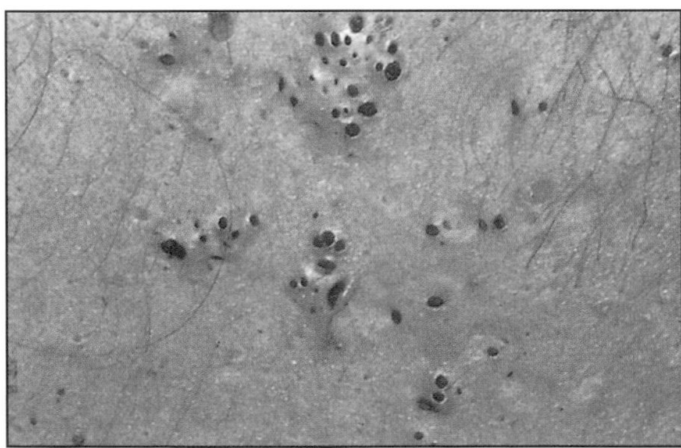

Fig. 28.4. Acne conglobata; fistulated comedones

The SAPHO syndrome is an acronym for synovitis, acne conglobata, palmoplantar pustulosis, hyperostosis and osteitis (Chap. 14). Sterile osteomyelitis is seen in patients with both severe acne and pustular psoriasis, hence the somewhat overlapping terminology.

Histopathology. Biopsies are almost never employed in acne, except for investigative purposes. They usually demonstrate the features discussed under etiology.

Course and Prognosis. As mentioned above, the course of acne vulgaris can be prolonged and frustrating. Even if a teenager has an average course, the 2–3 years of problems seems a long time. The unfortunate patients with more severe and more persistent disease are invariably frustrated.

Therapy

Acne almost always heals spontaneously in young adult life. This fact should not lead the physician to be complacent. Modern therapy can reduce the course and severity of the disease, reduce scarring and improve the psychosocial well-being of the patient. Many of the most grateful dermatologic patients are young adults with acne who find a dermatologist interested in helping them. In addition, more severe types of acne may last for many years and require repeated therapeutic intervention. Another fact of acne therapy is that there is no single agent that treats all aspects of the disease, with the possible exception of oral isotretinoin. Thus the available topical and systemic agents must be chosen based on the severity of the acne and the type of lesions predominating. What works for one patient may not work for the next, so a degree of trial and error is involved; the patient should be aware of this and become an active member of the therapeutic team, making suggestions about what has helped and what has been less successful. Finally, the patient's underlying skin type should always be kept in mind. The unfortunate patient with atopic dermatitis and acne will tolerate topical retinoids and other peeling agents far less well than an individual with seborrhea.

General Measures

Cleansing Agents. Despite the protestations of parents (and especially grandparents), acne is not a cleanliness problem. In fact, excessively aggressive washing may cause enough dryness to interfere with effective therapeutic agents. On the other hand, most acne patients have oily skin and wish to reduce their facial sheen. Alcoholic wipes or simply repeated use of absorbent paper towels are the best approach. Syndets (synthetic detergents) are popular for acne patients in Europe. They allow maintenance of a relatively specific pH, which can reduce the bacterial flora of the skin, especially *Propionibacterium acnes*. In addition, lotions and bars containing benzoyl peroxide are effective adjuncts.

Diet. There is no valid scientific evidence that any diet helps acne in the majority of patients. Unfortunately, many adults suffered acne diets as teenagers and seem disappointed when their children do not receive the same punishment. Prohibiting foods such as French fries, hamburgers, ice cream, cola beverages, chocolate or nuts is simply not warranted. The patient (not the parents) should be encouraged to be observant; if he or she notices that a given food product causes acne flares, then this should be avoided. The only common dietary trigger for acne is iodine; while iodinated table salt does not generally produce high enough levels to cause problems, it should not be used to excess. Some studies suggest that "McDonald's acne" is actually normal acne worsened by the excessive salt in the unlimited food available to employees rather than any exogenous worsening of acne from cooking fats. Kelp diets and other unusual diets may also contain excessive iodides.

Emotional Support. While only a rare acne patient needs professional psychiatric help, almost every one of them needs emotional support and a friendly helping physician. Simple inquiries about school and social life, encouragement that the disease is getting better, and other evidence that the physician cares about the patient are of great help to the often unhappy young adults. Patients with acne excoriée des jeunes filles and rare other patients with extreme anxiety about their acne and usually about their life may benefit from more professional counseling. Patients always ask if acne is caused by stress. Clearly every dermatologist daily sees patients with flares of acne during periods of stress; the problem is that both acne and stress are so common that a connection is hard to identify.

Phototherapy. Most acne patients report improvement in the summer months. Both UVB radiation and to a lesser extent combined UVA/UVB therapy were used for acne. Ultraviolet radiation seems to work by its antiinflammatory action and by causing peeling; there is no comedolytic action. The downside of phototherapy for acne is that middle-aged adults often present with more severe photodamage than their skin type or life style would suggest, because of extensive UV radiation treatments as teenagers. There are so many other effective treatments for acne that phototherapy has lost its once dominant position.

Cosmetics. Many women and some men with acne may wish to mask their lesions. Any light water-based cosmetic that can be easily washed off is usually effective; often a green make-up base reduces the erythema. Stage-type make-up should be avoided since its repeated use and removal damage the skin. Medicated cover-up products are usually not any more effective than ordinary cosmetics.

Zinc. Zinc is somewhat controversial. It has been recommended both topically, often combined with erythromycin, and orally (50 mg t.i.d.) for inflammatory acne. The topical agent is harmless; the oral products can cause gastrointestinal distress. We have seen little benefit from zinc and do not employ it.

Medical Management. Table 28.1 lists the major agents available for treating acne, subdivided by their likely mechanism of action. Representative products available in Europe and the USA are mentioned.

Comedolytic Agents. The mainstay is topical tretinoin, which causes peeling but also has a specific comedolytic action normalizing keratinization in the infundibulum. Since all acne lesions arise out of a comedo, it makes sense to treat all acne patients with tretinoin or other comedolytic agents. Tretinoin is available as Retin-A cream 0.025%, 0.5% and 1%; Retin-A Gel 0.01% and 0.025%; and Retin-A liquid 0.05%, as well as under many other brand names around the world. Two newer products are Avila, a 0.025% cream or gel formulated in a liquid polymer vehicle, and Retin-A Micro, in which the tretinoin is contained in microspheres for better release.

One must be careful with the various vehicles and their percentages. For example, the mildest agent is 0.025% cream and the second strongest 0.025% gel, so if the gel is mistakenly prescribed for an atopic dermatitis patient with mild comedonal acne, problems are bound to ensue. The liquid is only for very severe acne, usually of the trunk. Patients should be instructed to use tretinoin sparingly at night and to avoid skin folds and creases such as the nasolabial fold or corner of the mouth. Less irritating topical retinoids are isotretinoin (Isotrex), adapalene (Differin), and tazarotene (Tazorac); in our experience they are also slightly less effective. Patients should be warned about photosensitivity, irritation and the possibility of initial worsening before improvement occurs. Concern has been expressed about using topical retinoids in pregnancy; so little systemic absorption occurs that the theoretical risk is nil.

Table 28.1. Principles of acne therapy

Indication	Medication/approach	Examples[a]
Cleansing	Syndets	Dermowas, Eubos, Seba med
Antiseborrheic	**Systemic**	
	Estrogens	Oral contraceptives
	Chlormadinone acetate	Neo-Eunomin, Eunomin, Gestramestrol N
	Cyproterone acetate	Diane-35, Dianette
	Isotretinoin	Accutane, Roaccutan
	Topical	
	Alcoholic solutions, other lotions, emulsions and cleansers	
Comedolytic	**Systemic**	
	Isotretinoin	Accutane, Roaccutan
	Topical	
	Various retinoids	Tretinoin (many brands), isotretinoin (Isotrex, Accutane), adapalene (Differin), tazarotene (Tazorac).
	Benzoyl peroxide	Many brands, both water-based and alcohol-acetone-based; also washes
	Azelaic acid	Skinoren, Azelex
	α-Hydroxy acids	Many available
	Salicylic acid	0.5–3.0% in ethanol 50% or isopropanol 20–30%
	Removal of comedones	Comedonal extraction
Antimicrobial	**Systemic**	
	Tetracyclines	See Table 28.2
	Erythromycin	See text
	Many others	See text
	Topical	
	Erythromycin	Many products
	Clindamycin	Sobelin, Cleocin
	Tetracycline	Imex, Topicycline, Meclan, many other
	Benzoyl peroxide	Many forms (see above)
	Azelaic acid	Skinoren, Azelex
Antiinflammatory	**Systemic**	
	Corticosteroids	Intralesional, rarely systemic in severe flares, often combined with isotretinoin
	Antibiotics	See above
	Dapsone	See text
	Isotretinoin	Accutane, Roaccutan
	Topical	
	UV radiation	Sunlight or artificial sources
	CO_2-acetone slush	Also peeling

[a] Representative European and North American products

Another major peeling agent is benzoyl peroxide, which is also bactericidal. It effectively reduces levels of *Propionibacterium acnes* by over 95% over 2 weeks and thus lowers levels of free fatty acids. It causes some erythema and peeling and may bleach dark-colored skin or hair. Benzoyl peroxide is available in a variety of concentrations (2.5–10.0%) as both gels (alcohol or acetone-based) and creams (water-based). The latter are less drying. The percentage makes surprisingly little difference. Alternating benzoyl peroxide and topical antibiotics may reduce the risk of bacterial resistance. Other products with the same active ingredient include bar soaps, washing lotions and even shaving creams.

Azelaic acid (Skinoren, Azelex) is used as a 20% cream. It is somewhat antibacterial and antiinflammatory but causes little peeling or comedolysis. Thus azelaic acid is a good choice for acne patients with atopic dermatitis; its onset of action is rather slow, so the patient must be warned.

Other comedolytic agents include salicylic acid solutions, gels or soaps, and light chemical peels.

It is sometimes reasonable to perform comedo extraction early in the treatment of a patient with marked comedonal acne until the other measures begin to take hold. A range of older peeling agents, including sulfur, resorcinol and abrasive soaps containing either aluminum oxide or polyethylene granules, are rarely employed. The most comedolytic agent of all is oral isotretinoin but it is only rarely employed for comedonal acne. Oral vitamin A has an even less desirable riskbenefit ratio than isotretinoin and should not be employed. At levels above 10,000 IU/day, vitamin A is also a teratogen.

Antimicrobials. Sometimes when marked inflammation is presence, one must first attack this aspect and then add a comedolytic agent. The mainstays of antiinflammatory therapy are topical and systemic antibiotics, as well as benzoyl peroxide. Most patients prefer to first try topical antibiotics, viewing them as safer. The onset of action of systemic agents is so much more rapid that one should consider a combined therapy initially.

The standard topical antibiotics are erythromycin and clindamycin; each is available in a variety of vehicles that can be tailored to the patient's skin type. They can be applied daily or b.i.d., often combined with peeling agents. Gram-negative folliculitis and the selection of resistant strains of *Propionibacterium acnes* are the main complications. Combining erythromycin with benzoyl peroxide reduces the incidence of resistance. Although topical antibiotics are often combined with systemic antibiotics, this approach also increases the likelihood of resistant bacterial strains. Absorption of clindamycin is minimal, but measurable. Patients with inflammatory bowel disease should not use topical clindamycin, and all should be warned about possible gastrointestinal side effects.

Tetracycline (Imex) and meclocycline (Meclan) are available as creams. These are the least drying topical antibiotics, but perhaps less effective. Topicycline is a tetracycline solution that gives the skin a slight yellowish tint but more interestingly fluoresces with black lights, such as those often used in discotheques.

Patients with more severe pustular disease should be started on systemic antibiotics. It is especially futile to attempt to treat severe acne of the back with topical antibiotics. The tetracyclines are the mainstay of systemic therapy. The choice of a given tetracycline involves a risk-benefit evaluation (Table 28.2). At maximum dosage, all three agents are equally effective. In Europe, minocycline or doxycycline 50–100 mg daily have widely replaced tetracycline hydrochloride. Compliance is so much better with daily dosing independent of meals that the slightly increased cost is considered acceptable.

All the tetracyclines should be avoided in pregnancy and in young children because they tend to be deposited in growing bones and teeth, where they cause discoloration. After the age of about 12 years, the only likely site of deposition is the wisdom teeth (third molars), so the risks are minimal. Minocycline may also be deposited in acne lesions, scars, bones and even the thyroid, causing a blue-gray discoloration. About 10% of patients develop oral hyperpigmentation as the bones of the oral cavity become discolored and can be seen through the mucosa (black bone disease). Severe reactions associated with minocycline include a serum sickness-like disease, autoimmune hepatitis and drug-induced lupus erythematosus. Doxycycline causes a phototoxic reaction that is inexplicably less common in acne patients than in those taking the medication as prophylaxis against travelers' diarrhea. Concerns about tetracyclines reacting with oral contraceptives are overstated. There may be a direct chemical reaction because tetracyclines are chelating agents but this can be easily avoided. In addition, the antibiotics stimulate

Table 28.2. Comparison of different tetracyclines

Medication	Usual daily dose	Strengths and weaknesses
Tetracycline	500–1500 mg	+ Cheap, little photosensitivity – Must be taken on empty stomach, poor compliance, binds with other products
Doxycycline	50–100 mg	+ Inexpensive, good absorption – Photosensitivity
Minocycline	50–100 mg	+ Reaches sebaceous glands well, good absorption, no photosensitivity – More expensive

the hepatic metabolism of the hormones, slightly lowering serum levels, but not enough to cause clinical concern. Patients should be made aware of the interaction to avoid later medicolegal problems.

In patients who do not tolerate any of the tetracyclines, or who fail to improve, one can employ erythromycin 500–1000 mg daily, or the newer derivatives, azithromycin 250 mg daily, roxithromycin 150–300 mg b.i.d. or clarithromycin 250–500 mg b.i.d. In our experience, erythromycin is less effective than the tetracyclines and associated with more side effects, primarily gastrointestinal distress. Enteric-coated or time-release forms are available but they increase the expense. In addition, erythromycin cannot be used in conjunction with astemizole or terfenadine, as serious cardiovascular complications may result.

The issue of antibiotic resistance developing during acne therapy has assumed new importance in recent years. In the past, resistance of *Propionibacterium acnes* was uncommon, but in some studies today over 60% of organisms are resistant to erythromycin. Topical is just as likely as systemic treatment to select resistant strains. Fortunately, resistant *Propionibacterium acnes* has few public health implications. Of greater concern is the identification of resistant coagulase-negative staphylococci, including *Staphylococcus epidermidis*. Vancomycin resistance has not been documented in strains harvested from acne patients, but dermatologists must finally accept the reality of this problem. The adjunctive use of benzoyl peroxides (against which no resistance has evolved) and resisting the temptation to frequently switch antibiotics are the best prophylactic measures.

We tend not to use other oral antibiotics, but acknowledge that they may have a role, especially if isotretinoin is not a practical consideration. Ampicillin, clindamycin, trimethoprim-sulfamethoxazole, trimethoprim, various cephalosporins and even other agents have their supporters. Dapsone has also been employed, primarily for acne conglobata and acne fulminans. It probably has both antimicrobial and antiinflammatory actions, but in the dosages needed to be effective, it almost always induces methemoglobinemia.

Systemic Retinoids. While one generally starts with topical and systemic antibiotics, many patients with severe acne are candidates for oral isotretinoin (13-*cis*-retinoic acid, known as Accutane or Roaccutan). The standard treatment is 0.2–1.0 (usually 0.5) mg/kg daily for 12–16 weeks. Some patients are then cured; relapses occur in perhaps a quarter of cases, usually after months or years and milder in form. Isotretinoin has many mechanisms of action; the main one is its reduction of sebum production. The patient rapidly develop dry skin and mucosa. The sebaceous glands are reduced in size by up to 90%; in contrast antiandrogens such as cyproterone acetate achieve only a 20–35% reduction. In addition, isotretinoin is comedolytic; microcomedones and larger, more developed lesions disappear. Finally an antiinflammatory action is apparent. In addition, presumably by altering the microenvironment and nutrient factors for the microbes, isotretinoin is antibacterial even though it does not have a direct effect on microorganisms.

Isotretinoin has a number of side effects, some annoying and some catastrophic. Every patient experiences dry skin, dry lips and dry eyes. They must simply be convinced to lubricate their skin and use a lip balm and, if needed, artificial tears. Contact lens wearers may experience problems. Rarely, mucosal involvement may lead to dysuria, dyspareunia or mild bleeding after bowel movements. About 10–20% of patients have myalgia; this problem may be more severe in competitive athletes, who probably should not be treated during their season. Minor changes in liver function tests may occur, but the levels return rapidly to normal when therapy is stopped. Thus hepatic function should be monitored.

More serious complications include alterations in cholesterol and triglyceride levels. Fasting pretreatment levels should be obtained and then checked every 2–4 weeks until they have stabilized. Triglycerides are somewhat more likely to be affected. One should be cautious in patients with preexisting abnormalities of lipid metabolism, especially if they require higher dosages of isotretinoin. All changes are readily reversible when therapy is concluded. Pseudotumor cerebri has been described but is rare; one should not use tetracycline along with isotretinoin since both may lead to increased intracranial pressure. Impaired night vision may also result; patients should be cautioned about driving at night. Finally, higher dosages (>1.0 mg/kg daily) for many months may lead to skeletal changes, including hyperostosis of the vertebral processes and spinal ligaments. This has been described as the DISH (disseminated idiopathic skeletal hyperostosis) syndrome. In acne patients who require short-term treatment, this problem can be ignored, but it must be monitored in patients with disorders of keratinization requiring long-term therapy.

Contraindication: The final side effect of isotretinoin is catastrophic. Isotretinoin is a well-established teratogen, causing primarily CNS and cardiovascular defects. Retinoid embryopathy also includes abnormalities of the external ear and microphthalmia. Thus isotretinoin cannot be prescribed for women who may become pregnant without a series of precautions. We adhere to the following guidelines when employing isotretinoin. The patient should have severe acne, primarily acne conglobata and acne fulminans, that has failed to respond to standard therapy. Often experienced clinicians must ignore the latter caution, since they know the acne is so explosive and severe that standard therapy will fail and thus immediately choose isotretinoin. Other uses of isotretinoin in mild acne, seborrhea, rosacea and a variety of other settings are not officially approved in the USA. Thus the physician is accepting some personal responsibility in these settings.

Next, the patient must be appropriately cautioned about the side effects. Women require special instructions about contraception. In the USA the manufacturer provides extensive literature and will pay for a gynecologic consultation. The patient must sign a permit in which she acknowledges the contraceptive counseling, and accepts the risks, since no contraception is perfect. Patients under the legal age of consent must be accompanied by a parent who signs the form. Do not assume that a 14-year-old girl is not sexually active and ignore this question; embarrassment at the time of initiating therapy is preferable to later legal action. Generally speaking, oral contraception is the method of choice; intake should be commenced 1 month before the use of isotretinoin and continued for 1 month after completing therapy, i.e., 6 months of oral contraception for a 4 month course of isotretinoin.

A serum pregnancy test should be performed prior to therapy. The patient should start the drug on the 2nd or 3rd day of the next menstrual cycle. Any abnormalities in menses should be reported promptly to the dermatologist, who will almost certainly want to refer the patient to her gynecologist.

Hormonal Therapy. We tend not to employ any of these methods often for acne alone. They are discussed in greater detail in the chapter on hair disorders (Chap. 31), for the same approach is used in hirsutism and androgenetic alopecia in women. The main methods of reducing sebum production are retinoids and hormonal therapy. Ordinary oral contraceptives may have some effect, but today most are low in estrogens and may have progestational agents with an androgenic role in the skin, such as norgestrel and norethindrone. The number of choices in each country are so variable that the dermatologist must acquaint himself with the nature of the products available to his patients. In Europe, two antiandrogens are available. We use primarily cyproterone acetate combined with an estrogen (Diane 35, Dianette), although chlormadinone acetate is also available, both as a single product and combined with estrogens. We prefer to work with our colleagues in gynecology when prescribing either oral contraceptives or antiandrogens.

Several other approaches have been endorsed. In the USA, spironolactone, an antihypertensive aldosterone antagonist, is used for its secondary antiandrogen properties, usually in dosages of 50–100 mg daily. Because spironolactone is not approved for this use in Europe, we have no experience with this product. On rare occasion, either prednisone or dexamethasone can be used to suppress adrenal production of androgens. We prefer to have endocrinologists or gynecologists direct such therapy, once laboratory evaluation has confirmed hormonal dysfunction.

Surgical Management. Scarring is the fear of every acne patient, so scar correction becomes an important issue. Fortunately, almost all acne scars improve with time. Inflammatory nodules or keloids can be injected with intralesional corticosteroids or treated with cryotherapy. Cysts, fistulated comedones, ice-pick scars and deep or atrophic scars can often be excised. For almost all the remaining damage, dermabrasion offers the best prospects for improvement.

Comedonal extraction refers to the removal of comedones by extrusion; it is often erroneously called acne surgery. Open comedones can simply be expressed with a comedo extractor; closed lesions must first be opened with a lancet or a no. 11 blade. The comedones are better described as disturbed rather than removed. Histologic studies show that in most cases the follicular lumen refills and the comedo reappears. The improvement in appearance is thus relatively short-lived.

Acne Fulminans

(Windom et al. 1961; Plewig and Kligman 1975)

Synonym. Acute febrile ulcerative acne conglobata (with polyarthritis and leukemoid reaction)

Definition. Rare severe illness that affects almost exclusively boys in their midteens with papulopustular acne.

Clinical Findings. Acne fulminans is characterized by the sudden appearance of confluent abscesses leading to hemorrhagic necrosis. Often a jelly-like material can be curetted from the lesions. The face, neck and back are most often involved. At the same time, the patient is febrile with leukocytosis, joint pain and swelling (primarily involving iliosacral, iliac and knee joints). The patient tends to walk in a stiff bent-forward position. Additional findings may include a sterile osteomyelitis, especially involving the sternoclavicular joint. Occasionally erythema nodosum is present.

Histopathology. Frank hemorrhage and leukocytoclastic vasculitis are seen. Vasculitis is not a finding in other acne forms, suggesting that here an immunologic reaction is involved.

Laboratory Findings. The neutrophil count is usually elevated, sometimes strikingly, as is the erythrocyte sedimentation rate. Circulating immune complexes can be found. In addition, anemia and proteinuria are often present.

Course and Prognosis. Even with prompt and aggressive treatment, scarring is a major factor.

Differential Diagnosis. Tropical acne is the main differential point. Patients have explosive worsening of acne upon exposure to the high heat and humidity of a tropical climate. This was a major problem among US troops in the Vietnam War, resulting in a significant number of medical evacuations. The osteomyelitis and other systemic problems are not seen. Acne conglobata is also similar but patients usually lack systemic findings and have a more gradual course.

Therapy. Systemic isotretinoin is the mainstay. It is wise to initially treat the patient with prednisone 1.0 mg/kg daily for 7–10 days and then taper off rapidly, as isotretinoin therapy is started. This reduces the intense inflammation and provides a more prompt response. We usually use oral roxithromycin 150–300 mg b.i.d. or clarithromycin 250–500 mg b.i.d for 7–10 days. Often pyogenic granuloma-like vegetating lesions may form; they can be treated with high-potency corticosteroid creams for about 10 days. Usually a total treatment period of 8–12 weeks is required.

Acne Inversa

(Plewig and Steger 1989)

Synonyms. Hidradenitis suppurativa, intertriginous acne, acne triad, acne tetrad, perifolliculitis capitis abscedens et suffodiens (Hoffmann 1908), deep folliculitis decalvans (Nobel 1905)

Definition. Severe acne in the inverse body regions, such as scalp, axillae and groin.

Epidemiology. Men are more often affected than women. The disease is uncommon before puberty. We suspect that when mild forms are considered, such as patients with just a few lesions, acne inversa is somewhat more common than most sources suggest.

Etiology and Pathogenesis. Acne inversa is a disease of the hair follicles and sebaceous glands, not of the apocrine glands as was previously thought (hence the old name hidradenitis suppurativa). The apocrine glands are innocent bystanders involved secondarily by the massive inflammation. While bacteria can be cultured from lesions, it is agreed they play no primary role in chronic disease. In some women, there appear to be menstrual flares. Increased sweating, friction from clothes, irritation from shaving or epilating hairs and excess weight are all at least cofactors.

Clinical Findings. The tetrad of acne inversa includes:

- Acne conglobata of the chest, back and face. Often only scars of previous acne are present
- Chronic inflammatory lesions in the intertriginous areas (Fig. 28.5)
- Perifolliculitis and abscesses of the nape and scalp
- Pilonidal sinus or cyst (Chap. 53)

The unifying clinical feature is the presence of chronic furuncle-like nodules that lead to scars, sinuses and fistulas. The most common site is the axillae, but the inframammary folds and breasts,

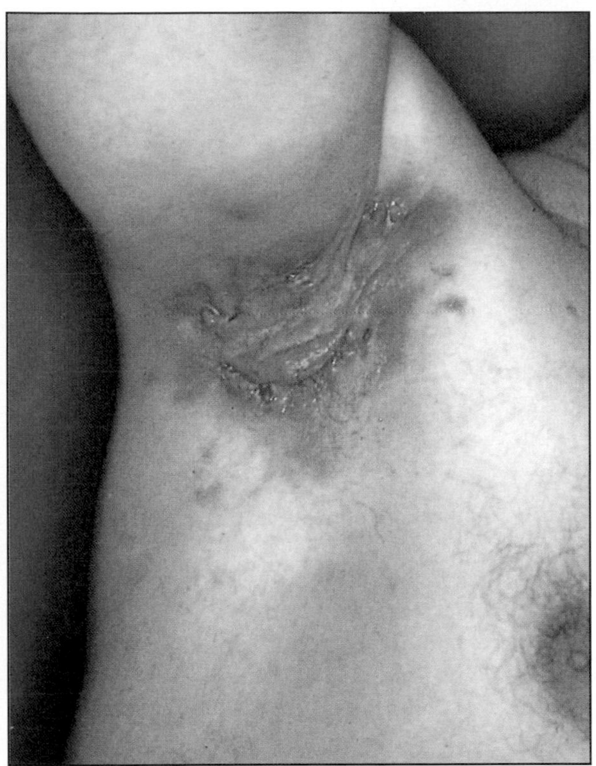

Fig. 28.5. Acne inversa

inguinal folds, scrotum, mons pubis and labia majora can all be involved. Other sites include the perineum, perianal area, buttocks and even the antecubital and popliteal fossae. The initial lesion is a superficial painful red nodule resembling a furuncle that enlarges, spreads downward and eventually ruptures with formation of sinuses, fistulas and scarring. Only small superficial lesions heal without scarring. Secondary comedones may be seen, but primary ones are not present. The tracts can extend to the deep fascia, while the scarring involves all the adnexal structures and can cause contractures. The combination of acute and chronic pain, systemic symptoms and foul-smelling drainage makes acne inversa an unpleasant disease.

On the scalp the situation is slightly different. Perifolliculitis capitis abscedens et suffodiens is a tongue-twister but accurate. The inflammation begins on the nape usually but spreads to involve much of the scalp. Almost all patients are adult men. A classic clinical finding is the presence of tufted or paintbrush hairs, where multiple hairs emerge from a single dilated follicle. Rare patients have nevoid tufted hairs; they are perhaps predisposed to the problem. The painful draining nodules, sinus tracts and scarring are all present. The sinus tracts may extend to the fascia. The process is often very widespread; when one presses on the scalp, serous fluid drains out not only at the expected sinus opening, but at distant points. The resultant alopecia is described as moth-eaten. The process is chronic and very unpleasant.

The relationship of the other clinical problems to acne and to each other often eludes the clinician. Typically, the patient with only axillary involvement is treated for years for "boils", before acne inversa is diagnosed. If appropriately cultured, the lesions are sterile or contain mixed flora including both gram-positive and gram-negative bacteria. Only later, if the disease process worsens or spreads, are other diagnoses considered. Acne inversa patients are truly sick; they may have fever, malaise and elevated erythrocyte sedimentation rate as well as leukocytosis and other laboratory markers of chronic disease.

Some unfortunate individuals are disabled by the disease as huge, confluent, fluctuant and then later indurated masses develop in the axillae, groin or buttocks. They invariably heal with massive scarring and sinus tracts. Contractures may develop. The persistent drainage in the inguinal and perianal region may require the patient to wear adult diapers. At the top of the anal fold multiple hairs may protrude from a scarred tract. Often the patients have had surgery for a pilonidal sinus or cyst in the past, so only an operative scar is present. The psychologic and social implications of this disease are enormous. Many patients develop emotional problems, as they are rejected by their friends and family because of unsightly appearance, odor and other hygienic issues. Alcoholism and difficulty in retaining steady employment are common problems.

Histopathology. While biopsy is seldom performed, abundant histologic material is available because surgery plays such a role in treatment. Deep abscesses are found, centered around follicles but also involving other adnexal structures as well as the intervening dermis. Inflammation may extend to the fascia, especially with scalp lesions. Foreign body granulomas are present, often associated with remnants of hairs.

Course and Prognosis. The course is long and frustrating. Chronic problems include the development of secondary amyloidosis and of squamous cell carcinoma in areas of chronic inflammation and ulceration (Marjolin ulcer: MARJOLIN 1823).

Differential Diagnosis. Acute bacterial infections of the flexural areas do occur and can also be designated hidradenitis suppurativa. It is almost impossible to separate a bacterial lesion from the onset of the long process of acne inversa.

Granuloma inguinale, Crohn disease, vegetating or blastomycotic pyoderma, actinomycosis, sporotrichosis and tuberculosis may also cause chronic draining abscesses. On the scalp, a deep *Trichophyton* infection should be excluded, as well as other forms of folliculitis. While the scarring on the nape can resemble acne keloidalis, the latter process is associated with much less inflammation.

Therapy

Surgical. The mainstay of therapy is surgery, rather than medical management. If small lesions are excised, often the disease course can be arrested. Thus while an axillary, nuchal or inguinal incision is not a simple procedure, in the long run, it offers patients the best outlook. If severe disease is present, we often treat with isotretinoin for several months prior to surgery. Incision and drainage may help relieve acute pain but produces an effect similar to that of the natural disease – scarring with tract formation.

Systemic. Oral retinoids alone bring improvement during the time of treatment, but relapse is almost inevitable, in contrast to ordinary acne. Systemic antibiotics may help acute lesions but lead to the presence of resistant strains of bacteria and do not alter the long-term course. When inflammation is extreme, short courses of systemic corticosteroids are also helpful. In the past, some women were treated with oral contraceptives of the antiandrogen type because of the alleged phenomenon of premenstrual flares. We do not recommend this approach.

Topical. Patients immediately report the futility of topical treatment once lesions have developed. Nonetheless, routine use of antibacterial scrubs, such as chlorhexidine, and disinfectant solutions or lotions may reduce the bacterial load and play a minor role in reducing the number of lesions or the degree of secondary infection.

Bodybuilding Acne

The use of androgenic steroids to increase muscle mass and improve athletic function may lead to papulopustular acne, acne conglobata and, in the particularly unfortunate patient, acne fulminans. Typically the patient has had mild acne prior to embarking upon androgen misuse; in other instances, an increase in the dose of the hormone leads to a dramatic change in the acne (Fig. 28.6). Not surprisingly, similar changes can occur when androgens are administered for medical purposes, such as speeding up the closing of the epiphyses in a rapidly growing individual.

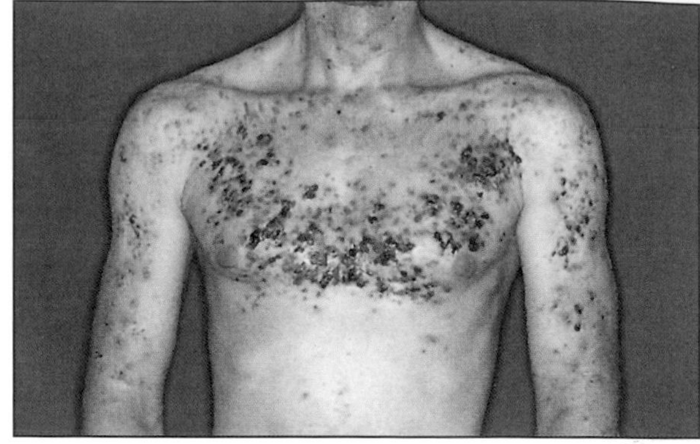

Fig. 28.6. Bodybuilding acne

Acne Mechanica

(Mills and Kligman 1975)

Mechanical factors can worsen an otherwise mild or moderate acne. The best example in the USA is acne of the shoulders and forehead in football players. Hippie acne describes the exacerbation of acne beneath a head band. Other triggering factors may include suspenders, belts, other items of clothing and back packs. In mechanical acne inflammation of microcomedones occurs and then secondarily larger comedones may develop.

Another special type of mechanical acne is the violinist's or fiddler's bump, which develops where the violin is pressed against the mandible and neck. Here ingrown hairs are also a problem, especially in males.

Acne Venenata

Synonym. Contact acne

When acne is clinically atypical or develops in patients of the "wrong" age group, one should think clinically of contact acne or acne venenata (*venenum* = poison). Patients with seborrhea, large skin pores, and previous or current acne are more predisposed to this problem. A wide variety of substances, including many occupational exposures, may lead to comedones, papules, pustules and even more severe acne forms. Many different variations of contact acne have been described.

Cosmetic Acne

Typically women past their teens are involved. They develop primarily small closed comedones, although occasionally open comedones may be seen (Fig. 28.7). The most common sites are the cheeks, zygomatic arch, forehead and chin. The offending agents are usually thick ointments, although consistency alone is not the determining factor. In the past, many cosmetics were comedogenic, but careful testing has eliminated most offenders. Occasionally the comedones become inflamed and even scar. A variant is the toxic or follicular reaction, in which a patient over a period of days develops a blend between folliculitis and acne, produced by an acute irritation of the follicle rather than by comedo formation.

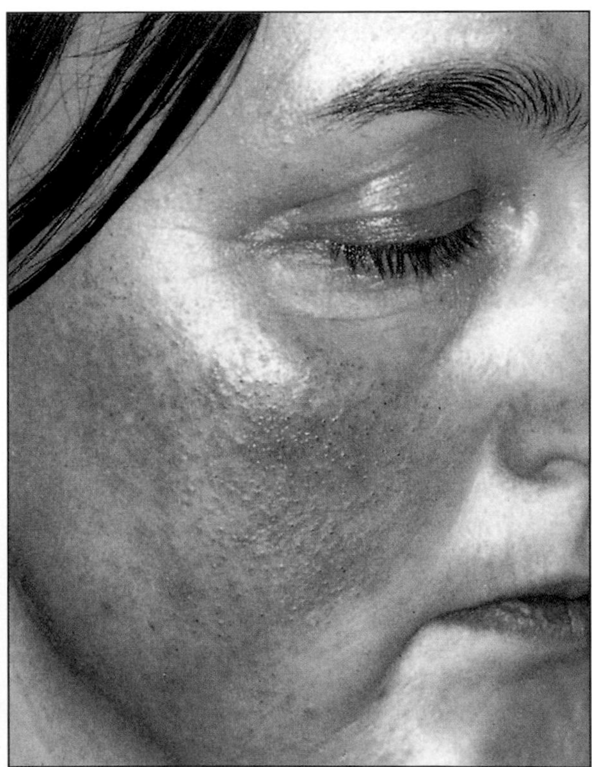

Fig. 28.7. Acne cosmetica

Pomade Acne

(PLEWIG et al. 1970)

Patients with curly hair who employ greasy hair care products (pomades) to make hair care easier and relieve dryness may develop a comedonal acne of the forehead. The hair care products almost invariably also reach this area; occasionally lesions are also seen on the cheeks. The history usually yields the correct diagnosis.

Oil, Tar and Pitch Acne

Cuttings oils, other petroleum products, tars in refineries and road construction and pitch can cause a chronic comedonal acne. Both direct contact with the chemical and indirect contact through soiled work clothes play a role. While grinders typically have oils sprayed onto the face and upper part of the chest, other workers, such as lathe operators and mechanics, may have soiled clothing, especially the upper pants legs, leading to acne of the thighs. The initial lesion is a comedo, which is often discolored by the oil or tar. Chronic exposure to pitch coupled with light exposure in road construction workers can lead to chronic pitch dermatitis, a recognized occupational skin disease in Germany. Patients typically have comedones, gray-brown hyperpigmentation of the eyelids, yellow sclerae, cutane-ous atrophy and elastosis and multiple skin tumors. Rarely, ingestion or inhalation of tar products may occur, but this is a greater problem in the next group.

Chloracne

Halogenated hydrocarbons, especially cyclic products, are likely to produce a variety of toxic changes. Prototypic agents include penta- and hexachloronaphthalene as well as halogenated biphenyl and polyhalogenated dibenzofurans, dioxins, azobenzenes and azoxybenzenes. While topical effects are possible, systemic absorption is held responsible for most of the changes. Best known in the USA is Agent Orange, a pesticide used during the Vietnam war. Patients typically develop a severe acne conglobata-like eruption initially, along with severe liver and bone marrow changes. If the exposure is massive, death may result. The acne characteristically involves not only the face, neck and retroauricular area, but also sites such as the axilla, groin or lower leg that are not involved by acne vulgaris. As the exposure is removed and the disease process improves, comedones often remain the only stigmata (Fig. 28.8).

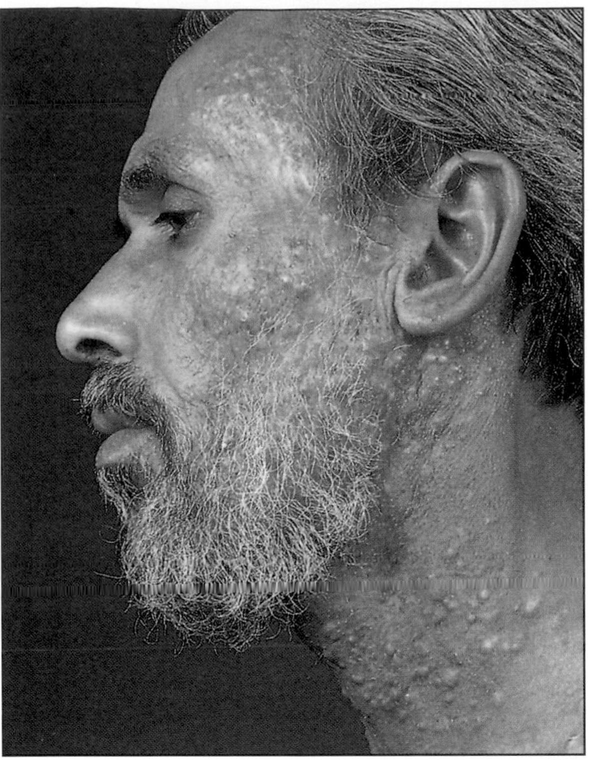

Fig. 28.8. Chloracne

A number of accidents have provided the best examples of chloracne, including Basel disease (presumably through exposure in the extensive chemical industry in that city), perna illness (from perchlornaphthalene exposure) following an explosion at the BASF chemical plant in Ludwigshafen, Germany, in 1953, Yusho illness from contaminated cooking oil in Japan, and the Seveso, Italy, accident in 1976 in which 2,3,78-tetrachloro-dibenzo-*p*-dioxin (TCDD) was released. Chloracne was seen once again in the war between Iraq and Iran, presumably from chemical warfare.

Comedones from Ionizing Radiation

The comedo reaction may occur following therapeutic radiation, including X-rays, cobalt and radium treatments. The lesions are almost exclusively comedones and they are limited to the area of irradiation.

Androgenic Syndromes

Acne is one of the characteristics seen in women with excessive androgen secretion. Other signs of virilization include hypertrichosis, male pattern alopecia, altered secondary hair patterns, menstrual abnormalities, clitoromegaly and deepened voice. Often a preexisting mild acne may suddenly become much more severe. The most likely causes are tumors or hyperplasias of either the adrenal cortex or ovary, whose metabolic pathways are deranged, leading to production of hormones with predominantly androgen function. The most common example is Stein-Leventhal syndrome with polycystic ovaries. Another well-defined entity is the functioning androluteoma of pregnancy.

Premenstrual and Postmenstrual Acne; Postmenopausal Acne

Many women experience a flare around the time of menses, usually featuring deep nodules most likely to involve the chin. Similar problems may arise after discontinuing oral contraceptives, after delivery, and during menopause. This is best viewed as a phenomenon, not a disease entity; some patients have almost no acne except for their flares; others have significant acne which then becomes worse. Clearly the changing hormone levels must be involved, but an exact physiologic explanation is not available.

Acne Neonatorum and Acne Infantum

(Crocker 1884)

Some children have acne at the time of birth or develop it shortly thereafter. Infants with acne tend to have both comedones and papulopustular lesions, but rarely nodules. The forehead and cheeks are most often involved (Fig. 28.9). The disease tends to regress spontaneously. The high levels of androgens produced by the adrenal cortex and an increased responsiveness of the sebaceous glands to androgens are felt to be key factors. This form is known as acne neonatorum and it must be carefully distinguished from acne infantum, which develops later in life and is more severe and more persistent.

Typically acne infantum starts after 1 year of life and involves the cheeks; usually deep, often confluent, nodular lesions are present in addition to papules and pustules. Comedones are often difficult to find, just as in acne conglobata, and acne infantum may be so severe that it is designated acne conglobata of infancy. Scarring is often seen, and the course may be protracted. The cause is unclear, but one must search for elevated androgen levels, produced either by the adrenal gland or by the gonads.

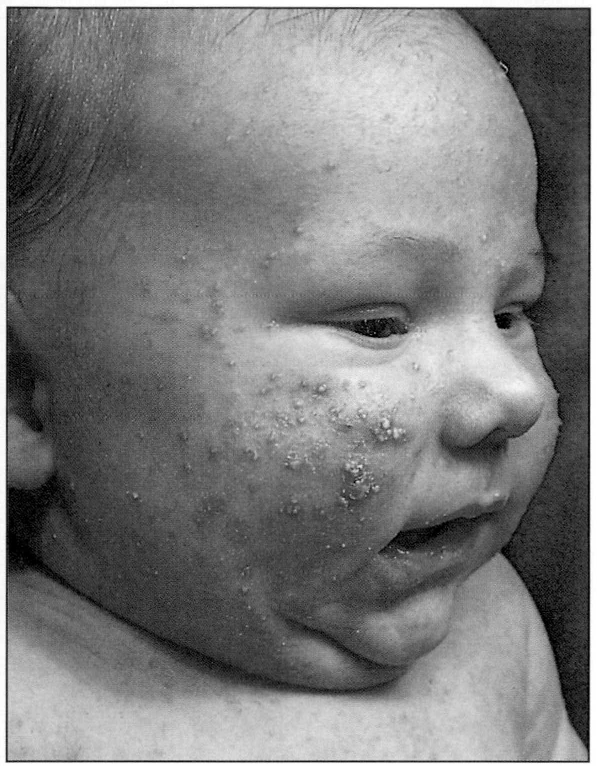

Fig. 28.9. Acne neonatorum

In contrast to acne neonatorum, treatment is necessary. We usually employ topical benzoyl peroxide initially, but are often forced to advance through the entire spectrum of teenage acne medications including systemic erythromycin. We have seen rare cases of acne infantum requiring systemic retinoids.

Both of these forms of childhood acne must be distinguished from contact acne of infancy. Infants are frequently overtreated with ointments and creams by anxious parents and develop a cosmetic acne. The forehead and cheeks are most commonly involved, often with large numbers of comedones. Once the comedogenic care products are stopped, the acne tends to resolve rapidly.

Acne Excoriée des Jeunes Filles

Some girls and young women, as well as an occasional male patient, are so distressed by what an outside observer perceives as minimal acne that they literally attack their lesions. Using either fingernails or instruments, they attempt to squeeze out or scratch away the disturbing spot, usually producing a hemorrhagic crusted excoriation or superficial ulcer. Such lesions invariably heal with scarring and hypo- or depigmentation. Common sites are the forehead, cheeks, chest and especially the hairline. Along the hairline the differential diagnosis includes acne necrotica. Even after the patient is told that her manipulation of minor lesions is producing far more scarring than the natural disease would, she is usually unable to stop picking.

Treatment includes a careful and sensitive psychosocial approach to the patient. One's treatment should be verbal, not prescriptional. The patient must be somehow sufficiently reassured that she is able to stop picking. Topical or systemic acne therapy is warranted only if true acne lesions are present. In some cases, professional counseling becomes essential.

Solid Facial Edema of Acne

(Connelly and Winkelmann 1985)

Synonyms. Persistent facial swelling in acne, persistent facial induration in acne, Morbihan disease

Definition. Firm indurated symmetric swelling, usually of the midface, in acne patients; not edema but instead fibrosis of the dermal connective tissue.

Etiology and Pathogenesis. The cause of this rare problem remains a mystery. It is different from persistent facial lymphedema recurrent herpes simplex and erysipelas, which tends to be unilateral. The exact relationship to acne is unclear; often the acne is quite mild and the swelling most distressing. The dermal fibrosis is often accompanied by numerous mast cells, which may play an etiologic role.

Clinical Findings. Swelling of the forehead, upper lids, cheeks, nasolabial folds or bridge of the nose alters the patient's appearance. The changes are often so subtle that one must compare the current appearance with old photographs to appreciate them. Otherwise the patient's complaints may be ignored. The swellings cannot be indented or blanched; erythema and scaling are not present. The swelling tends to be persistent, often lasting years.

Histopathology. Massive subcutaneous fibrosis is found without edema. Numerous mast cells are present, especially around vessels. No granuloma formation, as seen in rosacea with edema, occurs.

Differential Diagnosis. Melkersson-Rosenthal syndrome may present with persistent upper lip swelling; granulomas are found on biopsy. Elephantiasis nostras, or persistent lymphedema following recurrent erysipelas, is usually unilateral and has a different course with waxing and waning. Persistent facial edema is also seen in rosacea patients and has been described in patients without acne or rosacea.

Therapy

Systemic. Isotretinoin 0.1–0.5 mg/kg daily combined with an H1-antagonist such as ketotifen 1.0 mg b.i.d. has produced the best results. Therapy must be continued for many months. Clofazimine 100 mg daily has also been used with success in single cases.

Table 28.3. Causes of acneiform drug reactions

Common
Corticosteroids
Hydantoin
Lithium
Less common
Oral contraceptives
Androgens
Halides
Isoniazid, ethionamide, rifampin
Tetracyclines
Disulfuram
PUVA
Barbiturates
Cyclosporine
Vitamins B2, B6, B12

Acneiform Disorders

There are a number of diseases that clinically resemble acne and are often called acne but differ significantly. The primary lesion in acne is the microcomedo; in the acneiform disorders, the primary lesion is follicular inflammation and comedones are generally fewer in number and secondary.

Acneiform Drug Reactions

A wide variety of medications may lead to an acneiform exanthem. Just as with acne vulgaris, the most common sites of involvement are the face, chest and back, where large sebaceous follicles are present. The exanthem tends to be monomorphous, arise rapidly and have relatively few comedones. Possible causative agents are shown in Table 28.3 (Fig. 28.10).

The most common cause of iatrogenic acne are corticosteroids; at a therapeutically useful dosage, almost every patient gets some degree of steroid acne, especially those with seborrheic skin. Topical corticosteroids can also produce an acneiform exanthem. In steroid acne, comedones are common. Even if corticosteroids can be stopped, comedones may persist. Topical tretinoin therapy is useful (Fig. 28.11).

Differential Diagnosis. Bacterial folliculitis and *Pityrosporum* folliculitis must be excluded. In the normal host, this is fairly easy, as bacterial culture and biopsy suffice. In immunosuppressed patients, one must search diligently for eosinophilic pustulosis and other more exotic infectious forms of folliculitis.

Mallorca Acne

(Hjorth et al. 1972)

Synonym. Acne aestivalis

This acne-like eruption usually begins in the spring, peaks in early summer and then heals without scarring but is likely to recur. Hjorth and colleagues

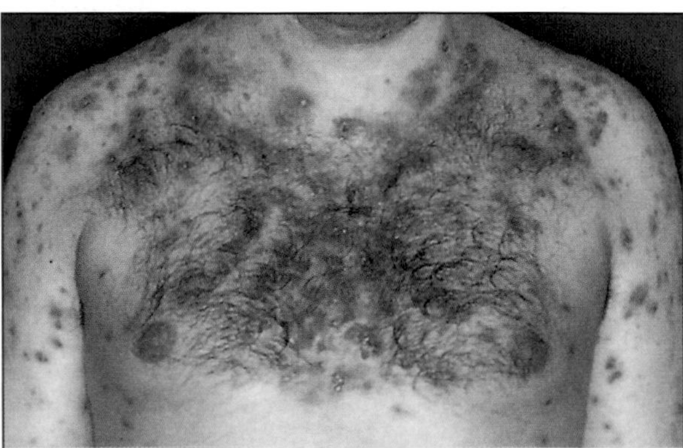

Fig. 28.10. Acneiform drug eruption caused by doxycycline

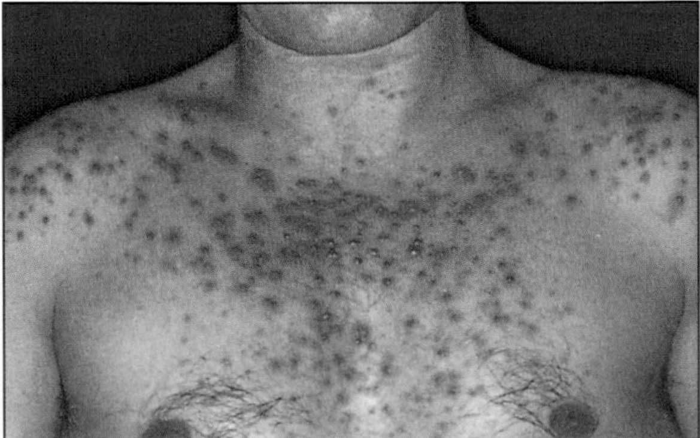

Fig. 28.11. Steroid acne following systemic corticosteroids

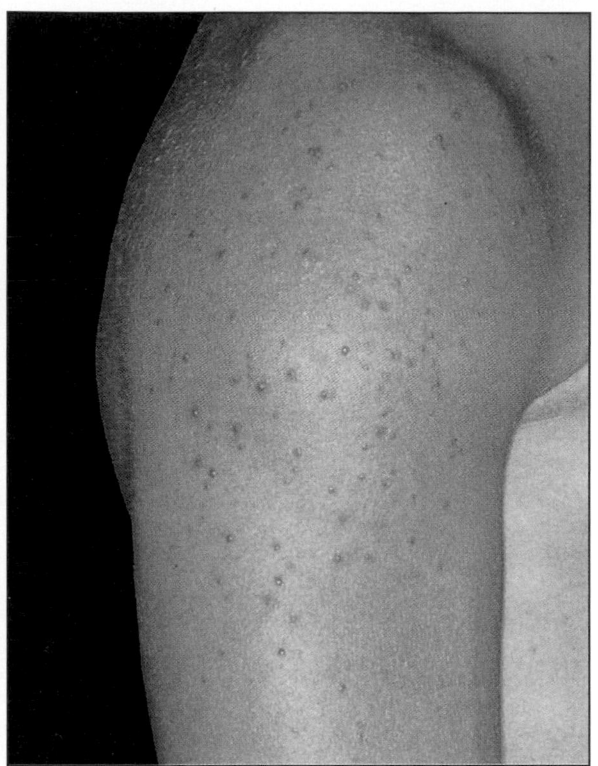

Fig. 28.12. Majorca acne

noticed it among patients from Scandinavia who traveled to Majorca, one of the Spanish Balearic Islands in the Mediterranean Sea. Typical areas of involvement include the lateral upper aspects of the arms and décolletage, although the face and back may also be affected. The lesions are monomorphous small reddish follicularly oriented keratotic papules; comedones and pustules are not seen (Fig. 28.12). Histologic examination reveals follicular hyperkeratotic plugs. Some have blamed oily sunscreens, suggesting Majorca acne is a variant of acne cosmetica, but it occurs in patients who use no sunscreens or lubricants. Similar reactions have been seen in patients treated with PUVA. Thus it is plausible that Majorca acne represents a follicular photosensitivity eruption, i.e., a variant of polymorphic light eruption. In any event, topical tretinoin or benzoyl peroxide provide the most effective therapy.

Halogen Acne

We distinguish between halogen acne and halogenoderma (iododerma or bromoderma). Halogen acne is most often an acute inflammatory exacerbation of an existing milder acne although it can arise de novo, as mentioned under acneiform drug reactions. Typical triggering agents are expectorants, sleeping pills, sedatives and other over-the-counter products. A special form is kelp acne, which develops when patients eat a diet rich in kelp or other seaweed that contain iodides.

Iododerma and Bromoderma

Longer exposures to higher amount of iodides or bromides may lead to a more dramatic clinical picture. Patients tend to develop indurated pustulonodular lesions on the face and extremities. The lesions may ulcerate or weep. They are often confused with a deep fungal infection. The clinical picture should lead one to ask about ingestion of medications, especially over-the-counter products, and measure serum or urine bromide and iodide levels. The only treatment is stopping the offending medication.

Trichostasis Spinulosa

(Landany 1954)

Trichostasis spinulosa only resembles acne clinically. Numerous small vellus hairs are retained in a sebaceous follicle. The brush-like accumulation may appear dark like a blackhead. Typical locations include the nose, cheek, forehead and neck. Trichostasis spinulosa is more common in older patients and in sun-exposed skin. The lesions can be expressed with a comedo extractor. Topical tretinoin may also be of some benefit.

Rosacea

Definition. Disorder primarily involving the midface in which papules and pustules develop on a congestive erythematous, telangiectatic background. There may be accompanying sebaceous gland hyperplasia and fibrosis, sometimes eventuating in circumscribed hypertrophy, i.e., rhinophyma.

Epidemiology. Rosacea is a common disorder. It usually starts after age 30 and peaks between age 40 and 60 years. While women are more often affected than men, the more extreme cases with rhinophyma are mainly seen in men.

Etiology and Pathogenesis. The cause of rosacea is unclear. It is not acne; the primary site of action is not the follicle. Since acne and rosacea are both so common, in some patients both diseases are present simultaneously, as rosacea gradually replaces acne. While many patients have seborrhea, others do not. Over the years many possible etiologies have been proposed including genetic predisposition, associated internal diseases, especially gastrointestinal problems, hypertension and *Demodex* infestation. None of these has been proven beyond doubt, but each has at least a grain of truth. Rosacea is very common in Ireland. Patients with hypertension may display flushing. *Demodex* folliculitis is now felt to be a separate disease. In recent years, increased emphasis has been placed on a possible gastrointestinal association, perhaps with *Helicobacter pylori*; this might explain the therapeutic success often achieved with topical or systemic antibiotics. There is an increased vascular response to warmth; warm drinks (not necessarily caffeinated drinks as previously thought) evoke flushing. Sunlight is a cofactor; almost all rosacea arises against the background of actinically damaged skin, as histologic studies confirm.

Clinical Findings. Early signs of rosacea may be discerned in young adults, but are often ignored. There may be a persistent dusky erythema, especially of the nose, as well as recurrent and then persistent facial erythema (flushers and blushers). Rosacea is a centrofacial disease that characteristically goes through stages of evolution. The most typical sites of involvement are the nose, cheeks, forehead and chin; less common sites include the retroauricular region, the décolletage, the upper aspect of the back, the side of the neck and the scalp. The natural course of the disease is slow progression. The stages typically include:

Transitory Erythema. Numerous stimuli produce a transitional erythema of the midface; typical triggers include heat, sunlight, emotional stress and warm beverages. Blushing is erythema in response to emotional stress; flushing is a general term for all such transitory erythema.

Persistent Erythema and Telangiectases (Grade I Rosacea). Later the erythema may become more persistent, lasting days or even becoming permanent. Many telangiectases arise, typically on the cheeks. They tend to be cosmetically disturbing.

Papules and Pustules (Grade II Rosacea). Gradually small, succulent, often grouped papules appear, primarily on the nose, medial aspects of the cheeks, chin, and forehead. They may have a fine scale. At the same time, some pustules develop; they are typically sterile or contain the normal facial flora (Figs. 28.13, 28.14). Edema is also a feature of this stage, as the patient may complain of fullness or thickening of the skin. No comedones are seen. The lesions tend to heal without scarring over weeks. Rarely the lesions may spread from the typical midfacial involvement to other areas of the head, neck and upper parts of the trunk.

Nodules and Plaques (Grade III Rosacea). The inflammatory lesions may become larger and coalesce. At the same time, fibrosis and sebaceous glands hyperplasia may create diffuse enlargement of a region of skin, known as a phyma.

There are also a number of other subsets that differ from classic rosacea. They include the following lesions.

Persistent Edema of Rosacea

The almost invariable edema may progress along with fibrosis to produce a nonpitting solid facial

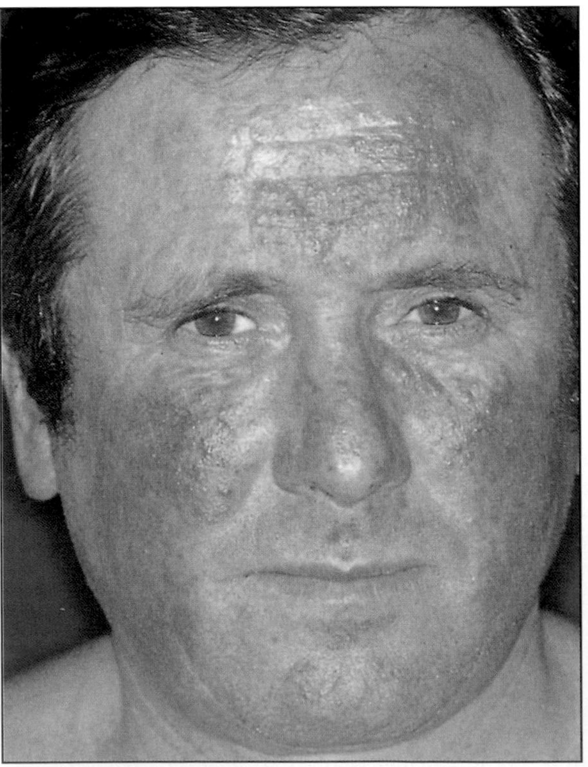

Fig. 28.13. Rosacea

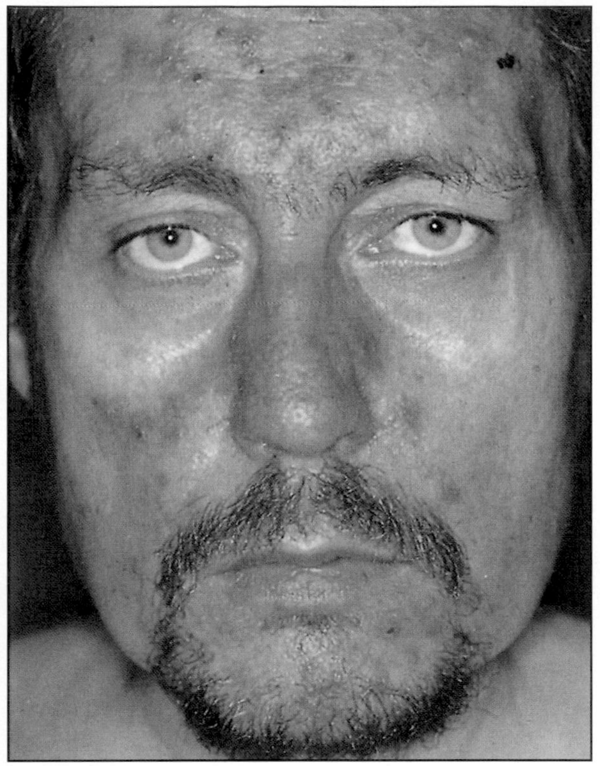

Fig. 28.14. Rosacea

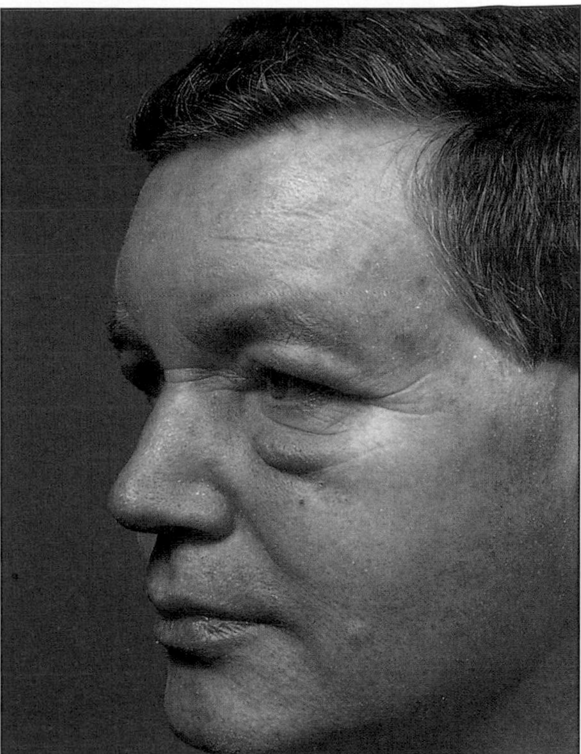

Fig. 28.15. Facial edema in rosacea

edema, just as discussed under acne vulgaris. Typically the forehead, glabella or cheeks are involved (Fig. 28.15). The diagnosis may be overlooked, as occasionally the other manifestations of rosacea are not prominent.

Lupoid Rosacea

Some patients develop numerous small red-brown papules or nodules which on diascopy have the apple-jelly color of cutaneous tuberculosis. Typical sites of involvement are the eyelids and the perioral region. Histologically the granulomatous changes are more prominent. The course is chronic. A series of confusing differential diagnostic issues are raised. Steroid rosacea can be identical, but should improve when treatment is stopped. Sarcoidosis can be excluded by histologic examination (sarcoid granulomas) and general evaluation. Lupoid perioral dermatitis tends to be more severe around the mouth and shows follicular changes under the microscope. Finally, lupus miliaris disseminatus faciei (Chap. 4) can be identical; most authors today feel that this alleged tuberculid is a rosacea variant, or lupoid perioral dermatitis.

Steroid Rosacea

(Leyden et al. 1974)

If rosacea patients are treated over long periods of time with topical corticosteroids, they may develop even more erythema, coupled with atrophy, pustules and even comedones. Typically, when the corticosteroid is stopped, the underlying disease flares. A rosacea-like picture may also develop in patients with other skin diseases treated with mid- to high-potency topical corticosteroids.

Ocular Rosacea

Synonyms. Ophthalmic rosacea, "rabbit eyes"

Rosacea is one of the few skin diseases with well-defined ocular findings. Up to 58% of rosacea patients have ocular abnormalities, including blepharitis, conjunctivitis, iritis, iridocyclitis, hypopyon or keratitis (Fig. 28.16). The skin and ocular diseases tend not to correlate well. Many patients are treated by ophthalmologists for a period of time before the possibility of ocular rosacea is raised; conversely, dermatologists may fail to question rosacea patients about ocular problems and thus overlook a serious

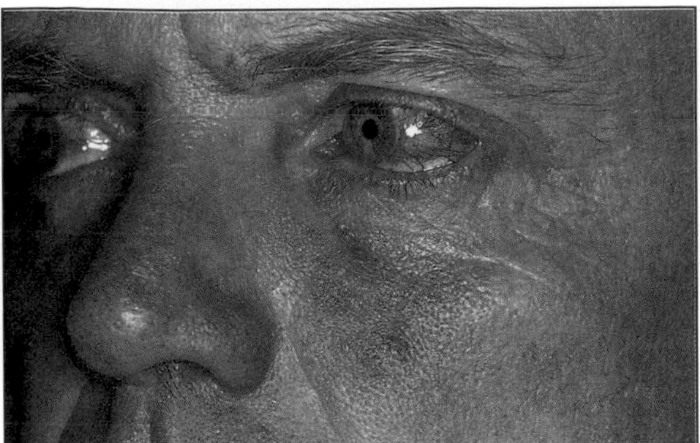

Fig. 28.16. Ocular rosacea

complication. We refer almost all patients with rosacea for baseline ophthalmologic evaluation. The most feared problem is rosacea keratitis, which can lead to blindness and necessitate a corneal transplant. Far more common are blepharitis and keratoconjunctivitis with photophobia and a foreign body sensation.

Rhinophyma

The localized tissue enlargement associated with rosacea is known as a phyma. The classic example is rhinophyma, producing a bulbous, sometimes grotesque nose (Fig. 28.17), perhaps best known in the comedian W. C. Fields. Such a nose was formerly known as drinker's nose, but that is an unwarranted stigma that only adds to the burden of this distressing cosmetic change. Other rarer sites include the forehead (mentophyma), chin (gnathophyma) and ears (otophyma) and eyelids (blepharophyma).

The bulbous changes of the nose develop as a result of fibrosis, sebaceous gland hyperplasia and telangiectases. The nose may enlarge asymmetrically, with nodules of varied size and orientation. While typical changes of rosacea are also usually present, they may be lacking. Rhinophyma is almost exclusively a disease of men.

Rosacea Conglobata

Sometimes rosacea becomes more severe; necrotic hemorrhagic nodules and plaques appear. Just as in the more common acne conglobata, the lesions fuse together with sinus tracts and often drain. The changes are usually confined to the typical areas of facial involvement, i.e., the medial aspects of the cheeks and the forehead.

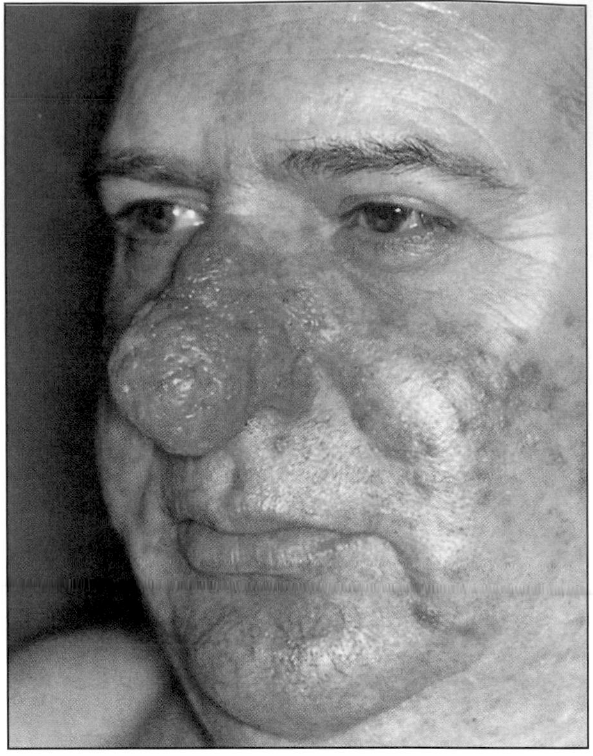

Fig. 28.17. Rhinophyma

Histopathology. While rosacea is usually a clinical diagnosis, the histopathology can help and is often instructive. In the early phase, only dilated blood vessels are seen. As the disease progresses, lymphectasias, actinic elastosis, edema and a perivascular and perifollicular lymphohistiocytic infiltrate appear. Small, poorly organized granulomas may be seen; in lupoid rosacea they are more common and better defined. Later the follicles are more definitely involved with spongiosis, while dermal fibrosis and sebaceous gland hyperplasia are also found. The infundibula are widely dilated and course through the altered dermis; they are filled with debris and often contain *Demodex folliculorum* mites.

In the phymas, each of the excess components may predominate. In the glandular form, there is marked sebaceous gland hyperplasia and prominent follicular filaments (debris from the enlarged follicles). In the fibrous form, the nose is quite firm and more uniformly enlarged, usually with marked actinic elastosis. Sometimes the actinic changes dominate; then one speaks of actinic rhinophyma. In the fibroangiomatous form, the persistent erythema and papulopustular lesions are most evident.

Differential Diagnosis. Usually rosacea is a straightforward diagnosis. In younger patients, there may be an overlap with acne vulgaris. Furthermore, perioral dermatitis and steroid acne may cause confusion. *Demodex folliculorum* infestations must also be excluded. When rhinophyma is present, one may consider sarcoidosis, leukemic infiltrates, and the leonine facies of cutaneous T cell lymphoma. Biopsy usually provides a rapid answer.

Therapy

Systemic. Oral tetracyclines as discussed under acne are effective in roughly the same dosages. We usually start with minocycline or doxycycline 50 mg b.i.d.; after clinical improvement is seen, we reduce the dose to 50 mg daily or even q.o.d. Usually treatment must be continued over many months, but at this dosage level problems are uncommon. The mechanism of action of tetracyclines in rosacea is unknown, but probably reflects their antiinflammatory properties. Tetracyclines also provide the best treatment for ocular rosacea, where they are strikingly antiinflammatory. The ophthalmologist may want to add artificial tears and topical corticosteroid eye drops as adjunctive therapy.

A second antibiotic that is generally effective is metronidazole, which can be used in dosages of 250–500 mg daily over a period of 2–3 weeks. There is an antabuse-like effect, so alcohol consumption must be avoided. Because of this and many other side effects, long-term therapy is not possible. Systemic metronidazole is not approved for rosacea in either the USA or Germany.

The most effective systemic therapy is isotretinoin, used in dosages of 0.2–1.0 mg/kg daily for 3–4 months. Long-term remissions can often be achieved. Isotretinoin is the treatment of choice for rosacea conglobata. Treatment smoothes the rest of the face, reduces sebaceous gland hyperplasia, lessens oiliness and eliminates edema. In other words, the entire face is somewhat rejuvenated as the rosacea is treated. Exactly the same precautions discussed under acne must be followed.

If *Helicobacter pylori* infection in the stomach can be documented, and especially if there are additional gastrointestinal signs or symptoms, then a course of therapy to eradicate this organism is well worth considering.

Topical. Irritating cleansing agents and alcoholic solutions should be avoided as they may provoke flushing. Topical antibiotics are usually effective; topical metronidazole (Metrogel 0.75 % gel or cream in the USA) is perhaps better than topical erythromycin. In some studies, a higher concentration of metronidazole (up to 2.0 %) has been employed; it can be compounded easily in a cream base. Azelaic acid 20.0 % cream and topical imidazoles, such as ketoconazole (Nizoral 2.0 % cream), can also be tried. Older rosacea creams, lotions and pastes usually contained sulfur or ichthyol; they are minimally effective and we no longer use them.

Topical corticosteroids should be avoided; with chronic use, even products of relatively low potency may cause steroid rosacea. The initial reduction in erythema through vasoconstriction is not maintained. The only exception is in treating rosacea fulminans.

Other Measures. While a rosacea diet has been recommended for many years, it has no scientific basis. Patients should simply avoid agents known to cause flushing, such as warm beverages and, in some cases, alcohol. If the patient is not a flusher, then no dietary instruction is needed.

An adjunct sometimes useful in the erythematous phase is facial massage, as described by Sobye. The patient is encouraged to spend 2–3 min each evening massaging the cheeks, nose and forehead to reduce edema. While controlled studies are not available, this harmless technique may help and gets patients involved in their disease care. Patients should be encouraged to use a broad-spectrum (UVB and UVA) sunscreen regularly, as sunlight is often a cofactor.

Surgical. Rhinophyma is a surgical problem. The excessive tissue can be shaved off with a blade or disposable razor, sanded away with a dermabrader, cut off with a hot loop or vaporized with a CO_2 laser. The choice of techniques depends on the individual skills and preferences of the surgeon. The hot loop tends to produce more scarring than the other forms. In general, parts of the deep prominent follicular infundibulum are left behind and serve as the nidus for reepithelialization. We recommend treatment with isotretinoin 0.5–1.0 mg/kg daily for 4 weeks before and 4 weeks after the surgical procedure.

Telangiectases can be treated with electrosurgery or a variety of lasers. Nodular lesions sometimes respond to cryotherapy.

Rosacea Fulminans
(Plewig et al. 1992)

Synonym. Pyoderma faciale (O'Leary and Kierland 1940)

This illness typically appears suddenly on the midface of young women; we interpret it as the maximum variant of rosacea and have thus named it rosacea fulminans in analogy to acne fulminans (Fig. 28.18). We believe it is identical to pyoderma faciale. Patients typically have almost an eruption of draining erythematous plaques with pustules involving their cheeks, chin and forehead. We have seen such patients later develop typical rosacea. The main differential diagnosis is acne fulminans, which occurs almost exclusively in young men who usually have some other stigmata of acne. Androgen-producing tumors, bromoderma and iododerma must be excluded, but tend to have a slower onset.

Therapy. Short courses of oral prednisone (20–40 mg daily) for 1–2 weeks can speed resolution of severe rosacea. Corticosteroids can be given for several weeks prior to institution of isotretinoin therapy in rosacea conglobata and rosacea fulminans.

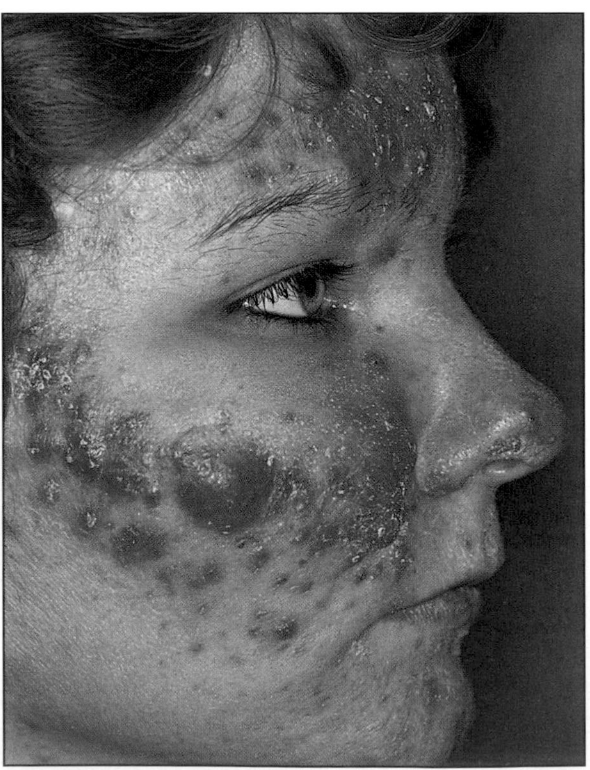

Fig. 28.18. Rosacea fulminans

Rosacea-like Disorders

Demodicosis

Synonyms. Demodex folliculitis, *Demodex* rosacea, pityriasis folliculorum

Etiology and Pathogenesis. In adults, especially the elderly, many hair follicles contain *Demodex folliculorum* mites; under some conditions, they can be pathogenic. The presence of the mites, eggs and feces leads to an inflamed spongiotic follicle which then leaks its contents into the surrounding dermis, causing a foreign body reaction. Other animal species such as dogs (*Demodex canis*) and cattle suffer severe demodectic mange.

Clinical Findings. Demodicosis is more common in elderly patients. *Demodex folliculorum* causes a rosacea-like appearance in humans. There are typically follicular papules and pustules, especially on the cheeks (Fig. 28.19). Unilateral distribution speaks for *Demodex folliculorum* and against rosacea. There may also be a fine scale and pruritus. The eyelids are also likely to be involved (*Demodex* blepharitis). There is scaling and crusting along the lid edge, while the organisms are found in the lid hair follicles (cilia) and meibomian glands. The infestation tends to be chronic and is often overlooked.

Histopathology. The mite must be identified. In addition, some degree of quantification is needed, as an occasional mite is often seen in facial follicles. The follicular contents can be extruded with a comedo extractor or using the cyanoacrylate technique. In the latter, a drop of rapidly drying glue is placed on the lesion and then touched with a glass slide. After the glue has dried, the slide is pulled off, removing the stratum corneum and follicular contents. If the material is examined under the microscope within 10 min, moving mites are seen. The mites can be quantified by counting the number of organisms per dislodged sebaceous filament in 1 cm^2 of skin surface. Often three to six mites per follicle plug are found.

Histologic examination is also helpful. A spongiotic follicle is seen, filled with mites whose heads are typically pointed towards the follicular opening. There is associated inflammation and occasionally a foreign body reaction in the adjacent dermis.

Therapy
Systemic. No specific internal therapy is available. Isotretinoin often leads to improvement by reduc-

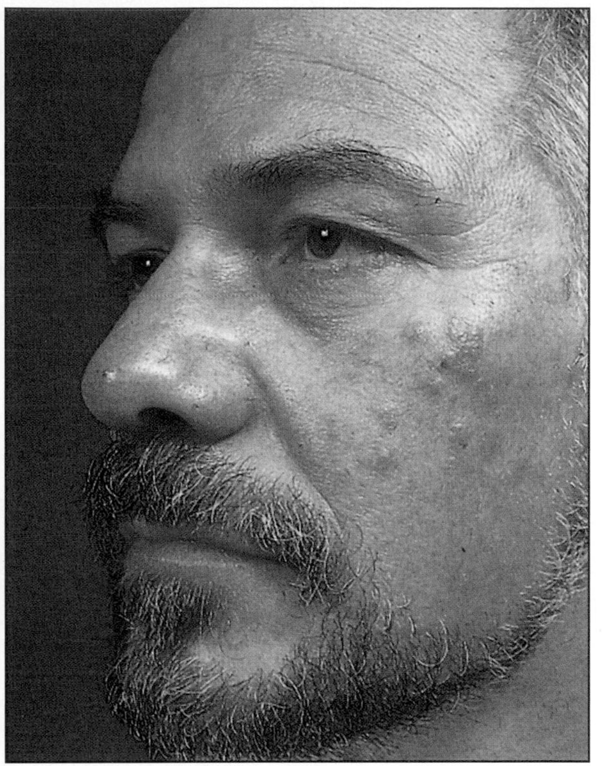

Fig. 28.19. Demodicosis

ing the sebum and narrowing the follicular canal, making the follicular microenvironment less hospitable for the mite.

Topical. Any of the standard antiscabetic treatments, such as lindane, crotamiton or permethrin, can be tried. Their effectiveness is debated. They can be applied once or twice weekly for several weeks. Topical pastes containing precipitated sulfur (5–10%) are also useful. The management of the lid problems is more challenging; the ophthalmologist can remove many of the mites directly under slit-lamp visualization. The permethrins are probably the least irritating topical product for this area.

Haber Syndrome

(Sanderson and Wilson 1965)

Henry Haber tragically died before he could publish his syndrome.

Synonym. Familial rosacea-like dermatitis with intraepidermal epithelioma

Definition. Very uncommon genodermatosis, probably inherited in autosomal dominant pattern, with persistent rosacea-like facial eruption and keratotic truncal lesions.

Clinical Findings. The disorder typically starts in childhood. Most patients are men. The facial skin is erythematous and often warm. The patient may complain of burning and photosensitivity. Telangiectases, dilated follicles, pustules, induration, characteristic perioral pitted scars and occasionally brown hyperpigmentation are seen. The second major feature is numerous verruciform papules and nodules, primarily on the neck and in the axillae, but also involving the trunk. The pattern in the axillae resembles Dowling-Degos disease (Chap. 26). In addition, hyperkeratotic plaques on the knees and elbows or even a diffuse ichthyosis-like hyperkeratosis may develop.

Histopathology. The facial lesions show dilated capillaries, edema and occasionally inflammation. The trunk lesions resemble pigmented seborrheic keratoses and may show intraepidermal clonal proliferations (Borst-Jadassohn phenomenon).

Differential Diagnosis. The facial lesions look like rosacea, while the trunk lesions are identical with seborrheic keratoses. The combined clinical picture should point to the correct diagnosis.

Therapy. Sunscreens are recommended. Individual seborrheic keratoses can be curetted or excised. The facial lesions are reported to respond to standard rosacea therapy; we have no personal experience of treating this disorder.

Perioral Dermatitis

(Mihan and Ayres 1964)

Synonyms. Light-sensitive seborrheid (Frumess and Lewis 1957), rosacea-like dermatitis (Steigleder and Strempel 1968), stewardess disease

Definition. Chronic often recurrent rosacea-like dermatitis, typically located around the mouth of young women.

Etiology and Pathogenesis. While its etiology is unknown, perioral dermatitis is a new disease, not found in older textbooks, that has been increasing in prevalence over the past 30 years. Many interesting theories regarding its cause have been proposed, including the following.

Irritant Reactions. One theory is that individuals with dry skin, such as atopic dermatitis patients, overuse moisturizing agents and develop follicular occlusion and irritation. Some preservatives, such as isopropylmyristate, have also been incriminated, as have fluorinated toothpastes, mouthwashes, soaps, perfumed disposable handkerchiefs, and even the partner's facial hair.

Topical Corticosteroids. There is no question that topical corticosteroids can both cause and, more often, exacerbate perioral dermatitis. The typical story is that an unclear facial condition is treated with a low-potency corticosteroid, improves, but then flares again. A higher-potency corticosteroid is then employed, and finally the patient develops full-blown perioral dermatitis. Some patients, however, develop perioral dermatitis without any use of corticosteroids. In the few men with the disease, the history of corticosteroid use is almost always obtained.

Ultraviolet Radiation. Sun exposure may also be a cofactor. Many patients describe worsening in the summer, but just as many present in the winter with relatively little light exposure.

Hormones. Because almost all patients are women, hormones and especially oral contraceptives have been blamed for perioral dermatitis. However, many patients who are not taking contraceptives develop the disorder. Some notice premenstrual flares, just as with acne vulgaris.

Miscellaneous. An infectious origin has not been established; implicated organisms include *Demodex folliculorum*, *Candida albicans,* and mixed infections. Similarly, gastrointestinal candidiasis and malabsorption have been postulated as causes, but we consider them unlikely factors.

This potpourri of alleged causes demonstrates clearly that we do not understand the etiology of perioral dermatitis. Some physicians reject perioral dermatitis as a single disorder, maintaining that it is a variant of rosacea or seborrheic dermatitis. We disagree; perioral dermatitis is a unique follicular disease.

Clinical Findings. The typical patient has numerous small red to red-brown succulent papules beginning around the mouth. Peri-perioral dermatitis would be a more accurate (but silly) name, for there is typically a spared pale area adjacent to the vermilion, then come the papules (Fig. 28.20). There may be an erythematous background and the lesions may become confluent. The lesions may burn slightly. Tiny pustules often develop; nodules are rare.

In addition to the area around the mouth, the nasolabial folds, the chin and the lateral periorbital region are typically involved. The disease occasionally involves the rest of the face, the scalp, the neck, and even the perianal region and genitalia. With extrafacial involvement, one should be most suspicious of corticosteroid use.

Lupoid or granulomatous perioral dermatitis is a clinical variant of ordinary perioral dermatitis, but the papules acquire a red-brown color, made more clear by diascopy (Fig. 28.21). They may be limited to the periorbital region. In such cases, there is almost always a history of corticosteroid use.

Histopathology. There is spongiosis and a lymphohistiocytic infiltrate, both of which involve the

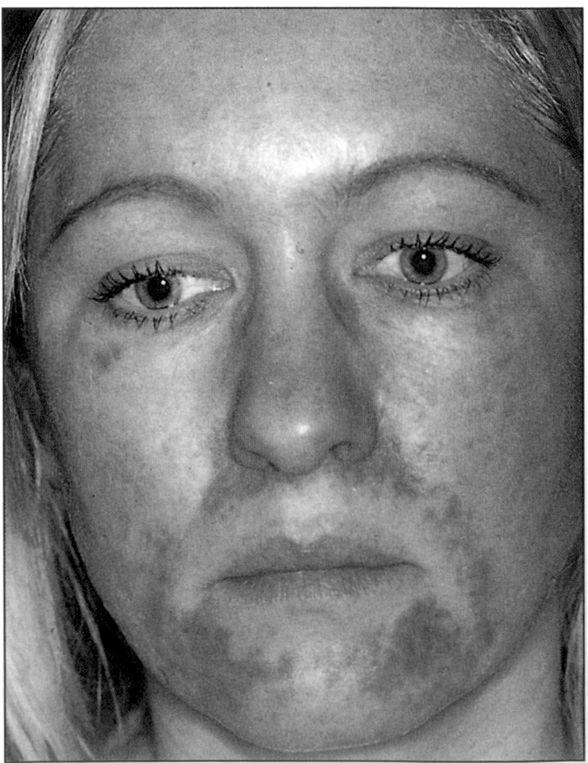

Fig. 28.20. Perioral dermatitis

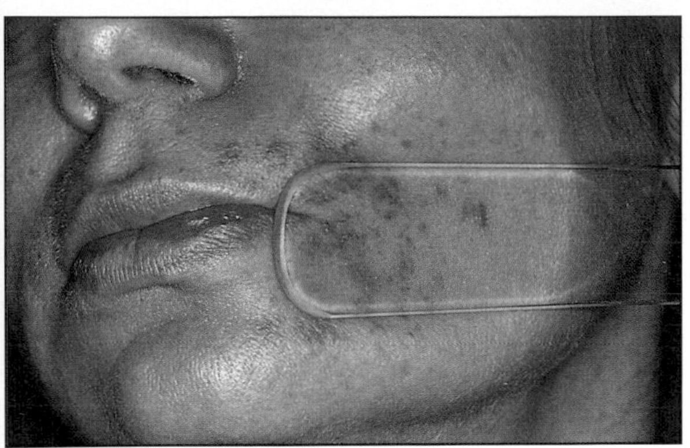

Fig. 28.21. Lupoid perioral dermatitis

vellus hair follicles. In the lupoid variant, there are granulomas located around the follicles, presumably as a response to leakage. Typical features of rosacea such as actinic elastosis, telangiectases and *Demodex folliculorum* are absent.

Course and Prognosis. The disease is chronic. It typically waxes and wanes from day to day. Topical corticosteroids produce a brief improvement and then a flare when they are discontinued. If left untreated, the disease may evolve into the lupoid form. Following treatment, the lesions resolve without scarring.

Differential Diagnosis. Perioral dermatitis is usually a straightforward clinical diagnosis. Rosacea involves a different age group and another part of the face, as does demodicosis. The main problem is to exclude side effects of topical corticosteroids used to treat atopic dermatitis, seborrheic dermatitis and even rosacea or acne.

Therapy

Systemic. Usually the tetracyclines produce prompt resolution. A typical regimen is minocycline or doxycycline 50 mg daily for about 4–6 weeks. On rare occasions, such as with more severe disease, a higher initial dose, such as 50 mg b.i.d., may be needed for 1–2 weeks. Often patients can control their disease with extremely low levels, such as 50 mg q.o.d. or even twice weekly. In very severe cases, especially associated with long-term corticosteroid use or disease of the lupoid type, isotretinoin can be considered; extremely low dosages (0.05–0.2 mg/kg daily) for 8–12 weeks are effective. Almost all patients are young women of childbearing age so the precautions become even more important.

Topical. "Zero therapy" is the goal. The patient should avoid all possible irritants, washing with just water. It is often impossible to get the patient to use nothing, and often one harmless nonocclusive moisturizing agent is better than a slew of possibly harmful ones. The patient must be forbidden to use topical corticosteroids. If the patient is unwilling or unable to take oral antibiotics, topical erythromycin or metronidazole in a gel or cream base can be used.

Miscellaneous Sebaceous Disorders

Sebaceous Hyperplasia

Many older adults develop multiple lesions of sebaceous hyperplasia, which has unfortunately been called senile sebaceous hyperplasia. The individual lesions are yellow nodules with a central pore, most common on the forehead (Chap. 57).There are several other settings in which sebaceous hyperplasia may have a different appearance.

- Organ Transplant Patients. Sebaceous hyperplasia is more common in recipients of heart or renal transplants than in age-matched controls. In Hispanic patients, this discrepancy is even more striking.
- Premature Sebaceous Hyperplasia. Some individuals develop marked sebaceous hyperplasia starting at puberty. There are multiple yellow small slightly elevated dimpled papules involving the main acne areas of the face, neck and upper aspects of the trunk. While the eruption superficially resembles acne, no comedones are present. In some instances, a positive family history is obtained, but more detailed genetic studies are lacking. Systemic isotretinoin has been effective.
- Diffuse Sebaceous Hyperplasia. Hundreds of tiny waxy papules stud the cheeks or forehead. The main differential diagnoses are eruptive vellus haircysts, milia or trichodiscomas. Systemic isotretinoin in low doses (10 mg daily) is often helpful.

Sebaceous Adenitis

(Renfro et al. 1993)

Synonyms. Neutrophilic sebaceous adenitis

In this rare disorder, annular boggy plaques are seen on the face. They resemble a pseudolymphoma, lupus erythematosus or erythema annulare centrifugum. Biopsy shows a neutrophilic infiltrate concentrated around sebaceous glands. This condition is more common in dogs, in which it is known as granulomatous sebaceous adenitis. In most human cases, resolution is spontaneous. Similar lesions have also been described as drug reactions.

Bibliography

General

Cunliffe WJ (1989) Acne. Dunitz, London

Marks R, Plewig (eds) (1989) Acne and related disorders. Dunitz, London

Plewig G, Kligman AM (2000) Acne, 3rd edn. Springer, Berlin

Stewart ME (1992) Sebaceous gland lipids. Semin Dermatol 11:100–105

Thody AJ, Shuster S (1989) Control and function of sebaceous glands. Physiol Rev 69:383–416

Acne

Brown SK, Shalita AR (1998) Acne vulgaris. Lancet 351: 1871–1876

Connelly MG, Winkelman RK (1985) Solid facial edema as a complication of acne vulgaris. Arch Dermatol 121: 87–90

Caputo R, Monti M, Ermacora E et al. (1988) Cutaneous manifestations of tetrachlorodibenzo-*p*-dioxin in children and adolescents: follow-up 10 years after the Seveso, Italy, accident. J Am Acad Dermatol 19:812–819

Driscoll MS, Rothe MJ, Abrahamian L et al. (1993) Long-term oral antibiotics for acne: is laboratory monitoring necessary? J Am Acad Dermatol 28:595–602

Eady EA, Cove JH, Jones DN et al. (1990) Topical antibiotics for the treatment of acne vulgaris: a critical evaluation of the literature on their clinical benefit and comparative efficacy. J Dermatol Treat 1:215–226

Eady EA, Jones CE, Tipper JL et al. (1993) Antibiotic resistant propionibacteria in acne: need for policies to modify antibiotic usage. Br Med J 306:555–556

Heydenreich G (1989) Testosterone and anabolic steroids and acne fulminans. Arch Dermatol 125:571–572

Jansen T, Burgdorf WHC, Plewig G (1997) Pathogenesis and treatment of acne in childhood. Pediatr Dermatol 14: 17–21

Jansen T, Plewig G (1997) Acne vulgaris. In: Demis DJ, Thiers BH, Burgdorf WHC, Raimer SS (eds) Clinical dermatology, vol 2, chap 10-2. Lippincott-Raven, Philadelphia, pp 1–37

Jansen T, Plewig G (1997) Miscellaneous acne disorders. In: Demis DJ, Thiers BH, Burgdorf WHC, Raimer SS (eds) Clinical dermatology, vol 2, chap 10-3. Lippincott-Raven, Philadelphia, pp 1–13

Jansen T, Plewig G (1997) Advances and perspectives in acne therapy. Eur J Med Res 2:321–334

Jansen T, Plewig G (1998) Acne inversa. Int J Dermatol 37:96–100

Jansen T, Plewig G (1998) Acne fulminans. Int J Dermatol 37:254–257

Jungfer B, Jansen T, Przybilla B et al. (1993) Solid persistent facial edema of acne: successful treatment with isotretinoin and ketotifen. Dermatology 187:34–37

Karvonen SL (1993) Acne fulminans: report of clinical findings and treatment of twenty-four patients. J Am Acad Dermatol 28:572–579

Kokelj F (1992) Occupational acne. Clin Dermatol 10:213–217

Lever L, Marks R (1990) Current views on the aetiology, pathogenesis and treatment of acne vulgaris. Drugs 39: 681–692

Leyden JJ (1997) Therapy for acne vulgaris. N Engl J Med 336:1156–1162

Meynadier J, Alirezai M (1998) Systemic antibiotics for acne. Dermatology 196:135–139

Noble WC (1990) Topical and systemic antibiotics: is there a rationale? Semin Dermatol 9:250–254

Plewig G, Steger M (1989) Acne inversa (alias acne triad, acne tetrad or hidradenitis suppurativa). In: Marks R, Plewig G (eds) Acne and related disorders. Dunitz, Dunitz, pp 345–357

Plewig G, Jansen T (1998) Acneiform dermatoses. Dermatology 196:102–107

Plewig G, Fulton JE, Kligman AM (1970) Pomade acne. Arch Dermatol 101:580–584

Plewig G, Nikolowski J, Wolff HH (1982) Action of isotretinoin in acne, rosacea, and gram-negative folliculitis. J Am Acad Dermatol 6:766–785

Seukeran DC, Cunliffe WJ (1999). The treatment of acne fulminans: a review of 25 cases. Br J Dermatol 141:307–309

Shaw JC (1996) Antiandrogen and hormonal treatment of acne. Dermatol Clin 14:803–811

Somech R, Arav-Boger R, Assia A et al. (1999) Complications of minocycline therapy for acne vulgaris: case reports and review of the literature. Pediatric Dermatology 16 (6) 469–472

Strauss JS (1990) The pathogenesis and treatment of acne. J Dermatol Treat 1 [Suppl 3]: S15–S17

Sykes NL Jr, Webster GF (1994) Acne: a review of optimum treatment. Drugs 48:59–70

Toyoda M, Morohashi M (1998) An overview of topical antibiotics for acne treatment. Dermatology 196:130–134

Webster GF (1995) Inflammation in acne vulgaris. J Am Acad Dermatol 33:247–255

Windom RE, Sanford JP, Ziff M (1961) Acne conglobata and arthritis, Arthr Rheum 4:632–635

Mallorca Acne

Hjorth N, Sjolin KE, Sylvest B et al. (1972) Acne aestivalis – Mallorca acne. Acta Derm Venereol (Stockh) 52:61–63

Mills OH Jr, Kligman AM (1975) Acne aestivalis. Arch Dermatol 111:891–892

Sjolin KE (1979) Acne aestivalis: a histopathological study. Acta Derm Venereol (Stockh) 59 [Suppl 85]:171–176

Trichostasis Spinulosa

Harford RR, Cobb MW, Miller ML (1996) Trichostasis spinulosa: a clinical simulant of acne open comedones. Pediatr Dermatol 13:490–492

Ladany E (1954) Trichostasis spinulosa. J Invest Dermatol 23:33–41

Lazarov A, Amichai B, Cagnano M et al. (1994) Coexistence of trichostasis spinulosa and eruptive vellus hair cysts. Int J Dermatol 33:858–859

Rosacea
Bleicher PA, Charles JH, Sober AJ (1987) Topical metronidazole therapy for rosacea. Arch Dermatol 123:609–614
Browning DJ, Proia AD (1986) Ocular rosacea. Surv Ophthalmol 31:145–158
Dupont C (1986) How common is extrafacial rosacea? J Am Acad Dermatol 14:839
Ertl GA, Levine N, Kligman AM (1994) A comparison of the efficacy of topical tretinoin and low-dose oral isotretinoin in rosacea. Arch Dermatol 130:319–324
Helm KF, Menz J, Gibson LE et al. (1991) A clinical and histopathologic study of granulomatous rosacea. J Am Acad Dermatol 25:1038–1043
Hoting E, Paul E, Plewig G (1986) Treatment of rosacea with isotretinoin. Int J Dermatol 25:660–663
Jansen T, Plewig G (1997) Rosacea. In: Demis DJ, Thiers BH, Burgdorf WHC, Raimer SS (eds) Clinical dermatology, vol 2, chap 10-7. Lippincott-Raven, Philadelphia, pp 1–11
Jansen T, Plewig G (1997) Miscellaneous rosacea disorders. In: Demis DJ, Thiers BH, Burgdorf WHC, Raimer SS (eds) Clinical dermatology, vol 2, chap 10-8. Lippincott-Raven, Philadelphia, pp 1–6
Jansen T, Plewig G (1997) Rosacea conglobata. In: Demis DJ, Thiers BH, Burgdorf WHC, Raimer SS (eds) Clinical dermatology, vol 2, chap 10-9. Lippincott-Raven, Philadelphia, pp 1–4
Jansen T, Plewig G (1997) The treatment of rosaceous lymphoedema. Clin Exp Dermatol 22:57
Jansen T, Plewig G (1997) Rosacea: classification and treatment. J R Soc Med 90:144–150
Leyden JJ, Thew M, Kligman AM (1974) Steroid rosacea. Arch Dermatol 110:619–622
O'Leary PA, Kierland RR (1940) Pyoderma faciale. Arch Dermatol 41:451–462
Persi A, Rebora A, Burton JL et al. (1985) Metronidazole in the treatment of rosacea. Arch Dermatol 121:307–308
Plewig G, Jansen T, Kligman AM (1992) Pyoderma faciale – a review and report of 20 additional cases: is it rosacea? Arch Dermatol 128:1611–1617
Quarterman MJ, Johnson DW, Abele DC et al. (1997) Ocular rosacea: signs, symptoms, and tear studies before and after treatment with doxycycline. Arch Dermatol 133:49–54
Rebora A (1987) Rosacea. J Invest Dermatol 88 [Suppl 1]: 56s–60s
Wiemer DR (1987) Rhinophyma. Clin Plast Surg 14:357–365
Wilkin JK (1994) Rosacea: pathophysiology and treatment. Arch Dermatol 130:359–362

Demodicosis
Ayres S (1930) Pilyriasis folliculorum (*Demodex*). Arch Dermatol 21:19–24
Bonnar E, Eustace P, Powell FC (1993) The Demodex mite population in rosacea. J Am Acad Dermatol 28: 443–448
Forton F, Seys B (1993) Density of *Demodex folliculorum* in rosacea: a case-control study using standardized skin-surface biopsy. Br J Dermatol 128:650–659
Shelley WB, Shelley ED, Burmeister V (1989) Unilateral demodectic rosacea. J Am Acad Dermatol 20:915–917

Haber Syndrome
McCormack CJ, Cowen P (1997) Haber's syndrome. Aust J Dermatol 38:82–84
Sanderson KV, Wilson HT (1965) Haber's syndrome. Familial rosacea-like eruption with intraepidermal epithelioma. Brit J Dermatol 77:1–8

Perioral Dermatitis
Frumess GM, Lewis HM (1957) Light-sensitive seborrheid. Arch Dermatol 75:245–248
Hogan DJ (1995) Perioral dermatitis. Curr Probl Dermatol 22:98–104
Manders SM, Lucky AW (1992) Perioral dermatitis in children. J Am Acad Dermatol 27:688–692
Mihan R, Ayres S (1964) Perioral dermatitis. Arch Dermatol 89:803–805
Steigleder GK, Strempel A (1968) Rosaceaartige Dermatitis des Gesichts. Periorale Dermatitis. Hautarzt 19:492–494
Veien NK, Munkvad JM, Nielsen AO et al. (1991) Topical metronidazole in the treatment of perioral dermatitis. J Am Acad Dermatol 24:258–260
Wells K, Brodell RT (1993) Topical corticosteroid "addiction": a cause of perioral dermatitis. Postgrad Med 93: 225–230

Sebaceous Gland Hyperplasia
Kumar P, Barton SP, Marks R (1988) Tissue measurements in senile sebaceous gland hyperplasia. Br J Dermatol 118: 397–402
Luderschmidt C, Plewig G (1978) Circumscribed sebaceous gland hyperplasia: autoradiographic and histoplanimetric studies. J Invest Dermatol 70:207–209
Schirren CG, Jansen T, Lindner A et al. (1996) Diffuse sebaceous gland hyperplasia: a case report and an immunohistochemical study with cytokeratins. Am J Dermatopathol 18:296–301

Sebaceous Adenitis
Martins C, Tellechea O, Mariano A et al. (1997) Sebaceous adenitis. J Am Acad Dermatol 36:845–846
Renfro L, Kopf AW, Gutterman A, et al. (1993) Neutrophilic sebaceous adenitis. Arch Dermatol 129:910–911

CHAPTER 29

Diseases of the Apocrine Sweat Glands

Contents

Basic Science Aspects

Figure 29.1 demonstrates the apocrine sweat glands as well as the eccrine glands covered in the next chapter. The apocrine sweat glands develop as part of the system of hair and sebaceous and apocrine glands. They are common in the axilla, anogenital region, periumbilical region, and on the nipples, and are occasionally found on the head and trunk. The hormonal changes during puberty stimulate the apocrine glands, which increase in size and begin to function more actively. Thus, disorders of these glands usually become clinically apparent after this event. Apocrine glands are larger and more active in men than women as well as in blacks as compared to whites or Orientals. The apocrine glands develop with the hair germ in the fourth to fifth months of fetal life. In the embryo, they are present over the entire body but disappear before birth, except in the favored locations.

Anatomically, the apocrine gland consists of a coiled, twisted, secretory apparatus resembling a ball of yarn in the lower part of the dermis or fat. The gland drains into a duct which empties into the terminal hair follicle just above the sebaceous duct.

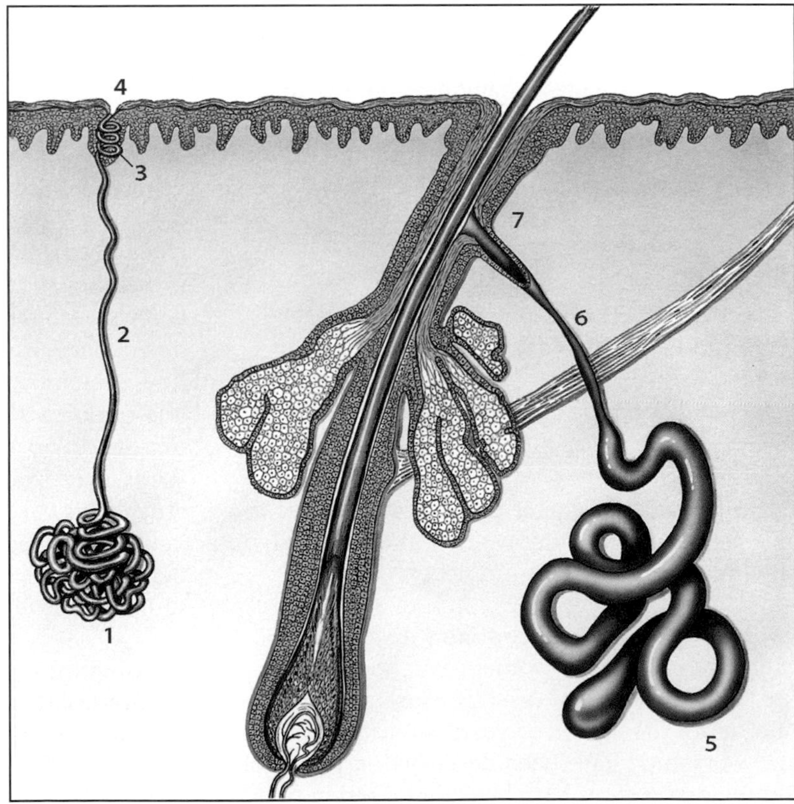

Fig. 29.1. The eccrine sweat glands (*1*) are coiled in the dermis; their product reaches the epidermis via a relatively straight duct (*2*) and then traverses the epidermis in the acrosyringium (*3*) to reach the surface (*4*). The apocrine glands (*5*) are connected via a short duct (*6*) to the hair follicle (*7*)

The mechanism of secretion is primarily decapitation, since the apical part of the cell appears to be pinched off before falling into the lumen. Viewed microscopically, decapitation or apocrine secretion is highly suggestive of the apocrine origin. Occasionally, merocrine and holocrine secretion is noticed. How apocrine secretion is controlled remains unclear. Nerve fibers containing cholinesterase and catecholamines can be demonstrated supplying the apocrine glands. In vitro investigations on isolated apocrine glands suggest that cholinergic stimulation is the most important factor, but β-adrenergic and, to a lesser extent, α-adrenergic stimuli are also effective. Apocrine function is also dependent on androgenic activity.

Following stimulation, a small amount of a viscous, opaque, yellowish white secretion is produced. The material is sterile and odorless; it consists of cholesterol (75%), triglycerides and fatty acids (20%), and small amounts cholesterol esters, wax esters, and squalene (5%) (These percentages refer to the lipid component of the apocrine secretion). In addition, small amounts of androgens such as dehydroepiandosterone and androsterone are found. Bacterial decomposition on the skin surface alters the apocrine secretion to produce the typical, penetrating odor of sweat or body odor; modified androgens seem to be responsible for most of the smell.

The apocrine glands have no clear function. In animals, they are a source of pheromones or hormones that instigate behavior responses to their odor; the classic examples are sexual attractants and territorial markers. Perhaps they play a similar role in humans, but their main effect now is to support a large deodorant market.

Fox-Fordyce Disease

(Fox and Fordyce 1902)

Synonym. Apocrine miliaria (Shelley and Levy 1956)

Definition. Chronic pruritic papular disorder usually occurring in young women and primarily involving the axillae.

Epidemiology. This uncommon disease is almost exclusively limited to women; over 90% of patients are female. Problems usually start after puberty but before the age of 40 years. Both improvement and worsening have been described in pregnancy. Simultaneous cases have been described in twins.

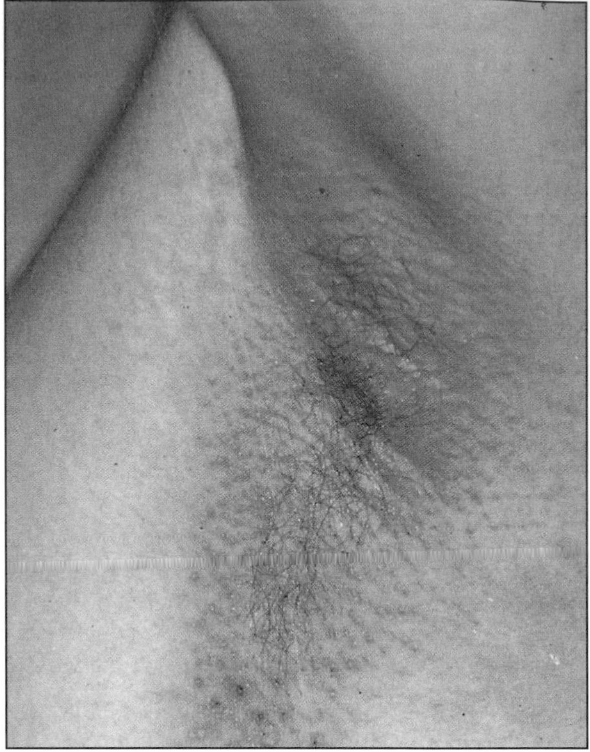

Fig. 29.2. Fox-Fordyce disease

Etiology and Pathogenesis. Functional hormonal changes presumably lead to occlusion of the apocrine ducts, producing so-called apocrine miliaria. The blocked secretions then leak into the surrounding tissue, producing inflammation and pruritus.

Clinical Findings. Many small, flat-topped skin-colored papules are typically found grouped closely together in the axillae (Fig. 29.2). The key feature is the intense pruritus; because of this, the axillary hairs are often irritated and broken off. Lichenification and excoriations are not seen. The patient may find shaving intolerable. Similar lesions are seen less often in the inguinal region, about the umbilicus, or on the nipple. Physical and emotional stress may exacerbate the problem. Occasionally, other physical signs of virilization or a history of menstrual irregularities are present, but most patients are normal in this respect. There is often spontaneous improvement following menopause.

Histopathology. Careful sectioning may reveal a keratinous plug of the apocrine duct where it enters the hair follicle. The overlying epidermis may show spongiosis, acanthosis, and hyperkeratosis. The glands themselves are either normal or somewhat dilated and surrounded by a chronic inflammatory infiltrate which spills into the adjacent dermis; there may be a granulomatous tissue response. The apocrine secretions stain positively with PAS stain.

Therapy

Systemic. Hormonal therapy with oral contraceptives may be helpful. In Germany, products containing an antiandrogen (cyproterone acetate, Diane 35 or Dianette) are often employed.

Topical. Corticosteroid cremes or lotions may provide some relief. In some instances, intralesional corticosteroids are also used; 2.5 mg/ml of triamcinolone acetonide is sufficient. Simple antipruritic therapy with distracters or topical anesthetics can also be tried. Occasionally, retinoids may help, especially if they are pushed to the point of irritation to induce peeling. Antiperspirants are also recommended but have little influence on the disease other than reducing maceration and other secondary changes.

Acne Inversa

Hidradenitis suppurativa was formerly felt to be a disease of the apocrine glands. Today we feel it is a variant of acne, best labeled acne inversa, primarily involving the hair follicles. While it does occur in areas rich in apocrine glands, these structures are probably just innocent bystanders (Chap. 28).

Bromhidrosis

Definition. Presence of unpleasant or unusual body odor as a result of excess or abnormal apocrine or eccrine secretions coupled with bacterial decomposition of sweat.

Etiology and Pathogenesis. Both apocrine and eccrine sweat is odorless. The apocrine sweat is altered by a variety of bacteria, especially *Corynebacteria*. These bacteria convert the androgens in apocrine sweat into odoriferous compounds. The role of *Micrococci* and *Staphylococci* is less specific, producing merely a sour smell. Additional odors may come from substances in foods (for example, garlic) or medications (dimethylsulfoxide, DMSO) which are excreted in the eccrine sweat.

Clinical Findings. Friends, coworkers, or parents often complain about a patient's intense body odor; less often, the patient calls attention to the problem himself. Problems start typically during puberty and may resolve in late adult life. Inappropriate body hygiene worsens the condition. Occasionally, erythrasma or trichomycosis axillaris are found.

Another less serious variant of unusual odors are those associated with foods and medications. Garlic is perhaps the most notorious offender, but topical DMSO can be absorbed in sufficient amounts to produce similarly disturbing odors. Such odors are harder to classify, as they may involve not only perspiration but also the breath.

Therapy. The most effective treatment is to limit eccrine sweat using aluminum chloride solutions or gels (Chap. 30). In addition, antimicrobial soaps, deodorants, and antiperspirants are helpful, but it is a rare patient who has not already tried these measures. Shaving the axillary hair is advisable. Most of the offending odors are trapped in shoes or garments, intimate apparel such as underwear or shirts, or sweaters or jackets that are difficult to launder. Diligent washing and dry cleaning measures are crucial.

Pseudobromhidrosis

Synonym. Bromhydrophobia

While some unfortunate individuals emit an unpleasant odor even with appropriate body hygiene and laundry measures, most patients who present to a physician complaining of unusual body odors actually smell quite normal and are suffering from pseudobromhidrosis. These individuals tend to be more concerned with axillary or genital odors or even those emanating from unusual sites such as the ear canals. This is a form of a monosymptomatic psychosis similar to acarophobia and delusions of facial asymmetry. Patients typically isolate themselves, become fanatic washers, and change clothes excessively. Psychiatric therapy is recommended; occasionally, pimocide or related compounds are helpful (Chap. 25).

Trimethylaminuria

(Humbert et al. 1970; Shelley and Shelley 1984)

Synonym. Fish odor syndrome

In this uncommon syndrome, patients develop body odor that resembles rotten or spoiled fish. The problem is not primarily apocrine but is included here because of the clinical overlap with bromhidrosis. The patients are unable to metabolize foul-smelling trimethylamine correctly. This substance is formed in the bowel by bacterial digestion of choline- and lecithin-rich foods. There may be a deficiency in hepatic trimethylamine oxidase or other perturbations in hepatic demethylization of trimethylamine. For whatever reason, the trimethylamine remains unchanged and imparts its terrible odor to urine, eccrine and apocrine sweat, and even expired air. The same substance is responsible for the unpleasant odor associated with vaginal *Gardnerella* infections. Some patients present with an altered sense of smell or taste. The diagnosis can be confirmed by identifying trimethylamine in the urine with gas chromatography. Avoiding foods rich in the precursor substances, such as fish, milk, eggs, and liver provides some relief.

Chromhidrosis

Synonym. Colored sweat

Uncommonly, sweat may assume unusual colors including yellow, blue, green, and black. Usually, small areas of skin are affected and the cause is exogenous. Nonetheless, chromhidrosis is considered an apocrine disorder because in the animal kingdom there are dramatic examples of colored apocrine sweat, such as the red secretions of hippopotamus. Pseudochromhidrosis refers to the application of exogenous chemicals which are interpreted as reaching the skin via sweat. The scare of red chromhidrosis among stewardesses was tracked down to dyes used for labeling the life vests which they put on at the start of each flight to demonstrate their use. In other instances, the patient may purpose fully apply color to the skin. Colored axillary sweat is generally the result of pigment production by bacteria; some of the *Corynebacteria* produce porphyrin-like materials. This superficial alteration of sweat color has also been designated pseudochromhidrosis. In what might be called true chromhidrosis, there is a focal area of hyperpigmented sweat which clogs the follicle orifices, in line with its apocrine origin. The color comes from the rich lipofuchsin content of apocrine sweat, but why localized areas are involved so often remains a mystery.

Bibliography

General Reading

Sato K, Kang WH, Saga K et al. (1989) Biology of sweat glands and their disorders. I. Normal sweat gland function. J Am Acad Dermatol 20:537–563

Shelley WB, Hurley HJ (1953) The physiology of the human axillary apocrine sweat gland. J Invest Dermatol 20: 285–297

Fox-Fordyce Disease

Fox GH, Fordyce JA (1902) Two cases of a rare papular disease affecting the axillary region. J Cutan Genito Urinary Dis 20: 1–5

Ranalletta M, Rositto A, Drut R (1996) Fox-Fordyce disease in two prepubertal girls: histopathologic demonstration of eccrine sweat gland involvement. Pediatr Dermatol 13:294–297

Shelley WB, Levy EJ (1956) Apocrine sweat retention in man. II. Fox-Fordyce disease (apocrine miliaria). Arch Dermatol 73:38–49

Bromhidrosis

Bang YH, Kim JH, Paik SW et al. (1996) Histopathology of apocrine bromhidrosis. Plast Reconstr Surg 98:288–292

Labows JN, McGinley KJ, Kligman AM (1982) Perspectives on axillary odor. J Soc Cosmet Chem 34:193–202

Leyden JJ, McGinley KJ, Hölzle E et al. (1981) The microbiology of the human axilla and its relationship to axillary odor. J Invest Dermatol 77:413–416

Strauss JS, Kligman AM (1956) The bacteria responsible for apocrine odor. J Invest Dermatol 27:67–71

Wang HJ, Cheng TY, Chen TM (1996) Surgical management of axillary bromhidrosis – a modified skoog procedure by an axillary bipedicle flap approach. Plast Reconstr Surg 98:524–529

Trimethylaminuria

Brand JM, Galask RP (1986) Trimethylamine: the substance mainly responsible for the fishy odor often associated with bacterial vaginosis. Obstet Gynecol 68:682–685

Humbert JR, Hammond KB, Hathaway WE et al. (1970) Trimethylaminuria: the fish odor syndrome. Lancet II: 770–771

Koblenzer CS (1985) The dysmorphic syndrome. Arch Dermatol 121:780–784

Leopold DA, Preti G, Mozell MM et al. (1990) Fish odor syndrome presenting as dysosmia. Arch Otolaryngol Head Neck Surg 116:354

Shelley ED, Shelley WB (1984) The fish odor syndrome: trimethylaminuria. JAMA 251:253–255

Chromhidrosis

MacSween RM, Millard LG (2000) A green man. Arch Dermatol 136:113–118

Mail-Gerrits MMG, van de Kerkhof P, Mier P et al. (1988) Axillary apocrine chromhidrosis. Arch Dermatol 124: 494–496

Marks JG, Hershey MD (1989) Treatment of apocrine chromhidrosis with topical capsaicin. J Am Acad Dermatol 21:418–420

Saff DM, Owens R, Kahn TA (1995) Apocrine chromhidrosis involving the areolae in a 15-year-old amateur figure skater. Pediatr Dermatol 12:48–50

CHAPTER 30

Diseases of the Eccrine Sweat Glands

Contents

Basic Science Aspects

The eccrine glands are free-standing adnexal structures that have no relationship to the hair follicle. They are distributed over the entire body, but are especially numerous on the palms, soles and forehead. The total number of eccrine glands is 2–3 million. The secretory part of the gland is a coiled structure lying deep in the dermis, often at the border with the subcutaneous fat. A straight duct leads to the epidermis, where the intraepidermal portion of the eccrine duct is known as the acrosyringium. The acrosyringium is corkscrew-like, usually with three clockwise turns in the epidermis and several additional turns in the stratum corneum. On most skin the orifice of the eccrine gland is slit-like and not noticeable; on the palms and soles, the openings are more funnel like and arranged along the dermatoglyphic ridges so they can be seen on close examination.

The innervation of the eccrine glands is accomplished by postganglionic sympathetic fibers. Nonetheless the main mediator is acetylcholine. In vitro studies show that α- and β-adrenergic fibers can also stimulate some secretion. Eccrine sweat is a clear, odorless watery substance, rich in sodium, potassium, calcium, magnesium and chloride ions, as well as uric acid, lactate and traces of amino acids, biogenic amines and vitamins. Many medications are also found in eccrine sweat. Two classic examples are the antifungal agents griseofulvin and ketoconazole.

Eccrine secretion requires energy; the glandular cells remain intact and secrete across their cell membrane into the lumen. Their main function is temperature regulation. Patients with a congenital or an acquired absence or diminution of eccrine glands dramatically demonstrate this, as they tolerate warm temperatures and increased physical activity poorly and may suddenly develop a heat stroke. When eccrine glands are not functioning, the cooling evaporative action of sweat is missing and the body has little chance to compensate. Under maximum thermal stimulation, an adult can lose up to 3 l/h through sweating.

The eccrine glands on the hands, feet and in the axillae are more likely to be influenced by emotional factors. Thus when one is nervous or upset, sweaty palms are a typical symptom. Otherwise, the eccrine glands of the palms and soles keep the thick stratum corneum lubricated to insure fine tactile skills and mobility. In the axillae, eccrine sweat dilutes the odoriferous apocrine products to insure their evaporation and spread.

Hyperhidrosis

Definition. Generalized or localized excess function of eccrine glands.

There are many different types of hyperhidrosis. The most common is physiologic. Persons who are adjusting to a warmer or more humid climate will initially sweat a great deal. Similarly, obese individuals, ones performing extensive manual labor and anyone exposed to very high temperatures will also sweat excessively. Marked perspiration also accompanies the hot flashes of menopause.

A variety of disease states are also associated with excessive sweating, which is then known as symptomatic hyperhidrosis. Most troubling to patients is idiopathic, genuine or emotional hyperhidrosis, in which there is no obvious explanation for the problem. Localized hyperhidrosis also occurs; the most uncommon is the so-called eccrine gland nevus which causes localized increased sweating. The term nevus may not be entirely appropriate, assometimes there is a localized increase in the number of eccrine glands, but in other instances there is a localized overfunction of a normal number of glands. Neurologic abnormalities are also associated with localized sweating.

Primary Hyperhidrosis

Synonyms. Emotional hyperhidrosis, genuine hyperhidrosis

Definition. Excessive eccrine sweating, either generalized or localized, without evident physical cause.

Etiology and Pathogenesis. The immediate cause of hyperhidrosis is often emotional stress, although there are many patients who simply sweat or even drip without obvious triggers. The underlying cause, i.e., which neurologic factors are responsible for the increased eccrine gland activity, remains a puzzle. Pain, fever, fear, stage fright or even joy may be the immediate trigger. Caffeine, hot spices and nicotine may contribute to the problem, as may increased ambient temperature.

Clinical Findings. Hyperhidrosis typically appears in puberty, although it can start earlier. The problem improves with time, as it is uncommon in middle-aged patients and rare in the elderly. The main sites of involvement are the palms, soles and axillae (Figs. 30.1–30.3); these are the three areas where eccrine glands are densest and where sweating seems to be most under emotional control. Less often, the face, especially the forehead and tip of the nose, as well as the nape, sternum, back and perianal region may be involved. As a result of the increased sweating, there is often maceration and

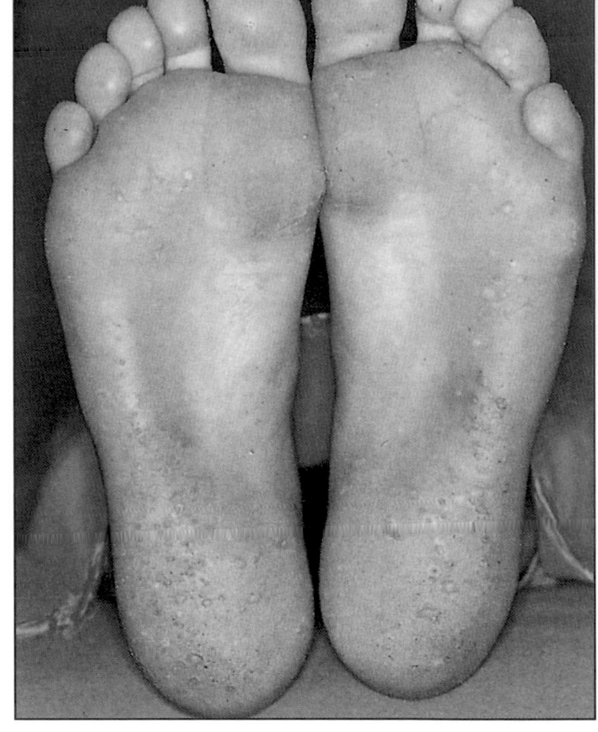

Fig. 30.2. Plantar hyperhidrosis with maceration and pitted keratolysis

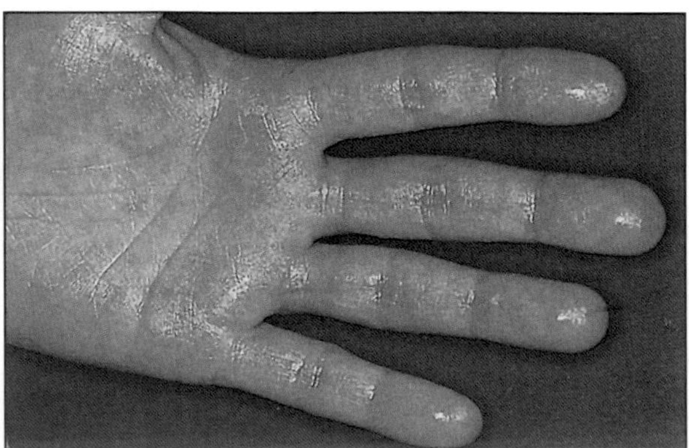

Fig. 30.1. Palmar hyperhidrosis

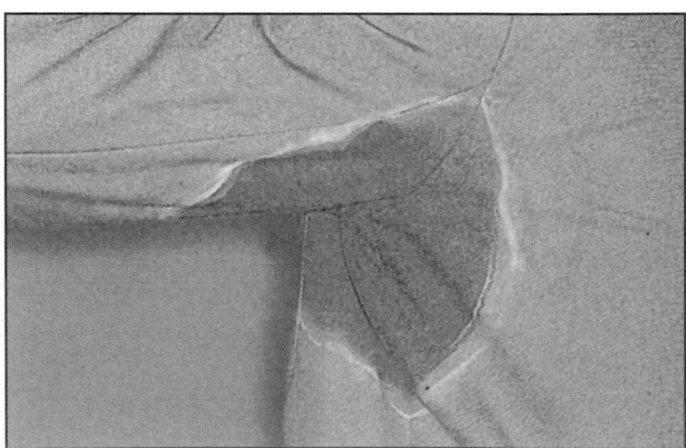

Fig. 30.3. Axillary hyperhidrosis with staining of garment

secondary bacterial or fungal infections. There may be other clinical signs of vasomotor instability, such as acrocyanosis or pseudoleucoderma angiospasticum.

Correct diagnosis is rarely a problem. One must attempt to exclude the secondary causes of hyperhidrosis, but this can usually be achieved through the history. Only rarely are screening laboratory tests needed. The excessive sweating can be quantified by gravimetry, weighing a sheet of blotting paper before and after a defined period of skin contact. The regional variations of hyperhidrosis are considered below.

Axillary Hyperhidrosis. Patients often experience almost explosive massive sweating, which sometimes has an emotional trigger but may also be spontaneous. The axillae immediately become soaking wet, sweat runs down their bodies and their clothing is instantly soaked. Garments are often discolored or damaged and typically a white band of salt is seen at the edge of the sweat line on dark cloth. The size of the sweat marks on the clothes is a good measure of the severity of the problem. Maceration is often marked and there may be a secondary irritant or even allergic contact dermatitis caused by excessive soap or antiperspirant use.

Palmar Hyperhidrosis. The palms are usually red but cool, secondary to evaporation. The epidermis may be swollen and macerated. Drops of sweat may appear on the lateral and even dorsal aspects of the fingers. In extreme cases sweat constantly drips from the hands. Such patients may complain that they constantly smear or soil papers or that, when they handle metal objects, corrosion occurs. Thus sometimes these unfortunate individuals are identified as rusters. Patients with hereditary palmar-plantar keratoderma also often have increased sweating.

Plantar Hyperhidrosis. On the feet the problems are exacerbated because of the occlusive effect of socks and shoes. Thus maceration is more extreme. The soles may have a livid color while the stratum corneum has a yellowish hue. The patients may complain of pain; walking short distances makes their feet uncomfortable. Often there are tiny pits and erosions in the horny layer; this phenomenon, known as pitted keratolysis, is caused by mixed infections with *Corynebacteria* and *Micrococci*. Other gram-negative bacterial infections and tinea pedis are also common, especially in the macerated toe webs. The mixture of moisture, occlusion, dead skin and microorganisms often produces a penetrating odor. Patients may complain of sweating through their shoes which are rapidly destroyed.

Therapy

The function of the eccrine glands can be theoretically interrupted at many levels:

- Removal of the sweat from the skin surface (soaps, powders, absorbent clothes)
- Mechanical interference with the secretory ducts (antiperspirants, primarily aldehydes and aluminum chloride salts)
- Functional alteration of the secretory cells through ionic flow (iontophoresis)
- Pharmacological blockage of the neurotransmitters (systemic anticholinergic agents, injection of botulinum toxin)
- Blocking the sympathetic nerves (sympathectomy or injection)
- Excision of the sweat glands (only practical in the axillae)

Systemic. No convincing systemic therapy for hyperhidrosis has been developed. Anticholinergic agents have undesirable side effects, such as dry mouth, dry eyes, mydriasis, urinary retention, or bradycardia. In addition, a specific antiperspirant effect is often difficult to prove. A number of products are available; in the United States glycopyrrolate 1.0 mg (Robinul) three to four times daily is recommended but not FDA approved for hyperhidrosis. In Germany, two combination products containing atropine, barbiturates and ergotamine are on the market but scarcely used; in addition, several natural products containing sage extracts are sold. We advise against any form of systemic therapy of hyperhidrosis, except in the occasional patient who is so anxious that a mild tranquilizer may be of benefit.

Topical. A long list of topical agents have been tried:

- Aluminum chloride salts. In the United States, 20% aluminum chloride in absolute alcohol (Drysol) is available. Similar products can also be readily compounded by the pharmacist. For the feet and axillae we like to add 1% methyl cellulose to the formulation to thicken the product. The mixture is then provided in a roll-on bottle.

A typical solution consists of the following:

Aluminum chloride	10–20
Methyl cellulose	1
Absolute alcohol (95%)	100

Alternatively, one can simply mix the salts with absolute alcohol, if the patient prefers a thinner product, such as one to be used on the hands. The products are applied every night or every other night depending on irritation. If no effect is seen after a week, the treated area can be occluded. The hands or feet are occluded with plastic gloves or plastic bags placed under socks. In the axillae, plastic wrap can be taped into place, an awkward but occasionally successful approach. Clothing may be damaged by higher concentrations of the aluminum chloride solution. Thus, ordinary high potency antiperspirants containing aluminum chloride salts should be used during the day.

The mechanism of action of aluminum salts is unclear. They appear to cause a plug to develop in the acrosyringium through their toxic action on adjacent epidermal cells and through formation of complexes with mucopolysaccharides in the stratum lucidum. Changes in the secretory cells may also occur. Efficacy correlates with concentration, but higher concentrations are more irritating and may lead to discontinuation of therapy. Allergic contact dermatitis is very uncommon. Zirconium salts were also employed, but they occasionally led to the formation of deodorant or axillary granulomas when they penetrated into the dermis. They are no longer used.

- Aldehydes. Either formaldehyde or glutaraldehyde may be used for the palms and soles. Both are usually too irritating for the axillae. These products are widely used in industry but often difficult to prescribe; usually the pharmacist must get the chemical from laboratory or hospital supply firms. Pharmaceutical grade products are not necessary and are very expensive. Formaldehyde is best avoided today because of all the environmental concerns. A 10% glutaraldehyde solution can be used nightly on the feet but will produce a mild discoloration; a lower concentration is less effective but does not stain. Methenamine breaks down on the skin to form ammonia and formaldehyde; it can be mixed as a 10% solution and is available as a 5% stick in the USA. Both allergic contact and irritant dermatitis may develop from the use of all these products.
- Acids. Tannic acid may denature keratin and temporarily block the acrosyringium. It is available in Germany as Tannolact for the preparation of foot baths and as a cream; similar products are not sold in the USA. Tannic acid powders can also be used as an adjunctive measure.
- Anticholinergic Agents. There is sufficient absorption that many of the side effects listed above for systemic therapy also apply here. Occasionally, topical scopolamine or similar products maybe tried but they are generally disappointing.
- Miscellaneous. Other topical measures have usually been tried by the patient and alone are not sufficient. Frequent washing, antibacterial soaps or syndets, absorbent powders (such as Zeasorb), absorbent clothes, frequent changes of clothes and shoes that breathe (i.e. leather, not rubber or plastic) are desirable but not very effective.

Other Measures

Iontophoresis. Tap water iontophoresis is the treatment of choice for the hands and feet. Weak direct current (10–15 mA) is directed through water baths to treat the hands or feet. Since its introduction by Levit in 1968, tap water iontophoresis has proven to be a safe and effective treatment. A wide variety of devices are available, many of which can be used for home therapy. Exact regimens obviously depend on which machines are available to the patient.

Botulinum Toxin. Recently this agent, which is primarily known for its spasmolytic activity, has been successfully used for the treatment of focal hyperhidrosis. Botulinum toxin-A inhibits the release of acetylcholine, which serves as neurotransmitter at the neuromuscular junction and in those sympathetic fibers enervating sweat glands. As all other sympathetic effects are mediated by epinephrine and norepinephrine, intradermal injections of botulinum toxin-A can effectively and specifically block sweating.

Although the drug is a powerful poison, it can be used safely within a pharmacologically defined dose range. While it is approved by the FDA only for the treatment of spastic muscular disorders, botulinum toxin-A appears to be a promising and valuable option in severe cases of axillary hyperhidrosis. Likewise, palmoplantar injections have been tried, but are far more painful for the patient and should be preceded by regional nerve blocks of the median and ulnar nerves. Palmar injections in particular pose the risk of impeding fine muscular movements of the fingers. Although this potential side effect is generally reversible within 3–6 months, it should be discussed explicitly with the patient. While ample long-term experience is not available yet, the duration of symptom-free intervals monitored in our patients after a single treatment with botulinum toxin-A has already exceeded 1 year (Fig. 30.4).

Biofeedback. Some patients are able to learn to control their sweating via biofeedback or autogenous training.

Surgical. The eccrine glands in the axilla lend themselves to surgical intervention. Often a relatively small area in the axillary vault is responsible for the bulk of the sweat production. It can be removed relatively simply after being identified via the starch-iodine test or similar sweat tests. In addition, wider areas can be removed through subcutaneous curettage.

Surgical sympathectomy is rarely employed, but can be considered the treatment of last resort for selected cases. Endoscopic surgery allows better visualization of small nerve branches and thus a relatively selective sympathectomy. When working in the cervical area, the list of complications includes gustatory hyperhidrosis, compensatory hyperhidrosis elsewhere and even Horner syndrome. In addition, occasionally the sympathetic supply to the hands can be effectively blocked by local injection of anesthetics, producing a short-term improvement.

Regional Approaches. One must approach the different areas with hyperhidrosis slightly differently. We generally prefer the following methods.

- Axilla: Aluminum chloride salts; if not successful, botulinum toxin, later surgical intervention
- Hands: Tap water iontophoresis, aluminum chloride salts, botulinum toxin, biofeedback training, sympathetic blockade as last resort
- Feet: Tap water iontophoresis, aluminum chloride salts, botulinum toxin

Secondary Hyperhidrosis

Synonym. Symptomatic hyperhidrosis

The underlying disorders associated with hyperhidrosis are legion. One must consider neurologic

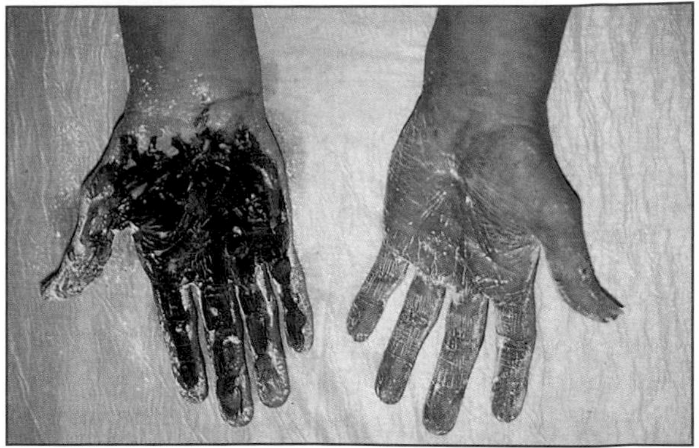

Fig. 30.4. Status 3 months after treatment with botulinum toxin-A on the right side. With the starch-iodine sweat test, the left hand is dark while the right hand fails to darken, indicating absence of sweating

problems, such as spinal cord and peripheral nerve injuries, rare CNS problems, Riley-Day syndrome and Parkinson disease. A variety of neurologic disorders with partial involvement of sympathetic tracts can also produce deranged sweating, including cervical rib syndrome, carpal tunnel syndrome and spinal cord lesions such as tabes dorsalis, syringomyelia and tumors. With such lesions the sweating may be localized or unilateral. Any acral vascular disturbance, such as Raynaud syndrome, may also be accompanied by increased sweating. Patients with hyperthyroidism are classically troubled by hyperhidrosis. Pituitary disorders, diabetes mellitus, pheochromocytoma and a whole host of other endocrine problems should also be considered. Night sweats are part of the staging criteria for Hodgkin disease and are often associated with tuberculosis. Mercury poisoning (acrodynia or pink disease) also leads to sweating disturbances, as do some antidepressants, most notably fluoxetine.

Riley-Day Syndrome

Synonym. Familial dysautonomia

Hyperhidrosis is one of the leading symptoms of this autosomal recessive inherited disorder, which has a frequency of around 1:4000 in Ashkenazi Jews. Apparently there is defective maturation of unmyelinated sensory and sympathetic nerves with a variety of autonomic abnormalities. Typical cutaneous findings include not only hyperhidrosis but also transient erythematous patches, often triggered by excitement or eating, cold extremities and a lack of pain sensation which leads to burns and other injuries. Tearing is reduced while salivation is increased. There are a wide variety of other more serious gastrointestinal, pulmonary and CNS problems; descriptions of these can be found in specialized sources.

Gustatory Hyperhidrosis

Many patients experience localized sweating involving the nose or forehead when eating certain foods, especially spicy or sour ones. While most gustatory sweating is normal, if the phenomenon is unilateral it may be a sign of an underlying disease process. Gustatory hyperhidrosis occurs in over two-thirds of patients who have had a dorsal sympathectomy. It is also associated with metastatic tumor spread to the sympathetic trunk (Pancoast syndrome), syringomyelia, diabetic neuropathy and other neurologic problems.

Frey Syndrome

(Frey 1923)

Synonym. Auriculotemporal syndrome

Auriculotemporal syndrome is a special variant of gustatory hyperhidrosis. It develops following surgery to the parotid gland or other structures in close vicinity, or following trauma or inflammation in the area. The auriculotemporal nerve contains parasympathetic fibers that supply the gland and sympathetic fibers to the overlying eccrine glands in the skin. Following trauma, there is a short circuit so that when salivation is stimulated, sweating also occurs in the overlying skin (Fig. 30.5).

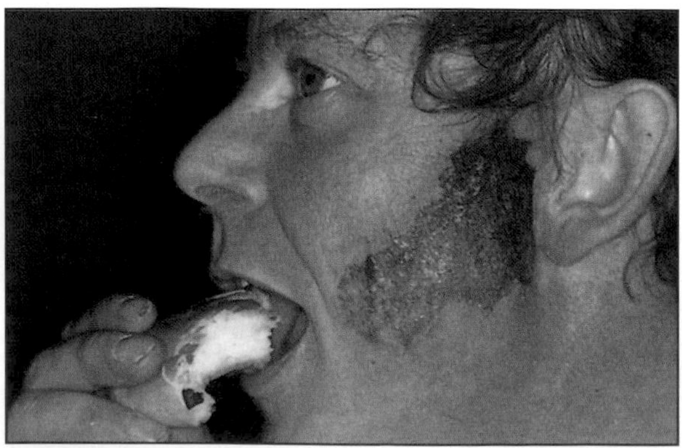

Fig. 30.5. Frey syndrome with positive starch-iodide sweat test

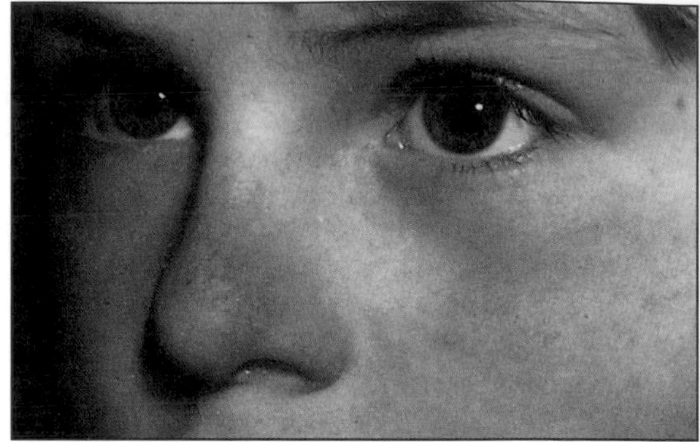

Fig. 30.6. Granulosis rubra nasi

Most patients do not require treatment, but topical aluminum chloride salts are often effective.

Granulosis Rubra Nasi

(Jadassohn 1901)

This extremely rare disorder of childhood features tiny papules of the cheeks and tip of the nose, associated with hyperhidrosis (Fig. 30.6). Blisters and pustules have also been reported. The nose may be somewhat blue or cyanotic. Acrocyanosis has also been described. Zinc shake lotions applied in the evening may be useful. The disease tends to resolves spontaneously in puberty.

Hypohidrosis and Anhidrosis

Reduced sweating is associated with a variety of disorders. There is no sharp line between hypohidrosis and anhidrosis; many patients designated as anhidrotic do have some eccrine glands. Scarred or burned skin may be truly anhidrotic but otherwise some eccrine glands are usually present. Reduced sweating poses a problem primarily because of impaired temperature control. Disorders associated with hypohidrosis include:

- Systemic disorders such as renal failure, hypothyroidism, Addison disease and diabetes insipidus
- Dehydration following severe diarrhea, vomiting, starvation, malnutrition and other chronic diseases
- Neurologic lesions involving either the central or peripheral nervous system. A classic example is the failure of patients with leprosy to sweat in involved areas

- Mechanical damage to the acrosyringium in inflammatory dermatoses such as atopic dermatitis, psoriasis and blistering disorders
- Direct inflammation of the acrosyringium in miliaria
- Blocked acrosyringia in some of the ichthyoses
- Medications such as quinacrine which directly damage the eccrine glands

In addition, there is a long list of genodermatoses associated with hypohidrosis including Bazex syndrome, Cockayne syndrome, EEC (ectrodactly-ectodermal dysplasia-clefting) syndrome and Franceschetti-Jadassohn syndrome. Usually the sweat glands are reduced in number, no totally absent.

Ross Syndrome

(Ross 1958)

The Ross syndrome is an unusual symptom complex consisting of a unilateral constricted pupil and areflexia (Holmes-Adie syndrome) coupled with progressive segmental anhidrosis and compensatory hyperhidrosis elsewhere. A wide variety of autonomic dysfunctional problems such as orthostatic hypotension, palpitations, vasovagal syncope, dyspnea, headaches, reflux esophagitis, irritable bowel and other psychosomatic complaints may be encountered. While the pathogenesis is unclear, Ross syndrome is felt to probably be a form of polyneuritis multiplex involving the autonomic nervous system. In most cases, the patient does not complain of segmental hypo-hidrosis but instead of the compensatory hyperhidrosis in other body regions. Some patients have been successfully treated with tap water iontophoresis to control the hyperhidrosis, but the multiple associated problems are not influenced.

Hypohidrotic Ectodermal Dysplasia

(Christ 1913)

Synonyms. Anhidrotic ectodermal dysplasia, Christ-Siemens-Touraine syndrome

Etiology and Pathogenesis. Hypohidrotic ectodermal dysplasia shows X-linked recessive inheritance in almost all cases. The gene has been localized to Xq11-21.1, allowing prenatal diagnosis.

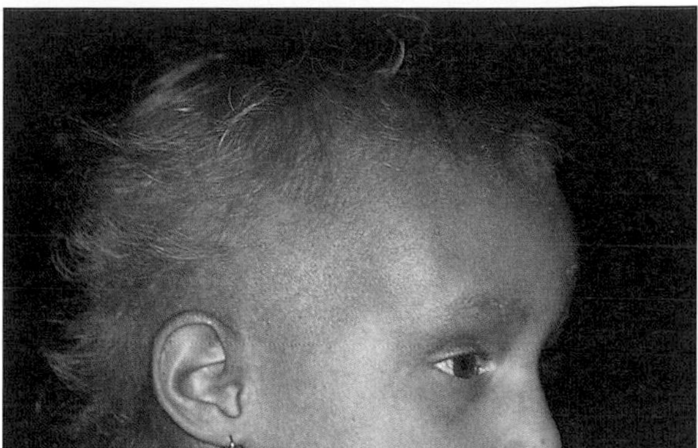

Fig. 30.7. Hypohidrotic ectodermal dysplasia

Clinical Findings. Patients have manifestations at birth with diffuse scaling and impaired temperature regulation. Later they have partial anodontia, conical teeth, wrinkling of the periorbital skin, fine sparse scalp hair, eyebrows and eyelashes, and reduced to absent sweat glands and mucous glands (Fig. 30.7). Additional features include a typical facies, which unfortunately has led to patients being compared to the cartoon character Popeye, with prominent forehead, depressed nasal bridge and the lack of lip support producing a characteristic speech pattern.

When the skin is examined with dental impression material, a reduced number of eccrine ducts can be demonstrated along the ridges of the palms and soles. Sweat function tests also demonstrate a marked diminution in eccrine glands. Mothers of the patients and other obligate carriers show patchy hypohidrosis, as well as hair and teeth defects. The main problem is temperature intolerance. Infants may have febrile convulsions. Because of lack of secretions in the upper airway, chronic respiratory problems are common. While patients need not avoid physical activity, they must be careful about the ambient temperature and take due precautions.

Laboratory Findings. In the absence of a genetic diagnosis, dental X-rays in small infants with febrile seizures may help suggest the correct diagnosis. Sweat testing may also be performed.

Differential Diagnosis. Several other ectodermal dysplasias may appear similar. The Rapp-Hodgkin syndrome (Rapp and Hodgkin 1968) is characterized by sparse hair, hypohidrosis, dental anomalies, chronic crusted scalp dermatitis, cleft lip and/or palate, shortened columnella, cup-shaped ears. Inheritance is probably autosomal dominant.

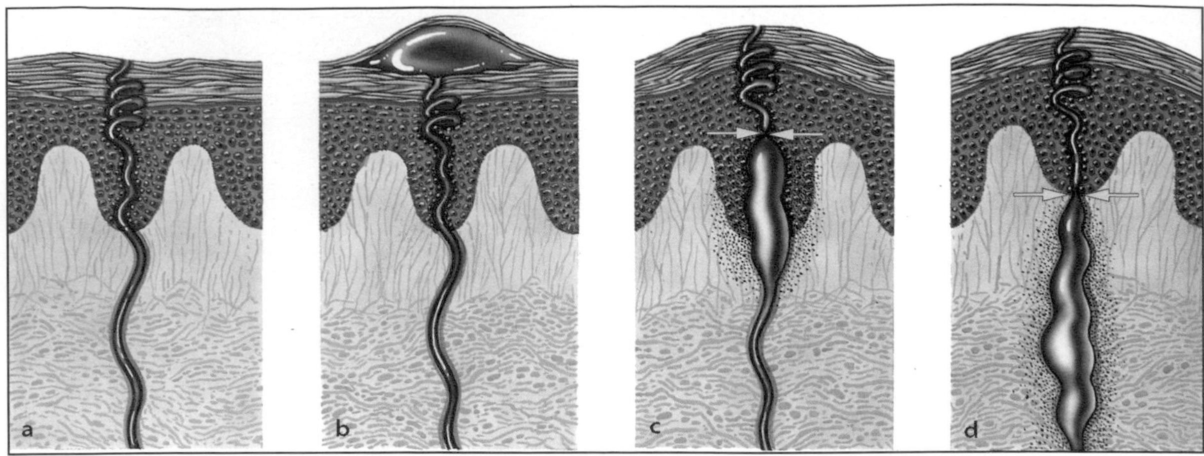

Fig. 30.8 a–d. Types of miliaria. **a** Normal eccrine gland; **b** miliaria crystallina; **c** miliaria rubra; **d** miliaria profunda

Hidrotic ectodermal dysplasia (Clouston syndrome; CLOUSTON 1929) is common in French Canadian pedigrees, but the disease should cause confusion only in name. Patients have sparse hair, leukoplakia, nail dystrophy, mental retardation, palmoplantar keratoderma, but normal sweating. The relevant gene is located at 13q11–q12 but its function is unknown.

Therapy. Avoidance of excessive activity during hot weather and constant attention to thermoregulation are crucial. Expert dental care early in life should improve not only appearance and eating, but also speech.

Other Eccrine Gland Disorders

Miliaria

Definition. Occlusion of the eccrine ducts, often triggered by heat, produces small often pruritic papules.

Etiology and Pathogenesis. The types of miliaria are classified based on the level of occlusion of the eccrine duct (Fig. 30.8). The condition typically occurs in the summer months, often when the patient enters a warmer or more tropical area. Use of a sauna may be another trigger. When occlusion is coupled with sweating, such as under wet suits, occlusive diapers or when febrile hospitalized patients lie on mattresses protected by plastic covers, the risk is great. Infants seem to be especially susceptible and often no obvious predisposing factor can be identified.

Miliaria Crystallina

Synonyms. Superficial miliaria, sudamina (ROBINSON 1884)

Etiology and Pathogenesis. Here the duct is closed within the stratum corneum. The causes include:

- Excessive sweating with swelling of the cells surrounding the opening
- Disorders of keratinization such that the duct is plugged by keratinous debris
- Inflammatory dermatoses in which the duct is sheared, such as in sunburn
- Use of topical agents that denature the stratum corneum and close the ducts, as discussed under the therapy of hyperhidrosis

Clinical Findings. Patients with miliaria crystallina seldom find their way to the doctor. The lesions are relatively transient and often asymptomatic. The history of sweating sometimes with occlusion is as outlined above. Hundreds of tiny small clear vesicles are seen, most often on the trunk (Fig. 30.9). On first glance, they resemble drops of sweat. The vesicles either rupture spontaneously or can be wiped away by the patient's hand. The lesions last for several hours and then resolve.

Therapy. Avoidance is the best therapy. Drying lotions, such as rubbing alcohol or zinc oxide shake lotion, suffice if treatment is demanded.

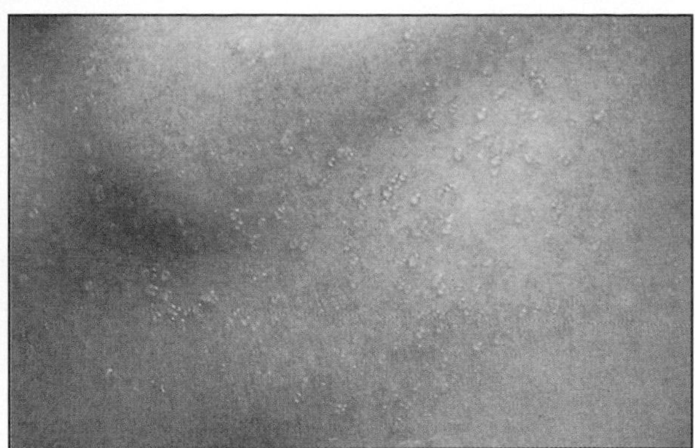

Fig. 30.9. Miliaria crystallina

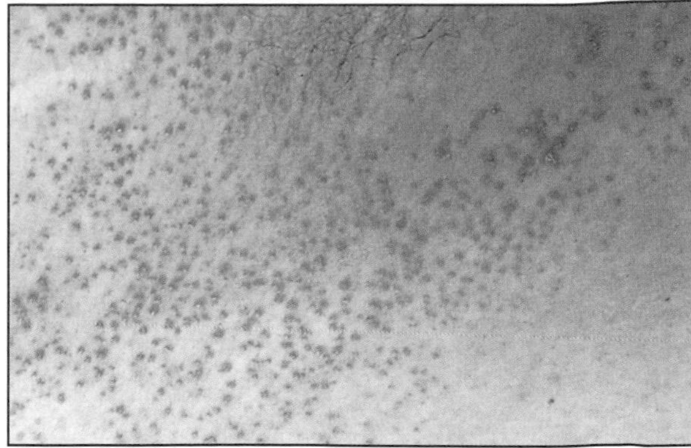

Fig. 30.10. Miliaria rubra

Miliaria Rubra and Miliaria Profunda

Synonyms. Deep miliaria, prickly heat, heat rash

Etiology and Pathogenesis. In miliaria rubra, the occlusion occurs within the intraepidermal acrosyringium, while in miliaria profunda it occurs in the upper dermal part of the eccrine duct. Eccrine sweat may leak into the interstitial space, attracting an inflammatory infiltrate and causing pruritus. The etiologic factors are similar but more extreme. Infants, the chronically ill and obese persons are far more likely to be affected. Possible causes include:

- Marked excess heat and humidity, such as experienced by soldiers serving in jungle areas or gold miners in South Africa
- Pronounced occlusion, such as in athletes exercising in occlusive suits to lose weight or divers in wet suits on warm days
- Bacterial toxins, after excessive sweating and maceration have provided a favorable milieu for bacterial growth. The toxins may enter eccrine ducts and elicit a more severe inflammatory response

Clinical Findings. Multiple tiny pruritic red papules develop, often in the diaper area or on the back where excessive sweating is coupled with occlusion, as in a truck driver (Fig. 30.10). The lesions tend to be symmetrical and spare the face, palms and soles. The papules may evolve into blisters or pustules, occasionally coalesce in the groin or axilla, and can become secondarily infected.

In contrast to the superficial form, deep miliaria can last for many days. Sometimes patients have to be evacuated from a tropical environment or placed in an air-conditioned area. If enough glands are involved, thermoregulatory problems can develop leading to a heat stroke (tropical anhidrotic asthenia). If secondary bacterial infection occurs, the patient may dramatically worsen, as can be seen among infants.

Histopathology. If a biopsy is carefully sectioned, an occluded eccrine duct surround by a neutrophilic infiltrate can occasionally be found. Sometimes an intraepidermal vesicle will be seen. Miliaria is rarely biopsied, but it is easy to overlook under the microscope.

Differential Diagnosis. In many cases, the hardest task is to convince the patient of the diagnosis. Patients tend to dislike being given what they perceive of as a lay diagnosis, such as heat rash.

Often deep miliaria is confused with folliculitis. If one looks closely, the follicles are not involved in miliaria. Some drug reactions with many tiny papules can cause confusion.

Therapy. Once again, avoidance is the best treatment. Putting the patient in a cooler environment, using drying lotions and treating secondary bacterial infections with topical or systemic antibiotics are all appropriate.

Neutrophilic Eccrine Hidradenitis

(Harrist et al. 1982)

Definition. Inflammation of eccrine glands and ducts presenting as multiple papules and nodules.

Epidemiology. Neutrophilic eccrine hidradenitis is seen in two main settings, in cancer chemotherapy patients and associated with infections including HIV/AIDS.

Etiology and Pathogenesis. In the case of chemotherapy patients, it is felt that various toxic compounds are excreted in the eccrine sweat and cause a local irritant reaction. Sometimes there may be an associated proliferation of the ductal cells, known as eccrine squamous syringometaplasia. In some instances bacteria have been cultured from the lesions, but this is an exception.

Clinical Findings. Erythematous papules and nodules develop, primarily in the axilla and on the extremities. The trunk and face may also be involved. Tiny pustules may be present, so that the lesions are generally considered to represent a folliculitis in an immunocompromised host and treated with often unnecessary antibiotics. Larger purpuric plaques may evolve. Spontaneous resolution is the rule. In rare cases, neutrophilic eccrine hidradenitis has been documented histologically in biopsies taken from chemotherapy-induced acral erythema.

Histopathology. The eccrine glands and duct are laced by a dense neutrophilic infiltrate.

Differential Diagnosis. Folliculitis and other infectious processes must be excluded. The larger plaques may suggest a hemorrhagic disorder.

Therapy. Resolution is usually spontaneous so that no therapy is needed. Drying shake lotions can be used.

Eccrine Squamous Syringometaplasia

In some patients with chemotherapy-related neutrophilic eccrine hidradenitis a proliferation of the eccrine ductal cells can be seen histologically. This is almost certainly triggered by the accumulation of toxins in the sweat. Clinically the two processes are identical. Syringometaplasia may also be found as an incidental, reactive histologic finding associated with tumors, scars, keratoacanthoma, pyoderma gangrenosum, panniculitis and undoubtedly other processes.

Palmoplantar Hidradenitis

Synonyms. Recurrent palmoplantar hidradenitis, idiopathic plantar hidradenitis, neutrophilic eccrine hidradenitis of childhood

In children, red papules and nodules may occasionally develop on the soles and less often the palms. They are tender and generally resolve spontaneously over 7–12 days, although recurrences are common. The patients may be unable to walk without marked pain. The etiology is unclear. Biopsy shows a deep, nodular neutrophilic infiltrate involving the eccrine glands which typically extend more deeply on the palms and soles. The differential diagnosis includes traumatic or pressure urticaria, which usually follows strenuous activity such as dancing or sports, and panniculitis. Resolution is spontaneous.

Bibliography

General Reading

Christophers E, Plewig G (1973) Formation of the acrosyringium. Arch Dermatol 107:378–382

Pinkus H (1939) Notes on the anatomy and pathology of the skin appendages. I. The wall of the intra-epidermal part of the sweat duct. J Invest Dermatol 2:175–186

Sato KT (1989) Biology of sweat glands and their disorders. I. Normal sweat gland function. J Am Acad Dermatol 20:537–563

Sato K, Kang WH, Saga K et al. (1989) Biology of sweat glands and their disorders. II. Disorders of sweat gland function. J Am Acad Dermatol 20:713–726

Watanabe S, Ichikawa E, Takanashi S (1993) Immunhistochemical localization of cytokeratins in normal eccrine glands with monoclonal antibodies in routinely processed, formalin-fixed, paraffin-embedded sections. J Am Acad Dermatol 28:203–212

Wenzel FG, Horn TD (1998) Non-neoplastic disorders ot the eccrine glands. J Am Acad Dermatol 38:1–17

Hyperhidrosis

Chan P, Kao GF, Pierson DL et al. (1985) Episodic hyperhidrosis on the dorsum of hands. J Am Acad Dermatol 12:937–942

Edmondson RA, Banerjec AK, Rennie JA (1992) Endoscopic transthoracic sympathoectomy in the treatment of hyperhidrosis. Ann Surg 215:289–293

Heckmann M, Ceballos-Baumann A, Schaller M et al. (1997) Botulinum beyond wrinkles. Dermatol Surg 23: 1221–1222

Heckmann M, Schaller M, Ceballos-Baumann A et al. (1998) Optimizing botulinum toxin therapy for hyperhidrosis. Br J Dermatol 138:553–554

Heckmann M, Breit S, Ceballos-Baumann A et al. (1999) Side-controlled intradermal injection of Botulinum toxin A in recalcitrant axillary hyperhidrosis. J Am Acad Dermatol 41:987–990

Hölzle E, Neubert U (1982) Antimicrobial effects of antiperspirant formulation containing aqueous aluminium chloride hexahydrate. Arch Dermatol Res 272:321–329

Hölzle E, Alberti N (1987) Long-term efficacy and side effects of tap water iontophoresis of palmoplantar hyperhidrosis – the usefulness of home therapy. Dermatologica 175:126–135

James WD, Schoomaker EB, Rodman OG (1987) Emotional eccrine sweating. A heritable disorder. Arch Dermatol 123:925–929

Jensen O, Nielsen E (1979) "Ruster". The corrosive action of palmar sweat. II. Physical and chemical factors in palmar hyperhidrosis. Acta Derm Venereol (Stockh) 59:139–143

Lillis PJ, Coleman W (1990) Liposuction for treatment of axillary hyperhidrosis. Dermatol Clin 8:479–482

Orteu CH, McGregor JM, Almeyda JR et al. (1995) Recurrence of hyperhidrosis after endoscopic transthoracic sympathectomy – case report and review of the literature. Clin Exp Dermatol 20:230–233

Schnider P, Binder M, Auff E et al. (1997) Double blind trial of botulinum A toxin for the treatment of focal hyperhidrosis of the palms. Br J Dermatol 136:548–553

Shelley WB, Talanin NY, Shelley ED (1998) Botulinum toxin therapy for palmar hyperhidrosis J Am Acad Dermatol 38:227–229

Sloan JB, Soltani K (1986) Iontophoresis in dermatology. A review. J Am Acad Dermatol 15:671–684

Watkins PJ (1973) Facial sweating after food: a new sign of diabetic autonomic neuropathy. Br Med J 1:583–587

Frey Syndrome

Dobrik C, Laskawi R (1995) Frey's syndrome: treatment with botulinum toxin. Acta Otolaryngol (Stockh) 115:459–461

Frey L (1923) Le syndrome du nerf auriculo-temporal. Rev Neurol (Paris) 2:98–104

Hypohidrotic Ectodermal Dysplasia

Advisory Board of the National Foundation for Ectodermal Dysplasia (1989) Scaling skin in the neonate: a clue to the early diagnosis of X-linked hypohidrotic ectodermal dysplasia (Christ-Siemens-Touraine syndrome). J Pediatr 114:600–602

Cambiaghi S, Restano L, Pääkkönen K et al. (2000) Clinical findings in mosaic carriers of hypohidrotic ectodermal dysplasia. Arch Dermatol 136:217–224

Christ J (1913) Über die kongenit. ektodermalen Defekte und ihre Beziehung zu einander; vikariirendes Pigment für Haartbildung. Arch Dermatol Syph 116:685–703

Clouston HRA (1929) A hereditary ectodermal dystrophy. Canad Med Assoc J 21:18–31

Kere J, Srivastava AK, Montonen O et al. (1996) X-linked anhidrotic (hypohidrotic) ectodermal dysplasia is caused by mutation in a novel transmembrane protein. Nat Genet 13:409–416

Rapp RS, Hodgkin WE (1968) Anhidrotic ectodermal dysplasia: autisomal dominant inheritance with palate and lip anomalies. J Med Genet 5:269–272

Ross Syndrome

Reinauer S, Schauf G, Hölzle E (1993) Ross syndrome: treatment of segmental compensatory hyperhidrosis by a modified iontophoretic device. J Am Acad Dermatol 28:308–312

Ross AT (1958) Progressive selective sudomotor denervation. Neurol 8:808–817

Miliaria

Dobson RL, Lobitz WC Jr (1957) Some histochemical observations on the human eccrine sweat glands. II. The pathogenesis of miliaria. Arch Dermatol 75:653–666

Hölzle E, Kligman AM (1978) The pathogenesis of miliaria rubra. Role of the resident microflora. Br J Dermatol 99:117–137

Robinson AF (1884) Miliaria and sudamina. J Cutan Venereol Dis 2:362–365

Shelley WB, Horvath PN (1950) Experimental miliaria in man. II. Production of sweat retention. Anhidrosis and miliaria crystallina by various kinds of injury. J Invest Dermatol 14:19–20

Shelley WB, Horvath PN (1950) Experimental miliaria in man. III. Production of miliaria rubra (prickly heat). J Invest Dermatol 14:193–204

Sulzberger MB, Emik LO (1946) Studies on prickly heat. I. Clinical and statistical findings. J Invest Dermatol 7:53–59

Sulzberger MB, Griffin TB (1969) Induced miliaria, postmiliarial hypohidrosis, and some potential sequelae. Arch Dermatol 99:145–151

Sulzberger MB, Griffin TB, Wiley HS (1967) Miliaria and anhidrosis. I. Experimental production in volunteers. Dermatologica 135:414–420

Neutrophilic Eccrine Hidradenitis

Brehler R, Reimann S, Bonsmann G et al. (1997) Neutrophilic hidradenitis induced by chemotherapy involves eccrine and apocrine glands. Am J Dermatopathol 19:73–78

Gross PR, Margolis D (1999) Neutrophilic dermatosis versus neutrophilic eccrine hidradenitis (letter). N Engl J Med 340:1371

Harrist TJ, Finde JD, Berman RS et al. (1982) Neutrophilic eccrine hidradenitis. A distinct type of neutrophilic dermatosis associated with myelogenous leukemia and chemotherapy. Arch Dermatol 118:263–266

Krischer J, Rutschmann O, Roten SV et al. (1998) Neutrophil eccrine hidradenitis in a patient with AIDS. J Dermatol 25:199–200

Eccrine Squamous Syringometaplasia

King DT, Barr RJ (1979) Synringometaplasia: mucinous and squamous variants. J Cutan Pathol 6:284–291

Munoz E, Valks R, Fernandez HJ et al. (1997) Herpetic syringitis associated with eccrine squamous synrigometaplasia in HIV-positive Patients. J Cutan Pathol 24:425–428

Valks R, Fraga J, Porras LJ et al. (1997) Chemotherapy-induced eccrine squamous syringometaplasia. A distinctive eruption in patients receiving hematopoietic progenitor cells. Arch Dermatol 133:873–878

CHAPTER 31

Diseases of Hair

Contents

Introduction

Hairs have little biological value in humans. Probably their main function today is as a sensory organ, measuring fine touch. If one simply tries to move an individual hair, the incredible sensitivity of the hair as a sensory organ will be noticed. In many individuals, the scalp hairs protect against sunburn and perhaps provide some insulation. But for the most part, hairs are a cosmetic appendage. The importance of the hairs in a person's self-image means that for some individuals, minor changes in number, color, texture or distribution cause great personal concern and may lead to a visit to the physician. Hair diseases are often associated with nail diseases as well as widespread skin disorders such as lichen planus or lupus erythematosus. Thus every patient presenting with hair problems should have their nails carefully examined and be offered a complete skin examination. From the physician's perspective, hair problems are very hard to treat. In addition the hair cycle often lasts many years. Even if one can influence the hair growth or structure, it may take many months before the patient notices any change.

Basic Science Aspects

Anatomy

The primitive hair germs arise along the basal layer of the epidermis in the 9th embryonic week. They grow down into the dermis, interacting with thickened clumps of fibroblasts known as the hair papillae. Interactions between the epidermal and mesenchymal components are critical to the development of the hair. The hair germ envelops the papillae, while at the same time the sebaceous and apocrine glands and arrector pili muscle form. No new follicles develop after birth.

The fully developed follicle consists of both epithelial and connective tissue components. The most important epithelial component is the hair matrix which lies in close contact with the dermal papillae. Through keratinization the outer layers of the hair – the medulla, cortex, cuticle and inner root sheath – are formed. The matrix also contains melanocytes which impart color to the hair. The follicular opening or infundibulum is similar to the adjacent skin, showing the same type of keratinization. The latter connective tissue components include dermal papillae, outer root sheath, nutrient vessels and sensory nerves. Destruction of the papillae leads to permanent hair loss.

Structure and Chemistry

The developed hair or hair shaft has a number of variable features. Thicker hairs have a central cavity or medulla; this feature is absent in thinner lanugo and vellus hairs. The bulk of the hair consists of longitudinally arranged spindle-shaped pigmented keratinocytes. These cells are surrounded by a cuticle which consists of overlapping scales similar to roof shingles or a pine cone. The scales are cornified cells.

The chemistry of hairs is well understood because of the commercial importance of wool, which is the best-studied hair. Keratin is the main structural component of hair. In contrast to the keratin of the stratum corneum, hair keratin contains about 20 % cysteine, a sulfur-rich amino acid. The keratin molecules are connected via a wide variety of bonds, of which the disulfide bonds are most important, and thus form a stable chemical and mechanical structure. Ultrastructural examination of the cortex shows 8-nm keratin filaments bound together by an osmiophilic cement substance into fibrils and fibrillar bundles. The thin keratin filaments of the cuticle are more randomly arranged.

Types of Hairs

Newborns are covered with nonmedullated, fine, usually nonpigmented lanugo hairs. These are soon replaced by vellus hairs, which are similar but more likely to have some pigment. During childhood there is a gradual transition of the scalp hairs from vellus to intermediate to terminal forms. Terminal hairs are always medullated, thicker, longer and in most instances more heavily pigmented. During puberty the vellus hairs of the hormonally sensitive body regions such as the axillae and genital area, as well as those of the beard, trunk and extremities in men, are replaced by terminal hairs.

Hormonal Influences

The simply observed cycle in male scalp hair growth (lanugo at birth, vellus in early childhood, then terminal and perhaps vellus again if male pattern baldness occurs) suggests that hormones influence hairs. Based on their response to androgens, hairs can be divided into three groups:

Sexual Hairs. These hairs are dependent on androgens in concentrations usually reached only in men. They include both beard hairs and body hairs especially those between the pubic triangle and the umbilicus, as well as those of the external ear.

Ambisexual Hairs. These hairs are also androgen-dependent, but respond to concentrations typically seen in women as well as men. They include the axillary and pubic hairs.

Nonsexual Hairs. Some hairs do not respond to androgens. Included in this group are the eyebrows and eyelashes.

Androgens are produced in the testes in men and in the ovaries and adrenal gland in women. The main androgen is testosterone, which is transported in the blood attached to a variety of binding or transport hormones. At its site of action in the hair matrix, it is converted within the keratinocytes by 5α-reductase into dihydrotestosterone and transferred via a cytoplasmic receptor to the nucleus. The receptor attaches to DNA and induces mRNA which then codes essential proteins, primarily keratins. Androgens are also responsible for the degenerative changes, or regression from terminal to vellus hair, as seen in male pattern baldness.

Hair Growth

Hair Cycle

Hairs do not grow continuously as do, for example, fingernails. Instead, each hair undergoes a cyclic rhythm of growth and rest. In some rodents, hair growth is synchronized, but in humans each hair cycles independently of its neighbors. At the end of the rest period the hair is shed, paving the way for a new hair. The shedding is also sporadic. While there is some seasonal variation, marked shedding in the spring and fall as shown by some fur-bearing animals is not seen. The following three phases are seen (Figs. 31.1, 31.2):

- Anagen or growing phase
- Catagen or transitional phase
- Telogen or resting phase

The anagen phase lasts years, the catagen lasts days, and the telogen lasts months. Normally on the scalp about 85% of hairs are in anagen, < 1% in catagen and 15% in telogen.

Anagen Phase. The hair root of the mature follicle lies deep in the dermis or subcutaneous fat. The matrix cells are extremely active, dividing every 24 h, and producing the growing hair with medulla, cortex, cuticle and inner root sheath. This outermost layer becomes hyalinized and is lost at the level of the sebaceous duct. The growing anagen hair is firmly attached to the hair root and can only be removed by force with accompanying pain. Hair growth averages about 0.35 mm daily, while the anagen period on the scalp may last from 2 to 6 years.

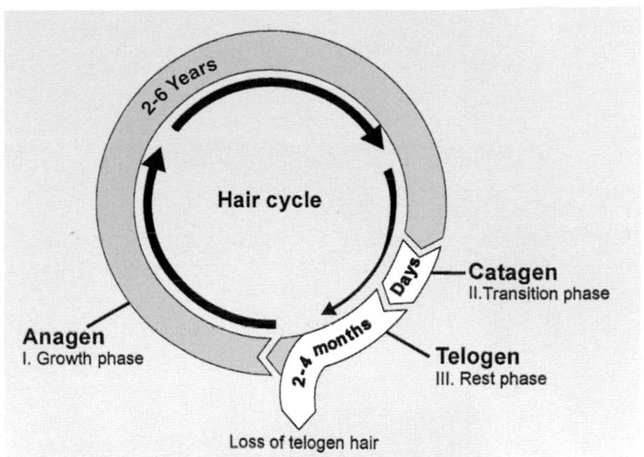

Fig. 31.1. Hair cycle

Catagen Phase. This phase is quite short, lasting only a few days. Growth suddenly stops, the bulb keratinizes and moves towards the epidermis. Only a small nest of epithelial cells remains nonkeratinized; it may form the basis for the next hair.

Telogen Phase. During this phase the distal end of the follicle is just below the opening of the sebaceous glands and contains club-shaped hairs surrounded by an epithelial sac. A fibrous tract extends from beneath this sac to the deeper site where the growing hair had been situated. The telogen phase lasts 3–4 months on the scalp. The eyebrows have a telogen phase lasting years (they are not affected by chemotherapy regimens). At the end of telogen, the hair is lost either by combing or spontaneously and the residual epithelial or stem cells move deeper into the dermis where they interact with the papillae and begin a new anagen phase. Thus all hairs that are normally lost are club-shaped hairs often with an epithelial sac. Patients may describe these hairs as having roots and are often reassured to learn that such hairs are normal.

The stem cells are located in the outer root sheath at the level of the bulge or attachment of the arrector pili muscles; they are not found in the hair matrix. The bulge activation hypothesis suggests that the continuous germ line cells in this region do not go through cyclic involution and are responsible for the new epithelial cells that descend to

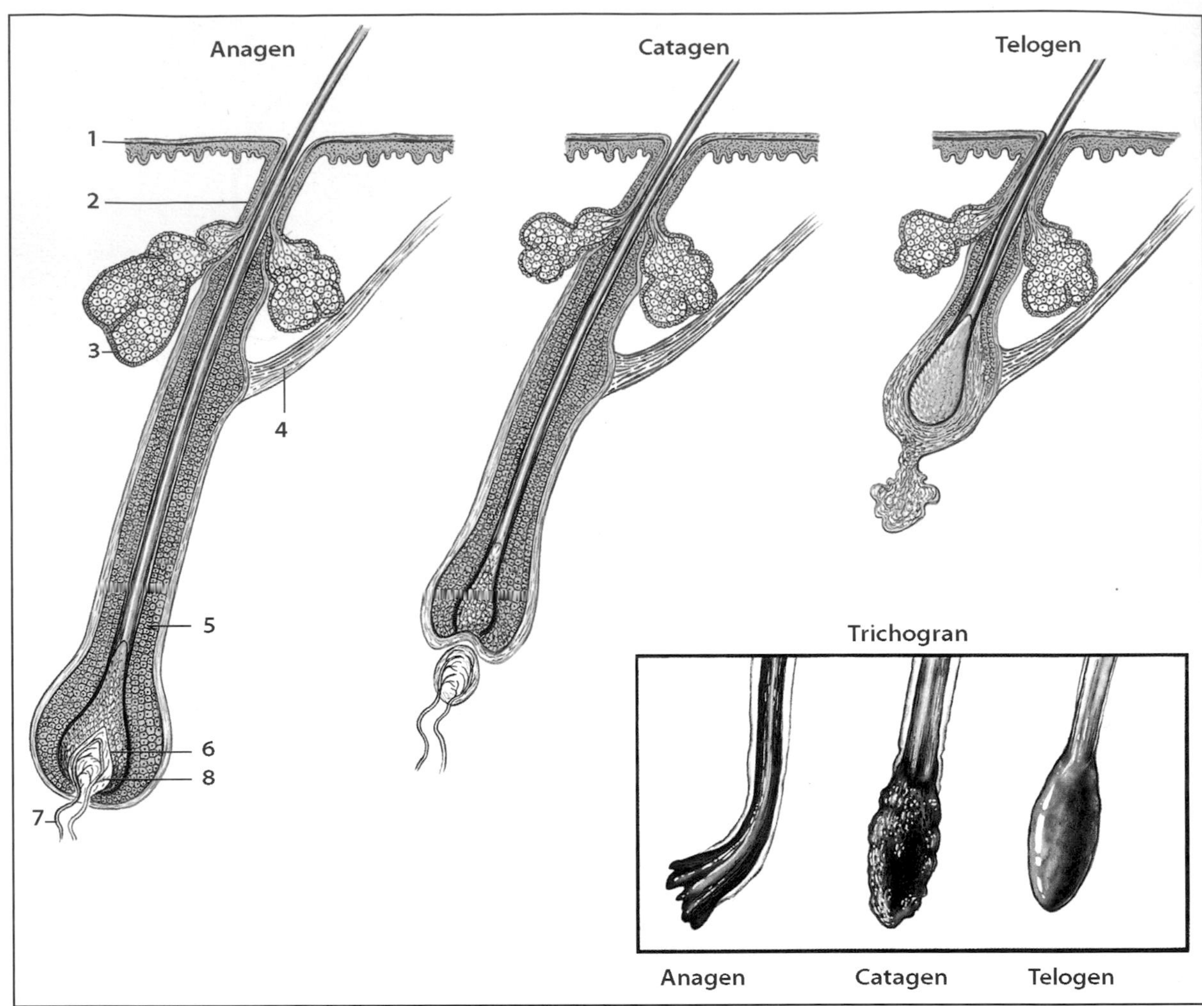

Fig. 31.2. Histological diagrams of the hair follicle in various stages (*1* epidermis, *2* infundibulum, *3* sebaceous gland, *4* arrector pili muscle, *5* hair shaft, *6* hair matrix, *7* blood vessel, *8* hair papilla). The *box* shows the appearance of the various stages in a trichogram

form the new hair. The keratinocytes of the hair matrix and lower part of the hair shaft disappear during catagen and telogen, to be replaced by new hairs from the bulge. The bulge hypothesis is a controversial area. Other workers feel that the matrical cells are not entirely lost and are responsible for the cyclic effect.

The hair cycle is under genetic control and varies in different body regions. The principle of donor dominance is what makes hair transplantation for male pattern baldness possible. Hair follicles taken from the back of the scalp and transplanted to the bald frontal area retain the growth characteristics of the donor region and continue to produce terminal hairs.

Trichogram

When a patient experiences hair loss, it is often helpful to study a group of hairs to assess the relationship between the different phases. In many cases, a light pull test is all that is necessary. One simply grasps a group of hairs between the thumb and forefinger and lightly pulls. The vast bulk of hairs in such a setting are telogen. Normally one gets up to two hairs with each light pull. The epithelial sacs and club shape can be identified with the naked eye. In telogen effluvium a greater number will be obtained, confirming the clinical diagnosis.

In more complicated cases, a heavy pull test combined with an exact analysis of hairs (trichogram) is needed. The procedure must be performed in a standardized way to get meaningful results. No cosmetic treatment such as hair dying or permanent waving is allowed in the preceding 2 weeks. Patients must not wash their hair for 5 days prior to the examination. Forceps covered with rubber tubing are using to remove a bundle of approximately 30–50 hairs which are pulled out sharply in the direction they naturally point. We usually recommend removing two samples. In diffuse hair loss, specimens are taken from the frontal region (2 cm behind the frontal hair line laterally) and occipital region. If circumscribed hair loss is present, a specimen is taken from the border and from the contralateral normal region. The hairs can be placed in physiologic saline between two glass slides, or mounted on a glass slide with Permount or another mounting medium. Then the roots are examined microscopically. The following hair types are identified and quantified:

Anagen Hairs. These hairs usually break off in the middle to upper part of the bulb. They contain a light region between the dark shaft and the dark bulb. Both inner and outer root sheath may be present. Anagen hairs can sometimes be badly damaged by epilation, broken off or extracted without a root sheath. Dystrophic anagen hairs reflect a major damage to the growing hair, as from cancer chemotherapy or poisoning. They are always pathologic. The hair breaks off with a bayonet tip.

Catagen Hairs. The entire club-shaped bulb is removed along with parts of the inner and outer root sheath. The dark keratogenous zone is still present.

Telogen Hairs. These hairs have lost the dark keratogenous zone and the root sheaths. The club is sometimes surrounded by an epithelial sack.

A normal trichogram will show at least 80% anagen hairs and up to 20% telogen hairs; the number of catagen hairs is very small (0.5–1.0%). In telogen effluvium these percentages can be almost reversed. Normal hair loss from the scalp ranges from 50–100 telogen hairs daily, depending on the patient and the method of study.

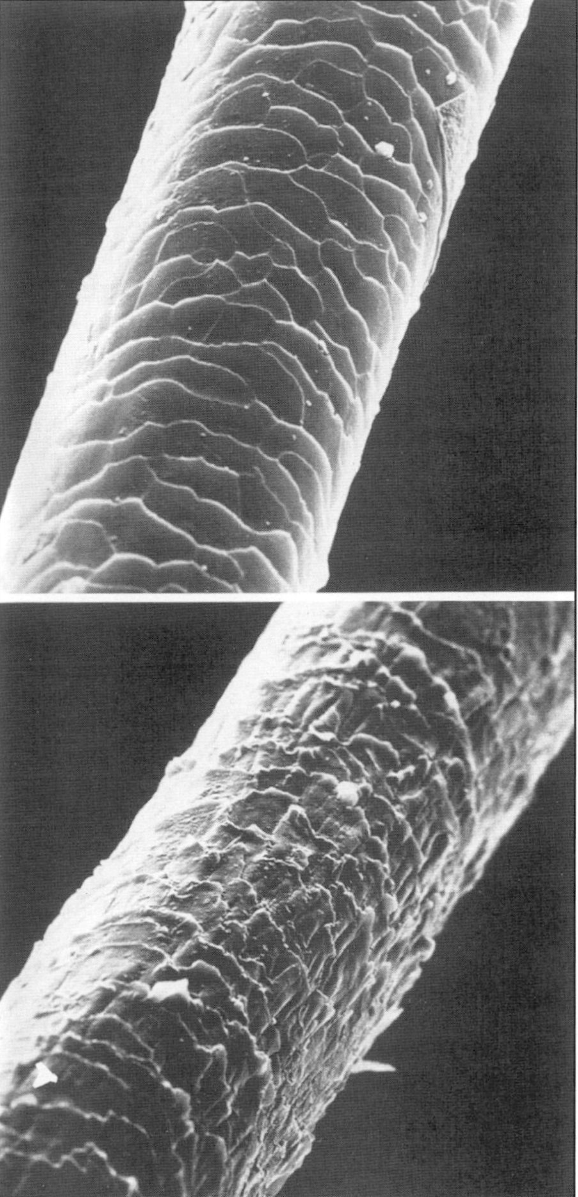

Fig. 31.3. Scanning electron micrograph showing a normal hair and one damaged by a permanent wave. The scales overlap to cover the hair

Structural Changes

Exogenous Causes of Mechanical Damage

Excessive or too-forceful combing and brushing can damage the cuticle and even the rest of the hair (Fig. 31.3). Patients with very curly hair, such as blacks, are more likely to produce such damage; they may induce trichorrhexis nodosa. Excessive washing of the hair can lead to brittleness and dryness, although this is uncommon with modern shampoos. Conditioners are substances such as animal proteins that are left on the hairs to increase their thickness and make them smoother, while rinses contain ionic compounds designed to make the hairs more manageable. Both are very useful in avoiding hair-care trauma.

On the other hand, dyes and permanent waves may cause structural problems. Hair dyes contain a wide range of substances some of which simply coat the hair and are totally harmless, while others alter the hair color more permanently and may at the same time damage the hair. Bleaches such as hydrogen peroxide oxidize the melanin the hair, but also weaken it structurally.

Temporary hair styling with a blow dryer and a variety of sprays and gels does not alter the hairs. On he other hand, permanent waves break disulfide bonds and other chemical connections important to the final three-dimensional structure of the hair and then reform them in a new position. In the past, many permanent waves were coupled with heat, but today almost all are done without heat. Some black patients may still have their hair straightened with heat and hot oils, leading to an irritation of the follicle (hot comb or hot oil folliculitis). This change is most rare and most cases probably reflect idiopathic follicular degeneration syndrome.

The standard permanent wave today uses 8% ammonium thioglycolate at a pH of 9.5 either at room temperature or at body temperature to break or reduce the disulfide bonds. After the bonds are reduced, the hairs are styled into the new form and then oxidized (fixed) with a 0.5–2.5% hydrogen peroxide solution. Then the basic agents are neutralized with a mild acid rinse. Today thioglycolic acid esters are often used as a reducing agent; they are felt to be milder. If a permanent wave is left on too long, if the concentrations of active agents are too high, or if the patient has especially sensitive or fragile hair, damage can occur (Fig. 31.4). In rare cases, many of the hairs will break off. Even if everything is done correctly, repeated dying, bleaching and waving of hair can cause cumulative damage.

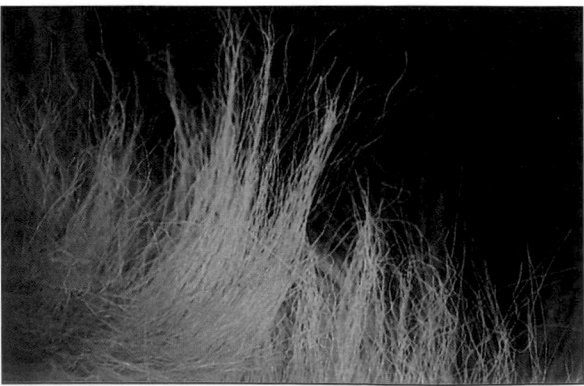

Fig. 31.4. Hair damaged by a permanent wave

Occasionally trichorrhexis nodosa will develop. Normally the follicles are not involved, so that as the new hairs grow out, they are entirely normal. In addition bleaches, dyes and permanent waves may cause allergic or toxic contact dermatitis in the patient or the hairdresser.

Diagnosis of Structural Changes

Structural changes caused by exogenous agents are often difficult to document. The hairs may appear dull, without spring and break easily. Under the light microscopic, broken hairs (trichoclasia) and split hairs (trichoptilosis) may be seen. The scanning electron microscope may reveal cuticular changes ranging from the destruction of several scales to total loss, as well as changes in the shaft. It is important to try to document the changes in cases where cosmetic care is felt by the patient to be responsible for the changes. Such cases often wind up in legal processes where documentation is crucial.

Congenital and Acquired Structural Abnormalities

There are a wide variety of diseases associated with hair shaft abnormalities. A logical classification is not available. Many overlaps occur, for a single metabolic problem may lead to multiple structural changes. A good working rule is that no structural abnormality is totally pathognomonic. Many patients with structural changes will show considerable variation over time. With these cautions in mind, we will consider the various structural abnormalities (Fig. 31.5).

Pili Annulati

(Karsch 1846)

Synonym. Ringed hair

Etiology and Pathogenesis. The cause is unknown. The disorder may be familial. The changes are noted shortly after birth.

Clinical Findings. The hairs show alternating 1–3 mm long light and dark bands (Fig. 31.5b). The light bands seem to result from an increased light reflex allegedly caused by air-filled spaces in the cortex. These clinically light bands are darker under microscopic examination, a puzzling paradox.

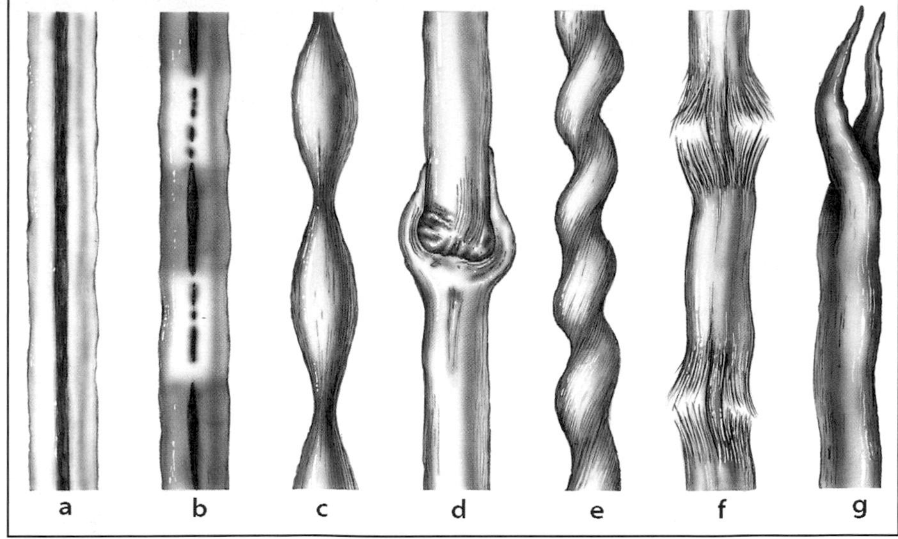

Fig. 31.5. *a* Normal hair, *b* pilus annulatus, *c* monilethrix, *d* trichorrhexis invaginata, *e* pilus tortus, *f* trichorrhexis nodosa, *g* trichoptilosis

There may also be variation in melanin content. Scanning electron microscopic evaluation may show fine splitting and folding in the dark areas.

Differential Diagnosis. Pili pseudoannulati (incorrectly called pseudopili annulati; PRICE 1968) also present with bands of light and dark, but have a different mechanism. Patients with fine blond hair develop periodic twisting and flattening of the shaft, which reflects light in such a way as to show banding.

Therapy. Neither condition is treatable, but most patients find the changes attractive and accept them.

Pili Torti

(SCHULZ 1900)

Synonym. Twisted hair

Etiology and Pathogenesis. Pili torti are usually inherited in an autosomal dominant fashion. They may be associated with a wide variety of other disorders. The disease may rarely be acquired, following cosmetic shaft damage.

Clinical Findings. The hairs are fragile and twisted along their longitudinal axis. They may thus appear either thick and thin, or light and dark, depending on the light reflection (Fig. 31.5e). The problem starts usually in infancy with fragile hairs and alopecia, but often the classical twisted hairs are not found for a year or two. Women and blondes are more often involved. There may be improvement at puberty. The patient's main problem is the fragility not the appearance.

Differential Diagnosis. Pili torti are a marker for a wide variety of disorders including Menkes syndrome (Chap. 46), Björnstad syndrome (deafness), citrullinemia, Basex syndrome (follicular atrophoderma, basal cell carcinoma), Crandall syndrome (deafness, hypogonadism), and many other ectodermal dysplasias, and are associated with a variety of other hair-shaft abnormalities, most reliably Netherton syndrome. Because of the association with deafness in so many different settings, hearing tests are recommended for all infants with suspected pili torti.

Therapy. None available. Gentle grooming and use of conditioners may help to reduce fragility. Permanent waves should be avoided.

Woolly Hair

(GOSSAGE 1908)

Occasionally white patients present with diffuse curly or woolly hair, resembling the normal hair of blacks, but not necessarily black in color. The hairs are difficult to comb, ellipsoid (as in blacks) but with splitting, breaks and rotation along the long axis. Woolly hair does not represent a single problem. The literature is full of descriptions of woolly, kinky and uncombable hair in single patients or single pedigrees. Both autosomal dominant and autosomal recessive pedigrees have been identified, and a Scottish family has been reported whose members had both straight and woolly hair intermixed. When the hairs become altered later in life, the diagnosis is acquired progressive kinking of the hair (Wise and Sulzberger 1932).

Woolly Hair Nevus

Some patients have a localized patch of woolly hair. When this is present at birth, it is termed nevoid (Wise 1927) and has been associated with an epidermal nevus on the same side of the body.

Whisker Hairs

(Norwood 1979)

Whisker hairs are curly hairs that develop around the ears in young adult men. Norwood, a hair transplant surgeon, has identified this finding as a sign that such individuals are likely to develop severe androgenetic alopecia and should be approached cautiously as surgical candidates. The curly hairs improve with time, probably because they are lost and never regrow.

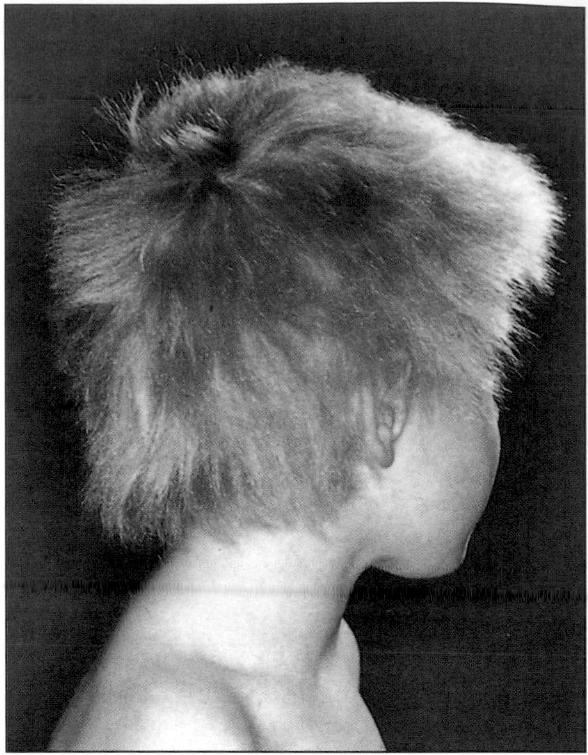

Fig. 31.6. Uncombable hair syndrome

Uncombable Hair Syndrome

(Dupré et al. 1973)

Synonyms. Cheveux incoiffables, pili canaliculi, pili trianguli et canaliculi, spun glass hair (Stroud and Mehregan 1974), unruly hair syndrome

Etiology and Pathogenesis. Most cases show autosomal dominant inheritance, but autosomal recessive inheritance has also been described and sporadic cases are seen. The underlying defect is unknown.

Clinical Findings. The hairs are usually blond, dry and unruly. The mother typically complains that she cannot comb the child's hair (Fig. 31.6). The hairs grow very slowly but are not fragile. Usually the hairs are normal at birth, but change over the first few years of life. Occasionally only part of the scalp will contain abnormal hairs. Other body hairs are usually not involved. Patients may also have pili torti or a diffuse alopecia. An association with atopic dermatitis has also been described. Improvement over time may occur.

Laboratory Findings. Histopathologic examination may show a premature keratinization of the inner root sheath. The hairs look surprisingly normal under the light microscope, but scanning electron microscopic evaluation reveals them to be triangular in shape with a central linear invagination or groove along one side. Examination under polarized light may show the groove as a dark line.

Differential Diagnosis. Menkes syndrome patients are so profoundly retarded that the diagnosis can be made in other ways. Woolly hair syndrome may appear similar, but does not have the characteristic ultrastructural changes.

Therapy. None available. Conditioners and styling greases or gels produce only minimal changes.

Monilethrix

(Smith 1879)

Synonyms. Beaded hair, nodose hair, spindle-shaped hair, aplasia pilorum intermittens (Virchow)

Etiology and Pathogenesis. Most cases are inherited in an autosomal dominant fashion, as would be expected of a structural abnormality. While the follicle appears normal, there is a cyclic perturbation of the anagen phase roughly every other day.

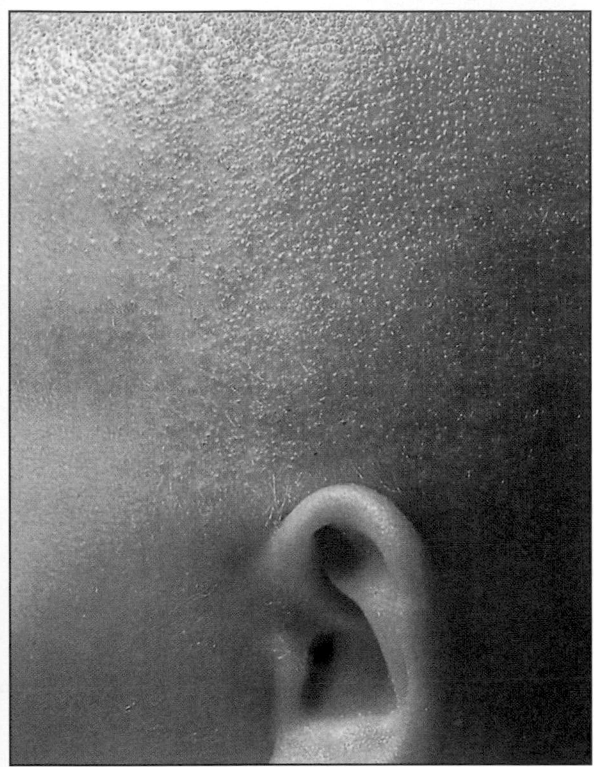

Fig. 31.7. Monilethrix

Clinical Findings. Patients typically have normal hair at birth, but it is soon replaced by fragile hairs which break off, so the typical patient has a diffuse alopecia (Fig. 31.7). The hairs are characteristic, alternating between nodular dark pearl-like thickened areas and thin light areas that are easily broken (Fig. 31.5 c). They may be retained in the follicles, producing a goose bump appearance. Keratosis follicularis may also be seen. While improvement has been reported in adult life, most patients are not so lucky.

Therapy. None available. Most patients wind up wearing a wig or toupee.

Pseudomonilethrix

(Bentley-Phillips and Bayles 1973)

Pseudomonilethrix has not stood the test of time. It was initially described in association with pili torti in several families showing autosomal dominant inheritance. The structural changes are somewhat nodose, but much more irregular than in monilethrix and the hairs are not fragile. It is probably either a variant of pili torti or may represent traumatic hair damage.

Trichorrhexis Nodosa

(Beigel 1855; Wilks 1857)

Definition. Hairs with macroscopic nodules which under the microscope resemble two paint brushes pushed into each other (Fig. 31.5 f).

Etiology and Pathogenesis. Congenital trichorrhexis nodosa is associated with a wide variety of other structural hair abnormalities and has been found in patients with arginosuccinic aciduria. Most cases of trichorrhexis nodosa are acquired and secondary to trauma.

Clinical Findings. There are two distinct types of acquired trichorrhexis nodosa: proximal and distal.

Proximal trichorrhexis nodosa is almost exclusively a disease of blacks, involving the scalp hairs. The typical complaint is "I used to have an Afro but now my hair won't grow out here and I had to cut it shorter". When hairs from the nongrowing region are examined, the typical paint-brush sign is found. If closely questioned, the patient may admit to having noticed broken off or short hairs. Constant picking, combing and straightening the hairs over years are felt to most likely induce the structural changes.

Distal trichorrhexis nodosa is a disease of whites and Asians. A typical location is the beard or mustache for whites, while in Asians the scalp is usually involved. Less often a history of trauma is obtained, and on the mustache, distal trichorrhexis nodosa is usually spontaneous. Breakage is much less common, so the little beads can be better seen clinically.

Differential Diagnosis. Hair casts, nits and trichomycosis axillaris have to be excluded when examining distal trichorrhexis nodosa. Proximal trichorrhexis nodosa is usually an easy clinical diagnosis, but other forms of hair breakage should be excluded. Congenital trichorrhexis nodosa is very rare and a difficult diagnosis. Often it is associated with other hair shaft abnormalities, so one should be reluctant to make the diagnosis and should examine a large number of hairs to exclude other findings.

Therapy. Proximal trichorrhexis nodosa will generally resolve spontaneously over a period of 2–4 years if the patients are gentle with their hair, avoid picks and straighteners, and use conditioners. The other forms are more chronic and no therapy is available.

Trichorrhexis Invaginata

(NETHERTON 1958)

Synonyms. Bamboo hair, Netherton syndrome

Trichorrhexis invaginata is a rare problem. The hairs have a typical microscopic appearance of a ball and cup invagination as seen in bamboo; another analogy is a collapsible telescope (Fig. 31.5 d). They tend to break off at a length of 3–4 cm. Usually only a small number of hairs show the dramatic structural changes, so that multiple examinations may be needed to confirm the diagnosis. Often pili torti are seen in the same patient. No treatment is available.

Netherton syndrome is an autosomal recessive inherited disorder which features atopic dermatitis, trichorrhexis invaginata and ichthyosis, usually ichthyosis linearis circumflexa (COMÈL 1949). Patients may also have a variety of immune defects with recurrent infections. Other types of ichthyosis have also been reported in Netherton syndrome. Some speak of Comèl-Netherton syndrome when ichthyosis linearis circumflexa is present and Netherton syndrome when other types of ichthyosis are seen (Chap. 17).

Bubble Hair

(BROWN et al. 1986)

Bubble hair appears to be the result of excessive use of blow dryers and electric curlers, as well as of bleaches and other chemicals. Most patients are women, who complain of localized hair breakage or loss. The texture of the remaining hairs changes to become straight and stiff. Light microscopic examination of the hairs reveals bubble-like areas within the hair shaft. Sometimes the hair shafts are also curved (boomerang deformity). If the hair is treated gently, it regrows normally.

Trichonodosis

(MICHELSON 1884)

Occasionally patients with curly hair develop knots in their hairs. Rarely the same problem occurs in patients with straight hairs. Usually the cause is excessive combing or intense rubbing and scratching because of an itchy scalp disorder. Microscopic examination identifies the knot. Knotted hairs can be cut and regrowth will be normal.

Trichoptilosis

Synonym. Split hairs

In trichoptilosis there are longitudinal splits in the hair, starting at the free end (Fig. 31.5 f). Only rarely do the splits reach to the mid-portion of the shaft. Other associated structural abnormalities such as pili torti, monilethrix, and trichorrhexis invaginata may be found. The cause is usually trauma, whether it be excessive combing, permanent waves or tugging and twisting by the patient. Sometimes tight braiding may produce the same effect. Avoidance of trauma will allow regrowth of normal hairs.

Trichoschisis

Trichoschisis is a nonspecific term for a variety of structural changes including both longitudinal and transverse splits and breaks. It is occasionally used as a synonym for trichothiodystrophy but may be also applied to some patients with various forms of ichthyosis and hair changes.

Trichothiodystrophy

(PRICE 1979)

Synonyms. Sulfur deficiency hair. A long list of associated syndromes, listed below, are not true synonyms. Trichoschisis is sometimes used as a synonym, but incorrectly.

Definition. Brittle hairs which result from a defect in sulfur metabolism.

Etiology and Pathogenesis. Most cases are associated with a variety of other disorders, most of which have autosomal recessive inherited enzyme defects, presumably involving sulfur metabolism.

Clinical Findings. Problems usually start in early childhood. The normally colored hairs are very brittle and break off easily. Patchy alopecia may be seen. Other associated findings are included in the listing below.

Laboratory Findings. Light microscopic examination may reveal an absent cuticle. Polarization microscopy shows characteristic dark and light stripes – the tiger tail sign. Scanning electron microscopic evaluation confirms the absence of the cuticle and reveals longitudinal grooves, known as fluting, along with marked folding. Biochemical studies show a striking decrease in sulfur-containing amino acids such as cystine and cysteine, and indeed the hair's sulfur content may be reduced 50–90%. Urine and serum sulfur levels are usually normal. In acquired partial trichothiodystrophy, patients have no biochemical abnormalities, suggesting that repeated manipulation or other external forces can produce similar hair changes.

Therapy. None is available.

Syndromes Associated with Trichothiodystrophy

There is a long list of overlapping syndromes, many described by an alphabet soup of puzzling initials, which have been associated with trichothiodystrophy. They all appear to be inherited in an autosomal recessive pattern and are considered in Chapter 13. A partial listing includes:

- BIDS syndrome: Brittle hair, intellectual impairment, decreased fertility and short stature (also known as Amish brittle hair syndrome).
- IBIDS: Ichthyosis+BIDS; also known as Tay syndrome (Tay 1971; Crovato and Rebora 1985; Jorizzo et al. 1982).
- PIBIDS: Photosensitivity+IBIDS. Several variants are present here. The form PIBI[D]S is used to indicate that fertility may not be decreased. Some patients have DNA repair defects similar to group D xeroderma pigmentosum; of this group, some develop skin cancers but some do not.
- Sabinas syndrome: Patients come from a small area of Mexico (Sabinas Hidalgo) and have brittle hair, nail dysplasias, mental retardation and retinal pigment defects (very similar to BIDS).
- Marinesco-Sjögren syndrome (Marinesco 1931; Sjögren 1950): profound retardation, failure to thrive, ataxia, brittle hair, nail defects, cataracts, dental abnormalities and many other problems.

Other Causes of Structural Changes

A wide variety of metabolic disorders can also lead to abnormal hairs. Thin, easily broken hairs are seen in patients with malabsorption, starvation, eating disorders and wasting. Often the hairs acquire a reddish hue, often described in kwashiorkor. Cancer chemotherapy usually leads to dystrophic anagen hairs (bayonet hairs) which are lost in great numbers. Textural and color changes (racoon hairs: alternating bands of light and dark hair) may also occur. Patients with disorders of amino acid metabolism (phenylketonuria and others) as well as Chédiak-Higashi syndrome may have pale fragile hair. Patients with hypothyroidism have dull thin hair which may be brittle.

Curved Hairs

There are two common conditions in which hairs grow in a curved shape, producing clinical changes.

Pili Recurvati

Synonyms. Pseudofolliculitis barbae, ingrown hairs

In some individuals hairs exit the skin surface but re-enter growing back down into the skin. This is most common in the beard area and the nape. It is seen primarily among blacks and other individuals with curly hair, but can occur in those with straight hairs. In the beard area of blacks, the problem is so common that is has a separate name: pseudofolliculitis barbae. The ingrown hair excites a foreign body response much as does a splinter. Sometimes postinflammatory comedones and small keloidal scars form (Chap. 66).

Rolled Hairs

This harmless condition is known to everyone, although there is not a universally accepted name in English. Sometimes hairs are trapped in the stratum corneum and then appear as a dark coiled ring around a plug (Fig. 31.8). The problem is most com-

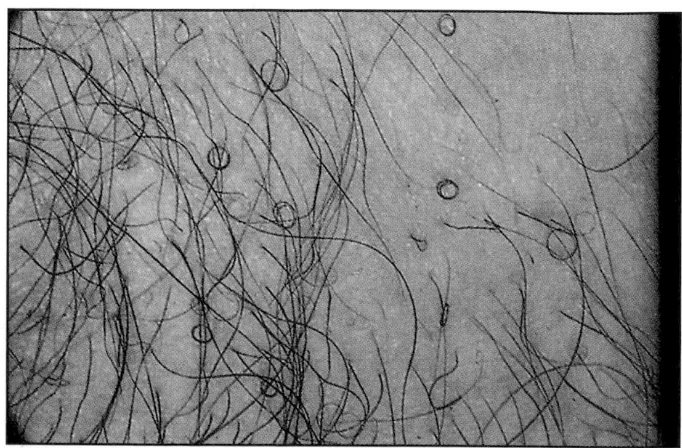

Fig. 31.8. Rolled hairs

mon on the abdomen of heavy people, suggesting that friction from clothing may play a role. It usually occurs in older patients. In younger individuals, it may be associated with keratosis pilaris or even with ichthyosis. The hair and the plug can be extracted from the follicle with a pointed tweezers.

Color Changes

Hair color depends on the proportion of eu- and pheomelanin, the number, size and shape of the melanin granules, and their distribution in the hair shaft. Each of these factors is probably influenced by multiple genes, explaining the wide range of normal hair colors. Celts with red hair and freckles have almost exclusively pheomelanin, blacks and Asians have high amounts of melanin, and whites have varying amounts of both melanins producing a range from blond to brunette to black hair. The color of the hair can be influenced by congenital factors. Acquired changes may be related to endogenous or exogenous factors.

Heterochromia

The presence of hairs of two different colors in the same individual is not unusual. Often there is a discrepancy between scalp and beard hair, or scalp and pubic hair. Most often bleaching or dyeing of scalp hair is the explanation, but not always. In addition, some patients may have natural streaks of a second color highlighting their hair, and sometimes a melanocytic nevus may be found at the base of the streak. In other instances the scalp appears normal and one must postulate a mosaic composition.

A different type of heterochromia has been reported in Japanese patients with iron deficiency anemia. The patients had hairs with alternating dark (normal color) and light bands. A uniform dark color regrew when iron was given. The term canities segmentata sideropenica has been proposed for the phenomenon.

Albinism and Piebaldism

Patients with albinism have a variety of defects in melanin synthesis. In true tyrosinase-negative albinism they totally lack melanin and have totally colorless hair. In the other types of albinism there may be small amounts of melanin producing light yellow to light brown hair. In piebaldism, there is a localized area of absence of melanin, often in the paramedian frontal region, resulting in a white forelock. Waardenburg syndrome has the same hair changes as piebaldism but other associated findings. Families with occipital locks of white hair have also been described.

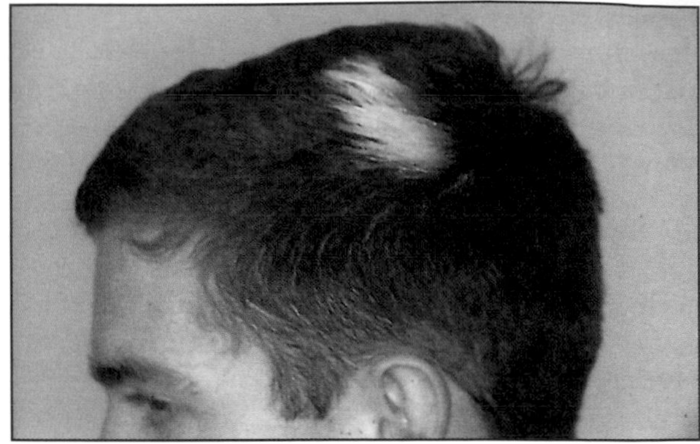

Fig. 31.9. Circumscribed poliosis

Poliosis

Definition. Acquired localized depigmented area of hair. Some schemes include piebaldism under poliosis; we separate them.

Clinical Findings. A sharply defined white patch of hair stands out among the normal darker hairs (Fig. 31.9). Probably the most common cause is vitiligo. Similar changes appear in the regrown hairs following alopecia areata, inflammatory processes (such as zoster), trauma, burns or X-ray radiation. In the latter situation, the hairs may also grow back darker, resulting in a focal hyperpigmentation. Other less common causes of circumscribed poliosis include neurofibromatosis I (often overlying a scalp neurofibroma), tuberous sclerosis and Vogt-Koyanagi syndrome. Dyeing the discolored hairs to match the normal ones is the simplest therapy.

Canities

Definition. Physiologic graying or whitening of the hair

Etiology and Pathogenesis. Gray hairs do not exist. The impression of gray hair comes from a mixture of varying amounts of white hairs and normal darker hairs. This is easier to ascertain in people with dark hair, who initially have a salt and pepper appearance. In those with light hair shades, the transition to gray is more subtle. Initially there is decreased tyrosinase activity in the hair bulb and degenerative changes in the melanocytes. Later the melanocytes disappear and no more melanin is deposited in new hairs, leaving them white. There are several different types of canities.

Physiologic Canities. Almost every individual eventually develops canities. The age of onset varies markedly, from the early 20s to the 60s or even 70s. The average age of onset is in the 40s. Typically the hair of the temples changes first, and then the process spreads to the rest of the scalp. The beard hair can become gray earlier than the scalp hair, or remain pigmented years afterwards. Axillary, pubic and eyebrow hair change last. In an unusual twist, some gray-haired individuals experience repigmentation when they develop Addison disease or porphyria cutanea tarda. The only courses of action are either to enjoy the distinguished look or to dye the hair. Pantothenic acid can reverse gray hair in some rodent models but has no effect in humans.

Premature Graying (Canities Praecox). When graying occurs before the age 20 years in whites or 30 years in blacks, one speaks of premature graying. Often this phenomenon is inherited in an autosomal dominant pattern. In the Böök syndrome, premature graying is associated with hyperhidrosis and dental anomalies. In many of the syndromes of premature aging, graying is an early sign.

Canities Symptomatica. Graying may be seen with hyperthyroidism, malnutrition, pernicious anemia, chemotherapy and following high fever, such as in malaria. Emotional stress has also been blamed for graying. Sometimes one reads of the hairs turning white over night or in a short period of time. Since it takes many months for gray hairs to grow out, the only plausible explanation is that dark-colored normal hairs rapidly fall out, leaving behind the more resistant white hairs. This unusual phenomenon is felt to occur as part of a diffuse alopecia areata, although often the physician is as puzzled as the patient by the sudden change in appearance.

Medication-Induced Canities. Chloroquine may cause lightening of already light-blond or red hair, but has little influence on black hair. Hydroxychloroquine does not share this action. Other possible drugs include retinoids, mephenesin and triparanol.

Exogenous Heterochromia

Sometimes a hair dyeing job is unsatisfactory or the individual changes his or her mind and desires yet a different color. Attempts to bleach or re-dye can produce most unusual colors which will puzzle every observer. White haired individuals who smoke a great deal may acquire a yellow tint to their hair.

Copper in swimming pool water can impart a green color to the hair of frequent swimmers (Fig. 31.10). The copper can occur naturally in the water supply, be added in algaecides or be leached from copper piping. The same problem occurs occasionally in homes with copper plumbing and subsequent leaching. Gray or blond individuals are at risk. They can be treated with a variety of chelating agents including EDTA and penicillamine used in shampoo-like formulations. Sometimes home water systems will acquire increased levels of copper either as a result of a lowering of the water pH from fluoridation leading to leaching of copper or from improperly grounded electrical devices driving copper into the water. Industrial exposure to copper may also impart a green tinge to the hair. Occupational exposure to cobalt and indigo may

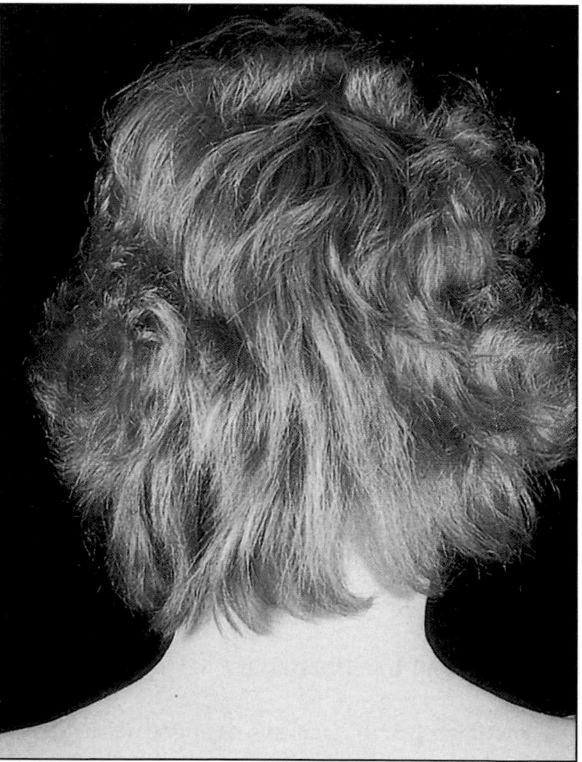

Fig. 31.10. Green hair from copper in swimming-pool water

give a blue color, while picric acid produces yellow tones. Anthralin and resorcinol both stain light-colored hair blue-brown, while benzoyl peroxide may bleach darker hair. Rarely microorganisms may discolor hair; the two best examples are piedra and trichomycosis axillaris.

Excessive Hair Growth

The density of the hairs on the scalp and body is highly variable. It is often impossible to determine if a given condition in a patient is within the normal range or represents an abnormal condition. A careful history and perhaps evaluation of previous records or photographs is most useful in deciding if too much or too little hair is present. A number of terms are used to describe apparent increase in hair number. They include:

- Hypertrichosis. Excess hairs appear to be present, but in every instance pale vellus hairs have been transformed into dark, thick terminal hairs. There is tremendous individual, family, age, sex, and ethnic group variation in what constitutes excess hair. Dark hairs on the upper lip of a Mediterranean woman are much more common than the same finding in a Celt. Hypertrichosis is often familial without any trace of hormonal abnormalities.
- Hirsutism. When women or children develop male pattern hair growth under the influence of androgens, we speak of hirsutism. Typically the upper lip, chin, cheeks, breasts, linea alba, and the upper part of the pubic triangle are involved. The cause may be either excess androgen production or increased end organ sensitivity of the hair apparatus to the hormone. In any event, once again vellus hairs in specific sites are converted to terminal hairs.
- Virilization. When hirsutism is accompanied by other signs of masculinization, we speak of virilization. Once again, androgens are always involved. Typical changes include acne, male pattern baldness, clitoral hypertrophy, deepening of the voice, breast atrophy, development of a male habitus and amenorrhea.

Hypertrichoses

Congenital Hypertrichosis

The fine coat of lanugo hairs is usually shed in utero during the eighth month of pregnancy. The discarded hairs form part of the vernix which covers the newborn. Some premature infants are born with their lanugo hair coat, which is then shed in the first postnatal month or two. This is a normal condition among premature infants and should not be confused with the much rarer congenital hypertrichosis lanuginosa.

Congenital Hypertrichosis Lanuginosa

Synonyms. Trichostasis lanuginosa, hypertrichosis universalis congenita, generalized familial hypertrichosis

In this very rare condition, infants present with excessive lanugo hairs, which are long, fine, usually lack pigment, and under the microscope lack a medulla (Fig. 31.11). They are either born with excess hairs (retention of fetal lanugo hairs) or in

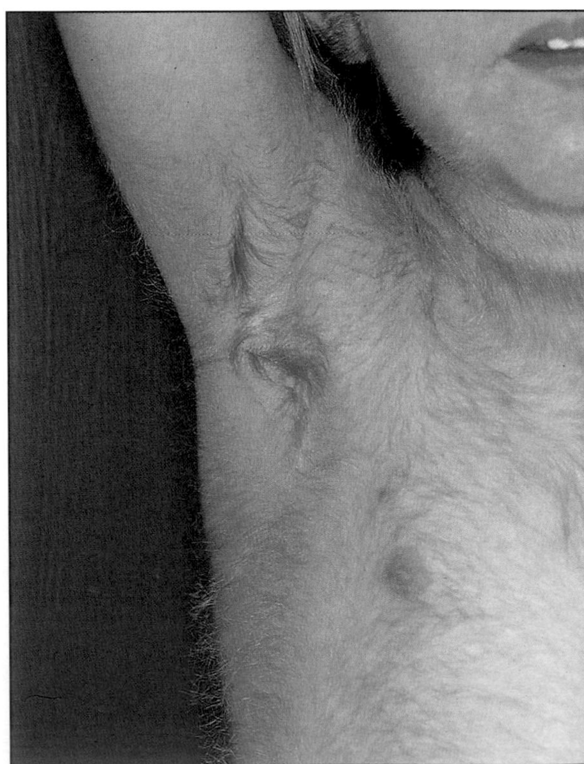

Fig. 31.11. Congenital hypertrichosis lanuginosa

some cases the extra hairs become apparent during the first weeks of life. In some cases, the hairs may acquire some terminal characteristics, such as pigment. Cases may either be sporadic or familial, inherited in an autosomal dominant pattern. Terrible names have been applied to such unfortunate individuals, such as "monkey men" or "dog-faced men", and they are occasionally featured in circus side shows. Both sporadic and familial cases have been reported with a wide range of associated disorders.

Acquired Hypertrichosis Lanuginosa

(Le Marquand and Bohn 1950)

Synonyms. Hypertrichosis lanuginosa acquisita. Herzberg-Potjan-Gebauer (1968) syndrome.

Acquired hypertrichosis lanuginosa is an almost invariable marker for an internal malignancy. It is usually associated with a carcinoma, often metastatic. In contrast to the congenital form, the hairs tend to be pigmented. Prominent papillae on the distal part of the tongue have been described as an associated finding.

Nevoid Hypertrichosis

A number of unrelated conditions are included under this heading. Probably the most common is the faun tail or a patch of long hairs over the sacrum. This may be a sign of an underlying spinal defect, such as spina bifida. Similar changes have been described in the cervical region associated with familial scoliosis. Congenital melanocytic nevi are often associated with hairs; sometimes the underlying nevus may be subtle. Becker nevus typically develops excess hairs during puberty. Hypertrichosis may also be associated with hypertrophy of body parts such as in congenital hemihypertrophy or Klippel-Weber-Trenaunay syndrome. In nevoid circumscribed hypertrichosis, there is a patch or tuft of hair, often dark and long, arising on clinically normal skin. The diagnosis of hair follicle nevus is a pathologic one. Usually the lesion is a pale to red nodule on the head or neck without excessive hairs but microscopically there is a collection of many normal follicles.

Acquired Circumscribed Hypertrichosis

Chronic low-grade trauma, radiation therapy, heat (such as from chronic heating pad use) and other stimuli may induce a localized hypertrichosis. One of the side effects of topical corticosteroid use is also localized hypertrichosis. While the pathogenesis in most cases is unclear, if the stimulus is removed improvement can be expected.

Hypertrichosis as a Sign of Internal Disease

Patients with several types of porphyria tend to develop hypertrichosis especially of the temples and cheeks. While facial hypertrichosis is common in porphyria cutanea tarda, more diffuse changes are seen in some of the congenital porphyrias. Postencephalitic hypertrichosis has become uncommon for unclear reasons. Multiple sclerosis patients may also have excess hairs. A long list of endocrine abnormalities can lead to excess hairs. They include acromegaly, hypothyroidism, and POEMS syndrome. In pretibial myxedema, there may be localized hypertrichosis over the mucinous plaques. Malnutrition and especially anorexia nervosa are also associated. Hypertrichosis is also a feature of dermatomyositis and epidermolysis bullosa acquisita.

Drug-Induced Hypertrichosis

Medications cannot induce new hairs. Instead, they may convert vellus hairs to terminal hairs, making them much more apparent (Figs. 31.12, 31.13). Table 31.1 lists some of the drugs implicated in causing hypertrichosis. Topical corticosteroids may cause localized erythema and hypertrichosis. In an attempt to utilize this side effect positively, the antihypertensive minoxidil is now used as a topical solution to treat male pattern baldness and other forms of alopecia. The hair growth induced by hormones is usually considered hirsutism, since it is androgen-mediated.

Table 31.1. Medications causing hypertrichosis

Benoxaprofen	Minoxidil
Cyclosporine	D-Penicillamine
Diazoxide	Phenytoin
Fenoterol	Psoralens (± UVA)
Hexachlorobenzene	Streptomycin
Interferons	Metyrapone

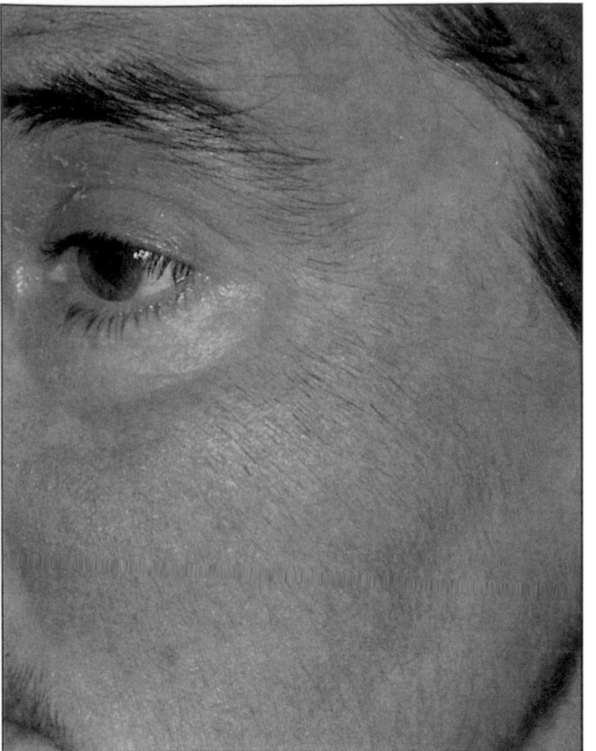

Fig. 31.12. Hypertrichosis from topical corticosteroids

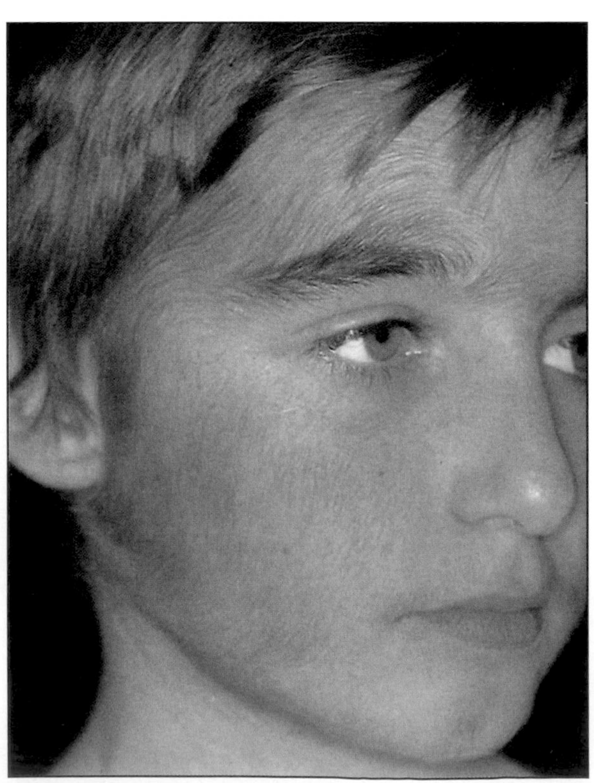

Fig. 31.13. Hypertrichosis from systemic minoxidil

Hirsutism

Hirsutism is increased hair growth in a male pattern in women or children, either caused by abnormal hormone levels or by increased end organ sensitivity to hormones. A woman stimulated with androgens may develop increased body hair, altered pubic hair pattern, facial hairs and even male pattern baldness (Figs. 31.14, 31.15). If other signs of masculinization are present, the diagnosis is virilization.

Hirsutism is typically caused by endocrine disturbances or by medications with androgenic actions, or may be idiopathic (Table 31.2). The typical endocrine causes involve secretion of androgens or androgen-stimulating mediators by the pituitary, ovaries or adrenal glands. There are a number of inherited disorders in which hirsutism is present. Almost all are variants of congenital adrenal hyperplasia in which cortisone production is hampered by a missing enzyme leading to increased ACTH levels and excess androgen produc-

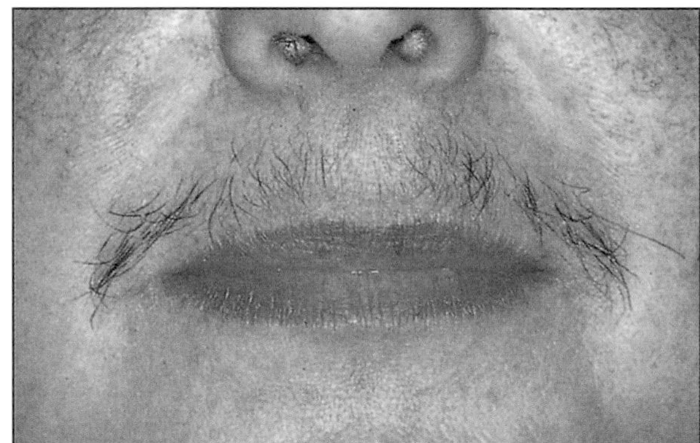

Fig. 31.14. Mustache hairs in a hirsute woman

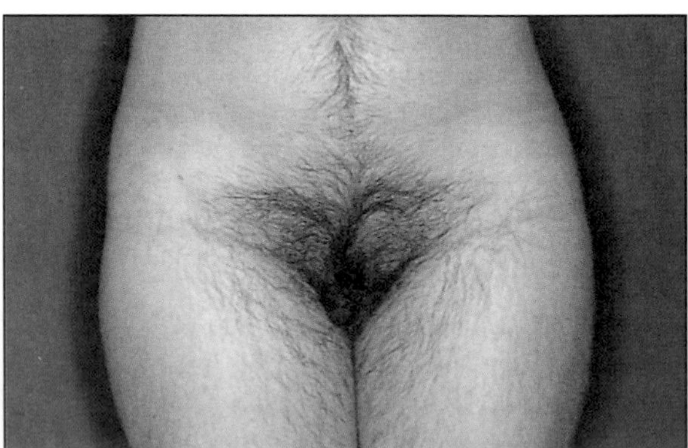

Fig. 31.15. Hirsutism in a woman

Table 31.2. Causes of hirsutism

Endocrine	Medications
Polycystic ovary syndrome (Stein-Leventhal syndrome)	ACTH
Ovarian tumors	Anabolic steroids
Adrenogenital syndrome (including female pseudo-hermaphroditism)	Androgens
Cushing syndrome and disease	Danazol
HAIR-AN syndrome (*h*yper*a*ndrogenism, *i*nsulin *r*esistance and *a*canthosis *n*igricans)	Progesterones
Adrenal tumors	Spironolactone
Acromegaly	Idiopathic
Hyperprolactinemia-hypogonadism syndrome	

tion. In the early-onset variants, female children will be born with ambiguous or masculine genitalia (female pseudohermaphroditism). In milder, later-onset cases, patients may present with hirsutism.

Two acquired syndromes typically involve hirsute women. In the Stein-Leventhal syndrome (Stein and Leventhal 1935), polycystic ovaries are associated with hirsutism, male pattern baldness, obesity and amenorrhea. The Achard-Thiers syndrome (Achard and Thiers 1921) is seen in postmenopausal women who develop hirsutism (especially facial hair), diabetes mellitus, obesity, frontal bone hyperostosis and occasionally virilization. They have an overproduction of adrenal androgens, which is no longer counteracted by their estrogens.

Idiopathic Hirsutism

Idiopathic hirsutism is a diagnosis of exclusion. In the past, it was often made, but as the sensitivity of endocrine testing improves, slight defects are found in more and more patients making idiopathic hirsutism far less common. There are tremendous individual, familial and even ethnic variations in the sensitivity of the hair follicle to androgens, as reflected by the varying degrees of "hairiness" seen among the earth's people. Apparently the variation lies in how individual hair follicles process androgens. Thus if an individual is clinically hirsute and has no detectable hormonal abnormalities, one can speak of idiopathic hirsutism.

Diagnostic Criteria

History. The following aspects should be explored: ethnic background, appearance of relatives, onset and progression of hair growth, variations at puberty, during pregnancy and at menopause, medications.

Clinical Findings. Exact description of localization and degree of excess hair growth, search for signs of virilization, gynecologic evaluation (usually in consultation).

Laboratory Findings. A laboratory evaluation is needed if one is not convinced that the excessive hair is normal for the patient, i.e. within the range seen in her family and in other members of her ethnic group. If the patient is taking a medication which could be responsible, it should be stopped first. The expense of doing a hormonal workup make it important to be aware of what individual tests cost and how screening can be most economically accomplished.

We employ testosterone and dihydroepiandrosterone sulfate (DHEA-S) as the most reasonable screens for ovarian and adrenal androgen production. If the patient has a long history, no virilization and a normal gynecologic examination, one can stop here. If these criteria are not met, one can proceed to more advanced testing in collaboration with a gynecologist or endocrinologist. Imaging of the ovaries and adrenal glands can also be accomplished in a variety of ways.

Therapy. If an underlying defect is found, it must be addressed by the appropriate specialist. Most tumors are amenable to surgery. Most dermatologic therapy consists of epilation of excess hairs and administration of antiandrogens.

Systemic. The medical treatment of hirsutism is almost always hormonal. Even idiopathic hirsutism is treated with antiandrogens. The patient must be patient; therapy cannot begin to be evaluated for at least 12 months. Many patients become discouraged or cannot tolerate the side effects and stop sooner. Two basic approaches are employed:

- Suppression of both ovarian and adrenal androgen production by replacement with estrogen/progesterone combinations (either oral contraceptives or any number of regimens described in the literature) and dexamethasone (0.5–1.0 mg/day). It is quite difficult to convince patients to take corticosteroids, so this approach is hard to employ. More acceptable is the use of oral contraceptives that are relatively estrogen-dominant and have a progestational agent without androgen activity. Unfortunately, in the movement towards lower estrogen levels to avoid thromboembolic problems, there are no longer any estrogen-dominant contraceptives available in the USA and few in western Europe.
- Use of antiandrogens. In Europe, cyproterone acetate is available both in combination with ethinylestradiol (Diane 35, Dianette) and alone (Androcur). It is the most widely used antiandrogen. The main indications are acne, hirsutism and male pattern baldness in women. For mild to moderate hirsutism, we often employ Diane 35. For more severe problems, we may employ Androcur along with ethinylestradiol. By not using combination tablets, we can adjust the dosages better, either to reduce side effects or to match the degree of hirsutism. One scheme is:
- Days 5–25 ethinylestradiol 0.04 mg
- Days 5–14 cyproterone acetate 10–20 mg

The level of cyproterone acetate is adjusted to match the severity of the hirsutism and increased if the response to therapy is unsuccessful. Because of potential damage to a fetus, cyproterone acetate must be used in combination with contraceptives. Conversely, menopausal patients or those who have experienced surgical menopause can be treated with cyproterone acetate alone in dosages of 10–20 mg. If improvement is achieved, one can move back to lower levels of medications or even switch to Diane. If all therapy is stopped, the excess hair growth usually reappears.

The main contraindications for cyproterone acetate are varicose veins and other risk factors for thromboembolic disease, uterine leiomyomas, smoking and cardiovascular disease. Side effects include fatigue, headaches, depression, weight gain, loss of libido, breast pain and menstrual irregularities. There is a theoretical risk of hepatic tumors, documented primarily in laboratory animals, but it is not a clinical problem.

The second antiandrogen available in Europe is chlormadinone acetate. Its mechanism is similar to that of cyproterone acetate. Several different brand names are available. In Germany one can choose between chlormadinone 2.0 mg or combination products – either 2.0 mg combined with 0.05 mg mestranol (Gestamestrol N) or 1.0 mg with 0.05 mg ethinylestradiol (Neo-Eunomin). Usage guidelines are similar to those for Diane 35 and Dianette. Both products are approved for hirsutism, as well as acne, marked seborrhea and androgenetic alopecia.

There are a number of other agents which are used to treat hirsutism, even though they are not officially approved for that use. In the USA spironolactone, an aldosterone antagonist, is often employed for its antiandrogen activity. Dosages of 50–100 mg/day usually suffice but some patients require 200 mg daily. Since potassium excretion is altered, electrolyte levels should be monitored until a stable pattern is seen. Side effects are similar to those with cyproterone acetate, and include menstrual problems and breast tenderness. Contraception should be practiced since male fetuses may be adversely affected.

In addition, a number of potent new antiandrogens have been introduced, primarily for treating hormonally responsive tumors. Flutamide is a very potent antiandrogen used in prostatic cancer. Finasteride is a 5α-reductase inhibitor with some specificity for the hair follicle. It is approved in several countries for treating androgenetic alopecia in males, as well as for benign prostatic hypertrophy.

Other Measures. Permanent epilation involves destroying the hair follicle with an electric current. Currently a number of lasers are being developed which promise better results in epilation. The main problems with electric epilation are pain, scarring and lack of effectiveness. It is estimated that in experienced hands only one-third of the treated follicles are permanently destroyed, requiring multiple treatments.

Temporary removal of hair can be done with chemical depilatories or simply by shaving or plucking. Chemical depilatories contain thioglycolates, but in a higher concentration than in permanent waves. They simply dissolve the hair, but invariably cause an irritant dermatitis. The question is – how irritated will the skin become? Another approach is the application of hot wax which is allowed to harden and then removed, ripping out the hairs. There is no scientific evidence that frequent shaving stimulates hair growth, but it is most difficult to convince a patient of this. It is at least plausible that vellus hairs may be stimulated towards terminal hairs by repeated manipulation. There are also newer electrical devices that epilate or pluck hairs by trapping them in a rotating spring-like device. Finally, many patients are best served by simply bleaching the excess hairs with hydrogen peroxide (3–5% solution); this makes them less noticeable.

Alopecia

The terminology used to describe a reduction in the amount of hair is even more confusing than that used to describe excess terminal hairs. Key terms include:

- Effluvium. The process of hair loss.
- Alopecia. The result of effluvium; the absence or reduction in number of hairs from areas where it is normally present. We distinguish between localized or diffuse alopecia, as well as partial or total complete alopecia. In alopecia the hair follicles may be retained, reduced in size (miniaturization) or replaced by scarring. In the most common alopecia, terminal hairs change into vellus-like hairs.
- Atrichia. Although not linguistically correct, atrichia is generally taken to mean alopecia because of the congenital absence of hair follicles. For example, in aplasia cutis congenita, no follicles are seen.
- Hypotrichosis. The presence of reduced numbers of hair. It is easier to reserve hypotrichosis for congenital disorders, just as with atrichia. Hypotrichosis can be diffuse or circumscript. The diffuse form is often associated with a long list of other ectodermal dysplasias. If one does not reserve hypotrichosis for congenital abnormalities, then hypotrichosis and alopecia are identical. We have not changed any of the standard names so both terms can be found throughout the chapter.

Yet another way to divide alopecias is into permanent, progressive and reversible. We will follow this categorization, since it reflects the major concern of patients and not our linguistic skills.

The patient with alopecia usually is most interested in knowing if the hair loss is temporary or permanent. Even temporary hair loss will take months to years to be corrected, for the average scalp hair in a woman is probably several years in growing. Permanent alopecia can result in a number of ways. In rare situations, the hair follicles are not present to begin with. In other situations, they are destroyed by infections, inflammatory infiltrates, tumors or exogenous factors such as trauma or X-rays. The transition from terminal hairs to vellus hairs in male pattern baldness is also a form of permanent alopecia, although there are many current efforts to change this trend.

Congenital Hypotrichosis

Reduced hair growth is associated with a long list of disorders discussed throughout this book. Many features can combine to produce the clinical picture of reduced hairs: decreased number of follicles, decreased hair growth and increased hair fragility. A decreased number of follicles is usually combined with other ectodermal defects. Decreased hair growth is seen in Rothmund-Thomson syndrome, Netherton syndrome, dyskeratosis congenita, many forms of ectodermal dysplasia and a wide variety of other disorders. Many of the structural hair shaft changes discussed earlier in the chapter present with hypotrichosis, such as monilethrix or pili torti. No therapy is generally available for congenital hypotrichosis. A search for associated defects, genetic counseling and encouraging the parents or patient to use a wig are the best we can offer.

Atrichia Universalis

(Lundbäck 1944)

These rare patients have a mutation in the human equivalent of the hairless gene of the mouse. This gene is a zinc finger transcription factor that controls a number of cytokines and growth factors just in the hair follicle. The disease is inherited in an autosomal recessive pattern. The best known pedigree traces the defect through a large inbred Pakistani family. The patients are born with hair, but lose it in the first months of life. They may also lose other hairs, such as eyebrows and eyelashes. Microscopic studies show the absence of hair follicles. Since hairs were at one time present, at least some scarring or follicular remnants should be present. This demonstrates once again the problems in linguistically distinguishing between hypotrichosis and atrichia.

Hypotrichosis Congenita Simplex
(Marie Unna 1925)

Synonym. Marie Unna syndrome

This is probably not a single disease but several different disorders, all inherited in an autosomal dominant pattern. The patients have hairs at birth but lose them either in the first months of life or as children. In Marie Unna's patients, the hairs were coarse and twisted, while in the descriptions of Jeanselme and Rime they were structurally normal. In another pedigree, affected members had very light-colored hair and multiple milia.

Atrichia Congenita with Papular Lesions
(Damsté 1954)

This disorder is inherited in an autosomal recessive pattern. While the infants are born with hairs, they lose them in the first months of life. Later as young adults they tend to develop numerous milia or epidermoid cysts. The latter are most common on the scalp and neck. Follicles may also be plugged, leading to atrophodermia vermiculata. The condition in such patients tends to overlap with keratosis follicularis spinulosa decalvans and even ichthyosis follicularis, atrichia and photophobia (IFAP) syndrome (Chap. 17).

Cartilage-Hair Hypoplasia
(McKusick 1964)

Synonym. Metaphyseal chondrodysplasia, type McKusick

McKusick described a type of chondrodysplastic dwarfism among the Amish with an increased susceptibility to infections and sparse blond hair. The scalp hairs are thin and silky, while the eyebrows and eyelashes are sparse. Other body hair is variable and the nails are normal. The patients have persistent lymphopenia and are especially susceptible to severe varicella infections.

Onychotrichodysplasia and Neutropenia Syndrome
(Cantú et al. 1975; Hernandez et al. 1979)

Synonym. ONMR syndrome (onychotrichodysplasia, neutropenia, mild retardation)

In this even rarer disorder, also inherited in an autosomal recessive pattern, patients have neutropenia, recurrent bacterial infections and mental retardation. Their hairs are sparse and they tend to have trouble with ingrowing eyelashes leading to keratitis. In some instances, trichothiodystrophy has been identified. In addition, they have hypoplastic brittle nails.

Congenital Triangular Alopecia
(Sabouraud 1905)

Synonym. Alopecia triangularis congenita

These patients have permanent triangular alopecia in the frontotemporal region. The cause is unknown. Parents often blame obstetric manipulation but this is not correct. No familial pattern has been described, but girls may be more often affected. There is a 2–4-cm hairless area, usually in the shape of a triangle whose base is along the frontal hair line and whose apex extends posteriorly. While the changes are present at birth, they are often not fully appreciated until the child is several years old. The changes are stable throughout the patient's life. While usually unilateral, congenital triangular alopecia may be bilateral. Hair follicles are markedly reduced or absent. The skin is otherwise normal. There is no scarring. If first recognized at a later age, this problem may be misdiagnosed as alopecia areata. The triangular shape, typical location and lack of follicles on biopsy are distinguishing features. Traction alopecia may produce similar clinical changes but the follicles are distorted or atrophic, not absent. There is no treatment.

Scarring Alopecia

All scarring processes are capable of damaging the hair follicle, leading to hair loss and by definition irreversible alopecia. The causes of scarring alopecia are listed in Table 31.3. Extensive inflammation, infections, tumors and trauma are the main causes. While scarring anywhere on the body can lead to

Table 31.3. Causes of scarring alopecia[a]

Genetic disorders	Physical damage	Tumors	Infectious disorders	Miscellaneous disorders
Darier disease Keratosis follicularis spinulosa decalvans Epidermolysis bullosa (primarily dystrophic forms) Ichthyosis (various forms) Chondrodysplasia punctata (X-linked dominant form, Conradi-Hünerman syndrome) Incontinentia pigmenti	Ionizing radiation Thermal burns Chemical injuries Mechanical trauma	Metastatic tumors Basal cell carcinoma Adnexal tumors Squamous cell carcinoma Hemangioma Lymphocytic infiltrate and lymphoma	Furuncles and carbuncles Leprosy Tertiary syphilis Lupus vulgaris Perifolliculitis abscedens et suffodiens Deep dermatophyte infections Zoster	Amyloidosis (mainly nodular forms) Cicatricial pemphigoid Eosinophilic pustulosis Erosive pustular dermatitis of the scalp Graft versus host disease Lichen sclerosus et atrophicus Lichen planus (lichen planopilaris) Lupus erythematosus (primarily discoid) Sarcoidosis Scleroderma and morphea Pityriasis amiantacea

[a] This list refers to true scarring alopecia and does not include the subcategory of atrophic alopecia or pseudopelade, shown in Table 31.4

alopecia, patients usually complain only when the scalp or face is involved.

Histologically, scarring alopecias are characterized by dermal scarring, often relatively deep, along with absent or reduced hair follicles and reduced numbers of arrector pili muscles.

In Europe, atrophic alopecias are considered a subcategory of scarring alopecias. Here the damage is caused by an inflammatory infiltrate. Clinically the skin is thinned and the follicle openings are reduced or absent. Very typical for atrophic alopecias is the retention of bundles of hair, often called the paint brush sign. While most atrophic alopecias are localized, occasionally they become diffuse. The histology shows reduced to absent hair follicles and retained arrector pili muscles. Pseudopelade of Brocq is taken as the prototype of atrophic alopecia, along with the alopecias associated with lichen planus and lupus erythematosus. A new classification of scarring of alopecias proposed by Sperling and colleagues is conceptually attractive and may lead to clarification of this puzzling topic.

Lichen Planus

At least one-third of patients with inflammatory and scarring alopecia have lichen planus (Chap. 14). While most patients have clues to lichen planus elsewhere on the skin or mucosa, some have disease confined to the scalp. There is generally a patchy alopecia, but individual follicular papules or hyperkeratotic plugs may be present. Frontal fibrosing alopecia (Kossard 1994) may be a variant. It typically involves the frontal hairline in postmenopausal women with perifollicular erythema. Cases have been described with typical lichen planus elsewhere.

Lupus Erythematosus

In discoid lupus erythematosus, the typical lesion has an erythematous border and a central white scarred area. In systemic lupus erythematosus, there is often a more diffuse alopecia, perhaps combining elements of telogen effluvium and diffuse or atrophic scarring alopecia.

Morphea and Systemic Sclerosis

Morphea, especially the en coup de sabre form, usually causes obvious alopecia. In systemic sclerosis the hair loss is more often diffuse and more subtle. There is a thickened dermis with entrapment and atrophy of follicles, but with no scarring, as shown by normal elastic fiber stains.

Graft Versus Host Reaction

Chronic graft versus host reaction has both sclerodermoid and lichenoid features, so it is not surprising that both types of alopecia may be seen.

Sarcoidosis

In sarcoidosis, the hair loss is focal and scarring, as sarcoidal granulomas destroy the follicles. It is more common in black women.

Pseudopelade

(Brocq 1885)

Synonym. Alopecia areata atrophicans

Definition. Chronic localized irreversible hair loss in which clinically or histologically atrophy can be identified. It is contrasted to alopecia areata or pelade which has no scarring or atrophy. In Germany pseudopelade is taken as an inclusive term, to describe all types of inflammatory scarring alopecia, including lupus erythematosus and lichen planus. In the USA, it is a diagnosis of exclusion, once other diseases have been ruled out. This fundamental difference makes comparing the literature confusing.

Etiology and Pathogenesis. It is unclear whether pseudopelade represents a separate disease or simply the end-point of a number of dermatoses. In our experience, in about half the cases we find no cause, while in the rest historical, clinical or histologic clues point towards an associated diagnosis (Table 31.4).

Table 31.4. The differential diagnosis of pseudopelade

Common causes	Uncommon dermatoses
Folliculitis decalvans	Necrobiosis lipoidica diabeticorum
Lichen planus	Granuloma annulare
Lupus erythematosus	Sarcoidosis
Morphea	Metastases
	Favus (and rarely other dermatophyte infections)
	Ulerythema ophryogenes

Clinical Findings. Pseudopelade is an uncommon disorder, primarily seen in middle-aged women. It begins with one or several small patches of alopecia, usually in the parietal region. Most often there are no symptoms. For this reason, the patches are sometimes quite large before the patient comes to the doctor. The areas of alopecia slowly expand. Initially they are round but later quite irregular. They may coalesce but also have a sharp border. Eventually the skin becomes shiny, yellow-white, thinned (cigarette paper-like) and lacks follicular orifices. Signs of inflammation or follicular plugging are not seen. Often small bundles of hairs remain (Fig. 31.16). As the disease progresses and no definite diagnosis or effective treatment is found, the patients often become emotionally upset. They almost never have pruritus.

Histopathology. By definition there is no obvious scarring. The epidermis is atrophic. Follicles are reduced in number or absent. In their place, naked arrector pili and fibrous sheaths perpendicular to the epidermis are found. A lymphocytic perivascular infiltrate may be seen. A perifollicular infiltrate should raise questions about an associated disorder. Stains for elastin reveal a loss of elastic fibers. The PAS stain shows a normal basement membrane, as contrasted to the thickened one seen in lupus erythematosus.

Course and Prognosis. The course is unpredictable. Some patients progress to diffuse alopecia; others have focal hair loss for many years. Degos (1951) used the term état pseudopéladique to describe the final appearance of pseudopélade, suggesting that in the late stages it is impossible to separate idiopathic and disease-associated forms.

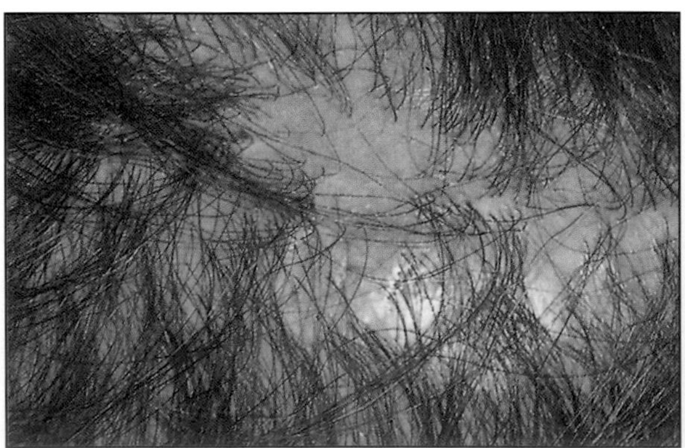

Fig. 31.16. Pseudopelade

Differential Diagnosis. The main step is to exclude the disorders listed in Table 31.4 before making the diagnosis of idiopathic pseudopelade. It is especially important to search for signs of lichen planus or lupus erythematosus elsewhere on the patient. In addition one should try to exclude alopecia areata, which has a much better prognosis for regrowth. Typically in alopecia areata hair follicle openings are still visible and exclamation point or pelade hairs as well as cadaverized hairs are visible at the active border. A biopsy will show a lymphocytic infiltrate about at least some follicles and may also reveal clues towards the underlying cause.

Therapy

Systemic. Many systemic approaches have been tried, including antimalarials, isoniazid, dapsone and nonsteroidal antiinflammatory drugs. Systemic corticosteroids, usually prednisone 40–80 mg daily for 2 weeks, then tapered rapidly over another 2 weeks, is a worthwhile attempt to arrest the process.

Topical. High-potency topical corticosteroids under occlusion are the best choice. Intralesional corticosteroids are another approach, but they too often fail. Triamcinolone acetonide 2.5 mg/ml can be injected at the periphery. If there is dramatic regrowth of hair, the initial diagnosis was probably wrong.

Lipedematous Alopecia

(Cornbleet 1935)

This unusual alopecia is most common in black women. The scalp hairs are short and require infrequent cutting, but are otherwise normal. The key finding is a boggy scalp – the first patient complained that it felt as if she had cotton padding between her skull and her scalp. The scalp thickness is about double that of normal individuals (12 mm versus 6 mm) when measured with ultrasound. Histologic examination reveals the abnormally thick subcutaneous fat layer. There is no treatment.

Mechanical Alopecia

Both acute and chronic pressure and traction can produce hair loss. Acute traction is either traumatic or intentional, as in a trichogram. Acute pressure alopecia usually occurs following a major surgical procedure when the patient's head was not moved or adjusted for many hours. The problem occurs more often in children. Thus the most typical location is on the occiput. In both situations, a few follicles may be destroyed but the vast majority will produce new hairs.

Chronic pressure alopecia occurs in localized areas and is often an occupational stigma. For example, it has been described in nuns being caused by their caps, and in individuals who carry heavy loads with the aid of a head strap. The most common mechanical alopecia is chronic traction alopecia. The first official description was probably that of Sabouraud (1931) who used the term chignon (French for bun) alopecia. Here the alopecia develops on the occipital region where the hair is pulled up into a bun. In Germany, one speaks of alopecia hassica, where hassica is the Latin word for Hessen, a German state where some old regional costumes also required the hair to be pulled up tightly (Fig. 31.17). Braids or pony tails where the hair is pulled back tightly cause hair loss along the anterior marginal hair line. The multiple tiny braids or corn rows often seen in blacks produce widespread alopecia in some individuals. Finally, long-term use of extremely tight hair curlers can also cause alopecia. The prognosis in chronic me-

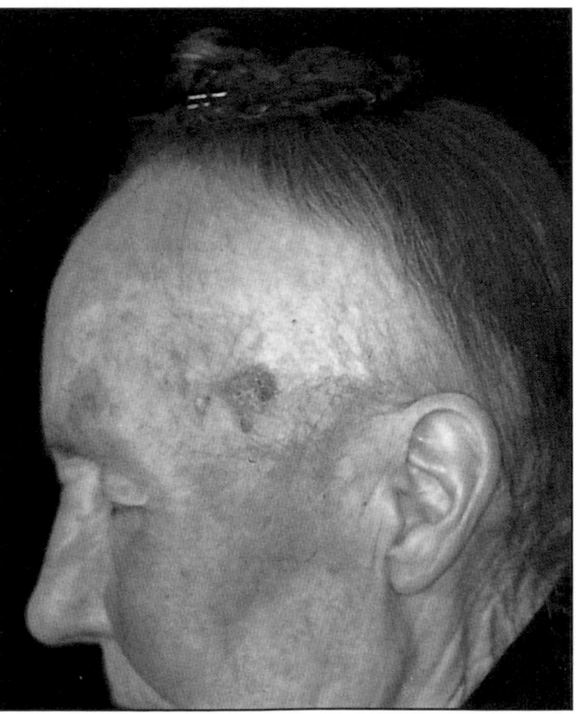

Fig. 31.17. Traction alopecia (alopecia Hessica) with an actinic keratosis on the temple as an additional finding

chanical alopecia is uncertain. If the problem is recognized and the mechanical forces removed, regrowth can be expected. If the patient or parent does not correct the problem, regressive follicular changes will occur, leading to either cessation of hair production or production of thin, short vellus-like hairs.

Progressive Non-scarring Alopecia

Androgenetic Alopecia

Synonym. Male pattern baldness

Definition. Androgen-dependent hair loss in men with a characteristic pattern.

Etiology and Pathogenesis. The three major factors are genetic predisposition, age and level of androgens. Orentreich has proposed the term androchronogenetic alopecia to encompass all three factors. Androgenetic alopecia is the most common alopecia of all, comprising 95% of cases. Almost every white man winds up with some degree of male pattern baldness. Racial and familial factors play a key role. The likelihood of a given man developing male pattern baldness is related to the number of first and second degree relatives with a bald head; if his mother or sister has androgenetic alopecia, the outlook is worse. Clearly the incidence of male pattern baldness increases with age. Finally, androgens are a must. As is well known, eunuchs do not become bald. Conversely, castrated men who are treated with androgens do develop hair loss.

The response of a given follicle in a given region at a given time is programmed. Aristotle raised the question – why do androgens stimulate beard and body hair but at the same time cause loss of hair on the scalp? We still cannot answer his question. But there seem to be important differences in the way follicles in different areas metabolize testosterone. The most important enzyme is 5α-reductase which converts testosterone to dihydrotestosterone, which is then transferred to the nucleus via a variety of receptors and binding proteins. There it can influence mRNA production. Another important enzyme appears to be 3-β-hydroxysteroid-dehydrogenase. In any event, some follicles metabolize androgens to stimulate hair growth, and others to inhibit growth.

Under the influence of these hormones the hair follicles undergo regressive metamorphosis. In each cycle the telogen phase becomes longer and thus more follicles are found in telogen. The following anagen phase is shorter and the new hair is shorter, thinner and less pigmented. Eventually pale fuzzy vellus-like hairs are the result. The trichogram is not necessary but shows primarily telogen hairs with many smaller less pigmented forms. The key concept is donor dominance. This means that hairs from the posterior-lateral regions, such as those remaining in stage 4 loss, are unlikely to ever fall out even if they are transferred to bald areas.

Clinical Findings. Androgenetic alopecia usually begins in the frontotemporal area and follows relatively well-defined patterns. Figure 31.18 is modified from the classification of Hamilton (1951)and Norwood (1975). Hair loss is gradual and rarely shows sharp borders as it progresses. In advanced stages, there is a sharp division between the hairs that remain and the smooth bald skin with vellus hairs. While the bald skin is not technically atrophic, it may feel thinned because so few hair bulbs are present. Since sebaceous glands are retained, they may appear clinically prominent as yellow bulbs or more often they may function too well, producing an oily scalp. When hairs are present, the sebum is spread over a far greater surface area than when they are absent.

Sometimes telogen effluvium can lead to an apparent worsening of male pattern baldness. Basically one can view this phenomenon as one telogen cycle of many being passed through extremely rapidly. Thus it plays almost no long-term role, but may explain why some patients complain of rapid baldness after a major traumatic or emotional event. Some patients with seborrheic dermatitis seem to have less hair loss if the dermatitis is treated aggressively. In the past, too-tight headgear and local circulatory problems were also considered cofactors for male pattern baldness, but there is little scientific support for these concepts.

Histopathology. There is a relative increase in telogen follicles and miniaturized follicles are found relatively higher up in the dermis. There is no scarring. The absolute number of hair follicles remains unchanged.

Course and Prognosis. The course is relentless, but it is impossible to predict the rapidity of hair loss or the final extent of the baldness.

Fig. 31.18. Male pattern hair loss,
a Stage 0
b Stage 1
c Stage 2
d Stage 2 (advanced)
e Stage 3
f Stage 4
(based on Orfanos and Happle 1990)

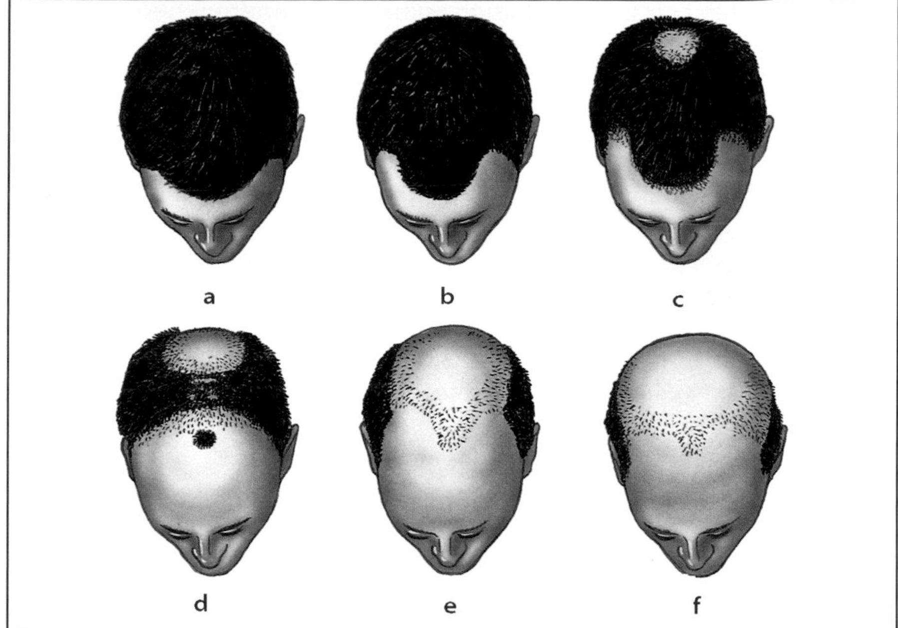

Simplified classification of androgenetic alopecia in men

Stage 0	Normal pattern
Stage 1	Loss in the frontotemporal areas
Stage 2	Loss in the occipital area (tonsure), as well in the frontal region; bridge of hair between the two zones
Stage 3	Confluence of the anterior and posterior areas of loss
Stage 4	Widespread loss with a horseshoe-shaped band of hair laterally and posteriorly

Therapy. Treatment of androgenetic alopecia is very difficult since the three major factors cannot be influenced. Male pattern baldness is often such a disturbing problem, causing emotional distress and distorted self-image, that not only physicians but also a wide variety of other healers have for centuries recommended an amazing list of ineffective therapies. Only in the past decades have several legitimate, but not ideal, approaches been developed.

Systemic. The only systemic therapy that works is chemical castration, that is the use of antiandrogens. Finasteride is an inhibitor of type II 5α-reductase which is approved in both Europe and USA but for which clinical experience is limited. The enzyme 5α-reductase converts testosterone to dihydrotestosterone. The type I form is most common in the skin including that of the scalp, while the type II form predominates in hair follicles as well as the prostate. Men with a genetic deficiency in type II 5α-reductase do not develop androgenetic alopecia. Oral finasteride lowers the serum, prostate and scalp levels of dihydrotestosterone. It shows good selectivity for the hair follicles and has few side effects. In patients treated for 2 years with 1 mg daily, there was increased hair growth, as assessed by hair counts, as well as improvement based on evaluator and patient assessments. The incidence of erectile dysfunction and decreased libido was around 1%; only the placebo group showed increased body hair growth. All other systemic treatments, such as vitamins, gelatin, amino acids (cystine, cysteine) and the like, are without benefit.

Topical. The only approved topical therapy in the USA is minoxidil 2% solution (Rogaine). Minoxidil was the subject of intensive research after it became clear that patients given systemic minoxidil often develop hypertrichosis. It appears that the best approach is twice-daily application of the 2% solution. The addition of topical retinoids seems to enhance the effect. The action is not dramatic. We tell patients that, if they are lucky, the minoxidil will arrest the further hair loss. In addition, some hairs may revert back towards more terminal characteristics. If the treatment is stopped, hair loss starts again, often at an increased rate (catch-up effect). Other than irritation, side effects are minimal. The product is very expensive: $ 60–100 per month with no support from most insurance plans. In the USA it is now an over-the-counter product.

Other topical treatments for male pattern baldness are ineffective. Estrogens are frequently prescribed. It is unclear if they ever help, but enough can be absorbed to have systemic side effects such as gynecomastia. The search goes on for an effective topical antiandrogen. Many products are in testing but none is currently commercially available.

Surgical. Hair transplantation is based on the principle of donor dominance. It is an effective method of producing permanent correction of male pattern baldness. The surgical procedures take a number of months, are painful, and are expensive. By combining a variety of techniques, an experienced hair surgeon can obtain remarkable result. The basic procedure is harvesting punch grafts; using special, very sharp, thin-walled punches, plugs are harvested from the occiput and transferred to bald areas, much as one plants a new lawn with plugs of grass. To provide wider coverage, flaps are sometimes used. In addition, scalp reduction may be employed to reduce the total area requiring coverage. Today, the uses of mini- and micrografts containing as few as one or two hairs, are used to create a more natural hairline. Some operators use a laser to make the incision in the recipient site; this decreases the bleeding. Further discussion of the many interesting approaches to hair transplant surgery is best sought in the specialized literature.

In some countries, the insertion of artificial hairs is still practiced. No matter what material is used for the replacement hairs, it eventually elicits a foreign body reaction, leading to intense inflammation, rejection of the hairs and massive scarring. We mention this approach only to condemn it.

Other Measures. Patients should be encouraged to consider wearing a wig or employing other nonsurgical hair replacement techniques where artificial hairs are woven into the hairs, rather than sewn into the scalp. Skilled hair stylists can also produce amazing improvement.

Androgenetic Alopecia of Women

Synonyms. Chronic diffuse alopecia, female "male pattern baldness"

This disorder is in need of a less derogatory name; no woman likes to hear that she has male pattern baldness or too many androgens. Chronic diffuse alopecia has never caught on, but it is the most natural, least-disturbing term.

Definition. Androgen-dependent alopecia in women which appears in a different clinical pattern from that in men and may be associated with underlying endocrine abnormalities.

Etiology and Pathogenesis. While androgenetic alopecia is not an illness in men, it is both a cause of great emotional distress and also a potential marker for internal disease in women. The same genetic factors apply to women as to men. While excess androgens in women tend to cause hirsutism and virilization, they may also cause hair loss on the scalp. Selected scalp hair follicles in some women show an exquisite androgen sensitivity, for many patients do not show elevated serum androgen levels. Conversely, only about one-quarter of women with virilization and proven elevated androgen levels have androgenetic alopecia. Both the ovaries and the adrenal glands may produce androgens.

Clinical Findings. Two relatively distinct patterns of hair loss can be seen: the female pattern which is more common before menopause, and the male pattern. Some patients have overlapping features. Most patients with the female pattern are between 20 and 40 years of age, have either no or minimal elevations in androgens and diffuse hair loss which can be staged in a way analogous to male pattern baldness. A valuable clinical sign is that even if the hair appears normal, when the patient makes a parting, it is wider than expected (Fig. 31.19). After menopause, about one-third of women have at least some frontotemporal loss. Although this alone is not unusual, other signs of virilization should be sought.

Histopathology. The histologic features are identical to those in male pattern baldness. The biopsy may be helpful in excluding a diffuse alopecia areata or even pseudopelade.

Laboratory Findings. The trichogram will show a telogen alopecia, just as with men. Free testosterone

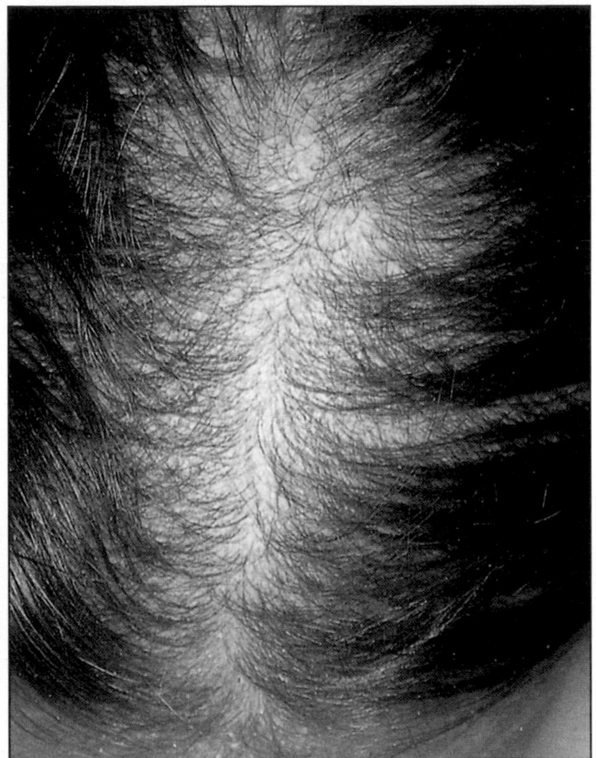

Fig. 31.19. Broad parting in a woman with androgenetic alopecia

and DHEA-S should be measured. Two additional tests may be valuable:

- If the testosterone/estrogen ratio is increased, less sex hormone-binding globulin (SHBG) is available and more active or free androgen will be circulating.
- The 3-α-17-α-androstendione/SHBG ratio is also often raised.

If other clinical signs are present, more extensive endocrine evaluation including measurement of prolactin, luteinizing hormone, and follicle stimulating-hormone levels should be considered.

Course and Prognosis. The development of complete baldness is uncommon. No matter what the age of onset, the alopecia can be expected to progress after menopause, as the counteraction of estrogens is lost.

Differential Diagnosis. Some patients feel they have marked loss, but clinically it is difficult to see much. One can speak of psychogenic pseudoalopecia. Such patients may be reassured by daily hair counts for 4 weeks, a trichogram and even a scalp biopsy. The loss of 50–100 hairs daily is normal. Other possible causes include medication-induced alopecia (Table 31.5), diffuse alopecia areata and pseudopelade. Syphilis can present with diffuse alopecia so a serology should be considered. Iron deficiency anemia and hypothyroidism are also associated with diffuse hair loss, which may be identical to some forms of androgenetic alopecia in women.

Therapy

Systemic. The therapy is very similar to that of hirsutism. Both oral contraceptives and antiandrogens can be employed using the same regimens outlined in detail.

Topical. Minoxidil solution, as discussed under male pattern baldness, is also approved for women. It should not be used during pregnancy or nursing. In Germany, a long list of topical tinctures and

Table 31.5. Medications and chemicals implicated in temporary hair loss

Anticoagulants	Anticonvulsants	Heavy metals
Heparin	Carbamazepine	Lead
Heparin derivatives	Cytostatic agents [a]	Mercury
Coumarin	Azathioprine	Selenium
β-Blockers	Cyclophosphamide	Thallium
Nadalol	Methotrexate	Arsenic
Propanolol	Vinca alkaloids	Thyroid inhibitors
Hormones	Miscellaneous	Thiamazole
Danazol	Colchicine	Propylthiouracil and other thiouracils
Androgens	Allopurinol	Vitamins
Lipid-lowering agents	Cimetidine	Retinoids
Fibrates (Clofibrate and others)	Levodopa	Vitamin A
Butyrophenone	Tricyclic antidepressants	

[a] Almost all cause hair loss in sufficient dosages; listed are a few common offenders.

lotions containing estrogens and corticosteroids are prescribed. No proof of their efficacy is available. Routine care of problems such as seborrheic dermatitis is also helpful.

Reversible Alopecia

Reversible hair loss or effluvium occurs following either endogenous or exogenous damage to anagen hair follicles; the resulting alopecia is usually diffuse. The two main diffuse reversible alopecias are anagen effluvium and telogen effluvium. In anagen effluvium there is acute damage to the follicle resulting in sudden loss of structurally damaged hairs. In telogen effluvium the damage is less severe and shifts more hairs into the telogen phase, so that after 2–5 months there is an increased loss of normal telogen hairs. In most cases only scalp hair is lost following damage to the hair follicle. The explanation may be that 85 % of scalp hairs are in anagen, actively growing, and readily damaged; only 15 % are in telogen. In other body areas, anagen is shorter and telogen longer, so that most hairs are in telogen and relatively resistant. The numbers (percent in telogen) are: eyebrows 80–90 %, axillary hairs 70 %, pubic hairs 60–80 % and terminal body hairs 60–80 %.

Anagen Effluvium

Definition. Sudden loss of dystrophic hairs secondary to acute toxic effects on the follicles.

Epidemiology. Diffuse anagen effluvium is common in cancer chemotherapy patients but otherwise rare.

Etiology and Pathogenesis. The difference between anagen and telogen effluvium is one of degree; the same agent that causes anagen effluvium usually cause telogen effluvium in lower doses. All the chemotherapy agents can cause anagen effluvium (Fig. 31.20). Colchicine is the most common nonchemotherapy agent to cause anagen effluvium. This is not surprising since it inhibits the mitotic spindle and arrests cell growth. Poisoning is another uncommon cause; thallium insecticides and pesticides were a common cause until banned commercially in the USA. Other heavy metals, arsenic, boric acid and some plant toxins are also occasionally incriminated. Radiation (3–10 Gy) produces reliable anagen effluvium; a half-century ago radiation was used to induce alopecia when treating tinea capitis. Marked starvation may also cause anagen effluvium, although telogen effluvium is more often seen with nutritional difficulties.

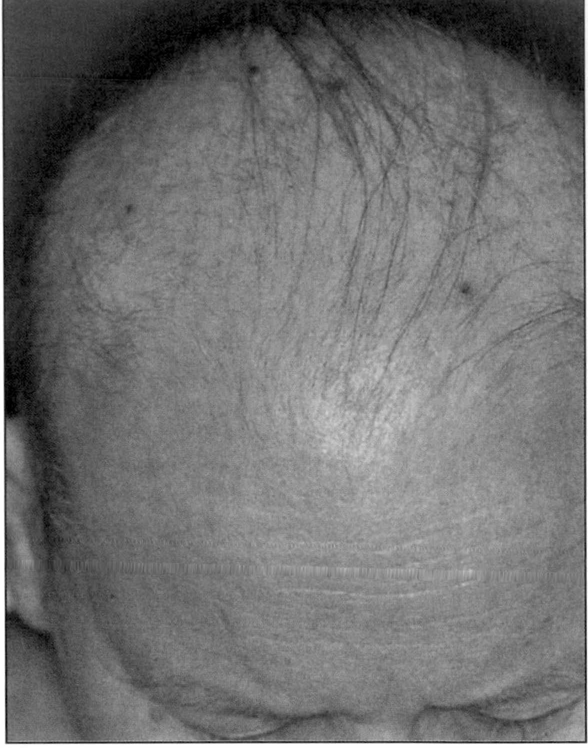

Fig. 31.20. Anagen effluvium associated with cancer chemotherapy

Severe damage to the growing anagen hairs leads to the development over a period of days of dystrophic hairs. When the rapid growth in the hair matrix is inhibited, the hair becomes thin at its base, breaks and falls out. The telogen cycle is skipped over. Thus there may be a rapid diffuse loss of hair immediately associated with the traumatic event.

With more severe toxic damage, the entire matrix is damaged. Hairs break off just above the zone of keratinization. The necrotic matrix forms plugs consisting of melanin, keratin and inner root sheath which are extruded through the follicular opening. These comedo-like plugs are known as cadaverized hairs. They are also common in alopecia areata. Another name for this process is trichomalacia. Despite the massive changes, the follicular unit is usually capable of forming new hairs.

Clinical Findings. The hair loss is sudden, rapid and may be very extensive. Patients may lose 90 % of their hairs in a matter of weeks. The hairs are often found in abundance on the patient's pillow, especially in chemotherapy wards.

Laboratory Findings. Examination with a hand lens will show the pointed or bayonet appearance of the proximal end of the hair. A trichogram confirms the presence of large numbers of dystrophic anagen hairs. The proximal end is tapered and lacks a clubbed root sheath. Pigment may be seen; it is usually absent in telogen hairs. A 1.0 % solution of 4-dimethylaminocinnamaldehyde (DACA) tends to selectively stain the inner root sheath and may make it easier to separate anagen and telogen hairs.

Course and Prognosis. If the toxin or outside agent is removed, in most cases regrowth is complete. Some chemotherapy patients regrow hairs in different colors or even textures, such as with curls when formerly the hair was straight, or just the opposite.

Differential Diagnosis. The main differential diagnostic consideration is severe telogen effluvium. Usually the history guides one in the right direction. The loose anagen syndrome is uncommon but should be considered in children with anagen effluvium.

Therapy. There is no good therapy. Ice caps have been used during chemotherapy but they are only appropriate for the treatment of solid tumors with little metastatic risk, as the cooled scalp offers a haven for circulating tumor cells.

Telogen Effluvium

Definition. Diffuse hair loss because of disturbance in hair cycle with disproportionate number of telogen hairs.

Epidemiology. Diffuse telogen effluvium is almost exclusively seen in women. While there is no reason to think the same process does not occur in men, the clinical hair loss is apparently not noticeable for men with generally shorter hair styles.

Etiology and Pathogenesis. The anagen hairs are rapidly growing and are sensitive to a variety of noxious agents. Telogen hairs in their resting state are relatively uninfluenced. Relatively minor damage to the anagen hair leads to a premature but otherwise physiologic ending of the anagen phase with subsequent develop of more telogen hairs than would have normally occurred. The time between the induced end of anagen and the loss of a telogen hair is about 2–5 months.

There is a long list of agents which have been incriminated as causing telogen effluvium. If a patient is exposed to a high fever or emotional or traumatic shock, delivers a baby, undergoes major surgery, or experiences similar events, a diffuse hair loss may occur several months later.

Infections. Any disease with a high fever can produce a telogen effluvium. Common causes are typhoid fever, malaria, and many viral illnesses. Even erysipelas may produce later hair loss.

Medications and Chemicals. Table 31.5 lists the common exogenous causes of telogen effluvium. The follicles seem to adjust to some medications. Patients may initially experience hair loss and then on the same dosage later experience total regrowth. The list of drugs in which hair loss has been described is endless; we have just chosen a few well-documented examples. It is often difficult in a single case to decide if the underlying disease or the medication has triggered the hair loss.

Hormonal Changes. The most common form of telogen effluvium is postpartum alopecia. It usually occurs 2–4 months after delivery and resolves spontaneously after a few months. The explanation is that during pregnancy the anagen phase is prolonged setting the patient up to lose telogen hairs later. A puzzling scenario is the transition from a telogen effluvium postpartum into a diffuse androgenetic alopecia in genetically predisposed women.

Either starting or stopping oral contraceptives may also trigger telogen effluvium. Usually the hair loss occurs in the first four to six cycles, but it may resolve even if the medication is continued. As in postpartum alopecia, hair loss may occur a few months after stopping oral contraceptives.

Both hypo- and hyperthyroidism can be associated with hair loss. It is usually telogen effluvium. Neither hormonal condition tends to present with hair loss; there are usually other symptoms. Ovarian, pituitary and adrenal tumors can all lead to hair loss. The clinical picture is mixed, based on stressed follicles and androgen influence. Prolactin-secreting tumors are particularly likely to cause a diffuse alopecia.

Acute and Chronic Illnesses. Almost any severe illness, including malignancies, connective tissue disorders, eating disorders, malabsorption, HIV/AIDS and many others, can lead to telogen effluvium. Some dermatologic disorders may also be responsible. Erythroderma is the most usual associations. Marked protein loss may occur in weeping skin disease or because of an associated enteropathy.

Iron Deficiency. Iron deficiency is an overrated cause of telogen effluvium. The problem is that 20–30% of women are deficient in iron at some time while menstruating and having children. Thus, random testing for iron and serum iron-binding levels in patients with any type of alopecia yields many positive results, but iron replacement helps the hair loss of very few patients.

Other Nutritional Deficiencies. In rare cases zinc, essential fatty acid and biotin deficiencies may lead to telogen effluvium. This rare association is often twisted to justify prescribing zinc, essential fatty acids (or even nonessential ones) and biotin (called vitamin H for *Haut* or skin in German) for telogen effluvium; they are of little benefit.

Acute Stress. Stress, be it physical (accident, major surgery) or mental (divorce, loss of loved one, war) may lead to either anagen effluvium or more often telogen effluvium, perhaps depending on the degree of stress (obviously impossible to quantify).

Physiologic Neonatal Hair Loss. Newborn infants may often lose large amounts of hairs in the first weeks of life, causing their parents great concern. A high percentage of hairs are in telogen at birth, so the loss should not be a surprise. Localized loss may also occur. When the infant lies on a pillow or mattress, increased friction and pressure over the back of the head may lead to bald spots. While most mothers can make the diagnosis themselves, some may need reassurance.

Clinical Findings. In most instances, one cannot see any evidence of hair loss at the same time as the woman explains how extensive her problem is and how many hairs she is loosing daily. Two factors appear to be at play. A woman must loose about 25% of scalp hairs before others can notice thinning. In addition, hair loss is a very emotional event for the victim, who is often further distressed when her problem is not taken seriously. If the patient says she is losing hair, the physician should accept her perception as valid.

In some patients one may see focal or diffuse of thinning. In general, if obvious thinning is present, one should wonder about the diagnosis of telogen effluvium It is helpful to examine the scalp carefully, looking for focal areas of total alopecia, short hairs of normal thickness (regrowing hairs) and checking the width of the parting in several areas.

Laboratory Findings. In the light pull test, increased numbers of hairs are removed. Most are telogen hairs with the typical epithelial sac. The trichogram confirms this impression, as the percentage of telogen hairs is markedly increased. More than 25% telogen hairs in a trichogram also strongly suggests telogen effluvium.

Hair counts can be done by the patient. The average individual loses 50–100 hairs daily. This number may double in telogen effluvium. If the diagnosis is clear, hair counts may keep the patient occupied and provide some reassurance if they gradually start to diminish. On the other hand, they may get the patient over-interested in her disease and make management more difficult, not less.

If the problem has persisted for many months, one can consider hormonal screening tests, thyroid function tests and routine hematologic tests to exclude iron deficiency. The yield of such testing is extremely low.

Differential Diagnosis. The differential diagnosis is usually clear. Several diseases must be excluded:

Diffuse Alopecia Areata. This is a difficult diagnosis, but sometimes alopecia areata does present rapidly and acutely. Usually the correct diagnosis is initially overlooked. Associated immune phenomena (vitiligo, for example) and fingernail changes are helpful clues. Often a scalp biopsy showing a lymphocytic perifollicular infiltrate provides the final answer.

Chronic Diffuse Alopecia of Women. Such patients usually have androgenetic alopecia. When the androgen levels are normal, an end-organ hypersensitivity to normal hormonal levels is postulated. But no matter which phrase one chooses, many patients with diffuse alopecia are women with widespread, distressing hair loss and no exact laboratory explanation. Another subset are the patients with psychogenic pseudoalopecia. These patients feel they have hair loss, but the hair counts, trichogram, scalp biopsy and even laboratory values are normal. Reassurance helps some, but others go on to haunt a host of physicians.

Therapy
Systemic. There is no treatment available to halt hair loss or speed regrowth. The patient should be reassured that the hair will eventually regrow and that she will not become bald. Oral gelatin, biotin and multivitamin preparations are often recommended. Kindly speaking, they are harmless.

Documented hormonal problems should be corrected, working with an endocrinologist or gynecologist. If medications are suspected, the product should be stopped remembering that it may take months before one is even able to hint at an improvement.

Topical. The patient should be encouraged to be gentle with her hair. Conditioners can add bulk while rinses reduce the number of hairs lost with brushing. Underlying scalp disorders, such as seborrheic dermatitis, should be treated. All other topical measures lack proof of efficacy and simply cost money and time. Some patients are so desperate to be doing something to their hair that hormonal tinctures and lotions are often prescribed.

Chronic Telogen Effluvium

The exact nature of this disorder is unclear. Some middle-aged women have a long fluctuating course of telogen effluvium, often producing widespread thinning and lasting for many years. There may be bitemporal recession, so that androgenetic alopecia is the main differential diagnostic consideration. Hormonal studies are normal and scalp biopsies show a normal terminal/vellus hair ratio and much less inflammation and fibrosis than in patients with androgenetic alopecia. There is no question that some patients with telogen effluvium do not satisfactorily regrow hairs. We suspect most have early or mild androgenetic alopecia.

Reversible Circumscribed Alopecia

Circumscribed areas of hair loss may develop following either endogenous or exogenous damage to hair follicles. Mechanical trauma, physical or chemical damage and local inflammation are the three main causes.

Loose Anagen Hair Syndrome
(ZAUN 1984)

Synonym. Short anagen hair syndrome

Definition. Presence of many easily removed anagen hairs in children.

Etiology and Pathogenesis. The cause is unknown. The cycle of hair growth is somehow distorted.

Clinical Findings. Most patients are children with blond hair. Typical age of onset is between 2 and 5 years. Girls are affected more often than boys. Often the child or parent notices that slight tugging produces a bundle of hairs which are easily and painlessly extracted. The children have generally short dry dull hairs which rarely require cutting. Facial and body hairs are not affected. The hairs regrow normally. The progress may continue for a number of years, but resolves spontaneously.

Laboratory Findings. The hair bulbs tend to be deformed and the inner root sheath may be reduced or show premature keratinization. Scanning electron microscopy reveals hairs with longitudinal grooves and irregular shapes on cross section. The trichogram reveals almost exclusively anagen hairs (> 95%), many of which are dystrophic.

Therapy. None is available. Obviously traction should be avoided.

Trichotillomania
(HALLOPEAU 1899)

Definition. Self-induced traction alopecia, in which the hairs are either purposely or unknowingly removed.

Clinical Findings. Trichotillomania is a relatively common disorder. It is about six times more common in women than men. About one-third of patients are children less than 10 years old, another one-third are teenagers, and the final one-third adults. The most typical finding is a localized area of hair loss in the frontotemporal region. If the patient is right handed, the lesion is usually on the left side, and vice-versa. Typically the hairs are twisted around the fingers and then pulled. The bald area is irregularly shaped and shows new hairs of varying lengths which can only be removed when they reach a certain graspable length. Often

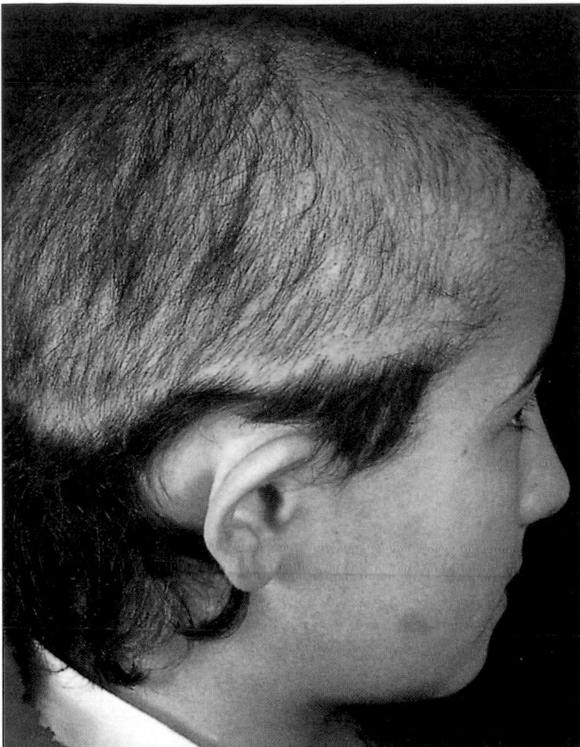

Fig. 31.21. Trichotillomania

fresh hemorrhage is seen in the follicles – an almost specific clinical sign. In more extreme cases, wider areas may be bald. The extreme example is the monsur or Friar Tuck look, in which a band of hair is retained peripherally, but the rest of the scalp is epilated (Fig. 31.21).

In all ages, trichotillomania may be a sign of underlying emotional disturbances. In children, the outlook is comparable to that of thumb sucking, nail chewing or similar habits. In teenagers and adults, trichotillomania is a form of obsessive-compulsive behavior which may merge into a psychosis. Sometimes the patients do regrow hairs but may simultaneously develop more severe emotional problems. Adults are also more likely to epilate other hairs, including pubic, axillary and facial hairs and especially eyelashes and eyebrows. Associated disorders often include trichophagia (eating hairs), trichobezoars (hair balls in GI tract) and bulimia.

Histopathology. The most typical feature is intra- and perifollicular hemorrhage. Other features include distorted worm-like or "pushed up shirt sleeve" follicles, many of which are empty and others of which show catagen features. Atrophic follicles are filled with degenerative products from the matrix including pigment, keratin and remnants of the inner root sheath. This histologic finding is known as trichomalacia. A nonspecific lymphocytic infiltrate may be seen about the follicle and adjacent dermal vessels.

Laboratory Findings. The trichogram shows almost no telogen hairs and often many catagen hairs – a most unusual finding. In clinically normal regions, the trichogram is normal. In children up to 95% of hairs may be anagen. Parents or patients often bring "lost" hairs; these tend to be broken off or dystrophic.

Therapy. Children can generally be managed by an understanding team of parents and a dermatologist or pediatrician. A good trick is to cut the hair very short; by the time it is once again "pullable", many patients have moved on to other habits. Direct confrontation is almost never effective. In many instances, the parents as well as the children refuse to accept the diagnosis. Mild shampoos or an antipruritic scalp lotion may serve as distracters and give the patient a graceful way out of the problem.

In teenagers and adults, the situation is grimmer. In most cases, psychological or psychiatric help will be required. Even if the dermatologist feels motivated to work with such patients, time will generally be the limiting factor. A small group of antidepressants seem to be relatively specific for obsessive-compulsive behavior, and indeed they were tested in trichotillomania first. Included in this group are clomipramine and fluoxetine. The dermatologist probably should get assistance in using these unfamiliar drugs, but they often are quite helpful.

Trichotemnomania

(Braun-Falco and Vogel 1968)

In this variant of trichotillomania, patients cut their hairs off in certain areas but deny doing so. This very rare disease usually affects postmenopausal women with psychiatric problems. In some instances, there may be an underlying organic brain syndrome associated with cerebral vascular problems.

Circumscript Postinfectious Alopecia

A variety of local infections, including impetigo, furuncles and carbuncles and dermatophyte infections can temporarily damage the hair follicles, producing localized alopecia. Regrowth is usually expected. Sometimes, especially with deep granulomatous dermatophyte infections of the follicle (Majocchi granuloma), scarring and thus irreversible alopecia may occur. We typically see this in children from Turkey or the Middle East who did not receive prompt treatment for a bacterial or fungal scalp infection.

Circumscript Inflammatory Alopecia

Similarly, a number of disorders may lead to local hair follicle damage. Common examples include psoriasis and atopic dermatitis. Patches of lichen simplex chronicus usually lack hair. One question is whether the inflammatory process has damaged the hair follicles or whether the rubbing and scratching secondary to pruritus is responsible.

Alopecia Areata

Definition. Inflammatory, usually circular, reversible hair loss of unknown cause.

Etiology and Pathogenesis. The cause of alopecia areata is a great mystery. While many facts point to an immunologic origin, neither the common triggers nor the pathogenic mechanism are clear. It has been proposed that the patient's hair follicle keratinocytes are abnormally sensitive to some endogenous or exogenous stimulus. A number of factors increase the likelihood of alopecia areata, including Down syndrome, Vogt-Koyanagi syndrome, emotional stress, endocrine problems such as thyroid disease, and atopic dermatitis. Neither autoimmune disorders nor autoantibodies are more common in alopecia areata patients. In addition, the presence of nail changes indicates that alopecia areata is not just a scalp problem.

The inflammatory response in the hair follicle is a vicious circle, whose starting point has eluded us. The keratinocytes release cytokines such as tumor necrosis factor (TNF)-α, interleukin (IL)-1β, IL-8) which activate endothelial cells. T cells and macrophages then accumulate about the follicle, releasing more cytokines, driving the inflammatory reaction further. T cells infiltrate the matrix. In addition, Langerhans cells are found in the lower part of the follicle. The degree of infiltration determines the degree of hair follicle damage, which can range from dystrophic changes and immediate hair loss or conversion to telogen hairs with eventual loss. When the inflammation has resolved, the hair follicles begin to function normally again.

Clinical Findings. The patient typically presents with one or more round or oval patches of sudden and complete hair loss (Figs. 31.22–31.26). The skin

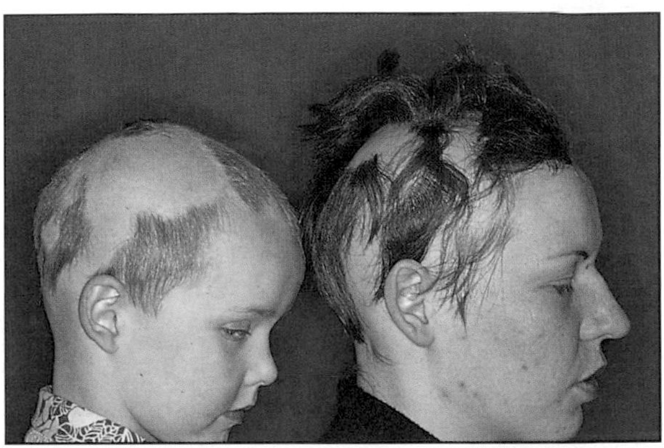

Fig. 31.22. Alopecia areata in siblings

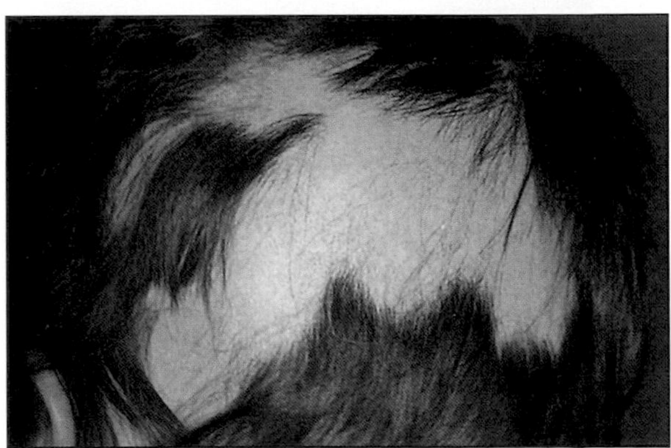

Fig. 31.23. Alopecia areata

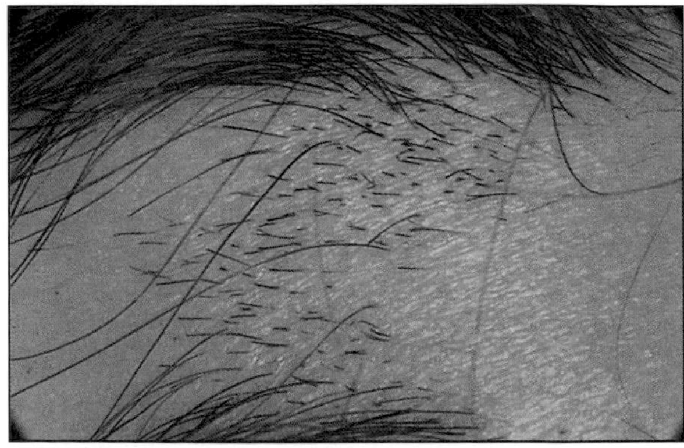

Fig. 31.24. Alopecia areata with exclamation point hairs

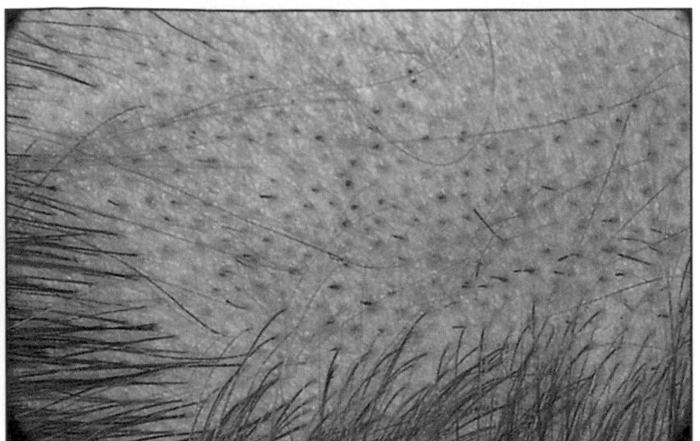

Fig. 31.25. Alopecia areata with both exclamation point and cadaverized hairs

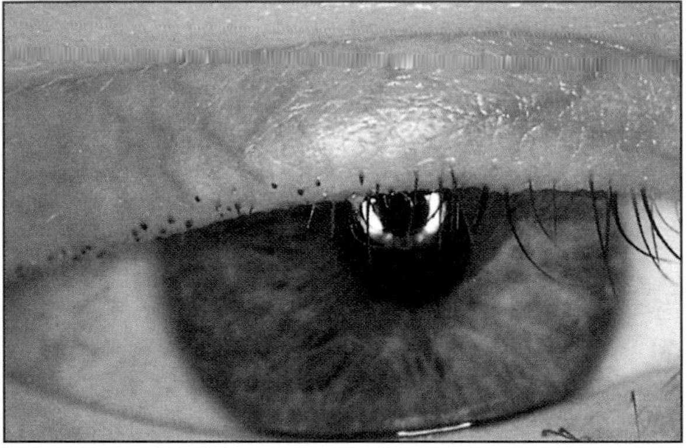

Fig. 31.26. Alopecia areata of eyelashes

in the hairless region is often slightly sunken because of the loss of the mass of the hair bulbs. There may be minimal erythema, but most often the color is ivory white. The follicle openings are preserved and there is no atrophy.

It is important to carefully examine the hairs at the border. If they are easily removed with a light pull, then further spread of the patch can be expected. If they are not easily removed, the disease process may have already slowed. When the extracted hairs are examined, they have a pointed proximal end and lack any root sheath. The shorter the point, the more intense the matrical damage. Two other phenomena may be noticed in this region.

- Exclamation point hairs are 0.2–0.7 cm long, minimally pigmented, often split on their distal end (trichorrhexis) and pointed on their proximal end.
- Cadaverized hairs look like comedones but contain necrotic matrix remnants.

Both exclamation point hairs and cadaverized hairs suggest the disease is likely to progress and help confirm the diagnosis of alopecia areata.

Another peculiar finding in alopecia areata is the Renbök phenomenon. Patients with inflammatory diseases such as psoriasis or seborrheic dermatitis involving the scalp may have regrowth of their hair in inflamed patches. Happle and colleagues proposed the new word Renbök which is Köbner spelled backwards.

The location of the disease is highly variable. On the scalp, the occipital and temporal regions are most often involved. Other body areas can also be affected, including the beard, eyebrows, eyelashes and other hairy areas. The only common associated clinical finding is a variety of nail changes, which are present in about 20% of patients. Pitted nails are most common but other structural changes can be seen. Spotted lunulae are also seen, while red lunulae have been described in severe forms. There are several special types of alopecia areata.

Alopecia Areata Diffusa. Sometimes there is diffuse hair loss without any localized patch. Such cases are most difficult to diagnosis. The trichogram will show primarily telogen hairs, while a biopsy will show typical changes of alopecia areata.

Ophiasis. Galen first used this term for baldness. It means a snake-like (oph-) condition (-iasis). Today the term is used to describe alopecia areata along the side of the head, especially in the temporal region and nape. There may be progression so that only a clump of hairs on the top of the scalp remains (lion's mane). Many patients have atopic dermatitis. This variant is notoriously persistent and difficult to treat.

Alopecia Totalis and Universalis. In extreme cases, either the entire scalp hairs are lost (totalis; Fig. 31.27) or the entire scalp and body hairs are lost (universalis). In the latter situation, the pubic and axillary hairs, as well as the eyelids and eyelashes are lost. The prognosis is dismal, although in rare instances spontaneous regrowth occurs.

Histopathology. The microscopic findings are often very helpful, especially when dealing with a diffuse alopecia. We generally take two adjacent biopsies, one for sectioning vertically (standard fashion) and the other horizontally. In bald areas, the follicles are normal in number but smaller

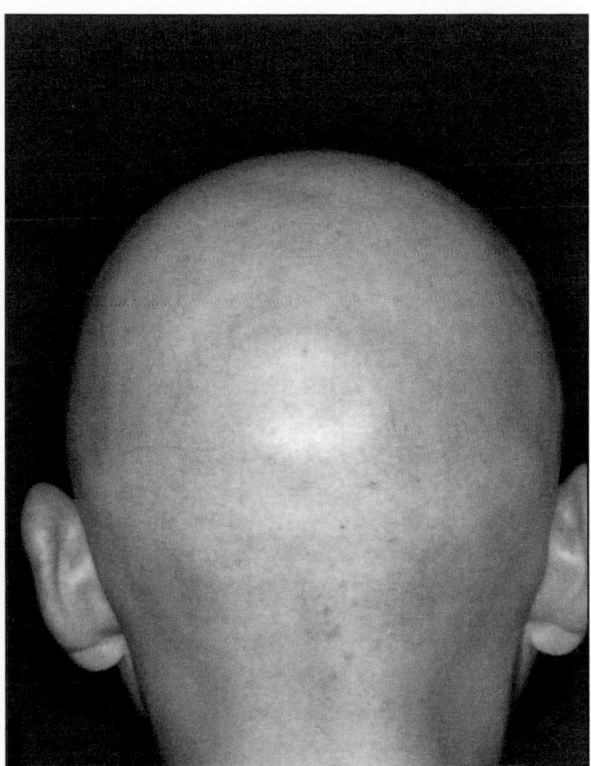

Fig. 31.27. Alopecia totalis

(miniature follicles), lie higher in the dermis and produce a parakeratotic keratin. The papillae are much larger than the accompanying matrix. The abnormal hairs often only reach the infundibulum, and sometimes the hairs are absent entirely. Some follicles will be plugged with matrix debris. The hair bulbs are surrounded early in the disease by clusters of lymphocytes (swarms of bees), which may also involve the papillae.

Laboratory Findings. The trichogram will show either a normal distribution or an increase in telogen hairs in slowly progressing cases. With more rapid disease progression, dystrophic anagen hairs may be found. The trichogram may be abnormal in clinically normal hair in 60 % of patients.

Often a wide variety of other laboratory tests are ordered, searching for an underlying disease or associated immune disorder. Such tests rarely help the patient and are usually unnecessary.

Course and Prognosis. The course of alopecia areata is very unpredictable. Regrowth occasionally occurs with hairs of a different color, usually lighter but occasionally darker than the normal hairs. In gray-haired patients, occasionally the pigmented hairs fall out and the white hairs remain. When this process is widespread, a patient can turn gray overnight (or at least very rapidly). In some cases, new areas continue to appear as old ones are regrowing hair.

In about one-third of patients regrowth occurs in 6 months, and in another one-third regrowth occurs in the next 6 months. In other words, the last one-third still have hair loss after 1 year. Less than half of the patients have effective regrowth and then a cure – that is, no recurrence in 5 years. The remainder will experience a recurrence within 5 years, although often the interval is only a matter of weeks.

Adults with a single patch of alopecia areata have the best outlook. Poor prognostic factors include age at first manifestation (worse when younger), severity of disease, speed of spread and duration of findings. Patients with atopic dermatitis tend to have more chronic disease. The outlook in ophiasis, alopecia totalis and alopecia universalis is also poor.

Differential Diagnosis. Syphilis can be excluded by serologic testing. Multiple lesions or an associated fever and lymphadenopathy should prompt such testing. Patients with secondary syphilis and hair loss always have positive serologic tests. Tinea capitis can be excluded with KOH examination and culture. Trichotillomania should show some broken off hairs, while pseudopelade may be very difficult to exclude without a biopsy. Diffuse alopecia areata is an extremely difficult diagnosis which can usually be made only with a biopsy after excluding other causes of diffuse alopecia.

Therapy. There is no specific curative therapy for alopecia areata. In addition, the highly variable course of the disease makes it difficult to objectively evaluate any therapy.

Systemic. Systemic corticosteroids can occasionally be helpful. They should be used in the first month of the disease, but only in very rapidly progressive or widespread disease. We start with prednisone 60 mg daily and taper to 20 mg daily over 3 weeks, after which low-dose maintenance therapy or alternate-day therapy can be continued for a maximum of 8 weeks. Frequently, when the corticosteroid therapy is stopped, the hair loss starts again. Others have recommended monthly intravenous corticosteroid pulse therapy. We estimate that less than 20 % of patients obtain satisfactory results from systemic corticosteroids.

Many other products have been recommended but none is effective. Oral zinc for 6–8 months is sometimes recommended but unproven. Since in two-thirds of patients the hair regrows in a year, any treatment which is safe enough to be continued for 8 months is likely to seem effective. Dapsone also has its advocates but the evidence is anecdotal. High-dose cyclosporine also seems helpful but is not medically justified. Experience is lacking with low-dose safer regimens. Mycophenolate mofetil also shows promise in early testing but the risk/benefit ratio remains unclear.

Topical. High-potency topical corticosteroids can be tried. One should prescribe lotions or gels which are easier to use on the scalp; they should be applied extending about 1 cm into the normal hair. When treating wider areas, such as alopecia totalis, with topical corticosteroids, one must be very sensitive to steroid side effects, both local (acne, atrophy) and systemic (because of absorption over a wide area).

Intralesional triamcinolone acetonide (2.5–5.0 mg/ml) mixed with a topical anesthetic is worth employing for solitary or few lesions. The border is generally infiltrated, usually requiring less than 5 ml. Injections can be repeated at 3–4-week intervals for a total of three injections in most cases. Patients should be warned that their scalp will become bumpy as some steroid atrophy occurs. Permanent changes do not develop. One should be careful when injecting over the frontal and temporal regions since early reports indicate the risk of intraarterial injection of steroid crystals leading to retinal artery emboli and blindness (Hoigné syndrome; Hoigné and Schoch 1959). Present-day corticosteroids have much smaller crystals so the risk is very low, but the fear persists. Lost eyebrows are cosmetically so distressing that the patient support group for alopecia areata in the USA recommends injections in this "dangerous" area.

Topical immunotherapy is the treatment of choice for selected alopecia areata patients. A variety of agents are used which reliably induce an allergic contact dermatitis. The patient is sensitized to a given agent and then a low-grade inflammatory reaction is maintained on the scalp using a lower concentration of the product. Early work in this field used dinitrochlorobenzene (DNCB), but this product is today no longer employed because of mutagenicity in vitro, although no problems in treated patients have been observed. No product has been officially approved for sensitization but today either squaric acid dibutylester or diphencyprone is used. The reader should become acquainted with the locally available product and seek detailed guidance in the literature. In brief, the patient is sensitized and then a low concentration is applied once weekly. Irritation must occur, as the idea is to induce a low-grade contact dermatitis. The exact mechanism of action is unknown. Skeptics claim that one is simply irritating the skin, but the ratio of helper to suppressor T cells is reduced and other immunologic parameters altered. If no improvement is seen after 6 months, not only has the patient failed immunotherapy but he or she is unlikely to respond to any other methods. Occasionally regional lymph nodes, especially in the nape, may become swollen. Vitiligo has also been described as a complication of immunotherapy.

The skin can also be irritated without relying on an immunologic reaction. Often anthralin is employed. We start with a 0.1% creme and work up to whatever concentration is required to produce irritation. Minoxidil solution can also be tried. The results reported in the literature have been highly variable, ranging from little benefit to response rates of over 50%. In our experience, cosmetically acceptable improvement with minoxidil is uncommon. Tretinoin has been added to both anthralin and minoxidil regimens. It may increase irritation or it may have some other unexplained mechanism. We have not seen striking benefits. Topical cyclosporine does not seem to help.

PUVA therapy may also be helpful. It seems to influence the ratio between helper and suppressor T cells. If one wishes to try topical PUVA, then a dilute psoralen solution should be prepared, as for PUVA bath therapy (Chap. 70), and then applied using a moist turban.

Other Measures. Most important is to be a friend to the patient. Alopecia areata is an amazingly distressful problem for patients, especially women and children. None of the therapies is simple or sure to work. One should not falsely raise hopes which are unlikely to be realized, or use treatments which cause hairs to regrow but have marked systemic side effects. One must remember that the problem is cosmetic, no matter how distressing it is. Often it is better to spend one's emotional energy convincing the patient to wear a wig, which has no side effects and is usually paid for by insurance companies.

Miscellaneous Disorders

Trichodynia

(Rebora 1996)

Synonym. Scalp dysthesia

There is a broad spectrum of patients with painful scalp disorders in whom there are no distinctive physical findings. In one survey, over 30% of patients with hair loss acknowledged the presence of scalp pains. It is not surprising that hairs could be tender when moved, as they are richly supplied with nerves. In some of these patients the scalp appears to have elevated levels of the neurotransmitter substance P. In extreme cases, the scalp pain is the presenting complaint; these patients are similar to those with vulvodynia or burning mouth syndrome.

Trichostasis Spinulosa

In this disorder multiple vellus hairs are retained in a follicle. The lesions resemble a comedo and are discussed in Chapter 28.

Trichomegaly

The presence of very long eyelashes and bushy eyebrows is known as trichomegaly. Many normal individuals have very bushy, thick eyebrows, as witness the famous American labor leader John L. Lewis, but long lashes are unusual. Today they are most often seen as an unexplained manifestation of HIV/AIDS. In the Oliver-McFarlane syndrome they are associated with retinal pigmentary degeneration and dwarfism.

Hair Casts

(Crocker 1932; Kligmann 1957)

Synonym. Peripilar keratin casts

Hair casts are extremely uncommon. They are rings of keratin, probably representing a shed cylinder of inner root sheet, which can often be slid along the hair shaft. Most patients have no associated disease. The differential diagnoses include nits, trichomycosis and remnants of hair sprays and gels which have hardened on the hairs. The other conditions do not produce sliding cylinders. Brushing with a fine brush will usually remove the casts.

Scalp Whorls

The study of hair directional patterns is trichoglyphics. Every mother is an expert as she assesses her child's scalp for a cowlick – the lay term in English for a normal scalp whorl. Multiple whorls or unusual patterns, such as the ridgeback anomaly with a band of hair resembling that of the Rhodesian ridgeback dog, may be markers for underlying disorders of skull or brain development.

Whorled Eyebrows

(Virchow 1912)

Virchow identified a family in which several members over two generations had a whorl in their eyebrows. The eyebrows showed a complete whorl. This has become accepted as an autosomal dominant inherited disorder. Similar tented or upswept eyebrows have been reported in several families; here the whorl was not complete. No associated diseases have been reported. Patients with thyroid-associated orbital disease may have acquired elevation of their lids.

Synophyrs

The tendency of eyebrows to be thick and grow together is known as synophyrs, which is Greek for meeting of the eyebrows. It is a classic sign of Waardenburg syndrome but is seen in several other rare genodermatoses including Cornelia de Lange syndrome and the mucopolysaccharidoses.

Barbula Hirci

The tufts of thick terminal hairs that grow on the tragi of adult men are known as barbula hirci – Latin for the little beard of the goat. In elderly men, the hairs sometimes become quite long and worrisome, interfering with hearing aid use. Hairy ears was for years reputed to be the only disorder transmitted on the Y chromosome, based on a study in India. More modern genetics has not substantiated this claim.

Bibliography

General

Camacho F, Montagna W (1997) Trichology. Diseases of the pilosebaceous follicle. Aula Medica Group, Madrid

Dawber R (ed) (1997) Diseases of the hair and scalp, 3rd edn. Blackwell Science, Oxford

Orfanos CE, Montagna W, Stüttgen G (eds) (1981) Hair research. Springer

Orfanos CE, Happle R, eds. (1990) Hair and hair diseases. Springer, Berlin

Proceedings of the 41st Annual Symposium on the Biology of the Skin: Fundamentals of Hair Biology (1993). J Invest Dermatol 101:(Suppl) 4:1S–148S

Sperling LC (1991) Hair anatomy for the clinician. J Am Acad Dermatol 25:1–17

Basic Science Aspects

Barman JM, Astore I, Pecoraro V (1965) The normal trichogram of the adult. J Invest Dermatol 44:233–236

Braun-Falco O, Heilgemeir GP (1985) The trichogram. Structural and functional basis, performance, and interpretation. Semin Dermatol 4:40–52

Chatenay F, Courtois M, Loussouarn G et al. (1996) Phototrichogram: an entirely automated method of quantification by image analysis. In: Neste D van, Randall VA (eds) Hair research for the next millenium. Elsevier, Amsterdam, pp 105–108

Commo S, Bernard BA (1997) Immunohistochemical analysis of tissue remodelling during the anagen-catagen transition of the human hair follicle. Br J Dermatol 137:31–38

Corcuff P, Roguet R, Kermici M (1989) A method for measuring the various constituents of the human hair follicle. J Microsc 156:115–123

Cotsarelis G (1998) The hair follicle. Dying for attention. Am J Pathol 151:1505–1509

Courtois M, Loussouarn G, Hourseau S et al. (1996) Periodicity in the growth and shedding of hair. Br J Dermatol 134:47–54

Eicheler W, Huth A, Happle R et al. (1996) RNA-levels of 5α-reductase and androgen receptor in human skin, hair follicles and follicle-derived cells. In: Neste D van, Randall VA (eds) Hair research for the next millenium. Elsevier, Amsterdam, pp 327–331

Elston DM, McCollough ML, Angeloni VL (1995) Vertical and transverse sections of alopecia biopsy specimens: combining the two to maximize diagnostic yield. J Am Acad Dermatol 32:454–457

Hamada K, Thornton MJ, Laing I et al. (1996) The metabolism of testosterone by dermal papilla cells cultured from human pubic and axillary hair follicles concurs with hair growth in 5-alpha-reductase deficiency. J Invest Dermatol 106:1017–1022

Kligman AM (1961) Pathologic dynamics of human hair loss. I. Telogen effluvium. Arch Dermatol 83:175–198

Maguire HC, Kligman AM (1964) Hair plucking as a diagnostic tool. J Invest Dermatol 43:77–79

Paus R, Cotsarelis G (1999) The biology of hair follicles. NETM 341:491–497

Randall VA, Ebling FJG (1991) Seasonal changes in human hair growth. Br J Dermatol 124:146–151

Sawaya ME, Price VH (1997) Different levels of 5α-reductase type I and II, aromatase, and androgen receptor in hair follicles of women and men with androgenetic alopecia. J Invest Dermatol 109:296–300

Tobin DJ, Hagen E, Botchkarev VA et al. (1998) Do hair bulb melanocytes undergo apoptosis during hair follicle regression (catagen)? J Invest Dermatol 111:941–947

Van Neste DJ, Brouwer B de, De Coster W (1994) The phototrichogram: analysis of some technical factors of variation. Skin Pharmacol 7:67–72

Whiting DA (1993) Diagnostic and predictive value of horizontal sections of scalp biopsy specimens in male pattern androgenetic alopecia. J Am Acad Dermatol 28:755–763

Structural Changes

Al-Harmozi SA, Mahmoud SF, Ejeckam GC (1992) Woolly hair nevus syndrome. J Am Acad Dermatol 27:259–260

Bentley-Phillips B, Bayles MAH (1973) A previously undescribed hair anomaly (pseudo-monilethrix). Br J Dermatol 89:159–167

Björnstad R (1965) Pili torti and sensory-neural loss of hearing. Proceedings of the 17th meeting of the Northern Dermatological Society, Copenahgen, May 1965

Brodin MB, Porter PS (1980) Netherton's syndrome. Cutis 26:52–68

Brown VM, Crounse RG, Abele DC (1986) An unusual new hair shaft abnormality: "bubble hair". J Am Acad Dermatol 15:1113–1117

Camacho F (1997) Hair shaft dysplasias. General concept and classification of the dysplasias. In: Camacho F, Montagna W (eds) Trichology. Aula Medica Group, Madrid, pp 179–202

Camacho F, Jorquera E (1995) Pili bi-bifurcati. Eur J Dermatol 5:88–89

Camacho-Martinez F (1989) Localized trichorrhexis nodosa. J Am Acad Dermatol 20:696–X697

Comél M (1949) Ichthyosis linearis circumflexa. Dermatologica 98:133–136

Crounse RG (1962) Trichorrhexis nodosa and amino acid metabolism. Arch Dermatol 86:391

Crovato F, Rebora A (1985) PIBI(D)S syndrome: an entity with defect of DNA excision repair system. J Am Acad Derm 13:363–366

Cullen SI, Fulghum DD (1989) Acquired progressive kinking of the hair. Arch Dermatol 125:252–255

Danks DM, Campbell PE, Stevens BJ (1972) Menkes' kinky hair syndrome. An inherited defect in copper absorption with widespread effects. Pediatrics 50:188–201

Dawber RPR (1974) Knotting of hair scalp. Br J Dermatol 91:169–173

DeBerker DAR, Ferguson DJP, Dawber RPR (1993) Monilethrix: a clinicopathological illustration of a cortical defect. Br J Dermatol 128:327–331

Detwiler SP, Carson JL, Woosley JT et al. (1994) Bubble hair. Case caused by an overheat-ing hair dryer and reproducibility in normal hair with heat. J Am Acad Dermatol 30:54–60

Dupré A, Bonafé JL (1978) A new type of pilar dysplasia. The uncombable hair syndrome with pili trianguli et canaliculi. Arch Dermatol Res 261:217–218

Dupré A, Rochiccioli P, Bonafé JL (1973) "Cheveux incoiffables": anomalie congénitale des cheveux. Bull Soc Fr Dermatol Syphiligr 80:111–112

Elston DM, Bergfeld WF, Whiting DA et al. (1992) Bubble hair. J Cutan Pathol 19:439–444

Esterly NB, Lavin MP, Garancis JC (1989) Acquired progressive kinking of the hair. Arch Dermatol 125:813–815

Ferrando J (1997) Uncombable hair syndrome (Pili canaliculi). In: Camacho F, Montagna W (eds) Trichology. Aula Medica Group, Madrid, pp 209–218

Ferrando J, Fontarnau J, Rodríguez-Pichardo A (1993) Is pseudomonilethrix an artifact? Int J Dermatol 29:380–381

Forslind B, Thomsen K, Anderson B (1985) Spun glass hair: two cases investigated with SEM and TEM. Acta Dermato Venereol (Stockh) 65:348–351

Gossage AM (1908) The inheritance of certain human abnormalities. Q J Med 1:331–347

Greene SL, Müller SA (1985) Netherton's syndrome. Report of a case and review of the literature. J Am Acad Dermatol 13:329–337
Guidetti MS, Fanti PA, Piraccini BM et al. (1995) Diffuse partial woolly hair. Acta Derm Venereol (Stockh) 75:141–142
Gummer CL (1994) Bubble hair: a cosmetic abnormality caused by brief, focal heating of damp hair fibres. Br J Dermatol 131:901–903
Gummer CL, Dawber RPR (1981) Pili annulati: electron histochemical studies on affected hairs. Br J Dermatol 105:303–309
Hutchinson PE, Wells RS (1973) Woolly hair. Br J Dermatol 81: 17
Hutchinson PE, Cairns RJ, Wells RS (1974) Woolly hair. Clinical and general aspects. Trans St John's Hosp Dermatol Soc 60:160–177
Itin PH, Pittelkow MR (1990) Trichothiodystrophy: review of sulfur-deficient brittle hair syndromes and association with the ectodermal dysplasias. J Am Acad Dermatol 22:705–717
Itin PH, Bühler U, Büchner SA et al. (1993) Pili trianguli et canaliculi: a distinctive hair shaft defect leading to uncombable hair. Dermatology 187:296–298
Itin PH, Schiller P, Mathys D et al. (1997) Cosmetically induced hair beads. J Am Acad Dermatol 36: 260–261
Ito M, Ito K, Hashimoto K (1984) Pathogenesis in trichorrhexis invaginata (bamboo hair). J Invest Dermatol 83:1–6
Ito M, Hashimoto K, Sakamato F et al. (1988) Pathogenesis of pili annulati. Arch Dermatol Res 280:308–318
Jorizo JL et al. (1982) Ichthyosis, brittle hair, impaired intelligence, decreased fertility and short stature (IBIDS) syndrome. Brit J Derm 106:705–710
Kaler SG (1994) Menkes disease. Adv Pediatr 41:263–304
Karsch A (1846) De Capillitiri humani coloiebus quardan. In: Landois L (1866) Das plötzliche Ergrauer der Haupthaare. Archiv für pathologische Anatomie und Physiologie 35:575
Krafchik BR (1992) Netherton's syndrome. J Am Acad Dermatol 13:329–331
Kuhn CA, Helm TN, Bergfeld WF et al. (1993) Acquired uncombable hair. Arch Dermatol 129: 1061–1062
Marinesco G et al. (1931) Nouvelle maladie familiale caractérisés par une cataracte congénitale et une arrêt du développement somato-neuro-psychique. Encéphale 26: 97–109
Mehregan AH, Thompson WS (1979) Pili multigemini. Report of a case in association with cleidocranial dysostosis. Br J Dermatol 100:315–322
Menkes JH, Alter M, Steigleder GK et al. (1962) A sex-linked recessive disorder with retardation of growth, peculiar hair, and focal cerebral and cerebellar degeneration. Pediatrics 29:764–779
Netherton EW (1958) A unique case of trichorrhexis nodosa: "bamboo hairs". Arch Dermatol 78:483–487
Norwood OT (1979) Whisker hair. Arch Dermatol 115:930
Ormerod AD, Main RA, Ryder ML et al. (1987) A family with diffuse partial woolly hair. Br J Dermatol 116: 401–405
Papa CM, Mills OH Jr (1972) Seasonal trichorrhexis nodosa: role of cumulative damage in frayed hair. Arch Dermatol 106:888–892
Pollit RJ, Jenner FA, Davies M (1968) Sibs with mental and physical retardation and trichorrhexis nodosa with abnormal amino acid composition of the hair. Arch Dis Child 43:211–216
Price VH, Thomas RS, Jones Ft (1970) Pseudopili annulati. An unusual variant of normal hair. Arch Dermatol 102: 354–358
Price VH (1979) Trichothiodystrophy. A defect in transcription. In: Camacho F, Montagna W (eds) Trichology. Aula Medica Group, Madrid, pp 237–242
Price VH, Odom RB, Ward WH et al. (1980) Trichothiodystrophy. Sulfur-deficient brittle hair as a marker for neuroectodermal symptom complex. Arch Dermatol 116: 1375–1384
Reda AM, Rogers RS III, Peters MS (1990) Wooly hair nevus. J Am Acad Dermatol 22:377–380
Rest EB, Fretzin DF (1990) Quantitative assessment of scanning electron microscope defects in uncombable-hair syndrome. Pediatr Dermatol 7:93–96
Ronchese F (1932) Twisted hairs (pili torti). Arch Dermatol Syphilol 26:98–109
Rushton DH, Norris MJ, James KC (1990) Amino-acid composition in trichorrhexis nodosa. Clin Exp Dermatol 15:24–28
Schütz J (1900) Pili moniliformis. Arch Dermatol Syphilol 53:69
Shieh X, Yi X (1992) Hair casts: a clinical and morphologic control study. Arch Dermatol 128:1553–1554
Sjögren T (1950) Hereditary congential spinocerebellar ataxia accompanied by congenital cataract and oligophrenia. A genetic and clinical investigation. Confinia Neur 10:293–308
Smith W (1879) A rare nodose condition of the hair. Br Med J 2:291–292
Steranovic DV, Dakovic Z, Minic S (1992) Pathogenesis in trichorrhexis invaginata (Bamboo hairs). Eur J Dermatol 2:15–20
Stroud JD, Mehegan AH (1974) "Spun glass" hair: a clinicopathologic study of an unusual hair defect. In: Proceedings, 1st human hair symposium. Atlanta, 1973. Medcom, New York, pp 103–107
Takayama K, Salazar EP, Broughton BC et al. (1996) Defects in the DNA repair and transcription gene ERCC2 (XPD) ind trichothiodystrophy. Am J Hum Genet 58:263–270
Tay CH (1971) Ichthyosiform erythroderma, hair shaft abnormalities, and mental and growth retardation. A new recessive disorder. Arch Dermatol 104:4–13
Tumer Z, Horn N, Tonnesen T et al. (1996) Early copper-histidine treatment for Menkes disease. Nat Genet 12: 11–13
Weary PE, Hendricks AA, Warner F et al. (1973) Pili bifurcati: new anomaly of hair growth. Arch Dermatol 108: 403–407
Whiting DA (1987) Structural abnormalities of the hair shaft. J Am Acad Dermatol 16:1–25
Whiting DA (1997) Fractures of the hair shaft. In: Camacho F, Montagna W (eds) Trichology. Aula Medica Group, Madrid, pp 203–208
Winter H, Rogers MA, Langbein L et al. (1997) Mutations in the hair cortex keratin hHb6 cause the inherited hair disease monilethrix. Nat Genet 16:372–374
Winter H, Labrèze C, Chapalain V et al. (1998) A variable monilethrix phenotype associated with a novel mutation, Glu402Lys, in the helix termination motif of the type II hair keratin hHb1. J Invest Dermatol 111: 169–172

Wise F (1927) Wooly hair nevus. A peculiar form of birthmark of hair of the scalp, hitherto undescribed, with report of two cases. Med J Rec 125:545–547

Wise F, Sulzberger MB (1932) Acquired progressive kinking of the scalp hair accompanied by changes in its pigmentation. Arch Dermatol Syphilol 25:99–110

Zhu WY, Xia MY (1993) Trichonodosis. Pediatr Dermatol 10:392–393

Zitelli JA (1986) Pseudomonilethrix. An artifact. Arch Dermatol 122:688–690

Color Changes

Dawber RPR (1997) Hair colour. In: Camacho F, Montagna W (eds) Trichology. Aula Medica Group, Madrid, pp 179–242

Kerker B, Hood A (1989) Chemotherapy-induced cutaneous reactions. Semin Dermatol 8:173–181

Levantine A, Almeyda J (1973) Drug induced changes in pigmentation. Br J Dermatol 116:485–489

Mosher DB, Fitzpatrick TB (1988) Piebaldism. Arch Dermatol 124:346–349

Melnik BC, Plewig G, Daldrup T (1986) Green hair: guidelines for diagnosis and therapy. J Am Acad Dermatol 15:1065–1068

Nanda A, Alsaleh Q (1994) Hair discoloration caused by etretinate. Dermatology 188:172

Excessive Hair Growth

Archard EC, Thiers J (1921) Le virilisme piliaire et son association à l'insufficiance glycolytique (diabéte des femme à barbe). Bull Acad Med Paris 86:51–66

Bumb RA, Makkar RK, Sulemani AA (1995) Acquired hypertrichosis singularis. Arch Dermatol 131:617

Camacho F(1997) Hypertrichosis. In: Camacho F, Montagna W (eds) Trichology. Aula Medica Group, Madrid, pp 243–264

Castello R, Tosi F, Perrone F et al. (1996) Outcome of long-term treatment with the 5-alpha-reductase inhibitor finasteride in idiopathic hirsutism: clinical and hormonal effects during a 1-year course of therapy and 1-year follow-up. Fertil Steril 66:734–740

Cusan L, Dupont A, Belanger A et al. (1990) Treatment of hirsutism with the pure antiandrogen flutamide. J Am Acad Dermatol 23:462–469

Dierickx CC, Grossman MC, Farinelli WA et al. (1998) Permanent hair removal by normal-mode ruby laser. Arch Dermatol 134:837–842

Erenus M, Yücelten D, Durmusoglu F et al. (1997) Comparison of finasteride versus spironolactone in the treatment of idiopathic hirsutism. Fertil Steril 68:1000–1003

Grossman MC, Dierickx C, Farinelli W et al. (1996) Damage to hair follicles by normal-mode ruby laser pulses. J Am Acad Dermatol 35:889–894

Herzberg JJ, Protjan K, Gebauer D (1968) Hypertrichosis languinosa (et terminalis) als paraneoplastisches Syndrom. Arch Klin Exp Dermatol 232:176–186

Kelestimur F, Sahin Y (1998) Comparison of Diane 35 and Diane 35 plus spironolactone in the treatment of hirsutism. Fertil Steril 69:66–69

Kvedar JC, Gibson M, Krusinsky PA (1985) Hirsutism: evaluation and treatment. J Am Acad Dermatol 24: 423–425

Lin TYD, Manuskiatti W, Dierickx CC et al. (1998) Hair growth cycle affects hair follicle destruction by ruby laser pulses. J Invest Dermatol 111:107–113

le Marquand HS, Bohn GI (1950) Recurrent peptic ulcers with general hypertrichosis including growth of hair on the bald scalp and later development of signs suggesting adrenal failure, Proc R Soc Med 44:155–157

Mortola JF (1999) Drugs used in reproductive endocrinology and infertility. In: Korting HC, Schäfer-Korting M (eds) The benefit/risk ratio. A handbook for the rational use of potentially hazardous drugs. CRC Press, Boston, pp 287–306

Nanni CA, Alster TS (1997) Optimizing treatment parameters for hair removal using a topical carbon-based solution and 1064-nm Q-switched neodymium:YAG laser energy. Arch Dermatol 133:1546–1549

Olsen EA (1999) Methods of hair removal. J Am Acad Dermatol 40:143–155

Patridge JW (1987) Congenital hypertrichosis lanuginosa: neonatal shaving. Arch Dis Child 62:623

Peluso AM, Misciali C, Vincenzi C et al. (1997) Diffuse hypertrichosis during treatment with 5% topical minoxidil. Br J Dermatol 136:118–120

Richards RN, McKenzie MA, Mehrag GE (1986) Electroepilation (electrolysis) in hirsutism. J Am Acad Dermatol 15:693–697

Sommer S, Render C, Burd R et al. (1998) Ruby laser treatment for hirsutism: clinical response and patient tolerance. Br J Dermatol 138:1009–1014

Sperling LC, Heimer WL (1993) Androgen biology as a basis for the diagnosis and treatment of androgenic disorders in women. I. J Am Acad Dermatol 28:669–683

Sperling LC, Heimer WL (1993) Androgen biology as a basis for the diagnosis and treatment of androgenic disorders in women. II. J Am Acad Dermatol 28:901–916

Stein IF, Leventhal ML (1935) Amenorrhea associated with bilateral polycystic ovaries. Am J Obst Gyn 29:181–191

Sudduth SL, Koronkowski MJ (1993) Finasteride: the first 5 alpha-reductase inhibitor. Pharmacotherapy 13:309–325

Tolino A, Petrone A, Sarnacchiaro F et al. (1996) Finasteride in the treatment of hirsutism: new therapeutic perspectives. Fertil Steril 66:61–65

Wheeland RG (1997) Laser-assisted hair removal. Dermatol Clin 15:469–477

Zemtsov A, Wilson L (1997) Successful treatment of hirsutism in HAIR-AN syndrome using flutamide, spironolactone, and birth control therapy. Arch Dermatol 133:431–433

Alopecia

Congenital Hypotrichosis

Ahmad W, Faiyaz-ul-Haque M, Brancolini V et al. (1998) Alopecia universalis associated with a mutation in the human hairless gene. Science 279:720–724

Cantú JM, Arias J, Foncerrada M et al. (1975) Syndrome of onychotricho-dysplasia with chronic neutropenia in an infant from consanguinous parents. Birth Defects 11/12:63–66

Damsté TJ, Prakken JR (1954) Atrichia with papular lesions: a variant of congenital ectodermal dysplasia. Dermatologica 108:114–121

Hernández A, Olivares F, Cantú JM (1979) Autosomal recessive onychotrichodysplasia, chronic neutropenia, and

mental retardation. Delineation of the syndrome. Clin Genet 15:147–152
Lündback H (1944) Total congenital hereditary alopecia. Acta Dermato Venereol (Stockh) 25:189
Mc Kusick VA et al. (1965) Dwarfism in the Amish. II. Cartilage-hair hypoplasia. Bull Johns Hopkins Hosp 116: 285–326
Sabouraud R (1905) Manuel élémentaire de dermatologie topographique régionale. Masson, Paris
Sabouraud R (1931) De l'alopécie liminaire frontale. Ann Dermatol et de Syphiligr 2:446
Unna M (1925) Hypotrichosis congenita hereditaria. Derm Wschr 81:1167–1178

Scarring Alopecia

Braun-Falco O (1986) Pseudopelade of Brocq. Dermatologica 172:18–23
Cornbleet T (1935) Cutis verticis gyrata? lipoma? Arch Deramtol Syphilol 32:688
Degos R, Rabut R, Duperrat B et al. (1951) A propos de 111 cas d'alopécies cicatricielles en petites aires (teignes exclues). L'etat pseudo-péladique. Bull Soc Fr Dermatol Syphiligr 58:451–452
Kossard S, Lee MS, Wilkinson B (1997) Postmenopausal frontal fibrosing alopecia: a frontal variant of lichen planopilaris. J Am Acad Dermatol 36:59–66
Kunte C, Löser C, Wolff H (1998) Folliculitis spinulosa decalvans: successful therapy with dapsone. J Am Acad Dermatol 39:891–893
Luelmo-Aguilar J, Gonzalez-Castro U, Castells-Rodellas A (1993) Tufted hair folliculitis. A study of four cases. Br J Dermatol 128:454–457
Matta M, Kibbi AG, Khattar J et al. (1990) Lichen planopilaris: a clinicopathologic study. J Am Acad Dermatol 22: 594–598
Mehregan DA, Hale HM van, Muller SA (1992) Lichen planopilaris: clinical and pathologic study of forty-five patients. J Am Acad Dermatol 27:935–942
Nayar M, Schomberg K, Dawber RP et al. (1993) A clinicopathological study of scarring alopecia. Br J Dermatol 128:533–536
Powell JJ, Dawber RPR, Gatter K (1999) Folliculitis decalvans including tufted folliculitis: clinical, histological and therapeutic findings. Br J Dermatol 140:328–333
Scerri L, Williams HC, Allen BR (1996) Dissecting cellulitis of the scalp: response to isotretinoin. Br J Dermatol 134:1105–1108
Schewach-Millet M, Ziv R, Shapira D (1986) Perifolliculitis capitis abscedens et suffodiens treated with isotretinoin (13-cis retinoic acid). J Am Acad Dermatol 15: 1291–1292
Siemens HW (1926) Keratosis follicularis spinulosa decalvans. Arch Dermatol Syphilol 151:384–386
Silver H, Chargin L, Sachs PM (1953) Follicular lichen planus (Lichen planopilaris). Arch Dermatol Syphilol 67: 346–354
Silvers DN, Katz BE, Young AW (1993) Pseudopelade of Brocq is lichen planopilaris: report of four cases that support this nosology. Cutis 51:99–105
Sperling LC, Solomon AR, Whiting DA (2000) A new look at scarring alopecia. Arch Dermatol 136:235–242
Suter L (1983) Folliculitis decalvans. Hautarzt 32:429–431
Tong AKF, Baden HP (1989) Tufted hair folliculitis. J Am Acad Dermatol 21:1096–1099
Wilson CL, Burge SM, Dean D et al. (1992) Scarring alopecia in discoid lupus erythematosus. Br J Dermatol 126: 307–314
Zinkernagel MS, Trüeb RM (2000) Fibrosing alopecia in a pattern distribution. Arch Dermatol 136:205–211

Androgenetic Male Alopecia

Bingham KD, Shaw DA (1973) The metabolism of testosterone by human male scalp skin. J Endocrinol 57: 111–121
Canfield D (1996) Photographic documentation of hair growth in androgenetic alopecia. Dermatol Clin 14: 713–721
Courtois M, Loussouarn G, Hourseau S et al. (1996) Periodicity in the growth and shedding of hair. Br J Dermatol 134:47–54
Dallob AL, Sadick NS, Unger W et al. (1994) The effect of finasteride, a 5α-reductase inhibitor, on scalp skin testosterone and dihydrotestosterone concentrations in patients with male pattern baldness. J Clin Endocrinol Metab 79:703–706
De Groot A, Nater JP, Herxheimer A (1987) Minoxidil: hope for the bald? Lancet 329:1019–1022
Diani AR, Mulholland MJ, Shull KL et al. (1992) Hair growth effects of oral administration of finasteride, a steroid 5α-reductase inhibitor, alone and in combination with topical minoxidil in the balding stumptail macaque (*Macaca actoides*). J Clin Endocrinol Metab 74:345–350
Drake LA, Dinehart SM, Farmer ER et al. (1996) Guidelines of care for androgenetic alopecia. J Am Acad Dermatol 35:465–469
Hamilton JB (1942) Male hormone stimulation is a prerequisite and an incitant in common baldness. Am J Anat 71:451–480
Hamilton JB (1951) Patterned loss of hair in man: types and incidence. Ann N Y Acad Sci 53:708–728
Kaufman KD, Olsen EA, Whiting D et al. (1998) Finasteride in the treatment of men with androgenetic alopecia (male pattern hair loss). J Am Acad Dermatol 36:578–589
Küster W, Happle R (1984) The inheritance of common baldness: two B or not two B? J Am Acad Dermatol 11:921–926
Leyden J, Dunlap F, Miller B et al. (1999) Finasteride in the treatment of men with frontal male pattern hair loss. J Am Acad Dermatol 40:930–937
Liang T, Rasmusson GH, Brooks JR (1983) Biochemical and biological studies with 4-aza-steroidal 5alpha-reductase inhibitors. J Steroid Biochem 19:385–390
Norwood OT (1975) Male pattern baldness: classification and incidence. South Med J 68:1359–1365
Orentreich N (1959) Autografts in alopecias and other selected dermatologic conditions. Ann N Y Acad Sci 83: 463–479
Price VH (1999) Treatment of hair loss. NETM J 41:964–973
Rittmaster RS (1994) Finasteride. N Engl J Med 330:120–125
Rushton DH, Ramsay ID, Norris MJ et al. (1991) Natural progression of male pattern baldness in young men. Clin Exp Dermatol 16:188–192
Savin RC, Atton AV (1993) Minoxidil. Update on its clinical role. Dermatol Clin 11:55–64
Schweikert HU, Wilson JD (1974) Regulation of human hair growth by steroid hormones. I. Testosterone meta-

bolism in isolated hairs. J Clin Endocrinol Metab 38:811–819
Unger W (1995) Hair transplantation. Dekker, New York

Androgenetic Female Alopecia

Georgala S, Gourgiotou K, Kassouli S et al. (1992) Hormonal status in postmenopausal androgenetic alopecia. Int J Dermatol 31:858–859
Ludwig E (1977) Classification of the types of androgenetic alopecia (common baldness) occurring in the female sex. Br J Dermatol 97:247–254
Rushton DH, Ramsay ID, James KC et al. (1990) Biochemical and trichological characterization of diffuse alopecia in women. Br J Dermatol 123:187–197
Sperling LC, Heimer WL (1993) Androgen biology as a basis for the diagnosis and treatment of androgenic disorders in women. I. J Am Acad Dermatol 28:669–683
Sperling LC, Heimer WL (1993) Androgen biology as a basis for the diagnosis and treatment of androgenic disorders in women. II. J Am Acad Dermatol 28:901–916
Venning VA, Dawber RPR (1988) Patterned androgenic alopecia in women. J Am Acad Dermatol 18:1073–1077

Reversible Alopecia

Braun-Falco O, Vogel PG (1968) Trichotemnomanie. Eine besondere Hautmanifestation eines hirnorganischen Psychosyndroms. Hautarzt 19:551–553
Cuozzo DW, Benson PM, Sperling LC et al. (1995) Essential syphilitic alopecia revisited. J Am Acad Dermatol 28:96–98
Hallopeau M (1889) Alopécie par grattage (trichomanie ou trichotillomanie). Ann Dermatol Syphiligr 10:440–441
Hamm H, Traupe H (1989) Loose anagen hair of childhood: the phenomenon of easily pluckable hair. J Am Acad Dermatol 20:242–248
Headington JT (1993) Telogen effluvium. Arch Dermatol 129:356–363
Muller SA (1990) Trichotillomania: a histopathologic study in sixty-six patients. J Am Acad Dermatol 23:56–62
Price VH, Gummer CL (1989) Loose anagen syndrome. J Am Acad Dermatol 20:249–256
Tosti A, Peluso AM, Misciali C et al. (1997) Loose anagen hair. Arch Dermatol 133:1089–1093
Whiting DA (1996) Chronic telogen effluvium: increased scalp hair shedding in middle-aged women. J Am Acad Dermatol 35:899–906
Zaun H (1984) Differential diagnosis of alopecia in children. In: Happle R, Grosshans E (eds) Pediatric dermatology. Springer, Berlin, pp 157–166

Alopecia Areata

Bergner T, Donhauser G, Ruzicka T (1992) Red lunulae in severe alopecia areata. Acta Derm Venereol (Stockh) 72:203–205
Coleman MD (1993) Dapsone: modes of action, toxicity and possible strategies for increasing patient tolerance. Br J Dermatol 129:507–513
Cunliffe WJ, Hall R, Stevenson CJ et al. (1969) Alopecia areata, thyroid disease, and autoimmunity. Br J Dermatol 81:877–881
Duhra P, Foulds IS (1990) Persistent vitiligo induced by diphencyprone. Br J Dermatol 123:415–416
Fiedler VC (1992) Alopecia areata. A review of therapy, efficacy, safety, and mechanism. Arch Dermatol 128:1519–1529
Friedli A, Labarthe MP, Engelhardt E et al. (1998) Pulse methylprednisolone therapy for severe alopecia areata: an open prospective study of 45 patients. J Am Acad Dermatol 39:597–602
Gordon PM, Aldridge RD, McVittie E et al. (1996) Topical diphencyprone for alopecia areata: evaluation of 48 cases after 30 months of follow-up. Br J Dermatol 134:869–871
Gupta AK, Ellis CN, Cooper KD et al. (1990) Oral cyclosporine for the treatment of alopecia areata. A clinical and immunohistochemical analysis. J Am Acad Dermatol 22:242–250
Happle R (1991) Topical immunotherapy in alopecia areata. J Invest Dermatol 96:715–745
Happle R, Steen PHM van der, Perret CM (1991) The Renbök phenomenon: an inverse Köbner reaction observed in alopecia areata. Eur J Dermatol 1:228–230
Healy E, Rogers S (1993) PUVA treatment for alopecia areata does it work? A retrospective review of 102 cases. Br J Dermatol 129:42–44
Hoting E, Boehm A (1992) Therapy of alopecia areata with diphencyprone. Br J Dermatol 127:625–629
MacDonald-Hull S, Pepall L, Cunliffe WJ (1991) Alopecia areata in children: response to treatment with diphencyprone. Br J Dermatol 125:164–168
Mitchell AJ, Krull EA (1984) Alopecia areata: pathogenesis and treatment. J Am Acad Dermatol 11:763–775
Olsen EA, Carson SC, Turney EA (1992) Systemic steroids with or without 2% topical minoxidil in the treatment of alopecia areata. Arch Dermatol 128:1467–1473
Peereboom-Wynia JDR, Beek CH, Mulder PGH et al. (1993) The trichogram as a prognostic tool in alopecia areata. Acta Dermato Venereol (Stockh) 73:280–282
Schmoeckel C, Weissmann I (1979) Treatment of alopecia areata by anthralin-induced dermatitis. Arch Dermatol 115:1254–1255
Taylor CR, Hawk JLM (1995) PUVA treatment of alopecia areata partialis, totalis and universalis: audit of 10 years' experience at St John's Institute of Dermatology. Br J Dermatol 133:914–918
Tosti A, Guidetti MS, Bardazzi F et al. (1996) Longterm results of topical immunotherapy in children with alopecia totalis or alopecia universalis. J Am Acad Dermatol 35:199–201
Van der Steen PHM, van Baar HM, Happle R et al. (1991) Prognostic factors in the treatment of alopecia areata with diphenylcyclopropenone. J Am Acad Dermatol 24:227–230
Weise K, Kretzschmar L, John SM et al. (1996) Topical immunotherapy in alopecia areata: anamnestic and clinical criteria of prognostic significance. Dermatology 192:129–133

Miscellaneous Disorders

Galewsky E Haaresser (haireater) of Crocker (1932) In: Jadassohn's Handbuch der Haut und Geschlechtskrankheiten, XIII/1, p. 215, Springer, Berlin
Kligmann AM (1957) Hair casts. Arch Dermatol 75:509
Rebora A, Semino MT, Guarrera M (1996) Trichodynia. Dermatology 192:292–293

CHAPTER 32

Diseases of the Nails

Contents

Basic Science Aspects

The nail unit (unguis, onyx = nail) consists of the nail matrix, the nail plate, the nail bed and the periungual skin or paronychium (Fig. 32.1). The nail matrix is the area of growth; it extends 3–6 mm proximally under the proximal nail fold. The nail matrix has two parts: the proximal nail matrix contributes to the dorsal part of the nail plate, while the distal nail matrix provides the ventral part of the plate. The nail plate continuously grows distally over the nail bed. At the distal end it becomes free, lying over the hyponychium. The proximal nail fold and cuticle mark the proximal end of the nail, while to the sides it is bordered by the lateral nail folds. The proximal end of the nail often has a half-moon shaped whitish area, the lunula. The bulk of nail has a faint red to pink color and often contains longitudinal ridges. At the distal end, where the nail is not attached, a 0.2–2.0 mm wide transverse white band (onychodermal band) is present.

The nail is usually between 0.5–0.7 mm in thickness; it is built up from 100–150 layers of nail plate corneocytes (cornified keratinocytes) piled irreg-

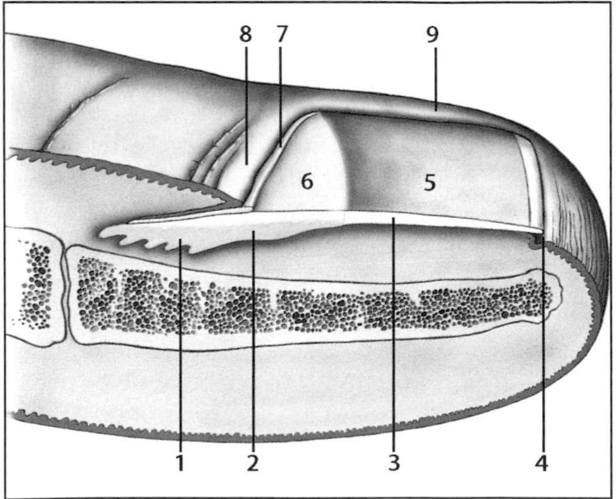

Fig. 32.1. Overview and cross-section of nail organ. *1* Nail matrix; *2* keratinizing zone; *3* nail bed; *4* hyponychium; *5* nail plate; *6* lunula; *7* cuticle; *8* proximal nail fold; *9* lateral nail fold

ularly atop one another. Individual corneocytes can be peeled off with cellophane tape and studied; they lack nuclei and have an irregular configuration. The size of the flat cell increases from about 600 μm² in infancy to 800 μm² in adults to 900–1100 μm² in older individuals. The same changes with age are also seen in the skin.

The nail grows about 0.9 mm/week. There are marked variations with season, use of nail and age. The nails of the middle fingers grow fastest; often nails grow faster on the dominant hand. In some skin diseases, such as psoriasis, the nails grow more rapidly; in others, for example lichen planus, their growth is slowed. The nail fold capillaries can be viewed through the transparent nail; their characteristic pattern can help in the diagnosis of dermatomyositis, progressive systemic sclerosis and even psoriasis. Changes in color, such as subungual hemorrhage, glomus tumors and pigmented lesions, such as melanocytic nevi and malignant melanoma, can be observed through the nail itself. The nail transmits light; the degree of transmission is very dependent on wave length. Thus 1–3% of UVB, 5–10% of UVA and 10–20% of visible light passes through. This is enough to make photo-onycholysis possible. In this situation, the combination of sunlight and a medication such as doxycycline or psoralens leads to loosening of the nail plate from the nail bed. In addition, actinic elastosis can be seen in the nail bed. Another surprising fact is that transepidermal water loss is about 100-fold greater through the nail than through adjacent skin.

The form of the nail varies greatly from person to person. The shape of the nail is dependent on that of the distal phalanx. Many nails have a gentle convex surface when viewed from the side; a concave silhouette is abnormal. The thickness also varies and is to some extent influenced by use or trauma. In older individuals, the longitudinal ridging is more common and the shingle-like pattern of the corneocytes may be more apparent.

Nails serve a number of purposes. Closely related to the claws of other animals, the nails may still be used as weapons by a small number of humans. But their main function is to facilitate fine actions of the fingers. Without nails, such tasks as picking up a thin needle or buttoning a button are difficult. Thus, patients with nail disorders often have problems with such activities. In addition the nails protect the digits and at least with the big toe, serve to help counteract the pressure generated by walking. Because the digits are so richly enervated, most subungual tumors and many other nail disorders are disproportionately painful.

Diseases of the Nail Plate

Onychoschisis

Synonyms. Onychoschizia, lamellar dystrophy

Often the distal end of the nail splits into two or more horizontal layers (Fig. 32.2). The cause is unknown, but it appears that the dorsal and ventral components of the nail plate are separated. Trauma, such as from playing a stringed instrument, is often mentioned as a cause. A second probably more important factor is dryness of the nail, often secondary to too much hand washing or use of harsh soaps. As mentioned above, the nail loses fair amounts of water and is easily dried out. Patients find this hard to believe. Use (or overuse) of nail polish and nail polish remover aggravate the problem. The lipid solvents in polish remover are especially damaging.

Therapy. Patients must avoid trauma and drying procedures. After bathing or washing, they should apply an ointment to their nails, just as they would treat dry skin. We also sometimes have patients soak their fingers for 5–10 min daily in olive oil or a similar oil. Such nails seem to do better with filing than with cutting.

Onychorrhexis

Onychorrhexis technically means longitudinal ridging of the nails. It is often associated with split-

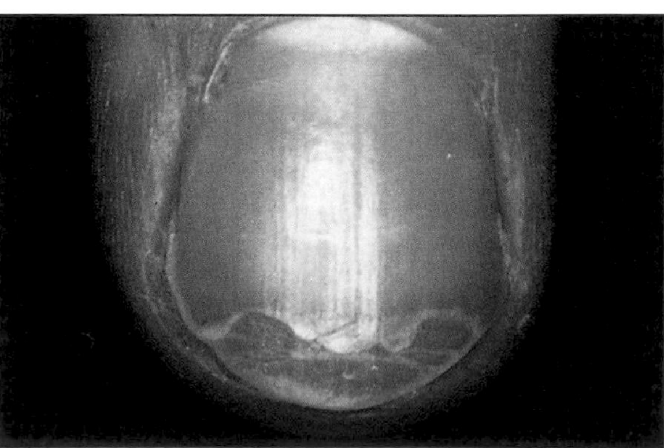

Fig. 32.2. Onychoschisis

ting or breaking and is loosely taken as a synonym for brittle nails. It thus overlaps with onychoschisis. Longitudinal ridging may be congenital and occur in families. It also appears in many older patients, so it is difficult to say when it is abnormal. Once again, dryness of nail, be it from repeated washing or use of nail polish removers appears to be a factor. Any chronic damage to the matrix area, such as repeated trauma to the cuticle, can also produce ridges. In addition, onychorrhexis is often cited as a sign of iron deficiency (associated with koilonychia), hyperthyroidism, malnutrition and even some vitamin deficiencies. In our judgment, it is almost a normal variant and rarely a specific clue.

Therapy. Gentle care as discussed under onychoschisis is all we have to offer. Gelatin, biotin, cystine, and other vitamins have been employed with little success. In Germany, biotin is the latest fashion and a few studies show possible benefit but we remain skeptical.

Onycholysis

Onycholysis or partial separation of the nail plate is a relatively common phenomenon; onychomadesis or total separation is uncommon. There are many possible causes listed in Table 32.1. The most important ones are minor trauma from long nails with leverage exerted against the nail, damage from nail care products, and maceration. Often one suspects one or more of these causes but the patient denies all possibilities and one diagnoses idiopathic onycholysis.

The most common clinical finding is distal onycholysis, also known as half-moon onycholysis (Fig. 32.3). It most commonly occurs when the nail unit is frequently exposed to water, such as in housewives or dishwashers. The free edge of the nail takes up fluid by capillary action and retains it. The resultant maceration loosens the nail. Minor repetitive trauma also helps. Sometimes the semicircular areas of loosening may coalesce, producing more widespread separation of the entire distal portion of the nail. In other instances, the separation proceeds proximally to the nail matrix, either in 3–4-mm stripes or via a single funnel-shaped or canal-like passage. The main differential diagnostic problem is leukonychia.

Therapy. Once again therapy is frustrating. Underlying disorders should be sought for and treated. If an underlying skin disease is present, it can be treated. Most happen to be corticosteroid-respon-

Table 32.1. Causes of onycholysis

Trauma
Acute: hammer blow to nail
Chronic: excessively long nails
Excessive use of nail polish, polish remover and hardeners
Maceration
Infections
Dermatophytes
Candida
Bacteria
Viruses
Medications
"Regular" onycholysis
Photoonycholysis
Dermatologic disorders
Psoriasis
Lichen planus
Contact dermatitis
Toxic epidermal necrolysis
Erythroderma
Genodermatoses
Pachyonychia congenita
Palmoplantar keratodermas
Systemic disorders
Severe systemic infections
Diabetes mellitus
Thyroid disease
Pregnancy
Porphyria
Iron deficiency
Vitamin deficiencies
Nail bed tumors (when solitary)
Subungual exostosis
Verruca
Squamous cell carcinoma (including kerato acanthoma, carcinoma in situ)
Idiopathic

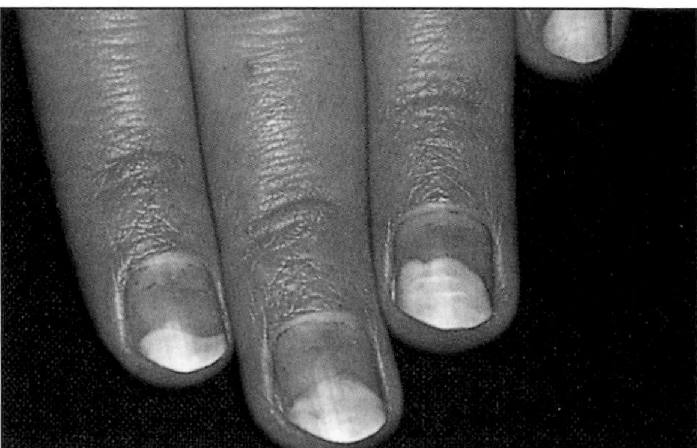

Fig. 32.3. Distal onycholysis

sive, so sometimes a corticosteroid lotion or solution is employed, even in the absence of a clear diagnosis. Avoidance of moisture and trauma is most crucial, as with all nail diseases.

Onychomadesis

Onychomadesis is simply an extreme form of onycholysis. The more dramatic causes of onycholysis, such as toxic epidermal necrolysis, erythroderma, scarlet fever and phototoxic reactions are most often associated with complete nail loss. Occasionally, psoriasis, lichen planus or alopecia areata may also be responsible.

Onychotillomania
(ALKIEWICZ 1934)

This is the nail equivalent of trichotillomania. The patient is almost always emotionally disturbed and destroys his or her nails with scissors, tweezers, a pen knife or even more bizarre tools. Occasionally a patient will preserve two or more opposing nails and use them to destroy all the rest. The only possible treatment is psychiatric.

Onychodystrophy

Synonym. Nail dystrophy

Transverse lines across the nails have been called "storytellers" They reflect damage to the nail matrix and become apparent as the nail grows distally. A number of different names have been applied. REIL (1792), BEAU (1846) and MEES (1919) all described basically the same phenomenon. We tend to use the term Mees lines to describe color changes and Beau lines to describe transverse ridging. The two patterns may overlap.

Mees lines or transverse leukonychia are actually not white; they usually have the same color as the lunula. They extend across the entire nail plate as a horizontal stripe (Fig. 32.4). The snow-white stripes of horizontal leukonychia rarely extend from nail fold to nail fold and often have pointed or irregular lateral borders. They were first described with arsenic poisoning and then later with thallium ingestion, but are the result of sudden nail matrix damage. If the insult is repeated, as in multiple attempts at poisoning, a row of stripes may be seen. Mees lines may follow a severe infectious disease, usually with high fever, malnutrition, and other acute illnesses. In such a case there is always just one band per nail.

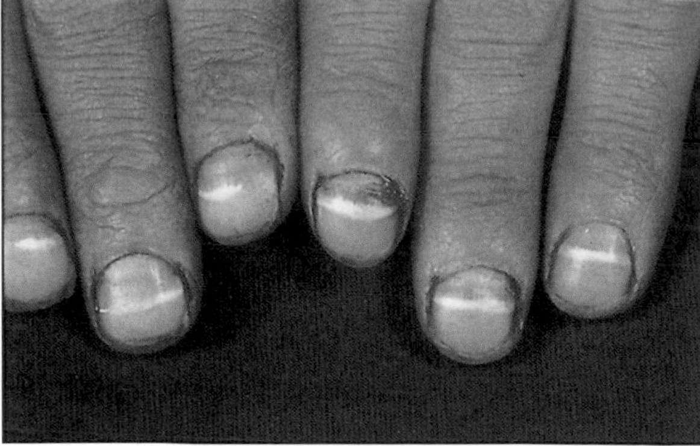

Fig. 32.4. Mees lines

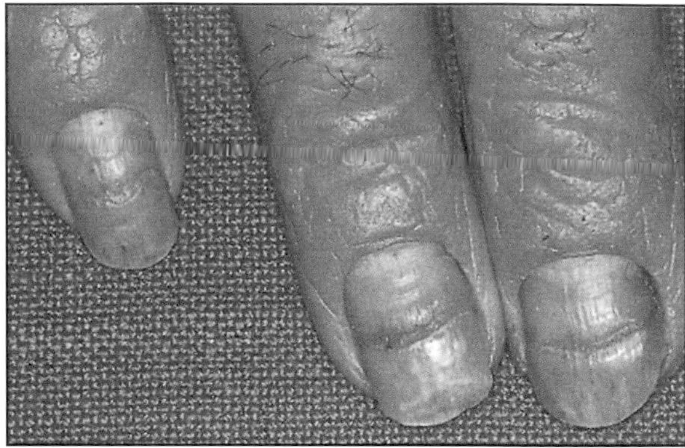

Fig. 32.5. Beau lines

If the damage is more severe, transverse ridges or Beau lines develop. One or more convex transverse lines run across the nail (Fig. 32.5). Usually some color change is also apparent. The causes are the same as with Mees lines. Acute dermatologic disorders involving the nail unit, such as psoriasis or erythroderma, usually lead to transverse ridges, not just color changes. In either event, the cause is often not apparent.

Minor repetitive trauma to the nail fold and cuticle can produce horizontally ridged nails. The term washboard nail is often employed, because multiple ridges are the rule. Typical causes include chronic manipulation of the cuticle, recurrent paronychial infections and repetitive manipulation as the result of a nervous tic.

No treatment is available. If the presumed causative event is not repeated, the lines should grow out spontaneously. If this does not occur, be suspicious of repeated mechanical trauma.

Leukonychia

White spots are probably the most common nail change. They may have many different patterns ranging from a totally white nail, which is most uncommon, to white spots or stripes, both of which are often seen. Because they are often associated with structural changes, such as bands or pits, white lesions are considered here, as well as under color changes below.

Why nails become white remains unclear. One suggestion is that air becomes trapped between the stacked corneocytes, but this seems unreasonable to us. More likely leukonychia reflects a disordered keratinization, similar to parakeratosis of the skin. The parakeratosis found in the normal white lunula seems to also reflect parakeratosis. Trauma also plays a rule; manipulation of the cuticle may often produce not only ridges but also white areas.

The most common form is leukonychia punctata, in which multiple small white spots up to 1–2 mm in size are scattered over the nails. No indentations are present.

Transverse leukonychia overlaps with Mees lines and Muehrcke lines, as discussed below. In leukonychia striata, longitudinal white stripes arise at the lunula and extend distally. They vary greatly in width and may taper at their distal end (Fig. 32.6). In leukonychia totalis, the entire nail is chalky white and brittle; usually all nails are involved (Fig. 32.7). Leukonychia totalis may show autosomal dominant inheritance; a variety of associated syndromes have been described, including Bart-Pumphrey syndrome (autosomal dominant inheritance, knuckle pads, sensory-neural deafness and leukonychia) and the Bushkell-Gorlin syndrome (autosomal dominant inheritance, multiple "sebaceous cysts", renal calculi and leukonychia).

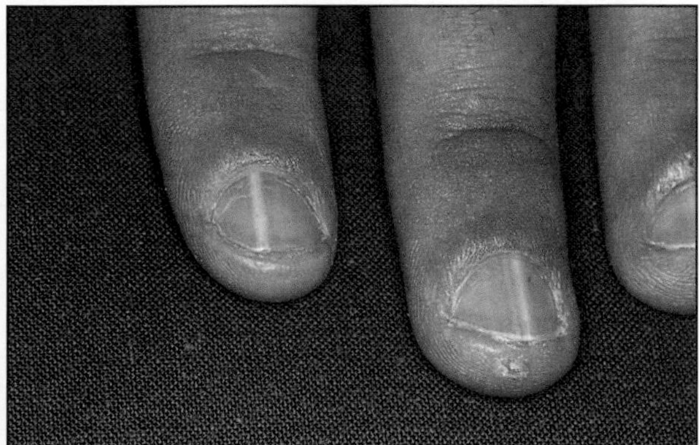

Fig. 32.6. Leukonychia striata

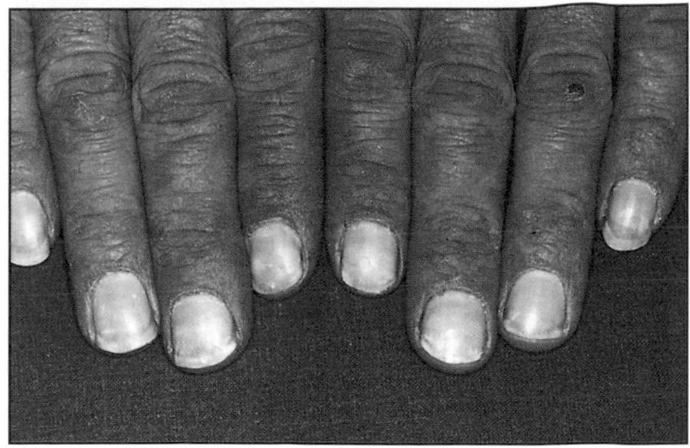

Fig. 32.7. Leukonychia totalis

The main differential diagnostic point is white tinea unguium. One unifying feature of leukonychia is that except for fungal disease treatment is hopeless. Some patients may be helped by avoidance of trauma and especially by less manipulation of the cuticle.

Onychogryphosis

Onychogryphosis refers to claw or talon nails, in other words, to markedly thickened and distorted nails. Such changes are uncommon on the hands, but often seen on the great toes and other toes especially of elderly patients. While patients always deny it, to a certain extent an inability to cut and trim the nails is always a factor. In addition, long term pressure on the nail from shoes, thus making the problem more common in women. Fungus infection of the nails is often diagnosed but rarely truly present. Chronic venous insufficiency and anatomic anomalies such as hallux valgus are clearly predisposing factors. Onychogryphosis may also be associated with some disorder of keratinization.

Clinically, the nails are thickened, hard and rounded along their longitudinal axis, thus resembling a claw or talon (Fig. 32.8). The are also almost invariably deviated laterally when involving the great toe, or otherwise pointed towards the midline of the foot. While the normal nail is slightly curved in a convex fashion and closely attached to the nail bed, the talon nail is distorted at the level of the nail matrix and grows away from the nail bed. This produces a hollow space beneath the nail which is filled with keratotic debris, blocking nail growth. Eventually a thick hard nail folded about its long axis and filled with debris results. Often it is almost impossible to cut.

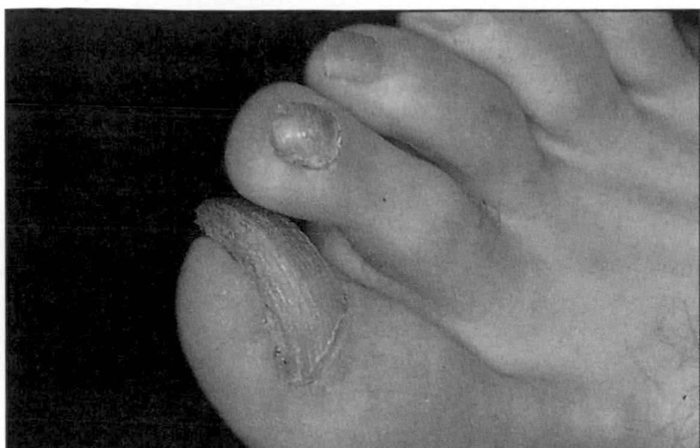

Fig. 32.8. Onychogryphosis

Therapy. The nails can be sanded down with a rotary file or stone, similar to performing a dermabrasion. Often podiatrists or cosmetologists perform this procedure. The operator should always wear a mask as some nails are infected or contaminated with Candida species or other fungi. When they are sanded away, a fine, potentially infectious dust is created. If such care is either unobtainable or ineffective, then removal of the nail with destruction of the matrix is the best approach. If the nail is simply removed, abnormal regrowth usually occurs.

Onychoauxis

Onychoauxis refers to a nail that is hypertrophic but normal in shape and direction of growth. It may follow chronic trauma; psoriasis and tinea unguium should be excluded.

Onychoatrophy

Onychoatrophy is a collective and not very useful term. Nails that are thin, small or even partially absent can be referred to as atrophic. Vascular insufficiency (such as in Raynaud syndrome or disease, Buerger disease and elderly patients) or neurologic impairments involving the extremities, systemic disorders (hyperthyroidism, malnutrition, chemotherapy, retinoid therapy, starvation and eating disorders), congenital disorders of keratinization, and dermatologic diseases (especially lichen planus) can all produce thinned nails. Trachyonychia shows marked overlaps with onychoatrophy; the two are not mutually exclusive.

Trachyonychia
(ALKIEWICZ 1950)

Synonym. Twenty nail dystrophy

In this condition, the surface of the nail is rough, as it is covered by many small fine scales (Fig. 32.9). Any disease process involving the nail matrix can produce such an end product. When all finger and toe nails are involved, one speaks of 20 nail dystrophy. The most common causes, which vary somewhat depending on the age, include atopic dermatitis, alopecia areata, psoriasis, and lichen planus. If the general examination does not show stigmata of any of these diseases, a nail biopsy should be performed. A biopsy from the matrix and proximal nail bed usually shows nonspecific spongiosis along with shingle-like parakeratosis; sometimes, lichen planus or psoriasis can be unequivocally diagnosed, even in the absence of disease elsewhere. If no associated disease is found, one speaks of idiopathic trachyonychia.

Therapy. No therapy is very successful. Since all the major associated disorders are responsive to corticosteroids, we usually try high potency topical corticosteroids, usually under occlusion.

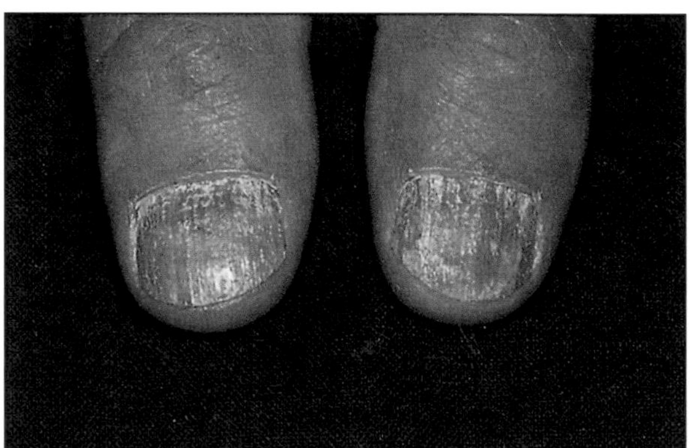

Fig. 32.9. Trachyonychia

Perionychitis Exfoliativa

Synonym. Neidnagel is the German word, meaning a nail that attracts attention or envy.

In this disorder the cuticle is the problem. Instead of being firmly attached to the nail, it becomes raised up with a transverse tear between the adherent and loose parts. This tear may extend into the proximal nail fold, is often painful and serves as a potential entry site for bacterial infections and verrucae.

Therapy. The entire cuticle should be pushed back and cut. The area should lubricated with an ointment several times daily and perhaps under occlusion at night.

Pincer Nails

(Cornelius and Shelley 1968)

Synonyms. Unguis in turriculo, tube nails, tower nails, parrot nails

Some adults spontaneously developed multiple rolled or tube nails. The nails pinch off or trap part of the nail plate and are painful (Fig. 32.10). The cause is unknown. Most commonly the great toe and thumb nails are involved. Many times the great toe also shows hallux valgus. The problem is more common in older women; it shares features with onychogryphosis. Paronychia may develop and there may be changes in the distal phalanxes, perhaps secondary to vascular restriction. In congenital pincer nails, most often all nails are involved. Sometimes a onychomycosis may produce a single pincer nail, so this should be excluded.

Therapy. If the changes are not too severe and are attacked early, it may be worth trying softening and removing the nail with a 40% urea product. A podiatrists can attach a spring-like device to the nail, designed to gradually straiten the curvature; this is very effect. If conservative measures fail, the nail can be removed and the matrix destroyed.

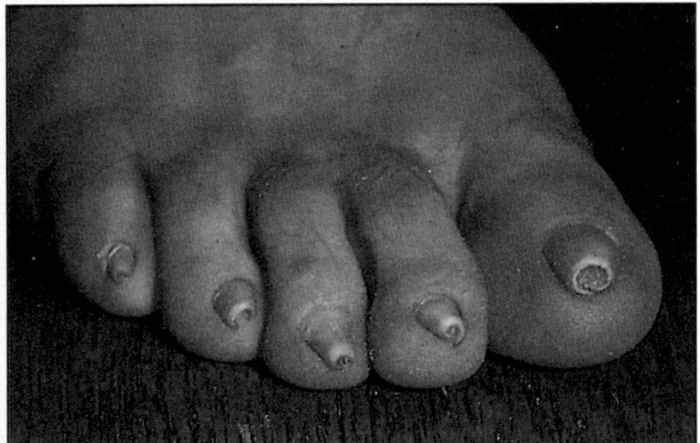

Fig. 32.10. Pincer nails

Neapolitan Nail

Synonym. Kantennagel in German refers to a nail with edges.

Sometimes the nails of older individuals acquire longitudinal ridges; in this special variant, the nail is divided into three flat surfaces, so that in cross-section it resembles a trapezoid. Such nails are sometimes called Neapolitan nails, in reference to the stripes of Neapolitan ice cream. The color may range from gray-white to opaque yellow. Often the lunula is not visible.

Platonychia

In this care, the nail is perfectly flat, neither concave nor convex. Often there is hyperkeratosis under the central part of the nail. Platonychia can be the result of trauma, as in chronic nail biters, but is also associated with a variety of disorders, such as Turner syndrome, thyroid disease and perhaps some vitamin deficiencies. Many view it as a transitory stage between a normal nail and koilonychia.

Koilonychia

(Heller 1898)

Synonym. Spoon nail

Concave nails are more common on the hands than the feet. Often multiple or even all nails are involved. The spoon-shaped depression is more likely to be somewhat distal. In addition, the nail plate may be thin and tends to split at its periphery (onychorrhexis). Spoon nails may be seen in nutritional deficiencies (especially iron deficiency), inherited as an isolated finding in an autosomal dominant pattern, associated with Raynaud disease and other peripheral vascular problems or follow mechanical damage. Lengthy exposure to moisture, especially combined with soaps or harsh chemicals, as well as repetitive trauma, such as in hand workers or typists, may also produce such changes. Hyperthyroidism, nail-patella syndrome and a long list of other problems may perhaps also produce spoon nails.

Therapy. Obviously, if an underlying cause is suspected, it should be corrected as well as possible. Otherwise, avoidance of mechanical trauma and

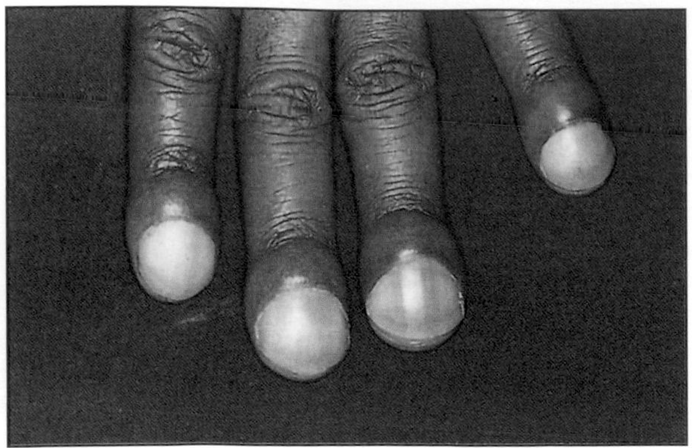

Fig. 32.11. Clubbed nails

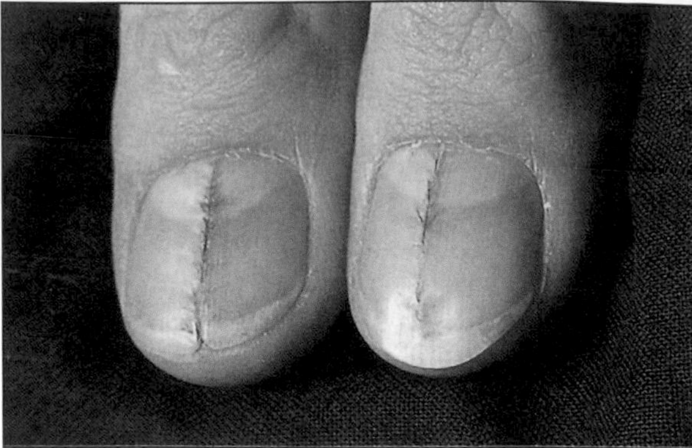

Fig. 32.12. Median canal dystrophy

prevention of drying are important. The nails can be massaged with an ointment after washing, or they can be soaked in olive oil or bath oil. In addition, nail polish may reduce splitting and maceration, but nail polish remover exacerbates it.

Clubbed Nails

Synonyms. Hippocratic nails, watch glass nails, *Trommelschlegelfinger* in German describes a finger shaped like a drum stick.

Hippocrates is generally credited with describing this changes in patients with chronic pulmonary disease. The stroma about the distal phalanx is fibrotic and hypertrophic. As a result, the nail is changed. Lovibond angle is the angle between the proximal nail fold and nail plate; it is normal about 160°, but with clubbed nails it exceeds 180°. The nail is enlarged and in all directions rounded or convex; another designation is hour glass nail (Fig. 32.11).

Clubbing is most often a sign of chronic pulmonary disease. But is it by no means a specific marker, as it may be idiopathic, familial or associated with a range of disorders, including cardiovascular and endocrine abnormalities. Clubbed nails are often found in pachydermoperiostosis. When limited to one or two digits, one should search for local changes, such as vascular insufficiency, digital tumors, chronic infections and other trauma. Pseudoclubbing refers to broad distal phalanxes without nail changes; Apert syndrome is the prototype of this change.

Therapy. No treatment is available.

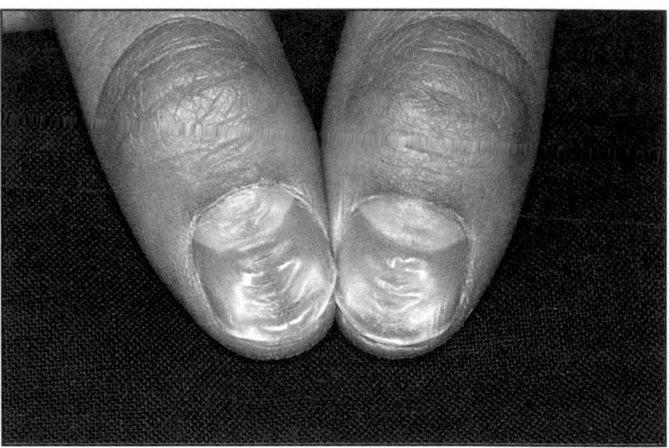

Fig. 32.13. Repetitive trauma mimicking median canal dystrophy

Median Canal Dystrophy
(Heller 1928)

Synonym. Onychodystrophia mediana canaliformis

A longitudinal canal or pit divides a nail, almost always the thumb nail. The process is usually idiopathic and may be inherited (Fig. 32.12). Repetitive trauma to the nail matrix may produce similar changes (Fig. 32.13). Recurrent minor trauma to the nail fold, such as in patients with a repetitive tic, produces a similar clinical picture but usually the changes are more superficial and irregular. If trauma is a potential factor, it should be avoided. Otherwise, there is no promising therapy.

Changes in Nail Color

When nails are discolored, the changes may occur on the nail surface, within the nail, or beneath the nail. The spectrum of colors is enormous; most lack specificity.

Brown longitudinal bands are very common in blacks. They usually reflect a freckle-like change in the nail matrix; that is, there is increased pigment with an increase in melanocytes. Multiple stripes, involving several nails, are not uncommon. In whites, a dark nail stripe usually reflects a melanocytic nevus or lentigo of the nail matrix, nail fold or nail bed (Fig. 32.14). In some instances, there is only an increase in melanin, analogous to a freckle. If the stripe is irregular, if pigment leaks from the edge, especially proximally to involve the cuticle (Hutchinson sign), or if the patient is an older adult, one should do an excisional biopsy to exclude an acral lentiginous malignant melanoma.

Diffuse brown nails may reflect Addison's disease or even diffuse melanosis in patients with metastatic malignant melanoma. More often, the pigment is exogenous and can be scraped off with a nail file; anthralin, silver nitrate, photo processing chemicals and many others can be responsible.

Green discoloration may result from infection with *Pseudomonas aeruginosa*, which can gain access to the subungual space following onycholysis (Fig. 32.15). The pigment will fluoresce with a Wood light. Other fungi and bacteria may produce other discolorations; *Aspergillus niger* can cause a brown-black tone.

A blue hue should suggest argyria. Usually the lunulae are prominently involved; the light-exposed finger nails are more discolored than the toenails, which are rarely involved (Fig. 32.16). The problem is caused by the systemic absorption of silver, usually from medications used to treat nasal problems or chronic leg ulcers. Cyanotic patients may also have a blue tone, but their more crucial problem should be obvious. Similar changes can be observed in methemoglobinemia, whether caused by carbon monoxide poisoning or dapsone therapy, and during busulfan therapy. Dark nails may also be seen in Wilson disease (copper), ochronosis (homogentistic acid) and hemochromatosis (melanin and to a lesser extent iron). The use of henna as a hair dye may produce reddish nails; obviously many other hair dyes may also discolor the nails.

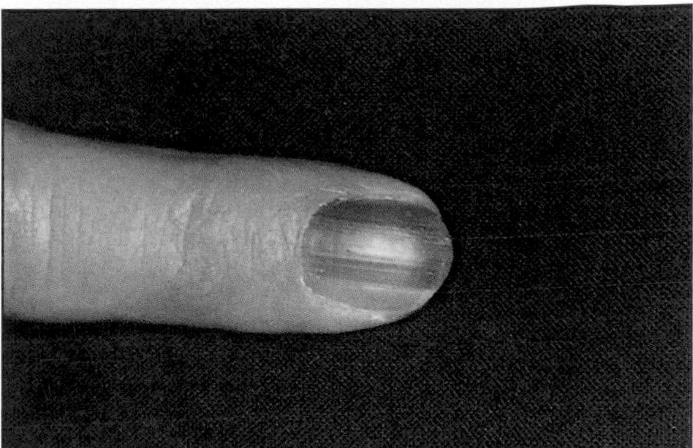

Fig. 32.14. Melanocytic nevus of nail fold

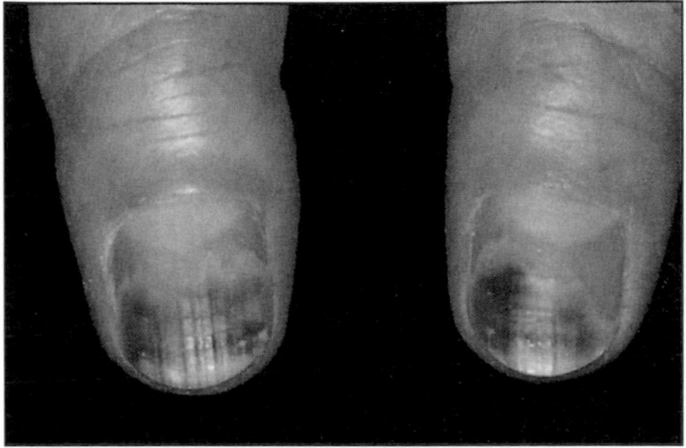

Fig. 32.15. *Pseudomonas* infection with onycholysis

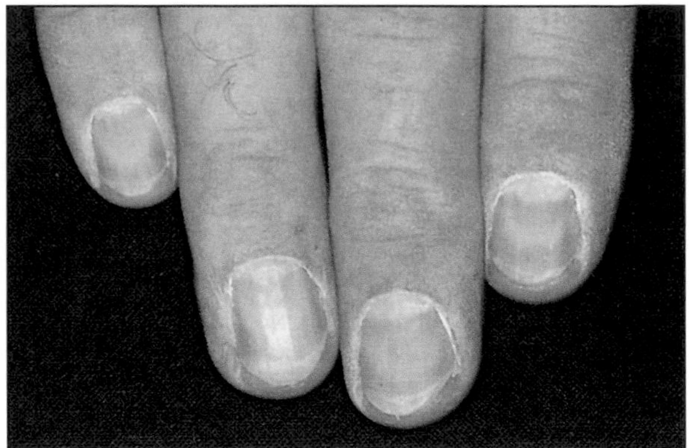

Fig. 32.16. Argyria

A number of medications also lead to discolored nails. Antimalarials, gold, mercury and phenolphthalein all produce dark nails, as do a variety of chemotherapy regimens (Fig. 32.17). Radiation therapy may lead to melanonychia, while trauma

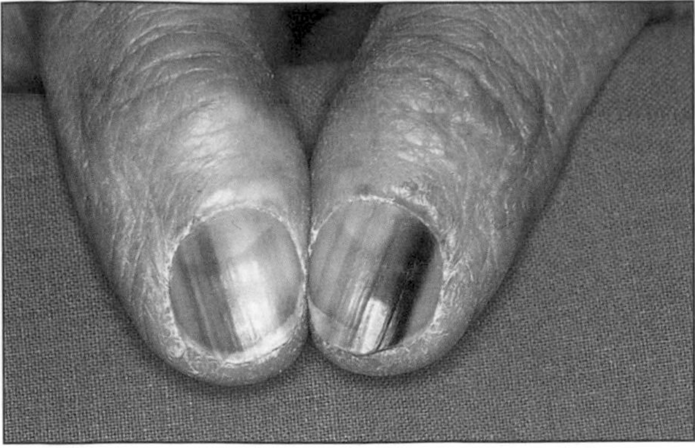

Fig. 32.17. Longitudinal stripes following chemotherapy, most likely representing focal increase in melanin

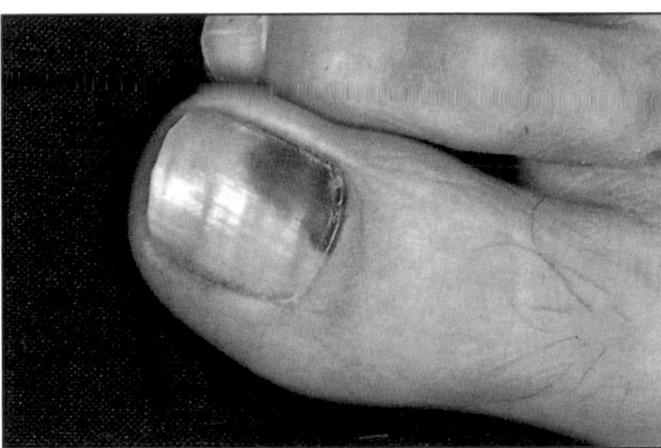

Fig. 32.18. Subungual hematoma

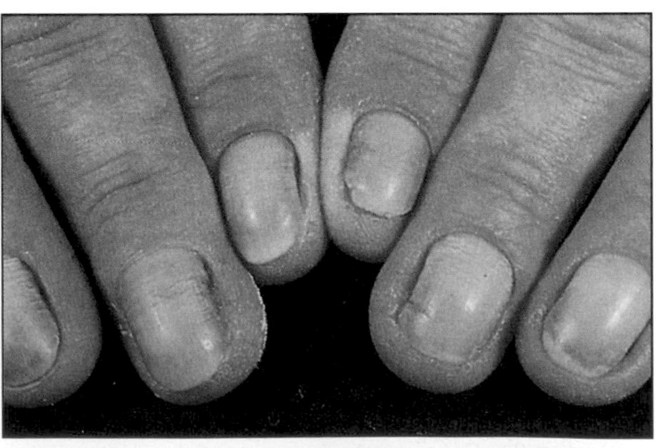

Fig. 32.19. Yellow nail syndrome

can produce a subungual hematoma. The latter may be very dark and suggest a melanocytic lesion but usually the history of sports, hiking or actual trauma (dropping something on the foot) leads one in the right direction (Fig. 32.18).

Yellow Nail Syndrome

(SAMMAN and WHITE 1964)

The yellow nail syndrome is uncommon but spectacular. One, many or all nails may become thick, yellow and grow very slowly (Fig. 32.19). The lunulae disappear and onycholysis may begin distally. Chronic pulmonary disease, including bronchiectasis, chronic bronchitis and sinusitis, as well as lymphedema are often found. α1-antitrypsin deficiency has been reported. Both penicillamine therapy and HIV/AIDS have also been associated with yellow nails. While the nail problems may improve spontaneously, the underlying disorders are all chronic. No effective therapy is available.

Muehrcke Bands

(MUEHRCKE 1956)

Muehrcke bands are a series of white transverse stripes that are parallel to the distal edge of the lunula. They involve the entire breadth of the nail plate. While Muehrcke bands are cited as a sign of hypoalbuminuria, they are neither specific or sensitive. They are also commonly associated with cancer chemotherapy and probably are best visualized as a nonspecific reflection of systemic nail matrix alterations.

Half and Half Nail

(BEAN 1963)

Nails that are white proximally and red-brown distally should suggest renal failure. They are seen about 25 % of this patient group. If the chronic renal disease is treated, the nails tend to improve.

Terry Nail

(TERRY 1954)

The proximal nail is chalky white, obscuring the lunula, while the distal nail has a normal pink color. While these changes were first described in chronic cirrhosis and hypoalbuminemia, they are not specific.

Laugier-Hunziker-Baran Syndrome

(LAUGIER and HUNZIKER 1970; BARAN 1979)

Rare patients may develop hyperpigmented macules of the lips, oral and genital mucosa, along with longitudinal hyperpigmented nail streaks. Thus when confronted with such nail changes, one should examine the mucosa. The condition is acquired, not familial, and totally harmless.

Circumscribed Color Changes

When a patient presents with a single circumscribed nail discoloration, one should think of a subungual tumor. Often such lesions, regardless of their origin, are painful, simply because they are space occupying lesions in a richly innervated area. Typical benign tumors that usually do not distort the nail include glomus tumor, hemangioma, neurofibroma, and similar processes. Verruca vulgaris, keratoacanthoma, subungual osteoma, epidermoid cyst and digital mucous cyst are more likely to damage the nail. A subungual verruca vulgaris may begin as a brown spot, identical to the oil spot in psoriasis; it is typically painful and may be multiple. Usually other periungual or palmarplantar warts are seen. In more chronic lesions, the nail may be badly damaged and the distal phalanx may show pressure damage. In addition, the subungual area is one region where human papilloma virus may be a carcinogen.

Congenital Nail Disorders

Most congenital nail abnormalities when inherited are associated with other ectodermal defects, thus being associated with the long list of ectodermal dysplasias. Some are solitary and represent spontaneous malformations.

Supernumerary Digit

Synonyms. Accessory digit, rudimentary digit

Supernumerary digits are usually located on the lateral side of the fifth digit. They are present at birth, may be bilateral, and are somewhat more common in blacks. They are a tiny finger and may have nerves, bone, cartilage, nails and dermatoglyphics. They are usually excised during infancy.

Differential Diagnosis. The differential diagnosis is confusing, primarily because of overlapping terminology.

- Polydactyly describes patients with additional fingers or toes; here there is a question simply of degree; a relatively complete skeletal structure is probably the simplest differential point. The best known polydactyly syndrome is Ellis-van Creveld syndrome; it is inherited in an autosomal recessive pattern, common among the Pennsylvania Amish, and features acromesomelic dwarfism, hair, nail and tooth abnormalities, as well as cardiac and genital problems.
- Infantile digital fibroma (Reye tumor) occurs on the distal parts of the phalanxes, arising during the first years of life as a broad-based smooth papule adjacent to the nail. Microscopic evaluation shows a fibrous proliferation with characteristic eosinophilic inclusions in the fibroblasts and abundant collagen.
- In some instances there is only an ectopic nail (Fig. 32.20).

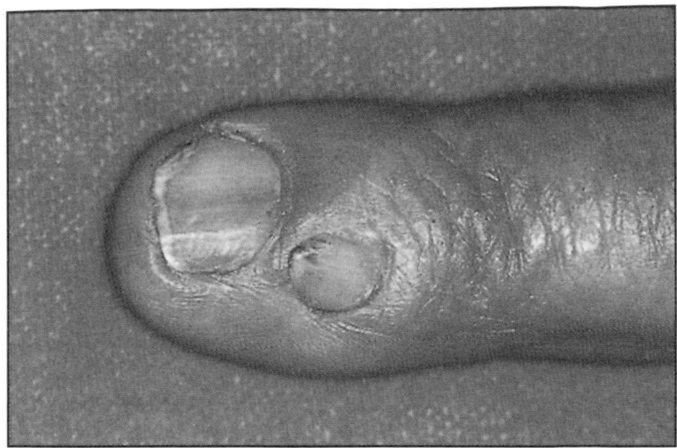

Fig. 32.20. Ectopic nail

Racket Nails

The distal phalanx is shortened and widened, producing a shorted, almost rectangular nail. The

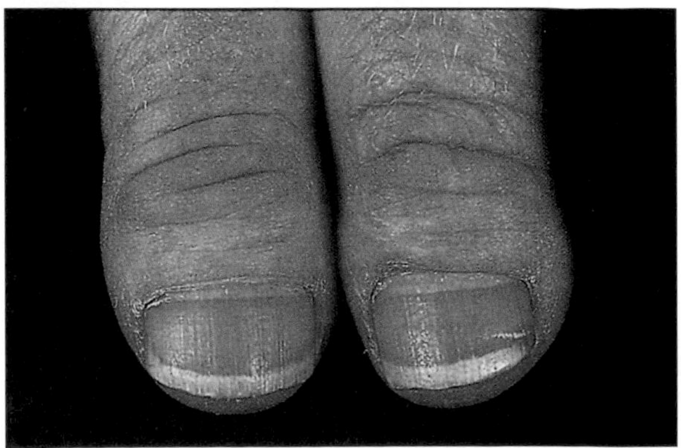

Fig. 32.21. Racket nails

condition usually involved both thumbs, is more common in females, and can be inherited in an autosomal dominant pattern (Fig. 32.21). Racket nails are not associated with any significant problems, although the affected individual may consider them a cosmetic disturbance.

Longitudinal Pachyleukonychia

(MOULIN et al. 1996)

In this variant of leukonychia, there are permanent thickened longitudinal white streaks. In one family, the disorder appeared to be inherited in an autosomal dominant pattern, involving three generations. There were no other ectodermal defects. The nail is thickened beneath the white ridge or band and on biopsy the nail bed is hyperplastic with papillomatosis and even apparent sebaceous-like cells.

Pachyonychia Congenita

(MUSEUS 1716; JADASSOHN and LEWANDOWSKY 1906)

Definition. Group of unrelated disorders featuring thickened nails and a wide variety of other ectodermal defects.

Epidemiology. All forms of pachyonychia congenita are extremely rare.

Etiology and Pathogenesis. Most forms of pachyonychia congenita are inherited in an autosomal dominant pattern, suggesting abnormalities of structural proteins; an autosomal recessive form has also been described. Individual mutations in various keratin molecules have been identified that allow a more precise understanding of the various types and a more accurate diagnosis. The most common Jadassohn-Lewandowsky type has mutations in either the keratin 16 or keratin 6A genes, while the less common Jackson-Lawler-Sertoli variant involves the keratin 17 or 6B genes. Other mutations have also been suggested and in the near future, we suspect pachyonychia congenita will be defined entirely on the basis of keratin mutations.

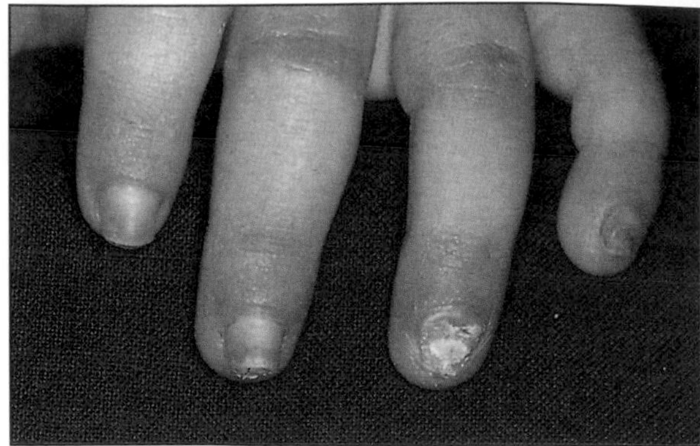

Fig. 32.22. Pachyonychia congenita

Clinical Findings. The hallmark clinical features are dystrophic nails, palmoplantar keratoderma, follicular hyperkeratotic plugs and oral leukokeratosis (Fig. 32.22). The various clinical features of the different subtypes are shown in Table 32.2. Only type I and II are clinically well-established. The nails are typically thickened, hard and claw-like. Usually all nails are involved and the abnormalities are apparent at birth or soon thereafter. They grow irregularly and are elevated. The nail

Table 32.2. Types of pachyonychia congenita

Type	Inheritance	Nails	Skin	Mucosa	Eyes	Comment
JADASSOHN-LEWANDOWSKY (I) (1906)	AD	+	+	+	–	Nails usually normal at birth; ocular and CNS changes rare
JACKSON-LAWLER-SERTOLI (II) (1951, 1949)	AD	+	+	–	–	Steatocystoma, epidermoid cysts, bullae, palmoplantar hyperhidrosis, natal teeth
SCHAFER-BRUNAUER (III) (1923, 1925)	AD	+	+	+	+	Corneal dyskeratosis and cataracts
TIDMAN-WELLS-MACDONALD (1987)	AD	+	+	–	–	Macular amyloidosis
HABER-ROSE (1986)	AR	+	+	+	–	Frequent blisters

AD autosomal dominant; AR autosomal recessive

changes are the unifying feature of the group and are relatively similar, although all forms are so rare that most clinicians never have the chance to compare two types. The skin may show follicular hyperkeratotic papules, most often on the extremities, knees, elbows and buttocks. In addition, palmar-plantar hyperkeratosis may be present, either in a diffuse or linear fashion. The combination of abnormal nails and hyperkeratotic palms usually interferes with the patient manual dexterity to a significant extent. Some forms show a tendency to blistering, with subsequent callus formation. The presence of steatocystoma multiplex strongly suggests the Jackson-Lawler-Sertoli variant, which is also more likely to have dental abnormalities.

The oral mucosal lesions are thick white plaques that simply show regular hyperkeratosis histologically and have no malignant potential. They are found on the tongue, labial and buccal mucosa and gingiva. Involvement of the nasal mucosa (dryness, discomfort), larynx (hoarseness), and tympanic membrane (deafness) has been described. Ocular changes include corneal opacities and cataracts, both of which can lead to blindness. A long and confusing list of associated symptoms probably reflects an attempt to group many disorders together and even include some of the epidermolysis bullosa family.

Histopathology. The various types of pachyonychia congenita cannot be separated microscopically. The hyperkeratotic skin and mucosal lesions show acanthosis and hyperkeratosis with parakeratosis; dyskeratosis or other premalignant changes are not seen. The dermis or lamina propria shows varying degrees of inflammation. In the Tidman-Wells-MacDonald type, the diffuse hyperpigmented areas show deposits of keratin-related amyloid in the dermal papillae and incontinence of pigment, typical for macular amyloidosis.

Course and Prognosis. All are persistent and range between inconvenient and disabling in their effects on the patient.

Differential Diagnosis. One should consider dyskeratosis congenita with oral changes but usually atrophic nails, psoriasis, other forms of palmoplantar keratoderma, and perhaps mild forms of epidermolysis bullosa with callus formation.

Therapy

Systemic. In some cases, systemic retinoids, usually acitretin, may be helpful.

Topical. The nails may be sanded or filed with a variety of devices; some patients are more comfortable without nails following removal and destruction of the matrix. Local keratolytics usually help the cutaneous lesions; blisters should be treated with an antibacterial preparation such as silver sulfadiazine. Topical retinoids have been tried for the oral lesions, but with little benefit.

Congenital Onychodysplasia

(Iso 1969; Kikuchi 1974)

Synonyms. Congenital onychodysplasia of the index fingers, Iso-Kikuchi syndrome

Some cases are inherited in an autosomal dominant pattern; most are sporadic. Ischemic damage in utero has been postulated, but then the involvement of just two digits is hard to explain. The nails of the index fingers and occasionally the corresponding 2nd toes are involved. The radial side is more often affected than the ulnar. Rarely are other nails involved. The changes range from micronychia or anychia through a variety of dystrophies. Syndactyly and changes in the distal phalanxes may also be seen. The Iso-Kikuchi syndrome should be considered whenever nail changes are symmetrical, involving the index fingers. No treatment is available.

In other instances, different nails are involved but the syndromes have not been exactly defined. The clinical picture is similar with micronychia (Fig. 32.23) or anychia.

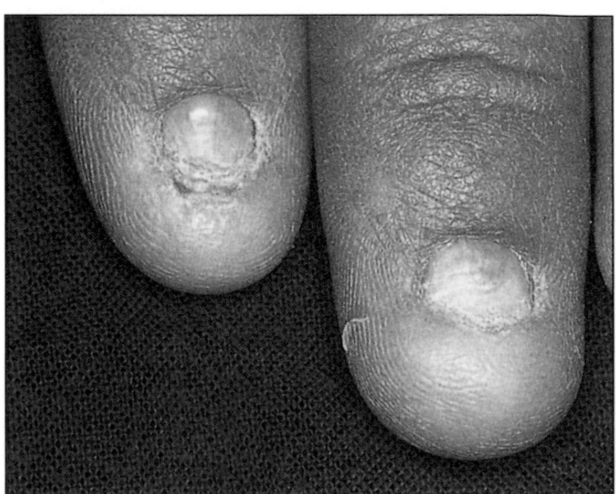

Fig. 32.23. Microonychia

Nail-Patella Syndrome

(Chatelain 1824; Little 1897)

Synonyms. Osteoonychodysplasia, Turner (1933)-Kieser (1939) syndrome

The nail-patella syndrome consists of onychodystrophy, palmarplantar hyperhidrosis, aplasia or hypoplasia of the patella, hypoplasia of the radial head with frequent subluxation of the radius, iliac horn, renal abnormalities ($^1/_3$ have chronic glomerulonephritis) and a long list of other associated findings. The syndrome is inherited in an autosomal dominant pattern. The causative gene is located on chromosome 9q34. The characteristic skeletal changes often allow a prenatal diagnosis via ultrasound or radiologic examination.

The nails may be absent or small and frequently show onychoschisis (horizontal splitting). A pathognomonic sign is triangular lunulae. The thumbs and index fingers are most often involved. Another clue is an irregularly pigmented iris; when the pupillary border is hyperpigmented, it is known as Lester sign. The knee and elbow problems are usually symptomatic, with abnormal gait and increased carrying angle of the elbow. The orthopedic problems may be amenable to surgery. The renal status should be monitored. The nails are not treatable.

In the trisomy 8 syndrome, patients may also have absent patella and absent or deformed nails, so a cytogenetic evaluation is reasonable in suspected cases.

Congenital Malalignment of the Great Toenails

(Samman 1978)

This rare problem is apparently inherited in an autosomal dominant pattern. Children are born with or soon develop abnormal great toe nails, resembling onychogryphosis. The nails are gray-yellow and twisted or folded along both their axes. Often they are narrowed distally and may be attached to the nail bed in only their proximal portion. Deviated growth is not seen, in contrast to onychogryphosis. The cause is unknown. The only treatment is surgical destruction of the nail matrix.

Pterygium Inversum Unguis

(Caputo and Prandi 1973)

This uncommon, occasionally familial condition is characterized by proliferation of the hyponychium or distal zone of the nail bed, corresponding to the *Sohlenhorn* of hoofed animals, which normally show distal keratinization. The distal nail proliferates, often covers the tip of the finger and is painful. The distal subungual sulcus is lost. Similar changes can be seen in patients with progressive systemic sclerosis and marked acral involvement.

Nail Changes Associated with Dermatologic and Systemic Disorders

Many skin diseases are associated with nail changes. Some of the most important ones are discussed below; others are mentioned in the relevant chapters.

Chronic Dermatitis. Chronic hand or foot dermatitis of any type – irritant or allergic contact – may lead to damaged nails. As soon as the cuticle and the lateral nail folds are damaged, the nail is likely to show riding, pitting, splitting and thickening. One can speak of eczema nails. If the underlying disease is treated, the nails can be expected to improve slowly.

Psoriasis. Classic changes include pitting, oil s pots and distal subungual debris, often leading to onycholysis. (Chap. 14) Other changes include trachyonychia and splinter hemorrhages. The dystrophic nails are frequently very distressing to the patient; clinically they resemble onychomycotic nails and the differentiation can be problematic. A significant percent of psoriasis patients (10–50%) have nail changes; thus any patient who presents with nail changes should be checked for psoriasis. Patients with severe pustular psoriasis and Reiter syndrome may also have nail involvement; typically because of more acute and severe disease, onycholysis is produced.

Alopecia Areata. Fine pits, longitudinal ridges and a rough surface are classically seen (Fig. 32.24). The lunula may be speckled. Leukonychia, onychomadesis, trachyonychia and onycholysis may also be present.

Lichen Planus. The diagnosis of lichen planus should not be made without examining the nails. Some cases of 20 nail dystrophy represent lichen planus. In more extreme cases, multiple nails may

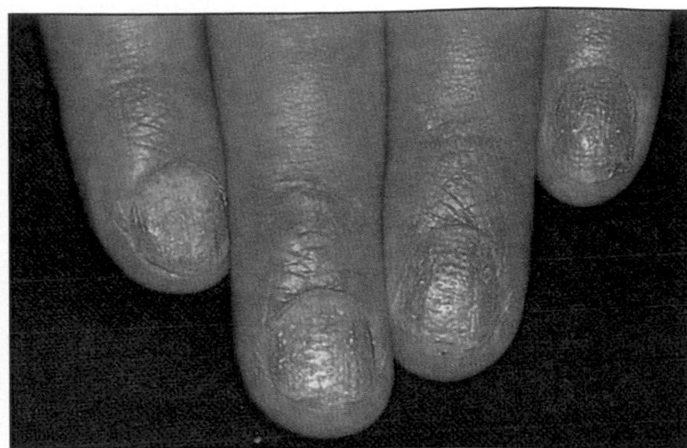

Fig. 32.24. Pitted nails in alopecia areata

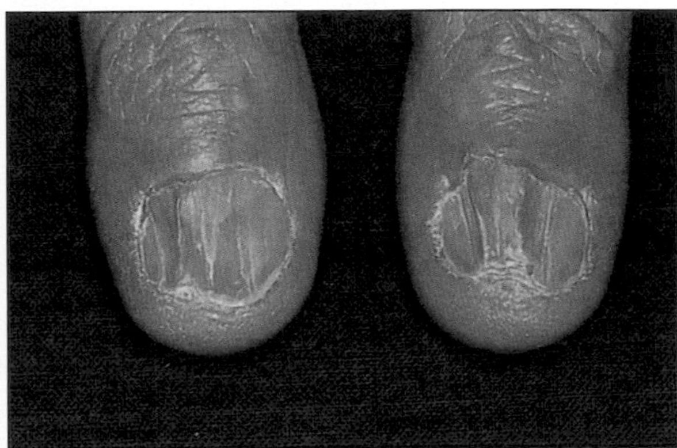

Fig. 32.25. Pterygium and nail dystrophy in lichen planus

be absent or partially lost. A pterygium is especially typical; here the nail is lost, and the nail bed atrophic and pulled together, producing a pterygium or wing (Fig. 32.25).

Dyskeratosis Congenita. The nails are often either absent or develop pterygium.

Epidermolysis Bullosa. The scarring or dystrophic types of epidermolysis bullosa may eventuate in the loss of multiple nails. Those that do survive may be small or dystrophic.

Toxic Epidermal Necrolysis. Just as broad sheets of skin are shed, multiple nails may be lost. Usually they regrow normally, but sometimes atrophic nails are a long-term sequel.

Blistering Diseases. Both pemphigus vulgaris and bullous pemphigoid may cause nail loss. Regrowth is to be expected.

Tuberous Sclerosis. One characteristic feature are the periungual fibromas (Koenen tumors). They may produce a painful disturbance of nail growth.

Darier Disease. Typically patients have dark and light colored stripes, covering most of the nail, even the lunula. Curiously, where such a stripe reaches the distal end, a V-shaped notch is usually formed. Markedly dystrophic nails can result from subungual hyperkeratosis.

Pityriasis Rubra Pilaris. Massive subungual hyperkeratosis with nail loss is another feature of pityriasis rubra pilaris that closely resembles psoriasis.

Scabies. In crusted scabies, what appears to be hyperkeratosis under the nails may actually be thousands of mites and scale scratched from other skin areas. Microscopic scrapings from beneath the nail of a "psoriasis" patient who is itching may provide a quick and dramatic diagnosis.

Lupus Erythematosus and Dermatomyositis. Both may have erythema of the proximal nail fold with telangiectases. Often the nail folds are painful. The nail plate may be brittle or contain transverse stripes.

Systemic Sclerosis. The finger tips become atrophic and the distal part of the nail plate tend to grow over them (pterygium inversum unguis-like). In addition nail fold telangiectases and nail atrophy may be seen.

Raynaud Disease. All conditions with impaired vascular supply to the digits may feature a variety of nail changes, including very commonly thin, brittle nails, as well as longitudinal stripes, koilonychia and many other changes.

Chronic Pulmonary Disease. Clubbing may be a feature.

Gastrointestinal Disease. All forms of malabsorption leading to relative malnutrition may produce horizontal ridges or alternating bands of color on the nail as well as absent lunulae. Other severe gastrointestinal disease, such as acute hepatitis, may also produce bands.

Renal Disease. The half and half or Lindsay nail is classic for chronic renal disease, but neither specific or sensitive. About 30% of dialysis patients have no lunula.

Acquired Nail Changes

Trauma

One of the most common causes of nail changes is trauma. Acute trauma is usually obvious, but chronic trauma may be less apparent. In addition, it is difficult to convince the patient of the diagnosis in such cases. The types of trauma are numerous, as listed below.

Hematoma. Following either frank blunt trauma (something being dropped on the toe, hitting the thumb with a hammer), blood collects under the nail (Fig. 32.18). While it is initially red, by the time the patient presents, the color is usually blue black. When no history of trauma is available, one should inquire about hiking (especially lengthy down hill hikes), other sports activities, dancing, and new or tightly fitting shoes.

Since the main differential diagnosis concern is a subungual acral lentiginous malignant melanoma, sometimes further evaluation is necessary. Removing a small part of the discoloration for histologic examination and iron stain is often recommended; even if positive, it should not provide false reassurance. In recent years, dermatoscopic examination has improved the clinical diagnostic accuracy in this setting. When questions remain, removing the nail and doing an adequate longitudinal incisional biopsy is preferred.

Repetitive Occupational Trauma. Typists were formerly the prototype for multiple horizontal ridges reflecting repeated insults to the tips of the nails. Word processors have reduced the amount of "hitting" needed and reduced this problem. Nonetheless, typists with long nails may still create damage. Other repetitive tasks, such as jack hammer use, may cause shortened, thickened nails. Auto mechanics often have subungual hemorrhages.

Tic Artifact. Some patients continuously manipulate their nails, especially the thumb. The flexed thumb is rubbed with the index or middle finger, producing a central groove (Fig. 32.13). Since the proximal nail fold is damaged, paronychia develop.

Nail Biting. Chewing or biting ones' nails is a relatively harmless trait in childhood but often persists into adult life. Chronic paronychia and transfer of digital warts to other digits or the oral cavity are two typical complications. Some emotionally disturbed patients bite, chew or extract their nails or damage them in what appears to be extremely painful ways. Such patients can be spotted quickly in the examining room; in our experience they almost invariably manipulate or remove their nails while explaining their "disease".

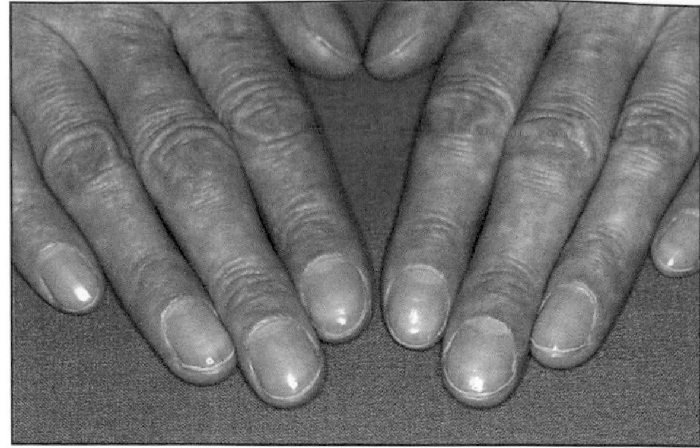

Fig. 32.26. Polished nails

Polished Nails. Some patients who rub rather than scratch pruritic dermatoses such as atopic dermatitis produce very smooth, shining nails. If they use lotions containing fine particles, such as zinc oxide lotion, the particles may serve as a sanding compound, giving the nails a polish-like shine. Other occupational challenges, such as extensively handling fabrics, may also smooth the nails (Fig. 32.26).

Shoe Trauma. Poorly fitting shoes may contribute to hallux valgus and thus indirectly to onychogryphosis. They may also lead to subungual hematomas.

Chemicals. Solvents, cleaning materials, oils and many other substances may directly damage the nail and more likely damage the cuticle and lateral nail fold, loosening the nail and exposing it to infections and further trauma. Patients exposed to polyvinyl chloride may develop acquired acro-osteolysis with shortened thickened nails; here the effects are probably systemic.

Infections. Bacteria, yeasts, fungi and viruses all may damage the nail. These problems are covered in the respective chapters.

Medications. A number of medications cause changes in nail or nail bed color. All antimetabolites have the potential to inhibit nail growth, producing either horizontal bands or ridges, as well as thin or brittle nails. Oral retinoids used to treat acne, psoriasis or disorders of keratinization, may cause dry, thin nails with multiple pyogenic granulomas along the nail folds.

Ingrown Nail

Synonym. Unguis incarnatus

Ingrown nails are a common problem. The lateral portion of the nail grows (or is forced) down into the paronychium, where it acts as a foreign object, eliciting an inflammatory response with granulation tissue (Fig. 32.27). Predisposing factors include anything that tends to force the nail out of its normal growth pattern poorly fitting shoes, poorly trimmed nails and any other chronic trauma. Ingrown nails are most common on the great toes and far more likely to be medial than lateral, supporting the role of trauma. The nail penetrates the lateral nail fold, making bacterial infections very common.

Therapy. Conservative therapy consists of appropriately trimming the nail, and forcing rolled strands of cotton balls, soaked in an antiseptic solution under the nail. This elevates the nail, reducing the foreign body action and also enables it to grow out over the distal nail fold. We have also had good luck forcing a small, longitudinally slit plastic tube over the edge of the nail; this reduces the foreign body reaction and enhances healing. Another approach, most often employed by podiatrists, is to attach a metallic spring or brace to the nail. This is designed to gradually straighten and lift the nail.

If these measures fail, a surgical procedure may be needed. A wide number of techniques are available. In the standard Emmert procedure, a wedge-shaped excision is carried out, excising a part of the entire lateral nail apparatus, including matrix. This produces a narrower nail. In another procedure, the lateral part of the nail is removed and the lateral matrix destroyed with caustics. Simply removing the nail rarely corrects the problem. If a bit of matrix is left behind, it may produce a nail spur, creating persistent problems.

Subungual and Periungual Tumors

Subungual Exostosis

(Dupuytren 1847)

The terminal phalanx may develop an osseous overgrowth that protrudes upward displacing the nail. While such lesions have been called osteomas, radiologic evaluation almost always shows a connection to the underlying bone. The overlying tissue may be ulcerated, callused or in the case of the nail, simply pushed aside. The most common site is the medial side of the great toe, once again suggesting a role for trauma (Fig. 32.28). While lesions are often misdiagnosed as ingrown nails, they can usually be distinguished clinically and the diagnosis confirmed with a X-ray. Other painful subungual tumors, such as glomus tumor, may also enter into the differential diagnosis. Occasionally, the pathologic examination will reveal cartilage and not bone; then the term subungual chondroma (or enchondroma) is used; the two processes are probably identical. The underlying bony defect must be corrected surgically; the cutaneous changes will generally resolve rapidly.

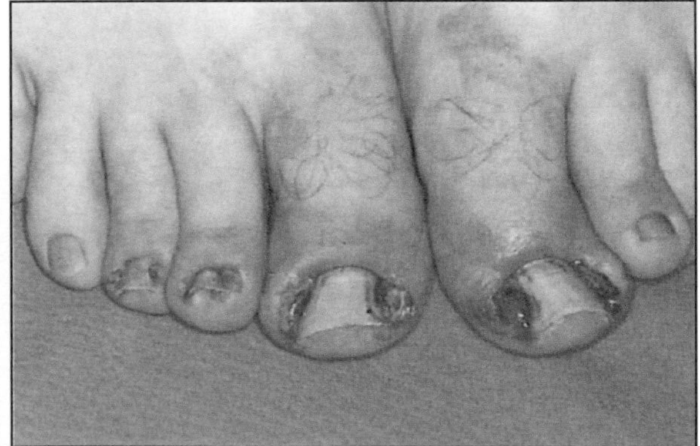

Fig. 32.27. Ingrown nails

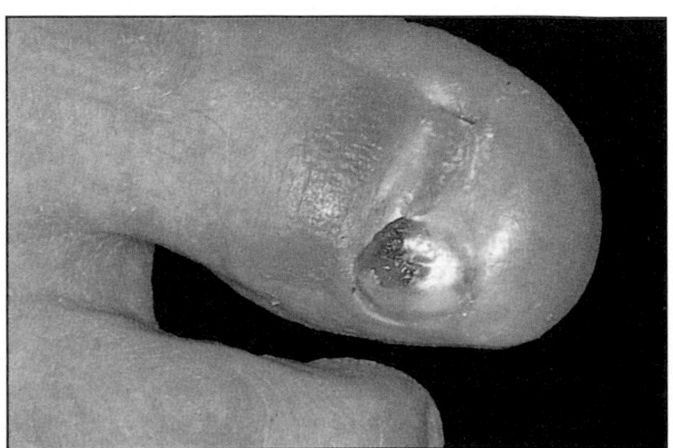

Fig. 32.28. Subungual exostosis

Epidermal Inclusion Cyst

Trauma can implant epidermal tissue into the skin of a digit, producing a true epidermal inclusion cyst. Sometimes the time interval between the injury and the appearance of the cyst is so long that no history of trauma is obtained. Ingrown nails may also push epidermis down producing trapped remnants and then cysts. Excision is curative.

Verrucae

The most common sub- and periungual tumors are verrucae. They are usually painful and associated with verrucae elsewhere. Children may have transferred the human papilloma virus to their mouth. True subungual verrucae are uncommon but present as a discoloration and later a painful tumor. The periungual lesions are more typical of warts.

Acquired Digital Fibrokeratoma

These slowly growing tumors arise from the nail bed or proximal nail fold. They most often are on the side of the finger. Both clinically and histologically they have a prominent epidermal collarette; their surface is smoother than a wart. The nail is often displaced. Microscopic examination shows a compact fibrous proliferation. Surgical excision is curative.

Bowen Disease

Bowen disease or squamous cell carcinoma in situ is often a subtle finding in the nail region. Usually older patients are involved and the typical sites are the thumbs and great toes. Often only a minimal erythema and onycholysis are identified. Thus, it is important to do a biopsy of any such nail change which is chronic and of unclear origin. If not identified, the tumor may develop into a frank squamous cell carcinoma. Fortunately, these malignancies are not extremely aggressive. Radiation exposure to the finger, such as in dentists, radiologists and surgeons years ago and arsenic exposure are two documented risk factors. Surgical excision is required; often microscopically controlled surgery or CO_2 laser excision bring advantages.

Keratoacanthoma

The exact nature of subungual keratoacanthoma is unclear. While traditional keratoacanthomas are follicular tumors, the subungual keratoacanthoma arises where no hair follicles are found. It may be a variant of a subungual wart. While ordinary keratoacanthomas are painless, the subungual variety is typically quite painful, as it grows rapidly and destroys not only the nail, but also the soft tissue and even bone. Bony destruction by a subungual tumor as seen with radiologic examination favors keratoacanthoma. The histology is also not typical of keratoacanthoma in other sites, but closer to a squamous cell carcinoma. Treatment is surgical.

Acral Lentiginous Malignant Melanoma

The early stages of acral lentiginous malignant melanoma are also very subtle and easily overlooked. Often there is a vague discoloration of the nail; one should search carefully for minimal discoloration of the proximal or lateral nail fold (Hutchinson sign), which suggests a melanocytic process, most likely acral lentiginous malignant melanoma, is present. Once again, the thumbs and great toes are most often involved and most patients are elderly. Dermatoscopy usually suggests the diagnosis, which is confirmed by biopsy. Definitive treatment is surgical. Often amputation of the digit is required.

Glomus Tumor

The glomus tumor is discussed in greater detail under vascular tumors (Chap. 59). It is often subungual, presenting as a painful red nodule. Glomus tumors are classically sensitive to touch and even temperature change. Excision is curative.

Bibliography

Basic Science Aspects

Achten G, André J, Laporte M (1991) Nails in light and electron microscopy. Semin Dermatol 10:54–64

Alves GF, Poon E, John J et al. (1999) Circumferential fingernail. Br J Dermatol 140:960–962

Baran R, Tosti A (1999) Nails. In: Freedberg JM, Eisen AZ, Wolff K, Austen KF, Goldsmith LA, Katz SJ, Fitzpatrick TB (eds) Dermatology in general medicine. McGraw Hill, New York, pp 752–768

Barnett JM, Scher RK (1992) Nail cosmetics. Int J Dermatol 31:675–681

De Berker DAR, Baran R, Dawber RPR (1995) Handbook of diseases of the nails and their management. Blackwell Science, Oxford
Clark RE, Madani S, Bettencourt MS (1998) Nail surgery. Dermatol Clin 16:145–64
Cohen PR (1996) The lunula. J Am Acad Dermatol 34: 943–953
Dawber RPR, Baran R, de Berker DAR (1999) Disorders of nails. In: Champion RH, Burton JL, Burns DA, Breathnach SM (eds) Rook/Ebling/Wilkinson textbook of dermatology. Blackwell Science, Oxford, pp 2815–2868
Goldminz D, Bennett RG (1992) Mohs micrographic surgery of the nail unit. J Dermatol Surg Oncol 18:721–726
Johnson M, Shuster S (1993) Continuous formation of nail along the bed. Br J Dermatol 128:277–280
Drake LA, Dinehart SM, Farmer ER et al. (1996) Guidelines of care for nail disorders. J Am Acad Dermatol 34: 529–533
Rich P (1992) Nail biopsy. Indications and methods. J Dermatol Surg Oncol 18:673–682
Sinclair RD, Wojnarowska F, Leigh IM et al. (1994) The basement membrane zone of the nail. Br J Dermatol 131: 499–505
Zaias N (1990) The nail in health and disease. Appleton and Lange, East Norwalk

Diseases of the Nail Plate

Onychoschisis

Wallis MS, Bowen WR, Guin JR (1991) Pathogenesis of onychoschizia (lamellar dystrophy). J Am Acad Dermatol 24:44–48

Onychorrhexis

Colombo VE, Gerber F, Bronhofer M et al. (1990) Treatment of brittle fingernails and onychoschizia with biotin: scanning electron microscopy. J Am Acad Dermatol 23: 1127–1132

Onycholysis

Baran R, Jeanmougin M, Cesarini JP (1997) Spontaneous photo-onycholysis in a west Indian type V skin. Acta Derm Venereol 77:169–170
Burden AD, Kemmett D (1996) The spectrum of nail involvement in palmoplantar pustulosis. Br J Dermatol 134: 1079–1082
Daniel CR III (1991) Onycholysis: an overview. Semin Dermatol 10:34–40
Daniel CR III, Daniel MP, Daniel CM et al. (1996) Chronic paronychia and onycholysis: a thirteen-year experience. Cutis 58:397–401
Makris A, Mortimer P, Powles TJ (1996) Chemotherapy induced onycholysis. Eur J Cancer 32:374–375

Onychomadesis

Bodman MA (1995) Miscellaneous nail presentations. Clin Podiatr Med Surg 12:327–346
Faber EM, Nall L (1992) Nail psoriasis. Cutis 50:174–178
Fleming CJ, Hunt MJ, Barnestin RS (1996) Mycosis fungoides with onychomadesis. Br J Dermatol 135:1012–1013
Tosti A, Morelli R, Bardazzi F (1994) Prevalence of nail abnormalities in children with alopecia areata. Pediatr Dermatol 11:112–115

Onychotillomania

Alkiewicz J (1934) Über Onychotillomanie. Dermat Wochenschr 98:519–521
Colver GB (1987) Onychotillomanie. Br J Dermatol 117: 397–399
Scott MJ Jr, Scott MJ III (1997) Dermatophagia: "wolf-biter". Cutis 59:19–20

Onychodystrophy

Beau JHS (1846) Note sur certains caractères de séméiologie rétrospective présentés par les ongles. Arch Générales de Médecine 11:447
De Berker DAR (1994) What do Beau's lines mean? Int J Dermatol 33:545–546
Hepburn MJ, English JC III, Meggert JJ (1997) Mees' lines in a patient with multiple parasitic infections. Cutis 59: 321–323
Huddleston HAT, Dunnihoo DR (1994) Beau's lines on Terry's nail? South Med J 87:867
Itin PH, Pittlekow MR (1990) Trichothiodystrophy: review of sulphur-deficient brittle hair syndromes and association with the ectodermal dysplasias. J Am Acad Dermatol 22:705–712
Marino MT (1990) Mees' lines. Arch Dermatol 126:827–828
Mees RA (1919) Een Verchijnsel bij Polyneuritis Arsenicosa. Nederl T Geneesh 1:391
Tolmie JL, de Berker DAR, Dawber R (1994) Syndromes associated with trichodystrophy. Clin Dysmorphology 3:1–14

Leukonychia

Baran R, Perrin C (1995) Transverse leukonychia of toenails due to repeated microtrauma. Br J Dermatol 133:267–269
Grossman M, Scher RK (1990) Leukonychia: review and classification. Int J Dermatol 29:535–541
Jemec GBE, Kollerup G, Jensen LB et al. (1995) Nail abnormalities in nondermatologic patients: prevalence and possible role as diagnostic aids. J Am Acad Dermatol 32:977–981
Ramer JC, Vasily DB, Ladda RL (1994) Familial leuconychia, knuckle pads, hearing loss, and palmoplantar hyperkeratosis: an additional family with Bart-Pumphrey syndrome. J Med Genet 31:68–71
Stevens KR, Leis PF, Peters S et al. (1998) Congenital leukonychia. J Am Acad Dermatol 39:509–512
Van Gelderen de Komaid A, Borges de Kestelman I, Duran EL (1997) Etiology and clinical characteristics of mycotic leukonychia. Mycopathologia 136:9–15

Onychogryphosis and Onychoauxis

Cohen PR, Scher RK (1992) Geriatric nail disorders: diagnosis and treatment. J Am Acad Dermatol 26:521–531

Onychoatrophy

Kitmaya Y, Tsukada S (1983) Congenital onychodysplasia: report of 11 cases. Arch Dermatol 119:8–11

Trachyonychia

Alkiewicz J (1950) Trachyonychie. Ann Dermatol Syphiligr 10:136–140
Tosti A, Bardazzi F, Piraccini BM et al. (1994) Idiopathic trachyonychia (twenty-nail dystrophy): a pathological study of 23 patients. Br J Dermatol 131:866–872

Tosti A, Fanti PA, Morelli R et al. (1991) Spongiotic trachyonychia. Arch Dermatol 127:584–585

Tosti A, Fanti PA, Morelli R et al. (1991) Trachyonychia associated with alopecia areata: a clinical and pathologic study. J Am Acad Dermatol 25:266–270

Pincer Nails

Cornelius CE, Shelley WB (1968) Pincer nail syndrome. Arch Surg 96:321–322

Jemec GBE, Thomsen K (1997) Pincer nails and alopecia as markers of gastrointestinal malignancy. J Dermatol 24:479–481

Greiner D, Schöfer H, Milbraft R (1998) Reversible transverse overcurvature of the nails (pincer nails) after treatment with a β-blocker. J Am Acad Dermatol 39:486–487

Neapolitan Nail

De Berker DAR, Baran R, Dawber RPR (1995) Apparent leuconychia. In: De Berker DAR, Baran R, Dawber RPR (eds) Handbook of diseases of the nails and their management. Blackwell Science, Oxford, pp 28–29

Koilonychia

Alanko K, Kanerva L, Estlander T et al. (1997) Hairdresser's koilonychia. Am J Contact Dermatol 8:177–178

Murdoch D (1993) Koilonychia in Sherpas. Br J Dermatol 128:39–40

Solomon LM, Keuer EJ (1980) Ectodermal dysplasias. Problems of classification and some newer syndromes. Arch Dermatol 11:1295

Clubbed Nails

Boonen A, Schrey G, Van der Linden S (1996) Clubbing in human immunodeficiency virus infection. Br J Rheumatol 35:292–294

Dickinson CJ (1993) The aetiology of clubbing and hypertrophic osteoarthropathy. Eur J Clin Invest 23:330–338

Michel C, Cribier B, Sibilia J (1997) Nail abnormalities in rheumatoid arthritis. Br J Dermatol 137:958–962

Sridhar KS, Lobo CF, Altman RD (1998) Digital clubbing and lung cancer. Chest 114:1535–1537

Median Canal Dystrophy

Heller J (1928) Dystrophia unguium mediana canaliformis. Dermatol Z 51:416

Zelger J, Wohlfarth P, Putz R (1974) Dystrophia unguium mediana canaliformis Heller. Hautarzt 25:629–631

Changes in Nail Color

Agger WA, Mardan A (1995) *Pseudomonas aeruginosa* infections of intact skin. Clin Infect Dis 20:302–308

Kwong YL (1996) Hydroxyurea-induced nail pigmentation. J Am Acad Dermatol 35:275–276

Morrow Gl, Abbott RL (1998) Minocycline-induced scleral, dental and dermal pigmentation. Am J Ophthalmol 125: 39–47

Plewig G, Lincke H, Wolff HH (1977) Silver-blue nails. Acta Derm Venereol (Stockh) 57:413–419

Yellow Nail Syndrome

Bull RH, Fenton DA, Mortimer PS (1996) Lymphatic function in the yellow nail syndrome. Br J Dermatol 134: 307–312

De Coste S, Imber MJ, Badeb HP (1990) Yellow nail syndrome. J Am Acad Dermatol 22:608–611

Hershko A, Hirshberg B, Nahir M et al. (1997) Yellow nail syndrome. Postgrad Med J 73:466–468

Samman PD, White WF (1964) The "yellow nail" syndrome. Br J Dermatol 76:710–711

Muehrcke Bands

Muehrcke RC (1956) The fingernails is chronic hypoalbuminemia. Brit Med J 116:875–878

Schwartz RA, Vickerman CE (1979) Muehrcke's lines of the fingernails. Arch Intern Med 139:242

Half and Half Nail

Bean WB (1963) A discourse on nail growth and unusual fingernails. Trans Am Clin Climat Assoc 74:152–167

Lindsay PG (1967) The half and half nail syndrome. Arch Intern Med 119:583–587

Mazuryk HA, Brodkin RH (1991) Cutaneous clues to renal disease. Cutis 47:241–248

Pico MR, Lugo Somolinos A, Sanchez JL et al. (1992) Cutaneous alterations in patients with chronic renal failure. Int J Dermatol 31:80–83

Sahin AA, Kalyoncu AF, Selcuk ZT et al. (1990) Behcet's disease with half and half nail and pulmonary artery aneurysm. Chest 97:1277

Terry's Nail

Huddleston HAT, Dunihoo DR (1994) Beau's lines on Terry's nail? South Med J 87:867

Terry RC (1954) White nails in hepatic cirrhosis. Lancet 1:757–759

Laugier-Hunziker-Baran Syndrome

Baran R (1979) Longitudunal melaotic streks as a clue to Laugier-Hunziker syndrome. Arch Dermatol 115:1448–1449

Baran R, Bariere H (1986) Longitudinal melanonychia with spreading pigmentation in Laugier-Hunziker syndrome: a report of 2 cases. Br J Dermatol 115:707–710

Gerbig AW, Hunziker T (1996) Idiopathic lenticular mucocutaneous pigmentation or Laugier-Hunziker syndrome with atypical features. Arch Dermatol 132:844–845

Laugier P, Hunziker N (1970) Pigmentation mélanique lenticulaire, essentielle, de la munqueuse jugale et des lévres. Arch Belg Dermatol Syphiligr 26:391–399

Mignogna MD, Lo-Muzio L, Ruoppo E et al. (1999) Oral manifestations of idiopathic lenticular mucocutaneous pigmentation (Laugier-Hunziker syndrome): a clinical, histopathological and ultrastructural review of 12 cases. Oral Dis 5:80–86

Veraldi S, Cavicchini S, Benelli C et al. (1991) Laugier-Hunziker syndrome: a clinical, histopathologic, and ultrastructural study of four cases and review of the literature. J Am Acad Dermatol 25:632–636

Circumscribed Color Changes

Gallais V, Lacour JPH, Perrin CH (1992) Acral hyperpigmented macules and longitudinal melanonychia in AIDS patients. Br J Dermatol 126:387–391

Tosti A, Baran R, Piraccini BM et al. (1996) Nail matrix nevi: a clinical and histopathologic study of twenty-two patients. J Am Acad Dermatol 34:765–771

Congenital Nail Disorders

Supernumerary Digit

Miura T, Nakamura R, Horii E et al. (1990) Three cases of syndactyly, polydactyly, and hypoplastic triphalangeal thumb: (Haas malformation). J Hand Surg Am 15:445–449

Racket Nails

Ronchese F (1973) The racket thumb-nail. Dermatologica 146:199–202

Longitudinal Pachyleukonychia

Moulin G, Baran R, Perrin CH (1996) Epidermal hamartoma presenting as longitudinal pachyleukonychia: a new nail genodermatosis. J Am Acad Dermatol 35:675–677

Pachyonychia Congenita

Brünauer SR (1923) Zur Vererbung des Keratoma hereditarium palmare et plantare. Acta Derm Venerol 4:489–509

Brünauer SR (1925) Zur Symptomatologie und Histologie der kongentialen Dyskeratosen. Dermatol Zschr 42:6

Covello SP, Smith FJ, Sillevis Smitt JH et al. (1998) Keratin 17 mutations cause either steatocystoma multiplex or pachyonychia congenita type 2. Br J Dermatol 139:475–480

Feinstein A, Friedman J, Schwach-Millet M (1988) Pachyonychia congenita. J Am Acad Dermatol 19:705–711

Haber RM, Rose TH (1986) Autosomal recessive pachyonychia congenita. Arch Dermatol 122:919–923

Hohl D (1997) Steatocystoma multiplex and oligosymptomatic pachyonychia congenita of the Jackson-Sertoli type. Dermatology 195:86–88

Jadassohn J, Lewandowski F (1906) Pachyonychia congenita: keratosis disseminata circumscripta (follicularis), Tylomata,Leukokeratosis linguae. In: Neisser A, Jacobi E (eds) Ikonographia dermatologica. Urbach & Schwarzenberg, Berlin, pp 29–31

Jackson ADML SD (1951) Pachyonychia congenita: a report of six cases in one family with a note on linkage data. Ann Eugen 16:141–146

Kansky A, Basta-Juzbasic A, Videnic N et al. (1993) Pachyonychia congenita (Jadassohn-Lewanowsky syndrome) – evaluation of symptoms in 36 patients. Arch Dermatol Res 285:36–37

Mouaci Midoun N, Cambiaghi S, Abimelec P (1996) Pachyonychia congenita tarda. J Am Acad Dermatol 35:334–335

Novice FM, Collison DW, Burgdorf WHC et al. (1994) Pachyonychia congenita. In: Handbook of genetic skin disorders. Saunders, Philadelphia, pp 427–431

Paller AS, Moore JA, Scher R (1991) Pachyonychia congenita tarda. Arch Dermatol 127:701–703

Schäfer E (1925) Zur Lehre von den congenitalen Dyskertosen. Arch Dermatol Syph 148:425–432

Schönfeld PHIR (1980) The pachyonychia congenita syndrome. Acta Dermato Venereol (Stockh) 60:45–49

Sertoli P (1949) Sopra una disonichia ereditaria familiare. Dermo-sifolografo 24:268

Tidman MJ, Wells RS, MacDonald DM (1987) Pachyonchia congenita with cutaneous amyloidosis and hyperpigmentation: a distinct variant. J Am Acad Dermatol 16:935–940

Congenital Onychodysplasia

Iso R (1969) Congenital nail defects of the index fingers and reconstructive surgery. Orthop Surg 20:1383–1384

Kameyoshi Y, Iwasaki Y, Hide M et al. (1998) Congenital onychodsyplasia of the index fingers in identical twins. Br J Dermatol 139:1120–1122

Kikuchi I (1974) Congenital onychodysplasia of the index fingers. Arch Dermatol 110:743–746

Nail-Patella Syndrome

Kieser W (1939) Die sog. Flughaut beim ihre Beziehung zum Status dysgraphicus und ihre Erblichkeit. Z Menschl Vererb 2:594–619

Letts M (1991) Hereditary onycho-osteodysplasia (nail-patella syndrome). A three generation familial study. Orthop Rev 20:267–272

Little EM (1897) Congenital absence or delayed development of patella. Lancet 2:781–784

McIntosh I, Clough MV, Schaffer AA et al. (1997) Fine mapping of the nail-patella syndrome locus at 9q34. Am J Genet 60:133–142

Turner JW (1933) hereditary arthrodysplasia associated with hereditary dystrophy of nails. JAMA 100:882–884

Congenital Malalignment of the Great Toenails

Baran R, Haneke E (1998) Etiology and treatment of nail malalignment. Dermatol Surg 24:719–721

Baran R (1996) Significance and management of congenital malalignment of the big toenail. Cutis 58:181–184

Dyall-Smith D (1996) Congenital malalignment of the great toenails. Aust J Dermatol 37:54

Samman PD (1978) Great toe nail dystrophy. Clin Exp Dermatol 3:81–82

Pterygium Inversum Unguis

Caputo R, Prandi G (1973) Pterygium inversum unguis. Arch Dermatol 108:817–818

Caputo R, Cappio F, Rigoni C (1993) Pterygium inversum unguis. Report of 19 cases and review of the literature. Arch Dermatol 129:1307–1309

Guidetti MS, Stinchi C, Vezzani C et al. (1996) Subungual exostosis of a finger resembling pterygium inversum unguis. Dermatology 193:354–355

Nail Changes Associated with Dermatologic and Systemic Disorders

De Berker DAR, Baran R, Dawber RPR (1995) The nail in dermatological disease. In: De Berker DAR, Baran R, Dawber RPR (eds) Handbook of diseases of the nails and their management. Blackwell Science, Oxford, pp 64–84

Bruckner-Tuderman L, Schnyder U, Baran R (1995) Nail changes in epidermolysis bullosa. Clinical and pathological considerations. Br J Dermatol 132:339–344

Clayton BD, Jorizzo JL, Hitchcock MG et al. (1997) Adult pityriasis rubra pilaris: a 10-year case series. J Am Acad Dermtol 36:959–964

Dhawan SS, Zaias N, Pena N (1990) The nail fold in pemphigus vulgaris. Arch Dermatol 126:1374–1375

Itin PH, Winkelmann RK (1991) Cutaneous manifestations in patients with essential thrombocytopenia. J Am Acad Dermatol 24:59–63

Jemec GB, Kollerup G, Jensen LB (1996) Nail abnormalities in nondermatologic patients: prevalence and possible role as diagnostic aids. J Am Acad Dermatol 35:136–137

Mehregan DA, Van-Hale HM, Muller SA (1992) Lichen planopilaris: clinical and pathologic study of forty-five patients. J Am Acad Dermatol 27:935–942

Milligan A, Graham-Brown RAC (1990) Lichen planus in childhood. Arch Dermatol 91:347–350

Ohtsuka T (1998) The relation between nailfold bleeding and capillary microscopic abnormality in patients with connective tissue diseases. Int J Dermatol 37:23–26

Rivera Diaz R (1996) Nail involvement in pemphigus vulgaris. Int J Dermatol 35:581–582

Tosti A, Peluso AM, Fanti PA et al. (1993) Nail lichen planus: clinical and pathologic study of twenty-four patients. J Am Acad Dermatol 28:724–730

Tosti A, Ghetti E, Piraccini BM et al. (1998) Lichen planus of the nails and fingertips. Eur J Dermatol 8:447–448

Acquired Nail Changes

Bouscarat F, Bouchard C, Bouhour D (1998) Paronychia and pyogenic granuloma of the great toes in patients treated with indinavir. N Engl J Med 338:1776–1777

Cribier B, Mena ML, Rey D et al. (1998) Nail changes in patients infected with human immunodeficiency virus. A prospective controlled study. Arch Dermatol 134: 1216–1220

Fisher AA, Baran R (1991) Adverse reactions to acrylate sculptured nails with particular reference to prolonged paraesthesia. Am J Contact Dermat 2:38–42

Gallais V, Lacour JPH, Perrin C (1992) Acral hyperpigmented macules and longitudinal melanonychia in AIDS patients. Br J Dermatol 126:387–391

Guy RJ (1990) The etiologies and mechanisms of nail bed injuries. Hand Clin 6:9–20

Prose NS, Abran KG, Scher RK (1992) Disorders of the nail and hair associated with human immunodeficiency virus infection. Int J Dermatol 31:453–457

Russo F, Collantes C, Guerrero J (1999) Severe paronychia due to zidovudine-induced neutropenia in a neonate. J Am Acad Dermatol 40:322–324

Schulte KW, Neumann NJ, Ruzicka T (1998) Surgical pearl: nail splinting by flexible tube – a new noninvasive treatment for ingrown toenails. J Am Acad Dermatol 39:629–630

Subungual and Periungual Tumors

Ashinoff R, Li JJ, Jacabson M et al. (1991) Detection of human papillomavirus DNA in squamous cell carcinoma of the nail bed and finger determined by polymerase chain reaction. Arch Dermatol 127:1813–1818

Baran R, Kechijian P (1996) Hutchinson's sign: a reappraisal. J Am Acad Dermatol 34:87–90

Baran A, Tosti A (1994) Metastatic bronchogenic carcinoma to the terminal phalanx with review of 116 non-melanoma metastatic tumours to the distal digit. J Am Acad Dermatol 31:311–316

Belanger SM, Weaver TD (1993) Subungual glomus tumor of the hallux. Cutis 52:50–52

Blessing K, Kernohan NM, Park KGM (1991) Subungual malignant melanoma – clinicopathological features of 100 cases. Histopathology 19:425–429

Davis DA, Cohen PR (1996) Subungual exostosis: case report and review of the literature. Pediatr Dermatol 13:212–218

Dawber RPR, Colver GB (1991) The spectrum of malignant melanoma in the nail apparatus. Semin Dermatol 10: 82–88

Drape JL, Idy-Peretti L, Goettmann S et al. (1996) Standard and high resolution magnetic resonance imaging of glomus tumors of toes and fingertips. J Am Acad Dermatol 35:550–555

Koenen J (1932) Eine familiäre hereditäre Form von tuberöser Sklerose. Acta Psychiat (Kbh) 1:813–821

Lemon B, Burns R (1998) Malignant melanoma: a literature review and case presentation. J Foot Ankle Surg 37:48–54

Rigby HS, Briggs JC (1992) Subungual melanoma: a clinicopathological study of 24 cases. Br J Plast Surg 45: 275–278

Sau P, McMarlin SL, Sperling LC et al. (1994) Bowen's disease of the nail bed and periungual area. A clinicopathologic analysis of seven cases. Arch Dermatol 130:204–209

Tosti A, Morelli R, Fanti PA, et al. (1993) Carcinoma cuniculatum of the nail apparatus: report of three cases. Dermatology 186:217–221

Van Geertruyden J, Lorea P, Goldschmidt D et al. (1996) Glomus tumor of the hand. A retrospective study of 51 cases. J Hand Surg Br 21:257–260

Warso M, Gray T, Gonzalez M (1997) Melanoma of the hand. J Hand Surg Am 22:354–360

Wiemers S, Stengel R, Schopf E et al. (1994) Subunguales Keratoakanthom. Hautarzt 45:25–28

CHAPTER 33

Diseases of the Lips and Oral Mucosa

Contents

Basic Science Aspects

The oral mucosa is derived from ectoderm and has many similarities with skin. Nonetheless there are significant differences. Structurally the oral mucosa undergoes a different type of keratinization; in some sites, parakeratosis is normal, and in most others no granular layer is seen. The epithelial surface is capable of regenerating very rapidly, replacing the cells lost through the trauma of eating and drinking. The salivary glands coat the epithelium in saliva, which has a protective role, as well as facilitating ingestion of food. The subepithelial connective tissue in the gastrointestinal tract, of which the mouth is a part, is known as lamina propria, not dermis. In some regions, such as the gingiva and hard palate, the lamina propria is directly attached to bone.

Many well-known cutaneous disorders also involve the oral mucosa. Classic examples include pemphigus vulgaris and lichen planus, both of which may begin in the mouth or remain confined to the mouth. The clinical picture is usually different in the mouth than on the skin. For example in lichen planus the polygonal violaceous papules are not seen in the mouth; instead, erythema, erosions, and lacy hyperkeratotic streaks are typical. In general, blisters in the mouth are short-lived, so the examiner is usually confronted with erosions.

The appearance of the mouth is often an aid to diagnosis. A young child with the vesicular eruption of chicken pox almost always has tiny erosions surrounded by erythema on the palate. Conversely, a patient with a subepidermal blistering disease of the buttocks who has oral lesions probably does not have dermatitis herpetiformis, but instead bullous pemphigoid or linear IgA disease.

The oral examination is part of the complete dermatologic examination. In any diffuse or complicated case, the physician should not ignore the possible clues hidden in the mouth. For this reason, he must be acquainted with normal anatomic and physiologic variants and with diseases confined to the mouth. In this chapter we cover the important primary oral findings and refer the reader to relevant sections elsewhere in the book for discussions of diseases that often involve the mouth (Table 33.1).

Diseases of the Lips

Ectopic Sebaceous Glands

(Fordyce 1896)

Synonyms. Fordyce glands, Fordyce spots, free sebaceous glands

Definition. Normal variant in which sebaceous glands are present on lips or other mucosal surfaces, not in association with hair follicles.

Clinical Findings. Small, 2–3-mm yellow papules are found on the upper and lower lip as well as buccal mucosa (Fig. 33.1). Although ectopic sebaceous glands are a developmental abnormality, the patient usually presents with the history that they appeared suddenly. Most often the explanation is the patient has examined their lips closely for the first time, often because of concern about a sexually transmitted disorder. Occasionally lesions along the vermilion border become inflamed.

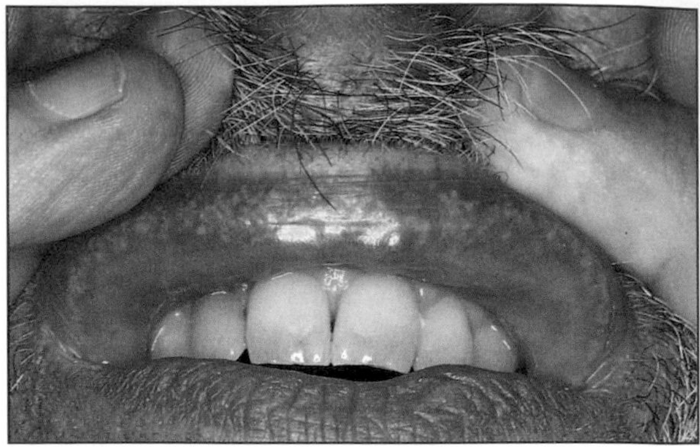

Fig. 33.1. Ectopic sebaceous glands

Histopathology. Small, normal sebaceous glands are seen beneath transitional or mucosal epithelium. They are called free sebaceous glands as they are not associated with hair follicles.

Therapy. No treatment is needed; one must simply convince the patient that the lesions are harmless and did not occur overnight.

Table 33.1. Cutaneous diseases commonly seen on lips and oral mucosa

Genodermatoses	Epidermolysis bullosa, Darier disease, Osler-Weber-Rendu disease
Viral diseases	Herpes simplex, zoster, varicella, hand-foot-moth disease, verrucae, oral hairy leukoplakia in HIV/AIDS
Bacterial diseases	Chancre in primary syphilis, other lesions in secondary, tertiary syphilis, tonsillitis in gonorrhea, actinomycosis, erysipelas, some forms of tuberculosis, leprosy
Fungal infections	Candidiasis, histoplasmosis
Bullous dermatoses	Pemphigus vulgaris, bullous pemphigoid, cicatricial pemphigoid, linear IgA disease
Connective tissue disorders	Lupus erythematosus, systemic sclerosis
Allergic reactions	Angioedema, fixed drug reaction, erythema multiforme, allergic contact dermatitis (stomatitis)
Benign tumors	Melanocytic nevi (often blue nevi), neurofibroma, granular cell tumor, pyogenic granuloma, hemangioma, lymphangioma
Malignant tumors	Squamous cell carcinoma, malignant melanoma, lymphoma, lethal midline granuloma, leukemic infiltrates
Miscellaneous	Lichen planus

Congenital Lip Pits or Sinuses

Definition. Congenital abnormality in which the lower lips fail to fuse properly.

Clinical Findings. The lower lip is almost always involved and the pits are usually bilateral and paramedian (Fig. 33.2). They may lead into sinuses that end in the orbicularis oris muscle. Frequently a mucoid material drains from the sinuses. Some cases show autosomal dominant inheritance (Van der Woude syndrome); these may be associated with cleft lip and cleft palate.

Therapy. Excision after the sinus tracts have been identified with a dye or probe.

Mucocele

Synonyms. Mucous retention cyst, traumatic mucous cyst

Definition. Traumatic lesion that follows the disruption or obstruction of a minor salivary gland duct.

Etiology and Pathogenesis. No matter what name one applies, most mucoceles are not true cysts. They result from the traumatic interruption of a minor salivary gland duct, usually from biting. Mucin leaks into the loose tissue of the lip and sometimes elicits a granulomatous reaction. Rarely true retention cysts arise when the duct is blocked and then mucin builds up behind the obstruction.

Clinical Findings. Both traumatic and retention mucoceles are clinically identical. They almost always occur on the lower lip (Fig. 33.3), but can be seen on the upper lip or buccal mucosa. Often

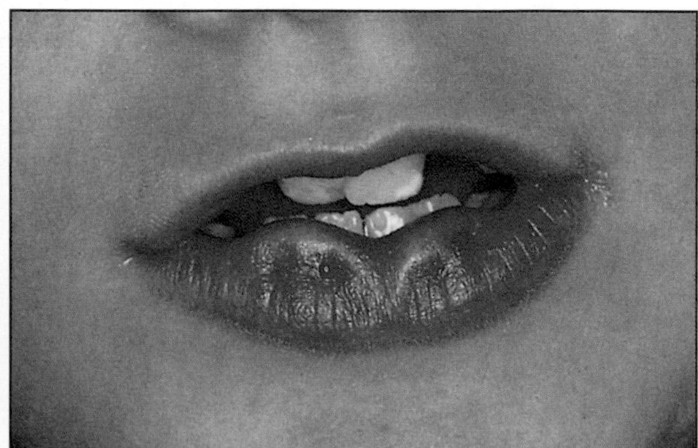

Fig. 33.2. Congenital lip pits

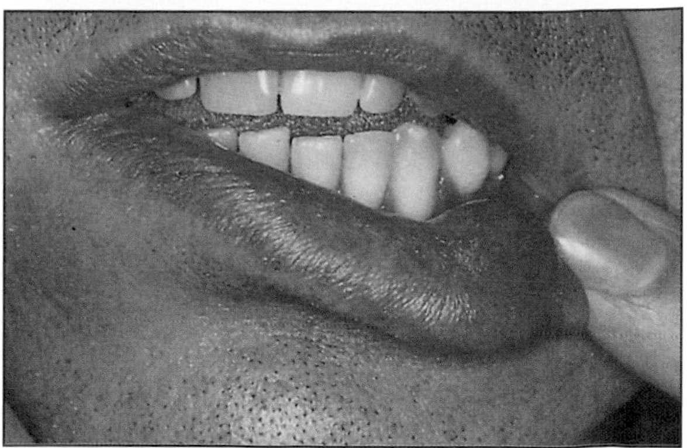

Fig. 33.3. Mucocele

there is a history of trauma and then the complaint that the nodule varies in size and interferes with chewing.

Histopathology. Sometimes one only sees a foreign body reaction; in other cases it is associated with mucin. In order to diagnose a retention cyst, one must identify the expanded duct wall.

Therapy. Simple excision is curative.

Cheilitis

Cheilitis is a general term for inflammation of the lips. There are many different types, having variable etiologies and a wide variety of clinical manifestations.

Angular Cheilitis

Synonyms. Cheilitis angularis, perlèche

Definition. Chronic or less often acute inflammation at the corner of the mouth.

Etiology and Pathogenesis. There are a number of causes of angular cheilitis. All have the same mechanism: saliva accumulates in the folds at the corner of the mouth and causes an irritant reaction; often secondary infection with *Candida albicans* or bacteria occurs. In infants, drooling is usually the answer. Individuals with disorders involving macroglossia such as congenital hypothyroidism and Down syndrome are at special risk. In older children, especially those with atopic dermatitis, a streptococcal infection may be responsible. In teenagers and adults, usually those patients with deep folds at the corner of their mouth are at greatest risk. Licking the area worsens the problem. In the elderly, both poorly fitted dentures and natural relaxation of the perioral skin lead to drooling, especially at night.

Acute angular cheilitis often results after major dental procedures during which the mouth has been held wide open for a long period of time and the angle traumatized by the dentist and his instruments. Such lesions are frequently unilateral, while in other cases angular cheilitis is more often bilateral.

While extreme vitamin and mineral deficiencies can lead to angular cheilitis, one should exclude mechanical causes and *C. albicans* before making this diagnose. The long list of nutritional problems associated with angular cheilitis makes it clear that it is not a sensitive clue. Angular cheilitis is more common in bulimia because of trauma to the mouth than it is in anorexia nervosa where starvation alone is the problem.

Clinical Findings. Erythema and small fissures are seen at the corner of the mouth (Fig. 33.4). Gradually the erythema spreads and the fissures deepen. Eventually an eroded, crusted plaque develops, usually crossed by deep fissures. A yellowish crust suggests impetigo, while a white coat points towards *C. albicans.*

Laboratory Findings. Bacterial cultures to exclude streptococci should be done in children. While it is appropriate to culture for *C. albicans*, most chronic lesions will be secondarily colonized and thus positive. Usually mechanical factors are still the answer. Extensive laboratory evaluation of nutritional status should only be done in resistant, unexplained cases, especially if other clues suggest a dietary problem.

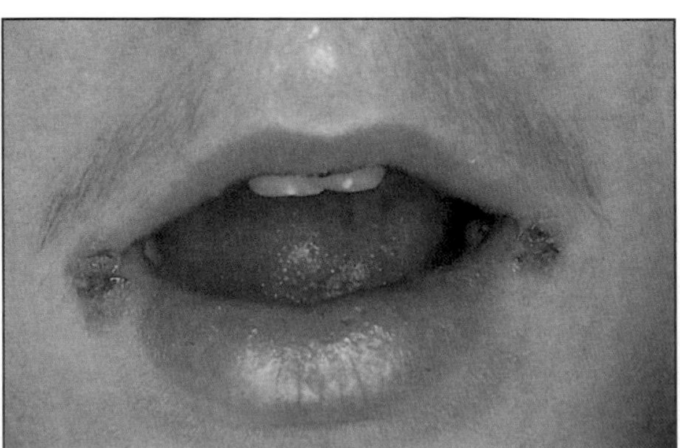

Fig. 33.4. Angular cheilitis

Differential Diagnosis. In secondary syphilis, there may be rhagadiform papules at the corner of the mouth. In acute cases, if the history fits, dark field examination and serologic testing are appropriate.

Therapy. Mechanical factors have to be corrected; unfortunately this is usually impossible. Dental consultation should be obtained for patients wearing dentures; often corrections can reduce the nature of the folds at the corner of the mouth and also reduce drooling. Treatment with protective pastes, often containing anticandidal agents, are most useful, especially at night. Creams containing low-potency corticosteroids and clioquinol may also be helpful. Painting the area with 2% aqueous silver nitrate solution at night helps to close the fissures and dry the area. If impetigo is diagnosed, either topical or systemic antibiotics should be employed.

Cheilitis Simplex

Synonym. Cheilitis

Definition. Acute or chronic inflammation of the lips, analogous to dermatitis of the skin.

Etiology and Pathogenesis. Most cheilitis is exogenous in nature. Probably the most common cause is dryness or chapping. Acute sun exposure, such as when skiing, is also a factor. Many patients with atopic dermatitis have cheilitis, often as the only active manifestation of their disease. Allergic contact cheilitis and irritant cheilitis are similar to their skin equivalents, allergic contact dermatitis and irritant dermatitis. Causes of contact allergy include lip sticks, dental products and medications, especially products used to treat herpes simplex infections. Toxic reactions usually result from aggressive attempts to dry the lips or from using materials on the lips that are not designed for this region. Both photoallergic and phototoxic reactions may be seen.

Many patients are lip lickers, continuously licking their lips to keep them moist. Paradoxically this leads to irritation and dryness. Eventually the lips split or crack. Some children are lip chewers, pulling in their lip, usually the lower one, sucking and biting the skin adjacent to the lip. This process produces a classic combination of cheilitis and a sharply marginated circumoral erythema with a

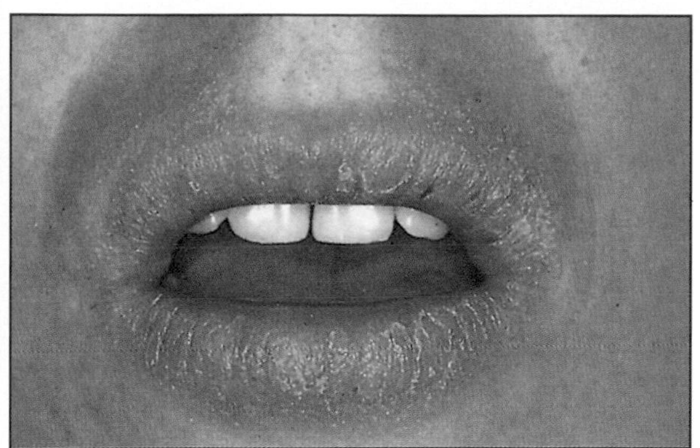

Fig. 33.5. Cheilitis simplex

free zone in between. While this is a relatively harmless form of artifactual cheilitis, patients may find an unbelievable variety of ways to damage their lips from spitting fire (spewing out lighter fluid which they ignite) to sucking unusual foreign objects.

Clinical Findings. All cheilitis looks similar. The lips are red, often split and crusted (Fig. 33.5). They may be painful. When marked exfoliation is present, one speaks of exfoliative cheilitis, which can be associated with any cause.

Differential Diagnosis. One should search for associated clinical features especially atopic dermatitis. If the process has slowly spread past the lips, allergic contact cheilitis is a good bet and should be excluded with patch testing and even photopatch testing.

Therapy. Acute cheilitis can be treated with low potency corticosteroid ointments, as well as frequent lubrication with petrolatum, available as a lip balm. Because of the risk of allergic contact dermatitis, one should initially avoid medicated lip balms. Most "Chap-Sticks" and related products today contain a sun screen, which is commendable, but may be the cause of allergic contact dermatitis.

Acute Actinic Cheilitis

Synonym. Solar cheilitis

Clinical Findings. The lower lip receives a great deal of sun, when compared to the upper lip, simply because of the shadowing of the face. It has been called the sun terrace of the face. In addition, the lips lack pigmentary protection. Thus in darker skinned patients actinic cheilitis may be seen without any sign of sunburn, while in lighter skinned individuals, the two tend to go together. Patients with acute sun damage to the lip present with redness and swelling; occasionally blisters develop. A typical history is skiing, mountain climbing or a day at the beach. The latent period is just several hours. Patients with atopic dermatitis may be at increased risk. Actinic cheilitis is a common finding in Native Americans with actinic prurigo (also known as polymorphic light eruption of Native Americans); it is less common in other forms of photosensitivity, but may be seen in lupus erythematosus.

Therapy. Low- to mid-potency corticosteroid ointments and then lip sticks with sunscreens are usually quite effective.

Chronic Actinic Cheilitis

Clinical Findings. While the etiology is once again sun exposure, the problem is quite different. Chronic actinic cheilitis is similar to actinically damaged skin and is a fertile ground for the development of squamous cell carcinoma. On the lower lip, squamous cell carcinoma arising from photodamage has a significant risk of metastasis, as compared to the low rate on the skin.

The same risk groups are involved; farmers, sailors and outdoor workers, especially individuals with fair skin and long-term exposure, such as in the tropics. The lower lip usually shows an indistinct vermilion border, atrophy, a white sheen, and then distinct hyperkeratotic or eroded areas (Fig. 33.6). When erosions are prominent, the term cheilitis abrasiva praecancerosa (Manganotti 1934)

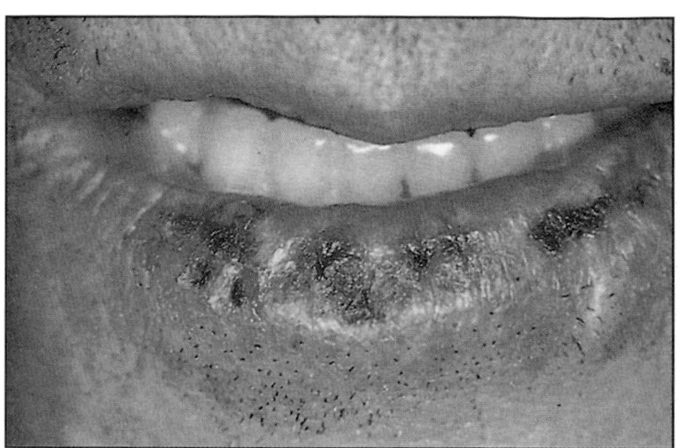

Fig. 33.6. Chronic actinic cheilitis

is often employed. It is a bit misleading because erosions and induration are the two best clues that the lesion has evolved into a squamous cell carcinoma.

Histopathology. Microscopic evaluation is essential. Initially there is epithelial atrophy without cytological atypia. Adjacent skin shows solar elastosis. Later squamous cell carcinoma in situ develops, with cytological atypia, epithelial atrophy or hyperplasia and then strands of epithelium growing down into the lamina propria.

Therapy. If the disease process is identified early, and no lesions suspicious of squamous cell carcinoma in situ are seen, compulsive sun protection and biannual follow-up are sufficient. Discrete small lesions can either be biopsied or treated with cryotherapy; if they persist, then biopsy is mandatory. The toluidine blue test can be employed to identify suspicious sites, but false negative and false positive results often occur. Diffuse or multiple lesions can be treated by cryotherapy, topical 5-fluorouracil or laser vaporization. The standard procedure in advanced situations is a vermilionectomy or lip shaving, in which the entire surface is removed and then covered by an advancement flap of epithelium from the inner lower lip. Squamous cell carcinomas should be treated by excision and the patient carefully evaluated for other oral lesions and lymph node involvement.

Cheilitis Glandularis

The presenting symptom is usually a swollen lip, as the disease activity centers around the minor salivary glands of the lip, rather than the epithelium.

Cheilitis Glandularis Simplex
(Volkmann 1870; Sutton 1909)

In this very uncommon disorder, the minor salivary glands of the lips, especially the lower lip, become inflamed. Tiny red papules are seen; they represent the duct orifices and may contain a drop of mucin or a concretion. The lips may feel sticky to the patient or examiner. Gradually the inflammation leads to a swollen lip or macrocheilia. The glands can be removed or destroyed via electrosurgery, laser or excision.

Cheilitis Glandularis Apostematosa
(Volkmann 1870)

In this variant, secondary staphylococcal infections develop in the minor salivary glands. Apostema is a synonym for abscess. There tends to be severe pain, crusting, draining of pus, fever and other systemic signs. Excision of the involved area of lip, usually through a long full-thickness wedge, is the only treatment. Preoperative antibiotic therapy may be helpful; macrolides such as spiramycin offer some advantages because they accumulate in salivary glands.

Cheilitis Granulomatosa
(Miescher 1945)

Synonym. Granulomatous cheilitis

Definition. Chronic granulomatous lip swelling of unknown etiology; often part of the Melkersson-Rosenthal syndrome.

Epidemiology. Uncommon in childhood, the disorder usually starts in young adult life and affects both sexes equally.

Etiology and Pathogenesis. The cause of granulomatous cheilitis is unknown. Occasionally other idiopathic granulomatous disorders such as Crohn disease may be seen. Granulomatous cheilitis is not a feature of tuberculosis or sarcoidosis.

Clinical Findings. Initially there is episodic inflammation and swelling of the lip, later the changes becomes persistent (Fig. 33.7). Enlarged or swollen lips are known as macrocheilia. The upper lip is involved more often than the lower; often the swell-

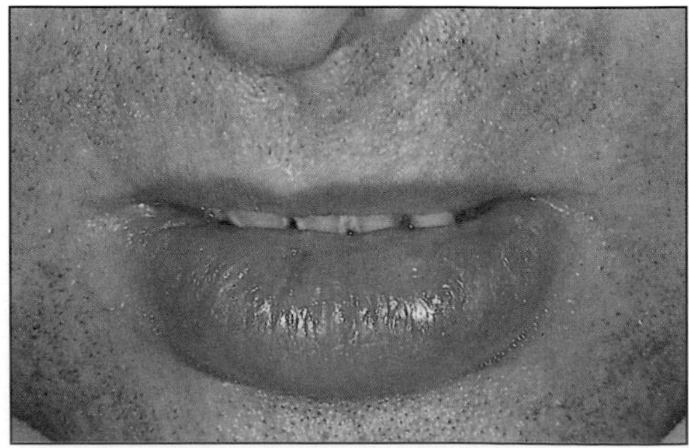

Fig. 33.7. Cheilitis granulomatosa

ing is asymmetric. In extreme cases the lips form into a small snout (tapir mouth). On palpation the lips are firm. There may be associated lymphadenopathy. Sometimes during episodes of swelling, the patient also experiences fever and malaise.

Histopathology. Biopsies from early lesions show only edema and a sparse infiltrate. Later there is a more intense infiltrate with small sarcoidal granulomas. Often one must do multiple biopsies and search diligently to find granulomatous changes.

Differential Diagnosis. The causes of macrocheilia are shown in Table 33.2. Probably the most important is elephantiasis nostras, the persistent edema that follows recurrent herpes simplex virus infection or recurrent erysipelas. Histologically there is often confusion with sarcoidosis or tuberculosis but lip swelling is not a part of these disorders.

Therapy. This is discussed under Melkersson-Rosenthal syndrome.

Melkersson-Rosenthal syndrome

(Melkersson 1928; Rosenthal 1931)

Definition. Triad of granulomatous cheilitis, facial nerve palsy and plicated tongue.

Etiology and Pathogenesis. Melkersson-Rosenthal syndrome is just as much as mystery as granulomatous cheilitis.

Clinical Findings. The lip changes are those discussed under granulomatous cheilitis. In addition there may be swelling of the cheeks, eyelids, forehead and gingiva with a similar clinical course. Some patients present with facial palsy first without any swelling. The paralysis is usually unilateral and may be recurrent (Fig. 33.8). The plicated tongue has usually been present for many years, but ignored as a normal variant.

Histopathology. The same changes seen in granulomatous cheilitis are seen. Lymph node involve may occur; the histologic changes are similar to sarcoidosis so diagnostic confusion may arise.

Table 33.2. Causes of macrocheilia

Congenital disorders
Idiopathic, familial macrocheilia
Ascher syndrome
Lymphangioma
Hemangioma
Trauma
Hematoma
Organized thrombus
Infections
Recurrent herpes simplex virus infections
Recurrent erysipelas (often combined with HSV)
Leprosy
Cheilitis glandularis
Angioedema, including hereditary angioneurotic edema
Tumors
Advanced squamous cell carcinoma with lymphatic involvement
Neurofibroma (especially in neurofibromatosis 1)
Lymphoma and lymphocytic infiltrates
Sarcomas
Miscellaneous
Crohn disease
Sarcoidosis
Melkersson-Rosenthal syndrome and cheilitis granulomatosa

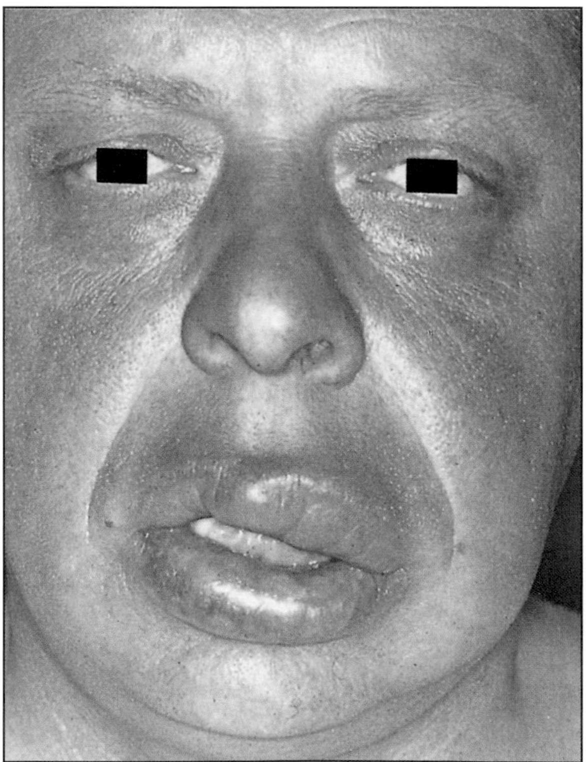

Fig. 33.8. Melkersson-Rosenthal syndrome with facial paralysis

Course and Prognosis. The course is highly variable; some patients clear entirely but more have persistent problems.

Differential Diagnosis. If the triad is present, the diagnosis is easy. If only isolated changes are found, one cannot make the diagnosis until other features appear. Persistent facial edema (Morbihan disease) should be considered.

Therapy. Intralesional corticosteroids are effective but not permanent treatment. Triamcinolone acetonide 2.5–5.0 mg/ml can be injected at 3- to 6-week intervals. One rarely needs more than 2–3 ml. Oral corticosteroids can also be employed, but are less effective and are associated with more side effects. Plastic surgery to reduce the bulk of the lip is also effective, particularly if the disease seems quiescent.

A number of other systemic agents have been recommended. We have had the most success with clofazimine 100 mg/day for 10 days and then 100 mg twice weekly for several months. Dapsone 100–150 mg daily as well as azathioprine 100 mg daily have also been employed.

Diseases of the Tongue

Lingual Tonsils
(LEVINSTEIN 1912)

Synonyms. Tonsilla heterotopica, heterotopic tonsils

Definition. Residual tonsillar tissue found at the base of the tongue.

Clinical Findings. The lingual tonsils are bilateral, several millimeter red nodules found at the base of the tongue. They have a convoluted surface just as regular tonsils. They are remnants of Waldeyer ring and participate in the inflammatory response. When a patient has tonsillitis, the lingual tonsils may also be swollen. Occasionally only the heterotopic lingual glands become inflamed. When they are inflamed, movement of the tongue is painful.

Histopathology. Typical lymphoepithelial tissue is found. Normally no biopsy is needed.

Therapy. Usually only reassurance is required. With recurrent infections, the same lengthy arguments for and against ordinary tonsillectomy can be advanced.

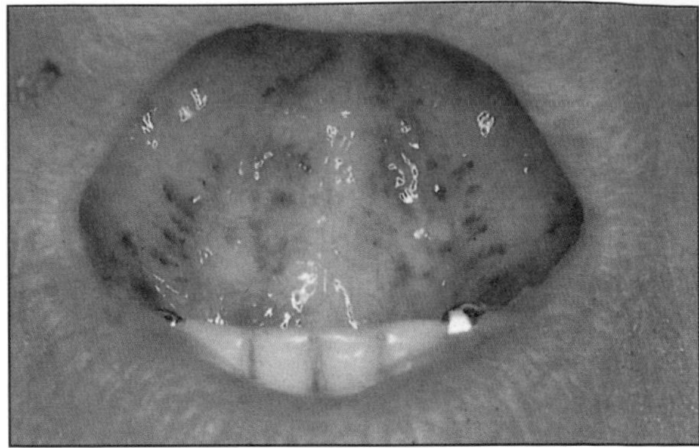

Fig. 33.9. Lingual varices

Lingual Varices

Every person has enlarged veins under the tongue (Fig. 33.9). Most children delight in showing them to their friends or viewing them in the mirror. Occasionally a patient becomes convinced that the varices have drastically changed and seeks reassurance. In older patients, they may be more prominent. Lingual varices are normal and require no treatment.

Plicated Tongue

Synonyms. Lingua plicata, furrowed tongue, scrotal tongue

Definition. Increased furrowing of the tongue's surface.

Etiology and Pathogenesis. This normal variant is present in 10–15% of population. It may be inherited in some cases.

Clinical Findings. Changes in the surface of the tongue are frequently a cause of concern to patients but rarely a clinical problem. Some patients become concerned about the normal taste papillae, while others worry about furrowing. The most common change is a central furrow, which can then develop side branches (Fig. 33.10). More complex furrowing was formerly designated scrotal tongue, a vivid description that understandingly upset patients and which has fallen into disrepute (Fig. 33.11). About 20% of patients also have migratory glossitis.

Differential Diagnosis. Plicated tongue may be associated with Melkersson-Rosenthal syndrome,

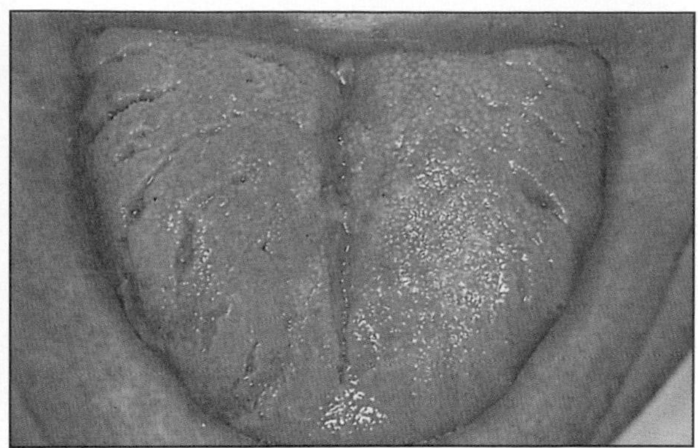

Fig. 33.10. Plicated tongue

but is usually a harmless finding that is clinically unmistakable.

Therapy. No therapy is needed.

Migratory Glossitis

Synonyms. Exfoliato linguae areata, geographic tongue

Definition. Idiopathic migratory inflammatory change involving both the tongue and oral mucosa.

Epidemiology. Migratory glossitis is seen in about 1–2% of the population, but in 40% of this group plicated tongue is also present.

Etiology and Pathogenesis. Migratory glossitis is usually isolated and without obvious cause. It is relatively uncommon but often associated with plicated tongue. Occasionally a familial pattern may be seen, as well as an association with HLA B5 and DR7. Migratory glossitis and especially migratory stomatitis are often associated with psoriasis; they may appear during flares of the disease.

Clinical Findings. The tongue is marked by distinctive bright red patches and plaques that lack any of the usual white epithelial coating (Fig. 33.12). These red areas gradually enlarge and resolve, creating a map-like picture, hence the name geographic tongue. Their borders are sharply defined and often the white coating of the normal areas is more prominent at the edge, as if it were piled up. Most patients are asymptomatic, although some complain of burning, often when they eat spicy foods. The changes tend to come and go, without obvious triggers.

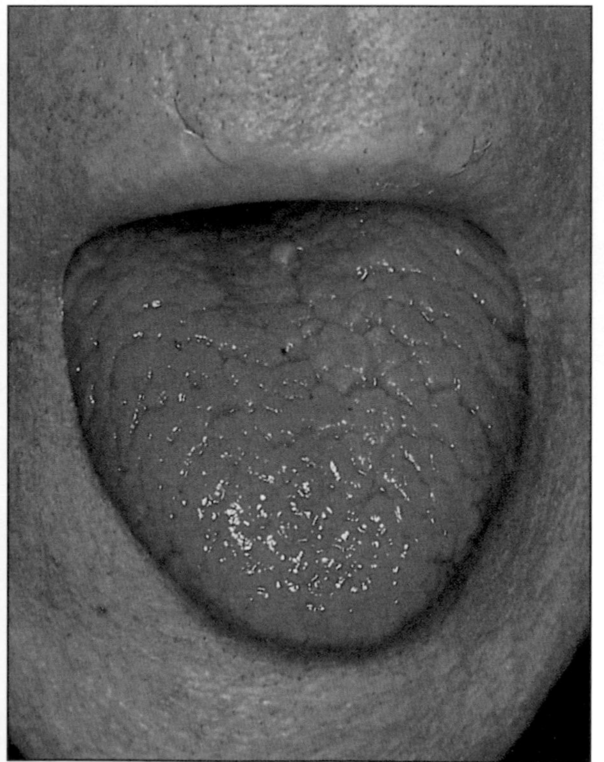

Fig. 33.11. Furrowed tongue

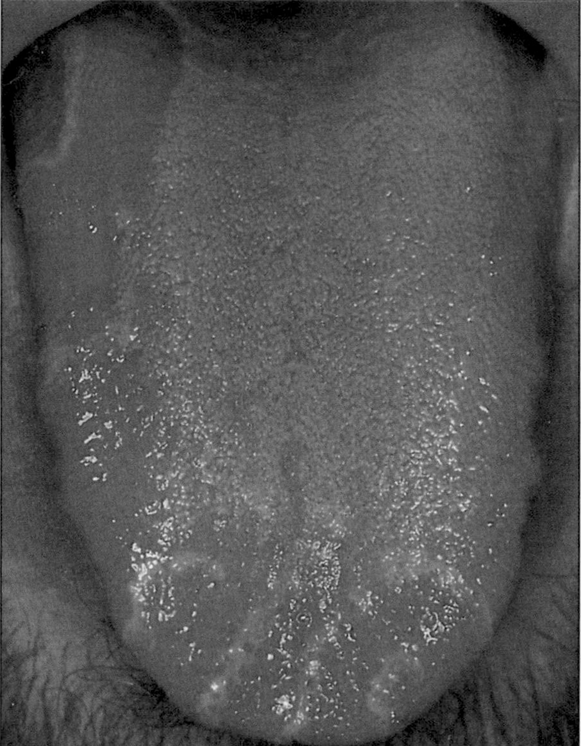

Fig. 33.12. Migratory glossitis

Histopathology. There is a striking resemblance to psoriasis, with spongiosis, migration of neutrophils into the epithelium and occasionally tiny spongioform pustules.

Course and Prognosis. The disease waxes and wanes, but rarely disappears.

Differential Diagnosis. The changes are so distinct that a differential diagnosis is hard to propose. In addition, the tongue is quite resistant to inflammation so that other forms of stomatitis rarely are found in this site.

Therapy. Usually none is needed; if burning is a problem, mild anesthetic mouth rinses are frequently recommended, but they seldom produce any positive change.

Median Rhomboid Glossitis

(Brocq and Pautrier 1914)

Definition. Sharply defined persistent rhomboid erythematous patch on the posterior midline of the tongue.

Epidemiology. Median rhomboid glossitis is a disease of men (3:1) and often involves the elderly.

Etiology and Pathogenesis. Two factors seem important. The posterior midline tongue is formed from the tuberculum impar which is covered by medial growth of the lateral embryologic contributions to the tongue. When this area is not completely covered, then it remains exposed and more easily irritated. In addition, the region is almost always colonized by *C. albicans*. In fact, some feel that the disease is exclusively a yeast infection and that the embryologic factors simply provide a more fertile ground for the yeast.

Clinical Findings. Median rhomboid glossitis is almost always asymptomatic. Patients are usually older men who discover the lesion and then begin to worry about tongue cancer. A sharply defined red patch, often arranged as a rhomboid, lies along the long axis of the tongue posteriorly. Sometimes the area is also depressed or even slightly verrucous in addition to the color difference (Fig. 33.13).

Histopathology. The epithelium is hyperplastic and usually separated from deeper strikers by a fibrous band in the upper lamina propria. In the parakeratotic layer *C. albicans* can usually be found.

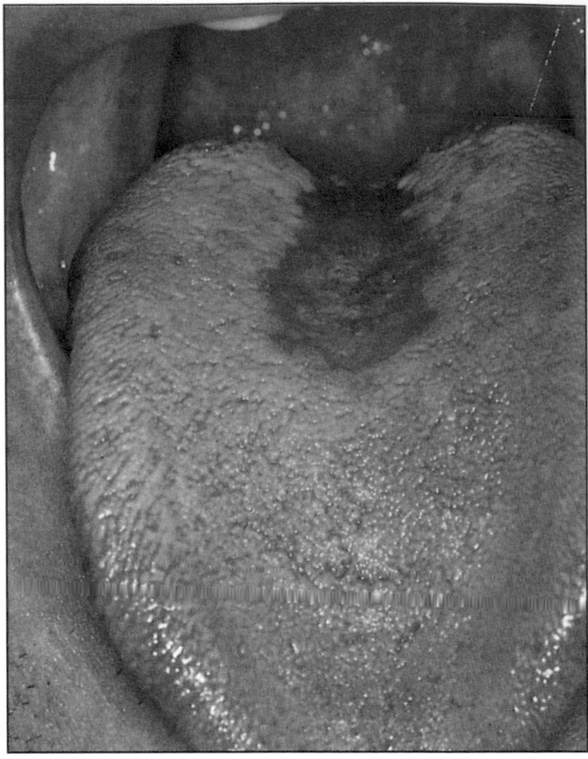

Fig. 33.13. Median rhomboid glossitis

Differential Diagnosis. Occasionally concern arises over the possibility of erythroplasia (squamous cell carcinoma in situ). This possibility can usually be clinically excluded, since carcinoma of the tongue usually spares the posterior dorsal location. If questions exist, a biopsy can be performed.

Therapy. A trial of topical anticandidal therapy, usually with imidazole troches is the simplest approach. Short courses of systemic imidazoles, such as fluconazole 50–100 mg daily for 1 week, or topical imidazole pastes can also be tried. Mild anesthetic mouthwashes are also helpful. In many instances, all that is needed is reassurance.

Black Hairy Tongue

Definition. Presence of dark, thread-like hyperkeratotic structures on the posterior dorsal aspects of the tongue.

Etiology and Pathogenesis. The filiform papillae of the posterior tongue are normally slightly hyperkeratotic. They serve as a nidus for bacterial growth, especially if influenced by systemic antibiotic therapy or topical irritation such as from tobacco. Many other topical and systemic causes have been suggested, but they serve to underline that we do not understand how black hairy tongue develops.

Clinical Findings. The dorsal surface of the tongue, especially posteriorly and medially, is covered by hyperkeratotic strands or threads that are typically 5–20 mm long (Fig. 33.14). They tend to lie flat on the tongue, pointing anteriorly, as if combed in place; thus one speaks of hairs, although of course this is incorrect. The threads tend to be dark, often black but also brown, red or yellow. The color is determined primarily by the bacterial organisms colonizing the region. The changes are usually asymptomatic; occasionally an unpleasant taste may develop.

Laboratory Findings. Candidal and bacterial cultures are frequently done, but rarely shed any light. In the mouth it is most difficult to correlate a positive culture with pathogenicity.

Therapy. Brushing the tongue with a soft tooth brush several times daily often suffices. One can use an antibacterial mouthwash such as chlorhexidine, perhaps applying it with a tooth brush directly to the site. Topical tretinoin applied sparingly once daily may help to remove the hyperkeratoses. Imidazole creams may also be helpful as they are both anticandidal and antibacterial. Eating hard food that requires aggressive chewing, such as a hard piece of bread may have a cleansing action, just as crunchy dog food is recommended as a way to keep canine mouth parts cleaner. The lesions can also be curetted away.

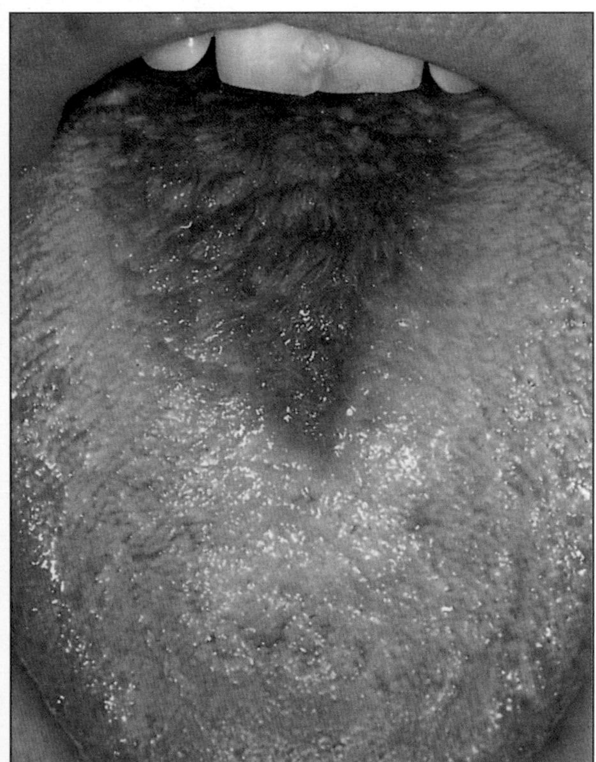

Fig. 33.14. Black hairy tongue

Eosinophilic Ulcer

The eosinophilic ulcer is a rare mucosal lesion that primarily involves the tongue. Its name is often confused with eosinophilic granuloma, the localized form of Langerhans cell histiocytosis, but the diseases are totally unrelated. The eosinophilic ulcer can present at any age and shows no sexual predilection. A large nodular infiltrate that is most often ulcerated and quite painful appears relatively rapidly. Multiple lesions may be present. A dense cellular infiltrate, rich in eosinophils and lymphocytes, extends deeply into the muscle bundles. The differential diagnosis includes squamous cell carcinoma clinically, as well as lymphoma and other eosinophilic infiltrates histologically. The lesions heal spontaneously, so only supportive care is needed.

Möller-Hunter Glossitis

(Möller 1851; Hunter 1909)

Synonym. Atrophic glossitis

Definition. Möller-Hunter glossitis, when used precisely, describes the inflammation and loss of surface features of the tongue that are associated with vitamin B_{12} deficiency and pernicious anemia. The term has become synonymous with atrophic glossitis, describing similar changes in many disorders (Chap. 49).

Etiology and Pathogenesis. Atrophic glossitis may be seen with a wide range of nutritional problems, including many vitamin B deficiencies, folic acid deficiency, iron deficiency, chronic inflammatory bowel disease, other vitamin deficiencies and eating disorders. In most instances, the patient suffers from multiple deficiencies and the exact etiologic connections are hard to identify. The exception is pernicious anemia, in which the deficiency is quite precise and the Möller-Hunter glossitis specific.

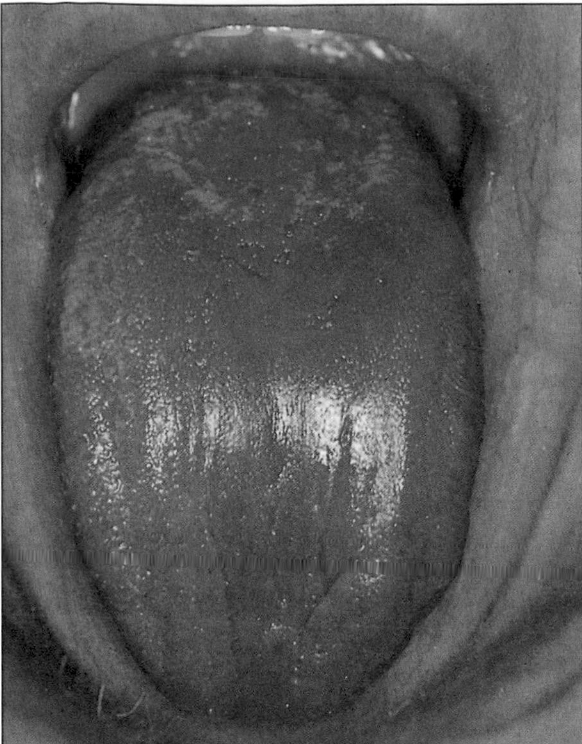

Fig. 33.15. Möller-Hunter glossitis

Clinical Findings. The tongue typically burns, is erythematous and smooth (Fig. 33.15). It has been compared to a piece of raw meat. Often only small areas are denuded and others, relatively normal. When the patient sticks the tongue out, small white areas of decreased perfusion may become apparent (Arndt sign). Eating hard, crisp or spicy foods may be painful. At the same time the patient may complain of distorted taste, a dry mouth and paresthesias.

Differential Diagnosis. All the deficiencies discussed under etiology should be considered. In Plummer-Vinson syndrome, atrophic glossitis occurs along with esophageal atrophy and web formation as a result of iron deficiency anemia. In addition, *C. albicans* may cause an atrophic glossitis rather than the usual white plaques of thrush. In many patients, no obvious etiology is found.

Therapy. If an underlying disorder is found, it must be treated. When a patient has a sore tongue and megaloblastic anemia, then it is reasonable to assume the two belong together and start appropriate treatment. For pernicious anemia, monthly vitamin B_{12} intramuscular injections are the usual course.

Macroglossia

A number of different disorders can produce an enlarged tongue. Sometimes the patient will complain of this problem, something to the effect of "my tongue doesn't fit in my mouth anymore" or more likely, feel that his teeth or dentures are at fault. Possible causes are shown in Table 33.3. They are discussed throughout this chapter and in other parts of the book.

A biopsy is often helping in narrowing the diagnosis in acquired macroglossia. However, biopsy of the tongue can be dangerous both because of bleeding problems and sudden swelling, leading to airway obstruction. Thus tongue biopsies should only be performed by physicians or dentists with appropriate training and facilities.

Table 33.3. Causes of macroglossia

Congenital disorders
Cavernous hemangioma or lymphangioma
Down syndrome
Hypothyroidism
Lipoid proteinosis
Episodic problems
Trauma
Angioedema, including hereditary angioneurotic edema
Acquired disorders
Hypothyroidism with myxedema
Acromegaly
Amyloidosis
Actinomycosis
Melkersson-Rosenthal syndrome
Sarcoidosis
Syphilis
Carcinoma
Mesenchymal tumors

Glossodynia

Synonyms. Glossopyrosis, burning tongue, burning mouth

Definition. Burning, pain or dysesthesias of the tongue or oral mucosa without clinically apparent changes.

Epidemiology. Glossodynia is primarily a disease of perimenopausal women.

Etiology and Pathogenesis. The etiology of the burning tongue or burning mouth syndrome is unclear. The patients are often depressed or have a pronounced fear of cancer.

Clinical Findings. By definition, one does not find anything abnormal. Occasionally the patient points out physiologic variants, such as prominent papillae, median rhomboid glossitis, geographic tongue and insists the changes are new and painful. More often, the patient acknowledges that there is little to see but emphasizes the severity of the symptoms. Nonetheless one should examine the mouth carefully, looking for subtle clues to the presence of an underlying disease.

Differential Diagnosis. Glossodynia is a diagnosis of exclusion and one which leaves most patients disappointed and ready to visit the next doctor. If any clues are seen, they should be tracked down. Possible causes of glossodynia are shown in Table 33.4. A biopsy of an inflamed area is wise; it can be combined with immunofluorescent examination to exclude blistering disorders. Patch testing can be done to investigate the possibility of allergic contact stomatitis. Cultures are often positive for *C. albicans*, just as they can be in people with a normal mouth. *C. albicans* is simply not the cause of burning without physical changes.

Table 33.4. Causes of glossodynia

Psychological factors
Anxiety
Depression
Cancerophobia
Dermatologic nondisease (Cotterill 1996)
Local Factors
Lichen planus, usually atrophic
Early stages of pemphigus vulgaris or bullous pemphigoid, before blisters are apparent
Allergic contact dermatitis, often from dental prostheses or mouth washes
Galvanic phenomenon between gold and amalgam fillings
Plicated tongue [a]
Migratory glossitis (geographic tongue) [a]
Systemic factors
Sicca syndrome (dry mouth)
Vitamin B_{12} deficiency
Plummer-Vinson syndrome (iron deficiency)
Other nutritional deficiencies

[a] Common almost normal variants that only rarely cause problems.

Therapy. If the mouth is dry, artificial saliva is often helpful, as are topical anesthetics. It is reasonable to try multivitamins with the idea that they will do no harm, but one should explain to the patient that a burning mouth as the sole sign of vitamin deficiency is very rare. Some practitioners also try an empirical course of anticandidal therapy, but this often serves to convince the patient they have untreatable oral and even systemic candidiasis and is no more helpful than placebo. Reassurance is probably most important. If the patient has other signs of depression, enlisting the aid of a psychologist or psychiatrist may be helpful. Antidepressant medication may tremendously improve the symptoms.

Diseases of the Gingiva

Gingivitis

Definition. Chronic gingival inflammation; the first step in periodontal disease.

Epidemiology. Virtually every adult has some degree of gingivitis.

Etiology and Pathogenesis. A number of factors interact to produce inflammation of the gingiva. The two key factors are the presence of plaque and the age of the patient. A healthy gingiva is sealed to the tooth, maintaining a line of defense against microorganisms. As dental plaque builds up on teeth, the nature of the participant organisms changes, producing more inflammation, which is reflected as redness of the gingiva. As the plaque then extends into the gingival sulcus, periodontal disease begins, eventually leading to lost support of the teeth and edentulism.

Clinical Findings. There is mild erythema of the gingival margins. When a blunt probe is inserted into the gingival sulcus, small pockets can be identified. When they extend below the cement-enamel junction, loss of attachment has occurred.

Therapy. Plaque removal is most important. Thus daily home dental care, following the guidance of a dental hygienist, and periodic dental examinations are critical.

Hyperplastic Gingivitis

Synonym. Gingivitis hyperplastica

Definition. Chronic inflammation and hyperplasia of the gingiva.

Etiology and Pathogenesis. There are many causes of hyperplastic gingivitis. Probably the most common are poor dental hygiene, pregnancy and medications. One common type of hyperplasia is known as mouth breather gingivitis. Here the drying of the gingiva through mouth breathing while sleeping causes irritation and swelling. Gingivitis may also be seen in association with xerostomia.

Phenytoin is the best known trigger for gingival hyperplasia but cyclosporine, diltiazem and nifedipine, as well as many other medications may cause similar problems. The hyperplasia that develops with medications is often called fibrous hyperplasia, because there is a marked proliferation of the lamina propria connective tissue. Similar changes can be seen in various forms of idiopathic and hereditary gingival hyperplasia, some of which have extraoral manifestations.

Patients with leukemia or Wegener granulomatosis may present with fragile, bleeding gums. In some genodermatoses, such a tuberous sclerosis, gingival changes are common. In addition, granulomatous disorders such as Melkersson-Rosenthal syndrome or Crohn disease may involve the gingiva and lead to enlargement.

Clinical Findings. Hyperplastic gingivitis is characterized by a chronic sponge-like swelling, dusky red color and gradual overgrowth of the gingiva (Fig. 33.16). In extreme cases, the teeth may be partially or totally obscured. In mouth breather's gingivitis, there is often a sharp line of distinction as the proximal gingiva covered by the lips remain normal and the distal, particularly anterior palatal, gingiva are swollen.

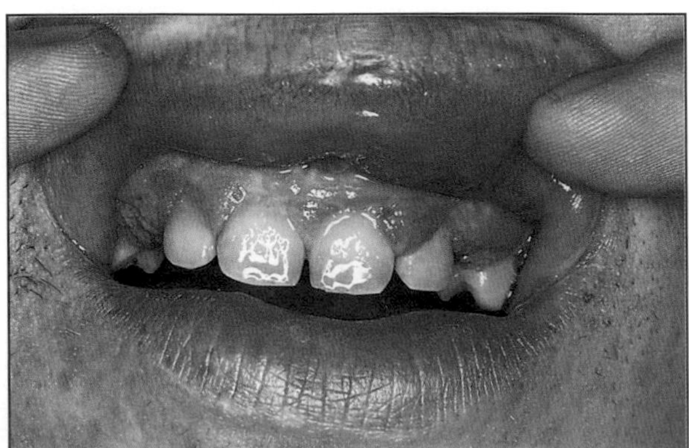

Fig. 33.16. Hyperplastic gingivitis

Therapy. Attention to proper oral hygiene and correction of triggering factors are most important. Gingival reduction can be accomplished surgically, but recurrences are likely. Plaque control is the most important factor to prevent worsening of the condition.

Acute Necrotizing Ulcerative Gingivitis

Acute necrotizing ulcerative gingivitis (ANUG) is an uncommon, fulminant destructive gingivitis, usually starting with the tips of the papillae and typically involving the lower anterior teeth initially. Usually a combination of bacteria are identified but the process does not appear to be primarily infective. Instead, it represents a unique host reaction to normal bacteria. It may progress rapidly, is typically painful and bleeds. Acute necrotizing ulcerative gingivitis was formerly known as trench mouth, for it occurred in soldiers in the trenches who had little or no opportunity to brush their teeth. This variant of gingivitis has become better known in the past decade for it is a not-uncommon finding in patients with HIV/AIDS. Other known trigger factors include smoking. Acute necrotizing ulcerative gingivitis involves an older age group than herpetic gingivostomatitis and is almost always confined exclusively to the gingiva.

Therapy. Initial debridement by a dentist or dental hygienist followed by meticulous home dental care is required. Chlorhexidene mouth washes are often a helpful adjunct. Oral antibiotics are often prescribed, but alone they constitute inadequate care.

Marginal Gingivitis

Synonym. Gingivitis marginalis

Marginal gingivitis is also more common in HIV/AIDS. There is a narrow band of erythema along the gingival margin, very similar to ordinary gingivitis. However, routine dental hygiene scarcely improves the problem. Some cases appear to be caused by *C. albicans*, while in other patients the findings are interpreted as a specific inflammatory manifestation of the underlying disease.

Rare Syndromes with Gingivitis

Papillon-Lefèvre Syndrome

Chronic gingivitis at an early age leads to tooth loss in these patients, who also have palmoplantar keratoderma (Chap. 17).

Acatalasia

(TAKAHARA 1952)

In this autosomal recessive inherited disorder, most common among Japanese, patients lack catalase and are especially susceptible to bacteria that produce hydrogen peroxide. Severe gingivitis often coupled with bone destruction is the major clinical feature. For uncertain reasons, many patients are asymptomatic. A simple test is to add H_2O_2 to the patient's blood, which then turns black.

Tuberous Sclerosis

Papular hyperplasia of the gingiva is a common finding; true gingivitis is usually lacking.

Tumors

There are a number of clinically simple growths that present as a pale to red swelling of a single interdental papillae. In the past, they were all known as epulis, a term that Virchow defined as a small tumor of the gums. Today one speaks of four separate conditions, all of which start with the letter P in English and are thus for mnemonic purposes known as the 4 Ps.

Pyogenic Granuloma

Pyogenic granulomas are common on the gingiva, often secondary to trauma or associated with pregnancy (tumor of pregnancy or epulis of pregnancy).

Peripheral Giant Cell Granuloma

Usually found between the incisors and the first molars, these reactive lesions contain hyperplastic granulation tissue and giant cells.

Peripheral Fibroma

Peripheral fibroma represents a reactive fibrous process, probably the gingival equivalent of a bite fibroma. Histologically it may contain bone (peripheral ossifying fibroma) or odontogenic epithelium (peripheral odontogenic fibroma).

Parulis

Synonyms. Periodontal abscess, gum boil

Gingival or periodontal pockets may become infected with bacteria. A painful red or yellow lump develops in the gingiva; when incised, it yields pus. In contrast to the other lesions, this finding is more common in children.

The treatment for the first three conditions is simple excision. A pyogenic granuloma may arise somewhat more rapidly than the other two, but differences are minimal. A parulis requires dental evaluation, radiologic studies to exclude a periapical abscess and then drainage and systemic antibiotic treatment.

Tori and Exostoses

Synonyms. Torus palatinus, torus mandibularis

Definition. Harmless nodular protuberances of mature bone.

Etiology and Pathogenesis. Tori are very common. It is estimated that 20% of people have a palatal torus and about 5% a mandibular torus. The lesions are more common in women than men. While the cause is unknown, in some isolated populations, autosomal dominant inheritance has been shown. Others have suggested that the tori represent a bony response to increased occlusive stresses.

Clinical Findings. The palatal torus is a broad-based firm mass of bone along the midline of the hard palate. They typically are first noticed in the third decade. The mandibular tori are almost always bilateral and grow on the lingual side of the mandible. Exostoses are isolated bony growths in other sites and are much less common. Usually the overlying mucosa is normal, but it can become ulcerated. Tori usually are asymptomatic unless they interfere with the wearing of a dental prosthesis.

Laboratory Findings. Microscopically, they consist of normal bone which can be visualized on radiologic examination.

Differential Diagnosis. The lesions are so unique that there is no differential. On first glance, other tumors may be considered.

Therapy. None is needed, but the tori can be removed if necessary when fitting a prosthesis.

Diseases of the Buccal and Palatal Mucosa

Leukoplakia and Other White Lesions

Leukoplakia is a term that has been justifiably damned as being very imprecise and causing far more confusion than illumination. We use it out of tradition as a inclusive term for localized white, not easily removed (to exclude *C. albicans*), lesions of the oral mucosa. Most hyperkeratotic oral lesions are white. Leukoplakia is also sometimes used to describe white hyperkeratotic lesions of other mucosal surfaces, such as in the anogenital region, which furthers the confusion. We will first discuss some of the other causes of white oral lesions and then consider leukoplakia.

Congenital White Lesions

There are a number of genodermatoses in which oral hyperkeratoses are a common finding. As with most structural disorders, i.e., disorders featuring an abnormal protein, they are transmitted in an autosomal dominant fashion. They include:

- Darier Disease. Cobblestoning of the palate is a frequent finding (Chap. 17).
- White Sponge Nevus (Cannon 1935). The disorder is inherited in an autosomal dominant pattern; there are mutations in the keratin 4 or 13 genes. Thick folded white plaques are seen, which are usually bilateral, and most often involve buccal mucosa, although other areas such as the vaginal and anal mucosa can be involved. The onset is in childhood or young adult life. Microscopic examination shows marked acanthosis and premature keratinization. There is no risk of malignant change.
- Hereditary Benign Intraepithelial Dysplasia (Witkop et al. 1960; Von Sallmann and Paton 1960). Identified among patients of a triracial (white, black and Native American) isolate in North Carolina, this rare condition has been traced back to a single patient who lived almost 150 years ago. The oral lesions are identical to white sponge nevus, but there are associated conjunctival lesions. The disease is inherited in an autosomal dominant pattern. On microscopic examination, there is individual cell keratinization or dyskeratosis.
- Hereditary Mucoepithelial Dysplasia (Witkop 1979). Patients have striking erythema of the oral mucosa as well as many other mucosal surfaces. They also have an increased susceptibility to respiratory infection and may develop blindness from the recurrent ocular inflammation. The pattern of inheritance is usually autosomal dominant. Histopathology shows striking acantholysis and dyskeratosis. This disorder is frequently confused with hereditary benign intraepithelial dyskeratosis because of the similarity in names and because both were described by Carl Witkop, an American dentist and human geneticist.
- Pachyonychia Congenita. Patients have thick white oral plaques, identical to white sponge nevus, thickened nails and hyperkeratotic cutaneous lesions (Chap. 32).
- Dyskeratosis Congenita. In addition to poikiloderma, nail dystrophies and tearing because of inadequate lacrimal ducts, these individuals have hyperkeratotic oral lesions that often evolve into squamous cell carcinoma. Early lesions simply are hyperkeratotic but later lesions show carcinoma in situ (Chap. 18).

Frictional Hyperkeratosis

Synonym. Morsicatio buccarum

Hyperkeratosis of the oral mucosa secondary to chronic trauma tends to produce white lesions. The best example is the bite lines along the buccal mucosa, present in most individuals, but more prominent in those with malocclusion or those who bite or chew their cheeks. Typically there are symmetric, linear, poorly defined opaline ridges. Asymmetric lesions suggest a local mechanical trigger. One can view this as the oral equivalent of a callus. Other sites include the lips and the edentulous ridges, when a denture fits poorly. The only treatment is to reduce or eliminate the trauma which usually represents an impossible task.

Nicotine Stomatitis
(Laun 1928)

Synonym. Leucokeratosis nicotina palati

Definition. Gray-white cobblestone-like patches on the roof of the mouth in long-term smokers.

Etiology and Pathogenesis. Irritant factors in tobacco smoke appear to damage the palatal mucosa as the patient is invariably a heavy smoker. The changes are far more common among cigar and pipe smokers and correlate well with pack-years in cigarette smokers. When part of the palate is covered by a prosthesis, then only the exposed region is involved. There are scattered reports of other forms of trauma causing the same changes; both hard candies and chewing gum have been vaguely incriminated.

Clinical Findings. The gray-white plaques are typically arranged in a cobblestone pattern. The most dramatic finding is the presence of central red puncta which represent the opening of a minor salivary gland duct (Fig. 33.17).

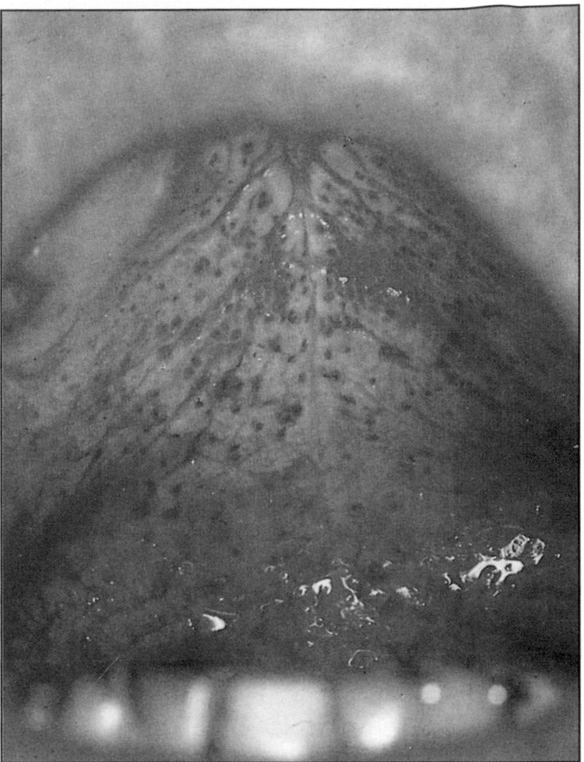

Fig. 33.17. Nicotine stomatitis

Course and Prognosis. There is a very small risk of malignant conversion. The palate is not a high-risk area for squamous cell carcinoma in smokers.

Therapy. Stop smoking. Some spontaneous reversal occurs.

Leukoplakia

Some physicians equate leukoplakia with carcinoma (or carcinoma in situ) of the oral mucosa. This is incorrect for two reasons. First, as documented above, there are many other types of white oral lesions with no connection to carcinoma. Second, many mucosal carcinomas begin with either an erythroplasia, a velvety red patch, or as a speckled red and white area, sometimes called speckled leukoplakia. Leukoplakia is generally reactive, associated with trauma but also with exposure to carcinogens such as tobacco. While the location and course may hint at whether a white lesion represents a malignancy, histologic evaluation is usually required.

Epidemiology. There are considerable differences worldwide in the prevalence of leukoplakia. When one excludes the congenital disorders, most patients are middle aged or older. The male : female ratio is about 3:1, but among younger patients it is almost 1:1. In a German study, among 4000 dermatology patients, 3% had leukoplakia. Of the 123 patients, biopsies revealed seven carcinoma in situ and six invasive carcinomas. The incidence of leukoplakia and the likelihood of conversion to squamous cell carcinoma are culturally influenced. In India, where much tobacco is chewed or simply held in the mouth and betel nut is also commonly used, squamous cell carcinoma of the mouth is an almost epidemic problem. The use of smokeless tobacco in the USA in young adults has resulted in an increase in leukoplakia of the lower labial mucosa, and in the development of squamous cell carcinomas in this site at a much earlier age.

Etiology and Pathogenesis. Actinic exposure, smoking and especially smokeless tobacco may lead to typical reactive changes that are white. In early lesions it may be difficult to tell whether tobacco or trauma has induced a lesion. Human papilloma viruses may also play a role, as in florid oral papillomatosis and verrucous carcinoma.

Clinical Findings. The lesions of leukoplakia are usually solitary. They are typically asymptomatic; one should not wait for lesions to become painful to be suspicious. The individual lesions may range from a subtle vague whiteness on a normal base to thickened leathery lesions often with fissuring (Figs. 33.18, 33.19). Several clinical variants have been described:

- Proliferative Verrucous Leukoplakia. These lesions are hyperkeratotic and become verrucous. They are persistent, may become multifocal and have a higher risk of malignant change.
- Erosive Leukoplakia. Ulcerations in a patch of leukoplakia suggest either acute trauma or malignant change.
- Speckled Leukoplakia. To repeat, speckled areas of mixed leukoplakia and erythroplasia are the best clinical marker for carcinoma, as they are premalignant in about 90 % of cases

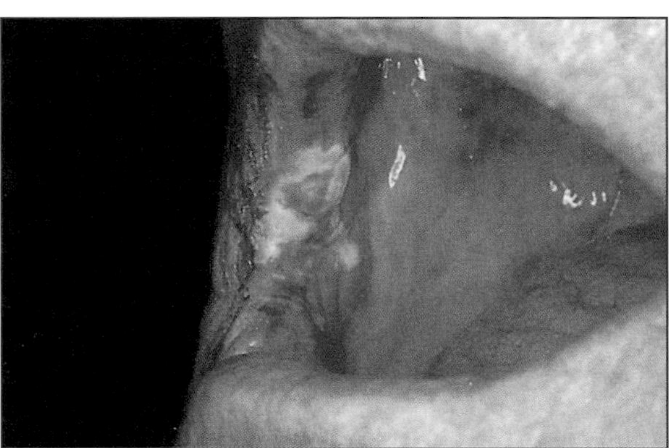

Fig. 33.18. Leukoplakia, presumably associated with chronic trauma

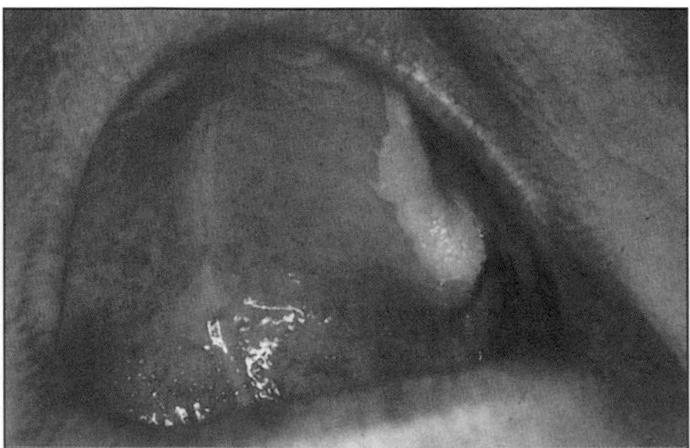

Fig. 33.19. Leukoplakia caused by denture-related trauma

Leukoplakia is most common on the mandibular and buccal mucosa. If leukoplakia is present on the floor of the mouth, it represents a carcinoma in situ or frank malignancy in about 40 % of cases. Other danger sites are the tongue and lower lip. In the retromolar area only 10 % of lesions are premalignant. Thus, if a lesion is verrucous, eroded or speckled, and located in a high-risk area, such as the floor of the mouth, one should be reluctant to make the diagnosis of reactive leukoplakia and should anticipate carcinoma in situ or carcinoma.

Histopathology. The biopsy will either reveal reactive changes or atypia. Just as in other epithelial tissues, there is little agreement on the criteria for diagnosing early carcinoma in situ in the mouth. Individual cell keratinization, nuclear atypia and mitoses are suggestive. When the tumor enters the lamina propria, then the diagnosis is squamous cell carcinoma. Papillomatous lesions can be either exophytic or less commonly endophytic, just as with inverted papillomas of the bladder. In rare cases, changes of lichen planus, lupus erythematosus or even Darier disease may appear, causing a change in diagnosis. Verrcuous carcinoma and other squamous cell carcinomas of the mouth are considered in Chapter 56.

Course and Prognosis. Idiopathic reactive lesions tend to wax and wane. Premalignant and malignant lesions are persistent, expand and thicken.

Differential Diagnosis. All the changes discussed in this section must be excluded before one diagnoses reactive leukoplakia.

Therapy. Reactive lesions can be followed. The patient should stop smoking. Either excision or cryotherapy can be employed. Both oral and topical retinoids may be useful. If the biopsy shows premalignant changes, then the lesion should be destroyed, usually by surgery. Laser destruction and radiation therapy are also effective.

Other White Lesions

- Oral Hairy Leukoplakia (Chap. 2).
- Hypertrophic Lichen Planus. While oral lichen planus is usually erythematous and atrophic, it may be hypertrophic. In such cases, it mimics many of the other lesions discussed above but tends to burn and be more troublesome (Chap. 14).

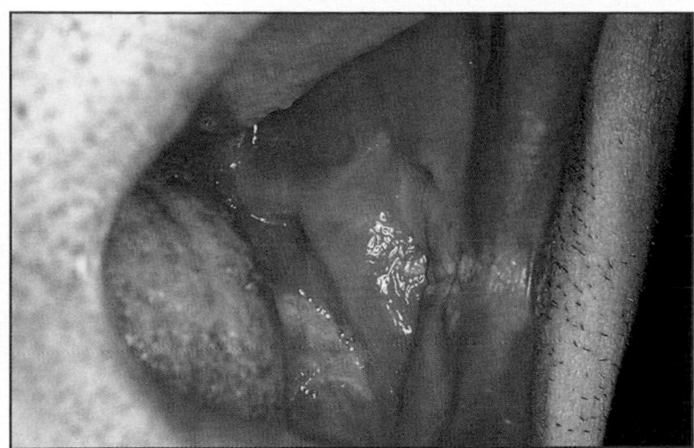

Fig. 33.20. Leukoedema

- Leukoedema. It is unclear if this finding is even abnormal. It is estimated that 90% of American blacks have leukoedema; the buccal mucosa is opaline or glossy but opaque (Fig. 33.20). Histologic examination reveals acanthosis and marked intracellular edema.
- Submucosal Fibrosis. Chronic use of betel nut and perhaps also chili peppers produce thickening of the soft palate or buccal mucosa with a white-yellow surface discoloration. Most patients are from the Indian subcontinent or southeast Asia.

Verruciform Xanthoma

(Shafer 1971)

Definition. Warty-like mucosal tumor that is also occasionally seen on the skin.

Etiology and Pathogenesis. While verruciform xanthoma resembles a wart, no human papilloma virus has been identified in the tumor. It appears to be a peculiar reaction to trauma or chronic inflammation. Despite the presence of numerous foam cells, no underlying lipid abnormality has been identified. The foam-laden histiocytes are not Langerhans cells.

Clinical Findings. In the oral mucosa, the verruciform xanthoma is a sharply bordered, generally exophytic tumor. It is most common on the palate, but is also seen on the lips and in other sites. On occasion, it may be ulcerated. Similar lesions have been described on the genitalia and on keratinizing skin in CHILD syndrome and a variety of inflammatory dermatoses including psoriasis and lupus erythematosus.

Histopathology. The histologic findings are striking. There is elongation of the rete ridges in the pattern of a verruca, usually with prominent parakeratosis. In the tips of the lamina propria are accumulations of foamy lipid-laden cells.

Differential Diagnosis. The initial differential diagnosis includes verruca and squamous cell carcinoma.

Therapy. Excision

Hyperpigmentation

Focal areas of hyperpigmentation of the lips or oral mucosa are not uncommon. They are often a racial variant; almost all blacks have some oral hyperpigmentation (Fig. 33.21). An amalgam tattoo as a result of the inadvertent implantation of amalgam filling into the mucosa is probably the most common cause of a single, hyperpigmented blue-gray macule (Fig. 33.22). While oral malignant melanoma is a feared diagnosis, it is actually very uncommon. As Table 33.5 shows, if one pays attention to the localization of the lesions, duration, color, underlying diseases and medications, one can usually form a reasonable differential diagnosis.

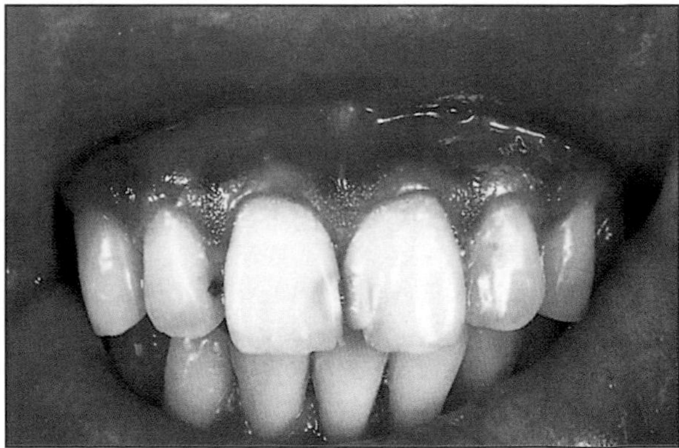

Fig. 33.21. Gingival hyperpigmentation in dark-skinned individual

Stomatitis

Stomatitis or acute inflammation of the oral mucosa overlaps heavily with gingivitis, and frequently the term gingivostomatitis is employed. Under gingivitis, we have discussed processes that are

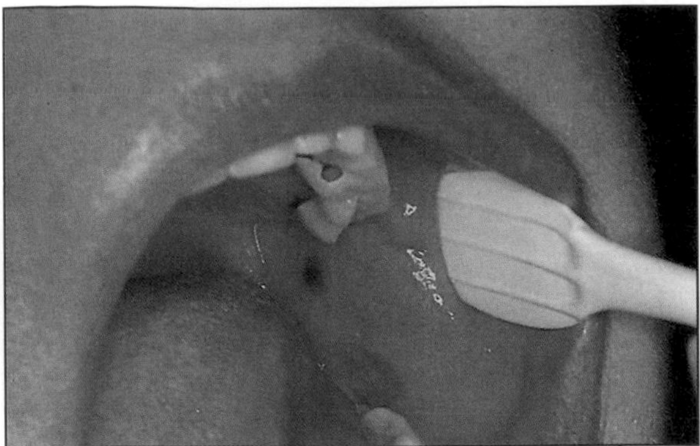

Fig. 33.22. Amalgam tattoo

usually limited to the gingiva, while here we consider more widespread diseases.

There are many causes for gingivostomatitis, including poor dental hygiene, allergic and toxic contact stomatitis and infections. Contrary to popular belief, both bacterial infections and nutritional deficiencies are relatively uncommon factors. Varying degrees of stomatitis are seen with many viral infections, including varicella, herpangina, hand-foot-and-mouth disease; the oral mucosa resist most bacteria.

Allergic Contact Stomatitis

Oral contact allergies are much less common than allergic contact dermatitis. Marion B. Sulzberger, the father of scientific dermatology in the USA, when working with Jules Chase, an immunologist, pointed out that one can induce tolerance to many potentially sensitizing chemicals when they are applied to the oral mucosa (Sulzberger-Chase phenomenon). Typical sensitizers include dental prostheses, mouth washes, tooth pastes and some spices, especially cinnamon. Standard patch testing may fail to identify suspected allergens, but mucous patch testing is awkward, time-consuming and only of minimal additional benefit.

Amalgam "Allergy"

The most common question of allergic contact stomatitis facing German dermatologists today is that of amalgam reactions. Dentists and insurance

Table 33.5. Focal hyperpigmentation of the oral mucosa

Idiopathic factors	
Racial hyperpigmentation	More common in blacks, Asians; symmetric, no cutaneous changes
Melanocytic lesions	
Oral melanotic macule	Usually on lips, probably an oral ephelis
Laugier-Hunziker-Baran syndrome	Labial, oral and subungual lentigines
Melanocytic nevi	In mouth, blue nevi most common, but all types possible
Malignant melanoma	Usually maxillary ridge or palate; appear in adults; usually detected late by dentists
Hemangiomas	Frequently mistaken for melanocytic lesions in mouth
Systemic disorders	
Addison disease	
Hyperthyroidism	
Neurofibromatosis	
Albright syndrome	
Peutz-Jeghers syndrome	
Acanthosis nigricans	
Hemochromatosis	
Malnutrition	
Exogenous agents	
Smoking	Hyperpigmentation of gingiva, especially in women
Amalgam	Amalgam tattoo; amalgam introduced into mucosa during dental procedure; typically blue-gray, focal and adjacent to filling
Decorative tattoo	
Heavy metal poisoning	Lead, mercury, bismuth, arsenic cause marginal hyperpigmentation of gingiva
Medications	Silver, chloroquine, minocycline, contraceptives
Fixed drug reaction	Usual causes (Chap. 10)

companies frequently call upon dermatologists to perform patch testing on patients who are reportedly intolerant of amalgam. If a patient tests positively to amalgam or mercury salts, then most German insurance companies will pay for more expensive gold fillings. Some patients are convinced that extraoral problems such as depression, insomnia or similar vague disorders are caused by amalgam. Their dentist may convince them that removing all amalgam is the answer to these problems, but the dentist obviously stands to benefit financially from such a decision.

While there is no question that amalgam and gold fillings may interact, producing an unpleasant electric current (battery effect), all other amalgam issues are cloudy. Elevated oral mercury levels are measurable during the first days after a filling is placed or removed, but soon the levels from amalgam are far beneath those from the environment.

If a patient has observable stomatitis directly adjacent to an amalgam filling, then testing for allergic contact stomatitis may be appropriate. Lichen planus-like lesions are occasionally seen adjacent to amalgam fillings. In the absence of any local physical findings in the mouth, amalgam is unlikely to be responsible for other complaints.

Drug-Related Stomatitis

True allergic reactions can be limited to the mouth. One may see a condition resembling oral lichen planus as a lichenoid oral drug reaction. More commonly, toxic effects, as from antimetabolites, are seen because the oral mucosa turns over rapidly and is quite sensitive. Oral ulcerations are one of the first signs of possible methotrexate toxicity in psoriasis therapy. Gold salts also cause a toxic reaction in the mouth, often as the first sign of pending intolerance. Drugs that reduce saliva production also cause stomatitis. Finally, antibiotics may create problems by damaging the normal oral flora. Unfortunately all stomatitis looks about the same: there is erythema and swelling. The dental impressions on the tongue may be more visible. Rarely, erosions and ulcerations develop. Soothing symptomatic care and a search for triggers are all that can be done.

Herpetic Gingivostomatitis

Primary herpes simplex virus infections of the oral mucosa usually have widespread involvement, in contrast to the recurrent disease which involves primarily the lips (Chap. 2).

Chronic Ulcerative Stomatitis

(Jaremko et al. 1990; Parodi and Carolda 1990)

In chronic ulcerative stomatitis (CUS) superficial erosions and ulcers are frequently mistaken for lichen planus. The immunologic findings are diagnostic. While anti-nuclear antibodies (ANA) testing is negative, direct and indirect immunofluorescent examination reveals SES (*s*tratified *s*quamous *e*pithelium) antibodies which react with a 70-kDa epithelial antigen. Sera from normal individuals and patients with systemic lupus erythematosus do not react with this antigen. The response to antimalarial agents is often dramatic.

Plaut-Vincent Stomatitis

Synonym. Gingivostomatitis Plant-Vincenti

Plaut-Vincent or fusospirochetal stomatitis is the mucosal equivalent of acute necrotizing ulcerative gingivitis. There is usually a large ulcer usually covered by a shaggy necrotic gray membrane. It is rare in the absence of gingival damage. The extreme form is known as noma or gangrenous stomatitis, in which there is widespread destruction of many oral structures, leading to disfigurement. (Chap. 48). Many clinicians feel that the mixed bacterial growth found in most lesions is a trigger for an abnormal host response, rather than a highly aggressive infection.

Xerostomia

Synonyms. Dry mouth, cotton mouth

Definition. Reduced salivary production or flow leading to a dry oral epithelium.

Etiology and Pathogenesis. Xerostomia or a dry mouth is not only a cause of patient distress, leading to difficulties in eating, speaking and other oral functions, but is also a major risk factor for caries. Typical causes include medications (atropine-like agents, antidepressives, antihistamines and many others), radiation therapy, dehydration, diseases associated with polyuria (diabetes mellitus, diabetes insipidus), Sjögren syndrome and related disorders. Viral and bacterial infections of the salivary glands may lead to reduced flow and even obstruction of one or more ducts, but there is usually sufficient reserve that dryness does not occur or is not the major complaint. Despite this list of associated disorders, most xerostomia is caused by medications, mouth breathing or anxiety.

Clinical Findings. Clinically one may see dry mucosa with erythema of gingival margins. Surprisingly often one sees a relatively normal mouth with no explanation for the problems.

Therapy. Artificial saliva is available and should be used generously, especially in the evenings. Sugar-free chewing gum or sugar-free lemon drops are sialogogues and may increase saliva flow. We often suggest that the patient put a few drops of lemon juice in water or tea to achieve the same effect. Increased dental care, often combined with the prophylactic use of fluoride-containing gels, may reduce the inevitable caries associated with a dry mouth.

Sjögren Syndrome

(Gougerot 1925; Sjögren 1933)

Synonym. Sicca syndrome

Definition. Multisystem disease of the exocrine glands that typically includes keratoconjunctivitis sicca (dry eyes), xerostomia and polyarthritis. The syndrome may occur in isolation (primary Sjögren syndrome) or in association with other autoimmune diseases (secondary Sjögren syndrome).

Epidemiology. Over 90% of patients are women, usually in the fourth to sixth decade of life. Sjögren syndrome affects about 1% of the adult population, although it is frequently underdiagnosed. About 10% of patients with rheumatoid arthritis have symptomatic Sjögren syndrome, as do a similar number of patients with lupus erythematosus and a much smaller percentage of systemic sclerosis patients. In other patients, there is serologic evidence for Sjögren syndrome but not the clinical findings.

Etiology and Pathogenesis. Sjögren syndrome is considered an autoimmune disorder but the triggering agents are unknown. Typically there are specific HLA markers (HLA-B8, -DR3, -DRw52) especially in primary and familial cases. HLA-DR4 is more often found in secondary cases. There appears to be polyclonal B cell activation associated with a lack of T cell regulation by the predominantly CD4-positive infiltrates. A viral etiology has Sjögren-like been suggested, because of the increased incidence of Sjögren syndrome in HIV/AIDS. Both retroviruses and Epstein-Barr virus have been incriminated, but the evidence is weak.

Clinical Findings

Mucosal Findings. Dryness of the eyes, mouth and other mucosal surfaces is usually the presenting complaint. Ocular dryness can be documented with the Schirmer test, in which a strip of filter paper is touched to the conjunctiva and the distance to which the tears flow is measured (normal is >10 mm in 5 min). Patients often complain that they cannot cry. Corneal damage may be so severe that strands hang from the surface (keratitis filiformis). The oral problems are considered above under xerostomia. Both taste and smell may be impaired. Some individuals may have dry genital mucosa or chronic interstitial cystitis. The dry respiratory mucosa may predispose the patient to frequent infections.

Cutaneous Findings. The skin may also be very dry. The reduced sweating may be more neural in nature rather than associated with eccrine gland dysfunction. In addition so-called inflammatory vascular disease has been described, presenting as petechiae, palpable purpura, chronic urticaria or urticarial vasculitis. A diffuse nonscarring alopecia may be present. Cryoglobulinemia may also lead to the development of leukocytoclastic angiitis. In Japanese patients with Sjögren syndrome, an unusual annular erythema is relatively common. Similar changes can be seen in infants of mothers with Sjögren syndrome.

Systemic Findings. The other hallmark of Sjögren syndrome is lymphocytic proliferations and infiltrates. Most patients have salivary gland enlargement, usually of the parotid gland. Gastrointestinal effects are also usually related to lymphocytic infiltrates, as is hepatobiliary disease, pancreatitis and thyroid disease. Pericarditis can be seen, as can a variety of renal problems. Peripheral neuropathies, especially of the facial nerve, are found. The polyarthritis is usually mild, relapsing and nonerosive, not fitting the requirements for rheumatoid arthritis. In addition, patients may have a wide range of nonspecific complaints such as fever, malaise and myalgias, so they are often misdiagnosed as having chronic fatigue syndrome or depression.

Other systemic problems, such as destructive arthritis, Raynaud syndrome, and esophageal dysfunction are usually signs of an associated, secondary connective tissue disorder.

Histopathology. When minor salivary glands are studied on a biopsy from the lower lip, a dense lymphocytic infiltrate is seen about them. Biopsy specimens of the skin lesions may show either leukocytoclastic angiitis or lymphocytic perivascular infiltrates, but they offer no clues as to the presence of Sjögren syndrome.

Laboratory Findings. A whole range of abnormal values are seen. Most patients show antibodies against rheumatoid factor, Ro (SS-A) and often La (SS-B). The estimated percentages of positivity are 90%, 70% and 50%, respectively. Ro and La antibodies are also seen in lupus erythematosus, especially subacute lupus erythematosus. In some instances, other ANA are found. In addition, there may be elevated immunoglobulin levels, a panoply of other antibodies, and often an anemia.

Course and Prognosis. The course and prognosis of primary Sjögren syndrome is determined by the very high risk of developing malignant lymphoma – one study showed a 44 fold increased risk. The B cell lymphomas tend to secrete IgM. While the salivary glands are most often affected by lymphocytic infiltrates, most lymphomas develop in the lymph nodes of the head and neck. Pseudolymphomas of lymph nodes may also develop. Patients with Ro and La antibodies are at risk of having infants with complete heart block and neonatal lupus erythematosus. The prognosis of secondary Sjögren syndrome is usually determined by the severity of the associated disorder.

Differential Diagnosis. The differential diagnosis of Sjögren syndrome is complicated by identifying primary and secondary variants. Usually the clinical and serologic findings point one in the right direction, but exact classification may be troublesome. All patients should have HIV testing, as the diffuse, infiltrative lymphocytosis syndrome seen in HIV/AIDS mimics Sjögren syndrome. HIV/AIDS patients typically do not have ocular findings. There are also subtle immunologic differences; for example, in HIV/AIDS CD8-positive cells dominate the infiltrates.

Therapy. The eye and mouth findings are treated with artificial tears and salvia. Often the systemic disease requires either corticosteroids or immunosuppressive agents. No single agent or regimen has distinguished itself.

Oral Ulcerations

There are many different causes of oral ulceration. Any damage to the surface epithelium may evolve rapidly from a minor erosion into an ulcer. Some are diseases well-known to dermatologists and are discussed elsewhere in the text, such as the whole range of bullous disorders including pemphigus vulgaris, bullous pemphigoid, erythema multiforme, lichen planus and lupus erythematosus. Oral drug reactions may occasionally ulcerate. Viral infections such as herpes simplex virus and bacterial diseases, most notably syphilis and actinomycosis, may ulcerate. Reiter syndrome may have oral erosions and ulcers. In addition, Wegener granulomatosis can present with oral, often gingival, ulcerations. Finally, patients with reduced immunity, whether it be from AIDS, chemotherapy, or rare problems such as chronic granulomatous disease, may present with ulcerations.

Sometimes the term aphthae is used to refer to any oral ulceration. Thus, herpetic gingivostomatitis is called stomatitis aphthosa, while a severe variant is known as aphthoid of Pospischill-Feyrter. These terms just cause confusion, as true aphthae are not herpetic. So-called solitary aphthae are simply oral ulcers usually caused by trauma as discussed below.

Aphthae

(Mikulicz 1888)

Synonym. Aphthous ulcers

Definition. Painful recurrent erosions and ulcers of the oral mucosa.

Epidemiology. Aphthae are extremely common. Almost everyone has an occasional lesion. Incidence estimates range from 20% to 60%. Aphthae are more common among professional people and those in higher income groups. They typically start appearing in young adult life and are more prevalent in women.

Etiology and Pathogenesis. The etiology of aphthae is unknown. They are definitely not associated with a viral infection, although many patients call them herpes. True, recurrent intraoral herpes simplex virus infections are very rare. Most studies suggest that aphthae reflect a cellular immune disturbance, perhaps with T cell cytotoxicity directed against epithelial antigens. Most patients learn that minor trauma is often a trigger. When one inadvertently bites the cheek, the chances of an aphthous ulcer developing are reasonable. Larger aphthae may appear in patients with bruxism who bite and chew their buccal mucosa, mostly at night. Nicorandil, a cardiac medication, has also been associated with larger aphthae. While a long list of triggering factors has been discussed, the most honest answer is that we do not know the cause. Table 33.6 lists many of the suspected triggers and associations.

Table 33.6. Findings associated with aphthae

Behçet syndrome	
Gastrointestinal disease	Crohn disease; ulcerative colitis; pernicious anemia; celiac disease
Hematologic disorders	Iron deficiency; folic acid deficiency; pernicious anemia
Immunodeficiency	HIV/AIDS; iatrogenic immunosuppression
Microbial factors	Adenoviruses; pleomorphic streptococci (?)
Miscellaneous factors	Trauma; emotional disorders; food intolerance (spicy or acid foods); medications (nicorandil)

Clinical Findings. Aphthae are recurrent, usually small, 2–5-mm circular or oval ulcerations with a sharply defined erythematous rim. The initial lesion is a red macule that evolves into a tiny, fragile blister which is rarely seen. As the blister disappears, the ulcer is coated by an adherent yellow-white fibrinous material. Small aphthae heal without scarring in 1–2 weeks. Aphthae typically involve the mobile oral mucosa, such as the labial and buccal mucosa, soft palate, tip of the tongue, frenulum, floor of the mouth and tonsillar pillars. They are not found on the vermilion, fixed gingiva or hard palate (Figs. 33.23, 33.24). Three subtypes are recognized.

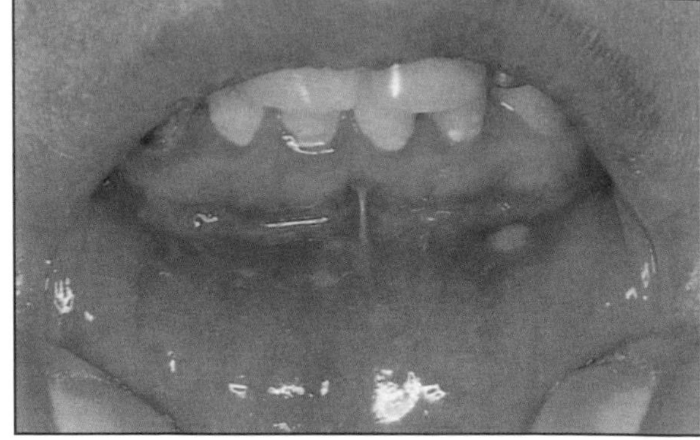

Fig. 33.23. Multiple aphthae

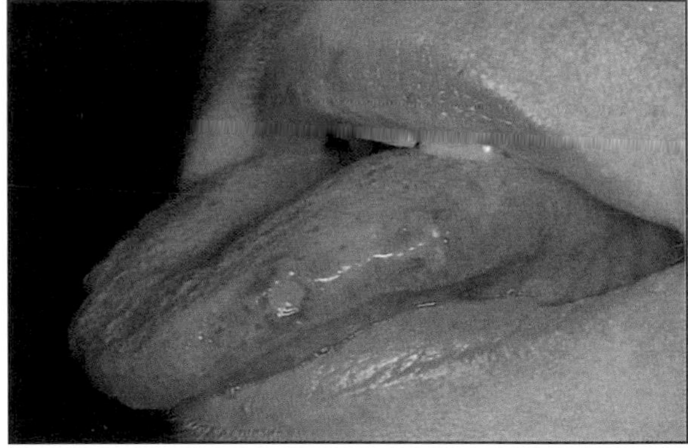

Fig. 33.24. Solitary aphthous ulcer

- Minor: Common problem; ulcers are solitary or few in number, small, and heal rapidly without scarring.
- Major (Sutton aphthae, periadenitis mucosa necrotica recurrens; Sutton 1941): Larger, deeper, often multiple, extremely painful lesions that heal over 4–6 weeks and scar. They typically have a ragged border.
- Herpetiform: Ulcers appear in crops or groups and are somewhat more likely to involve the palate. In some instances herpes simplex virus may be found.

Diagnostic Criteria. Aphthae are a clinical diagnosis; neither a histologic study nor other laboratory findings can confirm the diagnosis.

Course and Prognosis. Minor aphthae are a chronic, recurring but usually just annoying problem. Because of their multiplicity, herpetiform lesions may be more troublesome. With major aphthae the pain can be almost disabling and in any event interfere with eating, drinking and speaking.

Differential Diagnosis. In rare cases aphthae may be the presenting feature of Crohn disease or Behçet syndrome. Thus, a search for other signs of these disorders should be performed in more severe cases.

Therapy

Systemic. In more extreme cases, systemic therapy as discussed below under Behçet syndrome may be useful.

Topical. There is no good therapy. Most patients do fine with simple drying measures, including many over-the-counter products containing camphor or tincture of benzoin. Numbing agents, including topical anesthetics or mixtures of antihistamine elixirs with antacids (Benadryl Elixir and Maalox 50:50), are also useful. Topical corticosteroids, such as Lidex Gel or Kenalog in Orabase, may be helpful if applied early. Similarly, topical antibiotic solutions such as 5% tetracycline solutions may be useful, as may chlorhexidine solution 12% (Peridex).

Behçet Syndrome

(Adamantiades 1931; Behçet 1937)

Synonym. Aphthosis Behçet

Definition. Chronic multisystemic disease with ulcerations of the oral and genital mucosa and iridocyclitis as its main features.

Epidemiology. Behçet syndrome is most common in the Middle East (especially Turkey) and Asia, primarily Japan and Korea. One Korean study group follows over 2000 patients with Behçet syndrome. In Europe and the USA, Behçet syndrome is very rare and usually seen among Turkish, Persian or Asian individuals.

Etiology and Pathogenesis. The etiology of Behçet syndrome is unknown. Autoimmunity and perhaps a viral trigger are the best working explanations. The various HLA associations are striking: Mucocutaneous Behçet syndrome is associated with HLA-B12, arthritic with HLA-B27, and ocular with HLA-B5,-DR7. The neurologic type probably has no distinct associations.

Clinical Findings. The classic triad of oral and genital ulcerations and ocular problems is often not present, especially early in the course of the disease. In countries where Behçet syndrome is relatively common, complex classifications have been devised to reflect the many possible combinations. A simplified classification includes:

- Mucocutaneous type: Only oral and genital ulcerations are present. This type is also known as bipolar aphthae and may not progress to the full-blown disease.
- Arthritic type: Joint involvement plus two or more mucocutaneous findings.
- Neurologic type: CNS involvement with either mucocutaneous or arthritic changes.
- Ocular type: Iridocyclitis with one or more other cardinal features.

Patients with multiple recurrent aphthae should be questioned about genital and ocular problems. The ulcers in Behçet syndrome may also be larger (Fig. 33.25). Often they are minimal and raise no suspicion; ordinary aphthae are so common that they have little discriminatory value.

Cutaneous Findings. Genital ulcers typically involve the scrotum, penis and labia. Vaginal ulcers may also be present. Patients may also have erythema nodosum, superficial thrombophlebitis and pathergy, in which minor trauma such as from drawing blood or injecting sterile saline produces a pustular lesion. Rarely spontaneous pustules may be seen, sometimes presenting as a pseudofolliculitis. While microscopic examination reveals leukocytoclastic angiitis in many cases, typical palpable purpura is uncommon.

Systemic Findings. Behçet syndrome is a chronic disease, often coming in bursts and shifting from one organ to another. It is most feared because of

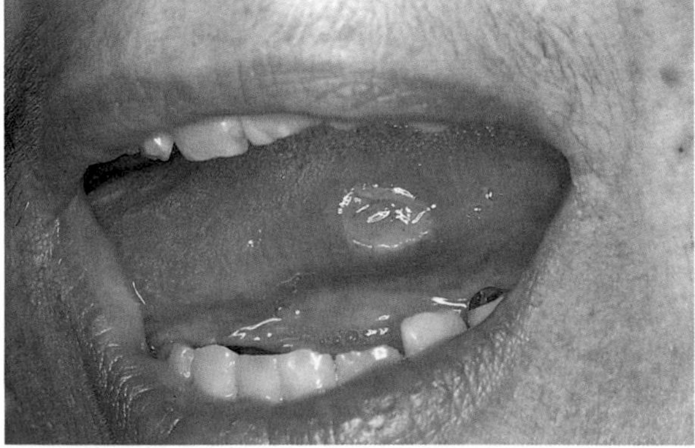

Fig. 33.25. Large aphthous ulcer in Behçet syndrome

blindness, as well as serious CNS problems. Most patients have fever, malaise, and an elevated erythrocyte sedimentation rate.

- Vascular System. Small vessel vasculitis is a unifying feature, found in many organs and responsible for a broad palette of problems. Aneurysms of both large (aorta) and small (renal and mesenteric arteries) vessels are dangerous, as is thrombophlebitis when it involves deeper vessels such as the vena cava.
- Eyes. The eye is the most commonly involved internal organ. A severe uveitis or iridocyclitis is most often seen; the patient may complain of visual problems, pain or photophobia. Hypopyon (pus in the anterior chamber) may occur. The uveitis may progress to blindness. Chorioretinitis, retinal vessel damage and vitreous body hemorrhage also occur
- Central Nervous System. About 20 % of patients have CNS disease, which represents a poor prognostic sign. Brainstem and spinal cord lesions, meningoencephalitis and psychiatric symptoms may all be found.
- Gastrointestinal Tract. While some patients have severe inflammatory bowel disease, similar to Crohn disease, less dramatic and less specific findings such as dysphagia or vague abdominal discomfort are more likely.
- Musculoskeletal System. The arthritis associated with Behçet syndrome is usually mild, symmetric and favors large joints. Some patients have sacroiliac disease, just as with all the other rheumatoid variants. The MAGIC syndrome refers to a form of relapsing polychondritis-Behçet syndrome overlap: *m*outh *a*nd *g*enital ulcers with *i*nflamed *c*artilage.
- Genitourinary System. The vasculitis presents as a focal glomerulonephritis. Inflammation of the testis and epididymitis is also seen.

Diagnostic Criteria. An International Study Group for Behçet Disease offered the following diagnostic criteria:

- Recurrent oral ulcerations, with at least three attacks of aphthae of any type in a 12-month period
- Plus two of the following:
  - Genital ulcerations
  - Ocular changes
  - Skin changes
  - Positive pathergy test

Another scheme that we employ uses slightly different criteria:

- **Major criteria**
  Oral and genital aphthae
  Iridocyclitis, uveitis or hypopyon
  Cutaneous vasculitis
- **Minor criteria**
  Polyarthritis
  Gastrointestinal symptoms
  Neurologic symptoms
  Vascular abnormalities (thrombophlebitis, aneurysms)
- **Diagnosis:** three major criteria, or two major criteria and two minor criteria

Differential Diagnosis. The problem is that everything has to start somewhere, so patients with only one or two features of Behçet syndrome simply cannot be diagnosed with certainty. The differential diagnostic list includes most of internal medicine.

Therapy. Systemic therapy is almost always necessary. Systemic corticosteroids are the mainstay of therapy, often combined with immunosuppressive agents such as azathioprine. Colchicine and dapsone may be helpful for treating the cutaneous vascular lesions. The ocular findings and by extrapolation the entire disease process are favorably influenced by cyclosporine therapy, which is thus the treatment of choice for impending blindness or other severe disease manifestations. Systemic interferon-α is also helpful. The usual regimen is 9×10^6 units three times weekly for 3 months, followed by maintance therapy with 3×10^6 units three times weekly. Thromboses should be treated with anticoagulants.

Pyostomatitis Vegetans

(McCarthy 1949)

Definition. Extremely rare, chronic, pustular oral mucosal disease usually associated with Crohn disease or ulcerative colitis.

Clinical Findings. The mucosa is erythematous, edematous, deeply folded and speckled by numerous small pustules that may evolve into ulcers. Thus, it is very similar to the appearance of the bowel in Crohn disease. Some have suggested it is the oral equivalent of pyoderma gangrenosum.

Histopathology. Intraepithelial pustules, often rich in eosinophils, are associated with pseudoepitheliomatous hyperplasia.

Differential Diagnosis. Aphthae and pemphigus vegetans must be excluded.

Therapy. Ideally, one treats the underlying disorder. In the rare situation in which none is found, systemic corticosteroids are usually tried.

Other Causes of Oral Ulcerations

Trauma

While the mouth is very resistant to trauma, occasionally damage does occur. Pizza burns on the hard palate or aspirin burns on the buccal mucosa when an aspirin is sucked, not swallowed, are two common examples. Traumatic lesions may also be iatrogenic; during dental procedures, removal of adherent cotton rolls or suction from a saliva ejector may induce damage, as may intraoral bleaching, etching and disinfecting materials, if they reach the mucosa. Radiation mucositis is almost expected during radiation therapy for head and neck cancers if the mucosa is traversed by the rays. In addition, some tooth pastes induce dentifrice-associated slough. The mechanisms are unclear, but allergic contact stomatitis is not involved. The patient notes a whitish discoloration and then a painless superficial slough or peel. Switching tooth paste usually effects a cure. Factitial lesions are difficult to diagnose in the oral cavity but do occur, either through biting or with more aggressive trauma.

Bednar aphthae are ulcerations found in the mouths of infants, presumably related to trauma from cleaning the mouth or from pacifiers and nipples. They are superficial, often quite broad, and described as butterfly-like. A pseudofactitial lesion is Riga-Fede sign, in which neonates with natal teeth may have tongue and lip ulcers.

Necrotizing Sialometaplasia

(Abrams et al. 1973)

This benign palatal ulcer appears suddenly, following ischemic necrosis of a minor salivary gland, often following trauma or a dental procedure. It typically occurs at the junction of the soft and hard palate as an erythematous swelling that rapidly ulcerates. Patients are surprisingly asymptomatic and healing is spontaneous over weeks to months.

Histopathology shows pseudoepitheliomatous hyperplasia, salivary gland necrosis and proliferation of the salivary gland ducts. Because of the epidermal reaction, the lesion may be mistaken for a squamous cell carcinoma.

Neurotic Cheek Ulcer

Some patients may chew so aggressively that they produce an ulceration along the buccal mucosa. One must exclude ill-fitting dentures and a sharp edge to the facing tooth, as well as oral blistering diseases such as giant aphthae, lichen planus, lupus erythematosus and pemphigus vulgaris. The buccal mucosa is an unusual spot for a squamous cell carcinoma in the absence of other risk factors. The same patients often have glossodynia.

Pharyngitis

Synonyms. Angina, tonsillitis

Literally, angina means a narrowing and refers to the painful swallowing associated with pharyngitis. Since the inflammation of the pharynx usually involves more than the tonsils, one speaks of pharyngitis, although tonsillitis is also acceptable. While there are many different causes of tonsillitis, the dermatologist requires at least a superficial knowledge in order to diagnose or exclude syphilitic pharyngitis. Reflecting the roots of dermatology, syphilitic angina has been called angina specifica.

Viral Pharyngitis

Many viral infections (Chap. 2) involve the pharynx. Often the common cold and influenza feature pharyngitis. Usually the pharynx is red, but not as swollen or covered with pus as typically seen in bacterial pharyngitis. Other viruses included in the group are:

- HIV: The initial infection with HIV often features a severe pharyngitis associated with malaise and an morbilliform exanthem.
- Herpangina: Caused by a Coxsackie virus, herpangina has small gray vesicles and ulcers usually on the tonsillar pillars, soft palate and uvula.
- Herpes simplex: Acute herpes simplex virus infections may be limited to the pharynx; in immunosuppressed patients chronic ulcerative pharyngitis may be a life-threatening problem. Patients with long-standing, therapy-resistant oral ulcerations in blistering disorders such as pemphigus vulgaris should be evaluated for a secondary herpes simplex infection. Often PCR

is the best way to identify the virus. Acyclovir produces amazing improvement in such unfortunate patients.

- Pharyngoconjunctival fever: Some adenoviruses cause both pharyngitis and conjunctivitis. Sufficient pharyngeal edema and exudate may be present to mimic bacterial pharyngitis.
- Epstein-Barr virus: Infectious mononucleosis typically presents with pharyngitis, which is frequently misdiagnosed as bacterial. Patients with infectious mononucleosis who are treated with antibiotics, especially ampicillin and amoxicillin, develop a characteristic macular exanthem.

Bacterial Pharyngitis

Many bacteria also cause pharyngitis (Chap. 4) including:

- Streptococcal Pharyngitis. Group A β-hemolytic *Streptococcus* (also known as *Streptococcus pyogenes*) infections typically involve pharynx. The patients are febrile and have a swollen, dusky red pharynx often covered with pus. The strains of streptococci that cause pharyngitis may also cause scarlet fever. Other streptococcal strains are also involved. Unfortunately, one cannot make a clinical diagnosis, so cultures and then antibiotic treatment are the usual approach to pustular pharyngitis.
- Plaut-Vincent Angina. A mixed infection with anaerobes and spirochetes is often incriminated in pharyngitis, in contrast to its unclear role in gingivostomatitis. Typically the tonsils are covered with gray exudates (Fig. 33.26) and there is a foul smell. Three unusual complications are septicemia, jugular vein septic thrombosis and peritonsillar abscess (formerly known as quinsy and frequently fatal prior to antibiotics).

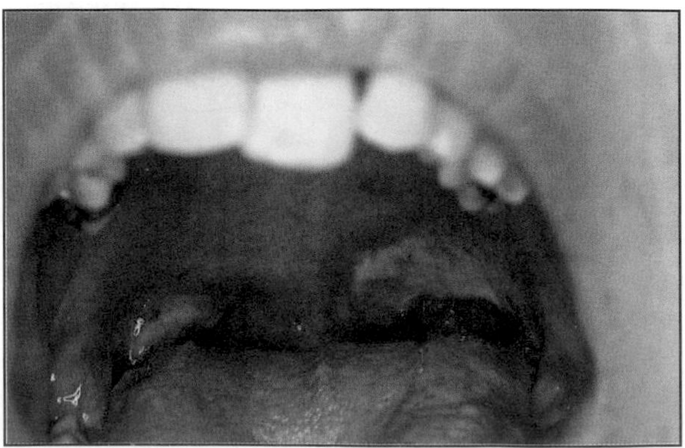

Fig. 33.26. Plaut-Vincent angina

- Diphtheria. *Corynebacterium diphtheriae* is a gram-positive bacillus. Despite the availability of vaccines, there have been several outbreaks of diphtheria in Eastern Europe causing casualties, but the disease is extremely rare in the USA. Pharyngitis is usually the first manifestation. Patients typically have bad breath and a gray pseudomembranous covering of their swollen tonsils. The bacteria produce a variety of toxins leading to cardiac and neurologic disease. In addition, cutaneous diphtheria may be seen. It is rare in the USA but has been described among homeless individuals, especially Native Americans and most often in the Pacific Northwest. Typically, slowly healing cutaneous ulcerations are seen; their relation to systemic diphtheria is unclear.
- Gonorrhea. While the pharynx is often involved in gonorrhea and may be culture-positive, clinical symptoms are rare.
- Syphilis. Mucous patches may develop in the pharynx in secondary syphilis. They tend to be asymptomatic gray erosions, often with an erythematous periphery. The lesions are teeming with spirochetes.
- Ludwig Angina. Also known as submandibular space infection, Ludwig angina is a potentially fatal, rapidly spreading cellulitis of the sublingual and submaxillary regions. It often follows dental work or periodontal infections. The causative organisms are anaerobes, usually very sensitive to penicillin. Often it is necessary to establish an airway because of the rapidity of the disease process.

Foetor ex ore and Halitosis

Synonym. Bad breath

Definition. One must distinguish between foetor ex ore, or an unpleasant smell in the mouth arising from oral changes, and halitosis or true bad breath, arising from the lungs, airways or gastrointestinal tract.

Etiology and Pathogenesis. Both problems have a long list of causes, as shown in Table 33.7. In a multidisciplinary breath odor clinic, about 87% of patients had oral causes for their problems (tongue coating, periodontitis, gingivitis); 8% had otorhinolaryngologic disorders (usually chronic tonsillitis) and in 5% no cause was found.

Table 33.7. Causes of foetor ex ore and halitosis (bad breath)

Foeter ex ore
Poor oral hygiene
Residual pieces of food in mouth
Necrotic tissue
Severe caries, periodontal disease
Improperly cleaned prostheses
Infections
Pharyngitis
Rhinitis
Sinusitis
Necrotic tumors
Hemorrhage
Xerostomia
Drugs
Sjögren syndrome
Others
Nasal foreign body
Tobacco
Other aromatic materials that are ingested or inhaled
Halitosis
Necrotic tissue and food particles
Diseases of the airways
Bronchiectasis
Bronchitis
Lung abscesses
Foreign body in upper GI tract
Necrotic tumors of esophagus and stomach
Motility disturbances
Achlasia
Stenosis
Reflux
Aromatic foodstuffs
Garlic
Low chain fatty acids
Systemic disorders
Diabetes mellitus
Liver failure
Uremia

Clinical Findings. In both instances, the patient complains of bad breath or an unpleasant odor emanating from the mouth. Often family members or close associates complain, or the physician simply notices the problem during the examination.

Therapy. If a specific cause is identified, it should be treated. Sometimes this is easy; in other instances, impossible. Symptomatic therapy with mouth washes, chewing gum or lozenges helps only in mild cases.

Bibliography

Basic Science Aspects

Bork K, Hoede N, Korting GW et al. (1996) Diseases of the oral mucosa and lips. Saunders, Philadelphia

Gartner LP (1994) Oral anatomy and tissue types. Semin Dermatol 13:68–73

Hornstein OP (1996) Erkrankungen des Mundes. Kohlhammer, Stuttgart

Lotti TM, Parish LC, Rogers RS (eds) (1998) Oral diseases. Textbook and atlas. Springer. Berlin

Scully C, Flint SR, Porter SR (eds) (1996) Oral diseases. An illustrated guide to diagnosis and management, 2nd edn. Dunitz, London

Diseases of the Lips

Allen CM, Camisa C, Hamzeh S et al. (1990) Cheilitis granulomatosa: report of six cases and review of the literature. J Am Acad Dermatol 23:444–450

Challacombe SJ (1997) Oro-facial granulomatosis and oral Crohn's disease: are they specific diseases and do they predict systemic Crohn's disease? Oral Dis 3:127–129

Daley TD (1993) Intraoral sebaceous hyperplasia. Diagnostic criteria. Oral Surg Oral Med Oral Pathol 75:343–347

Dufresne RG Jr, Curlin MU (1997) Actinic cheilitis. A treatment review. Dermatol Surg 23:15–21

Fordyce J (1896) A peculiar affection of the mucous membrane of the lips and oral cavity. J Cutan Dis 14:413–419

Fox PC (1997) Management of dry mouth. Dent Clin North Am 41:863–875

Greene RM, Rogers RS III (1989) Melkersson-Rosenthal syndrome: a review of 36 patients. J Am Acad Dermatol 21:1263–1270

Hornstein OP (1997) Melkersson-Rosenthal syndrome – a challenge for dermatologists to participate in the field of oral medicine J Dermatol 24:281–296

Kuno Y, Sakakibara S, Mizuno N (1992) Actinic cheilitis granulomatosa. J Dermatol 19:556–562

Melkersson E (1928) Ett fall av recidiverande facialispares i samband med angioneurotisk ödem. Hygiea 90:737–741

Mesrobian AZ (1974) Swellings of the salivary glands.I. Non-neoplastic enlargements. J Oral Med 29:79–83

Miescher G (1945) Über essentielle granulomatöse Makrocheilie (Cheilitis granulomatosa). Dermatologica 91:57–85

Ord RS, Sowray JH (1985) Congenital lip pits and facial clefts. Br J Oral Maxilofac Surg 23:391–397

Piscaia DD, Robinson JK (1987) Actinic cheilitis: a review of the etiology, differential diagnosis, and treatment. J Am Acad Dermatol 17:255–264

Rogers RS III, Bekic M (1997) Diseases of the lips. Semin Cutan Med Surg 16:328–336

Rosenthal C (1931) Klinisch-erbbiologischer Beitrag zur Konstitutionspathologie. Gemeinsames Auftreten von (rezidivierender familiärer) Fazialislähmung, angioneurotischem Gesichtsödem und Lingua plicata in Arthritismus-Familien. Z Neurol 131:475–500

Sutton RL (1909) Cheilitis glandularis apostematosa (with case report). J Cutan Dis 27:151–154

Swerlik RS, Cooper PH (1984) Cheilitis glandularis: a reevaluation. J Am Acad Dermatol 10:466–472

Volkmann R (1870) Einige Fälle von Cheilitis glandularis apostematosa (Myxadenitis labialis). Virchows Arch Pathol Anat 50:142–144

Diseases of the Tongue

Cotterill JA (1996) Dermatologic nondisease. Dermatol Clin 14:439–445

Gonzaga HF, Torres EA, Alchorne MM et al. (1996) Both psoriasis and benign migratory glossitis are assiciated with HLA-Cw6. Br J Dermatol 135:368–370

Itin PH, Lautenschlager S, Flickiger R et al. (1993) Oral manifestations in HIV-infected patients: diagnosis and management. J Am Acad Dermatol 29:749–760

Kolokotronis A, Kioses V, Antoniades D et al. (1994) Median rhomboid glossitis: an oral manifestation in patients infected with HIV. Oral Surg Oral Med Oral Pathol 78:36–40

Langtry JA, Carr MM, Steele MC et al. (1992) Topical tretinoin: a new treatment for black hairy tongue (lingua villosa nigra). Clin Exp Dermatol 17:163–164

Manabe M, Lim HW, Winzer M et al. (1999) Architectural organization of filiform papillae in normal and black hairy tongue epithelium: dissection of differentiation pathways in a complex human epithelium according to their patterns of keratin expression. Arch Dermatol 135:177–181

McGregor JM, Hay RJ (1993) Oral retinoids to treat black hairy tongue. Clin Exp Dermatol 18:291

Miyaoka H, Kamijima K, Katayama Y et al. (1996) A psychiatric appraisal of "glossodynia". Psychosomatics 37:346–348

Mezei MM, Tron VA, Stewart WD et al. (1995) Eosinophilic ulcer of the oral muosa. J Am Acad Dermatol 33:734–740

Murty GE, Fawcett S (1990) The aetiology and management of glossodynia Br J Clin Pract 44:389–392

Sigal MJ, Mock D (1992) Symptomatic benign migratory glossitis: report of two cases and literature review. Pediatr Dent 14:392–396

Storb LA, Pliskin ME (1991) Burning mouth syndrome. Gen Dent 39:31–32

Whitaker SB Singh BB (1996) Cause of median rhomboid glossitis. Oral Surg Oral Med Oral Pathol Oral Radiol Endod 81:379–380

Zhu JF, Kaminski MJ, Pulitzer DR et al. (1996) Psoriasis: pathophysiology and oral manifestations. Oral Dis 2:135–144

Diseases of the Gingiva

Anneroth G, Sigurdson A (1983) Hyperplastic lesions of the gingiva and alveolar mucosa. A study of 175 cases. Acta Odontol Scand 41:75–86

Bergman R, Friedman-Birnbaum R (1988) Papillon-Lefèrvre syndrome: a study of the long-term clinical course of recurrent pyogenic infections and the effects of etretinate treatment. Br J Dermatol 119:731–736

Daley TD, Nartey NO, Wysocki GP (1991) Pregnancy tumor: an analysis. Oral Surg Oral Med Oral Pathol 72:196–199

Daley TD, Wysocki GP (1994) Peripheral odontogenic fibroma. Oral Surg Oral Med Oral Pathol 78:329–336

Glick M, Muzyka BC, Salkin LM et al. (1994) Necrotizing ulcerative periodontitis: a marker for immune deterioration and a predictor for the diagnosis of AIDS. J Periodontol 65:393–397

Horning GM, Cohen ME (1995) Necrotizing ulcerative gingivostomatitis, periodontitis, and stomatitis: clinical staging and predisposing factors. J Periodontol 66:990–998

Israelson H, Binnie WH, Hurt WC (1981) The hyperplastic gingivitis of Wegener's granulomatosis. J Periodontol 52:81–87

Mighell AJ, Robinson PA, Hume WJ (1995) Peripheral giant cell granuloma: a clinical study of 77 cases from 62 patients, and literature review. Oral Dis 1:12–19

Nolte A, Schirren CG (1997) Torus mandibularis. Hautarzt 48:414–416

Ogata M (1991) Acatalasemia. Hum Genet 86:331–340

Riviere GR, Wagoner MA, Baker-Zander SA et al. (1991) Identification of spirochetes related to Treponema pallidum in necrotizing ulcerative gingivitis and chronic periodontitis. N Engl J Med 325:539–543

Seah YH (1995) Torus palatinus and torus mandibularis: a review of the literature. Aus Dent J 40:318–321

Takahara S (1952) Progressive oral gangrene probably due to lack of catalase in the blood (acatalasemia). Report of nine cases. Lancet ii:1101–1104

Diseases of the Buccal and Palatal Mucosa

Brickert SL (1994) Oral lichen planus: a review. Semin Dermatol 13:87–90

Cannon AB (1935) White sponge nevus of the mucosa (naevus mucosus albus mucosae). Arch Derm Syphilol 3:365–370

Chorzelski TP, Olszewska M, Jarzabek-Chorzelska M et al. (1998) Is chronic ulcerative stomatitis an entity? Clinical and immunological findings in 18 cases. Eur J Dermatol 8:261–265

Church LF Jr, Schosser RH (1992) Chronic ulcerative stomatitis associated with stratified epithelial specific antinuclear antibodies. A case report of a newly described disease entity. Oral Surg Oral Med Oral Pathol 73:579–582

Dorey JL, Blasberg B, Conklin RJ et al. (1984) Oral leukoplakia. Current concepts in diagnosis, management, and malignant potential. Int J Dermatol 23:638–642

Eisele DW, Inglis AF Jr et al. (1990) Noma and noma neonatorum. Ear Nose Throat J 69:119–123

Fischman SL (1994) Oral ulcerations. Semin Dermatol 13:74–77

Greenspan D, Greenspan JS (1996) HIV-related oral disease. Lancet 348:729–733

Huang W, Rothe MJ, Grant-Kels JM (1996) The burning mouth syndrome. J Am Acad Dermatol 34:91–98

Husak R, Garbe C, Orfanos CE (1996) Oral hairy leukoplakia in 71 HIV-seropositive patients: clinical symptoms, relation to immunologic status, and prognostic significance. J Am Acad Dermatol 35:928–934

Jainkittivong A, Langlais RP (1994) Allergic stomatitis. Semin Dermatol 13:91–101

Jaremko WM, Beutner EH, Kumar V et al. (1990) Chronic ulcerative stomatitis associated with a specific immunologic marker. J Am Acad Dermatol 22:215–220

Martin JL (1992) Leukoedema: a review of the literature. J Natl Med Assoc 84:938–940

Pang BK, Freeman S (1995) Oral lichenoid lesions caused by allergy to mercury in amalgam fillings. Contact Dermatitis 33:423–427

Parodi A, Caroda PP (1990) Patients with erosive lichen planus may have antibodies directed to a nuclear antigen of epithelial cells: a study on the antigen nature. J Invest Dermatol 94:689–693

Richard G, de Laurenzi V, Didona B et al. (1995) Keratin 13 point mutation underlies the hereditary mucosal epithelial disorder white sponge nevus. Nat Genet 11:453–455

Rugg EL, McLean WH, Allison WE et al. (1995) A mutation in the mucosal K4 is associated with oral white sponge nevus. Nat Genet 11:450–452

Shafer WG (1971) Verruciform xanthoma. Oral Surg Oral Med Oral Pathol 31:784–789

Siegel MA, Balciunas BA (1994) Oral presentation and management of vesiculobullous disorders. Semin Dermatol 13:78–86

Silverman S (1994) Oral cancer. Semin Dermatol 13:132–137

Virgili A, Corazza M, Trombelli L et al. (1996) Burning mouth syndrome: the role of contact hypersensitivity. Acta Derm Venereol (Stockh) 76:488–490

Von Sallmann L, Paton D (1960) Hereditary benign intraepithelial dyskeratosis. I. Ocular manisfestations. Arch Ophthalmol 63:421–429

Witkop CJ Jr et al. (1960) Hereditary benign intraepithelial dyskeratosis. II. Oral manifestations and hereditary transmission. Arch Pathol 70:696–711

Witkop CJ Jr, White JG, Sauk JJ Jr et al. (1978) Clinical, histologic, cytologic, and ultrastructural characteristics of the oral lesions from hereditary mucoepithelial dysplasia. A disease of gap junction and desmosome formation. Oral Surg Oral Med Oral Pathol 46:645–657

Witkop CJ Jr, White JG, King RA et al. (1979) Hereditary mucoepithelial dysplasia: a disease apparently of desmosome and gap junction formation. Am J Hum Genet 31:414–427

Wörle B, Wollenberg A, Schaller M et al. (1997) Chronic ulcerative stomatitis. Br J Dermatol 137:262–265

Yiannias A, el-Azhary R, Hand H et al. (2000) Relevant contact sensitivities in patients with the diagnosis of oral lichen planus. J Am Acad Dermatol 42:177–182

Sjögren Syndrome

Alexander E, Provost TT (1987) Sjögren's syndrome. Association of cutaneous vasculitis with central nervous disease. Arch Dermatol 123:801–810

Font J, Ramos-Casals M, Cervera R et al. (1998) Antineutrophil cytoplasmic antibodies in primary Sjögren's syndrome: prevalence and clinical significance. Br J Rheumatol 37:1287–1291

Fox RI, Tornwall J, Maruyama T et al. (1998) Evolving concepts of diagnosis, pathogenesis, and therapy of Sjögren's syndrome. Curr Opin Rheumatol 10:446–456

Fuji K, Fujimoto W, Ueda M et al. (1998) Detection of anti-type VII collagen antibody in Sjögren's syndrome/lupus erythematosus overlap syndrome with transient bullous systemic lupus erythematosus. Br J Dermatol 139:303–306

Gougerot H (1925) Insuffisance progressive et atrophie des glandes salivaires et muqueuses de bouche, conjonctives. Bull Soc Fr Dermatol Syphiligr 32:376

Markusse HM, Schoonbrood M, Oudkerk M et al. (1994) Leukocytoclastic vasculitis as presenting feature of primary Sjögren's syndrome. Clin Rheumatol 13:269–272

Mitchell J, Greenspan J, Daniels T et al. (1987) Anhidrosis (hypohidrosis) in Sjögren's syndrome. J Am Acad Dermatol 16:233–235

Oxholm P, Asmussen K (1995) Classification of disease manifestations in primary Sjögren's syndrome: present status and new proposal. Clin Rheumatol 14 [Suppl]:3–7

Royer B, Cazals-Hatem D, Sibila J et al. (1997) Lymphomas in patients with Sjögren's syndrome are marginal B-cell neoplasms, arise in diverse extranodal and nodal sites, and are not associated with viruses. Blood 90: 766–775

Sais G, Admella C, Fantova MJ et al. (1998) Lymphocytic autoimmune hidradenitis, cutaneous leukocytoclastic vasculitis and primary Sjögren's syndrome. Br J Dermatol 139:1073–1076

Sjögren HSC (1933) Zur Kenntnis der Keratoconjunctivitis sicca (Keratitis filiformis bei Hypofunktion der Tränendrüsen). Acta Ophthalmol [Suppl] (Copenh) 2:1–151

Wu AJ, Fox PC (1994) Sjögren's syndrome. Semin Dermatol 13:138–143

Aphthae and Behçet Syndrom

Adamantiades B (1931) Sur un cas d'iritis à hypopyon. Ann Oculist (Paris) 168:271–278

Azilerli G, Aksungur VL, Sarica R et al. (1994) The association of HLA-B5 antigen with specific manifestations of Behçet's disease. Dermatology 188:293–295

Behçet H (1937) Über rezidivierende, aphthöse, durch einen Virus verursachte Geschwüre am Mund, am Auge und an den Genitalien. Dermatol Wochenschr 105:1152–1157

Balabanova M, Calamia KT, Perniciaro C et al. (1999) A study of the cutaneous manifestations of Behçet's disease in patients from the United States. J An Acad Dermatol 41:540–545

Dega H, Petit A, Gaulier A et al. (1996) Mucocutaneous criteria for the diagnosis of Behçet's disease. J Am Acad Dermatol 35:789–790

Demiroglu H, Özcebe OI, Barista I et al. (2000) Interferon alfa-2b, colchicine, and benzathine penicillin versus colchicine and benzathine penicillin in Behçet's disease: a randomised trial. Lancet 355:605–609

Dündar SV, Gencalb U, Simsek W (1985) Familiar cases of Behçet's disease. Br J Dermatol 113:319–321

Fain O, Mathieu E, Lachassinne E et al. (1995) Neonatal Behçet's disease. Am J Med 98:310–311

Firestein GS, Gruber HE, Weisman MH et al. (1985) Mouth and genital ulcers with inflamed cartilage: MAGIC syndrome. Am J Med 79:65–72

Ghate JV, Jorizzo JL (1999) Behçet's disease and complex aphthosis. J Am Acad Dermatol 40:1–18

International study group of Behçet's disease (1990) Criteria for diagnosis of Behçet's disease. Lancet 335:1078–1080

Kaklamani VG, Vaiopoulos G, Kaklamanis PG (1998) Behçet's disease. Semin Arthritis Rheum 27:197–217

Mangelsdord HC, White WL, Jorizzo JL (1996) Behçet's disease. Report of twenty-five patients from the United States with prominent mucocutaneous involvement. J Am Acad Dermatol 34:745–750

Sakane T, Takeno M, Suzuki N et al. (1999) Behçet's disease. N Engl J Med 341:1284–1291

Sutton RL Jr (1941) Recurrent, scarring painful aphthae. Amelioration with sulfathiazole in two cases. JAMA 117:175–176

Yazici H, Yurdakul S, Hamuryudan V (1999) Behçet's syndrome. Curr Opin Rheumatol 11:53–57

Zouboulis CC, Orfanos EO (1998) Treatment of Adamantiades-Behçet's disease with systemic Interferon-α. Arch Dermatol 134:1010–1016

Pyostomatitis Vegetans

Ballo FS, Camisa C, Allen CM (1989) Pyostomatitis vegetans. Report of a case and review of the literature. J Am Acad Dermatol 21:381–387

McCarthy FP (1949) Pyostomatitis vegetans: report of three cases. Arch Dermatol Syph 60:750–764

Mehravaan M, Kemény L, Husz S et al. (1997) Pyodermatitis-pyostomatitis vegetans. Br J Dermatol 137:266–268

Other Causes of Oral Ulceration

Abrams AM, Melrose RJ, Howell FV (1973) Necrotizing sialometaplasia. A disease simulating malignancy. Cancer 32:130–135

Imbery TA, Edwards PA (1996) Necrotizing sialometaplasia: literature review and case reports. J Am Dent Assoc 127:1087–1092

Pharyngitis

Bisno AL (1996) Acute pharyngitis: etiology and diagnosis. Pediatrics 97:949–954

Bisno AL, Gerber MA, Gwaltney JM Jr et al. (1997) Diagnosis and management of group A streptococcal pharyngitis: a practice guideline. Clin Infect Dis 25:574–583

Huovinen P, Lahtonen R, Ziegler T et al. (1989) Pharyngitis in adults: the presence and coexistence of viruses and bacterial organisms. Ann Intern Med 110:612–616

Lapins J, Lindback S, Lidbrink P et al. (1996) Mucocutaneous manifestations in 22 consecutive cases of primary HIV-1 infection. Br J Dermatol 134:257–261

Peter JR, Haney HM (1996) Infections of the oral cavity. Pediatr Ann 25:572–576

Foetor ex ore and Halitosis

Ratcliff PA, Johnson PW (1999) The relationship between oral malodor, gingivitis, and periodontitis. A review. J Periodontol 70:485–489

Van Steenberghe D (1997) Breath malodor. Curr Opin Periodontol 4:137–143

Diseases of the Male Genitalia

Contents

The diagnosis and treatment of diseases involving the glans and prepuce (foreskin) present formidable clinical problems. First, the number of primary disorders is large. In addition, many common dermatoses, such as psoriasis, lichen planus and scabies, may have genital involvement. Examination of the genitalia can provide clues to the diagnosis of a puzzling dermatosis, such as psoriasis. Third, a variety of urethral disorders may also secondarily involve the penile skin. Finally, venereal disease must always be factored into the equation. The patient needs to be counseled adequately, correctly treated and referred to public health sources if a sexually transmitted disease is present. Almost as importantly, if the disorder is not sexually transmitted, the patient needs to be explicitly reassured. The approach to penile disease differs in Germany and America for two major, completely unrelated reasons. German dermatologists have considerably more training in sexually transmitted diseases and andrology, so they see patients who otherwise might go to urologists or sexually transmitted disease clinics. Another difference is that the average patient in Germany is not circumcised, while the typical American patient is.

Basic Science Aspects

There are many unique anatomic features of the penis. In an uncircumcised patient, the space between the glans penis and the inner aspect of the foreskin is a closed or capillary space. The inner aspect of the foreskin is very similar to the outer surface, also covered by keratinizing epithelium. The dermis is very loose and rich in vessels so it can expand rapidly when traumatized or involved in an allergic reaction. In addition, there are few other body regions where two sheets of skin lie in direct opposition to one another but yet slide freely. Thus the area under the foreskin is an intertriginous site subject to all the changes seen in other such areas, including raised temperature, increased moisture, more alkaline surface pH, microbial colonization, minor mechanical trauma and the accumulation of shed scales, sweat and sebum, known as smegma. In some experimental models, smegma acts as a carcinogen. The main human data supporting such a role is the rarity of penile cancers in circumcised individuals. In addition, cervical carcinoma is more common among partners of uncircumcised men, but here the role of human papilloma virus may be more important.

The normal bacterial flora of this area is highly variable. Coagulase-negative staphylococci, *Propionibacterium acnes* and *Bacteroides melanogenicus* are all found. The latter is fairly common beneath the foreskin, but its pathologic role is unclear. Occasionally coagulase-positive staphylococci, *Escherichia coli, Proteus mirabilis* or *Pseudomonas aeruginosa* are found. In circumcised individuals, far fewer bacteria are found. Patients who wash with alkaline antibacterial soaps or syndets may selectively favor Gram-negative organisms. These organisms, coupled with smegma, produce a fertile environment in which other bacteria, viruses and fungi can grow. Inadequate hygiene also plays a role, as does phimosis.

Circumcision

While a dermatology text is not the place to decide the issues surrounding circumcision, it is more convenient to discuss them in one place, rather than with each disease process where the presence of a foreskin plays a role. The arguments against circumcision in infants are that it is painful and probably unnecessary for most individuals. In patients with a family history of a bleeding disorder or hypospadias it is contraindicated. The main argument for universal circumcision is a reduced incidence of penile cancer in circumcised individuals. There may be less likelihood of trauma producing tiny defects that serve as a portal for bacteria, viruses and yeasts. In addition, in those individuals whose foreskin does not easily retract, hygiene may be less than ideal. Many of the disorders discussed below serve as the main indications for circumcision in adult life.

Congenital Abnormalities

The main congenital abnormalities in this area are the various forms of hypospadias, which we will leave to urology texts. Surprisingly, the two most common congenital problems, heterotopic sebaceous glands and pearly penile papules, are rarely noticed at birth but discovered later, often when the patient is concerned about the possibility of a sexually transmitted disease and subjects his penis to close scrutiny. Thus, in contrast to most other congenital lesions, they frequently form the basis of an urgent consultation.

Heterotopic Sebaceous Glands

The inner aspect of the foreskin is the most common site for the penile equivalent of the Fordyce glands of the lips. Tiny 1- to 3-mm yellow papules are present (Fig. 34.1). Slightly larger sebaceous glands on the frenulum are known as Tyson glands. Both are free sebaceous glands, not connected to hairs. When inflamed, they may be larger and more prominent. Since they are harmless, the patient needs only to be reassured. Such lesions can be mistaken for condylomata and unnecessarily treated.

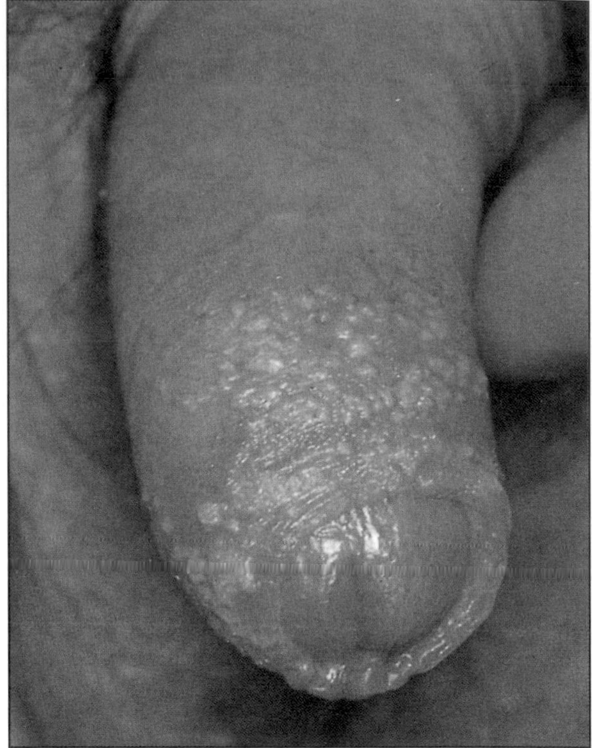

Fig. 34.1. Heterotopic sebaceous glands

Pearly Penile Papules

(Buschke 1909; Glicksman and Freeman 1966)

Synonyms. Papillae coronae glandis, hirsuties papillaris penis

These tiny white papules are located at the junction between the glans and the coronal sulcus (Fig. 34.2). They may occasionally be elongated, mimicking tiny hairs, hence the name hirsuties. Some patients may have only a few lesions, others hundreds, sometimes in multiple rows. They may have a red tint or appear telangiectatic. Microscopic examination is not necessary but reveals most lesions to be angiofibromas. Once again, no treatment is needed. Some extremely concerned patients insist on therapy; careful laser ablation is the best approach.

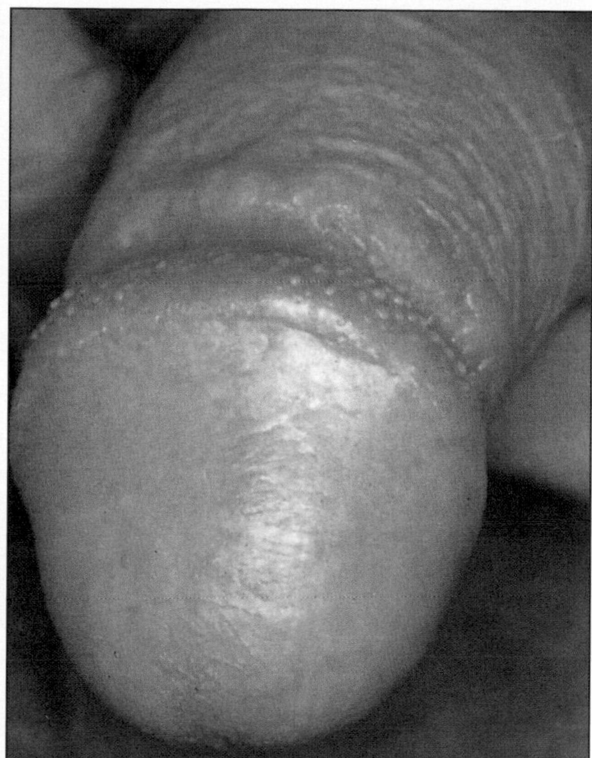

Fig. 34.2. Pearly penile papules

Penile Lesions

Penile Melanotic Macule

Synonyms. Penile lentigo

Definition. Local increase in pigment in basal layer keratinocytes. Identical to labial melanotic macule and vulvar melanotic macule.

Clinical Findings. The penile melanotic macule is a flat, tan or brown, often irregular lesion that is usually noticed in adolescence or young adult life. Often multiple lesions are present. They tend to slowly enlarge and increase in number. They are limited almost exclusively to the glans, but may extend to involve the inner aspect of the foreskin.

Histopathology. There is hyperkeratosis and acanthosis with increased melanin in the keratinocytes of the basal layer. There is no increase in the number of melanocytes, as in a true lentigo. Electron microscopic evaluation reveals larger solitary melanosome complexes, as typically seen in normal black skin.

Differential Diagnosis. The penile melanotic macule is only of interest because it is confused with a malignant melanoma. The latter lesion usually has a much shorter course, starts later in life and is far more irregular. If any question exists, a biopsy should be performed.

Therapy. Usually no therapy is needed. Superficial destruction with cryotherapy or a variety of lasers is possible. Surgical excision leaves a troublesome scar and is not recommended.

Nonvenereal Sclerosing Lymphangitis

Synonym. Lymphangiectasis penis

Definition. Inflammation of lymphatic channel proximal to glans, producing a cord-like thickening.

Etiology and Pathogenesis. The most typical cause of nonvenereal sclerosing lymphangitis is sexual intercourse. Apparently the trauma incurred produces inflammation and thickening of lymphatic vessels just proximal to the glans, usually involving the inner aspect of the prepuce. The disorder can, however, be seen slightly more proximally in uncircumcised individuals. Sometimes the lesions are coupled temporally with various forms of urethritis or prostatitis, but an infectious cause has not been identified.

Clinical Findings. The patient presents with the acute onset of a 1- to -2-cm-long, sausage-shaped, skin-colored cord. It is usually arcuate or semicircular and perpendicular to the long axis of the penis, but can run diagonally (Fig. 34.3). When the skin is stretched over it, it has a glassy appearance and resembles any other vascular ectasia. The lesion is usually not red, inflamed or painful, and the overlying skin is freely moveable. There may be associated edema of the foreskin. The lesion usually resolves spontaneously over weeks; rarely it may ulcerate, especially if further traumatized.

Histopathology. Biopsy is not recommended because of the risk of marked posttraumatic edema. In addition, the cord is often missed as it is quite mobile. An enlarged lymphatic vessel with minimal inflammation is found. In later lesions, the vessel may show fibrosis (lymphangiofibrosis thrombotica occlusiva).

Differential Diagnosis. The lymphangitis in primary syphilis is usually associated with a chancre, runs along the dorsal surface of the penis and is much harder. Nonetheless, it is wise to exclude syphilis. Sclerosing

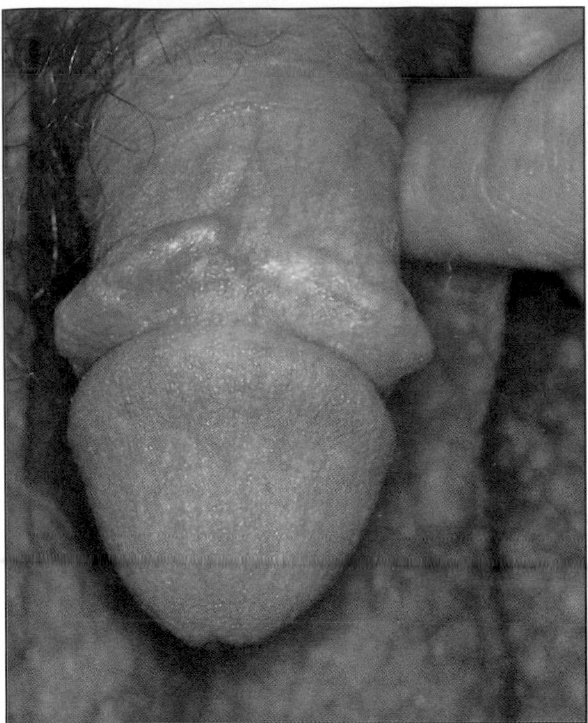

Fig. 34.3. Sclerosing lymphangitis

phlebitis usually is characterized by a larger, thicker cord that does not have a glassy appearance.

Therapy. None needed, but nonsteroidal antiinflammatory drugs can be given for pain. Heparin ointments are recommended in Europe, but their efficacy is poorly documented.

Nonvenereal Sclerosing Phlebitis

(Braun-Falco 1953)

Etiology and Pathogenesis. Unknown, but factors similar to those in nonvenereal sclerosing lymphangitis (trauma, chronic infection) have been postulated.

Clinical Findings. True phlebitis of the penis is uncommon. It may occur in association with Mondor disease of the thoraco-epigastric vein and with spontaneous phlebitis in other veins. It is very similar to nonvenereal sclerosing lymphangitis, but the lesion is firmer, longer, and does not have a glassy appearance when the foreskin is peeled back over it (Fig. 34.4). Resolution is spontaneous.

Histopathology. Biopsy shows an inflamed vein with fibrosing obliteration of the lumen. Elastic stains can help separate a vein from a lymph vessel.

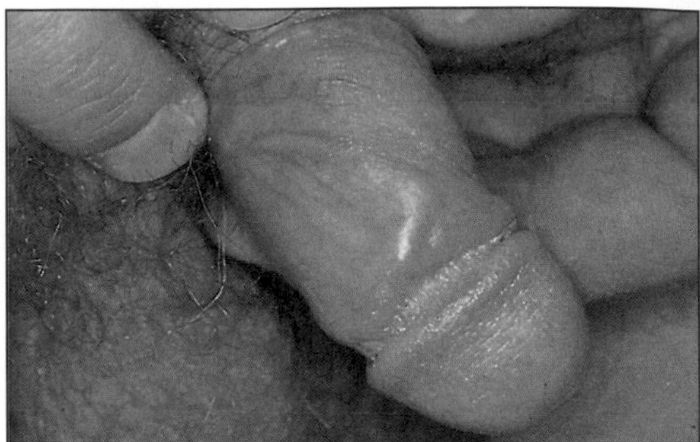

Fig. 34.4. Sclerosing phlebitis

Differential Diagnosis. The main differences between sclerosing lymphangitis and sclerosing phlebitis are: the latter is firmer, not glassy; there may be phlebitis elsewhere; and the histology is different.

Therapy. No therapy is needed; heparin ointments are often recommended.

Penile Rupture

This uncommon event occurs when the erect penis is damaged during sexual intercourse or exposed to other types of trauma. Sometimes the patient himself is responsible, by forcing objects into the urethra and then manipulating them. The tunica albuginea is damaged and a massive hematoma develops. It can be confined to the penis, or spread to involve the scrotum and adjacent abdominal and perineal skin.

Hematuria suggests that the urethra has also been damaged. Sonographic examination allows one to delineate the damage to the various erectile components of the penis (corpora cavernosa and corpus spongiosum).

Therapy. The patient should be immediately referred to a urologist for definitive evaluation and repair. Conservative treatment usually results in unsatisfactory scarring and, if the urethra is involved, may lead to many problems.

Phimosis

Definition. Condition in which the foreskin can be retracted only with difficulty or not at all.

Phimosis makes ordinary hygiene impossible and smegma accumulates. Smegmaliths are concretions of smegma that form under the foreskin. Inflammation also occurs; in the circumcised, it is called balanitis, while in the uncircumcised, it is designated balanoposthitis to reflect the involvement of the inner foreskin. Phimosis may also be a precancerous condition, predisposing to penile carcinoma, perhaps through the action of smegma. Complete phimosis means that the foreskin cannot be slid back at all. In partial phimosis, the foreskin can be retracted, but not when the penis is erect. Such patients are at risk of paraphimosis. Patients with a foreskin that is difficult to retract or only partially retractable may develop further problems later in life as a result of a variety of inflammatory and degenerative changes. The end result may then be complete phimosis.

Physiologic Phimosis

Normally the glans and inner aspect of the foreskin are adherent at birth. This physiologic condition has also been called pseudophimosis. The two surfaces tend to separate during the first year of life as both keratinize. Apoptosis appears to play a key role. Tiny epithelial pearls are formed from the keratinizing surfaces, help separate the two surfaces and are shed. Sometimes the separation occurs later in life, such as in puberty when more rapid penile growth occurs. When no separation occurs, the diagnosis of adhesive phimosis is made.

Therapy. Physiologic phimosis can be improved by gently retracting the foreskin during bathing and cleansing. Both facing surfaces should then be lightly lubricated to prevent adherence. If spontaneous separation does not occur, surgical correction may be needed.

Congenital Phimosis

Here there are structural differences in the foreskin that make retraction impossible. Sometimes it is long and thin, or trunk-like, or too bulky to be rolled back. This condition is known as hypertrophic phimosis. Other infants have a short tight foreskin and a very small preputial opening, so that once again retraction is not achievable. Both urination and erection are hampered by such phimosis. The urine stream can not be aimed, and urine collects under the foreskin, causing balanoposthitis. The risk of penile carcinoma appears higher than in those with easily retracted foreskins.

Therapy. Circumcision is the only logical treatment and should be performed promptly.

Acute Phimosis

The cause is almost always an acute infection of the glans and foreskin. The condition is usually painful and the patient alarmed, presenting as an emergency. The foreskin becomes edematous, giving the end of the penis a pear-like appearance. Often there is a discharge of pus. Possible causes include:

- Acute bacterial balanoposthitis (usually mixed infections)
- Acute gonorrhea with balanoposthitis
- Primary syphilis with chancre and secondary swelling
- Chancroid
- Herpes simplex, especially with primary infection
- Fixed drug eruption
- Irritated condylomata acuminata
- Superinfection of preexisting dermatoses, e.g., psoriasis

Therapy. The diagnosis is often impossible to make because the answer is hidden behind the swollen foreskin. Under local anesthesia a dorsal incision is made, releasing the pressure and exposing the area for physical examination and culture. Later, circumcision must be performed. Sometimes injections of hyaluronidase cause a reduction in edema and eliminate the need for a dorsal incision. Until culture results and other laboratory information is available, coverage with a broad-spectrum antibiotic is recommended. Later, more specific therapy is required. Antiseptic soaks, sparing use of a local disinfectant and perhaps inserting coated gauze between the glans and foreskin may provide short-term relief.

Chronic Phimosis

In this case, chronic inflammation or, more often, sclerosis is involved. The most common cause is lichen sclerosus et atrophicus, as shown by histologic examination of adult circumcisions. Often the lichen sclerosus et atrophicus is clinically overlooked. On the male genitalia, it is also called balanitis xerotica obliterans. Systemic sclerosis may also cause phimosis, but not in the absence of other symptoms. When chronic inflammation is the answer, the phimosis is often annular or ring-shaped (Fig. 34.5). Typically, older men, often with diabetes or inadequate hygiene, develop a chronic candidal balanoposthitis, which leads to induration and fibrosis. Painful fissures or rhagades may develop in the transitional zone from the external to the internal aspect of the prepuce. This predisposes the patient to

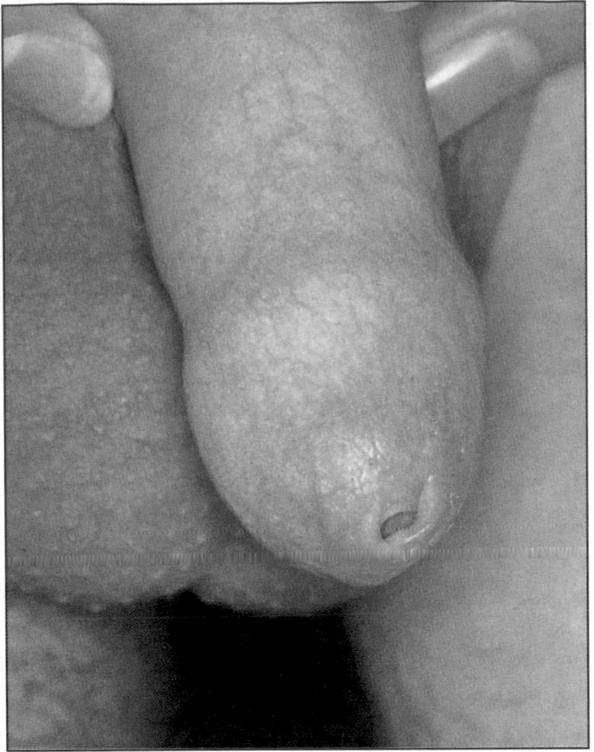

Fig. 34.5. Phimosis

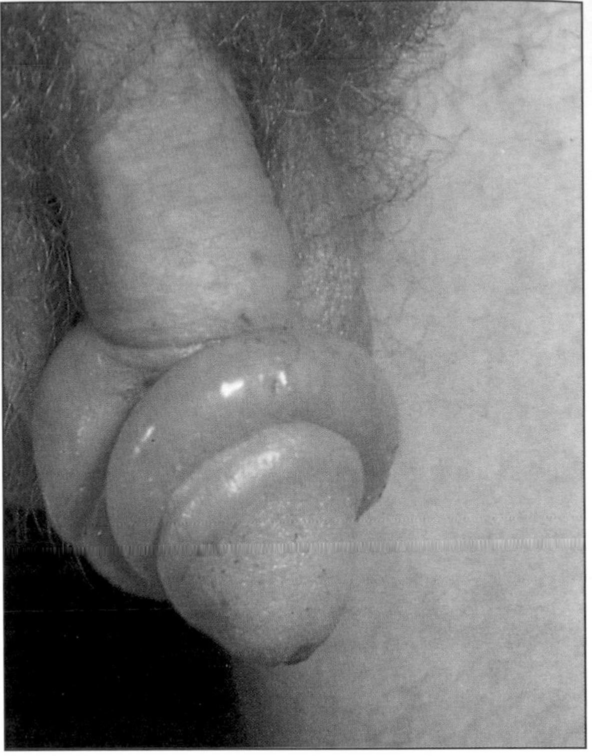

Fig. 34.6. Paraphimosis

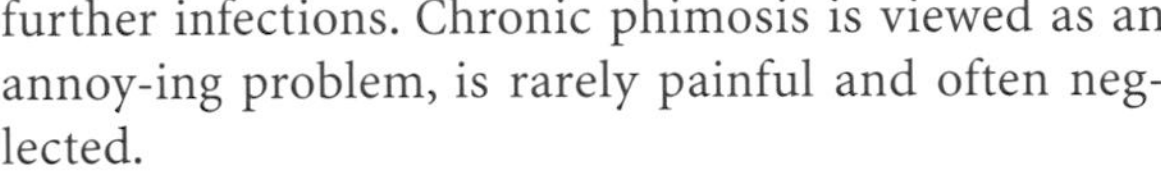

further infections. Chronic phimosis is viewed as an annoy-ing problem, is rarely painful and often neglected.

Therapy. The approach is circumcision, which also provides material for a histologic diagnosis. In young patients with lichen sclerosus et atrophicus and phimosis, high-potency topical corticosteroids can avoid the need for circumcision, but usually the latter is simpler.

Paraphimosis

Definition. Paraphimosis is an acute medical emergency when the foreskin becomes retracted and swollen, but can then not be replaced by the patient.

Etiology and Pathogenesis. Paraphimosis is usually the result of a somewhat tight foreskin and then varying degrees of manipulation during intercourse or other sexual activity. The foreskin is pushed back and the preputial ring forms a tight circle just posterior to the sulcus. This serves as a tourniquet, causing swelling of the glans and the trapped anterior part of the foreskin, which now cannot be retracted. The vicious circle continues.

Clinical Findings. The glans is usually blue-red and swollen. Behind it is the so-called Spanish collar or folded, edematous trapped portion of the foreskin (Fig. 34.6). Paraphimosis is very painful. The impaired circulation can lead to penile necrosis and gangrene, otherwise a rare event in the highly vascular organ. The preputial ring may also become necrotic.

Therapy. Sometimes, if the paraphimosis has not been present too long, it can be manually reduced by a physician. After administration of a minor tranquilizer, the penis is manually compressed moving proximally, attempting to reduce the swelling. Sometimes the so-called doorbell approach is sufficient to push the glans back through the opening. One holds the end of the penis between the second and third fingers and uses the thumb to push the glans proximally. Hyaluronidase injections may ease the task.

If this is unsuccessful, local anesthesia should be administered; usually a nerve block is preferable. Then, under sterile conditions, large-bore needles can be used to attempt to relieve the congestion and edema. Otherwise, the preputial ring must be surgically split and then later a circumcision performed. Because of the manipulation of already damaged tissue, broad-spectrum systemic antibiotic therapy is usually recommended.

Balanitis and Balanoposthitis

Definition. Balanitis is an inflammation of the glans; posthitis, one of the inner aspect of the foreskin. In uncircumcised men, usually the two tissues are simultaneously involved, thus balanoposthitis.

Phimosis, inadequate hygiene, trauma from clothing, diabetes mellitus and reduced resistance, such as in HIV infection, all play predisposing roles. Allergic contact dermatitis may develop, as patients try a variety of medications in the search for relief. Patients who are circumcised have many fewer problems. Regardless of the cause, it is convenient to speak of acute and chronic balanoposthitis. While we will primarily use the term balanoposthitis, all the statements apply equally well to balanitis. The principal difference is that the presence of a foreskin predisposes to maceration and prolongs the healing phase, even with appropriate treatment.

Acute Balanoposthitis

Acute balanoposthitis usually starts in the region of the coronal sulcus and spreads to involve the glans and inner aspect of the foreskin. Erythema and swelling occur, often associated with a serous discharge if infection is the cause (Fig. 34.7). Both phimosis and paraphimosis may result. There are many causes, including trauma, irritating material, smegma retention, allergic contact dermatitis and infections.

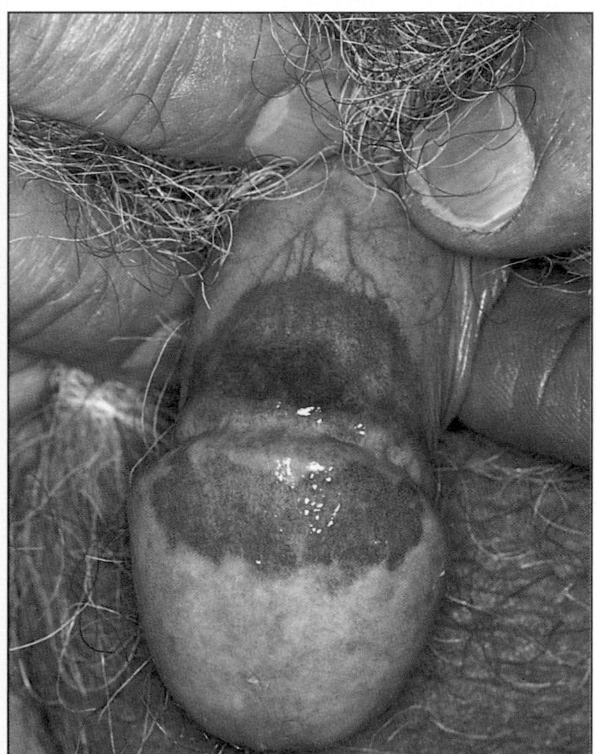

Fig. 34.7. Acute balanoposthitis

Injuries or simply mechanical friction can cause erythema and minor abrasions, predisposing to infections. Soaps, detergents, vaginal hygiene products and even vaginal secretions can accumulate and cause primary irritation. Not only inadequate washing but also overaggressive hygiene can cause irritation. An amazing variety of substances are applied to the penis, especially in association with sexual activity. Local irritants, such as Spanish fly (cantharidin) or mustard oil, are employed as aphrodisiacs in some cultures. In addition, podophyllin, when used to treat condylomata acuminata, can cause severe toxic balanoposthitis if not removed appropriately.

Allergic Contact Balanoposthitis

While this situation is uncommon, it should be considered when potential sensitizers are employed on the penis. Possible causes include contraceptives (spermicides, vehicle), deodorants and feminine hygiene sprays (disinfectant, perfume, vehicle), antiseptic agents (formaldehyde, quaternary ammonium compounds, salicylanilide, hexachlorophene), antibiotics (often used by partner) and condoms (latex, other rubber products, lubricants, preservatives). Most often the glans and foreskin are involved, but the inflammation can spread to the shaft.

Acute Infectious Balanoposthitis

Etiology and Pathogenesis. Infectious balanoposthitis is often a secondary phenomenon, following an episode of urethritis with the accumulation of secretions under the foreskin causing irritation and maceration. The moist microenvironment and minor breaks in the epithelial integrity also play a role in triggering balanoposthitis. Infections usually involve multiple organisms, as the normal flora of the prepuce is extensive and variable. Gram-negative organisms also are associated with more severe or eroded lesions. Staphylococci and streptococci may also be found.

Clinical Findings. Acute infectious balanoposthitis typically develops acutely, is associated with burning or pain, has a serous discharge and may produce enough swelling to cause phimosis or paraphimosis. Often the balanoposthitis is secondary to an established infection with discharge, which itself is irritating and causes a secondary problem. The classic example is the irritating "drip" in acute gonorrhea, but other forms of urethritis can produce the same result. Syphilis and chancroid may also present initially with an acute inflammation, so one should search carefully for the primary lesion, which is sometimes hidden behind the foreskin. Trichomonal infections can also produce balanoposthitis, so vaginal problems in the partner should be excluded. In older men, an infected carcinoma of the penis must be ruled out.

Different terms are employed for more severe forms of balanoposthitis:

- Anaerobic Erosive Balanitis. A mixed infection with anaerobic organisms and nontreponemal spirochetes is the most common cause of ulcerative balanitis. Erosions usually involve the glans, although they may affect the frenulum or the sulcus. Almost all patients are uncircumcised; edema of the prepuce is common. Orogenital contact is the usual source of transmission. When ulcerations are marked, obviously pain is a prominent feature. Gangrenous changes can develop. One should check the patient's immune status, especially HIV status, as reduced resistance is frequently found. Metronidazole is the treatment of choice.
- Phagedenic Balanitis (Balanitis Gangraenosa Phagedaenica). This even more advanced form of acute ulcerative balanitis is characterized by more marked swelling, lymphadenopathy, fever and penile gangrene.

Laboratory Findings. When cultures are taken, the laboratory should be notified of the source of the culture; otherwise, potential pathogens may be ignored. If urethral discharge is present, it should be cultured separately.

Differential Diagnosis. It is crucial to examine the entire glans and foreskin in every case of balanitis. This sounds easy but is hard to achieve in an uncircumcised patient with pain and swelling. Otherwise, valuable clues may be overlooked. Tiny grouped erosions of herpes simplex virus are usually painful and often polycyclic. The patient may give a history of a prodrome. Severe necrotic herpes simplex virus infections should suggest HIV infection. The primary chancre in syphilis is painless and often eroded, while the ulcer in chancroid is usually larger and painful. If the lesion has recurred several times in the same location or has a red-brown color and is not ulcerated, fixed drug eruption should be considered.

Therapy

Systemic. If a specific organism is identified, it is should be treated. Ulcerated and erosive forms are more likely to require antibiotic coverage. When *Trichomonas* is identified, both the patient and the partner should be treated.

Topical. The mainstay of therapy is eliminating the predisposing conditions. Basic measures include good hygiene, wet to dry soaks and then appropriate topical medications. For soaks, one can employ tap water or very mild disinfectants, such as 1:1000 chinosol, remembering that stronger disinfectants may injure the sensitive tissues. The penis can be soaked directly in a container or wrapped with wet clothes and rags that are allowed to almost dry. This has a cooling and débriding effect. Gentian violet 0.1–0.3% in water is a messy but effective drying solution that can be painted on the penis after soaking. A strip of gauze about 1–2 cm wide can be placed in the coronal sulcus and the foreskin pulled over it. This wicking action is helpful.

One should use lotions or very light creams. Fatty ointments or pastes tend to simply accumulate under the foreskin or on the glans and offer little advantage. Powders are frequently suggested, but if the lesions are weeping, they simply clump. Often anticandidal creams, sometimes mixed with low-potency corticosteroid creams, are useful. As soon as the lesion is no longer weeping, powders or lotions are easier to use. Uncircumcised patients will require far longer to get their balanitis under control. They need to treat the region each time they urinate.

Chronic Balanoposthitis

Once again, there are many possible causes. Many of the diseases associated with acute balanoposthitis (herpes simplex virus, syphilis) do not usually cause chronic problems, but acute bacterial balanoposthitis can merge into a chronic disorder. One should consider the following causes of chronic balanoposthitis.

Diabetic Balanoposthitis

Patients with diabetes mellitus are more likely to have all types of intertriginous skin disease. It is felt that the increased sugar levels in the skin are responsible, coupled with diminished hygienic measures. Thus some diabetics will have chronic balanitis without any secondary infection. Typically the glans and inner prepuce have a dusky red color. Most often, however, cultures identify either *Candida albicans* or a variety of bacteria.

Candidal Balanoposthitis

Candidal balanoposthitis has become more common in recent years. In the past it was considered a disease of elderly diabetics. Today it is frequently seen in sexually active younger men whose partner has a chronic vaginal candidiasis, perhaps secondary to oral contraceptives. Other predisposing factors include:

- Phimosis, reduced hygiene
- Any other type of balanitis
- Urethral discharge
- Underlying disorders such as diabetes mellitus, leukemia, HIV infection and other forms of immune deficiency
- Topical corticosteroids over a period of time
- Long-term therapy with oral contraceptives, oral corticosteroids, immunosuppressive agents or chemotherapeutic drugs

Clinical Findings. Candidal balanitis is usually a clinical diagnosis. There are often white-yellow pustules or erythematous macules with collarette scale and central white plaques. Similar plaques are found in the coronal sulcus. Sometimes larger white masses of hyphae, similar to oral thrush, may be seen. In other instances, there is similar erythema with superficial erosions, similar to atrophic oral candidiasis.

Laboratory Findings. Microscopic examination reveals hyphae and spores typical for *Candida albicans*. Cultures can be done by pressing the glans directly onto a culture dish and checking after 48–96 h for growth. A given percentage of asymptomatic males will have positive candidal cultures. Stool cultures are even harder to interpret, for about 50 % of people have some *Candida* species in their stool, and many have *Candida albicans*. Quantitative stool cultures may be helpful, as more massive infections are more likely to be pathogenic.

Therapy

Systemic. Oral imidazoles can be given for a short period of time. Fluconazole 150 mg either as a single dose or daily for 2–3 days may speed up resolution.

Topical. Usually anticandidal creams coupled with the general care measures discussed under acute balanoposthitis are sufficient. Aqueous gentian violet solutions are also anticandidal.

Surgical. Sometimes, even in older men who have lived many years with no problems, it becomes necessary to recommend circumcision when one simply can not get a chronic balanitis under control.

Circinate Balanitis

(Bataille and Berdal 1889)

Synonym. Balanitis circinata

Definition. Chronic usually circinate balanitis that is a marker for Reiter syndrome.

Etiology and Pathogenesis. Most often circinate balanitis is a marker for, or associated with, Reiter syndrome. In other instances it is one of the penile manifestations of psoriasis, especially in HIV patients, in whom Reiter syndrome and psoriasis tend to overlap. Many patients are HLA-B27 positive. Sometimes the term balanitis circinata parakeratotica is used to describe the scalier lesions seen in psoriasis. Ordinary bacterial and candidal balanitis may also occasionally appear circinate.

Clinical Findings. Circinate balanitis is usually very distinct clinically. Patients are usually young adults, following the age distribution for Reiter syndrome and psoriasis. Their balanitis begins with pinhead-sized gray-white papules that evolve into small beef-red erosions with a gray border. Typically the lesions start in the coronal sulcus and then involve the glans and inner aspect of the prepuce. The lesions are always sharply bordered but tend to coalesce, producing map-like lesions (Fig. 34.8). The distal or periurethral glans is usually spared. Occasionally there will be enough edema to produce phimosis. Most lesions are asymptomatic, but sometimes burning or itching is present. Even in florid Reiter syndrome, the balanitis is rarely persistent, but tends to come and go.

Differential Diagnosis. Bacterial and candidal balanitis should be excluded. The patient should be examined for other signs and symptoms of Reiter syndrome and/or psoriasis.

Therapy. Low-potency corticosteroid creams applied 1–2 times daily usually produce a prompt response. If not, mid- to high-potency versions can be used once daily for a week.

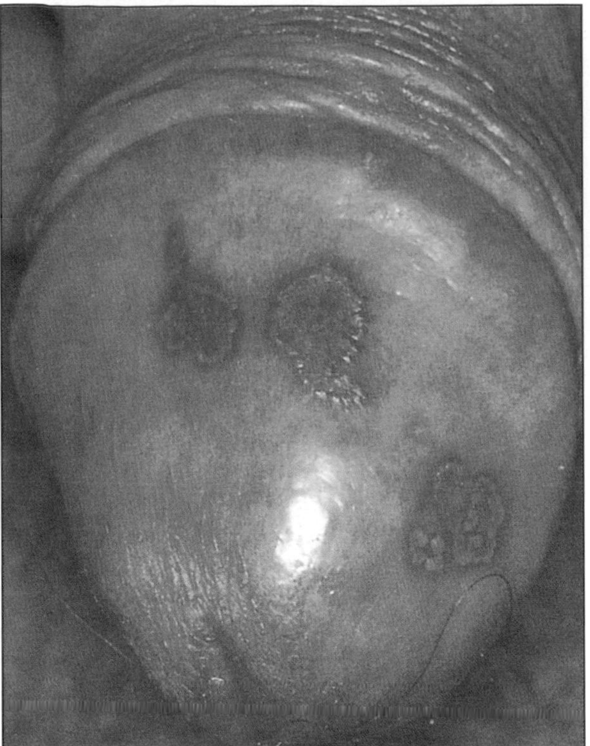

Fig. 34.8. Circinate balanitis

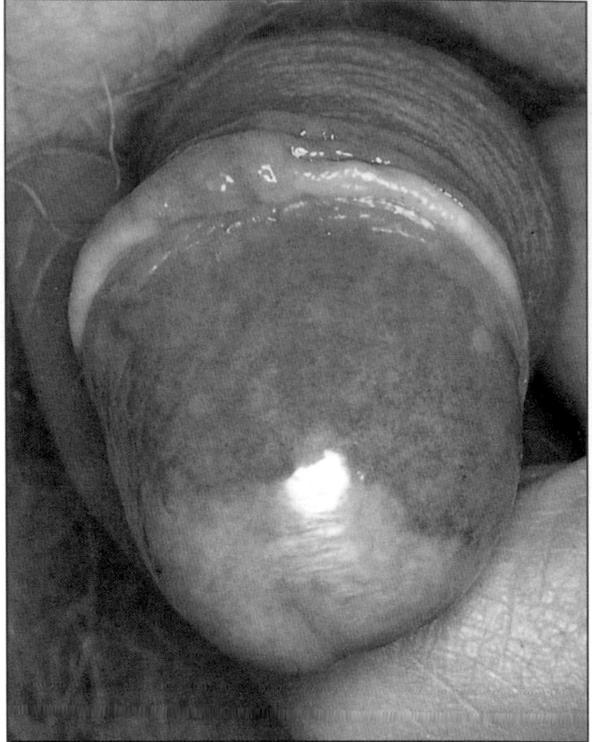

Fig. 34.9. Zoon balanitis

Zoon Balanitis

(Zoon 1972)

Synonyms. Balanoposthitis chronica circumscripta benigna plasmacellularis, plasma cell balanitis

Definition. Chronic circumscribed balanitis in elderly characterized by a plasma cell infiltrate.

Etiology and Pathogenesis. While there are many theories, the etiology of Zoon balanitis remains a mystery. No microorganism has been identified. Plasma cell infiltrates are common in the mouth and on the genitalia, so a deep immunologic explanation for the participation of plasma cells may not be forthcoming.

Clinical Findings. Patients tend to be in the fifth to eighth decade. The lesions are most often on the glans, but can involve the prepuce. They are invariably asymptomatic. Typically there is a sharply bordered patch that has a varnished appearance and red-brown color (Fig. 34.9). The lesions are flat or just barely palpable. Tiny petechial hemorrhages can be seen with diascopy. Swelling, discharge, crusting and similar signs of inflammation are absent. The lesions are chronic, but not premalignant.

Similar lesions can be found on the labia minora, in the mouth (palate, buccal mucosa, lips) and on the conjunctiva. In the latter two sites, they tend to be moister and somewhat more swollen. To avoid a long list of tongue-twister names, the group name of plasma cell mucositis has been suggested.

Histopathology. The epidermis is atrophic and may have occasional dyskeratotic cells. In the papillary dermis is a dense infiltrate of plasma cells, along with dilated vessels and minimal hemorrhage.

Differential Diagnosis. Erythroplasia of Queyrat (squamous cell carcinoma in situ) should be excluded; it is usually much redder has a granular surface and is usually slightly raised. If questions exist, biopsy should be performed.

Therapy. No therapy is very satisfactory. Usually low- to mid-potency corticosteroid creams are used. When circumcision is performed, often the involved areas not removed by the procedure also resolve.

Pseudoepitheliomatous Keratotic and Micaceous Balanitis

(Lortat-Jacob and Civatte 1961)

Synonym. Balanitis keratotica et pseudoepitheliomatosa

Definition. Chronic extremely hyperkeratotic form of balanitis.

Etiology and Pathogenesis. Human papilloma virus has been implicated as a factor, but not identified with recent sophisticated methods. We suspect some of these lesions are early or low-grade squamous cell carcinoma, such as verrucous carcinoma. The thick scale may be the mucocutaneous equivalent of a cutaneous horn. Lack of cleansing and protection by the foreskin may predispose to the accumulation of scale.

Clinical Findings. The original French description emphasizes micaceous crusts and laminated white-gold plaques on the glans. Sometimes warty excrescences are seen, especially in the sulcus. Often the glans itself appears atrophic. Usually the course is chronic over many years without malignant change.

Histopathology. There is massive hyperkeratosis and pseudoepitheliomatous hyperplasia. Because of the location, biopsies are frequently superficial. It is important to sample the lamina propria beneath the lesion to exclude carcinoma.

Differential Diagnosis. One must exclude verrucous carcinoma and ordinary squamous cell carcinoma. Even if the initial biopsy is normal, there may be sampling defects or progression of disease, so close clinical follow-up is essential.

Therapy. The lesion, including its base, must be destroyed. Possibilities include surgery, destruction with a CO_2 or neodymium-YAG laser or even electrocautery. If excision is performed in an uncircumcised patient, the foreskin can be used as a graft to cover the surgical defect. The possibility of recurrence is considerable, especially in those cases where human papilloma virus is present.

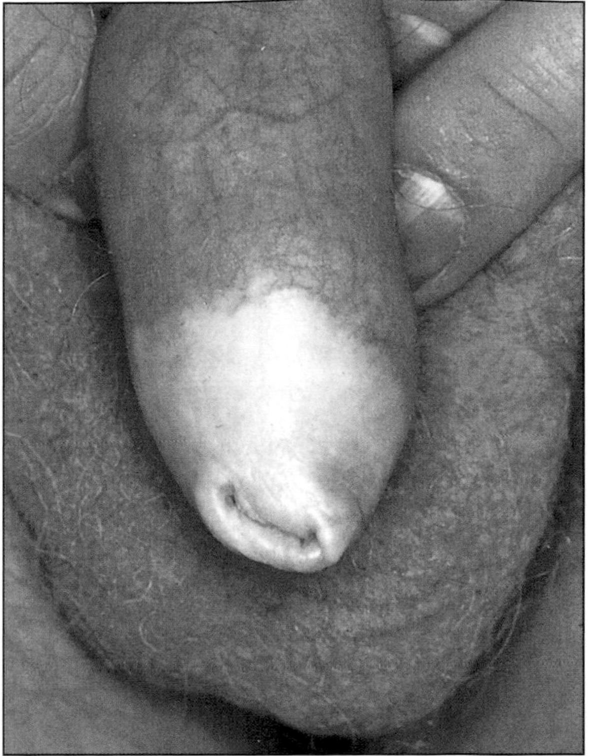

Fig. 34.10. Balanitis xerotica obliterans

Balanitis Xerotica Obliterans

(Stühmer 1928)

Synonym. Lichen sclerosus et atrophicus, kraurosis penis

While lichen sclerosus et atrophicus of the female genitalia is a well-known disorder, the equivalent problem in males has been overlooked. Most often the presenting complaint is phimosis and the diagnosis is first made histologically. Sometimes the diagnosis is obvious as the ivory to white indurated lesions are associated with phimosis (Fig. 34.10). Even in the USA, where circumcision in adults is uncommon, over half of those procedures reveal lichen sclerosus et atrophicus. Lichen sclerosus et atrophicus is a premalignant condition, although the risk is minimal. Squamous cell carcinoma is occasionally described, and both melanocytic nevi and, extremely rarely, malignant melanoma have been reported. Kraurosis penis is an obsolete term that refers to the sclerotic, phimotic stage of penile lichen sclerosus et atrophicus.

Bowenoid Papulosis

(Kopf and Bart 1977)

Synonym. Pigmented penile papules

Etiology and Pathogenesis. Bowenoid papulosis is usually caused by human papilloma virus. Often identified are the subtypes 16 and 18, which tend to be associated with squamous cell carcinoma in situ. In women there is often an association with carcinoma of the cervix and even rectum; the latter involvement can also be seen in men, especially homosexuals. Sometimes human papilloma virus is not identified; the question then is how to designate the lesions.

Clinical Findings. Two types of lesions are seen. On the glans there are typically small lichenoid papules, previously described as lichen planus-like warty lesions. On the shaft, the lesions are often somewhat larger, flat and pigmented, resembling clinically an irritated seborrheic keratosis (Fig. 34.11). They have been called pigmented penile papules. The same lesions are common in the perianal region and on the vulva. Overlaps between the two types of lesions occur. The lesions may regress.

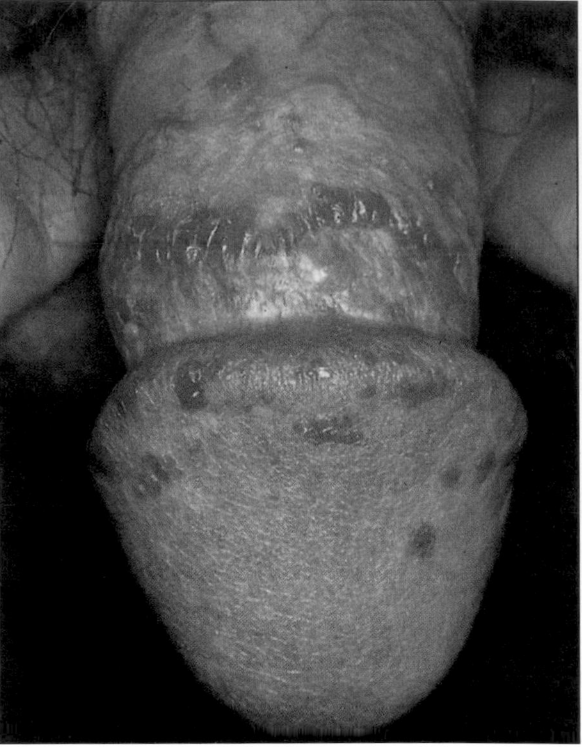

Fig. 34.11. Bowenoid papulosis

Histopathology. The hallmark is the presence of carcinoma in situ. Initially, the term "bowenoid changes" was used, suggesting that the microscopic picture only resembled carcinoma in situ. Today there is almost universal agreement that it actually is carcinoma in situ. Mitoses, large dyskeratotic cells and changes at all levels of the epidermis are present. In some lesions, there is a lichenoid dermal infiltrate; in others, accumulations of melanin both in the keratinocytes and in dermal melanophages.

Course and Prognosis. A small number of cases may progress to squamous cell carcinoma. Others may regress. The human papilloma virus can be identified with PCR and other molecular biologic techniques. It may be worthwhile subtyping the virus to identify patients and partners at particular risk for developing carcinoma. Modern concepts of oncology have identified a number of tumors in which a multiple hit approach to carcinogenesis is involved. Early lesions may be conquered by the immune system and regress; later ones may no longer be reversible.

Differential Diagnosis. If the patent is young and no carcinoma in situ changes are found on biopsy, the answer is probably verruca vulgaris or verruca plana. On the glans, lichen planus is another possibility,

Table 34.1. Carcinoma in situ of the male genitalia

Disease	Clinical features	Location	Histology
Bowenoid papulosis: lichenoid lesions	Lichenoid papules	Glans	Carcinoma in situ, lichenoid infiltrates
Bowenoid papulosis: pigmented lesions	Pigmented seborrheic keratosis-like lesions	Shaft	Carcinoma in situ, increased melanin
Bowen disease	Red scaly patch	Shaft	Carcinoma in situ
Erythroplasia of Queyrat	Red moist patch	Glans, prepuce	Carcinoma in situ
Leukoplakia	White patch	Glans, prepuce	Many patterns; rarely carcinoma in situ

so one should search for other signs. On the shaft, occasionally one finds an epidermal nevus or melanocytic nevus. In older individuals, one may encounter seborrheic keratoses, but these are very uncommon in younger people and on the glans, so this diagnosis should be made with reluctance. Table 34.1 expands on the differential diagnosis of carcinoma in situ in this area.

Therapy. Local destructive measures, such as cryotherapy, laser destruction or electrocautery, are effective. When many lesions are present, topical 5-fluorouracil or podophyllin can be employed. Just as with all other human papilloma virus disorders, recurrences are likely. Both interferon-α and oral retinoids have been recommended to reduce the risk of recurrence, but they are usually not needed. Careful clinical follow-up is essential.

Penile Gangrene

(Fournier 1883)

Synonym. Fournier gangrene

Definition. Acute infectious gangrene with rapid destruction of the penis and scrotum.

Etiology and Pathogenesis. The etiology of penile gangrene is unclear. A single consistent infectious agent has not been identified. Today it is considered a localized variant of necrotizing subcutaneous infections or synergistic necrotizing cellulitis (Chap. 4). Because the penis has such thin loose skin and subcutaneous tissue, infections of any type tend to spread rapidly and become necrotic.

Occasionally *Streptococcus pyogenes* alone may cause erysipelas which becomes gangrenous on the penis. In most instances, however, a mixture of bacteria are identified, including aerobic and anaerobic species. Often there is predisposing trauma or surgery; the latter is especially true with perineal involvement, which can secondarily affect the genitalia. The small vessels are often occluded. The combination of ischemia, edema and inflammation facilitates the growth of anaerobic organisms. Patients with diabetes mellitus are at particular risk, as are those with HIV infection or undergoing immunosuppressive therapy.

Clinical Findings. Penile gangrene usually begins spontaneously, probably following a minor injury, in a predisposed host. There is usually no preexisting balanitis. Suddenly the patient experiences massive scrotal and penile edema associated with fever and chills. Within 24 h the swollen penis, often compared to the clapper of a bell, has blue-black or white necrotic areas, which rapidly expand and ulcerate, causing marked tissue destruction. The tissue may be crepitant. Often so much skin is destroyed that the penis and scrotum blend together in a necrotic mass. The testicles may lie exposed. The corpora cavernosa and corpus spongiosum may be involved. The destruction may expand into the perineum or onto the abdominal wall.

Laboratory Findings. There is marked leukocytosis. Cultures are essential to direct therapy; pus should be aspirated from a swollen but not exposed area to improve accuracy. Radiologic examination may show soft tissue gas.

Course and Prognosis. The mortality is about 30% when all such infections are considered. Precise information on mortality from penile disease is not available. The vascular involvement may progress to arterial thromboses. In any event, survivors can count on destructive scars and may require plastic surgery to re-cover the testicles or corpora.

Differential Diagnosis. At the least suspicion, one must make the working diagnosis of penile gangrene. There is no time for differential diagnostic considerations. Phagedenic balanitis begins as balanitis and may spread and become destructive, but is rarely this severe.

Therapy. Initially one should treat with gentamicin and clindamycin, or a similar appropriate regimen, to cover both anaerobic and aerobic organisms while awaiting culture results. These can then direct a more specific antibiotic therapy. Even exactly the right agent is often not sufficient alone. Débridement is usually required to remove the necrotic tissue in which the anaerobes are thriving. When the genitalia are involved, one can not débride as aggressively as on the extremities, but it is nevertheless crucial. In most instances such patients are managed by urologists and infectious disease specialists.

Dequalinium and Chloroquinaldole Necrosis

(Wilkinson 1963)

Definition. Intertriginous necrosis secondary to use of medications, often corticosteroids, that contain dequalinium or chloroquinaldole as disinfectants.

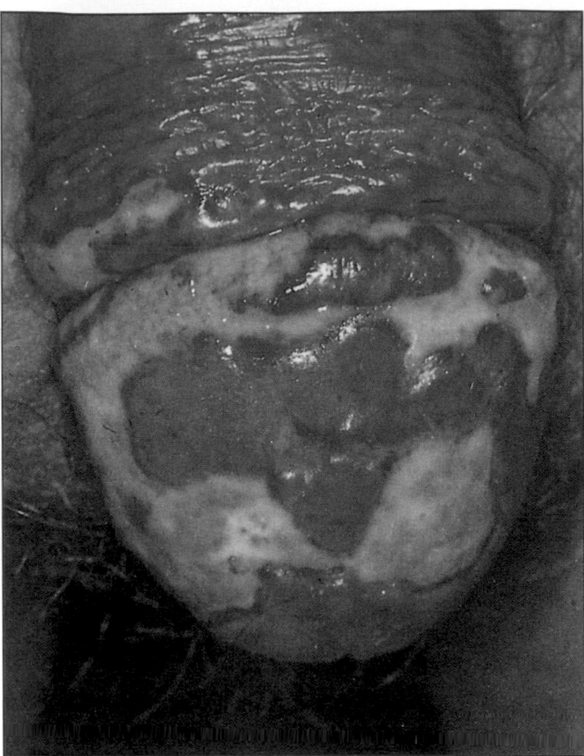

Fig. 34.12. Dequalinium necrosis

Etiology and Pathogenesis. Most patients have used the combination of a corticosteroid and dequalinium or chloroquinaldole for a long period of time. Often there has been preexisting chronic balanitis. The reaction is toxic, not allergic. Most patients are elderly, but we have also seen the problem in infants. While the glans and foreskin are most typically involved, the same changes can be seen on the vulva. In addition, we have seen similar changes in diaper dermatitis treated with the same combination of agents.

Clinical Findings. The typical clue is the presence of white necrotic areas that are separated from the rest of the glans by a narrow inflamed peripheral ring (Fig. 34.12). The lesions are relatively asymptomatic and systemic features such as fever or lymphadenopathy are rare. In other intertriginous regions, the changes are not as distinctive. When the responsible medication is stopped, healing occurs slowly over a period of weeks.

Histopathology. Microscopically one simply sees necrosis with no clues as to the etiology.

Differential Diagnosis. Other penile erosions and ulcerations are quite different. Aphthae are usually yellow, more ulcerated and very painful. Phagedenic balanitis has a more acute course. The lesions of syphilis and chancroid are clinically quite different. Occasionally a neglected squamous cell carcinoma may show such an uneven picture.

Diagnostic Approach to Other Penile Disorders

There are a number of diseases that may involve the glans and foreskin, but frequently occur elsewhere. We approach these by dividing them into three categories:

- Leukoplakias. Chronic disorders with white patches or plaques.
- Erythroplasias. Chronic disorders with red, or red and white patches or plaques. Many more carcinomas in situ present as erythroplasia than as leukoplakia.
- Melanoplakias. Chronic disorders with dark patches or plaques.

In most cases, a biopsy is needed to make an accurate diagnosis. Table 34.2 lists the disorders that one should consider. All are discussed in greater detail throughout the text.

Diseases of the Scrotum

Pruritus Scroti

Etiology and Pathogenesis. The skin of the scrotum, together with that of the eyelid, is the thinnest on the body. Thus the scrotal skin is easily damaged by friction, moisture and minor trauma. The itch-scratch cycle is very difficult to interrupt on the scrotum, so many patients with a wide variety of disorders present with a complaint of scrotal itching. While the intact scrotal skin is quite resistant to infection, minor damage may predispose to candidal infections. Rarely, tinea cruris may extend onto the scrotal skin. Atopic dermatitis, seborrheic dermatitis, psoriasis and contact dermatitis are also common on the scrotum. In our experience, most of these patients with an identifiable cause have atopic dermatitis. In many patients, no trigger for the pruritus is found.

Clinical Findings. Often one simply sees an erythematous, slightly swollen scrotum with minor erosions, scratches and even lichenification. In longstanding cases, the scrotum is enlarged with thickened exaggerated skin folds; this is the scrotal equivalent

Table 34.2. Diagnostic approach to chronic penile lesions

Clinical sign	Differential diagnosis
Leukoplakia	Carcinoma in situ Lichen sclerosus et atrophicus Candidiasis Bowen disease, keratotic variant Verrucae Lichen planus Psoriasis, rarely Discoid lupus erythematosus Vitiligo Speckled leukoplakia (carcinoma in situ)
Erythroplasia	Carcinoma in situ (erythroplasia of Queyrat) Bowen disease Bowenoid papulosis Squamous cell carcinoma Extramammary Paget disease Psoriasis Balanitis circinata (Reiter syndrome) Zoon balanitis Other types of chronic balanitis Langerhans cell histiocytosis Fixed drug reaction
Melanoplakia	Penile melanotic macule (common but not raised) Melanocytic nevus Blue nevus Malignant melanoma Angiokeratoma Hemangioma, especially if thrombosed

of severe lichen simplex chronicus. One should search for clues of other diseases in the inguinal folds or elsewhere on the body. Sometimes the erythema may be exaggerated and tiny papules or pustules present; this suggests prolonged treatment with topical corticosteroids, which results in rosacea-like changes. The patients are often very anxious, sometimes worried about the possible presence of a sexually transmitted disease and difficult to reassure. Some patients may have persistent redness of the scrotum associated with the pruritus (red scrotum syndrome).

Laboratory Findings. Fungal and yeast cultures should be performed if scaling is present or there are other clues to suggest this diagnosis.

Course and Prognosis. Pruritus scroti in the absence of an underlying disorder is a chronic frustrating problem for both patient and physician. Patch testing is useful to exclude allergic contact dermatitis.

Differential Diagnosis. The differential diagnosis includes all the disorders mentioned above. The question always is: can a disease be diagnosed, or does the patient have idiopathic pruritus scroti?

Therapy. Most patients have already been treated with topical corticosteroids and antimycotic agents. Neither is likely to be effective. The corticosteroids induce atrophy and rosacea-like changes; when they are stopped, many patients flare. The patient should be encouraged to wash the scrotum only when it is dirty, use only tap water or bath oil when bathing, rinse thoroughly, dry gently (perhaps with a hair dryer) and then apply a bland lotion or cream. We favor zinc oil in this setting. Topical anesthetics such as polidocanol 1–3% can be added.

Scrotal Lesions

Several harmless tumors are more common on the scrotum.

Scrotal Cysts

Ordinary epidermoid cysts (Chap. 53) tend to be multiple on the scrotum and often calcify. They may become ulcerated, infected and drain. Often they are painful, and many patients are very self-conscious about the numerous bumps in this private area.

Angiokeratomas

The scrotum is a common site for multiple angiokeratomas. Most patients are elderly. Usually numerous tiny 2- to 4-mm dark red papules are present. Occasional larger lesions may thrombose and be mistaken for a melanocytic tumor. The lesions are harmless but can be easily destroyed with electrocautery or lasers.

Common Disorders of the Genital Region

In addition to the changes considered above, which are either limited to or common on the penis and scrotum, a number of other processes are likely to be seen in this area.

In addition to all the sexually transmitted diseases (Chap. 5), dermatophyte infections, erythrasma, candidiasis, herpes simplex, molluscum and verrucae are often seen. Both psoriasis and lichen planus may be limited to the genital area. All of the blistering disorders can present in this area and sometimes are limited to the genitalia for a certain period of time. Among the ulcerative disorders, not only aphthae but also Behçet syndrome and Crohn syndrome can present with genital findings. Acne inversa may extend from the inguinal creases into the genital skin. The perianal and inguinal region is the most common site for extramammary Paget disease.

Bibliography

General

English JC III, Laws RA, Keough GC et al. (1997) Dermatoses of the glans penis and prepuce. J Am Acad Dermatol 37:1–24

Gross G, Jablonska S, Pfister H et al. (eds) (1990) Genital papillomavirus infections – modern diagnosis and treatment. Springer, Berlin

Lynch PJ, Edwards L (1994) Genital dermatology. Churchill Livingstone, New York

Micali G, Innmocenzi D, Nasca MR et al. (1996) Squamous cell carcinoma of the penis. J Am Acad Dermatol 35:432–451

Heterotopic Sebaceous Glands

Buschke A (1909) Über die Bedeutung der Papillen der Corona glandis. Med Klin 5:1621–1623

CarsonHJ, Massa M, Reddy V (1996) Sebaceous gland hyperplasia of the penis. J Urol 156:1441

Hyman AB, Guiducci AA (1963) Ectopic sebaceus glands. In: Montagna W, Ellis RA, Silver AF (eds) Advances in biology of skin, vol 4. Pergamon, London, pp 78–93

Kumar A, Kossard S (1999) Band-like sebaceous hyperplasia over the penis. Aust J Dermatol 40:47–48

Pearly Penile Papules

Ackerman AB, Kronberg R (1973) Pearly penile papules. Acral angiofibromas. Arch Dermatol 108:673–675

Glicksman JM, Freeman RG (1966) Pearly penile papules. A statistical study of incidence. Arch Dermatol 93:56–59

Magid M, Garden JM (1989) Pearly penile papules: treatment with the carbon dioxide laser. J Dermatol Surg Oncol 15:552–554

Ocampo Candiani J, Cueva Rodriguez JA (1996) Cryosurgical treatment of pearly penile papules. J Am Acad Dermatol 35:486–487

Vesper JL, Messina J, Glass LF et al. (1995) Profound proliferating pearly penile papules. Int J Dermatol 34:425–426

Penile Melanotic Macule

Barnhill RL, Albert LS, Shama SK et al. (1990) Genital lentiginosis: a clinical and histopathologic study. J Am Acad Dermatol 22:453–460

Landthaler M, Stolz W, Braun Falco O (1989) Lentigo der Glans penis. Hautarzt 40:222–225

Lenane P, Keane CO, Connell BO et al. (2000) Genital melanotic macules: Clinical, histologic, immunohistochemical and ultrastructural features. J Am Acad Dermatol 42:640–644

Revuz J, Clerici T (1989) Penile melanosis. J Am Acad Dermatol 20:567–570

Sclerosing Lymphangitis

Broaddus SB, Leadbetter GW (1982) Surgical management of persistent, symptomatic nonvenereal sclerosing lymphangitis of the penis. J Urol 127:987–988

Gharpuray MB, Tolat SN (1991) Nonvenereal sclerosing lymphangitis of the penis. Cutis 47:421–422

Lassus A, Niemi KM, Valle SL et al. (1972) Sclerosing lymphangitis of the penis. Br J Vener Dis 48:545–548

Marsch WC, Stuttgen G (1981) Sclerosing lymphangitis of the penis: a lymphangiofibrosis thrombotica occlusiva. Br J Dermatol 104:687–695

Sclerosing Phlebitis

Aloi FG, Tomasini CF, Molinero A (1989) Railway track-like dermatitis: an atypical Mondor's disease? J Am Acad Dermatol 20:920–923

Braun-Falco O (1953) Über strangförmige, oberflächliche Phlebitiden (Gleichzeitig ein Beitrag zur Kenntnis der Mondor'schen Krankheit). Dermatol Wochenschr 127: 506–518

Findlay GH, Whiting DA (1977) Mondor's phlebitis of the penis. A condition miscalled "non-venereal sclerosing lymphangitis". Clin Exp Dermatol 2:65–67

Tanii T, Hamada T, Asai Y et al. (1984) Mondor's phlebitis of the penis: a study with factor VIII related antigen. Acta Derm Venereol (Stockh) 64:337–340

Penile Rupture

McAninch JW, Kahn RI, Jeffrey RB et al. (1984) Major traumatic and septic genital injuries. J Trauma 24: 291–298

Orvis BR, McAninch JW (1989) Penile rupture. Urol Clin North Am 16:369–375

Rahmouni A, Hoznek A, Duron A, et al. (1995) Magnetic resonance imaging of penile rupture: aid to diagnosis. J Urol 153:1927–1928

Wespes E, Libert M, Simon J et al. (1987) Fracture of the penis: conservative versus surgical treatment. Eur Urol 13:166–168

Phimosis and Paraphimosis

Broadhurst N, Davey B (1984) Circumcision. A review of the literature and survey of current practice. Aust Fam Physician 13:731–733

Larsen GL, Williams SD (1990) Postneonatal circumcision: population profile. Pediatrics 85:808–812

Balanitis und Balanoposthitis

Edwards S (1996) Balanitis and balanoposthitis: a review (see comments). Genitourin Med 72:155–159

Hamdy FC, Hastie KJ (1990) Treatment for paraphimosis: the "puncture" technique. Br J Surg 77:1186

Vohra S, Badlani G (1992) Balanitis and balanoposthitis. Urol Clin North Am 19:143–147

Williams JC, Morrison PM, Richardson JR (1995) Paraphimosis in elderly men. Am J Emerg Med 13:351–353

Zoon Balanitis

Baldwin HE, Geronemus RG (1989) The treatment of Zoon's balanitis with the carbon dioxide laser. J Dermatol Surg Oncol 15:491–494

Davis DA, Cohen PR (1995) Balanitis circumscripta plasmacellularis. J Urol 153:424–426

Nishimura M, Matsuda T, Muto M et al. (1990) Balanitis of Zoon. Int J Dermatol 29:421–423

Zoon JJ (1972) Balanoposthite chronique circonscrite bénigne à plasmocytes. Dermatologica 105:1–7

Balanitis Keratotica et Pseudoepitheliomatosa

Irvine C, Anderson JR, Pye RJ (1987) Micaceous and keratotic pseudoepitheliomatous balanitis and rapidly fatal fibrosarcoma of the penis occurring in the same patient. Br J Dermatol 116X:719–725

Krunic AL, Djerdj K, Starcevic Bozovic A et al. (1996) Pseudoepitheliomatous, keratotic and micaceous balanitis. Case report and review of the literature. Urol Int 56: 125–128

Lortat-Jacob E, Civatte J (1961) Balanite pseudo-épithéliomaeuse, kératosique et micacée. Bull Soc Fr Dermatol 68:164–167

Read SI, Abell E (1981) Pseudoepitheliomatous, keratotic and micaceous balanitis. Arch Dermatol Syph 156:613–623

Balanitis Xerotica Obliterans

Aynaud O, Piron D, Casanova JM (1999) Incidence of preputial lichen sclerosus in adults: Histologie study of circumcision specimens. J Am Acad Dermatol 41:923–926

Bart RS, Kopf AW (1978) Squamous-cell carcinoma arising in balanitis xerotica obliterans. J Dermatol Surg Oncol 4:556–558

Howard B, Pride MD, Miller OF et al (1993) Penile squamous cell carcinoma arising from balanitis xerotica obliterans. J Am Acad Dermatol 29:469–473

Ledwig PA, Weigand DA (1989) Late circumcision and lichen sclerosus et atrophicus of the penis. J Am Acad Dermatol 20:211–214

Meyrick-Thomas RH, Ridley CM et al. (1987) Clinical features and therapy of lichen sclerosus et atrophicus affecting males. Clin Exp Dermatol 12:126–128

Nasca MR, Innocenzi D, Micali G (1999) Penile cancer among patients with genital lichen sclerosus. J Am Acad Dermatol 41:911–914

Pride HB, Miller F III, Tyler WB (1993) Penile squamous cell carcinoma arising from balanitis xerotica obliterans. J Am Acad Dermatol 29:469–473

Stühmer A (1928) Balanitis xerotica obliterans (post-operationem) und ihre Beziehungen zur Kraurosis glandis et praeputii. Arch Dermatol Syph 156:613–623

Bowenoid Papulosis

Gross G, Hagedorn M, Ikenberg H et al. (1985) Bowenoid papulosis. Presence of human papillomavirus (HPV) structural antigens and of HPV 16-related DNA sequences. Arch Dermatol 121:858–863

Knoll LD, Segura JW, Benson RC, et al. (1988) Bowenoid papulosis of the penis: successful management with neodymium:YAG laser. J Urol 139:1307–1309

Kopf AW, Bart RS (1977) Multiple bowenoid papules of the penis: a new entity. J Dermatol Surg Oncol 3: 265–269

Obalek S, Jablonska S, Beaudenon S et al. (1986) Bowenoid papulosis of the male and female genitalia: risk of cervical neoplasia. J Am Acad Dermatol 14:433–444

Schwartz RA, Janniger CK (1991) Bowenoid papulosis. J Am Acad Dermatol 24:261–264

Wade TR, Kopf AW, Ackerman AB (1978) Bowenoid papulosis of the penis. Cancer 42:1890–1903

Penile Gangrene

Efem S (1994) The features and aetiology of Fournier's gangrene. Postgrad Med J 70:568–571

Lamb RC, Juler GL (1983) Fournier's gangrene of the scrotum. A poorly defined syndrome or a misnomer? Arch Surg 118:38–40

Stein M, Anderson C, Ricciardi R et al. (1994) Penile gangrene associated with chronic renal failure: report of 7 cases and review of the literature (see comments). J Urol 152: 2014–2016

Weiner DM, Lowe FC (1996) Surgical management of ischemic penile gangrene in diabetics with end stage atherosclerosis. J Urol 155:926–929

Dequalinium Necrosis

Braun-Falco O, Lukacs I (1970) Dequalinium necrosis. Dtsch Med Wochenschr 95:1115–1117

Wilkinson DS (1963) Necrotizing ulcers of the penis. Br J Dermatol 75:16–20

Pruritus Scroti

Fischer BK (1997) The red scrotum syndrome. Cutis 60: 139–141

Kantor GR (1990) What to do about pruritus scroti. Postgrad Med 88:95–96, 99–102

CHAPTER 35

Diseases of the Female External Genitalia

Contents

Evaluation of the female genitalia involves many of the same problems discussed in the preceding chapter on the male genitalia. Common disorders such as psoriasis and seborrheic dermatitis may be most prominent on, or initially limited to, the genitalia. Another feature is the frequent association between vaginal discharge and secondary inflammation of the external genitalia.

Basic Science Aspects

The labia majora represent the border between the female genitalia and the adjacent skin. On their outer aspects, they have trichosebaceous units and apocrine glands and keratinize just as the rest of the skin does, with orthokeratosis. One distinctive feature is the abundant subcutaneous fat and relatively loose connective tissue, which allow dramatic swelling when the labia majora become inflamed. Their inner aspects represent the transition from skin to mucosa, much like the vermilion border of the lips. The surface is smooth without hairs, but contains free sebaceous glands. The labia minora are mucosal and have large numbers of free sebaceous glands, which can be seen as tiny yellow dots. Apocrine glands are abundant in both tissues, but most prominent on the mons pubis and in the outer aspects of the labia majora, perhaps explaining the propensity of extramammary Paget disease for these regions.

Several distinctive glands are found in the female genitalia. Bartholin glands are mucus-secreting glands in the vestibule (inner aspect of the labia minora) whose ducts empty into the groove between the hymen and the inner aspect of the labia minora. These glands may become infected and swollen, but are normally not noticeable. Skene glands are mucinous periurethral glands that may also become infected. Finally, the labia are rich in mammary-like glands (Van der Putte glands) that have a fibrous stroma and branch into lobuli, just like mammary glands. While there are snouts with decapitation secretion, the glands are not simple apocrine glands.

Another distinctive feature is the close proximity of the vaginal mucosa, which secretes moisturizing and lubricating fluids, to the external genitalia. Any vaginal inflammation or vaginitis is likely to lead to secondary vulvar irritation (vulvovaginitis). The vagina is lined by keratinizing squamous epithelium, when frequently contains clear cells and shows parakeratosis. Normal vaginal secretions contain cervical mucous secretions and shed epithelial cells, have a pH of 4.0–4.5 and may be watery, mucoid or, occasionally, milky. The Bartholin, apocrine and mammary-like gland secretions also end up in the vestibule. Invariably a variety of bacteria, especially corynebacteria and lactobacilli, are present. The type of microflora in the female genital tract varies with age, menses, pregnancy and contraception. Thus, the nature of the normal discharge may vary with the same factors. The transition between normal physiologic secretion to maintain lubrication and pathologic vaginal discharge is gradual; what is abnormal for one patient is normal for the next. In any case, discharge and draining lead rapidly to vulvar irritation, helped by the rubbing of garments and scratching. Similarly, urethral drainage, as in stress incontinence or urethritis, also reaches the exterior easily and causes irritation. Thus intertrigo is common in the region of the vulva and one must always search for internal predisposing factors.

Congenital Abnormalities

Heterotopic Sebaceous Glands

The multiple normal sebaceous glands of the labia minora and inner aspects of the labia majora may be quite prominent. When the tissue is stretched, one can see many small yellow papules that may be as large as several millimeters in diameter. They are harmless and analogous to the Fordyce glands of the lips or the same glands on the foreskin.

Hirsuties Papillaris Vulvae

Synonyms. Vestibular papillae, pseudocondyloma of the vulva

Similar to pearly penile papules, these lesions are found distal to the hymenal ring, and can form a fimbriated fringe. When less prominent, they are often mistaken for condylomata.

Vulvovaginitis

Definition. Inflammation of the vagina and vulva, usually evolving from vaginal discharge and secondary external irritation.

Epidemiology. Vulvovaginitis is extremely common. Almost every women has at least one bout of vulvovaginitis during her lifetime, and for many it is a chronic problem.

Etiology and Pathogenesis. Vulvovaginitis is very common and has many possible causes (Table 35.1). No one classification can logically cover all these disorders, which encompass vast sections of dermatology, gynecology and infectious disease. Many sexually transmitted diseases (Chap. 5) may present as vulvovaginitis, and conversely almost all infectious forms of vulvovaginitis can be sexually transmitted. Acute problems are most often infectious; chronic ones suggest predisposing factors or an exaggerated physiologic response. In all instances, a vaginal or cervical cause of the problem should be excluded. Treating an ulcerated, draining cervical neoplasm topically as a vulvar dermatitis is a tragic mistake. In menstruating women, most vulvovaginitis is infectious; in children and postmenopausal women, this is less likely. While one can speak of vulvitis, most physicians use the term vulvar dermatitis. All of the common forms of dermatitis – atopic, allergic contact and irritant contact – can involve the vulvar skin. Often there is an interplay

Table 35.1. Causes of vulvovaginitis

Infectious vulvovaginitis
Common
Bacterial vaginosis (*Gardnerella vaginalis*)
Candida albicans
Trichomonas vaginalis
Less common
Escherichia coli (in children)
Neisseria gonorrhoeae (with cervicitis)
Chlamydiae (with cervicitis, urethritis)
Staphylococci and streptococci
Gram-negative bacteria
Fusospirochetal organisms
Herpes simplex virus
Other viruses
Pinworms (*Enterobius vermicularis*)
Other types of vulvovaginitis
Physiologic
Atrophic vaginitis
Diabetes mellitus (predisposes to *Candida albicans*)
Immunodeficiency states (predispose to *Candida albicans*)
Excessive or inadequate hygiene
Contact allergy
Foreign body
Cervical or vaginal tumors
Cervical or vaginal adenosis secondary to diethylstilbestrol
Psychosomatic

of two or more factors. A patient with diabetes mellitus may have increased discharge, which predisposes to candidal infection. Prescribing a cream containing sensitizers may add allergic contact dermatitis to the existing problem.

Clinical Findings. Some patients complain of vaginitis or a vaginal discharge and have few skin findings. They are unlikely to come to a dermatologist. In others, the external skin irritation is more severe than the vaginal discharge. Finally, there may be only cutaneous disease, such as in allergic contact dermatitis or severe inverse psoriasis.

Typically there is a vaginal discharge, while the introitus and vulva are swollen and red. The nature of the discharge – cheesy, frothy or fishy – is often a valuable clue, as shown in Table 35.2. Scale, erosions, pus and crusting on the adjacent intertriginous skin may complete the picture. Ulcerations are uncommon but suggest either a severe infection or perhaps an underlying host immunodeficiency. Pruritus is almost always present; pain may also be problem, especially if ulcers are present, and dyspareunia is a frequent presenting complaint.

One should not ignore the possibility of an ascending cervical infection leading to tubal or adnexal inflammation. This constellation of findings is known as pelvic inflammatory disease (PID). The main causative organisms are *Neisseria gonorrhoeae*, *Chlamydia trachomatis* and mixed aerobic-anaerobic infections. Thus, a clinician treating one of these causes of vulvovaginitis must be aware of its potential to ascend, causing cervicitis, endometritis and salpingitis. The clinical diagnosis of PID is notoriously difficult and the sequelae of a missed infection are serious, including chronic PID, chronic pelvic pain, infertility and tubal pregnancy. Thus, a high index of suspicion must be maintained and such patients evaluated in cooperation with a gynecologist.

Differential Diagnosis. We will consider the different infectious causes of vulvovaginitis, discussing the therapy under each agent. The diagnostic approach includes physical examination; microscopic evaluation of the discharge looking for clue cells, hyphae, bacteria and inflammatory cells; measurement of pH; identification of chlamydiae; and culture to exclude *Neisseria gonorrhoeae*.

One should exert every effort to arrive at an exact diagnosis enabling specific treatment. Table 35.2 lists the common causes. The history should include what hygiene products are used, sexual activity and problems in the partner. The initial examination in every patient should include a search for localized lesions, foreign objects and lymphadenopathy. A Papanicolaou smear should also be performed.

Therapy

Systemic. Specific, systemic antiinfectious agents are the ideal approach, once a specific diagnosis is obtained. Sometimes, when the inflammation is severe, even with an infectious trigger, short courses of systemic corticosteroids must be employed along with conservative topical measures.

Table 35.2. Common infectious causes of vaginal discharge

Disease	Discharge	Most likely sites	Diagnostic tools
Bacterial vaginosis	White, clear, watery	Vaginal wall	pH > 5.5 Fishy odor worsened when KOH added Direct observation of clue cells
Candidiasis	White, milky, cheesy or lumpy	Vaginal wall	Direct observation culture
Trichomoniasis	White, frothy, thin	Posterior vault, cervical os	Direct observation of *Trichomonas vaginalis* in wet mount
Chlamydia	Yellow-white, mucopurulent	Urethra, cervix, rectum	Direct identification of chlamydiae, culture
Gonorrhea	Yellow, purulent	Urethra, Bartholin glands, cervix, rectum, blood	Methylene blue or Gram stain, culture

Topical. Many of the infectious agents can also be treated topically. When no specific cause is identified, then bland topical management is required. The patient should avoid all irritating and sensitizing products. Wet-to-dry dressings with tap water or saline are good for cooling and débridement. If erosions are present, 0.1–0.3% gentian violet in water is effective. Zinc oil is soothing, nonsensitizing and often effective. External lesions generally can be treated with a low-potency corticosteroid cream or lotion, perhaps with 0.5% clioquinol added. Sitz baths or povidone-iodine douches may also be a nonspecific way to control the vaginal aspects of the problem.

Infectious Vulvovaginitis

Bacterial Vaginosis

Synonym. Nonspecific vaginitis

Definition. Common vaginal discharge, associated with variety of organisms and altered host response.

Causative Organisms. *Gardnerella vaginalis*, *Bacteroides* spp. and *Mobiluncus* spp.

Epidemiology. Bacterial vaginosis is the most common cause of vaginal discharge.

Etiology and Pathogenesis. All of the organisms that can be identified are also present in the normal vaginal flora, so they cannot be viewed as true pathogens. Quantitatively, they may be increased in certain cases. *Gardnerella vaginalis* is the most common member of the group, but other quasi-pathogens have also been studied. *Mobiluncus curtisii* is a comma-shaped anaerobe that forms ammonia; it was first identified in 1895 in vaginal secretions and has gone through many name changes.

Clinical Findings. The patients usually have minimal discharge but complain of the odor, which indeed is penetrating. On examination, the vaginal discharge tends to be gray and rich in small bubbles, also strongly suggesting the correct diagnosis. The clue cells are found on a wet mount; they are normal vaginal epithelial cells studded with bacteria, giving the cells a granular appearance. Mixed infections are common; cervical involvement suggests the presence of a second pathogen. In rare instances, *G. vaginalis* may be associated with genitourinary infections and postpartum fever. Several studies suggest an increased risk of preterm births in women with bacterial vaginosis, and others have shown that antibiotic therapy may reduce the risk of preterm labor in women with asymptomatic vaginal infections.

Laboratory Findings. Bacterial vaginosis is identified by the following characteristics:

- Thin, homogeneous milky discharge
- pH > 4.5 (> 6.0 highly suggestive)
- Fishy odor from the biogenic amines; altered by addition of 10% KOH
- Clue cells in native preparation

G. vaginalis is easily cultured, either on chocolate agar or Totten medium. A positive culture is of little value in making a diagnosis since the organism is part of the normal vaginal flora.

Therapy. Metronidazole 500 mg orally b.i.d. for 7 days is preferred. Clindamycin cream 2%, 5 g intravaginally nightly for 7 days or metronidazole cream or gel 0.75%, 5 g intravaginally b.i.d. for 5 days are also recommended. Suppositories or a vaginal gel designed to lower pH are other alternatives.

In pregnancy, bacterial vaginosis may be associated with premature delivery, so treatment is recommended using a lower dosage of metronidazole 250 mg t.i.d. for 7 days.

Candidiasis

Candidal vaginitis or, more often, vulvovaginitis is most common during pregnancy, in patients with diabetes mellitus and in those on long-term antibiotic therapy or oral contraceptives. Almost every woman has had at least one encounter with candidal vulvovaginitis. Most patients can recognize the cottage cheese-like discharge, with associated redness and burning. A partner with candidiasis can be the source of reinfection, although usually *Candida* is transferred from women to men. Because of the close proximity between the anus and female genitalia, sometimes reinfections occur from the gastrointestinal tract. This may provide a rationale for systemic therapy, but attempting to purge the bowel of *C. albicans*, a normal part of the intestinal flora, is controversial. Diagnosis is based on the cheesy discharge, positive KOH examination and normal pH; culture provides confirmation.

Over 90% of cultures reveal *C. albicans*, although *Candida glabrata* has also been identified.

Therapy. Imidazole creams or suppositories may be used once or twice daily for 1 week. Oral therapy with fluconazole 150 mg in a single dose is effective, as is treatment with short courses of itraconazole or ketoconazole. Weekly or bi-monthly systemic therapy may be considered for prophylaxis in persistent cases or in immunosuppressed patients.

Trichomoniasis

Trichomoniasis is a common infections discussed in greater detail in Chapter 6. The frothy discharge associated with *Trichomonas vaginalis* is distinctive. Pruritus is massive, and physical examination reveals tiny petechiae on the vaginal wall, the so-called strawberry spots. The male partner is also infected in about 40% of cases. In both sexes urethritis may occur. Direct examination of a wet mount using reduced-light, phase-contrast or dark-field techniques allows one to see the motile flagellated protozoa. The pH is 5.0–6.0, and many neutrophils are seen in the smear.

Therapy. Metronidazole 250 mg t.i.d. to 500 mg b.i.d. for 1 week or 2.0 g in a single dose is standard therapy. Oral tinidazole or nimorazole are also effective. A variety of antibiotic-antifungal combination creams have been employed, but are not as effective. The oral therapy is needed to eliminate foci of infection in the urethra and Skene glands.

Gonorrhea

Women often have asymptomatic gonorrhea, or develop proximal spread to produce salpingitis or even intraabdominal disease. They are at risk of disseminated disease, especially during pregnancy and menses. When a discharge is present, it is purulent and thick, just as with the urethral discharge in men. In small children, gonorrhea is particularly likely to cause vaginitis because the immature vaginal cells are more susceptible. Treatment is outlined in Chapter 5.

Chlamydial Vaginitis

Chlamydia trachomatis is a common cause of cervical infections, but rarely evolves into vulvovaginitis. The urethra and Bartholin glands are often involved. Ascending infection in women accounts for about half of all cases of pelvic inflammatory disease and may lead to infertility. Direct immunofluorescent examination of smears with monoclonal antibodies provides quick identification that is almost as accurate as culture.

Therapy. Tetracycline 250 mg q.i.d. or erythromycin 250 mg q.i.d. for 10 days is the standard treatment.

Vulvovaginitis in HIV/AIDS

Both trichomoniasis and bacterial vaginosis are more common in HIV/AIDS. While candidiasis is clearly more common in this patient group, studies have not supported routine HIV testing in patients with chronic candidal vulvovaginitis and no other risk factors. Prophylactic treatment with oral imidazoles is appropriate; it is usually already being used for oral candidiasis. The imidazoles interact with many of the antiretroviral agents, so caution is warranted. Large genital ulcers, similar to severe oral aphthae, are also a marker of HIV/AIDS and may respond to thalidomide.

Other Infections

A wide variety of other organisms can cause vaginitis. Primary bacterial infections caused by a single organism are uncommon. Desquamative inflammatory vaginitis has been described in perimenopausal women, with marked desquamation of vaginal cells and a purulent discharge rich in gram-positive cocci. Such patients may respond to topical clindamycin, but the exact nature of their disorder is unclear. In children *Escherichia coli* may be found, while in adults streptococcus, staphylococcus and mycoplasma are occasionally incriminated.

Noninfectious Vulvovaginitis

Chronic Vulvovaginitis

Chronic vulvovaginitis is not a primary infection but usually represents an interplay of many factors. Many older often overweight patients with diabetes mellitus have chronic genital pruritus. Incontinence or improper hygiene may play a contributing role. These postmenopausal patients also have a somewhat more resistant vaginal mucosa, so they too tend to have primarily vulvar problems. *C. albicans* is very often the most important cofactor. There may be tiny pustules with a collarette scale, extending to the mons pubis or the inner aspects of the thighs as a sign of the yeast infection. *C. albicans* may also be found in the vaginal secretions or feces. The pruritus and resultant scratching may produce a secondary bacterial folliculitis. Generally the most important step is a topical anticandidal therapy, either with an imidazole lotion or with a drying solution such as 0.1–0.3% gentian violet in water. In resistant cases, oral imidazoles may be used weekly for prophylaxis; a typical regimen is fluconazole 150 mg once weekly. Control of the diabetes mellitus is also important.

Vulvovaginitis in Infants

In children the two most common causes are foreign objects and *N. gonorrhoeae*. The vaginal epithelium in children is more easily infected with *N. gonorrhoeae* than in adults. Other causes may include irritating bubble baths, *Escherichia coli* and *Enterobius vermicularis*. Acute inflammation in this age group may produce labial adhesions, which should be separated. The physical examination may be difficult. Most often the vagina can not be viewed without causing the patient extreme physical and emotional distress. Sonography can exclude a foreign object. One should search for signs of sexual abuse, including tears, abrasions or even a lax anal sphincter. Cultures for *N. gonorrhoeae* and perhaps *E. coli* are appropriate. Treatment is as in adults.

Atrophic Vaginitis

Following menopause the vagina undergoes several changes, as the epithelium becomes thinner and the pH rises. This favors a shift towards primarily gram-negative bacteria, so some clinicians consider this a bacterial disorder. Most patients are asymptomatic, but some may experience discharge, dyspareunia and spotting. The discharge is usually watery, with a pH of 5.0–7.0, while smears show neutrophils. There is often associated vulvar atrophy.

Therapy. Topical estrogen creams are the simplest approach. Applying a small amount with a vaginal applicator nightly for 2 weeks usually brings relief. Recurrences may suggest the need for systemic estrogen replacement.

Irritant Vulvovaginitis

Even when no infection is present, there may be marked vaginal discharge, burning, pain and irritated vulvar skin. In children, foreign objects must be excluded. In the elderly, a forgotten pessary may be the problem, but more often it is an overlooked tumor. A wide variety of products designed for vaginal use are potentially irritating; they include povidone-iodine, other douches, spermicides, topical antimycotic agents, soaps, perfumes, tampons, sanitary napkins and many other products. In children, bubble baths are often incriminated. Allergic contact dermatitis may develop; the most likely causes are latex condoms and topical medications.

Psychosomatic Vaginitis

Some patients who complain of a chronic vaginal discharge either have excessive physiologic secretions or have normal secretions to which they are reacting in an abnormal way. In either case, the physical examination and laboratory evaluation are normal. Both vulvar pruritus and vulvodynia may be complaints. These problems are considered in more detail below.

Other Vulvar Diseases

Aphthae

(Lipschütz 1918)

Synonym. Ulcus vulvae acutum

Etiology and Pathogenesis. Lipschütz blamed these lesions on *Bacillus grassus*, which was later identified as the Döderlein bacillus. Today, it is more honest to say we do not know the cause or causes of aphthae (Chap. 33). In some instances, they may be one of the manifestations of Behçet disease.

Clinical Findings. Several types of genital aphthae have been described. The gangrenous lesions are today still occasionally called Lipschütz disease. Large very painful rapidly growing ulcerations with a gray necrotic crust develop on the labia minora and may cause perforation. They are associated with fever and lymphadenopathy and may scar. Recurrence is unlikely. It seems reasonable to continue searching for an infectious cause of this type of ulceration and to separate it from the other types.

In the chronic form, small yellow ulcers with a red periphery arise on the mucosa of the introitus, labia minora and inner aspect of the labia majora. They tend to be associated with relatively few symptoms other than local pain and to recur. The lesions may become larger and have undermined edges (Fig. 35.1). In contrast, in the miliary form, the lesions are 2–3 mm in size, rarely expand and are more likely to involve the labia majora. They are equivalent to oral aphthae.

Histopathology. Biopsies are a disappointing approach. They may on occasion show signs of herpes simplex virus infection, aiding in the differential diagnosis.

Differential Diagnosis. When dealing with genital aphthae, attempts at isolation of viral and bacterial agents are worthwhile. Herpes simplex infections should be excluded, as their treatment is totally different. Occasionally acute genital ulcers may be associated with bacterial infections such as typhoid fever, viral infections such as Epstein-Barr virus, hand-foot-and-mouth disease and *Mycoplasma* as part of an erythema multiforme reaction. In addition, one should exclude inflammatory bowel disease and search for other signs of Behçet syndrome. A biopsy will help if individual lesions are persistent, in order to exclude an ulcerated tumor or Langerhans cell histiocytosis.

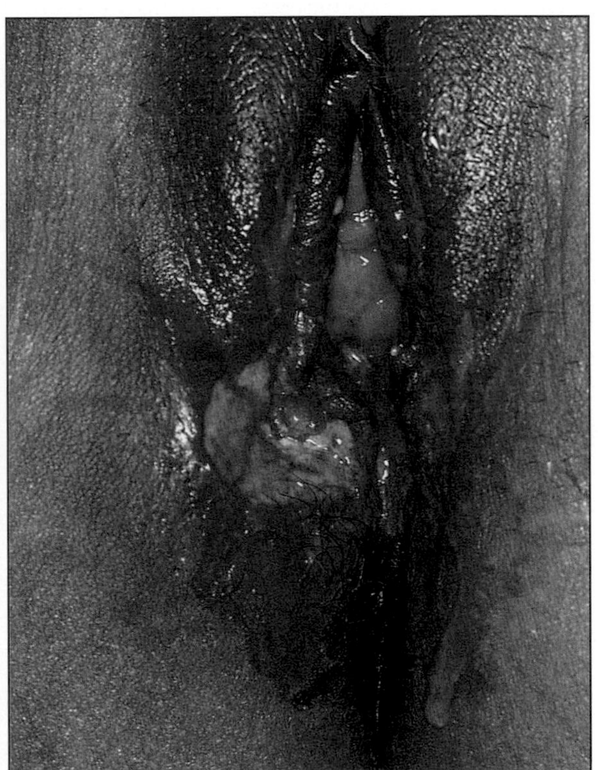

Fig. 35.1. Behçet disease

Therapy. Our approach to aphthae is discussed in Chapter 33. Vulvar lesions are often more severe and more painful, so that systemic corticosteroids may be necessary. Topical measures may include drying lotions or solutions, topical anesthetics and mild topical antibiotics such as zinc paste with clioquinol.

Blistering Disorders

Bullous diseases (Chap. 15) may have prominent vulvar involvement. In rare instances, patients may present with vulvar erosions or, less often, blisters. More often they present with pruritus, pain, crusts and secondary infections. Pemphigus vegetans almost always affects the vulva, while pemphigus vulgaris may also do so. The possibility of vaginal involvement should be considered. Herpes gestationis may also produce vulvar lesions. In addition, childhood bullous diseases frequently affect the genital region. Darier disease and Hailey-Hailey disease (Chap. 17) typically include vulvar lesions. Localized acantholytic and dyskeratotic disease of the vulva may be a variant of one of these disorders. Finally, both lichen planus and erythema multiforme may also have vulvar blisters or erosions.

Vulvar Edema

Swelling of the vulva may present diagnostic difficulties. Acute swelling may represent angioedema, perhaps caused by trauma or triggered by sensitivity to semen or latex. Crohn disease occasionally presents with vulvar edema. Acute infections such as herpes simplex may initially lack ulcerations and only produce swelling. Lymphedema may be associated with recurrent erysipelas, primary syphilis (edema indurativum), lymphogranuloma venereum, granuloma inguinale, filariasis or other infections.

Senile Vulvar Atrophy

Etiology and Pathogenesis. About 15% of postmenopausal or postoopherectomy women develop hormone-dependent genital atrophy. It is an exaggeration of the normal physiologic changes that occur in all hormone-dependent tissues.

Clinical Findings. The clitoris, labia minora and inner aspects of the labia majora shrink. There is no sclerosis. While labial adhesions may develop, they are not pronounced. White areas are not present. While the vaginal epithelium is usually perceived as dry, sometimes there may be vaginal discharge, known as atrophic vaginitis. The pubic hairs may turn gray and are usually diminished in number. Sometimes the cutanous dryness leads to pruritus.

Histopathology. The epithelium shows thinning and the connective tissue is also atrophic, although this is harder to see on a routine biopsy. The main purpose of the biopsy is to exclude lichen sclerosus et atrophicus.

Differential Diagnosis. One must be aware of normal or almost normal atrophy in order to sensibly interpret the vulvar dystrophies.

Therapy. One should work together with the patient's gynecologist. Topical estrogen products are helpful for both the external genitalia and the vagina. In some instances, systemic replacement therapy is more practical.

Vulvar Dystrophies

The standard terminology for localized vulvar lesions (Table 35.3) adopted by the International Society for the Study of Vulvar Diseases (ISSVD) reflects gynecologic attitudes and is rarely used by dermatologists. One should be aware of the terms and attempt to use them, perhaps as synonyms, when communicating with nondermatologists. The dermatologic terms of chronic dermatitis, lichen simplex chronicus, lichen sclerosus et atrophicus and carcinoma in situ are just as accurate. One can also use leukoplakia, erythroplasia and melanoplakia to describe individual lesions (Chap. 34; see Table 34.2)

Lichen Sclerosus et Atrophicus

Synonyms. Lichen sclerosus, kraurosis vulvae

Lichen sclerosus et atrophicus is discussed in Chapter 18. Only the gynecologic aspects will be repeated here.

Clinical Findings. The wide variety of names reflects the varying presentations: as white patches, as vulvar atrophy with adhesions, or as shrinkage and hardening of the introitus with dyspareunia. The disease is most common in premenarchal and postmenopausal women, but can affect all ages. Young patients tend to have white lesions, often in an hourglass pattern involving the genitalia, perineum and perianal area (Fig. 35.2). There may be hemorrhage or tears; these suggest child abuse. In older patients, atrophy and sclerosis are more prominent. Fine hemorrhagic lesions and telangiectases are common; occasionally bullous lesions will have larger hemorrhagic areas, especially after trauma. Sometimes the underlying fat becomes more apparent, imparting a yellow tone. Just as lichen sclerosus et atrophicus is often overlooked as a cause of phimosis, it may not be appreciated in patients complaining of dyspareunia, narrowing of the introitus, labial atrophy or adhe-

Table 35.3. Vulvar dystrophies

ISSVD[a] terminology	Equivalent dermatologic terminology
Lichen sclerosus	Lichen sclerosus et atrophicus
Other dermatoses	The many disorders discussed in this book
Squamous cell hyperplasia	
Benign (hyperplasia without atypia)	Most closely corresponds to lichen simplex chronicus
Mixed	Combination of two or more of the above
Neoplastic (hyperplasia with atypia)	Carcinoma in situ or vulvar intraepithelial neoplasia (VIN)

[a] International Society for the Study of Vulvar Diseases

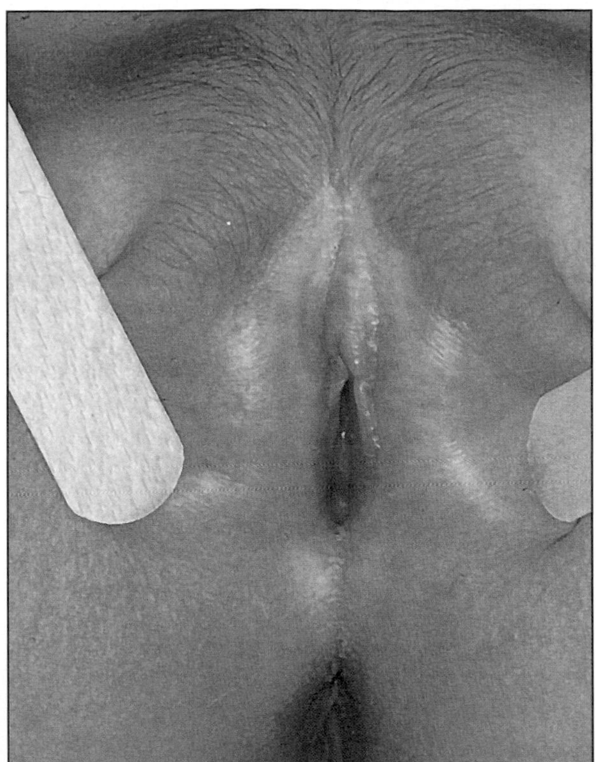

Fig. 35.2. Lichen sclerosus et atrophicus

sions. Because of dryness and pruritus, secondary lichenification is common. In chronic cases, thickened areas may represent premalignant change; this was formerly known as kraurosis. In both adults and children, melanocytic nevi and even rare malignant melanomas have been described in areas of lichen sclerosus et atrophicus.

Histopathology. The epidermis is atrophic. In the dermis there is initially a lichenoid infiltrate and marked hyalinization of the upper dermis. The main purposes of biopsy are to confirm the presence of lichen sclerosus et atrophicus and to exclude premalignant or malignant change.

Differential Diagnosis. All the forms of vulvar dystrophy and senile vulvar atrophy should be considered.

Therapy. There is no totally satisfactory treatment. High-potency topical corticosteroids or intralesional corticosteroids are probably the most effective agents, although they potentially can exaggerate the atrophy. Intralesional injections of triamcinolone acetonide 2.5–5.0 mg/ml in a local anesthetic give the most rapid relief, although they are painful. Topical hormone-containing products are more popular in the genital region. Both topical estrogen and testosterone are occasionally successful, but their use has not been supported by a large study. In Europe, heparincontaining creams are also tried.

Chronic Vulvar Dermatitis

Synonym. Hypertrophic vulvar dystrophy

Etiology and Pathogenesis. A number of dermatoses may be more severe in, or largely limited to, the vulvar region. Atopic dermatitis is the most common disorder, but psoriasis, seborrheic dermatitis, lichen planus and others should be considered. In addition, patients with pruritus vulvae may show similar changes in the absence of a clearly defined underlying disorder.

Clinical Findings. The normal vulvar skin is thin and easily injured. The itch-scratch cycle is particularly difficult to break in this region. Lichenification occurs readily with both localized hyperkeratotic plaques and diffuse change (Fig. 35.3). One should search carefully for clinical stigmata of atopic dermatitis or other inflammatory skin diseases. In atopic dermatitis, the vulva is usually red and the inflammation may spread to involve the inner aspects of the upper thighs. The anal and perineal regions may also be involved. The labia majora can become very thickened, edematous and slightly everted; in French this variant is known as *lichénification géante*. When the labia minora are exposed, they lose some of their mucosal features, becoming enlarged, dry and partially keratinized. Recurrent erysipelas, sometimes associated with herpes simplex, may produce similar changes. While the lichen simplex chronicus changes are included as vulvar dystrophy, they are not premalignant. One must distinguish between annoying but harmless diffuse lichenification and a focal hyperkeratotic plaque, which can represent carcinoma in situ.

Histopathology. The epidermis is hyperkeratotic and acanthotic but without atypia. There may be spongiosis and parakeratosis. In the dermis there is a lymphocytic perivascular infiltrate with exocytosis. The main purpose of the biopsy is, in the early stages, to exclude specific inflammatory

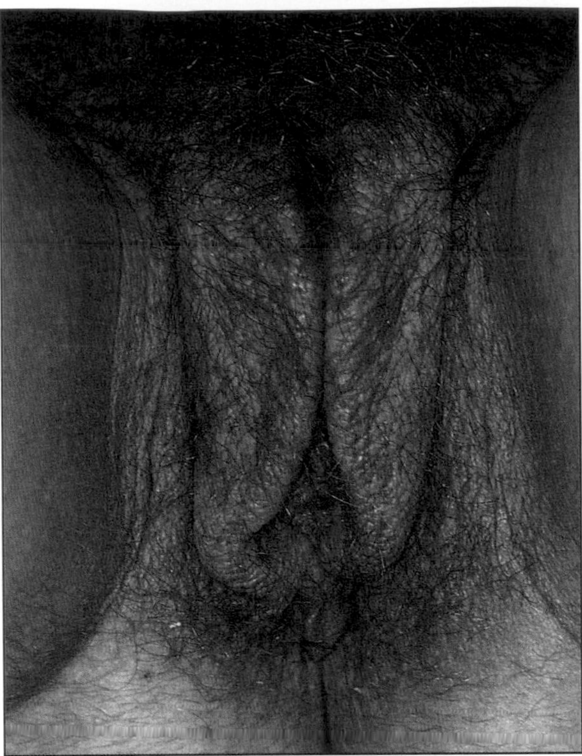

Fig. 35.3. Chronic atopic vulvar dermatitis

disorders and, in late forms, to rule out malignant changes.

Differential Diagnosis. Fungal infections of the groin are most uncommon in women, but can be excluded by KOH examination and culture. Erythrasma may also involve the groin and external genitalia; Wood light examination is helpful. Allergic contact dermatitis can be excluded via patch testing, paying particular attention to female hygiene products, condoms, spermicides and similar products.

Therapy. Treatment is discussed below under pruritus vulvae and in the various sections dealing with the individual dermatoses.

Vulvar Carcinoma In Situ

The diagnosis of vulvar carcinoma is often made at a late stage. This is inexcusable, since most women have a yearly genital examination. Carcinoma in situ can take several forms, listed in Table 35.4. The considerations are identical to those discussed for men (Chap. 34) and will not be repeated in detail. Bowenoid papulosis of the female genitalia is illustrated in Figure 35.4. Any persistent red, white or dark patch or plaque should be biopsied, if any clinical questions exist.

Other Vulvar Lesions

Human Papilloma Virus Infections

Human papilloma virus (HPV) infections of the female genitalia are common and in some instances quite serious. As discussed in Chapter 2, certain HPV types (especially 16 and 18) are clearly carcinogenic when they infect the cervix. There are several fairly distinct clinical patterns. When the labia majora are infected, the lesions are identical to cutaneous warts. If the mucosal surfaces of the labia minora are involved, then typically condylomata accuminata, soft moist velvety lesions, are seen. They may extend to the perineum and perianal region, or into the vagina. As discussed above, some people consider hirsuties papillaris vulvae to be microcondylomata and not an anatomic variant. HPV has not been convincingly demonstrated in these tiny lesions, also called microwarts. Some clinicians feel that their ablation is helpful in treating vulvodynia.

Table 35.4. Carcinoma in situ of the female genitalia

Disease	Clinical features	Location	Histology
Bowenoid papulosis, lichenoid lesions	Lichenoid papules	Labia minora	Carcinoma in situ, lichenoid infiltrates
Bowenoid papulosis, pigmented lesions	Pigmented seborrheic keratosis-like lesions	Labia majora	Carcinoma in situ, increased melanin
Bowen disease	Red scaly patch	Labia majora, adjacent skin	Carcinoma in situ
Erythroplasia of Queyrat	Red moist patch	Labia minora, introitus	Carcinoma in situ
Leukoplakia	White patch	Labia minora, introitus	Many patterns; rarely carcinoma in situ

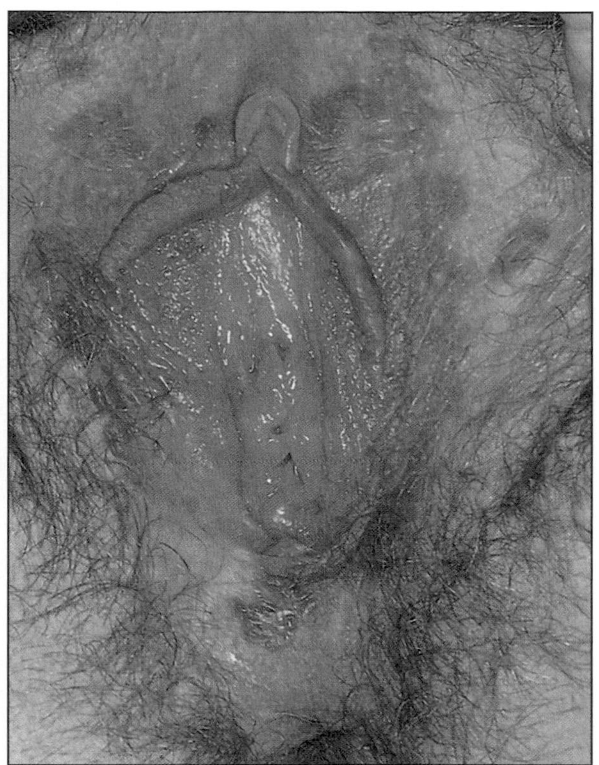

Fig. 35.4. Bowenoid papulosis, pigmented lesions

Plasma Cell Vulvitis

Synonym. Zoon vulvitis. See Chapter 34 for a discussion of the many terms used for this disorder.

The moist red patch of plasma cell mucositis may involve the inner aspect of the labia majora, the labia minora or even the vaginal mucosa. It rarely has specific clinical features and is frequently mistaken for erythroplasia. The diagnosis is made on biopsy. The therapy is as unrewarding as for Zoon balanitis. Some clinicians equate this entity with chronic vestibulitis.

Vulvar Melanotic Macule

Genital melanotic macules are more common in women than men and cause far more alarm. They are usually identified by family physicians or gynecologists who are not familiar with the entity and immediately suggest malignant melanoma. The most common location is the labia minora, often extending to the vestibule. Typically the macule is tan to brown, several centimeters in diameter and irregular in shape. Multiple lesions can be seen. Microscopic examination shows increased melanin in the basal layer and no melanocytic proliferation.

Angiokeratomas

Multiple small dark papules on the labia majora are usually angiokeratomas (Chap. 59). Sometimes a large or thrombosed angiokeratoma can be mistaken for a malignant melanoma. Histologic examination clarifies the situation.

Vulvar Pruritus and Pain

The entire topic of vulvar pruritus, burning and pain is a confusing one. Only in the past few years has any attempt been made to systemically study the disorders. Their classification is in its infancy. Some authors separate pruritus vulvae and vulvodynia, but we find the conditions frequently overlap. Pruritus vulvae involves itching of the external genitalia, the labia majora and perineum. In contrast, vulvodynia describes chronic vulvar pain or burning. One could consider the name introitodynia, for when one takes an accurate history, often there is a tender spot in the vestibule or on the labia minora or there is severe pain when the penis is inserted in intercourse.

Pruritus Vulvae

Definition. Pruritus of the female external genitalia with an itch-scratch cycle.

Etiology and Pathogenesis. There are many causes of pruritus vulvae, as shown in Table 35.5. We have discussed these problems under chronic vulvar dermatitis. We prefer to use the term pruritus vulvae to refer to the difficult cases in which there are no physical findings. Many such patients are depressed or have other emotional problems.

Clinical Findings. The unifying feature is the itch-scratch cycle, often producing lichen simplex chronicus. Almost all patients complaining of pruritus vulvae have some visible changes involving their labia majora. Most often, by the time the patient comes to the dermatologist the labia majora are at least somewhat swollen and lichenified and few clues as to the underlying disorder are seen. The labia minora may be thickened and dry; they are converted from mucosal structures to

Table 35.5. Selected causes of pruritus vulvae

Category	Examples
Pruritic dermatoses	Mycotic infections, especially candidiasis Irritant and allergic contact dermatitis Atopic dermatitis Infestations (scabies, pediculosis pubis) Lichen sclerosus et atrophicus Lichen simplex chronicus
Vaginal discharge	An forms of vulvovaginitis
Anal disorders	Pinworms Hemorrhoids Irritating foods
Underlying disorders	Diabetes mellitus Renal disease Many others
Excessive cleansing	
Vulvodynia	
Psychologic causes	

transitional ones. One should search carefully for other signs of an underlying disease. Often other body regions can offer clues: the antecubital fossae in atopic dermatitis or the oral mucosa in lichen planus.

Histopathology. Biopsy may disclose an overlooked disorder. In addition, it may reassure a patient that there is no sign of malignancy. In most cases, there is simply epidermal acanthosis and hyperkeratosis with nonspecific dermal perivascular infiltrates.

Therapy. The most important aspect of therapy is taking the patient's problem seriously. One should take a complete history, do a complete physical examination searching diligently for clues, order reasonable laboratory tests and try to display sympathy and understanding. If one immediately says, "Oh, there is nothing seriously wrong. Here is a prescription for something to stop the itching," most patients will be disappointed and the emotional component of their disease exacerbated.

If an underlying disorder is identified, it should be treated. If not, the first rule is to stop all topical treatments. Only tap water should be used for cleansing. If the patient claims this is too irritating, then mineral oil or zinc oil can be suggested. All feminine hygiene products, douches, bubble baths and soaps should be discontinued. The patient should be encouraged to wear loose-fitting, absorbent, perhaps cotton, undergarments. To reduce the risk of irritation from laundry products, a double-rinse cycle can be recommended.

If the patient has not been treated with topical corticosteroids, it is worth trying a mid- to high-potency corticosteroid cream or lotion, once daily for a maximum of 2 weeks, using a bland emollient the rest of the time. One can then switch to a low-potency corticosteroid such as hydrocortisone for another limited period. Most patients have already been treated with corticosteroids. Many will have evidence of corticosteroid-induced rosacea-like changes and will experience a rebound in their pruritus when the products are stopped.

Topical anesthetics are useful, but one should avoid the entire "caine" family, both because they have so often already been used and because of their potential to cause allergic contact dermatitis. We usually recommend pramoxine (in the USA) or polidocanol (in Europe); both can be combined with low-potency corticosteroids. Empirical topical and systemic anticandidal therapy is often tried but rarely brings lasting relief.

Systemic antihistamines can be prescribed, preferably an old soporific product, not a new non-sedating version. The patient should be encouraged to take this medication each evening for at least a week to see whether any benefit is obtained. Depending on the dermatologist's training, he may want to prescribe antidepressive agents or work with a another physician to accomplish this.

Vulvodynia

Definition. Vulvar burning, irritation or pain, usually associated with dyspareunia.

Etiology and Pathogenesis. A long list of causes for vulvodynia is presented in many textbooks. Clearly one should exclude potentially painful dermatologic disorders, such as herpes simplex infection, aphthae, blistering diseases and lichen planus. But in most cases, vulvodynia is a primary complaint without any accompanying physical findings. Rare patients with urticaria and dermographism have vulvodynia, so this should be checked. In our experience, such patients are unlikely to have dermatologic disease and far more likely to have emotional or psychosomatic problems.

Clinical Findings. The patient complains of burning or pain. The patient will almost always correct a remark such as "How long have you been itching?", sometimes quite impatiently. One should examine the introitus and vestibule painstakingly, searching for tiny erosions or ulcers, as well as erythematous patches. Usually nothing is found. If there is exquisite tenderness in the vestibule coupled with a history of pain on entering during intercourse, vestibulitis should be suspected. In pudendal neuralgia and other perineal pain syndromes, there are no skin findings.

Histopathology. Biopsy may once again reveal an overlooked diagnosis. Some clinicians recommend performing a direct immunofluorescent examination as well, in order to identify a latent bullous disorder, but we suspect that biopsy primarily serves to reassure.

Course and Prognosis. The outlook is dismal. Patients with vulvodynia bounce from doctor to doctor, desperately seeking aid.

Therapy. The general guidelines suggested above for pruritus vulvae also apply here, but topical treatment is rarely helpful and is often refused by the patient. The anxiolytic antidepressive agent amitriptyline, 30–50 mg daily, is occasionally helpful, as are benzodiazepines.

Vulvar Vestibulitis

Etiology and Pathogenesis. The causes of vulvar vestibulitis are poorly categorized. Many physicians do not consider this a diagnostic entity. Firm believers often list trauma, HPV infection and candidiasis as causes, but therapy directed at HPV and *Candida* rarely produces a cure. Most designate vestibulitis as an idiopathic disorder.

Clinical Findings. Features of vestibulitis include pain on entry during intercourse, tenderness to touch and focal erythema. The erythema may be confined to the orifices of the Bartholin, Skene and/or minor vestibular glands. In many instances, it is unclear whether minor variations in mucosal color play a pathophysiologic role. The pain may also be reproduced by other trauma, such as riding a bicycle or wearing tight pants.

Histopathology. There are normally only minimal inflammatory changes, sometimes centered around the vestibular glands. No epithelial changes are found. If an intense plasma cell infiltrate is present, then plasma cell mucositis (Zoon vulvitis) should be considered. The inner aspect of the labia minora is the most common site for Zoon disease in women. Some gynecologists equate plasma cell mucositis and chronic vestibulitis.

Therapy. Treating HPV and *C. albicans* rarely brings lasting relief. Topical anesthetics, including EMLA, have been recommended. Some patients have responded to intralesional interferon or laser ablation, but others have developed worse symptoms. Even limited excision of the vestibule has been recommended. There is no good solution.

Pudendal Neuralgia

Etiology and Pathogenesis. Nerve damage, such as that following zoster, related to nerve injuries or perhaps associated with small tumors or vascular lesions pressing upon the pudendal nerve, seems to be the unifying feature. In most cases there is no clear history of injury or of zoster. Imaging studies are frequently negative.

Clinical Findings. There are no cutaneous findings. The pain is unprovoked, often associated with extreme tenderness, typically involving the perineum and the inner aspects of the thighs. This corresponds to the distribution of the pudendal nerve. When the patients are examined, they have pain responses out of proportion to the stimulus. Just touching the pubic hairs may evoke exquisite pain. Light touch with a cotton-tipped applicator may lead to prolonged diffuse pain. Allodynia or burning pain may also be present; the clitoris is frequently so involved.

Differential Diagnosis. Other types of perineal pain may have muscular and neurologic components, but lack the sensory changes described with pudendal neuralgia.

Therapy. Most dermatologists will not be diagnosing or treating pudendal neuralgia. A wide variety of psychotherapeutic and antiseizure medications have been employed. In addition, nerve blocks, biofeedback techniques, acupuncture and transepidermal nerve stimulation have helped individual patients.

Endometriosis

Definition. Presence of ectopic endometrial mucosa

Epidemiology. Endometriosis is common, present in at least 25% of infertile women and many others. Cutaneous endometriosis is rare, seen in less than 1% of patients.

Etiology and Pathogenesis. Most endometriosis is confined to the genital tract, as ectopic tissue migrates into the Fallopian tubes and even ovaries. The same tissue may spread to the rest of the abdominal cavity and even appear in the umbilicus as cutaneous nodules. There may also be vascular or lymphatic spread. Following gynecologic surgery, there may be seeding to the abdominal cavity or cutaneous scars.

Clinical Findings. The typical cutaneous finding is a blue tender nodule, often in the vicinity of the umbilicus (Fig. 35.5), which varies in size or tenderness with the menstrual cycle. Menstrual pain, dyspareunia and infertility are the most common gynecologic complaints.

Histopathology. Biopsy of a cutaneous lesion shows typical glandular and stromal tissue of the endometrium lying within the dermis.

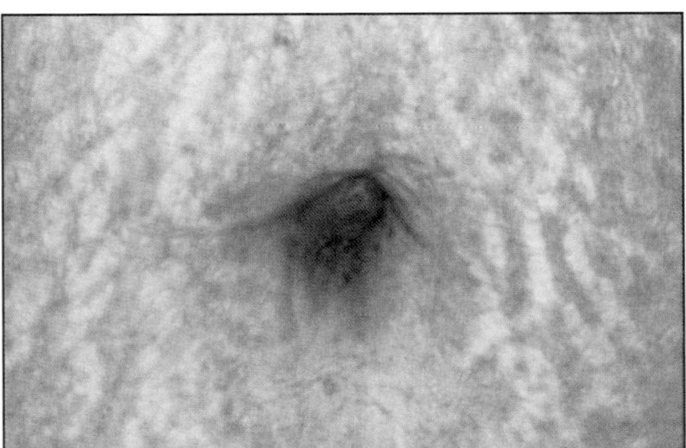

Fig. 35.5. Endometriosis involving umbilicus

Course and Prognosis. The cutaneous lesions continue to wax and wane until identified. More widespread involvement is a significant cause of pain and distress.

Differential Diagnosis. The cutaneous differential diagnosis includes almost any painful tumor, but the key feature is the monthly variation, which is almost diagnostic.

Therapy. Individual cutaneous lesions can be excised. With widespread disease, the choice lies between surgery and suppression of endometrial function. Danazol is the most commonly employed agent; it is usually used in dosages of 400–800 mg daily for 6 months.

Bibliography

Review Articles

Heller DS, Randolph P, Young A et al. (1997) The cutaneous-vulvar clinic revisited: a 5-year experience of the Columbia Presbyterian Medical Center Cutaneous-Vulvar Service. Dermatology 195:26–29

Leibowitch M, Staughton R, Neill S et al. (eds) (1997) An atlas of vulval disease, 2nd edn. Dunitz, London

Kamarashev JA, Vassileva SG (1997) Dermatologic diseases of the vulva. Clin Dermatol 15:53–65

Mardh PA (1991) The vaginal ecosystem. Am J Obstet Gynecol 165:1163–1168

Ridley CM (ed) (1988) The vulva. Churchill Livingstone, London

Turner ML (1992) Vulvar manifestations of systemic diseases. Dermatol Clin 10:445–458

Congenital Abnormalities

Hyman AB, Guiducci AA (1963) Ectopic sebaceous glands. In: Montagna W, Ellis RA, Silver AF (eds) Advances in biology of the skin, vol 4. Pergamon, London, pp 78–93

Khoda H, Hino Y, Fukuda H (1986) Hirsutoid papillomas of vulva. J Dermatol 13:154–156

Moyal-Barraco M, Leibowitch M, Orth G (1990) Vestibular papillae of the vulva. Arch Dermatol 126: 1594–1598

Vulvovaginitis

Easmon CS, Hay PE, Ison CA (1992) Bacterial vaginosis: a diagnostic approach. Genitourin Med 68:134–138

Elmer GW, Surawicz CM, McFarland LV (1996) Biotherapeutic agents. A neglected modality for the treatment and prevention of selected intestinal and vaginal infections. JAMA 275:870–876

Elsner P, Maibach HI (1989) Microbiology of specialized skin: the vulva. Semin Dermatol 8:300–304

Hay PE (1998) Therapy of bacterial vaginosis. J Antimicrob Chemother 41:6–9

Hay PE, Taylor-Robinson D (1996) Defining bacterial vaginosis: to BV or not to BV, that is the question. Int J STD AIDS 7:233–235
McKay M (1989) Vulvitis and vulvovaginitis: cutaneous considerations. Am J Obstet Gynecol 165:1176–1182
Sobel JD (1998) Vulvovaginitis. When *Candida* becomes a problem. Dermatol Clin 16:763–768
Sobel JD (1997) Vaginitis. N Engl J Med 337:1896–1903
Taylor-Robinson D, Furr PM (1998) Update on sexually transmitted mycoplasmas. Lancet 351 [Suppl 3]:12–15

Senile Vulvar Atrophy

Samsioe G (1998) Urogenital aging – a hidden problem. Am J Obstet Gynecol 178:S245–S249

Other Vulvar Diseases

Lampert A, Assier-Bonnet H, Chevailler B et al. (1996) Lipschütz's genital ulceration: a manifestation of Epstein-Barr virus primary infection. Br J Dermatol 135: 663–665
Lipschütz B (1918) Über Ulcus vulvae acutum. Wien Klin Wochenschr 31:461–464
Wong KK, Lin HP, Looi LM (1992) Histiocytosis X and vulvar ulceration. Int J Gynaecol Obstet 39:131–134
Vettraino IM, Merritt DF (1995) Crohn's disease of the vulva. Am J Dermatopathol 17:410–413

Vulvar Dystrophies

Ambros RA, Malfetano JH, Carlson JA et al. (1997) Non-neoplastic epithelial alterations of the vulva: recognition, assessment and comparisons of terminologies used among the various specialties. Mod Pathol 10: 401–408
Ayhan A, Tuncer ZS, Kaya H (1997) Vulvar dystrophy: an evaluation of 285 cases. Eur J Gynaecol Oncol 18: 139–140
Leibowitch M, Neill S, Pelisse M et al. (1990) The epithelial changes associated with squamous cell carcinoma of the vulva: a review of the clinical, histological and viral findings in 78 women. Br J Obstet Gynaecol 97: 1135–1139
Lewis FM (1998) Vulval lichen planus. Br J Dermatol 138: 569–575
Voet RL (1994) Classification of vulvar dystrophies and premalignant squamous lesions. J Cutan Pathol 21: 86–90

Lichen Sclerosus et Atrophicus

Bert-Jones, Graham-Brown RA, Barns DA (1991) Lichen sclerosus et atrophicans – a review of 15 cases in young girls. Clin Exp Dermatol 16:14–17
Fischer G, Rogers M (1997) Treatment of childhood vulvar lichen sclerosus with potent topical corticosteroid. Pediatr Dermatol 14:235–238
Hallel-Halevy D, Grunwald MH, Yerushalmi J et al. (1998) Bullous lichen sclerosus et atrophicus. J Am Acad Dermatol 39:500–501
Kartamaa M, Reitamo S (1997) Treatment of lichen sclerosus with carbon dioxide laser vaporization. Br J Dermatol 136:356–359
Marren P, Walkden V, Mallon E et al. (1996) Vulval cicatricial pemphigoid may mimic lichen sclerosus. Br J Dermatol 134:522–524
Thomas RH, Ridley CM, McGibbon DH et al. (1996) Anogenital lichen sclerosus in women. J R Soc Med 89: 694–698
Wakelin SH, Marren P (1997) Lichen sclerosus in women. Clin Dermatol 15:155–169

Vulvar Dermatitis

Kint B, Degreef H, Dooms-Goossens A (1994) Combined allergy to human seminal plasma and latex: case report and review of the literature. Contact Dermatitis 30: 7–11
Lewis FM, Shah M, Gawkrodger DJ (1997) Contact sensitivity in pruritus vulvae: patch test results and clinical outcome. Am J Contact Dermat 8:137–140
Lucke TW, Fleming CJ, McHenry P et al. (1998) Patch testing in vulval dermatoses: how relevant is nickel? Contact Dermatitis 38:111–112
Marren P, Wojnarowska F (1996) Dermatitis of the vulva. Semin Dermatol 15:36–41
Pincus SH (1992) Vulvar dermatoses and pruritus vulvae. Dermatol Clin 10:297–308

Vulvar Carcinoma

Crum CP, McLachlin CM, Tate JE et al. (1997) Pathobiology of vulvar squamous neoplasia. Curr Opin Obstet Gynecol 9:63–69
Lewis FM, Harrington CI (1994) Squamous cell carcinoma arising in vulval lichen planus. Br J Dermatol 131:703–705
Wagner W, Prott FJ, Weissmann J et al. (1999) Vulvar carcinoma: a retrospective analysis of 80 patients. Arch Gynecol Obstet 262:99–104
Wilkinson EJ (1992) Normal histology and nomenclature of the vulva, and malignant neoplasms, including VIN. Dermatol Clin 10:283–296
Zaki I, Dalziel KL, Solomonsz FA et al. (1996) The under-reporting of skin disease in association with squamous cell carcinoma of the vulva. Clin Exp Dermatol 21: 334–337

Plasma Cell Vulvitis

Kavanagh GM, Burton PA, Kennedy CT (1993) Vulvitis chronica plasmacellularis (Zoon's vulvitis). Br J Dermatol 129:92–93
Salopek TG, Siminoski K (1996) Vulvitis circumscripta plasmacellularis (Zoon's vulvitis) associated with autoimmune polyglandular endocrine failure. Br J Dermatol 135:991–994

Pruritus Vulvae and Vulvodynia

Baggish MS, Miklos JR (1995) Vulvar pain syndrome: a review. Obstet Gynecol Surv 50:618–627
Fischer G, Spurrett B, Fischer A (1995) The chronically symptomatic vulva: aetiology and management. Br J Obstet Gynaecol 102:773–779
Metts JF (1999) Vulvodynia and vulvar vestibulitis: challenges in diagnosis and management. Am Fam Physician 59:1547–1556, 1561–1562
McKay M (1992) Vulvodynia. Diagnostic patterns. Dermatol Clin 10:423–433
Mroczkowski TF(1998) Vulvodynia – a dermatovenereologist's perspective. Int J Dermatol 37:567–569

Ridley CM (1998) Vulvodynia. Theory and management. Dermatol Clin 16:775–778
Paavonen J (1995) Vulvodynia – a complex syndrome of vulvar pain. Acta Obstet Gynecol Scand 74:243–247

Endometriosis

Brosens IA (1998) Endometriosis. Current issues in diagnosis and medical management. J Reprod Med 43:281–286
Reddy S, Rock JA (1998) Treatment of endometriosis. Clin Obstet Gynecol 41:387–392
Sampson JA (1921) Perforating hemorrhagic (chocolate) cysts of the ovary. Their importance and especially their relation to pelvic adenomas of endometrial type ("adenomyoma" of the uterus, rectovaginal septum, sigmoid etc.). Arch Surg 3:245–323
Schenken RS (1998) Modern concepts of endometriosis. Classification and its consequences for therapy. J Reprod Med 43:269–275

Skin Diseases in Pregnancy

Contents

During pregnancy, there are multiple significant metabolic, hormonal, and immunologic changes that produce cutaneous manifestations. When evaluating a pregnant patient with skin findings, one should remember several rules. Most skin disorders during pregnancy represent either physiologic changes or other skin diseases that have simply appeared in pregnancy. All therapies, topical and systemic, should be reconsidered in light of the pregnancy. The evaluation of all papulosquamous eruptions should include serologic testing for syphilis; to miss secondary syphilis in pregnancy would be a major error.

Physiologic Changes

The most common change is hyperpigmentation involving the areolae, labia minora, and especially the linea alba, which turns grayish black and is then called the linea nigra or linea fusca. Areas of marked friction such as the axillae, perineum, and medial aspects of the thighs also darken. Melasma is common. The increased estrogen and progesterone levels are most likely responsible for these changes; melanocyte-stimulating hormone (MSH) levels are not elevated, as was previously suggested. The most disturbing change for patients is striae gravidarum, or stretch marks. Both striae and the pigmentary changes are generally permanent.

A variety of vascular changes also occur, including palmar erythema and spider angiomas. Both tend to regress or disappear after pregnancy. Occasionally, more permanent vascular proliferations may also appear, including telangiectases and small hemangiomas. Pregnancy gingivitis is common and often associated with pyogenic granulomas of the gingiva, which are common enough to be known as pregnancy tumors. Varicosities are more common, both on the legs and in the perineum. While the increased intraabdominal pressure, with compression of veins and lymphatics, is the major cause, hormonal relaxation must also play a role, since some changes are seen before the uterus is large enough to exert pressure.

Hair changes are also prominent. Many patients complain of hypertrichosis, usually involving the face and pubic hairs. These changes may be reversible. The scalp hair is usually unaffected or even thicker during pregnancy because of the prolonged anagen phase; after delivery, telogen effluvium is thus quite common.

Therapeutic Considerations

Most women prefer to avoid any systemic therapy during pregnancy. It is very difficult to convince a young couple that a congenital abnormality in their child is not the result of some therapeutic intervention. In fact, in some societies, skin therapy for the mother is considered a likely cause of skin disorders in the infant. In addition, one should probably try to avoid all therapy in the first trimester, as the fetus is the most susceptible during this time and almost anything taken or absorbed by the mother can eventually cross the placenta. When systemic medications are required, such as in patients with systemic lupus erythematosus or bullous disorders, they should be carefully discussed with the patient and father and the conversation well documented. Most countries have lists of systemic drugs which are acceptable in pregnancy; no matter what the dermatologist's personal opinions are, he should follow the recommendations exactly. Traditional antihistamines such as diphenhydramine and chlorpheniramine are probably preferable to the newer forms, whose safety is less well documented. Vitamin supplements should be left to the obstetrician or mother; for example, both vitamin A and vitamin D derivatives are proven to have deleterious effects on the fetus.

Even topical medications should be bland. For example, in treating acne in pregnancy, we rely on topical erythromycin, since systemic erythromycin, excluding erythromycin estolate, is considered safe in both the USA and Germany. The topical retinoids are generally not used, even though the minuscule amount that can be absorbed is not teratogenic. Podophyllin is also contraindicated in pregnancy. Topical corticosteroids should be used carefully. If high potency steroids are used over broad areas, effects on the fetus are possible.

Nonspecific Dermatologic Disorders

There is no skin disease against which pregnant patients are protected. Thus, every disorder listed in this book which is not limited to men can arise. Fortunately, most of the rashes and other skin changes of pregnancy involve common problems. There is a long list of skin disorders which may worsen during pregnancy, as shown in Table 36.1. Some disorders such as acne and psoriasis tend to improve in pregnancy, but one should not emphasize this to the patient, because in other instances they can worsen dramatically. Diseases which are often influenced favorably by increased estrogen levels, such as Fox-Fordyce disease or sarcoidosis, may also improve. Diseases with abnormal elastic fibers such as pseudoxanthoma elasticum and some types of Ehlers-Danlos syndrome may be associated with placental problems and premature labor. In a prospective study of almost 3200 women, only 51 (1.6 %) developed cutaneous problems. Most clinicians would probably place the risk slightly higher, but one should not overestimate the severity of the problem.

Erythema nodosum is very common among young women, but it may be even more common in pregnancy (erythema nodosum gravidarum) (Bombardieri et al. 1977). The lesions are clinically identical to those in nonpregnant patients, but no history of drug exposure or infection is obtained. The lesions may recur in subsequent pregnancies or when oral contraceptives are taken. Usually no treatment is needed, but in case of extreme pain the measures discussed under erythema nodosum can be considered.

Several tumors also change during pregnancy. The most troublesome clinical problem is the changes in melanocytic nevi and malignant melanomas during pregnancy. The eruption and rapid growth of melanocytic nevi is a well known event; more recent studies have shown estrogen receptors on a variety of melanocytic lesions, including melanocytic nevi and malignant melanomas. Patients with dysplastic nevus syndrome should be monitored more closely when pregnant. The management of malignant melanoma during pregnancy is complex. In general, if the clinical suspicion is of malignant melanoma and not simply a changing or irritated melanocytic nevus, then the same diagnostic and therapeutic approaches should be followed as for any other presentation. Metastatic malignant melanoma in pregnancy poses a risk for the fetus and thus becomes a controversial issue.

The other tumors that become more common are far less significant. Skin tags frequently increase, perhaps coupled with the same frictional changes that induce hyperpigmentation in the axillae and groin. There may well be a hormonal basis, since small skin tags arise before the same background as acanthosis nigricans and may reflect a similar

Table 36.1. Diseases which tend to worsen or be more severe during pregnancy

Infections	Candidal vaginitis Trichomoniasis Condylomata acuminata Herpes simplex Varicella Zoster HIV/AIDS Leprosy *Pityrosporum* folliculitis Scabies
Autoimmune disorders	Systemic lupus erythematosus Systemic sclerosis Dermatomyositis Pemphigus vulgaris
Metabolic disorders	Porphyria cutanea tarda Acrodermatitis enteropathica
Elastic tissue disorders	Ehlers-Danlos syndrome Pseudoxanthoma elasticum
Other diseases	Pityriasis rosea Mycosis fungoides Metastatic malignant melanoma Neurofibromatosis

problem, while larger ones may be more closely related to nevi. Another tumor which may be more common is dermatofibroma. Multiple dermatofibromas can be associated with systemic lupus erythematosus, which may worsen in pregnancy.

Specific Dermatologic Disorders

Over the past century, a large number of diseases have been reported to be associated with pregnancy. Only a few of them are clinically distinct and have reproducible criteria. Many present with itching and have been designated as types of prurigo.

Cholestasis of Pregnancy

Synonyms. Pruritus gravidarum, benign recurrent intrahepatic cholestasis, obstetric cholestasis

Definition. Diffuse pruritus usually appears in the last trimester and is associated with elevated liver enzymes, occasionally jaundice, and no primary skin lesions. It disappears after delivery.

Epidemiology. Jaundice occurs in one out of every 1000–2000 pregnancies. One must remember that viral hepatitis is a more common cause of obstetric jaundice than cholestasis of pregnancy. Most patients are not jaundiced but are identified on laboratory testing. The incidence of cholestasis of pregnancy ranges from 1–3% in various European countries to as high as 14% in Chilean Indios. Much of the variance is probably explained by different diagnostic criteria.

Etiology and Pathogenesis. The etiology of cholestasis of pregnancy is unclear and probably multifactorial. Bile secretion is blocked, but it is unclear how estrogens and other steroids cause this malfunction. One suggestion is that reduced hepatic blood flow leads to reduced clearance of toxins, including estrogens, which then increase biliary cholesterol levels and reduce excretion of bile salts.

Clinical Findings. The patients have intense pruritus, usually starting in the late second or early third trimester. No primary skin lesions are seen, just excoriations and lichenified areas. Most often, the abdomen is symptomatic first, but the problem generalizes rapidly. Symptoms persist for the rest of the pregnancy and are typically worse at night. Some women complain of almost unbearable itching of the palms.

In about 50% of patients, hepatic symptoms develop, including nausea, vomiting, right upper quadrant tenderness or pain, dark urine, light stools, or even jaundice.

Laboratory Findings. Neither skin nor liver biopsy is helpful. markedly elevated serum bile acids are the hallmark. Bilirubin may be found in the urine, with serum levels of 2–5 mg/dl and other hepatic parameters relatively normal. Since all the liver function tests may be aberrant in pregnancy, interpretation is difficult, but high bilirubin values or marked elevations, especially of aspartate aminotransferase, should suggest the possibility of other diagnoses. Vitamin K absorption may be reduced, leading to prolonged prothrombin time; this should be monitored so as to avoid hemorrhagic problems in the fetus.

Course and Prognosis. The outlook is good. Fetal risk is controversial; there may be an increase in premature labor and meconium staining. Patients should be carefully monitored. There is no fetal hepatic disease.

The pruritus tends to resolve within days after delivery and the jaundice over a few weeks. In rare cases, the problem may persist for weeks after delivery. Recurrence in subsequent deliveries is common, as is triggering by oral contraceptives. The risk is higher in twin pregnancies. One must exclude any exposure to hepatotoxic medications or other agents.

Differential Diagnosis. Viral hepatitis should be excluded by appropriate serologic studies. Any primary skin lesions suggest a different cause, as do major systemic symptoms or marked evidence of hepatic dysfunction. Many women have unexplained itching during pregnancy; this should not be equated with pruritus gravidarum.

Therapy

Systemic. Both cholestyramine and ursodeoxycholic acid have been recommended but should be employed by the obstetrician. Antihistamines are not very helpful. Vitamin K should be given intramuscularly, as suggested by hematologic studies.

Topical. Bland drying lotions such as zinc oxide lotion can be employed. In Europe, polidocanol is often added in concentrations of 2–5%. Topical distraction with phenol, thymol, and menthol is best avoided. Treatment with UVB radiation may also be helpful; several treatments with suberythemal doses weekly usually suffice.

Herpes Gestationis

This is the most specific dermatosis of pregnancy. Because of its many clinical and immunologic associations with bullous pemphigoid, it is discussed in the text on bullous disorders (Chap. 15). Patients with herpes gestationis may present only with pruritus or erythematous lesions. Sometimes, immunofluorescent evaluation is the only way to make the diagnosis, even before blisters have been identified.

Impetigo Herpetiformis

(Hebra 1872)

Impetigo herpetiformis is a serious illness which occurs during pregnancy; the discussion concerns whether it is a disease sui generis. Patients present with fever, chills, vomiting, diarrhea, and abdominal cramps. They have widespread sterile pustules and are in a miserable state. Often there are associated parathyroid abnormalities with hypocalcemia. We view such cases as variants of generalized pustular psoriasis occurring most often in pregnancy but sometimes in nonpregnant women and even in men (Chap. 14).

Pruritic Urticarial Papules and Plaques of Pregnancy

(Lawley et al. 1979)

Synonyms. PUPPP, toxic erythema of pregnancy, polymorphic eruption of pregnancy, toxemic rash of pregnancy (Bourne 1962), late onset prurigo of pregnancy (Nurse 1968).

Definition. Intensely pruritic dermatosis on the abdomen, especially in striae, starting typically in the last trimester and disappearing after delivery.

Epidemiology. PUPPP is without question the most common specific dermatosis of pregnancy. The incidence is around 1:200. It most often involves primiparas and tends not to recur in subsequent pregnancies.

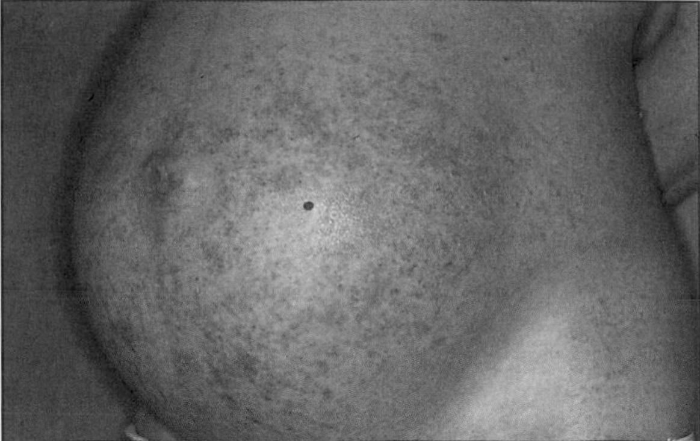

Fig. 36.1. Pruritic urticarial papules and plaques of pregnancy

Etiology and Pathogenesis. The etiology is unknown. Many factors have been excluded, such as HLA associations, liver disease, and immune deposits in the skin. Twinning remains a risk factor; some have suggested that the stretching of the abdominal skin is the direct trigger.

Clinical Findings. The pruritic erythematous edematous papules and plaques appear almost invariably first in the striae (Fig. 36.1). The absence of striae is very rare. The lesions spread to the buttocks, thighs, lateral part of the trunk, and arms. The face is almost never involved. Occasionally vesicles develop, but bullae do not evolve. The onset is usually in the last 2–3 weeks of pregnancy and resolution occurs shortly after delivery. Other than pruritus, there are no symptoms and no associated systemic diseases.

Histopathology. The epidermis shows modest spongiosis and parakeratosis. In the dermis, there are intense lymphocytic perivascular infiltrates, often admixed with eosinophils and associated with edema. While the papillary dermis is almost invariably involved, the infiltrates can extend more deeply. Immunofluorescent examination is negative, except that complement is found around the vessels on rare occasions. Deposition at the basement membrane zone suggests herpes gestationis.

Laboratory Findings. No other laboratory findings are helpful. Liver status is normal.

Course and Prognosis. Both mother and fetus do well. After delivery, the lesions disappear rapidly.

Differential Diagnosis. The differential diagnosis list is long, including erythema multiforme, atopic dermatitis, scabies, and drug eruptions. In addition, the other forms of prurigo in pregnancy can be considered, but usually this is a matter of semantics, not clinical judgment.

Therapy

Systemic. Systemic therapy is usually not needed, but soporific antihistamines can be employed, as the mature fetus is at almost no risk. Systemic corticosteroids have been prescribed for severe cases, usually in ranges of 20–40 mg daily of prednisone, but are controversial and usually not needed.

Topical. Topical distracters such as zinc oxide lotion or anesthetics such as polidocanol lotion can be employed. Low potency corticosteroid creams or lotions may also be of some benefit.

Prurigo of Pregnancy

Synonyms. Prurigo gestationis (Besnier 1904), papular dermatitis of pregnancy, Spangler disease (Spangler and Emerson 1971), early onset prurigo of pregnancy (Nurse), and many others.

Definition. Prurigo of pregnancy is the working name for a series of rare disorders described during pregnancy and otherwise inconsistently defined. They have been defined on the basis of response to therapy, of laboratory tests, of histopathology, and of physical findings alone.

Etiology and Pathogenesis. The etiology is unknown, although many suggestions have been made. As the vagueness of the following description will show, it is likely that many different, still poorly understood diseases have been lumped together and split apart so many times that they defy recognition. It might be more honest to say that there are rare pruritic papular eruptions in pregnancy that we simply do not understand. We suspect that some of these patients have papular atopic dermatitis.

Clinical Findings. These patients present in the second or third trimester with pruritus and papules, usually on the extensor surfaces, which are usually not exaggerated on the stretched abdomen and may involve the face. Just as in prurigo simplex subacuta, a seropapule or urticarial papule with a tense, tiny blister may be seen, if it is not scratched away first. Some lesions are follicular. The problem may persist for weeks to months after delivery, and recurrences in subsequent pregnancies are possible.

Prurigo Gestationis of Besnier. These patients were clinically defined as having pruritic papules of the extremities and trunk, with no further diagnostic details offered. Besnier felt the patients represented a variant of prurigo simplex subacuta, but he excluded papular atopic dermatitis.

Papular Dermatitis of Pregnancy. These patients were defined on the basis of elevated urine chorionic gonadotropin levels and a high fetal risk. Facial involvement and postinflammatory hyperpigmentation were emphasized, but both are clearly not specific.

Histopathology. The histologic changes are not specific and reflect the clinical findings. If folliculitis is identified, then the diagnosis should be changed to folliculitis of pregnancy.

Laboratory Findings. Other laboratory tests are only helpful for excluding cholestasis and ruling out other disorders. Spangler's reliance on urine chorionic gonadotropin levels has not stood the test of time.

Differential Diagnosis. One should exclude scabies, dermatitis herpetiformis, drug reactions, herpes gestationis and PUPPP and then consider the other variants, which may not be specific diseases.

Therapy. Symptomatic care is all that is available.

Other Dermatoses of Pregnancy

Many other dermatoses have been described as specific. Some fit clinically into prurigo of pregnancy but have alleged variations in histology or immunofluorescence studies. It is unfortunate that all of these are so rare that a single study looking for all the alleged biochemical and histologic parameters has not been performed. We suspect that such an effort would unify this field considerably.

Autoimmune Progesterone Dermatitis in Pregnancy

(Bierman 1973)

Etiology and Pathogenesis. Bierman described a single case, and a few other reports have trickled into the literature. The role of progesterone was defined using intracutaneous injections of progesterone and estrogen. The former elicited a delayed hypersensitivity response which progressed to an abscess. In the initial patient, the premenstrual spikes of progesterone caused no problems, but oral contraceptives did.

Clinical Findings. The clinical hallmark is an acne-like eruption appearing very early in pregnancy. Comedones, papules, and pustules are seen favoring the extremities and buttocks but not the face. The papules are small, firm, and often grouped. They may appear to be arranged around follicles. Pruritus is minimal. Joint pains have also been described.

In the initial patient, the skin findings occurred in two consecutive pregnancies, both of which ended in spontaneous abortion in the first trimester. Oral contraceptives have caused recurrences of the eruption and associated polyarthritis.

Histopathology. A dense perifollicular lymphocytic and eosinophilic infiltrate has been described. Epidermal involvement may occur as well as extension into the fat.

Laboratory Findings. There are no diagnostic findings, but the sedimentation rate may be raised and elevated levels of IgG and IgM were described in one case.

Course and Prognosis. The outlook for the mother is good but allegedly dismal for the infant.

Differential Diagnosis. The main differential diagnosis is acne vulgaris and other acneiform eruptions such as bromoderma, drug eruptions, and polymorphic light eruption. The acneiform nature and the lack of pruritus separate this disorder from prurigo variants.

Therapy. Both UVB radiation and mild topical acne therapy may be helpful.

Pruritic Folliculitis of Pregnancy

(Zoberman and Farmer 1981)

Clinical Findings. The key finding is eroded papules in a follicular pattern. Onset is at about the fourth month of pregnancy. The lesions are intensely pruritic and favor the trunk, although they may be generalized. Some patients simultaneously have cholestasis of pregnancy. This may simply be a variety of prurigo of pregnancy which has been histologically well studied.

Histopathology. Biopsy reveals folliculitis, often located relatively high in the follicle (ostiofolliculitis). Organisms are not identified with special stains or on culture. Immunofluorescent examinations have been negative.

Course and Prognosis. There is no evidence of fetal risk. The mothers tend to clear after delivery but may develop problems in subsequent pregnancies.

Differential Diagnosis. Other forms of folliculitis should be considered.

Therapy. Topical drying and antipruritic measures suffice.

Bibliography

Reviews

Black MM (1992) The specific dermatoses of pregnancy: the British perspective. Adv Dermatol 7:105–126

Harahap M, Wallach RC (eds) (1995) Skin changes and diseases in pregnancy. Dekker, New York

Shornick JK (1998) Dermatoses of pregnancy. Semin Cutan Med Surg 17:172–181

Winton GB (1989) Skin diseases aggravated by pregnancy. J Am Acad Dermatol 20:1–13

Wong RC, Ellis CN (1989) Physiologic skin changes in pregnancy. Semin Dermatol 8:7–11

Nonspecific Dermatologic Disorders

Bombardieri S, Munno OD, Di Punzio C et al. (1977) Erythema nodosum associated with pregnancy and oral contraceptives. Br Med J 1:1509–1510

Cholestasis of Pregnancy

Gillespie DA, Vickers CR (1993) Pruritus and cholestasia: therapeutic options. J Gastroenterol Hepatol 8:168–173

Reyes H (1997) Review: intrahepatic cholestasis. A puzzling disorder of pregnancy. J Gastroenterol Hepatol 12: 211–X216

Javitt NB (1998) Cholestasis of pregnancy: ursodeoxycholic acid therapy. J Hepatol 29:827–828

Herpes Gestationis

Yancey KB (1990) Herpes gestationis. Dermatol Clin 8: 727–735

Morrison LH, Anhalt GJ (1991) Herpes gestationis. J Autoimmun 4:37–45

Shornick JK (1993) Herpes gestationis. Dermatol Clin 11: 527–533

Varner MW (1991) Autoimmune disorders and pregnancy. Semin Perinatol 15:238–250

Impetigo Herpetiformis

Alli N, Lenk N (1996) Twins with impetigo herpetiformis. Int J Dermatol 35:149–150

Breier-Maly J, Ortel B, Breier F et al. (1999) Generalized pustular psoriasis of pregnancy (impetigo herpetiformis). Dermatology 198:61–64

Trevisan G, Kokelj F (1996) Impetigo herpetiformis and RhE isoimmunization: a case report. Cutis 58:87–89

Pruritic Urticarial Papules and Plaques of Pregnancy

Aronson IK, Bond S, Fiedler VC et al. (1998) Pruritic urticarial papules and plaques of pregnancy: clinical and immunopathologic observations in 57 patients. J Am Acad Dermatol 39:933–939

Bourne G (1962) Toxaemic rash of pregnancy. Proc R Soc Med 55:462–464

Carli P (1994) Skin immune system activation in pruritic urticarial papules and plaques of pregnancy. Int J Dermatol 33:884–885

Lawley TJ, Hertz KC, Wade TR et al. (1979) Pruritic urticarial papules and plaques of pregnancy. JAMA 241: 1696–1699

Trattner A, Ingber A, Sandbank M (1991) Antiepidermal cell surface antibodies in a patient with pruritic urticarial papules and plaques of pregnancy. J Am Acad Dermatol 24:306–308

Vaughan Jones SA, Dunnill MG, Black MM (1996) Pruritic urticarial papules and plaques of pregnancy (polymorphic eruption of pregnancy): two unusual cases. Br J Dermatol 135:102–105

Prurigo of Pregnancy

Nurse DS (1968) Prurigo of pregnancy. Australas J Dermatol 9:258–267

Shanmugam S, Thappa DM, Habeebullah S (1998) Pruritus gravidarum: a clinical and laboratory study. J Dermatol 25:582–586

Spangler AS, Emerson K Jr (1971) Estrogen levels and estrogen therapy in papular dermatitis of pregnancy. Am J Obst Gynecol 110:534–537

Roger D, Vaillant L, Fignon A et al. (1994) Specific pruritic diseases of pregnancy. A prospective study of 3192 pregnant women. Arch Dermatol 130:734–739

Autoimmune Progesterone Dermatitis in Pregnancy

Biermann SM (1973) Autoimmune progesterone dermatitis in pregnancy. Arch Dermatol 107:896–901

Pruritic Folliculitis of Pregnancy

Ford MJ, Gammon WR, Kilpatrick TM (1992) Pustular eruption of the striae in a primigravida. Cutis 50:225–228

Heymann WR, Wolf DJ (1986) Malassezia (*Pityrosporon*) folliculitis occurring during pregnancy. Int J Dermatol 25:49–51

Wilkinson SM, Buckler H, Wilkinson N et al. (1995) Androgen levels in pruritic folliculitis of pregnancy. Clin Exp Dermatol 20:234–236

Zoberman E, Farmer ER (1981) Pruritic folliculitis of pregnancy. Arch Dermatol 117:20–22

CHAPTER 37

Disorders of Lipoprotein and Lipid Metabolism

Contents

Basic Science Aspects

Abnormalities of lipid metabolism are one of the major health problems facing most developed countries. The combination of genetic factors, overeating, inappropriate balance of diet, lack of physical activity, smoking and alcohol consumption have led to an almost epidemic increased in cardiovascular disease, primarily coronary artery disease. In the USA, coronary artery disease is the leading cause of death, even though mortality is decreasing because of more effective medical and surgical treatment.

The main dietary lipids are cholesterol and triglycerides. Serum cholesterol levels >180–200 mg/dl are clearly associated with an increased risk of coronary artery disease. While triglyceride levels exceeding 250 mg/dl are considered abnormal, they correlate poorly with cardiac risk. Much higher levels, in the range of 1000–2000 mg/dl, are strongly associated with pancreatitis. Dermatologists may play a role in identifying patients at risk because cutaneous xanthomas are one of the few physical signs of lipid disorders.

Lipids and Lipoproteins

The body has developed a complex system of checks and balances to attempt to maintain lipid homeostasis. Lipids are relatively nonsoluble and are transported around the body in the blood by lipoproteins, combinations of lipids and proteins (Table 37.1). The lipoproteins create microemulsions that consist of small spherical particles. The central core of a lipoprotein contains the unipolar triglycerides and cholesterol esters, while the peripheral shell is made up of polar phospholipids, free fatty acids and apolipoproteins.

The apolipoproteins are not only structurally important but are also essential to the regulation of lipid metabolism. Apolipoproteins function both as enzyme co-factors and as ligands. While we will briefly discuss some of these functions, Table 37.2 is primarily designed to show the many important roles that these key components play, as genetic de-

Table 37.1. Types of apolipoproteins

Lipid	Apolipoprotein
Free cholesterol	A-I, A-II, A-IV
Cholesterol esters	B-48, B-100
Triglycerides	C-I, C-II, C-III
Phospholipids	D, E

Table 37.2. Types of apolipoproteins

Apolipoprotein	Major functions
A-I	Activates LCAT; part of HDL
A-II	Part of HDL
A-IV	?
B-48	Essential for chylomicron structure
B-100	Essential for VLDL, present in IDL, LDL; ligand for LDL receptor
C-I	?
C-II	Activates lipoprotein lipase
C-III	Involved in inhibiting hepatic uptake of chylomicron and VLDL remnants; may also inhibit lipo protein lipase
D	May be co-factor for cholesterol ester transfer protein
E	Ligand for hepatic chylomicron remnant receptor and LDL receptor

VLDL, very low density lipoprotein; IDL, intermediate density lipoprotein; LDL, low density lipoprotein; HDL, high density lipoprotein.

fects in apolipoprotein structure can wreak havoc with the system. Most of the apolipoproteins are very water soluble and interchangeable with other lipoproteins. The large B-lipoproteins (B-100, B-48) are less water soluble and also less interchangeable.

Lipoproteins are divided into five classes based on their density as determined by ultracentrifugation and their electrophoretic rate of migration. We will refer to them for the balance of the text by the standard initials given in Table 37.3. Previously, the hyperlipoproteinemias were classified using the 1967 system of FREDERICKSON et al., which considered lipoprotein electrophoretic motility and cholesterol and triglyceride levels to define six phenotypes, listed as I, IIa, IIb, III, IV and V. However, some specific disorders may show several phenotypes, and several phenotypes include multiple disorders. For these reasons, although electrophoretic screening is still useful to identify certain disorders, such as the dysbetalipoproteinemia (broad-β disease), the phenotypes are no longer employed, even by Frederickson.

There are three major enzymes involved in lipoprotein metabolism: lipoprotein lipase, hepatic lipase and lecithin-cholesterol acyl transferase (LCAT). Lipoprotein lipase is manufactured in striated muscle and fatty tissue and found along the endothelial surface of capillaries. It is responsible for the vast bulk of hydrolysis of triglycerides in the chylomicrons and very low density lipoproteins (VLDL). The enzyme is activated by apolipoprotein C-II, which is found in the triglyceride-rich lipoproteins. Hepatic lipase is produced in the liver, where it lines the hepatic endothelial cells. It facilitates the conversion of the VLDL and intermediate density lipoproteins (IDL) into low density lipoproteins (LDL). LCAT is also made in the liver. It synthesizes the bulk of the cholesterol esters by hastening esterification of high density lipoprotein (HDL)-cholesterol with lecithin. These cholesterol esters are transferred to IDL and LDL via a cholesterol transfer protein.

Lipid Transport Systems

Each day the average Westerner consumes about 400 mg of cholesterol and produces another 500–1000 mg in the liver. In addition a similar amount is secreted in the bile but then reabsorbed. Thus 1–2 g

Table 37.3. Classification of lipoproteins

Lipoprotein	Diameter (Å)	Electrophoresis	Density (g/ml)	Predominant lipids	Apolipoproteins
Chylomicrons	800–5000	No motion	<0.95	Dietary triglycerides	A-I, A-II, A-IV, B-48, C-I, C-I, C-III, E
VLDL	300–800	Pre-β	0.95–1.006	Endogenous triglycerides	B-100, C-I, C-II, C-III, E
IDL	250–350	Pre-β to β	1.006–1.019	Cholesterol esters, triglycerides	B-100, E
LDL	200–240	β	1.019–1.063	Cholesterol esters	B-100
HDL	50–120	α	1.063–1.210	Cholesterol esters	A-I, A-II, C-I, C-II, C-III, D, E

VLDL, very low density lipoprotein; IDL, intermediate density lipoprotein; LDL, low density lipoprotein; HDL, high density lipoprotein.

of cholesterol circulate in the plasma and are transferred to peripheral sites to manufacture cell membranes and steroid hormones, as well as being converted to bile salts. Triglycerides are primarily devoted to energy production and considerably more, probably over 100 g, enter and leave the circulation daily. To move cholesterol and triglycerides around, the body has several transport systems. The two major ones are the exogenous and endogenous pathways; in addition there is reverse cholesterol transport in the liver and lipoprotein-(a) transport.

Exogenous Pathway

The intestinal cells esterify fatty acids and cholesterol into triglycerides and cholesterol esters, which then form chylomicrons containing predominately triglycerides but also cholesterol esters. The chylomicrons go through the intestinal lymphatics and eventually the thoracic duct to reach the circulation. Along the way they pick up apolipoprotein C-II, which activates lipoprotein lipase in the endothelial cells of muscle and fat cells. This enzyme hydrolyzes the triglycerides back to free fatty acids, which are used for energy in the muscles and stored in the fat. Through a series of complex reactions, HDL are formed from cholesterol, phospholipids and apolipoproteins. Chylomicron remnants, relatively rich in cholesterol and marked with apolipoprotein E, bind to a liver receptor via apolipoprotein E receptor and provide cholesterol for the endogenous pathway and bile synthesis.

Endogenous Pathway

VLDL are manufactured in the liver and contain both cholesterol and triglycerides, much like chylomicrons. They too interact with lipoprotein lipase in the endothelial cells, once again triggered by apolipoprotein C-II. The triglycerides are broken down to provide fatty acids for energy and storage. They also yield smaller IDL particles, which are then converted to cholesterol ester-rich LDL, while their triglycerides are hydrolyzed by hepatic lipases. The rest of the VLDL (also called VLDL remnants) are taken up by hepatic LDL receptors (apo B, E receptors).

LDL is the main transporter of cholesterol, delivering it to peripheral sites to manufacture and repair cell membranes and synthesize steroid hormones. Apolipoprotein B-100 is the ligand for the uptake of LDL, binding to specific LDL receptors. The LDL is processed by receptor-mediated endocytosis, so that cholesterol ester is delivered to the lysosomes. Nonspecific macrophage scavenger systems complete the metabolism of LDL contents.

As cholesterol builds up in cells, several inhibitory pathways are brought into play. First, there is reduced synthesis of HMG-CoA reductase, the rate-limiting enzyme in endogenous cholesterol synthesis. Second, free cholesterol is more rapidly converted to its storage form, cholesterol esters. Finally, the synthesis of new LDL receptors is slowed, so that less LDL and thus less cholesterol can be taken up.

Reverse Cholesterol Transport

HDL removes cholesterol from peripheral sites and returns it to the liver, which is the only site of cholesterol excretion. HDL particles take up free cholesterol, which is esterified by LCAT. The free cholesterol on HDL may be returned directly to the liver, while the cholesterol esters follow a more complicated route via VLDL and IDL.

Lipoprotein-(a) Transfer

Lipoprotein-(a) is a large abnormal molecule consisting of LDL and a glycoprotein known as apolipoprotein-(a) which is unrelated to the normal apolipoproteins. It attaches poorly to the LDL receptor and is correlated with coronary artery disease but otherwise little is known about its function.

Hyperlipoproteinemias and Dyslipoproteinemias

Technically the term dyslipoproteinemia is more appropriate, since there may be both reductions and increases in lipoproteins as well as structural variations. It is easy to see how LDL has become known as the bad lipoprotein and HDL as the good member of the family. In patients with coronary artery disease and levels of cholesterol less than 200 mg/dl, often one finds low levels of HDL.

One must distinguish between the primary and secondary hyperlipoproteinemias. The primary hyperlipoproteinemias are covered in Table 37.4 and discussed individually. The far more common secondary causes are listed in Table 37.5. The mechanisms of the secondary hyperlipoproteinemias are amazingly complex, as multiple aspects of lipoprotein metabolism may be disrupted. In diabetes mellitus, VLDL production is increased and lipoprotein lipase activity drops. Hypothyroidism results in reduced LDL receptor activity and reduced lipoprotein lipase activity. In obesity the main defect is increased VLDL production. In the nephrotic syndrome there is reduced lipoprotein lipase activity and increased apolipoprotein B-100 secretion leading to increased VLDL. The regurgitation of bile into the plasma in primary biliary cirrhosis and other obstructive disorders results in high cholesterol levels through the formation of a unique lipoprotein designated lipoprotein X. Hepatic lipase activity is also reduced. Alcohol raises HDL and VLDL levels; thus if the HDL effect dominates, alcohol can have a positive effect on lipid levels, forming the basis for the current theory that a small amount of alcohol (one glass of beer or wine daily) may have a cardiovascular protective effect. The treatment of all the secondary hyperlipoproteinemias is control of the underlying disease or eliminating the trigger factor or medication. When these approaches fail, then secondary hyperlipoproteinemias may be treated just as the primary disorders.

The main clinical symptoms or risk factors that suggest dyslipoproteinemia are:

- Coronary artery disease
- Peripheral vascular disease
- Pancreatitis or unexplained abdominal pain
- Diabetes mellitus
- Obesity
- Alcoholism

Conversely, the three major risk factors for arteriosclerotic vascular disease are dyslipoproteinemia, hypertension and smoking. While all of the above disorders may produce a variety of signs and symptoms, sometimes the cutaneous and ophthalmologic examination can reveal signs of dyslipoproteinemia even in asymptomatic patients. These signs include:

- Xanthomas including xanthelasma
- Arcus lipoides and lipemia retinalis
- Gouty tophi and gouty arthritis

Laboratory Findings. Increasingly often, patients are detected by routine screening or directed screening because of a family member with coronary artery disease. In other instances, they may present with coronary artery disease or pancreatitis. The mainstay of diagnosis is assessment of the serum values for cholesterol, HDL-cholesterol and triglycerides. The patient should have been fasting for at least 12 h and not have recently eaten a diet rich in carbohydrates, saturated fats or alcohol. Either serum or plasma can be used. The specimen should be stored refrigerated overnight; the following steps should then be undertaken:

- Inspection of the serum: Both of the larger particles, VLDL and chylomicrons, impart a cloudy or turbid appearance to the serum, while only chylomicrons tend to float on top, like fat on homemade soup or cream on nonhomogenized milk. If the remainder of the serum sample is cloudy, this indicates the pres-

Table 37.4. The primary lipoproteinemias

Type of hyperlipoproteinemia	Lipoproteins ↑	Frequency/ 10,000 individuals	Atherogenic risk
Familial combined hyperlipidemia	VLDL	30–50	High
Familial hypercholesterolemia	LDL	10–20 (0.01 for homozygotes)	Very high; in homozygotes, extraordinary
Familial apolipoprotein B-100 defect	LDL	20	Very high
Familial dysbetalipoproteinemia	β-VLDL	2–4	High; also peripheral vascular disease
Familial lipoprotein lipase deficiency	CM	0.01	Normal; pancreatitis
Familial apolipoprotein C-II deficiency	CM	0.01	Normal; pancreatitis
Familial hypertriglyceridemia	CM	10	Normal

CM, chylomicrons

Table 37.5. Major causes of secondary hyperlipoproteinemia

Underlying disease or cause	Major elevated lipoproteins
Hormonal alterations	
Noninsulin-dependent diabetes mellitus	VLDL, CM
Insulin-dependent diabetes mellitus	VLDL, LDL, CM
Hypothyroidism	LDL, VLDL
Pregnancy	VLDL, LDL
Nutritional factors	
Obesity	VLDL, LDL, CM
Alcoholism	VLDL, HDL, CM
Anorexia nervosa	LDL
Hepatic disease	
Primary biliary cirrhosis	Lp-X
Extrahepatic biliary obstruction	Lp-X
Acute hepatitis	VLDL
Chronic hepatitis	VLDL, LDL
Renal disease	
Nephrotic syndrome	VLDL, LDL
Chronic renal disease	VLDL
Miscellaneous disorders	
Nicotine abuse	VLDL, LDL, HDL
Pancreatitis	CM, VLDL
Paraproteinemia	VLDL, LDL, CM
Glycogenosis type Ia (von Gierke)	VLDL
Lupus erythematosus	CM, VLDL, LDL
AIDS	VLDL
Medications	
Corticosteroids	VLDL, LDL, CM
Estrogens	VLDL, LDL, HDL
Androgens, progesterone	LDL
Retinoids	VLDL, LDL
β-blockers (lacking intrinsic sympathetic activity)	VLDL
Thiazides	VLDL, LDL
Cimetidine	VLDL
Tamoxifen	VLDL

CM, chylomicrons. These may be present if there is associated hypertriglyceridemia.

ence of VLDL. If it is clear, other lipoproteins may still be present.

- Measurement of serum lipids: Cholesterol levels <180 mg/dl and triglyceride levels <200 mg/dl are usually considered healthy
- Measurement of HDL-cholesterol and calculation of LDL-cholesterol. If the serum triglyceride is less than 400 mg/dl, then the Friedewald formula can be employed: *LDL-cholesterol = total cholesterol–HDL-cholesterol–triglycerides/5*. LDL-cholesterol <150 mg/dl is desirable. HDL-cholesterol <35 mg/dl is undesirable.
- Lipoprotein electrophoresis is useful for broad characterizations but has largely been replaced by measurement of LDL and HDL levels and the following specialized tests, which can be carried out in appropriately equipped laboratories:
  - Lipoprotein fractionation with ultracentrifugation
  - Measurement of lipoprotein lipase, hepatic lipase and LCAT activity
  - Measurement of apolipoprotein levels

If a secondary form of hyperlipoproteinemia is suspected, then the standard tests to exclude the various likely contributing factors should be performed.

Xanthomas

Xanthomas represent deposits of various lipids in the skin. There are many types of xanthomas (Table 37.6); in some instances, their presence allows the clinician to make a fairly specific diagnosis and institute prompt therapy in patients at risk for cardiovascular disease. For example tuberous xanthomas and tendon xanthomas together strongly suggest familial hypercholesterolemia, while xanthomas in the palmar creases point towards familial dysbetalipoproteinemia. Xanthomas are typically yellow papules or nodules that result from the leakage of lipoproteins through the blood vessel wall into the tissues and their subsequent uptake by macrophages. The distribution of lipids in xanthomas is similar to that in atheromatous plaques, suggesting that they have a similar pathophysiology. Because of the excessive uptake of lipids, the macrophages evolve into foam cells and multinucleated giant cells of the Touton type. In the early stages of xanthoma formation, the process can be limited if the lipid disturbances are improved or corrected. Later, the lesions become more permanent.

Many xanthomas can be identified clinically with a fair degree of certainty. This often allows one to make an educated guess about the most likely underlying lipid abnormality, although biochemical and, increasingly, genetic tests are employed to obtain a definitive answer.

Table 37.6. Types of xanthomas and their associated disorders

Type	Associated disorders	
Plane		
Palmar striae	Primary	Familial dysbetalipoproteinemia
	Secondary	Cholestasis
Intertriginous	Primary	Homozygous familial hypercholesterolemia
Diffuse	Primary	None
	Secondary	Paraproteinemia
Tuberous	Primary	Familial hypercholesterolemia Familial apolipoprotein B-100 deficiency Familial dysbetalipoproteinemia Cerebrotendinous xanthomatosis
	Secondary	Paraproteinemia
Tendinous	Primary	Familial hypercholesterolemia Familial B-100 apolipoprotein deficiency Familial dysbetalipoproteinemia Cerebrotendinous xanthomatosis Phytosterolemia
Subcutaneous	Primary	Familial hypercholesterolemia Phytosterolemia
	Secondary	Paraproteinemia
Eruptive	Primary	Familial lipoprotein lipase deficiency Familial apolipoprotein C-II deficiency Familial hypertriglyceridemia
	Secondary	Diabetes mellitus Cholestasis Some types of lipodystrophy Glycogenosis type I (von Gierke disease) Paraproteinemia
Tuberoeruptive	Primary	Familial hypertriglyceridemia Familial dysbetalipoproteinemia
	Secondary	Cholestasis Paraproteinemia
Arcus lipoides	Primary	Familial hypercholesterolemia Familial B-100 apolipoprotein deficiency Phytosterolemia
Tonsilar	Primary	Tangier disease
Xanthelasma	Primary	Familial hypercholesterolemia Familial dysbetalipoproteinemia Cerebrotendinous xanthomatosis Phytosterolemia
	Secondary	Paraproteinemia

Plane Xanthomas

Plane xanthomas take several forms. The rarest but most specific is the development of hundreds of tiny yellow plaques in the intertriginous spaces, strongly suggesting homozygosity for familial hypercholesterolemia. Diffuse plane xanthomas, often covering a large area of the body, such as both sides of the trunk or the thighs, are typically seen with monoclonal gammopathies (Fig. 37.1).

Tuberous Xanthomas

Tuberous xanthomas are symmetrical nodules that are typically found on the knees, elbows, hands, and feet (Fig. 37.2). They are often associated with tendi-

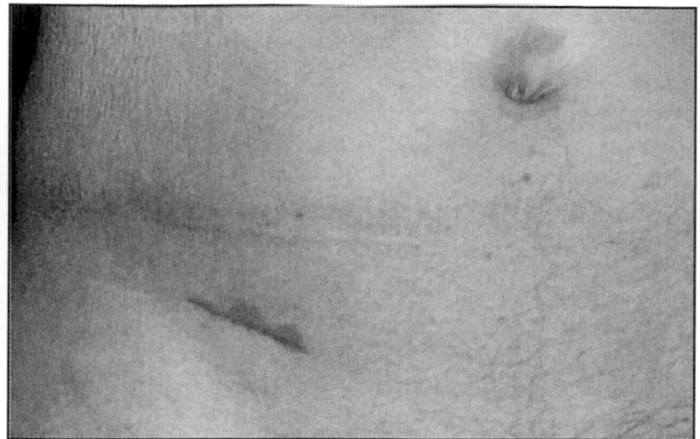

Fig. 37.1. Diffuse plane xanthomas

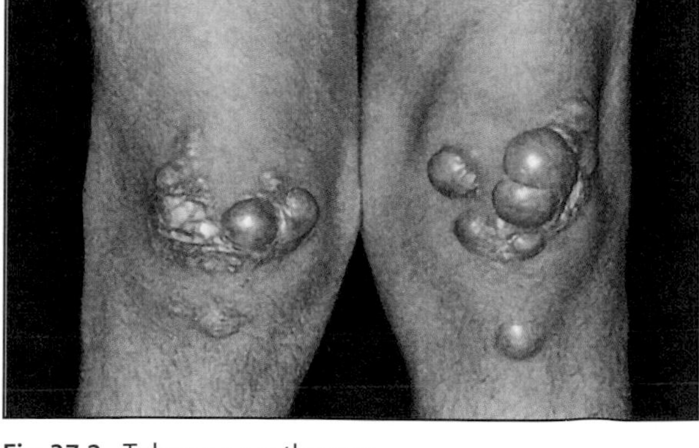

Fig. 37.2. Tuberous xanthomas

nous xanthomas, especially involving the Achilles tendons. While they develop slowly, they tend to be permanent. They are most often a sign of familial hypercholesterolemia and familial dysbetalipoproteinemia.

Tendinous and Articular Xanthomas

The combination of xanthomas involving the tendons, especially the Achilles tendons and the insertions of the patellar tendons, and the small joints on the dorsal aspects of the hands strongly suggests familial hypercholesterolemia or familial apolipoprotein B-100 deficiency (Fig. 37.3). The hand lesions should not be confused with gouty tophi or rheumatoid nodules.

Subcutaneous Xanthomas

These most uncommon lesions are clinically nonspecific, presenting as firm subcutaneous masses. They are most often seen in phytosterolemia and familial hypercholesterolemia.

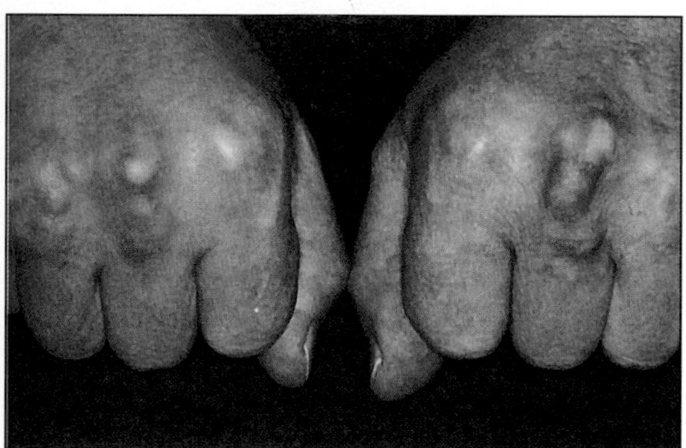

Fig. 37.3. Tendinous xanthomas

Eruptive Xanthomas

These xanthomas are very small, yellow dome-shaped papules that often are surrounded by a red ring (Fig. 37.4). They appear suddenly over days or weeks but also tend to regress if the lipid problem is corrected. The most typical sites are the buttocks and the extensor surfaces of the extremities. They are most closely associated with elevations in the triglyceride-rich lipoproteins (↑VLDL, ↑chylomicrons), so they are particularly associated with familial hypertriglyceridemia and familial lipoprotein lipase deficiency. Patients with poorly controlled diabetes mellitus may also have such xanthomas.

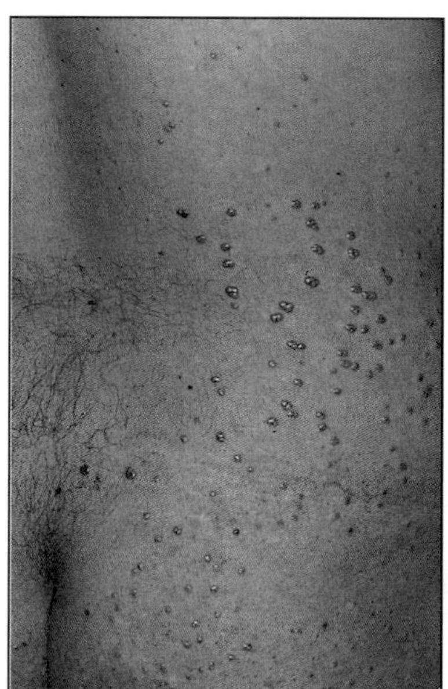

Fig. 37.4. Eruptive xanthomas

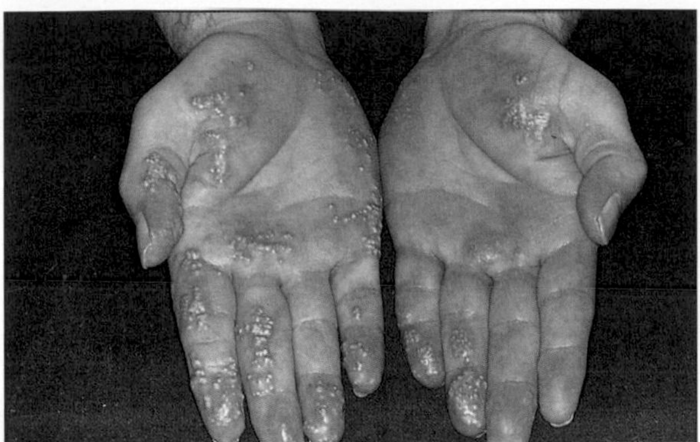

Fig. 37.5. Tuberoeruptive xanthomas

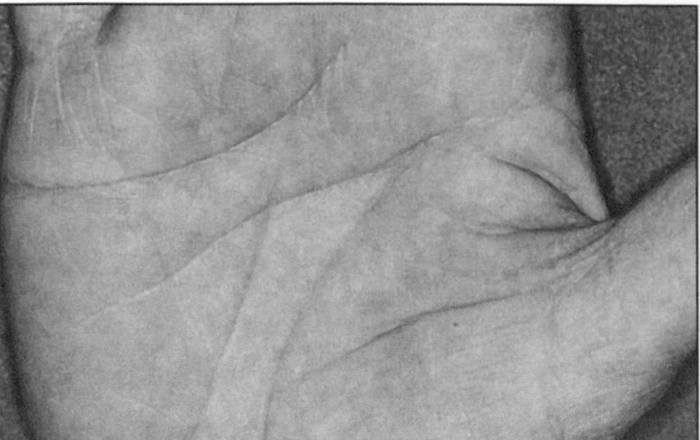

Fig. 37.6. Palmar crease xanthomas

Tuberoeruptive Xanthomas

These xanthomas are eruptive but appear more slowly and favor the knees and elbows. They are typically associated with familial dysbetalipoproteinemia (remnant particle disease) or familial hypertriglyceridemia (Fig. 37.5).

Palmar Crease Xanthomas

Synonyms. Xanthochromia palmaris, xanthoma palmare striatum, xanthoma palmare papulosum

Small xanthomas running in the palmar creases are very typical of dysbetalipoproteinemia. They impart a yellow striped appearance to the palms. The flexural surfaces may also develop tiny yellow papules. The palmar xanthomas associated with primary biliary cirrhosis are larger plaques which often extend beyond the creases (Fig. 37.6).

Related Ocular Findings

Lipemia retinalis is a marker of significantly increased triglyceride levels, often 1000–3000 mg/dl. The serum is creamy and the retinal vessels appear white against a pale background. Arcus lipoides or arcus juvenilis refers to the deposition of cholesterol and phospholipids in a ring just central to the corneal limbus (Fig. 37.7). While such rings are almost normal in the elderly (arcus senilis), in younger individuals they suggest lipid disturbances, primarily LDL elevation. Typically arcus lipoides only involves the lower half of the limbus, while arcus senilis may encircle the structure. If a patient has xanthelasma, which may or may not be a sign of systemic problems, one should search for an arcus lipoides, which strongly suggests a lipoprotein abnormality.

Histopathology. The microscopic picture of a xanthoma is distinctive, but not specific, for the given type of lesion. Often secondary clues, such as thin skin and striated muscle suggesting eyelid and thus xanthelasma, or a stratum lucidum suggesting palmar skin and therefore palmar xanthoma, are far more valuable than the actual appearance of the xanthoma. The lipids leak out of the dermal vessels and elicit an host inflammatory response which usually becomes granulomatous. Sometimes the inflammatory response is so extensive that one sees little lipid, as in eruptive xanthomas; in other cases, there is almost no host response, as seen with xanthelasmas. Foam cells are macrophages filled with lipid materials. They are the main components of xanthomas. In addition, giant cells are found, most commonly the Touton giant cell, containing a wreath of nuclei about a lipid-filled cytoplasm.

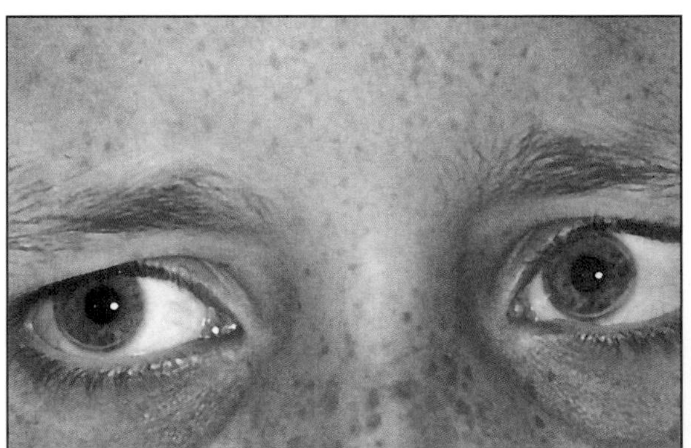

Fig. 37.7. Arcus lipoides

Older xanthomas, especially larger ones such as tuberous xanthomas, often show marked fibrosis and relatively few foam cells.

The lipid material is dissolved when the specimen is formalin-fixed and paraffin-embedded, leaving behind foamy shadows. The lipids can be demonstrated on frozen tissue using a Sudan stain and are also preserved in processing for electron microscopic examination. Here one sees lipoproteins, doubly refractile cholesterol crystals and the myelin figures of phospholipids. Fatty acids and neutral fats are also identified. The contents of the xanthoma do not correlate well with the biochemical abnormalities in the patient. Some eruptive xanthomas may contain urate crystals, even though the patients do not have gout.

Differential Diagnosis. Xanthomatization is used to describe the clinical presence of yellow infiltrates or the histologic identification of foamy cells and Touton giant cells in conditions in which there is no hyperlipoproteinemia. Many of these disorders are designated histiocytoses by convention (Chap. 64). Juvenile xanthogranuloma, reticulohistiocytoma and multicentric reticulohistiocytosis often are xanthomatous. Less often, Langerhans cell histiocytosis may have papular xanthoma-like lesions; often the CNS and bone lesions are foamy. Sarcoidosis can occasionally be very foamy, as can cutaneous T cell lymphoma.

Therapy. The therapy of xanthomas is that of the underlying disorder. Individual lesions can be excised.

Xanthelasmas

(Rayer 1835)

Definition. Flat, soft yellow plaques, usually on the upper eyelids, which are the most common xanthomas, occurring both in normolipemic individuals and patients with lipid abnormalities.

Etiology and Pathogenesis. The exact etiology of xanthelasmas is unclear. They tend to be associated with elevated LDL and cholesterol levels, not being seen in hypertriglyceridemia. But 50% of patients, especially older individuals, have no detectable lipoprotein abnormalities. While some may later develop systemic problems, many do not. The familial occurrence of xanthelasmas suggests an underlying lipid disturbance. In any event, there is local deposition of cholesterol and other lipids in the loose tissue about the eyes, followed by uptake by macrophages with little inflammation.

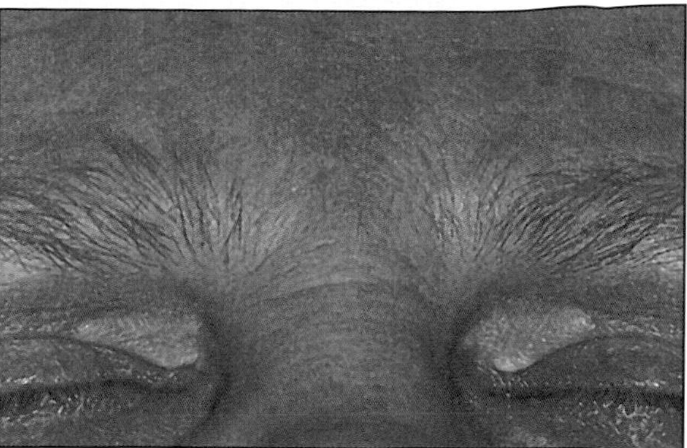

Fig. 37.8. Xanthelasmas

Clinical Findings. The most common location is the medial aspect of the upper lid, but the lower lid and skin of the inner canthus can also be involved (Fig. 37.8). The lesions are typically symmetrical. Initially one sees small yellow papules, which raise a umber of differential diagnostic questions. Later the papules coalesce into elongated soft yellow plaques that tend to run parallel to the skin creases, suggesting a role for microtrauma. The lesions are permanent and slowly progressive. They tend not to regress with lipid-lowering therapy.

Occasionally tiny cysts and comedones are found within xanthelasmas; this is known as xanthelasma cysticum. The combination of these changes and hyperpigmentation of the lids is one of the many Hutchinson syndromes; it was formerly felt to be a marker for liver disease.

Histopathology. Xanthelasmas are characterized by large foamy deposits with few giant cells or associated inflammatory response. The lipids appear to have diffused through the loose periorbital tissue. Good clues to the diagnosis are the presence of relatively superficial striated muscle with the thin skin.

Diagnostic Criteria. The diagnosis of xanthelasmas is easy. The challenge is how far to pursue the underlying diagnosis. We suggest:

- Detailed family history regarding lipid disorders, coronary artery disease and the presence of xanthelasmas or other xanthomas

- Search for other signs of lipid disorders (arcus lipoides, other xanthomas)
- Routine screening of lipids

Differential Diagnosis. Early lesions can be mistaken for syringoma, other adnexal tumors, plane warts, milia and Favre-Racouchot disease. Later, the findings are quite specific, but large xanthelasmas may overlap clinically with small necrobiotic xanthogranuloma.

Therapy. In contrast to all the other xanthomas, xanthelasmas are often treated. This phenomenon is explained by their prominent location and ease of treatment. Surgical excision, laser destruction or application of 35–50% trichloracetic acid all produce acceptable results. Recurrences are common.

Familial Hyperlipoproteinemia

There are a variety of single gene and polygenic disorders that feature disturbed lipoprotein metabolism. They were alluded to briefly in the earlier part of this chapter, but are now discussed as disease entities. Defects include abnormal biosynthesis and secretion of lipoproteins, defects in apolipoproteins, enzymatic defects and abnormal lipoprotein receptors.

The same agents are available for all the treatment of these disorders. Few dermatologists will actively manage such problems in their patients but they should be aware of these drugs and their profiles of action and side effects. Different recommendations are made depending on the number of risk factors and the presence of coronary artery disease. Diet is always the first therapeutic measure and consultation with a dietitian is usually productive.

Bile sequestration resins, such as cholestyramine and colestipol, are ion-exchange resins that bind bile acids in the intestine, preventing their reabsorption. Thus more cholesterol must be used for bile acid synthesis, more LDL receptors become free and the cholesterol and LDL levels drop. The main side effects are gastrointestinal problems and malabsorption of a variety of medications and vitamins.

Nicotinic acid is a vitamin (Chap. 49) that inhibits fat lipolysis, lowers VLDL and LDL levels and raises HDL levels. It causes flushing; more serious effects include pruritus and exanthems. In addition, hepatotoxicity and decreased glucose tolerance may appear. Nicotinamide does not cause flushing, but has no effect on lipid metabolism.

The statins, technically known as HMG-CoA reductase inhibitors, inhibit cholesterol biosynthesis and increase LDL receptor activity. The first agent was lovastatin; many more are available. They cause primarily gastrointestinal problems, which are usually mild and improve with time. The most serious side effect is myopathy, whose risk may be increased when the statins are combined with fibric acid derivatives or nicotinic acid.

Fibric acid derivatives increase lipoprotein lipase activity, lowering levels of VLDL and increasing HDL levels. Gemfibrozil is the most widely used, along with clofibrate. Both cause gastrointestinal problems, exanthems, hepatic dysfunction and increase the risk of gallstones.

Probucol is rarely used. It is an antioxidant which enhances LDL clearance, but unfortunately also blocks HDL synthesis, an undesirable effect. It too has primarily gastrointestinal side effects.

Polygenic Hypercholesterolemia

Before discussing the rare genetic disorders, we should mention the common problem. Most individuals with elevated cholesterol and LDL do not have one of the following problems. They tend to have a less striking family history; thus it is even more crucial to rule out secondary factors. They may have xanthelasmas and arcus lipoides but rarely have any other xanthomas. Efforts should be made to lower cholesterol to 180–200 mg/dl, maintain LDL below 150 mg/dl and strive to raise HDL levels that are <35 mg/dl. Initial studies showed benefits in reducing subsequent coronary artery disease in patients who had already had a myocardial infarction, but several recent studies show benefit for individuals identified because of family history or screening who have no history of cardiovascular disease.

Familial Combined Hyperlipidemia

Synonyms. Mixed hypertriglyceridemia, combined exogenous and endogenous hypertriglyceridemia, hyperprebetalipoproteinemia with chylomicronemia, multiple-type hyperlipoproteinemia

Etiology and Pathogenesis. This is the most common genetic disturbance (3–5/1000) of lipid metabolism but it is heterogeneous. There is a positive family history of coronary artery disease. Autosomal dominant inheritance appears most likely. Probably a number of genetic defects are currently grouped together under this rubric.

Clinical Findings. Typically, several different lipoprotein profiles are found within one family, reflecting individual variability in the response to elevated VLDL levels. About one-third of patients have isolated elevated triglycerides, another third elevated cholesterol and the balance elevated levels of both. Typical skin findings may include arcus lipoides and xanthelasmas; other xanthomas are not seen. Such patients often have diabetes mellitus and are obese.

Laboratory Findings. The serum may be cloudy or milky. Patients have elevated levels of VLDL, LDL or both, probably secondary to increased hepatic production of VLDL. The individual lipoprotein phenotype may change over time. Apolipoprotein B levels are also usually elevated.

Course and Prognosis. The risk of coronary artery disease is high. This combined pattern is so common that it accounts for about 10–20% of all myocardial infarctions.

Therapy. Diet and weight loss are the mainstays. If no improvement is seen, the patient should be treated according to the overriding lipid defect. If hypercholesterolemia predominates, then HMG-CoA reductase inhibitors are usually employed. If hypertriglyceridemia predominates, then the fibrates (fibric acid derivatives) or nicotinic acid are tried.

Familial Hypercholesterolemia

(Thannhauser and Magendantz 1939; Brown and Goldstein 1974)

Synonyms. Familial hyperbetalipoproteinemia, essential hypercholesterolemia, familial idiopathic hypercholesterolemic xanthomatosis

Etiology and Pathogenesis. Familial hypercholesterolemia is inherited in an autosomal dominant pattern. It involves a mutation in the LDL receptor on chromosome 19. Four different allelic mutations have been described.

The lack of an efficiently functioning LDL receptor system results in increased circulating levels of LDL cholesterol. Since the normal feedback does not work, the body uses other tricks, such as packaging the excess cholesterol in xanthomas.

Clinical Findings. The clinical findings vary radically between homozygotes and heterozygotes. Homozygosity occurs with a frequency of about 1/1,000,000. These more severely affected individuals have hypercholesterolemia at birth, may already have coronary artery disease in the first years of life and rarely survive beyond 30 years of age. Tendon xanthomas are virtually pathognomonic of this disorder. Patients also have typical intertriginous and digital web plane xanthomas, as well as arcus lipoides, subperiosteal xanthomas and even cardiac valve xanthomas. Some may also have sudden painful attacks of polyarthritis and tenosynovitis.

In contrast, heterozygosity is very common, with a frequency of 1/500. Affected individuals also have hypercholesterolemia at birth, but the levels are lower and coronary artery disease usually develops later, in the third decade. At least half the male patients have had a myocardial infarct by 60 years of age; in women, the curve is shifted somewhat, presumably because of estrogen's protective effects. The main cutaneous findings are similar to those in homozygotes but occur later. About 70% of adults have tendon xanthomas.

Laboratory Findings. The serum is clear. Homozygotes have cholesterol levels up to 1200 mg/dl with LDL levels also raised. Heterozygotes have levels ranging from 300–600 mg/dl. In both, triglycerides and HDL are close to normal. The specific LDL receptor defects can be identified in specialized laboratories.

Course and Prognosis. Homozygotes have a poor outlook, dying at an early age. About 25% of male heterozygotes (and 2% of female heterozygotes) are dead from coronary artery disease by 50 years of age.

Therapy. The most important step is to screen first degree relatives so they too can be followed. It is very difficult to produce much improvement with diet. Cholesterol intake should be held to a minimum, unsaturated fatty acids used and bulky foods that bind fats (such as oats, beans, pectins) employed. Heterozygotes are usually treated with HMG-CoA reductase inhibitors and a bile acid sequestrant. This combination stimulates expression of the LDL receptor coded by the normal gene. Some are treated with LDL apheresis, removing the LDL during plasma exchange. Ileal bypass operations, portocaval shunts and even liver transplants are also possibilities.

Familial Defective Apolipoprotein B-100

Etiology and Pathogenesis. In this rare autosomal dominant disorder, a point mutation in the apolipoprotein B-100 gene replaces arginine with glutamine. This interferes with the ability of the apolipoprotein and thus LDL to bind to the LDL receptor. The resulting disease is therefore similar to familial hypercholesterolemia. All patients have been heterozygotes thus far; the homozygote state is perhaps not compatible with life.

Clinical Findings. These patients are clinically very similar to heterozygotes with familial hypercholesterolemia. Both the clinical features, such as tendon xanthomas, arcus lipoides and xanthelasmas, and the prognosis are comparable.

Laboratory Findings. The serum is clear. The general laboratory pattern is identical to that of familial hypercholesterolemia. If LDL receptor studies are normal, then one should search for the apolipoprotein B-100 point mutation.

Therapy. Same as for familial hypercholesterolemia.

Familial Dysbetalipoproteinemia

(Gofmann 1954; Utermann et al. 1975)

Synonyms. Remnant particle disease, broad-β disease

Epidemiology. The disease has a prevalence of about 1:3000. The genetic defect is more common but cofactors must be present for it to become clinically apparent.

Etiology and Pathogenesis. Familial dysbetalipoproteinemia is caused by association of the apolipoprotein genotype E2/E2 with some other primary or secondary cause of hyperlipidemia. Diabetes mellitus, hypothyroidism, alcohol abuse and obesity are common triggers. Patients have VLDL that migrate at the β position, rather than at the normal pre-β position; these particles are remnants of both chylomicrons and VLDL. The mutant apolipoprotein E genes lead to impaired conversion of VLDL and to impaired hepatic uptake of remnants. The β-VLDL accumulate and form xanthomas and atherogenic deposits.

Clinical Findings. The first manifestations are usually in adult life. The most typical clinical finding is multiple tiny xanthomas in the palmar creases. There may be a variety of other xanthoma, including tuberoeruptive lesions and tendinous lesions. Arcus lipoides is also common. Diabetes mellitus is frequently present.

Laboratory Findings. The serum is cloudy and after refrigeration a band of chylomicrons can be seen. Cholesterol, triglyceride and VLDL levels are elevated, while LDL and HDL are usually within normal limits. In this case, the electrophoretic pattern is very helpful showing a broad β-band, composed of β-VLDL. The E2/E2 genotype can be confirmed in specialized laboratories.

Prognosis. These patients are at risk for coronary artery disease and also have significant peripheral vascular disease.

Therapy. Dysbetalipoproteinemia is quite therapy-responsive. If a secondary factor is found, it should be treated. Weight reduction and appropriate diet are usually sufficient. If not, fibric acid derivatives, nicotinic acid and HMG CoA reductase inhibitors are all effective.

Familial Lipoprotein Lipase Deficiency

(Bürger and Grütz 1932)

Synonyms. Familial hyperchylomicronemia, idiopathic hyperlipidemic xanthomatosis, exogenous hypertriglyceridemia, Bürger-Grütz syndrome

Etiology and Pathogenesis. The disorder is inherited in an autosomal recessive pattern, like most enzyme defects. Patients lack lipoprotein lipase and are unable to break down the chylomicrons in their exogenous pathway. Thus there is a massive accumulation of chylomicrons. A lack of apolipoprotein C-II produces the same effect since this apolipoprotein activates lipoprotein lipase.

Clinical Findings. Most patients present before 10 years of age with acute abdominal pain. They may simply have colicky pain, but often the answer is acute pancreatitis because of the high triglyceride levels. They develop eruptive xanthomas which may also involve the oral mucosa. Lipemia retinalis is also present. Hepatosplenomegaly is another common finding because of massive deposits of fat-laden macrophages.

Laboratory Findings. Triglyceride levels may range from 2000–12,000 mg/dl, spiking with fatty meals.

The milky or cloudy serum shows a chylomicron cap and electrophoresis reveals a massive nonmigratory collection of chylomicrons. Cholesterol levels are normal. Absent lipoprotein lipase activity can be demonstrated in adipose tissue biopsies.

Course and Prognosis. The main risk to these patients is recurrent pancreatitis. If the serum triglyceride values are over 1000 mg/dl, abdominal colic is likely. The xanthomas disappear when the triglyceride levels drop. There is no increased risk of coronary artery disease.

Therapy. Dietary measures are the only effective treatment. Fat must be reduced to under 20 g daily and should account for less than 15% of the daily caloric intake.

Familial Apolipoprotein C-II Deficiency

In this equally rare, autosomal recessive inherited disorder, apolipoprotein C-II is lacking. The patients are similar to familial lipoprotein lipase deficiency patients but develop less severe symptoms and at a later age. They can be identified by the high triglyceride levels, chylomicronemia and the absence of apolipoprotein C-II. Similarly, their defect is corrected in vitro when exogenous apo C-II is added. Treatment is dietary. Acute abdominal attacks can be treated with infusions of normal plasma or purified apolipoprotein C-II. Heterozygotes, that is, individuals with one normal gene, may have mild hypertriglyceridemia but are asymptomatic.

Familial Hypertriglyceridemia

This common, autosomal dominant inherited disorder has yet to be explained. The triglyceride and VLDL levels are elevated but HDL, LDL and cholesterol are normal. Patients are usually asymptomatic, unless they develop very high triglyceride levels. Diagnosis is based on the laboratory findings and similar findings in about 50% of first degree relatives. Treatment is dietary.

Tangier Disease

(Frederickson et al. 1961)

Synonyms. Familial HDL deficiency, analphalipoproteinemia

This disease was first described in the triracial isolate (Black, American Indian, Caucasian) on Tangier Island, an isolated fishing island in Chesapeake Bay, Maryland, USA. It is inherited in an autosomal recessive pattern. Apo-AI is in one way or another defective so that no HDL is formed. Patients have elevated triglyceride levels and abnormal chylomicron remnant particles. The most reliable clinical finding is yellow xanthomatous tonsils. Also typical are peripheral neuropathies, hepatosplenomegaly and, rarely, plane xanthomas. Cardiovascular disease is not a problem.

Watson-Alagille Syndrome

(Watson and Miller 1973; Alagille et al. 1975)

Synonyms. Alagille syndrome, arteriohepatic dysplasia

Watson-Alagille syndrome is inherited in an autosomal dominant pattern; the gene is located on chromosome 20p. The main problem is congenital hypoplasia of the intrahepatic bile ducts with resultant cholestasis and pruritus. The cholesterol and triglycerides are markedly elevated and lead to a variety of cutaneous xanthomas, which may improve with age or following liver transplantation. Other skin findings include steatocystoma multiplex, nevus comedonicus, palmar erythema, photosensitivity and, rarely, secondary amyloidosis. The face has been described as triangular with deeply set eyes and a long nose. Peripheral pulmonary artery stenosis is very common. Other features include thickened digits, mental retardation, ocular anomalies and a variety of skeletal defects, especially involving the vertebral arch.

Normolipemic Xanthomatoses

This term refers to a wide variety of totally unrelated disorders. By definition, they feature cutaneous or subcutaneous xanthomas but are not associated with lipoprotein abnormalities. They can be divided into several categories including noncholesterol sterol deposits and histiocytic disorders. Some authors include xanthelasmas here.

Noncholesterol Sterol Deposits

Cerebrotendinous Xanthomatosis

(van Bogaert et al. 1937)

Synonym. Van Bogaert syndrome

Etiology and Pathogenesis. In this very rare, autosomal recessive disorder, cholestanol (or dihydrocholesterol), a cholesterol metabolite, is deposited in the skin, CNS and bile. Missing is a hepatic mitochondrial enzyme CYP27, which is needed to hydroxylate bile acids, especially chenodeoxycholic acid. Because of faulty feedback control, an intermediate, cholestanol, accumulates.

Clinical Findings. The xanthomas are large tendinous lesions clinically identical to those associated with familial hypercholesterolemia and related disorders. While cholesterol is present in the deposits, serum levels are normal. The presence of a wide range of CNS problems should suggest the diagnosis; progressive cerebellar ataxia, spinal paresis and dementia are the usual outcome in untreated patients, with trouble most often starting in young adult life. Cataracts also develop, as does coronary artery disease. Diagnosis can be confirmed by serum cholestanol levels; imaging studies reveal the CNS deposits.

Therapy. The treatment is replacement of chenodeoxycholic acid, which inhibits the normal bile synthesis, reducing both cholestanol and cholesterol, and hopefully stabilizing the patient.

Phytosterolemia

(BHATTACHARYYA and CONNOR 1974)

Synonym. Sitosterolemia

Etiology and Pathogenesis. The etiology is not clear, but there appears to be increased absorption of the plant sterols sitosterol and campesterol. The disorder is inherited in an autosomal recessive pattern.

Clinical Findings. The cutaneous finding include large, subcutaneous tuberous and tendon xanthomas, just as in familial hypercholesterolemia. The patients also are at risk for coronary artery disease.

Laboratory Findings. The erythrocytes show fatty inclusions. Serum phytosterol levels are elevated, along with cholesterol and even cholestanol levels.

Therapy. The major treatment is a diet avoiding all vegetable oils. In addition, bile sequestrants increase the output of bile acids and bind plant oils in the intestine.

Histiocytic Disorders

There are a number of diseases which are arbitrarily classified as histiocytic (Chap. 64) but may present with or feature xanthomas. Included in this list are Langerhans cell histiocytosis, in which xanthomatous lesions are common in the CNS and bone but rare in the skin. Some of the macrophage disorders may also present with foamy or xanthomatous lesions. Patients with xanthoma disseminatum have multiple lesions which are clinically and histologically true xanthomas. Papular xanthomas may be solitary or multiple, while patients with progressive nodular histiocytomas may occasionally have foamy lesions. Several normolipemic diseases that are designated both as xanthomatoses and histiocytoses are discussed here.

Verruciform Xanthoma

(SHAFER 1971)

Verruciform xanthomas are most often found on the oral mucosa (Chap. 33), usually associated with trauma, and are often grouped with the non-Langerhans cell histiocytoses. They must be distinguished from human papilloma virus infections and squamous cell carcinoma. When present in the skin, they usually are found in epidermal nevi, CHILD syndrome and damaged skin, as in lupus erythematosus, lichen planus, chronic dermatitis and similar disorders. Histologically, they show markedly elongated rete ridges with foam-laden dermal papillae. The treatment is excision.

Trauma-Induced Xanthomas

Verruciform xanthoma can be taken as the prototype of a trauma-induced xanthoma. It usually arises in areas of direct skin or mucosal damage, or in skin which has been altered by chronic inflammation, such as in epidermal nevi and chronic inflammatory dermatoses, e.g., stasis dermatitis or lymphedema. Similar scenarios include the appearance of multiple xanthomas in atopic dermatitis, chronic sun-damaged skin and a variety of other inflammatory settings. The injection of oily or fatty substances into the skin may also induce xanthoma-like lesions. Another scenario is the leakage of lymphatic fluid in lymphedema leading to reactive xanthoma formation.

Diffuse Normolipemic Plane Xanthomas
(Altman and Winkelmann 1962)

Synonym. Xanthelasma corporis

Definition. Large, flat or patchy xanthomas usually associated with hematologic disease.

Clinical Findings. In diffuse normolipemic plane xanthomas, patients typically have yellow-orange papules that may coalesce in patches or even large sheets, covering the entire thorax, for example. The periorbital area is most often involved; initial lesions may be identical to xanthelasma, but the disease then progresses. The trunk is the second most common site of involvement. The lesions may initially present as urticarial papules and plaques. As the name suggests, the patients are normolipemic without lipid abnormalities.

Almost all patients have hematologic disease; paraproteinemias are most common, but benign monoclonal gammopathy (usually IgA), multiple myeloma, cryoglobulinemia and Castleman disease have been described. The skin disease may proceed the hematologic problem by many years.

Histopathology. The lesions are identical to xanthelasmas, infiltrates rich in foam cells without any other distinguishing features. The disorder is so rare that more detailed immunohistochemical studies are lacking.

Differential Diagnosis. The differential diagnosis is confusing, mainly because of the terminology. We diagnose diffuse normolipemic plane xanthoma when sheets of lesions are present, especially if periorbital involvement is present or the patient has a hematologic problem. Multiple papular xanthomas are probably the preferred diagnosis when lesions develop in an area of previous skin disease. The distinction between diffuse normolipemic plane xanthoma and necrobiotic xanthogranuloma is equally confusing. Both are typically periorbital and associated with paraproteinemia; necrobiotic xanthogranuloma is discussed in Chapter 50.

Therapy. No reliable therapy has been described. The underlying hematologic problem may require treatment with cytotoxic agents, which can produce some improvement in the skin condition.

Miscellaneous Disorders

A number of other disorders can present with xanthomatous lesions. All the granulomatous diseases, including sarcoidosis and lepromatous leprosy, can also occasionally have lesions that are so foamy under the microscope that one thinks of xanthomas. Rare dermatofibromas will be rich in lipids. A wide range of metabolic disorders in which unusual lipid products are deposited in various tissues can conceivably produce xanthomatous skin lesions. Some of these are discussed in Chapter 38.

Bibliography

Basic Science Aspects

Borgia MC, Medici F (1998) Perspectives in the treatment of dyslipidemias in the prevention of coronary heart disease. Angiology 49:339–348

Davignon J, Genest J Jr (1998) Genetics of lipoprotein disorders. Endocrinol Metab Clin North Am 27:521–550

Fredrickson DS, Levy RI, Lees RS (1967) Fat transport in lipoproteins – an integrated approach to mechanisms and disorders. N Eng J Med 276:34–42

Scriver CR, Beaudet AL, Sly WS et al. (eds) (1995) The metabolic and molecular bases of inherited disease, 7th edn. McGraw-Hill, New York

Xanthomas

Ahrens EH, Kunkel HG (1949) The relationship between serum lipids and skin xanthoma in eighteen patients with primary biliary cirrhosis. J Clin Invest 28:1565–1575

Braun-Falco O (1973)Origin, structure and function of the xanthoma cell. Nutr Metab 15:68–88

Braun-Falco O, Keller C, Zöllner N (eds) (1973) Xanthoma formation and other tissue reactions to hyperlipidemias. Karger, Basel

Cruz PD Jr, East C, Bergstresser PR (1988) Dermal, subcutaneous and tendon xanthomas: diagnostic markers for specific lipoprotein disorders. J Am Acad Dermatol 19:95–111

Miller DM, Brodell RT (1995) Eruptive xanthomatosis with linear koebnerization. J Am Acad Dermatol 33:834–835

Miwa N, Kanzaki T (1992) The Koebner phenomenon in eruptive xanthoma. J Dermatol 19:48–50

Parker F (1985) Xanthomas and hyperlipidemias. J Am Acad Dermatol 13:1–30

Xanthelasmas

Bergman R (1994) The pathogenesis and clinical significance of xanthelasma palpebrarum. J Am Acad Dermatol 30:236–242

Douste-Blazy P, Marcel YL, Cohen L et al. (1982) Increased frequency of Apo E-ND phenotype and hyperapobetalipoproteinemia in normolipidemic subjects with xanthelasmas of the eyelids. Ann Intern Med 96:164–169

Eedy DJ (1996) Treatment of xanthelasma by excision with secondary intention healing. Clin Exp Dermatol 21:273–275

Familial Hyperlipoproteinemia

Alagille D, Odievre M, Gautier M et al. (1975) Hepatic ductular hypoplasia associated with characteristic facies, vertebral malformations, retarded physical, mental, and sexual development, and cardiac murmur. J Pediatr 86: 63–71

Brown MS, Goldstein JL (1974) Expression of the familial hypercholesterolemia gene in heterozygotes: mechanism for a dominant disorder in man. Science 185:61–63

Bürger M, Grütz O (1932) Über hepatosplenomegale Lipoidose mit xanthomatösen Veränderungen in Haut und Schleimhaut. Arch Dermatol Syph 166:542–575

Frederickson DS, Altrocchi PH, Avioli LV et al. (1961) Tangier disease – combined clinical staff conference at the National Institutes of Health. Ann Intern Med 55:1016–1031

Innerarity TL, Weisgraber KH, Arnold KS et al. (1987) Familial defective apolipoprotein B-100: low density lipoproteins with abnormal receptor binding. Proc Natl Acad Sci USA 84:6919–6923

Knopp RH (1999) Drug treatment of lipid disorders. NEJM 341:498–511

Thannhauser SJ, Magendantz H (1939) The different clinical groups of xanthomatous diseases: a clinical physiological study of 22 cases. Ann Intern Med 11:1662–1746

Utermann G, Jaeschke M, Menzel J (1975) Familial hyperlipoproteinemia type III: deficiency of a specific apolipoprotein (apo E-III) in the very-low-density lipoproteins. FEBS Lett 56:352–355

Watson GH, Miller V (1973) Arteriohepatic dysplasia: familial pulmonary arterial stenosis with neonatal liver disease. Arch Dis Child 48:459–466

Weston CF, Burton JL (1987) Xanthomas in the Watson-Alagille syndrome. J Am Acad Dermatol 16:1117–1121

Normolipemic Xanthomatosis

Bhattacharyya AK, Connor WE (1974) β-Sitosterolemia and xanthomasosis. A newly described lipid storage disease in two sisters. J Clin Invest 53:1033–1043

Parker F (1986) Normocholesterolemic xanthomatosis. Arch Dermatol 122:1253–1257

van Bogaert L, Scherer HJ, Epstein E (1937) Une forme cérébrale de la cholesterinose généralisée. Masson and Cie, Paris

Verruciform Xanthoma

Kimura S (1984) Verruciform xanthoma of the scrotum. Arch Dermatol 120:1378–1379

Kraemer BB, Schmidt WA, Foucar E et al. (1981) Verruciform xanthoma of the penis. Arch Dermatol 117:516–518

Meyers DC, Woosley JT, Reddick RL (1992) Verruciform xanthoma in association with discoid lupus erythematosus. J Cutan Pathol 19:156–158

Neville B (1986) The verruciform xanthoma. A review and report of eight new cases. Am J Dermatopathol 8:247–253

Nowparast B, Howell FV, Rick GM (1981) Verruciform xanthoma: A clinicopathologic review and report of fifty-four cases. Oral Surg Oral Med Oral Pathol 51:619–625

Shafer WG (1971) Verruciform xanthoma. Oral Surg Oral Med Oral Pathol 31:784–789

Yamamoto T, Katayama I, Nishioka K (1995) Verruciform xanthoma in a psoriatic patient under PUVA Therapy. Dermatology 191:254–256

Diffuse Normolipemic Plane Xanthomas

Altman J, Winkelmann RK (1962) Diffuse normolipidemic plane xanthoma. Arch Dermatol 85:633–640

Ginarte M, Peteiro C, Toribio J (1997) Generalized plane xanthoma and idiopathic Bence-Jones proteinuria. Clin Exp Dermatol 22:192–194

Lynch PJ, Winkelmann RK (1966) Generalized plane xanthoma and systemic disease. Arch Dermatol 93:639–646

CHAPTER 38

The Sphingolipidoses

Contents

Basic Science Aspects

The lipid storage disorders are a very complex group of disorders. The lipid disorders that lead to xanthomas and an increased risk of coronary artery disease and pancreatitis are discussed in the preceding chapter (Chap. 37). Another major group are the lipid disorders associated with ichthyosis (Chap. 17). In this chapter we concentrate on the sphingolipidoses, listed in Table 38.1. In these extremely rare disorders, some of which have unique dermatologic findings, a missing lysosomal enzyme leads to the accumulation of a sphingo- or glycolipid in a variety of cells.

Sphingolipids are complex membrane lipids with three major components: (1) the C_{18} amino alcohol sphingosine; (2) a long-chain fatty acid attached to the C-2 amino group; (3) various polar molecules attached to the C-1 -OH group via a β-glycosidic linkage.

The prototype molecule is ceramide. Three basic types of sphingolipids are formed by a variety of replacements at C-1:

- Cerebroside: Sugar is attached at C-1
- Sphingomyelin: Phosphorylcholine or related molecule is attached at C-1

Table 38.1. The sphingolipidoses

Disease	Metabolic defect	Accumulated product	Skin findings
Fabry (1898)	α-Galactosidase deficiency	Globotriaosylceramide	Angiokeratomas
Gaucher (1882)	Glucocerebrosidase deficiency	Glucosylceramide	Hyperpigmentation
Niemann-Pick I	Sphingomyelinase deficiency	Sphingomyelin, cholesterol	Xanthomas, waxy infiltrates, hyperpigmentation
Niemann-Pick II	Sphingomyelinase deficiency, abnormal cholesterol esterification	Sphingomyelin, cholesterol, glycosphingolipids,bis(monoacylglycero)phosphate	None
Farber (1952)	Acid ceramidase deficiency	Ceramides	Subcutaneous nodules
Schindler	α-*N*-acetylgalactosaminidase deficiency	Glycosphingolipids	Angiokeratomas
Fucosidosis	α-l-fucosidase deficiency	Fucose-containing glycolipids	Angiokeratomas
Sialidosis (mucolipidosis type I)	α-Neuraminidase deficiency	Oligosaccharides	Angiokeratomas
Galactosialidosis	α-Neuraminidase, β-galactosidase deficiencies	Oligosaccharides	Angiokeratomas
Multiple sulfatase deficiency (Chap. 17)	Deficiencies of arylsulfatase-A, steroid sulfatase, mucopolysaccharide sulfatase	Multiple sulfolipids	Ichthyosis

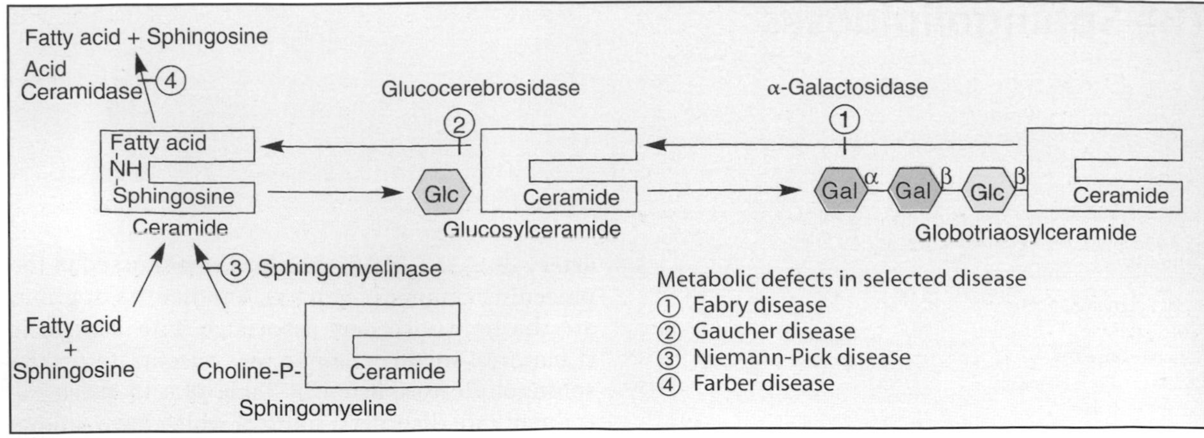

Fig. 38.1. Sphingolipid metabolism

- Gangliosides: The most complex; they contain several sugars and one or more sialic acid residues (G_M refers to monosialoganglioside)

The fatty acids may also vary but they do not determine the basic classes.

Lysosomal hydrolases are required to break down the sphingolipids. Their deficiency, usually inherited in an autosomal recessive (or occasionally X-linked recessive) pattern, leads to the accumulation of various sphingolipids, hence the terms storage disorder, lysosomal storage disorder, or sphingolipidosis. The sphingolipids are structural proteins, primarily involved in membrane formation and repair. Depending on the compound, the storage problem may make itself prominent in the CNS, liver, bone marrow or many other sites. Figure 38.1 provides an overview of sphingolipid metabolism. We will only consider those disorders which have cutaneous manifestations. The classic text *The Metabolic and Molecular Bases of Inherited Disease* (Scriver et al. 1995) should be consulted for further details on all these disorders.

Fabry Disease

(Fabry 1898; Anderson 1898)

Synonym. Angiokeratoma corporis diffusum

Definition. X-linked disorder with defect in α-galactosidase, characterized by angiokeratomas in the skin.

Epidemiology. Fabry disease is inherited in an X-linked recessive pattern; its incidence is estimated at 1:40,000.

Etiology and Pathogenesis. The defective gene is located on chromosome Xq21–22 and codes for α-galactosidase. Specific point mutations in the gene have been identified. Glycolipids, mainly globotriaosylceramide (ceramide trihexosidase), accumulate in a variety of cells. Endothelial, perithelial and vascular smooth muscle cells are most prominently involved, but myocytes, a variety of ocular cells, autonomic ganglion cells and renal glomerular epithelial cells are all involved. The female carriers have some level of the α-galactosidase but may have minor problems, depending on the Lyon effect.

Clinical Findings. The major organs of involvement are the renal and cardiovascular systems. In addition, significant ocular and autonomic nervous system problems arise, while the skin findings are an important marker.

Cutaneous Findings. Angiokeratomas are the classic finding in Fabry disease. They are small dark red papules, usually less than 5 mm in size, which blanch poorly on diascopy (Fig. 38.2). While the lesions are called angiokeratomas, they are no more keratotic that ordinary telangiectases or tiny hemangiomas. They initially appear before puberty and are first identified around the umbilicus, the buttocks or the genitalia. Later they may cover broad areas, coalesce and even become cosmetically disturbing. While the face is generally spared, there may be perioral

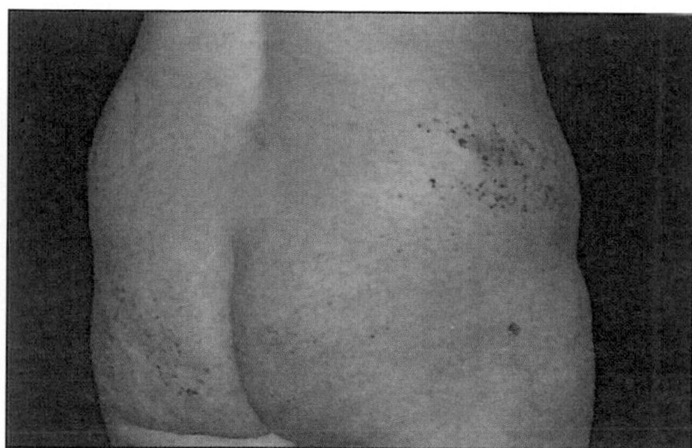

Fig. 38.2. Fabry disease

lesions, as well as involvement of the oral mucosa and conjunctiva.

Systemic Findings

Autonomic Nervous System. Often the presenting complaint is painful paresthesias involving the palms and soles. Typically the children are treated as "whiners" or "disturbed", unless a family history is available or until other findings appear. The pains may become so severe and persistent that they markedly hamper the patient's lifestyle. Typically they become worse with warmth, in contrast to erythromelalgia. The hands do not change color. Other signs of autonomic dysfunction include hypohidrosis and subsequent fever with marked physical activity in warm climates.

Cardiac, CNS and Renal Problems. With increasing age, the deposits in the heart, coronary vessels, brain and kidneys cause significant problems. There may be cardiac myopathy, cardiac valvular defects, conduction defects and coronary artery disease. Early or multiple strokes, as well as transient ischemic episodes, can lead to neurologic defects. Renal failure may also occur through a variety of mechanisms, often requiring renal transplantation, which may produce an improvement in many of the other problems.

Ocular Problems. The most classic finding is corneal lipid deposits known as cornea verticillata which are best seen with slit-lamp evaluation. They are diagnostically useful and may be found in heterozygous female carriers as well as affected males. Similar changes are seen following long-term chloroquine or amiodarone therapy. In addition, more serious problems include cataracts and retinal vascular damage.

Histopathology. Microscopic examination reveals small superficial ectatic vascular structures in the papillary dermis. When they impinge on the epidermis, there may be hyperkeratosis. Sometimes the vessel wall appears vacuolated even on hematoxylin-eosin examination. The lipid inclusions can be better appreciated if frozen tissue is examined, because they are doubly refractile, or if toluidine blue staining is used. Electron microscopic examination reveals the characteristic lamellated electron-dense sphingolipid inclusions in a variety of structures, including the cutaneous vessels.

Laboratory Findings. Examination of urine reveals birefringent lipid globules, the Maltese crosses, in shed epithelial cells. Similar changes can be found in bone marrow macrophages and in small vessels in skin or renal biopsies. Enzyme levels can be assayed in many tissues and the excess ceramides identified in the plasma or urine.

Course and Prognosis. The outlook is not favorable. The severe coronary, CNS and renal problems combine to reduce life expectancy to less than 50 years.

Differential Diagnosis. Many different types of angiokeratomas can be seen (Chap. 59). Older individuals may have scrotal or vulvar angiokeratomas without any underlying disease, which may be confused with Fabry disease until a history is taken. The other cutaneous variants are only confusing histologically. Several different metabolic disorders may also feature angiokeratomas. They include fucosidosis, sialidosis, galactosialidosis, Schindler disease and aspartylglucosaminuria. All have different clinical and biochemical markers. Finally, the telangiectatic vessels in hereditary hemorrhagic telangiectasia (Osler-Weber-Rendu syndrome) are similar, as are cherry or senile hemangiomas.

Therapy. The angiokeratomas, when disturbing, can be removed with lasers or other destructive therapy. Phenytoin and/or carbamazepine are the best treatment for the acral paresthesias. Hemodialysis or renal transplantation is often needed. The other problems are treated symptomatically. Substitution therapy with purified α-galactosidase as well as attempts to reinsert the gene with somatic cell therapy are in early development.

Gaucher Disease

(Gaucher 1882)

Synonyms. Glucosylceramide lipidosis, cerebroside lipidosis

Definition. Acute, subacute or chronic disease resulting from a defect in glucocerebrosidase with deposition of cerebrosides.

Epidemiology. Gaucher disease is uncommon but is the most common of the sphingolipidoses. The incidence of the adult type among Ashkenazi Jews is around 1:1000. It is inherited in an autosomal recessive pattern.

Etiology and Pathogenesis. The defect in glucocerebrosidase is found on chromosome 1q21. As a result, glucosylcerebrosidases accumulate in the lysosomes of macrophages primarily in the liver, spleen and bone marrow. These lipid-laden macrophages are known as Gaucher cells. They are 20–100 μm in diameter, may be multinucleated, stain positively with acid phosphatase and their cytoplasm has a "crumpled tissue-paper" appearance, as the ceramide-protein complexes form a woven network of fine fibers.

Clinical Findings. Three different types of Gaucher disease have been described. They presumably involve various mutations in the same locus.

Type I, Adult or Chronic. This is the most common and least-damaging variant because the nervous system is spared. There apparently is adequate enzyme activity in the neuronal tissue, suggesting perhaps a mutation in some part of the gene essential to tissue distribution. Onset is usually in adulthood but may start in the first decade. The main problems are hepatosplenomegaly, bone damage and pain and hematologic problems, including anemia, leukopenia and thrombocytopenia.

The typical skin finding is diffuse hyperpigmentation, often patchy and concentrated on the face. It can be mistaken for melasma. On the legs, the lesions tend to be more striped. The conjunctiva are also darkened. Both iron and melanin are deposited in the skin. If hematologic and liver problems are severe, petechiae, hemorrhages and telangiectases may be present.

Type II, Infantile or Acute. These patients have massive hepatosplenomegaly, mental retardation, numerous other CNS problems and usually die in the first 2 years of life. The cause of death is usually aspiration pneumonia or another infection. They may have pigmentary changes of the skin and conjunctiva.

Type III, Juvenile or Subacute. While similar to Type II, these patients have a slower course, often living into adolescence. They too may be hyperpigmented early in life and tend to darken.

Histopathology. No Gaucher cells are found in the skin. Instead hemosiderin, melanin and lipofuchsin are identified.

Laboratory Findings. The enzyme may be assayed in leukocytes or fibroblasts. Serum acid phosphatase is usually elevated. The Gaucher cells are easily found in the bone marrow. Prenatal diagnosis is possible, involving either enzyme assays or DNA analysis.

Course and Prognosis. While the type I patients do relatively well, the others have a less favorable outlook.

Differential Diagnosis. The main clinical differential is Niemann-Pick disease, as well as other even rarer metabolic disorders. The dermatologic findings are a curiosity and play no role in the diagnosis. The differential diagnosis of hyperpigmentation is discussed in Chapter 26.

Therapy. Type I patients may benefit from bone marrow transplantation, as well as splenectomy and skilled orthopedic management. Enzyme substitution with a modified glucocerebrosidase that is taken up selectively by macrophages has proven helpful. Type II and type III patients will probably only benefit from genetic procedures designed to return the missing gene to their body via manipulated hematopoietic stem cells.

The hyperpigmentation can be bleached like any other hyperpigmentation but results are uneven. Usually the skin is the least of the patient's problems.

Niemann-Pick Disease

(Niemann 1914; Pick 1926)

Synonyms. Sphingomyelin-cholesterol lipidosis, sphingomyelinosis

Etiology and Pathogenesis. Unfortunately for all students, Niemann-Pick Disease is not one disease but many and has been regrouped several times. The most workable classification involves:

- Niemann-Pick type I: Sphingomyelinase deficiency
- Niemann-Pick type II: Sphingomyelinase normal; variety of other cholesterol defects, including esterification

All forms are inherited in an autosomal recessive pattern. Type I involves several allelic mutations on chromosome 11p15. Most of these patients are Ashkenazi Jews. At least one form of type II involves a defect on chromosome 18p, the largest pedigree of which involves French Canadians. In type I, sphingomyelin and cholesterol are stored, while in type II sphingomyelin accumulation is less severe and cholesterol, glycosphingolipids and bis(monoacylglycero)phosphate also build up. The main sites of accumulation in both forms are the spleen, lymph nodes and CNS. There is no storage in the skin. The typical foamy Niemann-Pick macrophages in the bone marrow and other organs are 20–90 µm in diameter and described as mulberry cells, as they are packed with many small globules of sphingomyelin.

Clinical Findings. In the type I patients, there are acute, subacute and chronic forms. The acute form presents with hepatosplenomegaly, CNS problems, deafness and blindness in infancy. Often the first finding is vomiting and failure to thrive, associated with jaundice. Ocular examination reveals the cherry red spots, also seen in Tay-Sachs disease and other metabolic disorders. There is also diffuse lymphadenopathy. The patients with this form usually die in the first 2–3 years of life. Other patients may have a less progressive course or even first present in adolescence or adult life. The type II forms also are classified as acute, subacute or chronic, but only the acute form is well studied. No cutaneous findings are commonly described.

Of interest to the dermatologist are a variety of lesions which are of little importance to the tragically afflicted patients and their families. Remotely, one could include Niemann-Pick disease as a normolipemic xanthomatosis, since about 25% of the acute type I patients develop xanthomas in the axillae and on the face. In addition, the abdomen and extremities may acquire a waxy indurated appearance. Both of these changes are caused by deposits of sphingomyelin. There may also be diffuse hyperpigmentation, café-au-lait macules, Mongolian spots (dermal melanosis) and oral mucosal hyperpigmentation.

Histopathology. Usually only increased basal melanin is seen. If a nodular xanthomatous lesion is biopsied, foam cells may be seen. Electron microscopy of lymphocytes seen in the skin reveals lysosomal inclusions.

Laboratory Findings. The enzyme may be assayed and the characteristic cells found on bone marrow biopsy. Prenatal diagnosis is possible for type I disease, via sphingomyelinase assays. DNA analysis is also possible.

Course and Prognosis. The outlook is poor, but varies with the exact form of the disease.

Differential Diagnosis. Severe forms of Gaucher disease and Tay-Sachs disease are the main problems. It is unlikely that even the most enthusiastic individual could confuse Niemann-Pick with the lipid disorders discussed in Chapter 37. The lipid-related xanthomas generally appear later in life.

Therapy. Supportive care and bone marrow transplantation are all that is available.

Farber Disease

(Farber 1952)

Synonyms. Disseminated lipogranulomatosis, familial lipogranulomatosis, ceramidase deficiency

Definition. Rare storage disease with ceramide deposition and frequent skin involvement.

Epidemiology. Farber disease is inherited in an autosomal recessive pattern. Fewer than 50 patients have been reported.

Etiology and Pathogenesis. There is a defect in acid ceramidase; the gene is located at 8p22. Thus ceramides accumulate in many organs, especially the liver, lungs and CNS, as well as the skin. The cutaneous deposits probably arise because of the ceramides synthesized for the epidermal lipid barrier.

Clinical Findings. The classic triad is hoarseness from laryngeal infiltration, painful and restricted joint motility, and multiple subcutaneous brown

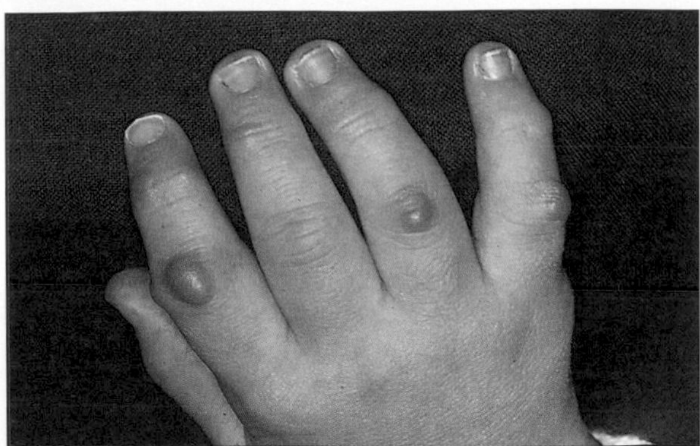

Fig. 38.3. Farber disease. (Courtesy of Christian Schmoeckel, MD, Munich, Germany)

nodules, most often located near joints (Fig. 38.3). The typical sites of skin involvement are the fingers, elbows, knees, ears and nape. Later the liver, spleen, lungs, heart and brain are infiltrated. Patients usually die in childhood. Those who live longer tend to develop more prominent and disabling skin and joint lesions.

Histopathology. The subcutaneous and periarticular nodules display granulomatous inflammation. Lipid-laden macrophages are common. In older lesions, there may be more lymphocytes, multinucleated giant cells and fibrosis. If frozen sections are examined, lipids can be identified. The diagnosis can be made on electron microscopy as typical, worm-like inclusions (zebra bodies or Farber bodies) are found in a variety of cells.

Laboratory Findings. The enzyme defect can be demonstrated. In addition, chromatographic studies can document the presence of ceramides in the skin nodules. The enzyme defect can also be assayed prenatally.

Differential Diagnosis. The cutaneous lesions can be confused with multicentric reticulohistiocytosis, which should not appear so early. Familial histiocytic dermatoarthritis (disabling arthritis, multiple red-brown nodules) and dermochondrocorneal dystrophy or Francois syndrome (corneal opacities, multiple skeletal abnormalities, skin and gingival nodules) are also similar. The classic zebra bodies are pathognomonic.

Therapy. None is available. Bone marrow transplantation or gene replacement seem the only reasonable approaches.

Other Sphingolipidoses and Related Disorders

Schindler Disease

There are several clinical patterns seen with α-*N*-acetylgalactosaminidase deficiency, all inherited in an autosomal recessive pattern. Some patients are mentally retarded and severely disabled. One variant has been described by the major group interested in Fabry disease. They used the alternative term angiokeratoma corporis diffusum with glycopeptiduria to describe an adult patient with angiokeratomas who was otherwise normal.

Sialidosis

Synonym. Mucolipidosis type I

The least-severe form of glycoprotein sialidase deficiency is also known as Spranger syndrome (Spranger et al. 1977). Patients have a course facies, dysostosis multiplex, myoclonus, mental retardation and angiokeratomas. Inheritance is in an autosomal recessive pattern.

I Cell Disease

Synonym. Mucolipidosis type II

This condition resembles severe mucopolysaccharidosis (Chap. 43) with dwarfism, skeletal abnormalities, hypertrichosis, gingival hyperplasia and severe retardation. The patients often have tight or thickened skin at birth and may be confused with those with the stiff skin syndrome (Chap. 18). Their fibroblasts and lymphocytes contain large prominent inclusions.

Galactosialidosis

These patients lack a protective protein and develop deficiencies in α-neuraminidase and β-galactosidase. Once again, inheritance is in an autosomal recessive pattern. They have mental retardation, course facial features, dysostosis multiplex, cherry-red macular spots and in the Japanese pedigrees, angiokeratomas.

Fucosidosis

Fucosidosis is either a very heterogeneous disorder or a group of several disorders. The largest pedigrees gave been described among the Navajo and Hispanics of the southwestern USA, as well as in Calabria. All forms are inherited in an autosomal recessive pattern. Because of a lack of α-L-fucosidase, glycolipids containing fucose accumulate in many cells. The facial features are coarse, and the patients, small with dysostosis multiplex. Multiple cutaneous and oral angiokeratomas are another prominent feature.

All of these disorders are so rare that they play little role in ordinary dermatologic diagnosis. On rare occasions, the dermatologist may be involved in diagnosing and biopsying the angiokeratomas but there are always other more prominent features. Today the diagnosis is made either by enzyme analysis or genetic methods and the only feasible long-term therapy will involve enzyme replacement perhaps via bone marrow transplantation or gene transfer techniques.

Bibliography

Basic Science Aspects

Chen CS, Patterson MC, Wheatley CL et al. (1999) Broad screening test for sphingolipid-storage diseases. Lancet 354:901

Meikle PJ, Hopwood JJ, Clague AE et al. (1999) Prevalence of lysosomal storage disorders. JAMA 281:249–254

Scriver CR, Beaudet AL, Sly WS et al. (1995) The metabolic and molecular bases of inherited disease, 7th edn. McGraw-Hill, New York

Angiokeratoma Corporis Diffusum

Anderson W (1898) A case of angio-"keratoma". Br J Dermatol 10:113–117

Chesser RS, Gentry RH, Fitzpatrick JE (1990) Perioral telangiectases: a new finding in Fabry's disease. Arch Dermatol 126:1655

Eng CM, Desnick RJ (1994) Molecular basis of Fabry disease: mutations and polymorphisms in the human α-galactosidase A gene. Hum Mutat 3:103–111

Fabry J (1898) Ein Beitrag zur Kenntnis der Purpura haemorrhagica nodularis (Purpura papulosa haemorrhagica Hebrae). Arch Dermatol Syph 43:187–200

Kang WH, Chun SI, Lee S (1987) Generalized anhidrosis associated with Fabry's disease. J Am Acad Dermatol 17:883–887

Lacour M, Lake BD (1995) Rapid laboratory confirmation of Fabry's disease: a reminder. Br J Dermatol 133:329–347

Lapins J, Emtestam L, Marcusson JA (1993) Angiokeratomas in Fabry's disease and Fordyce's disease: successful treatment with copper vapour laser. Acta Dermato Venereol (Stockh) 73:133–135

Nakamura T, Kaneko H, Nishino I (1981) Angiokeratoma corporis diffusum (Fabry disease): ultrastructural studies of the skin. Acta Derm Venereol (Stockh) 61:37–41

Peters FP, Sommer A, Vermeulen A et al. (1997) Fabry's disease: a multidisciplinary disorder. Postgrad Med J 73: 710–712

Wallace HJ (1973) Anderson-Fabry disease. Br J Dermatol 88:1–21

Gaucher Disease

Beaudet E (1992) Gaucher's disease. N Engl J Med 316: 619–621

Elstein D, Abrahamov A, Hadas-Halpern I et al. (1999) Recommendations for diagnosis, evaluation, and monitoring of patients with Gaucher disease. Arch Intern Med 159:1254–1255

Gaucher PCE (1882) De l'epitheliome primitif de la ratc. These, Paris. In: Rappeport JM, Barranger JA, Ginns EI (1986) Bone marrow transplantation in Gaucher disease. Birth Defects 22:101–109

Goldblatt J, Beighton P (1984) Cutaneous manifestations in Gaucher disease. Br J Dermatol 111:331–334

Mistry PK, Smith SJ, Ali M et al. (1992) Genetic diagnosis of Gaucher's disease. Lancet 339:889–892

Niemann-Pick Disease

Boustany RN, Kaye E, Alroy J (1990) Ultrastructural findings in skin from patients with Niemann-Pick disease, type C. Pediatr Neurol 6:177–183

Niemann A (1914) Ein unbekanntes Krankheitsbild. Jahrb Kinderheilkd 79:1–10

Touissant M, Worret WI, Drosner M et al. (1994) Specific skin lesions in a patient with Niemann-Pick disease. Br J Dermatol 131:895–897

Farber Disease

Chanoki M, Ishii M, Fukai K et al. (1989) Farber's lipogranulomatosis in siblings: light and electron microscopic studies. Br J Dermatol 121:779–785

Farber S (1952) A lipid metabolic disorder – disseminated "lipogranulomatosis" – a syndrome with similarity to, and important difference from, Niemann-Pick and Hand-Schüller-Christian disease. Am J Dis Child 84: 499–500

Schmoeckel C (1980) Subtle clues to diagnosis of skin diseases by electron microscopy. "Farber bodies" in disseminated lipogranulomatosis (Farber's disease). Am J Dermatopathol 2:153–156

Schindler Disease

Diggelen OP van, Schindler D, Klijer WJ et al. (1987) Lysosomal α-*N*-acetylgalactosaminidase deficiency: a new inherited metabolic disease. Lancet 2:804

Kanzaki T, Wang AM, Desnick RJ (1991) Lysosomal α-*N*-acetylgalactosaminidase deficiency, the enzymatic defect in angiokeratoma corporis diffusum with glycopeptiduria. J Clin Invest 88:707–711

Wang AM, Schindler D, Desnick R (1990) Schindler disease: the molecular lesion in the α-*N*-acetylgalactosaminidase gene that causes an infantile neuroaxonal dystrophy. J Clin Invest 86: 1752–1756

Sialidosis

Bonten E, Spoel A van der, Fornerod M et al. (1996) Characterization of human lysosomal neuraminidase defines the molecular basis of the metabolic storage disorder sialidosis. Genes Dev 10:3156–3169

Federico A, Cecio A, Battini GA et al. (1980) Macular cherry-red spot and myoclonus syndrome. Juvenile form of sialidosis. J Neurol Sci 48:157–169

Spranger J, Gehler, Cantz M (1977) Mucolipidosis I – a sialidosis. Am J Med Genet 1:21–29

Galactosialidosis

Okamura-Oho Y, Zhang S, Callahan JW (1994) The biochemistry and clinical features of galactosialidosis. Biochim Biophys Acta 1225:244–254

Fucosidosis

Breier F, Hobisch G, Fang-Kirchner S et al. (1995) Histology and electron microscopy of fucosidosis of the skin. Subtle clues to diagnosis by electron microscopy. Am J Dermatopathol 17:379–383

Cragg H, Williamson M, Young E et al. (1997) Fucosidosis: genetic and biochemical analysis of eight cases. J Med Genet 34:105–110

Fleming C, Rennie A, Fallowfield M et al. (1997) Cutaneous manifestations in fucosidosis. Br J Dermatol 136:594–597

Willems PJ, Gatti R, Darby JK et al. (1991) Fucosidosis revisited: a review of 77 patients. Am J Med Genet 38:111–131

CHAPTER 39

Disorders of Amino Acid Metabolism

Contents

Introduction

The inherited disorders of amino acid metabolism usually result from a missing enzyme or coenzyme which is essential for the breakdown or transport of an amino acid or a group of related amino acids. Some of the disorders have quite specific cutaneous changes, as a variety of amino acids are essential for various skin functions, such as the manufacture of melanin (Chap. 26). In other amino acid disorders, the cutaneous signs are less specific, so that the patient may present with dermatitis and failure to thrive. It is often hard to decide to what extent the skin changes are related to a specific amino acid defect and to what extent they are secondary to malnutrition. Most often the precursor compound that is not adequately converted spills over into the urine, rather than being stored in tissues. Thus, some designate these disorders aminoacidurias.

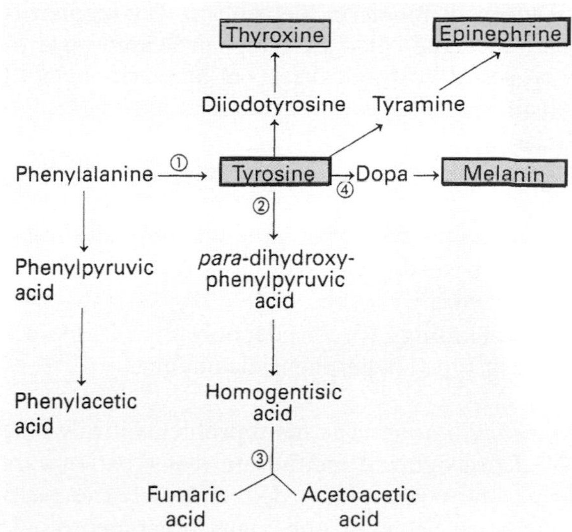

Fig. 39.1. Disturbances in tyrosine metabolism with blocks caused by genetic defects in various enzymes (*1* phenylketonuria, *2* tyrosinemia, *3* alkaptonuria, *4* albinism)

Phenylketonuria

(FÖLLING 1934)

Synonyms. Phenylalanine hydroxylase deficiency, hyperphenylalaninemia type I, Fölling disease, PKU

Epidemiology. The incidence in Western populations is about 1:10,000.

Etiology and Pathogenesis. The name phenylketonuria is not scientifically sound but generally accepted. This disorder is inherited in an autosomal recessive pattern; the gene lies on chromosome 12q22–24. There is a deficiency in phenylalanine hydroxylase or its cofactor tetrahydrobiopterin, so that the body is flooded with phenylalanine. The normal phenylalanine to tyrosine ratio is around 1:1. In these patients, the ratio is usually >3:1. There are alternate pathways so that excretion of phenylalanine metabolites is also increased, resulting in the presence of phenylketones and phenylamines in the urine which can then be detected. The elevated phenylalanine level has a number of effects, primarily on the CNS. Transport across the blood-barrier barrier is blocked, protein synthesis is inhibited and production of serotonin, dopamine and norepinephrine is reduced. The competitive inhibition of tyrosinase and the relative deficiency in tyrosine lead to reduced production of melanin (Fig. 39.1).

There are a variety of mutations responsible for phenylalanine hydroxylase deficiency. It seems that every patient has a unique mutation, making prenatal diagnosis difficult. There are several other scenarios which may lead to neonatal hyperphenylalaninemia. They include:

- Maternal Phenylketonuria. The pregnant phenylketonuria patient must pay particular attention to their special diet. Their children are at risk for mental retardation, microcephaly, cardiac defects and a variety of other problems.
- Defects of Biopterin Metabolism. The biopterins are essential cofactors for phenylalanine hydroxylase. At least four defects of biopterin metabolism may also lead to accumulations of phenylalanine.
- Secondary Causes. Prematurity, liver disease, high protein diets and certain medications especially methotrexate may produce findings similar to the basic disease.

Clinical Findings. We consider only phenylketonuria or classic type I hyperphenylalaninemia.

Systemic Findings. The main problems involve the CNS. Unrecognized and thus untreated patients are invariably severely retarded with seizures, self-destructive behavior and many other neurologic abnormalities. Early identification has made such patients a rarity.

Cutaneous Findings. The lack of melanin leads to a pale complexion. Patients have blue eyes, blond hair and pale nevi. Patients with phenylketonuria whose parents are fair may be as pale as an albino. Such patients are very light-sensitive. As the metabolic defect is corrected, the hairs are the first to darken. About 20–50% of the patients have a mild atopic dermatitis-like picture, often involving the cheeks and usually not too severe. They may also have sclerodermoid thickening of their skin, acrocyanosis and hyperhidrosis.

Histopathology. The biopsy can document the dermal thickening in sclerodermoid areas and perhaps reveal the decreased basal layer melanin. Little information is available.

Laboratory Findings. The key laboratory test is the mandatory blood screening in neonates to identify early cases. The urine has a mousy odor and was formerly screened for phenylamines and phenylketones (Guthrie test) but false-negative tests can occur in infancy. Prenatal diagnosis remains difficult because of the variety of mutations and the lack of enzyme expression in amniocyte cultures. Use of PCR to measure amniotic fluid enzyme levels seems promising.

Prognosis. The outlook for untreated individuals is poor. Those who are identified and treated may have minor CNS problems but do well. Even in the most severe variants, the risk of mental handicap in treated individuals is around 5% (compared to 2% in the general population).

Differential Diagnosis. The true differential diagnosis is the various disorders discussed under etiology. Remotely one may think of albinism, but the screening answers the question.

Therapy

Systemic. The treatment is diet, but a very special, foul-tasting diet which contains synthetic proteins and low levels of phenylalanine. The patient should be followed by a pediatrician experienced in this area, since low protein levels are undesirable and some phenylalanine is required. Usually the strict diet can be modified in late childhood or adolescence, but should be reinstated during pregnancy.

Topical. Sunscreens and routine care suffice.

Tyrosinemia Type II

(Richner 1938; Hanhart 1947)

Synonyms. Keratosis palmoplantaris circumscripta seu areata, Richner-Hanhart syndrome, oculocutaneous tyrosinemia

Etiology and Pathogenesis. This very rare disorder is inherited in an autosomal recessive pattern. The missing enzyme is hepatic tyrosine aminotransferase which is coded on chromosome 16q22–q24. The failure to metabolize tyrosine leads to elevated serum and urine levels. Tissue damage apparently results from the activation of lysosomal enzymes by tyrosine crystals.

Clinical Findings

Cutaneous Findings. Most typical are palmoplantar keratoses that appear in the first year of life. They favor the weight-bearing areas of the feet (heel, metatarsal heads), the finger tips, thenar and hypothenar eminences and occasionally the knees and elbows. The keratoses are generally quite exophytic and irregular. They can be associated with bullae and erosions. Hyperhidrosis is often present.

Systemic Findings. The eye findings usually precede the cutaneous changes. In the cornea, the tyrosine crystals seem to elicit an inflammatory reaction, manifested by conjunctivitis, photophobia and tearing. Later they produce severe dendritic keratitis with corneal ulcerations, neovascularization and blindness. Some patients may be mentally retarded.

Histopathology. Routine light microscopy shows hyperkeratosis, acanthosis and parakeratosis which are not specific. Epidermolytic hyperkeratosis has been reported. Electron microscopic studies may show lipid droplets in the epidermis, as well as cytoplasmic granules which hint at the diagnosis.

Laboratory Findings. Elevated plasma tyrosine and urinary tyrosine metabolite levels clinch the diagnosis.

Differential Diagnosis. The other forms of palmoplantar keratoderma should be considered (Chap. 17).

Patients with tyrosinemia type I are similar in name only. They have failure to thrive and later hepatic disease, but no skin findings.

Therapy. A low-phenylalanine/low-tyrosine diet is helpful. Once again, the patient should be managed by a physician with experience in this area. The ocular problems may require corneal transplantation if dietary therapy is not instituted promptly enough. The cutaneous problems may respond to systemic retinoids but lifelong treatment is required. In rare cases, the ocular and skin problems respond but mental retardation still occurs.

Hartnup Syndrome

(Baron et al. 1956)

Synonym. Pellagra-cerebellar ataxia-renal aminoaciduria syndrome

Epidemiology. The family described by Baron and colleagues was named Hartnup. The disease has been best studied in Massachusetts where it is included in routine natal screening and has an incidence of around 1:15,000.

Etiology and Pathogenesis. While Hartnup syndrome is inherited in an autosomal recessive pattern, it does not reflect an established enzyme defect. Instead, it is an inherited defect of amino acid transport at the cell membrane level. In such cases, there is selective renal aminoaciduria, as the involved amino acids are increased in the urine and reduced in the body. In Hartnup disease the urine and stool contain elevated levels of a wide range of amino acids, but tryptophan deficiency appears responsible for the cutaneous findings. The nonabsorbed tryptophan is metabolized to indole products in the gastrointestinal tract, so that urinary indican and indole levels may also be elevated. Since tryptophan is essential for production of niacin (nicotinic acid), it is not surprising that the clinical features resemble pellagra or nicotinic acid deficiency (Chap. 49).

Clinical Findings. Hartnup disease in most western countries is rarely symptomatic, as the dietary levels of amino acids are high enough to drive the system and adequate amounts of niacin and oligosaccharides bound to tryptophan are also present. In underdeveloped countries, the full-blown manifestations may be seen.

Cutaneous Findings. The skin changes usually precede the CNS problems. They start in early childhood often between 3 and 9 years of age, but may be delayed depending on the diet. The main feature is photosensitivity, often seasonal in nature and thus more obvious in the spring. Typically there is an erythematous sunburn-like rash without atrophy or scarring involving the nose and cheeks. Similar changes are seen on the backs of the hands and perhaps the knees (Fig. 39.2). In addition, stomatitis and glossitis may occur. Thus the resemblance to pellagra is striking; one can speak of a pellagroid picture.

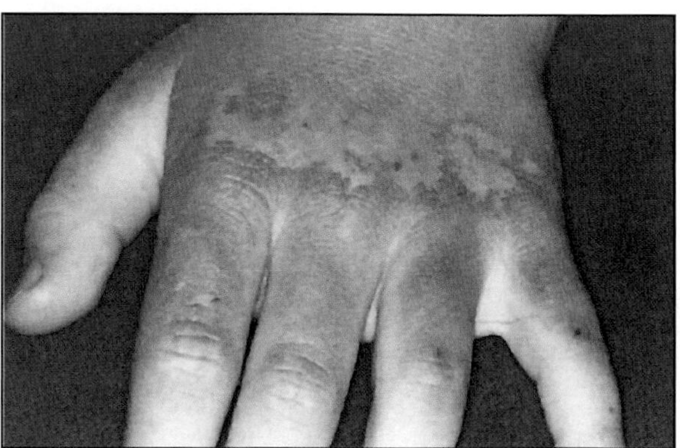

Fig. 39.2. Hartnup syndrome

Systemic Findings. Hartnup syndrome causes cerebellar ataxia, coupled with migraine headaches, psychiatric problems and perhaps mild mental retardation.

The CNS findings also vary with light exposure and may be triggered by fever, illness or dietary problems. Both the CNS and skin problems tend to improve over time.

Histopathology. A skin biopsy may be helpful to exclude lupus erythematosus, but otherwise is nonspecific.

Laboratory Findings. The excessive neutral amino acids in the urine and low levels in the blood confirm the diagnosis. An oral load of tryptophan will lead to increased amounts of indicans and indoles in the urine. Prenatal diagnosis is not currently available.

Differential Diagnosis. The whole spectrum of photosensitivity disorders should be considered. Acute CNS problems associated with photosensitivity may be confused with some of the porphyrias. Pellagra should also be excluded. Furthermore, Hartnup syndrome may be confused with various congenital poikilodermas and Cockayne syndrome.

Therapy

Systemic. Nicotinamide (niacinamide) therapy is simple and produces prompt responses. Daily dosages of 50–300 mg suffice. Using nicotinamide avoids the unpleasant vasodilatory responses associated with nicotinic acid. A diet adequate in protein is also helpful, as many other amino acids are somewhat deficient.

Topical. Sunscreens covering both UVA and UVB should be employed. The dermatitis can be treated with corticosteroids if severe.

Alkaptonuria

(Virchow 1866; Garrod 1901)

Synonym. Ochronosis

History. Alkaptonuria was one of the first metabolic diseases to be clinically described, as the famous German pathologist Virchow identified the dramatic pigmentary deposits in autopsies in the 1860s. Garrod described the metabolic defect in 1901.

Epidemiology. Alkaptonuria is a very uncommon disorder with an incidence of 1:300,000. In some regions, the incidence is much higher. For example, in parts of Slovakia it is estimated at 1:25,000.

Etiology and Pathogenesis. Alkaptonuria is inherited in an autosomal recessive pattern. The missing enzyme is homogentisic acid oxidase, the gene for which is found on chromosome 3q2. Homogentisic acid (2,5-dioxyphenylacetic acid) is an intermediary in the degradation of phenylalanine and tyrosine. It forms pigmented polymers which accumulate especially in fibrous and cartilaginous tissues. In the skin and cartilage, the polymers are oxidized to benzoquinone acetic acid, which imparts the final brown to blue-black color. The classic darkening of the urine results from an insoluble dark polymer originally called alkaptone. The urinary changes are usually noticed while the child is still in diapers.

Clinical Findings. The clinical triad described by Garrod was black urine, joint problems and darkening of the skin.

Cutaneous Findings. The skin usually develops dyschromic changes in middle age. The skin of the ears is thickened and has a blue-gray tint. The tip of the nose may also be discolored, as well as the cheeks, forehead, axillae and the skin over joints, especially the knuckles. The main discoloration arises from the pigments deposited in underlying superficial cartilage such as in the ears and distal part of the nose (Fig. 39.3).

Many other peculiar color changes may occur. Sometimes dark tendons or bones may also be seen through the skin. The sweat and cerumen may be darkened. The clothing may thus be soaked with alkaptonuric sweat, which darkens when the clothes are washed in an alkaline laundry product. The sclerae are also discolored.

Systemic Findings. The other major change is a destructive arthritis involving the larger joints and spine with intervertebral disc calcification. While the patient is likely to have severe and often disabling problems, life expectancy is otherwise normal. Cardiac involvement has been described.

Histopathology. The deposition of black pigment in cartilage and tendons is macroscopically visible and very dramatic. In the dermis, the

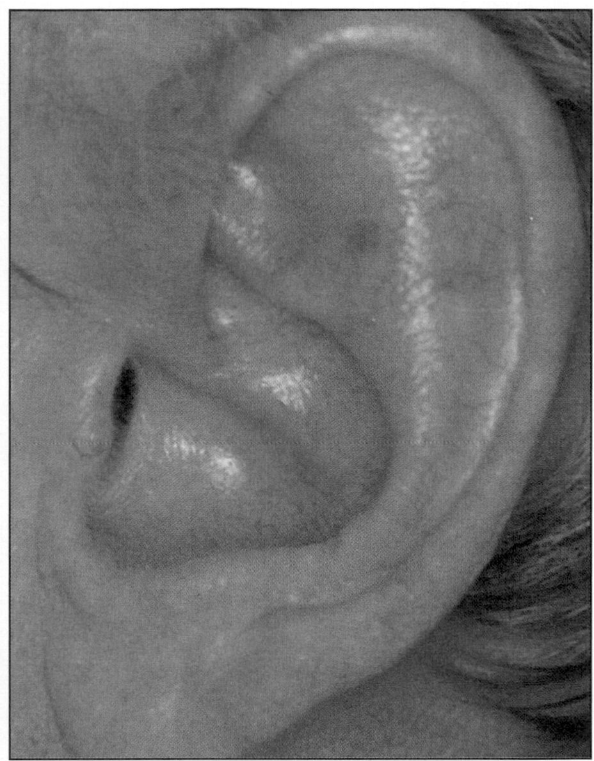

Fig. 39.3. Ochronosis in patient with alkaptonuria

changes in alkaptonuria are not as dramatic as in exogenous ochronosis. But the connective tissue fibers may be clumped and darkly stained. Methylene blue stains these alkaptonuric fibers black, helping to distinguish their pigment from melanin.

Laboratory Findings. Identification of homogentisic acid in the urine can be tentatively made by adding NaOH to make it alkaline thus turning it dark. A variety of enzymatic and chromatographic tests can confirm the diagnosis.

Differential Diagnosis. Usually the diagnosis is made in infancy, when the black diapers are noticed. Otherwise, it is important to question any patient with skin discoloration about arthritis and to examine the external ears in patients with unexplained arthritis. Often the diagnosis is first made by the orthopedic surgeon who discovers discolored bones during joint replacement.

Exogenous ochronosis is discussed in Chap. 27. It is a response to overuse of hydroquinone bleaching creams which damage the dermal collagen and produce a similar discoloration, most commonly on the cheeks without any articular or cartilaginous changes.

Therapy. There is no good therapy. Restrictive diets do not help because phenylalanine and tyrosine are essential amino acids. Standard rheumatologic care is indicated. Often replacement of a hip or knee is required. Masking cosmetics may be satisfactory for some patients.

Argininosuccinicaciduria

(Allen et al. 1958)

Epidemiology. The incidence is about 1:70,000.

Etiology and Pathogenesis. Argininosuccinicaciduria is inherited in an autosomal recessive pattern while the responsible gene is located on chromosome 7cen-q11. Multiple mutations have been identified. The missing enzyme is argininosuccinase which converts argininosuccinic acid to arginine and fumaric acid in the urea cycle. As a result there are elevated blood and urine levels of argininosuccinic acid, along with elevated blood ammonia and citrulline levels.

Clinical Findings

Cutaneous Findings. The major abnormalities are found in the hair. About half the patients have abnormal hair at birth. The nape is usually most severely involved. Typically it is dull, dry and very fragile. It may be difficult to groom but often haircuts are not needed. The most typical structural abnormality is trichorrhexis nodosa (Chap. 31) which resembles two paint brushes being pushed together to produce a nodule in the shaft. Other hairs, including eyebrows, eyelashes and body hairs, as well the nails, can also be fragile and slow growing. In adolescence there is generally some improvement.

Systemic Findings. As with so many of the amino acid disorders, there are neonatal and late-onset forms. The neonates usually die of failure to thrive with CNS problems, hepatosplenomegaly and other problems. The infantile form is associated with profound mental retardation and ataxia.

Histopathology. Typical structural changes can be seen in the hairs. In addition to trichorrhexis nodosa, the cuticle appears very irregular. In other cases, pili torti have been described.

Laboratory Findings. Levels of argininosuccinic acid in the urine are markedly elevated. Prenatal diagnosis through amniocentesis and DNA analysis is possible.

Differential Diagnosis. The many causes of trichorrhexis nodosa are reviewed elsewhere. The combination of fragile hair and profound retardation also suggests Menkes syndrome and perhaps monilethrix, although mental retardation is rare in the latter. In citrullinemia, argininosuccinic acid synethetase is absent. This enzyme is involved one step earlier in the urea cycle, making argininosuccinic acid from citrulline and aspartic acid. These patients tend to have weeping erosive plaques on the buttocks and genitalia but may also have the same hair and CNS abnormalities.

Therapy. Arginine supplementation coupled with protein restrictions may produce some improvement. Arginine tends to drive the urea cycle, increasing the excretion of nitrogen but also building up levels of argininosuccinic acid and citrulline. While this seems illogical, the goal is to increase nitrogen excretion and reduce blood ammonia levels. In addition, benzoate is added as it removes equimolar amounts of nitrogen as hippuric acid. Arginine deficiency may be responsible for the hair defects, as they tend to improve with replacement therapy.

Homocystinuria

(Carson and Neil 1962)

Epidemiology. Homocystinuria has an incidence of about 1:300,000 individuals.

Etiology and Pathogenesis. The most common cause of homocystinuria is a deficiency in cystathionine-β-synthetase. This autosomal recessive defect is located on chromosome 21q22. In this situation, the conversion of homocysteine and serine to cystathionine is blocked. In methionine metabolism, homocysteine is the link between the transmethylation and transsulfuration cycles, so there are many enzymes involved and a number of alternate pathways. In general homocysteine accumulates, is converted to homocystine and is then excreted in the urine. In addition, methionine levels climb and this amino acid is also found in the urine and serum. Homocysteine appears to cause abnormal collagen cross-linkages. Elevated homocystine levels are a risk factor for thrombotic disease.

Clinical Findings

Cutaneous Findings. The patients have a malar flush which is usually the first sign. They also are at risk for increased thrombophlebitis and other thrombotic events. Additional clinical findings include livedo racemosa, leg ulcers and fine atrophic scars. Some patients may have sparse or friable hair.

Systemic Findings. The systemic findings are more dramatic. The patients typically have a marfanoid appearance. Their major problem is the risk of early severe thrombotic problems, with subsequent emboli to the lungs or brain. Even individuals with minimally elevated homocystine levels, from any cause, appear to have increased risk of thrombotic problems. Ocular findings include lens dislocation, myopia and glaucoma. Orthopedic manifestations include osteoporosis at an early age, coupled with scoliosis and a tendency to pathologic fractures and vertebral collapse. Most of the skeletal changes seen in Marfan syndrome are also present, but instead of joint laxity, there is usually restricted motion. In addition to mental retardation and seizures, patients may have a wide range of other psychiatric problems.

Laboratory Findings. The elevated urine homocystine can be identified by the cyanide-nitroprusside reaction. Chromatographic studies can document the elevated homocystine and methionine levels in the blood and urine. Prenatal diagnosis is possible through amniotic cell fluid enzyme assays and DNA analysis.

Differential Diagnosis. The main differential diagnosis is Marfan syndrome. Usually the approach is to do the urine studies in any suspicious patient to rule out homocystinuria. Some of the clinical differences are shown in Table 39.1. Multiple endocrine neoplasia type 2b (MEN 2b) syndrome patients may be marfanoid and have mild retardation, but are otherwise quite different. Congenital contractural arachnodactyly presents with limited joint motion and elongated hands, but lacks the major systemic problems. In a totally different vein, there are many acquired causes of homocystinuria, including isoniazid therapy and vitamin B_{12} deficiency.

Therapy. The enzyme cystathionine-β-synthetase has pyridoxine (vitamin B_6) as a cofactor. In about half the patients, giving pyridoxine 200–500 mg daily drives the enzyme levels up enough to produce marked clinical improvement. This suggests that the enzymatic defect is a mutation that causes a

Table 39.1. Differences between homocystinuria and Marfan syndrome

Feature	Homocystinuria	Marfan
Arachnodactyly	Yes	Yes
Height	Tall	Taller
Joint motion	Restricted	Lax
Lens dislocation	Downward	Upward
Hairs	May be sparse	Normal
Malar flush	Yes	No
Psychiatric problems	Yes (50%)	No ("normal" levels)
Mental retardation	Yes	No
Thromboses	Yes	No
Defect	Homocysteine/homocystine	Fibrillin

minor functional problem which in some cases can be corrected. Those patients who respond have a relatively good outlook. The others tend to do poorly and die with thrombotic episodes and suffer from severe mental retardation. Additional treatment includes a low-methionine, high-cystine diet.

Prolidase Deficiency

Etiology and Pathogenesis. This rare disorder has been reported in fewer than 50 patients. It involves a defect in an exopeptidase known as prolidase or peptidase D. The responsible gene is located on chromosome 19p. As with most enzyme defects, this disorder is inherited in an autosomal recessive pattern. The defect is an inability to remove proline or hydroxyproline from the N-terminal region of dipeptides, leading to their accumulation in the urine. This is known as imidodipeptiduria.

Clinical Findings. About 75% of the reported patients have had clinical problems, and all had skin involvement. Nonetheless, 25% of those identified with the metabolic defect were asymptomatic. The onset of skin findings is between birth and 20 years of age. Typically there are severe, widespread therapy-resistant ulcerations often limited to the legs below the knees. The patients have no predisposing risks for leg ulcers such as chronic venous insufficiency or obesity. Occasionally there may be small ulcers elsewhere. In several reported cases, once the legs were amputated below the knees, admittedly a drastic therapy, the ulcerations stopped. Some patients have mild mental retardation or are emotionally labile, so the ulcers are often falsely diagnosed as factitial. Some patients have had an increased number of infections.

Laboratory Findings. The imidodipeptides can be identified in the urine and the enzyme deficiency confirmed in fibroblast cultures or homogenates of leukocytes.

Differential Diagnosis. The many causes of leg ulcers are discussed in Chapter 22. If one has a young patient with severe leg ulcers and no good explanation, even though prolidase deficiency is extremely rare, one should consider it.

Therapy. Topical glycine and proline have been successful in a few cases and are worth trying. Manganese is a cofactor for the enzyme and can also be tried. Skin grafts tend not to work and often amputation is needed.

Bibliography

Phenylketonuria

Burton BK (1998) Inborn errors of metabolism in infancy: a guide to diagnosis. Pediatrics 102:E69

De Freitas O, Izumi C, Lara MG et al. (1999) New approaches to the treatment of phenylketonuria. Nutr Rev 57:65–70

Fölling A (1934) Über Ausscheidung von Phenylbrenztraubensäure in den Harn als Stoffwechselanomalie in Verbindung mit Imbezilität. Hoppe Seylers Z Physiol Chem 227:169–176

Nogva MP, Kaufmann M, Halperin A (1992) Scleroderma-like skin indurations in a child with phenylketonuria: a clinicopathologic correlation and review of the literature. J Am Acad Dermatol 26:329–333

Penrose LS (1998) Phenylketonuria – a problem in eugenics. Ann Hum Genet 62:193–202

Tyrosinemia

Al-Hemidan AI, al-Hazzaa SA (1995) Richner-Hanhart syndrome (tyrosinemia type II). Case report and literature review. Ophthalmic Genet 16:21–26

Dubois J, Garel L, Patriquin H et al. (1996) Imaging features of type 1 hereditary tyrosinemia: a review of 30 patients. Pediatr Radiol 26:845–851

Hanhart E (1947) Neue Sonderformen von Keratosis palmoplantaris, u.a. eine regelmäßig-dominante mit systematisierten Lipomen, ferner zwei einfach-rezessive mit Schwachsinn und z.T. Hornhautveränderungen des Auges (Ektodermalsyndrom). Dermatologica 94:286–303

Holme E, Lindstedt S (1995) Diagnosis and management of tyrosinemia type I. Curr Opin Pediatr 7:726–732

Rabinowitz LG, Williams LR, Anderson CE et al. (1995) Painful keratoderma and photophobia: hallmarks of tyrosinemia type II. J Pediatr 126:266–269

Richner H (1938) Hornhautaffektionen bei Keratoma palmare et plantare hereditarium. Klin Monatbl Augenheilkd 10:580–588

Tanguay RM, Jorquera R, Poudrier J et al. (1996) Tyrosine and its catabolites: from disease to cancer. Acta Biochim Pol 43:209–216

Hartnup Syndrome

Baron DN, Dent CE, Harris H et al. (1956) Hereditary pellagra-like skin rash with temporary cerebellar ataxia, constant renal aminoaciduria and other bizarre biochemical features. Lancet II:421–428

Galadari E, Hadi S, Sabarinathan K (1993) Hartnup disease. Int J Dermatol 32:904

Milovanovic DD, Milovanovic L, Stankovic B et al. (1991) D-Tryptophan and its metabolites in a family with Hartnup disease. Adv Exp Med Biol 294:669–674

Oakley A, Wallace J (1994) Hartnup disease presenting in an adult. Clin Exp Dermatol 19:407–408

Schmidtke K, Endres W, Roscher A et al. (1992) Hartnup syndrome, progressive encephalopathy and allo-albuminaemia. A clinico-pathological case study. Eur J Pediatr 151:899–903

Alkaptonuria and Ochronosis

Albers SE, Brozena SJ, Glass LF et al. (1992) Alkaptonuria and ochronosis: case report and review. J Am Acad Dermatol 27:609–614

Dom K, Pittevils T (1997) Ochronotic arthropathy: the black hip. Case report and review of the literature. Acta Orthop Belg 63:122–125

Gutzmer R, Herbst RA, Kiehl P et al. (1997) Alkaptonuric ochronosis: report of two affected brothers. J Am Acad Dermatol 37:305–307

Kneebone TS, Selner AJ (1995) Ochronosis and alkaptonuria. Case report and literature review. J Am Podiatr Med Assoc 85:554–555

Reddy DR, Prasad VS (1998) Alkaptonuria presenting as lumbar disc prolapse: case report and review of literature. Spinal Cord 36:523–524

Touart DM, Sau P (1998) Cutaneous deposition diseases, part II. J Am Acad Dermatol 39:527–544, 545–546

Virchow R (1866) Ein Fall von allgemeiner Ochronose der Knorpel und knorpelähnlichen Teilen. Arch Pathol Anat 37:212

Argininosuccinic Aciduria

Allen JD, Cusworth CD, Dent CE et al. (1958) Disease, probably inhereditary, characterized by severe mental deficiency and constant growth abnormality of aminoacidic metabolism. Lancet I:182

Asai K, Ishii S, Ohta S et al. (1998) Fatal hyperammonaemia in argininosuccinic aciduria following enflurane anaesthesia. Eur J Pediatr 157:169–170

Mandell R, Packman S, Laframboise R et al. (1996) Use of amniotic fluid amino acids in prenatal testing for argininosuccinic aciduria and citrullinaemia. Prenat Diagn 16:419–424

Worthington S, Christodoulou J, Wilcken B et al. (1996) Pregnancy and argininosuccinic aciduria. J Inherit Metab Dis 19:621–623

Homocystinuria

De Franchis R, Sperandeo MP, Sebastio G et al. (1998) Clinical aspects of cystathionine beta-synthase deficiency: how wide is the spectrum? The Italian Collaborative Study Group on Homocystinuria. Eur J Pediatr 157:67–70

Dettmeyer R, Varchmin-Schultheiss K, Madea B (1998) Intracranial plasma cell granuloma and homocystinuria. Pathol Res Pract 194:205–208

Carson NAJ, Neill D (1962) Metabolic abnormalities detected in a survey of mentally backward individuals in Northern Ireland. Arch Dis Child 37:505–513

Pietrzik K, Bronstrup A (1997) Causes and consequences of hyperhomocyst(e)inemia. Int J Vitam Nutr Res 67:389–395

Singh H (1997) Selections from current literature: homocysteine: a modifiable risk factor for cardiovascular disease. Fam Pract 14:335–339

Townend J, O'Sullivan J, Wilde JT (1998) Hyperhomocysteinaemia and vascular disease. Blood Rev 12:23–34

Prolidase Deficiency

Arata J, Umemura S, Yamamoto Y et al. (1979) Prolidase deficiency. Arch Dermatol 114:62–67

Arata J, Hatakenaka K, Oono T (1986) Effect of topical application of glycine and proline on recalcitrant leg ulcers of prolidase deficiency. Arch Dermatol 122:626–627

Milligan A, Graham-Brown RAC, Burns DA et al. (1989) Prolidase deficiency. A case report and literature review. Br J Dermatol 121:405–409

Gammopathies

Contents

Basic Science Aspects

Hypergammaglobulinemia is the pathological increase in serum proteins of the γ-globulin type. There are two basic causes. A monoclonal gammopathy results from the clonal proliferation of a single B cell. The abnormal protein is called M (monoclonal) or paraprotein. The diseases associated with such a clonal proliferation have also been called plasma cell dyscrasias, immunoglobulinopathies or dysproteinemias. In contrast, in a polyclonal gammopathy, a number of different B cells are stimulated, producing a mixture of abnormal proteins. In most instances, a polyclonal gammopathy reflects an associated lupus erythematosus, rheumatoid arthritis, sarcoidosis or Sjögren syndrome. Chronic infections with repeated but variable antigenic stimulation can produce a similar picture. Only a few polyclonal gammopathies are clinically distinct.

These two different processes not surprisingly have different serum electrophoretic patterns. A monoclonal gammopathy results in identical proteins that produce a sharp spike or peak that most often lies in the γ-range but may also be found in the β- or α-2 range. A polyclonal gammopathy has many proteins without a peak, yielding a broad based increase in the γ range. Quantitative increases in γ-globulins usually occur with a polyclonal gammopathy but may be absent in the monoclonal form.

The historical designation of paraprotein and paraproteinemia for a monoclonal gammopathy is usually incorrect. The proteins are normal; they are just increased in amount. For this reason, the term M protein is preferred. In some cases the excess immunoglobulins are biologically active, damaging red blood cells, activating mast cells or performing similar tasks. In other instances, they are truly "para" or altered; in such instances incomplete immunoglobulin molecules are present, as is the case when excessive light chains (Bence-Jones proteins) or heavy chains (heavy chain disease) are formed. Perhaps half the patients with a monoclonal gammopathy excrete Bence-Jones proteins in their urine.

The standard diagnostic approach is serum protein electrophoresis and immunoelectrophoresis of serum or urine. One can identify the light and heavy chain types and decide if a gammopathy is IgG, IgM, IgA, IgE or IgD in type. Quantitative immunoglobulins are also usually obtained. Various diseases show associations with different immunoglobulin types and chain subtypes. The Bence-Jones proteins are also best identified with electrophoresis.

Monoclonal Gammopathies

In the typical monoclonal gammopathy, there is a malignant transformation of a B cell with subsequent uncontrolled proliferation and immunoglobulin synthesis. One speaks of a primary monoclonal gammopathy when no associated disease is identified. Patients with a wide variety of hematologic disorders, such as a B cell lymphoma, may also have a monoclonal gammopathy; in this instance other features of the disease are more dominating and troublesome. Some cryoglobulinemias, as well as cold agglutinins, are associated with a clonal proliferation, but other clinical signs of a tumor are absent. The only abnormal activity is the production of aberrant excessive proteins. Neoplastic T cells can also induce a monoclonal B cell proliferation. Finally, monoclonal gammopathies are seen in association with nonhema-

Table 40.1. Types of monoclonal gammopathy and their frequency

Type	Frequency (%)
Multiple myeloma	60
Benign monoclonal gammopathy	5
Waldenström macroglobulinemia	10
Lymphoma, lymphoid leukemia	10
Primary amyloidosis	5
Other disorders	10

tologic malignancies, infections and a variety of skin disorders, such as necrobiotic xanthogranuloma in which it is unclear how the two problems are related.

Table 40.1 shows the relative frequencies of the main monoclonal gammopathies. IgG gammopathy is usually related to multiple myeloma, as is IgA although the latter can be seen with pyoderma gangrenosum, subcorneal pustular dermatosis, Sweet syndrome and non-Hodgkin lymphoma. IgM gammopathy is clinically different enough that it is considered separately as Waldenström macroglobulinemia. IgD gammopathy is very rare but seen with multiple myeloma, while the equally rare IgE gammopathy may be seen with non-Hodgkin lymphoma and plasma cell leukemia. All of the disorders discussed below are potential markers for a gammopathy but may be present without any evidence of paraproteinemia. In each instance, the patient should be followed closely for the development of multiple myeloma and other hematologic malignancies.

Multiple Myeloma

Definition. Multiple myeloma is a low-grade non-Hodgkin B cell lymphoma involving the proliferation of a clone of plasma cells (Chap. 61).

Epidemiology. Multiple myeloma is a disease of older adults. Most patients are over 60 years of age. It has an incidence of 2–3/100,000 per year.

Etiology and Pathogenesis. The cause is unknown. The plasma cell clone expands so slowly that it has been estimated that the insult triggering the clone dates back 5–10 years prior to symptoms. Radiation, chemical mutation and perhaps an out-of-control antibody response have been suggested as possible triggers. About half the patients have an IgG gammopathy; 25% IgA, 20% only Bence-Jones proteins, while IgM and IgE peaks are quite rare. If the cells lose their ability to make heavy chains, then hypogammaglobulinemia may result along with Bence-Jones proteins.

Multiple myeloma causes trouble in a variety of ways. The normal bone marrow elements are replaced by plasma cells, leading to varying degrees of pancytopenia. Bones, particularly of the spinal column, are eroded and destroyed, both by the production of osteoclast-stimulating factor and other cytokines as well as by replacement of the bone by plasmacytomas (accumulations of tumoral plasma cells). The presence of the excessive immunoglobulins is usually a nuisance; hyperviscosity may result but it is more common in multiple myeloma variants. Excessive light chains may also produce amyloid deposits and cryoglobulinemia.

Clinical Findings

Cutaneous Findings. The most specific cutaneous finding is a cutaneous plasmacytoma, but it is very uncommon and occurs late in the disease. The typical cutaneous plasmacytoma is a blue dermal or subcutaneous mass. It may extend to the skin from the bone or be truly unattached. The other cutaneous manifestations of multiple myeloma are viewed as secondary, although in most instances their pathophysiology remains a mystery. Table 40.2 lists the disorders that are frequently associated with a monoclonal gammopathy and in which multiple myeloma should be excluded. In many instances, such as in the case of amyloidosis or pyoderma gangrenosum, the cutaneous findings may precede the systemic problems.

Systemic Findings. The classic findings in multiple myeloma include bone pain and destruction, anemia and renal disease. Hypercalcemia is common because of the bone destruction. The renal disease has many causes, including the abnormal calcium levels, toxic effects of light chains on kidneys, plasma cell infiltrates and protein deposition. Sometimes a solitary plasmacytoma with or without M protein will be found in the bone or other organs; this may be a precursor of multiple myeloma.

Histopathology. If a plasma cell infiltrate is identified in the skin, appropriate studies should be done to see if it is monoclonal, that is, if only κ or λ light chains are present. On occasions, crystals of protein causing an obstructive vasculitis are found.

Laboratory Findings. M protein should be sought in the serum and urine. On occasion, a single light chain will be associated with two different heavy chains,

Table 40.2. Cutaneous findings associated with monoclonal gammopathy

Disorder	Comments	Chapter
Primary or AL amyloidosis	Variety of gammopathies can produce amyloid	41
Cryoglobulinemia	Mono- or polyclonal forms	This chapter
Lichen myxedematosus/ scleromyxedema	Usually IgGλ	43
Scleredema adultorum		18
Pyoderma gangrenosum	Usually IgA, often comes first	22
Sweet syndrome	Usually IgA, overlaps with pyoderma gangrenosum	14
Subcorneal pustulosis	Usually IgA	16
Erythema elevatum diutinum	IgA > IgG, sometimes multiple myeloma	14
POEMS syndrome	Usually IgG > IgA	This chapter
Necrobiotic xanthogranuloma	IgG	37
Diffuse normolipemic plane xanthoma	Overlaps with necrobiotic xanthogranuloma	64
Xanthoma disseminatum	Rare	64
Hyperkeratotic spicules	Spicules may contain immunoglobulin	This chapter
Schnitzler syndrome	IgM	11
Capillary leak syndrome	IgG	This chapter
Acquired angioedema	Many causes, usually B cell proliferation, occasionally with monoclonal peak	11
Leukocytoclastic vasculitis	Uncommon, caused by vessel blockage or complement activation	22

producing a biclonal or double gammopathy. The patient should also be evaluated as any other lymphoma patient. The erythrocyte sedimentation rate is often very high. Bone marrow examination is mandatory, as well as a complete hematologic evaluation. Calcium levels and renal function should be checked. β-2 microglobulin levels may be elevated. Serum viscosity should be determined. Some type of baseline bone survey should be performed; in some situations CT scans and MRI offer advantages over a skeletal survey.

Course and Prognosis. The average survival is about 40 months. Some cases, called smoldering multiple myeloma, stumble along for many years, but the 10-year survival is 2%. The main problems include renal failure, CNS complications and infections.

Differential Diagnosis. The differential diagnosis is considered throughout this chapter and in Chapter 61.

Therapy. The therapy of multiple myeloma is frustrating. The course is slow, but relentless and difficult to influence. The disease is usually staged based on hemoglobin, serum calcium level, bone damage, and size of M protein, as well as presence or absence of renal disease. The standard therapy is melphalan and prednisone, but many more aggressive schemes are available. Localized bone lesions can be treated with radiation therapy and/ or surgery.

Cutaneous Plasmacytosis

This rare entity has been almost exclusively diagnosed among Japanese patients. They present with multiple, red-brown truncal nodules that show hyperplasia of mature, polyclonal plasma cells. Some patients have other signs and symptoms such as fever, anemia and lymphadenopathy, in which case one can argue for the diagnosis of systemic plasmacytosis. Rarely there may be progression to malignant lymphoma. The disease appears sufficiently different from multiple myeloma that it should be considered as a separate entity. Plasmacytosis is a smoldering disease, not responsive to therapy.

In very rare cases, patients present with a single cutaneous plasmacytoma. The diagnosis of primary extramedullary plasmacytoma should be made with caution, as several such patients have progressed to multiple myeloma or malignant lymphoma. A polyclonal cutaneous plasma cell infiltrate may mimic a recurrence when a basal cell carcinoma or other tumor is treated with destructive measures or following other skin trauma.

Benign Monoclonal Gammopathy

Synonym. Monoclonal gammopathy of unknown significance

Benign monoclonal gammopathy is defined by the presence of a monoclonal protein, usually IgM, in the serum or urine without convincing evidence for multiple myeloma. About 3% of patients over age 70 have such findings. Careful long-term studies have shown that this problem is not so benign; over 10 years about 40% receive other diagnoses including multiple myeloma, Waldenström macroglobulinemia, other lymphomas and amyloidosis.

Waldenström Macroglobulinemia

(Waldenström 1944)

Definition. Proliferation of a malignant plasma cell clone producing IgM and often causing hyperviscosity.

Etiology and Pathogenesis. The monoclonal IgM proliferation usually reflects an underlying immunocytoma (lymphoplasmacytoid lymphoma). When other immunoglobulins are present, then one simply speaks of a lymphoma-associated gammopathy. The increased amounts of IgM lead to hyperviscosity and interferes with clotting and platelet function. In addition, there appears to be vessel wall damage. A variety of autoimmune disorders including Sjögren syndrome, epidermolysis bullosa acquisita and idiopathic thrombocytopenic purpura can be associated with immunocytoma.

Clinical Findings. The hyperviscosity leads to a whole range of clinical problems. Urticaria, livedo racemosa and vasculitis can be seen. There may also be cutaneous infiltrates of plasma cells, usually juicy red to violet papules and plaques with focal petechiae. The periorbital region is a typical site. In other instances, there are translucent papules containing IgM, known as storage papules. Finally, immunoglobulin deposition at the basement membrane zone may lead to bullous lesions.

The problems in other organs are more severe, with retinal vascular damage, epistaxis, CNS bleeding, cardiac failure, renal failure and a whole host of other changes. Lymphadenopathy, edema secondary to hypoproteinemia and hepatosplenomegaly may also be seen.

Histopathology. Occasionally dermal vessels will be filled with the macroglobulins. When the infiltrate is specific, then the small lymphoplasmacytoid cells will fill the dermis in a monotonous pattern.

Laboratory Findings. In addition to the IgM peak, one may find an elevated erythrocyte sedimentation rate, prolonged bleeding time and anemia. Bone marrow examination should always be done to search for an underlying lymphoma or multiple myeloma.

Course and Prognosis. The disease is indolent but not curable. The hyperviscosity symptoms can usually be controlled, but once signs of lymphocyte proliferation occur, the life expectancy is a few years.

Differential Diagnosis. Other causes of petechiae should be excluded, but usually the patient has so many other problems that it is obvious something else is going on. The main issue is to identify the type of underlying lymphocytic proliferation. Primary cutaneous immunocytoma is a cutaneous marginal zone lymphoma that has nothing to do with Waldenström macroglobulinemia (Chap. 61).

Therapy. The hyperviscosity is treated with plasmapheresis. IgM is usually intravascular and the easiest antibody to remove with plasmapheresis. Cytotoxic agents, typically chlorambucil or cyclophosphamide, are used if plasmapheresis is ineffective or there are clear signs of a rapidly progressing lymphoma.

Heavy Chain Disease

The heavy chain disorders are all rare and have few cutaneous findings. In all, there is a proliferation of heavy chains without any light chains. The most common is α-heavy chain disease, which is also known as immunoproliferative small intestine disease or Mediterranean lymphoma because it usually involves the bowel where IgA plays a major role and is more common in patients of Mediterranean origin. Patients tend to present with diarrhea, malabsorption and weight loss. Early cases may be cured with antibiotics, suggesting an infectious trigger, as with mucosa-associated lymphoid tissue (MALT) lymphomas. The γ-heavy chain disease is characterized by heavy chain fragments in the urine, which can be missed when screening for Bence-Jones proteins. Problems include fever, lymphadenopathy, multiple infections and hemolytic anemia. The extremely rare μ-heavy chain disease is probably a variant of chronic lymphocytic leukemia. In all three, skin involvement is so rare that no pattern has been noted. Hemorrhagic macules and lymphocytic infiltrates have been described.

Other Diseases Associated with Gammopathies

Waldenström Purpura

(Waldenström 1948)

Synonym. Hyperglobulinemic purpura

Definition. Purpura of the lower aspects of the legs associated with polyclonal gammopathy. Waldenström described both macroglobulinemia and hyperglobulinemic purpura. Unfortunately, these two unrelated diseases are routinely confused.

Epidemiology. One expert stated that more papers had been published on Waldenström purpura than the total number of patients with the extremely rare disease.

Etiology and Pathogenesis. The cause is unknown. The increased amounts of immunoglobulins cause vessel damage and interfere with hemostasis.

Clinical Findings. There are typically crops of small, punctate or slightly larger purpuric lesions, usually on the legs. Urticarial lesions may also develop. As crops of lesions come and go, typical yellow-brown hemosiderin deposition is seen, just as in the progressive pigmented purpuras. The Rumpel-Leede test is positive. Rarely, there may be small papules reflecting vascular dilatation and proliferation, similar to pseudo-Kaposi disease. Sometimes there is marked edema localized to the ankles, rather than the entire foot. Pruritus or burning may occur.

Histopathology. Leukocytoclastic vasculitis may occasionally be seen. In addition, sludging of erythrocytes in the vessels may be found. Most often, however, there is exocytosis of erythrocytes without any obvious vessel damage.

Laboratory Findings. Marked elevation of γ-globulins is present without evidence of monoclonality. Serum albumin levels are often reduced. The erythrocyte sedimentation rate may be elevated and acute phase reactants present. Many patients are somewhat anemic.

Course and Prognosis. The course typically waxes and wanes, but is chronic. The patient should be monitored for the development of an underlying autoimmune or lymphoproliferative disorder.

Differential Diagnosis. Clinically, the appearance is that of a progressive pigmented purpura. One must exclude the presence of an underlying autoimmune disease with associated hypergammaglobulinemia, such as lupus erythematosus, systemic sclerosis or Sjögren syndrome. In chronic cirrhosis, there is also a polyclonal hypergammaglobulinemia but other signs of liver disease are present, such as thrombocytopenia and reduced levels of the liver-dependent clotting factors (II, VII, IX, X). Cryoglobulinemia should also be ruled out.

Therapy. There is no good therapy. Systemic corticosteroids are not effective. Some patients respond to azathioprine and other immunosuppressive agents, but the issue is when to employ such relatively risky medications for a harmless disorder.

Cryoglobulinemia

(Landsteiner 1903; Lerner and Watson 1947)

Definition. Cryoglobulins are circulating immunoglobulins often complexed with other proteins that precipitate reversibly in the cold. They may be either monoclonal or polyclonal.

Epidemiology. Cryoglobulinemia is relatively uncommon. Its frequency depends on the prevalence of the possible triggers, such as hepatitis.

Etiology and Pathogenesis. Cryoglobulinemia is not one disease but many. It may represent a monoclonal or polyclonal proliferation of proteins. One distinguishes between three types, as Table 40.3 shows. In type I cryoglobulinemia, the underlying disorder is a B cell proliferation producing the monoclonal protein, often yielding substantial amounts. The type II and III forms usually feature smaller amounts of protein and are more likely to be associated with immune disorders or infections. Essential mixed cryoglobulinemia in many instances is associated with hepatitis C infec-

Table 40.3. Types of cryoglobulinemia

Type	Mono- or polyclonal	Cases (%)	Immunologic features	Associated diseases
I	Mono	25	IgM or IgG monoclonal proliferation; rarely IgA or Bence-Jones	B cell proliferations
II	Both	25	Two components: one mono-, the other, polyclonal. Often monoclonal IgM rheumatoid factor coupled with polyclonal IgG	Autoimmune disorders, occasionally B cell proliferations
III	Poly	50	Wide range of mixtures, including immunoglobulins, complement, viral antigens, others	Autoimmune disorders, infections (hepatitis, infectious mononucleosis, cytomegalovirus), "essential"

tions. There are some patients in whom no underlying disease is found; they are almost invariably type III.

There are a number of ways in which tissue damage can occur. If a large amount of cryoprotein is present, it can form gels or even crystals in tissue, occluding vessels and producing necrosis. In other instances immune complexes are formed and activate complement, causing inflammation. Clotting factors can be consumed, leading to a coagulopathy.

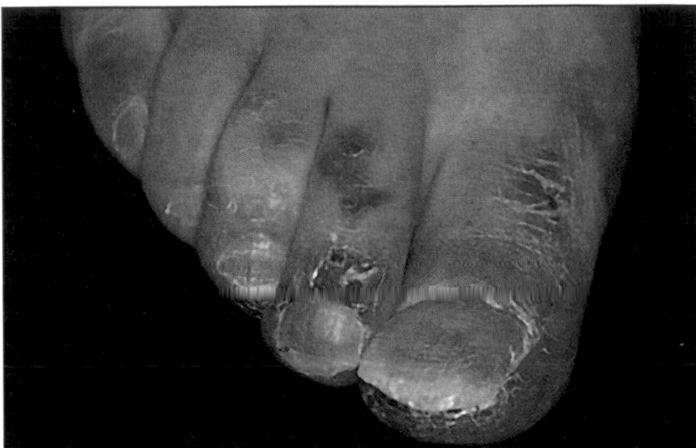

Fig. 40.1. Cryoglobulinemia

Clinical Findings

Cutaneous Findings. A unifying feature is the onset of symptoms when exposed to cold. Often only a minimum cooling is required. The patient has more problems in the spring or fall with rapidly changing temperatures than in the winter; perhaps this also reflects the increased caution shown in truly cold months. Another scenario is an individual coming into an air-conditioned building on a hot summer day and experiencing problems. A number of different patterns can be seen.

Pseudo-Raynaud Syndrome. Acrocyanosis develops on the fingers, nose and ears, usually immediately with cold exposure. With repeated exposure, there may be extreme pain and ulcerations. The typical three-phase reaction of Raynaud syndrome with erythema on warming is not seen.

Purpura. Following cold exposure, there may be purpura on the hands and feet, often associated with larger hemorrhages and focal necrosis (Fig. 40.1). A hallmark of type I cryoglobulinemia is non-inflammatory purpura. Inflammatory vascular lesions are most often seen in type II and III disease, mimicking leukocytoclastic vasculitis. Mucosal lesions with bleeding are also common, as in the nose or mouth.

Ulcerations. The leg ulcers with cryoglobulinemia are sometimes so distinctive that one can diagnose them clinically. There are usually multiple-grouped, quite superficial lesions in a patient with no other risk factors for arterial or venous ulcerations (Fig. 40.2). A similar picture can be seen when a patient with cryoglobulinemia is treated with cryotherapy for acral verrucae vulgares.

Urticaria. Cryoglobulins are a rare cause of cold urticaria. They appear to bind with mast cells and cause degranulation.

Panniculitis. Sometimes the action is deeper, so that a panniculitis develops. Deep subcutaneous nodules develop that often ulcerate.

Systemic Findings. The systemic findings are far more serious. In type I disease, retinal damage and arterial thrombosis are the main risks. In types II and III, renal disease, neurologic problems and arthritic changes are more typical. In one series, over 50% of patients with essential mixed cryoglobulinemia

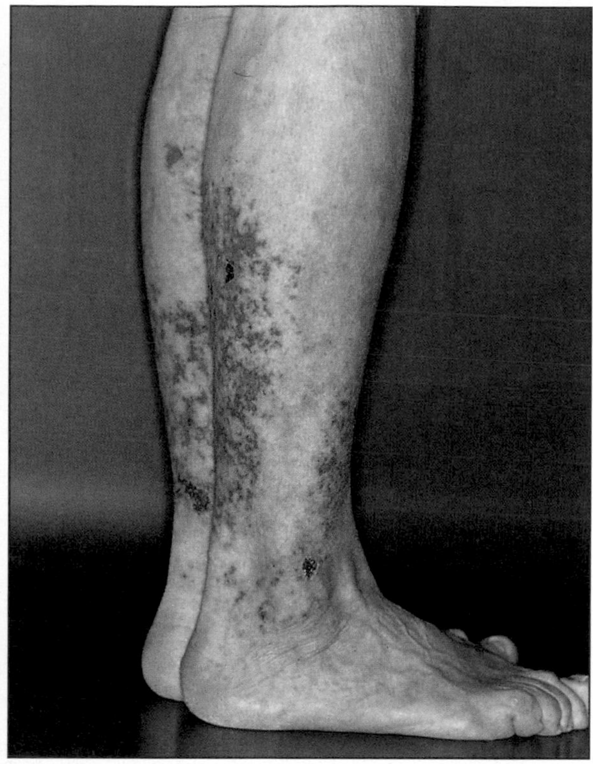

Fig. 40.2. Cryoglobulinemia with vasculitis and ulcerations

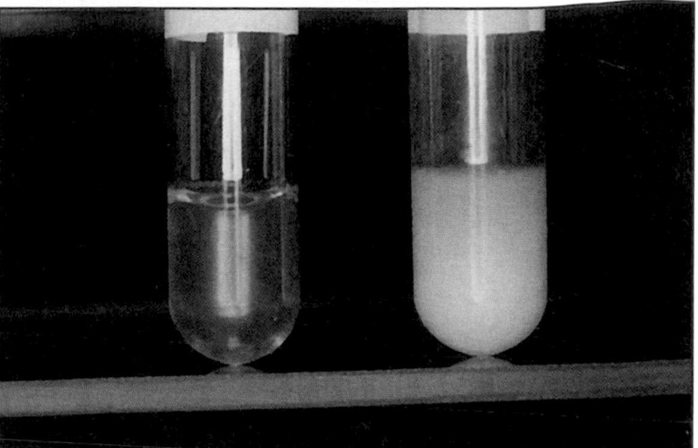

Fig. 40.3. Cryoprecipitate on right after specimen was held in the refrigerator

developed renal disease. In any such discussion, it is difficult to separate problems associated with the underlying disorder from those "caused" by the cryoglobulins.

Histopathology. The dermal vessels may be occluded by amorphous protein deposits; in addition, small vessels may show thrombi. Sometimes, there is leukocytoclastic vasculitis and one is lucky to see any evidence at all for the cryoglobulins.

Laboratory Findings. The evaluation of suspected cryoglobulinemia requires close cooperation between the physician and the laboratory. The blood must be drawn in a warmed syringe and the red cells removed using a warmed centrifuge. If the blood is not drawn in the laboratory, then it should be immediately taken there; one trick is to place the tubes in a deep pocket or under the arm. The plasma is then refrigerated for more than 24 h at 4 C and then centrifuged. A cryocrit can be determined and the cryoprecipitate analyzed in a variety of ways (Fig. 40.3).

Course and Prognosis. The outlook depends on the underlying disorder. As mentioned, even the so-called essential mixed cryoglobulinemia patients have a considerable risk of renal disease and may develop autoimmune problems.

Differential Diagnosis. The protean clinical manifestations of cryoglobulinemia mean that many patients must be studied to find the occasional, elusive positive case. There are other cold-sensitive materials in the serum that can be confused with cryoglobulins; they are summarized in Chapter 13.

Therapy. All approaches hinge on treating the underlying disorder or gammopathy when possible. Cold avoidance can reduce symptoms. Plasmapheresis can remove the guilty protein; this helps more in type I disease, inwhich the problem tends to be mechanical, than it does in types II and III, which are more inflammatory.

POEMS Syndrome

Synonym. Crow-Fukase syndrome

POEMS is an acronym for *p*olyneuropathy, *o*rganomegaly, *e*ndocrine disorders, *M* protein and *s*kin changes. The gammopathy is IgG or IgA, usually with λ-chains. The most disturbing problem is the neuropathy, which is usually a peripheral sensorimotor disturbance similar to Guillain-Barré syndrome. In addition, there may be neuropathic involvement of the respiratory muscles leading to pneumonia and inadequate ventilation. A long list of endocrine abnormalities have been reported, including gonadal dysfunction and thyroid disease. Organomegaly is usually hepatosplenomegaly. When bony lesions are present, they are osteosclerotic. The skin changes include scleroderma-like plaques, often hyperpigmented and typically over the sternum, as well as unusual hemangiomas. Under the microscope the latter lesions show a glomeruloid pattern and are somewhat distinct. Other skin findings including hyperpigmentation, hypertrichosis and sclerodactyly. Treatment of the underlying B cell proliferation produces only minimal improvement in the polysystemic disease.

Hyperkeratotic Spicules

Hyperkeratotic spicules are tiny follicular plugs most commonly involving the larger follicles about the nose and on the scalp. They can occur anywhere on the body. In the case of multiple myeloma and other gammopathies, they consist of plugs of the abnormal immunoglobulin or even cryoglobulin. In some cases, increased numbers of *Demodex folliculorum* have been found in the spicules. The same changes have been seen in normal individuals and in patients with chronic renal disease, inflammatory bowel disease and other disorders. In each instance, it is wise to check the patient for a gammopathy and to follow up carefully.

Systemic Capillary Leak Syndrome

In this extremely rare disorder, an IgG monoclonal gammopathy produces a functional protein that causes capillary leakage. The mechanism is unknown. Patients typically present with profound leakage of fluid into the extracellular space, producing hypovolemia as well as angioedema. Patients may be in shock because of the rapid shift. Serum albumin is low and the hematocrit and hemoglobin high. Rapid fluid replacement may also cause trouble, as there is a dramatic reuptake of the leaked fluids, often producing a rebound pulmonary edema and fluid overload. Typically there are recurrent attacks. The capillary leak associated with interleukin (IL)-2 administration in cancer chemotherapy is slightly different, because profound pulmonary edema occurs early in the process. A similar phenomenon has been described in severe pustular psoriasis. The 5-year survival is about 20 %; either the fluid disturbances or the underlying B cell proliferation is the cause of death.

Cold Agglutinin Disease

Cold agglutinin disease features high titers of IgM antibodies directed against erythrocytes. There is a postinfectious polyclonal form in young adults, usually associated with infectious mononucleosis or *Mycoplasma pneumoniae* infection, which is usually mild and self-limited. The more common variant is monoclonal and may be idiopathic or associated with a lymphoproliferative disease. The antibodies are most active at 4 °C , directed against the Ii antigens of erythrocytes and activate complement. In some patients the resulting hemolytic anemia dominates, while in other patients, when exposed to cold, the acral signs and symptoms are most prominent. The latter group of patients have pseudo-Raynaud phenomenon and other acral changes triggered by cold. The titers of IgM are often so high that their blood is viscous and difficult to draw. The best treatment is moving to a warmer climate. Exchange transfusions and plasmapheresis maybe helpful; a highly successful chemotherapeutic regimen is not available.

Paroxysmal Cold Hemoglobulinuria

This uncommon problem is often confused with cryoglobulinemia and cold agglutinin disease. It was formerly of great interest to dermatologists because the most common cause was syphilis, although today it is less common and associated with several viral diseases. The offender is an IgG antibody directed against the red blood cell P antigens. The main symptoms are those of intravascular hemolysis and anemia; there are no typical skin findings.

Bibliography

Monoclonal Gammopathies

Bluefarb SM (1955) Cutaneous manifestations in multiple myeloma. Arch Dermatol 72:506–23

Daoud MS, Lust JA, Kyle RA et al. (1999) Monoclonal gammopathies and associated skin disorders. J Am Acad Dermatol 40:507–535

Herrinton LJ (1996) The epidemiology of monoclonal gammopathy of unknown significance: a review. Curr Top Microbiol Immunol 210:389–395

Kois JM, Sexton FM (1991) Lookingbill DP. Cutaneous manifestations of multiple myeloma. Arch Dermatol 127:69–74

Kyle RA (1978) Monoclonal gammopathy of undetermined significance: natural history in 241 cases. Am J Med 64:814–26

Kyle RA, Lust JA (1989) Monoclonal gammopathies of undetermined significance. Semin Hematol 26:176–200

Kyle RA (1994) The monoclonal gammopathies. Clin Chem 40:2154–61

Lust JA (1994) Role of cytokines in the pathogenesis of monoclonal gammopathies. Mayo Clin Proc 69: 691–697

Mascaro JM, Montserrat E, Estrach T et al. (1982) Specific cutaneous manifestations of Waldenström's macroglobulinaemia: a report of two cases. Br J Dermatol 106: 217–22

Morgan G (1999) Advances in the biology and treatment of myeloma. Br J Haematol 105:4–6

Patel TC, Moore SB, Pineda AA et al. (1996) Role of plasmapheresis in thrombocytopenic purpura associated with Waldenstrom's macroglobulinemia. Mayo Clin Proc 71: 597–600

Shimizu S, Tanaka M, Shimiyz H et al. (1997) Is cutaneous plasmacytosis a distinct clinical entity? J Am Acad Dermatol 36:876–880

Tuting T, Bork K (1996) Primary plasmacytoma of the skin. J Am Acad Dermatol 34:386–390

Wagner DR, Eckert F, Gresser U et al. (1993) Deposits of paraprotein in small vessels as a cause of skin ulcers in Waldenström's macroglobulinemia. Clin Invest 72:46–49

Waldenström J (1944) Incipient myelomatosis of "essential" hyperglobulinemia with fibrogenopenia – a new syndrome? Acta Med Scand 117:216–247

Wong KF, Chan JK, Li LP et al. (1994) Primary cutaneous plasmacytoma: report of two cases and review of the literature. Am J Dermatopathol 16:392–397

Waldenström Purpura

Finder KA, McCollough ML, Dixon SL et al (1990) Hypergammaglobulinemic purpura of Waldenstrom. J Am Acad Dermatol 23:669–676

Waldenström J (1948) Zwei interessante Fälle mit Hyperglobulinämie. Schweiz Med Wochenschr 78:927–928

Cryoglobulinemia

Brouet JC, Clauvel JP, Danon F et al. (1974) Biologic and clinical significance of cryoglobulins: a report of 86 cases. Am J Med 57:775–788

Cohen SJ, Pittelkow MR, Su WDP (1991) Cutaneous manifestations of cryoglobulinemia: Clinical and histopathologic study of seventytwo patients. J Am Acad Dermatol 25:21–27

Cuellar ML, Garcia C, Molina JF (1995) Cryoglobulinemia and other dysproteinemias, familial Mediterranian fever, and POEMS syndrome. Curr Opin Rheumatol 7:58–64

Lerner AB, Watson CJ (1947) Studies of cryoglobulins. II. The spontaneous precipitation of protein from serum at 5 °C in various disease states. Am J Med Sci 214: 410–427

POEMS

Bardwick PA, Zvaifler NJ, Gill GN et al. (1980) Plasma cell dyscrasia with polyneuropathy, organomegaly, endocrinopathy, M protein, and skin changes: the POEMS syndrome. Report on two cases and a review of the literature. Medicine (Baltimore) 59:311–322

Crow RS (1956) Peripheral neuritis in myelomatosis. Br Med J 2:802–804

Feddersen RM, Burgdorf W, Foucar K et al. (1989) Plasma cell dyscrasia: A case of POEMS syndrome with a unique dermatologic presentation. J Am Acad Dermatol 21:1061–1068

Hitoshi S, Suzuki K, Sakuta M (1994) Elevated serum interleukin-6 in POEMS syndrome reflects the activity of the disease. Intern Med 33:583–587

Soubrier MJ, Dubost JJ, Sauvezie BJ (1994) POEMS syndrome: a study of 25 cases and a review of the literature. French Study Group on POEMS Syndrome. Am J Med 97: 543–553

Takanishi T, Sobue I, Toyokura Y (1984) The Crow-Fukase syndrome: A study of 102 cases in Japan. Neurology (Cleveland) 34:712–720

Other Diseases Associated with Gammopathies

Amoura Z, Papo T, Ninet J et al. (1997) Systemic capillary leak syndrome: report on 13 patients with special focus on course and treatment. Am J Med 103:514–519

Bork K, Böckers M, Pfeifle J (1990) Pathogenesis of paraneoplastic follicular hyperkeratotic spicules in multiple myeloma. Arch Dermatol 126:509–513

Kaplan MJ, Ellis CN, Bata-Csorgo Z et al. (1999) Systemic toxicity following administration of sirolimus (formerly rapamycin) for psoriasis. Arch Dermatol 135: 553–557

Requena L, Sarasa JL, Ortiz-Masllorens F et al (1995) Follicular spicules of the nose: a peculiar cutaneous manifestation of multiple myeloma with cryoglobulinemia. J Am Acad Dermatol 32:834–839

CHAPTER 41

The Amyloidoses

Contents

Basic Science Aspects

The amyloidoses are a group of uncommon disorders in which a fibrillar protein, amyloid, is deposited in tissue. There are localized and generalized forms of amyloidosis; both types may affect the skin. Virchow first described amyloid as a starch-like substance, not realizing how many forms it could take. As Table 41.1 makes clear, amyloid is not one substance but many. The main types of amyloid in the skin are primary or light-chain amyloid (AL), secondary or wear-and-tear amyloid (AA) and keratin-related or skin amyloid (AK). In tissue amyloid appears as a homogeneous,

Table 41.1. Types of amyloid

Type	Characteristics
AA	Amyloid A fibrillar protein. The precursor is serum amyloid A protein (SAA), an acute phase protein. AA is associated with longstanding disorders (secondary amyloid) and in several hereditary disorders including familial Mediterranean fever and Muckle-Wells syndrome.
AL	Amyloid from immunoglobulin light chains. The precursor proteins are produced by a monoclonal proliferation of either κ or λ light chains, such as associated with benign monoclonal gammopathies and a variety of malignant monoclonal B cell proliferations.
ATTR (AF)	Hereditary amyloid. Fibrillar proteins derived from genetically altered transthyretin and associated with a variety of polyneuropathies.
ATTR (ASc1)	Senile cardiovascular amyloid, also derived from transthyretin, but without mutations. It accumulates in older individuals in the heart, lungs, large vessels and joints.
ASc2	Senile atrial amyloid, derived from atrial natriuretic protein. One of the most common amyloids, found in almost everyone over 90 years of age.
A β_2M (AB)	Hemodialysis-associated amyloid, derived from β_2-microglobulin. Stored mainly about large joints, in the cartilage, connective tissue and even bones where amyloidomas (tumoral collections) can erode the bony structures and cause pathologic fractures.
A β	β or A4 protein is found in Alzheimer disease and congophilic angiopathy. It may lead to massive CNS bleeding and is in general associated with dementia; also in Down syndrome.
AC	Derived from a cytokine C altered and found in familial Icelandic apoplexy.
AE_T	Endocrine amyloid derived from thyrocalcitonin in medullary carcinoma of the thyroid.
AIAPP AE_I	Endocrine amyloid derived from a calcitonin-like hormone in the pancreatic islets known as IAPP and seem mainly in adult-onset diabetes mellitus.
ASAF or APrp	Scrapie-associated fibrillary protein or prion protein. Associated with Jacob-Kreutzfeld disease, scrapie, mad cow disease and related human and animal disorders. Prions are small proteins that can reproduce themselves via a poorly understood modeling pattern independent of nucleic acids.
AK (AD)	Keratins or their precursors are the most likely source of amyloid in primary cutaneous amyloidosis, as supported by electron microscopic, monoclonal antibody and amino acid sequencing studies.

Table 41.2. Staining characteristics of amyloid

Stain	Characteristics
Hematoxylin-eosin	Amorphous eosinophilic extra-cellular deposits
PAS	Usually purple
Methyl and crystal violet	Red metachromasia
Thioflavine T	Yellow fluorescence
Congo red	Faint red in light microscopy. With polarized light, apple green birefringence known as dichroism

amorphous almost translucent material with a variety of special staining characteristics, as shown in Table 41.2. Amyloid is typically deposited just below the basement membrane zone, about vessels or along collagen fibers. One cannot always distinguish amyloid histologically from other similar deposits, such as those in porphyria cutanea tarda, lipoid proteinosis and colloid milium. Usually the clinical features allow a distinction.

Structure

The unifying features of all the different amyloid proteins is their fibrillar structure with antiparallel β-pleated sheets. This structure is very stable and resistant, which explains why amyloid is so persistent once deposited in tissues. Most proteins have an α-helix structure. In these twisted molecules, hydrogen bonds stabilize one or two polypeptides. In the β-pleated sheet, the polypeptides are arranged side by side in parallel rows so a checkerboard of cross-linking with hydrogen bonds is formed. Depending on the directions of alternate rows of proteins, one speaks of parallel or antiparallel β-pleated sheets. Feathers, hooves and silk are also β-pleated sheets.

When examined under the electron microscope, all the different amyloids are quite similar. They are composed of fine, nonbranching fibrils ranging in length from 100 to 300 nm and in diameter from 7.5 to 10 nm. These fibrils are comprised of many smaller filaments and aggregated together in a loose network. They are probably responsible for the birefringence and help determine the other staining characteristics. The various amyloids have more amino acids and carbohydrates than do the ordinary structural proteins of the dermis, namely collagen and elastin. They are separated from each other primarily on the basis of biochemical, biophysical and immunologic techniques.

About 10% of all amyloids are nonfibrillar, consisting primarily of the P components. These structures are derived from a glycoprotein, the serum amyloid P protein (SAP), a pentraxin or doughnut-shaped pentagon that is closely related to C-reactive protein. They are felt to cause the PAS positivity of amyloid. With immunohistochemical methods, the P components can be identified in tissue amyloid deposits. They also appear to be present in normal skin. Antibodies against the P components attach to the basement membrane of capillaries and sweat glands, as well to elastic fibers. Surprisingly they are not located in the epidermal-dermal junction area.

Etiology and Pathogenesis

The pathogenesis of the amyloidoses remains unclear. In general, the deposition of amyloid appears to be an active process, not just the result of leakage or filtration of inert substances into the skin or other tissues. Amyloid is often found in association with macrophages, suggesting that they may alter or modify the protein prior to tissue binding. In addition, plasma cells may be seen, probably reflecting their role in the production of AL. The P component is bound to amyloid in a calcium-dependent manner and also binds mucopolysaccharides, but its normal role is unclear. It seems that abnormal proteins or prolonged stimulation or both are required for the deposition of amyloid. In the skin, amyloid may be deposited along the basement membrane zone and the reticulin fibers. This is known as perireticular amyloidosis and is usually seen with AA and in macular amyloidosis and lichen amyloidosus. In contrast, deposition along the collagen fibers, especially around blood vessels, known as pericollagenous amyloidosis, is typical of AL.

Classification

The exact classification of the amyloidoses is probably best made by identifying the precursor protein involved, as shown in Table 41.1. Most clinicians are used to approaching amyloid disorders slightly differently. The systemic amyloidoses are

Table 41.3. Types of cutaneous amyloidosis

Primary cutaneous amyloidosis	Lichen amyloidosus Macular amyloidosis Nodular amyloidosis Rare variants
Secondary cutaneous amyloidosis	Associated with epithelial tumors (basal cell carcinoma, seborrheic keratosis, actinic keratosis) Associated with actinic elastosis or PUVA therapy
Cutaneous amyloidosis associated with systemic amyloidosis	AL amyloid with light-chain proliferation AA amyloid with reactive, systemic diseases (rheumatoid arthritis, tuberculosis, and many others) AA amyloid in hereditary disorders

most often arranged on the basis of the underlying disorder. Table 41.3 shows the usual dermatologic approach, including primary cutaneous amyloidosis, secondary cutaneous amyloidosis and cutaneous amyloidosis associated with systemic amyloidosis. The hereditary forms of systemic amyloidosis are most often subdivided on the basis of the organs involved and the pattern of inheritance.

Cutaneous Amyloidoses

Primary Cutaneous Amyloidoses

Lichen Amyloidosus

Definition. Intensely pruritic papular dermatosis mostly commonly over the shins with superficial amyloid deposits.

Epidemiology. It is uncommon in most of the world but very common in Malaysia and China.

Etiology and Pathogenesis. The amyloid appears to be derived from keratinocytes. It contains keratins, immunoglobulins, complement proteins and the P component. The suggestion is that the basal layer keratinocytes undergo apoptosis and release keratin bodies into the dermis where they are coated by antikeratin autoantibodies and the P component. After phagocytosis by macrophages, this concoction is deposited as AK. Skeptics suggest that simple rubbing and itching traumatizes the skin, releasing keratin or other materials into the dermis.

Clinical Findings. The most typical location is over the shins. Many small flat-topped or slightly round hard papules with a lichenoid shine and pink to red-brown color are arranged close to one another (Figs. 41.1, 41.2). They may have fine scale, become hyperkeratotic or even verrucous and develop nodular areas. Often there are several groups of papules, with skipped areas in between. The lesions are typically highly pruritic, in contrast to most other forms of amyloidosis. The problem tends to be chronic.

Histopathology. There are small deposits of a pale-pink amorphous material in the tips of the dermal

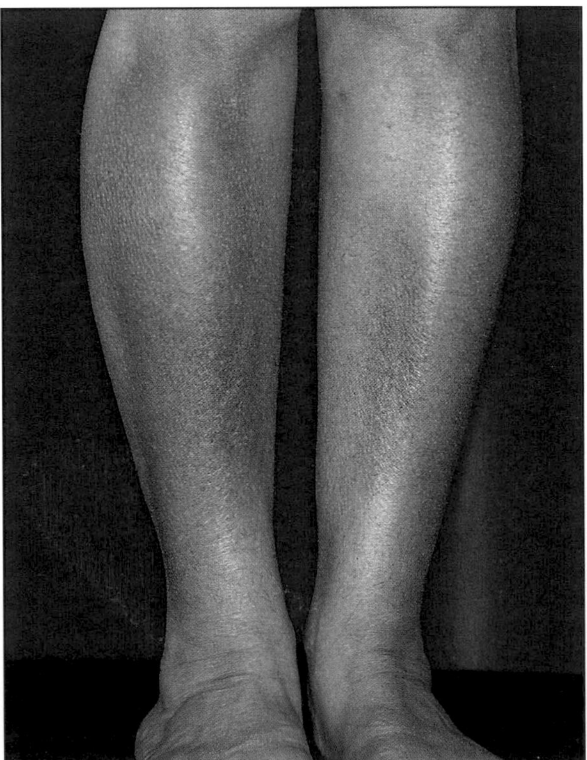

Fig. 41.1. Lichen amyloidosus

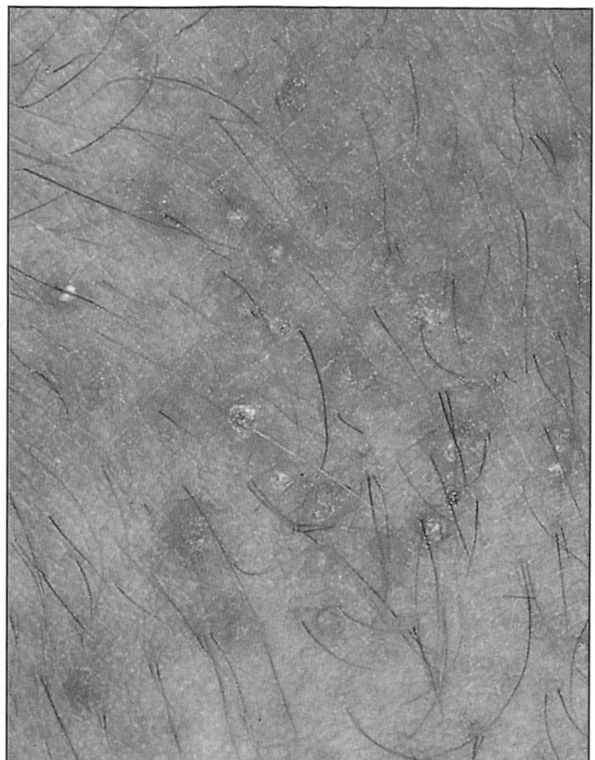

Fig. 41.2. Lichen amyloidosus

papillae. The epidermis may be slightly acanthotic and hyperkeratotic. Occasionally there are inflammatory cells associated with the deposits, but a true lichenoid band is uncommon. The material should stain faintly with Congo red or thioflavine T, but often this is most difficult to observe because of the paucity of amyloid. Antisera against multiple keratins or against amyloid P component usually provide positive staining.

Differential Diagnosis. Clinically one thinks of lichen planus, but lesions are not found elsewhere. Lichen planus is also more pink, has more flat-topped papules and usually has hyperkeratotic striate lines (Wickham striae) rather than scale. When considering the more nodular lesions, hypertrophic lichen planus is often identical. Lichen simplex chronicus does not usually have as many discrete small lesions. If the patient is Asian, one's index of suspicion should be much higher. A biopsy is decisive.

Therapy. There is no good therapy. Mid- to high-potency corticosteroids, perhaps under occlusion at night, are the best bet. Intralesional steroids are also appropriate. If the lesions are localized, surgery is a possibility. Dermabrasion may also be tried. Some sporadic reports indicate benefit from aromatic retinoids, but the long-term course is unclear.

Macular Amyloidosis

(Palitz and Peck 1952)

Synonyms. Intrascapular amyloidosis

Definition. Pruritic often hyperpigmented papules or patches, typically located on the upper aspects of the back.

Epidemiology. Intrascapular macular amyloidosis was first described in Israel, and most of the cases have been reported from Asia, and Central and South America. Most patients are 40–70 years old and women are far more often affected than men.

Etiology and Pathogenesis. Macular amyloidosis probably arises in a similar fashion to lichen amyloidosus. Localized trauma appears to play a role. The transition from notalgia paresthetica to macular amyloidosis is a gradual one, probably hastened by rubbing (Chap. 25). Japanese bath brush dermatitis is also macular amyloidosis, as are nylon brush amyloidosis and frictional amyloidosis. Finally macular amyloidosis may develop following a chronic inflammatory dermatosis on the back. The intrascapular localization remains a mystery, as does the racial variation.

Clinical Findings. The two most specific findings are the location in the intrascapular region and the blue-gray color (Fig. 41.3). Even though the legs, arms or other parts of the trunk can be involved,

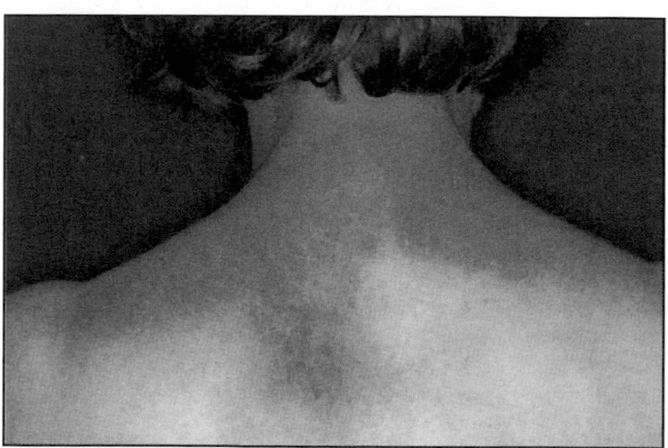

Fig. 41.3. Macular amyloidosis

almost all cases start between the scapulae. Often a patient will point to this region early in the course of their first visit and the alert clinician can make a diagnosis before even looking. Initially an irregular, poorly defined oval patch with a blue-gray or brown sheen is seen. More inflamed or chronic lesions may have firm small papules or even infiltrated plaques, resembling a lichenified atopic dermatitis (which may well be a precursor of macular amyloidosis). In other instances, manipulating the upper back with a bath brush or even back scratcher may hasten the development of the amyloidosis. There is usually mild pruritus coupled with an urge to manipulate the area. Most often the patients complain of the discoloration, not the itch. The disorder is chronic.

Histopathology. The deposits may be even more subtle than in lichen amyloidosus. They should be approached in the same way. If the location and discoloration are consistent, one can make the diagnosis reluctantly in the presence of widened dermal papillae, perhaps with an amorphous appearance, even though amyloid cannot be unequivocally demonstrated.

Differential Diagnosis. The most difficult problem is postinflammatory hyperpigmentation, which may be a variation on the same theme but without the immunologic reaction against keratin. Atopic dermatitis may appear similar, as may lichen simplex chronicus. Notalgia paresthetica may be a precursor to macular amyloidosis. When hyperpigmentation arises in notalgia paresthetica, it is macular amyloidosis. Sometimes fixed drug reactions appear on the back with the same color tones, but they usually consist of one or several larger lesions, waxing and waning with drug exposure.

Therapy. The topical measures discussed for lichen amyloidosus are appropriate. Distracters, such as mentholated lotions or creams, may also help. Topical capsaicin also appears useful, reinforcing the possible relation to notalgia paresthetica.

Nodular Amyloidosis

(Gottron 1950)

Synonyms. Amyloidosis cutis nodularis atrophicans, tumoral cutaneous amyloidosis, plaque-like tumoral cutaneous amyloidosis

Definition. Large plaques and nodular infiltrates of immunoglobulin-derived amyloid primarily on the trunk and legs.

Epidemiology. This form is very rare and more common among the elderly, supporting its relationship to primary systemic amyloid.

Etiology and Pathogenesis. Nodular amyloidosis breaks the rules. It is associated with a monoclonal proliferation of immunoglobulin light chains, just like primary systemic amyloidosis. In some instances, it represents the first stage of more widespread disease, while in other instances, the lesions remain confined to the skin for many years.

Clinical Findings. Clinically nodular amyloidosis is not easy to diagnose. While the legs are the most common site, the trunk may also be involved. Lesions on the head, penis and vulva have also been reported. Usually there is a red-brown, plate-like nodule that is elevated or papular at its border. Centrally, there may be atrophy or ulceration. Sometimes the epidermis is thin and wrinkled; in other cases, the underlying fat imparts a yellowish tone. Hemorrhagic areas may also be found. In yet other cases, the nodule is deep enough to offer no surface clues as to its etiology and is compatible with a variety of infiltrates and mesenchymal tumors. There may be a higher than expected incidence of diabetes mellitus.

Histopathology. The amorphous deposits occupy most of the dermis, usually sparing the epidermal-dermal junction. They can reach the subcutaneous fat and involve the vessels or adnexal structures. The overlying epidermis may be atrophic. Inflammatory infiltrates are often present, containing plasma cells.

Differential Diagnosis. When the typical surface atrophy is present, then nevus lipomatosus, anetoderma and atrophoderma should be considered. A red-brown infiltrate suggests lymphoma or leukemia. A cutaneous plasmacytoma is a variation on the same theme, with an abundant plasma cell infiltrate but no amyloid. If the lesion is firm, it may be mistaken for a fibrous tumor such as dermatofibrosarcoma protuberans. Deeper lesions have an endless differential diagnosis and can be diagnosed only on biopsy.

Therapy. Solitary or few lesions can be excised. Destruction with the CO_2 laser may also be helpful. Otherwise, intralesional corticosteroids are worth a try.

Secondary Cutaneous Amyloidosis

Amyloid deposits associated with cutaneous tumors are probably the most common cause of amyloid in the skin. When basal cell carcinomas are diligently examined, some observers have found amyloid in about 50% of them. The frequency with which amyloid is readily visible on routine hematoxylin-eosin sections is of course much lower. Amyloid may also be found associated with squamous cell carcinoma, seborrheic keratosis and many other tumors. The amyloid is AK in type, derived from epithelial cells.

Amyloid also has a propensity to attach to elastic fibers, mediated by the P component. Thus in solar elastosis, there may be both elastotic material and amyloid. As in skin treated with PUVA, there may be amyloid along the elastic fibers. This too is usually AK, although in so-called elastotic amyloidosis, the deposits are AL. Probably all amyloid with sufficient P components can bind to elastic fibers.

Systemic Amyloidoses

Primary Systemic Amyloidosis

(Virchow 1854; Lubarsch 1929)

Synonyms. AL amyloidosis, amyloidosis associated with lymphoproliferative disorders, idiopathic systemic amyloidosis, immunocyte-derived amyloidosis, paramyloidosis

Definition. Amyloidosis associated with the monoclonal production of light chains; rarely diagnosed by cutaneous findings.

Epidemiology. Patients tend to be older, in the same pattern as multiple myeloma.

Etiology and Pathogenesis. AL amyloidosis is associated with a monoclonal light-chain proliferation. Included among the underlying B cell disorders are multiple myeloma, Waldenström macroglobulinemia, Bence-Jones plasmacytoma, heavy-chain disease, and other malignant lymphomas. In addition, patients with benign monoclonal gammopathy develop AL amyloidosis. Individuals who present with AL amyloid with no other sign of immunocyte proliferation are labeled as primary amyloid by some, but they are likely to develop any one of the underlying disorders over the years.

In normal immunoglobulins, the κ/λ ratio is 2 : 1; in AL amyloid, it is 1 : 2, with the λ_{VI} type most common. Since the AL proteins are smaller than the normal light chains, it appears that some λ chains are especially susceptible to being taken up by macrophages and degraded into AL amyloid. Bence-Jones proteins are also an overproliferation of light chains, but these tend to wind up in the urine, rather than being deposited in tissues. Occasionally, local plasma cell tumors (plasmacytomas) also secrete AL. When the immunocytes remain localized and the amyloid accumulates, one finds nodular amyloidosis.

Clinical Findings.
Cutaneous Findings. In 30–50% of patients the skin or mucosa is involved. However, these problems are rarely either the presenting sign or symptom, nor are they a cause of significant morbidity. The most common cutaneous manifestation is vessel fragility from the perivascular amyloid infiltrates (Figs. 41.4, 41.5). This problem is usually most common in the region drained by the superior vena cava. Typical changes include small hemorrhages in the skin folds, such as of the eyelids or periorbital tissue, known as squint or pinch purpura. If the intravascular pressure is raised via the Valsalva maneuver, then more hemorrhage is seen. The alliterative term postproctoscopic pinch purpura describes one cause of the problem.

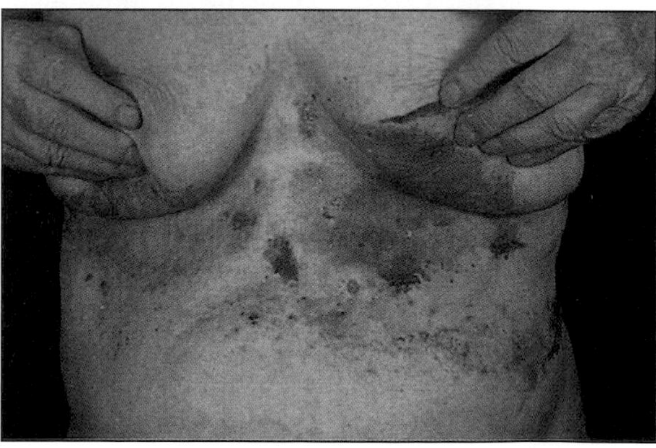

Fig. 41.4. Purpura in patient with primary systemic amyloidosis

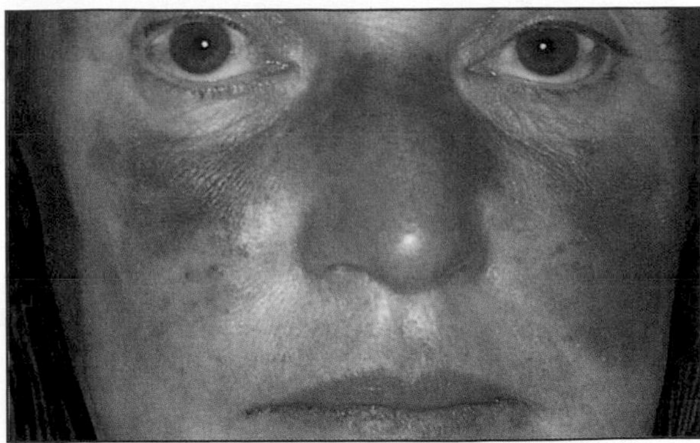

Fig. 41.5. Facial purpura in patient with multiple myeloma

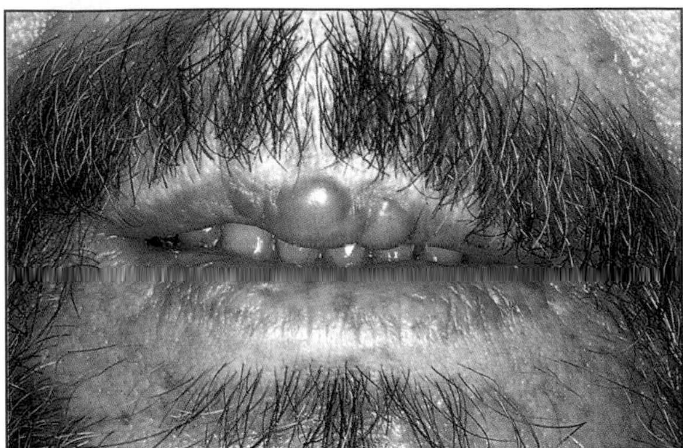

Fig. 41.6. Nodule in patient with multiple myeloma

When actual lesions are present, they are usually waxy or glassy infiltrated plaques, usually with a smooth or undulating surface (Fig. 41.6). The early lesions may be papular but they tend to coalesce. Typically the color is off-white or light-yellow. The face is once again the most common site; other possibilities include the scalp and genitalia. A sclerotic picture is created when the digits are infiltrated; this is known as scleroderma amyloidosum (Gottron).

Bullous amyloidosis results from the separation of the epidermis from the diffusely infiltrated dermis. It is typically associated with hemorrhage and can also occur in nodular amyloidosis. Finally, there is an elastotic variant of amyloidosis (amyloid elastosis Winkelmann 1985), in which the elastic fibers of the skin and other tissues are coated with amyloid. Presumably the P component is responsible for the binding to the elastin fibers. The cutaneous lesions are somewhat different, consisting of white or yellow firm papules and nodules on the shoulders, neck and upper trunk. Gastrointestinal and neurologic problems appear more common with this variant.

Mucosal Findings. The oral cavity and rectum are frequently involved. In the mouth, the most frequent problem is painful macroglossia, followed by difficulty in swallowing. The tongue may acquire a pale or waxy sheen, and often the teeth indent the expanded tissue. Infiltrated plaques, similar to those on the skin, can appear anywhere on the mucosa. The vocal cords may be damaged, causing hoarseness. In the perianal region, nodular lesions can be mistaken for condylomata acuminata, while rectal plaques also develop.

Systemic Findings. The other clinical manifestations of AL amyloid are protean. While AL infiltrates organs, the situation is more complicated than simply the insertion of foreign material. Usually the organ's function is distorted in other ways. If a patient has bilateral carpal tunnel syndrome, one should think of AL amyloid. Retrospective studies where surgically excised tissue from carpal tunnel release operations was more closely studied for amyloid have revealed that this diagnosis is frequently overlooked. More serious problems center around the heart and kidneys. In the heart, there are conduction disturbances and often a constrictive pericarditis. Such patients are hypersensitive to digitalis which should be avoided. Renal involvement may lead to the nephrotic syndrome. Pulmonary and bone nodules known as amyloidomas (analogous to nodular amyloidosis of the skin) may occur. Hemorrhagic problems may result from weakened blood vessels, trapping of factor X in the amyloid material and increased fibrinolysis. Other problems are listed in Table 41.4.

Histopathology. When a cutaneous lesion is biopsied, the findings are usually distinctive. There is a perivascular accumulation of amyloid, coupled with amorphous dermal deposits and perhaps separation at the epidermal-dermal junction. Some degree of hemorrhage is seen, along with an occasional plasma cell. Significant infiltrates do not develop. In the elastotic form, the elastic fibers are seemingly normal but coated by amyloid. When infiltrated mucosal plaques or the tongue are biopsied, there is massive infiltration which is easy to recognize.

The problem occurs when a skin, mucosal or rectal biopsy is done to rule in or out amyloidosis in the absence of obvious involvement, i.e., a blind

Table 41.4. Signs and symptoms of systemic amyloidosis

Signs and symptoms
Proteinuria (more often in AA amyloid)
Carpal tunnel syndrome, often bilateral
Cardiomyopathy, therapy-resistant with variety of conduction defects
Pericarditis
Diarrhea, constipation, malabsorption
Hypertension
Peripheral neuropathy
Autonomic dysfunction (postural hypotension, impotence)
Arthritis, especially of large joints
Splenomegaly
Endocrine gland infiltrates
Difficulty swallowing
Nonspecific findings (fatigue, headache, paresthesias, edema, weight loss)

biopsy of normal tissue. First, the yield is lower and second, the changes may be extremely subtle, limited to sparse perivascular deposits. In this situation, aspiration of abdominal wall fat coupled with Congo red staining has the highest yield.

Diagnostic Criteria. Two problems exist. One is the diagnosis of amyloid, which is usually made as discussed under histology. Rarely a cardiac or renal biopsy will provide the first sign. The next equally important step is the search for an underlying hematologic disorder and delineation of which organs are involved. Appropriate investigations include serum protein electrophoresis and immunoelectrophoresis, bone marrow examination, radiologic screening of the skeleton, urinalysis (looking especially for Bence-Jones proteins) and cardiac evaluation (EKG, echo).

Course and Prognosis. The prognosis depends on two factors: the underlying hematologic disorder and which organs are involved and how severely. The median survival of patients with primary systemic amyloidosis is worse than in multiple myeloma; it is about 1 year.

Differential Diagnosis. The cutaneous lesions present a variety of differential diagnostic points, as shown in Table 41.5. The differential diagnosis of systemic amyloidosis encompasses an entire internal medicine textbook.

Therapy. No dermatologic therapy is effective. The underlying hematologic disorders are notoriously therapy-resistant. Melphalan and prednisone has been shown superior to colchicine. If the patient's levels of urine or serum M component drop during therapy, the survival improves markedly to about 4 years. Colchicine should be reserved for familial Mediterranean fever and perhaps secondary amyloidosis.

Table 41.5. Differential diagnosis of cutaneous lesions in primary amyloidosis

Finding	Differential diagnosis
Purpura	Hematologic disorders, hemorrhage into solar elastosis
Waxy plaques	Colloid milium, some forms of porphyria, lichen myxedematosus, lipoid proteinosis
Bullous, hemorrhagic plaques	Lichen sclerosus et atrophicus, nodular solar elastosis
Elastotic nodules	Dermatofibrosis lenticularis disseminata, connective tissue nevus

Secondary Systemic Amyloidosis

Synonyms. AA amyloid, wear-and-tear amyloid

Definition. Amyloid deposits associated with an underlying chronic disease.

Etiology and Pathogenesis. AA amyloid is secondary to chronic underlying inflammatory and/or infectious processes. Thus the chief causes have waxed and waned over the past century. Typical causes include:

- Chronic infections: tuberculosis, lepromatous leprosy and previously tertiary syphilis
- Chronic draining abscesses: chronic bronchiectasis, empyema, osteomyelitis, severe forms of acne (acne inversa)
- Chronic inflammation: rheumatoid arthritis (probably most common today), severe psoriasis, ankylosing spondylitis, inflammatory bowel disease, connective tissue disorders, Behçet disease
- Tumors: renal cell carcinoma, occasionally Hodgkin disease and other hematologic disorders (usually associated with AL amyloid)
- Familial disorders: familial Mediterranean fever, Muckle-Wells syndrome (Muckle 1979) and many rare or noncutaneous disorders

- Miscellaneous: intravenous drug abuse, paraplegia (chronic infections and perhaps draining sores)

The precursor protein serum amyloid A (SAA) is produced in the liver as an acute-phase protein. In all these chronic disorders, there is overproduction of SAA. The acute-phase protein has a molecular weight of over 80,000 Da; an apparent monomer weighs about 10,000 Da. The AA protein is degraded by macrophages to a fiber with a molecular weight of around 8000 Da and deposited in tissues. In rheumatoid arthritis, those patients with high levels of SAA and C-reactive protein are most likely to develop AA.

Clinical Findings. The skin is almost never involved. Even blind biopsies have a lower yield than in AL amyloid. Specific cutaneous lesions do not occur. Neither the erysipelas-like lesions of familial Mediterranean fever nor the urticarial lesions of Muckle-Wells syndrome have amyloid deposits. Rheumatoid arthritis patients may develop extremely fragile skin with purpura, often from corticosteroid therapy.

The most likely organ to be involved is the kidney. Here deposition of amyloid along the basement membranes of the glomeruli leads to the nephrotic syndrome, which is the most common serious clinical finding. In amyloidosis associated with chronic renal failure and dialysis, the amyloid is derived from β_2-microglobulin, so the process is slightly different. The liver, spleen, adrenal glands, gastrointestinal tract and CNS may also be affected.

Histopathology. On occasion, a skin biopsy may show amyloid about blood vessels or diffusely in the dermis. We have seen this most commonly in the very thin skin of rheumatoid arthritis patients.

Laboratory Findings. While SAA can be measured in the serum, the diagnosis is usually made on renal or liver biopsy.

Prognosis. If the renal involvement is not life-threatening, then patients tend to do about as well as their underlying disease would suggest.

Therapy. The only therapy is treating the underlying disease and the renal involvement. The oral use of dimethyl sulfoxide to mobilize the amyloid has been proposed in AA amyloid but its efficacy is unclear. Colchicine produces clinical improvement in Behçet disease and familial Mediterranean fever. In animal models, it blocks the development of amyloid, but it is unclear if it achieves the same long-term effect in humans.

Table 41.6. Hereditary disorders with cutaneous amyloidosis

Disorder	Inheritance	Clinical findings	Cutaneous findings	Type of amyloid
Familial Mediterranean fever	AR	Febrile attacks with abdominal pain, synovitis, pleuritis, renal amyloidosis, mostly Arabs, Sephardic Jews, Armenians	Erysipelas-like eruption	ATTR (not in skin)
Muckle-Wells syndrome	AD	Episodic flu-like attacks, deafness, renal amyloidosis	Large urticarial lesions with attacks	ATTR (not in skin)
Multiple endocrine neoplasia 2A	AD	Parathyroid hyperplasia, pheochromocytoma, medullary thyroid carcinoma	Lichen amyloidosus in some kindreds	AK or AE_T
Pachyonychia congenita, Tidman type	AD	None	Nail dystrophy and palmarplantar keratoderma, diffuse mottled hyperpigmentation that is macular amyloidosis	AK
Familial lichen amyloidosus	AD	None	Lichen amyloidosus, earlier onset, more severe, more hyperpigmentation	AK

AD, autosomal dominant; AR, autosomal recessive

Hereditary Amyloidosis Syndromes

Very few of the hereditary amyloidosis syndromes involve the skin. The amyloid is usually derived from transthyretin, an α-globulin made in the liver that has many interesting functions. It binds with retinol-binding protein to transport retinol. In addition, it is a secondary transporter of T3 and T4. It has been called prealbumin, but this is misleading since it only refers to its electrophoretic mobility. In the genetic disorders there is usually a point mutation in the gene for transthyretin. For example, in the relatively common Portuguese type amyloidosis with polyneuropathy there is a point mutation at position 30 where valine replaces methionine. There are a few familial disorders with cutaneous amyloidosis. They are shown in Table 41.6.

Bibliography

Akpolat I, Akpolat T, Danaci M et al. (1997) Behçet's disease and amyloidosis. Review of the literature. Scand J Rheumatol 26:477–479

Al-Hoqail I, Naddaf H, Al-Rikabi A et al. (1997) Systemic lupus erythematosus and amyloidosis. Clin Rheumatol 16:422–424

Alster TS, Manaloto RM (1999) Nodular amyloidosis treated with a pulsed dye laser. Dermatol Surg 25:133–135

Bieber T, Ruzicka T, Linke RP et al. (1988) Hemorrhagic bullous amyloidosis. A histologic, immunocytochemical, and ultrastructural study of two patients. Arch Dermatol 124:1683–1686

Bonar L, Cohen AS, Skinner MM (1969) Characterization of the amyloid fibril as a cross-beta protein. Proc Soc Exp Biol Med 131:1373–1375

Breathnach SM (1988) Amyloid and amyloidosis. J Am Acad Dermatol 18:1–16

Carrell RW, Lomas DA (1997) Conformational disease. Lancet 350:134–138

Chang YT, Liu HN, Wong CK et al. (1997) Detection of Epstein-Barr virus in primary cutaneous amyloidosis. Br J Dermatol 136:823–826

Chang YT, Wong CK, Chow KC et al. (1999) Apoptosis in primary cutaneous amyloidosis. Br J Dermatol 140: 210–215

Cohen AS, Calkins E (1959) Electron microscopic observations on a fibrous component in amyloid of diverse origins. Nature 183:1202–1203

Falk RH, Comenzo RL, Skinner M (1997) The systemic amyloidoses. New Engl J Med 337:898–909

Gillmore JD, Hawkins PN, Pepys MB (1997) Amyloidosis: a review of recent diagnostic and therapeutic developments. Br J Haematol 99:245–256

Glenner GG, Terry W, Harada M et al. (1971) Amyloid fibril proteins: proof of homology with immunoglobulin light chains by sequence analyses. Science 172: 1150–1151

Goller MM, Cohen PR, Duvic M (1997) Lichen amyloidosis presenting as a papular pruritus syndrome in a human-immunodeficiency-virus-infected man. Dermatology 194:62–64

Gottron HA (1950) Amyloidosis cutis nodularis atrophicans diabetica. Dtsch Med Wochenschr 75:19–24

Goulden V, Highet AS, Shamy HK (1994) Notalgia paraesthetica – report of an association with macular amyloidosis. Clin Exp Dermatol 19:346–349

Hagari Y, Mihara M, Hagari S (1996) Nodular localized cutaneous amyloidosis: detection of monoclonality of infiltrating plasma cells by polymerase chain reaction. Br J Dermatol 135:630–633

Harahap M, Marwali MR (1998) The treatment of lichen amyloidosis. A review and a new technique. Dermatol Surg 24:251–254

Hashimoto K, Ito K, Kumakiri M et al. (1987) Nylon brush macular amyloidosis. Arch Dermatol 123:633–637

Helander I, Hopsu-Havu VK (1986) Treatment of lichen amyloidosus by etretinate. Clin Exp Dermatol 11:574–577

Holzman TF, Krafft GA (1996) The nanometer-scale structure of amyloid-beta visualized by atomic force microscopy. J Protein Chem 15:193–203

Horiguchi Y, Fine JD, Leigh IM et al. (1992) Lamina densa malformation involved in histogenesis of primary localized cutaneous amyloidosis. J Invest Dermatol 99: 12–18

Humphreys F, Spencer J, Mclaren K et al. (1996) An histological and ultrastructural study of the "dirty neck" appearance in atopic eczema. Clin Exp Dermatol 21: 17–19

Inazumi T, Hakuno M, Yamada H et al. (1994) Characterization of the amyloid fibril from primary localized cutaneous nodular amyloidosis associated with Sjögren's syndrome. Dermatology 189:125–128

Iwasaki K, Mihara M, Nishura S et al. (1991) Biphasic amyloidosis arising from friction melanosis. J Dermatol 18:86–91

Konig A, Wennemuth G, Soyer HP et al. (1999) Vulvar amyloidosis mimicking giant condylomata acuminata in a patient with multiple myeloma. Eur J Dermatol 9:29–31

Kousseff BG, Espinoza C, Zamore GA (1991) Sipple syndrome with lichen amyloidosis as a paracrinopathy: pleiotropy, heterogeneity, or a contiguous gene? J Am Acad Dermatol 25:651–657

Kyle RA, Gertz MA, Greipp PR et al. (1997) A trial of three regimens for primary amyloidosis: colchicine alone, melphalan and prednisone, and melphalan, prednisone, and colchicine. N Engl J Med 336:1202–1207

Lee DD, Huang CY, Wang CK (1998) Dermatopathologic findings in 20 cases of systemic amyloidosis. Am J Dermatopathol 20:438–442

Lien MH, Railan D, Nelson BR (1997) The efficacy of dermabrasion in the treatment of nodular amyloidosis. J Am Acad Dermatol 36:315–316

Lomakin A, Teplow DB, Kirschner DA et al. (1997) Kinetic theory of fibrillogenesis of amyloid-beta protein. Proc Natl Acad Sci U S A 94:7942–7947

Lubarsch O (1929) Zur Kenntnis ungewöhnlicher Amyloidablagerungen. Virchows Arch Pathol 271:867–889

Macsween RM, Saihan EM (1997) Nylon cloth macular amyloidosis. Clin Exp Dermatol 22:28–29

Masouyé I (1997) Diagnostic screening of systemic amyloidosis by abdominal fat aspiration: an analysis of 100 cases. Am J Dermatopathol 19:41–45
Muckle TJ (1979) The "Muckle Wells" syndrome. Br J Dermatol 100:87–92
Ogiyama Y, Hayashi Y, Kou C et al. (1996) Cutaneous amyloidosis in patients with progressive systemic sclerosis. Cutis 57:28–32
Ozkaya Bayazit E, Kavak A, Gungor H et al. (1998) Intermittent use of topical dimethylsulfoxide in macular and papular amyloidosis. Int J Dermatol 37:949–954
Palitz LL, Peck S (1952) Amyloidosis cutis: a macular variant. Arch Dermatol 65:451–457
Reider N, Sepp N, Fritsch P (1997) Remission of lichen amyloidosus after treatment with acitretin. Dermatology 194:309–X311
Robert C, Aractingi S, Prost C et al. (1993) Bullous amyloidosis. Report of 3 cases and review of the literature. Medicine (Baltimore) 72:38–44
Rocken C, Schwotzer EB, Linke RP et al. (1996) The classification of amyloid deposits in clinicopathological practice. Histopathology 29:325–335
Romero LS, Kantor GR, Lewin MW et al. (1997) Localized cutaneous amyloidosis associated with mycosis fungoides. J Am Acad Dermatol 37:124–127
Rubenow A, Cohen AS (1978) Skin involvement in generalized amyloidosis: a study of clinically involved and uninvolved skin in 50 patients with primary and secondary amyloidosis. Ann Intern Med 88:781–785
Ruzicka T, Schmoeckel C, Ring J et al. (1985) Bullous amyloidosis. Br J Dermatol 113:85–95
Sumitra S, Yesudian P (1993) Friction amyloidosis: a variant of an etiologic factor in amyloidosis cutis? Int J Dermatol 32:422–423
Tay CH, Dacosta JL (1970) Lichen amyloidosis: clinical study of 40 cases. Br J Dermatol 82:129–136
Tiitinen S, Kaarela K, Helin H et al. (1993) Amyloidosis – incidence and early risk factors in patients with rheumatoid arthritis. Scand J Rheumatol 22:158–161
Valentin R, Gurtler KF, Schaker A (1997) Renal amyloidosis and renal failure – a novel complication of the SAPHO syndrome. Nephrol Dial Transplant 12:2420–2423
Vestey JP, Tidman MJ, Mclaren KM (1994) Primary nodular cutaneous amyloidosis – long-term follow-up and treatment. Clin Exp Dermatol 19:159–162
Wang CK (1987) Cutaneous amyloidosis. Int J Dermatol 26:273–277
Wang CK (1990) Mucocutaneous manifestations in systemic amyloidosis. Clin Dermatol 8:7–12
Wang CK, Lin CS (1988) Friction amyloidosis. Int J Dermatol 27:302–307
Wang CK, Lee JY (1996) Macular amyloidosis with widespread diffuse pigmentation. Br J Dermatol 135:135–138
Wang WJ, Lin CS, Wong CK (1986) Response of systemic amyloidosis to dimethylsulfoxide. J Am Acad Dermatol 15:402–405
Westermark P, Noren P (1986) Two different pathogenetic pathways in lichen amyloidosis and macular amyloidosis. Arch Dermatol Res 278:206–213
Westermark P, Ridderstrom E, Valquist A (1996) Macular posterior pigmentary incontinence: its relation to macular amyloidosis and notalgia paresthetica. Acta Derm Venereol (Stockh) 76:302–304
Weyers W, Weyers I, Bonczkowitz M et al. (1997) Lichen amyloidosus: a consequence of scratching. J Am Acad Dermatol 37:923–928
WHO-IUIS Nomenclature Sub-Committee (1993) Nomenclature of amyloid and amyloidosis. Bull World Health Organ 71:105–112
Winkelman RK, Peters MS, Venencie PY (1985) Amyloid elastosis. A new cutaneous and systemic pattern of amyloidosis. Arch Dermatol 121:498–502

CHAPTER 42

The Hyalinoses

Contents

Basic Science Aspects

Hyalin is a poorly understood and even poorly defined word. It means "glassy or translucent substance" and has been applied to proteins that are amorphous and stain in such a fashion but lack other distinguishing characteristics. Hyaline is the corresponding adjective. In the skin, a hodgepodge of different materials have been identified. Some authors include amyloid and gouty tophi under hyalins; others specifically exclude these substances. The overproduction of carbohydrate-rich glycoproteins is the usual explanation for their genesis. Several exceedingly rare disorders are traditionally considered "hyalinoses".

Lipoid Proteinosis

(WIETHE 1924; URBACH 1933)

Synonyms. Hyalinosis cutis et mucosae, Urbach-Wiethe syndrome

Definition. Uncommon genodermatosis with deposits of hyalin in the skin and mucosa.

Epidemiology. This rare disease is present in large, somewhat inbred populations such as among the Afrikaans in South Africa and also in isolated areas of Sweden. Most American patients are of European origin.

Etiology and Pathogenesis. Lipoid proteinosis is a classic, autosomal, recessive inherited disorder. The gene has not been identified. The hyaline material in lipoid proteinosis is richer in lipids than other forms of hyalin, but there is no clear lipoprotein abnormality. The stored fats probably settle secondarily in the amorphous protein. Other features of the protein are discussed under histology. The pathogenesis is unknown.

Clinical Findings

Cutaneous Findings. The most typical site for hyaline deposits is the face. Multiple small waxy yellow papules are found along the eyelids (string of pearls sign or blepharosis moniliformis; Fig. 42.1) and the same lesions may be seen on the lips and over the knuckles, sides of the hand (Fig. 42.2), knees, elbows, and axillae. In the latter sites, the lesions may eventually become hyperkeratotic and verrucous. Early on, there may be bullous lesions,

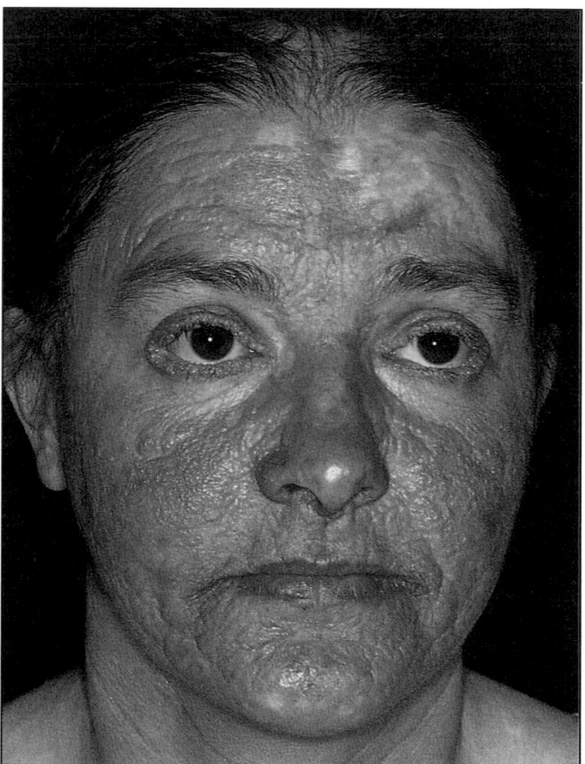

Fig. 42.1. Lipoid proteinosis with involvement of eye lids

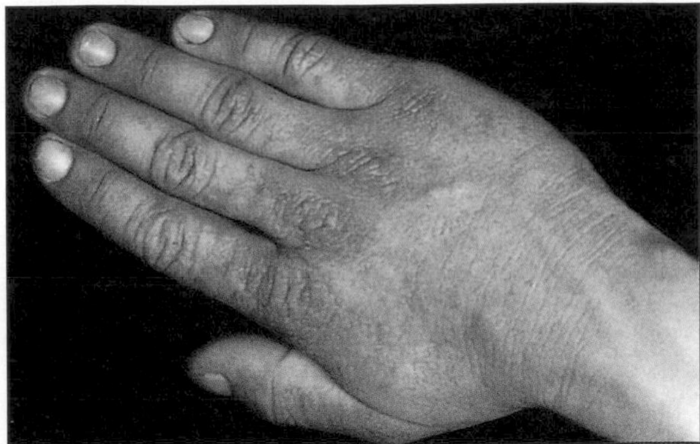

Fig. 42.2. Lipoid proteinosis with verruciform acral papules

especially on the cheeks, neck, and limbs; these heal with atrophic scars. In more extreme cases, the entire face is infiltrated, producing a leonine facies with numerous confluent yellow nodules and plaques. The facial hardening may lead to a fixed expression. Areas of infiltration may develop alopecia; the eyebrows and eyelashes are often missing, while patchy alopecia of the scalp and beard area may also occur.

Mucosal Findings. The mucosal findings are often responsible for the first symptom – a hoarse voice in a young child resulting from the waxy white or yellow infiltrates on the vocal cords. Similar papules, nodules and plaques may develop on the buccal mucosa, the tonsils, and the pharynx. The tongue and lips may be enlarged, thickened, and not very mobile (Fig. 42.3). The frenulum is often involved, further restricting tongue motion and therefore speech. The parotid duct may be obstructed.

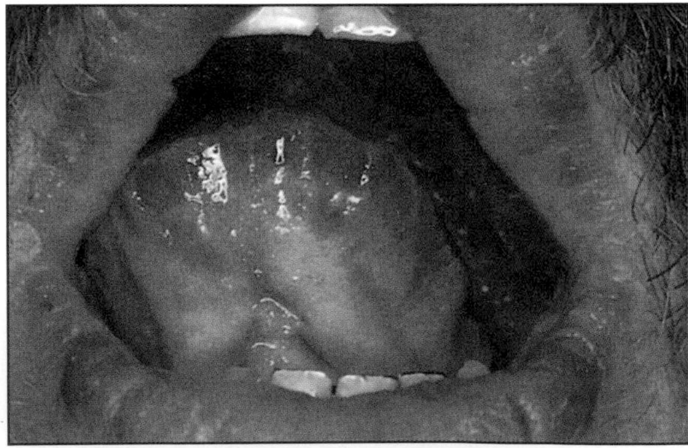

Fig. 42.3. Oral involvement in lipoid proteinosis

Systemic Findings. The same infiltrated plaques can involve the entire gastrointestinal tract, including most often the esophagus and rectum. Vaginal plaques also occur. The most characteristic systemic feature is symmetric calcifications just lateral and superior to the sella turcica. Other parts of the brain may also be calcified; at least 70 % of patients develop this finding. In this group, seizures or mild mental retardation have occasionally been described.

Histopathology. The epidermis tends to be normal or acanthotic and hyperkeratotic in the verruciform lesions. The hyaline material accumulates around blood vessels, sweat glands, and arrector pili muscles. Bundles of hyaline protein are found coursing through the papillary dermis, usually perpendicular to the epidermis. Sometimes the entire dermis is replaced by the amorphous masses.

The hyaline protein is completely different from amyloids; it does not show metachromasia or dichroism and is markedly PAS-positive and diastase-resistant. Fat stains may show droplets of lipid scattered throughout the amorphous background; hence the name of the disorder. Electron microscopic examination reveals a woven mat of small, 4–6 nm filaments which appear to contain reduplicated basement membranes. Collagen (most often type IV), glycoproteins, mucopolysaccharides (most often keratan sulfate), and many other substances have been identified, but all may be innocent bystanders. Mucin stains are usually negative.

Laboratory Findings. No specific laboratory test is helpful.

Course and Prognosis. The outlook is good. The disease tends to slow down in adult life, so that the main problems are hoarseness and cosmetic considerations.

Differential Diagnosis. Patients with erythropoietic protoporphyria develop very similar cutaneous lesions but lack mucosal changes. Hyalinosis has also been described in association with a plasmacytoma and IgG gammopathy. Colloid milium is also very similar, especially microscopically, but usually the plaques are larger and softer. When they are incised, as when doing a biopsy, a jelly-like material oozes out. Colloid milium is also usually associated with sun exposure, although juvenile colloid milium is not related to light. The scars on the neck may resemble pseudoxanthoma elasticum. The papules may also suggest xanthomas. When the infiltrative lesions enlarge and coalesce, other disorders such as scleromyxedema may be considered. Multiple infiltrative amyloid plaques may also be similar, especially when associated with mucosal involvement, but amyloid mainly enters into the histologic differential diagnosis.

Therapy. For a genodermatosis, there is a surprising number of treatment options. The laryngeal lesions should be removed to reduce hoarseness and the threat of obstruction. Laser or surgical correction are both possible; patients rarely require tracheotomy. The cutaneous lesions may be dermabraded or excised. In addition, oral retinoids may produce some improvement, and several reports endorse oral dimethyl sulfoxide, although other studies show it to be of no benefit.

Juvenile Hyaline Fibromatosis

(MURRAY 1873)

Synonyms. Murray-Puretic-Drescher syndrome, mesenchymal dysplasia

Etiology and Pathogenesis. This rare disorder is poorly understood and inherited in an autosomal recessive pattern. The gene is unknown and the underlying defect totally obscure.

Clinical Findings

Cutaneous Findings. In childhood, patients begin to develop multiple dermal and subcutaneous fibrous papules and nodules, some of which may become very large, reaching a size of many centimeters and eroding or ulcerating (Fig. 42.4). The face, scalp, knees, and elbows are most often involved. The lesions are painless but cosmetically unacceptable, and they often disturb normal joint function. While some lesions may resolve and others remain, for the most part they are permanent. A second finding is numerous small white papules, especially on the neck, ears, nose, and upper lip. Verrucous perianal lesions also may occur

Systemic Findings. Most patients have gingival hyperplasia. The biggest problem is flexion contractures, which result in most adults being bedridden. The lack of mobility leads to weakness, scoliosis, osteoporosis, and reduced height and weight. Osteolytic bone lesions are common, especially in the long bones and phalanxes. Similar deposits have been identified in many other organs. Most patients are of normal intelligence.

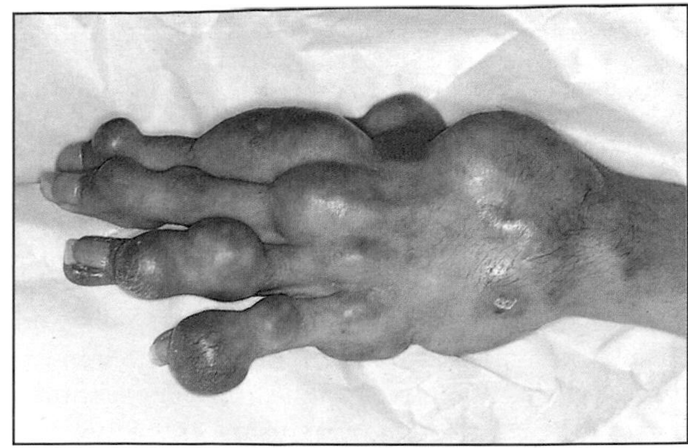

Fig. 42.4. Juvenile hyaline fibromatosis

Histopathology. The nature of the hyaline material is unclear. It is more mucoid and chondroid than the hyaline of lipoid proteinosis. In addition, spindle-shaped fibroblasts are still present in the matrix material. A variety of acid mucopolysaccharides have been identified.

Course and Prognosis. The outlook is dismal.

Differential Diagnosis. Infantile hyaline fibromatosis and the related Winchester syndrome are similar but lack the large disfiguring tumors. There are other disorders with multiple disfiguring tumors (neurofibromatosis, Proteus syndrome, and many others), but none has the disabling contractures seen here.

Therapy. There is not even palliative therapy. The lesions are not radiation-sensitive. While individual lesions can be excised, they are often intermingled with tendons and not easy to remove.

Infantile Hyaline Fibromatosis

(LANDING and NADORRA 1986)

This autosomal, recessive inherited disorder is either a severe form of juvenile hyaline fibromatosis or closely related. Once the genes are identified, the relationship should become clearer. Patients die of widespread hyaline infiltrates at an early age. They have severe joint contractures, gingival hyperplasia, and cutaneous infiltrates. The disfiguring tumors of the juvenile form either do not develop or have no time to develop.

Winchester Syndrome

(Winchester et al. 1969)

This disorder is also inherited in an autosomal recessive pattern. It is exceedingly rare and has some similarities to the hyaline fibromatoses. The facies are coarse and there are joint contractures, diffuse skin thickness, hyperpigmentation over the joint, and hypertrichosis. Gingival hypertrophy and corneal opacities are common. Thus, the clinical findings lie between the hyaline fibromatoses and a mucopolysaccharidosis. Confusing the issue are reports of abnormal urine oligosaccharides.

Bibliography

Breier F, Fang-Kirchner S, Wolff K et al. (1997) Juvenile hyaline fibromatosis: impaired collagen metabolism in human skin fibroblasts. Arch Dis Child 77:436–440

Chaudhary SJ, Dayal PK (1995) Hyalinosis cutis et mucosae. Review with a case report. Oral Surg Oral Med Oral Pathol Oral Radiol Endod 80:168–171

Fayad MN, Yacoub A, Salman S et al. (1987) Juvenile hyaline fibromatosis: two new patients and review of the literature. Am J Genet 26:123–131

Fleischmajer R, Krieg T, Dziadek M et al. (1984) Ultrastructure and composition of connective tissue in hyalinosis cutis et mucosae skin. J Invest Dermatol 82:252–258

Gilaberte Y, Gonzalez-Mediero, Lopez Barrantes V et al. (1993) Juvenile hyaline fibromatose with skull-encephalic anomalies: a case report and review of the literature. Dermatology 187:144–148

Glover MT, Lake BD, Atherton DJ (1991) Infantile systemic hyalinosis: newly recognized disorder of collagen. Pediatrics 87:228–234

Gruber F, Manestar D, Stasic A et al. (1996) Treatment of lipoid proteinosis with etretinate (letter). Acta Derm Venereol (Stockh) 76:154–155

Harper JI, Duance VC, Sims TJ et al. (1985) Lipoid proteinosis: an inherited disorder of collagen metabolism? Br J Dermatol 113:145–151

Hausser I, Biltz S, Rauterberg E et al. (1991) Hyalinosos cutis et mucosae (Morbus Urbach-Wiethe) – ultrastrukturelle und immunologische Merkmale. Hautarzt 42:28–33

Hofer PA, Larsson PA, Ek B et al. (1974) A clinical and histopathological study of twenty-seven cases of Urbach-Wiethe disease. Dermatologic, gastroenterologic, neurophysiologie, ophthalmologie, and Roentgen-diagnostic aspects, as well as the results of some clinicochemical and histochemical examinations. Acta Pathol Microbiol Scand [A] Suppl 245:1–87

Iwata S, Horiuchi R, Maeda H et al. (1980) Systemic hyalinosis or juvenile hyaline fibromatosis. Ultrastructural and biochemical study of cultured skin fibroblasts. Arch Dermatol Res 267:115–121

Kan AE, Rogers M (1989) Juvenile hyaline fibromatosis: an expanded clinicopathologic spectrum. Pediatr Dermatol 6:68–75

Konstantinov K, Kabakchiev P, Karchev T et al. (1992) Lipoid proteinosis. J Am Acad Dermatol 27:293–297

Landing BH, Nadorra R (1986) Infantile systemic hyalinosis: report of four cases of a disease, fatal in infancy, apparently different from juvenile systemic hyalinosis. Pediatr Pathol 6:55–79

Leheup BR, Jeandel C, Guedenet JC et al. (1986) Hyalinosis cutis and mucosae. Ultrastructural histochemical aspects indicating intracellular accumulation of glycosaminoglycans. Ann Pathol 6:53–59

Lubec B, Steinert I, Breier F et al. (1995) Skin collagen defects in a patient with juvenile hyaline fibromatosis. Arch Dis Child 73:246–248

Moy LS, Moy RL, Matsuoka LY et al. (1987) Lipoid proteinosis: ultrastructural and biochemical studies. J Am Acad Dermatol 16:1193–1201

Muda AO, Paradisi M, Angelo C et al. (1995) Lipoid proteinosis: clinical, histologic, and ultrastructural investigations. Cutis 56:220–224

Murray J (1873) On three peculiar cases of molluscum fibrocum in children. Med Chir Trans 38:235–253

Navarro C, Fachal C, Rodríguez C et al. (1999) Lipoid proteinosis. A biochemical and ultrastructural investigation of two new cases. Br J Dermatol 141:326–331

Newton JA, Rasbridge S, Temple A et al. (1991) Lipoid proteinosis – new immunopathological observations. Clin Exp Dermatol 16:350–354

Olsen DR, Chu ML, Uitto J (1988) Expression of basement membrane zone genes coding for type IV procollagen and laminin by human skin fibroblasts in vitro: elevated alpha 1 (IV) collagen mRNA levels in lipoid proteinosis. J Invest Dermatol 90:734–738

Ozkaya-Bayazit E, Ozarmagan G, Baykal C et al. (1997) Oral DMSO therapy in three patients with lipoidproteinosis. Results of long-term therapy. Hautarzt 48:477–481

Paller AS (1994) Histology of lipoid proteinosis. JAMA 272:564–565

Urbach E (1933) Kutane Lipoidosen. Dermatol Z 66:371–386

Urbach E, Wiethe C (1929) Lipoidosis cutis et mucosae. Virchows Arch Pathol Anat Physiol 273:285–319

Wiethe C (1924) Kongenitale, diffuse Hyalinablagerungen in den oberen Luftwegen, familiär auftretend. Z Hals Nasen Ohrenheilkd 10:359–362

Winchester P, Grossman H, Lim WN et al. (1969) A new acid mucopolysaccharidosis with skeletal deformities simulating rheumatoid arthritis. Am J Roentgenol Radium Ther Nucl Med 106:121–128

Mucinoses

Contents

Basic Science Aspects

The extracellular matrix of the dermis is composed of collagen fibers, elastic fibers, microfibrils and the amorphous interfibrillar ground substance, which contains a variety of protein-carbohydrate conjugates, water and various salts. The terms used to describe the ground substance proteins are shown in Table 43.1.

The most important components of the ground substance are the proteoglycans. These are predominantly proteins, with the protein component providing a backbone or core. Along the backbone are attached a number of glycosaminoglycans, which themselves consist of multiple heterosaccharides, assembling in repeating units with hexose and N-hexosamine groups attached and sulfated to varying degrees. Thus the entire proteoglycan molecule resembles a laboratory bottle brush. Glycosaminoglycans account for 0.1–1.0 mg/g of dried skin, so they are relatively common. The most prevalent ones are hyaluronic acid, dermatan sulfate, chondroitin-4-sulfate and chondroitin-6-sulfate. Heparin sulfate and heparin are also found, although heparin is free and not part of the proteoglycan structure. The composition of the glycosaminoglycans varies according to age, sex and body region. The skin of the adult contains relatively little hyaluronic

Table 43.1. Types of ground substance constituents

Term	Definition
Glycoproteins	Proteins conjugated with one or more covalently linked carbohydrate residues which account for less than 4% of weight. Sometimes used generically to include mucoproteins and proteoglycans
Mucoproteins	Proteins conjugated with polysaccharides containing many hexosamine residues and accounting for 4–30% of weight; usually found in mucous secretions
Proteoglycans	Proteins conjugated with large number of polysaccharides, particularly glycosaminoglycans, attached to a small protein backbone. Often multiple units attached to hyaluronic acid backbone to create "bottle brush" appearance. Always more than 30% carbohydrates. Main constituent of cartilage and connective tissue matrix
Glycosaminoglycans	High molecular weight, linear acidic heteropolysaccharides with multiple hexose and hexosamine groups attached. Examples include chondroitin sulfates, dermatan sulfates, heparan sulfate, heparin, keratin sulfates and hyaluronic acid. All except heparin are found in proteoglycans
Mucopolysaccharides	Synonym for glycosaminoglycans (acid mucopolysaccharides)
Glycolipids	Sphingosine-based lipids with carbohydrate groups (glycosphingolipids)

acid and more of the sulfated structures, while Wharton jelly in the umbilicus contains almost only hyaluronic acid. In studies on the treatment of photoaging, reversal of glycosaminoglycan distribution patterns and production of new glycosaminoglycans are taken as signs of "reversed aging".

Glycosaminoglycans and proteoglycans are essential in maintaining the balance of water and various ions in the skin. They are hydrophilic, negatively charged and form hydrated gels that bind large amounts of water and cations. Glycosaminoglycans expand to fill the extracellular spaces of the skin, providing resistance against pressure and allowing gradual deformation, while collagen and elastin fibers provide elasticity and resistance to sheering and tearing forces. The glycosaminoglycans also allow rapid diffusion of water soluble molecules through the dermis. Hyaluronic acid appears to play a special role in wound healing and cell migration. Injections of hyaluronidase are used to allow other agents to diffuse more easily, since the enzyme weakens the ground substance. Ground substance metabolism is under hormonal influence, as the deposition of glycosaminoglycans in some thyroid disorders demonstrates.

Fibroblasts are responsible for the secretion of glycosaminoglycans; in disorders of glycosaminoglycan synthesis or production, the fibroblasts may show accumulations of various metabolic products, many of which are also discharged into the dermis. The materials are degraded in lysosomes, so that when selected lysosomal enzymes are missing, there are pathologic accumulations in the target organs. We have already discussed the sphingolipidoses in Chapter 38; here we will consider other lysosomal disorders.

Mucopolysaccharidoses

Etiology and Pathogenesis. The mucopolysaccharidoses are a very diverse group of disorders involving defects in enzymes essential to the breakdown of glycosaminoglycans. Mucopolysaccharide is simply an older synonym for glycosaminoglycan but it has been retained as a clinical term. All these disorders are inherited in an autosomal recessive pattern, except for Hunter syndrome, which is inherited in a X-linked recessive pattern. The abnormal glycosaminoglycans not only accumulate in lysosomes but also within connective tissues throughout the body and are excreted in the urine.

Clinical Findings. Unifying features are small stature, a coarse or gargoyle facies, multiple skeletal abnormalities known as dysostosis multiplex, corneal clouding, organomegaly and varying degrees of mental retardation. The classification and specific clinical features of these rare disease should be sought in a genetics or pediatrics text.

The dermatologist will almost never be called upon to make the diagnosis of mucopolysaccharidosis. However there are cutaneous features. The skin is typically thickened because of excess deposits of various glycosaminoglycans. Acral infiltrates can mimic a sclerotic process. The most common finding is hirsutism, which is also associated with other mucinoses. The excess hairs are especially common on the face and legs. Often, pubic and axillary hair development does not occur in those few patients who reach puberty.

Hunter (1917) syndrome patients very often have cobblestone plaques over the scapulae extending to the posterior axillary fold. They represent local infiltrates of glycosaminoglycans. The papules are ivory in color, range in size from 1 to 10 mm and may coalesce. Occasionally, similar lesions are seen elsewhere on the body. Such changes have occasionally been described in other variants, but they are almost specific for Hunter disease. The clinical differential diagnosis includes connective tissue nevus and dermatofibrosis lenticularis disseminata.

Laboratory Findings. The disorders can be diagnosed by enzyme analysis of leukocytes, cultured fibroblasts or lymphocytes. Sometimes the white blood cells show metachromasia as a result of the glycosaminoglycans, which can also be visualized in a variety of cells using electron microscopy. In the past, mucopolysaccharidoses were also diagnosed by analysis of the excessive glycosaminoglycans present in the urine, but this screening test does not allow exact classification. Prenatal diagnosis is possible in all the disorders using either chorionic villi or amniocyte cultures.

Differential Diagnosis. The differential diagnosis of the mucopolysaccharidoses is beyond our scope. Most dermatologists would be happy to recognize the general family of disorders. One should consider other lysosomal disorders such as the sphingolipidoses, mucolipidoses, glycoprotein storage disorders, Winchester syndrome, and infantile hyaline fibromatosis.

Therapy. Early attempts at treatment with bone marrow transplantation and enzyme replacement therapy are underway; eventually gene transfer will offer the best hope. In general the life expectancy is reduced. Depending on the enzyme disorder, some patients die in childhood and others reach adulthood but are severely disabled.

Cutaneous Mucinoses

Mucinosis refers to the deposition of mucin in a skin. A variety of substances can be considered as mucins. In general they are slimy, tenacious materials that can be drawn into threads or strands; the Greek word translates as slime, while the Latin word is *mucus*. Most of the cutaneous mucins are proteoglycans. The constituent glycosaminoglycans are variably sulfated. As the number of sulfur molecules increases, the glycosaminoglycan becomes more acidic. Formerly one spoke of acidic and neutral mucopolysaccharides; today the equivalent terms are sulfated or nonsulfated glycosaminoglycans. Heparin, dermatan sulfate and chondroitin-6-sulfate are markedly sulfated and more acidic, while hyaluronic acid is not sulfated and more neutral.

These chemical aspects of the glycosaminoglycans determine to a great extent the staining characteristics of the cutaneous mucins. The weakly sulfated glycosaminoglycans are PAS-positive, while hyaluronic acid is only slightly positive and heparin and dermatan sulfate are negative. The Hale and alcian blue stains identify all the sulfated glycosaminoglycans. Most of the acid mucins show metachromasia with toluidine blue staining. Hyaluronic acid can be digested with both bacterial and testicular hyaluronidase; dermatan sulfate is sensitive to only the testicular hyaluronidase. In addition to the mucins made by fibroblasts, there may also, on rare occasions, be epithelial mucins in the skin. These are richer in sialic acid and may be found in sweat glands, hairs, salivary gland tumors and cysts, and metastatic glandular tumors. They tend to have a slightly different staining pattern, which on occasion may be important.

Because the glycosaminoglycans are so rich in water, they appear quite differently in fixed tissue. Much of the stringy or vacuolated appearance is a result of what is left behind when the glycosaminoglycans are dried out. In addition formalin-fixed, paraffin-embedded tissue loses a great deal of its glycosaminoglycans; when one is specifically searching for mucins, a fixative consisting of absolute alcohol with 1% formalin is preferable.

There is no widely accepted classification of cutaneous mucin deposits. Our version is shown in Table 43.2.

Dermal Mucinoses

There is an overproduction of various glycosaminoglycans or other related substances, triggered either by thyroid abnormalities, immunologic disturbances or for unknown reasons. The

Table 43.2. Types of cutaneous mucinosis

I. Dermal mucinosis

Associated with thyroid disease
1. Associated with hypothyroidism
   a. Diffuse myxedema
   b. Localized myxedema
2. Associated with hyperthyroidism
   a. Pretibial myxedema

Not associated with thyroid disease
1. Lichen myxedematosus (papular mucinosis)
2. Scleromyxedema
3. Scleredema
4. Focal cutaneous mucinosis
   Acral persistent papular mucinosis
   Reticulated erythematous mucinosis
   Rare miscellaneous disorders
      Mucinosis of the lip
      Self-healing juvenile cutaneous mucinosis
      Infantile cutaneous mucinosis
      Mucinous nevus
      Plaque-like erythema with milia

II. Epithelial mucinosis
1. Follicular mucinosis
2. Urticarial follicular mucinosis

III. Secondary mucinosis

Secondary dermal mucinosis
1. Inflammatory dermatoses (atopic dermatitis, psoriasis)
2. Connective tissue disorders (lupus erythematosus, dermatomyositis)
3. Infections (especially cryptococcosis)
4. Digital mucous cyst
5. Mesenchymal tumors (wide variety)
6. Miscellaneous (Degos disease)

Secondary epithelial mucinosis
1. Epithelial tumors (especially within and around basal cell carcinoma, mucinous carcinoma, other adnexal tumors, metastatic glandular tumors)
2. Mucinous syringometaplasia

histologic picture is of focal deposits of an amorphous stringy material that displaces the collagen fibers of the dermis, but does not alter the epidermis. Thus the picture is similar to that seen in the umbilicus with Wharton jelly – massive deposits of locally made mucin.

Mucinoses Associated with Thyroid Disease

Thyroid diseases and the skin are discussed in detail in Chapter 48. The causes of thyroid problems, the laboratory evaluation and the therapy are briefly mentioned there or can be sought in internal medicine texts.

Hypothyroidism

Diffuse Myxedema

(ORD 1878)

Synonyms. Myxedema, true myxedema

Etiology and Pathogenesis. The lack of thyroid hormone function leads to the deposition of mucins in the dermis. There are many causes of hypothyroidism. How the thyroid hormones control glycosaminoglycan synthesis in the skin remains unclear.

Clinical Findings. The skin tends to be dry, pale, waxy and swollen. Typically the facial involvement is most distinctive, with swollen lids and puffy cheeks. The extremities can also be affected. When one attempts to press into puffy myxedematous skin, no pitting or depression is produced because the glycosaminoglycans are not easily displaced. Papular lesions are occasionally present. The mucinous deposits tend to disappear with thyroid replacement therapy.

Often the skin of the face, especially the nasolabial region, and the palms and soles are slightly yellow; this is a result of secondary carotenemia. Sebum production is reduced and both follicular keratoses and ichthyosis-like changes are seen. There is often alopecia with dry, brittle straw-like hairs. Patients may complain of acral paresthesias.

Histopathology. The dermis is often surprisingly normal. Only in severe myxedema is there obvious infiltration of the dermis by mucin. The most likely sites are about hair follicles and blood vessels. Mucin stains will usually reveal sparse amounts of positively staining material in these sites.

Therapy. Appropriate thyroid replacement therapy.

Localized Myxedema

(JADASSOHN and DÖSSEKKER 1916)

Synonyms. Circumscript myxedema, myxedema tuberosum

Some hypothyroid patients present with this very rare variant of diffuse myxedema, in which localized, sometimes exaggerated swelling is found. Either soft skin-colored plaques or more nodular accumulations are present. Sometimes the lesions are erythematous and mistaken for cellulitis. In other cases, there is localized swelling of a limb or the genitalia, resembling elephantiasis. Finally, solitary facial edema may occur, but this is usually considered as part of diffuse myxedema. The other aspects of the problem including treatment are identical to the diffuse disorder.

Hyperthyroidism

The causes of hyperthyroidism are multiple, although Graves disease is most common.

Pretibial Myxedema

(TROTTER and EDEN 1942)

Synonyms. Myxodermia circumscripta praetibialis, myxedema circumscriptum thyreotoxicum

Etiology and Pathogenesis. The cause of pretibial myxedema is a fascinating story. It is most often associated with Graves disease, in which autoantibodies (TRab) against the thyroid stimulating hormone (TSH) receptor are present. These immunoglobulins were formerly known as LATS (long acting thyroid stimulator) because they remained in the serum longer than TSH. Some may stimulate the TSH receptor; others simply block it. While the TRab are felt to be pathogenic, it is unclear how they influence the overproduction of mucin, both in the skin and in the retroorbital space. Perhaps fibroblasts in these tissues are stimulated in the same way. In some cases, pretibial myxedema has been associated with hypothyroidism, usually after thyroidectomy, and other forms of thyroid disease.

Clinical Findings. The most likely location for pretibial myxedema should be obvious. Initially there is simply swelling or edema over the shins, often transient and subtle. Next, generally symmetrical, slowly growing, puffy plaques appear (Fig. 43.1). Their color varies between pink-white and yellow-gray. The superficial deposits of mucin displace the sebaceous glands downwards, making the hair follicle openings more funnel-like and producing a characteristic peau d'orange (orange skin) or pig skin appearance. Hypertrichosis is also common. As the plaques persist, they may darken and enlarge. Erosion or ulceration is very rare.

Lesions may occur in other parts of the body. The next most common site is the dorsal aspect of the foot, where verrucous nodules or diffuse swelling can occur, producing an elephantiasis-like picture. In other cases, small inflamed nodules resembling erythema nodosum may appear, while in yet other cases the lesion may be inflamed and resemble cellulitis. Keloids may develop following trauma or even a punch biopsy.

Histopathology. The epidermis is often atrophic and the dermis replaced by sheets of stringy pale-staining material, which is mucin, primarily hyaluronic acid. Only a few collagen fibers and fibroblasts lie in lakes of mucin, just as with Wharton jelly of the umbilicus. The degree of infiltration is far more extreme than in diffuse myxedema and impossible to overlook. Often the clinician performing the biopsy has noticed the gelatinous nature of the dermis.

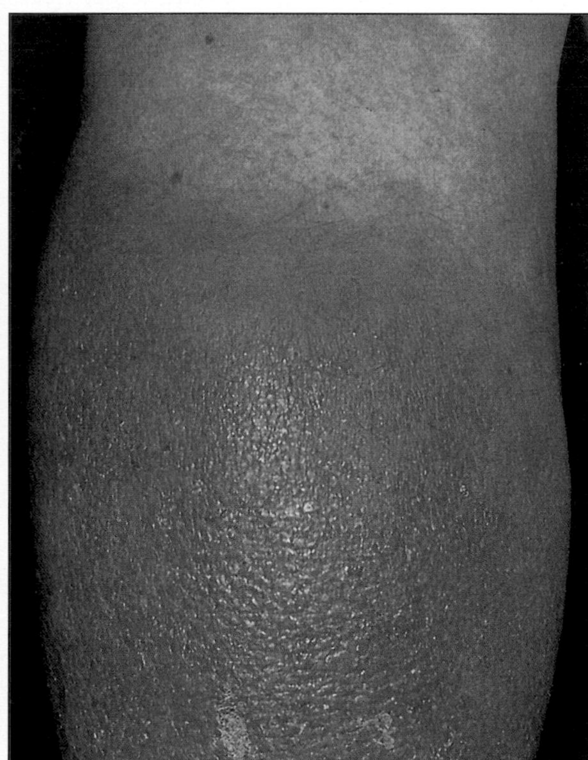

Fig. 43.1. Pretibial myxedema

Course and Prognosis. The lesions may persist despite appropriate systemic therapy for the underlying thyroid disease.

Differential Diagnosis. Some patients with severe stasis dermatitis will also develop mucinous deposits, as has also been described in Japanese Sjögren syndrome patients.

Therapy. High potency topical or intralesional corticosteroids are probably the best approach. The pretibial surface lends itself well to occlusion, which may be achieved with impermeable kitchen wraps or more elegant silicone sheeting. Hyaluronidase can also be injected with the corticosteroid to ease injection and perhaps dissolve some mucin. In the early stages, compression dressings or stockings are useful.

Systemic therapy is most often employed when orbital involvement is prominent. In addition to treating the underlying thyroid disorder, one should consider systemic corticosteroids especially when exophthalmos is prominent. Cyclosporine has also been employed.

EMO Syndrome

(Thomas 1933)

Synonyms. Diamond syndrome (1959), thyroid acropachy, ophthalmic Graves disease and many others. EMO is an acronym proposed by Braun-Falco and Petzoldt (1967) for exophthalmos, myxedema and osteoarthopathy.

Etiology and Pathogenesis. The mucin deposition is related to the TRab discussed above. The same or other autoantibodies may be directed against ocular muscle antigens, leading to not only mucin production but also intense lymphocytic inflammation about the eye. The mechanism of the skeletal changes is unclear.

Clinical Findings. The typical patient has all three aspects of the syndrome: pretibial myxedema, exophthalmos and thyroid acropachy. Some patients may present with dysthyroid eye disease without other diseases of hyperthyroidism; this has been called ophthalmologic Graves disease. Thyroid acropachy is a swelling of the digits, most commonly involving the thumb and index finger, due to infiltration with mucin. The end effect is clubbing of the fingers and toes. Radiologic examination may show focal subperiosteal bone formation.

Course and Prognosis. The changes respond poorly to therapy. In all other aspects, the EMO syndrome is similar to pretibial myxedema.

Lichen Myxedematosus

(Montgomery and Underwood 1953)

Synonym. Papular mucinosis

Definition. Discrete, often disseminated, deposition of mucin in the skin.

Etiology and Pathogenesis. The exact etiology is unclear but there is a deposition of mucin in the skin often associated with a monoclonal gammopathy. The aberrant protein is almost always IgG, usually with λ-light chains, but rarely with κ chains or other immunoglobulins. Presumably the immunoglobulin stimulates not only the production of mucin but also of collagen, as both are increased. Not all patients with lichen myxedematosus have a gammopathy. In some it may appear later in the disease course; in others, there must be another mechanism.

Clinical Findings. Typically there are small skin-colored or ivory papules, usually found on the nape, forehead, arms, thighs or lower trunk (Fig. 43.2). The lesions are rarely more than several millimeters in size, but they may be grouped or confluent. Sometimes they have a white tone and appear more lichenoid. The papules may be arranged in a linear (moniliform) pattern or resemble the working surface of an old-fashion kitchen grater. They may be pruritic but often are asymptomatic.

Histopathology. The papular lesions simply show a focal deposit of mucin in the dermis. There is also an increased number of fibroblasts and collagen fibers, reflecting the dual nature of the proliferation. Plasma cell infiltrates may be seen and the collagen fibers often appear swollen.

Laboratory Findings. Serum protein electrophoresis and immunoelectrophoresis should be performed as part of the diagnostic approach. If positive, then bone marrow examination is essential.

Course and Prognosis. The skin problems are very troublesome, but the nature of the gammopathy and its response to therapy dictate the course, which is usually dismal. Those patients without a gammopathy may even experience some regression of the cutaneous lesions. Lichen myxedematous may evolve into scleromyxedema in some patients.

Differential Diagnosis. Papular mucinosis is usually used as a synonym for lichen myxedematosus. We prefer to use the term for other idiopathic papular mucinoses. In lichen myxedematosus, the papules are flat-topped or lichenoid, while in the other disorders the papules are more dome-shaped. Rarely papular mucinosis can be seen in both hypo- and hyperthyroidism, as well as associated with HIV infection and borelliosis.

Therapy

Systemic. The treatment of the underlying plasma cell proliferation is most important, but very difficult. Melphalan and prednisone is the standard approach, but a hematologist should direct treatment. A patient with stable lichen myxedematosus and no gammopathy worsened when treated with interferon-α for chronic active hepatitis C.

Topical. The lesions may be treated with topical or intralesional corticosteroids. Radiation therapy, CO_2 laser, PUVA, PUVA bath therapy and a variety of other modalities have been recommended but none are dramatically effective.

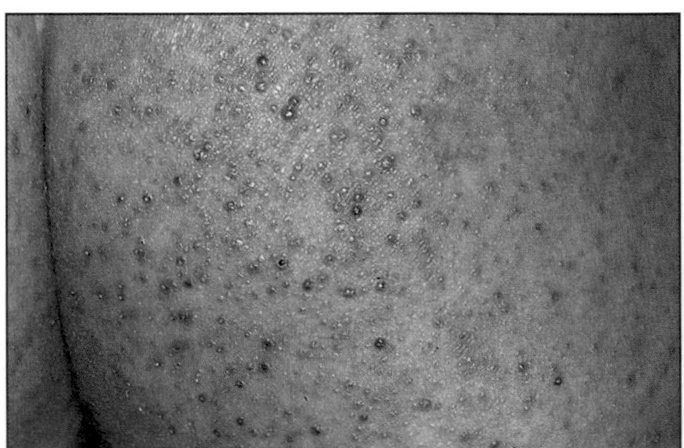

Fig. 43.2. Lichen myxedematosus

Scleromyxedema
(GOTTRON 1954)

Synonym. Arndt-Gottron syndrome

Definition. Chronic sclerotic skin disease with thickened skin, lichenoid papules and associated gammopathy.

Etiology and Pathogenesis. Scleromyxedema is closely related to lichen myxedematosus. There is always a plasma cell proliferation and gammopathy. The deposition of the aberrant immunoglobulins may lead to synthesis of both collagen and glycosaminoglycans. The serum of patients with scleromyxedema in vitro can stimulate fibroblast DNA synthesis and proliferation.

Clinical Findings. Scleromyxedema is characterized by lichenoid papules and thickened or elephant-like skin with distinctive folds. The lichenoid papules are similar to those in lichen myxedematosus, but tend to become more numerous and densely grouped together especially on the nape and forehead (Fig. 43.3). The skin becomes thickened in these areas, but also on the trunk. It becomes very difficult to pick up or pinch together and can only be compressed into large coarse folds (Fig. 43.4). At the same time, there may be acral sclerosis with tightening of the fingers and toes. The face may be thickened and expressionless similar to systemic sclerosis (Fig. 43.5). At this stage, pruritus is more common. A diffuse hyperpigmentation may develop. Systemic signs in addition to the gammopathy and its underlying hematologic disorder may include damage to the cerebral, coronary, renal and retinal vessels. A myopathy may also develop.

Histopathology. The skin biopsy may be dominated by either deposition of mucin, usually sulfated glycosaminoglycans, or proliferation of collagen, although usually evidence of both features is found. If papular lesions are biopsied, they are rich in mucin. In specimens from sclerotic skin, the increased mucin may be very subtle, present in fine strands between thickened collagen fibers. Plasma cells are often increased. Mucin deposition and plasma cells may also be found in other organs, especially the muscles. The nature of the systemic changes remains unclear. In some instances mucin has been found in the coronary, cerebral, renal or other visceral vessels.

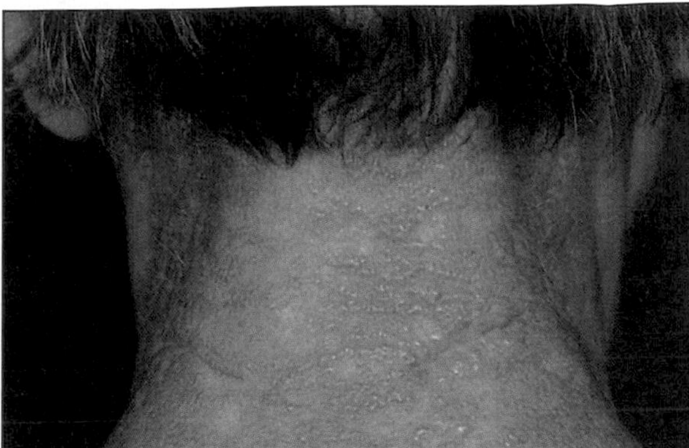

Fig. 43.3. Scleromyxedema

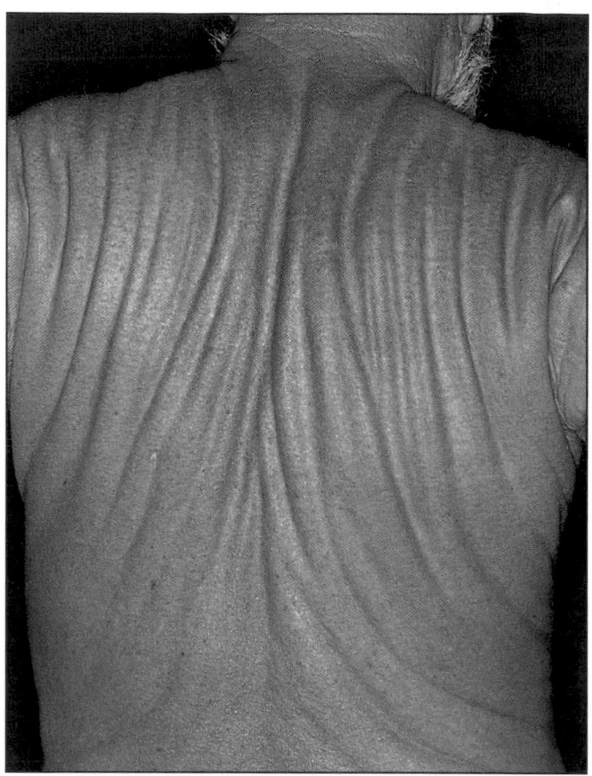

Fig. 43.4. Scleromyxedema

Course and Prognosis. The course is long but the outlook poor, as patients succumb to infections, cardiac or cerebral disease. In some instances, they may develop multiple myeloma.

Differential Diagnosis. The more diffuse changes evoke the entire differential diagnosis of systemic sclerosis (Chap. 18), but the associated presence of papules and the pronounced skin thickening on the nape and back should point one in the right direc-

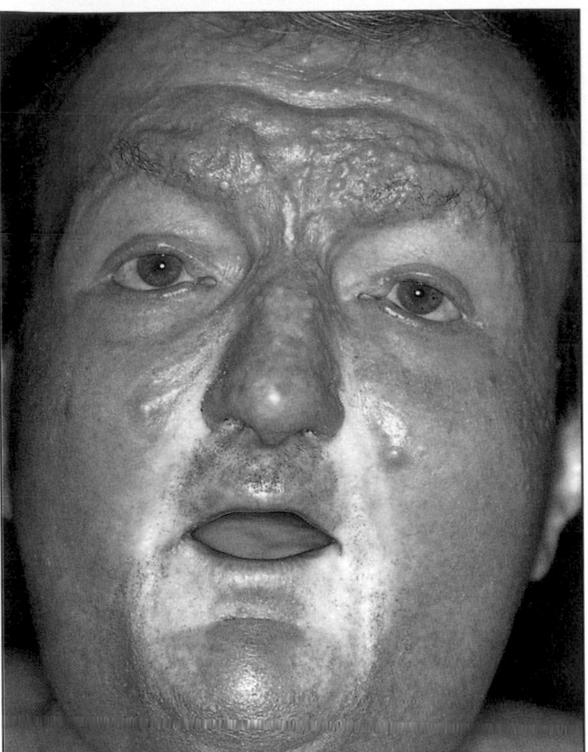

Fig. 43.5. Scleromyxedema

tion. Scleredema may appear similar, but has no papular or sclerotic changes and is often associated with diabetes mellitus.

Therapy

Systemic. Treatment is very difficult and there is no reliably effective approach. Systemic corticosteroids and antimetabolites are usually employed, just as in lichen myxedematosus. The usual choices are melphalan or cyclophosphamide. Retinoids and plasmapheresis have also been endorsed, as well as photopheresis. PUVA and PUVA bath therapy have also helped some patients.

Topical. Electron beam therapy has been recommended. Other external measures have little to offer.

Scleredema

(Buschke 1900)

Synonyms. Scleredema adultorum, scleredema of Buschke

Epidemiology. Scleredema shows two peaks; it is more common among children and younger women, and then again among older men. Thus the name adultorum does not fit well.

Etiology and Pathogenesis. There appear to be two causes or perhaps two diseases. Among children and young women, scleredema appears to be a postinfectious event, sometimes associated with a streptococcal infection, occasionally following viral infections and often with no triggering event. In adults, it is typically associated with diabetes mellitus. In these patients there may be abnormalities of the aldose reductase system just as in diabetic stiff hand syndrome.

Massive amounts of acid mucopolysaccharides are deposited in the dermis; the most typical materials are hyaluronic acid and less sulfated glycosaminoglycans. Rare associations with a monoclonal gammopathy and even multiple myeloma have been described, but this feature is far more common in scleromyxedema.

Clinical Findings. The typical finding is a diffuse, rather sudden hardening of the skin. In younger patients, the face is most often involved, along with the neck and the patient may complain of being squeezed or choked. There may be problems with eating and swallowing. In older individuals the trunk is usually first involved. The follicular openings tend to be prominent (orange peel skin) and the infiltration often causes a blanching. The skin is pale, tight, firm and one cannot pinch it into folds; it has been compared to a fully inflated rubber inner tube (Fig. 43.6). In both age groups there is relative sparing of the extremities, with no distal disease and no Raynaud phenomenon.

The list of associated systemic problems is long but there is no unifying pattern. The tongue, eso-

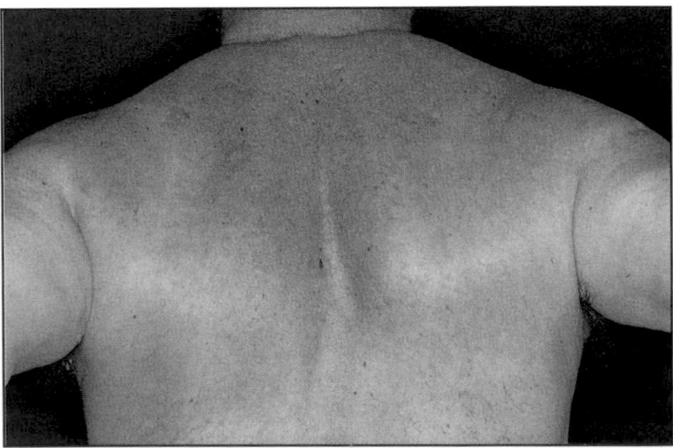

Fig. 43.6. Scleredema

phagus, pericardium, pleura, heart, skeletal muscle, liver and salivary glands have been involved, in addition to the possibility of a gammopathy.

Histopathology. The swollen and edematous collagen fibers in the dermis and subcutaneous tissues are pushed apart by increased amounts of acid mucopolysaccharides, especially hyaluronic acid. Therefore metachromatic mucin stains often reveal surprisingly little material. The elastic fibers are normal. There is often a sparse lymphocytic perivascular infiltrate that may feature plasma cells and mast cells.

Laboratory Findings. There are no specific laboratory tests; depending on the clinical signs of internal involvement, appropriate tests should be chosen.

Course and Prognosis. The postinfectious form usually resolves over 12–24 months. The diabetic form may improve when the disease is brought under better control. Sometimes the process persists for many years.

Differential Diagnosis. Initially one may think of early scleroderma or eosinophilic fasciitis, but the disease course and biopsy results soon point out the correct diagnosis. Scleromyxedema may also have papules and acral changes, as well as an associated gammopathy. Other forms of edema and mucin deposition can usually be easily excluded.

Therapy. If the infection has not been treated, then antibiotics are of course employed. Sometimes, high-dose intravenous penicillin therapy for 3–4 weeks is tried, just as in systemic sclerosis, even in the absence of a documented infection. Systemic corticosteroids have also been employed but are not dramatically successful. Both PUVA and in particular PUVA bath therapy seem most promising at this time.

Focal Mucinoses

A number of entirely unrelated rare disorders have been described, with nothing unifying them except the presence of mucin in the skin. Generically one can speak of cutaneous focal mucinosis when a group of papules or a solitary plaque is identified, mucin demonstrated under the microscope and no systemic disease found. On occasion, the location or age of the patient may lead to another term being used.

In all such cases, thyroid disease, diabetes mellitus, lupus erythematosus, and a gammopathy must be excluded before one can confidently speak of cutaneous mucinosis. Most often the diagnosis of cutaneous focal mucinosis suffices. Several diseases in this category appear clinically distinct. The two best examples are acral persistent papular mucinosis and reticulated erythematous mucinosis.

We do not use papular mucinosis as a synonym for lichen myxedematosus, although many groups do. It is not a single disease, but a collection of poorly understood entities. Patients present with one or many papules, nodules or plaques containing mucin. By definition, they do not have thyroid disease or a gammopathy. Some may have borreliosis or HIV/AIDS. In rare instances, there is an association with lupus erythematosus. These conditions can almost always be separated from lichen myxedematosus, except perhaps in the earliest days of the disease course.

Acral Persistent Papular Mucinosis

(Rongioletti et al. 1986)

This may be a variant of lichen myxedematosus, as associated gammopathies have on occasion been identified. Most patients, however, are adult women who are otherwise well. The disease is characterized by disseminated, soft skin-colored or red papules on the dorsal aspects of the hands and extensor surfaces of the forearms. Occasionally the equivalent locations on the feet may be affected. The course is generally chronic.

Reticular Erythematous Mucinosis

(Steigleder et al. 1974)

Synonyms. Mucinosis erythematosa reticularis, plaque-like mucinosis, midline mucinosis, REM syndrome (reticular erythematous mucinosis)

Definition. Erythematous disseminated infiltrate on the chest and back with deposition of mucin.

Epidemiology. Most patients are young or middle-aged women.

Etiology and Pathogenesis. The cause of REM syndrome is unknown. Light may play an etiologic role.

Clinical Findings. Typically there are almost flat, erythematous plaques either in the mid-chest or

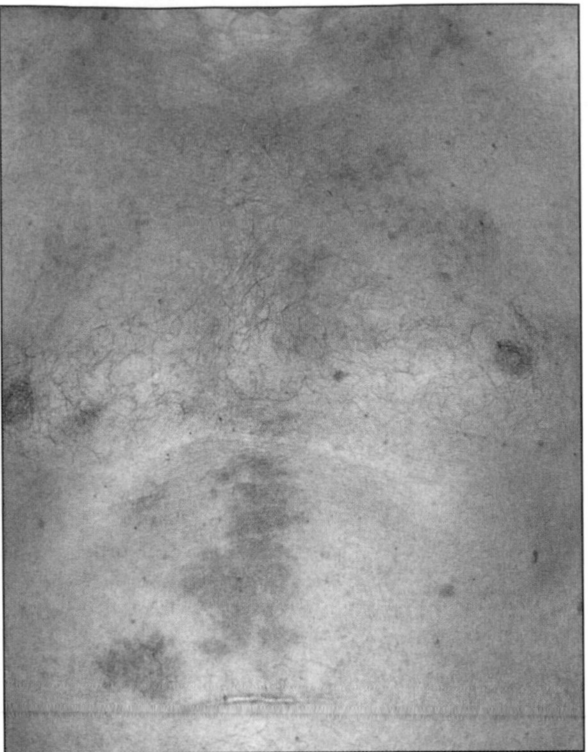

Fig. 43.7. Reticular erythematous mucinosis

mid-upper back (Fig. 43.7). They lack scale or other surface changes and are slightly palpable. The erythema may be reticulated or more irregular, but is always sharply separated from the normal skin. There is no atrophy. Occasionally the lesions are pruritic. Some lesions may be thicker and have scattered papules; these were described by PERRY (1960) as plaque-like cutaneous mucinosis.

Histopathology. The epidermis is either normal or may show minimal vacuolar change. In the reticular dermis are sparse mucin deposits associated with a lymphocytic perivascular infiltrate. These deposits are positive with Hale or alcian blue stain and PAS-negative. Periadnexal lymphocytic infiltrates are not seen. Immunofluorescent evaluation is negative.

Course and Prognosis. The REM syndrome often persists for months or years and then resolves. Rare cases have developed into lupus erythematosus.

Differential Diagnosis. At first glance, the lesions look like seborrheic dermatitis, but the scale is lacking. Serologic and direct immunofluorescent examination should be performed to exclude lupus erythematosus. In addition, the experimental production of lesions with UV radiation and then another biopsy may help to separate the two conditions.

Therapy. Some patients have responded to systemic antimalarial agents. The rarity of the disease and its tendency to spontaneous resolution make therapeutic recommendations troublesome. Often, topical corticosteroid creams suffice.

Rare Forms of Focal Mucinosis

Many other types of focal mucinosis have been described. They include:

Mucinosis of the Lip (NÖDL and ZAUN 1983). Local infiltration of the upper lip can produce erysipelas-like changes.

Self-Healing Juvenile Cutaneous Mucinosis (BONERANDI et al. 1980). Numerous flesh-colored papules, often in a linear pattern, are found on the face, trunk and especially the periarticular regions. The lesions are associated with arthralgias and resolve spontaneously. Some cases have been familial.

Infantile Cutaneous Mucinosis (LUM 1980). Tiny papules rich in mucin can be present at birth or appear in the first months of life. They are asymptomatic and fade away.

Mucinous Nevus (REDONDO-BELLÓN et al. 1993). This term overlaps with infantile cutaneous mucinosis. Some patients have been described with persistent papular lesions grouped in a linear fashion.

Plaque-Like Erythema with Milia (CARRINGTON et al. 1998). Described in immunosuppressed patients, especially those on cyclosporine, this disorder sounds like an overlap between REM syndrome and follicular mucinosis. On biopsy there is diffuse mucin deposition.

Epithelial Mucinoses

There are a limited number of disorders where the mucin accumulates within epithelial structures. While many other epithelia, such as those of the lungs and gastrointestinal tract, normally secrete mucins, the cutaneous structures do not. The most common histologic example of epithelial mucinosis is syringometaplasia. Eccrine sweat ducts show reticular degeneration and mucin deposition, presumably as a reactive change. Many such lesions have been acral verrucous papules, but others have lacked distinctive clinical features. Braun-Falco suggested the term mucophanerosis, phanerosis being defined as the setting free of substances that have been previously bound and invisible. In this case, normal cutaneous epithelial cells contain mucopolysaccharides which could be released. Others feel that the epithelial cells dedifferentiate and produce mucin.

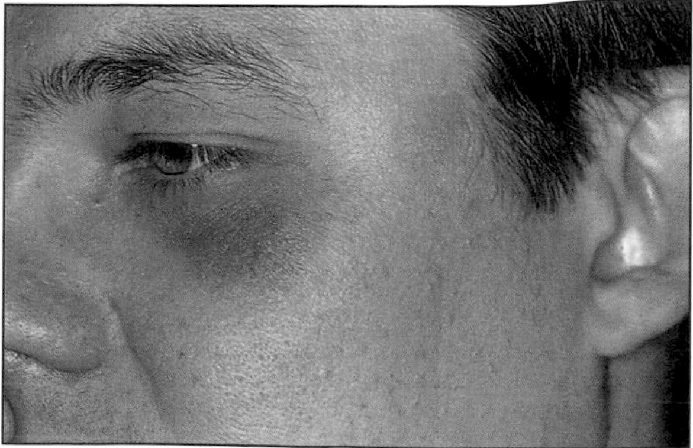

Fig. 43.8. Follicular mucinosis

Follicular Mucinosis

(Kreibich 1926)

Synonyms. Alopecia mucinosa (Pinkus 1957), mucophanerosis intrafollicularis et seboglandularis (Braun-Falco 1957), mucinosis follicularis (Jablonska et al. 1959)

Etiology and Pathogenesis. We view follicular mucinosis as a reaction pattern. A number of inflammatory dermatoses may occasionally show deposition of mucin in the outer root sheath, sebaceous glands and rarely the epidermis adjacent to the follicular ostia. In our experience, over 80 % of cases of follicular mucinosis are associated with a lymphocytic proliferation. Radiolabeled ^{35}S studies have failed to show the new synthesis of glycosaminoglycans, supporting the concept of mucophanerosis. Whether associated with a lymphoma or an inflammatory infiltrate, the mucin is a secondary change.

Clinical Findings. The clinical picture is frequently not characteristic, so the diagnosis is often made histologically. Usually one finds one or more, relatively sharply bordered, slightly elevated, edematous erythematous plaques (Fig. 43.8). Most often there is a fine adherent scale. The most frequent locations are the scalp, nape and shoulders but the balance of the trunk and occasionally the extremities may be involved. Sometimes multiple papular and nodular lesions are present, involving wider areas of the body. The follicular orifices may be prominent; sometimes they are filled with keratotic plugs (Fig. 43.9). When gentle pressure is applied from the sides, a stringy sticky material may ooze out of the openings. The hairs are usually lost; thus lesions in a region with terminal hair may present as alopecia mucinosa, while those in other areas may not be noticed as soon. More diffuse hair loss has also been described. The lesions may be pruritic.

Traditionally one has identified idiopathic and lymphoma-associated follicular mucinosis. Unfortunately, the two forms are not distinct and cannot be separated with certainty on clinical grounds. In general, when children and young adults are involved, the process is more likely to be reactive, while in older patients the chance of malignant lymphoma is higher. We have seen severe mycosis

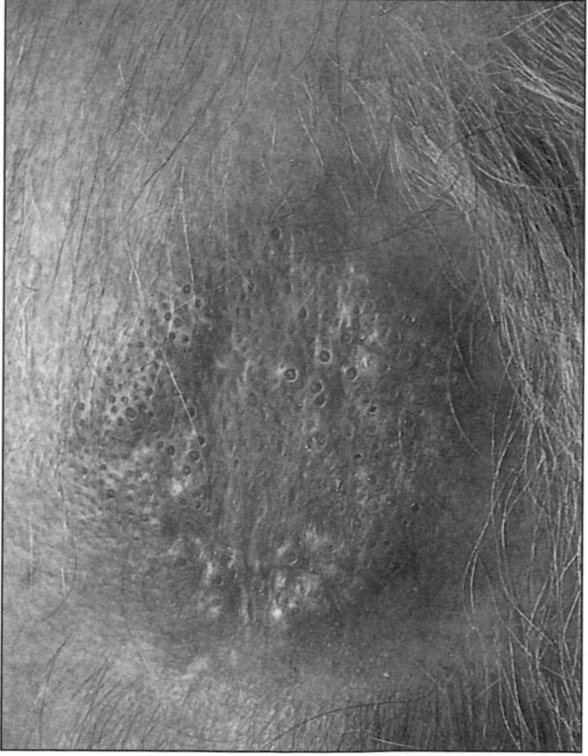

Fig. 43.9. Follicular mucinosis showing plugged follicles. This case was in a patient with mycosis fungoides

fungoides evolve out of follicular mucinosis in teenagers, so age should not be too reassuring and repeated biopsies are needed.

Sometimes the lesions heal after a period of weeks or months. No atrophy develops and the hairs regrow. In such a case, one can assume that the changes were reactive, perhaps associated with atopic dermatitis or another inflammatory dermatosis. If the lesions persist, develop into succulent plaques or subcutaneous nodules and slowly spread, then one must worry about a malignant lymphoma. The persistent lesions are most common on the shoulders. Some patients have widespread disease for years without developing any systemic problems.

Because so many cases do evolve into lymphoma, we view follicular mucinosis as a preneoplastic disorder. That is, if the lesions persist and there is no other explanation (severe dermatitis, lupus erythematosus elsewhere), one must follow the patient. The most common malignant lymphoma is mycosis fungoides although other T cell lymphomas, Hodgkin disease, angioimmunoblastic lymphadenopathy and other lymphoproliferative disorders have been found.

Histopathology. The typical sites of involvement are the outer root sheath of the hair follicle, and less often the sebaceous glands or epidermis. There is a lymphocytic infiltrate associated with reticular degeneration of the epithelium. Splits and cystic spaces appear, filled with mucin. The basophilic, often thread-like material is metachromatic, Hale-positive and PAS-negative. In the idiopathic form, eosinophils may be admixed with the lymphocytes. Sophisticated analysis of the infiltrative cells includes a search for clonal T cell receptor rearrangements, which may help to decide earlier in the disease course if a malignant lymphoma is present. Sometimes atypical lymphocytes, such as the cerebriform cells of mycosis fungoides can be found, but this is unusual.

Course and Prognosis. The prognosis is of course determined by whether or not a malignant lymphoma is present or will develop. The patient should be followed with repeated biopsies.

Differential Diagnosis. In hairy areas, one must think of tinea capitis, inflammatory alopecia areata, metastatic carcinoma (especially breast) and other causes of alopecia. Lichenified dermatitis on the scalp may also be without hair, but there should be more epidermal inflammation and scaling. In other parts of the body, the lesions are even less specific and harder to recognize.

Therapy. If a malignant lymphoma is identified, it must be treated in the standard fashion. If clinical signs of an associated disorder are present, then the follicular mucinosis should be treated just as the basic problem. If no clues are available, topical corticosteroids may be tried. Larger or thicker lesions respond poorly, so that intralesional or systemic corticosteroids may be needed. In the latter instance, we use prednisone 20 – 40 mg daily tapered gradually. Dapsone, PUVA, soft X-rays (3–4 × 1 Gy, delivered in weekly dosages) and interferon-α have also been tried.

Urticarial Follicular Mucinosis

(Crovato et al. 1985)

This rare disorder is difficult to categorize. Most patients have been middle-aged men who developed transient urticaria-like lesions of the head and neck areas. On biopsy, there was a lymphocytic infiltrate about follicles in which mucin could be visualized. The lesions resolved spontaneously and never showed chronic changes such as alopecia or follicular plugging. No association with lymphoma has been identified.

Secondary Mucinoses

Several of the secondary types of mucinosis deserve a brief mention. All are diagnosed histologically and have little direct clinical relevance. Many inflammatory dermatoses may secondarily show mucin deposition, especially in their chronic stages. In a routine dermatopathology practice, mucin is often identified without any clear explanation for its presence other than inflammation. Lupus erythematosus is associated with mucin in a number of ways. Some cases of papular mucinosis are associated with systemic lupus erythematosus; males are more often affected, and there may be vasculitis in the same lesions. Lupus profundus may present as a plaque or nodule that on biopsy exudes mucin and shows only dermal mucin on histologic examination. In addition, lupus erythematosus and REM syndrome can overlap. But most often mucin is detected microscopically in lesions of discoid and systemic lupus erythematosus where it is often a clue to the correct diagnosis, along with the other changes. Among infections, cryptococcosis is notorious for clinically forming lesions that may be stringy or gelatinous on biopsy. The mucinous capsule of *Cryptococcus neoformans* is probably responsible for this change. Degos disease frequently has dermal mucin deposits associated with necrosis; the exact nature of the ground substance changes is unclear.

A number of lesions often designed as mucinous tumors actually have more complex etiologies. A digital mucous cyst (Chap. 53) reflects the accumulation of mucin material resembling synovial fluid in the skin, usually about the nail fold. Many mesenchymal tumors contain mucin, as the neoplastic or altered fibroblasts secrete ground substance in abnormal amounts or of abnormal composition. In almost all cases, the primary tumor can still be recognized, whether it be a dermatofibroma, progressive nodular histiocytoma, acquired digital fibrokeratoma or any other fibrous tumor (Chap. 59). When a tumor has only mucinous deposits and scattered fibroblasts, it can be designated a myxoma but there are no criteria for separating myxomas from plaques of focal cutaneous mucinosis. In Carney syndrome (Chap. 65), the term cutaneous myxoma seems justified, as cardiac myxomas are also present. Cutaneous emboli from an atrial myxoma may also present as localized mucin deposits, although in such cases the mucin is very hard to find. Dermatologists may occasionally encounter an intramuscular myxoma as a soft tissue mass.

Secondary epithelial mucinosis also occurs. Many epithelial tumors may also contain mucins; once again the mechanism of phanerosis appears likely. Basal cell carcinomas with mucin deposition are not uncommon. The eccrine mucinous carcinoma has small islands of carcinoma cells admixed with lakes of mucin (Chap. 57). Metastatic adenocarcinomas may also have mucin. An oral mucocele arises when a salivary gland duct is interrupted or dilated (Chap. 33); thus it too contains epithelial mucin. Mucinous syringometaplasia is a reactive change in eccrine ducts in which mucin is present. While the list of diseases and processes where mucin has been reported is almost endless, these are the most important disorders.

Bibliography

Mucopolysaccharidoses

Finlayson LA (1990) Hunter syndrome (mucopolysaccharidosis II). Pediatr Dermatol 7:150–152

Hunter CA (1917) A rare disease in two brothers. Proc Roy Soc Med 10:104–116

Neufeld EF, Muenzer J (1995) The mucopolysaccharidoses. In: Scriver CR, Beaudet AV, Sly WS, Valle D (eds) The metabolic and molecular bases of herited disease, 7th edn. McGraw-Hill, New York, pp 2465–2494

Mucinoses

Rongioletti F, Rebora A (1991) The new cutaneous mucinoses: a review with an up-to-date classification of cutaneous mucinoses. J Am Acad Dermatol 24:265–270

Rongioletti F, Rebora A (1993) Les mucinoses cutanees. Ann Dermatol Venereol 120:75–87

Truhan AP, Roenigk HM (1986) The cutaneous mucinoses. J Am Acad Dermatol 14:1–18

Mucinoses Associated with Thyroid Disease

Braun-Falco O, Petzoldt D (1967) E.M.O.-Syndrom. Exophthalmus, Myxoedema circumscriptum praetibiale und Osteoarthropathia hypertrophicans (E.M.O.-Syndrom). Münch Med Wochenschr 79:1523–1529

Derrick EK, Tanner B, Price ML (1995) Successful surgical treatment of severe pretibial myxedema. Br J Dermatol 133:317–318

Diamond MT (1959) The syndrome of exopthalmus, hyperthrophic osteoarthropathy and localized myxedema: a review of the literature and report of a case. Ann Intern Med 50:206–213

Doyle L (1991) Myxoedema: some early reports and contributions by British authors, 1873–1898. J R Soc Med 84: 103–106

Fatourechi V, Pajouhi M, Fransway AF (1994) Dermatopathy of Graves' disease (pretibial myxedema). Review of 150 cases. Medicine 73:1–7

Heymann WR (1992) Cutaneous manifestations of thyroid disease. J Am Acad Dermatol 26:885–902

Ishizawa T, Sugiki H, Anzai S et al. (1998) Pretibial myxedema with Graves' disease: a case report and review of Japanese literature. J Dermatol 25:264–268

Kato N, Ueno H, Matsubara M (1991) A case report of EMO syndrome showing localized hyperhidrosis in pretibial myxedema. J Dermatol 18:598–604

Koshiyama H, Mori S, Fujiwara K et al. (1993) Successful treatment of hypothyroid Graves' disease with a combination of levothyroxine replacement, intravenous high-dose steroid and irradiation to the orbit. Intern Med 32: 421–423

Kiljnski J, Nebes V, Wall JR (1996) Significance of tissue specific and tissue non specific autoimmune reactions of Graves'disease. Clin Exp Rheumatol 14 [Suppl 15]:69–79

Lynch PJ, Maize JC, Sisson JC et al. (1973) Pretibial myxedema and nonthyreotoxic thyreoid disease. Arch Dermatol 129:1152–1156

Omohundro C, Dijkstra JWE, Camisa C et al. (1996) Early onset pretibial myxedema in the absence of opthalmopathy: a morphologic evolution. Cutis 58:211–214

Reuter MJ (1931) Histopathology of the skin in myxedema. Arch Dermatol Syph 24:55–71

Signore RJ, von Weiss J (1991) Alopecia of myxedema: clinical response to levothyroxine sodium. J Am Acad Dermatol 25:902–904

Somach SC, Helm TN, Lawlor KB et al. (1993) Pretibial mucin. Arch Dermatol 129:1152–1156

Thomas HM Jr. (1933) Acropachy. Secondary subperiosteal new bone formation. Arch Int Med 51:571–588

Wright AL, Buxton PK, Menzies D (1990) Pretibial myxedema localized to scar tissue. Int J Dermatol 29:54–55

Lichen Myxedematosus

Dominguez Aunon JD, Postigo-Llorente C, Llamas-Martin R et al. (1997) Lichen myxoedematosus associated with human immunodeficiency virus infection – report of two cases and review of the literature. Clin Exp Dermatol 22:265–268

Hardie RA, Hunter JAA, Urbaniak S et al. (1979) Spontaneous resolution of lichen myxedematosus. Br J Dermatol 100:727–730

Hill TG, Crawford JN, Rogers CC (1976) Successful management of lichen myxedematosus. Arch Dermatol 112: 67–69

Kaymen AH, Nasr A Grekin RC (1989) The use of carbon dioxide laser in lichen myxedematosus. J Dermatol Surg Oncol 15:862–865

Montgomery H, Underwood LJ (1953) Lichen myxedematosus (differentiation from cutaneous myxedemas of mucoid state). J Invest Dermatol 20:213–216

Tarantini G, Zerboni R, Muratori S et al. (1996) Lichen myxoedematosus in a patient with AIDS. Br J Dermatol 134:1122–1124

Wieder JM, Barton KL, Baron JM et al. (1993) Lichen myxedematosus treated with chlorambucil. J Dermatol Surg Oncol 19:475–476

Yamazaki S, Fujisawa T, Yanatori A et al. (1995) A case of lichen myxedematosus with clearly exacerbated skin eruptions after UVB irradiation. J Dermatol 22:590–593

Scleromyxedema

Braun-Falco O, Weidner I (1970) Skleromyxödem Arndt-Gottron mit Knochenmarks-Plasmocytose und Myositis. Arch Belg Dermatol (Suppl) 26:193–217

Dinneen AM, Dicken CH (1995) Scleromyxedema. J Am Acad Dermatol 33:37–43

Elliott MP, Dooley P (1998) Scleromyxedema (papular mucinosis). A surgical perspective. Ann Plast Surg 41:436–439

Farr PM, Ive FA (1984) PUVA treatment of scleromyxedema. Br J Dermatol 110:347–350

Godby A, Bergstresser PR, Chaker B et al. (1998) Fatal scleromyxedema: report of a case and review of the literature. J Am Acad Dermatol 38:289–294

Gottron HA (1954) Skleromyödem (Eine eigenartige Erscheinungsform von Myxthesaurodermie.) Arch Dermatol Syph 199:71–91

Harris RB, Perry HO, Kyle RA et al. (1979) Treatment of scleromyxedema with melphalan. Arch Dermatol 115: 295–X299

Hisler BM, Savoy LB, Hashimoto K (1991) Improvement of scleromyxedema associated with isotretinoin therapy. J Am Acad Dermatol 24:854–857

Keong CH, Asaka Y, Fukuro S et al. (1990) Successful treatment of scleromyxedema with plasmaphoresis and immunosuppression. J Am Acad Dermatol 22:824–844

Lowe NJ, Dufton PA, Hunter RD et al. (1982) Electrobeam treatment of scleromyxoedema. Br J Dermatol 106: 449–454

McFarlane AW, Davenport A, Verbov JL et al. (1987) Scleromyxedema-successful treatment with plasma exchange and immunosuppression. Br J Dermatol 117:653–657

Taschen JA, Chang JR (1999) Scleromyxedema: treatment with interferon alfa. J Am Acad Dermatol 40:303–307

Verma UN, Singh RR, Misra R et al. (1992) Scleromyxoedema with features of systemic sclerosis. Ann Rheum Dis 51:1159–1161

Webster GF, Matsuoka LY, Burchmore D (1993) The association of potentially lethal neurologic syndromes with scleromyxedema (papular mucinosis). J Am Acad Dermatol 28:105–108

Scleredema

Angeli Besson C, Koeppel MC, Jacquet P et al. (1994) Electron beam therapy in scleredema adultorum with associated monoclonal hypergammaglobulinaemia. Br J Dermatol 130:394–397

Basarab T, Burrows NP, Munn SE et al. (1997) Systemic involvement in scleredema of Buschke associated with IgG-kappa paraproteinaemia. Br J Dermatol 136:939–942

Buschke (1900) Verhandlungen der Berliner Dermatologischen Gesellschaft. Arch Dermatol Syph 53:383–386

Cole HG, Winkelmann RK (1990) Acid mucopolysaccharide staining in scleredema. J Cutan Pathol 17:211–213

Cron RQ, Swetter SM (1994) Scleredema revisited. A poststreptococcal complication. Clin Pediatr (Phila) 33:606–610

Hager CM, Sobhi HA, Hunzelmann N et al. (1998) Bath-PUVA therapy in three patients with scleredema adultorum. J Am Acad Dermatol 38:240–242

Hwang JH, Cho KH, Park KC et al. (1998) A case of congenital scleredema. Clin Exp Dermatol 139:139–140

Sansom JE, Sheehan Al, Kennedey CT et al. (1994) A fatal case of scleredema Buschke. Br J Dermatol 130:669–670

Seyger MM, van-den-Hoogen FH, de Mare S et al. (1999) A patient with a severe scleroedema diabeticorum, partially responding to low-dose methotrexate (letter). Dermatology 198:177–179

Young Woo R, Ki Beom S, Jeung Hoon L et al. (1998) A clinical observation of scleredema adultorum and its relationship to diabetes. J Dermatol 25:103–107

Papular Mucinosis

Coulson ICH, Malett RB, Holden CA (1992) Acral persistent papular mucinosis. Br J Dermatol 126:283–285

Flowers SL, Cooper PH, Landes HB (1989) Acral persistent papular mucinosis. J Am Acad Dermatol 21:293–397

Rongioletti F Rebora A (1992) Acral persistent papular mucinosis. Arch Dermatol 122:1237–1239

Yen A, Samchez RL, Raimer SS (1997) Papular mucinosis associated with AIDS: Response to isotretinoin. J Am Acad Dermatol 37:127–128

Reticular Erythematous Mucinosis

Braddock SW, Davis CS, Davis RB (1988) Reticular erythematous mucinosis and thrombocytopenic purpura, report of a case and review of the world literature, including plaque-like cutaneous mucinosis. J Am Acad Dermatol 19:859–868

Bulengo-Ransby SM, Ellis CN, Griffiths CEM et al. (1992) Failure of reticular erythematous mucinosis to respond to cyclosporine. J Am Acad Dermatol 27:825–828

Cohen PR, Rabinowitz AD, Ruszkowski AM et al. (1990) Reticular erythematous mucinosis Syndrome: review of the world literature and report of the syndrome in a prepubertal child. Pediatr Dermatol 7:1–10

Izumi T, Tajima S, Harada R et al. (1996) Reticular erythematous mucinosis syndrome: glycosaminoglycan synthesis by fibroblast and abnormal response to interleukin-1 beta. Dermatology 192:41–45

Perry HO, Kierland RR, MOntgomery H (1960) Plaque-like formation of cutaneous mucinosis. 82:980–985

Steigleder GK, Gartmann H, Linker U (1974) REM syndrome: reticular erythematous mucinosis (round-cell erythematosis), a new entity? Br J Dermatol 91:191–199

Velasco JA, Santos JC, Villabona V et al. (1992) Reticular erythematous mucinosis and acral papulokeratotic lesions associated with myxoedema due to Hashimoto thyroiditis. Dermatology 184:73–77

Rare Forms of Focal Mucinosis

Bonerandi JJ, Andrac L, Follana J et al. (1980) Self-healing juvenile cutaneous mucinosis. Clinical, histological and ultrastructural study. Ann Dermatol Venereol 107: 51–57

Carrington PR, Nelson-Adesokan P, Smoller BR (1998) Plaque-like erythema with milia: a noninfectious dermal mucinosis mimicking cryptococcal cellulitis in a renal transplant recipient. J Am Acad Dermatol 39:334–337

Crovato F, Nazzari G, Nunzi E et al. (1985) Urticaria-like follicular mucinosis. Dermatologica 170:133–135

Gonzalez-Enseat MA, Vicente MA, Castella N et al. (1997) Self-healing infantile familial cutaneous mucinosis. Pediatr Dermatol 14:460–462

Lum D (1983) Cutaneous mucinosis of infancy. Arch Dermatol 116:198–200

Nödl F, Zaun H (1983) Euthyreote zirkumskripte symmetrische Myxodermie der Oberlippe. Hautarzt 34:27–30

Redondo Bellón P, Vázquez-Doval J, Idoate M et al. (1993) Mucinous nevus. J Am Acad Dermatol 28:797–798

Velho GC, Oliveira M, Alves R et al. (1998) Childhood cutaneous mucinosis. J Eur Acad Dermatol Venereol 10: 164–166

Follicular Mucinosis

Abajo P, Martin R, Dauden E (1998) Follicular mucinosis associated with cutaneous leishmaniasis (letter). Acta Derm Venereol (Stockh) 78:315

Braun-Falco O (1957) Mucophanerosis intrafollicularis et seboglandularis. Dermatol Wochenschr 136:1289–1303

Emmerson RW (1969) Follicular mucinosis. A study of 47 patients. Br J Dermatol 81:395–413

Guerriero C, De Simone C, Guidi B et al. (1999) Follicular mucinosis successfully treated with isotretinoin. Eur J Dermatol 9:22–24

Jablonska S, Chorzelski T, Lanucki J (1959) Mucinosis follicularis. Hautarzt 10:27–33

Jackow CM, Papadopulos E, Nelson B et al. (1997) Follicular mucinosis associated with scarring alopecia, oligonal T cell receptor V beta expansion, and Staphylococcus aureus: when does follicular mucinosis become mycosis fungoides? J Am Acad Dermatol 37:828–831

Kreibich C (1926) Mucin bei Hauterkrankung. Arch Dermatol Syph 150:243–248

Mehregan DA, Gibson LE, Muller SA (1991) Follicular mucinosis: histopathologic review of 33 cases. Mayo Clin Proc 66:387–390

Pinkus H (1957) Alopecia mucinosa. Arch Dermatol 76: 419–426

Meissner K, Weyer U, Kowalzick L et al. (1991) Successful treatment of primary progressive follicular mucinosis with interferons. J Am Acad Dermatol 24:848–850

Sumner WT, Grichnik JM, Shea CR et al. (1998) Follicular mucinosis as a presenting sign of acute myeloblastic leukemia. J Am Acad Dermatol 38:803–805

Walchner M, Messer G, Rust A et al. (1998) Follicular mucinosis in association with squamous cell carcinoma of the tongue. J Am Acad Dermatol 38:622–624

Wittenberg GP, Gibson LE, Pittelkow MR et al. (1998) Follicular mucinosis presenting as an acneiform eruption: report of four cases. J Am Acad Dermatol 38:849–851

Secondary Mucinosis

Kaufmann R, Greiner D, Schmidt P et al. (1998) Dermatomyositis presenting as plaque - like mucinosis. Br J Dermatol 138:889–892

Maruyama M, Miyauchi S, Hashimoto K (1997) Massive cutaneous mucinosis associated with systemic lupus erythematosus. Br J Dermatol 137:450–453

Rongioletti F, Ghigliotti G, De Marchi R et al. (1998) Cutaneous mucinoses and HIV infection. Br J Dermatol 139:1077–1080

CHAPTER 44

The Porphyrias

Contents

Basic Science Aspects

There are two tetrapyrroles of extraordinary biologic importance. One is chlorophyll which is responsible for photosynthesis in plants and thus is crucial for life on earth. In animals, the porphyrin derivative heme is required for the transport and metabolism of oxygen. The porphyrias are uncommon. They are primarily hereditary disturbances in the synthesis of heme, involving well-defined enzymatic defects. Figure 44.1 shows the process of heme synthesis involving multiple intermediates and at least eight enzymes. Defects in each of these enzymes can lead to a clinical disease. Thus porphyrin metabolism provides a fascinating interplay which has interested biochemists, hematologists, geneticists and dermatologists.

Heme Synthesis

The biosynthesis of porphyrin occurs both in mitochondria and in the cytoplasm. The first step, the synthesis of δ-aminolevulinic acid from glycine and succinyl coenzyme A (CoA) occurs in the mitochondria. Then in the cytoplasm two molecules of δ-aminolevulinic acid are combined to make a monopyrrole ring, porphobilinogen. Then four porphobilinogen molecules are combined to make a tetrapyrrole, hydroxymethylbilane. Here the pathway splits. Uroporphyrinogen-III cosynthetase (also known as isomerase) locks the ring to make uroporphyrinogen III, while in the absence of the enzyme, uroporphyrinogen I is formed. Both of the uroporphyrinogens are then converted to their respective coproporphyrinogens by the oxidative decarboxylation of acetate groups to methyl groups. Only coproporphyrinogen III participates further, being oxidized to protoporphyrinogen IX which is returned to the cytoplasm. It is then oxidized to protoporphyrin IX. In the final step, iron is added to make heme.

Biochemical Attributes

A most interesting aspect of the porphyrias is that they are enzyme defects but almost all are inherited in an autosomal dominant pattern. This means that when only 50% of the enzyme is missing, clinical problems can arise, showing the importance and intricacy of heme synthesis. In addition, although the enzyme defect is genetic and permanent, the symptoms are often intermittent and often do not appear until after puberty. This is particularly true in porphyria cutanea tarda, acute intermittent porphyria and variegate porphyria. The explanation here is found in δ-aminolevulinic acid synthetase, the rate-limiting enzyme which is inhibited by heme in a feedback loop. Hepatic δ-aminolevulinic acid synthetase is highly inducible. The main factors can be viewed as the four Ms: *m*edications, *m*enses, *m*alnutrition (both starvation and extreme diets) and *m*edical illness. As δ-aminolevulinic acid synthetase is induced, then the system is flooded with precursors and enzyme inadequacies become more apparent. In addition, if heme is bound or lost, the feedback loop is less effective and derepression of δ-aminolevulinic acid synthetase occurs.

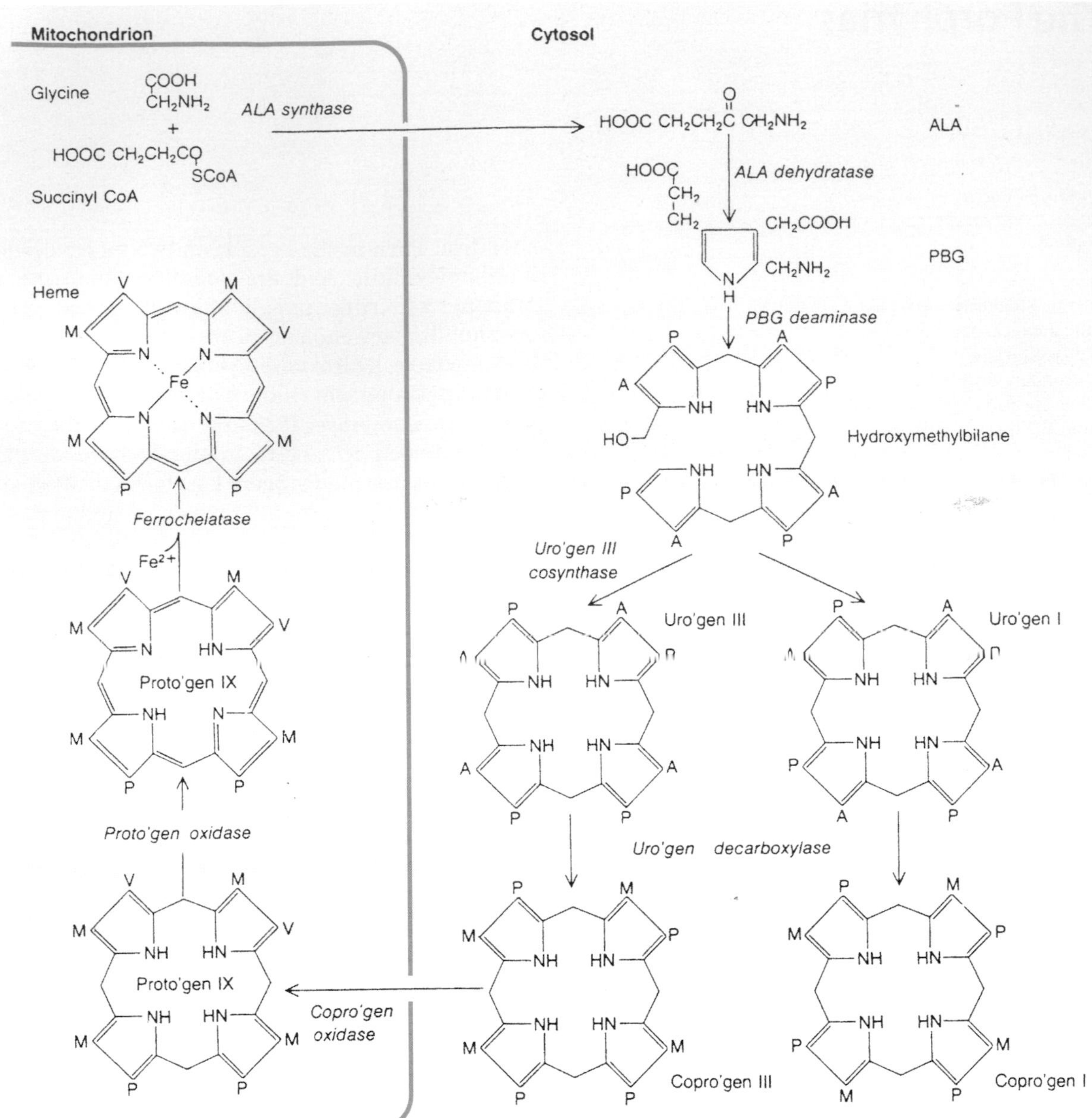

Fig. 44.1. Porphyrin biosynthesis

Another important structure is cytochrome P450 as about 40% of the hepatic heme is incorporated into this enzyme. Medications which are metabolized by cytochrome P450 tend to induce this enzyme, increasing its production, reducing heme and reducing the inhibition of δ-aminolevulinic acid synthetase. This longer process seems to be more important in porphyria cutanea tarda, as toxins including alcohol, metals, hexachlorobenzene and many other materials are metabolized in the liver. Hepatitis C virus also plays a role, especially in AIDS patients. Finally, increased iron loads predispose to porphyrias.

The porphyrins have many other interesting characteristics. All the porphyrinogens are spontaneously oxidized to their respective porphyrins. Their solubility changes as they are metabolized. Coproporphyrin and protoporphyrin are much less soluble and are found in the stool, while δ-aminolevulinic acid, porphobilinogen and uroporphyrin are excreted in the urine. In addition, the porphyrins show a red fluorescence when exposed to UV radiation in the Soret band (400–410 nm). This is useful in their diagnosis as urinary porphyrins can be identified by fluorescence as a screening test. In addition, patients with some severe forms of porphyria may develop fluorescence of bones and other tissues. When enough energy is absorbed by the erythrocytes, photohemolysis occurs and the oxidized porphyrins are released. The most phototoxic of them is protoporphyrin, responsible for the extreme photosensitivity of many patients. Protoporphyrin acts in tissues to create free radicals and singlet oxygen which damage a variety of structures. Because of the peak activation at 400 nm, sunscreens must protect against UVA and the lower ranges of visible light to be helpful in photosensitivity associated with porphyria.

Classification

A simplified classification of the porphyrias is shown in Table 44.1. Traditionally, the porphyrias have been divided into erythropoietic and hepatic. Reticulocytes are capable of responding to blood loss, hypoxia and erythropoietin secretion by turning on their metabolism. The peripheral erythrocytes are no longer responsive. Only one disorder is purely erythropoietic, congenital erythropoietic porphyria, and it is an autosomal recessive variant, suggesting that all the reticulocytes have to be missing the needed enzyme for an influence to be seen. In erythropoietic protoporphyria (also known as erythrohepatic porphyria), both red cell and hepatic defects are identified, while in the other porphyrias, the main problem

Table 44.1. The porphyrias: the defects are listed in the order of the appearance of the enzymes during heme synthesis.

Disease	Inheritance	Gene location	Enzyme	Type	Photosensitivity	Acute symptoms
Congenital sideroblastic anemia	XLR		δ-Aminolevulinic acid synthetase	No porphyria; defect appears before cyclic structures present	No	No
Doss porphyria	AR		δ-Aminolevulinic acid dehydratase (porphobilinogen synthetase)	Hepatic	No	Yes
Acute intermittent porphyria	AD	11q24	Hydroxymethylbilane synthetase (porphobilinogen deaminase, uroporphyrinogen I synthetase)	Hepatic	No	Yes
Congenital erythropoietic porphyria (Günther)	AR	10q25	Uroporphyrinogen III cosynthetase	Erythropoietic	Yes	No
Porphyria cutanea tarda	AD	1p34	Uroporphyrinogen decarboxylase	Hepatic	Yes	No
Hepatoerythropoietic porphyria	AD	1p34	Uroporphyrinogen decarboxylase (homozygous)	Hepatic	Yes	No
Hereditary coproporphyria	AD		Coproporphyrinogen oxidase	Hepatic	Yes	Yes
Variegate porphyria	AD	1q23	Protoporphyrinogen oxidase	Hepatic	Yes	Yes
Erythropoietic protoporphyria	AD	18q21	Ferrochelatase	Erythrohepatic	Yes	No

is in the liver. The porphyrias have long been classified by clinicians as acute or chronic. Acute porphyrias are associated with sudden attacks of abdominal pain and neuropsychiatric symptoms, often with known triggers; they are also hepatic.

Secondary Porphyrias

There are also secondary porphyrias. The best known one is acute lead poisoning, in which δ-aminolevulinic acid dehydratase is blocked and massive amounts of δ-aminolevulinic acid are excreted in the urine leading to symptoms of acute intermittent porphyria, along with a profound anemia. Chronic liver disease and hemolysis, as well as some tumors, are associated with increased urinary coproporphyrin excretion, but clinical symptoms are rare and the levels are comparable to those of porphyria patients in between attacks. Patients with chronic renal disease undergoing dialysis also develop porphyria cutanea tarda like changes. Apparently some highly carboxylated porphyrins, mainly uroporphyrin, accumulate in the serum as the dialysis does not remove them as efficiently as the kidney. Identifying these uncommon porphyrins requires a highly specialized laboratory.

Identification of Porphyrins

There are a number of ways to diagnose the porphyrias. The individual laboratory findings are discussed under each disease and summarized in Table 44.2. The three best known tests are the least useful:

- Wood light examination of urine: Many of the porphyrins fluoresce, so this is very nonspecific and if levels are too low, may also give a false-negative result.
- Urine color: While δ-aminolevulinic acid is colorless, porphobilinogen is converted non-enzymatically to a dark-brown pigment, porphobilin, which imparts a port-wine stain color to urine during acute attacks of acute intermittent porphyria. The conversion normally takes place in the bladder but also occurs if the urine is allowed to stand, especially if exposed to light.
- Watson-Schwartz test: This chromogen test using Ehrlich's reagent can be used to screen the urine

Table 44.2. Laboratory diagnosis of the porphyrias

Disease	Urine				Feces			RBC		
	ALA	PBG	Uro	Copro	Uro	Copro	Proto	Uro	Copro	Proto
Doss porphyria	+++	+/–	++	+++						++
Acute intermittent porphyria	+++ (++)	+++ (++)	++	++ (+)	++	+				
Congenital erythropoietic porphyria (GÜNTHER 1912)			+++	+++	++	+++	+	+++	++	++
Porphyria cutanea tarda			+++	+	++	++	+			
Hepatoerythropoietic porphyria			+++	+	++	++				++
Hereditary coproporphyria	+++ (+)	+++ (+)	++	+++ (+)	+	++++ (+++)	+			
Variegate porphyria	+++ (+)	+++ (+)	++	+++ (+)	+	++ (+)	+++			
Erythropoietic protoporphyria						+/–	+++		+	++++

ALA, δ-aminolevulinic acid; PBG, porphobilinogen. Values in parentheses are values during remission. Based on table in FERNANDES et al. (1995) p 334 for porphobilinogen. The Hoesch test is similar. Neither is reliable enough to be used alone without confirmatory testing.

The best established diagnostic approaches today include:

- Urine: δ-Aminolevulinic acid and porphobilinogen are measured using ion-exchange resins and chromatographic photometric measuring techniques (Doss-Schmidt method). The total urine porphyrins can also be measured in this way, while high-pressure liquid chromatography is needed to identify the various molecules, as developed by SEUBERT and SEUBERT (1986).
- Erythrocytes: Erythrocyte fluorescence can help identify erythropoietic protoporphyria and congenital erythropoietic porphyria. Porphobilinogen deaminase can be measured in erythrocytes. High-pressure liquid chromatography is needed to separate the various porphyrin products in the urine.
- Feces: In this source only high-pressure liquid chromatography has proven effective.

Clinical Aspects

In the following pages, each of the disorders will be considered as an individual entity. We will use the same sequence as in Table 44.1 following the steps involved in heme production. The locations of the involved genes are also shown in Table 44.1 and not in the text.

X-Linked Sideroblastic Anemia

Defective Enzyme. δ-aminolevulinic acid synthetase

These patients do not have any of the features of porphyria. The disorder is inherited in an X-linked recessive pattern. The affected men have a refractory hemolytic anemia, apparent early in life. Iron overload is common, as they are unable to incorporate the mineral. Thus hypersplenism and hemosiderosis develop. They have a hyperchromic microcytic anemia. Pyridoxine is an essential cofactor for δ-aminolevulinic acid synthetase and some patients may respond to large dosages of the vitamin. If not, then repeated transfusions and iron chelation are the best approaches.

Doss Porphyria

(Doss et al. 1980)

Synonym. Lead porphyria

Defective Enzyme. δ-aminolevulinic acid dehydratase (porphobilinogen synthetase)

This is a very rare form of porphyria – fewer than ten cases have been reported. It is inherited in an autosomal recessive pattern. Once again there are no cutaneous problems, only gastrointestinal and neurologic symptoms. The diagnosis is based on elevated δ-aminolevulinic acid in the urine, associated with elevated urinary and fecal porphyrins.

Acute Intermittent Porphyria

(WALDENSTRÖM 1937)

Synonym. Swedish porphyria

Defective Enzyme. Hydroxymethylbilane synthetase (porphobilinogen deaminase, uroporphyrinogen I synthetase)

History. Acute intermittent porphyria has played an interesting role in history. It seems clear that the House of Hanover, British monarchs reigning in the 1700s, had some form of hepatic porphyria. There are references to acute abdominal attacks, neuropsychiatric symptoms, especially in George III, and dark urine. A cottage industry has developed among medical historians around the argument as to whether the illness was acute intermittent porphyria, variegate porphyria or another mysterious porphyria. Since skin findings do not feature in most descriptions, acute intermittent porphyria seems most likely.

Epidemiology. Acute intermittent porphyria is one of the most common porphyrias. In most countries, including Germany and the USA, it is the second most common after porphyria cutanea tarda. Even though it is inherited in an autosomal dominant pattern, there is a female predominance: almost two-thirds of patients and three-fourths of those with acute attacks are women. The first signs of the disease usually appear during young adult life, between 20 and 40 years of age. When populations are screened, as in Lapland where the incidence is about 1:1000, it become clear that up to 40% of people with the aberrant gene are latent carriers never having any problems.

Table 44.3. Drugs and the hepatic porphyrias[a]

Sedatives	Barbiturates, glutethimide, carbromal
Antiinflammatory agents	Phenylbutazone and pyrazolone derivatives
Anesthetic agents	Halothane, ketamine, pentazocine, many others
Psychotropic agents	Diazepam, meprobamate, imipramine, micethamide, many others
Anticonvulsants	Phenytoin, trimethadione
Steroids	Estrogens, oral contraceptives, danazol
Antibiotics	Sulfonamides, chloramphenicol, griseofulvin
Antidiabetic agents	Tolbutamide, chloropropamide
Others	Ergotamine, methyldopa, theophylline

[a] The medications are likely to precipitate acute attacks in acute intermittent porphyria, variegate porphyria and hereditary coproporphyria. Anesthetic agents, barbiturates and sulfonamides (and related amides) are probably the most dangerous.

Etiology and Pathogenesis. The enzyme defect is well known, but the rest of the pathogenesis is more complicated. A number of different mutations have been identified. Although the enzyme defect can be shown in all cells, the problems arise primarily in the liver. The defect alone is not sufficient to cause problems. A long list of trigger factors are known, and in over half of the cases medications are responsible. The reactions to medications can be immediate, dramatic and even fatal. We offer a selected list (Table 44.3), emphasizing that many other drugs may trigger the hepatic porphyrias and that one should use all medications with caution in this group. As is discussed under porphyria cutanea tarda, medication reactions in that disorder involve a slightly different list, are much less common and are never acute. Although they are rarely triggers, steroid hormones seem of particular importance, perhaps explaining why women are more likely to be symptomatic. δ-Aminolevulinic acid and other porphyrin precursors interact with the peripheral benzodiazepine receptors, helping to explain the neuropsychiatric symptoms.

Clinical Findings. There are no cutaneous findings. The patients are not photosensitive and their internal symptoms are not provoked by sunlight exposure. On occasion, hyperhidrosis may occur during acute attacks, as a sign of autonomic dysfunction. A wide variety of other organ systems may be involved in an acute attack. The most common physical findings are red urine, abdominal tenderness, tachycardia and hypertension.

- Abdominal Symptoms. The most common symptoms of an acute attack are abdominal pain and tenderness. Constipation, nausea and vomiting are also common. Usually the pain is colicky and may be misdiagnosed as acute appendicitis, biliary colic or pancreatitis. This produces a vicious circle since anesthetics are notorious triggers and an operation can have fatal consequences. About 75% of patients with an acute attack will have darkened urine.
- Cardiovascular Symptoms. Hypertension and tachycardia are each present in about half the patients.
- Neurologic Symptoms. Peripheral neuropathies are most common, and some can be life-threatening including paralysis of the respiratory muscles, laryngeal muscles and cranial nerves. About half of acute attacks involve some muscle paralysis. In other cases, distal paresthesias are all that occurs. In addition, a similar proportion of patients have psychiatric symptoms ranging from behavioral changes and depression to frankly psychotic behavior.
- Other Problems. Urinary retention may occur, as well as pains in other parts of the body than the abdomen. Amenorrhea and nipple discharge also are found.
- Hepatic Problems. Despite being the site of the action, the liver is not damaged. Liver function tests are not abnormal.

Laboratory Findings

Acute Attacks

- Urine: The urine is usually dark and fluoresces. Watson-Schwartz or Hoesch test is positive. The urine δ-aminolevulinic acid and porphobilinogen levels are markedly elevated, as are the uroporphyrin and coproporphyrin levels.

- Feces: Fecal porphyrins may be minimally elevated but they play no diagnostic role.
- Erythrocytes: No fluorescence. Hydroxymethylbilane synthetase deficiency can be identified.
- Serum: Normal porphyrin values but electrolyte disturbances are common.

Latent Period. Erythrocyte hydroxymethylbilane synthetase levels are the most reliable way to confirm the diagnosis between attacks and to screen family members. If the enzyme level is $<50\%$ of normal, the diagnosis is certain. Urine δ-aminolevulinic acid and porphobilinogen as well as fecal coproporphyrins may be elevated, but may also be in the normal range.

Prognosis. In an acute attack, the biggest risk is inappropriate anesthesia. Respiratory paralysis is fatal in about 50 % of cases. Otherwise, the outlook is good if triggering factors can be avoided. The major points are to carefully counsel the patient about dangerous medications, suggest safe alternatives, be sure she carries a Medi-Alert bracelet or tag to warn anesthesiologists, and screen first-degree relatives so they too can avoid triggering factors.

Differential Diagnosis. The main differential diagnosis is the other porphyrias. Lead poisoning is similar but erythrocyte δ-aminolevulinic acid synthetase is reduced and serum lead levels elevated. The manifestations of acute intermittent porphyria are so diverse than almost any diagnosis can be considered. Many patients are misdiagnosed as neuropsychiatric patients with functional bowel problems.

Therapy. Once again, the best approach is intelligent supportive care using safe medications. For example, opiates should be used for pain and phenothiazines for nausea. Intravenous fluids should be rich in glucose (400–500 g/day) as glucose inhibits δ-aminolevulinic acid synthetase and may short circuit the cycle. Beta-blockers may help with the tachycardia and hypertension. Respiratory assistance and parenteral nutrition may be required.

An interesting therapy is the use of hematin, the iron form of heme. Hematin is a powerful suppressor of hepatic δ-aminolevulinic acid synthetase. About 250–500 mg daily of hematin can be infused for 4–7 days. Sometimes this helps prevent the onset of respiratory paralysis. Both local thrombophlebitis at the infusion site and a coagulopathy, perhaps involving factor XII, are associated with hematin use.

Preventive therapy, other than avoidance, is hardly available. Oral contraceptives may fall into this category. While they can raise δ-aminolevulinic acid and porphobilinogen levels and trigger attacks, they usually do not, and their role in preventing menses may outweigh the other risk. Hematin has also been used prophylactically.

Congenital Erythropoietic Porphyria

(Günther 1911)

Synonyms. Günther disease, congenital porphyria

Defective Enzyme. Uroporphyrinogen III cosynthetase (isomerase)

Epidemiology. This extremely rare disease has attracted more than its share of attention because it is so dramatic. The mythical werewolves may well have been patients with congenital erythropoietic porphyria. The combination of only night-time activity, extreme hypertrichosis, fluorescent teeth and mutilating skin lesions is suggestive. It is inherited in an autosomal recessive pattern.

Etiology and Pathogenesis. Although the defect is present in all cells, congenital erythropoietic porphyria predominantly involves erythrocytes. The lack of uroporphyrinogen cosynthetase throws the entire pathway into the I-isomer series, leading to massive accumulations of uro-, copro- and protoporphyrins in the erythrocytes, urine and feces.

Clinical Findings

Cutaneous Findings. The hallmark is extreme photosensitivity in infancy. Along with xeroderma pigmentosum, these patients show light intolerance during the first summer of their life. The reaction is a phototoxic one, similar to a burn. They are sensitive to both visible light and UVA radiation, so the reaction occurs through window glass, as when riding in an automobile. Another early sign is the red urine staining the diapers.

Even minimal light exposure leads to pruritus, burning and pain in the exposed areas. A sunburn develops with prominent blisters which rapidly ulcerate and heal with scarring. After a series of such burns, mutilating changes frequently appear, resembling an unfortunate third-degree burn pa-

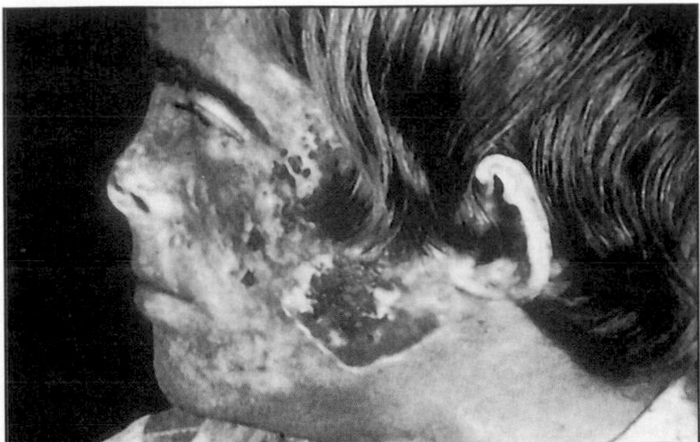

Fig. 44.2. Congenital erythropoietic porphyria with marked mutilation

tient. The nose loses its tip and scars down, as do the ears. In addition there is marked hyper- and hypopigmentation. The scarred skin is a facultative precancerous condition. Such patients may develop multiple squamous cell carcinomas and basal cell carcinomas, as well as malignant melanoma, if they live long enough. The nonexposed skin is normal. Another finding is marked hypertrichosis which is not limited to the light-damaged areas (Fig. 44.2).

Systemic Findings. The erythrodontia or fluorescent teeth are a most reliable but extraordinary finding; bones are similarly effected (Fig. 44.3). The orbital region is also scarred, producing ectropion, as well as ocular inflammation in the form of keratoconjunctivitis. The most troublesome systemic finding is the marked hemolysis which leads to anemia, hypersplenism and hepatosplenomegaly. There may be bone marrow hyperplasia of the erythrocyte series displacing leukocyte and platelet precursors.

Histopathology. The acute phototoxic reaction is not unique. The epidermis is damaged and there is minimal dermal inflammation. In skin which has already been damaged, dermal scarring occurs associated with amorphous hyaline deposits about the vessels and in the papillary dermis. Sometimes a subepidermal blister may be seen. The mechanisms of blistering are discussed under porphyria cutanea tarda.

Laboratory Findings

- Urine: The urine is dark and always fluoresces (Fig. 44.4). δ-Aminolevulinic acid and porphobilinogen are normal, but the other porphyrins (uro-, copro-, protoporphyrin) are as much as 100-fold elevated, with I-isomers dominating.
- Feces: The same changes are seen, but the less-soluble copro- and protoporphyrins dominate.
- Erythrocytes: The erythrocytes fluoresce; they are called fluorocytes. Blood can be dried on a filter paper, protected from ambient light and sent to a specialized laboratory where the fluorescence can be assessed. The erythrocyte precursors in the bone marrow fluoresce even better. Once again, copro- and protoporphyrins are most common but a wide variety can be identified by high-pressure liquid chromatography.

Prognosis. The prognosis is grim. At the very best, the patient must spend their entire life in the dark or under specially filtered lights. Only rich, intelligent parents can provide these conditions. The average patient, if such an individual exists, gets enough light to develop hideous scarring, eventual cutaneous malignancies, hepatosplenomegaly and hematologic problems.

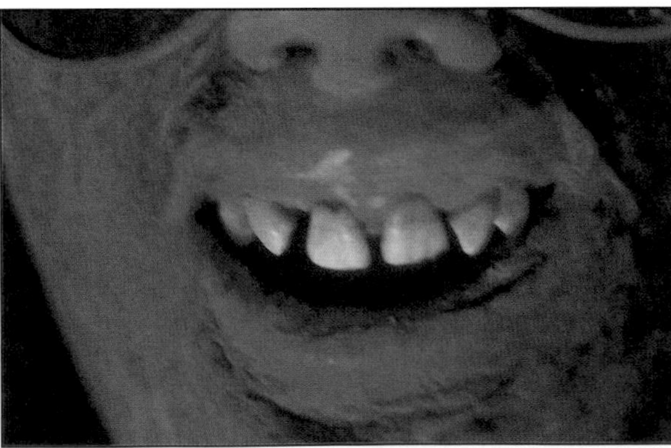

Fig. 44.3. Fluorescent teeth in congenital erythropoietic porphyria

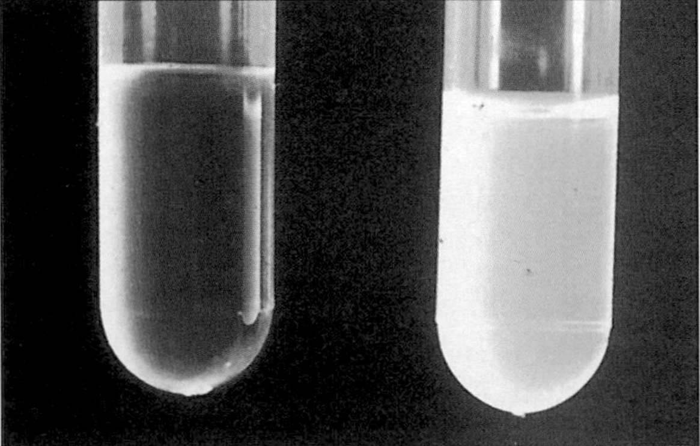

Fig. 44.4. Fluorescent urine from congenital erythropoietic porphyria patient on the left; normal urine is on the right and appears blue under UV radiation

Differential Diagnosis. In infants with extreme photosensitivity, one must also consider xeroderma pigmentosum. Extremely severe hepatoerythropoietic porphyria may appear similar. The Turkish porphyria caused by hexachlorobenzene also causes mutilating skin changes.

Therapy. Total light avoidance is required; no sunscreen protects these patients. Oral β-carotene has been suggested but is ineffective, in contrast to erythropoietic protoporphyria where it is useful. Transfusions are usually needed. The role of splenectomy is debated. Hematin infusions can also help. Charcoal and cholestyramine may absorb porphyrins from the gut, reducing the load. Liver transplantation has been employed in some cases, but its merits are hard to assess.

Porphyria Cutanea Tarda

(GÜNTHER 1922; WALDENSTRÖM 1937; IPPEN 1959)

Defective Enzyme. Uroporphyrinogen decarboxylase

Epidemiology. Porphyria cutanea tarda is the most common porphyria. In a typical dermatology clinic, it comprises 80–90% of the porphyria patients, if not more. The incidence has been estimated at 1:25,000. The epidemiology is less clear than in the other porphyrias, because more than a single enzyme defect is involved. There are both inherited and acquired forms of porphyria cutanea tarda. In the rare inherited form, the male/female ratio is 1:1, but in the acquired form, men are far more often affected, perhaps reflecting the higher rate of male alcoholism in the past. Over the past three decades, this ratio has also started to approach 1:1 as women have been exposed to more estrogens and also perhaps increased their alcohol intake.

Etiology and Pathogenesis. Hereditary porphyria cutanea tarda involves a mutation of the uroporphyrinogen decarboxylase gene. The disease is inherited in an autosomal dominant pattern. The enzyme levels are reduced to about 50% of normal in all tissues. In the acquired form, the hepatic enzyme activity is reduced by 50%, although the structural protein is present. In extrahepatic locations, both the structure and function are normal. The familial cases tend to have a somewhat earlier onset in the first two decades, while acquired cases typically appear after age 30 years. In all, about 20% of patients have a positive family history of porphyria cutanea tarda.

In both forms, usually a triggering agent is present. The most common ones are alcohol abuse (60%), estrogens (25%) and liver disease (20%). Medications and hepatomas each account for some cases while in about 10% of patients, no cause is identified. In recent years hepatitis C has been found in a fair number of patients with porphyria cutanea tarda, especially in HIV-positive individuals. Thus a hepatitis screen is always appropriate. Other HIV/AIDS patients may have porphyria cutanea tarda for as-yet-unclear reasons.

The role of medications is quite different in porphyria cutanea tarda than in acute intermittent porphyria, variegate porphyria and hereditary coproporphyria. While some lists include most of the same medications as triggers for these diseases, this is perhaps an oversimplification. First, drug reactions are responsible for fewer than 5% of flares of porphyria cutanea tarda, as compared to 60% of the acute reactions in the hepatic porphyrias. Almost all the involved medications are capable of inducing cytochrome P450 isoenzyme in the liver. In addition, the reactions in porphyria cutanea tarda, even if clearly drug-related, are usually quite gradual and never involve acute abdominal or neuropsychiatric problems. Thus for all practical purposes, the medications in the hepatic porphyria lists can be employed for routine use in porphyria cutanea tarda patients, but it is wise to avoid any potentially hepatotoxic medications. Two drugs that have been reported to cause acute reactions are the antimalarial agents, chloroquine and hydroxychloroquine. But severe reactions must be rare; they have not been often documented among either soldiers or tourists taking these medications. In fact, both can be used in very low dosages as an alternate form of therapy.

The other triggering agents in porphyria cutanea tarda are of both medical and social interest. They include:

- Alcohol. Chronic alcohol use is the major risk factor in porphyria cutanea tarda, but alcohol acts at so many levels of heme synthesis that it is unclear what mechanisms are responsible.
- Estrogens. Once again the mechanisms are not clear, but oral contraceptives, replacement estrogens and estrogens given to males with prostate cancer have all triggered porphyria cutanea tarda.
- Iron. Hepatic iron stores are elevated in almost all porphyria cutanea tarda patients, often to twice normal. Alcohol and iron seem to interact,

but porphyria cutanea tarda is uncommon in patients with hemochromatosis where the iron overload is manyfold that of porphyria cutanea tarda. Patients with iron overload should be screened for both hemochromatosis and porphyria cutanea tarda.

- Hexachlorobenzene. In a region of southeastern Turkey, wheat seeds treated with hexachlorobenzene sent for planting were used for food. Over 4000 individuals, including many children, developed a porphyria cutanea tarda-like illness. The classic studies of Cripps and colleagues over 30 years have shown that over two-thirds of the patients have chronic skin changes of porphyria cutanea tarda, arthritis, neurologic problems and elevated fecal and urine porphyrins.
- Dioxin. The dioxin family of chemicals are most well known for producing chloracne, but porphyria cutanea tarda is a another side effect in experimental animals and was accepted as a service-connected manifestation of Agent Orange exposure by the US government when Vietnam War veterans were evaluated.

Clinical Findings. The cutaneous findings in porphyria cutanea tarda are multiple and distinctive. Gastrointestinal and neuropsychiatric problems do not occur. Many different types of lesions may develop.

Bullous Lesions. The blisters of porphyria cutanea tarda are the classic example of a noninflamed subepidermal blister. They are in sun-damaged skin most often on the back of the hand, cheeks or temples (Fig. 44.5). The blisters range in size from a few millimeters to several centimeters, and are quite stable and painless. Occasionally they may be

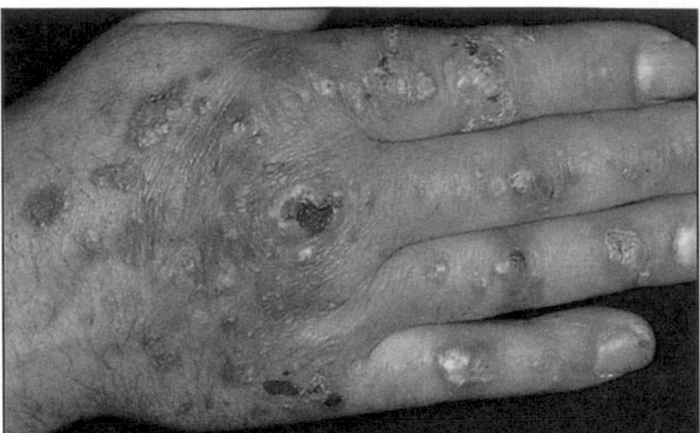

Fig. 44.6. Erosions, milia, and atrophic scars in porphyria cutanea tarda

hemorrhagic and crusted. When they do rupture, scarring, hypo- and hyperpigmentation and milia may all develop, producing a varied clinical picture (Fig. 44.6). Another typical aspect is increased skin fragility. Many patients complain that the slightest trauma will damage their sun-exposed skin and that wound healing is delayed. In contrast, patients almost never associate their blisters with acute light exposure and they often deny photosensitivity.

Other Reversible Changes. Hypertrichosis is also a common sign. It most often involves the temples, connecting the eyebrows to the hair line and cheeks (Fig. 44.7). In addition, many patients have facial hyperpigmentation resembling melasma. A particularly subtle but interesting finding is the heliotrope discoloration and swelling of the mid face, often associated with lid swelling and conjunctivitis. Similar findings have been described in polycythemia vera, but also may be seen in chronic alcoholism, so their exact significance is unclear.

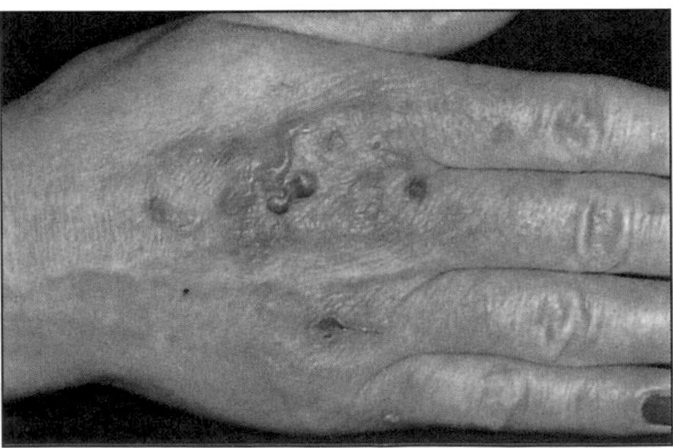

Fig. 44.5. Blisters on the hand in porphyria cutanea tarda

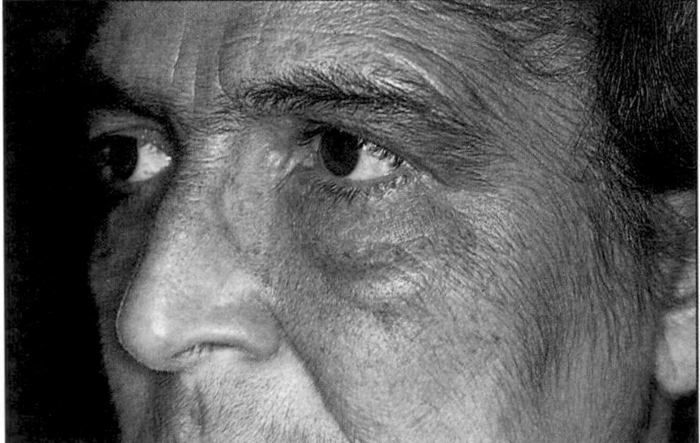

Fig. 44.7. Patient with porphyria cutanea tarda and hirsutism

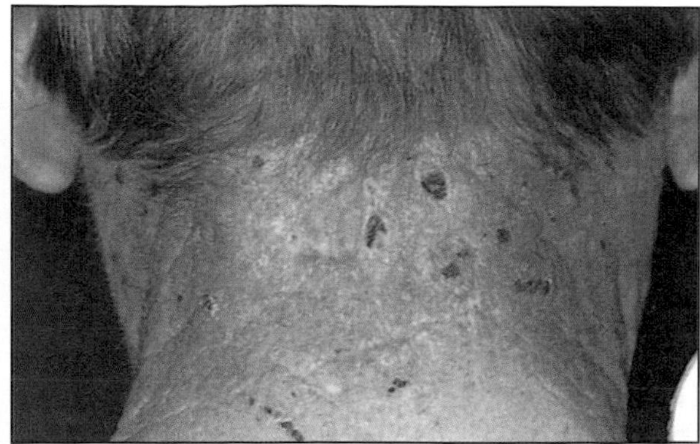

Fig. 44.8. Chronic actinic damage on the nape in porphyria cutanea tarda

Chronic Actinic Damage. Porphyria cutanea tarda patients often have Favre-Racouchot disease, diffuse actinic elastosis, deep furrows and wrinkles and other signs of chronic actinic damage (Fig. 44.8). The presence of marked actinic damage in a young patient should suggest the possibility of porphyria cutanea tarda (Borda sign). In contrast to congenital erythropoietic porphyria, they have no more trouble with actinic keratoses and cutaneous malignancies than the general sun-exposed population.

Sclerodermoid Changes. Porphyria cutanea tarda is one of the classic causes of pseudoscleroderma. Most often the skin of the lateral aspects of the face and neck is involved, although nonexposed areas such as the chest may also be involved (Fig. 44.9). Clinically the skin is firm and indurated. Possible clues that porphyria cutanea tarda is the answer, and not systemic sclerosis, are the presence of small erosions, hemorrhagic areas, crusts or varioliform scars. The sclerodermoid plaques may calcify and then ulcerate. Sclerodermoid changes can also be seen in hepatoerythropoietic porphyria.

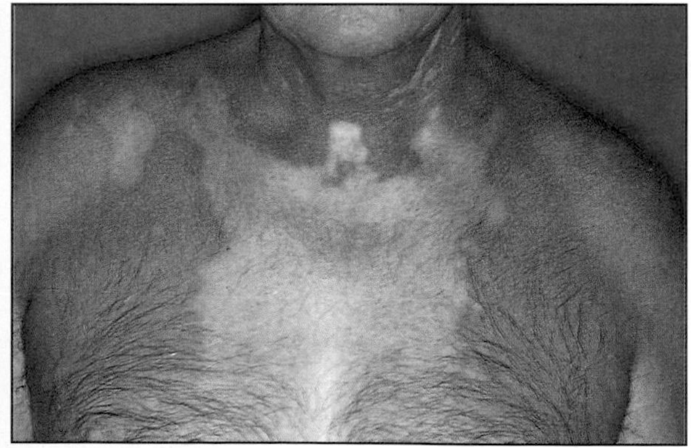

Fig. 44.9. Sclerodermoid porphyria cutanea tarda; the normal skin is erythematous and the central white areas are sclerotic

Lupus Erythematosus. A number of patients have been reported with both porphyria cutanea tarda and lupus erythematosus. If a patient with lupus erythematosus has blisters, one should think of porphyria cutanea tarda and if a porphyria cutanea tarda patient has acute photosensitivity, one should think of lupus erythematosus. This overlap is clinically important, as the dose of chloroquine used in lupus erythematosus is too high for porphyria cutanea tarda patients.

Histopathology. The typical subepidermal blister in porphyria cutanea tarda is well-preserved. The dermal papillae are often still intact, described as naked papillae, projecting into the blister space. Inflammatory cells are usually sparse. In addition, the basement membrane zone at the epidermal-dermal junction and around vessels is thickened and usually stains PAS-positive. One distinctive clue is the presence of amorphous eosinophilic globules known as caterpillars in the blister roof.

As discussed in Chapter 15, the level of blistering in porphyria cutanea tarda is not as exactly defined as for many of the immunologic blistering disorders. The PAS-positive material may be on either side of the separation. Electron microscopic studies indicate that separation occurs mainly in the lamina lucida. Direct immunofluorescent examination shows deposition of broad linear deposits of IgG, other immunoglobulins and complement components in the basement membrane area of both the vessel walls and the epidermis. The immune reactants are presumably passively trapped in the thickened structures. Indirect immunofluorescent examination is negative.

One should always keep an eye out for possible changes of associated lupus erythematosus. While the sclerodermoid lesions look the same as scleroderma, occasionally one will find separation at the epidermal-dermal junction or amorphous perivascular material, suggesting porphyria cutanea tarda. In addition, there is usually actinic elastosis or other elastic fiber changes, while in scleroderma the elastic fibers are maintained.

Laboratory Findings

- Urine: The most appropriate test is a 24-h urine evaluation; screening tests on spot urines are unreliable. There is a massive increase in all

urine porphyrins but coproporphyrins usually dominate. The urine may be discolored.
- Feces: Fecal analysis is not needed but also shows elevated levels of the porphyrins. The presence of isocoproporphyrin is taken as diagnostic.
- Serum: The porphyrins can also be identified in the serum; this is of particular importance in renal dialysis patients.
- Erythrocytes: The uroporphyrinogen decarboxylase levels are used to separate the acquired form (normal levels) from the familial form (50 % reduction).
- Other Tests: Liver function tests may show modest elevations. Serum iron and total iron-binding capacity should be measured, and hepatitis, HIV and ANA screening carried out.

Differential Diagnosis. The differential diagnosis of porphyria cutanea tarda includes several problems. Most traditional is the issue of pseudoporphyria, implying the typical firm blisters on the hands and face. Several disorders should be considered if a patient's disorder looks like porphyria cutanea tarda but porphyrin studies are negative:

Bullous Disease of Renal Dialysis. Patients with chronic renal disease, most often dialysis patients, may develop blisters. Many of these patients have porphyria cutanea tarda (or a close relative thereof). As more sophisticated techniques have become available, serum porphyrin levels have been found to be raised in such individuals.

Epidermolysis Bullosa Acquisita. Epidermolysis bullosa acquisita may be identical to porphyria cutanea tarda. They can be identified by the presence of antibodies to type VII collagen (Chap. 15).

Drug-Induced Pseudoporphyria. A variety of medications including furosemide, nonsteroidal anti-inflammatory drugs, nalidixic acid and tetracycline have been reported to cause an eruption clinically similar to porphyria cutanea tarda. This problem is different than drug-induced porphyria cutanea tarda as the patients have normal porphyrin values, but the mechanism is unclear. It most likely represents a variation on a phototoxic drug reaction. The blisters are usually large and not associated with an inflammatory infiltrate; they have been called reactionless (Fig. 44.10).

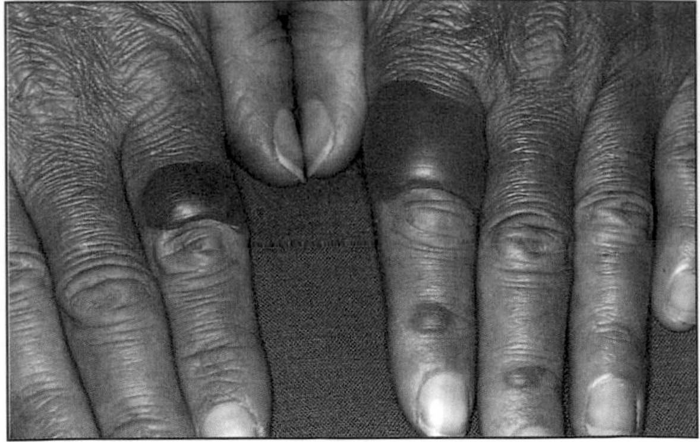

Fig. 44.10. Pseudoporphyria secondary to a diuretic

Tanning Devices. Excessive use of tanning beds and booths has been reported to cause blisters and increased skin fragility independent of burning.

Prognosis. The outlook is good if the patient does not have permanent liver damage and avoids future hepatic insults. A small percentage of patients either have a hepatoma or may develop one, so some consider porphyria cutanea tarda a paraneoplastic marker. This is perhaps an over-reaction, but close monitoring is required.

Therapy. The standard therapy is repeated phlebotomy, as popularized by Ippen in the 1950s. Usually 250–500 ml of blood can be withdrawn every 2 weeks for several months and then the frequency decreased. The iron load is nowhere near as high as in hemochromatosis so that the aggressive regimens described for this disease are not usually needed. The hemoglobin or hematocrit levels should not be driven below 12 g/dl or 36 %, respectively. Serum iron and urine porphyrin levels slowly drop, as the clinical findings improve. Blistering and skin fragility improve first, often after several months, while over years hypertrichosis and the sclerodermoid changes may get better. Patience is the key word, as rapid improvement is not seen, but phlebotomy is usually effective.

Oral antimalarial agents are also quite effective. The mechanism is a minor hepatotoxic reaction with release of porphyrins which are excreted in the urine. Some physicians use them as first-line therapy. They are also useful in patients who are anemic, have HIV infection or for other reasons cannot tolerate phlebotomy. Chloroquine is usually used in very low dosages, as at higher dosages severe hepatotoxic responses may be seen. A dosage of 125 mg twice weekly has become standard. In this approach, liver function must be monitored carefully, especially at the beginning of therapy. Ocular toxicity is a possibility but unlikely at such low dosages. We prefer to combine chloroquine 125 mg twice weekly with more modest phlebotomies, usually 250 ml every other week.

Other approaches include the use of iron-binding chelating agents, both orally and intravenously, and combining erythropoietin with phlebotomy in anemic patients. Topical treatments are usually not needed, except for routine wound care for the eroded blisters. Sunscreens may reduce the chronic actinic changes but seem to help little against blistering.

Hepatoerythropoietic Porphyria

(PINOL AGUADE 1969; GÜNTHER 1967)

Synonyms. Hepatoerythrocytic porphyria, erythropoietic porphyria, porphyrin hepatitis

Defective Enzyme. Uroporphyrinogen decarboxylase

Etiology and Pathogenesis. Hepatoerythropoietic porphyria is another rare form which results when an individual is homozygous for the loss of uroporphyrinogen decarboxylase, the defective enzyme in porphyria cutanea tarda. In contrast to porphyria cutanea tarda, these patients also have erythrocyte porphyrin accumulations. Both parents are at risk for porphyria cutanea tarda, although one or both may be asymptomatic.

Clinical Findings. The cutaneous changes can be viewed as being between those of porphyria cutanea tarda and congenital erythropoietic porphyria. Onset is usually in early childhood, without exposure to any triggering factors. The patients are photosensitive, have fragile skin, develop blisters in sun-exposed areas and later develop sclerosis. The face and back of the hands are most often involved. Hypertrichosis also occurs. The Turkish porphyria patients described under porphyria cutanea tarda could also be viewed as closer to this disorder. Ocular changes similar to those in congenital erythropoietic porphyria develop. Hemolytic anemia and splenomegaly may occur, but iron storage does not appear to be such a problem.

Histopathology. Little experience is available, but the blisters are identical to those of porphyria cutanea tarda and the dermis may show either perivascular hyaline changes as in porphyria cutanea tarda or more diffuse hyalinosis cutis-like changes as in congenital erythropoietic porphyria and erythropoietic protoporphyria.

Laboratory Findings

- Urine: The urine is always dark and fluoresces. The porphyrins are massively elevated. δ-Aminolevulinic acid and porphobilinogen are normal.
- Feces: Porphyrin levels are elevated but not needed for diagnosis.
- Erythrocytes: Total porphyrins are markedly elevated. The uroporphyrinogen decarboxylase levels are below 10 % of normal, and both parents should have a 50 % level.

Prognosis. The degree of internal involvement determines the outlook. There is insufficient experience with the disease to make any sweeping conclusions.

Differential Diagnosis. The only serious differential is congenital erythropoietic porphyria.

Therapy. Photoprotection or avoidance of sunlight is crucial. It might be worthwhile to try β-carotene and antimalarial agents. Phlebotomy is not an option because of the hemolytic anemia.

Hereditary Coproporphyria

(WATSON 1949; BERGER and GOLDBERG 1955)

Defective Enzyme. Coproporphyrinogen oxidase

Etiology and Pathogenesis. Hereditary coproporphyria is another rare disease, with over 100 patients reported. Harderoporphyria appears to represent the homozygous version of hereditary coproporphyria, just as hepatoerythropoietic porphyria relates to familial porphyria cutanea tarda.

Clinical Findings. The patients have a mild version of acute intermittent porphyria, with occasional attacks which are not as severe but subject to the same triggering agents. Skin changes are present in perhaps one-fourth of patients, and include both photosensitivity and mild porphyria cutanea tarda-like changes. Many patients are asymptomatic.

Laboratory Findings
- Feces: The diagnosis is based on elevated fecal coproporphyrin levels even during latent or stable periods.
- Urine: In acute attacks, δ-aminolevulinic acid, porphobilinogen, and uro- and coproporphyrins are elevated, but they are often normal in between.
- Erythrocytes: Normal

Differential Diagnosis. The other forms of porphyria are the only considerations. If someone with apparent acute intermittent porphyria has cutaneous findings, the fecal coproporphyrin levels should be investigated.

Therapy. Photoprotection in addition to the treatment discussed under acute intermittent porphyria.

Variegate Porphyria

(Barnes 1951; Dean and Barnes 1959)

Synonyms. Hereditary protocoproporphyria, mixed hepatic porphyria, South African porphyria, hereditary porphyria cutanea tarda (Waldenström)

Defective Enzyme. Protoporphyrinogen oxidase

Epidemiology. Variegate porphyria is an autosomal dominant inherited disorder in which large pedigrees have been studied in South Africa and Sweden. Barnes initially identified the disease. He was not a physician but later worked together with Dean to develop huge pedigrees tracing variegate porphyria in South Africa back to two early Dutch settlers in the late seventeenth century. The incidence in South Africa among whites is about 1 : 300. In contrast, porphyria cutanea tarda is more common among black South Africans.

Etiology and Pathogenesis. Patients usually first have trouble in young adult life when exposed to triggering agents. The porphyrin pathway is blocked quite late at the level of conversion from protoporphyrinogen to protoporphyrin, so when production is increased all the precursors can accumulate.

Clinical Findings. Variegate porphyria is even more of an overlap between porphyria cutanea tarda and acute intermittent porphyria. About 30 % of the patients have only cutaneous findings, which are identical to those in porphyria cutanea tarda but perhaps milder. The skin lesions start earlier than in porphyria cutanea tarda and do not correlate with the acute attacks. A typical feature is the presence of central facial papular lymphangiectases. Men seem to have more skin changes while women have more systemic problems. The acute attacks are identical to those in acute intermittent porphyria, with the same triggers. About 15 % of patients identified in pedigrees or with enzyme testing are asymptomatic.

Laboratory Findings
- Urine: During attacks the urine is dark and fluoresces. δ-aminolevulinic acid, porphobilinogen and porphyrins are found, especially coproporphyrin. Findings are normal in between.
- Feces: The fecal levels of proto- and coproporphyrins are elevated, even between attacks. This is the best way to distinguish variegate porphyria from acute intermittent porphyria. An especially insoluble molecule, porphyrin X, is most often found in specimens from variegate porphyria but can occur in other porphyrias.
- Serum: A special porphyrin that fluoresces with a 626 nm emission peak when stimulated with 405 nm radiation is pathognomonic of variegate porphyria. Occasionally porphyrin levels are elevated during attacks.
- Erythrocytes: Normal

Differential Diagnosis. If an acute intermittent porphyria patient has skin findings, one must think of hereditary coproporphyria and variegate porphyria. If a porphyria cutanea tarda patient has early onset of disease or systemic problems, variegate porphyria should be ruled out, especially if the patient is of Swedish or South African descent.

Therapy. The same treatment as discussed under acute intermittent porphyria is needed for acute attacks. The systemic management used for porphyria cutanea tarda is not effective, so patients are left with sunlight avoidance or protection and wound care.

Erythropoietic Protoporphyria

(Magnus 1961; Kosenow and Treibs 1966 et al.)

Synonyms. Erythrohepatic protoporphyria, protoporphyria

Defective Enzyme. Ferrochelatase

Epidemiology. Erythropoietic protoporphyria is probably the third most common porphyria after porphyria cutanea tarda and acute intermittent porphyria. About 5–10% of patients screened for photosensitivity have erythropoietic protoporphyria.

Etiology and Pathogenesis. The genetics of erythropoietic protoporphyria are more confusing than the other porphyrias. One ferrochelatase gene has been located but there may be other genes or multiple mutations. Evidence for both autosomal dominant and autosomal recessive inheritance has been presented using sensitive ferrochelatase assays. In most patients the pattern is autosomal dominant.

Ferrochelatase is responsible for adding iron to protoporphyrin to produce heme. This process occurs almost exclusively in the red blood cells, but also involves the liver. Protoporphyrins are released from erythrocytes, and perhaps the liver, as a result of normal turnover. Following photohemolysis they are deposited in the tissues, especially the skin. They lead to the production of singlet oxygen and other free radicals, perhaps explaining the skin damage. In lead poisoning, erythrocyte protoporphyrins are also markedly elevated but bound to zinc and globulin chains, so they cannot diffuse into the dermis. Thus patients with lead poisoning are not photosensitive. Protoporphyrins are excreted primarily in the bile. This leads to two consequences: possible development of gall stones at an early age and in about 10% of the patients cirrhosis, which often develops at an early age.

Clinical Findings. Most patients have only cutaneous findings. The initial complaint is burning or stinging upon sun exposure, accompanied by sunburn, and occurring in early childhood (Fig. 44.11). The parents may report that the child screams when exposed to sunlight. Often there is swelling and erythema after several hours. The same reaction can be elicited through window glass. While most problems are in the summer in temperate climates, winter ski trips can also produce flares. Some patients only experience acute reactions, while others develop permanent changes.

Several different types of skin changes have been described within light-exposed areas:

Pruritic Type. Some patients have no skin findings but complain of burning or stinging when exposed to light. These symptoms are often ignored and these children or young adults are only rarely diagnosed.

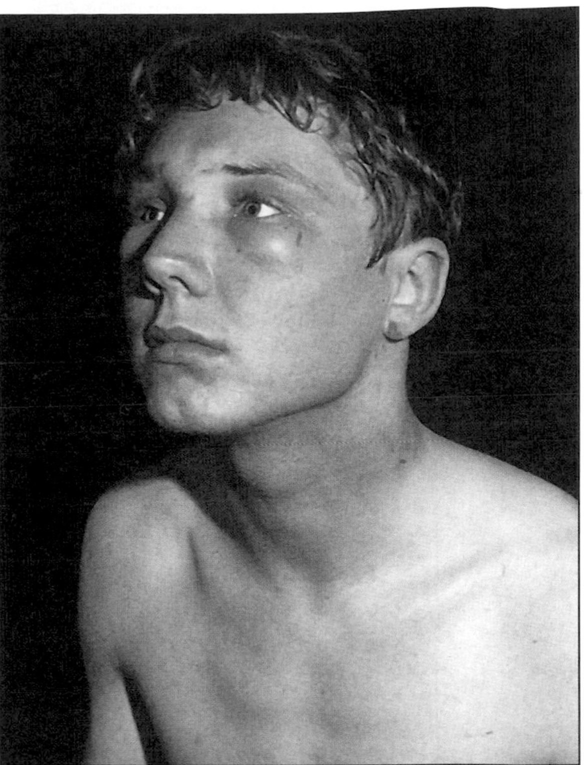

Fig. 44.11. Acute phototoxicity in patient with erythropoietic protoporphyria

Dermatitic Type. In this group, erythema develops on the nose, cheeks, chin and tips of the ears, as well as the back of the hands. It is associated with modest swelling and is more persistent than ordinary sunburn. Blisters, especially on the tip of the nose, often develop and heal with distinctive varioliform scars. Finally there may be an exaggeration of the skin markings producing verruciform changes (Fig. 44.12).

Urticarial Type. In addition to burning or pain, patients develop acute urticaria. Erythropoietic protoporphyria must be ruled out in all cases of solar urticaria.

Angioedematous Type. Following sun exposure, deep subcutaneous swellings develop on the backs of the hands, about the eyes and on the cheeks. They resemble angioedema and usually lack overlying surface changes. Any patient with sunlight-induced angioedema is very likely to have erythropoietic protoporphyria (Fig. 44.13).

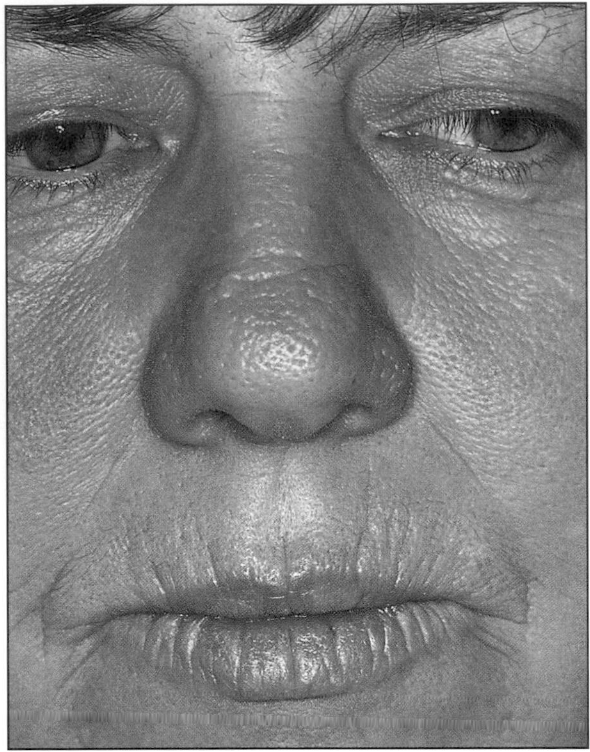

Fig. 44.12. Mild erythema and typical scars on nose in erythropoietic protoporphyria

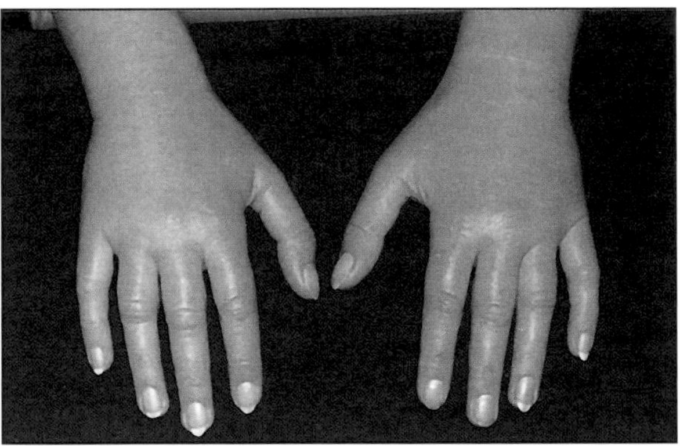

Fig. 44.13. Angioedema in erythropoietic protoporphyria

Other Chronic Findings. Hypertrichosis may occur, as may exaggerated perioral skin folds known as pseudorhagades.

Pseudo-Lipoid Proteinosis. As a result of the chronic, repeated sun damage, some patients develop chronic persistent dermal thickening, especially on the backs of the hands, the ears, the upper lip and nose (Fig. 44.14). These skin-colored plaques with exaggerated skin markings resemble the changes

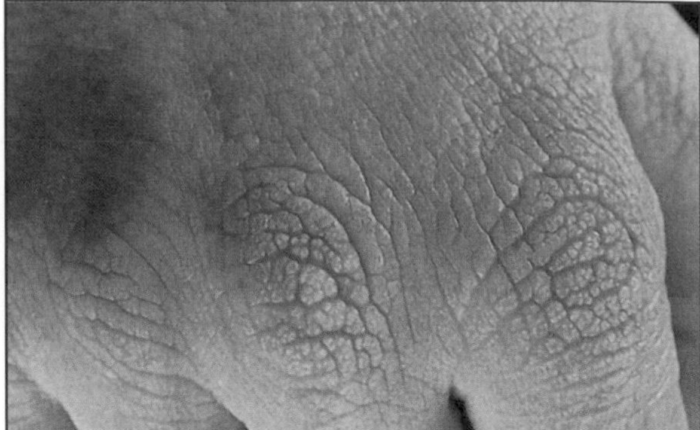

Fig. 44.14. Verruciform changes on backs of hands in erythropoietic protoporphyria

in lipoid proteinosis (Chap. 42) and are identical histologically.

Patients with erythropoietic protoporphyria should be followed for possible liver problems and development of gall stones, but in general they have few systemic problems. Why some have hepatic disease, even fulminant hepatic disease, may become clear when the various genetic possibilities are better delineated.

Histopathology. Initial changes are centered around the dermal blood vessels and the epidermal-dermal junction where hyaline material accumulates. It is strongly PAS-positive and contains heterogeneous basement membrane fragments containing laminin and type IV collagen, as well as amyloid P component. Around the vessels the changes have been compared to onion skin. While similar changes are seen in porphyria cutanea tarda and other porphyrias, they are most dramatic in erythropoietic protoporphyria. As the disease progresses, the hyaline deposits become more massive and widespread.

Laboratory Findings

- Erythrocytes: While fluorescence occurs, it is often mild or transient, and does not involve all cells. The key to diagnosis is measuring the erythrocyte protoporphyrin levels.
- Feces: Both proto- and coproporphyrin levels are raised.
- Urine: Normal, as the proto- and coproporphyrins are relatively insoluble and wind up in the bile.

Prognosis. The prognosis is excellent except for the small percentage who develop liver disease. Generally photosensitivity decreases with age, or perhaps the patients get smart and stay out of the light.

Differential Diagnosis. Erythropoietic protoporphyria is often overlooked. When a patient complains of burning on light exposure, worse in the summer, occurring through glass and relieved by cooling, i.e., cold water, one should exclude this disease. Red cell protoporphyrin levels should be checked in all photosensitivity evaluations. Congenital erythropoietic porphyria and hepatoerythropoietic porphyria have far more severe photosensitivity and positive urine. Polymorphic light eruptions are usually more papular, more widely distributed, not associated with burning, uncommon in small children and improve over the summer. The actinic prurigo of Native Americans may involve small children, but is dermatitic and associated with cheilitis. When the dermal thickening with folds develops, one should think of lipoid proteinosis, but the lack of hoarseness and eyelid lesions usually allows a clinical distinction.

Therapy

Systemic. β-Carotene appears effective. Dosages of 60–300 mg daily are usually employed, leading to orange skin and stools but no other side effects. Treatment should be started about 1 month before the sunny season is expected and continued until the fall. Not every patient responds, but most report increased sun tolerance. The β-carotene does not function as a sunscreen but interacts somehow with free protoporphyrin.

Topical. Sunscreens are an essential life-long requirement. They must protect against UVA radiation and the lower ranges of visible light.

Bibliography

Reviews

Elder GH (1990) The cutaneous porphyrias. Semin Dermatol 9:63–69

Elder GH (1998) Update on enzyme and molecular defects in porphyria. Photodermatol Photoimmunol Photomed 14:66–XX69

Fernandes J, Saudubray J-M, Berghe G van den (eds) (1995) Inborn metabolic diseases. Diagnosis and treatment, 2nd edn. Springer, Berlin

Lim HW, Murphy GM (1996) The porphyrias. Clin Dermatol 14:375–387

Lim HW, Cohen JL (1999) The cutaneous porphyrias. Semin Cutan Med Surg 18(4):285–292

Moore MR (1993) Biochemistry of porphyria. Int J Biochem 25:1353–1368

Murphy GM (1999) The cutaneous porphyrias: a review. Br J Dermatol 140:573–581

Nordmann Y, Puy H, Deybach JC (1999) The porphyrias. J Hepatol 30:12–16

Scarlett YV, Brenner DA (1998) Porphyrias. J Clin Gastroenterol 27:192–198

Seubert A, Seubert S (1986) High-performance liquid chromatographic analysis of porphyrins and their isomers with radial compression columns. Methods Enzymol 123:346–352

Touart DM, Sau P (1998) Cutaneous deposition diseases, part I. J Am Acad Dermatol 39:149–171

Young JW, Conte ET (1991) Porphyrias and porphyrins. Int J Dermatol 30:399–406

Doss Porphyria

Doss M, Tiepermann R, Look D et al. (1980) Hereditäre und nicht-hereditäre Form der chronischen hepatischen Porphyrie: unterschiedliches Verhalten der Uroporphyrinogen-Decarboxylase in Leber und Erythrozyten. Klin Wochenschr 58:1347–1356

Jacob K, Egeler E, Gross U et al. (1999) Investigations on the formation of urinary coproporphyrin isomers I-IV in 5-aminolevulinic acid dehydratase deficiency porphyria, acute lead intoxication and after oral 5-aminolevulinic acid loading. Clin Biochem 32:119–123

Acute Intermittent Porphyria

Grandchamp B (1998) Acute intermittent porphyria. Semin Liver Dis 18:17–24

Sassa S (1996) Diagnosis and therapy of acute intermittent porphyria. Blood Rev 10:53–58

Schreiber WE (1995) Acute intermittent porphyria: laboratory diagnosis by molecular methods. Clin Lab Med 15: 943–956

Congenital Erythropoietic Porphyria

Deybach JC, Verneuil H de, Boulechfar S et al. (1990) Point mutations in the uroporphyrinogen III synthase gene in congenital erythropoietic porphyria (Günther's disease). Blood 75:1763–1765

Freesemann AG, Bhutani LK, Jacob K et al. (1997) Interdependence between degree of porphyrin excess and disease severity in congenital erythropoietic porphyria (Günther's disease). Arch Dermatol Res 289:272–276

Freesemann AG, Hofweber K, Doss MO (1997) Coexistence of deficiencies of uroporphyrinogen III synthase and decarboxylase in a patient with congenital erythropoietic porphyria and in his family. Eur J Clin Chem Clin Biochem 35:35–39

Fritsch C, Bolsen K, Ruzicka T et al. (1997) Congenital erythropoietic porphyria. J Am Acad Dermatol 6: 594–610

Goerz G, Bunselmeyer S, Bolsen K et al. (1996) Ferrochelatase activities in patients with erythropoietic protoporphyria and their families. Br J Dermatol 134: 880–885

Günther H (1911) Die Hämatoporphyrie. Dtsch Arch Klin Med 105:89–146

Poh-Fitzpatick MB (1986) The erythropoietic porphyrias. Dermatol Clin 4:291–300

Todd DJ (1998) Molecular genetics of erythropoietic protoporphyria. Photodermatol Photoimmunol Photomed 14:70–73

Porphyria Cutanea Tarda

English JC III, Peake MF, Becker LE (1996) Hepatitis C and porphyria cutanea tarda. Cutis 57:404–408

Boisseau AM, Couzigou P, Forestier JF et al. (1991) Porphyria cutanea tarda associated with human immunodeficiency virus infection. A study of four cases and review of the literature. Dermatologica 182:155–159

Chuang T-Y, Brashear R, Lewis C (1999) Porphyria cutanea tarda and hepatitis C virus: A case-control study and meta-analysis of the literature. J Am Acad Dermatol 41:31–36

Cohen DJ, McKay M (1996) Porphyria cutanea tarda: a clinical review. Compr Ther 22:175–178

Mansourati FF, Stone VE, Mayer KH (1999) Porphyria cutanea tarda and HIV/AIDS: a review of pathogenesis, clinical manifestations and management. Int J STD AIDS 10:51–56

Rich MW (1999) Porphyria cutanea tarda. Don't forget to look at the urine. Postgrad Med 105:208–210, 213–214

Sampietro M, Fiorelli G, Fargion S (1999) Iron overload in porphyria cutanea tarda. Haematologica 84:248–253

Waldenström J (1937) Studien über Porphyrie. Acta Med Scand (Stockh) [Suppl] 82:1–254

Hepatoerythropoietic Porphyria

Castano Suarez E, Zamarro Sanz O, Guerra Tapia A et al. (1996) Hepatoerythropoietic porphyria: relationship with familial porphyria cutanea tarda. Dermatology 193:332–335

Elder GH (1997) Hepatic porphyrias in children. J Inherit Metab Dis 20:237–246

Günther H (1912) Die Hämataporphyrie. Deut Arch Klin Med 105:89–146

Gunther WW (1967) The porphyrias and erythropoietic porphyria. Aust J Dermatol 9:23–29

Pinol Aquade J, Herrero C, Almeida J et al. (1969) A case of biochemically unclassifiable hepatic porphyria. Br J Dermatol 81:270–X275

Roberts AG, Elder GH, De Salamanca RE et al. (1995) A mutation (G281 E) of the human uroporphyrinogen decarboxylase gene causes both hepatoerythropoietic porphyria and overt familial porphyria cutanea tarda: biochemical and genetic studies on Spanish patients. J Invest Dermatol 104:500–502

Hereditary Coproporphyria

Berger H, Goldberg A (1955) Hereditary coproporphyria. BMJ 2:85–92

Elder GH, Evans JO, Thomas N et al. (1976) The primary enzyme defect in hereditary coproporphyria. Lancet II: 1217–1219

Günther WW (1967) The porphyrias and erythropoietic protoporphyria: an unusual case. Aust J Dermatol 9: 23–30

Martasek P (1998) Hereditary coproporphyria. Semin Liver Dis 18:25–32

Watson CJ, Schwartz S, Schultze W et al. (1949) Studies of coporphyrin III: idiopathic coporphyrinuria, a hitherto unrecognized form characterized by lack of symptoms in spite of the excretion of large amounts of coporphyrin. J Clin Invest 28:465

Variegate Porphyria

Barnes HD (1951) Further South African cases of porphyrinuria. S Afr J Clin Sci 2:117–169

Dean G, Barnes HD (1959) Porphyria in Sweden and South Africa. S Afr Med J 33:246–253

Frank J, Jugert FK, Kalka K et al. (1998) Variegate porphyria: identification of a nonsense mutation in the protoporphyrinogen oxidase gene. J Invest Dermatol 110:449–451

Kirsch RE, Meissner PN, Hift RJ (1998) Variegate porphyria. Semin Liver Dis 18:33–41

Tidman MJ, Higgins EM, Elder GH et al. (1989) Variegate porphyria associated with hepatocellular carcinoma. Br J Dermatol 121:503–505

Timonen K, Niemi KM, Mustajoki P et al. (1990) Skin changes in variegate porphyria. Clinical, histopathological, and ultrastructural study. Arch Dermatol Res 282:108–114

Erythropoietic Protoporphyria

Braun-Falco O, Burg G, Schmidt D (1970) Protoporphyrinämische Lichtdermatose vom Typ des Quinckeschen Ödems. Münch Med Wochenschr 112:1443–1447

Cox TM (1997) Erythropoietic protoporphyria. J Inherit metab Dis 20:258–269

Kosenow W, Treibs A (1966) Lichtüberempfindlichkeit und Porphyrinämie. Z Kinderheilkd 73:82–92

Magnus IA, Jarret A, Prankard TAJ et al. (1961) Erythropoietic protoporphyria: a new porphyria syndrome with solar urticaria due to protoporphyrinaemia. Lancet (ii); 448–451

Todd DJ (1994) Erythropoietic protoporphyria. Br J Dermatol 131:751–766

Todd DJ (1998) Clinical implications of the molecular biology of erythropoietic protoporphyria. J Eur Acad Dermatol Venereol 11:207–213

Treatment of Porphyrias

Bickers DR, Merk H (1986) Treatment of porphyrias. Semin Dermatol 5:186–197

Freesemann A, Frank M, Sieg I et al. (1995) Treatment of porphyria cutanea tarda by the effect of chloroquine on the liver. Skin Pharmacol 8:156–161

Gorchein A (1997) Drug treatment in acute porphyria. Br J Clin Pharmacol 44:427–434

Rogers PD (1997) Cimetidine in the treatment of acute intermittent porphyria. Ann Pharmacother 31:365–367

CHAPTER 45

Cutaneous Calcification

Contents

Basic Science Aspects

The regulation of serum calcium levels is a delicately balanced homeostatic process. Derangements can lead to metabolic bone disease, renal disease, and a variety of other problems. Calcium is involved in most cell membrane message transmission, so its levels are of crucial importance. The skin is often involved, but only rarely in a significant fashion.

The average diet provides 0.5–1.0 g of calcium daily; a disturbing trend in Western countries is the fall in calcium intake, which leads to skeletal problems in younger individuals. In developed countries, calcium deficiency is usually secondary to inappropriate diets, while in less developed countries it is one of the many problems associated with malnutrition.

There are two major factors controlling calcium metabolism: parathyroid hormone and vitamin D. Parathyroid hormone is secreted by the parathyroid chief cells in response to decreased extracellular fluid calcium levels. It raises the levels by increasing bone reabsorption, renal phosphate excretion, and renal tubular calcium reabsorption and by stimulating renal conversion of vitamin D to its most active form.

Vitamin D is a provitamin which can be provided in the diet or manufactured in the skin from 7-hydrocholesterol in the presence of sunlight. It is converted in the liver to 25-hydroxy vitamin D and then in the kidneys to 1.25-dihydroxy vitamin D. The key enzyme in the second step is 1-α-hydrolase, which is stimulated by parathyroid hormones, low phosphate levels, and many other hormones such as growth hormone and prolactin. Vitamin D increases intestinal calcium absorption and stimulates calcium release from bone tissue as well as increasing intestinal phosphate absorption. Vitamin D plays many other roles in cutaneous differentiation; these are utilized in the topical treatment of psoriasis with vitamin D analogs.

There are many other factors complicating the entire calcium-phosphate balance. Calcitonin blocks bone resorption by osteoclasts and thus lowers calcium levels. A whole host of other hormones, including estrogens, androgens, and corticosteroids, influence calcium and bone metabolism, and interact with a variety of mediators.

Bone is the major storage site for calcium. It is formed out of type I collagen, secreted by the osteoblasts, mesenchymal cells, and calcium- and phosphate-containing crystals such as hydroxyapatite. The crystals provide a rigid structure. Many other proteins are involved, including other mesenchymal cells such as osteocytes and the osteoclasts, which are hematopoietic cells that remodel bone. When calcium is stored in the skin, it may be incorporated into bony structures; but this is the exception. Instead, it is most often deposited as

Table 45.1. Types of cutaneous calcification

Feature	Metastatic	Dystrophic	Idiopathic
Calcium level	Elevated	Normal	Normal
Prior tissue damage	No	Yes	No
Internal involvement	Likely	Unlikely	Unlikely
Pattern	Diffuse	Localized or diffuse	Localized or diffuse

amorphous calcium phosphate and calcium carbonate salts. Most cutaneous ossification is reactive and not tumoral; this problem is discussed in Chapter 59.

Only a small proportion of the body's calcium is physiologically active. About 99 % is stored in hydroxyapatite crystals; the remaining 1 % is in extracellular fluids and soft tissues. Of this small percentage, only the ionized form of calcium in the serum is involved in the various signaling processes. About 50 % of serum calcium is ionized and active; the balance is bound to phosphate and other ions (10 %) or proteins (40 %). Most multiple channel analyzers provide only the total serum calcium; this must be corrected for albumin levels, since albumin is the major calcium-binding protein.

Today, virtually all hypercalcemic patients are discovered during routine screening and are asymptomatic. The main causes of hypercalcemia are primary hyperparathyroidism and malignancies. In the former, parathyroid hormone is elevated, while in the latter, parathyroid hormone-related protein is present in increased amounts. The principal causes of hyperparathyroidism are parathyroid hyperplasia and the closely-related solitary adenoma. Multiple adenomas should suggest a multiple endocrine neoplasia (MEN) syndrome. Carcinomas are very uncommon. In those patients who are symptomatic, the main clinical findings are skeletal and renal; skin calcification is unlikely.

Secondary hyperparathyroidism is a different story. It develops in renal failure patients; both hypocalcemia and hyperphosphatemia trigger increased production of parathyroid hormone, which leads to bone reabsorption and restores calcium levels to near normal but maintains high phosphate levels. These patients may develop cutaneous problems as discussed below. In tertiary hyperparathyroidism, the persistent stimulation of the parathyroid gland with inadequate feedback loops leads to autonomous parathyroid hormone release.

Traditionally, cutaneous calcification has been divided into three types (Table 45.1):

- Metastatic Calcification. The serum calcium and/or phosphate levels are abnormal and calcium salts are deposited in apparently normal tissues.
- Dystrophic Calcification. The serum calcium and phosphate levels are normal and calcium salts are deposited in abnormal tissues.
- Idiopathic Calcification. The serum calcium and phosphate levels are normal and calcium salts are deposited in apparently normal tissues.

Obviously, idiopathic calcification is a faulty concept: something has to be abnormal or the calcification would not occur. Finally, some authors prefer the term cutaneous mineralization because of the essential role of phosphate ions and the contributions of other ions. We will retain calcification because its use is so widespread.

Metastatic Calcification

Synonym. Calcinosis metastatica

Etiology and Pathogenesis. In metastatic calcification there are elevated levels of calcium and usually phosphate ions in the serum. Local factors also play a role; calcification is more likely to occur in acidic tissues such as the kidneys, lungs, and stomach, usually as calcium phosphate. In addition, trauma plays a role, so that cutaneous changes are often located periarticularly and especially around the

Table 45.2. Causes of metastatic calcification

Primary and, especially, secondary hyperparathyroidism
Other forms of renal osteodystrophy (rickets, osteomalacia, aluminum intoxication)
Malignancy-associated hypercalcemia, usually mediated by PTH-like protein in carcinomas and by various cytokines in lymphoma/leukemia
Destructive bone disease (osteomyelitis, bone tuberculosis, multiple myeloma, Paget disease of bone, bone metastases)
Sarcoidosis
Medications: excess vitamin D, lithium, thiazides, aminophylline
Familial hypocalciuric hypercalcemia
Milk-alkali syndrome
Excessive calcium ingestion

knees and elbows. The site of the intracellular mineralization is usually the mitochondria; tiny crystals form and propagate, killing the cell.

Years ago, Selye proposed the concept of calciphylaxis as similar to anaphylaxis. He suggested that when calcium and phosphate levels are abnormal, other factors such as mast cell degranulation could trigger rapid deposition of calcium in a variety of tissues. While Selye's animal models turned out to be more reproducible than his human model, rapid calcification in the human skin is nonetheless called calciphylaxis.

The main associated disorders are those which produce hypercalcemia (Table 45.2). Occasionally, one can have normal serum calcium levels and dystrophic calcification. In chronic renal failure and primary hypoparathyroidism, the calcium levels may be reduced, but the phosphate values are quite high. The more chronic forms of hypercalcemia, especially secondary hyperparathyroidism, are most likely to have metastatic calcification. Malignancy-related calcinosis is sudden in onset and often associated with such a poor outlook that cutaneous problems rarely occur.

Clinical Findings. Secondary hyperparathyroidism can be taken as a prototype disorder. The most common finding is of firm, symmetrical, often linear white papules or subcutaneous plaques around large joints. The calcium salts tend to elicit an inflammatory or foreign-body type of reaction, so erythema may be present. Over the elbows, ulceration often occurs with the discharge of chalky material. In other instances, large nodules will form which can be mistaken for subcutaneous granuloma annulare or even cysts. The deposits may decrease in size as the serum phosphate levels are brought under control through renal dialysis.

A second more dramatic finding is calciphylaxis. The chief target is the media of the deep dermal and subcutaneous blood vessels, which become occluded and produce peripheral vascular insufficiency and gangrene. Extensive necrosis may develop (Fig. 45.1). In some patients, the subcutaneous injection of erythropoietin triggers the process. At the same time, there is deposition of calcium in other tissues such as fat and the lungs. The differential diagnosis for calciphylaxis is lengthy, including coumarin necrosis, vasculitis, and panniculitis.

A third and probably the most common effect of calcium is the role it plays in pruritus (Chap. 25).

Histopathology. Calcium is readily identified on routine hematoxylin-eosin stains by its blue color. Usually the pattern is amorphous, although calcium sometimes outlines other structures such as vessels, collagen fibers, glands, or muscles. Because the presence of calcium salts in the skin is so nonspecific, the histologic features will not be repeated for each type. One should pay particular attention to the presence of calcium in vessel walls.

Several stains can confirm the presence of calcium. The von Kossa stain is actually a silver reduction stain that identifies anionic salts such as phosphate and carbonate salts. Because almost all such material is bound to calcium, the von Kossa is an indirect but specific calcium stain. A true calcium stain is the dye lake reaction with alizarin red S which, at 4.2 pH, complexes only with calcium.

Course and Prognosis. Prognosis is related to the underlying disease. In most cases, the systemic process is chronic and the cutaneous calcification is an annoying, persistent problem.

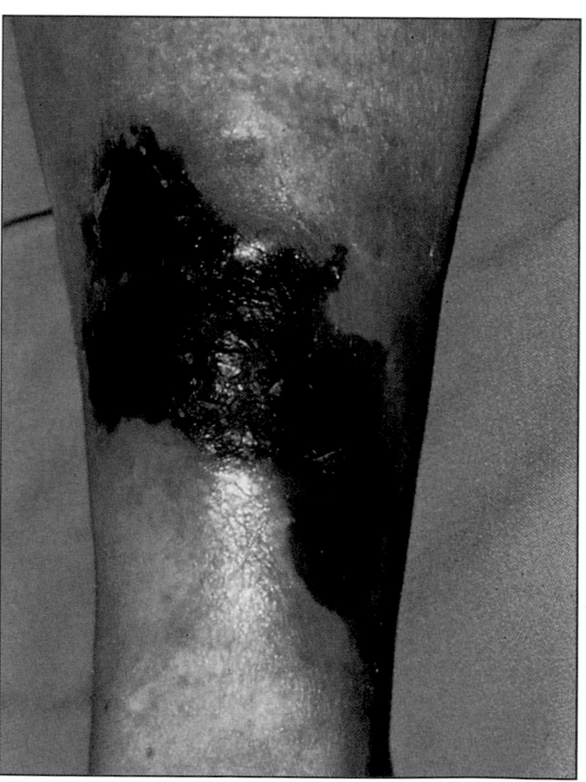

Fig. 45.1. Calciphylaxis with extensive necrosis. (From Hafner et al. 1995, with the permission of Dr. Hafner and the publishers)

Therapy. The treatment of the underlying diseases should be sought in a standard medicine text. Parathyroidectomy is often helpful for the most common scenario: secondary hyperparathyroidism and renal disease. Individual cutaneous lesions can be excised if they are troublesome.

Dystrophic Calcification

Etiology and Pathogenesis. The list of diseases in which cutaneous calcification in damaged skin may occur is lengthy. The microscopic process may be slightly different, in that the damaged dermal collagen may simulate the microenvironment set up by collagen I in bone and thus lead to mineralization. One should consider localized and generalized forms of dystrophic calcification, as shown in Table 45.3.

A number of tumors typically calcify; two which show calcification in over 50% of cases are pilomatricoma and trichilemmal or pilar cyst. Pilomatricomas are particularly likely to ulcerate and discharge chalky granules. Among malignant tumors, basal cell carcinomas may occasionally calcify. This is perhaps more common in nevoid basal cell carcinoma syndrome. Other adnexal tumors and a variety of mesenchymal tumors may also calcify.

Table 45.3. Types of dystrophic calcification

Trauma	Exposure to calcium salts via EEG electrodes, extravasation of calcium-rich infusions Industrial exposure to calcium salts in mines, fertilizer, ice cream manufacture Subcutaneous fat necrosis, other fatty damage Abrasions, scars, hematomas, minor trauma (heel sticks in neonates) with no exposure to calcium Chronic inflammatory diseases such as stasis dermatitis, tuberculosis, leprosy, severe acne
Degenerative disorders	Pseudoxanthoma elasticum, Ehlers-Danlos syndrome, Rothmund-Thomson syndrome, Werner syndrome Porphyria cutanea tarda Acrodermatitis chronica atrophicans
Connective tissue disease	Dermatomyositis CREST syndrome Lupus erythematosus
Tumors	Pilomatricoma, trichilemmal cyst, basal cell carcinoma, many others

Localized trauma, especially if combined with exposure to calcium, is another trigger. In many instances, it is iatrogenic. For example, in newborns and especially premature infants, repeated heel sticks may trigger calcification and present with many tiny white papules on the heels. Subcutaneous fat necrosis of the newborn also may evolve into a group of calcified nodules which tend to resolve slowly. The trauma from EEG electrodes may produce a similar effect, as the contact paste often contains calcium salts; the extravasation of intravenous fluids containing calcium is another trigger. Periocular calcification following corticosteroid injection in infantile hemangiomas has also been reported.

Occupational exposure to calcium salts combined with trauma is another scenario; miners and farmers using calcium nitrate fertilizer are at special risk. Many individuals have tiny calcified nodules in the superficial veins over their tibias; trauma is presumably the main cause of these phleboliths, which may develop in other veins following intravenous drug abuse or therapy. Resolving hematomas also tend to calcify. Petrified ear describes idiopathic or post-traumatic calcification of the auricular cartilage. In wrestlers' and boxers' ears, repeated trauma produces multiple hematomas which may then calcify. Finally, a wide variety of scars may calcify; keloids usually contain calcium microscopically, but this is rarely clinically evident. Burn scars are particularly likely to undergo such changes. The development of tiny nodules in a scar should suggest either calcification or scar sarcoidosis, as well as recurrence of the underlying problem in the event that a neoplasm has been excised.

Chronic inflammation provides another fertile ground. Cutaneous tuberculosis frequently calcifies and ulcerates. Severe acne conglobata may also evolve into firm calcified masses, particularly on the cheeks. The ulcers associated with chronic venous insufficiency may show calcification at their peripheries, especially in the adjacent vessels. Sometimes, acute cutaneous infections such as those from varicella zoster and herpes simplex viruses, cytomegalovirus, and molluscum contagiosum virus can produce dystrophic calcification. Worms and other parasites that die in the skin may also calcify; such changes can sometimes be identified radiologically.

Among the causes of diffuse dystrophic calcification, connective tissue disorders are the best known. Childhood dermatomyositis calcifies often, early in the disease course, and severely. Sheets of calcified tissue develop in the fascial planes between muscles, producing an exoskeleton. Such patients are also at risk of cutaneous vasculitis and do poorly, as their growth and mobility are restricted by the calcium deposits. This variant of dermatomyositis was formerly known as universal calcinosis until the features of the connective tissue disorder were better appreciated. In systemic sclerosis, the calcification occurs as a late sequel of the disease and is associated with a better prognosis. In systemic and discoid lupus erythematosus, calcification is quite uncommon.

Other disorders of connective tissue also show cutaneous calcification. In pseudoxanthoma elasticum, calcification is always present, although it may not be clinically obvious. The vascular calcification is more significant and may be seen on radiologic examination, which may show diffuse subcutaneous calcified plaques as a secondary finding. In some types of Ehlers-Danlos syndrome, the abnormal collagen serves as a nidus for calcification, usually as firm small nodules or spherules on the lower extremity. In Werner syndrome, the dystrophic calcification is usually arterial, involving the legs; calcified nodules may also appear around the knees and ankles. Finally, sclerodermoid porphyria cutanea tarda may also have deposition of calcium salts in the thickened skin.

Clinical Findings. The clinical findings were alluded to in the etiologic description. Usually there is obvious skin disease in other sites to guide the diagnosis or there is a history of trauma or inflammation with some type of nodular change. White, firm papules or nodules, especially if inflamed, or discharged chalky grains or concretions should raise clinical suspicion of calcification.

Therapy. The therapy is that of the underlying disorder. If the lesions are localized or particularly painful or troublesome, they may be excised. Healing is often delayed but, in the end, satisfactory results can be obtained. Acral lesions typically heal poorly and should be approached with caution, no matter what the cause.

CREST Syndrome

(THIBIERGE and WEISSENBACH 1911; WINTERBAUER 1964)

Synonyms. Thibierge-Weissenbach syndrome

Clinical Findings. CREST is an acronym for ***c***alcification of skin, ***R***aynaud syndrome, ***e***sophageal dysmotility, ***s***clerodactyly, and ***t***elangiectases.

The serologic hallmark is the presence of anticentromere antibodies. Clinically, the patients have a localized, relatively limited form of acral systemic sclerosis. The calcification is typically acral and associated with the trophic changes and ulcerations seen in Raynaud syndrome. White papules and nodules develop on the fingers, toes, ankles, wrists, knees, and elbows (Figs. 45.2, 45.3). Perforation, ulceration, and discharge of calcified material is almost the rule. Such ulcerated lesions are very painful and heal slowly. Calcium deposits may also develop in tendons, muscles, and fascia. There is no

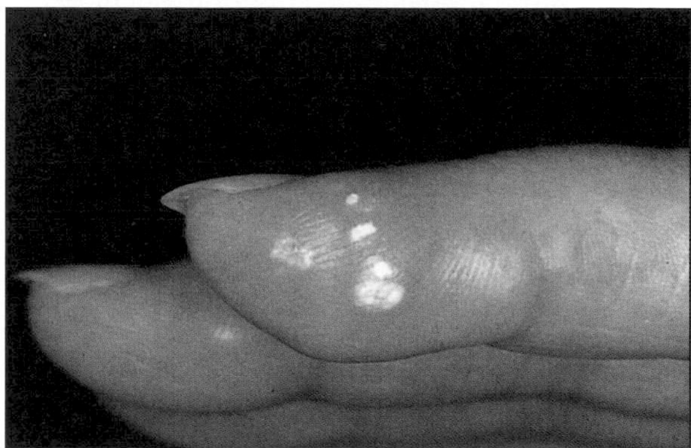

Fig. 45.2. Acral calcification in a patient with CREST syndrome

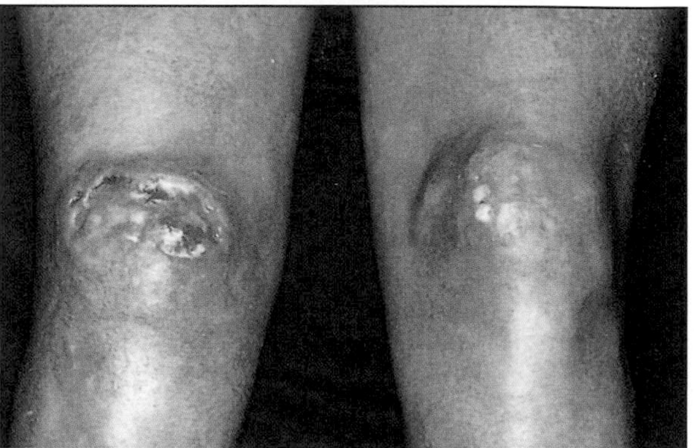

Fig. 45.3. More extensive calcification in a different patient with CREST syndrome

satisfactory treatment. The acral lesions do poorly when excised. Further aspects of the disorder are discussed under systemic sclerosis (Chap. 18).

Idiopathic Calcification

Synonym. Metabolic calcification

The term metabolic does little to advance our understanding of this puzzling group. The disseminated forms of idiopathic calcification are all so rare that classification is difficult. The localized forms of idiopathic cutaneous calcification bear a plethora of names and are also poorly understood.

Tumoral Calcinosis

(Teutschländer 1935)

Synonyms. Teutschländer syndrome, universal metabolic calcinosis, lipocalcinogranulomatosis

Etiology and Pathogenesis. Tumoral calcinosis is probably misclassified here. It may well be a form of metastatic calcification. Patients tend to have elevated phosphate levels and relatively normal calcium levels, just as in secondary hyperparathyroidism. Urinary calcium excretion is often decreased. While the basic defect is unknown, the process is inherited in an autosomal recessive pattern affecting mainly children and young adults. Blacks are affected more often. Tumoral calcinosis has been described in association with a number of disorders including pseudoxanthoma elasticum.

Clinical Findings. Typically there are large, symmetrical, subcutaneous deposits of calcium phosphate complexes located primarily around joints. Muscle calcification may also occur. The skin may have papules and nodules but more often is secondarily affected by the upward expansion of deeper masses. As the skin becomes involved, it turns red, becomes tender, and eventually ulcerates with discharge of necrotic, creamy, calcified material. Other organs are not involved. The massive calcifications interfere greatly with mobility and the patients are often bedridden from an early age. The disease is chronic and progressive.

Histopathology. The cutaneous histology typically reveals a combination of massive calcium deposits associated with fat cells and a granulomatous tissue response, explaining many of the older names.

Differential Diagnosis. One must exclude myositis ossificans, which has even deeper involvement and severe dermatomyositis with calcification and has also been called Teutschländer syndrome.

Therapy. There is no good therapy. Both ion-exchange resins and hormonal regimens have failed to mobilize the subcutaneous calcium. Individual lesions can be excised.

Subepidermal Calcified Nodule

(Winer 1952; Woods and Kellaway 1963)

Synonyms. Calculus cutaneous, localized idiopathic calcinosis

Etiology and Pathogenesis. The etiology is unclear. In some cases, a precursor lesion such as a melanocytic nevus, cyst, or sebaceous gland has been identified histologically, but in most cases there is no clue.

Clinical Findings. Most often there is a single or small number of dermal or subcutaneous nodules. They are usually pale in color, although they may be inflamed, hyperkeratotic, or even ulcerated. Winer described lesions in infants or children, occasionally congenital in nature, while Woods and Kellaway reported on lesions in both children and adults. Typical locations include the face and digits.

Histopathology. Usually the lesion is submitted as a cyst or dermatofibroma, but the histology shows nests or clusters of amorphous calcified masses. Multiple sections should be taken to see if a preexisting lesion has been calcified.

Therapy. Excision.

Idiopathic Scrotal Calcinosis

Etiology and Pathogenesis. This name is probably also incorrect. Most patients have multiple scrotal cysts which tend to calcify. In other instances, eccrine milia appear to serve as the nidus.

Clinical Findings. Usually, multiple nodules are found on the scrotum. They range from a few millimeters to several centimeters in size. Some are yellowish white and resemble epidermoid cysts. Others are inflamed and may ulcerate with discharge of chalky material. Most patients present as adolescents or young adults. They complain either of pain or simply are disturbed by the increasing number of bumps on their scrota. In rare cases, patients have only single lesions.

Histopathology. We suspect that idiopathic scrotal calcinosis is in most cases truly a dystrophic calcification. If multiple sections are taken and several lesions studied, one can usually find remnants of an epidermoid cyst or blocked eccrine duct associated with granulomatous inflammation. In other patients, multiple epidermoid cysts will be present along with several calcified lesions.

Therapy. Excision.

Auricular Calcinosis

Clinically, one or more small, white papules are noticed on the free edge of the helix. Often the edge appears beaded, like a rosary chain. The papules are painless, although they may occasionally ulcerate. They usually follow some form of trauma such as auricular pernio, frostbite, ochronosis, acromegaly, and perhaps even relapsing polychondritis. Most often however, the patient has no idea of the trigger.

Elastotic nodules of the ear are very similar and may be precursor lesions. In chondrodermatitis nodularis helicis, the lesion is usually solitary, painful, and not located directly on the edge of the helix. In addition, some scale or crust is present, often with a central dell. The lesions from gout are larger. Other considerations include basal cell carcinoma and granuloma annulare. No therapy is needed, but individual lesions can be easily excised.

Bibliography

Calcinosis Cutis

Basis Science and Reviews

Bucko AD, Burgdorf WC (1997) Cutaneous calcification. In: Demis JD (ed) Clinical dermatology, vol 2 (12.12). Lippincott-Raven, Philadelphia, pp 1–18
Hussmann J, Russell RC, Kucan JO et al. (1995) Soft-tissue calcifications: differential diagnosis and therapeutic approaches. Ann Plast Surg 34:138–147
Mehregan AH (1984) Calcinosis cutis: a review of the clinical forms and report of 75 cases. Semin Dermatol 3:53–61
Orlow SJ, Watsky KL, Bolognia JL (1991) Skin and bones. I. J Am Acad Dermatol 25:205–221
Orlow SJ, Watsky KL, Bolognia JL (1991) Skin and bones. II. J Am Acad Dermatol 25:447–462
Touart DM, Sau P (1998) Cutaneous deposition diseases, part II. Am Acad Dermatol 39:527–544
Walsh JS, Fairley JA (1995) Calcifying disorders of the skin. J Am Acad Dermatol 33:693–706
Walsh JS, Perniciaro C, Randle HW (1999) Calcifying basal cell carcinomas. Dermatol Surg 25:49–51

Metastatic Calcification

Cockerell CJ, Dolan ET (1992) Widespread cutaneous and systemic calcification (calciphylaxis) in patients with the acquired immunodeficiency syndrome and renal disease. J Am Acad Dermatol 26:559–562
Hafner J, Keusch K, Wahl C, Sauter B et al. (1995) Uremic small-artery disease with medial calcification and intimal hyperplasia (so-called calciphylaxis): a complication of chronic renal failure and benefit from parathyroidectomy. J Am Acad Dermatol 33:954–962
Kerr DN (1997) Hypercalcemia and metastatic calcification. Cardiovasc Res 36:293–297
Oh DH, Eulau D, Tokugawa DA et al. (1999) Five cases of calciphylaxis and a review of the literature. J Am Acad Dermatol 40:979–987
Selye H (1962) Calciphylaxis. University of Chicago Press, Chicago
Winkelmann RK, Keating FR Jr (1970) Cutaneous vascular calcification, gangrene, and hyperparathyroidism. Br J Dermatol 83:263–268
Zouboulis CC, Blume-Peytavi U, Lennert T et al. (1996) Fulminant metastatic calcinosis with cutaneous necrosis in a child with end-stage renal disease and tertiary hyperparathyroidism. Br J Dermatol 135:617–622

Dystrophic Calcification

Azón-Masoliver A, Ferrando J, Navarra E et al. (1989) Solitary congenital nodular calcification of Winer located on the ear: report of two cases. Pediatr Dermatol 6:191–193
Christensen OB (1978) An exogenous variety of pseudoxanthoma elasticum in old farmers. Acta Derm Venereol (Stockh) 58:319–321
Goldminz D, Barnhill R, McGuire J, Stenn KS (1988) Calcinosis cutis following extravasation of calcium chloride. Arch Dermatol 124:922–925
Johnson RC, Fitzpatrick JE, Hahn DE (1993) Calcinosis cutis following electromyographic examination. Cutis 52:161–164
Kanda A, Uchimiya H, Ohtake N et al. (1999) Two cases of gigantic dystrophic calcinosis cutis caused by subcutaneous and/or intramuscular injections. J Dermatol 26:371–374
Marzano AV, Kolesnikova LV, Gasparini G et al. (1999) Dystrophic calcinosis cutis in subacute lupus. Dermatology 198:90–92
Mills CM, Knight AG (1993) Cutaneous calcinosis. An unusual complication of intravenous phosphate administration. Clin Exp Dermatol 18:370–372
Pitt AE, Ethington JE, Troy JL (1990) Self-healing dystrophic calcinosis following trauma with transepidermal elimination. Cutis 45:28–30
Sahn EE, Smith DJ (1992) Annular dystrophic calcinosis cutis in an infant. J Am Acad Dermatol 26:1015–1017

Sell EJ, Hansen RC, Struck-Pierce S (1980) Calcified nodules on the heel: a complication of neonatal intensive care. Pediatrics 96:473

Song DH, Lee KH, Kang WH (1988) Idiopathic calcinosis of the scrotum: Histopathologic observations of 51 nodules. J Am Acad Dermatol 19:1095–1101

Swinehart JM, Golitz SE (1982) Scrotal calcinosis: dystrophic calcification of epidermoid cysts. Arch Dermatol 118:985–988

Walsh JS, Fairley JA (1995) Calcifying disorders of the skin. J Am Acad Dermatol 33:693–706

Wang WJ, Lo WL, Wong CK (1988) Calcinosis cutis in juvenile dermatomyositis: remarkable response to aluminium hydroxide therapy. Arch Dermatol 124:1721–1722

Wheeland RG, Roundtree JM (1985) Calcinosis cutis resulting from percutaneous penetration and deposition of calcium. J Am Acad Dermatol 12:172–175

Wiley HE III, Eaglstein WE (1979) Calcinosis cutis in children following electroencephalography. JAMA 242:455–456

Idiopathic Calcification

Abraham Z, Rozner I, Rozenbaum M (1996) Tumoral calcinosis: report of a case and brief review of the literature. J Dermatol 23:545–550

Gormally S, Dorman T, Powell FC (1992) Calcinosis of the scrotum. Int J Dermatol 31:75–79

Harwood CA, Cook MG, Mortimer PS (1996) Tumoral calcinosis: an unusual cause of cutaneous calcification. Clin Exp Dermatol 21:163–166

Rodriguez-Cano L, Garcia-Patos V, Creus M et al. (1996) Childhood calcinosis cutis. Pediatr Dermatol 13:114–117

Shmunes E, Wood MG (1972) Subepidermal calcified nodules. Arch Dermatol 105:593–597

Teutschländer O (1935) Über progressive Lipogranulomatose der Muskulatur. Zugleich ein Beitrag zur Pathogenese der Myopathia osteoplastica progressiva. Klin Wochenschr 14:451–453

Thibierge G, Weissenbach RJ (1911) Concrétions calcaires sous-cutanées et sclérodermie. Ann Dermatol Syphil 2:129–155

Velayos EE, Masi AT, Stevens MB et al. (1979) The 'CREST' syndrome. Comparison with systemic sclerosis (scleroderma). Arch Intern Med 139:1240–1244

Winer LH (1952) Solitary congenital nodular calcification of the skin. Arch Dermatol 66:204–211

Winterbauer RH (1964) Multiple telangiectasia, Raynaud's phenomenon, sclerodactyly and subcutaneous calcinosis. Bull Johns Hopkins Hosp 114:361–383

Woods B, Kellaway TD (1963) Cutaneous calculi. Subepidermal calcified nodules. Br J Dermatol 75:1–11

CHAPTER 46

Disorders of Mineral Metabolism

Contents

Iron

Iron is a common but crucial element in the body. The average adult has 4–5 g of iron, absorbing about 1 mg daily and losing a similar amount. Iron is absorbed from the gastrointestinal tract and attached to transferrin. It is then distributed to the peripheral tissues. About two-thirds of the iron is involved in red cell production, either in the bone marrow or in circulating erythrocytes. The rest is incorporated into myoglobin, bound in hepatocytes or attached to the two iron storage proteins ferritin and hemosiderin. The latter two proteins are stored in the liver, spleen and bone marrow, where they offer iron stores that can be readily mobilized. Ferritin consists of ferric salts and apoferritin; it is water soluble. Hemosiderin is insoluble, dark brown and usually found in macrophages; it consists of altered ferritin complexes. Hemosiderin is seen in the skin following leakage of blood into the dermis, because the dermal scavengers only slowly and inefficiently remove iron stores.

Iron Deficiency

The most common causes of iron deficiency are increased blood loss from the gastrointestinal or genitourinary tracts, increased iron demand as in pregnancy, inadequate intake, for example in vegetarian diets and impaired gastrointestinal absorption either following surgery or because of various types of malabsorption. In menstruating females, iron deficiency is generally ascribed to menses, although occasionally several factors may interplay. Patients with severe skin disease, such as widespread psoriasis or erythroderma of any cause, are also often iron deficient. They typically lose iron as a part of the massive epidermal turnover and also typically have a degree of enteropathy.

The best known manifestation of iron deficiency is microcytic anemia. There are also a number of mucocutaneous features, discussed in Chapter 33. None are truly specific for iron deficiency and a large number of patients, especially women, lack iron, so often associations are drawn that are not entirely rigorous. Perlèche and glossitis are the two most cited features of iron deficiency, but both are more common in patients with multiple nutritional deficits. Diffuse alopecia is a possible marker for iron deficiency, while burning of the tongue is almost never a solitary marker. Two far less common but more specific signs are koilonychia (Chap. 32) and dysphasia from esophageal web formation (Plummer-Vinson syndrome). If iron deficiency is discovered during routine screening, the patient should have a hematologic evaluation before iron is administered. Once replacement has been started, further hematologic studies are more complicated. Mucocutaneous problems respond only slowly to iron replacement.

Hemochromatosis

Synonyms. Bronze diabetes, siderosis, Troisier-Hanot-Chauffard syndrome (1872, 1882)

Definition. Inherited disorder in which body iron stores are increased caused multisystem damage.

Epidemiology. Hemochromatosis is one of the most common genetic disorders. About 10% of adults are heterozygous carriers, while 3–4/1000 are homozygotes and have the disease. Onset is in adult life; problems start about a decade earlier in men (>50 years) than in women (> 60 years) and tend to be more severe.

Etiology and Pathogenesis. The responsible gene is known as HLA-H and is located on chromosome 6p21.3 near the HLA-A locus. The gene's function is unclear, but the main defect appears to reside in the gastrointestinal cells, which absorb too much iron. Heterozygotes or carriers may store excess iron, but only homozygotes become symptomatic. The onset of problems is accelerated in those with marked alcohol intake and delayed in women because of the iron loss associated with menstruation. The iron stimulates the production of free radicals, which lead to cell damage, fibrosis (especially in the liver as cirrhosis) and cell death. In some models iron is also a carcinogen, perhaps helping to explain the risk of hepatic carcinoma in hemochromatosis.

Secondary hemochromatosis is the result of multiple blood transfusions, as in sickle cell anemia or thalassemia. It can also be caused by excessive ingestion of iron, either as foods or medications. Alcohol ingestion appears to be a cofactor, as many symptomatic patients also have alcoholic liver disease. Patients with porphyria cutanea tarda also develop iron overload and may carry the gene for hemochromatosis, but their levels of iron are much lower than in hemochromatosis. The Bantu in southern Africa brew their local beer in iron pots and are thereby afflicted with hemochromatosis, cirrhosis and porphyria cutanea tarda.

Clinical Findings. Iron is deposited in a variety of tissues, leading to a whole spectrum of problems.

Cutaneous Findings. The skin acquires a slate gray or gray-brown discoloration, which in severe cases may take on the a bronze tone. Light-exposed areas are most prominently involved, involving the face and back of the hands. The increased pigment is melanin, not iron. The patient's skin is also dry and may even be ichthyosis-like. Many patients lose secondary sexual hairs as a result of pituitary insufficiency. Koilonychia can be seen and spotty intraoral pigmentation may be found.

Systemic Findings. The systemic findings are more dramatic.

- Liver disease: Hepatic deposition is often the main problem, especially in alcoholic patients. There is hepatosplenomegaly, cirrhosis and a significant risk of hepatocellular carcinoma. Esophageal varices are also a complication.
- Pancreas: The infiltration leads to reduced insulin production, known as bronze diabetes.
- Pituitary: Many different problems arise including hypogonadism, impotence, gynecomastia, loss of axillary and pubic hairs and hypothyroidism.
- Heart: Arrhythmias and cardiac failure can be seen.
- Joints: Polyarthritis with chondrocalcinosis may develop mimicking osteoarthritis or leading to an erosive arthropathy. The function of iron overload in this process is unclear.

Histopathology. The skin shows increased basal layer melanin and deposition of hemosiderin in the dermis. Sometimes the pigment is concentrated around sweat glands and endothelial cells. In patients with both vitiligo and hemochromatosis, the areas that are clinically white show abundant iron but no increase in melanin under the microscope.

Laboratory Findings. Serum ferritin is markedly increased, often exceeding 1000 µg/l. Serum iron is also elevated. Liver function tests may be normal, so a liver biopsy should be performed to assess the degree of cirrhosis, which is the most important prognostic factor. At this time, liver iron levels can be measured; usually more than 180 µg/g of dry liver are present. All first degree relatives should be screened for abnormal serum ferritin and iron levels. In most pedigrees, the gene can be identified, usually via other HLA linkages.

Course and Prognosis. The prognosis is dependent on the time of diagnosis and the patient's ability to avoid further liver disease, i.e., to quit drinking alcohol. About 10% of patients develop hepatocellular carcinoma but they are most often those with severe cirrhosis. In young patients, there may be a fulminant course with cardiac complications.

Differential Diagnosis. The many causes of diffuse hyperpigmentation are discussed in Chapter 26. Argyria, arsenic pigmentation, Addison disease, ochronosis, Gaucher disease and perhaps porphyria cutanea tarda should be considered.

Therapy. The mainstay is phlebotomy. Large amounts of iron are present, so the bleeding must be quite aggressive, often requiring removal of 500 ml weekly for several years, and then decreasing the frequency once ferritin levels are normal. A diet low in iron is helpful but insignificant in comparison to phlebotomy. Chelating agents, such as deferoxamine, can be used in anemic individuals. The other problems are treated in standard fashion.

Zinc

Zinc is required for a variety of metalloenzymes (carbonic anhydrase, alcohol dehydrogenase, lactate dehydrogenase, alkaline phosphatase and many others), is an important component of many DNA transcription factors (known as zinc fingers) and is required for the synthesis of many proteins. The body contains 1.0–2.5 g of zinc, distributed among many organs including skin and hair (which can be used to measure zinc levels). In the plasma, about one-third is bound to albumin and the rest to globulins. Measuring plasma zinc levels is quite an art, because red cells are rich in zinc and many blood drawing systems also contain zinc.

Zinc Intoxication

Zinc is used therapeutically in hepatic encephalopathy and occasionally, with less data, for other problems, such as impaired wound healing, acne and alopecia areata. While its efficacy is sometimes controversial, zinc sulfate is a very safe drug and toxicity is almost unheard of. Excess zinc does bind copper, producing a relative copper deficiency with a microcytic anemia. Neurologic symptoms have been observed following industrial exposure; this is known as metal fume fever or zinc shakes. Sometimes when beverages are brewed in a galvanized container, zinc levels may be high enough to cause nausea and vomiting.

Zinc Deficiency

There are many ways to become zinc deficient including:

- Inadequate dietary zinc, as in fad diets, eating disorders, certain infant formulas, diets with high phytate (green leaf) content, alcoholism
- Failure to absorb zinc, as in inflammatory bowel disease, malabsorption, other causes of chronic diarrhea, pancreatitis, chronic renal disease
- Increased zinc usage, as in pregnancy and lactation, burns, post-operatively and in any severe disease, such as a malignancy

In a rare disorder, acrodermatitis enteropathica, patients are unable to absorb zinc. They are described in more detail below, but patients with acquired zinc deficiency have virtually identical clinical changes. In some instances zinc deficiency may cause skin changes similar to necrolytic migratory erythema, which is usually associated with a pancreatic glucagonoma.

Zinc deficiency is characterized by acral and periorificial skin disease, diarrhea (producing a vicious cycle), growth retardation, photophobia and CNS changes. In infants, the skin changes usually are most striking, but in adults with perhaps less severe degrees of deficiency, mood changes, impaired wound healing, hypogeusia (impaired sense of taste) and other rarer manifestations may be seen. Zinc seems essential for a wide variety of immunologic functions, as both impaired cellular and humoral responses can be identified. Zinc deficiency should be suspected in burn patients as well as in those with inflammatory bowel disease, on parenteral nutrition or with metastatic malignancies. The term marginal zinc deficiency has been applied to patients with chronic, slightly below normal zinc levels; a wide variety of problems have been blamed on reduced zinc levels but much controversy remains.

Zinc appears to play a role in wound healing. Patients with leg ulcers and low zinc levels show improved healing rates with replacement therapy. The role of zinc in speeding healing in patients with already normal levels is unclear. Zinc replacement has been suggested in acne, atopic dermatitis and alopecia areata, but there is little evidence of a deficiency.

In the animal world, zinc deficiency is known as parakeratosis, seen primarily in calves and piglets. It is inherited in an autosomal recessive pattern. The animals have psoriasiform skin changes especially acrally and periorificially as well as skin fragility. They tend to die of severe infections and failure to thrive.

Acrodermatitis Enteropathica

(Brandt 1936; Danbolt and Closs 1942)

Definition. Inherited disorder with impaired intestinal zinc absorption leading to acral and periorificial skin changes, as well as diarrhea.

Epidemiology. This disorder is extremely rare; an incidence of 1:500,000 has been estimated in Denmark.

Etiology and Pathogenesis. While inheritance is in an autosomal recessive pattern, the genetic defect is unknown. The patients are unable to absorb zinc in the gastrointestinal tract. Human milk contains zinc-binding proteins that facilitate transfer. Two dermatologists, Moynahan in the UK and Neldner in the USA, were instrumental in establishing zinc deficiency as the cause of acrodermatitis enteropathica.

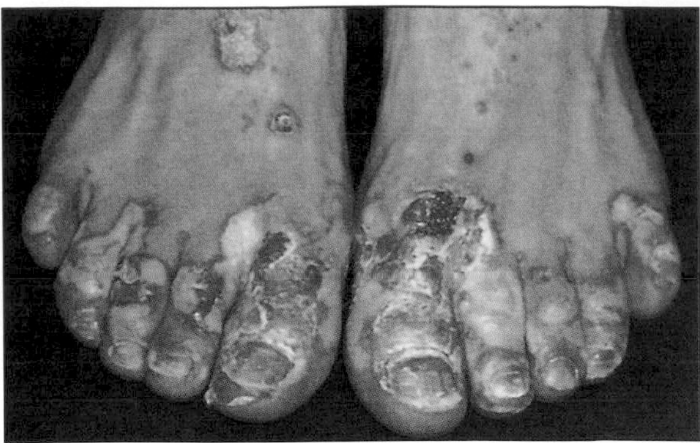

Fig. 46.2. Acrodermatitis enteropathica

Clinical Findings

Cutaneous Findings. The clinical problems start days after birth or weaning. The typical sites of involvement are periorificial (about the mouth, nostrils and perianal region) and acral (fingers, toes, palms, soles) (Figs. 46.1, 46.2). The typical lesion is an eroded, crusted, sharply bordered erythematous patch with central crust and peripheral vesicles or pustules. The chronic, rather polymorphic eruption is often psoriasiform. The perianal and perioral lesions are almost invariably initially diagnosed as *Candida albicans* and so treated. Often the yeast can be cultured as part of the spectrum of secondary infections. In addition, the patient's immune status is weakened, so more significant *C. albicans* infections are possible.

The adnexal structures are also involved. Almost every child has diffuse alopecia and paronychiae leading to dystrophic nails. In some cases zebra hairs with light and dark bands may develop, presumably reflecting varying zinc levels. There may also be glossitis and stomatitis. Women with acrodermatitis enteropathica tend to have difficulties in pregnancy. Prior to zinc replacement, they often had catastrophic problems. Today they simply must be sure to increase their zinc ingestion.

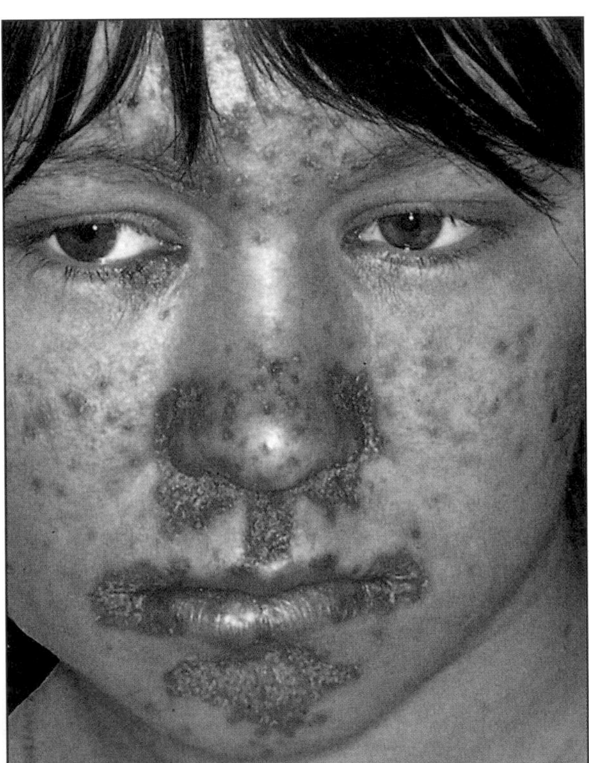

Fig. 46.1. Acrodermatitis enteropathica

Systemic Findings. Failure to thrive is the most consistent finding. Patients have varying degrees of diarrhea, which can be severe. They may also have a variety of mood changes, irritability, blepharitis, photophobia, chronic otitis media and many other problems.

Histopathology. In the early lesions there is striking parakeratosis overlying a spongiotic acanthotic epidermis with basket-weave hyperkeratosis. The upper layers of the epidermis are necrotic and pale. Intraepidermal clefts may also be found. In the latter lesions, the distinctive pallor is replaced by psoriasiform hyperplasia and crust. In the papillary dermis there is a lymphohistiocytic perivascular infiltrate. The changes in necrolytic migratory erythema are similar.

Laboratory Findings. The plasma zinc levels are very low. Normal values are 70–110 μg/dl. Serum levels are somewhat higher. If the plasma is not separated immediately, its zinc levels will be falsely elevated. Many aspects of blood collection and analysis involve zinc-containing compounds, so contamination is a potential problem. There are significant diurnal variations in zinc levels, as well as fluctuations during severe illness, burns and similar events. Urinary zinc levels are vary variable but do decline as the serum zinc levels drop.

Course and Prognosis. If the problem is not recognized and treated, most patients die young or suffer greatly. Today all do well with zinc replacement therapy.

Differential Diagnosis. Seborrheic dermatitis and atopic dermatitis usually do not appear in the first days of life, but come into question when severe dermatitis follows weaning. Multiple carboxylase deficiency (biotin deficiency) is clinically identical. Widespread candidiasis is often diagnosed, but usually incorrectly. When severe blistering occurs, epidermolysis bullosa should be considered. Necrolytic migratory erythema, while similar, is a disease of adults. The many causes of secondary zinc deficiency discussed above should be excluded in adult cases.

Therapy. Oral zinc therapy is miraculous. The skin lesions begin to improve within 1–2 days and are clear within a week. Replacement should be lifelong. The usual dose is 30–150 mg daily.

Copper

Copper is an essential enzyme cofactor. It is transported in the plasma bound to ceruloplasmin. Copper is required for cytochrome oxidase or mitochondrial energy utilization, tyrosinase and thus melanin production, as well as for lysyl oxidase, which is a key enzyme in elastin production. Acquired copper deficiency is most uncommon, although dietary deficiencies and malabsorption can produce reduced serum levels. However, there are two inherited disorders of copper metabolism that have dermatologic manifestations, as discussed below. Copper toxicity can result from ingestion of large amounts of the metal, producing hemolytic anemia and abdominal problems but no skin findings.

Menkes Syndrome

(Menkes et al. 1962)

Synonyms. Kinky hair syndrome, trichopoliodystrophy

Definition. Inherited disorder in which the intestinal absorption of copper is inadequate leading to primarily cutaneous and CNS problems.

Epidemiology. Menkes syndrome is a very rare, X-linked recessive inherited disorder. The incidence ranges from 1/35,000–1/100,000.

Etiology and Pathogenesis. The gene is located at Xq12–q13 and encodes a copper transport ATPase. There is faulty intestinal uptake of copper leading to low serum copper and ceruloplasmin levels. Metallothioneine, an important transport protein, is apparently a key factor in copper uptake and it appears to be abnormal. The impaired lysyl oxidase and tyrosinase functions lead to cutaneous findings caused by elastin and melanin defects, but the entire enzymatic system of the patient is virtually on arrest because copper is such an essential cofactor.

Clinical Findings

Cutaneous Findings. The classic feature is hypopigmented, brittle steel wool-like hairs. The scalp hairs are broken off and short; they also show a variety of structural defects including pili torti, trichorrhexis nodosa and monilethrix. The eyebrows and eyelashes may also be broken off. The skin is hypopigmented, reflecting the decreased melanin, and puffy or doughy because of defective elastin. The upper lip may have a characteristic "cupid's bow" pucker to it. Focal hypopigmentation has been described in female carriers.

Systemic Findings. The infant is profoundly ill. Mental retardation coupled with seizures, hypotonia and lethargy are the most dramatic finding. The CNS problems are progressive. The arteries are tortuous, as may be observed in the retina or even the skin, as they lack adequate elastin. More importantly, there may be large vessel disease or skin hemorrhages that can be mistaken for child abuse. Radiologic examination may reveal metaphyseal widening in the long bones and wormian bones, which are free bones in the skull suture lines named after Worm, a 16th century Danish anatomist. Multiple genitourinary defects also occur.

Laboratory Findings. Serum copper and ceruloplasmin levels are dramatically reduced. Prenatal diagnosis has been done via assessment of amniotic cell copper metabolism but genetic diagnosis is on the way. This will be a reliable way to screen carriers, who may have minor hair problems.

Course and Prognosis. Dismal; patients succumb within 2–3 years.

Differential Diagnosis. Björnstad syndrome presents with congenital pili torti and deafness but no CNS defects. Argininosuccinic aciduria and other amino acid defects are also similar but can be separated quickly via laboratory testing.

Therapy. Copper supplementation even with massive intramuscular doses has been shown not to help. When it was employed, sometimes the hair or skin became darker, but the more serious problems remained unaffected.

Wilson Disease

(WILSON 1912)

Definition. Inherited disorder in which copper excretion is abnormal causing primarily hepatic disease.

Epidemiology. Wilson disease is inherited in an autosomal recessive pattern. The incidence is about 1:50,000.

Etiology and Pathogenesis. The gene is located on chromosome 13q14.2 and its product is also involved in copper transport. The patients are unable to combine copper with ceruloplasmin in the liver and excrete it in the bile in a normal fashion, so the metal accumulates in a variety of tissues. The genetic defect in Wilson disease has DNA homology to that in Menkes syndrome, even though two different chromosomes are involved.

Clinical Findings

Cutaneous Findings. The skin changes are minor and few patients find their way to the dermatologist. The most striking finding is the blue lunulae of the nails. In addition, there may be gray-brown hyperpigmentation, often limited to the pretibial region. In patients treated with penicillamine, elastosis perforans serpiginosa may develop.

Systemic Findings. The best known finding is the Kayser-Fleischer ring, a yellow-brown ring that results from copper deposition in the cornea. This change is best seen with slit-lamp examination. One must be suspicious of Wilson disease in any infant with unexplained liver disease or CNS findings. The liver changes can progress to cirrhosis and liver failure, while the CNS problems include decreased coordination, ataxia and dementia. Copper deposition is marked in the basal ganglia and cortical areas. A variety of renal problems may develop, presumably from toxic copper deposits.

Laboratory Findings. Serum ceruloplasmin levels are reduced while serum and urinary copper levels are elevated. Radioisotope-labeled copper is poorly incorporated into ceruloplasmin.

In some cases all laboratory tests are normal and a liver biopsy must be done to determine hepatic copper levels. Siblings of known patients should be carefully screened and followed.

Course and Prognosis. The prognosis is good if the diagnosis is made before significant CNS problems have developed. The other problems tend to reverse more easily with therapy than do the neurologic changes.

Differential Diagnosis. The various causes of hyperpigmentation are considered in Chapter 26. The regional localization may provide a clue. Gaucher disease may have hepatic disease, CNS disease and hyperpigmentation. The presence of blue lunulae is so rare that one should immediately think of Wilson disease.

Therapy. Chelation of the copper with penicillamine is helpful, as the excess copper is excreted in the urine. However, penicillamine has a host of side effects and is poorly tolerated over a lifetime. Trientene hydrochloride is an even more toxic alternative chelator. Thus, Wilson disease patients have become leading candidates for liver transplantation, as the new liver is able to make the appropriate transport protein and excrete the copper. Lowered dietary copper and use of oral zinc to block copper absorption are two useful adjuncts.

Sulfur

Sulfur is another essential element. It is a component of several amino acids that are important in the skin including cystine, cysteine and methionine. These amino acids are required for keratinization, especially of the hairs, and are also involved in synthesis of the dermal ground substance, primarily chondroitin sulfate. Sulfur deficiency is most likely to cause trouble with the hair and nails, but pure sulfur or sulfate deficits are extremely rare. In exfoliative dermatoses, sulfur may be lost along with many other elements. In trichothiodystrophy (Chap. 31) the sulfur content (more exactly the cysteine and cystine levels) of the hairs is greatly reduced, leading to short, rough hairs.

Mercury

Exposure to mercury can occur through industrial fumes, exposure to significant amounts of metallic liquid mercury, and formerly through both systemic (mercury diuretics) and topical (ammoniated mercury) medications. Methylmercury accumulates in fish, which are an additional source of the element. The two exposures patients most often fear – from a broken thermometer and from merthiolate used for wound care – are only rarely a source of problems. Mercury has become a very controversial element in Europe because of the arguments over the toxicity of amalgam (Chap. 33).

Mercury Poisoning

Acute mercury poising usually presents with gastrointestinal distress, abdominal pain and often renal disease or even failure. Chronic mercury poisoning is characterized by CNS disturbances and gingival hyperpigmentation. Because of the frequency of chronic mercury poisoning in the hat industry in the past, the saying "mad as a hatter" came about. This is beautifully described in Carroll's *Alice in Wonderland.*

A special form of mercury poisoning of interest to dermatologists is acrodynia or pink disease. Patients are typically children with CNS disease and cold, clammy swollen reds hands and feet with hyperhidrosis and desquamation. If the disease is not diagnosed promptly, they may develop alopecia, nail loss, teeth damage, burning and pain in their extremities and more severe neurologic findings. Pink disease has been reported in patients with no history of mercury exposure except a recent broken thermometer with the mercury dispersed in the carpet or bedding. Urine mercury levels of 10 µg/l are normal, but patients with much lower levels may have dramatic rises in excretion when treated treated with a chelating agent such as 2,3-dimercaptosuccinic acid.

Lead

Epidemiology. Lead is a ubiquitous poison that causes a variety of problems. Lead poisoning is known as plumbism. There are many possible ways to be exposed to lead. Probably the most common is the ingestion of chips of lead-containing paint by children. The habitual ingestion of nonnutritive substances is known as pica; all such children should be checked for possible lead toxicity. Other individuals may ingest lead-containing objects such as shot, fishing weights and similar materials; the stomach acids slowly leach out the mineral. Acidic beverages that are stored in either ceramic or metal containers containing lead may become contaminated. This was a particular problem for consumers of moonshine in rural areas of the Southeastern USA. Fumes from leaded gasoline or lead-painted wood burned in fireplaces may also be a source. A variety of folk medicines also contain lead salts.

Etiology and Pathogenesis. Most of the effects of lead are toxic, affecting a variety of tissues directly. In the brain, cerebral edema appears to be the main problem. Lead inhibits δ-amino levulinic acid dehydrase. This may explain some of the overlaps between lead and acute intermittent porphyria.

Clinical Findings

Systemic Findings. The most disturbing findings are cognitive problems, hematologic disease and chronic renal damage. In adults, the onset of trouble tends to be slow, while in children it may be abrupt or insidious. Patients present with intestinal colic, headache. In children there are behavioral problems, ataxia and seizures. Chronic exposure leads to accumulation of lead in the kidneys with tubulointerstitial damage. The CNS and renal problems may nonetheless persist after lead exposure is stopped and therapy instituted.

Cutaneous Findings. Lead poisoning should be diagnosed before cutaneous changes appear. Lead may cause hyperpigmentation of the gingiva, often appearing as a peripheral blue-black line. There may also be patchy mucosal hyperpigmentation or, rarely, generalized cutaneous hyperpigmentation.

Laboratory Findings. The diagnosis is made based on lead and free erythrocyte protoporphyrin (FEP) levels. The latter is a good screening test, as FEP is a sensitive indicator of the effect of lead on heme synthesis.

Therapy. Stopping exposure and aggressive chelation are required. Usually both dimercaprol (BAL) and edetate calcium disodium (calcium EDTA) are employed.

Iodine

Iodine is required for normal thyroid function (Chap. 48). Some 80 % of the body's iodine is contained in thyroglobulin. Iodine deficiency can result when the local soil and thus drinking water is low in the element. For this reason, many countries insist on the use of iodinated salt (NaCl) in the food industry and recommend it for home use. Iodine deficiency usually results in a goiter in adults but can cause cretinism in infants and children. Iodides are used in the form of supersaturated potassium iodide (SSKI) in the treatment of sporotrichosis and occasionally other granulomatous diseases, including some forms of panniculitis. Excess iodides or other halogens can cause halogenoderma and exacerbate acne and dermatitis herpetiformis. Individuals eating kelp or seaweed diets, as well as those who consume too much salt, may also develop halogenoderma.

Selenium

Selenium is metabolically closely related to vitamin E and is involved in a variety of essential glutathione reactions. Its deficiency has been well-established in some regions of China where it causes Keshan disease, a childhood cardiomyopathy. Muscle pain and tenderness, as well as whitening of the nail beds, have been described to improve with replacement therapy. However, in other regions of China, selenium toxicity has been identified with hair and nail loss, flaking skin and neurologic findings. Selenosis is better established in animals. Since the margin of safety between too little and too much selenium is unclear, selenium supplements for nail growth or oxidative protection are questionable at this time.

Bibliography

Iron Metabolism and Iron Deficiency

Blankship MI (1971) Dysplastic hairs in iron deficiency anemia. Cutis 7:467

Hard S (1963) Non-anemic iron deficiency as an aetiological factor in diffuse loss of hair of the scalp in woman. Acta Dermato Venereol (Stockh) 43:652–659

Sato S (1991) Iron deficiency: structural and microchemical changes in hair, nails and skin. Semin Dermatol 10: 313–319

Weijmer M, Neering H, Welten C (1990) Preliminary report: furuncolosis and hypoferaemia. Lancet 336:464–466

Hemochromatosis

Bothwell Th, Charlton RW, Motulsky AG (1995) Hemochromatosis. In: Scriver CR, Beaudet AL, Sly WS et al. (eds) The metabolic and molecular bases of inherited disease, 7th end, McGraw-Hill, New York, pp 2237–2270

Cartwright GE, Edwards CQ, Kravitz K et al. (1979) Hereditary hemochromatosis. Phenotypic expression of the disease. N Engl J Med 301:175–179

Chevrant-Breton J, Simon M, Bourel M et al. (1977) Cutaneous manifestations of idiopathic hemochromatosis: study of 100 cases. Arch Dermatol 113:161–165

Hanot VC, Chauffard AM (1882) Cirrhose hypertrophique pigmentaire dans le diabète sucré. Rev Méd 2:385–403

Mildner MS, Cook JD, Straay S et al. (1980) Idiopathic hemochromatosis, an interim report. Medicine (Baltimore) 59:34–49

Nichols GM, Bacon BR (1989) Hereditary hemochromatosis: pathogenesis and clinical features of a common disease. Am J Gastroenterol 84:851–862

O'Reilly FM, Carby C, Fogarty J et al. (1997) Screening of patients with iron overload to identify hemochromatosis and porphyria cutanea tarda. Arch Dermatol 133:1098–1101

Roberts AG, Whatley SD, Morgan RR et al. (1997) Increased frequency of the haemo-chromatosis Cys282Tyr mutation in sporadic porphyria cutenea tarda. Lancet 349: 1025–1025

Santos M, Clevers HC, Marx JJM (1997) Mutation of hereditary hemochromatosis candidate gene HLA-H in porphyria cutanea tarda. N Engl J Med 336:1326–1327

Troisier CE (1871) Diabète sucré. Bull Soc Anat 16:231

Sulfur

Alapetite C, Benoit A, Moustacchi E et al. (1997) The comet assay as a repair test for prenatal diagnosis of xeroderma pigmentosum and trichothiodystrophy. J Invest Dermatol 108:154–159

Bracun R, Hemmer W, Wolf-Abdolvahab S et al. (1997) Diagnosis of trichothiodystrophy in 2 siblings. Dermatology 194:74–76

Chen E, Cleaver JE, Weber CA et al. (1994) Trichothyodystrophy: Clinical spectrum, central nervous system imaging, and biochemical characterization of two siblings. J Invest Dermatol 103:154S–158S

Hersh JH, Klein LR, Joyce MR et al. (1993) Trichothiodystrophy and associated anomalies: a variant of SIBIDS or new symptom complex? Pediatr Dermatol 10:117–122

Itkin PH, Pittelkow MR (1990) Trichothiodystrophy: review of sulfur-deficient brittle hair syndromes and association with the ectodermal dysplasia. J Am Acad Dermatol 22:705–717

McCuaig C, Marcoux D, Rasmussen JE et al. (1993) Trichothiodystrophy associated with photosensitivity, gonadal failure, and strikking osteosclerosis. J Am Acad Dermatol 28:820–826

Roe DA (1969) Sulphur metabolism in relation to cutaneous disease. Br J Dermatol 81 [Suppl]:49–69

Tolmie JL, Berker de D, Dawber R et al. (1994) Syndromes associated with trichothio-dystrophy. Clin Dysmorphol 3:1–14

Zinc

Brandt T (1936) Dermatitis in children with disturbance of the general condition and the adsorption of food elements. Acta Derm Venereol (Stockh) 17:513–546

Cochran RJ, Tucker SB, Flannigan SA (1985) Typical zinc therapy in acne vulgaris. Int J Dermatol 24:188–190

Danbolt N, Closs K (1942) Akrodermatitis enteropathica. Acta Derm Venereol (Stockh) 23:127–169

Delaporte E, Catteau B, Piette E (1997) Necrolytic migration erythema-like eruption in zinc deficiency associated with alcoholic liver disease. Br J Dermatol 137:1011–1031

Fraker PJ, Jardieu P, Cook J (1987) Zinc deficiency and immune function. Arch Dermatol 123:1699–1701

Krasovec M, Frenk E (1996) Acrodermatitis enteropathica secondary to Crohn's disease. Deramtology 193:361–363

Kumar SP, Anday EK (1984) Edema, hypoproteinemia, and zinc deficiency in low-birth-weight infants. Pediatrics 73:327–329

Kuramoto Y, Igarashi Y, Tagami H (1991) Acquired zinc deficiency in breast-fed infants. Semin Dermatol 10: 309–312

Moynahan EJ, Barnes PM (1972) Zinc deficiency and a synthetic diet for lactose intolerance. Lancet 1:676

Prasad AS (1995) Zinc: an overview. Nutritition 11 [Suppl]: 93–99

Sawai T, Sugiura H, Danno K et al. (1996) Acquired acrodermatitis enteropathica during chemotherapy for acute lymphocytic leukemia in a child with Down syndrome. Br J Dermatol 135:652–668

Sinclair SA, Reynolds NJ (1997) Necrolytic migratory erythema and zinc deficiency. Br J Dermatol 136:783–785

Strobel CT, Byrne WJ, Abramovits W et al. (1978) A zinc deficiency dermatitis in patients on total parenteral nutrition. Int J Dermatol 17:575–581

Copper

Menkes Syndrome

Danks DM (1995) Disorders of copper metabolism. In: Scriver CR, Beaudet AL, Sly WS et al. (eds) The metabolic and molecular bases of inherited disease, 7th end, McGraw-Hill, New York, pp 2211–2236

Gerdes AM, Tonnesen T, Pergament E et al. (1988) Variability in clinical expression of Menkes' syndrome. Eur J Pediatr 148:132–135

Harris ED (1993) Menkes' disease: perspective and update on a fatal copper disorder. Nutr Rev 51:235–238

Harris ED, Reddy MC, Quian Y et al. (1999) Multiple forms of the Menkes' Cu-ATPase. Adv Exp Med Biol 448:39–51

Hart DB (1983) Menkes' syndrome: an update review. J Am Acad Dermatol 9:145–152

Martins C, Goncalves C, Moreno A et al. (1997) Menkes' kinky hair syndrome: ultrastructural cutaneous alterations of the elastic fibers. Pediatr Dermatol 14:347–350

Menkes JH, Alter M, Steigleder GK et al. (1962) A sexlinked recessive disorder with retardation of growth peculiar hair, and focal cerebral and cerebellar degeneration. Pediatrics 29:764–779

Mortimer PS, Gummer D, English J et al. (1985) Acquired progressive kinking of hair. Report of six cases and review of literature. Arch Dermatol 121:1031–1033

Nadal D, Baerlocher K (1988) Menkes' disease: long-term treatment with copper and D-penicillamine. Eur J Pediatr 147:621–625

Wilson Disease

Arima M, Takeshita K, Yoshino K et al. (1977) Prognosis of Wilson's disease in childhood. Eur J Pediatr 126:147–154

Bacon BR, Schilsky ML (1999) New knowledge of genetic pathogenesis of hemochromatosis and Wilson's disease. Adv Intern Med 44:91–116

Dobyns WB, Goldstein NP, Gordon H (1979) Clinical spectrum of Wilson's disease. Hepatolenticular degeneration. Mayo Clin Proc 54:35–44

Ferlan-Marolt V, Stepec S (1999) Fulminant Wilsonian hepatitis unmasked by disease progression: report of a case and review of the literature. Dig Dis Sci 44:1054–1058

Hoogenraad TU, van der Hamer CJA, Hattum JV (1984) Effective treatment of Wilson's disease with oral zinc sulphate: two case reports. Br Med J 289:273–276

Kemppainen R, Palatsi R, Kallioninen M et al. A (1998) A homozygous nonsense mutation and a combination of two mutations of the Wilson's disease gene in patients with different lysyl oxidase activities in cultured fibroblasts. J Invest Dermatol 108:35–39

Miyagawa S, Yoshioka A, Hatoko M et al. (1987) Systemic sclerosis-like lesions during long-term penicillamine therapy for Wilson's disease. Br J Dermatol 116:95–100

Rodeck B (1999) Treatment of copper associated liver disease in childhood. Eur J Med Res 28:253–256

Schaefer M, Gitlin JD (1999) Genetic disorders of membrane transport. IV. Wilson's disease and Menkes' disease. Am J Physiol 276:311–314

Strickland GT, Leu ML (1975) Wilson's disease. Clinical and laboratory manifestations in 40 patients. Medicine (Baltimore) 54:113–137

Sturniolo GC, Mesteriner C, Irato P et al. (1999) Zinc therapy increases duodenal concen-trations of metallothionein and iron in Wilson's disease patients. Am J Gastroenterol 94:334–338

Wilson SAK (1912) Progressive lenticular degeneration: a familial nervous disease associated with cirrhosis of the liver. Brain (London) 34:295–509

CHAPTER 47

Disorders of Purine Metabolism

Contents

Introduction

Purine and pyrimidine nucleotides are important cellular constituents involved in energy transfer and metabolic control, as well as the synthesis of DNA and RNA. Purine metabolism can be divided into three parts: biosynthesis, catabolism to uric acid, and salvage to recover purine bases provided by the diet or catabolism (Fig. 47.1). There are many rare enzymatic defects involving these three steps. We consider only the Lesch-Nyhan syndrome, a dramatic problem centered around the salvage cycle. The only common defect involving purine metabolism is gout, in which the catabolism is deranged.

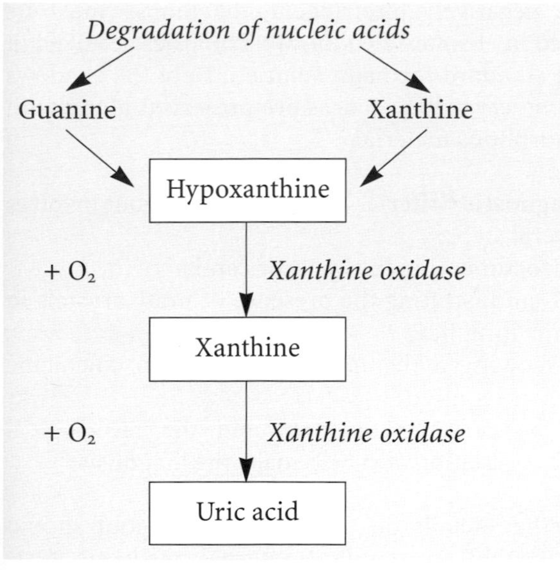

Fig. 47.1. Purine metabolism

Gout

Synonym. Podagra

Definition. Disorder with abnormal purine catabolism leading to hyperuricemia and then possible tissue deposition of urate crystals.

Epidemiology. Hyperuricemia is very common; between 2% and 12% of the population have elevated uric acid levels. The vast bulk of patients with gout are men (more than 95%); this is explained by a higher baseline or normal uric acid level. The upper limit of the normal value is 7.0 mg/dl in men and 6.0 mg/dl in women. The few women who develop gout are usually postmenopausal or have a predisposing factor.

Etiology and Pathogenesis. Gout is not a single disease. While a small number of patients are lacking a specific enzyme in the purine cycle, most do not have a defined problem but suffer from hyperuricemia. While most hyperuricemia is idiopathic or unexplained, sometimes it may be secondary to a high turnover of cells, such as in leukemia, in other myeloproliferative disorders, in polycythemia vera, following cancer chemotherapy with marked cell death, and even in proliferative skin disorders such as psoriasis. In all these cases, the system is confused with too many nucleic acids to recycle or salvage. Another mechanism for hyperuricemia is reduced renal excretion in lead poisoning, with alcohol abuse during diuretic therapy (especially with thiazides). Other medications such as low-dose aspirin may also drive up uric acid levels. A number of other disorders such as hyper- and hypoparathyroidism, hypothyroidism, chronic renal disease, myocardial infarction and obesity are also associated with hyperuricemia and gout through a variety of mechanisms. While in the past, dietary factors were considered important in hyperuricemia, modern investigations suggest they play less of a role. On the other hand, gout is rare in patients with eating disorders or malnutrition.

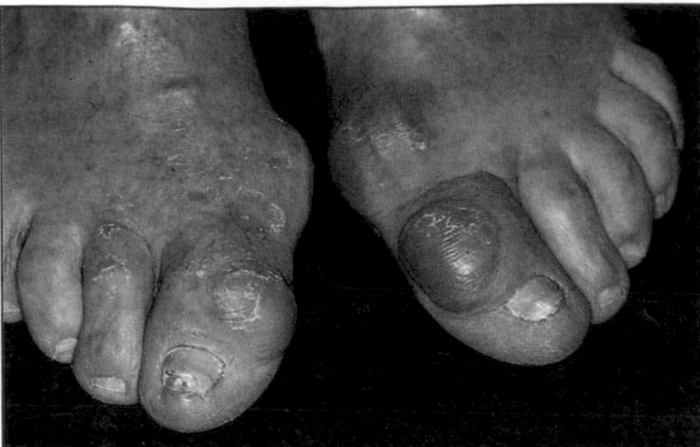

Fig. 47.2. Podagra

Hyperuricemia does not equal gout. Only a small percentage of people with elevated uric acid levels ever develop clinical gout. The key factor is the limited solubility of monosodium urate crystals in body fluids and tissue. The main sites of deposition are the kidneys and joints. In both situations the pH is acidic, leading to more rapid crystal deposition. In the kidneys, calculi are common along with parenchymal deposition. In the joints, the crystals cause damage by themselves but also elicit a brisk inflammatory reaction that is the major problem.

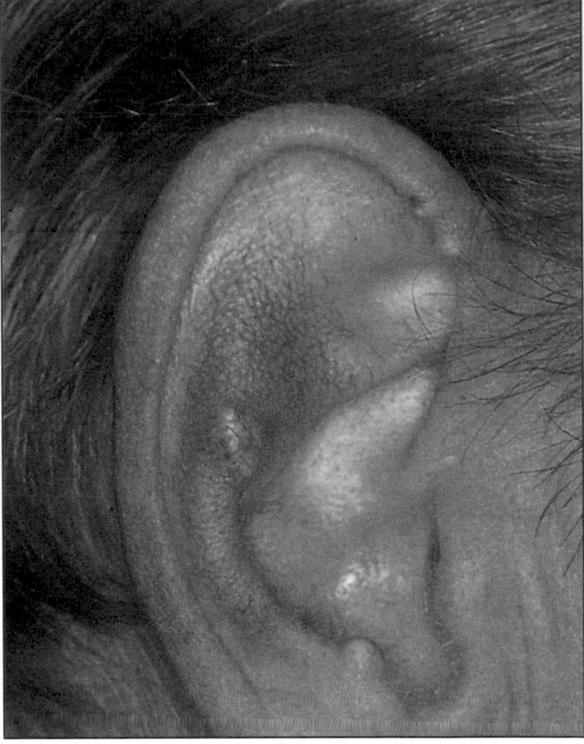

Fig. 47.3. Gouty tophus

Clinical Findings. Acute gout typically involves the distal joints of the extremities. All of a sudden the patient experiences a swollen, inflamed exquisitely painful joint. When the great toe is involved, one speaks of podagra (from the Greek for grip or seize) (Fig. 47.2). The acute attack may last several days and is accompanied by fever and chills. Another acute manifestation of gout is acute renal colic. Between attacks of gout in the inter-critical period, the patient is asymptomatic, but the frequency of attacks increases. In chronic gout, there is either destructive arthritis, chronic renal disease or both.

The main skin finding is a tophus or an accumulation of uric acid crystals in the subcutaneous tissue. Typical sites include the involved digital joints, the elbows, Achilles tendons and the helix of the ear (Fig. 47.3). The early tophi are small white to yellow movable nodules. Later the masses may enlarge, become fixed and ulcerate, draining gravel-like material which contains urate crystals. Tophi may develop in hyperuricemic patients before they have symptoms of gout.

Histopathology. Microscopic examination reveals a dermal or subcutaneous mass of urate crystals surrounded by an intense inflammatory infiltrate. On the extremities, the clinical diagnosis is usually obvious and few biopsies are performed. Often the ear tophi are not so obvious and may be biopsied. To best preserve the crystals and allow their identification by polarization microscopy where they are negatively birefringent, the biopsy must be fixed in absolute alcohol. Most biopsies are fixed in the standard formalin solution. Here the shadows of the crystalline spaces are preserved along with amorphous material.

Diagnostic Criteria. The diagnosis of gout involves several steps:

- Documenting the hyperuricemia
- Demonstrating the presence of urate crystals in the joint fluid
- Showing a therapeutic response to colchicine (not required)

  The presence of tophi and the radiological examination also help make the diagnosis.

Further details on the diagnosis of gout should be sought in standard internal medicine textbooks.

Differential Diagnosis. The differential diagnosis of gout can be divided into several groups.

- Ear tophi. One must consider chondrodermatitis nodularis chronica helicis, elastotic or calcified nodules of the ear, granuloma annulare and a variety of tumors including basal cell carcinoma.
- Distal tophi. Rheumatoid nodules, subcutaneous granuloma annulare, Heberden nodes, giant cell tumor of tendon sheath and other mesenchymal tumors come into question.
  In both of these cases, the biopsy readily clarifies the diagnosis.
- Amorphous dermal deposits. Sometimes gouty tophi and nodular amyloid can be similar. Since gout is common and amyloid rare, it is usually worthwhile to check the uric acid level in supposed cases of nodular amyloid. In rare instances, urate crystals may be found in the skin in patients without gout. Transepidermal elimination of these crystals has been described. Nodular foci of calcification may represent calcified tophi; often the calcification obscures other details.

The differential diagnosis of an acute joint is beyond our expertise. One must consider infections, trauma and other crystalline disorders. In pseudogout, the patient's uric acid levels are normal, larger joints are usually involved, tophi are uncommon, and the crystalline material consists of positively birefringent calcium pyrophosphate dihydrate crystals. In addition, radiological examination usually shows articular calcifications, especially of the knees.

Therapy

Systemic. The systemic therapy of gout includes treating the acute episodes, preventing recurrent disease and using hypouricemic agents. Further details should be sought elsewhere. In general, colchicine or nonsteroidal antiinflammatory drugs are used in acute attacks, while lower daily doses of colchicine are the most effective way to prevent recurrent attacks. Unfortunately, colchicine does not relieve the hyperuricemia or elute crystals from the joints and kidney. To accomplish this, one must employ uricosuric agents such as probenecid or sulfinpyrazone or block uric acid synthesis with allopurinol. Both can be combined. Salicylates antagonize the action of both uricosuric agents and should be avoided. Acetaminophen is acceptable.

Weight loss, adequate fluid intake and a reasonable diet are important adjunctive measures. The approach to asymptomatic hyperuricemia is unclear; most experts recommend treatment with either uricosuric agents or allopurinol only in special risk groups (chemotherapy patients, family history of renal stones, extremely high uric acid values).

Topical. A tophus which is painful, ulcerated or otherwise troublesome can be excised. Slow healing and drainage is the rule, rather than the exception.

Lesch-Nyhan Syndrome

[Lesch and Nyhan 1964]

Definition. Hypoxanthine-guanine phosphoribosyltransferase (HGPRT) deficiency associated with mental retardation and self-mutilation.

Epidemiology. Lesch-Nyhan syndrome is very rare. The gene is located at Xq27, so both Lesch-Nyhan syndrome and partial HGPRT deficiency are inherited in an X-linked recessive pattern.

Etiology and Pathogenesis. While it is simple enough to say that patients with Lesch-Nyhan syndrome lack HGPRT, we do not understand how this leads to neurological disturbances and self-mutilation. Partial HGPRT deficiency may be seen in a very small subset of patients with gout. A number of different point mutations in the gene have been identified.

Clinical Findings. The main dermatologic finding is the peculiar tendency to self-mutilation. The unfortunate usually institutionalized patients destroy their lips by biting them away (Fig. 47.4). They

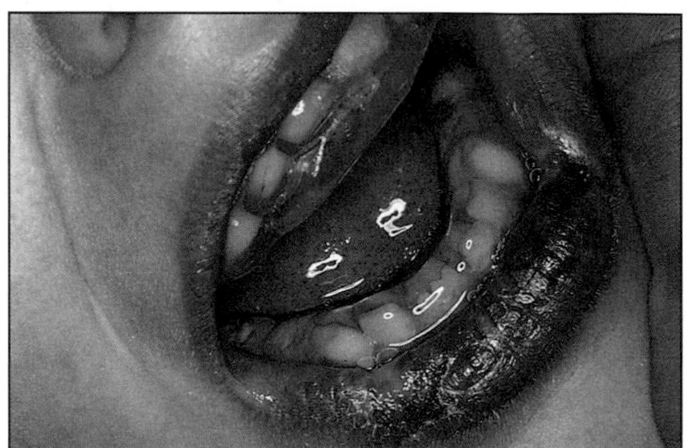

Fig. 47.4. Lesch-Nyhan syndrome with lip mutilation

also damage their hands, feet and any other body parts they can reach. The neurologic problems are multiple and profound. Patients with Lesch-Nyhan syndrome often excrete uric acid crystals in their urine at an early age; mothers may describe yellow-orange crystals or grains in the diapers. They almost all develop renal uric acid deposits and calculi, but gout is uncommon. Conversely, patients with partial HGPRT deficiency usually have gout.

Laboratory Findings. Elevated uric acid levels, and an increased ratio of uric acid to creatinine are the standard screening tests. Red blood cell HGPRT can be measured. The gene can be identified.

Differential Diagnosis. Some patients show self-mutilation and neurologic problems, but do not lack HGPRT. The exact classification of this condition remains unclear, but it is called pseudo-Lesch-Nyhan syndrome. Self-mutilation may also be seen in a number of patients with various types of mental retardation but it is rarely as dramatic as in Lesch-Nyhan syndrome. Similar problems have been described in Cornelia de Lange syndrome and Möbius syndrome.

Therapy. Allopurinol can prevent urate nephropathy but does not influence the neurologic symptoms. Bone marrow transplantation can restore erythrocyte HGPRT levels to normal but also does not favorably influence the neurologic situation.

Bibliography

Gout

Abramson SB (1992) Treatment of gout and crystal arthropathies and uses and mechanisms of action of nonsteroidal anti-inflammatory drugs. Curr Opin Rheumatol 4:295–300

Agudelo CA, Wise CM (1998) Crystal-associated arthritis. Clin Geriatr Med 14:495–513

Becker MA, Roessler BJ (1995) Hyperuricemia and gout. In: Scriver CR, Beaudet AL, Sly WS, Valle D (eds) The metabolic and molecular bases of inherited disease, 7th edn. McGraw-Hill, New York, pp 1655–1678

Eng AM, Schmidt K, Bansal V (1994) Finger pad deposits. Gout. Arch Dermatol 130:1435–1438

Fam AG, Assaad D (1997) Intradermal urate tophi. J Rheumatol 24:1126–1131

Touart DM, Sau P (1998) Cutaneous deposition diseases, part II. J Am Acad Dermatol 39:527–544

Koh WH, Seah A, Chai P (1998) Clinical presentation and disease associations of gout: a hospital-based study of 100 patients in Singapore. Ann Acad Med Singapore 27:7–10

Peters TD, Ball GV (1992) Gout and hyperuricemia. Curr Opin Rheumatol 4:566–573

Veerapen K, Schumacher HR Jr, Linthoudt van D, et al. (1993) Tophaceous gout in young patients with systemic lupus erythematosus. J Rheumatol 20:721–724

Wernick R, Winkler C, Campbell S (1992) Tophi as the initial manifestation of gout. Report of six cases and review of the literature. Arch Intern Med 152:873–876

Lesch-Nyhan Syndrome

Erhard U, Herkenrath P, Benz-Bohm G, et al. (1997) Lesch-Nyhan syndrome. Clinical diagnosis and confirmation by biochemical and genetic methods. Pediatr Nephrol 11:124–125

Lesch M, Nyhan WL (1964) A familial disorder of uric acid metabolism and central nervous system function. Am J Med 36:561–570

Lucke TW, Fallowfield ME, Evans A et al. (1999) Transepidermal elimination of urate-like crystals: a new perforating disorder? Br J Dermatol 141:310–314

Schepis C, Greco D, Siragusa M, et al. (1996) What syndrome is this? Lesch-Nyhan syndrome. Pediatr Dermatol 13:169–170

Rossiter BJF, Caskey CT (1995) Hypoxanthine-guanine phosphoribosyltransferase deficiency: Lesch-Nyhan syndrome and gout. In: Scriver CR, Beaudet AL, Sly WS, Valle D (eds) The metabolic and molecular bases of inherited disease, 7th edn. McGraw-Hill, New York, pp 1679–1706

CHAPTER 48

Nutritional, Metabolic and Endocrine Disorders

Contents

Nutritional Disorders

A well-balanced diet with sufficient protein and calories is essential for normal skin. Patients with malnutrition, inappropriate diets or malabsorption often have cutaneous signs reflecting their inadequate nutrition. Such problems are, not surprisingly, most common in the Third World, but they may also occur in the poor, elderly, alcoholics, drug abusers, individuals with chronic diseases and those with psychosomatic eating disorders or more severe psychiatric illnesses. Initially a variety of nutritional deficiencies were seen in postoperative patients or chronic bowel disease patients who received long-term parenteral nutrition. Today, however, the parenteral diets are so carefully monitored that deficiencies are the exception. In an experiment at the University of Minnesota volunteers received a 1570 calorie diet for 23 weeks. Their skin showed changes also associated with aging, as it became thinner, drier and less elastic. Lack of protein and inadequate caloric intake lead to a variety of illnesses; while the spectrum is broad, one usually speaks of marasmus and kwashiorkor although the two frequently overlap.

Marasmus

Definition. State of general malnutrition in which both proteins and calories are insufficient.

Epidemiology. Starvation is a problem across much of the world. World Health Organization estimates vary but a staggering number of people around the globe go hungry. In western countries, malnutrition is a more appropriate designation; seriously and terminally ill patients, the elderly, and the poor are all at risk.

Etiology and Pathogenesis. While one can write a great deal, the cause is simple. Starvation leads to marasmus.

Clinical Findings. Patients with marasmus generally weigh less than 60% of their ideal body weight and have no edema. In developing countries, marasmus is frequently seen as food supplies are simply inadequate, especially during periods of drought, pestilence or war. In western countries, marasmus is almost only seen in dying patients, generally those with widespread cancer. Intake of proteins, calories and vitamins is inadequate. Many patients, especially children, have sunken cheeks through loss of the buccal fat. What is typically absent is the edema associated with protein loss alone – also known as "hunger edema." In addition, the patients are hungry and eager to eat, not apathetic.

Cutaneous signs are numerous. Most typically the skin is very dry and may show excessive folds, as the subcutaneous fat is markedly reduced. For the same reason, some muscles may appear more prominent, although in truth most are reduced in size, especially those of the neck and gluteal region. Follicular hyperkeratoses may develop. The hairs tend to be an early marker, as they become thin, pale, fragile and grow slowly. Telogen effluvium is almost an invariable component of malnutrition, especially if the nutritional problem is of sudden onset. Similarly, the nails become more brittle and may be split.

Therapy. An adequate diet is all that is needed.

Kwashiorkor

Definition. Kwashiorkor is a Ghanaian tribal word meaning (roughly paraphrased) "the first child gets it, when the second is on the way." Kwashiorkor typically appears in small children after nursing is stopped, as they receive insufficient proteins and too much of their caloric intake (which is usually adequate or even excessive) is made up of starches or sugars.

Epidemiology. Kwashiorkor is probably more common than marasmus, but limited to societies in which adequate amounts of starch are available. When only maize products are on hand, pellagra may develop simultaneously with kwashiorkor.

Etiology and Pathogenesis. The primary cause is protein deficiency. Thus kwashiorkor is most common in those primarily tropical lands where the diet is comprised mostly of beans, rice or corn. Vitamin deficiency, infections and bowel diseases may predispose or exacerbate kwashiorkor. Dark-skinned races are more often involved, but this probably reflects economic and social factors rather than racial predisposition.

Clinical Findings. Kwashiorkor usually develops in children older than 6 months, generally when they cease to nurse. Not all patients have cutaneous involvement, but it may be very characteristic.

Pigmentary abnormalities are quite common. There may be hypopigmentation about the mouth and on the legs, which are also generally swollen and scaly. Hyperpigmentation may also be seen, especially following inflammatory changes, such as impetigo. The skin also shows discrete erythematous, hyperkeratotic lesions, which typically spare sun-exposed areas, in contrast to pellagra. The lesions have been compared to peeling paint; they are irregular, sharply bordered and can be diffuse. Deep fissures may develop around the joints and the mouth. Mucosal surfaces may be dry and irritated; the lips and genital mucosa are most often involved.

The hair may also be characteristic. Typically it is dry, lusterless, and has a pale red-brown color. Very characteristic is the flag sign, in which there are bands of normally colored and hypopigmented hair. In contrast, in the flag sign of chemotherapy, the bands of abnormal hair are darker than the normal color. The hairs are fine and easily broken. A trichogram may reveal reduced numbers of anagen hairs which appear atrophic.

The clinical manifestations of kwashiorkor are often made more obvious by concomitant infections. Because of the protein deficiency, not only is growth deficient but there may be mental retardation as well. Muscle atrophy, fatty infiltration of the liver, and a moon-like facies are also seen. A secondary kwashiorkor may be associated with bowel surgery and resultant malabsorption or inadequate nutrition.

If the nutritional defects are corrected, the systemic findings as well as the skin and hair changes are reversible. If the protein malnutrition continues, the process may be lethal or at a minimum destroy the child's prospects for normal development.

Histopathology. The epidermis shows parakeratosis and necrotic basal cells. The changes are not specific.

Diagnosis and Differential Diagnosis. The diagnosis is made when children achieve only 60–80% of their normal weight and at the same time have edema and/or hypoalbuminuria. The skin and hair changes aid in the diagnosis. As mentioned, there are often associated vitamin deficiencies. Pellagra may lead to hyperpigmented, scaly skin changes, but they are typically in sun-exposed areas.

Therapy. A diet with the appropriate amount of protein is required. Vitamin and mineral supplements should also be instituted.

Essential Fatty Acid Deficiency

Definition. Shortage of essential fatty acids secondary to nutritional deficiencies.

Etiology and Pathogenesis. There is no natural essential fatty acid deficiency. Patients fed a diet too low in linoleic and linolenic acid can develop skin findings, growth failure and impaired wound healing. A large study three decades ago evaluated over 400 infants who were maintained on diets low in linoleic acid for many months. In addition, patients on parenteral nutrition and following major gastrointestinal resections and otherwise healthy individuals on bizarre diets may develop essential fatty acid deficiency. Premature infants also seem to be at risk. The essential fatty acids are needed for prostaglandin synthesis but are also involved in many membrane processes. They are a major constituent of triglycerides and are also bound to sterol esters in the epidermis.

Clinical Findings. The skin becomes dry, leathery and flaky but with an underlying erythema. The flexural areas are often eroded and weeping. In the large study, the findings were more striking in black children. While the severity of skin changes correlates with low serum levels of linoleic acid, many deficient individuals have no skin findings.

Course and Prognosis. The outlook is that of the underlying disorder.

Differential Diagnosis. In patients on an inadequate diet who present with erythema and scaling, often acrally or periorifically, one should consider zinc deficiency, biotin disorders, cystic fibrosis and free fatty acid deficiency, as well as the most likely diagnosis of a mixed deficiency state.

Therapy. Systemic linoleic and linolenic acid supplements rapidly reverse the problem. Sunflower seed oil is a ready source. In some experimental studies, topical sunflower seed oil helped the skin problems, but systemic administration is more reasonable.

Noma

Synonyms. Cancrum oris, gangrenous stomatitis

Noma comes from the Greek and refers to an ulcer or tumor that eats itself, as the root word is closest to a meadow where animals graze.

Definition. Rare destructive disease involving the orofacial tissues, most often of sick children.

Epidemiology. Noma is rarely seen in the United States or western Europe but more often in countries where malnutrition is a problem. It is most common in sub-Saharan Africa.

Etiology and Pathogenesis. Many factors combine to produce noma. Most patients are children with malnutrition, infections, immune disorders or debilitating diseases. Actual tissue necrosis occurs as a result of invasion by a variety of anaerobic bacteria including Vincent spirochetes and fusiform bacilli. Noma shares many features in common with the less severe acute necrotizing ulcerative gingivitis, including its occurrence in AIDS patients.

Clinical Findings. The disorder usually begins with a painful ulceration, either involving the gingiva or the buccal mucosa. It may spread rapidly to produce massive destruction involving soft tissue, teeth and bones. The entire mid-face may be destroyed. Rarely, noma may start in other sites, such as the nose or genitalia. The disease may be fatal if not treated promptly.

Differential Diagnosis. Noma is primarily a clinical diagnosis. The culture findings may guide therapy but are not diagnostically specific. Sometimes other causes of severe oral ulceration, such as major aphthae or myeloproliferative disease, can produce a milder but similar picture.

Therapy
Systemic. Broad-spectrum antibiotics are necessary but not sufficient treatment. Restoration of good nutrition, intravenous fluids, and general supportive measures are equally important.

Topical. Débridement may be helpful, as well as expert oral hygiene which usually must be supervised by a health care provider. Topical antiseptics and anesthetics may provide some relief but are clearly adjunctive measures.

Surgery. Reconstructure facial surgery is of great benefit for severely afflicted children.

Tropical Ulcer

Synonyms. Desert ulcer, tropical phagedena

Definition. Mixed bacterial infection, usually involving traumatic wounds of the legs, often in patients with malnutrition.

Etiology and Pathogenesis. As the name suggests, tropical ulcer is usually seen in warm, damp climates, primarily in adults. Epidemics may occur in military troops or plantation workers, such as those on rubber or banana plantations. But natives suffering from malnutrition and chronic diseases seem to be at greater risk. They are predisposed to progressive, severe mixed cutaneous infections. Staphylococci, streptococci and a variety of gram-negative organisms can be cultured. The same organisms found in noma may also be identified.

Clinical Findings. The most common site is the lower aspects of the legs, just above the ankles, usually following minor injuries. Initially the lesion is an ecthyma, often with blisters and bloody fluid. Untreated the disease progresses to produce massive tissue necrosis, often involving subcutaneous structures, fat, muscle or even periosteum. A serious complication is the destruction of larger blood vessels leading to dangerous hemorrhage. Scarring is expected and may produce such severe contractures that amputation is needed. Typically the scarred tissue has a hyperpigmented periphery. Minor injuries may lead to recrudescence in the damaged skin.

Differential Diagnosis. The ulcers caused by *Mycobacterium ulcerans* (Chap. 4) are equally extensive but not associated with malnutrition.

Therapy

Systemic. Broad-spectrum antibiotics, rationally adjusted to culture results, have made the prognosis much better. While penicillin is most often used because of its price and availability in poor regions, cephalosporins, aminoglycosides and ciprofloxacin have also been recommended. Once again, adequate nutrition, vitamins and good supportive care are essential.

Topical. Surgical debridement may be needed. Moist wound care is helpful.

Eating Disorders

Eating disorders have become a fashionable disease in the past decade and much public attention has been focused on such patients, both because of the number of celebrities suffering from an eating disorder and because of the difficulty in treating the problems. Eating disorders are primarily a disease of women.

Bulimia

Definition. Eating disorder characterized by binge eating and purging, either with self-induced vomiting, laxatives and/or diuretics.

Epidemiology. Bulimia has a prevalence of 2–5% in young women in the USA, but a far higher number have at least occasionally indulged in bingeing and purging.

Etiology and Pathogenesis. The cause of bulimia is unclear. The increasing emphasis on a thin body, as typified by the Barbie doll, has exerted unusual pressure on young women. Once one enters the cycle of bingeing and purging, then a vicious cycle results. Attempts at caloric restriction trigger more binges and more purging.

Clinical Findings. Bulimic patients tend to be healthier than those with anorexia nervosa. The typical patient is a young, often depressed woman. These individuals are underweight but have on average less weight loss than anorexia nervosa patients, are rarely amenorrheic and may have normal sexual relations. Their skin is usually normal, but they often have angular stomatitis or perlèche because they stretch and damage the corners of their mouths as they induce vomiting. They may also develop calluses on their knuckles and the backs of their fingers because of contact with the upper teeth during the same process

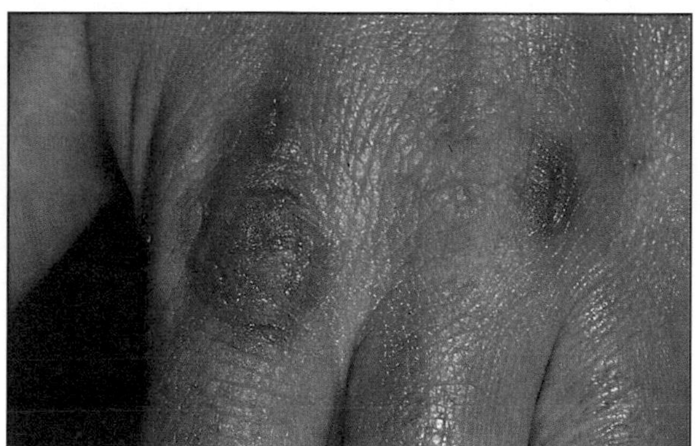

Fig. 48.1. Knuckle calluses in a patient with bulimia. (Courtesy of Johnannes Ring, M.D., Munich, Germany)

(Fig. 48.1). They tend to have marked caries and periodontal disease, both from their inclination to eat sweets and the repeated exposure of their oral cavity to stomach acids.

Course and Prognosis. Bulimia patients may have problems for many years that tend to wax and wane and sometimes respond very well to therapy.

Differential Diagnosis. Other patients eat in binges but do not purge. Not surprisingly they tend to be obese. Men are affected about as often as women and the onset of problems tends to be after 40 years of age.

Therapy. Both antidepressant medications and psychosocial or behavioral therapy can be beneficial.

Anorexia Nervosa

Definition. Eating disorder characterized by marked dietary restrictions, extreme weight loss and amenorrhea.

Epidemiology. Anorexia nervosa is much rarer than bulimia. Its prevalence is around 0.2% for women and much less for men. Several studies suggest that its incidence may be increasing.

Etiology and Pathogenesis. The same factors that play a role in bulimia are important here. The patient has a weight phobia, with a desire for thinness but an unrealistic assessment of her own status. Depression is also associated and there is a familial tendency to the problem.

Clinical Findings. Anorexia nervosa is characterized by extreme weight loss (more than 25% of body weight), a distorted body image and often amenorrhea. The patients live in fear of becoming fat and show signs as of starvation. Often there is a history of obesity or excessive exercise. Their skin is prematurely aged, thin and pale. It is usually dry and scaly, mimicking a mild ichthyosis. Similarly their hair tends to be sparse, brittle and often light colored. The axillary and pubic hair is usually normal. The edema of kwashiorkor may occur but is uncommon as they tend to be starving themselves and lack calories as well as proteins. They tend to suffer from cold skin and especially acrocyanosis. The clinical picture may be complicated by vitamin deficiencies. Some patients simply starve themselves, while others starve, occasionally binge and purge.

Course and Prognosis. Anorexia nervosa patients do poorly as their disease progresses relentlessly, while they have little insight into their problem. It is estimated that 5% of anorexia nervosa patients die of their disease or associated psychiatric problems, including suicide. Often they express concern about getting fat as they are literally wasting away.

Another 20–30% remain abnormally thin despite therapy, while the rest show some improvement but are rarely normal.

Differential Diagnosis. Panhypopituitarism and severe psychiatric disorders must be excluded, but usually the diagnosis is obvious.

Therapy. Aggressive therapy, most often in special clinics or with special support groups, offers the best hope of interrupting the disease course and allowing the patient to lead a normal life. A variety of techniques are used to encourage eating and reward weight gain. Antidepressants are less helpful than in bulimia patients are they further suppress the appetite. The skin requires only routine care.

Metabolic Disorders

Cystic Fibrosis

(Andersen 1938)

Synonym. Mucoviscidosis

Definition. Inherited disorder with abnormal transmembrane ion transport causing primarily pulmonary and pancreatic problems.

Epidemiology. Cystic fibrosis is one of the most common genetic disorders. It has an incidence of 1/2000 in northern Europeans, but drops to 1/100,000 in Asians. The frequency of heterozygotes or carriers among Europeans is about 1 in 22.

Etiology and Pathogenesis. The cystic fibrosis gene is on chromosome 7q31.3. It is a very large gene in which many different mutations have been identified, but a single mutation δ-F508 accounts for about 70 % of all cases. The gene product, cystic fibrosis transmembrane regulator (CFTR) protein, controls the chloride channel in the cell membrane. Its absence leads to a high sodium content in the sweat and a reduced water content in the respiratory and intestinal mucus.

Clinical Findings. Onset of problems is usually early in life. Patients present with repeated respiratory infections, malabsorption, steatorrhea and, in about 10 % of patients, meconium ileus. As the disease progresses, bronchiectasis, pancreatic insufficiency with diabetes mellitus, gallstones, mucoid intestinal obstruction and infertility are problems. The vas deferens fails to develop in over 95 % of men. Heterozygous males (1/22 in Europe) may be infertile for the same reason (Chap. 67). Women may be fertile, but their limited life expectancy threatens their chances to rear a family. Heterozygous individuals may also be at increased risk for chronic pancreatitis.

Striking skin findings occasionally can be seen, primarily in the small subset of cystic fibrosis patients presenting with malnutrition. Erythematous scaly papules and patches can be found on the distal aspects of the often edematous extremities, perineum and periorificial areas. Erythroderma and alopecia can develop. The skin findings stem from the secondary deficiencies in zinc, proteins and essential fatty acids.

Laboratory Findings. The diagnosis is based upon measuring sweat chloride levels. The normal value is usually less than 60 mmol/l. False-positive results have occasionally been reported in atopic dermatitis patients, who may have similar skin changes.

Course and Prognosis. The outlook has improved for cystic fibrosis patients. Fifty years ago 80 % died in the first year. Today the average age at death is around 30 years. The main cause of death is pulmonary failure. Some patients have been treated with lung transplants.

Differential Diagnosis. The rare infant presenting with skin disease should be examined for acrodermatitis enteropathica, free fatty acid deficiency, biotin disorders and inadequate nutrition. The rest of the differential diagnosis is beyond our scope.

Therapy. The essence of therapy is pancreatic replacement and attentive pulmonary care with appropriate and early treatment of infections. Recombinant human DNAse is used as an aerosol to thin the respiratory mucus. Inhaled gene therapy has also been tried, but with less success. The skin problems resolve if dietary measures are undertaken, supporting their secondary nature.

Prophylaxis. Prenatal diagnosis is possible, but carrier screening tests are still in developmental stages.

Endocrine Disorders

In the German edition of this book, there is no specific section dealing with the cutaneous manifestations of endocrine diseases. Instead, the various skin disorders are mentioned throughout the book; for example, myxedema is discussed under the mucinoses. In this section, we will review the various endocrine disorders briefly, discuss their cutaneous findings and make extensive cross-references to the relevant chapters. The basic science aspects of the endocrine disorders will be discussed in barest detail, while the laboratory diagnosis and treatment will not be covered.

Pituitary Gland

The pituitary gland was formerly described as the "master gland" but this is incorrect. It secretes a number of hormones which direct the function of other organs, but is regulated to a great extent by the hypothalamus, which serves as a control center for processing the many neural stimuli and then redirecting the body's hormonal response. The hypothalamic releasing hormones reach the anterior pituitary by a vascular route; they stimulate the release of growth hormone, thyroid stimulating hormone (TSH), luteinizing hormone (LH), follicle stimulating hormone (FSH), growth hormone, prolactin and adrenocorticotropic hormone (ACTH). The ACTH story is more complex, as a prohormone, pro-opiomelanocortin (POMC) is broken down into both ACTH, which is then split to α-melanocyte stimulating hormone (α-MSH) and corticotrophin-like peptide (CLIP), and β-lipotropin which yields β-MSH endorphins and encephalins. These hormones have few direct actions on the skin, but can be identified by abnormal function of their target glands. The hypothalamus also manufactures antidiuretic hormone (ADH, vasopressin) and oxytocin, which pass directly down the neural stalk to the posterior lobe of the pituitary.

Hypopituitarism

The main causes of reduced pituitary function include tumors, postpartum ischemia (Sheehan syndrome), injury (radiation, trauma), granulomatous disease (sarcoidosis, tuberculosis, Langerhans cell histiocytosis) and in children developmental defects. The tumors and granulomas may also cause space-occupying defects, such as visual field disturbances and headache. Usually the clinical findings are the result of reduced production and release of several hormones. Thus there may be varying signs of hypogonadism, hypothyroidism and adrenal insufficiency. Prolactin is rarely affected and growth hormone (GH) deficiency is not clinically detectable in adults, although it causes dwarfism in children. The overall cutaneous picture includes loss of body hair, usually first involving the axillae, pallor, and dry perhaps slightly puffy skin. The relative loss of pigmentation is blamed on the lack of melanocyte-stimulating hormone (MSH), but exactly what role MSH plays in melanocyte stimulation is controversial. The various hormones which are lacking can be replaced.

Hyperpituitarism

While most pituitary tumors are not functional, some produce increased levels of the various hormones, causing a variety of cutaneous findings. Almost all pituitary tumors are benign. Different morphologic types of tumors have different secretion patterns.

Acromegaly

Acromegaly is the result of oversecretion of GH in an adult. In a child, the same tumor causes gigantism, but if the problem is not corrected, the individual also develops features of acromegaly. Coarse facial features and enlarged hands and feet are the most common findings. In adults the changes are so gradual that diagnosis is often long delayed; studying older photographs often demonstrates how long the facial features have been changing. The skin becomes thickened and furrowed; the unfortunate expression of a "basset hound look" is descriptive. Some patients may develop cutis verticis gyrata. About 10 % of patients have acanthosis nigricans or increased skin tags. Other skin findings such as hypertrichosis, onychodystrophy and increased oiliness may reflect overlaps with other hormonal disturbances. Treatment is generally surgical; if it is unsuccessful, bromocriptine, a dopamine antagonist, is usually tried.

Prolactinoma

In women, prolactinomas are detected fairly early because they lead to amenorrhea, infertility and often galactorrhea. The main later problem is osteoporosis. In men, the changes are more subtle, but include impotence, infertility and perhaps gynecomastia and galactorrhea. The eruption of cherry angiomas has been described with prolactinomas. In addition, elevated prolactin levels can cause hyperandrogenism, producing androgenetic alopecia and hirsutism. It appears that prolactin enhances the end-organ response to normal androgen levels. Phenothiazines and estrogens may also stimulate increased prolactin levels. The usual treatment is bromocriptine, with surgery reserved for medical failures.

Cushing Disease

Isolated excess secretion of ACTH is true Cushing disease. Cushing was a neurosurgeon who described an ACTH-secreting pituitary tumor. Cushing syndrome refers to any patient with the clinical features produced by excessive corticosteroids, as discussed below. Interestingly, one of Cushing's first patients, Minnie G., appears to have had Carney syndrome (Chap. 65), with an autoimmune type of Cushing syndrome, not a tumor. In Nelson syndrome, a secreting pituitary tumor develops after bilateral adrenalectomy for adrenal hyperplasia. These patients have very high ACTH levels because of reduced feedback inhibition, are invariably hyperpigmented and often have evidence for other hormonal problems.

Diabetes Insipidus

Secretion of ADH creates no cutaneous changes. Diabetes insipidus is primarily of interest to dermatologists because of its association with Langerhans cell histiocytosis (in which infiltrates in the pituitary saddle damage the posterior lobe) and xanthoma disseminatum (in which the foam cells damage the connection between the hypothalamus and pituitary).

Thyroid Gland

The thyroid gland takes up iodides out of the diet, converts them to iodine and combines them with tyrosine to make iodotyrosines, which are complexed into thyroxine (T_4) or triiodothyronine (T_3). These hormones are combined with thyroglobulin in the proteinaceous colloid of the thyroid gland. The complexes are released into the circulation, primarily bound to thyroid-binding globulin, but only the free form (1%) is active. The thyroid hormones influence many aspects of carbohydrate, protein and fat metabolism. Their classic role is increasing the basal metabolic rate, but their function is much more finely tuned, as thyroid hormones alter membrane function and regulate transcription of various receptor proteins and enzymes.

Hypothryoidism

The main cause of hypothryoidism in western countries is autoimmune disease, usually Hashimoto thyroiditis with destruction of the gland. About 90% of patients are women. Previous treatment for hyperthyroidism, whether surgical or with radioactive ^{131}I is also a common factor. In endemic regions, lack of iodine may also play a major role. Rarely, lack of TSH or even lack of hypothalamic factors may be responsible.

The symptoms of hypothyroidism are protean and include weight gain, cold intolerance, fatigue and constipation. The skin findings are also numerous. Typically the skin is puffy, waxy, cool and dry. The most striking effect of this is a lack of facial expression. The diffuse puffiness is secondary to increased deposits of mucin in the skin, known as myxedema. On rare occasion, there may be localized myxedema. (Chap. 43). The hair is dry, brittle and grows slowly. There may be diffuse or patchy hair loss; if the hypothyroidism is sudden, telogen effluvium may result. Another suggestive finding is loss of lateral third of the eyebrows (Hertoghe sign). The nails grow slowly and may also be brittle. The tongue is thickened and enlarged, often interfering with articulate speech. A puzzling feature is the yellowish tint that the skin frequently acquires; there is carotenemia but secondary apparently to hepatic alterations, not increased ingestion of carrots.

Many of the skin findings, and systemic findings, are relatively nonspecific. This works to the patient's disadvantage in two ways. The diagnosis of hypothyroidism may be delayed, as fatigue or hair loss maybe interpreted as physiologic. Conversely, hypothyroidism may diagnosed incorrectly, or even worse, thyroid replacement may be used in women with normal thyroid function who have hair loss, brittle hair, fatigue or obesity. The index of suspicion for hypothyroidism should be high, but the diagnosis should only be made with absolute laboratory confirmation. Replacement therapy reverses all the signs and symptoms.

Congenital Hypothyroidism

Most patients with congenital hypothryoidism or cretinism have embryonic thyroid gland defects or inborn errors in thyroid hormone production. In endemic cretinism, there is a dietary lack of iodine in the mothers. Rare causes are use of antithyroid medications by the mother and the presence of maternal antithyroid antibodies. The main effects of congenital hypothryoidism are on the CNS, the infants are docile or inactive. In addition, they may have an enlarged tongue, a puffy face, dry cool skin, brittle hair and a long list of other problems Although they surely have myxedema, it is the least of the problems and rarely plays a role in the diagnosis. In many countries, neonatal screening is performed, because thyroid replacement can correct all of the problems, while an untreated infant may experience irreversible CNS changes prior to diagnosis.

Hashimoto Thyroiditis

Hashimoto thyroiditis features an intense lymphocytic infiltrate. Initially the patients may be hyperthyroid, but as the disease burns out and the gland is destroyed, they become hypothyroid. The main symptom is pain. Hashimoto thyroiditis is associated with a variety of other autoimmune diseases.

Hyperthryoidism

The most common cause of hyperthyroidism is Graves disease. Once again, 90% of patients are women. Other causes include toxic multinodular goiter, toxic adenoma, surreptitious ingestion of thyroid hormones, acute stages of thyroiditis and, rarely, pituitary tumors producing TSH. Important symptoms include anxiety, heat intolerance, palpitations, weight loss, weakness and eye problems. On physical exam, there is often tachycardia, thyroid enlargement and a tremor.

The cutaneous findings are also dramatic. The skin tends to be warm, moist and smooth. Patients complain of sweaty palms, often with striking erythema. Flushing and urticaria can occur. There may be diffuse alopecia, while nails often show distal onycholysis in which the free edge curves upward (Plummer nail). Hyperpigmentation can develop in those rare patients with overproduction of TSH via overlaps with ACTH/MSH.

Graves Disease

(Graves 1835; von Basedow 1840)

Synonyms. Basedow disease, diffuse toxic goiter

Definition. Autoimmune thyroid disease often in association with exophthalmos, pretibial myxedema and acropachy. EMO is an acronym proposed by Braun-Falco and Petzoldt (1967) for exophthalmos, myxedema and osteoarthopathy, as first described by Thomas (1933). Von Basedow, a physician in Merseburg, Germany described the Merseburg triad – exophthalmos, diffuse goiter and tachycardia.

Etiology and Pathogenesis. There are a variety of immune phenomena present in Graves disease. Autoantibodies (TRab) react with the TSH receptor; most stimulate it but some block it. Antibodies may also be directed against thyroglobulin and microsomes. In addition, there can be a diffuse lymphocytic infiltrate which is mild in the thyroid gland but can be more severe in the ocular muscles. The relationship of the TRab to the periorbital and cutaneous deposits is poorly established. Presumably fibroblasts are stimulated to secrete mucin which accumulates in the skin. The antibodies can cross the placenta and cause transient neonatal hyperthyroidism.

Clinical Findings. Patients with Graves disease have all the metabolic findings associated with thyroid disease, but also a series of additional problems.

Systemic Findings. The thyroid gland is diffuse, enlarged and smooth. There is usually a fine tremor, tachycardia and an increased pulse pressure. Most disturbing to the patient is the ophthalmic involvement. Early on they may complain of swollen lids, foreign body sensation, tearing and erythema. Later the more classic changes of exophthalmos occur. The combination of mucin deposition and lymphocytic inflammation appear responsible. The conjunctival vessels are prominent and the lids may become red and thickened (chemosis). Visual disturbances are common, both from the impaired lid mobility and involvement of the ocular muscles.

Cutaneous Findings. The cutaneous findings of pretibial myxedema and acropachy, as well as EMO syndrome, are discussed in Chapter 43. Both vitiligo and alopecia areata are somewhat more common in Graves disease, with an incidence of about 5%.

Course and Prognosis. The thyroid disease, ocular changes and cutaneous involvement generally run hand in hand. In some patients the mucin deposition is relatively independent of the thyroid disease, so that they may have exophthalmos without thyroid disease or their eye problems may persist or worsen even as the thyroid disease is being treated. The same relationship exists for the other types of deposition but is not as clinically -important.

Differential Diagnosis. In the clinical setting of hyperthyroidism, any hint of lid swelling or exophthalmos usually means Graves disease. If the changes are unilateral, one should make the diagnosis with great caution after excluding all the other possible causes.

Thyroid Tumors

While functional adenomas can cause hyperthyroidism, most thyroid carcinomas are not functional and are identified as masses in the neck. Patients with multiple endocrine neoplasia (MEN) 2B have multiple mucosal neuromas and medullary thyroid carcinoma (Chap. 65).

Parathyroid Gland

The parathyroid glands secrete parathormone (PTH), which is mainly involved in calcium metabolism. The normal role of PTH and the problems associated with hyperparathyroidism are discussed in Chapter 45. Hyperparathyroidism is usually discovered through routine blood chemistries revealing an elevated calcium. It is caused by functioning adenomas in most cases. Jellinek sign refers to darkening of the eyelids in hyperparathyroidism; the so-called raccoon eyes can also be seen with neuroblastoma and lupus erythematosus.

The usual cause of hypoparathyroidism is surgical removal of the parathyroid glands during thyroidectomy. They may also be involved in several rare polyendocrinopathies. There are no skin changes. Pseudohypoparathyroidism is associated with osteoma cutis (Chap. 59).

Adrenal Glands

Most of the diseases of the adrenal gland relate to excessive, inappropriate or deficient secretion by the adrenal cortex. The adrenal medulla is the source of pheochromocytomas. Lack of the adrenal medulla does not produce any significant clinical problems.

Hyperadrenalism

Dermatologists are intimately familiar with the effects of excess amount of glucocorticosteroids because of the frequent occurrence of iatrogenic Cushing syndrome in patients with pemphigus vulgaris and other corticosteroid-dependent disorders. The problems associated with adrenocortical hyperplasia are many, depending on what types of hormones are produced in excess. There are frequently overlaps. Excessive mineralocorticoid production has no specific skin findings.

Cushing Syndrome
(Cushing 1912)

Definition. Disorder caused by excessive levels of glucocorticosteroids.

Epidemiology. Cushing syndrome is extremely rare, except as an iatrogenic disorder. The incidence of the noniatrogenic forms is estimated at one per million.

Etiology and Pathogenesis. There are many causes, including:

- Cushing disease, in which a pituitary adenoma secretes ACTH. This accounts for 75% of cases. In rare instances there may be hypothalamic overproduction of corticotrophin releasing factor (CRF) rather than a pituitary tumor.
- Autoimmune Cushing disease, in which autoantibodies stimulate the adrenal ACTH receptors. This is extremely rare but occurs in Carney syndrome (Chap. 65).
- Functional adrenal adenomas or carcinomas can also produce excess levels of hormones. While they are the most common cause of Cushing syndrome in children, these tumors account for only a small group in adults.
- Ectopic secretion of either ACTH or even CRF by a carcinoma, most often small cell tumors of the lung.
- Long-term administration of corticosteroids is the most common cause. While the usual route is systemic, overuse of potent topical corticosteroids, especially in children, can also cause Cushing syndrome.

Clinical Findings

Systemic Findings. The most common systemic findings include diabetes mellitus, hypertension, osteoporosis, and hypogonadism. They are present in over 75% of patients. Almost as common are hemorrhagic problems secondary to vessel wall weakness, muscle weakness and emotional disturbances.

Cutaneous Findings. The full plethoric facies is known as moon facies. It appears early in the disease and continues to worsen. The fat is redistributed, leading to truncal obesity and the formation of an intrascapular clump of fat, known as a buffalo hump. Other changes include acne (often worse on the trunk; Chap. 28), hirsutism (Chap. 31), purpura (especially on the forearms and associated with trauma; Chap. 23) hyperpigmentation (Chap. 26) and marked striae distensae (Chap. 18). Wound healing is also often impaired.

Laboratory Findings. The diagnostic steps are complex and should be sought in an internal medicine text.

Therapy. Treatment depends on the underlying cause but is usually surgical. In some instances, even with a pituitary tumor, adrenal surgery and hormone replacement are chosen. Pharmacologic blockers of corticosteroids are available but quite toxic.

Hypoadrenalism

The failure of the adrenal gland to produce normal amounts of gluco- and mineralocorticosteroids may be either primary, known as Addison disease, or secondary, due to lack of appropriate ACTH secretion. The latter may be the result of pituitary or hypothalamic disease.

Addison Disease

(Addison 1855)

Epidemiology. Addison disease has a prevalence of around 50 per million; thus it is more common than non-iatrogenic Cushing syndrome. It occurs more often in women.

Etiology and Pathogenesis. Autoimmune damage to the adrenal cortex is responsible for 75% of. Most of these patients have circulating antibodies against adrenal cortical structures. Tuberculosis accounts for about 20% while a variety of rare destructive processes accounts for the balance. Systemic fungal infections and malignant lymphomas are included in this group. Waterhouse-Friderichsen syndrome is caused by fulminant meningococcal infection (Chap. 4) with extensive purpura (Chap. 22); hemorrhage into the adrenal gland may cause an acute Addisonian crisis. Occasionally there is a family history of Addison disease or other autoimmune endocrine disorders.

Clinical Findings

Systemic Findings. The early systemic findings are vague, so that the diagnosis is often overlooked. The patients may complain of fatigue, dizziness or lethargy. Later there may be weight loss and abdominal complaints. Often the disorder is first identified when an Addisonian crisis is triggered by a second problem such as a severe infection, trauma or even elective surgery.

Cutaneous Findings. The main skin finding is hyperpigmentation (Chap. 26). The high ACTH level produced as a response to the lack of corticosteroid production is primarily responsible for the hyperpigmentation, which is greatest in sun-exposed areas, in scars and over pressure points. There may also be hyperpigmentation of the oral mucosa and lips.

Histopathology. There is increased melanin but not an increased number of melanocytes.

Laboratory Findings. The diagnosis is usually made on the 9 A.M. plasma cortisol level and its response to an injection of ACTH. More complicated endocrinologic and imaging tests can be employed depending on the clinical setting.

Therapy. Lifelong hormonal treatment is required with a glucocorticosteroid, e.g., hydrocortisone 20 mg in the morning and 10 mg in the afternoon and a mineralocorticosteroid, e.g., fludrocortisone 0.1–0.2 mg daily. In the event of surgery, trauma or other metabolic stress, the dosages must be increased. An Addisonian crisis is a medical emergency requiring intravenous hydrocortisone and generous fluid replacement.

Excessive Androgen Production

The adrenal gland can produce excessive amounts of androgens. The main adrenal processes involved are secretory tumors in adults and congenital adrenal hyperplasia in children. In adults, the tumors, both adenomas and carcinomas, have abnormal production pathways so that androgens may be overproduced. In infants, there may enzymatic defects, usually 21-hydroxylase deficiency, so that glucocorticosteroids are not produced, ACTH levels increase and the androgen precursors that occur along the synthetic pathway before the step involving the enzymatic defect are overproduced. Depending on the defect, the problem may appear in infancy or later on, even in adult life. Functional adrenal tumors can also be seen in children.

The main clinical findings in women include acne (Chap. 28), hirsutism (Chap. 31), cliteromegaly, frontal baldness, deepened voice and amenorrhea. In men, there may be decreased testicular volume. In infants and children, girls experience masculinization (pseudohermaphroditism), while boys show signs of precocious puberty. The diagnosis is usually based on finding elevated levels of both testosterone and dihydroepiandrosterone sulfate (DHEA-S) in the serum. Treatment is either surgical or, if this is not possible, then with adrenal blockers such as mitotane. In the 21-hydroxylase deficiency, glucocorticosteroids can be administered and the integrity of the feedback loop thereby restored.

Pheochromocytoma

Epidemiology. Pheochromcytomas are rare tumors. They are present on autopsies in perhaps 1:5000–10,000 cases but when one looks at series of hypertensive patients, they account for several per thousand.

Etiology and Pathogenesis. The adrenal medulla is one of the sites responsible for the production of epinephrine, which it manufactures from dopamine. Epinephrine has numerous effects on intermediate metabolism and cardiac function; surprisingly, it does not need to be replaced in patients following surgical adrenalectomy. The medulla may be destroyed in Addison disease, but once again no problems result.

Most pheochromocytomas are adrenal, but 10–20% are extraadrenal, found throughout the abdomen and even the thorax. The most common sites are along the vertebrae or in the organ of Zuckerkandl (paraaortic bodies). Bilateral pheochromocytomas are seen in neurofibromatosis, MEN-2 and several other syndromes. About 10–15% of pheochromocytomas are malignant, although it is hard to distinguish sometimes between a metastasis and multifocal primary tu-mors.

Clinical Findings. While many pheochromocytomas are asymptomatic, those that cause clinical problems almost always cause hypertension. While classically one reads of pheochromocytomas causing paroxysmal hypertension, they are about as likely to cause sustained hypertension. Other problems may include headache, palpitations, hyperhidrosis, anxiety and a tremor. Skin findings are minimal. In contrast to carcinoid syndrome, flushing does not occur; instead there may be facial pallor. The features of Raynaud phenomenon are occasionally triggered or worsened. Treatment is surgical removal under careful medical control to avoid hypertensive crisis.

Testes

The diseases of the testes relevant to dermatologic practice are discussed in Chap. 67.

Ovaries

A discussion of the many endocrine actions of the ovaries is beyond the scope of this text. Several cutaneous diseases have been identified as hormonally sensitive because of their tendency to flare with menses. In many cases, this is probably not a firm association but still a worthwhile clue. Chap. 36 considers the wide range of changes associated with pregnancy. The ovaries are the other main source of androgens, so they play a role in both hirsutism (Chap. 31) and acne (Chap. 28).

Pancreas

The main problems associated with pancreatic disease are diabetes mellitus and necrolytic migratory erythema, usually associated with a glucagon-secreting tumor (Chap. 14).

Diabetes Mellitus

Definition. Clinical syndrome representing an interaction between genetic and environmental factors that is characterized by elevated blood sugar values and a variety of end organ changes. Two basic types have been identified: insulin dependent diabetes mellitus (IDDM or type I) and noninsulin-dependent diabetes mellitus (NIDDM or type II).

Epidemiology. The prevalence in the USA is around 2–3%. Certain small populations such as the Pima Indians have much higher rates, supporting a genetic component. Type I disease frequently appears before the age of 30 years, while the more common type II disease usually starts later.

Etiology and Pathogenesis. Diabetes mellitus does not have a single cause, but many causes. IDDM preferentially involves patients with selected HLA types. In these individuals viral infections may trigger an autoimmune response against the pancreatic islet cells with resultant failure to manufacture insulin. This usually occurs in children; without insulin, such patients die.

In type II disease the peripheral cells appear to lose their sensitivity to insulin. In this group, most patients are adults and over 90% are obese. While they may require insulin for proper management, they can live without it. There are also genetic disorders with abnormalities of the insulin receptors; such patients may also have other endocrine abnormalities and often have acanthosis nigricans. Pregnancy may trigger a temporary or gestational diabetes mellitus, while a variety of medications may also derange the glucose control mechanisms.

Many end organs are involved. One unifying feature is small vessel disease, or diabetic microangiopathy, which may lead to retinal and renal glomerular disease as well as skin changes. While small vessel disease is most common in IDDM, large vessel disease or accelerated arteriosclerosis is a common finding in NIDDM. Peripheral neuropathy is also frequently found and may contribute to skin changes.

Clinical Findings. Diabetes mellitus has a number of cutaneous manifestations, which are discussed below. Unfortunately, they do not allow themselves to fall into any easy grouping. It is uncommon to diagnose diabetes mellitus because of skin findings, although occasionally the skin may be the first site of involvement.

- Infections: Diabetics are more susceptible than normal individuals to a variety of bacterial and fungal disorders. The disease-specific neuropathy and vascular disease may predispose the skin to minor injuries and to inadequate healing. The latter is more common in NIDDM where obesity is so common. In the preantibiotic era, severe staphylococcal infections such as furuncles or carbuncles could produce massive gangrenous necrosis and even death. Similarly, streptococcal erysipelas was often severe and recurrent, producing marked lymphedema. Even today, recurrent folliculitis or erysipelas should prompt a search for diabetes mellitus.
  Of the fungal diseases, *Candida albicans* is the most common infectious agent. In addition to its typical sites of the mouth and genitalia, candidiasis may also involve normal skin in diabetic patients, presenting as folliculitis or intertrigo. The latter is more common in obese patients with NIDDM. While diabetics may not have more tinea pedis, they have more trouble with the disease, as the minor crevices between the toes can easily become infected by a variety of bacteria. In addition, erythrasma is more common in diabetics. Some far more serious fungal disorders, such as rhinocerebral phycomycosis (mucormycosis, zygomycosis), also show a predilection for diabetes mellitus patients.
- Vascular Disease. A variety of skin findings are associated with diabetic microangiopathy. They include Binkley spots or diabetic shin spots, tiny brown macules found on the shins of many normal patients but of almost all diabetics. A perhaps extreme variant of the diabetic shin spot is the acral erythema of diabetics, which presents as a sharply circumscribed erythematous patch on the shin or foot. It mimics erysipelas but the skin is not warm and the patient is not ill. In addition, it is a permanent change. Rubeosis diabeticorum is a dusky facial erythema that is similar to acral erythema. In addition, necrobiosis lipoidica diabeticorum (Chap. 50) is an uncommon but highly suggestive sign of diabetes mellitus. Patients typically have a sharply bordered, yellow atrophic patch usually on the shin. Histologically small vessel disease and the characteristic necrobiosis of collagen are found. Disseminated granuloma annulare is another necrobiotic disorder that may be a marker for diabetes mellitus. Patients with severe arteriosclerotic disease may develop diabetic gangrene with necrotic regions on their extremities secondary to arterial obstruction.
- Neuropathy. The lack of sensation in the feet predisposes to many minor injuries which can evolve into diabetic neurotrophic ulcers (Chap. 25). Bacterial infections complicate neuropathic injuries. It is essential for diabetic patients to be carefully instructed in foot care; they should inspect their feet daily for injuries and report promptly to their physician with any suspicious lesions. Comfortable, often specially fitted shoes are helpful, as is routine podiatric care. It is often better for the podiatrist to cut the patient's toe nails, to minimize the risk of injury.

There are a number of disorders which do not fit into the above categories but which are commonly seen in diabetics.

- Bullous disease of diabetes: This poorly understood disorder, also known as bullosis diabeticorum, typically involves elderly diabetics. Large, relatively stable bullae develop on the extremities, last for several weeks and then resolve. Histologic examination shows a subepidermal blister with little inflammation. Immunofluorescent evaluation has not identified any immunoglobulin deposition, in contrast to bullous pemphigoid which is the main differential diagnostic consideration. Topical antibiotics, such as silver sulfadiazine, are usually sufficient therapy.
- Diabetic thick skin: Some diabetics develop thickened waxy skin, especially of the hands, as-

sociated with limited joint motility. They typically cannot press their palms together, as the hands remain slightly flexed (Fig. 48.2). Sometimes numerous small papules are seen. Most patients have antibodies to glutamic acid dicarboxylase in their serum. Very similar antibodies are found in the stiff man syndrome, a neurologic disorder often associated with polyendocrine disorders. There appears to be increased glycosylation and cross-linking of collagen. The main differential diagnostic consideration is scleroderma, but the patient has diabetes mellitus and lacks other stigmata. Treatment with aldose reductase inhibitors appears promising.

- Scleredema adultorum: A thick brawny induration of the nape and back is a rare but almost pathognomonic sign (Chap. 43). The dermis is thickened because of increased glycosylation of collagen, just as in diabetic stiff skin syndrome.
- Acanthosis nigricans: In diabetics, acanthosis nigricans is generally associated with one of the syndromes of insulin resistance and hyperinsulinemia. Type A insulin resistance usually reflects a mutation of the insulin receptor, making effective binding impossible. Type B disease is associated with circulating antibodies against parts of the insulin receptor; they block the attachment of insulin and may be a paraneoplastic sign. Type C disease is less well defined, but seems to involve signal transduction problems after insulin has successfully bound. In patients with unexplained acanthosis nigricans, one must think of diabetes mellitus as well as the possibility of an underlying malignancy.
- Skin tags (soft fibromas): Skin tags are histologically quite similar to acanthosis nigricans, so it seems theoretically possible that they too could be a marker for diabetes mellitus. However, they are so common in obese people that it is hard to document any special association.
- Yellow skin: Some patients have increased levels of carotene, as well as of glycosylated collagen, but no evidence of increased ingestion of carotene, liver disease or other risk factors for carotenemia. Their skin is identical to that of patients who eat too many carrots (Chap. 19).

In addition the disease has been associated with a long list of dermatologic disorders (Table 48.1).

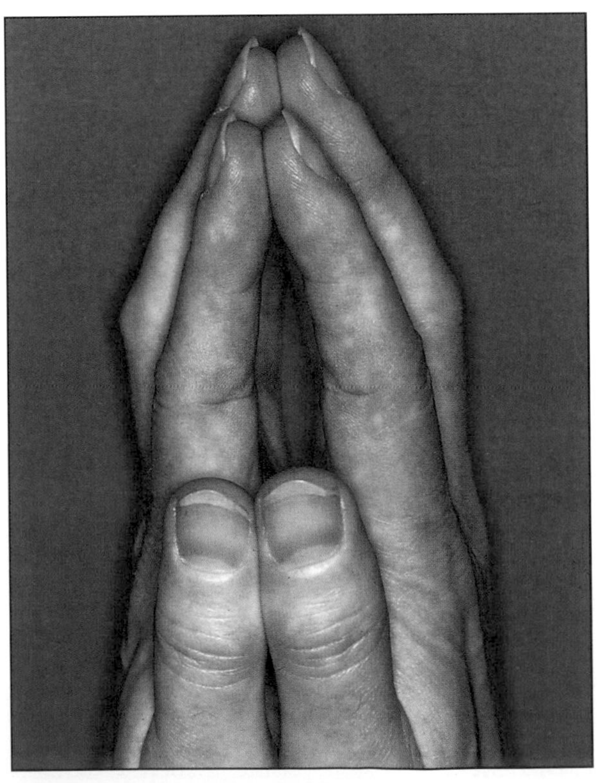

Fig. 48.2. Diabetic stiff skin syndrome

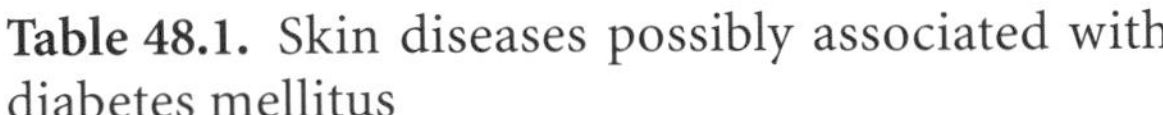

Table 48.1. Skin diseases possibly associated with diabetes mellitus

Disseminated granuloma annulare
Pruritus
Lichen simplex chronicus
Prurigo nodularis
Vitiligo
Lichen planus, especially oral lichen planus
Perforating disease of renal failure/dialysis
Fibromatoses
Lipodystrophy

- Cutaneous complications of therapy: Either insulin or oral hypoglycemic agents can be employed. Insulin is likely to cause a variety of allergic reactions. When insulin from an animal source is used, many patients have a local, immediate, usually IgG-mediated reaction. Delayed reactions are more likely to be cell-mediated, while generalized reactions are often caused by IgE. Some patients have both IgG and IgE antiinsulin antibodies with a biphasic reaction. In all such cases, the easiest solution is to switch to human recombinant insulin. With this agent, reactions are rare and probably reflect changes in the tertiary structure of the new protein, making it antigenic.

Injections of insulin may also cause lipoatrophy or lipodystrophy (Chap. 21), producing either a depressed or bumpy area at the injection site. Insulin may be lipolytic, but changes in the fat probably reflect a wide variety of immunologic reactions, just as in the skin.

The oral hypoglycemic agents cause several problems, including phototoxic and photo-allergic reactions, as well as a macular exanthem. It is often possible to simply treat the latter reaction. Chlorpropamide may produce flushing by release of endogenous opioids; over 10 % of individuals cannot tolerate the medication for this reason. The predisposition appears to be inherited in an autosomal dominant pattern.

The further aspects of diabetes mellitus, such as pathology, laboratory evaluation, diagnostic criteria and therapy, are beyond the scope of this book.

Polyendocrine Disorders

There are a group of disorders that frequently occur together, involving several endocrine glands and many other organs. There are two basic groups: polyendocrine deficiency syndromes and multiple endocrine neoplasia.

Polyendocrine Deficiency Disorders

This group of autoimmune disorders is characterized by lymphocytic infiltrates and autoantibodies. One major group is hypoadrenalism, hypoparathyroidism and mucocutaneous candidiasis, usually occurring in childhood. Another is Schmidt syndrome with hypoadrenalism, Hashimoto thyroiditis and often diabetes mellitus with onset in young adult life. Patients may present with vitiligo or alopecia totalis. Many combinations are possible, as seen in Table 48.2: one can combine one or more of the diseases from each column. The presence of any one disease should prompt the physician to search for or at least be alert to the other problems. In this way, early diagnosis and more effective treatment will be possible.

Multiple Endocrine Neoplasia

There are two separate syndromes with totally separate defects in which multiple endocrine tumors can be found. Both are inherited in an autosomal dominant pattern. In each case both adenomas and carcinomas can develop; many are functional but some are silent.

MEN 1 (Wermer syndrome) is caused by a defect on chromosome 11q13. Typical tumors include parathyroid, pancreatic islet cell and pituitary adenomas. The most common finding is hypercalcemia; gastrointestinal problems and diabetes mellitus may also occur. Cushing syndrome (from ACTH-secreting tumors), acromegaly and prolactinomas are also found. Both mutiple facial angiofibromas and connective tissue nevi have been described, even though the gene is not related to either of the tuberous sclerosis genes.

MEN 2 involves mutations in the *ret* oncogene on chromosome 10q11. Two syndromes whose relationship has been argued for years have been shown to have slightly different mutations in the same gene. (1) MEN 2A (Sipple syndrome) features medullary thyroid carcinoma, parathyroid adenomas and pheochromocytomas. (2) MEN 2B (mul-

Table 48.2. Features of polyendocrine deficiency syndromes

Endocrine diseases	Associated diseases
Graves disease	Vitiligo
Hashimoto thyroiditis	Alopecia areata
Idiopathic hypothyroidism	Dermatitis herpetiformis
Idiopathic Addison disease	Gluten sensitive enteropathy
Idiopathic hypoparathyroidism	Chronic mucocutaneous candidiasis
Diabetes mellitus	Myasthenia gravis
Primary gonadal insufficiency	Sjögren syndrome
Pituitary insufficiency (hypophysitis)	Chronic atrophic gastritis
	Pernicious anemia
	Autoimmune hepatitis
	Primary biliary cirrhosis

tiple mucosal neuroma syndrome) is discussed in Chapter 65. The patients have distinctive mucosal neuromas, a marfanoid facies, medullary thyroid carcinomas and pheochromcytomas.

Bibliography

Nutritional Disorders

Miller SJ (1989) Nutritional deficiency and the skin. J Am Acad Dermatol 21:1–30

Prendeville JS, Manfredi LN (1992) Skin signs of nutritional disorders. Semin Dermatol 11:88–97

Telfer NR, Moy RL (1993) Drug and nutrient aspects of wound healing. Dermatol Clin 11:729–737

Marasmus

Barbul A, Purtill WA (1994) Nutrition in wound healing. Clin Dermatol 12:133–140

Briend A, Lacsala R, Prudhon C et al. (1999) Ready-to-use therapeutic food for treatment of marasmus. Lancet 353:1767–1768

Souba WW (1997) Nutritional support. N Engl J Med 336: 41–48

Kwashiorkor

Albers SE, Brozena SJ, Fenske NA (1993) A case of kwashiorkor. Cutis 51:445–446

Eastlack JP, Grande KK, Levy ML et al. (1999) Dermatosis in a child with kwashiorkor secondary to food aversion. Pediatr Dermatol 16:95–102

Jelliffe DB, Jelliffe EF (1992) Causation of kwashiorkor: toward a multifactorial consensus. Pediatrics 90:110–113

Lathham MC (1991) The dermatosis of Kwashiorkor in young children. Semin Dermatol 10:270–272

Lipschitz DA (1991) Malnutrition in the elderly. Semin Dermatol 10:273–281

McLaren DS (1985) Aetiology of kwashiorkor. Lancet (i):55

McLaren DS (1987) Skin in protein energy malnutrition. Arch Dermatol 123:1674–1676

Essential Fatty Acid Deficiency

Burton JL (1989) Dietary fatty acids and inflammatory skin diseases. Lancet 7:27–30

Cederholm TE, Berg AB, Johansson EK et al. (1994) Low levels of essential fatty acids are related to impaired delayed skin hypersensitivity in malnourished chronically ill elderly people. Eur J Clin Invest 24:615–620

Isseroff RR (1988) Fish again for dinner! The role of fish and other dietary oils in the therapy of skin disease. J Am Acad Dermatol 19:1073–1080

Ozsoylu S (1998) Clinical importance of essential fatty acid deficiency. Eur J Pediatr 157:779

Ziboh VA (1989) Implications of dietary oils and polyunsaturated fatty acids in the management of cutaneous disorders. Arch Dermatol 125:241–245

Noma

Adolph HP, Yugueros P, Woods JE (1996) Noma: a review. Ann Plast Surg 37:657–668

Enwonwu CO, Falkler WA Jr, Idigbe EO et al. (1999) Pathogenesis of cancrum oris (noma): confounding interactions of malnutrition with infection. Am J Trop Med Hyg 60:223–232

Enwonwu CO (1995) Noma: a neglected scourge of children in sub-Saharan Africa. Bull World Health Organ 73:541–545

Lin JY, Wang DW, Peng CT et al. (1992) Noma neonatorum: an unusual case of noma involving a full-term neonate. Acta Paediatr 81:720–722

Valadas G, Leal MJ (1998) Cancrum oris (noma) in children. Eur J Pediatr Surg 8:47–51

Tropical Ulcer

Adriaans B, Hay R, Drasar B et al. (1987) The infectious aetiology of tropical ulcer – a study of the role of anaerobic bacteria. Br J Dermatol 116:31–37

Robinson DC, Adriaans B, Hay RJ et al. (1988) The clinical and epidemiologic features of tropical ulcer (tropical phagedenic ulcer). Int J Dermatol 27:49–53

Webb J, Murdoch DA (1992) Tropical ulcers after sports injuries. Lancet 339:129–130

Eating Disorders

Becker AE, Grinspoon SK, Klibanski A et al. (1999) Eating disorders. N Engl J Med 340:1092–1098

Halmi KA (1996) Eating disorder research in the past decade. Ann N Y Acad Sci 789:67–77

Kaye WH (1997) Persistent alterations in behavior and serotonin activity after recovery from anorexia and bulimia nervosa. Ann N Y Acad Sci 817:162–178

Marcos A (1997) The immune system in eating disorders:an overview. Nutrition 13:853–862

Walsh BT, Devlin MJ (1998) Eating disorders: progress and problems. Science 280:1387–1390

Yager J (1994) Psychosocial treatments for eating disorders. Psychiatry 57:153–164

Cystic Fibrosis

Andersen DH (1938) Cystic fibrosis of the pancreas and its relation to celiac disease. A clinical and pathological study. Am J Dis Child 56:344–399

Darmstadt GL, Schmidt CP, Wechsler DS et al. (1992) Dermatitis as a presenting sign of cystic fibrosis. Arch Dermatol 128:1358–1364

Hansen RC, Lemen R, Revsin B (1983) Cystic fibrosis manifesting with acrodermatitis enteropathica-like eruption. Association with essential fatty acid and zinc deficiencies. Arch Dermatol 119:51–55

Laufer P, Laufer R (1985) Contact dermatitis in cystic fibrosis. Cutis 35:557

Phillips RJ, Crock CM, Dillon MJ et al. (1993) Cystic fibrosis presenting as kwashiorkor with florid skin rash. Arch Dis Child 69:446–448

Rosenstein BJ, Zeitlin PL (1998) Cystic fibrosis. Lancet 351:277–282

Schmidt CP, Tunnessen W (1991) Cystic fibrosis presenting with periorificial dermatitis. J Am Acad Dermatol 25: 896–897

Stern RC (1997) The diagnosis of cystic fibrosis. N Engl J Med 336:487–491

Endocrine Disorders

Thiboutot DM (1995) Clinical review 74: Dermatological manifestations of endocrine disorders. J Clin Endocrinol Metab 80:3082–3087

Pituitary Gland

Shimon I, Melmed S (1998) Management of pituitary tumors. Ann Intern Med 129:472–483

Veznedaroglu E, Armonda RA, Andrews DW (1999) Diagnosis and therapy for pituitary tumors. Curr Opin Oncol 11:27–31

Acromegaly

Colao A, Lombardi G (1998) Growth-hormone and prolactin excess. Lancet 352:1455–1461

Melmed S (1990) Acromegaly. N Engl J Med 322:966–977

Melmed S, Jackson I, Kleinberg D, Klibanski A (1998) Current treatment guidelines for acromegaly. J Clin Endocrinol Metab 83:2646–2652

Prolactinoma

Colao A, Lombardi G (1998) Growth-hormone and prolactin excess. Lancet 352:1455–1461

Molitch ME (1999) Diagnosis and treatment of prolactinomas. Adv Intern Med 44:117–153

Diabetes Insipidus

Baylis PH, Cheetham T (1998) Diabetes insipidus. Arch Dis Child 79:84–89

Robinson AG, Verbalis JG (1997) Diabetes insipidus. Curr Ther Endocrinol Metab 6:1–7

Shimizu H, Obi T, Miyajima H (1997) Anhidrosis:an unusual presentation of diabetes insipidus. Neurology 49:1708–1710

Singer I, Oster JR, Fishman LM (1997) The management of diabetes insipidus in adults. Arch Intern Med 23 157:1293–1301

Thyroid Gland

Baker JR Jr (1997) Autoimmune endocrine disease. JAMA 278:1931–1937

Braun-Falco O, Petzoldt D (1967) E.M.O.-Syndrom. Exophthalmus, Myxoedema circumscriptum praetibiale und Osteoarthropathia hypertrophicans (E.M.O.-Syndrom). Münchn Med Wochenschr 79:1523–1529

Hamlet KR, Stevens SR, Gushurst C et al. (1995) Juvenile pemphigus vulgaris associated with Graves' disease. J Am Acad Dermatol 33:132–134

Missner SC, Ramsay EW, Houck HE et al. (1998) Graves' disease presenting as localized myxedema in a thigh donor graft site. J Am Acad Dermatol 39:846–849

Nagai Y, Ishikawa O, Miyachi Y (1996) Multiple eccrine hidrocystomas associated with Graves' disease. J Dermatol 23:652–654

Omohundro C, Dijkstra JW, Camisa C et al. (1996) Early onset pretibial myxedema in the absence of ophthalmopathy: a morphologic evolution. Cutis 58:211–214

Peacey SR, Flemming L, Messenger A et al. (1996) Is Graves' dermopathy a generalized disorder? Thyroid 6:41–45

Priestley GC (1994) Skin fibroblast activity in pretibial myxoedema and the effect of octreotide (Sandostatin) in vitro. Br J Dermatol 131:52–56

Somach SC, Helm TN, Lawlor KB et al. (1993) Pretibial mucin. Histologic patterns and clinical correlation. Arch Dermatol 129:1152–1156

Thomas HM Jr (1933) Acropachy. Secondary subperiosteal new bone formation. Arch Int Med 51:571–588

Wortsman J (1996) Graves' dermopathy. Thyroid 6:655–657

Cushing Disease

Bornstein SR, Stratakis CA, Chrousos GP (1999) Adrenocortical tumors: recent advances in basic concepts and clinical management. Ann Intern Med 130:759–771

Cushing H (1912) The pituitary body and its disorders. Lippincott, Philadelphia

Freda PU, Wardlaw SL, Bruce JN et al. (1995) Differential diagnosis in cushing syndrome. Use of corticotropin-releasing hormone. Medicine 74:74–82

Stratakis CA, Mastorakos G, Mitsiades NS et al. (1998) Skin manifestations of Cushing disease in children and adolescents before and after the resolution of hypercortisolemia. Pediatr Dermatol 15:253–258

Addison Disease

Addison T (1855) On the constitutional and local effects of the suprarenal capsula. Samuel Highley, London

Babich DJ (1996) Clinical problem-solving: identifying Addison's disease. N Engl J Med 334:1403–1404

Kong MF, Jeffcoate W (1994) Eighty-six cases of Addison's disease. Clin Endocrinol (Oxf) 41:757–761

Schloot N, Eisenbarth GS (1995) Isohormonal therapy of endocrine autoimmunity. Immunol Today 16:289–294

Pheochromocytoma

Bravo EL (1991) Diagnosis of pheochromocytoma. Reflections on a controversy. Hypertension 17:742–744

Bravo EL (1997) Pheochromocytoma. Curr Ther Endocrinol Metab 6:195–197

McGrath PC, Sloan DA, Schwartz RW et al. (1998) Advances in the diagnosis and therapy of adrenal tumors. Curr Opin Oncol 10:52–57

Walther MM, Keiser HR, Linehan WM (1999) Pheochromocytoma: evaluation, diagnosis, and treatment. World J Urol 17:35–9

Diabetes Mellitus

Eaglstein WH (1998) Dermagraft treatment of diabetic ulcers. J Dermatol 25:803–804

Jelinek JE (1994) Cutaneous manifestations of diabetes mellitus. Int J Dermatol 33:605–617

Joshi N, Caputo GM, Weitekamp R (1999) Infections in patients with diabetes mellitus. NEJ Med 19/2:341

Goodfield MJ, Millard L (1988) The skin in diabetes mellitus. Diabetologia 31:567–575

Jelinek JE (1995) Cutaneous manifestations of diabetes mellitus. J Am Acad Dermatol 32:143–144

Mathur SK, Bhargava P (1997) Insulin resistance and skin tags. Dermatology 195:184

O'Toole EA, Kennedy U, Nolan JJ et al. (1999) Necrobiosis lipoidica: only a minority of patients have diabetes mellitus. Br J Dermatol 140:283–286

Perez MI, Kohn SR (1994) Cutaneous manifestations of diabetes mellitus. J Am Acad Dermatol 30:519–531

Requena L, Sarasa JL, Pique E et al. (1997) Clear-cell porocarcinoma: another cutaneous marker of diabetes mellitus. Am J Dermatopathol 19:540–544

Rosenbloom AL (1989) Diabetic thick skin and stiff joints. Diabetologia 32:74–76

Shemer A, Bergman R, Linn S et al. (1998) Diabetic dermopathy and internal complications in diabetes mellitus. Int J Dermatol 37:113–115

Polyendocrine Disorders

Betterle C, Volpato M, Greggio AN et al. (1996) Type 2 polyglandular autoimmune disease (Schmidt's syndrome). J Pediatr Endocrinol Metab 1:113–123

Betterle C, Greggio NA, Volpato M (1998) Autoimmune polyglandular syndrome type 1. J Clin Endocrinol Metab 83:1049–1055 (Clinical review, vol 93)

Chung AD, English JC III (1997) Cutaneous hyperpigmentation and polyglandular autoimmune syndrome type II. Cutis 59:77–80

Garty B (1998) Erythema annulare centrifugum in a patient with polyglandular autoimmune disease type 1. Cutis 62:231–232

Torrelo A, Espana A, Balsa J, Ledo A (1992) Vitiligo and polyglandular autoimmune syndrome with selective IgA deficiency. Int J Dermatol 31:343–344

Multiple Endocrine Neoplasia

Darling TN, Skarulis MC, Steinberg SM et al. (1997) Multiple facial angiofibromas and collagenomas in patients with multiple endocrine neoplasia type 1. Arch Dermatol 1333: 853–857

Kousseff BG (1995) Multiple endocrine neoplasia 2 (MEN 2)/MEN 2A (Sipple syndrome). Dermatol Clin 13:91–97

Marx S, Spiegel AM, Skarulis MC et al. (1998) Multiple endocrine neoplasia type 1: clinical and genetic topics. Ann Intern Med 129:484–494

Pacini F, Fugazzola L, Bevilacqua G et al. (1993) Multiple endocrine neoplasia type 2A and cutaneous lichen amyloidosis: description of a new family. J Endocrinol Invest 16:295–306

Pujol RM, Matias-Guiu X, Miralles J et al. (1997) Multiple idiopathic mucosal neuromas: a minor form of multiple endocrine neoplasia type 2B or a new entity? J Am Acad Dermatol 37:349–352

Vitamin Disorders

Contents

Introduction

Vitamins are micronutrients. They are essential for health, are consumed in small amounts, usually function as enzyme cofactors and in other catalytic roles and are excreted relatively unchanged. Vitamins are subdivided into fat-soluble (A, D, E, K) and water-soluble (the rest). The fat-soluble ones and vitamin B_{12} tend to be stored in the body. Thus states of vitamin excess or hypervitaminosis may occur. The water-soluble vitamins are excreted through the kidneys and rarely accumulate.

Vitamin deficiencies arise when insufficient vitamins are present in the diet. While clinical vitamin deficiencies are most often seen in malnourished patients, the two phenomena are not automatically associated. Causes of vitamin deficiencies include alcoholism, fad diets, inadequate parenteral nutrition and inadequate absorption because of gastrointestinal abnormalities. Vitamin dependency refers to patients who require many times the normal requirement of a vitamin to function as a coenzyme because of a mutation in their basic enzyme. Vitamin excess is more common than deficiency and is almost always associated with some type of megavitamin therapy, whether it be administered by the physician or the patient.

There are some basic principles that enable one to rationally approach vitamin-related diseases. In Western countries, one rarely sees isolated vitamin deficiencies. Most inadequately nourished patients are lacking several vitamins. Often one deficiency may be more apparent clinically. Second, since vitamins influence enzyme action, their absence or excess is usually apparent in many organs, not just the skin. Third, one should be reluctant to diagnose vitamin deficiency based on clinical signs, such as perlèche, hair breakage, fatigue or other nonspecific symptoms. Vitamins are not harmless and almost all have an upper margin of safety, which is often not as generous as patients believe. For example, it now seems clear that more than 10,000 IU of vitamin A daily should not be used in pregnancy because of the risk of teratogenicity. Thus vitamins should be used in replacement dosages for documented deficiency. Megadosages should be avoided except in cases of vitamin-dependent disorders which require massive or pharmacologic dosages. These disorders are rare, never involve just the skin and require careful monitoring to avoid vitamin toxicity.

Vitamin A

Vitamin A refers to a group of fat-soluble vitamins of considerable importance in dermatology. The main active substances include retinol, retinal and retinoic acid. Many synthetic modifications of vitamin A also exist; some have been employed in dermatologic and cancer therapy. The entire family of vitamin A derivatives is known as the retinoids. Retinol is only found in animals; milk, eggs, butter, liver, kidney and fish oils are rich sources. Leafy green and yellow vegetables contain alpha- and beta-carotene (also known as carotenoids) which are split in the intestine and then esterified to retinol. Vitamin A is stored in the liver (body pool 300–900 μg) and released to the circulation as retinol, bound to retinol binding protein (RBP). It is then taken up by cells, attached to carrier molecules and transferred to the nucleus where it regulates a variety of processes. The two most active forms are retinol and retinoic acid. Retinal (11-*cis*-vitamin A aldehyde) is bound to opsin to form the essential photoreceptor pigment rhodopsin.

Vitamin A is essential for the normal development of many tissues, including the skin. It helps control mitotic activity in the skin, may produce a mucoid transformation of keratinizing epithelium and destabilizes lysosomal membranes, setting enzymes free. This action on lysosomes fits together with the role of vitamin A in keratinization, as the action of lysosomal enzymes is a key part of the cellular changes in the granular layer which lead to cornification. Because retinoids are so essential to cellular differentiation, they have been employed in tumor therapy, for example in some leukemias, to cause immature tumor cells to differentiate properly. In addition, in the skin they not only profoundly alter keratinization, but may also play an antitumor role. On the other hand, all retinoids are to some extent teratogenic, which limits their role in many diseases.

Vitamin A Deficiency

Clinical Findings. Vitamin A deficiency is common in parts of Southeast Asia where the diet consists primarily of rice. Secondary vitamin deficiency may occur with a variety of intestinal malabsorption disorders, as well as biliary and hepatic diseases. Infants who are felt to be allergic to milk and receive a milk-free supplement such as soy without supplemental vitamin A are also at risk.

Vitamin A deficiency is a major cause of blindness in children in many Third World countries. The earliest clinical sign is usually impaired night vision. Xerosis of the cornea and conjunctiva may occur. If the deficiency persists, patients may develop xerophthalmia and then keratomalacia. Bitot spots are small gray conjunctival lesions with a foamy surface which may aid in the diagnosis. Growth retardation and abnormalities of many other epithelia have been described.

In children, the skin is generally dry and scaly. In adults, the changes may be more extreme with marked hyperkeratoses, especially involving hair follicles. This more severe condition is called phrynoderma. In adults, sweat and sebaceous gland activity is reduced.

Histopathology. The epidermis shows hyperkeratosis and often a degree of follicular plugging is seen. The sebaceous glands may be noticeably decreased in size.

Diagnostic Criteria. The clinical diagnosis may be apparent in children in endemic areas. Often the plasma retinol levels are normal early in the disease until the liver stores are depleted. Normal levels are 20–50 μg/dl; less than 10 μg/dl represents a marked deficiency. One should not diagnose vitamin A deficiency based on the presence of dry skin or follicular plugging; they are too nonspecific. In addition, vitamin C deficiency may also contribute to follicular changes.

Therapy

Systemic. Vitamin A should be given in therapeutic doses initially and then in maintenance amounts. Care should be taken in pregnancy and during lactation not to exceed recommended levels and one should be wary of megadosages leading to hypervitaminosis A.

Prophylaxis. Children at risk should receive oral vitamin A every 3–6 months. Individuals with intestinal absorption problems and infants on milk-free diets also require supplements.

Vitamin A Excess

Acute effects of excessive vitamin A ingestion include nausea, vomiting and headache. There may also be widespread desquamation after several days. Chronic vitamin A toxicity affects a wide variety of organs. While it is seldom seen today, many of the same features are seen when retinoids or vitamin A derivatives are employed. The skin is a major target organ; it frequently becomes dry and scaly. The mucosal surfaces, especially the lips and nasal mucosa, may dry out and desquamate or crack. Both the nares and skin may be more readily colonized with *Staphylococcus aureus*. Both follicular hyperkeratotic plugs and palmoplantar keratoderma may develop. Such conditions were also previously treated with vitamin A, demonstrating nicely how the effects of decreased and excessive vitamin A resemble each other. A diffuse hair loss, generally a telogen effluvium, may occur. Night vision may be impaired. The conjunctivae tend to be very dry. Musculoskeletal pain is also common, and in children cortical hyperostoses may develop; this is known as the DISH syndrome (Chap. 28). There may also be pain in the fascia, especially the plantar fascia and the lumbosacral spine, as well as subtle changes such as anorexia, weight loss and lethargy.

Rarer complications include pseudotumor cerebri and hypercalcemia with vascular calcification. In addition, vitamin A is a potent teratogen. Doses exceeding more than 10,000 IU/day are potentially teratogenic and should be avoided in pregnancy.

The problem can usually be diagnosed clinically. There are often increases in the hepatic enzymes, especially the transaminases and alkaline phosphatase. Only rarely does structural liver damage occur. Similarly, the triglycerides and cholesterol levels generally increase. Pancreatitis is possible if triglycerides rise enough. Radiologic examination may lead to identification of early changes such as cortical hyperostoses. All changes are reversible when the exogenous vitamin A is stopped.

Vitamin A Therapy

Acute vitamin A toxicity was until recently a therapeutic problem in dermatology. Massive doses (or overdoses) of vitamin A, in the range of 300,000–500,000 IU/day were employed for psoriasis, pityriasis rubra pilaris and Darier disease, while doses of 50,000–100,000 IU/day were common in the treatment of acne. The desquamation following vitamin ingestion was one reason for its therapeutic use. In the past three decades a series of synthetic vitamin A derivatives or retinoids have assumed a major role in treating acne, disorders of keratinization and many other dermatologic problems.

Initially, topical therapy was employed, using *all-trans*-retinoic acid (tretinoin, Retin-A). Topical retinoic acid corrects the infundibular keratinization defect in acne, leading to a reduction in the number of comedones. It also produces mild skin inflammation but is free of any systemic effects. In recent years, retinoic acid has also been approved for the topical treatment of photoaging or photodamaged skin. Here it seems to favorably influence epithelial differentiation and dermal composition, but long term data are lacking. Additional topical retinoids have become available in recent years including 13-*cis*-retinoic acid (Isotrex), adapalene (Differin) and tazarotene (Zorac).

The first major systemic retinoid was 13-*cis*-retinoic acid (isotretinoin, Accutane, Roaccutane) which was approved for the treatment of severe nodulocystic acne in the early 1980s. Its range of indications has been expanded to include less severe acne, rosacea, psoriasis and disorders of keratinization. Two aromatic retinoids, initially etretinate (Tegison, Tigason) and now acitretin (Soriatane, Neotigason), are also available. They are most often employed in psoriasis therapy. All the systemic retinoids have similar side-effects to those discussed under vitamin A toxicity. They are teratogenic, which prohibits their use in women at risk for pregnancy unless contraceptive measures are employed, and also cause dry skin and mucous membranes, musculoskeletal symptoms and distortions of hepatic enzymes, cholesterol and triglycerides. Their use is discussed in more detail in Chapters 14 and 28.

Vitamin B

The B vitamins include a variety of water-soluble compounds of great biologic importance. Neither acute nor chronic ingestion of excessive amounts of a single B vitamin leads to skin disease. Chronic ingestion of large amounts of multivitamins may be one cause of acne medicamentosa. Deficiencies of B vitamins are usually complex. In animal experiments it is possible to provide a diet deficient in a single vitamin but this is extremely difficult in humans. The studies alleging to achieve this were all done before the days of human experimentation rules and fraught with ethical as well as methodologic problems. Nonetheless, deficiencies of riboflavin (vitamin B_2), nicotinic acid (vitamin B_3) and pyridoxine (vitamin B_6) were often described as causing fairly specific skin findings. The cutaneous and mucosal changes of these deficiency states tend to overlap, and also share many features with zinc deficiency (acrodermatitis enteropathica) and glucagonoma syndrome. In addition, the histology of the various vitamin B deficiencies is similar. In the acute and subacute state, there are striking clear cells in the damaged spinous layer, while older lesions are more psoriasiform.

Vitamin B_1 (Thiamine)

Thiamine is found in many cereal grains including rice, wheat, barley and rye, as well as in beer yeast and bakers' yeast. When the grain is rolled or ground, much of the thiamine is lost. Thiamine pyrophosphate is an important coenzyme for a variety of enzymes involved in carbohydrate metabolism, the citric acid cycle and the pentose phosphate cycle.

Beriberi, a deficiency in thiamine, occurs mostly in Southeast Asia, and results from eating an unbalance diet dominated by polished rice. If the rice is boiled before the husk is removed, then the vitamin is dispersed throughout the grain. Secondary beriberi may occur in patients with malabsorption, liver disease or increased requirements, such as in hyperthyroidism or pregnancy. Many of these factors often combine in alcoholics. Beriberi is characterized by massive edema, cardiac symptoms, CNS problems (Wernicke-Korsakoff syndrome) and peripheral neuropathies. The edema is most massive acrally and in the face. Generally, multiple vitamin B supplements are effective in reversing the problem. Critically ill patients may require specific therapy with thiamine 20–100 mg/day and magnesium supplements.

Vitamin B_2 (Riboflavin)

Riboflavin is present in many animal and plant tissues. A major human source is dairy products. The yellow color of whey is caused by its high riboflavin levels. In the form of flavin mononucleotide or flavin adenine dinucleotide, riboflavin serves as an essential coenzyme in many oxidation and reduction reactions of carbohydrate metabolism. The same pathways also involve other B vitamins, including pyridoxine, tryptophan and folic acid, explaining perhaps why the clinical features of the vitamin B deficiencies overlap.

While a pure deficiency in riboflavin is most uncommon, it may occur in patients who avoid milk and other animal proteins. In addition, chronic gastrointestinal problems, alcoholism and inadequate parenteral nutrition may play a role. The skin and mucous membranes appear to be often involved. The term "oral-oculo-genital syndrome" has been proposed for riboflavin deficiency.

Angular stomatitis or perlèche is one of the alleged hallmarks of riboflavin deficiency. It has many other, more common causes (Chap. 33) and one should be very reluctant to diagnose vitamin deficiency when perlèche is the only clinical finding. There may also be cheilitis and glossitis, so that the patient complains of pain when eating hot, spicy or acidic foods. Secondary involvement with *Candida albicans* may also occur. In the skin, a seborrheic dermatitis-like rash occurs involving the nasolabial folds, periorbital and periauricular folds, and genitalia with an erythematous scaly rash. For unclear reasons, this has been called shark skin. Most patients who fit this picture have seborrheic dermatitis, not riboflavin deficiency. The nails may also show chronic paronychia.

The most serious and dramatic findings involve the eyes. An angular blepharitis, analogous to seborrheic blepharitis, may be seen. Furthermore, corneal neovascularization, keratitis and amblyopia may occur.

The diagnosis can be confirmed by measuring urinary excretion of riboflavin or levels of erythrocyte glutathione reductase. Therapy with riboflavin 10–30 mg/day is quite effective, as is restoration of a normal diet. In patients with a documented restricted diet or predisposing factors, a trial of therapy may be appropriate.

Vitamin B_3 (Nicotinic Acid, Niacin)

Niacin is an important cofactor for a long list of enzymes. Niacinamide or nicotinamide is part of NAD (nicotine-adenine dinucleotide) and NADP (nicotine-adenine dinucleotide phosphate), and thus is involved in many reactions of intermediate metabolism. Most organisms including humans can synthesize niacin out of tryptophan, so it is theoretically not a vitamin. Consequently, however, patients who are unable to absorb tryptophan may develop secondary niacin deficiency, resembling Hartnup syndrome. The synthesis of niacin from tryptophan is partially dependent on thiamine and pyridoxine which helps to explain why there are so many overlaps in vitamin B deficiencies.

Pellagra

(Casál 1762)

Definition. Clinical constellation of features which result from deficiency of niacin.

Etiology and Pathogenesis. In the past pellagra was most common in countries where corn was the mainstay of the diet. The main regions were the southeastern United States, Italy and the Balkan peninsula. The lack of tryptophan in corn was the problem. In India, the consumption of millet with its high content of leucine also seems to predispose to pellagra. Today pellagra is much less common and is seen among people who eat one-sided diets, often coupled with psychiatric problems or alcoholism, and those with chronic malabsorption problems. Hartnup syndrome involves a hereditary abnormality of renal tryptophan transport, clinically resembles pellagra and may also respond to niacin. Some medications may also produce pellagra either by interfering with absorption or by directly competing with niacin to form NAD, as does the major offender isoniazid (INH). Finally, rare patients with carcinoid syndrome divert tryptophan to form 5-hydroxytryptamine and develop pellagra.

Clinical Findings. Pellagra is traditionally known to medical students under the four Ds: dermatitis, diarrhea, dementia and death.

Cutaneous Findings. The skin changes generally appear first. The patients are photosensitive and develop dermatitis on sunlight-exposed areas, especially the face, neck (Casál necklace), and back of the hands (Figs. 49.1, 49.2). The changes initially are symmetrically bordered edematous red patches and plaques that resemble sunburn. Over time they acquire a mahogany or violaceous color, a parchment texture and fine scales which often desquamate in the middle leaving a collarette. The lesions may develop blisters or even ulcers. Similar lesions may develop in areas of trauma and sweating, such as the axillae and groin, showing that light is not absolutely required. Chronic lesions may become lichenified with thicker scales or even hemorrhagic crusts. Palmoplantar hyperkeratoses and painful fissures about the joints can also be seen.

Mucosal Findings. Mucosal lesions are less specific, perhaps reflecting the frequent occurrence of several vitamin B deficiencies together. The lips tend to be hyperkeratotic and cracked, while the tongue becomes red, swollen and painful. Increased salivation occurs and oral ulcerations may develop. Patients may also complain of a burning mouth. Similar changes can be seen on the vaginal and urethral mucosa.

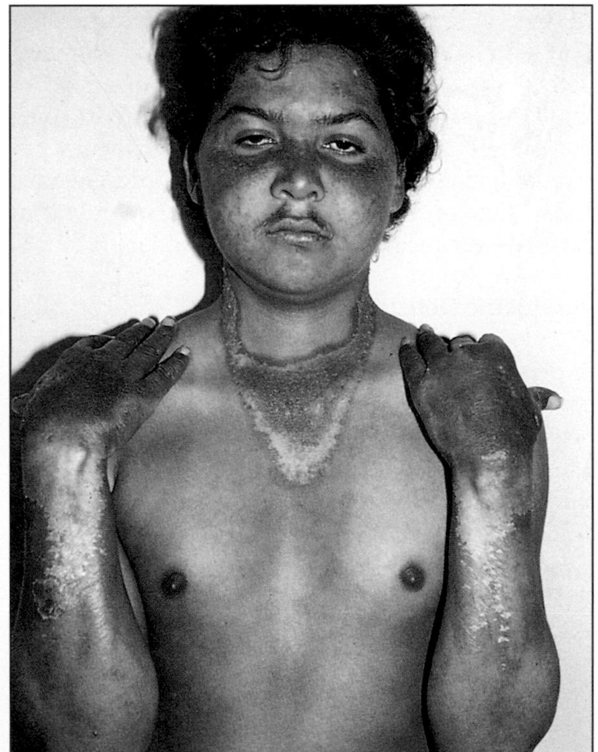

Fig. 49.1. Pellagra showing Casál necklace

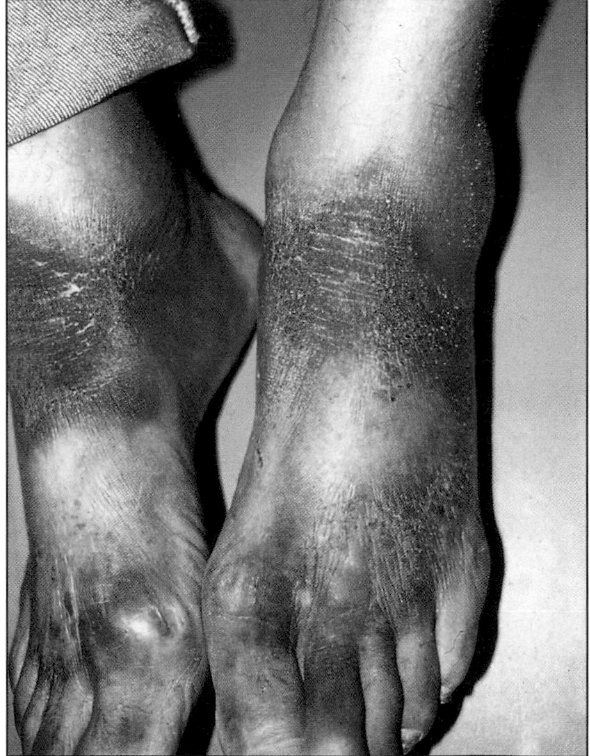

Fig. 49.2. Pellagra. (Courtesy of Juan J. Ochoa, MD, Chihuahua, Mexico)

Gastrointestinal Findings. The most common complaints are diarrhea and abdominal pain. The diarrhea may be bloody.

CNS Findings. Two major types of reactions are seen:

- Psychosis characterized by confusion, memory loss, confabulation and a wide range of other symptoms
- Encephalopathy with clouded consciousness, peripheral rigidity and pathologic reflexes

As a dramatic documentation of the severity of the CNS findings in pellagra, many residents of mental institutions in the southeastern US in the early part of the 20th century were found to have pellagra. The cutaneous findings tend to show seasonal variation, supporting the role of light. The more serious systemic findings are slower to develop but then more constant. They may lead to death in the absence of treatment. Often the changes seen today are limited to the skin; then one may speak of pellagroid changes.

Histopathology. While pellagra is rarely biopsied, dramatic changes can be seen. There is parakeratosis, hyperkeratosis, pallor of the upper layers of the epidermis and a lymphocytic infiltrate in the upper dermis. Follicular plugging and sub- or intraepidermal blisters may be seen. Thus, features of necrolytic migratory erythema, acrodermatitis enteropathica and lupus erythematosus are all present.

Laboratory Findings. Urinary levels of *N′*-methylniacinamide and pyridone are typically decreased.

Differential Diagnosis. The main considerations are porphyrias (porphyria cutanea tarda and variegate porphyria), Hartnup syndrome and drug-induced pellagroid reactions. While kwashiorkor can appear similar, pellagra tends to involve adults and spare the hair and nails. Some chronic photoallergic reactions and persistent light reactions may appear similar.

Therapy. Usually the treatment of choice is niacinamide (nicotinamide) in dosages of 100–300 mg/day. Niacin (nicotinic acid) is usually avoided because of its marked vasodilatatory action which causes unpleasant flushing. The skin findings respond much better than the gastrointestinal and CNS problems. Often patients with such problems are treated with a high-protein (100–150 g daily) diet and supplemental B vitamins.

Niacinamide has been tried in a whole host of other photosensitivity dermatoses, such as lupus erythematosus, with little effect. When combined with antibiotics, it may have an immunoregulatory role and be beneficial in bullous pemphigoid.

Vitamin B_3 Excess

Natural vitamin B_3 excess does not occur, because the body has too many alternate pathways. Patients who are treated with niacin (nicotinic acid) for hyperlipoproteinemia receive 3–6 g/day. This dosage not only causes flushing but may lead to a variety of other signs and symptoms, including urticaria, dry skin, hyperpigmentation and acanthosis nigricans. All changes are reversible when therapy is stopped.

Vitamin B_6 (Pyridoxine)

Pyridoxine is the main component of vitamin B_6. Closely related compounds include pyridoxal and pyridoxamine. All are phosphorylated to form pyridoxal phosphate which functions as a coenzyme in many processes including decarboxylation and transamination of amino acids, metabolism of essential fatty acids and conversion of linoleic acid to arachidonic acid (the main component of prostaglandins), and conversion of tryptophan to niacin. Vitamin B_6 is present in a wide range of foods and is especially abundant in carrots, liver, meat, fish, eggs and grain.

Pyridoxine Deficiency

A primary deficiency in vitamin B_6 is most unusual. An epidemic of vitamin B_6 deficiency has been described in children fed with powdered milk which had been denatured by overheating. They showed similar findings to those in experimental animals deprived of the vitamin: growth retardation, convulsions and anemia. A more usual occurrence is pyridoxine deficiency secondary to malabsorption, or caused by medications (isoniazid, hydralazine, penicillamine, and others).

Clinical Findings. Cutaneous findings are uncommon. They include chronic cheilitis and glossitis, as well as seborrheic dermatitis. The latter is thought to reflect the altered fatty acid metabolism. The clinical changes resemble those seem with riboflavin deficiency. Systemic findings are more common and include peripheral neuropathy, normoblastic anemia and lymphopenia. There are also a number of pyridoxine dependency states described, in which apoenzymes are genetically altered so that the patient requires excessive amounts of the vitamin to function normally.

Therapy. The replacement dose of 50–100 mg/day should be prescribed for patients taking drugs likely to cause deficiency and for those with severe malabsorption. Primary deficiency is so rare that one can almost ignore it; there is no accepted laboratory test to confirm the diagnosis. Pyridoxine should not be used to treat cheilitis, glossitis or seborrheic dermatitis in the absence of other findings. A pyridoxine toxicity state has been described with a variety of neurologic findings. It occurs only after megadosages are taken for months.

Vitamin B_{12} (Cyanocobalamin)

Vitamin B_{12} is a complex cyanocobalamin, a ring structure resembling the porphyrins with a cobalt atom in the center. Vitamin B_{12} is found primarily in animal tissue such as meat, liver, milk and eggs (it was once known as animal protein factor). Some legumes, contain microorganisms which also manufacture the vitamin. It is absorbed in the ileum after binding to intrinsic factor in the stomach; a neutral pH and adequate calcium are also required. Its main role in the body is in the early stages of nucleic acid synthesis.

Vitamin B_{12} Deficiency

Primary vitamin B_{12} deficiency is rare. It may occur in vegetarians and in children nursed by vegetarian mothers, as well as rarely in alcoholics and people on fad diets. Secondary deficiency is far more common. The best known primary cause is pernicious anemia in which there is an absence of intrinsic factor, but other problems including achlorhydria, malabsorption, tapeworms, blind loop syndrome and celiac sprue may also produce a deficiency. Because the body stores are relatively large, it usually takes some months for problems to develop.

Clinical Findings. The hallmarks are a macrocytic anemia and neurologic symptoms. The anemia is similar to that in folic acid deficiency. The neurologic problems are complex and refer to diffuse degenerative changes. The older names of combined system disease and subacute combined degeneration of the spinal cord are best replaced simply by vitamin B_{12} deficiency. There have also been reports of the cyanide in tobacco smoke leading to a depletion of the cobalamin structures and causing "tobacco" amblyopia. Infants may show growth retardation in addition to the neurologic and hematologic problems.

The integumentary changes are only a small part of the problem. In children, hyperpigmentation of the extremities has been described. Both glossitis (Hunter-Möller glossitis) and buccal mucosal lesions occur with pernicious anemia. Initially the lesions are hypertrophic, deep-red and tender, but they may evolve to both smooth or atrophic.

Laboratory Findings. Vitamin B_{12} deficiency can be documented by measuring the serum levels using a variety of assays. Usually gastric analysis demonstrates achlorhydria. The Schilling test measures the uptake of radioactively labeled vitamin B_{12} with and without intrinsic factor.

Therapy. Vitamin B_{12} must be given by intramuscular injection. The usual regimen is 1000 µg several times weekly until the hematologic parameters are restored, which usually takes several weeks. Then monthly injections suffice. The neurologic problems may take several years to improve. The skin and mucosal changes also take months to change.

Vitamin B_{12} injections should only be used in patients with documented deficiency or with underlying diseases that suggest that they are quite likely to become deficient. Injections for nonspecific oral changes such as a burning tongue or mouth are not helpful and may be harmful. Injections have been recommended for postherpetic neuralgia but their effectiveness is unproved.

Folic Acid

Folic acid is widely available in green vegetables and liver. It is easily destroyed by cooking. Considerable amounts of folic acid are also manufactured by intestinal bacteria. Tetrahydrofolates are essential coenzymes for a number of one-carbon unit transfers, such as in the synthesis of purines and pyrimidines and the manufacture of amino acids. Folic acid deficiency is usually the result of a poor diet or total parenteral nutrition. It is also more common in alcoholics as alcohol may also interfere with folate metabolism. Among dermatologic patients, the administration of methotrexate is the most common cause of folic acid deficiency. Agents that interfere with folic acid metabolism include trimethoprim, barbiturates, phenytoin and primidone. Folic acid absorption may also affected by other drugs, such as cyclosporine and oral contraceptives, and in malabsorption syndromes and blind loop syndrome. Folic acid may also be inappropriately or excessively consumed by the body. For example, in widespread erythroderma, there are often lowered folic acid levels. The acid requires adequate levels of vitamin B_{12} and vitamin C to function properly.

Folic Acid Deficiency

Clinical Findings. Folic acid deficiency produces a macrocytic anemia similar to that in vitamin B_{12} deficiency. Other findings such as glossitis and stomatitis, as well as an intestinal mucosal defect leading to further malabsorption, are less common. Acral hyperpigmentation has been described, but it is neither common nor definitely associated with folic acid deficiency.

Laboratory Findings. Both red blood folate levels and plasma tetrahydrofolate levels can be measured.

Therapy. The usual oral dose is 1 mg/day. Patients with documented deficiency or those at risk, such as patients taking methotrexate, should be treated. It is crucial to rule out vitamin B_{12} deficiency before instituting therapy with folic acid, otherwise the folic acid may mask the anemia of vitamin B_{12} deficiency allowing the neurologic damage to progress.

Pantothenic Acid

Pantothenic acid is a component of coenzyme A and is thus crucial to the metabolism of carbohydrates and fatty acids. It is available in a wide variety of foods including liver, egg yolk, yeast and grain, so that deficiency does not naturally occur. Volunteers fed a diet deficient in pantothenic acid develop burning feet and abdominal problems.

Prisoners of war in the Far East in World War II developed the so-called burning feet syndrome with acral paresthesias and distal motor impairment. This problem has never been adequately explained, but it is unlikely that pantothenic acid was responsible. Many patients, not prisoners of war, with distal paresthesias were treated with pantothenic acid with no clear benefit. Similarly, it has been employed for burning mouth and burning tongue syndrome, hair loss and impaired wound healing without marked success. Today there are no definite systemic indications for pantothenic acid.

Dexpanthenol, a D-isomer alcoholic form of pantothemic acid, is widely employed topically in Europe. It is used in wound salves as well as in products for diaper rash.

Vitamin C (Ascorbic Acid)

Vitamin C is present in all fruits and vegetables; citrus fruits are an especially good source. Other less publicized sources include berries, parsley, cabbage, peppers and even rosehips. Vitamin C is present either as L-ascorbic acid or D-dehydroascorbic acid. It is easily oxidized and thus forms a cellular redox system.

Vitamin C is essential for collagen synthesis as it helps in the hydroxylation of protocollagen proline and lysine to collagen hydroxyproline and hyroxylysine. It is also needed for elastin synthesis, and for the intracellular cement in various epithelia. It is involved in a number of other mesenchymal structures, such as osteoid of bones and dentin of teeth, as well as in wound healing and recovery from thermal burns. Vitamin C also plays a role in tyrosine and phenylalanine synthesis, so it may produce pigmentary changes. Finally, it interacts with both folic acid and iron, so it can lead to anemia. Linus Pauling, the Nobel Laureate, recommended megadosages of vitamin C to treat the common cold, but most physicians today feel that this approach is not helpful. In addition, undesirable side effects such as renal stones and iron overload may occur.

Scurvy

Scurvy or vitamin C deficiency is a disease which has been well known for many years. It takes two distinctive courses, depending on whether it develops in adults or children. Vitamin C deficiency usually results from an inadequate diet. Adult male alcoholics who prepare their own meals are at greatest risk. Burns, extensive wounds, hyperthyroidism and pregnancy can increase the requirement for vitamin C, while intestinal problems can lead to malabsorption.

Clinical Findings. In adults clinical findings develop after months of deprivation. The typical cutaneous finding is follicular hyperkeratoses in association with corkscrew hairs and perifollicular hemorrhage, most commonly seen on the shins. In addition, there may be other hemorrhagic lesions, including bulbar conjunctival hemorrhage. The oral changes are similar. There is a hemorrhagic gingivitis, as the gums become red, swollen, friable and bleed easily. Eventually teeth may become loose and fall out. Wound healing may become noticeably impaired. The reason for the hemorrhage in so many areas is a loss of support for the vessel walls because of mesenchymal changes. The systemic findings are numerous. They include malaise, irritability, myalgias, arthritis from bleeding about a joint, cardiomyopathy, neurologic findings and a host of other problems.

In children, the situation is different; the disorder is known as Möller-Barlow disease (Möller 1859; Barlow 1873). Today vitamin C deficiency in infants is rare, but may occur if they are fed a restricted diet of just milk or if they have chronic gastroenteritis and malabsorption. They, too, have gingival changes, with hemorrhage and disruption of dentition. The cutaneous hemorrhages are more likely to involve the head and neck region, and the conjunctival hemorrhages more common. Intestinal hemorrhage can lead to both bloody stools and microcytic anemia. Hematuria may also occur. Especially characteristic of childhood scurvy are the extremely painful subperiosteal hemorrhages, which are only rarely seen in adults. In German, one speaks of the Hampelmann sign (jumping jack sign): even the slightest manipulation of the leg leads the child to retract the leg in pain, just as the beloved wooden toy's leg retracts when one pulls on the string. In contrast, follicular changes are rare.

Laboratory Findings. Ascorbic acid is best measured in the white blood cell layer of centrifuged blood. Plasma and urine levels can also be used but are not as reliable.

Therapy. Vitamin C 150–300 mg/day in children and 500–1000 mg/day in adults leads to a rapid reversal of the signs of scurvy. In patients at risk, 100 mg/day is fully protective. Vitamin C has been employed for a variety of cutaneous hemorrhagic problems including pigmented purpura and senile purpura with no documented effectiveness.

Vitamin D

Vitamin D consists of a number of closely related sterols. Vitamin D_2 (ergocalciferol) is produced by irradiated yeasts. Vitamin D_3 (cholecalciferol) is manufactured in the skin by the irradiation of 7-dehydrocholesterol, which is found in eggs and fish oils. Milk is fortified with one or both forms of the vitamin. Vitamin D_3 is then carried to the liver bound to vitamin D_3-binding protein. There it is hydroxylated to 25-hydroxy D_3. Further processing occurs in the liver where the most active form, 1,25-dihydroxy D_3, is synthesized.

The scope of action of vitamin D is enormous and can only be briefly covered. It is essential for regulation of calcium metabolism, increasing intestinal absorption and stimulating bone formation and mineralization. Hydroxylation of vitamin D_3 is controlled to an extent by parathyroid hormone. Phosphate levels also play a crucial role. Vitamin D_3 plays an important regulatory role in many other organs besides the bone, modulating a number of cell growth processes.

Vitamin D Deficiency

Patients with inadequate diets and insufficient exposure to sunlight are likely to develop vitamin D deficiency. In childhood, the disorder is known as rickets. It was formerly a common disease of poor city children. Today it may be seen in poor refugee populations where diets are inadequate and children kept covered or indoors, such as the Asian immigrants in the United Kingdom and Turkish immigrants in Germany. Typically the infants have specific skeletal defects, such as bowing of the legs, that can be identified easily by radiologic examination. In addition, they may have growth retardation and even tetany. Adults with inadequate vitamin D_3 develop osteomalacia with bone pain and stress fractures. There has been concern that elderly patients using sunscreens might block the first step in the formation of active vitamin D, but this is not clinically relevant.

There are many types of secondary vitamin D deficiency. Patients with malabsorption syndromes fail to take up the precursors. Those with severe renal or hepatic disease may not hydroxylate well enough. Barbiturates and phenytoin may increase catabolism of the precursors. In addition, there are patients with vitamin D-dependent rickets with congenital defects in hydroxylation (type I) or defect or absent cellular 1,25-dihydroxy D3 receptors (type II). The latter patients typically have diffuse non-scarring alopecia. Otherwise, skin changes are few and far between in vitamin D deficiency.

Laboratory Findings. The diagnosis of rickets or osteomalacia is quite complex because of the many forms and the multiple compensatory actions inherent in the regulatory system. Radiologic examination is helpful. In the laboratory, measuring the specific metabolites in the blood is possible and can be combined with calcium and phosphate levels.

Therapy. Fortified milk provides adequate levels for almost everyone. If questions exist, a single 3000-IU (75-μg) capsule of vitamin D_3 weekly is more than enough. Other food products can also be fortified. Higher levels or intramuscular injections may be used in severe deficiency.

Vitamin D Excess

Vitamin D toxicity occurs relatively easily. Dosages of 40,000 to 100,000 IU daily are not uncommonly employed and may lead to hypercalcemia and clinical problems in a matter of months. Nausea, vomiting, malaise and then renal disease with metastatic calcification are the most common features. There are many more active forms of vitamin D available which are more effective but also more toxic. Vitamin D excess most typically occurs when treating patients with hypoparathyroidism and/or renal disease with hypocalcemia. In addition, some fad vitamin users simply abuse the vitamin, taking massive doses.

Vitamin D Therapy

Previously, patients with sarcoidosis, psoriasis and lupus vulgaris were treated with massive dosages of vitamin D, but this is no longer done. Sarcoidosis patients (Chap. 50) tend to get hypercalcemia. Sarcoidal granulomas may secrete vitamin D. In addition, marked sun exposure is felt to increase the risk of elevated calcium levels in patients with sarcoidosis. Topical forms of vitamin D analogs are immunomodulatory and alter cell cycle dynamics. Calcipotriene and tacalcitol are used topically to treat psoriasis; they can cause hypercalcemia but rarely produce significant clinical problems (Chap. 14)

Vitamin E (Tocopherol)

Vitamin E includes a variety of tocopherols (α, β, γ, δ); the α-form is most active. All serve as antioxidants preserving membrane stability. Vitamin E is present in grains, colostrum, and to a lesser extent in vegetables, plant oils and margarine. Vitamin E deficiency may develop in infants, especially if their diets are limited and rich in unsaturated oils. Some malabsorption syndromes in adults may also lead to deficiency.

The clinical manifestations of vitamin E deficiency are unclear. Children may develop anemia, elevated creatinine levels and neurologic findings. Peripheral edema and a resultant scaly dermatitis may be associated but are clearly non-specific. Other cutaneous signs of vitamin E deficiency have not been described.

Vitamin E toxicity is probably a more common problem than deficiency. In children, increased sepsis and thrombocytopenia may be seen, while in adults both cardiac and hemorrhagic problems have been described. Vitamin E has been recommended for a long list of dermatologic problems, including among many others epidermolysis bullosa. There is no proof of its efficacy in any of these disorders and we rarely employ it. Vitamin E can be used to treat retrolental fibroplasia but it is unclear if a deficiency causes the problem. It has been employed in recent years in a variety of trials as cancer preventive agent because of its antioxidant, free radical scavenger status. At the time of writing, it is difficult to assess the effectiveness of such regimens.

Biotin (Vitamin H)

Biotin is also known in Europe as vitamin H; the H stands for *Haut* (German for skin). Biotin is a water-soluble coenzyme essential in fat and carbohydrate metabolism. It is found in yeasts, egg yolk, milk and liver, and can be synthesized by the intestinal flora. Thus biotin deficiency is rare, although it may be seen during total parenteral nutrition, in starvation or in patients who eat large amounts of egg white, which contains avidin, a substance that tightly binds to biotin and blocks its action. This affinity is the basis of avidin-biotin stains used as markers in immunohistochemistry.

Patients with biotin deficiency develop primarily neurologic symptoms, although glossitis and a dermatitis involving the extremities and neck have been described. More dramatic is the cutaneous picture in infants with inherited defects in biotin-dependent carboxylases. A number of different defects have been described, including holocarboxylase synthetase deficiency and biotinidase deficiency. Such patients may develop an acrodermatitis enteropathica-like picture which responds to large doses of biotin (10 mg/day). Biotin is frequently prescribed in Germany for nail problems, such as brittle nails. There are no convincing studies supporting this use.

Vitamin K

Vitamin K consists of a group of phylloquinones. Vitamin K_1 is found in green plants and vitamin K_2 is synthesized by bacteria. The most active form is menadione or 2-methyl-1,4-naphthoquinone. Vitamin K is both acquired through the diet and manufactured by intestinal bacteria. It is essential for the synthesis of the clotting factors II (prothrombin), VII, IX and X in the liver. All these structures contain γ-carboxylglutamic acid, which is also found in a wide variety of other organs, suggesting a broader role for vitamin K.

Vitamin K deficiency may develop because of intestinal problems or hepatic disease. True dietary deficiencies occur only rarely because of the role of the intestinal bacteria. Infants are at special risk because of immature liver capacity and lack of intestinal flora. Treatment with antibiotics also may exacerbate the problem. In adults, liver disease (especially in alcoholics), malabsorption and long-term antibiotic therapy may lead to a deficiency, but the most common cause is the therapeutic use of coumarin anticoagulants which competitively inhibit vitamin K. Thus in this setting vitamin K "deficiency" is known to every physician. The clinical features are those of impaired coagulation, including petechiae, hemorrhages and more frank bleeding such as ecchymoses and deep hematomas.

The most reliable laboratory test is the prothrombin time; vitamin K deficiency will always lead to prolongation of this value. The usual therapy is phytonadione, which is given for prophylaxis in newborns and used to reverse coumarin toxicity. It is usually given intramuscularly. Rare patients have been described with an allergic reaction to vitamin K injections. They develop dramatic erythematous hemorrhagic circular lesions. Vitamin K_1 appears to be responsible. In even rarer cases, indurated sclerodermatous plaques may develop (Texier disease).

Bibliography

General

Keller KL, Fenske NA (1998) Uses of vitamins A, C, and E and related compounds in dermatology: a review. J Am Acad Dermatol 39:611–625

Lupulescu AP (1996) Hormones, vitamins, and growth factors in cancer treatment and prevention. A critical appraisal. Cancer 78:2264–2280

Rackett SC, Rothe MJ, Grant-Kels JM (1993) Diet and dermatology. The role of dietary manipulation in the prevention and treatment of cutaneous disorders. J Am Acad Dermatol 29:447–461

Ryan AS, Goldsmith LA (1996) Nutrition and the skin. Clin Dermatol 14:389–406

Vitamin A

Chandraratna RA (1998) Future trends: a new generation of retinoids. J Am Acad Dermatol 39:S149–S152

DiGiovanna JJ, Sollitto RB, Abangan DL et al. (1995) Osteoporosis is a toxic effect of long-term etretinate therapy. Arch Dermatol 131:1263–1267

Orfanos CE, Zouboulis CC, Almond-Roesler B et al. (1997) Current use and future potential role of retinoids in dermatology. Drugs 53:358–388

Van den Berg H (1996) Vitamin A intake and status. Eur J Clin Nutr 50:S7–S12

Vitamin B

Bradford GS, Taylor CT (1999) Omeprazole and vitamin B_{12} deficiency. Ann Pharmacother 33:641–643

Juhlin L, Olsson MJ (1997) Improvement of vitiligo after oral treatment with vitamin B12 and folic acid and the importance of sun exposure. Acta Derm Venereol (Stockh) 77: 460–462

Metz J (1999) What's the use of oral vitamin B_{12}? Med J Aust 170:407–408

Stolzenberg R (1994) Possible folate deficiency with post-surgical infection. Nutr Clin Pract 9:247–250

Pellagra

Hampl JS, Hampl WS (1997) Pellagra and the origin of a myth: evidence from European literature and folklore. J R Soc Med 90:636–639

Hendricks WM (1991) Pellagra and pellagralike dermatoses: etiology, differential diagnosis, dermatopathology and treatment. Semin Dermatol 10:282–292

Isaac S (1998) The "gauntlet" of pellagra. Int J Dermatol 37: 599

Vitamin C

Fain O, Mathieu E, Thomas M (1998) Scurvy in patients with cancer. BMJ 30:1661–1662

Paoletti R, Sies H, Bug J et al. (1998) Vitamin C. The state of the art of disease prevention sixty years after the Nobel prize. Springer, Berlin

Puntis J (1997) The battle with scurvy. Arch Dis Child Fetal Neonatal Ed 77:F158

Weber P, Bendich A, Schalch W (1996) Vitamin C and human health – a review of recent data relevant to human requirements. Int J Vitam Nutr Res 66:19–30

Vitamin D

Blank S, Scanlon KS, Sinks TH et al. (1995) An outbreak of hypervitaminosis D associated with the overfortification of milk from a home-delivery dairy. Am J Public Health 85:656–659

Haddard JG (1992) Vitamin-D solar rays, the milky way, or both? N Engl J Med 326:1213–1215

Holick MF, Chen ML, Kong XF (1996) Clinical uses for calciotropic hormones 1,25-dihydroxyvitamin D_3 and parathyroid hormone-related peptide in dermatology: a new perspective. J Invest Dermatol Symp Proc 1:1–9

Kang S, Li XY, Voorhees JJ (1996) Pharmacology and molecular action of retinoids and vitamin D in skin. J Invest Dermatol Symp Proc 1:15–21

Kragballe K (1997) The future of vitamin D in dermatology. J Am Acad Dermatol 37:S72–S76

Vitamin K

Filkenstein H, Champion MC, Adam JE (1987) Cutaneous hypersensitivity to vitamin K_1 injection. J Am Acad Dermatol 16:540–545

Janin-Mercier A, Mosser C, Souteyrand P et al. (1985) Subcutaneous sclerosis with fasciitis and eosinophilia after phytonadione injections. Arch Dermatol 121:1421–1423

Newman P, Shearer MJ (1998) Vitamin K metabolism. Subcell Biochem 30:455–488

Sanders MN, Winkelmann RK (1988) Cutaneous reactions to vitamin K. J Am Acad Dermatol 19:699–704

Zipursky A (1999) Prevention of vitamin K deficiency bleeding in newborns. Br J Haematol 104:430–437

CHAPTER 50

Granulomatous Diseases

Contents

Introduction

In this chapter a number of unrelated disorders are considered. All are described as granulomatous because they display granulomas in the skin and other organs. A cutaneous granuloma is defined as a localized primarily dermal area with chronic cellular inflammation containing giant cells and macrophages. The classification of granulomas is confusing because various authors employ clinical appearance, etiologic agents and microscopic features to divide up the family of disorders. When one considers clinical appearance, most granulomas are nodular lesions, often with a red-brown color, although deeper granulomas may have overlying normal skin. If one considers etiologic agents, infections and foreign bodies are well-established causes, while most of the other granulomatous processes are idiopathic in nature.

Two of the most usable histologic classifications are those of Weedon and Ackerman. Both identify four basic patterns, which are also summarized in Table 50.1.

- Sarcoidal granuloma: Naked granuloma, sharply defined, usually sparse accompanying lymphocytic inflammation, no necrosis.
- Tuberculoid granuloma: Less sharply defined than sarcoidal granuloma, more lymphocytes, lesions merge together, necrosis seen. Langhans giant cell is prototypical.
- Necrobiotic or palisading granuloma: Histiocytes and giant cells are arranged in a palisade fashion at the periphery of a necrobiotic area of collagen. Necrobiosis literally means a dead (necro-) condition of life (-biosis). It is used to describe the pale-staining somewhat altered collagen seen in granuloma annulare, rheumatoid nodules and similar disorders.
- Suppurative granuloma: In addition to giant cells, there are abundant neutrophils and frank tissue necrosis. Often there is pseudoepitheliomatous hyperplasia, as well as abscesses both in the dermis and occasionally within the epidermis. Most suppurative granulomas reflect an underlying infection.

Two other categories, not used in either of the schemes are:

- Foreign body granuloma: Foreign objects can cause all of the above granulomas, so this category introduces overlaps and repetitions but is clinically common.
- Xanthogranuloma: Here both foamy macrophage and giant cells usually of the Touton type are seen (Chap. 64).

In addition, a variety of giant cells can be seen. Giant cells result from the interaction of macrophages with lymphocytes, cytokines and often infectious agents or foreign objects. Most contain multiple nuclei and many have ingested lipids, foreign objects or other substances. No given giant cell is specific for a single disorder or even family of granulomas. The three best known types are:

Table 50.1. Common types of granulomas

Histological pattern	Examples
Sarcoidal	Sarcoidosis Melkersson-Rosenthal syndrome (Chap. 33) Foreign bodies (zirconium, beryllium, silica, tattoo)
Tuberculoid	Infections (tuberculosis, leprosy, tertiary syphilis) Rosacea, perioral dermatitis, lupus miliaris disseminatus faciei Crohn disease Foreign bodies (rare)
Palisading or necrobiotic	Necrobiosis lipoidica diabeticorum Granuloma annulare Annular elastolytic giant cell granuloma Necrobiotic xanthogranuloma Rheumatoid nodule Rheumatic fever nodules Neutrophilic and palisaded granulomatous dermatitis (Churg-Strauss granuloma) Lichen nitidus (also lichenoid pattern) Foreign bodies, especially bovine collagen Many rare variants
Suppurative	Infections (bacterial, fungal, algal) Ruptured cysts and damaged follicles Foreign bodies Pyoderma gangrenosum, especially superficial variants
Miscellaneous	Myospherulosis Malakoplakia Granuloma faciale (not a true granuloma) Granuloma gluteale infantum (not a true granuloma) Granulomatous lymphoma, especially granulomatous slack skin (Chap. 61) Sclerosing lipogranuloma or paraffinoma (Chap. 21)

- Foreign body giant cell: Numerous nuclei are scattered haphazardly throughout eosinophilic cytoplasm of the macrophage.
- Touton giant cell: A wreath of nuclei surrounds a central zone, while at the periphery the cytoplasm is foamy. Such cells are typical of xanthogranulomas and xanthomas.
- Langhans giant cell: Most common in tuberculoid granulomas, the Langhans giant cell has a horseshoe-shaped rim of nuclei at the periphery of an eosinophilic cytoplasm.

There are many cautions and tricks when interpreting granulomas. First, one must always include an infectious etiology. Culturing a fresh piece of tissue is the best approach. In most granulomas, routine bacterial and fungal special stains on formalin-fixed tissue have a low yield, although specific monoclonal antibodies, especially one against mycobacteria cell wall components, and polymerase chain reaction (PCR) are very helpful. In addition, multiple sections should be taken searching for a foreign body. Polarization may help and more sophisticated physical-chemical analysis may be useful when searching for evidence of small particles such as silica. Most granulomas have a lifecycle, so that early lesions may show a nonspecific cellular infiltrate and late lesions have fibrosis, while only occasionally does one find the classically described features. In addition, there are many processes that are rich in macrophages but are sometimes focal and sometimes more diffuse. No classification has adequately come to grips with this phenomenon.

Sarcoidosis

(Hutchinson 1877; Besnier 1889; Boeck 1899; Schaumann 1936)

Synonyms. Boeck disease, Boeck sarcoid

Definition. Multisystemic disorder of unknown cause characterized by noncaseating epithelioid granulomas.

History. HUTCHINSON first mentioned the cutaneous findings of sarcoidosis. BESNIER described lupus pernio in 1889; the clinical picture resembled pernio and the histologic picture tuberculosis. BOECK in 1899 used the German term *benignes Miliarlupoid*, or benign miliary lupoid, describing the disease as widespread and benign, i.e., not as severe as tuberculosis but resembling the latter histologically. SCHAUMANN further expanded knowledge about the disease concentrating on the pulmonary findings and histologic picture. He suggested the name "benign lymphogranulomatosis" for he suspected a lymphatic disorder. JÜNGLING in 1920 identified the bone changes in the fingers, which he called ostitis tuberculosa multiplex cystica. The many contributions of these early workers and hundreds of later ones help to document just how many organ systems are involved in sarcoidosis.

Epidemiology. While sarcoidosis is found worldwide, its distribution is variable. The prevalence of pulmonary sarcoidosis is highest in the Scandinavian countries, northern Europe, parts of the USA and Uruguay. It is uncommon in Russia, Saudi Arabia and the Near East. In the USA, the disease is more common in the Southeast; it is uncommon in the Southwest. The prevalence in Germany is around 50/100,000 inhabitants. In the USA the prevalence is lower among whites, but approaches 100/100,000. The lifetime risk for blacks in USA is 2.5%. Blacks also tend to have more severe disease. There seems to be a female predisposition for cutaneous sarcoidosis. Most aspects of sarcoidosis such as incidence, severity and pattern of organ involvement vary from country to country.

Etiology and Pathogenesis. The cause of sarcoidosis is unknown. Genetic factors have long been discussed. A number of reports of familial sarcoidosis are found in the literature. HLA studies have created more confusion than unity. Different preferred patterns have been found in different population groups. HLA-B8, -B13, and -DR5 seem to be most important.

Granulomas are complex immunologic structures. Three steps are required: exposure to antigen, development of a cellular immune response against the antigen and then summoning of diverse inflammatory responses by immune effector cells. An antigen is processed by macrophages and presented to T cells. The T cells through their cytokines direct macrophage accumulation and differentiation. The macrophages evolve into larger epithelioid cells and may become multinucleated giant cells. CD4-positive, helper T cells are admixed with the macrophages, as are some CD8-positive suppressor-cytotoxic T cells. The same cells that cause granuloma formation may also stimulate fibrosis. Macrophages and mast cells both stimulate pulmonary fibrosis, one of the unfortunate events in sarcoidosis.

All data suggest that sarcoidosis represents an immune response to a persistent antigen. The question is: what is the antigen? A wide variety of infectious agents have also been blamed. Community outbreaks and case contact tracing suggest a possible infectious cause. For many years, mycobacteria were suspected because of the histologic and to some extent clinical similarities between sarcoidosis and tuberculosis. Although mycobacteria were not identified with traditional methods, mycobacterial DNA has been found in sarcoidal lesions. Other implicated antigens include chlamydia, corynebacteria, *Yersinia* enterocolitica, viruses bacteriophages, fungi, dust, tumor cells and many others. The definitive interpretation of the newer molecular biologic studies is awaited with great interest.

Clinical Findings. Sarcoidosis involves so many organs (Fig. 50.1) that it is difficult to describe all the features. About 40–50% of patients have cutaneous involvement. It is useful to consider two phases of sarcoidosis: early and late. In early sarcoidosis, the changes are often reversible, perhaps representing an acute immune response to the exiting antigens. The main cutaneous sign is erythema nodosum. Hilar lymphadenopathy, arthralgias and iridocyclitis are other early signs. While spontaneous regression may occur, many cases become more chronic.

In the late or chronic phase, pulmonary fibrosis leads to impairment of function. Many other organs may be involved, either directly with granulomas or as a result of metabolic changes induced by the granulomas and their cytokines. The cutaneous lesions in the late phase tend to be more persistent. They are typically red-brown, have an apple jelly color on diascopy (just as in lupus vulgaris) and cannot be explored with a probe (unlike those of lupus vulgaris). Acute sarcoidosis generally resolves. Patients with more chronic disease have a highly variable course.

The features of acute and chronic sarcoidosis are compared in Table 50.2.

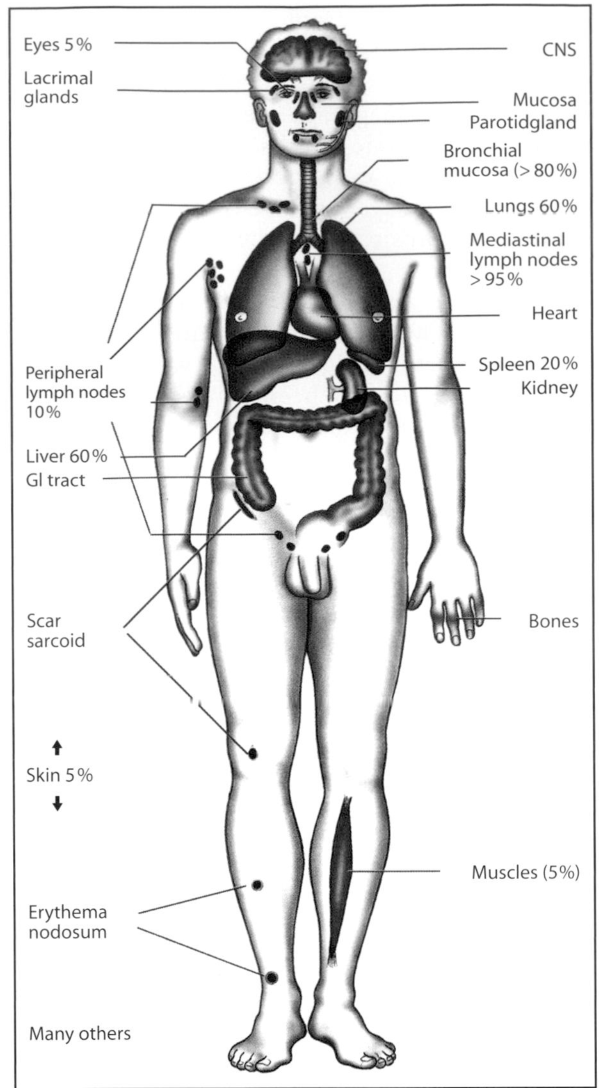

Fig. 50.1. Manifestations of sarcoidosis. (Modified from Reusch 1982)

Cutaneous Findings. Every patient with cutaneous sarcoidosis should be evaluated for possible systemic sarcoidosis. Various cutaneous findings may have prognostic significance. Erythema nodosum is the most common cutaneous finding, but often described as nonspecific because it does not reveal sarcoidal granulomas upon microscopic examination. The other forms of cutaneous sarcoidosis do contain granulomas. Erythema nodosum is almost always associated with acute disease with a benign course. Lupus pernio and plaques are markers of chronic disease with a tendency towards more severe internal manifestations.

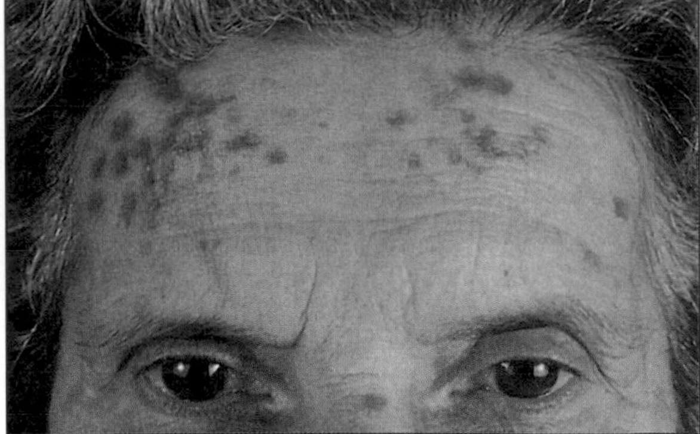

Fig. 50.2. Miliary sarcoidosis

Erythema Nodosum. This is one of the most typical findings in acute or subacute sarcoidosis, present in 30–40% of cases. In most parts of the world, it is necessary to exclude sarcoidosis when erythema nodosum is diagnosed in adults (Chap. 21). Erythema nodosum is more likely to represent sarcoidosis in Germany than in USA.

Angiolupoid Sarcoidosis (Brocq and Pautrier 1913). This form of chronic cutaneous sarcoidosis features red-brown papules, nodules and plaques. The nomenclature is somewhat confusing and many overlaps exist. Soft plaques with prominent telangiectases tend to involve the mid-face of women. The lesions are stubborn; they may improve with topical or intralesional corticosteroids but tend to recur. The differential diagnosis includes lupus vulgaris, pseudolymphoma, and facial granuloma.

Miliary Sarcoidosis (Benign Miliary Lupoid). The typical lesion is red-brown, 2–5 mm in diameter and macular, papular or nodular. Lesions may be few in number but are usually multiple and either diffuse or locally grouped (Fig. 50.2). Some appear lichenoid. Secondary changes such as scale, crust or ulceration are very rare. The most common sites are the face, extensor surfaces of the extremities and the trunk. Mucosal surfaces can be involved. Some larger lesions show central clearing, producing an annular variant. Both hyper- and hypopigmentation may occur. Annular facial lesions are particularly common in black patients. Patients with this type often have no internal involvement and in general have a relatively benign course.

Circinate Sarcoidosis. Yellow-red band-like, usually slightly raised lesions show circular or gyrate patterns and are typically found on the forehead,

Table 50.2. Comparison between acute and chronic sarcoidosis

	Acute sarcoidosis	Chronic sarcoidosis
Course	Transitory	Persistent
Average age (years)	30	40
Onset	Abrupt	Gradual
Skin changes	Erythema nodosum, small lesions	Lupus pernio, large lesions
Eye changes	Iritis, conjunctivitis, conjunctival granulomas	Uveitis, glaucoma, cataracts, keratoconjunctivitis sicca
Lymphadenopathy, facial paralysis, parotid disease	Common and transitory	Uncommon
Bone cysts	None	Present
Chest X-ray	Bilateral hilar lymphadenopathy	Diffuse changes
Cardiac changes	Arrhythmias	Cor pulmonale
Histology	Granulomas with epithelioid cells and giant cells	Fibrosis
Calcium metabolism	Hypercalcemia, hypercalcuria	Nephrocalcinosis
Urinary hydroxyproline	Elevated	Normal
Bronchoalveolar lavage	Increased lymphocytes	Usually normal
Serum angiotensin-converting enzyme	May be elevated	Usually normal
Prognosis	Favorable	Less favorable, depends on organ involvement

cheeks or nape (Fig. 50.3). There may be minimal scale. The lesions spread peripherally with central clearing, depigmentation and atrophy. The lesions are very similar to Miescher granuloma and necrobiosis lipoidica diabeticorum.

Nodular Sarcoidosis. Large, red-brown telangiectatic nodules can be seen, often involving the nose, ear lobes or cheeks. The lesions may show central regression (Fig. 50.4). A particular variant of nodu-

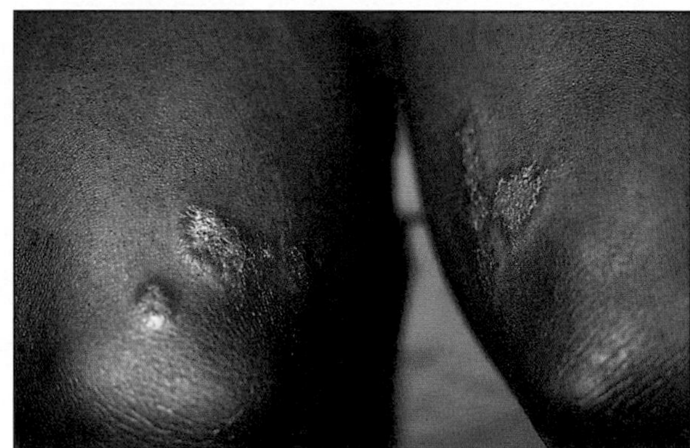

Fig. 50.3. Circinate sarcoidosis. (Courtesy of Robert Swerlick, MD, Atlanta, Georgia)

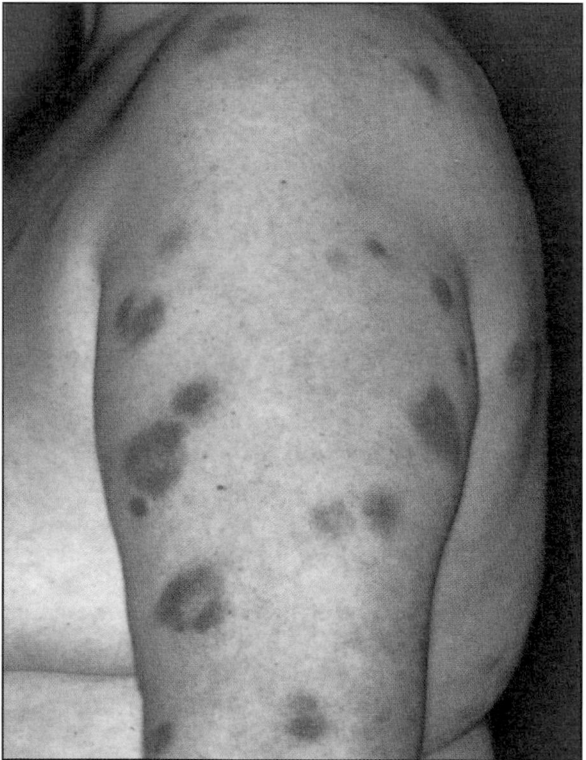

Fig. 50.4. Nodular sarcoidosis

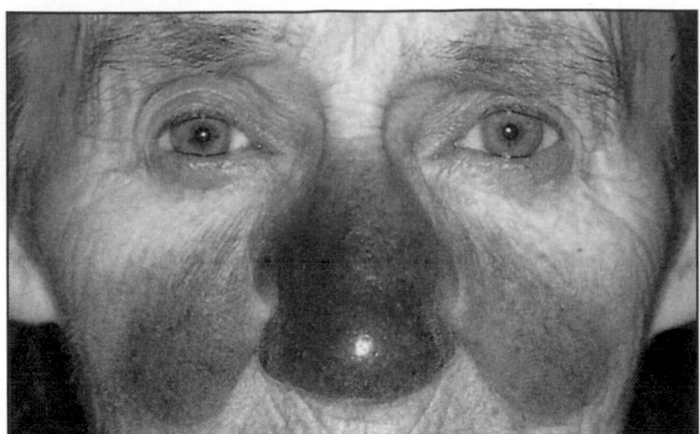

Fig. 50.5. Sarcoidosis – lupus pernio

lar sarcoidosis is lupus pernio. Here the nose and cheeks are involved, mimicking true pernio or a cold injury (Fig. 50.5). Such patients are usually women who often have sarcoidal bone disease that is clinically manifested by swellings of the digits and distinctive bone cysts on radiologic examination.

Subcutaneous Sarcoidosis. When the granuloma is situated somewhat deeper, the classic red-brown color may not be seen. Instead, the overlying skin may be normal or slightly red. One can palpate a deeper nodule. In other cases, the infiltrative process may mimic nodular or subcutaneous morphea. The inflammation may extend to the subcutaneous fat, causing a granulomatous panniculitis. The term Darier-Roussy sarcoidosis (Darier and Roussy 1906) is sometimes equated with panniculitis in sarcoidosis. Unfortunately, it is unclear what Darier and Roussy were describing, as granulomatous panniculitis can be associated with many disorders. Today the term is no longer used.

Scar Sarcoidosis. Patients with sarcoidosis apparently are able to react to a variety of traumatic events with granuloma formation. This may be clinically useful. Patients who develop tiny red-brown nodules along operative scars or even venepuncture sites may well have sarcoidosis. When surgical patients are studied for scar changes, some patients with undiagnosed sarcoidosis are found. Conversely, when sarcoidosis patients are surveyed for changing scars, the yield is also striking. The presence of a foreign body in a granuloma does not exclude sarcoidosis entirely. Many cases of scar sarcoidosis arise following car accidents with exposure to glass and dirt. Explosion of landmines may also drive powder, metal fragments or dirt into the skin. The pathologic diagnosis of sarcoidal foreign body granuloma mandates a search for other signs of sarcoidosis.

Ulcerated Sarcoidosis. The cutaneous lesions of sarcoidosis very rarely ulcerate. When they do, the most common site is the lower extremities, so that an ulcerated necrobiosis lipoidica diabeticorum must also be considered. However, most patients with ulcerative sarcoidosis have systemic involvement making the diagnosis easier.

Other Forms of Cutaneous Sarcoidosis. The scalp may rarely be involved with either nodules or a scarring alopecia. A variety of nail changes have been described, but none is specific. If the pulmonary involvement is severe, and clubbing may be seen. Nasal and conjunctival mucosa may also be involved with granulomas. The nasal disease may lead to septal perforation and sinus disease.

Systemic Findings. The systemic problems associated with sarcoidosis are numerous and beyond the scope of this text. We will just mention a few selected problems. Most patients have general symptoms, such as malaise, fever and weight loss. Night sweats may also occur.

Pulmonary Disease. The lungs are probably the most often involved systemic organ. The chest X-ray is often a valuable tool to diagnosis, showing hilar lymphadenopathy and often parenchymal disease, even in asymptomatic patients. The hilar node enlargement is usually bilateral, but may be unilateral. The parenchymal involvement may present as diffuse ground-glass change, multiple small lesions or larger nodules resembling metastases. Pulmonary disease may have minimal symptoms; cough and dyspnea are most common. Severe fibrosis and cor pulmonale are the possible end results.

Ocular Disease. About 15–25% of patients have eye involvement. The most common problem is granulomatous uveitis, which may lead to secondary glaucoma and blindness, if not treated. Lacrimal gland involvement, leading to keratitis sicca, retinal bleeding and neovascularization, and chorioretinitis may all occur. Acute iridocyclitis may present with pain, light sensitivity and distorted vision. We refer all patients with cutaneous sarcoidosis to an ophthalmologist to search for involvement and establish a baseline.

Table 50.3. Syndromes associated with sarcoidosis

Specific for sarcoidosis	Löfgren syndrome	Bilateral hilar lymphadenopathy, arthritis (typically in ankles) and erythema nodosum
	Heerfordt syndrome (uveoparotid fever)	Facial nerve palsy, iridocyclitis, and parotid gland swelling
	Jüngling syndrome (ostitis multiplex cystoides)	Multiple cysts in distal phalanges
Occur in sarcoidosis	Mikulicz syndrome	Parotid gland swelling and pain, often with sicca syndrome
	Sicca syndrome	Reduction in saliva and tear flow with dry eyes and/or mouth (but without obvious parotid swelling)
	Parinaud syndrome (oculoglandular syndrome)	Conjunctivitis (usually unilateral) with lymphadenopathy; more often seen with cat scratch fever and other infections

Neurologic Disease. Either the CNS or peripheral nerves are involved in about 10% of patients. Changes usually appear early in the disease course. Cranial nerve palsies, especially facial nerve palsy, are most common and have a relatively good outlook. Other peripheral neuropathies and CNS disease, including encephalitis, meningitis and space-occupying granulomatous lesions, have a less favorable outlook.

Renal Disease. The macrophages in the sarcoidal granulomas produce 1,25-dihydroxy vitamin D and related compounds. Thus hypercalcemia and hypercalcuria may occur, producing renal stones and even nephrocalcinosis leading to renal failure. In addition, sarcoidal granulomas may occur in the renal interstitium. Fortunately, systemic corticosteroid therapy has reduced the likelihood of progressive renal disease. In addition, CNS granulomas may involve the pituitary, producing diabetes insipidus.

Bone Disease. Most often the phalanges are involved, especially in patients with lupus pernio. The bony destruction is also mediated by vitamin D analogs produced by the granulomas. In addition an osteoclast-activating factor is produced. The involvement of the digits is known as ostitis multiplex cystoides (Jüngling disease). The radiologic examination reveals multiple circular radiolucent lesions – the punched-ticket sign. Often the patient is unable to abduct the digits, but this is not a reliable sign. Long bone involvement is less common. In addition sarcoidal granulomas can directly involve the bones.

Arthritis. About 40% of sarcoidosis patients present with joint disease. It occurs in association with other early inflammatory reactions, such as erythema nodosum and hilar lymphadenopathy. The main sites of involvement are the knees, ankles and to a lesser extent, the hands and feet. Muscular involvement, both acute and chronic, is very rare.

Hepatic Disease. The liver contains granulomas in over 70% of patients, so that a liver biopsy is a fruitful diagnostic tool. On the other hand, only 10–20% of patients have abnormal hepatic function and even fewer are symptomatic with hepatomegaly or jaundice.

Childhood Sarcoidosis. Young patients with sarcoidosis tend to have extensive skin involvement, arthritis and uveitis. The Blau-Jabs syndrome is similar but perhaps inherited in an autosomal dominant fashion.

Associated Syndromes. Sarcoidosis is associated with a number of syndromes, or perhaps better, disease constellations which are listed in Table 50.3.

Löfgren Syndrome (Löfgren 1946). Arthritis, often involving the ankles, erythema nodosum and bilateral hilar lymphadenopathy is known as Löfgren syndrome. Most patients have fever and malaise. This is a typical pattern for acute sarcoidosis, usually involving women 20–40 years old with every expectation of spontaneous resolution.

Heerfordt Syndrome (Heerfordt 1909). Uveoparotid fever is a another name for the combination of acute parotid swelling, facial nerve palsy and ocular disease. Other salivary glands may be involved, as may be the similar lacrimal glands. Some patients develop a sicca syndrome. Once again, the combination occurs acutely, usually involves younger patients and has a good outlook.

Mikulicz Syndrome (Mikulicz-Radecki 1892). It is unclear what Mikulicz-Radecki was describing. His patient had bilateral parotid and submandibular gland swelling with xerostomia. While this constellation is traditionally attached to sarcoidosis, most such individuals have Sjögren syndrome.

Histopathology. The typical sarcoidal granuloma consists of epithelioid macrophages, giant cells and a sparse lymphocytic infiltrate. The naked granulomas are sharply defined and may be found throughout the skin, ranging from abutting onto the epidermis to involving the deep fat. Caseation necrosis is not seen. The two main differential diagnostic problems are tuberculoid leprosy and foreign body granulomas. The systemic granulomas are similar, but the range of systemic pathologic findings is beyond our scope.

Laboratory Findings. A single reliable marker for sarcoidosis does not exist. Probably the most often employed test is measurement of serum angiotensin-converting enzyme (ACE) which is produced by macrophages. Unfortunately, serum levels are also elevated in other granulomatous processes, making ACE a poor diagnostic tool, but often a useful way to follow documented sarcoidosis.

Alkaline phosphatase and other hepatic enzymes may be elevated, but this too is nonspecific. Calcium levels should be measured. Uric acid levels may be high, but gout is only rarely seen.

Diagnostic Criteria. The diagnosis of sarcoidosis mandates combining a number of other diagnostic approaches. One needs histologic evidence of a sarcoidal granuloma coupled with proof of involvement of various organs. One begins with a chest X-ray. If the pattern is typical and the patient asymptomatic, one can still make the diagnosis. In a small percentage of symptomatic patients, the radiograph will be normal. Other imaging studies can also be used to search for lymphadenopathy. The next step is a search for histologic confirmation. Usually the skin or lymph nodes are most accessible, but if none is identified, a transbronchial lung biopsy, a mediastinal lymph node biopsy or a liver biopsy is recommended.

The Kveim-Siltzbach test has a long and interesting history. Most dermatologists have encountered the name when preparing for their specialty examination but have never performed the procedure. The test was based on the intradermal injection of extracts from the spleen or lymph nodes of patients with acute sarcoidosis. Because of the risk of transferring viruses and other biologic agents, the material is unavailable in both the USA and Germany. The material is injected, and after a period of 4–6 weeks, a red-brown papule or nodule may develop resembling cutaneous sarcoidosis and revealing sarcoidal granulomas when excised. The test is unreliable (a negative test says nothing), possibly dangerous, time-consuming and expensive; it should be viewed as a relic of historical interest.

Many patients with sarcoidosis are relatively anergic. This is puzzling since both cellular and humoral immunity is in many ways stimulated. Tuberculin testing should be carried out. A negative second strength reaction excludes tuberculosis, which may mimic sarcoidosis or occur simultaneously. Anergy towards other standard test materials such as trichophytin, *Candida albicans*, other fungal antigens or 2,4-dinitrochlorobenzene (DNCB) can be documented, if desired.

Two other potentially helpful diagnostic tools are bronchoalveolar lavage and gallium scanning. Pulmonary lavage reveals a relative lymphocytosis, but unfortunately this is not very sensitive or specific. Lymphocyte levels have been used to determine the need for systemic corticosteroids and to monitor their effectiveness but this approach is expensive and probably unnecessary. Radionucleotide scanning using gallium-67 is a sensitive way to identify granulomas, but it is not specific for sarcoidosis. It can help to identify an active disease site when planning a biopsy or to help distinguish between persistent granulomas and fibrosis.

Course and Prognosis. Race and extrapulmonary disease both correlate with outcome. In the USA, the rough 10-year likelihood of recovery in whites and blacks, respectively, are as follows: 90% and 75% for those with pulmonary disease alone, and 70% and 45% for those with extrapulmonary disease.

About 10% of patients with sarcoidosis have chronic serious disease. The main problems are ocular and pulmonary. Pulmonary fibrosis is the leading cause of death.

Differential Diagnosis. The differential diagnosis of sarcoidosis in the skin includes the entire range of granulomatous reactions. Whenever red-brown nodules are identified, one must think of sarcoidosis, tuberculoid leprosy, tuberculosis, leishmaniasis, syphilis, foreign body reactions, granulomatous or lupoid rosacea, pseudolymphoma, lymphoma and leukemic infiltrates. Patients with several types of immunodeficiency may develop sarcoidal granulomas in the skin, lungs and other organs. The biopsy should point one in the correct direction, but one must also search for other systemic clues. The differential diagnosis of the systemic aspects of sarcoidosis includes most of internal medicine.

Therapy
Systemic. Oral corticosteroids are the mainstay of therapy in sarcoidosis, but one should carefully consider the risk/benefit ratio. Not every patient with sarcoidosis requires treatment. While corticosteroids increase the rate of clearance of pulmonary symptoms and produce radiologic improvement, they provide no overwhelming long-term benefits. Corticosteroids should be reserved for severe inflammatory disease in dangerous (eye involvement) or painful (arthritis, fever) situations. NSAIDs may be sufficient for symptom relief in acute sarcoidosis. Pulmonary distress, cardiac arrhythmias, CNS disease and hepatic dysfunction all are indications for systemic therapy. Hypercalcemia responds very well to corticosteroids and should be considered almost an absolute indication. Usually relatively low dosages work well. One can start with prednisone 40 mg daily, but usually control can be achieved with 15–20 mg every other day or 5–10 mg daily. One risk of corticosteroid therapy is the possible reactivation of tuberculosis.

When corticosteroids are ineffective, the situation becomes more difficult. Methotrexate, chlorambucil, cyclophosphamide, azathioprine and thalidomide all have been employed as alternative agents. They have mainly been employed to retard pulmonary fibrosis or for disfiguring skin lesions. Antimalarials are occasionally employed to treat cutaneous sarcoidosis and may help pulmonary disease. The presence of cutaneous lesions should usually not be the determining factor in the choice of systemic agents.

Topical. High-potency topical corticosteroids are usually quite effective in controlling the cutaneous disease. They can be used under occlusion or injected intralesionally. We use 2.5 mg/cc of triamcinolone acetonide, usually in a local anesthetic. PUVA has been useful in some cases; we have had good success recently with PUVA bath therapy (Chap. 13).

Necrobiotic Diseases

Granuloma Annulare

(Colcott Fox 1895)

Definition. Benign granulomatous disease of unknown etiology, that usually presents with papules arranged in a ring. Histologically, it features necrobiosis or partial death of collagen.

Epidemiology. Granuloma annulare is a disease of the young. The solitary lesions frequently affect children, while more disseminated disease affects young adults with a heavy female predominance.

Etiology and Pathogenesis. While many possible causes for granuloma annulare have been postulated, it is simplest to say that the cause is unknown. Trauma, sunlight, PUVA therapy, arthropod bites and medications have been incriminated. Vitamin D in the levels used to treat tuberculosis was often blamed years ago (granuloma vigantolicum; Vigantol was the brand name of the vitamin D). While generalized granuloma annulare is associated with diabetes mellitus in about 20 % of cases, no pathophysiologic association has been established. The nature of necrobiosis is also not understood, but it is found in a number of granulomatous processes. Histologically, the abnormal collagen is pale staining, associated with mucin and glycogen and often surrounded by histiocytes.

Clinical Findings. The typical lesion of granuloma annulare involves the extremities of a young child. The most typical location is the back of hand or foot, but the fingers, toes and elbows are also likely sites (Fig. 50.6). Granuloma annulare is often over a joint. More diffuse lesions may involve the face or

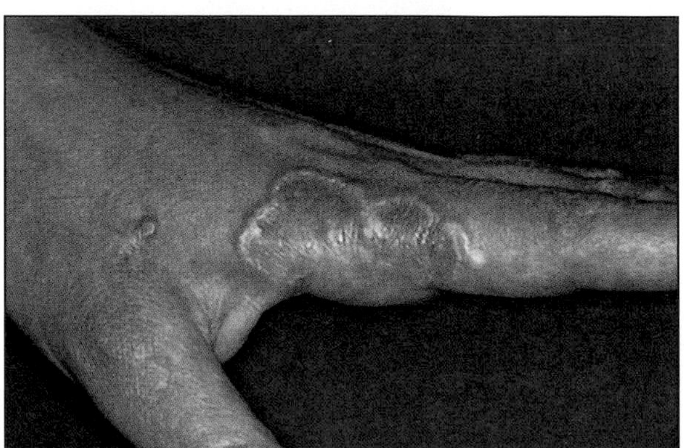

Fig. 50.6. Granuloma annulare

trunk. The acral lesion starts as a firm pale-red papule, which slowly grows with central clearing. The border becomes circular, comprised of multiple small, often flat-topped papules that are sharply bordered. The lesions can become several centimeters in diameter. The border is usually palpable. The cleared area is not atrophic. Scale is almost always lacking. The lesions are not pruritic. Granuloma annulare has several other distinct forms that are less typical:

- Erythematous form: Initially widespread, often complex areas of erythema are present. With time, these become indurated and individual papules may be appreciated.
- Plaque form: Large, flat infiltrated plaques may be found. They typically are red-brown in color and resemble necrobiosis lipoidica diabeticorum or annular elastolytic giant cell granuloma.
- Subcutaneous form: Deep dermal nodules, often over joints, involving the fingers or toes, or on the skull are common in children but also seen in adults. These lesions are clinically similar to rheumatoid nodules. Children with juvenile rheumatoid arthritis rarely have rheumatoid nodules.
- Perforating form: Granuloma annulare belongs to the perforating dermatoses. The acral nodules are most likely to ulcerate, discharging necrotic collagen and other debris. While the ulcerated nodule may cause clinical concern, a biopsy usually allows one to easily make the diagnosis.
- Disseminated form: When numerous typical annular lesions are present, the diagnosis is easy. Sometimes disseminated erythematous papules without a hint of annularity are present (Fig. 50.7). Even in such patients, annular lesions can often be found on the extremities, especially the feet. Adult patients are usually affected, most often younger women. About 20% of patients have diabetes mellitus.

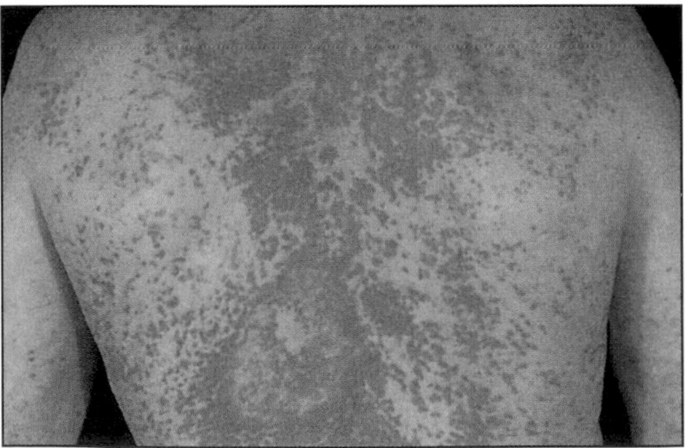

Fig. 50.7. Disseminated granuloma annulare

Histopathology. Granuloma annulare is characterized by necrobiosis, palisading histiocytes and a limited number of giant cells. There is usually some mucin and glycogen between the strands of collagen, and in some cases the mucin may dominate the picture. The process is usually centered in the mid-dermis, but in the subcutaneous variant may involve the fat. In early or diffuse lesions, sometimes no necrobiosis is found; only a perivascular lymphocytic infiltrate and histiocytes infiltrating between bundles of collagen are seen. This incomplete form of granuloma annulare represents a most difficult histologic diagnosis. While much has been made of vasculitis in granuloma annulare, in our experience it is uncommon and not helpful.

Course and Prognosis. Typical childhood granuloma annulare almost always resolves spontaneously after 1–2 years. The other forms, especially disseminated granuloma annulare, are more persistent and therapy-resistant. Puzzling, but nonetheless a relief, is the tendency of a lesion to disappear after a biopsy.

Differential Diagnosis. The clinical differential diagnosis varies greatly with the form of granuloma annulare. The typical annular lesions in children are almost pathognomonic. The pale color is quite districtive in contrast to other deeper red granulomas. Dermatophyte infections, especially when treated with topical corticosteroids, and annular lichen planus may cause problems. Many other diseases may occasionally be annular, such as papular mucinosis and erythema elevatum diutinum. Nodules may be confused with sarcoidosis, basal cell carcinoma and other tumors. Disseminated disease should be separated from sarcoidosis, lichen planus and other infiltrates. The overlaps between granuloma annulare and both necrobiosis lipoidica diabeticorum and rheumatoid nodule are discussed below.

Therapy

Systemic. Generally systemic therapy is both unnecessary and unrewarding. A variety of agents have been proposed for disseminated granuloma annulare, including dapsone, antimalarials and of course systemic corticosteroids. The risk/benefit ratio rarely favors therapy. Antimetabolites have also been recommended, but appropriately discarded in recent years. Some patients have benefited from retinoids and/or PUVA therapy.

Topical. Intralesional corticosteroids, such as triamcinolone acetonide 2.5–5.0 mg/ml, are the simplest therapy. Any given lesion, even subcutaneous nodules, can be eliminated. The problems are that sometimes there are too may lesions or the procedure is too painful for a child. Occlusive therapy using corticosteroid creams and Saran Wrap or occlusive tapes impregnated with corticosteroids are a good second choice. For widespread disease, we have had good success with topical bath-PUVA therapy. Even scarification has been recommended because of the tendency of granuloma annulare to regress following minor trauma.

Annular Elastolytic Giant Cell Granuloma

(O'Brien 1975; Hanke et al. 1979)

Synonyms. Actinic granuloma, actinic granuloma annulare, facial Miescher granuloma, facial necrobiosis lipoidica diabeticorum

Definition. Necrobiotic process usually appearing on sun-exposed skin with large annular lesions.

Etiology and Pathogenesis. The etiology of this confusing entity is unclear. As the befuddling list of synonyms shows, some consider it to be a variant of granuloma annulare, simply appearing on the face or other sun-exposed skin. Others have classified it as necrobiosis lipoidica diabeticorum away from the shins. Often the giant cells in annular elastolytic giant cell granuloma contain elastotic or sun-damaged collagen and elastin. This has been taken as a possible defining criterion, but may just reflect the location.

Clinical Findings. Typically there are large annular red-brown plaques, often with bizarre shapes, found on the face, neck and arms of older adults (Fig. 50.8). The borders are not as papular as in granuloma annulare, and the central cleared areas seem more atrophic, but once again this may simply reflect the age of the patients and the location. The lesions tend to spread slowly and are persistent.

Histopathology. Microscopic examination reveals solar elastosis, relatively little necrobiosis and multinucleate giant cells. Usually strands of elastotic material can be found in some of the giant cells; an elastic stain may help to make this finding more obvious.

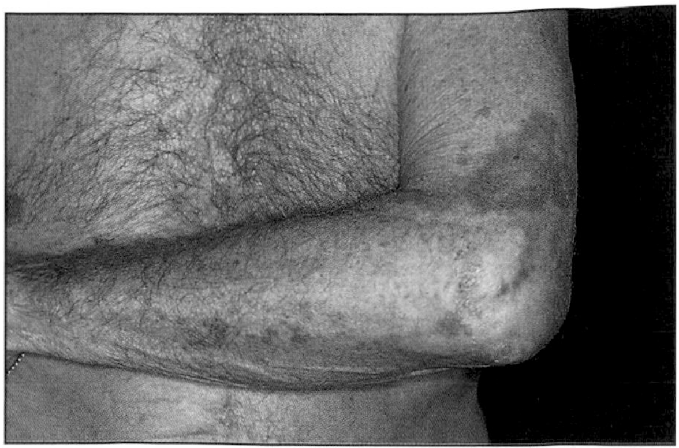

Fig. 50.8. Annular elastolytic giant cell granuloma

Therapy. There is no satisfactory therapy. The same approaches as discussed under granuloma annulare have been tried, but with little success. Intralesional corticosteroids probably are most effective. Antimalarials, dapsone and clofazimine have all been tried systemically.

Granuloma Multiforme

(Leiker et al. 1964)

Synonym. Mkar disease

This uncommon annular eruption has been described primarily in central Africa. It probably represents a variant of granuloma annulare or annular elastolytic giant cell granuloma. Typically the face, arms and trunk are involved. The large annular lesions may develop central hypopigmentation. The disease tends to be chronic. Microscopic examination reveals necrobiosis and a histiocytic infiltrate, perhaps with more giant cells than typically seen in granuloma annulare.

Actinic Granuloma Annulare

This disease is most often seen in Saharan Africa and the Middle East. It may represent granuloma multiforme in a different ethnic group. The lesions are typically located on the hands, face and sun-exposed aspects of the neck. They may be solitary or multiple and tend to be large annular lesions with central hypopigmentation. The differences between this disorder and annular elastolytic giant cell granuloma are primarily microscopic.

Necrobiosis Lipoidica Diabeticorum

(Oppenheim 1930; Urbach 1932)

Synonyms. Necrobiosis lipoidica, granulomatosis disciformis chronica et progressiva of Miescher, granulomatosis tuberculoides pseudosclerodermiformis of Gottron. While the name necrobiosis lipoidica is preferable since many patients do not have diabetes mellitus, the longer name of necrobiosis lipoidica diabeticorum has become established.

Definition. Chronic granulomatous process usually involving the shins of patients with diabetes mellitus.

Epidemiology. Necrobiosis lipoidica diabeticorum is an uncommon disease. Fewer than 1% of patients with diabetes mellitus have these changes. Conversely, about 40% of patients with necrobiosis lipoidica diabeticorum have diabetes mellitus.

Etiology and Pathogenesis. An etiologic role involving abnormal glucose metabolism has long been sought but never found. Necrobiosis lipoidica diabeticorum may appear prior to the development of diabetes mellitus, but appears to be independent of the severity of the metabolic disturbance. Most patients have late-onset or type II diabetes mellitus. Middle-aged women are most often affected. Similar HLA patterns as in diabetes mellitus are found; HLA-B8, -Cw3 and -DR4 are increased in frequency. Small vessel damage is frequently observed, suggesting an association with diabetic microangiopathy. Vasculitis may be observed microscopically, and primarily perivascular deposition of C3, IgG, IgM and IgA occurs. Hypohidrosis may be found; it has been blamed on local nerve damage. In addition, abnormalities of collagen metabolism have been described. Finally, an association appears to exist between necrobiosis lipoidica diabeticorum and familial β-lipoproteinemia.

Clinical Findings. Most lesions are found on the extensor aspects of the legs. The most typical site is the shins, but the ankle and dorsal part of the foot can also involved (Fig. 50.9). Less often the calf or thigh is involved. About 15% of lesions are estimated to appear elsewhere on the body. The lesions are usually yellow to red-brown irregular, sharply bordered plaques which range between slightly indurated and atrophic. The border tends to be darker than the central region, which usually has a yellow tone. Prominent telangiectases may be present, especially centrally. Diascopy will usually reveal the yellow color and the prominent vessels. The yellow color suggests a similarity to lupus vulgaris, while the progressive red-brown border resembles morphea. Thus Gottron coined the name granulomatosis tuberculoides pseudosclerodermiformis.

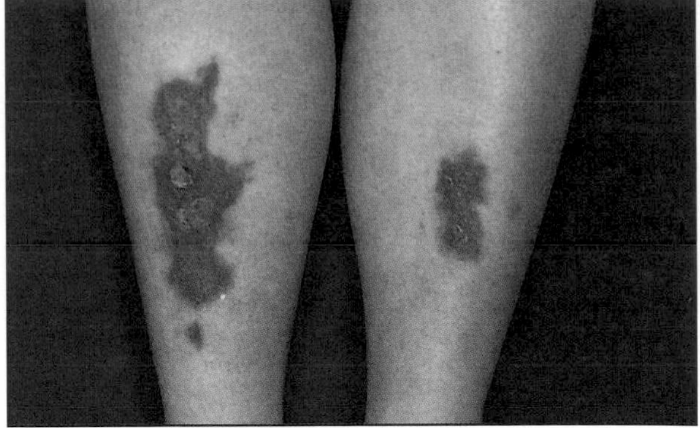

Fig. 50.9. Necrobiosis lipoidica diabeticorum

While the initial lesion is often unilateral, symmetric involvement of both shins is the rule. Small plaques frequently coalesce. About one-third of lesions become ulcerated; the yellow ulcers with a fatty base heal very slowly. Even minor trauma or a small punch biopsy may produce a nonhealing ulcer. When the ulcer is directly over the tibia, a painful infection of the periosteum may arise. As necrobiosis lipoidica diabeticorum heals, atrophy results with destruction of hair follicles and sweat glands.

There are many clinical variants of necrobiosis lipoidica diabeticorum, each of which causes problems in differential diagnosis and nomenclature, especially if the patient has no diabetes mellitus and no shin involvement.

- Disseminated Form. Multiple plaques, several centimeters in size and red to red-brown in color, are dispersed over the extremities and trunk. The lesions are similar to those of disseminated granuloma annulare. If necrobiosis lipoidica diabeticorum is present on the shin, then one diagnoses disseminated necrobiosis lipoidica diabeticorum. If not, one can try to employ histologic differences, but the distinction is clinically unimportant.
- Facial or Actinic Form. We consider this the same as annular elastolytic giant cell granuloma or actinic granuloma annulare.

- Scalp Form. Scalp lesions are typically bizarre and circinate, resembling circinate sarcoidosis. There may be atrophy and hair loss, so that necrobiosis lipoidica diabeticorum is one of the causes of pseudopelade.
- Granulomatosis Disciformis Chronica et Progressiva (Miescher and Leder 1948). This tongue twister, usually shortened to Miescher granuloma, is sometimes incorrectly used as a synonym for annular elastolytic giant cell granuloma. Miescher described bilateral shin lesions in nondiabetic patients with a more prominent giant cell reaction and without lipid deposits.
- Associated with Ataxia-Telangiectasia (Chap. 13). Patients with the rare genodermatosis ataxia-telangiectasia tend to develop atrophic ulcerated plaques with prominent borders that resemble necrobiosis lipoidica diabeticorum. While an infectious trigger appears intuitively likely, none has been found.

Histopathology. The principal changes are necrobiosis, accumulations of macrophages and giant cells, and perivascular groups of lymphocytes. Sometimes plasma cells are common. Sudan stain usually demonstrates the presence of lipids. True vasculitis is uncommon but extravasation of red blood cells may occur. The disease process typically involves the entire dermis and may extend into the subcutaneous fat. Sometimes palisading macrophages about necrobiotic zones predominate; this correlates somewhat with the presence of diabetes mellitus. In older patients, the giant cell response predominates; one could describe this as the Miescher pattern. Thus, while there are distinct differences, histologic overlaps between granuloma annulare, annular elastolytic giant cell granuloma and necrobiosis lipoidica diabeticorum can rarely occur.

Differential Diagnosis. The differential diagnosis is lengthy in unusual forms. Typical necrobiosis lipoidica diabeticorum of the shin is a one-look diagnosis. When necrobiosis lipoidica diabeticorum involves other body areas, one must think of granuloma annulare and annular elastolytic giant cell granuloma. Often the correct diagnosis is simply a question of preferred nomenclature. Scalp involvement is very similar to that seen in sarcoidosis. In addition, lupus vulgaris and morphea occasionally appear similar. These three diseases can be confidently excluded with a biopsy, but at the risk of a shin ulcer. Ulcerated lesions mimic a tuberous-serpiginous lesion of tertiary syphilis.

Therapy. There is no good therapy, so many approaches have been recommended. Surprisingly, since necrobiosis lipoidica diabeticorum tends to be atrophic, treatment with high-potency topical corticosteroids under occlusion or even intralesional corticosteroids can be effective. Pulse therapy with high-dose intravenous corticosteroids has also been employed. Attempts to improve the microcirculation with agents such as pentoxifylline or aspirin plus dipyridamole are occasionally successful but usually fail.

Rheumatoid Nodule

(Hilliers 1868)

Definition. Firm subcutaneous masses usually found over bony prominences in patients with rheumatoid arthritis (Chap. 18).

Epidemiology. Rheumatoid nodules are found in about 20% of patients with rheumatoid arthritis. They are more common in patients with severe disease. Rarely they are described in patients with no evidence of rheumatoid arthritis, but we tend to classify these as subcutaneous granuloma annulare.

Etiology and Pathogenesis. The association between severe rheumatoid arthritis, high titers of rheumatoid factor and evidence of either cutaneous or systemic vasculitis has made the blood vessel a focus for those seeking the cause of rheumatoid nodules. Trauma also appears to play a role. Interactions between heat shock proteins, T cells and macrophages offer a plausible explanation. While rheumatoid nodules are occasionally described in other connective tissue diseases, in many cases other types of granulomas have been incorrectly classified.

Clinical Findings. Rheumatoid nodules are firm hard subcutaneous masses that are frequently painful. The sites of predilection are the elbows and ulnar aspect of the arm, supporting the possible role of trauma as a trigger (Fig. 50.10). Other common sites include the fingers, knees, feet and occasionally ears. Multiple lesions are usually present. Sometimes the nodules will ulcerate and drain; trauma may trigger the ulceration. Many variants of rheumatoid nodule have been described:

- Linear, papular and ulcerative: All three of these variants have similarities, including grouped smaller lesions, an association with vasculitis and possible ulceration. In many cases, the more

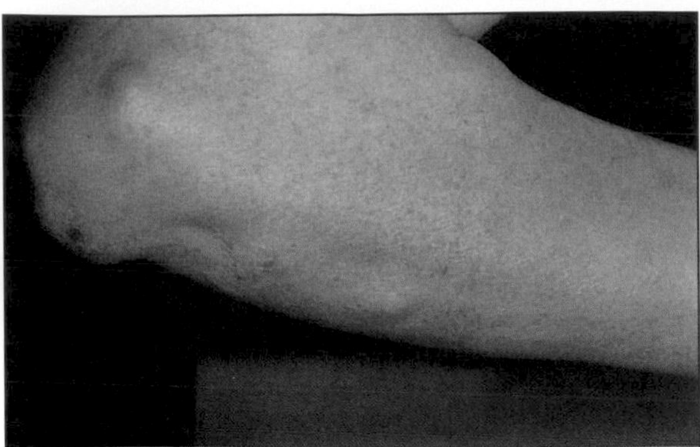

Fig. 50.10. Rheumatoid nodules

accurate description may be neutrophilic and palisaded granulomatous dermatitis.

- Rheumatoid nodulosis: Multiple subcutaneous nodules and no evidence of rheumatoid arthritis.
- Palindromic or recurrent rheumatism: These patients have multiple rheumatoid nodules, minimal arthritis not meeting the criteria for rheumatoid arthritis and a benign course highlighted by recurrent flares.

Histopathology. Massive necrobiosis is the hallmark. The zone of abnormal collagen is surround by palisading histiocytes and giant cells. The nodules are rich in fibrin, which can be identified with immunofluorescent examination if desired. In addition, immunoglobulins are deposited at the periphery and about vessels. In contrast to granuloma annulare, mucin is usually not present. Larger lesions may have a pseudocapsule so that they can be shelled out.

Course and Prognosis. Rheumatoid nodules are permanent and often painful and troublesome. In addition, they are a marker for more severe rheumatic disease. Ulceration is the most feared complication.

Differential Diagnosis. Heberden nodules of chronic osteoarthritis are often suggested as a differential point, but they are more numerous, smaller and involve the digits. The fibrous nodules of acrodermatitis chronica atrophicans, tendinous xanthomas, gouty tophi, cutaneous calcinosis, giant cell tumor of tendon sheath and other soft tissue tumors can be excluded clinically, histologically or serologically.

Therapy. Small lesions can be treated with intralesional corticosteroids. Larger or nonresponsive lesions should only be excised if painful or draining, as healing is often poor.

Neutrophilic and Palisaded Granulomatous Dermatitis

(Finan and Winkelmann 1983)

Synonyms. Churg-Strauss granuloma, interstitial granulomatous dermatitis with arthritis, rheumatoid papules

Clinical Findings. The Churg-Strauss syndrome is a type of granulomatous vasculitis with prominent asthma and pulmonary granulomas (Chap. 22). Rarely patients with rheumatoid arthritis and other systemic disorders may have cutaneous granulomas that share similarities with granuloma annulare and rheumatoid nodule but appear distinct. In most cases the lesions are papules. Sometimes they may be crusted or umbilicated. In other instances they may be arranged as annular lesions or as linear subcutaneous cords. Associated diseases also include lupus erythematosus, other forms of systemic vasculitis and both carcinomas and hematologic malignancies. Even in patients with features of rheumatoid arthritis, the serologic findings may be initially negative.

Histopathology. The most common microscopic appearance is what has been described as interstitial or incomplete granuloma annulare. A neutrophilic infiltrate extends between strands of collagen (interstitial) as well as about vessels. The infiltrate is bottom heavy and also rich in lymphocytes, eosinophils and histiocytes. The collagen may be somewhat basophilic. In some fields, there may be tiny palisading granulomas arrayed about degenerated collagen. Mucin is far less common than in granuloma annulare and is distributed more diffusely.

Therapy. Therapy is directed at the underlying disease. Individual lesions can be treated just as outlined for granuloma annulare.

Necrobiotic Xanthogranuloma

(Kossard and Winkelmann 1980)

Synonym. Necrobiotic xanthogranuloma with paraproteinemia

Definition. Granulomatous disorder usually involving periorbital region and associated with paraproteinemia.

Epidemiology. This disorder is extremely rare with about 100 cases described.

Etiology and Pathogenesis. The cause is unknown. But almost all patients have or develop a paraproteinemia. Presumably the abnormal proteins bind to lipids that are then deposited in the skin. Patients may have necrobiotic xanthogranuloma and diffuse normolipemic plane xanthoma (Chap. 37) simultaneously, suggesting a relationship between the two marker disorders. Possible associations with Hodgkin disease and HTLV-1 infection have also been reported.

Clinical Findings. Most patients are elderly; the average age is around 65 years. The most typical site of involvement is the periorbital region; over 90% of patients have red-yellow infiltrative plaques in this area. Early lesions can be mistaken for xanthelasmas. Larger lesions may also extend into the subcutaneous tissue. More advanced lesions may show central atrophy and ulcerations. There may be infiltrates behind or about the eyes; true ocular involvement is also seen. Typical additional sites include the rest of the face, neck, trunk and rarely the proximal extremities. Similar changes have been described in a variety of internal organs.

Histopathology. The term xanthogranuloma simply means that both foamy cells and giant cells are present. The histopathologic pattern is striking. There is a combination of massive necrobiosis, numerous multinucleated giant cells and clusters of lymphocytes. The macrophages are typically foamy and Touton giant cells are present. Occasionally plasma cells are prominent. The disease process often involves the subcutaneous fat where it has been described as xanthogranulomatous panniculitis.

Laboratory Findings. Usually the immunoglobulin is IgG and κ-light chains are more common than λ-chains.

Patients should be evaluated and then followed for the development of multiple myeloma, cryoglobulinemia and hematologic malignancies.

Course and Prognosis. The outlook is based on the severity of the periocular disease and the nature of the underlying hematologic disorder.

Differential Diagnosis. Early lesions resemble xanthelasmas. As they continue to grow or appear on other body areas, the diagnosis becomes clear. There is an overlap with diffuse normolipemic plane xanthoma, but the necrobiotic xanthogranulomas are always larger and redder. Granuloma annulare and necrobiosis lipoidica diabeticorum have histologic similarities but are clinically quite different. Sarcoidosis may be clinically similar but never shows massive necrobiosis.

Therapy. The lesions can be excised or treated with intralesional corticosteroids. If an underlying hematologic disorder is found, it should be treated in cooperation with the hematologists. Both oral prednisone 20–40 mg daily and chlorambucil 2–6 mg daily have led to improvement in the cutaneous lesions.

Cutaneous Crohn Disease

(Crohn et al. 1932)

Synonym. Metastatic Crohn disease

Definition. Granulomatous skin reaction in patients with Crohn disease.

Etiology and Pathogenesis. Since the etiology of Crohn disease of the intestine is unclear, the cause of the skin changes must also remain obscure. If we assume that Crohn disease is caused by an infectious agent or some other antigen that initiates a granulomatous response, then either the same antigen or a cross-reacting antigen in the skin could elicit the same reaction.

Clinical Findings. The clinical features are highly variable. Most often lesions arise in the perianal region, or around stomas or fistulas. Other lesions may appear at more distant sites in entirely normal skin. Typically there is erythema, induration and often ulceration. Oral lesions include not only granulomatous lesions, but also aphthae and pyostomatitis vegetans.

Histopathology. The hallmark of Crohn disease and thus of its cutaneous lesions is granulomatous inflammation. Usually the process is centered about vessels in its early stages. Granulomatous vasculitis may be seen, but more often the advanced lesions are ulcerated and less specific. Giant cells may seen.

Differential Diagnosis. The differential diagnosis is very long, since all inflammatory conditions, such as infections, acne inversa and artifactual damage, must be considered. The key is the history of Crohn disease; only rarely do cutaneous manifestations precede gastrointestinal.

Therapy. The only therapy is adequate control of the underlying gastrointestinal disease.

Foreign Body Granuloma

The most common group of granulomas is foreign body granulomas, where the body evokes a variety of defense mechanisms to destroy, eliminate or isolate either exogenous or endogenous material that has wound up in the skin (Table 50.4).

Table 50.4. Examples of foreign body granulomas

Exogenous causes	Insect parts, especially tick mouth parts Hairs (hairdressers, farmers) Cactus spines Sea urchin spines Splinters Glass fragments (rare reactions) Zirconium, beryllium, silica Silicone Foreign collagen Tattoos Vaccines Other injections Exogenous ochronosis
Endogenous causes	Calcium salts Gouty tophi Oxalate crystals Keratin (hairs, cysts, ingrown nails)

Foreign body granulomas can have a wide range of histologic patterns, ranging from sarcoidal lesions from zirconium to necrobiotic lesions caused by injected collagen, often bovine, to suppurative lesions associated with vegetable or animal material. Inert objects such as glass splinters elicit little reaction and show more of a fibrotic response, as the body attempts to simply isolate the material. When the material is retained, it can often be identified with dark field or polarization microscopy if it has the property of double refraction. Some examples of foreign body granuloma are considered below.

Zirconium Granuloma

(Pinkus and Botvinick 1957)

Synonyms. Axillary granuloma, deodorant granuloma

Zirconium salts were formerly a component of some aerosol-based deodorants. They are capable of eliciting a granulomatous tissue response after entering the skin along hair follicles, sweat glands or through minor injuries. The main problem was associated with aerosol-based zirconium products, which the FDA banned in 1977. Nonaerosol zirconium salts in concentrations less than 20% are still legal but rarely encountered. Zirconium granulomas are still seen in miners and other industrial workers, occasionally forming the basis for workmen's compensation complaints.

Multiple red papules and nodules were seen in the axilla. They tended to be small and to disappear over a period of years once the zirconium exposure was ended. In the dermis numerous small granulomas consisting primarily of multinucleated giant cells with few inflammatory cells were found. Zirconium salt crystals do not polarize. While spontaneous resolution was the rule, sometimes topical corticosteroids were employed. Particularly troublesome lesions could be easily excised.

Silicone Granuloma

Silicone refers to complex organic silicon polymers which may be gels, liquids or even solids. The liquid form was formerly injected directly into the skin for re-contouring or tissue augmentation. In the 1950s to 1960s, it was the main material for cosmetic breast enlargement. In recent years highly purified silicone liquids and gels have been employed in sealed silicone rubber elastomer bags for breast reconstruction or enlargement. Some silicone leaks out of the bags, causing a local granulomatous responses. In cases where the implant ruptures, then there is massive exposure to silicone. Silicone also may migrate to distant sites such as the skin of the arm or lymph nodes. Perforation of the skin with discharge of oily silicone has been described. The solid forms are used in artificial joints and release tiny particles via routine wear and tear. The typical microscopic picture is pseudocystic vacuoles of varying size surrounded by histiocytes and giant cells. There is usually some fibrosis. The silicone itself may be retained in the tissue, depending on its consistency. The solid particles tend to evoke a more ordinary foreign body granulomatous response. In the last few years, great controversy has surrounded silicone implants. Some feel that the immune response to leaking silicone may trigger connective tissue diseases, but convincing evidence is lacking.

Collagen Implant

Bovine collagen is used extensively for correcting tissue defects. Both Zyderm, which is non-cross-linked, and Zyplast, which has glutaraldehyde-induced cross-linking have been employed. Initially the injected collagen can be seen between the strands of human collagen as a finely fibrillar material with slightly different tinctorial properties. Lymphocytes and especially eosinophils maybe seen in the early response. It apparently stimulates the production of new collagen by the fibroblasts, but on occasion may cause abscesses, urticarial reactions and granulomatous changes, including both foreign body giant cell reactions and lesions similar to granuloma annulare.

Bioplastique Implants

Bioplastique is a combination of a biologically derived carrier gel and popcorn-like polymethylsiloxane particles that can be injected for correction of defects. The larger size of the particles impedes their migration. If the material is injected too superficially, an erythematous cutaneous nodule may develop. Microscopically there are irregularly shaped holes containing the siloxanes, as well as fibrosis and foreign body giant cells.

Lipogranuloma

Injection of oily materials such as liquid paraffin produces a lipid-rich granuloma, as discussed in Chapter 21. Such lesions are also known as paraffinomas.

Hair Granuloma

There are several settings in which hairs are driven into the skin. Hairdressers and also people milking animals are likely to have hairs introduced into the skin. A particularly common site is between the fingers. Here the hair elicits a foreign body response (trichogranuloma). Endogenous hairs can achieve a similar effect, such as in a pilonidal sinus, persistent acne nodule, dermal melanocytic nevus or pseudofolliculitis barbae (Chap. 72).

Tattoo Reactions

Tattoos elicit a range of reactions (Chap. 27). In most instances the material simply sits in the corium. In some instances, a sarcoidal granuloma may develop; this is analogous to scar sarcoidosis and the patient should be investigated. Other patients respond with a pseudolymphoma (Chap. 60). Still others may develop allergic contact dermatitis to one of the metal salts producing, for example, a weeping red eye on a dramatic eagle, usually caused by cinnabar (mercury) allergy. Finally, some patients may develop a foreign body response. This is more common in the case of accidental or amateur tattoos when larger particles are introduced.

Miscellaneous Granulomatous Disorders

In this section are included peculiar granulomatous responses to several infections or alleged infections, as well as several processes that are called granulomas although they histologically have other patterns.

Myospherulosis

Myospherulosis was originally described as an unusual infection. Various investigators found large spherules containing small endobodies. The initial cases where found in the skin and the paranasal sinuses. Multiple attempts at culture proved unsuccessful. Rosai (1978) then convincingly showed that the spherules were accumulations of altered red blood cells rather than the more exotic suggestions. In most cases, the cells have been exposed to antibiotics, forming antibiotic-hematin complexes. Most cases in the skin occur following attempts at intramuscular antibiotic injection while those in the upper airway occur following packing with antibiotic ointments or impregnated gauzes. In a unique case, a patient with multiple steatocystoma developed a myospherule within a cyst, presumably from the action of the oily cyst contents on hemorrhaged blood.

Malakoplakia

(Michaelis and Gutmann 1902)

Malakoplakia is a peculiar response to chronic infection. It most typically occurs in the urinary tract, gastrointestinal tract and retroperitoneum. A small number of cases have occurred in the skin. The most usual site is the perianal region or genitalia, as well as the groin and axillae, although isolated lesions have been reported on glabrous skin. Clinically the lesion is a weeping plaque or polypoid mass that is usually chronic.

On biopsy, sheets of histiocytes (von Hansemann cells) are found, some of which contain distinctive target-like spherules of calcified material known as Michaelis-Gutmann bodies. The latter stain positively with the van Kossa stain for calcium salts. Plasma cells may also be found. No single bacteria has been identified, but in most cases there appears to be a poorly defined defect in the disposal of phagocytosed bacteria such as *Escherichia coli* or *Staphylococcus aureus*. Either surgical removal or long-term treatment with ciprofloxacin (500 mg twice daily for 4–6 months) have been recommended.

Granuloma Faciale

(Pedace and Perry 1966)

Synonyms. Granuloma eosinophilicum faciei (Wigley 1945), eosinophilic facial granuloma. This disease is not granulomatous, but is discussed here because of its name.

Definition. Chronic inflammatory cutaneous disorder characterized by red-brown facial nodules and plaques. The granulomatous infiltrate usually is rich in eosinophils.

Epidemiology. Granuloma faciale is a disease of adults. Most patients are men 40–60 years of age. Most patients are white.

Etiology and Pathogenesis. The cause is unknown. Early lesions sometimes show vasculitis but the course is atypical for vessel disease. While an infectious etiology has often been suggested, no organisms have been reliably identified. Sun exposure has also been suggested as a trigger.

Clinical Findings. Initially, one or more sharply bordered minimally infiltrated nodules or plaques are seen (Fig. 50.11). Sometimes the lesions are polycyclic. As they progress, they become more indurated, often with orange skin surface markings. The typical color is red-brown. Sometimes telangiectases are observed. The sites of predilection are the cheeks, temples, nose, earlobes and scalp, although any part of the face can be involved. Most lesions are asymptomatic, but occasionally burning or pruritus is described. Most patients are white adults. There is no systemic involvement. Spontaneous healing may occur, but more often the lesions are chronic.

Histopathology. Microscopic examination reveals a normal epidermis and a Grenz zone of normal papillary dermis. At first there are accumulations of neutrophils and eosinophils around the vessels. Giant cells or foamy macrophages are uncommon. In very early lesions leukocytoclastic vasculitis may be present. In more advanced lesions, fewer eosinophils are found and lymphocytes, plasma cells and mast cells may be seen, as well as hemosiderin and fibrosis. Direct immunofluorescent examination may reveal nonspecific deposits of immunoglobulins and complement in the basement membrane zone.

Differential Diagnosis. Sarcoidosis, fixed drug eruption, lupus erythematosus profunda, lympho-

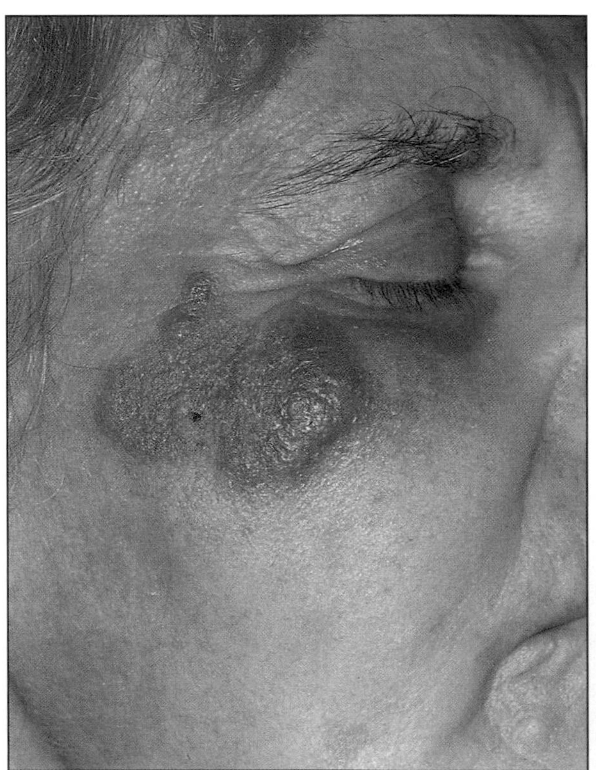

Fig. 50.11. Granuloma faciale

cytic infiltrates, lymphoma and leukemia are the most realistic disorders to be excluded. Erythema elevatum diutinum is similar histologically but most often has smaller brown-red acral lesions.

Therapy

Systemic. There is no satisfactory solution. Probably the most reliable systemic agent is dapsone; antimalarials can also be tried.

Topical. Intralesional corticosteroids or corticosteroid-impregnated tapes are probably the best approach. Corticosteroid creams and ointments rarely producc improvement.

Surgical. A wide variety of destructive methods, including dermabrasion, cryotherapy and several different laser treatments have been employed with occasional good results.

Granuloma Gluteale Infantum

(Tappeiner and Pfleger 1971)

Definition. Inflammatory nodules arising in an area of diaper dermatitis or other exudative dermatitis treated with topical corticosteroids. While this lesion clinically resembles other granulomas, it does not have granulomatous inflammation.

Epidemiology. While granuloma gluteale infantum was initially described in diaper-wearing infants, its distribution has changed. Similar changes are frequently sent in incontinent elderly patients who either wear diapers or are not receiving ideal care.

Etiology and Pathogenesis. The chronic use of fluorinated corticosteroids in treating a diaper dermatitis is felt to be the most likely trigger. However, some patients with diaper dermatitis develop typical lesions without exposure to corticosteroids. *Candida albicans* may also play a rolc.

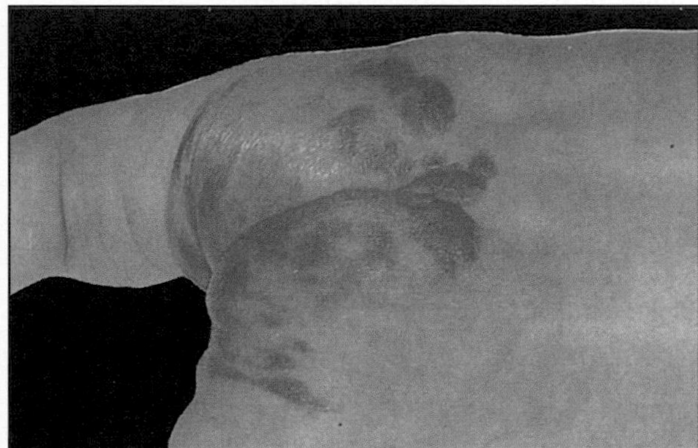

Fig. 50.12. Granuloma gluteale infantum

Clinical Findings. Multiple blue-red nodules and plaques are seen. They tend to be firm, round or oval and often lie in the skin folds. The typical sites of involvement are the buttocks and the inguinal creases (Fig. 50.12). The surface may be eroded. Often there is a background of diaper dermatitis. The same patient may also have other signs of *C. albicans* infection, such as white patches or red erosions.

Histopathology. The dermis shows a mixed inflammatory infiltrate with neutrophils, eosinophils, plasma cells and giant cells.

Differential Diagnosis. In most cases, the diagnosis is clear. Sometimes a biopsy is needed to exclude mast cell tumors, pseudolymphoma, lymphoma and leukemic infiltrates.

Therapy. Drying measures usually suffice. Frequent diaper changes, the use of cloth diapers and allowing the child periods without diapers usually suffice. In adults, nursing efforts must be intensified. A drying lotion such as zinc oxide lotion can be employed. Topical corticosteroids should be avoided.

Bibliography

General Reading

Rabinowitz LO, Zaim MT (1996) A clinicopathologic approach to granulomatous dermatoses. J Am Acad Dermatol 35:588–600

Strutton G (1997) The granulomatous reaction pattern. In: Weedon D (ed) Skin pathology. Churchill Livingstone, Edinburgh, pp 161–184

Sarcoidosis

Besnier E (1889) Lupus pernio de la face. Ann Dermatol Syph 10:333

Blau EB (1985) Familial granulomatous arthritis, iritis and rash. J Pediatr 107:689–693

Boeck C (1899) Multiple benign sarkoid of the skin. J Cutan Genitourin Dis 17:543

Brechtel B, Haas N, Henz BM et al. (1996) Allopurinol: a therapeutic alternative for disseminated cutaneous sarcoidosis. Br J Dermatol 135:307–309

Brocq L, Pautrier LM (1913) L'angio-lupoide. Ann Dermatol Syphil: 1–16

Cox N, Gawkrodger D (1988) Nail dystrophy in chronic sarcoidosis. Br J Dermatol 118:697–701

Gupta AK, Haberman HF, From GL et al. (1987) Sarcoidosis with extensive cutaneous ulceration. Dermatologica 174: 135–139

Hanno R, Needelman A, Eiferman RA et al. (1981) Cutaneous sarcoidal granulomas and the development of systemic sarcoidosis. Arch Dermatol 117:203–207

Heerfordt CF (1909) Über eine "Febris uvea-parotidea subchronica", an der Glandula parotis und an der Uvea des Auges lokalisiert und häufig mit Paresen cerebrospinaler Nerven kompliziert. Arch Ophthalmol 70:254–273

Hetherington S (1982) Sarcoidosis in young children. Am J Dis Child 136:13–15

Hruza GJ, Kerdel FA (1986) Generalized atrophic sarcoidosis with ulcerations. Arch Dermatol 122:320–322

Hutchinson J (1877) Case of livid papillary psoriasis. In: Illustrations of clinical surgery. Churchill, London, p 42

James DG (ed) (1994) Sarcoidosis and other granulomatous disorders. Dekker, New York

Jones E, Callen JP (1990) Hydroxychloroquine is effective therapy for the control of cutaneous sarcoidal granulomas. J Am Acad Dermatol 23:487–489

Jüngling O (1920) Ostitis tuberculosa multiplex cystica. Fortschr Röntgenstr 27:375

Kerdel FA, Moschella SL (1984) Sarcoidosis. An update review. J Am Acad Dermatol 11: 1–19

Kveim A (1941) En ny ogspesifikk kirtan reaksjon ved Boecks sarcoid. Nord Med 9:169

Li N, Bajoghli A, Kubba A et al. (1999) Identification of mycobacterial DNA in cutaneous lesions of sarcoidosis. J Cutan Pathol 26:271–278

Löfgren S (1946) Erythema nodosum. Studies on etiology and pathogenesis in 185 adult cases. Acta Med Scand [Suppl] 174:1–197

Mana J, Marcoval I, Graells J et al. (1997) Cutaneous involvement in sarcoidosis. Arch Dermatol 133:882–888

Mangiapan G, Hance AJ (1995) Mycobacteria and sarcoidosis: an overview and summary of recent molecular biological data. Sarcoidosis 12:20–37

Matarasso SL, Bruce S (1991) Ichthyosiform sarcoidosis: report of a case. Cutis 47:405–408

Mikulicz J (1892) Über eine eigenartige symmetrische Erkrankung der Tränen- und Mundspeicheldrüsen. Beitr Chir Fortschr, Stuttgart, pp 610–630

Newman LS, Rose CS, Maier LA (1997) Sarcoidosis. N Engl J Med 336:1224–1234

Pitt P, Hamilton E, Innes E et al. (1983) Sarcoid dactylitis. Ann Rheum Dis 42:634–639

Rasmussen JE (1981) Sarcoidosis in young children. J Am Acad Dermatol 5:566–570

Reusch G (1982) Clinical course of sarcoidosis. Internist (Berl) 23:314–324

Saxe N, Benatar SR, Bok L et al. (1984) Sarcoidosis with leg ulcera and annular facial lesions. Arch Dermatol 120:93–96

Siltzbach LE (1961) The Kveim test in sarcoidosis: a study of 750 patients. J Am Med Assoc 178:476

Thestrup-Pedersen K, Rømer FK, Jensen JH et al. (1985) Serum angiotensin-converting enzyme in sarcoidosis and psoriasis. Arch Dermatol Res 277:16–18

Vainsencher D, Winkelmann RK (1984) Subcutaneous sarcoidosis. Arch Dermatol 120:1028–1032

WASOG (1994) Consensus conference: activity of sarcoidosis. 3rd WASOG Meeting, Los Angeles, 8–11 Sept 1993. Eur Respir J 7:624–627

Zic JA, Herowitz DH, Arzubiaga C et al. (1991) Treatment of cutaneous sarcoidosis with chloroquine. Review of the literature. Arch Dermatol 127:1034–1040

Granuloma Annulare

Allen T (1966) Granuloma annulare-like reaction to sunlight. Aust J Dermatol 8:252

Andersen BL, Verdich J (1979) Granuloma annulare and diabetes mellitus. Clin Exp Dermatol 4:31–37

Bardach HG (1977) Granuloma annulare with transfollicular perforation. J Cutan Pathol 4:99–104

Barksdale SK, Perniciaro C, Halling KC et al. (1994) Granuloma annulare in patients with malignant lymphoma: clinicopathologic study of thirteen new cases. J Am Acad Dermatol 31:42–48

Colcott Fox T (1895) Ringed eruption of the fingers. Br J Dermatol 7:91–92

Cox NH, McQueen A, Evans TJ (1987) An annular erythema of infancy. Arch Dermatol 123:510–513

Dabski K, Winkelmann RK (1989) Generalized granuloma annulare: histopathology and immunopathology. J Am Acad Dermatol 20:28–39

Dabski K, Winkelmann RK (1989) Generalized granuloma annulare: clinical and laboratory findings in 100 patients. J Am Acad Dermatol 20:39–47

Filotico R, Vena GA, Coviello C et al. (1994) Cyclosporine in the treatment of generalized granuloma annulare. J Am Acad Dermatol 30:487–488

Kossard S, Winkelmann RK (1978) Response of generalized granuloma annulare to alkylating agents. Arch Dermatol 114:216–220

Krahl D, Hartschuh W, Tilgen W (1993) Granuloma annulare perforans in herpes zoster scars. J Am Acad Dermatol 29: 859–862

Muhlbauer JE (1980) Granuloma annulare. J Am Acad Dermatol 3:217–230

Ratnavel RC, Norris PG (1995) Perforating granuloma annulare: response to treatment with isotretinoin. J Am Acad Dermatol 32:126–127

Salomon RJ, Gardepe SF, Woodley DT (1986) Deep granuloma annulare in adults. Int J Dermatol 25: 109–112

Steiner A, Pehamberger H, Wolff K (1980) Sulfone treatment of granuloma annulare. J Am Acad Dermatol 13: 1004–1008

Umbert P, Winkelmann RK (1977) Histologic, ultrastructural and histochemical studies of granuloma annulare. Arch Dermatol 113:1681–1686

Wolff HH, Maciejewski W (1977) The ultrastructure of granuloma annulare. Arch Dermatol Res 259:225–234

Annular Elastolytic Giant Cell Granuloma

Barnhill RL, Goldenhersh MA (1989) Elastophagocytosis: a non-specific reaction pattern associated with inflammatory processes in sun-protected skin. J Cutan Pathol 16: 199–202

Hanke CW, Bailin PL, Roenigk HH Jr (1979) Annular elastolytic giant cell granuloma: a clinicopathologic study of five cases and a review of similar entities. J Am Acad Dermatol 1:413–421

Kato H, Kitajima Y, Yaoita H (1991) Annular elastolytic giant cell granuloma: an unusual case with papular lesions. J Dermatol 18:667–670

Kurose N, Nakagawa H, Iozumi K et al. (1992) Systemic elastolytic granulomatosis with cutaneous, ocular, lymph nodal and intestinal involvement. J Am Acad Dermatol 26:359–363

McGrae JD Jr (1986) Actinic granuloma. A clinical, histopathologic and immunocytochemical study. Arch Dermatol 122:43–47
O'Brien JP (1975) Actinic granuloma. An annular connective tissue disorder affecting sun- and heat-damaged (elastotic) skin. Arch Dermatol 111:460–466
Ragaz A, Ackerman AB (1979) Is actinic granuloma a specific condition? Am J Dermatopathol 1:43–50
Schwarz T, Lindlbauer R, Gschnait F (1983) Annular elastolytic giant cell granuloma. J Cutan Pathol 10:321–326
Sina B, Wood C, Rudo K (1992) Generalized elastophagocytic granuloma. Cutis 49:355–357
Yanagihara M, Kato F, Mori S (1987) Extra- and intracellular digestion of elastic fibers by macrophages in annular elastolytic giant cell granuloma. An ultrastructural study. J Cutan Pathol 14:303–308

Granuloma Multiforme

Allenby CF, Jones WE (1969) Granuloma multiforme. Trans St Johns Hosp Dermatol Soc 55:88–98
Browne SG (1966) Granuloma multiforme in eastern Nigeria. Int J Lepr Other Mycobact Dis 34:27–29
Cherian S (1990) Granuloma multiforme in India. Int J Lepr Other Mycobact Dis 58:719–721
Cherian S (1994) Is granuloma multiforme a photodermatosis? Int J Dermatol 33:21–22
Leiker DL, Ziedses des Plantes M (1967) Granuloma multiforme in Kenya. East Afr Med J 44:429–436
Leiker DL, Kok SH, Spaas JJ (1964) Granuloma multiforme. A new disease resembling leprosy. Int J Lepr Other Mycobact Dis 32:368–370

Necrobiosis Lipoidica Diabeticorum

Beck HI, Bjerring P, Rasmussen I et al. (1985) Treatment of necrobiosis lipoidica with low-dose acetylsalicylic acid. A randomized double-blind trial. Acta Derm Venereol (Stockh) 65:230–234
Gotz A, Eckert F, Landthaler M (1994) Ataxia-telangiectasia (Louis-Bar syndrome) associated with ulcerating necrobiosis lipoidica. J Am Acad Dermatol 31:124–126
Heymann WR (1996) Necrobiosis lipoidica treated with topical tretinoin. Cutis 58:53–54
Huntley AC (1982) The cutaneous manifestations of diabetes mellitus. J Am Acad Dermatol 7:427–455
Kavanagh GM, Novelli M, Hartog M et al. (1993) Necrobiosis lipoidica – involvement of atypical sites. Clin Exp Dermatol 18:543–544
Littler CM, Tschen EH (1987) Pentoxifylline for necrobiosis lipoidica diabeticorum. J Am Acad Dermatol 17:314–315
Lowitt MH, Dover JS (1991) Necrobiosis lipoidica. J Am Acad Dermatol 25:735–748
McDonald L, Zanolli MD, Boyd AS (1996) Perforating elastosis in necrobiosis lipoidica diabeticorum. Cutis 57: 336–338
Miescher G, Leder M (1948) Granulomatosis disciformis chronica et progressiva. Dermatologica 97:25–34
Miller RAW (1980) Koebner phenomenon in a diabetic with necrobiosis lipoidica diabeticorum. Int J Dermatol 29: 52–53
Oppenheim M (1930) Eigentümlich disseminierte Degeneration des Bindegewebes der Haut bei einem Diabetiker. Zentralbl Dermatol 32:179
Petzelbauer P, Wolff K, Tappeiner G (1992) Necrobiosis lipoidica: treatment with systemic corticosteroids. Br J Dermatol 126:542–545
Ullman S, Dahl MV (1977) Necrobiosis lipoidica. An immunofluorescence study. Arch Dermatol 113:1671–1673
Urbach E (1932) Eine neue diabetische Stoffwechseldermatose: Necrobiosis lipoidica diabeticorum. Arch Dermatol Syph 166:273–285

Rheumatoid Nodule

Beatty EC (1959) Rheumatic-like nodule occurring in nonrheumatic children. Arch Pathol 68:154–159
Bennett GA, Zeller JW, Bauer W (1940) Subcutaneous nodules of rheumatoid arthritis and rheumatic fever. A pathologic study. Arch Pathol 30:70–89
Higaki Y, Yamashita H, Sato K et al. (1993) Rheumatoid papules: a report on four patients with histopathologic analysis. J Am Acad Dermatol 28:406–411
Lowney ED, Simons HM (1963) "Rheumatoid" nodules of the skin. Arch Dermatol 88:853–858
Wolf P, Gretler J, Aglas F et al. (1994) Anticardiolipin antibodies in rheumatoid arthritis: their relation to rheumatoid nodules and cutaneous vascular manifestations. Br J Dermatol 131:48–51

Neutrophilic and Palisaded Granulomatous Dermatitis

Chu P, Connolly MK, LeBoit PE (1994) The histopathologic spectrum of palisaded neutrophilic and granulomatous dermatitis in patients with collagen vascular disease. Arch Dermatol 130:1278–1283
Finan MC, Winkelmann RK (1983) The cutaneous extravascular necrotizing granuloma (Churg-Strauss granuloma) and systemic disease: a review of 27 cases. Medicine (Baltimore) 62:142–158

Necrobiotic Xanthogranuloma

Barzilai A, Trau H, Shipro D et al. (1996) Necrobiotic xanthogranuloma with paraproteinemia. Cutis 57:320–322
Finan MC, Winkelmann RK (1986) Necrobiotic xanthogranuloma with paraproteinemia: a review of 22 cases. Medicine (Baltimore) 65:376–388
Finan MC, Winkelmann RK (1987) Histopathology of necrobiotic xanthogranuloma with paraproteinemia. J Cutan Pathol 14:92–99
Finelli LG, Ratz JL (1987) Plasmapheresis, a treatment modality for necrobiotic xanthogranuloma. J Am Acad Dermatol 17:351–354
Gibson LE, Reizner GT, Winkelmann RK (1988) Necrobiosis lipoidica diabeticorum with cholesterol clefts in the differential diagnosis of necrobiotic xanthogranuloma. J Cutan Pathol 15:18–21
Hernandez-Martin A, Baselga E, Drolet BA et al. (1997) Juvenile xanthogranuloma. J Am Acad Dermatol 36: 355–367
Johnston KA, Grimwood RE, Meffert JJ (1997) Necrobiotic xanthogranuloma with paraproteinemia: an evolving presentation. Cutis 59:333–336
Kossard S, Winkelmann RK (1980) Necrobiotic xanthogranuloma with paraproteinemia. J Am Acad Dermatol 3:257–270
Mehregan DA, Winkelmann RK (1992) Necrobiotic xanthogranuloma. Arch Dermatol 128:94–100

Novak PM, Robbins TO, Winkelmann RK (1992) Necrobiotic xanthogranuloma with myocardial lesions and nodular transformation of the liver. Hum Pathol 23: 195–196

Plotnick H, Taniguchi Y, Hashimoto K et al. (1991) Periorbital necrobiotic xanthogranuloma and stage I multiple myeloma. Ultrastructure and response to pulsed dexamethasone documented by magnetic resonance imaging. J Am Acad Dermatol 25:373–377

Reeder CB, Connolly SM, Winkelmann RK (1991) The evolution of Hodgkin's disease and necrobiotic xanthogranuloma syndrome. Mayo Clin Proc 66:1222–1224

Valentine EA, Friedman HD, Zamkoff KW et al. (1990) Necrobiotic xanthogranuloma with IgA multiple myeloma: a case report and literature review. Am J Hematol 35:283–285

Venecia PY, Le Bras P, Toan ND et al. (1995) Recombinant interferon alpha-2b treatment of necrobiotic xanthogranuloma with paraproteinemia. J Am Acad Dermatol 32:666–667

Winkelmann RK, Litzow T, Umbert I et al. (1997) Giant cell granulomatous pulmonary and myocardial lesions in necrobiotic xanthogranuloma with paraproteinemia. Mayo Clin Proc 72:1028–1033

Cutaneous Crohn Disease

Buckley C, Bayoumi AHM, Sarkany I (1989) Metastatic Crohn's disease. Clin Exp Dermatol 15:131–133

Burgdorf W (1981) Cutaneous manifestations of Crohn's disease. J Am Acad Dermatol 5:689–695

Crohn BB, Ginzburg L, Oppenheimer GD (1932) Regional ileitis. JAMA 99:1323–1329

Greenstein AJ, Janowitz HD, Sachar DB (1976) The extra-intestinal complications of Crohn's disease and ulcerative colitis: a study of 700 patients. Medicine (Baltimore) 55:401–412

Lebwohl M, Fleischmajer R, Janowitz H et al. (1984) Metastatic Crohn's disease. J Am Acad Dermatol 10:33–38

Peltz S, Vestey JP, Ferguson A et al. (1993) Disseminated metastatic cutaneous Crohn's disease. Clin Exp Dermatol 18:55–59

Shum DT, Guenther L (1990) Metastatic Crohn's disease. Case report and review of the literature. Arch Dermatol 126:645–648

Talbot T, Jewell L, Schloss E et al. (1984) Cheilitis antedating Crohn's disease: case report and literature update of oral lesions. J Clin Gastroenterol 6:349–354

Worsaae N, Christensen KC, Bondesen S et al. (1980) Melkersson-Rosenthal syndrome and Crohn's disease. Br J Oral Surg 18:254–258

Foreign Body Granulomas

Hirsh BC, Johnson WC (1984) Pathology of granulomatous diseases. Foreign body granulomas. Int J Dermatol 23: 531–538

Maas CS, Papel ID, Greene D et al. (1997) Complications of injectable synthetic polymers in facial augmentation. Dermatol Surg 23:871–877

Montemarano AD, Sau P, Johnson EB et al. (1997) Cutaneous granulomas caused by an aluminum-zirconium complex: an ingredient of antiperspirants. J Am Acad Dermatol 37:496–498

Overholt MA, Tschen JA, Font RL (1993) Granulomatous reaction to collagen implant: light and electron microscopic observations. Cutis 51:95–98

Pinkus H, Bortvinick I (1957) Deodorant stick eruption (zirconium granuloma) of axillae. Arch Dermatol 75: 756–757

Shelley WB, Hurley HJ (1958) The allergic origin of zirconium deodorant granulomas. Br J Dermatol 70:75–101

Terzakis JA, Shustak SR, Stock EG (1978) Talc granuloma identified by X-ray microanalysis. JAMA 239:2371–2372

Granuloma Faciale

Apfelberg DB, Druker D, Maser M et al. (1983) Granuloma faciale. Treatment with the argon laser. Arch Dermatol 119:573–576

Guill MA, Aton JK (1982) Facial granuloma responsive to dapsone therapy. Arch Dermatol 118:332–335

Nieboer C, Kalsbeek GL (1978) Immunofluorescence studies in granuloma eosinophilicum faciale. J Cutan Pathol 5: 68–75

Pedace FJ, Perry HO (1966) Granuloma faciale. A clinical and histopathologic review. Arch Dermatol 94:387–395

Perrin C, Lacour JP, Michiels JF et al. (1992) Facial granuloma. Ann Dermatol Venereol 119:509–516

Pinkus H (1952) Granuloma faciale. Dermatologica 105: 85–99

Sears JK, Gitter DG, Stone MS (1991) Extrafacial granuloma faciale. Arch Dermatol 127:742–743

Wigley JE (1945) Sarcoid of Boeck – eosinophilic granuloma. Br J Dermatol 57:68–69

Myospherulosis

Lazarov A, Avinoach I, Giryes H et al. (1994) Dermal spherulosis (myospherulosis) after topical treatment for psoriasis. J Am Acad Dermatol 30:265–267

McClatchie S, Warambo MW, Brenner AD (1969) Myospherulosis: a previously unreported disease? Am J Clin Pathol 51:699–704

Patterson JW, Kannon GA (1998) Spherulocystic disease ("myospherulosis") arising in a lesion of steatocystoma multiplex. J Am Acad Dermatol 38:274–275

Rosai J (1978) The nature of myospherulosis of the upper respiratory tract. Am J Clin Pathol 69:475–481

Malakoplakia

McClure I (1983) Malakoplakia. J Pathol 140:275–330

Michaelis M, Gutmann C (1902) Über Einschlüsse in Blasentumoren. Z Klin Med 47:208–215

Palazzo JP, Ellison DJ, Garcia IE et al. (1990) Cutaneous malakoplakia simulating relapsing malignant lymphoma. J Cutan Pathol 17:171–175

Granuloma Gluteale Infantum

Bluestein J, Furner BB, Phillips D (1990) Granuloma gluteale infantum: case report and review of the literature. Pediatr Dermatol 7:196–198

Maekawa Y, Sakazaki Y, Hayashibara T (1978) Diaper area granuloma of the aged. Arch Dermatol 114:382–383

Tappeiner S, Pfleger L (1971) Granuloma gluteale infantum. Hautarzt 22:383–388

CHAPTER 51

Disorders with Hypereosinophilia

Contents

Basic Science Aspects

Paul Ehrlich first described the eosinophil in 1879, choosing the name because of the cell granules' affinity for eosin. Eosinophils are bone marrow-derived cells formed from colony forming unit and granulocyte macrophage (CFU-GM) precursor cells. They account typically for 1–5% of the peripheral leukocytes. In normal individuals, the absolute count ranges between 0.015 and 0.65 × 10^9/l. The eosinophil level shows a circadian rhythm, dropping in the morning, when serum cortisol values are highest. Treatment with systemic corticosteroids also suppresses the eosinophil count. However, eosinophils are primarily tissue cells; the ratio of tissue cells to circulating cells is about 100 : 1.

The functions of eosinophils are complex and poorly understood. The many factors controlling eosinophil activation, migration, and apoptosis are a current focus of research. Eosinophils work in close connection with IgE. They are often found in tissue sites where IgE immune reactions occur, such as in nasal polyps. Eosinophils are activated by the eosinophil chemotactic factor and many other local mediators; mast cells coated with IgE and stimulated by antigen release many such mediators. The eosinophil granules contain a variety of enzymes that can deactivate mediators of immediate hypersensitivity, so they may play a modulating or positive role in this setting. In the skin, the role of eosinophils in the late phase reaction has been best demonstrated. When an allergen is injected intradermally, eosinophils can be easily identified in the skin after 24 hours. It appears that eosinophils in patients with atopic dermatitis are impaired in apoptosis or programmed cell death. Thus, the cells are present for longer periods of time, which may partially explain their role in the disease.

Another apparent role is to defend against helminths and other multicellular parasites. The eosinophils are attracted to parasites coated with immunoglobulin or, in some instances, complement. They release a number of toxic proteins, including major basic protein, lysophospholipase (which forms Charcot-Leyden crystals), and many others. Antibodies against major basic protein are often used to identify a role of eosinophils in cutaneous reactions. The eosinophils may cluster around the parasite, releasing the toxic materials from their granules and eventually damaging the invader. Some interleukins, namely IL-3, enhance this function, but there are many other complex control mechanisms.

Many systemic disorders and dermatologic diseases are associated with elevated blood eosinophilia. Tables 51.1 and 51.2 list examples of both these situations. Eosinophils are most commonly seen in cutaneous drug reactions, arthropod bites and infestations. In this chapter we discuss disorders with increased tissue and/or blood eosinophil levels which are not covered elsewhere.

Idiopathic Hypereosinophilic Syndrome

(Griffin 1919; Hardy and Anderson 1968)

Synonyms. Eosinophilic leukemoid (Schmidt-Weyland 1925), eosinophilic reticulosis (Gottron 1956)

Definition. Multisystem, potentially fatal disorder with peripheral blood eosinophilia and infiltration of heart, bone marrow, and other organs.

Epidemiology. The disorder is extremely rare. Most patients are men; a male : female ratio of 9 : 1 has been described. The typical age of onset ranges from 20 to 50 years.

Table 51.1. Internal disorders with peripheral blood eosinophilia

Infestations (worms)
Allergic disorders
Atopy (asthma, rhinitis, conjunctivitis, atopic dermatitis)
Urticaria and angioedema
Food allergies
Bronchopulmonary aspergillosis
Drug reactions
Connective tissue disorders
Eosinophilia myalgia syndrome
Polyarteritis nodosa
Churg-Strauss syndrome
Parasitic disorders
Malignancies
Hodgkin's disease
Mycosis fungoides
Leukemia
Immune deficiencies
HIV infection
Wiskott-Aldrich syndrome
Hyper IgE syndrome
Selective IgA deficiency
Miscellaneous
Graft versus host disease
Sarcoidosis
Toxic oil syndrome
Idiopathic hypereosinophilic syndrome and its variants

Table 51.2. Dermatoses with tissue and/or peripheral blood eosinophilia

Atopic dermatitis
Urticaria and angioedema
Mast cell diseases
Parasitic infestations
Drug reactions
Bullous diseases
Dermatitis herpetiformis
Bullous pemphigoid
Pemphigus vulgaris
Erythema multiforme
Kimura disease
Angiolymphoid hyperplasia with eosinophilia
Granuloma faciale
Eosinophilic cellulitis (Wells syndrome)
Eosinophilic fasciitis (Shulman syndrome)
Eosinophilic pustular folliculitis (Ofuji syndrome)
Eosinophilic histiocytosis
Eosinophilic tongue ulcer
Hypereosinophilic dermatitis (variant of hypereosinophilic syndrome)

Etiology and Pathogenesis. The etiology is unclear. A number of different disorders are probably included under this rubric. In general, eosinophil survival appears to be prolonged. Eosinophil granule proteins such as major basic protein appear to be responsible for the direct cardiac injury. Some patients wind up with leukemia or lymphoma, as the synonyms suggest.

Clinical Findings. Patients with idiopathic hypereosinophilic syndrome usually present with nonspecific findings such as fever, malaise, cough, or night sweats. In other cases, the elevated peripheral eosinophilia is detected on routine screening.

Systemic Findings. The most common site of systemic involvement is the heart. Cardiac and related thromboembolic disease is the main cause of morbidity and mortality. The cardiac disease process has been divided into three stages: the acute necrotic stage with active endomyocarditis, the thrombotic stage, and the fibrotic stage with restrictive cardiomyopathy and valvular dysfunction. The bone marrow is rich in eosinophils; as many as three-quarters of the cells may be eosinophils in varying stages of maturation. In contrast, in eosinophilic leukemia the dominant cell is an immature eosinophil. Many other organs may be involved, including the lymph nodes, nervous system, gastrointestinal tract, kidneys, eyes, lungs, liver, and musculoskeletal system.

Cutaneous Findings. The skin is involved in about 50% of these patients. The spectrum of involvement is highly variable; lesions include urticaria, urticarial dermographism, angioedema, infiltrated plaques, vasculitis, nodules, and marked pruritus. A wide variety of nonspecific papular and lichenified dermatoses have also been described. Less frequent manifestations include blisters, acral necrotic lesions, erythema annulare centrifugum, and erythroderma. A poor clinical sign is the presence of oral ulcerations, which suggests an unfavorable disease course.

Histopathology. Microscopic examination reveals perivascular and periadnexal inflammatory infiltrates which are usually rich in eosinophils, although the characteristic cell may sometimes be not so obvious. Deposition of major basic protein and other eosinophil granule proteins may be extensive.

Diagnostic Criteria. The diagnostic criteria as proposed by Chusid include: (1) a peripheral blood eosinophilia count of 1500/mm^3 for at least 6 months, (2) no evidence of other causes of eosinophilia, and (3) organ system dysfunction due to the eosinophilia, usually of the heart and/or bone marrow.

Course and Prognosis. Survival ranges from several months to many years. The absolute eosinophil count is a reasonable predictor; when it is very high, such as 100,000/mm^3, the outlook is grim. Cardiac or neurologic dysfunction is also an unfavorable sign.

Differential Diagnosis. The diseases listed in Tables 51.1 and 51.2 should be excluded. One of the most difficult diagnoses is to differentiate between eosinophilic myocarditis, eosinophilic gastroenteritis or eosinophilic pulmonary disease, and the hypereosinophilic syndrome. In the other disorders, usually only one organ is involved. One must exclude neoplasms, parasitic infestations, drug reactions, and other allergic processes in each case.

Therapy. The therapy for hypereosinophilic syndrome is best left in the hands of physicians with considerable experience. In general, systemic corticosteroids are the initial treatment for patients with minor organ dysfunction, except for cardiac involvement. Patients with cardiac diseases or those who fail to respond to corticosteroids are usually treated with hydroxyurea. If this fails, one must consider other cytotoxic regimens or the use of biological response modifiers. Recent reports have shown a promising role for interferon-α. Psoralen plus ultraviolet A (PUVA) therapy may be helpful for the cutaneous lesions. Also, anticoagulation is often necessary.

Hypereosinophilic Dermatitis

(Nier and Westfried 1981)

Definition. Part of the spectrum of hypereosinophilic syndrome with cutaneous but no internal involvement.

Etiology and Pathogenesis. Radiaton therapy may occasionally produce similar changes.

Clinical Findings. In contrast to the cutaneous findings in hypereosinophilic syndrome, which are extremely variable, here the situation is more homogenous. Patients tend to have generalized polymorphous eruptions with pruritic, reddish brown papules and nodules as well as erythematous macules. The head, palms, soles, and glans are usually spared. Systemic involvement is absent except for peripheral blood eosinophilia, which is usually about 20 %, with an absolute count of around 3000/mm^3. The bone marrow also shows an increase in mature eosinophils. The disease ends to be chronic, with waves of new lesions appearing. Electrocardiographic abnormalities have rarely been reported.

Histopathology. There is a superficial and deep perivascular and periappendageal lymphohistiocytic infiltrate. Numerous eosinophils and plasma cells may be seen. The infiltrate may be denser than in hypereosinophilic syndrome.

Diagnostic Criteria. The patient must have peripheral blood eosinophilia and cutaneous lesions with eosinophils but no evidence of other systemic involvement. However, the diagnosis should be made with reluctance and the patients followed closely.

Course and Prognosis. The course tends to wax and wane. Some of these cases will eventuate into hypereosinophilic syndrome; others may remain stable for many years.

Differential Diagnosis. The same differential diagnostic points suggested in Tables 51.1 and 51.2 also apply here.

Therapy

Systemic. Low dose systemic corticosteroids can be employed. The other more drastic agents discussed under hypereosinophilic syndrome are not appropriate. Ketotifen and dapsone may both also be tried.

Topical. Corticosteroids may prove helpful. In some cases, PUVA has also been effective.

Nodular Eosinophilic Infiltration with Immunoglobulin Isotype Imbalance

(Hauser and Saurat 1991)

This rare disease, described only once to our knowledge, is probably best viewed as a variant of hypereosinophilic dermatitis. Patients have infiltrated plaques involving the hands and face and tend to suffer from chronic infections. The lesions are rich in eosinophils and there is also a peripheral blood eosinophilia, but other systemic manifestations have not been described. The unusual name reflects the presence of elevated levels of IgE and IgG_4, with reduced levels of IgM and IgG_{1-3}. It is unclear how reliably one can define an entity with such restricted findings.

Eosinophilic Myositis/Perimyositis

In this group of rare, diverse inflammatory muscle disorders with peripheral or tissue eosinophilia, there may also be cutaneous findings. About one-third of the patients have cutaneous infiltrates, urticaria, and angioedema. In contrast to idiopathic hypereosinophilic syndrome, the infiltrates tend to be deeper and often subcutaneous. Patients with peripheral eosinophilia, deep subcutaneous infiltrates, and muscle symptoms should be suspected of having eosinophilic myositis/perimyositis, which carries a better prognosis than idiopathic hypereosinophilic syndrome. In addition, focal muscle changes and primarily perimysial accumulations of eosinophils suggest a good outlook. In most cases, systemic corticosteroid therapy is effective.

Eosinophilic Cellulitis

(Wells 1971)

Synonyms. Wells syndrome, recurrent granulomatous dermatitis with eosinophilia, acute eosinophilic infiltrate of the skin with facial nerve paralysis and eosinophilia (Miescher 1952).

Definition. Chronic inflammatory condition in which the dermal infiltrate is rich in eosinophils and collagen bundles are surrounded by eosinophilic granules, producing so-called flame figures.

Etiology and Pathogenesis. The etiology is unknown. While flame figures are frequently taken as synonymous with an indication of eosinophilic cellulitis, they can occur anytime there is an exuberant tissue eosinophilia. The eosinophils then release their granules and damage the collagen minimally, producing the typical flame figure. Probably there are many causes for these histologic changes, including arthropod bites, drug reactions, infections, and idiopathic hypereosinophilic syndrome.

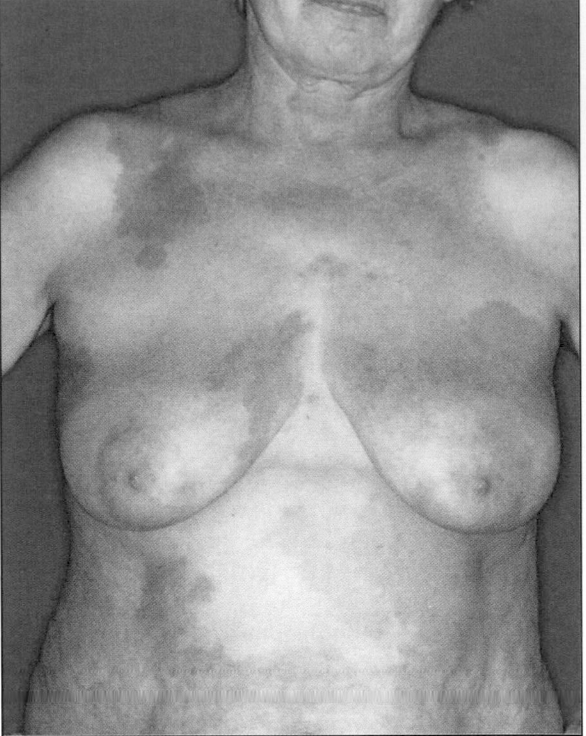

Fig. 51.1. Eosinophilic cellulitis

Clinical Findings. The clinical features can be divided into two stages. The initial acute phase is what has been termed eosinophilic cellulitis, for the lesions do resemble a cellulitis. There is erythema, circumscribed edema, and warmth. The edema may lead to blisters. Lesions may be solitary or multiple and become large, exceeding 10–15 cm in diameter. The limbs and trunk are the most common sites (Fig. 51.1). The lesions may be pruritic. Ordinary urticarial lesions may appear at the same time. The acute lesions last 2–3 days; then there is the late or granulomatous phase, in which the lesions are less erythematous but still infiltrated and pruritic. These gradually heal over months but may recur, often in the same location.

In general, there are few systemic findings. Facial paralysis has been described, perhaps simply from a deep infiltrate and/or edema pressing on the superficial facial nerve. Many patients have fever and arthralgias; pulmonary and cardiac symptoms have rarely been described. About half the patients show a peripheral blood eosinophilia. Bone marrow evaluation should be performed; patients with eosinophilic infiltrates are more likely to have a chronic, more serious course.

Histopathology. Early on, there is edema and a rich eosinophilic infiltrate. Subepidermal blisters occur sometimes, as well as infiltration of the subcutaneous fat. In later lesions, the typical flame figures are identified. The collagen in the middle of a flame figure is slightly modified so that it stains a brighter or deeper red with hematoxylin-eosin. At the periphery, nuclear debris, eosinophilic granules, macrophages, and foreign body giant cells are seen. Vasculitis is not seen. In late lesions, the damaged collagen may appear necrobiotic. A wide variety of direct immunofluorescent findings have been reported, but none are specific. Immunoglobulins and fibrinogen may be deposited in the dermis and subcutaneous fat; immunoglobulins have occasionally been described at the epidermal-dermal junction. Eosinophilic granule protein can be identified around the flame figures.

Course and Prognosis. The disease is usually chronic and lasts months to years, although spontaneous remissions can be seen. This course is hard to fit in with an acute insult as listed above.

Differential Diagnosis. Eosinophilic cellulitis raises a long differential diagnostic list. Early lesions may resemble erysipelas, bacterial cellulitis, or an insect bite (which may be the trigger). Larger lesions with active borders are similar to those in morphea. Since urticarial lesions are often associated, the entire process may be taken as severe urticaria (which, once again, may be correct.) When blisters are present, bullous pemphigoid should be excluded. Later lesions resemble those from granuloma annulare or erythema elevatum diutinum.

Therapy

Systemic. Corticosteroids form the mainstay of therapy. Moderate doses of prednisone over a period of weeks to months are usually needed, often in alternate-day regimens. A suitable alternative is dapsone, perhaps combined with corticosteroids when the latter have failed alone. Many other agents have been employed, but clear benefits have not been shown, perhaps because the disease is so rare. While antihistamines have not been helpful, cetirizine is a new H1 blocker with antieosinophilic activity which seems promising.

Topical. Antipruritics and topical corticosteroids can be tried. Usually they are inadequate.

Eosinophilic Histiocytosis

(McLeod and Winkelmann 1985)

This rare condition is probably a variant of pityriasis lichenoides et varioliformis acuta (PLEVA) or lymphomatoid papulosis. Patients have multiple chronic or recurrent papules and nodules which often ulcerate and heal with scarring. No systemic findings are present. Microscopic examination reveals a perivascular lymphocytic infiltrate, often with large prominent cells but also admixed with eosinophils.

Bibliography

Basic Science Aspects

Liesveld JL, Abboud CN (1991) State of the art; the hypereosinophilic syndromes. Blood Rev 5:29–37

Oliver JW, Deol I, Morgan DL et al. (1998) Chronic eosinophilic leukemia and hypereosinophilic syndromes. Proposal for classification, literature review, and report of a case with a unique chromosomal abnormality. Cancer Genet Cytogenet 107:111–117

Trüeb RM, Pericin M, Winzeler B et al. (1997) Eosinophilic myositis/perimyositis: Frequency and spectrum of cutaneous manifestations. J Am Acad Dermatol 37:385–391

Idiopathic Hypereosinophilic Syndrome

Butterfield JH, Gleich GJ (1994) Response of six patients with idiopathic hypereosinophilic syndrome to interferon-alfa. J Allergy Clin Immunol 94:1318–1326

Griffin HZ (1919) Persistent eosinophilia with hyperleukocytosis and splenomegaly. Am J Med 158:618–629

Hardy WR, Anderson RE (1968) The hypereosinophilic syndrome: clinical features, laboratory findings and treatment. Ann Intern Med 68:1220–1229

Leiferman KM (1995) Hypereosinophilic syndrome. Semin Dermatol 14:122–128

Malbrain ML, Van den Bergh H, Zachee P (1996) Further evidence for the clonal nature of the idiopathic hypereosinophilic syndrome: complete hematologic and cytogenetic remission induced by interferon-α in a case with a unique chromosomal abnormality. Br J Haematol 92:176–183

May LP, Kelly J, Sanchez M (1990) Hypereosinophilic syndrome with unusual cutaneous manifestations in two men with HIV infection. J Am Acad Dermatol 23:202–204

Mezei MM, Tron VA, Stewart WD et al. (1995) Eosinophilic ulcer of the oral mucosa. J Am Acad Dermatol 33:734–740

Shelley WB, Shelley ED (1985) Erythema annulare centrifugum as the presenting sign of the hypereosinophilic syndrome: Observations on therapy. Cutis 35:53–55

Trüeb RM (1997) Idiopathische Eosinophilie. Hautarzt 48:153–156

van den Hoogenband HM (1982) Skin lesions as the first manifestation of the hypereosinophilic syndrome. Clin Exp Dermatol 7:267–271

Weller PF, Dvorak AM (1996) The idiopathic hypereosinophilic syndrome. Arch Dermatol 132:583–585

Wemmer U, Thiele B, Steigleder GK (1988) Hypereosinophilie-Syndrom (HES)-erfolgreiche PUVA-Therapie. Hautarzt 39:42–44

Hypereosinophilic Dermatitis

Jacyk VVK, Simson LW, Slater DN et al. (1996) Pachydermatous eosinophilic dermatitis. Br J Dermatol 134:469–474

Nier MA, Westfried M (1981) Hypereosinophilic dermatitis. A distinct manifestation of the hypereosinophilic syndrome with response to dapsone. Dermatologica 162:444–450

Rueda RA, Valencia IC, Covelli C et al. (1999) Eosinophilic, polymorphic, and pruritic eruption associated with radiotherapy. Arch Dermatol 135:804–810

Nodular Eosinophilic Infiltration with Immunoglobulin Isotype Imbalance

Hauser C, Saurat JH (1991) A syndrome characterized by nodular eosinophilic infiltration of the skin and immunoglobulin isotype imbalance. J Am Acad Dermatol 24:352–355

Eosinophilic Cellulitis (Wells Syndrome)

Aberer W, Konrad K, Wolff K (1988) Wells' syndrome is a distinctive disease entity and not a histologic diagnosis. J Am Acad Dermatol 18:105–114

Anderson CR, Jenkins D, Tron V et al. (1995) Wells' syndrome in childhood: case report and review of the literature. J Am Acad Dermatol 1995:857–864

Brehmer Andersson E, Kaaman T, Skog E et al. (1986) The histopathogenesis of the flame figure in Wells' syndrome based on five cases. Acta Derm Venereol (Stockh) 66:213–219

Fisher GB, Greer KE, Cooper PH (1985) Eosinophilic cellulitis (Wells' syndrome). Int J Dermatol 24:101–107

Melski JW (1990) Wells' syndrome, insect bites, and eosinophils. Dermatol Clin 8:287–293

Perret C (1988) Eosinophilic Zellulitis unter dem Bild einer Prurigo diabetica. Aktuel Dermatol 14:61–63

Schorr WF, Tauscheck AL, Dickson KB et al. (1984) Eosinophilic cellulitis (Wells' syndrome): Histologic and clinical features in arthropod bite reactions. J Am Acad Dermatol 11:1043–1049

Wells GC (1971) Recurrent granulomatous dermatitis with eosinophilia. Trans St John's Hosp Dermatol Soc 57:46–56

Wells GC, Smith NP (1979) Eosinophilic cellulitis. Br J Dermatol 100:101–109

Eosinophilic Histiocytosis

Helton JL, Maize JC (1996) Eosinophilic histiocytosis. Histopathology and immunohistochemistry. Am J Dermatopathol 18:111–117

McLeod WA, Winkelmann RK (1985) Eosinophilic histiocytosis: a variant form of lymphomatoid papulosis or a disease sui generis? J Am Acad Dermatol 13:952–958

Tuneu A, Moreno A, Pujol RM et al. (1988) Eosinophilic histiocytosis. A subset of lymphomatoid papulosis. Dermatologica 176:95–100

Nevi

Contents

A generally accepted definition of a nevus has not been achieved. The term nevus has been used to describe neoplastic and nonneoplastic, congenital and acquired, and hereditary and nonhereditary disorders. Happle has defined a nevus as a "visible, circumscribed long-lasting lesion of the skin or neighboring mucosa". In most cases nevi reflect genetic mosaicism. With the exception of melanocytic nevi, they do not grow other than to keep pace with the patient's growth. While some melanocytic nevi are precursors of malignant melanomas, other nevi do not show malignant transformation. Most nonmelanocytic nevi are congenital but not hereditary. Sometimes they are first identified in the first years of life or at puberty. A nevus may consist of melanocytes, keratinocytes, adnexal structures, vessels, nerves, muscles, fat cells or any combination thereof. Further confusing the issue is the use of the term nevoid, meaning resembling a nevus. When a definition is as unclear as that of nevus, then almost anything can be taken as resembling a nevus. We avoid the term nevoid except where it is an accepted part of the name of a disorder.

Confusing the matter is the Anglo-Saxon and German tendency to call a melanocytic nevus a nevus. We too will employ this second less-precise usage; when we say nevus in dealing with pigmented lesions, we mean melanocytic nevus. We discuss melanocytic nevi in Chapter 58, but consider all other nonmelanocytic nevi here.

Epidermal Nevi

Epidermal nevi are congenital lesions with a circumscribed alteration in the arrangement or quantitative composition of otherwise normal cutaneous elements. Separation between an epidermal nevus and a benign epidermal tumor (Chap. 54) may be difficult. Epidermal nevi usually reflect genetic mosaicism following a somatic mutation (Chap. 1). They are often distributed along the lines of Blaschko, but can also be arranged in other patterns, such as zosteriform or even involving one half or one quarter of the body, as in CHILD syndrome. One can divide epidermal nevi into pure epidermal nevi and organoid nevi.

Pure Epidermal Nevi

Definition. Epidermal nevi having an abnormal epidermal pattern without significant dermal changes.

Etiology and Pathogenesis. Epidermal nevi are caused by somatic mutations producing mosaicism. Changes in any gene whose product is involved in keratinization or other epidermal processes can theoretically produce an epidermal nevus. This was first shown for the epidermolytic epidermal nevus, where gonadal as well as cutaneous mosaicism can lead to the unfortunate scenario of a patient with such an epidermal nevus having a child with congenital bullous ichthyosiform erythroderma. Identical defects in keratin 1 or 10 have been shown in both disorders.

Clinical Findings. While epidermal nevi are present at birth, they may initially appear as a localized area of hyperpigmentation and not become clinically apparent as raised or warty lesions until later in life. The hyperpigmentation is a result of subtle hyperkeratosis.

Larger epidermal nevi generally have a patterned distribution. Most often they are linear, following Blaschko lines. In addition, segmental distribution may be seen. Smaller lesions may resemble both clinically and histologically a seborrheic keratosis or verruca. Epidermal nevi tend to grow with the patient and are permanent without change or regression. The old term nevus unius lateris is not helpful; all epidermal nevi can be unilateral. This clinical finding simply suggests a relatively late somatic mutation.

The following types of epidermal nevi have been identified. Since epidermal nevi are characterized by both clinical and histologic features, both aspects will be discussed together. This classification is by no means exclusive as an epidermal nevus may be hard, linear and inflamed.

Soft Epidermal Nevus. Such nevi are often hyperpigmented with a velvety surface. Individual papules are similar to small acrochordons but many such lesions are grouped together. Microscopically they have papillomatosis with minimal hyperkeratosis, the so-called church spire effect (Fig. 52.1).

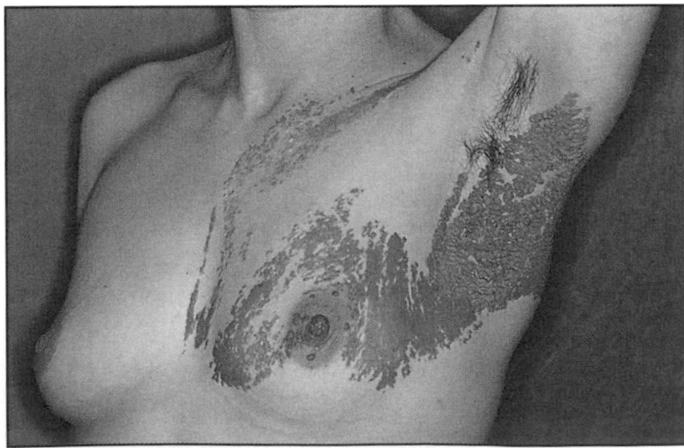

Fig. 52.1. Epidermal nevus following Blaschko lines

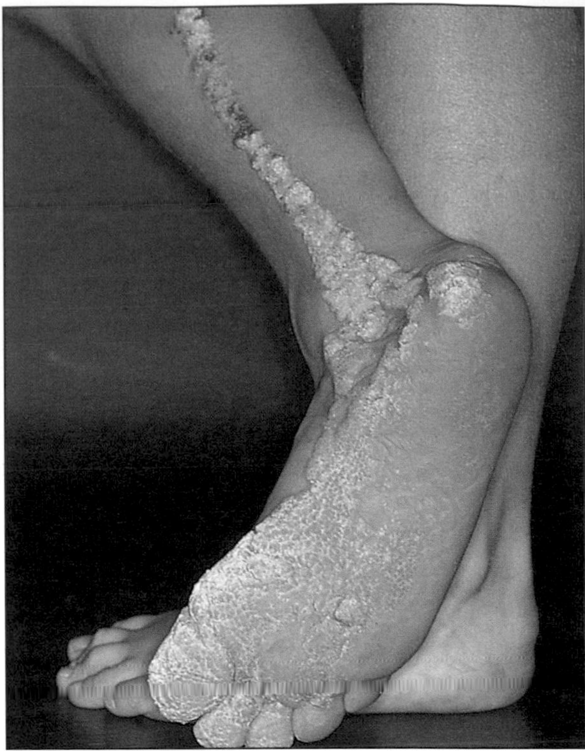

Fig. 52.2. Hyperkeratotic epidermal nevus

Hard Epidermal Nevus. This form is clinically thicker and often has heavy scale (Fig. 52.2). Under the microscope it may resembled a seborrheic keratosis, but usually has dramatic hyperkeratosis.

Epidermolytic Epidermal Nevus. This form is typically thick and scaly. Microscopically the picture is that of epidermolytic hyperkeratoses or bullous congenital ichthyosiform erythroderma (Chap. 17). Mutations in keratin 1 or 10 genes are responsible.

Segmental Darier Disease. Even though the name is different, segmental Darier disease is an epidermal nevus with the same mutation as seen in Darier disease (Chap. 17). Just as the lesions of Darier disease may improve or worsen, this nevus may also vary. The histologic picture is that of acantholysis and dyskeratosis. Some patients with Darier disease have a segmental loss of heterozygosity and then an epidermal nevus in which the changes are far more severe than the surrounding heterozygous skin.

Segmental Hailey-Hailey Disease. Because the changes in Hailey-Hailey disease (Chap. 17) are normally more subtle than in the others in this group, it is suspected that loss of heterozygosity is more often responsible for these epidermal nevi. In other words, many individuals with segmental Hailey-Hailey disease actually have true Hailey-Hailey disease which can be identified if they are examined carefully and followed.

Nevus Corniculatus. This type is the rarest form of epidermal nevus, as only a few cases have been described. Corniculatus means covered with horns, and the lesions are very hyperkeratotic with both thick warty excrescences and filiform lesions. Microscopically there is focal acantholysis along with epidermal depressions filled with compact keratin. The generalized equivalent of nevus corniculatus has not be identified and may be lethal.

Inflammatory Linear Verrucous Epidermal Nevus (ILVEN). Here there is a lesion with erythema, scale and pruritus, reflecting persistent inflammation not associated with trauma or infection (Fig. 52.3). ILVEN may wax and wane. Thus they are clinically different from other members of this group. One could imagine a region of skin with a mosaic change which would predispose to the development of psoriasis or lichen planus or any of a list of disorders. Just as common psoriasis clears, the psoriatic ILVEN could clear, even though the underlying mutation remains. Alternatively, an ILVEN could be another variety of epidermal nevus in a patient predisposed to psoriasis or another inflammatory process.

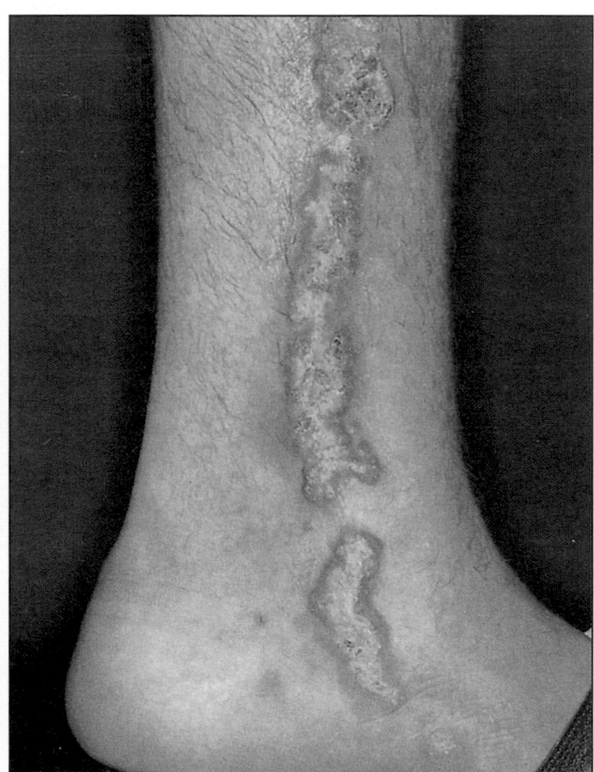

Fig. 52.3. ILVEN

CHILD Epidermal Nevus. CHILD is an acronym for *c*ongenital *h*emidysplasia, *u*nilateral *i*chthyosiform erythroderma and *l*imb *d*efects. While most often a CHILD nevus is associated with the underlying disorders implied in the name, occasionally only the cutaneous changes may be present. CHILD syndrome is discussed in Chapter 17. A CHILD nevus is quite different from all the others in this group. Almost all patients are women, as the gene is located on the X chromosome and lethal in men. The lesions do not follow Blaschko lines, but instead are patchwork, respecting the midline and also favor the flexural areas (ptychotropism). Some of the nevi may improve with time, although the flexural lesions are more persistent. On histologic examination the lesions resemble psoriasis, but may also have the changes of verruciform xanthoma with lipids stored in the dermal papillae (Chap. 37).

Course and Prognosis. Epidermal nevi are permanent. They may wax and wane, but they do not disappear. In addition, they do not change types, despite occasional reports in the literature suggesting this.

Differential Diagnosis. The differential diagnosis includes other organoid nevi, as well as the various members of the group.

Therapy. The only effective approach is surgical excision. Often the size of the lesion mandates a staged excision. Widespread lesions clearly cannot be excised, but often the most disturbing part or parts can be removed. The soft epidermal nevus is relatively responsive to superficial destruction, such as laser therapy. Dermabrasion or split-thickness excision produces excellent temporary improvement. Despite the normal appearance of the dermis, it must produce abnormal growth factors for as re-epithelialization occurs, often the epidermal changes redevelop.

Topical treatment with retinoids or keratolytics may also produce some improvement. Such therapy can be combined with some sort of abrasion using a pumice stone, masonry-type sandpaper or even a small power sanding device. Motivated parents and patients can often obtain satisfactory results although the process is lifelong. Systemic retinoids have been employed in widespread cases. Depending on the exact nature of the epidermal defect, they may bring about dramatic but only temporary responses.

Organoid Nevi

Both Jadassohn (1895) and Pinkus (1965) struggled with the definition of organoid nevi. We use the term to describe segmental mosaicism in which not only epidermal but also adnexal and dermal components are altered. Thus the etiology is exactly the same as with epidermal nevi, except that the mutation involves a gene that affects adnexal structures or their interaction with dermal elements. Many different types have been described.

Nevus Sebaceus

(Jadassohn 1895)

Definition. Organoid nevus usually involving the scalp with prominent proliferation of sebaceous glands.

Etiology and Pathogenesis. Familial cases of nevus sebaceus have been described, probably representing paradominant inheritance (Chap. 1).

Clinical Findings. Nevus sebaceus is usually recognized in infancy as a localized area of alopecia. While it can be located anywhere, the scalp, especially the frontal-temporal region, and cheek are the most common sites. Often it has a hint of yellow or pink and shows velvety papillomatosis at this stage (Fig. 52.4). During childhood, it grows with the patient but at puberty, becomes verrucous and more yellow. Later in adult life, patients may identify a changing nodule or crust within the nevus sebaceus which reflects the development of a tumor. While at least 30% develop such changes, most lesions are trichoblastomas or syringocystadenoma papilliferum, not basal cell carcinomas as previously suggested.

Histopathology. Early lesions are very similar to epidermal nevi, but contain numerous hair germs. Biopsies taken in infancy often show no changes in the sebaceous glands. Later there are not only the expected increased number of sebaceous glands but also increased numbers of apocrine and eccrine structures. In addition, the epidermal changes such as acanthosis, hyperkeratosis and papillomatosis become more prominent.

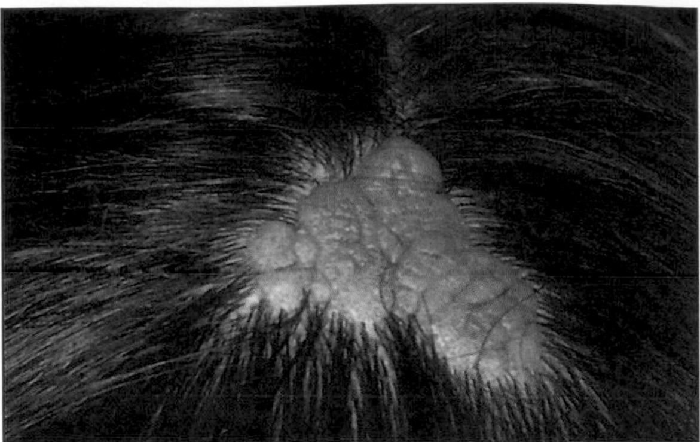

Fig. 52.4. Nevus sebaceus

Differential Diagnosis. Early lesions may be mistaken for aplasia cutis congenita, but the latter is usually on the vertex of the scalp and shows erosions and atrophy. More mature nevus sebaceus can be confused with a papillomatous melanocytic nevus but the histology rapidly provides a distinction.

Therapy. Nevus sebaceus may be excised for cosmetic reasons. The idea that the removal of such a lesion is necessary under the umbrella concept of tumor prophylaxis is exaggerated. Most of the tumors that develop are entirely benign, and if a basal cell carcinoma should develop, it can be easily treated.

Nevus Comedonicus

(Kofmann 1895)

Clinical Findings. Nevus comedonicus is an uncommon and often misunderstood lesion. Patients present with a localized grouping of comedones which are better described as dilated plugged follicles (Fig. 52.5). Usually no hairs are present. In most cases, the lesions are asymptomatic, but sometimes they may become inflamed and be confused with acne.

Histopathology. The epidermis shows dilated patulous plugged hair follicles and small cysts. The latter probably reflect tangential sections. Acne comedones typically have a small orifice while the

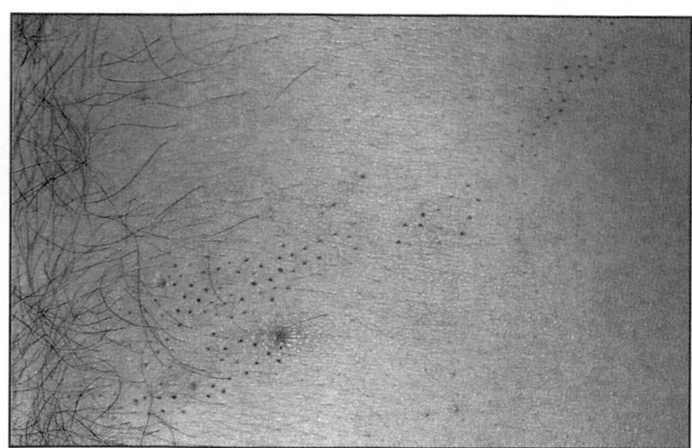

Fig. 52.5. Nevus comedonicus

lesions in nevus comedonicus are barrel shaped and contain almost no coryneform bacteria. This perhaps explains why they are less likely to become inflamed.

Differential Diagnosis. Usually the diagnosis is obvious and specific. Acne or acneiform changes in a limited area may reflect occupational exposure to comedogenic agents, such as cutting fluids, or may be seen in a Becker nevus.

Therapy. Excision is the only successful therapy. The lesions are often on the trunk and cause few cosmetic problems, so many patients choose to have no therapy. Standard acne therapy can be employed in the rare cases that develop inflammatory changes.

Other Types of Organoid Nevi

Becker Nevus. Because this form of organoid nevus is often confused with a café-au-lait macule or melanocytic nevus, it is considered in Chap. 58. Biologically it is especially interesting as there is often an associated proliferation of smooth muscles, identical to a smooth muscle hamartoma (Chap. 59). This suggests a mutation in a gene involved in the organization of the hair follicle and its interaction with the mesenchyme to form the arrector pili muscles.

Hair Follicle Nevus. Many so-called hair follicle nevi are actually accessory tragi. There are numerous vellus hairs but the cartilage core is not captured in the biopsy specimen. True hair follicle nevi are flat to pebbly patches usually following Blaschko lines and containing terminal hairs. In most cases the hairs become apparent after puberty and are more readily seen in men, just as with a Becker nevus. Woolly hair nevus is discussed in Chap. 31.

Apocrine Nevus. Apocrine nevi are extremely rare because apocrine glands arise embryologically from the hair germ, so excessive apocrine glands usually accompany hair follicle or sebaceous proliferations. Apocrine nevi have been described in focal dermal hypoplasia (Chap. 19).

Eccrine Nevus. Pure eccrine nevi are also very rare. They typically are plaques with no distinct clinical features except localized hyperhidrosis.

Porokeratotic Eccrine Nevus (Abell and Reed 1986)

Also known as porokeratotic eccrine ostial and dermal duct nevus, this unusual lesion can mimic a hard epidermal nevus when it occurs on glabrous skin. It is often found on the palms and soles, where multiple small horn-filled pits and filiform hyperkeratoses are seen. On biopsy cornoid lamellae are seen in the ostia of the eccrine ducts, rather than arising from the intervening epidermis as is usually the case (Chap. 17).

Eccrine Angiomatous Hamartoma. These typically linear lesions have an increase in both blood vessels and eccrine glands. There may be associated hair follicles. In most instances, there is localized hyperhidrosis.

Eccrine Acrosyringeal Nevus. These lesions are typically linear or plaque-like. They may be seen in association with Schöpf syndrome. Linear anastomosing strands of acrosyringeal epithelium extend down into the dermis from the underside of a thickened epidermis. There are often dermal plasma cells. The microscopic picture is thus similar to that in the syringofibroadenoma of Mascaro (Chap. 57).

Palmar Cutaneous Hamartoma. This rare malformation contains increased amounts of several tissue elements normally found in palmoplantar skin, including eccrine glands, fat and neurovascular bodies, similar to Sucquet-Hoyer canals. While only palmar lesions have been described, plantar lesions should also occur.

Munro Nevus (Munro and Wilkie 1998). Also known as an acneiform nevus, the Munro nevus is completely different from a Becker nevus or nevus comedonicus. Munro studied a patient with modest facial acne but severe inflammatory acne with comedones following Blaschko lines on the upper arm. Apert syndrome is a skeletal malformation syndrome in which patients have severe acne; the defect lies in a mutation in fibroblast growth factor 2. Munro found the same mutation in the linear lesion of his patient, but not in the normal skin.

Phakomatosis Pigmentokeratotica. Twin spotting appears to be the explanation for this unusual association of nevus sebaceus and nevus spilus.

Differential Diagnosis. All of the organoid nevi must be separated from epidermal nevi, based on the histologic picture. In addition, they have to be separated from solitary adnexal tumors; presence at birth and distribution following Blaschko lines are most helpful. Some melanocytic nevi are relatively pale at birth and may have dark hairs. They may be clinically confused with a hair nevus, but histologic examination reveals the correct diagnosis.

Therapy. All the organoid nevi have a degree of dermal involvement, so they are difficult to treat with superficial measures. In most instances, the only approach is excision.

Epidermal Nevus Syndromes

(Solomon et al. 1968)

Both pure epidermal nevi and organoid nevi can be associated with a constellation of underlying defects.

Etiology and Pathogenesis. In such instances the somatic mutation causing the syndrome must occur slightly early earlier in embryonic life, so that mesenchymal and endodermal structures are also involved. While often the underlying changes are ipsilateral with the skin changes, they may be contralateral or even bilateral, depending on the timing of the mutation. It is not surprising that a wide variety of changes can be seen and that there is much confusion over the naming of these disorders. We follow the classification of Happle.

Clinical Findings. Once again, there are a number of different syndromes with only partially distinctive clinical features. Note that the most common ordinary soft or hard linear epidermal nevi are rarely if ever associated with underlying defects.

Proteus Syndrome. The Proteus syndrome (Chap. 19) features soft epidermal nevi, as well as hemihypertrophy, cerebriform palmoplantar connective tissue nevi and many other malformations. It is probably caused by a gene which is lethal when present in all cells, so that only mosaic patients can survive.

CHILD Syndrome. This is another unusual epidermal nevus syndrome. Almost all patients are women who in addition to the typical CHILD nevi have ipsilateral skeletal, CNS, pulmonary, cardiac and renal anomalies. In our estimation, patients with ILVEN and systemic defects have CHILD syndrome.

Schimmelpenning-Feuerstein-Mims Syndrome (Schimmelpenning 1957; Feuerstein and Mims 1962). Also known as nevus sebaceus syndrome, this disorder features one or more patches of nevus sebaceus associated with underlying CNS, ocular, cardiac and skeletal defects. Once again, a lethal mutation appears to be responsible, one which can only be manifested clinically in the mosaic state. Patients with more widespread nevi sebacei are probably at a greater risk of having underlying disease. Usually the internal problems are obvious, so that extensive evaluation of otherwise healthy children with nevus sebaceus is not necessary.

Nevus Comedonicus Syndrome. Rare patients with nevus comedonicus may also have ipsilateral skeletal or ocular problems.

Becker Nevus Syndrome. The hallmark of Becker nevus syndrome is ipsilateral breast hypoplasia. For this reason, the syndrome is most often described in women, just as paradoxical as the fact that Becker nevi are more often identified in men where the terminal hairs are more visible. Both the isolated nevus and the syndrome are equally common in both sexes. Additional changes may include ipsilateral skeletal changes, usually hypoplastic in nature. Becker nevus syndrome may be seen in families; the explanation is predominant inheritance (Chap. 1).

Phakomatosis Pigmentokeratotica Syndrome. The original patient with this combination of nevus sebaceus and nevus spilus had a variety of other problems. Associated findings may include hemiatrophy, segmental dysesthesias or hyperhidrosis, and several types of CNS and ocular malformations. Loss of heterozygosity is the usual explanation for the almost-mirror image pairing of two unrelated defects, presumably caused by genes which are close together on a given chromosome.

Differential Diagnosis. The differential diagnosis once again primarily includes the various members of this family.

Therapy. The skin lesions may be amenable to surgery. The underlying skeletal defects and ocular defects such as cataracts and lid anomalies can usually be surgically repaired. The CNS defects may lead to epilepsy which should be treated appropriately.

Connective Tissue Nevi

Definition. Localized region with increased elastin and/or collagen in the dermis; a mesenchymal nevus.

There are many different types of connective tissue nevi. They have been classified based on associated disorders (such as tuberous sclerosis), on the predominance of elastin or collagen in histologic sections, on whether familial and on whether solitary or multiple. Since these categories are not mutually exclusive, the situation is confusing. In our experience, determining unequivocally whether elastin or collagen is altered in a biopsy specimen is very difficult. Molecular genetic studies of collagen and elastin gene expression have begun to provide clarification, but we tend to lump together collagen-rich (collagenomas) and elastin-rich (elastomas) connective tissue nevi.

Connective Tissue Nevus

Synonyms. Shagreen patch, cobblestone nevus

Clinical Findings. These asymptomatic lesions are usually lumbosacral and may be a marker for tuberous sclerosis. While they are present at birth, they often are more apparent later in life. Usually grouped firm hyperkeratotic nodules or a plaque are seen (Fig. 52.6). Shagreen patch and facial fibrous plaque in tuberous sclerosis are variants (Chap. 19). Linear, grouped or segmental lesions can be seen. Occasionally multiple lesions are seen. As is so often the case, single lesions are usually sporadic while multiple lesions frequently are inherited, usually in an autosomal dominant pattern. Familial cutaneous collagenoma has been used to describe multiple lesions in several generations of a family. The trunk is the most common site for multiple nevi.

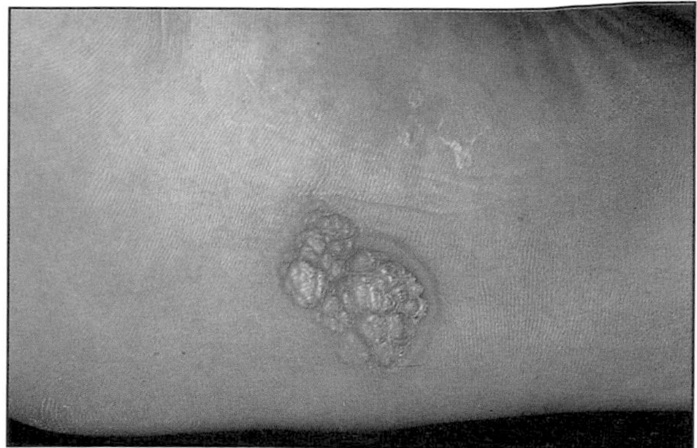

Fig. 52.6. Connective tissue nevus

Histopathology. The epidermis is normal and the dermis is thickened with dense, coarse hypocellular fibers which are interwoven. The parallel arrangement of a scar or keloid is absent.

Therapy. Excision is the only reasonable approach.

Nevus Elasticus

(Lewandowsky 1921)

Both solitary and multiple lesions have been described in terms identical to connective tissue nevus. The region about the nipple is a common site, but some of these lesions may represent leiomyomas that have been misinterpreted. In addition, Lewandowsky's lesion about the nipple shows fragmented and reduced elastin, so some have designated it as nevus anelasticus. Nevus elasticus or juvenile elastoma (Weidmann et al. 1933) is usually applied to a single plaque rich in elastin while elastomas refer to the multiple, often familial lesions. Both are typically present at birth.

Buschke-Ollendorff Syndrome

(Buschke and Ollendorff 1928)

Synonym. Dermatofibrosis lenticularis disseminata

Clinical Findings. Patients have multiple yellow-tan plaques and nodules which are usually not identified at birth, but develop during early childhood. While the trunk is the most common site, the limbs may also be involved. In addition, the patients have osteopoikilosis, asymptomatic calcified sclerotic lesions in their long bones. Both the skin and bone lesions are harmless.

Histopathology. The lesions resemble a dermatofibroma but special stains in the original cases revealed thickened, branching elastic fibers. The elastin matrix appears increased while the microfibrils are reduced in number. Other studies have also documented increased collagen, reflecting the above-mentioned confusion.

Therapy. Large or troubling cutaneous lesions can be excised. The skeletal changes require no treatment.

Fat Nevi

Definition. Focal circumscribed increase of fat tissue.

Fat nevi are both rare and hard to define. The lipoma is perhaps the most common adult tumor, but in many ways in meets the criteria for a fat nevus. Other fat accumulations such as a hibernoma or residual brown fat are also considered tumors.

Nevus Lipomatosus Superficialis

(Hoffmann and Zurhelle 1921)

Typically several soft, easily indented papules or nodules are seen on the buttocks or flanks (Fig. 52.7). Most patients are female. Clinically, neurofibroma and papillomatous melanocytic nevus are the usual considerations. Excisional biopsy reveals a normal epidermis, a thinned dermis, and lobular accumulations of fat close to the epidermal surface. A similar histologic picture can be seen in focal dermal hypoplasia (Chap. 19). If treatment is desired, smaller lesions can be excised.

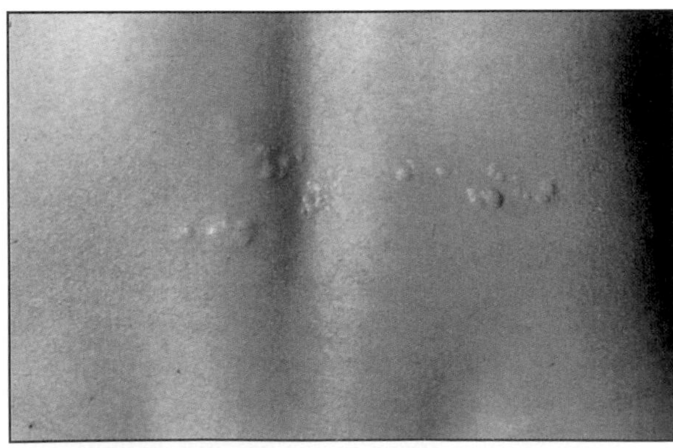

Fig. 52.7. Nevus lipomatosus

Nevus Psiloliparus

(Happle and Küster 1998)

The name psiloliparous is derived from the Greek words for hairless and fatty. These rare lesions are found on the scalp and have a smooth surface without hair follicles. They are typically found in patients with encephalocranial lipomatosis (Chap. 59) or Proteus syndrome (Chap. 19), but can appear as an isolated finding. Microscopic examination reveals a thin dermis, isolated arrector pili muscles and abundant fat. The arrector pili help to distinguish nevus psiloliparous from nevus lipomatosus superficialis. Excision is the only treatment.

Michelin Tire Baby Syndrome

(Ross 1969)

The Michelin tire baby is not a single syndrome, but a descriptive term applied to rare unfortunate infants with excess folds of skin, just like the Michelin icon. In the initial report and some of the subsequent descriptions, biopsy revealed increased and high dermal fat. Other patients simply had fibrosis and one had spontaneous keloid-like lesions. Most cases have been sporadic but autosomal dominant inheritance has been reported. A wide range of associated abnormalities including profound mental retardation have been found.

Vascular Nevi

Vascular nevi are the most common congenital malformation, occurring in about 40% of infants. There are two basic types of lesions: hemangiomas and vascular malformations. Hemangiomas are endothelial proliferations that tend to grow during infancy but eventually regress. Thus they are not nevi and are discussed under vascular tumors (Chap. 59). Vascular malformations are permanent localized excesses of vessels, often associated with other malformations, and thus true nevi.

Port-Wine Stain

Synonyms. Nevus flammeus, Unna-Pollitzer nevus, salmon patch, stork-bite nevus, nevus telangiectaticus

Etiology and Pathogenesis. Most port-wine stains probably also reflect somatic mosaicism, as they too often follow Blaschko lines and may be associated with underlying skeletal or CNS problems. Familial cases have been described, perhaps reflecting paradominant inheritance.

Clinical Findings. These lesions tend to be deep red when fully developed, but may present at birth as pink to pale red patches or plaques, ranging in size from several millimeters to covering a large body segment (Fig. 52.8). The larger lesions frequently follow Blaschko lines and are more likely to be associated with underlying abnormalities. The nuchal region is a particular common site; such lesions are known as Unna-Pollitzer nevi. They may be inflamed in infants with weeping, scaling and crusting, but without infection. In rare cases, bilaterally symmetric port-wine stains have been described as Rorschach ink-blot stains and butterfly stains.

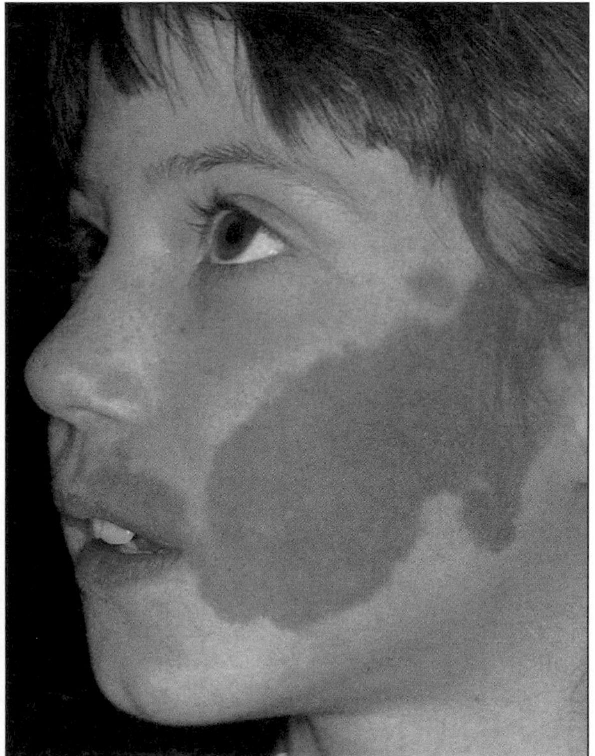

Fig. 52.8. Nevus flammeus

Another variant is the telangiectatic nevus which has more distinct individual vessels, is usually midline and frequently involves the face, nape or sacrum. All the malformations fade when examined with diascopy. Most are permanent and grow in proportion to the child. In adults, small nodules may appear within the port-wine stains, usually representing hemangiomas or other vascular tumors. Malignant change does not occur.

One of the common clinical variants is the salmon patch or stork-bite nevus which tends to involve areas of embryonic fusion such as the glabella, upper eye lids or nuchal region. The lesions are pink or pale red macules or patches without underlying enlarged vessels. In several large surveys the prevalence at 1 year of age has found to be as high as 80–90%, dropping to less than 5% at puberty. Peculiarly, the prevalence rises again in adult life, suggesting that the salmon patches fade, but do not truly disappear, and then reappear.

Histopathology. The lesions are so clinically distinct that biopsies are rarely performed. They simply reflect the clinical impression, revealing dilated small upper dermal vessels for the pale-pink lesions and larger deeper vessels in the dark-red plaques.

Therapy. The tunable dye and copper lasers (Chap. 70) have revolutionized the treatment of those port-wine stains that are not expected to fade spontaneously. Argon lasers were previously popular, but worked best for deep-colored lesions and were used in adults when the risk of scarring is reduced. In contrast, the tunable dye lasers and copper lasers can be employed in earliest infancy, and indeed the first treatment is often given before the newborn infant leaves the hospital. The light waves at 577–585 nm penetrate to a depth of about 0.75 mm, reaching the vessels where they are absorbed by hemoglobin. The short pulses are matched to the vessel's thermal relaxation time, so that necrosis is avoided. Thus, scarring is usually minimal.

Other treatments including cryotherapy, surgery and radiation therapy are no longer appropriate for ordinary cases. Small lesions can be covered very well with special make-ups such as Covermark and similar brands.

Disorders Associated with Port-Wine Stains

Port-wine stains are associated with a variety of other cutaneous, ocular, soft-tissue and CNS abnormalities. In many instances, they appear to represent somatic mosaicism. Multiple genes are probably involved. In some cases a lethal gene which can only exist in the mosaic state may be responsible, while in other instances there is paradominant inheritance and loss of heterozygosity.

Sturge-Weber Syndrome

(Luschka 1854; Sturge 1879; Weber 1907)

Synonyms. Encephalofacial angiomatosis, encephalotrigeminal angiomatosis

Definition. Vascular malformation in region served by trigeminal nerve, often with ocular and CNS involvement.

Etiology and Pathogenesis. Most cases of Sturge-Weber syndrome are sporadic, but rare familial cases exist. Predominant inheritance appears the best explanation for these families, in which other members may have increased numbers of nevi flammei but no systemic malformations.

Clinical Findings. Most often there is a unilateral port-wine stain involving the first or second branch of the trigeminal nerve (Fig. 52.9). In about 15% of cases, the lesions are bilateral. The oral cavity may be involved. The port-wine stains tend to be traversed by large palpable vessels and there may be a palpable thrill, reflecting arteriovenous malformations. In addition, there may be congenital or acquired glaucoma, so all patients should have their intraocular pressures monitored. If both the first and second branches of the trigeminal nerve are involved, the risk of glaucoma is considerably higher. About 50% of patients eventually develop elevated intraocular pressure.

The second serious associated problem is the possibility of dilated leptomeningeal vessels which may calcify and lead to a variety of CNS problems including seizures, motor dysfunction and mental retardation. A variety of imaging approaches are satisfactory to monitor this aspect. Over 75% of patients have seizures, and mental retardation is estimated at about 50%. Motor problems, including hemiplegia, arise in about 25%.

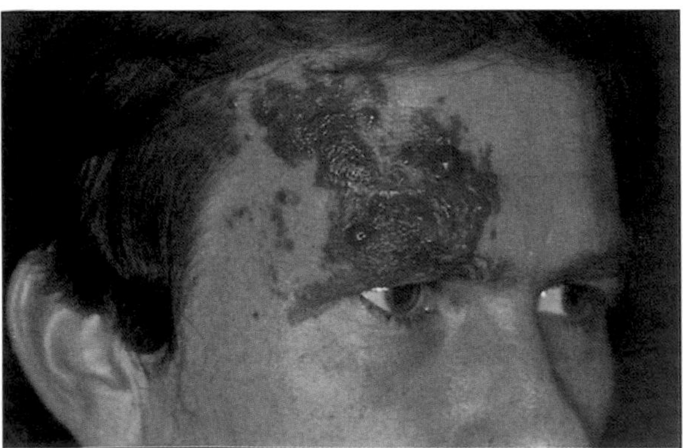

Fig. 52.9. Sturge-Weber syndrome

Histopathology. Biopsies are rarely performed. Large thickened vessels, both arterial and venous, may be identified, along with the expected capillary proliferation.

Therapy. The skin lesions can be treated best with tunable dye or copper lasers. A pediatrician or neurologist and an ophthalmologist should be involved in the continuing care of the patient.

Klippel-Trénaunay-Weber Syndrome

(Klippel and Trénaunay 1900; Weber 1922)

Synonyms. Angio-osteohypertrophy syndrome, osteohypertrophic angioectasia

Definition. Vascular malformation of limb associated with bone and soft tissue hypertrophy.

Etiology and Pathogenesis. Just as with Sturge-Weber syndrome, this vascular malformation is usually sporadic. The same genetic explanations can be evoked for the rare familial cases. The only difference is the location of the vascular malformation.

Clinical Findings. Usually a single limb is covered to a great extent by a port-wine stain. Rarely two limbs may be involved or there may be simultaneous facial involvement (Fig. 52.10). Large thickened vessels can be seen or palpated underlying the discolored skin. Varicose veins are also often present. Occasionally a nevus anemicus is present within the malformation. In adults, multiple hemangiomas or other vascular tumors may arise, presumably from persistent angiogenic stimulation.

The underlying bone and soft tissue is hypertrophic resulting in gigantism of the involved limb.

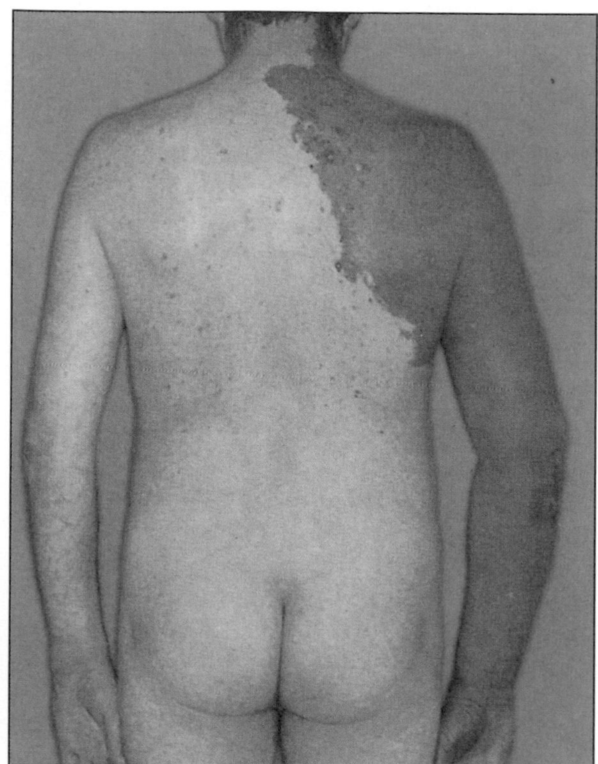

Fig. 52.10. Klippel-Trénaunay-Weber syndrome

While the limbs may be of unequal size at birth, more often this becomes apparent as the child grows. A thrill may be palpated or a bruit heard, as arteriovenous malformations are present. There may be high-output cardiac failure because of shunting. The involved limb is often painful and may become edematous or even ulcerate. Recurrent cellulitis is also a problem. The bone may even be weakened. Other associated abnormalities may include visceral vascular malformations, polydactyly and syndactyly. In rare cases, the skin is normal but underlying problems are present; some designate this scenario as Parkes Weber syndrome. There is an overlap in some patients between Klippel-Trénaunay-Weber syndrome and cutis marmorata telangiectatica congenita (Chap. 22).

Therapy. The port-wine stain can be treated as discussed above. The patient should be evaluated by a radiologist or vascular surgeon to assess the degree of arteriovenous shunting and other malformations. Compression stockings or more elaborate home compression devices may help to minimize the disproportionate limb growth and edema. Sometimes arteriovenous shunts can be closed surgically or obstructed via intravascular embolization techniques.

Cobb Syndrome

(Berenbruch 1890; Cobb 1915)

Synonym. Cutaneomeningeal angiomatosis

Cobb syndrome features a cutaneous vascular lesion, usually a port-wine stain, on the back overlying meningeal or dural vascular malformations. While the description is usually of dermatomal lines, in most published pictures Blaschko lines are followed. In some families, other members have had multiple hemangiomas. Lymphangiomas and angiokeratomas have also been described. The Valsalva maneuver may often make the cutaneous lesions more prominent, indicating that the malformations are connected and that shunting occurs.

Von Hippel-Lindau Syndrome

The von Hippel-Lindau syndrome is rarely seen by dermatologists. The main features are vascular malformations of the retina and cerebellar leptomeninges. On occasion, there may be a port-wine stain, most often of the face (Chap. 19).

Other Vascular Nevi and Malformations

Venous Malformations

(Servelle 1948)

Synonyms. Venous angioma, Servelle-Martorell syndrome

Epidemiology. Pure venous malformations are much less common than mixed arteriovenous malformations. They have been underdiagnosed or misdiagnosed, even though they have distinctive features.

Etiology and Pathogenesis. Venous malformations are hemodynamically inactive, feature slow blood flow and often have thromboses or subclinical intravascular coagulation.

Clinical Findings. The pure venous malformations typically are blue even at room temperature and tend to swell with activity or when an involved limb is in a dependent position (Fig. 52.11). The ectatic veins can be seen in the dermis. Usually a single limb is involved. More extensive malformations often extend to the trunk and very extensive mal-

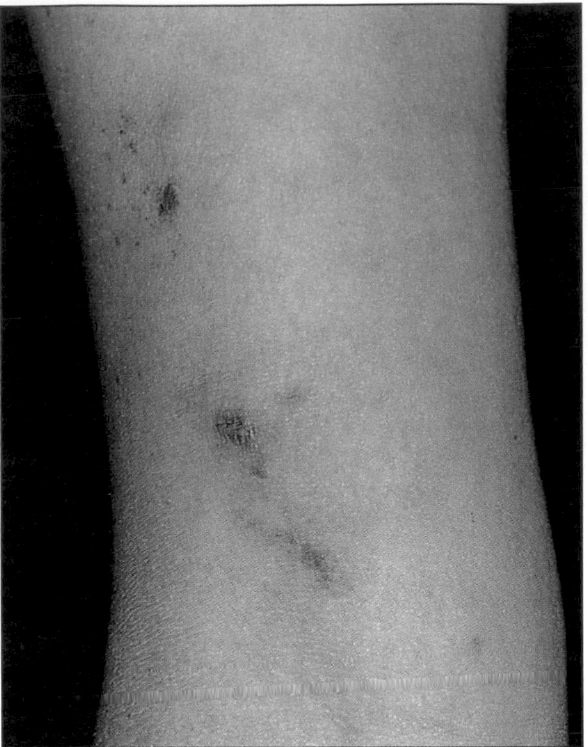

Fig. 52.11. Venous malformation with several thromboses

formations may involve several limbs. Sometimes deeper lesions have no cutaneous changes, presenting only with swelling and other complications.

Because of the slow flow, coagulation disturbances are common, even though marked hemorrhage is rare. More common is the development of thromboses in the ectatic veins, leading to painful nodules which often calcify into phleboliths. In addition, small vascular tumors may develop on the background of the venous bed; their exact nomenclature remains unclear. Almost all patients have muscle involvement and about two-thirds show bony abnormalities. The limb length and girth are either normal or decreased. Hypertrophy as seen in Klippel- Trénaunay-Weber syndrome is very uncommon. When a leg is involved, both pain and hemorrhage in the knee joint is almost expected. In adults bone thinning, demineralization and even osteolysis may be seen.

Histopathology. Microscopic evaluation is a poor way to make the diagnosis. Irregular vascular channels are seen infiltrating through connective tissue and muscles. Although endothelial cells can usually be found lining the vascular spaces, exact classification of the vessels is difficult.

Laboratory Findings. The patient's coagulation parameters should be monitored prior to surgery. Both ultrasonography and magnetic resonance imaging are effective in displaying the extent of the malformations and monitoring progression.

Course and Prognosis. The lesions continue to expand, but the main chronic problems involve the affected joints and muscles.

Differential Diagnosis. The main differential diagnosis is Klippel-Trénaunay-Weber syndrome. Most patients are misdiagnosed, but the history of thromboses, decrease in limb size and abnormal clotting studies are good clues.

Therapy. Compression stockings are a must. Sclerotherapy may be useful, especially for genital involvement where compression therapy is impossible. Excision usually leads to extensive scarring. Knee joint involvement may require synovectomy or reconstructive surgery. In any surgical setting, low molecular weight heparin should be considered to interrupt the smoldering intravascular coagulation process.

Phakomatosis Pigmentovascularis

(Ota et al. 1921)

This tongue twister refers to a variety of clinically unusual patients who present with a combination of vascular and epidermal or melanocytic abnormalities. The disorders are very rare and have been most often described in Japanese patients and appear in a sporadic fashion. Twin spotting may be the explanation for this group of patients. The vascular lesions are nevi flammei, while a variety of other changes can be found. The vascular lesions typically have a patchwork pattern or follow Blaschko lines and stand in contrast to other, generally contralateral, malformations. The usual clinical categories are shown in Table 52.1. Standard methods of therapy can be employed for cosmetic reasons. The vascular lesions are generally amenable to laser treatment while the associated changes are harder to treat.

Nevus Anemicus

(Vörner 1906)

Etiology and Pathogenesis. In contrast to all the other malformations listed above, nevus anemicus is unique. It is the prime example of a pharmaco-

Table 52.1. Types of phakomatosis pigmentovascularis

Type[a]	Synonym	Vascular lesion	Associated features
I	Adamson-Best syndrome	Nevus flammeus	Epidermal nevus
II	Takano-Krüger-Doi syndrome	Nevus flammeus	Aberrant Mongolian spots ± nevus anemicus
III	Kobori-Toda syndrome	Nevus flammeus	Nevus spilus ± nevus anemicus
IV		Nevus flammeus	Aberrant Mongolian spots, nevus spilus ± nevus anemicus

[a] Sometimes the suffixes "A" (no systemic involvement) and "B" (systemic involvement) are also used.

logic nevus. The vessels in a given area are exquisitely sensitive to catecholamines and remain constricted producing a pale color. There is donor dominance, so when parts of a nevus anemicus are transplanted to a normal region, the area remains pale. Injection of α-receptor blockers produces vessel widening and erythema.

Clinical Findings. Nevus anemicus has many interesting clinical features. The lesions are highly irregular sharply bordered white patches that are always asymptomatic (Fig. 52.12). While most patients have a single patch on the trunk, widespread multiple lesions may also be seen. Often they are difficult to see against the background color of the patient's skin, but if a sunburn develops, then the white area stands out prominently. Similarly, if the skin is rubbed or irritated, there is no reflex reddening in the nevus anemicus.

Nevus anemicus may also be seen within a vascular malformation such as a port-wine stain; in this case, it is easily recognized. Nevus anemicus may also occur in all the variants of phakomatosis pigmentovascularis.

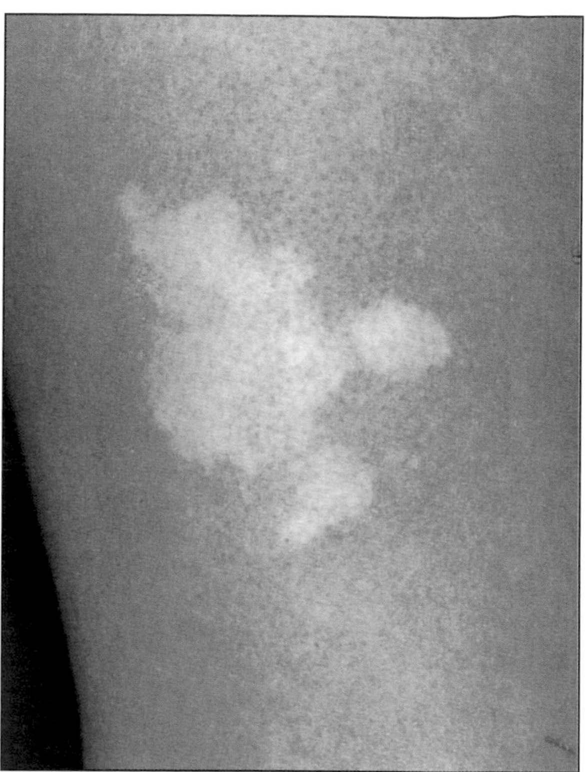

Fig. 52.12. Nevus anemicus

Histopathology. The skin is entirely normal. Nevus anemicus is thus one of the classic disorders in which microscopic examination offers no clue to the disease.

Differential Diagnosis. There is no significant differential diagnostic spectrum. Occasionally vitiligo and nevus depigmentosus are considered, but the physical findings are so classic that the diagnosis soon becomes obvious. A search for associated abnormalities is more important.

Therapy. There is no treatment other than excision which is rarely needed.

Nevus Vascularis Mixtus

(Fischer 1909; Hamm and Happle 1986)

The association of a telangiectatic nevus and a nevus anemicus in close proximity is too common to be left to chance. Once again twin spotting may be the explanation for nevus vascularis mixtus. If a gene for vascular tone control was present in the heterozygous state and then somatic recombination occurred, one patch would have too much vascular constriction (nevus anemicus) and the other, too little (nevus telangiectaticus).

Nevus Oligemicus

(Davies et al. 1981)

In this disease, there is a persistant livid erythema, localized in a pattern similar to nevus anemicus. The skin is often cooler than the adjacent areas and seems to have reduced blood flow. It has been suggested that nevus oligemicus is caused by constriction of deeper dermal vessels with a form of localized stasis in the superficial vessels producing lividity. The border is much less sharply defined than nevus anemicus and the pharmacology is unclear.

Bibliography

Review

Brown TJ, Friedman J, Levy ML (1998) The diagnosis and treatment of common birthmarks. Clin Plast Surg 25:509–525

Happle R (1995) What is a nevus? A proposed definition of a common medical term. Dermatology 191:1–5

Epidermal Nevi and Epidermal Nevus Syndrome

Happle R (1995) Epidermal nevus syndromes. Semin Dermatol 14:111–121

Losee JE, Serletti JM, Pennino RP (1999) Epidermal nevus syndrome: a review and case report. Ann Plast Surg 43:211–214

Olivares JL, Ramos FJ, Carapeto FJ et al. (1999) Epidermal naevus syndrome and hypophosphataemic rickets: description of a patient with central nervous system anomalies and review of the literature. Eur J Pediatr 158:103–107

Solomon LM, Fretzin DF, Dewald RL (1968) The epidermal nevus syndrome. Arch Dermatol 97:273–285

Segmental Darier Disease

Happle R (1997) A rule concerning the segmental manifestation of autosomal dominant skin disorders. Review of clinical examples providing evidence for dichotomous types of severity. Arch Dermatol 133:1505–1509

Happle R, Itin PH, Brun AM (1999) Type 2 segmental Darier disease. Eur J Dermatol 9:449–451

O'Malley MP, Haake A, Goldsmith L et al. (1997) Localized Darier disease. Implications for genetic studies. Arch Dermatol 133:1134–1138

Nevus Corniculatus

Happle R, Steijlen PM, Kolde G (1990) Naevus corniculatus: a new acantholytic disorder. Br J Dermatol 122:107–112

ILVEN

Altman J, Mehregan AH (1971) Inflammatory linear verrucose epidermal nevus. Arch Dermatol 102:253–259

Hodge SJ, Barr JM, Owen LG (1978) Inflammatory linear verrucose epidermal nevus. Arch Dermatol 114:436–438

Kawaguchi H, Takeuchi M, Ono H et al. (1999) Adult onset of inflammatory linear verrucous epidermal nevus. J Dermatol 26:599–602

Morag C, Metzker A (1985) Inflammatory linear verrucous epidermal nevus: report of seven new cases and review of the literature. Pediatr Dermatol 3:15–18

Oprsalova K, Filo V, Danilla T et al. (1996) Unilateral perianogenital papulokeratotic lesion. Inflammatory linear verrucous epidermal nevus (ILVEN). Arch Dermatol 132:1508–1509, 1511–1512

Zhuang L, Zhu W (1996) Inflammatory linear verrucose epidermal nevus coexisting with lichen amyloidosus. J Dermatol 23:415–418

CHILD Nevus

Fink-Puches R, Soyer HP, Pierer G et al. (1997) Systematized inflammatory epidermal nevus with symmetrical involvement: an unusual case of CHILD syndrome? J Am Acad Dermatol 36:823–826

Happle R (1996) CHILD nevus: a need for a name. Pediatr Dermatol 13:78–80

Happle R, Mittag H, Kuster W (1995) The CHILD nevus: a distinct skin disorder. Dermatology 191:210–216

Organoid Nevi

Buescher L, DeSpain JD, Diaz-Arias AA et al. (1991) Keratoacanthoma arising in an organoid nevus during childhood: case report and literature review. Pediatr Dermatol 8:117–119

Gordon CJ (1991) Proliferating trichilemmal cyst in an organoid nevus. Cutis 48:49–52

Kanekura T, Kawahira M, Kanzaki T (1994) Three cases of organoid nevus on the trunk and extremity. J Dermatol 21:771–775

Romer JC, Taira JW (1994) Mucinous eccrine nevus. Cutis 53:259–261

Rongioletti F, Rebora A (1996) Mucinous nevus. Arch Dermatol 132:1522–1523

Suhr KB, Ro YW, Kim KH et al. (1997) Mucinous nevus: report of two cases and review of the literature. J Am Acad Dermatol 37:312–313

Nevus Sebaceus

Cribier B, Scrivener Y, Grosshans E (2000) Tumors arising in nevus sebaceus: A study of 596 cases. J Am Acad Dermatol 42:263–268

Jadassohn J (1895) Bemerkungen zur Histologie der systematisierten Naevi und über „Talgdrüsen-Naevi". Arch Dermatol Syphilol 88:355–394

Wilson Jones E, Heyl T (1970) Naevus sebaceus. A report of 140 cases with special regard to the development of secondary malignant tumours. Br J Dermatol 82:99–117

Palazzi P, Artese O, Paolini A et al. (1996) Linear sebaceous nevus syndrome: report of a patient with unusual associated abnormalities. Pediatr Dermatol 13:22–24

Pinkus H (1965) Zur Begriffbestimmung der Naevi, Organnaevi, und Tumoren. Hautarzt 16:184–190

Warrenburg BP van de, Gulik S van, Renier WO et al. (1998) The linear naevus sebaceus syndrome. Clin Neurol Neurosurg 100:126–132

Nevus Comedonicus

Barsky S, Doyle IA, Winkelmann RK (1981) Nevus comedonicus with epidermolytic hyperkeratosis. Arch Dermatol 117:86–88

Patrizi A, Neri I, Fiorentini C et al. (1998) Nevus comedonicus syndrome: a new pediatric case. Pediatr Dermatol 15:304–306

Vasiloudes PE, Morelli JG, Weston WL (1998) Inflammatory nevus comedonicus in children. J Am Acad Dermatol 38: 834–836

Eccrine Nevus and Apocrine Nevus

Imai S, Nitto H (1983) Eccrine nevus with epidermal changes. Dermatologica 166:84–88

Pippione M, Depaoli MA, Sartoris S (1976) Eccrine-nevus (in French). Dermatologica 152:40–46

Valks R, Abajo P, Fraga J et al. (1996) Porokeratotic eccrine ostial and dermal duct nevus of late onset: more frequent than previously suggested? Dermatology 193:138–140

Becker Nevus Syndrome

Happle R, Koopman RJ (1997) Becker nevus syndrome. Am J Med Genet 68:357–361

Munro Nevus

Munro CS, Wilkie AO (1998) Epidermal mosaicism producing localised acne: somatic mutation in FGFR2. Lancet 352:704–705

Schimmelpenning Feuerstein Mims and Proteus Syndrome

Feuerstein R, Mims L (1962) Linear nevus sebaceus with convulsions and mental retardation. Am J Dis Child 104: 675–697

Hamm H (1999) Cutaneous mosaicism of lethal mutations. Am J Med Genet 85:342–345

Schimmelpennig GW (1957) Klinischer Beitrag zur Symptomatologie der Phakmatosen. Fortschr Roentgen 87:716–720

Schworm HD, Jedele KB, Holinski E et al. (1996) Discordant monozygotic twins with the Schimmelpenning-Feuerstein-Mims syndrome. Clin Genet 50:393–397

Phakomatosis Pigmentokeratotica

Ota M, Kawamura T, Ito N (1947) Phacomatosis pigmentovascularis (Ota). Jpn J Dermatol 52:1–3

Torrelo A, Zambrano A (1998) What syndrome is this. Phakomatosis pigmentokeratotica (Happle). Pediatr Dermatol 15:321–323

Nevus Elasticus

Lewandowsky F (1921) Über einem eigentümlichen Nevus der Brustgegend. Arch Dermatol Syphilol 87:5–25

Sanchez Yus E, Aguilar A, Requena L et al. (1990) Nevus elasticus and lichen sclerosus et atrophicus on the vulva. Cutis 45:252–255

Weidmann FD, Anderson NP, Ayres S (1933) Juvenile elastoma. Arch Dermatol Syphilol 28:182–189

Buschke-Ollendorff Syndrome

Buschke A, Ollendorf H (1928) Ein Fall von Dermatofibrosis lenticularis disseminata und Osteopathia condensans disseminata. Dermatol Wochenschr 86:257–262

Schirren H, Schirren CG, Stolz W et al. (1994) Papular elastorrhexis: a variant of dermatofibrosis lenticularis disseminata (Buschke-Ollendorff syndrome)? Dermatology 189:368–372

Schnur RE, Grace K, Herzberg A (1994) Buschke-Ollendorff syndrome, otosclerosis, and congenital spinal stenosis. Pediatr Dermatol 11:31–34

Trattner A, David M, Rothem A et al. (1991) Buschke-Ollendorff syndrome of the scalp: histologic and ultrastructural findings. J Am Acad Dermatol 24:822–824

Fat Nevi

Eng W, Cohen PR (1998) Nevus with fat: clinical characteristics of 100 nevi containing mature adipose cells. J Am Acad Dermatol 39:704–711

Happle R, Kuster W (1998) Nevus psiloliparus: a distinct fatty tissue nevus. Dermatology 197:6–10

Hoffman E, Zurhelle E (1921) Über einen Naevus lipomatodes cutaneus superficialis der linken Glutalgegend. Arch Dermatol Syphilol 130:327–333

Jones EW, Marks R, Pongsehirun D (1975) Naevus superficialis lipomatosus. A clinicopathological report of twenty cases. Br J Dermatol 93:121–133

Mehregan AH, Tavafoghi V, Ghandchi A (1975) Nevus lipomatosus cutaneus superficialis (Hoffmann-Zurhelle). J Cutan Pathol 2:307–313

Orteu CH, Hughes JR, Rustin MH (1996) Naevus lipomatosus cutaneous superficialis: overlap with connective tissue naevi. Acta Derm Venereol (Stockh) 76:243–245

Park HJ, Park CJ, Yi JY et al. (1997) Nevus lipomatosus superficialis on the face. Int J Dermatol 36: 435–437

Ross CM (1972) Generalized folded skin with underlying lipomatous nevus: the Michelin tire baby. Arch Dermatol 106:320–323

Uitto J, Santa-Cruz DJ, Eisen AZ (1979) Familial cutaneous collagenoma: genetic studies on a family. Br J Dermatol 101:185–195

Vascular Nevi and Malformations

Atiyeh BS, Musharrafieh RS (1995) Klippel-Trenaunay-type syndrome: an eponym for various expressions of the same entity. J Med 26:253–260

Bean WB (1958) Vascular spiders and related lesions of the skin. Thomas, Springfield

Cobb S (1915) Haemangioma of the spinal cord associated with skin naevi at the same metamere. Ann Surg 62: 641–649

Enjolras O, Ciabrini D, Mazoyer E et al. (1997) Extensive pure venous malformations in the upper or lower limb: a review of 27 cases. J Am Acad Dermatol 36:219–225

Hagiwara K, Uezato H, Nonaka S (1998) Phacomatosis pigmentovascularis type IIb associated with Sturge-Weber syndrome and pyogenic granuloma. J Dermatol 25:721–729

Hippel E von (1895) Vorstellung eines Patienten mit einem sehr ungewöhnlichen Aderhautleiden, Ber 24. Versamml Ophthalm Ges 269

Katugampola GA, Lanigan SW (1996) The clinical spectrum of naevus anaemicus and its association with port wine stains: report of 15 cases and a review of the literature. Br J Dermatol 134:292–295

Klippel M, Trénaunay P (1900) Du naevus variqueux ostéohypertrophique (in French). Arch Gen Med (Paris) 641–642

Krabbe KH (1934) Facial and meningeal angiomatosis associated with calcifications of the brain cortex, a clinical and anatomopathologic contribution. Arch Neurol Psychiatry 32:737–755

Meine JG, Schwartz RA, Janniger CK (1997) Klippel-Trenaunay-Weber syndrome. Cutis 60:127–132
Mirowski GW, Liu AA, Stone ML et al. (1999) Sturge-Weber syndrome. J Am Acad Dermatol 41:772–773
Miteva LG, Dourmishev AI, Schwartz RA et al. (1998) Oral vascular manifestations of Klippel-Trenaunay syndrome. Cutis 62:171–174
Requena L, Sangueza OP (1997) Cutaneous vascular anomalies. Part I. Hamartomas, malformations, and dilatation of preexisting vessels. J Am Acad Dermatol 37:523–549
Servelle M (1948) Stase veneuse et croissance osseuse. Bull Acad Nat Med (Paris) 132:471–474
Sturge WA (1879) A case of partial epilepsy apparently due to a lesion of one of the vasomotor centres of the brain. Cin Soc Trans 12:162
Truhan AP, Filipek PA (1993) Magnetic resonance imaging. Its role in the neuroradiologic evaluation of neurofibromatosis, tuberous sclerosis, and Sturge-Weber syndrome. Arch Dermatol 129:219–226
Waner M, Suen JY (eds) (1999) Hemangiomas and Vascular Malformation of the Head and Neck. John Willey, New York
Weber FP (1907) Angioma formation in connection with hypertrophy of limbs and hemihypertrophy. Br J Dermatol 19:231–235
Weber FP (1922) Right-sided hemihypotrophy resulting from right-sided congenital spastic hemiplegia, with morbid condition of left side of brain, as revealed by radiogram. J Neur Psychopath 3:134–139

Nevus Anemicus

Ahkami RN, Schwartz RA (1999) Nevus anemicus. Dermatology 198:327–329
Bielsa I, Paradelo C, Ribera M et al. (1998) Generalized nevus spilus and nevus anemicus in a patient with a primary lymphedema: a new type of phakomatosis pigmentovascularis? Pediatr Dermatol 15:293–295
Fischer W (1909) Über Naevus anaemicus. Arch Dermatol Syph 96:47–58
Greaves MW, Birkett D, Johnson C (1970) Nevus anemicus: a unique catecholamine-dependent nevus. Arch Dermatol 102:172–176
Montcastle EA, Diestelmeier MR, Lupton GP (1986) Nevus anemicus. J Am Acad Dermatol 14:628–632
Vörner H (1906) Über Naevus anaemicus. Arch Dermatol Syph 82:391–398

Nevus Oligemicus

Davies MG, Greaves MW, Coutts A et al. (1981) Nevus oligemicus: a variant of nevus anemicus. Arch Dermatol 117:111–113
Plantin P, Leroy JP, Guillet G (1992) Nevus oligemicus: a new case. J Am Acad Dermatol 26:268–269

Cysts and Sinuses

Contents

Introduction

Cysts in the skin are tumors or tumor-like growths that clinically or histologically appear to have a capsule and a central fluid or semisolid content. They may be divided into:

True Cysts. A true cyst consists of a space surrounded by an epithelial cell wall. The cyst contents may be fluid, semisolid or solid. The cyst may be entirely enclosed, but often has a pore or other surface connection, usually reflecting a follicular origin (Fig. 53.1). Cysts may develop either from keratinizing (skin, hair) or glandular (sweat glands) epithelium. The size may vary from minuscule (a 1–2 mm milium) to enormous (trichilemmal scalp cysts may be as large as a fist). Some cysts may be posttraumatic, such as a true epidermal inclusion cyst arising after a piece of skin is jabbed or pushed into the dermis during an accident, such as an injury from an awl. Other cysts may develop after superficial trauma, such as milia following dermabrasion or porphyria cutanea tarda. Some cysts reflect the embryologic misplacement of epithelial structures. Multiple epithelial cysts are often associated with genodermatoses and usually reflect autosomal dominant inheritance. Two examples of the latter are Gardner syndrome and steatocystoma multiplex. Cysts are named to reflect the nature of the epithelial lining.

Pseudocysts. These resemble cysts clinically but lack an epithelial lining. One common examples is a mucocele (Chap. 33), which usually results from the rupture of a minor salivary gland duct and consists of extravasated mucin surrounded by an accumulation of histiocytes. Similarly, a digital mucous cyst also contains extravasated mucin, perhaps from a synovial structure, without a cyst wall.

Cystic Tumors. Many tumors appear clinically cystic and contain a liquid or semisolid material. The classic example is a cystic basal cell carcinoma. Many eccrine tumors are also cystic. Other tumors may appear clinically solid but show cystic spaces under the microscope. Yet other tumors, such as benign adnexal tumors, protrude out of the skin as if encapsulated, but microscopic examination reveals no true cyst wall.

Table 53.1 lists many of the true cysts, pseudocysts and cystic tumors of the skin. Many of the latter disorders will be covered in subsequent chapters, as many adnexal tumors may occasionally present

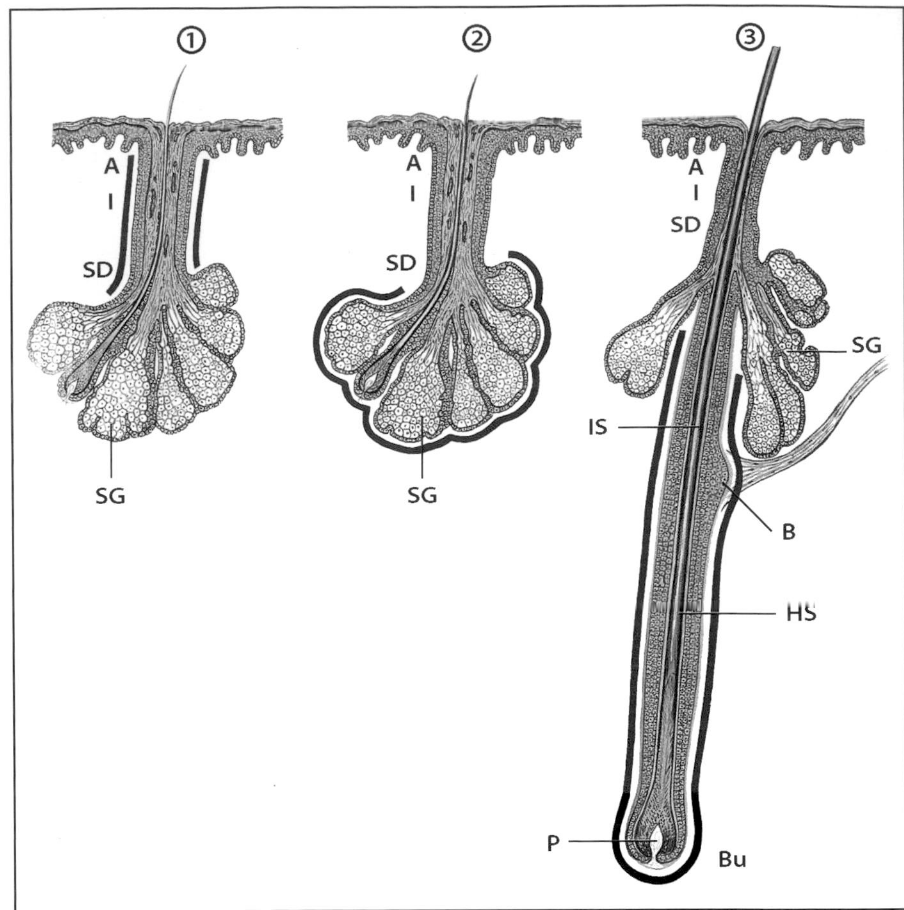

Fig. 53.1. Histogenesis of various cysts. Sebaceous follicle; cysts may develop from the infundibulum (epidermoid cyst ①) or from the sebaceous glands (steatocystoma ②). Mature hair follicle; cysts can develop from the isthmus or other parts of deeper follicle ③. Pilomatricomas have features of the matrix as found in the bulb.
A, acroinfundibulum
I, infrainfundibulum
SD, sebaceous duct
SG, sebaceous gland
Is, isthmus
B, bulge
HS, hair shaft
Bu, hair bulb
P, dermal papillae

clinically as cysts but are better considered with their companion tumors. Clearly the distinction between an epidermoid cyst and a cystic tumor derived from the hair follicle, such as a pilomatricoma, is somewhat artificial.

Epithelial Cysts

Epidermoid Cyst

Synonyms. Follicular cyst, infundibular type; epidermal inclusion cyst, "sebaceous" cyst

Definition. Common cyst with wall resembling follicular infundibulum.

To most Americans this lesion is known as a "sebaceous" cyst, although this designation is incorrect. While Ackerman's term of follicular cyst, infundibular type is preferable, it has taken decades for epidermoid cyst to win gradual acceptance and we are skeptical if another change is likely.

Etiology and Pathogenesis. While some sort of follicular obstruction leads to a cyst, the mechanisms are unclear in most cases, although sometimes preceding comedo formation may predispose to cyst formation.

Clinical Findings. Epidermoid cysts are typically 3–20 mm in diameter, usually round or egg-shaped and almost invariably connected to the epidermal surface by a pore – the residuum of the precursor hair follicle (Fig. 53.2). The pore is usually small, so that the cyst is closed at the top. Sometimes the pore may be slightly open with the same dark color as an open comedo. The overlying skin may be stretched or slightly erythematous; the dermal vessels may be

Table 53.1. Cutaneous cysts and related structures

Type of cyst	Differentiation	Example	Histologic features	Class
Epithelial	Interfollicular epidermis	Traumatic inclusion cyst	Stratum granulosum, fibrosis, scarring	C
	Hair follicle	Milium	Small sub- or intraepithelial keratin filled cyst, no bacteria	C
		Epidermoid cyst	Stratum granulosum	C
		Scrotal cyst	Usually calcified, scarred	C
		Acne comedo	Stratum granulosum, sebaceous glands	C
		Giant comedo	Stratum granulosum, no sebaceous glands	C
		Trichilemmal cyst	Trichilemmal keratinization, no stratum granulosum	C
		Proliferating trichilemmal cyst	Marked proliferation of cyst wall keratinocytes	C>Tu
		Pilomatricoma	Shadow cells, calcification (Chap. 57)	C>Tu
		Steatocystoma	Sebaceous cells, hairs	C
		Vellus hair cyst	Multiple vellus hairs	C
Glandular	Eccrine glands	Eccrine hidrocystoma	Eccrine cyst wall	C
	Apocrine glands	Apocrine hidrocystoma	Apocrine cyst wall	Tu
	Salivary glands	True retention cyst	Dilated salivary duct, often with sialolith	C
		Mucocele	Ruptured duct with mucin, inflammation	PC
	Endometrial glands	Endometriosis	Endometrial lining (Chap. 35)	C
Synovial	Joint space or tendon sheath	Ganglion	Synovial lining	C
		Metaplastic synovial cyst	Synovial lining, fibrosis	PC
Developmental	Ectoderm, along lines of fusion	Dermoid	Keratinizing epithelium, multiple adnexal structures	C
	Median raphe (ventral midline perineum and penis)	Median raphe cyst	Columnar epithelium	C
	Müllerian duct	Ciliated cyst	Ciliated cuboidal epithelium	C
	Ventral midline of chest	Bronchogenic cyst	Ciliated, mucin-producing epithelium	C
	2nd branchial cleft	Branchial cleft cyst	Stratified squamous and ciliated epithelium	C
	1st branchial cleft	Preauricular cyst	Stratified squamous and ciliated epithelium, also cartilage	C
	Thyroglossal duct	Thyroglossal duct cyst	Stratified squamous or ciliated epithelium, thyroid tissue	C
	Lymphatics	Cystic hygroma (Chap. 24)	Endothelium	C
Pseudocyst		Digital mucous cyst	Mucin, perhaps from synovium	PC
		Auricular pseudocyst (Chap. 20)	Cavity within cartilage	PC
Sinus	Follicular epithelium	Pilonidal sinus	Epithelial-lined tracts, fibrosis	S
		Dental sinus tract	Inflammation, fibrosis	S

Cyst (C), pseudocyst (PC), cystic tumor (Tu), C>Tu (early lesions cystic, later usually solid), sinus (S)

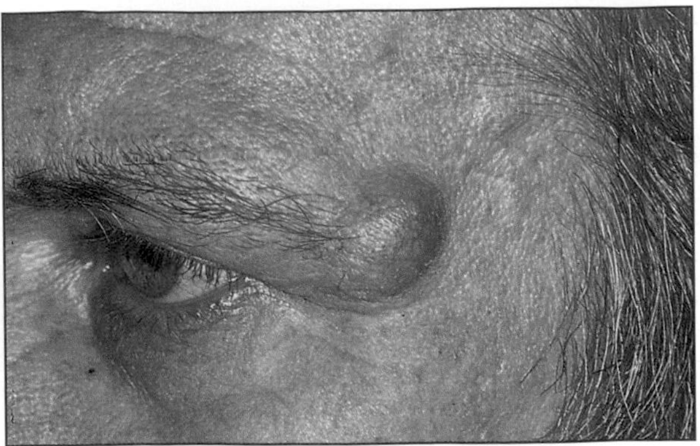

Fig. 53.2. Epidermoid cyst

visible. These cysts are most common on the face, behind the ears, on the neck and on the back, but may arise anywhere where sebaceous or terminal hair follicles are present. The lining continues to produce keratin so that the cyst may slowly expand. Sometimes the cyst is pigmented, because the cyst wall contains considerable amounts of melanin. Occasionally one or many hairs may be found in the cyst.

Because of the surface connection, epidermoid cyst may become infected. In such cases, they expand rapidly, filling with pus and becoming red, tender and malodorous. While they usually contain the normal follicular bacteria (*Micrococci, Propionibacterium acnes*) and fungi (*Pityrosporum ovale*), the infection is caused by surface staphylococci or streptococci. The lesion may burst and drain spontaneously, then heal with fibrosis and scarring. Once a lesion has been infected, recurrent infections are the rule rather than the exception.

There are a number of variants of epidermoid cysts:

- True epidermal inclusion cysts arise when a tiny piece of skin is implanted into the dermis where it forms a cyst. The typical scenario is a sewing needle, awl or nail injury on the hand; the palmar and plantar epithelium appear particularly vulnerable to this process. Cysts may also result from surgical procedures; not only operative scars but also drainage sites and similar areas may heal with inclusions of skin that become cystic.
- Epidermoid cysts can develop in acne, presumably secondary to follicular occlusion and resultant dermal expansion of the follicle. These cysts typically arise along the eyebrows, behind the ears, and on the chest and back. The more typical cystic lesions in acne are pseudocysts – succulent inflamed nodules following destruction of most of the follicular structure.
- Human papilloma virus(HPV)-related cysts have also been described. The most common is a plantar cyst containing HPV 60, which apparently enters the skin through an eccrine duct. In the verrucous epidermal cyst, other HPV types produce verrucous changes in the cyst lining including koilocytes and keratohyaline granules.
- Most patients with several epidermoid cysts have no associated disease. Multiple cysts suggest Gardner syndrome or the closely related Turcot and Oldfield syndromes (Chap. 65). Acral epidermoid cysts should raise the question of Gardner syndrome or nevoid basal cell carcinoma syndrome. In the latter disorder, on rare occasions the cutaneous cysts may have the same corrugated lining as the odontogenic keratocysts of the jaw.

Histopathology. Epidermoid cysts are surrounded by an epithelium that is undergoing infundibular keratinization, which is similar to that of the skin. There is a granular layer and basket-weave hyperkeratosis. If the cyst keratin is more compacted, it can acquire a layered onion-skin pattern. Hairs are rarely seen and other adnexal structures such as sebaceous and apocrine glands are almost never found, although they must be present at the start of the process. Frequently the cell wall shows different types of keratinization, such as trichilemmal or pilomatricomal in addition to infundibular; such cysts are designated as hybrid or mixed.

If the cyst has not ruptured, the overlying epidermis may show atrophy and the surrounding dermis thinning and prominent vessels. Following rupture, there is dermal fibrosis and often a granulomatous inflammatory infiltrate. Fragments of keratin may be seen in giant cells where they polarize nicely. The cyst contents may calcify. Rarely, there may be proliferation of the epithelial elements of the cyst wall, but this phenomenon is more common in trichilemmal cysts. Squamous cell carcinomas have been described as arising from a proliferating epidermal cyst, but this must be an extremely rare event.

Differential Diagnosis. Sometimes an epidermoid cyst and a trichilemmal cyst can be difficult to distinguish. The latter is usually firmer and located on the scalp. On rare occasions, a cystic adnexal tumor, cystic basal cell carcinoma or even a cutaneous metastasis may resemble an epidermoid cyst, but the histology provides the correct diagnosis.

Therapy. Most epidermoid cysts require no therapy. Common indications for removal are cosmetic complaints and recurrent infections. When a cyst has never been inflamed, it can often be removed intact through a relatively small incision, producing the best cosmetic results. If the cyst is quite large, it can be opened and emptied and then the cyst wall removed through blunt dissection and traction. Scarred cysts usually need to be excised en bloc.

An acutely infected cyst can be opened and drained. Sometimes the cyst wall can be extracted at this time. It is generally best not to suture such a lesion, but instead to place a wick and allow secondary closure. Alternatively, one can suture the opening shut after the infection has resolved. Oral antibiotics such as macrolides or cephalosporins are usually prescribed for 5–7 days. Attempts to treat infected cysts with antibiotics alone without drainage are usually unsuccessful.

Milium

Definition. Tiny epidermoid cyst. Milium is Latin for millet, a tiny variety of grain. The plural is milia.

Clinical Findings. Primary milia present as 1–3 mm yellow-white papules, typically on the cheeks, about the eyes and on the temples (Fig. 53.3). Milia are very common in infants and may appear in great numbers in young girls; the latter phenomenon is known as eruptive milia. Milia have no apparent connection to the skin surface and rarely become infected, in contrast to comedones which are otherwise similar.

Secondary milia are caused by superficial trauma of all types such as dermabrasion, chemical peels, burns and radiation therapy. In addition blistering dermatoses may also heal with blisters; this often occurs with porphyria cutanea tarda on the backs of the hands and is a clinical sign of junctional or subepidermal disease in epidermolysis bullosa. Milia are also associated with bullous pemphigoid. Even diseases without blisters such as lichen sclerosus et atrophicus may resolve with milia, as may granulomatous dermatoses such as sarcoidosis and lupus vulgaris. While primary milia tend to be permanent, secondary milia may spontaneously improve.

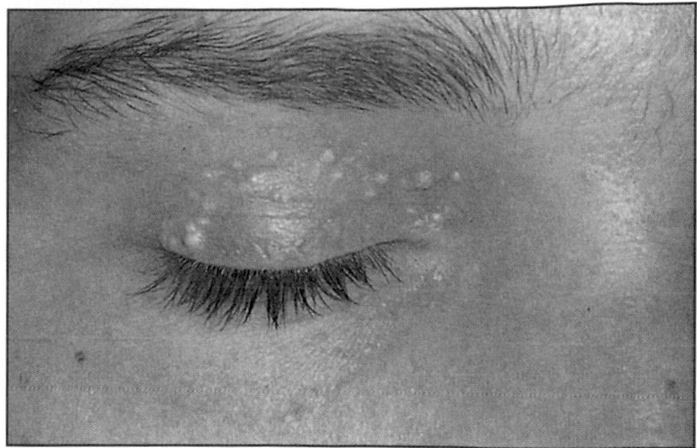

Fig. 53.3. Multiple milia

Histopathology. Primary milia arise from a hair follicle, as do almost all secondary milia. The latter may also develop from the injured interfollicular epidermis or an eccrine duct. Sometimes the milium is still attached to its precursor structure but histologic sectioning often fails to reveal this feature. One finds instead a small accumulation of keratin, often with an onion-skin pattern, surrounded by epithelium. A granular layer is usually visible. Bacteria are noticeably absent.

Differential Diagnosis. Tiny adnexal tumors, such as syringomas, may appear similar but can be separated histologically. Colloid milium are larger plaques usually found in sun-damaged skin. Xanthelasmas may appear similar.

Therapy. Milia can be easily extruded or extracted. The roof of the lesion can be opened with an #11 blade or a large injection needle and then the contents easily squeezed out manually or with a comedo extractor.

Multiple Eruptive Milia
(MIESCHER 1957)

In some patients many milia develop suddenly often over wide areas of the face and trunk. This rare condition can occur in three settings, spontaneously or inherited in an autosomal dominant pattern, either alone or associated with multiple other adnexal tumors, such as Brooke syndrome (Chap. 57). The spontaneous multiple eruptive milia in older individuals are probably triggered by the same factors discussed above, including medications, hyperhidrosis and bullous diseases.

Scrotal Cyst
(BLASCHKO and GUMPERT 1924)

Definition. Variant of epidermoid cyst on the scrotum with frequent calcification.

Clinical Findings. Scrotal cysts are most often multiple, 5–10 mm and yellow. Because the scrotal skin is so thin, their yellow color is prominent and they are usually raised above the skin surface (Fig. 53.4). On close examination, some have central pores and their caseous contents can be at least partially extruded. Scrotal cysts become easily infected and then may heal with fibrosis and calcification, producing painful scarred lesions. Often the inflammation obliterates the cyst wall, making both removal and histopathologic interpretation difficult. Occasionally multiple epidermoid cysts will be seen on the labia, but in this location one must consider several other possible cyst types (Chap. 35).

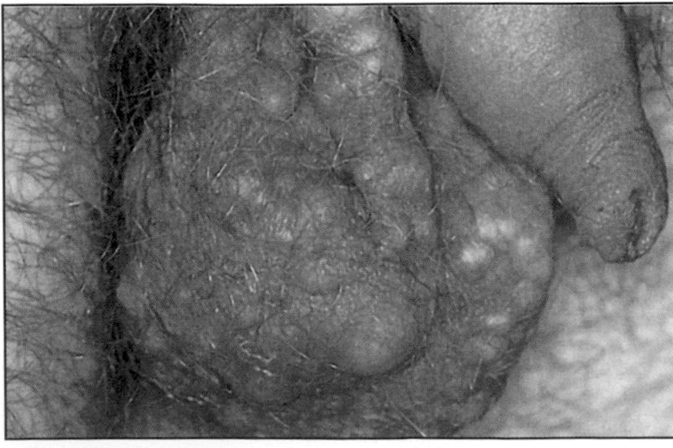

Fig. 53.4. Scrotal cysts

Histopathology. Initially scrotal cysts were felt to be true sebaceous cysts, perhaps because of their clinical similarity to steatocystoma multiplex, but histologic examination does not reveal sebaceous glands. Some investigators have suggested that scrotal cysts represent primary calcifications without a precursor cyst or other structure. Both of these explanations are wrong. When noninflamed scrotal cysts are evaluated, they show the typical features of an epidermoid cyst. Mixed cysts may be slightly more common on the scrotum.

Therapy. Excision of large or painful cysts will produce a grateful patient. Scrotal cysts seem to cause more concern and anguish than an equivalent number of cysts elsewhere.

Giant Comedo

A giant comedo is a small cyst associated with a relatively large opening. Thus the keratin plug is almost always dark, just as with an open comedo in acne. Comedones in acne are always associated with abundant sebaceous glands, but giant comedones typically lack this feature. Many giant comedones are posttraumatic, reflecting an epidermal invagination with continuous production of keratin into a semi-closed space. The overlap between small cysts and giant comedones is also seen in Favre-Racouchot disease (Chap. 18). While large comedones certainly develop in acne, especially on the back, they are not generally included in this category. The treatment is excision, for extruding the keratin plug produces no permanent improvement.

An unusual variation on this theme is the omphalith or navel stone, in which the natural contours of the umbilicus, perhaps associated with less than ideal cleanliness, lead to keratin concretions. The giant pore of Winer is a benign hair follicle tumor; it has no connection with a giant comedo.

Trichilemmal Cyst
(OSTERMAYER 1897)

Synonyms. Follicular cyst, isthmus-catagen type; pilar cyst, wen, atheroma

Definition. Common cyst usually found on the scalp.

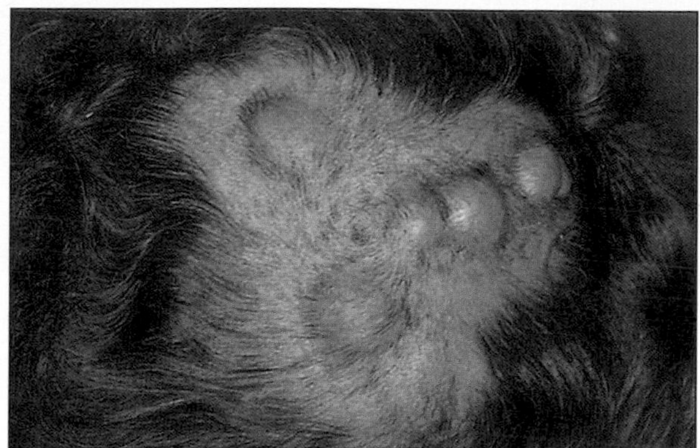

Fig. 53.5. Multiple trichilemmal cysts

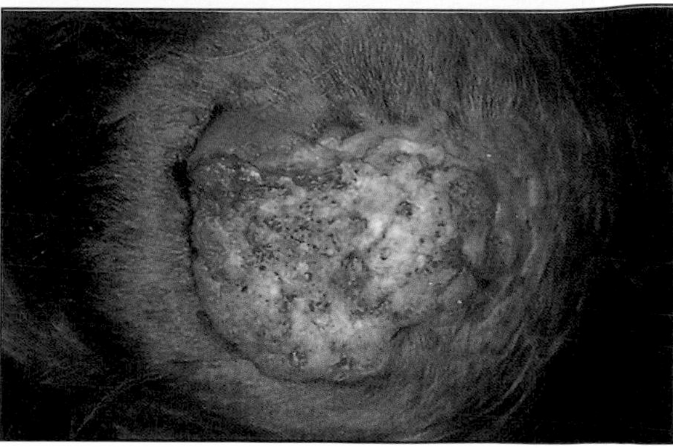

Fig. 53.6. Proliferating trichilemmal cyst; we do not have clinical follow-up but suspect this may have become squamous cell carcinoma

Etiology and Pathogenesis. Once again Ackerman's term of follicular cyst, isthmus-catagen type, most clearly describes the pathogenesis of these common cysts. Their lining resembles a slightly deeper level of the hair follicle than that of an epidermoid cyst. The trichilemmal sheath contains several different patterns of keratinization, so this term is less than perfect but established.

Clinical Findings. In about 90% of case, trichilemmal cysts are found on the scalp; in 30% of cases, they are solitary and in 70%, multiple (Fig. 53.5). Most patients with multiple trichilemmal cysts give a history of family members with similar cyst, suggesting autosomal dominant inheritance. The cysts are usually 1–2 cm in size but can become much larger. Because they are located between the skull and the skin without any fat layer in which to hide, they are easily palpated and often mobile. The overlying hairs may be thinned. Sometimes several cysts will be grouped together. Perhaps reflecting their deeper follicular origins, trichilemmal cysts do not have a visible pore and they are less often inflamed or infected.

Histopathology. The cyst is often removed intact, appearing grossly as a glistening white marble. The cyst wall shows trichilemmal keratinization; that is, the epithelial cells show no flattening and there is no granular layer. Instead, there is an abrupt transition between epithelial cells and compact keratin. Most show microscopic calcification, and ectopic bone is occasionally seen. Often, both epidermal and trichilemmal keratinization are present in the same cyst.

Differential Diagnosis. A proliferating trichilemmal cyst is usually larger and more irregular. Sometimes an adnexal tumor, most often a cylindroma or eccrine poroma, can appear clinically similar. Epidermoid cysts cannot be separated with clinical certainty, but the distinction is rarely of significance, as the prognosis and therapy are identical.

Therapy. Excision is easy because of the firm, usually intact cyst wall. The lesions can be removed through a simple incision.

Proliferating Trichilemmal Cyst

(Wilson Jones 1966)

Synonym. Pilar tumor

Definition. Large rapidly growing cyst with histologic features of a squamous cell carcinoma.

Etiology and Pathogenesis. Proliferating trichilemmal cysts are most likely derived from ordinary trichilemmal cysts, but they display striking clinical and histologic differences. Their occurrence in patients with multiple trichilemmal cysts supports the close connection.

Clinical Findings. A proliferating trichilemmal cyst is usually a large, growing, often inflamed and ulcerated scalp tumor (Fig. 53.6). About 85% arise in women, who are usually elderly. Only 10% occur away from the scalp; the back is the second most common site. They may become quite large if untreated and overlying alopecia is even more common than in trichilemmal cysts. While most often the proliferating trichilemmal cyst is clinically benign, there are rare tumors which spread locally or metastasize to lymph nodes. They are so uncommon that no reliable criteria exist to identify them either clinically or histologically.

Histopathology. Proliferating trichilemmal cysts are probably a variant of squamous cell carcinoma. They show a wide range of microscopic patterns. Often an otherwise unremarkable trichilemmal cyst may have focal areas in its wall with keratinocytes in disorderly array. In the more typical case, the pattern is dominated by accumulations of atypical keratinocytes and little if any cyst wall or residual trichilemmal keratinization is retained. Usually the aggressive or proliferating component is directed into the cyst. Mitoses may be identified, as well as individual cell keratinization. The surrounding stroma usually shows fibrosis and granulomatous inflammation.

Differential Diagnosis. The clinical differential diagnosis includes ordinary trichilemmal cysts and other adnexal tumors, including pilomatricomas and basal cell carcinomas. A confusing consideration is trichilemmal carcinoma, which is the rare malignant version of a trichilemmoma, is not cystic and arises on sun-damaged skin, it is similar in name only.

Therapy. Surgical excision is required. Sometimes the lesions are so large that the defect must be covered with a flap or graft. Since the histologic distinction between benign and malignant forms remains unclear, it is wise to excise the lesion in toto.

Steatocystoma

Definition. Steatocystomas are the closest lesion to true sebaceous cysts. They are almost always multiple and develop from the region of the hair follicle where the sebaceous duct enters the lumen.

Steatocystoma Multiplex
(Pringle 1899)

Etiology and Pathogenesis. Steatocystoma multiplex is inherited in an autosomal dominant pattern, as are so many of the syndromes with multiple adnexal tumors. They may be associated with pachyonychia congenita type II (Chap. 32), in which case mutations in keratin 6B and 17 are usually found.

Clinical Findings. The lesions are present at birth, but often not noticed until puberty when they become more apparent (Fig. 53.7). The cysts are usually 3–5 mm in size, often fluctuant and with a blue tinge. Some patients may have hundreds of cysts; others, just a few. Occasional lesions may become quite large. The most typical site is the chest, although the axillae, back, genital area and even forehead may be involved. Patients often attempt to express the cyst contents, obtaining a lipid-rich fluid but also producing infections and scarring. Otherwise, inflammation is rare, as the cysts have no epidermal connection and are sterile. Associated systemic findings are most rare; natal teeth have been described.

Histopathology. The cyst is lined by thin epithelium that has a crenulated or wavy cornified layer. No granular layer is present. Usually one or more flattened sebaceous glands can be found in the cyst wall. The cyst contains lipids and keratin. Vellus follicles maybe found in the cyst wall and vellus hairs admixed in the contents.

Differential Diagnosis. The main differential diagnostic consideration is eruptive vellus hair cysts. The two closely related lesions cannot be separated clinically or histologically with certainty. Occasionally, multiple adnexal tumors, especially if cystic, such as hidrocystomas, may be identical. Acne cysts and scars over the sternum may also be very similar, but comedones and a history of acne elsewhere usually answer the question.

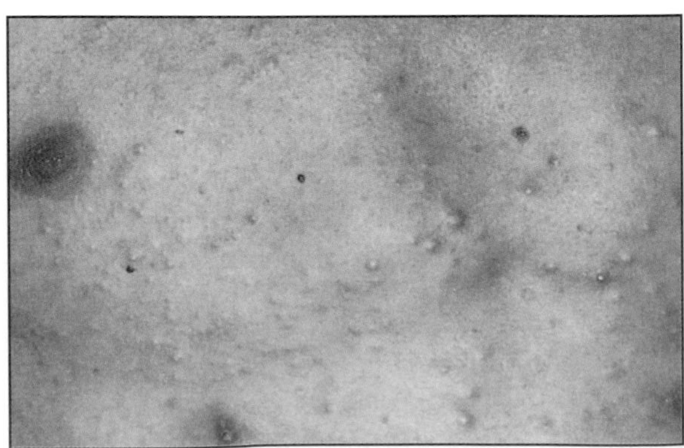

Fig. 53.7. Steatocystoma multiplex

Therapy. Individual lesions can be excised. This is difficult and may lead to significant scarring, especially over the sternum. Systemic therapy with isotretinoin produces temporary improvement, especially in those patients whose cysts are rich in sebaceous glands, but permanent improvement is uncommon.

Steatocystoma Multiplex Conglobatum

(PLEWIG et al. 1982)

Sometimes, patients with steatocystoma multiplex will develop severe, persistent inflammation with scarring and sinus tracts. We described this in a group of men who had striking involvement of the axilllae and over the sternum. Mechanical factors such as pressure, rubbing and sweating probably play a role. The lesions look identical to acne conglobata but residual steatocystoma structures can be found histologically. Treatment is surgical excision.

Steatocystoma Simplex

(BROWNSTEIN 1982)

The solitary version of steatocystoma is not clinically distinct and usually a histologic surprise. Most are excised and submitted as epidermoid cysts or adnexal tumors. The patients are usually adults and the same regions rich in sebaceous follicles are favored. Treatment is excision.

Eruptive Vellus Hair Cysts

(ESTERLY et al. 1977)

Definition. Cysts containing multiple vellus hairs.

Etiology and Pathogenesis. Eruptive vellus hair cysts are closely related to steatocystoma multiplex, but we still separate them. Autosomal dominant inheritance has been documented in some cases.

Clinical Findings. Eruptive vellus hair cysts are multiple, small 1–3 mm papules which are typically found on the chest and back, although the face and proximal aspects of the extremities may also be involved. They do not erupt, but are present at birth and appear gradually, in some cases becoming more prominent at puberty. Sometimes they are inflamed, which makes them more noticeable. The larger flaccid cysts seen with steatocystoma are usually not present, although patients have been described with both types of lesions.

Histopathology. Typically one finds a small cyst filled with keratin and containing by definition one or more vellus hairs. No granular layer is present. Sebaceous glands may also be found in the cyst wall. If the cyst is incised, often a clump of vellus hairs can be extracted.

Differential Diagnosis. Other adnexal tumors, comedones and other types of follicular plugging should be considered. The diagnosis is based on the predominant histologic feature – vellus hairs.

Therapy. Individual lesions can be excised but the result are unsatisfactory. Laser destruction has been employed. Systemic isotretinoin is often less successful than in steatocystoma multiplex, perhaps because the sebaceous component is much less or absent.

Glandular Cysts

Cysts can develop from a variety of glandular epithelia. In the skin such cysts develop from apocrine and eccrine structures. Steatocystomas or true sebaceous cysts have been discussed above because of their close relationship to vellus hair cysts. In the oral cavity, salivary glands form mucoceles and true cysts.

Eccrine Hidrocystoma

(ROBINSON 1893)

Synonym. Hidrocystome noire

Etiology and Pathogenesis. The existence of eccrine hidrocystoma has been challenged in recent years. Its etiology is presumably a dilated obstructed eccrine.

Clinical Findings. Eccrine hidrocystomas are almost limited to the periorbital region, but may occur on other parts of the face or even trunk. Most often they are solitary lesions located on the border of the lid (Fig. 53.8). Women are affected more often than men. Typically there is a several millimeter, soft translucent cyst which may have a blue or black tinge (hidrocystome noire; Fig. 53.9). If it is lanced,

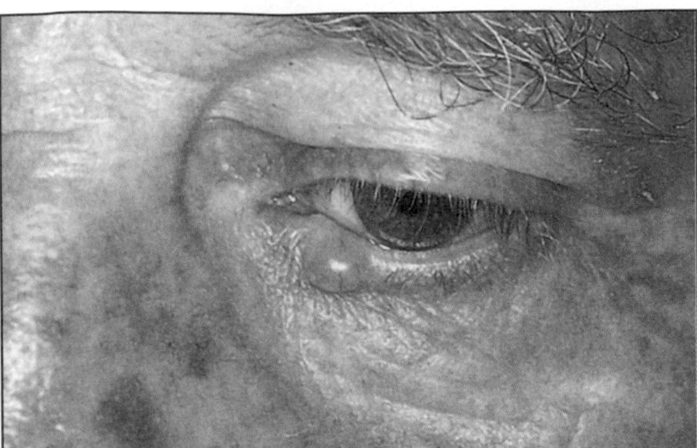

Fig. 53.8. Hidrocystoma

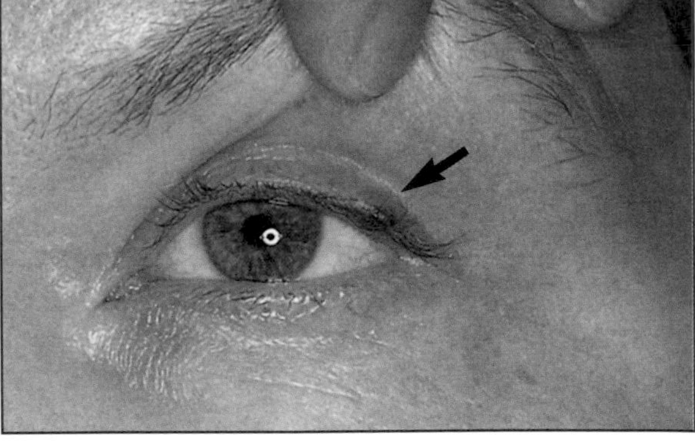

Fig. 53.9. Pigmented hidrocystoma

a thin, watery sweat-like fluid comes out. Eccrine hidrocystomas may enlarge in the summer months and regress with atropine therapy.

Histopathology. The epidermis is normal or thinned. In the dermis there is a collapsed cyst perhaps containing eosinophilic material. The cyst wall contains one to two layers of cuboidal cells without myoepithelial elements. No apocrine decapitation secretion or sebaceous elements are seen.

Differential Diagnosis. See discussion under apocrine hidrocystoma below.

Therapy. Surgical excision

Apocrine Hidrocystoma

(Mehregan 1964)

Synonym. Apocrine cystadenoma

Etiology and Pathogenesis. The apocrine hidrocystoma is regarded as a cystic tumor, not a dilated duct. Both their association with organoid nevi and the presence of solid tumor areas support this view.

Clinical Findings. Apocrine hidrocystomas are almost invariably solitary and most common in the periorbital region. While also occurring in other areas, they are uncommon in the apocrine-rich groin and axillary regions. Clinically these cysts are very similar to eccrine hidrocystomas, presenting as cystic translucent papules which may also be blue or black in color. They can develop within an organoid nevus

Histopathology. The lining of the cyst in the dermis shows decapitation secretion; myoepithelial elements may be present. The cysts may be unilocular or multilocular.

Differential Diagnosis. Eccrine and apocrine hidrocystomas cannot be distinguished clinically. Both may be mistaken for basal cell carcinoma, blue nevus and other melanocytic nevi, as well as for vascular lesions such as a venous lake.

Therapy. Surgical excision

Salivary Gland Cysts

In the mouth, both true cysts and mucoceles may arise in association the minor salivary glands and their ducts. A mucocele develops when a duct is severed by trauma and the mucin secretions accumulate in the lamina propria without a cyst wall, while a retention cyst most often forms behind an obstructive stone (Chap. 33).

Synovial Cysts

Ganglion

A ganglion is a synovial cyst which develops in the vicinity of a joint. An extreme example is the Baker cyst of the knee and popliteal space. Most ganglions encountered by dermatologists are about the wrist.

They develop as herniations of the synovial lining of a joint, so by definition, all are connected to an underlying space. They are always subcutaneous, usually soft and somewhat moveable and vary greatly in size. Occasionally they may mimic a rheumatoid nodule, subcutaneous granuloma annulare, giant cell tumor of tendon sheath and other tumors related to tendons and joints. The treatment is surgical, with attention paid to the probable underlying connection.

Metaplastic Synovial Cyst

These cysts or sinuses arise following surgery or trauma. They have a lining resembling hyperplastic synovium but show no connection to joints or other synovial structures.

Developmental Cysts

A number of cysts arise as minor variations in embryologic migration and development. They typically occur in location where lines of fusion are present or migration occurs. Several contain ciliated epithelium, which is not normally found in the skin. We discuss several examples that may be encountered by dermatologists.

Dermoid Cyst

Definition. Uncommon subcutaneous cyst of ectodermal origin that often arises in lines of embryologic fusion, contains multiple ectodermal structures and may also contain mesodermal and endodermal elements.

Clinical Findings. Dermoid cysts are present at birth, typically involving the eyelids, bridge of the nose, anterior aspect of the neck or genital region. They range in size from 1 cm to 5 cm. Those on the bridge of the nose often have a sinus tract and a tuft of hairs protruding out. When dermoid cysts present in adult life, the scenario is usually an overlooked congenital lesion that has become inflamed.

Histopathology. A dermoid by definition contains multiple ectodermal structures. The predominant feature is keratinous or cornified debris, often exuding out as a cheesy mass when the cyst is opened. The cyst wall may contain hairs, sebaceous, apocrine and eccrine glands.

Differential Diagnosis. Epidermoid cysts are similar but usually not present at birth. A subcutaneous hemangioma may not immediately be identified as a vascular lesion. Nasal gliomas and other congenital malformations of the CNS may present as nasal masses. All congenital midline cysts should be evaluated with modern imaging techniques to exclude deep, especially intracranial, connections. If nerves, bony fragments or other mesenchymal and endodermal elements are found, the designation cystic teratoma has been suggested.

Therapy. While dermoid cysts are best excised, the approach should be a careful one. Any midline cystic lesion in a child should be approached recognizing the possibility that deeper connections may be found. It is wise to have neurosurgical operative assistance available before embarking on such an excision.

Median Raphe Cyst

Etiology and Pathogenesis. The median raphe extends from the urethra to the anus. Defects in its closure can produce a cystic inclusion anywhere along the line.

Clinical Findings. Median raphe cysts are most common on the ventral part of the penis just posterior to the urethra, although they can be found along the entire line to the anus (Fig. 53.10). In women they are restricted to the perineum. They are typically small translucent papules that may drain or become inflamed following trauma.

Histopathology. A dermal cyst is found whose wall consists of squamous epithelium and which occasionally contains mucous glands.

Therapy. Surgical excision

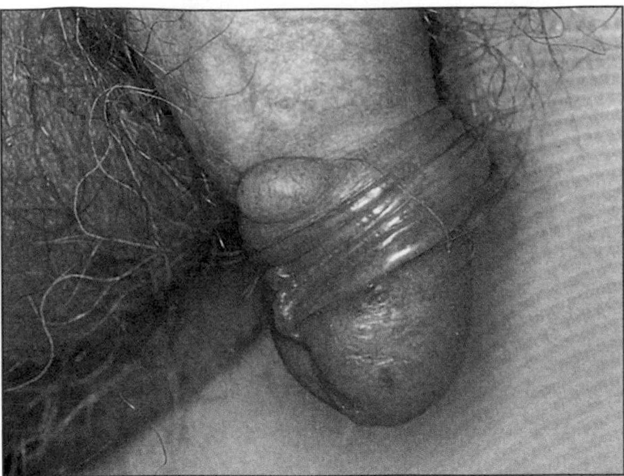

Fig. 53.10. Median raphe cyst

Ciliated Cyst

(HESS 1890)

Etiology and Pathogenesis. While all cutaneous ciliated cysts reflect abnormal embryologic development, it is unclear just how and why the aberrant tissue winds up in the skin. The sites where ciliated epithelium occurs normally include the respiratory tract, uterine and fallopian tube epithelium, efferent ductules of the testis, middle ear and ependyma of the brain.

Clinical Findings. Only the location and the presence since birth or early life gives a clue to the diagnosis. Ciliated cysts occur primarily in women and usually on the leg, which is an uncommon site for epidermoid cysts. Sometimes they are first noticed during puberty. Perineal ciliated cysts can be found in both sexes; they may represent a persistent primitive tailgut. The cysts are typically subcutaneous swellings, without a central pore.

Histopathology. Ciliated cysts tend to have a firm wall and contain a clear to oily fluid on gross examination. They lie in the dermis or subcutaneous fat. The wall is lined by ciliated cells. The surrounding stroma is unremarkable, but may contain a sparse lymphohistiocytic infiltrate.

Differential Diagnosis. Ciliated cysts are never diagnosed clinically. They are too rare and are usually mistaken for an epidermoid cyst or some other benign process.

Therapy. Surgical excision

Bronchogenic Cyst

Etiology and Pathogenesis. Bronchogenic or foregut cysts are usually seen in the mediastinum but can be found in the skin and subcutaneous tissue. Perhaps as the mesenchymal bars of the sternum fuse, outpouchings of the primitive bronchi and trachea are trapped in the skin.

Clinical Findings. Bronchogenic cysts are usually mediastinal and situated at the sternal notch; in one review over 80 % were located there. They have also been described as subcutaneous masses all over the chest and back, as well as on the chin. They, too, are subcutaneous masses, usually in children.

Differential Diagnosis. All of the embryologic cysts of the head and neck region should be considered when evaluating subcutaneous masses in a young patient. Bilateral lesions present since birth and associated defects, such as skin tags or pits, are good clues that one is dealing with a developmental defect.

Histopathology. Bronchogenic cysts are derived from respiratory epithelium, so their lining contains columnar ciliated epithelium and goblet cells. In addition, they may be accompanied by smooth muscle, seromucous glands and cartilage as well as an inflammatory infiltrate.

Therapy. Surgical excision, with careful attention to potential underlying connections and structures

Branchial Cleft Cyst

Synonym. Lateral cervical cyst

Etiology and Pathogenesis. These cysts arise through aberrant development of the second branchial arch. They lie along the anterior border of the sternocleidomastoid muscle. In addition to subcutaneous cysts, sinuses or pits may be found. Often bilateral lesions are present. Occasionally a skin tag, sometimes with cartilage, may be found along with the pit or sinus.

Histopathology. Branchial cleft lesions contain a variety of epithelial structures almost invariably associated with lymph node tissue including germinal centers. The same lesion in the floor of the mouth is known as a lymphoepithelial cyst.

Therapy. Surgical excision, once again with careful attention to potential associated problems

Preauricular Cyst

Synonym. Preauricular sinus

Etiology and Pathogenesis. These lesions result from inappropriate development of the first branchial arch. They are less common than those arising from the second arch.

Clinical Findings. The most common finding is an accessory tragus (Chap. 19) – a small skin tag-like lesion that often has a cartilaginous core. In more severe cases there may be a cyst, often with a connecting sinus, anterior to the ear at the superior anterior border of the sternocleidomastoid muscle. Malformations of the entire ear may also be present, since it develops primarily from the first branchial arch.

Histopathology. The cyst is similar to branchial cleft cysts.

Therapy. Surgical excision. Even when excising an accessory tragus, one should be aware of the possibility of an underlying cyst.

Thryoglossal Duct Cyst

Etiology and Pathogenesis. Thryoglossal duct cysts result when the embryonic thyroglossal duct, connecting the back of the tongue and the thyroid, fails to close.

Clinical Findings. These cysts are always midline and most often near the hyoid bone. Sometimes the entire duct may remain patent, so that the patient can "spit out of his neck", that is, force saliva through the patent duct to the opening on the neck. The cysts are typically small and move with swallowing or sticking out the tongue.

Histopathology. Usually thyroglossal duct cysts contain thyroid follicles and do not usually have muscle or cartilage. They are lined by either stratified squamous epithelium or, if below the hyoid bone, may have ciliated epithelium.

Differential Diagnosis. A thymic cyst and an ectopic or accessory thyroid gland must be excluded. The presence of other functioning thyroid tissue should be insured before a midline cyst is removed from the neck; sometimes the aberrant thyroid tissue is all that the patient has.

Therapy. Surgical excision

Pseudocysts

A number of structures are cystic but do not have a true cyst wall microscopically. The most common example is the mucocele mentioned above. Auricular pseudocyst (Chap. 20) is another common example. Pseudocysts usually have a fibrous capsule of connective tissue so they may excavated just like a cyst during surgery. Many benign adnexal tumors, while not clinically cystic, share this propensity.

Digital Mucous Cyst
(Hyde 1897)

Synonyms. Mucous digital cyst, myxoid cyst, myxoid pseudocyst

Etiology and Pathogenesis. The origin of a digital mucous cyst has been long disputed. One school holds that all arise as synovial extrusions, that is, as mini-versions of a ganglion with a tiny duct connecting the cyst space to a joint. An alternative viewpoint is that they simply represent a degenerative change in the digital collagen, reflecting trauma and perhaps osteoarthritis. While this issue has never been resolved, it is of no clinical importance.

Clinical Findings. Digital mucous cysts are typically translucent nodules arising over the proximal nail fold or the distal interphalangeal joint (Fig. 53.11). They may be 5–10 mm in size and can be painful. While they do occur on the toes, they are far more common on the fingers. Those arising on the nail fold are almost invariably associated with a longitudinal furrow in the nail. Radiologic examination may reveal osteophytic changes.

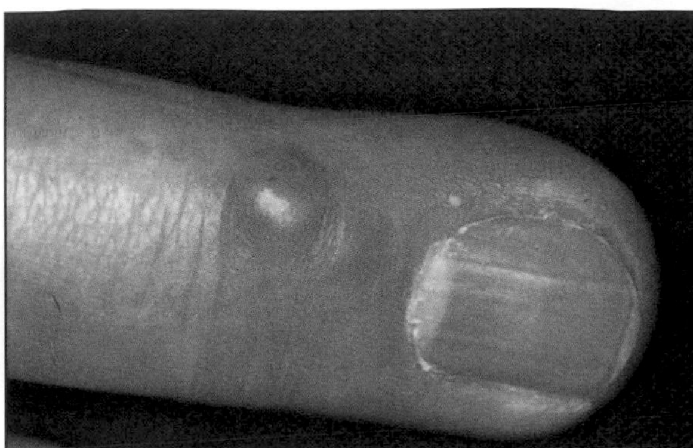

Fig. 53.11. Digital mucous cyst

When the cyst is ruptured or pierced, a clear gelatinous material oozes out, confirming the clinical diagnosis.

Histopathology. The overlying epidermis shows changes typical of acral skin, offering a clue to the diagnosis of the mucinous deposits in the dermis. A cyst wall is not present, but when a digital mucous cyst is completely excised, a duct (presumably synovial in origin) may occasionally be found at the base. Often there is a histiocytic or granulomatous inflammatory response at the periphery of the mucin, along with a fibrous capsule. While seldom needed, Hale or alcian blue stain can be used to confirm the presence of mucin.

Differential Diagnosis. When the localization is typical and the gelatinous material found, then there is no differential diagnosis. Otherwise, one can consider other digital tumors such as old warts and acquired digital fibrokeratoma.

Therapy. When a digital mucous cyst is incised, it rapidly refills. The best treatment is excision. Alternatively one can try cryotherapy or injection with triamcinolone acetonide 2 mg/ml followed by a pressure dressing.

Infectious Cysts

Infectious organisms can be walled off by the body producing a cystic structure. The best example is cysticercosis (Chap. 9), in which the larval form of *Taenia solium* forms subcutaneous cysts. Some of the subcutaneous fungi (Chap. 7) can produce a cyst or sinus, often centered about a splinter or other foreign object that has served to introduce the infection.

Sinuses

A sinus is technically a cavity or space, such as the familiar frontal and maxillary sinuses of the face. An alternative meaning is a channel often allowing drainage of fluid or pus. Dermatologists are most likely to encounter the second situation following chronic infection of a cyst, in severe acne, in destructive infections such as osteomyelitis or tuberculosis and in similar settings. Here we discuss two common and well-defined disorders that are usually referred to as sinuses.

Pilonidal Sinus

Synonym. Pilonidal cyst

Etiology and Pathogenesis. A pilonidal sinus arises from chronic inflammation and pressure involving a hair-bearing region. A tract develops connecting the skin surface with a collection of hairs, cell debris and keratinizing epithelial tissue. Often, many interconnected tracts form, resembling the burrow of a rabbit or fox. Thus a pilonidal sinus can be viewed as a large complicated scar with epithelium-lined tracts.

Clinical Findings. A pilonidal sinus most often arises in or just above the gluteal cleft, where the prerequisites of hair-bearing skin, maceration and pressure are most readily found (Fig. 53.12). Typically the lesions become clinically apparent in teenagers or young adults. If the sinus opening is small or blocked, the patient may present with a fluctuant swelling. Sometimes the lesions are infected, red and tender. A variant is the motorcyclist's or j eep driver's nodule, in which the source of the trauma is more obvious. Patients with acne inversa or acne conglobata are also very likely to have pilonidal sinuses. Pilonidal sinuses can also develop in other body regions. Chronic pilonidal sinuses can serve as a site for the development of squamous cell carcinoma, similar to an osteomyelitis sinus, but the risk is much less.

A variant of pilonidal sinus is the digital sinus of the barber, beautician or animal trimmer. Here, foreign hairs are driven into the interdigital web space, stimulating a granulomatous response.

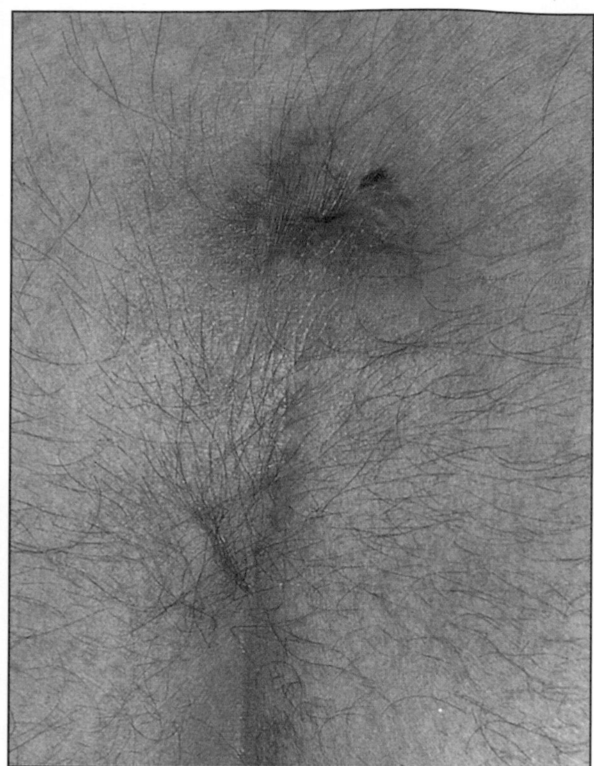

Fig. 53.12. Pilonidal sinus

Histopathology. The main finding is fibrosis and chronic often granulomatous inflammation. Depending on what type of specimen is obtained, one may see a keratinizing epithelial wall, hairs and perhaps a duct or sinus opening to the skin surface.

Therapy. The only definitive therapy is wide and deep local excision, followed either by primary closure or often by secondary healing. Temporarily, one can drain an acutely inflamed, infected sinus and treat with systemic antibiotics, but this is only a stop-gap measure and should be followed by surgery.

Dental Sinus

Synonyms. Dental fistula, periapical abscess with sinus tract

Etiology and Pathogenesis. In this situation there is no question about the etiology. The patient has a periapical abscess, usually involving one of the mandibular teeth. The abscess drains externally through the skin.

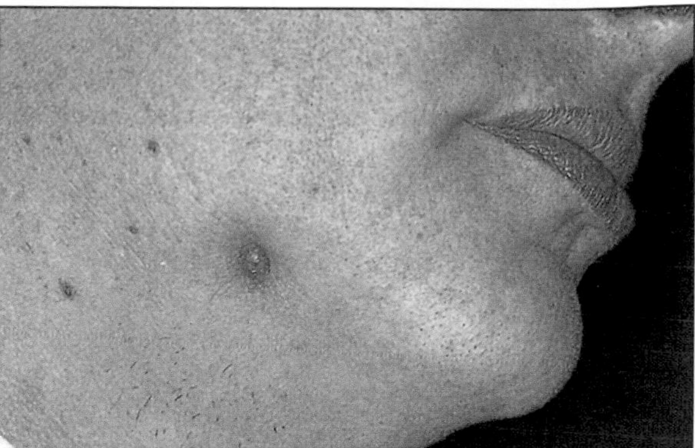

Fig. 53.13. Dental sinus

Clinical Findings. Initially there is almost always some tooth pain, if one takes a careful history. The cutaneous lesion may present as a warm, inflamed abscess, in the past known as Ludwig angina when it was submandibular. Later, a sinus tract or granulomatous pseudocyst may develop. The most likely location is along the jaw line or the anterior part of the neck; occasionally a lesion may arise on the cheek (Fig. 53.13). Most maxillary periapical abscesses drain internally. Palpation may reveal an indurated tract extending from the mandible to the site of inflammation. The diagnosis can be best confirmed by dental examination and radiologic evaluation of the appropriate teeth.

Histopathology. The biopsy shows varying degrees of acute or chronic inflammation. It is never diagnostic of a dental sinus, but allows one to exclude other possibilities.

Differential Diagnosis. The usual differential diagnosis is an abscess, or an epidermoid cyst, but without considering the dental origin. A good rule is to consider dental sinus for any recurrent cyst on the jaw or neck, no matter what a biopsy report says.

Therapy. The periapical abscess must be treated first. Usually the skin then heals spontaneously, but occasionally a sinus tract must be excised.

Bibliography

Epidermoid Cysts

Akasaka T, Imamura Y, Kon S (1997) Pigmented epidermal cyst. J Dermatol 24:475–478

Brook I (1989) Microbiology of infected epidermal cysts. Arch Dermatol 125:1658–1661

Diven DG, Dozier SE, Meyer DJ et al. (1998) Bacteriology of inflamed and uninflamed epidermal inclusion cysts. Arch Dermatol 134:49–51

Egawa K, Honda Y, Inaba Y et al. (1995) Detection of human papillomaviruses and eccrine ducts in palmoplantar epidermoid cysts. Br J Dermatol 132:533–542

Fisher BK, Macpherson M (1986) Epidermoid cyst of the sole. J Am Acad Dermatol 15:1127–1129

Meyer LM, Tyring SK, Little WP (1991) Verrucous cyst. Arch Dermatol 127:1810–1812

Pavlidakey GP, Mehregan A, Hashimoto K (1986) Pigmented follicular cysts. Int J Dermatol 25:174–177

Soyer HP, Schadendorf D, Cerroni L et al. (1993) Verrucous cysts: histopathologic characterization and molecular detection of human papillomavirus-specific DNA. J Cutan Pathol 20:441–417

Milium

Combemal P, Faisant M, Dupin M (1995) Milia en plaque in the supraclavicular area. Dermatology 191:262–263

Langley RGB, Walsh NMG, Ross JB et al. (1997) Multiple eruptive milia: report of a case, review of the literature, and a classification. J Am Acad Dermatol 37:353–356

Losada-Campa A, de la Torre-Fraga C, Cruces-Prado M (1996) Milia en plaque. Br J Dermatol 134:970–972

Miescher VG (1957) Eruptive milien und epithelioma adnoides cysticum Brooke. Dermatologica 115:712–716

Scrotal Cyst

Blaschko H, Gumpert M (1924) Verkalkte Scrotalxanthome. Arch Dermatol Syphilol 146:323–329

Dare AJ, Axelsen RA (1988) Scrotal calcinosis: origin from dystrophic calcification of eccrine duct milia. J Cutan Pathol 15:142–149

Swinehart JM, Golitz LE (1982) Scrotal calcinosis. Dystrophic calcification of eperidermoied cysts. Arch Dermatol 118:985–988

Wrigth S, Navsaria H, Leigh IM (1991) Idiopathic scrotal calcinosis is idiopathic. J Am Acad Dermatol 24:727–730

Trichilemmal Cyst

Leppard BJ, Sanderson KV, Wells RS (1977) Hereditary trichilemmal cysts. Clin Exp Dermatol 2:23–32

Leppard BJ, Sanderson KV (1976) The natural history of trichilemmal cysts. Br J Dermatol 94:379–390

Pinkus H (1969) "Sebaceous cysts" are trichilemmal cysts. Arch Dermatol 99:544–553

Proliferating Trichilemmal Cyst

Brownstein MH, Arluk DJ (1979) Proliferating trichilemmal cysts. Arch Dermatol 115:1347

Requena L, Sanches Yus E (1991) Follicular hybrid cysts. Am J Dermatol 13:228–233

Sau P, Graham JH, Helwig EB (1995) Proliferating epithelial cysts. Clinicopathological analysis of 96 cases. J Cutan Pathol 22:394–406

Sleater J, Beers B, Stefan M et al. (1993) Proliferating trichilemmal cyst. Report of four cases, two with nondiploid DNA content and increased proliferation index. Am J Dermatol 15:423–428

Weiss J, Heine M, Grimmel M et al. (1995) Malignant proliferating trichilemmal cyst. J Am Acad Dermatol 32: 870–873

Wilson Jones (1966) Proliferating epidermoid cysts. Arch Dermatol 94:11–19

Steatocystoma

Brownstein MH (1982) Steatocystoma simplex. A solitary steatocystoma. Arch Dermatol 118:409–411

Covello SP, Smith FJD, Sillevis Smitt JH et al. (1998) Keratin 17 mutations cause either steatocystoma multiplex or pachyonychia congenita type 2. Br J Dermatol 139:475–480

Holmes R, Black MM (1980) Steatocystoma multiplex with unusually prominent cysts on the face. Br J Dermatol 102:711–713

Kanekura T, Kawamura K, Nishi M et al. (1995) A case of steatocystoma multiplex with prominent cysts on the scalp treated successfully using a simple surgical technique. J Dermatol 22:438–440

Keefe M, Leppard BJ, Royle G (1992) Successful treatment of steatocystoma multiplex by simple surgery. Br J Dermatol 127:41–44

Kiene P, Hauschild A, Christophers E (1996) Eruptive vellus hair cysts and steatocystoma multiplex. Variants of one entity? Br J Dermatol 134:365–367

Ohtake K, Kubote Y, Takayama O et al. (1992) Relationship between steatocystoma multiplex and eruptive vellus hair cysts. J Am Acad Dermatol 26:876–878

Plewig G, Wolff HH, Braun-Falco O (1982) Steatocystoma multiplex: anatomic reevaluation, electron microscopy and autoradiography. Arch Dermatol Res 272:363–380

Eruptive Vellus Hair Cysts

Esterly NB, Fretzin DF, Pinkus H (1977) Eruptive vellus hair cysts. Arch Dermatol 113:500–503

Grimalt R, Gelmetti C (1992) Eruptive vellus hair cysts: case report and review of the literature. Pediatr Dermatol 9:98–102

Kiene P, Hauschild A, Christophers E (1996) Eruptive vellus hair cysts and steatocystoma multiplex. Variants of one entity? Br J Dermatol 134:365–367

Ohtake K, Kubote Y, Takayama O et al. (1992) Relationship between steatocystoma multiplex and eruptive vellus hair cysts. J Am Acad Dermatol 26:876–878

Pavlidakey GP, Mehregan A, Hashimoto K (1986) Pigmented follicular cysts. Int J Dermatol 25:174–177

Piepkorn MW, Clark L, Lombardi DL (1981) A kindred with congenital vellus hair cysts. J Am Acad Dermatol 5:661–665

Sánchez-Yus E, Aguilar-Martinez A, Cristobal-Gil MC et al. (1988) Eruptive vellus hair cyst and steatocystoma multiplex: two related conditions? J Cutan Pathol 15: 40–42

Sandoval R, Urbina F (1994) Pigmented follicular cyst. Br J Dermatol 131:130–131

Weedon D (1992) Cysts and Sinuses. In: Weedon D (ed) The skin. Churchill Livingston, Edingburgh, pp 483–498

Eccrine and Apocrine Hidrocystoma

Armstrong DKB, Walsh MY, Corbett JR (1998) Multiple facial eccrine hidrocystomas: effective topical therapy with atropine. Br J Dermatol 139:558–559

Bures FA, Kotynck J (1982) Differentiating between apocrine and eccrine hidrocystoma. Cutis 29:616–620

de Viragh PA, Szeimies RM, Eckert F (1997) Apocrine cystademoma, apocrine hidrocystoma, and eccrine hidrocystoma: three distinct tumors defined by expressions of keratins and human milk fat globulin 1. J Cutan Pathol 24:249–255

Glusac EJ, Hendrickson MS, Smoller BR (1994) Apocrine cystadenoma of the vulva. J Am Acad Dermatol 31:498–499

Hashimoto K, Zagual-Mally ZW, Youngberg G et al. (1987) Electron microscopic study of Moll's gland cyst. J Cutan Pathol 14:23–26

Hassan MO, Khan MA (1979) Ultrastructure of eccrine cystadenoma. A case report. Arch Dermatol 115:1217–1221

Holder WR, Smith JD, Mocega EE (1971) Giant apocrine hidrocystoma. Arch Dermatol 104:522–523

Kruse TV, Khan MA, Hassan MO (1979) Multiple apocrine cystadenomas. Br J Dermatol 100:675–681

Langer K, Konrad K, Smolle J (1989) Multiple apocrine hidrocystomas on the eyelids. Am J Dermatopathol 11:570–573

Mehregan AH (1964) Apocrine cystadenoma. Arch Dermatol 90:274–279

Smith JD, Chernosky ME (1974) Apocrine hidrocystoma. Arch Dermatol 109:700–702

Veraldi S, Gianotti R, Pabisch S et al. (1991) Pigmented apocrine hidrocystoma – a report of two cases and review of the literature. Clin Exp Dermatol 16:18–21

Dermoid Cyst

Kimura T, Miyazawa H, Aoyagi T et al. (1991) Folliculosebaceous cystic hamartoma. A distinctive malformation of the skin. Am J Dermatol 13:213–220

Saito H, Ogonuki R, Yanadori A et al. (1994) Congenital dermal sinus with intracranial dermoid cyst. Br J Dermatol 130:235–237

Templeton SF (1996) Folliculosebaceous cystic hamartoma: a clinical pathologic study. J Am Acad Dermatol 34:77–81

Median Raphe Cyst

Asarch RG, Golitz LE, Sausker WF et al. (1979) Median raphe cysts of the penis. Arch Dermatol 115:1084–1086

Claudy AL, Dutoit M, Boucheron S (1991) Epidermal and urethroid penile cyst. Acta Derm Venereol (Stockh) 71:61–62

Paslin D (1983) Urethoid cysts. Arch Dermatol 119:89–90

Romaní J, Barnadas MA, Miralles J et al. (1995) Median raphe cyst of the penis with ciliated cells. J Cutan Pathol 22:378–381

Sharkey MJ, Grabski WJ, McCollough ML et al. (1992) Postcoital appearance of a median raphe cyst. J Am Acad Dermatol 26:273–274

Ciliated Cyst

Cortes-Franco R, Carrasco D (1995) Cutaneous ciliated cyst. Int J Dermatol 34:32–33

Farmer ER, Helwig EB (1978) Cutaneous ciliated cysts. Arch Dermatol 118:70–73

Hess K (1890) Über eine subcutane Flimmerzyste. Beitr Pathol 8:98–108

Kang IK, Kim YJ, Choi KC (1995) Ciliated cyst of the vulva. J Am Acad Dermatol 32:514–515

Le Gall F, Patoux-Pibouin M, Le Normand I et al. (1994) Cutaneous ciliated cyst with associated apocrine-like cells. Eur J Dermatol 4:459–462

Tachibana T, Sakamoto F, Ito M et al. (1995) Cutaneous ciliated cyst: a case report and histochemical, immunohistochemical, and ultrastructural study. J Cutan Pathol 22:33–37

Bronchogenic Cyst

Ambiavagar PC, Rosen Y (1979) Cutaneous ciliated cyst of the chin. Probable bronchogenic cyst. Arch Dermatol 115:895–896

Fraga S, Helwig EB, Rosen SH (1971) Bronchogenic cyst in the skin and subcutaneous tissue. Am J Clin Pathol 56:230–238

Jona JZ (1995) Extramediastinal bronchogenic in children. Pediatr Dermatol 12:304–306

Patterson JW, Pittman DL, Rich JD (1984) Presternal ciliated cyst. Arch Dermatol 120:240–242

Pul N, Pul M (1994) Bronchogenic cyst of the scapular area in an infant: case report and review of the literature. J Am Acad Dermatol 31:120–122

Shareef DS, Salm R (1981) Ectopic vestigial lesions of the neck and shoulders. J Clin Pathol 34:1155–1162

van der Putte SCJ, Toonstra J (1985) Cutaneous "bronchogenic" cyst. J Cutan Pathol 12:404–409

Branchial Cleft Cyst

Betti R, Lodi A, Palvarini M et al. (1992) Branchial cyst of the neck. Br J Dermatol 127:195

Coleman WR, Homer RS, Kaplan RR (1989) Branchial cleft heterotopia of the lower neck. J Cutan Pathol 16:353–358

Digital Mucous Cyst

Goldman JA, Goldman L, Jaffe MS et al. (1977) Digital mucinous pseudocysts. Arthritis Rheum 20:997–1002

Newmeyer WL, Kilgore ES Jr, Graham WP (1974) Mucous cysts: the dorsal distal interphalangeal joint ganglion. Plast Reconstr Surg 53:313–315

Salasche SJ (1984) Myxoid cysts of the proximal nail fold: a surgical approach. J Dermatol Surg Oncol 10:35–39

Auricular Pseudocyst

Delvin J, Harrison CJ, Whitby DJ et al. (1990) Cartilaginous pseudocyst of the external auricle in children with atopic eczema. Br J Dermatol 122:699–704

Fukamizu H, Imaizumi S (1984) Bilateral pseudocysts of the auricles. Arch Dermatol 120:1238–1239

Glamb R, Kim R (1984) Pseudocysts of the auricle. J Am Acad Dermatol 11:58–63

Gonzalez M, Raton JA, Manzano D et al. (1993) Pseudocyst of the ear. Acta Derm Venereol (Stockh) 73:212–213

Grabski WJ, Salasche SJ, McCollough ML et al. (1989) Pseudocyst of the auricle associated with trauma. Arch Dermatol 118:528–530

Pilonidal Sinus

Matter I, Kunin J, Schein M et al. (1995) Total excision versus non-resectional methods in the treatment of acute and chronic pilonidal disease. Br J Surg 82:752–753

Patel MR, Bassini L, Nashad R et al. (1990) Barber's interdigital pilonidal sinus of the hand: a foreign body hair granuloma. J Hand Surg Am 15:652–655

Sagi A, Rosenberg L, Grief M et al. (1984) Squamous cell carcinoma arising in a pilonodal sinus: a report of a case and review of the literature. J Dermatol Surg Oncol 10:210–212

CHAPTER 54

Benign Epithelial Tumors

Contents

Introduction

A wide variety of cutaneous tumors have epithelial elements. In this chapter we discuss neoplasms which appear to show epidermal differentiation. The tumors of apparent adnexal differentiation are covered in Chapter 57. Epidermal tumors can be identified with antibodies against specific cytokeratins or against a cocktail of such molecules, but this is seldom needed. Many of the neoplasms discussed here have histologic patterns which can also be seen in keratinization disorders (Chap. 17) and epidermal nevi (Chap. 52).

Seborrheic Keratosis

Synonym. Verruca seborrhoica senilis, senile keratosis, seborrheic wart

Definition. Common superficial hyperkeratotic tumor with a variety of clinical and histologic patterns.

Epidemiology. Seborrheic keratoses are almost certainly the most common tumor. Every adult has one or two and many people have a great number.

Etiology and Pathogenesis. The origin of seborrheic keratoses is unknown. While they often have the same gross and microscopic patterns as a common wart, human papilloma virus particles are usually not present. Eruptive seborrheic keratoses may well be triggered by growth factors released by tumors, while acanthosis nigricans, which microscopically is similar to a seborrheic keratosis, is often related to insulin resistance.

Clinical Findings. Seborrheic keratoses are invariably benign but cosmetically disturbing, easily irritated, and occasionally confused with a host of malignant tumors, including malignant melanoma. They are most common on the trunk but also appear on the face, especially the hairline, neck, and upper aspects of the arms and legs. Some patients have hundreds of lesions (Fig. 54.1) and often report that other family members have the same problem. The lesions are found in varying sizes and stages of development on any given patient. The early lesions are small, skin-colored or tan, sharply bordered papules. They are often overlooked or the patient may notice them simply as an uneven spot. Frequently they are scratched or rubbed off when drying after a bath. As they grow larger, they become darker, more elevated, and more papillomatous. The retained cornified material gives them a waxy feeling; larger, thicker lesions have been

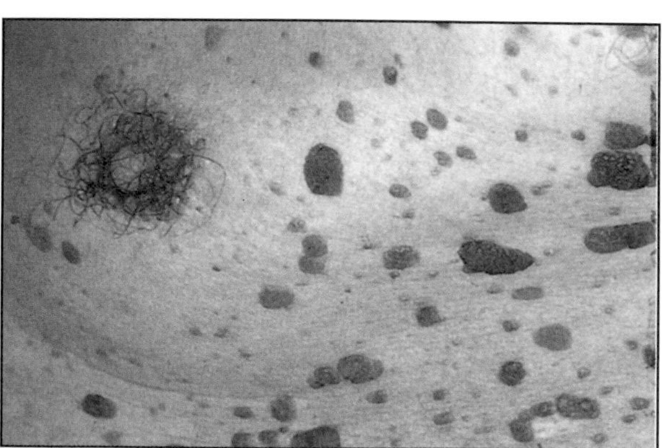

Fig. 54.1. Multiple seborrheic keratoses

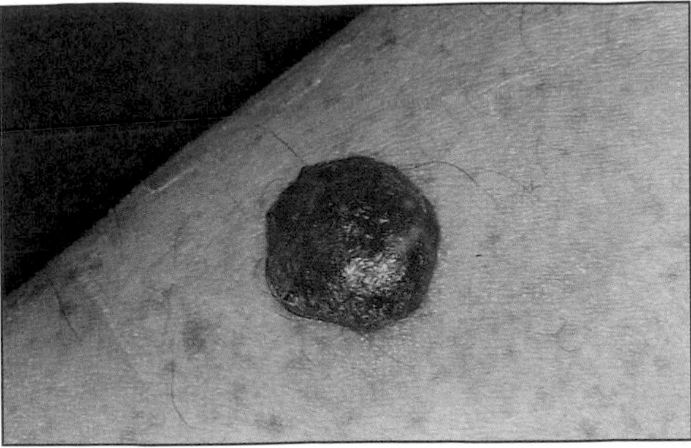

Fig. 54.2. Irritated seborrheic keratosis

compared to a drop of wax on a table because of their texture and appearance of being stuck onto the skin surface. The convoluted surface yields plugs of retained cornified material which can easily be seen with a dermatoscope but are often appreciated with the naked eye or a hand lens, readily helping to confirm the diagnosis.

There are many clinical and histologic variants of seborrheic keratoses. Some lesions become inflamed, most often through trauma. Then they may become red and even eroded (Fig. 54.2). Often the changes are more subtle. In our view, benign lichenoid keratosis is an irritated flat seborrheic keratosis most commonly found on the neck and upper part of the trunk. Flat seborrheic keratoses are often designated as age spots or liver spots by patients and as solar lentigines by physicians. Other thicker lesions, especially in the groin and axilla, are rubbed smooth and lack the typical surface texture. There is an overlap between seborrheic keratoses and acrochordons, especially on the neck. Acral lesions may lack pigment; others may be so dark as to resemble melanocytic lesions.

Histopathology. The unifying feature of seborrheic keratoses is a proliferation of entirely benign basaloid epithelial cells that typically appear to lie on the skin surface. Most seborrheic keratoses are removed by curettage, so one is confronted with basaloid tumor fragments. When one is excised, a line drawn along its base usually lies at the level of the adjacent epidermis. Another common feature is the pseudocysts, which are the crypts with their keratin plugs and usually sectioned tangentially. Much attention has been devoted to the histologic variants of seborrheic keratosis. Thick or acanthotic lesions are most likely to be rich in pseudocysts. The reticulated variant breaks the rule of upward growth, as long lacy fingers, often only several cells wide, extend down into the dermis. When accompanied by deeper pseudocysts, the same pattern is designated adenoid or glandular. The amount of melanin both in the basaloid tumor cells and in the upper dermis is highly variable.

Several histologic changes can cause confusion. Thicker lesions, especially if irritated, may develop whorls or swirls of basaloid cells resembling the squamous eddies of a squamous cell carcinoma; such changes have been called pseudosquamous eddies. Some dermatopathologists diagnose lesions rich in these structures as irritated or activated seborrheic keratoses. One must distinguish between lesions that are clinically irritated and those that are histologically irritated, since the correlation is not perfect. Another striking change is the proliferation of compact nests of basaloid cells that are often somewhat paler than the adjacent cells. This change has been designated the Borst-Jadassohn effect (Borst 1904; Jadassohn 1926) and ascribed to the clonal proliferation of a different population of cells within the epidermis. The Borst-Jadassohn effect is most often seen with seborrheic keratoses but may also occur with eccrine tumors, Bowen disease, and malignant melanoma in situ. Another puzzling tumor which has some histologic features of a seborrheic keratosis is inverted follicular keratosis, which may represent the same process as a seborrheic keratosis but is associated with a hair follicle.

Differential Diagnosis. Most seborrheic keratoses are easy to identify. Solitary nonpigmented lesions may be clinically and microscopically similar to verrucae. The term verruciform acanthoma has been applied to such in-between lesions. When irritated, they may be confused with a basal cell carcinoma and especially its pigmented variant. Benign lichenoid keratosis may resemble a superficial basal cell carcinoma. Smooth lesions, especially if heavily or irregularly pigmented, may be confused with malignant melanoma, but dermatoscopic examination to identify the plugged crypts allows a ready distinction. Large, flat, irregularly pigmented seborrheic keratoses in areas exposed to sun often can only be separated from lentigo maligna via biopsy.

Therapy. Most seborrheic keratoses are removed by curettage because they are so superficial. Flat lesions are also easily treated with cryotherapy. Destruction with a variety of lasers, e.g., pulsed CO_2 or erbium, is also possible. A superficial tangential excision is also appropriate, but deeper excisions and electrosurgical destruction often lead to s carring. The same agents used for chemical peels when applied in higher concentrations by experienced operators can also easily remove seborrheic keratoses. Multiple lesions can be dermabraded.

Variants of Seborrheic Keratosis

There are many lesions which clinically or microscopically resemble a seborrheic keratosis. In different countries, some are viewed as distinct entities, but the similarities far exceed the differences.

Stucco Keratosis

(Unna 1898; Kocsard et al. 1958)

Epidemiology. Stucco keratoses are almost always acral. Peculiarly, they are more common in patients with marked light exposure but often appear on the legs, which presumably receive less light than other body parts. Patients with dry skin also appear predisposed.

Clinical Findings. Acral seborrheic keratoses are often small and pale. When multiple lesions are present, most often on the distal aspects of the legs, one speaks of stucco keratoses (Fig. 54.3). Less common sites of involvement are the dorsal aspects of the feet, the ankles, and occasionally the dorsal aspects of the hands and distal part of the forearm. The individual lesions resemble small dabs or drops of plaster as might be splattered when stucco is applied. They invariably have a rough surface and are harmless.

Histopathology. Stucco keratoses are typically very hyperkeratotic and may have a papillomatous pattern. They lie above the level of the adjacent skin.

Therapy. As for seborrheic keratosis.

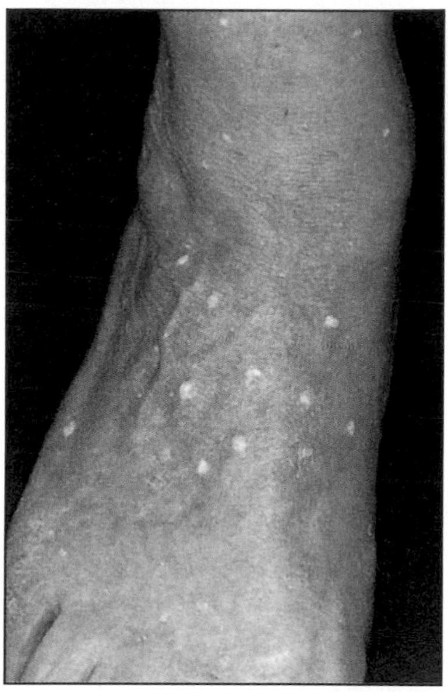

Fig. 54.3. Stucco keratoses

Verruca Plana-Like Seborrheic Keratosis

(Keining and Halter 1949)

Heavily pigmented acral seborrheic keratoses are often difficult to diagnose correctly. These lesions are most common on the backs of the hands and distal parts of the forearm. They overlap with larger flat seborrheic keratoses. Individual lesions are very similar to verruca plana; if pseudocysts are present, one can make a confident diagnosis. They are relatively difficult to treat but respond to the same methods as ordinary seborrheic keratoses.

Melanoacanthoma

(Mishima and Pinkus 1960)

Solitary large pigmented seborrheic keratoses have been designated melanoacanthomas (Fig. 54.4). While one may think clinically of a malignant melanoma, the presence of horn pseudocysts firms the diagnosis. Observed microscopically, not only is there abundant pigment in the basaloid cells, but there also may be rich deposits in the upper dermis. Melanoacanthomas are often excised because of concern about malignant melanoma, but if the clinical diagnosis is clear, they can be treated just as all other seborrheic keratoses.

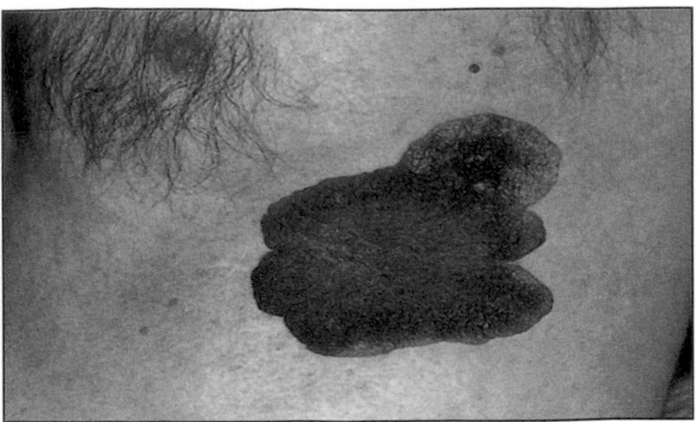

Fig. 54.4. Melanoacanthoma

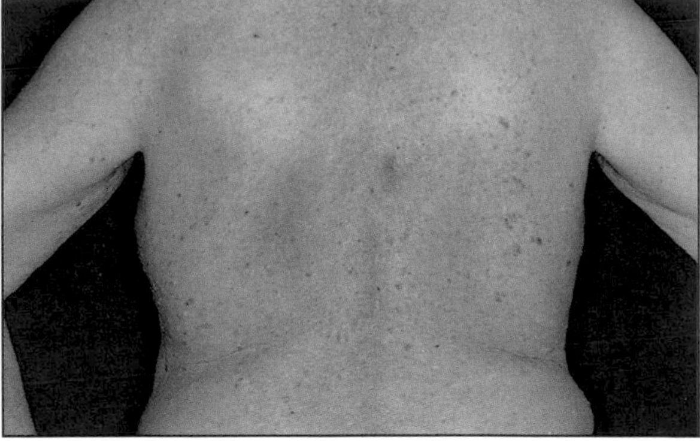

Fig. 54.5. Leser-Trélat sign. The patient complained about multiple new seborrheic keratoses and was found to have a previously undiagnosed renal cell carcinoma

Leser-Trélat Sign

(Leser and Trélat 1890)

Definition. The sudden appearance of multiple seborrheic keratoses as a sign of internal malignancy.

Etiology and Pathogenesis. Some internal malignancies, primarily adenocarcinomas, are apparently capable of secreting growth factors which stimulate the proliferation of seborrheic keratoses, acrochordons, acanthosis nigricans, and oral papillomas. All these lesions look similar microscopically and all may appear in various patterns in the same patient.

Clinical Findings. Since so many adults have hundreds of seborrheic keratoses, the diagnosis of Leser-Trélat sign must be made reluctantly. There should be reliable historic or photographic evidence that the patient has experienced the explosive growth of multiple, usually small seborrheic keratoses (Fig. 54.5). The presence of other changes such as acanthosis nigricans or eruptive acrochordons clinches the diagnosis. If there is no history of underlying malignancy, then a search is mandated. In contrast to other seborrheic keratoses, these eruptive lesions may regress or wax and wane as the underlying tumor is treated or recurs.

Histopathology. The histopathology is identical to that of seborrheic keratosis. The lesions themselves have no malignant potential.

Other Epidermal Tumors

Dowling-Degos Disease

(Dowling 1938; Degos and Ossipowski 1954)

Synonyms. Reticulated pigment anomaly of the flexures, verrucosis seborrhoica (Cramer 1969)

Definition. Macular reticulated hyperpigmentation, especially of the axillae and other flexural areas.

Clinical Findings. Dowling-Degos disease is an uncommon disorder which may be more common in Asians. There are numerous hyperpigmented macules in flexural areas that often blend together in a reticulated pattern. Larger lesions are identical to small seborrheic keratoses. Some patients have pigmented pits of the perioral and acral areas. Many cases are familial, inherited in an autosomal dominant fashion. Basal cell carcinomas may develop in the pigmented areas.

Histopathology. There is increased basal layer melanin associated with an epidermal hyperplasia similar to that of an adenoid seborrheic keratosis. The rete ridges are elongated and form a lacy pattern which may also be seen along follicle walls (in contrast to seborrheic keratoses). Pseudocysts are seen. The melanocytes are normal in size and number, but melanin may be increased.

Differential Diagnosis. The terminology of Dowling-Degos disease is befuddling. Two other disorders are very similar:

Haber Syndrome. Autosomal dominant disorder with multiple pigmented seborrheic keratoses, facial erythema, and hyperpigmentation, also associated with basal cell carcinomas (Chap. 28).

Kitamura Reticulate Acropigmentation. Reticulate acral lesions, especially on the dorsal aspects of hands and feet and the palmoplantar pit.

The hyperpigmentation in all three disorders is associated with the same lacy epithelial down growths associated with small plugged follicles. The clinical features may allow separation. Acanthosis nigricans and variants of Leser-Trélat sign may appear similar but arise more suddenly. Individual lesions must be separated from ordinary seborrheic keratoses.

Therapy. Individual lesions can be removed just as any other seborrheic keratosis. Changing larger lesions should be excised, as basal cell carcinomas may develop.

Clear Cell Acanthoma

(DEGOS et al. 1962)

Synonyms. Pale cell acanthoma, Degos tumor

Clinical Findings. Clear cell acanthoma is an uncommon benign tumor which usually presents as a solitary lesion on the leg of an older adult. It is typically a slowly growing, sharply bordered exophytic tumor that may appear somewhat inflamed. Hemorrhagic puncta may be seen and there is often a crusted collarette scale at the periphery. Lesions occasionally appear elsewhere on the body. Rare patients with multiple lesions have been described; such cases may be familial.

Histopathology. The microscopic findings are distinctive. Centrally, the epidermis is acanthotic and dominated by large pale cells which replace all but the basal layer. These cells are typically rich in glycogen, as demonstrated by a PAS stain. The transition between the central acanthotic pale tumor and the adjacent normal epidermis is abrupt. In the dermis there are telangiectases and often a sparse inflammatory infiltrate. The rete ridges are often elongated in a psoriasiform pattern.

Differential Diagnosis. The differential diagnostic list is endless. Most often one thinks of an irritated seborrheic keratosis, pyogenic granuloma or basal cell carcinoma. Dermatofibroma, eccrine poroma and other adnexal tumors, should also be considered, along with melanotic malignant melanoma. Once one has seen this uncommon tumor, the clinical diagnosis is usually easy the second time.

Therapy. Surgical excision.

Large Cell Acanthoma

(PINKUS 1970)

Clinical Findings. The large cell acanthoma is poorly understood. It is not identified clinically, but histologically. Most are described as a sharply bordered, pale flat tumors in areas exposed to the sun. Histologically, there is a flat or slightly papillomatous, minimally acanthotic epidermal tumor with sharp lateral borders. The striking feature is the predominance of very large keratinocytes, at least twice the size of their normal counterparts, but without mitoses or other atypia. It remains unclear whether large cell acanthoma is a variant of actinic keratosis, seborrheic keratosis, or a unique entity. Treatment is simple excision or curettage.

Focal Acantholytic Dyskeratosis

Synonyms. Papular acantholytic dyskeratoma, dyskeratotic acanthoma (solitary lesions), papular acantholytic dyskeratosis, acquired dyskeratosis acanthosis (multiple lesions).

The combination of acantholysis and dyskeratosis typifies Darier disease but may also be seen in many other settings including Grover disease, epidermal nevi (Chap. 52), and palmoplantar keratoderma (Chap. 17). Occasionally, actinic keratoses (Chap. 55) may also have such a pattern. Sometimes the changes are an incidental finding.

Finally, there are rare tumors that may have the histologic features of Darier disease. While their etiology is unknown, one can speculate that they represent clonal mutations involving the same defect in keratinization. Another possibility is that human papilloma virus induces this defect.

Both solitary and multiple papules and nodules may occasionally be seen. The solitary lesions are similar to warty dsykeratoma but are acanthotic and more exophytic. They are most commonly seen on the trunk. The multiple lesions are most common on the vulva but also appear on the penis, in the perianal region, and on the trunk. They may be eroded or ulcerated, perhaps because of maceration. Mucosal lesions are also seen.

Warty Dyskeratoma

(Szymanski 1957)

Synonyms. Dyskeratosis follicularis isolata (Nikolowski 1959), dyskeratoma segregans, isolated Darier disease

Etiology and Pathogenesis. In many cases, warty dyskeratomas involve hair follicles. They may represent a unique human papilloma virus infection of the follicular epithelium leading to acantholytic dyskeratosis.

Clinical Findings. A warty dyskeratoma is rarely diagnosed clinically, although an astute clinician may suggest the diagnosis when confronted by a solitary warty lesion on the scalp, cheek, or neck of an older adult. The lesion is typically crusted, not otherwise distinct, and may bleed when traumatized. Warty dyskeratomas are entirely benign and may regress.

Histopathology. Warty dyskeratomas show the histologic changes of Darier disease but confined to a single follicle wall or small cyst. Dyskeratotic cells with corps ronds, grains, and acantholysis are seen in the follicular or cyst wall. Often the lesions are removed by tangential excision; another clue to diagnosis is the marked focal parakeratosis in the excised cap.

Differential Diagnosis. Usually one thinks of a wart, irritated seborrheic keratosis, or hypertrophic actinic keratosis.

Therapy. Surgical excision

Acantholytic Acanthoma

Clinical Findings. Some patients have solitary or multiple papules dominated by acantholysis, reproducing the histologic pattern of Hailey-Hailey disease (Chap. 17). The lesions may be solitary or multiple. Solitary lesions are most commonly found on the trunk. Vulvar and mucosal lesions may occur. Multiple lesions have been described in renal transplant patients and rarely in others.

Histopathology. Flat lesions are identical with those of Hailey-Hailey disease. The more nodular lesions have marked acanthosis and hyperkeratosis, which is usually not seen in Hailey-Hailey disease.

Differential Diagnosis. The histologic differential diagnosis includes not only Hailey-Hailey disease, but also Grover disease and even pemphigus vulgaris for mucosal lesions. The clinical situation is easier. Solitary lesions resemble verruca vulgaris, while the multiple lesions may be confused with verrucae or seborrheic keratoses.

Epidermolytic Acanthoma

Once again, either solitary or multiple papules and nodules are found. Their histology mimics epidermolytic hyperkeratosis (Chap. 17). The solitary form resembles a wart. The multiple form is usually truncal and may be triggered by exposure to the sun. In many instances, epidermolytic hyperkeratosis is an incidental finding in another lesion such as a cyst wall or actinic keratosis.

Waxy Keratoses

Waxy keratoses appear in childhood, usually on the trunk, and have a shiny, yellow, waxy sheen. Similar lesions on the hand are known as acral mosaic keratoses. They may represent a variant of confluent and reticulated papillomatosis, as the microscopic picture is similar, except for marked compact hyperkeratosis.

Bibliography

Seborrheic Keratosis

Borst M (1904) Über die Möglichkeit einer ausgedehnten intraepithelialen dermalen Verbreitung des Hautkrebses. Verh Dtsch Ges Pathol 7:118–123

Braun-Falco O (1963) Zur Histogenese der Verruca seborrhoica. I. Mitteilung: Einleitung, histologische und histochemische Befunde. Arch Klin Exp Dermatol 216:615–649

Braun-Falco O (1964) Zur Frage der Entartung von Verrucae seborrhoicae seniles. Hautarzt 15:645–650

Jadassohn J (1926) Demonstration von selteneren Hautepitheliomen. Bruns Beitr Klein Chir 136:345–358

Li J, Ackerman AB (1994) "Seborrheic keratoses" that contain human papillomavirus are condylomata acuminata. Am J Dermatopathol 16:398–405

Sanderson KV (1968) The structure of seborrheic keratoses. Br J Dermatol 80:588–593

Stucco Keratosis

Braun-Falco O, Weissmann I (1987) Stukkokeratosen. Übersicht und eigene Beobachtungen. Hautarzt 29:573–577

Kocsard E, Ofner F (1966) Keratoelastoidosis verrucosa of the extremities (stucco keratoses of the extremities). Dermatologica 133:225–235

Kocsard E, Carter JJ (1971) The papillomatous keratoses. The nature and differential diagnosis of stucco keratosis. Aust J Dermatol 12:80–88

Kocsard E, Ofner F, Coles JL et al. (1958) Senile changes in the skin and visible mucous menbranes of the Australian male. Aust J Dermatol 4:216–223

Scott O, Ward J (1971) Stucco keratosis. Br J Dermatol 84:376–379

Willoughby C, Soter NA (1972) Stucco keratosis. Arch Dermatol 105:859–861

Verruca Plana-Like Seborrheic Keratosis

Keining E, Halter K (1949) Verrucae planae-artige seborrhoische Warzen. Arch Dermatol Syphil 188:482–489

Melanoacanthoma

Lambert WC, Lambert MW, Mesa ML et al. (1987) Melanoacanthoma and related disorders. Simulants of acrallentiginous (PPSM) melanoma. Int J Dermatol 26:508–510

Mishima Y, Pinkus H (1960) Benign mixed tumor of melanocytes and malpighian cells. AMA Arch Dermatol 81:539–550

Prince C, Mehregan AH, Hashimoto K et al. (1984) Large melanoacanthomas: A report of five cases. J Cutan Pathol 11:309–317

Leser-Trélat Sign

Holländer E (1900) Beiträge zur Frühdiagnose des Darmcarcinoms (Hereditätsverhältnisse und Hautveränderungen). Deutsch Med Wochenschr 26:483–485

Schwartz RA (1996) Sign of Leser-Trelat. J Am Acad Dermatol 35:88–95

Leser E (1901) Über ein die Krebskrankheit beim Menschen häufig begleitendes, noch wenig gekanntes Symptom. MMW 51:2035–2036

Dowling-Degos Disease

Cliff S, Otter M, Cook MG et al. (1997) Dowling Degos disease in association with multiple seborrhoeic warts. Clin Exp Dermatol 22:34–36

Cramer HJ (1969) Verrucosis seborrhoica. Hautarzt 20:31–34

Dowling GB, Freudenthal W (1938) Acanthosis nigricans. Br J Dermatol 50:467–471

Degos R, Ossipowski B (1954) Dermatose pigmentaire reticulée des plis. Ann Dermatol Syphil 81:147–151

Kim YC, Davis MD, Schanbacher CF et al. (1999) Dowling-Degos disease (reticulate pigmented anomaly of the flexures): A clinical and histopathologic study of six cases. J Am Acad Dermatol 40:462–467

Milde P, Goerz G, Plewig G (1992) Morbus Dowling-Degos mit ausschließlich genitaler Manifestation. Hautarzt 43:369–372

Clear Cell Acanthoma

Degos R, Delort J, Civatte J et al. (1962) Tumeur épithelial d'aspect particulier: Acanthome à cellules claires. Ann Dermatol Syphil 89:361–371

Degos R, Civatte J (1970) Clear cell acanthoma. Experience of 8 years. Br J Dermatol 83:248–254

Goette DK, Diakon NC (1983) Multiple clear cell acanthomas. Arch Dermatol 119:359–361

Large Cell Acanthoma

Pinkus H (1970) Epidermal mosaic in benign and precancerous neoplasia (with special reference to large-cell acanthomas). Acta Dermatol 65:75–81

Rabinowitz AD (1983) Multiple large cell acanthomas. J Am Acad Dermatol 8:840–845

Rahbari H, Pinkus H (1978) Large cell acanthoma. One of the actinic keratoses. Arch Dermatol 114:49–52

Sanchez Yus E, del Rio E, Requena L (1992) Large-cell acanthoma is a distinctive condition. Am J Dermatopathol 14:140–147

Weinstock MA (1992) Large-cell acanthoma. Am J Dermatopathol 14:133–134

Focal Acantholytic Dyskeratosis

DiMaio DJ, Cohen PR (1998) Incidental focal acantholytic dyskeratosis. J Am Acad Dermatol 38:243–247

Roten SV, Bhawan J (1995) Isolated dyskeratotic acanthoma. A variant of isolated epidermolytic acanthoma. Am J Dermatopathol 17:63–66

Zunt SL, Tomich CE (1990) Oral focal acantholytic dyskeratosis. J Dermatol Surg Oncol 16:510–515

Warty Dyskeratoma

Azuma Y, Matsukawa A (1993) Warty dyskeratoma with multiple lesions. J Dermatol 20:374–377

Griffiths TW, Hashimoto K, Sharata HH et al. (1997) Multiple warty dyskeratomas of the scalp. Clin Exp Dermatol 22:189–191

Nikolowski W (1959) Dyskeratosis follicularis isolata. Arch Klin Exp Dermatol 208:174–180

Szymanski FJ (1957) Warty dyskeratoma. A benign cutaneous tumor resembling Darier's disease microscopically. Arch Dermatol 75:567–572

Acantholytic Acanthoma

Brownstein MH (1988) Acantholytic acanthoma. J Am Acad Dermatol 19:783–786

Megahed M, Scharffetter-Kochanek K (1993) Acantholytic acanthoma. Am J Dermatopathol 15:283–285

Epidermolytic Acanthoma

Knipper JE, Hud JA, Cockerell CJ (1993) Disseminated epidermolytic acanthoma. Am J Dermatopathol 15:70–72

Miyamoto Y, Ueda K, Sato M, Yasuno H (1979) Disseminated epidermolytic acanthoma. J Cutan Pathol 6:272–279

Waxy Keratosis

Coleman R, Malone M, Handfield-Jones S et al. (1994) Waxy keratoses of childhood. Clin Exp Dermatol 19:173–176

CHAPTER 55

Premalignant Epithelial Tumors

Contents

Introduction

The term precancerous as introduced by Dubreuilh in 1896 is admittedly outdated after 100 years of service. Nonetheless we have retained it, for many physicians and patients clinically consider lesions such as actinic keratoses precancerous, i.e. they have the potential to turn into skin cancers. Histologically, these lesions are carcinoma in situ; pre-invasive lesions might be a better term. Another fertile ground for cancer is some types of chronic inflammation with associated epithelial hyperplasia, such as burn scars, acne inversa and tuberculous sinus tracts. One can speak of carcinoma in situ as an obligate precancerous lesion. If the patient lives long enough, at least some of the lesions can be expected to progress to invasive carcinoma. The hyperplastic inflammatory lesions are considered facultative precancerous lesions for they only rarely develop into malignancies.

Precancerous lesions have many possible etiologies and often reflect an interaction between nature and nurture. Probably the most precancerous of all lesions is the genodermatosis xeroderma pigmentosum. Every patient develops a large number of cutaneous malignancies, including basal cell carcinoma, squamous cell carcinoma and malignant melanoma, because they are unable to correctly repair sunlight-induced DNA damage. Other genetic factors, such as degree of skin pigmentation, also determine how much sunlight damage occurs. Viruses, primarily human papillomavirus (HPV), also play a role. Patients with another rare genodermatosis, epidermodysplasia verruciformis, develop infections with multiple HPV types. Some of the HPV types are especially likely to cause warty lesions which evolve into squamous cell carcinoma. In addition to sunlight and HPV, exposure to other exogenous substances such as tars, arsenic and other forms of irradiation may also cause precancerous lesions.

Actinic Keratosis

(Neumann 1869)

Synonym. Solar keratosis

Definition. Scaly lesions in sunlight-exposed skin that usually appear in adults and may evolve into squamous cell carcinoma.

Epidemiology. Prevalence. Very common. Increasing in Europe, probably because of increased leisure time and increased travel to sunny lands.

- Age: Usually begin after age 40 years of age
- Sex: More common in men, presumably reflecting outdoor work
- Race: Far more common in whites, and among whites, Celts and others with skin type I have many more lesions
- Occupation: Far more common in outdoor workers. Sunlight-damaged skin is known in different cultures as farmer's skin, seaman's skin or today as sun-worshipper's skin.
- Genetics: Probably many factors involved. Variants of xeroderma pigmentosum have been postulated as one explanation.
- Geography: More common in sunny lands closer to the equator or higher in elevation

Etiology and Pathogenesis. As the name and the epidemiology clearly show, the main factor is the sunlight. But there is a complex interaction between solar irradiation and the skin which eventually leads to the development of actinic keratoses and then skin cancers. In brief, the UV radiation not only damages the DNA of keratinocytes but it also diminishes the immune response in the skin and reduces the patient's ability to repair deleterious changes. The most dangerous wavelengths of light are those of UV-B (280–320 nm). The cells in which DNA damage has occurred continue to grow and divide. Typically they show disordered keratinization which is clinically reflected as a rough area. As long as the changes are above the basement membrane zone, the lesion is a squamous cell carcinoma in situ. At some point, malignant cells may enter the dermis producing an invasive squamous cell carcinoma. The latency period is estimated at 10–20 years and probably no more than 5% of all actinic keratoses develop into squamous cell carcinoma.

Exogenous immunosuppression, such as from cancer chemotherapy, may facilitate the more rapid progression of actinic keratoses into squamous cell carcinoma. Most squamous cell carcinomas arising from actinic keratoses have a good prognosis. On the scalp and lower lip, the risk of aggressive behavior is greater. Metastatic disease is rare. If the lesions have been exposed to or treated with ionizing radiation, progression is more likely.

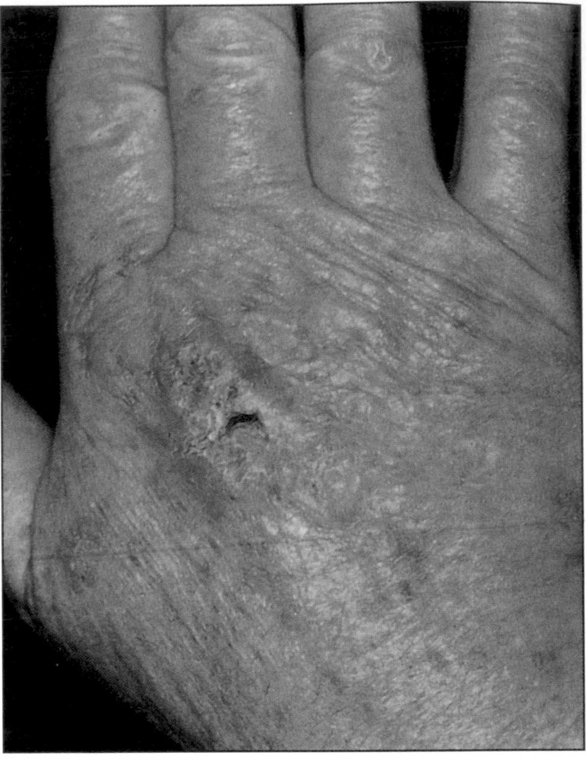

Fig. 55.2. Large actinic keratosis which evolved into squamous cell carcinoma

Clinical Findings. Actinic keratoses are found wherever chronic sunlight exposure has occurred. Thus the most common locations are the face (Fig. 55.1) and the back of the hands (Fig. 55.2). On the face, there are also striking differences. The scalp of a bald-headed man is at particular risk (Fig. 55.3), as are the forehead, nose, tops of the ears, cheeks, forearms and lower lip. The chin, upper lip and eyelids are only rarely involved. Actinic keratoses are also found almost anywhere on the body. One should inspect the trunk and occasionally one may find lesions on the legs.

Early actinic keratoses are best identified by palpation, not visual inspection. Actinic keratoses are identified as tiny rough macules or patches long before they acquire any striking clinical features. They are usually asymptomatic, although occasional lesions may itch when inflamed. The patient often notices the actinic keratoses when shaving, washing or otherwise caring for the skin. A clinician experienced in treating actinic keratoses almost always searches the at-risk areas via light palpation.

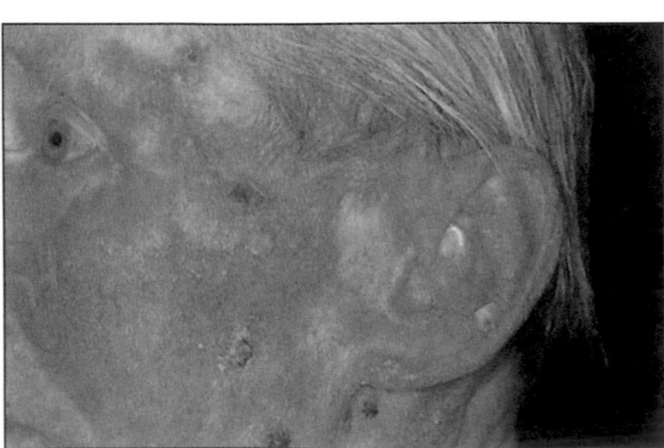

Fig. 55.1. Multiple actinic keratoses

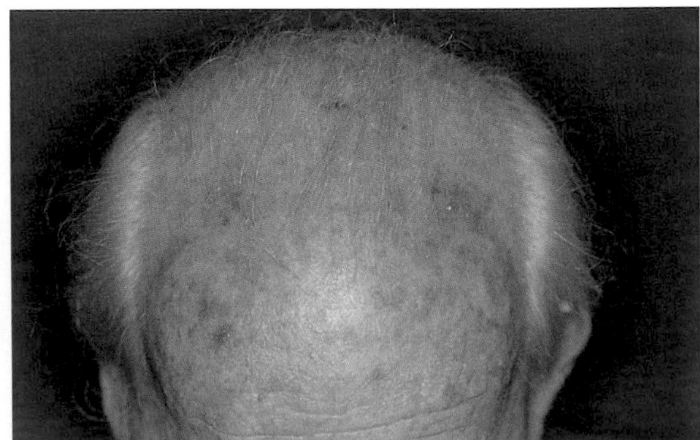

Fig. 55.3. Multiple actinic keratoses

In addition, the presence of other signs of sunlight-damaged skin such as solar elastosis or irregular pigmentation should suggest a fertile field for actinic keratoses. Magnifying glasses of some type and excellent light also help in finding early lesions. As the actinic keratoses become somewhat more prominent, they may assume a variety of clinical patterns. The type does not correlate with biologic behavior. The following types have been identified.

Erythematous. Early lesions frequently have a pink or red tint, presumably reflecting the limited inflammatory response. Patients may scratch the lesions off, producing minor bleeding.

Keratotic. This is the most common variant. As lesions grow, the normal process of cornification is disrupted and scales accumulate. The color then switches from pink to dirty yellow or brown. When such lesions are removed, such as by brisk drying after a soaking bath, the base is red and irregular often with tiny bleeding points and a thin inflamed border.

Cutaneous Horn. A cutaneous horn represents the massive accumulation of keratin over an epidermal lesion, producing a clinical horn. Actinic keratoses are one of the most common precursors of a cutaneous horn. The typical locations are the rim of the ear and the forehead.

Lichen Planus-Like. Some lesions, especially on the dorsal aspect of the forearms, may have a purple tint and resemble lichen planus. Histologically they show a lichenoid infiltrate.

Pigmented. The most common site for this variant is the face, especially the temples and cheeks. It is usually light-brown reflecting both a thickened stratum corneum and increased melanin. Changes in melanocytes are not seen. It is very difficult to separate pigmented actinic keratosis, flat seborrheic keratosis and senile lentigo. Often a biopsy is needed. if the pigmentation is irregular then this recommendation is especially appropriate as a lentigo maligna must be excluded.

Cheilitis. Actinic cheilitis is an actinic keratosis of the lip, almost always the lower lip. The risk of malignant change is somewhat greater than with cutaneous lesions (Chap. 33).

Histopathology. The actinic keratosis is a classic example of carcinoma in situ. Thus the most important change is the presence of abnormal keratinocytes confined to the epidermis. But many different patterns may be seen, reflecting the great clinical variability. Typical features include focal areas of parakeratosis alternating with hyperkeratosis (the pink and blue sign), frequent sparing of the follicular structures, and budding of the basal layer with pegs of atypical cells fingering down into the papillary dermis. Most atypical cells are seen in the basal layer, reflecting damage to the level where cell division occurs. The dermis invariably shows at least some degree of solar elastosis and may contain a sparse inflammatory infiltrate and telangiectases. As an actinic keratosis grows, it not only tends to grow downwards, but also spreads within the epithelium, invading hair follicles and even sweat gland ducts.

A variety of special names have evolved to describe variations in the histologic picture. When the atypia involves all levels of the epidermis, one speaks of a bowenoid actinic keratosis. If there is a localized or clonal proliferation of abnormal cells, then a Borst-Jadassohn effect or Borst-Jadassohn actinic keratosis can be identified. Very thick lesions are described as acanthotic and very thin as atrophic. Marked thickening of the stratum corneum typifies hypertrophic actinic keratosis or a cutaneous horn associated with an actinic keratosis. When a cleft (Freudenthal lacuna) develops just above the basal layer with minimal acantholysis, an acantholytic actinic keratosis is the preferred term. Pigmented actinic keratoses show increased melanin in the basal layer and often the upper dermis. Sometimes the atypical keratinocytes are rich in glycogen and clear; this form is known as clear-cell actinic keratosis. When a lichenoid infiltrate is present, the diagnosis of lichen planus-like actinic keratosis can be made. We diagnose this when parakeratosis and cytologic atypia are accompanied by a lichenoid infiltrate; otherwise we favor a diagnosis of benign lichenoid keratosis (Chap. 54). When an atrophic actinic keratosis has an intense lichenoid infiltrate, one is often confronted with a picture identical to that seen in lupus erythematosus. Here one must be quite careful, since the lesions of lupus erythematosus also occur in sunlight-damaged skin.

The histologic question always is – when does a lesion stop becoming an actinic keratosis and start to become a squamous cell carcinoma? Dermatopathologists work out their own solution to the problem. Often the submitted material is a curettage specimen, so the dermis is either poorly sampled or cannot be adequately assessed. In addition, the change from actinic keratosis to squamous cell carcinoma is very gradual. Terms such as early or microinvasive squamous cell carcinoma arising in an actinic keratosis are probably the best solution when only occasional malignant cells are in the papillary dermis, telling the clinician that this particular lesion requires special attention. When islands or strands of malignant keratinocytes are present in the dermis, then the diagnosis should be squamous cell carcinoma.

Course and Prognosis. The basic clinical question when dealing with actinic keratoses is – how many will convert to squamous cell carcinoma? Studies done many years ago suggest that 10–20% convert. More detailed studies in Australia have caused us to reassess these numbers. Regression of many actinic keratoses occurs, with about 25% disappearing in one year especially in patients who alter their sunlight exposure. Furthermore, it seems that about 0.25% of actinic keratoses undergo malignant change in a given year and that only 60% of squamous cell carcinomas develop from actinic keratoses. Almost every patient with a squamous cell carcinoma in sunlight-exposed skin also has actinic keratoses. Unfortunately, these fascinating data were developed just as insurance companies in many countries were looking for ways to save money. Thus it has become an issue whether or not to treat actinic keratoses. We tell our patients that some of the actinic keratoses may turn into squamous cell carcinomas over a period of years. We feel that the treatment of actinic keratoses is still not only medically correct but also cost effective.

Differential Diagnosis. When one is evaluating a single lesion, one can consider a lightly pigmented seborrheic keratosis or a verruca, as well as Bowen disease, superficial basal cell carcinoma and other tumors. Most seborrheic keratoses are on the trunk and readily distinguished. In many instances, one is assessing hundreds of lesions in several minutes and simply assumes all are actinic keratoses, recognizing that a few may be something else, but equally harmless.

Therapy. The mainstay of therapy in the USA is cryotherapy with liquid nitrogen. One can treat many lesions rapidly when using a cryospray device. Typically one freezes lesions for 3–6 s; thicker lesions or those that have proven resistant to therapy can be frozen longer or twice in one sitting. One rapidly develops great facility with this technique, and experienced patients help identify the lesions and return for repeat treatments every 3–12 months depending on the number of keratoses. When fewer lesions are present, one can also use peeling agents, such as trichloroacetic acid or 25% podophyllin in alcohol, but the degree of inflammation is greater, the number of treatments required larger and patient satisfaction lower.

Thick, resistant or suspicious lesions should be removed surgically. Most are removed by curettage, since actinic keratoses are usually superficial. Sometimes when curetting one notices that the dermis is soft or mushy; this should suggest the presence of an invasive tumor. Individual lesions can also be excised. Electrosurgical removal produces an unsatisfactory histologic specimen and also creates an unsatisfactory scar. Ionizing radiation is effective, but should be avoided except in very special cases because it increases the risk of later development of squamous cell carcinomas. When very large numbers of lesions are present, another therapeutic option is dermabrasion. The hyperkeratotic lesions on the backs of the hands and the scalp can be effectively treated this way.

Topical 5-fluorouracil (5FU) is another favorite approach for multiple actinic keratoses. During the early days when 5FU was being tested for systemic use, it was noticed that patients' actinic keratoses flared during systemic treatment. Topical 5FU creams and ointments were promptly developed. The patient treats the entire area of sunlight-damaged skin once or twice daily for 3–6 weeks. Not only do the previously recognized actinic keratoses become inflamed, eroded and eventually disappear, but also small, often overlooked lesions are highlighted and cured. Scarring is not expected. The trick is to keep the lesions inflamed for several weeks. For lesions on the face, 2 weeks suffices, but for those on the arms and scalp, much longer times are needed. The patients are miserable, look quite unsightly and compliance may be a problem.

To speed the process, topical 5FU may be combined with systemic isotretinoin. We give 10–20 mg of isotretinoin daily simultaneously and have designated this combination as the "turbo technique." After maximum inflammation has been obtained in about 3 weeks, the isotretinoin and 5FU are stopped and topical corticosteroids are usually used to more rapidly dampen the irritation. For maintenance care bland emollients are prescribed. On the scalp this has become our treatment of choice.

In theory, the use of sunscreens is the most important therapeutic approach. In fact, things are more complicated. If a patient is less than 60 years old, one surely should insist on diligent use of sunscreens, telling the patient that this will first make a difference in 10–20 years, as it takes actinic keratoses a good while to develop. The issue comes when an 80-year-old person starts to worry about sunscreens; they are probably not needed.

Radiation Keratosis

Definition. Keratosis arising in skin damaged by ionizing radiation following radiation therapy or accidental exposure.

Etiology and Pathogenesis. Following exposure to all types of ionizing radiation, there is a dose-response curve for the development of chronic radiation dermatitis and then keratoses and carcinomas (Chap. 13). Usually about 10 Gy of exposure is required. Both a single large dose, such as an from an industrial accident (Chernobyl) or atomic bomb explosion (Hiroshima or Bikini Atoll), and multiple small doses, such as previously acquired by dentists who held X-ray film in patients' mouths during exposure, can lead to damage. In contrast to actinic damage, direct cell damage appears more important than the associated immunologic effects.

Clinical Findings. Radiation keratoses develop on a background of chronic radiation damage, with atrophy, telangiectases and pigmentary changes. There may also be chronic ulcerations, which sometimes reflect malignant change themselves. The radiation keratoses are typically sharply circumscribed and more keratotic than most actinic keratoses (Fig. 55.4).

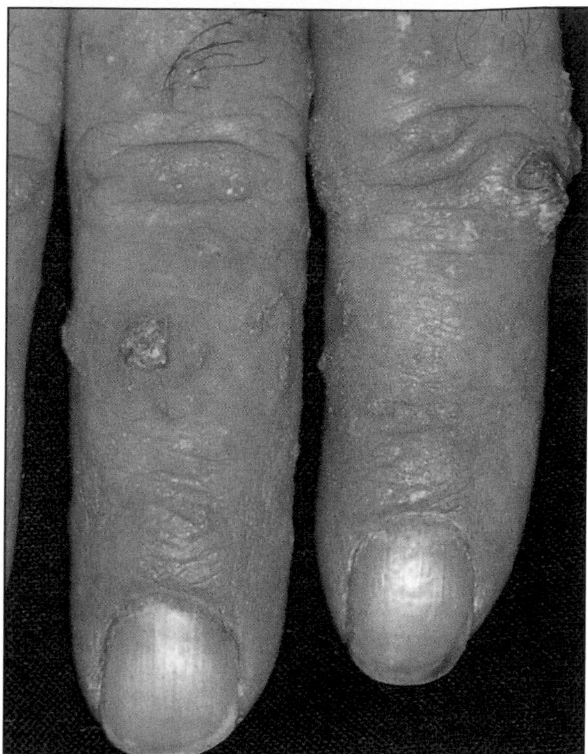

Fig. 55.4. Radiation keratoses

Histopathology. The dermis may show the amorphous changes with large fibroblasts and dilated vessels that typify chronic radiation damage. The keratoses themselves are carcinomas in situ and identical to hypertrophic actinic keratoses.

Differential Diagnosis. The history and overall clinical appearance provide the diagnosis. An individual lesion is identical to an actinic keratosis.

Therapy. Surgical excision is preferable. Often skin grafting is needed because of the poor healing tendency of radiation-damaged skin. Since the risk of malignant change is considerably higher in radiation keratoses, all should be removed as soon as possible. Further radiation therapy is contraindicated.

Arsenical Keratosis

Etiology and Pathogenesis. Patients who have been exposed to inorganic arsenical compounds for a long period of time are at risk for both internal and cutaneous malignancies. The type of internal tumor varies greatly depending on which arsenical compounds are involved. There is invariably a long latency period, usually 10–30 years. There are a number of ways in which an individual can be exposed to arsenic. They include:

- Ground water naturally containing arsenic: Most common in parts of Taiwan and Argentina (Cordoba region).
- Ground or surface water contaminated with arsenic: Most common in mining regions, such as in German Erzgebirge and Polish/German Riesengebirge. Such problems have been almost eliminated by increased regulations about dumping of byproducts and reduced mining.

- Other industrial exposure: Vine growers in Germany used arsenic-containing insecticides until the 1930s. The home-made brandy from the contaminated pressings caused many cases of chronic arsenic poisoning.
- Medical therapy: Fowler solution was formerly used for psoriasis and was recommended for asthma as late as the 1960s in the USA and for psoriasis in Germany at the same time. "Asiatic pills" (Pilulae asiaticae) also contained arsenic. Arsenic is still available in various countries as a medication. The organic arsenical compounds used for so many years to treat syphilis did not induce chronic arsenicism.
- Poisoning: A clever poisoner aims for acute arsenic poisoning and death, but now and again patients appear with chronic arsenic intoxication and it is found that someone is poisoning them.

Clinical Findings

Cutaneous Findings. The cutaneous hallmarks of chronic exposure to inorganic arsenicals include palmoplantar keratoses, multiple cutaneous malignancies, especially superficial basal cell carcinoma and Bowen disease, and a diffuse mottled hyperpigmentation. The marvelous descriptive term "rain drops on a dusty road" has enabled generations of dermatologists to envisage the small islands of normal, light-colored skin, amidst a background of irregular gray-black hyperpigmentation (Fig. 55.5). While arsenic salts are deposited in the skin, most of the color comes from disturbances in the production and distribution of melanin with incontinence of pigment.

The punctate keratoses are typically small hard 1–2-mm papules, barely arising above the skin surface. As they grow, they acquire a thick, adherent hyperkeratotic horn. On the palms and soles, they may be associated with more diffuse hyperkeratosis, especially prominent on pressure areas such as the heel. The acral changes may be painful and fissured. In addition, keratoses can be found on the head, neck and trunk. The trunk is the most common site for the cutaneous malignancies. Superficial basal cell carcinoma and Bowen disease are most common. It is usually impossible to determine if a keratosis was the precursor lesion or not. Keratoses are more common on the palms and soles; cancers more common on the trunk. Thus arsenical keratoses are probably more often tumor markers than tumor precursors.

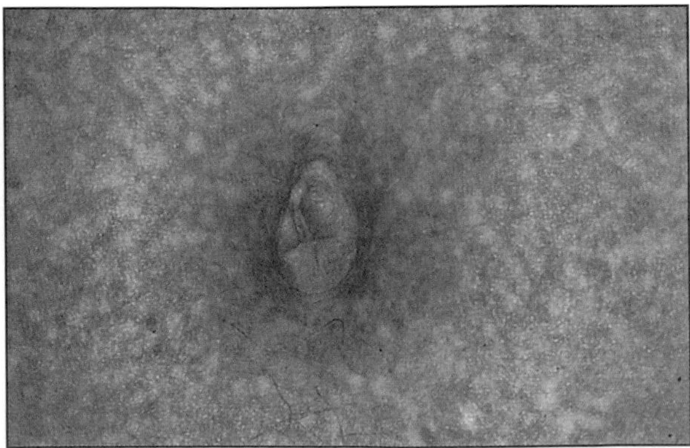

Fig. 55.5. Pigmentary changes associated with chronic arsenic use

Systemic Findings. The patients are at risk for a wide range of internal malignancies, which vary somewhat depending on exactly which arsenic salt is involved. Tumors of the lungs, for example, are most common among miners exposed to bismuth-arsenic salts. Other organs commonly involved include the liver, kidneys and pancreas. In Taiwan, blackwater fever is a complication of chronic arsenic exposure; patients suffer renal and peripheral vascular disease.

Histopathology. Arsenical keratoses are also carcinomas in situ but have more cytologic atypia on average than actinic keratoses. In areas where numerous arsenical keratoses are evaluated such as Taiwan, different grading schemes have been employed. The bowenoid lesions with full-thickness epidermal atypia are more likely to progress than the lesions that mimic a hypertrophic actinic keratosis. The unequivocal histologic diagnosis of arsenical keratosis is not possible. When an invasive squamous cell carcinoma develops, it is often associated with an intense inflammatory infiltrate. The discolored skin shows deposition of melanin in the papillary dermis.

Differential Diagnosis. The punctate forms of palmoplantar keratoderma must be excluded. A personal and family history usually suffices to make the distinction. Plantar warts and keratotic lichen planus may also appear similar on the palms and soles. On other sites actinic keratoses must be considered.

Therapy. If arsenical keratoses are diagnosed, a thorough systemic evaluation and monitoring to exclude cutaneous and internal malignancies are most important. Arsenical keratoses are difficult to treat, just as are all keratodermas. Mechanical debridement, perhaps coupled with topical or even systemic retinoids may be tried. Oral retinoids, usually acitretin, have been employed for tumor-preventive therapy. Since it is impossible to treat the hundreds of lesions, it is most crucial to watch for signs of malignant changes such as rapid growth or ulceration, not just on the palms and soles but also on the rest of the body.

Tar Keratosis

Synonym. Tar wart

Etiology and Pathogenesis. Sir Percival Pott's description of scrotal cancer in chimney sweeps in 18th century England is acknowledged as the first report of chemical carcinogenesis. The polycyclic aromatic hydrocarbons are a large family of chemicals derived from coal tar, creosote, oil, other petroleum products, shale oil and many other sources. Many are reliable carcinogens in a variety of animal models. They appear to function best as tumor promoters in association with UV radiation. Today industrial exposure is widespread including those working in the extractive industries, refineries, road construction and still chimney sweeps. Medical exposure to tars also occurs, best typified by the Goeckerman regimen in which coal tar and UV-B irradiation are combined in the treatment of psoriasis. Patients previously treated with tars appear to have a greater risk of developing PUVA-related skin cancer, and even scrotal squamous cell carcinomas. The use of tar in dermatologic practices is considered safe, as the benefit usually far outweighs the small risk.

Clinical Findings. Usually the first change is a photosensitization reaction, involving the face, neck and often arms. Many years later poikilodermatous changes appear and then much later the tar warts. They are tiny hyperkeratotic papules most common on the cheeks and neck, but also seen on the dorsal aspect of the forearms and hands. The risk of malignant change is relatively low.

Therapy. The tar keratoses can be easily removed by curettage or excision. Anyone with tar-induced skin changes should be checked for scrotal cancer and encouraged to use sunscreens.

Cutaneous Horn

Synonym. Cornu cutaneum

Definition. Cutaneous horn is a clinical diagnosis for the localized compact accumulation of cornified material.

Clinical Findings. A cutaneous horn is just what the name suggests – a projection of cornified material from the skin. Usually a solitary lesion is found, most often on the temples, cheeks or ears. It is typically yellow brown and arises vertically as a cylinder or pyramid from the skin (Fig. 55.6). Lesions may be as large as 15 cm, although 2–4 cm is more typical. The horn may have longitudinal or transverse grooves and larger lesions are almost invariably curved. The base is typically uninflamed. By definition, one can not clinically identify the underlying lesion, for if one could, then one would not diagnose cutaneous horn. One can guess based on the location, age of the patient and neighboring lesions, but it is hard to be sure. For example, a horn on the cheek of a 70-year-old farmer with hundreds of actinic keratoses is likely to cover either an actinic keratosis or a squamous cell carcinoma.

Histopathology. Microscopic examination is required to obtain a final diagnosis. The horn itself is unexciting – a mass of cornified material. At the base there are many possibilities including actinic keratosis, squamous cell carcinoma, keratoacanthoma, verruca vulgaris, Bowen disease, other malignancies, other keratoses, inflammatory lesions such as discoid lupus erythematosus and even virtually no change as in tinea amiantacea.

Therapy. A tangential excision is the usual first step. Further treatment is then based on the biopsy results.

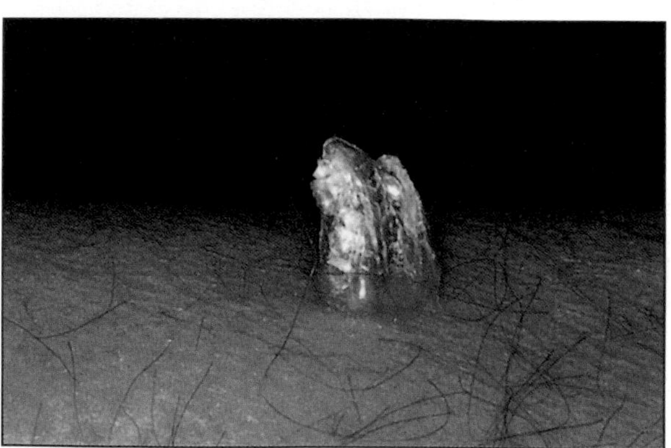

Fig. 55.6. Cutaneous horn

Bowen Disease

(Bowen 1912)

Definition. Full-thickness epidermal carcinoma in situ, often with a typical clinical appearance, not related to sunlight exposure.

Etiology and Pathogenesis. In the past arsenic exposure was probably the most common cause of Bowen disease. Today evidence has been accumulating that many lesions are caused by HPV. In bowenoid papulosis (Chap. 34), HPV16 and 18 have been found. HPV has been identified to a lesser extent in extragenital Bowen disease and is probably involved in Bowen disease of the nailbed. Sunlight can also induce bowenoid lesions, but we refer to them as bowenoid actinic keratoses. Chronic ionizing radiation can also produce bowenoid-like lesions.

Clinical Findings

Cutaneous Findings. Bowen disease is typically a slowly growing psoriasiform patch or plaque in an older adult. It may occasionally be pruritic. While the trunk is the most common location, Bowen disease can also be seen on the face (Fig. 55.7), genital region, fingers (Fig. 55.8) and on mucosal surfaces where it is known as erythroplasia of Queyrat. Bowen disease certainly also develops on sunlight-exposed skin of the face and trunk. It is just extremely difficult to distinguish it from an actinic keratosis. In about 60% of patients there is a solitary lesion; the remaining 40% have multiple lesions described as multicentric Bowen disease. In the latter group, one should search diligently for exposure to a carcinogen.

The lesions are sharply bordered, initially flat, erythematous and with a fine crust. Occasionally annular lesions or more bizarre patterns evolve as central regions may appear to involute. Adjacent lesions can intersect and form polycyclic designs. When the scale is removed, a moist red eroded surface, often slightly papillomatous, is found. The presence of an ulceration or nodule suggests the development of an invasive tumor. If the patient lives long enough, conversion to an invasive squamous cell carcinoma (Bowen carcinoma) is expected in most untreated cases. These carcinomas tend to be aggressive and metastasize more often than other cutaneous squamous cell carcinomas. Bowen disease is most common in elderly individuals, so it is unclear how often nature has a chance to follow this course.

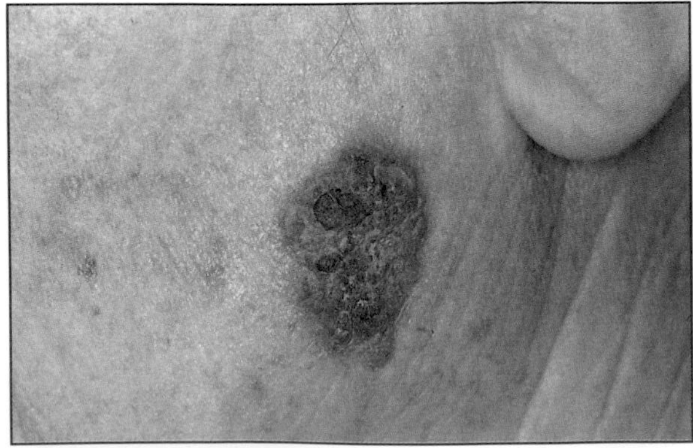

Fig. 55.7. Bowen disease

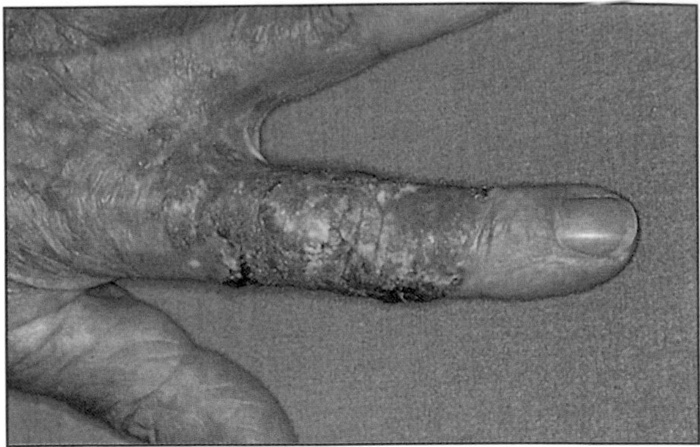

Fig. 55.8. Bowen disease

An unusual variant of Bowen disease is that involving the finger or nailbed. The finger lesions in the past were most common in dentists and radiologists, reflecting occupational exposure. There was also an epidemic of digital Bowen disease in the USA in the 1970s. Gold radon seeds had been recycled into gold-class rings many years before and then began producing malignant changes. Nailbed involvement is often overlooked. It most often involves the thumb and great toe and may be associated with HPV.

Systemic Findings. The association of Bowen disease and internal malignancy has long been controversial. In the past there was clearly an association but it was via exposure to inorganic arsenic. In addition, Bowen disease patients are older, so they are at risk for a wide variety of internal malignancies. If Bowen disease today is a marker for systemic cancers, it must be regarded as a very weak one. In addition, it only appears plausible for patients with multiple lesions of Bowen disease.

Histopathology. The diagnostic feature is the presence of atypical keratinocytes at all levels of the epidermis. In addition, the epidermal pattern is altered. There is acanthosis and the rete ridges are larger and more bulbous. Dyskeratotic cells, multinucleated cells and mitoses are easily found. There may be a brisk inflammatory response in the dermis consisting of lymphocytes and plasma cells. One unusual variant is clear-cell Bowen disease in which many of the abnormal keratinocytes are rich in glycogen. Multiple sections should be checked to insure that the tumor has not expanded across the basement membrane zone into the dermis. The invasive squamous cell carcinoma that develops in this situation is called a Bowen carcinoma.

Differential Diagnosis. The classic differential diagnosis for a patch of "dermatitis" or "psoriasis" that slowly expands and never regresses includes Bowen disease, superficial basal cell carcinoma and in the right locations Paget disease and extramammary Paget disease. Lesions such as bowenoid actinic keratosis, bowenoid papulosis and erythroplasia of Queyrat are separated more by definition than by clinical or histologic features. Rarely discoid lupus erythematosus and lupus vulgaris can also appear similar.

Therapy. There are many possibilities for treating Bowen disease. Surgical excision, curettage, electrocautery, cryotherapy or laser ablation are all appropriate. In more difficult patients with large lesions or poor general health, topical 5-FU cream used twice daily for 4–6 weeks may be helpful. Such treatment is more effective when dealing with a nonhair-bearing area, since the tumor cells which extend along follicles are harder to reach with 5-FU. Radiation therapy may also be used in older patients. We recommend a total dose of 40–60 Gy in daily divided doses of about 3–4 Gy, using a half-value layer of 2.0–3.0 mm. Electron beam therapy can also be used.

Erythroplasia of Queyrat

(Queyrat 1911)

Definition. Squamous cell carcinoma in situ on mucosal or transitional surfaces.

Etiology and Pathogenesis. HPV 16 and 18 are probably responsible for a significant percentage of cases.

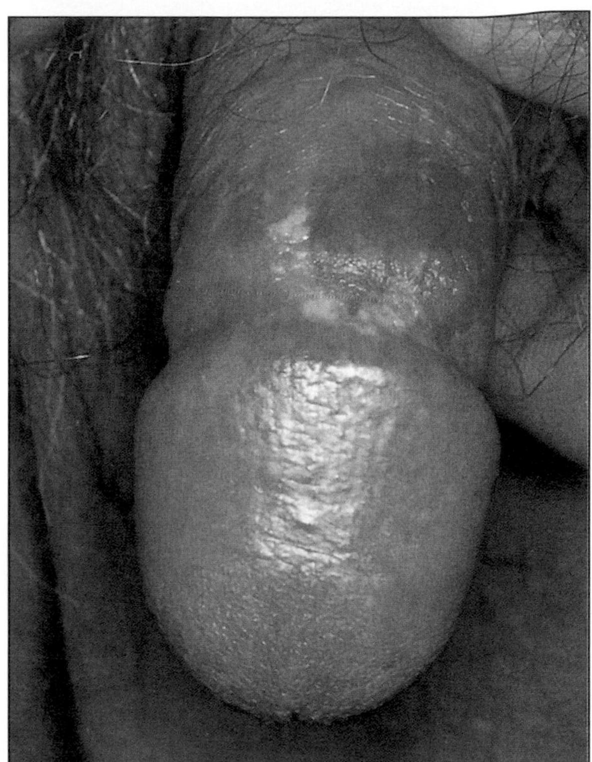

Fig. 55.9. Erythroplasia of Queyrat

Clinical Findings. Carcinoma in situ appears different on mucosal surfaces. It is typically a red velvety patch or plaque. While the classic location for erythroplasia of Queyrat is the penis (Fig. 55.9), similar lesions are found on the female genitalia, about the anus and in the mouth. Most patients are older adults. On the penis, most lesions occur around the inner prepuce or glans in uncircumcised individuals. There is a sharply bordered irregular red plaque which has often been treated as dermatitis, psoriasis or candidiasis but failed to respond. The surface resembles that of Bowen disease after the scale has been removed. Infiltration, nodularity or ulceration suggest conversion to an invasive squamous cell carcinoma. In the mouth, erythroplasia is often admixed with leukoplakia (white areas). So-called speckled leukoplakia is the type of leukoplakia most likely to evolve into invasive squamous cell carcinoma (Chap. 33). Because erythroplasia of Queyrat is clinically so different from Bowen disease and may have a worse prognosis, we have chosen to retain it is a separate entity.

Histopathology. The constant feature is the presence of full-thickness epidermal atypia but the mucosal or transitional location produces several other clues. The rete ridges are enlarged and the epithelium is eroded. Thus the superficial vessels are very close to surface. In French the lesion is called *épithéliome papillaire nu* meaning an epithelioma with naked papillae. There is less dyskeratosis than in Bowen disease and more inflammation usually rich in plasma cells.

Differential Diagnosis. One must exclude balanitis, candidiasis, psoriasis, plasma cell balanitis of Zoon, lichen planus, fixed drug eruption and bowenoid papulosis. All except bowenoid papulosis can be excluded easily on biopsy. Bowenoid papulosis tends to be in young individuals who have multiple lesions, often involving skin as well as mucosa, but the distinction is not absolute as overlap lesions are seen. A good rule is to biopsy any genital patch which does not respond promptly to topical therapy. The differential diagnosis of oral lesions is considered in Chap. 33.

Therapy. All of the treatments discussed under Bowen disease are appropriate. Topical 5-FU can be used with somewhat more enthusiasm since the area by definition is not hair-bearing. We prefer surgical excision with control of margins whenever possible. The patient should be monitored with particular attention paid to the regional lymph nodes.

Paget Disease

(Paget 1874)

Definition. Chronic dermatitis-like change involving nipple and adjacent skin of the breast as a manifestation of an underlying carcinoma of the breast. While Paget disease is not carcinoma in situ, it clinically and histologically mimics such lesions and is thus included in the group.

Epidemiology. Paget disease is uncommon. It is almost always unilateral and usually in women older than 40 years of age. It has been reported in men.

Etiology and Pathogenesis. The cutaneous changes in Paget disease reflect the spread (or metastasis) of adenocarcinoma cells from the breast into the epidermis. Thus it is viewed as an epidermotropic adenocarcinoma. The cause of the underlying breast carcinoma remains unclear. In most cases, the tumor is intraductal in location. In rare cases no breast tumor is found. There are two explanations: either the intraductal carcinoma was small and missed, or the malignant cells arose from epidermal structures, such as sweat glands, as is the case with extramammary Paget disease.

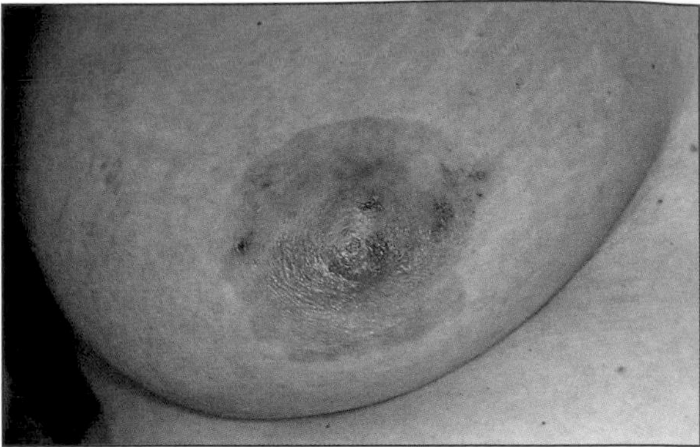

Fig. 55.10. Paget disease of the nipple

Clinical Findings. Initially minimal changes are noticed involving one nipple. There may be erythema or mild crusting, often associated with pruritus. Thus, nipple dermatitis is usually the first diagnosis, if the patient even bothers to report the change to her doctor. As the lesion slowly expands, it also becomes more distinct with a sharp border, eroded and covered with scales and crusts (Fig. 55.10). The nipple may become distorted. Ulcerations or nodules suggest that the underlying breast carcinoma has already spread from its intraductal location.

Histopathology. The Paget cells or breast carcinoma cells are large clear cells with an edematous or swollen-appearing cytoplasm and large oval nuclei. They simply sit in the nipple epidermis, eliciting little inflammatory response. The basal layer is usually spared, and dyskeratotic changes are not seen. Thus most of the action is in the spinous layer. The epidermis typically is somewhat eroded and there is a variable dermal inflammatory response.

The cells are PAS-positive and contain mucin. They stain positively with carcinoembryonic antigen (CEA), epithelial membrane antigen (EMA) and selected antikeratin stains.

Diagnostic Criteria. Every persistent nipple dermatitis should be biopsied. If the clinical features or biopsy suggest Paget disease, the patient must be evaluated just as any other breast cancer patient with complete physical examination (with particular attention to regional lymph nodes).

Differential Diagnosis. The clinical differential diagnosis is nipple dermatitis, which is usually bilateral, common in younger women, often those with atopic dermatitis who are nursing, and sometimes a reflection of allergic contact dermatitis. Other possibilities include scabies, erosive adenomatosis of the nipple, psoriasis and both superficial basal cell carcinoma and Bowen disease. Despite the fact that Bowen disease is far more common than Paget disease, on the nipple one should diagnosis Bowen disease with extreme reluctance.

Histologically Paget disease may be confused with a malignant melanoma in situ and Bowen disease. An amelanotic malignant melanoma is particularly hard to separate with routine examination. Immunohistochemistry usually allows a rapid distinction, as S100 staining allows one to identify melanoma cells while CEA and EMA are relatively specific for Paget disease. The biopsy should be completely sectioned. Often a ductal structure with carcinoma cells is found, clinching the diagnosis. On the eyelid, sebaceous carcinoma typically also has a pagetoid pattern.

In additional, there are clear cells in the normal nipple epithelium (Toker 1970) in perhaps 10% of individuals. These nonmelanocytic cells are perhaps aberrant sweat gland ductal cells. Perhaps some cases of Paget disease without underlying breast carcinoma reflect malignant proliferation of the usually harmless clear cells of the nipple.

Therapy. The treatment is that appropriate for the breast carcinoma diagnosis. Small intraductal tumors may be treated by lumpectomy, often with irradiation, but in many cases a mastectomy is recommended. In the rare cases where no underlying breast carcinoma is found, an experienced breast cancer surgeon should still be consulted.

Extramammary Paget Disease

Definition. Adenocarcinoma involving skin which clinically and histologically resembles Paget disease but does not feature underlying carcinoma of the breast.

Etiology and Pathogenesis. The nature of extramammary Paget disease is confusing. There are probably several disorders that all are grouped together. In perhaps 10% of cases, an underlying adenocarcinoma is found which has extended to the skin, in an analogous manner to Paget disease. The most common associated tumors are those of the rectum, prostate, bladder and cervix. In the vast majority of cases, no underlying tumor is found, so one is confronted with a primary adenocarcinoma of the skin. Most favor an apocrine origin, in which a scenario exactly opposite from Paget disease arises. Cells move down from the epidermis to populate the ducts and follicles. Others suggest that epidermal stem cells evolve into malignant glandular cells.

Clinical Findings. Extramammary Paget disease is similar to Paget disease of the nipple. The most common location for this extremely uncommon disorder is the anogenital region where a slowly expanding, erythematous crusted patch or plaque is found. Other sites include the axilla (Fig. 55.11), umbilicus, groin and even the external ear (which is rich in apocrine-like glands). While women are more often affected than men, we have seen larger lesions in men, spreading to involve groin, anus and scrotum. Multifocal lesions are not uncommon, in contrast to Paget disease. Ulcerations and nodules are more common when an underlying malignancy is present, but the two modes of development cannot be separated clinically in most cases. In extramammary Paget disease without an underlying

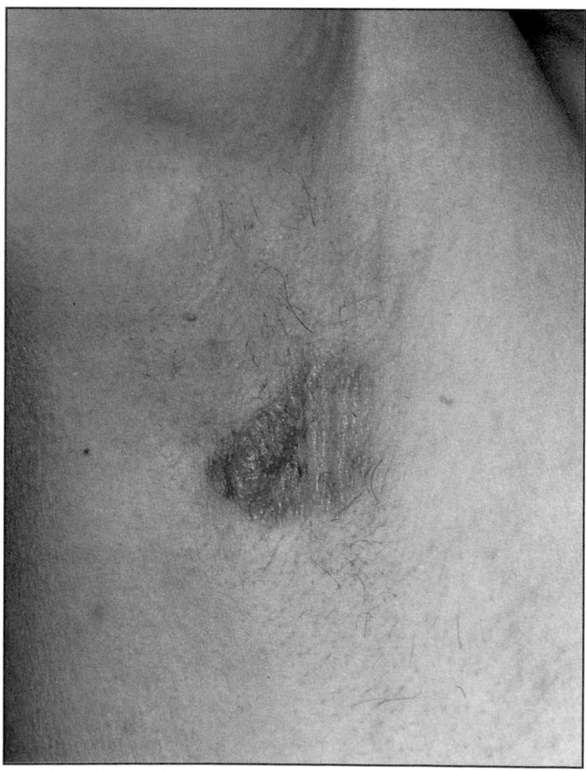

Fig. 55.11. Extramammary Paget disease

tumor, the cells tend to remain in the epidermis, spreading laterally, although rarely more aggressive behavior may be seen.

Histopathology. The microscopic picture is identical to that in Paget disease. There may be immunohistochemical differences, such as the presence of acidic mucins, in contrast to the neutral mucins found in Paget disease. Signet ring cells in which mucin has pushed the nucleus to the cell periphery are far more common in extramammary Paget disease. Usually one can neither separate Paget disease and extramammary Paget disease nor identify the source of the intraepidermal cells on biopsy.

Differential Diagnosis. The most common considerations are chronic nummular dermatitis, inverse psoriasis and candidiasis. Usually the lesions are so large that one does not immediately think of a tumor such as Bowen disease or superficial basal cell carcinoma. The histologic differential diagnosis is the same as for Paget disease.

Therapy. Therapy is determined by whether or not an underlying tumor is found. If so, then the case is best handled by an oncologic surgeon. If no underlying tumor is found, then the cutaneous lesion should be excised generously with rigid margin control. Micrographic surgery has proven very useful in this setting. Almost invariably, skin grafting is required for coverage. The large specimen should also be carefully analyzed microscopically searching for extension downwards or signs of an adjacent tumor.

In addition, the lymph nodes must be evaluated. If there is a documented underlying malignancy, the need for lymph node dissection will be determined by the surgeon. If an enlarged node is found, or if the surgical specimen shows dermal invasion by the epidermal adenocarcinoma, then a lymph node biopsy is warranted.

Clear Cell Papulosis

(Kuo et al. 1987)

Clear cell papulosis has only been described among young Taiwanese children who present with multiple hypopigmented macules and papules on abdomen and trunk, generally along the milk line. It is not a precancerous condition but may be confused histologically with Paget disease. Microscopically there are large solitary clear cells within the epidermis, primarily in the basal layer, along with a decrease in melanin. The clear cells stain with antibodies against keratin and carcinoembryonic antigen and probably represent altered sweat gland cells. They thus have the same features as the clear cells of Toker seen in the nipple.

Facultative Precancerous Lesions

There is a long list of lesions in which a malignancy may develop but usually does not. These facultative precancerous conditions are often reactive with a potential for reversal. The most typical setting that of chronic irritation and inflammation. Two classic examples in the past were the draining ulcers and sinuses associated with tuberculosis and osteomyelitis. Even a chronic ulcer in stasis dermatitis has a small risk of malignant conversion. Thus, the advice is often given to biopsy the edge of a poorly healing ulcer. The more common scenario is that a basal cell carcinoma has been overlooked and treated as an ulcer, but in any event, caution is appropriate. Chronic inflammation such as acne inversa, psoriasis following ionizing radiation especially in the groin and gluteal cleft, and lichen planus of the mouth and soles may very rarely evolve into a squamous cell carcinoma.

Skin that is atrophic or scarred is also more likely to develop malignant changes. The classic example is a burn scar or chronic radiation dermatitis. Healed lupus vulgaris and even chronic discoid-lupus erythematosus may also undergo change. Another prototypical example is the dermis defective in type VII collagen in dystrophic epidermolysis bullosa, where almost every patient develops first mitten-type scars and then malignancies (Chap. 15). Acrodermatitis chronica atrophicans, lichen sclerosus et atrophicus and other atrophic conditions may also very rarely undergo malignant change.

The pathologic term of pseudoepitheliomatous hyperplasia is used to describe the microscopic findings of hyperplastic but cytologically benign epithelial strands extending further into the dermis than do normal epidermal elements. These changes are typically seen at the edge of a chronic ulcer but also found in many other settings. One unusual location is over a granular cell tumor of the oral cavity. In lichen simplex chronicus and prurigo nodularis, reactive epidermal hyperplasia is invariably present. It also often accompanies dermatofibromas. The wide variety of clinical and histologic situations in which reactive epidermal hyperplasia occurs renders the pathologic term pseudoepitheliomatous hyperplasia relatively unhelpful in describing clinical entities.

In Europe, papillomatosis cutis carcinoides (GOTTRON 1932) has been used to describe the thickened, proliferative changes that occur on the lower leg or dorsal foot, sometimes in association with an underlying disorder and sometimes on seemingly normal skin. We consider Gottron's term as synonymous with verrucous carcinoma and consider it further in Chapter 56.

A final category is the scenario when benign tumors undergo malignant change. The most common example is the development of a malignant melanoma in a melanocytic nevus. It is estimated that about 25 % of malignant melanoma have a nevus as a precursor. Another such situation is that of nevus sebaceus, in which tumors frequently develop. Most are trichoblastoma or syringocystadenoma papilliferum but occasionally a genuine basal cell carcinoma arises. Patients with multiple trichoepitheliomas (Brooke syndrome) also develop basal cell carcinomas. It is unclear if the carcinomas arise from or adjacent to the follicular neoplasms.

Bibliography

Actinic Keratosis

Brash DE, Ziegler A, Jonason AS et al. (1996) Sunlight and sunburn in human skin cancer: p53, apoptosis, and tumor promotion. J Invest Dermatol Symp Proc 1:136–142

Braun-Falco O, Schmöckel C, Geyer C (1986) Pigmentierte aktinische Keratosen. Hautarzt 37:676–678

Callen JP, Bickers DR, Moy RL (1997) Actinic keratoses. J Am Acad Dermatol 36:650–653

Feldman SR, Fleischer AB Jr, Williford PM et al. (1999) Destructive procedures are the standard of care for treatment of actinic keratoses. J Am Acad Dermatol 40:43–47

Kaugars GE, Pillion T, Svirsky JA et al. (1999) Actinic cheilitis: a review of 152 cases. Oral Surg Oral Med Oral Pathol Oral Radiol Endod 88:181–186

Marks R (1995) An overview of skin cancers. Incidence and causation. Cancer 75:607–612

Neumann J (1869) Sitzungsbericht der Akademischen Wissenschaften Wien, mathematisch-naturwissenschaftliche Klasse

Neumann J (1880) Lehrbuch der Hautkrankheiten, 5. Aufl, Vienna

Picascia DD, Robinson JK (1987) Actinic cheilitis: a review of the etiology, differential diagnosis, and treatment. J Am Acad Dermatol 17:255–264

Prieto VG, Casal M, McNutt NS (1993) Lichen planus-like keratosis. A clinical and histological reexamination. Am J Surg Pathol 17:259–263

Sander CA, Pfeiffer C, Kligman AM et al. (1997) Chemotherapy for disseminated actinic keratoses with 5-fluorouracil and isotretinoin. J Am Acad Dermatol 36: 236–238

Schwartz RA (1996) Premalignant keratinocytic neoplasms. J Am Acad Dermatol 35:223–242

Schwartz RA (1997) The actinic keratosis. A perspective and update. Dermatol Surg 23:1009–1019

Sober AJ, Burstein JM (1995) Precursors to skin cancer. Cancer 75:645–650

Subrt P, Jorizzo JL, Apisarnthanarax P et al. (1983) Spreading pigmented actinic keratosis. J Am Acad Dermatol 8: 63–67

Suchniak JM, Baer S, Goldberg LH (1997) High rate of malignant transformation in hyperkeratotic actinic keratoses. J Am Acad Dermatol 37:392–394

Unis ME (1995) Short-term intensive 5-fluorouracil treatment of actinic keratoses. Dermatol Surg 21:162–163

Radiation Keratoses

Braun-Falco O, Lukacs S, Goldschmidt H (1976) Dermatoradiotherapy. Springer, Berlin

Kurban AK, Farah FS (1969) Effects of X-irradiation of the skin. Acta Derm Venereol (Stockh) 49:64–71

Martin H, Strong E, Spiro RH (1970) Radiation induced cancer of the head and neck. Cancer 25:61–71

Arsenic Keratosis

Maloney ME (1996) Arsenic in dermatology. Dermatol Surg 22:301–304

Schwartz RA (1997) Arsenic and the skin. Int J Dermatol 36: 241–250

Wong SS, Tan KC, Goh CL (1998) Cutaneous manifestations of chronic arsenicism: review of seventeen cases. J Am Acad Dermatol 38:179–185

Tar Keratosis

Götz H (1976) Tar keratosis. In: Andrade R, Gumport SL, Popkin GL et al. (eds) Cancer of the skin. Biology-diagnosis-management. Saunders, Philadelphia, pp 492–523

Schwartz RA (1996) Premalignant keratinocytic neoplasms. J Am Acad Dermatol 35:223–242

Cutaneous Horn

DiMaio DJ, Cohen PR (1998) Trichilemmal horn: case presentation and literature review. J Am Acad Dermatol 39: 368–371

Gould JW, Brodell RT (1999) Giant cutaneous horn associated with verruca vulgaris. Cutis 64:111–112

Thappa DM, Garg BR, Thadeus J et al. (1997) Cutaneous horn: a brief review and report of a case. J Dermatol 24: 34–37

Bowen Disease

Bell HK, Rhodes LE (1999) Bowen's disease – a retrospective review of clinical management. Clin Exp Dermatol 24: 338–339

Bowen JT (1912) Precancerous dermatoses: a study of two cases of chronica atypical epithelial proliferation. J Cutan Dis 30:241–255

Landthaler M, Haina D, Brunner R et al. (1986) Laser therapy of bowenoid papulosis and Bowen's disease. J Dermatol Surg Oncol 12:1253–1257

Lee MM, Wick MM (1993) Bowen's disease. Clin Dermatol 11: 43–46
McGrae JD Jr, Greer CE, Manos MM (1993) Multiple Bowen's disease of the fingers associated with human papilloma virus type 16. Int J Dermatol 32:104–107

Erythroplasia of Queyrat

Goette DK (1974) Erythroplasia of Queyrat. Arch Dermatol 110:271–273
Goette DK (1976) Review of erythroplasia of Queyrat and its treatment. Urology 8:311–315
Goette DK, Carson TE (1976) Erythroplasia of Queyrat: treatment with topical 5-fluorouracil. Cancer 38:1498–1502
Queyrat M (1911) Erythroplasie du gland. Bull Soc Fr Dermatol Syph 22:378–382

Paget Disease

Evans AT, Neven P (1991) Invasive adenocarcinoma arising in extramammary Paget's disease of the vulva. Histopathology 18:355–360
Markopoulos C, Gazet JC (1988) Paget's disease of the nipple occurring after conservative management of early breast cancer. Eur J Surg Oncol 14:77–78
Ojeda VJ, Heenan PJ, Watson SH (1987) Paget's disease of the groin associated with adenocarcinoma of the urinary bladder. J Cutan Pathol 14:227–231
Paget J (1874) On disease of the mammary areola preceding cancer of the mammary gland. St Bartholomew's Hosp Rep 10:87–89
Toker C (1970) Clear cells of the nipple epidermis. Cancer 25:601–610

Extramammary Paget Disease

Cappuccini F, Tewari K, Rogers LW et al. (1997) Extramammary Paget's disease of the vulva: metastases to the bone marrow in the absence of an underlying adenocarcinoma – case report and literature review. Gynecol Oncol 66:146–150
Koh KB, Nazarina AR (1995) Paget's disease of the scrotum: report of a case with underlying carcinoma of the prostate. Br J Dermatol 133:306–307
Kurzl RG (1996) Paget's disease. Semin Dermatol 15:60–66
Mazoujian G, Pinkus GS, Haagensen DE Jr (1984) Extramammary Paget's disease – evidence for an apocrine origin. An immunoperoxidase study of gross cystic disease fluid protein-15, carcinoembryonic antigen, and keratin proteins. Am J Surg Pathol 8:43–50
Morgan JM, Carmichael AJ, Ritchie C (1996) Extramammary Paget's disease of the axilla with an underlying apocrine carcinoma. Acta Derm Venereol 76:173–174

Clear Cell Papulosis

Kuo TT, Huang CL, Chan HL et al. (1987) Clear cell papulosis: a new entity with histogenetic implications for cutaneous paget's disease. Am J Surg Pathol 11:827–834. J Am Acad Dermatol 33:230–233
Lee JY, Chao SC (1998) Clear cell papulosis of the skin. Br J Dermatol 138:678–683

CHAPTER 56

Malignant Epithelial Tumors

Contents

Introduction

The lifetime risk of skin cancer in the USA has been estimated as 1 in 5. More than one-third of all cancers originate in the skin. Over 97% of these are non-melanoma cutaneous cancers, i.e., basal cell carcinoma and squamous cell carcinoma. The correct incidence is probably much higher. Many of these lesions are removed in clinical settings such as a dermatologic practice where reporting is not routine. In addition, histologic confirmation may be performed by the dermatologist, so that the diagnoses are not reflected in pathology records.

Some of the lesions in this chapter are discussed in the German text as pseudomalignancies. The entire family of verrucous carcinoma is confusing, as the lesions are very chronic, histologically bland and only rarely become aggressive squamous cell carcinomas. We have chosen to include them here.

Verrucous Carcinoma

Synonyms. There are many synonyms which vary with the location and are considered below

Definition. Low-grade squamous cell carcinoma with a verrucous clinical appearance, minimal cytologic atypia and a low risk of metastasis.

Etiology and Pathogenesis. Verrucous carcinoma is a puzzling entity. It is a squamous cell carcinoma with relatively indolent behavior, minimal cytologic atypia and pushing margins. In recent years human papillomavirus has been found in a number of the variants, reconfirming the clinical suspicions voiced over the years. In the mouth, tobacco use (chewing tobacco, snuff and betel) is a second clear risk factor, while on the sole trauma appears important. There are four common sites for verrucous carcinoma: the oral cavity, the genitalia, the leg and the sole. Each is covered separately after discussing the microscopic appearance which is the unifying factor.

Histopathology. The epidermis (or epithelium) is hyperplastic and often has rounded projections pushing into the dermis (or lamina propria). In some instances, especially on the sole, there may be marked hyperkeratosis. Typical changes associated with verruca vulgaris such as granular layer inclusions and koilocytes are usually lacking. Mitoses, individual cell keratinization and pleomorphism are all uncommon. Any significant degree of atypia should prompt the diagnosis of ordinary squamous cell carcinoma. Beneath the epithelium, there is usually a brisk inflammatory response which in the mouth and on the genitalia is dominated by plasma cells. Early on, it is very hard to separate a verrucous carcinoma from pseudoepitheliomatous hyperplasia, so multiple biopsies may be required.

Oral Verrucous Carcinoma

(Ackerman 1948)

Synonyms. Carcinoma verrucosum, florid oral papillomatosis (Rock and Fisher 1960), papillomatosis mucosae carcinoides

Epidemiology. In the mouth, verrucous carcinoma accounts for 5–10% of squamous cell carcinomas. The lesions typically arise in older men (60–80 years of age) who have been heavy smokers. The use of smokeless tobacco and chewing tobacco appears to be even more dangerous.

Clinical Findings. Two-thirds of cases involve the buccal mucosa and most of the rest affect the gingiva. Early lesions are white patches or plaques. As they grow, they thicken with protuberant papules and irregular, indurated borders, fancifully resembling a head of cauliflower (Fig. 56.1). Sometimes multiple lesions are present initially and they may coalesce. Very large lesions can interfere with eating or speaking.

Course and Prognosis. About 30% develop into an invasive squamous cell carcinoma, and the number would probably be higher if an old patient population was not involved. Even following treatment, the lesions are likely to recur.

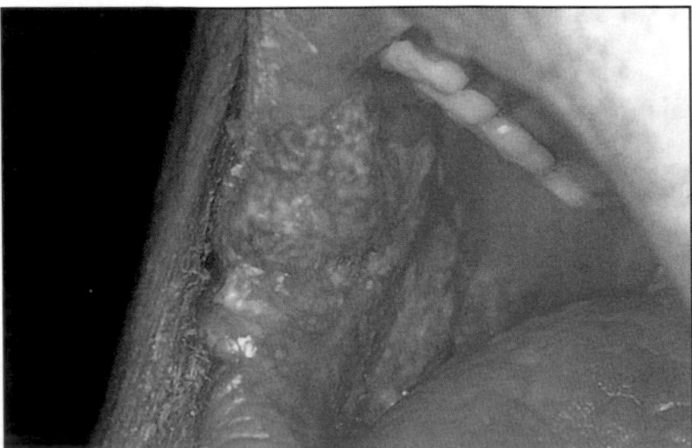

Fig. 56.1. Verrucous carcinoma of mouth

Differential Diagnosis. The differential of leukoplakia is considered in Chapter 33. In most instances, a biopsy is required and the microscopic picture provides the answer. Reactive leukoplakia at one end and speckled erythroplasia or squamous cell carcinoma in situ at the other encompass the spectrum.

Therapy. Surgical excision is preferred when technically possible. Radiation therapy and laser destruction are other possibilities along with photodynamic therapy. Treatment with systemic retinoids and interferons, as well as chemotherapy agents (bleomycin, methotrexate), has been recommended for inoperable lesions.

Papillomatosis Cutis Carcinoides

(Gottron 1932)

Epidemiology. This disease is also more common among the elderly and it almost always presents on the shins. Tumors may develop de novo but more often appear in association with chronic ulcerated lesions such as lupus vulgaris, halogenoderma, deep fungal infections and chronic pyodermas. Verrucous carcinoma is often the type of squamous cell carcinoma that develops in any other chronic ulcer or area of long-standing inflammation.

Clinical Findings. Lesions may be unilateral or bilateral. Large cauliflower-like vegetating masses develop over the shins or the dorsal aspect of the feet and may reach a size of 10–15 cm (Fig. 56.2). Only rarely have tumors on the arms been described. They are typically covered with crust and debris, but tend not to ulcerate. There may be small islands of hyperkeratotic papules or granulation tissue dispersed across the eroded tumor. Often the margin is rolled up or elevated. The tumors bleed easily and may be an entry site for recurrent erysipelas. The inguinal lymph nodes should be routinely evaluated by palpation and ultrasonography.

Course and Prognosis. The tumors slowly expand and thicken. Over many years with repeated biopsies, it is usually possible to identify a verrucous carcinoma.

Differential Diagnosis. The differential diagnosis includes all the many causes for leg ulcers, as well as the predisposing factors listed above.

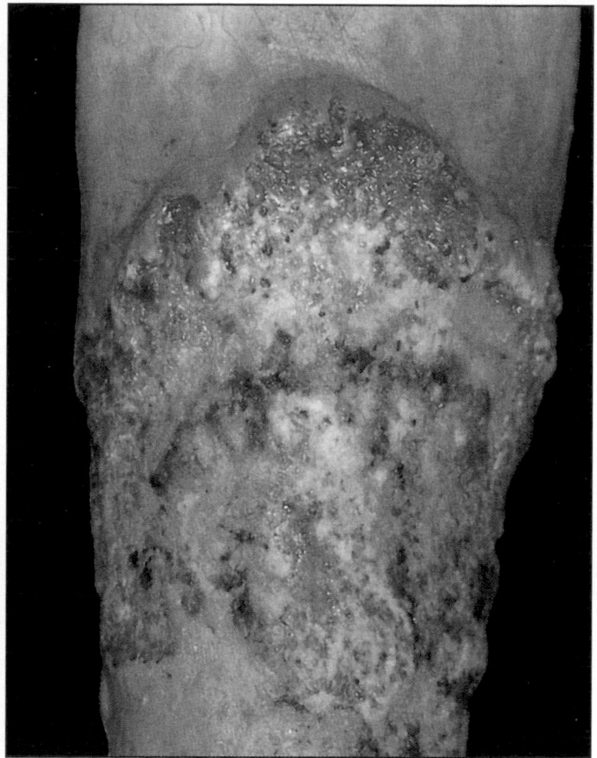

Fig. 56.2. Papillomatosis cutis carcinoides

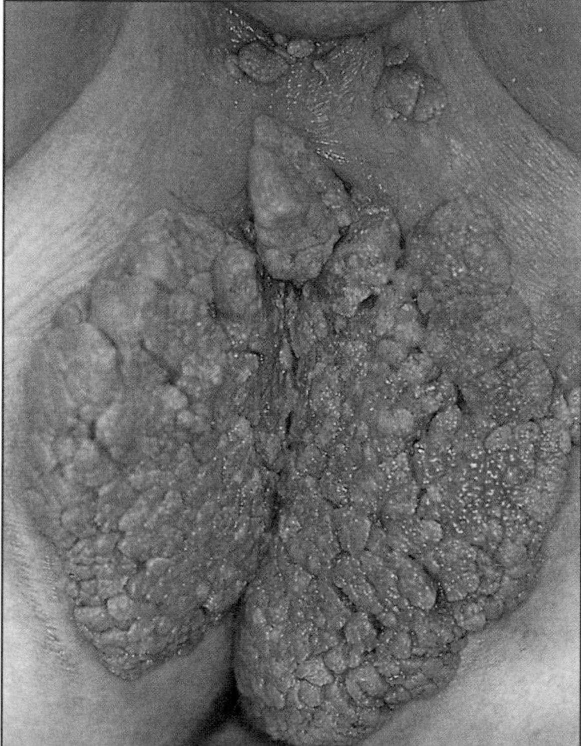

Fig. 56.3. Giant genital wart

Therapy. Surgical excision with graft coverage is the best approach. The same alternatives discussed under oral verrucous carcinoma apply here.

Giant Genital Wart

Synonyms. Condyloma giganteum, Buschke-Löwenstein tumor

This giant verrucous lesion of the genitalia can be grotesque in appearance. HPV6 and HPV11 have been identified in these lesions, making them the most clearly viral members of the verrucous carcinoma family (Chap. 2). The lesions are more common in men, usually involving the distal part of the penis. The groin and perianal area may also be affected (Fig. 56.3).

Epithelioma Cuniculatum
(Aird et al. 1954)

Etiology and Pathogenesis. Epithelioma cuniculatum also appears to be associated with various HPV. It is unclear if the propensity towards persistent growth and malignant change reflects the nature of the virus or the repeated trauma.

Clinical Findings. Epithelioma cuniculatum is a rare tumor found only on the sole. Its name is derived from the Latin word *cuniculus* meaning a rabbit or its burrow. For these large often exophytic lesions typically have crevices and even sinuses. Often there is discharge of pus, blood or cornified debris. The border is callused, just like a plantar wart. Most patients give a history of having had a smaller wart present for many years, which then began to grow and become painful, interfering with walking.

Course and Prognosis. After many years, an invasive growth phase may begin, resulting in a rapidly expanding very painful tumor.

Differential Diagnosis. The question for many years is if a large wart or an early verrucous carcinoma is present. Later when the tumor begins to grow more rapidly, it may resemble an amelanotic malignant melanoma.

Therapy. Generous surgical excision with grafting is usually the best approach, as it will allow earlier ambulation. The same alternatives discussed under oral verrucous carcinoma apply here.

Keratoacanthoma

(Hutchinson 1889; Dupont 1930)

Synonyms. Molluscum sebaceum, molluscum pseudocarcinomatosum

Definition. Quickly growing tumor that develops from a hair follicle, mimics a squamous cell carcinoma microscopically but regresses spontaneously in most cases.

Epidemiology. Most patients are over 60 years of age and men are more often affected than women.

Etiology and Pathogenesis. Almost all keratoacanthomas arise from hair follicles. In many ways, a keratoacanthoma recapitulates the story of the deeper part of the hair follicle, which develops anew from the hair germ, grows rapidly with many mitoses, is then stable for the balance of the hair cycle and finally regresses with marked mesenchymal fibrosis. Occasionally keratoacanthomas are seen on hairless areas, such as the nailbed or oral cavity. One can postulate that epithelial germ cells have differentiated toward a follicular structure.

Its tendency towards spontaneous regression makes keratoacanthoma fascinating tumors. The nature of a keratoacanthoma has long been disputed. In the German version of this book, keratoacanthomas are included as pseudomalignancies. In almost all instances they behave in a benign fashion. Because they so resemble a squamous cell carcinoma microscopically and occasionally behave in an aggressive manner, many view them as low-grade squamous cell carcinomas which the body can usually but not always control.

In several syndromes with multiple keratoacanthomas, there are clearly defined genetic factors. It remains to be determined whether they play a role in sporadic solitary tumors. In at least some instances, mutations in DNA mismatch repair genes, typical of the Muir-Torre syndrome (Chap. 65), have been identified in solitary keratoacanthomas.

In experimental settings, hair-bearing animals can be treated topically with tars and similar agents to reliably produce keratoacanthomas. Sunlight, trauma and industrial exposure all appear to play a role in humans. Smokers have more keratoacanthomas than nonsmokers. In some cases HPV has been identified. Type 25 was first found but many others have been subsequently documented. Immunosuppression also is important as patients receiving cancer chemotherapy or immunosuppressed for other reasons may develop crops of keratoacanthomas. In such immunosuppressed patients, HPV is more likely to be found and play a role. Patients treated with suramin in antineoplastic dosages have developed more keratoacanthomas than expected.

Clinical Findings. A solitary keratoacanthoma has a distinctive history and clinical appearance. The patient describes a rapidly growing nodule that has been initially interpreted as a boil or pimple. Over weeks to months a dome-shaped nodule with a central dell filled by a keratotic plug develops (Fig. 56.4). If the lesion continues to grow, a wide shallow central crater with a peripheral ring evolves. Sometimes waxy debris is extruded; hence the old name molluscum sebaceum. The color is usually pale-red to red-violet with many telangiectases coursing along the wall.

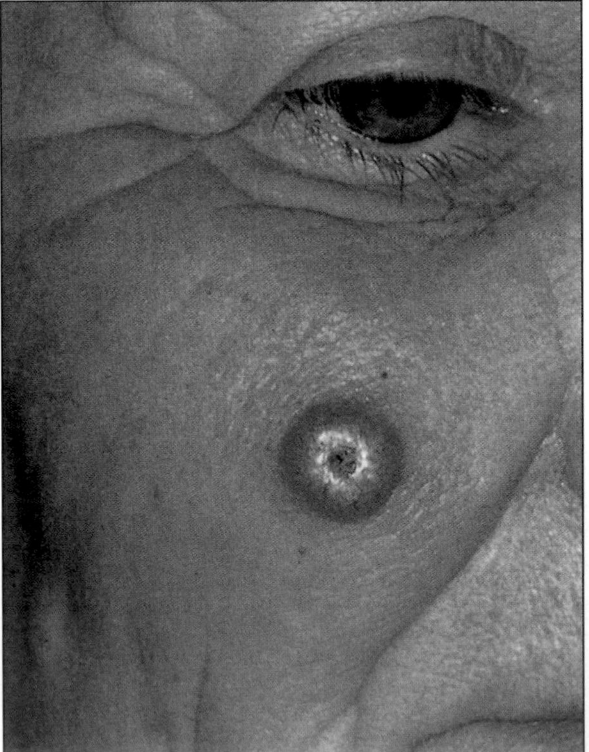

Fig. 56.4. Keratoacanthoma

After a period of months, the keratoacanthoma regresses usually leaving an irregular depressed scar, sometimes with pits and sinuses. Probably the average life of a keratoacanthoma is 6 months. Local recurrences may occur. It is impossible to identify with certainty the rare keratoacanthomas that will not regress but instead behave aggressively and even metastasize.

There are many clinical variants of keratoacanthoma, representing a host of different processes. There is no single unifying feature; some resemble a keratoacanthoma clinically, others, histologically. Included in this group are.

Giant Keratoacanthoma

Synonym. Keratoacanthoma giganteum

An initially typical keratoacanthoma just keeps growing. The most common locations are the nose, eyelids and backs of the hands. Here the distinction between keratoacanthoma and squamous cell carcinoma is most difficult. The tumors may be destructive and even metastasize. They may initially be confused with blastomycosis-like pyoderma or tuberculosis cutis verrucosa. Not all lesions regress, and those that do invariably cause scarring.

Keratoacanthoma Centrifugum Marginatum

(Heid et al. 1979)

In this case, a giant keratoacanthoma just keeps on expanding and never regresses. The clinical picture would never be confused with a solitary keratoacanthoma. Instead there is an elevated peripheral wall that moves outwards, leaving behind an atrophic center (Fig. 56.5). In other words, the keratoacanthoma regresses centrally as it moves peripherally. The lateral wall may have keratotic plugs, resembling that seen in an ordinary keratoacanthoma. The typical locations are the back of the hand and occasionally the legs. Lesions as large as 20 cm may be seen.

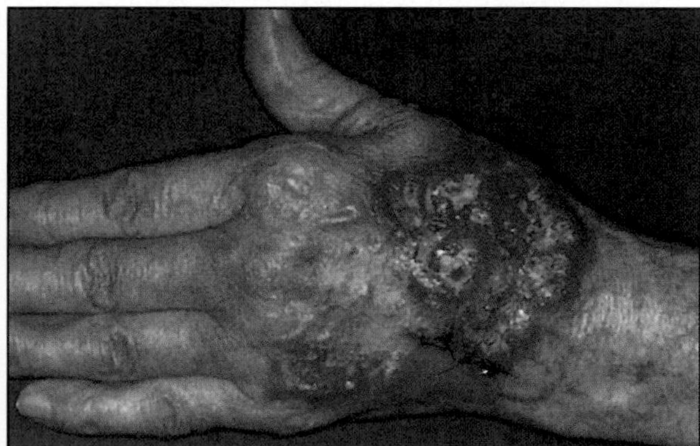

Fig. 56.5. Keratoacanthoma centrifugum marginatum

Multiple Keratoacanthomas

Patients with a particularly unlucky industrial exposure, such as roofers exposed to tar and pitch may over years develop many lesions. They differ from the groups discussed below in that the occurrence is not eruptive and there is not a positive family history.

Generalized Eruptive Keratoacanthomas

(Grzybowski 1950; Witten and Zak 1952)

These patients develop hundreds of lesions, typically involving the face, trunk and often the oral mucosa. In some cases, autosomal dominant inheritance has been shown. The lesions may be nodular without a central crater. In some schemes, Gryzbowski-type refers to those without crateriform lesions and Witten-Zak to those with both types of lesions. In other schools, Gryzbowski is eruptive while Witten-Zak is not. Some of these patients show little tendency to spontaneous regression; in others, regression can be expected. Immunosuppressed patients may also suddenly develop many keratoacanthomas, mimicking the spontaneous disorder.

Muir-Torre Syndrome

Patients with the Muir-Torre syndrome develop multiple keratoacanthomas, multiple sebaceous neoplasms and a wide variety of internal malignancies, inherited in an autosomal dominant pattern. The frequent overlaps between keratoacanthoma and sebaceous neoplasm in these patients suggest that their lesions arise from that part of the follicle where the sebaceous duct empties (Chap. 65).

Ferguson-Smith Syndrome

(Ferguson-Smith 1934)

Synonym. Multiple self-healing epitheliomata

Ferguson-Smith in the 1930s identified several Scottish families in which multiple keratoacanthomas were transmitted in an autosomal dominant fashion. The gene has been localized to chromosome 9q22-q31 but its function is unclear. Typically, Ferguson-Smith patients have striking facial involvement, deep crater-like scars around the mouth and onset at an early age. The tumors are more likely to show perineural involvement than ordinary keratoacanthomas. While almost all their tumors regress, these patients are likely to have at least one aggressive squamous cell carcinoma over their lifetime.

Histopathology. The classic histologic pattern of a fully developed keratoacanthoma is quite distinctive. But there are many problems associated with the pathologic study of keratoacanthomas. First, a biopsy which allows the dermatopathologist to view a transverse section of the entire lesion, studying its architecture, edge and depth, is essential. Small or superficial biopsies are to be discouraged. A keratoacanthoma evolves histologically just as it does clinically. The observer must be able to identify very early and resolving keratoacanthomas. Finally, microscopic study does not allow one to identify those rare tumors that will behave aggressively.

The classic picture is that of a cup-shaped tumor arising from one or a small number of adjacent follicles. Columns of well-differentiated epidermis encase or lip the central plug which is filled with cornified debris. At the base the keratinocytes are enlarged, rich in glycogen and often described as having ground-glass cytoplasm. They cornify without much of a granular layer. At the base, most of the tumor islands are rounded or blunted and create a smooth curved line. Plugs of keratin, often associated with small abscesses, are encased by the pale cytoplasm. Inflammatory cells are also found in the dermis, including neutrophils, histiocytes and plasma cells. Occasionally the infiltrate is rich in eosinophils. In some areas, there may be strands of epithelium infiltrating into the dermis, described as pseudocarcinomatous infiltration. In addition mitoses and cytologic atypia are the rule, not the exception. As the lesion regresses, a thin epidermis is found, often with just a few irregular projections. The cup is less invaginated, so that the lesion is more exophytic and keratotic.

Each dermatopathologist will develop his own approach to reporting keratoacanthomas. Most have some sort of standard text saying "keratoacanthoma, but squamous cell carcinoma cannot be entirely ruled out." One is justified to diagnose a keratoacanthoma when an adequate specimen is available and the above criteria are met. The stumbling block is that almost all, but not all, keratoacanthomas regress.

Differential Diagnosis. An early lesion may be mistaken for molluscum contagiosum or furuncle. Later on, one may consider basal cell carcinoma which grows more slowly, has a pearly border and is firmer to palpation, or squamous cell carcinoma, which tends to arise on sunlight-damaged skin, grows more slowly and is rarely dome-shaped or crateriform.

Therapy. Theoretically, no therapy is needed but few trust themselves to observe such a dramatic lesion. In addition, an excisional biopsy is the only way to confirm the diagnosis. All recommended therapies are hard to evaluate because so many keratoacanthomas involute spontaneously. We prefer excision. Larger keratoacanthomas or those in areas where recurrence is common, such as the nose, should always be excised. Small lesions can be tangentially excised or curetted, especially when dealing with patients with hundreds of lesions.

Radiation therapy is also a possibility: 20–40 Gy suffices, given in eight to ten divided doses. Intralesional 5-fluorouracil (0.5–1.0 ml of 10 mg/ml) can also be used. Roughly one-half of the dose is injected into the tumor and the balance injected at the base. The procedure usually must be repeated one or two additional times. Other reports endorse intralesional bleomycin, methotrexate and even triamcinolone acetonide; we have no experience with these modalities.

The patient should be aware that the lesion in most cases is easily removed and does not come back. But it is smart to warn him that one cannot always separate this lesion from a squamous cell carcinoma, so that follow-up is mandatory and in rare cases, additional therapy will be needed.

Squamous Cell Carcinoma

Definition. Malignant epithelial tumor which in the skin usually arises from an actinic keratosis or other form of carcinoma in situ.

Epidemiology. The same epidemiologic factors discussed under actinic keratoses (Chap. 55) apply to squamous cell carcinoma. In Germany the incidence is 6:100,000 for women and 12:100,000 for men. In the southwestern USA and in Australia the incidence rages from 30–60:100,000. The ratio of basal cell carcinoma to squamous cell carcinoma ranges from 5:1 to 10:1 in white populations. In blacks and other darker-skinned races, the ratio is lower, i.e., squamous cell carcinoma is more common.

Etiology and Pathogenesis. The etiology of squamous cell carcinoma is covered under the discussions of actinic keratoses, other carcinomas in situ and verrucous carcinomas. Table 56.1 summarizes some of the pathogenic factors.

Irradiation. In addition to sunlight, which leads to actinic keratoses and then rarely squamous cell carcinomas, other forms of irradiation are important. Squamous cell carcinomas are common in skin damaged by therapy with ionizing radiation. In addition, both long-term UV and PUVA therapy increase the risk of squamous cell carcinoma. Heat, in the absence of light, is also a factor, as shown by the kangri ulcers of the abdomen in Tibet and other parts of Asia where heated coals are held against the body. Another example is the presence of squamous cell carcinomas on the legs in patients with erythema ab igne, following chronic exposure to open fires.

Table 56.1. Pathogenic factors for squamous cell carcinoma

Cause	Date	Author(s)
Scrotal cancer in chimney sweeps	1775	Pott
Arsenic	1822	Paris
Tight or abnormal scars	1828	Marjolin
Burn scars	1860	Hertreux
Coal tar	1876	Volkmann
Petroleum oil	1876	Bell
Sunlight	1894	Unna
Ionizing radiation	1902	Frieben
Creosote	1930	Heller
Iatrogenic immunosuppression	1970	Penn
PUVA therapy	1979	Stern et al.
HPV (oncogenic viruses)	1982	Ostrow et al.

Chronic Degenerative and Inflammatory Processes. A wide variety of scars may predispose to squamous cell carcinoma, including burn scars, healed lupus vulgaris, radiation dermatitis, acrodermatitis chronica atrophicans and even discoid lupus erythematosus. Tight or bound-down scars are at far greater risk than scars in loose skin, such as a typical appendectomy scar. A ulcer in such a scar is known as a Marjolin ulcer (Marjolin 1828) and the possible subsequent tumor as a Marjolin tumor. Draining sinuses or fistulas, such as from osteomyelitis or acne inversa, also pose a risk, as do chronic leg ulcers. On mucosal surfaces, chronic inflammation such as in erosive lichen planus may rarely evolve into squamous cell carcinoma.

Chemical Carcinogenesis. The most common causes are petroleum products, a variety of other hydrocarbons and in the mouth, tobacco products. In a study of more than 600 tar refinery workers in Germany, there was a long latency period between tar exposure and skin cancers. About 20% of the workers developed keratoacanthomas, while the ratio of squamous cell carcinoma to basal cell carcinoma was 1.7:1. Arsenic is a factor in several parts of the world because of both industrial exposure and groundwater rich in or contaminated by the chemical.

Oncogenic Viruses. Human papillomavirus is the most common human oncogenic virus, best documented with types 16 and 18 in carcinoma of the cervix. HPV has been identified in a variety of genital, anal and oral squamous cell carcinomas, as well as occasionally in skin tumors.

Immunosuppression. The tendency to squamous cell carcinomas was first clearly shown in renal transplant patients, in whom the ratio of squamous cell carcinoma to basal carcinoma is closer to 1:1. Similar observations have been made in HIV/AIDS patients. All immunosuppressed patients are more susceptible to oncogenic viruses. Patients with kidney and heart transplantation are at greater risk of both cutaneous and lip squamous cell carcinomas.

Personal Habits. Both alcohol and tobacco use are significant factors. Many oral and upper airway tumors are far more common in patients consuming these products.

Clinical Findings. Since most squamous cell carcinomas evolve from a precursor lesion, they rarely have a distinct clinical picture. The question always is: has this actinic keratosis, large persistent plantar wart or thickened ulcer rim progressed to a squamous cell carcinoma? Unfavorable signs include rapid growth, induration, ulceration and bleeding (Fig. 56.6). At some point the tumor becomes so abnormal that it is identified. Thus classic descriptions of squamous cell carcinomas deal with a late stage. Typically one sees a hard exophytic, often inflamed nodule (Fig. 56.7). Sometimes when one presses on the nodule, masses of keratin are extruded (*vermiottes* in French, or little worms). The tumor may outgrow its blood supply and become ulcerated and necrotic. The growth is more destructive than a basal cell carcinoma and more likely to produce metastases.

The risk of metastasis varies greatly depending on the precursor lesion and location of the squamous cell carcinoma, as well as on its degree of differentiation. Those that evolve from actinic keratoses, especially located on the hands, almost never metastasize. Facial lesions are also usually content to spread locally, but we have seen a number of fatal squamous cell carcinomas evolve out of hypertrophic actinic keratoses on bald scalps in elderly men. Another possible site is the finger or nailbed, especially of the thumb or great toe. Typically the precursor lesion is Bowen disease. Lip lesions have a higher risk, somewhere in between that for skin and that for oral mucosa. Genital lesions also have a poor prognosis. Squamous cell carcinomas arising in radiation dermatitis or tuberculosis scars are most likely to metastasize. In our patient collection, the total rate of metastasis is about 2.5%.

There are a number of clinical locations in which a squamous cell carcinoma either looks or behaves a bit differently. We have thus chosen to consider some of these lesions separately.

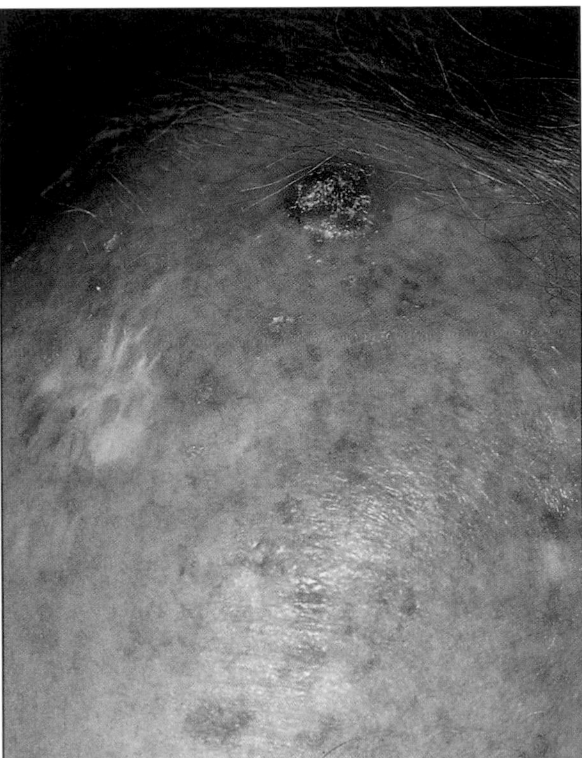

Fig. 56.6. Squamous cell carcinoma of scalp arising amidst actinically damaged skin and multiple actinic keratoses

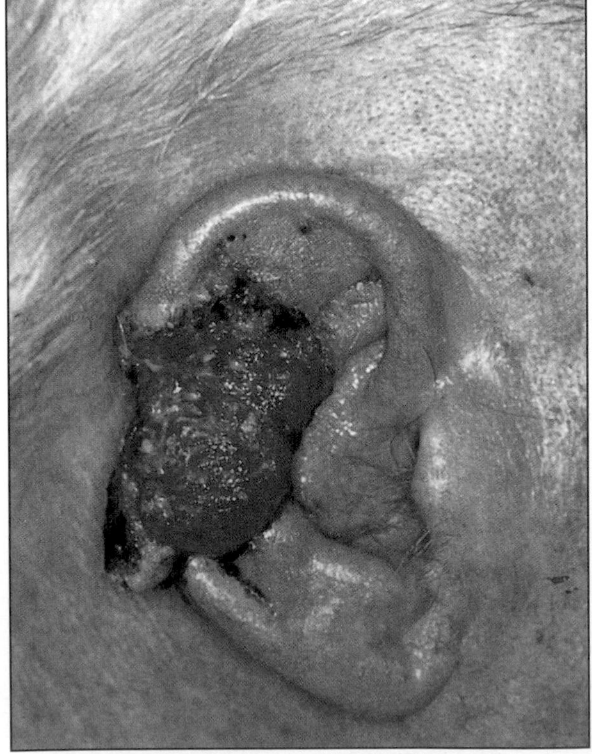

Fig. 56.7. Advanced squamous cell carcinoma of ear

Labial Squamous Cell Carcinoma

On the lip a squamous cell carcinoma has a worse prognosis than the same tumor arising a few centimeters away on the forehead. About two-thirds of the squamous cell carcinomas seen by dermatologists involve the lip. The male to female ratio is at least 20:1 and usually the lower lip of older patients is affected (Fig. 56.8). In German one speaks of the lower lip as one of the "sun terraces" of the face. Both the vermilion and the adjacent skin may show sunlight-induced damage.

There are almost always precursor lesions such as either actinic cheilitis or damage from smoking, primarily pipe smoking. Smokeless tobacco affects the buccal mucosa, not the lip. Initially the patient may just notice the slightest crusting. As the diseases progresses, the patient acquires a multicolored lip with subtle small areas of red, white, yellow and brown, reflecting varying degrees of hyperkeratosis, vascular proliferation and inflammation.

The two most disturbing signs are ulceration and induration. While a tiny erosion may be the first sign, on palpation there is usually minimal thickening and hardening. Sometimes a tiny nodule will first arise and then ulcerate. The erosions or ulcerations are almost always painless and often overlooked.

One can think of an early squamous cell carcinoma of the lip as growing in all directions. Patients and physicians tend to be reassured as long as there is no exophytic growth, but this is a false hope. Downward indurated growth is far more common and more worrying. In addition, there may be lateral spread, which coupled with the multicentricity of actinic cheilitis, means several tumors may be present at the same time. If the lip is thickened or distorted by the tumor, the stage is usually quite advanced. Any time that squamous cell carcinoma of the lip is suspected, a careful search for regional lymph nodes should be made by palpation and with ultrasonography.

Differential Diagnosis. The differential diagnosis may also include a painless chancre, verruca vulgaris, verrucous carcinoma, lichen planus and other forms of leukoplakia (Chap. 33). Basal cell carcinoma is uncommon about the lower lip and almost never extends onto the vermilion.

Lingual Squamous Cell Carcinoma

This is the second most common oral tumor after lip carcinoma. It too is far more common in older men than women or younger individuals. The greatest risk factor is tobacco. Pipe and cigar smoking is worse than cigarette smoking, except in those countries where reverse smoking is practiced. Here, the proximity of the burning cigarette tip to the tongue causes considerable problems. Other major risk factors include chronic inflammation, especially ulcerative lichen planus, and HPV. Syphilitic gumma also may evolve into squamous cell carcinoma. About 50% of lesions arise on the posterior lateral border of the tongue and another 30% on the posterior portion or base. Thus painless tongue carcinomas are easily overlooked (Fig. 56.9). The most classic presentation is a nonhealing ulcer; occasionally a white patch of leukoplakia may be seen. The tongue is difficult to biopsy and the dermatologist is well-advised to refer the patient to an oral surgeon or otorhinolaryngologist. A search for

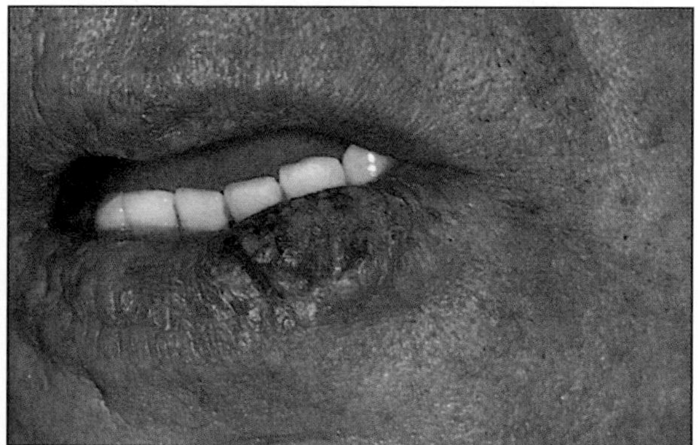

Fig. 56.8. Squamous cell carcinoma of lower lip

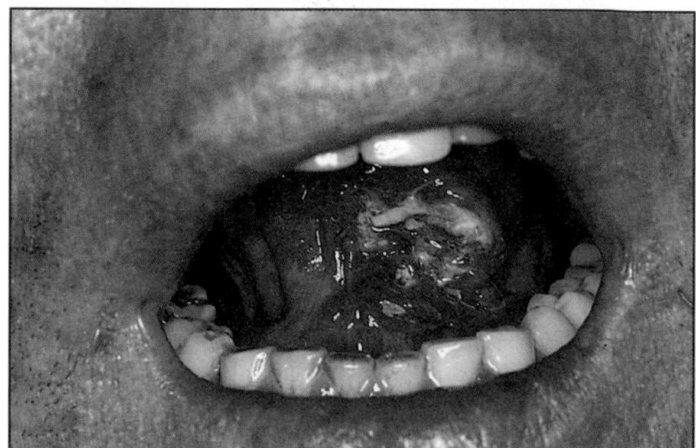

Fig. 56.9. Squamous cell carcinoma of base of tongue

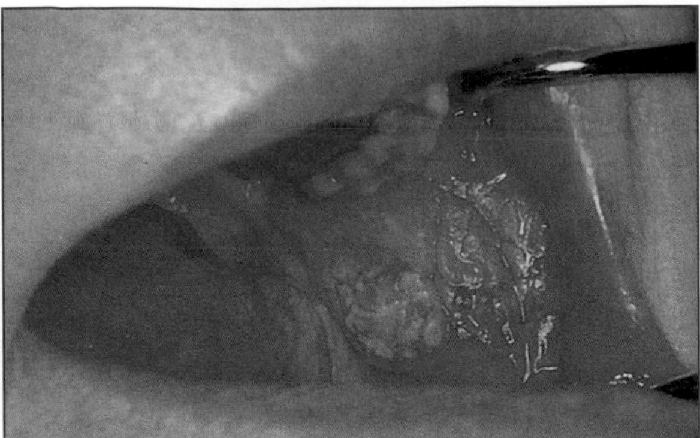

Fig. 56.10. Squamous cell carcinoma arising in area of leukoplakia

regional lymph node enlargement including ultrasonography is mandatory. Unfortunately, metastases are common, even at the time of first diagnosis.

Other oral carcinomas may present as areas of leukoplakia or erythroplasia (Chap. 33). Mixed lesions, often designated speckled leukoplakia, are more likely to evolve into a squamous cell carcinoma. Thickening or development of nodules in an area of leukoplakia often indicates malignant change (Fig. 56.10).

Penile Squamous Cell Carcinoma

This is a tumor of older, uncircumcised individuals. Risk factors appear to include poor hygiene perhaps leading to smegma accumulation, HPV and chronic inflammation. In horses, the risk among castrated geldings is tenfold greater than among stallions. The role of erections in cleansing the space under the foreskin is felt to be decisive. It is not a trivial problem as over 20% of all cancers in male horses involve the penis. Human smegma has been show to be carcinogenic in mice. In addition, chronic balanitis may rarely evolve into squamous cell carcinoma, as may lichen sclerosus et atrophicus. Erythroplasia of Queyrat is a squamous cell carcinoma in situ, often involving the penis, so its malignant potential should come as no surprise.

Almost all tumors are found on the glans (Fig. 56.11). The most common sites are the dorsal surface and the coronal sulcus. Occasionally lesions will develop on the inner side of the foreskin. As with so many tumors on transitional sites, the two

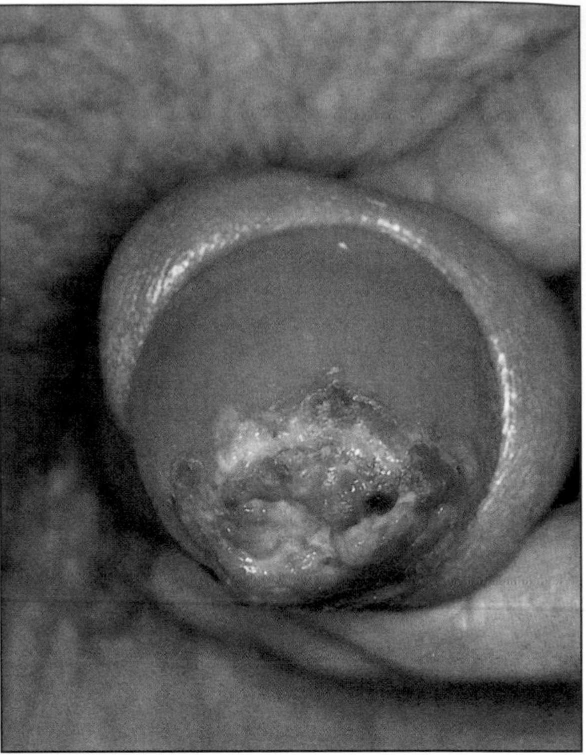

Fig. 56.11. Penile squamous cell carcinoma

main presentations are an indurated erosion or an exophytic verrucous papule or nodule. The induration on palpation is remarkable and pathognomonic. Unfortunately the erosions are often ignored. The risk of metastasis is considerable, so one should be eager to biopsy, as it is a fair assumption that the patient will have delayed in presenting. We transfer our patients immediately to the urologists. Lesions on the shaft are often related to HPV and do not carry the same risk as carcinoma of the glans.

Vulvar Squamous Cell Carcinoma

This too is a tumor of older individuals, usually involving the transition between the labia majora and labia minora. One again, one can identify predisposing factors, such as lichen sclerosus et atrophicus, as well as precancerous lesions, such as Bowen disease and extramammary Paget disease. Erosions and verrucous lesions may be seen. Indurated or infiltrated lesions often suggest that the diagnosis has been made too late (Fig. 56.12).

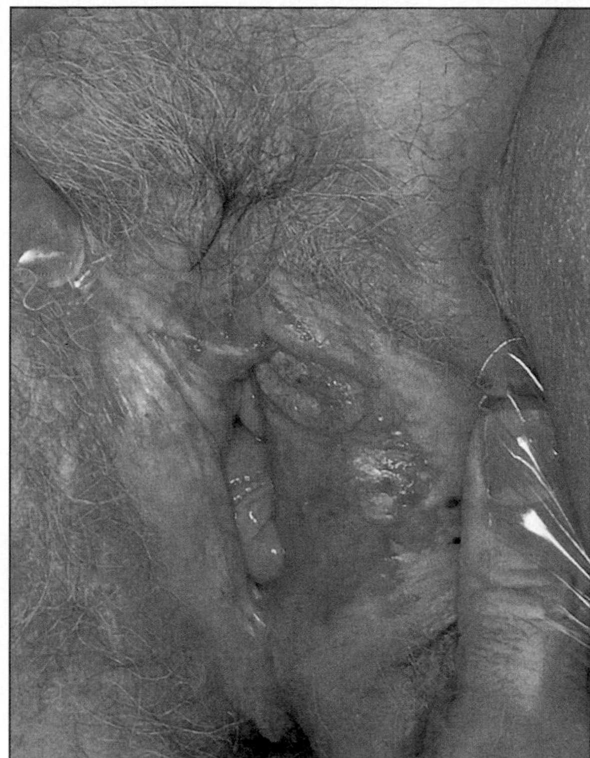

Fig. 56.12. Vulvar squamous cell carcinoma arising in area of erythroplasia of Queyrat

Histopathology. A squamous cell carcinoma consists of a proliferation of atypical keratinocytes that extends into the dermis and perhaps beyond. The transition between actinic keratosis (and other carcinomas in situ) and squamous cell carcinoma is just as hard to identify under the microscope as it is clinically. The standard is the presence of tumor cells in the dermis. When one or two small islands are found beneath an actinic keratosis, most dermatopathologists hedge a bit, with terms such as "squamous cell carcinoma arising in an actinic keratosis" or "microinvasive squamous cell carcinoma."

Squamous cell carcinomas in the skin are not too different from those in other organs. There is an infiltrative proliferation of atypical epithelial cells, in this case keratinocytes that show varying degrees of differentiation or keratinization. Mitoses, including abnormal mitoses, are common; the cells are frequently large and bizarre. Well-differentiated lesions may show individual cell keratinization or even more organoid changes such as small concentric lamellated accumulations of cornified debris, surrounded by strands of tumor cells and known as either squamous eddies or horn pearls. Less-differentiated lesions show no keratinization but still show the intercellular bridges or spinous processes so typical of keratinocytes. Poorly differentiated lesions lack all these features and are anaplastic with frequent mitoses. There is almost always a prominent host response, consisting of both inflammatory cells, primarily lymphocytes and plasma cells, occasionally eosinophils, and dermal fibrosis.

Broders' grading of squamous cell carcinomas (Broders 1921) is not as useful in the skin as in other organs, but it is still of prognostic value. It is based on the percentage of cells that show no sign of keratinization, a hard feature to unambiguously identify. The grades are:

Grade I	< 25 % undifferentiated cell
Grade II	< 50 % undifferentiated cells
Grade III	< 75 % undifferentiated cells
Grade IV	> 75 % undifferentiated cells

Other probably more valuable prognostic factors include the diameter and the thickness of the lesion, as well as the level of invasion. Lesions less than 1 cm in diameter have over a 99 % cure rate. As the diameter increases both the risk of local recurrence and distant metastases increases. A tumor thickness of greater than 4 mm and penetration through the dermis into the fat are also associated with a greater likelihood of recurrence and metastasis. Perineural involvement is also an unfavorable sign.

There are several histologic variants of squamous cell carcinoma which have few if any distinct clinical correlates and do not affect prognosis. A spindle cell squamous cell carcinoma must be separated from a malignant melanoma with immunohistochemistry. The former is positive for keratin; the latter for S100. In the past, when one relied on intercellular bridges, mistakes were common. An atypical fibroxanthoma without much atypia can also appear similar, but a failure to identify this tumor has fewer consequences.

Desmoplastic squamous cell carcinomas have narrow strands of atypical squamous epithelium, sometimes with foci of keratinization, infiltrating through or surrounded by a thickened stroma. There may be perineural or perivascular infiltration or extensive cutaneous spread which may not be clinically apparent. In a large German series, about 8 % of squamous cell carcinomas had desmoplastic features. These tumors showed over 20 % local recurrence and 20 % metastases, even when treated with micrographic surgery.

The acantholytic and clear-cell variants of squamous cell carcinoma are analogous to and develop from the similarly named actinic keratosis variants. Even less common is the signet-ring squamous cell carcinoma, a type of clear-cell squamous cell carcinoma in which the nuclei are pushed to the side, mimicking a signet ring, as is seen in breast and gastric carcinomas. An adenoid squamous cell carcinoma is quite uncommon. It has a very glandular pattern and may be mistaken for either a basal cell carcinoma or a metastasis.

Course and Prognosis. The prognosis is dependent on the location, size, thickness and degree of differentiation of the tumor. Patients with squamous cell carcinomas arising from actinic keratoses on sunlight-damaged skin have an excellent outlook as metastases are rare. Intermediate-risk lesions are those of the ear, lip and nonexposed sites such as the sole or perineum. Tumors with the highest malignant potential are those arising in scars, especially burn scars, chronic inflammation, previously irradiated sites or Bowen disease. Patients with tumors greater than 2 cm in diameter, 4 mm in thickness, reaching the fat, or showing lack of differentiation, have a progressively worse outlook, with recurrences and metastases ranging from 5–10% in various studies. Once regional lymph node involvement has occurred, the 5-year survival is around 20–25%. Squamous cell carcinomas in transitional areas, such as the lip, penis and vulva have a worse outlook, while intraoral disease is the least favorable of those conditions considered above.

Differential Diagnosis. Squamous cell carcinoma must be distinguished from all the precursor lesions discussed above and in Chapter 55. In addition, a wide variety of benign and malignant adnexal tumors, as well as an amelanotic malignant melanoma must be excluded. An irritated seborrheic keratosis may also be confused with a squamous cell carcinoma. In brief, any nodular, indurated or ulcerated lesion in a clinical risk setting should be biopsied to exclude squamous cell carcinoma.

Therapy. Treatment is not dissimilar to that of basal cell carcinoma, as discussed below in more detail. The British Association of Dermatologists has issued guidelines for treating squamous cell carcinoma which we find helpful. The recommended approach considers the size of the tumor, the location and other risk factors. Therapy must also be adjusted to the age and general condition of the patient.

The mainstay is excision. For low-risk tumors less than 2 cm in diameter a minimum 4-mm margin is recommended and can be expected to completely remove 95% of all tumors. For larger or higher-risk tumors, microscopically controlled surgery or larger margins are suggested. In the special locations, additional techniques may be useful. On the lip, invasive tumors are treated by wedge-shaped excisions; up to one-third of the lip can be removed and the wound closed primarily. Larger lesions require flaps or other procedures. Tongue, penile and vulvar lesions are best referred to other specialists. Some invasive lesions require more aggressive surgery, such as removal of a finger for an invasive subungual squamous cell carcinoma or penectomy for selected tumors.

For small low-risk tumors less than 1 cm in diameter that have been histologically confirmed, both deep cryotherapy and curettage and electrodesiccation produce cure rates over 95%, comparable to those achieved by surgery. We are hesitant to recommend these therapies when excision is feasible, but instead reserve them for special cases.

Radiation therapy is also appropriate. A cumulative dose ranging from 50 to 80 Gy is employed with fractionated doses of 3–5 Gy daily. Once again, older patients who are poor operative risks are the best candidates. Rapidly growing tumors also are effectively treated with radiation therapy. Lesions involving the eyelids and lips are especially suitable. Ear lesions, with the underlying cartilage, and hand lesions do less well; they may be treated with a lower voltage to reduce penetration. Considerably different regimens are used for squamous cell carcinoma of the tongue, where often aggressive radiation therapy can provide a life-saving cure and still preserve function.

Sentinel lymph node dissection (Chap. 58) may also be appropriate for high-risk squamous cell carcinoma. Both lymph node dissections and chemotherapy may be necessary in selected cases. The dermatologist is unlikely to be involved in either of these procedures, but should be aware of what is being done to his patient.

Follow-up may involve many physicians. In Germany, patients receive a wallet-sized "follow-up record" which facilitates the interaction. We prefer to see our patients every 3 months for the first year and then every 6 months. In addition to observing the tumor site, one must examine the regional lymph nodes and search for new primary lesions. Ultrasonography is useful both for monitoring the operative scar and the regional lymph nodes. The follow-up also leads to earlier detection of other tumors, as most patients have significant risk factors.

Basal Cell Carcinoma

(KROMPECHER 1900)

Synonyms. Basal cell epithelioma, basalioma, rodent ulcer

Definition. Common slowly growing locally aggressive tumor which rarely if ever metastasizes. For this reason it is also designated "epithelioma", suggesting a lower grade of malignancy.

Epidemiology.

- Incidence. In sunny areas inhabited by white people, the incidence is very high. The incidence in Europe is 40–80/10,000; in the southern USA, 300/10,000 and in Australia over 1600/10,000. The incidence has doubled in all these areas over the past 15 years. In the USA, over 500,000 basal cell carcinomas are reported yearly; many more probably are treated but escape statistical analysis. Basal cell carcinomas are about ten times as common as squamous cell carcinomas in the USA.
- Age. More common in patients over 60 years of age.
- Gender. More common in men than women, probably because of increased sunlight exposure in the past.
- Race. Much less common in darker-skinned individuals, in whom squamous cell carcinomas are proportionately more common.
- Occupation. Outdoor exposure favors their development.
- Geography. More common in patients living at higher altitudes and closer to the equator.

Etiology and Pathogenesis. Many different clues to the origin of basal cell carcinoma exist.

Genetics. In recent years many insights into both the molecular biology and embryologic source of basal cell carcinoma have been obtained. The gene in nevoid basal cell carcinoma syndrome is located on chromosome 9q22.3; it has been designated as the PTCH gene, a homologue of the patched gene in *Drosophila.* The patched gene is important in the segmental development of the insect, controlling growth and regulating form. Mutations in the PTCH gene have also been identified in sporadic basal cell carcinoma. Other genetic factors also play a role. Clearly skin color is a very important factor. Even in nevoid basal cell carcinoma syndrome, black patients have very few basal cell carcinomas. This phenomenon is explained by the increased solar protection offered by dark skin.

Sunlight. The best-established extrinsic risk factor for the development of a basal cell carcinoma is sunlight exposure. But basal cell carcinomas occur on non-sun-damaged skin, while actinic keratoses do not. Finally, they are uncommon on the back of the hand, where sunlight damage is common.

Ionizing Radiation. A dose of about 10 Gy is sufficient to markedly increase the risk of developing a basal cell carcinoma. The average latency period is about 25–35 years, although tumors have appeared within a few years. Just as with sunlight, ionizing radiation may produce basal cell carcinomas without the dramatic chronic radiation damage, although they also arise in chronic radiation dermatitis.

Carcinogens. Chronic ingestion of or exposure to inorganic arsenic compounds may induce basal cell carcinomas along with other cutaneous and internal malignancies. Many of the basal cell carcinomas are of the superficial type.

Chronic Skin Damage. Basal cell carcinomas may develop in damaged skin, but this is more typical of squamous cell carcinoma. Basal cell carcinomas have been described in immunization scars, traumatized scars and beneath prostheses. Persistent ulcers, such as in severe stasis dermatitis, may also develop basal cell carcinoma, although often the correct answer is an ulcerated basal cell carcinoma that was misdiagnosed.

Other Factors. Immunosuppressed patients have a greater risk of developing basal cell carcinomas but exact immunologic factors have not been determined.

Surprisingly, for years, the source of the most common human tumor remained a mystery. The name basal cell carcinoma suggests that the tumor arises from the epidermal basal cells and for years this was accepted, since the tumor cells are small, round, basophilic and with any imagination can be thought of as basal cells. Recent immunohistochemical studies suggest that the basal cell carcinomas develop from pluripotential epidermal cells either in the basal layer or in the outer root sheath of the hair follicle. The cytokeratin patterns of basal cell carcinomas and tumors of hair follicle origin show striking similarities. For example, most basal cell carcinomas express keratins 5 and 14, typical of the basal layer of the epidermis and follicle, but fail to express keratins 1 and 10 which are found in the spinous layer. Basal cell carcinomas also express keratins associated with follicular differentiation. Thus one can argue scientifically that a basal cell carcinoma is an adnexal tumor, but we have chosen to retain it in this chapter.

Clinical Findings. The vast bulk of basal cell carcinomas are found on the face. In about 80% of patients they occur above a line connecting the corners of the mouth to the bottom of the ears. The lower part of the face, the scalp and the upper part of the trunk are less common sites. Basal cell carcinomas typically arise on normal skin and are painless. Actinic keratoses may be markers for basal cell carcinoma, but are not precursors. Basal cell carcinomas have a large number of both histologic and clinical variants. Because they are such common tumors, one must be aware of all these variants to avoid overlooking a basal cell carcinoma. The differential diagnosis will be discussed with each variant as it changes from type to type.

Initial Basal Cell Carcinoma

Early basal cell carcinomas are very subtle. Often one may seen only a tiny indurated pearly area with a few telangiectases. The patient may complain of a crusted or scabbed area, perhaps one that bleeds after shaving, and never heals. Lesions about the cheek and nose are often first blamed on irritation from eyeglasses. Thus, any nonhealing spot on the face should be suspected of being a basal cell carcinoma, no matter what the history nor how innocent the appearance.

Nodular Basal Cell Carcinoma

This variant is the most common. There is a nodular tumor with a pearly or waxy border, prominent telangiectases (Fig. 56.13) and sometimes a central dell or ulceration with crust. The tumor may bleed when the crust is removed by the patient or physician. The differential diagnosis include adnexal tumors and minimal pigmented melanocytic nevi, although once the typical central ulceration occurs, the answer is easier. A keratoacanthoma also has a telangiectatic border, but is more elevated and grows more rapidly.

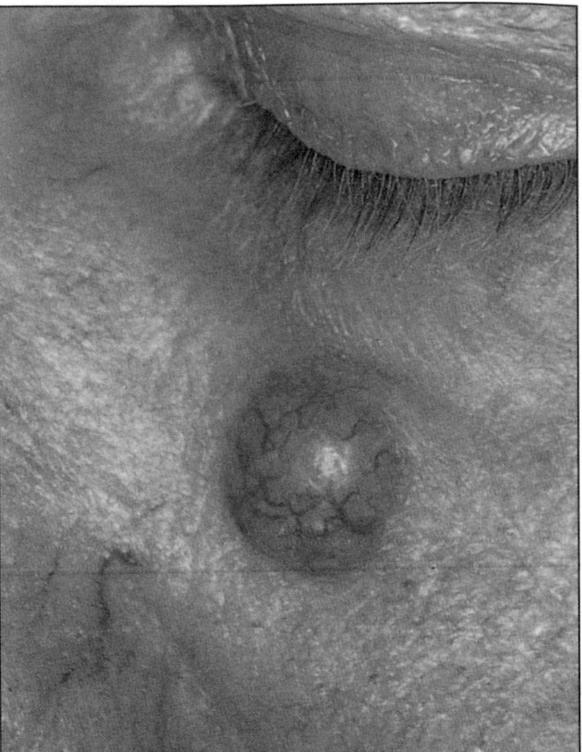

Fig. 56.13. Nodular basal cell carcinoma

Ulcerated Basal Cell Carcinoma

The old term of ulcus rodens or rodent ulcer is no longer applied, out of respect for our patients. A large destructive basal cell carcinoma can have such a ragged border that one can imagine a rodent created the lesion by gnawing. Such lesions are most common in the nasolabial fold, medial canthus and about the ear (Fig. 56.14). On the lower aspect of the legs, such tumors may frequently be mistaken for a stasis or traumatic ulcer and ignored, so that they reach giant proportions. They are surprisingly painless, frequently bleed, and can best be distinguished from traumatic ulcers by their pearly border.

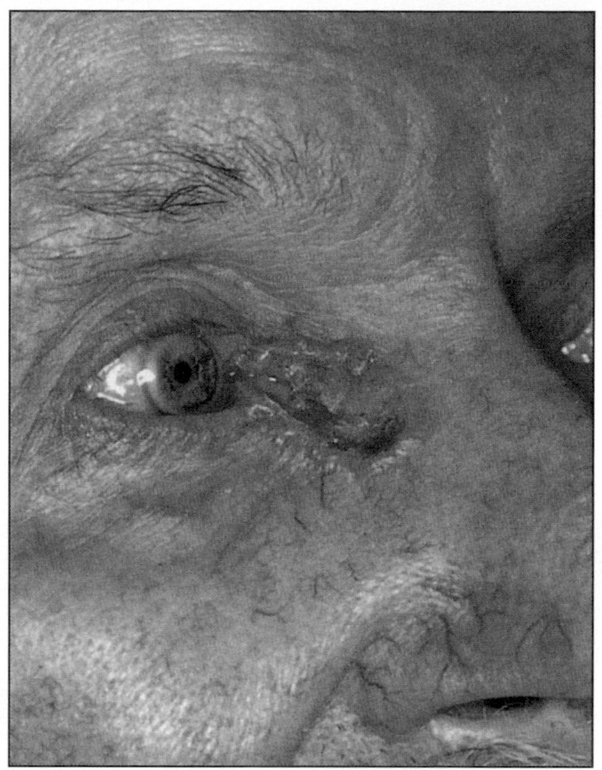

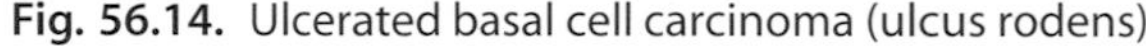
Fig. 56.14. Ulcerated basal cell carcinoma (ulcus rodens)

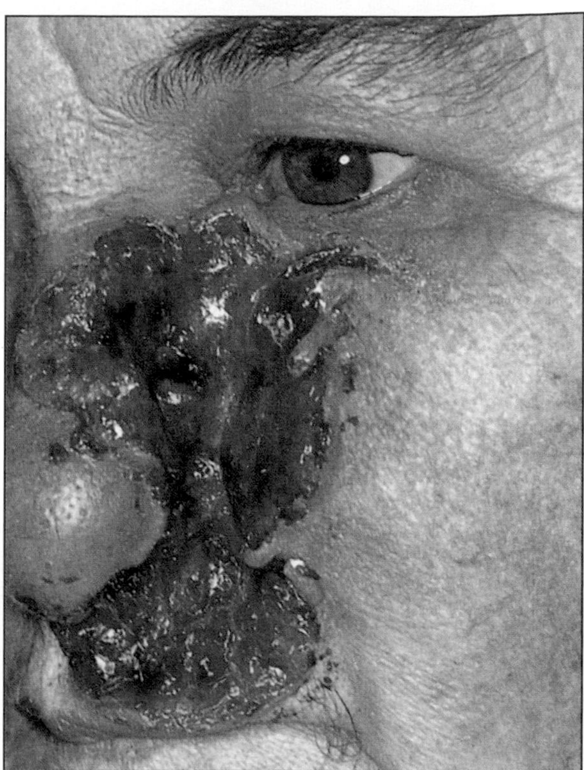

Fig. 56.15. Ulcerated basal cell carcinoma (ulcus terebrans)

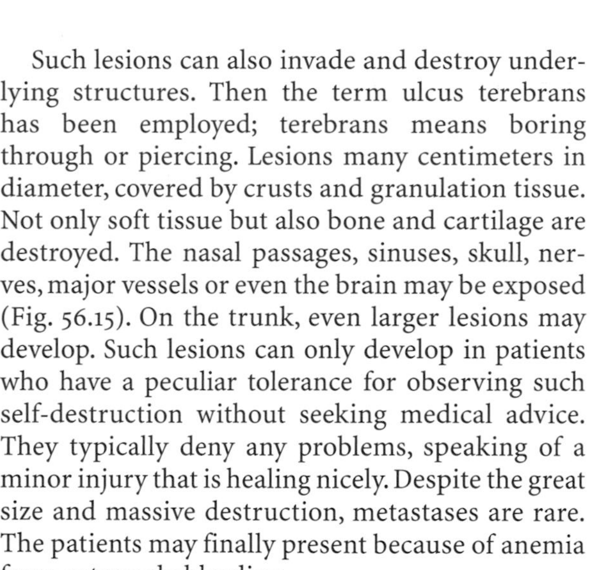
Such lesions can also invade and destroy underlying structures. Then the term ulcus terebrans has been employed; terebrans means boring through or piercing. Lesions many centimeters in diameter, covered by crusts and granulation tissue. Not only soft tissue but also bone and cartilage are destroyed. The nasal passages, sinuses, skull, nerves, major vessels or even the brain may be exposed (Fig. 56.15). On the trunk, even larger lesions may develop. Such lesions can only develop in patients who have a peculiar tolerance for observing such self-destruction without seeking medical advice. They typically deny any problems, speaking of a minor injury that is healing nicely. Despite the great size and massive destruction, metastases are rare. The patients may finally present because of anemia from extremely bleeding.

The differential diagnosis initially may include all the different types of ulcers. But on the face, one should always suspect a basal cell carcinoma as a likely cause of ulceration. Factitial ulcers are about the only other facial ulceration that may occasionally mimic a large ulcerated basal cell carcinoma. The trick is to observe and biopsy the border, because tumor cells may be hard to find in the central part of the ulcer.

Pigmented Basal Cell Carcinoma

Pigmented basal cell carcinomas are most commonly found in blacks, Hispanics, Native Americans and Orientals. All these individuals have very few basal cell carcinomas, but when they do develop one, it is likely to be pigmented. Because so many more basal cell carcinomas are seen in whites, one will also encounter a fair number of pigmented basal cell carcinomas in these patients. While it has been stated that pigmented basal cell carcinomas are not seen in blue-eyed patients, we have seen this rule often broken. The tumor is typically papular or nodular and has a slate-blue to black color. The pearly border and telangiectases are present but hard to appreciate (Figs. 56.16, 56.17). The differential diagnosis includes melanocytic nevus, blue nevus, malignant melanoma, vascular lesions (angiokeratoma, hemangioma) and irritated or heavily pigmented seborrheic keratosis. Dermatoscopic examination usually can clarify the diagnosis, but a histologic diagnosis is mandatory.

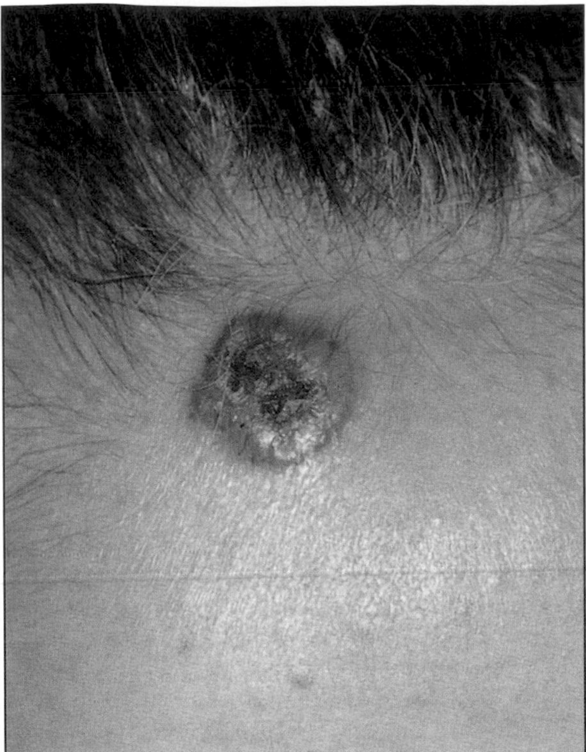

Fig. 56.16. Pigmented partially ulcerated basal cell carcinoma

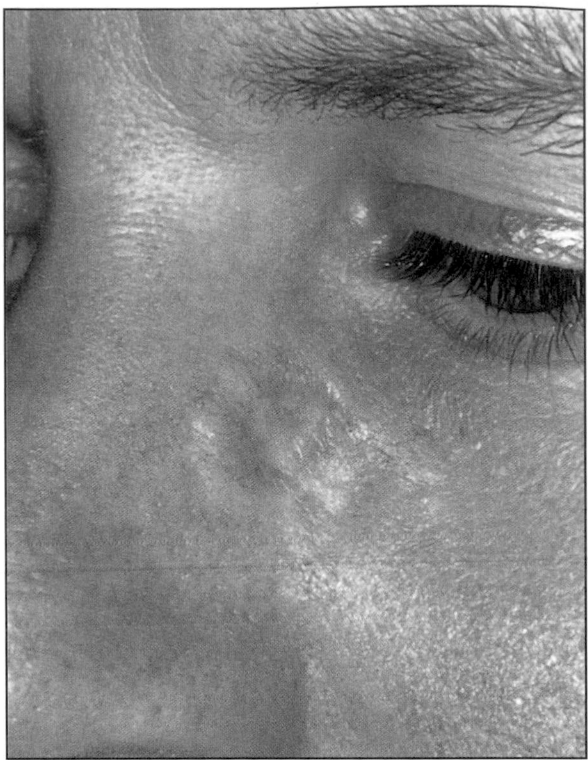

Fig. 56.18. Sclerosing basal cell carcinoma

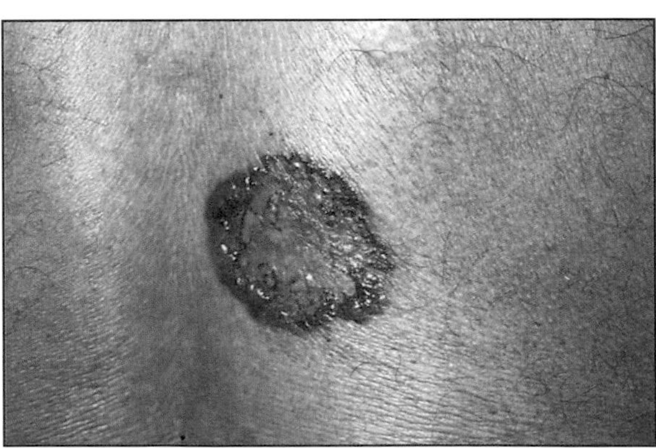

Fig. 56.17. Pigmented superficial basal cell carcinoma in a Hispanic (courtesy of Juan J. Ochoa, MD, Chihuahua, Mexico)

Sclerosing Basal Cell Carcinoma

Synonym. Morpheaform basal cell carcinoma

This variant is particularly important to recognize as it is often overlooked and requires more aggressive therapy. Typically an atrophic scar with a few telangiectases is found on the face, most often about the nose or on the forehead or cheeks (Fig. 56.18). Lesions can be quite large without ulcerating. Sometimes they will rise above the skin surface, mimicking a keloid. The patient often describes them as a scar, following some minor trauma. Any sclerotic or keloidal lesion in which there is not a reasonable history of trauma should be suspected of being a sclerosing basal cell carcinoma. Dermatofibrosarcoma protuberans may also present as a spontaneous scar, but it is usually more elevated, occurs in younger patients and only rarely occurs on the face. Sclerosing basal cell carcinomas are more clinically aggressive, often involve deeper structures and should not be treated by curettage. We employ micrographic surgery for all tumors of this type.

Cystic Basal Cell Carcinoma

A cystic basal cell carcinoma is a soft, translucent papule, usually about the eyes. It cannot be clinically separated from a hidrocystoma, as it too has a broad base, fine telangiectases and a blue tint. Other adnexal tumors may also have such an appearance. Any cyst or inflammatory lesion of the eyelid which does not resolve within a reasonable period should be examined histologically.

Superficial Basal Cell Carcinoma

Synonyms. Multicentric basal cell carcinoma, pagetoid basal cell carcinoma, eczematoid basal cell carcinoma

Superficial basal cell carcinomas look so different from the other forms that they are often misinterpreted. The typical lesion is an erythematous crusted patch that grows slowly and is mistaken for dermatitis or psoriasis (Figs. 56.19, 56.20). It may even be pruritic. Both Bowen disease and extramammary Paget disease look similar. Lesions may range in size from several millimeters to several centimeters. Except in very large patches, ulceration is uncommon. Very close examination may reveal several pearly papules or a fine band of hypopigmentation at the periphery. Superficial basal cell carcinomas are more likely than other forms to be pigmented, although the color is often light-brown, not blue-black.

The most common location is the trunk, although tumors may also be found on the extremities and face. Most patients have multiple superficial basal cell carcinomas, providing a clue (Fig. 56.21). One very difficult clinical situation is the patient with psoriasis who has been treated with UV radiation, tar or arsenic. It is very difficult to sort out the tumors from the psoriasis. In addition to arsenic, chronic sunlight exposure and ionizing radiation are possible causes of superficial basal cell carcinomas, but the relative sparing of the face remains unexplained.

The lesions are so superficial that therapy is easier. They never invade the deeper reaches of the dermis and can thus be more readily and successfully treated. Because of the tendency to multiple lesions, it is often difficult to tell if a new lesion is a recurrence or not. Similarly, if a lesion is excised generously, tiny tumor buds may still be found at the periphery, reflecting the multicentricity.

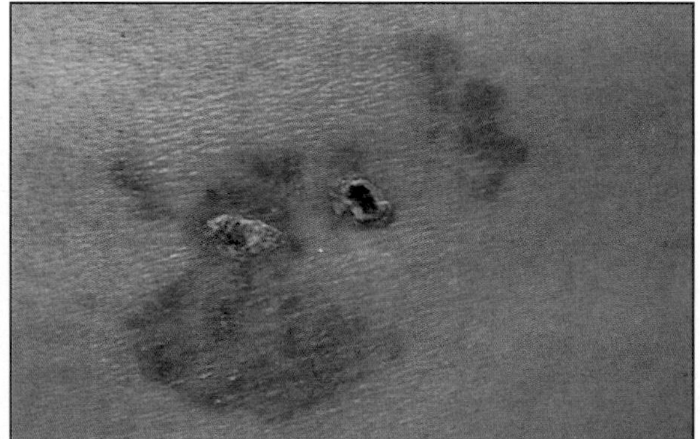

Fig. 56.19. Superficial basal cell carcinoma

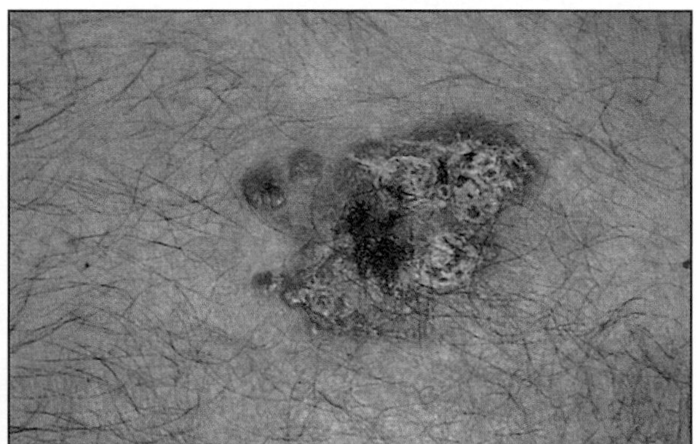

Fig. 56.20. Crusted and nodular superficial basal cell carcinoma

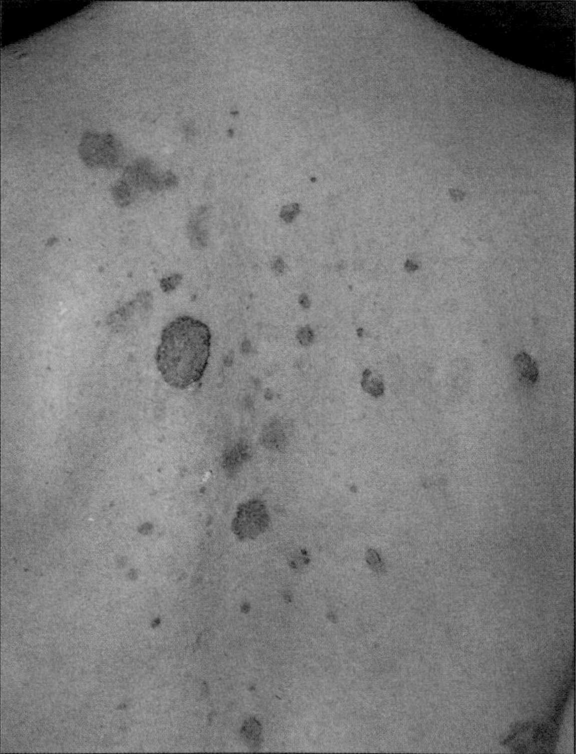

Fig. 56.21. Multicentric basal cell carcinomas

Fibroepithelioma

(PINKUS 1953)

Synonym. Pinkus tumor

Fibroepitheliomas are usually soft pink or flesh-colored nodules or plaques on the trunk, usually the lumbosacral region. They are extremely rare on sunlight-exposed sites and do not ulcerate. The usual clinical diagnosis fibroma or nevus lipomatosus. Histopathologic findings include lacy strands of basaloid cells extending into a fibrous stroma. Only rarely will one find areas of the tumor with more classic findings for basal cell carcinoma. In other cases the lesion may recur as a more typical basal cell carcinoma. Some consider fibroepithelioma as a benign tumor, while others view it as a very low-grade basal cell carcinoma.

Metatypical Basal Cell Carcinoma

Synonyms. Keratinizing basal cell carcinoma, basosquamous carcinoma, epithélioma pavimentaux métatypique mixte (DARIER and FERRAND 1922), epithélioma pavimentaux intermédiaire (DARIER)

Considering how rare these basal cell carcinoma variants are, it is unfortunate that so much has been written about them and so many names proposed. The issues are: what diagnosis should one make when a tumor shows microscopic differentiation towards both a basal cell carcinoma and squamous cell carcinoma and does this have clinical significance? We see several possibilities:

- Collision Tumor. Since both basal cell carcinoma and squamous cell carcinoma are common and arise in sunlight-damaged skin, it is not surprising that two independent tumors should collide. Histologically one sees two distinct types of cells that abut or mingle slightly.
- Keratotic Basal Cell Carcinoma (epithélioma pavimentaux métatypique mixte). Since some basal cell carcinomas have a follicular origin, it seems logical that some show keratinization. Such tumors do not differ clinically from ordinary basal cell carcinomas.
- Adenoid Squamous Cell Carcinoma. Some tumors have a glandular pattern but otherwise fulfill the histologic and immunohistochemical criteria for squamous cell carcinoma. They are easily confused with an adenoid basal cell carcinoma and maybe viewed as overlap tumors.
- Metatypical Basal Cell Carcinoma (epithélioma pavimentaux intermédiaire). This variant is perhaps a unique tumor, but it is very rare and may simply be a subset of basal cell carcinoma that is radiation-resistant. Under the microscope one cannot differentiate between a poorly differentiated basal cell carcinoma and squamous cell carcinoma. Clinically they tend to be large aggressive tumors that usually have been unsuccessfully irradiated. For that reason, they have become less common as more basal cell carcinomas are treated surgically. Two typical locations are the back and the nose. Almost all true metastatic basal cell carcinomas arise from this type.

Basal Cell Carcinoma in Scars

Two clinical scenarios are seen. As mentioned above, basal cell carcinomas may arise in scarred or damaged skin. Here one typically finds an ulcer, not a typical telangiectatic nodule. A second situation is distinguishing between a recurrent basal cell carcinoma and a scar. When a tumor 1 cm or larger is treated by curettage, typically an erythematous nodule develops after 3–6 weeks. This has no English name but in French is known as a pseudorecurrence. It usually flattens out and causes no problem. When a papule or erosion develops in the scar of a basal cell carcinoma, it should be biopsied or excised to exclude a recurrence.

Metastatic Basal Cell Carcinoma

While we tell our patients with a basal cell carcinoma that metastases do not occur, rarely they do. The two rare settings have both become even more rare. Metatypical basal cell carcinomas recurring following radiation therapy can lead to bloodborne metastases. Pseudometastases can spread from large ulcerated basal cell carcinomas in the mid-face when tumor fragments are aspirated and seed the lungs where they grow with difficulty. Since tumors are treated earlier, more aggressively and more often surgically, the chance of both of these scenarios has become less. Even more rarely ordinary looking, but almost always large, basal cell carcinomas may metastasize, usually in elderly or immunosuppressed hosts.

Histopathology. While many histologic patterns are seen in basal cell carcinomas, they all consist of both a basaloid tumor with at least some epidermal connections and a dermal component forming the tumor stroma. Typically there is clefting or separation between the tumor and its stroma, in contrast to trichoblastoma in which the clefts form between the stroma and the normal dermis. The basement membrane about the tumor islands is usually retained at least in part. Both PAS staining and identification of laminin and type IV collagen confirm this. Sometimes, the basement membrane can be strikingly thickened, just as with a cylindroma. In more aggressive basal cell carcinomas, the basement membrane zone may be lacking.

The epidermis is usually atrophic and may be ulcerated. The adjacent dermis may show signs of sunlight damage. Nests and strands of basaloid tumor cells are seen. They are darker than the normal epidermal cells, have little cytoplasm and frequent mitoses. Necrosis is occasionally seen, in contrast to benign adnexal tumors where it is rare. The peripheral cells in a nodule are arranged in a picket fence or palisade fashion. Thus, most pathology reports concerning a basal cell carcinoma speak of "a basaloid tumor with peripheral palisading and clefting."

There is a slight inflammatory response in the dermis. When one is searching for a basal cell carcinoma microscopically and only finds small clusters of lymphocytes, one should cut further into the block. The inflammation is the halo of the tumor. This is of special importance to micrographic surgeons.

The histologic patterns to some extent correlate with the clinical appearance. Some nodular tumors may have multiple small nodules (micronodular variant) or jagged irregular cords and strands in a thickened stroma (infiltrative pattern). The micronodular form tends to do poorly, both because the tumor is endophytic and because its margins are difficult for the surgeon to identify. The sclerosing form has pronounced dermal fibrosis, thin tumor strands and often no apparent epidermal connection. In the fibroepithelioma, the stroma is far more prominent than the lacy epidermal strands. In the superficial form, multiple basaloid buds are found along the dermoepidermal junction with occasional deeper larger nodules. The infundibulocystic type is typically a small keratotic tumor with cysts and hair germs, which some consider a hamartoma and not a true tumor.

The nodular tumors themselves may have a variety of histologic features which are of uncertain importance. Pigmented tumors contain melanin which is increased both within keratinocytes and in the tumor stroma; no proliferations of melanocytes are seen. They can be very glandular (adenoid type) with abundant stromal mucin mimicking an adenocarcinoma. The Hale and alcian blue stains are positive. Another variant is the adamantinoid basal cell carcinoma which resembles an ameloblastoma with a single row of peripheral basaloid cells surrounding cells that are identical to the stellate reticulum of the enamel organ. Rarely eccrine, apocrine or sebaceous differentiation may be seen. Keratotic changes are also possible, as discussed under metatypical basal cell carcinoma above. Marked clear-cell change has also been described. While this resembles trichilemmal keratinization, the cells show a variety of degenerative changes. Sometimes the mesenchyme will show metaplasia with islands of bone or cartilage.

Course and Prognosis. A cure rate of more than 95% should be obtainable. Most local recurrences can be easily handled. While it is appropriate to reassure the patient that such cancers never spread, one should be alert to the occasional large ulcerated tumor which may be more aggressive. The risk of additional basal cell carcinomas is far greater than the risk of any problems with a given tumor. In German, there is a saying that one never sees a basal cell carcinoma alone, but that the tumor is almost always followed by others. The sclerosing, infiltrative and micronodular types have been viewed as aggressive basal cell carcinomas. They appear to be increasing in incidence in the older population of the USA.

Differential Diagnosis. The differential diagnosis has been discussed above with the different clinical variants. While basal cell carcinoma is usually a straightforward diagnosis, featuring a telangiectatic nodule with a pearly border and a central dell, many other patterns are possible and present entirely different problems. Fortunately, a biopsy always provides an unambiguous answer.

Therapy. There are many different ways to treat a basal cell carcinoma. To some extent, the best method of treatment is determined by the size, location and subtype of the tumor, and in many cases, it is a question of physician and patient preference. With all the standard forms, the recurrence rate is less than 5%, meaning that the outlook is good but that follow-up examinations are needed, both to watch for recurrences and to identify additional basal cell carcinomas and other tumors at an early stage.

The following methods are all useful and are discussed in more detail in Chapter 71. Their advantages and disadvantages when dealing with basal cell carcinomas are highlighted here.

Excision. We prefer excision for the majority of patients. A basal cell carcinoma should be excised with a 5-mm margin. Larger or sclerotic lesions probably need a 1.0 cm margin. Microscopic control of the surgical margins is essential. Because of the jagged, irregular outline of a basal cell carcinoma, occasionally tumor strands and fingers will be missed, no matter how carefully the pathologist works. The cure rate should be 98% when the surgical margins are free. Even if excision is incomplete, the resultant inflammation and fibrosis apparently destroy some residual tumor cells, as the cure rate is about 70%.

Micrographic Surgery. This technique offers the highest cure rate, well over 99%. Both the Mohs and Tübingen sectioning methods, illustrated in Chapter 71, offer extremely reliable margin control. We use this technique for large, complicated and recurrent tumors. It has a very high degree of patient satisfaction because recurrence rates are so low. It is the method of choice for sclerosing basal cell carcinoma.

Cryotherapy. Tumor cryotherapy is different from that employed for verrucae or actinic keratoses. Usually two deep freeze-thaw cycles reaching below the tumor are performed with a thermocouple monitor placed beneath the tumor so one can be sure of achieving sufficient cooling to kill the tumor cells. The tumor base should reach –20°C. Initially the lesion ulcerates and often bleeds, but the final cosmetic result is usually good. Histologic control is not possible. In skilled hands, this is a valuable approach for selected, mostly elderly patients.

Curettage and Electrodesiccation. Lesions less than 1 cm in diameter and superficial basal cell carcinomas can be treated by curettage and then electrodesiccation. Some perform the procedure twice in one sitting; others, three times. Others find the electrodesiccation unnecessary. Histologic control of the margins is not possible, sclerotic tumors are inadequately treated, the healing time is prolonged and the cosmetic results are less acceptable than with other methods. We rarely employ this method, but recent surveys in Europe show that it is still widely used.

Radiation Therapy. Fractionated doses of 3–5 Gy, delivered four or five times weekly to a total dose of 50–60 Gy provide the best cosmetic results while still insuring a tumor-killing dose. Earlier regimens were less fractionated and caused relatively more skin damage. Usually the margin for the field is planned as 0.5–1.0 cm larger than the visible or palpable tumor margin. The depth can be assessed on the biopsy or with ultrasonography so that an appropriate half-value layer is chosen.

There are also some techniques that are less standard but occasionally useful. Topical 5-fluorouracil can be used on multiple superficial truncal lesions, but recurrences are common. We avoid it because we have seen patients treated with topical 5-fluorouracil develop deep tumors while the surface following treatment appears relatively normal. In addition, patients given 5-fluorouracil for home use tend to be less faithful about follow-up, which is frequently disastrous in nevoid basal cell carcinoma syndrome or xeroderma pigmentosum. Intralesional injection of a 5-fluorouracil/epinephrine gel appears promising, while several protocols have employed intralesional IFN α-2b. Photodynamic therapy is still experimental, but offers promise. At present, it is reserved for problematic tumors, using research protocols.

How does one choose the right therapy? The following are simple guidelines, designed to be broken but hopefully useful:

- Excision is appropriate for almost all tumors.
- Microscopically controlled surgery is probably not needed for simple, small tumors. It is useful for recurrent tumors, lesions which will need to be closed by a flap or graft, lesions which invade bone, lesions in high-risk areas such as the nasolabial fold, eye and ear, and lesions such as sclerosing basal cell carcinoma where the margins are difficult to determine.
- Cryotherapy is particularly effective about the eye, on the nose and for superficial lesions.
- Curettage and electrodesiccation is useful for small or superficial tumors, avoiding high-risk areas such as the nasolabial fold, eye and about the ear.

- Radiation therapy is best for older patients, where the risk of radiation-induced tumors then becomes meaningless, and for those who cannot or will not tolerate surgery. It is especially useful for lid tumors.

Systemic. Oral retinoids have been employed for chemoprophylaxis in patients with nevoid basal cell carcinoma syndrome, xeroderma pigmentosum and severe carcinogen exposure (ionizing radiation accident victims, for example). Both acitretin and isotretinoin have been employed. The doses needed are higher than those employed for acne or ichthyosis and the therapy must be lifelong, so side effects can be expected. Tumors are not prevented but reduced in number. Occasionally a tumor may appear to regress, but this should be confirmed histologically and the oral medication not considered a treatment but a prophylactic measure.

There is no established systemic treatment for inoperable locally invasive basal cell carcinoma or the rare metastatic basal cell carcinoma. The few patients requiring chemotherapy are treated with whatever protocol is available that seems to offer the most hope for malignant epithelial tumors.

Prophylaxis. Far more important than the retinoid therapy discussed under systemic therapy is the prophylaxis offered by routine follow-up examinations. We prefer to see patients at 2, 6 and 12 months and then yearly. A complete skin examination should be performed, since once a patient has had a basal cell carcinoma, the risk of developing a second tumor is considerable. Particular attention should be paid to the area covered by a flap or graft, as in this setting a deep recurrence is hard to detect.

Patients should also be strongly encouraged to regularly use sunscreens and wear protective clothing. The benefits to young and middle-aged adults are indisputable, but in the very elderly, the benefits are probably minimal, because of the delay in developing a basal cell carcinoma following exposure.

Nevoid Basal Cell Carcinoma Syndrome

(Jarisch 1894; Gorlin and Goltz 1960)

Synonyms. Basal cell nevus syndrome, Gorlin syndrome, Gorlin-Goltz syndrome

Etiology and Pathogenesis. Nevoid basal cell carcinoma syndrome is inherited in an autosomal dominant pattern. The responsible PTCH gene is on chromosome 9q22.3. The homologue in *Drosophila* is the patched gene, important in the segmental development of the insect, controlling growth and regulating form. This may explain why nevoid basal cell carcinoma syndrome features both developmental abnormalities and tumors.

Clinical Findings. Patients develop many basal cell carcinomas. Early in life, in the nevoid phase, most of the tumors do not look at all like basal cell carcinomas. Instead they resemble small melanocytic nevi or acrochordons, typically most numerous on the nape but scattered over the entire body. Later, in the oncogenic phase, more typical basal cell carcinomas appear with ulceration and scarring. About 10 % of patients with nevoid basal cell carcinoma syndrome have no basal cell carcinomas.

There are other cutaneous signs of disease. Patients typically have tiny palmoplantar pits, which may be the first sign, often identified in early childhood. In addition, acral epidermoid cysts should alert one to the possible diagnosis. The face is also abnormal with an exceptionally large skull (without hydrocephalus), frontal bossing, hypertelorism and an enlarged mandible (Fig. 56.22). The mandible and less often the maxilla contain a single or more often multiple cysts, known as odontogenic keratocysts, which can be identified on radiologic examination. While over 80 % of patients have at least one cyst, the lesions are usually asymptomatic and never undergo malignant change. The falx cerebri may also be calcified; this too can be identified on radiologic examination.

Systemic malignancies are also associated with nevoid basal cell carcinoma syndrome, so it is often considered a cancer-associated genodermatosis or paraneoplastic syndrome. Some children present with medulloblastoma prior to any other signs of disease. If they are treated with ionizing radiation, they tend to develop hundreds of basal cell carcinomas in the radiation portals. Ovarian fibromas are also present. They usually appear in adolescence

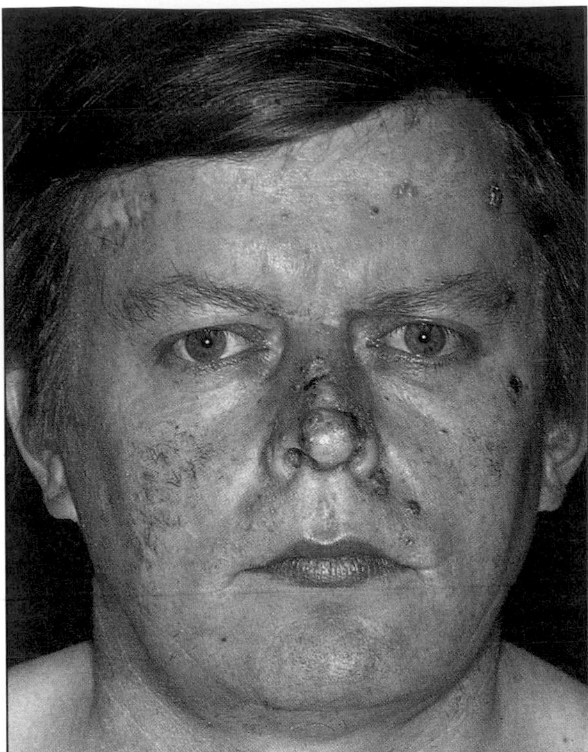

Fig. 56.22. Nevoid basal cell carcinoma syndrome with multiple tumors and frontal bossing

as bilateral calcified pelvic masses identifiable with ultrasound or radiologic evaluation and only rarely undergo malignant change.

Histopathology. The basal cell carcinomas cannot be distinguished with certainty from ordinary tumors. But sometimes clues may be present. The infundibulocystic variant is far more common in nevoid basal cell carcinoma syndrome. In addition, the acrochordon-like lesions with tiny buds of tumor in a pedunculated papule should suggest the answer, especially in the absence of any sunlight damage. Tumors in nevoid basal cell carcinoma syndrome patients may be more likely to calcify and ossify.

The histopathology of the palmoplantar pits is confusing. Some studies have shown associated basal cell carcinomas, others have not. Clinically normal skin from such patients often shows totally unexpected small basal cell carcinomas, so a random association cannot be excluded.

Course and Prognosis. The patients tend to have a modestly shortened life expectancy because of the risk of systemic tumors. While they may develop hundreds of basal cell carcinomas with subsequent scarring, the skin tumors can usually be identified early and controlled.

Therapy. All of the traditional treatment methods are appropriate except for radiation therapy, which tends to induce multiple new tumors in its fields. The multiple small lesions may be treated with curettage, cryotherapy, dermabrasion or tangential excision. While topical 5-fluorouracil and topical retinoids are often endorsed, we have found them relatively ineffective. In addition, they may induce surface healing but allow a tumor to grow downward. Chemoprevention with oral retinoids may also be of some value. Sunscreens are useful as UV radiation, although a minor factor, is one which can be ameliorated.

Other Syndromes Associated with Multiple Basal Cell Carcinomas

There are several exceedingly rare syndromes in which multiple basal cell carcinomas are found.

Multiple Hereditary Infundibulocystic Basal Cell Carcinomas (Requena et al. 1999). These patients have multiple basal cell carcinomas but no palmar pits or jaw cysts.

Bazex Syndrome (Bazex et al. 1966). This autosomal dominantly inherited disorder features follicular atrophoderma associated with multiple basal cell carcinomas, hypohidrosis and hypotrichosis.

Rombo Syndrome (Michaelsson et al. 1981). The main features of this autosomal dominantly inherited syndrome are facial milia, atrophodermia vermiculata, acral cyanosis, alopecia and multiple trichoepitheliomas and basal cell carcinomas in adult life.

Multiple Eccrine-Pilar Hamartoma Syndrome (Peyrí et al. 1981). These patients have multiple adnexal neoplasms with features of follicular and eccrine differentiation, as well as milia and hypotrichosis. The original patient has also developed basal cell carcinomas, many in association with the follicular tumors. While inheritance in an autosomal dominant pattern is presumed, studies are lacking.

Syndromes with Multiple Adnexal Neoplasms. Patients with multiple trichoepitheliomas (Chap. 58) also develop basal cell carcinomas. The same phenomenon may rarely be seen in other patients with multiple adnexal tumors, especially with follicular differentiation.

Cutaneous Metastases

Definition. Spread of an internal malignancy to the skin.

Etiology and Pathogenesis. A cutaneous metastasis is almost invariably a poor prognostic sign. It may represent the first sign of a tumor, the first sign of the tumor's spread from its primary organ, or the first sign of recurrence of a hopefully cured tumor. Various studies suggest that between 3% and 10% of cancer patients have cutaneous metastases. The numbers vary somewhat depending if patients with cancer or patients with metastatic cancer are evaluated.

While tumors from any organ can spread to the skin, there are some clear patterns. The most common tumors are the most common sources of metastases. In men, the three most frequent are malignant melanoma and carcinomas of the lung and colon. Squamous cell carcinoma of the oral cavity, renal cell carcinoma and gastric adenocarcinoma are also important. Even though prostate cancer is very common and responsible for over 10% of cancer deaths in men, it rarely metastasizes to the skin. In women, far and away the most common source is carcinoma of the breast, followed by malignant melanoma. Much less common are tumors from the ovary, lung, oral cavity and colon. Note that metastatic malignant melanoma is a common source of metastasis in both sexes; in some series, it is the overall leader.

Malignant tumors can spread to the skin in at least three ways. The simplest is direct spread, where, for example, a neglected carcinoma of the breast infiltrates the skin locally and ulcerates. When lymphatic spread occurs, it is usually late in the disease and involves skin overlying the tumor or within its lymphatic drainage pattern. Lymphatic spread is often associated with an inflammatory or fibrotic reaction occasionally producing a distinctive clinical picture. Finally, hematogenous spread may occur, producing many lesions often at distant sites. Some metastatic tumors home in on the epidermis (epidermotrophic metastasis). Malignant melanoma does this most often, but some breast and prostate cancers can also mimic primary skin tumors. The reasons for this attraction are not known.

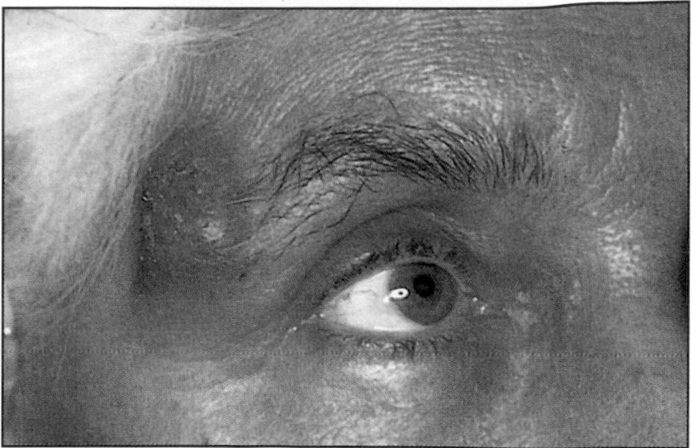

Fig. 56.23. Nodular metastasis from an adenocarcinoma

Clinical Findings. Usually a cutaneous metastasis is not clinically unique. Typically there may be one or several skin-colored or red nodules which may be subcutaneous or more often involve both the skin and fat (Fig. 56.23). The location of the cutaneous metastasis may give a clue as to its origin. Malignant melanoma may be found in the regional lymphatics or it may spread hematogenously, showering the body with small dark papules and nodules. Breast cancer usually spreads to the skin of the chest wall, back or head and neck; it is rarely found below the level of the breasts. Renal cell carcinoma has a propensity for the skin of the head and neck region, while the skin of the thorax is the favored sites for lung carcinomas. Intestinal tumors involve the skin of the abdominal wall or lower part of the back, while ovarian tumors are often found in the perineal region. Tumors of the oral cavity and upper airways typically spread to the skin of the upper part of the chest and neck. But the main clinical problem is that any tumor can appear anywhere from the top of the head to the tip of the toes.

Some metastases are quite distinct clinically and so can be recognized.

Sister Mary Joseph Nodule. Tumors of the stomach, colon and pancreas may metastasize to the umbilicus. Sister Mary Joseph was an operating room nurse for the Mayo brothers at The Mayo Clinic. She is credited with noticing that patients with an umbilical nodule, which she often identified while prepping the patient for surgery, usually had intraabdominal metastases (Fig. 56.24).

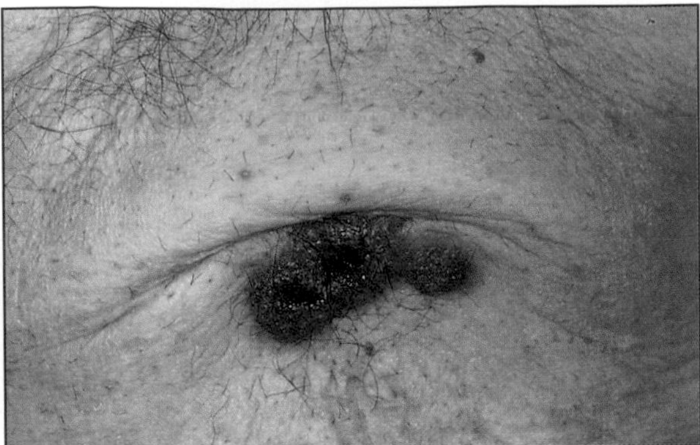

Fig. 56.24. Sister Mary Joseph's nodule

Cancer en Cuirasse. Breast carcinoma and to a less extent other head and neck tumors can elicit a massive fibrotic response. The German term is *Panzerkrebs* or armored cancer. The skin becomes indurated resembling scleroderma. There may be telangiectases and locally dilated lymphatics producing a pebbly or warty skin surface. When these lymphatic spaces are large enough, they can appear bullous or ulcerated. When the upper chest wall or arm is involved, there is usually peripheral edema as lymphatic return is obstructed.

Peau d'Orange. Breast cancer is notorious for producing local induration and edema so that the follicular openings on the skin become very prominent, resembling fancifully the skin of an orange. This change is probably the same as cancer en cuirasse, but involving a more expandable tissue, the breast.

Carcinoma Erysipelatoides. Superficial lymphatic metastases, once again usually from a breast cancer, elicit an intense inflammatory response mimicking erysipelas (Fig. 56.25). Typically there are irregular erythematous bands. Biopsy reveals the lymphatics occluded by tumor cells producing an infarct. The patient is not febrile and the disease only slowly changes. After weeks, the skin may acquire a yellow hue and become fibrotic, overlapping with cancer en cuirasse.

Other Inflammatory Lesions. Breast carcinoma frequently involves the skin of the eyelids. Here the early red nodule is usually mistaken for a infectious process, such as a sty.

Melanomatosis. Patients with metastatic malignant melanoma may produce so much melanin, usually from massive internal metastases, that it is carried by the blood to all areas of the skin, producing a slate-gray skin color as well as discolored urine.

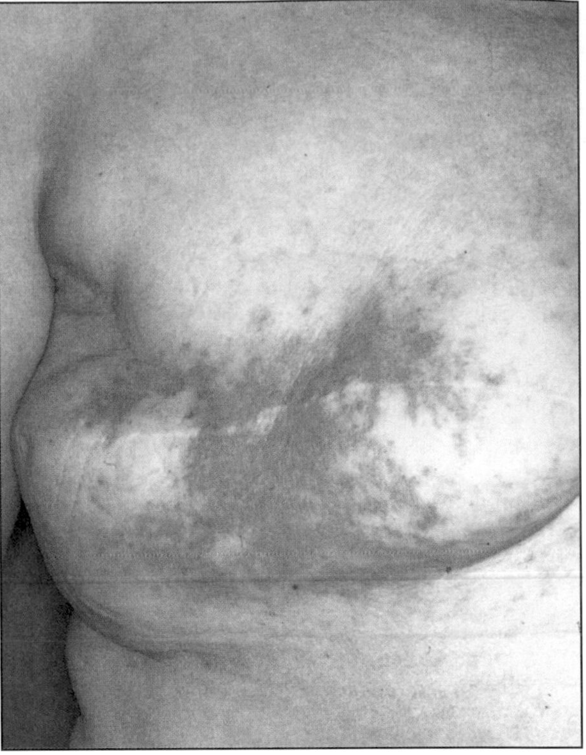

Fig. 56.25. Carcinoma erysipelatoides

Alopecia. Carcinoma of the breast often spreads to the scalp where it may produce a small minimally indurated area of hair loss which is often mistaken for alopecia areata.

Hemangioma-like lesions. Metastatic renal cell carcinoma is quite vascular and mimics a hemangioma or pyogenic granuloma. It is most common on the scalp.

Histopathology. The histologic identification of a cutaneous metastasis can be a challenging problem. First, early lesions may be very subtle with just a few malignant cells and thus overlooked with unfortunate consequences. Early sclerotic breast carcinoma metastases are notorious for the paucity of metastatic cells. Next, one must be sure one is dealing with a metastasis. The diagnosis of malignant sweat gland tumor can only be made after excluding the possibility of a cutaneous metastasis. Metastases are far more common than primary sweat gland carcinomas. An epidermotropic metastatic malignant melanoma may exactly mimic a primary malignant melanoma; the history is essential. Sometimes while the dermatopathologist is laboring over the question as to whether the lesion is a metastasis or a primary tumor, the patient will develop additional lesions, confirming the diagnosis.

Once one has identified the lesion as a metastasis, then one is confronted with trying to identify the source of the tumor cells. In many cases, the primary is already known and the pathologist's task is straightforward – simply to confirm that the metastasis is compatible with the original primary. Most metastatic adenocarcinomas are from the breast, gastrointestinal tract or lung, while metastatic squamous cell carcinomas usually arise from the lung, oral cavity, upper airways or esophagus. Signet ring cells arise from the gastrointestinal tract. Clear-cell tumors are most likely malignant melanoma or renal cell tumor, while neuroendocrine tumors are usually Merkel cell tumors or small-cell (oat-cell) lung tumors.

When tumors are poorly differentiated and show no typical pattern, or when the patient has no known underlying malignancy, then a series of immunohistochemical stains and electron microscopy can be employed to determine the origin of the tumor cells. Occasionally it is impossible to identify the likely source of the metastasis histologically. For example, some malignant melanomas metastatic to the skin simply do not have any residual structural features of a melanoma, but they usually retain histochemical markers such as S100 or HMB45. More puzzling is the situation in which despite intensive investigations, no internal tumor is identified. Even in research cancer centers, this occurs in 3–5% of patients who present with metastases. Then one must unfortunately await the evolution of the clinical situation.

Course and Prognosis. Cutaneous metastases are a bad prognostic sign. Their presence always leads to the patient being included in a less-favorable prognostic category and in many cases, is the first signal that the patient will eventually succumb to a tumor.

Differential Diagnosis. As discussed under clinical appearance, a metastasis can mimic a wide variety of lesions. One must continuously be alert to the possibility, for failure to consider a cutaneous metastasis can have disastrous consequences.

Therapy. Individual lesions can be excised or irradiated. More widespread metastases may respond to chemotherapy. The real question is how the presence of cutaneous metastases will influence the patient's overall treatment program. Usually treating individual skin lesions is of little importance, except for patient comfort.

Bibliography

Verrucous Carcinoma

Ackerman LV (1948) Verrucous carcinoma of the oral cavity. Surgery 23:670–678

Arid I, Johnson HD, Lennox B et al. (1954) Epithelioma cuniculatum. A variety of squamous carcinoma peculiar to the foot. Br J Surg 42:245–250

Buschke A, Löwenstein L (1925) Über carcinomähnliche Condylomata acuminata des Penis. Klin Wochenschr 4: 1726–1728

Florin EH, Kolbusz RV, Goldberg LH (1994) Verrucous carcinoma of the oral cavity. Int J Dermatol 33:618–622

Gottron HA (1932) Ausgedehnte, ziemlich symmetrisch angeordnete Papillomatosis cutis beider Unterschenkel bei einem 59jährigen Kranken. Dermatol Z 63:409–410

Grussendorf-Conen EI (1997) Anogenital premalignant and malignant tumors (including Buschke-Löwenstein tumors). Clin Dermatol 15:377–388

Kao GF, Graham JH, Helwig EB (1982) Carcinoma cuniculatum (verrucous carcinoma of the skin). A clinicopathologic study of 46 cases with ultrastructural observations. Cancer 49:2395–2402

Lubbe J, Kormann A, Adams V et al. (1996) HPV-11- and HPV-16-associated oral verrucous carcinoma. Dermatology 192:217–221

Masih AS, Stoler MH, Farrow GM et al. (1992) Penile verrucous carcinoma: a clinicopathologic, human papillomavirus typing and flow cytometric analysis. Mod Pathol 5:48–55

Noel JC, Pery MO, Goldschmidt D et al. (1993) Human papillomavirus type I DNA in verrucous carcinoma of the leg. J Am Acad Dermatol 28:1036–1038

Rock JA, Fisher ER (1960) Florid papillomatosis of the cavity and larynx. Arch Otolaryngol 72:480–593

Schwartz RA (1990) Buschke-Loewenstein tumor: verrucous carcinoma of the penis. J Am Acad Dermatol 23:723–727

Schwartz RA (1995) Verrucous carcinoma of the skin and mucosa. J Am Acad Dermatol 32:1–21

Spiro RH (1998) Verrucous carcinoma, then and now. Am J Surg 176:393–397

Keratoacanthoma

Beham A, Regauer S, Soyer HP et al. (1998) Keratoacanthoma: a clinically distinct variant of well differentiated squamous cell carcinoma. Adv Anat Pathol 5:269–280

Dangoisse C, Meyvisch K, Ledoux M (1993) Multiple eruptive keratoacanthoma and immunity disorders. Dermatology 186:313–316

Dupont A (1930) Kyste sebace atypique. Bull Soc Belge Dermatol 177–179

Ferguson-Smith J (1934) A case of multiple primary squamous-celled carcinomata of the skin in a young man with spontaneous healing. Br J Dermatol 46:267–272

Frank TL, Maguire HC Jr, Greenbaum SS (1996) Multiple painful keratoacanthomas. Int J Dermatol 35:648–650

Gassenmaier A, Pfister H, Hornstein OP (1986) Human papillomavirus 25-related DNA in solitary keratoacanthoma. Arch Dermatol Res 279:73–76

Grine RC, Hendrix JD, Greer KE (1997) Generalized eruptive keratoacanthoma of Grzybowski: response to cyclophosphamide. J Am Acad Dermatol 36:786–787

Grob JJ, Suzini F, Weiller M, et al. (1993) Large keratoacanthomas treated with intralesional interferon alfa-2a. J Am Acad Dermatol 29:237–241

Grzybowski M (1950) A case of peculiar generalized epithelial tumours of the skin. Br J Dermatol Syph 62:310–313

Heid E, Grosshans E, Lazrak B et al. (1979) Keratoacanthoma centrifugum marginatum. Ann Dermatol Venereol 106:367–370

Hutchinson J (1889) Morbid growths and tumours. I. The "crateriform ulcer of the face," a form of acute epithelial cancer. Trans Pathol Soc Lond 40:275–281

Jaber PW, Cooper PH, Greer KE (1993) Generalized eruptive keratoacanthoma of Grzybowski. J Am Acad Dermatol 29:299–304

Keeney GL, Banks PM, Linscheid RL (1988) Subungual keratoacanthoma: report of a case and review of the literature. Arch Dermatol 124:1074–1076

Richards FM, Goudie DR, Cooper WN et al. (1997) Mapping the multiple self-healing squamous epithelioma (MSSE) gene and investigation of xeroderma pigmentosum group A (XPA) and PATCHED (PTCH) as candidate genes. Hum Genet 101:317–322

Rook A, Whimster I (1979) Keratoacanthoma – thirty year retrospect. Br J Dermatol 100:41–47

Schaller M, Korting HC, Wolff H et al. (1996) Multiple keratoacanthomas, giant keratoacanthoma and keratoacanthoma centrifugum marginatum: development in a single patient and treatment with oral isoretinoin. Acta Derm Venereol (Stockh) 76:40–42

Tamir G, Morgenstern S, Ben-Amitay D et al. (1999) Synchronous appearance of keratoacanthomas in burn scar and skin graft donor site shortly after injury. J Am Acad Dermatol 40:870–871

Torre C de la, Losada A, Cruces MJ (1997) Keratoacanthoma centrifugum marginatum: treatment with intralesional bleomycin. J Am Acad Dermatol 37:1010–1011

Witten VH, Zak FG (1952) Multiple, primary self-healing prickle-cell epithelioma of the skin. Cancer 5:539–550

Wright AL, Gawkrodger DJ, Branford WA et al. (1988) Self-healing epitheliomata of Ferguson-Smith: cytogenetic and histological studies, and the therapeutic effect of etretinate. Dermatologica 176:22–28

Squamous Cell Carcinoma

Broders AC (1921) Squamous cell epithelioma of the skin. Ann Surg 73:114–160

Cubilla AL (1995) Carcinoma of the penis. Mod Pathol 8:116–118

Dinehart SM, Nelson-Adesokan P, Cockerell C et al. (1997) Metastatic cutaneous squamous cell carcinoma derived from actinic keratosis. Cancer 79:920–923

Dupree MT, Boyer JD, Cobb MW (1998) Marjolin's ulcer arising in a burn scar. Cutis 62:49–51

Gray DT, Suman VJ, Su WP et al. (1997) Trends in the population-based incidence of squamous cell carcinoma of the skin first diagnosed between 1984 and 1992. Arch Dermatol 133:735–740

Guenthner ST, Hurwitz RM, Buckel LJ et al. (1999) Cutaneous squamous cell carcinomas consistently show histologic evidence of in situ changes: a clinicopathologic correlation. J Am Acad Dermatol 41:443–448

Micali G, Innocenzi D, Nasca MR et al. (1996) Squamous cell carcinoma of the penis. J Am Acad Dermatol 35:432–451

Miller CS, White DK (1996) Human papillomavirus expression in oral mucosa, premalignant conditions, and squamous cell carcinoma: a retrospective review of the literature. Oral Surg Oral Med Oral Pathol Oral Radiol Endod 82:57–68

Ong CS, Keogh AM, Kossard S et al. (1999) Skin cancer in Australian heart transplant recipients. J Am Acad Dermatol 40:27–34

Ostrow RS, Bender M, Niimura M et al. (1982) Human papillomavirus DNA in cutaneous primary and metastasized squamous cell carcinomas from patients with epidermodysplasia verruciformis. Proc Natl Acad Sci USA 79:1634–1638

Paz IB, Cook N, Odom-Maryon T et al. (1997) Human papillomavirus (HPV) in head and neck cancer. An association of HPV 16 with squamous cell carcinoma of Waldeyer's tonsillar ring. Cancer 79:595–604

Penn I (1978) Tumors arising in organ transplant recipients. Adv Cancer Res 28:31–61

Rowe DE, Carroll RJ, Day CL Jr (1992) Prognostic factors for local recurrence, metastasis, and survival rates in squamous cell carcinoma of the skin, ear, and lip. Implications for treatment modality selection. J Am Acad Dermatol 26:976–990

Stern RS, Thibodeau LA, Parrish JA et al. (1979) Skin cancer after PUVA treatment. N Engl J Med 301:555

Yuspa SH (1998) The pathogenesis of squamous cell cancer: lessons learned from studies of skin carcinogenesis. J Dermatol Sci 17:1–7

Basal Cell Carcinoma

Altman A, Rosen T, Tschen JA et al. (1987) Basal cell epithelioma in black patients. J Am Acad Dermatol 17:741–745

Caro MR, Howell JB (1951) Morphea-like epithelioma. Arch Dermatol Syphilol 63:53–69

Cott RE, Wood MG, Johnson BL Jr (1987) Use of curettage and shave excision in office practice. Microscopic confirmation of removal. J Am Acad Dermatol 16:1243–1251

Cox NH (1992) Basal cell carcinoma in young adults. Br J Dermatol 127:26–29

Darier J, Ferrand M (1922) L'épithéliome pavimenteux mixte et intermédiaire. Forme métatypique du cancer malpighien de la peau et des orifices muqueux. Ann Dermatol Syphiligr VI (3):385–406

Dinehart SM, Dodge R, Stanley WE et al. (1992) Basal cell carcinoma treated with Mohs surgery. J Dermatol Surg Oncol 18:560–566

Domarus H von, Stevens PJ (1984) Metastatic basal cell carcinoma. Report of five cases and review of 170 cases in the literature. J Am Acad Dermatol 10:1043–1060

Drake LA, Ceilley RI, Cornelison RL et al. (1992) Guidelines of care for basal cell carcinoma. J Am Acad Dermatol 26:117–120

Dubin N, Kopf AW (1983) Multivariate risk score for reoccurrence of cutaneous basal cell carcinomas. Arch Dermatol 119:373–377

Farmer ER, Helwig EB (1980) Metastatic basal cell carcinoma: a clinicopathological study of 17 cases. Cancer 46:748–757

Goldberg LH (1996) Basal cell carcinoma. Lancet 347: 663–667

Goldschmidt H, Breneman JC, Breneman DL (1994) Ionizing radiation therapy in dermatology. J Am Acad Dermatol 30:157–182

Leffell DJ, Haedington JT, Wong DS et al. (1991) Aggressive-growth basal cell carcinoma in young adults. Arch Dermatol 127:1663–1667

LeSueur BW, Silvis NG, Hansen RC (2000) Basal cell carcinoma in children. Arch Dermatol 136:370–372

Lo JS, Snow SN, Reizner GT et al. (1991) Metastatic basal cell carcinoma: report of twelve cases with a review of the literature. J Am Acad Dermatol 24:715–719

Lowe L, Rapini RP (1991) Newer variants and simulants of basal cell carcinoma. J Dermatol Surg Oncol 17:641–648

Maloney ME, Jones DB, Sexton FM (1992) Pigmented basal cell carcinoma: investigation of 70 cases. J Am Acad Dermatol 27:47–78

Marghoob A, Kopf AW, Bart RS et al. (1993) Risk of another basal cell carcinoma developing after treatment of a basal cell carcinoma. J Am Acad Dermatol 28:22–28

Miller SJ (1991) Biology of basal cell carcinoma, part I. J Am Acad Dermatol 24:1–13

Miller SJ (1991) Biology of basal cell carcinoma, part II. J Am Acad Dermatol 24:161–175

Pinkus H (1953) Premalignant fibroepithelial tumors of skin. Arch Dermatol Syphilol 67:598–615

Pinkus H (1965) Epithelial and fibroepithelial tumors. Arch Dermatol 91:24–37

Salasche SJ, Amonette RA (1981) Morpheaform basal-cell epitheliomas. A study of subclinical extensions in a series of 51 cases. J Dermatol Surg Oncol 7:387–394

Silverman MK, Kopf AW, Bart RS et al. (1992) Recurrence rates of treated basal cell carcinomas. Surgical excision. J Dermatol Surg Oncol 18:471–476

Stern JB, Haupt H, Smith RRL (1994) Fibroepithelioma of Pinkus. Eccrine duct spread of basal cell carcinoma. Am J Dermatopathol 16:585–587

Torre D (1986) Cryosurgery of basal cell carcinoma. J Am Acad Dermatol 16:917–929

Wilder RB, Shimm DS, Kittelson JM et al. (1991) Recurrent basal cell carcinoma treated with radiation therapy. Arch Dermatol 127:1668–1672

Wolf DJ, Zitelli JA (1987) Surgical margins for basal cell carcinoma. Arch Dermatol 123:340–344

Other Syndromes Associated with Multiple Basal Cell Carcinomas

Bazex A, Dupré A, Christol B (1966) Atrophodermie folliculaire proliférations baso-cellulaires et hypotrichose. Ann Dermatol Syphiligr 93:241–254

Michaëlsson G, Olsson E, Westermark P (1981) The rombo syndrome: A familial disorder with vermiculate atrophoderma, milia, hypotrichosis, trichoepitheliomas, basal cell carcinomas and peripheral vasodilation with cyanosis. Acta Derm Venerol (Stockh) 61:497–503

Plosila M, Kiistala R, Niemi K-M (1981) The Bazex syndrome: follicular atrophoderma with multiple basal cell carcinomas, hypotrichosis and hypohidrosis. Clin Exp Dermatol 6:31–41

Peyri J, Ferrandiz C, Pinol Aguade J et al. (1981) Multiple eccrine-pilar hamartoma. Med Cutan Ibero Lat Am 9: 45–49

Requena L, Fariña MdC, Robledo M et al. (1999) Multiple hereditary infundibulocystic basal cell carcinomas. Arch Dermatol 135:1227–1235

Nevoid Basal Cell Carcinoma Syndrome

Bale AE (1997) The nevoid basal cell carcinoma syndrome: genetics and mechanism of carcinogenesis. Cancer Invest 15:180–186

Gailani MR, Bale AE (1997) Developmental genes and cancer: role of patched in basal cell carcinoma of the skin. J Natl Cancer Inst 89:1103–1109

Gorlin RJ, Goltz RW (1960) Multiple nevoid basal-cell epithelioma, jaw cysts and bifid rib. A syndrome. N Engl J Med 262:908–912

Gorlin RJ (1987) The nevoid basal cell carcinoma syndrom. Medicine 66:98–113

Gorlin RJ (1995) Nevoid basal cell carcinoma syndrome. Dermatol Clin 13:113–125

Howell JB, Freeman RG (1980) Structure and significance of the pits with their tumors in the nevoid basal cell carcinoma syndrome. J Am Acad Dermatol 2:224–238

Jarisch W (1894) Zur Lehre von den Hautgeschwulsten. Arch Dermatol Syph 28:163–222

Peck GL, Gross EG, Butkus D et al. (1982) Chemoprevention of basal cell carcinoma with isotretinoin. J Am Acad Dermatol 6:815–823

Cutaneous Metastases

Lookingbill DP, Spangler N, Helm KF (1993) Cutaneous metastases in patients with metastatic carcinoma: a retrospective study of 4020 patients. J Am Acad Dermatol 29: 228–236

Schwartz RA (1995) Histopathologic aspects of cutaneous metastatic disease. J Am Acad Dermatol 33:649–657

Adnexal Tumors

Contents

Introduction

Adnexal tumors are a confusing aspect of dermatology. They are relatively uncommon yet occupy at least 10 % of the pages of almost all the current dermatopathology texts. In most instances, they are a solitary skin-colored to red nodule, often on the head, with a differential diagnosis of melanocytic nevus, epidermoid cyst and basal cell carcinoma. Excision is curative. Most adnexal tumors are benign; frequently they have a fibrous pseudocapsule and shell out easily when removed surgically. Microscopically the benign tumors are symmetrical, have a vertical growth pattern and sharp borders. There are frequent histologic overlaps. We will not repeat these basic facts for each tumor, but only point out where they differ from the trend.

The distinction between a nevus, hamartoma and benign adnexal neoplasm is often a linguistic problem or, microscopically, almost impossible. Lesions present at birth or in early childhood that consist of an excess of normal skin structures and which tend to be stable are often called nevi or hamartomas. While the distinctions are arbitrary, we have included a discussion of many such lesions in Chapter 52, while larger embryologic malformations, such as an accessory nipple, are described in Chapter 19.

Some malignant adnexal tumors, if overlooked, can be fatal; however, the difficulty is that, frequently, at least at first glance, they are not dissimilar from their benign counterparts. There are several categories of malignant adnexal tumors. The most common is carcinoma ex adenoma, i. e., a tumor that resembles a benign lesion such as a poroma but which has the histologic features of malignancy and behaves aggressively. The most common example is eccrine porocarcinoma. Most chemotherapy protocols that deal with malignant adnexal tumors are based on porocarcinomas, which are more common than metastatic basal cell carcinomas. Another major category are the sclerosing sweat duct tumors, in which the fibrous stroma may make accurate margin identification difficult, just as with a sclerosing basal cell carcinoma. The most common member of this group is the microcytic adnexal carcinoma. Finally there are a few, unique malignant adnexal tumors, such as the mucinous eccrine carcinoma. Some adnexal neoplasms, although entirely benign, may be rich in mitoses and thus mistaken for a malignancy. In almost every case, when a carcinoma is metastatic to the skin, the differential diagnosis is adnexal neoplasm.

There are a number of disorders with multiple adnexal tumors, often with associated disorders. For example, a solitary sebaceous neoplasm has little meaning, while multiple keratoacanthomas and sebaceous neoplasms suggest Muir-Torre syndrome, with defects in DNA mismatch repair and a high lifetime risk of internal malignancy. The suspicion is that the same mutation in the germ line that leads to a syndrome can be seen sporadically in the solitary tumors; this has been shown to be the case in both Muir-Torre syndrome (Chap. 65) and nevoid basal cell carcinoma syndrome (Chap. 56) and is undoubtedly true for other tumors.

There is no simple classification of adnexal tumors. Under the microscope, they may resemble various epidermal and adnexal structures. In recent years, many monoclonal antibodies have been employed in elegant studies to show the relationships between the various, normal cutaneous structures and the corresponding tumors. The tumors may resemble the interfollicular epidermis (Chap. 56), hair follicle, eccrine, apocrine or sebaceous glands and are so classified. Such schemes should not be taken as suggesting a given tumor arises from a given structure. It is often very difficult to determine the direction of differentiation, especially because the eccrine and apocrine ducts are almost identical, so that tumors with ductal features are hard to classify. It is just as likely that a more primitive epithelial cell has gone astray and differentiated in the direction of an adnexal structure. Finally, the most common adnexal tumor is not discussed in this chapter but in Chapter 56. Basal cell carcinoma is a malignant tumor that, at least in its nodular forms, has striking histologic and immunohistochemical similarities with tumors of hair follicle origin, especially trichoblastomas. Tradition demands that basal cell carcinoma be considered along with other epidermal neoplasms.

If there is a heaven for lumpers and splitters, it is the study of adnexal tumors. We are lumpers and will concentrate on those tumors that are common and that have distinct clinical features. We also call to the reader's attention the four, detailed profusely illustrated texts by Ackerman and his colleagues on adnexal neoplasms.

Hair Follicle Tumors

Benign Hair Follicle Tumors

Hair follicle tumors are most common on the face and scalp. They resemble part of the hair follicle or the perifollicular mesenchyme. Immunohistochemical studies using monoclonal antibodies directed against cytokeratins have been most helpful in establishing the relationship between normal follicular elements and various tumors.

Trichoblastoma

(Headington 1976; Ackerman et al. 1993)

Synonyms. Trichoblastic fibroma, immature trichoepithelioma, giant trichoepithelioma

Definition. Benign follicular tumor containing follicular germinative cells.

Clinical Findings. Trichoblastomas are uncommon except in nevus sebaceus (Chap. 52) where they are the most common secondary tumor. In this setting, they have been confused with a basal cell carcinoma both clinically and histologically. Trichoblastomas tend to be fairly large tumors, 1–2 cm in size, and occupy both the dermis and subcutaneous tissue. While they may be both endophytic and exophytic, they rarely ulcerate. Any area of the body may be involved. Multiple lesions are extremely uncommon.

Histopathology. Many histologic patterns may be seen. Headington divided all follicular tumors into epithelial, mesenchymal-epithelial and purely mesenchymal. This classification has been for the most part replaced, but it emphasizes a crucial feature of most hair follicle tumors – dermal interaction just as seen between the hair germ and papilla. The typical nodular trichoblastoma is a large, symmetrical vertically growing tumor with a sharp border. It has an adherent fibrous capsule, presumably induced by the hair germ elements. Connections to the epidermis are uncommon. Clefts arise between this capsule and the normal dermis, while in a basal cell carcinoma clefts arise between the tumor cells and the dermis. Hair germs must be present; they are usually common but on occasion one must search.

Ackerman has identified five patterns that frequently overlap. They are: large nodular, small nodular, racemiform (like an elk's antlers), cribiform (like a sieve) and retiform (like a net.) Larger lesions often are cystic; the space contains amorphous cell debris. Mucin may be present. Since hair follicles are rich in mitoses, follicular tumors also may contain abundant dividing cells, but atypical mitoses, marked cellular pleomorphism, necrosis and ulceration are all rare. A pigmented trichoblastoma has abundant melanin in the tumor cells and in dermal melanophages but is otherwise identical. Cutaneous lymphadenoma appears to be an adamantinoid or clear cell trichoblastoma with a generous lymphocytic infiltrate.

Differential Diagnosis. The differential diagnostic considerations include basal cell carcinoma, dermal melanocytic nevus, epidermoid cyst and other adnexal tumors.

Therapy. Surgical excision

Trichoepithelioma

(Brooke 1892)

Synonyms. Superficial trichoblastoma; when multiple, Brooke syndrome, Brooke-Spiegler syndrome, epithelioma adenoides cysticum, epithelioma papulosum multiplex, Brooke tumor

Definition. Superficial variant of trichoblastoma, also containing hair germs, but often with multiple lesions.

Etiology and Pathogenesis. Brooke syndrome is inherited in an autosomal dominant fashion. Brooke-Spiegler syndrome refers to patients with multiple trichoepitheliomas, cylindromas and spiradenomas. Gene studies show the relationship between these two disorders. One relevant gene is located on chromosome 16q12–q13. Families have been described in which one member has multiple trichoepitheliomas and the other, multiple spiradenomas and cylindromas.

Clinical Findings. In contrast to trichoblastoma, trichoepithelioma is usually multiple. The typical patient has numerous small papules in the nasolabial folds or periorbital region, but also may have occasional larger or ulcerated lesions and may have involvement of other parts of the face (Fig. 57.1). The individual lesions are usually several millimeters in diameter, translucent or pearly and grouped together. There is often a family history of similar changes in a parent or child. The lesions usually appear in childhood, become more prominent in puberty and remain stable. A changing lesion, especially one that is ulcerated, may represent a basal cell carcinoma and should be biopsied. It is unclear if trichoepitheliomas evolve into basal cell carcinoma or if both tumors arise on the same background. Some patients may simultaneously have cylindromas and milia.

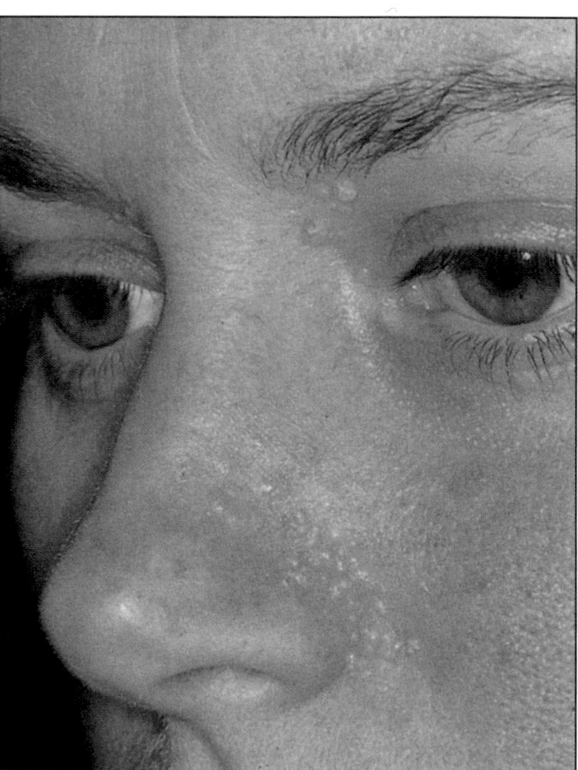

Fig. 57.1. Multiple trichoepitheliomas

Histopathology. Basaloid tumor strands arise from the epidermis and connect in complex patterns. Cysts containing lamellated accumulations of keratin are common, as are primitive hair germs.

Differential Diagnosis. The multiple adenoma sebaceum (probably better designated angiofibroma) of tuberous sclerosis are clinically similar, so one should search for other stigmata of tuberous sclerosis and do a biopsy.

Therapy. Therapy is very difficult. Both dermabrasion and a variety of laser destructive methods have been employed. Often multiple treatments are needed, as the trichoepitheliomas usually slowly recur. The patient should be followed closely since basal cell carcinomas also develop and can be obscured by laser or dermabrasion, presenting later as a larger, deeper tumor.

Desmoplastic Trichoepithelioma

(Brownstein and Shapiro 1977)

Synonym. Sclerosing epithelial hamartoma, although clearly an acquired tumor.

Definition. Benign follicular tumor with prominent mesenchymal component.

Clinical Findings. Even though it is uncommon, a desmoplastic trichoepithelioma can often be diagnosed clinically, especially when one sees it for the second time. The lesions are invariably on the face, usually in young women and on the chin or cheek. They are large, flat-topped or form plaques, which may be centrally depressed. Patients with multiple desmoplastic trichoepitheliomas have been reported; as expected, the disorder is inherited in an autosomal dominant pattern.

Histopathology. The broad-based nature of the tumor can be appreciated and serves as a clue. The dermis contains small cysts with lamellated keratin as well as strands of basaloid cells, both surrounded by a fibrous stroma that is sharply separated from the adjacent normal dermis. The basaloid strands resemble a sclerosing basal cell carcinoma but other features are not seen. The tiny cysts suggest a microcystic adnexal carcinoma but they contain keratin; this is not true in the carcinoma, which also invariably extends far deeper.

Differential Diagnosis. Most lesions are diagnosed as basal cell carcinoma, dermatofibroma or scar.

Therapy. Surgical excision

Trichilemmoma

(Headington and French 1962)

Synonym. Tricholemmoma

Definition. Benign follicular tumor resembling the outer root sheath.

Etiology and Pathogenesis. Ackerman has suggested that trichilemmomas are the end stage of human papilloma virus (HPV) infections of the hair follicle. While there are clinical and histologic overlaps between trichilemmoma and verruca, HPV has not been consistently identified in trichilemmoma.

Clinical Findings. A solitary trichilemmoma is uncommon, but probably often not biopsied. The lesions are typically exophytic verrucous papules, most often on the nasolabial folds, about the mouth and eyes and also seen over the entire head and neck region. Multiple trichilemmomas are a cardinal clinical sign of Cowden syndrome (Chap. 65).

Histopathology. A symmetric basaloid tumor is vertically oriented around a follicle, with acanthotic proliferation of the follicle wall. While the basal layer of this epithelium is normal, the balance is altered by a clear cell change. The large clear cells are PAS-positive. The basal membrane is often prominent. Clefts are not seen. Pseudosquamous eddies may be found, as there is a microscopic overlap with irritated seborrheic keratosis.

Differential Diagnosis. A solitary lesion is invariably confused with a verruca vulgaris. Multiple verrucae, tuberous sclerosis and multiple trichoepitheliomas should be considered in the case of Cowden syndrome.

Therapy. Surgical excision. Multiple lesions can be treated with dermabrasion or laser destruction. Patients with Cowden syndrome must be monitored for the development of breast carcinoma (life time risk $>50\%$ in women) and other malignancies.

Trichilemmal Horn
(Brownstein 1979)

Synonym. Trichilemmal keratosis

This lesion is probably a variant of actinic keratosis and will not be confused clinically or histologically with an adnexal tumor, but its name is misleading. Usually a thickened keratosis or horn is found on sunlight-exposed skin in an older adult. The epidermis may be delled and resembles the follicular isthmus, while the horn is similar to the contents of a pilar cyst.

Pilomatricoma
(Malherbe and Chenantais 1880; Forbis and Helwig 1961)

Synonyms. Pilomatrixoma, Malherbe tumor, calcifying epithelioma of Malherbe

Definition. Benign follicular tumor with features of the follicle matrix.

Clinical Findings. Pilomatricoma is typically a tumor of childhood. It is the second most common "lump and bump" (cutaneous or subcutaneous tumor) in children, following only epidermoid cyst. It is also seen in adults. In addition to being common, a pilomatricoma can often be recognized clinically. It appears as a bone-hard, often inflamed cystic structure, usually on the face, shoulder or upper aspect of arm (Fig. 57.2). The eyebrows and temple are especially common sites. There may be a history of rupture with discharge of grains or pebbles. When not inflamed, a pilomatricoma is clinically identical to an epidermoid cyst.

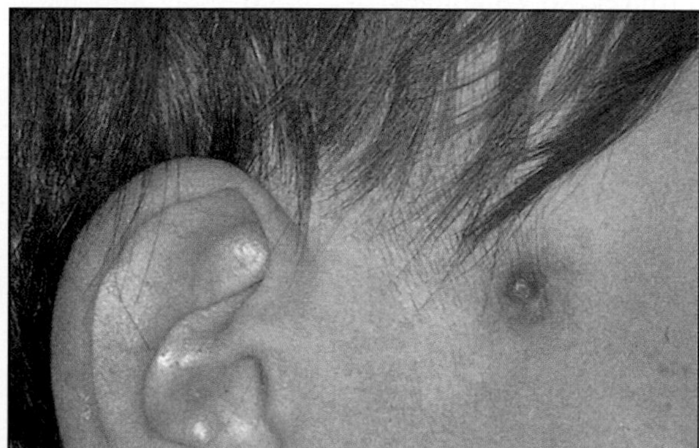

Fig. 57.2. Pilomatricoma

Multiple and eruptive pilomatricomas have been described. Some patients with multiple pilomatricomas have myotonic dystrophy (Curschmann-Steinert syndrome). This disorder is inherited in an autosomal dominant pattern. Other features include myotonia (inability to relax muscles after use), premature frontal alopecia, cataracts and testicular atrophy.

Histopathology. There are several classic histologic markers for pilomatricoma. They include sheets of basaloid cells with a transition to amorphous keratinous sheets with empty spaces (shadow cells or cornified hair matrix cells), foci of calcification and even ossification, and an intense foreign body inflammatory response. Similar patterns of keratinization may be seen within epidermoid cysts, especially in Gardner syndrome.

Differential Diagnosis. The main consideration is epidermoid cysts and other cystic lesions. A ruptured discharging lesion may be mistaken for a foreign body granuloma. A deep noninflamed lesion is clinically identical to subcutaneous granuloma annulare or rheumatoid nodule, but quite different under the microscope.

Therapy. Surgical excision. Patients with multiple pilomatricomas should be referred to a neurologist to exclude myotonic dystrophy.

Follicular Cysts

The two most common cysts are both also technically hair follicle tumors. Epidermoid and trichilemmal cysts, including proliferating trichilemmal cysts, are covered in Chapter 53.

Trichoadenoma
(Nikolowski 1958)

Clinical Findings. This rare tumor is usually found on the face or buttocks. It is usually 1 – 2 cm in size, nodular and firm.

Histopathology. Multiple cystic spaces resembling the infundibular portion of the follicle are seen. The cysts are usually connected by basaloid strands and hair germs may be present.

Tumor of the Follicular Infundibulum

(MEHREGAN and BUTLER 1961)

Synonyms. Infundibuloma, isthmicoma

Clinical Findings. Tumor of the follicular infundibulum is usually a solitary papule or, more often, a plaque on the head and neck of older patients. Multiple lesions have been described in Cowden syndrome (Chap. 65).

Histopathology. The microscopic picture of this clinically banal tumor is striking. There is a plate of isthmic epithelium running parallel to the skin surface and occasionally connected to it via the intervening follicles.

Differential Diagnosis. Microscopically the lesions can be confused with superficial basal cell carcinoma or reticular seborrheic keratosis.

Therapy. Surgical excision

Trichofolliculoma

(GRAY and HELWIG 1962)

Synonym. Most lesions described as hair follicle nevi are either trichofolliculomas or accessory tragi (Chap. 20).

Clinical Findings. Trichofolliculomas are often clinically distinct. They are one of the few hair follicle tumors that usually feature hairs. The typical lesion is a firm papule on the face of an adult with a wisp of white hair emerging from a central dell (Fig. 57.3).

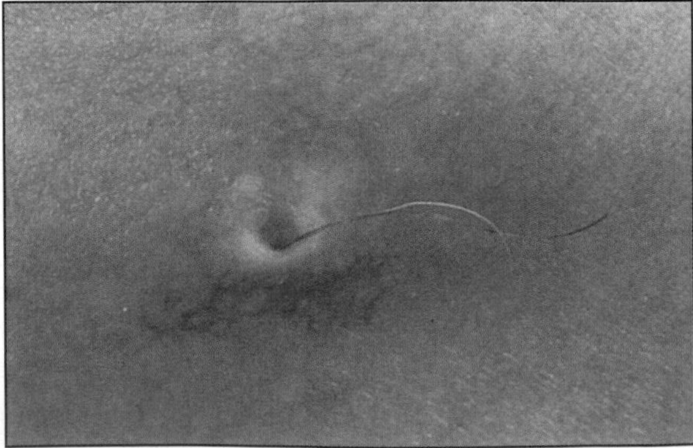

Fig. 57.3. Trichofolliculoma

Histopathology. Typically there is a dilated follicle or cystic lesion containing hairs. Branching out from the central cavity are many incomplete follicular structures. When many sebaceous glands are present, one can diagnose folliculosebaceous cystic hamartoma.

Therapy. Surgical excision

Folliculosebaceous Cystic Hamartoma

(KIMURA et al. 1991)

Synonyms. Sebaceous folliculoma (PLEWIG 1980)

Etiology and Pathogenesis. Just as the normal hair follicle shows a cycle of growth and regression, sometimes the follicles in a adnexal neoplasm may also change. This appears to be the mechanism linking trichofolliculoma, sebaceous trichofolliculoma and folliculosebaceous cystic hamartoma. All are clinically identical.

Clinical Findings. Folliculosebaceous cystic hamartoma is usually a solitary cystic tumor on the bridge of the nose. There is a central pore that often contains terminal or vellus hairs. The tumor occurs primarily in men.

Histopathology. There is a central dilated pore surrounded by numerous sebaceous glands, all of which empty into the space. Both hair germs and hairs may be seen, but there are usually signs of regression of the follicular epithelium. Thus, microscopically, folliculosebaceous cystic hamartoma appears to represent a trichofolliculoma in a late stage.

Differential Diagnosis. Dermoid cysts and nasal gliomas may also be found on the nose, but they are present early in life, are larger, usually lack a central pore and have a strikingly different histologic picture.

Therapy. Surgical excision

Pilar Sheath Acanthoma

(MEHREGAN and BROWNSTEIN 1978)

Clinical Findings. Pilar sheath acanthomas are uncommon benign tumors that usually present as solitary lesions in sun-exposed skin. They may be clinically identifiable, as they typically are broad-based skin colored papules with a central depression that is filled with a cornified plug. Sometimes the plug can be extruded just as with a comedo. The most common sites are the forehead, upper lip and lateral side of the neck. Most patients are older and there is no sexual preference.

Histopathology. There is a central cystic invagination that arises from the epidermis and involves a hair follicle. The cyst wall is acanthotic and the cells of the basal layer may be hyperpigmented. The mass of compact cornified material is easily seen, but often multiple sections are required to find a terminal or perhaps a vellus hair.

Differential Diagnosis. Giant pore of Winer, trichofolliculoma, Favre-Racouchot disease and giant comedo must all be considered. The histologic examination makes the distinction, although admittedly sometimes the clinical importance of the diagnosis is minimal.

Therapy. Surgical excision

Giant Pore of Winer

(WINER 1954)

Synonym. Dilated pore

Clinical Findings. A giant pore is usually found on the face, neck or upper part of the chest of older adults, just as with a pilar sheath acanthoma. A large dilated follicle is present, which is usually dark and typically located beneath the skin surface, sometimes expanded into a cystic structure that may undermine the skin laterally (Fig. 57.4). In contrast, an acne comedo is usually dome-shaped and arises above the skin level. Once again, the keratinous plug can occasionally be extruded but the lesion reforms.

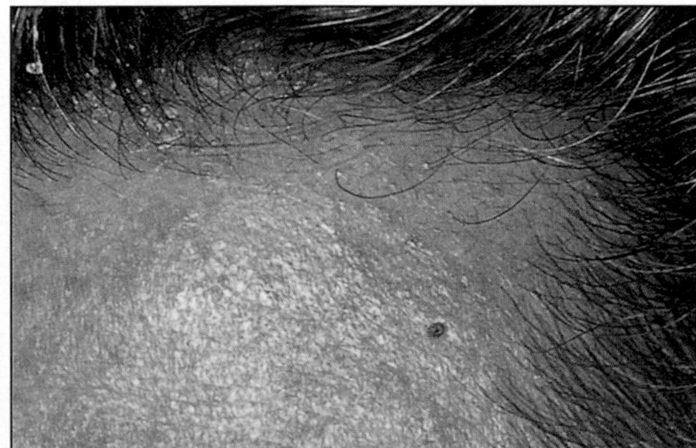

Fig. 57.4. Giant pore of Winer

Histopathology. A large, dilated sebaceous follicle is identified. The central cavity is filled with cornified material while the wall may show minimal thickening, sometimes in a papillomatous pattern and with increased melanin. Hair germs and sebaceous glands are usually absent, and perifollicular fibroses are not seen.

Differential Diagnosis. A dilated pore and pilar sheath acanthoma are clinically identical and can only be separated under the microscope. They probably are minimal variants of the same theme. The rest of the differential is as discussed under pilar sheath acanthoma.

Therapy. Surgical excision

Inverted Follicular Keratosis

Etiology and Pathogenesis. The existence of inverted follicular keratosis is challenged, so it is not surprising that the etiology is unclear. Some investigators feel that inverted follicular keratosis represents a follicular variant of verruca vulgaris, and others consider it a follicular or downward-growing type of seborrheic keratosis. We tentatively include it as a follicular tumor.

Clinical Findings. Inverted follicular keratosis is a solitary tumor usually seen in older men and almost always on the face. It is often crusted.

Histopathology. The tumor involves a follicle; the walls of the expanded follicle resemble a seborrheic keratosis with basaloid hyperplasia and pseudosquamous eddies. The lesion can best be thought of as a seborrheic keratosis pointed in the wrong direction, vertical not horizontal.

Differential Diagnosis. Usually the clinical diagnosis is verruca or seborrheic keratosis.

Therapy. Surgical excision

Fibrofolliculoma and Perifollicular Fibroma

Synonym. Mantleoma

Etiology and Pathogenesis. We view fibrofolliculoma, perifollicular fibroma and trichodiscoma as

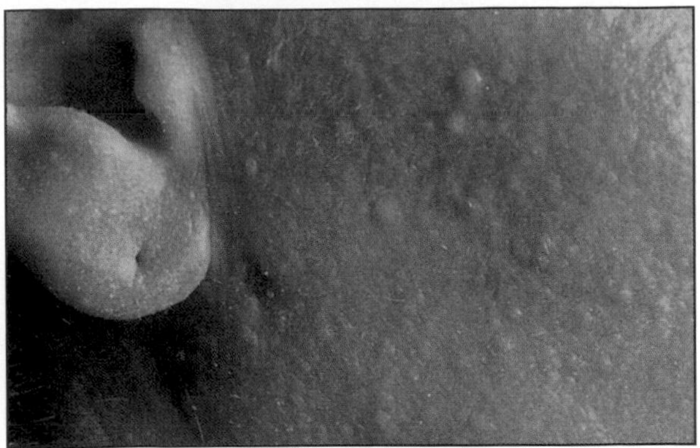

Fig. 57.5. Multiple fibrofolliculomas and trichodiscomas

the same tumor in different stages of evolution. All three lesions represent a proliferation of the dermal perifollicular mesenchyme, probably associated with the follicular mantle which gives rise to the sebaceous glands. For this reason the term mantleoma has been proposed to cover all three tumors. The age of the lesion and even the method of sectioning may determine which features are most prominent.

Clinical Findings. Small papules are found, sometimes with a central pore; they may resemble acne scars (Fig. 57.5). Occasionally a large, solitary exophytic tumor may be seen. The combination of multiple fibrofolliculomas, perifollicular fibromas and trichodiscomas is known as the Birt-Hogg-Dubé syndrome, which may be a marker for internal malignancies, especially renal cell carcinoma (Chap. 65).

Histopathology. A perifollicular fibroma shows a normal or dilated follicle with fibrosis of the adjacent dermis. In a fibrofolliculoma, there are long lacy strands of follicular epithelium, sometime with sebaceous cells, extending into a more nodular fibrous stroma. The lacy pattern recapitulates the downward growth of the follicular mantle cells to form the sebaceous glands. This is the usual pattern of the solitary tumors.

Differential Diagnosis. The many, tiny follicular-based lesions are often misdiagnosed as acne scars.

Therapy. Solitary or disturbing lesions can be excised. The multiple tumors are difficult to treat; dermabrasion and laser destruction are most useful.

Trichodiscoma

(Pinkus et al. 1974)

Etiology and Pathogenesis. The tumor known as the trichodiscoma has no clear relationship to the hair disc, which is a sensory organ most common in animals and rich in Merkel cells. Trichodiscoma is a proliferation of the mantle cells that are the precursors of the sebaceous gland and duct. Trichodiscomas are part of the same clinical and histologic spectrum as fibrofolliculoma and perifollicular fibroma.

Clinical Findings. Trichodiscomas are small, flat-topped flesh-colored papular usually on the face or trunk. The ears are a typical location. The lesions are usually multiple and can be inherited in an autosomal dominant fashion.

Histopathology. The epidermis is slightly raised and flattened, covering a fibrous proliferation with scattered mucin. While these spindle cells were long held to be neural, they are definitely fibrous.

Therapy. Surgical excision

Malignant Hair Follicle Tumors

Malignant hair follicle tumors are very uncommon, other than the exception discussed in the introduction – basal cell carcinoma. There is a malignant equivalent of the pilomatricoma known as a pilomatrical carcinoma. It is seen in adults, in contrast to the young age group affected by pilomatricoma. The tumor is usually quite large, often ulcerated and diagnosed only histologically by the increased number of mitoses and pleomorphism. Since the hair matrix is an active area, mitoses are also found in ordinary pilomatricomas, so this distinction may be extremely difficult and easily overlooked. The trichilemmal carcinoma bears the same relationship to a trichilemmoma. In other instances, the term trichilemmal carcinoma is used to describe a squamous cell carcinoma arising out of a trichilemmal keratosis. While proliferating pilar cyst (Chap. 53) is usually considered a mimic of squamous cell carcinoma, we suspect it may be a low-grade variant, for there are rare reports of such lesions metastasizing.

Sweat Gland Tumors

Benign Sweat Gland Tumors

The terminology of eccrine and apocrine tumors is also a confusing story. While it is usually easy to decide that a given tumor is of sweat gland origin, distinguishing between eccrine and apocrine elements is difficult. There are several reasons for this problem. First, the eccrine and apocrine ducts are almost identical, so that ductal tumors cannot be reliably differentiated. Second, apocrine tumors have a classic morphologic marker – decapitation secretion; eccrine tumors have no such marker. Immunohistochemical studies have begun to bring order to this complex area. We have attempted to identify those tumors that seem to have specific eccrine or apocrine features, but expect many changes in the years to come.

Cylindroma

(Ancell 1842; Spiegler 1899)

Synonyms. Turban tumor, Spiegler tumor

Definition. Benign adnexal tumor usually on the scalp and often multiple.

Etiology and Pathogenesis. One can find convincing arguments suggesting that cylindromas show eccrine, apocrine and hair follicle differentiation. Clinically the location on the scalp and the frequent association with other follicular tumors add support to the follicular origin of cylindroma. We await definitive studies.

Clinical Findings. The most typical location for cylindromas is the scalp; hence the name turban tumors. Multiple lesions are common. Since cylindromas become larger than other hair follicle tumors, often the unfortunate patient does look as if he is wearing a form of turban. The individual lesions are flesh-colored to red, hairless, rather soft and often covered with telangiectases (Fig. 57.6). Lesions may be found on the rest of the face, but the smaller ones are often trichoepitheliomas. Lesions usually begin to appear in childhood. While the large lesions may ulcerate, malignant change does not occur.

Patients with multiple cylindromas, spiradenomas, trichoepitheliomas and milia have been designated as having Brooke-Spiegler syndrome, which is inherited in an autosomal dominant pattern.

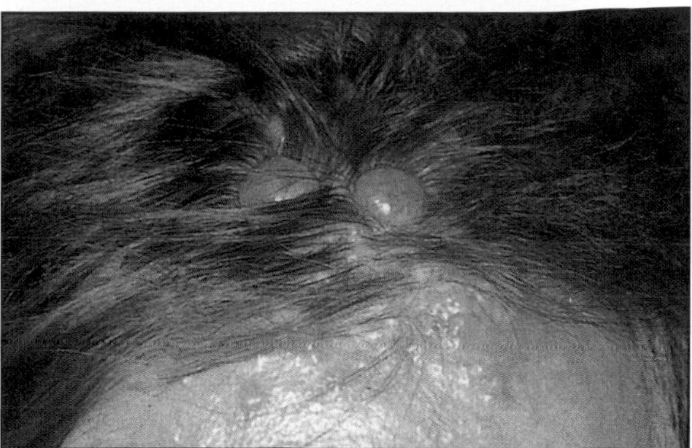

Fig. 57.6. Multiple cylindromas, including smaller paler lesions on forehead

Histopathology. The pattern of cylindroma is striking. There are dermal nests of basaloid tumor cells that contain PAS-positive hyaline inclusions and are surrounded by a dense hyaline (or amorphous) membrane. The pattern formed by these almost interlocking nests has been compared to a jigsaw puzzle. This striking membrane appears to be of epithelial, not mesenchymal, origin. In the early days of pathology, tissue probes were often macerated before being examined; when cylindromas were treated in this manner, the hyaline tubes or cylinders remained relatively unchanged.

Differential Diagnosis. The large tumors may suggest neurofibromatosis. A solitary lesion can be confused with a basal cell carcinoma or variety of cysts. Usually the physician can make a confident clinical diagnosis.

Therapy. Surgical excision of individual disturbing lesions

Hidrocystoma

Hidrocystomas are traditionally divided into eccrine and apocrine forms, although today most are held to be apocrine in nature. They are translucent cystic lesions usually about the eyes and are discussed in Chapter 53.

Syringoma

Clinical Findings. Syringomas are probably the most common adnexal tumor. They typically occur below the eyes of young women and are almost always multiple (Fig. 57.7). They are small skin-colored or pale papules. A much less common form

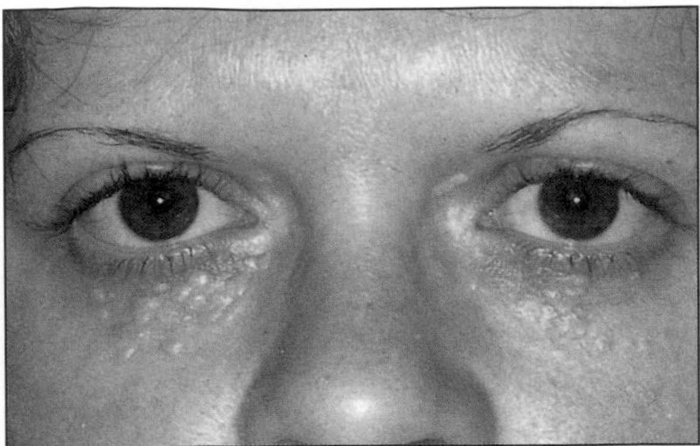

Fig. 57.7. Multiple syringomas

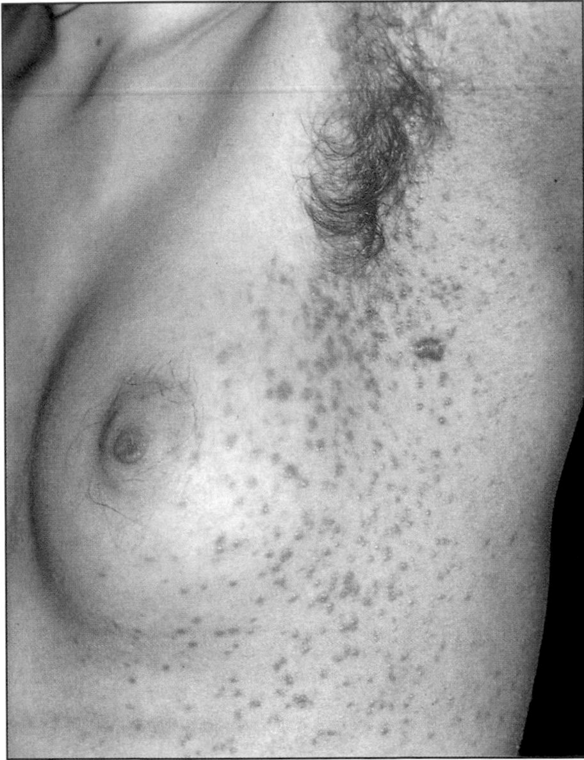

Fig. 57.8. Eruptive disseminated syringomas

is the eruptive or disseminated syringomas, which also involve primarily young women. These patients over a short period of time develop hundreds of papules and nodules, typically involving the face, midchest or vulva, but occurring in any site where eccrine glands are found (Fig. 57.8). The individual lesions tend to be somewhat darker on the trunk. They do not itch. Malignant change does not occur.

Histopathology. The epidermis is normal. In the dermis, multiple, small, round or elongated cystic or ductal structures are seen, along with strands of basaloid cells. The colorful terms comma-shaped and tadpole have been used to describe the shape of the glandular elements. The cyst wall consists of two layers of epithelial cells and surrounds amorphous, pale PAS-positive material. Larger lesions may have considerable fibrosis. Some syringomas show striking clear cell change (clear cell syringoma), but they are clinically not different from other syringomas.

Differential Diagnosis. The facial lesions may be confused with plane warts, milia and xanthelasmas. The truncal lesions are very similar to eruptive vellus hair cysts and disseminated granuloma annulare; all three of these disorders typically involve young women. On first glance, they may also resemble an exanthem, such as secondary syphilis.

Therapy. There is no good treatment for the multiple lesions. They can be destroyed with a laser or dermabrasion but invariably recur. Individual lesions can be excised or otherwise destroyed.

Eccrine Poroma

(Pinkus et al. 1956)

Clinical Findings. Eccrine poromas are typically mistaken for vascular tumors. They are typically red-brown sharply demarcated nodules that occur either on the feet or the scalp. Only rarely are other body regions involved. They may be crusted or eroded and are always included in the list of painful tumors, but in our experience, the foot lesions are painful, the others, not.

Histopathology. A basaloid tumor arises from the epidermis and extends as a broad plate-like process into the dermis. There is a sharp transition between the normal epidermis and the tumor. The tumor cells are small basaloid cells with a pink cytoplasm. PAS staining not only highlights their cytoplasm but aids in identifying the small ductal structures that can often be found.

Two histological variants are:

- Hidroacanthoma Simplex. The tumor nests are confined to the epidermis, producing the picture of intraepithelial clones or the Borst-Jadassohn phenomenon.
- Dermal Duct Tumor. No epidermal connections are seen.

Differential Diagnosis. The typical eccrine poroma is mistaken for a pyogenic granuloma or other vascular tumor. Histologically, it may be confused with clear cell acanthoma.

Therapy. Surgical excision

Clear Cell Hidradenoma

(KEASBEY and HADLEY 1954; KERSTING 1963)

Synonyms. Eccrine acrospiroma (JOHNSON and HELWIG 1969), nodular hidradenoma, solid-cystic hidradenoma, clear cell myoepithelioma

Clinical Findings. Clear cell hidradenomas are simply dermal nodules; they cannot be recognized clinically. If they are superficial enough, they may have a red tint. They often become quite large (Fig. 57.9).

Histopathology. The dermis contains multiple lobules containing two cell populations and surrounded by a fibrous capsule. There is usually no epidermal connection. Ductal structures and small cysts are invariably present and larger tumors may be very cystic. The clear cell is the most prominent feature; it represents an eccrine secretory cell, is usually columnar and may contain mucin. The smaller basaloid cells represent ductal cells. In some clear cell hidradenomas apocrine decapitation secretion can occasionally be found.

Differential Diagnosis. Histologically one should think of metastatic renal cell carcinoma and metastatic malignant melanoma. When clear cells are uncommon and the cystic spaces are large, a glomus tumor may be suggested.

Therapy. Surgical excision

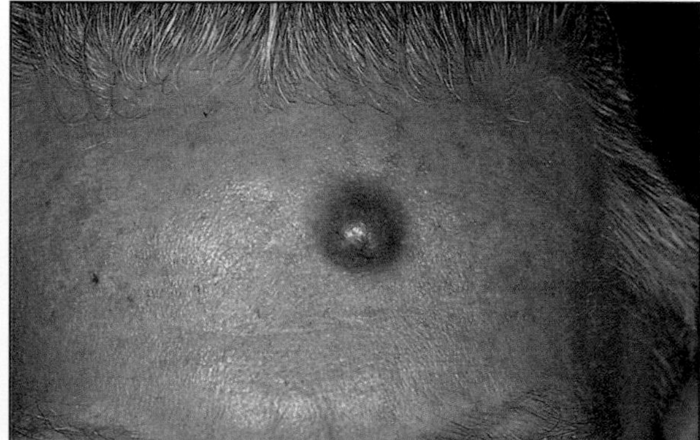

Fig. 57.9. Clear cell hidradenoma

Eccrine Spiradenoma

(KERSTING and HELWIG 1956)

Clinical Findings. Once again, the clinical findings – dermal nodules – are not helpful. The nodules are often painful upon palpation. There are patients with multiple eccrine spiradenomas, which are inherited in an autosomal dominant pattern and often associated with other adnexal tumors.

Histopathology. The pattern of eccrine spiradenoma is that of rosettes contain two distinct cell populations. Forming the rosettes are larger cells with vesicular nuclei; intermixed are small, dark basaloid cells with little cytoplasm. Ductal elements may be found. There is a thick basement membrane surrounding the tumor, similar to a cylindroma, but the jigsaw pattern of the latter is not seen.

Differential Diagnosis. There are no notorious mimics. One should think of the other painful tumors, listed with glomus tumors in Chapter 59.

Therapy. Surgical excision

Mixed Tumor of Skin

(LENNOX et al. 1952)

Synonym. Chondroid syringoma (HIRSCH and HELWIG 1961)

Clinical Findings. Mixed tumor of skin is usually a firm dermal or subcutaneous lesion on the head or neck of an elderly man.

Histopathology. A wide variety of structures may be found in a mixed tumor of skin, as the name suggests. Both eccrine and apocrine forms occur. Either small, round eccrine tubules or larger branching apocrine tubules are found in a fibrous stroma. Another striking change is the development of amorphous cartilaginous areas that are relatively acellular and rich in mucin. Chondrocytes are seen and myofibroblasts may be common.

Differential Diagnosis. There may be small chondroid areas in otherwise ordinary clear cell hidradenomas and acrospiromas.

Therapy. Surgical excision

Papillary Eccrine Adenoma
(Rulon and Helwig 1977)

Clinical Findings. These tumors are either solitary papules or nodular and usually located on the arms.

Histopathology. Dilated tortuous ducts are embedded in a fibrous stroma. The ductal epithelium has two cell layers and marked papillary changes.

Therapy. Surgical excision

Aggressive Digital Papillary Adenoma
(Kao et al. 1987)

Clinical Findings. These rare tumors usually present as an enlarging mass involving a fingernail bed. The toes, palms and soles may also be involved. The tumors are usually not painful.

Histopathology. An epidermal connection is usually not present. In the dermis are numerous nodules in a fronded or papillary pattern, comprised of small blue cells and larger eosinophilic myoepithelial cells. The name aggressive reflects the difficulties in separating this tumor from its malignant equivalent – digital papillary adenocarcinoma. There is probably a continuum beginning with papillary eccrine adenoma and extending to a carcinoma; mitoses and necrosis are the best clues to malignancy.

Differential Diagnosis. The main differential point is a glomus tumor (Chap. 59).

Therapy. Because of the problems in determining the biologic nature of such tumors, a wider excision is often recommended but usually hard to achieve on the digit.

Eccrine Syringofibroadenoma
(Mascaro 1963)

Synonym. Mascaro tumor

Clinical Findings. This rare tumor is typically located on the extremities and presents as a solitary hyperkeratotic nodule in adults. Microscopically there are thin, anastomosing epithelial strands extending from the base of the epidermis down through a fibrous stroma. Small ducts are seen among the tumor cords.

The same microscopic picture can be seen in several settings.

- Multiple papules and nodules that may be associated with Schöpf syndrome (Chap. 17).
- Eccrine acrosyringeal nevus, which tends to be linear and present at birth (Chap. 52).
- Erosive erythematous plaques of the palmoplantar skin in patients with hidrotic ectodermal dysplasia (Chap. 30) and in those with severe inflammatory disorders involving the same region, such as bullous pemphigoid. Presumably chronic inflammation and damage to the sweat ducts causes reactive changes. In the case of hidrotic ectodermal dysplasia, there could also be structural defects in the eccrine glands predisposing to this problem. Other investigators have suggested that some of these lesions may be caused by HPV.

Differential Diagnosis. The solitary lesions may be confused with eccrine poroma, verruca vulgaris or even malignant tumors.

Therapy. Surgical excision

Syringocystadenoma Papilliferum
(Elliott 1893; Werther 1913)

Clinical Findings. Syringocystadenoma papilliferum is typically a verrucous nodule on the scalp, temple or occasionally the cheek. There are usually no hairs over the tumor; there may be a central fistulous tract draining a brown fluid, which produces a crust. After trichoblastoma, it is the most common tumor developing in nevus sebaceus.

Histopathology. The dermis contains a complex cystic structure with many invaginations and finger-like projections. There is a surface connection, which often is only seen after multiple sections have been obtained. The epidermis is usually hyperkeratotic and crusted. The cystic spaces are lined by two layers of cells, the innermost of which invariably displays decapitation secretion. This is the tumor in which it is easiest to find this unequivocal sign of apocrine differentiation. The stroma is also rich in plasma cells, another reliable clue.

Differential Diagnosis. The tumor is often mistaken for a basal cell carcinoma, especially in the background of a nevus sebaceus. Otherwise one may think of a verruca vulgaris or irritated seborrheic keratosis.

Histologically, one must consider cutaneous endometriosis and exclude an adenocarcinoma by means of the normal cytologic appearance of the cells.

Therapy. Surgical excision.

Hidradenoma Papilliferum
(Werth 1878)

Synonym. Vulvar hidradenoma

Clinical Findings. The tumor is almost exclusively limited to women and found almost only in the genital region, typically the labia. It most commonly appears during young adulthood and is confused with other labial masses such as a Bartholin gland cyst. There is no epidermal change.

Histopathology. Hidradenoma papilliferum can be thought of as a syringocystadenoma papilliferum without plasma cells or an epidermal connection.

Therapy. Surgical excision

Tubular Apocrine Adenoma
Landry and Winkelmann 1972)

This tumor is typically a large, lobulated scalp nodule found in older individuals. The microscopic pattern reveals multiple tubular structures with distinct decapitation secretion extending deep into the dermis. The stroma is fibrotic and does not contain inflammatory cells. There are histologic overlaps with papillary eccrine tumors.

Therapy. Surgical excision

Tumors of Modified Apocrine Glands

There are a number of modified apocrine glands associated with benign and malignant tumors. The best known modified apocrine-like gland is the breast. One could even speak of an accessory nipple (Chap. 19) as an apocrine hamartoma, but this is somewhat misleading.

Papillary Adenoma of the Nipple

Synonyms. Erosive adenomatosis of the nipple, pseudo-Paget disease of the nipple

Clinical Findings. This uncommon tumor presents as a unilateral nipple lesion with an inflamed, crusted surface and an underlying tumor. Thus the resemblance to Paget disease is unmistakable. The lesion involves women of all ages. Men are seldom affected. Despite the name, erosions or ulcerations are uncommon.

Histopathology. Erosive adenomatosis is a benign proliferation of the secretory ducts of the nipple, which are of apocrine origin. Microscopically the tumor resembles hidradenoma papilliferum with a benign ductal proliferation, fibrous stroma and plasma cell infiltrate.

Differential Diagnosis. Nipple dermatitis is often bilateral and occurs in patients with atopic dermatitis. Paget disease is excluded by the biopsy.

Therapy. Surgical excision

Glands of Moll

The glands of Moll are modified apocrine glands in the eyelids. Both adenomas and adenocarcinomas involving these structures have been described. Thus, if an inflammatory eyelid lesion fails to resolve in a reasonable period of time, a biopsy should be performed.

Ceruminous Glands

The ceruminous glands are located in the external auditory gland and produce ear wax. They may give rise to benign and malignant tumors. While the term ceruminoma is often employed, it is best forgotten, since it has been employed for almost all tumors of the ear canal.

Anogenital Mammary-Like Glands
(van der Putte 1991)

These glands are common in the anogenital region and are generally associated with a fibrous stroma, much like the mammary glands. Both eccrine and apocrine type secretions have been morphologically identified. Tumors such as perianal apocrine fibroadenoma and other fibrous apocrine lesions probably involve these intermediate glands.

Malignant Sweat Gland Tumors

Microcystic Adnexal Carcinoma
(Goldstein et al. 1982)

Synonym. Sclerosing sweat duct carcinoma, malignant syringoma

Clinical Findings. Microcystic adnexal carcinomas can occasionally be recognized clinically. They typically are slowly growing deep nodules or plaques found in the nasolabial fold or on the cheek or chin, mainly in older women. In rare instances they may involve other parts of the body, including the axillae. When the skin is stretched over the tumor, there is often a yellow tint. The lesion may be adherent to underlying structures.

Histopathology. The appearance of microcystic adnexal tumor is surprisingly bland, leading to many missed diagnoses. Usually there are no epidermal connections. The dermis is diffusely filled by nests and strands of keratinocytes admixed with both small ducts and cystic structures, suggesting both eccrine and follicular differentiation. Mitoses are few in number and necrosis does not occur. Perineural involvement is typical. Thus it is easy to diagnose a superficial biopsy from a microcystic adnexal carcinoma as a syringoma; the diagnosis of solitary syringoma should be made reluctantly and if the disease process extends to the base of the specimen, a reexcision should be encouraged.

Therapy. The tumor margins are both deep and indistinct. This feature coupled with the ability to spread along nerves produces a high recurrence rate and occasional metastases. Micrographic surgery is considered particularly valuable in dealing with such tumors. The patient should be warned before surgery that the defect will be far out of proportion to the innocent, preoperative clinical appearance.

Mucinous Carcinoma

Mucinous carcinomas typically present on the face of older men. More than half involve the eyelids. When the lesion is excised, the gelatinous nature of the tumor is apparent. Microscopically, nests and cords of epithelial cells float in lakes of mucin. The cells are not highly atypical, but if the tumor is not completely excised, recurrences are expected and local spread may occur.

Carcinoma ex Adenoma

Porocarcinomas are the most common adnexal carcinoma. They arise on the extremities or scalp of elderly patients, distributed just as are poromas. Porocarcinomas histologically may be confined to the epidermis in a clonal or Borst-Jadassohn pattern, which is thus a carcinoma in situ. If untreated, they spread to involve the dermis and may resemble squamous cell carcinoma. Ductal differentiation is the most reliable clue. Treatment is wide local excision. Malignant variants of cylindromas and spiradenomas have occasionally been described, as well as many rarer forms.

Aggressive Digital Papillary Carcinoma

The ambiguity of this tumor's name reflects the problem. There is a spectrum of acral eccrine tumors that microscopically have a complex folded papillary pattern and range from harmless (adenoma) to locally aggressive (destroying bone, for example) to frankly malignant. Since there is great variation within a given tumor, it is wise to insure that all acrally located, papillary eccrine tumors are completely excised.

Adenoid Cystic Carcinoma
(Boggio 1975)

Synonyms. Eccrine epithelioma, basal cell carcinoma with eccrine differentiation

The adenoid cystic carcinoma has no distinguishing clinical features. It is a red or skin-colored nodule, often on the nose, which shows a distinctive cribriform or sieve-like pattern microscopically. The tumor cells are small basaloid cells that may also be arranged in sheets and tubules. The ductal spaces may contain mucin. Therapy consist of wide local excision. The tumor also shows a predilection for the inner ear, but here it is often hard to decide if it represents local spread of a parotid tumor or a primary skin tumor.

Apocrine Carcinoma

Apocrine adenocarcinomas occur in the axillae or inguinal region, where apocrine glands are most densely found. They are usually solitary nodules in older adults. The tumor may spread to regional lymph nodes but is relatively nonaggressive. The histologic picture combines apocrine features such as ductal elements and decapitation secretion with solid, poorly differentiated pleomorphic areas.

Extramammary Paget Disease

In many instances this is also an apocrine or even eccrine ductal neoplasm that presents clinically as dermatitis and histologically with intraepidermal tumor cells. For the latter reason it is discussed in Chap. 55.

Lymphoepithelioma-Like Carcinoma
(SWANSON et al. 1988)

This rare tumor histologically resembles a nasopharyngeal tumor of the same name. Its etiology is unclear, as some authors classify it as an epidermal tumor and others, as adnexal. Clinically there is usually a facial or scalp nodule in an older adult, so a metastatic lesion often must be excluded. Microscopically there are islands or strands of atypical epithelium surrounded by a dense, mixed lymphocytic infiltrate. Both local recurrences and metastases have been described, so wide local excision is recommended.

Sebaceous Gland Tumors

Benign Sebaceous Gland Tumors

Sebaceous gland differentiation is usually identified by the presence of foamy, lipid-laden epithelial cells, known as sebocytes. There are no reliable immunohistochemical markers for sebaceous differentiation; thus, poorly differentiated sebaceous neoplasms remain a problem.

Sebaceous Hyperplasia

Synonym. Senile sebaceous hyperplasia

Etiology and Pathogenesis. Sebaceous hyperplasia is an extremely common finding in seborrheic sun-damaged skin. Some have suggested it represents a combination of sebaceous gland growth and diminution of the adjacent dermal tissues. Patients on renal dialysis may also have prominent sebaceous hyperplasia.

Clinical Findings. The individual lesion is distinctive; it is a papule or small nodule with a central depression surrounded by several small white-yellow nodules (Fig. 57.10). The most common sites are the forehead and cheek. Men are more frequently involved than women. Multiple lesions are the rule. The lesions are reactive, may regress and have no malignant potential (Chap. 28). Areolar sebaceous hyperplasia may also occur.

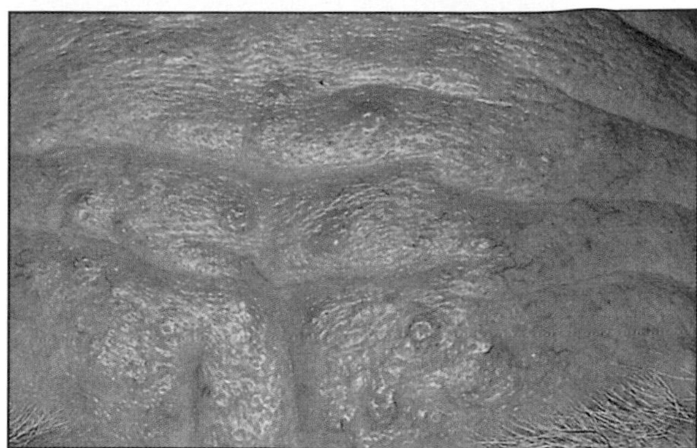

Fig. 57.10. Sebaceous hyperplasia

Histopathology. The microscopic picture exactly recapitulates the clinical one. There is a sebaceous follicle surrounded by an excess of very large sebaceous lobules. The balance of the epidermis and dermis usually shows sun damage.

Differential Diagnosis. If no pore is present and there is only a single lesion, one may think of a basal cell carcinoma or small cyst.

Therapy. Sebaceous hyperplasia should either be excised or ignored. The lesions are deep enough that shave excisions or other destructive measures usually produce a pitted scar. Very small lesions can be treated with cryotherapy. If there are dozens of lesions, especially in patients with marked seborrhea, low dose isotretinoin, (10 mg daily) may bring marked improvement.

Sebaceous Adenoma

Clinical Findings. Sebaceous adenomas are typically solitary, perhaps yellow or tan, nodules arising on the head and neck of adult patients. They may occur in nevus sebaceus. When multiple sebaceous adenomas or sebaceomas are present, one must rule out the Muir-Torre syndrome, which is associated with multiple keratoacanthomas and multiple internal malignancies.

Histopathology. There is usually an epidermal connection, representing a sebaceous follicle. The corium is replaced by a lobular tumor centered around the follicle. The individual lobules show an increased number of basaloid or peripheral cells and fewer foamy cells. When the basaloid cells predominate or when the lobular arrangement is not present, then one should diagnose a sebaceoma. One can think of sebaceous adenoma as a large, slightly disorganized sebaceous hyperplasia.

Cystic sebaceous adenomas are larger lesions with a well-defined central cyst and focal areas of sebaceous differentiation. They are almost exclusively limited to Muir-Torre syndrome.

Differential Diagnosis. Most lesions are submitted as basal cell carcinomas.

Therapy. Surgical excision

Sebaceoma

(Troy and Ackerman 1984)

Clinical Findings. A sebaceoma is just as indistinct clinically as a sebaceous adenoma.

Histopathology. In sebaceoma, basaloid cells predominate. Sometimes one will find only a smattering of foamy cells, making identification very hard. Some individuals have called such tumors sebaceous epitheliomas but that term is unwise. There are no agreed upon criteria and sebaceomas are benign, whereas sebaceous epithelioma suggests a behavior similar to basal cell carcinoma. Basal cell carcinoma with sebaceous differentiation is an uncommon event; most such cases also represent sebaceoma.

Therapy. Surgical excision

Malignant Sebaceous Tumors

Sebaceous Carcinoma

Sebaceous carcinomas present on the eyelid about 50% of the time. Other lesions are simply solitary nodules occurring anywhere on the body where sebaceous glands are found. While sebaceous carcinomas may develop in Muir-Torre syndrome, they are surprisingly rare. The eyelid lesions are frequently misdiagnosed as an infectious process, so that the correct treatment is delayed until the tumor has progressed to involve other ocular structures. Sebaceous carcinomas also present histologic problems, as they have a carcinoma in situ pattern with large clear cells dispersed through the epidermis, mimicking malignant melanoma in situ, Paget disease or Bowen disease. Treatment is generous local surgery with careful margin control. A S-100 stain should be employed to exclude a melanocytic lesion.

Bibliography

Abenoza P, Ackerman B (1990) Neoplasms with eccrine differentiation. Lea and Febiger, Philadelphia

Ackerman AB, Viragh PA, Chongchitnant N (eds) (1993) Neoplasms with follicular differentiation. Lea and Febiger, Philadelphia

Hashimoto K, Mehregan AH, Kumakiri M (1987) Tumors of skin appendages. Butterworths, Boston

Requena L, Ackerman B, Kiryu H (1998) Neoplasms with apocrine differentiation. Lippincott-Raven, Philadelphia

Steffen C, Ackerman B (1994) Neoplasms with sebaceous differentiation. Lea and Febiger, Philadelphia

Wick MR, Swanson PE (1991) Cutaneous adnexal tumors. ASCP press, Chicago

Trichoblastoma

Aloi F, Tomasini C, Pippione M (1992) Pigmented trichoblastoma. Am J Dermatopathol 14:345–349

Headington JT (1976) Tumors of the hair follicle. A review. Am J Pathol 85:479–514

Rosen LB (1990) A review and proposed new classification of benign acquired neoplasms with hair follicle differentiation. Am J Dermatopathol 12:496–516

Schirren CG, Rütten A, Sander C et al. (1995) Trichoblastom. Ein Tumor mit follikulärer Differenzierung. Hautarzt 46: 81–86

Trichoepithelioma

Brooke HG (1892) Epithelioma adenoides cysticum. Br J Dermatol 4:269–286

Gray HR, Helwig EB (1963) Epithelioma adenoides cysticum and solitary trichoepithelioma. Arch Dermatol 87:102–114

Johnson SC, Bennett RG (1993) Occurrence of basal cell carcinoma among multiple trichoepitheliomas. J Am Acad Dermatol 28:322–326

Puig L, Nadal C, Fernandez-Figueras MT et al. (1998) Brooke-Spiegler syndrome variant: segregation of tumor types with mixed differentiation in two generations. Am J Dermatopathol 20:56–60

Schirren CG, Worle B, Kind P et al. (1995) A nevoid plaque with histological changes of trichoepithelioma and cylindroma in Brooke-Spiegler syndrome. An immunohistochemical study with cytokeratins. Cutan Pathol 22:563–569

van der Putte SC (1995) The pathogenesis of familial multiple cylindromas, trichoepitheliomas, milia, and spiradenomas. Am J Dermatopathol 17:271–280

Weyers W, Nilles M, Eckert F et al. (1993) Spiradenomas in Brooke-Spiegler syndrome. Am J Dermatopathol 15: 156–161

Desmoplastic Trichoepithelioma

Brownstein MH, Shapiro L (1977) Desmoplastic trichoepithelioma. Cancer 40:2979–2986

Hunt SJ, Abell E (1991) Malignant hair matrix tumor ("malignant trichoepithelioma") arising in the setting of multiple hereditary trichoepithelioma. Am J Dermatopathol 13:275–281

Lazorik FC, Wood MG (1982) Multiple desmoplastic trichoepitheliomas. Arch Dermatol 118:361–362

Takei Y, Fukushiro S, Ackerman AB (1985) Criteria for histologic differentiation of desmoplastic trichoepithelioma (sclerosing epithelial hamartoma) from morphea-like basal-cell carcinoma. Am J Dermatopathol 7:207–221

Tricholemmoma

Ackerman AB (1978) Trichilemmoma. Arch Dermatol 114: 286

Ackerman AB, Wade TR (1980) Tricholemmoma. Am J Dermatopathol 2:207–224

Brownstein MH, Shapiro L (1973) Trichilemmoma. Analysis of 40 new cases. Arch Dermatol 107:866–869

Brownstein MH, Mehregan AH, Bikowski JB et al. (1979) The dermatopathology of Cowden's syndrome. Br J Dermatol 100:667–673

Headington JT, French AJ (1962) Primary neoplasms of the hair follicle. Arch Dermatol 86:430–431

Hunt SJ, Kilzer B, Santa Cruz DJ (1990) Desmoplastic trichilemmoma: histologic variant resembling invasive carcinoma. J Cutan Pathol 17:45–52

Rohwedder A, Keminer O, Hendricks C et al. (1997) Detection of HPV DNA in trichilemmomas by polymerase chain reaction. J Med Virol 51:119–125

Trichilemmal Horn

Brownstein MH (1979) Trichilemmal horn: cutaneous horn showing trichilemmal keratinization. Br J Dermatol 100:303–309

DiMaio DJ, Cohen PR (1998) Trichilemmal horn: case presentation and literature review. J Am Acad Dermatol 39:368–371

Poblet E, Jimenez-Reyes J, Gonzalez-Herrada C et al. (1996) Trichilemmal keratosis. A clinicopathologic and immunohistochemical study of two cases. Am J Dermatopathol 18:543–547

Pilomatricoma

Berberian BJ, Colonna TM, Battaglia M et al. (1997) Multiple pilomatricomas in association with myotonic dystrophy and a family history of melanoma. Am Acad Dermatol 37:268–269

Behnke N, Schulte K, Ruzicka T et al. (1998) Pilomatricoma in elderly individuals. Dermatology 197:391–393

Forbis RSM, Helwig EB (1961) Pilomatrixoma (calcifying epithelioma). Arch Dermatol 83:606–618

Geh JL, Moss AL (1999) Multiple pilomatrixomata and myotonic dystrophy: a familial association. Br J Plast Surg 52:143–145

Graells J, Servitje O, Badell A et al. (1996) Multiple familial pilomatricomas associated with myotonic dystrophy. Int J Dermatol 35:732–723

Julian CG, Bowers PW (1998) A clinical review of 209 pilomatricomas. J Am Acad Dermatol 39:191–195

Lopansri S, Mihm MC Jr (1980) Pilomatrix carcinoma or calcifying epitheliocarcinoma of Melherbe. A case report and review of literature. Cancer 45:2368–2373

Malherbe A, Chenantais J (1880) Note sur l'épithélioma calcifié des glandes sébacées. Bull Soc Anat Paris 5:169–176

Trichoadenoma

Nikolowski W (1958) Tricho-Adenom (organoides Follikel-Hamartom). Arch Klin Exp Dermatol 207:34–35

Rahbari H, Mehregan A, Pinkus H (1977) Trichoadenoma of Nikolowski. J Cutan Pathol 4:90–98

Yamaguchi J, Takino C (1992) A case of trichoadenoma arising in the buttock. J Dermatol 19:503–506

Tumor of the Follicular Infundibulum

Cribier B, Grosshans E (1995) Tumor of the follicular infundibulum: a clinicopathologic study. J Am Acad Dermatol 33:979–984

Kolenik SA III, Bolognia JL, Castiglione FM Jr et al. (1996) Multiple tumors of the follicular infundibulum. Int J Dermatol 35:282–284

Mehregan AH (1971) Tumor of follicular infundibulum. Dermatologica 142:177–183

Mehregan AH (1984) Infundibular tumors of the skin. J Cutan Pathol 11:387–395

Mehregan AH, Butler JD (1961) A tumor of follicular infundibulum. Arch Dermatol 83:924–927

Trichofolliculoma

Gray HR, Helwig EB (1962) Trichofolliculoma. Arch Dermatol 86:619–625

Labandeira J, Peteiro C, Toribio J (1996) Hair follicle nevus: case report and review. Am J Dermatopathol 18:90–93

Miescher G (1944) Un cas de trichofolliculome. Dermatologica 89:193–194

Folliculosebaceous Cystic Hamartoma

Kimura T, Miyazawa H, Aoyagi T et al. (1991) Folliculosebaceous cystic hamartoma. A distinctive malformation of the skin. Am J Dermatopathol 13:213–220

Plewig G (1980) Sebaceous trichofolliculoma. J Cutan Pathol 7:394–403

Schulz T, Hartschuh W (1998) Folliculo-sebaceous cystic hamartoma is a trichofolliculoma at its very late stage. J Cutan Pathol 25:354–364

Simon RS, de Eusebio E, Alvarez-Vieitez A, Sanchez Yus E (1999) Folliculo-sebaceous cystic hamartoma is but the sebaceous end of tricho-sebo-folliculoma spectrum. J Cutan Pathol 26:109

Pilar Sheath Acanthoma

Mehregan AH, Brownstein MH (1978) Pilar sheath acanthoma. Arch Dermatol 114:1495–1497

Giant Pore of Winer

Klövekorn G, Klövekorn W, Plewig G et al. (1983) Riesenpore und Haarscheidenakanthom. Klinische und histologische Diagnose. Hautarzt 34:209–216

Winer LH (1954) The dilated pore, a trichoepithelioma. J Invest Dermatol 23:181–188

Inverted Follicular Keratosis

Lund HZ (1983) The nosologic position of inverted follicular keratosis is still unsettled. Am J Dermatopathol 5:443–445

Mehregan AH (1983) Inverted follicular keratosis is a distinct follicular tumor. Am J Dermatopathol 5:467–470

Fibrofolliculoma and Perifollicular Fibroma

Birt AR, Hogg GR, Dube WJ (1977) Hereditary multiple fibrofolliculomas with trichodiscomas and acrochordons. Arch Dermatol 113:1674–1677

De la Torre C, Ocampo C, Doval IG et al. (1999) Acrochordons are not a component of the Birt-Hogg-Dube syndrome: does this syndrome exist? Case reports and review of the literature. Am J Dermatopathol 21:369–374

Junkins-Hopkins JM, Cooper PH (1994) Multiple perifollicular fibromas: report of a case and analysis of the literature. J Cutan Pathol 21:467–471

Pinkus H (1979) Perifollicular fibromas. Pure periadnexal adventitial tumors. Am J Dermatopathol 1:341–342

Scully K, Bargman H, Assaad D (1984) Solitary fibrofolliculoma. J Am Acad Dermatol 11:361–363

Starink TM, Brownstein MH (1987) Fibrofolliculoma: solitary and multiple types. J Am Acad Dermatol 17:493–496

Zackheim HS, Pinkus H (1960) Perifollicular fibromas. Arch Dermatol 82:913–917

Trichodiscoma

Pinkus H, Coskey R, Burgess GH (1974) Trichodiscoma. A benign tumor related to haarscheibe (hair disk). J Invest Dermatol 63:212–218

Weinstein M, Berger RS, Bancila E (1990) Multiple hypopigmented papules. Trichodiscoma. Arch Dermatol 126: 1093–1096

Malignant Hair Follicle Tumor

Herrero J, Monteagudo C, Ruiz A et al. (1998) Malignant proliferating trichilemmal tumours: an histopathological and immunohistochemical study of three cases with DNA ploidy and morphometric evaluation. Histopathology 33:542–546

Cylindroma

Ancell H (1842) History of a remarkable case of tumours, developed on the head and face, accompanied with a similar disease in the abdomen. Med Chir Trans 25:227–246

Delfino M, D'Anna F, Ianniello S et al. (1991) Multiple hereditary trichoepithelioma and cylindroma (Brooke-Spiegler syndrome). Dermatologica 183:150–153

Spiegler E (1899) Über Epitheliome der Haut. Arch Dermatol Syph 50:163–176

Syringoma

Janniger CK, Brodkin RH (1990) Eruptive syringomas. Cutis 46:247–249

Patrizi A, Neri I, Marzaduri S et al. (1998) Syringoma: a review of twenty-nine cases. Acta Derm Venereol 78:460–462

Pruzan DL, Esterly NB, Prose NS (1989) Eruptive syringoma. Arch Dermatol 125:1119–1120

Eccrine Poroma

Harvell JD, Kerschmann RL, LeBoit PE (1996) Eccrine or apocrine poroma? Six poromas with divergent adnexal differentiation. Am J Dermatopathol 18:1–9

Pinkus H, Rogin JR, Goldman P (1956) Eccrine poroma. Tumors exhibiting features of the epidermal sweat duct unit. Arch Dermatol 74:511–521

Clear Cell Hidradenoma

Gianotti R, Alessi E (1997) Clear cell hidradenoma associated with the folliculo-sebaceous-apocrine unit. Histologic study of five cases. Am J Dermatopathol 19:351–357

Johnson BL Jr, Helwig EB (1969) Eccrine acrospiroma. Cancer 23:641–657

Keasby LE, Hadley GG (1954) Clear-cell hidradenoma: report of three cases with widespread metastases. Cancer 7:934–952

Kersting DW (1963) Clear cell hidradenoma and hidradenocarcinoma. Arch Dermatol 87:323–333

Requena L, Kiryu H, Ackerman AB (1998) Apocrine hidradenoma. In: Requena L, Kiryu H, Ackerman AB (eds) Neoplasms with apocrine differentiation. Lippincott-Raven, Philadelphia, pp 243–325

Eccrine Spiradenoma

Kersting DW, Helwig EB (1956) Eccrine spiradenoma. Arch Dermatol 73:199–227

Revis P, Chyu J, Medenica M (1988) Multiple eccrine spiradenoma: case report and review. J Cutan Pathol 15:226–229

Mixed Tumor of Skin

Hirsch P, Helwig EB (1961) Chondroid syringoma. Arch Dermatol 84:835–847

Lennox B, Pearse AGE, Richards HGH (1952) Mucin-secreting tumours of the skin: with special reference to the so-called mixed salivary tumour of the skin and its relation to hidradenoma. J Path Bact 64:865–880

Virchow R (1863) Die krankhaften Geschwülste, vol 1. Hirschwald, Berlin, p 481

Papillary Eccrine Adenoma

Megahed M, Holzle E (1993) Papillary eccrine adenoma. A case report with immunohistochemical examination. Am J Dermatopathol 15:150–155

Mizuoka H, Senzaki H, Shikata N et al. (1998) Papillary eccrine adenoma: immunohistochemical study and literature review. J Cutan Pathol 25:59–64

Rulon DB, Helwig EB (1977) Papillary eccrine adenoma. Arch Dermatol 113:596–598

Aggressive Digital Papillary Adenoma

Ceballos PI, Penneys NS, Acosta R (1990) Aggressive digital papillary adenocarcinoma. J Am Acad Dermatol 23: 331–334

Kao GF, Helwig EB, Graham JH (1987) Aggressive digital papillary adenoma and adenocarcinoma. A clinicopathological study of 57 patients, with histochemical, immunopathological, and ultrastructural observations. J Cutan Pathol 14:129–146

Eccrine Syringofiboadenoma

Mascaro JM (1963) Considérations sur les tumeurs fibro-épithéliales. Le syringofibroadénome eccrine. Ann Dermatol Syphiol 90:146–153

Starink TM (1997) Eccrine syringofibroadenoma: multiple lesions representing a new cutaneous marker of the Schopf syndrome, and solitary nonhereditary tumors. J Am Acad Dermatol 36:569–576

Syringocystadenoma Papilliferum

Elliot GT (1893) Adeno-cystoma intracanaliculare occurring in a nevus unius lateris. J Cutan Genitourin Dis 11:168–173

Helwig EB, Hackney VC (1955) Syringadenoma papilliferum: lesions with and without naevus sebaceous and basal cell carcinoma. Arch Dermatol 71:361–372

Mammino JJ, Vidmar DA (1991) Syringocystadenoma papilliferum. Int J Dermatol 30:763–766

Werther L (1913) Syringadenoma papilliferum (naevus syringadenomatosus papilliferus. Arch Dermatol Syph 116:865–870

Hidradenoma Papilliferum

Vang R, Cohen PR (1999) Ectopic hidradenoma papilliferum: a case report and review of the literature. J Am Acad Dermatol 41:115–118

Werth R (1878) Zur Anatomie der Cysten der Vulva. Zentralbl Gynakol 22:513–516

Tubular Apocrine Adenoma

Landry M, Winkelmann RK (1972) An unusual tubular apocrine adenoma: Histochemical and ultrastructural study. Arch Dermatol 105:869–879

Tellechea O, Reis JP, Marques C et al. (1995) Tubular apocrine adenoma with eccrine and apocrine immunophenotypes or papillary tubular adenoma? Am J Dermatopathol 17:499–505

Toribio J, Zulaica A, Peteiro C (1987) Tubular apocrine adenoma. J Cutan Pathol 14:114–117

Papillary Adenoma of the Nipple

Brownstein MH, Phelps RG, Magnin PH (1985) Papillary adenoma of the nipple: analysis of fifteen new cases. J Am Acad Dermatol 12:707–715

Anogenital Mammary-Like Glands

Van der Putte SC et al. (1991) Anogenital "sweat" glands. Histology and pathology of a gland that may mimic mammary glands. Am J Dermatopathol 13:557–567

Microcystic Adnexal Carcinoma

Burns MK, Chen SP, Goldberg LH (1994) Microcystic adnexal carcinoma. Ten cases treated by Mohs micrographic surgery. J Dermatol Surg Oncol 20:429–434

Friedman PM, Friedman RH, Jiang SB et al. (1999) Microcystic adnexal carcinoma: collaborative series review and update. J Am Acad Dermatol 41(2/1):225–231

Goldstein DJ, Barr RJ, Santa Cruz DJ (1982) Microcystic adnexal carcinoma: a distinct clinicopathologic entity. Cancer 50:566–572

Sebastien TS, Nelson BR, Lowe L et al. (1993) Microcystic adnexal carcinoma. J Am Acad Dermatol 29:840–845

Mucinous Carcinoma

Santa Cruz DJ, Prioleau PG (1984) Adnexal carcinomas of the skin. J Cutan Pathol 11:450–456

Snow SN, Reizner GT (1992) Mucinous eccrine carcinoma of the eyelid. Cancer 70:2099–3104

Carcinoma ex Adenoma

Girishkumar H, Kamineni S, Hwang RR et al. (1997) Eccrine porocarcinoma. Dermatol Surg 23:583–584

Landa NG, Winkelmann RK (1991) Epidermotropic eccrine porocarcinoma. J Am Acad Dermatol 24:27–31

Aggressive Digital Papillary Adenocarcinoma

Ceballos PI, Penneys NS, Acosta R (1990) Aggressive digital papillary adenocarcinoma. J Am Acad Dermatol 23:331–334

Kao GF, Helwig EB, Graham JH (1987) Aggressive digital papillary adenoma and adenocarcinoma. A clinicopathological study of 57 patients, with histochemical, immunopathological, and ultrastructural observations. J Cutan Pathol 14:129–146

Adenoid Cystic Carcinoma

Boggio RR (1985) Primary adenoid cystic carcinoma of the skin. Arch Pathol Lab Med 109:707

Chang SE, Ahn SJ, Choi JH et al. (1999) Primary adenoid cystic carcinoma of skin with lung metastasis. J Am Acad Dermatol 40:640–642

Headington JT, Teears R, Niederhuber JE et al. (1978) Primary adenoid cystic carcinoma of skin. Arch Dermatol 114:421–424

Lymphoepithelioma-Like Carcinoma

Dozier SE, Jones TR, Nelson-Adesokan P et al. (1995) Lymphoepithelioma-like carcinoma of the skin treated by Mohs micrographic surgery. Dermatol Surg 21:690–694

Requena L, Sanchez Yus E, Jimenez E et al. (1994) Lymphoepithelioma-like carcinoma of the skin: a light-microscopic and immunohistochemical study. J Cutan Pathol 21:541–548

Swanson SA, Cooper PH, Mills SE et al. (1988) Lymphoepithelioma-like carcinoma of the skin. Mod Pathol 1:359–365

Sebaceous Hyperplasia

Prioleau PG, Santa Cruz DJ (1984) Sebaceous gland neoplasia. J Cutan Pathol 11:396–414

Sebaceous Adenoma

Yus ES, Simon P (1999) About benign neoplasms with sebaceous differentiation. Am J Dermatopathol 21:298–300

Sebaceous Carcinoma

Nelson BR, Hamlet KR, Gillard M et al. (1995) Sebaceous carcinoma. J Am Acad Dermatol 33:1–15

Sebaceoma

Troy JL, Ackerman AB (1984) Sebaceoma: a distictive benign neoplasm of adnexal epithelium differntiating toward sebaceous cells. Am J Dermatopathol 6:7–13

Sanchez Yus E, de Diego Polo V, Sanz Vico MD (1985) Sebaceoma. Am J Dermatopathol 7:198–199

Melanocytic Lesions

Contents

Introduction

Melanotic spots, melanocytic nevi, and malignant melanomas are one of the most important areas of dermatology. Melanomas are the only common, potentially life-threatening disorder that involves the skin and thus are worthy of careful attention. While most nevi as defined in Chapter 52 are stable and only rarely undergo change, the same cannot be said of melanocytic nevi. About 20–30% of malignant melanomas arise from melanocytic nevi; in addition, these nevi typically change throughout the life of the patient, being subject to genetic, hormonal, environmental (sunlight), and many other less well-understood factors. For the balance of the chapter, the term nevus will be equated with melanocytic nevus. We will not employ the terms nevus cell or nevocyte; the cells in a melanocytic nevus are in fact melanocytes, and the use of this historic term is confusing.

While there are many ways to subdivide melanocytic lesions, we will use three major categories: melanotic spots, melanocytic nevi, and malignant melanomas. Melanotic spots are epidermal lesions containing increased melanin and perhaps increased melanocytes. Melanocytic nevi are benign proliferations of melanocytes, while malignant melanomas are their malignant counterparts. There are frequent overlaps between all of these artificial categories, primarily because of the tendency of melanocytic lesions to evolve during a patient's lifetime.

Another potential category is lentigo, typically defined as a lesion with an increase in melanocytes in the basal layer but with no nests of melanocytes. Many patients with multiple lentigines syndromes have freckles. Patients with Carney syndrome have both small, dark permanent lentigines and lighter freckles that show seasonal variation. The most common lentigo of all, the solar or senile lentigo, is a seborrheic keratosis. Even the histologic distinction between a freckle and a lentigo is imperfect, except when flat sheets of skin are studied and the melanocytes quantitatively analyzed. The entire concept of lentigines is so confusing that we have chosen to include them under melanotic spots.

Another crucial point is the distinction between melanocytic and pigmented lesions. While we also tend to describe a nevus or malignant melanoma as a pigmented lesion, this is imprecise. There are many types of pigmented lesions. Sometimes there is an overproduction of melanin, but no increase in melanocytes. In Chapter 26, the pathophysiology of melanin production is reviewed and diffuse hyperpigmentation considered. Because lesions with a focal increase in melanin are often clinically confused with nevi, they are considered here. In addition, many other lesions can appear dark, but have no increase in either melanocytes or melanin. Included in the latter group are seborrheic keratoses, vascular proliferations, especially angiokeratomas and venous lakes, dermatofibromas, pigmented basal cell carcinoma, and traumatic or intentional tattoos.

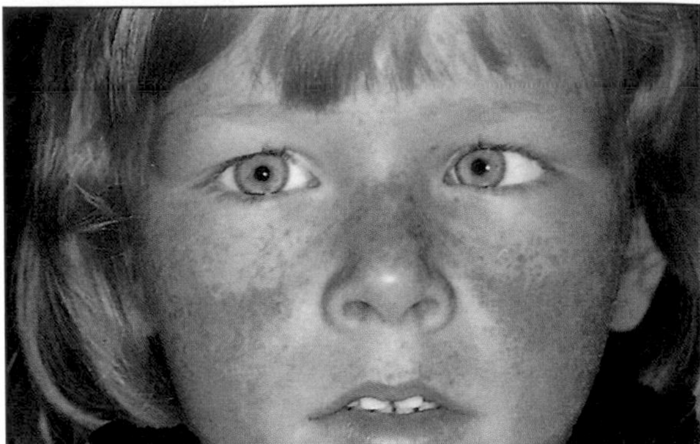

Fig. 58.1. Ephelides in a young, blue eyed, Celtic girl

Melanotic Spots

There are a wide variety of lesions, often erroneously referred to as nevi, that actually reflect increased production of melanin. These melanotic spots overlap with the diffuse hypermelanotic conditions described in Chapter 26; all of which are flat and tend to be less dark and less sharply defined than melanocytic nevi.

Ephelis

Synonym. Freckle

Definition. Local increase in melanin that varies with sunlight exposure.

Etiology and Pathogenesis. Fair-skinned patients, especially Celts with red hair, are particularly likely to be freckled. There is a strong familial tendency towards freckling, suggesting inheritance in an autosomal dominant pattern; no genes have been identified. The melanocytes in freckles differ from their normal counterparts in that they produce more melanin, package it in larger melanosomes, and transfer it more efficiently to keratinocytes. It is possible to induce freckles in these patients on almost any part of the body with UV radiation.

Clinical Findings. Freckles are flat tan-brown lesions, with irregular or even bizarre borders, that show a wide variation in size. The most typical location is the face (Fig. 58.1), although they are also seen on the arms, shoulders, and upper parts of the back. Some Celts are virtually covered from head to toes by freckles. While the lips are commonly involved, the oral mucosa and other unexposed locations are usually spared. Freckles almost invariably appear in childhood and become more prominent each summer. In older patients, freckles tend to regress. The same patients are particularly likely to experience sunburn and develop early signs of actinic damage; they also have an increased risk of malignant melanoma.

Histopathology. There is an increase of melanin in the basal layer with no increase in melanocytes. Incontinence of pigment is a rare feature.

Differential Diagnosis. The main differential diagnostic point involves the syndromes associated with multiple lentigines. In many instances, the distinction between a lentigo and a freckle is unclear, as the quantification of melanocytes is a difficult task. Patients with xeroderma pigmentosum develop so-called permanent freckles at an early age, often after the first summer, and often on the legs and even the gap between their diapers and T-shirt. The lesions are not freckles, but early lentigines, often with melanocytic atypia. Occasionally, multiple, small plane warts will be dark and mistaken for freckles.

Therapy. The best therapy is the sensible use of sunscreens. Attempts at bleaching are usually disappointing. Individual freckles can be removed with cryotherapy or light chemical peeling agents.

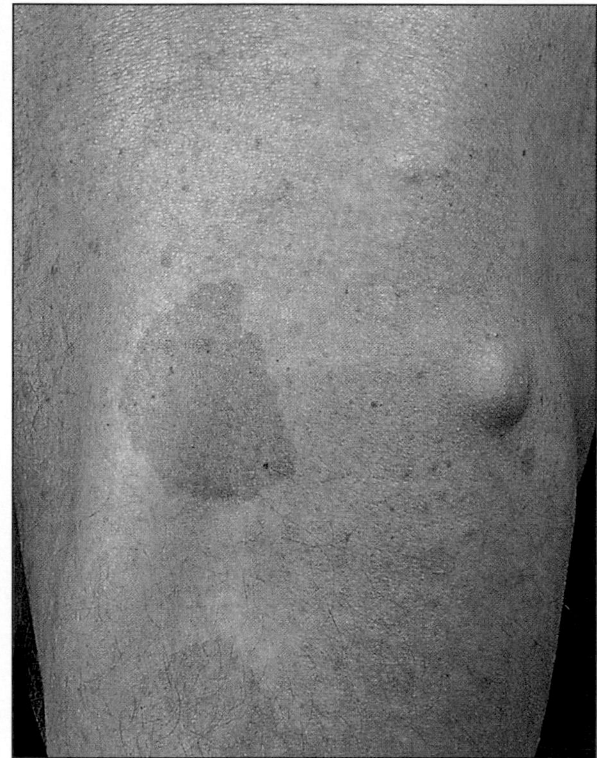

Fig. 58.2. Two café-au-lait macules on the left and a fleshy neurofibroma on the right in a patient with neurofibromatosis 1

Café-au-Lait Macule

Clinical Findings. These lesions are large, oval, generally light brown macules or patches ranging in size from several to many centimeters (Fig. 58.2). They tend to have a uniform color and a smooth, rounded "coast of California" border. While café-au-lait macules are the prototypic lesion in neurofibromatosis, they may also be seen in normal individuals. Furthermore, they are associated with an endless list of other disorders in which they are of uncertain importance. Café-au-lait macules are harmless and never undergo malignant change. They are seen in many other syndromes, which are discussed in Chapter 19 along with neurofibromatosis.

Histopathology. Melanin is increased in the keratinocytes of the basal layer. There may also be a slight increase in the number of melanocytes. Giant melanosomes are occasionally seen; they are most common in café-au-lait macules associated with neurofibromatosis but are not specific for this disorder.

Therapy. No treatment is needed. The lesions are only rarely facial and thus patients seldom seek treatment. If a particular café-au-lait macule is cosmetically disturbing, it can be covered with make-up.

Axillary Freckles

(Crowe 1964)

Axillary freckles or Crowe sign is one of the criteria for the diagnosis of neurofibromatosis 1. The lesions resemble tiny freckles in the axilla and groin, but do not have a chance to change with solar exposure. Histologically, they are freckles. In dark-skinned individuals, axillary freckles are common enough that they lose their utility as a diagnostic sign.

McCune-Albright Syndrome

(McCune and Bruch 1937; Albright et al. 1937)

Synonym. Polyostotic fibrous dysplasia

Etiology and Pathogenesis. McCune-Albright syndrome occurs in a sporadic fashion; it involves a postzygotic mutation of a lethal autosomal dominant gene located on chromosome 20q13 and encoding the G_S-α protein, which controls cyclic AMP activity. The mutations result in an upregulation of G_S-α.

Clinical Findings. The triad of pigmentary changes, bony defects, and precocious puberty characterizes McCune-Albright syndrome. The skin lesions are large tan patches that often are located over bony lesions. The most common sites are the trunk, buttocks, and extremities, but occasionally the scalp and nape are involved. The lesions are usually larger than café-au-lait macules, fewer in number, and have a more irregular "coast of Maine" border than the café-au-lait macules in neurofibromatosis. They are also more likely to follow the lines of Blaschko, suggesting a somatic mutation. Epidermal nevi and cutaneous myxomas can also be seen. The bony changes lead to pain, deformities, and pathologic fractures in childhood and may appear without skin or endocrine changes. The endocrinologic disturbances, especially precocious puberty, are more common in women.

Histopathology. The microscopic appearance is similar to a café-au-lait macule.

Course and Prognosis. Fractures and other bony changes cause pain and often require surgery. The endocrine problems are very difficult to manage. If the mutation also occurs in the germline and is passed on to children, they will die in utero.

Differential Diagnosis. The main differential diagnostic consideration is neurofibromatosis, but the nature of the skeletal changes and the qualities of the café-au-lait macules are usually quite different.

Becker Nevus

(Becker 1949)

Synonym. Melanosis naeviformis

Etiology and Pathogenesis. This relatively common lesion is a form of organoid nevus (Chap. 52) or hamartoma resulting from a postzygotic or somatic mutation. The gene is unknown. It is included in this chapter because it is usually mistaken for a café-au-lait macule or melanocytic nevus with hairs.

Clinical Findings. Becker nevus most often present as an asymptomatic patch on the shoulder of a young man. Other common sites are the arm and trunk (Fig. 58.3). At birth, the lesion is either unidentifiable or simply a slightly hyperpigmented patch. There may be prominent follicular papules caused by an underlying smooth muscle hamartoma (Chap. 59), resulting in a permanent state of cutis anserina (goose bumps). Smooth muscle hamartoma may also be present without any overlying pigmentary or hair changes. In puberty, the color becomes a darker brown, and prominent hairs develop, facilitating the diagnosis. The same androgen sensitivity may lead to acne lesions within the nevus. Peripheral satellite lesions are common. Often the lesion is first identified in summer, following sunlight exposure, as the lesion darkens more than the surrounding tissue. In women, there is less androgen sensitivity, and the lesions are thus paler, less hairy, and more likely to be overlooked. A wide variety of skeletal and CNS changes have been described in the Becker nevus syndrome, one type of epidermal nevus syndrome (Chap. 52).

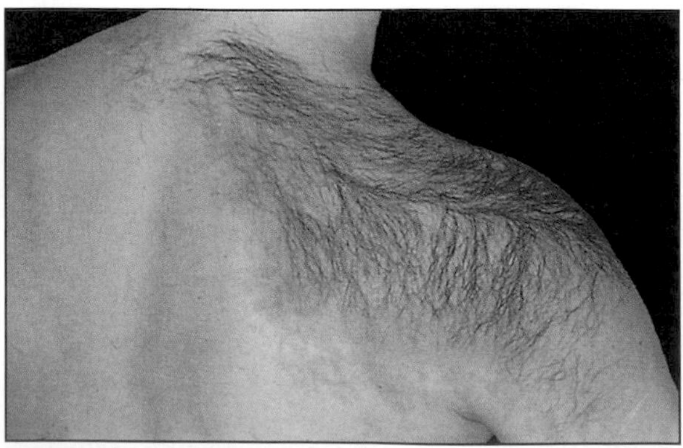

Fig. 58.3. Becker nevus

Histopathology. The rete ridges are elongated, and the increase in melanin may be subtle. The number of melanocytes is unchanged. There may be incontinence of pigment with melanin located in dermal melanophages. In the mid- to deep dermis, bundles of smooth muscles may be found. Electron microscopic studies suggest that the melanocytes are overactive in the production of melanin.

Course and Prognosis. The lesions may continue to darken and become more hairy, but they have no malignant potential.

Therapy. The lesions are usually too large for surgical excision. Shaving, bleaching, or epilation of the hairs is sometimes cosmetically helpful.

Mucosal Melanotic Macule

Synonyms. Labial melanotic macule, penile melanotic macule, vulvar melanotic macule

Clinical Findings. All of these mucosal lesions are similar. They present as tan, irregular, frequently multiple flat lesions on the lips or genitalia. The lip and penile lesions can be identified and monitored by the patient, but the lesions of the female genitalia are rarely known to the patient and frequently produce an emergency referral from a family physician or gynecologist who discovers them during a routine examination.

Histopathology. Biopsy shows transitional epithelium, rather than epidermis, with increased basal layer pigmentation. The lamina propria is more vascular than the dermis, offering another clue that one is dealing with a mucosal spot.

Therapy. Usually, no treatment is needed. Laser destruction is probably preferred. On the lips cryotherapy is often helpful. If clinical suspicion of malignant melanoma exists, then an excisional biopsy is appropriate.

Solar Lentigo

Synonyms. Lentigo senilis, senile lentigo, liver spot, age spot

These common lesions are not lentigines but epidermal proliferations. They are larger than simple lentigines, usually seen in sunlight-exposed skin, especially the face and lower arms, and more common in older patients (Fig. 58.4). If questions exist about the exact diagnosis, a biopsy can be performed. Histologically, there are elongated rete ridges with increased melanin at the tips. The number of melanocytes is not increased. Since they are early plane or reticulated seborrheic keratoses (Chap. 54), the dermatoscopic picture is also helpful. They may become inflamed and then are one precursor of benign lichenoid keratoses. Both cryotherapy and lasers (pulsed ruby, erbium, CO_2) offer elegant therapeutic approaches. Sometimes bleaching creams may be helpful for early lesions.

Ink Spot Lentigo

(BologNIA 1992)

Synonym. Reticulated melanotic macule

This clinically distinct and dramatic lesion appears on the trunk or back of adults as an irregular, dark brown or black reticulated macule that has been likened to an ink spot. On biopsy, the epidermis shows a slight increase in melanocytes with darkening of the tips of normal (not elongated) rete ridges. Solar elastosis is rarely present to any significant degree. Many such lesions are excised because of concern about malignant melanoma; once one has learned their clinical appearance, they can be readily diagnosed.

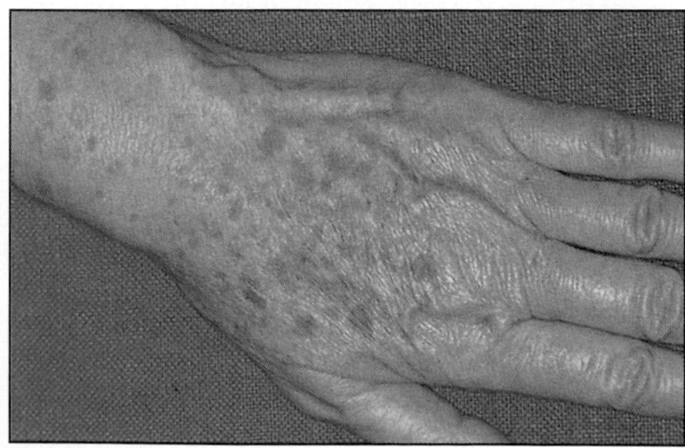

Fig. 58.4. Solar lentigines

PUVA Lentigo

Patients treated with psoralens and ultraviolet A radiation (PUVA) tend to develop small, irregular pigmented macules that are closest to a freckle or perhaps a mini-ink spot lentigo. As many of 50% of patients receiving long-term PUVA therapy develop some lentigines, especially on the trunk. Histologically, these lesions can be worrisome because of the presence of melanocytes above the basal layer, often with large dendrites. However, the melanocytes are relatively uniformly spaced and not greatly increased in number.

Lentigines Syndromes

There are a number of syndromes in which lentigines, freckles, or even melanocytic nevi are prominently featured. They have little else in common but are often grouped together.

Peutz-Jeghers Syndrome

(Peutz 1921; Jeghers et al. 1949)

Synonyms. Hamartomatous intestinal polyposis, periorificial lentiginosis

Etiology and Pathogenesis. Peutz-Jeghers syndrome is inherited in an autosomal dominant pattern. The gene has been localized to 19p34-p36 and is known as STK 11, a serine-threonine kinase involved in growth control regulation.

Clinical Findings

Cutaneous Findings. The usual cutaneous finding is multiple, often unnoticed freckles on the lips and buccal mucosa (Fig. 58.5). While the cutaneous lesions may fade, the buccal lesions tend to be more permanent. Acral and periorbital lesions may also be seen, as well as conjunctival pigmented macules. In several cases, the pigmented lesions have developed in areas of resolving psoriasis.

Systemic Findings. The hallmark of Peutz-Jeghers syndrome is hamartomatous polyps that may occur

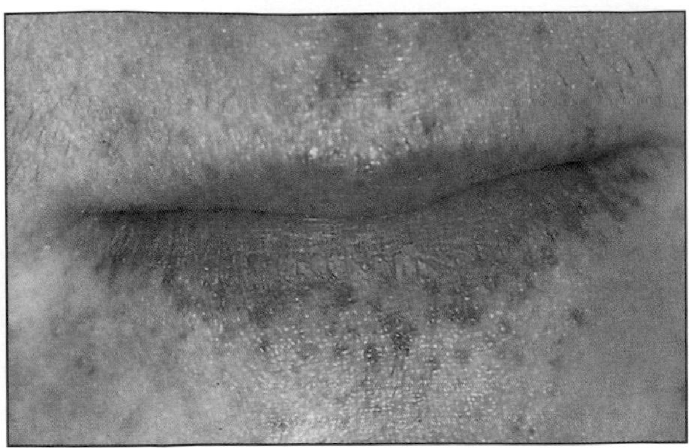

Fig. 58.5. Peutz-Jeghers syndrome

anywhere in the gastrointestinal tract but always involve the jejunum. Younger patients frequently present with intussusception and bleeding, triggered by one of their many polyps. While the malignant risk for a given hamartomatous polyp is small, the lifetime risk for gastrointestinal carcinoma is high, exceeding 50%. Pancreatic carcinomas have also been reported. Patients have an increased incidence of genital and mammary tumors; women are at far greater risk than men. The tumors are often bilateral, histologically unusual, and may secrete hormones.

Histopathology. The lesions have only rarely been analyzed, but more appear to be freckles than lentigines. They are perhaps closest to labial melanotic macules.

Therapy. The skin lesions require no therapy. The patients should be carefully followed by a gastroenterologist or surgeon with a special interest in their myriad problems.

Carney Syndrome

(Carney et al. 1985)

Synonyms. Myxoma, spotty pigmentation and endocrine overactivity syndrome; NAME syndrome (Atherton et al. 1980); LAMB syndrome (Rhodes et al. 1984)

- NAME: *N*evi, *a*trial myxoma, *m*yxoid neurofibromas, *e*phelides
- LAMB: *L*entigines, *a*trial myxoma, *m*ucocutaneous myxomas, *b*lue nevi

Etiology and Pathogenesis. The Carney syndrome is inherited in an autosomal dominant pattern; two genes (2p16, 17q23) have been identified but their functions are unknown.

Clinical Findings

Cutaneous Findings. Patients typically have spotty hyperpigmentation, including freckles, lentigines, and blue nevi. While the lips may be involved, buccal involvement is uncommon, in contrast to Peutz-Jeghers syndrome. In addition, patients have cutaneous myxomas, small flesh-colored or translucent papules often involving the external ear or eyelid. The cutaneous features are variable; some patients have no pigmented lesions; others are covered with multiple freckles, lentigines, and blue nevi.

Systemic Findings. The most intriguing change is pigmented nodular adrenal hyperplasia. The patients have circulating autoantibodies that stimulate the adrenal gland, producing Cushing disease without any elevation in ACTH. The adrenal gland contains numerous, small dark nodules. The most serious tumor in Carney syndrome is the cardiac myxoma; while it is benign, the operative mortality is around 20%. These cardiac tumors tend to be multiple and occur at an earlier age than sporadic cardiac myxomas, which are usually solitary right atrial lesions. Fragments of necrotic cardiac myxomas may break off and cause arterial emboli.

A second, potentially dangerous tumor is the psammomatous melanotic schwannoma which typically involves the subcutaneous tissues and may show malignant changes. Bilateral, large-cell, calcifying Sertoli cell testicular tumors are another unusual feature; they may cause sexual precocity. Pituitary adenomas that produce growth hormone may cause acromegaly. In addition, myxoid fibromas of the breast occur but are innocent.

Laboratory Findings. A patient with Cushing syndrome and a normal ACTH level may well have Carney syndrome.

Histopathology. The pigmented lesions have been designated as both freckles and lentigines. In our experience, patients have both. They are histologically indistinct. The blue nevi in some cases may be epithelioid. The myxomas not only have a mucinous stroma but may also show epithelial strands extending from a follicular structure, so that they may be designated epithelioid myxomas. The original descriptions of myxoid neurofibromas were in error.

Differential Diagnosis. On clinical appearance alone, Carney syndrome and LEOPARD syndrome have been confused. The associated problems are so different that distinction should be straightforward.

Therapy. The myxomas may be excised, as may be large or disturbing blue nevi or lentigines.

The host of troubling internal tumors and the adrenal disease require a skilled endocrinologist and surgeon to manage the patient jointly.

LEOPARD Syndrome

(ZEISLER and BECKER 1936; MOYNAHAN 1962)

Synonyms. Multiple lentigines syndrome, progressive cardiomyopathic lentiginosis, Moynahan syndrome

LEOPARD is an acronym for the major clinical features: *l*entiginosis, *e*lectrocardiographic abnormalities, *o*cular hypertelorism, *p*ulmonary stenosis, *a*bnormal genitalia, *r*etarded growth and *d*eafness.

Etiology and Pathogenesis. This rare disorder is inherited in an autosomal dominant pattern with variable expressivity. The genetic defect is unknown.

Clinical Findings. The lentigines tend to be most prominent on the neck, trunk, and abdomen. The oral mucosa is spared. The trunk may be covered entirely by thousands of closely packed lentigines (Fig. 58.6). Admixed among the smaller lentigines are larger lentigines (café-noir spots of Gorlin), café-au-lait macules, and melanocytic nevi. The skin changes are the least of these unfortunate patients' problems, although they frequently aid in the diagnosis.

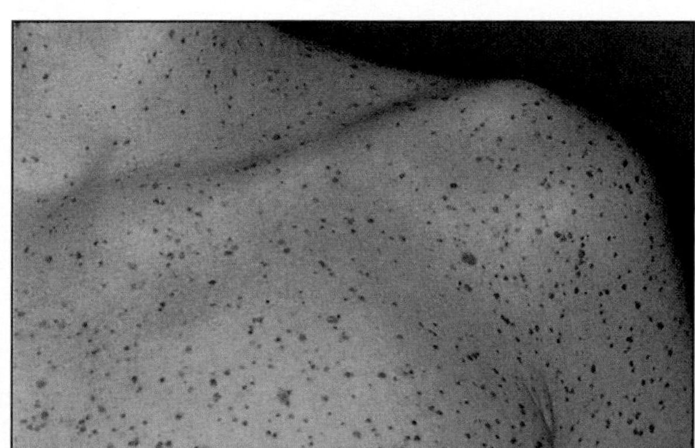

Fig. 58.6. LEOPARD syndrome

Lentiginosis and Arterial Dissection Syndrome

(SCHIEVINK et al. 1995)

The genetics are poorly worked out, but several families have been identified in which multiple lentigines track with arterial dissection at an early age.

Inherited Patterned Lentiginosis

Synonyms. Lentiginosis mediofacialis, mid-facial lentiginosis

Many blacks, especially those with red-brown hair, have prominent, flat, pigmented lesions concentrated in the mid-third of their face. Often several members of the same family will show these features, so that autosomal dominant inheritance has been postulated. The lesions are persistent and not seasonally variable, and the oral mucosa is not involved, although the lips may be affected.

Centrofacial Lentiginosis

(TOURAINE 1941)

Synonym. Lentiginosis centrofacialis

This very rare syndrome is inherited in an autosomal dominant pattern. As the name suggests, the patients have lentigines concentrated in the midface. The lateral aspects of the face tend to be free; the lentigines may become more prominent in summer. A wide variety of CNS and skeletal defects have also been reported, but the syndrome is so rare that a clear picture does not exist. Many of the skeletal defects appear to involve the midline, suggesting some form of fusion defect.

Other Multiple Lentigines Syndromes

- Laugier-Hunziker-Baran Syndrome. Acquired hyperpigmented macules of the lips and oral mucosa, along with longitudinal hyperpigmented nail streaks.
- Lentiginosis Profusa Perigenitoaxillaris (KORTING 1967). These patients have axillary and inguinal freckling; in some instances, they may have an incomplete form of neurofibromatosis known as type 3 (Chap. 19).
- Cantu Syndrome (CANTU et al. 1978). Multiple facial and acral lentigines associated with palmoplantar keratoderma.

Speckled Lentiginous Nevus

(Stewart et al. 1978)

Synonyms. Zosteriform lentiginous nevus, agminated lentigines, lentiginous mosaicism, segmental lentiginosis

Clinical Findings. As the multiple names suggest, this is a confusing concept. Patients occasionally present with a circumscribed grouping of lentigines. The most likely explanation is a mosaic variant of diffuse lentiginosis. The same term has been applied to a segmental nevus spilus, in which the background pigmentation is lentiginous and the speckles are nevi, not lentigines. The distinction is not crucial, but one should attempt to be accurate.

Melanocytic Nevi

Melanocytic nevi are benign proliferations of melanocytes. They are circumscribed macules or papules that may be skin-colored, blue, brown, or black. Both congenital and acquired melanocytic nevi are seen. Table 58.1 shows one classification of the different types of melanocytic nevi. The individual melanocytes may have a wide variety of cytologic features. Ackerman, Cerroni, and Kerl (1994) have identified ten types – all without nuclear atypia. They include small round, large round, pagetoid, wavy, balloon, oval, polygonal, spindle, dendritic, and multinucleate cells. Another histologic hallmark is the presence of nests of melanocytes either at the epidermal-dermal junction or in the dermis.

Table 58.1. Types of melanocytic nevi

Dermal melanocytoses
Classic blue nevus
Cellular blue nevus
Combined nevus (blue nevus + common nevus)
Deep penetrating blue nevus
Mongolian spot
Nevus of Ota and nevus of Ito
Common melanocytic nevi
Lentigo simplex
Clark nevus
Miescher nevus
Unna nevus
Spitz nevus
Congenital nevus (congenital hairy nevus, nevus pigmentosus et pilosus)
Nevus spilus
Halo nevus
Meyerson nevus
Dysplastic nevus and dysplastic nevus syndrome

Dermal Melanocytoses

These lesions are all characterized clinically by a blue-gray color and histologically by dendritic dermal melanocytes. The working explanation is that these melanocytes never reach the epidermis in their migration from the neural crest but instead are stopped in the dermis. The blue-gray color is due to the reflection and scatter of the shorter wavelengths of visible light by the dermal pigmentation; this is called the Tyndall (1872) effect.

Mongolian Spot

A high percentage (> 90%) of Asian, Hispanic, and black children have a diffuse blue-gray hyperpigmentation over their sacrum (Fig. 58.7). The discoloration tends to fade over a period of years. Similar lesions are seen in perhaps 10% of white infants; while they may be more prominent, they

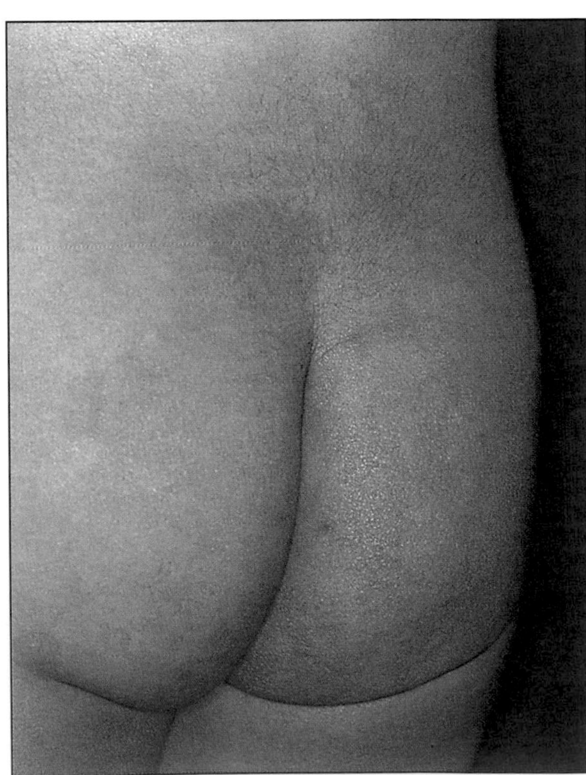

Fig. 58.7. Mongolian spot

are of no greater importance. Ectopic Mongolian spots are also common, especially in Native Americans. They may be found over the dorsal aspects of the hands and feet, as well as scattered over the body. Ectopic Mongolian spots tend to be more permanent. In generalized dermal melanocytosis (Bashiti et al. 1981), infants present with diffuse dermal melanosis. These rare children probably have an extreme variant of Mongolian spots. At first glance, a biopsy from a Mongolian spot looks like normal skin. On closer examination, there are scattered dermal dendritic cells that contain melanin. Melanophages may also be present. Malignant changes do not occur, and therapy is unnecessary because it is likely that Mongolian spots will fade in early childhood. Persistent lesions can be treated with any laser that selectively destroys melanin.

Nevus of Ota

(Ota 1939)

Synonyms. Nevus fuscocoeruleus ophthalmomaxillaris, oculodermal melanocytosis

Etiology and Pathogenesis. Once again, this form of dermal melanosis is also almost entirely limited to Asians. The female:male ratio is 3:1. Most cases are present at birth; others either appear at puberty or become more prominent as hormonal changes occur. Darkening in pregnancy or even with menses has been observed. Some cases are associated with a nevus flammeus; this variant is known as phakomatosis pigmentovascularis, and several subtypes have been identified (Chap. 19).

Clinical Findings. The lesions are usually unilateral and involve the first and second branches of the fifth cranial nerve. In children, flat blue lesions with an irregular border and occasional satellites are seen involving the ocular area and upper part of the cheek. About two-thirds of patients have a blue-gray discoloration of the sclera, occasionally extending to other parts of the eye (Fig. 58.8). The upper lip, palate, buccal and nasal mucosa may also be affected. In perhaps 5% of cases, bilateral changes are seen. Deafness is another complication. In adults, speckled hyperpigmentation is common, and small nodules may develop that usually represent blue nevi, although rarely malignant melanoma has been described. In addition, melanin-producing brain tumors can occur.

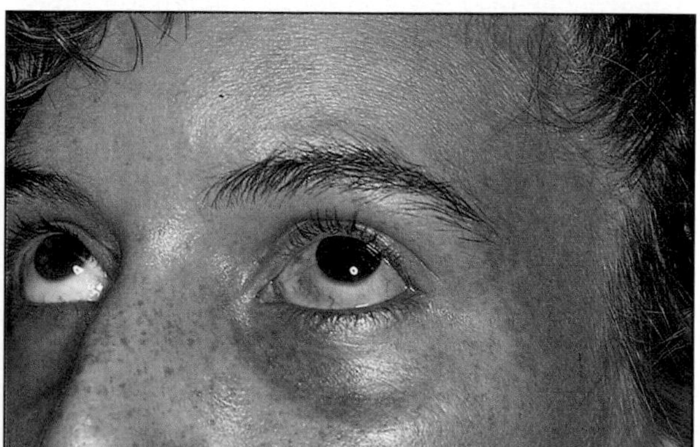

Fig. 58.8. Nevus of Ota with scleral involvement

Histopathology. The microscopic features are identical to those of Mongolian spot. Most nodules are blue nevi.

Therapy. Because of the permanent nature and facial location, treatment is often sought. Cover-up cosmetics are the standard approach; today a range of lasers offer very promising results.

Nevus of Ito

(Ito 1954)

Synonyms. Nevus fuscocoeruleus deltoideoacromialis, deltoideoacromial melanocytosis

The nevus of Ito is identical in every way to the nevus of Ota, except that it involves the shoulder region. Malignant change is even less common, and therapy is rarely needed because of the covered location.

Blue Nevus

(Tièche 1906; Jadassohn 1938)

Synonym. Nevus coeruleus

Definition. Blue nodule often present since birth or early childhood and characterized by dermal melanocytes.

Etiology and Pathogenesis. Most blue nevi are sporadic. Multiple blue nevi are seen in Carney syndrome. Rarely, other cases of familial blue nevi have been described.

Clinical Findings. The blue nevus is typically a small, sharply circumscribed papule (Fig. 58.9). The patient or parents usually describe the lesion as having been present for many years. The blue-

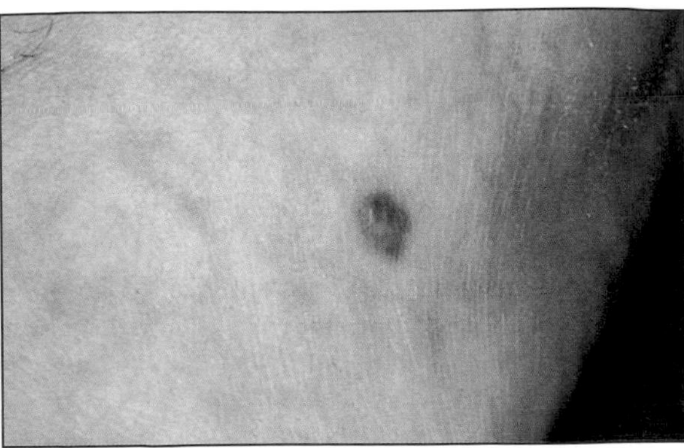

Fig. 58.9. Blue nevus

gray color derives from the dermal location of the melanin, producing the same tones as a dark tattoo. The lesions tend to be quite firm. Most are acrally located, but they can be found anywhere on the body.

Histopathology. Usually, there is a dermal proliferation of pigmented spindled melanocytes and melanophages often associated with a fibrous stroma. The epidermis is normal without the reactive changes seen in a dermatofibroma. Many histologic variants of blue nevus have been described including:

- Combined nevus, in which the spindle cells are associated with the melanocytes of a common nevus found both at the epidermal-dermal junction and in the superficial dermis.
- Deep penetrating nevus is a variant of combined nevus in which the spindle or blue nevus component may extend deeply into the dermis or even subcutaneous fat, showing some large and pleomorphic nuclei; thus, this type of nevus may simulate malignant melanoma.
- Cellular blue nevus is a designation reserved by purists for large lesions in which dermal melanocytes are combined with neuroid elements. Such lesions are usually nodules or plaques on the buttocks which are immediately identified as a blue nevi clinically. The term is more often used less precisely to describe any blue nevus that has a prominent cellular component.
- Malignant blue nevus can occur but is extremely uncommon. Unless there is unequivocal evidence of change from a long-standing blue nevus to a malignant melanoma, one suspects the answer is usually that a malignant melanoma was initially misdiagnosed as a blue nevus. Further confusion is added to the issue by the possibility that melanocytes from blue nevi, especially those on the scalp, may spread to local lymph nodes. This same phenomenon is seen with other nevi; it does not represent metastasis.

Differential Diagnosis. Clinically, a pigmented dermatofibroma is the most likely difficulty. Dermatoscopic examination is helpful. When a blue nevus is not prominently pigmented, it may be histologically identical to a dermatofibroma, but usually lacks the reactive epidermal changes. Metastatic malignant melanoma is also a serious diagnostic possibility; a blue nevus of recent onset in an adult should be regarded with concern. Rarely, a deep or predominantly venous vascular neoplasm, such as an arteriovenous fistula or venous lake, may also clinically mimic a blue nevus. The vascular lesions are usually less firm and may be compressible. A small pigmented dermatofibrosarcoma protuberans (Bednar tumor; Chap. 59) may also be confused with a blue nevus, particularly when only a small biopsy specimen is available.

Therapy. Surgical excision suffices.

Common Melanocytic Nevi

Definition. Pigmented tumor comprised of melanocytes, present at birth or developing later in life, with a variety of clinical and histologic patterns.

Etiology and Pathogenesis. Melanocytic nevi, known to most patients as moles, are surprisingly poorly understood, when one considers that every individual has at least several lesions. It has been estimated that the typical adult has 20 melanocytic nevi. While some melanocytic nevi are present at birth, most develop later, often appearing during puberty or young adulthood. In addition, they may grow or may develop into a malignant tumor, malignant melanoma. They may also regress in later adult life.

The most important etiologic factors are genetics, hormones, and sunlight exposure. The proliferation of nevi during puberty and especially during pregnancy underscores the hormonal role, while the increased number of nevi in light-exposed areas, especially following significant, intermittent UV radiation, is also important. Immunosuppression may also play a role, as shown by the almost explosive development of nevi in some children receiving chemotherapy for malignant tumors. Most congenital nevi are sporadic; some families show a tendency to multiple nevi or even multiple atypical nevi.

Nevi are often described as junctional, compound, or dermal. While one can guess at these histologic features during clinical evaluation, little is achieved by doing so. Flat lesions in younger patients tend to have melanocytes, either singly (lentigo) or in nests (junctional nevus), at the epidermal-dermal junction, while papular or nodular lesions are likely to have melanocytes in the dermis, either alone (dermal nevus) or combined with junctional changes (compound nevus). This constellation of clinical and histologic features led Unna (1893) to propose the theory of *Abtropfung* (German for dripping) to explain the pathogenesis of nevi. He suggested that the melanocytes were cells of epidermal origin that multiplied, producing first junctional nests and then sinking like drops into the dermis to form compound and eventually dermal lesions. Later, Masson (1951) postulated that melanocytes arise in the neural crest and migrate to the skin, and a generation of biologists has confirmed the theory. This suggests that blue nevi are lesions in which the melanocytes never reach the epidermis and thus retain their dendritic features. While Unna's theory is a convenient model, it should not be accepted as the sole possibility. Masson actually suggested that there was melanocyte traffic in both directions – to and from the epidermis. Problems such as the development of multiple nevi in dermabraded areas hint that, in adults, the epidermis can still be recolonized from below. In addition, the lentiginous melanocytic hyperplasia seen so often in light-damaged skin of adults, either alone or associated with a nevus probably has a completely different biology than the lentigines with a few small nests that are accepted as early nevi.

Clinical Findings. Nevi take a wide range of forms and shapes, from a flat 2-mm lesion to a large elevated plaque covering more than half the body surface. They may be papillomatous, pendulous, dark, pale, hairless, inflamed, irritated, surrounded by a halo or show countless other variations. (Figs. 58.10 – 58.12) Ackerman and colleagues proposed naming the melanocytic nevi after distinguished colleagues who originally described the variants. Using largely this terminology, one can speak of:

Lentigo Simplex. A simple or true lentigo is the most subtle type of melanocytic proliferation, that is, an increased number of normal melanocytes in the basal layer. Lentigo is derived from lentil and originally meant simply a small lesion. It has not yet received an eponym. A simple lentigo is a small, sharply bordered, flat dark lesion that can be a first step in the development of a melanocytic nevus. Histologically, the epidermis is normal except for an increase in melanocytes in the basal layer. There may also be melanin in the stratum corneum. Almost everyone has a number of simple lentigines. They are rarely a problem but can be easily removed if suspicions arise.

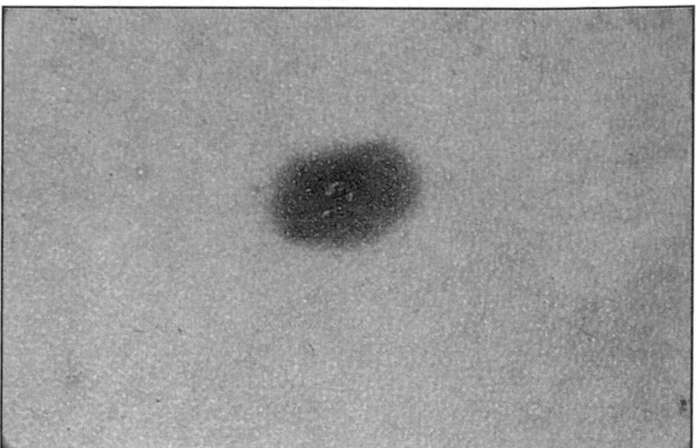

Fig. 58.10. Common flat nevus

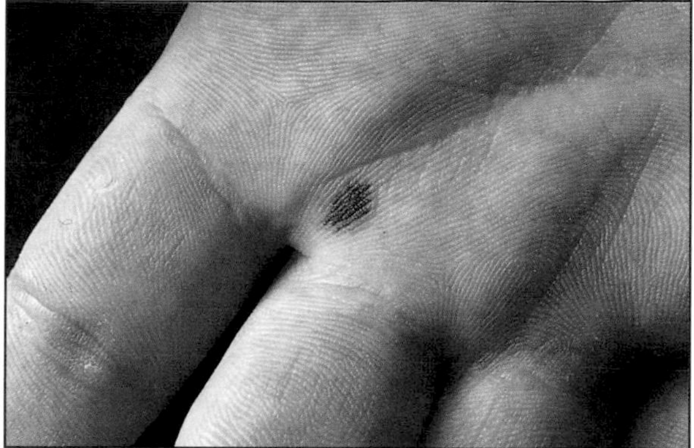

Fig. 58.11. Common nevus on palm with typical leakage of pigment

Eruptive lentigines occur most often in children, who occasionally develop hundreds of small lentigines in a short period of time. Sometimes the patients have been sunburned; in other cases, they are immunodeficient or iatrogenically immunosuppressed.

Clark Nevus (Clark et al. 1978). Ackerman has proposed the term Clark nevus for a slightly elevated, smooth, or subtly mamillated nevus that may have melanocytes at the epidermal-dermal junc-

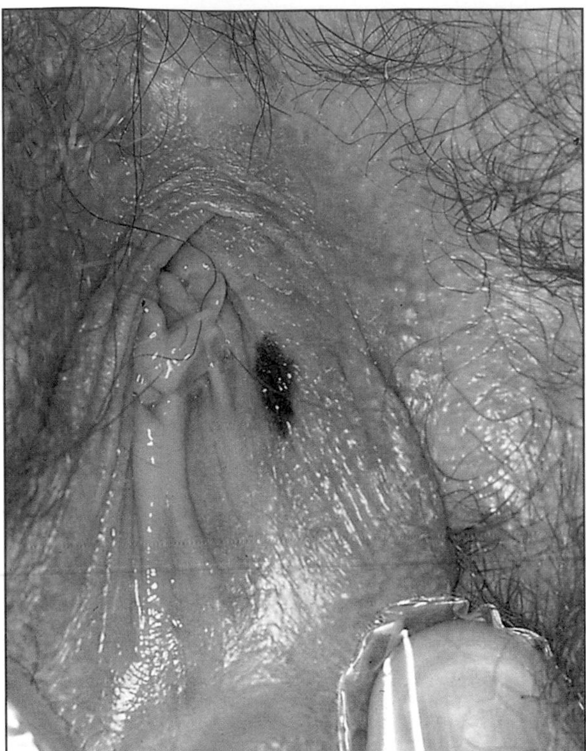

Fig. 58.12. Common nevus on female genital mucosa with irregular shape

tion and in the superficial dermis. While he suggested Clark nevus to replace dysplastic nevus, his definition includes considerably more nevi than the large irregular lesions Clark described. We describe a small, flat nevus as a common nevus and reserve the term dysplastic nevus for lesions with atypical clinical and histologic features.

Miescher Nevus (Miescher and von Albertini 1935). A broad-based nodular lesion, usually on the face, often only modestly pigmented and with a smooth surface.

Unna Nevus (Unna 1896). A protuberant, papillomatous, usually heavily pigmented nevus usually found on the trunk. Its surface may resemble that of a seborrheic keratosis with marked hyperkeratosis. In addition, it may be easily irritated by clothing or trauma and thus become directly swollen and inflamed.

Other Types of Common Melanocytic Nevi

- Molluscoid Nevus. Similar to an Unna nevus but with a smoother surface and less pigment. These lesions are often confused with large acrochordons or solitary neurofibromas.
- Divided Nevus (Fuchs 1919). Also known as a kissing nevus, the divided nevus is typically seen on both the upper and lower eyelids, showing that the change causing the nevus occurred prior to the embryologic step creating the lids (Fig. 58.13).
- Corymbiform Nevus (Löffler and Effendy 1998). Corymbiform means grape-like and describes a fleshy nevus made up of many, closely grouped pedunculated papules and nodules.
- Nevus Pigmentosus et Pilosus. Patients often express great concern about a nevus with terminal hairs. In general, this is a small congenital nevus, although on occasion such lesions first become apparent in childhood. A larger congenital hairy nevus is a straightforward diagnosis in the delivery room.
- Ancient Nevus (Kerl et al. 1998). This nevus is usually found on the face, especially the cheek or ear, of adults. The dome-shaped lesions has invariably been present for many years. It has the silhouette of a Miescher nevus but is asymmetric because of the presence of two populations of melanocytes as well as mesenchymal degenerative changes. There are focal, perhaps clonal, areas with striking atypia of melanocytes. The name is based on the analogy to ancient schwannoma (Chap. 59).

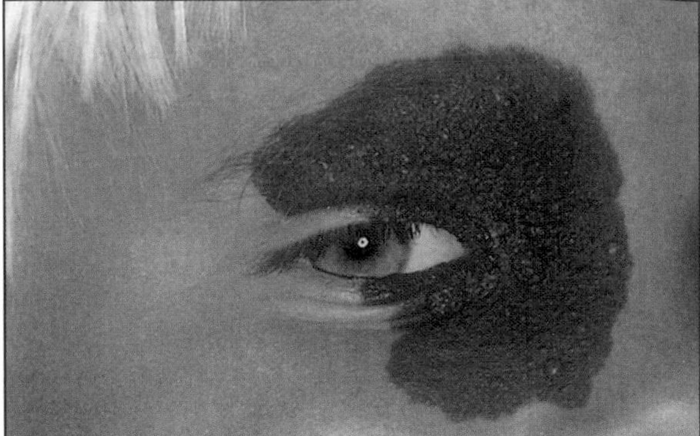

Fig. 58.13. Divided nevus

Histopathology. The histologic features have been discussed to an extent with the clinical features, as the two are so intertwined. The major challenge is to exclude malignant melanoma; this problem is discussed later. Fortunately, most nevi appear fairly banal under the microscope. The junctional melanocytes tend to be round or polygonal cells with large nuclei and obvious pigment. They are relatively uniformly dispersed along the basal layer and appear in small nests, often at the tip of elongated rete ridges. While melanocytes are rarely found in the upper layers of the epidermis, melanin is common and often deposited in the stratum corneum. The presence of irregularly sized nests also involving the papillary dermis, lymphocytic infiltrates, and melanophages has been termed junctional activity. Such changes are common in flat nevi and probably not worthy of a potentially alarming name.

Dermal melanocytes tend to have a variety of histologic patterns. Pigment is less common and when present is often confined to the cells that lie higher in the dermis. Miescher and von Albertini (1935) and Mishima (1965) described three types of dermal melanocytes: A, epithelioid, similar to the junctional cells; B, lymphocytoid, small, round dark cells usually without obvious pigment; and C, neuroid or spindled cells, almost invariably without pigment. In addition, other changes may be seen such as rosettes of nevus cells (also called erroneously nevus giant cells) or the replacement of melanocytes by fat cells. Balloon cell nevus is a histologic diagnosis for a clinically mundane nevus containing large clear melanocytes in which the nucleus is pushed to the side by accumulations of degenerating melanosomes. Balloon cell malignant melanomas are also seen.

Differential Diagnosis. In most cases the diagnosis of melanocytic nevus is obvious to the patient and physician. The differential diagnosis of ordinary melanocytic nevi includes all the variants already discussed, as well as the nevus variants and malignant melanoma. Dermatoscopic examination greatly facilitates the exclusion of nonmelanocytic lesions such as seborrheic keratoses and vascular growths and allows one to more precisely identify the few nevi that need excision to microscopically exclude malignant melanoma. The same diagnostic approach discussed under melanoma is used to assess nevi, since in almost all instances the question is: nevus versus malignant melanoma.

Course and Prognosis. The prognosis of nevi is by definition excellent. The challenge is to identify the small percentage of nevi that may evolve into malignant melanoma. This problem is further explored in the sections on congenital nevi, dysplastic nevi, and malignant melanoma. Patients with large numbers of ordinary nevi have a greater risk of developing malignant melanoma. In addition, histologically 20–30% of malignant melanoma reveal residual nevus cells; in yet other malignant melanomas, the nevus cells may have been destroyed. Thus, both patient and physician should be prepared to monitor nevi for change, as discussed under malignant melanoma.

Therapy. The treatment of choice for nevi is excision. The common reasons to decide to remove a nevus include cosmetic considerations, desire for a histologic diagnosis to exclude malignant melanoma, and the wish to eliminate nevi that are continually subjected to irritation such as from clothing or during physical activity. While many destructive methods can be employed, it is prudent to always obtain and submit a specimen for pathologic interpretation. Thus, electrocautery, cryotherapy, dermabrasion, and similar techniques are not recommended.

Many exophytic nevi can be removed by a simple tangential excision, especially if their base is relatively small. When larger lesions are tangentially excised, or when relatively flat nevi are removed by deep tangential excision or saucerization techniques, two problems arise. The large defect that is allowed to heal secondarily often produces an unacceptable scar and frequently the shave is not deep enough, so that the nevus is only partially removed. While large lesions, especially congenital nevi, are often removed by staged excisions, in general an excision is preferred over an incisional biopsy. While studies have not documented any worse prognosis for appropriately treated malignant melanomas diagnosed via incisional biopsy, we feel it is wise to avoid this approach.

Variants of Common Melanocytic Nevi

Some of the variants of common melanocytic nevus are clinically or histologically so distinct that they are usually discussed as separate lesions.

Spitz Nevus

(Spitz 1948)

Synonyms. Epithelioid cell and spindle cell nevus, spindle cell nevus, epithelioid cell nevus, benign juvenile melanoma (mentioned only for historical reasons and to be condemned)

Definition. Benign melanocytic tumor, primarily seen in children, with prominent spindle and epithelioid cells that may lead to confusion with malignant melanoma microscopically.

Etiology and Pathogenesis. There is nothing to suggest that a Spitz nevus is biologically different from other nevi. It appears to be acquired and not congenital, although it may be associated with a variety of congenital lesions.

Clinical Findings. The typical Spitz nevus is a red-brown, dome-shaped nodule seen most often on the face of a child (Figs. 58.14, 58.15). It is usually less than 1 cm in diameter and may have appeared over weeks to months. The surface may be telangiectatic. When examined with diascopy, it often has a lupoid appearance. While the face is the most common site for Spitz nevi in adults, they may also appear on the trunk and extremities.

There are many clinical variations of Spitz nevi. Some may appear in an eruptive fashion, or grouped (agminated Spitz nevi). This phenomenon may arise within a congenital nevus, on a background of a congenital café-au-lait macule-like lesion, or involve normal skin. Others may be sclerotic, resembling a dermatofibroma. The pigmented spindle cell nevus of Reed (1985) is a predominantly junctional, pigmented version of a Spitz nevus, usually seen on the upper chest of young adults.

Histopathology. The histopathology of a Spitz nevus is one of the real stumbling blocks in dermatopathology. Sophie Spitz initially thought she was describing a variant of malignant melanoma with a good prognosis (benign juvenile melanoma). While cytologically the large epithelioid and spindle cells of a Spitz nevus can be confused with those of malignant melanoma, the architectural features are usually different. A Spitz nevus sometimes has epidermal hyperplasia with hyperkeratosis. Melanocytes are gathered in nests within the thickened epidermis; these nests are often elongated and vertical. There may be clefts between the nests and the adjacent keratinocytes. Eosinophilic amorphous pink globules, known as Kamino bodies (Kamino et al. 1979), are found in the epidermis, and probably represent basement membrane material. The base of the sharply circumscribed lesion is usually clearly delineated; the cells at the bottom are often smaller and more closely resemble ordinary melanocytes.

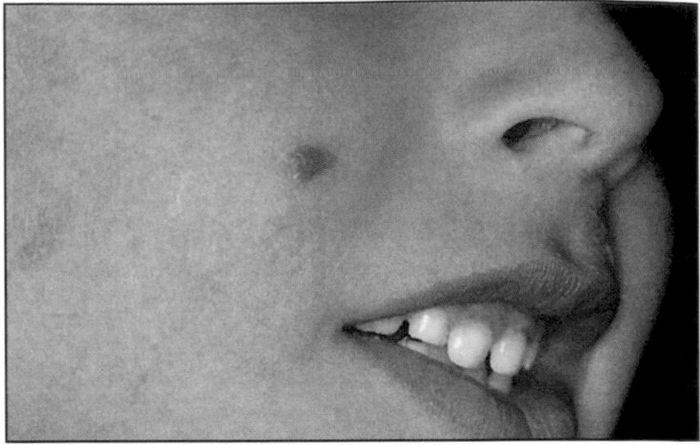

Fig. 58.14. Spitz nevus

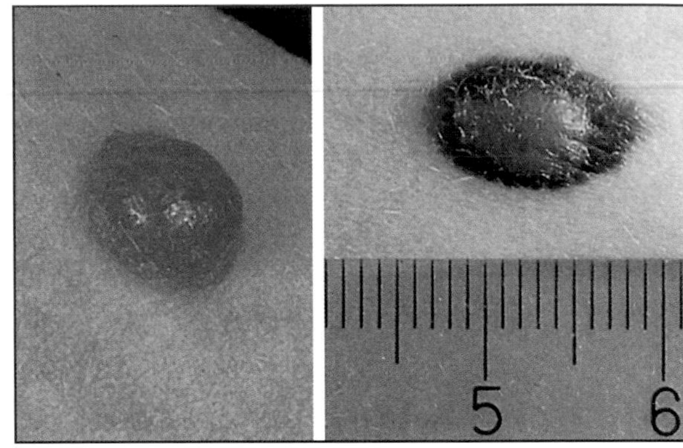

Fig. 58.15. Two Spitz nevi, one with little pigment and the other quite dark

A desmoplastic Spitz nevus often lacks junctional melanocytes and features a fibrotic dermis with isolated spindle and epithelioid cells. Often, S100 staining is needed to distinguish it from a fibrohistiocytic tumor. The spindle cell nevus of Reed contains nests of spindled melanocytes at the epidermal-dermal junction, often arranged in a horizontal fashion and richly pigmented. When the clinical features fit a Spitz nevus and the patient is a child, the microscopic diagnosis can usually be made comfortably. Conversely, the diagnosis of Spitz nevus in an adult is always a challenge and generally elicits a prompt call for consultation, even among experienced dermatopathologists.

Differential Diagnosis. In children, the most common differential diagnostic considerations are another type of melanocytic nevus, mast cell tumor, juvenile xanthogranuloma, lupus vulgaris, hemangioma, and pseudolymphoma. Hyperkeratotic or desmoplastic variants may resemble dermatofibromas.

Course and Prognosis. Experts in the field have strikingly different interpretations of Spitz nevus. Most regard them as morphologically unique but banal childhood nevi. At the other extreme, some groups recommend conservative reexcision of all lesions diagnosed as Spitz nevi. Melanocytes from a Spitz nevus may seed the regional lymph nodes, but this is not metastasis. We reject the concept of a malignant Spitz nevus, viewing such lesions as malignant melanomas. In addition, until better morphologic or molecular biological criteria are available, we refrain from the diagnosis of an atypical Spitz nevus.

Therapy. Surgical excision is the only therapy needed. There is no reason to require wide margins or conservative reexcision for a Spitz nevus.

Halo Nevus

(SUTTON 1916)

Synonyms. Leucoderma centrifugum acquisitum, Sutton nevus

Definition. Nevus surrounded by a halo of depigmentation, most likely undergoing regression.

Etiology and Pathogenesis. The accumulation of lymphocytes surrounding a nevus leads to a destruction of the melanocytes in the adjacent epidermis, producing a depigmented halo. At the same time, the melanocytes at the epidermal-dermal junction and in the upper dermis are also immunologically attacked and often destroyed, producing regression. Halo nevi are more common in patients with vitiligo and metastatic malignant melanoma; in these groups, circulating antimelanocyte antibodies can be identified, but the key damage seems to be lymphocyte-mediated.

Clinical Findings. The typical patient is a child with multiple nevi who suddenly develops a depigmented halo about one or more lesions (Fig. 58.16). Usually, no trigger is apparent. Sometimes a sunburn precedes the appearance of the halo nevus. In light-skinned individuals, Wood light examination makes the halo easier to see. The central nevus may disappear, or it may survive the immunologic attack. Later, the depigmented area tends to repigment. While a halo is alarming to the patient, it is usually of no concern. One should look for signs of vitiligo elsewhere and in an adult ask about previously removed nevi and malignant melanoma.

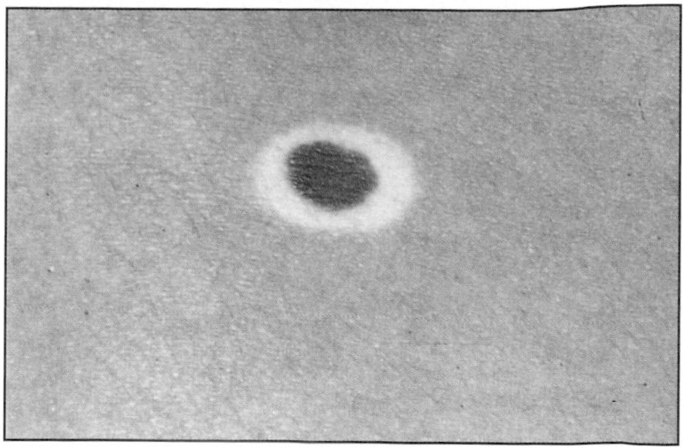

Fig. 58.16. Halo nevus

Other lesions that have a halo effect should also be searched for. By doing this, one may occasionally find a regressing melanoma.

Histopathology. When the original nevus is preserved, the diagnosis is fairly easy, as there is an intense infiltrate of lymphocytes and plasma cells. The halo is difficult to find on routine histology, unless the patient has relatively dark skin so that the contrast can be seen. Sometimes the destruction of the nevus is so complete that only a lichenoid infiltrate is present. In such a situation, one must hedge histologically, saying "compatible with halo nevus" but pointing out that a regressed malignant melanoma could look about the same microscopically.

Therapy. None is required. If clinical questions about the nature of the precursor melanocytic lesion exist, then excision should be performed.

Other Inflamed or Altered Nevi

- Meyerson Nevus (MEYERSON 1971). Nevus with associated acute inflammatory response, producing a peripheral ring of erythema and scale. Under the microscope, a junctional or compound nevus is seen admixed with a mixed infiltrate, spongiosis, and crust. Most inflamed nevi are the result of trauma and do not have the classic clinical features described by Meyerson. Another common type of inflamed nevus without a clinical name is the combination of an inflamed epidermoid cyst and a Miescher nevus.
- Cockade or Cockarde Nevus (HAPPLE 1974). Persistent inflammation may produce a target effect with a series of rings of pigment about a central junctional or compound nevus. Halo nevi may

also have a target pattern, as may malignant melanomas.

- Nanta Nevus (NANTA 1911). In this situation, a facial nevus, usually of the Unna type, is associated with cutaneous bone formation (osteoma cutis). The bone often serves as a nidus of irritation, leading to eventual removal of the lesion.
- Desmoplastic Nevus. Fibrosis in the papillary dermis is another aspect of the regression of nevi or melanomas; sometimes fibrosis dominates, producing a dermatofibroma-like lesion. A Spitz nevus may also be associated with extensive fibrosis, making the histologic diagnosis very difficult.
- Recurrent Nevus. Sometimes the fibrosis is a response to a surgical procedure or injury. When a compound or dermal nevus is removed by a tangential excision, it may recur as a flat, irregularly pigmented lesion, often with white areas in the center; such lesions were originally termed pseudomelanomas. The explanation is that, following the tangential excision, a junctional proliferation of melanocytes develops, associated with a papillary dermal scar and often the presence of residual deep melanocytes, producing a puzzling clinical and histologic picture if the history of a previous procedure is not available.

Nevus Spilus

Clinical Findings. Nevus spilus is a most distinctive lesion: many tiny, dark papules and nodules are scattered over a large light-brown patch (Fig. 58.17). Thus, nevus spilus represents a café-au-lait macule speckled with multiple nevi. The nevi may have a variety of histologic patterns, including ordinary junctional and compound nevi, as well as Spitz nevi. At birth, often no lesion is apparent or only a pigmented patch is noticed, but later the dark spots or speckles appear. The trunk is the most common location. Nevus spilus may be one of the components of phakomatosis pigmentovascularis. While nevus spilus is generally harmless, there are reports of malignant melanoma developing in the darker lesions, so that life-long clinical follow-up is needed. Sometimes nevus spilus occurs following the lines of Blaschko.

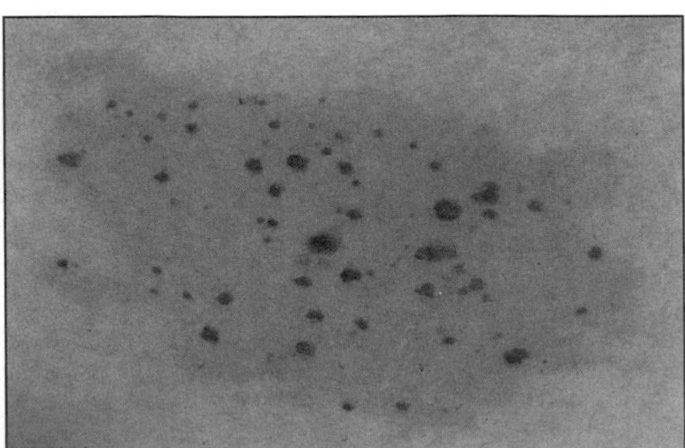

Fig. 58.17. Nevus spilus

Histopathology. If the tan background is biopsied, the findings are subtle with only slight hyperpigmentation. Giant melanosomes may be found. When a dark papule is biopsied, a junctional or compound nevus is usually identified, although sometimes Spitz nevi are also found.

Therapy. No treatment is needed; usually, the lesions are too large for surgery. If areas in a nevus spilus change, these should be biopsied to rule out malignancy.

Dysplastic Nevus and Dysplastic Nevus Syndrome

(CLARK et al. 1978; LYNCH et al. 1978)

Synonyms. B-K mole syndrome, familial atypical multiple mole melanoma (FAMMM) syndrome, atypical nevus-melanoma syndrome

Definition. Acquired melanocytic nevi, typically flat, often large, and with allegedly specific histologic features. Some groups prefer to use the term atypical nevi for lesions that attract clinical attention and reserve dysplastic nevus for those lesions with proven histologic changes.

Epidemiology. Dysplastic nevi are common. Some studies have shown that 60–90% of the population have at least one dysplastic nevus. In contrast, the dysplastic nevus syndrome, in which patients have many atypical nevi, is uncommon.

Etiology and Pathogenesis. An introductory textbook is not the place to resolve the issue of dysplastic or atypical nevi. The issue is too complex. There are some patients who have multiple, flat, irregular nevi and a personal or family history of malignant melanoma. These patients, referred to by the initial of the surnames of the first two families,

B and K, were identified simultaneously by Clark's and Lynch's groups as individuals or families at risk for malignant melanoma. Initially, autosomal dominant inheritance was postulated, but no single gene defect has been consistently identified, and most observers support the concept of multifactorial inheritance, that is, several genes being responsible.

The problem arose, in our judgment, when physicians made two illogical conclusions. First, they began to identify individual nevi on a wide range of patients clinically as dysplastic nevi, overlooking the fact that flat, irregular nevi are the most common acquired nevi on the trunk of adults. Similarly, some pathologists began to call all nevi with alleged dysplastic features dysplastic nevi and suggested a risk of malignant melanoma. By the mid-1980s, combining the skills of clinical dermatologists and dermatopathologists, it became possible to identify the dysplastic nevus syndrome in 50–90% of patients. This frequency is patently absurd.

Clinical Findings. The typical dysplastic nevus is a small, dark, flat, sharply bordered lesion that is usually only several millimeters in size (Figs. 58.18, 58.19). It is seen most commonly on the trunk and tends to increase in number during adolescence or pregnancy and following intense sun exposure or immunosuppression. Larger dysplastic nevi may be up to 10–15 mm in size, have several colors, contain a central elevated or dark nodule, and even show white areas of regression or have an erythematous border. Thus, they can be very difficult to distinguish from malignant melanoma.

The clinical features in patients with the dysplastic nevus syndrome are more striking. They tend to have many more nevi, many of which are quite large (Fig. 58.20). Estimates have been offered that the number of large atypical nevi ranges from 10 to more than 100. In addition, many smaller, flat, irregular nevi are also present. They often have multiple scars where suspicious nevi and malignant melanomas have been removed, and they give

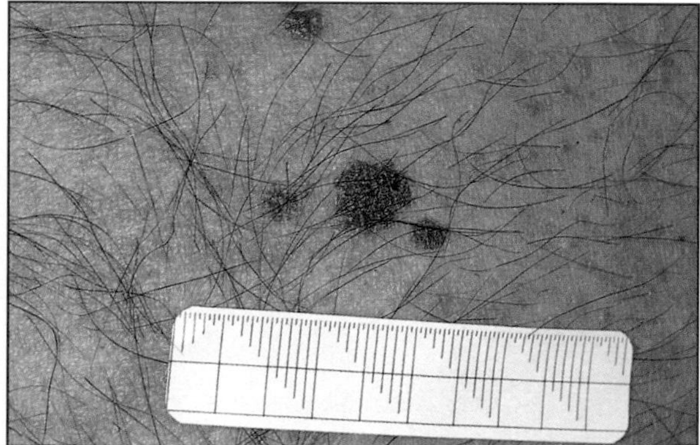

Fig. 58.18. Multiple dysplastic nevi

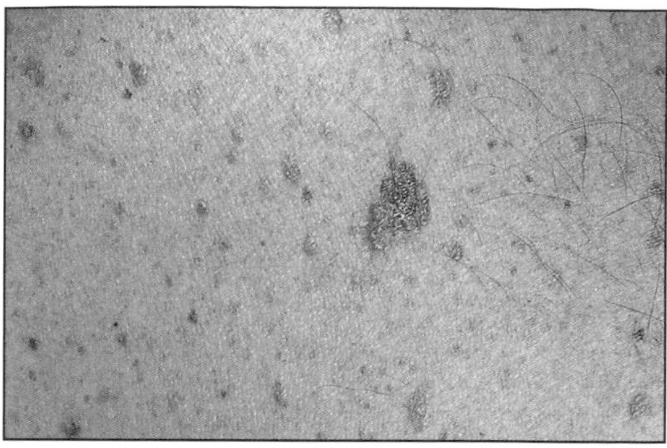

Fig. 58.19. Large dysplastic nevus with multiple smaller lesions, some of which are freckles and others probably early dysplastic nevi

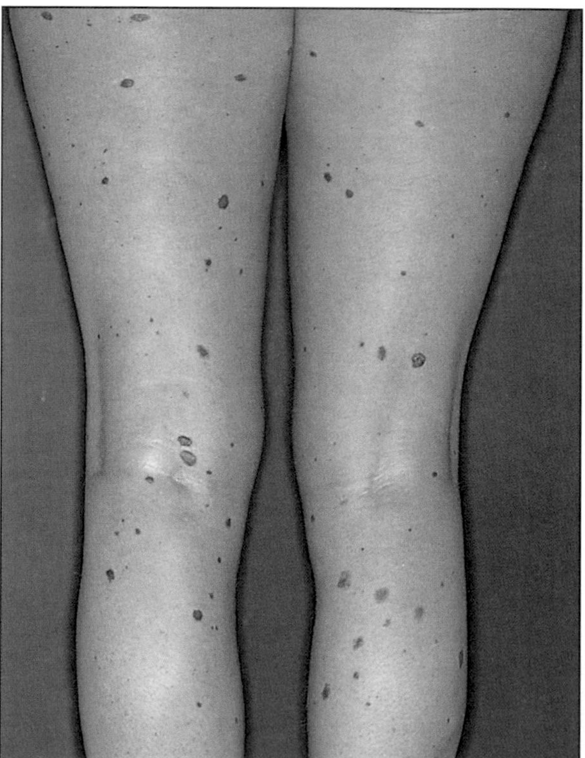

Fig. 58.20. Patient with dysplastic nevus syndrome, multiple nevi, and a scar on the right calf where a malignant melanoma was excised

a history of developing new nevi well into their adult life. The phenomenon of activation of nevi in pregnancy is probably due to lesions in patients with the dysplastic nevus syndrome being very sensitive to hormonal stimulation.

It is still unclear whether these multiple nevi are melanoma precursors or markers for melanoma susceptibility. We suspect both. Careful photographic studies, such as those of Clark, clearly show in some cases the evolution of a malignant melanoma from a preexisting nevus. In addition, malignant melanomas from such patients often show residual features of a dysplastic nevus. On the other hand, some patients develop new malignant melanomas, not arising in a preexisting, documented dysplastic nevus.

The nonhereditary dysplastic nevus syndrome refers to patients who fulfill the requirements for dysplastic nevus syndrome but have no positive family history. Until the genetics are clarified, there seems little reason or logic to separate the two groups.

Histopathology. The histopathologic features of dysplastic nevus are the basis of long and sincere controversy between many colleagues in dermatopathology. Suffice it to say no one has defined dysplasia in a manner that enables the ordinary dermatologist and dermatopathologist to reproducibly identify dysplastic nevi. Nevertheless, some features are relatively constant and worth mentioning. Dysplastic nevi have irregular borders, so that microscopically the shoulder effect is seen as melanocytes extend in small groups or nests within the epidermis past the borders of the main part of the nevi. The junctional melanocytes are often increased in number, fused into irregular nests, and occasionally show upward spread towards the stratum corneum. In the dermis, the nests of melanocytes are more ordinary, but there is often fibrosis in the papillary dermis, associated with a lymphocytic infiltrate. There may be increased dermal vascularity. Cytologic atypia is not a common feature of dysplastic nevi in our experience. Expert opinions range from "No atypia is ever found" to "Atypia is always found and can be easily graded."

All of these criteria were developed looking at nevi from patients with dysplastic nevus syndrome. Undoubtedly, some of the criteria were based on lesions which were early malignant melanomas, since for a number of years, vast numbers of lesions were excised from such patients. Unfortunately, relatively ordinary, flat nevi from patients without an unusual clinical appearance or positive family history may have exactly the same features.

Therapy. The therapy of a single dysplastic nevus is not different from that of any other nevus. It can be simply excised so that the patient and physician no longer have to worry about following it. Such surgery should not be viewed as melanoma prophylaxis. Patients with several large, flat nevi can simply be followed at 6- to 12-month intervals with measurement of lesions and dermatoscopic examination. They should be aware that there is a low risk of any one nevus becoming a malignant melanoma and know which of their nevi are particularly suspicious.

The patient with dysplastic nevus syndrome requires different management. We find photographic documentation helpful. Today, many clinicians are able to store the information in computers via digital cameras, making storage and retrieval much simpler. In addition, dermatoscopic evaluation also greatly helps in monitoring changes or identifying suspicious lesions. We prefer to see such patients every 6 months. We encourage them to avoid intense exposure to sunlight and sunburns. The use of oral contraceptives is controversial; we do not argue against their use.

Other Syndromes Associated with Melanocytic Nevi

While one typically thinks of sporadic congenital nevi and dysplastic nevus syndrome, there are a number of other syndromes in which congenital or acquired nevi are seen. Carney syndrome, although listed under multiple lentigines, also features multiple blue nevi. Patients with a variety of epidermal nevus syndromes (Chap. 52) may also have congenital melanocytic nevi. Turner syndrome and Noonan syndrome (Chap. 19) are also associated with numerous common melanocytic nevi.

Congenital Melanocytic Nevus

(Alibert 1832)

Synonyms. Congenital hairy nevus, giant nevus, bathing trunk nevus

Definition. Melanocytic nevus present at birth, often large and containing terminal hairs.

Etiology and Pathogenesis. The cause of congenital melanocytic nevi is unknown. They presumably represent a significant defect in the migration of melanocytes from the neural crest. The presence of matching nevi on both the upper and lower eyelids (Fig. 58.13) suggests that the defect occurs during embryonic development after eyelid fusion at 8–9 weeks but before eyelid reopening at 24–26 weeks. While familial reports of congenital melanocytic nevi exist, most cases are sporadic. The incidence is less than 1%, and most lesions are small. The incidence of the large, disfiguring, congenital melanocytic nevus is extremely low, in the range of 1/5,000–20,000 births.

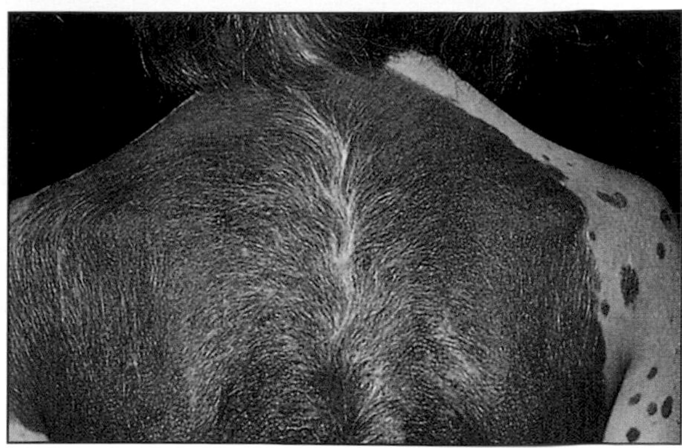

Fig. 58.22. Large bathing trunk congenital nevus with prominent hairs

Clinical Findings. There is a great variation in the clinical appearance of congenital nevi. Lesions may range in size from several millimeters to covering almost the entire body. Some may follow Blaschko lines, reflecting somatic mosaicism. While most are identified at birth, they maybe very pale and not apparent until later in infancy. Most contain terminal hairs, but some do not. Primarily in order to discuss prognosis, congenital melanocytic nevi have been subdivided according to size. Many schemes are available: none is perfect. A National Institutes of Health Consensus Conference in 1984 suggested the following classes: small < 1.5 cm, medium 1.5–20 cm, and large > 20 cm.

Most congenital nevi are oval, have a papillomatous surface, and a regular but often speckled coloring (Fig. 58.21). Early lesions may be pale tan, resembling a café-au-lait macule, but soon become darker and more easily identified. In larger lesions, the surface may be very irregular, and numerous dark macules and nodules may be distributed on a lighter background (Fig. 58.22). In addition, multiple, small, congenital melanocytic nevi may be associated with a larger lesion. On the scalp, deep, weakly pigmented congenital melanocytic nevi may present as cutis verticis gyrata.

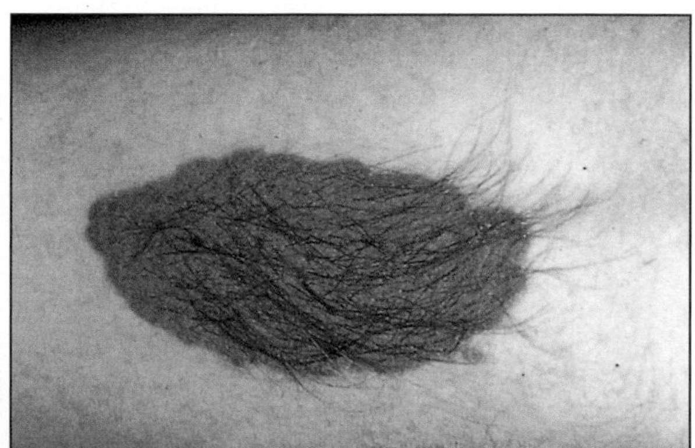

Fig. 58.21. Small congenital nevus

Congenital nevi may be associated with a wide variety of other defects. There is an association between congenital melanocytic nevi and neurofibromatosis 1. When the nevi involve the dorsal midline, the likelihood of melanocytic proliferations in the CNS is increased. In the most extreme example, neurocutaneous melanosis (Virchow 1859; Rokitansky 1861; Touraine 1949), patients are born with a large congenital melanocytic nevus, often involving the lumbosacral region, associated with multiple small nevi, and even involving the palms and soles. Usually, the lesions are heavily pigmented and rich in hairs (Fig. 58.23). The patients also have leptomeningeal proliferations of melanocytes, leading to hydrocephalus and other CNS defects. These individuals are at risk not only for cutaneous malignant melanoma but also for leptomeningeal melanoma. All patients with large congenital melanocytic nevi involving the dorsal midline should be investigated neurologically.

Histopathology. Microscopic examination is rarely needed to establish the diagnosis of congenital melanocytic nevus. The only exception is a pale tan lesion present at birth, which may also be a café-au-lait macule. In this situation, the presence of nests of melanocytes gives the answer. Lesions that are biopsied in infancy may show extremely bizarre and unusual nests of melanocytes at the epidermal-dermal junction. Not knowing that the biopsy is from an infant can lead the dermatopathologist to a false diagnosis.

A wide variety of patterns have been described. Probably the most reliable feature suggesting a

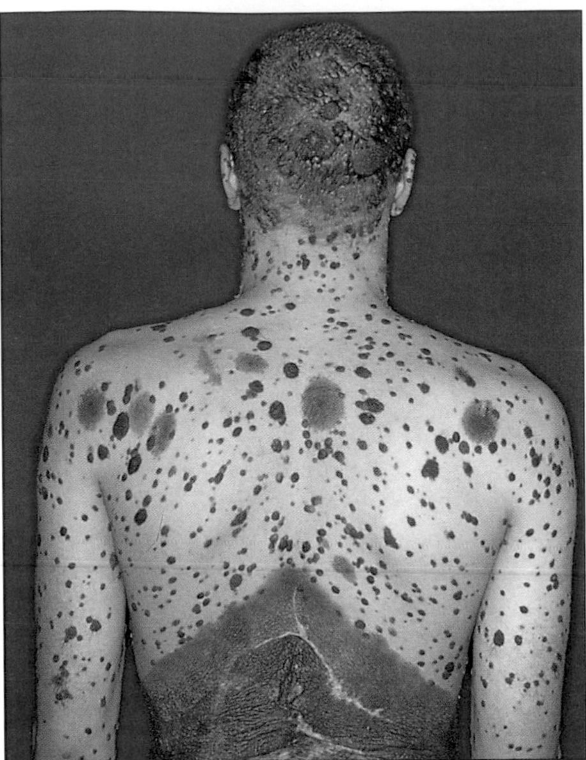

Fig. 58.23. Neurocutaneous melanosis

congenital nevus is infiltration of nevus cells along the adnexal structures into the deeper dermis. The presence of large numbers of terminal hairs is also a clue. Neuroid differentiation, sometimes with well-developed sensory structures, occurs. Rarely, congenital nevi may have spindle and epithelioid cell areas, or dermal dendritic elements, mimicking a Spitz nevus or blue nevus. In very large nevi, occasionally ectopic structures such as muscle, bone, and vessels may be seen.

The paradox is that large, clinically obvious congenital melanocytic nevi are likely to have distinctive histologic features, while the smaller (1.5–3.0 cm) congenital nevi are usually indistinguishable microscopically from a common dermal or compound nevus.

Diagnostic Criteria. When examining a child, it is easy to establish whether a nevus has been present since birth and is thus congenital. When dealing with adults, the patient often does not know. It is well worth having the individual ask their parents. In addition, photographic documentation using childhood pictures may be an effective tool.

Course and Prognosis. The exact prognosis of congenital melanocytic nevi is not known, which makes planning therapy a difficult problem. The most common clinical sign of malignant change is the development of a nodule, often deep in the nevus. The rare large or giant lesions have a definite risk of melanoma, with estimates ranging from 5% to 40%. This wide scatter shows how difficult it is to assess the problem. In large congenital melanocytic nevi, malignant melanoma may develop very early in life, even in infancy. Despite the scarcity of large congenital melanocytic nevi, they are responsible for almost all malignant melanomas in infancy, as the only other cause is metastasis from a mother with malignant melanoma.

The prognosis of smaller congenital melanocytic nevi is clearly better; the question is how much better. Small lesions probably have a lifetime risk of 1–5% of developing into malignant melanoma, and thus may be responsible for a not insignificant number of cases of adult malignant melanoma. Changes in childhood are rare in small lesions.

Differential Diagnosis. At birth, large, hairy, pigmented lesions have no differential diagnostic considerations. Paler lesions may be confused with café-au-lait macules or even epidermal nevi. A biopsy will rapidly provide the answer. Later in life, Becker nevus and nevus spilus are frequently confused with congenital melanocytic nevus, but they have different clinical and histologic features. Finally, in adults, the differential diagnosis includes noncongenital melanocytic nevi.

Therapy. The basic treatment of congenital melanocytic nevi is surgical excision. The stimulus towards therapy is to prevent the later development of malignant melanoma and to provide cosmetic improvement for what can be extremely distressing problems. Since the large congenital melanocytic nevi may evolve into malignant melanoma in the first year of life, excision should be undertaken as soon as the risks associated with anesthesia are acceptable. Often several staged excisions, combined with tissue expanders or skin grafting, are needed. The propensity of congenital melanocytic nevi to extend quite deep means that often some melanocytes are left behind. Sometimes extremely superficial, pale congenital melanocytic nevi are treated early in life with dermabrasion; this offers an easier and safer way to treat larger areas in a small child but also leaves behind deep melanocytes.

Smaller lesions can be excised later, perhaps after 8–10 years of age when local anesthesia usually suffices. Some patients and children may choose to observe the nevus; this, too, is acceptable.

Malignant Melanoma

Definition. Malignant cutaneous tumor arising from melanocytes with a propensity for metastasis.

Epidemiology

Incidence. Malignant melanoma is not only a common tumor, but its incidence has increased dramatically in the past 30 years, and the rate of increase shows little sign of leveling off. The incidence in Europe is about 12/100,000; in the Munich area it is 14/100,000. In Australia and the southwestern USA, the incidence is much higher, exceeding 40/100,000.

Prevalence. Using these incidence numbers, the lifetime risk is about 1/100 to 1/200 for white individuals in Europe and the USA.

Age. Malignant melanoma is a disease of middle-aged adults. The malignant melanomas that arise in congenital melanocytic nevi are more common in children, while lentigo maligna melanoma is a disease of the elderly.

Sex. Women are more often involved but have a better prognosis. The face and legs are most often involved in women, while the trunk is the most common site in men.

Race. Whites are at a far greater risk. Many studies have shown a much lower risk for blacks. In New Mexico, the incidence among Native Americans is far less than 1/100,000, while in Hispanics it is about 4/100,000. Similar data have been obtained all around the world.

Occupation. Outdoor work is a risk factor, but not as significant as when considering basal cell carcinoma and squamous cell carcinoma. Apparently, repeated short intense bursts of sunlight exposure and severe sunburns, especially in childhood, play a greater role.

Genetics. There are families with an increased incidence of malignant melanoma. Most but not all of them are those with dysplastic nevus syndrome. As many as 5% of all malignant melanomas arise in such families. Defects in a number of candidate genes have been identified. The best established is located at 9q21 and is known as the CDKN2A gene, also referred to as p16 gene or MTS1 (multiple tumor suppressor gene 1). The gene product interacts with cyclin-dependent kinases which interact with the retinoblastoma gene to control transcription. The CDKN2A proteins block the kinases and thus inhibit cell growth. When they are defective, growth control is impaired. Some somatic mutations in CDKN2A have been shown to be specific for ultraviolet-induced DNA damage. The most generous estimate is that CDKN2A is present in 30% of melanoma-prone families and associated with dysplastic nevus syndrome. Thus, many other genes must be involved.

Geography. The closer one is to the equator and the higher the altitude at which one lives, the greater the risk. For example, in the western USA, the incidence is higher in Albuquerque than in Denver; both are mile-high cities, but Albuquerque lies further south. Similarly, when one compares Albuquerque and Dallas which are at about the same latitude, Albuquerque lies much higher and has a greater incidence of malignant melanoma. Similar patterns are seen in Australia, as the incidence is higher in the north than the south. In other parts of the world, people living closer to the equator tend to be darker (perhaps an evolutionary trait to offer sun protection) so that the statistics are not as dramatic.

Etiology and Pathogenesis. The best established risk factor for developing malignant melanoma is sun exposure and sunburn. The development of malignant melanoma on the hands, feet, oral mucosa, and genitalia demonstrates that these are not the only factors, although some argue that sunlight could induce hematogenous factors that then cause malignant melanoma in unexposed skin. The second major risk is the presence of preexisting melanocytic lesions that may evolve into malignant melanoma. In contrast to all other nevi, melanocytic nevi are not stable, and a given percentage serve as precursors of malignant melanoma. The third major factor is the individual's genetic background. A final risk factor is immunosuppression or immunodeficiency. Table 58.2 shows a mnemonic (MMRISK) devised by Fitzpatrick to summarize the risk factors for malignant melanoma.

The principle problem with malignant melanoma is its tendency to metastasize. The melano-

Table 58.2. Mnemonic device for increasing malignant melanoma risk awareness

M	Moles: atypical or dysplastic?
M	Moles: how many common moles?
R	Red hair or freckles
I	Inability to tan (skin types I, II)
S	Sunburn: severe sunburn as child
K	Kindred: family history of malignant melanoma

cyte is a proven explorer, reaching the skin from the neural crest. It appears equally capable of moving once again under the right circumstances. Even normal melanocytes occasionally wind up in regional lymph nodes. The melanocytes in nevi and malignant melanoma have no intercellular adhesions or connections; thus, following cell division, new melanocytes are relatively free to migrate or wander. This may explain, albeit simplistically, the propensity of malignant melanoma to metastasize while still a relatively small tumor.

There is often a prominent host response against melanocytic lesions, including malignant melanoma. Lymphocytic infiltrates are seen in halo nevi, as well as in many malignant melanomas. Sometimes the host response is so successful that a patient presents with metastatic malignant melanoma as the primary tumor regresses. In major cancer centers, up to 5% of patients with malignant melanoma present with no known primary. When the immune response is hampered, such as with iatrogenic immunosuppression or in AIDS, the likelihood of malignant melanoma increases.

In 50–60% of patients, malignant melanomas develop in clinically normal skin. Since most adults do not continue to develop new melanocytic nevi, such an event should be brought to the physician's attention. In the past, it was common for patients to ignore such lesions, until such signs as marked increase in size, ulceration, bleeding, or pruritus developed. Often such lesions were so advanced that metastasis was almost to be expected. Today, thanks to public education programs and skin cancer screening efforts, most malignant melanomas are recognized at a relatively early stage.

The remainder of malignant melanomas arise from precursor lesions. The most common precursors are small congenital melanocytic nevi and dysplastic nevi, although more banal nevi can also show malignant change. The relative contribution of these two risk factors varies from population to population but probably accounts for about 30% of malignant melanomas. The risk of malignant melanoma in giant congenital melanocytic nevi is higher, but they are fortunately uncommon. Another well-established precursor is lentigo maligna. We view these lesions arising on light-damaged skin of older individuals as malignant melanoma in situ. They usually have a prolonged latent period, averaging about 15 years, before evolving into a lentigo maligna melanoma. They account for perhaps 5% of malignant melanomas.

All other scenarios are uncommon; acral lentiginous melanomas develop on the extremities, most often involving the great toe or thumb and account for about 2% of malignant melanomas. While these lesions can arise from preexisting acral nevi, in most cases they are malignant melanomas from the beginning but were initially overlooked or misdiagnosed. Malignant melanomas may also develop out of blue nevi, most often the larger cellular variant. They also develop on the oral and genital mucosa and even more rarely in internal organs. Finally, the clear cell sarcoma has been called a malignant melanoma of soft parts but has unique features and is considered in Chapter 59.

One recurrent question among both physicians and lay individuals is the role of trauma in causing malignant melanoma. Often one reads of how repeated trimming of a callus on the toe led to a malignant melanoma or how the constant irritation of a bra strap induced a malignancy. Such scenarios are unfortunate, but usually the correct explanation is that the early malignant melanoma was not diagnosed and thus ignored until it became clinically obvious. Clearly, repeated traumatization of nevi is not desirable, but it is not likely to be a major etiologic factor in malignant melanoma. Similarly, incomplete removal of a nevus, or even cutting into a nevus, is not a likely trigger of malignancy. Patients still labor under the impression that removing a melanocytic lesion may cause the melanocytes to spread. This reflects the futile attempts at surgery for large nodular malignant melanomas several generations ago.

Clinical Findings. Malignant melanomas are usually divided into several clinical subtypes. Table 58.3 shows the breakdown of over 30,000 patients in the German Melanoma Registry from 1983 to 1995. In the early papers of Clark, discussing the subtypes of malignant melanoma, a key biologic determinant is the relative length of the horizontal or radial growth phase, before the onset of the invasive or

Table 58.3. Clinical-histologic subtypes of malignant melanoma

Type	Percent	Median age (years)
Superficial spreading melanoma	57	51
Nodular melanoma	21	56
Lentigo maligna melanoma	9	68
Acral lentiginous melanoma	4	63
Unclassifiable melanoma	4	54
Other melanomas (amelanotic, mucosal, noncutaneous)	5	54

Based on 30,015 patients in German Melanoma Registry, 1983–1995

vertical growth phase. In the horizontal phase, the tumor is confined to the epidermis so that metastasis is unlikely and the outlook excellent. We will use the traditional subtypes of malignant melanoma as a convenient didactic tool. Except for lentigo maligna, the differential diagnosis and therapy will be considered at the end.

Lentigo Maligna and Lentigo Maligna Melanoma

(Hutchinson 1890; Dubreuilh 1912)

Synonyms. Melanosis circumscripta precancerosa (Dubreuilh), Hutchinson freckle

Definition. Lentigo maligna is a slowly growing, malignant melanoma in situ that can evolve into a frankly malignant melanoma, then designated lentigo maligna melanoma.

Etiology and Pathogenesis. Lentigo maligna is a tumor of older white individuals, almost always found on the face. Women are affected twice as often as men, and their average age is over 60 years. The lentigo maligna is usually present for about 15 years before the development of lentigo maligna melanoma. Lentigo maligna is the prototype of a horizontal growth phase of malignant melanoma; when atypical melanocytes begin to grow down into the dermis, the vertical growth phase has begun, representing lentigo maligna melanoma. Lentigo maligna is one variant of malignant melanoma in situ arising in sun-damaged skin; almost all malignant melanomas begin in the epidermis and are thus in situ for a period of time.

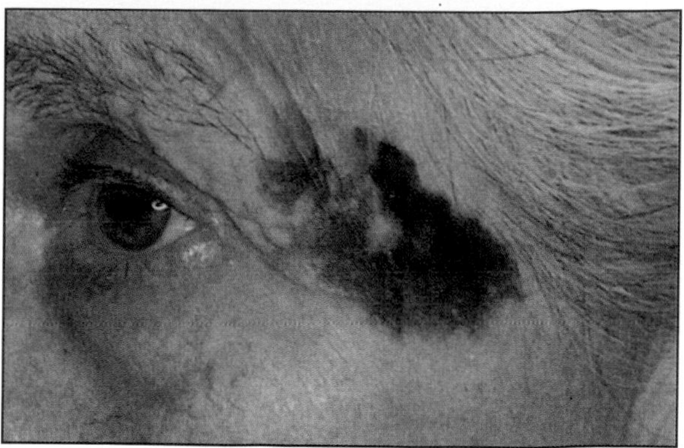

Fig. 58.24. Lentigo maligna

Clinical Findings. Lentigo maligna is typically an irregular brown to black macule that slowly enlarges to become a patch (Fig. 58.24). The most typical location is the cheek, as the part of the face that gets the most exposure to sunlight. A larger lentigo maligna almost invariably has multiple colors, including occasional white areas of regression as well as various dark hues. Its border is usually irregular. Sometimes the darker areas are spotted or reticulated. While the border is usually indistinct, sometimes it may be quite sharp and marked by rounded extensions. The skin markings are usually well-preserved. If a darker papule or nodule arises, or if the skin markings are destroyed, then a lentigo maligna melanoma is probably developing (Fig. 58.25). The nodules are usually darker, but need not be so, and can even be amelanotic. A lentigo maligna is usually asymptomatic; pruritus should also suggest the possible initiation of the vertical growth phase and a more prominent host response.

Histopathology. The hallmark of lentigo maligna is the proliferation of atypical melanocytes in the epidermal basal layer. There is an increased number of clear cells, many of which are large, irregular, or polygonal and which may have atypical nuclei. Sometimes nests of these cells may be seen, often located in a free space below the epidermis but not invading the dermis. In addition, the epidermis is usually thinned. Some dermatopathologists take the presence of nests as a criterion for the diagnosis of malignant melanoma in situ. The atypical melanocytes often extend down adnexal structures. In the dermis, there is almost always marked

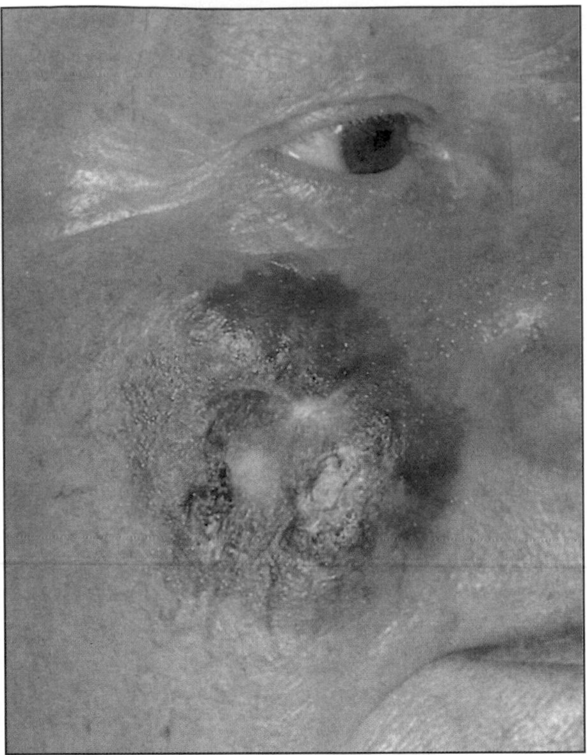

Fig. 58.25. Lentigo maligna melanoma

solar elastosis; the diagnosis of lentigo maligna is not tenable in the complete absence of elastosis. In the upper dermis, one often finds a scattered lymphohistiocytic infiltrate, occasionally admixed with plasma cells and melanophages. If tumor cells have clearly started to invade the dermis, the diagnosis is lentigo maligna melanoma.

It is often difficult to determine the borders of a lentigo maligna, especially when studying reexcision specimens. Actinically damaged skin contains scattered, large, atypical melanocytes; they may become more common in the skin adjacent to excision sites, perhaps stimulated by the healing process. Thus, one should be very careful in assessing the adequacy of excision of lentigo maligna and rely heavily on clinicopathologic correlation. A variety of monoclonal antibodies, such as HMB45 or S100, may help to identify the melanocytes but cannot assess their biologic role.

Diagnostic Criteria. The main features are facial location, age of patient, slow growth and microscopic evidence of sunlight-induced damage. Otherwise, the diagnosis of superficial spreading melanoma may be more appropriate, suggesting the likelihood of a somewhat more aggressive course. It is often wise to sample several areas, as the variability of the lesion is notorious. One should continue to monitor a suspected lentigo maligna carefully, even after receiving a reassuring pathologic report following an incisional biopsy.

Course and Prognosis. Lentigo maligna has a good prognosis. Its course is unpredictable, not only because of the biologic variability of the tumor, but also because of the age of the patient. Since lentigo maligna may be present for 10–20 years before developing an invasive component, many patients die with their lentigo maligna, rather than from their lentigo maligna melanoma. On the other hand, as patients live longer and longer, the incidence of lentigo maligna melanoma has increased. Perhaps a quarter of lentigo maligna cases evolve into lentigo maligna melanoma. Once lentigo maligna melanoma is present, it has about the same prognosis as any other malignant melanoma of the same thickness.

Differential Diagnosis. Lentigo maligna has a somewhat different differential diagnosis than the other malignant melanomas. A large, flat, irregularly pigmented lesion on the face may also be a flat, perhaps irritated seborrheic keratosis, a solar lentigo, or a pigmented actinic keratosis. These lesions usually do not have the variable color that a lentigo maligna has, but exceptions occur. The distinction with dematoscopy or biopsy is easy. A rare situation is the presence of an amelanotic lentigo maligna that is almost invariably clinically misdiagnosed as a basal cell carcinoma or actinic keratosis. Thus the correct diagnosis is usually made quite late.

Superficial spreading melanoma is more often slightly elevated and has sharper borders and more tongue-like extensions. It is also more likely to have multiple hues, including white areas of regression. It usually has been noticed for a shorter period of time. If a lesion is not typical for lentigo maligna or lentigo maligna melanoma, then the diagnosis of superficial spreading melanoma should be made.

Therapy. Excision is the treatment of choice for lentigo maligna. Because it has relatively indistinct borders, micrographic surgery has been recommended. Frozen sections are a difficult way to assess the borders of a lentigo maligna. Even under ideal circumstances, actinically damaged skin at the border of a lentigo maligna may show some melanocytic hyperplasia that may be exaggerated during the healing process after an incisional biopsy.

In contrast to other malignant melanomas, alternative therapy forms can be considered for lentigo maligna. There is considerable experience using radiation therapy, which is often a blessing for older patients. A typical regimen is 10–20 Gy daily for a total of 100 Gy using a tissue half-value layer of 1.0–2.0 mm. Marked erosions occur, but healing is usually excellent. There may be transient hyperpigmentation secondary to melanin in the papillary dermis, but it usually resolves after several months. This change should not be confused with a recurrence. The main problem is the possible presence of malignant melanocytes along adnexal structures. Other means of superficial removal include cryotherapy, dermabrasion, and superficial laser destruction; we do not recommend these approaches. Along with radiation therapy, they all suffer from the same lack of histologic control. There may be superficial resolution of the lesion but concurrent deep growth because of incomplete destruction.

If a lentigo maligna melanoma is diagnosed, then the same surgical criteria discussed at the end of the section should be employed. Sometimes complete excision is technically impossible, either because of the size or location of the lesion or because of the age and general health of the patient. Often a nodule of lentigo maligna melanoma is found within a much larger lentigo maligna. Our approach in this case is to surgically remove the nodular lesion and then irradiate the residual flat lesion.

Superficial Spreading Melanoma

Clinical Findings. Superficial spreading melanomas are most common in middle-aged individuals. In women, they are most often seen on the legs, while in men they are usually found on the upper aspects of the back. Often superficial spreading melanomas are mistaken for melanocytic nevi during their early stage, when they are small and may be relatively uniformly colored and sharply bordered (Fig. 58.26). The lesion has usually been present for a relatively short time, perhaps 1–5 years, when the patient comes to medical attention. The old story of a melanocytic nevus turning into a malignant melanoma probably hinges on failing to clinically identify the horizontal growth phase of a superficial spreading melanoma.

A typical superficial spreading melanoma is about 2–5 cm in size, round to oval, and usually sharply distinguished from the adjacent normal skin. It has rounded or polycyclic borders, sometimes with tongue-like projections. There may be a slight leakage of pigment across the border. Fitzpatrick described the superficial spreading melanoma as the „red, white and blue“ tumor. While the bulk of the lesion is represented with various nuances of brown and black, there are also white areas (regression), red areas (host inflammatory response), and blue to gray regions (mixture of deep pigment and regression; Fig. 58.27). Initially, superficial spreading melanomas are relatively flat, but

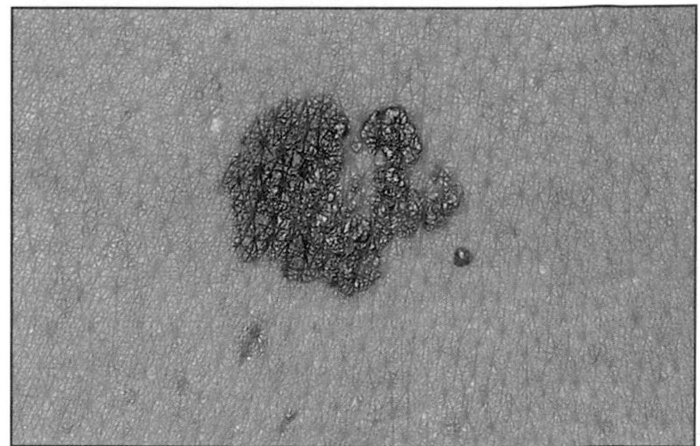

Fig. 58.26. Superficial spreading melanoma

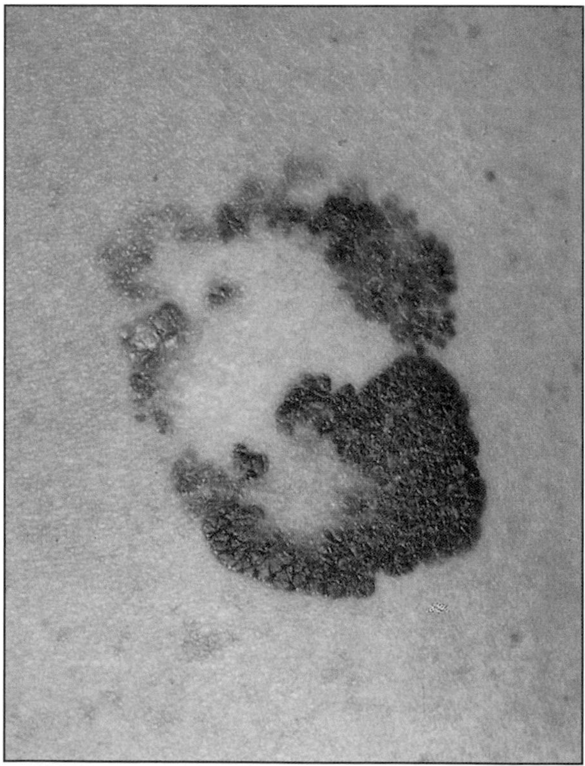

Fig. 58.27. More advanced superficial spreading melanoma with marked regression

they tend to become more bumpy and raised as they enter their vertical growth phase. Later, lesions are multicolored nodules, sometimes with a verrucous surface or even ulcerations.

Histopathology. The hallmark of superficial spreading melanoma is the initial spread of atypical melanocytes both singly and in nests throughout the slightly acanthotic epidermis; hence the alternative histologic name of pagetoid malignant melanoma. This intraepidermal spread of large cells with abundant cytoplasm is the horizontal growth phase. As the vertical growth phase is entered, cells begin to enter the dermis, often accompanied by an intense lymphocytic response. Typically, areas of regression with fibrosis and few obvious melanocytes are found in the papillary dermis.

Course and Prognosis. The outlook for superficial spreading melanoma has improved markedly over the past years, as patients and clinicians have become more adroit at distinguishing a small superficial spreading melanoma and a melanocytic nevus. Today, many thin lesions are identified with a relatively good outlook.

Nodular Melanoma

Clinical Findings. The nodular melanoma is an often intensely dark, rapidly growing nodule (Fig. 58.28). The history is usually relatively short, perhaps 1–2 years. Nodular tumors arising within lentigo maligna or well-documented nevi are not by definition nodular melanoma. In the past a nodular melanoma was defined as not having a horizontal growth phase. This is impossible, as the tumor also arises in the epidermis. The vertical growth phase starts very early and far outpaces the horizontal. Onc can distinguish between a true nodular lesion, which is typically very dark, shaped like a dome, and may undergo regression, and a flatter nodular tumor, which shows some horizontal growth at the same time it is invading.

A very difficult problem is presented by amelanotic nodular melanomas. They are usually misdiagnosed as pyogenic granulomas, presenting as red ulcerated masses. They are often found on the feet or hands. Because of the delay in diagnosis, their outlook is more dismal. Another unusual variant is the polypoid nodular melanoma, which has a stalk or narrow base. When this region is examined carefully, one may see an irregularly pigmented macular proliferation. In some ways one can view the polypoid tumor as the reverse of a typical nodular melanoma.

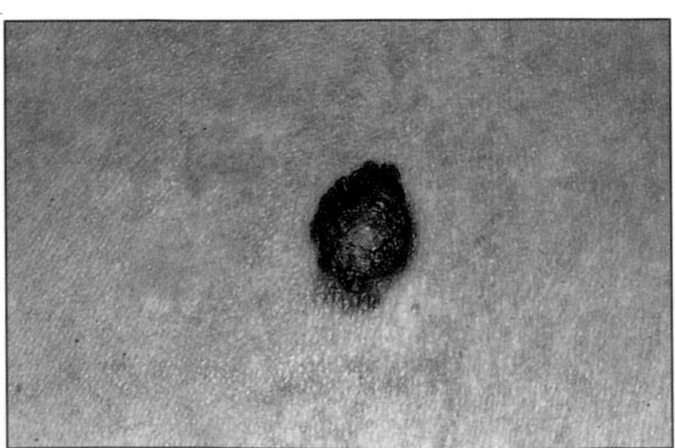

Fig. 58.28. Nodular melanoma

Histopathology. Microscopically, one sees a solid tumor comprised of large, often clear cells with a variety of microscopic patterns including spindle, epithelioid, and polymorphous cells. These cells invade into the dermis and sometimes into the fat. There is usually a prominent host response. The polypoid tumors rise above the skin surface, so they may not invade as deeply into the dermis. While some horizontal spread of melanocytes can be seen, it should be less than three rete ridges in width; otherwise, a superficial spreading melanoma is probably the better diagnosis.

Course and Prognosis. In general, nodular melanomas have the worst prognosis because of their propensity for rapid, invasive growth.

Acral Lentiginous Melanoma

Synonym. Melanotic whitlow

Clinical Findings. Acral lentiginous melanomas develop primarily on the digits, usually the great toe or thumb (Fig. 58.29). They usually arise from the nail matrix, or less often from the nail bed or nailfold. They may also appear on the palmar or plantar skin. Acral lentiginous melanomas are similar to lentigo maligna melanoma in that an irregularly pigmented macule is present for a long period of time. It tends to grow slowly, develop areas of regression, and eventually form a nodular component. Sometimes by this point the involved

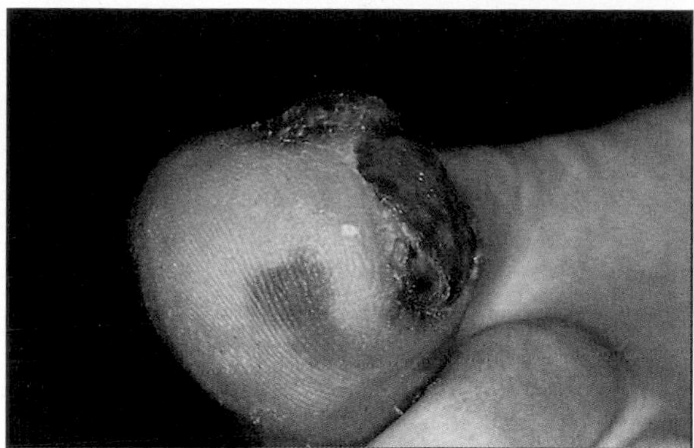

Fig. 58.29. Acral lentiginous melanoma

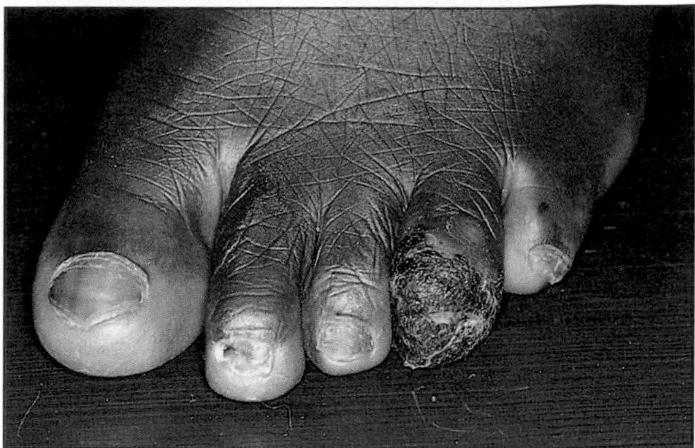

Fig. 58.30. More advanced acral lentiginous melanoma in a black

digit is swollen and enlarged. Often this lesion lies in the area of the nailfold, producing a discoloration of the nail. One should carefully search for the Hutchinson sign, the spread of pigment into the nailfold and more proximal areas of the finger, which suggests a malignant melanoma. Similarly, a sharply bordered stripe under the nail suggests a melanocytic nevus, while an irregular stripe is more likely to be an acral lentiginous melanoma.

Acral lentiginous melanomas are responsible for the bad reputation that nevi on the palms and soles have acquired. Current evidence suggests that a junctional nevus on a digit has exactly the same outlook as a junctional nevus on the trunk. When doubt exists, a biopsy is crucial. One should be very suspicious of new nevi in acral regions in adults, and never blame ulceration or bleeding of a nevus on trauma in this region. By following these hints, one can hopefully avoid missing acral lentiginous melanomas.

In black, Hispanic, and Asian patients, acral lentiginous melanomas are responsible for a much higher proportion of the malignant melanomas. They are not more common, but all the other types are so much less common that, proportionally, the acral lentiginous melanoma assumes a greater role. In some studies of blacks, over 20% of malignant melanoma involved the nails (Fig. 58.30). This phenomenon demonstrates that sunlight is not the only important factor in malignant melanoma development.

Histopathology. In order to rule out a malignant melanoma, an adequate excisional biopsy is essential. Tangential biopsies from acral lesions or inadequate punch biopsies from nailfolds often lead to mistaken diagnoses and medicolegal problems.

Initially, an acral lentiginous melanoma is very hard to identify under the microscope. There are large, highly dendritic melanocytes in the basal layer and often little else to see. As the tumor progresses, nests of atypical melanocytes are seen at the junction and then advancing into the corium.

Course and Prognosis. Once again, delayed recognition contributes to the relatively poor prognosis of acral lentiginous melanoma.

Differential Diagnosis. It is easy to miss an acral lentiginous melanoma; often the lesions acquire a reactive hyperkeratotic surface and can be mistaken for a verruca or callus, even to the point of being repeatedly trimmed or treated with cryotherapy or destructive acids. When the lesion is amelanotic, the likelihood of such a mistake multiplies.

Other Variants of Malignant Melanoma

There are many other variants of malignant melanoma; we have already alluded to many of them throughout this chapter but repeat them here for the purposes of clarity.

Malignant Melanoma Associated with Preexisting Melanocytic Nevus

The least common but most feared scenario is the presence of a nodule of invasive tumor cells in a giant congenital melanocytic nevus (Fig. 58.31). When a thick nodule develops in such a lesion, the outlook is grim. Often the nodule may be inflamed or amelanotic, so that the correct diagnosis is delayed, as one considers the possibilities of an abscess or infection. In smaller congenital melano-

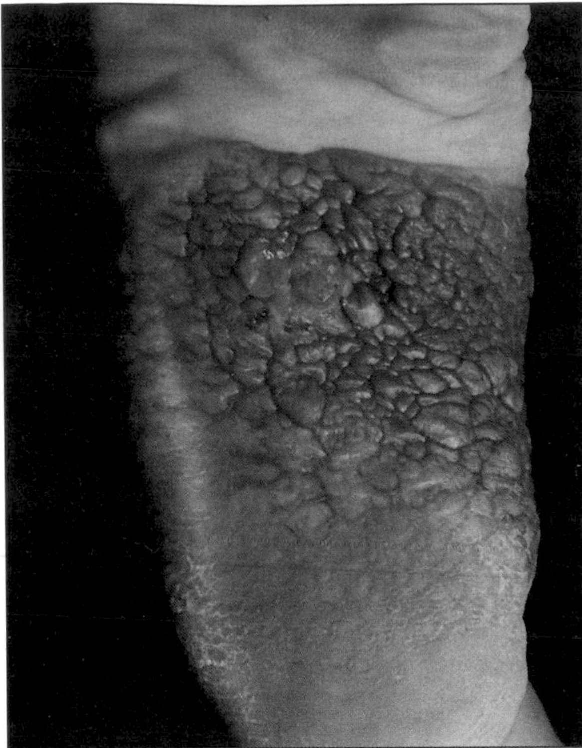

Fig. 58.31. Malignant melanoma arising on congenital nevus

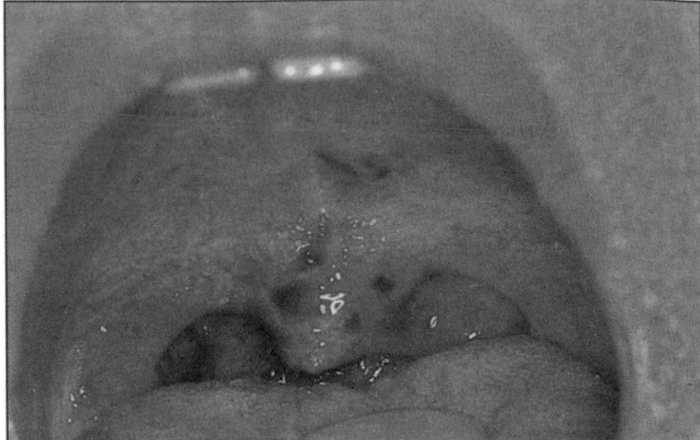

Fig. 58.32. Oral malignant melanoma with involvement of left tonsil

cytic nevi, the clinical and histologic identification of a precursor nevus is somewhat easier. Finally, other melanocytic nevi, especially large dysplastic nevi, may develop pigmented nodules, which usually can be identified clinically and histologically.

Amelanotic Malignant Melanoma

Without the clues of pigment, the diagnosis of a malignant melanoma is very difficult. The flat lesions are usually mistaken for actinic keratosis or superficial basal cell carcinoma; more nodular, ulcerated tumors are misidentified as basal cell carcinoma or pyogenic granuloma. Typically, the pathologic specimen is unsatisfactory so that staging is quite difficult.

Verrucous Malignant Melanoma

On the foot, it is easy to misinterpret the hyperplastic epidermal response associated with an acral lentiginous melanoma. Other, perhaps amelanotic, superficial spreading melanomas may also have a verrucous surface.

Polypoid Malignant Melanoma

Such lesions represent an extreme variant of nodular melanoma; they are unfortunately confused with large skin tags and other fibromas, especially if not darkly pigmented. When inflamed or ulcerated, they resemble pyogenic granulomas.

Mucosal Malignant Melanoma

Mucosal malignant melanomas are similar to acral lentiginous melanoma; sometimes the term acral lentiginous mucosal melanoma is used. The clinical features are so different that lumping these two forms accomplishes little. Oral malignant melanomas have an initial lentiginous appearance, which is frequently overlooked (Fig. 58.32). They too are over-represented in darker-skinned individuals, and may be more common in this population. The clinical diagnosis is made more complicated by the presence of benign hyperpigmented areas in the mouths of many dark-skinned individuals. Sometimes amalgam tattoos can also be confused with melanocytic lesions.

Similar malignant melanomas can develop on the genital mucosa (Fig. 58.33), more often of women, and in the rectum. The differential diagnosis includes melanotic macules as well as melanocytic nevi. Genital nevi are likely to have atypical histologic features and produce diagnostic problems. These malignant melanomas have a terrible prognosis, presumably because they are invariably discovered quite late, when invasion has already occurred.

Desmoplastic and Neurotropic Malignant Melanoma

While many malignant melanomas elicit a prominent host desmoplastic response, in some instances this is the dominant feature, often associated with a more marked perineural infiltration. Usually, the initial lesion is situated on the face or arm and is a

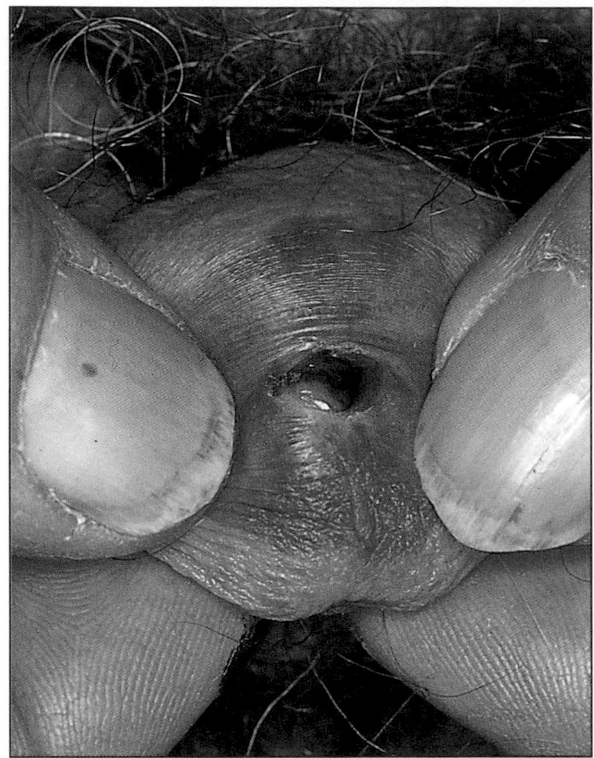

Fig. 58.33. Penile malignant melanoma with nodule in urethra

lentigo maligna or at least resembles a lentigo maligna clinically and histologically. After apparently adequate treatment, a nodule develops and is usually misdiagnosed as a hypertrophic scar; it may even be biopsied and falsely interpreted under the microscope. Many desmoplastic malignant melanomas wind up as lawsuits. As a clinician, one should be reluctant to make the diagnosis of hypertrophic scar in a melanoma excision site. It is probably wise to do S100 and HMB45 staining on all scar tissue associated with a treated nevus or malignant melanoma and to search carefully for atypical melanocytes in the fibrous stroma or along nerves. S100 is more likely to be positive than HMB45.

Ocular Malignant Melanoma

The terminology for melanocyte proliferations of the eye, its adnexal structures, and conjunctiva is very confusing, especially for dermatologists accustomed to a totally different set of terms. The most popular term is primary acquired melanosis (PAM), about as inadequate as lentigo to describe a flat, acquired, hyperpigmented lesion involving the conjunctiva and occasionally extending to the cornea or adjacent tissues. When atypical melanocytes are identified in PAM, the lesion is considered premalignant. Conjunctival melanomas most often arise in PAM but may also develop de novo or in association with conjunctival nevi (Fig. 58.34). Malignant melanoma of the uvea or retina may also occur, but comes within the realm of the ophthalmologist. Patients with dysplastic nevus syndrome seem to have an increased risk of ocular malignant melanoma and should have regular ophthalmologic evaluations.

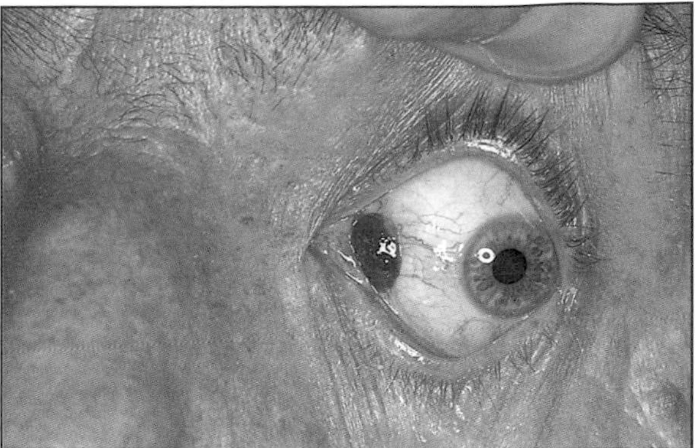

Fig. 58.34. Conjunctival malignant melanoma

Malignant Melanoma in Pregnancy

Melanocytes have been shown to have hormone receptors and to be hormone-responsive cells. It has long been suggested that pregnant patients are likely to develop new melanocytic nevi and experience enlargement and darkening of preexisting lesions. Many such patients probably have dysplastic nevus syndrome. Malignant melanomas also arise in pregnancy; they appear statistically to be thicker than lesions in nonpregnant women, but when this factor is taken into account, the prognosis is similar. The treatment of malignant melanoma in pregnancy is controversial. If a primary skin tumor is identified, it should be removed, as the risk to the mother of delayed treatment is greater than the minimal risk to the fetus from minor surgery. If metastatic disease is identified in a pregnant patient, the problems are immense. The infant is at risk for in utero metastases and is threatened by major operations or systemic treatment. On the bright side, there is no evidence that a treated malignant melanoma patient need avoid future pregnancies.

Malignant Melanoma in Children

About 2% of malignant melanomas occur in patients less than 20 years of age, but only 0.3% occur prior to puberty. The entire issue of congenital melanocytic nevi is primarily relevant to children. In addition, a mother with visceral metastases can transfer tumor cells transplacentally, producing a newborn with disseminated metastases. Children with xeroderma pigmentosum have an increased risk of malignant melanoma; about 5% develop a malignant melanoma, often in their teenage years. Children from families with dysplastic nevus syndrome should avoid sunburn or extensive exposure to the sun and be monitored closely as they enter puberty.

Table 58.5. Histologic simulators of malignant melanoma

Dysplastic nevus
Spitz nevus
Combined nevus
Recurrent/persistent nevus
Halo nevus
Nevus with partial regression
Acral nevus
Genital nevus in young adults
Congenital nevus in newborns and infants
Deep penetrating nevus
Ancient nevus
Nevus after ultraviolet irradiation
Traumatized nevi
Melanocytic proliferation in the epidermis
Above some dermal nevi
In severely sunlight-damaged facial skin
Within solar lentigines
Sometimes in clinically normal skin of eyelid

Clinical Approach to Malignant Melanoma

Diagnosis

Differential Diagnosis

The clinical diagnosis of malignant melanoma is coupled with a misdiagnosis rate of 10–20%. Thus, one must hope to be astute enough to identify all suspicious or atypical nevi, remove them, submit them for pathologic interpretation, and then live with a small degree of error in the pathologic interpretation. Most experienced dermatologists remove many more nevi to exclude malignant melanoma, than malignant melanomas. Dermatoscopy or skin surface microscopy has greatly improved the preoperative diagnostic accuracy for melanocytic lesions and often allows one to exclude nonmelanocytic lesions such as seborrheic keratosis, pigmented basal cell carcinoma, and vascular lesions. Automated picture analysis systems are available for the diagnosis and systemic follow-up of melanocytic lesions. Table 58.4 lists the major clinical differential diagnostic considerations, while Table 58.5 shows some of the benign histologic simulators of malignant melanoma.

Table 58.4. Clinical differential diagnosis of malignant melanoma

Melanocytic tumors
Common melanocytic nevi, especially dysplastic nevus and recurrent nevus
Spitz nevus
Blue nevus
Epithelial tumors
Pigmented basal cell carcinoma
Seborrheic keratosis, especially if irritated
Verruca with hemorrhage
Pigmented hidrocystoma
Pigmented actinic keratosis
Other adnexal tumors, especially if pigmented
Vascular tumors
Angiokeratoma
Hemangioma, especially if thrombosed or traumatized
Pyogenic granuloma
Venous lake
Kaposi sarcoma
Glomus tumor, especially if subungual
Other tumors
Dermatofibroma
Miscellaneous
Subungual or subcorneal hemorrhage (black heel)
Tattoo

Diagnostic Criteria

Early identification of flat lesions by patients and family members is a potential tool to find and treat thinner malignant melanomas. In the past, the American Cancer Society included a growing mole and a bleeding or ulcerated mole as two of the seven danger signs of cancer for nonphysicians. These signs develop far too late and usually indicate an advanced malignant melanoma. After the classic work of Clark and Fitzpatrick in accurately identifying the features of earlier, flatter, potentially curable malignant melanomas, the ABCD criteria (Table 58.6) became popular in the USA and have spread to other parts of the world. They are imperfect but allow one to separate nevi which might be melanomas from more banal nevi and then

Table 58.6. The A-B-C-D-E criteria

Criteria	Harmless	Suspicious
A = Asymmetry	Symmetric	Asymmetric
B = Border	Sharply defined	Poorly defined, leakage of pigment
C = Color	One color	Two or more colors; white areas
D = Diameter	<6 mm	>6 mm, growing
E = Elevation	No change	Increase in thickness

either excise or more carefully follow the suspicious lesions. They also suggest which lesions should be examined with dermatoscopy. These guidelines can also be effectively employed for screening by non-physicians. MacKie's group in Glasgow suggested adding pruritus as an important criterion. We also use E for elevation. Since an elevated papillomatous or dome-shaped nevus is almost always harmless, the key is change in elevation. Papules or nodules developing in flat or congenital nevi are danger signs. These changes can often be best recognized with serial clinical photographs or computerized collections of both clinical and dermatoscopic pictures that can be carefully compared.

The diagnostic approach to a lesion suspected of being a malignant melanoma is fairly straightforward. Almost all cases are diagnosed by biopsy, followed by evaluation of formalin-fixed, paraffin-embedded tissue. An excisional biopsy is always preferred to reduce the theoretical risk of causing a malignant melanoma to disseminate as a result of the trauma of the biopsy. Most large studies have not confirmed this risk; nonetheless, it is usually possible to avoid incisional biopsies. Large lesions such as a suspected lentigo maligna can be studied with one or more small biopsies of dark or thickened areas, but the risk of a sampling error remains. When a malignant melanoma is biopsied superficially, then the assessment of tumor thickness becomes impossible, and the staging is inaccurate. If the suspicion of malignant melanoma is reasonably high and is supported by dermatoscopic examination, it is appropriate to perform an excision with 1-cm margins initially. This is no more than a generous excisional biopsy for an atypical nevus and will provide appropriate treatment for a thin malignant melanoma.

In our opinion, the clinician's responsibilities begin, not end, with the performance of a procedure such as a biopsy. Many points deserve mention. First of all, if an incisional biopsy is performed and not interpreted as a malignant melanoma, this does not always exclude malignant melanoma, because of the possibilities of a sampling defect. If the diagnosis is pigmented seborrheic keratosis, then the approach is clear. However, if a large irregular lesion is biopsied and the pathology report reads "atypical nevus," one should not be falsely reassured. Instead, additional biopsies, or at very least clinical and dermatoscopic surveillance, is required. In addition, the tumor thickness may be underestimated in a biopsy; final tumor thickness must be based on examination of the entire tumor.

The clinician is responsible for assuring that an adequate pathology report is obtained and acted upon. For example, we have encountered patients in whom a lesion is interpreted as a malignant melanoma, but the pathology report is filed in the patient's chart and overlooked. In addition, in this age of managed care in the USA, many pathologists examining skin specimens are definitely not experts in the interpretation of pigmented lesions. If the clinician does not insist upon consultation in what he or she perceives as difficult cases, who will? Surely not the insurer. In our experience with a variety of malignant melanoma study groups, it has become clear that, even for experts, the diagnosis of malignant melanoma is a challenge. A good rule is that every malignant melanoma should be viewed by at least two dermatopathologists. In many studies, a disturbing discordance among expert observers has been identified. This means that to be careful, many borderline lesions must be treated as malignant melanoma in order not to jeopardize the patient through our own lack of skills.

Occasionally, other diagnostic approaches are appropriate. The use of frozen sections to evaluate a biopsy and guide the subsequent therapy in one sitting is acceptable, but rarely necessary. Most excisional biopsies are performed under local anesthesia, and the final excision carried out a few days later. Major malignant melanoma study groups have made extensive use of frozen sections with superb clinical results. One should approach lesions in a consistent fashion; if considerable experience with frozen sections exists, they offer a time-saving and perhaps cost-saving option. Cytologic examination of cells aspirated from a pigmented tumor can often confirm the diagnosis of malignant melanoma but provides no staging information.

Course and Prognosis

We have discussed the prognosis of malignant melanoma in general terms for each of the major variants but will consider it in more detail here. The prognosis of malignant melanoma is almost directly related to the degree to which the tumor has invaded the skin. The major independent risk factor is tumor thickness, type of malignant melanoma, sex of the patient, and the location of the primary lesion appear significant in some studies. A number of schemes have been proposed to classify malignant melanomas and offer prognostic information.

Clark Level (CLARK et al. 1969). It was obvious to Wallace Clark in the 1960s that the system so useful for other tumors left much to be desired when classifying malignant melanoma. Traditionally stage I lesions (those confined to the skin) included a wide range of tumors ranging from a lentigo maligna, with an almost 100% five year survival rate, to a deep nodular malignant melanoma penetrating to the subcutaneous fat, with a much lower survival rate. Clark thus suggested his levels (Table 58.7) to better stratify tumors confined to the skin. Note that staging today is more refined (Tables 58.10 and 58.11).

Even though Clark's levels were perhaps the most important advance in our understanding of the prognosis of malignant melanoma, there are nonetheless weaknesses which soon became apparent. Most importantly, they are not very reproducible, as the transition from the papillary to reticular dermis is not easily identified. In addition, they fail to help account for the thickness of skin; a level IV tumor on the eyelid may be much thinner than a level II tumor on the back. Finally, they also fail to assess rare polypoid tumors adequately, which may be level II–III but which are rapidly fatal.

Table 58.7. Clark levels

Level	Location of tumor cells
I	Confined to epidermis
II	Entering papillary dermis
III	Filling papillary dermis
IV	Entering reticular dermis
V	Filling reticular dermis, involving subcutaneous fat tissue

Breslow Tumor Thickness (BRESLOW 1970). Alexander Breslow made the next major contribution, using an ocular micrometer to measure the tumor thickness from the granular layer to the deepest reach of a tumor. His stratification is shown in Table 58.8. Breslow's approach allows one to measure polypoid tumors and to better predict the behavior of tumors found in very thin or thick skin. Most reports today give both the Breslow thickness and the Clark level. The exact break points in the Breslow scale have been manipulated statistically. The German melanoma registry uses 0.75, 1.50, and 4.00 mm. Other groups have other break points; each system has its advocates and advantages.

Table 58.8. Breslow tumor thickness

Thickness	Ten-year survival (%)
≤0.75 mm	97
0.76–1.50 mm	90
1.51–4.00 mm	65
>4.00 mm	50

Prognostic Index. SCHMOECKEL and BRAUN-FALCO (1978) coupled the mitotic index to the tumor thickness and called this the prognostic index, hoping to improve the assessment of the metastatic risk of mid-thickness malignant melanomas. The mitotic index is the number of mitoses per mm^2; it is not easily reproduced between observers which is a disadvantage to this refinement. The mitotic index is not an independent prognostic factor.

Independent Prognostic Factors. The most important of these are:

- Tumor Thickness. The Breslow tumor thickness is the most important independent prognostic factor. As far as Clark levels go, the difference between levels II and III is of prognostic importance, but also the most difficult distinction to make microscopically.
- Sex. Men have a worse prognosis than women.
- Location. Malignant melanomas in the BANS region (back, upper aspects of arms, neck, and scalp) may have a slightly worse prognosis than matched tumors elsewhere. Tumors in locations where they are invariably discovered late have a worse prognosis.
- Type of Malignant Melanoma. Nodular melanoma and acral lentiginous melanoma appear in some series to have a worse prognosis than

Table 58.9. TNM classification of malignant melanoma

pT	**Primary tumor**
pTX	Primary tumor cannot be evaluated
pT0	No primary tumor
pTis	Malignant melanoma in situ (Clark level I)
pT1	Tumor thickness ≤0.75 mm and/or Clark level II[a]
pT2	Tumor thickness 0.76–1.50 mm and/or Clark level III[a]
pT3	Tumor thickness 1.50–4.00 mm and/or Clark level IV[a]
pT4(a)	Tumor thickness > 4.00 mm and/or Clark level V[a]
pT4(b)	Satellites within 2 cm from primary tumor
N	**Regional lymph nodes**
NX	Regional lymph nodes cannot be evaluated
N0	No regional lymph nodes metastases
N1	Metastases ≤ 3 cm in size in any regional lymph nodes
N2	Metastases ≤ 3 cm in size in any regional lymph nodes and/or in-transit metastases[b]
N2(a)	Metastases ≥ 3 cm in size
N2(b)	In-transit metastases[b]
N2(c)	Metastases ≥ 3 cm in size and in-transit metastases
M	**Distant metastases**
MX	Distant metastases cannot be evaluated
M0	No distant metastases
M1(a)	Metastases in skin, subcutaneous tissue, or lymph nodes beyond the regional lymph nodes
M1(b)	Visceral metastases

Based on UICC Classification (HERMANEK et al. 1987).
[a] If there are discrepancies between the tumor thickness and the Clark level, the worse finding takes precedence.
[b] In-transit metastases are metastases that are more than 2 cm from the primary tumor but not beyond the regional lymph nodes.

Table 58.10. Staging of malignant melanoma

Stage	Primary tumor	Lymph nodes	Metastases
I	pT1, pT2	N0	M0
II	pT3	N0	M0
III	pT4	N0	M0
	Any PT	N1, N2	M0
IV	Any pT	Any N	M1

After UICC (HERMANEK) 1987

superficial spreading melanoma and lentigo maligna melanoma, even when tumors of the same thickness are compared.

- Ulceration. In some studies ulceration has been an independent risk factor.

Staging

The staging of a malignant melanoma patient is a controversial subject. The standard TNM (tumor-nodes-metastases) classification of malignant melanoma is shown in Table 58.9 and the resulting stages in Table 58.10. We employ the refined staging recommended by the German Dermatological Society, as shown in Table 58.11. Most patients today are identified with low-risk lesions, and there are no data that extensive staging is cost-effective or prolongs lives. On the other hand, in higher-risk patients, staging is essential so that treatment protocols, even if the given patient is not treated, can be scientifically evaluated. A complete physical examination with careful attention paid to the presence of other malignant melanomas or their precursors in the skin or mucous membranes, routine blood work, and radiologic evaluation including sonography and/or advanced imaging techniques should be used to identify or exclude brain, liver, lung, and

Table 58.11. Refined staging of malignant melanoma

Stage	Primary tumor	Lymph nodes	Metastases	Ten-year survival (%)
Ia	pT1 (≤ 0.75 mm)	N0	M0	97
Ib	pT2 (0.76–1.50 mm)	N0	M0	90
IIa	pT3 (1.51–4.00 mm)	N0	M0	67
IIb	pT4 (> 4.00 mm)	N0	M0	43
IIIa	pTa, pTb	N0	M0	28
IIIb	Any pT	N1, N2	M0	19
IV	Any pT	any N	M1	3

Recommendations of the German Dermatological Society (KAUFMANN et al. 1998); pTa, satellite metastases; pTb, in-transit metastases

Table 58.12. Staging techniques

Complete skin examination with dermatoscopic evaluation of suspicious lesions
Search for satellite and in-transit metastases
Regional lymph nodes examination (palpation, 7.5 MHz ultrasound)
Chest X-ray
Abdominal ultrasound or computed tomography (CT)
With tumor thickness > 1.50 mm, consider CT or magnetic resonance examination of skull
Laboratory – routine hematologic studies, liver function tests, serum S100 levels
Further specialized studies determined by signs and symptoms

other metastases. Our suggestions for a staging evaluation are shown in Table 58.12. The evaluation of possible lymph node involvement is so intricately connected with therapy that it is considered in further detail there.

Therapy

Surgical

The basis of therapy is surgical excision. In the past, 5-cm margins were recommended, but this was clearly overtreatment and is no longer tenable. While there is no universal consensus, the recommendations of the German Dermatological Society are shown in Table 58.13. Even for lesions > 4.0 mm, many groups are now using 2.0 mm margins. Smaller excisions can usually be closed primarily, while larger margins may necessitate closing with a flap or graft. Microscopically controlled surgery also has its advocates, but malignant melanoma surgery is not tissue-sparing to begin with, as definite margins of safety are recommended by all.

Table 58.13 Recommended excision margins for stage I malignant melanoma

Tumor thickness	Excision margin (cm)
Malignant melanoma in situ	0.5
≤ 1.00 mm	1.0
> 1.00 to ≤ 4.00 mm	2.0
> 4.00 mm	3.0

Recommendations of the German Dermatological Society. If additional risk factors are present (such as ulceration, regression), the next larger excision margin should be employed.

Elective Lymph Node Dissection

A major controversy in malignant melanoma therapy concerns the role of elective lymph node dissection. Patients with no clinical sign of lymph node enlargement have a relatively high risk of micrometastases, depending on the thickness of their tumor. Patients with clinically enlarged nodes should undergo surgery, but what should we recommend for those without obvious lymph node disease? Those patients with malignant melanomas ranging from 1.0 to 4.0 mm in thickness have an intermediate risk of metastasis. Recent large studies have shown little advantage in performing elective lymph node dissection in this group and an increase in morbidity because of surgical complications. More superficial lesions are so readily cured by surgery alone that lymph node dissection is not warranted. With lesions thicker than 4.0 mm, the chances of lymph node involvement are high enough that many groups proceed directly to lymph node dissection, although its benefits are also not clearly established.

Sentinel node dissection has shown promise in refining the need for elective lymph node dissection. Morton et al. (1992) found that the first, or sentinel, node in the regional lymph nodes draining a primary tumor could be identified in over 80% of cases. Often the thickness of a primary malignant melanoma can be accurately assessed preoperatively with ultrasound examination. Radioactive technetium, sometimes coupled with a vital blue dye, is injected around the primary tumor or the biopsy site. After several hours, the sentinel node can be identified, excised, and studied with step sections and special stains such as S100, HMB45, or molecular biological techniques to improve the diagnostic accuracy. The findings in the sentinel node predict the presence or absence of nodal disease in more than 95% of patients.

There are some problems with sentinel node biopsies. First of all, they should not be viewed as a standard procedure at this point because of the lack of information from controlled trials. We offer them to patients with malignant melanomas thicker than 1.0 mm. Randomized studies are in progress. If a positive sentinel node is identified, elective lymph node dissection is performed. In many patients, only the sentinel node is positive; such individuals often undergo surgery that is too extensive and thus suffer an unnecessary increase in morbidity. The likelihood of recurrent disease in the regional lymph nodes following a negative sentinel node biopsy is around 5 % at 3 years.

Lymph node dissection does not insure survival. Patients with tumor thickness > 1.0 mm, no clinically apparent nodes and micrometastases found after elective lymph node dissection have about a 50 % five year survival, while those who receive a therapeutic lymph node dissection for clinically apparent disease have a 30 % five year survival. Another large study involving patients with tumor thickness > 1.5 mm compared immediate elective lymph node dissection to observation and therapeutic lymph node dissection if enlarged nodes were found. There was no benefit to immediate surgery. Patients may have distant hematogenous or lymphatic metastases independent of regional lymph node disease, which may simply be a marker for a more aggressive primary tumor.

Adjuvant Chemo- and Immunotherapy

Adjuvant therapy is another controversial aspect of treating malignant melanoma. Intermediate-risk patients offer an attractive target group, as any intervention that could reduce the development of metastatic disease in this group would save lives. Malignant melanomas are known to be immunogenic tumors. They have a higher spontaneous remission than most other malignancies and often show areas of regression. The presence of a T cell infiltrate is the microscopic equivalent of regression. In addition, vitiligo is more common in malignant melanoma patients and is a good prognostic sign, suggesting an immune response directed against melanocytes. For all these reasons, immunotherapy appears attractive.

Many approaches have been tried, but there is no standard adjuvant therapy. Nonspecific immunostimulation with Bacillus Calmette-Guérin or *Corynebacterium parvum* failed to prolong life or the disease-free interval. There is also no evidence that any chemotherapy regimen offered prophylactically improves survival in mid- or high-risk patients. Another approach has been isolated limb perfusion, usually with melphalan, often combined with hyperthermia. The treatment is toxic and does not prolong survival, although it does reduce or delay local recurrences.

Very high-dose recombinant interferon (IFN)-α2b has been shown in one major study of high-risk patients to increase the 5-year survival from 37 % to 46 %, with improvement in the disease-free interval and other relevant parameters. The dosage was 20 million units/m^2 intravenously daily for 4 weeks and then 10 million units/m^2 subcutaneously three times weekly for 1 year. The toxicity was considerable, so a lower dose protocol with 10 million units/m^2 subcutaneously three times weekly for 2 years is being evaluated. In Europe, there are several studies in progress comparing IFN-β in both intermediate- and high-risk patients without lymph node disease to control groups. In another study, interleukin (IL)-2 is combined with IFN-α2b.

Follow-Up

The most important contribution a dermatologist can make is to monitor the patient for development of a second primary melanoma, as well as other tumors such as basal cell carcinoma and squamous cell carcinoma. The outlook for a second primary is far better than for a metastatic tumor. It is also important to check the operation site, in-transit area, and regional lymph nodes to identify local recurrences at an early time, when treatment may make a difference. Palpation alone is not sufficient; we routinely employing ultrasonography to evaluate the scars and regional nodes. Table 58.14 shows the recommendations for other follow-up procedures in the various stages. The yield from routine chest x-ray and blood work is very low, so these procedures have been dropped by many groups. One promising method is monitoring serum S100 levels. Following surgical treatment, rising levels correlate to some degree with disease recurrence or progression. Identifying and treating a solitary metastasis may both prolong survival and improve the patient's quality of life. Unfortunately, there is no

Table 58.14. Follow-up of patients with malignant melanoma

Stage	Recommendations
MM in situ	Yearly skin examinations
I, II a	Quarterly skin and lymph node examinations for 5 years; then biannually for 5 years, then yearly. Abdominal and lymph node ultrasonography and chest X-ray yearly. Routine hematology and liver function tests
II b, III	Same as above, but imaging studies biannually for 5 years
IV	Individually adjusted

evidence at this time that it helps a patient to know whether he or she has widespread visceral metastases. Because of the propensity for malignant melanoma to metastasize many years later and because of the 5–10% chance of second tumors, follow-up for malignant melanoma patients should be lifelong.

Prophylaxis

Having a high index of suspicion and removing lesions that are changing or develop in adult life and fulfill the ABCDE criteria have, in a generation, totally changed the average thickness of the removed malignant melanoma. The almost 100% cure rate for malignant melanoma < 0.75 mm in thickness speaks for itself. Removal of some melanocytic nevi can thus be viewed as prophylaxis. Excision of congenital melanocytic nevi, especially larger ones, should almost always be undertaken. Many patients choose to observe smaller congenital melanocytic nevi, but they should be counseled about their risk. Similarly excision or radiation therapy of lentigo maligna makes sense.

Excision of multiple dysplastic nevi is a more controversial issue. Individual patients may have several hundred lesions, all of which cannot be removed. It is appropriate to remove the most striking and largest nevi from such patients. In addition, lesions that show suspicious features on dermatoscopic examination or changes when compared to previous photographs or electronically stored images are candidates for excision.

Another indication for prophylactic excision is the presence of melanocytic nevi that are often traumatized, for example, those on the palms or soles, on the neck, at the belt line, or underneath bra straps. While there is no concrete evidence that such lesions are likely to change into malignant melanoma, it is easier to remove them than to worry and argue.

Metastatic Malignant Melanoma

Epidemiology. Metastatic malignant melanoma has some unique features, in contrast to metastases from other tumors. In 50–60% of patients with metastatic disease, the first site of involvement is the regional lymph nodes, while 30% present with distant metastases, and 10% with local recurrences. About 80% of metastases occur within the first 3 years after removal of the primary tumor. Another 15% occur during the next 2 years, but fully 5% of malignant melanoma metastases occur more than 5 years after removal of the primary tumor, and metastases 10–30 years later have been documented. Lymph node and systemic metastases typically spell the beginning of the end for a patient. As Table 58.11 shows, patients with lymph node involvement have a 19% ten year survival, while those with distant or visceral metastases have only a 3% ten year survival. Another important statistic is that about 5% of patients with a malignant melanoma develop a second primary malignant melanoma in their lifetime; since metastases can be confused with second primaries, which have a much better prognosis, one must always keep this tendency in mind.

Clinical Findings. Several types of metastases are seen; the skin is often involved. Satellite metastases are lesions that spread via the lymphatics and arise within 2 cm of the primary tumor. In-transit metastases involve the skin between the primary tumor and the regional lymph nodes, while distant metastases appear beyond the regional lymph nodes, and visceral metastases involve a variety of internal organs.

The skin metastases from malignant melanoma may be pigmented and clinically mimic melanocytic nevi or blue nevi (Fig. 58.35). Typical for metastases is their presence at many different levels of the skin and subcutaneous tissues. The sudden occurrence of many lesions should raise clinical suspicion, even in the those patients in whom a primary malignant melanoma has not been identified. Another complicating factor is the presence of amelanotic metastases, which then present as flesh-colored or red tumor nodules, not dissimilar

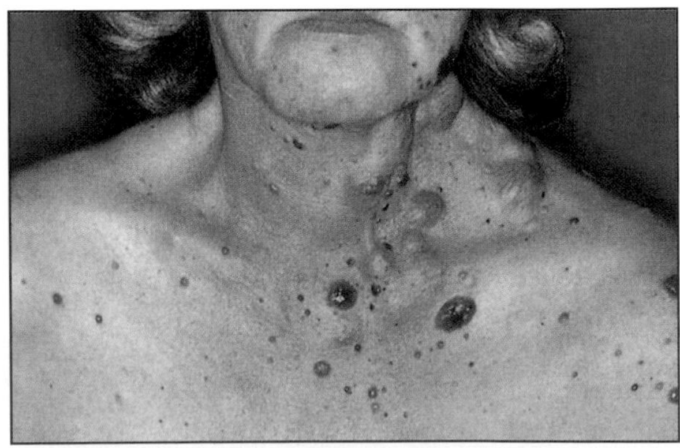

Fig. 58.35. Patient with widespread cutaneous metastases of malignant melanoma

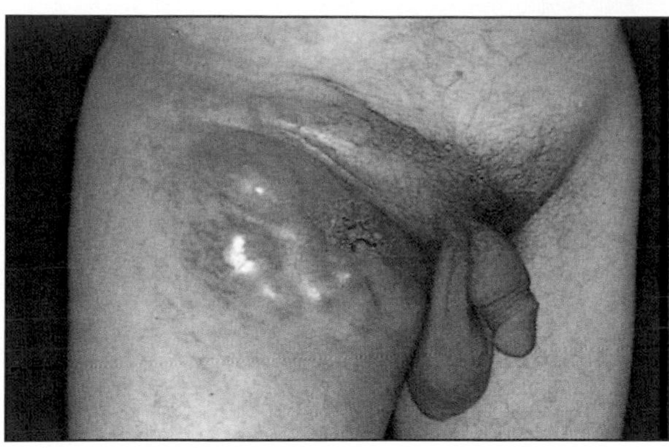

Fig. 58.36. Marked lymphadenopathy caused by metastatic malignant melanoma; the mass is superficially ulcerated. The patient had a malignant melanoma on the leg

from carcinoma metastases. In other instances the metastases may be hypomelanotic; that is, the skin around them may be depigmented. The presence of vitiligo in association with malignant melanoma metastases often suggests regression and a somewhat less dismal prognosis.

Lymph node metastases typically present as localized enlargement of nodes (Fig. 58.36). In more extreme cases, the tumor cells can spread to the overlying skin, producing necrosis and ulcerations. The hematogenous metastases are likely to reach the liver, lungs, CNS, heart, bones, and many other sites. They, too, may often lack melanin (leukometastases).

Some patients with advanced disease may develop a diffuse blue-gray pigmentation, reflecting the presence of melanin in their circulation with perivascular depositions in the dermis. The biopsy findings are subtle, as no melanoma cells are seen, just traces of melanin, both free and in melanophages. The urine may also be dark. At the last stage of the disease, patients with metastases develop cachexia, weight loss, and anemia just as with any other terminal metastatic disease.

In 5–10% of all metastatic malignant melanoma patients, the initial primary tumor remains undiscovered despite a total skin and mucous membrane examination, ophthalmologic examination and excisional biopsy of all potentially regressed lesions. The presumption is that the primary lesion regressed under the influence of an aggressive host response at the same time as vertical parts of the tumor were metastasizing.

In addition, some primary malignant melanomas arise in lymph nodes, while even less often malignant melanoma has been described as a primary tumor in any organ that has melanocytes, including the urogenital tract, gastrointestinal system, and CNS. Involvement of the latter tissues is particularly likely in individuals with large congenital melanocytic nevi involving the dorsal midline region. The same patients may often have hydrocephalus.

Histopathology. The microscopic diagnosis of a metastatic malignant melanoma is usually easy. An epidermotropic metastasis can be confused with a primary malignant melanoma or even an atypical melanocytic nevus, if the dermatopathologist is not warned. The cells in a metastasis are generally quite atypical.

Therapy. There is no satisfactory treatment for metastatic malignant melanoma, but advances in recent years give grounds for cautious optimism. When satellite or in-transit metastases are identified, all are removed along with therapeutic lymph node dissection. When technically possible, the dissection is usually done en bloc. Similarly, when lymph node involvement is present, radical lymph node dissection is recommended. Some groups do fine-needle aspiration of enlarged lymph nodes, while others feel the presence of enlarged lymph nodes is itself sufficient indication for therapeutic lymph node dissection. Patients with stage IIIb disease also benefit from adjuvant therapy with IFN-α, and probably from other adjuvant schemes discussed under prophylaxis. In the case of metastatic disease involving the limbs, hyperthermic perfusion with chemotherapeutic agents may be considered.

Solitary metastases should always be treated. We have seen patients with solitary cerebral, hepatic, and pulmonary metastases do well for a number of years after excision or radiation therapy. Clearly, all such patients should also be entered into a study with systemic chemo- and immunotherapy, as they are likely to have other visceral metastases. In addition, metastatic malignant melanoma is a very unpredictable tumor. Spontaneous remissions are occasionally reported, and often there is an aggressive immune response, primarily T cell in nature.

Radiation therapy is the treatment of choice for skeletal and cerebral metastases. Stereotactic convergence radiation, known as the γ-knife approach, is often recommended for brain lesions, sometimes combined with diffuse irradiation of the brain. Ionizing radiation is also employed sometimes for lymph node and soft-tissue involvement, usually combined with surgery. There is no convincing evidence that combined lymph node dissection and postoperative radiation therapy improved either the local recurrence or survival rate.

The only agent approved in the USA for systemic chemotherapy of metastatic malignant melanoma is dacarbazine or DTIC (dimethyl-triazen-imidazol-carboxamine). It typically produces responses but not cures. In Europe, DTIC, vindesin, and fotemustin are all employed as monochemotherapy with response rates of 15–30%. IL-2 has been approved in the USA for monotherapy for metastatic malignant melanoma. About 15% of the patients responded, and half of this group had a complete remission, lasting up to 6 years.

To improve these numbers, several polychemotherapy and combined immunochemotherapy regimens are under evaluation. Many have shown high response rates, some over 50%, but cures remain elusive, and the toxicity is considerable. We suggest that all our patients with metastatic malignant melanoma be treated within a protocol so that we can continue to gather information on the best approach. The reader should acquaint himself with the polychemotherapy and immunochemotherapy protocols available to his patients. They change too frequently to be listed in a standard textbook.

Active specific immunization is another approach for patients with advanced disease. All these medications are injected into the patient in an attempt to increase the immune reaction against a variety of melanoma antigens. Fragments of melanoma cells are combined with either bacterial proteins, inserted into nonpathogenic viruses such as vaccinia or injected in other ways. The combination of melanoma fragments and bits of *Mycobacterium tuberculosis* known as Melacine is awaiting approval in the USA. The National Cancer Institute has attempted to develop a vaccine that incorporates a particularly antigenic fragment of malignant melanoma and IL-2. At New York University, a polyvalent vaccine incorporating a variety of melanoma surface antigens encapsulated in liposomes also containing IL-2 is being developed. Yet other groups are injecting irradiated malignant melanoma cells. Many other immunotherapy schemes are also under investigation. It is too early to assess which ones, if any, will prove beneficial and be employed in daily practice.

Bibliography

General References

Hölzle E, Kind P, Plewig G et al. (1993) Malignant melanoma. Diagnosis and differential diagnosis. Schattauer, Stuttgart

Maize JC, Ackerman AB (1987) Pigmented lesions of the skin. Lea and Febiger, Philadelphia

Ephelis

Bliss JM, Ford D, Swerdlow AJ et al. (1995) Risk of cutaneous melanoma associated with pigmentation characteristics and freckling: systemic overview of 10 case-control studies. Int J Cancer 62:367

Breathnach AS, Wyllie LM (1964) Electron microscopy of melanocytes and melaosomes in freckled human epidermis. J Invest Dermatol 42:389

Crowe FW (1964) Axillary freckling as a diagnostic aid in neurofibromatosis. Ann Intern Med 61:1142–1143

Hölzle E (1992) Pigmented lesions as a sign of photodamage. Br J Dermatol 127 [Suppl 41]:48–50

Café-au-Lait Macule

Crowe FW, Schull WJ, Neel JV (1956) A clinical, pathological, and genetic study of multiple neurofibromatosis. Springfield, Thomas

Landau M, Krafchik BR (1999) The diagnostic value of cafe-au-lait macules. J Am Acad Dermatol 40:877–890

Nakayama J, Kiryu H, Urabe K et al. (1999) Vitamin D3 analogues improve cafe au lait spots in patients with von Recklinghausen's disease: experimental and clinical studies. Eur J Dermatol 9:202–206

McCune-Albright-Syndrome

Albright F et al. (1937) Syndrome characterized by osteitis fibrosa disseminata, areas of pigmentation and endocrine dysfunction, with precocious puberty in females. Report of five cases. N Engl J Med 216:727–746

McCune D, Bruch H (1937) Osteodystrophia fibrosa. Report of a case in which the condition was combined with precocious puberty, pathologic pigmentation of the skin and hyperthyroidism, review of the literature. Am J Dis Child 54:806–848

Riminucci M, Fisher LW, Shenker A et al. (1997) Fibrous dysplasia of bone in the McCune-Albright syndrome: abnormalities in bone formation. Am J Pathol 151:1587–600

Becker Nevus

Becker SW (1949) Concurrent melanosis and hypertrichosis in distribution of nevus unius lateris. Arch Dermatol 60:155–160

Hanecke E (1979) The dermal component in melanosis naeviformis Becker. J Cutan Pathol 7:404–409

Maessen-Visch MB, Hulsmans RF, Hulsmans FJ (1997) Melanosis naeviformis of Becker and scoliosis: a coincidence? Acta Derm Venereol (Stockh) 77:135–136

Jain HC, Hisher BK (1989) Familial Becker's naevus. Int J Dermatol 28:263–264

Mucosal Melanotic Macule

Cohen LM, Callen JP (1992) Oral and labial melanotic macules in a patient infected with human immunodeficiency virus. J Am Acad Dermatol 26:653–654

Gupta G, Williams RE, Mackie RM (1997) The labial melanoticmacule: a review of 79 cases. Br J Dermatol 136: 772–775

Weathers DR, Corio RL, Crawford BE et al. (1976) The labial melanotic macule. Oral Surg 42:196–205

Solar Lentigo

Braun-Falco O, Schocfinius HH (1971) Lentigo senilis. Übersicht und eigene Untersuchungen. Hautarzt 22:277–283

Hedblad MA, Borglund E (1995) Precursor lesion of malignant melanoma in xeroderma pigmentosum: reflections about solar lentigo as the precursor. J Am Acad Dermatol 32:680–682

Ortonne J-P (1990) Pigmentary changes of the aging skin. Br J Dermatol 122 [Suppl 35]:21–28

Ink Spot Lentigo

Bolognia JL (1992) Reticulated black solar lentigo (ink spot lentigo). Arch Dermatol 128:934–940

PUVA Lentigo

Abel EA, Reid H, Wood C et al. (1985) PUVA-induced melanocytic atypia: is it confined to PUVA lentigines? J Am Acad Dermatol 13:761–768

Rhodes AR, Stern RS, Melski JW (1983) The PUVA lentigo: an analysis of predisposing factors. J Invest Dermatol 81: 459–563

Peutz-Jeghers-Syndrome

Jeghers H, McKusick VA, Katz KH (1949) Generalized intestinal polyposis and melanin spots on the oral mucosa, lips and digits. A syndrome of diagnostic significance. N Engl J Med 241:993–1005

Jenne DE, Reimann H, Nezu J et al. (1998) Peutz-Jeghers syndrome is caused by mutations in novel serine threonine kinase. Nat Genet 18:38–43

Kitagawa S, Townsend BL, Hebert AA (1995) Peutz-Jeghers syndrome. Dermatol Clin 13:127–133

Peutz JL (1921) Over een zeer merkvaardige, gecombinerde familiaire polyposis van de slijmvliezen, van den tractus intestinales met die van de neuskeelholte en gepaard met eigenaardige pigmentaties van huiden slijmvliezen. Ned Mschr Genesk 10:134–146

Westerman AM, Entius MM, de Baar E et al. (1999) Peutz-Jeghers syndrome: 78-year follow-up of the original family. Lancet 353:1211–1215

Carney Syndrome

Atherton DJ, Pitcher DW, Wells RS et al. (1980) A syndrome of various cutaneous pigmented lesions, myxoid neurofibromata and atrial myxoma: the NAME syndrome. Br J Dermatol 103:421–429

Carney JA, Gordon H, Carpenter PC et al. (1985) The complex of myxomas, spotty pigmentation, and endocrine overactivity. Medicine (Baltimore) 64:270–283

Carney JA (1995) The Carney complex (myxomas, spotty pigmentation, endocrine overactivity, and schwannomas). Dermatol Clin 13:19–26

Rhodes AR, Silverman RA, Harrist TJ et al. (1984) Mucocutaneous lentigines, cardiomucocutaneous myxomas, and multiple blue nevi: the "LAMB" syndrome. J Am Acad Dermatol 10:72–82

LEOPARD Syndrome

Coppin BD, Temple IK (1997) Multiple lentigines syndrome (LEOPARD syndrome or progressive cardiomyopathic lentiginosis). J Med Genet 34:582–586

Gorlin RJ, Anderson RC, Blaw M (1969) Multiple lentigines syndrome. Am J Dis Child 117:652–662

Jozwiak S, Schwartz RA, Janniger CK (1996) LEOPARD syndrome (cardiocutaneous lentiginosis syndrome). Cutis 57:208–214

Moynahan EJ (1962) Multiple symmetrical moles with psychic and somatic infantism and genital hypoplasia. First male case of a new syndrome. Proc R Soc Med 55:959–960

Schepis C, Greco D, Siragusa M et al. (1998) An intriguing case of LEOPARD syndrome. Pediatr Dermatol 15: 125–128

Zeisler EP, Becker SW (1936) Generalized lentigo: ist relation to systemic nonelevated nevi. Arch Dermatol 33: 109–125

Lentiginosis and Arterial Dissection Syndrome

Schievink WI, Michels VV, Mokri B et al. (1995) Brief report: a familial syndrome of arterial dissections with lentiginosis. N Engl J Med 332:576–579

Lentigines Syndromes

Cantu JM, Sanchez-Corona J, Fragoso R et al. (1978) A "new" autosomal dominant genodermatosis characterized by hyperpigmented spots and plamoplantar hyerkeratosis. Clin Genet 14:165–168

Korting GW (1967) Lentiginosis profusa perigenito-axillaris. Z Haut Geschlechtskr 42:19–22

O'Neill JF, James WD (1989) Inherited patterned lentiginosis in blacks. Arch Dermatol 125:1231–1235

Stewart DM, Altman J, Mehregan AH (1978) Speckled lentiginous nevus. Arch Dermatol 1978:895–896

Touraine A (1941) Lentiginoses centro-faciale et dysplasies associées. Bull Soc Fr Dermatol Syphil 48:518–522

Uhle P, Norvell SS Jr (1988) Generalized lentiginosis. J Am Acad 18:444–448

Melanocytic Nevi

Marghoob AA, Orlow SJ, Kopf AW (1993) Syndromes associated with melanocytic nevi. J Am Acad Dermatol 29:373–388; quiz 388–390

Skender-Kalnenas TM, English DR, Heenan PJ (1995) Benign melanocytic lesions: risk markers or precursors of cutaneous melanoma? J Am Acad Dermatol 33:1000–1007

Mongolian Spot

Bashiti HM, Blair JD, Triska RA et al. (1981) Generalized dermal melanocytosis. Arch Dermatol 117:791–793

Carmichael AJ, Tan CY, Abraham SM (1993) Adult onset of Mongolian spot. Clin Exp Dermatol 18:72–74

Park KD, Choi GS, Lee KH (1995) Extensive aberrant Mongolian spot. J Dermatol 22:330–233

Nevus of Ota and Ito

Hidano A, Kajima H, Endo Y (1965) Bilateral nevus Ota associated with nevus Ito. A case of pigmentation on the lips. Arch Dermatol 36:133–154

Ito M (1954) Studies on melanin. XXII. Nevus fuscocaeruleus acromiodeltoideus.. Tohoku J Exp Med 60:10

Mishima Y, Mevorah B (1961) Nevus Ota and nevus Ito in American negroes. J Invest Dermatol 36:133–154

Ota M (1939) Nevus fusco-coeruleus ophtalmomaxillaris. Tokyo Med J 63:1243–1245

Ueda S, Isoda M, Imayama S (2000) Response of naevus of Ota to Q-switched ruby laser treatment according to lesion colour. Br J Dermatol 142:77–83

Blue Nevus

Blackford S, Roberts DL (1991) Familial multiple blue naevi. Clin Exp Dermatol 16:308–309

Connelly J, Smith JL Jr (1991) Malignant blue nevus. Cancer 67:2653–2657

Jadassohn J (1938) Dermatologie. Vienna, p 429

Kamino H, Tam ST (1990) Compound blue nevus: a variant of blue nevus with an additional junctional dendritic component. Arch Dermatol 126:1330–1333

Knoell KA, Nelson KC, Patterson JW (1998) Familial multiple blue nevi. J Am Acad Dermatol 39:322–325

Kuhn A, Groth W, Gartmann H et al. (1988) Malignant blue nevus with metastases to the lung. Am J Dermatopathol 10:436–441

O'Grady C, Barr RJ, Billman G et al. (1999) Epithelioid blue nevus occurring in children with no evidence of Carney complex. Am J Dermatopathol 21(5):483–486

Rodriguez HA, Ackerman LV (1968) Cellular blue nevus. Clinicopathologic study of forty-five cases. Cancer 21: 393–405

Tièche M (1906) Über Melanome ("Chromatophorome") der Haut. "Blaue Naevi". Virchows Arch 186:212–228

Common Melanocytic Nevus

Ackerman AB, Magana-Garcia M (1990) Naming acquired melanocytic nevi. Unna's, Miescher's, Spitz's, Clark's. Am J Dermatopathol 12:193–209

Ackerman AB, Milde P (1992) Naming aquired melanocytic nevi. Common and dysplastic, normal or atypical, or Unna, Miescher, Spitz and Clark? Am J Dermatopathol 14:447–453

Boyd AS, Rapini RP (1994) Acral melanocytic neoplasms: a histologic analysis of 158 lesions. J Am Acad Dermatol 31:740–745

Clark WH Jr, Reimer RR, Greene M et al. (1978) Origin of familial malignant melanomas from heritable melanocytic lesions. "The B-K mole syndrome". Arch Dermatol 114:732–738

Fallowfield ME, Collina G, Cook MG (1994) Melanocytic lesions of the palm and sole. Histopathology 24:463–467

Haupt HM, Stern JB (1995) Pagetoid melanocytosis. Histologic features in benign and malignant lesions. Am J Surg Pathol 19:792–797

Kerl H, Soyer HP, Cerroni L et al. (1998) Ancient melanocytic nevus. Semin Diagn Pathol 15:210–215

Löffler H, Effendy I (1998) Korymbiformer Nävuszellnävus. Hautarzt 49:730–732

Magana-Garcia M, Ackermann AB (1990) What are nevus cells? Am J Dermatopathol 12:93–102

Masson P (1965) My concept of cellular nevi. Cancer 4:9–38

Miescher G, von Albertini A (1935) Histologie de 100 as de naevi pigmentaires d'après les methodes de Masson. Bull Soc Fr Dermatol Syphil 42:1265–1273

Mishima Y (1965) Macromolecular changes in pigmentary disorders. Arch Dermatol 91:519–557

Unna PG (1893) Naevi und Naevocarcinome. Berl Klin Wochenschr 30:14–16

Unna PG (1896) Histopathology of diseases of the skin. Mac Millan, New York, pp 1129–1144

Spitz Nevus

Allen AC (1963) Juvenile melanomas. Ann NY Acad Sci 100: 29–48

Aloi F, Tomasini C, Pippione M (1995) Agminated Spitz nevi occuring within a congenital speckled lentiginous nevus. Am J Dermatopathol 17:594–598

Barnhill RL, Argenyi ZB, From L et al. (1999) Atypical Spitz nevi/tumors: lack of consensus for diagnosis, discrimination from melanoma, and prediction of outcome. Hum Pathol 30:513–520

Barnhill RL, Barnhill MA, Berwick M et al. (1991) The histologic spectrum of pigmented spindle cell nevus. Hum Pathol 22:52–58

Cramer SF (1998) The melanocyte differentiation pathway in spitz nevi. Am J Dermatopathol 20:555–570

Dawe RS, Wainwright NJ, Evans AT et al. (1998) Multiple widespread eruptive Spitz naevi. Br J Dermatol 138:872–874

Fabrizi G, Massi G (2000) Polypoid Spitz naevus: the benign counterpart of polypoid malignant melanoma. Br J Dermatol 142:128–132

Kamino H, Misheloff E, Ackerman AB (1979) Eosinophilic globules in Spitz's nevi. New findings and a diagnostic sign. Am J Dermatopathol 1:319–324

Piepkorn M (1995) On the nature of histologic observations: a case of the Spitz nevus. J Am Acad Dermatol 32:248–254

Reed RJ, Ichinose H, Clark WH et al. (1975) Common and uncommon melanocytic nevi and borderline melanomas. Semin Oncol 2:119–147

Reed RJ (1985) The histological variance of malignant melanoma: the interrelationsship of histological subtype, neoplastic progression, and biological behaviour. Pathology 17:301–312

Sabroe RA, Vaingankar NV, Rigby HS et al. (1996) Agminate Spitz naevi occurring in an adult after the excision of a solitary Spitz naevus-report of a case and review of the literature. Clin Exp Dermatol 21:197–200

Sau P, Graham JH, Helwig EB (1993) Pigmented spindle cell nevus: a clinicopathologic analysis of ninety-five cases. J Am Acad Dermatol 28:565–571

Spitz S (1948) Melanomas of childhood. Am J Pathol 24: 591–609

Wistuba I, Gonzalez S (1990) Eosinophilic globules in pigmented spindle cell nevus. Am J Dermatopathol 12: 268–271

Halo Nevus

Akasu R, From L, Kahn HJ (1994) Characterization of the mononuclear infiltrate involved in regression of halo nevi. J Cutan Pathol 21:302–311

Sutton RL (1916) An unusual variety of vitiligo (leukoderma acquisitum centrifugum). J Cutan Dis 34:797–801

Zeff RA, Freitag A, Grin CM et al. (1997) The immune response in halo nevi. J Am Acad Dermatol 37:620–624

Meyerson Nevus

Meyerson LB (1971) A peculiar papulosquamous eruption involving pigmented nevi. Arch Dermaol 103:510–512

Nicholls DSH, Mason GH (1988) Halo dermatitis around a melanocytic naevus: Meyerson's naevus. Br J Dermatol 118:125–129

Cockarde Nevus

Happle R (1974) Kokardennävus. Eine ungewöhnliche Variante des Nävuszellnävus. Hautarzt 25:594–596

Guzzo C, Johnson B, Honig P (1988) Cockarde nevus: a case report and review of the literature. Pediatr Dermatol 5:250–253

Nanta Nevus

Culver W, Burgdorf WHC (1993) Malignant melanoma arising in a nevus of Nanta. J Cutan Pathol 20:375–377

Moulin G, Souquet D, Blame B (1991) Naevus pigmentarires et ossifications cutanées. A propas de 125 cas d'osteno-naevus. Ann Dermatol Venereol 118:199

Nanta M (1911) Sur l'osteo – naevus. Ann Dermatol Syphil 2:562

Recurrent Nevus

Duve S, Schmoeckel C, Burgdorf WHC (1996) Melanocytic hyperplasia in scars. A histopathologic investigation of 722 cases. Am J Dermatopathol 18:236–240

Estrada JA, Pierard-Franchimont C, Pierard GE (1990) Histogenesis of recurrent nevus. Am J Dermatopathol 12:370–372

Nevus Spilus

Borrego L, Hernandez Santana J, Baez O et al. (1994) Naevus spilus as a precursor of cutaneous melanoma: report of a case and literature review. Clin Exp Dermatol 19:515–517

Dysplastic Nevus

Clark WH Jr, Reimer RR, Greene M et al. (1978) Origin of familial melanomas from heritable melanocytic lesions. "The B-K mole syndrome." Arch Dermatol 114:732–738

Clark WH Jr, Elder DE, Guerry D IV et al. (1984) A study of tumor progression: the precursor lesions of superficial spreading and nodular melanoma. Hum Pathol 15:1147–1165

Lynch HT, Frichot BC, Lynch JF (1978) Familial atypical multiple mole-melanoma syndrome. J Med Genet 15: 352–356

Murphy GF, Mihm MC (1999) Recognition and evaluation of cytological dysplasia in acquired melanocytic nevi. Hum Pathol 30:506–512

National Institutes of Health (1984) Precursors to malignant melanoma. NIH Consensus Development Conference Statement. J Am Acad Dermatol 10:683–688

Sagebiel RW, Banda PW, Schneider JS et al. (1985) Age distribution and histologic patterns of dysplastic nevi. J Am Acad Dermatol 13:975–982

Congenital Melanocytic Nevus

DeDavid M, Orlow SJ, Provost N et al. (1996) Neurocutaneous melanosis: clinical features of large congenital melanocytic nevi in patients with manifest central nervous system melanosis. J Am Acad Dermatol 35:529–538

DeDavid M, Orlow SJ, Provost N et al. (1997) A study of large congenital melanocytic nevi and associated malignant melanomas: review of cases in the New York University Registry and the world literature. J Am Acad Dermatol 36:409–416

Touraine A (1949) Les mélanoses neuro-cutaneées. Ann Dermatol Syphil 9:489–524

Malignant Melanoma

Ackerman AB, Cerroni L, Kerl H (1994) Pitfalls in histopathologic diagnosis of malignant melanoma. Lea & Febiger, Philadelphia

Balch CM, Sober AJ, Houghton AN et al. (1997) Cutaneous melanoma. Quality Medical, St. Louis

Brady MS, Coit DG (1997) Sentinel lymph node evaluation in melanoma. Arch Dermatol 133:1014–1020

Breslow A (1970) Thickness, cross-sectional areas and depth of invasion in the prognosis of cutaneous melanoma. Ann Surg 172:902–908

Breslow A (1979) Prognostic factors in the treatment of cutaneous melanoma. J Cutan Pathol 6:208–212

Brown TJ, Nelson BR (1999) Malignant melanoma: a clinical review. Cutis 63:275–284

Cerroni L, Kerl H (1998) Simulators of malignant melanoma of the skin. Eur J Dermatol 8:388–396

Clark WH Jr, From L, Bernardino EA et al. (1969) The histogenesis and biologic behavior of primary human malignant melanomas of the skin. Cancer Res 29:705–827

Dicker TJ, Kavanagh GM, Herd RM et al. (1999) A rational approach to melanoma follow-up in patients with primary cutaneous melanoma. Br J Dermatol 140:249–254

Dubreuihl MW (1912) De la melanose circonscrite precancereuse. Ann Dermatol Syphil 3:129–151

Garbe C, Schaumburg-Lever G (1997) Klinik und Histologie des malignen Melanoms. In: Garbe C et al. (eds) Dermatologische Onkologie. Springer, Berlin

Gilchrest A, Eller MS, Geller C et al. (1999) The pathogenesis of melanoma induced by ultraviolet radiation. N Eng J Med 340:1341–1348

Grant-Kels JM, Bason ET, Grin CM (1999) The misdiagnosis of malignant melanoma. J Am Acad Dermatol 40:539–548

Hermanek P, Scheibe O, Spiessl B et al. (eds) (1987) TNM Klassifikation maligner Tumoren, 4th edn. Springer, Berlin

Hutchinson J (1890) On senile moles and senile freckles and their relationship to cancerous processes. Arch Surg 2:218

Johnson TM, Yahanda AM, Chang AE et al. (1998) Advances in melanoma therapy. J Am Acad Dermatol 38:731–741

Kaufmann R, Tilgen W, Garbe C (1998) Malignes Melanom. Der Hautarzt 49:330–338 (Supplement)

Kirkwood JM (1998) Systemic adjuvant treatment of high-risk melanoma: the role of interferon alfa-2b and other immunotherapies. Eur J Cancer 34 [Suppl 3]: S12–17

Manci E, Balch CM, Murad TM (1981) Polypoid melanoma, a virulent variant of the nodular growth pattern. Am J Clin Pathol 75:810–815

Metcalf JS (1996) Melanoma: criteria for histological diagnosis and its reporting. Semin Oncol 23:688–692

Morton DL, Wen DR, Cochran AJ et al. (1992) Management of early stage melanoma by intraoperative lymphatic mapping and selective lymphadenectomy. Surg Oncol Clin North Am 1:247–259

National Institutes of Health (1992) Diagnosis and treatment of early melanoma. NIH Consensus Development Panel on Early Melanoma. JAMA 268:1314–1319

Orfanos CE, Garbe C (eds) (1998) Das maligne Melanom der Haut. W Zuckschwerdt, Munich

Patel BC, Egan CA, Lucius RW et al. (1998) Cutaneous malignant melanoma and oculodermal melanocytosis (nevus of Ota): report of a case and review of the literature. J Am Acad Dermatol 38:862–865

Piepkorn M, Weinstock MA, Barnhill RL (1997) Theoretical and empirical arguments in relation to elective lymph node dissection for melanoma. Arch Dermatol 133:995–1002

Schmöckel C, Braun-Falco O (1978) Prognostic index in malignant melanoma. Arch Dermatol 114:871–873

Volkenandt M, Plewig G (eds) (1999) Maligne Melanome. W Zuckschwerdt, Munich

Lentigo Maligna and Lentigo Maligna Melanoma

Cohen LM (1995) Lentigo maligna and lentigo maligna melanoma. J Am Acad Dermatol 33:923–936

Cohen LM (1997) Lentigo maligna and lentigo maligna melanoma. J Am Acad Dermatol 36:913

Kaufmann R, Nikelski K, Weber L et al. (1995) Amelanotic lentigo maligna melanoma. J Am Dermatol 32:339–342

Kelli RI, Cook MG, Mortimer PS (1994) Aggressive amelanotic lentigo maligna. Br J Dermatol 131:562–565

Weinstock MA, Sober AJ (1987) The risk of progression of lentigo maligna to lentigo maligna melanoma. Br J Dermatol 116:303–310

Acral Lentiginous Melanoma

Blessing K, Kernohan NM, Park KGM (1991) Subungual malignant melanoma: clinicopathologic features of 100 cases: Histopathology 19:425–429

Dwyer PK, MacKie RM, Watt DC et al. (1993) Plantar malignant melanoma in a white Caucasian population. Br J Dermatol 128:115–120

Saida T (1989) Malignant melanoma in situ on the sole of the foot. Ist clinical and histopathologic characteristics. Am J Dermatopathol 11:124–130

Other Malignant Melanomas

Farber M, Schutzer P, Mihm C Jr (1998) Pigmented lesions of the conjunctiva. J Am Acad Dermatol 38:971–978

Norris HJ, Taylor HB (1966) Melanomas of the vagina. Am J Clin Pathol 46:420

Rapini RP, Golitz LE, Greer RO (1985) Primary malignant melanoma of the oral cavity: a review of 177 cases. Cancer 55:1543

Desmoplastic and Neurotropic Malignant Melanoma

Anstey A, McKee P, Wilson Jones E (1993) Desmoplastic malignant melanoma: a clinicopathological study of 25 cases. Br J Dermatol 129:359–371

Baer SC, Schultz D, Synnestvedt M et al. (1995) Desmoplasia and neurotropism. Prognostic variables in patients with stage 1 melanoma. Cancer 76:2242–2247

Barnhill RL, Bolognia JL (1995) Neurotropic melanoma with prominent melanization. J Cutan Pathol 22:450–459

Malignant Melanoma in Children

Ceballos PI, Ruiz-Maldonado R, Mihm MC Jr (1995) Melanoma in children. N Engl J Med 332:656–662

Chun K, Vazquez M, Sanchez JL (1993) Malignant melanoma in children. Int J Dermatol 32:41–43

Mesenchymal and Neural Tumors

Contents

In this chapter, tumors of connective tissue, lymphatics, vessels, smooth muscle, cartilage, bone, fat, and nerves will be considered. This is a broad spectrum and the subject will, for the most part, not be reviewed in detail. We shall pay the most attention to common lesions that can be identified clinically. Those that are primarily of interest to dermatopathologists will receive less coverage. Many lesions included here are best defined as reactive processes, not tumors, but we have grouped them all together because there is so much overlap. The majority of the cutaneous lesions are benign; only a few sarcomas present in the skin.

Benign Fibrous Tumors

This is one of the most difficult groups of disorders to put into logical categories. Many problems are obvious. One is the relationship between fibroblasts and myofibroblasts. Many fibrous proliferations contain populations of both cells. A myofibroblast is a fibroblast that also contains smooth muscle elements. While one might intuitively expect such a cell to dominate in remodeling processes such as scar formation, where contractility might be an advantage, this is not always the case. Furthermore, a fibroblast or myofibroblast may manufacture collagen or elastin as part of a reactive process or as part of tumor growth. It is almost impossible to sort out the two possibilities under the microscope.

There is another group of cells in the dermis that appears to be involved in some fibrous proliferations. These are the dermal dendrocytes or antigen-processing cells. One subset is Factor XIIIa-positive and usually found in close proximity to vessels and mast cells. Another type is CD34-positive, much more common, and associated with vessels, adnexal structures, and found throughout the reticular dermis. Dermatofibromas often contain Factor XIIIa-positive cells, while CD34-positive spindle cells are very typical of dermatofibrosarcoma protuberans.

Some fibrous proliferations have been traditionally considered along with the connective tissue disorders in Europe. Included in this group are knuckle pads, Dupuytren contracture, Ledderhose disease, and Peyronie disease; all are covered in Chapter 18. Periadnexal fibrous proliferations are considered along with the adnexal neoplasms in Chapter 57.

Keloid

(Alibert 1816)

Definition. An exuberant scar that extends beyond the original boundaries of the injury.

Epidemiology. Keloids are far more common among blacks, and there is a familial tendency towards keloid formation. In some black groups in Africa, keloid formation is an integral part of ritual scarification. Children and young adults are more susceptible than older individuals, and women are at greater risk than men.

Etiology and Pathogenesis. The etiology is unknown. The risk factors mentioned above play a role, as well as the site on the body and the type of scar. For example, burn scars are at greater risk, as are acne scars and immunizations. Bacterial secondary infections appear to increase the risk. The sites of predilection include the presternal area, ear lobes, shoulder girdle, ankle, and face. Skin tension is also a factor, perhaps explaining the frequent occurrence over the sternum and about the ankle. Even clean, smooth operation scars under little or no tension and without infection can evolve into keloids. The same trauma may produce a keloid at one site and none at another.

Clinical Findings. A keloid develops weeks to months after an injury or operation. Thick firm nodules and plaques extend beyond the boundaries of the original wound. The growths can be several centimeters thick, extremely hard, and have a

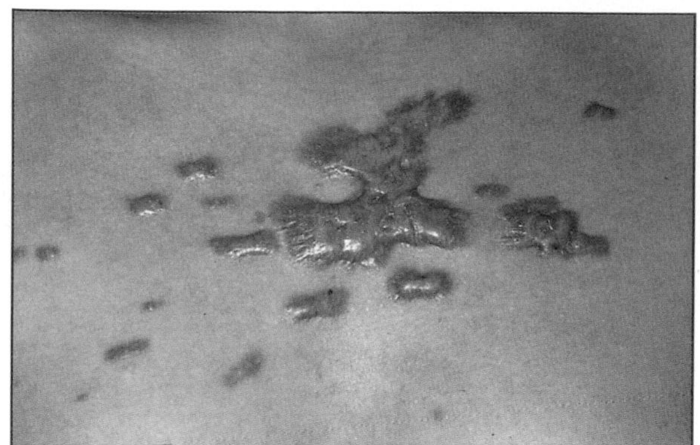

Fig. 59.1. Keloids

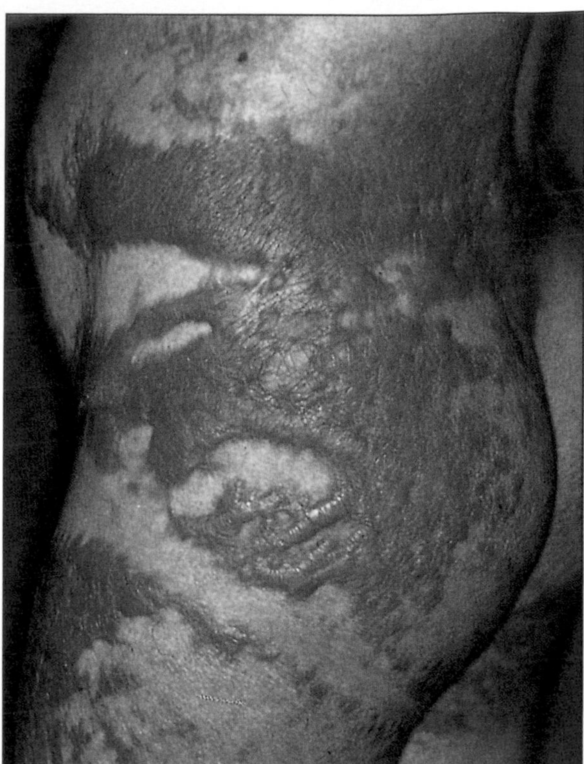

Fig. 59.2. Keloids in burn scar

smooth, mirror-like surface without appendages. The name keloid refers to the pincers of a crab and is appropriate because often claw-like extensions appear at the edge of a keloid (Figs. 59.1, 59.2). Fresh keloids are red-brown; later they pale and eventually become almost white, speckled by telangiectases.

When a keloid reaches a certain size, growth usually stops. Some regression may occur, leaving a softer but not more attractive lesion. In rare cases, the keloid may relentlessly progress. They are usually not painful but can itch. Larger ones may restrict the motion of a limb or the neck.

The keloids over the sternum associated with acne and folliculitis were formerly called spontaneous keloids. While the scarring is far out of proportion to the trauma, today such keloids are accepted as secondary to the minor trauma of follicular inflammation. Probably the most common keloids seen today are those associated with ear piercing, and occasionally with other types of piercing. They are unpredictable, not limited to blacks, and should serve as a warning to the patient to avoid further use of earrings designed for pierced ears.

Histopathology. A biopsy is rarely needed. The epidermis is normal or atrophic. Younger keloids may be hypercellular with numerous fibroblasts, ground substance, vessels, and even inflammatory cells. Developed lesions are relatively acellular with large, irregular bundles of homogenous collagen running in various directions. This is in contrast to the parallel bundles in hypertrophic scars. Atrophic trapped appendages may be present and elastic fibers are sparse.

Course and Prognosis. The lesions are chronic, hard to treat, and tend to recur. They also serve as a warning sign for those attempting future surgical procedures on the same patient.

Differential Diagnosis. The main differential diagnostic consideration is a hypertrophic scar, but here the distinction is a matter of degree. Occasionally, a dermatofibroma may be similar to a keloid. The very rare X-linked Goeminne (1968) syndrome features facial asymmetry, congenital torticollis, and numerous keloids, which are described as spontaneous and apparently associated with overlooked trauma.

Therapy. One should treat a keloid with healthy respect and use conservative measures. The confident surgeon who blames the keloid on the techniques used by his predecessor often produces a bigger keloid when he attempts reexcision. The long list of possible treatments underlines the fact that there is no one excellent approach.

Topical. Keloids are difficult to treat externally. High-potency corticosteroid creams under occlusion may help with very early lesions. Tretinoin may also be helpful; in vitro it inhibits fibroblast growth, and some studies have shown benefits from long-term application. Intralesional injection of interferon (IFN)-γ has been helpful in some studies, but is very expensive. In Europe, ointments containing heparin, ichthyol, and plant extracts in various combinations are available but probably ineffective. Since mechanical pressure helps reduce keloid growth, anything that is regularly massaged into the lesion is likely to have some positive effect.

Systemic. No good systemic approach has been identified. In high-risk patients, one can try isotretinoin for several months.

Surgical. Surgical excision is usually doomed to failure. When a lesion is small, tangential excision can be combined with intralesional corticosteroids and pressure. Laser destruction offers another method of superficial removal with perhaps less tendency to recurrence; both flashlight pumped dye lasers and neodymium:YAG lasers are effective.

Other Measures. Intralesional corticosteroids soften the keloid, reduce itching, and arrest growth, but do not produce true resolution. One should use triamcinolone acetonide in concentrations of 10–20 mg/ml. We usually dilute the standard 40 mg/ml preparation with a local anesthetic and inject every 3–4 weeks, as the aim is to induce the atrophy that is otherwise considered a side-effect. The first time one injects a keloid, it is very difficult to push the needle in but on subsequent attempts, it enters more easily. One can freeze the lesion first, let it thaw, and then inject to speed the process. Another alternative is the use of a pressure jet injector, such as a Derma-Jet.

A firm pressure dressing is very effective and should be considered. One can either make a dressing with a piece of foam rubber 1–2-cm thick, cut to the size of the lesion and compressed with an elastic bandage, or work with a medical device expert to produce a sleeve or cuff of rubber or another elastic material. When treating earlobe keloids, old-fashioned earrings with a screw-clamp fastening can be used to apply pressure to the back of the ear.

Silicone sheeting has also been claimed to be effective in several studies. Products such as Topigel, Sil-K, or Epiderm are cut to size and held in place without pressure; they are left on for 12–24 h daily for long periods. We have not been impressed and follow-up studies have not documented convincing results.

Radiation Therapy. Keloids are one of the benign conditions in which properly applied soft X-rays are still useful. Radiation is usually combined with a tangential excision of the keloid; intralesional corticosteroids can also be used simultaneously. A useful therapy plan is: half-value depth 1–15 mm, 20–50 kV or more, filter 0.4–2.0 mm Al, single dose 1–2 Gy, total dose 4–12 Gy, interval one week. We no longer employ this modality for keloids. UVA1 phototherapy may offer an acceptable alternative, but studies are still in the preliminary stage.

Prophylaxis. Every surgeon tries to avoid producing keloids. Meticulous operative technique that avoids skin tension and infection is helpful but offers no guarantee. In patients at risk, such as young black girls, one should only do surgery that is absolutely necessary. It is often better to leave a harmless lesion on the breast of a young lady. Tangential excisions are preferable to electrosurgical removal. In addition, aggressive treatment of acne may reduce the risk of keloid formation. In burn patients, the postoperative use of pressure suits has proven to be most effective when trying to avoid large, disabling keloids.

Acrochordon

Synonyms. Fibroma molle, skin tag, soft fibroma, fibroepithelial polyp

Definition. Harmless pedunculated or stalked outpouching of skin.

Etiology and Pathogenesis. One can distinguish between multiple acrochordons which may reflect obesity and endocrine disease and solitary larger lesions which may occasionally represent dermal melanocytic nevi in regression. Some studies showed a connection between multiple acrochordons and gastrointestinal polyps, but they were not epidemiologically sound.

Clinical Findings. A solitary lesion is usually skin-colored, has a folded surface, often a stalk, and ranges in size from several millimeters to in rare instances many centimeters (Fig. 59.3). Multiple lesions are usually much smaller, many only a few millimeters in size, found on the neck, axillae, groin, and submammary regions in predominantly overweight individuals. Occasional larger tags may be admixed with the small lesions. They have similarities to acanthosis nigricans, but only when they

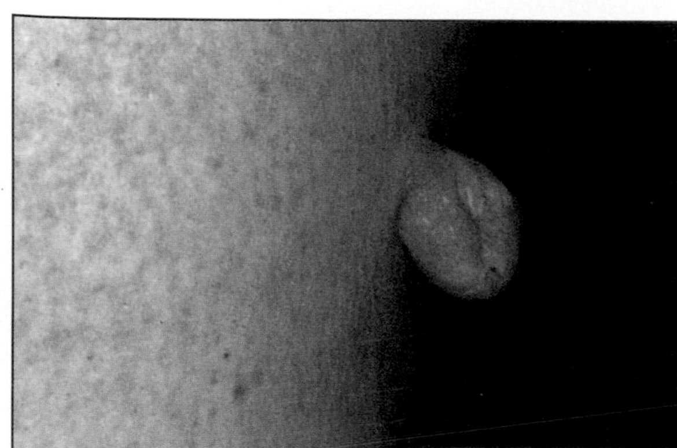

Fig. 59.3. Acrochordon

appear suddenly should one consider an underlying disorder.

Histopathology. The epidermis typically has a papillomatous acanthotic pattern, while the dermis is normal. One may find increased dermal fat or vessels in some instances. Elastic fibers are often reduced, suggesting that some lesions at least represent regression.

Differential Diagnosis. The only differential diagnostic point is a flesh-colored dermal nevus. Histology provides the answer.

Therapy. Tangential excision or scissors excision is the easiest. Other forms of destruction can also be employed but increase the risk of scarring.

Sclerotic Fibroma

(Rapini and Golitz 1989)

Sclerotic fibroma is one of the hallmarks of Cowden syndrome (Chap. 65). In addition, sporadic lesions may occur. They are typically flesh-colored papules or nodules. Histologically, the dermis is hypocellular with hyalinized bundles of collagen and prominent clefting, producing an unique image that has been compared to a sliced onion. Increased synthesis of type I collagen has been demonstrated in some lesions. Excision is curative.

Pleomorphic Fibroma

(Kamino et al. 1989)

This lesion is only diagnosed histologically. Clinically, it is a dome-shaped or polypoid nodule usually confused with a skin tag. Microscopically, the spindle-shaped dermal cells show striking pleomorphism. They express vimentin and actin, suggesting that they are fibroblasts or myofibroblasts. Excision is curative.

Dermatofibroma

Synonyms. Fibroma durum, histiocytoma, hard fibroma, nodular subepidermal fibrosis, dermatofibroma lenticulare, sclerosing hemangioma

Definition. Firm pigmented nodule usually on the legs.

Epidemiology. Dermatofibromas are extremely common. Many adults have at least one; they are more common in women and usually appear in young adult life.

Etiology and Pathogenesis. The etiology is unknown, but the two usual trigger factors are an arthropod bite and folliculitis. Experts disagree about whether dermatofibroma is a reactive process or a tumor. The many different names reflect the different theories about the cell of origin – fibroblasts, histiocytes, or even vascular elements. Most current research suggests that factor XIIIa-positive dermal dendrocytes are key cells, but their normal function remains poorly understood.

Clinical Findings. A dermatofibroma is firm, usually rises slightly above the skin surface and has a variety of colors ranging from red to brown to black (Fig. 59.4). The size is usually less than 1 cm. While the leg is the most common site, lesions may

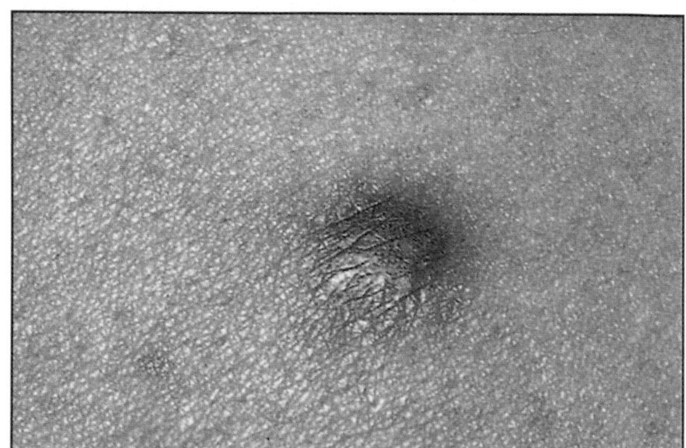

Fig. 59.4. Dermatofibroma

occur anywhere. The skin markings are usually retained. Dermatofibromas are painless, feel much like a button, and are freely moveable. When the adjacent skin is compressed, the dermatofibroma dimples or retracts, while normal skin or a melanocytic nevus bulges. This dimple sign is also known as Fitzpatrick sign. Most lesions are asymptomatic; some may itch.

There are several clinical variants of dermatofibroma that deserve attention. Multiple lesions especially in blacks have been associated with systemic lupus erythematosus. On the shoulder girdle, dermatofibromas may be depressed and telangiectatic, mimicking a basal cell carcinoma. Sometimes lesions will become very large. Others may be bright red, suggesting a prominent vascular component.

Histopathology. A number of histologic patterns can be seen in dermatofibroma. Most have no correlation to the clinical appearance. The epidermis is usually acanthotic and may show basaloid buds or sebaceous lobules that represent rudimentary hair germs. In rare instances, a true aggressive basal cell carcinoma may develop over a dermatofibroma. In the dermis, there may be a fibrous infiltrate, a cellular infiltrate, a lacy vascular pattern, or a mixture of all of the above. There is usually entrapment of normal collagen at the periphery. Sectioning through the tumor, one often finds multiple patterns, providing the most convincing argument that all these histologic variants represent the same lesion.

Differential Diagnosis. The differential diagnosis is lengthy. Nondermatologists and patients often confuse dermatofibromas with melanocytic nevi. The red-brown earlier lesions resemble Spitz nevus, mastocytoma, or juvenile xanthogranuloma. Leiomyomas may also appear similar, but are typically multiple and arranged in a follicular pattern. An atrophic dermatofibroma may suggest a basal cell carcinoma or scar.

Therapy. The best therapy is none. Dermatofibromas tend to occur in areas of skin tension, and frequently the scar is worse than the lesion. If the patient insists, surgery is acceptable. Cryotherapy or intralesional corticosteroids may soften the lesions, but rarely produce cosmetic improvement.

Calcifying Aponeurotic Fibroma

(Keasbey 1953)

Synonym. Juvenile aponeurotic fibroma

This painful mass is somewhat similar to Dupuytren contracture, usually involving the palms of teenagers or young adults. It may involve other aponeuroses. Histologically, it is quite distinct, with foci of calcification, nodules of cartilage, and sheets of fibroblasts. While spontaneous resolution can occur, excision is usually preferred.

Nuchal Fibroma

(Enzinger and Weiss 1988; Lister et al. 1988)

Synonym. Collagenosis nuchae

Despite the name, this process is probably reactive. A deep, poorly defined dermal plaque or nodule is typically found on the nape or on the upper back between the scapulae. The clinical differential diagnosis includes spindle cell lipoma and elastofibroma, as well as scar tissue. When nerve entrapment occurs, the lesions can be painful. Microscopically, there are strands of collagen infiltrating the fat septae and replacing fat. The collagen may merge with the ligamentum nuchae. Excision is curative.

Acquired Digital Fibrokeratoma

(Bart et al. 1968)

Clinical Findings. Acquired digital fibrokeratoma are usually found on the lateral or medial aspect of the fingers over an interphalangeal joint, but occasionally along the nailfold (Fig. 59.5). The toes can

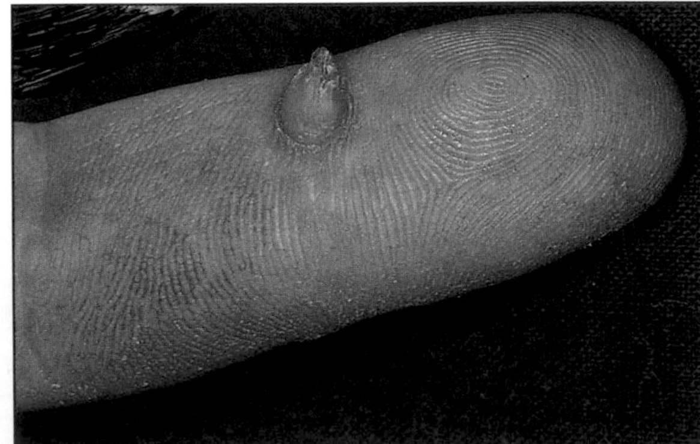

Fig. 59.5. Acquired digital fibrokeratoma

also be involved, and occasionally one sees a similar lesion elsewhere on the body. Clinically, they have normal skin surface markings (in contrast to warts), are usually less than 1 cm in size, and have a collarette scale.

Histopathology. Microscopic examination reveals an acanthotic, hyperkeratotic epidermis, often a peripheral invagination reflecting the collarette, and dermal fibrous proliferation with collagen bundles often vertically oriented and admixed with small vessels. Multiple familial acral mucinous fibrokeratomas have also been described; here the lesions have epithelial strands admixed with mucin and small vessels. Such lesions could also be considered angiomyxomas.

Differential Diagnosis. The differential diagnosis includes a rudimentary digit (which should have a different history and show nerves or bone under the microscope), an old wart, and perhaps a digital mucous cyst, based solely on location.

Therapy. Surgery is curative.

Fibroma of Tendon Sheath

(Geschickter and Copland 1949; Chung and Enzinger 1979)

Clinical Findings. This is a slowly growing, benign, often painful tumor which occurs on the hands of middle-aged men. The lesions are solitary, attached to a tendon sheath, and can be 1–2 cm in diameter.

Histopathology. The well-circumscribed nodules are subcutaneous but may impinge upon the dermis. They consist of a dense fibrous stroma with vascular slits, occasional cellular areas, and myxoid changes. The proliferative cell is a myofibroblast. In the pleomorphic variant, the myofibroblasts have more nuclear variability.

Therapy. Excision is the only option, if the lesions are painful. Recurrences are common.

Giant Cell Tumor of Tendon Sheath

(Chassiagnac 1852)

Clinical Findings. Giant cell tumor of tendon sheath is somewhat more common than fibroma of tendon sheath. The fingers are the most common site, especially the dorsal surface over the intraphalangeal joints (Fig. 59.6). Multiple lesions are not uncommon. Most patients are young adults, and women are more often affected than men. These tumors can also become quite large, as they are often several centimeters in size. They are usually painless.

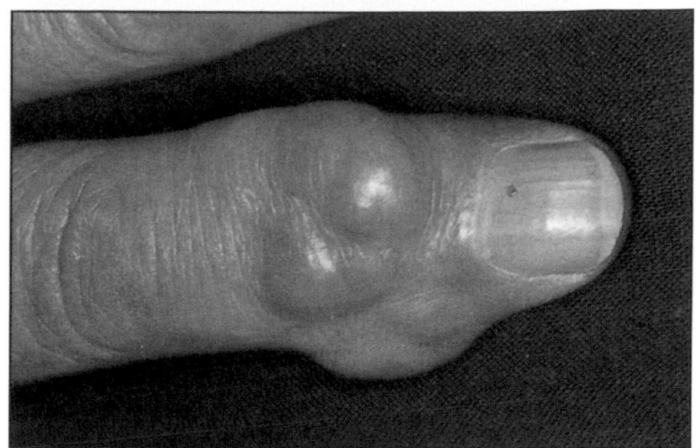

Fig. 59.6. Giant cell tumors of tendon sheath

Histopathology. The tumor is encapsulated and attached to a tendon sheath. There is an eosinophilic collagenous stroma with numerous multinucleate giant cells. Hemosiderin is usually present, as well as lipid-laden cells. The cell of origin is most likely synovium.

Therapy. If troublesome, the lesions can be excised. Recurrences are common.

Angiofibromas

A series of clinically different lesions that all have similar dermal changes and can best be considered together. All are felt to be derived from the papillary or periadnexal dermis, tend to be rich in factor XIIIa-positive cells, and are entirely benign. Two different angiofibromas are seen in tuberous sclerosis (Chap. 19): adenoma sebaceum and Koenen tumor (periungual fibroma). Pearly penile papules also belong to the group (Chap. 34).

Fibrous Papule of the Nose

(Graham 1965)

Synonyms. Fibrosis nodularis nasi, fibrous papule of the face

Etiology and Pathogenesis. The cause is unknown. Most lesions are rich in factor XIIIa-positive der-

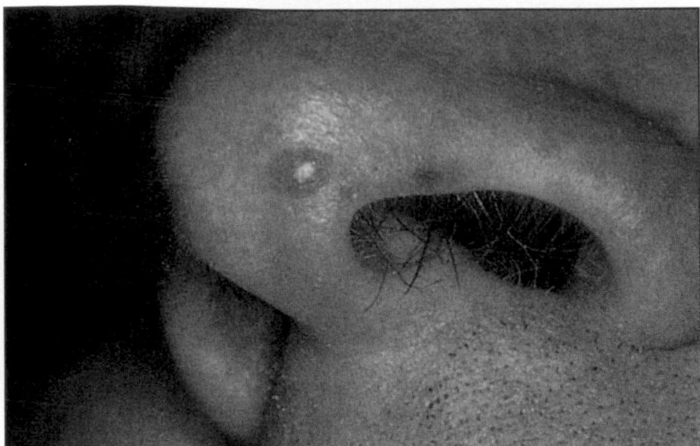

Fig. 59.7. Fibrous papule of the nose

mal dendrocytes. In some instances, residua of an intradermal nevus are found, but then the preferred diagnosis is nevus.

Clinical Findings. Most of these small papules are found on the nose, either the tip or the alae (Fig. 59.7). They range in color from normal skin shade to tan and are dome-shaped. Similar lesions may occur on the ears or anywhere else on the face.

Histopathology. Microscopy reveals a normal epidermis, sometimes with increased basal layer pigmentation, and proliferation of small vessels and fibroblasts in the dermis. The collagen may be arranged around the vessels, and often the fibroblasts are stellate or otherwise irregular. A granular cell variant has been described.

Differential Diagnosis. Both a small basal cell carcinoma and sebaceous hyperplasia can appear very similar, but are rapidly distinguished under the microscope.

Therapy. Tangential excision is curative.

Connective Tissue Nevus

These lesions are described in Chapter 52. They are most common in tuberous sclerosis, but are also seen in Buschke-Ollendorff syndrome. In addition, patients present with multiple or solitary fibrous papules and nodules that are rich in collagen and often elastin. A solitary lesion is often clinically called a fibroma.

Elastofibroma

(Järvi and Saxén 1961)

Synonym. Elastofibroma dorsi

Elastofibromas are slowly growing nodules located in the subscapular fascia. They probably represent a response to wear-and-tear; why the mesenchymal cells in this area can be induced to produce elastin is unclear. The lesions are almost always asymptomatic but, if large enough, may become clinically apparent. In autopsy series, many subclinical lesions have been found. Under the microscope, there is a poorly defined fibrous stroma rich in fragmented elastic fibers. Treatment consists of surgical removal.

Nodular Fasciitis

(Konwaler et al. 1955)

Synonym. Pseudosarcomatous fasciitis

Etiology and Pathogenesis. Nodular fasciitis is a disease of young adults. It often appears to be a response to trauma, and the predominant cell is the myofibroblast.

Clinical Findings. Most lesions are rapidly growing subcutaneous nodules on the forearm; other sites include the upper aspects of the arm and the leg. Tumors may reach several centimeters in size over a period of weeks, alarming the patient. Multiple lesions have been described. The rapid growth and presence of mitoses led early observers to call this lesion a pseudosarcoma. Cranial fasciitis is a variant seen in children with involvement of the deep fascia of the scalp and skull.

Histopathology. A fibrous capsule surrounds a myxoid stroma rich in spindle-shaped tumor cells. The spindle cells may be arrayed in a storiform pattern or scattered about. Mitoses are common, but atypical ones are rare. The tumors are vascular with frequent hemorrhage. Osteoid may be seen, especially in the cranial form. Many variants have been described, including intravascular fasciitis and proliferative fasciitis, which contains ganglion-like cells.

Therapy. Most lesions are excised because of their rapid growth. Recurrences are rare, even if the initial excision was not complete.

Fibrous Hamartoma of Infancy
(REYE 1956)

Clinical Findings. This nodule is usually present at birth or appears in the first year of life. The most common location is around the shoulder girdle, but many sites have been described. The tumor is usually subcutaneous and freely movable. Boys are more often affected.

Histopathology. There are three distinctive components to this poorly defined tumor: fat, trabeculae of fibrous tissue, and nests of immature mesenchymal cells. Myxoid changes are common.

Therapy. Excision is the only approach.

Fibromatoses

The fibromatoses have been defined as nonmetastasizing fibrous tumors that tend to recur and be locally aggressive. The best known members of the family are Dupuytren contracture, Ledderhose disease, and Peyronie disease (Chap. 18). Others are considered here.

Infantile Digital Fibromatosis
(FRANCK 1908; Reye 1965)

Synonyms. Recurring digital fibrous tumor of children, inclusion body fibromatosis, Reye tumor

Clinical Findings. This rare tumor typically involves the fingers or toes, but almost never the thumb or great toe (Fig. 59.8). The lesions are present at birth or appear early in life. Most lesions are solitary; occasionally, two lesions are found. Larger lesions may be painful or hamper use of the digit. In contrast to other fibrous tumors of childhood, girls are more often affected than boys.

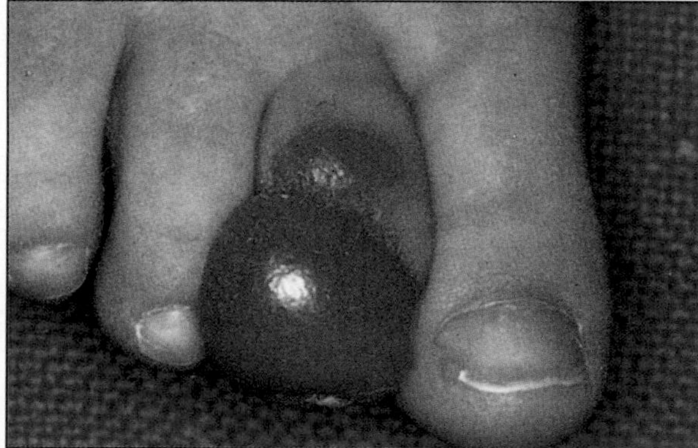

Fig. 59.8. Infantile digital fibromatosis

Histopathology. The tumor is nonencapsulated and extends irregularly into the subcutaneous fat. The interlacing spindle cells are myofibroblasts, being actin- and vimentin-positive, and have distinctive eosinophilic cytoplasmic inclusions. While these were originally suspected of being viral particles, they are now felt to be accumulations of actin. They stain red with Masson trichrome stain.

Juvenile Hyaline Fibromatosis

Patients with this rare disorder (Chap. 42) have multiple, often periarticular nodules that have a hyaline stroma.

Gingival Fibromatosis

Most gingival fibromatosis or hyperplasia is secondary to medications such as phenytoin or cyclosporine (Chap. 33). There are several rare syndromes in which infants develop gingival enlargement; sometimes this is the only change, while in other instances there are associated disorders. The best known dermatologic syndrome with gingival fibromatosis is Cowden syndrome (Chap. 65). The lesions are unlikely to be mistaken for other forms of fibromatosis.

Desmoid Tumor

Synonym. Musculoaponeurotic fibromatosis

Desmoid tumors arise from a muscular aponeurosis and tend to grow slowly, often infiltrating into the muscle. They may become quite large, displacing normal structures and hampering function. Most are solitary and found in the abdomen, usually arising from the rectus abdominis muscle following pregnancy. Extraabdominal desmoids may occur in any skeletal muscle. There may be a history of trauma or an operation. Thus, women undergoing Cesarean sections are at greater risk. Multiple desmoid tumors may occur in Gardner syndrome (Chap. 65). Microscopically, there are poorly circumscribed bundles and sheets of bland spindle cells with abundant collagen but regular nuclei and few mitoses. The best clue to the locally aggressive behavior is the invasion of adjacent muscle fibers.

Generous local excision is the best treatment for the solitary lesions; a variety of relatively ineffective measures including chemotherapy and cytokines have been tried in aggressive lesions and in Gardner syndrome patients.

Infantile Myofibromatosis

(Stout 1954)

Synonyms. Congenital generalized fibromatosis, juvenile fibromatosis, juvenile myofibroma (when solitary)

Etiology and Pathogenesis. This uncommon disorder is characterized by solitary or multiple plaques or nodules involving the skin, subcutaneous tissue, and viscera. While most feel the dominant cell is a myofibroblast, there are still uncertainties. Some suggest that the cell of origin is a smooth muscle cell. In addition, the relationship between infantile myofibromatosis and congenital fibrosarcoma remains unclear.

Clinical Findings. The most common clinical presentation is one or a small number of pale to red nodules involving the skin and subcutaneous tissue, as well as extending into muscles. About 50 % of such superficial lesions are present at birth, and over 90 % appear in the first two years of life. The most common location is the head and neck region. The outlook is good, with spontaneous regression often occurring and recurrence after excision uncommon.

In multicentric or generalized infantile myofibromatosis, the story is different. Most patients are affected at birth, have many cutaneous and soft tissue lesions, and may have pulmonary, cardiac, or gastrointestinal nodules. While most cases are sporadic, familial cases have been reported with both autosomal dominant and autosomal recessive patterns of inheritance. About one-third of patients with multiple cutaneous and subcutaneous lesions also have visceral involvement. Of this group, about three-fourths die, usually because of pulmonary complications.

Histopathology. Nodules of spindle cells are found in the dermis, as well as in the other tissues. The cells are plump and on routine microscopy resemble smooth muscle cells. They are frequently arranged about vessels. The cytologic picture is relatively bland with few mitoses. Vimentin and actin are positive, while desmin is usually negative, suggesting a myofibroblastic nature.

Therapy. In most superficial cases, the lesions will spontaneously regress, so no treatment is needed. In more aggressive tumors with visceral involvement, occasionally surgery is necessary but fraught with problems.

Adult Myofibroma

Adult myofibroma is a solitary, acquired tumor that usually appears on the extremities. Microscopically, the lesions are identical to juvenile myofibromas, with sharply circumscribed nodules consisting of both clumps of bland spindle cells as well as round or polygonal cells arranged around vessels. Spontaneous regression does not often occur, but excision is usually curative.

Dermatomyofibroma

(Cooper 1992; Kamino et al. 1992)

Synonym. Plaque-like dermal fibromatosis (Hügel 1991)

Clinical Findings. This lesion is typically a slowly growing plaque in the axillae of younger women. It is most often asymptomatic and may reach a large size, greater than 10 cm. The overlying skin may have a pebbly or pigskin-like surface.

Histopathology. The spindled tumor cells run parallel to the skin surface in the mid-dermis. The adnexal structures are spared. The cells may expand into the subcutaneous fat but do not infiltrate along septae. In most cases, immunohistochemistry reveals positive staining for vimentin and actin, suggesting that the cells are myofibroblasts. Hügel chose the designation fibromatosis because in some cases the myofibroblastic origin is difficult to prove.

Differential Diagnosis. The main differential diagnostic point is dermatofibrosarcoma protuberans. It too occurs in the shoulder girdle area, but is usually more nodular and has more nuclear atypia and downward extension on histologic examination.

Therapy. Excision is curative.

Infantile Desmoid-Type Fibromatosis

Synonyms. Fibrosarcoma-like fibromatosis, aggressive fibromatosis

This is biologically the most puzzling entity in the fibromatosis group. One could say that the diagnosis evolved to explain the fact that some microscopically aggressive fibrous tumors in infants do better than a similar tumor in an adult. In older patients, the diagnosis of fibrosarcoma would be made. The lesions are usually solitary, large, and may grow rapidly. Histologically, they show a variety of patterns, all featuring significant nuclear atypia. Generous surgical excision is usually the treatment of choice; amputation, radiation therapy, and chemotherapy are not often needed. Our advice is to leave the distinction between fibromatoses and fibrosarcomas in childhood to pediatric pathology and oncology referral centers.

Malignant Fibrous Tumors

Dermatofibrosarcoma Protuberans

(Darier and Ferrand 1924; Hoffmann 1925)

Clinical Findings. Dermatofibrosarcoma protuberans (DFSP) is an uncommon tumor, usually involving the shoulder girdle region of young to middle-aged adults. Often there is a history of trauma. The early lesion may be mistaken for a scar or keloid, as a firm red-brown plaque with associated protuberant nodules slowly develops (Fig. 59.9). At this stage, the lesion is freely movable. An uncommon variant is the atrophic form, which may be more common in childhood. Later, larger adherent nodules develop. The overlying epidermis becomes thinned, and telangiectases appear. Bleeding and ulceration are uncommon. Even when allowed to grow for many years, the tumors are usually asymptomatic.

Histopathology. The tumor consists of interwoven spindle cells with prominent nuclei and little collagen. They are often arranged in a cartwheel fashion with fascicles radiating out from an acellular area. Typically, the spindle cells insinuate along the fibrous septae of fat. The tumor bundles almost always extend into the subcutaneous fat, where they entrap fat and may surround muscles. The periphery of the tumor is poorly defined, making surgical check of the margins difficult. Mitoses are present, and large numbers may correlate with a risk of metastasis. The predominant cell is probably a poorly differentiated fibroblast. The best diagnostic marker is CD34, human progenitor cell antigen. In some instances, numerous melanocytes are also present. Other histologic variants include myxoid and granular cell forms, as well as those rich in giant cells.

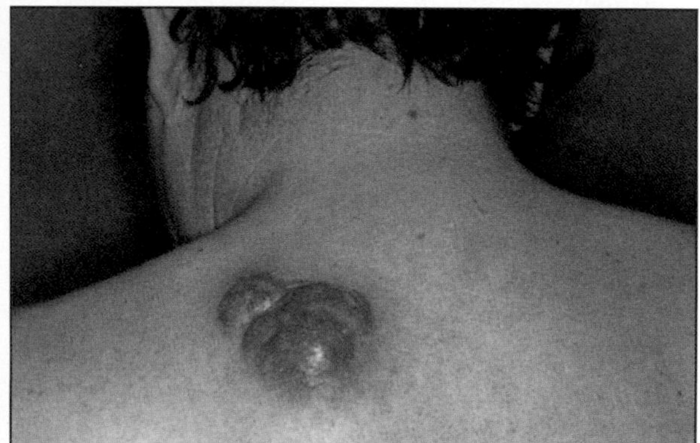

Fig. 59.9. Dermatofibrosarcoma protuberans

Course and Prognosis. Dermatofibrosarcoma protuberans is quite likely to recur locally. The rate has been estimated as 33%, but clearly depends on the surgical approach. Metastases are very uncommon; hematogenous spread is more often seen than lymphatic.

Differential Diagnosis. The clinical differential diagnosis includes keloid and dermatofibroma. Microscopically, the main problem is distinguishing a deep or cellular dermatofibroma; this tumor is usually Factor XIIIa-positive and CD34-negative and tends not to follow fat septae or entrap fat. In addition, mitoses are uncommon.

Therapy. Wide and deep local excision is required. The first excision offers the best chance for cure. Five-centimeter margins are usually suggested, but the deep extensions are hard to identify, even when one excises to the fascia. Mohs surgery is useful, and it may be helpful to perform a margin check with CD34 staining.

Pigmented Dermatofibrosarcoma Protuberans

(Bednar 1957)

Synonyms. Pigmented storiform neurofibroma, Bednar tumor

This tumor is a dermatofibrosarcoma protuberans that has been colonized by melanocytes. It is not a neurofibroma. The melanocytic component has no malignant potential. The lesion's biology is that of dermatofibrosarcoma protuberans.

Giant Cell Fibroblastoma

(Schmookler et al. 1989)

This rare tumor is probably a childhood dermatofibrosarcoma protuberans. It is more common in male infants, usually arising on the back or chest. Under the microscope, one finds a spindle cell tumor with multinucleated giant cells, sinusoidal spaces, and a myxoid stroma. Lesions have recurred as dermatofibrosarcoma protuberans, and focal areas of giant cell fibroblastoma may be found within ordinary dermatofibrosarcoma protuberans in adults. The treatment is surgery, but recurrence is very common.

Malignant Fibrous Histiocytoma

(O'Brien and Stout 1964; Weiss and Enzinger 1978)

Etiology and Pathogenesis. The only thing that most experts would agree upon when discussing malignant fibrous histiocytoma is that the tumor is not histiocytic, in the sense of being derived from the monocyte/macrophage lineage. It probably represents a primitive mesenchymal cell that differentiates in a variety of directions, showing fibroblastic, myofibroblastic and macrophagic features.

Clinical Findings. Malignant fibrous histiocytoma is the most common soft tissue sarcoma of adults. It is almost never a cutaneous tumor. The most common sites are the deep soft tissue and muscles of the proximal parts of the limbs, as well as the retroperitoneum. While subcutaneous lesions are not uncommon, they usually extend deeply, rather than involving the skin. Most patients are over 50 years of age, although the angiomatoid variant involves children and young adults. Occasionally, lesions may develop in the skin, either via direct spread, hematogenous metastasis, or, primarily, perhaps associated with trauma such as a vaccination or burn scar. The myxoid variant is somewhat more likely to be superficial. It can be confused with a cutaneous myxoma or mucinosis in its early stages, but will eventually evolve into a larger mass.

Histopathology. The microscopic appearance of malignant fibrous histiocytoma is beyond our scope. Five different patterns have been described: pleomorphic, myxoid, giant cell, inflammatory, and angiomatoid. They vary in terms of location, immunohistochemical features, and prognosis. The unifying feature is the presence of nuclear atypia with frequent mitoses.

Course and Prognosis. The 5-year survival rate is about 25%. Angiomatoid and myxoid lesions have a better prognosis. Small and superficial lesions do better than large and deep ones. Both aggressive local spread and metastases to the lungs and lymph nodes may occur.

Differential Diagnosis. The differential possibilities include the whole spectrum of soft tissue tumors.

Therapy. Wide local excision may be combined with radiation therapy and even chemotherapy.

Atypical Fibroxanthoma

(Helwig 1963)

Etiology and Pathogenesis. Atypical fibroxanthoma is probably a superficial variant of malignant fibrous histiocytoma. It was initially described as a pseudosarcoma because the patients did so well, but occasional adverse clinical experiences and histochemical similarities have led to the current view.

Clinical Findings. Most tumors arise in the sun-damaged skin of elderly patients. Usually, lesions are red-brown nodules that grow fairly rapidly to reach a size of 1–2 cm. They are often crusted, eroded, or ulcerated. Lesions occurring in younger patients or on unexposed sites should be regarded as malignant fibrous histiocytoma.

Histopathology. The epidermis usually shows atrophy or mild atypia, as expected in sun-damaged skin. The action is in the dermis, where there is a poorly defined accumulation of highly atypical cells, with striking nuclear pleomorphism. If one searches carefully, three cell types can usually be identified: spindle cells, foam cells, and giant cells. Multinucleated cells and mitoses, even atypical mitoses, are common. When the lesion was still considered a benign pseudosarcoma, it was often described as "too malignant for a malignancy."

Necrosis, invasion of vessels, and fat are all bad signs. The immunohistochemical staining patterns are highly variable, but S100 and keratin are negative.

Course and Prognosis. Following excision, about 5% recur, and over a dozen patients with metastases have been described.

Differential Diagnosis. The two main differential diagnostic points are squamous cell carcinoma, especially the spindle cell variant, and amelanotic malignant melanoma. The lack of staining for pankeratin and S100 markers has simplified this diagnosis. In the past, electron microscopy was required, but mistakes were common.

Therapy. Excision as for a basal cell carcinoma is usually curative. Large, deep, higher-risk lesions should be treated more aggressively.

Epithelioid Sarcoma

(ENZINGER 1970)

Etiology and Pathogenesis. The cell of origin of epithelioid sarcoma is disputed, but many experts consider it to be a synovial tumor. Occasionally, there is a history of trauma.

Clinical Findings. This rare tumor usually involves the extremities of young men. Occasionally, the genitalia are affected. While most tumors are situated in the subcutaneous fat and fascia, some may arise in the dermis. When the skin is involved, one or more slowly growing nodules are seen. Ulceration is a late feature. Cases may be mistaken for granuloma annulare or granulomatous inflammation.

Histopathology. Microscopically, the diagnosis can be quite difficult, as a superficial biopsy may only show necrobiosis or granulomatous inflammation. Typically, poorly defined nodules are seen in the deep dermis extending into the fat, invading along nerves and showing central necrosis. There is usually an inflammatory infiltrate about the nodules. The tumor cells range from oval to polygonal to spindle, but usually have nuclear atypia and mitoses. The hallmark of the cells is that they are usually positive for both keratin and vimentin, a most unusual combination. Some are CD34-positive, but macrophage markers are usually negative.

Therapy. Generous surgical excision is required. About 80% of cases recur locally, and over 30% metastasize. Because this indolent tumor is potentially fatal, aggressive reexcision is almost always called for after the histologic diagnosis is made.

Fibrosarcoma

Fibrosarcomas are not primary cutaneous tumors. As the fibromatoses have been better identified and malignant fibrous histiocytoma established as a diagnosis, fibrosarcomas have become rare. In the skin, they primarily develop by extension from deeper tissues or following burns or radiation therapy. Fibrosarcomas in children (infantile fibrosarcoma) have a better prognosis than those in adults. Most tumors develop from muscle, tendon, or deep fascia as an expanding nodule. Under the microscope, they classically have a herringbone pattern with interlaced fascicles of spindle cells. Mitoses are common, and there is no evidence of differentiation into other cell types; only vimentin is typically positive. Treatment consists of radical surgery combined with ionizing radiation. Chemotherapy is disappointing.

Benign Vascular Tumors

Some of the vascular tumors have been considered in Chapter 52 under vascular nevi. Others are considered in Chapter 22 where telangiectases are discussed. An area of confusion is the distinction between vascular tumors and hyperplasias. The hyperplasias should regress when the stimulating trigger is removed or damped. Most vascular lesions are benign; Kaposi sarcoma and angiosarcoma are both uncommon and relatively clinically distinct, so they should not be overlooked. The differential diagnosis is not emphasized for each lesion, as in essence, the entire spectrum of vascular proliferations and tumors serves as its own differential diagnostic list. In addition, eccrine tumors and metastatic tumors, especially renal cell carcinomas, may often appear clinically very similar.

Pyogenic Granuloma

(PONCET and DOR 1897)

Synonyms. Granuloma pyogenicum, granuloma teleangiectaticum, granuloma pediculatum

Definition. Reactive, often friable and bleeding vascular proliferation following trauma.

Etiology and Pathogenesis. Pyogenic granulomas are common in one specific clinical setting – the gingiva in pregnancy, where they are also known as epulis gravidarum or pregnancy tumor (Chap. 33).

In all other settings, they are uncommon, unpredictable responses to minor trauma. Some clinicians distinguish between an eruptive hemangioma and a pyogenic granuloma, but only rarely is there a history of hemangioma being present prior to trauma.

Clinical Findings. The typical pyogenic granuloma is a soft, friable, red papule or nodule less than 1 cm in diameter (Fig. 59.10). Typical locations in addition to the gingiva include the fingers, palms, face, and scalp, presumably because they are most often subject to trauma. The lesions are invariably friable, bleeding, and crusted. They often have a stalk. There is a pale epidermal collarette.

There is a blurred line of distinction between pyogenic granuloma and granulation tissue. For example, many patients with severe acne, especially when starting isotretinoin therapy, develop multiple friable red nodules in their most severe lesions. The almost gelatinous material can be curetted away. Such lesions are often called pyogenic granulomas, but are clearly related to the exuberant wound response seen about the umbilicus of infants or in other surgical wounds, if irritated or infected.

Histopathology. The main point is that a true granuloma with giant cells is rarely, if ever, seen. Instead, there is a crusted epidermis overlying a lobular vascular proliferation consisting of many small new capillaries arranged around a central vessel. This lobular pattern is frequently found in new vascular proliferations, because it is simply a recapitulation of the development of vessels in the embryo. If the epidermis is intact, an inflammatory infiltrate is rare; some prefer to call such lesions eruptive hemangiomas. Once ulceration arises, there are many neutrophils present.

There are several unusual variants of pyogenic granuloma:

- Intravascular pyogenic granulomas are almost never recognized clinically. They present as a dermal nodule, are discovered to be intravascular when they bleed excessively during surgery, and are identified by the pathologist.
- Satellite or recurrent pyogenic granulomas usually develop after the removal of a solitary pyogenic granuloma. Occasionally, they may erupt following excision of another type of lesion such as a melanocytic nevus. The dramatic changes worry all involved but are simply a reflection of the proliferative response.

Course and Prognosis. Most pyogenic granulomas regress spontaneously, but they are so annoying to the patient that they are usually removed.

Differential Diagnosis. A typical crusted, bleeding lesion can only be confused with an ulcerated tumor, but usually the history is different. Amelanotic malignant melanomas are often similar in appearance on the digits; another reason for removing the lesions is to exclude this serious differential diagnosis.

Therapy. Excision offers the lowest rate of recurrence, but often superficial destruction with electrosurgery, curettage, or chemical cautery is successful. Laser destruction is also effective. Potent topical corticosteroids applied under occlusion can be used to treat an initial lesion. In acne patients with disseminated pyogenic granulomas, a short course of systemic prednisone (1 mg/kg daily) is most useful.

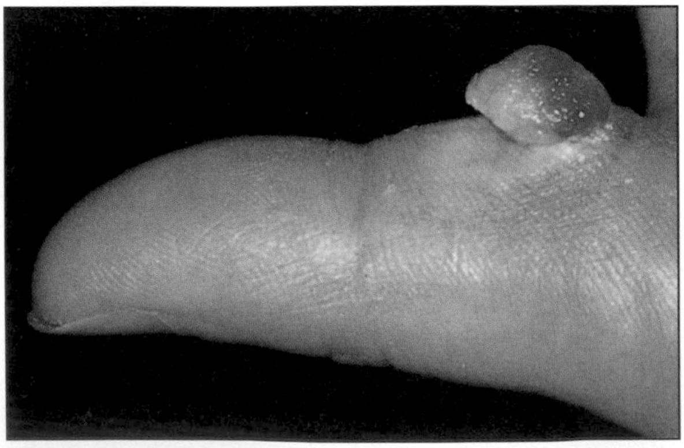

Fig. 59.10. Pyogenic granuloma

Thrombosed Capillary Aneurysm

(Epstein et al. 1956)

Another misnomer, this thrombosed venule presents suddenly as a dark macule or papule, raising the question of malignant melanoma. The excisional biopsy shows a dilated vascular space in the upper dermis with a thrombosis, answering all questions. Venous lakes, varicosities, angiokeratomas, and verrucous hemangiomas may also thrombose suddenly. The unifying feature is the presence of thin-walled vessels in the uppermost dermis.

Angiolymphoid Hyperplasia with Eosinophilia

(Wells and Whimster 1969)

Synonyms. Atypical pyogenic granuloma, pseudopyogenic granuloma, papular angioplasia, histiocytoid hemangioma, epithelioid hemangioma. In addition, some include Kimura disease as yet another synonym but this is incorrect.

Definition. Vascular proliferation with distinctive endothelial cells, admixed with a varying lymphocytic and eosinophilic response.

Epidemiology. This uncommon process is more often seen in women.

Etiology and Pathogenesis. The cause is unknown. Occasionally, there is a history of trauma, and in some surgical specimens, arteriovenous shunts have been identified.

Clinical Findings. The most typical location is the head and scalp (Fig. 59.11). Very often, multiple, grouped, red, dome-shaped nodules are found on the anterior aspect of the external ear, even filling the auditory canal. Another common site is the hair line of the temple. The skin surface is smooth and glistening. Erosions occasionally occur. Widespread lesions may be found, but are most unusual.

Histopathology. The microscopic findings are striking. There is a lobular proliferation of vessels with unusual plump endothelial cells that have been called histiocytoid or epithelioid. The term "hobnail" is apt, as the vessels are lined by multiple endothelial cells that protrude into the lumen. Others have described the vessels as having too many endothelial cells. Surrounding and often almost obscuring the vessels is a dense mixed lymphocytic infiltrate, often with admixed eosinophils. Lymphoid follicles can be seen at the periphery. Mucin can be present.

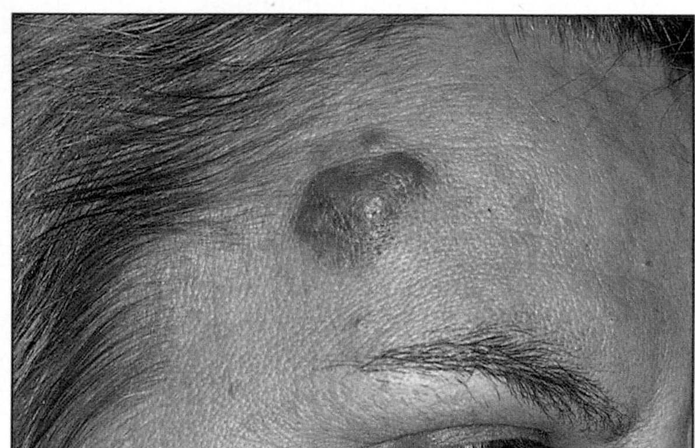

Fig. 59.11. Angiolymphoid hyperplasia with eosinophilia

Laboratory Findings. On occasion, primarily in patients with widespread disease, there may be an elevated eosinophil count.

Course and Prognosis. The lesions are persistent, speaking against their reactive nature. Following excision, recurrences are not unusual.

Differential Diagnosis. The differential diagnostic list is long, as any red bump on the face and scalp must be included. Pyogenic granuloma, other vascular tumors, lymphocytic infiltrates, facial granuloma, and adnexal tumors all must be considered. Kimura disease is different.

Therapy. Excision or laser destruction are the most certain methods. Intralesional corticosteroids may induce remission of smaller lesions. The lesions are sensitive to ionizing radiation.

Kimura Disease

(Kimura et al. 1948)

Synonym. Eosinophilic lymphofolliculosis

Kimura disease is a rare systemic disease, possibly an infection, which occurs almost exclusively in Asians. There are deep subcutaneous masses, involvement of lymph nodes, and massive peripheral eosinophilia. The head and neck are the most typical site; most patients are young men. Skin findings are very rare and the result of upward extension of deep tumors. The subcutaneous masses contain dense lymphocytic infiltrates with abundant eosinophils but without any vascular proliferation. Both peripheral eosinophilia and elevated IgE levels can be seen. There is no satisfactory treatment; most often systemic corticosteroids are employed, as well as surgery for localized masses. Most patients do well, and malignant degeneration has not been described.

Infectious Vascular Proliferations

Two bacterial infections produce lesions that clinically and histologically resemble pyogenic granuloma. Both bacillary angiomatosis and verruga peruana are caused by *Bartonella* spp. (Chap. 4.)

Reactive Benign Angioendotheliomatosis

(Pfleger and Tappeiner 1959)

Angioendotheliomatosis presents with bruise-like lesions on the trunk and extremities. For many years, benign and malignant forms were described, but surprisingly the latter turned out to be an intravascular lymphoma, despite the microscopic similarities (Chap. 61). Immunohistochemical studies using lymphocytic and vascular markers allow a ready distinction today. Reactive angioendotheliomatosis is usually associated with subacute bacterial endocarditis, and rarely with other types of sepsis. It may also be seen secondary to intravascular deposition of cryoproteins and to iatrogenic arteriovenous fistulas. There are dilated vessels filled with proliferating endothelial cells. Once the underlying infection is treated, the skin changes regress.

Acroangiodermatitis

This reactive process is associated with chronic venous insufficiency (Chap. 22). Its other name, pseudo-Kaposi sarcoma, is misleading, because while there may be fleeting clinical similarities, the histologic diagnosis is straightforward.

Stewart-Bluefarb Syndrome

(Stewart 1967; Bluefarb and Adams 1967)

Reactive vascular nodules may appear in patients with arteriovenous malformations. Usually one limb is involved, such as in the Klippel-Weber-Trenaunay syndrome. Similar changes have been described in paralyzed patients and following placement of an arteriovenous shunt in hemodialysis patients. The underlying malformation is usually apparent, with a thrill or bruit, warmth, limb enlargement, and swelling. The lesions usually appear on the dorsal surfaces of the toes or foot, starting as red-purple papules that evolve into nodules and plaques. Microscopic examination reveals numerous thick-walled vessels, extravasation of erythrocytes, and hemosiderin. Occasionally, an arteriovenous shunt may be found in the depths of a large specimen. Treatment is difficult as the underlying process is hard to reverse. Excision or laser destruction is probably the most reasonable option.

Intravascular Papillary Endothelial Hyperplasia

(Masson 1923)

Synonyms. Masson phenomenon, Masson pseudoangiosarcoma, vegetant intravascular hemangioendothelioma (Masson's term)

Two giants of pathology, Masson and Ewing, independently described unusual intravascular changes in thrombosed hemorrhoidal veins. Many subsequent authors have identified the same phenomenon in a variety of vascular lesions. Masson phenomenon is almost certainly an unusual type of recanalization of a thrombus. Under the microscope, there is an intravascular proliferation, with large vascular spaces with numerous hyalinized papillary blebs coated by endothelial cells. Once one has seen the histologic picture, confusion with angiosarcoma is inexcusable. The intravascular location, the papillary pattern, and the lack of mitoses, as well as the usual history of some preexisting vascular lesion, indicate the diagnosis.

Hemangioma

Definition. Benign vascular tumor that is present in infants and enlarges by proliferation of endothelial cells.

Epidemiology. Hemangiomas are quite common. They are found in 5–10% of all infants. While they may be present at birth, they typically appear in the first weeks of life and expand rapidly. There is a female dominance. They are more common in premature infants. In 15–20% of affected patients, multiple lesions are present. These infants are at greater risk of visceral hemangiomas.

Etiology and Pathogenesis. The cause of the endothelial proliferation is unknown. A number of angiogenic factors have been identified, and attempts to modulate them offer promise in therapy, but where they come from and how they function remain unclear.

Clinical Findings. Much has been made of the distinction between capillary and cavernous lesions. This distinction cannot be made clinically, and it is more reasonable to speak of superficial and deep hemangiomas. The former are bright red

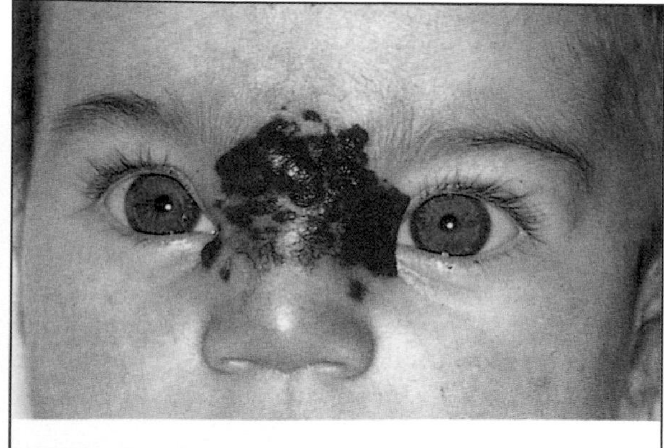

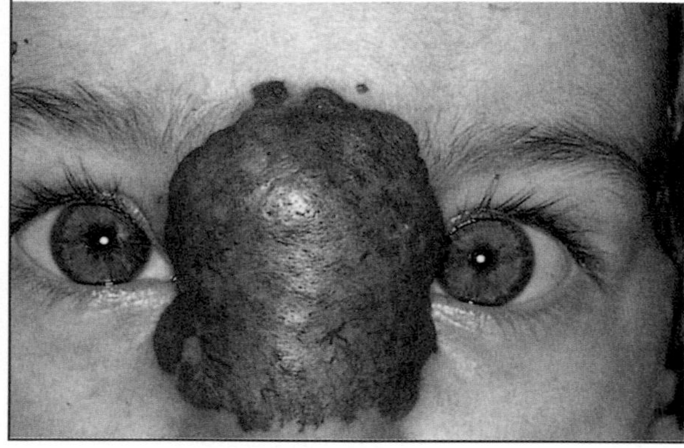

Fig. 59.12. Hemangioma; *lower picture* was taken 11 months later and shows both an increase in size and a gray sheen suggesting regression

lesions, the so-called strawberry hemangioma (Fig. 59.12). The latter is deeper, has overlying normal skin, and often a more bluish tone. Many tumors have both a superficial and deep component; some are iceberg-like with an innocent superficial lesion overlying large dermal nodules.

The most common site is the face and scalp, but any part of the body can be involved. Mucosal lesions are uncommon, although periorificial ones are not. Hemangiomas typically evolve through characteristic stages that include a growth phase, a stable period, and finally spontaneous regression. They usually present as a pink macule but rapidly become nodular with a smooth or lobulated surface, depending on the depth of the proliferation. They are often described as rubbery and can be compressed. Their color tends to darken with time. Growth is rapid, and lesions 5–10 cm in size are not uncommon. They tend to expand out of proportion to the child's growth. Careful measurements or clinical pictures should be used to document the changes in size, as the various therapeutic approaches are often based on a rough estimate of the growth rate.

A variety of systemic defects can be associated with cutaneous hemangiomas. They may be markers for underlying hemangiomas or other developmental defects. Large midline lesions or multiple hemangiomas are most likely to be markers for such problems. Other midline malformations such as sternal cleft or abdominal raphe defects are common. PHACES syndrome refers to posterior fossa defects, hemangiomas, coarctation of the aorta, cardiac defects, eye defects, and sternal malformations. Hemangiomas in the lumbosacral region may be markers for spinal cord or skeletal problems, as well as for gastrointestinal and genitourinary abnormalities. Hemangiomas in the beard region may reflect underlying airway problems. Recently, families have been described in which multiple hemangiomas and vascular malformations have been inherited in an autosomal dominant pattern; further studies are needed to identify the target genes, the products of which will perhaps clarify the relationship between hemangiomas and vascular malformations.

Histopathology. Very few hemangiomas are biopsied. Only atypical or unusual lesions are likely to be sampled, because of the obvious problems with bleeding. Early lesions are very cellular, with few vascular channels; such lesions are particularly common about the orbit, usually with a deep component, and have been called cellular angiomas. Mitotic figures and mast cells may be prominent. Later, vessel lumina become apparent. As regression occurs with fibrosis of the cellular areas, the vessels can further dilate, producing a cavernous pattern.

Course and Prognosis. There are a number of complications of hemangiomas. They include:

- Obstruction of Vital Functions. A large tumor blocking one eye can lead to serious visual problems, such as amblyopia. Similarly, nasal, oral, or aural obstruction presents difficulties in breathing, eating, or hearing, but these are usually not as troublesome.
- Ulceration. Even though parents are understandably afraid of ulceration, it is relatively common and not usually associated with bleeding problems. Hemangiomas in the diaper area are particularly likely to be traumatized and then become eroded. In other instances, there is deep necrosis and secondary ulceration, followed by regression.
- Kasabach-Merritt Syndrome. A consumptive coagulopathy has been described in large hem-

angiomas, but more detailed studies suggest that it is most common in kaposiform hemangioendothelioma and tufted angioma. Any young infant with a large vascular tumor who shows bruising or bleeding at other sites should be evaluated for this possibility.

- Visceral Involvement. In addition to the syndromes discussed above, some infants will have cutaneous and systemic hemangiomas without evidence of other problems. We prefer the term diffuse neonatal hemangiomatosis to describe such children. The mortality rate is relatively high in the growth phase of the process, with high output cardiac failure and gastrointestinal bleeding being the main culprits. Any child with multiple cutaneous hemangiomas should be studied with imaging techniques to search for internal lesions. Those infants with simply many skin lesions and no internal involvement have been designated as having benign neonatal hemangiomatosis. In both settings, the same tendency towards spontaneous regression exists.

The first sign of regression is usually gray streaks on the surface of the lesion. A rough rule of thumb for regression is that 30% will resolve within 3 years, 50% by 5 years, and 70% by 7 years. Regression does not mean disappearance; there is usually redundant skin and perhaps telangiectases.

Differential Diagnosis. The main challenge is distinguishing between vascular malformations and hemangiomas. The former are permanent and do not grow rapidly during the first weeks of life. The deeper lesions may be confused with other soft tissue tumors, but only rarely.

Most hemangiomas not present at birth have slightly different clinical or microscopic appearances than congenital hemangiomas. Occasionally, a deep hemangioma may first become apparent later in life. In general, the term acquired hemangioma is imprecise and usually can be replaced by a more accurate diagnosis.

Therapy. Because of the well-established tendency towards spontaneous regression, all therapeutic measures are difficult to evaluate. In the past, most physicians took a wait-and-see attitude. Today, with the effectiveness of laser therapy, many children are being treated earlier, to eliminate the lesion before it completes its growth phase, thus reducing scarring.

Lasers. The flash lamp-pulsed dye laser (Chap. 70) is probably the best choice for treating superficial hemangiomas. It can be used under anesthesia, or with EMLA topical anesthetic. In about 75% of cases, there is a reduction in size, and 25–50% of the lesions disappear entirely after several treatments. The deeper component is not influenced by this laser. The continuous wave neodymium:YAG laser, used through an ice cube, is probably the best approach to the deeper vessels. Argon lasers are another option but usually reserved for adults, as the treatment is more painful and may cause more scarring in infants.

Cryotherapy. Early contact cryotherapy is another preferred approach. Standard spray cryotherapy does not work well. Instead, one must use a cooled metallic plate or a special contact cryotherapy unit. The lesion is frozen for 10–15 s. One or two treatments spaced 4 weeks apart usually produce satisfactory improvement. Ulceration may occur but is not a problem. Again, deeper vessels are not influenced.

Corticosteroids. Both systemic and intralesional corticosteroids have been used in severe cases. A small amount of triamcinolone acetonide (2.5–10.0 mg/ml) can be injected safely into troublesome lesions; this is not as effective as lasers or contact cryotherapy, and we no longer employ it.

Ophthalmologists developed the first guidelines for using systemic corticosteroids in infants who were developing visual problems because of a periorbital hemangioma blocking their sight. The usual dosage is 2–3 mg/kg prednisone daily. Within several weeks, tumor growth is usually arrested. There are no firm rules for length of therapy and how to taper the dosage.

Interferon-α. Used in dosages of 3 million IU/m^2 daily, usually injected subcutaneously, this cytokine appears effective. It is not approved for this indication, is expensive, and the duration of treatment has not been well worked out.

Other Methods. Ionizing radiation is also effective, but has been replaced by other methods. Surgical excision, injection of sclerosing agents, and compression are also occasionally recommended. Excision is usually reserved for lesions that repeatedly bleed or show no sign of regression.

Verrucous Hemangioma
(Imperial and Helwig 1967)

Verrucous hemangiomas present in early life but tend not to resolve. Often the first finding is a cluster of small red papules without epidermal changes. Later there is reactive epidermal hyperplasia producing verrucous plaques or bands. The lesions may be larger than 5 cm. The most common site is the legs. Histologically, there are dilated vessels in the deep and superficial dermis. The uppermost changes mimic an angiokeratoma, but the latter lesion has no cavernous component. Surgical excision is the best treatment; it is often wise to perform this in childhood to avoid problems with increasing expansion and ulceration. Sometimes grafting is needed.

Mafucci Syndrome
(Mafucci 1881; Kast and von Recklinghausen 1889)

Synonyms. Dyschondroplasia with hemangiomas syndrome, Kast syndrome

Mafucci syndrome is a sporadic malformation in which cavernous hemangiomas are combined with enchondromas of the hands and feet. Enchondromas are islands of nonossifying cartilage that persist in metaphyses of growing bone. The vascular lesions are highly variable and perhaps better considered as malformations. Nonetheless, the most common change is a compressible cavernous hemangioma, present in infancy but unlikely to regress. Over half of these patients die from malignant mesenchymal tumors such as chondrosarcomas, angiosarcomas, or fibrosarcomas.

Blue Rubber Bleb Nevus Syndrome
(Bean 1958)

The blue rubber bleb nevus syndrome is a rare disorder; it is sometimes inherited in an autosomal dominant pattern, although most cases are sporadic. Multiple cavernous hemangiomas are present; they are often tender or painful and associated with local hyperhidrosis (Fig. 59.13). Under the microscope, the vascular channels are often associated with increased eccrine sweat glands. The patients also have multiple gastrointestinal hemangiomas leading to pain, blood loss, and melena. Rarely, other internal organs such as the liver may be involved. Presentation is usually in adult life, in contrast to diffuse neonatal hemangiomatosis. The main differential diagnostic consideration is multiple glomus tumors; the distinction is based on histology. Osler-Weber-Rendu syndrome has smaller cutaneous lesions and almost always nasal involvement. While the cutaneous lesions can be removed, the gastrointestinal ones are difficult to handle.

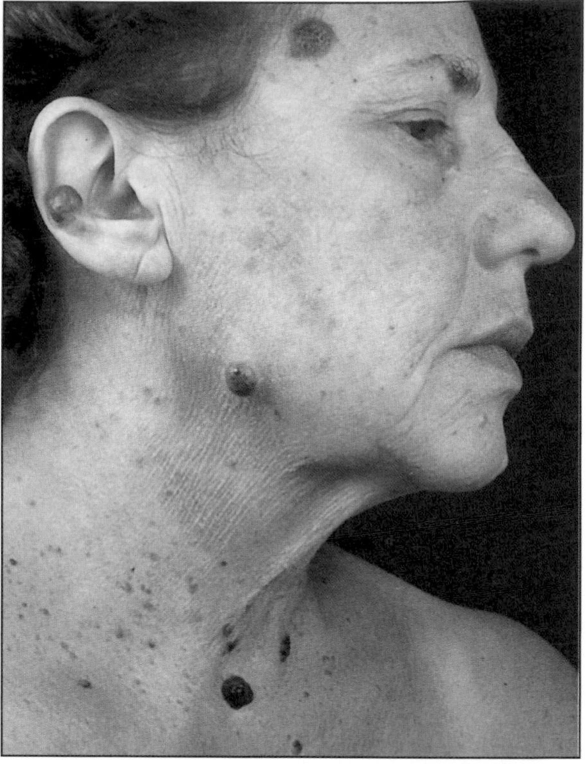

Fig. 59.13. Blue rubber bleb nevus syndrome

Acral Arteriovenous Hemangioma
(Girard et al. 1974)

Synonyms. Cirsoid aneurysm, arteriovenous aneurysm, arteriovenous fistula

These acral or scalp lesions are typically solitary, firm or pulsating, purple nodules. They may be associated with trauma, in which case they are also called posttraumatic arteriovenous fistulas. Microscopically, they are characterized by an accumulation of very thick-walled vessels in the superficial dermis. Often a deep feeder vessel is seen.

None of the names is truly correct, as the lesion is not an aneurysm and is often not acral. Simple excision is curative.

Racemose Angioma

This extremely rare vascular malformation is composed of multiple arteriovenous fistulas, often arranged in a branching pattern. Racemose means resembling a bunch of grapes. The lesions clinically resemble varicosities, occur usually on the head or upper part of the trunk, and appear early in life. The individual lesions may be pulsatile. Under the microscope, they resemble an arteriovenous hemangioma, although other histologic patterns may be seen.

Cherry Angioma

(DE MORGAN 1872)

Synonyms. Senile angioma, ruby spot, de Morgan spot

These extremely common lesions also lack an appropriate name. While they appear in adult life, they are definitely not associated with senility. They have little in common with cherries, since they are much smaller, and not all cherries have the deep red color responsible for the association. Almost every adult has several cherry angiomas, and many have hundreds (Fig. 59.14). In some instances, there is a familial predilection. In other cases, there may be a sudden eruption of cherry angiomas associated with pregnancy or prolactin-secreting tumors. Microscopically, they consist of a proliferation of capillaries. Since they can be diagnosed with certainty and are usually multiple, electrosurgical or laser destruction is most practical, if removal is desired. Sometimes, worried patients are relieved to learn that the spots are harmless and have the same color as a high quality ruby, a gemstone associated with good luck.

Venous Lake

(BEAN and WALSH 1956)

This soft, blue, easily compressible papule is usually found on the lips or ears (Fig. 59.15). Both solitary and multiple lesions are common. It may be mistaken by a novice for a pigmented lesion when on the lips or thrombosed. Microscopically, there is a single, irregular, large vascular space filling the upper dermis. Excision or destruction is curative.

Targetoid Hemosiderotic Hemangioma

(SANTA CRUZ and ARONBERG 1988)

This rare form of hemangioma is often clinically puzzling, but usually distinct once one has encountered an example. There is a central, red-brown papule surrounded by a pale ring with an erythematous border. The peripheral changes resolve, but the central papule remains. Under the microscope, the central part of the lesion usually shows a preexisting hemangioma with thrombus formation and papillary projections. At the periphery, there are dissecting, thin-walled, vascular spaces associated with hemosiderin deposits, mimicking patch-stage Kaposi sarcoma. The clinical pattern usually allows differentiation.

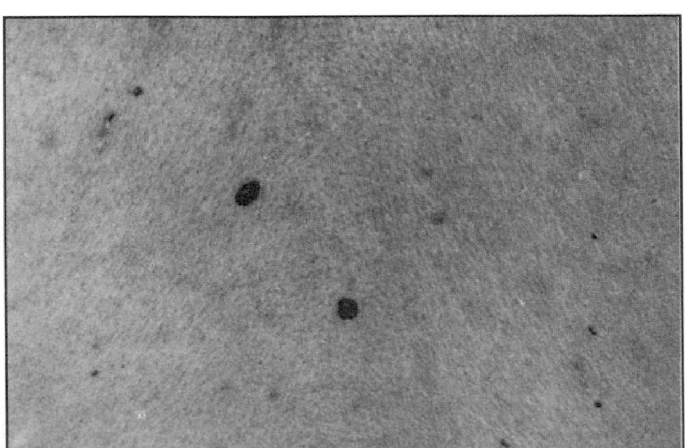

Fig. 59.14. Cherry angiomas

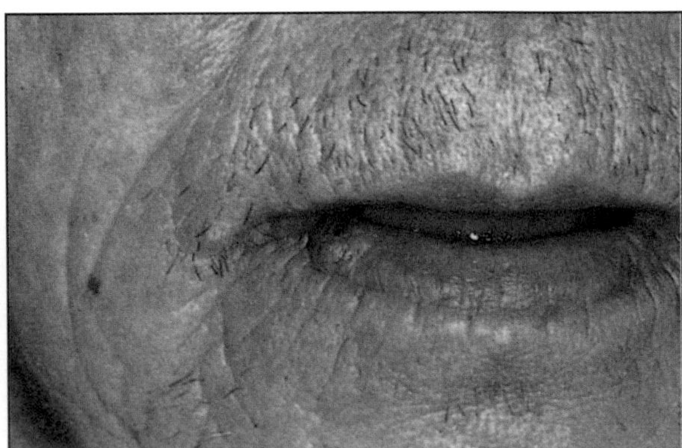

Fig. 59.15. Venous lake

Microvenular Hemangioma

(BANTEL et al. 1989; HUNT et al. 1991)

Synonym. Microcapillary hemangioma

This very rare tumor was probably overlooked until the explosion in the incidence of Kaposi sarcoma caused dermatopathologists to more carefully classify hemangiomas. It presents typically as a small, red-brown nodule, usually on the forearm. Histologic examination reveals an extensive proliferation of small, uniform vessels with inconspicuous lumina filling the dermis. There is usually an associated dermal fibrosis. Such lesions were in the past probably diagnosed as fibrosed hemangioma or even sclerosing hemangioma (vascular dermatofibroma).

Tufted Angioma

(MACMILLAN and CHAMPION 1971; WILSON JONES 1976)

Synonym. Progressive capillary angioma

Tufted angiomas are vascular tumors of children that usually appear in the shoulder girdle area. Initially, they are flat, red-brown patches that resemble a bruise but which slowly expand and may develop papules. Occasionally, they are painful. There is no tendency to spontaneous regression. Microscopically, there is a lobular pattern just as in pyogenic granuloma but without surface changes. Treatment is a problem because of the large size of the lesions in a location not amenable to extensive surgery. For this reason, laser destruction seems most logical, although a series of cases will probably never be collected.

The angioblastoma of Nakagawa (1949) has only been described in Asian infants; it is clinically similar, but our colleagues in the East tell us that the age of onset and subtle histologic features allow distinction.

Multinucleate Cell Angiohistiocytoma

(SMITH and WILSON JONES 1986)

While it is unclear whether this lesion is a variant of hemangioma or a histiocytic process, clinically it presents as red-violet papules, usually on the legs of middle-aged women. Thus, clinically, it may be confused with Kaposi sarcoma. Microscopically, there is an increased number of small vessels in the upper dermis associated with large multinucleated giant cells.

Glomeruloid Hemangioma

(CHAN et al. 1990)

Glomeruloid hemangiomas have only been reported in POEMS syndrome (Chap. 40). POEMS is an acronym for polyneuropathy, organomegaly, endocrinopathy, monoclonal gammopathy, and skin lesions. The main skin changes include hypertrichosis, scleroderma-like thickening, and hemangiomas. While a variety of vascular lesions has been described, the most distinctive is the glomeruloid hemangioma. Clinically, the lesions are simply red papules; microscopically, they contain proliferations of small capillaries within a larger vascular space, resembling a renal glomerulus. They are morphologically closely related to intravascular pyogenic granuloma or to the intravascular proliferation seen in cryoglobulinemia. Perhaps the monoclonal protein stimulates endothelial proliferation.

Bossed Hemangioma

(MARTINEZ-PEREZ et al. 1995)

This most unusual variant of a congenital hemangioma features a raised mass with numerous central telangiectases and peripheral pallor. Most have been seen on the legs, and all have regressed rapidly after birth. The microscopic picture is a capillary hemangioma.

Angiokeratomas

Angiokeratomas are traditionally separated from hemangiomas, although there are overlaps. The cardinal feature of an angiokeratoma is the presence of large vascular spaces located just beneath the epidermis, which often shows papillomatosis and hyperkeratosis. Often there is only a thin trace of dermis, and, if sections are cut tangentially, there may appear to be intraepidermal vessels, a biological impossibility. The different types of angiokeratomas have little in common but are considered together for convenience. The histology is so similar that it will not be repeated. The larger lesions can be removed surgically or with electrosurgical

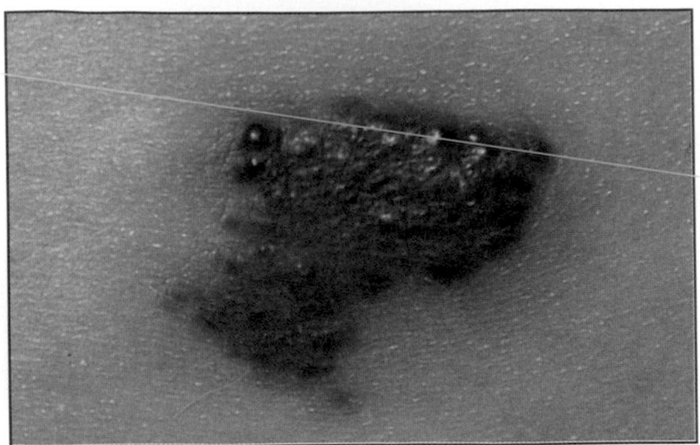

Fig. 59.16. Angiokeratoma

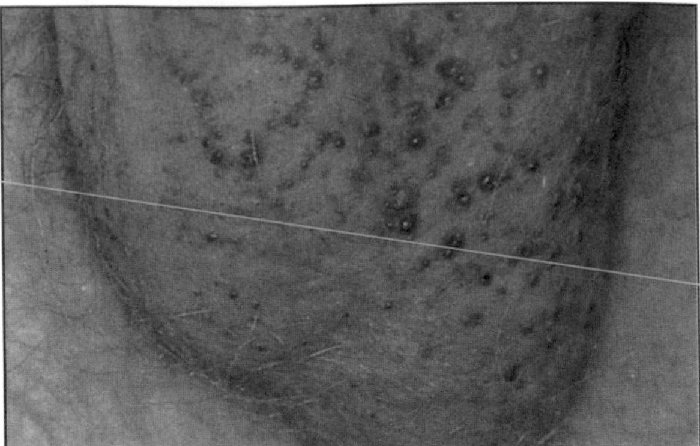

Fig. 59.17. Scrotal angiokeratomas

or laser destruction. The smaller lesions usually do not require therapy.

Solitary Angiokeratoma

(Imperial and Helwig 1967)

This lesion is most closely related to a traumatic aneurysm. It presents as a single, dark, red-brown papule that is often mistaken for a melanocytic lesion (Fig. 59.16). Most lesions are located on the limbs, and there is often a history of trauma.

Angiokeratoma of Mibelli

(Mibelli 1889)

Synonym. Angiokeratoma acroasphycticum digitorum

This very uncommon lesion is almost exclusively limited to the acral areas and breasts of young girls with cold intolerance. Numerous dark, red-gray papules appear and develop hyperkeratotic verrucous surface changes. They tend to progress slowly but can be surgically removed or destroyed with a laser.

Angiokeratoma Circumscriptum. These large, verrucous lesions are present at birth or soon thereafter. They are often linear or band-like and located on a limb. Other vascular malformations, such as Klippel-Weber-Trenaunay syndrome, may involve the same limb. We suspect most such lesions have a deep cavernous component and are best considered verrucous hemangiomas.

Fordyce Angiokeratoma. Multiple, small, 3–5-mm papules appear on the scrotum or labia majora in middle-aged or elderly adults (Fig. 59.17). They are totally harmless. Except for their location, they are very similar to cherry angiomas and may represent the same process on an unusual site with exceptionally thin skin.

Metabolic Angiokeratomas. Fabry syndrome (Chap. 38) is also known as angiokeratoma corporis diffusum. The tiny angiokeratomas are often the first clue to the diagnosis. A number of other, even less common metabolic disorders may also be associated with angiokeratomas, as discussed under Fabry syndrome.

Pseudolymphomatous Angiokeratoma. This entity is covered in Chapter 60; it is most commonly seen on the extremities of children.

Glomus Tumor

(Masson 1924)

Synonym. Glomangioma

Definition. Benign vascular tumor arising from the contractile cells about the Sucquet-Hoyer canals.

Epidemiology. Solitary glomus tumors are uncommon, while the presence of multiple glomus tumors is usually inherited in an autosomal dominant pattern and is extremely rare.

Etiology and Pathogenesis. While the cause of glomus tumors is unknown, their smooth muscle origin fits with many of their clinical features. They are typically painful to touch, presumably because of contraction, reflecting their neuromuscular origins. Most are acral, since this is where Sucquet-Hoyer canals are most commonly found. The diffuse nature and usual lack of pain in multiple glo-

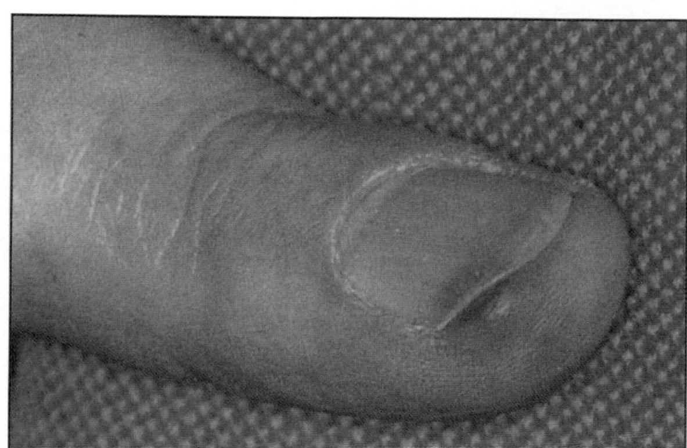

Fig. 59.18. Glomus tumor

mus tumors suggests that they may have a slightly different etiology.

Clinical Findings. The most common site for solitary glomus tumors is the digits, especially in a subungual location (Fig. 59.18). There is usually a 5 mm blue-violet nodule that is tender to touch and may be spontaneously painful. If subungual, there is frequently overlying nail dystrophy. The multiple lesions are usually larger, compressible, and not tender. Telangiectatic glomus tumors have also been described; they present as a plaque with matted telangiectases. Glomus tumors can be disseminated or follow Blaschko lines, and may appear on mucosal surfaces or in the gastrointestinal tract.

Histopathology. The epidermis is usually normal. In the dermis, a proliferation of cuboidal monotonous cells is arranged around a small vascular space. At first glance, one may also consider a melanocytic nevus or eccrine tumor. In solitary tumors, the vascular spaces may be subtle, while in the multiple form, there are usually large vascular channels; the latter form has also been designated glomangioma. Mast cells and nerve bundles may also be found. When prominent smooth muscle bundles abut the vessels, the term glomangiomyoma is used.

Differential Diagnosis. The clinical differential diagnosis includes all the painful tumors, reproduced as the mnemonic BENGAL in Table 59.1. Some nonpainful lesions may suggest a blue nevus or even a malignant melanoma. The main differential diagnosis for the multiple lesions is blue rubber bleb nevus syndrome; the distinction is histologic, but many suspect that the two disorders are quite similar.

Therapy. Excision is curative.

Table 59.1. Painful cutaneous tumors

B	Blue rubber bleb nevus
E	Eccrine tumors
N	Neural tumors
G	Glomus tumor
A	Angiolipoma
L	Leiomyoma

Benign Lymphatic Tumors

There are a series of related benign lymphatic proliferations all of which are more common in childhood and once again represent an overlap between a neoplasm and a malformation.

Superficial Lymphangioma

(Morris 1889)

Synonyms. Lymphangioma circumscriptum, lymphangioma circumscriptum cysticum

Etiology and Pathogenesis. Superficial lymphangioma is more common in girls and most often present at birth. It has been suggested that the lesion results because cutaneous lymphatics fail to acquire their essential deep connection. Sometimes the term lymphangiectasia is used when there is an underlying lymphatic obstruction. However, many extensive lymphangiomas in infancy show dilation or other abnormalities of the deep lymphatics, so this distinction may be artificial.

Clinical Findings. The most common locations are the oral mucosa, especially the tongue, and the proximal aspects of the limbs, groin, axillae, and trunk. The lesions are often compared to frog spawn, as they consist of many tiny, often clear vesicles, often in a herpetiform pattern. Larger lesions usually have at least some red-brown areas, suggesting either hemorrhage or an overlap with arteriovenous lesions (Fig. 59.19). Such lesions can be designated hematolymphangiomas. There may be verrucous secondary changes, once again reflecting the location of the vessels high in the dermis. Limb lesions may be associated with enlargement and other signs of severe vascular malformations, and thus such patients should be followed closely. Vulvar lymphangiomas have been described following recurrent cellulitis, Crohn disease, and radiation therapy, as well as lymphedema. Occasionally, small, otherwise typical

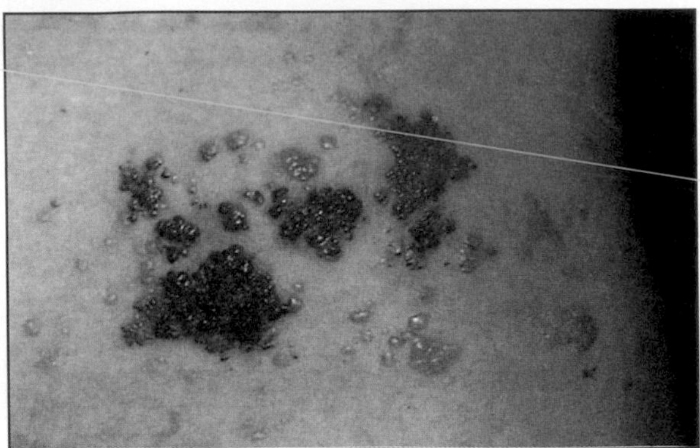

Fig. 59.19. Superficial hematolymphangioma

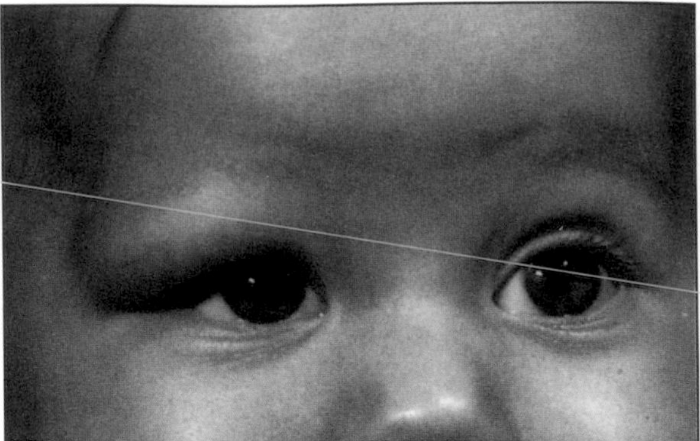

Fig. 59.20. Deep lymphangioma

lesions will develop spontaneously in an adult without any evidence of underlying lymphatic problems.

Histopathology. The key finding is the presence of large, dilated vascular spaces containing few erythrocytes but often thick proteinaceous material. The endothelial cells are variably positive for endothelial markers, so it is difficult to unequivocally separate a lymphatic from a dilated venule.

Differential Diagnosis. The main considerations are angiokeratomas and verrucous hemangiomas. The lesions may morphologically resemble herpes simplex or zoster but the course is different.

Therapy. Smaller lesions can be surgically excised. Larger lesions, especially those of the oral cavity, are extremely difficult to treat. Despite their name, most superficial lymphangiomas have a deep component that is responsible for the high recurrence rate.

Deep Lymphangioma

Synonyms. Lymphangioma cavernosum subcutaneum, cavernous lymphangioma

Etiology and Pathogenesis. These lesions arise from the deeper lymphatic cisterns but are otherwise similar to the more superficial forms. Cystic hygroma describes a deep lymphangioma of the neck, apparently representing failure of the jugular lymphatic sack to connect with the jugular vein. Cystic hygromas are more common in patients with Turner syndrome (XO females).

Clinical Findings. There is usually a compressible subcutaneous mass, most often present early in life. The most common site is the neck, but oral, periorbital, and other body sites may be involved (Fig. 59.20). Very large lesions can be transilluminated or punctured with a needle to aspirate lymphatic fluid. The overlying skin is usually normal. Once again, the feeder lymphatic channels may be abnormal, leading to hypertrophy of a limb.

Histopathology. The deep lymphangiomas have larger cavities, often associated with strands of smooth muscle. They may have a spongy appearance, with many small vessels, or be cystic.

Differential Diagnosis. If the lesions are large and translucent, one can guess at the diagnosis. Otherwise, the entire spectrum of soft tissue masses in children comes into play.

Therapy. Surgery is the only proven approach, although it is difficult. Attempts at intraluminal occlusion or destruction are worth considering if local expertise is available.

Lymphangiomatosis

In this rare condition, patients have multiple deep lymphangiomas involving not only the skin and soft tissue, but also bones and internal organs. The outlook depends on which organs are involved and how severe the changes are.

Acquired Progressive Lymphangioma

(Wilson Jones 1976)

Synonym. Lymphangioendothelioma

This rare disorder usually presents as a single, red-brown, slowly expanding macule or papule. It does not have the clinical features of other lymphangiomas and more closely resembles tufted angioma. Some cases appear in childhood. Rarely, radiation therapy has been identified as a triggering factor. Microscopic examination reveals an accumulation of thin-walled vascular spaces that dissect between bundles of collagen, closely resembling Kaposi sarcoma. Nonetheless, the clinical behavior is benign. We suspect it is a proliferation of vessels, having features of both venules and lymphatics, that awaits further clarification. Smaller lesions can be surgically excised; larger ones are problematic. Perhaps laser destruction is worth a try.

Malignant Vascular Tumors

We will first discuss the two major malignant vascular tumors and then list a number of much rarer tumors that appear to represent low-grade vascular malignancies.

Kaposi Sarcoma

(Kaposi 1872)

Synonym. Sarcoma idiopathicum multiplex hemorrhagicum

History. The story of Kaposi sarcoma is one of the most fascinating in recent medical history. In the past three decades, it has advanced from an odd indolent tumor on the extremities of elderly Mediterranean men to an aggressive, perhaps infectious childhood tumor in tropical Africa to a complication of iatrogenic immunosuppression to one of the most reliable cutaneous markers for HIV/AIDS.

Epidemiology. Table 59.2 summarizes the epidemiology of Kaposi sarcoma. Today, clearly HIV/AIDS is the main risk factor, but even within this patient group there are striking variances, as Kaposi sarcoma is common in homosexual men and rare in all other risk groups. In classic Kaposi sarcoma, there is at least a 15:1 male:female predilection, and most patients are Jews or Mediterranean Europeans.

Etiology and Pathogenesis. The exact cause of Kaposi sarcoma remains puzzling, but at least in HIV/AIDS patients, human herpes virus-8 plays a very important role. An infectious cause for Kaposi sarcoma has been suspected since Templeton's classic work in Africa documented the acute childhood form. The indolent changes in classic Kaposi sarcoma raised little suspicion of infection and still remain hard to explain. Another cause of puzzlement is the long-running argument regarding whether Kaposi sarcoma is a tumor or reactive process, since it can appear in several sites almost simultaneously and may regress, as for example when immunosuppression is reduced in a renal transplant patient. While intuitively we lean towards a reactive process, recent studies have shown clonality in many cases, supporting the diagnosis of malignancy. Finally, the arguments about whether Kaposi sarcoma arises from lymphatics or venules remains unclear. As with so many other vascular tumors, there appear to be too many overlaps to allow one to speak with certainty.

Table 59.2. Types of Kaposi sarcoma

Type	Risk group	Age group (years)
Classic	Elderly men of Jewish, Mediterranean extraction	50–80
Endemic	Blacks in Africa	
Nodular, aggressive, and florid	Adults	25–40
Lymphadenopathic	Children	2–15
Iatrogenic	Solid organ transplantation patients, rarely other types of immunosuppression	20–60
Epidemic (HIV/AIDS)	Homosexual men (95%)	20>

Clinical Findings

Classic Kaposi Sarcoma. The typical lesions of classic Kaposi sarcoma are innocent, slowly growing, livid macules and papules, almost always on the feet or shins (Fig. 59.21). Initially, there are red-brown macules that may be associated with edema. They slowly thicken, become indurated, and form coalescent plaques and nodules. New papules and nodules develop at the periphery, and the edema may become severe, producing elephantiasis-like changes. There are frequent hemorrhages, imparting a bruised color to some regions, while other areas are deep red to blue-black. Those on the soles are painful. The lesions may ulcerate, especially when exposed to trauma.

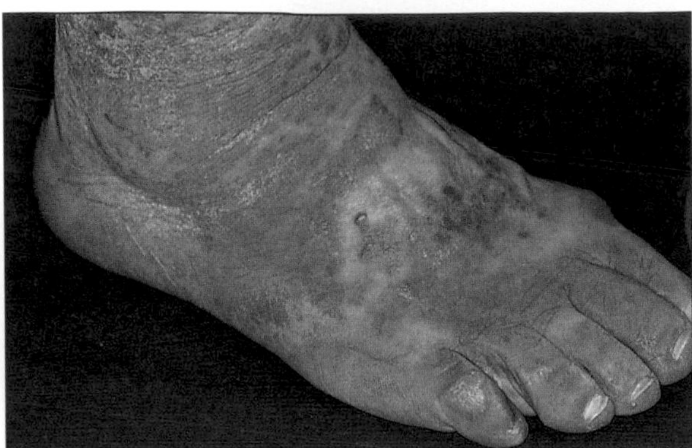

Fig. 59.21. Kaposi sarcoma

Over years or decades, lesions may appear on the thighs, genitalia, trunk, and even face. Mucosal lesions are distinctly rare, although internal involvement, primarily of the gastrointestinal tract, has been occasionally described. In addition, hepatic and splenic infiltrates may be seen. While most patients with classic Kaposi sarcoma die with their disease, those with internal involvement are at risk of dying from the process.

Endemic Kaposi Sarcoma. Kaposi sarcoma is probably the most common tumor in equatorial Africa, accounting for over 10 % of the malignancies in the few tumor registries. In adults, it is often considerably more aggressive than classic Kaposi sarcoma and takes three forms:

- Benign nodular: Similar to classic Kaposi sarcoma, but the lesions are likely to grow more rapidly and to be nodular.
- Aggressive: These patients suffer involvement not only of skin but also of underlying bone and muscle.
- Florid or disseminated: This resembles HIV/AIDS Kaposi sarcoma, with mucosal and systemic involvement.

In addition, there is the lymphopathic childhood Kaposi sarcoma, presenting with rapid onset of extensive cervical lymphadenopathy, not dissimilar to Burkitt lymphoma, and disseminating, which leads to a fatal outcome.

Surprisingly, Kaposi sarcoma is not a major problem in the many African and Asian patients now suffering from HIV/AIDS. Occasionally, patients in Mediterranean countries such as Israel or Greece are described who are HIV-negative but have aggressive mucocutaneous and internal Kaposi sarcoma. Their classification remains unclear.

Iatrogenic Kaposi Sarcoma. Patients who undergo solid organ transplantation and aggressive immunosuppression, usually with corticosteroids, azathioprine, and cyclosporine, may develop widespread Kaposi sarcoma. The lesions are usually macular and widespread, rather than being limited to the legs. They may appear months to years after starting immunosuppression and tend to regress or resolve if the medications can be reduced.

HIV/AIDS Kaposi Sarcoma. This problem is discussed and illustrated in detail in Chapter 2. Special attention should be paid to the frequent involvement of the oral mucosa and the numerous facial lesions, uncommon in other forms.

Histopathology. Until the early 1980s, histologic descriptions had concentrated on the nodular lesions of classic Kaposi sarcoma, which feature a dermal accumulation of spindle-shaped cells about vascular slits with intra- and extravascular erythrocytes, hemosiderin, and fibrosis. The spindle cells may have mitoses and other features of atypia, but these are generally scant and hard to identify. Usually, there is an associated plasma cell infiltrate. Often hyaline globules are seen, probably representing degenerated erythrocytes. Fortunately, Ackerman, a dermatopathologist with a special interest in Kaposi sarcoma, was involved in studying many of the early patients with HIV/AIDS Kaposi sarcoma. He and his colleagues pointed out the features of early Kaposi sarcoma including tenuous vascular slits insinuating about preexisting vessels, adnexal structures, and between strands of collagen. Plasma cells and hemosiderin-laden macrophages also appear early. In some instances, the periphery of definite lesions of Kaposi sarcoma may mimic pyogenic granuloma with a lobular pattern or lymphangioma with large dilated spaces.

Laboratory Findings. A variety of techniques have been utilized to search for internal involvement in Kaposi sarcoma. Endoscopy, computed tomography, and a variety of nucleotide scans, often using technetium, appear most helpful.

Course and Prognosis. The outlook varies with the clinical setting. Classic Kaposi sarcoma is usually just a nuisance, unless extensive internal involvement develops. Endemic Kaposi sarcoma is generally fatal, while the HIV/AIDS form may be disfiguring and interfere with eating.

Differential Diagnosis. The differential diagnosis is extensive. Classic Kaposi sarcoma can be mistaken for dermatofibromas, severe stasis dermatitis, acroangiodermatitis (pseudo-Kaposi sarcoma), and other benign hemangiomas. In the event of extensive limb edema, the clinical appearance may be identical to Stewart-Treves syndrome. The multiple lesions of iatrogenic Kaposi sarcoma can be mistaken for multiple leiomyomas because of the grouping and red-brown color.

Therapy. Therapy is detailed in Chapter 2. The same principles can be applied to any type of disseminated Kaposi sarcoma. Local lesions can be treated with surgery, low-dose ionizing radiation (20–30 Gy in ten divided doses), or intralesional alkaloids. X-ray works especially well for plantar lesions.

Angiosarcoma

(Livingston and Klemperer 1926; Stewart and Treves 1948)

Synonyms. Hemangiosarcoma, lymphangiosarcoma, malignant hemangioendothelioma

Epidemiology. Angiosarcomas are extremely rare. There are three clinical settings in which they involve the skin.

- Spontaneous: Insidious tumor on the face or scalp of elderly individuals, most often men.
- Edematous postmastectomy limbs: This is known as Stewart-Treves syndrome and occurs in perhaps 0.5% of women with postsurgical lymphedema who survive for at least 5 years after their breast carcinoma. The malignant change may appear long after the initial surgery, sometimes after two decades. Rarely, lesions arise in other lymphedematous limbs.
- Postradiation: Angiosarcomas are an extremely rare complication of ionizing radiation. They have most often been described in irradiated hemangiomas but presumably can occur in any clinical setting.

In addition, there are angiosarcomas of the deep soft tissue and female breast. The latter are particularly subtle and rapidly fatal.

Etiology and Pathogenesis. The term angiosarcoma is preferred, as it is impossible in most cases to determine the exact origin of such tumors, and all appear similar microscopically. They are usually sufficiently dedifferentiated that special marker studies do not resolve the issue of cell of origin. In addition to the two most obvious triggers of lymphedema and ionizing radiation, angiosarcomas have been associated with DNA repair defects (for example, xeroderma pigmentosum), immunosuppression, chronic trauma (such as persistent ulcers or burn scars), radioactivity (use of Thorotrast, an obsolete radioactive contrast material containing thorium), and chemical carcinogens (arsenic among others).

Clinical Findings. The classic angiosarcoma of the face and scalp is often diagnosed quite late because initially it appears so innocent. It presents as a slowly expanding, red or violet patch which may be mistaken for a bruise or hemangioma (Fig. 59.22). For years it continues to expand and develops nodular areas and even ulcerations.

In Stewart-Treves syndrome, there is diffuse persistent edema of the involved limb, making a diagnosis difficult. Once again, livid macules are usually seen first, and by the time they have become clinically apparent nodules, the disease is usually widespread (Fig. 59.23). In angiosarcomas associat-

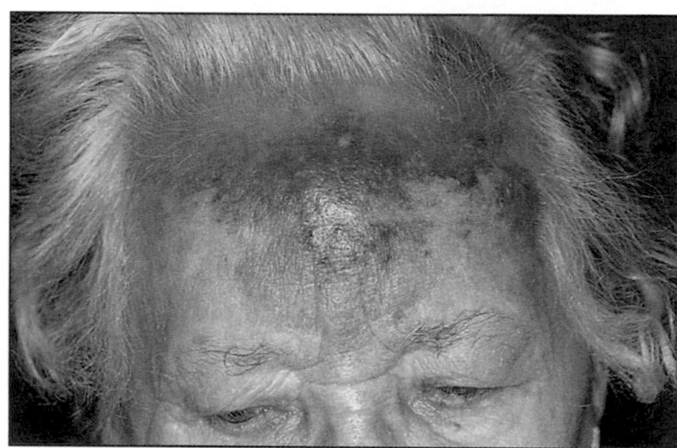

Fig. 59.22. Angiosarcoma

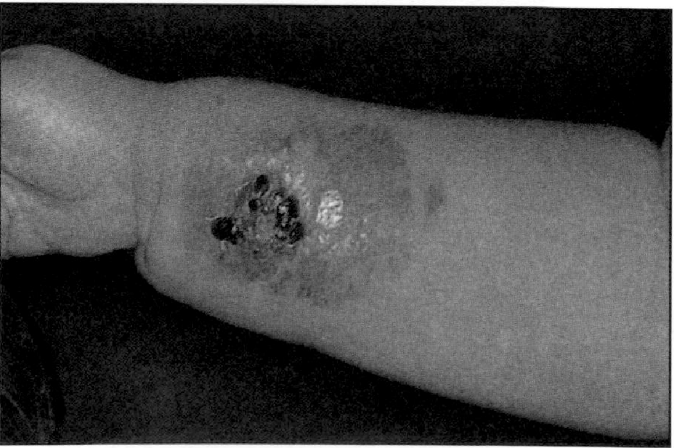

Fig. 59.23. Stewart-Treves syndrome; angiosarcoma in edematous limb postmastectomy

ed with radiation or trauma, there is a nodular reactive change in a radiation, surgical, or burn scar.

Histopathology. Angiosarcomas can have many appearances under the microscope. There may be cellular areas that are obviously malignant with pleomorphic cells, multiple mitoses, and irregular vascular channels. Some tumor cells may have cytoplasmic vacuoles recapitulating primitive lumen formation. Often at the periphery there are irregular vascular channels insinuating between strands of collagen with atypical but scarce endothelial cells. Other regions may resemble Kaposi sarcoma or pyogenic granuloma.

Course and Prognosis. The outlook is dismal in all cases.

Differential Diagnosis. Angiosarcoma of the face and scalp is often mistaken early on for a bruise or benign vascular proliferation. In Stewart-Treves syndrome, the main differential diagnostic consideration is metastatic breast carcinoma. Kaposi sarcoma may also be associated with extensive edema.

Therapy. The lesions of the head usually extend far beyond the clinically visible or palpable margins. Thus, extensive surgery is required, but often clear margins simply cannot be obtained. Radiation therapy and complex chemotherapy regimens may buy time but are rarely curative. In Stewart-Treves syndrome, there is little hope; sometimes amputation is performed, along with radiation and chemotherapy, but these patients often have already undergone both for their breast carcinoma and may tolerate therapy poorly.

Other Malignant Vascular Tumors

There are a series of probably malignant vascular tumors, all of which are rare, which we will only mention briefly. Hemangioendothelioma has become accepted as a designation for vascular tumors with a low risk of malignant behavior. There is no logical linguistic explanation for this choice. Probably, all these tumors should have originally been designated low-grade angiosarcomas.

Spindle Cell Hemangioendothelioma
(Weiss and Enzinger 1986)

This tumor usually arises in Mafucci syndrome or Klippel-Weber-Trenaunay syndrome. Thus, in most instances it probably represents a reactive process associated with abnormal local blood flow. When the underlying vascular process is treated, regression may occur. The tumors have spindle cell areas resembling Kaposi sarcoma but without atypia or hyaline globules. In addition, there are usually larger vascular spaces often with thrombi and associated with smooth muscle. The one often reported example of malignant degeneration occurred in a patient with Mafucci syndrome, who already had an underlying risk of malignancy and was irradiated.

Endovascular Papillary Hemangioendothelioma
(Dabska 1969)

Synonym. Dabska tumor

This rare low-grade angiosarcoma is seen almost exclusively in children. It is often present at birth as a deep soft tissue tumor but may also involve the skin. The hallmark of the tumor is extensive vascular channels lined by prominent endothelial cells with papillary projections into the lumen. Lymphocytes are usually associated with the tumors. Although lymph node metastases have been described, no deaths have been reported.

Epithelioid Hemangioendothelioma
(Weiss and Enzinger 1982)

These lesions usually involve soft tissue and bone, but may occur in the skin. The solitary primary skin tumors appear benign, while those associated with bone tumors are usually locally aggressive. Although metastases have been reported, the tumors are less virulent than a conventional angiosarcoma. The tumor is often not diagnosed immediately as a vascular lesion because of the presence of plump epithelioid cells in a fibrous or myxoid stroma. Vascular spaces are uncommon, but cytoplasmic vacuole formation (primitive vascular channels) may be seen.

Retiform Hemangioendothelioma
(Calonje et al. 1994)

This tumor usually involves the skin or subcutaneous tissue, presenting with slowly growing plaques or nodules. Some cases have been associated with chronic lymphedema or ionizing radiation. Microscopically, there are complex arborizing vascular patterns resembling the rete testis. In addition, the endothelial cells are prominent, often projecting into the lumen in the hobnail pattern. Again, there is often an intense lymphocytic infiltrate.

Glomangiosarcoma

Malignant glomus tumors are extremely rare. They may arise in glomus tumors or de novo. The usual course is locally aggressive behavior, sometimes associated with an infiltrative pattern under the microscope. In rare instances, distant metastases have been reported.

Kaposiform Hemangioendothelioma
(TSANG and CHAN 1991)

This rare, distinctive, vascular neoplasm occurs in children. It is usually found in the deep soft tissues, especially the retroperitoneum, but may be seen in the skin. The tumor can be locally aggressive but has not been reported to metastasize. Most cases of Kasabach-Merritt syndrome actually arise in this rare neoplasm. There may be associated lymphangiomatosis, but the lesions are clinically separate. Under the microscope, there is once again a nodular pattern with spindled endothelial cells lining slit-like spaces. In the absence of an appropriate history, it may be hard to exclude Kaposi sarcoma, but the latter is very rare in children (except in the endemic African form in which it presents with lymphadenopathy).

Hemangiopericytoma
(STOUT and MURRAY 1942)

If there is a tumor more confusing than hemangiopericytoma, we have yet to encounter it. We mention it only for the sake of completeness. The original concept of hemangiopericytoma was a low-grade malignant tumor arising from the pericytes. Two forms were described: an adult form arising in the deep soft tissues of young adults, and an infantile form found in the subcutaneous tissues of the head and neck. The latter lesions have been reclassified as part of the spectrum of infantile myofibromatosis. Many experts feel that a variety of sarcomas in adults may have a hemangiopericytoma-like pattern. The key microscopic features are dense accumulations of poorly defined tumor cells surrounding highly irregular, often stag horn-like, vessels. Our advice is to leave this diagnosis to soft tissue tumor experts and to not expect to find such lesions in the skin.

Tumors of Fat

Lipoma

Epidemiology. Ordinary lipomas are one of the most common tumors. Almost every individual has one or more. They account for over 99% of the fatty tumors seen in most practices. Often there is a positive family history of lipomas. In some pedigrees, multiple lipomas appear to be inherited in an autosomal dominant pattern.

Etiology and Pathogenesis. The cause of lipomas is unknown. They tend not to respond to ordinary metabolic fat control; that is, when a patient starves, they only poorly mobilize their lipoma fat stores. Thus, one can view lipomas as poorly regulated areas of fat, rather than as true tumors. Lipomas can also develop after systemic corticosteroid or anti-retroviral therapy, but in this instance the fatty growths are usually mediastinal, pericardial, or epidural.

Clinical Findings. Lipomas are poorly defined tumors usually lying between the skin and subcutaneous fascia. They are most common on the shoulders, over the ribs, on the back, and on the extensor surfaces of the forearms. Some patients may have multiple lesions (Fig. 59.24). Lipomas have a thin capsule and a lobular or slightly bumpy surface, which distinguishes them from cysts. They are usually compressible and can be pushed about slightly. Some lesions, usually larger ones, are painful, perhaps because they trap a nerve. In addition, angiolipomas are usually painful, so this histologic diagnosis can be suspected clinically. Lesions may achieve an enormous size; the litera-

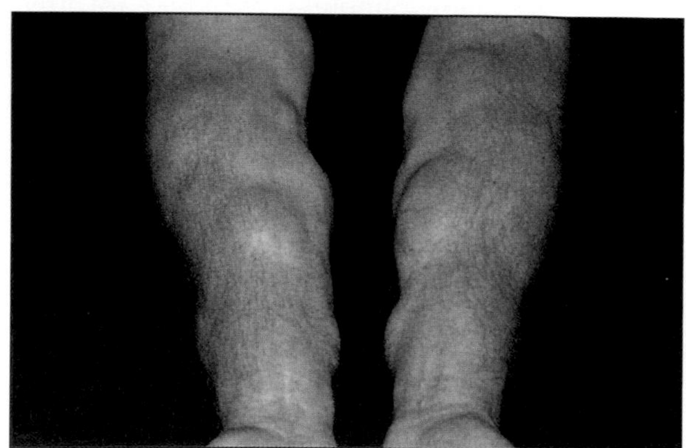

Fig. 59.24. Multiple lipomas

ture describes tumors weighing more than 25 kg. When lipomas are present over the spinal column, one should suspect an underlying defect and proceed accordingly.

Histopathology. Microscopically, one finds a thin or fragmented connective tissue capsule surrounding normal fat cells. Often the capsule is lost during surgery, and one is confronted simply with normal fat. There are several histologic variants described below.

Differential Diagnosis. While any subcutaneous tumor can be confused with a lipoma, usually they are clinically distinct. Cysts have a central pore if one searches carefully and a smoother surface; in addition, they have a capsule. Deep neurofibromas may be quite similar, as may myxoid tumors. Occasionally, metastases are confused, but they arise suddenly and are usually multiple. If any questions exist, excision and microscopic study will settle the question.

Therapy. Surgery is the answer. Often a small lipoma can be teased through a modest incision. In addition, liposuction can be employed. Tumescent anesthesia is a convenient way to approach a large number of lipomas.

Lipoma Variants

There are a number of variants of lipomas, identified either clinically or histologically. In all instances, the differential diagnosis is that of subcutaneous masses, and surgery is curative.

Angiolipoma

The hallmark of angiolipomas is that they are often painful. In addition, they are usually located on the extremities or trunk. Quite often multiple lesions are present. Microscopic examination reveals normal fat admixed with groups of small vessels, some of which usually contain fibrin thrombi. Mast cells are also increased in number.

Mobile Encapsulated Lipoma

Some lipomas, usually located on the extensor surfaces of the forearms, are small, firm, marble-like lesions that can be moved several centimeters, sliding along between the skin and subcutaneous tissue. Under the microscope, they have a distinct capsule and may show necrosis.

Subfascial Lipoma

Lipomas on the forehead, just along the hairline, often penetrate or lie beneath the fascia. They are difficult to diagnose and to remove. Because of their deep location and lack of mobility, they are often interpreted as bony lesions. When confronted by fascia, the unsuspecting surgeon may be reluctant to explore more deeply, but this is required to remove such lipomas.

Spindle Cell Lipoma

Most of these lipomas are found on the nape of older men. There is a fibrous stroma admixed with small foci of fat and scattered spindle cells. Some lesions may be quite vascular.

Pleomorphic Lipoma

A tumor of adults, pleomorphic lipoma is also more common in the shoulder girdle area. Microscopically, it contains mature fat, myxoid stroma, multinucleated giant cells with marginally placed nuclei (floret giant cell cells), and foci of lymphocytes. The unusual cytologic features may suggest a liposarcoma, but mitoses are uncommon.

Other Fatty Tumors

Nevus Lipomatosus

Nevus lipomatosus is considered among nevi (Chapter 52). It is characterized by high dermal accumulations of fat, usually presenting as a grouping of nodules about the buttocks of young women.

Painful Piezogenic Papule

These painful nodules are herniations of fat between the fascia along the sides of the heels (Chap. 19).

Hibernoma

Hibernoma are fatty tumors of young adults, usually found about the axillae or scapula. They consist of brown fat which microscopically has mulberry-like cells with multiloculated cytoplasm. Brown fat is more commonly found in hibernating mammals and neonates. The exact relation of this tumor to normal brown fat is unclear.

Lipoblastoma

(JAFFE 1926; VELLIOS et al. 1958)

This rare tumor of infants and small children is felt to be derived from fetal white fat. It may be localized or more diffuse (lipoblastomatosis). Under the microscope, mature fat is found admixed with lipoblasts and a myxoid or fibrous stroma. Lipoblasts may have multiple fat vacuoles and are more likely to have central rather than eccentric nuclei.

Lipomatosis

There are a number of conditions in which multiple lipomas are found. In most cases, a patient simply has lots of lipomas without associated diseases. Multiple lipomas are more common in men than in women and can be inherited in an autosomal dominant pattern. In some instances, the multiple lipomas may reflect a hamartomatous disease such as Gardner syndrome or Proteus syndrome.

Dercum Disease

(DERCUM 1888)

Synonym. Adipositas dolorosa, adiposalgia, lipalgia

Etiology and Pathogenesis. The cause of Dercum disease is unknown. In some instances, the lipomas represent herniations of fat through fascial defects with secondary incarceration and necrosis. More superficial true lipomas can become painful, but there is no good explanation for this.

Clinical Findings. Dercum disease is usually seen in menopausal women, who have multiple, exquisitely painful lipomas. The most common sites are the trunk and distal parts of the extremities. The pain tends to follow a cyclic pattern. The overlying skin can be slightly discolored, with a violet tint. The pain may be disabling. Most patients also have psychological problems, but it is difficult to say which aspect appeared first.

Histopathology. The fat deposits are normal; only rarely are inflammatory changes seen.

Therapy. Individual lesions can be excised. Otherwise the patient is a good candidate for a pain control clinic as few individual practitioners have the fortitude to manage such a difficult and demanding problem.

Benign Symmetric Lipomatosis

(MADELUNG 1888; LAUNOIS and BENSAUDE 1898)

Synonyms. Madelung disease, Launois-Bensaude disease

Definition. Localized striking increase in fat deposits leading to altered body habitus.

Epidemiology. Benign symmetric lipomatosis is primarily a disease of middle-aged men, often suffering from alcoholism. The age of onset ranges from 30 years to 60 years, and the male:female ratio is about 13:1.

Etiology and Pathogenesis. The cause is unknown, but there appear to be definite disturbances in lipocyte metabolism, as lipolysis is inhibited.

Clinical Findings. There is a striking increase in the fatty tissue about the neck, shoulder girdle, or abdomen in patients who are otherwise not obese. The increase may be so severe as to be disfiguring and cause great emotional damage. Three subtypes have been described, according to the location of the fat.

- Type I: Neck (Madelung disease; known in German as *Fetthals* or fat neck)
- Type II: Shoulders (pseudoathletic type; Fig. 59.25)
- Type III: Abdomen (gynecogenic)

In addition, many patients have hepatic disease, diabetes mellitus, polyneuropathy, gynecomastia, hyperuricemia, and lipid abnormalities. It is always difficult to determine the cause and effect relationship.

Therapy. Liposuction or surgery can be tried, but gradual recurrences are the rule. Particularly distressing to patients is the need for specially tailored clothes to help conceal the grotesque body contours.

Encephalocraniocutaneous Lipomatosis

This may be a variant of Proteus syndrome (Chap. 19) or a distinct entity. Patients present in infancy with facial and scalp lipomas, CNS lipomas, mental retardation, and many other problems.

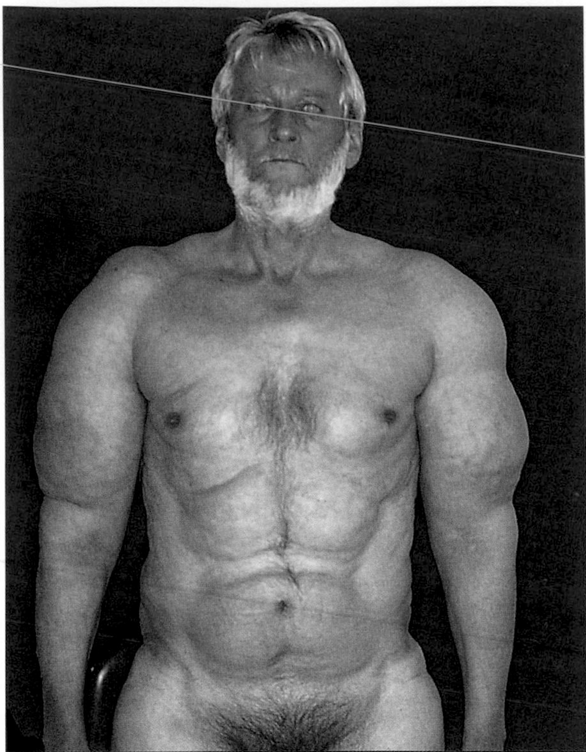

Fig. 59.25. Benign symmetric lipomatosis; pseudoathletic type

Liposarcomas

Liposarcomas are among the most common soft tissue sarcomas, but they are found increasingly rarely in the skin. They typically arise in the soft tissue of the thighs and pelvic girdle. When they involve the skin, it is usually by upward spread. They do not appear to develop from preexisting lipomas. Four histologic patterns have been described: well-differentiated, myxoid, round cell, and pleomorphic. The former two are more likely to be seen in the skin. They can be bland and easily overlooked under the microscope. Once the diagnosis has been made, generous surgical excision is the major treatment. Postoperative radiation and chemotherapy may be considered for high-risk lesions.

Tumors of Muscle

Muscle tumors are relatively uncommon in the skin. Most contain smooth muscle, which is not surprising as there are numerous normal smooth muscle bundles associated with cutaneous structures. In contrast, striated muscle is found only near the skin of the face, in the muscles of facial expression and lids.

Leiomyoma

Etiology and Pathogenesis. Leiomyomas may arise from the smooth muscle of the hair (arrector pili), scrotum (dartos), nipple and blood vessels.

Clinical Findings. Pilar leiomyomas (or piloleiomyomas) are more often multiple than single. They may be inherited in an autosomal dominant fashion. Typically, they are small, oval, red-brown tumors distributed in a follicular pattern, most common on the extensor surfaces of the limbs, as well as the face and trunk (Fig. 59.26). They may be painful and are often tender when touched or stroked, as muscle contraction is initiated. Most are about 1 cm in size. Sometimes they are confined to a segmental pattern, suggesting a somatic mutation. The less common solitary lesion is often larger and deeper, but less likely to be painful. In some studies, an association has been made with uterine leiomyomas. A fascinating complication is that some of the tumors produce erythropoietin, causing polycythemia. The genital lesions are quite uncommon, presenting as nodules on the scrotum, or less often the labia majora or nipple. They are usually solitary and not painful.

Histopathology. All lesions are identical, consisting of nonencapsulated bundles of spindle-shaped cells centered in the mid-dermis. The cells have cigar-shaped nuclei with blunt ends, as compared to the cells of a neural tumor. The fascicles interlace, and those cut in cross-section often have a vesicular cytoplasm. In the piloleiomyomas, hair follicle rem-

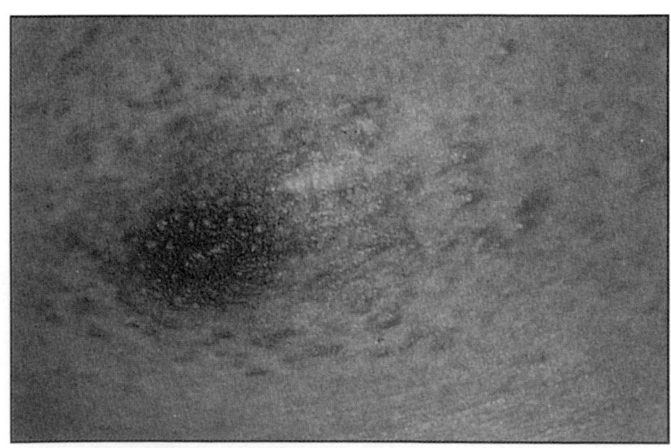

Fig. 59.26. Multiple leiomyomas

nants may be found among the tumor cells. The diagnosis can be confirmed by immunohistochemistry, as smooth muscle actin and desmin may be positive, while neural stains are negative.

Differential Diagnosis. Multiple lesions are usually clinically distinct. An individual lesion may be confused with a Spitz nevus or mast cell tumor if the red-brown color is present. In the absence of the pigmentary changes, one should consider the list of painful tumors.

Therapy. Excision is the best treatment. When multiple lesions are present and painful, calcium channel blockers or α-adrenergic blockers can be tried.

Angioleiomyoma

These tumors are usually solitary nodules found on the legs of middle-aged patients; women are more commonly involved than men. They, too, may be painful or tender when stroked. They appear to arise from the smooth muscle of a vein in most cases. Under the microscope, there is a well-circumscribed or encapsulated tumor; the capsule is the original vessel wall. The bulk of the tumor consists of interlacing sheets and strands of smooth muscle cells, admixed with small blood vessels. Excision is curative.

Smooth Muscle Hamartoma

This rare congenital lesion presents as a flesh-colored or hyperpigmented plaque on the trunk or extremities. When the lesion is stroked, goose bumps may arise through the contraction of the muscle fibers; this is known as pseudo-Darier sign. In some instances, hairs are prominent; we consider smooth muscle hamartoma and Becker nevus (Chap. 58) as part of a spectrum. In one instance, widespread smooth muscle hamartomas were associated with the Michelin tire baby syndrome (Chap. 52). Microscopic evaluation reveals discrete, clearly defined bundles of smooth muscle fibers admixed with the dermal stroma. In contrast to leiomyoma, the bundles are better organized and more closely resemble normal arrector pili. The presence of basal layer hypermelanosis supports the overlap with Becker nevus. The lesions are usually too large to be conveniently excised, but have no malignant potential.

Leiomyosarcoma

Etiology and Pathogenesis. Dermal leiomyosarcomas presumably arise from the arrector pili muscles, although malignant change in leiomyomas must be extremely rare. Other subcutaneous and deep leiomyosarcomas may reach the skin by upward spread, but are rarely diagnosed by dermatologists.

Clinical Findings. The superficial leiomyosarcoma is usually a slowly growing, often red-brown nodule on the extremities or trunk. It may be painful and usually is larger than a leiomyoma, frequently reaching several centimeters in diameter. Some may be painful, and most have spread into the subcutaneous tissue by the time of diagnosis.

Histopathology. Leiomyosarcomas are more cellular than leiomyomas, more likely to enter the fat, and have an increased mitotic rate.

Course and Prognosis. Superficial leiomyosarcomas have a good prognosis. They may recur locally but do not metastasize. In contrast, subcutaneous and deep leiomyosarcomas behave like all other sarcomas and are potentially fatal.

Therapy. Local excision with generous margins is usually curative. If anatomic considerations allow, a 2–3 cm margin is probably wise.

Rhabdomyoma

Cutaneous tumors with skeletal muscle differentiation are very rare. Striated muscle may be found in congenital malformations, such as associated with accessory tragi (Chap. 19) or other branchial arch anomalies (Chap. 53). Rarely, solitary papules or nodules composed of striated muscle will appear in adults, usually on the face where relatively superficial striated muscles are normally present. Cardiac rhabdomyomas are the most common deep rhabdomyomas and a marker for tuberous sclerosis (Chap. 19). Diagnosis is based on the presence of striated muscle fibers, as well as positive staining for muscle-specific actin but negative staining for smooth muscle actin. Simple excision suffices for the cutaneous lesions.

Striated Muscle Hamartoma

Synonym. Rhabdomyomatous mesenchymal hamartoma

Most striated muscle hamartomas are solitary, dome-shaped or pedunculated nodules on the face clinically identified as congenital skin tags. They usually appear in sites where normal skeletal muscle is superficially located, such as around the mouth or over the platysma. A unique feature is that they may show spontaneous motion. Under the microscope, striated muscle is found admixed with normal cutaneous structures. Patients with multiple hamartomas of this type may have oculocerebrocutaneous syndrome (Chap. 19).

Rhabdomyosarcoma

Malignant striated muscle tumors are the most common sarcoma of childhood. They usually involve the head and neck region, retroperitoneum, genitalia, or pelvic girdle. The most common subtype is the embryonal form, seen in infants and young children, usually found on the head and neck region. The botryoid form is an exophytic variant of the embryonal rhabdomyosarcoma involving the genitourinary tract. The alveolar type in adolescents and the pleomorphic type in adults favor the trunk and extremities. In rare cases, rhabdomyosarcomas may present in the skin as dermal nodules often on the face. Treatment with surgery, radiation therapy, and often chemotherapy has improved the outlook.

Cutaneous Ossification

Cutaneous bone formation is an unusual event. Bone may form in the skin in the absence of an explainable cause; this is referred to as a primary osteoma cutis. More often, it develops in an area of trauma, chronic inflammation, and scarring, presumably as a result of altered fibroblast differentiation, known as secondary osteoma cutis. Often a nidus of calcification serves as the trigger. Bone in the skin is frequently associated with fat and even with hematopoietic elements, thus often resembling bone marrow. Probably the term heterotopic ossification is more accurate, suggesting that the skin can be a suitable location for bone formation when mesenchymal cells receive the wrong signals regarding bone manufacture. Therapy will not be discussed here, as it is similar in all cases – surgical removal.

Primary Ossification

Albright Hereditary Osteodystrophy
(Albright 1942)

Synonym. Pseudohypoparathyroidism

This is not a single disorder, but probably a group of diseases. Many different patterns of inheritance have been described; the best documented is autosomal dominant transmission. There is a defect in the G-protein system encoded by the gene *GNAS1* on chromosome 20q13. This mutation leads to end-organ lack of responsiveness to parathyroid hormone (PTH) and occasionally other hormones. The patients have short stature, brachydactyly (especially of the fourth and fifth digits, knuckle-knuckle-dimple-dimple sign), hypocalcemia, elevated PTH levels, and parathyroid gland hyperplasia. They may present with subtle morphologic changes and cutaneous osteomas prior to having metabolic problems. The osteomas are small, movable, subcutaneous masses that can be identified with imaging studies, ultrasonography, or biopsy. In addition, the deranged calcium and phosphorus metabolism may predispose patients to cutaneous calcification. In pseudopseudohypoparathyroidism, the same morphologic changes are present, but the parathyroid disease is absent, and the calcium metabolism is normal. Thus, the calcium disorder is not a sine qua non for the formation of osteomas.

Plate-Like Cutaneous Osteoma
(Worret and Burgdorf 1978)

This rare problem is usually seen in infants but can occur later in life. A sheet of bone develops between the skin and subcutaneous tissue. It is clinically distinct and can be easily identified on radiologic examination. Often the plate of bone lies over a joint and may restrict motion. The term progressive osseous heteroplasia has been used to describe this change by orthopedic surgeons who have encountered patients literally encased in an exoskeleton of membranous bone. No satisfactory treatment exists.

Fibrodysplasia Ossificans Progressiva

Synonym. Myositis ossificans

This rare disorder is inherited in an autosomal dominant pattern. Aggressive fibroblast proliferation is associated with heterotopic bone formation. Patients develop multiple tender nodules attached to tendons and ligaments, as well as within muscles. The nodules may appear at sites of trauma but are usually spontaneous. The lesions calcify and then go on to become bony nodules or plates. Hallus valgus present at birth is often the first clue. Antiinflammatory regimens such as systemic corticosteroids or interferons may reduce the inflammatory phase, while biphosphonates appear to help prevent new bone formation. Plate-like cutaneous osteomas may represent a superficial mild variant of this severe disease.

Ossifying Fasciitis

(DaRoca et al. 1982)

This rare disorder has been viewed as an ossifying variant of nodular fasciitis or a superficial variant of fibrodysplasia ossificans progressiva. Typically, there is a single nodule located in the subcutaneous tissue with an admixture of myofibroblastic cells and new bone. Excision is curative.

Subungual Exostosis

Although it is often designated as an osteoma, the subungual exostosis (Chap. 37) is almost always connected to the underlying bone, usually on the great toe. Surgical removal, including curettage of the digit to remove the bony protuberance, is curative. Elements of both cartilage and mature bone are typically found in the surgical specimen.

Idiopathic Osteoma Cutis

Rarely, an osteoma will appear in normal skin in a patient with no metabolic disturbances or history of trauma. Most such cases are congenital, but occasionally the process will occur in an adult.

Secondary Cutaneous Ossification

The main causes of secondary ossification are tumors, trauma, chronic inflammation, and scarring. Of the tumors, pilomatricoma, basal cell carcinoma, and melanocytic nevus are most likely to ossify. Such nevi are known as a nevus of Nanta; for unknown reasons, they appear almost exclusively on the face. A long list of other adnexal and fibrous tumors may also ossify. Bone found in scars is peculiar. Among surgical scars, the highest risk is in vertical midline scars; the chunks of bone develop invariably either near the xiphoid or the pubic bone, not somewhere in the middle.

Multiple tiny osteomas develop in some acne patients. They appear as small white nodules that are initially mistaken for milia. If the patient is on minocycline, the lesions may have a bluish discoloration and fluoresce under Wood light examination. Rare patients with multiple facial osteomas deny having had acne; their problem awaits explanation. Patients with chronic venous insufficiency may develop phleboliths which then ossify. Bone formation has also been described in morphea and CREST syndrome and may be seen in any disorder with cutaneous calcification (Chap. 45).

Tumors of Bone and Cartilage

All tumors of bone and cartilage only extremely rarely involve the skin. Extraskeletal chondromas are usually acral and benign. Both chondroblastomas and osteoblastomas, although usually benign, may occasionally involve the skin directly or very rarely as metastases. Chondrosarcomas only reach the skin as metastases. Similarly, osteosarcomas are also very rare in the skin, although scattered primary cutaneous osteosarcomas have been described. They may develop in heterotopic bone after many years. If one identifies bone in a cutaneous metastasis, the most likely explanation is secondary ossification in a metastatic carcinoma, rather than an osteosarcoma.

Chordoma

(Luschka 1856)

Chordomas are rare soft tissue tumors that arise from notochord remnants. They are most common in the sacral region or at the base of the skull. They are tumors of adults, typically slowly growing, painful, and locally destructive. Skin involvement is almost always the result of direct local spread and thus limited to the regions of predilection. Rarely, distant metastases may arise, and they too may involve the skin. Microscopically, the cells are large, polygonal, and often vacuolated in a mucoid matrix. The term physaliphorous is used to describe these cells; it comes from the Greek for bubble-bearing. Chordomas are usually positive for S100, keratin, and vimentin. A parachordoma is similar but develops adjacent to tendon, synovium, or bone in a site where the notochord was not present; it presumably represents dedifferentiation of a mesenchymal stem cell. Parachordoma has the same staining profile and behavior pattern. Radical wide excision is the recommended therapy.

Benign Neural Tumors

The exact classification of neural tumors remains confusing. Most are felt to arise from the nerve sheath, but the relative contribution of Schwann cells and perineural cells remains under discussion. In true neuromas, axons also appear. Both S100 and myelin basic protein stains are positive, but they do not help to clarify the histogenesis. Congenital malformations with ectopic nerves include nasal glioma and cutaneous meningioma (Chap. 19).

Neuroma

A neuroma is a nerve sheath tumor in which both axons and Schwann cells are roughly equally represented. They are uncommon but may be associated with trauma, rudimentary polydactyly, or even multiple endocrine neoplasia (MEN) IIB. Traumatic neuromas are most common; they are found as painful nodules in amputation stumps or at sites of injury. Neuromas on the lateral aspect of the hand or foot at the base of the fifth digit are felt to represent rudimentary digits that have undergone autoamputation. The mucosal neuromas in MEN IIB may have ganglion cells (large polyhedral cells with vesicular nuclei); in addition, the facial skin may contain thickened nerves (dermal hyperneury).

Pacinian Corpuscle Hyperplasia

Synonym. Pacinioma

These painful digital lumps may be confused with digital neuromas. They too may be associated with trauma. There may be either enlarged Pacinian corpuscles or an increased number of the mechanoreceptors. Simple excision is curative. Other neural tumors may also have the sliced onion appearance of a Pacinian corpuscle along with varying degrees of myxoid change. They have received a bewildering array of names, which we will avoid listing here.

Palisaded and Encapsulated Neuroma

(Reed et al. 1972)

This uncommon tumor usually presents as a solitary mass on the face of middle-aged patients. It has a fine capsule or is at least well-separated from the adjacent dermis. Fascicles of neurons intertwine together. There is palisading or orderly arrangement of the nuclei in some areas of the tumor. The bundles when cut in cross-section do not show the cytoplasmic clarity seen in leiomyoma.

Neurilemmoma

(Stout 1935)

Synonym. Schwannoma

Most neurilemmomas are solitary tumors found on the limbs of adults. Many are painful. In rare instances, multiple lesions may be present; this condition has been diagnosed as neurilemmomatosis or schwannomatosis (Chap. 19). On gross examination, the well-encapsulated tumor often shows signs of attachment to a fragment of nerve. The hallmark of the tumors is the presence of two distinct tissue types: Antoni A tissue is cellular with palisading of nuclei and eosinophilic masses known as Verocay bodies, while Antoni B tissue is myxoid with scattered neural cells. Prominent thick-walled vessels are also a clue to the diagnosis. Many histologic variants of neurilemmomas have been described but are of limited clinical utility, since most refer to changes found in deeper neurilemmomas associated with major nerve trunks. The psammomatous melanotic schwannoma is a marker for Carney syndrome (Chap. 58).

Neurofibroma

Epidemiology. Neurofibromas are the most common cutaneous neural tumors. When multiple, they are one of the striking markers for neurofibromatosis (Chap. 19). Solitary neurofibromas carry no such diagnostic significance.

Clinical Findings. Neurofibromas are usually molluscoid nodules that rise above the skin surface but which can be pushed back into the skin, much like a lesion of anetoderma. In other instances, they may be large, firm, or pedunculated nodules. In neurofibromatosis, some lesions feel like a bag of worms in the subcutaneous tissue; these plexiform neurofibromas are histologically distinct and have a malignant potential.

Histopathology. Typical neurofibromas have a loose arrangement of spindle cells in a pale stroma. The cells have wavy, sharply pointed nuclei. The tumors are not encapsulated, but there is usually a distinct Grenz zone beneath the epidermis. The stroma is often rich in mast cells. Many different morphologic variants have been reported. The most significant is the plexiform, in which distinct large nerves are seen at the base of the tumor. One should always search for overlying melanocytes at the junction or in the upper dermis, since the main differential diagnostic point is a neural nevus.

Differential Diagnosis. The differential diagnosis of multiple lesions is limited. A solitary neurofibroma in an adult should cause no alarm. The two main possibilities are a large acrochordon or a melanocytic nevus that has undergone neural change.

Neurothekeoma
(Harkin and Reed 1967)

Synonym. Nerve sheath myxoma

These uncommon tumors are found mostly on the face of young adults, usually women. They present as small, dome-shaped papules. Under the microscope, one sees spindle cells arranged in a myxoid stroma with a lobular pattern. A cellular variant has been reported. In all instances, surgical excision is curative.

Perineurioma
(Pulitzer and Reed 1985)

Synonyms. Storiform perineural fibroma, perineural myxoma

Perineuriomas are benign, circumscribed, noncapsulated tumors that typically appear as nodules on the fingers and palms of young adults. They contain elongated spindle cells, often arranged in fascicles, and sometimes with a storiform pattern. In other instances, myxoid changes or psammoma bodies (calcified spherules) are found. The cells are typically positive for epithelial membrane antigen and vimentin.

Malignant Neural Tumors

Malignant Peripheral Nerve Sheath Tumor

Synonyms. Malignant schwannoma, neurofibrosarcoma

Malignant peripheral nerve sheath tumor is a rare, highly aggressive, soft tissue tumor with differentiation towards Schwann cells, perineural cells, and fibroblasts. About 50 % arise in patients with neurofibromatosis 1, usually in the deep soft tissues of the thighs or shoulder girdle. They are generally associated with a major nerve or a plexiform neurofibroma. The age of onset in neurofibromatosis patients is about 30 years of age, while the sporadic variant appears much later. The skin is occasionally involved, almost always by spread from a deeper site. Histologically, the lesions may have epithelioid features or contain glandular or muscular elements (Triton tumor). Aggressive surgery and chemotherapy offer the only chance for cure; the mean survival rate is several years.

Neuroblastoma

Etiology and Pathogenesis. Neuroblastoma is a malignant tumor derived from primitive neural crest cells. It is the most common tumor of infancy and one of the most common childhood neoplasms. Most tumors arise as abdominal masses. Over 50 % of cases occur in infants, and they are particularly likely to have widespread disease.

Clinical Findings. There are a number of unusual cutaneous findings. About one-third of infants with widespread disease have cutaneous lesions, and many present with skin signs. The raccoon eyes sign refers to the periorbital ecchymoses secondary to orbital involvement. Some patients have heterochromia irides. Most distinctive is the blanching that occurs in the overlying skin when the firm blue-gray metastatic nodules are stroked. This is the result of catecholamine release and persists for some time.

Differential Diagnosis. The differential diagnosis includes leukemic infiltrates, Ewing sarcoma, other peripheral neuroendocrine tumors, Langerhans cell histiocytosis, TORCH lesions (blueberry muffin sign), and hemangiomas. If questions exist, a biopsy will settle the issue.

Course and Prognosis. The infants with widespread disease paradoxically do quite well, with about 80% survival and some spontaneous regression. In older children, the degree of organ involvement determines the outlook.

Therapy. Both surgery for localized disease and chemotherapy are usually employed.

Merkel Cell Carcinoma

(Toker 1972)

Synonyms. Neuroendocrine carcinoma, trabecular carcinoma

Etiology and Pathogenesis. This uncommon cutaneous neoplasm shares many features in common with the Merkel cell, an intraepithelial neuroendocrine cell. Nonetheless, it has not been established with certainty that the tumor arises from Merkel cells. Only in rare instances have intraepidermal Merkel cell tumors with a pagetoid pattern been described. PUVA therapy appears to be a risk factor.

Clinical Findings. Merkel cell carcinoma is a tumor of the elderly, seen most commonly on the face and more often in women (Fig. 59.27). The tumors are dome-shaped nodules, often with a red-brown color. They are usually several centimeters in size, rapidly growing, and perhaps already ulcerated by the time the diagnosis is made.

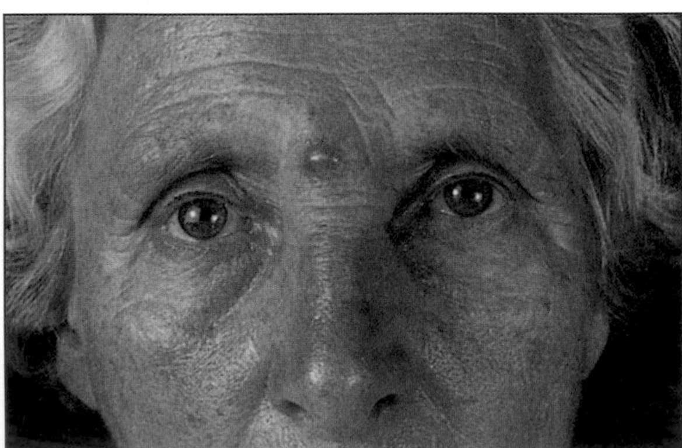

Fig. 59.27. Merkel cell tumor

Histopathology. The tumor consists of small blue cells with smudged or indistinct borders and usually arranged in sheets, although occasionally a trabecular pattern is seen. Mitoses are common. The cells typically extend into the subcutaneous fat and may also impinge upon the epidermis. The diagnosis can be confirmed by the unusual staining pattern of cytokeratins, especially cytokeratin 20, which produce a punctate perinuclear staining. Neuron-specific enolase and neurofilaments are also positive, while leukocyte common antigen and other hematologic markers are negative. Electron microscopic examination confirms the presence of neurosecretory granules.

Course and Prognosis. The outlook is gloomy. The statistical analysis results are highly variable, but the local recurrence rate and incidence of regional lymph node involvement in the first year following surgery are each at least 50%. Almost all the patients with lymph node involvement die in a matter of months to years.

Differential Diagnosis. The main clinical and histologic differential diagnostic considerations include lymphoma, metastatic small cell carcinoma of the lung, other rarer peripheral neuroectodermal tumors, eccrine carcinoma, and malignant melanoma.

Therapy. Generous surgical excision often supplies the best chance of a cure. If clear margins cannot be obtained because of anatomic considerations, postoperative radiation therapy can be considered. In the case of recurrences or metastases, chemotherapy is required.

Myxoid Tumors

There are two major problems with cutaneous myxomas. First, many tumors may show mucinous deposits, sometimes to the extent that it is difficult to identify the underlying tumor. Neural and sweat gland tumors, as well as metastatic adenocarcinomas, are particularly likely to show this change, but many other tumors may also be laden with mucin. Second, the distinction between a focal deposit of mucin, interpreted as a metabolic or degenerative change, and a myxoma, in which the mucin represents tumor stroma, is a philosophical one. Cutaneous mucinous deposits are discussed in Chapter 43.

Cutaneous Myxoma

Synonyms. Superficial myxoma, angiomyxoma, epithelioid myxoma

Many cutaneous myxomas are associated with Carney syndrome (Chap. 58). Some have many small vessels dispersed through the mucin. In others, there are lacy epithelial strands or even small cysts. In some instances, the tumors are sporadic and not associated with any underlying disorder.

Miscellaneous Mesenchymal Tumors

Granular Cell Tumor

(Abrikossoff 1926)

Synonyms. Abrikosoff tumor, granular cell myoblastoma

Etiology and Pathogenesis. The origin of a granular cell tumor is unclear. There may well be several different tumors included under this umbrella heading. Current evidence suggests that most lesions have a neural origin, so the term myoblastoma should be dropped.

Clinical Findings. The most common sites for granular cell tumors are the oral cavity and skin. On the tongue, they often present as a verrucous papule or nodule. On the skin, they rarely have distinctive clinical findings but may be verrucous (Fig. 59.28). A few patients may have multiple or internal lesions. A perhaps related condition is congenital epulis, found on the anterior alveolar ridge of newborns, which tends to regress spontaneously but is microscopically identical. Malignant granular cell tumors are very rare and more common in deeper locations.

Histopathology. The two key features are the presence of pseudoepitheliomatous hyperplasia and of sheets of polyhedral tumor cells with a granular cytoplasm. The striking reactive hyperplasia on the oral mucosa, when coupled with an inadequate

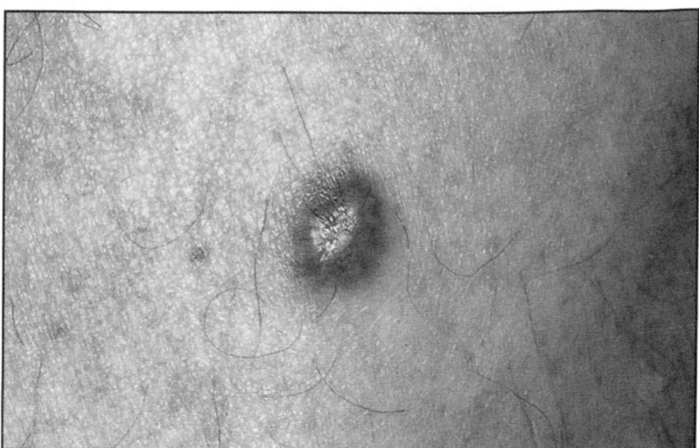

Fig. 59.28. Granular cell tumor

biopsy, may lead to the diagnosis of squamous cell carcinoma. Many other tumors may present with granular cell change, so one should search carefully for other clues before settling on the diagnosis.

Therapy. Excision is curative.

Clear Cell Sarcoma

(Enzinger 1965)

Synonym. Malignant melanoma of soft parts

This rare tumor may involve the skin secondarily. It is a soft tissue tumor, usually of the extremities and most often affecting young adults. The tumor is generally intimately connected with tendons or aponeuroses. While this is not a site where melanocytes are routinely encountered, the pale-staining fusiform tumor cells arranged in nests and strands are often positive for S100 or HMB-45 and contain melanin in most cases. Generally, there is a translocation involving chromosome 12, a feature not seen in cutaneous malignant melanomas. The course is locally aggressive with frequent recurrences and occasional metastases.

Bibliography

General

Enzinger FM, Weiss SW (1995) Soft tissue tumors, 3rd edn. Mosby, St. Louis

Niemi KM (1970) The benign fibrohistiocytic tumours of the skin. Acta Derm Venereol (Stockh) 50 [Suppl 63]: 1–66

Weedon D (1997) Skin pathology. Churchill Livingstone, Edinburgh

Keloid

Alibert JLM (1806) Description des maladies de la peau observeés à l'Hopital Saint-Louis et exposition des meilleures methodes suiviés pour leur traitment. Paris, Banoid L'Ainé, Paris, p 113

Alibert JLM (1816) Note sur la kéloide. J Univ Sc Med 2:207–216

Alster TS, West TB (1997) Treatment of scars: a review. Ann Plast Surg 39:418–432

Alster TS (1997) Laser treatment of hypertrophic scars, keloids, and striae. Dermatol Clin 15:419–429

English RS, Shenefelt PD (1999) Keloids and hypertrophic scars. Dermatol Surg 25:631–638

Goeminne L (1968) A new probably X-linked inherited syndrome: congenital muscular torticollis, multiple keloids cryptorchidism and renal dysplasia. Acta Genet Med Gemellol (Roma) 17:439–467

Murray JC (1994) Keloids and hypertrophic scars. Clin Dermatol 12:27–37

Niessen FB, Spauwen PH, Schalkwijk J et al. (1999) On the nature of hypertrophic scars and keloids: a review. Plast Reconstr Surg 104:1435–1458

Acrochordon

Beitler M, Eng A, Kilgour M et al. (1986) Association between acrochordons and colonic polyps. J Am Acad Dermatol 14:1042–1044

Kahana M, Grossman E, Feinstein A et al. (1987) Skin tags: a cutaneous marker for diabetes mellitus. Acta Derm Venereol 67:175–177

Margolis J, Margolis LS (1976) A frequent sign of diabetes mellitus. N Engl J Med 294:1184

Sclerotic Fibroma

Chapman MS, Perry AE, Baughman RD (1998) Cowden's syndrome, Lhermitte-Duclos disease, and sclerotic fibroma. Am J Dermatopathol 20:413–416

McCalmont TH (1994) Sclerotic fibroma: a fossil no longer. J Cutan Pathol 21:82–85

Rapini RP, Golitz LE (1989) Sclerotic fibromas of the skin. J Am Acad Dermatol 20:266–271

Pleomorphic Fibroma

Kamino H, Lee JY, Berke A (1989) Pleomorphic fibroma of the skin: a benign neoplasm with cytologic atypia. A clinicopathologic study of eight cases. Am J Surg Pathol 13:107–113

Dermatofibroma

Kamino H, Salcedo E (1999) Histopathologic and immunohistochemical diagnosis of benign and malignant fibrous and fibrohistiocytic tumors of the skin. Dermatol Clin 17:487–505

Kuniyuki S, Shindow K (1996) Multiple dermatofibromas accompanied by eruptive benign keratoses in a patient with systemic lupus erythematosus. J Dermatol 23:619–622

Nestle FO, Nickoloff BJ, Burg G (1995) Dermatofibroma: an abortive immunoreactive process mediated by dermal dendritic cells? Dermatology 190:265–268

Requena L, Farina MC, Fuente C et al. (1994) Giant dermatofibroma. A little-known clinical variant of dermatofibroma. J Am Acad Dermatol 30:714–718

Sharata H, Hashimoto K, Fernandez-Madrid F (1994) Multiple hyperpigmented nodules. Multiple dermatofibromas in a patient with systemic lupus erythematosus (SLE). Arch Dermatol 130:650–653

Calcifying Aponeurotic Fibroma

Fetsch JF, Miettinen M (1998) Calcifying aponeurotic fibroma: a clinicopathologic study of 22 cases arising in uncommon sites. Hum Pathol 29:1504–1510

Keasbey LE (1953) Juvenile aponeurotic fibroma (calcifying fibroma): a distictive tumor arising in the palms and soles of young children. Cancer 6:338–346

Nuchal Fibroma

Abraham Z, Rozenbaum M, Rosner I et al. (1997) Nuchal fibroma. J Dermatol 24:262–265

Balachandran K, Allen PW, MacCormac LB (1995) Nuchal fibroma. A clinicopathological study of nine cases. Am J Surg Pathol 19:313–317

Lister DM, Graham-Brown RA, Burns DA et al. (1988) Collagenosis nuchae – a new entity? Clin Exp Dermatol 13: 263–264

Shek TW, Chan AC, Ma L (1996) Extranuchal nuchal fibroma. Am J Surg Pathol 20:902–903

Acquired Digital Fibrokeratoma

Bart RS, Andrade R, Kopf AW et al. (1968) Acquired digital fibrokeratomas. Arch Dermatol 97:120–129

Berger RS, Spielvogel RL (1988) Dermal papule on a distal digit. Acquired digital fibrokeratoma. Arch Dermatol 124:1559.1560, 1562–1563

Kint A, Baran R, De Keyser H (1985) Acquired (digital) fibrokeratoma. J Am Acad Dermatol 12:816–821

Fibroma of Tendon Sheath

Chung EB, Enzinger FM (1979) Fibroma of tendon sheath. Cancer 44:1945–1954

Geschickter CF, Copland MM (1949) Tumors of bone, 3rd edn. Lippincott, Philadelphia

Maluf HM, DeYoung BR, Swanson PE et al. (1995) Fibroma and giant cell tumor of tendon sheath: a comparative histologic and immunohistologic study. Mod Pathol 8: 155–159

Giant Cell Tumor of Tendon Sheath

Ciattaglia G, Filosa G, Bugatti L (1991) Giant cell tumor of tendon sheath. J Am Acad Dermatol 25:728–729

Chassaignac CME (1852) Cancer de la gaine des tendons. Gaz Hosp Civ Milit 47:185

Vogrincic GS, O'Connell JX, Gilks CB (1997) Giant cell tumor of tendon sheath is a polyclonal cellular proliferation. Hum Pathol 28:815–819

Angiofibromas

Requena L, Sangueza OP (1998) Cutaneous vascular proliferations, part III. Malignant neoplasms, other cutaneous neoplasms with significant vascular component, and disorders erroneously considered as vascular neoplasms. J Am Acad Dermatol 38:143–175

Fibrous Papule of the Nose

Ackerman AB, Viragh PA, Chongchitnant N (1993) Fibrous papule. In: Ackerman AB, Viragh PA, Chongchitnant N

(eds) Neoplasms with follicular differentiation. Lea and Febiger, Philadelphia, pp 207–229
Cerio R, Rao BK, Spaull J et al. (1989) An immunohistochemical study of fibrous papule of the nose: 25 cases. J Cutan Pathol 16:194–198
Cerio R, Spaull J, Oliver GF et al. (1990) A study of factor XIIIa and MAC 387 immunolabeling in normal and pathological skin. Am J Dermatopathol 12:221–233
Graham JH, Sanders JB, Johnson WC et al. (1965) Fibrous papule of the nose: a clinicopathological study. J Invest Dermatol 45:194–203

Elastofibroma

Järvi OH, Saxén E (1961) Elastofibroma dorsi. Acta Pathol Microbiol Scand 51:83–84
Madri JA, Dise CA, LiVolsi VA et al. (1981) Elastofibroma dorsi: an immunochemical study of collagen content. Hum Pathol 12:186–190
Palmer CH, Burgdorf WHC (1990) Elastofibroma dorsi. In: Demis DJ (ed) Clinical dermatology, vol 4. Lippincott-Raven, Philadelphia, pp 24–16

Nodular Fasciitis

Bernstein KE, Lattes R (1982) Nodular (pseudosarcomatous) fasciitis, a nonrecurrent lesion: clinicopathologic study of 134 cases. Cancer 49:1668–1678
Graham BS, Barrett TL, Goltz RW (1999) Nodular fasciitis: response to intralesional corticosteroids. J Am Acad Dermatol 40:490–492
Haas AF (1999) Nodular fasciitis of the forehead. Dermatol Surg 25:140–142
Konwaler BE, Keasby L, Kaplan L (1955) Subcutaneous pseudosarcomatous fibromatosis (fasciitis). Am J Clin Pathol 25:241–255
Krasovec M, Burg G (1999) Nodular fasciitis (pseudotumor of the skin). Dermatology 198:431–433

Fibrous Hamartoma of Infancy

Mitchell ML, di Sant'Agnese PA, Gerber JE (1982) Fibrous hamartoma of infancy. Hum Pathol 13(6):586–588
Paller AS, Gonzalez-Crussi F, Sherman JO (1989) Fibrous hamartoma of infancy. Eight additional cases and a review of the literature. Arch Dermatol 125:88–91
Reye RDK (1956) A consideration of certain subdermal "fibromatous tumors" of infancy. J Pathol Bact 72:149–154
Scott DM, Pena JR, Omura EF (1999) Fibrous hamartoma of infancy. J Am Acad Dermatol 41:857–859

Infantile Digital Fibromatosis

Frank A (1908) Ein Fall von angeborenen Fibromen am Finger nebst Beiträgen zur Kasusitik von Fingertumoren. Wien Klin Rundsch 22:659
Hayashi T, Tsuda N, Chowdhury PR et al. (1995) Infantile digital fibromatosis: a study of the development and regression of cytoplasmic inclusion bodies. Mod Pathol 8:548–552
Kawaguchi M, Mitsuhashi Y, Hozumi Y et al. (1988) A case of infantile digital fibromatosis with spontaneous regression. J Dermatol 25:523–526
Reye RDK (1965) Recurring digital fibrous tumors of childhood. Arch Pathol 80:228
Yun K (1988) Infantile digital fibromatosis. Immunohistochemical and ultrastructural observations of cytoplasmic inclusions. Cancer 61:500–507

Gingival Fibromatosis

Takagi M, Yamamoto H, Mega H et al. (1991) Heterogeneity in the gingival fibromatoses. Cancer 68:2202–2212

Desmoid Tumor

Pereyo NG, Heimer WL Jr (1996) Extraabdominal desmoid tumor. Am Acad Dermatol 34:352–356
Rodriguez-Bigas MA, Mahoney MC, Karakousis CP et al. (1994) Desmoid tumors in patients with familial adenomatous polyposis. Cancer 74:1270–1274

Infantile Myofibromatosis

Giannakopoulou C, Hatzidaki E, Giannakopoulos K et al. (1999) Infantile myofibromatosis: a case study and review of literature. J Dermatol 26:595–598
Goldberg NS, Bauer BS, Kraus H et al. (1988) Infantile myofibromatosis: a review of clinicopathology with perspectives on new treatment choices. Pediatr Dermatol 5:37–46
Stout AP (1954) Juvenile fibromatoses. Cancer 7:953

Adult Myofibroma

Requena L, Kutzner H, Hugel H et al. (1996) Cutaneous adult myofibroma: a vascular neoplasm. J Cutan Pathol 23:445–457
Smith KJ, Skelton HG, Barrett TL et al. (1989) Cutaneous myofibroma. Mod Pathol 2:603–609

Dermatomyofibroma

Cooper PH (1992) Dermatomyofibroma: a case of fibromatosis revisited. J Cutan Pathol 19:81–82
Hügel H (1991) Die plaqueförmige dermale Fibromatose. Hautarzt 42:223–226
Kamino H, Reddy VB, Gero M et al. (1992) Dermatomyofibroma. A benign cutaneous, plaque-like proliferation of fibroblasts and myofibroblasts in young adults. J Cutan Pathol 19:85–93

Infantile Desmoid-Type Fibromatosis

Keltz M, DiCostanzo D, Desai P et al. (1995) Infantile (desmoid-type) fibromatosis. Pediatr Dermatol 12(2):149–151

Dermatofibrosarcoma Protuberans

Cohen PR, Rapin RP, Farhood AI (1994) Dermatofibroma and dermatofibrosarcoma protuberans: differential expression of CD34 and factor XIIIa. Am J Dermatopathol 16:573–574
Darier J, Ferand M (1924) Dermato-fibromes progressifs et récidivants ou fibro-sarcomes de la peau. Ann Dermatol Syphil 5:545–562
Gloster HM Jr (1996) Dermatofibrosarcoma protuberans. J Am Acad Dermatol 35:355–374
Haycox CL, Odland PB, Olbricht SM et al. (1997) Immunohistochemical characterization of dermatofibrosarcoma protuberans with practical applications for diagnosis and treatment. J Am Acad Dermatol 37:438–444
Hoffmann E (1925) Über das knollentreibende Fibrosarkom der Haut (Dermatofibrosarkoma protuberans). Dermatol Zeitschr 43:1–28
Mentzel T, Beham A, Katenkamp D et al. (1998) Fibrosarcomatous ("high-grade") dermatofibrosarcoma protuberans: clinicopathologic and immunohistochemical study

of a series of 41 cases with emphasis on prognostic significance. Am J Surg Pathol 22:576–587

Pigmented Dermatofibrosarcoma Protuberans

Bednar B (1957) Storiform neurofibromas of the skin, pigmented and nonpigmented. Cancer 10:368–375

Elgart GW, Hanly A, Busso M et al. (1999) Bednar tumor (pigmented dermatofibrosarcoma protuberans) occurring in a site of prior immunization: immunochemical findings and therapy. J Am Acad Dermatol 40:315–317

Giant Cell Fibroblastoma

Diaz-Cascajo C, Borrego L, Bastida-Inarrea J et al. (1996) Giant cell fibroblastoma. New histologic observations. Am J Dermatopathol 18:403–408

Perry DA, Schultz LR, Dehner LP (1993) Giant cell fibroblastoma with dermatofibrosarcoma protuberans-like transformation. J Cutan Pathol 20:451–454

Shmookler BM, Enzinger FM, Weiss SW (1989) Giant cell fibroblastoma. A juvenile form of dermatofibrosarcoma protuberans. Cancer 64:2154–2161

Malignant Fibrous Histiocytoma

Kamino H, Salcedo E (1999) Histopathologic and immunohistochemical diagnosis of benign and malignant fibrous and fibrohistiocytic tumors of the skin. Dermatol Clin 17:487–505

O'Brien JE, Stout AP (1964) Malignant fibrous xanthomas. Cancer 17:1445

Weiss SW, Enzinger FM (1978) Malignant fibrous histiocytoma: an analysis of 200 cases. Cancer 41:2250–2266

Atypical Fibroxanthoma

Fretzin DF, Helwig EB (1973) Atypical fibroxanthoma of the skin. A clinicopathologic study of 140 cases. Cancer 31(6):1541–1552

Helwig EB (1963) Case 6-atypical fibroxanthoma. In: 18th annual tumor seminar of the San Antonio Society of Pathologist. Tex Med 59:664

Starink TH, Hausman R, Van Delden L et al. (1977) Atypical fibroxanthoma of the skin. Presentation of 5 cases and a review of the literature. Br J Dermatol 97:167–177

Epitheloid Sarcoma

Enzinger FM (1970) Epitheloid sarcoma. A sarcoma simulating a granuloma or a carcinoma. Cancer 26:1029–1041

Fibrosarcoma

Mark RJ, Sercarz JA, Tran L et al. (1991) Fibrosarcoma of the head and neck. The UCLA experience. Arch Otolaryngol Head Neck Surg 117:396–401

Vascular Tumors

Prieto VG, Shea CR (1999) Selected cutaneous vascular neoplasms. A review. Dermatol Clin 17:507–520

Requena L, Sangueza OP (1997) Cutaneous vascular proliferations, part II. Hyperplasias and benign neoplasms. J Am Acad Dermatol 37:887–920

Requena L, Sangueza OP (1998) Cutaneous vascular proliferations, part III. Malignant neoplasms, other cutaneous neoplasms with significant vascular component, and disorders erroneously considered as vascular neoplasms. J Am Acad Dermatol 38:143–175

Pyogenic Granuloma

Cooper PH, McAllister HA, Helwig EB (1979) Intravenous pyogenic granuloma: a study of 18 cases. Am J Surg Pathol 3:221–228

Coskey RJ, Mehregan AH (1967) Granuloma pyogenicum with multiple satellite recurrences. Arch Dermatol 96:71–73

Mills SE, Cooper PH, Fechner RE (1980) Lobular capillary hemangioma: the underlying lesion of pyogenic granuloma. Am J Surg Pathol 4:471–479

Mooney MA, Janniger CK (1995) Pyogenic granuloma. Cutis 55:133–136

Patrice SJ, Wiss K, Mulliken JB (1991) Pyogenic granuloma (lobular capillary hemangioma): a clinicopathologic study of 178 cases. Pediatr Dermatol 8:267–276

Poncet A, Dor L (1897) Botromycose humaine. Rev Chir Orthop 18:996

Shah M, Kingston TP, Cotterill JA (1995) Eruptive pyogenic granulomas: a successfully treated patient and review of the literature. Br J Dermatol 133:795–796

Strohal R, Gillitzer R, Zonzits E et al. (1991) Localised vs generalised pyogenic granuloma: a clinicopathologic study. Arch Dermatol 127:856–861

Thrombosed Capillary Aneurysm

Epstein E et al (1956) Melanoma-simulating nodules due to capillary aneurysms. Calif Med 85:22

Epstein E, Novy FG Jr, Allington HV (1965) Capillary aneurysms of the skin. Arch Dermatol 91:335–341

Angiolymphoid Hyperplasia with Eosinophilia

Bonnetblanc JM, Bernard P, Malinvaud G (1985) Treatment of angiolymphoid hyperplasia with eosinophilia. J Am Acad Dermatol 13:668–669

Helander SD, Peters MS, Kuo TT et al. (1995) Kimura's disease and angiolymphoid hyperplasia with eosinophilia: new observations from immunohistochemical studies of lymphocyte markers, endothelial antigens, and granulocyte proteins. J Cutan Pathol 22:319–326

Olsen TG, Helwig EB (1985) Angiolymphoid hyperplasia with eosinophilia in the skin. Am J Acad Dermatol 12:781–796

Rosai J (1982) Angiolymphoid hyperplasia with eosinophilia of the skin. Its nosological position in the spectrum of histiocytoid hemangioma. Am J Dermatopathol 4:175–184

Rosai J, Gold J, Landy R (1979) The histiocytoid hemangiomas: a unifying concept embracing several previously described entities of the skin, soft tissue, large vessels, bone and heart. Human Pathol 10:707–730

Wells GC, Whimster IW (1969) Subcutaneous angiolymphoid hyperplasia with eosinophilia. Br J Dermatol 81:1–14

Kimura Disease

Kimura T, Yoshimura S, Ishikawa E (1948) Unusual granulation combined with hyperplastic change of lymphatic tissue. Trans Soc Pathol Jpn 37:179–180

Kung ITM, Gibson JB, Bannatyne PM (1984) Kimura's disease: a clinicopathological study of 21 cases and its distinction from angiolymphoid hyperplasia with eosinophilia. Pathology 16:39–44

Kuo TT, Shih LY, Chan HL (1988) Kimura's disease: involvement of regional lymph nodes and distinction from angiolymphoid hyperplasia with eosinophilia. Am J Surg Pathol 12:843–854

Reactive Benign Angioendotheliomatosis

Krell JM, Sanchez RL, Solomon AR (1994) Diffuse dermal angiomatosis: a variant of reactive cutaneous angioendotheliomatosis. J Cutan Pathol 21:363–370

Lazova R, Slater C, Scott G (1996) Reactive angioendotheliomatosis: case report and review of the literature. J Dermatopthol 16:63–69

Pfleger L, Tappeiner J (1959) Zur Kenntnis der systemisierten Endotheliomatose der cutanen Blutgefäße. Hautarzt 10:359

Requena L, Farina MC, Renedo G et al. (1999) Intravascular and diffuse dermal reactive angioendotheliomatosis secondary to iatrogenic arteriovenous fistulas. J Cutan Pathol 26:159–164

Stewart-Bluefarb Syndrome

Bluefarb SM, Adams LA (1967) Arteriovenous malformation with angiodermatitis. Stasis dermatitis simulating Kaposi's disease. Arch Dermatol 96:176–181

Goldblum OM, Kraus E, Bronner AK (1985) Pseudo-Kaposi's sarcoma of the hand associated with an acquired, iatrogenic arteriovenous fistula. Arch Dermatol 121:1038–1040

Landthaler M, Stolz W, Eckert F et al. (1989) Pseudo-Kaposi's sarcoma occurring after placement of arteriovenous shunt: a case report with DNA analysis. J Am Acad Dermatol 21:499–505

Stewart WM (1967) Fausse angiosarcomatose de Kaposi par fistules arterioveineuses multiples. Bull Soc Fr Dermatol Syphil 74:664–665

Intravascular Papillary Endothelial Hyperplasia

Kuo TT, Sayers CP, Rosai J (1976) Masson's "vegetant intravascular hemangioendothelioma": a lesion often mistaken for angiosarcoma. Cancer 1227–1236

Masson P (1923) Hemangioendothelioma vegetant intravasculaire. Bull Soc Anat 93:517

Miyamoto H, Nagatani T, Mohri S et al. (1988) Intravascular papillary endothelial hyperplasia. Clin Exp Dermatol 13:411–415

Rosai J, Ackerman LR (1974) Intravascular atypical vascular proliferation. Arch Dermatol 109:704–717

Hemangioma

Boulinguez S, Teillac-Hamel D, Bedane C et al (1998) Cervicofacial hemangioma and a minor sternal malformation: inclusion in PHACES syndrome? Pediatr Deramatol 15:119–121

Drolet BA, Esterly NB, Frieden IJ (1999) Hemangiomas in children. N Engl J Med 341:173–181

Edgerton MT (1976) The treatment of hemangiomas: with special reference to the role of steroid therapy. Ann Surg 183:517–532

Enjolras O, Mulliken JB (1997) Vascular tumors and vascular malformations (new issues). Adv Dermatol 13:375–423

Enjolras O, Wassef M, Mazoyer E et al (1997) Infants with Kasbach-Merritt syndrome do not have "true" hemangiomas. J Pediatr 130:631–640

Enjolras O, Mulliken JB, Wassef M et al. (2000) Residual lesions after Kasabach-Merritt phenomenon in 41 patients. J Am Acad Dermatol 42:225–235

Esterly NB (1983) Kasbach-Merritt syndrome in infants. J Am Acad Dermatol 8:504–513

Esterly NB (1996) Cutaneous hemangiomas, vascular stains and malformations, and associated syndromes. Curr Probl Pediatr 26:3–39

Garzon MC, Enjolras O, Frieden J (2000) Vascular tumors and vascular malformations: Evidence for an association. J Am Acad Dermatol 42:275–279

Kasbach HH, Merritt KK (1940) Capillary hemangioma with extensive purpura: report of a case. Am J Dis Child 59:1063–1070

Mulliken JB, Young AE (eds) (1988) Vascular birthmarks: hemangiomas and malformations, WB Saunders, Philadelphia

van de Kerkhof PC, de Rooij M, Steijlen PM (1998) Spontaneous course of hemangiomas: facts and speculations. Int J Dermatol 37:101–102

Warner M, Suen JY (1999) Hemangiomas and vascular malformations of the head and neck. Wiley, New York

Wirth FA, Lowitt MH (1998) Diagnosis and treatment of cutaneous vascular lesions. Am Fam Physician 57:765–773

Verrucous Hemangioma

Imperial R, Helwig EB (1967) Verrucous hemangioma. A clinicopathologic study of 21 cases. Arch Dermatol 96:247–253

Mafucci Syndrome

Loewinger RJ, Lichtenstein JR, Dodson WE et al. (1977) Maffucci's syndrome: amesenchymal dysplasia and multiple tumour syndrome. Br J Dermatol 96:317–322

Maffuci A (1881) Di un caso encendroma ed angioma multiplo. Movimento Medico-Chirurgico 3:399

Blue Rubber Bleb Nevus Syndrome

Bean WB (1958) Blue rubber bleb nevi of the skin and gastrointestinal tract. In: Vascular spiders and related lesions of the skin. Thomas Springfield, pp 178–185

Garen PD, Sahn EE (1994) Spinal cord compression in blue rubber bleb nevus syndrome. Arch Dermatol 130:934–935

Acral Arteriovenous Hemangioma

Connelly MG, Winkelmann RK (1985) Acral arteriovenous tumor. A clinicopathologic review. Am J Surg Pathol 9:15–21

Girard C, Graham JH, Johnson WC (1974) Arteriovenous hemangioma (arteriovenous shunt). A clinicopathological and histochemical study. J Cutan Pathol 1:73–87

Cherry Angioma

De Morgan C (1872) The Origin of Cancer considered with reference to the treatmerment of the disease. Churchill, London

Tuder RM, Young R, Karasek M et al. (1987) Adult cutaneous hemangiomas are composed of nonreplicating endothelial cells. J Invest Dermatol 89:594–597

Venous Lake

Bean WB, Walsh JR (1956) Venous lakes. Arch Dermatol 74:459–463

Targetoid Hemosiderotic Hemangioma

Carlson JA, Daulat S, Goodheart HP (1999) Targetoid hemosiderotic hemangioma- a dynamic vascular tumor: report of 3 cases with episodic and cyclic changes and comparison with solitary angiokeratomas. J Am Acad Dermatol 41:215–224

Mentzel T, Partanen TA, Kutzner H (1999) Hobnail hemangioma ("targetoid hemosiderotic hemangioma"): clinicopathologic and immunohistochemical analysis of 62 cases. J Cutan Pathol 26:279–286

Santa Cruz DJ, Aronberg J (1988) Targetoid hemosiderotic hemangioma. J Am Acad Dermatol 19:550–558

Microvenular Hemangioma

Aloi F, Tomasini C, Pippione M (1993) Microvenular hemangioma. Am J Dermatopathol 15:534–538

Hunt SJ, Santa Cruz DJ, Barr RJ (1991) Microvenular hemangioma. J Cutan Pathol 18:235–240

MacMillan A, Champion RH (1971) Progressive capillary haemangioma. Br J Dermatol 85:492–493

Tufted Angioma

McMillan A, Champion RH (1971) Progressive capillary hemangioma. Br J Dermatol 85:492–493

Nakagawa K (1949) Case report of angioblastoma of the skin. Nippon Hifuka Gakkai Zasshi 59:92–94

Padilla RS, Orkin M, Rosai J (1987) Acquired "tufted" angioma (progressive capillary hemangioma). A distinctive clinicopathological entity related to lobular capillary hemangioma. Am J Dermatopathol 9:292–300

Wilson Jones E (1976) Dowling oration 1976: malignant vascular tumors. Clin Exp Dermatol 1:287–312

Multinucleate Cell Angiohistiocytoma

Annessi G, Girolomoni G, Giannetti A (1992) Multinucleate cell angiohistiocytoma. Am J Dermatopathol 14:340–344

Chang SN, Kim HS, Kim SC et al. (1996) Generalized multinucleate cell angiohistiocytoma. J Am Acad Dermatol 35:320–322

Smith NP, Wilson-Jones E (1986) Multinucleate cell angiohistiocytoma: a new entity. J Cutan Pathol 13:77

Smolle J, Auboeck L, Gogg-Retzer I et al. (1989) Multinucleate cell angiohistiocytoma: a clinicopathological, immunohistochemical and ultrastructural study. Br J Dermatol 121:113–121

Glomeruloid Hemangioma

Chan JK, Fletcher CD, Hicklin GA et al. (1990) Glomeruloid hemangioma. A distinctive cutaneous lesion of multicentric Castleman's disease associated with POEMS syndrome. Am J Surg Pathol 14:1036–1046

Rongioletti F, Gambini C, Lerza R (1994) Glomeruloid hemangioma. A cutaneous marker of POEMS syndrome. Am J Dermatopathol 16:175–178

Bossed Hemangioma

Martinez-Perez D, Fein NA, Boon LM et al. (1995) Not all hemangiomas look like strawberries: uncommon presentations of the most common tumor of infancy. Pediatr Dermatol 12:1–6

Patrizi A, Neri I, Marzaduri S et al. (1998) Tumor of the right shoulder in a newborn. Bossed hemangioma with telangiectasia and peripheral pallor. Arch Dermatol 134:1146–1149

Angiokeratomas

Imperial R, Helwig EB (1967) Angiokeratoma. A clinicopathological study. Arch Dermatol 95:166–175

Kaddu S, Cerroni L, Pilatti A et al. (1994) Acral pseudolymphomatous angiokeratoma. A variant of the cutaneous pseudolymphomas. Am J Dermatopathol 16:130–133

Mibelli V (1889) Di una nuova forma di cheratosis angiocheratoma. G Ital Mal Vener 30:285–301

Schiller PI, Itin PH (1996) Angiokeratomas: an update. Dermatology 193:275–282

Glomus Tumor

Landthaler M, Baun-Falco O, Eckert F et al. (1990) Congenital multiple plaque-like glomus tumor. Arch Dermatol 126:1203–1207

Masson P (1924) Le glomus neuro-myo-arteriel des regions tactiles et ses tumeurs. Lyon Chir 20:257–280

Nuovo MA, Grimes MM, Knowless DM (1990) Glomus tumors: clinicopathologic and immunohistochemical analysis of forty cases. Surg Pathol 3:31–40

Parsons ME, Russo G, Fucich L et al. (1997) Multiple glomus tumors. Int J Dermatol 36:894–900

Taafe A, Barker D, Wyat EH et al. (1980) Glomus tumors: a clinicopathological survey. Clin Exp Dermatol 5:219–225

Yang J-S, Ko J-W, Suh K-S et al. (1999) Congenital multiple plaque-like glomangiomyoma. Am J Dermatopathol 21(5):454–457

Superficial Lymphangioma

Eliezri YD, Sklar JA (1988) Lymphangioma circumscriptum: review and evaluation of carbon dioxide laser vaporization. J Dermatol Surg Oncol 14:357–364

Flanagan BP, Helwig EB (1977) Cutaneous lymphangioma. Arch Dermatol 113:24–30

Requena L, Sangueza OP (1997) Cutaneous vascular proliferation, part II. Hyperplasias and benign neoplasms. J Am Acad Dermatol 37:887–919

Deep Lymphangioma

Harwood CA, Mortimer PS (1995) Causes and clinical manifestations of lymphatic failure. Clin Dermatol 13:459–471

Acquired Progressive Lymphangioma

Grunwald MH, Amichai B, Avinoach I (1997) Acquired progressive lymphangioma. J Am Acad Dermatol 37:656–657

Kato H, Kadoya A (1996) Acquired progressive lymphangioma occurring following femoral arteriography. Clin Exp Dermatol 21:159–162

Meunier L, Barneon G, Meynadier J (1994) Acquired progressive lymphangioma. Br J Dermatol 131:706–708

Watanabe M, Kishiyama K, Ohkawara A (1983) Acquired progressive lymphangioma. J Am Acad Dermatol 8:663–667

Kaposi Sarcoma

Antman K, Chang Y (2000) Kaposi's Sarcoma. N Engl J Med 342:1027–1038

Cesarman E, Knowles DM (1999) The role of Kaposi's sarcoma-associated herpesvirus (KSHV/HHV-8) in lymphoproliferative diseases. Semin Cancer Biol 9:165–174

Chor PJ, Santa Cruz DJ (1992) Kaposi's sarcoma: a clinciopathologic review and differential diagnosis. J Cutan Pathol 19:6–20

Fenig E, Brenner B, Rakowsky E et al. (1998) Classic Kaposi sarcoma: experience at Rabin Medical Center in Israel. Am J Clin Oncol 21:498–500

Friedman-Kien E, Saltzman BR (1990) Clinical manifestations of classical, endemic, African and epidemic AIDS-associated Kaposi's sarcoma. J Am Acad Dermatol 22: 1237–1250

Gottlieb GJ, Ackerman AB (1988) Kaposi's sarcoma: a text and atlas. Lea and Pebiger, Philadelphia

Kaposi M (1872) Idiopathisches multiples Pigmentsarkom der Haut. Arch Dermatol Syph 4:265–278

Neipel F, Fleckenstein B (1999) The role of HHV-8 in Kaposi's sarcoma. Semin Cancer Biol 9:151–164

Reitz MS Jr, Nerurkar LS, Gallo RC (1999) Perspective on Kaposi's sarcoma: facts, concepts, and conjectures. J Natl Cancer Inst 91:1453–1458

Schwartz RA (1996) Kaposi's sarcoma: advances and perspectives. J Am Acad Dermatol 34:804–814

Swift PS (1996) The role of radiation therapy in the management of HIV-related Kaposi's sarcoma. Hematol Oncol Clin North Am 10:1069–1080

Tappero JW; Conant MA, Wolfe SF, Berger TG: Kaposi's sarcoma: epidemiology, pathogenesis, histology, clinical spectrum, staging criteria and therapy. J Am Acad Dermatol 28:371–395

Templeton AC (1972) Studies in Kaposi's sarcoma. Cancer 30:854–867

Tur E, Brenner S (1996) Treatment of Kaposi's sarcoma. Arch Dermatol 132:327–331

Angiosarcoma

Bolin DJ, Lukas GM (1996) Low-grade dermal angiosarcoma of the breast following radiotherapy. Am Surg 62:668–672

Caldwell JB, Ryan MT, Benson PM et al. (1995) Cutaneous angiosarcoma arising in the radiation site of a congenital hemangioma. J Am Acad Dermatol 33: 865–870

Cooper PH (1987) Angiosarcoma of the skin. Semin Diagn Pathol 4:2–17

Girard C, Johnson WC, Graham JH (1970) Cutaneous angiosarcoma. Cancer 26:868–883

Hodgkinson DJ, Soule EH, Woods JE (1979) Cutaneous angiosarcoma of the head and neck. Cancer 44:1106–1113

Stewart FW, Treves N (1948) Lymphangiosarcoma in postmastectory lymphedema. Cancer 1:64–81

Spindle Cell Hemangioendothelioma

Perkins P, Weiss SW (1996) Spindle cell hemangioendothelioma. An analysis of 78 cases with reassessment of its pathogenesis and biologic behavior. Am J Surg Pathol 20:1196–1204

Weiss SW, Enzinger FM (1986) Spindle cell hemangioendothelioma. A low-grade angiosarcoma resembling a cavernous hemangioma and Kaposi's sarcoma. Am J Surg Pathol 10:521–530

Endovascular Papillary Hemangioendothelioma

Dabska M (1969) Malignant endovascular papillary angioendothelioma of the skin in childhood. Clinicopathologic study of 6 cases. Cancer 24:503–510

Morgan J, Robinson MJ, Rosen LB et al. (1989) Malignant endovascular papillary angioendothelioma (Dabska tumor). A case report and review of the literature. Am J Dermatopathol 11:64–68

Quecedo E, Martinez-Escribano JA, Febrer I et al. (1996) Dabska tumor developing within a preexisting vascular malformation. Am J Dermatopathol 18:302–307

Epitheloid Hemangioendothelioma

Palsson B (1999) Epitheloid hemangioendothelioma. Acta Oncol 38:659–661

Weiss SW, Enzinger FM (1982) Epithelioid hemangioendothelioma: a vascular tumor often mistaken for a carcinoma. Cancer 50:970–981

Retiform Hemangioendothelioma

Calonje E, Fletcher CD, Wilson-Jones E et al. (1994) Retiform hemangioendothelioma. A distinctive form of low-grade angiosarcoma delineated in a series of 15 cases. Am J Surg Pathol 18:115–125

Fletcher CD (1998) Recent developments in soft tissue tumors. Verh Dtsch Ges Pathol 82:33–46

Kaposiform Hemangioendothelioma

Tsang WY, Chan JK (1991) Kaposi-like infantile hemangioendothelioma. A distinctive vascular neoplasm of the retroperitoneum. Am J Surg Pathol 15:982–989

Vin-Christian K, McCalmont TH, Frieden IJ (1997) Kaposiform hemangioendothelioma. An aggressive, locally invasive vascular tumor that can mimic hemangioma of infancy. Arch Dermatol 133:1573–1578

Hemangiopericytoma

Spitz FR, Bouvet M, Pisters PW et al. (1998) Hemangiopericytoma: a 20-year single-institution experience. Ann Surg Oncol 5:350–355

Stout AP, Murray MR (1942) Hemangiopericytoma: a vascular tumor Featuring Zimmermann's pericytes. Ann Surg 116:26

Lipoma

Digregorio F, Barr RJ, Fretzin DF (1992) Pleomorphic lipoma. Case reports and review of the literature. J Dermatol Surg Oncol 18:197–202

Duve S, Müller-Hocker J, Worret WI (1995) Spindle-cell lipoma of the skin. Am J Dermatopathol 17:529–533

Fanburg-Smith JC, Devaney KO, Miettinen M et al. (1998) Multiple spindle cell lipomas: a report of 7 familial and 11 nonfamilial cases. Am J Surg Pathol 22:40–48

Grosshans EM (1990) Subfascial lipoma of the forehead. J Am Acad Dermatol 23:153–154

Hurt MA, Santa Cruz DJ (1989) Nodular-cystic fat necrosis. A reevaluation of the so-called mobile encapsulated lipoma. J Am Acad Dermatol 21:493–498

Kikuchi I, Okazaki M, Narahara S (1984) The so-called mobile encapsulated lipoma. J Dermatol 11:410–412

Meis JM, Enzinger FM (1993) Chondroid lipoma. A unique tumor simulating liposarcoma and myxoid chondrosarcoma. Am J Surg Pathol 17:1103–1112

Puig L, Moreno A, de Moragas JM (1986) Infiltrating angiolipoma: report of two cases and review of the literature. J Dermatol Surg Oncol 12(6):617–619

Sanchez MR, Golomb FM, Moy JA et al. (1993) Giant lipoma: case report and review of the literature. J Am Acad Dermatol 28:266–268

Hibernoma

Rigor VU, Goldstone SE, Jones J et al. (1986) Hibernoma. A case report and discussion of a rare tumor. Cancer 57: 2207–2211

Lipoblastoma

Mentzel T, Calonje E, Fletcher CD (1993) Lipoblastoma and lipoblastomatosis: a clinicopathological study of 14 cases. Histopathology 23:527–533

Miller GG, Yanchar NL, Magee JF et al. (1998) Lipoblastoma and liposarcoma in children: an analysis of 9 cases and a review of the literature. Can J Surg 41: 455–458

Vellios F, Baez J, Shumaker HB (1958) Lipoblastomatosis: a tumor of fetal fat different from hibernoma. Am J Pathol 34:1149–1159

Dercum Disease

Brenner S, Politi Y (1995) Dermatologic diseases and problems of women throughout the life cycle. Int J Dermatol 34:369–379

Dercum FX (1888) A subcutaneous connective tissue dystrophy of the arm and the neck, associated with symptoms resembling myxedema. Univ Med Gaz Philadelphia 1:140–150

Held JL, Andrew JA, Kohn SR (1989) Surgical amelioration of Dercum's disease: a report and review. J Dermatol Surg Oncol 15:1294–1296

Lipomatosis

Comings DE, Glenchur H (1968) Benign symmetric lipomatosis. JAMA 203:305

Launois PE, Bensaude R (1898) Del'adéno-lipomatose symmétrique. Bull Soc Med Hop Paris 1:298–318

Leffell DJ, Braverman IM (1986) Familial multiple lipomatosis. Report of a case and a review of the literature. J Am Acad Dermatol 15:275–279

Madelung O (1888) Über den Fetthals (diffuses Lipom des Halses). Arch Klin Chir 37:106–130

Ruzicka T, Vieluf D, Landthaler M et al. (1987) Benign symmetric lipomatosis Launois-Bensaude. Report of ten cases and review of the literature. J Am Acad Dermatol 17:663–674

Smith PD, Stadelmann WK, Wassermann RJ et al. (1998) Benign symmetric lipomatosis (Madelung's disease). Ann Plast Surg 41:671–673

Uhlin SR (1979) Benign symmetric lipomatosis. Arch Dermatol 115:94–95

Liposarcoma

Azumi N, Curtis J, Kempson RL et al. (1987) Atypical and malignant neoplasms showing lipomatous differentiation. A study of 111 cases. Am J Surg Pathol 11:161–183

Saunders JR, Jaques DA, Casterline PF et al. (1979) Liposarcomas of the head and neck: a review of the literature and addition of four cases. Cancer 43:162–168

Leiomyoma

Fernandez-Pugnaire MA, Delgado-Florencio V (1995) Familial multiple cutaneous leiomyomas. Dermatology 191: 295–298

Heffernan MP, Smoller BR, Kohler S (1998) Cutaneous epithelioid angioleiomyoma. Am J Dermatopathol 20: 213–217

Raj S, Calonje E, Kraus M et al. (1997) Cutaneous pilar leiomyoma: clinicopathologic analysis of 53 lesions in 45 patients. Am J Dermatopathol 19:2–9

Thyresson HN, Su WP (1981) Familial cutaneous leiomyomatosis. J Am Acad Dermatol 4:430–434

Smooth Muscle Hamartoma

Gagne EJ, Su WP (1993) Congenital smooth muscle hamartoma of the skin. Pediatr Dermatol 10:142–145

Grau-Massanes M, Raimer S, Colome-Grimmer M et al. (1996) Congenital smooth muscle hamartoma presenting as a linear atrophic plaque: case report and review of the literature. Pediatr Dermatol 13:222–225

Tsambaos D, Orfanos CE (1982) Cutaneous smooth muscle hamartoma. J Cutan Pathol 9:33–42

Leiomyosarcoma

Davidson LL, Frost ML, Hanke CW et al. (1989) Primary leiomyosarcoma of the skin.Case report and review of the literature. J Am Acad Dermatol 21:1156–1160

Fletcher CD, McKee PH (1985) Sarcomas – a clinicopathological guide with particular reference to cutaneous manifestation. II. Malignant nerve sheath tumour, leiomyosarcoma and rhabdomyosarcoma. Clin Exp Dermatol 10: 201–216

Headington JT, Beals TF, Niederhuber JE (1977) Primary leiomyosarcoma of skin: a report and critical appraisal. J Cutan Pathol 4:308–317

Rhadomyoma

Kapadia SB, Meis JM, Frisman DM et al. (1993) Fetal rhabdomyoma of the head and neck: a clinicopathologic and immunophenotypic study of 24 cases. Hum Pathol 24: 754–765

Kapadia SB, Meis JM, Frisman DM et al. (1993) Adult rhabdomyoma of the head and neck: a clinicopathologic and immunophenotypic study. Hum Pathol 24:608–617

Kilpatrick SE, Mentzel T, Fletcher CD (1994) Leiomyoma of deep soft tissue. Clinicopathologic analysis of a series. Am J Surg Pathol 18:576–582

Striated Muscle Hamartoma

Sanchez RL, Raimer SS (1994) Clinical and histologic features of striated muscle hamartoma: possible relationship to Delleman's syndrome. J Cutan Pathol 21: 40–46

Scrivener Y, Petiau P, Rodier-Bruant C et al. (1998) Perianal striated muscle hamartoma associated with hemangioma. Pediatr Dermatol 15:274–276

Rhabdomyosarcoma

Chang Y, Dehner LP, Egbert B (1990) Primary cutaneous rhabdomyosarcoma. Am J Surg Pathol 14:977–982

Dagher R, Helman L (1999) Rhabdomyosarcoma: an overview. Oncologist 4:34–44

Lee HH, Farhat W, Prasad A et al. (1999) Pediatric genitourinary tumors. Curr Opin Oncol 11:218–25

Merlino G, Helman LJ (1999) Rhabdomyosarcoma – working out the pathways. Oncogene 18:5340–5348

Cutaneous Ossification

Bucko AD, Burgdorf WHC (1997) Cutaneous ossification in Clinical Dermatology (Demis DJ ed) Vol. 2 Unit 24-13 Philadelphia JB Lippincott

Burgdorf W, Nasemann T (1977) Cutaneous osteomas: A clinical and histopathologic review. Arch Dermatol Res 260:121–135

Orlow SJ, Watsky KL, Bolognia JL (1991) Continuing medical education. Skin and bones II. J Am Acad Dermatol 25:447–462

Roth SI, Stowell RE, Helwig EB (1963) Cutaneous ossification: Report of 120 cases and review of the literature. Arch Pathol 76:56–66

Albright Hereditary Osteodystrophy

Albright F, Burnett CH, Smith CH et al. (1942) Pseudohypoparathyroidism-example of "Seabright bantam syndrome": Report of three cases. Endocrinology 30:922–932

Eyre WG, Reed WB (1971) Albright's hereditary osteodystrophy with cutaneous bone formation. Arch Dermatol 104:634–642

Farfel Z, Bourne HR, Iiri T (1999) The expanding spectrum of G protein diseases. N Engl J Med 340:1012–1020

Fitch N (1982) Albright's hereditary osteodystrophy: a review. Am J Med Genet 11:11–29

Trueb RM, Panizzon RG, Burg G (1993) Cutaneous ossification in Albright's hereditary osteodystrophy. Dermatology 186:205–209

Plate-Like Cutaneous Osteoma

Monroe AB, Burgdorf WHC, Sheward S (1987) Platelike cutaneous osteoma. J Am Acad Dermatol 16:481–484

Tressera L, Tressera F, Grases PJ et al. (1998) Congenital platelike osteoma cutis of the forehead: an atypical presentation from. J Craniomaxillofac Surg 26:102–106

Worret W-I, Burgdorf W (1978) Angeborenes plattenartiges Osteoma cutis bei einem Säugling. Hautarzt 29:590–596

Fibrodysplasia Ossificans Progessiva

Bridges AJ, Hsu KC, Singh A et al. (1994) Fibrodysplasia (myositis) ossifications progressiva. Semin Arthritis Rheum 24:155–164

Buyse G, Silberstein J, Goemans N et al. (1995) Fibrodysplasia ossificans progessiva: still turning into wood after 300 years? Eur J Pediatr 154:694–699

Jouve JL, Cottalorda J, Bollini G et al. (1997) Myositis ossificans: report of seven cases in children. J Pediatr Orthop B 6:33–41

Kaplan FS, Craver R, MacEwen GD et al. (1994) Progressive osseous heteroplasia: a distinct developmental disorder of heterotopic ossification: two new case reports and follow-up of three previously reported cases. J Bone Joint Surg Am 76:425–436

Kaplan FS, Hahn GV, Zasloff MA (1994) Heterotopic ossification: two rare forms and what they can teach us. J Am Acad Orthop Surg 2:288–296

Miller ES, Esterly NB, Fairley JA (1996) Progressive osseous heteroplasia. Arch Dermatol. 132:787–791

Ossifying Fasciitis

DaRoca PJ Jr, Pulitzer DR, LoCicero J III (1982) Ossifying fasciitis. Arch Pathol Lab Med 106:682–685

Innocenzi D, Giustini S, Barduagni F et al. (1997) Ossifying fasciitis of the nose. J Am Acad Dermatol 37:357–361

Idiopathic Osteoma Cutis

Gfesser M, Worret WI, Hein R et al. (1998) Multiple primary osteoma cutis. Arch Dermatol 134:641–643

Lilga HV, Burns DC (1942) Osteomatosis cutis: Report of a case. Arch Dermatol Syph 46:872–874

Nakamura S, Imai T, Nakayma K et al. (1987) Primary osteoma cutis. J Dermatol 14:85–88

Tumors of Bone and Cartilage

Chung EB, Enzinger FM (1978) Chondroma of soft parts. Cancer 41:1414–1424

Dahlin DC, Salvador AH (1974) Cartilaginous tumors of the soft tissues of the hands and feet. Mayo Clin Proc 49:721–726

Holmes HS, Bovenmeyer DA (1976) Cutaneous cartilaginous tumor. Arch Dermatol 112:839–840

Kobos JW, Yu GH, Varadarajan S et al. (1995) Primary cutaneous osteosarcoma. Am J Dermatopath 17:53–57

Kuo T-t (1992) Primary osteosarcoma of the skin. J Cutan Pathol 19:151–155

Chordoma

Cesinaro AM, Maiorana A, Annessi G et al. (1995) Cutaneous metastasis of chordoma. Am J Dermatopathol 17:603–605

Gagne EJ, Su WP (1992) Chordoma involving the skin: an immunohistochemical study of 11 cases. J Cutan Pathol 19:469–475

Miller SD, Vinson RP, McCollough ML et al. (1997) Multiple smooth skin nodules. Chordoma cutis. Arch Dermatol 133:1579–1580, 1582–1583

Peramezza C, Cellini A, Berardi P et al. (1993) Chordoma with multiple skin metastases. Dermatology 186:266–268

Neuroma

Argenyi ZB (1993) Recent developments in cutaneous neural neoplasms. J Cutan Pathol 20:97–108

Requena L, Sangueza OP (1995) Benign neoplasms with neural differentiation: a review. Am J Dermatopathol 17:75–96

Pacinian Corpuscle Hyperplasia

Jones NF, Eadie P (1991) Pacinian corpuscle hyperplasia in the hand. J Hand Surg [Am] 16:865–869

Reznik M, Thiry A, Fridman V (1998) Painful hyperplasia and hypertrophy of pacinian corpuscles in the hand: report of two cases with immunohistochemical and ultrastructural studies, and a review of the literature. Am J Dermatopathol 20:203–207

Palisated and Encapsulated Neuroma

Argenyi ZB, Penick GD (1993) Vascular variant of palisaded encapsulated neuroma. J Cutan Pathol 20:92–93

Reed RJ, Fine RM, Meltzer HD (1972) Palisaded, encapsulated neuromas of the skin. Arch Dermatol 106:865–870

Neurilemmoma

Megahed M, Ruzicka T (1994) Cellular schwannoma. Am J Dermatopathol 16:418–421

Megahed M (1994) Plexiform schwannoma. Am J Dermatopathol 16:288–293

Reith JD, Goldblum JR (1996) Multiple cutaneous plexiform schwannomas. Report of a case and review of the literature with particular reference to the association with types 1 and 2 neurofibromatosis and schwannomatosis. Arch Pathol Lab Med 120:399–401

Stout AP (1935) The peripheal manifestations of the specific nerve sheath tumor (neurolemmoma). Am J Cancer 19: 24:751–796

Neurofibroma

Reed ML, Jacoby RA (1983) Cutaneous neuroantomy and neuropathology. J Am Dermatopathol 5:335–362

von Recklinghausen FD (1882) Über die multiplen Fibrome der Haut und ihre Beziehung zu den multiplen Neuromen. Hirschwald, Berlin

Neurothekeoma

Argenyi ZB, LeBoit PE, Santa Cruz D et al. (1993) Nerve sheath myxoma (neurothekeoma) of the skin: light microscopic and immunohistochemical reappraisal of the cellular variant. J Cutan Pathol 20:294–303

Chang SE, Lee TJ, Ro JY et al. (1999) Cellular neurothekeoma with possible neuroendocrine differentiation. J Dermatol 26:363–367

Harkin JC, Reed RJ (1969) Tumors of the peripheral nervous system. In: Atlas of tumor pathology series 2, fascicle 3. Washington DC: Armed Forces Institute of Pathology, pp 60–64

Tomasini C, Aloi F, Pippione M (1996) Cellular neurothekeoma. Dermatology 192:160–163

Zelger BG, Steiner H, Kutzner H et al. (1998) Cellular 'neurothekeoma': an epithelioid variant of dermatofibroma? Histopathology 32:414–422

Perineurioma

Mentzel T, Dei Tos AP, Fletcher CD (1994) Perineurioma (storiform perineurial fibroma): clinico-pathological analysis of four cases. Histopathology 25:261–267

Pulitzer DR, Reed RJ (1985) Nerve-sheath myxoma (perineurial myxoma). Am J Dermatopathol 7:409–421

Tsang WY, Chan JK, Chow LT et al. (1992) Perineurioma: an uncommon soft tissue neoplasm distinct from localized hypertrophic neuropathy and neurofibroma. Am J Surg Pathol 16:756–763

Malignant Peripheral Nerve Sheath Tumor

Reith JD, Goldblum JR (1996) Multiple cutaneous plexiform schwannomas. Report of a case and review of the literature with particular reference to the association with types 1 and 2 neurofibromatosis and schwannomatosis. Arch Pathol Lab Med 120:399–401

Rasbridge SA, Browse NL, Tighe JR et al. (1989) Malignant nerve sheath tumour arising in a benign ancient schwannoma. Histopathology 14:525–528

Reznik M (1991) Cutaneous neuropathology: neurofibromas, schwannomas and other neural neoplasms with cutaneous and extracutaneous expressions. Clin Neuropathol 10:225–231

Robson DK, Ironside JW (1990) Malignant peripheral nerve sheath tumour arising in a schwannoma. Histopathology 16:295–297

Neuroblastoma

Klapman MH, Chun D (1991) Cutaneous and subcutaneous neuroblastoma in children and adults: case reports and population study. J Am Acad Dermatol 24:1025–1027

Van Nguyen A, Argenyi ZB (1993) Cutaneous neuroblastoma. Peripheral neuroblastoma. Am J Dermatopathol 15: 7–14

Merkel Cell Carcinoma

Brown TJ, Jackson BA, Macfarlane DF et al. (1999) Merkel cell carcinoma: spontaneous resolution and management of metastatic disease. Dermatol Surg 25:23–25

Hanly AJ, Elgart GW, Jorda M et al. (2000) Analysis of thyroid transcription factor-1 and cytokeratin 20 separates Merkel cell carcinoma from small cell carcinoma of lung. J Cutan Pathol 27:118–120

Skelton HG, Smith KJ, Hitchcock CL et al. (1997) Merkel cell carcinoma: analysis of clinical, histologic, and immunohistologic features of 132 cases with relation to survival. J Am Acad Dermatol 37:734–739

Toker C (1972) Trabecular carcinoma of the skin. Arch Dermatol 105:107–110

Cutaneous Myxoma

Gardner SS, Solomon AR (1991) Cutaneous and cardiac myxomas: an important association. Semin Dermatol 10:148–151

Wilk M, Schmoeckel C, Kaiser HW et al. (1995) Cutaneous angiomyxoma: a benign neoplasm distinct from cutaneous focal mucinosis. J Am Acad Dermatol 33:352–355

Granular Cell Tumor

Abrikosoff A (1926) Über Myome, ausgehend von der quergestreiften, willkürlichen Muskulatur. Virchows Arch Pathol Anat 260:215–233

Apisarnthanarax P (1981) Granular cell tumor. An analysis of 16 cases and review of the literature. J Am Acad Dermatol 5:171–182

Ordonez NG (1999) Granular cell tumor: a review and update. Adv Anat Pathol 6:186–203

Ordonez NG, Mackay B (1999) Granular cell tumor: a review of the pathology and histogenesis. Ultrastruct Pathol 23:207–222

Sahn EE, Dunlavey ES, Parsons JL (1997) Multiple cutaneous granular cell tumors in a child with possible neurofibromatosis. J Am Acad Dermatol 36:327–330

Clear Cell Sarcoma

Chung EB, Enzinger FM (1983) Malignant melanoma of soft parts. A reassessment of clear cell sarcoma. Am J Surg Pathol 7:405–413

Deenik W, Mooi WJ, Rutgers EJ et al. (1999) Clear cell sarcoma (malignant melanoma) of soft parts: a clinicopathologic study of 30 cases. Cancer 86:969–975

Enzinger FM (1965) Clear cell sarcoma of tendons and aponeuroses: an analysis of 21 cases. Cancer 18:1163

Graadt van Roggen JF, Mooi WJ, Hogendoorn PC (1998) Clear cell sarcoma of tendons and aponeuroses (malignant melanoma of soft parts) and cutaneous melanoma: exploring the histogenetic relationship between these two clinicopathological entities. J Pathol 186:3–7

Pseudolymphomas

Contents

Introduction

Cutaneous pseudolymphomas are reactive lymphocytic proliferations that appear in the skin and resemble a malignant lymphoma. Many different terms have been used to describe such disordered infiltrates. No one term is ideal. The problem is that a number of unrelated inflammatory disorders may resemble lymphomas, either because of clinical or histologic features. The number of names attached to these disorders is baffling, as shown in Table 60.1. We feel that pseudolymphoma is the simplest and most satisfactory.

The accuracy of the diagnosis pseudolymphoma in the past when one relied exclusively on clinical and histologic features left much to be desired. Today the assessment of the malignant potential of a lymphocytic infiltrate is entrusted to special laboratories where the various surface markers and clonality of the cells can be assessed. Clonality cannot be taken as an unequivocal marker for malignancy. Confusing the picture is the fact that some cutaneous lymphomas have such a slow or benign course that biologic behavior may be misleading unless very long-term follow-up is available. Thus the diagnosis of pseudolymphoma or lymphoma should be continuously reassessed as the patient is followed. There is no single reliable histologic or molecular biologic procedure to unequivocally identify a lymphocytic infiltrate as benign.

There is no widely agreed classification. The division into B cell and T cell types does not greatly aid one's understanding, although it is most widely used. We prefer to speak of idiopathic and reactive pseudolymphomas. Most important is to identify those pseudolymphomas in which the etiology is clear. In our area a common cause of pseudolymphoma is *Borrelia burgdorferi*. Borrelial pseudolymphomas respond to antibiotic therapy so it is crucial to diagnose them.

Table 60.1. Terms used to describe benign cutaneous lymphocytic infiltrates

Term	First described Author	Year
Sarcomatosis cutis	Kaposi	1891
	Spiegler	1894
	Fendt	1900
Sarcoid of Spiegler-Fendt	Darier	1910
Lymphadenosis cutis circumscripta	Burckhardt and Arndt	1911
Lymphocytoma cutis	Biberstein	1923
Lymphadenosis cutis benigna	Bäfverstedtstedt	1943
Lymphocytic infiltration of the skin	Jessner and Kanof	1953
Pseudolymphoma syndrome	Saltzstein and Ackerman	1959
Pseudolymphoma	Hirsch and Lukes	1965
Cutaneous lymphoid hyperplasia	Caro and Helwig	1969

B Cell Pseudolymphomas

Synonyms. The two terms most often employed for this group are lymphadenosis cutis benigna and lymphocytoma cutis

Epidemiology. Most patients are young adults with a female dominance. Children can also be affected. The age and sex distribution is heavily dependent on how much borreliosis is included in the study group.

Etiology and Pathogenesis. The most common identified cause for B cell pseudolymphoma is infection with *B. burgdorferi*. Other well-established causes include tattoo reactions, immunizations or allergen desensitization injections, ear-piercing reactions and infections with herpes simplex and zoster. Presumably all these other uncommon triggers elicit a localized B cell response through poorly understood mechanisms. In most B cell pseudolymphomas not related to borreliosis, the precipitating antigens remain obscure.

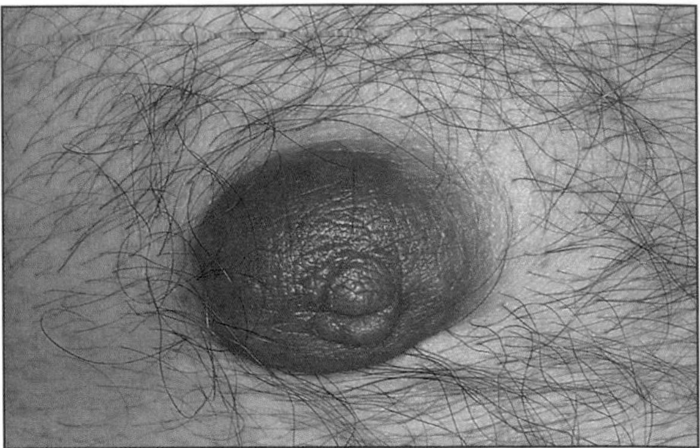

Fig. 60.1. Borrelial pseudolymphoma of nipple

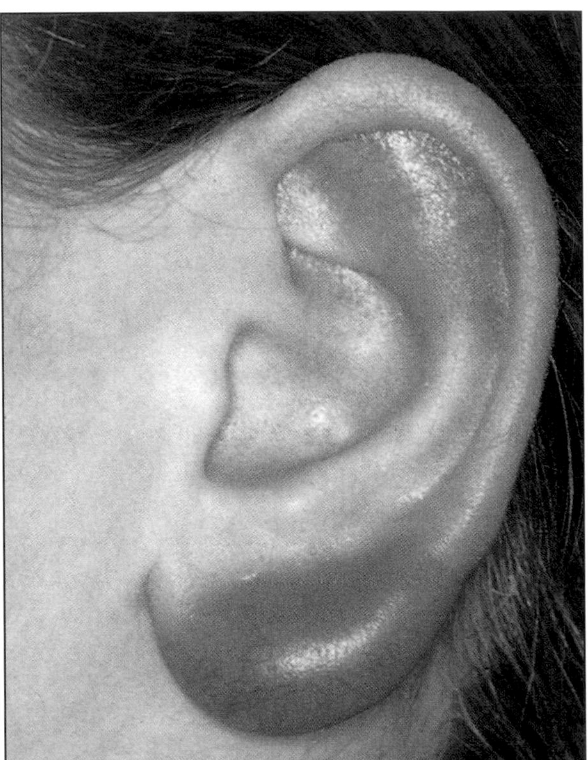

Fig. 60.2. Borrelial pseudolymphoma of earlobe

Clinical Findings. The clinical variation is considerable. The most common type was described by Bäfverstedt as lymphadenosis cutis benigna solitaria. This category is somewhat of a misnomer as both solitary and multiple lesions may be seen. Most patients have a single large nodule or a limited number of smaller nodules which are sharply bordered, soft, red to blue-red, dome-shaped and covered by thinned skin. When the infiltrate is examined via diascopy, a yellow-gray often lupoid infiltrate is seen. The sites of predilection are the ear lobes, nape, nipple and areola, axillae, scrotum and dorsum of the foot. The nipple and ear lobe are especially common locations for borrelial pseudolymphoma (Figs. 60.1, 60.2). Pseudolymphomas are usually asymptomatic. If lymphadenopathy is present, one should suspect malignant lymphoma or another underlying cause, such as an infection.

Other even rarer clinical forms have also been described. All were identified before modern techniques for studying lymphocytic infiltrates became available. In general, widespread lesions, patches or plaques should clinically increase the suspicion that a malignant lymphoma is present. The other forms include:

- Widespread: These patients have many lesions distributed over the entire body and are almost always adults.
- Disseminated miliary: These patients have numerous symmetric small blue-red papules and nodules which favor the face and trunk. These lesions also show a yellow-gray lupoid infiltrate upon diascopic examination.
- Patch-like or infiltrative: In these individuals there are larger patches and plaques, often with telangiectases and hemosiderin deposition. These larger lesions are most often on the legs and also have a lupoid diascopic appearance.

Plaques of pseudolymphoma on the eyelids may resemble xanthelasma. Mucosal pseudolymphomas have also been identified. Probably conjunctival involvement is most common with multiple small pink papules. In the oral mucosa, the problem is even more confusing as normal lymphoid aggregates are present. They are felt to represent ectopic tonsillar tissue and often diagnosed as oral tonsils. In addition, papules and nodules may appear on the palate.

Histopathology. The epidermis is normal and there is usually a Grenz zone in the upper dermis. The balance of the dermis is involved either diffusely or more often in a nodular fashion by a sharply demarcated polymorphic infiltrate of small lymphocytes admixed with plasma cells and eosinophils. The infiltrate is likely to be top-heavy. Often there are follicular structures with germinal centers. Just as in lymph nodes, these structures contain centroblasts, centrocytes, germinal center (tingible body) macrophages and numerous mitoses. Dendritic reticulum cells can be identified with immunohistochemical stains. Eosinophils and plasma cells are found at the periphery of the follicle. In some instances, follicular structures are not seen. The lymphocytes are polyclonal containing both κ- and λ-light chains. Other common findings include sparing of adnexal structures and a prominent vascular patterns with plump endothelial cells in the venules of the dermis.

A histologic variant has been identified as large cell lymphocytoma. There is a dense often deep infiltrate of centroblasts and centrocytes with many mitoses, but still with tingible body macrophages, eosinophils and plasma cells.

Course and Prognosis. The outlook is good. There is often spontaneous regression and those pseudolymphoma associated with *B. burgdorferi* respond well to treatment. While expansion of individual lesions or appearance of new lesions may occur, such a course always mandates a reevaluation.

Differential Diagnosis. A number of conditions appear clinically similar but are easily excluded histologically. Included in this list are sarcoidosis, lupus vulgaris, granuloma faciale and lupus erythematosus profundus.

The main problem is excluding a malignant lymphoma. The hallmarks of a B cell pseudolymphoma are a mixed cell population and germinal centers with tingible body macrophages. A follicular B cell lymphoma is more likely to have naked germinal centers with less of a lymphocytic band about them, poor circumscription, uniform size and lack of inflammatory cells. In addition, the B cells are more likely to have only one light-chain type and be positive for CD10, a marker of follicular differentiation. If the pseudolymphoma lacks follicles, then immunohistochemical means are usually needed to exclude B cell lymphoma and chronic lymphocytic leukemia.

Therapy. The treatment for borreliosis is detailed in Chapter 4. Other lesions can be treated by excision, injection with intralesional corticosteroids (triamcinolone acetonide 2.5–5.0 mg/ml in several divided doses), cryotherapy or irradiation with low dosages of ionizing radiation. Soft x-rays with a half-value layer of 0.2–0.4 mm Al and a target skin distance of 15–30 cm are employed. A typical regimen is 3 Gy every 3–4 weeks for a total of 9–12 Gy, although smaller dosages such as 1–2 Gy may also be effective. Grenz rays can also be used.

T Cell Pseudolymphomas

The spectrum of T cell pseudolymphoma is perhaps even more confusing than that of B cell pseudolymphoma. A wide variety of triggering agents are associated producing somewhat different clinical patterns. Histologically there may be a band-like or nodular T cell infiltrate. In addition, some of the conditions traditionally designated as T cell pseudolymphomas are potentially premalignant.

Drug-Induced Pseudolymphoma

Epidemiology. There are several clinically distinct settings in which drug reactions may mimic lymphoma. The best established is the anticonvulsant reaction usually caused by phenytoin, related products or carbamazepine, with lymphadenopathy, fever and erythroderma. The only other medications reliably associated with this process are the angiotensin-converting enzyme (ACE) inhibitors. Patients have a pseudolymphoma but it usually involves the lymph nodes, not the skin. Confusing the situation is the fact that patients on long-term phenytoin therapy have an increased risk of true lymphoma. Other cutaneous drug reactions may be associated with lymphadenopathy.

Table 60.2. Medications associated with pseudolymphoma

Common	Phenytoin and related agents Carbamazepine ACE inhibitors	
Rare	Allopurinol Atenolol Azathioprine Cyclosporine Diltiazem Etretinate Filgrastim Hydroxychloroquine	Nitrofurantoin Phenothiazines Penicillamine Penicillin Pyrazolone Pyrimethamine Razoxane Sulfasalazine

In other instances, although there is no clinical question of the diagnosis, histology may reveal some of the features of mycosis fungoides. Localized nodular pseudolymphoma, as described under B cell pseudolymphoma, may occur following injections. The list of products associated at least once with a pseudolymphoma is show in Table 60.2. We emphasize that this is an anecdotal list.

Clinical Findings. There are actually no typical clinical features. The pseudolymphomatous reaction to anticonvulsants or ACE inhibitors is a systemic illness. The skin findings may include a widespread maculopapular eruption or erythroderma. Nodules are rare.

Histopathology. There is usually a band-like infiltrate of lymphocytes. Both nuclear atypia and even cerebriform nuclei may be present. True Pautrier microabscesses are rare. Often there are intraepidermal accumulations of lymphocytes with an inverted vase pattern. In other instances, there is a nodular dermal infiltrate of atypical lymphocytes. Marker studies indicate the cells are T cells with no hint of monoclonality.

Differential Diagnosis. The problem is distinguishing drug eruptions histologically from mycosis fungoides. Other inflammatory dermatoses may also cause the same problem. The presence of atypical lymphocytes, solitary lymphocytes in the epidermis in the absence of spongiosis, or groups of lymphocytes clustered in the epidermis or along the basal layer suggest mycosis fungoides. In addition, there may be larger lymphocytes in the epidermis than the dermis and a fine sclerosis of the papillary dermis.

Therapy. If the answer is drug eruption, then stopping the medication and avoiding cross-reacting products solves the problem.

Lymphomatoid Contact Dermatitis

In very rare instances, persistent allergic contact dermatitis may produce histologic changes mimicking mycosis fungoides. This phenomenon has been infrequently described and no one agent has distinguished itself as a likely cause. Just as with any other unexplained dermatitis, it is probably wise to do patch testing if the biopsy suggests a T cell pseudolymphoma and no other obvious explanation is available.

Persistent Arthropod Bite Reaction

Etiology and Pathogenesis. The most common cause is scabies, but any arthropod bite can lead to a persistent nodular response.

Clinical Findings. In this case, the pseudolymphoma is always nodular. One or more red-brown papules or nodules occur. In the case of scabies, the most common sites are the axilla and male genitalia. Other frequently involved areas include the elbows, forearms and abdomen.

Histopathology. There is a highly mixed lymphocytic infiltrate. A distinguishing feature is the frequent presence of abundant eosinophils. In most cases T cells dominate but in some instances, the infiltrate is primarily comprised of B cells. There is often overlying pseudoepitheliomatous hyperplasia.

Acral Pseudolymphomatous Angiokeratoma

(Crow 1980)

Synonym. APACHE is a fantasy-laden acronym for the usual title

This rare problem has been described in a handful of children and one adult. Patients develop multiple red-violet discrete papules usually on the hands. In several instances, the lesions were felt to be persistent arthropod bite reactions. There is often a collarette scale or overlying hyperkeratosis. Microscopically, there is a nodular accumulation of lymphocytes associated with dilated vessels high in the dermis. Most cases have been dominated by T cells. There are many settings in which lymphocytes and vessels proliferate in unison, and some prefer to classify this entity among the angiokeratomas.

Actinic Reticuloid

Persistent light reaction or actinic reticuloid is discussed in detail in Chapter 13. Patients with persistent light reactions may on occasion have lymphocytic atypia on biopsy. At least some of these patients advance to malignant lymphoma.

Lymphomatoid Papulosis

We have chosen to cover this complex but fascinating entity along with malignant lymphomas, but recognize that many authors consider it a pseudolymphoma. In any case, the infiltrate is predominantly T cell and only a small percentage of patients develop malignant lymphoma.

Other Pseudolymphomas

There is a list of other diseases that are often called pseudolymphomas. They do not truly resemble a lymphoma either clinically or histologically but have a dense lymphocytic infiltrate when examined microscopically.

Lymphocytic Infiltration of the Skin

(Jessner and Kanof 1953)

Synonyms. Lymphocytic infiltration of Jessner-Kanof, Jessner-Kanof disease

Epidemiology. This uncommon disease has a striking male dominance (10:1) and is usually seen in young adults.

Etiology and Pathogenesis. The nature of lymphocytic infiltration of the skin is unclear. Some group it as a T cell pseudolymphoma while others consider it a variant of lupus erythematosus or polymorphic light eruption. It appears most often on sunlight-exposed skin.

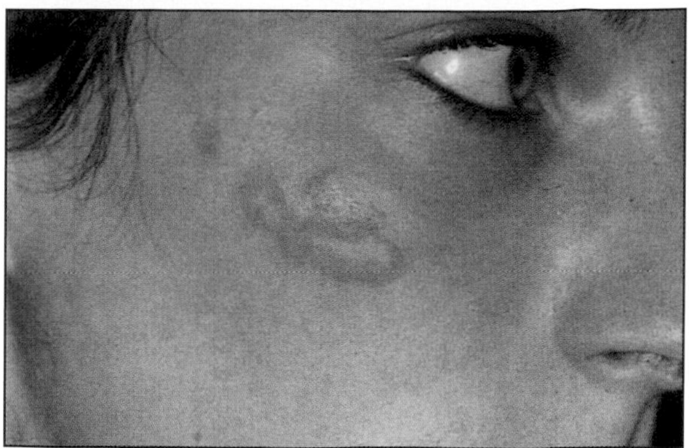

Fig. 60.3. Lymphocytic infiltration of the skin with typical annular facial lesions

Clinical Findings. The most common sites are the cheeks, forehead, and nape. On occasion the trunk may be involved. One or more symmetrically distributed sharply bordered red-brown papules appear. The papules tend to evolve into plaques which often become circinate or annular with central clearing (Fig. 60.3). Scale, follicular plugging, atrophy and scarring do not occur. The lesions are asymptomatic.

Histopathology. The epidermis is normal. In the dermis is a monotonous dense infiltrate of small lymphocytes arranged about the vessels and adnexal structures. The infiltrates are nodular and sharply separated from the adjacent dermis. Immunologic analysis confirms that they are predominantly T cells. Mucin is not present and immunofluorescent analysis does not reveal an lupus erythematosus band.

Course and Prognosis. In most instances, the disease waxes and wanes. Some individuals clear entirely.

Differential Diagnosis. The obvious differential diagnostic considerations are lupus erythematosus, especially the profundus form, and polymorphic light eruption. We suspect that lymphocytic infiltration of Jessner-Kanof and lupus erythematosus are either closely related or extremely difficult to separate. Erythema annulare centrifugum may also be suggested but is rarely so infiltrated and moves more rapidly. Drug reactions may also appear similar; a detailed drug history should be taken.

Therapy. Both sunscreens and antimalarial drugs may help, supporting the overlap with polymorphic light eruption. In addition, intralesional corticosteroids, cryotherapy and radiation therapy as discussed under B cell pseudolymphoma above can be employed.

Palpable Migratory Arciform Erythema

(Clark et al. 1974)

Synonym. Erythema migrans arciforme et palpabile

The nature of this entity is even more confusing than the last. Clark described patients with infiltrated blue-violet nodules which had unusual morphologic features. The lesions are typically arcuate with raised, sharp borders. Centrally they show clearing. They are chronic but slowly migrate. The sites of predilection are the trunk, arms and thighs rather than light-exposed areas. Under the microscope there is a dense periadnexal and perivascular infiltrate of uniform small lymphocytes. It is not known whether T cells or B cells predominate. The main task is to exclude a malignant lymphoma.

Angiolymphoid Hyperplasia with Eosinophilia

This entity is covered under vascular proliferations in Chapter 59. It is another example of the intimate way in which lymphocytes and blood vessels proliferate together. The key feature is the presence of vessels with very prominent endothelial cells. In some specimens, these structures may be obscured by an intense lymphocytic infiltrate, occasionally with follicular centers. In most instances, eosinophils are abundant, but they too can be scarce. When the vessels and eosinophils are not obvious, then the diagnosis is likely to be a B cell pseudolymphoma.

Dermatopathic Lymphadenopathy

(Pautrier and Woringer 1932)

Synonyms. Lipomelanotic reticulosis, Pautrier-Woringer disease

Definition. Non-specific reactive lymphadenopathy associated with widespread inflammatory dermatoses and mycosis fungoides.

Epidemiology. Lymph node enlargement is common in many widespread skin disorders such as psoriatic erythroderma. It is also a prominent feature of mycosis fungoides and other malignant lymphomas.

Etiology and Pathogenesis. The lymphatics drain the skin and present antigens from the skin to the regional lymph nodes. When there is skin inflammation and damage, a variety of products such as melanin, hemosiderin and lipids are transported to the lymph nodes. There they elicit a reactive response which includes proliferation of paracortical histiocytes and occasionally of lymphoid follicles.

Modern molecular biologic studies have cast some doubt on the nature of dermatopathic lymphadenopathy. Puzzling is the observation that the presence or absence of enlarged lymph nodes in mycosis fungoides correlates better with prognosis than the presence of dermatopathic lymphadenopathy or a malignant infiltrate in the nodes. In some patients with mycosis fungoides, small numbers of malignant cells can be found in the enlarged nodes. These malignant cells may help trigger the reactive response.

Clinical Findings. The clinical features are similar, no matter what the nature of the skin disorder. The unifying aspect is that the skin disease is usually extensive. Typically there are enlarged cervical, axillary or inguinal nodes. Every patient with Sézary syndrome has some degree of lymphadenopathy, but in mycosis fungoides it is rare in the early stages. In drug-induced erythroderma, there may also be lymphadenopathy. In addition, patients with erythroderma associated with psoriasis, pityriasis rubra pilaris, extensive lichen planus or atopic dermatitis also have enlarged lymph nodes.

Histopathology. The diagnosis of dermatopathic lymphadenopathy is a microscopic issue. The paracortical histiocytes are increased in number and often contain lipids, melanin and hemosiderin (lipomelanotic reticulosis). A rich mixture of lymphocytes of various lineages, plasma cells and eosinophils are usually present. In addition, there are large reactive germinal centers. Molecular biologic methods, including searching for rearrangement of the T cell receptor gene, should be undertaken in difficult cases.

Course and Prognosis. If the nodes are truly reactive, they regress as the underlying skin disease is treated. Even if a biopsy shows dermatopathic lymphadenopathy in a patient with mycosis fungoides, one should be aware that this is a negative prognostic sign.

Differential Diagnosis. The differential diagnosis includes the entire spectrum of lymphadenopathy. The most difficult distinction involves a follicle center lymphoma (Brill-Symmers disease).

Therapy. The only treatment is that of the associated skin disease.

Castleman Disease

(CASTLEMAN 1956)

Synonym. Giant lymph node hyperplasia

Castleman disease is another disease of lymph nodes that overlaps with malignant lymphoma but is usually benign. Solitary Castleman disease is apparently a reactive B cell and plasma cell proliferation, although the triggers are unknown. There is follicular hyperplasia associated with endothelial hyperplasia and vascular proliferation. In the most common hyaline-vascular form, young patients present with a localized mediastinal mass, and surgery is usually curative. The rarer plasma cell form comprises about 10 % of cases and may be associated with a variety of systemic symptoms.

Multicentric Castleman disease is a different process. It is viewed as a lymphoproliferative process with morphologic features of Castleman disease. Patients are usually older men who have multiple areas of lymph node involvement, hepatosplenomegaly and a wide range of systemic signs and symptoms. Cutaneous infiltrates can be seen; they are usually red-brown plaques or nodules. About one-third of patients develop malignancies, including non-Hodgkin lymphoma, Kaposi sarcoma and even carcinomas. Castleman disease is of interest to dermatologists because of its association with POEMS syndrome (Chap. 40) and paraneoplastic pemphigus (Chap. 15).

Bibliography

Ablele DC, Anders KH, Chandler FW (1989) Benign lymphocytic infiltration (Jessner-Kanof): another manifestation of borreliosis? J Am Acad Dermatol 21:795–797

Albrecht AS, Hofstadter S, Artsob H et al. (1991) Lymphadenosis benigna cutis resulting from *Borrelia* infection (Borrelia lymphocytoma). J Am Acad Dermatol 24: 621–625

Bouloc A, Delfau-Larue MH, Lenormand B et al. (1999) Polymerase chain reaction analysis of immunoglobulin gene rearrangement in cutaneous lymphoid hyperplasias. Arch Dermatol 135:168–172

Brady SP, Magro CM, Diaz-Cano SJ et al. (1999) Analysis of clonality of atypical cutaneous lymphoid infiltrates associated with drug therapy by PCR/DGGE. Hum Pathol 30:130–136

Caro WA, Helwig HB (1969) Cutaneous lymphoid hyperplasia. Cancer 24:487–502

Castleman B et al. (1956) Localised mediastinal lymph node hyperplasia resembling thymoma. Cancer 46:822–830

Clark WH, Mihm MC Jr, Reed RJ et al. (1974) The lymphocytic infiltrates of the skin. Hum Pathol 5:25–43

Crow KD (1980) Case for diagnosis. Br J Dermatol [Suppl] 18:78

De Diego J, Berridi D, Saracibar N et al. (1998) Cutaneous pseudolymphoma in association with molluscum contagiosum. Am J Dermatopathol 20:518–521

Egan CA, Patel BCK, Morschbacher R et al. (1997) Atypical lymphoid hyperplasia of the eyelids manifesting as xanthelasma-like lesions. J Am Acad Dermatol 37:839–842

Hirsch P, Lukes R (1965) Reactive pseudolymphoma, nodular type. Arch Dermatol 91:408–409

Jessner M, Kanof NB (1953) Lymphocytic infiltration of the skin. Arch Dermatol 68:447–449

Kaddu S, Cerroni L, Pilatti A et al. (1994) Acral pseudolymphoma angiokeratoma. A variant of the cutaneous pseudolymphomas. Am J Dermatopathol 16:130–133

Kobayashi Y, Nanko H, Nakamura J et al. (1992) Lymphocytoma cutis induced by gold pierced earrings. J Am Acad Dermatol 17:457–458

Kuflik AS, Schwartz RA (1992) Lymphocytoma cutis: a series of five patients successfully treated with cryosurgery. J Am Acad Dermatol 26:449–452

Landa NG, Zelickson BD, Peters MS et al. (1993) Lymphoma versus pseudolymphoma of the skin: gene rearrangement study of 21 cases with clinicopathologic correlation. J Am Acad Dermatol 29:945–953

Nathan DL, Belsito DV (1998) Carbamazepin-induced pseudolymphoma with CD-30 positive cells. J Am Acad Dermatol 38:806–809

Pautrier LM, Woringer F (1932) Note préliminaire sur un tableau histologique particulier de lésions ganglionnaires accompagnant des éruptions dermatologiques généralisées prurigineuses, de types cliniques différentes. Bull Soc Fr Dermatol Syphilol 39:947–955

Ploysagam T, Breneman DL, Mutasim DF (1998) Cutaneous pseudolymphoma. J Am Acad Dermatol 38:877–905

Rijlaarsdam U, Bakels V, Oostveev JW van et al. (1992) Demonstration of clonal immunoglobulin gene rearrangements in cutaneous B cell lymphomas and pseudolymphomas: differential diagnostic aspects. J Invest Dermatol 99:749–754

Toonstra J, Wildschut A, Boer J et al. (1989) Jessner's lymphocytic infiltration of the skin. Arch Dermatol 125: 1525–1530

Van Hale HM, Winkelmann RK (1985) Nodular lymphoid disease of the head and neck: lymphocytoma cutis, benign lymphocytic infiltrate of Jessner, and their distinction from malignant lymphoma. J Am Acad Dermatol 12:455–461

CHAPTER 61

Malignant Lymphomas

Contents

Introduction

Malignant lymphomas are neoplastic proliferations of lymphoid tissue. The term lymphoma is used as a synonym for malignant lymphoma; not only is it shorter but just as accurate. We will compromise, writing malignant lymphoma but also saying B cell lymphoma or mantle cell lymphoma without attaching the understood malignant. While lymphomas typically involve lymph nodes, they may also be found in many other organs. Among these extranodal sites is the skin; it is the second most common extranodal site after the gastrointestinal tract.

Lymphomas recapitulate the normal development of lymphocytes. The first major division is into B cells involved with humoral immunity and manufacture of immunoglobulins and T cells concerned with cellular immunity. Neither B cells nor T cells represent a homogenous population. Both develop from primitive stem cells, go through defined stages of differentiation for which various cellular markers are available and populate different parts of lymph nodes. For example, one can speak of follicle center, mantle or marginal zone lymphocytes. The wide variety of normal lymphocytes translates into a great array of malignant lymphomas whose classification remains one of the major challenges in medicine. The cellular features of most nodal and extranodal malignant lymphomas are so similar that the same schemes can be used to describe both tumors.

Cutaneous involvement in malignant lymphomas can be primary or secondary. Many malignant lymphomas appear first in the skin and remain a cutaneous problem for many years. Lymphocytes that are normally present in the skin may, even during neoplastic transformation and expansion, retain these homing properties. The best example is mycosis fungoides. In other instances, the lymphoma may present in the lymph nodes or other internal organs and then spread to involve the skin. While immunologic and molecular biological techniques are required today for the exact diagnosis of lymphomas, the clinical features and light microscopic evaluation are still essential to even begin the diagnostic process.

Classification

Traditionally malignant lymphomas have been classified into Hodgkin disease and non-Hodgkin lymphoma. Among the non-Hodgkin lymphomas, various classifications attach different weight to clinical features, morphologic appearance, immunologic markers and prognosis. The basic premise is that each lymphoma has a normal equivalent somewhere along the pathway of lymphocyte differentiation with which it shares morphologic, immunologic and molecular biological features. Many different classifications have been proposed; many have been accepted, used for years and modified as the tools for cell analysis have improved. The traditional classifications include the Rappaport, Lukes-Collins and Working Formulation in the USA and the Kiel in Europe. To simplify matters, we will only employ the Revised European-American Lymphoma classification (REAL), but we have indicated the Kiel classification equivalents in Tables 61.1 and 61.2. The Working Formulation uses the categories of low-, intermediate- and high-grade lymphomas, while the Kiel classification, which was initially strictly morphologic, evolved to use the terms low-grade and high-grade. Such distinctions are missing in the REAL scheme. The cutaneous lymphoma project group of the European Organization for the Research and Treatment of Cancer (EORTC) has suggested a separate classification for primary cutaneous lymphomas, emphasizing that neoplasms which appear in the skin and remain confined there for long periods of time have a different outlook than tumors of the same cell type which start in nodes and secondarily involve the skin. While we will incorporate the observations of this group, we will not use their scheme.

Clinical Considerations

When evaluating a patient with a suspected cutaneous lymphoma, there are several equally important factors. The first step is to decide with certainty if a lymphoma is present or not. Occasionally this is impossible, such as in very early mycosis fungoides; then the patient should be carefully followed. Second, the malignant lymphoma should be classified. This will provide information on the prognosis and therapeutic approach. Finally, staging is essential. Even with apparent cutaneous lymphomas, a thorough work-up to rule out systemic disease or delineate where it is found is mandatory. Usually the staging is accomplished by working with oncologists, radiologists and pathologists. Interdisciplinary clinics often make such evaluations more efficient.

The following procedures are usually required:

- History and physical examination with special attention paid to lymph nodes, spleen, liver, tonsils, and the skin.
- A skin biopsy should be performed. An excisional or incisional biopsy is usually best; it should be generous and done with a sharp instrument to avoid artifactual damage. Similarly, the specimen should not be handled with a forceps

Table 61.1. Classification of T cell lymphomas

REAL classification	Kiel classification
Precursor T cell neoplasms	
Precursor T lymphoblastic lymphoma/ leukemia	T lymphoblastic lymphoma
Peripheral T cell neoplasms	
T cell chronic lymphocytic leukemia/ prolymphocytic leukemia	T cell chronic lymphocytic leukemia, T cell prolymphocytic leukemia
Mycosis fungoides/Sézary syndrome	Small cell, cerebriform lymphoma (mycosis fungoides, Sézary syndrome)
Peripheral T cell lymphomas, unspecified	T zone lymphoma, lymphoepithelioid cell lymphoma, pleomorphic small, medium and large cell lymphoma, T cell immunoblastic lymphoma
Subcutaneous panniculitic T cell lymphoma	No equivalent
Angioimmunoblastic T cell lymphoma	Angioimmunoblastic lymphoma
T/NK cell lymphoma, nasal and nasal type (angiocentric lymphoma)	No equivalent
Intestinal T cell lymphoma	No equivalent
Adult T cell lymphoma/leukemia	Pleomorphic small, medium and large cell (HTLV1+) lymphoma
Anaplastic large cell ($CD30^+$) lymphoma	Large cell anaplastic lymphoma

Table 61.2. Classification of B cell lymphomas

REAL classification	Kiel classification
Precursor B cell neoplasms	
Precursor B lymphoblastic leukemia/lymphoma	B lymphoblastic lymphoma
Peripheral B cell neoplasms	
B cell chronic lymphocytic leukemia/prolymphocytic leukemia/small lymphocytic leukemia	B lymphocytic, chronic lymphocytic leukemia; B lymphocytic, prolymphocytic leukemia
Lymphoplasmacytoid lymphoma/immunocytoma	Lymphoplasmacytic immunocytoma
Mantle cell lymphoma	Centrocytic lymphoma; centroblastic lymphoma, centrocytoid subtype
Follicle center cell lymphoma	Centroblastic-centrocytic lymphoma, follicular; centroblastic-centrocytic lymphoma, diffuse; centroblastic lymphoma, follicular
Marginal zone lymphoma, extranodal type (MALT type)	No equivalent
Hairy cell leukemia (Chap. 62)	Hairy cell leukemia
Plasmacytoma/plasma cell myeloma (Chap. 40)	Plasmacytic lymphoma
Diffuse large B cell lymphoma	Centroblastic lymphoma (with subtypes)
Burkitt lymphoma	Burkitt lymphoma

but gently lifted with a skin hook or the fingers. Crush artifact makes interpreting the biopsy most difficult. The specimen should be divided, so that part can be fixed in formalin and the rest, quick-frozen in liquid nitrogen.

If the clinical examination and biopsy suggest the possibility of lymphoma, then the rest of the evaluation should be completed.

- Routine laboratory procedures includes routine hematologic studies, liver function tests, renal status and measurement of uric acid levels.
- Serum protein electrophoresis and immunoelectrophoresis may be helpful in studying B cell processes.
- If lymphadenopathy is identified, a lymph node biopsy is appropriate. Often a bone marrow examination will also be done.
- Imaging studies should include a routine chest film as well as ultrasonography and computerized tomography to evaluate the liver, spleen and lymph nodes that are not palpable.

A paradox in the clinical approach will become apparent as we allude to high-grade or aggressive lymphomas and then suggest that they are responsive to therapy. High-grade malignant lymphomas such as a lymphoblastic leukemia/lymphoma are curable with aggressive systemic chemotherapy, sometimes combined with bone marrow transplantation or stem cell transfusions. Low-grade malignant lymphomas that are better differentiated, such as systemic immunocytoma, smolder along and have a much better 5-year survival rate than high-grade tumors but never plateau and are not usually curable.

Lymphocyte Characterization

The clinical and histologic criteria and the relevant immunohistochemical and molecular biological tests will be mentioned under the discussion of the various malignant lymphomas. Most of the important B and T cell antigens have been standardized, carry a cluster designation (CD) number (Table 61.3), and can be shown on formalin-fixed, paraffin-embedded tissue. While the light microscopic appearance will usually suggest the possibility of a lymphoma, in most instances the final diagnosis is only made after appropriate marker studies.

The search for clonality is another important clue to the presence of a malignancy. The immunoglobulin molecules on B cells may have either κ or

Table 61.3. Commonly used lymphocyte markers

Marker	Comments
CD2	Pan-T cell antigen
CD3	Pan-T cell antigen
CD4	Helper-inducer T cell antigen
CD5	Pan-T cell antigen, expressed by B cells in CLL
CD7	Majority T cell antigen, present in most peripheral blood T cells, usually lost in mycosis fungoides and may be present in inflammatory infiltrates
CD8	Suppressor-cytotoxic T cell antigen
CD10	B cell antigen; also known as CALLA (see text) but widely expressed, even on immature T cell neoplasms
CD19	B cell antigen
CD20	Pan-B cell antigen not expressed by plasma cells
CD22	Pan-B cell antigen
CD23	B cell antigen, not expressed by mantle cell lymphoma
CD25	Activation marker that detects α-chain of interleukin-2 receptor (Tac)
CD30	Activation marker (Ki-1), characteristic for Hodgkin disease, large cell anaplastic lymphoma
CD45	Leukocyte common antigen, positive in both leukemias and lymphomas
CD45R	Pan-T cell marker
O	
CD56	NK cell marker
CD79a	Pan-B cell marker
CD103	$\alpha E\beta 7$ integrin; involved in epidermotropism
TdT	Terminal deoxynucleotidyl transferase; marker for lymphoblasts
TCR	T cell receptor; used in clonal restriction
Ig	κ or λ chain analysis; used in clonal restriction
Ki-67	Proliferation marker

λ light chains; if only one type is present, a clone of B cells is likely. Analyzing T cells for clonality is more complex, but one can analyze part of the T cell receptor (TCR), such as the β-chain or γ-chain. Either Southern blot analysis or PCR can be used to show clonality of the TCR molecule. A word of caution is appropriate: while clonality usually means malignancy, clonal proliferations of T cells have been found in a variety of benign cutaneous infiltrates.

Hodgkin Disease

(Hodgkin 1832)

Definition. Hodgkin disease is a primarily nodal lymphoma that almost never involves blood or bone marrow. The characteristic cell is the multinucleated Reed-Sternberg giant cell. The standard classification is the Rye classification, which is now included in the REAL classification.

Epidemiology. There is a 2:1 male dominance and most patients are young adults. There is a second smaller peak at about 60 years of age. Primary cutaneous Hodgkin disease is extremely rare.

Etiology and Pathogenesis. While there are many clues, the etiology of Hodgkin disease remains unclear. Even the predominant cell is the source of disagreement. The cells in lymphocyte-rich Hodgkin disease appear to be B cells, but both B and T cell origins have been proposed for the Hodgkin cells and Reed-Sternberg cells. The latter also stain with some macrophage markers. Most likely, Hodgkin disease is really Hodgkin syndrome, including a variety of different proliferative processes. There is occasionally clustering of Hodgkin disease, suggesting an environmental or infectious cause. The risk to other family members is greater, suggesting a specific HLA association. The Epstein-Barr virus genome can be identified in the malignant cells of about half the patients.

The cells overexpress CD30, which is a growth factor receptor. Hodgkin disease is associated with two other CD30-positive processes that are common in the skin – lymphomatoid papulosis and anaplastic large cell lymphoma. There is no usual order of process; any of the disorders can come first.

Clinical Findings

Systemic Findings. The typical presentation is painless lymphadenopathy, most often involving the cervical, supraclavicular and axillary nodes. When the diaphragm is crossed, the spleen is the next most likely site, followed by the abdominal nodes. Rarely, the disease may start in the inguinal nodes. About one-third of the patients present with type B or systemic symptoms including night sweats, fever, weight loss and pruritus. Less than 5% of cases present in extranodal sites. In advanced disease, the liver, lungs, bone marrow and bone may be affected.

Cutaneous Findings. About 50% of patients have non-specific skin findings but less than 1% have Hodgkin disease of the skin. The specific lesions are almost always related to the areas of nodal involvement. Direct extension from lymph nodes to the overlying skin may also occur, producing massive indurated plaques. Because of their rapid growth, ulceration is common. Sometimes the deeper infiltrates mimic erysipelas. In other cases, papules, nodules or subcutaneous masses appear, unrelated to patterns of lymph node involvement (Fig. 61.1). The disease process may also involve the tonsils, producing a necrotic angina. In contrast to acute myelogenous leukemia and agranulocytosis, the gingiva are not involved.

The rarest of all forms is primary cutaneous Hodgkin disease. Occasionally, patients have been described with cutaneous nodules that morphologically fulfilled the requirements for Hodgkin disease; however, extensive evaluation failed to reveal any lymph node disease. Such patients probably all develop Hodgkin disease at some point; otherwise, the appropriate diagnosis is probably lymphomatoid papulosis or anaplastic large cell lymphoma.

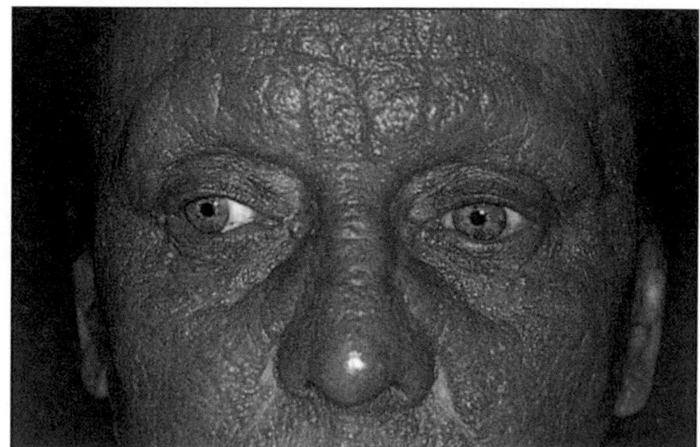

Fig. 61.1. Specific cutaneous infiltrate in Hodgkin disease producing a leonine facies; this is an extremely rare occurrence

There are many secondary or nonspecific cutaneous problems in patients with Hodgkin disease.

- Pruritus and hyperpigmentation: Intense pruritus may be the presenting feature of Hodgkin disease. It usually starts on the legs and does not respond to routine therapy. Excoriations, secondary infections and lichenification frequently appear. At the same time the patients may develop a diffuse hyperpigmentation.
- Prurigo: Hodgkin disease is one of causes of prurigo (Chap. 25). Tiny, transient pruritic papules appear, are destroyed by scratching and evolve into hyperpigmented crusted papules and nodules, sometimes progressing to prurigo nodularis.
- Ichthyosis-like dermatitis: Most patients have dry skin. In some, this problem is more severe and may mimic ichthyosis vulgaris.
- Viral infections: Almost every patient with Hodgkin disease suffers from zoster, which may be generalized or recurrent. Many have troubles with refractory warts or mollusca contagiosa.

Histopathology. The histopathology of the lymph nodes forms the basis for the classification and eventual therapy and prognosis of Hodgkin disease. The Reed-Sternberg and mononuclear Hodgkin cell are the malignant cells, but they compromise a small minority of the infiltrate, which is mixed and rich in other lymphocytes, plasma cells, fibroblasts and even fibrous tissue. In the skin atypical mononuclear Hodgkin cells may be seen; they often have large nuclei and prominent nucleoli. The Reed-Sternberg cells are rare in the skin but are 15–60 μm with abundant cytoplasm, multiple nuclei and eosinophilic nucleoli. In addition, necrotic areas may develop within the infiltrates.

Laboratory Findings. The number of abnormal laboratory findings is lengthy, but one can expect a normocytic anemia with leukocytosis and eosinophilia. Routine staging as discussed above should be performed.

Course and Prognosis. The various histologic subcategories of Hodgkin disease cannot be identified in the skin. They, as well as the extent of disease and presence of associated signs and symptoms, correlate with survival, as shown in the Ann Arbor classification (Table 61.4) The overall cure rate is about 75%, but approaches 90% for localized disease involving one group of lymph nodes. While patients with skin involvement are officially put

Table 61.4 Staging of Hodgkin disease: Ann Arbor classification

Stage	Features
I	Involvement of single lymph node group
I_E	Single extranodal site
II	Involvement of two or more nodal groups on same side of diaphragm
II_E	Involvement of one lymph node group and one extranodal site on same side of diaphragm
III	Involvement of lymph nodes on both sides of diaphragm along with spleen (III_S), extranodal site (III_E) or both (III_{ES})
IV	Diffuse involvement including liver, bone marrow and skin
A	No systemic signs or symptoms
B	Systemic signs (fever, night sweats, weight loss, pruritus)

into group IV, skin involvement is nowhere as serious as bone marrow or liver disease. Many patients with skin involvement respond well to therapy. The gloomy news for all treated Hodgkin disease patients is the risk of second malignancies, such as leukemia, many years after treatment.

Differential Diagnosis. The clinical differential diagnosis includes all the causes of lymphadenopathy. Procedures to examine the lymph nodes are required to distinguish between Hodgkin disease and non-Hodgkin lymphoma. In the skin, the differential diagnosis includes large cell anaplastic lymphoma, which has a more monotonous appearance, and lymphomatoid papulosis, which consists of smaller lesions that tend to come and go.

Therapy. The mainstays of therapy for the systemic disease are radiation therapy and combination chemotherapy regimens. In stages IA and IIA ionizing radiation alone may be employed, usually with a total dose of about 40 Gy, directed to the involved lymph nodes and immediately contiguous structures. Hodgkin disease tends not to skip nodal areas, making this therapy reasonable. With B symptoms or more advanced disease, chemotherapy and wider-field radiation therapy is employed, often in combination. A staging laparotomy is usually done in such patients if radiation therapy alone is planned.

The main dermatologic problem is the pruritus. Irradiation with UVB or PUVA can be tried, as well as the standard antipruritic measures including topical distracters or polidocanol and systemic antihistamines. Isolated cutaneous infiltrates can also be treated with X-rays or electron beam therapy.

T Cell Lymphomas

In the following discussion of T cell and then B cell lymphomas, we will use the REAL name and give only the Kiel name as a synonym. Hopefully this will simplify matters.

T Lymphoblastic Leukemia/Lymphoma

Synonym. Kiel: T lymphoblastic lymphoma

Etiology and Pathogenesis. The normal counterpart is precursor T cells, either prothymocytes or thymocytes. No consistent genetic abnormalities have been identified.

Clinical Findings. Most patients are adolescent and young adult males. This disease accounts for 40% of childhood lymphomas and inevitably converts into acute lymphoblastic leukemia. Most patients present with thymic masses and lymphadenopathy. CNS involvement is common. About 20% of patients have skin lesions and, in rare instances, the skin may be the first site of involvement. The most common sites are the head and neck. The lesions are highly variable, including purpuric plaques, red-violet nodules and deeper infiltrates.

Histopathology. The responsible cells are small lymphoblasts with round or convoluted nuclei, few nucleoli, dispersed chromatin and little cytoplasm. They are CD7-, CD3- and TdT-positive and should be negative for immunoglobulins and B cell antigens. The rare skin infiltrates contain monomorphic infiltrates of such cells. The main microscopic differential diagnosis is precursor B cell neoplasms, which are morphologically identical but have different markers.

Therapy. Aggressive chemotherapy can produce cures.

T Cell Chronic Lymphocytic Leukemia (T-CLL)/Prolymphocytic Leukemia (T-PLL)

Synonym. Kiel: T cell chronic lymphocytic leukemia/prolymphocytic leukemia

Etiology and Pathogenesis. This rare aggressive tumor comprises less than 5% of chronic lymphocytic leukemias (Chap. 62). The normal counterpart is the circulating T cell.

Clinical Findings. This neoplasm usually presents with lymphadenopathy and elevated leukocyte counts. The bone marrow, spleen and liver may also be involved. Both cutaneous and mucosal infiltrates are common. The skin lesions are usually red-brown, soft large nodules or plaques, which may be the first manifestation. Erythroderma has also been described.

Histopathology. The cells resemble normal circulating T cells. In most instances, they have some nuclear irregularity and are thus classified as prolymphocytic, but the markers of the two variants are identical. Typically, CD7 and CD2, 3 and 5 are positive. There is usually a clonal rearrangement of the TCR.

Differential Diagnosis. When patients have erythroderma early in their disease course, separation from Sézary syndrome can be difficult. The cutaneous infiltrate is usually deeper and not epidermotropic, and the circulating cells different.

Therapy. The outlook is gloomy; most such patients do not respond to chemotherapy.

Mycosis Fungoides

(Alibert 1806)

Synonym. Kiel: small cell, cerebriform lymphoma

Cutaneous T cell lymphoma is often used as a synonym, but we feel this is unwise as there are so many T cell lymphomas involving the skin.

Definition. Low-grade, peripheral T cell lymphoma with primary cutaneous involvement and distinct clinical features.

Epidemiology. Mycosis fungoides is the most common cutaneous lymphoma. The incidence is about 0.5–1.0/100,000. Most patients are adults, with the onset around 40 years of age. There is usually a long delay in diagnosis, casting doubt on such numbers. A definite male dominance exists and the disease is more common among patients with chronic industrial exposure to chemicals.

Etiology and Pathogenesis. The nature of mycosis fungoides has been the subject of intense debate and research for many years. The gist of the argument is: are the early lesions already lymphoma or does a lymphoma develop in chronically inflamed skin? The normal counterpart is the peripheral epidermotropic T cell. Because of their complex cutaneous homing mechanisms, these cells are confined to the skin for long periods. Molecular biological studies have identified clonal T cell populations in the very early lesions of mycosis fungoides and follow-up studies have shown that these clones expand as the tumor progresses. Perhaps persistent allergic contact dermatitis or other immune stimulation plays a role in triggering this clonal expansion. Retroviruses such as HTLV have also been implicated but the evidence is underwhelming.

Clinical Findings. The clinical spectrum of mycosis fungoides is very broad. Most patients go through the classical disease progression we will describe, but others do not follow the rules. Bazin, a student of Alibert, was the first to identify the different stages of mycosis fungoides with their changing clinical and microscopic appearances. One should remember that, as the disease advances, the patient may show early, intermediate and late lesions simultaneously. Classification is based on the most severe changes.

Patch Stage. Mycosis fungoides develops slowly over many years and can remain clinically and histologically indistinct. The lesions are slowly growing, round, oval, serpiginous or polycyclic red-violet patches that have a distinct border. They may also have a fine wrinkling centrally that can be mistaken for atrophy. Pruritus is quite variable; some patients are asymptomatic while others have uncontrollable itching. Either fine pityriasiform

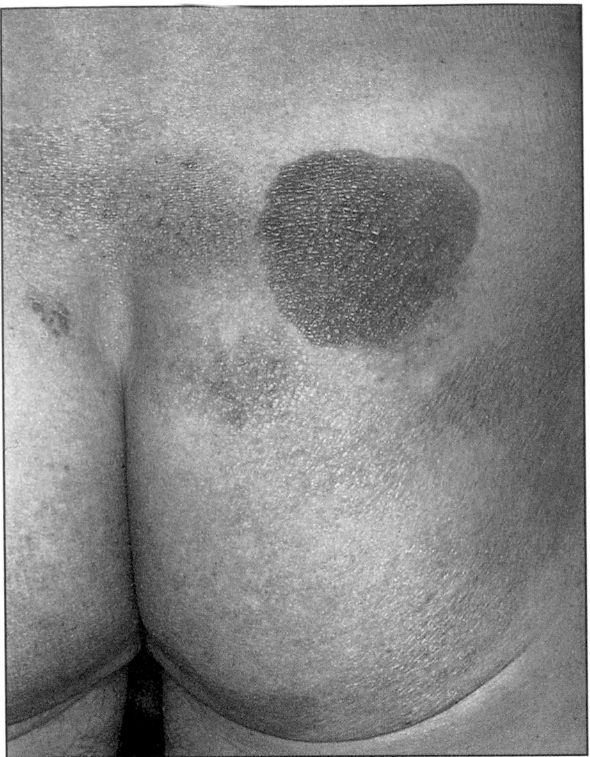

Fig. 61.2. Thickened darker plaque of mycosis fungoides arising amidst large-patch parapsoriasis

scale or more prominent psoriasiform changes can be seen. The most common sites are the trunk and buttocks although any part of the body can be involved (Fig. 61.2). This description should remind the reader of that given for large-patch parapsoriasis in Chapter 14. We will not repeat the arguments again here, but simply state that large-patch and especially poikilodermatous parapsoriasis are the same as early mycosis fungoides, while the relationship of small-patch parapsoriasis to lymphoma remains unclear.

Early mycosis fungoides may take many other forms. In blacks, the initial presentation may be with hypopigmented patches, confused with vitiligo (Fig. 61.3). Often there is striking loss of hairs, perhaps associated with follicle destruction by tumor cells or follicular mucinosis (Fig. 61.4). Localized verrucous lesions may develop, as discussed below under pagetoid reticulosis. In other instances, the eruption may resemble vasculitis, pigmented purpura or folliculitis. In rare instances, vesicular or pustular lesions have been identified.

The clinical diagnosis is difficult in this stage. Often one has a working diagnosis of atopic dermatitis, psoriasis or chronic irritant dermatitis. The failure of the lesions to respond to therapy may be the first clue that a different diagnosis should be considered. The slow gradual growth, frequent recurrences and improvement with UV radiation may suggest mycosis fungoides. Multiple lesions should be biopsied and the patient followed at routine intervals once this possibility has been considered. Patients with a single lesion tend to do better.

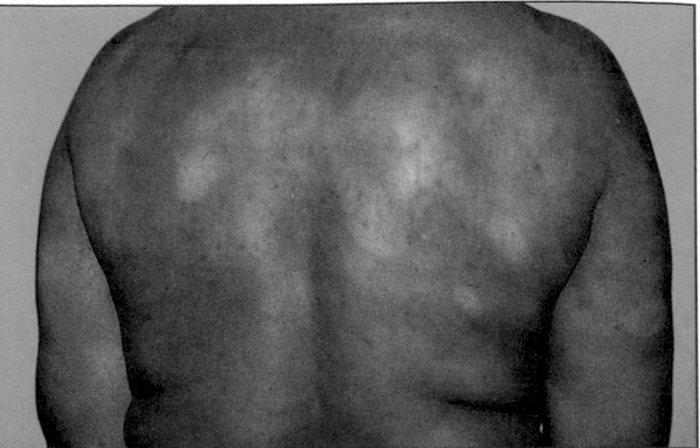

Fig. 61.3. Hypopigmented mycosis fungoides in blacks. (Courtesy of Roselyn E. Epps, M. D., Washington, D. C.)

Infiltrative Stage. At this stage mycosis fungoides should be diagnosable. Either the preexisting patches become infiltrated or new, thicker lesions arise de novo. Now sharply bordered, slightly elevated irregular plaques are present, with colors ranging from red to violet to red-brown (Fig. 61.5). Many patients experience pruritus at this stage. All the plaques slowly expand and increase in thickness. Often, sharply defined islands of normal skin may be skin within a plaque; these are known as nappes claires. A similar change is the sparing of

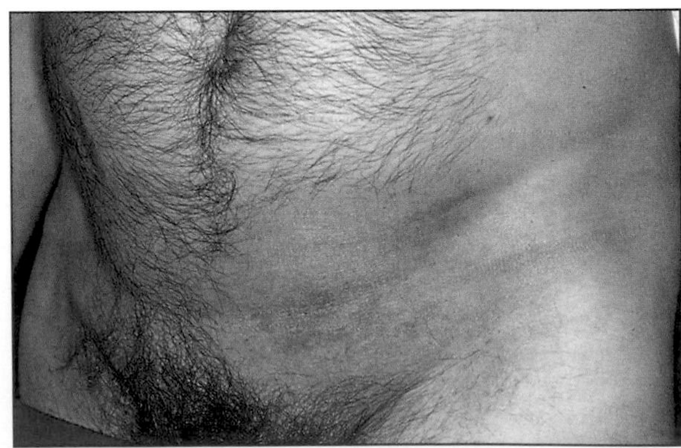

Fig. 61.4. Patch stage mycosis fungoides with prominent hair loss

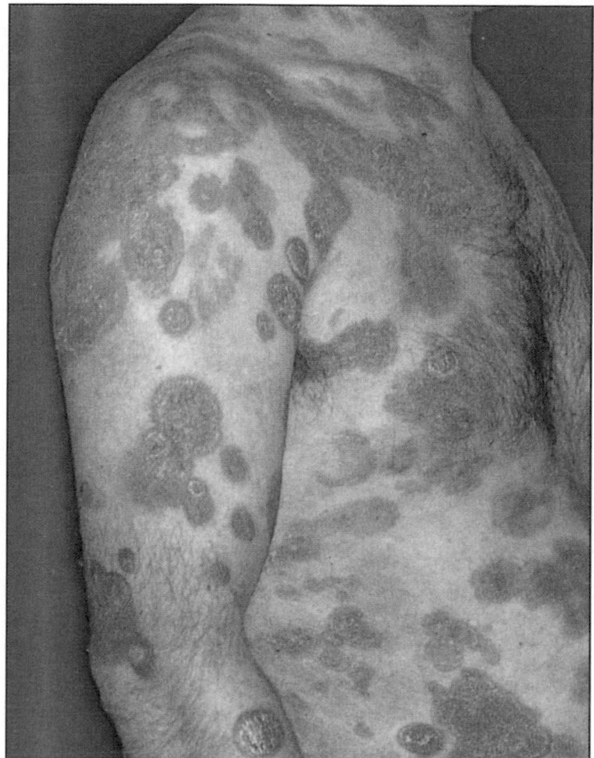

Fig. 61.5. Infiltrative stage mycosis fungoides

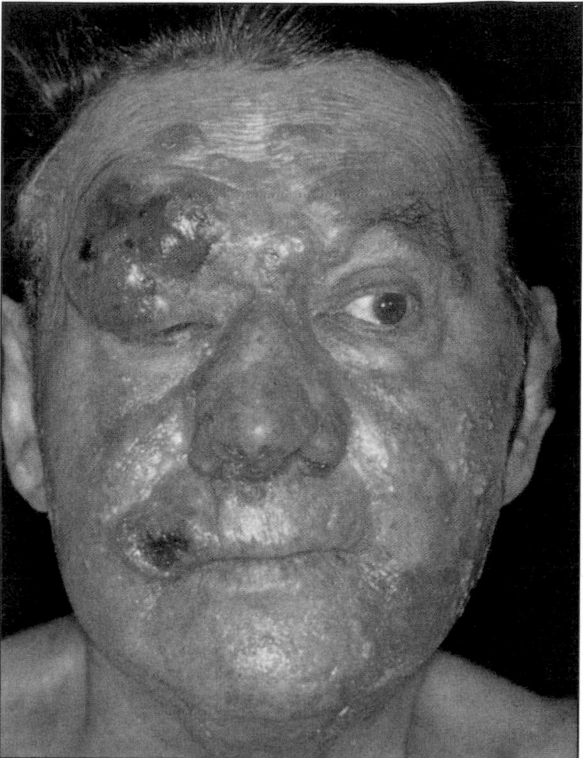

Fig. 61.6. Tumor stage mycosis fungoides with leonine facies and marked disfigurement

skin folds, such as behind the knees; this is called the deck chair sign. Often the areas show alopecia, reflecting follicular involvement or even follicular mucinosis. In this stage, there may be lymphadenopathy, but it is often dermatopathic.

Tumor Stage. This is the end stage of mycosis fungoides. Large thick tumors develop, once again either within preexisting lesions or de novo. Facial involvement can lead to a leonine facies. The tumors often grow rapidly, are red-brown ulcerated and reminded the Alibert of mushrooms, hence the name (Fig. 61.6). Most patients at this stage show signs of systemic disease.

There are several other forms or precursor stages of mycosis fungoides that do not fit into the above schemes.

Mycosis Fungoides D'Emblee (Vidal and Brocq 1885). These patients rapidly develop large tumors without showing any signs of the earlier stages of mycosis fungoides. Today it is felt that almost all such patients have other high-grade lymphomas, as born out by modern marker studies.

Mycosis Fungoides Erythroderma (Hallopeau and Besnier 1891). Some patients present with widespread erythroderma. As the disease progresses, the infiltrate turns out to be that of mycosis fungoides. A typical clinical feature is the small islands of sparing. Other patients may develop erythroderma during the evolution of their mycosis fungoides. While most such cases are Sézary syndrome, erythroderma may develop without circulating Sézary cells or lymphadenopathy.

Follicular Mucinosis. This change (Chap. 43) may be the first sign of mycosis fungoides or other T cell lymphomas. Patients present with boggy patches of alopecia, which on biopsy show a mucinous infiltrate of the hair follicles or sebaceous glands. In some instances, follicular mucinosis is idiopathic, but one must always be alert to the risk of malignant lymphoma. We have seen mycosis fungoides develop in patients with follicular mucinosis in all age groups, even though childhood follicular mucinosis is usually not associated with tumors. In addition, follicular mucinosis may develop during the course of otherwise typical mycosis fungoides.

Granulomatous Slack Skin. In this rare form, patients have a destructive granulomatous infiltrate associated with their mycosis fungoides. Typical sites of involvement are the axillae, groin and breasts. The damage to the elastic fibers produces a drooping sagging skin, much like acquired cutis laxa. Other patients may have granulomatous changes microscopically without any clinical evidence of slack skin. The disease of these patients seem particularly likely to evolve into anaplastic T cell lymphoma. Occasionally granulomatous slack skin has been described with other malignant lymphomas.

Papuloerythroderma of OFUJI (1984). This rare but distinct clinical entity (Chap. 14) features intense pruritus and red-brown flat-topped papules that frequently coalesce and yet leave islands of sparing. It affects primarily older men and may have associated eosinophilia and lymphopenia. Some patients may later develop mycosis fungoides.

Pityriasis Rotunda (Chap. 14). Patients typically have large, scaly hyperpigmented patches on their buttocks, not dissimilar from a giant lesion of large-patch parapsoriasis. The acquired form is more common in blacks and Orientals and may evolve into mycosis fungoides.

Systemic Findings

Lymphadenopathy is the key change. In the infiltrative stage, enlarge lymph nodes typically show dermatopathic lymphadenopathy, as discussed below. Paradoxically, the presence of lymphadenopathy, rather than the presence of specific lymphoma infiltrates in the nodes, is a better predictor of a severe course. Rapid develop of lymphadenopathy can be a sign of the conversion of mycosis fungoides into a more aggressive T cell lymphoma.

Other organs may also be infiltrated in the later stages. The tonsillar region, liver, spleen, lungs, gastrointestinal tract and CNS may also be involved. Many patients have systemic symptoms such as weight, malaise or weight loss.

Histopathology. In its early stages, mycosis fungoides is difficult to diagnose with certainty. The classic features of atypical epidermotropic lymphocytes and Pautrier abscesses are not seen. There is usually a modest lymphocytic infiltrate in the upper dermis, occasionally band-like, and admixed with eosinophils and plasma cells. Clues to the correct diagnosis may be lymphocytes in the epidermis without spongiosis, clusters of lymphocytes in the epidermis or along the basement membrane zone, larger lymphocytic cells in the epidermis than the dermis, interface dermatitis, and fine fibrosis of the papillary dermis. Marker and molecular biological studies also often fail at this stage because of the paucity of atypical cells in the skin. In addition, treatment with topical corticosteroids may suppress the development of Pautrier microabscesses.

The diagnosis can be made in the infiltrative stage. The characteristic cerebriform lymphocytes can usually be found, in the dermal infiltrate and in the epidermis, both isolated and in small clusters; these are known as Pautrier microabscesses. The infiltrate is usually denser but still polymorphic and there tend to be reactive epidermal changes, with hyperkeratosis and elongated rete ridges mimicking psoriasis. Adnexal structures may also be infiltrated; there may be follicular mucinosis or infiltrates limited to just the follicles. The lymphoma cells have a large, usually cerebriform nucleus that can be seen better with ultra-thin sections or using electron microscopy. These cells usually have a T helper phenotype and are positive for CD4, 2, 3 and 5. Some cells are CD8-positive and CD4-negative. CD7 is absent. Clonal TCR rearrangements can usually be shown.

In the tumor stage, the diagnosis of malignancy is obvious, as there are sheets of tumor cells. Often there is a loss of epidermotropism. The main task is to identify the switch to a large cell lymphoma. The anaplastic tumor cells may appear identical to and acquire some of the markers associated with anaplastic large cell lymphoma or other high-grade lymphomas, but often TCR analysis shows that they are still part of the same clonal proliferation identified earlier in the disease course.

Laboratory Findings. Occasionally the atypical lymphocytes can be found in the blood; this problem is discussed under Sézary syndrome. Otherwise, routine laboratory studies are required to monitor the possibility of internal organ involvement.

Diagnostic Criteria. Patients with mycosis fungoides should be staged as outlined in Table 61.5. The most important criteria are the degree of cutaneous disease and the presence or absence of lymph node, blood and internal organ involvement.

Table 61.5. TNM classification of cutaneous T cell lymphomas

Stage	Description
Skin (T)	
T0	Possible involvement
T1	< 10% involvement
T2	> 10% involvement
T3	Tumors
T4	Erythroderma
Lymph nodes (N)	
N0	No involvement
N1	Clinically involved nodes, pathology negative
N2	No clinically enlarged nodes; pathology positive
N3	Clinically involved nodes; pathology positive
Viscera (M)	
M0	No involvement
M1	Involvement

Stage	Skin	Lymph nodes	Other organs
I A	T1	N0	M0
I B	T2	N0	M0
II A	T1, T2	N1	M0
II B	T3	N0, N1	M0
III	T4	N0, N1	M0
IV A	T1 – T4	N2, N3	M0
IV B	T1 – T4	N0 – N3	M1

Course and Prognosis. The prognosis of mycosis fungoides is hard to state. The premycotic stage can last for decades. Some experts propose following mycosis fungoides patients with a 25-year survival rate. If many early cases of mycosis fungoides are included in a series, then the outlook will be better, as some cases will never progress. Probably a 7–10-year survival rate is reasonable for infiltrative disease involving less than 10% of body surface area, with a 2–3-year survival rate for tumor stage. The patients usually die because of systemic organ involvement or infections.

Differential Diagnosis. The early lesions can mimic many different dermatoses, as discussed above. In the tumor stage, one must exclude other types of pseudolymphoma, malignant lymphoma and leukemia, but usually the history of precursor lesions points the way.

Therapy. The treatment of mycosis fungoides is extremely difficult to assess because of the long period during which the patients do well. The age-old question is: Does early diagnosis and treatment of mycosis fungoides, perhaps with very aggressive measures, lead to cure? If the early stages are reactive, then aggressive therapy makes little sense; if they represent a malignant lymphoma with just a few cells in action, then attacking seems reasonable. While this question cannot be answered with certainty, the answer appears in most cases to be "No". We treat stages I A – II B primarily with external measures, but lean towards chemotherapy for stages III – IV. Another practical aspect of mycosis fungoides therapy is that, once a therapy form has been employed, the likelihood is that later stages will be relatively resistant to the same approach.

Topical. Very early lesions often respond to relatively bland measures. Topical corticosteroids may control small lesions for a period of time. UV radiation is frequently helpful; sunlight, UVB and PUVA are all effective. We tend to employ PUVA and PUVA bath therapy most often, as they quickly induce remission and then can be used periodically for maintenance.

When these two measures are ineffective, many choose to use topical nitrogen mustard. This approach is more popular in the USA and Scandinavia than in Germany. It is probably best reserved for individuals who either have no access to PUVA or fail to respond to it. The standard mechlorethamine used for systemic chemotherapy comes in 10 mg vials that are reconstituted with 60 ml of water. This must be done daily to insure a fresh solution. An alternative is to mix the chemical in 60 g of Eucerin; this preparation is more stable and less sensitizing but harder to apply. The mechlorethamine must be applied to the entire body surface daily. Whoever applies the medication should wear plastic gloves and a mask, as allergic contact dermatitis is an invariable side effect. The main complication are irritant and allergic reactions; in such cases, a more dilute mixture can be used. As the lesions begin to resolve, the frequency of application can be tapered. Many patients end up apply mechlorethamine weekly for long periods of time. The main long-term problems are recurrent disease, hypo- and hyperpigmentation, and an increased risk of cutaneous malignancies.

A similar approach with which we have less experience is topical carmustine (BCNU), as popularized by Zackheim. This product is easier to use since 50 mg can be mixed into 200 ml of 95% alcohol, a solution that is stable in the refrigerator. It is applied daily or every other day for several months. Enough absorption occurs that 30% of patients experience hematologic changes. An irritant reaction also develops, and many have allergic contact dermatitis. For this reason, treatment is usually stopped after 6–8 weeks. Few patients tolerate long-term use. Posttreatment telangiectases are common.

Radiation therapy plays an important role in treating mycosis fungoides. While total body X-ray therapy was formerly employed, today most protocols recommend total skin electron beam therapy. Because the electrons only penetrate the dermis, there are no systemic effects. Dosages of greater than 30–36 Gy should be employed, as the remission rates and disease-free survival intervals are better. The entire body must be treated, including palms, soles, scalp, axillae and groin. Usually the dose is highly fractionated, so the therapy takes many months, is expensive and is subject to geographic restrictions. Generally, a second course of 30–36 Gy can be given in the case of relapse. About two-thirds of patients may have long disease-free intervals; some of these individuals are cured while others relapse late. Complications include dry skin, pruritus, atrophy, alopecia and radiation dermatitis with an increased risk of cutaneous malignancies.

Localized lesions that are stubborn can be easily treated with soft X-rays. Typically 20–30 Gy given in five to ten divided doses will eliminate almost any infiltrative lesion.

The 5-year survival rates following PUVA, topical nitrogen mustard and total-body electron therapy appear comparable. When these localized or relatively simple measures fail, one must consider more aggressive forms of treatment.

Extracorporeal photopheresis may be an effective therapy. The patient ingests psoralens, just as for PUVA therapy, but then his blood is irradiated outside the body. A device separates out the leukocytes and irradiates them with UVA. It is also possible to add the psoralens to the leukocyte mixture. Initially it was thought that the undesired cells were being killed, but this is not true. Instead, inactivated lymphoma cells are recirculated in the body, where they are exposed to the immune system but are unable to secrete cytokines or carry out other functions. Presumably the body is then better able to mount an immune response against the aberrant cells. Patients are usually treated on two consecutive days biweekly or monthly. There may be a febrile response, but the procedure is surprisingly well-tolerated and is not immunosuppressive. While extracorporeal photopheresis was initially touted for Sézary syndrome, it is also effective in the early stages of mycosis fungoides.

Many different systemic chemotherapy regimens have been tried, the simplest being prednisone and chlorambucil. A typical daily regimen involves 20–40 mg of prednisone and 4–6 mg of chlorambucil. The latter is gradually increased with hematologic monitoring. Often 8–10 mg can be tolerated. As improvement is seen, the prednisone is tapered to 15–20 mg q.o.d. and the chlorambucil adjusted to hematologic parameters. It is doubtful if any patient is cured with this approach, but many are helped. The long-term risks include marrow suppression and the development of acute myelogenous leukemia.

Many other regimens can be employed. The choice will probably depend more on local preferences and the wishes of the oncologists. Methotrexate can be used either in relatively low dosages, such as 15–30 mg once a week in three doses over 24 h, or in large monthly intravenous doses, up to 200 mg/m^2, with citrovorum factor rescue. Other regimens include interferon-α, fludarabine monophosphate, and etoposide. Both interferon-α and oral retinoids have been combined with PUVA therapy. Finally, many of the complex, multiagent chemotherapy regimens used for other malignant lymphomas can be employed for patients with advanced stage III disease or evidence of visceral involvement.

Two extremely new approaches have not been adequately tested but are exciting. Bexarotene is an oral retinoid, while denileukin diftitox is a monoclonal antibody directed against CD25, the IL-2 receptor. Both have been approved for treating refractory cutaneous T cell lymphomas.

Sézary Syndrome

(Sézary and Bouvrain 1938)

Synonyms. Kiel: small cell, cerebriform lymphoma, T cell erythroderma (Winkelmann 1974)

Definition. Combination of erythroderma, lymphadenopathy and circulating, cerebriform atypical lymphocytes in the blood, rather than confined to the skin as in ordinary mycosis fungoides.

Epidemiology. Sézary syndrome is extremely rare. Most patients are elderly.

Etiology and Pathogenesis. The etiology is unknown. There is a monoclonal proliferation of T cells, just as in mycosis fungoides.

Clinical Findings. The early course of the disease is usually misdiagnosed. The patient presents with erythematous scaly patches, often with islands of sparing. Initially, one considers seborrheic dermatitis, psoriasis or allergic contact dermatitis. Over a long period of time, the entire integument becomes involved producing the characteristic erythroderma (in Sézary's French, l'homme rouge). The skin is also thickened, with scaling, weeping and marked pruritus (Fig. 61.7). There is often striking, sometimes rapid hyperpigmentation; thus the older name of melanoerythroderma (Fig. 61.8). Edema is prominent and a leonine facies may result.

The patients typically shiver and complain of the cold. The marked scaling causes shedding of debris all over their bedding and their room. Alopecia is common and involves all hair-bearing sites including the scalp, eyebrows, eyelashes, axillae and groin. The palms and soles are typically hyperkeratotic and deeply fissured; nail dystrophies often develop.

The other classic finding is lymphadenopathy. There are typically many swollen boggy nodes involving multiple sites. While early microscopic examination often reveals only dermatopathic lymphadenopathy, molecular biological studies have shown the same clonal T cells identified in the

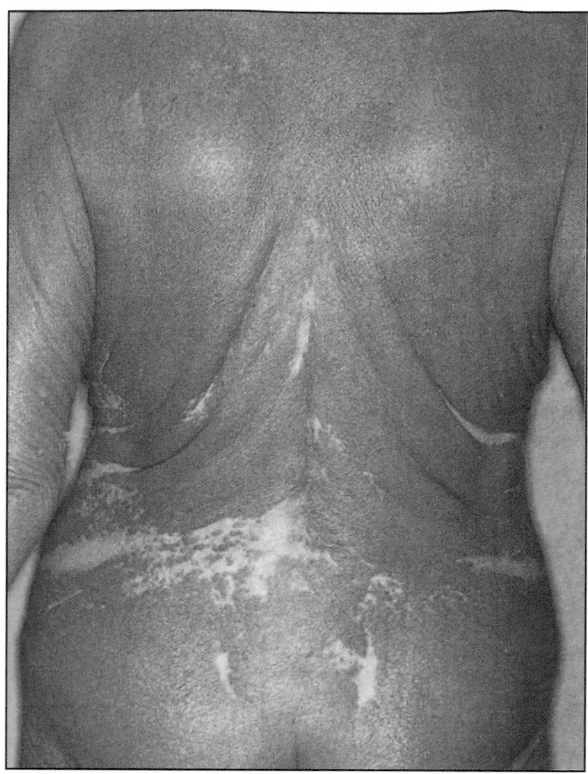

Fig. 61.7. Sézary syndrome

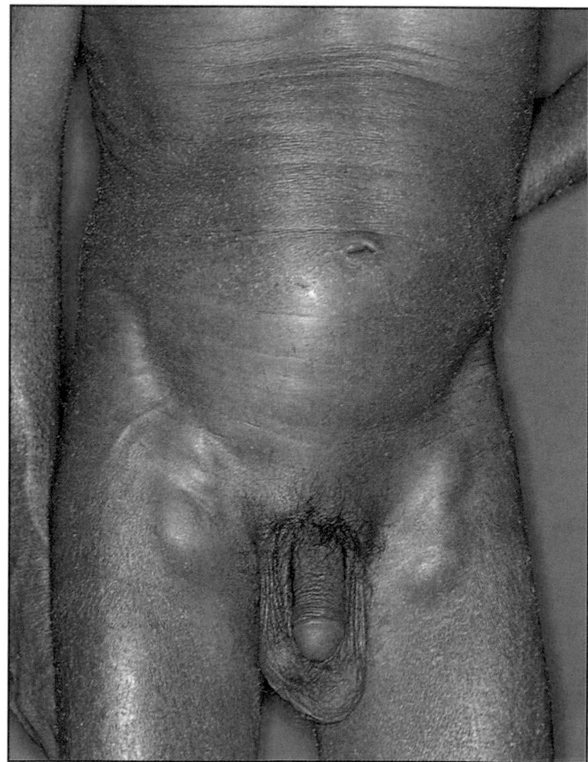

Fig. 61.8. Sézary syndrome – melanoerythrodermic form with striking lymphadenopathy

skin and blood present in small numbers in the nodes but overwhelmed by reactive processes. Later, the lymph nodes are effaced by large numbers of malignant lymphocytes.

A key difference between mycosis fungoides and Sézary syndrome is that the latter patients are more severely immunosuppressed. As the blood accumulates both Sézary cells and other malignant lymphocytes, the number of normal functional cells may be sharply diminished and immune function is impaired. Recurrent infections, both cutaneous and systemic, are common and responsible for much of the morbidity associated with the disease. In addition, in Sézary syndrome there may be a protein-losing enteropathy that further weakens the patient.

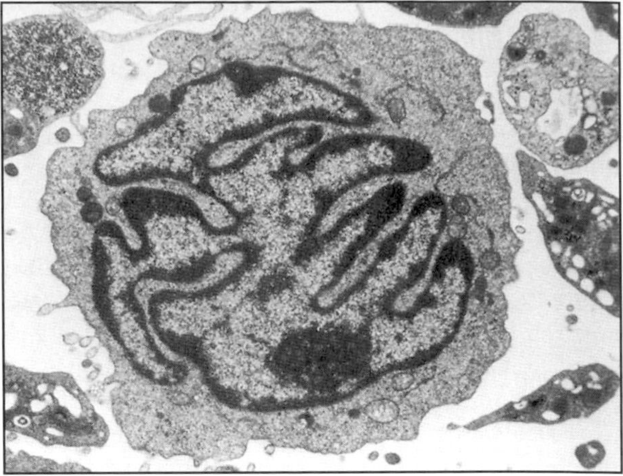

Fig. 61.9. Sézary cell

Histopathology. A skin biopsy is often a hard way to diagnosis Sézary syndrome. In the early erythrodermic stage, there may be a sparse perivascular infiltration of lymphocytes which are not at first glance atypical. Spongiosis may be present. Later on, the findings are identical to mycosis fungoides except that there are more of the atypical cerebriform lymphocytes.

Laboratory Findings. The key finding is identification in the peripheral blood of the almost-specific atypical lymphocytes, with cerebriform nuclei (Fig. 61.9). These cells have been called either Sézary cells or Lutzner cells, as the latter investigator described the complex nuclear invaginations seen so well on electron microscopy. While most Sézary cells are relatively small, some are as large as 10 µm. Although Sézary cells in the appropriate clinical setting strongly suggest Sézary syndrome, they are not diagnostic. A number of problems arise. The cells can be found in the peripheral blood in other lymphomas and leukemias and in inflammatory dermatoses such as atopic dermatitis. In our laboratory, counts of greater than 1000 cells/mm^3 are taken as diagnostic. Other groups suggest more than 30% of total circulating lymphocytes should be Sézary cells to allow the diagnosis. Yet others have done computerized studies of the nuclear contour ratio or the nuclear: cytoplasmic ratio to separate malignant from benign Sézary cells, as there is frequent disagreement between skilled observers over what constitutes a Sézary cell. The immunophenotyping is identical to that of mycosis fungoides.

Course and Prognosis. The average survival time with Sézary syndrome is 2–3 years. The usual cause of death is either a severe infection or conversion of the disease into a more aggressive, anaplastic large cell lymphoma.

Differential Diagnosis. The differential diagnosis of erythroderma usually includes exacerbation of underlying dermatosis and drug reactions. There may also be erythroderma associated with mycosis fungoides or other lymphomas without evidence of circulating Sézary cells. A pre-Sézary syndrome can be diagnosed when the white blood cell count is less than 1000/mm^3 but all the other symptoms fit. Melanoerythroderma with lymphadenopathy and cachexia in the elderly has been described but where it fits into the spectrum of Sézary syndrome is unclear.

Therapy. In the acute stage of Sézary syndrome systemic corticosteroids may produce rapid improvement in the patient's well-being. We usually use prednisone 1 mg/kg daily for 3–5 days and then taper. A bolus of intravenous corticosteroids (1000 mg methylprednisolone) is also helpful. The patient must be in a warm room and receive the same kind of medical attention given to any other erythrodermic patient (Chap. 14).

The treatments discussed under mycosis fungoides are also useful here. The chlorambucil and prednisone regimen is a convenient way to buy time for the patient. Many may respond to PUVA, PUVA bath or electron beam therapy, although photosensitivity can be a limiting factor. Because of the circulating malignant cells, most oncologists prefer a more aggressive chemotherapy regimen. Extracorporeal photopheresis was first used for

Sézary syndrome and may still be its best indication. Finally, ordinary leukopheresis may be a method to reduce the number of Sézary cells in the blood.

Pagetoid Reticulosis

(Woringer and Kolopp 1939; Braun-Falco et al. 1973)

Synonyms. Woringer-Kolopp disease, epidermotropic reticulosis, localized mycosis fungoides

Definition. Low-grade, localized, often acral T cell lymphoma. Reticulosis refers to the extinct term reticulum cell sarcoma, which was used for some high-grade malignant lymphomas.

Epidemiology. Pagetoid reticulosis is extremely rare and occurs mostly in men.

Etiology and Pathogenesis. The cause is unknown. The cell of origin was debated for years but now appears in most cases to be an atypical T cell.

Clinical Findings. Localized pagetoid reticulosis is known as Woringer-Kolopp disease. The typical lesion is a persistent, sharply localized scaly patch, usually on the extensor surface of the hand or foot (Fig. 61.10). The color is typicallyred-brown and the border may be prominent. The lesion is asymptomatic, often mistaken for psoriasis or a fungal infection, and usually ignored. Over many years the lesion slowly expands. Occasionally, several small grouped lesions may fuse together, producing a complex series of rings.

Disseminated pagetoid reticulosis is known as Ketron-Goodman (1931) disease. There are no criteria to separate diffuse, rapidly progressive pagetoid reticulosis from mycosis fungoides and we do not employ this diagnosis.

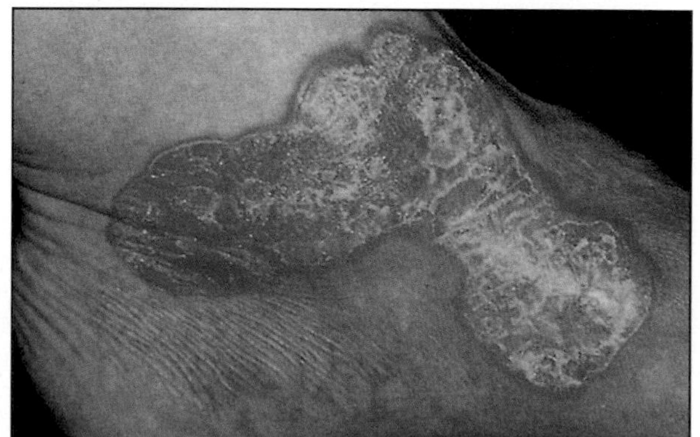

Fig. 61.10. Pagetoid reticulosis (Woringer-Kolopp disease)

Histopathology. The striking microscopic feature is pagetoid change. Large clear cells are seen scattered through an epidermis that is acanthotic and hyperkeratotic. Hair follicles and eccrine glands can also be infiltrated by pagetoid cells. The dermal infiltrate may be quite innocent, containing only small lymphocytes. The polymorphic picture seen in mycosis fungoides with eosinophils and plasma cells is not found. Analysis of the cells shows that they are T cells, with many similarities to mycosis fungoides but with some differences. Most are CD3- and CD4-positive but some may display CD8.

Laboratory Findings. Circulating Sézary cells are not found.

Differential Diagnosis. The clinical differential diagnosis is usually psoriasis, hypertrophic lichen planus, chronic dermatitis or dermatophyte infection. Mycosis fungoides may also have hyperkeratotic lesions, but usually multiple other changes are present. The histologic differential diagnosis includes amelanotic malignant melanoma, Paget disease and Bowen disease. On occasion, mycosis fungoides is also pagetoid; this feature is enough to explain away Ketron-Goodman disease.

Therapy. Excision, radiation therapy, PUVA or PUVA bath are usually helpful.

Lymphomatoid Papulosis

(Dupont 1965; Verallo and Haserick 1966; Macaulay 1968)

Synonym. No Kiel equivalent

Definition. Heterogeneous group of patients with clinically benign or spontaneously regressing cutaneous infiltrates that microscopically resemble a lymphoma and whose disease occasionally evolves into Hodgkin disease or non-Hodgkin malignant lymphoma.

Epidemiology. Lymphomatoid papulosis has been described in infants and octogenarians. Most patients are adults between 30 and 40 years of age. Men are more often affected.

Etiology and Pathogenesis. The cause of lymphomatoid papulosis is unknown and its very nature is highly controversial. In about 10–20% of cases, the patient eventually develops a definite lymphoma. Hodgkin disease and primary cutaneous anaplastic large cell lymphoma may both show overlaps; other patients may have mycosis fungoides. Most puzzling is that there is no logical time sequence or progression; any of the related diseases can appear before, simultaneously with or following lymphomatoid papulosis. Even in the cases of lymphomatoid papulosis that do well or regress, molecular biological studies have shown evidence of one or more clones of T cells.

Clinical Findings. There are two basic patterns. Most patients have multiple small papules and nodules that develop scales, hemorrhages and crusts, thus closely resembling pityriasis lichenoides et varioliformis acuta or pityriasis lichenoides chronics (Fig. 61.11). The asymptomatic lesions come and go in crops over cycles of 1–3 months and heal with varioliform scars. At the same time, larger dermatitis-like patches and solitary tumors may appear (Fig. 61.12). In the other group, a much smaller number of lesions appear, with sharply bordered, violet to red-brown papules that clinically suggest pseudolymphoma or lymphoma. The lesions regress over weeks to months but tend to recur. Signs of systemic disease such as lymphadenopathy are rare and suggest a wrong diagnosis.

Histopathology. The Dutch cutaneous lymphoma group has described several histologic categories of lymphomatoid papulosis that partially correspond to the clinical ones. In short, there is typically a wedge-shaped, initially nonepidermotropic mixed infiltrate with large atypical lymphocytes. These are associated with eosinophils, small lymphocytes, neutrophils and histiocytes. In other instances, the infiltrate may be band-like or nodular. Immunohistochemical studies fail to clarify the situation. The large lymphocytes resemble those seen in anaplastic large cell lymphoma; they are CD30-positive, and may also be positive for CD2, 3, 4 and 5 and the proliferation marker Ki-67. Other infiltrates will mark in patterns similar to mycosis fungoides, reflecting the heterogeneity of lymphomatoid papulosis.

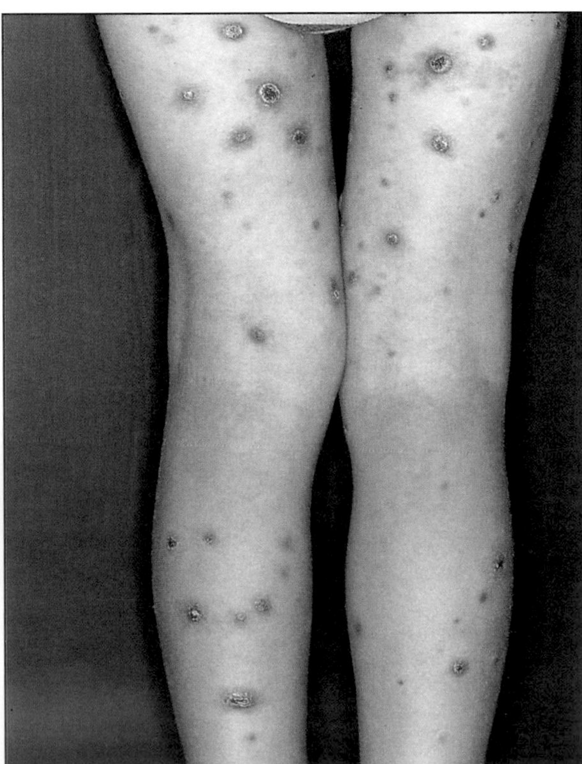

Fig. 61.11. Lymphomatoid papulosis with primarily papules and some ulcers

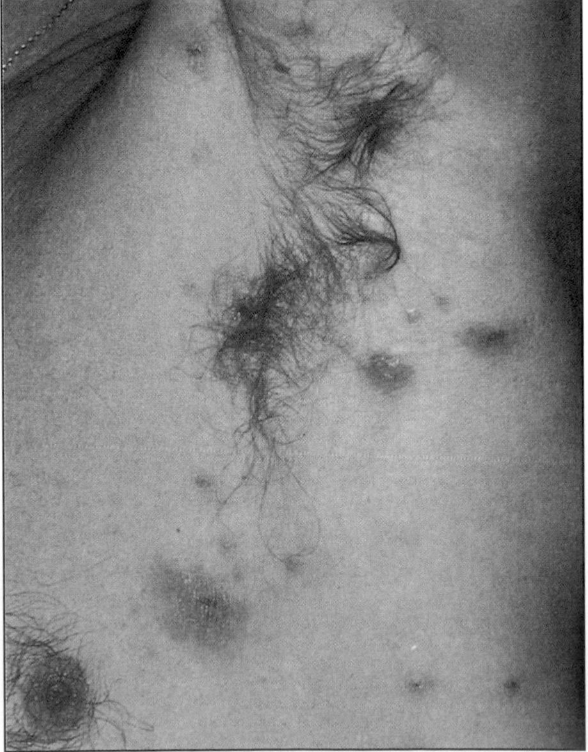

Fig. 61.12. Lymphomatoid papulosis with several larger lesions

Laboratory Findings. No evidence for circulating atypical cells is found. Elevated lymphocyte counts and hypergammaglobulinemia may be seen.

Course and Prognosis. The course is chronic, often lasting over decades. In one large registry, the 5-year survival rate was 100% for 70 patients. Only those few patients (10–20%) whose disease evolved into lymphoma then had a reduced life expectancy. Clinical signs that suggest a likely progression to malignancy include large or ulcerated tumors and papulonecrotic lesions in a dermatomal or localized distribution.

Differential Diagnosis. The multiple lesions must be distinguished from pityriasis lichenoides et varioliformis acuta, pityriasis lichenoides chronica, secondary syphilis, syphilis maligna, papulonecrotic tuberculid and widespread lesions of malignant lymphoma or leukemia. The history is usually decisive. The solitary tumors must be separated from pseudolymphoma, malignant lymphoma and other malignant infiltrates.

Therapy. There is no curative therapy. For patients with widespread lesions, PUVA bath therapy has been the most effective in our hands. Often low-dose methotrexate regimens such as 7.5–15 mg weekly will be effective. However, even these dosages cause concern in patients with a problem that may not truly require any therapy. PUVA and topical corticosteroids may also help some individuals. Aggressive regimens are not appropriate.

Peripheral T Cell Lymphoma, Unspecified

Synonyms. Kiel: T zone lymphoma, lymphoepithelioid lymphoma, pleomorphic small cell lymphoma, pleomorphic medium cell lymphoma, pleomorphic large cell lymphoma, T immunoblastic lymphoma

As the title suggests, this is a very mixed group. It brings together a number of lymphomas that were separated out based on light microscopic features in the Kiel classification. Several more specific subsets of peripheral T cell lymphoma are discussed below.

Clinical Findings. Nodal origin is the rule and patients typically have generalized disease with eosinophils, hemophagocytosis, pruritus and evidence of internal organ involvement. About 25–50% of patients have cutaneous lesions. The cutaneous findings are highly variable and can occasionally be the first sign of disease. Cutaneous infiltrates may be papular, nodular or sometimes plaque-like. The tumors tend to grow rapidly and may have a hemorrhagic or bruised color.

Histopathology. Microscopically, there is a broad range of atypical small- and medium-sized lymphocytes, sometimes admixed with eosinophils and epithelioid histiocytes. Lennert lymphoma (lymphoepithelioid lymphoma) rarely has skin involvement, but falls into this category. Thus, not all granulomatous lymphomas are mycosis fungoides. The cells have a variety of T cell markers, lack B cell markers and usually show clonal TCR rearrangement.

Therapy. Peripheral T cell lymphomas tend to be aggressive tumors but usually respond to multiple drug chemotherapy regimens. The skin lesions are probably best treated with electron beam or ionizing radiation, if they do not respond to the usual chemotherapy regimens.

Angioimmunoblastic T Cell Lymphoma

Synonyms. Kiel: T cell angioimmunoblastic lymphoma, angioimmunoblastic lymphadenopathy with dysproteinemia (AILD; Frizerra et al. 1974), lymphogranulomatosis X (Radaskiewicz and Lennert 1973)

Etiology and Pathogenesis. This rare disease was initially described as an abnormal immune reaction, often felt to be triggered by medications. Both the clinical course of the patients and clonality studies have shown that it is a malignant lymphoma.

Clinical Findings. Patients typically present with nodal disease and type B symptoms. They may also have hepatosplenomegaly. Skin involvement is seen in 30–40% of patients. The most common change is pruritus usually associated with a widespread, livid, maculopapular eruption. Clinically the lesions may resemble urticaria, although not transient, or even vasculitis. Nodules and plaques are unlikely to occur.

Histopathology. The lymph node changes are characteristic. The nodal architecture is effaced, with proliferation of small nodule vessels, called high endothelial venules, associated with follicular dendritic cells. The lymphocytic infiltrate is relatively sparse and mixed; the tumor cell is a mid-sized lymphocyte with a somewhat clear cytoplasm that is usually CD4-positive, carries other T cell markers and usually displays clonality. In some cases evidence for Epstein-Barr virus genomic material is found. In the skin, accumulations of tumor cells are few and far between. Most commonly one sees a lymphocytic perivascular infiltrate or even vasculitis.

Laboratory Findings. There is usually a polyclonal gammopathy, along with marked anemia.

Course and Prognosis. Angioimmunoblastic lymphoma is a slow smoldering disease. Infectious complications are common, and occasionally progression to high-grade T cell (or rarely B cell) lymphoma occurs.

Therapy. Many patients experience prolonged remissions with systemic corticosteroids. Nonetheless, recognizing that a true lymphoma is present, it may be more appropriate to use multidrug chemotherapy regimens or interferon-α.

Subcutaneous Panniculitic T Cell Lymphoma

(Gonzalez et al. 1991)

Synonym. No Kiel equivalent

Clinical Findings. This unusual variant of lymphoma presents clinically as panniculitis, with erythematous, firm subcutaneous infiltrates. Just as with inflammatory panniculitis, the legs are most commonly involved.

Histopathology. The infiltrate spares the dermis. In the fat, there is lobular involvement with necrosis, nuclear debris and occasionally erythrophagocytosis. The latter finding of macrophages laden with erythrocytes (bean bag sign) is very typical and regularly seen in the bone marrow. The aberrant cells have T cell markers including TIA-1, may show clonality and in some instances have a γ–δ TCR.

Differential Diagnosis. The main differential is cytophagic panniculitis (Chap. 21), which can be viewed as subcutaneous involvement in the hemophagocytic syndrome. Some cases have been identified with Epstein-Barr virus and they seem to be less likely to evolve into malignant lymphoma. The nature of the lymphocytes in the panniculitis is the most helpful clue; if they are cytologically normal and polyclonal, then perhaps an inflammatory process is present.

Therapy. This is a very aggressive lymphoma. Most patients succumb. The only hope is early multidrug chemotherapy regimens.

T/NK Cell Lymphoma, Nasal and Nasal Type

(Liebow et al. 1972)

Synonyms. Kiel: no equivalent. Angiocentric lymphoma, lymphomatoid granulomatosis, angiocentric immunoproliferative lesion, lethal midline granuloma, polymorphic reticulosis. We will use the older term angiocentric lymphoma for convenience, recognizing that all such malignant lymphomas are not angiocentric.

Definition. Systemic often angiocentric destructive process, long held to be reactive, but today considered a lymphoma.

Etiology and Pathogenesis. This definition must still be viewed as a working classification. The Epstein-Barr virus plays an important role in many of these lesions, especially in Asians. Most cases classically described as lymphomatoid granulomatosis appear to be T cell proliferations induced by Epstein-Barr virus. The normal counterpart is either a poorly defined T cell subset or NK (natural killer) cells. It appears that T cells handle Epstein-Barr virus infection less well than B cells.

Clinical Findings. The classic angiocentric lymphoma is a highly destructive tumor that frequently arises in extranodal sites, especially the nose or palate. CNS and renal involvement is also common, while lymph node, spleen and bone marrow involvement are rare. The old term lethal midline granuloma adequately describes these often horrific tumors. Skin involvement may also occur; usually red-brown nodules appear rapidly and soon ulcerate. Primary cutaneous angiocentric lymphomas have also been reported. Aggressive T/NK leukemia may be a very similar disease but with a primary leukemic phase. Patients present with widespread disease and skin involvement is common.

In contrast, lymphomatoid granulomatosis most typically involves the lungs. Skin involvement is also common; erythematous macules and papules as well as vasculitic lesions may be seen. Annular vesicular and bullous lesions on the legs have been described, mimicking necrobiosis lipoidica diabeticorum.

Another possible variant of angiocentric lymphoma is the hydroa vacciniforme-like malignant lymphoma of childhood, reported primarily in Mexico and Japan. The children have edema, vesicles, blisters and scars on the face, dorsal hands and forearms, but they are not photosensitive.

Histopathology. Nodal involvement is uncommon, so the diagnosis must almost always be made on other tissues. A key feature is accumulations of lymphocytes about vessels in the target tissue. The vessel walls may be invaded by a polymorphic mixture of small normal-appearing lymphocytes, occasional large atypical cells, eosinophils and plasma cells. When vessel occlusion or destruction occurs, the result is necrosis of the adjacent tissue. In some instances there is no predilection for vessels. Despite the older name of lymphomatoid granulomatosis, granulomas are not reliably seen and macrophages are uncommon.

In the skin, the diagnosis can be very difficult. Often, the atypical cells are few in number and not identifiable. There may be concentric fibrosis about vessels, fibrin deposits and, most importantly, lymphocytes in the vessel wall. Some infiltrates are more nodular and extend into the subcutaneous fat.

The atypical cells appear to be either peripheral T cells or NK cells, expressing most reliably CD2 along with either CD4, 5, 7 or 8, usually CD3-negative and often CD56-positive. In the cases with extensive pulmonary disease, B cell markers are found. Depending on the cell line, both TCR and immunoglobulin genes are usually germ-line.

Epstein-Barr virus is found in most cases of systemic angiocentric lymphoma and in the hydroa vacciniforme-like variant but is uncommonly present in the primary cutaneous form in adults.

Course and Prognosis. The outline for the nasal lymphomas is dismal. Almost all patients die within 2–3 years, despite aggressive chemotherapy and radiation therapy. The pulmonary form is a more chronic disease, often responsive to systemic corticosteroids. It took over a decade for Liebow and colleagues to recognize that their original description was incorrect and that clinical evidence indicated a malignant lymphoma.

Anaplastic Large Cell Lymphoma

(Stein et al. 1985)

Synonyms. Kiel: large cell anaplastic lymphoma, T and null types, regressing atypical histiocytosis, malignant histiocytosis (some cases)

Definition. Lymphoma comprised of distinctive, large pleomorphic T cells that were originally identified as CD30-positive.

Etiology and Pathogenesis. There are two distinct forms of anaplastic large cell lymphoma: (1) a primary nodal form and (2) a primary cutaneous form, which has a far better outlook. The primary cutaneous form is more common in adults, while the more aggressive systemic form has a bimodal distribution in children and adults.

CD30 is a sign of activation and may be positive in many other malignant lymphomas. Today this category is identified based on both CD30 positivity and morphologic features. CD30 also serves as a unifying feature between anaplastic large cell lymphoma, lymphomatoid papulosis and Hodgkin disease, as the tumor cells in all three disorders are often positive and clinical overlaps are seen. Most of the anaplastic lymphomas seen late in mycosis fungoides are CD30-positive although Sézary cells are negative.

Clinical Findings. Adults with primary cutaneous disease typically have one or more red-brown plaques or nodules. Ulceration is common and regression occurs in about 25% of patients, confirming the overlaps with lymphomatoid papulosis. In the systemic form, many of the patients are younger. They may present with skin disease but almost always have systemic involvement at the time. Thus it is essential to intensely scrutinize any patient with anaplastic large cell lymphoma of the skin before categorizing him.

Histopathology. The cutaneous lesion is composed of cohesive sheets of large pleomorphic cells often with horseshoe-shaped nuclei. On occasion, multinucleate cells are seen, resembling Reed-Sternberg cells. The cells are larger and more variable than in other large cell lymphomas. In the skin, there are less anaplastic variants; about 20% of such tumors are described as large cell rather than anaplastic. The tumor cells must be CD30-positive. There is generally some evidence for T cell differentiation, often with CD positivity but with a loss of pan-T cell antigens.

Course and Prognosis. The 5-year survival rate for primary cutaneous anaplastic large cell lymphoma is about 90%, with no difference between frankly anaplastic and large cell forms. The cutaneous anaplastic lymphomas arising in mycosis fungoides or Sézary syndrome have a poor prognosis. The systemic form is an aggressive lymphoma but is potentially curable.

Differential Diagnosis. Separating out tumors of lymphomatoid papulosis or the extremely rare, primary cutaneous Hodgkin disease has been an almost philosophical task. The clinical picture and course determine the diagnosis. The presence of rapidly growing, ulcerated nodules and the large atypical cells with puzzling marker characteristics (prior to discovery of CD30) led to a variety of mistaken diagnoses, including malignant histiocytosis, regressing atypical histiocytosis, metastatic carcinoma or even malignant melanoma.

Therapy. The cutaneous form is best treated by localized radiation therapy. Excision is also reasonable for a solitary lesion. The systemic form and that arising in mycosis fungoides require multiple-drug chemotherapy regimens.

Intestinal T Cell Lymphoma

This tumor involves intestinal intraepithelial T cells and usually presents with jejunal ulcerations or a mass. It is the most common type of lymphoma to arise in patients with a gluten-sensitive enteropathy, including patients with dermatitis herpetiformis. Although this malignant lymphoma was long described as "intestinal malignant histiocytosis", there is a clonal proliferation of T cells that are CD3-, 7- and 103-positive. The outlook is poor because of the refractory intestinal ulcers.

Adult T Cell Lymphoma/Leukemia

Synonyms. Kiel: pleomorphic small, medium and large cell lymphoma (HTLV-1-positive)

This disease, caused by a retrovirus, HTLV-1, more often presents with leukemic features and is discussed in Chapter 62.

B Cell Lymphomas

B cell lymphomas are less common in the skin. They may have a follicular pattern, thus often making the distinction from pseudolymphomas difficult. Their clonality is easier to determine, as one can study light chains rather than the TCR.

B Cell Lymphoblastic Leukemia/Lymphoma

Synonym. Kiel: lymphoblastic B cell lymphoma

Epidemiology. Children are more often involved. Most cases present as leukemia rather than lymphoma.

Clinical Findings. Lymphoblastic leukemia/lymphoma is a very aggressive systemic disease. The B cell form is somewhat more likely to involve the skin. The head and neck region is usually involved; solitary or multiple scalp nodules are especially common. Rare cases present with cutaneous disease. Even if there is no lymphadenopathy or bone marrow involvement at this time, it will soon appear, so all such cases should be regarded as systemic from the start.

Histopathology. There is a monotonous nodular infiltrate of lymphoblasts; the cells, which are larger than normal lymphocytes, have a fine chromatin and scant cytoplasm. T and B cell lymphoblasts are identical and must be separated by marker studies. The cells are TdT-, CD19-, CD79a- and, often, CD10-positive. Immunoglobulins are usually not expressed, in contrast to more mature B cell lymphomas, but heavy chain rearrangement is usually present.

Therapy. Aggressive multidrug chemotherapy is frequently successful in curing this high-grade lymphoma.

B Cell Chronic Lymphocytic Leukemia

Synonyms. Kiel: B cell chronic lymphocytic leukemia; B cell prolymphocytic leukemia; immunocytoma, lymphoplasmacytoid type

These chronic smoldering B cell proliferations behave as leukemias and are discussed in Chapter 62.

Lymphoplasmacytoid Lymphoma/ Immunocytoma

Synonym. Kiel: immunocytoma, lymphoplasmacytic type

The REAL classification limits the spectrum of lymphoplasmacytoid lymphoma/ immunocytoma. While many B cell lymphomas show some degree of plasma cell differentiation, this diagnosis is limited to a lymphoma that lacks features of any other B cell lymphoma and almost always has a monoclonal IgM peak, resulting in the clinical disorder of Waldenström macroglobulinemia (Chap. 40). Cutaneous infiltrates are uncommon, but usually consist of diffuse papules or nodules. The cells have both surface and cytoplasmic immunoglobulin, usually prominent, and are CD5-negative, allowing separation from B cell chronic lymphocytic leukemia (B-CLL). Other B cell antigens are usually positive (CD19, 79a) but CD10 is negative. The proliferation is monoclonal.

Marginal Zone B Cell Lymphoma

Synonyms. Kiel: no specific term, closest to monocytoid B cell lymphoma, cutaneous immunocytoma, MALT lymphoma

Etiology and Pathogenesis. The B cells of the marginal zone of the follicle are the normal counterparts; they tend to home to certain tissue compartments such as gut or skin and can differentiate into plasma cells. MALT (mucosa-associated lymphoid tissue) refers to intestinal lymphoid tissue, usually a rich source of B cells. MALT lymphomas are frequently extranodal; the gastrointestinal tract is most commonly involved. There is an association with Sjögren syndrome, Hashimoto thyroiditis and *Helicobacter pylori* infections. Some early MALT lymphomas have apparently cleared with anti-bacterial therapy directed against *Helicobacter pylori*, suggesting that there is an early reversible lymphocytic proliferation that at some point turns into a lymphoma.

The cutaneous equivalent of a MALT lymphoma is known as a cutaneous immunocytoma; it is not related to the lymphoplasmacytoid lymphoma/immunocytoma discussed above. We have suggested a relationship with *Borrelia burgdorferi* for the skin variant.

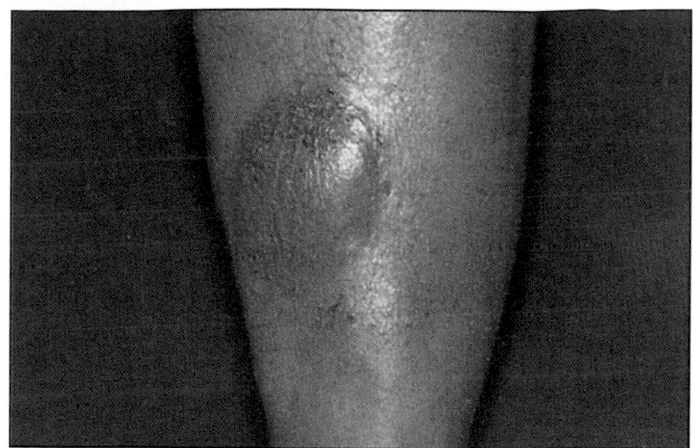

Fig. 61.13. Marginal zone B cell lymphoma

Clinical Findings. While most tumors are extranodal, some later appear in the lymph nodes. For example, this is the type of nodal lymphoma associated with Sjögren syndrome. Rarely there may be a primary nodal MALT lymphoma.

In the skin, most lesions occur on the extremities. One or more papules or nodules are found (Fig. 61.13). Sometimes larger plaques are seen with a red-brown color, mimicking the early stage of acrodermatitis chronica atrophicans. Ulcerations are rare. Local recurrence or spread is common but involvement of lymph nodes or bone marrow is very rare.

Histopathology. The characteristic microscopic features are a heterogeneous infiltrate with marginal zone or centrocytic cells, larger monocytoid B cells, small lymphocytes, plasmacytoid cells and germinal centers. The cells express surface immunoglobulin and about half have cytoplasmic immunoglobulin. The B cell associated antigens (CD19, 20, 79a) are positive; the plasmacytoid cells lack CD20; neither CD5 nor CD10 is found. Clonal rearrangement of immunoglobulin genes can be observed.

Laboratory Findings. There is no evidence of circulating immunoglobulins.

Course and Prognosis. The 5-year survival rate is 100% for patients with cutaneous lesions only. The nodal and other extranodal lymphomas are indolent but not usually curable.

Therapy. Cutaneous immunocytomas can be treated with radiation therapy or excised. Although chemotherapy has been tried for systemic MALT lymphomas, the results were disappointing. As mentioned above, some intestinal lymphomas have responded to antibiotic treatment for *Helicobacter pylori* infection.

Mantle Cell Lymphoma

Synonym. Kiel: centrocytic lymphoma

Mantle cell lymphoma is a cytologically innocent but clinically aggressive lymphoma that is usually widespread at diagnosis. It is a disease of older adults and favors men. Common sites include lymph nodes, spleen, tonsils, gastrointestinal tract, bone marrow and blood. Skin involvement is extremely rare; red papules, nodules and plaques have been described. The mantle cell is a B cell in the mantle zone of the lymphoid follicle. It is usually has surface IgM and IgD and B cell associated antigens. CD23 is negative, in contrast to B-CLL; CD5 is positive, in contrast to follicle center cell and marginal zone lymphomas.

Follicle Center Cell Lymphoma

Synonyms. Kiel: centroblastic/centrocytic lymphoma, centroblastic lymphoma

Epidemiology. Follicle center cell lymphoma is one of the most common lymphomas of adults, affecting both sexes equally.

Etiology and Pathogenesis. There is a common translocation [t(14;18)] involving the *bcl*-2 gene. This gene is an anti-apoptosis gene; when it is regulated by those genes responsible for immunoglobulin synthesis, it is expressed at higher levels, allowing long-lived centroblasts. The translocation appears to occur prior to antigenic stimulation; the cell is then by chance triggered and expands clonally. This translocation is found in 75–95% of nodal lymphomas but is only rarely found in primary cutaneous follicle center cell lymphomas.

Clinical Findings. Follicule center cell lymphoma is primarily a nodal disease. It is usually widespread at presentation, involving multiple nodal groups, as well as perhaps the spleen. Skin involvement is most often about the head and neck, with firm solitary or multiple nodules. In addition, there is often extensive cervical and axillary lymph node involvement, with secondary induration of the skin. Reactive erythroderma has also been described.

There is also a primary cutaneous follicule center cell lymphoma. These patients present with grouped papules, plaques or nodules, once again on the head and neck, or occasionally on the trunk. Scalp involvement frequently causes alopecia. The lesions may be surrounded by erythematous rings or bands.

Histopathology. The follicle centers contain small centrocytes that mature to centroblasts. In the REAL classification these lymphomas are graded cytologically. In addition, a diffuse variant has tentatively been recognized in which the same cells are seen, but the follicles are missing. In the skin, the follicles can usually be seen, thus mitigating against the old adage that germinal centers mean pseudolymphoma. The infiltrate is focal, bottom-heavy and almost never impinges on the epidermis.

The cells in the skin are positive for CD10 and B cell associated antigens and have surface immunoglobulins. CD10 positivity helps exclude marginal zone lymphoma while the lack of CD5 tends to rule out mantle cell lymphoma. Peculiarly the primary cutaneous follicle center cell lymphomas usually lack surface immunoglobulins, even though they are monoclonal; they do not have the *bcl*-2 translocation.

Course and Prognosis. The primary cutaneous lesions have an excellent prognosis, with a 5-year survival rate over 95%. The systemic form is indolent but not usually not curable.

Therapy. The primary form should be treated with radiation therapy, either soft X-rays or electron beam. Polychemotherapy has been employed for systemic disease but with little success.

Diffuse Large B Cell Lymphoma

Synonyms. Kiel: centroblastic lymphoma, immunoblastic B cell lymphoma, large cell anaplastic B cell lymphoma

The REAL classification groups the large B cell tumors formerly described as centroblastic, immunoblastic and anaplastic together. Several tumors of special interest to dermatologists fall in this group and will be discussed separately.

Epidemiology. Diffuse large B cell lymphomas are the other common adult lymphoma, also accounting for 30–40% of all non-Hodgkin lymphomas. While the peak age of onset is in the sixth decade, the range is broad.

Clinical Findings. Patients usually present with a rapidly enlarging, often painful or otherwise symptomatic mass at a single nodal or extranodal site. About one-third of these masses are extranodal. The skin may be primarily involved. Once again, there is usually a single nodule or cluster of lesions most often on the head and neck region (Fig. 61.14). Two clinical variants have been described:

- Reticulohistiocytoma (Crosti 1951). This nodular infiltrate on the back of adult men has a relatively good prognosis. Some cases may have also represented follicle center cell lymphomas.
- Large B Cell Lymphoma of the Leg. The Dutch lymphoma group has noticed that these large cell lymphomas tend to affect women over the age of 70 years. The patients present with red-blue nodules on one or both shins or calves. They do less well than younger patients with lesions on the trunk or head.

In this day of immunologic diagnoses, it seems dangerous to assign a prognosis based on body location, but one should keep in mind the trends shown by these two variants.

Histopathology. The cells of a diffuse large B cell lymphoma are at least twice the size of a normal lymphocyte. Most of the cells are centroblasts without a cleaved nucleus or immunoblasts with a cleaved nucleus (buttocks nucleus). Because the interobserver variation in identifying these two cells is so great, the REAL classification has put the two together. In the skin there is typically a nodular infiltrate of large lymphocytes with little subtlety. It tends to be deep and only rarely impinges upon the epidermis. The cells tend to stain with B cell associated antigens and CD45, but lack T cell antigens. Immunoglobulins are usually not expressed. Rearrangement of the *bcl*-2 gene is also seen in some cases.

An interesting histological variant is the T cell-rich B cell lymphoma. Although the neoplastic cell is a large B cell, the infiltrate is dominated by normal T cells which presumably are attracted to the site by B cell related cytokines.

Course and Prognosis. The patients with strictly cutaneous lesions do fairly well, as progression is uncommon. The patients with nodules on the legs and thus a slightly worse prognosis still have a 60% 5-year survival rate. The lymphomas involving nodal or other extranodal sites are also fairly therapy-responsive as long as they are localized.

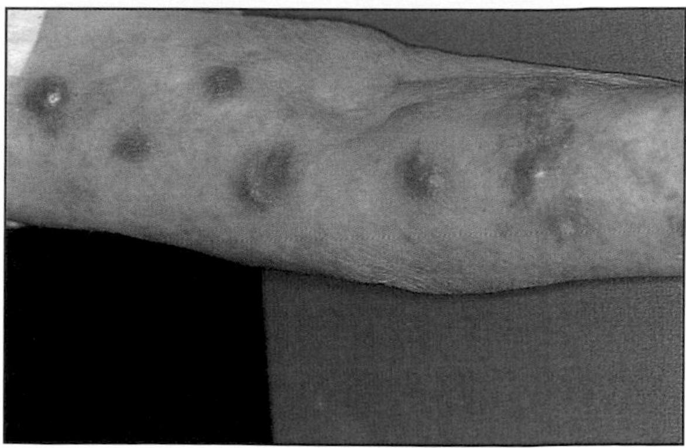

Fig. 61.14. Diffuse large B cell lymphoma with multiple nodules

Therapy. The local cutaneous lesions should be irradiated. Systemic disease requires aggressive multidrug chemotherapy. The monoclonal antibody rituximab is directed against CD20 and has been employed both systemically and intralesionally to treat CD20-positive B cell lymphomas.

Intravascular Large B Cell Lymphoma

(Tappeiner and Pfleger 1959)

Synonyms. Kiel: no equivalent. Malignant angioendotheliomatosis, angioendotheliomatosis proliferans systematisata, angiotrophic large cell lymphoma

Definition. Unique large cell lymphoma, usually of B cell origin, that remains confined to the vessel lumina but is disseminated in many organs. A second, histologically identical disease is caused by an endothelial cell proliferation and is known as reactive benign angioendotheliomatosis (Chap. 59).

Etiology and Pathogenesis. There is a defect in lymphocytic trafficking so that the cells cannot reliably escape from the vessels. Apparently, some vascular homing receptors are expressed on the lymphocyte surface. Careful analysis of tissue specimens usually identifies a few extravascular lymphoma cells.

Clinical Findings. The cutaneous lesions are identical in the benign and malignant forms of angioendotheliomatosis. There are red-blue infiltrated plaques that frequently resemble bruises. In addition, papules and nodules may be present and often ulcerate. The patients are usually chronically ill, feverish, may have signs of recurrent infections and frequently have CNS or lung involvement. Lymph node disease is uncommon.

Histopathology. In the dermis, the blood vessels are filled by nests and clumps of large cells that may cause occlusion. Exocytosis of erythrocytes is common and occasional tumor cells may leak. Once again, the reactive changes are identical in the benign and malignant forms, even though the endothelial cells are proliferating, and a distinction can only be made with immunohistochemical studies. In the cases of intravascular lymphoma, the tumor cells stain with CD45 and B cell associated antigens (CD19, CD20, CD22, CD79a). Rare cases may show T cell markers.

Course and Prognosis. The outlook is usually dismal. If the patient has lung and CNS involvement, the survival is measured in months. Some patients have primarily skin involvement and their disease smolders for longer periods.

Differential Diagnosis. Clinically, patients may be mistaken for HIV/AIDS patients, with the combination of red skin nodules, weakness and diffuse disease. HIV serology is negative. Similarly, polyarteritis nodosa may have clinical overlaps but it has a different histology. Microscopically, there is also room for error, as intravascular metastatic carcinomas and malignant melanomas can appear very similar.

Therapy. Aggressive polychemotherapy is the only hope, but usually does not offer much improvement.

Burkitt Lymphoma

(Burkitt 1958)

Synonym. Kiel: Burkitt lymphoma

Definition. Aggressive small B cell neoplasm that is common in equatorial Africa and usually associated with Epstein-Barr virus.

Epidemiology. Endemic Burkitt lymphoma is the most common childhood tumor in equatorial Africa, where it is ten times as frequent as the next tumor. It is also endemic in parts of North Africa, South America and New Guinea. The peak age of onset is about 5 years and the male : female ratio is 2 : 1. It tends to be most common in areas where malaria is also endemic. Sporadic Burkitt lymphoma is responsible for about 2% of lymphomas in the USA, where it is the most common form of malignant lymphoma in patients with HIV/AIDS and one of the most common in those with iatrogenic immunosuppression.

Etiology and Pathogenesis. The molecular biology of Burkitt lymphoma is well-understood. There is a translocation involving the c-*myc* oncogene from chromosome 8 to an immunoglobulin gene. The most common change involves the immunoglobulin heavy chain region on chromosome 14 [t(8; 14)]. Less often, light chain regions on chromosomes 2 or 22 are involved. The translocation lead to uncontrolled expression of c-*myc*, a growth factor. The exact location of the translocation is different in the endemic and sporadic forms. Epstein-Barr virus can be demonstrated in almost all African cases, in about one-third of HIV/AIDS cases, and rarely in sporadic disease. In HIV/AIDS and posttransplantation malignant lymphomas, the latent membrane protein 1 of Epstein-Barr virus appears to mimic tumor necrosis factor (TNF) receptors and transmit growth messages. In the endemic cases, the virus can be found but this growth control pathway is not seen.

Clinical Findings. African children with Burkitt lymphoma almost always have involvement of the facial bones, especially the jaw and orbit. They thus present with marked distortions of these structures. In sporadic cases, abdominal involvement is most common. Lymph nodes are uncommonly affected and skin changes are very rare.

Histopathology. The diagnosis is usually made on tissues other than lymph nodes. There is a diffuse infiltrate of small lymphocytes with histiocytes scattered through the tumor, producing clear spaces or the starry sky pattern. B cell markers are positive, as is Ki-67 since the malignant lymphoma is very aggressive and grows rapidly.

Course and Prognosis. The cure rates are very high in the endemic form, being well over 80%. For sporadic Burkitt lymphoma the prognosis is somewhat dependent on the underlying disease.

Differential Diagnosis. The differential diagnosis includes other high-grade lymphomas when confronted with a sporadic Burkitt lymphoma in a nonimmunosuppressed patient. In the endemic form, Kaposi sarcoma should also be considered.

Therapy. Polychemotherapy and surgical debulking are both recommended. The response rate is very high.

Plasmacytoma/Plasma Cell Myeloma

Most plasmacytomas present as a disseminated disease process known as multiple myeloma (Chap. 40). Solitary bone plasmacytomas tend to progress to multiple myeloma, but the rare, solitary extramedullary plasmacytomas have a better prognosis. Primary cutaneous plasmacytomas are quite uncommon; they present as red-brown nodular dermal infiltrates comprised of mature plasma cells. While most lesions are solitary, multiple lesions are occasionally seen. Among Japanese patients, and rarely in patients in other countries, both cutaneous plasmacytosis and systemic plasmacytosis involving two or more organ systems have been described. The tumor cells have cytoplasmic immunoglobulins and other B cell markers. Many cases reported in the past as cutaneous plasmacytomas were either less mature B cell lymphomas with plasmacytoid features or were reactive processes. For example, polyclonal plasma cell infiltrates may develop in curettage sites or following arthropod bites. Once the diagnosis of cutaneous plasmacytoma is established, either surgery or radiation therapy is appropriate and the cure rate is 100%.

Bibliography

Introductory and Review Articles

Bachelez H (1999) The clinical use of molecular analysis of clonality in cutaneous lymphocytic infiltrates. Arch Dermatol 135:200–202

Burg G, Braun-Falco O (eds) (1983) Cutaneous lymphomas, pseudolymphomas and related disorders. Springer-Verlag, Berlin Heidelberg New York

Burg G, Dummer R, Kerl H (1994) Classification of cutaneous lymphomas. Dermatol Clin 12:213–217

Burg G, Kempf W, Haeffner AC et al. (1997) Cutaneous lymphomas. Curr Probl Dermatol 9:137–204

Cerroni L, Kerl H, Gatter K (eds) (1998) An illustrated guide to skin lymphoma. Blackwell Science, Oxford

Cerroni L, Kerl H (1999) Diagnostic immunohistology: cutaneous lymphomas and pseudolymphomas. Semin Cut Med Surg 18:64–70

Harris LH, Jaffe SE, Stein H et al. (1994) A revised European-American classification of lymphoid neoplasms: a proposal from the international lymphoma study group. Blood 84:1361–1392

Isaacson PG, Norton AJ (eds) (1994) Extranodal lymphomas. Churchill Livingstone, Edinburgh

Knowles DM (ed) (1992) Neoplastic hematology. Williams and Wilkins, Baltimore

Küppers R, Klein U, Hansmann M-L et al. (1999) Cellular origin of human B cell Lymphomas. NEJM 341:1520–1529

Sander CA, Kind P, Kaudewitz P et al. (1997) The revised European-American classification of lymphoid neoplasms (REAL): a new perspective for the classification of cutaneous lymphomas. J Cutan Pathol 24:329–341

Sander CA, Flaig MJ, Kaudewitz P et al. (1999) The revised European-American classification of lymphoid neoplasmas (REAL): a preferred approach for the classification of cutaneous lymphomas. Am J Dermatopathol 21:274–278

Weinberg JM, Rock AH, Lessin SR (1993) Molecular diagnosis of lymphocytic infiltrates of the skin. Arch Dermatol 129:1491–1500

Willemze N, Belijaards RC, Meijer CJCN et al. (1994) Classification of primary cutaneous lymphomas. Historical overview and perspectives. Dermatology 189 [Suppl 2]: 8–15

Willemze R, Kerl H, Sterry W et al. (1997) EORTC classification for primary cutaneous lymphomas: a proposal from the Cutaneous Lymphoma Study Group of the European Organisation for Research and Treatment of Cancer. Blood 90:354–371

Willemze R, Meijer CJLM (1999) EORTC Classification for primary cutaneous lymphomas: the best guide to good clinical management. Am J Dermatopathol 21:265–273

Wood G (1992) Benign and malignant cutaneous lymphoproliferative disorders including mycosis fungoides. In: Knowles DM (ed) Neoplastic hematology. Williams and Wilkins, Baltimore, pp 917–952

Hodgkin Disease

Cerroni L, Beham-Schmid C, Kerl H (1995) Cutaneous Hodgkins's disease: an immunohistochemical analysis. J Cut Pathol 22:229–235

Hayes TG, Rabin VR, Rosen T et al. (1990) Hodgkins's disease presenting in the skin: case report and review of the literature. J Am Acad Dermatol 22:944–947

Hodgkin T (1832) On some morbid appearances of the absorbent glands and spleen. Med Chir Tr 17:68–114

Kaudewitz P, Stein H, Plewig G et al. (1990) Hodgkin's disease followed by lymphomatoid papulosis. J Am Acad Dermatol 22:999–1006

Morretti S, Pimpinelli N, Di Lollo S et al. (1989) In situ immunologic characterization of cutaneous involvement in Hodgkins's disease. Cancer 63:661–666

Sioutos N, Kerl H, Murphy SB et al. (1994) Primary cutaneous Hodgkin disease: unique clinical, morphologic and immunophenotypic findings. Am J Dermatopathol 16:2–8

Smith JL, Butler JJ (1980) Skin involvement in Hodgkins's disease. Cancer 45:354–361

White RM, Patterson JW (1985) Cutaneous involvement in Hodgkins's disease. Cancer 55:1136–1145

Mycosis Fungoides and Sézary Syndrome

Alibert JLM (1806) Tableau du pian fongoide. Description des maladies de la peau, observées à l'Hôpital Saint Louis et exposition des meilleurs méthodes suivies pour le traitment. Barrois L'Ainé, Paris

Anagnostopoulos J, Hummel M, Kaudewitz P et al. (1996) Low incidence of Epstein-Barr virus presence in primary cutaneous T cell lymphoproliferations. Br J Dermatol 134:276–281

Argenyi ZB, Goeken JA, Piette WW et al. (1992) Granulomatous mycosis fungoides. Clinicopathologic study of two cases. Am J Dermatopathol 14:200–210

Bakels V, van Oostveen JW, Gordijn RLJ et al. (1992) Frequency and prognostic significance of clonal T cell receptor β-gene rearrangements in the peripheral blood of patients with mycosis fungoides. Arch Dermatol 129: 1602–1607

Barcos M (1992) Mycosis fungoides. Diagnosis and pathogenesis. Am J Clin Pathol 99:452–458

Basarab T, Fraser-Andrews EA, Orchard G et al. (1998) Lymphomatoid papulosis in association with mycosis fungoides: a study of 15 cases. Br J Dermatol 139:630–638

Boehncke WH, Krettek S, Parwaresch MR et al. (1992) Demonstration of clonal disease in early mycosis fungoides. Am J Dermatopathol 14:95–99

Breneman DL, Nartker AL, Ballman EA et al. (1991) Topical mechlorethamine in the treatment of mycosis fungoides. J Am Acad Dermatol 25:1059–1064

Cerroni L, Rieger E, Hödl S et al. (1992) Clinicopathologic and immunologic features associated transformation of mycosis fungoides to large cell lymphoma. Am Surg Pathol 16:543–552

Cerroni L, Fink-Puches R, El-Shabrawi-Caelen et al. (1999) Solitary skin lesions with histopathologic features of early mycosis fungoides. Am J Dermatopathol 21(6): 518–524

Chinn DM, Chow S, Kim YH et al. (1999) Total skin electron beam therapy with or without adjuvant topical nitrogen mustard or nitrogen mustard alone as initial treatment of T2 and T3 mycosis fungoides. Int J Radiat Oncol Biol Phys 43:951–958

Delfau-Larue MH, Dalac S, Lepage E et al. (1998) Prognostic significance of polymerase chain reaction-detectable dominant T-lymphocyte clone in cutaneous lesions of patients with mycosis fungoides. Blood 92:3376–3380

Diamandidou E, Cohen PR, Kurzrock R (1996) Mycosis fungoides and Sezary syndrome. Blood 88:2385–2409

Diamandidou E, Colome M, Fayad L et al. (1999) Prognostic factor analysis in mycosis fungoides/Sezary syndrome. J Am Acad Dermatol 40:914–924

Duncan K, Heald P (1998) Cutaneous T cell lymphoma: centuries of controversy. Semin Cut Med Surg 17:133–140

Duvic M, Hester JP, Lemak NA (1996) Photopheresis therapy for cutaneous T cell lymphoma. J Am Acad Dermatol 35: 573–579

Giuatard J, Kaul K (1999) A new polymemerase chain reaction-based method for the detection of T cell clonality in patients with possible cutaneous T cell lymphoma. Arch Dermatol 135:158–162

Gottlieb SL, Wolfe JT, Fox FE et al. (1996) Treatment of cutaneous T cell lymphoma with extracorporeal photopheresis monotherapy and in combination with recombinant interferon alpha: a 10-year experience at a single institution. J Am Acad Dermatol 35:946–957

Grevelink SA, Fuller GN, Olsen EA (1991) Central nervous system involvement by cutaneous T cell lymphoma. J Am Acad Dermatol 25:542–549

Hallopeau H, Besnier E (1892) The forms of erythrodermia of mycosis fungoides. Br J Dermatol 4:318

Heald P, Rook A, Perez M et al. (1992) Treatment of erythrodermic cutaneous T cell lymphoma with exreacorporeal photochemotherapy. J Am Acad Dermatol 27:427–433

Heald PW, Glusac EJ (2000) Unilesional cutaneous T-cell lymphoma: Clinical features, therapy, and follow-up of 10 patients with a treatment-responsive mycosis fungoides variant. J Am Acad Dermatol 42:283–285

Holloway KB, Flowers FP, Ramos-Caro FA (1992) Therapeutic alternatives in cutaneous T cell lymphoma. J Am Acad Dermatol 27:367–378

Jürg B, Kerl H, Thiers B et al. (1994) Therapeutic approaches in cutaneous lymphoma. Dermatol Clin 12:433–441

Kamarashev J, Burg G, Kempf W et al. (1998) Comparative analysis of histological and immunological features in mycosis fungoides and Sezary syndrome. J Cut Pathol 25: 407–412

Kern DE, Kidd PG, Moe R et al. (1998) Analysis of T cell receptor gene rearrangement in lymph nodes of patients with mycosis fungoides. Prognostic implications. Arch Dermatol 134:158–164

Kikuchi A, Naka W, Harada T et al. (1993) Parapsoriasis en plaques: its potential for progression to malignant lymphoma. J Am Acad Dermatol 29:419–422

Kim YH, Chow S, Varghese A et al. (1999) Clinical characteristics and long-term outcome of patients with generalized patch and/or plaque (T2) mycosis fungoides. Arch Dermatol 135:26–32

Koch SE, Zackheim HS, Williams ML et al. (1987) Mycosis fungoides beginning in childhood and adolescence. J Am Acad Dermatol 17:563–570

Kuzel TM, Roenigk HH, Samuelson E et al. (1995) Effectiveness of interferon alpha-2a combined with phototherapy for mycosis fungoides and the Sezary syndrome. J Clin Oncol 13:257–263

Lacour JP, Castanet J, Perrin C et al. (1993) Follicular mycosis fungoides. A clinical and histologic variant of cutaneous T cell lymphoma: report of two cases. J Am Acad Dermatol 29:330–334

Mainguene C, Picard O, Audouin J et al. (1993) An unusual case of mycosis fungoides presenting as sarcoidosis or granulomatous mycosis fungoides. Am J Clin Pathol 99:82–86

Ofuji S, Furukawa F, Miyachi Y et al. (1984) Papuloerythroderma. Dermatologica 169:125–130

Olerud JE, Kulin PA, Chew DE et al. (1992) Cutaneous T cell lymphoma. Evaluation of pretreatment skin biopsy specimens by a panel of pathologists. Arch Dermatol 128: 501–507

Pereyo NG, Requena L, Galloway J et al. (1997) Follicular mycosis fungoides: a clinicohistopathologic study. J Am Acad Dermatol 36:563–568

Russell-Jones R (2000) Extracorporeal photopheresis in cutaneous T-cell lymphoma. Inconsistent data underline the need for randomized studies. Br J Dermatol 142: 16–21

Sézary A, Bouvrain Y (1938) Erythrodermie avec présence de cellules monstrueuses dans le derme et le sang circulant. Bull Soc Fr Dermatol Syphiligr 45:254–260

Simon M, Flaig MJ, Kind P et al. (2000) Large plaque parapsoriasis: clinical and genotypic correlations. J Cutan Pathol 27:57–60

Stadler R, Otte HG, Luger T et al. (1999) Prospective randomized multicenter clinical trial on the use of interferon alpha 2a plus Acitretin versus interferon alpha-2a plus PUVA in patients with cutaneous T cell lymphoma stages I and II. Blood 92:3578–3581

Sterry W, Siebel A, Mielke V (1992) HTLV-1-negavtive pleomorphic T cell lymphoma of the skin: the clinicopathological correlations and natural history of 15 patients. Br J Dermatol 126:456–462

Tan RSH, MacLeod TIF, Dean SG (1987) Pagetoid reticulosis, epidermotropic mycosis fungoides and mycosis fungoides: a disease spectrum. Br J Dermatol 116:67–77

Toyo JR, Stoll HL, Stomper PC et al. (1997) Prognostic factors and evaluation of mycosis fungoides and Sézary syndrome. J Am Acad Dermatol 37:58–67

Van Haselen CW, Diederen PVMM, Toonstra J et al. (1997) The small cell variant of mycosis fungoides: a clinicopathological and quantitative electron microscopic study on 14 patients. Arch Dermatol Res 290:583–590

Vidal E, Brocq L (1885) Etude sur le mycosis fungoide. la france Médical 2:946–1019

Wakelin SH, Stewart EJC, Emmerson RW (1996) Poikilodermatous and verrucous mycosis fungoides. Clin Exp Dermatol 21:205–208

Weinstock MA, Reynes JF (1999) The changing survival of patients with mycosis fungoides: a population-based assessment of trends in the United States. Cancer 85: 208–212

Wieselthier JS, Koh HKM (1990) Sézary syndrome: diagnosis, prognosis, and critical review of treatment options. J Am Acad Dermatol 22:381–401

Winkelman RK (1974) Clinical studies of T cell erythroderma in the Sézary's syndrome. Mayo Clin Proc 49:519–525

Winkelman RK, Buecher SA, Diaz-Perez JL et al. (1984) Pre-Sezary syndrome. J Am Acad Dermatol 10:992–999

Wood GS (1999) Using molecular biologic analysis of T cell receptor gene rearrangements to stage cutaneous T cell-lymphoma. Arch Dermatol 134:221–223

Zackheim HS, Epstein EH (1989) Low-dose methotrexate for the Sézary syndrome. J Am Acad Dermatol 21:757–762

Zackheim HS, Epstein EH, Crain WR (1990) Topical carmustine (BCNU) for cutaneous T cell lymphoma: a 15-year experience in 143 patients. J Am Acad Dermatol 22:802–810

Zackheim HS, Amin S, Kashani-Sabet M et al. (1999) Prognosis in cutaneous T cell lymphoma by skin stage: long-term survival in 489 patients. J Am Acad Dermatol 40: 418–425

Zic JA, Stricklin GP, Greer JP et al. (1996) Long-term follow up of patients with cutaneous T cell lymphoma treated with extracorporeal photochemotherapy. J Am Acad Dermatol 35:935–945

Other T Cell Lymphomas

Amagai M, Kawakubo Y, Tsuyuki A et al. (1995) Lymphomatoid papulosis followed by Ki-1 positive anaplastic large cell lymphoma: proliferation of a common T cell clone. J Dermatol 22:743–746

Beljaards RC, Willemze R (1992) The prognosis of patients with lymphomatoid papulosis associated with malignant lymphomas. Br J Dermatol 126:596–602

Beljaards RC, Kaudewitz P, Bert DE et al. (1993) Primary cutaneous CD30-positive large cell lymphoma: definition of a new type of cutaneous lymphoma with a favorable prognosis. A European multicenter study of 47 patients. Cancer 71:2097–2104

Berti E, Cerri A, Cavicchini S, et al. (1991) Primary cutaneous gamma/delta T cell lymphoma presenting as disseminated pagetoid reticulosis. J Invest Dermatol 96:718–723

Braun-Falco O, Marghescu S, Wolff HH (1973) Pagetoide Retikulose (Morbus Woringer-Kolopp). Hautarzt 24: 11–21

Burns MK, Chan LS, Cooper KD (1995) Woringer-Kolopp disease (localized pagetoid reticulosis) or unilesional mycosis fungoides? Arch Dermatol 131:325–329

Davis TH, Morton CC, Miller-Cassman R et al. (1992) Hodgkin's disease, lymphomatoid papulosis, and cutaneous T cell lymphoma derived from a common T cell clone. N Engl J Med 326:1115–1122

Dupont A (1965) Langsam veralufende und klinische gutartige Reticulopathie mit höchst maligner histologischer Struktur. Hautarzt 16:284–286

el-Azhary RA, Gibson LE, Kurtin PJ et al. (1994) Lymphomatoid papulosis: a clinical and histopathologic review of 53 cases with leukocyte immunophenotyping, DMA flow cytometry, and T cell receptor gene rearrangement studies. J Am Acad Dermatol 30:210–218

Frizzary G, Moran EM, Rappaport H (1974) Angioimmunoblastic lymphadenopathy with dysproteinaemia. Lancet I:1070–1073

Giuatard J, Kaul K (1999) A new polymemerase chain reaction-based method for the detection of T cell clonality in patients with possible cutaneous T cell lymphoma. Arch Dermatol 135:158–162

Gonzalez CL, Medeiros JL, Braziel RM et al. (1991) T cell lymphoma involving subcutaneous tissue. Am J Surg Pathol 15:17–27

Herbst H, Sander C, Tronnier M et al. (1997) Absence of anaplastic lymphoma kinase (ALK) and Epstein-Barr virus gene products in primary cutaneous anaplastic large cell lymphoma and lymphomatoid papulosis. Br J Dermatol 137:680–686

Hirakawa S, Kuyama M, Takahashi S et al. (1999) Nasal and nasal-type natural killer/T cell lymphoma. J Am Acad Dermatol 40:268–272

Karp DL, Horn TD (1994) Lymphomatoid papulosis. J Am Acad Dermatol 30:397–395

Kaudewitz P, Stein H, Dallenbach F et al. (1989) Primary and secondary cutaneous Ki-1^{+} (CD30^{+}) anaplastic large cell lymphomas. Am J Pathol 135:359–367

Ketron LW, Goodman MH (1931) Multiple lesions of the skin apparently of epithelial origin resembling clinically mycosis fungoides. Arch Dermatol 24:758–777

Kumar S, Krenacs L, Medeiros J et al. (1998) Subcutaneous panniculitic T cell lymphoma is a tumor of cytotoxic T lymphocytes. Hum Pathol 29: 397–403

Liebow AA, Carrington CB, Friedman PJ (1972) Lymphomatoid granulomatosis. Hum Pathol 3:457–558

Macaulay WL (1968) Lymphomatois papulosis. A continuing self-healing eruption. Clinically benign – histologically malignant. Arch Dermatol 97:23–30

Mandojana RM, Helwig EB (1993) Localized epidermotropic reticulosis (Woringer Kolopp disease). J Am Acad Dermatol 8:813–829

Mielke V, Wolff HH, Winzer M et al. (1989) Localized and disseminated pagetoid reticulosis. Arch Dermatol 125: 402–406

Perniciaro C, Zalla MJ, White W Jr et al. (1993) Subcutaneous T cell lymphoma. Report of two additional cases and further observations. Arch Dermatol 129:1171–1176

Radaskiewicz T, Lennert K (1975) Lymphogranulomatosis X. Dtsch Med Wochenschr 100:1157–1163

Sander CA, Medeiros LJ, Abruzzo LV et al. (1991) Lymphoblastic lymphoma presenting in cutaneous sites. J Am Acad Dermatol 25:1023–1031

Schmoeckel C, Burg G, Hoffmann-Fezer G et al. (1982) Cutaneous immunoblastic T cell lymphoma. Arch Dermatol Res 274:141–154

Stein H, Mason DY, Gerdes J et al. (1985) The expression of the Hodgkin's disease antigen Ki-1 in reactive and neoplastic lymphoid tissue: evidence that Reed-Sternberg cells and histiocytic malignancies are derived from activated lymphoid cells. Blood 66:848–858

Than RSH, MacLeod TIF, Dean SG (1987) Pagetoid reticulosis, epidermotropic mycosis fungoides and mycosis fungoides: a disease spectrum. Br J Dermatol 116:67–77

Verallo VM, Haserick JR (1966) Mucha-Habermann's disease simulating lymphoma cutis. Arch Dermatol 94: 295–299

Weiss LM, Wood GS, Trela M et al. (1986) Clonal T cell populations in lymphomatoid papulosis. N Engl J Med 315:475–479

Whittaker S (1996) T cell receptor gene analysis in cutaneous T cell lymphomas. Clin Exp Dermatol 21:81–87

Willemze R (1985) Lymphomatoid papulosis. Dermatol Clin 3:735–747

Willemze R, Beljaards RC (1993) Spectrum of primary cutaneous CD30 (Ki-1) positive lymphoproliferative disorders: a proposal for classification and guidelines for management and treatment. J Am Acad Dermatol 28: 973–980

Woringer F, Kolopp P (1939) Lésion érythématosquameuse polycyclique de l'avant-bras évoluant depuis 6 ans chez ungarçonnet de 13 ans. Ann Dermatol Syphilol 10:945–958

Zackheim HS, LeBoit PE, Gordon BI et al. (1993) Lymphomatoid papulosis followed by Hodgkin's lymphoma. Differential response to therapy. Arch Dermatol 129:86–91

Zirbel GM, Gellis SE, Kadin ME et al. (1995) Lymphomatoid papulosis in children. J Am Acad Dermatol 33:741–748

B Cell Lymphomas

Bailey EM, Ferry JA, Harris NL et al. (1996) Marginal zone lymphoma (low-grade B cell lymphoma of mucosa-associated lymphoid tissue type) of skin and subcutaneous tissue. A study of 15 patients. Am J Surg Pathol 20: 1011–1023

Berti E, Alessi E, Caputo R et al. (1988) Reticulohistiocytoma of the dorsum. J Am Acad Dermatol 19:259–272

Burkitt D (1958) A sarcoma involving the jaws in African children. Br J Surg 46:218–223

Cerroni L, Volkenandt M, Rieger E et al. (1994) bcl-2 protein expression and correlation with the interchromosomal 14;18 translocation in cutaneous lymphomas and pseudolymphomas. J Invest Dermatol 102:231–235

Cerroni L, Zöchling N, Pütz B, Kerl H (1997) Infection by Borrelia burgdorferi and cutaneous B cell lymphoma. J Cut Pathol 24:457–461

Cerroni L, Signoretti S, Häfler G et al. (1997) Primary cutaneous marginal zone B cell lymphoma. A recently described entity of low-grade malignant cutaneous B cell lymphoma. Am J Surg Pathol 21:1307–1315

Chang YT, Wong CK (1994) Primary cutaneous plasmacytomas. Clin Exp Dermatol 19:177–180

Crosti A (1951) Micosi fungoide e reticolo-istiocitomi cutanei maligni. Minerva Dermatol 26:3–11

Duncan LN, LeBoit PE (1997) Are primary cutaneous immunocytoma and marginal zone lymphoma the same disease? Am J Surg Pathol 21:1368–1372

Garbe C, Stein H, Dienemann D et al. (1991) Borrelia-burgdorferi-associated cutaneous B cell lymphoma: clinical and immunohistologic characterization of four cases. J Am Acad Dermatol 24:584–590

Garcia CF, Weiss LM, Warnke RA et al. (1986) Cutaneous follicular lymphoma. Am J Surg Pathol 10:454–463

Gianotti B (1993) Skin-associated lymphoid tissue (SALT)-related B cell lymphoma (primary cutaneous B cell lymphoma): a concept and a clinicopathologic entity. Arch Dermatol 129:353–355

Heinzerling L, Dummer R, Kempf W et al. (2000) Intralesional therapy with anti-CD20 monoclonal antibody rituximab in primary cutaneous B cell lymphoma. Arch Dermatol 136:374–378

Kerl H, Cerroni L (1996) The morphologic spectrum of cutaneous B cell lymphomas. Arch Dermatol 132:1376–1377

Kerl H, Cerroni L (1997) Primary B cell lymphomas of the skin. Annals of Oncology 8 [Suppl 2]:29–32

LeBoit PE, McNutt NS, Reed JA et al. (1994) Primary cutaneous immunocytoma. A B cell lymphoma that can easily be mistaken for cutaneous lymphoid hyperplasia. Am J Surg Pathol 18:969–978

Perniciaro C, Winkelmann RK, Daoud MS et al. (1995) Malignant angioendotheliomatosis is an angiotropic intravascular lymphoma. Immunohistochemical, ultrastructural, and molecular genetics studies. Am J Dermatopathol 17:242–248

Petroff N, Koger OW, Fleming MG et al. (1989) Malignant angioendotheliomatosis: an angiotropic lymphoma. J Am Acad Dermatol 21:727–733

Pfleger L, Tappeiner J (1959) Zur Kenntnis der systemisierten Endotheliomaose der cutanen Blutgefässe (Reticuloendotheliose?). Der Hautarzt 10:359–363

Rijlaarsdam JU, Meijer CJLM, Willemze R (1990) Differentiation between lymphadenosis benigna cutis and primary cutaneous follicular center cell lymphomas: a comparative clinicopathologic study of 57 patients. Cancer 65:2301–2306

Rijlaarsdam JU, van der Putte SCJ, Berti E et al. (1993) Cutaneous immunocytomas: a clinicopathologic study of 26 cases. Histopathology 23:117–125

Rijlaarsdam JU, Toonstra J, Meijer CJLM et al. (1996) Treatment of primary cutaneous B cell lymphomas of follicle center cell origin: a clinical follow-up study of 55 patients treated with radiotherapy or polychemotherapy. J Clin Oncol 14:549–555

Sander CA, Flaig MJ (1999) Morphologic spectrum of cutaneous B cell lymphomas. Dermatol Clin 3:593–599

Santucci M, Pimpinelli N, Arganini L (1991) Primary cutaneous B cell lymphoma: a unique type of low-grade lymphoma. Clinicopathologic and immunologic study of 83 cases. Cancer 67:2311–2326

Schmid U, Eckert F, Griesser H et al. (1995) Cutaneous follicular lymphoid hyperplasia with monotypic plasma cells. A clinicopathologic study of 18 patients. Am J Surg Pathol 19:12–20

Sepp N, Schuler G, Romani N et al. (1990) "Intravascular lymphomatosis" (angioendotheliosis): evidence for a T cell origin in two cases. Hum Pathol 21:1051–1058

Slater DN (1994) MALT and SALT. the clue to cutaneous B cell lymphoproliferative disease. Br J Dermatol 131: 557–561

Slater DN (1994) Cutaneous B cell lymphoproliferative diseases: a centenary celebration classification. J Pathol 172:301–305

Torne R, Su WPD, Winkelmann RK et al. (1990) Clinicopathologic study of cutaneous plasmacytoma. Int J Dermatol 29:562–566

Tüting T, Bork K (1996) Primary plasmacytoma of the skin. J Am Acad Dermatol 34:386–390

Vermeer MH, Geelen FAMJ, van Haselen CW et al. (1996) Primary large cutaneous B cell lymphomas of the legs. A distinct type of cutaneous B cell lymphoma with an intermediate prognosis. Arch Dermatol 132:1304–1308

Volkenandt M, Cerroni L, Rieger E et al. (1992) Analysis of the 14; 18 translocation in cutaneous lymphomas using the polymerase chain reaction. J Cutan Pathol 19: 353–356

Wick MR, Rocamora A (1988) Reactive and malignant 'angioendotheliomatosis': a discriminant clinicopathological study. J Cut Pathol 15:260–271

Willemze R, Meijer CJLM, Sentis HJ et al. (1987) Primary cutaneous large cell lymphomas of follicular center cell origin: a clinical follow-up study of 19 patients. J Am Acad Dermatol 16:518–526

Willemze R, Meijer CJLM, Scheffer E et al. (1987) Diffuse large cell lymphomas of follicular center cell origin presenting in the skin: a clinicopathologic and immunologic study of 16 patients. Am J Pathol 126:325–333

Wong KF, Chan JKC, Li LPK et al. (1994) Primary cutaneous plasmacytoma. Report of two cases and review of the literature. Am J Dermatopathol 16:392–397

CHAPTER 62

Cutaneous Aspects of Leukemia

Contents

Introduction

Normally the various mature leukocytes of the peripheral blood develop in a series of regulated steps from the primitive or pluripotential hematopoietic stem cells in the bone marrow. If a cell undergoes malignant transformation somewhere along this path of differentiation, then a leukemia develops. By definition leukemia is a systemic hematologic malignancy which primarily involves the bone marrow and peripheral blood. Malignant lymphomas are tumors which may involve the same cell lines but have predominantly lymph node involvement. Hematologists and hematopathologists include many diseases which are designated leukemia, such as chronic lymphocytic leukemia, in their classification of malignant lymphoma. This causes confusion among the uninitiated but is done because the lymph node (lymphoma) and blood (leukemia) involvement may vary. Many of the leukemias are alluded to in Chapter 61. Table 62.1 shows the classification of the acute leukemias. We will first discuss the types of cutaneous involvement, then briefly describe the different forms of leukemia mentioning their likely skin changes.

Cutaneous Signs of Leukemia

The skin is frequently involved in leukemia. This is not surprising since the leukemic cells in the peripheral circulation pass through the skin and have the chance at least to leave the circulation and remain in the dermis. When the leukemic cells can be identified in the skin, one speaks of leukemia cutis or a specific leukemic infiltrate. A very puzzling concept is the leukemid. Some patients with leukemia develop diffuse maculopapular eruptions. These exanthems were thought to be allergic reactions to circulating leukemic cells but most are probably true leukemic infiltrates with very few malignant cells. Leukemid is used imprecisely to refer to the nonspecific cutaneous findings seen in leukemia patients.

Table 62.1. FAB (French-American-British) classification of acute leukemias

Class	Description
Myeloid	
M0	Acute myeloid leukemia with minimal differentiation
M1	Acute myeloblastic leukemia without maturation
M2	Acute myeloblastic leukemia with maturation
M3	Acute promyelocytic leukemia (including hypergranular form)
M4	Acute myelomonocytic leukemia (including abnormal eosinophils)
M5	Acute monocytic leukemia
M6	Erythroleukemia
M7	Acute megakaryoblastic leukemia
Lymphoid	
L1	Acute lymphocytic leukemia (childhood form)
L2	Acute lymphocytic leukemia (adult forms)
L3	Acute lymphocytic leukemia (Burkitt cell type)

Leukemia Cutis

Leukemic infiltrates can present as widespread macules and papules, infiltrated plaques or nodules. The lesions are typically firm dome-shaped papules or nodules that have a distinctive blue-violet or red-brown color (Fig. 62.1). Nodules are frequently ulcerated and some may be bullous (Fig. 62.2). The lesions are often associated with purpura or ecchymosis. The thin skin of the eyelids and scrotum appears predisposed to leukemic infiltrates (Fig. 62.3). Other common locations include sites of trauma, such as in scars of zoster or in intravenous access sites. Leukemic paronychia has also been reported. Subcutaneous infiltrate may mimic a panniculitis. Infiltrates involving the gingivae and tonsillar region are common in acute leukemias (Fig. 62.4). Often a patient has several different types of infiltrate. It is important to diagnose a leukemic infiltrate for several reasons. In several types of leukemia, the cutaneous changes may appear first in a small percentage of patients; this is known as aleukemic leukemia cutis. In addition, the development of cutaneous infiltrates during therapy usually mandates a switch in the therapeutic regimen. Finally, it is not unusual for leukemia cutis to herald a relapse.

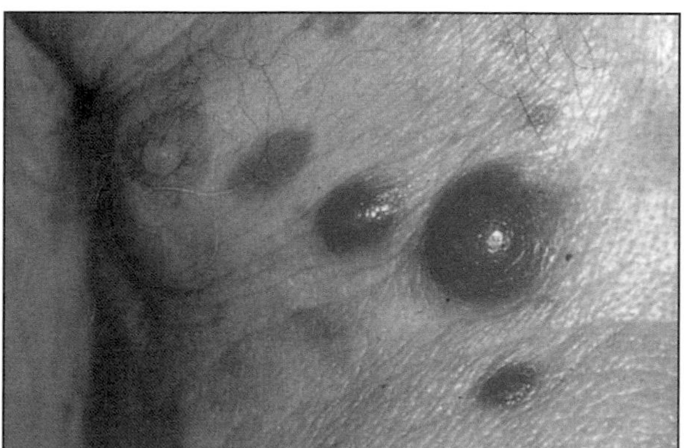

Fig. 62.1. Nodular infiltrates of acute monocytic leukemia, formerly called reticulosarcomatosis of Gottron

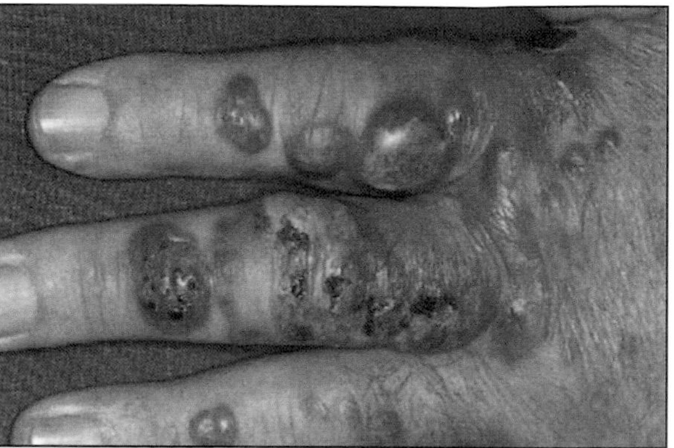

Fig. 62.3. Acute myeloid leukemia with bullous and ulcerated infiltrates

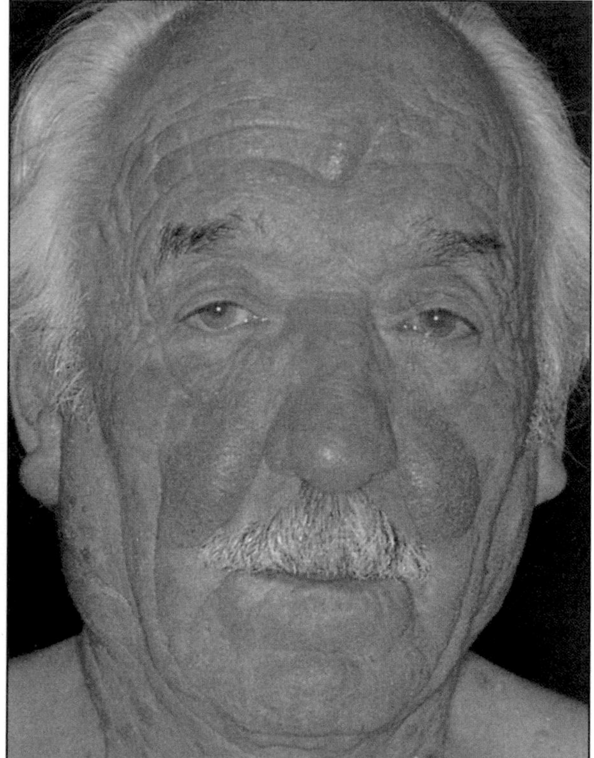

Fig. 62.2. Chronic lymphocytic leukemia with leonine facies and distinctive nodular infiltrates of cheeks

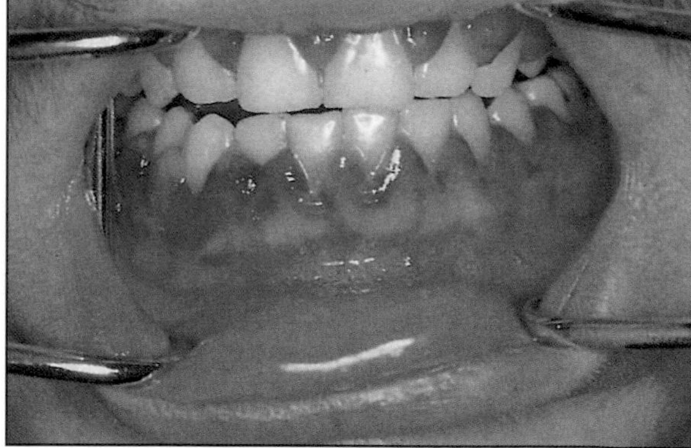

Fig. 62.4. Acute myeloid leukemia with gingival infiltrates

Nonspecific Lesions

Almost all patients with leukemia have cutaneous lesions at some point. Most of these nonspecific changes relate to the impaired bone marrow function. Hemostasis is usually abnormal so purpura, hemorrhage and ecchymosis are almost invariable. Prolonged bleeding after dental extraction may be another clue. Most patients are anemic, so they tend to be pale. In addition, the excessive leukocytes are usually not functional, so the individuals have impaired immunity, leading to a broad spectrum of infections including herpes simplex, zoster, warts, *Candida albicans*, dermatophytes and deep fungi.

Sweet syndrome and pyoderma gangrenosum are also associated with leukemia. Bullous Sweet syndrome, which may actually be a variant of pyoderma gangrenosum, has been most often described with hairy cell leukemia and acute myelogenous leukemia. The lesions, no matter what name is attached, are superficial bullae with a blue-gray halo which ulcerate easily. Another bullous lesion is the severe necrotic arthropod bite reaction seen in chronic lymphocytic leukemia.

Many other skin changes can be seen. Pruritus is less common with leukemia than with lymphoma, but may occur. Some individuals may have diffuse pruritic, often urticarial, maculopapular exanthems for which no other explanation can be found. Others may develop erythroderma or generalized gray-brown hyperpigmentation which is usually associated with chronic leukemias. Follicular mucinosis, while usually associated with mycosis fungoides, may also be a marker for acute leukemia.

Drug reactions are another problem. Leukemia patients are on complex chemotherapy regimens, often pushed to toxicity, and they develop many toxic and allergic reactions. For example, many cases of acral erythema of chemotherapy develop in leukemic patients (Chap. 10). The rash of lymphocyte recovery is a transient maculopapular eruption which appears as the lymphocytes begin to repopulate the body after aggressive chemotherapy. It is easily confused with a drug reaction. The standard problems of mucositis, hair loss and nail changes are seen in most patients. In addition, every patient receives many antibiotics which are the agents most likely to cause skin reactions. The possibilities are limitless.

Histopathology. The microscopic findings in leukemic infiltrates can be highly variable. Sometimes there is a subtle perivascular accumulation of malignant cells which can be easily overlooked if one is not warned. In more advanced changes, there are more extensive infiltrates, usually monotonous and often extending into the subcutaneous tissues. The epidermis is usually spared but adnexal structures and vessels may be damaged. Some degree of tissue hemorrhage is expected. In such settings, one immediately realizes the infiltrate is abnormal, but the classification is frequently difficult. The individual cells reflect the underlying disease. Leukemia by definition has bone marrow and peripheral blood involvement, so the diagnosis is made in these this tissues. In the rare cases of aleukemic leukemia cutis and granulocytic sarcoma, standard hematologic techniques are employed to identify the infiltrating cells and tentatively classify the leukemia.

Differential Diagnosis. The differential diagnosis is lengthy. Considering just papular and nodular infiltrates, one must think of Langerhans cell histiocytosis, Kaposi sarcoma, malignant lymphoma, pseudolymphoma, mast cell tumors and sarcoidosis.

Therapy. The therapy is that of the underlying leukemia. Individual worrisome cutaneous lesions can be irradiated if ulcerated or painful. The regimens recommended for pseudolymphoma (Chap. 60) are appropriate for this palliative treatment.

Acute Leukemias

Epidemiology. The acute leukemias present with proliferation of hematologic stem cells in the bone marrow with obvious peripheral blood involvement. Two major categories exist: acute myeloid leukemia (AML) and acute lymphocytic leukemia (ALL). In some systems, AML is called acute nonlymphocytic leukemia. Acute leukemias have an incidence of about 4/100,000. There is a sharp distinction between children and adults. AML is a disease of adults except for the neonatal period while ALL is a disease of children. Table 62.1 shows a simplified classification of the acute leukemias. The lymphocytic leukemias are divided in a variety of ways in addition to the simple morphologic classification. Most L1 leukemias carry the common ALL antigen (CD10, CALLA), while L3 lesions are almost all B cell in origin. The L2 group includes T cell, B cell and null cell types. The morphologic, immunologic and chromosomal findings are combined to characterize the disease.

Etiology and Pathogenesis. Acute leukemias may develop following exposure to ionizing radiation, as in industrial accidents (Chernobyl) or nuclear attacks (Hiroshima), chemicals (benzene) or alkylating agents, or result from genetic factors (Down syndrome), and evolve out of the myelodysplastic disorders. The human T cell leukemia virus, a retrovirus, causes a T cell ALL in parts of the Caribbean and Japan. In addition, patients treated successfully for lymphoma face a considerable risk of developing leukemia. In Hodgkin disease, for example, over 5% of cured patients die of leukemia within 10 years. Chromosome aberrations are found in many forms of acute leukemia and often have a prognostic significance.

Clinical Findings

Systemic Findings. The clinical features of acute leukemia usually reflect the displacement of the normal hematologic cells, so they include anemia, thrombocytopenia and granulocytopenia with fever and infections.

Cutaneous Findings. Leukemia cutis is seen in more than 10% of patients with AML; it is uncommon in ALL. Those with M4 and M5 are most likely to have skin lesions; perhaps as many as one-third are affected. The skin changes are highly variable, ranging from a single nodule or plaque to a diffuse rash. The papules and nodules are typically dome-shaped, firm, sharply bordered lesions with a range of colors from livid red to violet. Sometimes bullae develop. The face, scalp and trunk are the most common sites. In more unusual cases the conjunctiva, scrotum and traumatized or scarred lesions may be involved.

Occasionally a limited number of large nodules are found, especially in M4 and M5. These lesions were formerly diagnosed as a reticulum cell sarcoma (or reticulosarcomatosis of Gottron) and classified with lymphomas, but today they are accepted as leukemic infiltrates. They may precede the diagnosis of leukemia.

Granulocytic Sarcoma. Extramedullary tumors containing AML cells, usually M1-M3, often show a green cut surface in the laboratory because they are so rich in myeloperoxidase. Thus they are also known as chloromas (green tumors). These lesions are seen almost exclusively in children, may arise in the skin, periorbital region, bones, sinuses or other sites, and often precede the development of leukemia by many months. In Africa, about 25% of children with AML have granulocytic sarcoma, and almost all have a specific 8;21 translocation. Granulocytic sarcoma may also appear during a blast crisis when a chronic myelogenous leukemia is converting into its acute form.

Mucosal Findings. Oral manifestations are very common early in AML. In both M4 and M5, over 75% of patients have gingival changes at the time of diagnosis and often these are the presenting factor. In M1–M3, oral changes are present in more than 50% of new patients. The infiltrates typically grow over the teeth, sometimes even covering the crowns. They tend to bleed, ulcerate and be painful. Sometimes teeth will be loosened by the periodontal infiltrates. Tonsillar infiltrates may also be painful and bleed. All combine to cause a bad odor. The salivary glands may be involved, leading to painful enlargement and decreased secretions. The resulting dry mouth offers a fertile ground for candidiasis.

Laboratory Findings. The peripheral blood usually shows thrombocytopenia, a mild anemia and highly variable numbers of leukocytes ranging from decreased to strikingly elevated in number. The neutrophils are decreased in number and immature forms may be seen. Bone marrow examination reveals over 50% immature cells, confirming the diagnosis. Immunophenotyping is used to identify the cell of origin.

Therapy. Aggressive chemotherapy to induce remissions, combined with consolidation and maintenance regimens, cures about 20% of adults and 40% of children. Bone marrow transplantation is employed for some high-risk younger patients in remission. In acute promyelogenous leukemia systemic retinoids have been surprisingly effective, reversing the differentiation defect in many cases. Usually the systemic form of tretinoin is employed.

Adult T Cell Leukemia/Lymphoma

Epidemiology. This disease in endemic in parts of Japan and the Caribbean. In Europe it is seen primarily in immigrants from the Caribbean. Sporadic cases have been described in the USA.

Etiology and Pathogenesis. The human T cell leukemia virus (HTLV1) is a retrovirus which is found in all cases. Many patients in endemic areas are infected without disease. Transmission is via blood, breast feeding or other body fluids. It has been suggested that HTLV1 may play a role in mycosis fungoides, but despite occasionally histologic similarities, the virus is usually not found in mycosis fungoides lesions by PCR.

Clinical Findings

Systemic Findings. The most common presentation is with an acute leukemic form with marked leukocytosis. The acronym HOTS has been suggested (hypercalcemia, osteolytic bone lesions, T cell malignancy and skin involvement). Hepatosplenomegaly may been seen, as well as opportunistic infections. There may be noncompressive spinal cord deficits (tropical spastic paresis). Other cases are more chronic or even smoldering, while in rare cases the disease is confined to lymph nodes.

Cutaneous Findings. About two-thirds of patients have skin findings. The lesions are usually red-brown infiltrated papules or nodules without scales. Patches, as seen in mycosis fungoides, are not described. Plaques, purpura, subcutaneous nodules and a variety of other lesions have been described. In children infective dermatitis is frequently seen. Despite the rather nondescript name, this severe generalized chronic and relapsing dermatitis with associated lymphadenopathy has been well documented in Jamaican children with HTLV1 infection.

Histopathology. There are usually dense superficial infiltrates of small lymphocytes. The infiltrates may be band-like with single or clustered lymphocytes found in a hyperplastic epidermis. The cells may be more anaplastic, especially in larger nodules. The cells carry typical T cell markers (CD2, 3 and 5); most are CD4-positive and often express the interleukin (IL)-2 receptor (CD25). In the peripheral blood multilobulated (clover leaf) nuclei and marked eosinophilia are usually seen, but these features are hard to appreciate in the skin.

Therapy. While chemotherapy may be tried, the disease is usually rapidly fatal. A combination of acyclovir and interferon-α appears most promising. Monoclonal antibodies against the IL-2 receptor have also been tried. Opportunistic infections and CNS disease are responsible for considerable morbidity.

Childhood Acute Leukemias

Specific cutaneous infiltrates have been described in congenital monoblastic leukemia as well as other myeloid forms. While congenital leukemia is rare, about 50% of patients have cutaneous lesions which are often the first sign. The red-violet nodules can be confused with Langerhans cell histiocytosis, mast cell tumors, neuroblastoma and blueberry muffin syndrome (extramedullary hematopoiesis secondary to congenital infections). Granulocytic sarcomas are also most common in children. Cutaneous infiltrates in ALL are rare; they may be seen late in the course of the disease.

Chronic Leukemias

Chronic Lymphocytic Leukemia

Epidemiology. Chronic lymphocytic leukemia (CLL) is the most common chronic leukemia. It has an incidence of about 3/100,000, but among octogenarians, the incidence rises to 30/100,000.

Etiology and Pathogenesis. The etiology is unclear. The factors discussed under acute leukemias appear to play no role. Over 95% of CLL are B cell in origin. The leukemic cells are small and normal-appearing but have a prolonged life, accumulating in blood, bone marrow spleen and lymph nodes.

Clinical Findings

Systemic Findings. The course is slow but relentless. About 25% of patients are diagnosed while they are asymptomatic. Typical complaints include fever, fatigue, lymphadenopathy and recurrent infections. One possible complication is conversion to a large B cell lymphoma (Richter syndrome).

Cutaneous Findings. Cutaneous infiltrates are common in CLL. Often they involve the face with symmetric nodular lesions producing a leonine facies. Erythroderma has also been described. There may be associated infiltration and obstruction of the salivary glands. A unique change in CLL is an exaggerated arthropod bite reaction. Patients develop indurated papules and nodules that may become vesicular, bullous or necrotic. The infiltrate is mixed and rich in eosinophils. Immunofluorescent examination is negative. Leukemic cells are difficult to identify. In rare patients, the history of exaggerated response to arthropod bites precedes or facilitates the diagnosis of CLL.

Laboratory Findings. The diagnosis is based on the presence of elevated numbers, up to 200,000/µl, of small lymphocytes which almost always have B cell markers, including surface immunoglobulin, B cell-associated antigens (CD19, -20, -79a), CD5 and CD23. There may be a small serum M spike. The neutropenia often leads to impaired immunity and increased infections.

Differential Diagnosis. The usual question is – what type of leukemia is present? The cutaneous infiltrates usually occur in patients in whom the diagnosis has already been made. Morphologically they resemble malignant lymphomas, pseudolymphoma, sarcoidosis, lupus vulgaris tumidus and lupus erythematosus.

Therapy. Chemotherapy, usually with alkylating agents, is used when symptoms are severe, not to treat the lymphocyte count. Aggressive therapy brings little benefit and is usually reserved for those patients with Richter syndrome. A preferred regimen for B-CLL has not been developed. The cutaneous lesions can be irradiated if troublesome. The pruritus often responds well to PUVA or PUVA bath therapy, as may the erythroderma. Electron beam therapy has also been employed for refractory erythroderma in this setting.

Chronic Myeloid Leukemia

Epidemiology. Most patients are adults. It has an incidence of 1/100,000. A rare juvenile form also exists.

Etiology and Pathogenesis. Both radiation exposure and chemicals, especially benzene, have been implicated but in most cases there are no clues. Chronic myelogenous leukemia is of special interest because it is the first human cancer in which a chromosomal abnormality was discovered. The Philadelphia chromosome represents a 9;22 translocation with oncogene activation (*bcr-abl*) and is present in almost all cases. In juvenile chronic myeloid leukemia, the Philadelphia chromosome is not present. The age of onset is less than 2 years and there is an association between neurofibromatosis 1 and juvenile xanthogranuloma.

Clinical Findings
Systemic Findings. In the early phases of this disease, patients are anemic and often have purpura but have few other signs or symptoms. Splenomegaly is often present. This chronic phase lasts months to years. At some point their diseases accelerates and evolves into a blast crisis. Fever, infections, a tender spleen, bleeding and weight loss are the main problems.

Cutaneous Findings. Leukemic infiltrates are relatively uncommon in chronic myeloid leukemia. Bullous Sweet syndrome may be associated with the blast phase, as may leukemia cutis and even granulocytic sarcomas. In children, the combination of juvenile xanthogranuloma and stigmata of neurofibromatosis should prompt a hematologic evaluation. Leukemic infiltrates are rare in this group.

Laboratory Findings. The diagnosis is suspected when immature myeloid cells and increased basophils are present in the peripheral blood. The cells fail to stain for leukocyte alkaline phosphatase. The Philadelphia chromosome or the specific translocation can be found in almost all cases; it is the usual way to exclude a chronic myelomonocytic leukemia.

Therapy. Chemotherapy is palliative. In children and young adults, allogeneic bone marrow transplantation offers a chance of cure.

Hairy Cell Leukemia

Synonym. Leukemic reticuloendotheliosis

Clinical Findings
Systemic Findings. Hairy cell leukemia is a disease somewhere between leukemia and lymphoma. The patients are adults who usually have splenomegaly and bone marrow involvement, but few circulating cells, in contrast to classic leukemias, and little lymphadenopathy, in contrast to malignant lymphomas. The bone marrow damage and increased splenic function lead to pancytopenia and reduced resistance to infection. Along with HIV/AIDS patients, they appear especially susceptible to atypical mycobacterial infections.

Cutaneous Findings. Skin infiltrates in hairy cell leukemia are most uncommon. Small blue-red firm papules may be seen. Bullous Sweet syndrome or pyoderma gangrenosum is also associated with hairy cell leukemia. Both leukocytoclastic angiitis and polyarteritis nodosa have been described.

Laboratory Findings. The diagnosis is usually made on bone marrow biopsy, as this site is always involved. The hairy cell is a B cell which in hematologic smear preparations shows a bean-shaped nucleus and multiple villi or hairs. The classic stain is tartrate-resistant acid phosphatase, but the most specific stain to separate out hairy cells from other B cells is CD103.

Therapy. The treatment of choice is 2-CDA (2-chlorodeoxyadenosine). While in the past, one waited until the patients became ill to initiate any therapy, the success of 2-CDA means that patients should be treated as early as possible. Interferon-α is also effective therapy, but not as promising as 2-CDA. Either cures or very long term remissions with tumor-free bone marrow can be expected.

Large Granular Lymphocyte Leukemia

This is another rare overlap between lymphoma and leukemia. Most patients present with lymphocytosis and neutropenia. Some are anemic. In Asians, there is often an association with Epstein-Barr virus and a worse outlook. Splenomegaly may be seen, but lymph node enlargement is uncommon. The disease is so named because the circulating malignant cells in the peripheral blood have large eccentric nuclei, pale-blue cytoplasm and azurophilic granules. Two subtypes are identified, carrying T cell and NK markers.

In one large study, fewer than 5% of patients had cutaneous infiltrates, but they had a less favorable progress. The disease is indolent, but not curable. The anemia and neutropenia cause most of the morbidity.

Myelodysplastic Syndromes

A group of patients tend to fall somewhere in between acute and chronic myeloid leukemia. Most are older men with some type of cytopenia and associated functional problems. There may be a long period before the disease declares itself. The classification is beyond our scope. Some patients have refractory anemia with less than 5% blasts in their bone marrow while others have a higher percentage of blast forms and evolve over months into AML. Chronic myelomonocytic leukemia falls into this group. Patients tend to die from anemia, bleeding, infections or their leukemia. There are no specific cutaneous findings other than purpura and hemorrhage. Infiltrates are rare. Treatment is ineffective.

Myeloproliferative Disorders

The myeloproliferative disorders include a number of related problems in which there is relatively uncontrolled proliferation of the normal elements of the bone marrow. There is a monoclonal proliferation of a bone marrow stem cell in each case; the exact nature of the stem cell determines which cell lines will be clinically most affected. The erythrocytes, leukocytes and megakaryocytes may all be effected. It is often difficult to separate the individual disorders. In all there may be increased levels of basophils. They include:

- Chronic myeloid leukemia.
- Primary thrombocythemia (Chap. 23): These patients tend to have more bleeding than clotting problems. They often have erythromelalgia.
- Osteomyelofibrosis: Here there is a combination of early proliferation of all marrow cell lines, coupled later with marrow fibrosis and extramedullary hematopoiesis especially in the spleen. There are no special skin features.
- Polycythemia vera.

There is no satisfactory treatment for any of the myeloproliferative disorders but all tend to smolder.

Polycythemia Vera

Etiology and Pathogenesis. Polycythemia vera is a monoclonal proliferation of a marrow stem cell in which increased erythrocyte counts dominate. Other causes of secondary polycythemia include compensatory production of erythropoietin, for example as a result of chronic cardiovascular disease, chronic obstructive pulmonary disease, heavy smoking or living at high altitude), inappropriate secretion of erythropoietin, for example as a result of renal carcinoma, other carcinomas or leiomyomas (even from cutaneous lesions). Some professional athletes, especially bicycle racers (e.g., the 1998 Tour de France), are suspected of misusing erythropoietin. In polycythemia vera, there are elevated levels of leukocytes and platelets as well, while in the secondary disorders only the red cell mass is increased.

Clinical Findings. The patients have marked hyperviscosity with increased cardiac workload. They may be hypertensive and because of red cell turnover, often have elevated uric acid levels. Typical complaints include headache, dizziness and acral paresthesias. A unique complaint is intense pruritus after a warm bath. Erythromelalgia may also be seen. Their skin especially on the face is cyanotic, but often almost plethoric with a blue-red tone. The conjunctival vessels may be full and prominent. The oral mucosa is also often darkened and the vessels beneath the tongue may be noticeably engorged. The hyperviscosity may lead to cutaneous ulcerations. As the disease progresses, both bleeding and thromboses may become problems.

Laboratory Findings. Simply measuring the hemoglobin and hematocrit does not suffice for diagnosing polycythemia vera. While elevated levels suggest the problem, bone marrow examination is needed to confirm the diagnosis.

Therapy. The main therapy is repeated withdrawal of blood. If this fails, hydroxyurea can be considered.

Bibliography

Aractingi S, Bachmeyer C, Dombret H et al. (1994) Simultaneous occurrence of two rare cutaneous markers of poor prognosis in myelodysplastic syndrome: erythema elevatum diutinum and specific lesions. Br J Dermatol 131:112–117

Aractingi S, Bachmeyer C, Miclea JM et al. (1995) Unusual specific cutaneous lesions in myelodysplastic syndromes. J Am Acad Dermatol 33:187–191

Baer M (1993) Management of unusual presentations of acute leukemia. Hematol Oncol Clin North Am 7:275–292

Baer MR, Barcos M, Farrell H et al. (1989) Acute myelogenous leukemia with leukemia cutis. Eighteen cases seen between 1969 and 1986. Cancer 63:2192–2200

Baksh FK, Nathan D, Richardson W et al. (1998) Leukemia cutis with prominent giant cell reaction. Am J Dermatopathol 20:48–52

Barzilai A, Shpiro D, Goldberg I et al. (1999) Insect bite – like reaction in patients with hematologic malignant neoplasms. Arch Dermatol 135:1503–1507

Benucci R, Annessi G, Signoretti S et al. (1996) Minimally differentiated acute myeloid leukemia revealed by specific cutaneous lesions. Br J Dermatol 135:119–123

Buescher L, Anderson PC (1990) Circinate plaques heralding juvenile chronic myelogenous leukemia. Pediatr Dermatol 7:122–125

Burg G, Braun-Falco O (1983) Leukemic lymphomas and leukemias. In: Burg G, Braun-Falco O (eds) Cutaneous lymphomas, pseudolymphomas and related disorders. Springer, Berlin, pp 341–376

Campbell DC, Grippaudo FR, Lewandowski R (1997) Congenital leukemia cutis: an unusual manifestation of a rare disease. Plast Reconstr Surg 100:1809–1811

Chen MJ, Huang ML, Hung HJ et al. (1997) Leukemia cutis as the initial manifestation of acute nonlymphocytic leukemia in a young child. Cutis 60:263–264

Desch JK, Smoller BR (1993) The spectrum of cutaneous disease in leukemias. J Cutan Pathol 20:407–410

Gottesfeld E, Silverman RA, Coccia PF et al. (1989) Transient blueberry muffin syndrome of a newborn with congenital monoblastic leukemia. J Am Acad Dermatol 21:347–351

Hahn WC, Jones D, Leavitt P et al. (1997) Leukemia cutis. J Clin Oncol 15:2170–2171

Horlick HP, Silvers DN, Knobler EH et al. (1990) Acute myelomonocytic leukemia presenting as a benign-appearing cutaneous eruption. Arch Dermatol 126:653–656

Jones D, Dorfman DM, Barnhill RL et al. (1997) Leukemic vasculitis: a feature of leukemia cutis in some patients. Am J Clin Pathol 107:637–642

Kaddu S, Zenahlik P, Beham-Schmid C et al. (1999) Specific cutaneous infiltrates in patients with myelogenous leukemia: a clinicopathologic study of 26 patients with assessment of diagnostic criteria. J Am Acad Dermatol 40:966–978

Klapman MH (1989) Cutaneous diseases preceding diagnosis of lymphoreticular malignancies. J Am Acad Dermatol 20:583–586

Koizumi H, Kumakiri M, Ishizuka M et al. (1991) Leukemia cutis in acute myelomonocytic leukemia: infiltration to minor traumas and scars. J Dermatol 18:281–285

La Grenade L, Manns A, Fletcher V et al. (1998) Clinical, pathologic, and immunologic features of human T-lymphotrophic virus type I – associated infective dermatitis in children. Arch Dermatol 134:439–444

Longacre TA, Smoller BR (1993) Leukemia cutis: analysis of 50 biopsy-proven cases with emphasis on occurrence in myelodysplastic syndromes. Am J Clin Pathol 100: 276–284

Macfarlane AW, Parry DH, Caslin AW et al. (1996) Cutaneous lesions in a case of acute megakaryoblastic leukemia. Clin Exp Dermatol 21:201–204

Manns A, Hisada M, La Grenade L (1999) Human T-lymphotropic virus type I infection. Lancet 353:1951–1958

Nagao K, Kikuchi A, Kawai Y et al. (1997) Skin infiltration in acute promyelocytic leukemia. Dermatology 194:168–171

Ohno S, Tadashi Y, Ohta M et al. (1990) Aleukemic leukemia cutis. J Am Acad Dermatol 22:374–377

Ratnam KV, Khor CJL, Su WPD (1994) Leukemia cutis. Dermatol Clin 12:419–431

Ratnam KV, Su WPD, Ziesmer SC et al. (1992) Value of immunohistochemistry in the diagnosis of leukemia cutis: study of 54 cases using paraffin-section markers. J Cutan Pathol 19:193–200

Resnik KS, Brod BB (1993) Leukemia cutis in congenital leukemia. Analysis and review of the world literature with report of an additional case. Arch Dermatol 129:1301–1306

Richert S, Bloom EJ, Flynn K et al. (1996) Widespread eruptive dermal and atypical melanocytic nevi in association with chronic myelocytic leukemia: case report and review of the literature. J Am Acad Dermatol 35: 326–329

Richter MN (1928) Generalized reticular cell sarcoma of lymph nodes associated with lymphatic leukemia. Am J Pathol 4:285–292

Sepp N, Radaszkiewicz T, Meijer CJLM et al. (1993) Specific skin manifestations in acute leukemia with monocytic differentiation: a morphologic and immunohistochemical study of 11 cases. Cancer 71:124–132

Smoller BR (1997) Leukemic vasculitis: a newly described pattern of cutaneous involvement. Am J Clin Pathol 107: 627–629

Su D (1994) Clinical, histopathological, and immunohistochemical correlations in leukemia cutis. Semin Dermatol 13:223–230

Su WPD, Buechner SA, Li CY (1984) Clinicopathologic correlations in leukemia cutis. J Am Acad Dermatol 11:121–128

Sumner W, Grichnik JM, Shea CR et al. (1998) Follicular mucinosis as a presenting sign of acute myeloblastic leukemia. J Am Acad Dermatol 39:803–805

Suzuki Y, Kuroda K, Kojima T et al. (1995) Unusual cutaneous manifestation of myelodysplastic syndrome. Br J Dermatol 133:483–486

Taniguchi S, Hamada T, Kutsuna H et al. (1996) Lymphocytic aleukemic leukemia cutis. J Am Acad Dermatol 35:849–850

Tomasinis C, Quaglino P, Novelli M et al. (1998) "Aleukemic" granulomatous leukemia cutis. Am J Dermatopathol 20: 417–421

Vestey JP, Turner M, Biddlestone L et al. (1993) Disseminated cutaneous granulomatous eruptions associated with myelodysplastic syndrome and acute myeloid leukemia. Clin Exp Dermatol 18:559–563

Wong TY, Suster S, Bouffard D et al. (1995) Histologic spectrum of cutaneous involvement in patients with myelogenous leukemia including the neutrophilic dermatoses. Int J Dermatol 43:323–329

Yen A, Sanchez R, Oblender M et al. (1996) Leukemia cutis: Darier's sign in a neonate with acute lymphoblastic leukemia. J Am Acad Dermatol 34:375–378

Zengin N, Kars A, Özisik Y et al. (1998) Aleukemic leukemia cutis in a patient with acute lymphoblastic leukemia. J Am Acad Dermatol 38: 620–621

Mastocytoses

Contents

The term mastocytoses or mast cell disorders includes a number of probably unrelated conditions, all of which are characterized by increased tissue mast cells. Most of the benign mastocytoses involve only the skin and about 75% present before 2 years of age. Systemic mastocytoses are usually reactive but may rarely evolve into a malignant process, usually described as mast cell leukemia. The crucial event appears to be the presence of mast cells in the peripheral blood. Table 63.1 shows a working classification of the mastocytoses.

Basic Science Aspects

Mast cells were first described by Paul Ehrlich in 1877. They are 8–20 µm in diameter, may be cuboidal or spindled and have a "stuffed" or "filled" appearance because of their abundant cytoplasmic granules (Fig. 63.1). ("Mast" is the German word for "stuffed", such as in *Mastgans*, a force-fed goose.) Because of their high content of negatively charged acid glycoproteins, the granules stain metachromatic with basic dyes such as toluidine blue or alcian blue. Another excellent stain is the Giemsa stain. The most sensitive and specific way of identifying mast cells is immunohistochemical staining for the proteinase tryptase, the major protein of the cell. The granules are electron-dense and easy to identify with electron microscopy.

Along with the lungs and gastrointestinal tract, the skin is relatively rich in mast cells, containing about 7000 cells/mm^3. They are most common about the vessels of the papillary dermis, but are also found near nerves and the adnexal structures. As many of these structures are rich in laminin, mast

Table 63.1. Classification of the mastocytoses

Cutaneous mastocytoses
Solitary lesion
Mastocytoma
Multiple lesions
Disseminated mastocytomas
Urticaria pigmentosa
Telangiectasia macularis eruptiva perstans
Diffuse disease
Diffuse mastocytosis
Bullous mastocytosis
Mast cell erythroderma
Systemic mastocytoses
Involvement of the bone marrow and other organs (liver, spleen, lymph nodes, gastro-intestinal tract, bones) as well as secondary skin involvement. No circulating mast cells.
Malignant mastocytoses
Mast cell leukemia: similar pattern of involvement as with systemic mast cell disease but also with circulating, often atypical mast cells

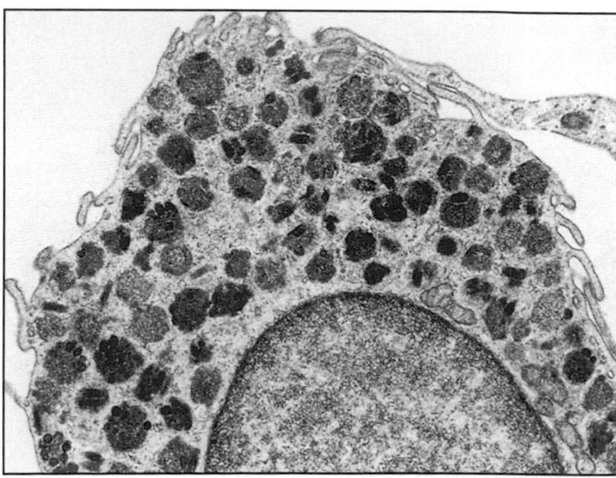

Fig. 63.1. Electron microscopic view of a mast cell showing dense granules

cells may adhere to them with their laminin receptors. The close relationship between mast cells and nerves may be of functional importance, in that mast cells may be activated by neuropeptides such as vasoactive intestinal peptide (VIP), substance P or calcitonin gene-related peptide (CGRP).

Mast cells arise in the bone marrow as CD34-positive, pluripotential precursor cells. They differentiate both in the bone marrow and in the peripheral organs such as the skin under the influence of an array of growth factors, particularly the so-called stem cell factor, c-*kit* ligand or mast cell growth factor. Why mast cells accumulate in the skin remains unclear.

Three types of mast cells have been identified based on their protease composition, containing either tryptase and chymase (MC_{TC}), tryptase alone (MC_T) or rarely chymase alone (MC_C). MC_{TC} are also known as connective tissue-type mast cells and often contain lattice-like granules. MC_T or mucosal mast cells typically contain scroll-like granules. Mast cells, as well as Langerhans cells and basophils, express the high-affinity IgE receptor, $Fc_\varepsilon RI$, on their surface. This receptor binds to the Fc portion of the IgE. When attached IgE molecules bind with antigen and form bridges, the mast cell releases mediators. These may be synthesized in response to the stimuli or preformed and stored in the granules. Release of the latter mediators is known as degranulation and is followed by a lag phase. Mast cells appear to mediate a wide variety of physiologic actions such as vascular permeability, coagulation, inflammatory responses and tissue remodeling processes. They may act in conjunction with cutaneous nerves and may recruit and interact with leukocytes.

The major preformed mediators are biogenic amines (primarily histamine), proteases (tryptase, chymase, carboxypeptidase and others), proteoglycans (especially heparin) and a cathepsin G-like enzyme. The de novo synthesized mediators are primarily part of the arachidonic acid cascade (especially prostaglandin D_2). Mast cells also produce cytokines; the pattern of production is similar to that of helper T cells of the TH2 type. Skin mast cells seem to produce primarily tumor necrosis factor (TNF)-α and interleukins-4 and -8. There are significant differences in how different mast cells respond to stimuli. Cutaneous mast cells are less sensitive to IgE stimulation than pulmonary mast cells, but more sensitive to mediators such morphine. Both the type of mast cell and the type of stimulus may determine which mediators are released.

In addition to antigen-induced or allergic mast cell activation, there are a number of other stimuli that, in selected individuals, can cause release of mediators by nonallergic mechanisms. The clinical features are similar to an allergic reaction; one often speaks of histamine liberators or degranulators, as primarily the preformed mediators are released. Included in the group are:

- Physical Factors. Heat, cold, pressure, vibration, light, water
- Medications. Codeine, morphine, aspirin, nonsteroidal antiinflammatory drugs, quinine, vancomycin, curare, succinylcholine, radiologic contrast materials and many others. General anesthesia may also pose a risk.
- Biologic Substances. Snake poisons, wasp and bee toxins, bacterial toxins, some helminths (*Ascaris*), compound 48/80, neural mediators (substance P), hormones (e.g., estrogens, gastrin), alcohol and many others. Scombroid fish poisoning, usually caused by mackerel, tuna or albacore, causes mast cell degranulation signs and symptoms, but this is because the meat itself is rich in histamine-like products, a result of bacterial decomposition.

The physical factors that induce the many variants of physical urticaria are also responsible for Darier's sign. When a cutaneous mast cell lesion is rubbed, it may develop an urticarial reaction or even a blister. In addition, ordinary dermographism, common near mast cell tumors and also in patients with atopic dermatitis, is best explained by physical degranulation. The systemic agents can lead to massive histamine release and anaphylactic shock.

Cutaneous Mastocytoses

The etiology of the cutaneous mastocytoses is unclear. Recent observations have shown a soluble form of stem cell factor in the skin of patients with mastocytosis, as well as mutations in its cDNA in patients with associated hematologic disorders, suggesting an etiologic role for derangements in the networking of this growth factor and its receptor. The pathophysiology of the clinical signs and symptoms is clear, as mast cell stimulation produces an exaggeration of the normal reaction, as would be expected when an excessive number of cells are present. Even though a number of different diseases are discussed separately below, there is a broad continuous spectrum of cutaneous mast cell disorders, ranging from one nodule to multiple nodules to hundreds of macules or papules to diffuse skin infiltration. Therapy is discussed at the end of the chapter, since it is similar for all the various disorders described.

Mastocytoma

(TILBURY FOX 1883)

Synonym. Mast cell nevus

Definition. Focal accumulation of mast cells in the skin.

Epidemiology. Most patients are less than 2 years of age; many times the lesions are present at birth or identified shortly thereafter. Nonetheless, mastocytomas also appear in older children and even adults.

Clinical Findings. Typically one identifies one or several, red to red-brown minimally infiltrated nodules or plaque (Fig. 63.2). Occasionally the lesion is so dark that it is mistaken for a melanocytic nevus. One characteristic clinical feature is the tendency of the lesion to swell and even blister, either spontaneously or following mechanical stimulation (a self-induced Darier sign). The lesions may itch, especially when stimulated, and the adjacent skin usually shows urticarial dermographism. Sufficient mediator release to cause systemic symptoms is rare. The lesions usually resolve spontaneously over months to years. In patients with disseminated mastocytomas, there are many, often widely spread papules or nodules, but each individual lesion is a mastocytoma (Fig. 63.3).

Histopathology. The dermis contains a dense infiltrate of mast cells that are usually cuboidal. Some edema may be present. Mast cell stains, such as Giemsa or toluidine blue, are positive. So many mast cells are present that the diagnosis is straightforward.

Course and Prognosis. Spontaneous resolution over months to years is the rule.

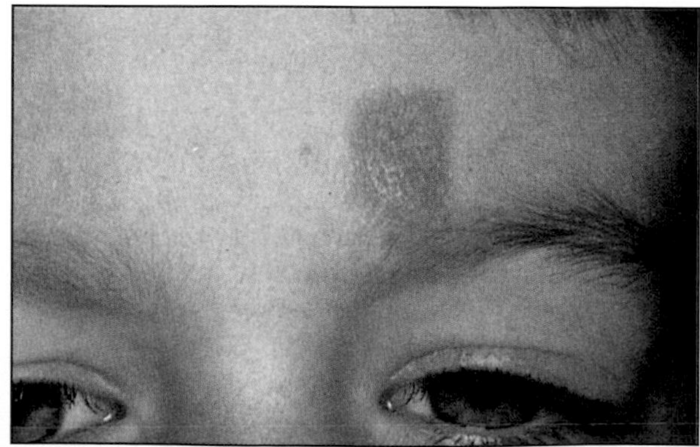

Fig. 63.2. Solitary mastocytoma

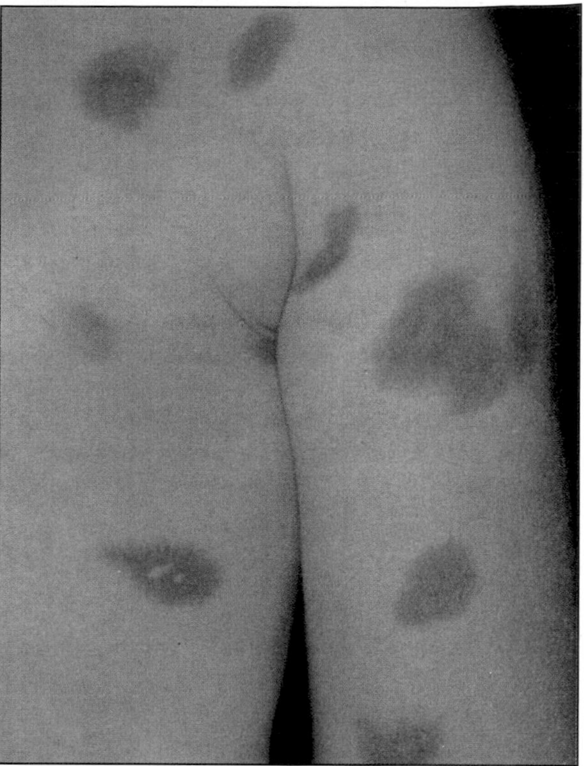

Fig. 63.3. Disseminated mastocytomas

Differential Diagnosis. The standard differential diagnosis for a red-brown nodule in a child includes mastocytoma, Spitz nevus and juvenile xanthogranuloma. A solitary lesion may be mistaken for a persistent bite reaction, perhaps with blistering. Some lesions have a yellowish hue and are mistaken for xanthomas; TILBURY FOX initially used the term xanthelasmoidea.

Urticaria Pigmentosa

(NETTLESHIP 1869; SANGSTER 1878)

Definition. Multiple macules and occasionally tiny papules containing mast cells and resembling an exanthem.

Epidemiology. Most patients are infants and children. While the disorder usually occurs in the first 6 months of life, adults may also be involved. There is no sex predilection. No pattern of inheritance has been identified.

Clinical Findings. Patients have many hundreds of characteristically hyperpigmented macules, patches and occasionally papules which tend to urti-

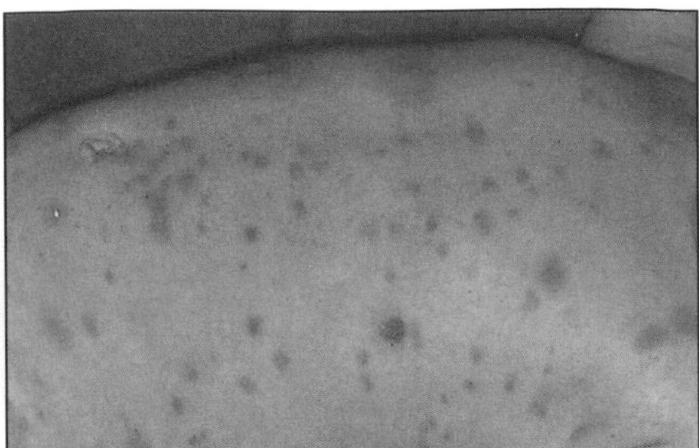

Fig. 63.4. Urticaria pigmentosa

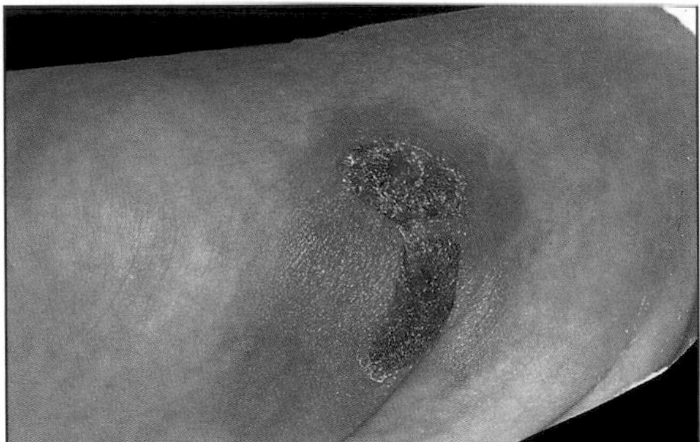

Fig. 63.5. Bullous urticaria pigmentosa

cate either following manipulation or spontaneously (Fig. 63.4). The lesions vary greatly in size and are not sharply defined. The trunk is the most common site; the palms, soles, and face are usually spared. Oral involvement has been reported but must be very rare. Nodules are uncommon. In contrast to solitary mast cell tumors, the hyperpigmentation is more prominent. Melanocytes at the epidermal-dermal junction are stimulated, perhaps by mast cell mediators or simply by the recurrent episodes of edema.

The same symptoms as mentioned under mastocytoma are more often present in urticaria pigmentosa because of the greater number of lesions. Pruritus may be intense. Following rubbing or scratching, urticarial lesions appear and blisters may form because of subepidermal edema. A positive Darier sign and urticarial dermographism are expected. About 10% of patients have evidence of internal involvement, but even these patients are usually asymptomatic, except for the intense pruritus.

Two variants of urticaria pigmentosa have been described. Hemorrhagic urticaria pigmentosa is uncommon. Sometimes there is sufficient vessel permeability that red blood cells leak out into the skin. Despite the alarming appearance, no permanent vessel damage occurs and the only sequel is hyperpigmentation from hemosiderin. The lips and oral mucosa are somewhat more likely to be involved.

Bullous urticaria pigmentosa is best viewed as an extreme form of urticaria pigmentosa that overlaps with bullous mastocytosis. If the basic lesions are multiple pigmented papules, one speaks of bullous urticaria pigmentosa; if only diffuse changes are present, the preferred term is bullous mastocytosis. Only young infants are affected and spontaneous resolution is the rule, despite the alarming appearance. Marked mediator release leads to recurrent blister formation (Fig. 63.5).

Histopathology. The mast cell infiltrate tends to be somewhat more sparse than in mastocytoma. Mast cells are usually perivascular in location. The basal layer generally shows increased melanin; incontinence of pigment (melanin dropping into the papillary dermis) is not the explanation for the hyperpigmentation.

Course and Prognosis. The lesions resolve spontaneously, often over a number of years.

Differential Diagnosis. Multiple leiomyomas can appear quite similar and may also show Darier sign; in this case, there is pain and swelling as the arrector pili smooth muscles contract. Leukemic infiltrates, lymphomas and multiple adnexal tumors may also appear similar but usually do not urticate. Urticarial Langerhans cell histiocytosis has been reported. Sometimes in ordinary chronic urticaria, the individual lesions will resolve with postinflammatory hyperpigmentation; this situation is known as urticaria cum pigmentatione.

Telangiectasia Macularis Eruptiva Perstans

(Weber and Hellenschmied 1936)

Synonym. Urticaria pigmentosa adultorum. The correct Latin name – teleangiectasia macularis eruptiva perstans – has been altered in English.

Definition. Widespread cutaneous mast cell proliferation in adults, characterized by brown macules.

Epidemiology. This very uncommon disorder is usually diagnosed in adult life.

Clinical Findings. Patients are usually covered with thousands of asymptomatic flat brown macules, often associated with telangiectases (Fig. 63.6). The trunk is most typically involved. Usually the patient has ignored the lesions, believing them to be freckles or melanocytic nevi. Often a history of aspirin or codeine allergies is obtained; there is no allergy but medication-induced release of histamine and other mediators. Both medications and mechanical stimulation may lead to a shock-like picture if degranulation is massive enough. Almost every patient has some pruritus and urticarial dermographism. Rarely, telangiectases dominate; in other cases, there is pruritus without any skin findings. Blisters do not occur. Scattered papules or nodules similar to those of urticaria pigmentosa may also be present. The disease tends to be chronic, and if resolution occurs, the patient is lucky. The risk of internal organ involvement is greater than in the childhood forms. The combination of telangiectasia macularis eruptiva perstans with hepatosplenomegaly (from mast cell infiltration) and multiple xanthomas (secondary to hepatic-induced hyperlipoproteinemia) has been described.

Histopathology. Microscopic examination reveals subtle changes; often there are only a few mast cells present. They may have few granules and be spindle-shaped, in contrast to the more cuboidal cells seen in mastocytoma. Dilated capillaries and basal layer pigmentation are two good clues to the right diagnosis. Occasionally a blind biopsy of normal skin in a patient with intense pruritus will reveal a number of mast cells. Unfortunately, the quantification of cutaneous mast cells is not well worked out, so the question always arises, "How many mast cells must one find to suggest an abnormality?"

Course and Prognosis. The disease is chronic and disturbing, due to both the cosmetic aspects and the pruritus. Rare patients may go on to develop systemic mast cell disease.

Differential Diagnosis. The cutaneous findings are usually misinterpreted as melanocytic lesions of some type. When telangiectases predominate, essential progressive telangiectasia or a connective tissue disease may be considered.

Diffuse Cutaneous Mastocytosis

Some patients have excessive numbers of mast cells involving their entire skin (Fig. 63.7). While children are most often involved, the same problem

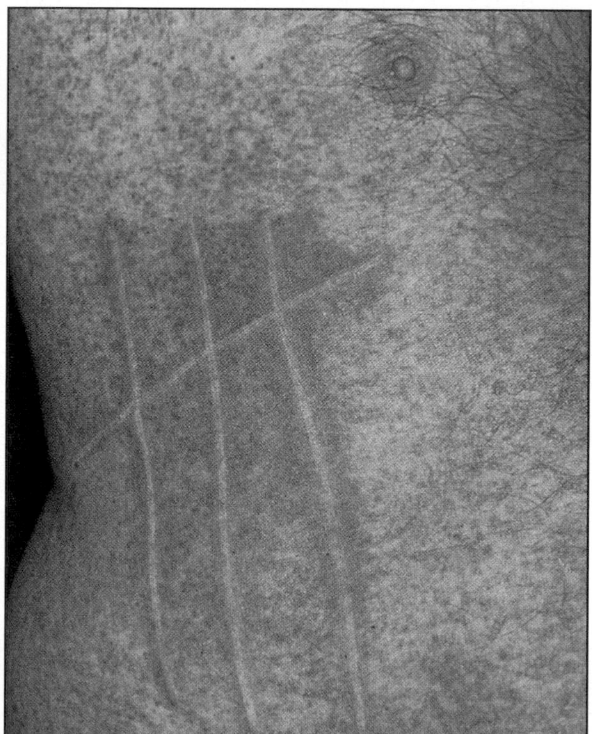

Fig. 63.6. Telangiectasia macularis eruptiva perstans with dermographism

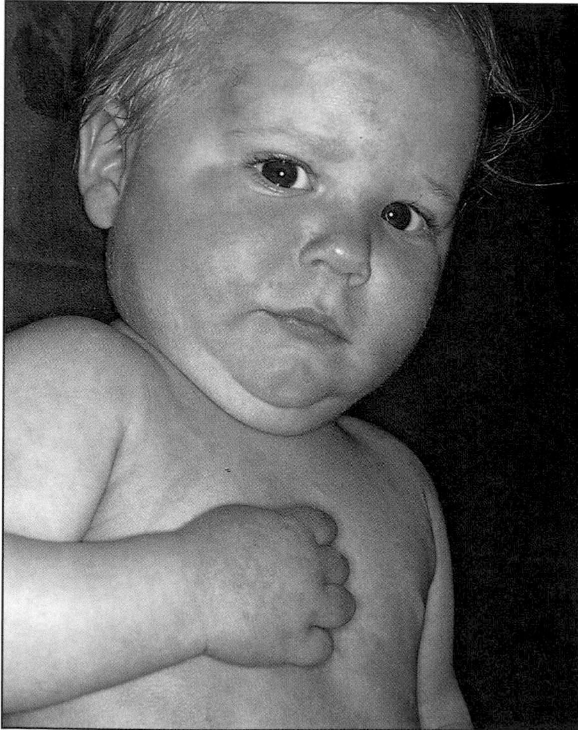

Fig. 63.7. Diffuse mastocytosis in an infant

may also be seen in adults. In children, spontaneous resolution is the rule; in adults, persistent disease and probable systemic involvement are expected. The skin becomes thickened and has been compared to elephant skin; the mechanism is presumably the repeated episodes of edema with eventual fibrosis. The skin may acquire a yellow hue; the skin folds are prominent and the surface markings resemble pigskin. Hyperpigmentation generally develops, especially in the intertriginous areas and pressure points. Pruritus is invariable and extreme; dermographism is also present. Rubbing of clothes or scratching may cause blisters as well as systemic symptoms such as bronchospasm or diarhea.

Two clinical variants of diffuse mastocytosis have been described; they reflect which aspect of excessive degranulation dominates in a given patient and do not represent different disease processes. In both, the risk of systemic involvement is high.

Bullous Mastocytosis

This problem has been alluded to under bullous urticaria pigmentosa. Some patients do not have individual lesions, but instead a diffuse infiltrate with massive subepidermal blisters and erosions. Initially, blistering disorders such as epidermolysis bullosa, staphylococcal scalded skin syndrome or childhood bullous pemphigoid may be considered. The thickened edematous skin and the biopsy showing a dermis full of mast cells provide the correct diagnosis.

Erythrodermic Mastocytosis

In this situation, patients have marked vasodilatation resulting in erythroderma with little blister formation. Pruritus is intense.

Histopathology. Histopathologic findings include edema, fibrosis and usually a dense infiltrate of mast cells. When internal organs are involved, they too are characterized by a mast cell infiltrate and fibrosis.

Systemic Mastocytosis

Clinical Findings. Mast cell infiltrates can involve a variety of organs, producing a spectrum of symptoms. In patients with mastocytomas or urticaria pigmentosa, the likelihood of systemic involvement is minimal, symptoms are extremely rare and spontaneous resolution is the rule. In telangiectasia macularis eruptiva perstans and especially diffuse mastocytosis, the risk of systemic involvement is about 40 %. Systemic involvement also occurs without skin involvement; such patients have pruritus and may have increased numbers of cutaneous mast cells without physical findings. Almost all patients with systemic mastocytosis have the symptoms of mast cell mediator release, ranging from pruritus to urticaria to flushing to gastrointestinal distress. Some of the typically involved organs include the following:

Skeletal System. Localized defects arise through mast cell infiltration. Vertebral involvement and collapse may lead to loss of height. Other pathologic fractures may occur. Osteoporosis and osteofibrosis may also be seen.

Gastrointestinal Tract. Most symptoms are the result of excessive mediator release, not local infiltration. Diarrhea, abdominal pain and peptic ulcers are most common.

Bone Marrow. Mast cell proliferation in the bone marrow is common; by definition, the mast cells are normal, but they may cause pain or anemia by crowding out normal elements. Patients may develop mast cell disease in association with other hematologic malignancies, such as leukemias, myeloproliferative disorders, myelodysplastic disorders or even lymphomas. True isolated mast cell leukemia is rare.

Liver. Infiltration, fibrosis and even portal hypertension may occur. Rarely, hyperlipoproteinemia has been described.

Lymph Nodes and Spleen. Both may be infiltrated by mast cells; the infiltration of lymph nodes is a poor sign, suggesting a trend towards malignant disease.

Cardiovascular System. Once again, the symptoms are explained by mediator release; hypertension, tachycardia, arrhythmias and shock symptoms occur.

Lungs. Despite the large number of mast cells in the lungs, pulmonary involvement in systemic mastocytosis is quite rare.

Neuropsychiatric. Headaches, depression and a wide variety of indistinct problems have been reported. Many patients with systemic mastocytosis suffer from a delayed diagnosis and from being told for years that they are imagining their gastrointestinal or cardiac problems. Their neuropsychiatric status improves dramatically when they receive a correct diagnosis, even if their general health does not change.

Other. The patients are at risk for degranulation, especially when given general anesthesia or when desensitized, especially against bee and wasp toxins. Extreme hypotension and even shock may occur.

Malignant Mastocytosis

The main risk is the development of mast cell leukemia or the proliferation of immature, atypical mast cells in the bone marrow. In this situation, mast cells eventually wind up in the peripheral blood; this change is taken as the defining event for malignant mast cell disease. The prognosis is dismal. The cause of death is usually bleeding from thrombocytopenia.

Diagnosis

When skin involvement is present, clinical examination, search for Darier's sign and dermographism, and evaluation of a biopsy usually provide the diagnosis. Mast cell mediators can also be identified in the serum and urine. Serum tryptase levels are probably the most sensitive test. Urine histamine metabolites and prostaglandin D_2 metabolites can also be determined. These tests are only needed if the clinical picture suggests systemic mastocytosis. At the same time, carcinoid syndrome and pheochromocytoma should be excluded. A symptom-directed search for internal involvement may include peripheral blood and bone marrow evaluation, skeletal evaluation, abdominal sonography, and perhaps intestinal biopsy.

Therapy

Solitary lesions rarely require therapy. Topical antipruritic agents may be prescribed. High-potency topical corticosteroids seem to stabilize or inhibit the mast cells, especially if applied under occlusion. Individual lesions can also be excised.

Patients with more diffuse disease should be counseled about likely degranulating agents and encouraged to avoid mechanical stimuli, such as jumping into a cold lake or hot tub. If they have widespread involvement and are at risk for anaphylaxis, they should wear a medical alert tag or bracelet and carry epinephrine. They should inform anesthesiologists about their disease because of the possibility of problems with general anesthesia. In addition, desensitization to allergens should probably be avoided (or approached very carefully).

The mainstay of active therapy is systemic antihistamines. H_1 receptor antagonists are most useful; they help block cardiac and gastrointestinal symptoms, as well as reducing itch and flush. Often it is helpful to alternate two different antihistamines. If the patient does not respond well to H_1, one may add H_2 blockers; the latter agents may be required if peptic ulcer disease is present. Severe intestinal symptoms can be treated with oral sodium chromoglycate; absorption is so poor that other symptoms are rarely influenced. Ketotifen is not only an H_1 antagonist but also inhibits activation of some mast cells; it provides another option.

Systemic corticosteroids are not very effective, but are sometimes employed in severe diffuse cutaneous mastocytosis or in patients with malabsorption. Recent reports also show some improvement with systemic interferon-α.

The treatment of choice for widespread cutaneous mast cell disease, that is, urticaria pigmentosa and telangiectasia macularis eruptiva perstans, is PUVA. Amazing results have been achieved in a disease which is otherwise hard to influence. PUVA bath therapy is even more effective and safer, so that in our clinic we prefer it.

The treatment of patients with malignant mast cell disease is not encouraging. No clearly beneficial chemotherapy regimen has been found. In simplistic terms, the malignant mast cells are not very abnormal and are thus hard to influence. Sometimes splenectomy is recommended to improve thrombocytopenia.

Bibliography

Mast Cells

Braun-Falco O, Salfeld K (1959) Leucine aminopeptidase activity in mast cells. Nature (London) 183:51–52

Eady RAJ, Cowen T, Marshall TF et al. (1979) Mast cell population density, blood vessel density and histamine in normal human skin. Br J Dermatol 100:623–633

Foreman JC (ed) (1993) Immunopharmacology of mast cells and basophils. Academic, London

Galli SJ (1993) New concepts about the mast cell. N Engl J Med 328:257–265

Goldstein SM (1995) Mast cell carboxypeptidase: structure and regulation of gene expression. In: Caughey GH (ed) Mast cell proteases in immunology and biology. Dekker, New York, pp 109–126

Irani AM, Schechter NM, Craig SS et al. (1986) Two types of human mast cells with distinct neutral protease compositions. Proc Natl Acad Sci USA 83:4464–4468

Irani AM (1995) Tissue and developmental variation of protease expression in human mast cells. In: Caughey GH (ed) Mast cell proteases in immunology and biology. Decker, New York, pp 127–143

Rottem M, Okada T, Goff JP et al. (1994) Mast cells cultured from the peripheral blood of normal donors and patients with mastocytosis originate from a $CD34^+$/Fc epsilon RI cell population. Blood 84:2489–2496

Weidner N, Austen KF (1993) Heterogeneity of mast cells at multiple body sites. Fluorescent determination of avidin binding and immunofluorescent determination of chymase, tryptase, and carboxypeptidase content. Pathol Res Pract 189:156–162

Whitaker-Menezes D, Schechter NM, Murphy GF (1995) Serine proteases are regionally segregated within mast cell granules. Lab Invest 72:34–41

Clinical Disease

Azana JM, Torrelo A, Mediero IG et al. (1994) Urticaria pigmentosa: a review of 67 pediatric cases. Pediatr Dermatol 11:102–106

Akaiyama M (1990) A clinical and histological study of urticaria pigmentosa: relationships between mast cell proliferation and the clinical and histological manifestations. J Dermatol 17:347–355

Christophers E, Hönigsmann H, Wolff K et al. (1978) PUVA-treatment of urticaria pigmentosa. Br J Dermatol 98: 701–702

Emanuel PD, Barton JC, Gualtieri RJ et al. (1991) Urticaria pigmentosa and preleukemia: evidence for reactive mast cell proliferation. J Am Acad Dermatol 24:893–897

Friedmann BS, Santiago ML, Berkebile C et al. (1993) Comparison of azaelastine and chlorphen-hydramine in the treatment of mastocytosis. J Allergy Clin Immunol 92: 520–526

Golkar L, Bernhard JD (1997) Mastocytosis. Lancet 349: 1379–1385

Godt O, Proksch E, Streit V et al. (1997) Short- and long-term effectiveness of oral and bath PUVA therapy in urticaria pigmentosa and systemic matocytosis. Dermatology 195: 35–39

Horny HP, Ruck P, Krober S et al. (1997) Systemic mast cell disease (mastocytosis). General aspects and histopathological diagnosis. Histol Histopathol 12:1081–1089

Katoh N, Hirano S, Yasuno H (1996) Solitary mastocytoma treated with tranilast. J Dermatol 23:335–339

Kettelhut BV, Metcalfe DD (1991) Pediatric mastocytosis. J Invest Dermatol 96:15S–18S

Kors JW, van Doormaal JJ, de Monchy JG (1993) Anaphylactoid shock following hymenoptera sting as a presenting symptom of systemic mastocytosis. J Intern Med 233:255–258

Kors JW, Van-Doormaal JJ, Breukelman H et al. (1996) Long-term follow up of indolent mastocytosis in adults. J Intern Med 239:157–164

Kurosawa M, Amano H, Kanbe N et al. (1997) Heterogeneity of mast cells in mastocytosis and inhibitory effect of ketotifen and ranitidine on indolent systemic mastocytosis. J Allergy Clin Immunol 100:S25–S32

Lazarus GS (1996) Mastocytosis: new understandings in cutaneous pathophysiology. J Dermatol 23:769–772

Longley J (1994) Is mastocytosis a mast cell neoplasia or a reactive hyperplasia? Clues from the study of mast cell growth factor. Ann Med 26:115–116

Longley J, Duffy TP, Kohn S (1995) The mast cell and mast cell disease. J Am Acad Dermatol 32:545–561

Mackey S, Pride HB, Tyler WB (1996) Diffuse cutaneous mastocytosis. Treatment with psoralen plus UV-A. Arch Dermatol 132:1429–1430

McDonagh AJ, Messenger AG, Priestley BL (1991) Bullous eruption in an infant. Bullous mastocytosis. Arch Dermatol 127:1049–1050

Park YM, Cha MK, Kim TY et al. (1994) Pseudoxanthomatous mastocytosis (xanthelasmoidea) treated with PUVA therapy. Ann Dermatol 7:253–258

Parker RI (1991) Hematologic aspects of mastocytosis I: bone marrow pathology in adult and pediatric systemic mast cell disease. J Invest Dermatol 96:52S–53S

Parker RI (1991) Hematologic aspects of mastocytosis II: management of hematologic disorders in association with systemic mast cell disease. J Invest Dermatol 96: 47S–51S

Schwartz LB, Metcalfe DD, Miller JS et al. (1987) Tryptase levels as an indicator of mast cell activation in systemic anaphylaxis and mastocytosis. N Engl J Med 316:1622–1626

Soter NA (1991) The skin in mastocytosis. J Invest Dermatol 96:32S–38S

Tharp MD (1997) Understanding mast cells and mastocytosis. J Invest Dermatol 108:698–699

Topar G, Staudacher C, Geisen F et al. (1998) urticaria pigmentosa. A clinical, hematopathologic, and serologic study of 30 adults. Am J Clin Pathol 109:279–285

Valent P (1996) Biology, classification and treatment of human mastocytosis. Wien Klin Wochenschr 108:385–397

Van Gysel D, Oranje AP, Vermeiden I et al. (1996) Value of urinary N-methylhistamine measurements in childhood mastocytosis. J Am Acad Dermatol 35:556–558

Weidner N, Horan RF, Austen KF (1992) Mast cell phenotype in indolent forms of mastocytosis. Ultrastructural features, fluorescence detection of avidin binding, and immunofluorescent determination of chymase, tryptase and carboxypeptidase. Am J Pathol 140:847–857

Original Papers

Ehrlich P (1877) Beiträge zur Kenntnis der Anilinfärbungen und ihrer Verwendung in der mikroskopischen Technik. Arch Mikr Anat 13:263–264

Fox WT (1883) On urticaria pigmentosa or xanthelasmoidea. Med Chir Trans 66:329–347

Nettleship E (1869) Rare forms of urticaria. Br Med J 2: 323–324

Sangster A (1878) An anomalous mottled rash accompanied by pruritus, factitious urticaria and pigmentation, "urticaria pigmentosa?" Trans Clin Soc Lond 11:161–163

Weber FP, Hellenschmied R (1936) Teleangiectasia macularis eruptiva perstans. Br J Dermatol 42:374–382

CHAPTER 64

Histiocytoses

Contents

Basic Science Aspects

The histiocytoses are diseases characterized by the proliferation of histiocytic cells. Today histiocytes are divided into two groups: dendritic cells and macrophages. Both cell types arise in the bone marrow and populate the skin, but they show considerable morphologic and functional differences.

The macrophage is a professional phagocyte. It is identified as a monocyte in the peripheral blood and then as a macrophage in tissue. Depending on the organ where it serves, the macrophage acquires a variety of specialized names. Structurally, it is a metabolically active cell, rich in phagosomes and containing a number of digestive enzymes. It may evolve into a number of different giant cells, including foreign body, epithelioid, Touton and Langhans types. The enzymes were previously used to identify the cell; antibodies against lysozyme, trypsin and chymotrypsin were among the early macrophage markers. Today a more elegant series of markers is available, including Ki-M1P, KP1 and HAM 56.

The dendritic cells are antigen-presenting cells that interact with T cells. The prototype dendritic cell in the skin is the Langerhans cell. The Langerhans cell is located within the epidermis. It is a clear cell in hematoxylin-eosin sections and was initially confused with a melanocyte. It typically has a large almost kidney-shaped nucleus. Electron microscopy reveals the characteristic cytoplasmic organelle, the Langerhans or Birbeck granule (Birbeck et al. 1961), a bilaminar tennis racket-shaped structure that is involved in pinocytosis (Fig. 64.1). Langerhans cells move to the dermis and then the regional lymph nodes where they present antigen to T cells. Cells whose maturation and progression is interrupted may remain in the dermis; they are identified as indeterminate cells and often have both Langerhans cell and macrophage markers. Langer-

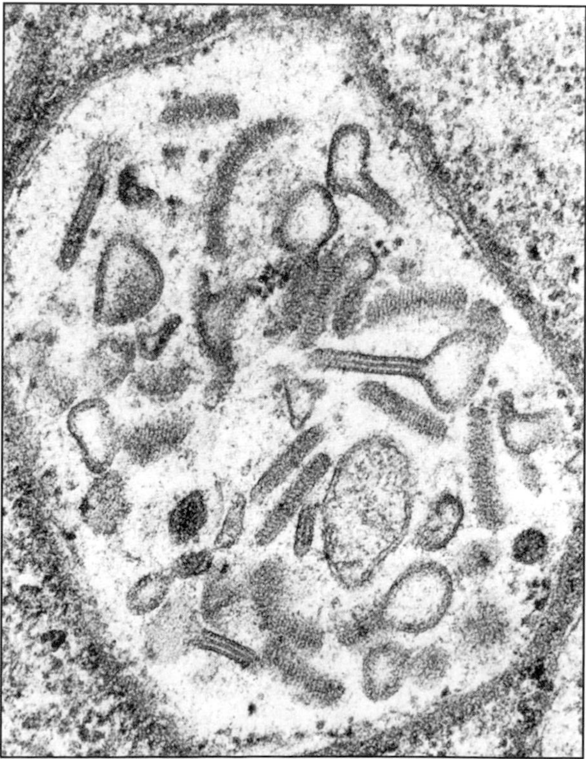

Fig. 64.1. Langerhans cell with typical tennis racket-shaped Birbeck granules (× 70,000)

Table 64.1. Morphologic classes of cutaneous histiocytoses

Disease	Marker			
	S100	CD1a	Birbeck	Macrophage[a]
Langerhans cell histiocytosis	+	+	++	–
Congenital self-healing reticulohistiocytosis	+	+	+	–
Indeterminate cell histiocytosis	+	+	–	+
Sinus histiocytosis with massive lymphadenopathy	+	–	–	+
Macrophage disorders	–	–	–	+

[a] Any of a number of macrophage markers

hans cells are S100- and CD1a-positive, along with many other markers that are less generally available. Other dendritic cells found in the lymph node include interdigitating dendritic cells (old name: interdigitating reticulum cell) which present antigens to T cells in the cortex, and the follicular dendritic cells (old name: dendritic reticulum cell) which react with B cells. Their exact relation to Langerhans cells is unclear.

There is a third population of histiocytes in the dermis, known as the dermal dendrocytes. These cells are found in a perivascular location primarily and stain best with Factor XIIIa. They may be the predominant cell in dermatofibroma or histiocytoma, a reactive tumor-like process considered in Chap. 59. Other possible populations of dermal dendrocytes have been identified, using markers such as MS-1, but their exact role is unclear. In the past, it was felt that some phagocytic cells might arise from fibroblasts in the dermis, not the bone marrow. Such cells have not been identified with modern techniques.

Today the histiocytoses are best classified based on their cell of origin, as Table 64.1 shows. A number of disorders that clearly feature macrophages are not included in this chapter but are discussed elsewhere in the book. Many infections, such as tuberculosis and leprosy, are dominated by histiocytes; sarcoidosis is a histiocyte disorder. The predominant cell in many of the necrobiotic disorders, such as granuloma annulare, annular elastolytic giant cell granuloma, necrobiosis lipoidica diabeticorum and necrobiotic xanthogranuloma is an activated histiocyte. The dermatofibroma or histiocytoma has already been discussed. Malignant fibrous histiocytoma and its cutaneous variant atypical fibroxanthoma lack macrophage markers and are probably fibrosarcomas. All xanthomas result from the ingestion of lipids or lipoproteins by histiocytes which are then transformed into foam cells; those associated with lipid abnormalities are covered in Chap. 37. There is an unusual and rare group of normolipemic xanthomas. These are disorders that clinically and histologically appear as xanthomas but where the patient's cholesterol and triglyceride levels are normal. Some of these lesions are covered under xanthomas, and those for which there is evidence that they are closely related to more traditional histiocytic disorders are included in this chapter. Table 64.2 shows a list of the disorders covered in this chapter, arranged on the basis of the predominant cell.

Table 64.2. The cutaneous histiocytoses

Langerhans cell histiocytosis (CD1a⁺, S100⁺)
Letterer-Siwe disease
Hand-Schüller-Christian disease
Eosinophilic granuloma
Congenital self-healing reticulohistiocytosis
Non-Langerhans cell histiocytoses
Overlap disorders (CD1a⁻, S100⁺)
Indeterminate cell histiocytosis
Sinus histiocytosis with massive lymphadenopathy
Macrophage disorders (CD1a⁻ S100⁻, macrophage marker⁺)
Xanthogranuloma (juvenile and adult)
Benign cephalic histiocytosis
Generalized eruptive histiocytomas
Xanthoma disseminatum
Papular xanthoma
Reticulohistiocytoma
Multicentric reticulohistiocytosis
Progressive nodular histiocytosis
Diffuse normolipemic plane xanthoma (Chap. 37)
Normolipemic xanthomas (Chap. 37)
Necrobiotic xanthogranuloma (Chap. 50)

Langerhans Cell Histiocytoses

Definition. Several overlapping clinical disorders are included today as Langerhans cell histiocytoses

(LCH). Lichtenstein first used the term histiocytosis X in the 1950s to identify Letterer-Siwe disease, Hand-Schüller-Christian disease and eosinophilic granuloma, as he recognized that the same cell was involved in all three disorders. Basset et al., in 1973, discovered that the cell was a Langerhans cell. For all practical purposes, the cell of LCH is identical to the normal Langerhans cell; there are minor functional and laboratory differences that we can ignore. The presence of such cells, identified by immunohistochemical markers such as S100 and CD1a, as well as electron microscopic visualization of Birbeck granules, defines the disorders.

Epidemiology. All the LCH are rare disorders. Their age distribution will be discussed for the various clinical patterns.

Etiology and Pathogenesis. Initially LCH was considered a metabolic disturbance because many of the cells, especially in internal organs, are xanthomatized. Later it was felt to be a neoplastic disease, although the highly variable course led others to consider LCH a reactive process. Recent data suggest that the cells are clonal for a number of X-linked polymorphisms, but clonality does not prove malignancy. No etiologic factors have been identified; the cause of the disease remains a mystery.

Clinical Findings. An ideal clinical classification for LCH does not exist. There are marked overlaps between the various clinical types. While the Histiocyte Society has proposed new, somewhat more scientific sounding names, they do not resolve the problem with overlaps. The old names have stood us in good stead and we continue to use them. The following terms are roughly equivalent; we will discuss each disease separately, fully aware of the overlaps.

- Acute disseminated LCH: Letterer-Siwe disease
- Chronic multifocal LCH: Hand-Schüller-Christian disease
- Chronic focal LCH: Eosinophilic granuloma

Letterer-Siwe Disease

(Letterer 1924; Siwe 1933; Abt 1936)

Synonyms. Abt-Letterer-Siwe disease (the standard name in Germany), acute disseminated LCH

Definition. Acute multisystem involvement by Langerhans cells, usually present in infants.

Clinical Findings. Most patients are infants less than 2 years of age. Their primary lesion is a small, transparent pink papule that rapidly develops a crust. The lesions may be purpuric. Generally widespread scale develops as lesions coalesce (Fig. 64.2). The flexural and seborrheic areas are the most common sites (Fig. 64.3). Lesions may appear in crops, with a tendency towards self-healing. Nodules may occur. Petechiae on the hands and feet are common. Gingival involvement with bleeding may occur. Sometimes jaw defects lead to loose teeth. Xanthomatized lesions are rarely seen; they occur more often in localized and internal LCH. Similar findings may be seen in patients well into adult life. About 80 % of patients have cutaneous findings.

Many unusual forms of cutaneous LCH have been described. They do not fit conveniently into the conventional patterns but are included here. For example, vesicular, bullous, ulcerated and even urticarial variants have been described. All may create diagnostic havoc. In addition nail-bed involvement is not uncommon, but when solitary or the initial sign, almost always overlooked.

Most patients are seriously ill with fever, lymphadenopathy, hepatosplenomegaly, and pulmonary infiltrates. Bone involvement is uncommon, except for the mastoid bones, where it causes at first otitis media and then otitis externa. In general, about 10 % of patients with Letterer-Siwe disease die, one-third clear and the rest have a chronic, difficult course. Some patients have only skin involvement and a much better prognosis.

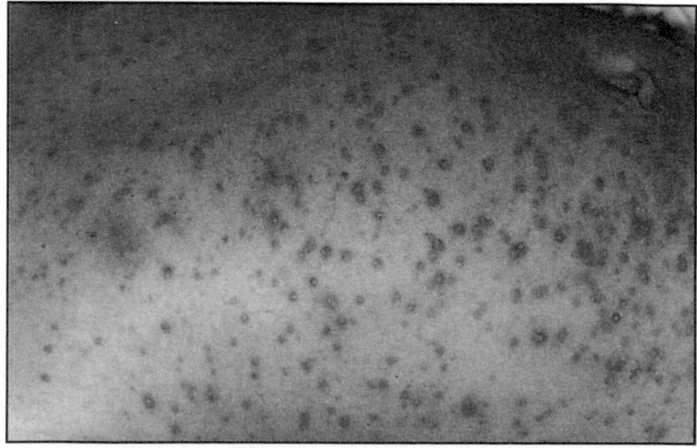

Fig. 64.2. Langerhans cell histiocytosis (Letterer-Siwe disease) with multiple scaly papules

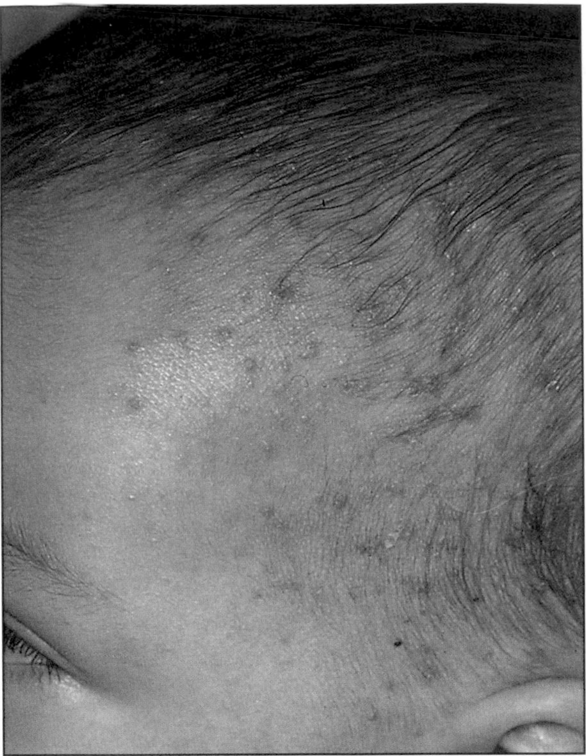

Fig. 64.3. Langerhans cell histiocytosis (Letterer-Siwe disease) with typical scalp involvement

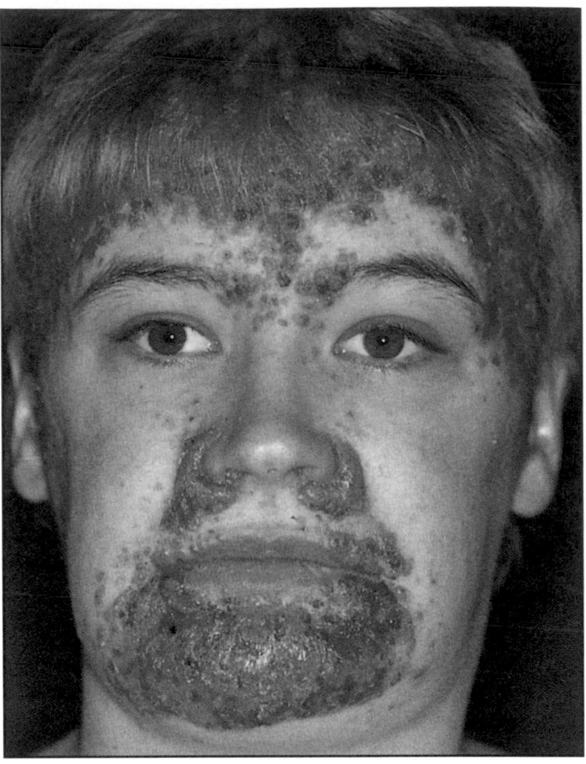

Fig. 64.4. Langerhans cell histiocytosis (Hand-Schüller-Christian disease) in adult with extensive crusting and scaling, as well as nodules.

Hand-Schüller-Christian Disease

(Hand 1893; Schüller 1915; Christian 1920)

Synonym. Chronic multifocal LCH

Definition. LCH with the classic triad of bony defects, diabetes insipidus and exophthalmos.

Clinical Findings. Patients with Hand-Schüller-Christian disease are usually older than those with Letterer-Siwe disease. Patients with only the classic triad are rare; many variations are seen. While the skin lesions may resemble those in Letterer-Siwe disease, they are more often papulonodular and xanthomatized, involving the axillae, groin and perineum. Approximately 30% of patients have skin involvement. A diffuse scaly seborrheic dermatitis-like eruption may be present, but it is seldom so severe or hemorrhagic as in small children. However, as Fig. 64.4 shows, such eruptions do occur. Mucosal disease is common; not only the mouth but also the genitalia are likely to be involved.

Many patients have bone involvement on skeletal surveys. The characteristic skeletal change is caused by a histiocytic proliferation that produces punched out defects on radiography and cause trouble as space-occupying lesions. The frequent involvement of the calvarium with punched out lesions has given rise to the term map-like skull. Histologically, such areas are usually xanthomatized. About 50% of the patients have diabetes insipidus from involvement of the pituitary saddle, which can be visualized by radiography and other imaging techniques. The peculiar propensity of the infiltrate for this region remains unexplained. Middle ear involvement and orbital infiltrates leading to proptosis may be seen. Jaw involvement may lead to floating or loose teeth.

Eosinophilic Granuloma

Synonym. Chronic focal LCH

Definition. Localized, but often multiple, infiltrates of Langerhans cells, often associated with eosinophils.

Clinical Findings. The most common sites of involvement are the bones. Patients have one or more focal lesions that can be easily treated and progression into more severe disease is rare. Most typical is a single lesion in the mandible or maxilla leading to a single loose tooth. Spontaneous fractures, diabetes insipidus and otitis media are three other common presentations. Patients tend to be older adolescents and adults. Solitary pulmonary LCH is not uncommon. In addition, lymphadenopathy and hepatosplenomegaly may occur. Cutaneous disease is usually nodular, since diffuse or widespread disease would place the patient in another category. Nodules resembling juvenile xanthogranuloma with yellow hues are most common, but they may be ulcerated. In addition, solitary ulcerated plaques occur. Once again oral and anogenital disease may be seen.

Congenital Self-Healing Reticulohistiocytosis

(Hashimoto and Pritzker 1973)

Synonym. Hashimoto-Pritzker disease

Definition. Variant of cutaneous LCH featuring lesions present early in life with a tendency to regression.

Clinical Findings. Congenital self-healing reticulohistiocytosis is often presented as a separate disease but it is not one; self-healing is a feature of all forms of LCH but is more common among the congenital forms. Classic patients, as described by Hashimoto and Pritzker, are newborns with one or several erythematous to red-brown nodules, which are often superficially ulcerated (Fig. 64.5). They may be scattered over the body, but the head and neck are the most common sites. In about 25% of cases a solitary lesion is found. The classic tiny crusted papules of Letterer-Siwe disease are not present. The nodules tend to regress over weeks to years, leaving behind atrophic scars. Systemic involvement by definition is not present.

But real life is not as crystal clear as this classic definition. Some patients develop one or more nodules shortly after birth, so the lesions are not congenital but neonatal. Some patients with nodules early in life do not show regression but go on to develop Letterer-Siwe disease. Some children develop multiple skin lesions but otherwise do well. Their disease has been designated infantile LCH (Bonifazi et al. 1982). Yet other patients may have one or two skin nodules and a solitary bony defect (detected perhaps only by skeletal survey but asymptomatic). They too do well but officially they have Hand-Schüller-Christian disease. One cannot always separate congenital self-healing reticulohistiocytosis from Letterer-Siwe disease; one must await the clinical course – regression or progression.

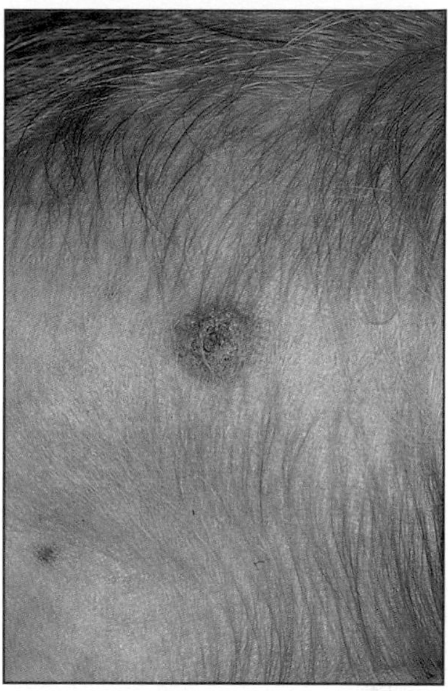

Fig. 64.5. Congenital self-healing histiocytosis; solitary nodule that resolved spontaneously

Histopathology. Not surprisingly, the histopathology of LCH varies with the type of clinical lesion. The unifying feature is the large histiocytes with kidney-shaped nuclei that are found in all forms and stages of the disease; they do not exhibit marked cellular atypia or mitoses. Sometimes, almost pure "cultures" of such cells are seen; that is, uniform sheets of Langerhans cells. Their identity is confirmed with S100 and CD1a staining, both of which can now be performed on formalin-fixed, paraffin-embedded tissue. Antibodies against peanut agglutinin antigen (PAN) and proliferating cell nuclear antigen (PCNA) can also stain the cells but are of limited utility. Finally, electron microscopic examination can be used to find the Birbeck granules. Earlier reports emphasized that congenital self-healing reticulohistiocytosis often have fewer Birbeck granules and a variety of other ultrastructural markers, including laminated bodies and dense bodies. The latter structures may reflect the involution that the histiocytes are undergoing. There are, however, sufficient overlaps so that ultrastructure is not used to separate out the self-healing form of LCH.

Four types of microscopic lesions have been described: proliferative, xanthomatous, granulomatous and fibrous. The individual lesions have characteristic changes reflecting their clinical variability. The scaly papules of Letterer-Siwe disease typically show hemorrhages and crust with an infiltrate of histiocytes in the upper dermis often impinging on the epidermis; they typify the proliferative form. Touch preparations taken from such lesions also nicely demonstrate the typical cells. These slides can also be stained with S100 and CD1a antibodies. The granulomatous pattern is seen in bony lesions and larger cutaneous nodules. Here sheets of histiocytes are found, often admixed with numerous eosinophils. Lymphocytes and even lymphoid aggregates may be seen. In the xanthomatous form, foamy histiocytes are seen. Such lesions are rare in the skin and very difficult to distinguish from ordinary xanthomas. This pattern is more common in the pituitary and mastoid lesions. The fibrous lesions are old and represent scarring.

Laboratory Findings. Individual organ involvement should be sought and documented with traditional methods. Peripheral blood involvement does not occur and no special tests are necessary.

Diagnostic Criteria. The diagnostic criteria involve demonstrating the presence of the classic cell in the appropriate clinical setting. The Histiocyte Society considers the presence of typical cells in the appropriate clinical setting as sufficient for a "presumptive diagnosis". S100 positivity produces a "diagnosis", and CD1a positivity or presence of Birbeck granules advances one to a "definite diagnosis".

The prognosis in LCH in based on three factors:

- Age of the patient
- Number of organs involved
- Degree of dysfunction of bone marrow, liver or lungs

A puzzling paradox is that disease at birth is generally a good sign, but disease in early infancy a bad sign. Later, increasing age suggests a better prognosis, although octogenarians with severe fatal Letterer-Siwe disease have been described.

Differential Diagnosis. The differential diagnosis of LCH reflects the many different clinical patterns. Examples include:

- Letterer-Siwe Disease. Severe or especially petechial seborrheic dermatitis should always prompt a biopsy, especially in infants. Chronic unresponsive otitis media and externa is another differential point. In older patients, the lesions appear almost identical to those of Darier disease or Hailey-Hailey disease. Scabies in infants can appear similar, with widespread crusted areas and infiltrated nodules. Crusted or ulcerated lesions suggest persistent herpes simplex virus infection or other chronic infections. In addition, many forms of congenital immunodeficiency, such as familial hemophagocytic lymphohistiocytosis and Omenn syndrome (congenital reticuloendotheliosis with eosinophilia and immunodeficiency), should be considered. Infection-associated hemophagocytic syndrome may also appear similar; however, erythrophagocytosis is not a feature of LCH.
- Hand-Schüller-Christian Disease. The nodules suggest juvenile xanthogranuloma or even a mast cell tumor. When xanthomatous lesions are present, then the entire differential diagnosis of such infiltrates must be considered. The massive genital involvement suggests severe, therapy-resistant herpes simplex virus infection, as seen in HIV/AIDS and other immunodeficiency disorders.
- Eosinophilic Granuloma. The bony lesions have the long list of differential diagnostic possibilities of osteolytic or radiolucent lesions, as found in any radiology text. The skin lesions are identical to those of Hand-Schüller-Christian disease.
- Congenital Self-Healing Reticulohistiocytosis. The differential diagnostic possibilities for congenital tumors include leukemia, neuroblastoma, choriocarcinoma and malignant melanoma. In addition, the blueberry muffin lesions, representing extramedullary hematopoiesis, as seen in congenital infections (TORCH syndrome) and hemolytic disease, must be excluded.

Therapy

Systemic. The rule of "do no harm" is especially important in confronting LCH. The disease in all its forms is unpredictable, but often shows regression and is not relentlessly fatal. Systemic therapy should be considered for widespread disease with internal organ dysfunction. The trend in recent years is towards less-aggressive therapy. The mainstay of most regimens is corticosteroids; typical dosages are prednisone 1–2 mg/kg daily. The most commonly employed cytostatic agent is vinblastine, although many others have been tried. In addition, prednisone and vinblastine can be combined.

Etoposide (epipodophyllotoxin, VP-16) has shown promise as a monoagent, but cases of acute myelogenous leukemia have been described in LCH patients in whom it was employed. Thalidomide is also a promising agent, producing remarkable responses in a few patients.

More drastic combination chemotherapy regimens, such as those employed in leukemias and lymphomas, have not been shown to be of clear benefit. In patients refractory to traditional therapy, high-dose chemotherapy and then bone marrow transplantation has been used. Patients with hepatic failure and otherwise good prognostic parameters have been treated with liver transplantation.

Diabetes insipidus, present in 50% of Hand-Schüller-Christian disease patients, is not an insignificant problem. A variety of synthetic vasopressin agents, some administered transnasally, have improved control of this aspect.

Topical. The best-established topical therapy is topical nitrogen mustard, as discussed in the treatment of mycosis fungoides. Both Grenz ray and PUVA therapy can also been employed. Symptomatic relief for weeping crusting lesions can be provided with antibacterial agents, drying lotions such as zinc oxide lotion and perhaps topical corticosteroid lotions and milks.

Surgical. Solitary lesions such as in congenital self-healing reticulohistiocytosis are usually excised, both for diagnostic and therapeutic purposes. Other worrisome individual lesions can also be excised. Bone lesions use usually treated satisfactorily by curettage; amputation is not employed.

Other Measures. Radiation therapy is often employed for bone lesions, usually combined with curettage. In addition, solitary cutaneous lesions can be irradiated. Langerhans cells are relatively radiosensitive and 3–6 Gy suffices.

Non-Langerhans Cell Histiocytoses

The rest of the histiocytoses either feature poorly defined cells or macrophages. In any event, they do not represent a proliferation of Langerhans cells. While this is an awkward way to define a group of diseases, it is clinically useful especially in children as LCH has a less favorable outlook.

Overlap Histiocytoses

Two diseases, indeterminate cell histiocytosis and sinus histiocytosis with massive lymphadenopathy, represent the borderline between LCH and non-Langerhans cell histiocytosis. Both disorders contain histiocytes that are S100-positive but lack the other defining features.

Indeterminate Cell Histiocytosis

(Wood et al. 1985)

Indeterminate cell histiocytosis is a very uncommon disorder. It is defined by the presence of cells that have features of both Langerhans cells and macrophages. The cells are thus typically S100-positive, may be CD1a-positive and display one or more macrophage markers. Clinically patients may present with a solitary red-brown nodule or with multiple disseminated papules. These are the two common presentations for all the non-Langerhans cell histiocytoses. The disorder is too uncommon to draw any clinical conclusions.

The indeterminate cells are presumably epidermal Langerhans cells that have migrated to the dermis but are arrested there and do not reach the regional lymph nodes. Just as Langerhans cells can be manipulated in vitro to acquire macrophage characteristics and become somewhat phagocytic, for example by the use of various cytokine combinations, these arrested Langerhans cells also acquire phagocytic markers and perhaps function.

Microscopic examination reveals an infiltrate of round cells without distinct characteristics. Electron microscopy does not reveal Birbeck granules, but may show phagocytic structures. Thus the diagnosis is made by immunohistochemistry. No center has enough experience with the disease to propose therapy. Disseminated disease should probably be treated as LCH.

Sinus Histiocytosis with Massive Lymphadenopathy

(Destombes 1965; Rosai and Dorfman 1969)

Synonym. Rosai-Dorfman disease

Definition. Massive benign lymph node proliferation of unknown etiology that may involve the skin.

Clinical Findings. Typical patients are children and young adults, more often blacks, who present with fever, chills and other signs of systemic illness. The most striking finding is massive lymphadenopathy, usually involving the cervical lymph nodes. Inguinal and mediastinal nodes are also frequently involved and about 10% of patients have hepatosplenomegaly. A wide variety of internal organs can be also be affected. The disease resolves spontaneously after a period of months to years in most cases. In the large Rosai-Dorfman registry, only a few patients died from their disease while another group had persistent problems.

About 10% of patients have cutaneous lesions, once again red-brown papules and nodules (Fig. 64.6). Panniculitis may also occur. When the lymphadenopathy is present, the cutaneous lesions present no diagnostic problem. A far more difficult situation arises when sinus histiocytosis with massive lymphadenopathy presents in the skin, either as a solitary subcutaneous nodule or as multiple lesions. These cutaneous changes can be a precursor to full-blown disease or they can be the only finding, even after a long follow-up.

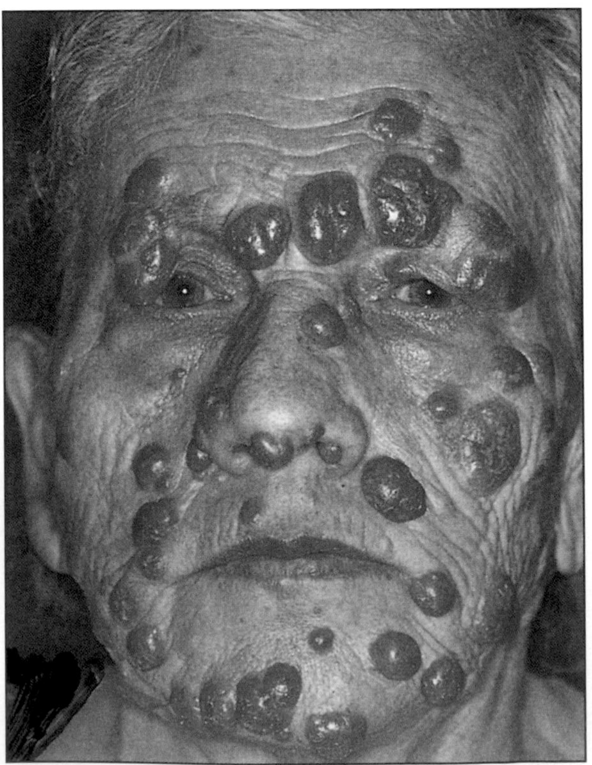

Fig. 64.6. Extensive cutaneous involvement in sinus histiocytosis with massive lymphadenopathy

Histopathology. The lymph node pathology is characteristic: the sinuses are dilated and crowded with inflammatory cells, primarily histiocytes. These cells have a foamy cytoplasm and display emperipolesis or the uptake of lymphocytes. They have been fancifully compared to a bean-bag, for the lymphocytes are taken into the cell, but not digested as in phagocytosis.

In the skin, there is a generous perivascular lymphohistiocytic infiltrate that may coalesce into sheets of cells. The histiocytes are usually foamy, may be multinucleated, and at least some should show emperipolesis. Red cells may also be taken up (erythrophagocytosis). Neutrophils and plasma cells may also be found.

Immunohistochemistry reveals the cells to be S100-positive and CD1a-negative. A wide spectrum of macrophage markers are variably positive. In addition, proliferation markers such as CD30 are positive in about 50% of cases. Staining for factor XIIIa has also been described, but its significance is unclear. Electron microscopy shows no Birbeck granules and evidence of phagocytosis or emperipolesis.

Therapy. Solitary nodules can be excised. No satisfactory therapy is available for disseminated disease.

Macrophage Disorders

A wide variety of seemingly disparate disorders are grouped under this heading. Recent work by Zelger, Wilson-Jones and colleagues provides a unifying approach that simplifies the understanding of this disease group. They have identified different types of histiocytes in the prototype lesion – juvenile xanthogranuloma – and then used histiocyte morphology to subcategorize the diseases. While many of these disorders may feature foamy cells, all are normolipemic. In all instances the etiology and pathogenesis are unknown.

Juvenile Xanthogranuloma
(McDonagh 1912)

Synonyms. Xanthogranuloma, nevoxanthoendothelioma, juvenile xanthoma, juvenile giant cell granuloma

Definition. Lesion composed of macrophages that lack S100 positivity and contain no Birbeck granules. A wide range of clinical and histologic patterns are possible. While the term juvenile xanthogranuloma is misleading, because xanthogranulomas can be found in adults, we have chosen to retain it. Xanthogranuloma in general pathology refers to any infiltrate with both foamy cells and giant cells, so it lacks precision.

Clinical Findings. Juvenile xanthogranulomas present as red-brown papules or nodules, often with a yellow hue (Fig. 64.7). They can range in size from several millimeters to many centimeters. While juvenile xanthogranuloma can be present at birth, no genetic influence has been identified. Most lesions appear in the first several years of life. The head, axilla, groin and extensor surfaces of the extremities are the most common sites. While solitary lesions occur, most commonly the patient has several tumors. Some authors distinguish between micronodular and macronodular forms, although the distinctions are not sharp. Patients with micronodular disease have large numbers of small juvenile xanthogranulomas and are more likely to have ocular involvement, while those with macronodular disease have fewer, larger nodules and perhaps a greater likelihood of internal involvement.

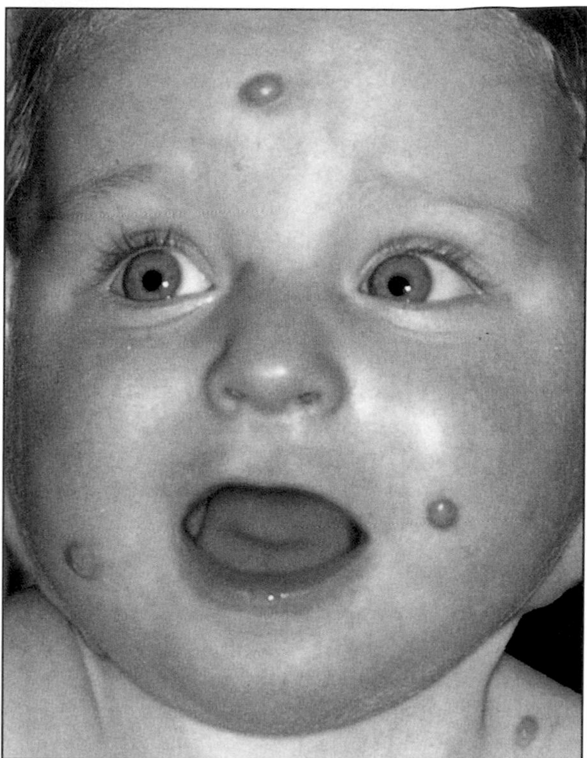

Fig. 64.7. Juvenile xanthogranulomas

Many clinical variants of juvenile xanthogranuloma have been described, including lichenoid papules, plaques, and subcutaneous lesions. The Cyrano form with disfiguring nasal and facial lesions refers to *Cyrano de Bergerac*, the long-nosed hero of the comedy by the dramatist Edmond Rostand. Most childhood lesions regress spontaneously over a period of months to years, usually leaving behind an atrophic scar. On the scalp, alopecia may result. Adult lesions are more likely to be solitary and less likely to regress.

Juvenile xanthogranulomas may be found in many internal organs. The most typical site is the eye. About 10% of patients have ocular lesions, usually glaucoma, bleeding into the anterior chamber or a space-occupying lesion. Thus ophthalmologic examination is recommended for all patients with juvenile xanthogranuloma. Oral mucosal involvement is very rare, but does occur. Changes have been described in many internal organs, but their significance is unclear. When accompanying cutaneous lesions are present, one can assume that the same idiopathic disease process is involved. But there are also many reports of strictly internal involvement by juvenile xanthogranuloma; in such a setting the terminology is less clear. For example, Erdheim-Chester disease is defined as subcutaneous xanthogranulomatous tumors and bone lesions; is it a variant of juvenile xanthogranuloma? Many associations have been reported for juvenile xanthogranuloma. The most significant is probably the triad of neurofibromatosis I, multiple juvenile xanthogranulomas and juvenile chronic myelogenous leukemia. Increased numbers of juvenile xanthogranulomas have also been reported in both urticaria pigmentosa and LCH.

Histopathology. The classic lesions contain a dermal macrophage infiltrate with a variety of prominent cells. Most obvious are the Touton giant cells, multinucleated giant cells with a wreath of nuclei enclosing a paler central region. Other less perfectly organized multinucleate giant cells are also present. Foamy cells are also common, as are eosinophils. Sometimes, most often in early lesions, one identifies only a monotonous vacuolated cell infiltrate; this histologic variant has been designated mononuclear cell xanthogranuloma.

The least distinct histologic variant is the spindle cell xanthogranuloma. These lesions, often seen in adults, are confused both clinically and histologically with dermatofibromas and may represent an overlap. The macrophages are predominantly spindle-shaped. Entrapment of collagen, fibrosis and epidermal hyperplasia, all clues to the diagnosis of dermatofibroma, are usually absent.

Immunohistochemistry reveals positive macrophage markers, which vary slightly depending on the predominant type of macrophage. S100 and CD1a are in general negative, but a number of authors have identified occasional positive S100 cells in clinically typical juvenile xanthogranuloma. These cells may be normal passengers. If a large proportion of the histiocytes are S100-positive, then one is more likely dealing with LCH or a variant thereof.

Differential Diagnosis. The classic differential diagnosis includes mastocytoma and Spitz nevus. Darier's sign may be positive, so a biopsy is essential. The other variants of non-Langerhans cell histiocytosis may all appear similar and often one is faced with a linguistic and not a scientific question. True xanthomas, of course, appear similar, but can be excluded by serum lipid studies if necessary. While many juvenile xanthogranulomas appear to be very yellow clinically, only rarely is the infiltrate as foamy as in a xanthoma.

Benign Cephalic Histiocytosis
(GIANOTTI et al. 1971)

Definition. Eruption of multiple small papules primarily on the cheeks of children.

Clinical Findings. Patients with this very rare disorder are typically children 2–3 years of age. They develop multiple yellow to red-brown papules, concentrated on their cheeks and forehead. The papules are often relatively flat. While other body sites such as the trunk or upper aspects of the arms can be involved, the bulk of lesions must be on the head. The lesions are asymptomatic and heal spontaneously over 2–5 years, often leaving small fine scars. No systemic or mucosal involvement has been described.

Histopathology. Microscopic examination reveals a relatively monotonous infiltrate of vacuolated or ground-glass histiocytes, usually in a perivascular pattern. Giant cells and eosinophils are uncommon. The cells stain with macrophage markers and lack Langerhans cell markers. Comma bodies are a possible electron microscopic clue, as they are especially common in this disorder. Occasional patients may clinically fit a diagnosis of benign cephalic histiocytosis but have many S100-positive cells. The disease in these patients is best interpreted as a self-healing papular variant of LCH.

Differential Diagnosis. Lesions are often confused with plane warts, but a biopsy is definitive. When nodular lesions or many noncephalic lesions are present, one is confronted with an overlap between multiple juvenile xanthogranulomas or generalized eruptive histiocytomas.

Therapy. None is effective, but fortunately none is necessary.

Generalized Eruptive Histiocytomas
(WINKELMANN and MULLER 1963)

Definition. Very rare, rapidly appearing, often self-healing disseminated papular histiocytosis.

Clinical Findings. Patients with generalized eruptive histiocytomas by definition have multiple lesions that appear relatively suddenly in crops. Typically hundreds of small red-brown papules appear on the trunk, face and proximal aspects of the extremities. Mucosal involvement may be seen. In most cases the lesions persist for months to years and then spontaneously disappear.

Generalized eruptive histiocytomas probably do not represent a single disease. The disease in some patients may represent an early or eruptive phase of multicentric reticulohistiocytosis, progressive nodular histiocytomas, xanthoma disseminatum, or multiple xanthogranulomas. In addition, the course of generalized eruptive histiocytoma may wax and wane with an underlying disease process or appear as a possible paraneoplastic marker. Nonetheless, the majority of patients are completely healthy.

Histopathology. There is a monomorphous vacuolated or round cell infiltrate. Macrophage markers are positive and Langerhans cell markers, negative. If giant cells, foamy cells or oncocytic cells are seen, then the disease must be reclassified as above.

Differential Diagnosis. All the various papular forms of histiocytoses must be considered, as well as urticaria pigmentosa, and a long list of papular dermatoses, since the disease may present so suddenly.

Therapy. None is available.

Xanthoma Disseminatum

(Ausset 1899; Montgomery and Osterberg 1938)

Synonym. Montgomery syndrome

Definition. Normolipemic, sporadic disorder with diffuse xanthomas in a clinically typical pattern as well as frequent oral mucosal involvement and diabetes insipidus.

Clinical Findings. Most patients begin to show manifestations of their disease between the ages 5 and 25 years. Initially they develop numerous red-brown papules that coalesce into nodules and plaques. The lesions are typically located in the flexural areas, such as the axillae and groin, as well the face, especially eyelids, and side of the neck (Fig. 64.8). The most common sites for the initial lesions are the eyelids. While most lesions are red-brown, some may become yellow. The facial lesions may be quite disfiguring.

About 50% of patients have mucosal involvement. Most often there are numerous yellow papules involving the lips or buccal mucosa, but the entire mouth can be involved with extension into the pharynx or even larynx. Some patients even require a tracheotomy because of upper airway disease. The conjunctiva and even cornea may be involved, leading to blindness. In addition, about 40% of patients have diabetes insipidus, which has led to confusion between xanthoma disseminatum and Hand-Schüller-Christian disease. In xanthoma disseminatum the diabetes insipidus is usually mild, often transitory and results from either infiltration of the hypothalamic-pituitary axis by xanthomatous cells or pressure on the hypophysis from meningeal xanthomas. In LCH there is usually a destructive lesion of the sella.

While a long list of other internal lesions, such as osteolytic lesions, pulmonary infiltrates and CNS lesions (mainly meningeal xanthomas) have been described, they are rare. Bone marrow, kidney, pancreas, uterus, lymph nodes and liver involvement have also been described. About 20% of patients at some time in their disease course show elevated cholesterol or triglycerides. These changes are transitory and unexplained. No familial lipoprotein or similar abnormalities have been identified.

In xanthosiderohistiocytosis, the skin is more diffusely infiltrated by foam cells that extend into the subcutaneous fat and muscle, producing a scleroderma-like pattern.

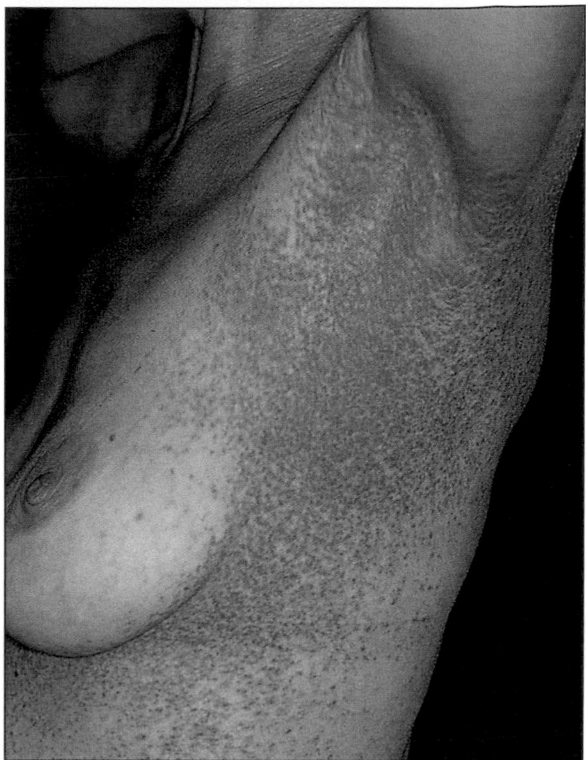

Fig. 64.8. Typical flexural involvement of xanthoma disseminatum

The skin lesions may appear sclerotic. Clinically similar cases have been described as disseminated dermal dendrocytomas. Caputo and colleagues suggest there are three clinical variants of xanthoma disseminatum.

- Self-healing form: Uncommon, with spontaneous resolution after a few years.
- Persistent form: Most common, facial disfigurement and mucosal damage may persist forever.
- Progressive form: Extremely rare. Five of the approximately 100 reported cases have had multi-organ involvement.

Histopathology. The early lesions have few if any foamy cells, but occasional scalloped histiocytes. The infiltrate may be quite mixed, containing eosinophils, neutrophils and lymphocytes as well. Later lesions are predominantly foamy and often cannot be separated from true xanthomas. They may contain Touton giant cells. Once again, no Birbeck granules are found and the histiocytes show macrophage markers, not S100 or CD1a.

Differential Diagnosis. There are overlaps among the different non-Langerhans cell histiocytoses, but one is entering a world of semantics, not science. The typical patient with flexural disease, oral mucosal disease and diabetes insipidus is unmistakable. When patients have multiple xanthomas, but not other findings and are normolipemic, then one speaks of multiple papular xanthomas. Multiple juvenile xanthogranulomas are not foamy. Multicentric reticulohistiocytosis may initially appear similar but has more acral cutaneous lesions and usually arthritis. LCH is excluded by immunohistochemistry and true xanthomas by blood lipid studies.

Therapy. There is no good therapy for this distressing condition. The diabetes insipidus can be treated with vasopressin or desmopressin products, usually as nasal sprays. The ocular and airway problems may require surgical intervention. Antimetabolites and lipid-lowering agents have been disappointing.

Papular Xanthoma

(Winkelmann et al. 1980)

Definition. Normolipemic xanthomas that appear singly or in groups but without an obvious histiocytic phase.

Clinical Findings. Patients may present with one, several or a large number of cutaneous nodules. Mucosal involvement has also been reported. The lesions may sometimes have a yellowish hue, suggesting that they contain lipids. Both children and adults are affected. Systemic abnormalities are not present and the patients are normolipemic. In most patients, the disease tends to regress after a number of years. Two possible variants are:

- Eruptive normolipemic xanthomas: These patients suddenly develop multiple lesions, analogous to the eruptive xanthomas associated with lipid abnormalities. The acral predilection of true eruptive xanthomas has not been reported.
- Diffuse papular xanthomas: These are associated with inflammatory skin diseases such as atopic dermatitis or even mycosis fungoides, as well as with chronic actinic dermatitis.

Histopathology. Clearly the original definition offered by Winkelmann is theoretically impossible. The primary cells are macrophages, as immunohistochemistry shows. However, they tend to rapidly phagocytose lipids and even in early lesions appear as foamy cells. Later giant cells may also be seen.

Therapy. Individual lesions can be excised.

Reticulohistiocytoma

(Caro and Senear 1952)

Synonyms. Reticulohistiocytic granuloma, giant cell histiocytoma

Definition. Solitary nodule clinically identical to juvenile xanthogranuloma but occurring in adults.

Clinical Findings. Usually a solitary hard brown nodules is present. The lesions range in size from 0.5 to 2.0 cm. The most common sites are the head and the distal aspects of the extremities, but any part of the body may be involved. Spontaneous resolution may occur. While several lesions may be present, decidedly unusual are multiple reticulohistiocytomas without evidence of systemic disease – that is, a separate disorder from multicentric reticulohistiocytosis.

Histopathology. Microscopic examination reveals a diffuse dermal infiltrate of multinucleated giant cells with abundant ground-glass cytoplasm. While these cells have been designated as oncocytic, they are not in any way related to the true oncocytes of various internal organs. An oncocyte is a large acidophilic cell rich in mitochondria. The histologic pattern is similar to that seen in multicentric reticulohistiocytosis but there may be subtle differences as discussed under that heading.

Differential Diagnosis. The potential list for solitary red-brown nodules is long. Dermatofibroma, mast cell tumor and juvenile xanthogranuloma must be considered. In our view a reticulohistiocytoma is a variant of juvenile xanthogranuloma in adults. There are frequently individual lesions that show overlaps between the two classic histologic patterns.

Therapy. Surgical excision

Multicentric Reticulohistiocytosis

(Targett 1897; Goltz and Laymon 1954)

Synonym. Lipoid dermatoarthritis

Definition. Very rare disorder with multiple cutaneous nodules, destructive arthritis and frequent association with systemic illnesses.

Epidemiology. The disease is much more common in women than men with about a 3:1 ratio. Most patients are adults, with an average age of onset of 45 years.

Clinical Findings

Cutaneous Findings. The primary lesions are small red-brown papules that may slowly both increase in size and coalesce. Even the larger lesions do not ulcerate, although they may develop a fine scale, which is unusual for histiocytic lesions in general. Both spontaneous remissions and recurrence of individual lesions are seen. The most typical locations are the hands, ears, lips and nares. The facial lesions may be so extreme as to produce a leonine facies. Multiple tiny papules along the nailfold are typical; this has been called the coral bead sign. The nailfold involvement frequently leads to longitudinal ridging, as well as hyperpigmentation. Intraoral lesions are uncommon except for the lips. For unexplained reasons, about one-third of patients have xanthelasmas.

Systemic Findings. The most common and reliable feature is the arthritis, which may be severe and destructive. In about half the patients, the joint pain and swelling is the first sign and in another third, it accompanies the cutaneous changes. The acute inflammatory arthritis may last for a number of years. Younger patients are more likely to develop destructive changes, such as the "opera glass" or "telescope" fingers when the interphalangeal joints are destroyed. The most typical sites of involvement are the hands, knees and shoulders, but the spine and pelvis can also be affected. Radiologic examination reveals rarefaction of bones as well as joint destruction, especially of the hands. Synovial fluid from the swollen joints may be bland or may be rich in neutrophils, while synovial biopsy reliably yields typical ground-glass giant cells.

A long list of other organs have been described as involved in rare instances, but their association with multicentric reticulohistiocytosis is unclear. The same giant cells have been found in virtually every organ, including the lungs, pleura, bone marrow, eye and muscles but no reproducible pattern is seen.

On the other hand, the association with systemic diseases of other types, especially immunologic disorders and malignancies, is about 25%. The list of associated diseases includes lupus erythematosus, primary biliary cirrhosis, dermatomyositis, Sjögren syndrome, systemic vasculitis and paraproteinemia. Tumors that have been identified include carcinomas of the colon, bronchi, breast, cervix and stomach, as well as a scattering of sarcomas, mesotheliomas and lymphomas. In 75% of cases, the multicentric reticulohistiocytosis is diagnosed first; in 25%, the tumor appears first.

Histopathology. Microscopic examination reveals an infiltrate of ground-glass multinucleated giant cells quite similar to that in reticulohistiocytoma. The macrophages have an eosinophilic homogeneous cytoplasm. Early lesions usually contain an associated lymphocytic infiltrate, while later lesions show fibrosis. A variety of phospholipids and neutral fats can be identified in the cells with special stains or electron microscopy; this led to the old name of lipoid dermatoarthritis. The same cells are seen in the synovia and occasionally in other organs. Morphologically, there may be differences between the giant cells in reticulohistiocytoma and multicentric reticulohistiocytosis, but they are subtle.

Laboratory Findings. Reflecting the increased incidence of xanthelasmas and the uptake of lipids in the giant cells, serum cholesterol levels are often elevated. The erythrocyte sedimentation rate is typically increased. Rheumatoid factor is negative and there are no specific tests that help in the diagnosis. Most of the associated diseases are diagnosed via laboratory testing.

Differential Diagnosis. The skin lesions are relatively specific. Early lesions of course may initially be identified as reticulohistiocytoma in the absence of arthritis. Sometimes granuloma annulare is also diagnosed, but the correct answer soon becomes apparent. When the patient presents with arthritis alone, the diagnosis is much more difficult. Rheumatoid arthritis may appear quite similar. Large nodules on the hands associated with joint pain can be confusing, but the histology should help. Gout, osteoarthritis and sarcoidosis may also be suggested.

In younger patients, Francois syndrome (familial dermochondrocorneal dystrophy), familial histiocytic dermatoarthritis and Farber syndrome (Chap. 38) may combine arthritis with skin nodules, but all three are even rarer than multicentric reticulohistiocytosis.

Therapy. In recent years, aggressive therapy of the arthritis has led to an apparent reduction in the destructive nature of the disease. Low-dose systemic corticosteroids, perhaps combined with antimalarials, seem to be the most reasonable starting point. Nonsteroidal antiinflammatory drugs appear to offer little. If joint destruction is marked or pain extreme, then a cytotoxic drug should be added or used alone. All alkylating agents, such as cyclophosphamide or chlorambucil, appear about as effective, but because of the rarity of multicentric reticulohistiocytosis, no controlled studies have been carried out. Individual skin lesions can be excised or treated with intralesional corticosteroids.

Progressive Nodular Histiocytosis

(Robinson et al. 1963)

Synonyms. Progressive nodular histiocytomas, multiple lipoidal histiocytomas

Definition. Multiple cutaneous nodules of two distinct types – superficial and deep – in patients without systemic disease.

Clinical Findings. Patients with progressive nodular histiocytosis are clinically distinct. They have hundreds of red-brown nodules of two distinct types. There are small superficial flat papules or nodules, as well as deeper larger tumors. The latter tend to have overlying telangiectases. They may become painful, usually because of hemorrhage or necrosis. A leonine facies may develop. No other systemic findings have been reported.

Histopathology. The superficial lesions are usually xanthomatous, containing foamy cells and giant cells. They tend to have an epidermal collarette. The deeper lesions are spindle cell xanthogranulomas, as described above. Thus, progressive nodular histiocytosis may well be viewed as a variant of multiple xanthogranulomas. A variant in which the tumors contain mucin has been described.

Differential Diagnosis. Most of the disorders discussed in this chapter may appear similar. Progressive mucinous histiocytosis (Bork and Hoede 1988) may be a variant. The presence of two distinct types of cutaneous lesions is the defining characteristic, along with the absence of systemic involvement.

Therapy. The disease is so rare that no therapy can be considered established. In a single case, both electron beam therapy and vinblastine seemed helpful. Individual deep lesions may become painful from hemorrhage; they can be easily excised.

Malignant Histiocytic Disorders

A number of diseases have been described that could fit in this category. Most if not all of them have turned out to be variations on malignant lymphoma and no longer belong in this section.

The problems with malignant LCH have been discussed above. There are solitary tumors for example involving the lymph nodes or gastrointestinal tract that are composed of histologically atypical dendritic cells. Rarely such tumors have been described in the skin. LCH itself occupies a puzzling position. Clonality studies suggest it is a neoplasm but the course is highly variable. Individual cases of LCH with cytologic atypia and a poor course have been described, but it is unclear if such patients can reliably be identified prospectively.

Malignant histiocytosis or histiocytic medullary reticulosis (Scott and Robb-Smith 1939) is almost always a T cell lymphoma. The best-established examples of true malignancy are childhood malignant histiocytosis with the 5q35 gene rearrangement and malignant hemophagocytic histiocytosis. True histiocytic lymphomas do occur, but the more lymphomas are studied, the rarer these tumors have become. Almost all cases of cytophagic histiocytic panniculitis and atypical regressing histiocytosis, two malignant histiocytoses added to the list in the 1980s, have been reclassified as T cell lymphomas. The only undisputed members of this family are the myelomonocytic and monocytic leukemias which may have skin involvement. In all cases, the diagnosis hinges on identifying a malignant tumor, either involving multiple organs or lymph nodes, that lacks both T and B cell markers but has macrophage markers. All these disorders are discussed in the chapters on lymphoma and leukemia, respectively.

Bibliography

Reviews and Basic Science Aspects

Birbeck MS, Breathnach AS, Everall JD (1961) An electron microscopic study of basal melanocyte and high level clear cell (Langerhans cell). J Invest Dermatol 37:51–63

Burg G, Braun-Falco O (1983) Cutaneous lymphomas, pseudolymphomas, and related disorders. Springer Berlin

Caputo R (1998) Text and atlas of histiocytic syndromes. A dermatological perspective. Martin Dunitz, London
Gianotti F, Caputo R (1985) Histiocytic syndromes: a review. J Am Acad Dermatol 13:383–404
Snow JL, Su WPD (1995) Histiocytic diseases. J Am Acad Dermatol 33:111–116
Winkelmann RK (1981) Cutaneous syndromes of non-X histiocytosis. A review of the macrophage-histiocyte diseases of the skin. Arch Dermatol 117:667–672
Wood GS, Haber RS (1993) Novel histiocytoses considered in the context of histiocyte subset differentiation (editorial). Arch Dermatol 129:210–214

Langerhans Cell Histiocytosis

Grosshans E, Illy G (1984) Thalidomide therapy for inflammatory dermatoses. Int J Dermatol 23:598–602
Helm KF, Lookingbill DP, Marks JG (1993) A clinical and pathologic study of histiocytosis X in adults. J Am Acad Dermatol 29:166–170
Kwong YL, Chan AC, Chan TK (1997) Widespread skin-limited Langerhans cell histiocytosis: complete remission with interferon alfa. J Am Acad Dermatol 36:628–629
Lichtenstein L (1953) Histiocytosis X. Integration of eosinophilic granuloma of bones, "Letterer-Siwe-disease" as related manifestations of a single nosologic entity. Arch Pathol 56:84–102
Mejia R, Dano JA, Roberts R et al. (1997) Langerhans' cell histiocytosis in adults. J Am Acad Dermatol 37:314–317
Papa CA, Pride HB, Tyler WB et al. (1997) Langerhans cell histiocytosis mimicking child abuse. J Am Acad Dermatol 37:1002–1004
Thomas L, Ducros B, Secchi T et al. (1993) Successful treatment of adult's Langerhans cell histiocytosis with thalidomide. Report of two cases and literature review. Arch Dermatol 129:1261–1264
Yu RC, Chu AC (1996) Langerhans cell histiocytosis clinicopathological reappraisal and human leukocyte antigen association. Br J Dermatol 135:36–41

Congenital Self-Healing Reticulohistiocytosis

Bernstein EF, Resnik KS, Loose JH et al. (1993) Solitary congenital selfhealing reticulohistiocytosis. Br J Dermatol 129:449–454
Bonifazi E, Caputo R, Ceci A et al. (1982) Congenital self-healing histiocytosis. Arch Dermatol 118:267–272
Hashimoto K, Pritzker MS (1973) Electron microscopic study of reticulohistiocytoma. An unusual case of congenital self-healing reticulohistiocytosis. Arch Dermatol 107:263–270
Hashimoto K, Bale GF, Hawkins HK (1986) Congenital self-healing reticulohistiocytosis (Hashimoto-Pritzker type). Int J Dermatol 25:516–523

Indeterminate Cell Histiocytosis

Contreras F, Fonseca E, Gamallo C et al. (1990) Multiple self-healing indeterminate cell lesions of the skin in an adult. Am J Dermatopathol 12:396–401
Levisohn D, Seidel D, Phelps A et al. (1993) Solitary congenital indeterminate cell histiocytoma. Arch Dermatol 129:81–85
Sidoroff A, Zelger B, Steiner H et al. (1996) Indeterminate cell histiocytosis – a clinicopathological entity with features of both X- and non-X histiocytosis. Br J Dermatol 134:525–532
Wood GS, Hu CH, Beckstead JH et al. (1985) The indeterminate cell proliferative disorder: report of a case manifesting as an unusual cutaneous histiocytosis. J Dermatol Surg Oncol 11:1111–1119

Sinus Histiocytosis with Massive Lymphadenopathy

Annessi G, Giannetti A (1996) Purely cutaneous Rosai-Dorfman disease. Br J Dermatol 134:749–753
Destombes P (1965) Adénite avec surcharge lipidique de l'enfant ou de l'adulte jeune, observées aux Antilles et au Mali. Quatre observations. Bull Soc Pathol Exot Filiales 58:1169–1182
Foucar E, Rosai J, Dorfman RF (1988) Sinus histiocytosis with massive lymphadenopathy (Rosai-Dorfman disease). Semin Diagn Pathol 7:74–82
Rosai J, Dorfman RF (1969) Sinus histiocytosis with massive lymphadenopathy. A newly recognized benign clinicopathological entity. Arch Pathol 87:63–70
Scheel MM, Rady PL, Tyring SK et al. (1997) Sinus histiocytosis with massive lymphadenopathy: presentation as giant granuloma annulare and detection of human herpesvirus 6. J Am Acad Dermatol 37:643–646

Juvenile Xanthogranuloma

Caputo R, Grimalt R, Gelmetti C et al. (1993) Unusual aspects of juvenile xanthogranuloma. J Am Acad Dermatol 29:868–870
Caputo R, Cambiaghi S, Brussasco A et al. (1998) Uncommon clinical presentations of juvenile xanthogranuloma. Dermatology 197:45–47
Cohen BA, Hood A (1989) Xanthogranuloma: report on clinical and histologic findings in 64 patients. Pediatr Dermatol 6:262–266
Hernadez Martin A, Baselga E, Drolet BA et al. (1997) Juvenile xanthogranuloma. J Am Acad Dermatol 36: 355–367
Kolde G, Bonsmann G (1992) Generalized lichenoid juvenile xanthogranuloma. Br J Dermatol 126:66–70
McDonagh JER (1912) A contribution to our knowledge of the naevoxantho-endotheliomata. Br J Dermatol 24:85–99
Morier P, Mérot Y, Paccaud D et al. (1990) Juvenile chronic granulocytic leukemia, juvenile xanthogranulomas, and neurofibromatosis. J Am Acad Dermatol 22:962–965
Tan HH, Tay YK (1998) Juvenile xanthogranuloma and neurofibromatosis 1. Dermatology 197:43–44
Yamashita JT, Rotta O, Michalany NS et al. (1990) Xanthogranulome juvénile du majeur chez un nourrisson. Ann Dermatol Venereol 117:295–296
Zelger BG, Zelger B, Steiner H et al. (1995) Solitary giant xanthogranuloma and benign cephalic histiocytosis – variants of juvenile xanthogranuloma. Br J Dermatol 133:598–604
Zvunov A, Barak Y, Metzker A (1995) Juvenile xanthogranuloma, neurofibromatosis, and juvenile chronic myelogenous leukemia. World statistical analysis. Arch Dermatol 131:904–908

Benign Cephalic Histiocytosis

Gianotti F, Caputo R, Ermacora E (1971) Singulière histiocytose infantile à cellules avec particules vermiformes intracytoplasmiques. Bull Soc Fr Dermatol Syphiligr 78:232–233

Gianotti R, Alessi E, Caputo R (1993) Benign cephalic histiocytosis: a distinct entity or a part of a wide spectrum of histiocytic proliferative disorders of children? A histopathological study. Am J Dermatopathol 15:315–319

Larralde de Luna M, Glikin I, Golberg J et al. (1989) Benign cephalic histiocytosis: report of four cases. Pediatr Dermatol 3:198–201

Generalized Eruptive Histiocytomas

Caputo R, Ermacora E, Gelmetti C et al. (1987) Generalized eruptive histiocytoma in children. J Am Acad Dermatol 17:449–454

Repiso T, Roca Miralles M, Kanitakis J et al. (1995) Generalized eruptive histiocytoma evolving into xanthoma disseminatum in a 4-year-old boy. Br J Dermatol 132:978–982

Stables Gl, Mackie RM (1992) Generalized eruptive histiocytoma. Br J Dermatol 126:196–199

Umbert I, Winkelmann RK (1989) Eruptive histiocytoma. J Am Acad Dermatol 20:958–964

Winkelmann RK, Muller SA (1963) Generalized eruptive histiocytoma: a benign papular histiocytic reticulosis. Arch Dermatol 88:586–597

Xanthoma Disseminatum

Bergman R, Kasif Y, Aviram M et al. (1996) Normolipidemic xanthelasma palpebrarum: lipid composition, cholesterol metabolism in monocyte-derived macrophages, and plasma lipid peroxidation. Acta Derm Venereol (Stockh) 76:107–110

Braun-Falco O, Braun-Falco F (1957) Zum Syndrom "Diabetes insipidus und disseminierte Xanthoma". Gleichzeitig ein histochemischer Beitrag zur Natur der gespeicherten Fettsubstanzen. Z Laryngol Rhinol Otol 36:378–387

Buezo GF, Porras JI, Fraga J et al. (1996) Coexistence of diffuse plane normolipaemic xanthoma and amyloidosis in a patient with monoclonal gammopathy. Br J Dermatol 135:460–462

Caputo R, Veraldi S, Grimalt R et al. (1995) The various clinical patterns of xanthoma disseminatum. Dermatology 190:19–24

Montgomery H, Osterberg AE (1938) Xanthomatosis: correlation of clinical, histopathologic and chemical studies of cutaneous xanthoma. Arch Dermatol Syphil 37: 372–402

Papular Xanthoma

Chen CG, Chen CL, Liu HN (1997) Primary papular xanthoma of children: a clinicopathologic, immunohistopathologic and ultrastructural study. Am J Dermatopathol 19:596–601

Goerdt S, Kretzschmar L, Bonsmann G et al. (1995) Normolipemic papular xanthomatosis in erythrodermic atopic dermatitis. J Am Acad Dermatol 32: 326–333

Winkelmann RK; Kossasrd S, Fraga S (1980) Eruptive histiocytoma of childhood. Arch Dermatol 116:565–570

Reticulohistiocytoma

Bauer A, Garbe C, Detmar M et al. (1994) Multizentrische Retikulohistiozytose und myelodysplastisches Syndrom. Hautarzt 45:91–96

Caro MR, Senear PE (1952) Reticulohistiocytoma of the skin. Arch Dermatol 65:701–713

Fedler R, Frantzmann Y, Schwarze EW et al. (1995) Die multizentrische Retikulohistiozytose. Therapie mit Azathioprin und Prednisolon. Hautarzt 46:118–120

Zelger B, Cerio R, Soyer HP et al. (1994) Reticulohistiocytoma and multicentric reticulohistiocytosis. Histopathologic and immunophenotypic distinct entities. Am J Dermatopathol 16:577–584

Multicentric Reticulohistiocytosis

Franck N, Amor B, Ayral X et al. (1995) Multicentric reticulohistiocytosis and methotrexate. J Am Acad Dermatol 33:524–525

Ginsburg WW, O'Duffy JD, Morris JL et al. (1989) Multicentric reticulohistiocytosis: response to alkylating agents in 6 patients. Ann Intern Med 111:384–388

Goltz RW, Laymon CW (1954) Multicentric reticulohistiocytosis of the skin and synovia. Arch Dermatol 69: 717–731

Olivier GF, Umbert I, Winkelmann RK et al. (1990) Reticulohistiocytoma cutis – review of 15 cases and an association with systemic vasculitis in two cases. Clin Exp Dermatol 15:1–6

Snow JL, Muller SA (1995) Malignancy-associated multicentric reticulohistiocytosis: a clinical, histological and immunophenotypic study. Br J Dermatol 133:71–76

Toporcer MB, Kantor GR, Benedetto AV (1991) Multiple cutaneous reticulohistiocytomas (reticulohistiocytic granulomas). J Am Acad Dermatol 25:948–951

Progressive Nodular Histiocytosis

Bork K, Hoede N (1988) Hereditary progessive mucinous histiocytosis in women. Arch Dermatol 124:1225–1229

Burgdorf WH, Kusch SL, Nix TE Jr et al. (1981) Progressive nodular histiocytoma. Arch Dermatol 117:644–649

Robinson HM Jr, Harmon LE (1963) Multiple lipoidal histiocytomas with regression. Arch Dermatol 88:660–667

Taunton OD, Yeshurun D, Jarrat M (1978) Progressive nodular histiocytoma. Arch Dermatol 114:1505–1508

Malignant Histiocytic Disorders

Egeler RM, Schmitz L, Sonneveld P et al. (1995) Malignant histiocytosis: a reassessment of cases formerly classified as histiocytic neoplasms and review of the literature. Med Pediatr Oncol 25:1–7

Levine EG, Hanson CA, Jaszcz W (1991) True histiocytic lymphoma. Semin Oncol 18:39–49

CHAPTER 65

Paraneoplastic Markers and Syndromes

Contents

Introduction

Paraneoplasia infers an association with malignancy. There are a number of syndromes familiar to dermatologists in which the patients have a higher risk of developing internal malignancies. These are summarized in Tables 65.1 and 65.2. Most of these syndromes have been discussed elsewhere in the text and are cross-referenced. The others are described in this chapter.

There are several genodermatoses which could be considered paraneoplastic. For example, many immunodeficiency disorders (Chap. 4) tend to have a much higher risk for hematologic malignancies. Some readers may miss xeroderma pigmentosum, but these unfortunate patients (Chap. 13) rarely develop systemic tumors, only cutaneous ones. Similarly, in both neurofibromatosis and tuberous sclerosis, there are a wide variety of systemic tumors, but they tend to be benign. We have attempted only to highlight some of the more fascinating examples and not to present an exhaustive list.

Probably of more interest to the practicing dermatologist are acquired cutaneous signs of internal malignancy. These are listed in Table 65.3 and only those not covered in detail elsewhere in the text are expanded upon.

Cancer-Associated Genodermatoses

There are three basic mechanisms by which a mutation can lead to a cancer-associated syndrome. There may be mutations in a tumor suppressor gene (Gardner syndrome), in a growth control gene (MEN 2B) or in a DNA repair gene (Muir-Torre syndrome). Each is discussed below. Unifying clinical features include appearance of tumors at an earlier age, often multiple tumors and a generally better survival chance than patients with solitary tumors. In addition, often the same mutation is found in sporadic tumors as in those associated with a syndrome. In almost all cases the cutaneous manifestations appear first, allowing an earlier diagnosis and better monitoring. Information on prenatal diagnosis changes constantly and we do not attempt to present more than an overview in Chap. 19.

Cowden Syndrome

(Lloyd and Dennis 1963)

Synonym. Multiple hamartoma syndrome (Weary et al. 1972)

Etiology and Pathogenesis. The gene for Cowden syndrome is located on chromosome 10q22-q23 and is known as PTEN (a phosphatase designated "ten" which is involved in tumor suppression). The disease is inherited in an autosomal dominant pattern. Several other overlapping syndromes are also caused by PTEN mutations:

- Riley-Smith syndrome: Macrocephaly, pseudopapilledema, hemangiomas.
- Bannayan-Zonana syndrome: Macrocephaly, pseudopapilledema, hemangiomas, lipomas, lymphangioma, meningioma.
- Ruvalcaba-Myhre-Smith syndrome: Macrocephaly, intestinal polyps, lipomas, acanthosis nigricans and penile melanotic macules; known in American slang as "speckled pecker" syndrome.
- Sotos syndrome: Large body size, mental retardation.

Table 65.1. Autosomal dominant tumor-associated genodermatoses

Syndrome	Cutaneous lesions	Systemic malignancies	Frequency of malignancies	Gene	Function	Chapter
Nevoid basal cell carcinoma	Multiple basal cell carcinomas, palmar pits	Medulloblastoma	~20%	PTCH, 9q22.3	Growth control	57
Carney	Lentigines, blue nevi, myxomas	Cardiac myxomas, testes, breast	>75%	2p16		58
Cowden	Trichilemmomas, oral and acral papules	Breast, thyroid, gastrointestinal tract	70%	PTEN, 10q22-q23	Growth control	
Gardner	Cysts, fibromas	Colon	100%	APC, 5q21-q22	Tumor suppressor	
Multiple endocrine neoplasia 2B	Mucosal neuromas	Thyroid (medullary), pheochromocytoma	>85%	RET, 10q11.2	Growth control	
Peutz-Jeghers	Lentigines	Testes, ovaries, gastrointestinal tract	Uncommon	STK 11, 1p36-p34	Growth control	58
Muir-Torre	Sebaceous tumors, keratoacanthomas	Gastrointestinal tract, lung, urogenital system	100%	Several genes at various sites	DNA mismatch repair	
Howel-Evans	Keratoderma, leukoplakia	Esophagus	100%	TOC, 17q23-qter	Unknown	17
Birt-Hogg-Dubé	Fibrofolliculomas, trichodiscomas	Kidney, thyroid gastrointestinal tract	?	?	?	
Dysplastic nevus syndrome	Multiple atypical melanocytic nevi	Eye, ?testes	Uncommon	?	?	58

Table 65.2. Autosomal recessive tumor-associated genodermatoses

Syndrome	Cutaneous lesions	Systemic malignancies	Frequency of malignancies	Gene	Function	Chapter
Bloom	Telangiectases, photosensitivity	Leukemia, lymphoma, gastrointestinal tract	Very high in those who reach adult life	BLM, 5q31	?	22
Ataxia-telangiectasia	Telangiectases	Leukemia, lymphoma, breast	Very high in those who reach adult life	ATM, 11q22-q23	Signal transduction	22
Dyskeratosis congenita	Dyspigmentation, leukoplakia, nail dystrophy	Squamous cell carcinoma, aplastic anemia	Very high in those who reach adult life	Xq28	?	18
Fanconi anemia	Dyspigmentation	Leukemia, lymphoma, ?? squamous cell carcinoma	Very high in those who reach adult life	UPRT, Xq26	DNA repair	18
Chédiak-Higashi	Hypopigmentation	Lymphoma	Common	1q42-q44, 10q2		26
Werner	Premature aging	Carcinomas, sarcomas	~10%	8p12-p11		18

It should be clear from this list that all these syndromes are actually variants on the same theme, probably caused by mutations at different sites in the same or a series of closely linked genes.

Clinical Findings
Cutaneous Findings. Patients with Cowden syndrome have multiple verrucous facial papules which histologically have been diagnosed as trichilemmomas. There is some evidence that both sporadic trichilemmomas and those in Cowden syndrome may be caused by human papillomavirus. In addition, there are mucosal papules and condylomata as well as acral papules. A variety of other changes including hemangiomas, lipomas and ephelis-like lesions have been reported.

Systemic Findings. The main malignancies associated with Cowden syndrome are carcinoma of the breast and thyroid, as well as hamartomatous intestinal polyps which have a low risk of malignant conversion. The signal case, Rachel Cowden, had massive breast hypertrophy and died of breast cancer. Patients also have macrocephaly, learning disabilities and a peculiar hamartomatous cerebellar proliferation known as Lhermitte-Duclos syndrome.

Therapy. Since almost all women have at least fibrocystic changes and about 50% develop cancer, prophylactic mastectomy has been recommended.

Gardner Syndrome
(Gardner 1950)

Synonyms. Familial adenomatous polyposis, familial polyposis of the colon, adenomatous polyposis coli

Etiology and Pathogenesis. Gardner syndrome is a variant of familial adenomatous polyposis (FAP) with cutaneous findings. Familial adenomatous polyposis is caused by a classic tumor repressor gene APC located on chromosome 5q21–q22. A normal patient has two functioning APC genes in each cell; a patient with Gardner syndrome has but one. Thus, any sporadic mutation in this gene leaves a cell with impaired surveillance and the potential to clonally expand into a malignancy. Inheritance is in an autosomal dominant pattern. Gardner is a college zoology teacher at Utah State University, not a physician. He identified pedigrees with a high incidence of colon cancer among his students and has published on this disorder over the past 50 years.

Clinical Findings
Cutaneous Findings. The main cutaneous finding is multiple epidermoid cysts (Fig. 65.1), occasionally with pilomatricoma-like changes on microscopic examination.

Systemic Findings. The classic finding is multiple adenomatous polyps of the colon and rectum. If untreated, the lifetime risk of developing carcinoma of the colon is 100%. Polyps and then carcinomas may also develop in the stomach and small bowel. There is also an increased risk of hepatoblastoma, otherwise a very rare tumor. Another troubling problem is the growth of abdominal desmoids or fibrous tumors. These are particularly likely to arise after cesarean section or other abdominal surgery and may reach massive size. Although histologically benign, they are clinically malignant because they compress vital structures in the pelvis and abdomen.

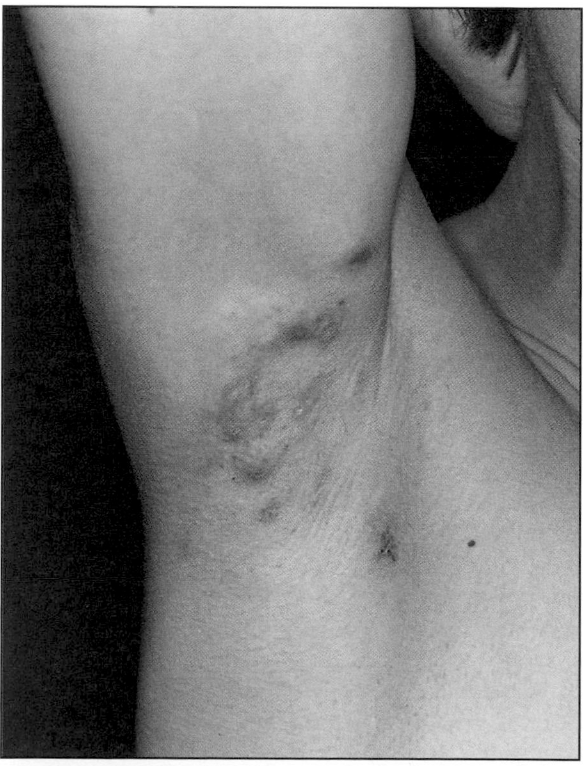

Fig. 65.1. Multiple epidemoid cysts in Gardner syndrome, mimic king acne inversa

Probably the earliest sign of Gardner syndrome is pigmented retinal lesions known as congenital hypertrophy of the retinal pigment epithelium (CHRPE). If bilateral dark retinal spots are identified in a patient at risk, the diagnosis is clinched. Unilateral lesions or a normal retina does not exclude the diagnosis. Most patients have osteomas of the jaws which can be occasionally seen as bulges through the skin and easily spotted on radiologic examination, such as a panoramic study.

Two syndromes show overlaps with Gardner syndrome:

- Oldfield syndrome (Oldfield 1954). These patients had gastrointestinal polyposis and true sebaceous cysts or steatocystomas (Chap. 54). No such patients have been identified in the intervening 60 years and the original family cannot be found, so the nature of this syndrome remains unclear.
- Turcot syndrome (Turcot 1959). Among patients with gastrointestinal polyps and CNS tumors, about half have a mutation in the APC gene and medulloblastomas. The rest, including Turcot's first patient, have mutations like that in Muir-Torre syndrome and glioblastomas.

Therapy. Once the diagnosis is made, prophylactic colectomy and careful monitoring of extracolonic sites is required. Nonsteroidal antiinflammatory drugs seem to decrease the development of polyps and are often administered. Cutaneous lesions may be excised.

Multiple Endocrine Neoplasia Syndrome Type 2B

(Wagenmann 1922; Froeboese 1923; Gorlin et al. 1968)

Synonyms. Multiple mucosal neuroma syndrome. Multiple endocrine neoplasia syndrome type 2B (MEN 2B) has also been called MEN 3 but since it has been shown that MEN 2A and 2B are allelic, type 3 has been dropped. Sipple syndrome is a synonym for type 2A.

Etiology and Pathogenesis. The gene for both MEN 2A and MEN 2B is a growth control gene RET located on chromosome 10q11.2. It is one of the classic oncogenes, as a mutation leads to overproduction of a growth stimulating gene. The RET gene product is apparently most crucial in neuroendocrine tissue. Inheritance is in an autosomal dominant pattern.

Clinical Findings

Cutaneous Findings. The major cutaneous finding is the presence of multiple neuromas of the lips and oral cavity, as well as occasionally other mucosal surfaces. The "inverted lid" sign is often seen. Because of thickened nerves in the upper eyelids, the structure may spontaneously evert.

Systemic Findings. Many patients have a Marfanoid habitus. There is about an 85% risk of medullary thyroid carcinoma and a 50% chance of pheochromocytoma. The thyroid tumors may metastasize and are the main reason for a life expectancy of only 20 years. Intestinal ganglioneuromatosis, similar to Hirschsprung disease, leads to megacolon and constipation. Enlarged corneal nerves can be identified.

Differential Diagnosis. In addition to Marfan syndrome and its other mimics, one is often confronted with the possibility of other forms of MEN. Only type 2B has mucosal neuromas.

- MEN 1: Almost all patients have hyperparathyroidism with overlaps between adenomas and carcinomas, as well as functioning pituitary and pancreatic tumors. The gene is located at 11q13 and appears to be a tumor suppressor. Patients may have multiple angiofibromas and connective tissue nevi.
- MEN 2A (Sipple syndrome; Sipple 1961): Medullary thyroid carcinoma and pheochromocytoma are seen. Macular amyloidosis has been described in some pedigrees.

Therapy. The thyroid gland should be removed and replacement therapy instituted. Older recommendations to monitor calcitonin are inappropriate. If hypertension or other relevant symptoms develop, pheochromocytoma should be suspected.

Muir-Torre Syndrome

(Muir 1967; Torre 1968)

Etiology and Pathogenesis. In Muir-Torre syndrome, which is inherited in an autosomal dominant pattern, there are a series of mutations in a variety of DNA mismatch repair genes with "alphabet soup" names and different chromosomal locations.

The genes are the same as those involved in the cancer family syndrome (Warthin 1913; Lynch 1966) confirming Lynch's speculation that Muir-Torre syndrome is the cutaneous part of his syndrome. These genes repair mistakes in DNA replication prior to cell division. When they are defective, a characteristic cytogenetic change known as microsatellite instability occurs. It has been found in tumors from Muir-Torre syndrome patients and in similar sporadic tumors.

Clinical Findings

Cutaneous Findings. Patients have multiple sebaceous tumors and keratoacanthomas. The lesions are clinically very similar, most common on the face and probably arise from a common site where the sebaceous duct enters the hair follicle. They tend to be 1–2 cm in size, often delled or with a horny plug.

Systemic Findings. The most common tumors are those that are most common in the general population. Thus pulmonary, gastrointestinal and urogenital neoplasms are most often seen. They tend to appear at an early age, but be less aggressive than the same tumor in a normal host.

Therapy. Oral retinoids may possibly inhibit the develop of the cutaneous tumors. A clear risk:benefit assessment is not available.

Birt-Hogg-Dubé Syndrome

(Birt et al. 1977)

Synonyms. Hornstein-Knickenberg (Hornstein and Knickenberg 1975) syndrome, multiple fibrofolliculoma-trichodiscoma syndrome

Etiology and Pathogenesis. The genetic defect in Birt-Hogg-Dubé syndrome is unknown although the disease is inherited in an autosomal dominant pattern.

Clinical Findings

Cutaneous Findings. The patients have hundreds of tiny white papules most common on the face and chest. We have seen several patients where the lesions were mistaken for acne scars. On biopsy, a variety of adnexal tumors are found. In some instances, there is perifollicular fibrosis. These lesions are known as fibrofolliculomas or perifollicular fibromas. In other lesions, there is compact fibrosis in the upper dermis. Such lesions are known as trichodiscomas, but they have nothing to do with Felix Pinkus' hair disc and represent more extensive fibrosis. The site of action appears to be the mantle of the hair follicle from which sebaceous glands develop.

Systemic Findings. Birt-Hogg-Dubé syndrome is identified in about 20 % of the members of families with renal cell carcinoma. In the initial Canadian pedigree, there was an increase in thyroid cancer, while in the first German family, gastrointestinal cancer appeared increased. In other patients and families, only the cutaneous changes are present.

Cutaneous Markers for Internal Malignancy

There are many cutaneous signs of internal malignancy. They are outlined in detail in Table 65.3 and discussed in the relevant chapters. The ideal paraneoplastic marker is one that is only seen with a tumor, disappears when the tumor is treated and may reappear should a recurrence or metastasis occur. Few meet these criteria. Only those of special interest are briefly expanded upon here.

Acanthosis Nigricans

It is a common but false belief that acanthosis nigricans is a genetic marker of malignancy. While the skin changes are associated with many genetic disorders, in relation to malignancy they are almost always acquired. The disease is discussed in greater detail in Chapter 17.

Etiology and Pathogenesis. It seems clear that some sort of epidermal growth factor is involved, presumably made by a tumor. In some cases, levels of growth factors correlate well with stage of the primary tumor and severity of the acanthosis nigricans.

Clinical Findings

Cutaneous Findings. Darker areas such as the axillae, groin, perianal region, nipples and nape are most often affected. Hundreds of tiny dark papules create a velvety pattern. Clinically there are no clear differences between the cutaneous changes in the different settings where acanthosis nigricans is seen. On the lips, oral, genital and rectal mucosa,

Table 65.3. Cutaneous markers of malignancy

Marker	Skin findings	Underlying malignancy	Degree of association	Chapter
Acanthosis nigricans	Velvety papillomatous changes in flexural areas	Adenocarcinoma (two-thirds stomach)	~100% in adult-onset, non-obese patients	14
Florid cutaneous papillomatosis	Diffuse acanthosis nigricans-like changes	Same as acanthosis nigricans	~100%	
Leser-Trélat sign	Eruptive seborrheic keratoses	Same as acanthosis nigricans	~100%	54
Tripe palms	Thickened papillomatous palms and soles	Same as acanthosis nigricans	~100%	
Palmoplantar keratoderma	Thickened keratotic palms and soles	Carcinomas	Rare (when Howel-Evans and tripe palms are excluded)	17
Bazex acrokeratosis	Psoriasiform changes on fingers, toes, ears, nose	Carcinoma, often upper airway	~100%	
Acquired ichthyosis	Dry scaly skin	Hodgkin disease, occasionally other lymphomas or carcinomas	Common	17
Dermatomyositis	Gottron papules, heliotrope eyelids, photosensitivity	Carcinoma, often ovarian	~15% in adults	18
Digital ischemia	Raynaud phenomenon or gangrene, other signs of cryoglobulinemia	Carcinomas, hematologic malignancies	Uncommon	22
Erythema gyratum repens	Migrating erythema and scales in wood-grain pattern	Carcinomas, often with inappropriate polypeptide secretion	~100%	14
Erythema annulare centrifugum	Slowly expanding annular erythema	Carcinoma, Hodgkin disease, other lymphomas	Very rare	14
Erythroderma	Diffuse erythema with scale	Lymphomas, rarely carcinomas	~25%	14
Follicular mucinosis	Boggy nodules or plaques	Lymphomas	Often associated in adults	43
Flushing	Diffuse sudden erythema	Carcinoid tumors and rarely other tumors with inappropriate secretion	Common	14
Hyperpigmentation	Diffuse or localized darkening	Metastatic malignant melanoma, also with bronchial, thyroid and pancreatic tumors	Uncommon	26, 58
Hypertrichosis lanuginosa acquisita	Widespread lanugo hairs, red lingual papules	Carcinomas	~100%	31
Necrolytic migratory erythema	Periorificial and acral erythema and erosions	Glucagonoma, rarely pancreatic disease, other chronic diseases	~90% with malignancy	14
Pachydermoperiostosis (acquired form)	Thickened digits, periosteosis	Often lung carcinomas	Common	19
Panniculitis	Painful nodules, often not limited to legs (also fat necrosis)	Pancreatic carcinomas and pancreatitis	Uncommon	21
Paraneoplastic pemphigus	Mucosal erosions, cutaneous lesions that overlap between lichen planus, erythema multiforme and pemphigus vulgaris	Non-Hodgkin lymphoma, less often Castleman tumor, thymoma and others	~100%	15

Table 65.3 (continued)

Marker	Skin findings	Underlying malignancy	Degree of association	Chapter
Pruritus	Itching without cutaneous lesions	Many malignancies, especially Hodgkin disease	Uncommon	25
Pyoderma gangrenosum	Aggressive ulcers without a clear etiology	Gammopathies, usually IgA, other hematologic disorders	~10–20%	22
Sweet syndrome	Succulent red nodules and plaques	Leukemia, especially hairy cell type, other hematologic malignancies	Uncommon	14
Trousseau sign	Recurrent migratory thrombophlebitis	Carcinomas	~30–40%	22
Diffuse plane xanthomas	Broad sheets of tiny xanthomas	Gammopathy	~100%	37
Necrobiotic xanthogranuloma	Red-yellow nodules, almost always periorbital	Gammopathy	~100%	37
Zoster	Severe or generalized zoster in young adult	Lymphoma (HIV infection)	Uncommon	2

multiple grouped papules appear. They tend to follow the skin markings, yielding a bark-like pattern. Florid cutaneous papillomatosis, Leser-Trélat sign (eruptive seborrheic keratoses), and tripe palms are all variants on the same theme. While multiple acrochordons or skin tags are quite common, if they appear suddenly, they too may overlap with acanthosis nigricans. Florid oral papillomatosis is not related. It is instead a low-grade squamous cell carcinoma.

Systemic Findings. A wide variety of tumors have been associated with acanthosis nigricans, but adenocarcinoma of the stomach accounts for two-thirds of cases.

Paraneoplastic Acrokeratosis

(Bazex et al. 1965)

Synonyms. Acrokeratosis neoplastica, Bazex syndrome. The latter should be avoided since Bazex also described several other syndromes

Clinical Findings. Almost all patients are men. They develop dirty scaly hyperkeratotic patches on the fingers, toes, ears and nose (Fig. 65.2). In addition nail dystrophies may be seen. The underlying tumor is usually of the upper airway or esophagus. If the tumor is successfully treated, the changes tend to improve.

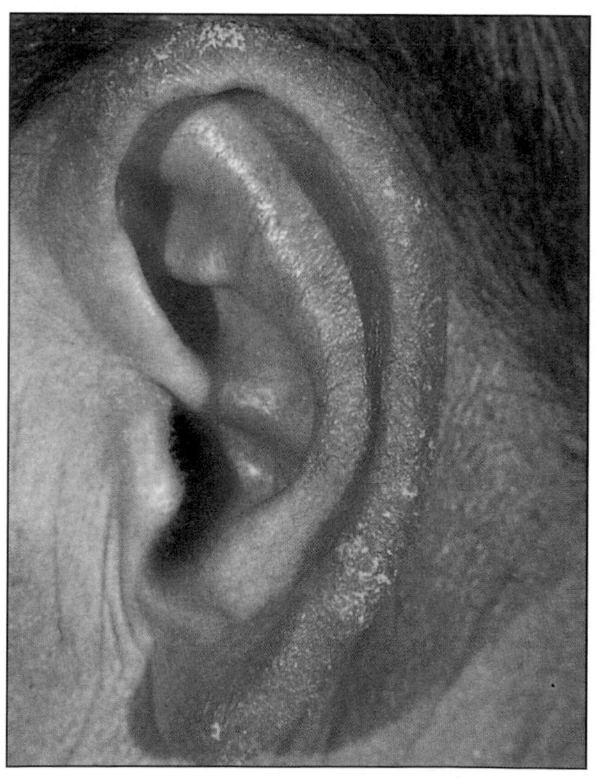

Fig. 65.2. Ear involvement in paraneoplastic acrokeratosis

Bibliography

General References

Andreev VC (1978) Skin manifestations of visceral cancer. Current problems in dermatology, vol 8. Karger, Basel

Burgdorf WH, Koester G (1992) Multiple cutaneous tumors: what do they mean? J Cutan Pathol 19:449–457

Braverman IM (1981) Skin signs of systemic disease, 2nd edn. Saunders, Philadelphia

Callen JP (1987) Skin signs of internal malignancy. Aust J Dermatol 28:106–114

Callen JP, Jorizzo JL (eds) (1995) Dermatological signs of internal disease, 2nd edn. Saunders, Philadelphia

Lynch HT, Fusaro RM (eds) (1982) Cancer-associated Genodermatoses. Van Nostrand Reinhold, New York

Poole, S, Fenske NA (1993) Cutaneous markers of internal malignancy. I. Malignant involvement of the skin and the genodermatoses. J Am Acad Dermatol 28:1–13

Worret WI (1993) Skin signs and internal malignancy. Int J Dermatol 32:1–5

Cowden Syndrome

Albrecht S, Haber RM, Goodman JC et al. (1992) Cowden syndrome and Lhermitter-Duclos disease. Cancer 70: 869–876

Chapman MS, Perry AE, Baughman RD (1998) Cowden's syndrome, Lhermitter-Duclos disease, and sclerotic fibroma. Am J Dermatopathol 20:413–416

DiLiberti JH (1998) Inherited macrocephaly-hamartoma syndromes. Am J Med Genet 79:284–290

Lloyd KM II, Dennis M (1963) Cowden's disease, a possible new symptom complex with multiple system involvement. Ann Intern Med 58:136–142

Perriard J, Saurat J-H, Harms M (2000) An overlap of Cowden's disease and Bannayan-Riley-Ruvalcaba syndrome in the same family. J Am Acad Dermatol 42:348–350

Weary PE, Gorlin RJ, Gentry WC (1972) Multiple hamartoma syndrome (Cowden's disease). Arch Dermatol 106:682

Gardner Syndrome

Gardner FJ, Stephens FE (1950) Cancer of the lower digestive track in one family group. Am J Hum Genet 2:41–48

Lynch PM (1999) Clinical challenges in management of familial adenomatous polyposis and hereditary nonpolyposis colorectal cancer. Cancer 86:1713–1719

Oldfield MC (1954) The association of familial polyposis of the colon with multiple sebaceous cysts. Brit J Surg 41:534–541

Perniciaro C (1995) Gardner's syndrome. Dermatol Clin 13:51–56

Turcot J et al. (1959) Malignant tumors of the central nervous system associated with familial polyposis of the colon. Dis Col Rectum 2465–2468

MEN Syndrome

Darling N, Skarulis MC, Steinberg SM et al. (1997) Multiple facial angiofibromas and collagenomas in patients with multiple endocrine neoplasia type 1. Arch Dermatol 133:853–857

Gorlin RJ, Sedano HO, Vickers RA et al. (1968) Multiple mucosal neuromas, pheochromocytoma, and medullary carcinoma of the thyroid: a syndrome. Cancer 22:293–299

Heath D (1998) Multiple endocrine neoplasia. J R Coll Physicians Lond 32:98–101

Heshmati HM, Hofbauer LC (1997) Multiple endocrine neoplasia type 2: recent progress in diagnosis and management. Eur J Endocrinol 137:572–578

Miller Ja, Norton JA (1997) Multiple endocrine neoplasia. Cancer Treat Res 90:213–225

Sipple JH (1961) The association of pheochromocytoma with carcinoma of the thyroid gland. Am J Med 31:163–166

Muir-Torre Syndrome

Cohen PR, Kohn SR, Davis DA et al. (1995) Muir-Torre syndrome. Dermatol Clin 13:79–89

Lynch HT, Shaw MW, Magnuson CW et al. (1966) hereditary factors in cancer. Study of two large midwestern kindreds. Arch Int Med 117:206–212

Muir EG, Bell AJY, Barlow KA (1967) Multiple primary carcinomata of the colon, duodenum, and larynx associated with kerato-acanthomata of the face. Br J Surg 54: 191–195

Rütten A, Burgdorf W, Hügel H et al. (1999) Cystic sebaceous tumors as marker lesions for the Muir-Torre syndrome: a histopathologic and molecular genetic study. Am J Dermatopathol 21:405–413

Schwartz RA, Torre DP (1995) The Muir-Torrre syndrome: a 25-year retrospect. J Am Acad Dermatol 33:90–104

Torre D (1968) Multiple sebaceous tumors. Arch Dermatol 98:549–551

Birt-Hogg-Dubé Syndrome

Birt AR, Hogg GR, Dubé WJ (1977) Hereditary mulitple fibrofolliculomas with trichodiscomas and acrochordons. Arch Dermatol 113:1674–1677

De la Torre C,Ocampo C, Doval IG et al. (1999) Acrochordons are not a component of the Birt-Hogg-Dubé syndrome: does this syndrome exist? Case reports and review of the literature. Am J Dermatopathol 21:369–374

Hornstein OP, Knickenberg M (1975) Perifollicular fibromatosis cutis with polyps of the colon – a cutaneo-intestinal syndrome sui generis. Arch Dermatol Res 253:161–175

Schulz T, Hartschuh W (1999) Birt-Hogg-Dubé syndrome and Hornstein-Knickenberg syndrome are the same. Different sectioning techniques as the cause of different histology. J Cutan Pathol 26:55–61

Toro JR, Glenn G, Duray P et al. (1999) Birt-Hogg-Dubé syndrome: a novel marker of kidney neoplasia. Arch Dermatol 135:1195–1202

Cutaneous Markers of Internal Malignancy

Bazex A et al. (1965) Syndrome para-néoplasique à type d'hyperkératose des extrémites. Guérison aprés le traitment de l'épithéliome larynge. Bull Soc Fr Derm Syph 72:182

de Boucaud JL (1904) Contribution à l'étude des naevi considérés comme un signe de malignité dans les tumeurs (Signe de Trélat). Thesis No. 118. Bordeaux, Faculté de Médecine et de Pharmacie de Bordeaux.

Leser E (1901) Ueber ein die Krebskrankheit beim Menschen häufig begleitendes, noch wenig bekanntes Symptom. München med Wchnschr 48:2035–2036

Poole, S, Fenske NA (1993) Cutaneous markers of internal malignancy. II. Paraneoplastic dermatoses and environmental carcinogens. J Am Acad Dermatol 28:147–164

Schwartz RA (1994) Acanthosis nigrans. J Am Acad Dermatol 31:1–19

Schwartz RA (1996) Sign of Leser-Trelat. J Am Acad Dermatol 35:88–95

Diseases of Black Skin

Roselyn E. Epps and John A. Kenney, Jr.

Contents

Introduction

Skin diseases in blacks and other peoples of color are often puzzling to physicians only experienced in diagnosing and treating white patients. The reasons for the problems are many. Many of the descriptions employed in dermatology, such as salmon-colored patches in pityriasis rubra pilaris or violaceous papules in lichen planus, are unintentionally racially exclusive, as the lesions almost never assume such colors in blacks. In addition, common skin diseases may be radically different in blacks. For example, pityriasis rosea in black patients is often acral, papular, pruritic and persistent – features only rarely seen in white patients. Some diseases are seen almost exclusively in blacks, such as dermatosis papulosa nigra. Others are more distressing to the patient because they are more easily seen, such as vitiligo. There are many physiologic variations that may confuse the uninformed observer. Finally, one must remember that many problems described as racial actually reflect availability of care, occupational patterns, economic status and other sociologic issues.

In this chapter we concentrate on the aspects of the various diseases that are most important when treating black patients. Almost all these topics are covered elsewhere in the text but with a different emphasis. This leads to some unavoidable repetition. Similar problems confront the physician treating Asian patients and other pigmented individuals such as Hispanics or Native Americans. Some of these problems are also alluded to in this chapter, as well as throughout this volume.

Anatomy of Black Skin

The structural differences between black and white skin are surprisingly small. The darker color results from different packaging and transfer of melanosomes, not from an increased number of melanocytes (Chap. 26). Eccrine, apocrine and sebaceous glands are similar in number and capacity. The hair shaft is quite different as it is elliptical in cross-section, and helical or spiral in configuration. This not only results in a different appearance, but hairs are more likely to exit the follicle improperly (ingrown hairs) or grow back into the skin (pseudofolliculitis barbae).

Pigmentary Changes

Normal Variants

Skin pigmentation in darker skin types often shows normal variation. Natural hyperpigmentation and hypopigmentation in specific patterns may be seen. Symmetrical lines of demarcation between lateral dark and medial light areas of the upper aspects of the arms are most common; they are known as Futcher, Voigt or Matsumoto lines. Similar lines may be found on the forearms and legs (Fig. 66.1). Paired median or paramedian chest lines with midline extension are more common in Japanese individuals. Posterior median lines as well as obliquely oriented, symmetrical, bilateral hypopigmented chest macules are less common. The lines usually appear in early childhood. About 75% of black adults showed at least one pigmentary demarcation line in one study.

Many blacks acquire a median infraumbilical hyperpigmented line, also known as linea nigra; while this change is well-known as a pregnancy-related change in whites, it is common in blacks of both sexes. Midline hypopigmentation, known as linea alba, is more common above the umbilicus. Infants may have hyperpigmentation of the scrotum, nipples, ears and other sites. Palmar and plantar hyperpigmented macules are common; they are present in more than 50% of blacks over age 50 and increase in incidence with age. They are not seen in infants.

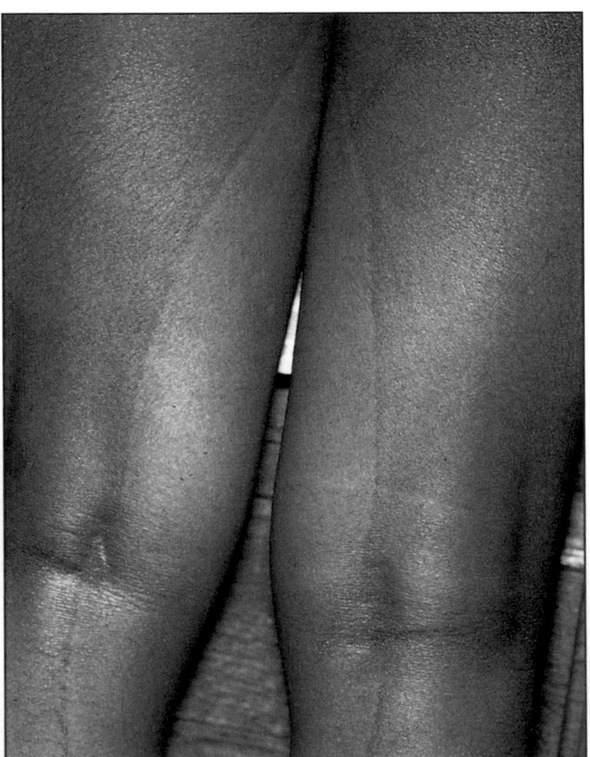

Fig. 66.1. Pigmentary demarcation lines on the legs. (Courtesy of Rebat M. Halder, M.D. Washington, D.C.)

Nails may also show physiologic hyperpigmentation. Dark streaks of pigmentation of some or all nails are not uncommon; the darker the skin pigmentation, the more diffuse the pattern tends to be. Subungual melanocytic nevi also occur and may be mistaken for melanonychia. The differential diagnosis of melanonychia is identical to that in white patients (Chap. 32) but in blacks, the likelihood of a physiologic variant is much higher. While a biopsy of the nail matrix may be required for the definitive diagnosis, it is less likely to be needed in a black patient.

Mucosal hyperpigmentation is also very common. Infants may have darkening of the inner aspects of both lips. In older individuals, over three-fourths of blacks have macular dark areas on their lips, and/or buccal or especially gingival mucosa. Most such hyperpigmentation represents increased melanin, although occasionally lentiginous change with increased melanocytes may be seen.

The most common pigmentary alteration in black and Asian infants is dermal melanosis. Over 90% have the lumbosacral Mongolian spot and many have similar patches on the trunk, buttocks and extremities. Multiple lesions may be seen. Most lesions disappear with time and all at least fade. Black infants may also have hair lines with dark lanugo hair on the lateral aspect of the arm and no visible hair on the medial aspect; these are clearly related to the later-appearing lines of demarcation.

Postinflammatory Hyperpigmentation

Postinflammatory hyperpigmentation is a frequent sequel of skin disease or trauma. Increased pigmentation may be more distressing to many patients than the underlying condition. Common problems such as acne or allergic contact dermatitis (Fig. 66.2) are often associated with hyperpigmentation. Leukotrienes and thromboxanes have been implicated in the induction of postinflammatory hyperpigmentation. Normal human melanocytes became more dendritic and showed increased tyrosinase immunoreactivity when cultured with leukotrienes; in addition they may proliferate more rapidly.

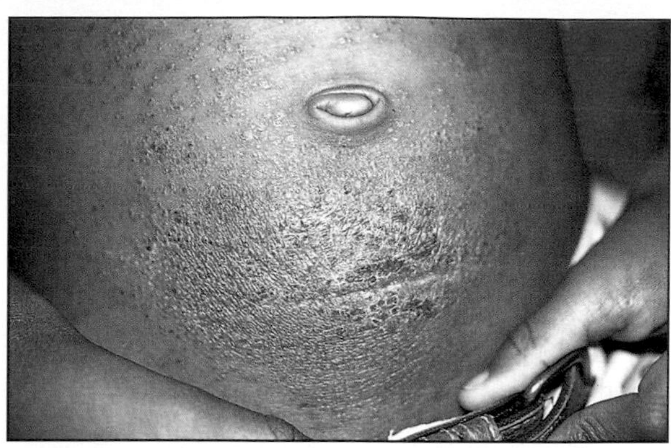

Fig. 66.2. Postinflammatory hyperpigmentation following allergic contact dermatitis to nickel in belt buckle. (Courtesy of Robert Swerlick, M.D., Atlanta, Georgia)

The degree of postinflammatory hyperpigmentation may correlate with the degree of inflammation and the amount of chemical mediators released during the inciting process. Ultraviolet radiation may also play a role by inducing melanophages that can activate T cell subpopulations and possess antigen-presenting ability. Diseases commonly associated with postinflammatory hyperpigmentation include acne, lichen planus and atopic dermatitis. Pityriasis rosea and pityriasis lichenoides et varioliformis acuta tend to more often lead to postinflammatory hypopigmentation. Often both hyper- and hypopigmented lesions may be seen, either occurring simultaneously or developing over time.

Therapy. Treatment of postinflammatory hyperpigmentation begins with addressing the underlying cause of inflammation. Topical and intralesional steroids are useful for treating some conditions. Tretinoin, α-hydroxy acid and hydroquinone, alone or compounded in various combinations, have been utilized to reduce pigmentation. Paradoxically, if irritation occurs with application of these agents, more hyperpigmentation may result. Sunscreen application is also useful adjunctive therapy. Physiologic variations in color are relatively refractory to treatment. In some cultures, lightening of dark skin is sought, and very high concentrations of hydroquinone are often employed, leading to acquired ochronosis (Chap. 39).

Melasma

Melasma is an acquired macular hyperpigmentation common in adult women of all races (Chap. 26). It is more common in Hispanics, Asians and blacks. Although melasma is usually seen in women, among darker-skinned races it also occasionally occurs in men. The major risk factors include elevated female hormones, exposure to sunlight and a racial or genetic predisposition. Treatment is similar to that of postinflammatory hyperpigmentation.

Vitiligo

Epidemiology. Vitiligo is a disease that often begins early in life and is frequently familial. The disease is found in all races and afflicts from 1% to 3% of the population. It may be slightly more common in blacks and is definitely more noticeable and distressing to the patient.

Etiology and Pathogenesis. While the cause of vitiligo is unknown, there are three principal theories commonly cited. The neural theory proposes that there is a chemical mediator liberated at nerve endings that may destroy melanocytes and/or inhibit melanin production. The self-destruction hypothesis suggests that melanocytes are destroyed by a toxic intermediate or metabolic product of melanin synthesis. The autoimmune theory is most popular. It was advanced because of the occurrence of so many autoimmune diseases in conjunction with vitiligo, the inflammatory changes found in the skin and the presence of many autoantibodies. It suggests that there is an aberration of immune surveillance that leads to melanocyte dysfunction or destruction. None of these theories explains all the features of vitiligo. Probably the final explanation will incorporate aspects of all these mechanisms (Chap. 26).

Clinical Findings. Vitiligo is characterized by the loss of melanocytes and the formation of progressive, well-circumscribed white macules (Fig. 66.3). Ocular abnormalities, autoantibodies and a high incidence of associated disorders, particularly thyroid disease and diabetes mellitus, are also seen. Most patients first note the appearance of white or depigmented macules on the face, hands, arms or legs. These lesions are usually asymptomatic although in some patients there may be mild pruritus. In many patients the depigmentation appears about body orifices such as the mouth, vulva or perianal areas. In some men, the depigmentation involves the glans penis. The depigmented lesions can range from a few millimeters to several centi-

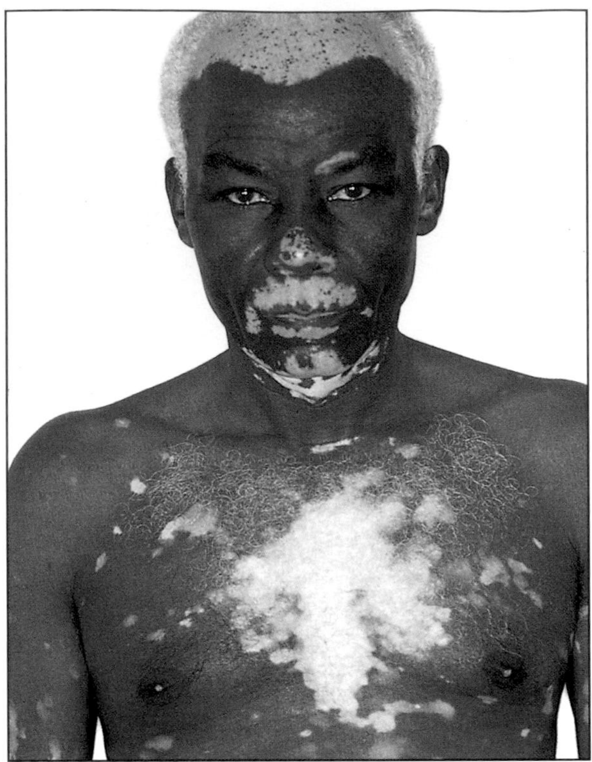

Fig. 66.3. Vitiligo with extensive whitening of hair

meters in size. Some patients, especially darker patients early in the disease course, will have normal dark skin, hypopigmented areas, and white depigmented areas; this constellation is known as trichrome vitiligo.

Vitiligo often involves the mucosal surfaces. At times the palms and soles can also be involved. Focal leukotrichia, prematurely gray hair and halo nevi are also associated with vitiligo. Alopecia areata may also occur in the same individuals or even the same spots, increasing the level of patient distress.

In whites or those of light complexion, the lesions are often not apparent until tanning occurs. Examination with a Wood light is a useful way to identify the full extent of involvement. In contrast, the disorder is often strikingly noticeable in those of dark complexion such as East Indians, blacks, and Asians. Physicians, health insurance officials, and others need to understand the impact of vitiligo on such individuals. For some it is catastrophic. Employers are often reluctant to hire the patient who has noticeable vitiligo lesions of the face or hands. Some in the public think vitiligo is contagious and are fearful of catching it; vitiligo patients report that upon sitting down on a train or bus, their neighbor will quickly get up and move to another seat.

Histopathology. The essential process in vitiligo is the loss of melanocytes. Well-established lesions of vitiligo reveal no melanocytes when examined with special staining techniques or electron microscopy.

Course and Prognosis. It is not possible to reliably predict the course of vitiligo. In some patients the lesions remain stationary with no progression. In others there is a continuous enlargement of the depigmented sites. In veloce vitiligo there is rapid spread of the depigmentation.

Differential Diagnosis. Usually vitiligo can be diagnosed by inspection. Wood light examination may help separate vitiligo from hypomelanotic disorders. Tinea versicolor may be confused with vitiligo, but is scaly and rich in microorganisms on KOH examination. Both lupus erythematosus and systemic sclerosis may occasionally present with hypo- or depigmented lesions, especially in blacks. If there is any hint of erythema at the border or induration, a biopsy should be performed. Vitiligo may be associated with diabetes mellitus and thyroid disease, so we exclude these disorders.

Therapy. If the patient has only a few lesions that do not involve the face or other cosmetically important areas, advice regarding the use of cosmetics or cover-ups and sunscreens may suffice. However if the vitiligo involves the face and extremities, or is more widespread, treatment is usually warranted. One must make it clear to the patient that the treatment is long-term, usually requiring many months of often weekly visits to the physician's office or clinic. Either topical or systemic psoralens can be combined with UVA radiation. If the area to be treated is less than 20% of the skin surface area, then painting the vitiligo sites with psoralen solution, followed after 30 min with UVA exposure is preferable. The psoralen solution should not be given to the patient, although requiring the patient to come to the office is inconvenient. Even when using dilute solutions of topical psoralens, phototoxic reactions can occur in patients allowed to paint their lesions at home and use either natural or artificial light sources. The UVA exposure time with topical psoralens is much less than it is with oral psoralens. The patient must apply a proper sunscreen before leaving the office. If larger areas are involved, then either PUVA or PUVA bath therapy is more practical. In addition, narrow-band 311 nm UVB radiation plus oral psoralens also appears to be effective (Chap. 70).

If a patient fails to improve after several months of psoralen therapy or has extensive disease (more than 50 % of their skin surface area affected), one should consider using topical monobenzyl ether of hydroquinone (monobenzone) to attempt to destroy the remaining normal areas. The patient then has only depigmented skin. Since this treatment turns a black patient white, informed documented consent is required, including parental consent if the patient is a minor. Often there are psychologic considerations that should be discussed with a psychiatrist before a final decision is made. The depigmentation is usually permanent and irreversible. The depigmented skin is much more liable to sunburn and the patient must be diligent about the use of sunscreens. Since monobenzone may not destroy every last melanocyte, sun exposure may cause pigmented spots to appear in the depigmented areas, requiring retreatment.

If a decision is made to treat by depigmentation, we first use a 10 % monobenzone cream, diluting the commercially available Benoquin cream, which has a 20 % concentration. The patient is directed to first apply a small amount under the chin or on the arm at night and allow it to remain on for 24 h, as a skin test to detect any allergy to the hydroquinone. If no allergy is present, the patient is instructed to apply the 10 % cream to the remaining, normally pigmented brown or black skin areas morning and night, and to use an SPF15 or stronger sunscreen daily. If he experiences no difficulties with the 10 % cream after 1 month, he may switch to the full-strength 20 % cream. Several months to more than a year may be required to achieve the desired depigmentation.

Postinflammatory Hypopigmentation

In other instances, cutaneous inflammation may heal with hypopigmentation. In the case of occupational hypopigmentation, as caused by various phenolic germicides or rubber gloves, there is toxic damage to melanocytes. When hypopigmentation follows inflammation and trauma, the explanation is more likely to be impaired transfer of melanin to keratinocytes. Pityriasis rosea, pityriasis lichenoides et varioliformis acuta and pityriasis alba are the most common causes of postinflammatory hypopigmentation seen in blacks. Pigmentation tends to return with time. There is no specific treatment.

Albinism

Albinism is not more common in blacks but more obvious. Depending on the enzymatic defect (Chap. 26), blacks with albinism may have café-au-lait to light yellow-brown skin, yellow to red hair and even freckling. Tyrosinase-negative black albinos tend to be as pale as their white counterparts; there is an increased incidence of this type of albinism among some Nigerian tribes, in whom multiple squamous cell and basal cell carcinomas develop because of inadequate sun protection.

Atopic Dermatitis

One of the most frequent dermatologic diseases seen in infants and children is atopic dermatitis. In some countries atopic dermatitis is more prevalent in blacks. When brown and dark-skinned persons are affected by atopic dermatitis, postinflammatory hyperpigmentation can be profound and persist for weeks to months, long after the other symptoms have subsided. These changes are often distressing to the patient. In addition, some aspects of atopic dermatitis are more prominent or noticeable in black skin. Often there is a follicular pattern with small flesh-colored to hypopigmented papules widely distributed over the chest and back, or clustered in small patches. This pattern may either coexist with more typical lesions or be the only manifestation of the condition. Inexperienced physicians often misinterpret the pruritic follicle papules as scabies or even dermatitis herpetiformis; both of these disorders are uncommon in blacks, while follicular atopic dermatitis is very common.

Hyperpigmented infraorbital creases may be a helpful finding in an individual patient, but they are also seen in nearly half of unaffected black children. Pityriasis alba features hypopigmented macules often with fine scale, usually located on the face. It is more common in patients with atopic dermatitis and more noticeable in darker-skinned patients but may also be seen in fair- skinned individuals, especially after tanning. If the hypopigmentation is significant, pityriasis alba may be mistaken for vitiligo; however, it is not accentuated under Wood light examination.

Keloids

Etiology and Pathogenesis. Keloids and hypertrophic scars are more frequently seen in black skin. Keloids extend beyond the original borders of the skin injury, while hypertrophic scars are confined to the area of damage. Keloids commonly develop after ear piercing, acne and burns, but may also arise following minor injuries, superficial excoriations or even varicella infection. While keloids are occasionally described as arising spontaneously, generally the explanation is subclinical inflammation. An example is secondary to mild acne in an area of great risk, such as over the sternum. The cause of keloids is unknown. While they are much more common in blacks, they are seen in all races. There is often a family history of similar problems. In blacks, however, a negative history is of no value, as the problem is too common.

Clinical Findings. Often the scars tend to remain red or violet, become thickened, bulbous or polypoid and may be painful or pruritic. Tongues or claws of scar tissue extend from the sides of the lesion, often along lines of tension. Sites of predilection include the mid-chest, shoulder girdle, ears, scalp and about the ankles. Sternal incisions made for cardiovascular surgery often lead to massive keloids.

Histopathology. The microscopic appearance of hypertrophic scars and keloids is often indistinguishable in the early stages. There is granulation tissue admixed with nodules containing bundles and whorls of thickened collagen. In hypertrophic scars, collagen bundles become less nodular and tend to be parallel to the skin surface. In keloids, nodules persist with bundles of collagen oriented in many directions.

Therapy. Although no treatment is required for small, asymptomatic lesions, keloids may become pruritic, painful and disfiguring. Potent corticosteroids may be used topically, under occlusion, or as impregnated tape. The mainstay of therapy is intralesional triamcinolone acetonide. Concentration of 20–40 mg/ml are used initially but decreased once softening or blanching is seen. Injections are performed every 3–4 weeks. In such concentrations, hypopigmentation may be an inevitable side effect in black patients. Silicone gel sheeting is a newer treatment to compress keloid and hypertrophic scars. Although results have been mixed, this approach may be helpful when treating newer scars. Keloids can be excised or debulked but rapid recurrence is possible. If a surgical approach is chosen, postoperative intralesional corticosteroids or even ionizing radiation should be considered.

Follicular Diseases

The thicker elliptical hairs of blacks are usually curly. They tend to rupture the follicular wall in the dermis or to reenter the skin after successfully exiting the follicle. Both changes produce considerable inflammation which, combined with the tendency towards keloid formation, cause dramatic clinical consequences.

Pseudofolliculitis Barbae

Clinical Findings. Pseudofolliculitis barbae is a recurrent, papular inflammatory condition of the face and neck due to shaving (Fig. 66.4). While most commonly seen on the face of young black men, this disease may occur in anyone with curly hair growth in any area, such as the axilla or genital area when pubic hairs are shaven. The typical patient is an individual who is required to shave daily. Shaving serves to sharpen the shaft of the curly hair

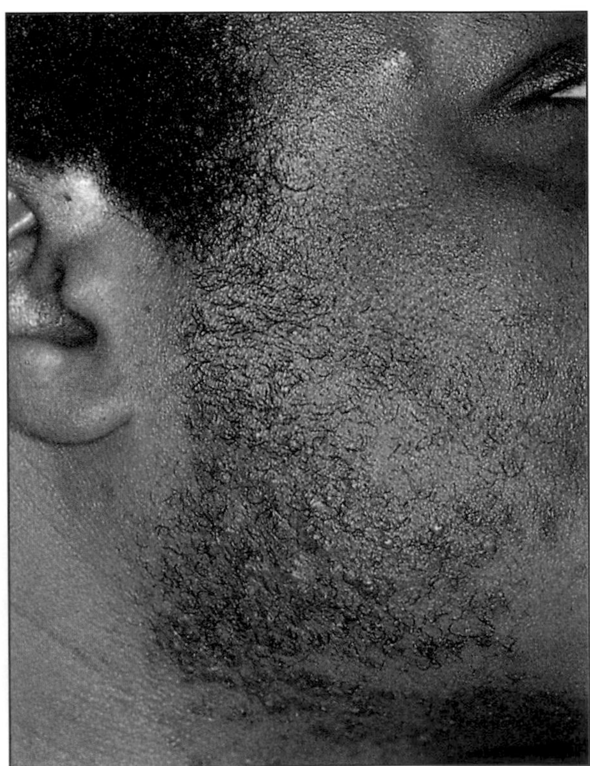

Fig. 66.4. Pseudofolliculitis barbae

so that it may penetrate the adjacent skin, resulting in a papular inflammatory reaction, usually with pustules. On close inspection, a hair is usually seen extending from a follicular opening into the inflamed area – hence the term pseudofolliculitis. There may be associated irritation and pruritus. Keloids and postinflammatory hyperpigmentation commonly develop. Continued shaving is uncomfortable and exacerbates the condition.

Therapy. For many men the best treatment is to stop shaving and allow beard growth. This solution is not possible for some professions requiring no facial hair; for example, the military is well-known for stipulating a clean-shaven appearance. If a razor is used, the individual should shave only with the grain of the hairs and not attempt to achieve an extremely close shave. Plucking hairs is not helpful, as the problem is not in the follicle. Hairs should be gently lifted out of the skin and then allowed to grow so they can be removed by shaving. Some patients do better with an electric razor or a fine hair clippers, leaving a "5-o'clock shadow". Others prefer chemical epilation, which may irritate the skin. It is often wise to recommend 0.5–1.0 % hydrocortisone cream to be used as an aftershave cream to reduce the risk of postinflammatory hyperpigmentation. Intralesional triamcinolone acetonide (2.5 mg/ml) may be used in early keloids to arrest their evolution; most pustules resolve spontaneously. Hair removal by laser may allow periods of remission; more studies of this approach are needed.

Other topical treatments are generally disappointing, as the problem is mechanical rather than infectious or inflammatory. Retinoids, glycolic and other α-hydroxy acids, benzoyl peroxide and salicylic acid all may occasionally help. Oral and topical antibiotics may reduce the inflammation. Oral isotretinoin has been less than successful in our hands.

Acne Keloidalis Nuchae

Etiology and Pathogenesis. Acne keloidalis nuchae is a chronic scarring condition frequently affecting blacks. It is most common in young black men but can be seen in women and members of other races. Increased fasting blood testosterone levels have been found in some men, but excess androgens have not been detected in women with this disorder. There is usually no associated personal or family history of keloids. Trauma from close haircuts or chemical hair treatments often serves as a trigger.

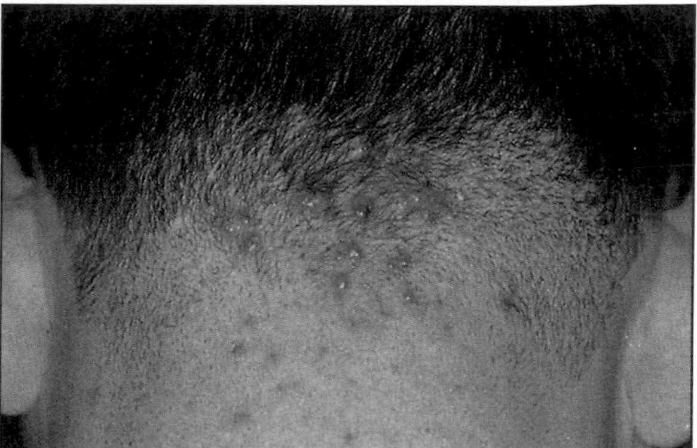

Fig. 66.5. Early acne keloidalis nuchae

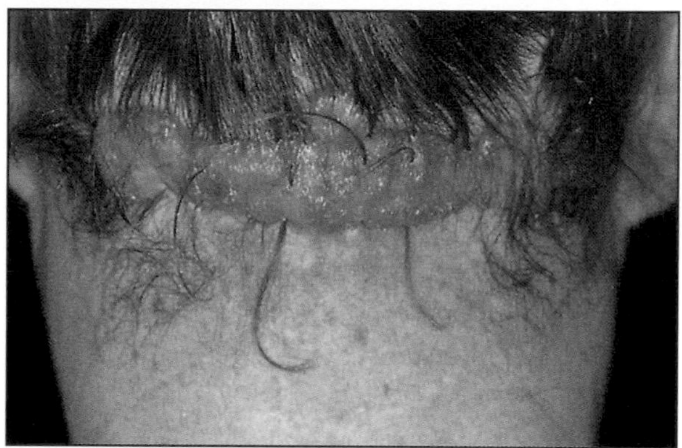

Fig. 66.6. More advanced acne keloidalis nuchae with massive keloid in white patient

Clinical Findings. The disease begins as folliculitis on the nape and adjacent areas of the scalp. With continued inflammation or infection, firm hyperpigmented follicular papules develop which may progress to hypertrophic scars or keloids (Fig. 66.5). In some cases, the keloids expand and coalesce into large disfiguring plaques (Fig. 66.6). Chronic abscesses and alopecia are also seen.

Histopathology. During the early phases, microscopic examination reveals acute folliculitis. The follicle wall is disrupted and the hair penetrates into the dermis with resultant perifolliculitis. Later, chronic inflammation and scarring develop. The older lesions are keloids.

Therapy. Treatment should begin as early in the process as possible. Oral and topical antibiotics, topical and intralesional steroids, and cryosurgery have been successfully utilized. In contrast to other keloids, surgery may be beneficial but must be individualized. Staged excision, tissue expansion and then excision, excision with grafting, and excision with healing by secondary intention may all achieve acceptable cosmetic results.

Perifolliculitis Capitis Abscedens et Suffodiens

Synonym. Dissecting scalp cellulitis

This rare chronic inflammation of the scalp usually affects young black men. Its etiology is unknown but it may be seen in association with acne conglobata and acne inversa. The process is suppurative, progressive, and may result in cicatricial alopecia. Clinical findings include comedones, pustules, abscesses, edema and erythema. Manipulation may express pus. Later, clusters of hairs may penetrate scarred or keloidal areas, producing the paintbrush or toothbrush sign. Treatment is difficult. Systemic antibiotics, corticosteroids and isotretinoin all may show some benefit. If no response is obtained, surgery should be considered. The course is often protracted, with multiple relapses and marked scarring alopecia even after resolution of the inflammatory process.

Other Hair Problems

Traction Alopecia

Many hair styles favored by blacks exert considerable pressure on the hair shaft and follicle. Pony tails, braids, corn rows, and hair weaves, when pulled too forcefully, result in thinning of the hair especially at the margins. Small papules and pustules may also be seen in the involved areas. If traction occurs over prolonged periods, hair loss may be permanent. Treatment must begin with loosening of the hairstyle. Topical corticosteroids may also be used if inflammation is present.

Hot Comb Alopecia

Previously, some blacks used chemicals or a hot comb and oil to straighten their hair. This approach produced striking damage to the shaft and, on occasion, injured the follicle leading to long-term or permanent alopecia. Because of current hair styling and a greater awareness of the problem, this type of hair loss has become less common. The process has also been called the follicular degeneration syndrome because it also occurs without any history of trauma.

Acquired Trichorrhexis Nodosa

Often blacks will complain of an area of scalp hair that no longer grows out to the desired length. In most instances, a pick or larger fork-like comb is used to fluff out or tease the hair. When the hairs are examined under the microscope, typical areas of trichorrhexis nodosa (Chap. 31) are seen. If the hairs are treated gently and combed after applying a conditioner or even water, the problem improves spontaneously over many months. As with all hair shaft abnormalities, there is no direct treatment.

Connective Tissue Diseases

Lupus Erythematosus

Both systemic and discoid lupus erythematosus are more common in black Americans than in white.

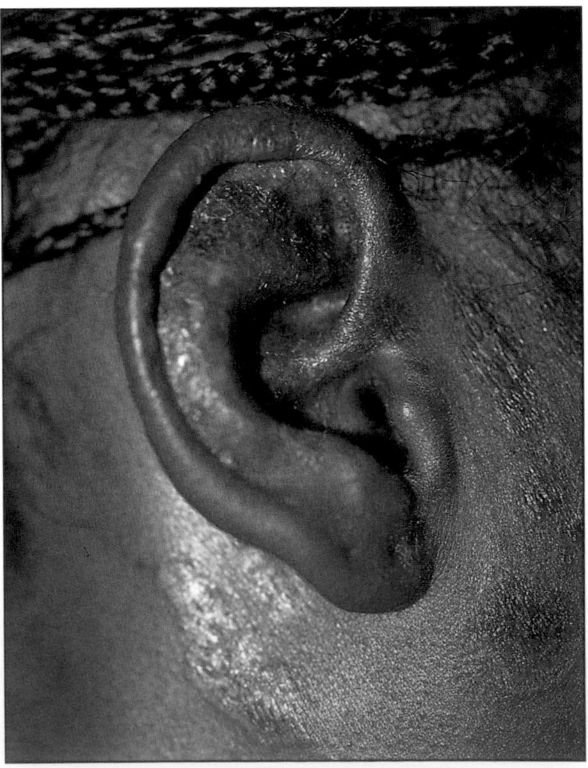

Fig. 66.7. Discoid lupus erythematosus with annular lesions and pigmentary change. (Courtesy of Robert Swerlick, M.D., Atlanta, Georgia)

The female predominance is maintained. The erythematous eruptions associated with acute systemic lupus erythematosus may be less apparent or even overlooked in blacks. The chronic lesions of discoid lupus erythematosus are often centrally hypopigmented with an erythematous or hyperpigmented border (Fig. 66.7). Scarring alopecia is often seen in blacks. Mucosal disease has been more often described in blacks, especially involving the lips and perianal region.

Systemic Sclerosis

While systemic sclerosis appears to be less common in blacks than whites, its presentation can be quite different. Hypopigmentation, often in a confetti-like pattern, can be the presenting sign. These changes are most often seen on the trunk and legs. In addition, the inflamed sclerotic areas may develop both hyper- and hypopigmentation.

Miscellaneous Diseases

Sarcoidosis

Sarcoidosis is a multisystem, chronic granulomatous disease of unknown etiology. American and West Indian blacks are up to ten times more likely to be affected than whites, and black women are more commonly affected than black men. Africans are less commonly diagnosed with the disorder, possibly due to a lower actual incidence, or inadequate diagnosis and misdiagnosis as tuberculosis. Cutaneous sarcoidosis may be the initial sign of disease.

Blacks usually have more extensive and severe skin involvement. Annular lesions are more common; they are typically on the face and consist of multiple small papules. These lesions may be mistaken for lupus, granuloma annulare, secondary syphilis, and leprosy. Larger plaques may also develop and tend to be hyperpigmented with a slightly elevated border. Hypopigmented macules may also be seen, representing active disease rather than a postinflammatory phenomenon. Ulcerative sarcoidosis may occur within preexisting lesions or de novo, usually on the legs. Sarcoidosis has also been known to develop in scars. Changes in longstanding scars or keloids may be an early sign of sarcoidosis. Ichthyosiform sarcoidosis, usually located on the shins, shows hyperpigmented scaly plaques reminiscent of ichthyosis and is also much more common in blacks. Subcutaneous nodular sarcoidosis may show hyperpigmentation overlying deeper nodules. Erythema nodosum is one of the most common findings associated with this disease; however, it is a more frequent presenting feature in whites than nonwhites. The mortality rate in blacks is higher than in whites, and higher in women than in men.

Treatment of the cutaneous lesions may include topical and intralesional steroids; oral corticosteroids, methotrexate or hydroxychloroquine may be required for ulcerative lesions and recalcitrant disease.

Pityriasis Rosea

Pityriasis rosea is a benign self-limited eruption thought to be viral in etiology. A large, solitary, round to oval patch with peripheral scale appears initially. This is followed by a more widespread eruption with smaller ovoid patches. In black skin, these patches are often hyperpigmented and may be violaceous to gray in color, with the darkest area centrally. Typically, the eruption is on the trunk and proximal extremities along the lines of cleavage. While pruritus is uncommon in whites, it is a frequent complaint among black patients. One pattern more commonly seen in blacks is inverse pityriasis rosea with acral lesions involving the hands, feet and nape. This atypical pattern must be differentiated from secondary syphilis. Micropapular forms may also be seen; instead of round to ovoid patches, numerous, follicular papules are commonly noted. Pityriasis rosea usually resolves after 6 weeks, but the inverse form generally lasts much longer. Annular lesions on the nape may persist longer and be mistaken for granuloma annulare. Postinflammatory hyperpigmentation often results but is not permanent.

Pomade Acne

Pomade acne is a form of acne cosmetica. When oily hair dressing or hair sprays are used on the scalp and for styling, the products often migrate onto the forehead, temples, and hairline areas. A comedonal eruption results. There are numerous closed comedones, which can be hyperpigmented. Once the oily hair products have been discontinued, standard topical therapy for comedones is generally successful.

Lichen Nitidus

The tiny white papules of lichen nitidus (Chap. 14) are common in blacks and more readily recognized.

Psoriasis

There is conflicting information on the prevalence of psoriasis in blacks. African surveys have shown a higher frequency in East Africans than in West Africans. Since many American blacks have West African roots, this may explain the apparent lower incidence in this population.

Sickle Cell Anemia

Sickle cell anemia and sickle cell trait are most common in blacks but also seen in individuals of Mediterranean background. Patients with the disease with homozygous expression of hemoglobin SS have a high incidence of leg ulcers; about half the patients have trouble with such ulcers during their life. In addition, infants with the disease have more severe atopic dermatitis or else an inflammatory dermatitis clinically indistinguishable from that associated with atopy. They also tend to have severe dactylitis. Individuals with the heterozygous trait have few clinical findings and no skin changes.

Tumors

Dermatosis Papulosa Nigra

Clinical Findings. Dermatosis papulosa nigra are tiny acquired lesions resembling seborrheic keratoses that are seen in about half of adult blacks and rarely in other dark skinned individuals. They are discrete dark papules most commonly found on the cheeks and neck (Fig. 66.8) While thc lesions are usually small, ranging in size from 1 to 5 mm, occasionally larger nodules will develop which are identical to a seborrheic keratosis. On the neck, there is no difference between a lesion of dermatosis papulosa nigra and a pigmented acrochordon or skin tag. Variations in epidermal growth factor production or receptor function, implicated in skin tags, may also be operative.

Histopathology. The microscopic picture is that of a pedunculated or acanthotic pigmented seborrheic keratosis.

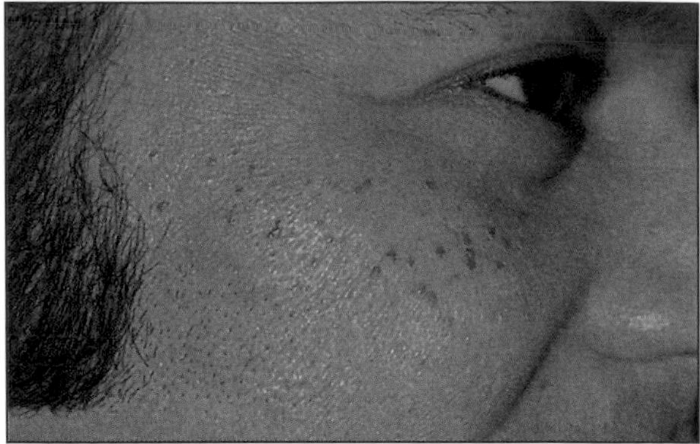

Fig. 66.8. Dermatosis papulosa nigra

Differential Diagnosis. When multiple lesions cluster in the nasal folds, then adenoma sebaceum of tuberous sclerosis and multiple trichoepitheliomas may be suggested. Otherwise, the pattern is distinct.

Therapy. Most cases require no therapy. Any destructive measure carries the risk of postinflammatory hypo- and hyperpigmentation. Curettage, electrodesiccation, cryotherapy and superficial laser destruction are all effective.

Squamous Cell and Basal Cell Carcinomas

The best established risk factor for squamous cell carcinoma, basal cell carcinoma and malignant melanoma is sunlight. Because black skin is far more resistant to UV radiation, skin cancers are much less common in blacks and other dark-skinned people. The presence of skin cancers in such individuals, however, demonstrates that UV radiation is not the only factor. Skin cancer accounts for 1–2% of all cancers in blacks; when one includes basal cell carcinoma, over 50% of all cancers in whites involve the skin.

Squamous cell carcinoma is the most frequent type of skin cancer in blacks, representing over 60% of cutaneous malignancies. This is contrast to whites, in whom basal cell carcinoma is most common. The most common locations in blacks are the legs, head and neck. Sun-protected areas, especially the groin area, are also frequently affected. Other risk factors in addition to UV radiation include burns, chronic ulcers and other scars. Squamous cell carcinoma may be a complication of chronic discoid lupus erythematosus scars. Basal cell carcinomas may be darkly pigmented and thus mistaken for malignant melanoma.

Melanocytic Lesions

Melanocytic nevi are less common in blacks than whites. In addition, freckling is rare. An exception is midfacial lentiginosis which is clinically distinct, common and poorly understood. Some relatively pale blacks with red hair have numerous lentigines of the face. While they are described as freckles, they are permanent and reflect increased numbers of melanocytes, according to the few available studies. While this trait has been described as a genodermatosis inherited in an autosomal dominant pattern, it may well reflect genetic heterogeneity.

Although uncommon in nonwhites, cutaneous malignant melanomas do occur. The most frequent type is acral lentiginous melanoma. The incidence of acral lentiginous malignant melanoma is nearly equally in blacks and whites; the paucity of other types of malignant melanoma explains the dominance of the acral type. Additionally, some malignant melanomas arise in preexisting nevi; the risk of malignant transformation of congenital melanocytic nevi in blacks was estimated to be 1 in 2000 in one study. Nonwhite patients with malignant melanoma tend to have a poorer prognosis than white patients. This increased mortality is probably explained by the frequent acral location with delayed diagnosis. When malignant melanomas are matched for other variables, race is not a significant independent variable in most series.

Mycosis Fungoides

An unusual hypopigmented form of mycosis fungoides has been described primarily in black patients. Hypo- or depigmented macules are seen, either alone or in conjunction with more advanced nodular lesions and lymphadenopathy. The macules are frequently located on the trunk, hips, and extremities. The differential diagnosis includes pityriasis alba, atopic dermatitis, and vitiligo. Histologically, the macules show epidermotropism, with moderate to profound exocytosis but little epidermal atrophy. The treatment of choice is PUVA therapy. Repigmentation is usually rapid and complete. Topical nitrogen mustard and BCNU treatment have also been used for successful repigmentation. Long-term follow-up is lacking, but it is assumed that these patients will have the same course as other mycosis fungoides patients.

Kaposi Sarcoma

Endemic Kaposi sarcoma is a problem of African blacks. There is a childhood or lymphadenopathic form which clinically mimics a lymphoma, as well as highly destructive variants in adults. In the USA, Kaposi sarcoma shows no predilection for blacks.

Bibliography

Pigmentary Variants

Henderson AL (1983) Skin variations in blacks. Cutis 32: 376–377

James WD, Carter JM, Rodman OG (1987) Pigmentary demarcation lines; a population survey. J Am Acad Dermatol 16:584–590

Selmanowitz VJ, Krivo JM (1975) Pigmentary demarcation lines. Comparison of Negroes with Japanese. Br J Dermatol 93:371–377

Tosti A et al. (1996) Nail matrix nevi: a clinical and histopathologic study of twenty-two patients. J Am Acad Dermatol 34:765–771

Postinflammatory Hyperpigmentatus

Bulengo-Ransby SM, Griffiths CE, Kimbrough-Green CK et al. (1993) Topical tretinoin (retinoic acid) therapy for hyperpigmented lesions caused by inflammation of the skin in black patients. N Engl J Med 328:1438–1443

Tomita Y, Maeda K, Tagami H (1992) Melanocyte-stimulating properties of arachidonic acid metabolites: possible role in postinflammatory pigmentation. Pigment Cell Res 5:357–361

Tomita Y, Maeda K, Tagami H (1988) Leukotrienes and Thromboxane B2 stimulate normal human melanocytes in vitro: possible inducers of postinflammatory pigmentation. Tohoku T Exp Med 156:303–304

Weiss JS, James WD, Cooper KD (1988) Melanophages in inflammatory skin disease demonstrate the surface phenotype of OKM5+ antigen-presenting cells and activated macrophages. J Am Acad Dermatol 19:633–641

Pseudofolliculitis Barbae

Friedman SJ (1987) Treatment of steatocystoma multiplex and pseudofolliculitis barbae with isotretinoin. Cutis 39:506–507

Hage JJ, Bouman FG (1991) Surgical depilation for the treatment of pseudofolliculitis or local hirsutism of the face; experience in the first 40 patients. Plast Reconstr Surg 88:446–451

Halder RM (1988) Pseudofolliculitis barbae and related disorders. Dermatol Clin 6:407–412

Acne Keloidalis Nuchae

Dinehart SM, Tanner L, Mallory SB et al. (1989) Acne keloidalis in women. Cutis 44:250–252

George AO, Aknji AO, Nduka EU et al. (1993) Clinical, biochemical and morphologic features of acne keloidalis in a black population. Int J Dermatol 32:714–716

Glenn MJ, Bennett RG, Kelly AP (1995) Acne keloidalis nuchae: treatment with excision and second-intention healing. J Am Dermatol 33:243–246

Herzberg AJ, Dinehart SM, Kerns BJ et al. (1990) Acne keloidalis. Transverse microscopy, immunohistochemistry, and electron microscopy. Am J Dermatopathol 12:109–121

Layton, AM, Yip J, Cunliffe WJ (1994) A comparison of intralesional triamcinolone and cryosurgery in the treatment of acne keloids. Br J Dermatol 130:498–501

Pestalardo CM, Cordero A Jr, Ansorena JM et al. (1995) Acne keloidalis nuchae. Tissue expansion treatment. Dermatol Surg 21:723–724

Perifolliculitis Capitis Abscendens et Suffodiens

Shaffer N, Billick RC, Srolovitz H (1992) Perifolliculitis capitis abscendens et suffodiens. Resolution with combination therapy. Arch Dermatol 128:1329–1331

Williams CN, Cohen M, Roman SG et al. (1986) Dissecting cellulitis of the scalp. Plast Reconstr Surg 77:378–382

Sarcoidoses

Edmondstone WM, Wilson AG (1985) Sarcoidosis in Caucasians, Blacks, and Asians in London. Br J Dis Chest 79: 27–36

Minus HR, Grimes PE (1983) Cutaneous manifestations of sarcoidosis in blacks. Cutis 32:361–363

Albertini JG, Tyler W, Miller OF (1987) 3rd Ulcerative sarcoidosis. Case report and review of the literature. Arch Dermatol 133:215–219

Alabi GO, George AO (1989) Cutaneous sarcoidosis and tribal scarification in West Africa. Int J Dermatol 28:29–31

Dermatosis Papulosa Nigra

Babapour R, Leach J, Levy H (1993) Dermatosis papulosa nigra in a young child. Pediatr Dermatol 10:356–358

Hairston MA Jr, Reed RJ, Derbes VJ (1964) Dermatosis papulosa nigra. Arch Dermatol 89:655–658

Michael JC, Searle ER (1929) Dermatosis papulosa nigra. Arch Dermatol Syphilol 20:629–640

Malignant Tumors

Altman A, Rosen T, Tschen JA et al. (1987) Basal cell epithelioma in black patients. J Am Acad Dermatol 17: 741–745

Amir H, Mbonde MP, Kitinya JN (1992) Cutaneous squamous cell carcinoma in Tanzania. Cent Afr J Med 38: 439–443

Caruso WR, Stewart ML, Nanda VK et al. (1987) Squamous cell carcinoma of the skin in black patients with discoid lupus erythematosus. J Rheumatol 14:156–159

Cress RD, Holly EA (1997) Incidence of cutaneous melanoma among non-Hispanic whites, Hispanics, Asians, and Blacks; an analysis of California Cancer registry data, 1988–1993. Cancer Causes Control 8:246–252

Dhir A, Orengo I, Bruce S et al. (1995) Basal cell carcinoma on the scalp of an Indian patient. Dermatol Surg 21:247–250

Di Landro A, Marchesi L, Naldi L et al. (1997) A case of hypopigmented mycosis fungoides in a young Caucasian boy. Pediatr Dermatol 14:449–452

Garsaud P, Boisseau-Garsaud AM, Ossondo M et al. (1988) Epidemiology of cutaneous melanoma in the French West Indies (Martinique). Am J Epidemiol 147:66–68

Hudson DA, Krige JE (1995) Melanoma in black South Africans. J Am Coll Surg 180:65–71

Kalter DC, Goldberg LH, Rosen T (1984) Darkly pigmented lesions in dark-skinned patients. J Dermatol Surg Oncol 10:876–881

Krishnamurthy S, Yeole B, Jooshi S et al. (1994) The descriptive epidemiology and trends in incidence of non-ocular malignant melanoma in Bombay and India. Indian J Cancer 31:64–71

Lambrosa E, Cohen SR, Phelps R et al. (1995) Hypopigmented variant of mycosis fungoides: demography, histopathology, and treatment of seven cases. J Am Acad Dermatol 32:987–993

Shpall S, Frieden I, Chesney M et al. (1994) Risk of malignant transformation of congenital melanocytic nevi in blacks. Pediatr Dermatol 11:204–208

Singh B et al. (1998) Presentation, course, and outcome of head and neck cancer in African Americans: a case control study. Laryngoscope 108:1159–1163

Weinstock MA (1993) Non-melanoma skin cancer mortality in the United States, 1969 through 1988. Arch Dermatol 129:1286–1290

Whitmore SE, Simmons-O'Brien E, Rotter FS (1994) Hypopigmented mycosis fungoides. Arch Dermatol 130: 476–480

Dermatologic Proctology

Contents

In many countries the diagnosis and therapy of anal diseases falls into the realm of dermatology. Problems in the perianal area and anus are common; in Germany it is estimated that 70 % of adults have complaints that refer to this region. Most common are hemorrhoids, but several other diseases are also seen. Many dermatologic diseases are either common in the perianal region or appear differently there. The diagnosis can usually be made with an exact history and relatively simply diagnostic procedures.

Diagnostic Approach

History

A careful history is of paramount importance. One should inquire about pruritus, burning, weeping, foul odor, cramps, pain and appearance of bright red blood or dark stools on defecation. It is also important to know if bowel movements are normal or if constipation, diarrhea, incontinence or laxative abuse come into play. One should also inquire about gastrointestinal problems, liver disease, metabolic disorders and unexplained weight loss. The family history should specifically cover hemorrhoids and varicose veins, as both are taken as signs of a relative connective tissue weakness. In addition, a family history of colorectal polyps and cancer may be important. Results of previous proctologic evaluations, including diagnostic procedures, surgical treatments and medications, all belong in the records.

Physical Examination

The patient's position is of great importance, as is adequate lighting. The traditional military pose of standing, bending over and separating the buttocks only suffices for an external examination. Either lying on the side with the legs drawn up (Sims position) or the lithotomy position, as for a routine pelvic examination, can be used for a better view. In some instances the knee-elbow position with the buttocks sticking in the air is best, but it is least tolerated by patients, unless a special examination table is available. By tradition, findings are described according to a clock face and with the patient in the lithotomy position, so the perineum is at 12 o'clock.

Inspection. When the buttocks are spread, one can examine the skin and mucosa. One may see maceration of intertrigo, peripheral pustules of candidiasis, lichenification and scale of a chronic dermatitis, fissures, fistula tracts, condylomata acuminata, condylomata lata, anal tags and other tumors. If the patient is asked to press gently, hemorrhoids, an anal fissure or even early anal prolapse may become apparent.

Digital Examination. The anus can be palpated with a gloved, lubricated finger to a distance of about 10 cm. One should observe the sphincter tone, gaps in the sphincter, the surface of the rectal mucosa (nodules, ulcerations, thickenings); the prostate and vagina should also be checked. Stage I or II hemorrhoids tend to disappear with pressure so they are hard to palpate. As the finger is withdrawn, the anus should firmly seal. In addition, one should check the examining finger for blood, mucous or pus. Often an anal fissure is so painful that the digital examination cannot be performed without local anesthesia. If a cotton wad is placed in the rectum, as it is withdrawn, a streak of blood may delineate the location of the fissure.

Proctoscopy and Rectoscopy. Proctoscopes and rectoscopes allow an illuminated view of the anus and rectum to a distance of 15 cm. They facilitate the diagnosis of hemorrhoids, inflammatory mucosal lesions and tumors, such as condylomata acuminata, polyps and carcinomas. If there is any question about higher lesions, sigmoidoscopy, colonoscopy and imaging examinations should be undertaken by a surgeon or gastroenterologist.

Hemorrhoids

Etiology and Pathogenesis. Hemorrhoids arise from the enlargement of the corpora cavernosa recti. These highly vascular bodies are situated in the cranial third of the rectal canal and play an important role in continence. They are similar to the erectile structures of the penis and are served by three arteries, at 3, 7 and 11 o'clock, that penetrate the rectal wall about 5 cm from the orifice at the level of the dentate line (Fig. 67.1).

Hemorrhoids are the most common proctologic disease. In addition to a genetic predisposition, many other factors play a role. Chronic constipation with prolonged pressing and raised sphincter tone, laxative abuse and, occasionally, chronic diarrhea are factors. A high-fat diet low in bulk food, prolonged sitting, alcohol abuse and the effects of pregnancy also may be important. If the cavernous bodies cannot empty as the stool passes and the sphincter tightens, they become swollen, hypertrophic and eventually subject to mild trauma that leads to bleeding.

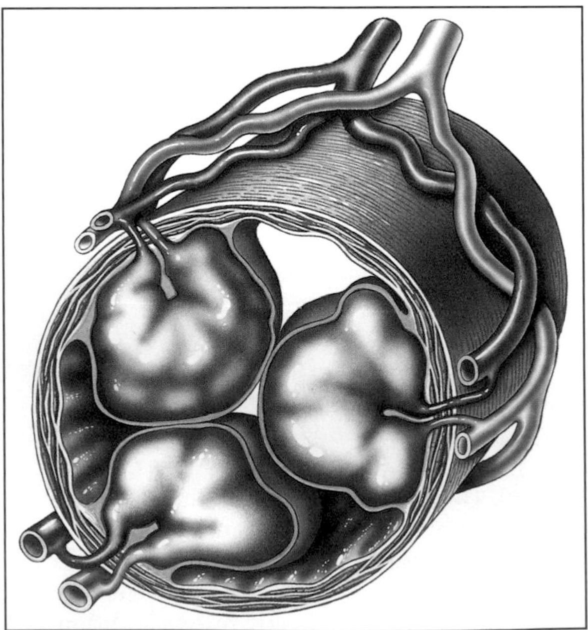

Fig. 67.1. The arterial supply to hemorrhoids from the superior rectal artery

Clinical Findings. Hemorrhoids are traditionally divided into four stages.

- Stage I. One or more nodules develop about the dentate line. They may be discovered on proctoscopy but are not palpable. Bright red blood on the stool or toilet paper is the most common symptom. Pain is uncommon.
- Stage II. The nodular vascular proliferations expand, extending down the anal canal and may extrude out when the patient is straining. However, they immediately retract. As they become thrombosed or fibrotic, they are easier to palpate. Bowel movements are often painful and spasms may occur.
- Stage III. The lesions are larger and noticeable in the anal canal. When they extend through the opening, they remain outside and must be manually repositioned. In addition to the pain, there may be leakage of stool onto the perianal skin (Fig. 67.2).
- Stage IV. There is permanent anal prolapse with the livid, red anal mucosa and fibrotic hemorrhoids protruding out of the rectum. The anal architecture is distorted and the closing mechanism impaired.

There are many complications of hemorrhoids. The leakage of stool and enzyme-rich mucus causes intertrigo and dermatitis. Since patients use so many creams and ointments, allergic contact dermatitis is a frequent problem. The main sensitizers are vehicle ingredients (wool wax alcohol, cocoa butter, balsam of Peru), anesthetics and distracters (menthol, phenol, benzocaine, witch hazel, tincture of benzoin), antimicrobial agents (neomycin, iodine, resorcinol), preservatives and medications administered per suppository. The maceration and excoriations can just as easily produce an irritant contact dermatitis. Secondary infection with *Candida albicans*, usually seeding from normal intestinal sources, is frequently a problem. The damaged skin offers a fertile home for human papilloma

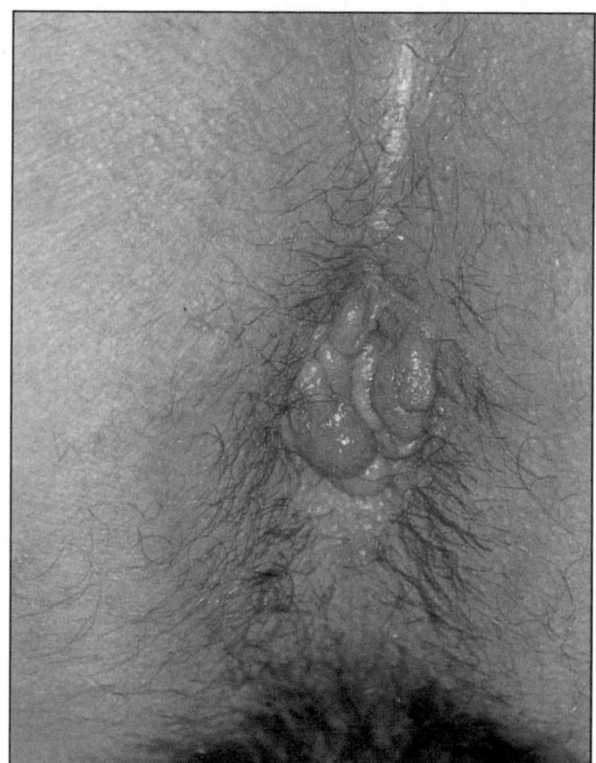

Fig. 67.2. Hemorrhoids and anal prolapse

virus, so condylomata acuminata are more common. Thrombosis of a hemorrhoid is extremely painful; a tender, blue-black swollen nodule protrudes into or out of the anal ring.

Differential Diagnosis. The main concern is not to dismiss the signs and symptoms of an anal or rectal carcinoma as hemorrhoids. The beefy nodules of condylomata lata in secondary syphilis should not be misdiagnosed; the dark field examination is always positive and other clues to syphilis are present. Gonorrhea can also present with anal inflammation, and the primary chancre of syphilis may be found on the anal mucosa. Inflammatory bowel disease, acne inversa and periorificial tuberculosis may present with similar signs and symptoms, but the exact localization is usually different. So-called external hemorrhoids or anal tags have nothing in common with true hemorrhoids, but are thrombosed, prolapsed external veins, as discussed below.

Therapy

Stool Control. A diet rich in fibers, fruits and vegetables, maybe combined with the addition of bran or bulking agents. Laxatives should be avoided.

Topical. Suppositories and ointments may produce temporary pain relief in milder cases. Chronic use causes the many problems discussed above. Corticosteroids are occasionally prescribed, but have even less of a role as they readily cause atrophy in this region and predispose to infections.

Sclerosing Therapy. Sclerosing therapy is useful for stage I and II disease. In Germany, 25% quinine dihydrochloride is usually used; lower concentrations are recommended in the USA. Following digital evaluation, a proctoscope is inserted and 0.2–0.8 ml of the medication is injected into the submucosal layer beneath the hemorrhoid. Initially only one site is treated to test how well the procedure is tolerated. Later, multiple sites can be injected. Usually a series of six to ten treatments is needed for satisfactory results. Occasionally retreatment is required. If the patient is allergic to quinine, as is the case in about 1% of individuals, then either 5% phenol in oil or materials used for sclerosing varicose veins (Chap. 22) can be employed.

Infrared Coagulation. Infrared light is induced via a laser with a special tip and applied to the mucosa. Up to four sites can be treated at one session. Except for minor postoperative bleeding, the procedure is almost painless.

Cryotherapy. Special sounds cooled with liquid nitrogen can be introduced through a proctoscope. The procedure is painful and postoperative bleeding common because of marked necrosis, just as when a hemangioma on the skin is so treated.

Rubber Band Ligation. This successful and safe approach involves ligating the hemorrhoid with a rubber band, using an instrument designed for that purpose. Stage I, II and occasionally III lesions can be treated. The result is a flat ulcer that heals with fibrosis.

Dilatation. Dilatation is an old method still used occasionally when painful hemorrhoids are associated with a markedly increased sphincter tone. It is understandably unpopular among patients.

Surgical. When stage III and IV hemorrhoids are present, a hemorrhoidectomy, often combined with a lateral subcutaneous sphincterotomy, offers the best chances of cure. The hemorrhoidal nodules are removed and the feeder vessels ligated. Many approaches have been devised. One crucial factor is to leave enough intervening tissue behind to avoid scarring stenosis and prolapse, which was a complication when a circumferential hemorrhoidectomy was performed. Such procedures are best left in the hands of a specialized surgeon.

Anal Dermatitis

Definition. In Germany, one speaks of *Analekzem* (anal eczema) as a specific diagnosis, defining the disorder as acute to chronic intertrigo with pruritus in the perianal region. In the USA, one tends simply to use the term intertrigo.

Etiology and Pathogenesis. The perianal region is intrinsically moist, dark and features skin surfaces that are in close contact. Any increase in moisture, whether from leakage because of anal sphincter problems (such as with hemorrhoids), increased sweating or decreased hygiene, leads to maceration and reduced barrier function. The many proteolytic enzymes found in stool and rectal mucoid secretions are also imitating. Obesity, excessive hair or variations in the nature of the anal anatomy contribute to the problem. The most distinctive change is the so-called *Trichteranus* (funnel anus); the name describes the situation adequately. Other changes about the anus such as deep or excessive skin folds, anal tags, fissures or fistulas obviously worsen the situation. Diabetes mellitus may be a predisposing factor.

Clinical Findings. A wide range of clinical changes can be appreciated depending on the chronicity of the problem. A unifying feature is intense pruritus. Initially there may be a weeping erythema, later crusts and scales and still later lichenification. The main secondary factors are allergic contact dermatitis, *Candida albicans* infection and condylomata acuminata, as discussed above under hemorrhoids (Fig. 67.3).

Histopathology. A biopsy is rarely helpful. It may aid in identifying *Candida albicans* as a pathogen and can exclude some of the entities listed under differential diagnosis.

Course and Prognosis. Perianal intertrigo is a difficult problem. Its prognosis depends on the nature of the predisposing factors, and how successfully they can be addressed.

Differential Diagnosis. Many common dermatoses lose their distinctive features in the perianal region, as they too are subject to maceration and frictional changes. Psoriasis is particularly likely to occur in this area, sometimes even presenting here or being confined to the site. One should search for psoriasis elsewhere (nails, scalp, knees, elbows) and inquire again about family members with psoriasis. If the perianal dermatitis extends into the gluteal cleft, psoriasis is a very good bet. Lichen planus may also be worse in this area. Sometimes lichen sclerosus et atrophicus can be confused with corticosteroid-induced atrophy or can present without the distinctive ivory color. Both extramammary Paget disease and Bowen disease can be overlooked at this site. Perianal Bowen disease has been described in psoriatic patients treated locally with ionizing radiation or with systemic arsenic.

Therapy. The first step is to attempt to treat any anal disease. The next most important factor is anal hygiene. The patient should be encouraged to wash the perianal region after each bowel movement; in Europe this is more easily accomplished with a bidet but the advice is sound everywhere. Most individuals can train themselves to have their bowel movements when at home, washing and then rinsing well. Thorough drying should be accom-

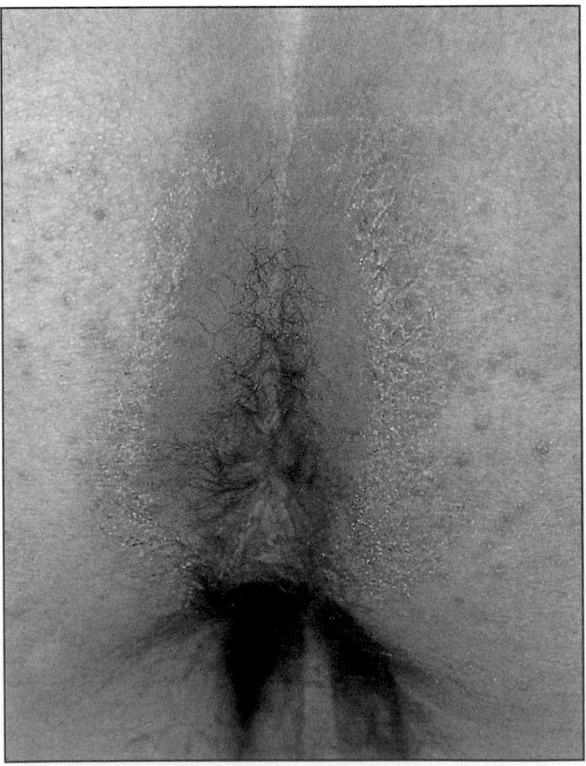

Fig. 67.3. Anal dermatitis

plished with gentle patting. Diaper wipes are often used but can cause irritation or even allergic contact dermatitis. Some patients do better when they place a gauze pad or cotton wad in the anal fold to absorb moisture.

Specific topical therapy must be adjusted to the stage of the dermatitis. When weeping lesions are present, wet-to-dry dressings and water-based 'disinfectant solutions (0.1–0.5% aqueous gentian violet) are effective but messy and hard to use at home. Corticosteroids bring rapid relief and it is easy to adjust the vehicle, starting with a lotion and later using a cream. For chronic changes, a corticosteroid paste is wisest. Because of the chronic nature of perianal dermatitis, some clinicians try to avoid any use of topical corticosteroids.

If candidiasis is suspected, topical imidazoles usually suffice. They are available in protective paste forms, designed for use in diaper dermatitis. Topical nystatin is also available in many useful vehicles. The role of *Candida albicans* in the stool is somewhat controversial. In the USA most physicians consider it part of the normal flora; in Germany quantitative stool cultures for the yeast are performed to try and assess the likelihood of it being responsible for disease. If stool cultures are repeatedly positive for *Candida albicans* and other treatments do not help, one can try a 2-week course of oral nystatin 500,000–1,000,000 units t.i.d. The drug is not absorbed and thus ideal for trying to reduce the stool load. Unfortunately dramatic or long-term improvement in perianal symptoms is the exception, not the rule.

Pruritus Ani

Definition. Perianal itching, occasionally in the absence of identified disease.

Etiology and Pathogenesis. There are many different causes of pruritus ani. They are listed in Table 67.1. The most difficult situation is the patient with extensive pruritus and no physical findings. While such patients are often diagnosed as having psychogenic pruritus ani, many are atopics who have a pruritic response to their stool. They benefit from increased hygienic measures as mentioned above. Unfortunately this is a two-edged sword, for such advice may induce a worried patient to devote too much effort to hygiene. In some cases psychologic guilt, such as over anal intercourse, plays a major role. In yet other cases, the patient is obviously depressed or anxious and has chosen pruritus ani as the preferred outlet.

Clinical Findings. The changes vary from none to finding any of the conditions listed in Table 67.1.

Course and Prognosis. All the complications discussed for hemorrhoids and perianal dermatitis also apply. In contrast to pruritus scroti and pruritus vulvae, the chances for improvement are greater. Often a specific diagnosis can be made.

Therapy. The underlying disease should be treated. If no clinical changes are identified, increased hygiene should be discussed and a topical antipruritic cream or corticosteroid cream prescribed. In Europe polidocanol is often used, while in the USA pramoxine, often combined with a low-potency corticosteroid, is a favorite. Long-term use of corticosteroids should be avoided.

Table 67.1. Causes of pruritus ani

Primary irritant dermatitis from leakage
Hemorrhoids
Anal tags
Anal fistula
Anal fissure
Inflammatory bowel disease
Diarrhea
Laxative abuse
Allergic contact dermatitis
Anal medications
Contents of suppositories
Cleansing products
Various dermatoses
Atopic dermatitis
Psoriasis
Lichen planus
Lichen sclerosus et atrophicus
Bowen disease
Extramammary Paget disease
Langerhans cell histiocytosis
Local infections
Candidiasis
Tinea glutealis
Oxyuriasis
Condylomata acuminata
Bowenoid papulosis
Condylomata lata
Benign and malignant anal tumors
Generalized pruritus
Hodgkin disease
Diabetes mellitus
Chronic renal and hepatic disease
Many others
Psychogenic or idiopathic

Proctalgia Fugax

Synonyms. Anorectal neuralgia, proctalgia nocturna

Some patients experience cramps and pain in the rectum. The typical scenario is a young adult who is awakened in the early morning hours with intense pain which lasts from a few minutes to a half hour. The attacks are irregular, often recurring after several months. The cause is unknown; vascular spasms and cramping of the pelvic musculature have been suggested as factors. While there are many other causes of sudden rectal pain, none have these fleeting quality. Most patients achieve some comfort with a warm water bottle or heating pad, changing their body position, trying to have a bowel movement or similar tricks. In some instances, nitroglycerin has been helpful, supporting a possible vascular etiology, perhaps a migraine equivalent.

Perianal Ergotismus

(Wienert and Grussendorf 1980)

Definition. Perianal ulcerations following long-term use of ergot suppositories.

Epidemiology. This problem develops primarily in women, because they are at greater risk for migraine headaches, which are treated with ergot suppositories.

Etiology and Pathogenesis. The locally applied ergot compounds cause marked vessel constriction, relative hypoxia and then cutaneous necrosis.

Clinical Findings. Ulcers can be found both in the immediate perianal region and in the distal part of the anus. They are typically painful, deep and often have a mucopurulent coating. Often they appear punched-out. Healing is achieved by stopping the suppositories.

Differential Diagnosis. Syphilis, granuloma inguinale, tuberculosis, herpes simplex and other infections should be excluded. Carcinomas and Langerhans cell histiocytosis may also present with perianal ulcerations.

Therapy. Standard wound care suffices.

Anal Fissure

Definition. Radial tear in the anal canal.

Etiology and Pathogenesis. The exact cause is unknown. One major factor is a tear in the anal mucosa from a hard or large stool. They are most common on the midline, suggesting an underlying weakness. The fissure extends to the internal sphincter causing it to contract, which then worsens the problem. Fissures may also develop secondary to hemorrhoids, thrombophlebitis, inflammatory bowel disease and surgical measures.

Clinical Findings. Most fissures are found at 6 o'clock although some arise at 12 o'clock. The defect is typically about 1 cm long and as much as 0.5 cm wide, extending from the dentate line to the skin, which is not involved. A fold of skin at the external end of the fissure is known as the sentinel pile. The main symptom is marked pain with defecation. The cramping pain can be so intense that the patient is afraid of a bowel movement, becomes constipated, worsening the situation, and may have psychiatric complaints. The anal ring is tightly shut and often an examination is only possible with local anesthesia.

Therapy. Early fissures may respond to stool softeners, sitz baths postdefecation and bland suppositories. If hemorrhoids are present, they should be treated. More advanced cases are approached with dilatation to stretch the internal sphincter or a sphincterotomy. Other measures that can be tried include injecting below the fissure with either sclerosing fluid or triamcinolone acetonide (2.5–5.0 mg/ml in an anesthetic solution), cryotherapy or excision of the fissure. Botulinum toxin injections relax the sphincter and also work well.

Perianal Thrombosis

Synonym. Acute anal vein thrombosis; often incorrectly designated as thrombosed hemorrhoid

Definition. Acute development of thrombosed, painful perianal vein.

Etiology and Pathogenesis. This common problem usually arises in patients who are constipated or have hemorrhoids. Extensive or forceful pressing on defecation leads to a tear in a perianal vein with a hematoma and then thrombosis.

Clinical Findings. The patient notices a painful swelling just exterior to the anal ring. The nodule may be several centimeters in diameter and has a blue-red to black color, depending on the age of the lesion (Fig. 67.4). Often an adequate examination is first possible with local anesthesia.

Therapy. The area should be anesthetized and then the nodule incised to remove the blood clot. It is wise to excise a bit of the overlying skin so that the wound does not spontaneously reseal too rapidly. Sitz baths and a bland ointment provide comfort during the postoperative period.

Anal Tags

Anal skin tags should not be confused with acrochordons or soft fibromas, as seen in the axillae, groin and neck. They are larger folds of skin, usually the result of a resolved perianal thrombosis. Anal tags may interfere with local hygiene and lead to perianal dermatitis. They can be easily excised, often with electrocautery, if deemed necessary. One should avoid extensive surgery at any one session to reduce the risk of postoperative stenosis.

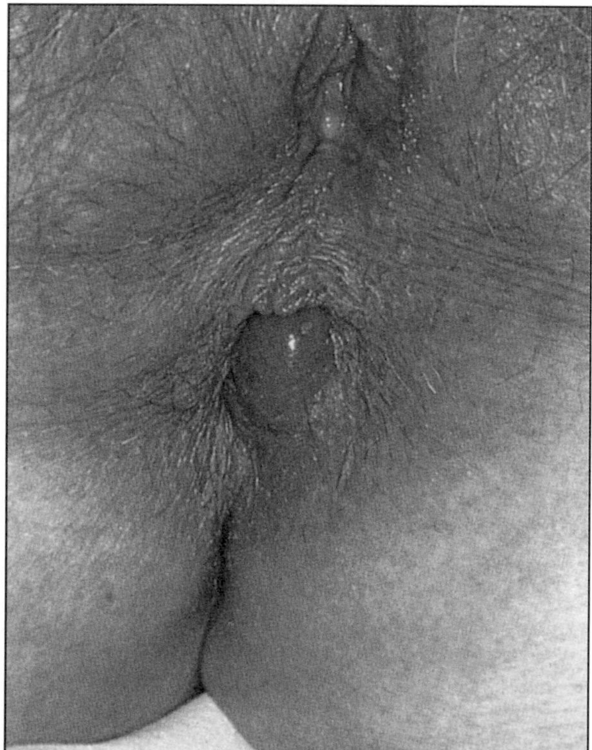

Fig. 67.4. Perianal thrombosis

Anal Fistula and Abscess

An anal fistula connects the anal canal and the skin. Often the end of the tunnel is difficult to find. An incomplete or blind fistula drains from the anal canal into the soft tissue but never reaches the skin. Very complex intertwined systems of fistulas can develop. A complete fistula results in the discharge of mucus, stool and even blood onto the skin surface, as typically seen on the underwear. This discharge contributes to perianal dermatitis and pruritus ani. In some instances, a complete fistula is quite painful. A blind fistula may lead to a perianal abscess. The approach to both problems is best left in the hands of surgeons.

Bibliography

Arabi Y, Alexander-Williams J, Keighley MRB (1977) Anal pressures in hemorrhoids and anal fissure. Am J Surg 134:608–610

Arnous J, Denis J (1971) Pathogenetic concepts on anal fissure. Am J Proctol 22:184–186

Beck DE (ed) (1997) Handbook of colorectal surgery. Quality Medical, St. Louis

Brühl W (1987) Differentialdiagnose und Therapie perianaler Knoten. Verdauungskrankh 5:188–194

Buchmann P (1994) Lehrbuch der Proktologie, 3rd edn. Huber, Bern

Delco F, Sonnenberg A (1998) Associations between hemorrhoids and other diagnoses. Dis Colon Rectum 41:1534–1541

Fazio VW, Tjandra JJ (1996) The management of perianal diseases. Adv Surg 29:59–78

Festen C, van Harten H (1998) Perianal abscess and fistula-in-ano in infants. J Pediatr Surg 33:711–713

Gordon N (ed) (1992) Principles and practice of surgery for the colon, rectum and anus. Quality Medical, St. Louis

Hamalainen KP, Sainio AP (1998) Incidence of fistulas after drainage of acute anorectal abscesses. Dis Colon Rectum 41:1357–1361

Hooker GD, Plewes EA, Rajgopal C et al. (1999) Local injection of bupivacaine after rubber band ligation of hemorrhoids: prospective randomized study. Dis Colon Rectum 42:174–179

Hyman N (1999) Anorectal abscess and fistula. Prim Care 26:69–80

Jones DJ (1992) ABC of colorectal diseases. Pruritus ani. BMJ 305:575–577

Jost WH, Schanne S, Mlitz H et al. (1995) Perianal thrombosis following injection therapy into the external anal sphincter using botulinum toxin. Dis Colon Rectum 38:781

Kaufmann HD (ed) (1981) The haemorrhoid syndrome. Abacus, Turnbridge Wells

Lentner A, Wienert V (1996) Long-term, indwelling setons for low transsphincteric and intersphincteric anal fistulas. Experience with 108 cases. Dis Colon Rectum 39: 1097–1101

Lowenstein B, Cataldo PA (1998) Treatment of proctalgia fugax with topical nitroglycerin: report of a case. Dis Colon Rectum 41:667–668

Lund JN, Scholefield JH (1998) A randomized, prospective, double-blind, placebo-controlled trial of glyceryl trinitrate ointment in treatment of anal fissure. Lancet 349: 11–14

Lundhus E, Gottrup F (1993) Outcome at three to five years of primary closure of perianal and pilonidal abscess. A randomised, double-blind clinical trial with a complete three-year followup of one compared with four days' treatment with ampicillin and metronidazol. Eur J Surg 159:555–558

Lunniss PJ, Barker PG, Sultan AH et al. (1994) Magnetic resonance imaging of fistula-in-ano. Dis Colon Rectum 37:708–718

Lysy J, Israelit-Yatzkan Y, Sestiere-Ittah M et al. (1998) Treatment of chronic anal fissure with isosorbide dinitrate: long-term results and dose determination. Dis Colon Rectum 41:1406–1410

MacRae HM, McLeod RS (1997) Comparison of hemorrhoidal treatments: a meta-analysis. Can J Surg 40:14–17

Makowiec F, Jehle EC, Becker HD et al. (1997) Perianal abscess in Crohn's disease. Dis Colon Rectum 40:443–450

Maria G, Brisinda G, Bentivoglio AR et al. (1998) Botulinum toxin injectios in the internal anal sphincter for the treatment of chronic anal fissure: long-term results after two different dosage regimens. Ann Surg 228:664–669

Marti M-C, Givel J-C (eds) (1990) Surgery of anorectal diseases. Springer, Berlin

Mazier WP (1994) Hemorrhoids, fissures, and pruritus ani. Surg Clin North Am 74:1277–1292

Moesgaard F, Nielsen ML, Hansen JB et al. (1982) High fiber diet reduces bleeding ans pain in patients with hemorrhoids. Dis Colon Rectum 25:454–456

O'Connor JJ (1979) Infrared coagulation of hemorrhoids. Pract Gastroenterol 10:8–14

Oliver DW, Booth MW, Kernick VF et al. (1998) Patient satisfaction and symptom relief after anal dilatation. Int J Colorectal Dis 13:228–231

Orkin BA, Schwartz AM, Orkin M (1999) Hemorrhoids: what the dermatologist should know. J Am Acad Dermatol 41:449–456

Robertson WG, Mangione JS (1998) Cutaneous advancement flap closure: alternative method for treatment of complicated anal fistulas. Dis Colon Rectum 41:884–886

Sailer M, Bussen D, Debus ES et al. (1998) Quality of life in patients with benign anorectal disorders. Br J Surg 85: 1716–1719

Savioz D, Roche B, Glauser T et al. (1998) Rubber band ligation of hemorrhoids: relapse as a function of time. Int J Colorect Dis 13:154–156

Shafik A (1990) An injection technique for the treatment of idiopathic pruritus ani. Int Surg 75:43–46

Smith LE, Henrichs D, McCullah RDJ (1982) Prospective studies on the etiology and treatment of pruritus ani. Dis Colon Rectum 25:358–363

Sommer B, Hagedorn M (1996) Development of squamous cell carcinoma in chronic anal eczema and therapeutic consequences. Hautarzt 47:850–853

Stein E (1998) Proktologie. Lehrbuch und Atlas, 3rd edn. Springer, Berlin

Stein E (1992) Diseases of the anus and perianal region. In: Demis DJ (eds) Clinical dermatology, vol 4. Lippincott-Raven, Philadelphia, pp 1–21

Thompson WC (1984) Proctalgia fugax. Am J Gastroenterol 79:450–452

Toglia MR (1998) Pathophysiology of anorectal dysfunction. Obstet Gynecol Clin North Am 25:771–781

Verbov J (1984) Pruritus ani and its management – a study and reappraisal. Clin Exp Dermatol 9:46–52

Vincent C (1999) Anorectal pain and irritation: anal fissure, levator syndrome, proctalgia fugax, and pruritus ani. Prim Care 26:53–68

Wienert V (1985a) Diagnose und Therapie des Analekzems. Hautarzt 36:232–233

Wienert V (1985b) Die Analfissur. Hautarzt 36:234–236

Wienert V, Grussendorf E-J (1980) Anokutaner Ergotismus gangraenosus. Hautarzt 31:668–670

Wienert V (1991) Peri-anal dermatopathies. Z Gastroenterol Verh 26:173–175

CHAPTER 68

Andrology

Hans Wolff and Wolf-Bernhard Schill

Contents

Introduction

Clinical andrology deals with diseases of the male genital organs (Fig. 68.1), focusing on male infertility and erectile dysfunction. In Germany, andrology has been mainly advanced by dermatologists and therefore is part of the German dermatology board certification. There is close cooperation with other disciplines such as urology, endocrinology, and gynecology.

Most often, andrologists are involved in the diagnostic workup of the male member of an infertile couple. Infertility is defined by the absence of pregnancy despite regular sexual intercourse for more than 12 months. In Western countries, approximately 15 % of all couples have infertility problems, with a male factor in up to 50 % of these couples.

Spermatogenesis and Sperm Transport

Hormones

The formation of spermatozoa starts in puberty and is dependent on hypothalamic, pituitary, and testicular hormones. In a pulsatile fashion, neurons of the hypothalamus secrete gonadotropin-releasing hormone (GnRH), a decapeptide that stimulates the anterior pituitary gland to produce the glycoproteins follicle-stimulating hormone (FSH) and luteinizing hormone (LH). Via the circulation, FSH and LH reach the testicles where FSH initiates spermatogenesis in the seminiferous tubules and LH stimulates interstitial Leydig cells to produce testosterone. Testosterone is essential for sexual differentiation, spermatogenesis, and erection. In addition, it helps to build up and maintain muscle and bone mass (Table 68.1).

Testis

The formation of spermatozoa occurs in the seminiferous tubules of the testicles. A healthy man has

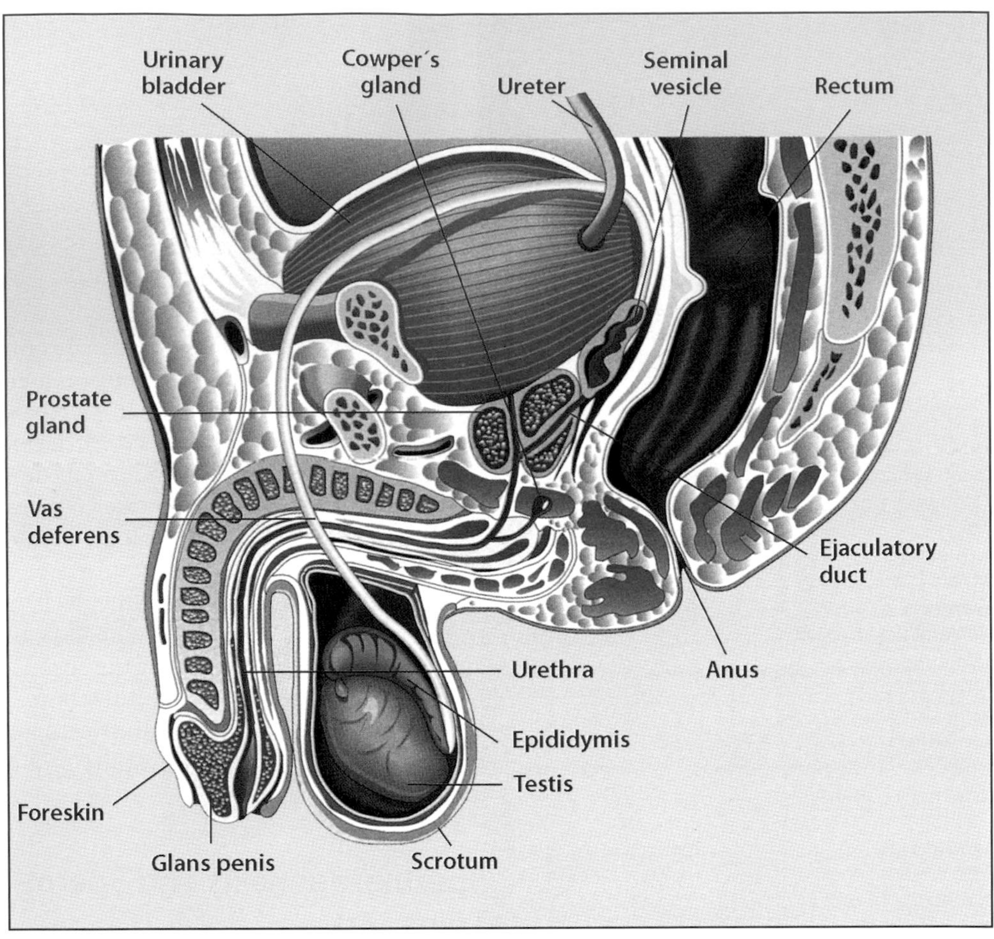

Fig. 68.1. The male genital tract organs (testes, epididymides, seminal vesicles, prostate, urethra, penis)

500–1000 seminiferous tubules with a total length of approximately 300 m. The walls of the seminiferous tubules are lined with Sertoli cells which closely interact with the germinative cell lineage. Sertoli cells provide important nutrients to the germ cells to support normal maturation.

The maturation of one spermatozoon (spermatogenesis) comprises two mitotic and two meiotic cell divisions and lasts approximately 60–75 days. The first step is the division of a primary (type A) spermatogonia. One of the two cells remains a primary spermatogonia with the potential of repeated divisions, while the other cell differentiates into a secondary (type B) spermatogonia. After another mitotic division, two primary sper-

Table 68.1. Hormones for the regulation of spermatogenesis and testosterone production

Origin	Hormone	Target organ	Function
Hypothalamus	GnRH	Pituitary	FSH and LH production
Pituitary	FSH	Seminiferous tubules	Spermatogenesis
Pituitary	LH	Leydig cells	Testosterone production
Leydig cells	Testosterone	Seminiferous tubules Bones, muscles Hypothalamus	Spermatogenesis Anabolic functions GnRH suppression
Sertoli cells	Inhibin	Pituitary	FSH suppression

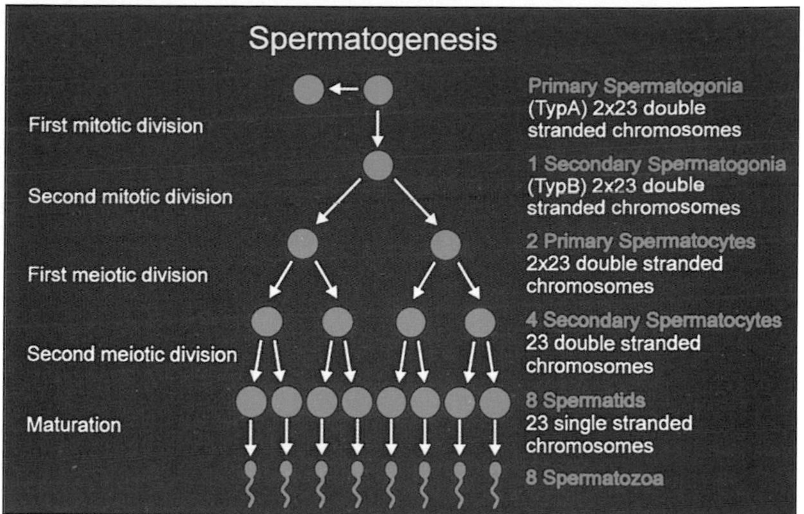

Fig. 68.2. Spermatogenesis

matocytes are produced. In the following meiotic cell division, two primary spermatocytes, still containing 46 double-stranded chromosomes each (diploidy), produce four secondary spermatocytes which now contain only 23 double-stranded chromosomes (haploidy). In the second meiotic division, the four secondary spermatocytes produce eight spermatids, each containing 23 single-stranded chromosomes (Fig. 68.2).

In the following weeks, the spermatids undergo three differentiation steps:

- Condensation of the DNA to fit into the small head of a spermatozoon
- Differentiation of the Golgi complex to form the acrosome
- Differentiation of the centrioles to generate the sperm tail

Finally, the mature spermatozoon is released from the germinal epithelium (spermiation) and is passively transported to the rete testis. From there, the spermatozoa enter the epididymis via approximately ten efferent ducts.

Epididymis

The epididymis is a tiny, heavily coiled tube. Uncoiled, its length is approximately 6 m. Starting in the head of the epididymis, spermatozoa undergo further maturation to improve sperm motility and acrosome function in order to increase their fertilizing capacity. It takes approximately 1–2 weeks until spermatozoa reach the tail of the epididymis where they are stored until ejaculation.

Ejaculation

During ejaculation, spermatozoa are pressed out of the epididymis into the spermatic cord. Under the control of sympathetic nerves, the smooth muscles of the spermatic cord perform coordinated contractions to advance spermatozoa into the posterior urethra. In the utriculus region, the secretions of the prostate and seminal vesicles join in. The ejaculate is expelled in a series of three to five muscular contractions.

Spermatozoa in the Female Genital Tract

From the posterior vagina, spermatozoa enter the cervical mucus which is least viscous at the time of ovulation. The cervical mucus is an impenetrable barrier for bacteria and low motility spermatozoa. After having passed through the uterine cavity, a small fraction of the spermatozoa is able to enter the fallopian tubes. During this ascent, capacitation of the spermatozoa occurs, a prerequisite for the acrosome reaction. In the ampulla, at the end of one fallopian tube, approximately 100–200 spermatozoa encounter the oocyte. By releasing hyaluronidase, the spermatozoon is able to penetrate the cell layer of the cumulus oophorus. Reaching the zona pellucida, the spermatozoon binds to specific glycoprotein receptors (zona pellucida protein ZP-3), by which the acrosome reaction is initiated. In this well-orchestrated exocytotic burst, the proteolytic enzyme acrosin is released, enabling the spermatozoon to penetrate the zona pellucida. When the first spermatozoon reaches the egg plasma membrane, the oocyte becomes impenetrable for other spermatozoa within milliseconds. Sperm and oocyte plasma membranes fuse, leading to mixture of the intracellular contents of both cells. Then, the highly compacted sperm chromatin is decondensed, and finally 23 chromosomes from the spermatozoon pair with 23 chromosomes from the oocyte. In the following days, a series of embryonic cell divisions takes place while the zygote is being transported down the fallopian tube to reach the uterine cavity after 3–4 days for implantation.

Clinical and Laboratory Evaluation

Medical History

The medical history can yield important clues for the presence and origin of fertility disorders. If there was hormonal or surgical treatment for undescended testicles in childhood (cryptorchidism), the patient is more likely to have reduced semen quality. Surgical hernia repair can lead to irreversible damage of the spermatic cord and the testicular artery. Mumps-associated autoimmune orchitis can lead to testicular atrophy. Although more frequently seen in the preantibiotic era, ascending gonorrheal or chlamydial infections can cause epididymitis with scarring occlusion of the epididymal ducts, resulting in azoospermia.

Chronic diseases can significantly impair male fertility. Long-standing diabetes mellitus can lead to erectile and ejaculatory dysfunction, the latter due to autonomic nerve damage. Men taking sulfasalazine for Crohn disease or ulcerative colitis often have reversible, drug-induced oligozoospermia. A history of cytostatic chemotherapy predisposes to reduced semen quality. Occupational factors such as inhalation of solvents in painters or chronic heat exposure in steel workers may lead to reduced sperm production. Excessive use of alcohol, nicotine or marihuana has also been associated with male infertility.

A brief gynecologic history of the female partner should also be obtained, including length and regularity of the menstrual cycle, history of STDs and previous therapeutic attempts to conceive. Finally, the frequency and timing of sexual intercourse during the menstrual cycle can be of crucial importance. By using basal temperature charts, the woman should know her fertile days. Daily intercourse is recommended before and after suspected ovulation.

Physical Examination

As the first step of the physical examination, the general appearance of the patient is evaluated. If the patient is taller than 190 cm, has broad hips, gynecomastia, and sparse body hair, Klinefelter syndrome can be suspected. Bilateral gynecomastia may indicate a prolactinoma of the pituitary, a hormone-secreting testicular cancer, or a side effect of a drug. In unilateral gynecomastia, a mammary cancer should be excluded by ultrasonography, mammography, or surgery.

During examination of the penis, the position of the urethral orifice should be checked to exclude epi- or hypospadia. In both cases, problems with the correct precervical deposition of semen may occur. If uncircumcised, the retractibility of the prepuce should be checked to exclude phimosis, which may also interfere with the precervical deposition of semen. The glans penis should be examined for condylomas, candidiasis, Zoon disease, and other dermatologic disorders.

The testicles should have a firm elastic consistency and be 15–30 ml in size. The volume of a testis can be estimated with the help of a Prader orchidometer, which is a string of elliptical spheres between 2 and 30 ml. Alternatively, testicular size and structure can be determined by ultrasonography. If there is a very firm, painless induration or enlargement, testicular cancer has to be excluded. The testicles should be located in the scrotum. In some men, they can be mobilized into the inguinal canal – a phenomenon called retractile testicles. Cryptorchidism is the term for testicles consistently present in the inguinal canal or in the peritoneal cavity.

The epididymides are attached to the cranial and posterior surfaces of the testicles. They should be soft. Induration may be indicative of chronic inflammation or obstruction of sperm outflow. Finally, the spermatic cords are identified to exclude uni- or bilateral absence of the vas deferens.

The testicular veins should be palpated for varicose enlargements. By asking the patient to perform the Valsalva maneuver, the functionality of the venous valves can be examined. In addition, Doppler ultrasonography should be performed to diagnose and grade a varicocele.

The prostate is palpated rectally. It should be soft and chestnut-sized. By rectal sonography the prostate and seminal vesicles can be visualized. Sonography of the seminal vesicles is particularly helpful if high obstruction of the seminal outlet is suspected. Here, both enlargement and complete absence of the seminal vesicles may hint at anatomic obstruction.

Semen Analysis

Semen is a mixture of secretions from different male genital tract organs. The testes and epididymides contribute only 5% to the final ejaculate volume, prostatic fluid 30–40%, and seminal vesicle secretions 50–60%. Seminal vesicle fluid has a basic pH and is rich in fructose and prostaglandins. Prostatic fluid has an acidic pH and is rich in zinc, acid phosphatase, citrate, and a serine protease, prostate-specific antigen (PSA). A very small fraction – sometimes emerging before ejaculation as a clear, viscous fluid – is contributed by the bulbourethral glands.

The analysis of semen is the central part of every male infertility workup. To obtain comparable results, the criteria defined by the World Health Organization (WHO) should be applied (Table 68.2).

Sexual Abstinence

A factor strongly affecting the number of spermatozoa is sexual abstinence before semen analysis. Therefore, the patient should abstain from ejaculation for 3–6 days. Usually, semen is obtained by masturbation. Due to spermiotoxic substances, condoms are not suitable for semen collection. For microbiologic examination, the urinary bladder should be voided before masturbation to flush the urethra. The ejaculate should be analyzed within 1–2 h. In cases of low sperm counts, it is recommended to analyze the postejaculatory urine to exclude retrograde ejaculation.

Table 68.2. Normal semen parameters (WHO 1992)

Liquefaction time	<60 min
Appearance of ejaculate	Milky
Volume	>2.0 ml
pH	7.2–8.0
Sperm number	$>20\times10^6$/ml $>40\times10^6$/ejaculate
Sperm motility	>50% motile sperm (WHO a+b) >25% progressively motile (WHO a)
Sperm morphology	>30% normal morphology
Round cells	$<5\times10^6$/ml
White blood cells	$<1\times10^6$/ml

Coagulation and Liquefaction

Immediately after ejaculation, seminal vesicle proteins cause clotting of the ejaculate. The evolutionary advantage of this coagulation is probably to prevent leakage of the semen from the vagina. Through the action of the prostatic serine protease, the semen liquefies again within 30–60 min. If not, the man suffers from hyperviscosity of the semen, which may prevent his spermatozoa from leaving the semen coagulum to ascend into the cervix. To liquefy hyperviscous semen, proteolytic enzymes such as chymotrypsin (150 U/ml) or bromelain (1 mg/ml) can be added to the ejaculate.

Ejaculate Volume

The normal volume of an ejaculate after a sexual abstinence of at least 2 days is 2.0–6.0 ml. Hypospermia, an ejaculate volume of less than 2.0 ml, may be a symptom of seminal vesicle dysfunction because these glands contribute most to the ejaculate. Further diagnostic workup should include measurement of seminal fructose, the classic seminal vesicle marker enzyme, and serum testosterone, because the seminal vesicles are strongly androgen-dependent. Small-volume, low-pH (<7.0), and low-fructose ejaculates indicate anatomic obstruction or atresia of the seminal vesicles. Here, rectal ultrasonography should be performed.

Sperm Motility

For microscopic semen analysis, 10 µl of the liquefied ejaculate are placed on a microscope slide and covered by a 22×22 mm coverslip. The temperature should be close to 37°C. Reliable assessment of sperm motility is difficult and requires continuous training. A total of 100 spermatozoa are classified according to the following WHO categories:
a = Rapidly progressive motile
b = Slowly progressive motile
c = Motile, but not progressive
d = Not motile

The motility assessment is repeated once. The final result is the percent mean of the two procedures. If less than 50 % of the spermatozoa are motile, or less than 25 % are progressively motile, the patient suffers from asthenozoospermia. If all spermatozoa are immotile, the patient may have an immotile cilia syndrome. As a supplement to conventional semen analysis, computer-assisted semen analysis (CASA) may be used. However, these machines are not more reliable than a trained technician and difficult to use with very low or high density sperm samples.

Sperm Count

Sperm numbers are crucial for male fertility assessment. A 50 μl sample of the ejaculate is mixed with 950 μl of distilled water. This 1:20 dilution allows for convenient counting in a hemocytometer because spermatozoa are immediately immobilized by the distilled water. Sperm numbers have a special nomenclature shown in Table 68.3.

If no spermatozoa are seen in the wet mount, the ejaculate should be centrifuged to examine the pellet. The occurrence of spermatogenic cells indicates the patency of the seminal duct system.

Sperm Morphology

The structure of the spermatozoon is assessed using special stains such as Giemsa, Papanicolaou, or Shorr for semen smears on microscope glass slides. At a 400 – 1000 × magnification, 100 spermatozoa are classified as morphologically normal or abnormal. This must be done by a technician with extensive experience and thorough training. A normal spermatozoon has an oval head of 4.0 – 5.5 μm and a tail of approximately 50 μm. The sperm acrosome should cover 40 – 70 % of the head. If all spermatozoa have small round heads without acrosomes, the man is suffering from globozoospermia. Because these spermatozoa are not able to penetrate the zona pellucida, men with globozoospermia are sterile.

Compared to animals such as stallions or boars, human ejaculate contains a high number of abnormal spermatozoa. Only if more than 70 % of the spermatozoa are morphologically abnormal is the ejaculate termed teratozoospermic.

Frequently, male infertility patients have combined disorders of sperm number, motility, and morphoplogy, called oligo-astheno-terato-zoospermia.

Table 68.3. Nomenclature of abnormal findings in semen analysis

Aspermia	No ejaculation (“dry orgasm”)
Hypospermia	< 2.0 ml ejaculate volume
Azoospermia	0×10^6 Sp/ml
Cryptozoospermia	$< 1 \times 10^6$ Sp/ml
Oligozoospermia	$< 20 \times 10^6$ Sp/ml
Polyzoospermia	$> 250 \times 10^6$ Sp/ml
Asthenozoospermia	< 50 % motile sperm (WHO a + b) < 25 % progressively motile sperm (WHO a)
Teratozoospermia	< 30 % normal sperm forms
Hematospermia	Blood in the ejaculate
Leukocytospermia	$> 10^6$ white blood cells/ml

White Blood Cells in Semen

Round cells in semen can be either immature germ cells or white blood cells. The latter are easily identified by a cytochemical peroxidase stain. For this purpose, a stock solution is prepared of 125 mg benzidine + 50 ml distilled water + 50 ml 96 % ethanol. To obtain the working solution, 5 μl of 30 % H_2O_2 is added to 4.0 ml of stock solution. To evaluate peroxidase-positive granulocytes in semen, 20 μl of ejaculate are mixed with 160 μl of distilled water and 20 μl of working solution. After 5 min at room temperature, the peroxidase-positive brown cells are assessed in a counting chamber. If the peroxidase-positive white blood cells exceed 10^6/ml, the ejaculate is termed leukocytospermic.

Biochemical Investigations

There are several biochemical markers in semen that provide information on different organ systems. The most important marker for seminal vesicle function is fructose, which should be above 13 mmol per ejaculate. Decreased fructose may hint at a lack of testosterone because the seminal vesicles are strongly androgen-dependent. Alternatively, there may be postinflammatory atrophy of the seminal vesicles. Prostatic function is reflected by normal levels of citric acid in the semen (> 52 mmol per ejaculate). An important marker for patency of the spermatic cord is neutral α-glucosidase in semen. If the level of this epididymal marker is below 20 mU per ejaculate, azoospermia is probably due to anatomic obstruction rather than to testicular insufficiency. If an inability of the spermatozoa to fertilize oocytes is suspected, the determination of acrosin in several fractions of semen may be helpful. In addition, sperm function assays, such as the triple-stain method to evaluate the acrosome reaction or the hemizona assay to assess the ability of spermatozoa to bind to the zona pellucida, may be useful in certain cases. Aniline blue staining of sperm DNA provides information about the nuclear maturity, which correlates well with the fertilizing ability of ejaculated spermatozoa.

Varicocele

Approximately 10–20% of all men and 20–40% of male infertility patients have valvular insufficiency of the testicular veins. This leads to varicose enlargement of the scrotal part of the vein, called varicocele (Fig. 68.3). The stasis and retrograde flow of blood cause overheating of the testicles, which is detrimental to spermatogenesis. In more than 95% of affected men, the varicoceles are left-sided because the left testicular vein goes up to the renal vein, which it enters at a hemodynamically unfavorable right angle. In contrast, the right testicular vein joins the inferior vena cava at a favorable small angle. Therefore, right sided varicoceles are additionally present in only 5–10% of affected men. Varicoceles can be classified both clinically and by Doppler ultrasonography. In both gradings, the Valsava maneuver plays an important role. The clinical varicocele grading is:

- Clinical grade I: Varicocele not visible but palpable on Valsalva pressing
- Clinical grade II: Varicocele not visible but always palpable
- Clinical grade III: Varicocele always visible (Fig. 68.3)

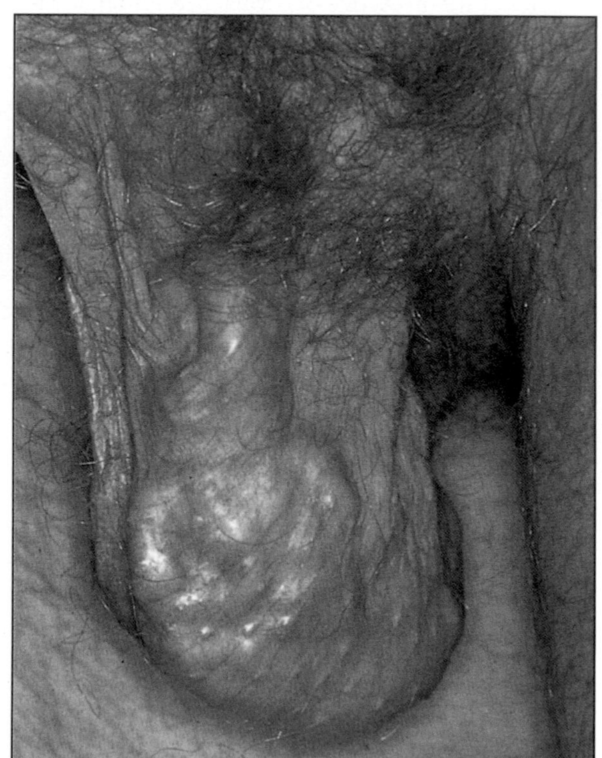

Fig. 68.3. Varicocele grade III

The functional examination of a varicocele is performed by Doppler ultrasonography. First, the pulsating testicular artery is localized at the base of the scrotum, along the spermatic cord. Then, the Doppler flow of the testicular vein is examined and graded:

- Sonography grade –: No reflux, even with Valsalva pressing
- Sonography grade +: Reflux only with Valsalva pressing
- Sonography grade ++: Spontaneous reflux without Valsalva pressing.

Therapy. Men with reduced semen quality may benefit from varicocele therapy. This can be done by radiologically controlled sclerosing of the testicular veins – in an expert's hands an effective and safe outpatient procedure. Very large varicoceles should be treated surgically. After 3–6 months, a significant improvement of semen quality can be expected in approximately two-thirds of the patients. In parallel, significant increases of pregnancy rates compared with untreated controls can be observed.

Oligo- and Azoospermia

A low sperm count is the most frequent finding in infertile men. It reflects either insufficient spermatogenesis or anatomic obstruction of sperm transport. Spermatogenesis can be disturbed for many reasons, as shown in Table 68.4.

Table 68.4. Reasons for oligo- and azoospermia

Congenital factors and syndromes
Cryptorchidism
Sertoli-cell-only syndrome
Kallmann syndrome
Klinefelter syndrome
Endocrinology
Hypothalamic dysfunction (GnRH deficiency, Kallmann syndrome)
Pituitary dysfunction (tumors, prolactinoma, FSH and LH deficiency)
Drugs
Cytostatic chemotherapy
Salazosulfapyridine
Anabolic steroids (body building)
Environmental factors (solvent exposure of painters)
Ionizing radiation
Overheating of testicles (varicocele, hot baths, excessive car seat heating)
Anatomic obstruction (postinflammatory, vasectomy)
Congenital absence of the vas deferens (cystic fibrosis gene)
Idiopathic (no known cause)

Congenital Factors

The most frequent congenital abnormality among infertile men is a history of undescended testes, in which the testicles are not correctly positioned in the scrotum after birth. Mostly, the gonads are located in the inguinal canal, sometimes still in the peritoneal cavity (cryptorchidism). Although undescended testes are not uncommon immediately after birth (>4%), in most boys the testicles spontaneously descend within the next few months. If not, hormonal therapy with human chorionic gonadotropin (HCG) or GnRH should be started by the pediatrician within the first year of life to induce testicular descent and to prevent further testicular damage by overheating. If unsuccessful, surgical therapy is necessary to bring the testicles into the scrotum (orchidopexy). Despite therapy, undescended testes in childhood are often associated with impaired spermatogenesis in the adult.

In the Sertoli-cell-only syndrome or Del Castillo syndrome, the seminiferous tubules contain exclusively Sertoli cells and no germ cells. In Kallmann syndrome, there is an association between hypogonadotropic hypogonadism and anosmia, both manifestations of a hypothalamic developmental abnormality. Because hypothalamic GnRH secretion is lacking, there is neither pituitary FSH nor LH secretion and thus neither spermatogenesis nor testosterone production. There are numerous other syndromes leading to infertility. Often the general disturbances are so serious that fertility is not relevant in these men. One example is the Prader-Labhart-Willi syndrome in which hypogenitalism and cryptorchidism is associated with reduced intelligence, dwarfism, obesity, and diabetes mellitus.

Side Effects of Drugs

There are a number of drugs that impair spermatogenesis. After chemotherapy with cytostatic drugs, spermatogenesis is arrested for several years in some patients forever. Approximately 20–30% of young men undergoing chemotherapy remain sterile. Therefore, cryopreservation of semen should be performed before chemotherapy. Sulfasalazine, a drug frequently used in Crohn disease and rheumatoid arthritis, can lead to reversible oligozoospermia.

Overheating of the Testicles

The ideal temperature for spermatogenesis is 32 °C. The most frequent reason for overheating of the testicles is the presence of a varicocele. Sometimes occupational reasons lead to increased heat exposure, for example in steel workers. Some people overheat their testicles by frequently taking hot baths, visiting saunas, or continuously using car seat heating.

Tumors and Malignancies

Testicular tumors are often associated with decreased semen quality. Tumors of the hypothalamus and the pituitary gland can lead to defective secretion of GnRH, FSH, and LH and consequently to disturbed spermatogenesis. Many men with Hodgkin and non-Hodgkin lymphomas have reduced sperm numbers, even before undergoing chemotherapy. Men with advanced HIV infection often develop testicular atrophy, leading to low sperm numbers and insufficient testosterone production.

Anatomic Obstruction

Anatomic obstruction of sperm transport is an important differential diagnosis in azoospermia. It can be congenital or acquired. In congenital

Table 68.5. Differential diagnosis of azoospermia

	Anatomic obstruction	Disturbed spermatogenesis
History	Epididymitis	Cryptorchism in childhood
Testis size	Normal (>15 ml)	Low (<10 ml)
FSH	Normal (<10 IU/ml)	Increased (>10 IU/ml)
α-Glucosidase	Low (<20 IU/ejaculate)	Normal (>20 IU/ejaculate)

absence of the vas deferens, a cystic fibrosis gene mutation should be suspected. Because these men can often be helped with modern methods of assisted reproduction, both partners should be given genetic counseling for the risk of giving birth to a child with cystic fibrosis. Acquired anatomic obstruction of sperm transport is most often due to postinflammatory occlusion of the epididymal ducts (Table 68.5). In men under 35 years old, *Chlamydia trachomatis* is the main culprit for epididymitis; in men over 35 years old, it is *Escherichia coli.*

Therapy

Often none of the factors mentioned above can be held responsible for the oligozoospermia – it is then termed idiopathic. There are a number of empirical therapies that can be tried in oligozoospermia, although they have not proven their efficacies in randomized, double-blind, placebo-controlled clinical trials. To monitor their efficacy, a therapeutic effort should be preceded by two baseline semen analyses. As one cycle of spermatogenesis takes 2.5 months, follow-up semen analyses should be performed every 3 months. Therapy should be given for at least 3–6 months. The empiric regimens listed in Table 68.6 are currently in use for idiopathic oligozoospermia.

There is no accepted definition for the effectiveness of andrologic drug therapy. However, if ingestion of the drug is accompanied by doubling of the sperm numbers, some effectiveness may be assumed. As none of the empirical therapies is able to correct idiopathic oligozoospermia permanently, the drugs have to be taken for as long as the positive effect is desired.

Endocrine Disorders

There are several indications for the measurement of serum hormones. In patients with hypoplastic testicles or severe oligozoospermia, a set of three hormones should be determined: FSH, LH, and testosterone. If the FSH and LH levels are below normal, a gonadotropin-releasing hormone (GnRH) test is warranted, in which 100 μg of LH-RH, a GnRH analogue, are injected intraveneously. Before and 30 min after injection, venous blood is drawn to monitor changes of FSH and LH levels. Table 68.7

Table 68.6. Empiric drug therapy for idiopathic oligozoospermia

Drug	Oral dosage per day	Type of drug
Kallikrein	3×200 IE	Kininogenase
Pentoxifylline	3×400 mg	Rheologic agent
Tamoxifen	2×10 mg	Antiestrogen
Testosterone undecanoate	3×40 mg	Androgen
Mesterolone	3×25 mg	Androgen
Folic acid	3×5 mg	Vitamin
Tocopherol	1×600 mg	Vitamin E

Table 68.7. Differentiation of hypogonadism by the GnRH test

FSH[a]	GnRH test	Site of pathology	Type of hypogonadism
High	–	Testis	Primary
Low	FSH and LH stay low	Pituitary	Secondary
Low	FSH and LH rise	Hypothalamus	Tertiary

[a] High FSH: >10 IU/ml; low FSH: <1.0 IU/ml

shows the possible results and their interpretations in reference to the type of hypogonadism.

Most frequently, low sperm numbers are due to primary, testicular hypogonadism, as indicated by high serum FSH levels. The increase of FSH is caused by a lack of testicular inhibin production which normally controls the pituitary's FSH secretion. The higher the FSH level in the serum, the more severe the testicular damage. In secondary hypogonadism, the pituitary is not able to produce FSH and LH, even with stimulation of LH-RH. Here, a pituitary tumor has to be excluded by computed tomography.

In tertiary hypogonadism, FSH and LH rise after injection of LH-RH, proving the functionality of the pituitary. The best known example of tertiary hypogonadism is Kallmann syndrome.

Therapy. In secondary and tertiary hypogonadism, low FSH and LH levels can be augmented pharmacologically to induce spermatogenesis. For this purpose, a fixed scheme of intramuscular injections is employed:

- Human menopausal gonadotropin (HMG), 3×150 IU per week
- Human chorionic gonadotropin (HCG), 2×2500 IE per week

In men with hypothalamic hypogonadism, missing GnRH can be administered subcutaneously by a pump in a pulsatile fashion (given continuously, GnRH does not stimulate but inhibits FSH and LH secretion).

If responsive, spermatogenesis starts after 3 months in both regimens. Due to the high costs of these therapies ($500–1000 per month), reproductive assistance should be given early with in vitro fertilization (IVF) or intracytoplasmic sperm injection (ICSI). In addition, spermatozoa should be cryopreserved for later trials.

Low serum testosterone levels should be investigated further. If pituitary LH is normal or elevated, the testicular Leydig cells are not working properly. Testosterone should be replaced pharmacologically to normalize sexual function and to avoid osteoporosis and loss of muscle mass. The most effective way to achieve reliable testosterone replacement is intramuscular injection of 250 mg testosterone enanthate every 2–4 weeks. In cases of less severe reduction, oral testosterone undecanoate (3×40 mg/day) or topically applied testosterone-releasing patches can be tried.

Genital Tract Infections

Most andrologic patients have no clinical signs of acute genital tract infection. Because chronic genital tract infections may be silent, microbiologic investigations of the ejaculate should be performed if there are signs of inflammation. These can come from the medical history, clinical findings, and semen analysis:

- A female partner with genital tract infection
- Urethral discharge
- Burning sensation during urination
- Perineal or rectal pain (prostatitis)
- Testicular or epididymal pain
- Many bacteria in the semen wet mount
- Many round cells in semen ($>5\times10^6$/ml)
- Leukocytospermia ($>1\times10^6$ WBC/ml)
- pH > 8.0
- Massive sperm agglomeration

Diagnosis. The ejaculate should be checked for gonococci, enterococci, *E. coli*, mycoplasma, *Ureaplasma urealyticum*, and *C. trachomatis*. Whereas in the preantibiotic era gonococci played an important role, today *C. trachomatis* may have the strongest impact on the fertility of a couple. In men, chlamydia can cause urethritis, prostatitis, and epididymitis. In women, chlamydia not only induce cervicitis but may ascend to cause salpingitis, which can lead to bilateral tubal occlusion. Chlamydial cultures of urethral scrapings on McCoy cell feeder layers are often negative because the urethra is not representative of the entire male genital tract. Although the ejaculate reflects all relevant genital tract organs, it cannot be used for McCoy cell cultures because the semen contains cytotoxic substances. Therefore, modern and sensitive methods such as the polymerase chain reaction (PCR) should be applied to detect *C. trachomatis* in semen. Seminal IgA and IgG antibodies against chlamydia appear to have a high sensitivity but low specificity. Because antibodies tend to persist even after antibiotic therapy, they are not suited for monitoring responses.

The clinical relevance of the presence of *E. coli*, enterococci, mycoplasma, and *U. urealyticum* is questionable in patients without signs of infection. However, to minimize potential infertility cofactors, one antibiotic course in both partners may be justified.

Some men have persistently increased numbers of white blood cells in their semen without evidence of microorganisms. If present in high numbers ($>4\times10^6$/ml semen), white blood cells may damage spermatozoa. For example, granulocytes can secrete large amounts of reactive oxygen species or proteases that may damage the sperm acrosome. One should always try to localize the origin of white blood cells in semen. Therefore, prostatic massage should be performed and further workup by an urologist is warranted to exclude rare reasons for sterile leukocytospermia such as genital tract tuberculosis.

Therapy. Male genital tract infections should be treated by antibiotic courses of no less than 10–15 days. Drugs widely used include doxycycline (2×100 mg/day), erythromycin (4×500 mg/day), roxithromycin (2×150 mg/day), ofloxacin (2×200 mg/day) or other broad-spectrum antibiotics. In severe leukocytospermia, antiinflammatory drugs such as indomethacin (100–150 mg/day) or antioxidative regimens with vitamins E and C (600 mg and 1000 mg/day, respectively) may be tried.

Sperm Antibodies

Approximately 10% of infertile men have antibodies against spermatozoa in their serum or seminal plasma. While serum antibodies against spermatozoa may indicate previous testicular and epididymal inflammation, obstruction, or trauma, they have no clinical relevance. In contrast, sperm antibodies in the seminal plasma may lead to agglutination and immobilization of spermatozoa. Sometimes spermatozoa coated by antibodies stick to the cervical mucus, which microscopically can be seen as a shaking phenomenon. Rarely, sperm antibodies may affect the acrosome reaction or lead to phagocytosis by granulocytes.

Diagnosis. There are several methods to detect sperm antibodies in semen. The MAR (mixed agglutination reaction) test can be performed within minutes using fresh ejaculate of the patient. In the immunobead test, spermatozoa are washed before being used. In both tests, sperm-bound antibodies are visualized by secondary anti-human IgA or IgG antibodies linked to red blood cells or latex beads. If more than 20–40% of spermatozoa participate in these mixed agglutinations, the ejaculate is classified as sperm antibody-positive.

Therapy. Corticosteroids are rarely given to suppress sperm antibody formation because of their side effects and lack of efficacy. Intrauterine insemination and intracytoplasmic sperm injection are now the therapies of choice for men with functionally relevant sperm antibodies.

Ejaculatory Disorders

The most frequent cause of blocked sperm transport is vasectomy, in which for contraceptive purposes the spermatic cords have been severed. Sometimes, there is congenital aplasia of the spermatic cords, especially in men carrying a cystic fibrosis gene mutation. Another reason for obstruction of the sperm outlet is postinflammatory occlusion of the epididymal ducts, for example as a result of gonococcal or chlamydial infection of the epididymis.

Functional disturbance of sperm transport may result from destruction of the paraaortic sympathetic nerves which are responsible for the smooth muscle contractions of the spermatic cord during ejaculation. In addition, sympathetic nerves may be damaged by autonomic neuropathy in diabetes mellitus or due to sympatholytic drugs used in psychiatry or antihypertensive therapy.

In patients with testicular tumors such as seminoma, it may be necessary to remove the paraaortic lymph nodes. In 10–30% of these men, the paraortic sympathetic nerves will be damaged, resulting in ejaculatory disorders. These can range from retrograde ejaculation into the urinary bladder to complete aspermia.

Diagnosis. In retrograde ejaculation, the postejaculatory urine contains more spermatozoa than the ejaculate. In aspermia, the patient has an orgasm but no emission of semen (dry orgasm); the postejaculatory urine also contains no sperm. The diagnosis of a functional ejaculatory disorder can be confirmed by a midodrin test, in which the patient receives intraveneously 5–15 mg of midodrin, an α-sympathomimetic drug for the treatment of hypotension. After 15 min, semen and postejaculatory urine samples are collected. If ejaculated spermatozoa are more numerous in the urine, a functional, midodrin-responsive defect of sperm transport may be suspected. Side effects of the midodrin test include increased blood pressure and a temporary inability to void urine.

Therapy. Sympathetic nerve activity can be substituted pharmacologically by giving either sympathomimetic or parasympatholytic drugs. In men without hypertension, 5–15 mg of midodrin, which stimulates α-receptors, can be given intravenously 15 min before ejaculation. Alternatively, the parasympatholytic drug imipramine can be taken orally, starting with 25 mg per day. If there is no improvement of aspermia or retrograde ejaculation, the imipramine dose can be increased to 50–75 mg/day. In diabetic patients with partial retrograde ejaculation, brompheniramine has been used with success.

Male Infertility Syndromes

Klinefelter Syndrome

(KLINEFELTER et al. 1942)

The most frequent genetic disorder related to male infertility, Klinefelter syndrome, is present in approximately 1 of 1000 unselected men and in up to 10% of men with hypogonadism. Klinefelter syndrome is caused by an additional X chromosome. The karyotype of affected men is 47,XXY. Combinations of the following findings should alert the clinician to suspect Klinefelter syndrome (Fig. 68.4):

- Tall height (>190 cm)
- Bilateral gynecomastia
- Leg ulcerations
- Small testicles (<10 ml)
- Low sperm counts
- Increased FSH (>10 U/ml)
- High-normal LH (≥10 U/ml)
- Low testosterone (<2.6 ng/ml)

The diagnosis is confirmed by karyotyping of peripheral blood mononuclear cells. It is important to note that some men with Klinefelter syndrome appear clinically normal except for small testicles. Therefore, genetic counseling including karyotyping should be performed in all men with small testicles. Men with Klinefelter syndrome who wish to have children can sometimes be helped with intracytoplasmic sperm injection. There should be lifelong monitoring of the serum testosterone levels and substitution of the hormone to prevent osteoporosis and loss of muscle mass.

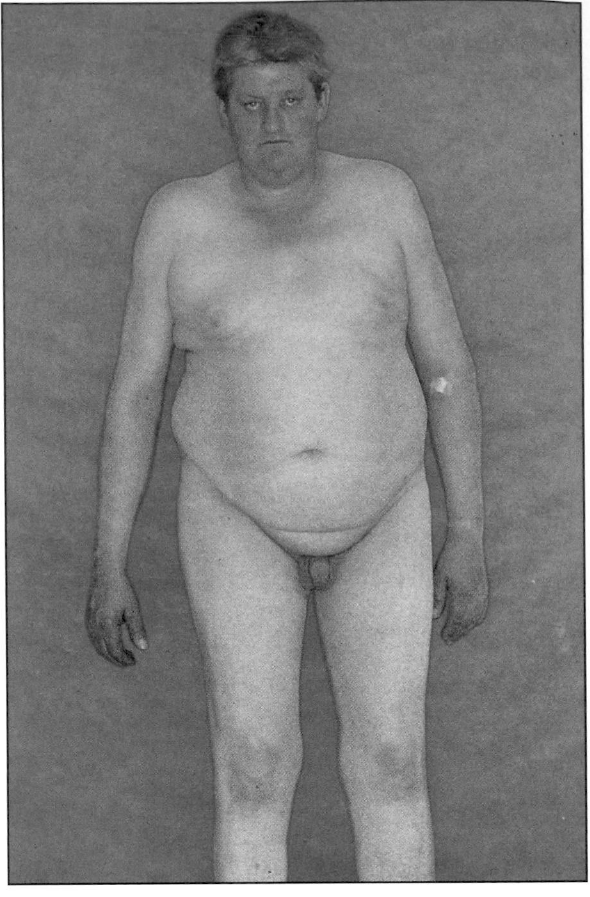

Fig. 68.4. Man with Klinefelter syndrome

Kallmann Syndrome

This disorder is characterized by tertiary hypogonadism and anosmia, both caused by congenital hypothalamic anomalies. In addition, there may be skull dysplasias, epilepsy, and sometimes mental retardation. Due to the hypothalamic malfunction, there is no GnRH to stimulate the pituitary to secrete FSH and LH. Subsequently, the testes remain small and show no spermatogenesis. Replacement of GnRH by a pulsatile pump or substitution of FSH and LH by HCG and HMG injections is sometimes able to induce spermatogenesis. If the serum testosterone level is low, replacement therapy is needed.

Congenital Bilateral Absence of the Vas Deferens

This defect is seen in all men homozygous for a cystic fibrosis gene mutation, mostly located at δF508.

Although these men have normal-sized testes and normal serum FSH, LH, and testosterone levels, they are azoospermic. As spermatozoa can be obtained surgically from the epididymis or testis and some men with congenital bilateral absence of the vas deferens (CBAVD) do not show symptoms of cystic fibrosis, all andrologic patients with CBAVD and their partners should be referred for genetic counseling prior to assisted reproduction. The probability that men with CBAVD are homozygous for a cystic fibrosis gene mutation is 42–77%.

Immotile Cilia Syndrome

If all spermatozoa are immotile, this uncommon syndrome should be suspected. Usually, there is a clearly defined defect of the sperm tail anatomy such as missing dynein arms or lack of central tubules (9+0 pattern instead of 9+2). Other ciliary structures may also be affected. In the Kartagener syndrome, there is a triad of situs inversus (heart on the right side), frequent bacterial infections of the bronchi leading to bronchiectases, and aplasia of the maxillary sinuses. Most of these disturbances are due to a lack of ciliary function. Men with immotile cilia syndrome are sterile but can be helped with intracytoplasmic sperm injection.

Globozoospermia

In this syndrome, the spermatozoa lack acrosomes. Microscopically, all of the spermatozoa have small, round heads. Despite normal motility, the gametes are not able to penetrate the zona pellucida of the oocyte. Men with globozoospermia are sterile but can be helped with intracytoplasmic sperm injection.

Assisted Reproductive Techniques

Severe andrologic disorders require modern methods of assisted reproduction. Therefore, the infertile couple should always be seen as a unit and should be treated by both the andrologist and a gynecologist specialized in reproductive medicine.

Intrauterine Insemination

This approach is often helpful in cases of moderate sperm motility impairment, provided the sperm number is normal. There are two factors determining the success of intrauterine insemination (IUI): good timing in relation to ovulation and optimal semen workup. In the andrologic laboratory, methods such as sperm swim-up or glass wool filtration can be used to obtain a pure fraction of highly motile sperm that are then inseminated into the uterus by a flexible catheter. Pretreatment of the woman with gonadotropins to induce multiple ovulations gives higher pregnancy rates but increases the risk of multiple gestations. Overall, the probability of obtaining a pregnancy by IUI is approximately 6–10% per cycle, provided that at least 10^6 highly motile sperm are inseminated.

In Vitro Fertilization

Although originally introduced in 1978 for women with tubal occlusions, it turned out that in vitro fertilization (IVF) is also able to circumvent andrologic problems such as severe oligo- and asthenozoospermia. To increase the number of oocytes available, the woman is given gonadotropins. By ultrasonography, the maturation of the follicles is monitored. Harvesting of the oocytes is done transvaginally under sonographic control. In vitro, the oocytes are added to highly motile sperm obtained by swim-up or other selective techniques. Upon fertilization, the zygote undergoes repeated cell divisions. After 2 days, a maximum of three 16-cell embryos are transferred into the uterus. Using a minimum of about 10^5 highly motile sperm, the pregnancy rate by IVF is approximately 15–25% per cycle.

Intracytoplasmic Sperm Injection

Introduced in 1993, intracytoplasmic sperm injection (ICSF) is similar to IVF except that the spermatozoa do not have to penetrate the zona pellucida of the egg. One motile spermatozoon is picked up by a micropipette and injected into the oocyte (Fig. 68.5). Spermatozoa from men with immotile cilia syndrome can also be used, provided a vital spermatozoon is selected. More than 80% of the oocytes survive the injection procedure and start to divide. After 2 days up to three fertilized eggs are transferred into the uterus. The great advantage over conventional IVF is that with ICSI one living spermatozoon is sufficient. The pregnancy rate is 20–30% per cycle. Because ICSI is very efficient,

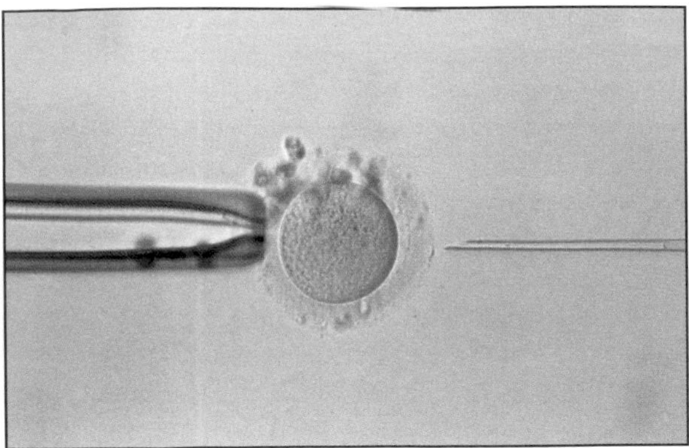

Fig. 68.5. Sperm-oocyte microinjection (ICSI)

surgically obtained epididymal and testicular spermatozoa can also be used. It is even possible to successfully microinject spermatids from men with incomplete spermatogenesis.

Microepididymal Sperm Aspiration

Men with obstructive azoospermia due to vasectomy, epididymal inflammation, or congenital bilateral absence of the vas deferens often have congested epididymal ducts from which spermatozoa can be aspirated. When used in combination with ICSI, these spermatozoa can fertilize an oocyte.

Testicular Sperm Extraction

In men with azoospermia of unknown origin, testicular sperm extraction (TESE) can combine the diagnostic method of a testicular biopsy with the therapeutic method of sperm injection (ICSI). Small pieces of the testicular tissue are enzymatically digested to release mature spermatozoa for sperm injection. Remaining spermatozoa can be cryopreserved for future attempts with ICSI.

Testicular Tumors

The symptoms of testicular tumors should be known to every andrologist. Testicular tumors are the most frequent malignancies among young men between 25 and 35 years. If diagnosed in time, approximately 90% can be cured. Men with Klinefelter syndrome or cryptorchidism have an increased risk of developing a testicular tumor. Germ cell tumors, which constitute more than 90% of all testicular tumors, are divided into seminomas (50%) and nonseminomatous tumors such as embryonal carcinoma, teratoma, choriocarcinoma, and yolk-sac carcinoma.

Diagnosis. Only few men present with the classic sign of a painless testicular mass. Most men have diffuse testicular pain, swelling, hardness, or a combination of these signs. There may be concomitant acute epididymitis and a testicular tumor. Ultrasonography of the testis may show discrete hypoechoic areas and microcalcifications. As testicular biopsies must not be performed to prevent spread of tumor cells, the only reliable diagnostic method for a testicular tumor is radical inguinal orchiectomy with ligation of the spermatic cord. Primary sites of lymphatic and vascular drainage include the retroperitoneal lymph nodes and renal or great vessels. Therefore, abdominal computed tomography and chest X-ray should be performed to check for metastases. Retroperitoneal lymph nodes between 1.0 and 2.0 cm in size have a 70% risk of being metastases. Approximately 15–20% of metastatic seminomas and 40–60% of metastatic nonseminomatous testicular tumors show increased serum HCG levels. α-Fetoprotein production is seen in 40–60% of metastatic embryonal carcinomas and yolk-sac tumors. In the USA, germ cell tumors are classified as follows.

Stage I Tumor limited to the testis, epididymis, or spermatic cord
Stage II Disease limited to the retroperitoneal lymph nodes
Stage III Supradiaphragmatic or visceral metastases

Therapy. Every testicular tumor is primarily treated by radical inguinal orchiectomy. Patients with seminomas in stages I and II also receive radiation to the retroperitoneal and ipsilateral pelvic lymph nodes. Further advanced stages (III) and relapses are treated with three or four cycles of chemotherapy; all of these regimens include cisplatin, a drug highly effective in germ cell tumors. Patients with stage I nonseminomatous tumors can be either surveyed or treated by a nerve-sparing retroperitoneal lymphadenectomy. In stage II, either retroperitoneal lymphadenectomy or cisplatin chemotherapy should be performed. In stage III, chemotherapy is always warranted. Overall, more than 90% of all patients with testicular germ cell tumors will be cured. Therefore, it is important to consider cryopreservation of their spermatozoa before therapy because retroperitoneal lymphadenectomy can lead to retrograde ejaculation in approximately 20% of the patients, and cisplatin chemotherapy may induce permanent azoospermia, especially if the cumulative cisplatin dose exceeds 400 mg.

Cryopreservation of Semen. Semen can be stored for many years at −196°C. To avoid rupture of the sperm membranes, a cryoprotective medium is added. Most of the cryoprotectants in use are based on glycerol and egg yolk. One of these media is:

Na-citrate	1.0 g
Fructose	0.5 g
Glycerol	10.0 ml
Egg yolk	30.0 ml
Distilled water ad	100.0 ml

Before cryopreservation, it should be ascertained that the man is not infected with hepatitis B or C, or HIV because these viruses can be transmitted by semen. Therefore, every patient should undergo antibody testing for these viruses. Upon thawing, cryopreserved spermatozoa usually lose a significant portion of their motility and ability to fertilize oocytes. Therefore, it is often better to use intracytoplasmic sperm injection than to inseminate these spermatozoa.

Erectile Dysfunction

Impotence or erectile dysfunction is a widely prevalent disorder. It is estimated that 30 million American men are affected. The management of erectile dysfunction requires a multidisciplinary approach involving andrologists, urologists, internists, and psychotherapists.

Etiology and Pathogenesis. The process of erection requires different systems to interact properly. Mechanically, it is mediated by the filling of the penile spongy tissues with blood. There are three anatomic structures involved: two large corpora spongiosa and the relatively small periurethral corpus spongiosum. In the flaccid condition, there is a high resistance and low-flow state of the cavernous tissues. Upon erection, relaxation of the arterial and sinus smooth muscles occurs, leading to the rapid filling of the corpora cavernosa. To stabilize erection, the venous outflow is minimized. An important chemical mediator of this process is nitric oxide, also called endothelium-derived relaxing factor.

Traditionally, a distinction has been made between erectile dysfunction due to psychologic disorders and organic causes. Today it is suspected that approximately 70–80% of cases have an organic cofactor. The latter can be classified into several categories:

- Hormonal (testosterone deficiency, hyperprolactinaemia)
- Neurogenic (autonomous neuropathy in diabetes mellitus)
- Vascular (arteriosclerosis, venous outflow insufficiency)
- Drug side effects (ranitidine, β-blockers, antipsychotic drugs)

Diagnosis. The medical history can give important hints as to the origin of erectile dysfunction. Diabetes mellitus and hypertension predispose towards this disorder. Drugs such as ranitidine, antihypertensives, or antipsychotics can cause erectile dysfunction as a side effect. The most important objective diagnostic method is the intracavernous injection of a smooth muscle relaxant such as prostaglandin E_1 or papaverine. A full erection achieved within minutes indicates normal arterial inflow. If the erection is maintained for at least 30 min, normal reduction of venous outflow can be assumed. In special cases, arteriography or cavernosography may be useful.

Therapy. The treatment of erectile dysfunction depends on the underlying cause. Medications potentially causing impotence should be changed. Hormonal disturbances are rare; if subnormal, testosterone should be substituted. Oral medications such as yohimbine seem to be beneficial for patients with mild or moderate erectile dysfunction or psychogenic factors. This effect has been shown in randomized, placebo-controlled clinical trials. Patients suffering from psychologic impotence or premature ejaculation may benefit from partner-assisted sexual therapy. Vacuum-induced erection stabilized by rubber constriction devices may be beneficial for some patients. One proven effective pharmacologic option is intracavernous self-injection of smooth muscle relaxants such as prostaglandin E_1, papaverine, or phentolamine. However, this method requires an educated patient and constant access to an urologic emergency unit for treatment of prolonged erection (priapism). An alternative to intracavernous self-injection is the intraurethral self-application of these substances. Penile prostheses have been placed in approximately 250,000 men in the USA. They are either constantly rigid, semi-rigid, or inflatable. Reoperations due to infections or loss of function are necessary in 10–15% of the men within 5–10 years.

By far the most effective and currently the most widely used drug to overcome erectile dysfunction is sildenafil (Viagra). This phosphodiesterase V-inhibitor helps the smooth muscle of the corpus cavernosum of the penis to relax and thus to prevent outflow of blood necessary to maintain erection. Taken orally as a tablet of 25, 50 or 100 mg, sildenafil restores the ability of having a full erection in approximately 70–80% of impotent men. Despite the very large number of men now regularly taking sildenafil, reports of side effects such as headaches or temporary blue-vision are rare. Sildenafil is contraindicated in men taking nitrate-containing heart medication.

Gynecomastia

Gynecomastia is a benign enlargement of the male breast. According to its etiology, several forms of gynecomastia can be differentiated (Table 68.8).

Physiologic gynecomastias are self-limited or clinically irrelevant. In newborns, maternal steroid hormones may lead to transient gynecomastia. Pubertal gynecomastia develops in approximately 40–50% of all boys and is preferentially left-sided. In adipose men, gynecomastia cannot be differentiated from fat. In elderly men, gynecomastia is due to declining testosterone levels leading to a relative increase of estrogens.

Table 68.8. Possible causes of gynecomastia

Physiologic	Newborns Puberty Obesity Advanced age
Symptomatic	Prolactinoma Klinefelter syndrome Hypogonadism Hormone-secreting tumors Hepatic diseases
Drug-related	Gonadotropins Androgens Estrogens Tamoxifen Spironolactone Ranitidine Digitalis Diazepam Vitamins A, D_2 Isoniazid Antipsychotic drugs Antihypertensives

More importantly, in young adults, gynecomastia may be due to a HCG-producing testicular germ cell tumor. In elderly men, HCG may be secreted by a bronchial carcinoma. Rarely, gynecomastia may be a symptom of systemic diseases such as leprosy, leukemia, malignant lymphoma, tuberculosis, or sarcoidosis. In one-sided gynecomastia, benign and malignant mammary tumors must be excluded by mammography or surgery, especially if there are nodular or cystic indurations.

Therapy. If no etiologic factors can be found, surgery is a simple and highly efficient method to treat gynecomastia. Using a perimamillary incision, mammary tissue and fat is removed, followed by careful remodeling of the breast.

Bibliography

Afzelius BA (1976) A human syndrome caused by immotile cilia. Science 193:317–319

Bosl GJ, Motzer RJ (1997) Testicular germ cell cancer. N Engl J Med 337:242–253

Chillon M, Casals T, Mercier B et al. (1995) Mutations in the cystic fibrosis gene in patients with congenital absence of the vas deferens. N Engl J Med 332:1475–1480

Comhaire FH (1996) Male Infertility. Clinical investigation, cause evaluation and treatment. Chapman and Hall Medical, London

Comhaire F, Verschraegen G, Vermeulen L (1980) Diagnosis of accessory gland infection and its possible role in male infertility. Int J Androl 3:32–45

Devroey P, Liu J, Nagy Z et al. (1995) Pregnancies after testicular sperm extraction and intracytoplasmic sperm injection in non-obstructive azoospermia. Hum Reprod 10:1457–1460

Goldstein I, Lue TF, Padma-Nathan H et al. (1998) Oral sildenadil in the treatment of erectile dysfunction. N Engl J Med 338:1397–1404

Goverde AJ, McDonnell J, Vermeiden JPW et al. (2000) Intrauterine insemination or in-vitro fertilization in idiopathic subfertility and male subfertilitiy: a randomized trial and cost-effectiveness analysis. Lancet 355:13–18

Hargreave TB (1994) Male infertility, 2nd edn. Springer, Berlin

Holstein AF, Roosen-Runge EC (1981) Atlas of human spermatogenesis. Grosse, Berlin

Holstein AF, Roosen-Runge EC, Schirren C (1988) Illustrated pathology of human spermatogenesis. Grosse, Berlin

Kamischke A, Nieschlag E (1999) Analysis of medical treatment of male infertility. Hum Reprod 14 [Suppl]:1–23

Klinefelter HF Jr, Reifenstein EC Jr, Albright F (1942) Syndrome characterized by gynecomastia, aspermato-genesis without A-leydigism, and increased excretion of follicle-stimulating hormone. J Clin Endocr 2:615–627

Koehn FM, Schill WB (1994) The alpha-sympathomimetic midodrin as a tool for diagnosis and treatment of sperm transport disturbances. Andrologia 26:283–287

Krane RJ, Goldstein I, de Tejada IS (1989) Impotence. N Engl J Med 321:1648–1659

Lewis RW (1995) „How prevalent is erectile dysfunction? What can be done to treat it?" In: Robaire B, Pryor JL, Trasler JM (eds) Handbook of andrology. American Society of Andrology, Lawrence, Kansas, pp 63–67

Ludwig G, Frick J (1996) Spermatology. Springer, Berlin

Mann T, Lutwak-Mann C (1981) Male reproductive function and semen. Springer, Berlin

Marshburn PB, Kutteh WH (1994) The role of antisperm antibodies in infertility. Fertil Steril 61:799–811

Mazumdar S, Levine AS (1998) Antisperm antibodies: etiology, pathogenesis, diagnosis, and treatment. Fertil Steril 70:799–810

Mortimer D (1994) Practical laboratory andrology. Oxford University Press, New York

Nieschlag E, Behre HM (1997) Andrology – male reproductive health and dysfunction. Springer, Berlin

Pont J, Albrecht W (1997) Fertility after chemotherapy for testicular germ cell cancer. Fertil Steril 68:1–5

Robaire B, Pryor JL, Trasler JM (1995) Handbook of andrology. American Society of Andrology, Lawrence

Sanger WG, Olson GH, Sherman JK (1992) Semen cryobanking for men with cancer – criteria change. Fertil Steril 58:1024–1027

Sellors JW, Mahony JB, Chernesky MA et al. (1988) Tubal factor infertility: an association with prior chlamydial infection and asymptomatic salpingitis. Fertil Steril 49:451–457

Silber S, van Steirteghem AC, Liu J et al. (1995) High fertilization and pregnancy rate after intracytoplasmic sperm injection with spermatozoa obtained from testicle biopsy. Hum Reprod 10:148–152

Silber SS, Nagy Z, Devroey P et al. (1997) Distribution of spermatogenesis in the testicles of azoospermic men: the presence or absence of spermatids in the testes of men with germinal failure. Hum Reprod 12:2422–2428

Tournaye H, Merdad T, Silber S et al. (1999) No differences in outcome after intracytoplasmic sperm injection with fresh or with frozen-thawed epididymal spermatozoa. Hum Reprod 14:90–95

Wolff H (1995) The biologic significance of white blood cells in semen. Fertil Steril 63:1143–1157

World Health Organization (1992) WHO laboratory manual for the examination of human semen and sperm-cervical mucus interaction. Cambridge University Press, Cambridge

Yavetz H, Yogev L, Hauser R et al. (1994) Retrograde ejaculation. Hum Reprod 9:381–386

Yoshida A, Miura K, Shirai M (1996) Chromosome abnormalities and male infertility. Assisted Reprod Rev 6:93–99

Topical Therapy

Contents

The treatment of skin diseases usually involves external therapy. There are many reasons for this. Appropriate topical treatment can often supplant or at least enhance systemic measures. Most patients and physicians have come to prefer topical measures. In addition there is psychologic value to having the patient care for their skin; an old saying is "busy hands are happy hands".

Many topical medications are available to treat the broad spectrum of skin diseases. Some are available in the USA without prescription. These include many wart medicines, 1% hydrocortisone cream, and an array of antimycotic agents. In Europe a number of phytopharmaceutical products are also available without prescription. There are also products that fall into the general category of cosmetics. Some are used to enhance the appearance of the skin (decorative cosmetics, such as make-up, eye shadow or lipstick); in other cases, they are intended to correct abnormal properties of the skin (skin care products such as antidandruff shampoos, moisturizers or keratolytics) or protect the skin (sunscreens or hand protection creams.)

The distinctions between cosmetics and medications have become blurred in recent years. In Germany, for example, cosmetics are regulated by the same board that controls food products, while medications are supervised by a pharmaceutical agency. As of 1998, European laws require cosmetics that make statements of efficacy, such as a sunscreen claiming a degree of protection or a facial cream claiming to reduce wrinkles, to have proof of this effect, much as has always been demanded for a medication.

The wise use of topical agents is different from the use of most systemic agents and is often a difficult skill for young dermatologists or colleagues in other specialties who attempt to treat skin disease. One must forget the idea that there is a single topical medication that will help every case of a given skin disease. This simply is not true. A medication may help a number of patients, but then may cause a flare in the next instance. The vehicle may be inappropriate, the patient may develop allergic contact dermatitis to the active ingredient or one of the vehicle components or the disease may be at a stage at which topical measures do not suffice. Thus one must consider dermatologic topical therapy as a new and important discipline, paying particular attention to three areas.

- Knowledge of the various vehicles and when to employ them
- Understanding of the active ingredients including their mechanism of action
- Clear appreciation of the appropriate indications for the various products

Basic Science Aspects

The skin, with its surface area of 1.6 – 2.0 m^2, offers an extensive region for the application and absorption of topical medications. The active ingredients penetrate the skin in two ways, either via transepidermal or transfollicular pathways. Once absorbed, the ingredients are taken up by the lymphatics or blood vessels and circulate through the organism. Almost every topically applied product can be detected in the blood; usually the levels are low. Under ideal situations, such as an occlusive patch and a special vehicle, medications can be administered through the skin. Antimotion sickness medications, hormones and antihypertensives, as well as nicotine, are all available in patch form. Toxicity from cutaneous application is also possible. This is a special risk in children, who have a relatively greater surface area and a less well-developed cutaneous barrier.

Some of the important parameters of cutaneous drug administration are considered individually.

Liberation. The first step is the release of the medication from the vehicle. If an active ingredient is more soluble in the vehicle than in the skin surface lipid film, then its action will be slow and minimal.

Adsorption. Various agents bind to different structures of the skin through a variety of physical-chemical bonds. Corticosteroids, for example, form a reservoir in the stratum corneum and are slowly released into the deeper layers of the skin.

Absorption. In this process the substances move from the vehicle through the different layers of the skin. In other words, adsorption describes the attachment of a molecule to a surface, while absorption refers to the process of uptake.

Penetration. A medication spreads through the stratum corneum into the epidermis. Some of the product remains on the outer surface. The stratum corneum is the main barrier. In addition to the percent of the material that is taken up, the form of the absorbed material is important. There are many enzymes in the outermost layer of living epidermal cells that can metabolize foreign molecules. For example, corticosteroids can be deesterified; the nonhalogenated double ester molecules such as prednicarbate are locally metabolized, reducing their topical and systemic side effects while allowing high local activity. Anthralin is metabolized in the upper layers of the epidermis so that systemic toxicity is almost unheard of.

Permeation. The entire process of passing through the skin via the transepidermal and transfollicular routes is known as permeation. It depends on many factors, including the nature of the lipid layer (containing sebum and epidermal lipids), the stratum corneum, the granular layer with the intracellular Odland or membrane-binding granules, the balance of the epidermis, the basement membrane zone, the dermal connective tissue and the lymphatic and blood vessels. In addition to these intrinsic factors, permeation is influenced by the size and charge of the active molecule, its concentration, relative solubility in its vehicle and the skin, and other complex physical-chemical factors.

Resorption. Once an agent has been taken up in the blood vessels, one speaks of resorption. Using radiolabeled molecules or similar techniques, one can exactly determine what percentage of an externally applied dose winds up in the blood stream.

All of these steps are influenced by a number of properties of the skin. These include:

Age of Patient. The skin of infants and children is more permeable than that of adults. In addition, the ratio of surface area to body weight is greater, so the risk of obtaining significant blood levels of externally applied materials is greater. Salicylic acid used for keratolytic purposes may produce salicylism and high-potency topical corticosteroids can cause Cushing syndrome; both of these problems are far more likely in infants. The cleansing product hexachlorophene and the antiscabetic lindane both may cause neurotoxicity in infants.

Area of the Body. The thinness of the skin and the density of hair follicles both facilitate uptake. A classic example is the scrotum, where penetration is very high. Some corticosteroid molecules show 40-fold (4000%) more absorption on the scrotum than on the forearm. The thickness of the stratum corneum also plays a role; thus uptake on the palms and soles is much lower than on the dorsal aspects of the hands and feet.

Pathologic Changes in the Skin. If the stratum corneum is tape-stripped (repeated application and removal of Scotch tape) or defatted, passage of medications into the skin is markedly increased. The skin of patients with atopic dermatitis also show increased uptake, while the same is true in patches of psoriasis.

Hydration of the Stratum Corneum and Skin Temperature. Both factors increase the permeation of active ingredients. When corticosteroid creams are occluded, such as with plastic wrap or an air-tight bandage, the resorption is increased 10- to 100-fold. Preparations that are well-tolerated on glabrous skin may be toxic in intertriginous areas. A good example is anthralin when used to treat psoriasis. If perspiration is blocked, the stratum corneum is further hydrated and penetration improved.

Vascular Supply. As blood flow through the skin increases, resorption is increased.

Role of Vehicle. The first factor is the relative affinity of the active ingredient for the vehicle as compared to the skin. In addition, the vehicle can by itself improve penetration if it has an occlusive effect. Sometimes salicylic acid or urea is added; the keratolytic role of these agents is thought to enhance penetration. The combination of low-potency corticosteroids and urea is as effective as slightly more potent corticosteroids.

Vehicles

In German, the role of the vehicle is described as indifferent treatment (*indifferente Behandlung*). An old truth is that an experienced dermatologist can often achieve more by skillfully manipulating the vehicle than a less-experienced colleague manipulating active ingredients. The different classes of vehicles and how they relate to each other is shown in Fig. 69.1. Correct choice of a vehicle may im-

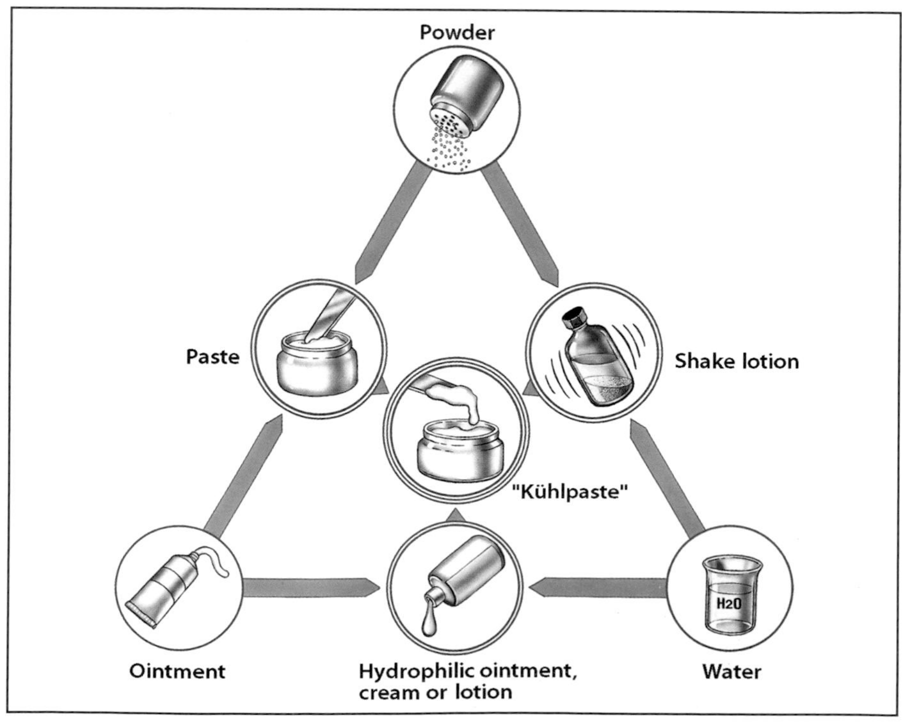

Fig. 69.1. Different dermatologic vehicles

prove a skin disease regardless of active ingredients, while an inappropriate vehicle may be counter-productive. The ingredients of vehicles, such as preservatives, perfumes, animal fats and similar products, may also cause allergic contact dermatitis. Thus not every case of a suspected allergic reaction to a topical medication should be blamed on the medication itself. The lists in Chap. 12 demonstrate the role of vehicle ingredients in testing for allergic contact dermatitis.

The pharmaceutical industry has firmly seized the concept of wise use of vehicles. Consider topical corticosteroids, which are available in a mind-baffling array of forms including creams, fatty creams, ointments, lotions, solutions, tinctures, pastes and impregnated tapes. In Germany, many of the vehicles used for favorite corticosteroid preparations are also available without the active ingredient. These tandem products are useful for two main purposes; they can be used as compounding bases and they can be employed for maintenance care. Such standardized vehicles have many advantages over spontaneously compounded mixtures; they have been carefully tested for stability, compatibility with a variety of active ingredients and resistance to bacterial contamination.

Water-Based Solutions

Definition. Liquid mixtures containing primarily water with dissolved active ingredients.

Solutions

Water-based solutions can be applied directly to the skin or mucous membranes. A common use of water-based solutions is to apply antimicrobials to mucous membranes. For example chlorhexidine 1–2% solutions are popular for oral hygiene. Solutions are also useful for treating open wounds and ulcers where an alcoholic product might burn. Water-based benzalkonium chloride solutions can be used for disinfecting skin prior to drawing blood or performing minor procedures.

Baths

Medicated baths are an inexpensive and effective way to treat the entire body surface. They can be used for hospitalized patients, in daycare centers and even at home. Either the entire body or limited areas, such as the hands or feet, can be treated. The water temperature can be varied. Table 69.1 shows some of bath additives used in Germany.

Advantages. Baths serve to clean the skin, removing crusts, scales and residual medications. If oils are added, they help to lubricate the skin. The stratum corneum is rehydrated, improving penetration. Active ingredients can be added, such as psoralens in PUVA bath therapy or tars in treating psoriasis.

Disadvantages. Baths can be irritating and dry out the skin, especially if overused.

Table 69.1. Examples of dermatologic baths and their active ingredients

Ingredient	Examples[a]	Effect	Indications
Tensides	Many	Cleansing	Weeping, crusting dermatoses
Disinfectants	Chinolinol, dyes, $KMnO_4$	Cleansing, disinfection	Weeping, secondarily infected dermatoses, may reduce odor as well
Astringents	Tannic acid	Drying, reduce inflammation	Weeping, blistering dermatoses, especially on hands and feet
Lipids	Many	Cleansing, lubrication	Dry skin, atopic dermatitis, ichthyosis; especially children
"Antiinflammatory"	Chamomile	Unclear	Chronic dermatitis, pruritus, prurigo, psoriasis
Antipruritic with lipids	Polidocanol, usually	Antipruritic	Pruritic diseases
Keratolytic	NaCl, usually with lipid	Removes scale	Psoriasis, ichthyosis, atopic dermatitis

[a] These are examples of types of products available in Germany

Wet Dressings

An absorbent cloth, either a cotton rag or a special dermatologic product, is laid over or wrapped about the affected area and then doused with a water-based solution. If the hands or feet are so treated, material should be intertwined between the digits to avoid maceration. Wet dressings are an effective way to cleanse and cool, so they are useful for crusted, infected conditions, as well as for cleaning ulcers. The skin can first be covered with an ointment or emollient cream and then treated with wet dressings. This reduces the drying effect and improves debridement. Similarly the patient may put on damp pajamas after applying the topical medication. In Germany this is known as the *Fett-feucht* (fat-wet) approach. Active ingredients such as corticosteroids can be used; the procedure enhances penetration.

Advantages. The moisture and evaporation provide cooling, which is often a relief to the patient. The crusts and scales are softened and can be more easily removed.

Disadvantages. Excessive or inappropriate use leads to drying out of the skin.

Alcoholic Solutions

Water-based solutions can be prepared with larger amounts of alcohol, such as ethanol (50–70%) or isopropanol (25–35%). This may allow active ingredients that are more soluble in alcohol to be better absorbed. Alcoholic solutions are especially useful for oily skin, the scalp and other hairy areas. A wide variety of organic dyes in alcoholic solutions were formerly used for their antimicrobial properties; they are effective for interdigital and intertriginous areas. One example is Castellani solution.

Advantages. Alcoholic solutions also have a direct disinfectant and defatting effect, as well as a marked cooling action.

Disadvantages. Alcoholic solutions produce marked dryness. They are not tolerated by patients with dry skin, may burn or otherwise cause pain if the skin is not intact.

Tinctures

Definition. Active ingredient dissolved in alcohol.

Advantages. Tinctures are a cosmetically elegant way to apply medications to the skin. As the alcohol evaporates, it cools and leaves behind a film of active ingredients. Tinctures are especially applicable for use on the scalp, as well as for applying high concentrations of relatively toxic materials to a tiny area.

Disadvantages. Tinctures tend to dry and can be irritating.

Examples. Podophyllin is prepared in a tincture for treating warts, condylomata acuminata and actinic keratoses. A wide variety of tinctures are available for use on the scalp; many are cosmetics but some may contain tar products or keratolytic agents. Several antimicrobials are also compounded as tinctures. For example, 0.5% chlorhexidine in 70% isopropyl alcohol is a popular surgical hand rinse. Tincture of benzoin is used as a vehicle for podophyllin and is employed by some athletes beneath adhesive tape to make the supportive wrap adhere better. In the latter setting it frequently leads to contact sensitization.

Varnishes or Films

There is not a good English name for this type of agent, a tincture which also contains flexible collodion. Thus as the alcohol evaporates, a very thin film of collodion or other plastic material is left on the skin surface. Most commercial wart remedies are films. Several such nail polishes containing antimycotic agents are available in Europe.

Sprays or Aerosols

Definition. Sprays pump fine droplets of a liquid onto the skin, while aerosols contain some type of propellant. The fluid they deliver may be water- or alcohol-based.

Advantages. Such products are cosmetically elegant and rapidly cover wide areas.

Disadvantages. For the most part, only low concentrations can be delivered. The products tend to be expensive, much waste occurs and there may be environmental concerns about the propellant gases in aerosols, as well as the risk of inhaling the product.

Examples. There are a number of disinfectant sprays, as well as some skin protective products. Antimycotic, antibacterial and antiparasitic agents are also available as sprays.

Powders

Definition. One or more products are ground into a fine powder for application to the skin. The materials may be shaken onto the skin or compressed into a firm mass. Such compact powders are familiar as cosmetics, for example, rouges and blushes. Some medicated compact powders are available for acne, as well as camouflage make-up for vitiligo and vascular anomalies.

Advantages. Powders absorb moisture and are thus cooling and drying. They can cover wide areas and reduce friction in skin folds or intertriginous areas.

Disadvantages. If the skin lesions show extensive weeping, the drying action of a powder is likely to be overwhelmed, producing a clumped mess. Medicated powders are an expensive way of delivering a product to the skin.

Examples. Most powders are mineral-based, such as talcum powder and zinc oxide powder. Talcum powder is very fine, reducing friction but absorbing poorly. Vegetable powders, such as corn starch or rice starch, absorb well but often turn into culture media. While they are still popular as folk remedies, they are rarely recommended by physicians. Zeasorb powder consists of microporous cellulose from corn cobs and is very absorbent.

Powders are also available containing both antibiotics and antimycotic agents. The latter are useful for prophylaxis against tinea pedis. Nystatin powder is popular for diaper dermatitis, but is expensive. It is more sensible to use an imidazole cream and a nonmedicated powder. When lactose is combined with active ingredients for application to wounds or ulcers, a self-dissolving powder is produced which dissolves in the wound secretions.

Shake Lotions

Definition. Suspensions of solids, usually powders, in water- or alcohol-based solutions.

Shake lotions have many other names. They have been called liquid powders; as the carrier solution dissolves, a film of powder is left on the skin. Since the powders are suspended, not dissolved, the two components always separate out, requiring vigorous shaking prior to application. In the hospital, such mixtures are often painted on the skin with a paint brush. Shake lotions are ideal for pruritic dermatoses that are not weeping and to dry out early blisters, as in zoster and dyshidrotic dermatitis. Thickeners such as glycerin or traganth can be added to make the residual powders stickier. Oils can be added to reduce drying; peanut oil is an old favorite. The term lotion refers to a very thin or liquid cream, as discussed below. Thus, although everyone says calamine lotion, one truly means calamine shake lotion.

Advantages. Shakes lotions are cooling, drying and antipruritic.

Disadvantages. These products can be too drying. If the underlying skin is moist, they form an unpleasant, messy artificial crust. The risk of secondary infection increases. Often a light oil must be used to remove the crust.

Examples. The two best known shake lotions are lotio alba and calamine lotion. Standard prescriptions include:

- Lotio alba (white shake lotion)
  Zinc oxide, talc $\overline{aa}$/ad 20.0
  Glycerin, distilled water $\overline{aa}$/ad 100.0

When ferric oxide is added, the shake lotion acquires flesh-colored tones. The mixture of zinc oxide and 0.5 % ferric oxide is known as calamine.

- Calamine lotion
  Calamine 8.0
  Zinc oxide 8.0
  Glycerin 2.0
  Bentonite magma 25.0
  Calcium hydroxide solution ad 100.0

Many items can be added to either base. Alcohols can be incorporated in place of water to make them more drying, or peanut oil added to produce a calamine liniment. In addition, menthol or camphor, usually in a concentration of 0.5 – 1.0 %, can be used as distracters. To increase the antipruritic effect, polidocanol 1 – 5 % can be added. Both liquor carbonis detergens 5% and ichthyol 5% can be prepared as shake lotions to treat seborrheic dermatitis.

Zinc Gels

This unfamiliar name refers to commonly used products. Gelatina zinci or zinc gel is the thick mixture used to impregnate Unna bandages. When these bandages are applied to the skin, usually as a wrapping about the ankle and lower aspect of the leg, they harden, producing a firm bandage, often called an Unna boot. The bandage material may have elastic properties as well. The main indications are chronic venous insufficiency, venous leg ulcers and to occlude suspected artifactual lesions to allow unimpaired healing. While most physicians will apply the finished bandage, the zinc gel is mixed as follows:

- Zinc gel
  Zinc oxide 10.0
  Glycerol 85% 40.0
  Gelatin 15.0
  Water 35.0

Plasters

Definition. A plaster was initially defined as a kneadable mass which adhered to the skin. Today it usually has a backing of plastic or fabric. The ordinary adhesive tape or adhesive dressing, i.e., Band-Aid, is also technically a plaster.

Advantages. Plasters deliver high concentrations of ingredients to a sharply defined area. They are occlusive and cause hydration of the stratum corneum, improving penetration. Nonmedicated wound coverings provide protection.

Disadvantages. Some patients may become allergic to various ingredients of a plaster or tape. In addition, the removal of a tape causes a degree of irritation.

Examples. Most plasters today are wound dressings or medicated products. The improvement in wound dressings over the past generation is striking. There are stretchable, thin and impermeable backings, coupled with easily removed adhesives of low sensitization potential. Many products are both waterproof and at the same time allow evaporation, containing membranes that work on the principle of Gore-Tex. Wound dressings are discussed further in Chap. 72.

Examples of medicated plasters include:

- Salicylic acid plaster: The standard concentration in the USA is 40% salicylic acid in a thick plaster with a moleskin backing. Stronger concentrations are available in Germany. The material is cut to size and applied to warts, calluses or clavi for a keratolytic action.
- Corticosteroid-impregnated tapes: Blenderm tape impregnated with 0.05% flurandrenolide is known in the USA as Cordran tape. It is a convenient way to deliver high concentrations of corticosteroids to small areas.

Gels

Definition. Gels are transparent semisolids that readily become liquids and spread easily.

The chemical definition of a gel is somewhat different than the clinical one given above. A gel is a compound containing a liquid bound in a macromolecular way to a polymer. Most gels are hydrogels, as the liquid is usually water, although acetone, alcohol and propylene glycol can all be employed. The macromolecule is agar, gelatin, methyl cellulose, pectin, polyethylene glycol or a similar bulk-forming agent. The key feature to a gel is its easy conversion from a semisolid to a liquid. The increase in temperature between the room and the body, coupled with the heat applied by rubbing the gel, effect the change.

A new type of a gel is a lipogel, in which the active ingredient is dispersed in liposomes throughout a traditional hydrogel. Oleogels contain lipids bound to polymers; they have little use in dermatology.

Advantages. Gels have a high degree of patient acceptance as they are cosmetically elegant and penetrate well. They are easily used in hairy areas. Patients with oily skin, such as those with acne, rosacea or seborrheic dermatitis, especially appreciate gels. Gels have a cooling action, so many antipruritic medications are combined in gels.

Disadvantages. Gels are more drying than creams or lotions. They are quite complex chemically and somewhat unstable; one should not attempt to add other ingredients to a gel.

Examples. There are many gels available, with active ingredients including retinoids, antibiotics, antimycotic agents and corticosteroids.

Oils

Definition. Oils are viscous liquids that may contain either dissolved or suspended active ingredients.

Oils can come from many different sources. These include:

- Minerals: Mineral oil is not a single ingredient, but refers to a wide variety of liquid hydrocarbons distilled from crude oil.
- Plants: Olive oil, almond oil, soy bean oil and peanut oil are widely used for their lubricating and emollient properties. Castor oil and burdock root oil are popular in hair tonics, while evening primrose oil and borrage oil are felt to perhaps help correct epidermal lipid abnormalities in atopic dermatitis and dry skin.

Advantages. Oils add fat to dry skin and make shake lotions less drying, producing liniments. Oils can be used to soften and remove crusts and scales, as well as for cleansing the remnants of pastes, ointments and shake lotions.

Disadvantages. The only disadvantage is that patients with oily skin do not benefit from such products.

Examples. One classic use of oils is to remove scales in psoriasis and severe seborrheic dermatitis. Commercial products are available that are somewhat easier to remove but this old standby is still very useful. A favorite mixture is:

- Salicylic acid oil
  Salicylic acid 3.0
  Olive oil ad 100.0

Another classic form is a mixture of a powder and oil:

- Zinc oil
  Zinc oxide
  Olive oil $\overline{aa}$ ad 100.0

This is an effective way to treat widespread dermatoses. It is messy and much of the material winds up on the bedclothes, so frequent applications are needed.

Modifications. Bath oils are also very popular. Both plant and mineral oils are available, often with additional ingredients such as polidocanol, tar or even sulfur. There are two principal types of bath oils. One has dispersal agents added so it is water-miscible; the other forms a film on the top of the water and coats the patients as he leaves the tub. Because of the risks associated with slippery tubs and the difficulties in cleaning such surfaces, some patients prefer to apply the oils after bathing.

Ointments and Creams

Definition. The chemical differences between ointments and creams are complicated and thus we recommend concentrating on the clinical characteristics. Patients tend to describe "greasy ointments" and "creams that rub in".

Table 69.2 simply compares the more accurate scientific terms and those in common use. In the USA one does not distinguish routinely between hydrophobic and hydrophilic ointments, although one should. We will use terms "true ointment or hydrophobic ointment" and "hydrophilic ointment." A salve in the USA usually means a paste, while a liniment is a shake lotion with oil added.

Table 69.2. Types of creams and ointments

American name	German name	Chemical composition	Consistency	Example
Ointment (hydrophobic)	*Fettsalbe*	Single phase, not water miscible	Semi-solid, spreadable	Vaseline, axle grease
Ointment (hydrophilic)	*Salbe*	Water in oil emulsion, water miscible	Semi-solid, spreadable	Eucerin, butter
Cream	*Creme*	Oil in water emulsion	Semi-solid, easily spreadable	Most creams
Lotion	*Milch*	Oil in water emulsion	Liquid	Milk, most liquid moisturizers

A hydrophobic ointment is a single phase, simply a grease or solid oil. Hydrophilic ointments, creams and lotions are emulsions. This means they contain a mixture of oils or oil-soluble substances and water or water-soluble substances. Hydrophilic ointments contain tiny droplets of water in a background of oil; thus they are known as water-in-oil emulsions. Creams are the reverse; they contain oils dispersed in water and are technically oil-in-water emulsions. A lotion is simply an oil-in-water emulsion with more water. Complex emulsions are possible; for example water droplets containing oils can be dispersed in a second oil; these are known as polyphase emulsions.

Hydrophobic Ointments

Advantages. In the USA it is sufficient to say Vaseline in order to give patients an idea of what awaits them. Such products resist water and are used for lubrication and protection. They are most useful for extremely dry skin, as in ichthyosis, and for chronic hyperkeratotic disorders of the palms and soles.

Disadvantages. Because they are occlusive, hydrophilic ointments can cause maceration, as they retain heat and water. Thus they are not well-suited for acute dermatoses. They should not be used in hairy areas.

Hydrophilic Ointments

These products are also called lipophilic creams and sometimes emollient creams. They are easily mixed with oil products, but also to a degree take up additional water. One hydrophilic ointment that takes up great amounts of water is Aquaphor; while it feels greasy, it can be mixed in equal parts with water to produce Eucerin. They are usually employed for subacute to chronic, often hyperkeratotic conditions.

Advantages. Hydrophilic ointments have the same advantages as hydrophobic ointments; in addition, they are somewhat easier to remove and to an extent can be mixed with water.

Disadvantages. While they are slightly less occlusive than hydrophobic ointments, the same problems are seen.

Creams

Creams are richer in water, less occlusive and can therefore be used more easily in acute conditions and on hairy areas. They are more easily contaminated than ointments and thus require a variety of conservatives. Emulgators or tensides are usually incorporated to produce a stable emulsion; these agents are amphophilic, having molecules with both lipophilic and hydrophilic domains. They reduce the surface or interface tension between the two components of the emulsion. Cetylstearyl alcohol is often used. Both conservatives and emulgators are possible causes of allergic contact dermatitis.

Advantages. Creams have a cooling effect, leave behind no greasy film and are well-accepted by patients. They are suited for use by those with oily skin.

Disadvantages. Creams are slightly drying and may exacerbate dry skin.

Lotions

Lotions are simply thin or liquid creams. They are not to be confused with shake lotions, which are entirely different. Lotions are widely employed as skin cleansers and moisturizers. When medications are added, they are appropriate for treating acute dermatoses.

Advantages. Lotions have all the features of creams, but are more easily spread and disappear more quickly. They can be used on hairy areas or mucosal surfaces. Another plus is the ease with which they allow one to cover large areas quickly.

Disadvantages. Lotions can be rather drying. They are not suited for treating ichthyosis and other disorders of keratinization.

Types of Ointment and Cream Bases

Just as with oils, there are many sources.

Minerals. When crude oil is distilled, two major types of hydrophilic ointments and oils are obtained. In one process, a series of saturated aliphatic hydrocarbons known as paraffins are extracted. Paraffin comes from the Latin *parum* (too little) and *affinis* (neighbor), indicating that these products are oils or greases with little affinity for other substances. In the USA one tends to think of paraffin as the hard white wax used to make candles. The British use the term correctly, describing solid paraffins as well as thick-liquid and thin-liquid forms. The temperature of separation determines which paraffin one obtains. Mineral oil is liquid paraffin.

A second product obtained by distillation is petrolatum or petroleum jelly, best known as Vaseline. Petrolatum contains methane and olefin hydrocarbons, is firm at room temperature and has a yellow color (vaselinum flavum); it can be bleached to produce vaselinum album. The white petrolatum is generally preferred; there is some concern over a carcinogenic role for the yellow product although the risk must be infinitesimal. In the USA, "yellow" Vaseline usually refers to carbolated Vaseline. Some individuals prefer this mixture of petrolatum and carbolic acid, which can be irritating or cause allergic contact dermatitis.

Plant Products. The same materials discussed under oils come into consideration here. Soybean oil can be most easily formed into semisolid products. Phospholipids such as lecithin, with its main ingredient phosphatidyl choline, are also well-incorporated. They are also used in liposomes.

Animal Products. Animal fats tend to be triglycerides with long-chain fatty acids or fatty alcohol esters. They are similar to human epidermal lipids in many ways and are somewhat less occlusive than mineral products, but tend to become rancid and may occasionally cause allergic contact dermatitis. Wool wax and wool wax alcohol are by-products obtained when sheep are shorn and the wool cleansed. Lanolin is a term attached to many different wool fat products; in the USA, hydrous wool fat (USP) is lanolin. This is a mixture of purified wool fat and 28% water which is capable of taking up large amounts of additional water. Wool wax alcohol works as a self-emulgator, allowing for the easy uptake of water.

In the past both whale oil and lard were used in compounding. The former has been dropped for environmental reasons. It was an excellent emulgator but has been replaced by cetylstearyl alcohol (Lanette N) and similar products. The latter is rarely used for esthetic reasons, as it rapidly becomes rancid unless saturated with preservatives.

Synthetics. A number of macromolecules have been synthesized that serve much as do the mineral products. Some are based on silica, such as dimethylpolysiloxane, which is present in many protective creams. Oleic acid esters, as well as isopropylmyristate and isopropylpalmitate, are also used. All have a very low likelihood of being allergens. Polyethylene glycols are long-chain molecules that can have a molecular weight ranging from 200 to 6000 and thus a consistency from thin liquid to hard wax. Most polyethylene glycols are extremely miscible with water and easy to wash off. The popular Cetaphil cleansing lotion is rich in these agents.

Examples. Many examples could be cited, but we will just list a few classic ones.

Hydrophobic Ointments. There are usually not mixed. The two best examples are petrolatum and mineral oil.

Hydrophilic Petrolatum. Less greasy than petrolatum, but greasier than hydrophilic ointments, this mixture can take up significant amounts of water.

- Hydrophilic petrolatum USP
  Cholesterol 3.0
  Stearyl alcohol 3.0
  White wax 8.0
  White petrolatum ad 100.0

Hydrophilic ointment is more complex and contains preservatives which may cause allergic contact dermatitis. It can be used with many water-soluble active ingredients.

- Hydrophilic ointment USP
  Methyl paraben 0.025
  Propyl paraben 0.025
  Sodium lauryl sulfate 1.0
  Stearyl alcohol 25.0
  White petrolatum 25.0
  Propylene glycol 12.0
  Polyoxyl 40 stearate 5.0
  Water ad 100.0

Cold Creams. These have many different formulas. Most are oil in water, but some approach water in oil. All contain significant amounts of water to achieve cooling by evaporation. While this cooling effect was formerly highly treasured, today it is realized that cooling may equal drying. Since the official America formula still contains spermaceti, we recommend the German standard. Another name for cold cream is rose water cream since so many of the preparations have added fragrances and rose water was one of the first.

- Cold cream (unguentum leniens DAB)
  Yellow wax 7.0
  Cetyl palmitate 8.0
  Peanut oil 60.0
  Water 25.0

Pastes

Definition. An ointment (or cream) containing a large amount of powder.

One can distinguish between different pastes depending on the relative amount of powder and the resulting consistency:

- Paste: Powder ≅ ointment (usual form)
- Hard paste: Powder 2 parts, ointment 1 part
- Soft paste: Powder 1 part, ointment 2 parts

Advantages. Pastes have both a protective effect and a cooling effect. The harder the paste, the more protection and less cooling. Pastes also tend to take up a bit of fluid, so they can be used on weeping areas. Hard pastes can be used to treat macerated areas, such as diaper dermatitis, or to protect normal skin around a leg ulcer. We often use a sandwich approach, applying a corticosteroid product first and then covering it with a paste, as when treating perianal intertrigo.

Disadvantages. Pastes tend to occlude and have lower patient acceptance. Hard pastes must often be applied with a wooden blade. Areas treated with pastes must be covered. They do not work well in hairy areas. Pastes are hard to remove; olive oil may be useful. Pastes do not lend themselves well to compounding, as little is known about the release of active ingredients and their desired pharmacologic actions. Pastes can also have water added to increase their spreadability and cooling effect. Such products are known as *Kühlpasten* in German; there is no equivalent English term.

Examples. There are several classic paste prescriptions:

- Zinc paste
  Zinc oxide 25.0
  Wheat starch 25.0
  White petrolatum 50.0
- Soft zinc paste
  Zinc oxide 30.0
  Thick paraffin 40.0
  White petrolatum 20.0
  Bleached wax 10.0

Some pastes containing active ingredients are available. These include corticosteroids, antimycotic and anticandidal agents.

Compounding

Compounding or prescribing special mixtures of active ingredients that a pharmacist must prepare enjoys varying degrees of popularity around the world. In the USA it is often almost impossible to find a pharmacist willing to compound at an affordable price. In Germany, in contrast, the pharmacist must compound, but the reimbursement is not very generous. Nonetheless, some compounded formulations are less expensive than the similar finished products.

The advantages of compounding are many. First, the physician can exactly choose the vehicle, the active ingredients and their concentrations. For example, a corticosteroid can be combined with a keratolytic agent for a hyperkeratotic hand dermatitis. Second, the dermatologist can work with vehicles known to be free of sensitizers or known to be well-tolerated by a given patient. Third, there may be cost-saving if the materials are mixed in bulk and then distributed to many patients, although physician dispensing is not legal in many countries. Table 69.3 shows some of the many possible products for compounding and if they work better in a hydrophilic or hydrophobic ointment.

There are many disadvantages to compounding. The final preparation of a topical product is very complicated, as industrial chemists and pharmacists hasten to tell us. The stability of a mixture, the dispersal of the active ingredient throughout the vehicle and the interaction between various active ingredients and vehicle components are hard to predict. In addition, an active ingredient must often be specially dissolved, buffered or otherwise manipulated before it is mixed into a cream or ointment base. In general, compounded products have a shorter shelf life and are more easily contaminated than finished products. Most chemists and pharmacists recommend that, if one chooses to compound, one use a neutral vehicle and add the active ingredients in raw form, rather than taking a

Table 69.3. Compatibility of various active ingredients

Hydrophobic ointment
Ammonium bituminosulfonate (Ichthyol)
Anthralin
Dexamethasone
Glycerol
Hydrocortisone
Peanut oil
Petrolatum
Polidocanol
Prednisolone acetate
Resorcinol
Salicylic acid
Zinc oxide
Hydrophilic ointment
Allantoin
Aluminum acetate
Aluminum chloride
Ammonium bituminosulfonate (Ichthyol)
Anthralin
Benzocaine
Chlorhexidine gluconate
Clioquinol
Clotrimazole
Dexamethasone
Erythromycin
Hydrocortisone
Lactic acid
Nystatin
Olive oil
Peanut oil
Prednisolone acetate
Salicylic acid
Urea
Zinc oxide

finished product such as a corticosteroid cream and then mixing in another finished product, such as an antibiotic cream. Physicians and pharmacists often find the latter approach simpler, but the stability and reliability of the mixture are often uncertain. As a general rule, one should never have more than two active ingredients in a compounded product; otherwise the interactions become impossible to sort out. Mistakes in choosing the nature and concentration of the ingredient occur with compounding and are almost unheard of when using commercial products. Finally, compounded products have no package insert.

We personally compound only when an equivalent commercial product is not available. The high standards and quality control of commercial products are almost impossible to equal in a compounded form. How should one proceed? We have the following suggestions. Work with reliable pharmacists who are knowledgeable about compounding and use a limited number of mixtures – those you know are stable and effective. Pick several basic vehicles, stick with them and only add active ingredients in an approved way. In many countries there are formularies outlining well-tested compounding mixtures. Some of the examples of compounded products are taken from two such sources, the United States Pharmacopoeia (USP) or the *Deutsche Arznei Buch* (DAB). In Germany, there are two excellent books with compounding information which we recommend in the references. Since the language of compounding is Latin, these books can be used by anyone with a smattering of German skills and a good imagination.

Choice of Vehicles

One must learn by experience how to choose the right vehicle. The three main determinants are:

- Patient's skin type
- Degree of acuity of the disease
- Nature of the lesions

When all else fails, it is often helpful to ask the patient or parent if the individual does better with a cream or lotion that rubs in or an ointment that sticks. We often prescribe two similar products differing only in vehicle, to be used on different body parts or at different times of day.

Skin Type. About 50% of individuals have oily skin or seborrhea. They do better with creams, lotions, solutions, shake lotions and powders, and usually dislike ointments of any type. The 30% of the population with dry skin do better with ointments, pastes and perhaps heavier creams for use during the day. The balance have more neutral skin and can usually use either creams or ointments.

Skin type is not absolute. In the summer, more people have oily skin. Someone practicing in Albuquerque, New Mexico, has more patients with dry skin than a colleague in Houston, Texas. Different racial groups have far different patterns of oiliness or dryness. Many teenagers complain of oily skin on the forehead and dry skin on the cheeks; other patients with seborrheic dermatitis have an oily scalp but a dry trunk. One must listen, look and adjust.

Degree of Acuity. Acute inflammatory processes are best treated with creams or lotions. If the lesions

Table 69.4. Choice of vehicles for different lesions

Lesion	Recommended	Best avoided
Acute erythema	Powder, shake lotion, lotion, cream	Paste, ointment
Vesicles	Powder, shake lotion, gel	Paste, ointment
Blisters	Wet dressing, shake lotion	Paste, ointment, powder
Erosions	Wet dressing, ointment	Powder, shake lotion
Crusts	Wet dressing, ointment, paste	Powder, shake lotion, cream, gel
Scales	Wet dressing, ointment, paste	Powder, shake lotion, cream, gel
Chronic inflammation	Paste, ointment	Powder, shake lotion, cream, gel

are weeping, then shake lotions are also fine. As the process resolves, thicker vehicles can be employed. For chronic hyperkeratotic disorders, ointments are better.

Types of Lesions. Table 69.4 suggests suitable vehicles for various clinical lesions.

Amount of Topical Medication

A common error of physicians inexperienced in treating the skin is to prescribe inappropriate amounts. If a patient has psoriasis covering 50% of body and receives a 30 g tube of corticosteroid cream for 1 week, the prescription is worthless. One can estimate that to treat the entire body one needs 30–60 g. A lotion or cream will go further than an ointment. The rule of nines, used in calculating the percent of surface area involved by burns (Chap. 13), can be used to estimate smaller areas. The hands, feet, face and genital area each require about 2 g, an arm 3 g, a leg 4 g and the trunk 6 g.

Initially one should prescribe a small amount to be sure the patient tolerates the product. Amazing saving are possible in bulk. Corticosteroid creams such as triamcinolone acetonide are available in the USA in 5-pound tubs; they are several hundred-fold cheaper than slightly stronger, newer corticosteroids in 30 g or 60 g tubes. In Germany, the physician can win by prescribing smaller tubes, in that his prescribing costs, monitored by a central agency, are then lower. In the USA, since most patients pay themselves for medications, this incentive is less common, although managed health care has introduced the concept.

Specific Topical Therapy

In the following sections, we will consider the many different categories of topical agents available. The following section should not be viewed as a formulary. We have not attempted to cover every agent discussed in the book. Products whose range of use is limited have been discussed under their specific indications. There is some repetition between the discussion here and in the rest of the text. For example, we have considered acne medications in detail in Chapter 28 and will only review them here. Conversely, we have mentioned topical corticosteroids hundreds of times in the text, but will discuss them in detail only here.

In most instances, it is relatively easy to pick the appropriate active ingredient in a suitable vehicle. Occasionally one may have to use an active ingredient that is not the first choice because of the lack of a suitable vehicle. For example, some high-potency corticosteroids are not available in vehicles suitable for scalp use, so one must choose a slightly weaker form for scalp psoriasis. Medications with two active ingredients were formerly quite popular; typical examples included antiinfective agents mixed with corticosteroids. The FDA now requires that the mixture be proven more effective than each individual component, rather than more effective than the vehicle. Combination products have become rare in the USA. Many are still available in Europe.

Antiinfective Agents

Antibiotics are often equated with the whole host of other products that can be used to treat infectious organisms. We have probably also made this error although we have tried to be precise. The first major distinction is between antibiotics and antiseptics. A antiseptic or disinfectant denatures or destroys the cell wall; thus it works rapidly, has a wide spectrum and resistance is rare. The down side is that the host cells are equally attacked. An antibiotic usually influences bacterial metabolism, such as DNA or protein synthesis; its onset of action is slower and its spectrum more specific. The host cells are spared, but both allergic contact dermatitis and resistance may be problems. Since surface levels of antibiotics can far exceed the usual in vitro levels, there is not absolute correlation between in vitro sensitivity and clinical effectiveness. There is no question that resistant strains can be selected out in vivo through the indiscriminate use of topical antibiotics. A true antibiotic is made by one organism to protect it against another organism; thus sulfonamides are not technically antibiotics, but we will not try to maintain this distinction.

Disinfectants

Synonym. Antiseptics

Definition. Agents that destroy bacteria by direct cell damage.

The main features of disinfectants are reviewed above. Disinfectants are used for simple wound care, to reduce the skin load of microorganisms, clean the skin prior to surgery, cleanse the hands of health care workers and treat the environs of an office or hospital. Gram-negative organisms are usually somewhat less affected. Blood, pus and serous discharges also tend to block antiseptics, as may soaps and detergents. Six major categories are available; they are summarized in Table 69.5.

Alcohols. There are many simple mixtures of alcohols, usually available as sprays or wipes. They are frequently used to prepare a site prior to a minor surgical procedure.

Halogens. The halogens and their salts have been used as disinfectants for centuries. The old standard is tincture of iodine, usually 3%. Polyvinylpyrolidone or povidone-iodine is an iodophor or water-soluble organic iodine complex that slowly releases iodine. The best known range of products in the USA is Betadine, available as surgical scrub solution, impregnated scrub brushes, skin cleanser, ointment, shampoo and even douche. Iodine is absorbed if wide areas are treated.

Chloride products are also popular. Hexachlorophene (pHisohex) was widely used for years for child care, as well as acne patients, but it causes a neuropathy and should not be used in infants or on large open areas. Chlorhexidine (Hibiclens) is the most widely used topical chloride compound, available in about as many forms as polyvinyl-

Table 69.5. Disinfectants

Agent	Concentration (%)	Indications
Alcohols	Variable	Gram-positive bacteria
Halogens		
Polyvinyl-pyrolidone	0.5–10	Bacteria, viruses, fungi, yeast
Hexachlorophene	0.5–3.0	Gram-positive bacteria
Chlorhexidine	1.0–2.0	Bacteria, fungi, yeast
Clioquinol	0.5–1.0	Bacteria, fungi, yeasts
Heavy metals		
Merbromin	0.1	Bacteria
Silver sulfadiazine	1.0	Bacteria, yeasts
Oxidants		
H_2O_2	1–10.0	Bacteria, fungi
Benzoyl peroxide	2.5–10.0	Bacteria
$KMnO_4$	<0.05	Bacteria
Dyes		
Gentian violet	0.1–1.0	Bacteria, yeasts
8-Chinolinol sulfate	0.1–1.0	Bacteria (weak)

pyrolidone, as well as an effective mouth wash that is useful both in acute necrotizing ulcerative gingivitis and in preventing plaque. It is inactivated by soaps. The final widely used member of this group is clioquinol or iodochlorhydroxyquin (Vioform), often mixed with topical corticosteroids and used for diaper dermatitis and other secondarily infected dermatoses. It too is potentially neurotoxic; formerly it was prescribed orally as an amebicide. Clioquinol compounds stain the skin and clothing yellow and occasionally cause allergic contact dermatitis. They are also incompatible with zinc oxide.

Heavy Metals. Mercury and silver are the two main metals used. Merbromin is the main ingredient of mercurochrome, while thiomersal is known as merthiolate. Both are widely used but should be confined to treating small wounds, such as a minor scrape, because of the absorption of mercury. Thiomersal often causes allergic contact dermatitis. The most widely used form of silver is silver sulfadiazine (Silvadene), known in the USA as "burn butter" because it comes in a very effective aqueous cooling vehicle. Siver nitrate ($AgNO_3$) can also be used in dilute (0.01–1.0%) aqueous solutions to disinfect. Silver nitrate sticks can be used to treat granulation tissue: they are known as lapis infernalis or, in German, *Höllensteinstift* (pencil of hell's stone) because of their caustic action. We no longer employ them. Argyria may result if any of these silver products are overused.

Oxidants. Hydrogen peroxide is capable of killing both bacteria and, at higher concentrations, fungi by releasing activated oxygen molecules or free radicals. It is available in a cream form (Microcid) in Germany. Benzoyl peroxide works in the same fashion; it is usually used for acne, but in higher concentrations can be used to stimulate granulation tissue and clean infected leg ulcers. Both resistance and allergic contact dermatitis are very uncommon. Potassium permanganate ($KMnO_4$) is also an oxidant but very messy to use as it discolors skin, nails and bath tubs. Low concentration solutions can be used for wet soaks or baths; higher concentrations are irritating and can cause burns. We do not use it any more.

Dyes. The use of antiseptic and astringent dyes has always been far more popular in Europe than America. There are two main categories in use, the triphenylmethane and the acridine dyes. The best known triphenylmethane representatives are methyl violet, crystal violet and brilliant green. Gentian violet is a mixture of several such dyes; still it is used in the USA. All these dyes are active against bacteria and *Candida albicans.* In children lower concentrations in aqueous vehicles should be used; otherwise necrosis can be seen (Chap. 10). While the necrosis is called pyoktanin (methyl violet) necrosis, it can result from any of the dyes. Among the acridine dyes, 8-chinolinol (Chinosol) is best known in Germany. It is often used to prepare a mild 1:1000 antiseptic solution for wet dressings.

The best known dye mixture is Castellani solution. It formerly contained boric acid but today is modified.

- Castellani solution
  Chlorocresol 0.1
  Resorcinol 10.0
  Sodium edetate 0.02
  Acetone 5.0
  Fuchsin 4% in ethanol 10.0
  Water ad 100.0

Castellani solution is still used for treating gram-negative toe web infections and weeping, secondarily infected dermatoses. While designed as an antimycotic, it is nowhere near as effective as the modern agents. Because many patients prefer not to have the intensive red color; a colorless version without fuchsin is also available but we have found it less effective. In addition, there are concerns about resorcinol, so that we rarely employ this mixture.

Miscellaneous. Benzalkonium chloride is a quaternary ammonium compound that is antibacterial. It can be used to disinfect the skin as well as surfaces in a clinical practice or laboratory. It is also used as a preservative in cosmetics and other formulations. Aluminum salts are very effective antiseptics and antiperspirants. We use 1:1000 aluminum chloride with wet compresses to treat oozing leg ulcers. In USA, Burow solution is most often employed for the same purpose; it consists of 5% aluminum diacetate diluted 1:20 or 1:40. The risk of contact sensitization is almost null.

Antibiotics

Definition. Agents that interfere with bacterial growth and function, often derived from other microorganisms.

Topical antibiotics are typically used for wound care, acne, rosacea and secondarily infected dermatoses. The main issues with topical antibiotics are the development of resistance and allergic contact dermatitis. One general rule is not to use as a topical agent any antibiotic that could later be life-saving when used internally. While there is not an exact correlation between in vitro resistance and the lack of effectiveness of topical antibiotics, as very high levels can be used on the skin surface, there is no question that topical antibiotics select out resistant strains in both patients and even family members. Many antibiotics, being complex large molecules, easily produce allergic contact dermatitis; penicillin is so likely to do this that is was rapidly dropped as a topical agent. For years, neomycin has been close to the top of the list among contact sensitizers.

The treatment of acne with topical erythromycin, tetracycline or clindamycin is discussed in detail in Chapter 28. Erythromycin is likely to select out resistant staphylococci but the clinical significance of this is unclear. While in the past resistant *Propionibacterium acnes* were uncommon, today they are often found. Clindamycin can be a life-saving drug so we use it topically with reluctance. It also tastes very bitter and is thus unpleasant to use around the mouth. The risk of pseudomembranous colitis with topical use is very low. Both erythromycin and clindamycin are available in a variety of vehicles, including solutions, gels, creams and even ointments. In some instances, erythromycin is combined with isotretinoin, benzoyl peroxide or zinc sulfate. Tetracycline is less widely used as a topical agent. In addition to these agents, topical metronidazole is also used in treating rosacea (Chap. 28).

Mupirocin. No doubt the most effective topical antibiotic, mupirocin, is about as useful against cutaneous staphylococci and streptococci as systemic antibiotics. It is widely used in treating impetigo and also to treat nasal carriers of *Staphylococcus aureus*. Its cost is the chief factor limiting its still wider use.

Fusidic Acid. While fusidic acid (Fucidine) is very widely used in Europe, it is not available in the USA. It is available as a cream, ointment, gel and in many other forms. Fusidic acid is also available mixed with a midpotency corticosteroid. It is most effective against gram-positive organisms including methicillin-resistant *S. aureus*.

Bacitracin. Very widely used in the USA, bacitracin has a wide gram-positive spectrum, although some staphylococci are resistant. It is most stable in an ointment base and may cause allergic contact dermatitis.

Tyrothricin. A mixture of gramicidin and tyrocidine, this agent has a spectrum similar to bacitracin and is equally safe.

Polymyxin B. Of all the widely used topical antibiotics, this agent is most active against gram-negative bacteria. In the same clinical setting, many antiseptics are cheaper and more effective.

Chloramphenicol. This agent continues to be widely used, accounting for over 3% of compounded dermatologic prescriptions in Germany. This trend persists despite the facts that extremely rare cases of aplastic anemia have been reported following topical use of chloramphenicol. It can also cause allergic contact dermatitis and its effectiveness as a topical agent is poorly documented.

Aminoglycosides. Many aminoglycosides are used topically, including gentamicin, neomycin and kanamycin. There is no defense for using topical gentamicin as it is often essential in treating gram-negative septicemia. Neomycin (framycetin) is widely used but is a potent sensitizer and can easily be replaced by other products. Kanamycin also has little going for it. Cross-resistance and cross-sensitivity may develop among family members, and both renal and aural damage may occur following absorption. The best advice is not to employ these popular drugs.

Sulfonamides. Sulfonamides are used for the treatment of burns, either as silver sulfadiazine or mafenide (Sulfamylon). Both are potential sensitizers, causing severe allergic contact dermatitis and systemic cross-reactions with diuretics and antidiabetic drugs with similar sulfonylurea structures. Sodium sulfacetamide is occasionally used in the USA to treat acne, usually combined with sulfur; we do not use it. It is also widely found in eye drops and in treating seborrheic blepharitis. Allergic contact dermatitis is somewhat less common, perhaps because extensive denuded areas found in burn patients are not seen in the latter setting.

Antiviral, Antimycotic and Antiparasitic Agents

The many topical and systemic agents available for treating viruses, dermatophytes and deep fungi and parasites are discussed in Chapters 2, 7 and 9, respectively, and will not be repeated here.

Sunscreens

Today people are exposed to sun light not only as an almost unavoidable occupational risk (farmers, sailors, other outdoor workers, life guards) but also intentionally during their leisure activities and vacations. A tan is a sign of health in may cultures, but the role of UV radiation in the development of basal cell carcinoma, squamous cell carcinoma and malignant melanoma, as well as the many diseases discussed in Chapter 13, has given sunscreens a central place in the modern cosmetic-pharmaceutical interface.

Sunscreens are rated by their sun protection factor (SPF) in the USA and *Lichtschutzfaktor (LSF)* in Germany. In simplest terms, these are expressions of the increased time required to develop radiation-induced erythema. For example if some one usually gets red in 10 min of noonday sun, an SPF 15 will allow him to stay out about 150 min. Technically the SPF is expressed as: SPF = MED protected skin/MED unprotected skin; MED = minimum erythema dose in minutes.

There are European (COLIPA), American and Australian standards for determination of the SPF which are quite similar and address the issue of protection against UVB satisfactorily. The main issues are if extremely high values such as SPF 50–60 are accurate and clinically relevant. An exact protocol for testing UVA protection is not available; most UVA SPF values are measured in complex in vitro systems. Some UVA is included in the solar stimulators recommended for use in determining the SPF, but some firms claim very high, differently or poorly documented UVA protection for their products.

While the vast majority of dermatologists and photobiologists endorse sunscreens, some groups worry about negative effects. One concern is that people with sunscreens will simply stay out longer and accumulate the same damage. Others suggest that if UVB is screened out, the more-penetrating UVA may cause deep damage without being detected. This theory is at least partially responsible for the fashionable status of UVA sunscreens. Yet others suggest that sunscreens may be responsible for the increasing incidence of malignant melanoma; little data are available to support this view. We continue to use and recommend sunscreens.

Active Ingredients

Blockers. Particles of metallic iron, titanium dioxide or zinc oxide physically block light and may reflect it. To a lesser extent barium sulfate and talcum are also used. The familiar white nose and lips of lifeguards in the beach movies of the 1950s is a vivid example of this effect, but today many elegant products are available achieving very satisfactory SPF values. Since these particles are inert, the risk of allergic contact dermatitis is almost zero, so most hypoallergenic sunscreens fall into this category. Furthermore these products cause little if any irritation around the eyes, of special importance in children and athletes. In addition, the same particulate material can be added to chemical sunscreens to achieve the very high values such as SPF 40–60. Variations in particle size can influence the degree of UVA and UVB protection, as smaller particles are more effective against the latter.

Chemical Filters. Such products absorb UV radiation which is given up as a weaker radiation after complex molecular interactions. Depending the on molecule, there is a spectrum of energy at which absorption is best. The main products used today and their ranges are:
Benzophenones: 250–365 nm
PABA esters: 280–320 nm
Arobenzones (Parsol 1789): 305–385 nm
Cinnamates: 290–320 nm
Salicylates: 290–320 nm

The following factors should be considered when making a suggestion about sunscreen use.

- SPF
- Vehicle
- Special properties

SPF. Most patients are well-served by a SPF 15. If one desires a quicker tan, an 8–12 can be used. Lower numbers may be chosen by individuals with relatively little risk of sunburn, such as those with types IV–VI skin. When exposure is more intense, then a higher SPF should be employed. Agents with an SPF > 15 are called sunblockers. Skiers and mountaineers benefit from SPF 30–50 products on their faces, as do others who spend long periods of time in the sun. Patients with photosensitivity also need to consider higher SPF products with UVA and UVB blockers.

Vehicle. Gels penetrate better and offer a more rapid onset of protection, but may be drying. They tend to burn around the eyes, even if carefully applied. Presumably sweat carries them down to this sensitive area. Lotions are the first choice of most individuals; creams are less drying but may be slightly occlusive for some. Special lipsticks are available; they can also be used to stripe a protective band around the lateral and inferior aspects of the eyes.

Special Properties. The main questions are UVA protection, substantivity (the ability of the sunscreen to remain on the skin when exposed to rubbing, sweating and especially water), water resistance and the risk of allergic contact dermatitis. The need for UVA protection for the average individual is unclear, but almost all drug-induced photosensitivity is caused by UVA radiation and many other photosensitive individuals also require such protection. While exact quantification remains controversial, the manufacturers' guidelines at least allow one to choose somewhat intelligently. Each of the SPF testing schemes incorporates some assessment of water resistance, since so much sunscreen use centers around swimming and sunbathing. As a rough rule, 50% of the protection should be maintained following a swim. Exactly how one documents this is a source of argument in the industry. Swimming, showering and rinsing the skin with a special shower are all possible, but the results vary greatly. A generation ago sunscreens were not considered a likely cause of allergic contact dermatitis. Today they are a major factor and any patient with a photosensitive dermatitis should be suspected of having an allergic contact dermatitis to sun screens (Chaps. 12, 13).

Protective Creams

When one considers the number of work days lost because of irritant and allergic contact dermatitis, then the need for good skin protection creams or barrier creams is obvious. Unfortunately, no product or group of products has established itself as effective. The required features are persistence and water resistance, but at the same time good penetration so that the hands do not remain greasy or sticky. In addition, recent elegant studies with labeled barrier creams have shown tremendous variation in how effectively users apply them to all exposed surfaces.

Silicone Products. The main stimulus for the development of silicone topical agents was the incidence of macerated feet among US Army ground troops during the Vietnam War. Tinea pedis and pyodermas were the second most common reason for medical evacuation after battle wounds. Silicone is available in creams, ointments, gels and sprays. All provide good water protection but lack permanence. The usual main ingredient is dimethicone.

Other Products. Special creams and ointments are available both in the USA and Europe, designed for use when the individual is exposed to water, solvents or dusts and grime. Recommendations should be made after consulting with the plant physician or nurse, who may have access to more detailed information. We have been disappointed with the efficacy of these products.

Cleansers

Both soaps and detergents are taken much for granted by patients and physicians but they can play an important role. Washing removes the surface lipid film, along with dirt, bacteria and residual cosmetics and medications. At the same time, washing by definition is drying. Thus patients with dry skin need to reduce the frequency of washing and lubricate their skin afterwards.

Soaps. Most soaps are alkaline, as they contain sodium or potassium salts of free fatty acids. Their alkalinity disturbs the normal acidity (acid mantle) of the skin, causes swelling of the stratum corneum and leads to dryness and often pruritus. Thus patients with sensitive skin, such as those with atopic dermatitis, may be well-advised to use a soap-free cleanser. Soaps to which an oil has been added may lubricate better, but for the most part this is difficult to document. In the USA, Dove consistently performs as well as more expensive soaps in tests of irritation. While patients often claim to be allergic to soaps, they are usually describing an irritant reaction. Some may develop true allergic contact dermatitis to a perfume, preservative or dye. The early antiseptics in deodorant soaps occasionally led to persistent photoallergic reactions but this risk has been almost eliminated (Chap. 13). The current antibacterial, deodorant soaps contain triclosan or tricloban, low risk sensitizers.

Soap-Free Cleanser or Syndet. There are a number of synthetic detergents available that clean as well as soaps but are adjusted so that they do not alter the skin surface pH. Some are combined with oils so that they lubricate the skin as they wash. Nonetheless, if one washes too often, dryness can also result with these products. Allergic contact dermatitis is almost unheard of.

Abrasive Cleansers. The old standard in the USA is Lava soap, a soap which contains particles of pumice. Many acne cleansers are still available with some type of abrasive particle, ranging from aluminum oxide granules to polyethylene granules to organic sources. Some of the granules dissolve; others do not. In general, such an approach to acne is no longer warranted and we do not recommend abrasive cleansers.

Shampoos

There are many shampoos that occupy a position between a medication and a cosmetic. This probably reflects the uncertain status of seborrheic dermatitis, which is so common that some question its designation as an illness. All of these shampoos are used primarily to treat dandruff or seborrheic dermatitis. There are some general observations that can be made. It has been shown in several studies that alternating shampoos is helpful; most patients accommodate to the product, better described as tachyphylaxis, if they regularly use the same shampoo. In addition, it seems reasonable to leave a medicated product on the scalp for a matter of minutes to increase its effectiveness.

Trial and error is the best way to determine which families of shampoos are most appropriate for a given individual. A physician or cosmetician who walks in the room and says "Product X is exactly the right product for your special scalp problem", is either poorly informed or trying to sell a given product. Finally, there have been a variety of scares about the toxicity of various shampoos, including tar, selenium and salicylic acid products. Tars are no longer available without prescription in Germany and full-strength selenium products require a prescription in the USA. It is unclear if the tentative evidence for toxicity in laboratory studies is relevant to the practical setting where shampoos are rinsed off promptly.

Shampoos consist of a collection of tensides that must lather well, remove dirt and not damage the hairs. In addition to the tensides, shampoos contain agents to alter their consistency, perfumes, dyes, tiny pearls (that reflect light and give a sheen to the product) and a long list of preservatives. Some shampoos are combined with conditioners or rinses. A conditioner must leave something behind on the hair, while a rinse usually imparts a slight ionic charge to the hairs so that they separate more easily. Baby shampoos are usually formulated with milder cleansing products but also have their pH carefully adjusted so it approximates that of the eyes, leading to less tearing on inadvertent exposure.

The following active ingredients are available. This list is not intended to be complete and many new formulations appear each year. The reader should determine which categories are available for his patients. In all cases except ketoconazole, medicated shampoos have not been accurately compared to their shampoo base, and their mechanism of action is unclear. Most of the active ingredients are contained in excellent, well-designed shampoos and the cleansing effect may be most important.

Salicylic Acid. This old standard is a proven keratolytic and is the mainstay of most American shampoos.

Tar. A wide variety of tars are available, many of which are combined with salicylic acid. The older tar products were dark, foul smelling and discolored blond or gray hair. Many elegant newer products avoid these problems. The tars may be derived from coal products, shale, juniper, birch and many other sources. Folliculitis may result from tar use but is uncommon with shampoos.

Ammonium Bituminosulfonate. Ichthyol is also combined into shampoos in Europe. It appears to function similarly to tar.

Zinc Pyrithione. Widely used worldwide, this antimicrobial product is not only useful for dandruff and seborrheic dermatitis, but also effective against tinea versicolor.

Selenium Sulfide. These products are better prescribed to treat tinea versicolor than for routine shampooing. Many patients experience a rebound oiliness if they regularly employ such products. The

2.5% suspension (Selsun) is a prescription item in the USA, but lower concentrations such as Selsun Blue are available as over-the-counter products. Similar products are also available in Europe but less widely used.

Imidazoles. Ketoconazole shampoo has been shown to reduce levels of *Pityrosporum ovale* on the scalp and to improve seborrheic dermatitis. Exactly how the two features interrelate is unclear. Several other imidazoles and other antimycotic agents are also available in shampoos and seem to be comparable. Usually such shampoos should be employed once or twice weekly.

Other Antimicrobials. In Europe piroctonolamine and related products are also widely employed.

Antiperspirants

These products are considered in Chapter 30.

Keratolytic Agents

The removal of a thickened stratum corneum layer or scales is a common problem in dermatology and many agents have been employed for this purpose. In some instances, such as with palmoplantar keratoderma, removal of massive hyperkeratoses is the issue. It is unclear how the keratolytics soften the stratum corneum; they may decrease adhesion between keratinocytes or add water to the stratum corneum. Thus some favor calling them keratoplastic agents.

Salicylic Acid. The most widely used keratolytic is clearly salicylic acid. Its chemical name is *o*-hydroxy benzoic acid. It may be used in films or plasters to remove thickened stratum corneum over warts or calluses. In somewhat lower concentrations, usually ranging from 5–10%, it is applied to the scalp, left on for a matter of hours or overnight and rinsed out to treat severe seborrheic dermatitis or psoriasis. In still lower concentrations, 2–5%, it can be used on glabrous skin to help remove scale such as in psoriasis. In addition, salicylic acid is added to anthralin as an antioxidant. One must always bear in mind that systemic absorption can occur and cause renal and CNS problems (salicylism), so caution should be used when treating larger areas in patients with impaired barrier function. Infants and small children should not be treated with this product.

Salt. Salts have become quite popular in recent years in Europe. Table salt (NaCl) is an old standard. It is often combined with urea, but may be used as a single ingredient. Industrial NaCl is far cheaper than table salt. Because of the success of psoriasis therapy at the Dead Sea, creative individuals have either packaged Dead Sea salt for sale or created their own special salt mixtures, none of which are proven better than NaCl and all of which are much more expensive.

Many clinics and offices use saline baths combined with phototherapy as an outpatient approach. Concentrations of $<5\%$ are used in atopic dermatitis, while 10–30% solutions are best for psoriasis. The higher salt solutions are a hazard to the plumbing of the building and the environment. Creative manufacturers have built recycling machines so that the same salt solution can be employed for a number of patients. The risk of gram-negative folliculitis from contaminated solutions means that a variety of antibacterial agents must be added if recycling is employed.

Urea. Technically urea is a humectant, in that it holds water in the skin. But the most useful corollary of this is a mild keratolytic effect that increases scaling and penetration, perhaps because it splits hydrogen bonds in keratin. Urea products may burn slightly on application, making their use in infants problematic. They are available in a wide range of prescription and over-the-counter products with concentrations ranging from 3% to 25%. If one is compounding, concentrations higher than 10% are hard to achieve. One favorite keratolytic prescription is urea-salt ointment:

- Urea-salt ointment
  Urea 5–10.0
  NaCl 5–10.0
  Hydrophilic ointment ad 100.0

α-Hydroxy Acids. There are many organic acids with an α-hydroxy group, including glycolic acid, citric acid and lactic acid. The latter has long been used for its keratolytic and hygroscopic properties, frequently employed in the same manner as urea. An especially effective product is LacHydrin, which is a 12%, buffered lactic acid product that avoids many of the problems of burning occurring at such high concentrations. It is useful in treating ichthyosis.

Today products containing α-hydroxy acids are hot-selling items. Their possible effectiveness was pointed out many years ago, both in low concentrations to treat aged skin and in higher concentrations to destroy superficial lesions such as seborrheic keratoses. They are widely available in antiaging products, as they produce a mild peeling and erythema, as well as some changes in the dermis. Higher concentrations are employed by physicians to produce the same peeling effects. Where the α-hydroxy acids fall into the regulatory scheme, i.e., cosmetic or medication, has not been sorted out and their effectiveness is unclear. In Germany, they are not considered a medication and the patient must pay for them directly.

Propylene Glycol. The combination of 40–60% propylene glycol and overnight occlusion is an extremely effective, nontoxic keratolytic method. Nonsterile propylene glycol is also relatively inexpensive, an important consideration when treating ichthyosis, where broad areas must be treated often and forever. Keralyt Gel is a combination of propylene glycol and salicylic acid in an optimized vehicle; it is useful for treating palmoplantar keratoderma, although in this condition mechanical debridement is also always required.

Retinoids

The retinoids do produce some irritation and peeling, but because their mechanisms of action are so complex, they are usually not lumped together with the keratolytics. Their main use is in acne, where they are the most effective comedolytic agents (Chap. 28). The old stand-by is tretinoin but two newer products, isotretinoin and adapalene, are also available and are somewhat less irritating. In addition, tazarotene is available for the treatment of psoriasis (Chap. 14).

Astringents and Caustics

The interface between astringents–antiperspirants and astringents–caustics is unclear in both cases. An astringent must cause some shrinkage of the skin tissues. Patients often apply so-called astringents, such as alcohol-based after shave products or tighteners, to reduce the size of their facial pores, but this is not mechanically possible. A mild irritation may cause the skin around the pores to swell, slightly leveling things out a bit. If a chemical such as an aluminum or zirconium salt causes a slight denaturing of the epidermal cells, it may interfere with eccrine sweating. Whether it achieves this by constriction of the duct is disputed. Tannic acid, available in many forms in Europe, is claimed to be an astringent and occasionally employed for treating hyperhidrosis. Low concentrations of $AgNO_3$ are also denaturing agents, thus astringents.

$AgNO_3$ is also an example of a caustic, an agent that destroys more tissue than the superficial damage of an astringent. When it is used in higher concentrations, such as on a stick applicator, it can destroy granulation tissue or normal skin. Trichloracetic acid is a better example of a caustic; in 30–50% concentrations it is used to destroy warts and xanthelasmas. Monsel solution is a ferric subsulfate solution that is dark brown and tends to stain the skin when used for hemostasis. We no longer employ it. If a topical hemostatic agent is desired, 30% aluminum chloride is just as effective and colorless. Finally the whole array of solutions used in chemical peeling are caustic.

Cytostatic Agents

A number of products are used to chemically remove warts and actinic keratoses. They function by a variety of different mechanisms and are discussed elsewhere in the text.

Podophyllin. Podophyllin is extracted from the May apple (*Podophyllum peltatum*) or related plants. One of the main active ingredients is podophyllotoxin. It inhibits mitosis in metaphase by its action on the cytoskeleton. Podophyllin is used in the office or clinic as a 10–25% mixture in either alcohol or tincture of benzoin. These mixtures have a limited shelf life because the alcohol evaporates. In addition, inappropriate use can lead to severe reactions. Inadvertent finger-to-eye contact can produce severe corneal reactions. We never prescribe them for home use. Because the plant extract is not well-standardized, even fresh mixtures can show great variability. Podophyllotoxin is available as a 0.5% solution for home use. Guidelines for using podophyllin in treating warts are discussed in Chapter 2. In Europe, higher concentrations of podophyllin (20–25%) are favorably used to treat actinic keratoses; multiple applications about 7–14 days apart are the rule.

5-Fluorouracil. The nucleoside analogue 5-fluorouracil (5FU) has an almost magical affect on actinic keratoses. It was first noticed that the actinic keratoses in patients treated with systemic 5FU became inflamed and often disappeared. Today 5FU is available in many forms for the topical treatment of actinic keratoses, including a ready-to-use tape (Actino-Hermal) (Chap. 55). After repeated application, the actinic keratoses become inflamed and gradually slough off, while the adjacent normal skin is spared. It is also used occasionally for removing warts, especially on mucosal surfaces, and for treating nails affected by psoriasis.

Antipsoriatic Agents

The treatment of psoriasis is detailed in Chap. 14, including tars, vitamin D analogues and topical retinoids. Topical corticosteroids are discussed below. In Germany, tar use has been restricted by federal health agencies. Today's residents no longer learn how to manage skin diseases with tar products, but this is no great loss as many other more effective measures are available.

Antipruritic Agents

These products are discussed in Chapter 25. Probably the most widely prescribed topical antipruritic medications are benzocaines and antihistamines. Both have such a high risk of allergic contact dermatitis that we employ neither. We favor polidocanol which can be compounded in a cream or lotion vehicle in concentrations of 2–5%. It is also a component of several European bath oils. Polidocanol does not seem to sensitize. EMLA (eutectic mixture of local anesthetics) is available as a cream or plaster. It can be used to numb the skin for venipuncture, spinal puncture, curettage of molluscum and even tangential excisions. In addition, it can be used to treat extremely itchy small areas, although its cost is the limiting factor.

Capsaicin

This product derived from chili peppers is approved in the USA for treatment of postherpetic neuralgia (Chap. 2) and fibromyalgia. It allegedly functions by depleting substance P but also has a definite counterirritative effect. In Germany a 3% solution also containing camphor and nicotinic acid is approved for treating a variety of rheumatic complaints but we do not employ it.

Corticosteroids

Chemistry

The importance of topical corticosteroids in dermatology cannot be underestimated. Since the introduction of topical hydrocortisone by SULZBERGER and WITTEN in 1952, there has been a slow evolution towards increasingly potent derivatives. The clinical effectiveness of a topical corticosteroid is determined by the chemical structure and the vehicle. The basic chemical structure is a pregnane ring, a cyclic hydrocarbon with four rings. A series of modifications have produced more potent molecules that penetrate the skin better and bind to receptors on epidermal cells. These steps include:

- Inserting double bonds
- Addition of halogen atoms, such as fluorine or chlorine
- Esterification by attaching acid side chains

A good example of an esterified, halogenated corticosteroid is betamethasone-17-valerate. It has an additional double bond at position 1, a fluorine atom at position 11 and a valeric acid ester at position 17. A double esterification produces betamethasone dipropionate, a molecule which provides maximum potency when incorporated in an optimized vehicle. Clobetasol propionate is the most potent topical corticosteroid molecule; it has three halogen atoms.

In general, it is difficult to separate potency and side effects in these molecules, i.e., the more effective a topical corticosteroid, the greater the side effects. In recent years, improvement in this area has been made. Several nonhalogenated molecules with multiple esters have been produced. These forms are metabolized in the skin and show fewer side effects than other, older molecules of comparable efficacy. Examples in this group include modifications of prednisolone, such as prednicarbate and 6-methylprednisolone aceponate. Hydrocortisone has been similarly altered to hydrocortisone aceponate and hydrocortisone buteprate.

Function

Corticosteroids bind to specific steroid receptors and exert an enormous range of actions. They are taken up into the cell, bound to transfer molecules and then attached to the nucleus where they influence messenger RNA synthesis and thus protein production. A number of different effects can be seen:

- Antiinflammatory: A family of proteins known as lipomodulins are produced that modify the production of prostaglandins and leukotrienes. In addition, cell membranes are stabilized.
- Antiproliferative: DNA synthesis can also be influenced, accounting somewhat for the effectiveness of corticosteroids in diseases with increased cell turnover, such as psoriasis. The inhibition of fibroblast metabolism probably also contributes to the cutaneous atrophy associated with these hormones.
- Vasoconstrictive: The prompt vasoconstriction caused by topical corticosteroids is both clinically relevant and used to assess the potency of the various molecules.
- Immunomodulatory: Both T cells and B cells are influenced, as well as many other immune functions.

Another important aspect of topical corticosteroid function is tachyphylaxis. If a product is repeatedly used, its effectiveness can become reduced in a reversible fashion. For this reason, it is wise not to apply topical corticosteroids more than once or twice a day and to consider interval therapy.

Classification

Topical corticosteroids are classified in Germany in classes I–IV, with I being weak and IV being very potent. The USA system is just the opposite; classes 1 through 7 are employed, but 1 is most potent and 7 the weakest. In both systems, the mainstay of rating is the vasoconstrictor assay of McKenzie and Stoughton (1962). It is important to note that the classification involves finished products, not specific molecules. Both vehicle and concentration play a role. In general, ointments are more effective than creams, and higher concentrations are more potent than lower ones. Readers should acquaint themselves with the agents available in their country and select a limited number of products to prescribe.

Tables 69.6 and 69.7 show modified forms of the European and American classifications. A brief study of the American table will reinforce many of the concepts discussed regarding vehicles. First of all, the concentration alone is meaningless; the least

Table 69.6. German classification of topical corticosteroids

Active ingredient	Concentration (%)	Brand names	Forms
Class I (weakest)			
Hydrocortisone	0.5–1.0	Many	L, C, O
Hydrocortisone-21-acetate	0.5–2.5	Many	C,O
Prednislone	0.4	Linola-H N, Linola-H Fett N	C, EC
Fluocortinbutylester	0.75	Vaspit	C, EC, O
Class II			
Methylprednisolone aceponate	0.1	Advantan	C, EC, O, T
Hydrocortisone aceponate	0.1	Retef	C, EC, O
Triamcinolone acetonide	0.025–0.1	Volon, many others	C, O
Fluprednidene-21-acetate	0.1	Decoderm	C,O, P
Hydrocortisone buteprate	0.1	Pandel	C, EC, O
Betamethasone-17-valerate	0.05	Betnesol-V mite	C, O, T
Prednicarbate	0.25	Dermatop	C, EC, O, T
Desoximetasone	0.05	Topisolon mite	O
Class III			
Betamethasone-17-valerate	0.1	Betnesol-V	C, O, L, T
Betamethasone-17,21-dipropionate	0.05	Diprosone	C, O, T
Diflucortolone-21-valerate	0.1	Nerisona	C, EC, O
Class IV (strongest)			
Diflucortolone-21-valerate	0.3	Nerisona forte	O
Clobetasol-17-propionate	0.05	Dermoxin	C, O, T

L, lotion; C, cream; O, ointment; EC, emollient cream or cream-ointment; T, tincture, scalp solution

Table 69.7. USA classification of topical corticosteroids

Active ingredient	Concentration (%)	Brand names	Forms
Class 1 (strongest)			
Betamethasone dipropionate	0.05	Diprolene (OV)	C, O
Clobetasol-17-propionate	0.05	Temovate (OV)	C, O
Diflorasone diacetate	0.05	Psorcon (OV)	O
Halbetosal propionate	0.05	Ultravate	C, O
Class 2			
Amicinonide	0.1	Cyclocort	O
Betamethasone dipropionate	0.05	Diprosone, Diprolene AF	C, O
Desoximetasone	0.25	Topicort	C, O
Desoximetasone	0.05	Topicort	G
Diflorasone diacetate	0.05	Fluorone	O
	0.05	Lidex	C, G, O
Halcinonide	0.1	Halog	C
Mometasone furoate	0.1	Elocon	O
Triamcinolone acetonide	0.5	Kenalog, others	O
Class 3			
Amicinonide	0.1	Cyclocort	C, L
Desoximetasone	0.05	Topicort LP	EC
Betamethasone dipropionate	0.05	Diprosone	C
Betamethasone valerate	0.1	Valisone	O
Diflorasone diacetate	0.05	Fluorone	C
Fluocinonide	0.05	Lidex E	EC
Halcinonide	0.1	Halog	O
Triamcinolone acetonide	0.1	Aristocort A	O
Triamcinolone acetonide	0.5	Aristocort HP	C
Class 4			
Betamethasone valerate	0.1	Valisone	L
Desoximetasone	0.05	Topicort	C
Flurandrenolide	0.05	Cordran	O
Fluocinolone acetonide	0.2	Synalar HP	C
Fluocinolone acetonide	0.025	Synalar	O
Halcinonide	0.025	Halog	C
Hydrocortisone valerate	0.2	Westcort	O
Mometasone furoate	0.1	Elocon	C
Triamcinolone acetonide	0.1	Aristocort, Kenalog	O
Class 5			
Betamethasone dipropionate	0.02	Diprosone	L
Betamethasone valerate	0.1	Valisone	C
Clocortalone	0.1	Cloderm	C
Fluocinolone acetonide	0.025	Synalar, Fluonid	C
Flurandrenolide	0.05	Cordran	C
Fluticasone propionate	0.05	Cutivate	C
Hydrocortisone butyrate	0.1	Locoid	C
Hydrocortisone valerate	0.2	Westcort	C
Prednicarbate	0.1	Dermatop	C
Triamcinolone acetonide	0.25	Aristocort	C
Class 6			
Aclometasone dipropionate	0.05	Aclovate	C, O
Betamethasone valerate	0.1	Valisone	L
Desonide	0.05	Tridesilon, Desowen	C, O
Fluocinolone acetonide	0.01	Synalar	C, T
Triamcinolone acetonide	0.1	Kenalog	C, L
Class 7 (weakest)			
Hydrocortisone	0.5–2.5	Many	C, O
Dexamethasone	0.1	Decadron	C
Methylprednisolone	1.0	Medrol	C

OV, optimal vehicle; L, lotion; C, cream; O, ointment; EC, emollient cream or cream-ointment; T, tincture, scalp solution.

effective products in class 7 have the highest concentrations (1.0–2.5%). Patients tend to read the concentration and, lacking knowledge of the relative potency of the various ingredients, they falsely assess the strength of their corticosteroid. Second, there are many instances in which a product falls into several classes, depending on whether an ointment or cream formulation is used. In most cases, the ointment is more potent, but notice that Halog cream is stronger than Halog ointment. In addition, almost all the class 1 products are in optimized vehicles; in the same concentration but in a conventional vehicle, they fall into a weaker class. For all these reasons, the best advice is to learn just a few agents and their intricacies. We find the American classification a bit too detailed and do very well choosing from just four groups.

Combination Products

Topical corticosteroids have been combined with a long list of other active ingredients. In most instances it is unclear if significant advantages are obtained. Keratolytic agents such as urea or salicylic acid are claimed to increase penetration and allow one to use lower potency corticosteroids. Corticosteroids are combined with both fusidic acid and clioquinol in Europe; the most popular product contains a midpotency corticosteroid and gentamicin, but we do not recommend this product because of the risk of sensitization and the need for gentamicin and its relatives for treating life-threatening infections. A medication combining a corticosteroid and an antimycotic is attractive for treating a diaper dermatitis or intertrigo where one expects to find *Candida albicans*. Unfortunately, many of the combination products contain a relatively potent corticosteroid which is not appropriate for the occluded diaper area of infants. In general, we prefer to use two separate agents; this allows more flexibility.

Indications and Usage

The indications for topical corticosteroid are almost endless, but the two main categories are inflammatory dermatoses and psoriasis. Treating moderate to severe atopic dermatitis or dyshidrotic dermatitis without topical corticosteroids is a real challenge. In psoriasis, topical corticosteroids are extremely useful, but usually should be combined with other modalities. Almost any condition with a lymphocytic infiltrate is somewhat responsive to topical corticosteroids; examples include lichen planus, lupus erythematosus and even pseudolymphomas. One should not view topical corticosteroids as antipruritic agents; they help itchy inflammatory dermatoses, but do almost nothing against pruritus or urticaria.

The wisest way to use topical corticosteroids is sparingly. Application once or twice a day usually suffices; some patients are well-served applying them every other day. The corticosteroids are partially stored in the stratum corneum so that there is a slow release over the course of the day. We frequently employ tandem therapy, applying the corticosteroid in the evening and the corresponding base or vehicle in the morning. This also helps reduce the incidence of tachyphylaxis. Another trick is interval therapy, in which the corticosteroid is used for perhaps a week and then the vehicle employed for the next week with the cycle repeated as needed. In Germany, many of the vehicles for topical corticosteroids are sold separately for this purpose but any cream or ointment can also be used.

While there are no clear rules, German class I corticosteroids are usually used for children, on the face and genitalia and for long-term use in atopic dermatitis. The class II agents usually suffice for flares of atopic dermatitis, while those in class III are needed for psoriasis, dyshidrotic dermatitis and lymphocytic processes. The superpotent class IV steroids should be reserved for disorders that have failed to respond to weaker agents. In addition to class, one must consider the cost of corticosteroids. Those available in bulk are a wise choice for patients with extensive, chronic disease such as psoriasis. Just as an example, take a patient with severe psoriasis covering 25% of the body. To treat for 1 week in the evening with clobetasol propionate cream in the USA would require at least 50 g, costing over $40.

One must also adjust the potency and vehicle for the location on the body. Absorption and side effects are much greater on the face, axillae, groin and genitalia. Maximum uptake occurs on the eyelids and scrotum. In addition, if the scalp is to be treated, a lotion, solution or gel is needed, not an ointment. A class III gel that reaches the scalp is more potent than a class IV ointment that remains on the hairs or is not even applied because it is so messy. Side effects are uncommon on the scalp.

Side Effects

The list of side effects from topical corticosteroids is long, but if they are used wisely, most problems can be avoided. Systemic side effects should never occur. If 50 g of a high potency product such as clobetasol propionate is applied over 1 week to an adult's skin, there will be measurable but not clinically relevant suppression of the adrenal axis. If wide areas need to be treated, if occlusion is used, or if the patient is young or small, systemic effects can occur. Cushing syndrome, osteoporosis, hypokalemia, diabetes mellitus and growth suppression can all occur. Every effort should be made to avoid this scenario. Other treatment methods should be chosen or systemic corticosteroids employed; they are much cheaper and easier to use.

Topical side effects are more common, often subtle and hard to avoid. Two problems that fall between topical and systemic reactions are glaucoma and steroid acne. They can result from systemic absorption but are more often a local phenomenon. Even short-term application of mid- to high-potency topical corticosteroids about the eyes can increase intraocular pressure. Steroid acne can occur from systemic absorption or at local sites. Acute problems with topical corticosteroids are uncommon but include irritant effects from a poorly chosen vehicle as well as allergic contact dermatitis. The latter is usually from a vehicle component, but some patients do develop corticosteroid allergy. This problem may be hard to detect because the antiinflammatory action of the offending agent has a masking effect (Chap. 12).

The chronic local effects of topical corticosteroids are well-known. They include the following.

Epidermis. Atrophy is produced but its clinical relevance is unclear.

Hair Follicles. Steroid acne is particularly like to occur in the sebaceus follicles of the acne-prone areas. Typically, there are many fine comedones and pustules. In addition, hypertrichosis may develop. We have seen comedones on the scalp.

Dermis. Dermal atrophy is one of the best-documented effects. In some efficacy models, the loss of dermal thickness is used to assess corticosteroid potency. The dermis usually recovers its original consistency once the applications are stopped. While usually there is subtle thinning, striae may develop. They are most common in the inner aspects of the thigh and axillae. Another common example is the often permanent depression seen after intralesional injection of corticosteroids, as for alopecia areata, or by inappropriate injection of intramuscular corticosteroids. Topical corticosteroids also exaggerate the stellate pseudoscars and purpura seen on the arms of older patients with extensive sunlight exposure.

Pigmentation. Hypopigmentation can be seen after intralesional injections; it has been described with corticosteroid-impregnated tape but must be very rare.

Vessels. Both erythema and telangiectases can occur, especially on the face. The combination of telangiectases and atrophy is known as rubeosis steroidica.

There are also a number of other phenomena associated with topical corticosteroids. Since they delay wound healing, they may have an adverse effect on leg ulcers. They also reduce the local defense mechanisms, making infections with bacteria, viruses, yeasts and fungi more common. Perioral dermatitis is often triggered by topical corticosteroids and almost invariably made worse. The rebound effect of corticosteroids can be dramatic. Patients with perioral dermatitis frequently describe marked improvement with topical corticosteroid but then worsening when the medication is stopped. In psoriasis, when the medication is stopped, there may be a severe or even pustular flare. Granuloma gluteale infantum is a peculiar nodular reaction in macerated areas such as under diapers, often caused or made worse by topical corticosteroids.

Nonsteroidal Antiinflammatory Agents

In many countries there is a considerable movement among patients against topical corticosteroids. For the most part, the fears are irrational, since, if topical corticosteroids are reasonably used, side effects need not be a problem. In our view, not treating a child with moderate to severe atopic dermatitis with topical corticosteroids has more risks than treating; secondary infections, uncontrolled itching, inadequate sleep and many more side effects of nontreatment can be listed. These arguments tend to fall on deaf ears and many parents and patients absolutely refuse topical corticosteroids. This has triggered interest in topical nonsteroidal antiinflammatory drugs.

Tacrolimus

Tacrolimus (FK506) is a macrolide immunosuppressant which appears quite useful topically. It has a molecular weight high enough that little penetration occurs through intact skin, although damaged skin can be easily entered. It is available in Japan and will be introduced in Europe and USA in 2000. It is available as Protopic ointment 0.03 % and 0.1 % to be used b.i.d. Acute atopic dermatitis responds very rapidly, while lichenified areas are slower to improve. The main acute side effect is burning on application, which tends to improve with continued use. Systemic absorption is minimal, contact dermatitis is rare and no corticosteroid-related side effects are seen.

True Nonsteroidal Antiinflammatory Agents

Among the true nonsteroidal antiinflammatory drugs, bufexamac is widely used topically in Germany. It is loved by pediatricians, who view it as equivalent to a low-potency corticosteroid. Its topical effectiveness has not been well-proven and many consider this category of agents as worthless. They are not approved for topical usage in the USA. Both allergic contact dermatitis and severe erythema multiforme-like reactions have been reported. We do not use these products.

Antiinflammatory Phytopharmaceuticals

This interesting group of agents allows one to offer "natural products" to patients or parents with a "fear of corticosteroids". Some of these agents have minimal but documented antiinflammatory actions and are often worth a try. In Europe commercial products are available with witch hazel, tannin, chamomile, arnica and pot marigold, just to cite a few examples. Most are harmless, although pot marigold is a potent topical sensitizer. Licorice and its relatives are often billed as "natural corticosteroids," as their main active ingredient has some mineralocorticoid properties; their topical role is totally unproved. In the USA, widely used topical phytopharmaceuticals include malaleuca or tea tree oil and aloe vera, both of which may also be sensitizers.

Bibliography

General Reading

Altmeyer P (eds) (1997) Therapielexikon Dermatologie und Allergie. Springer, Berlin

Arndt KA (1995) Manual of dermatologic therapeutics, 5th edn. Little Brown, Boston

Braun-Falco O, Korting HC, Maibach HI (eds) (1992) Liposome dermatics. Springer, Berlin Heidelberg New York

Boyd AS, Neldner KH (1991) Hydroxyurea therapy. J Am Acad Dermatol 25:518–524

de Groot AC, Weyland JW, Nater JP (1994) Unwanted effects of cosmetics and drugs used in dermatology, 3rd edn. Elsevier, Amsterdam

Garbe C, Reimann H, Sander-Bähr C (eds) (1996) Rationelle dermatologische Rezeptur. Thieme, Stuttgart

Hörmann HP, Korting HC (1994) Evidence for the efficacy and safety of topical herbal drugs in dermatology, part I. Anti-inflammatory agents. Phytomedicine 1:161–171

Korting HC, Schäfer-Korting M (eds) (1995) The benefit/risk ratio: a handbook for the rational use of potentially hazardous drugs. CRC Press, Boca Raton

Maddin S (1991) Current dermatologic therapy, 2nd edn. Saunders, Philadelphia

Merk HF, Bickers DR (1992) Dermatopharmakologie und Dermatotherapie. Blackwell, Berlin

Mukhtar H (ed) (1992) Pharmacology of the skin. CRC Press, Boca Raton

Orfanos CE, Garbe C (eds) (1995) Therapie der Hautkrankheiten. Springer, Berlin

Shelley WB, Shelley ED (1987) Advanced dermatologic therapy. Saunders, Philadelphia

Disinfectants, Antibiotics

Epstein ME, Amodio-Groton M, Sadick NS (1997) Antimicrobial agents for the dermatologists. I. β-Lactam antibiotics and related compounds. J Am Acad Dermatol 37:149–165

Espersen F (1998) Resistance to antibiotics used in dermatological practice. Br J Dermatol 139 [Suppl 53]:4–8

Hogan DJ (1991) Benzoyl peroxide: carcinogenicity and allergenicity. Int J Dermatol 30:467–470

Höger PH (1998) Topische Antibiotika und Antiseptika. Hautarzt 49:331–347

Korting HC, Kerscher MJ, Schäfer-Korting M et al. (1993) Influence of topical erythromycin preparations for acne vulgaris on skin surface pH. Clin Invest 71:644–648

Niedner R, Pfister-Wartha A (1990) Farbstoffe in der Dermatologie. Aktuel Dermatol 95:255–261

Veien NK (1998) The clinician's choice of antibiotics in the treatment of bacterial skin infection. Br J Dermatol 139:30–36

Sunscreens

Gasparro FP, Mitchnick M, Nash JF (1998) A review of sunscreen safety and efficacy. Photochem Photobiol 68 (3):243–256

Murphy GM (1999) Sunblocks: mechanisms of action. Photodermatol Photoimmunol Photomed 15:34–36

Naylor MF, Farmer KC (1997) The case for sunscreens. A review of their use in preventing actinic damage and neoplasia. Arch Dermatol 133:1146–1154

Skin Protection, Skin Cleaners

Estlander T, Jolanki R (1988) How to protect the hands. Dermatol Clin 6:105–114

Ortonne JP (1990) Skin cleansing: an important problem in occupational dermatology. Wien Med Wochenschr [Suppl] 108:19–21

Stoughton RB, Leyden JJ (1987) Efficacy of 4 percent chlorhexidine gluconate skin cleanser in the treatment of acne vulgaris. Cutis 39:551–553

Wigger-Alberti W, Maraffio B, Wernli M et al. (1997) Self-application of a protective cream. Pitfalls of occupational skin protection. Arch Dermatol 133:861–864

Cytostatics

Goette DK (1981) Topical chemotherapy with 5-fluorouracil. A review. J Am Acad Dermatol 4:633–649

Jansen GT (1992) Topical chemotherapy. Clin Dermatol 10:305–307

Knulst AC, De La Faille HB, Van Vloten WA (1995) Topical 5-fluorouracil in the treatment of Darier's disease. Br J Dermatol 133:463–466

Miller RA (1985) Podophyllin. Int J Dermatol 24:491–498

Schwartz RA (1996) Therapeutic perspectives in actinic and other keratoses. Int J Dermatol 35:533–538

Capsaicin

Breneman DI, Cardone JS, Blumsack RF et al. (1992) Topical capsaicin for treatment of hemodialysis-related pruritus. J Am Acad Dermatol 26:91–94

Hautkappe M, Roizen MF, Toledano A et al. (1998) Review of the effectiveness of capsaicin for painful cutaneous disorders and neural dysfunction. Clin J Pain 14:97–106

Norton SA (1998) Useful plants of dermatology. V. Capsicum and capsaicin. J Am Acad Dermatol 39:626–628

Corticosteroids

Ahluwalia A (1998) Topical glucocorticoids and the skin-mechanisms of action: an update. Mediators Inflamm 7:183–193

Drake LA, Dinehart SM, Farmer ER et al. (1996) Guidelines of care for the use of topical glucocorticosteroids. J Am Acad Dermatol 35:615–619

Korting HC, Kerscher MJ, Schäfer-Korting M et al. (1992) Topical glucocorticoids with improved benefit/risk ratio: do they exist? J Am Acad Dermatol 27:87–92

Maibach HI, Surber C (eds) (1992) Topical corticosteroids. Karger, Basel

McKenzie AW, Stoughton RB (1962) Method for comparing percutaneous absorption of steroids. Arch Dermatol 86:608–610

Sulzberger MB, Witten VH (1952) The effects of topically applied compound F in selected dermatoses. J Invest Dermatol 19:101–102

Tacrolimus

Ruzicka T, Bieber T, Schöpf E et al. (1997) A short-term trial of tacrolimus ointment for atopic dermatitis. N Engl J Med 337:816–821

Ruzicka T, Assmann T, Homey B (1999) Tacrolimus. Arch Dermatol 135:574–580

Systemic Therapy

Contents

Introduction

In many instances, systemic therapy is either more effective, quicker or cheaper than topical therapy. In this chapter we discuss medications such as systemic corticosteroids, which are recommended throughout the text. Oral medications used for limited purposes, such as antimycotic agents, are covered in the respective chapters. In addition, we concentrate on the dermatologic use of agents such as dapsone or antimalarial drugs whose cutaneous indications do not coincide with the recommendations usually found in pharmacology textbooks. In every instance when prescribing systemic drugs, the physician needs to be well acquainted with the agent, its side effects, its cross-reactions with other medications, its role in pregnancy and the patient's other underlying illnesses.

Corticosteroids

Pharmacology. Oral corticosteroids are absorbed in the jejunum, most of them rapidly and nearly completely. The presence of food in the gastrointestinal tract may delay the absorption but only minimally. Since peak plasma levels are obtained after 30–90 min, little consideration need be given to speed of action when choosing between oral forms.

The mechanisms of action of corticosteroids are numerous. In general, they bind to cortisol-binding globulin or transcortin thereby competing with endogenous cortisone molecules. The active agent is the free molecule, which attaches to intracellular cytosolic corticoid receptor and is then translocated into the nucleus where it influences DNA, RNA and protein synthesis.

Antiinflammatory and Immunosuppressive Action. Corticosteroids inhibit the production and release of cytokines, including interleukin (IL)-1, IL-6 and tumor necrosis factor (TNF)-α, from macrophages, Langerhans cells and monocytes. These cytokines are involved in the activation of T cells and in triggering the entire immunoreactive cascade (Chap. 1). Corticosteroids also interfere with phospholipase A2 and thus arachidonic acid metabolism so that prostaglandin and leukotriene levels are reduced. They cause vasoconstriction so that various blood cells have less access to the tissues, as do immunoglobulins and immune complexes. In addition, they cause a lymphocytopenia, primarily because of redistribution of the cells away from the peripheral blood.

Antiproliferative Action. Mitosis is inhibited so that cell growth and proliferation are reduced. Fibroblasts are particularly affected, producing less collagen and other matrix proteins.

From the vantage point of the dermatologist, all of the other physiologic actions of corticosteroids are exaggerated, becoming side effects of therapy, as discussed below.

Indications. Systemic corticosteroids are the most important single therapeutic agent for serious dermatologic diseases. They are used for both acute and chronic diseases, but one should carefully distinguish between these settings. In acute situations, such as severe urticaria, allergic contact dermatitis and perhaps drug reactions, the initial dose is high, the product is tapered rapidly over 1–2 weeks and the expected side effects are minimal. In the extreme acute example, anaphylaxis, corticosteroids are given intravenously in very large bolus doses. Other acute situations in which systemic corticosteroids may be useful include severe dyshidrotic dermatitis, Sweet syndrome, erythema multiforme and lichen planus.

When employed in the treatment of a chronic disease, corticosteroids must be used for months to years and side effects are inevitable. The main indications are autoimmune bullous diseases, lupus erythematosus, dermatomyositis, mixed connective tissue disease, pyoderma gangrenosum and some forms of vasculitis. While systemic corticosteroids are also effective for other disorders, such as atopic dermatitis and psoriasis, the risk/benefit ratio is generally unfavorable and we rarely employ them in such settings.

Available Products. While there are many different corticosteroids for oral therapy, one can do quite well using only a single agent. Table 70.1 shows the features of some of the available products. Depending on the standard of care in one's country, one can use either prednisone, prednisolone or 6-methyl prednisolone routinely. By becoming familiar with one drug, one can avoid errors in dosage. Rare patients fail to metabolize prednisone to prednisolone and should be treated with the latter product. Those with marked sodium or fluid retention may do better with triamcinolone, betamethasone or dexamethasone. The differences in serious side effects between these agents is insignificant.

The prescribed regimen is highly variable. For acute problems, we prefer a 2–3-week course. One reasonable regimen is prednisone 60 mg daily for 5 days, then 40 mg daily for 5 days and then 20 mg daily for 5 days. Thus a total of thirty 20 mg pills are required over 15 days. Many other schedules can be created, all starting with about 60 mg of prednisone or the equivalent and tapering over 2–3 weeks. While a number of unit dose packs are available, in which various corticosteroids are packaged much like oral contraceptives with detailed instructions for short-term use, most are only designed for 6 days. This is simply too short for treating severe allergic contact dermatitis or dyshidrotic dermatitis; once the six day course is complete, a flare is almost to be expected. Corticosteroids should be given in the morning; natural secretion shows a diurnal rhythm and is at its highest level at this time. Occasionally split doses may be needed for more rapid control, such as in vasculitis or lupus erythematosus with CNS involvement.

Table 70.1. Systemic corticosteroids

Product	Equivalent dose (mg)	Duration (h)	Cushing threshold (mg/day)	Sodium retention[a]
Prednisone	5	24–36	10	0.8
Prednisolone	5	24–36	10	0.8
6-Methyl prednisolone	4	24–36	8	0.5
Triamcinolone	4	36–48	8	0
Betamethasone	1	>48	2	0
Dexamethasone	1	>48	2	0

[a] Hydrocortisone taken as 1.0

When starting to treat a chronic disease, many factors must be considered. The initial dose must be high enough to control the disease. We try avoid exceeding 1.0 mg/kg daily, although rarely higher levels are needed to control pemphigus vulgaris or severe systemic lupus erythematosus. Alternate day administration of systemic corticosteroids spares the pituitary-adrenal axis somewhat and leads to fewer side effects. Typical regimens are prednisone 20–40 mg every other morning. Sometimes disease such as bullous pemphigoid can be brought under control initially with alternate day dosing, perhaps combined with other immunosuppressive agents. If a disease is severe, then it usually flares on the day without medication, making the approach of questionable value.

There are many other ways to use systemic corticosteroids. In dramatic situations, intravenous pulse therapy may be needed, usually with methylprednisolone in dosages of 500–1000 mg daily or b.i.d. for 3–5 days. This approach is most often employed in systemic lupus erythematosus for CNS disease, nephritis and thrombocytopenia. It is also used for vasculitis and has been employed for pyoderma gangrenosum.

The administration of intramuscular corticosteroids, usually triamcinolone acetonide, is recommended by some clinicians. When treating inflammatory conditions, a typical dose is 40 mg of triamcinolone acetonide. For more chronic conditions, the same dosage must be given IM every 4–8 weeks. The degree of adrenal suppression is somewhat greater with intramuscular products because the daily variation is eliminated. In addition, if the injection is too superficial, cutaneous atrophy and sometimes hypopigmentation may result. On the other hand, patient compliance is higher. We do not use intramuscular corticosteroids but respect their place in the armamentarium. Others prefer to use intramuscular ACTH, reasoning that, if the adrenal glands are overstimulated to produce excess corticosteroids, there will be less harm than with external administration. ACTH is somewhat antigenic so that allergic reactions can occur and the levels of corticosteroid production are variable. We do not use ACTH injections.

Side Effects. The side effects of administering systemic corticosteroids are both expected and predictable, as the normally produced hormones influence the body in so many ways.

Endocrine Effects. The pituitary-adrenal axis is suppressed, so ACTH levels are reduced. While sophisticated testing can detect abnormalities in the axis after just a few days, clinical effects take longer. If a patient who is taking long-term corticosteroids is confronted by a stressful situation, such as a car accident or emergency surgery, his body may fail to respond with the usual outpouring of adrenal hormones. Similarly if exogenous corticosteroids are too rapidly tapered, an Addisonian crisis may result.

A rare but related problem is the steroid withdrawal syndrome. Some patients, after receiving short bursts of high-dose corticosteroids, may experience diffuse problems including emotional lability, fatigue, nausea, vomiting and loss of appetite when the dosage is reduced rapidly. This diagnosis is hard to prove, as the serum cortisol levels are normal, but most patients improve dramatically when they receive a higher dosage and are then tapered very gradually.

In children, there may be growth retardation. Children with atopic dermatitis treated with systemic corticosteroids show slowing of their growth curves during the periods when they required systemic therapy, but the long-term effects are usually minimal.

Other endocrinologic problems are related to the diabetogenic effects of corticosteroids, which for this reason are also called glucocorticoids. Some patients may develop frank diabetes mellitus when treated with systemic corticosteroids; often they have had an abnormal glucose tolerance test prior to therapy. In rare cases, diabetic ketoacidosis and coma can result. There is also a catabolic effect because of impaired protein synthesis, leading to loss of tissue mass, especially muscle wasting. Finally, secondary amenorrhea is extremely common; even with short-term therapy, menstrual irregularities are to be expected.

Immunologic Effects. The influences on the immune system are protean. Many different infections tend to be more common during treatment with corticosteroids, including bacterial, viral and fungal diseases. Cellular immunity appears to be more affected than humoral and macrophage function. Tuberculosis occupies a special role, as corticosteroid therapy increases the risk of reactivation; thus, all patients should be screened for tuberculosis prior to long-term treatment. Systemic corticosteroid therapy alone does not increase the risk of malignancies, in contrast to many other forms of immunosuppression.

Skeletal System. Two of the most feared problems associated with systemic corticosteroids involve the skeleton. Almost every patient develops corticosteroid-induced osteoporosis. By contrast, aseptic necrosis of the neck of the femur is much more unpredictable. While it occasionally appears after relatively low dosages, the risk increases as the dose and duration of therapy increase. Myopathy also occurs.

Cardiovascular. Hypertension usually develops. The main factors are vasoconstriction, sodium retention and increased renin levels. Using products with less sodium retention reduces the problem. Fluid retention can lead to or exacerbate heart failure. Because of the hypokalemia, alkalosis may evolve.

Gastrointestinal. Peptic ulcers are somewhat more common, especially in patients simultaneously treated with aspirin or nonsteroidal antiinflammatory drugs. While there are conflicting recommendations, we suggest that proton pump inhibitors such as omeprazole be prescribed for patients with a history of peptic ulcer disease. Antacids alone may not be sufficient prophylaxis for those at risk. Fatty infiltration of the liver, pancreatitis and intestinal perforation also occur. It is unclear what direct influence the corticosteroids have on the pathogenesis of these disorders and to what extent they unmask underlying problems.

Central Nervous System. Both corticosteroid-induced psychosis and pseudotumor cerebri can be seen. Women are at greater risk. Distinguishing between CNS involvement in lupus erythematosus and corticosteroid-induced psychosis is a challenging task. Pseudotumor cerebri tends to occur when high doses are rapidly tapered; it presents with nausea, vomiting, headaches and visual disturbances.

Ocular. Glaucoma may occur, but it is more common with periorbital use of topical corticosteroids. When long-term therapy is employed, the risk of cataracts, usually bilateral posterior subcapsular lesions, is considerable. Every patient facing long-term systemic corticosteroid therapy should have baseline and interval ophthalmologic examinations.

Hematologic. The erythrocyte and leukocyte counts both go up, but the number of lymphocytes and eosinophils drops. The increased erythrocyte mass may predispose to thrombosis, but this is rarely a clinical issue.

Cutaneous. The many cutaneous changes are usually associated with Cushing syndrome. They include acne, facial erythema, telogen effluvium, hirsutism (often with lanugo hairs), striae distensae, fragile skin, purpura and rearrangement of subcutaneous fat to produce facial swelling (moon facies) and an accumulation over the nape and upper back (buffalo hump). Wound healing is also impaired. These changes are discussed in Chapter 48.

Pregnancy. Corticosteroids are neither teratogenic nor mutagenic. They have been used in many pregnancies because of the frequency of systemic lupus erythematosus in young women. A firm indication is required. The fetus may experience the same changes discussed above, as the medication crosses the placenta. Suppression of the hypophyseal-pituitary axis may make the fetus less capable of responding to the stresses of birth, thus increasing the risk at delivery.

Precautions and Prophylactic Measures. Although the long-term effects of corticosteroids are well known, occasionally, in the haste to get a disease under control, one forgets to institute appropriate prophylactic therapy to minimize the chronic problems down the road.

Osteoporosis is one such problem. Every patient embarking upon more than a 1–2-week course of systemic corticosteroids should have baseline bone densitometry measurements. Those with no evidence of preexisting osteoporosis should receive calcium 1000–1500 mg daily and vitamin D 400–800 IU daily, as well as being encouraged to eat a calcium-rich diet, get adequate exercise and avoid alcohol (reduces osteoblast function), nicotine (interferes with estrogen) and coffee (increases calcium diuresis). Postmenopausal females should receive hormonal replacement in consultation with a gynecologist. If a 24-h urine study after 2–3 weeks shows increased calcium excretion, a thiazide diuretic should be added. If the patient already shows evidence of osteoporosis, especially with a history of a fracture, then calcitonin, biphosphonates and sodium fluoride may be added to the regimen.

Ophthalmologic examination should be obtained as soon as practical so that corticosteroid-induced cataracts can be monitored. A baseline chest X-ray is needed, so that potential activation of tuberculosis can be assessed. If the patient has a history of peptic ulcer disease or is taking other ulcerogenic medication, a proton pump inhibitor should be prescribed. Other complications such as hypertension and diabetes mellitus require periodic monitoring. Finally, we encourage patients to wear a Medi-Alert tag alerting other physicians to their dependence on corticosteroids, so that they receive appropriate care if involved in an accident or require emergency surgery.

Drug Interactions. Systemic corticosteroids show surprisingly few drug interactions. They increase renal clearance of aspirin, so if they are tapered, the aspirin dose must be adjusted downwards. There is also an increased risk of gastrointestinal bleeding if a patient takes corticosteroids along with aspirin or nonsteroidal antiinflammatory drugs. Oral contraceptives prolong the half-life of corticosteroids, while a variety of medications, including phenobarbital, phenytoin, isoniazid and rifampin, increase their hepatic degradation. The hypokalemia may lead to digitalis toxicity.

Contraindications. Active untreated tuberculosis, systemic mycoses and ocular herpes simplex infections are taken as absolute contraindications. All of the problems alluded to under side effects present relative contraindications. Thus if a patient has diabetes mellitus, hypertension, a peptic ulcer, osteoporosis or congestive heart failure, one must use systemic corticosteroids with great care. Diverticulitis and recent intestinal surgery with a bowel anastomosis are also delicate situations, as the risk of perforation is increased.

Other Hormonal Agents

A number of other products that mimic or block hormones are also useful in dermatology.

Antiandrogens

Cyproterone Acetate. This antiandrogen is used in acne (Chap. 28) and hirsutism (Chap. 31). It is not available in the USA. In Germany, it is most often prescribed in combination with an estrogen (Diane 35 or Dianette) so that contraception is insured. We tend to use Dianette, which contains 2 mg of cyproterone acetate and 35 μg of ethinyl estradiol.

Chlormadinone. Another antiandrogen available in Europe, chlormadinone, comes as 2-mg tablets. It is used for similar indications and in similar ways as cyproterone acetate.

Spironolactone. This aldosterone antagonist is a potassium-sparing diuretic and has some antiandrogen effects. While it is not approved for these indications, it is sometimes prescribed in low dosages, i. e., 50–100 mg daily, for patients with acne or hirsutism. We do not use it because we have access to the approved antiandrogens listed above.

Finasteride. Newly approved for male pattern alopecia, finasteride inhibits the conversion of testosterone to 5-hydroxy testosterone by blocking the type II α-reductase enzyme, as discussed in Chapter 31.

Danazol and Stanozolol. These modified androgens are used in treating hereditary angioedema (Chap. 11). They both have a protean spectrum of action and should only be prescribed by physicians familiar with their properties.

Oral Contraceptives

We occasionally recommend estrogen-dominant oral contraceptives for young women with acne, but always work together with a gynecologist. Some women report that their acne flares with their menses; this subset may respond better to hormonal intervention (Chap. 28). Estrogens suppress sebum production in most cases. They may also be helpful in the treatment of severe rosacea or rosacea fulminans.

Cytostatic Agents

Many of the cytostatic agents used in cancer chemotherapy are employed in lower dosages in dermatology for their immunosuppressive effects. For example, methotrexate can be used in psoriasis where it interferes with the rapid epidermal turnover but more importantly has direct effects on lymphocytes. All of the cytostatic agents have some immunomodulatory effect, as they kill active cells, be they tumor cells, lymphocytes or any rapidly growing tissue (mucosa, hair matrix, testes or bone marrow.) The margin of safety with most such agents is small, although the lower dosages employed by dermatologists offer some advantages. All have some degree of bone marrow suppression. In addition, immunosuppression increases the risk of infections and of long-term tumor development. The most common use of the cytostatic agents in dermatology is as steroid-sparing agents in the treatment of autoimmune diseases. A discussion of the theoretical aspects of the immunomodulatory role of cytostatic and immunosuppressive agents is included in the immunology section (Chap. 1).

Alkylating Agents

These drugs cause DNA cross-linking and breakage. They may cause insterility and often lead to myelodysplastic syndromes or acute nonlymphocytic leukemia. The main members of the group are:

Cyclophosphamide. In dosages of 50–200 mg daily, cyclophosphamide is probably the most effective agent in this group, but it is somewhat toxic. It has some selectivity for plasma cells, and is widely used for treating Wegener granulomatosis. Major side effects include hemorrhagic cystitis, neutropenia, sterility and a 5–10% lifetime risk of malignancies, including malignant lymphomas, leukemias and solid neoplasms.

Chlorambucil. This agent has a fairly rapid onset of action and in dosages of 4–8 mg daily is a well-tolerated steroid-sparing agent which is also used in early Sézary syndrome (Chap. 61). The main side effect is mild myelosuppression.

Dacarbazine or DTIC. This is the only agent approved for treatment of metastatic malignant melanoma (Chap. 58). While it is an alkylating agent, it also appears to block the cell cycle.

Mechlorethamine (Nitrogen Mustard) and Carmustine (BCNU). These two drugs are used in a diluted form topically to treat early lesions of mycosis fungoides (Chap. 61). They are potent irritants and allergens in this setting.

Antimetabolites

These drugs act to inhibit various metabolic processes, often involving purine and pyrimidine metabolism. They usually displace a natural, structurally related product, thereby interrupting cell growth.

5-Fluorouracil (5FU). Topical 5FU is used to treat actinic keratoses. Systemic 5FU is widely used for solid gastrointestinal tumors but has on occasion been recommended for psoriasis. It frequently causes the acral erythema of chemotherapy reaction.

Methotrexate. The most common dermatologic use for methotrexate is in psoriasis. The usual limiting factor is either bone marrow suppression or mucosal damage. The main long-term concerns are liver damage and secondary malignancies. The usual dosage today for psoriasis is 10–15 mg once weekly (Chap. 14). Intravenous, intramuscular and oral regimens are possible. Methotrexate is also used for its steroid-sparing effects. Intralesional methotrexate has been employed for treating keratoacanthomas.

Antitumor Antibiotics

Most antibiotics interfere with tumor growth by hampering DNA and protein synthesis.

Bleomycin. Rarely used by dermatologists, bleomycin is of interest because of its side effects – pulmonary fibrosis, acral sclerosis and Raynaud phenomenon – which are similar to systemic sclerosis. It also causes dermatitis leading to unique flagellate or streaky hyperpigmentation. It has been used intralesionally to destroy warts, especially subungual warts, but acral ulcerations and pain are problems.

Alkaloids

The alkaloids vincristine and vinblastine disrupt microtubule assembly in mitosis. They are useful in the treatment of Kaposi sarcoma and Langerhans cell histiocytosis. In Kaposi sarcoma, they are also often used intralesionally (Chap. 2). Podophyllin is another member of this family; its relative etoposide (VP-16) is effective systemically in Langerhans cell histiocytosis, but long-term concerns about induction of other hematologic malignancies limit its use in this setting.

Other Agents

Hydroxyurea. This medication inhibits ribonucleotide reductase and is used in the treatment of hematologic malignancies. It is approved for sickle cell anemia and thrombocythemia. In dosages of

500 – 1500 mg daily, it can be used for psoriasis. The limiting factor is the development of a megaloblastic anemia.

Immunosuppressive Agents

These agents are immunomodulatory but are not primarily cytotoxic. The classic example are the corticosteroids, as discussed above. Many other agents also modulate the immune response, most often by having a toxic effect on certain effector cells at a level that does not produce much other toxicity. One can view immunosuppression occurring at three levels, blocking different signals (Chap. 1).

- Signal 1 is the activation of the T cell receptor, leading to stimulation of calcineurin and then promotion of IL-2 production. This signal is blocked by cyclosporine and tacrolimus.
- Signal 2 involves transcription of the IL-2 gene and is one of the many targets of corticosteroids.
- Signal 3 involves autocrine stimulation of the IL-2 receptor, which can be blocked by antibodies against this structure or by sirolimus, an experimental agent that inhibits the messenger signals directed towards cell cycle stimulation. De novo purine synthesis, the end result of this process, is blocked by azathioprine and mycophenolic acid.

Cyclosporine

This small, 11-amino acid polypeptide is the mainstay of solid organ transplantation. It was isolated from soil fungi and proved to be a disappointing antibiotic but an amazing immunosuppressive agent. It blocks the earliest stages of the immune response by binding to cyclophylin, thus inhibiting calcineurin. This is the first step in T cell activation following stimulation of the T cell receptor. Thus IL-2 production is blocked. The main effect is on helper T cells; cytotoxic and suppressor T cells are relatively unaffected. Bone marrow suppression does not occur.

Cyclosporine is available for intravenous and oral therapy. The initial oral product, Sandimmune, was poorly absorbed; it has been replaced by a more reliably absorbed oral preparation, Neoral, in most markets. The drug is absorbed from the gastrointestinal tract with varying degrees of efficiency and has a half-life of about 18 h. The main side effects are renal toxicity, hypertension and hepatic damage. It has a wide variety of drug interactions, once again involving the hepatic cytochrome P450 system. Agents that stimulate these enzymes, such as rifampin, phenobarbital, carbamazepine and phenytoin, lead to low levels of cyclosporine, while macrolide antibiotics, imidazoles and similar products can cause overdosage. Gingival hyperplasia and hypertrichosis are side effects of dermatologic interest.

Cyclosporine has proven to be very effective for treating severe psoriasis (Chap. 14). The usual dosage is 2.5 – 5.0 mg/kg; improvement is seen over 4 – 8 weeks. Once the dosage is tapered, the psoriasis usually reappears. There are many contraindications, including hepatic disease, renal disease and hypertension. Cyclosporine is usually not combined with PUVA therapy, oral retinoids or other immunosuppressive therapies.

Other indications include atopic dermatitis, pyoderma gangrenosum and Behçet syndrome, especially with ocular involvement. Lichen planus, particularly oral lichen planus, responds quite well. While there are many other dermatoses that are responsive, the expense and toxicity of cyclosporine have limited its role in dermatologic therapy.

Tacrolimus

This is a newer immunosuppressive drug that is replacing cyclosporine in many solid organ transplant settings. Tacrolimus (FK506) also inhibits calcineurin but does so by binding to a different receptor, FKBP (FK binding protein)-12. It appears effective for the treatment of atopic dermatitis and pyoderma gangrenosum, but has not been extensively studied or used in dermatologic patients. The usual dose for transplantation patients is 0.1 – 0.3 mg/kg daily in two divided doses. The side effects are similar to those of cyclosporine, but there is less hirsutism and gingival hyperplasia. The heart walls and septum may become thickened, so echocardiographic monitoring is recommended.

Azathioprine

Azathioprine's immunosuppressive role is complex. It is metabolized in the liver to its active metabolites, which inhibit purine interconversion enzymes and thus nucleic acid synthesis. In higher dosages, it has the same marrow suppressive effects as its relatives, as well as nausea, vomiting and cholestasis. Azathioprine is part of virtually every immunosuppressive regimen following solid organ transplantation. It plays a role in the frequency of squamous cell carcinoma in the sun-exposed skin of renal transplant patients.

In its usual dosage of 50–100 mg daily, azathioprine is used for the treatment of vasculitis, lupus erythematosus, dermatomyositis and bullous diseases, once again in an attempt to get by with lower levels of corticosteroids. Azathioprine may be helpful in both Behçet syndrome and pyoderma gangrenosum, leading some clinicians to recommend it for neutrophilic disorders. It is also effective for chronic actinic dermatitis (Chap. 13) and has been employed to treat psoriasis and pityriasis rubra pilaris.

Mycophenolate Mofetil

Mycophenolic acid, the active metabolite of mycophenolate mofetil, was used two decades ago to treat psoriasis but fell out of favor. Today it is replacing azathioprine in many immunosuppressive regimens, as it appears to be a more specific inhibitor of de novo purine synthesis in lymphocytes. It acts by blocking inosine monophosphate dehydrogenase. The main side effects in the usual dosage range of 1.0 g b.i.d. are diarrhea and hematologic suppression.

Antihistamines

This family of agents is highly effective for allergic rhinitis and conjunctivitis, and the best treatment for urticaria. When treating other pruritic disorders such as atopic dermatitis, it has been well-shown that the anti-pruritic action of antihistamines is roughly comparable to their soporific action. Several histamine receptors have been described. The major receptor on cutaneous mast cells is the H1 receptor, so that agents which competitively block this entity are of most importance in dermatology. The H2 receptors are clinically important because, when they are blocked, gastric acid secretion is reduced. H2 receptors are found in the skin; however, they play a minor role in cutaneous disease. While there are other mast cell receptors, including intracellular ones, their clinical relevance is unclear.

There is considerable variance in the onset of action and metabolism of antihistamines. Those with a relatively rapid onset, such as cetirizine, are ideal when the patient takes the medication as a response to allergic symptoms or hives. On the other hand, antihistamines that maintain an effective level for 24 h, such as fexofenadine, are more convenient for continuous use.

The major clinical actions are the opposite of those mediated by histamine. The bronchioles and small vessels dilate, vascular permeability is reduced, secretions dry up and histamine-mediated pruritus improves. As discussed in Chapter 25, histamine is only in part responsible for pruritus. Different antihistamines have additional beneficial actions; cyproheptadine blocks serotonin, cetirizine inhibits eosinophilic chemotaxis and mizolastin has an antiinflammatory action.

The main side effects of the classic antihistamines are sedation and associated CNS symptoms. Thus drink-and-drive precautions are both essential and of medical-legal importance. Some children have a paradoxical hyperactive reaction. Anticholinergic effects such as a dry mouth, dye eyes, accommodation problems and urinary retention may develop. There are some differences between the various chemical classes but most problems are discovered by trial and error.

The newer antihistamines have a different spectrum of problems, as they have cardiac side effects, especially when taken with other medications that are metabolized by hepatic enzymes dependent on cytochrome P450. A prolonged Q-T interval, torsades de pointes, ventricular arrhythmias and even sudden death have been described. For this reason, terfenadine is no longer available over-the-counter, and most physicians have replaced it with a modified form, fexofenadine, that is not metabolized in the liver. Drugs that should not be combined with antihistamines include imidazole antimycotic agents, macrolide antibiotics (especially erythromycin), cyclosporine, calcium channel blockers and oral contraceptives. Astemizole is associated with increased appetite and weight gain, and has been removed from the market in the USA because of its cardiac effects.

Other contraindications to antihistamine use include narrow-angle glaucoma, urinary retention as with prostatic hypertrophy, alcoholism and sedative abuse. The use of monamine oxidase inhibitors is also a contraindication. While no antihistamine is endorsed as safe during pregnancy or nursing, the classic drugs such as diphenhydramine are probably safe. In the USA it is a paradox that many of these older antihistamines are available over-the-counter but are not officially safe. In children, one must be alert to the paradoxical hyperactivity response.

One should have a logical approach to the use of antihistamines. It is reasonable to try agents from several different biochemical classes in order to find the medications that are best tolerated and most effective. The following classes are available, as shown in Table 70.2. The first seven groups include the traditional antihistamines, which are relatively nonspecific H1 blockers. Because they are lipophilic and cross the blood-brain barrier, they tend to cause drowsiness, which may be desirable when they are used at night. The nonsedating antihistamines have all been modified in some fashion so that they do not as readily cross the blood-brain barrier. The tricyclic antidepressant doxepin has both H1 and H2 action. The role of H2 blockers is less clear; they usually should be combined with a traditional H1 agent. Cyproheptadine is often endorsed for cold urticaria, and hydroxyzine for all forms of physical urticaria.

The patient should be counseled about side effects, as he may be taking the product for some time. Discuss drinking and driving precautions, as well as the many cross-reactions associated with some of the nonsedating agents that can cause cardiac rhythm disturbances. Terfenadine and astemizole should not be used with erythromycin or ketoconazole or in patients with a history of cardiac arrhythmias.

Table 70.2. Types of antihistamines

Class	Examples
Ethanolamines	Diphenhydramine Clemastine
Ethylenediamines	Tripelennamine Pyrilamine
Piperazines	Hydroxyzine
Alkylamines	Brompheniramine Chlorpheniramine
Piperidines	Cyproheptadine Ketotifen
Phenothiazines	Promethazine
Tricyclic agents	Doxepin
Nonsedating agents	Cetirizine Fexofenadine Loratadine Mizolastin (Astemizole) (Terfenadine)
H2 blockers	Cimetidine Ranitidine

Retinoids

The oral retinoids are modified vitamin preparations. While many different retinoids have been synthesized, only 13-*cis*-retinoic acid (isotretinoin) and the aromatic retinoids, acitretin and etretinate, are routinely used clinically. In Europe acitretin has replaced etretinate because it has a shorter serum half-life. Isotretinoin is used for the treatment of acne (Chap. 28), while etretinate and acitretin are employed for psoriasis (Chap. 14) and disorders of keratinization (Chap. 17). Other retinoids are used in treating leukemia. Some forms of myelogenous leukemia have translocations involving retinoid receptors and are responsive to these agents.

The main problem with retinoids is teratogenicity. Thus all female patients taking systemic retinoids must practice some form of contraception. Long-term effects on the skeletal system are another limiting factor when treating patients with disorders of keratinization for which treatment may be required over many years. All of these problems are discussed in detail in the respective chapters.

Nonsteroidal Antiinflammatory Drugs

The family of nonsteroidal antiinflammatory drugs is very large, ranging from aspirin to a number of elegant and expensive agents with considerable specificity. About 20 nonsalicylate agents are available in both Europe and USA. All interfere with some aspect of arachidonic acid metabolism. Arachidonic acid is released from tissue phospholipids by the actions of phospholipase; it is further metabolized by cyclooxygenases to prostaglandins and thromboxane, and by 5-lipoxygenase to leukotrienes (Chap. 1). Agents are available that inhibit either cyclooxygenase(COX) or 5-lipoxygenase.

Cyclooxygenase inhibitors are further subdivided into the traditional COX1 inhibitors and the new COX2 inhibitors. COX1 is found in all cells and is primarily responsible for the physiologic action of prostaglandins on the stomach, kidneys and bronchial system. In contrast, COX2 is induced during inflammatory reactions by a variety of cytokines. Most of the traditional nonsteroidal antiinflammatory drugs inhibit both COX enzymes. Those newer agents which primarily inhibit COX2 have less gastrointestinal side effects. Representative examples of nonsteroidal antiinflammatory drugs vary from country to country and further information should be sought in general texts.

The main role for nonsteroidal antiinflammatory drugs in dermatology is probably for pain relief. Aspirin is also used for treating a variety of platelet disorders (Chaps. 22 and 23). Because of its irreversible inhibition of platelets, aspirin should be discontinued well before embarking upon surgical procedures. Aspirin and other nonsteroidal antiinflammatory drugs are able to block the erythema induced by UV radiation, but this is rarely clinically practical. Most patients with psoriatic arthritis receive some form of nonsteroidal antiinflammatory drug. Erythema nodosum is another dermatologic indication.

In general this family of agents is far better known to dermatologists for its side effects. Both anaphylaxis and serious reactions such as Stevens-Johnson syndrome and toxic epidermal necrolysis can occur. In addition, gastrointestinal distress and bleeding, as well as renal damage, especially in the elderly, are major concerns. Up to 20% of chronic urticaria patients have aspirin sensitivity, and hypersensitivity reactions may occur in response to all the nonsteroidal antiinflammatory drugs. The spectrum of side effects varies greatly among the different agents. Our advice is to carefully study the properties of a limited number of these drugs and restrict their use to well-established indications such as pain or arthritis.

Antimalarials

The antimalarials are used extensively to treat lupus erythematosus and are occasionally employed for other dermatologic indications. Their mechanism of action is unclear but they appear to stabilize lysosomal enzymes. While all antimalarials have weak UV radiation screening effects, this does not explain their effectiveness.

There are two products available in the USA: hydroxychloroquine 200 mg (155 mg base) and chloroquine 250 mg (150 mg base). While hydroxychloroquine and chloroquine have similar actions, hydroxychloroquine has a better margin of safety and is almost universally recommended. Both are aminoquinolones with a two-ring structure.

The side effects are similar and include gastrointestinal distress, bone marrow toxicity, hemolysis with glucose-6-phosphate dehydrogenase (G6PD) deficiency, hepatic damage, and both reversible and irreversible ocular toxicity with retinal damage and corneal deposits. There are also cutaneous changes. About 20% of patients develop pruritus and a morbilliform rash, requiring discontinuation of therapy. In addition, blue-black hyperpigmentation may occur, as well as hypopigmentation, especially of the hairs.

We usually use hydroxychloroquine 200–400 mg daily for treating discoid lupus erythematosus patients who have failed to respond to topical corticosteroids and sunscreens. If the daily dose is kept below 6.5 mg/kg, toxicity from hydroxychloroquine is rare. The onset of action of antimalarials is slow; if no improvement is seen after 3–6 months, quinacrine can be added.

Quinacrine has a third benzene ring and is structurally closer to acridine. Quinacrine is also used for giardiasis, for staining chromosomes (Q bands) and for treating malignant pleural effusions and ascites. Quinacrine may cause lichen planus-like lesions. Quinacrine does not cause retinal toxicity, but does produce a harmless, reversible yellow discoloration of the skin and sclera.

Recent Royal College of Physician guidelines recommend pretreatment evaluation of renal and hepatic function, as well as G6PD levels in black or Mediterranean patients. One should ask about visual problems and screen near-vision prior to starting therapy. While visual problems should be queried at each visit and screening should be done yearly, ophthalmologic consultation is only recommended if problems or changes arise. There is no effective early screening test for hydroxychloroquine retinal damage.

One of the fascinating uses for chloroquine is in porphyria cutanea tarda, where its toxic hepatic effects are used to help flush porphyrins out of the system (Chap. 44.) A much lower dosage must be employed, usually 125 mg twice weekly.

Some patients with severe polymorphic light eruption and photosensitive dermatomyositis may also benefit from antimalarials. These agents are also effective for treating rheumatoid arthritis and systemic lupus erythematosus, which indicates that they do more than just block UV radiation. They have also been tried in granulomatous diseases, such as sarcoidosis, where they are quite helpful, and granuloma annulare, where we have not been impressed. Some pseudolymphomas also respond, even when lupus erythematosus has been completely ruled out.

Antibiotics

Antibiotics are products of microorganisms that can inhibit the growth of other microorganisms. Technically, synthetic antimicrobial agents such as sulfonamides are not antibiotics but we will not try to maintain this distinction. Entire textbooks are available on antibiotics; here, we will only review some general principles of antibiotic therapy, list the major classes of agents and briefly review their side effects. In Chapter 4, we offered general therapeutic guidelines in most cases. Detailed recommendations are impractical because of changing availability, costs and resistance profiles.

There are many factors to be considered when prescribing antibiotics.

- Mechanism of action: In most cases, antibiotics interfere with DNA and protein synthesis. Antibiotics can be bactericidal, as is penicillin, which interferes with bacterial cell wall synthesis. By contrast, the tetracyclines are bacteriostatic. Some drugs are bactericidal for one species and bacteriostatic for another.
- Indications: Suspected or diagnosed bacterial infections are the most obvious indication. However, in dermatology there are other possibilities.
  - Secondarily infected dermatitis, especially atopic dermatitis.
  - Diseases in which bacteria play a role but do not cause a primary infection, such as acne.
  - Diseases in which antibiotics are highly effective even though no organisms have been identified, such as rosacea and perioral dermatitis.
  - Peculiar uses, such as for immunosuppression: Some individuals recommend erythromycin for bullous pemphigoid, sometimes combined with nicotinamide.
- Initial therapy: The clinical picture usually allows one to institute appropriate therapy, perhaps bolstered by a Gram stain. One must be knowledgeable about local patterns of resistance, especially differences between community- and hospital-acquired infections. A culture should be taken and if positive, antibiotic susceptibility testing be performed. Storing an acute phase serum is always wise in a puzzling suspected infection.
- Status of patient: Some patients are clearly critically ill and require immediate empirical therapy. In dermatology, the best example is destructive soft tissue infections; occasional patients with meningitis and purpura may also be diagnosed by dermatologists. Patients who are neutropenic, asplenic or immunosuppressed require quick therapy. In our patient population, the major members of this group are HIV/AIDS patients and those with autoimmune dermatoses receiving immunosuppressive drugs. Bactericidal therapy is always preferable in such individuals. One must be aware of pregnancy, as well as underlying renal or hepatic disease. Often the dose of an antibiotic must be adjusted for a patient in renal or hepatic failure, depending on where the drug is metabolized.
- Route of administration: Seriously ill patients require intravenous antibiotics. In the USA this often takes them out of the hands of dermatologists when they are hospitalized.
- Drug interactions: Antibiotics have a wide range of drug interactions – just consider the innocent combination of systemic erythromycin for acne and a nonsedating antihistamine for allergic rhinitis. There is a risk of cardiac conduction abnormalities and sudden death. Each time a new antibiotic is used, one should check a reliable source for possible cross-reactions.
- Combination therapy: The main reason for using several antibiotics at once is to provide empirical coverage when a definite diagnosis is not available. Sometimes multiple organisms are present, as after a ruptured bowel. In the case of chronic treatment regimens, as for tuberculosis and leprosy, the complex combinations are designed to reduce the likelihood of resistance.
- Resistance: Bacterial resistance to antibiotics has become a major problem in recent years. One must use the antibiotic that has the narrowest possible spectrum to avoid selecting out primary resistant strains in the patient or the community. Acquired or secondary resistance is far more serious. In an organism that divides as often as bacteria do, mutations are common. When growth occurs in the presence of antibiotics, mutants may be selected out that have evolved a mechanism for avoiding the antibiotic's effect – either by altered cell wall properties, induction of a new enzyme or similar tricks. Worsening the problem is the extrachromosomal transfer of resistance by plasmids, which often simultaneously produce resistance against an entire series of agents. Methicillin-resistant *Staphylococcus aureus* (MRSA) has become a worldwide public health problem.

How can the dermatologist help? The most important factor is simply being aware of the problem. Long-term oral antibiotic treatment of acne was formerly considered harmless; today it is known that patients and even family members are more likely to harbor resistant bacteria. Acne treatment violates two rules of good antibiotic prescribing; the treatment is not only long-term, but it is also usually underdosed.

- Side effects: Probably no group of agents has a broader spectrum of side effects than antibiotics. Since antibiotics are often related, cross-reactions may occur. A patient with a documented penicillin allergy should not receive another penicillin and may even react with a cephalosporin. Many patients with alleged antibiotic allergies really are not allergic. In children antibiotics are often prescribed in the early stages of a viral infection and then the viral exanthem is misinterpreted as a drug reaction. Patients who experience a rash while taking ampicillin often do not react on rechallenge. Nonetheless, hypersensitivity reactions and toxic epidermal necrolysis both may result from antibiotics, so caution is warranted.
  Some side effects are dose-related and not allergic. For example, the otic and renal toxicity of the aminoglycosides is almost to be expected at higher dosages and with prolonged use. Some cephalosporins interfere with the synthesis of vitamin K-dependent clotting factors, producing a bleeding disorder. Antibiotics may disrupt the normal flora of the bowel, causing diarrhea or even pseudomembranous enterocolitis when growth by *Clostridium difficile* is promoted. Vaginal candidiasis often follows antibiotic treatment. Vancomycin may cause the red man syndrome by triggered marked histamine release. Other drugs cause phototoxic or even photoallergic reactions, even though they are harmless until the patient is exposed to UV radiation (Chap. 13). Finally, the Jarisch-Herxheimer reaction occurs when antibiotics are too effective, rapidly killing organisms that release large amounts of toxins. While this was first described with syphilis, it can be seen in other settings.

β-Lactams

This family of antibiotics interferes with bacterial cell wall synthesis. It includes penicillins, cephalosporins, monobactams and carbapenems.

Penicillins

Penicillins are among the least toxic of all drugs. One can administer massive dosages with little sign of damage. Penicillin is also completely safe in pregnancy. Nonetheless, penicillin allergy is very common, and it is estimated that about 5% of the population is allergic. While a number of immunologic mechanisms may be involved, the acute hypersensitivity reaction leading to anaphylaxis and serum sickness is the most important. The different penicillins have varying degrees of resistance to β-lactamase, acid resistance (allowing oral use) and spectrums of action. Many organisms make β-lactamases; that made by *S. aureus* is known as penicillinase.

Penicillin G (Benzyl Penicillin). This form is not active when taken orally. It is available in an aqueous form for intravenous and intramuscular use, as well as in two long-acting forms. Aqueous penicillin G has many indications but its main use in dermatology is to treat erysipelas. Benzathine penicillin releases low levels of penicillin for several weeks and is used in treating syphilis and streptococcal pharyngitis as well as for rheumatic fever prophylaxis. Procaine penicillin is another depot form that must be avoided in patents with procaine allergies. In Germany, clemizol-penicillin is available; the carrier molecule is an antihistamine, perhaps explaining this drug's effectiveness in rare cases of cold urticaria.

Penicillin V. The simplest oral form of penicillin, it is usually used for group A streptococci and other organisms that do not produce β-lactamase. Thus it is recommended for streptococcal pharyngitis, scarlet fever and rheumatic fever prophylaxis.

Penicillinase-Resistant Penicillins. Several well-known drugs are in this group. Dicloxacillin and cloxacillin are available for oral use, while oxacillin and nafcillin are parenteral forms. The prototype of the group, methicillin, is more nephrotoxic than the other members of the group and used less often. These agents are more toxic than ordinary penicillin, with renal, hepatic and bone marrow effects, and are less effective against organisms that do not produce penicillinase.

Amino Penicillins. Ampicillin and amoxicillin have extended gram-negative coverage. The latter is better absorbed orally and should be chosen. They are of interest to dermatologists primarily for the drug reactions they cause. Most of the exanthems the amino penicillins produce are not allergic. In addition, patients with infectious mononucleosis almost always get an ampicillin rash.

Broad-Spectrum Penicillins. A number of penicillins have been modified to have better gram-negative action. They include ticarcillin, temocillin, piperacillin and related agents. None plays a role in dermatologic therapy.

Cephalosporins

The cephalosporins also cause some hypersensitivity reactions and may cross-react with penicillins. The risk of a person with penicillin allergy reacting to one of these agents is about 5%. The cephalosporins are more resistant against β-lactamases, although some gram-negative bacteria produce enzymes that do attack the molecules. There are first-, second- and third-generation cephalosporins; in each group oral and parenteral agents are available. Marked variation in susceptibility, even within a generation of cephalosporins, has been observed, and many new agents become available each year, so a current antibiotic handbook should be checked before prescribing any of the newer agents. These play some role in dermatologic care.

First-Generation Cephalosporins. These agents are effective against gram-positive and -negative strains, and are not sensitive to β-lactamase. They are useful for mixed skin and soft tissue infections, even when penicillinase-producing *S. aureus* is expected. Cephalexin can be used in a b.i.d. regimen, such as 500–1000 mg b.i.d., for non-life-threatening pyodermas.

Second-Generation Cephalosporins. These drugs have a better gram-negative spectrum than the older agents. In the skin, they offer few advantages.

Third-Generation Cephalosporins. These agents often have less gram-positive coverage, but better gram-negative action and can be used for the treatment of meningitis. The main oral form, cefixime, is not effective against *S. aureus*. Cefixime 400 mg orally and ceftriazone 125 mg intramuscularly are effective against *Neisseria gonorrhoeae*. Ceftriaxone is used intravenously for 2–3 weeks to treat advanced Lyme borreliosis.

Other β-Lactam Agents

The monobactam aztreonam has primary gram-negative action, while the carbapenem agent imipenem is given with cilastin, which blocks its degradation. This combination has a very wide spectrum but should be saved for sepsis and severe mixed infections. Clavulinic acid blocks β-lactamases of many species; it can be combined with amoxicillin to produce an agent often recommended for human bite wounds, as well as many other infections.

Macrolides

The basic structure of this family is a lactone ring with a variety of sugars attached. These drugs tend to be bacteriostatic, inhibiting ribosomal protein synthesis. The macrolides produce good tissue levels and most can be given orally. They have a wide range of drug interactions because of their extensive hepatic metabolism. They may elevate levels of cyclosporine, coumarin, theophylline and many other agents, as well as interfere with the nonsedating antihistamines.

Erythromycin. The usefulness of erythromycin has changed in recent years. The likelihood of community based *S. aureus* to be resistant is high in many areas. Depending on the pattern of resistance, erythromycin should be considered for pyodermas in penicillin-allergic patients. It is also effective against *Legionella pneumophila* (Legionnaire disease), mycoplasma and chlamydia. Some time-release forms are less likely to cause gastrointestinal distress. Erythromycin base should be chosen over the estolate, as the latter has a higher incidence of cholestasis. While oral erythromycin is widely used in treating acne, rosacea and perioral dermatitis, topical formulations (Chap. 28) are favored as they cause fewer problems with resistant *S. aureus* and *Propionibacterium acnes*.

Clarithromycin and Azithromycin. These two, more stable variations on erythromycin can be taken orally usually for 5 days; clarithromycin (250–500 mg q. 12 h) and azithromycin (250–500 mg daily). They have roughly the same spectrum as erythromycin, are more expensive but produce fewer gastrointestinal side effects. Clarithromycin and azithromycin are useful when a patient is allergic to penicillin, as well as for situations in which erythromycin is often not effective because of resistance, such as staphylococcal infections or mixed secondary infections in atopic dermatitis and dyshidrotic dermatitis. Both drugs are occasionally used for acne in short courses. Clarithromycin is also effective against mycobacteria. It is not recommended in pregnancy. Azithromycin is useful in treating chlamydia infections. It can increase the activity of ergot alkaloids, causing ergotism.

Spiramycin. A weak sister of this family, it has action against *Toxoplasma gondii* and can be used for ocular toxoplasmosis, as so often seen in HIV/AIDS patients.

Lincosamides

The lincosamides have a spectrum similar to the macrolides. The two main agents are clindamycin and lincomycin. Systemic clindamycin was formerly used in treating acne, where it was effective. The risk of pseudomembranous colitis has dimmed the enthusiasm of dermatologists for these agents, although clindamycin is still useful against penicillinase-positive *S. aureus*. Topical clindamycin is still widely used for acne.

Glycopeptides

The main member of this group is vancomycin. It is poorly absorbed orally, but produces high enough intraluminal levels to be effective against *Clostridium difficile*-induced pseudomembranous colitis. The red man syndrome is the most dramatic side effect of intravenous vancomycin; it appears to be caused by histamine release and can be avoided by slow intravenous infusion over 90–120 min. Vancomycin and the closely related teicoplanin are used intravenously against MSRA; they are the last resort for this difficult problem. Rare cases of MSRA resistant to vancomycin have been identified.

Tetracyclines

There are a number of tetracyclines available, differing primarily with regard to degree of oral absorption and incidence of photosensitivity. The tetracyclines are napthene ring structures that are bacteriostatic, as they inhibit the formation of peptides on the ribosomes. The main agents are shown in Table 70.3.

The main indication for the tetracyclines in dermatology is still acne. Because they have a very wide spectrum, they are also the agent of choice for treating rickettsial, chlamydial and mycoplasma infections. In addition, they are effective against many gram-positive bacterial infections such as brucellosis, tularemia and even plague. The tetracyclines are a possible second line agent for skin and soft tissue infections, syphilis, gonorrhea and many others. Doxycycline is probably the best oral agent for *Borrelia burgdorferi*. It is also used for the prophylaxis and treatment of travelers' diarrhea; in this setting, its otherwise low photosensitizing capacity is often brought to fore.

Tetracyclines cause a fair amount of gastrointestinal distress. They should not be taken just before retiring because of the risk of esophagitis. Even though it is tempting to take them with milk or antacids, the tetracyclines are chelating agents and bind well to calcium or iron salts, thereby losing their effectiveness. Of the tetracyclines, doxycycline is least affected by concomitant food intake. Since these drugs are deposited in growing bone and teeth, they should not be used during pregnancy or in children whose visible permanent teeth have not formed; usually 12 years of age is safe. Because of their stimulation of hepatic metabolism, tetracyclines have a very slight effect on the serum levels of oral contraceptives; whether this is of clinical importance or not remains unclear. We consider them appropriate and safe in patients taking oral contraceptives.

Table 70.3. Tetracyclines

Agent	Absorption with food	Excretion	Gastrointestinal tolerance	Photosensitivity
Tetracycline[a]	Poor	Kidney	Fair	Low
Minocycline	Good	Kidney	Good	Very Low
Doxycycline	Good	Liver	Good	Occasional

[a] Tetracycline HCl or oxytetracycline

Aminoglycosides

The aminoglycosides are bactericidal agents that are usually used in combination regimens for life-threatening sepsis. For this reason, gentamicin cream should not be used topically, as an allergic reaction will deprive the patient of a possible life-saving drug later. In addition, resistant strains may appear. There are a number of agents including gentamicin, tobramycin, netilmicin, kanamycin and amikacin. The oldest aminoglycoside is streptomycin, which is still used for treating plague, tularemia, brucellosis and tuberculosis. The main side effects are renal and otic toxicity. Spectinomycin is given once 2–4 g intramuscular for gonorrhea.

Quinolones

The quinolones inhibit the DNA gyrase enzyme (topoisomerase II); in German they are known as gyrase blockers. Among the older quinolones, nalidixic acid is the best example. Today the fluoroquinolones are most widely employed. They cover a broad range of gram-positive and gram-negative organisms including some *S. aureus* strains. There are a number of agents available, but ciprofloxacin is most widely used in dermatology. It is recommended for *Neisseria gonorrhoeae* infections in a single oral dosage of 250 mg. In addition, it is an effective agent against cellulitis and other severe skin and soft tissue infections.

Folic Acid Inhibitors

Sulfonamides. This is the oldest group of antimicrobial agents. Not true antibiotics, they were synthesized in the 1930s by Domagk, who later received the Nobel Prize for this work. Because of the incidence of allergic reactions, frequently severe, the sulfonamides are used less often. They are still occasionally prescribed for uncomplicated urinary tract infections. Sulfadiazine is recommended for nocardiosis and toxoplasmosis. Sulfapyridine is a weak antibacterial agent that is used in treating dermatitis herpetiformis; it is not available in Germany and is almost an orphan drug in the USA. Sulfasalazine is used to treat inflammatory bowel disease; it breaks down to sulfapyridine and aminosalicylic acid.

Trimethoprim-Sulfamethoxazole. Trimethoprim has a minimal antibacterial action alone, but is usually combined with sulfamethoxazole. The combination drug is widely used for urinary tract infections, typhus and shigellosis. In dermatology, trimethoprim-sulfamethoxazole may be employed for wound infections, nonsevere gram-negative infections and for prophylaxis and treatment of *Pneumocystis carinii* pneumonia in HIV/AIDS. The risk of severe drug reactions, including toxic epidermal necrolysis, is considerable; almost all HIV/AIDS patients at some point develop a rash from this agent. Bone marrow suppression can be seen and the medication should not be used in pregnancy or in combination with methotrexate.

Dapsone. This sulfone is the mainstay of treatment for leprosy. In addition, dermatologists often employ dapsone for a variety of other indications, especially dermatitis herpetiformis (Chap. 15). Other indications include cicatricial pemphigus, subcorneal pustulosis, pyoderma gangrenosum and even severe acne. The mechanism of action of dapsone in these noninfectious conditions is totally unclear; some investigators consider it immunosuppressive and others feel it inhibits neutrophilic inflammation. Dapsone regularly causes methemoglobinemia and may cause hemolysis in patients deficient in G6PD, which should be screened for prior to therapy.

Miscellaneous Antibiotics

Metronidazole. This nitroimidazole is effective against a variety of anaerobic bacteria and protozoa infections. It is the treatment of choice for *Trichomonas vaginalis.* While metronidazole is effective in both systemic and topical forms for rosacea, it is only approved for topical use. It has a disulfuram-like effect and should not be used in pregnancy.

Rifampicin. This antimycobacterial agent can also be used for chronic or recurrent *S. aureus* infections in a variety of regimens where it is given for several weeks along with a more effective agent. It provides high tissue levels. Patients must be warned about red tears, sweat and urine, while physicians should be aware of the induction of cytochrome P450 enzymes, resulting in the increased metabolism and subtherapeutic concentrations of many other drugs.

Clofazimine. Another antimycobacterial drug, clofazimine has been tried for a variety of skin disorders. It has been reported effective in pyoderma gangrenosum, Melkersson-Rosenthal syndrome, Sweet syndrome and pustular psoriasis, but we rarely employ it.

Rheological Agents

Pentoxifylline

This dimethylxanthine derivative is thought to improve blood flow by reducing blood viscosity and increasing the flexibility of erythrocytes. The enhanced blood flow improves tissue oxygenation even in compromised tissues. In the USA it is only approved for intermittent claudication but it has been used for a wide spectrum of problems, ranging from cerebrovascular insufficiency to diabetic angiopathy. In the skin, it has been tried for leg ulcers, Raynaud phenomenon, granuloma annulare, necrobiosis lipoidica diabeticorum and many other diseases in which peripheral microcirculation is impaired. It has also been recommended for aphthous ulcers. While pentoxifylline is very safe in the usual dosage of 400 mg t.i.d., it has not been dramatically effective in our hands. We use it primarily in patients with systemic sclerosis and Raynaud phenomenon.

Prostaglandins

Several different prostaglandins are available in Europe and the USA in injectable forms for treating various vascular disorders.

- Prostacylin (epoprostenol or prostaglandin I_2) is the most potent available inhibitor of platelet aggregation and a powerful vasodilator. It is approved in the USA for long-term treatment of primary pulmonary hypertension. In Europe it is used for intraarterial injection in patients with severe peripheral arterial disease and impending occlusion.
- Prostaglandin E1 is also used for treating severe peripheral arterial disease in Europe. In addition it is approved for maintaining a patent ductus arteriosus and for injection into the corpora cavernosa in erectile dysfunction.

Photosensitizing Agents

The psoralens play a major role in dermatology. They are usually combined with UV radiation as PUVA. They are discussed both under psoriasis (Chap. 14) and phototherapy (Chap. 71).

Psychotherapeutic Agents

There are many interactions between skin and psyche, so psychotherapeutic agents may play a significant role in dermatologic therapy. Unfortunately there are a number of barriers to their usage by dermatologists. Most of us simply are not trained in psychiatric diagnosis and the monitoring of psychiatric patients on long-term medications. For example, patients with neurotic excoriations may have primarily depression or anxiety. One must have the right working diagnosis in order to choose an effective medication. On the other hand, many patients resent going to a psychiatrist and it is tempting to try and help them through a dermatology practice. Catastrophic side effects or problems with physical addiction are minimal, but in many instances dependency can occur. Our advice is to limit oneself to a few medications which one can learn well and use them initially under the guidance of a more experienced physician. In this vein we only discuss drugs which we have had a chance to use. Numerous new antipsychotic and antidepressants are available; many undoubtedly offer advantages for psychodermatologic care. Finally dermatologists should avoid treating patients in whom there is even a hint of suicidal or violent tendencies.

Antipsychotic Agents

Pimocide

The antipsychotic agent is a good choice for monosymptomatic psychoses, such as delusions of parasitosis, dysmorphophobia and abnormal body odor. Any one who has dealt with such patients realizes that while it is tempting to try and convince them of the errors of their ways, it is futile. Pimocide is often quite effective; as such patients inevitably decline psychiatric help, it is up to the dermatologist to initiate treatment. We frequently explain the medication as "something that has helped people with problems like yours." One can start at 1 mg daily and then increase the daily dose by 1 mg every 1–2 weeks. Most patients respond at 2–4 mg daily. The main side effects are extra-pyramidal symptoms, prolonged QT interval and anticholinergic effects, such as urinary retention, constipation and exacerbation of narrow-angle glaucoma. If a dosage of more than 4 mg daily is required, or if the extra-pyramidal symptoms such as tardive dyskinesia or restlessness require a second drug, we strongly recommend involving a psychiatrist.

Antidepressants

Depressed patients may present with self-induced skin disease such as neurotic excoriations, delusions of parasitosis, trichotillomania and similar findings. Pharmacological treatment is usually the best approach for these individuals. Severe dermatological disorders such as psoriasis or atopic dermatitis may lead to depression, simply because of their tremendous impact on a patient's life, interfering with outdoor activities, acceptance by public and relationship with loved one. Such patients usually respond best to aggressive dermatological management but may also require antidepressants.

Doxepin

Doxepin, a tricyclic antidepressant, is probably the most useful agent for dermatologists. In lower dosages it is used to treat chronic urticaria as it is a good blocker of H1 and H2 receptors at relatively modest levels. In this setting, we start a 25 mg in the evening and increase to 50 mg and then 75 mg, each time after one week. We rarely exceed 75 mg, which is about 50 % of the usual psychiatric dose. In patients with idiopathic pruritus, doxepin is also helpful, although higher levels are required. It seems that a more central analgesic effect is involved. Topical doxepin is also available in the USA as an anti-pruritic but is has proved itself to be a potent sensitizer.

When treating depression, the usual dose is between 100 – 300 mg in the evening. The dosage should only be increased every 5 – 7 days because of the long time required for serum doxepin levels to stabilize. Doxepin has the same spectrum of side effects as the other classic tricyclic antidressants including sedation, cardiac conduction problems (prolonged QT interval) and the potential for fatal overdosage or suicide. A less sedating but otherwise similar tricyclic antidepressant is desipramine, which can be used in dosages of 25 – 100 mg in the evening, increasing the dose in the same way as for doxepin.

Clomipramine

This tricyclic antidepressant is specifically approved in the USA for obsessive-compulsive disorders. Several of these fall into the realm of dermatology, such as trichotillomania, onychotillomania and obsessive hand washing. Such patients realize the absurdity of their action and are distressed by it, but still are only able to find relief by such activity. The usual starting dose is 25 mg daily of clomipramine. The daily dosage can be increased by 25 mg on a weekly basis. A non-psychiatrist should probably stop at 100 – 150 mg although psychiatrists go to higher levels. The dose should initially be divided, but once the patient is titrated, a single evening dose is fine. The main side effects are anti-cholinergic, so that one should once again worry about constipation, urinary retention, narrow angle glaucoma and orthostatic hypotension. Most patients get mucosal dryness. Other problems can include reversible liver damage, weight gain, and rarely either excitation or over-sedation.

Newer Antidepressants

Two newer non-tricyclic agents are also approved for obsessive-compulsive disorders. Fluoxetine is a selective serotonin uptake inhibitor which is used in depression at dosages of 20 – 40 mg daily; often slightly higher doses are needed for obsessive-compulsive patients. Side effects are minimal including diarrhea and agitation. The possibility has been raised that fluoxetine made increase suicidal tendencies. Fluvoxamine is another selective serotonin uptake inhibitor used in dosages up 100 – 300 mg daily given in two divided dosages. Its main side effect is nausea.

Antianxiety Agents

There are many situations where an antianxiety agent or minor tranquilizer may help a dermatologic patient. Psychophysiologic disorders refers to those diseases which frequently flare with situational stress or anxiety. Dermatologic members of this group include atopic dermatitis, chronic urticaria, acne (especially in adults), dyshidrotic dermatitis and psoriasis. In addition, if the skin disease is severe, it contributes to the stress. One can use the terms psychosomatic for stress affecting the skin and somatopsychic for skin disease affecting the psyche.

If one wishes to treat such anxious patients with a psychotherapeutic agent, alprazolam is often a good choice in dosages of 0.25 – 0.75 mg b. i. d. – t. i. d. The main side effect is sedation, which can be titrated. The unique thing about alprazolam is that it is an anti-anxiety drug that does not have a depressant effect in most patients. If the drug is used for 2–3 weeks for acute situational anxiety, the risk of dependency is almost nil. When terminating therapy, the patient must be gradually weaned off, not abruptly discontinued.

If a patient seems to require longer term antianxiety measures, then buspirone is worth considering. It is a non-sedating, non-dependency producing medication which can be used in dosages of 5–10 mg t.i.d. One disadvantage is its slow onset of action, which may be as long as 2–4 weeks, coupled with the fact that it cannot be taken on an as needed basis when anxiety flares. Low dose doxepin 10 mg b.i.d. is another possibility for the long term amelioration of anxiety.

Miscellaneous Medications

There are a group of drugs that do not nicely fit into the above categories but are often used in dermatologic care, usually for nonapproved indications.

Cytokines

A number of cytokines are available for special dermatologic indications. The list will undoubtedly change radically, before this book appears in print. Some of the products available in the USA and Europe in 2000 with selected indications include:

- Interferon-α2a and α2b: Hairy cell leukemia, Kaposi sarcoma, condyloma acuminata, laryngeal papillomatosis, chronic active hepatitis, hepatitis C, metastatic malignant melanoma, other metastatic tumors, mycosis fungoides, non-Hodgkin's lymphoma, multiple myeloma.
- Interferon-α3: Condyloma acuminata (usually intralesional).
- Interferon-β, β1a, β1b: Multiple sclerosis, Kaposi sarcoma, malignant melanoma, metastatic renal cell carcinoma, mycosis fungoides.
- Interferon-γ1b: Infections associated with chronic granulomatous disease.
- Interleukin-2: Metastatic malignant melanoma (Chap. 58).
- Growth factors: Granulocyte/macrophage colony-stimulating factor (GM-CSF), G-CSF – both used to stimulate bone marrow after aggressive chemotherapy. Erythropoietin is widely used in myelodysplastic disorders, the anemia associated with chronic renal disease and HIV/AIDS.

Of interest is the availability of a human fibroblast interferon-β gel in Germany for treatment of condylomata acuminata. The clinical effectiveness is not dramatic, while the price is.

Thalidomide

Even in Germany, with about 3000 victims of the thalidomide disaster, this drug is beginning to reawaken interest. It is the most effective agent for erythema nodosum leprosum and can be obtained for this purpose from appropriate public health agencies. In addition, it is the best drug for treating the severe aphthous ulcers seen in HIV/AIDS patients, and has been employed for the same problem in patients with Behçet disease and ordinary but severe aphthae. Puzzlingly, it is not very effective for Asian patients with Behçet disease. We have also seen dramatic responses in Langerhans cell histiocytosis, lupus erythematosus and chronic actinic dermatitis. The most obvious side effect is somnolence, as thalidomide was introduced as a sleeping pill. The usual limiting factor is the development of a non-reversible peripheral neuropathy, while clearly it cannot be used in women who are at risk of getting pregnant.

Colchicine

Colchicine is technically a cytostatic agent, as it interferes with microtubule formation inhibiting cell motility. Since colchicine accumulates in neutrophils, it especially inhibits their activities. It is used primarily in the treatment of gout and familial Mediterranean fever. The usual dosage is 0.5 or 0.6 mg b.i.d. or t.i.d. Gastrointestinal side effects are usually what determines the final dosage. Colchicine has been tried in Behçet disease, leukocytoclastic angiitis, pustular psoriasis, palmoplantar pustulosis, Sweet syndrome and many other problems. It cannot be used during pregnancy, and hematologic and hepatic parameters should be monitored. Colchicine is associated with severe cutaneous reactions, including toxic epidermal necrolysis, and often produces alopecia. In our experience it is most useful in Behçet syndrome and leukocytoclastic angiitis.

Gold Salts

Gold salts enjoyed a period of popularity as steroid-sparing agents in pemphigus vulgaris and other bullous diseases. Their safety profile sets them apart even from other drugs used for these serious problems. Hematologic toxicity, stomatitis, alopecia, severe skin reactions, pulmonary fibrosis and renal damage are all seen. Gold sodium thiomalate and auriothioglucose must be given intramuscularly; oral gold or auranofin is less toxic but also appears less effective. We do not employ the gold salts.

Bibliography

Introduction

Barranco V (1998) Clinically significant drug interactions in dermatology. J Am Acad Dermatol 38:599–612

Reed BR (1997) Dermatologic drugs, pregnancy, and lactation. Arch Dermatol 133:894–898

Singer MI, Shapiro LE, Shear NH (1997) Cytochrome P-450 3A: Interactions with dermatologic therapies. J Am Acad Dermatol 37:765–771

Corticosteroids

Fritz KA (1984) Systemic glucocorticosteroid therapy of skin disease in children. Pediatr Dermatol 1:236–245

Hirschmann JV (1986) Some principles of systemic glucocorticoid therapy. Clin Exp Dermatol 11:27–33

Werth VP (1993) Management and treatment with systemic glucocorticoids. Adv Dermatol 8:81–101

Other Hormonal Agents

Beylot C, Doutre MS, Beylot Barry M (1998) Oral contraceptives and cyproterone acetate in female acne treatment. Dermatology 196:148–152

Fruzzetti F, Bersi C, Parrini D et al. (1999) Treatment of hirsutism: comparisons between different antiandrogens with central and peripheral effects. Fertil Steril 71: 445–451

Glovsky MM (1998) C1 esterase inhibitor transfusions in patients with hereditary angioedema. Ann Allergy Asthma Immunol 80:439–440

Kaufman KD, Olsen EA, Whiting D et al. (1998) Finasteride in the treatment of men with androgenetic alopecia. Finasteride male pattern hair loss study group. J Am Acad Dermatol 39:578–589

Shaw JC (1996) Antiandrogen and hormonal treatment of acne. Dermatol Clin 14:803–811

Cytostatic and Immunosuppressive Agents

Dutz JP, Ho VC (1998) Immunosuppressive agents in dermatology. An update. Dermatol Clin 16:235–251

Lim KK, Su WP, Schroeter AL et al. (1996) Cyclosporine in the treatment of dermatologic disease: an update. Mayo Clin Proc 71:1182–1191

Lipsky JJ (1996) Mycophenolate mofetil. Lancet 348:1357–1359

Nousari HC, Sragovich A, Kimyadi-Asadi A et al. (1999) Mycophenolate mofetil in autoimmune and inflammatory skin disorders. J Am Acad Dermatol 40:265–268

Ruzicka T, Assmann T, Homey B (1999) Tacrolimus: the drug for the turn of the millenium? Arch Dermatol 135:574–580

Tan BB, Lear JT, Gawkrodger DJ et al. (1997) Azathioprine in dermatology: a survey of current practice in the U.K. Br J Dermatol 136:351–355

Younger IR, Harris DW, Colver GB (1991) Azathioprine in dermatology. J Am Acad Dermatol 25:281–286

Antihistamines

Seto A, Einarson T, Koren G (1997) Pregnancy outcome following first trimester exposure to antihistamines: meta analysis. Am J Perinatol 14:119–124

Gonzalez MA, Estes KS (1998) Pharmacokinetic overview of oral second-generation H1 antihistamines. Int J Clin Pharmacol Ther 36:292–300

Slater JW, Zechnich AD, Haxby DG (1999) Second-generation antihistamines: a comparative review. Drugs 57:31–47

Davies RJ, Bagnall AC, McCabe RN et al. (1996) Antihistamines: topical vs oral administration. Clin Exp Allergy 26:11–17

DuBuske LM (1999) Second-generation antihistamines: the risk of ventricular arrhythmias. Clin Ther 21:281–295

Ring J, Brockow K, Ollert M et al. (1999) Antihistmines in urticaria. Clin Exp Allergy 29:31–37

Retinoids

Bergfeld WF, Kligman AM, Wiegand UW et al. (1997) The evolving role of retinoids in the management of cutaneous conditions. J Am Acad Dermatol 39 [Suppl]:1–122

Cunliffe WJ, van de Kerkhof PCM, Caputo R et al. (1997) Roaccutane treatment guidelines: result of an international survey. Dermatology 194:351–357

Orfanos CE, Zouboulis CC, Almond-Roesler B et al. (1997) Current use and future potential role of retinoids in dermatology. Drugs 53:358–388

Ortonne JP (1997) Oral isotretinoin treatment policy. Do we all agree? Dermatology 195 [Suppl 1]:34–37

Saurat JH (1998) Systemic retinoids. What's new? Dermatol Clin 16:331–340

Nonsteroidal Antiinflammatory Drugs

Fivenson DP (1997) Nonsteroidal treatment of autoimmune skin diseases. Dermatol Clin 15:695–705

Antimalarials

Jones SK (1999) Ocular toxicity and hydroxychloroquine: guidelines for screening. Br J Dermatol 140:3–7

Parke AL, Rothfield NF (1996) Antimalarial drugs in pregnancy – the North American experience. Lupus 5S:67–69

Rynes RI (1998) Ophthalmologic considerations in using antimalarials in the United States. Lupus 5S:73–74

Tsakonas E, Joseph L, Esdaile JM et al. (1998) A long-term study of hydroxychloroquine withdrawal on exacerbations in systemic lupus erythematosus. The Canadian Hydroxychloroquine Study Group. Lupus 7:80–85

Antibiotics

Arbiser JL, Moschella SL (1995) Clofazimine: a review of its medical uses and mechanisms of action. J Am Acad Dermatol 32:241–247

Blondeau JM (1999) Expanded activity and utility of the new fluoroquinolones: a review. Clin Ther 21:3–40
Cleach LL, Bocquet H, Roujeau JC (1998) Reactions and interactions of some commonly used systemic drugs in dermatology. Dermatol Clin 16:421–429
Epstein ME, Amodio-Groton M, Sadick NS (1997) Antimicrobial agents for the dermatologist. I. Beta-lactam antibiotics and related compounds. J Am Acad Dermatol 37:149–165
Epstein ME, Amodio-Groton M, Sadick NS (1997) Antimicrobial agents for the dermatologist. II. Macrolides, fluoroquinolones, rifamycins, tetracyclines, trimethoprim-sulfamethoxazole, and clindamycin. J Am Acad Dermatol 37:365–381
Thestrup-Pedersen K (1998) Bacteria and the skin: clinical practice and therapy update. Br J Dermatol 53 [Suppl]:1–3
Veien NK (1998) The clinician's choice of antibiotics in the treatment of bacterial skin infection. Br J Dermatol 53 [Suppl]:30–36

Rheological Agents

Anaya JM, Espinoza LR (1995) Phosphodiesterase inhibitor pentoxifylline: an antiinflammatory/immunomodulatory drug potentially useful in some rheumatic disease. J Rheumatol 2:595–599
Bruynzeel I, Stoof TJ, Willemze R (1998) Pentoxifylline and skin inflammation. Clin Exp Dermatol 23:168–172
Ely H (1988) Pentoxifylline therapy in dermatology. A review of localized hyperviscosity and its effects on the skin. Dermatol Clin 6:585–608
McNamara DB, Champion HC, Kadowitz PJ (1998) Pharmacologic management of peripheral vascular disease. Surg Clin Nord Am 78:447–464
Pizarro A, Herranz P, Navarro A et al. (1996) Recurrent aphthous stomatitis: treatment with pentoxifylline. Acta Derm Venereol (Stockh) 76:79–80
Wu K (1997) Prostacyclin and nitric oxide-related gene transfer in preventing arterial thrombosis and restenosis. Agents Actions 48 [Suppl]:107–123
Yoshikawa Y, Mizutani H, Shimizu M (1996) Systemic lupus erythematosus with ischemic peripheral neuropathy and lupus anticoagulant: response to intravenous prostaglandin E1. Cutis 58:393–396

Psychtherapeutic Agents

Gupta MA, Gupta AK (1996) Psychodermatology: an update. J Am Acad Dermatol 34:1030–1046
Koo J (1995) Psychodermatology: a practice manual for clinicians. Curr Probl Dermatol 7:199–234
Sandor P, Baker B, Irvine J et al. (1998) Effectiveness of fluoxetine and doxepin in treatment of melancholia in depressed patients. Depress Anxiety 7:69–72
Strange PG (1999) Mechanisms of action of anti-psychotic drugs. Biochem Soc Trans 27:175–178

Cytokines

Asadullah K, Sterry W, Stephanek K et al. (1998) IL-10 is a key cytokine in psoriasis. Proof of principle by IL-10 therapy: a new therapeutic approach. J Clin Invest 101:783–794
Beutner KR, Spruance SL, Hougham AJ et al. (1998) Treatment of genital warts with an immune-response modifier (imiquimod). J Am Acad Dermatol 38:230–239
Gross G, Rogozinsky T, Schofer H et al. (1998) Recombinant interferon beta gel as an adjuvant in the treatment of recurrent genital warts: results of a placebo-controlled double-blind study in 120 patients. Dermatology 196: 330–334
Punt CJ (1998) The use of interferon-alpha in the treatment of cutaneous melanoma: a review. Melanoma Res 8: 95–104
Stadler R (1998) Interferons in dermatology. Present-day standard. Dermatol Clin 16:377–398

Thalidomide

Jacobson JM, Greenspan JS, Spritzler J et al. (1997) Thalidomide for the treatment of oral aphthous ulcers in patients with human immunodeficiency virus infection. National Institute of Allergy and Infectious Diseases AIDS Clinical Trials Group. N Engl J Med 336:1487–1493
Lee JB, Koblenzer PS (1998) Disfiguring cutaneous manifestation of sarcoidosis treated with thalidomide: a case report. J Am Acad Dermatol 39:835–838
Mangelsdorf HC, White WL, Jorizzo JL (1996) Behcet's disease. Report of twenty-five patients from the United States with prominent mucocutaneous involvement. J Am Acad Dermatol 34:745–750
Nightingale SL (1998) From the Food and Drug Administration. JAMA 280:872
Rouseau L, Beylot-Barry M, Doutre MS et al. (1998) Cutaneous sarcoidosis successfully treated with low doses of thalidomide. Arch Dermatol 134:1045–1046
Stirling DI (1998) Thalidomide and its impact in dermatology. Semin Cutan Med Surg 17:231–242
Wolkenstein P, Latarjet J, Roujeau JC et al. (1998) Randomised comparison of thalidomide versus placebo in toxic epidermal necrolysis. Lancet 352:1586–1589

Colchicine

Sullivan TP, King LE Jr, Boyd AS (1998) Colchicine in dermatology. J Am Acad Dermatol 39:993–999

Physical Methods of Therapy

Contents

There are many physical modalities of therapy that play a major role in dermatology. Some are discussed in Chap. 72 because they are best grouped together with operative dermatology. Included in this group are cryotherapy, electrosurgery and dermabrasion.

Cold Therapy

In addition to cryotherapy, cold packs may be used for pain relief. As best we can determine, the choice of when to use warm packs and when to use cold packs remains one of the most difficult, if least important, questions confronting modern medicine. If the practices of athletes are any indication, cold should be used initially and heat later on.

In dermatologic care, cold is often used for angioedema and postoperative swelling. Ice packs have been applied to the scalp during cancer chemotherapy to reduce the severity of posttreatment anagen effluvium from direct toxicity. The only problem is that the cooled scalp may provide a hiding place for tumor cells, so this technique is best used for solid tumors with no hint of metastasis.

Therapeutic cold may also be a source of injury. For example, an ice pack to the scrotum can damage the skin as well as the testes. Excessive cold during dermabrasion, usually achieved with evaporative sprays, can exaggerate the skin damage and prolong healing.

Heat Therapy

Warmth application, whether via a hot water bottle, heating pad or warm compresses, is useful for pain relief and for treating a deep infection. The theory is that heat increases blood flow and may speed healing. Patients speak of using warm compresses to bring a lesion "to a head", which may be just as accurate scientifically.

Diathermy is popular for pain relief and has also found applications in dermatology, treating postherpetic neuralgia and other pain syndromes. It has also been tried for pernio, as well as used as adjunctive therapy in treating deep infections (furuncles, carbuncles, acne inversa) and panniculitis.

Heat can also be used experimentally for tumor treatment. It has been employed for treating squamous cell carcinoma of the nose in cattle, a serious and expensive problem in pale breeds and is conceivably adaptable to cutaneous tumors. More likely, however, is its use for treating carcinoma of the prostate and other relatively accessible internal malignancies.

Light Therapy

The principles of photobiology and the diagnostic approach to clinical disorders triggered by sunlight are considered in Chapter 13 and not repeated here, where we will only concern ourselves with light as a therapeutic modality. As a reminder, therapeutic UV radiation includes UVB (280–320 nm) and UVA (320–400 nm). Many diseases respond well to UV radiation; the treatment of psoriasis without phototherapy is hard to imagine. In many instances, combined therapy with psoralens and UVA

Table 71.1. Measurements used in phototherapy

Parameter	Unit	Abbreviation
Frequency	Hertz	Hz
Time	Second	s
	Millisecond (10^{-3} s)	ms
	Nanosecond (10^{-9} s)	ns
Length	Meter	m
	Millimeter (10^{-3} m)	mm
	Micrometer (10^{-6} m)	µm
	Nanometer (10^{-9} m)	nm
	Ångstrom (10^{-10} m)	Å
Energy	Watt	W
Energy/unit time	Joule = W/s = watt-second	J or Ws
	Millijoule = milliwatt-second	mJ or mWs
	or Erg = 10^{-7} J	erg
	or electron volt = 1.6×10^{-19} J	ev
Dose (energy/time/unit area)	Joule/square meter	J/m^2 or Ws/m^2
	Millijoule/square centimeter	mJ/cm^2 or mWs/cm^2
Total dose (energy/unit area)	Watt/square meter	W/m^2
	or Joule/second-square meter	J/s × m^2
	Milliwatt/ square centimeter	mW/cm^2

radiation has proven more effective than radiation alone. The units used in phototherapy are shown in Table 71.1.

Sources of Light

Natural Light

Sunlight can be used for therapeutic purposes. It is more intense at higher altitudes, such as in the mountains, has higher reflectance on the beaches and from snow, and has a higher UVA content at depressions such as the Dead Sea. All of these factors can be used to influence sunlight therapy. In Europe, many patients go to the Dead Sea for their psoriasis, where the salt water baths appear to combine well with the slightly altered sunlight. Other patients go to the seashore or high in the mountains for light therapy.

Artificial Light Sources

The main artificial light sources in routine clinical use are shown in Table 71.2

Fluorescent Tubes. The tubes contain a variety of gases, often mercury, and are coated on the inside. The combination of the type of gas and the nature of the coating determines the emission spectrum. Both UVA and UVB fluorescent tubes are available.

High Pressure Mercury Lamps with Metal Halide Addition. The addition of various metal salts, such as iron salts, can enrich selected parts of the spectrum, such as UVA. Many modern UVA lamps are of this type.

UVB Phototherapy

UVB irradiation can be administered either as total body or localized therapy. There are several types of UVB radiation in clinical use:

- Traditional or broad band UVB lamps deliver radiation over 280–320 nm. We use them mainly for treating psoriasis, atopic dermatitis and pruritus.
- Selective UVB phototherapy (SUP) has peaks at 305 and 325 nm. While it has not proven as effective in treating psoriasis as originally hoped, SUP appears superior to ordinary UVB for the treatment of atopic dermatitis.
- Narrow band UVB lamps (Philips TL01) delivers almost exclusively 311 nm radiation. This source is clearly superior to traditional UVB in treating psoriasis and is comparable to PUVA therapy; it is also effective in treating atopic dermatitis.

Table 71.2. Recommended light sources for phototherapy

Source	Wavelengths (nm)	Main indications	Comments
UVB	280–320 nm	Psoriasis, atopic dermatitis, pruritus	Combine with salt water bath ≤5% for atopic dermatitis, 10–30% for psoriasis
SUP	Several peaks in 300–325 nm range	Atopic dermatitis, pruritus, psoriasis	Combine with salt water bath ≤5% for atopic dermatitis, 10–30% for psoriasis
311	311 nm	Psoriasis, atopic dermatitis, small-patch parapsoriasis, vitiligo, lichenoid graft versus host reaction	Combine with salt water bath ≤5% for atopic dermatitis, 10–30% for psoriasis
UVB-UVA	280–400 nm (two sets of bulbs)	Atopic dermatitis	Not clearly better than UVB or UVA
UVA	320–400 nm	Psoriasis, lichen planus, atopic dermatitis, palmo-plantar dermatitis, small-patch parapsoriasis, mycosis fungoides, graft versus host reaction, granuloma annulare	Only used in combination with photosensitizers Types: PUVA, PUVA bath, PUVA cream Hand and foot box useful
UVA 1	340–400 nm	Morphea, systemic sclerosis, atopic dermatitis, granuloma annulare	Hand and foot irradiation useful for systemic sclerosis; three dose ranges: Low: 20–30 J/cm^2 Medium: 40–60 J/cm^2 High: 90–120 J/cm^2

We also employ this source with success in small-patch parapsoriasis, vitiligo and lichenoid graft versus host reaction.

- The simultaneous administration of UVB and UVA radiation has been recommended for treating both atopic dermatitis and psoriasis; in our hands, this therapy is not better than either source alone. Because of the presence of UVA, one must pay particular attention to the use of photosensitizing medications.
- Saline baths are popular in Europe as part of a phototherapy regimen; they can be combined with UVB. Both industrial NaCl and various combinations designed to match Dead Sea water are used. Patients soak for 20 min and then are irradiated. We use 5% or weaker solutions for atopic dermatitis and 10–30% solutions for psoriasis. Oil can be added to the baths. Both SUP and 311 nm narrow band irradiation can also be combined with saline baths.
  The salt water must be disposed of carefully or recycled, as corrosion of plumbing and even phototherapy devices is a problem. By using a large plastic sheet in the tub, one can reduce the amount of saline solution needed. The tub is partially filled with water, then the large sheet placed over the tub, the patient lies on top of the sheet and the salt water is added.

We prefer cabinets over beds, which we only use for handicapped or elderly patients who cannot tolerate the required standing. Beds are available both as a bank of lights above a bed or, as is often seen in tanning parlors, with light sources on the top and bottom of the almost clam-like unit. All modern light sources have built-in dosimeters which must be calibrated regularly with a separate dosimeter. Patients are treated three to five times weekly. The eyes and male genitalia should be protected, and the face shielded if it is not involved. After the minimal erythema dose (MED) in minutes is determined, we start with about 80% of this dose and increase each time by 15–30%. A very modest erythema is required for maximum efficacy; if obvious redness develops, the dose is not increased. If treatments are missed, one must revert to the previous lower dose. Usually light therapy is continued until the lesions are entirely healed; the frequency of treatments can be reduced. Maintenance therapy is frequently beneficial, but raises risk: benefit questions. If patients are very light-sensitive, an effective dose level cannot be obtained because of burning, while if they are very dark-skinned, prolonged exposures may be required to have any effect. Except for the purpose of hardening, patients with photosensitive disorders are not treated with phototherapy.

UVA Phototherapy

In most instances UVA is combined with psoralens, as discussed below under photochemotherapy. Special UVA1 (340–400 nm) lamps were first shown effective in treating acute atopic dermatitis. We have found them more useful for treating morphea and systemic sclerosis, especially as hand and foot units. While this approach was initially labeled high-dose UVA1, because dosages of up to 120 J/cm^2 were employed, lower levels such as 20–30 J/cm^2 also are effective. In addition, UVA1 appears to help in generalized granuloma annulare. When UVA therapy is administered, one must pay attention to the use of any systemic photosensitizing medication.

Photochemotherapy

The essence of photochemotherapy is the ingestion or application of a photosensitizing chemical from the psoralen (P) family plus exposure to UVA radiation. Thus, the combination is also known as PUVA from P + UVA. The main indications for PUVA are psoriasis, mycosis fungoides, atopic dermatitis, vitiligo and to harden patients with polymorphic light eruption and other photosensitive disorders. Other indications and contraindications are shown in Tables 71.3 and 71.4. Different types of photochemotherapy are summarized in Table 71.5

- Psoralens. Usually 8-methoxypsoralen is used for treating psoriasis and cutaneous lymphomas; it can also be employed for vitiligo. It is available in 10 mg capsules, known as Oxsoralen in the USA, as well as in a 1% lotion, which should be used in a physician's office with great care and never given to the patient for home use. Trimethylpsoralen is more often used for vitiligo and in hardening. It comes in 5 mg pills known as Trisoralen in the USA. In Europe 5-methoxypsoralen is also available. It and trimethylpsoralen have a greater margin of safety but are not as effective as 8-methoxypsoralen in most instances. All the psoralens can cause nausea and vomiting as their main acute side effect.
- UVA Radiation. The usual fluorescent and metal halide UVA sources produce a broad spectrum of irradiation (320–400 nm) although there may be differences in the individual peaks. UVA1 sources are used without psoralens. The same careful frequent dosimetry is required for the UVA units.

Table 71.3. Uncommon indications for photochemotherapy

Actinic prurigo
Actinic reticuloid
Alopecia areata
Chronic actinic dermatitis
Erythropoetic protoporphyria
Graft versus host reaction
Granuloma annulare
Hydroa vacciniformia
Lichen planus
Solar urticaria
Lymphomatoid papulosis
Morphea
Parapsoriasis
Pityriasis lichenoides chronica
Pityriasis rubra pilaris
Prurigo nodularis
Urticaria pigmentosa

Table 71.4. Contraindications for photochemotherapy

Absolute contraindications
Bloom syndrome
Cockayne syndrome
Dermatomyositis
Dysplastic nevus syndrome
Malignant melanoma
Nevoid basal cell carcinoma syndrome
Systemic lupus erythematosus
Trichothiodystrophy
Xeroderma pigmentosum
Relative contraindications
Age < 10 years
History of basal cell carcinoma or squamous cell carcinoma
Immunosuppressive therapy, pregnancy or nursing
Treatment with X-rays, arsenic or cyclosporine
Use of photosensitizing medication

The minimal phototoxic dose (MPD) must be determined. The patient is given a weight-adjusted dose of 30–50 mg of 8-methoxypsoralen and a series of areas are exposed, just as with the UVB determination of MED. The main difference is that PUVA erythema is delayed and can first be read after 72 h. This same delayed erythema plays a

Table 71.5. Types of photochemotherapy

Type	Medication	Application	Irradiation
PUVA	8-Methoxypsoralen	Oral	UVA
	5-Methoxypsoralen	Oral	UVA
	Trimethylpsoralen	Oral	UVA
Local PUVA	8-Methoxypsoralen	Topical	UVA
(bath, hand-foot)	Trimethylpsoralen	Topical	UVA
Khellin	Khellin	Systemic	UVA

clinical role because a phototoxic reaction may not become apparent until 24–72 h after treatment.

Systemic Photochemotherapy. The usual dose of psoralens is 0.6–0.8 mg/kg of 8-methoxypsoralen or 1.2–1.4 mg/kg of 5-methoxypsoralen given 2 h prior to exposure. The newer capsules allow exposure 1 h after ingestion. It is crucial to maintain the same dosage of medicine and the same time interval; otherwise too many variables are introduced. Treatment is started with 50–80% of the MPD. Most patients are treated three to four times weekly (either Mo-We-Fr or Mo-Tu-Th-Fr). The dosage is first increased after 72 h; usually with jumps of 15–30%. If there is marked erythema, either the level of radiation is left unchanged or a treatment is skipped. Once the patient is clear, we usually treat twice weekly for 4 weeks and then once a week for 4 weeks. In addition, since the psoralens remain in the system, the patient must practice sunlight protection or avoidance for 8 h following treatment and during this time wear special sunglasses that block UVA, in order to reduce the risk of cataracts. PUVA can be combined with oral retinoids to increase its effectiveness, as discussed under psoriasis in Chapter 14.

A variation on systemic photochemotherapy in treating vitiligo is the use of khellin, a photosensitizer with almost no phototoxic properties and no carcinogenic risk. The patient takes 100 mg and is irradiated after 2 h just as with standard PUVA therapy. Another approach for treating vitiligo is psoralens plus sunlight, known as PUVASOL. This is not a recommended approach, but in the USA some patients simply live too far from a UVA unit. One can then prescribe modest doses of trimethylpsoralen 2 h before exposure to noonday sun. One can start with 10 mg and increase by 5 mg increments weekly with a maximum dosage of 0.6–1.0 mg/kg. Both of these methods are occasionally successful.

Topical Photochemotherapy. While it may be tempting to prescribe 8-methoxypsoralen lotion for home use, our advice is not to do this. The phototoxicity is considerable, sunlight is hard to monitor, home PUVA units have an unclear medical-legal position and the problems outweigh the benefits. Since one needs a prescription to buy many light units for home use, one can view this as a lifetime prescription with no physician control – a difficult situation. We have seen severe burns with the standard 1% solution and even with diluted forms.

In the office or clinic, one should use a 0.1–0.15% solution of 8-methoxypsoralen, applied directly to localized lesions, such as palmoplantar dermatoses or solitary plaques of mycosis fungoides, and followed in 30 min by 0.25 J/cm^2 UVA. Another possibility is the use of topical psoralens in a cream base; we have no personal experience with this new approach and prefer PUVA bath therapy to other forms of topical PUVA therapy.

PUVA Bath Therapy. This approach to photochemotherapy has greatly expanded the indications and reduced the side effects. Patients bathe for 20 min in 150 l of water at 37°C containing 0.5–1.0 mg/l of 8-methoxypsoralen or trimethylpsoralen. The UVA radiation is given immediately after the bath, as the desired phototoxic effect vanishes rapidly. One must start carefully, usually with 30–50% of the MPD. Once again, we use a three to four times weekly schedule with careful increases after 72 h periods. The advantages of the PUVA bath therapy include no systemic effects from psoralens, no need for sunglasses and a much lower total UVA dose. PUVA bath therapy is effective not only for treating all types of psoriasis, but also in the treatment of morphea, systemic sclerosis, granuloma annulare, atopic dermatitis, lichen planus, graft versus host reaction, small-patch parapsoriasis and mycosis fungoides.

Hand-Foot PUVA Therapy. Special units are available for irradiating just the palms, soles and nails. This is a very effective way to approach treatment of pustular psoriasis and other acral pustular disorders, as well as severe dyshidrotic or hyperkeratotic palmoplantar dermatitis. While one can use oral psoralens, topical psoralens or bath therapy with these special units, we strongly favor bath therapy because of the much lower side effect profile and comparable, if not greater, efficacy.

Psoriasis Phototherapy

Psoriasis patients still comprise the bulk of patients in most phototherapy units.

While ordinary UVB therapy is effective, narrow band 311 nm and PUVA are better. If the psoriatic lesions are treated with an ointment prior to irradiation, such as petrolatum, the UVB is more effective. Many different types of UVB combination therapy are employed.

- UVB + tar: The Goeckerman regimen is not clearly superior to UVB monotherapy and has lost acceptance in recent years.
- UVB + anthralin: The Ingram method uses UVB light (either broad band or narrow band) followed by topical anthralin. With either source, the healing is more rapid and the cumulative UVB dose less than with monotherapy. Most often the method is restricted to inpatients because it is so messy and time-consuming.
- UVB + topical corticosteroids: There is little benefit, other than an initial more rapid reduction in erythema.
- UVB + topical vitamin D derivatives: Both sources can be effectively combined with vitamin D analogues, which should be applied after irradiation as they have a UV filtering effect. This approach is not as effective as the Ingram method, but easier for outpatients.
- UVB + salt solutions: We use 10–30 % concentrations for psoriasis patients.
- UVB + systemic therapy: UVB light can be combined with retinoids, methotrexate or cyclosporine. Psoralens have been combined with 311 nm UVB.

Both systemic PUVA and PUVA bath therapy are very effective treatments for psoriasis. We increasingly tend to use PUVA bath therapy.

Phototherapy of Other Skin Diseases

The various skin diseases that can be treated with light are listed in the tables and in the discussion of the individual sources.

- Atopic Dermatitis. Most patients with atopic dermatitis are relatively UV-responsive. UVA1 is most effective; all types of UVB have been employed, as well as combination UVB-UVA and PUVA. The main problem with treating atopic dermatitis is that many of the patients are small children, so that parental reluctance and unclear safety guidelines offer discouragement.
- Pruritus. UVB is the best treatment for pruritus associated with renal failure. Some long-term dialysis units also irradiate their patients. UVB can also be tried for other types of pruritus such as seen in cholestasis, polycythemia vera and even chronic urticaria.

Photohardening

Hardening can be used in cases of polymorphic light eruption, solar urticaria, chronic actinic dermatitis and photo-aggravated atopic dermatitis. One can use very low dosages of either UVB or a combination of UVA (1 J/cm^2) and UVB (2–4 mJ/cm^2). Irradiation is given three to five times weekly, slowly increasing the dose. In the case of polymorphic light eruption, this is an effective and safe way to treat individuals if they come in 6–8 weeks prior to their expected intense light exposure. In the other disorders, it is much harder to use, and may even require initial coverage with systemic corticosteroids, as in the case of severe chronic actinic dermatitis.

Lasers

History. Einstein, in 1917, described the principle of stimulated emission which laid the basis for lasers. Schawlow and Towns, in the 1950s, made further basic science advances, while Maiman, in 1960, was the first to use a functioning laser. Goldman, in Cincinnati, was the main moving force in introducing dermatologists to lasers.

Basic Science Aspects. Laser is an acronym for *l*ight *a*mplification by *s*timulated *e*mission of *r*adiation. Stimulated emission leads to an increase in strength of radiation. Each photon of light has the potential to stimulate emission of another photon of the same energy. Mirrors are used to bounce the photons back and forth through the medium, amplifying the light while a small fraction is transmitted through a gap in one of the mirrors. The active medium of the laser is the substance into which the photons are introduced. It can be a solid (ruby crystal, neodymium: YAG crystal, alexandrite crystal), a liquid (such as rhodamine dye), a gas (argon, krypton, CO_2) or a semi-conductor (diode). There is also an electrical, chemical or optical pump that serves as the energy source for the system.

Laser light is monochromatic, meaning it has a very uniform wave length. For example, the width of emission from a helium-neon laser is only 0.002 nm. In addition, it is collimated, meaning that the photons run in parallel, and coherent. Finally, the light can be bundled, using lenses to produce very high energy levels. For example, a 50 W CO_2 laser can vaporize granite.

Lasers emit light either continuously or in pulses. Continuous wave (CW) lasers are used for coagulation, cutting and vaporization of tissue. In contrast, pulsed lasers allow selective photothermolysis. If the correct wave length and a very short pulse time are chosen, the heat injury can be confined to a very small site, such as a vessel, pigmented cell or clump of exogenous pigment. The thermal relaxation time of a target, such as a vessel, is the time this structure needs to release the heat acquired from irradiation to its surroundings. If the pulse time is less than this, then little heat will be accumulated and transferred, but instead the damage will be confined to the target, selectively destroying it. If a laser has a very high pulse rate and relatively little energy per pulse, it may be pulsed but behaves like a CW laser; this is known as a pseudo-CW or quasi-CW laser. The best example is the copper vapor laser. Q-switching refers to blocking light from the laser cavity and then suddenly releasing it, yielding short, high-intensity pulses.

The intensity (I) of the radiation delivered to the skin reflects the energy of the beam (P) and the surface area exposed (A), using the formula $I = P/A = W/\text{cm}^2$. The dose (D) is the product of $I \times t$, expressed in W-s/cm^2 or J/cm^2.

Clinical Applications. The major lasers used in dermatology are listed in Table 71.6 and discussed here briefly.

Argon Laser. Due to its good absorption by hemoglobin and melanin, the argon laser is well-suited for the coagulation destruction of superficial vascular and pigmented structures. The depth of coagulation is limited to about 1.0 mm. The light is led through a flexible light cable into a hand piece that has a lens, allowing variation in the width of the ray from 0.5–4.0 mm. The maximum energy is about 10 W. The removal of small facial telangiectases, venous lakes on the lips and ears and cherry angiomas is unproblematic. Tiny nodules arising in a nevus flammeus can also be simply destroyed. Among the nonvascular lesions, soft epidermal nevi, xanthelasmas and syringomas are easily treated.

Flashlamp-Pumped Dye Laser (FPDL). This laser produces a yellow light at a wave length of 585 nm. It is good for treating pale nevi flammei, especially in infants and children. The specific wave length and the short exposition time (0.45 ms) allow selective vascular destruction with little risk of scarring. In addition, the wider beam width (5–10 mm) makes therapy more rapid and efficient, and the procedure is not very painful. Thus FPDL has

Table 71.6. Lasers used in dermatology

Laser	Wave length(s) nm	Function	Main absorption by
Argon	488, 514	CW	Hgb, Mel
CO_2	10,600	CW, pulsed	H_2O
Nd:YAG	1064	CW, Q-switch	H_2O (Hgb, Mel)
	532	Q-switch	H_2O (Hgb, Mel)
Dye	577	CW	Hgb, Mel
	577, 585, 590, 595, 600	Pulsed	Hgb, Mel
Copper vapor	510, 578	Pseudo-CW	(Hgb, Mel)
Ruby	694	Q-switch	Mel, exogenous pigments
Er:YAG	2940	Pulsed	H_2O
Krypton	521, 530, 568	CW	Hgb
Alexandrite	755	Q-switch	Melanocytes

CW, continuous wave; Q-switch, quality-switched; Hgb, hemoglobin; Mel, melanin

become the treatment of choice for these vascular malformations. When lesions are darkened or have developed nodules, then the argon laser remains a good choice.

The FPDL also offers advantages in treating hemangiomas of infancy. Hemangiomas are proliferations of endothelial cells, experiencing a growth phase and later a regression phase in most cases. Using one or more treatments with FPDL, it is possible to completely remove about 20–50% of hemangiomas and reduce the size of over 75%. The main factor determining success of the laser therapy is the thickness of the lesion. Because this approach is relatively safe and almost free of side effects, one can reasonably suggest treating all disturbing or rapidly-growing hemangiomas in infancy. The deep vascular component, consisting of mature thick vessels is not influenced by the light and may proliferate further.

Finally, FPDL with a longer impulse time (1.5 ms), variable wave length (590–600 nm) and elliptical treatment area can be used to treat star-burst veins. In small lesions with a vessel diameter less than 1.0 mm, satisfactory results are obtainable.

Copper Vapor and Krypton Lasers. Both of these are used for superficial vascular changes. The copper vapor laser can reach energy levels of 5 W with relatively good absorption by hemoglobin, so that it can achieve similar results to argon or dye lasers for small lesions. Even though pulsed, it has a pseudo-CW nature and does not allow selective photothermolysis.

Q-Switched Ruby Laser. Maiman's first laser was a ruby laser, but only with Q-switching techniques did ruby become of interest again. With its 694 nm wave length and a pulse time in nanoseconds (ns), it vaporizes black or dark blue tattoo pigment. Other colors respond far less satisfactorily. In fact, with brown or skin-colored tattoos, an irreversible color change towards black may be caused. Traumatic tattoos can also be treated with this device if the foreign material has the right color.

Lesions with increased melanin also respond well. Lentigines, café-au-lait macules and both nevus of Ota and Ito all do fairly well. Since the latter are almost impossible to treat with other methods, the Q-switched ruby laser represents a real breakthrough. Ordinary melanocytic nevi should not be treated with lasers except as part of clinical studies with excellent follow-up. Non-pigmented cells and deeper cells are not destroyed, so that recurrences are expected and histologic control is lost.

Alexandrite Laser. This laser has been used to remove green, blue and purple tattoos when set at 755 nm with a pulse duration of 50–100 ns. It can also be used for epilation.

Q-Switched Neodymium:YAG Laser. YAG stands for yttrium-aluminum-garnet. When used in the Q-switched mode, the neodymium:YAG laser emits infrared radiation at 1064 nm, which is absorbed primarily by water. It has been used for treating pigmented skin lesions and black tattoos. By adding a potassium dihydrogenphosphate crystal, the frequency can be doubled producing 532 nm radiation, which can be used for epidermal melanin and red tattoo pigments.

CW-Neodymium:YAG Laser. The 1064 nm CW infrared radiation penetrates fairly deeply and can cause coagulation at a depth of 5–6 mm. It is often directed through an ice cube so that the skin surface is cooled to reduce scarring. The beam is coupled with a visible red pilot beam and the beam's thickness is varied by moving the hand piece towards or away from the skin. This is the most useful laser for treating deep vascular malformations or hemangiomas with a significant deep component.

The neodymium:YAG laser can be fitted with sapphire tips so that it can be used as a contact scalpel for cutting, vaporizing or coagulating. Quartz fibers (known as bare fibers) can be introduced through the skin into large hemangiomas or vascular malformations, allowing intralesional coagulation with direct or ultrasound visualization. The bare fibers can be sterilized and reused.

CO_2 Lasers. These devices emit very long infrared waves with a wave length of 10,600 nm. They are absorbed by water, producing relatively high energy levels that can be employed for coagulation, cutting or vaporization. Good indications for blood-free destruction with the CO_2 laser are condylomata acuminata, complicated verrucae (subungual for example), thicker epidermal nevi and actinic cheilitis.

Special scanner hand pieces or the use of a pulsed CO_2 laser allow superficial removal of the skin, in the fashion of a dermabrasion, with little thermal necrosis. Such lasers are used for treating scars, actinically damaged skin and, in recent years, for skin resurfacing or the destruction of superficial wrinkles. When wide areas are superficially abraded, problems such as milia, persistent erythema and bacterial and herpetic superinfections may occur, so precise counseling and close follow-up are essential.

Erbium:YAG Laser. The 2940 nm infrared rays also allow a superficial dermabrasion-like removal of skin, so this device has the same indications as the pulsed CO_2 laser.

Photodynamic Therapy

History. The first photodynamic therapy (PDT) was carried out in Munich, in 1903, by von Tappeiner and Jesionek. They painted facial tumors with a variety of photosensitizing dyes, usually eosin, and then exposed the patients to sunlight or artificial light sources with reportedly good results. The Renaissance of PDT occurred in the 1960s, when Lipson and colleagues at the Mayo Clinic used hematoporphyrin derivatives synthesized by Schwartz (of Watson-Schwartz fame) to identify tumors. The material was infused intravenously and then the patient irradiated. Dougherty, in the 1970s, successfully treated first animal and then human tumors with PDT. Today PDT is approved for the treatment of bladder, esophageal and lung cancers in the USA, but is still regarded as an experimental approach to skin tumors.

Basic Science Aspects. A number of factors are required for PDT. They include:

- A photosensitizing substance
- A light source that conforms to the absorption spectrum of the photosensitizing agent
- A tumor or other disorder that because of angiogenesis or rapid proliferation selectively takes up the photosensitizer
- An adequate supply of oxygen, as free radical formation is crucial

Light Source. The depth of penetration of radiation in the skin increases with increasing wave length up to about 1100 nm. The standard photosensitizing agent Photofrin absorbs maximally at 630 nm, so either an argon ion pumped dye laser (630 nm) or a gold vapor laser (628 nm) are used. With these sources, the maximum depth of penetration is 4 mm. The main advantage of laser sources is that fiber optics can be used for the endoscopic treatment of lesions within body cavities. In dermatologic applications, an incoherent light source can be used; the lamp generally used in Germany (Waldmann PDT 1200) irradiates over a spectrum of 580–740 nm, is much less expensive than a laser, covers a wider area, can be used with multiple photosensitizers and is effective.

Photosensitizers. Almost all photosensitizing agents are based on porphyrins. The only approved photosensitizer is Photofrin, an oligomeric mixture of modified hematoporphyrin molecules. It is given intravenously and causes generalized photosensitization for up to 8 weeks. Obviously it does not lend itself well to dermatologic applications. The photosensitizers being tested in dermatology have maximum absorption between 630 nm and 700 nm, allowing a penetration of just over 4 mm. Some are used intravenously, but many are being tested for topical application, some in liposome suspensions to enhance penetration. Another variable is the use of precursor molecules such as 5-aminolevulinic acid (ALA), which must be converted enzymatically to the sensitizing compound protoporphyrin IX in the target tissue.

Tumor Uptake. An ideal photosensitizer should be taken up selectively in more vascularized, more rapidly growing tumors or other lesions. Of the sensitizers under current investigation ALA shows the most selectivity, whether applied topically or administered systemically. Upon excitation with UV radiation, e.g., Wood light, the photosensitizers also fluoresce, emitting light at a longer wave length (usually red). This can be useful for the endoscopic identification of early neoplastic sites in the bladder or lung and may help to delineate tumor margins in clinically ill-defined cutaneous malignancies.

Photooxidative Reactions. The polycyclic porphyrin compounds absorb light and pass its energy along to molecular oxygen or other substrates. As a consequence, singlet oxygen and free radicals such as superoxide are formed. These highly reactive forms interact with adjacent molecules, such as cell membrane lipids or amino acid residues. Lipophilic photosensitizers tend to attack membranes while hydrophilic agents are taken up by pinocytosis and accumulate in lysosomes. Two major types of damage are produced. The primary cellular damage occurs early in the process, as the photooxidative reactions directly damage the tumor cells. Far more important are the secondary vascular effects, as endothelial cell damage leads to thrombosis, necrosis and occlusion of the tumor's vascular network.

Clinical Applications. Most studies have concentrated on using PDT in treating cancers and precancerous lesions. The most data are available for systemic PDT, usually using Photofrin. Not surprisingly, more superficial lesions, such as Bowen disease, superficial basal cell carcinoma and actinic keratoses respond best, although other tumors, such as basal cell carcinoma, squamous cell carcinoma, keratoacanthoma, Kaposi sarcoma, mycosis fungoides and even cutaneous metastases, have been treated. The lesions of psoriasis also accumulate porphyrins because of their vascularity, so this pathway has been explored. Finally, human papilloma virus-associated lesions, especially the multiple, sometimes premalignant lesions of epidermodysplasia verruciformis, can be treated.

While the large porphyrin molecules do not penetrate the epidermis, ALA is a much smaller molecule and can be applied topically. Within the skin, ALA is taken up more by epithelial than by mesenchymal structures. It is cleared rapidly, so generalized photosensitivity is minimal. Superficial malignancies, such as superficial basal cell carcinoma, Bowen disease and actinic keratosis, can be treated very effectively with ALA. Most lesions can be treated in a single session. While satisfactory cure rates have been reported for superficial basal cell carcinomas, as soon as the tumors become deeper, the cure rate drops. Pigmented basal cell carcinomas cannot be treated, as the melanin absorbs the light and blocks the photodynamic effect. Topical PDT with ALA can also be used for treating psoriasis; multiple sittings, up to five, are usually required.

The exact role of PDT in dermatology is difficult to assess at this time. Systemic PDT is rarely indicated because of the long-term photosensitivity that is induced; it may play a role in patients with large tumors who are not good surgical candidates. In contrast, topical PDT with ALA can be considered for superficial lesions; it is effective and compares to other methods. Furthermore, there is little pain other than a sunburn-like sensation, and the cosmetic results are quite good. We have avoided giving times, concentrations of photosensitizers and light dosages because all these parameters need to be better established. This exciting field is still in its experimental stages and the most useful indications for PDT are yet to be determined or agreed upon.

Ionizing Radiation

Treatment of a wide range of benign and malignant cutaneous diseases with ionizing radiation was for many years a major part of dermatologic practice. In both Germany and the USA, almost every dermatologic practice had one or more X-ray machines and every resident was taught the principles of radiation therapy. Today this situation has changed in the USA and is changing in Germany. Very few residents in the USA learn radiation therapy. The costs of the machines, their maintenance and the price of malpractice insurance have made radiation therapy a dying art. In addition, public opinion is strongly against administering X-rays for benign disorders and many are totally opposed to this modality, even when it is the best treatment available. Similar trends are starting to appear in Germany; the manufacturer of the most popular X-ray machine, the Siemens Dermopan, has discontinued production of the device.

Basic Science Aspects. X-rays are part of the electromagnetic spectrum, along with visible light, ultraviolet radiation, infrared radiation, gamma rays and radio waves. Electromagnetic waves are characterized by the following parameters:

$$c = \nu\lambda$$

where c is the velocity; in a vacuum it is the speed of light 300,000 km/s, ν is the frequency or number of waves passing a given point per second and λ is the wave length. Thus wave length and frequency are inversely related; as one increases, the other decreases.

The next crucial formula is:

$$E = \mathrm{h}\nu$$

where E is energy in ergs, h is Planck's constant, and ν is the wave frequency. Thus as the frequency increases, the energy of the wave increases. Visible light has a wave length of 400–760 nm and a photon energy of 1.6–3.0 eV. In contrast, X-rays have wave lengths of 1–0.01 Å and photon energies of 10–1000 keV.

Röntgen. The amount of X-radiation that is produced in 0.001293 g of dry air (1 cm^3 at 0 °C and 760 mm Hg) is a charge of 1 electrostatic unit of either sign. Thus a Röntgen is a measure of the radiation exposure.

Rad (radiation absorbed dose). An absorbed dose of 100 ergs/g. For skin at usual X-ray energy levels, a Röntgen and a rad are almost equal.

Gray (Gy). This term for the energy dose of a X-ray is roughly equal to 100 rads, although it is defined in a more complex way. In addition to the dosage in Gy, the quality of the X-rays is of great therapeutic importance.

Tube Kilovoltage. The higher the kilovoltage, the shorter the wave length and the higher the energy of the X-rays. The tube kilovoltage is used to define the "hardness" of the X-rays:

- Ultrasoft radiation, including Grenz rays (< 20 kV)
- Soft radiation (20 – 60 kV)
- Superficial radiation (60 – 150 kV)

Filters. The standard filter in dermatologic radiation therapy is aluminum. Filters can be used to alter the quality of the X-rays. In simplest terms, if a filter removes low-energy radiation, then the radiation that has passed through the filter consists of higher energy photons on average and the dose is correspondingly less.

Half-Value Thickness. The half-value thickness is the thickness of an aluminum filter (or other material) that reduces the intensity of the X-ray beam to 50 % of its given value.

Factors Affecting Radiation Quantity

$$I = \frac{\text{mA} \times \text{kV}^2 \times \text{time}}{\text{TSD}^2}$$

where I = intensity, mA = milliamperes, and kV = kilovoltage.

While this formula is not exactly correct and all devices today calculate the dose with complicated computer programs, it allows one to visualize how shifting several parameters can produce an X-ray with the ideal qualities for the given lesion.

- Target Skin Distance (TSD). If the distance between the radiation source and the target is doubled, then the intensity is reduced by a factor of four. A cone is usually used to precisely fix the target skin distance and increase protection. If the lesion is small, the TSD should be at least 15 cm. If the lesion is larger, the TSD should be double the size of the field. With this relationship, the periphery gets about 90 % of the central dose. If the skin surface is irregular, one selects a longer distance to reduce the variation in intensity between peaks and valleys.
- Milliamperes. This number is fixed by machine and not varied.
- Kilovoltage. As the voltage doubles, the dose increases by a factor of four.
- Time. If the exposure doubles, the dosage doubles.

Tissue Half-Value Depth ($D_{1/2}$). This crucial parameter is the depth in tissue at which 50 % of the surface dose is delivered. It should be equal to the depth of the lesion. One can alter it by increasing kilovoltage, adding filtration to deliver harder X-rays, altering the field size and increasing the TSD.

Biologic Effects of X-Rays. Whenever X-rays interact with tissues, they transfer energy by means of atomic excitation and ionization. Once the energy is absorbed, it must be dissipated and this in turn causes the biologic effects of X-rays. Probably the most significant effect is the ability of X-rays to damage vital cellular structures such as nucleic acids and proteins. This can lead to direct killing in high dosages; of the cells in the skin, lymphocytes are the most radiation-sensitive. In addition, ionizing radiation is well-known for its mutagenic, teratogenic and carcinogenic actions. But there are also a number of clinical changes in the skin that can be seen following ionizing radiation, ranging from erythema to sebum suppression to hair loss to long-term precancerous lesions (Chap. 13). X-rays are so effective at epilation that they were used to treat tinea capitis in the days before systemic antimycotic agents; 400 rad (4 Gy) was sufficient to cause complete alopecia with regrowth, hopefully without the dermatophytes, beginning in a few weeks.

Clinical Applications

Grenz Rays. Grenz rays, first introduced in 1928 by the Berlin dermatologist Bucky, are very low energy X-rays that only penetrate the epidermis and perhaps enter the upper dermis. A special window must be used, as the ordinary X-ray tube window would absorb these rays. Grenz rays cause erythema, hyperpigmentation and, with larger doses, even atrophy. They were formerly used for treating a variety of superficial disorders, perhaps being most effective for chronic hand dermatitis and pruritus, but they play little role today.

Soft X-Rays. The introduction of beryllium window tubes made the 20–50 kV tubes practical for dermatologic therapy. Beryllium has very low inherent filtration and allows soft X-rays to pass. Advantages of soft X-rays include: use of rays with limited penetration reducing damage to normal tissue; easy adjustment of $D_{1/2}$; high dose rates, allowing shorter exposure times and greater TSD for larger areas. The Siemens Dermopan had four standard kV-filter arrangements with automatic control allowing $D_{1/2}$ to be varied 0.2–20 mm. Most soft X-ray machines can also be used for with a TSD of 2.0 m (teleradiation) for total body irradiation, i.e., as for treating mycosis fungoides.

Superficial X-Rays. Superficial X-rays have a higher kV, usually in ranges of 50–100 kV. Most machines have a $D_{1/2}$ of 7–10 mm which results in more penetration and damage to normal skin than is needed. The indications are comparable, although deep or thick lesions can be better treated with these units.

Indications. The most established uses for soft and superficial X-rays are to treat basal cell carcinoma and squamous cell carcinoma. Typical regimens today employ ten treatments with 4–5 Gy on each exposure. Some physicians fractionate the dose even more, using 15 treatments. The greater the fractionation, the less scarring in most cases. In addition, pseudolymphomas, cutaneous malignant lymphomas and Kaposi sarcoma are quite radiation-sensitive and can be treated with lower dosages than basal cell or squamous cell carcinomas. Many other tumors are also responsive to radiation therapy. Lentigo maligna, especially if large, may often be best treated with this approach. Exact regimens should be sought in specialized texts and discussed with physicians who are experts in the field.

The indications for treating benign conditions with ionizing radiation are limited, not so much by any lack of effectiveness but by public fear and malpractice pressures. For example, severe acne vulgaris can be treated with a sebostatic dose of 6 Gy with immediate improvement, allowing time for other therapies to become effective. Acne inversa can be approached in a similar fashion. Radiation therapy is the most effective, but not the best, treatment for psoriatic onychodystrophy. It works so well that patients tend to seek too much treatment, get excessive cumulative radiation from several different unwitting doctors and eventually get chronic radiation dermatitis. Irradiation of the operative site after removing a keloid is perhaps the one still-accepted indication for treating a benign disorder with X-rays.

Particle Accelerators. Two types of accelerators are used for medical purposes.

- Linear Accelerator. Here, particles, usually electrons, are accelerated in alternating electrical fields. The particles are discharged from the device in high-energy pulses or bursts, usually with an energy of 4–25 MeV, occasionally as high as 40 MeV.
- Circular Accelerator. The electrons are accelerated in a circular magnetic field, reaching almost the speed of light. The best known device is the Betatron from Siemens.

The advantages of particle accelerators are many. They produce electron beams of a defined single energy and thus a defined depth of penetration in tissue. Beyond this depth, the dosage is nil. In addition, radiation is uniform in tissue to about half of the total depth. The destruction of tissues is thus very well-defined. The main indications for electron beam therapy are for both total body and spot irradiation in cutaneous malignant lymphomas, as well as for treating tumors overlying bone or cartilage, where damage to these structures should be avoided.

Safety Measures. Every country has very strict rules regarding radiation safety. They should be followed exactly, or else a practice or clinic runs the risk of serious administrative problems and fines. The requirements cover such factors as shielding of rooms in which X-ray therapy is provided, annual maintenance and calibration of such units, use of dosimeter badges by all personnel and exact documentation of therapeutic measures. All such considerations are deserving of detailed attention.

Bibliography

General Reading

Goldschmidt H (1978) Physical modalities in dermatologic therapy. Springer, Berlin

Cold

Johansen LV (1985) Scalp hypothermia in the prevention of chemotherapy-induced alopecia. Acta Radiol 24:113–116

Soukop M, Campell A, Gray MM et al. (1978) Adriamycin, alopecia, and the scalp tourniquet. Cancer Treat Rep 62:489–490

Heat

Dover JS, Philips TJ, Arndt KA (1989) Cutaneous effects and therapeutic uses of heat with emphasis on infrared radiation. J Am Acad Dermatol 20:278–286

Venning VA, Colver GB, Millard PR et al. (1987) Tattoo removal using infra-red coagulation: a dose comparison. Br J Dermatol 117:99–105

Light

Behrens-Williams S, Gruss C, Grundmann-Kollmann M et al. (2000) Assessment of minimal phototoxic dose following 8-methoxypsoralen bath: maximal reaction on average after 5 days. Br J Dermatol 142:112–115

Bethea D, Fullmer B, Syed S et al. (1999) Psoralen photobiology and photochemotherapy: 50 years of science and medicine. J Dermatol Sci 19:78–88

British Photodermatology Group (1994) British Photodermatology Group guidelines for PUVA. Br J Dermatol 130:246–255

British Photodermatology Group (1997) An appraisal of narrowband (TL-01) UVB phototherapy. British Photodermatology Group Workshop Report (April 1996). Br J Dermatol 137:327–330

Cox NH, Jones SK, Downey DJ et al. (1987) Cutaneous and ocular side-effects of oral photochemotherapy; results of an 8-year follow-up study. Br J Dermatol 116:145–152

Deleu H, Roelandts DH (1990) Protecting the eye from ultraviolet A radiation during photochemotherapy. Photodermatol Photoimmunol Photomed 7:233–236

Diffey BL, Roelandts R (1986) Status of ultraviolet A dosimetry in methoxsalen plus ultraviolet A therapy. J Am Acad Dermatol 15:1209–1213

Fain-Bell W (1985) Cutaneous photobiology. Oxford Medical, Oxford

Halpern SM, Anstey AV, Dawe RS et al. (2000) Guidelines for topical PUVA: a report of a workshop of the British Photodermatology Group. Br J Dermatol 142:22–31

Hannuksela A, Pukkala E, Hannuksela M et al. (1996) Cancer incidence among Finnish psoriasis patients treated with trioxsalen bath PUVA. J Am Acad Dermatol 35:685–689

Hannuksela-Svahn A, Pukkala E, Koulu L et al. (1999) Cancer incidence among Finnish psoriasis patients treated with 8-methoxypsoralen bath PUVA. J Am Acad Dermatol 40:694–696

Harber LC, Bickers R (1989) Photochemotherapie: Grundlagen-Klinik-Praxis-Forschung. Springer, Vienna

Henseler T, Christophers E, Hönigsmann H et al. (1987) Skin tumors in the European PUVA Study. J Am Acad Dermatol 16:108–116

Honig B, Morison WL, Karp D (1994) Photochemotherapy beyond psoriasis. J Am Acad Dermatol 31:775–790

Kerscher M, Volkenandt M, Plewig G et al. (1993) Combination phototherapy of psoriasis with calcipotriol and narrow-band UVB. Lancet 342:923

Kerscher M, Volkenandt M, Meurer M et al. (1994) Treatment of localised scleroderma with PUVA bath photochemotherapy. Lancet 343:1233

Kerscher M, Volkenandt M, Gruss C et al. (1998) Low-dose UVA1 phototherapy for treatment of localized scleroderma. J Am Acad Dermatol 38:21–26

Krutman J, Hönigsmann H (eds) (1997) Handbuch der dermatologischen Phototherapie und Photodiagnostik. Springer, Berlin

Lindelöf B, Sigurgeirsson B, Tegner E et al. (1991) PUVA and cancer: a large-scale epidemiologic study. Lancet 338:91–93

Lindelöf B, Sigurgeirsson B, Tegner E et al. (1992) Comparison of the carcinogenic potential of trioxsalen bath PUVA and oral methoxsalen PUVA. Arch Dermatol 126: 1341–1344

Lowe NJ, Weingarten D, Moly LS (1986) PUVA therapy for psoriasis: comparison of oral and bathwater delivery of 8-methoxypsoralen. J Am Acad Dermatol 14:754–760

Lüftl M, Degitz K, Plewig G et al. (1997) Psoralen bath plus UV-A therapy. Possibilities and limitations. Arch Dermatol 133:1597–1603

Morison WL, Baughman RD, Day RM et al. (1998) Consensus workshop on the toxic effects of long-term PUVA therapy. Arch Dermatol 134:595–598

Ortel B, Tanef A, Hönigsmann H (1988) Treatment of vitiligo with khellin and ultraviolet A. J Am Acad Dermatol 18:693–701

Stege H, Berneburg M, Humke S et al. (1997) High-dose UVA1, radiation therapy for localized scleroderma. J Am Acad Dermatol 36:938–944

Stern RS (1990) Genital tumors among men with psoriasis exposed to psoralens and ultraviolet A radiation (PUVA) and ultraviolet B radiation. The Photochemotherapy Follow-up Study. N Engl J Med 322:1093–1097

Stern RS, Nichols KT, Väkevä LH (1997) Malignant melanoma in patients treated for psoriasis with methoxsalen (psoralen) and ultraviolet A radiation (PUVA). N Engl J Med 336:1041–1045

Volc-Platzer B, Hönigsmann H, Hinterberger W et al. (1990) Photochemotherapy improves chronic cutaneous graft-versus host disease. J Am Acad Dermatol 23:220–228

Whitmore SE, Morison WL (1997) Melanoma after PUVA therapy for psoriasis. N Engl J Med 337:502–503

Lasers

Anderson RR (1996) Laser medicine in dermatology. J Dermatol 23:778–782

Dover JS, Arndt KA, Dinehart SM et al. (1999) Guidelines of care for laser surgery. J Am Acad Dermatol 41:484–495

Goldman L, Blaney DJ, Kindel DJ Jr et al. (1963) Effect of the laser beam on the skin: preliminary report. J Invest Dermatol 40:121–122

Hellwig S, Petzoldt D, König K, Raulin C (1998) Aktueller Stand der Lasertherapie in der Dermatologie. Hautarzt 49:690–704

Johnson TM, Sebastien TS, Lowe L et al. (1992) Carbon dioxide laser treatment of actinic cheilitis. J Am Acad Dermatol 27:737–740

Maiman T (1960) Stimulated optical radiation in ruby. Nature 187:493–494
Schawlow AL, Townes CH (1958) Infra-red and optical masers. Phys Rev 112:1940–1941
Steiner R, Kaufmann R, Landthaler M et al. (eds) (1991) Lasers in dermatology. Springer, Berlin

Photodynamic Therapy

Allison RR, Mang TS, Wilson BD (1998) Photodynamic therapy for the treatment of nonmelanomatous cutaneous malignancies. Semin Cutan Surg 17:153–163
Bissonnette R, Lui H (1997) Current status of photodynamic therapy in dermatology. Dermatol Clin 507–519
Dougherty TJ, Grindey GB, Fiel R et al. (1975) Photoradiation therapy. II. Cure of animal tumors with hematoporphyrin and light. J Natl Cancer Inst 55:115–121
Fritsch C, Goerz G, Ruzicka T (1998) Photodynamic therapy in dermatology. Arch Dermatol 134:207–214
Lipson RI, Baldes EJ (1960) The photodynamic properties of a particular haematoporphyrin derivative. Arch Dermatol 82:508–516
McCaughan JS Jr (1999) Photodynamic therapy: a review. Drugs Aging 15:49–68
Schwartz SK, Absolon K, Vermund H (1955) Some relationships of porphyrins, x-rays and tumours. Univ Minn Med Bull 27:7–8
Stender IM, Na R, Fogh H et al. (2000) Photodynamic therapy with 5-aminolaevulinic acid or placebo for recalcitrant foot and hand warts: randomised double-blind trial. Lancet 355:963–966
Szeimies R-M, Abels C, Bäumler W et al. (1997) Photodynamische Therapie in der Dermatologie. In: Krutmann J, Hönigsmann H (eds) Handbuch der dermatologischen Phototherapie und Photodiagnostik. Springer, Berlin, pp 196–233

Ionizing Radiation

Braun-Falco O, Lukacs S, Goldschmidt H (1976) Dermatologic radiotherapy. Springer, Berlin
Davis MM, Hanke CW, Zollinger TW et al. (1989) Skin cancer in patients with chronic radiation dermatitis. J Am Acad Dermatol 20:608–616
Edwards EK Jr, Edwards EK Sr (1990) Grenz ray therapy. Int J Dermatol 29:17–18
El-Akkad S, Bull CA, El-Senoussi MA et al. (1986) Kaposi's sarcoma and its management by radiotherapy. Arch Dermatol 122:1396–1399
Goldschmidt H (1986) Dermatologic radiotherapy. The risk-benefit ratio. Arch Dermatol 122:1385–1388
Goldschmidt H, Panizzon RG (1991) Modern dermatologic radiation therapy. Springer, Berlin
Goldschmidt H, Sherwin WK (1983a) Office radiotherapy of cutaneous carcinomas I. Radiation techniques, dose schedules, and radiation protection. J Dermatol Surg Oncol 9:31–46
Goldschmidt H, Sherwin WK (1983b) Office radiotherapy of cutaneous carcinomas II. Indications in specific anatomic regions. J Dermatol Surg Oncol 9:47–76
Goldschmidt H, Gorson RO, Lassen M (1983) Dermatologic radiotherapy and thyroid cancer. Arch Dermatol 119: 383–390
Goldschmidt H, Breneman JC, Breneman DL (1994) Ionizing radiation therapy in dermatology. J Am Acad Dermatol 30:157–182
Harwood AR (1982) Conventional radiotherapy in the treatment of lentigo maligna and lentigo maligna melanoma. J Am Acad Dermatol 6:310–316
Landthaler M, Lukacs S, Braun-Falco O et al. (1981) Röntgenweichstrahlentherapie der Lippenkarzinome. Hautarzt 32:80–83
Landthaler M, Hendel B, Schiele-Luftmann K et al. (1983) Röntgenweichstrahlentherapie von Lidbasaliomen. Hautarzt 34:118–122
Lindelöf B, Eklund G (1986) Incidence of malignant skin tumors in 14140 patients after Grenz-Ray treatment for benign skin disorders. Arch Dermatol 122:1391–1395
van Vloten WA, Hermans J, van Daal EAJ (1987) Radiation-induced skin cancer and radiodermatitis of the head and neck. Cancer 59:411–414

CHAPTER 72

Operative Dermatology

RAINER ROMPEL

Contents

General Aspects

Dermatology is both a medical and a surgical specialty. A broad knowledge of the biology and function of the skin and the pathology of dermatologic disorders enables the dermatologist to choose the best treatment modalities, either medical or surgical or the combination of both.

Operative dermatology is subject to the same rules and responsibilities as all other branches of surgery, including the pre-, intra-, and postoperative periods. The general condition of the patient must be taken into account as the surgical procedure is planned. Since nearly all procedures in dermatologic surgery are elective, one should consider the noninvasive techniques available when a patient appears to have operative risks.

Indications. A major part of dermatologic surgery is the removal of malignant and premalignant tumors. In addition, many benign tumors and malformations are removed both for aesthetic reasons and for prophylaxis to avoid malignant change. Another indication for surgery is the treatment of inflammatory and postinflammatory conditions e.g., acne inversa, acne scars, posttraumatic scars.

Surgery for skin cancer has certain advantages in comparison to nonsurgical methods:

- The treatment and recovery periods are short
- The three-dimensional histologic control of the excised specimen allows the most accurate determination of complete tumor removal
- Surgery avoids damage to underlying bone or cartilage, which may occur when inadequate radiation therapy or cryotherapy is employed on the nose, ears, cheeks and fingers
- Radiation therapy produces a scar that tends to worsen over time and has a risk of developing squamous cell carcinoma after a long latency period
- Some skin tumors respond poorly to radiation therapy
- Radiation therapy leads to hair loss, limiting its usefulness on the scalp

History and Preoperative Examination. The initial discussion with the patient should cover the past medical history with particular attention to allergies (for example to local anesthetics, antibiotics, analgesics, latex, tape, and others), cardiac problems, CNS diseases, endocrine disorders, and infectious diseases, e.g. hepatitis and HIV infection. In addition, a history of wound healing problems such as hypertrophic scars, keloids, or tendency towards dehiscence must be noted.

All medications that the patient is taking should be noted, including over-the-counter products. Anticoagulants are of obvious importance. Coumarin products should be discontinued and, if needed, replaced by heparin. Low-dose aspirin for platelet aggregation inhibition should be suspended 2 weeks preoperatively. Coagulation parameters should be assessed prior to surgery if the history suggests bleeding problems, or if the planned procedure involves marked blood loss.

In general, for larger operations the patient should be seen by both an internist and an anesthesiologist. This permits the patient's general health and suitability for anesthesia to be best evaluated and documented. Most dermatologic cases are less complicated and can be handled by the dermatologist alone. In complicated cases or when other problems are discovered, the preoperative evaluation must be expanded. Standard preoperative tests include red and white blood counts, platelet counts, liver function tests, creatinine and electrolytes, fasting blood sugar and electrocardiogram. Optional preoperative tests might be coagulation studies, blood typing, HIV status and hepatitis serology, thyroid evaluation, syphilis serology, chest X-ray, and peripheral vascular evaluation. Of course, one must determine whether the patient has had previous untoward reactions to local anesthetics. The possibility of allergy can be further evaluated with appropriate testing.

Informed Consent. The physician must conduct a thorough discussion with the patient, providing information on the expected benefits and possible risks of the proposed operation, and also of the alternative noninvasive methods. The reasons for the procedure, the planned approach, the expected results, and the risks entailed, must all be explained by the physician in terms that the patient can understand. The possible complications should be discussed in detail; they may include:

- Bleeding during operation
- Postoperative bleeding
- Wound infection
- Wound dehiscence
- Damage to sensory or motor nerves
- Unsatisfactory scars (hypertrophic scars, keloids)
- Recurrence of the tumor

It is particularly important to explain changes in the surgical approach which may become necessary intraoperatively, e.g., that a certain flap may prove impossible once the actual wound defect is established intraoperatively. Less common complications should also be discussed. Furthermore, one must discuss the "pros" and "cons" for alternative approaches such as radiation therapy or cryotherapy. In oncologic cases the patient should be informed of the prognosis and the possibility of recurrence or metastasis. Possible consequences resulting from the refusal of an operation should be mentioned. The preoperative discussion is even more crucial when a cosmetic procedure is being planned. Generally, weak indications for surgery require hard preoperative discussion and informed consent.

For medical-legal purposes it is essential that the preoperative discussion is carefully documented. A signed preprinted operative permit alone does not verify informed consent and must be supplemented by a chart note outlining the nature of the conversation. In general, individual notes including specific questions by the patient are more valuable than simply checking off boxes as "questions answered".

Postoperative care is essential and should be emphasized preoperatively so that the patient feels comfortable that the physician will have a lasting interest in his or her problem and will be available.

Perioperative Considerations

Preparing for the Operation. Preparations are naturally more complicated when general anesthesia is planned than in the case of a local procedure. The patient must not eat or drink during the 6 h preceding general anesthesia. Smoking during the preoperative period is also forbidden. The patient must realize the danger of violating these rules, for the danger of suffocation through an anesthetic accident is considerable. The administration of a preoperative sedative is not mandatory but is often helpful.

Antisepsis. The measures for antisepsis include all considerations for the prevention of wound infection. The aim of presurgical preparation of the skin is to remove the transient bacterial flora. Clean techniques may be sufficient for small operative procedures, but sterile technique is required for all medium or large operations. Hair should be removed because it can be a source of *Staphylococcus aureus*. Although it is impossible to completely sterilize the skin, it is possible to remove the transient and pathogenic bacteria and to decrease the resident flora. A mechanical scrub and an effective antiseptic agent are used. Iodophors, alcoholic solutions or chlorhexidine are preferred commonly. The operative field is prepared from the center to the periphery using a circular motion twice or more before the sterile drapes are applied. Sterile gloves and coats for the physician are the standard. Furthermore, antisepsis is supported by meticulous surgical technique including adequate hemostasis, atraumatic preparation, consideration of blood supply and optimal dressings and wound care.

Antibiotic Prophylaxis. For clean wounds systemic antibiotics have not shown a benefit in preventing wound infections. In the case of clean-contaminated conditions, e.g. in the oral cavity, genitoanal region or axillae, antibiotics may be useful. For contaminated or infected wounds the antibiotics are considered therapeutic and not prophylactic. However, the choice of the antibiotic should always made in consideration of the organism most likely to cause the infection, and appropriate therapeutic antibiotics should be administered according to the antibiogram. A special case for antibiotic prophylaxis is in patients who are in danger of endocarditis. The choice of the agent should be made according to current guidelines.

Thromboembolism Prophylaxis. Age, general condition, immobilization, thrombophilia, and concomitant internal disorders contribute to an enhanced risk for venous thromboembolism. The nature and the duration of the operation are factors contributing to the operative risk. Small operations usually do not require thromboembolism prophylaxis. For medium and large dermatologic operations usually low-dose heparin prophylaxis of 2–3×5000 IE/day is preferred. Alternatively, low molecular weight heparins once daily can be chosen. The thromboembolism prophylaxis is continued for 7–10 days postoperatively, or until complete mobilization of the patient.

Patient Positioning. The patient's position on the operation table is important. The physician must insure that no unusual pressure points are present which could lead to tissue or nerve damage. In addition, one must be sure that no joints are hyperextended. When operating in the head and neck region, particular attention must be paid to insuring that the neck is not overextended. Elderly patients are at particular risk, for they almost always have arthritis changes and may suffer cervical spine fractures if positioned improperly. One must be especially cautious if repositioning a patient under general anesthesia because both protective reflexes and normal muscle tension are missing. During operations under local anesthesia the patient should be comfortably positioned on the operation table throughout the procedure.

Planning the Operation

Excision Margins. Most benign and premalignant lesions can be treated with narrow surgical margins and maximal tissue conservation. Malignant tumors require wider surgical margins depending on the nature of the tumor. Stretching the skin enables one to best appreciate the margins of a tumor, the skin elasticity, and the course of the relaxed skin tension lines. All this should be done prior to injecting a local anesthetic as this distorts the anatomic structures to some extent. Micrographic surgery for squamous cell carcinoma and basal cell carcinoma provides the most tissue preservation and complete margin control. A punch or incisional biopsy should precede the surgical excision of the tumor. In case of malignant melanoma a complete diagnostic excision (excisional biopsy) is the first step. Incisional biopsy of melanoma should be avoided in order to insure accurate microstaging and to minimize the risk of local recurrence.

Incision Lines. A major point for the planning of the operation is the course of the scalpel incision. After the margin of the tumor excision has been determined, the incision lines for reconstruction must be carefully planned. Functional as well as aesthetic aspects should be considered. Generally, the line of the incision will be placed to follow the relaxed skin tension lines (Fig. 72.1). These do not always follow the primary folds and wrinkles of the skin, although they often overlap. When flaps are planned, the major final closure lines should follow these lines. The relaxed skin tension lines reflect the functional situation of the skin in body movement and facial expression. In any individual region the course of these lines can easily be checked by compressing the skin between the thumb and forefinger in order to check the tension. In the head and neck region the skin of older patients shows numerous folds and wrinkles, usually perpendicular to the muscles of facial expression but individually variable. Wrinkled skin provides a convenient place to hide scars and serves as a source of tissue for flaps. The best way to determine the wrinkle lines is to ask the patient to do certain mimic maneuvers.

Aesthetic Units. For surgical procedures of the face, the major aesthetic units of the face should be considered: scalp, forehead, temples, eyelids/eyebrows,

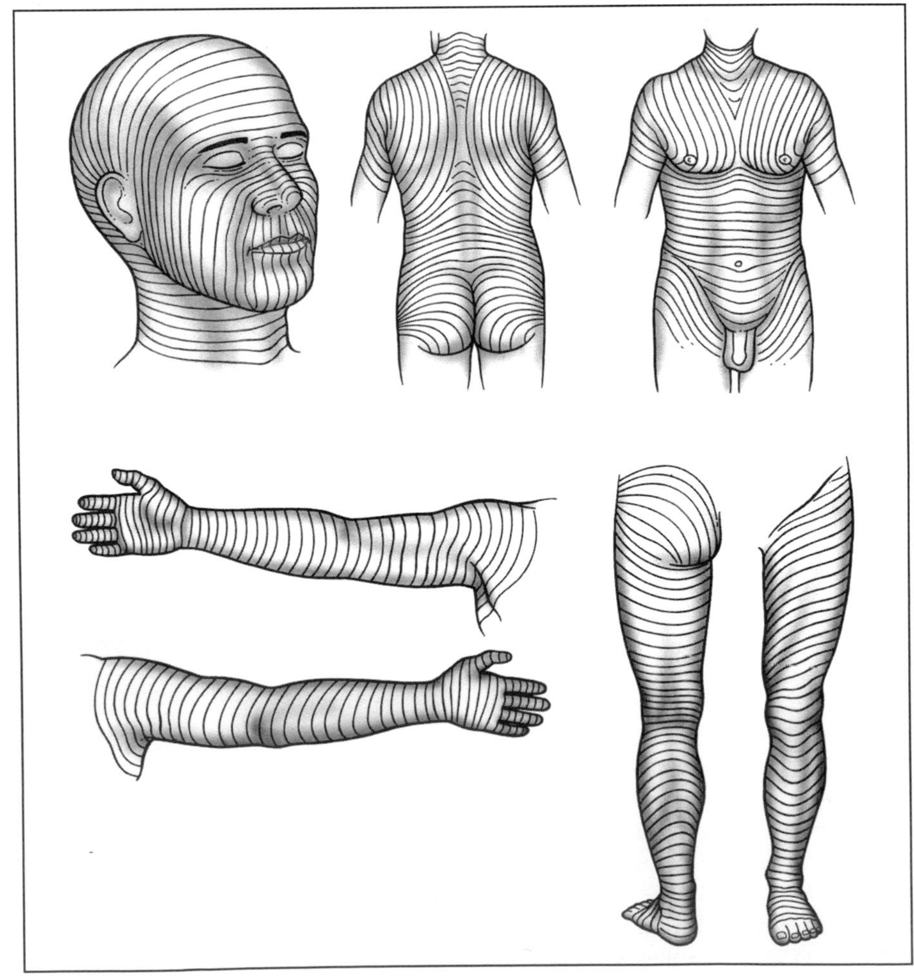

Fig. 72.1. Relaxed skin tension lines

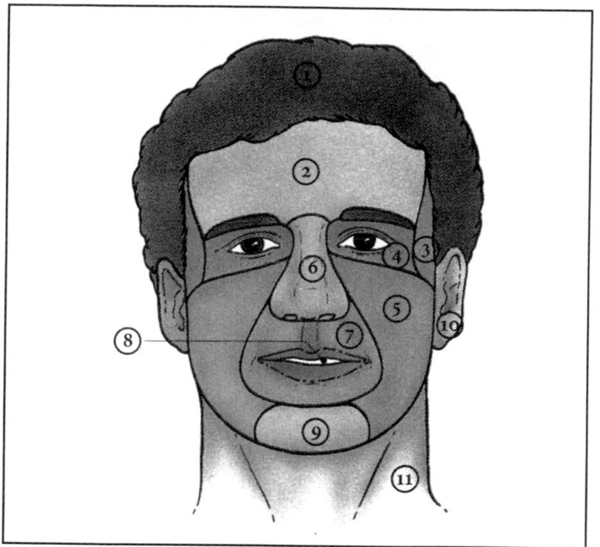

Fig. 72.2. Aesthetic units of the head and neck

cheek, nose, lips/perioral region, mouth, chin, ear and neck (Fig. 72.2). Within each of these regions, certain surface characteristics are similar, such as surface texture, pigmentation, pore size, hair quality, and the vascular reaction to autonomic innervation. Large excisions with undermining or large flaps will result in the best functional and aesthetic outcome when they involve only one aesthetic unit or just the neighboring unit that is of similar structure.

Surgical Instruments

The choice of appropriate surgical instruments and suture material plays a major role in determining the success of an operative procedure. Coarse or toothed forceps, awkward needle holders and scissors, and excessively large needles all contribute to wound edge trauma. Microthrombi and wound necrosis may result, leading to wide or gaping scars. Therefore special instruments are essential for delicate cutaneous surgery. A basic set consists of a scalpel handle, no. 11 and no. 15 disposable blades, biopsy punches (usually disposable in various sizes), curettes, needle holders, forceps, clamps, scissors, wound hooks and nail avulsion forceps. Small, rounded, slightly curved Metzenbaum scissors are essential for undermining and correctly preparing flaps. Delicate Adson forceps (dissecting and tissue forceps) as well as curved and straight mosquito clamps for bleeding sites are also needed. Wound edge adaptation, however, should be carried out with single- or double-pronged wound hooks, not with forceps. Naturally the choice of instruments must be appropriate to the site being treated.

Suture Material

The major choice is between resorbable material, employed for subcutaneous sutures and ligatures, and nonresorbable material, used for some subcutaneous work but primarily for approximating wound edges (Table 72.1). Resorbable material is digested or otherwise enzymatically destroyed over a period of time. The newer synthetic resorbable materials have much greater tensile strength than the classic catgut suture. As the wound becomes stronger, one can accept a diminution in the strength of the suture material. Determination of the appropriate resorbable suture involves a balancing of these two factors.

Monofilament sutures elicit minimal tissue reaction and are easy to use, but produce a knot which may work itself loose. On the other hand, woven sutures have greater tensile strength and knot security but may function with a sawlike effect when under tension in tissue. Some newer woven sutures are coated with a thin sheet of polyglactin, which

Table 72.1. Characteristics of various suture materials (++ very good, + good, (+) mediocre, – poor)

Material	Handling	Tear resistance	Knot safety	Tissue tolerance	Duration in tissue[a]
Silk	++	+	++	–/(+)	Permanent
Nylon, Perlon	+	++	–	++	Permanent
Polypropylene	(+)	++	–	++	Permanent
Polyester	+	++	+	(+)	Permanent
Catgut	–	–	+	(+)	70–90 days
Vicryl	(+)	+	+	+/++	75–90 days
Dexon	+	+	(+)/+	+/++	90–120 days
PDS	+	++	–	++	150–180 days

[a] Time until suture is completely resorbed

minimizes the sawing effect. One should be aware that resorbable sutures can lead to granuloma formation before they are absorbed.

Virtually all dermatologic surgeons use atraumatic needles already swedged onto the suture material as such needles create minimum damage at entry and exit sites. Cutting needles are preferred for the skin sutures, while the subcutaneous sutures can be placed with either a round or cutting needle. On mucosal surfaces better success will be achieved with round needles.

Postoperative Measures

Wound Dressings. There are a wide range of possibilities for covering a wound. The various recommendations in the literature are often confusing: occlude versus leave open, ointment versus no ointment, pressure versus no pressure. Each physician must develop his or her own approach to wound dressings that allows wounds to be effectively dressed on different body sites. A dry wound dressing is really practical only for small noncontaminated wounds, such as a simple closure or following a small transposition flap. Here a light pressure dressing is sufficient, fixed with a nonirritating adhesive tape. The therapeutic value of antibiotic creams, ointments, and powders is controversial. If creams do have a role, it is in the first 24 h, when occlusion seems to speed healing. If powders are used, they should not contain talc which carries the risk of granuloma formation. For larger wounds, such as those resulting from flaps, grafts, and dermabrasion, a moist wound dressing may be favorable. This reduces the danger of flap or graft necrosis and minimizes crusting. Moist dressings include an impregnated fatty gauze and an enzymatic ointment, and are fixed in place with soft pads and an elastic bandage. Following a skin graft, the dressing should insure some degree of immobilization and is left on for 5–8 days. In this situation the restriction of motion takes precedence over the other functions of the dressing. On the extremities further immobilization can be achieved with a simple plaster cast at the same time. Donor sites for split-thickness skin grafts can be covered with hydrocolloid, alginate or hydrogel sheetings.

Temporary Wound Covering. In the case of multistep procedures a temporary wound covering is necessary. Polyurethane sheetings or any other inert material may be applied. This produces a clean granulating wound, which can then be excised and closed as needed, or grafted after an adequate base has evolved.

Anesthesia

The choice of anesthetic technique for most dermatologic surgery cases is a matter of individual preference, both from the perspective of the patient and from that of the physician. One must consider not only the technical aspects of the operation but also the emotional status of the patient. In general, the increased convenience and greater margin of safety, especially in patients with cardiovascular or respiratory disease, lead us to favor local or regional anesthesia.

Local Anesthesia

One advantage of local anesthesia is that the physician can communicate with the patient during the operation. This becomes of special importance when operating near critical nerves, for the patient can help to insure that nerve function is retained. A technical disadvantage is that the injection of local anesthetic may lead to swelling of the tissues, making it more difficult to adapt the wound edges exactly.

Local Anesthetic Agents. Ideally, local anesthetic agents are characterized by rapid onset of action, sufficiently long duration of action to cover the operation, and minimum degree of toxicity and allergenicity. For the most part the amide types of local anesthetic meet these criteria. Lidocaine, mepivacaine and prilocaine are especially useful in dermatologic surgery because of the low doses required for prolonged action (Table 72.2). While the maximum dosage recommendations should be carefully followed, it is possible to reinject up to 25% of this amount after a 30-min interval, if additional anesthesia proves necessary.

The addition of vasoconstrictive agents such as epinephrine causes a transitory vasoconstriction and reduces intraoperative bleeding. This vasoconstriction also speeds the onset of action and prolongs the duration of the effect of the local anesthetic. In addition, somewhat higher tissue concentrations can be achieved since there is less agent carried away by the circulation. A disadvantage is that vasodilatation results when the epinephrine wears off, which may increase bleeding. In some body areas, vasoconstriction may be undesirable

Table 72.2. Classification and pharmacology of local anesthetics

Anesthetic	Type	Onset of action	Maximum dose		Duration of action (min)
			Adult (mg)[a]	Child (mg/kg)	
Procaine	Ester	Slow	500	2	15–30
Mepivacaine	Amide	3–5 min	300	4	30–120
Lidocaine	Amide	3–5 min	300	7	45–120
Prilocaine	Amide	<3 min	400	5.7	30–120
Etidocaine	Amide	3–5 min	300	4.2	120–180
Bupivacaine	Amide	3–5 min	175	2	120–180

[a] Maximum single dose for a 70-kg adult

and can lead to tissue damage. Traditionally it has been recommended that epinephrine-containing agents should not be used when anesthetizing digits or the penis; the nose and ears are other possible risk areas. It is probably more important to avoid epinephrine in patients with peripheral arterial disease, diabetes, and other vascular disorders. Even small amounts of added epinephrine may precipitate cardiovascular disease in susceptible patients, leading to tachycardia, angina and hypertension. Agents with epinephrine should also be avoided in glaucoma patients and in pregnant patients. Sodium bicarbonate can be added to the anesthetic solution to increase the pH value and subsequently reduce pain. Solutions containing sodium bicarbonate should be prepared fresh, at least on a daily basis.

Allergic reactions to local anesthetics are often feared and described by patients, but are actually uncommon when the amide type of agent is employed. The next most common cause of adverse reactions is simply exceeding the maximum recommended dosage and producing a toxic effect. Accidental intravenous injection, more rapid absorption or delayed metabolism in patients with hepatic disease may also lead to toxic changes. The symptoms of an overdose of amide anesthetic include paresthesias, sensitivity to light, hyperactivity and abnormal speech. In more severe cases, respiratory and cardiovascular collapse can occur, leading even to death. It is therefore crucial to adhere to the maximum recommended doses of the amide agents, especially in large or long cases. Other adverse effects are shown in Table 72.3.

Table 72.3. Possible side effects of local anesthetics

Nerve damage (traumatic or toxic)
Allergic reactions
Vascular injury
Pneumothorax (in plexus blocks)
Infection in area of injection
Intravascular injection
Tissue necrosis (when a vasoconstrictor is used)
Systemic toxic reactions
CNS reactions
Hyperventilation
Agitation
Cardiovascular reactions

Cryoanesthesia

Cryosprays produce a transient anesthesia for superficial procedures. Fluoroethyl is the most widely used cryoanesthetic agent. Although capable of freezing skin, it does not produce severe cryogenic injury. Spraying for 5–10 s produces about 1 min of partial anesthesia that is sufficient for curetting seborrheic keratoses, dermabrasion of small areas and performing shave and perhaps some punch biopsies. Potential side effects of the cryospray may be hyper- or hypopigmentation, freezing of underlying periosteum, and persistent erythema.

Topical Anesthesia

A commercial mixture of 2.5% lidocaine and 2.5% prilocaine in a special vehicle (EMLA cream) is a relatively effective topical anesthetic. It must be applied under occlusion for 45–60 min but then produces a good level of anesthesia. It is often used to remove molluscum contagiosum in children and for curetting seborrheic keratoses in adults. In addition, it is often all that is needed in many laser cases. Methemoglobinemia has been reported following the use of EMLA over large wide areas in children, but otherwise the product is very safe.

Infiltration Anesthesia

Local infiltration of the operative site is the most commonly employed form of anesthesia in cutaneous surgery. It produces safe and very rapid anesthesia. The injection is not done directly into the lesion but peripherally in a fan-shaped manner, utilizing several injection sites to entirely encompass the operative field. This approach also minimizes the theoretical risk of spreading a malignant tumor by traumatizing it with the needle and perhaps moving cells along the needle track lines. Furthermore, histologic evaluation of the excised tissue is facilitated by lack of dermal edema from the injection. Finally, intravascular injections will be avoided efficiently by aspirating when the needle is moved.

Tumescence Anesthesia

Definition and Principle. The tumescent technique for locoregional anesthesia was initially used for liposuction, but now is increasingly used in many cases of dermatologic surgery. The technique offers a regional anesthesia of large areas of skin and subcutaneous tissue. Large volumes of a dilute anesthetic are used in concentrations of 0.05–0.1% in saline solution, and epinephrine, sodium bicarbonate and triamcinolone are added. Various formulas for the tumescence solution have been suggested by different authors (Table 72.4). Commonly used anesthetic agents are lidocaine and prilocaine. For liposuction the maximal dose of 7 mg/kg lidocaine can be increased to 35 mg/kg, and also 32–35 mg/kg prilocaine seems to be safe. This is due both to the special pharmacokinetics of the tumescence solution that limit the systemic spread and to the removal of both local anesthetic solution and fat during the procedure. In all other types of procedures the maximal dosage recommendations of lidocaine and prilocaine should be followed.

Indications. Liposuction, phlebectomy, dermabrasion, large excisions, large flaps, grafts.

Technique. The solution is injected into the subcutaneous tissue to produce swelling and complete anesthesia of targeted areas. The infiltration can be done using a syringe or preferably an automated infusion system with a flow rate of 50–500 ml/h (for liposuction even higher). The tumescence of the tissue and the effect of the epinephrine allow a longstanding vasoconstriction that prevents marked bleeding during the operation. Typically, a blanche effect and marked swelling appear (Fig. 72.3). The swelling of the skin produces intraoperative tissue expansion that may be useful for special indications such as large excisions or flaps. In addition, the subcutaneous layers are divided and preparation may be easier.

Regional Anesthesia

An effective approach is to inject a long-acting local anesthetic proximal to the operative site around the major sensory nerve. One must avoid trauma-

Table 72.4. Tumescence solutions

Author	Ingredient	Amount
Klein (1987)	Lidocaine 1%	500–1000 mg
	Epinephrine	0.5–0.75 mg
	Sodium bicarbonate	10 mval
	Triamcinolone	10 mg
	Normal saline	1000 ml
Sattler (1997)	Prilocaine 1%	500 mg
	Epinephrine	0.75–1.0 mg
	Sodium bicarbonate	10 mval
	Triamcinolone	20 mg
	Normal saline	1000 ml
Mang and Arnold (1998)	Prilocaine 1%	330–400 mg
	Epinephrine	0.75–1.0 mg
	Sodium bicarbonate	10 mval
	Triamcinolone	10 mg
	Normal saline	1000 ml

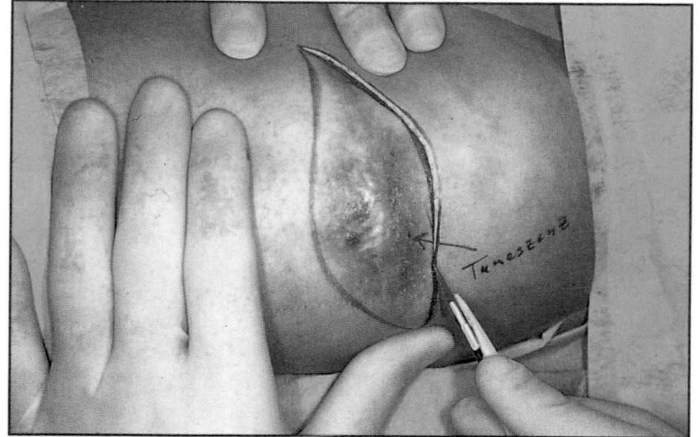

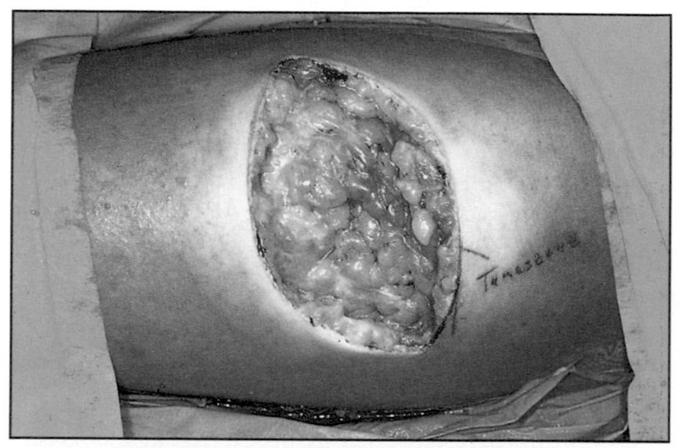

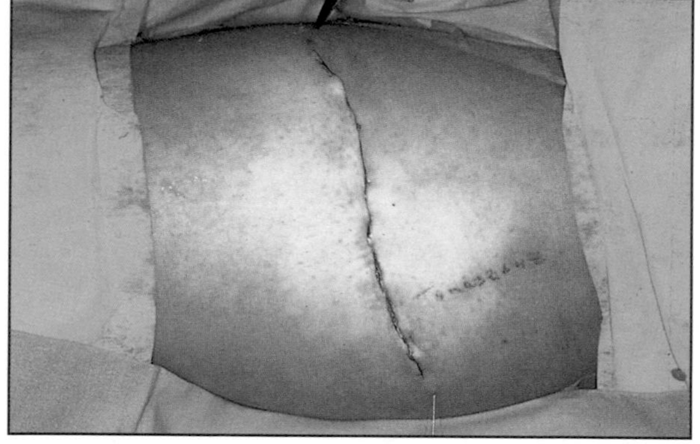

Fig. 72.3 a–c. Tumescence anesthesia. **a** Typical blanche effect surrounding the nevus to be excised. **b** Minimal bleeding after complete excision. **c** Wound closure

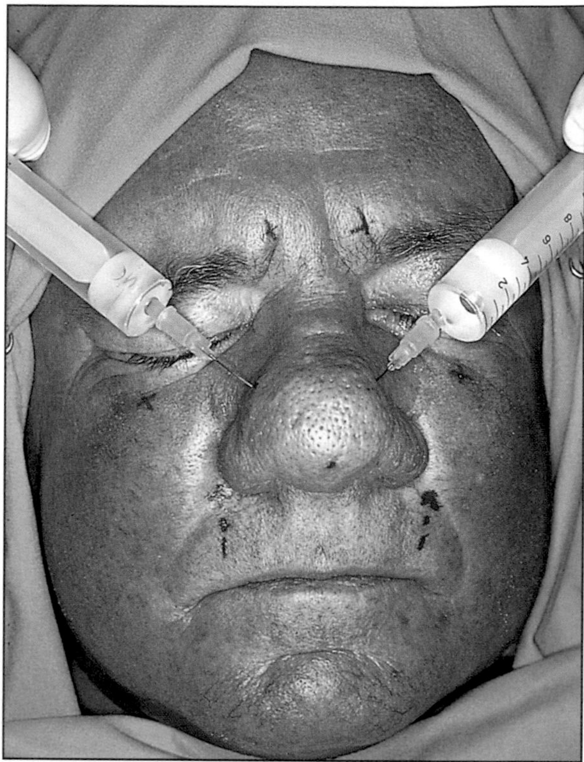

Fig. 72.4. Injection sites to block the branches of the trigeminal nerve (n. supraorbitalis; n. infraorbitalis; r. nasalis n. ethmoidalis anterior; gingival branches of n. infraorbitalis; not depicted n. submentalis)

tizing the nerve and instead surround it with 1–2 ml of anesthetic agent. This approach may be favorably used in the face, the digits, and the male genitalia. In the face the sensory branches of the trigeminal nerve can be blocked where they pass through the skull and into the skin (Fig. 72.4). When injecting the digits, the technique recommended by Oberst is used (Fig. 72.5). One begins dorsally and moves ventrally, injecting on both sides of the digit at its base. In this way, both the dorsal and palmar digital nerves are blocked. On the penis, one also begins dorsally, blocking the dorsal penile nerves on both sides. The needle can be moved just beneath the loose skin and above the penile fascia to accomplish a circumferential block. Hand and foot blocks are specialized methods to block the extremities, but are rarely used in dermatologic surgery.

General Anesthesia

General anesthesia is the field of the anesthesiologist. Considerably more dermatologic procedures are done under general anesthesia in Europe than in the USA, simply because in Europe many operations are performed in hospitals, while in North America most are carried out in the outpatient setting. The trend towards ambulatory or day surgery centers has made general anesthesia more attractive for some of the larger cutaneous cases.

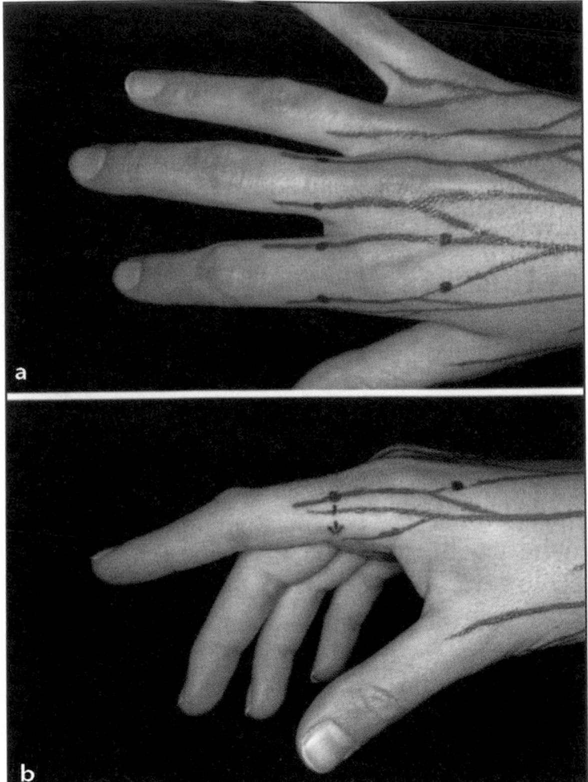

Fig. 72.5 a, b Injection sites for nerve blocks of the digits. **a** Injection sites at the base of the fingers and in the metacarpal region. **b** Injection from the dorsal aspect in the palmar direction

Basic Operative Techniques

Suturing Techniques

Along with the careful planning of the incision, attention to relaxed skin lines, natural skin folds and aesthetic regions, the surgeon's suture technique plays a major role in determining the final aesthetic results. The following points should be given particular attention:

- Since the subcutaneous sutures are primarily responsible for holding the wound edges in approximation, they should be placed extremely carefully. The skin sutures serve only for fine approximation.
- Wound tension should always be reduced by subcutaneous sutures and not by increasing the thickness and tension of the skin sutures.
- The knots of the skin sutures must not deform or squeeze the skin. This pressure leads to a ladder-type scar.
- Some operators use resorbable sutures for percutaneous stitches, but this practice is associated with problems: the sutures generally remain in place too long, so that their stitch canals tend to epithelialize, producing an unsatisfactory result.
- The thickness of the sutures for the skin may vary between 7-0 for the lids and 0-0 for the trunk and limbs. The dermatologist must choose the appropriate suture material based on both skin thickness and wound tension.

Subcutaneous Suture

Technique. Even when the wound tension is minimal, it is often wise to place a subcutaneous suture in order to achieve an optimal vertical adaptation. Vicryl or PDS sutures are generally used. Since they remain in the body for a relatively long period of time, a granulomatous reaction may occur. Therefore, a minimum number of subcutaneous sutures should be used. PDS is present for a much longer period of time and thus helps to prevent dehiscence when wound tension is considerable.

One generally chooses between 3-0 and 6-0 suture material depending on the body location and wound tension. While it is possible to insert running subcutaneous sutures, we prefer single sutures. In a simple buried suture the needle enters through the subcutaneous tissue, exits through the dermis, re-enters through the opposing dermis and exits through the subcutaneous fat. When tied, the knot is inverted at the base of the suture (Fig. 72.6 a). Thus the possibility of a visible reaction to this deeply placed suture is far less than with a more superficial placement.

Skin Suture

Simple Suture. One should choose as fine a suture as possible. We favor either monofil or coated woven polyester or polypropylene sutures. Alternatives are silk and PDS. The latter materials are all very well tolerated by the tissues and show minimal tissue reaction. On visible body parts, the sutures should enter and exit about 1–2 mm from the wound edge (Fig. 72.6 b). One should view the skin sutures as adapting the wound edges or placing them next to each other, rather than as "pulling them together". To minimize the risk that one wound edge may rise or sink in relation to the other, producing an unacceptable step scar, one must pay careful attention to

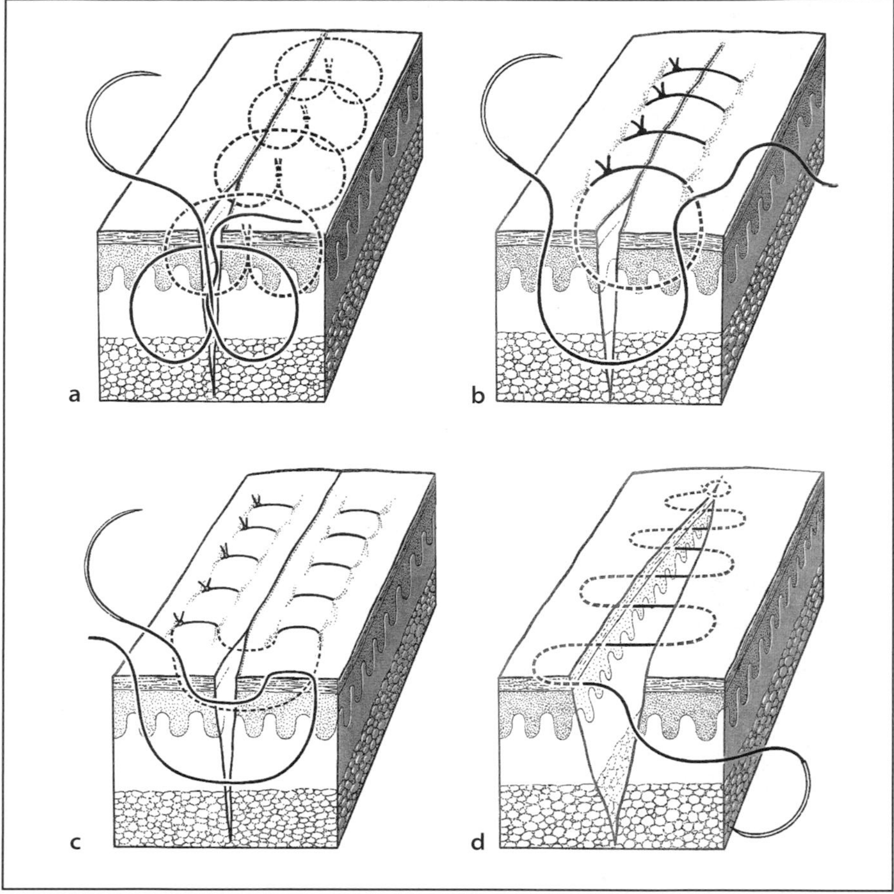

Fig. 72.6 a–d. Common types of sutures
a Subcutaneous suture
b Simple interrupted skin suture
c Vertical mattress suture
d Running intracutaneous suture

making a vertical incision and then to placing the suture to the same depth on both sides. Often a three-dimensional view of the wound helps in this task.

Horizontal Mattress. The first part of the stitch is identical to the simple interrupted suture. The suture is continued parallel to the wound, and a second stitch is placed in the reverse direction. The horizontal mattress is a convenient skin suture, as it is similar to single sutures but closes the wound more quickly, with the placement of fewer sutures.

Vertical Mattress. In the technique described by Donati, the initial entry and exit points are placed somewhat farther back from the wound edge and then the suture material re-enters the skin in line with the exit point but closer to the wound edge and similarly exits a second time closer to the opposite wound edge (Fig. 72.6 c). The vertical mattress is an excellent way to evert the skin, avoiding sunken wounds, and to improve approximation. The modification of Allgöwer includes an incomplete intracutaneous suture. The entry point is similar to that of the standard vertical mattress suture, but there is no exit on the opposite edge, but instead an intracutaneous stitch. The exit point is then placed exactly like the final exit point with a standard suture. This modified vertical mattress requires considerable experience.

Running Suture. There are many types of running sutures, such as the running overlapping suture and the running horizontal mattress. Each is far more rapid than the simple interrupted sutures and are thus favored by general surgeons who often need to close a large wound quickly. This may lead to a less perfectly adapted wound edge and result in an unacceptable scar.

Running Intracutaneous Suture. The running intradermal suture is an elegant suture that offers a good cosmetic outcome because there will be no stitch marks. After appropriately reducing wound tension through subcutaneous sutures, the wound is placed under longitudinal tension with two skin hooks, one at each end. The initial entry point is near the skin hook and the exit point in the dermis just at the beginning of the wound. Then the suture is placed horizontally across the wound, staying at exactly the same level in the skin (Fig. 72.6 d). Each entrance site in the dermis is backtracked slightly fom the opposite exit point. When the wound is closed, the suture exits the skin about 0.5 cm from the distal wound end. The ends may be fixed with knots or simply using adhesive tapes. A long-lived but resorbable suture such as PDS 3-0 to 5-0 is often used for this stitch. If this breaks during suture removal, resorption still occurs.

Skin Staple. A wound can also be closed with a variety of metal skin clips or staples. Today several systems are available, including some with staples that are fine enough for use in cosmetic skin surgery. Many staples are purchased loaded in a plastic stapler to simplify application. With a fine forceps the wound is approximated and the staples are inserted transcutaneously approximately every 0.7 – 1.0 cm. They are removed with a special forceps which simply opens them.

Suture Removal

Transcutaneous sutures should be removed as soon as possible to reduce the scarring at entry and exit sites, as well as pressure or ladder-type scars. Tied sutures are removed by cutting the suture beneath the knot and as close to the skin as possible with scissors or a scalpel and then removing the suture without pulling any exposed suture through the tissue. This technique is needed to avoid the possibility of stitch pathway infections. The timing of suture removal depends on the degree of wound tension and the body site, e.g. on the face, neck and nape on days 5 – 7, on the scalp and trunk on days 10 – 14, on the extremities on days 12 – 16, and on the genitalia on days 7 – 10. The physician must always balance the optimal timing according personal experience and wound appearance. It is often appropriate to remove some of the sutures or staples on one day and the rest a day or two later. After removal of the sutures, the patient should be instructed to protect the area.

Biopsy Techniques

Skin Biopsy

The use of a tissue biopsy to aid in the diagnostic process is far more common in dermatology than in any other specialty. The skin is readily accessible, a biopsy can be obtained easily, and it is often the only way to identify a malignancy with certainty or distinguish between two clinically similar dermatoses. Similarly, an accurate biopsy and tissue diagnosis is essential for planning an operation. Only when the margins that will be required are known exactly, can the approach for a given lesion be mapped out.

Three types of biopsies are generally performed:

- In the punch biopsy a cylindrical instrument sharpened on one end is used to excise a cylinder of tissue. The punches vary in diameter from 2 mm to 8 mm, and may be either disposable or autoclavable permanent instruments. The skin is stretched perpendicularly to the relaxed skin tension lines, and then the punch is twisted between the surgeon's fingers as it is pressed into the tissue (Fig. 72.7). Often one can pop the cylindrical tissue up out of the skin and snip of the base. The wound will easily heal by secondary intention or may be stitched with one skin suture.

- The spindle shaped or elliptical incisional biopsy is performed with a scalpel and closed with several skin sutures. In some situations an elliptical biopsy is preferable, especially if large and deep specimen across the edge of a lesion are required to establish the histologic diagnosis, as for example in keratoacanthoma.

- The tangential incisional biopsy (shave or saucer biopsy) yields a saucer-like specimen. Since only superficial tissue is biopsied, no histologic information about deep structures can be obtained. The procedure is done by lifting the center of the area using a small needle, and then the scalpel incision is made horizontally to the skin surface. The wound heals by secondary intention.

Lymph Node Biopsy

The diagnostic extirpation of an enlarged lymph node is of particular importance in mycosis fungoides or other cutaneous lymphomas, malignant melanoma or other metastasizing cutaneous tumors, and also in cases of underlying internal malignancies. The complete extirpation is the preferable method with a much higher specificity as compared to fine-needle biopsy. A skin incision is made over the palpable node, and the lymph node is approached using blunt preparation techniques. Supplying vessels should be carefully ligated and the lymph node

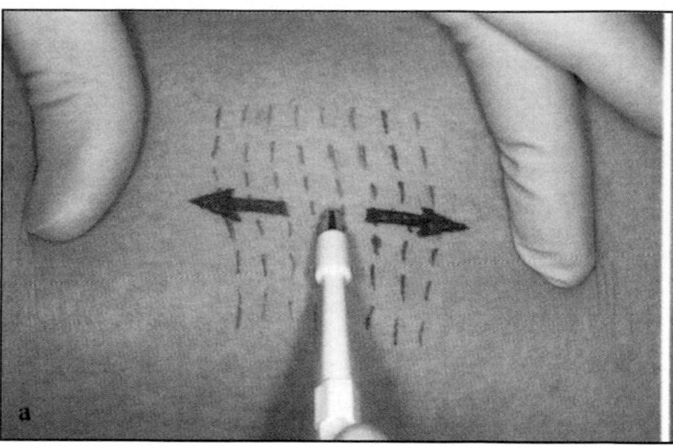

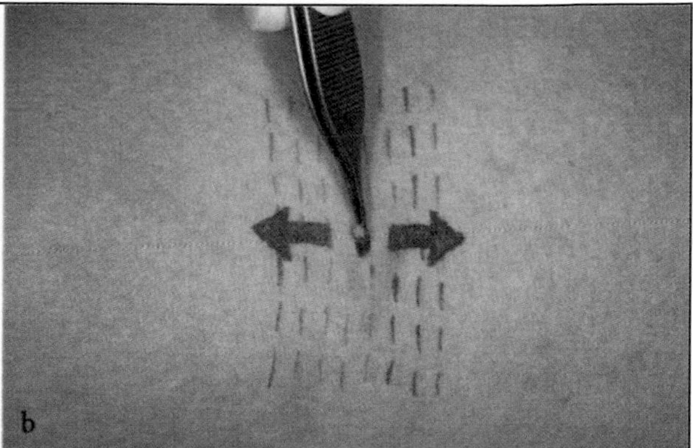

Fig. 72.7 a, b. Punch biopsy using a disposable punch. **a** Skin stretched perpendicular to tension lines and punch rotated. **b** Biopsy cylinder removed

can then be extirpated atraumatically. The wound is closed by subcutaneous and skin sutures.

Sentinel Lymph Node Biopsy

Definition and Principle. The method of sentinel lymph node biopsy was developed by Morton and coworkers (Morton et al. 1992). It is considered as a staging procedure in primary malignant melanoma enabling the initial draining lymph node (the sentinel node) of the regional lymph basin to be identified. The sentinel node is histologically examined by serial sections including immunohistologic methods. If occult metastasis is detected, a radical therapeutic regional lymph node dissection should follow the procedure.

Two methods have been described to identify the sentinel node: preoperative lymphoscintigraphy with intraoperative color-coded lymphatic mapping or preoperative lymphoscintigraphy plus the intraoperative use of a gamma probe. The combination of the two methods will result in the highest rate of identification of the sentinel node and the highest specificity and sensitivity.

Technique. On the day before the operation, a 99m-technetium-labeled colloid is injected intradermally around the primary melanoma site. Gamma camera imaging is then used to identify lymphatic drainage channels and locate sentinel nodes, whose positions are marked on the overlying skin. At the time of the operation another intradermal injection of 0.5–1.5 ml of blue dye (patent blue V or isosulfane blue) is done at the site of the primary tumor (Fig. 72.8). The incision is made where the sentinel node was located by lymphoscintigraphy.

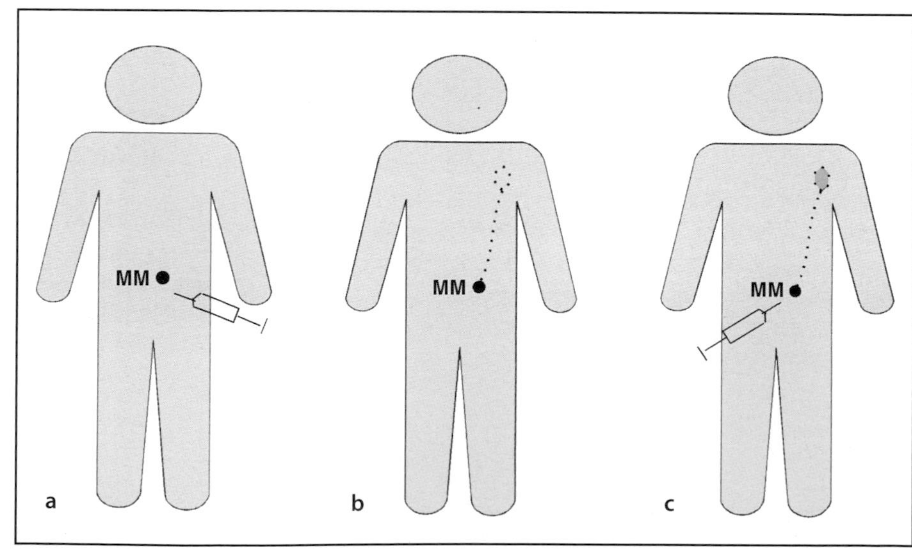

Fig. 72.8 a–c. Technique of lymphatic mapping
a Injection of 99m-technetium-colloid
b Scintigraphic mapping of the lymphatic drainage and the sentinel node
c Patent blue injection immediately prior to operation

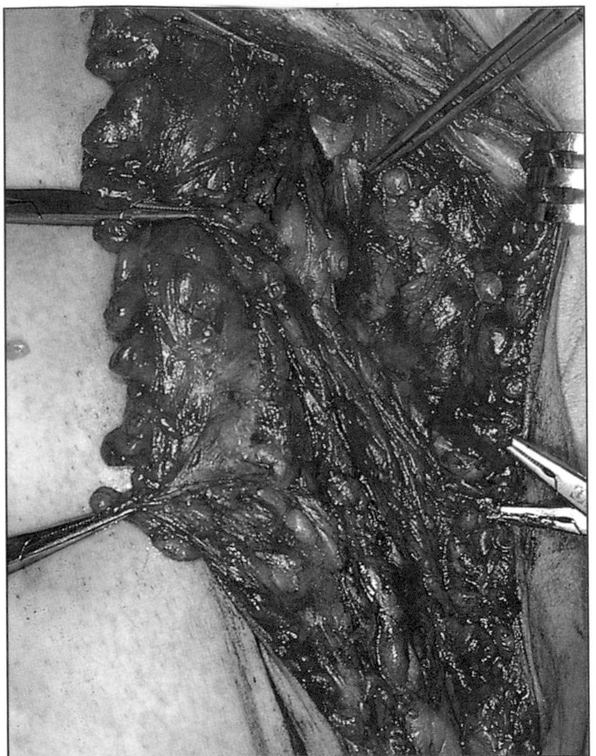

Fig. 72.9. Sentinel node including lymphatic vessels, both showing the typical blue stain

Blue-stained draining lymphatic channels lead to the sentinel nodes. An intraoperative gamma probe may also help to find the exact location of the sentinel node that shows the typical blue stain (Fig. 72.9). Using the combination of these two techniques the incision is small, while the procedure is rapid and sensitive.

Indications. Malignant melanoma, squamous cell carcinoma, Merkel cell carcinoma, adnex tumors, sarcomas.

Superficial Tissue Removal

Curettage

Curettage consists of the removal of superficial tissues with the use of a sharp curette. Convenient disposable ringed curettes are available. Epidermal proliferations such as verrucae, condylomata, seborrheic keratoses, molluscum contagiosum, and actinic keratoses are treated by this method. The curetted material should always be submitted for histologic evaluation. Although the pathologist does not receive an ideal specimen, interpretation is usually possible. If the diagnosis is unclear or if a malignant process seems likely, then a punch biopsy should be performed initially.

It is important to stretch the skin tightly during the procedure (Fig. 72.10). For larger lesions, such as large seborrheic keratoses, cryotherapy of the lesions prior to curettage is often helpful. As long as only superficial elements are curetted, the wound usually heals without scarring. There may be hypo- or hyperpigmentation but this change typically resolves over time. Bleeding is generally minimal, and simple pressure is therefore adequate for control. Light electrocautery or hemostatic solution may be used.

Small or superficial basal cell carcinomas are often treated by curettage combined with electro-

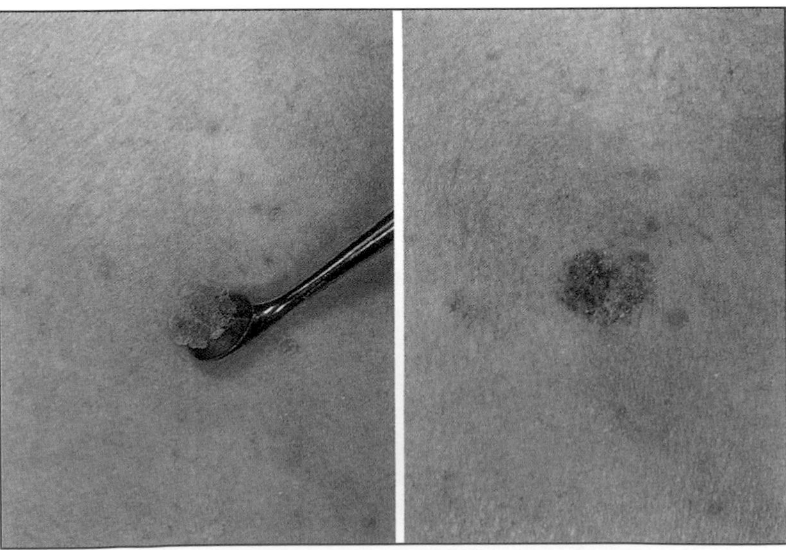

Fig. 72.10. Curettage of a seborrheic keratosis

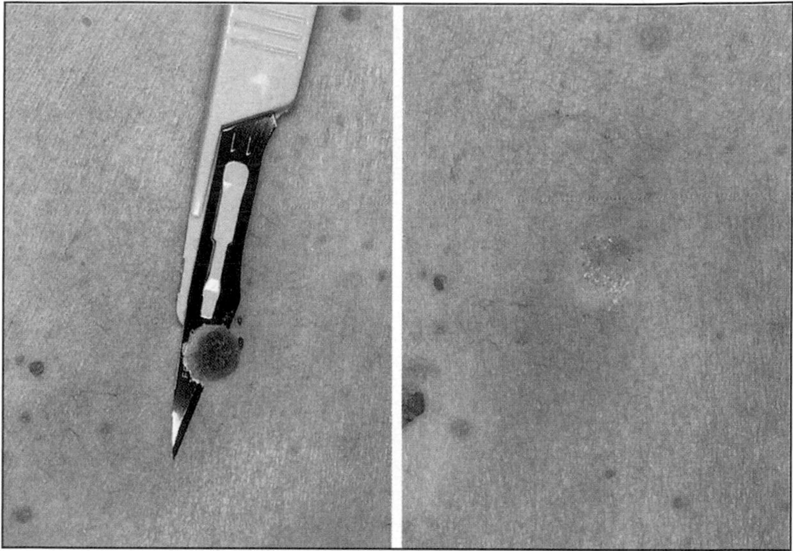

Fig. 72.11. Tangential excision of a seborrheic keratosis

desiccation or electrocautery. In the USA three such passes of treatment are traditionally employed in a single sitting. Although the cure rate for basal cell carcinomas smaller than 1 cm in size and for superficial basal cell carcinomas is quite good, the cosmetic results are less acceptable than excision in most cases.

Tangential Excision

A tangential excision (shave excision) is performed with a scalpel or double-edged razor blade. The cut is made roughly parallel to the skin surface, removing superficial tissues (Fig. 72.11). The procedure is ideal for small papillomatous melanocytic nevi, skin tags, and similar lesions. The wound is allowed to heal secondarily, and scarring is minimal. The use of shave biopsies or shave excisions with larger nevi with a dermal component is less desirable. A so-called deep shave, adequate to remove an entire nevus, leaves a defect which heals with a scar. In addition, superficial removal of a malignant melanoma compromises the histologic staging.

Scissors Excision

Scissors excision is simple and quick. A pedunculated lesion, usually a skin tag or small nevus, is grasped with forceps and snipped off at the base. Most defects are allowed to heal secondarily, but a skin suture may be helpful to speed healing after the removal of larger skin tags.

Dermabrasion

Definition. Erosion of the superficial layers of the skin by high-speed abrading devices.

Dermabrasion with high speed instruments (up to 60,000 rpm) was developed independently by Schreus and by Kurtin. Kromayer initiated the procedure using instruments of much lower speed. Dermabrasion today is a widely employed technique with many possible indications. Newly developed ablative lasers produce similar superficial tissue removal effects as dermabrasion.

Technique. The power driven systems for dermabrasion have foot pedals with which the speed can be easily controlled. The choice of the abrasive head is crucial to the success of the procedure. The standard instrument is a diamond fraise. Carborundum fraises, or wire or nylon brushes may be employed for special sites or problems. The dermabrasion procedure requires an experienced operator with a light touch. The skin must be stretched tight by an assistant. The physician must be aware of the direction in which the fraise is turning, so that mobile tissues such as the lower lip or eyelid do not become caught in the rotations. The skin must be cooled during the procedure with normal saline to avoid thermal tissue damage from the heat created by the fraise as it rotates. One must try to avoid going deeper than the epidermal-dermal junction to avoid scarring (Fig. 72.12). The depth of the procedure is controlled by the speed of the fraise and the pressure the surgeon generates between the fraise and the skin.

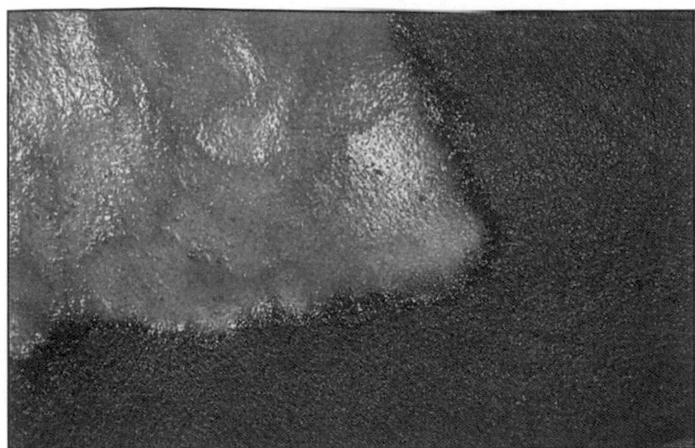

Fig. 72.12. Correct depth of dermabrasion. Close-up view of a partially removed congenital melanocytic nevus

In the postoperative care of dermabraded tissue, moist wound treatment or hydrocolloids are applied. Complications of dermabrasion may be milia, persistent erythema, hyper- or hypopigmentation, scarring, exacerbation of herpes simplex or bacterial infections, and hypertrichosis. Special care is needed to prevent dyspigmentation by using sunscreens with a high protection factor for some months.

Indications. Acne scarring, rhinophyma, congenital melanocytic nevus (in infancy), epidermal nevus, adenoma sebaceum, syringoma, lentigo, seborrheic keratosis, telangiectasia, Favre-Racouchot disease, scars, traumatic tattoos, decorative tattoos, superficial wrinkling (such as perioral), and amyloidosis.

In acne scars or accidental scars two or more abrasive treatments are often necessary for optimal results. Rhinophyma treatment often combines tangential excision for larger exophytic hypertrophies and dermabrasion for fine modeling of the nose. Large and giant congenital nevi cannot be completely excised by any operative technique. Dermabrasion will result in a good cosmetic removal of pigmentation if performed during the newborn period (Fig. 72.13). It has been suggested that the reduction in the amount of melanocytes and nevus nests following dermabrasion results in a lower lifetime risk of malignant transformation within the nevus.

Dermabrush

Dermabrush is used for prompt removal of superficial powder or dirt particles after an accident, such

Fig. 72.13 a, b. Giant congenital melanocytic nevus in a newborn. **a** Preoperative status. **b** Appearance after several dermabrasion procedures, now at age of 6 months

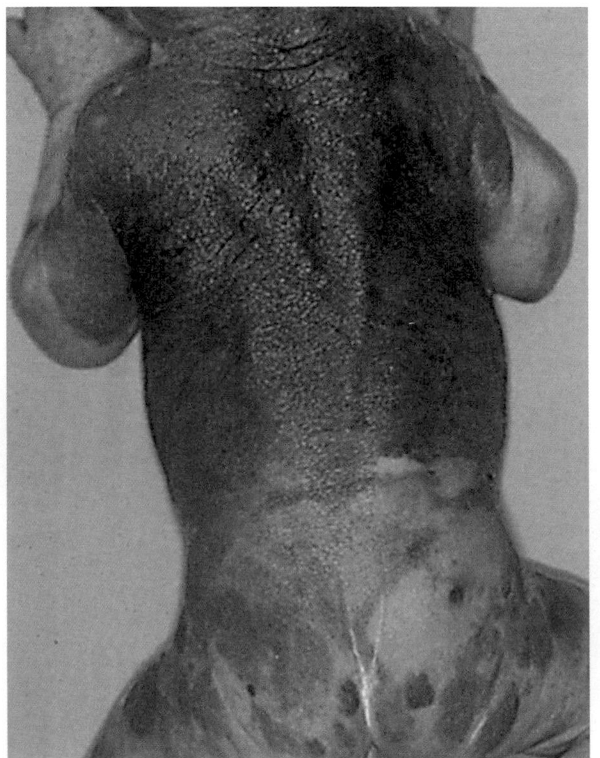

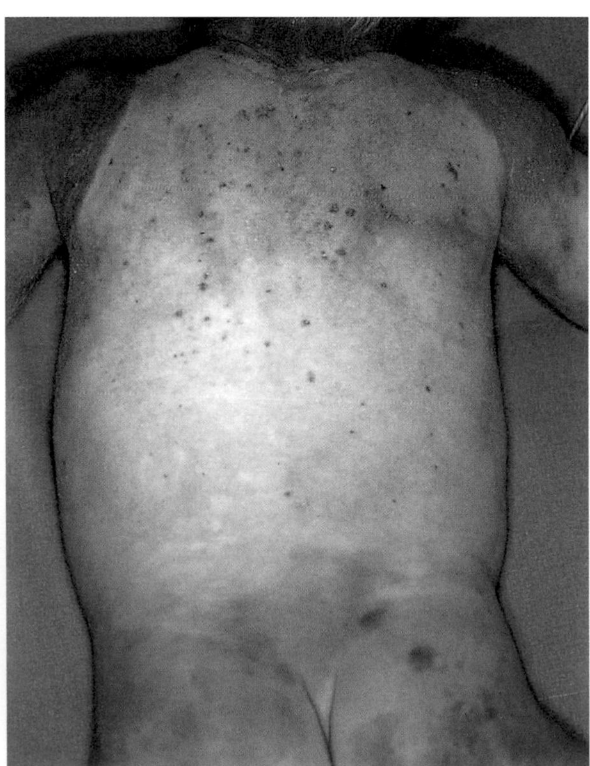

as misfire of a gun or explosion of a firecracker. Sterile toothbrushes and hand brushes are employed to perform the procedure. Both soft and hard brushes, made only out of nylon, should be used. Particles which are too deep to be reached with the brushes can be removed with a splinter forceps or excised with a small punch. The wound is rinsed with sterile saline and then the same dressings are applied as are used after dermabrasion.

Micrographic Excision Techniques

Principles. The fundamental principle of histographic controlled excision or micrographic surgery involves serial excision and microscopic study of tissue to identify malignant cells. All the modifications of the technique result in total ablation of the malignancy while sacrificing the least amount of uninvolved tissue.

Micrographic surgery is of significant value in the treatment of carcinomas of the centrofacial area, the periorbital region, and the auricles. Malignant epithelial tumors, especially basal cell carcinomas, invade in a surprisingly irregular and unpredictable manner, with a tendency to spread a great distance from the apparent clinical border. Basal cell carcinoma rarely invades cartilage of the nose or ear but tends to glide off and extend a considerable distance from its origin in a plane between cartilage and epidermis. The higher recurrence rate in special locations such as the auricular and retroauricular areas may have its origin in their embryologic development, and because these areas contain many different fusion planes and layers, the tumor may penetrate and disperse itself between the different planes. Cure rates for basal cell carcinomas are about 98% and 96% for primary and recurrent tumors, respectively.

Indications. Primary or recurrent basal cell carcinomas, Bowen disease, erythroplasia of Queyrat, squamous cell carcinoma, any malignant epithelial tumors with subcutaneous extensions, multicentric tumors, and tumors in areas where tissue needs to be conserved, such as the eyelids, the inner canthus, and the ala nasi.

Aggressive histopathologic types such as morphea-like, infiltrating and fibrotic basal cell carcinomas should be included in this high-risk group. Large tumors or those with poorly demarcated clinical borders represent additional indications for the use of micrographic surgery. Rare but useful indications are dermatofibrosarcoma protuberans, adnexal carcinoma and extramammary Paget disease.

Mohs Fixed Tissue Technique

Classical chemosurgery, or fixed tissue micrographic surgery, as originally developed by Frederick Mohs (Mohs and Guyer 1941) is rarely employed today. It is a modification of the technique of Schreus (Schreus 1950) for removing basal cell carcinomas with zinc chloride solution. Mohs' method involves fixation of tissue in situ without altering its architectural structure. The tumor is first debulked by a deep shave excision or curettage. Either dichloroacetic or trichloroacetic acid is then applied to increase tissue permeability, followed by 40% zinc chloride paste which is left on for 24 h. This paste is very painful. The tissue, fixed in vivo, is excised, carefully marked and examined histologically. If the tumor remains in certain areas of the excision, these areas are then refixed and excised until a tumor-free plane is obtained. The microscopic sections can be prepared as frozen sections or as permanent sections.

Mohs originally favored letting the resultant wound heal by secondary intention. The initial fear was that when treating high-risk tumors, a plastic closure would obscure the clinical evidence of a possible recurrence. The wound healing process was extremely long and the risk of recurrence turned out to be extremely low, so that almost all cases treated by this technique today are primarily repaired immediately.

Mohs Fresh Tissue Technique

Almost all Mohs surgery is performed today using frozen sections of fresh tissue. This eliminates the painful 24-h wait for zinc chloride fixation, allows multiple stages to be carried out on the same day, and produces a less-traumatized wound which can be more easily closed with a better aesthetic outcome. This refinement of Mohs technique using fresh tissue permits the same pinpoint precision to be achieved in eradication of skin cancer. The fresh-tissue technique was first employed when the chemosurgical procedure of Mohs was performed in the periorbital area, namely the medial canthus and the upper and lower lids. The tissue is excised under local anesthesia and without the use of chemicals. The application of this technique to other areas of the body was first described by TROMOVITCH and STEGMAN (1978).

The clinical extent of the tumor is first evaluated by gross examination. The area is anesthetized either regionally or locally. A curette may be used to debulk the tumor and remove any necrotic tissue. The essence of the technique is the removal of disc-shaped pieces of tissue. Thus the initial skin incision is performed at an angle of about 45° and then extended parallel to the skin surface at the base of the tumor. The excision specimen is removed, carefully mapped and then sectioned (Fig. 72.14). This is the crucial step. The first section must include the entire base and sides of the disc; in other words, the disc must be flattened at its base. The dermatologic surgeon interprets his own histologic sections. Careful mapping with multicolored tissue marking inks allows him to pinpoint any residual tumor at the side or base of the tumor site. Reexcision, if needed, is done using the same approach until the entire site is shown to be free of tumor. Finally, the sloping margins must be excised to allow a cosmetically acceptable wound closure.

Histographically Controlled Surgery

In Germany so-called histographically controlled surgery is widely used. It is a modification of Mohs technique and corresponds well with the aims and principles of Mohs micrographic technique. Generally, the excision is performed in a hospital or private office, and the specimen sent to a pathologist or dermatopathologist for interpretation, again using either frozen or fixed tissue sections. The tumor

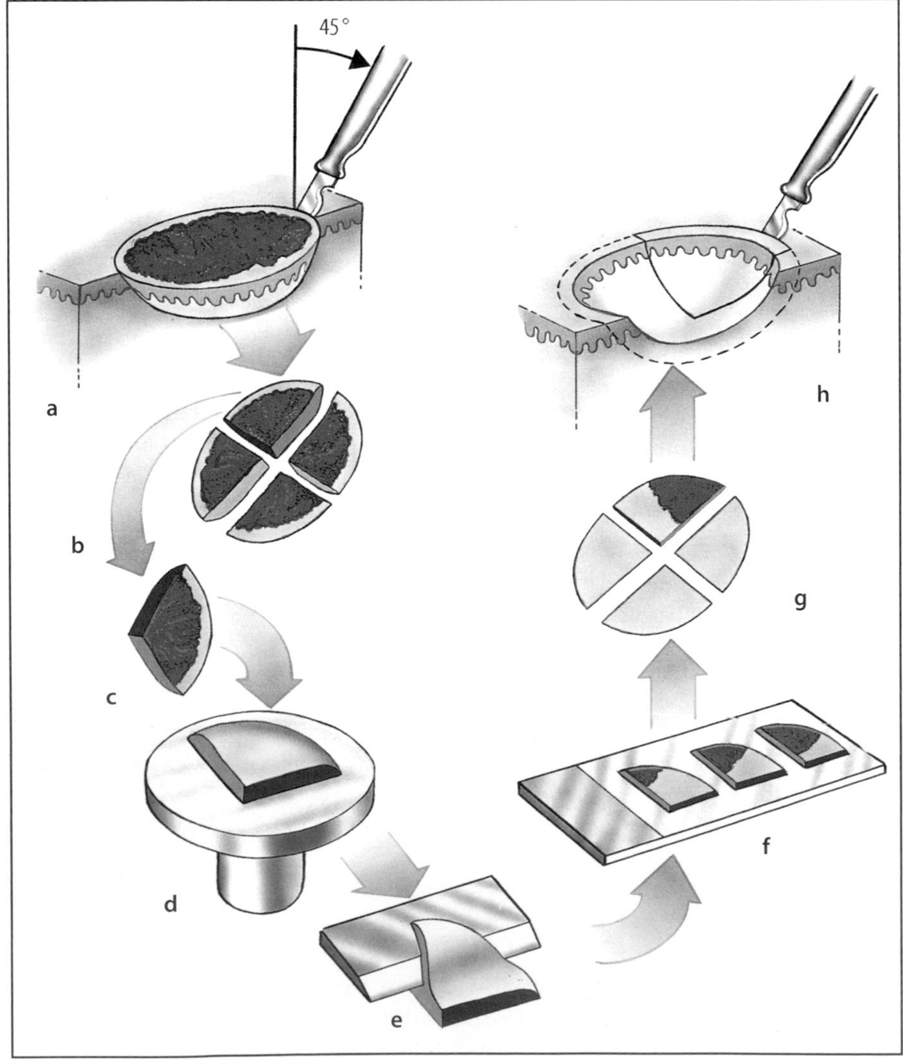

Fig. 72.14a–h. Mohs micrographic technique. **a** After debulking the tumor by curettage a thin disc of tissue is excised at an angle of 45° **b** The tissue is cut into sections and color-coded **c** The specimen is turned deep side up **d** Mounted specimen **e** Microtome **f** Histopathologic evaluation **g** Tumor-positive areas are noted on the scheme **h** Reexcision of the tumor-positive areas

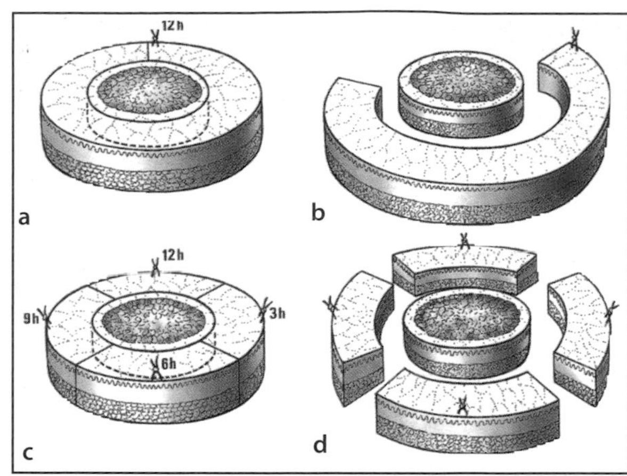

Fig. 72.15 a–d. Histographically controlled surgery. **a** Specimen marked at 12 h. **b** Circular border cut around the specimen. **c** Multiple points marked with sutures. **d** Multiple sections of the margins cut

is excised in the shape of a hockey puck or cake with vertical margins and color-coded or marked by sutures (Fig. 72.15). A strip is cut around the lateral periphery of the tumor and divided into conventionally sized pieces which are sectioned starting at the outer rim. In addition, a flat section is taken across the base of the tumor, and the central tumor is sectioned in routine fashion. During the time required for a histologic examination, the excision site is dressed temporarily, for example using polyurethane sheets. If tumor is found to extend to the margin of the excision, a further excision is performed in the involved areas. The process is repeated as often as needed to produce a tumor-free wound, which can then be closed using a variety of reconstructive procedures. Several other modifications of this method have been proposed, all resulting in complete three-dimensional tumor clearance.

Simple Excision and Repair Techniques

Elliptical Excision with Primary Closure

The defect created by a spindle-shaped or elliptical excision is closed by bringing the wound edges together with single or running skin sutures. The wound edges usually are easier to approximate accurately if subcutaneous stitches are first used. In some locations, accurate subcutaneous or intracutaneous butterfly stitches can be combined with superficial adhesive tapes, so that no skin sutures are needed. One should always attempt to create an optimal ellipse in order to prevent dog ears.

Elliptical Excision with Undermining

Larger elliptical excisions generally require undermining before closure can be attempted. The area adjacent to the wound is separated from its subcutaneous connections so that the skin moves freely over the fat (Fig. 72.16). Then the wound margins can be more easily approximated. Undermining allows a far more cosmetically acceptable wound to be produced that is less likely to stretch during the late stages of healing as the resorbable sutures weaken. The ellipse must be properly planned to lie along the relaxed skin tension lines and the undermining must be adequate. When undermining is optimally employed, relatively large defects can be successfully closed.

Modifications of Elliptical Excision

In the VY-plasty after a V-shaped excision of the lesion the tissue is undermined and then closed in a Y-shaped fashion. This flap is especially useful about orifices, such as around the mouth, eyes and female genitalia. Larger wedge-shaped excisions, such as of the lip, generally produce a long, vertical scar which is cosmetically unattractive. To improve the situation, one can perform an M- or W-shaped excision which, when closed, produces a Y-shaped scar which is shorter, more interrupted, and thus cosmetically more acceptable. The WY-plasty can be combined with a variety of other flap approaches to achieve the double goals of reducing the primary

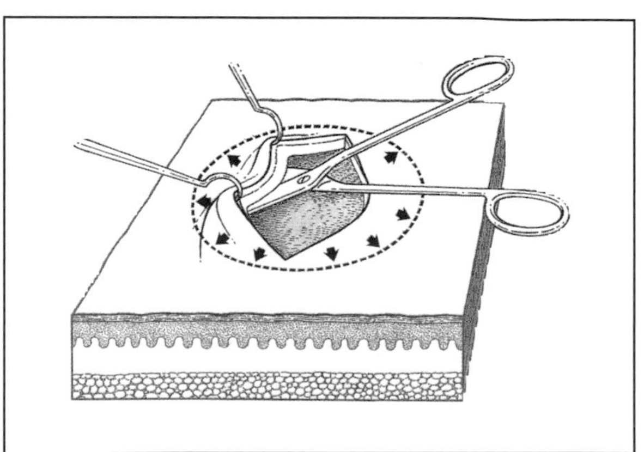

Fig. 72.16. Elliptical excision with undermining

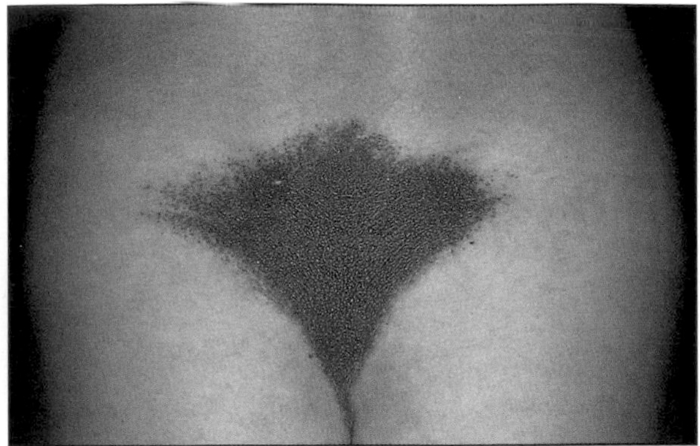
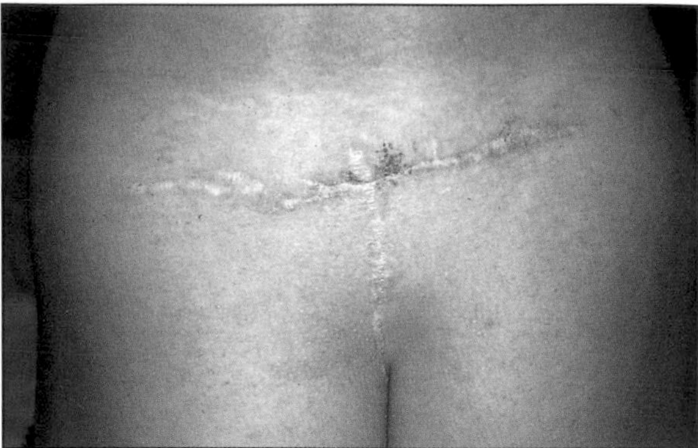

Fig. 72.17 a, b. Serial excision. a Large congenital nevus in the sacral region. b Appearance after four steps of serial excision

defect and avoiding lengthy uninterrupted scars. This WY-plasty is used commonly on the lower lip. The double WY-plasty is a combination of two M- or W-shaped excisions placed at opposite ends of the wound. They are each closed in a Y-shaped manner. This approach is employed in closing larger defects on the trunk, as well as on the back of the neck.

Serial Excision

Some benign skin lesions, for example congenital nevi and large cosmetic tattoos, sometimes cannot be removed in a single procedure with satisfactory cosmetic results. In such cases a partial excision or serial excision is performed. Part of the nevus is excised and the wound is closed and allowed to heal. After the skin has stretched (after about 9–12 months) another part of the wound including the old scar is excised. Closure is generally with undermining. The skin is very forgiving and amazingly large lesions can be removed with this approach (Fig. 72.17).

Dog Ear Repair

Occasionally after a wound is closed swellings or folds of tissue are created at one or both ends. These folds, called dog-ears, are usually the result of a wound which is too wide for its length, or the opposite sides are of unequal length. Dog ears are generally corrected by elevating the fold with a wound hook and then excising with a scalpel, lengthening the wound.

Excision of Cyst

Tiny cysts or milia can generally be removed by making a small incision in the overlying skin and simply squeezing the cyst out. Sutures are seldom necessary. With large cysts, one can excise a small ellipse to include the are of the central pore. It is important not to incise the cyst during this stage. Then the cyst is freed up by blunt dissection and removed. One can also remove smaller cysts by using a 3–5-mm punch to excise around the pore and then simply extrude the cyst wall and contents. An inflamed cyst is somewhat more difficult to handle. Often one must simply incise and drain the cyst to remove pus and infected cyst contents, treat the patient with antibiotics and await secondary wound healing. Such cysts tend to scar and often become reinfected, so that excision during a quiescent period is appropriate. Following an episode of inflammation, it is more difficult to extrude or pop out a cyst, so that one must usually perform a sharp surgical excision of the cyst and scarred surroundings.

Excision of Lipoma

Lipomas are generally simply to remove. A small incision is made over the tumor. It is then pressed from the sides and generally slides out through the incision. Sometimes the edges must be freed with blunt dissection. After closing the cavity with subcutaneous sutures, the skin edges are under little tension so that butterfly tapes generally are sufficient. Some lipomas lie within the subcutaneous muscles, such as over the masseters and zygomatic arch or along the rib cage, or under the muscle fascia, as on the forehead. Once one reaches the fascia, it should be separated with an incision parallel to the direction of the muscle fibers. The muscles themselves are generally separated by blunt dissection until the lipoma becomes apparent. It is then freed up by blunt technique.

Plastic Procedures

Local and Regional Flaps

Definition and Principle. When a defect cannot be closed using simple closure techniques, with or without undermining, some sort of plastic surgical repair must be undertaken. In most cases, tissue is moved about locally, generally in the form of a flap or advancement procedure. In a few cases, it is more appropriate to transfer tissue from a distant site, creating a graft. Flaps and grafts are most frequently used in repairing the defects created by the histographically controlled removal of skin cancers.

Flaps provide a multitude of ways to ideally close a wound achieving good cosmetic results with minimum risk for the patient. These are especially effective in the head and neck region. Here the donor and recipient areas, when considered as anatomic or aesthetic units, are generally quite good matches, so that a satisfactory cosmetic result is achieved more easily. Local flaps can be classified in terms of the blood supply and the major movement of the tissue. The pattern of blood supply distinguishes: (a) random pattern flaps with a randomized supply by the dermoepidermal vascular plexus, and (b) axial pattern flaps which have a specific vascular supply along the major axis of the flap. The latter can therefore have a higher length to width ratio. The major ways of moving tissue can be: (a) advancement flaps, (b) rotation flaps, and (c) transposition flaps (Fig. 72.18). Many variants of one of these basic types are known, and they have more or less one major pattern of blood supply or even mixed vascular supply.

Planning the Flap. An important point for planning the flap is that in general the longest incision should lie in one of the relaxed skin tension lines or preformed natural folds. In deciding which type of flap to use, the following factors must be weighed:

- The form of the surgical defect and the direction of the skin lines: Depending on the age of the patient, the incision is oriented along either the wrinkle lines or the lines of skin tension.
- Matching the skin texture and color according to the aesthetic units: The preferred technique is that which allows one to fill the defect with skin most closely matching the recipient site.
- Vascular supply: One should consider the regional variations in vascularity to minimize flap necrosis.
- Hair: When hair-bearing skin is moved, one must be aware of the consequences, being aware of the direction of hair growth, and where hairs are wished or to be avoided.

Fig. 72.18 a–c. Basic local flaps. **a** Advancement flap. **b** Rotation flap. **c** Transposition flap

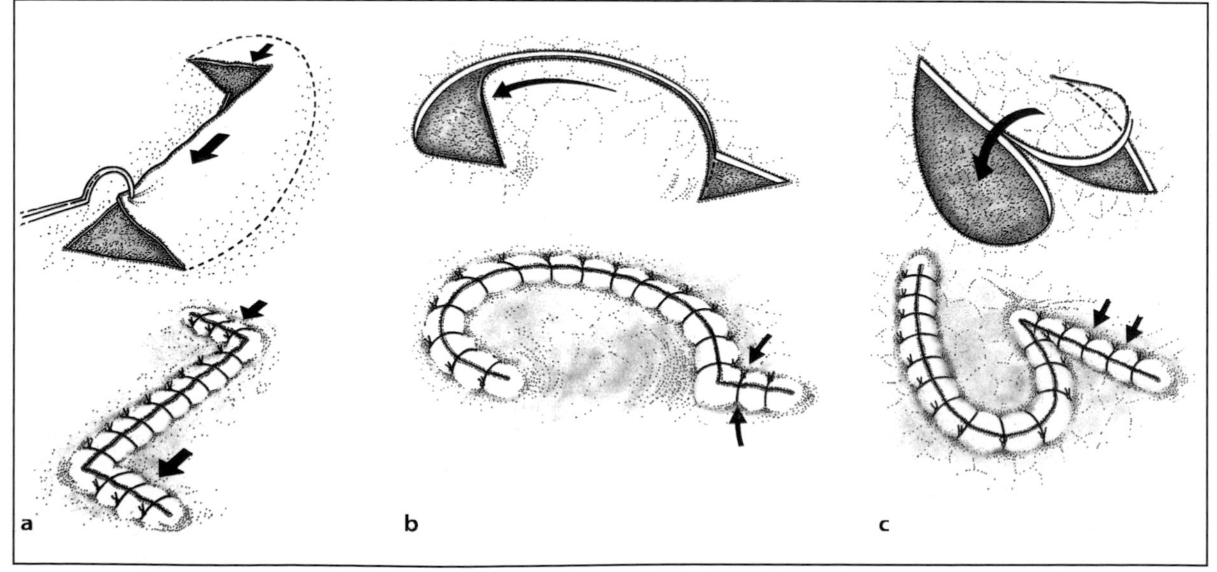

- Natural lines: Every effort should be made to place the major scar in a natural fold, such as the nasolabial fold, forehead wrinkle, or anterior to the ear, where it will be much less noticeable.

Advancement Flap

The lesion is excised in the shape of an equilateral triangle. Then one arm of the triangle is extended laterally, and a Burow triangle is excised on the contralateral side of the extension. After undermining the area between the main defect and the Burow triangle, the tissue can be advanced and the wound closed under relatively little tension.

A-to-T Flap

In a bidirectional advancement flap, the excision is extended in both directions along one side of the triangle, but then closed just as described above. This so-called A-to-T flap is most often used on the head and neck, as well as the trunk, when the incisions can be placed in tension or fold lines, or along natural anatomic boundaries to maximize the cosmetic result.

U-plasty, H-plasty

The U-plasty is variant of a Burow advancement flap. The defect is excised in a square or rectangular fashion and then the incision extended in the same direction on two opposing parallel sides of the defect. At the end of each extension, a small Burow triangle must be created. Then one frees up the U-shaped flap and undermines the adjacent tissue with special attention to the base of the flap, and moves the flap into the defect. U-plasty most commonly is used at the back of the nose, along the eyebrows, and lips. The H-plasty is actually a double U-plasty, or double advancement flap. It is especially effective on the forehead and when closing defects of the eyebrows. Two U-plasty flaps are created as mirror images of one another. Both the U-plasty and the H-plasty have mainly an axial pattern blood supply.

Rotation Flap

The rotation flap is a modification of Burow advancement flap as developed by Imre (1928). The incision is extended along the short edge of the triangular defect in a curved fashion, once again using Burow triangles on the contralateral side to allow further motion. After undermining and mobilisation, the flap is rotated into the primary defect. Areas in which the rotation flap works particularly well include the scalp, face, lateral neck and trunk.

Rotation or Advancement Flap with Back Cut

This flap is also known as an ax flap or a J-shaped rotation flap. By introducing an incision at the back end of an ordinary rotation or advancement flap, one can often avoid the use of a Burow triangle. This technique has two major advantages. First, there is a sparing of tissue since the triangles are not sacrificed. Second, the flap is significantly easier to move, since the back cut is placed in the direction in which the flap rotates.

Double Rotation Flap

Large round or oval defects can be effectively closed with this approach. Starting at two points which lie directly opposite each other on the wound edges, one creates two curved incisions going in opposite directions. The two flaps are rotated past each other (O-to-Z flap). Generally, one or more Burow triangles are needed to facilitate adapting the wound edges. This flap is commonly used on the scalp and trunk. In selected regions, such as the chin and the forehead, it is sometimes difficult to close larger triangular defects with a simple rotation flap. In such cases, a double rotation flap may be successful, placed on both sides of the base of the triangle (O-to-T flap). Undermining and closure is identical to that for a simple rotation flap.

Transposition Flap

The basic concept of a transposition flap or lobed flap is to cover a drop-shaped defect with a similar smaller drop-shaped flap. The flap is taken from nearby tissue and after appropriate undermining moved over the intervening normal tissue into the defect. The source of the flap is closed primarily. In planning the operation, particular attention should be payed to the lines of tension. In addition, the ratio between the length and breadth of the flap should be about 4:1. This relatively simple flap produces good results in the mid-facial region, around the ear and on the neck and trunk. It is most often used on the ala nasi where it is crucial to thin the flap by removing the subcutaneous fat. If this is not done, because of fear of flap necrosis, an irregular-

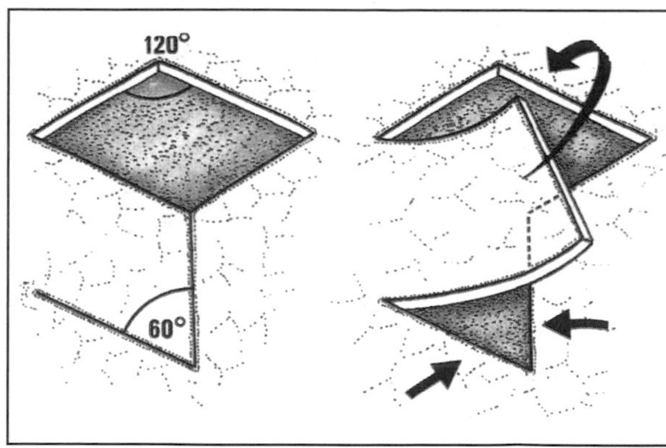

Fig. 72.19. Rhomboid flap

ly raised result on the nose, the so-called trap-door effect, is produced.

Bilobed Flap

This flap is similar to the transposition or lobed flap, but two successively smaller lobed flaps are created to close a defect. A flap is raised to cover the original defect, and then a second smaller flap is created to repair the defect left by the first flap. The defect left by the second flap is closed primarily. Both flaps share a common base.

Rhomboid Transposition Flaps

These two modifications of the transposition flap differ only slightly between themselves. They are used to close a round or oval defect. A rhomboid flap is created in the adjacent tissue. In the Limberg technique (LIMBERG 1966) the tip should have an angle of 50–60° (Fig. 72.19). In the Dufourmentel technique a modified angle is used. After undermining the flap and adjacent skin, the triangle is moved into the defect and the flap defect closed primarily (DUFOURMENTEL 1971). Both of these flaps can be used in closing small and large defects at almost any site.

Subcutaneous Pedicle Flap

This relatively new closure is created by completely separating a flap from the adjacent skin but leaving it attached to a subcutaneous pedicle (sliding flap). The flap is nourished solely through this subcutaneous connection (Fig. 72.20). The preparation of the subcutaneous pedicle is a delicate task. If the pedicle is too thick, the flap will not have the needed motility; if it is too thin, vascular supply will be inadequate, leading to necrosis. Because the flap can be cut to an exact size, it produces excellent cosmetic results, in the face as well as on the trunk and extremities. Sometimes, double pedicle flaps are employed to close larger wounds, moving one flap from each of two opposite sides to cover the defect.

Island or Tunnel Flap

This intriguing flap resembles the lobed flap, but the pedicle of the flap with its subcutaneous vascular supply is developed at a distance from the wound edge and tunneled under the normal skin into the defect (Fig. 72.21). If carefully prepared, the pedicle can be rotated by as much as 180° without producing necrosis. This flap is most often used around the nose, with the flap raised either on the forehead or in the nasolabial region.

Forehead Flap with Vascular Pedicle

This procedure involves a modified transposition flap that can be used to cover larger defects in the midfacial region. The flap is based on a specific axial vascular supply, i.e. the flap has only a temporary

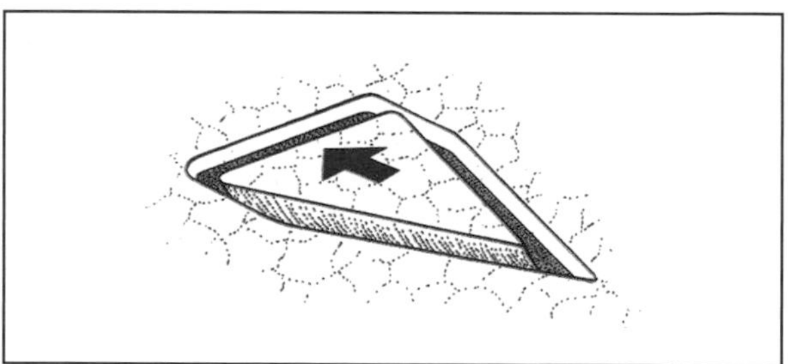

Fig. 72.20. Subcutaneous pedicle flap (sliding flap)

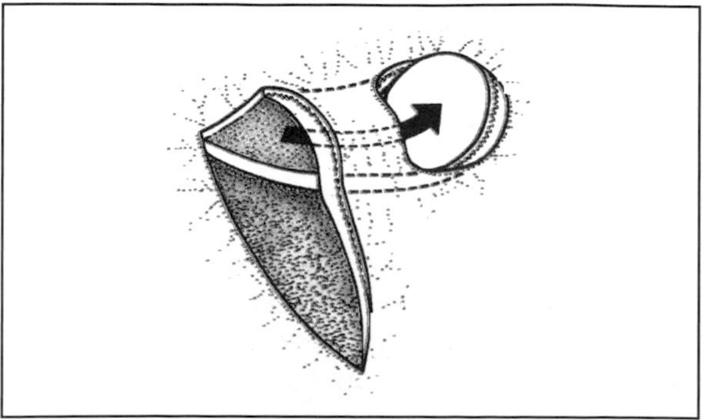

Fig. 72.21. Island or tunnel flap

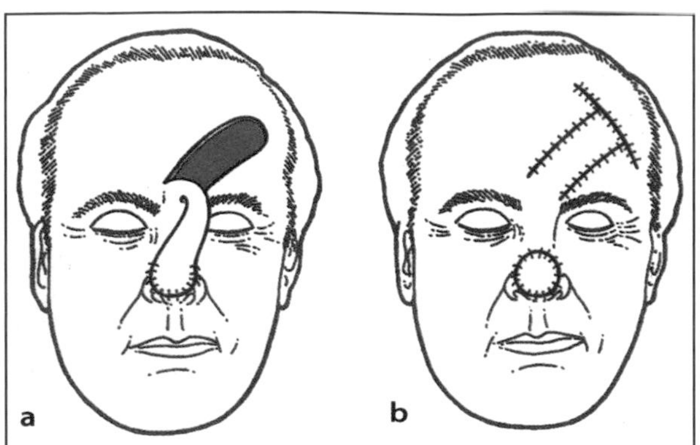

Fig. 72.22 a, b. Forehead flap. a Transposition of the flap to cover the defect of the nasal tip. b After 2 weeks the pedicle of the flap is returned to the donor site

pedicle (Fig. 72.22). It is placed in the midline or mediolaterally with its base at the glabella. Because the vascular supply is so critical, the vessels should be localized preoperatively using Doppler ultrasound. The flap can be rotated up to 180° because of its excellent vascularity. The operation is performed in two parts. In the first, the flap is developed and sewn into the defect. Then, after 2–3 weeks, the stem of the flap is divided and repositioned. At the same time, the transplanted flap must often be trimmed or remodeled. The donor defect created by the flap is generally closed primarily after undermining, or by a local flap or a free skin graft. The temporal flap with vascular pedicle is a similar procedure in which forehead skin serviced by the temporal artery and vein is used to cover a more central defect.

Other Two-Stage Flaps

The same principles can be employed in other anatomic regions. For example, a flap can be raised in the nasolabial area to repair a defect in the ala nasi. On the ear, pre- or retroauricular flaps can be used to cover defects in the concha or helix. The stalk of the flap is separated after about 14 days and either discarded or used to help close the donor site.

Advanced Flaps

A variety of more complicated flaps can be used to produce very acceptable cosmetic results in difficult situations. Included in this group are tubed flaps, myocutaneous flaps and microvascularized flaps. They all allow the surgeon to repair large and deep defects with tissue from a distant site. In general these flaps are beyond the needs and the capabilities of the dermatologist; they are best left to the plastic surgeon, ENT surgeon, and facial reconstructive surgeon.

Tissue Expansion

Definition. The aim of tissue expansion is to produce an artificial donor area close to a certain lesion by insertion of a pouch that will be filled over time and thereby expand the area.

Technique. In the first step, the tissue expander pouch is implanted in the vicinity of a lesion which is to be excised. The pouch is usually made of silicone or another material which elicits little tissue reaction. The expander is inflated initially with normal saline through a valve. Several instillations of normal saline are done in intervals of 8–12 days over a 6–8-week period. The skin expands and grows over the expander. Each instillation is made until the overlying tissue is compressed to produce mild ischemia. The skin gained by this technique is then used to close the defect (Fig. 72.23). Often a tissue expander is the only way by which the use of a skin graft in an area where such a procedure promises to be difficult or cosmetically compromising can be avoided. If the expander is too aggressively inflated, the vascular supply of the skin can be severely compromised and necrosis may occur.

Indications. Tissue expansion is indicated particularly in the removal of large benign lesions such as congenital nevi and scars, as well as in scalp reduction surgery for scarring alopecia. It is also commonly used in treating skin with chronic radiation damage. Tissue expanders are more difficult to use in infants and small children, because the pressure created by the expanded pouch may press upon and damage the underlying bone at the same time that it is stretching the skin.

Modifications. Immediate intraoperative tissue expansion uses the skin's ability to immediately stretch and increase in surface area; it thus represents a modification of the conventional technique. The expander is placed in a one-stage procedure and undergoes three or four expansion cycles before it is removed and the stretched skin used for reconstruction. The gain of additional tissue is much less than with the conventional tissue expansion technique.

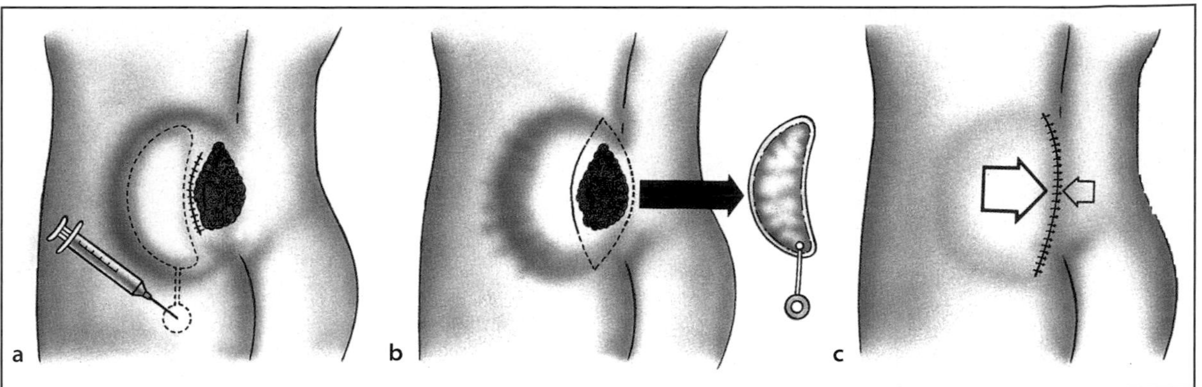

Fig. 72.23 a–c. Technique for use of the tissue expander. a The expander is inserted adjacent to the lesion, and the device is periodically expanded by injection of sterile saline through the subcutaneous valve. b Removal of the lesion and the expander. c The lateral skin reservoir created by the expander is used to close the defect

Grafts and Transfers

Definition. Autologous transfer of full-thickness or split-thickness skin from a donor site to a distant recipient region. The graft contains no vascular pedicle and healing is dependent on diffusion and ingrowing vessels.

Principle. Grafts are employed when simple wound closure or a local flap is impossible or is unlikely to produce satisfactory results. Free skin grafts require a healthy recipient site. It is preferable to precondition the graft site by covering it with polyurethane foam dressings for 8–14 days while dressings are changed every 1–2 days. This is called wound conditioning. Using this approach one creates a site composed of firm and vascularized granulation tissue which increases the likelihood of a successful graft. The postoperative dressing is also crucial. This must be designed to produce a gentle and uniform pressure across the entire graft to provide maximal contact between the transplanted tissue and its new vascular supply. When free grafts are used on the extremities, especially near joints, we prefer immobilization with a splint or cast for 7–10 days.

Split-Thickness Graft

Split-thickness grafts consist of epidermis and the superficial part of the dermis, thus containing few if any skin appendageal structures. The grafts are classified as thin (up to 0.3 mm), medium (0.4–0.5 mm), and thick (about 0.6 mm). One can harvest split skin grafts either with a manual device or with a motor driven electric dermatome. The latter is preferable because it produces a more uniform graft. The dermatome can be adjusted to produce grafts of thicknesses from 0.1 to 2.0 mm in steps of 0.05 mm and widths up to 8 cm. The graft is then cut somewhat generously based on the pattern made from the recipient site and sewed in under slight tension with resorbable sutures (Fig. 72.24). Alternatively, metal clips or tissue glue can be employed. Split-thickness grafts should preferably be taken from the thigh or buttocks. Generally the donor site heals spontaneously with minimal scarring.

The great advantage of split-thickness skin grafts is that they are more easily maintained so that necrosis is relatively unlikely. A disadvantage is the approximately 20% rate of shrinkage, which will occur even if the donor site is immobilized and the graft takes rapidly. In addition, split-thickness skin grafts are easily traumatized, so that they cannot be used in weight-bearing areas (soles) or when much manual pressure is expected (palms). Split-thickness skin grafts are rarely successful on the face, for the match in skin texture and color between the donor and recipient sites is usually cosmetically inferior. On the other hand, split-thickness skin grafts are ideal to cover leg ulcers and larger defects on the trunk and extremities, especially after the recipient site has been appropriately conditioned.

Mesh Graft

The meshing produces a donor graft capable of covering much larger areas than a simple split-

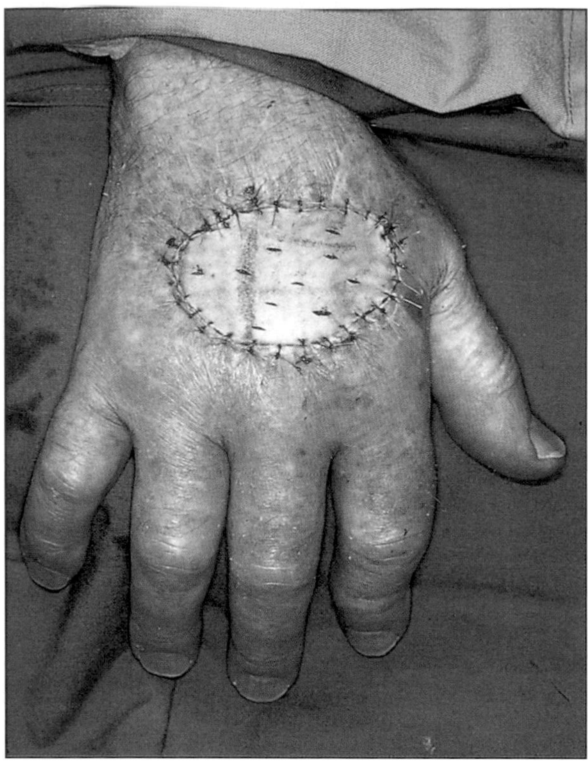

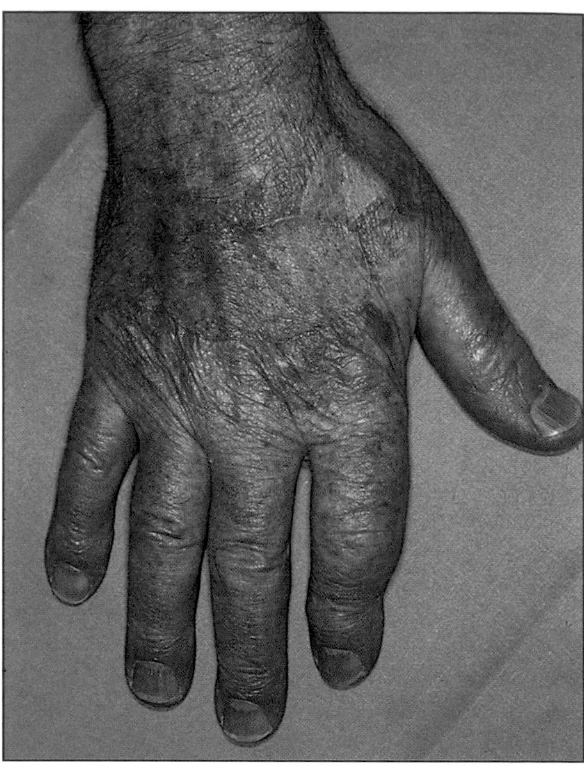

Fig. 72.24a, b. Split-thickness skin graft. **a** Graft sewn in place, after excision of a squamous cell carcinoma. **b** Appearance after 9 months

thickness graft (Fig. 72.25). This procedure has made possible the dramatic coverage often achieved in severely burned patients, but it has many other applications as well. After the mesh graft is applied, areas that are not covered reepithelialize by seeding from the graft.

A special instrument, the so-called skin graft mesher, is needed to cut mesh grafts. Initially a split-thickness graft is harvested and placed on a hard plastic sheet with a pattern for cutting a mesh. Then the skin and plastic sheeting are rolled through a cutting device to cut the pattern out. The skin graft mesher cuts the skin graft into a geometrically defined form, while the expansion ratio is predetermined by the plastic skin carriers (e.g. 1:1.5, 1:3, 1:6). Then the graft is tacked with resorbable sutures and dressed just like a split-thickness graft. The main advantage is that wide areas can be covered. Mesh grafts can only be used where cosmetic results are unimportant but rapid coverage is crucial, such as with large wounds on the trunk and extremities.

Full-Thickness Skin Graft

Full-thickness or whole-skin grafts contain the epidermis and entire dermis with appendages, extending down to the subcutaneous fat. Thus the donor site does not heal primarily but must be closed with a primary suture. The two main advantages of full-thickness grafts are that they do not shrink and can be used on weight- or pressure-bearing surfaces. They take longer to become vascularized and are more likely to undergo necrosis and failure, especially if there is bleeding from the recipient bed. Full-thickness grafts work best over flat bony surfaces and over firm, not too curved areas such as the skull, forehead, temples, and extremities.

Performing a full-thickness graft requires a careful operative technique. The recipient site should be well vascularized, but absolute hemostasis must be achieved. Preferable donor sites for full-thickness skin grafts are the retroauricular region or the medial surface of the upper arm. These donor sites have the advantage of not having been exposed to the sun, so that actinic damage is minimal. Other possible donor sites are the preauricular, supraclavicular or inguinal region. The nasolabial fold or the upper lid may serve as a

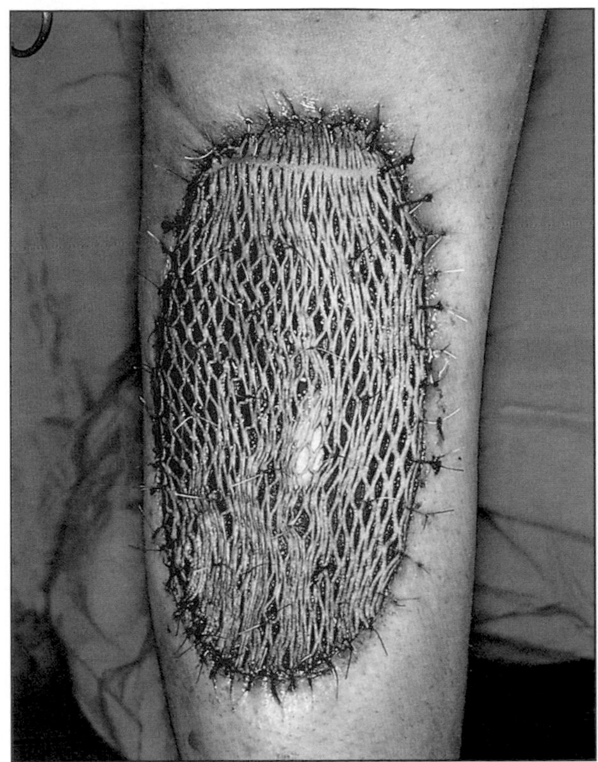

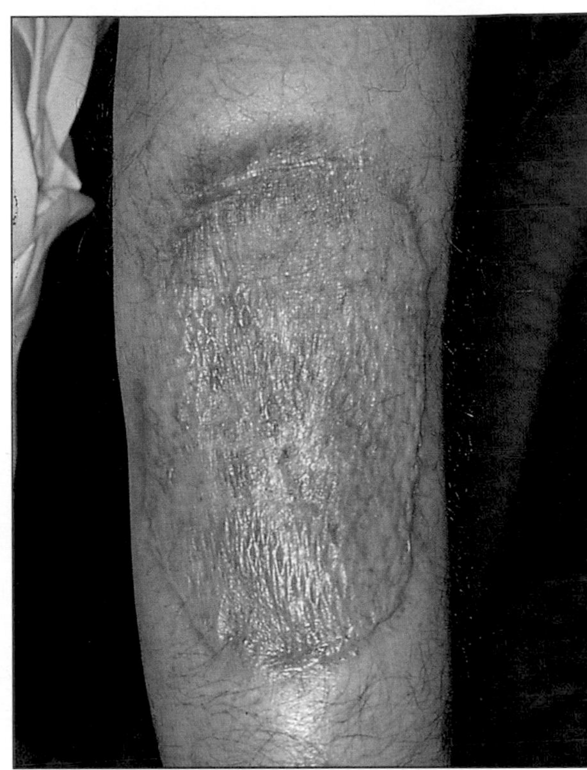

Fig. 72.25 a, b. Mesh graft. **a** Mesh graft to cover a large defect of a previously excised leiomyosarcoma of the lower leg. **b** Appearance after 10 months

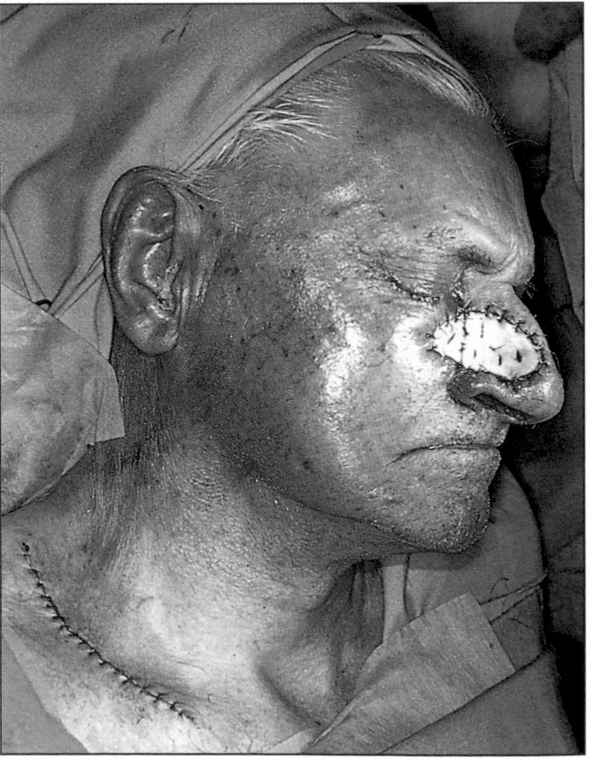

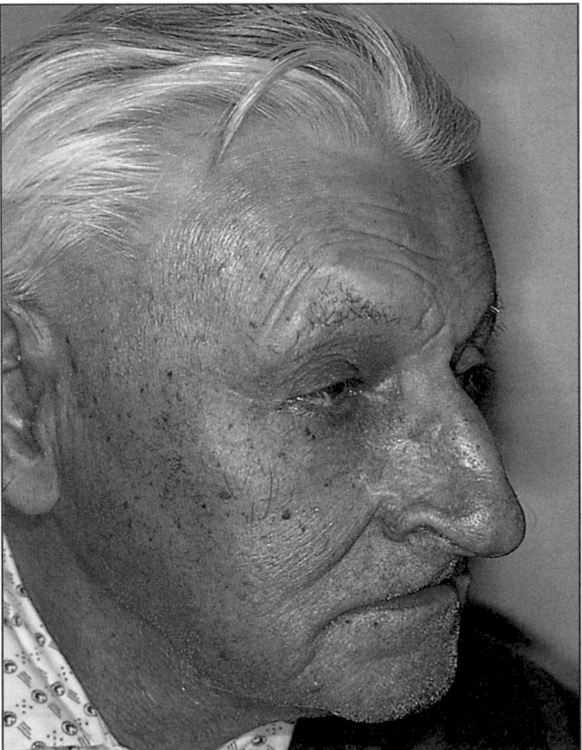

Fig. 72.26 a, b. Full-thickness skin graft. **a** After excision of a basal cell carcinoma of the nose the graft is harvested from the supraclavicular region. **b** Appearance after 6 months

donor site in cases where the graft must achieve high aesthetic similarity to the region of the recipient site. The graft is excised free-handedly with a scalpel, usually based on a pattern from the recipient site. The graft must be defatted and then is fixed in place under slight tension, using 5-0 or 6-0 sutures (Fig. 72.26). Sometimes it is helpful to place a few stitches in the center of the graft to improve fixation. Fibrin glues also improve fixation but can theoretically interfere with the diffusion of nutrients into the graft.

Composite Graft

Composite grafts contain two different tissues. The only composite graft commonly used in dermatologic surgery contains skin and cartilage. They are used to reconstruct the nose, ears and occasionally to repair lid damage. The donor sites are the ear for repairing the nose or the contralateral ear, and the healthy eyelid for repair of the contralateral eyelid. The composite graft is generally excised in a wedge-shaped form so that the defect can be closed in a primary fashion. Composite grafts are even more sensitive to vascular problems than full-thickness grafts. Minimal seepage can lead to necrosis, while a far longer period of time is needed for the cartilage to become vascularized.

Fat Transplantation

Technique. Fat can be relatively easily transferred to fill in defects. We use fat transplantation to treat conditions where there is a loss of skin volume such as in hemifacial atrophy and sunken scars following orthopedic procedures. The fat can be obtained by liposuction or simple excision, using the buttocks or abdomen as a donor site. Using a syringe the fat tissue is gently inserted into the subcutaneous recipient area. If necrosis of the fat transplant occurs, the final result may be compromising.

Electrosurgery

Definition and Principles. There are two basic types of electrosurgery: electrocautery and high-frequency electrosurgery. Electrocautery, or cautery, involves the use of a hot instrument to damage tissue. No electric current enters the patient, and the procedure is therefore safe for patients with pacemakers. Small battery-operated ophthalmologic units are currently in use for hemostasis. In addition, the Shaw scalpel is available for cautery cutting. All other electrosurgery involves high-frequency alternating current and must be used with a large neutral grounding electrode. The tip of the instrument is "cold", but the electric current delivered to the tissue encounters resistance, producing heat and tissue damage. The patient must be carefully positioned on the table so that there is no contact with metal table parts or anesthesia equipment. The presence of a pacemaker is a relative contraindication to high-frequency electrosurgery. There are four types of high-frequency electrosurgery: electrosection or electrocutting, electrocoagulation, electrodesiccation and electrofulguration (Table 72.5).

Electrosection or Electrocutting

Electrosection or electrocutting uses a high-voltage, high-amperage current to separate tissue. Since a pure cutting current provides almost no hemostasis, most devices produce a blend of cutting and coagulation current. Fine-needle or wire loop electrodes or very thin blade electrodes are used to produce a fine incision with minimal damage to ad-

Table 72.5. Electrosurgery

	Tip	Current	Mono- or biterminal	Tissue touched	Degree of damage
Electrocautery	Hot	Direct	Mono	+	++++
Electrocutting	Cold	Alternating HF	Bi	+	++++
Electrocoagulation	Cold	Alternating HF	Bi	+	+++
Electrodesiccation	Cold	Alternating HF	Mono	+	+
Electrofulguration	Cold	Alternating HF	Mono	–	+

HF, high frequency

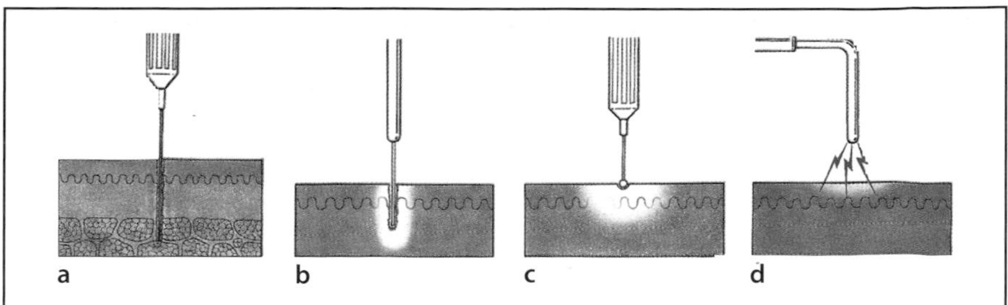

Fig. 72.27 a–d. Types of electrosurgery
a Electrosection or electrocutting
b Electrocoagulation
c Electrodesiccation
d Electrofulguration

jacent tissues (Fig. 72.27). The blade electrodes tend to produce too much heat. Since tissues handled with electrocutting have delayed healing, it is often wise to incise the skin with a scalpel and then switch to electrosection for the deeper, bloodier surgery, such as in the removal of a large tumor. When electrocutting is used to perform shave excisions of seborrheic keratosis or warts, one must be careful not to cut deep into the dermis as this produces unsatisfactory scars. Wire loop or sling electrocutting is frequently used to treat perianal condylomata. Because of the large amount of current used, particular attention must be paid to properly grounding the patient.

Electrocoagulation

Electrocoagulation uses a low-voltage, high-amperage bipolar current to thermally damage relatively deep tissue, especially vessels. One can employ bipolar forceps when coagulating vessels or clamp the bleeding vessel with a forceps which is then touched with the electrocoagulation needle. This technique works poorly with electrodesiccation/electrofulguration devices. The higher energy of electrocoagulation is more effective when working in a bloody field. A variety of active electrodes are available including needles, ball-shaped electrodes and flat blades. One must be sure to keep the electrode clean because a crust formed of blood and tissue fragments interferes with the transfer of current, leading to the formation of sparks.

Electrodesiccation

Electrodesiccation and electrofulguration differ only in degree. Both involve a monoterminal active electrode which transfers current to the skin where it is converted into heat. The low energy involved limits tissue damage. In electrodesiccation the electrode, usually a needle or ball-shaped electrode, comes into contact with the tissue. Disposable needles are available as well as adaptors to allow the use of metal hypodermic needles. In North America, electrodesiccation is often combined with curettage in the treatment of seborrheic keratoses, verrucae, molluscum contagiosum, actinic keratoses, small basal cell carcinomas, and occasionally other tumors. When basal cell carcinomas are treated, three cycles of curettage and electrodesiccation (or electrofulguration) are traditionally performed. The disadvantages of this technique are a lack of histologic control of the surgical margins and unsatisfactory scarring. Small vascular lesions, skin tags and other tiny lesions may also be treated effectively.

Electrofulguration

Here the electrode does not come into contact with the skin; instead high-energy sparks jump from the electrode to burn the tissue. Otherwise it is identical to electrodesiccation. In fact, most physicians employ both techniques in any given case, sometimes touching the tissue and sometimes letting a spark jump. Electrofulguration is slightly less easy to control precisely and produces even more superficial damage.

Cryotherapy

Principles of Cryobiology. The destruction of tissue through cold is a complex, poorly understood phenomenon. Water clearly plays a central role. As ice crystals are formed, the electrolyte concentration within the cell changes, and the membrane structure is altered. Both the rate of freezing and the rate of thawing contribute to the degree of tissue damage. When freezing is very rapid, crystals form both within and outside the cells simultaneously; this phenomenon is known as homogeneous nucleation. It results in collapsed dehydrated cells with a toxic increase of electrolyte concentrations. As the tissue is allowed slowly to thaw, multiple cycles of crystal formation and destruction occur, coupled with electrolyte changes, which all combine to cause cell death. Since not all cells die after the first freeze-thaw cycle, it is generally repeated.

The practical requirements for effective cell killing by cryotherapy are: (a) rapid freezing at a rate greater than 100 °C/min, (b) tissue temperature below –25 °C, (c) slow thawing at a rate of 10 °C/min or less, (d) two freeze-thaw cycles.

Indications. Actinic keratosis, verruca, keloid, granuloma annulare, hemangioma, keratoacanthoma, Bowen disease, basal cell carcinoma, squamous cell carcinoma, Kaposi sarcoma (early lesions), cutaneous metastases from malignant melanoma (palliative).

Cryotherapy is the treatment of choice in most cases of verrucae and actinic keratoses. The cryotherapy of cutaneous malignancies must be regarded as an alternative method, since surgical excision provides histologic control and a more rapidly healing wound. In addition, cryotherapy of tumors requires additional surgical experience and specialized equipment. Larger benign lesions such as keloids and hemangiomas usually heal with unsatisfactory scars. Granuloma annulare responds to many types of minor trauma including light freezing. The early flat lesions of Kaposi sarcoma in AIDS can often be most simply treated with cryotherapy.

Contraindications. Sclerosing basal cell carcinoma, scalp tumors, tumors of the nasal region in young patients, invasive and larger tumors of the periorbital region, invasive tumors of the external ear, connective tissue disorders, Raynaud syndrome or disease, cold urticaria, cryoglobulinemia.

Techniques

Both carbon dioxide ice (–78.9 °C) and liquid nitrous oxide (–89.7 °C) have been used in the past for cryotherapy, but they fail to achieve a sufficiently rapid freezing rate and are no longer used. Liquid nitrogen with a temperature of –195.8 °C has become the standard agent. While only one product is widely used, a multitude of devices are available to deliver it to the skin surface. The traditional method of dipping a cotton-tipped applicator in a cup of liquid nitrogen and then applying it rapidly to the skin is generally inadequate. Too little liquid is transferred, and freezing is therefore slow and superficial. This traditional technique is only applicable for small verrucae or similar lesions. One must choose between a spray device or contact probes or sounds. Spray units freeze the tumor rapidly, even when it has an irregular surface in which case a probe is ineffective. We rarely use copper sounds and then only in treating mucosal lesions, such as in the mouth or vagina.

One must have a biopsy diagnosis prior to embarking on the case. The dermatopathologist should measure the tumor depth. After completing a procedure and allowing healing to occur, a second biopsy as a follow-up confirms that a cure has been obtained. Thermal probes placed at the base help to assure that an adequate killing temperature has been achieved throughout the tumor. However, their placement is difficult to standardize. With spray devices, a temperature of –40 °C can be obtained to a depth of about 12 mm; contact freezing achieves this temperature only at a depth of about 4 mm.

The necessary rapid rate of freezing (100°C/min) is best obtained with the open spray technique. Initially one sprays continuously until a white pearly surface is obtained. Thereafter intermittent spraying is sufficient to maintain the effect for the duration of the freezing time. We freeze actinic keratoses for 1–2×15–20 s (Fig. 72.28); basal cell carcinomas require 2×40–60 s. These recommendations are not absolute; they must be adjusted depending on the size and depth of the tumor and on individual differences. Sometimes, a third freeze-thaw cycle is needed.

The neighboring tissue can be protected by forms or molds. These are needed only when critical structures such as the eye must be shielded. Otherwise it is sufficient to freeze with the open spray technique up to marked borders. This leads to the border of the scar being more diffuse, rather than sharply delineated by the form.

Tissue Reactions

The above methods allow a relatively exact application of cryogen with a predictable tissue damage

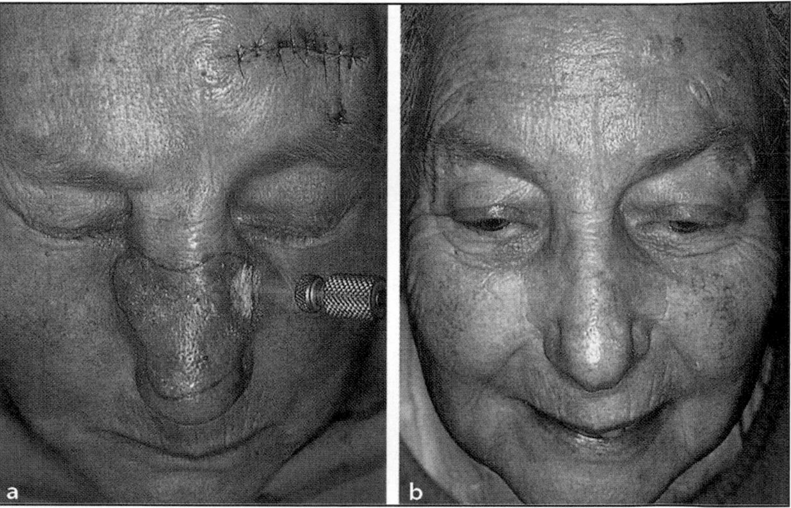

Fig. 72.28 a, b. Cryotherapy using the liquid nitrogen spray. **a** Large actinic keratosis at the back of the nose. **b** Appearance after 1 year

ranging from a blister healing without a scar to total tissue destruction with scarring. Short superficial freezing produces a subepidermal blister. This allows actinic keratoses to be removed with excellent, almost scar-free cosmetic results. Necrosis and loss of tissue are the goals in treating a basal cell carcinoma; here a scar is inevitable. Multiple freeze-thaw cycles are employed to protect adjacent and deeper structures. In granulomatous skin diseases, lymphocytic infiltrates, and keloids, the goal is to influence the tissue reaction without producing necrosis. The mechanism of this is unclear. Freezing can also be combined effectively with intralesional injection of corticosteroids.

The healing process following cryotherapy usually entails the following stages: (1) erythema, (2) edema, (3) blister and exudate, (4) crust and scale, and (5) scar. The time sequence is highly variable depending on the patient, site, and characteristics of the cryotherapy. The healing process following cryotherapy is far longer than following cold steel surgery, and this must be carefully explained to the patient prior to the procedure. The actual freezing process can be quite painful. For larger lesions and if multiple freeze-thaw cycles are required, it is often wise to administer a local anesthetic prior to treatment. The prolonged exudative phase is generally most bothersome to the patient. The resultant scar is generally hypopigmented and repigments only slowly; patchy hyperpigmented scars develop occasionally.

Complications

Causes

Incorrect clinical or histologic diagnoses can lead to inappropriate under- or overtreatment. However, overtreatment rarely if ever causes as much trouble as an undertreatment. If surgical margins are incorrectly assessed by the pathologist, or if a malignant melanoma is misdiagnosed as a nevus, inadequate surgical treatment may be provided. Only when a local recurrence or metastasis occurs, are the doctor and the patient aware of the dilemma.

The most important step in avoiding intraoperative complications is to choose the least complicated procedure to achieve the needed results. In addition, the physician is morally obliged to undertake only those operations in which he or she has expertise. During the operation complications can arise because of the physician's inexperience and lack of skill, inattention, frank sloppiness, or simple bad luck. The last of these is the most common cause of complications, which are postoperative bleeding, scar formation, keloids, and wound infections. In addition, the patient may have an underlying disease, such as diabetes mellitus or a collagen vascular disorder, the potential effects of which have been overlooked or underestimated. Only when wound healing is disappointing does the surgeon become fully aware of the severity of the patient's underlying condition. In this era of quality assurance, every surgical operation has a threshold of acceptable complications, supporting the simple fact that problems may arise even under the best of circumstances. Unfortunately, this reality is not widely accepted by patients and attorneys.

Intraoperative Changes in the Operation Plan

This awkward title reflects an awkward situation. The patient has been counseled in great detail about an operative plan, which must then be changed, resulting in a longer operation, bigger scar, longer hospital stay, or larger bill. The preoperative discussion and operative consent should include the possibility of a larger procedure based on intraoperative clinical or histologic findings, for example a basal cell carcinoma showing finger-like projections with Mohs surgery, or if the temporal artery is cut during a procedure on the forehead, it may be necessary to enlarge the excision to adequately control bleeding.

If the patient has specifically expressed opposition to a specific aspect of a procedure, only the previously planned procedure should be completed. The patient must then be recounseled and a second procedure performed if the patient consents.

Complications of Cosmetic Procedures

When planning procedures which are entirely cosmetic, the preoperative discussion should include all possible complications, even those which are quite uncommon. The patient must realize that the operative scar may be more disturbing than the preoperative problem, and that a hypertrophic scar or keloid is possible in every case, despite excellent technical efforts. Postoperative bleeding, wound infections, and necrosis all delay healing and lead to a less acceptable result.

Complications of Minor Procedures

Even relatively minor excisions can lead to cosmetically unacceptable scars. This is particularly true when operating on the back, especially over the scapula, shoulder, and extensor surfaces of the arms. On the extremities where there is often marked tension perpendicular to the scar, dehiscence may occur. Certain areas such as the ear lobes and décolletage are particularly prone to keloid formation. Failure to consider the skin tension lines can lead to a widened scar or to a distortion of normal structures.

Complications of Flaps

Ensuring adequate vascular supply is the key to avoiding complications of flaps and grafts. Seldom do local flaps contain a single crucial vessel; rather, they are generally served randomly by diffusion through the dermal-subcutaneous vascular plexus. If the base of the flap is too narrow in relation to its length, tip necrosis may occur (Fig. 72.29). One must also have a thorough knowledge of the vascular and nerve supply of the operative field. Especially the facial nerve can be easily damaged during a procedure anterior to the ear.

Meticulous control of bleeding is essential during the procedure. Locating vessels with a small clamp and then tying them off is more certain and less traumatic than using cautery. Postoperative bleeding and necrosis are usually more common when cautery is used to control bleeding as flaps are developed. If the flap covers a relatively large wound, a suction drain is very helpful to help insure that the flap takes, and that bleeding causes minimal problems.

Again, careful planning is crucial to avoid problems. When working around the eyes and mouth,

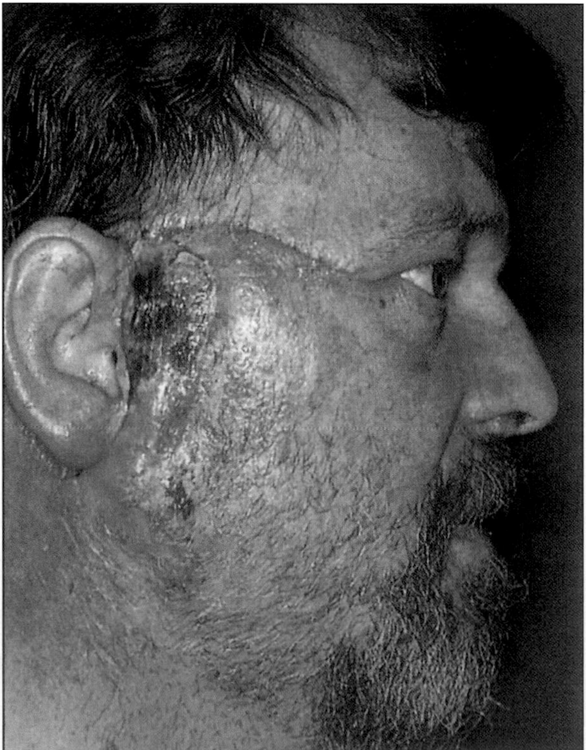

Fig. 72.29. Tip necrosis of a lobed flap as part of a complex flap procedure

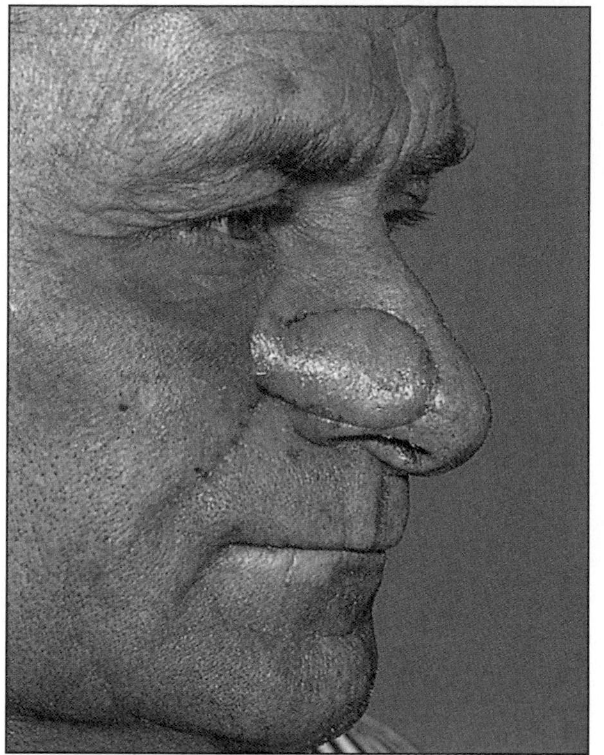

Fig. 72.30. Trapdoor effect of a transposition flap

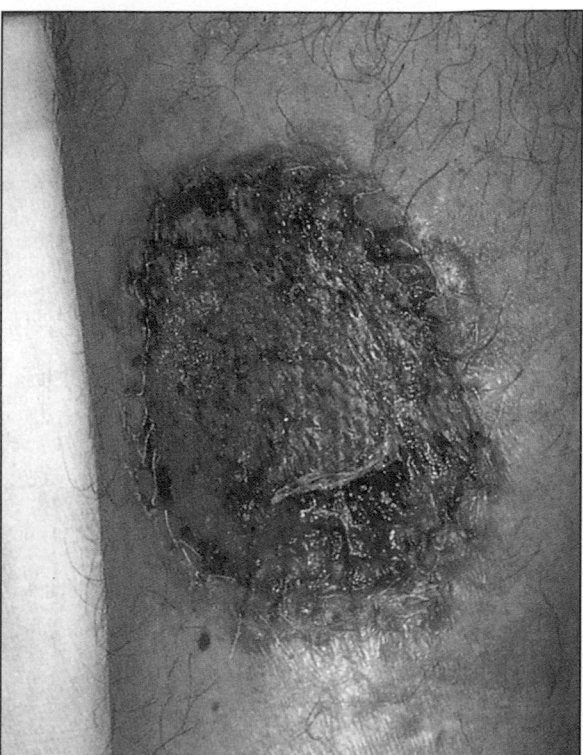

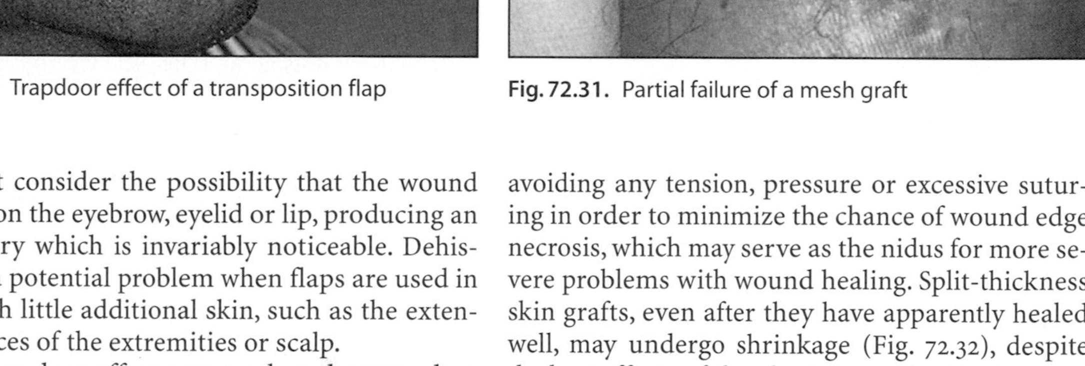

Fig. 72.31. Partial failure of a mesh graft

one must consider the possibility that the wound may tug on the eyebrow, eyelid or lip, producing an asymmetry which is invariably noticeable. Dehiscence is a potential problem when flaps are used in areas with little additional skin, such as the extensor surfaces of the extremities or scalp.

The trap-door effect occurs when the two edges of the wound are not at the same level. This may occur when the flap is not trimmed properly so that it remains thicker than the adjacent skin. Such a situation often occurs when nasolabial flaps are used to cover nasal defects (Fig. 72.30).

Complications of Grafts

The most important issue involving a graft is whether or not it takes (Fig. 72.31). Many factors are important, including where and how it is obtained, how well the host site is prepared and how good its vascular supply is. All grafts should be taken from healthy well-vascularized sites in as gentle and atraumatic a manner as possible. Full-thickness skin grafts must be defatted to avoid uneven edges and to allow more rapid diffusion of nutrients. The graft should be carefully fitted to the host site, avoiding any tension, pressure or excessive suturing in order to minimize the chance of wound edge necrosis, which may serve as the nidus for more severe problems with wound healing. Split-thickness skin grafts, even after they have apparently healed well, may undergo shrinkage (Fig. 72.32), despite the best efforts of the physician and patient.

Medical-Legal Aspects

Complications may arise in operative dermatology not only through problems during the surgery but also because of inadequate preoperative evaluation and planning or because of less than ideal postoperative care. In addition, underlying diseases may contribute to inadequate healing, bleeding or wound infections. In the eyes of the patient, the doctor is responsible for all these problems, and in most instances the law also takes this viewpoint.

Once a contract between the doctor and patient has been established, usually in the form of a patient visit, and once counseling and agreement to perform an operation have taken place, the physician is held responsible for adequately informing

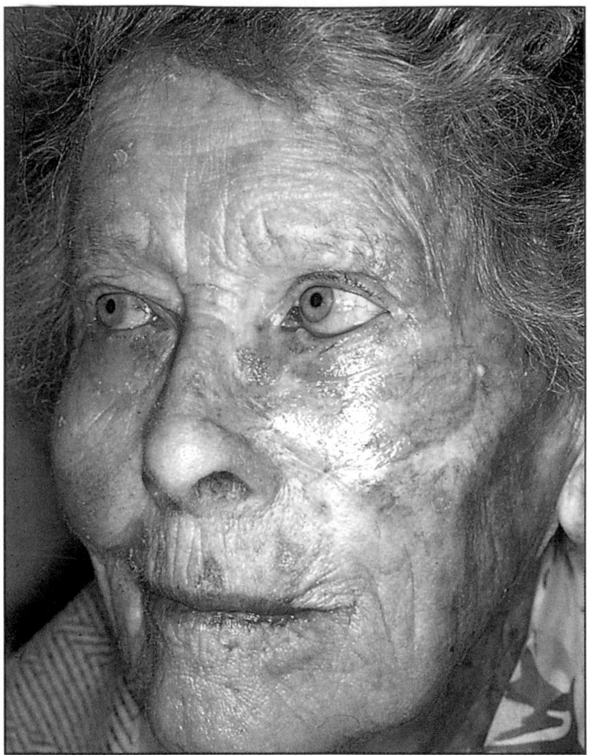

Fig. 72.32. Shrinkage of a split-thickness skin graft leading to ectropion of the lower lid

the patient about the benefits and risks of the procedure, for performing it according to the standards of care appropriate for his specialty and place of practice, and for being available for all postoperative care. Obviously many of these tasks may be delegated to assistants, but the physician is still ultimately responsible.

Bibliography

Books

Bennett RG (1988) Fundamentals of cutaneous surgery. Mosby, St. Louis

Fewkes JL, Cheney ML, Pollack SV (1992) Illustrated atlas of cutaneous surgery. Lippincott-Gower, Philadelphia

Kaufmann R, Landes E (1992) Dermatologische Operationen. Thieme, Stuttgart

Lask G, Moy RL (1996) Principles and techniques of cutaneous surgery. McGraw-Hill, New York

Petres J, Rompel R, Robins P (1996) Dermatologic surgery. Textbook and atlas. Springer, Berlin

Robinson JK, Arndt KA, LeBoit PE et al. (1996) Atlas of cutaneous surgery. Saunders, Philadelphia

Usatine RP, Moy RL, Tobinick EL et al. (1998) Skin surgery. A practical guide. Mosby, St. Louis

Wheeland RG (1994) Cutaneous surgery. Saunders, Philadelphia

General Aspects

Borges AF (1984) Relaxed skin tension lines (RSTL) versus other skin lines. Plast Reconstr Surg 73:144–150

Brown CD, Zitelli JA (1993) A review of topical agents for wounds and methods of wounding. Guidelines for wound management. J Dermatol Surg Oncol 19:732–737

Consensus Conference NIH (1986) Prevention of venous thrombosis and pulmonary embolism. JAMA 256: 744–757

Duncan KO, Leffell DJ (1997) Preoperative assessment of the elderly patient. Dermatol Clin 15:583–593

Dzubow LM, Zack L (1990) The principle of cosmetic junctions as applied to reconstruction of defects following Mohs surgery. J Dermatol Surg Oncol 16:353–355

Goldsmith SM, Leshin B, Owen J (1993) Management of patients taking anticoagulants and platelet inhibitors prior to dermatologic surgery. J Dermatol Surg Oncol 19: 578–581

Haas AF, Grekin RC (1995) Antibiotic prophylaxis in dermatologic surgery. J Am Acad Dermatol 32: 155–176

Joint American Academy of Dermatology/American Society of Dermatologic Surgery Liason Committee. (1999) Current issues in dermatologic office-based surgery. J Am Acad Dermatol 41:624–634

Leshin B, Whitaker DC, Swanson NA (1988) An approach to patient assessment and preparation in cutaneous oncology. J Am Acad Dermatol 19: 1081–1088

Macpherson DS (1993) Preoperative laboratory testing: should any tests be "routine" before surgery? Med Clin North Am 77: 289–308

Page CP, Bohnen JM, Fletcher JR et al. (1993) Antimicrobial prophylaxis for surgical wounds. Guidelines for clinical care. Arch Surg 128: 79–88

Partsch H, Blättler W (1996) Leitlinien zur Thromboembolie-Prophylaxe. Phlebologie 25:261–266

Perez M (1997) Advances in dermatologic surgery. Dermatol Clin 15:9–18

Rompel R, Petres J (1994) Wound healing in oncological dermatosurgery. In: Altmeyer P, Hoffmann K, el-Gammal S (eds) Wound healing and skin physiology. Springer, Berlin, pp 551–559

Sebben JE (1988) Sterile technique and the prevention of wound infection in office surgery, part I. J Dermatol Surg Oncol 14:1364–1371

Sebben JE (1989) Sterile technique and the prevention of wound infection in office surgery, part II. J Dermatol Surg Oncol 15:38–48

Singer AJ, Clark RAF (1999) Cutaneous wound healing. N Engl J Med 341:738–746

Anesthesia

Auletta MJ (1994) Local anesthesia for dermatologic surgery. Semin Dermatol 13:35–42

Dinehart SM (1994) Topical, local, and regional anesthesia. In: Wheeland RG (eds) Cutaneous surgery. Saunders, Philadelphia, pp 102–112

Elliott TG (1998) Tips for a better local anaesthetic. Australas J Dermatol 39:50–51

Klein JA (1995) Tumescent technique chronicles. Dermatol Surg 21:449–457

Lener EV, Bucalo BD, Kist DA et al. (1997) Topical anesthetic agents in dermatologic surgery. A review. Dermatol Surg 23:673–683

Mang WL, Arnold W (1998) Die Tumeszenztechnik in der plastisch-ästhetischen Chirurgie mit der Mang'schen Lösung. In: Mang WL, Kokoschka EM (eds) Ästhetische Chirurgie. Einhorn, Reinbek, pp 293–300

Sattler G, Rapprich S, Hagedorn (1997) Tumeszenz-Lokalanästhesie – Untersuchung zur Pharmakokinetik von Prilocain. Z Hautkr 72:522–525

Basic Operative Techniques

Benedetto AV, Griffin TD, Benedetto EA et al. (1992) Dermabrasion: therapy and prophylaxis of the photoaged face. J Am Acad Dermatol 27:439–447

Hill TG (1995) Dermal suturing technique. J Am Acad Dermatol 32:535

Kromayer E (1923) Die Behandlung der kosmetischen Hautleiden unter besonderer Berücksichtigung der physikalischen Heilmethoden und der narbenlosen Operationsweisen. Thieme, Leipzig

Landes E (1984) Dermabrasion, eine vielseitige Therapieform. In: Müller RPA, Friederich HC, Petres J (eds) Operative Dermatologie im Kopf-Hals-Bereich. Fortschritte der operativen Dermatologie, vol 1. Springer, Berlin, pp 295–302

Morton DL, Wen DR, Wong JH et al. (1992) Technical details of intraoperative lymphatic mapping for early stage melanoma. Arch Surg 127:392–399

Moy RL, Waldman B, Hein DW (1992) A review of sutures and suturing techniques. J Dermatol Surg Oncol 18: 785–795

Namiki Y, Fukuta K, Alani H (1992) The directions of static skin tensions in the face: their roles in facial incisions. Ann Plast Surg 28:147–151

Orozco-Covarrubias ML, Ruiz-Maldonado R (1999) Surgical facial wounds: simple interrupted percutaneous suture versus running intradermal suture. Dermatol Surg 25: 109–112

Petres J, Rompel R (1996) Dermabrasion. In: Mang WL, Bull HG (eds) Ästhetische Chirurgie. Einhorn, Reinbek, pp 383–386

Robinson JK (1986) Fundamentals of skin biopsy. Year Book Medical Publishers, Chicago

Rompel R, Möser M, Petres J (1997) Dermabrasion of congenital nevocellular nevi: experience in 215 patients. Dermatology 194:261–267

Schreus HT (1950) Hochtouriges Schleifen der Haut (ein neues Behandlungsverfahren). Z Haut Geschlechtskr 8: 151–156

Snow SN, Dortzbach R, Moyer D (1991) Managing common suturing problems. J Dermatol Surg Oncol 17:502–508

Wong NL (1993) Review of continuous sutures in dermatologic surgery. J Dermatol Surg Oncol 19:923–931

Zalla MJ (1994) Basic cutaneous surgery. Cutis 53:172–186

Zoltán J (1977) Atlas der chirurgischen Schnitt- und Nahttechnik. Karger, Basel

Micrographic Excision Techniques

Breuninger H (1984) Histologic control of excised tissue edges in the operative treatment of basal cell carcinomas. J Dermatol Surg Oncol 10:724–727

Burg G, Hirsch R, Konz B et al. (1975) Histographic surgery: accuracy of visual assessment of the margins of basal-cell epithelioma. J Dermatol Surg 1:21–24

Kopke LF, Konz B (1995) Mikrographische Chirurgie. Eine methodische Bestandsaufnahme. Hautarzt 46:607–614

Mikhail GR (1991) Mohs micrographic surgery. Saunders, Philadelphia

Miller PK, Roenigk RK, Brodland DG et al. (1992) Cutaneous micrographic surgery: Mohs procedure. Mayo Clin Proc 67:971–980

Mohs FE, Guyer MF (1941) Pre-excisional fixation of tissues in the treatment of cancer in rats. Cancer Res 1:49–51

Nelson BR, Railan D, Cohen S (1997) Mohs' micrographic surgery for nonmelanoma skin cancers. Clin Plast Surg 24:705–718

Schreus HT (1951) Chlorzinkschnellätzung des Epithelioms. Ein Beitrag zur Chemochirurgie. Hautarzt 2:317–319

Shriner DL, McCoy DK, Goldberg DJ et al. (1998) Mohs micrographic surgery. J Am Acad Dermatol 39:79–97

Tromovitch TA, Stegman SJ (1978) Microscopic-controlled excision of cutaneous tumors: chemosurgery, fresh tissue technique. Cancer 41:653–658

Simple Excision and Repair Techniques

Fabri PJ, Adams JR (1987) Simplified excision of lipomas. Surg Gynecol Obstet 165: 173–174

Frumkin A, Cottel WI, Swanson NA (1989) Basic principles of dermatologic surgery. J Am Acad Dermatol 20: 808–814

Hudson-Peacock MJ, Lawrence CM (1995) Comparison of wound closure by means of dog ear repair and elliptical excision. J Am Acad Dermatol 32:627–630

Scholz A, Sebastian G, Hackert I et al. (1992) Wann ist die Serienexzision von Naevi indiziert? In: Burg G, Hartmann AA, Konz B (eds) Onkologische Dermatologie. Neue Aspekte. Altersbedingte Besonderheiten. Fortschritte der operativen und onkologischen Dermatologie, vol 7. Springer, Berlin, pp 238–242

Zachary CB (1991) Basic cutaneous surgery. Churchill Livingstone, New York

Plastic Procedures

Baker SR (1994) Local cutaneous flaps. Otolaryngol Clin North Am 27:139–159

Dobke MK, Miller SH (1997) Tissue repair after Mohs surgery. A plastic surgeon's view. Dermatol Surg 23: 1061–1066

Dufourmentel C, Talaat SM (1971) The kite flap. Transactions of the 5th international congress on plastic reconstructive surgery. Butterworth, Melbourne, pp 1123–1134

Haneke E (1998) Surgical treatment of defects on the tip of the nose. Dermatol Surg 24: 711–717

Heniford BW, Bailin PL, Marsico RE Jr (1998) Field guide to local flaps. Dermatol Clin 16:65–74

Hill TG (1994) Skin grafts. In: Wheeland RG (eds) Cutaneous surgery. Saunders, Philadelphia, pp 318–328

Imre J (1928) Lidplastik und plastische Operation anderer Weichteile des Gesichtes. Studium, Budapest

Konz B, Wörle B, Sander CA (1997) Aesthetic reconstruction of nasal defects using forehead flaps. Facial Plast Surg 13: 111–117

Limberg AA (1966) Design of local flaps. Mod Trends Plast Surg 2:38–61

Menick FJ (1998) Facial reconstruction with local and distant tissue: the interface of aesthetic and reconstructive surgery. Plast Reconstr Surg 102:1424–1433

Petres J, Hundeiker M (1975) Korrektive Dermatologie. Springer, Berlin

Petres J, Rompel R (1994) Defektversorgung mittels lokaler und regionaler Lappenplastiken nach Tumorexzision im Gesicht. In: Mahrle G, Schultz HJ, Krieg T (eds) Wundheilung – Wundverschluß. Fortschritte der operativen und onkologischen Dermatologie, vol 8. Springer, Berlin, pp 69–74

Rompel R, Petres J (1992) Surgical treatment of lip cancer. Asian J Oral Maxillofac Surg 4:63–71

Rompel R, Petres J (1993) Reconstructive techniques in oncologic dermatosurgery of the auricular region. FACE 2: 171–177

Rompel R, Petres J (1995) Operative Akne-Therapie. Z Hautkr 70:700–704

Skouge JW (1991) Skin grafting. Churchill Livingstone, New York

Summers BK, Siegle RJ (1993) Facial cutaneous reconstructive surgery: facial flaps. J Am Acad Dermatol 29:917–941

Trevaskis AE, Rempel J, Okunski W et al. (1970) Sliding subcutaneous pedicle flaps to close a circular defect. Plast Reconstr Surg 46:155–157

Tromovitch TA, Stegman SJ, Glogau RG (1989) Flaps and grafts in dermatologic surgery. Mosby Yearbook, St. Louis

Whitaker DC (1994) Random-pattern flaps. In: Wheeland RG (ed) Cutaneous surgery. Saunders, Philadelphia, pp 329–352

Zimany A (1953) The bilobed flap. Plast Reconstr Surg 11: 424–434

Zoltán J (1984) Atlas der Hautersatzverfahren. Akadémiai Kiadó, Budapest

Electrosurgery

Hainer BL (1991) Fundamentals of electrosurgery. J Am Board Fam Pract 4:419–426

Le Vasseur JG, Kennard CD, Finley EM et al. (1998) Dermatologic electrosurgery in patients with implantable cardioverter-defibrillators and pacemakers. Dermatol Surg 24:233–40

Sebben JE (1988) Electrosurgery principles: cutting current and cutaneous surgery, part I. J Dermatol Surg Oncol 14: 29–31

Sebben JE (1988) Electrosurgery principles: cutting current and cutaneous surgery, part II. J Dermatol Surg Oncol 14: 147–150

Taylor KW, Desmond J (1970) Electrical hazards in the operating room, with special reference to electrosurgery. Can J Surg 13: 362–364

Cryotherapy

August PJ (1995) Cryotherapy of nonmelanoma skin cancer. Clin Dermatol 13: 589–592

Breitbart EW (1983) Kryochirurgie: Methodik und Ergebnisse. Hautarzt 34:612–619

Cajacob A (1982) Dermatologische Kryotherapie. Dermatologica 165:369–383

Dachow-Siwiec E (1985) Technique of cryotherapy. Clin Dermatol 3:185–188

Dawber RP (1990) Cryosurgery: complications and contraindications. Clin Dermatol 8:108–114

Graham GF (1993) Cryosurgery. Clin Plast Surg 20: 131–147

Kuflik EG (1994) Cryosurgery updated. J Am Acad Dermatol 31:925–944

Complications in Dermatologic Surgery

Campbell SP, Moss ML, Hugo NE (1992) When does a random flap die? Plast Reconstr Surg 89:718–721

Harahap M (1993) Complications of dermatologic surgery. Springer, Berlin Heidelberg New York

Hayes CM, Whitaker DC (1994) Complications of cutaneous surgery. Adv Dermatol 9:161–178

Kaufman AJ, Kiene KL, Moy RL (1993) Role of tissue undermining in the trapdoor effect of transposition flaps. J Dermatol Surg Oncol 19:128–132

Konz B, Braun-Falco O (1984) Komplikationen in der operativen Dermatologie. Springer, Berlin

Rompel R, Petres J (1993) Vermeidung von Komplikationen bei dermatochirurgischen Tumoreingriffen in der periorbitalen Region. In: Neumann HJ (ed) Ästhetische und plastisch-rekonstruktive Gesichtschirurgie. Einhorn, Reinbek, pp 160–169

Salasche SJ (1986) Acute surgical complications: cause, prevention, and treatment. J Am Acad Dermatol 15: 1163–1185

Scheflan M (1984) Complications of skin grafting. In: Greenfield LJ (eds) The unfavorable result in plastic surgery – avoidance and treatment. Little Brown, Boston, pp 143–149

Subject Index

C

D

G

H

J

K

L

M

N

O

P

Q

R

S

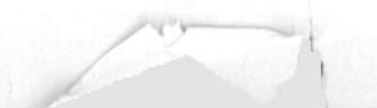

T

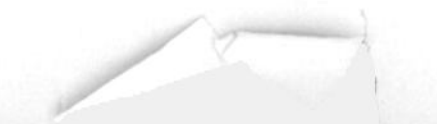

U

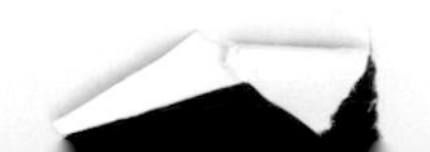

V

W

X

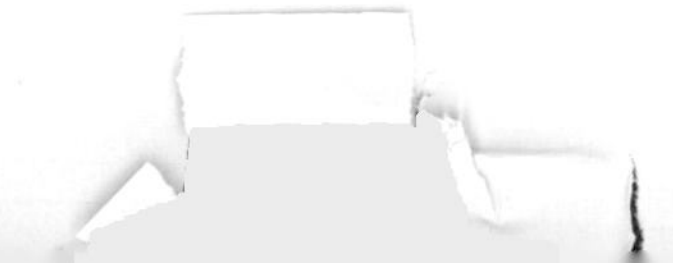